Brief Contents

P9-CDB-958

Fundamentals of Nursing

The Art and Science of Person-Centered Nursing Care

Fundamentals of Nursing

The Art and Science of Person-Centered Nursing Care

Eighth Edition

Carol Taylor, PhD, MSN, RN

Professor of Nursing
Georgetown University School of Nursing and Health Studies
Washington, DC

Carol Lillis, MSN, RN

Faculty Emerita
Delaware County Community College
Media, Pennsylvania

Pamela Lynn, MSN, RN

Instructor
Gwynedd Mercy University
Frances M. Maguire School of Nursing and Health Professions
Gwynedd Valley, Pennsylvania

Priscilla LeMone, DSN, RN, FAAN

Associate Professor Emerita
University of Missouri Sinclair School of Nursing
Columbia, Missouri
Adjunct Associate Professor
The Ohio State University College of Nursing
Columbus, Ohio

Philadelphia • Baltimore • New York • London
Buenos Aires • Hong Kong • Sydney • Tokyo

Publisher: Lisa McAllister
Executive Editor: Sherry Dickinson
Product Development Editor: Helen Kogut
Editorial Assistant: Dan Reilly
Development Editors: Tom Lochhaas, Sarah Kyle
Marketing Manager: Dean Karampelas
Production Project Manager: Cynthia Rudy
Design Coordinator: Holly Reid McLaughlin
Illustration Coordinator: Jennifer Clements
Manufacturing Coordinator: Karin Duffield
Prepress Vendor: Aptara, Inc.

8th Edition

Library of Congress Cataloging-in-Publication Data

Taylor, Carol (Carol R.), author.
  Fundamentals of nursing : the art and science of person-centered nursing care / Carol Taylor, Carol Lillis, Pamela Lynn. –Eighth edition.
      p. ; cm.
  Preceded by Fundamentals of nursing / Carol R. Taylor . . . [et al.]. 7th ed. c2011.
  Includes bibliographical references and index.
  ISBN 978-1-4511-8561-4 (alk. paper)
  I. Lillis, Carol, author. II. Lynn, Pamela (Pamela Barbara), 1961- author. III. Title.
  [DNLM: 1. Nursing Care. 2. Nursing Process. 3. Patient-Centered Care. WY 100.1]
  RT41
  610.73–dc23
                                                                                2014013308

*To all who labor to make health care "work" for all, especially
the most vulnerable!*

—Carol Taylor

*To my ten grandchildren, who bring so much laughter, love,
and enjoyment to my life.*

—Carol Lillis

*To past, present, and future nursing students and my family:
Each one of you helps me to continue learning and caring every day.*

—Pam Lynn

Contributors

Contributors for the Eighth Edition

Kerry H. Cheever, PhD, RN
Professor and Chairperson
Department of Nursing
Moravian College
Bethlehem, Pennsylvania
PICO in Practice: Asking Clinical Questions

Carrie Bowman Dalley, MS
Certified Registered Nurse Anesthetist (CRNA)
Georgetown University Nurse Anesthesia Program
Washington, DC
Chapter 39: Fluid, Electrolyte, and Acid–Base Balance

Elizabeth Genazzio, MA, BSN, RN, CNOR, RNFA
Perioperative Nurse and RNFA
Lankenau Medical Center
Wynnewood, Pennsylvania
Faculty Assistant
Delaware County Community College
Media, Pennsylvania
Chapter 29: Perioperative Nursing

Victoria M. Goode, PhD(c), MSNA, CRNA
Instructor
Nurse Anesthesia Program
Georgetown University School of Nursing and Health Studies
Washington, DC
Chapter 39: Fluid, Electrolyte, and Acid–Base Balance

Susan J. Hayden, PhD, MSN, BSN, BS, RN
Assistant Professor
College of Nursing
University of Southern Alabama
Mobile, Alabama
Chapter 32: Activity

Catherine Horvath, MSN, BSN, CRNA
Instructor
Nurse Anesthesia Program
Georgetown University School of Nursing and Health Studies
Washington, DC
Chapter 39: Fluid, Electrolyte, and Acid–Base Balance

Donna Marie Jasinski, PhD, CRNA
Associate Professor
Georgetown University School of Nursing and Health Studies
Washington, DC
Chapter 39: Fluid, Electrolyte, and Acid–Base Balance

Jane C. Rothrock, PhD, RN, CNOR, FAAN
Adjunct Professor, Perioperative Nursing
Delaware County Community College
Media, Pennsylvania
Chapter 29: Perioperative Nursing

Margaret Mary Thomas, BS, RN, CNOR
Bryn Mawr Hospital
Bryn Mawr, Pennsylvania
Chapter 29: Perioperative Nursing

Denise H. Tola, MSN, CRNA
Clinical Director
Nurse Anesthesia Program
Georgetown University School of Nursing and Health Studies
Washington, DC
Chapter 39: Fluid, Electrolyte, and Acid–Base Balance

Contributors for the Seventh Edition

Lynn Burbank, MSN, RN, CPNP
Learning Resource Coordinator
Dixon School of Nursing
Abington Memorial Hospital
Abington, Pennsylvania
Chapter 29: Medications

Kerry H. Cheever, PhD, RN
Professor and Chairperson
St. Luke's School of Nursing at Moravian College
Assistant Vice President
St. Luke's Hospital & Health Network
Bethlehem, Pennsylvania
PICO in Practice: Asking Clinical Questions

Joanne O'Brien, MSN, RN
Associate Professor
Delaware County Community College
Media, Pennsylvania
Concept Maps

Christine E. Smith, MSN, RN, CNOR
Perioperative Clinical Nurse Specialist
Lucile Packard Children's Hospital at Stanford
Palo Alto, California
Chapter 30: Perioperative Nursing

For a list of the contributors to the Student and Instructor Resources accompanying this book, please visit thePoint at http://thepoint.lww.com/Taylor8e.

Reviewers

Monique Bacher, MSN/Ed, BScN, RN
PN/PSW Clinical Coordinator, Professor
George Brown College
Toronto, Ontario

Kathy Batton, PhD, MSN
Nursing Instructor
Hinds Community College
Raymond, Mississippi

Mary Lee Berg, MS, RNC-MNN
Assistant Professor
Onondaga Community College
Syracuse, New York

Joanne Bonesteel, MS, RN
Faculty Program Director
ADN Programs, Excelsior College
Albany, New York

Dana M. Botz, MSN, RN
Nursing Faculty
North Hennepin Community College
Brooklyn Park, Minnesota

Diane C. Bridge, EdS, MSN, RN
Assistant Professor of Nursing
Liberty University
Lynchburg, Virginia

Lynn Burbank, MSN, RN, CPNP
Learning Resource Coordinator
Abington Memorial Hospital
Dixon School of Nursing
Willow Grove, Pennsylvania

Paula Burnett, DNP, RN, CNE
Assistant Professor
Salem State University
Salem, Massachusetts

Marinela Castaño, MSN
Professor of Nursing
Lone Star College—North Harris
Houston, Texas

Desiree A. Díaz, PhD, RN-BC, CNE, CHSE
Associate Clinical Professor
University of Connecticut School of Nursing
Storrs, Connecticut

Loree M. DuBose, MSN, RN
Clinical Assistant Professor
Texas A&M University—Corpus Christi
College of Nursing and Health Sciences
Corpus Christi, Texas

Mary A. Ehret, MS, RN
Director of Nursing
Brookdale Community College
Lincroft, New Jersey

Susan Lynn Estes, MSN, BSN, RN
Clinical Associate Professor
Mercer University
Georgia Baptist College of Nursing
Atlanta, Georgia

Janet Riga Goeldner, MSN
Professor
University of Cincinnati
Cincinnati, Ohio

Joan M. Hall, MS, APRN, BC
Lecturer/Clinical Instructor
San Diego State University
San Diego, California

Linda G. Harmon, MSN
Nursing Instructor
Antelope Valley College
Lancaster, California

Jeanne Heatlie, MSN
Assistant Professor
Madonna University
Livonia, Michigan

Lori Ann Huber, MSN, CNS
Program Coordinator
Portage Lakes Career Center
Cuyahoga Falls, Ohio

Denise Pruskowski Kavanagh, MSN, RN
Assistant Professor
LaSalle University
Philadelphia, Pennsylvania

Patricia T. Ketcham, MSN, RN
Director of Nursing Laboratories
Oakland University
Rochester, Michigan

Carol A. Kincaid, MSN, BSN
Instructor
Crouse Hospital College of Nursing
Syracuse, New York

Kara Lesher, MSN, RN
Nurse Educator
Reading Hospital School of Health Sciences
Reading, Pennsylvania

Sandi McCarthy, MSN, RN, CNE
Assistant Professor
University of Texas Medical Branch
Galveston, Texas

Megan McHugh, MSN/ED, MSIS, RN, CCRN, CNRN
Nursing Informaticist
MedStar Georgetown University Hospital
Washington, DC

Michelle Montpas, EdD, MSN, RN, CNE
Professor of Nursing
Mott Community College
Flint, Michigan

Cynthia K. Neff, MSN
Professor of Nursing
Allegany College of Maryland
Cumberland, Maryland

Virginia Ann Ousley, MSN, BSN, RN, AAS
Professor
Radford University
Radford, Virginia

Karen Parker, DNP, FNP, RN
Assistant Professor
St. John Fisher College
Rochester, New York

Jonni K. Pielin-Kircher, MSN, RN, CSN
Assistant Professor of Nursing
Westmoreland County Community College
Youngwood, Pennsylvania

Susan M. Randol, MSN, RN, CNE
Semester Coordinator and Master Instructor
University of Louisiana at Lafayette
Lafayette, Louisiana

Dana Reeves, MSN, RN
Assistant Professor
University of Arkansas–Fort Smith
Fort Smith, Arkansas

Wanda Jane Revis, MSN, BSN, RN
Associate Professor, Fundamentals Team Leader
Greenville Technical College
Greenville, South Carolina

Joscelyn A. Richey, MSN, ARNP, CDE
Nursing Faculty
Hillsborough Community College
Tampa, Florida

Wendy Robinson, PhD, FNP-BC, CNE
Associate Professor
Helene Fuld College of Nursing
New York, New York

Kari Sand-Jecklin, EdD, MSN, RN
Associate Professor and Vice Chair
West Virginia University School of Nursing
Morgantown, West Virginia

Joann Sands, DNP, RN, ANP-BC
Clinical Assistant Professor
SUNY–University at Buffalo
Buffalo, New York

Mary Susan Servey, MSN, MSA, RN, BC
Professor
Wayne County Community College District
Detroit, Michigan

Joyce A. Shanty, PhD, RN
Associate Professor
Indiana University of Pennsylvania
Indiana, Pennsylvania

Catherine Sikorski, MSN, RN
Professor
Macomb Community College
Warren, Michigan

Sharon Souter, PhD, RN, CNE
Dean and Professor
University of Mary-Hardin Baylor
Belton, Texas

Lorelei Stellwag, MSN, RN, NE-BC
Director of Technology Transformation
Nursing Administration
MedStar Georgetown University Hospital
Washington, DC

Twila Sterling-Guillory, PhD, MSN, BSN
Associate Professor of Nursing
McNeese State University
Lake Charles, Louisiana

Carmen G. Vela, MSN, BSN, RN
Nursing Instructor, Faculty
Covenant School of Nursing, Covenant Health
Lubbock, Texas

Sharon Stahl Wexler, PhD, RN, GCNS-BC, FNGNA
Assistant Professor
Pace University
Lienhard School of Nursing
New York, New York

Samantha S. Wilson, MSN, BSN
Associate Professor of Nursing
Germanna Community College
Locust Grove, Virginia

Kamomilani Anduha Wong, MSN, APRN, FNP-BC
Assistant Professor
Hawaii Pacific University
College of Nursing and Health Sciences
Kaneohe, Hawaii

For a list of the reviewers of the Test Generator accompanying this book, please visit thePoint at http://thepoint.lww.com/Taylor8e

Preface

Today's competitive, market-driven health care environment is challenging the very nature of professional nursing practice. *Fundamentals of Nursing: The Art and Science of Person-Centered Nursing Care, Eighth Edition*, promotes nursing as an evolving art and science, directed to human health and well-being. It challenges students to cultivate the Quality and Safety Education for Nurses (QSEN) and blended competencies they will need to serve patients and the public well. Our aim is to prepare nurses who combine the highest level of scientific knowledge and technologic skill with responsible, caring practice. We want to challenge students to identify and master the cognitive and technical skills as well as the interpersonal and ethical/legal skills they will need to effectively nurse the patients in their care. We refuse to allow accountability and caring relationships to become relics of a bygone era.

Those new to nursing can quickly become overwhelmed by the demands placed on the nurse's knowledge, technical competence, interpersonal skills, and commitment. Therefore, much care has gone into the selection of both the content in this edition and the manner of its presentation. We strive to capture the unique essence of both the art and science of nursing, distilling what the person beginning the study and practice of nursing needs to know. We invite students to identify with the profession, to share in its pride, and to respond to today's challenges competently, enthusiastically, and accountably.

LEARNING EXPERIENCE

This text and the entire Taylor Suite have been created with the student's experience in mind. Care has been taken to appeal to all learning styles. The student-friendly writing style ensures that students will comprehend and retain information. The updated art program and strong features enhance understanding of important concepts. Free video clips clearly demonstrate and reinforce important skill steps; as students watch and listen to the videos, comprehension increases. In addition, each element of the Taylor Suite, which is described later in the preface, coordinates to provide a consistent and cohesive learning experience.

ORGANIZATION

Fundamentals of Nursing: The Art and Science of Person-Centered Nursing Care, Eighth Edition, is organized into eight units. Ideally, the text is followed sequentially, but every effort has been made to respect the differing needs of diverse curricula and students. Thus, each chapter stands on its own merit and may be read independently of others.

Unit I, Foundations of Nursing Practice

Unit I opens with a description of contemporary nursing. Successive chapters introduce content foundational to nursing

practice: theory, research, and evidence-based practice; health and illness; health of the individual, family, and community; cultural diversity; values, ethics, and advocacy; and legal implications.

Unit II, Health Care Delivery

Unit II is completely revised in light of the continuing changes in health care delivery. The new content highlights nurses' expanding roles in care coordination as partnerships are forged with patients, families, and communities. Chapters address the variety of community-based health care settings; continuity of care as the patient enters a health care facility, is transferred within the facility, and is discharged into another setting within the community; and care provided within the home.

Unit III, Person-Centered Care and the Nursing Process

Unit III offers a detailed, step-by-step guide to each component of the nursing process with practical guidelines and examples included in each chapter. New NANDA International and NIC/NOC content has been added, along with a stronger emphasis on clinical decision making. Each chapter concludes with a section on "Reflective Practice Leading to Personal Learning" that invites readers to look at their experience with each step of the nursing process, understand it, and learn from it. The goal is always to invite reflection on how we can improve our thoughtful, person-centered practice.

Chapter 10 is completely revised and offers a careful introduction to thoughtful and person-centered practice with expanded content on theories of caring, clinical reasoning, judgment, decision making, and reflective practice. Separate chapters address the nursing process as a whole: Quality and Safety Education for Nurses (QSEN) and blended competencies, critical thinking, assessing, diagnosing, outcome identification and planning, implementing, and evaluating. Chapter 16 includes expanded content on privacy guidelines and standards for social media, electronic health records (EHRs), reporting, conferring, and using informatics.

Unit IV, Promoting Health Across the Lifespan

Unit IV provides the basis for understanding growth and development across the lifespan and acknowledges nursing's differing requirements arising from the various developmental stages and abilities to meet developmental tasks.

Unit V, Roles Basic to Nursing Care

Unit V describes major roles in which nurses function as they interact holistically with patients. Chapters focus on the communicator, teacher and counselor, and leader and manager roles of the nurse as caregiver.

Unit VI, Actions Basic to Nursing Care

Unit VI introduces the foundational skills used by nurses: maintaining asepsis, measuring vital signs, assessing health, promoting safety, incorporating complementary and alternative therapies, administering medication, and caring for surgical patients.

Unit VII, Promoting Healthy Physiologic Responses

Unit VII explores the nurse's role in helping patients meet basic physiologic needs: hygiene; skin integrity and wound care; activity; rest and sleep; comfort and pain management; nutrition; urinary elimination; bowel elimination; oxygenation and perfusion; and fluid, electrolyte, and acid–base balance. Chapter 38 now has expanded cardiovascular content that includes cardiac function and perfusion. In each chapter, guidelines are included for assessing and diagnosing unhealthy responses and for planning, implementing, and evaluating appropriate care strategies.

Unit VIII, Promoting Healthy Psychosocial Responses

Unit VIII uses the same format as Unit VII to focus on the psychosocial needs of patients: self-concept; stress and adaptation; loss, grief, and dying; sensory functioning; sexuality; and spirituality.

THEMES

The following themes are interwoven throughout the text to provide a broad knowledge base of nursing essentials while emphasizing holistic care.

Thoughtful Practice and Person-Centered Care

The change in our subtitle, the first title change since the first edition, reflects today's new emphasis on person-centered care. Readers will see the new emphasis on clinical reasoning, judgment, decision making, and reflective practice in every chapter.

Emphasis on Partnering With Patients, Family, and Professional Caregivers

Today, we have witnessed the health care "industry" transform patients to "customers," who buy health care (if they are able) as a commodity in the marketplace. We do not believe that a "customer orientation" serves patients or nurses well. One of our students shared her belief that she owes less to a "customer" and even to a "client" than she does to a "patient." We, therefore, use the term *patient*—in its most positive sense—to designate the recipient of nursing care.

Careful attention is paid to directing students to identify, value, and develop the interpersonal skills that will allow them to effectively partner with patients, family, and profes-

sional caregivers. This edition highlights collaborative practice and nursing strategies for actively engaging patients, family caregivers, and the public in the development of health goals and strategies to achieve these goals. Patients may be individuals, families, or communities.

Care has been taken to communicate that both nurses and patients may be male or female and that they come from every racial and ethnic background and socioeconomic group. Whenever possible, we have tried to avoid male/female distinctions in personal pronouns.

Integrated Nursing Process

After the nursing process is introduced in Unit III, it provides the organizational framework for successive chapters. Chapters in Units VII and VIII, which deal with physiologic and psychosocial responses, begin with a succinct background discussion of the concept, followed by identification of factors that influence how different individuals respond to these needs. Steps in the nursing process are used to describe related nursing responsibilities. Throughout these chapters, students will find numerous practical examples of how to conduct focused assessments; develop and write diagnostic statements; identify goals and outcomes; and select, implement, and evaluate appropriate nursing interventions. These examples will reinforce the student's mastery of nursing process skills. This edition highlights the Quality and Safety Education for Nurses (QSEN) competencies. Most chapters in Units VII and VIII conclude with a *Nursing Plan of Care* that illustrates each step of the nursing process and a sample documentation of nursing assessment or intervention. In addition, concept maps demonstrating the nursing process are included in several chapters.

Nursing as an Art and Science

Nursing as a science is characterized by a growing body of knowledge that links technical and interpersonal interventions to desired patient outcomes; as an art, nursing demands of its practitioners sufficient competency to creatively design individualized strategies to assist patients to reach personal health goals. A unique spirit of caring always must prevail.

New to this edition is the inclusion of *Delegation Considerations* in each skill. Delegation decision-making information is provided, using delegation guidelines based on American Nurses Association (ANA) and National Council of State Boards of Nursing (NCSBN) principles and recommendations (Appendix A). Appendix A, *Guidelines for Delegation Decision Making*, can be found on thePoint website.

Health and Health Disparities Orientation

A health rather than an illness orientation provides a framework for presentation of content. This edition includes expanded content on health literacy and health disparities. Special features such as *Promoting Health*, *Teaching Tips*, and *Health Literacy* boxes help to highlight this important content.

Holistic Care Across the Lifespan

A holistic orientation to basic human needs is essential across the lifespan. This orientation is emphasized through information about growth and development in Unit IV, *Promoting Health Across the Lifespan*; through age considerations in many *Skills*; and through developmental considerations in related tables and displays, as well as diverse ages and needs of patients represented in numerous features. Wherever appropriate, cultural considerations are included.

Attention to Special Needs of the Older Person

Because the age of the population is increasing, nurses encounter growing numbers of older patients in all practice settings. Chapter 19: *The Aging Adult,* the *Focus on the Older Adult* boxes, and general considerations for the older patient that appear within the text aim to sensitize students to the special nursing needs of this population. Readers of the eighth edition will find expanded information related to dementia, depression, and delirium; a discussion of cascade iatrogenics; the Fulmer SPICES tool used to identify common problems that lead to negative outcomes in older adults; and the American Geriatrics Society and ANA Position Statement on Restraint Use. The Hendrich II Fall Risk Model and other helpful reference materials are available on thePoint.

Critical Thinking and Clinical Reasoning

Unit III, *Person-Centered Care and the Nursing Process,* invites students to reflect on their ability to be the critical difference for recipients of their thoughtful practice. The revised *Reflective Practice* boxes, *Focused Critical Thinking Guides*, and *Developing Clinical Reasoning* material in each chapter challenge students to use new knowledge and experience to "think through" learning exercises designed to demonstrate how careful thinking can change outcomes.

Healthy Work Environments

This edition addresses current issues of incivility, nurse bullying, cyber terror, lateral violence, aggressive behavior, and nurses' use of social media to help readers understand what it takes to have a healthy work environment.

Focus on Nursing Skills

Skills are presented in a concise, straightforward, and simplified format that is intended to facilitate competent performance of nursing skills. A scientific rationale accompanies each nursing action; many color photographs and illustrations further reinforce mastery. *Delegation Considerations* assist students and graduate nurses in developing the critical decision-making skills necessary to transfer responsibility for the performance of an activity to another individual and to ensure safe and effective nursing care. *Special Considerations*, including modifications and age and home health care considerations, are given where appropriate. Unexpected situations and associated interventions are included to help students think critically about the skills they are performing. Also included are documentation guidelines and samples to help students learn what and how to document when performing skills.

Focus on Community and Expanded Nursing Roles

Patients today spend fewer days in the hospital, are frequently transferred both within the hospital and between health care institutions and home, and need to rely on rapidly proliferating community-based health care resources. New content on accountable care organizations, medical homes, and medical neighborhoods, as well as content on the new roles for nurses (nurse coach, clinical nurse leader, nurse navigator, and nurse care coordinator) highlight both traditional and innovative care in institutional and community-based practice settings.

Focus on Safety

New content highlights today's emphasis on patient safety, including expanded safety information related to children, adolescents, and older adults. The Institute of Medicine safety content, 2014 Joint Commission National Patient Safety Goals and Sentinel Event Statistics are highlighted, and new information is provided on health care–associated infections (HAIs). Safe Patient Handling and Movement Practices—based on guidelines from VISN 8 Patient Safety Center, 2006, 2007, and 2009—are included in this edition as well as expanded content on patient "hand-offs."

Research as a Strength to Practice

Content on research and evidence-based practice has been updated and is included in Unit I for increased emphasis early in the learning experience. The updated feature, *PICO in Practice: Asking Clinical Questions*, encourages readers to delve into research to solve a clinical question using the PICO format and guidelines. Updated *Research in Nursing: Bridging the Gap to Evidence-Based Practice* boxes, appearing throughout the book, promote the value of research and apply its relevance to nursing practice. Students are challenged to become informed participants in, or consumers of, clinical research. To that end, students can explore additional research in nursing journal articles provided for each chapter on thePoint website (http://thePoint.lww.com/Taylor8e).

Up-to-Date Clinical Information

Revisions in each clinical chapter will help educators and students remain current. Sample new content includes:

- Expanded information on genomics
- New information on SIDS and SUID (sudden unexplained infant death)
- Expanded discussion of childhood obesity
- Dangers associated with energy drinks, synthetic marijuana, and bath salts
- Expanded information on multiple drug–resistant organisms; use of care bundles or evidence-based protocols; the impact of staffing issues on HAIs

- Use of alcohol-based handrubs with *Clostridium difficile* (*C diff*)
- ANA recommendations on reducing use of restraints
- Periop: "never events," new guidelines for preop fasting and skin prep
- The Joint Commission (TJC) universal protocol and "time-out"
- Noise prevention in acute care and ICU
- TJC Sentinel Alert on fatigue in health care workers
- Role of Pain Resource Nurse
- New content on gender dysphoria and intersex
- Expanded content on sensory changes associated with aging
- TJC 2014 National Patient Safety Goals
- SBAR/SBARR communication to improve patient "hand-offs" from one professional caregiver to another
- Updated ANA Standards of Practice, International Council of Nurses (ICN) Definition of Nursing, and *Healthy People 2020*
- ANA Principles of Delegation
- Purnell Model of Cultural Competence
- Social media guidelines
- Updated content on "Do Not Use" Abbreviations, Institute for Safe Medication Practices (ISMP) error prone abbreviations
- Updated variance reports
- Enhanced content on impaired nurses
- Updated information on electronic medical records (EMRs), new information technologies, and privacy considerations
- Inclusion of PUSH tool to assess/document pressure ulcer healing
- Dietary Reference Intakes (DRIs)
- My Plate food guidance system

Self-Assessment Guides

Fundamentals of Nursing has always encouraged students to be independent learners. Checklists throughout the text (e.g., blended skills assessment, use of nursing process, health assessments) allow students to evaluate their personal strengths and limitations and develop related learning goals.

SPECIAL FEATURES

Many features appear throughout the text to help students grasp important content. Refer to the "How to Use *Fundamentals of Nursing*" section on pages xiv–xx to learn more about them.

A FULLY INTEGRATED COURSE EXPERIENCE

We are delighted to introduce an expanded suite of digital solutions and ancillaries to support instructors and students using *Fundamentals of Nursing: The Art and Science of Person-Centered Nursing Care, Eighth Edition*. To learn more about any solution with the Taylor suite, please contact your local Wolters Kluwer representative.

Lippincott **CoursePoint**

Lippincott CoursePoint: An Adaptive Learning Experience

Lippincott CoursePoint is a fully adaptive and integrated digital course solution for nursing education. CoursePoint synthesizes adaptive learning tools and content with an electronic version of the text and a wide array of integrated learning aids—all in one convenient location.

At the heart of CoursePoint is our adaptive learning system, powered by prepU. In numerous studies, prepU has demonstrated improved student performance in both nursing courses and on the NCLEX. CoursePoint extends prepU's adaptive tools by connecting students to the resources that will help them *understand* the correct answers, with quiz results linked to relevant sections of the *Fundamentals of Nursing* integrated eBook as well as videos, animations, interactive tutorials, and practice and learn case studies via SmartSense links.

As the instructor, you have everything you need to develop your course, with easily accessible resources, organized by type or chapter, including:

- **Lippincott Test Generator** (1,500 test items)
- **Pre-Lecture Quizzes** (and answers) in Microsoft Word
- **New Detailed Lesson Plans**
- **PowerPoint Presentations** with integrated multiple-choice questions
- **Textbook Image Bank**
- **Guided Lecture Notes**
- **Suggested Discussion Topics**
- **Assignments** (and answers)
- **Case Studies** (with questions and answers)
- **A sample Syllabus**
- **Articles from Wolters Kluwer journals**
- **QSEN Competency KSAs, mapped to the text**
- **Master Checklist for Skills Competency**

CoursePoint's instructor reporting tools enable you to monitor individual student and class progress and strengths and weaknesses.

Lippincott **CoursePoint+**

Lippincott CoursePoint+

Available in Fall of 2015, Lippincott CoursePoint+ takes learning one step further by integrating additional skills and simulation tools within the CoursePoint platform.

vSim for Nursing
SIMULATION, SKILLS, AND VIDEO RESOURCES

- *vSim for Nursing | Fundamentals*, a new virtual simulation platform (*available via thePoint*). Co-developed by Laerdal Medical and Wolters Kluwer, *vSim for Nursing |*

Fundamentals helps students develop clinical competence and decision-making skills as they interact with virtual patients in a safe, realistic environment. *vSim for Nursing* records and assesses student decisions throughout the simulation, then provides a personalized feedback log highlighting areas needing improvement.

- *Taylor's Video Guide to Clinical Nursing Skills* (*available via thePoint or DVD*). With more than 12 hours of video footage, this updated series follows nursing students and their instructors as they perform a range of essential nursing procedures. Institutions can purchase the videos on enhanced DVD or access them online.

- DocuCare **Lippincott DocuCare** (available via thePoint). Lippincott DocuCare combines web-based electronic health record simulation software with clinical case scenarios that link directly to many of the skills presented in Taylor's *Fundamentals of Nursing*. Lippincott DocuCare's nonlinear solution works well in the classroom, simulation lab, and clinical practice.

- *Skill Checklists for Fundamentals of Nursing: The Art and Science of Person-Centered Nursing Care, Eighth Edition* (*available in print or via Lippincott CoursePoint*). This workbook offers step-by-step summaries of all of the essential skills covered in the textbook, in an easy-to-use format.

- *Taylor's Clinical Nursing Skills, Fourth Edition*, by **Pamela Lynn, MSN, RN** (*available in print or eBook*) covers all of the *Skills* and *Guidelines for Nursing Care* identified in *Fundamentals of Nursing, Eighth Edition*—plus additional skills—at the basic, intermediate, and advanced levels, each following the nursing process format. Features include Skill Variations, which present alternate techniques; Documentation Guidelines and Samples; Unexpected Situations and Associated Interventions; Delegation Considerations; and Special Considerations.

- *Taylor's Handbook of Clinical Nursing Skills, Second Edition*, by **Pamela Lynn, MSN, RN** (*available in print*). This easy-to-use quick reference provides streamlined skills consistent with those in *Taylor's Clinical Nursing Skills, Fourth Edition*. Presented for quick reference or on-the-go review, skills are organized alphabetically by key word.

- *Skill Checklists for Taylor's Clinical Nursing Skills, Fourth Edition* (*available in print*). This collection of checklists with convenient perforated pages is designed to accompany *Taylor's Clinical Nursing Skills, Fourth Edition*, and promote proper technique while increasing confidence.

ADDITIONAL MEDIA AND PRINT RESOURCES

A wide variety of resources are available to enhance the learning experience. Visit http://www.lww.com for purchasing options.

- *Study Guide for Fundamentals of Nursing, Eighth Edition* contains a wealth of exercises and study review tools, including hundreds of NCLEX-style questions. ISBN: 978-1-4511-9272-8

- prepU **prepU for *Fundamentals of Nursing, Eighth Edition*** includes personalized, adaptive quizzes linked to Taylor's textbook content that fosters formative assessment for students and instructors. ISBN: 978-1-4698-8177-5

- NCLEX-RN PassPoint **Lippincott PassPoint for the NCLEX, powered by prepU** is an online, adaptive learning NCLEX preparation resource that allows students to take practice quizzes and comprehensive NCLEX-style exams. ISBN: 978-1-4698-0935-9

- thePoint **Student Web Site** (*Free to students who purchase a new copy of Fundamentals of Nursing, Eighth Edition*). Visit http://thepoint.lww.com/Taylor8e using the one time activation code in the front of your book to discover a wealth of information and activities, including chapter key concepts and NCLEX-style review questions. See the full listing of Student Resources available on thePoint in the front of your book.

Additional Instructor Assessment and Preparation Resources

The following teaching resources are available on thePoint for instructors who adopt Fundamentals of Nursing, Eighth Edition:

- Lippincott Test Generator (with 1,500 questions)
- New Lesson Plans
- Pre-Lecture Quizzes (and answers)
- PowerPoint Presentations
- Textbook Image Bank
- Suggested Discussion Topics (and answers)
- Assignments (and answers)
- Case Studies
- A sample Syllabus
- Articles from Wolters Kluwer journals
- QSEN Competency KSAs, mapped to the text
- Master Checklist for Skills Competency

Instructors may also download a Learning Management System cartridge for Blackboard Learn (ANGEL/WebCT/Blackboard) that includes all instructor materials for Taylor. Contact your sales representative or our product support team (1-800-468-1128 or techsupp@lww.com) for assistance.

How to Use *Fundamentals of Nursing*

Dear Student,

Congratulations on choosing an exciting and rewarding profession! All of us who have been part of the writing of this text welcome you warmly to our profession and prize our role as your guides to excellent practice. We have tried in this text to present in a readable and enjoyable format the scientific and technical knowledge you will need to design safe and effective nursing care. But we want to do more than prepare you intellectually and technically. You will also find narratives that will teach you valuable interpersonal skills and content specifically designed to prepare you to meet the ethical and legal challenges in today's practice. So take a deep breath and dig in. Your patients are counting on you and so are we!

Carol Taylor, Carol Lillis, and Pamela Lynn

HERE'S HOW TO GET STARTED!

FOLLOW THE STORY LINES!

Get to know your patients by reading the chapter opening **Case Scenarios**.

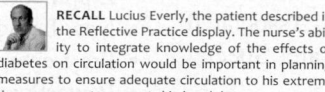

LUCIUS EVERLY

Lucius, a 52-year-old man who has a history of diabetes and circulatory problems, underwent abdominal surgery several days ago and is in the critical care unit. He is slouched down in bed; his abdominal dressing is moist and only part of the tape securing the dressing is adhering to the skin. His level of consciousness is decreased, and he responds only to moderate touch and pain. Further assessment reveals the pressure ulcer on his heel.

Narratives throughout the chapter refer back to these scenarios, helping you to consider how the chapter content applies to care of real patients.

healing. Circulation may be impaired in older adults and in people with peripheral vascular disorders, cardiovascular disorders, hypertension, or diabetes mellitus. Oxygenation of tissues is decreased in people with anemia or chronic respiratory disorders and in those who smoke.

RECALL Lucius Everly, the patient described in the Reflective Practice display. The nurse's ability to integrate knowledge of the effects of diabetes on circulation would be important in planning measures to ensure adequate circulation to his extremities as a means to prevent skin breakdown. ●

In addition, large amounts of subcutaneous and tissue fat (which has fewer blood vessels) in people who are obese may slow wound healing because fatty tissue is more difficult to suture, is more prone to infection, and takes longer to heal.

GET READY TO LEARN!

Before reading the chapter content, read the **Learning Objectives**. These roadmaps help you understand what is important and why. Create your own learning outline or use them for self-testing.

LEARNING OBJECTIVES

After completing the chapter, you will be able to accomplish the following:

1. Discuss the processes involved in wound healing.
2. Identify factors that affect wound healing.
3. Identify patients at risk for pressure ulcer development.
4. Describe the method of staging of pressure ulcers.
5. Accurately assess and document the condition of wounds.
6. Provide nursing interventions to prevent pressure ulcers.
7. Implement appropriate dressing changes for different kinds of wounds.
8. Provide information to patients and caregivers for self-care of wounds at home.
9. Apply hot and cold therapy effectively and safely.

Review the **Key Terms** lists to become familiar with new vocabulary presented throughout the narrative. Look for them in **bold type** throughout the chapter and use the Glossary at the end of the book to review their meaning.

KEY TERMS

bandage
biofilm
débridement
dehiscence
dermis
desiccation
dressing
epidermis
epithelialization
eschar
evisceration
exudate

fistula
friction
granulation tissue
ischemia
maceration
necrosis
negative-pressure wound therapy (NPWT)
pressure ulcer
purulent drainage

sanguineous drainage
scar
serosanguineous drainage
serous drainage
shear
sinus tract
subcutaneous tissue
wound

DEVELOP CRITICAL THINKING AND CLINICAL REASONING SKILLS!

Read **Reflective Practice** boxes and discover how other nursing students confront challenging situations (cognitive, technical, interpersonal, or ethical/legal). What course of action did the student take? Would you do the same? Reflect on how you would respond to similar situations while developing QSEN competencies.

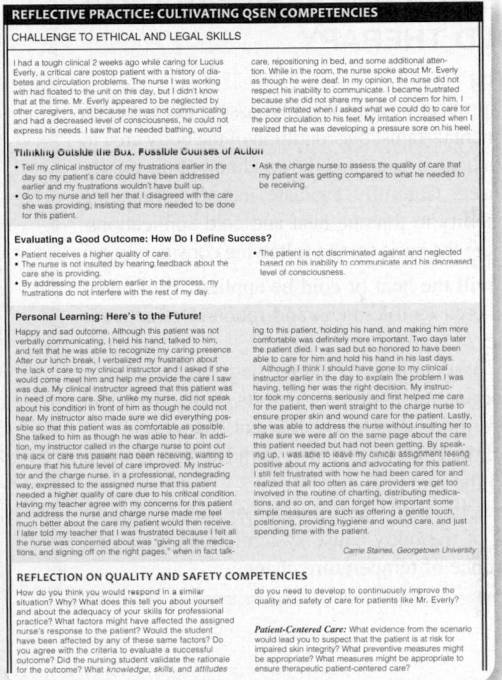

REFLECTIVE PRACTICE: CULTIVATING QSEN COMPETENCIES

CHALLENGE TO ETHICAL AND LEGAL SKILLS

I had a tough clinical 2 weeks ago when caring for Lucius Everly, a critical care postop patient with a history of diabetes and circulation problems. The nurse I was working with had floated to the unit on this day, but I didn't know that at the time. Mr. Everly appeared to be neglected by other caregivers, and because he was not communicating and had a decreased level of consciousness, he could not express his needs. I saw that he needed bathing, wound care, repositioning in bed, and some additional attention. While in the room, the nurse spoke about Mr. Everly as though he were deaf. In my opinion, the nurse did not respect his right to communicate. I became frustrated because she did not share my sense of concern for him. I became irritated when I asked what we could do to care for the poor circulation to his feet. My irritation increased when I realized that he was developing a pressure sore on his heel.

Thinking Outside the Box: Possible Courses of Action

- Tell my clinical instructor of my frustrations earlier in the day so my patient's care could have been addressed earlier and my frustrations wouldn't have built up.
- Go to my nurse and tell her that I disagreed with the care she was providing, insisting that more needed to be done for this patient.
- Ask the charge nurse to assess the quality of care that my patient was getting compared to what he needed to be receiving.

Evaluating a Good Outcome: How Do I Define Success?

- Patient receives a higher quality of care.
- The nurse is not insulted by hearing feedback about the care she is providing.
- By addressing the problem earlier in the process, my frustrations do not interfere with the rest of my day.
- The patient is not discriminated against and neglected based on his inability to communicate and his decreased level of consciousness.

Personal Learning: Here's to the Future!

Happy and sad outcome. Although this patient was not verbally communicating, I held his hand, talked to him, and felt that he was able to recognize my caring presence. After our lunch break, I verbalized my frustration about the lack of care to my clinical instructor and I asked if she would come meet him and help me provide the care I saw was due. My clinical instructor agreed that this patient was in need of more care. She, unlike my nurse, did not speak about his condition in front of him as though he could not hear. My instructor also made sure we did everything possible so that this patient was as comfortable as possible. She talked to him as though he was able to hear. In addition, my instructor called in the charge nurse to point out the lack of care this patient had been receiving, wanting to ensure that his future level of care improved. My instructor and the charge nurse, in a professional, nondegrading way, expressed to the assigned nurse that this patient needed a higher quality of care due to his critical condition. Having my teacher agree with my concerns for this patient and address the nurse and charge nurse made me feel much better about the care my patient would then receive. I later told my teacher that I was frustrated because I felt all the nurse was concerned about was "giving all the medications, and signing off on the right pages," when in fact talking to this patient, holding his hand, and making him more comfortable was definitely more important. Two days later the patient died. I was sad but so honored to have been able to care for him and hold his hand in his last days.

Although I think I should have gone to my clinical instructor earlier in the day to explain the problem I was having, telling her was the right decision. My instructor took my concerns seriously and first helped me care for the patient, then went straight to the charge nurse to ensure proper skin and wound care for the patient. Lastly, she was able to address the nurse without insulting her to make sure we were all on the same page about the care this patient needed but had not been getting. By speaking up, I was able to leave my clinical assignment feeling positive about my actions and advocating for this patient. I still felt frustrated with how he had been cared for and realized that all too often as care providers we get too involved in the routine of charting, distributing medications, and so on, and can forget how important some simple measures such as offering a gentle touch, positioning, providing hygiene and wound care, and just spending time with the patient.

Carrie Staines, Georgetown University

REFLECTION ON QUALITY AND SAFETY COMPETENCIES

How do you think you would respond in a similar situation? Why? What does this tell you about yourself and about the adequacy of your skills for professional practice? What factors might have affected the assigned nurse's response to the patient? Would the student have been affected by any of these same factors? Do you agree with the criteria to evaluate a successful outcome? Did the nursing student validate the rationale for the outcome? What knowledge, skills, and attitudes do you need to develop to continuously improve the quality and safety of care for patients like Mr. Everly?

Patient-Centered Care: What evidence from the scenario would lead you to suspect that the patient is at risk for impaired skin integrity? What preventive measures might be appropriate? What measures might be appropriate to ensure therapeutic patient-centered care?

FOCUSED CRITICAL THINKING GUIDE 31-1

WOUND CARE: PROMOTING ACCEPTANCE OF CHANGES IN BODY IMAGE

During both clinical days in 1 week, you (a female student) have been assigned to care for a middle-aged woman who has had a breast removed because of cancer. The patient, Mrs. Nola, is an attractive woman who is usually cheerful and eager to get better and return home. However, on both days, she turned her head away and would not look at the incision when her dressing was changed. She tells you that she "just can't stand to look at herself." Her husband has left the room during the dressing changes after telling you that "it makes me sick to see what happened to my wife." Mrs. Nola is to be discharged to her home the next day and needs to learn how to provide self-care for her wound. What do you do?

1. Identify goal of thinking

Determine the most effective way of ensuring wound care and at the same time assisting Mrs. Nola in accepting her altered self-image.

2. Assess adequacy of knowledge

Pertinent circumstances: The diagnosis of cancer was made only 1 day before the surgical removal of the breast. The patient is to be discharged to her home the next day. The wound from her mastectomy has not completely healed and will require dressing changes for another 3 or 4 days. Mrs. Nola has had a disfiguring surgery and is coping with not only a change in body image, but also the diagnosis of cancer. She has never been seriously ill or had surgery. She has a strong, loving relationship with her husband, but he is unable to deal with the physical disfigurement at this time.

Prerequisite knowledge: Before you decide what to do in this situation, you need to know at what level Mrs. Nola is in coping with the diagnosis of cancer. If she is still in denial about the disease, it is likely that she is also denying the surgical procedure and the changes in her body. You will need to review responses to the diagnosis of cancer as well as the stages of grief and loss. You will have to learn what her sources of support are and how she can best access and use them. You will need to assess how best to help her achieve wound care in the face of her continued refusal even to look at the wound.

Room for error: If she is forced to look at the wound or made to feel inadequate because of her inability to do so, she will feel threatened and most likely will become angry in response to the perceived threat.

Time constraints: Some decision about wound care must be made before her discharge the next day.

3. Address potential problems

There are several potential obstacles to critical thinking in this situation. As a student, you want to exhibit safe, knowledgeable care, and the importance of teaching for home care has been an emphasis in this course. As a woman, you have a sense of what the loss of a breast must mean. Having had a family member die of cancer, you find yourself wanting to do everything for Mrs. Nola. As a novice in nursing, you find it difficult to handle these emotional components of patient care and find yourself wanting to scold both the patient and her husband for being so silly about something as simple as a dressing.

4. Consult helpful resources

You must first understand the loss and grief Mrs. Nola is experiencing, and you must then relate that to her response to self-care of the wound. Your best source of information about her coping methods and sources of personal strength is Mrs. Nola herself. You also discuss the most effective way of providing wound care at home with your instructor and the case manager for Mrs. Nola.

5. Critique judgment/decision

After talking to Mrs. Nola, your instructor, and the case manager, you mutually agree that Mrs. Nola cannot be hurried into acceptance of her medical diagnosis or her body changes. The case manager consults with Mrs. Nola's physician, who writes an order for a home health care nurse to visit for the next 4 days and complete the dressing change. After talking with Mrs. Nola, you identify that she is still very much in denial. You discuss with her the possibility of having a visitor from "Reach to Recovery," a support group for women with breast cancer who have had a mastectomy. Mrs. Nola tells you that she thinks she would like to talk to someone with the same problem, and you call a referral for her. When you tell Mrs. Nola that a home health care nurse will be visiting her for the first few days at home to change her dressing, tears come into her eyes. She says "I am so scared, I just don't know what to do." You realize that insisting that Mrs. Nola do her own dressing would have been extremely stressful for her and that you would have considered the wound as more important than the patient. When you share the situation in post-conference, your clinical group supports your decision.

Learn how careful thinking can change patient outcomes. Like nursing care, careful thinking and reflective practice follow a process. Study the **Focused Critical Thinking Guides** to gain skill in working through the step-by-step critical thinking process.

Challenge yourself! Use the new knowledge you've gained to "think through" learning exercises in the **Developing Clinical Reasoning** section at the end of each chapter.

MASTER NURSING PROCESS!

Throughout the clinical chapters, you will find many ways to help you visualize and understand the nursing process.

THE NURSING PROCESS FOR HEAT AND COLD THERAPY
Assessing

Before initiating heat or cold therapy, assess the patient's physical and mental status, the condition of the body area to be treated with heat or cold, and the condition of the equipment to be used. Carefully evaluate factors influencing the patient's ability to tolerate heat and cold applications. These factors are the basis for the following considerations:

• How long will the heat or cold be applied? Prolonged exposure increases tolerance, and rebound effects are undesirable.
• What body part is involved? Some body areas, such as the neck, perineum, and inner aspects of the wrist and forearm, are more sensitive to thermal changes.
• Is the skin intact? Open tissue or abraded skin is more sensitive to thermal changes.
• How large is the area? Applications of heat or cold to large areas of the body cause systemic responses and lower tolerance of temperature change.

Follow the step-by-step organization of the **Nursing Process section** to understand nursing responsibilities.

Examine the **Nursing Plan of Care** box (derived from the chapter opener cases) to discover common health problems and the wide variety of independent and collaborative interventions that nurses manage.

NURSING PLAN OF CARE 31-1

for Mary Biesicker

Mary Biesicker, who is 84 years of age, has been cared for at home by her daughter since being hospitalized last year for a stroke. During the past several months, Mary has been confined to her bed, has had minimal appetite, and has occasionally been confused and disoriented. During the past week, she has had several episodes of bowel and bladder incontinence. Her daughter also reports that Mary has developed a "blister on her lower back at the end of her backbone." She is scheduled for an assessment visit by the nurse from a local home health care agency because her daughter is finding it increasingly difficult to care for her mother alone.

The nurse's initial assessment of Mary, relative to skin integrity, revealed the following:

Skin status: Presence of a nickel-sized open area on the sacrum (stage II pressure ulcer), 2 cm in diameter and 1 cm in depth. No abnormal pathways noted. Reddened area (0.5 cm) surrounding lesion. No drainage noted. Reddened area (2.5 cm) also noted on right elbow. Skin dry over all body surfaces.
Nutritional status: Daughter states, "usual weight is 115 to 120 lb, and she has definitely lost some weight." Poor skin turgor.
Elimination status: Wearing "adult diaper," diaper damp with urine and small amount of light brown liquid stool.
Activity status: Lying quietly in bed, moans when area around lesion is palpated.

NURSING DIAGNOSIS	Impaired Skin Integrity related to mechanical factors, inactivity, altered nutritional intake, and incontinence as manifested by stage II pressure ulcer on sacral area and reddened area on right elbow
EXPECTED OUTCOME	6/6/15—at weekly visit, the patient will: • Experience reduction of pressure on bony prominences (absence of any additional reddened areas)

NURSING INTERVENTIONS	RATIONALE	EVALUATIVE STATEMENT
Assess skin for development of any pressure areas (use agency tool).	Pressure results in poor circulation that causes skin breakdown.	6/13/15 Outcome met. Patient has been turned from side to side every 2 hours. Reddened area on right elbow measures 1.25 cm in diameter. No new reddened areas observed.
Avoid sitting or lying on a pressure ulcer.	This facilitates pressure relief in the area and allows blood to reenter capillaries and provide oxygen to the area.	
Reposition from side to side at least every 2 hours.	The duration of pressure is more devastating to skin than the amount of pressure.	*Recommendation:* Arrange for delivery of hospital bed with over-bed trapeze setup. Secure a home health care aide for limited period of time to assist with repositioning during the night and allow daughter time to rest.
Use pillows to maintain side-lying or oblique position in bed and support right elbow off bed surface.	Pillows relieve pressure on lesion and areas at risk and promote improved circulation to those areas.	
Place foam overlay mattress on bed.	Static device provides support and relieves pressure on skin surface.	M. Lieb, RN

EXPECTED OUTCOME	6/6/15—at weekly visit, the patient will: • Demonstrate a reduction in the size of the stage II pressure ulcer on sacrum

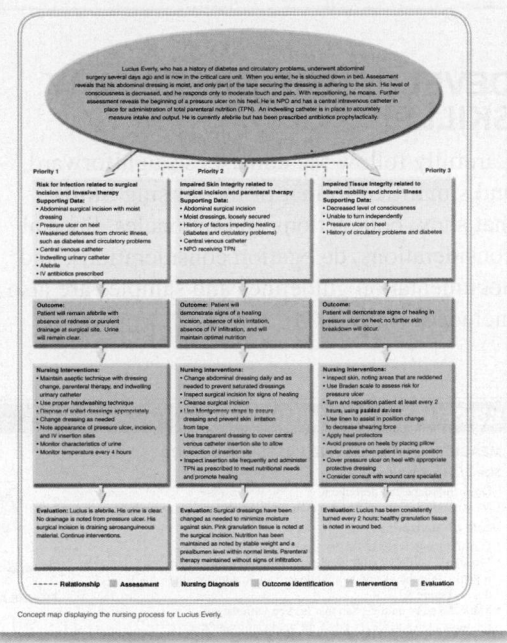

Concept map displaying the nursing process for Lucius Everly.

View the **Concept Map** (from selected chapter opener cases) to see how the nursing process can be visually represented when planning care for a patient.

Then use these tools to further develop your nursing process skills:

FOCUSED ASSESSMENT GUIDE 31-1

SKIN INTEGRITY

Factors to Assess	Questions and Approaches
Appearance of skin	• Do you have any skin areas that are discolored? • Do some areas of skin on your body feel warmer or colder than others? • Describe the moisture in your skin: is it damp, dry, oily? • Have you noticed that your skin seems to be thinner? Where? • Have you noticed any swelling in your feet, ankles, or fingers? • Tell me about how you take care of your skin. For example, do you take a tub bath or shower? How often? Do you use oils or lotions?
Recent changes in skin	• Do you have any sores on your body? If so, how many, and where are they? Have they changed in size? Do you have any drainage from them? • Have you noticed that the skin over your hips or backbone gets red if you sit or lie in one position for a long time? Does this disappear in a short time when you are up? • Have you gotten a piercing or tattoo recently?

Focused Assessment Guides with sample interview questions will help strengthen your assessment skills.

EXAMPLES OF NANDA-I NURSING DIAGNOSES

PATIENT WITH A WOUND OR PRESSURE ULCER

Nursing Diagnoses	Related Factors	Sample Defining Characteristics
Impaired Skin Integrity	Any condition that alters the dermis and/or epidermis, such as a surgical incision or traumatic wound; moisture, physical immobilization	• Presence of intentional or unintentional wound; disruption of skin surface • Presence of a pressure ulcer; destruction of skin layers
Risk for Infection	Any condition that interferes with the normal inflammatory healing process or provides an entry for infectious agents	Risk factors: • Disruption in skin integrity • Immunosuppression • Chronic disease (such as diabetes mellitus or obesity) • Extremes of age • Malnutrition • Presence of drains, tubes, or catheters

Examples of NANDA-I Nursing Diagnoses teach you how to develop and write diagnostic statements.

EXAMPLES OF NURSING INTERVENTIONS AND NURSING OUTCOMES CLASSIFICATIONS (NIC/NOC)

RISK FOR IMPAIRED SKIN INTEGRITY

Nursing Interventions	Nursing Outcomes
• Bed Rest Care • Incision Site Care • Wound Care • Pressure Management • Pressure Ulcer Prevention • Skin Surveillance	• Tissue Integrity: Skin and Mucous Membranes • Immobility Consequences: Physiological

Examples of Nursing Interventions and Nursing Outcomes Classifications (NIC/NOC) boxes help you select, implement, and evaluate appropriate nursing interventions and outcomes.

DEVELOP THE NECESSARY SKILLS!

Carefully follow the concise, straightforward, and simplified format of the nursing **Skills** that show both actions and rationales. Special considerations, delegation considerations, and documentation guidelines and samples are also included.

SKILL 31-1 CLEANING A WOUND AND APPLYING A DRY, STERILE DRESSING

DELEGATION CONSIDERATIONS	Wound care and procedures requiring the use of a sterile field and other sterile items are not delegated to nursing assistive personnel (NAP) or unlicensed assistive personnel (UAP). Depending on the state's nurse practice act and the organization's policies and procedures, these procedures may be delegated to licensed practical/vocational nurses (LPNs/LVNs). The decision to delegate must be based on careful analysis of the patient's needs and circumstances, as well as the qualifications of the person to whom the task is being delegated. Refer to the Delegation Guidelines in Appendix A (found on thePoint).
EQUIPMENT	• Sterile gloves • Clean disposable gloves • Additional PPE, as indicated • Gauze dressings • Surgical or abdominal pads • Sterile dressing set or suture set (for the sterile scissors and forceps) • Sterile cleaning solution as ordered (commonly 0.9% normal saline solution, or a commercially prepared wound cleanser) • Sterile basin (may be optional) • Sterile drape (may be optional) • Plastic bag or other appropriate waste container for soiled dressings • Waterproof pad and bath blanket • Tape or ties • Bath blanket or other linens for draping patient • Additional dressings and supplies needed or required by the primary care provider's order

GUIDELINES FOR NURSING CARE 31-1

MEASURING WOUNDS AND PRESSURE ULCERS

Size of the Wound
• Draw the shape and describe it.
• Measure the length, width, and diameter (if circular).

Depth of the Wound
• Perform hand hygiene. Put on gloves.
• Moisten a sterile, flexible applicator with saline and insert it gently into the wound at a 90-degree angle with the tip down (Figure A).
• Mark the point on the swab that is even with the surrounding skin surface, or grasp the applicator with the thumb and forefinger at the point corresponding to the wound's margin (Figure B).
• Remove the swab and measure the depth with a ruler (Figure C).

Wound Tunneling
• Use standard precautions; use appropriate transmission-based precautions when indicated.
• Perform hand hygiene. Put on gloves.
• Determine direction: Moisten a sterile, flexible applicator with saline and gently insert a sterile applicator into the site where tunneling occurs. View the direction of the applicator as if it were the hand of a clock (Figure D). The direction of the patient's head represents 12 o'clock. Moving in a clockwise direction, document the deepest sites where the wound tunnels.

FIGURE A

FIGURE B

FIGURE C

Guidelines for Nursing Care outline important points to remember in practice and will help you gain competence in performing nursing skills.

Many skills and guidelines have free accompanying video clips, indicated by the **Watch & Learn** icon, or free accompanying activities, indicated by the **Practice & Learn** icon. All of these are available on thePoint website at http://thePoint.lww.com/Taylor8e.

PROMOTE HEALTH AND WELLNESS!

Learn not only to treat illness but also to promote the health and wellness of your patients.

Check out the **Promoting Health** boxes, which include assessment checkpoints for specific health and wellness topics and suggestions for designing a self-care prescription.

Use the **Promoting Health Literacy** boxes to help identify patients and families at risk for poor health outcomes and discover the key questions that all patients should ask their providers.

Develop appropriate nurse–patient communication using **Teaching Tips** boxes to help improve your patient's and family's outcomes.

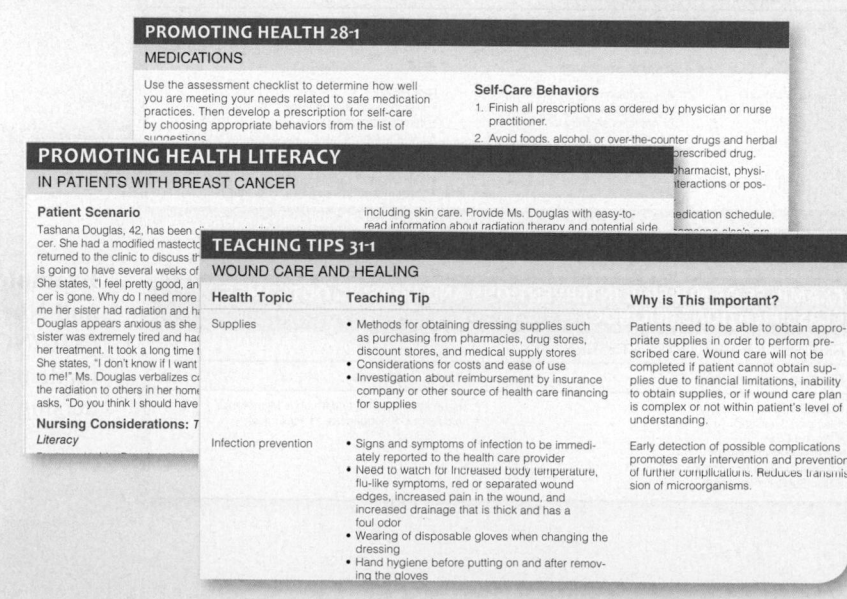

PROMOTING HEALTH 28-1

MEDICATIONS

Use the assessment checklist to determine how well you are meeting your needs related to safe medication practices. Then develop a prescription for self-care by choosing appropriate behaviors from the list of suggestions.

Self-Care Behaviors
1. Finish all prescriptions as ordered by physician or nurse practitioner.
2. Avoid foods, alcohol, or over-the-counter drugs and herbal ... prescribed drug. ... pharmacist, physi- ...teractions or pos- ... medication schedule. ...

PROMOTING HEALTH LITERACY

IN PATIENTS WITH BREAST CANCER

Patient Scenario
Tashana Douglas, 42, has been d... cer. She had a modified mastecto... returned to the clinic to discuss th... is going to have several weeks of... She states, "I feel pretty good, an... cer is gone. Why do I need more... me her sister had radiation and h... Douglas appears anxious as she... sister was extremely tired and ha... her treatment. It took a long time t... She states, "I don't know if I want... to me!" Ms. Douglas verbalizes co... the radiation to others in her home... asks, "Do you think I should have...

Nursing Considerations: T... Literacy

including skin care. Provide Ms. Douglas with easy-to-read information about radiation therapy and potential side ...

TEACHING TIPS 31-1

WOUND CARE AND HEALING

Health Topic	Teaching Tip	Why is This Important?
Supplies	• Methods for obtaining dressing supplies such as purchasing from pharmacies, drug stores, discount stores, and medical supply stores • Considerations for costs and ease of use • Investigation about reimbursement by insurance company or other source of health care financing for supplies	Patients need to be able to obtain appropriate supplies in order to perform prescribed care. Wound care will not be completed if patient cannot obtain supplies due to financial limitations, inability to obtain supplies, or if wound care plan is complex or not within patient's level of understanding.
Infection prevention	• Signs and symptoms of infection to be immediately reported to the health care provider • Need to watch for increased body temperature, flu-like symptoms, red or separated wound edges, increased pain in the wound, and increased drainage that is thick and has a foul odor • Wearing of disposable gloves when changing the dressing • Hand hygiene before putting on and after removing the gloves	Early detection of possible complications promotes early intervention and prevention of further complications. Reduces transmission of microorganisms.

BE A PATIENT ADVOCATE!

Read the scenarios in the **Nursing Advocacy in Action** boxes and learn how you can advocate for vulnerable individuals.

Consider the special needs of the older adult with the **Focus on the Older Adult** boxes

NURSING ADVOCACY IN ACTION

Patient Scenario

Alex is a 28-year-old man admitted to the surgical intensive care unit after undergoing a partial gastric bypass surgical procedure. He originally weighed 700 lbs but lost 100 lbs...

we take a risk of hurting ourselves when he obviously doesn't care?"
- "His mother told the charge nurse yesterday that caregivers were making comments related to his size and were ...ity of care as they gave to...

...Advocacy

...e Alex's nurse? Talk with your ...nurses about the questions

...Alex, what practical steps can ...ith outcomes?

...t of a student nurse, a gradu-...ed nurse in this situation?

...eeded to effectively respond to...

FOCUS ON THE OLDER ADULT

NURSING STRATEGIES TO ADDRESS AGE-RELATED CHANGES IN SKIN

Age-Related Changes	Nursing Strategies
Subcutaneous and dermal tissue become thin: • Skin is more easily injured. • Skin has less capacity to insulate. • Skin wrinkles more easily. • Sensation of pressure and pain is reduced.	• Do not apply tape to skin unless necessary. • Check skin frequently to observe for any signs of a pressure ulcer. • Pad bony prominences if necessary. • Assess pressure tolerance by checking pressure points for redness after 30 minutes.
Activity of the sebaceous and sweat glands decreases: • Skin becomes dryer. • Pruritus (itching) may occur.	• Clean perineal area daily but do not bathe full body on a daily basis. • Apply lotions as needed. • Encourage adequate hydration.
Cell renewal is shorter: • Healing time is delayed.	• Perform careful skin assessments, looking for signs of skin breakdown.
Melanocytes (cells that make the pigment that colors hair and skin) decline in number: • Hair becomes gray-white. • Skin may be unevenly pigmented.	• Assist patient with skin checks, observing for any signs of melanoma or other skin abnormalities.

THROUGH THE EYES OF A STUDENT

The first time I took care of a patient with "multiple tubes," I was horrified at the thought of actually touching the patient. I hadn't really been exposed to that many critically ill patients until my last semester as a student nurse. I remember being assigned a patient in the cardiothoracic intensive care unit. The patient was a "fresh heart"—a coronary artery bypass graft patient who had just been operated on that morning.

I remember walking into the room and thinking, "What do I do with all of these tubes?" and then with horror thinking, "What if one of them falls out?" Needless to say, I was overwhelmed and frightened but at the same time excited at the challenge that faced me. I asked my preceptor what

each tube was for and where it was hooked up and whether it would fall out if I touched it. She answered all my questions with patience and understanding and asked me if I wanted to handle the tubes. I looked at her as if she were insane, but went ahead and did it. Would you believe that nothing fell out! I must admit that the experience taught me a lot, but it also got me over the fear of tubes.

I now chuckle every time I see a nursing student's face with that same look of horror as I had, and I try to answer every question with the same degree of patience and understanding that my preceptor had for me.

—*Lynda L. Ullmer, RN, Gaithersburg, MD*

GAIN NEW INSIGHTS!

Students, patients, and family caregivers share their experiences in boxes entitled *Through the Eyes of a Student*, *Through the Eyes of a Patient*, and *Through the Eyes of a Family Caregiver*. These real-life stories demonstrate how nursing can make a difference in the lives of patients and their families.

EXAMINE THE EVIDENCE!

Gain insight into the "why" behind nursing care. Consider **Research in Nursing: Bridging the Gap to Evidence-Based Practice** boxes to discover recent findings in nursing care and relate their relevance to nursing practice.

Read the **PICO in Practice: Asking Clinical Questions** to think about how you can do a systematic search, formulate questions, and apply evidence-based answers in your practice by following the PICO model.

RESEARCH IN NURSING

BRIDGING THE GAP TO EVIDENCE-BASED PRACTICE

Accurate Assessment of Pressure Ulcers

Pressure ulcers are costly in terms of patient discomfort, disfigurement, decreased quality of life, fatalities, and health care expenditures. Nurses play an important role in accurate assessment of pressure ulcers, which is essential to providing appropriate and effective wound care.

Related Research

Alvey, B., Heard, H., & Hennen, N. (2012). Improving accuracy of

to test for differences between PU groups, including overall accuracy, accuracy in accepting the CCDS suggested stage, and accuracy when the override function was used. Nurses accurately staged PU photographs 64% of the time (79 of 123) during the simulation exercise by either accepting the CCDS-suggested stage or overriding the suggestion. Within the accurately staged PUs, nurses agreed with the CCDS-suggested stage 55% of the time (68 of 123). In the other 9% ...aged accurately by over-...n was based on incorrect ...gnificantly more accurate ...mpared to PU staged by ...concluded these findings ...g the CCDS to improve ...cause the characteristics ...d, the CCDS assigns the

PICO IN PRACTICE

ASKING CLINICAL QUESTIONS

Scenario: You are a staff nurse who works in a same-day surgery center. You are asked to serve as a preceptor for a newly hired nurse, Terri, who has just finished a nurses' refresher course at the local community college. Terri worked as a perioperative nurse for over 12 years, but her practice was on hiatus while she stayed at home to raise two children for the past 15 years. One day, Terri asks you why it is no longer standard practice to shave patients' surgical sites to prepare them for surgery. She notes to you that this was standard protocol for patients 15 years ago, and was thought to diminish the incidence of surgical site infections.

- POPULATION: Perioperative patients
- INTERVENTION: Surgical site shaving of hair
- COMPARISON: No surgical site shaving of hair
- OUTCOME: Lower rates of surgical site infections

PICO Question: Does preoperative shaving of the surgical site result in lower rates of surgical site infections?

Finding: From the Cochrane Collaboration: Tanner, J., Norrie, P., & Melen, K. (2011). Preoperative hair removal to reduce surgical site infections. *Cochrane Database of Systematic Reviews, 11,* CD004122.

Findings from this systematic review indicate that routine shaving of surgical sites is not associated with lower rates of surgical site infections and may pose a surgical site infection risk. If hair must be removed preoperatively from a surgical site, clippers are associated with lower rates of surgical site infections than razors.

Level of Evidence: Level I

Recommendation: You note to Terri that though shaving surgical sites may have been standard practice 15 years ago, this practice actually may pose a surgical site infection risk and is no longer advocated. If hair must be removed from a surgical site preoperatively, then clippers should be used rather than razors.

PREPARE FOR NCLEX!

Start preparing for NCLEX right from the beginning of your nursing education. The **Practicing for NCLEX** section at the end of each chapter uses the multiple-choice question format to test your knowledge of basic through complex concepts. Answers with rationales are provided for immediate reinforcement. Additional NCLEX-style Chapter Review Questions are available on thePoint website at http://thePoint.lww.com/Taylor8e.

Lippincott
NCLEX-RN PassPoint

You may also be interested in Lippincott PassPoint, our adaptive, online NCLEX-preparation tool. Through PassPoint, you can take quizzes accessing thousands of NCLEX-style questions and even take simulated NCLEX questions that adapt to your answers—just like the real exam. To learn more about PassPoint, visit thePoint.lww.com/PassPoint. ISBN: 978-1-4698-0935-9

PRACTICING FOR NCLEX

1. Thirty-six hours after having surgery, a patient has a slightly elevated body temperature and generalized malaise, as well as pain and redness at the surgical site. Which intervention is most important to include in this patient's nursing care plan?
   a. Document the findings and continue to monitor the patient.
   b. Administer antipyretics, as ordered.
   c. Increase the frequency of assessment to every hour and notify the patient's primary care provider.
   d. Increase the frequency of wound care and contact the primary care provider for an antibiotic order.

2. A nurse caring for patients in the PACU teaches a novice nurse how to assess and document wound drainage. Which statements accurately describe a characteristic of wound drainage? Select all that apply.
   a. Serous drainage is composed of the clear portion of the blood and serous membranes.
   b. Sanguineous drainage is composed of a large number of red blood cells and looks like blood.
   c. Bright red sanguineous drainage indicates fresh bleeding and darker drainage indicates older bleeding.
   d. Purulent drainage is composed of white blood cells, dead tissue, and bacteria.
   e. Purulent drainage is thin, cloudy, and watery and may have a musty or foul odor.
   f. Serosanguineous drainage can be dark yellow or green depending on the causative organism.

 Concept Mastery Alert

A helpful way to remember which technique to use for wound care is this:
   Surgery occurs under sterile conditions, so surgical wounds = sterile technique; pressure ulcers = clean technique.

Concept Mastery Alerts highlight and clarify the most common misconceptions in nursing fundamentals, as identified by Lippincott's online adaptive learning platform. Our team reviewed data from thousands of fundamentals students across North America to identify the points of confusion for most students to help you learn more effectively.

COORDINATE YOUR STUDY PLAN!

From traditional texts to video and interactive products, the Taylor Fundamentals suite is tailored to fit every learning style. This integrated suite of products offers students a seamless learning experience you won't find anywhere else. Look for the **Taylor Suite Resources** listed at the end of every chapter to see what other parts of the Taylor Suite can help you learn, review, and apply knowledge and skills related to the chapter.

TAYLOR SUITE RESOURCES

Explore these additional resources to enhance learning for this chapter:
- NCLEX-Style Questions and other resources on thePoint, http://thePoint.lww.com/Taylor8e
- *Study Guide for Fundamentals of Nursing, 8th edition*
- Adaptive Learning | Powered by prepU, http://thepoint.lww.com/prepu
- *Skill Checklists for Fundamentals of Nursing, 8th edition*
- *Taylor's Clinical Nursing Skills:* Chapter 8, Skin Integrity and Wound Care
- *Taylor's Video Guide to Clinical Nursing Skills:* Skin Integrity and Wound Care

---

Lippincott CoursePoint
LIPPINCOTT COURSEPOINT

Powered by prepU, Lippincott's adaptive learning engine, CoursePoint allows you to study more efficiently and access our digital course content precisely when you need it. With CoursePoint, you can access hundreds of quiz questions for each chapter, as well as a complete electronic version of the textbook and valuable reference and study resources.

Acknowledgments

This revision is the work of many talented and committed people; we wish to gratefully acknowledge the assistance of all who have contributed in any way to the completion of this project. Our first debt of gratitude is to all the nurse educators and students who have adopted the text and shared with us their experiences in using the teaching and learning package. We are deeply grateful for their revision suggestions and trust they will enhance the learning experiences of others.

The work of this revision was capably facilitated by our Product Development Editor, Helen Kogut. She worked tirelessly behind the scenes to make sure that a superb, state-of-the-art product was delivered on time! Our very special thanks to her; Christine Abshire, Product Development Editor; Sherry Dickinson, Executive Editor; and to Tom Lochhaas and Sarah Kyle, Development Editors, for their hard work and guidance throughout the project. Thank you to the members of the Creative Services department, who brought a fresh look to the entire Taylor Suite of products: Holly Reid McLaughlin, Design Coordinator; and Jennifer Clements, Illustration Coordinator. The Instructional Services Consultants also deserve special thanks for their focus on our products to provide curriculum guidance, instructional design, technology support, and training. We also want to thank Marilee LeBon, who works creatively on many aspects of the teaching/learning package to ensure that faculty and students alike are getting the best resources to facilitate learning.

We thank all who generously gave their time, ideas, and resources, and we gratefully acknowledge the special contributions of the following:

- Rick Brady, Joe Mitchell, Ken Kasper, Barbara Proud, Gates Rhodes, and Kathy Sloane, photographers
- Marie Clark, who developed the math problems and solutions in the "Medications" chapter
- Kathleen Lucente, RN, MT, CIC, Infection Control Manager at Paoli Hospital, Paoli, Pennsylvania, for advising and updating us on changing infection-control protocols.

We gratefully acknowledge the influence of our mentors and teachers who have influenced our thoughts and writing; each person we have been privileged to care for as nurses; our students, who continually challenge us to find more effective means to teach nursing; our professional colleagues; and perhaps most important, our families and friends, whose love sustained us through the long hours of research and writing.

Contents

**UNIT
IV**

Promoting Health Across the Lifespan

UNIT
VII

Promoting Healthy Physiologic Responses

U N I T
VIII

Promoting Healthy Psychosocial Responses

Resources Available on the Point

Research in Nursing: Bridging the Gap to Evidence-Based Practice

Guidelines for Nursing Care

Foundations of Nursing Practice

*N*ursing is both an art and a science. It is a profession that uses specialized knowledge and skills to promote wellness and to provide care for people in both health and illness in a variety of practice settings. Unit I introduces concepts that provide the foundation for nursing practice by defining nursing as a whole. Chapters in this unit introduce the profession of nursing; theory, research, and evidence-based nursing practice; cultural diversity; health and illness; basic needs and health of individuals, their families, and the community; and ethical and legal implications for nursing practice.

Historical perspectives, educational preparation, professional organizations, and guidelines for professional nursing practice serve as a base for understanding what nursing is and how it is organized. Nursing theories and nursing research provide a foundation for evidence-based nursing practice, defining the rationale for nursing actions and offering a focus for nursing care. The diverse society in which nurses care for others mandates the ability to provide culturally competent care. An understanding of basic human needs and the individualized definitions of wellness and illness prepare the nurse to integrate the human dimensions—the physical, intellectual, emotional, sociocultural, spiritual, and environmental aspects of each person—into nursing care to promote wellness, prevent illness, restore health, and facilitate coping with altered function or death. Knowledge of the varied methods of care delivery is necessary in today's complex health care system. An understanding of the influence of values on human behavior and of the ethical dimensions of nursing practice is essential to responsible and accountable patient care. Finally, sensitivity to the legal implications of professional nursing practice is imperative in today's culture.

Unit I explores the foundations for nursing practice from both the perspective of the nurse and a holistic understanding of the patient. Students of nursing are introduced to a challenging and rewarding profession, and are provided with a knowledge base to ground the development of caregiving skills and professional relationships and behaviors.

Basic to any philosophy of nursing seems to be these three concepts: (1) reverence for the gift of life; (2) respect for the dignity, worth, autonomy, and individuality of each human being; (3) resolution to act dynamically in relation to one's beliefs."

Ernestine Wiedenbach (1900–1996) a faculty member at Yale University School of Nursing, where she developed her model of nursing from years of experience in various nursing positions

1

Introduction to Nursing

ROBERTO PECORINI

Roberto is a 38-year-old man diagnosed with metastatic colon cancer. Having undergone radiation treatments and chemotherapy, he is extremely weak and malnourished. He is receiving intravenous fluids via a central venous catheter. He has two pressure ulcers on his sacrum, each approximately 1½" in diameter, requiring wound care. He also has a colostomy that he cannot care for independently.

MICHELLE FINE

Michelle, a 19-year-old first-time mother who was discharged with her healthy 7-lb 8-oz baby girl 2 days ago, calls the nursery. She reports, "My baby isn't taking to my breast and she hasn't had any real feeding for 24 hours."

AHMAD BASSHIR

Ahmad, a 62-year-old male who is at risk for heart disease, is being taught about lifestyle modifications, such as diet and exercise. He states, "Just save your breath. Why should I bother about all that? I'd be better off dead than living like I am now, anyway!"

What is nursing? Consider the following examples of who nurses are and what they do:

- Delton Nix, RN, graduated from an associate degree nursing program 3 years ago. He is now working full-time as a staff nurse in a hospital medical unit while attending school part-time toward a baccalaureate degree in nursing; his goal is to become a nurse anesthetist.
- Jeiping Wu, RN, MSN, FNP, specializes as an advanced practice family nurse practitioner. She has an independent practice in a rural primary health clinic.
- Samuel Cohen, LPN, decided to follow his life's dream to become a nurse after 20 years as a postal worker. After examining all his options and goals, he completed a practical nursing program and is now a member of an emergency ambulance crew in a large city.
- Amy Orlando, RN, BSN, graduated 2 years ago and recently began a new job in an urban community health service.
- Roxanne McDaniel, RN, PhD, with a doctorate in nursing, teaches and conducts research at a large university.

These examples show how difficult it is to describe nursing simply. If everyone in your class were asked to complete the sentence, "Nursing is...," there would be many different responses because each person would answer based on his or her own personal experience and knowledge of nursing at that time. As you progress toward graduation and as you practice nursing after graduation, your own definition will reflect changes as you learn about and experience nursing.

Nursing is a profession focused on assisting individuals, families, and communities to attain, recover, and maintain optimum health and function from birth to old age. Nurses act as a bridge between an often extremely vulnerable public and the health care resources that can literally make the difference between life and death, health and disease/disability, and well-being and discomfort. Nursing care involves a wide range of activities, from carrying out complicated technical procedures to something as seemingly simple as holding a hand. Nursing is a blend of science and art. The science of nursing is the knowledge base for the care that is given, and the art of nursing is the skilled application of that knowledge to help others achieve maximum health and quality of life.

This chapter introduces you to nursing, including a brief history of nursing from its beginnings to the present, and provides the definitions and aims of nursing. In examining nursing as a profession, educational preparation, professional organizations, and guidelines for professional nursing practice are discussed to help you better understand what nursing is and how it is organized. (For an example demonstrating the importance of licensure to nursing practice and responsibilities, see the accompanying Reflective Practice box (on page 6)). Because nursing is a part of an ever-changing society, current trends in nursing also are discussed.

HISTORICAL PERSPECTIVES ON NURSING

Caregivers for those who were ill or injured have always been a part of history. The roles, settings, and responsibilities, however, have changed over time, as is summarized in the following section.

Development of Nursing from Early Civilizations to the 16th Century

Most early civilizations believed that illness had supernatural causes. The theory of animism attempted to explain the cause of mysterious changes in bodily functions. This theory was based on the belief that everything in nature was alive with invisible forces and endowed with power. Good spirits brought health; evil spirits brought sickness and death. In providing treatment, the roles of the physician and the nurse were separate and distinct. The physician was the medicine man who treated disease by chanting, inspiring fear, or opening the skull to release evil spirits (Dolan, Fitzpatrick, & Herrmann, 1983). The nurse usually was the mother who cared for her family during sickness by providing physical care and herbal remedies. This nurturing and caring role of the nurse has continued to the present.

As ancient Greek civilizations grew, temples became the centers of medical care because of the belief that illness was caused by sin and the gods' displeasure (*disease* literally means "dis-ease"). During the same period, the ancient Hebrews developed rules through the Ten Commandments and the Mosaic Health Code for ethical human relationships, mental health, and disease control. Nurses cared for sick people in the home and the community and also practiced as nurse–midwives (Dolan et al., 1983).

REFLECTIVE PRACTICE: CULTIVATING QSEN COMPETENCIES

CHALLENGE TO ETHICAL AND LEGAL SKILLS

During nursing school, I was working as a nurse's aide on a busy oncology unit. It was here that I met Roberto Pecorini, a 38-year-old man diagnosed with metastatic colon cancer. He had undergone radiation treatments and chemotherapy, and was extremely weak and malnourished. He was receiving numerous intravenous fluids via a central venous catheter. In addition, he had developed two pressure ulcers on his sacrum, each approximately 1½″ in diameter, that required wound care. He also had a colostomy that he could not care for independently.

Although the staff was very helpful, the orientation I received to the unit was brief because they were very short staffed. During one occasion, shortly after I had been oriented to the floor, I was working a night shift and was the only nurse's aide on the unit. The nurses I was working with asked me to care for Mr. Pecorini, including performing several tasks and skills with which I was unfamiliar. In addition to my lack of familiarity with skills such as changing central line dressings and performing blood draws and wound care, I was not licensed to perform these tasks. I felt uncomfortable performing these skills on my own. However, the nurses were extremely busy and I wanted to help them as much as possible. If I performed these skills on my own, I could be putting the patient at risk. Moreover, I could be threatening the license of the nurses.

Thinking Outside the Box: Possible Courses of Action

- Perform the tasks requested despite the fact that I had little experience with them.
- Inform the nurses that I did not feel comfortable completing these skills on my own and ask that they assign me other tasks within my scope of duty.
- Ask the nurses to be present when I performed these tasks so that they could observe my skills and intervene if necessary.
- Refrain from performing these tasks and alert the nurse manager the following day that I was assigned to tasks outside my scope of duty.

Evaluating a Good Outcome: How Do I Define Success?

- The patient received safe, comprehensive care without being placed at risk.
- I performed tasks and skills within my scope of practice.
- The nurses understood my job duties and properly delegated the necessary tasks.
- The nurses' licensure was not put in jeopardy.
- I felt comfortable and competent in my job performance.

Personal Learning: Here's to the Future!

Since I felt uncomfortable in performing the duties assigned to me by the nurses, I confronted them and told them that I had recently been oriented to the floor and did not have experience with these skills. Although somewhat surprised that I didn't have the experience, they understood and did not want me to do anything I felt uncomfortable with. The nurses were used to having an LPN as a night aide, and the LPN's scope of practice was broader than mine. Throughout the night, I observed the nurses performing the skills and tasks, with the nurses walking me through several of the skills that I was allowed to perform but in which I did not feel proficient. In the morning, we spoke with the nurse manager, who realized the need for clarifying the job duties of the nurse's aides and the appropriate delegation of tasks. I feel that I made the right decision in speaking to the nurses because patient safety could have been compromised by my inexperience. The nurses' licensure also could have been put at risk. As a result of our conversation with the nurse manager, the orientation for new nurse's aides was reorganized, helping greatly to define the scope of duties for the aides.

Colleen Kilcullen, Georgetown University

REFLECTION ON QUALITY AND SAFETY COMPETENCIES

How do you think you would respond in a similar situation? Why? What does this tell you about yourself and about the adequacy of your skills for professional practice? How was the nursing student's action ethical? Legal? Please explain. What other *knowledge, attitudes* and *skills* do you need to develop to continuously improve the quality and safety of care for patients like Mr. Pecorini?

Patient-Centered Care: What role did the different members of the nursing team play in creating a partnership with Mr. Pecorini to best coordinate his care? What special talents do you bring to creating this partnership?

Teamwork and Collaboration/Quality Improvement: What communication skills do you need to improve to ensure that you function as a competent, caring, and responsible member of the patient-care team and ensure that you obtain assistance when needed? How would you have responded if nursing leadership did not address your concerns? What special talents do you bring to promoting a well-functioning interdisciplinary team?

Safety/Evidence-Based Practice: What priority did Mr. Pecorini's care team accord to his health, well-being, and safety? What evidence in the nursing literature supports adhering to the scope of practice and roles?

Informatics: Can you identify the essential information that must be available in Mr. Pecorini's electronic record to support safe patient care and coordination of care? Can you think of other ways to respond to or approach the situation?

In the early Christian period, nursing began to have a formal and more clearly defined role in society. Led by the idea that love and caring for others were important, women called "deaconesses" made the first organized visits to sick people, and members of male religious orders gave nursing care and buried the dead. Both male and female nursing orders were founded during the Crusades (11th to 13th centuries). Hospitals were built for the enormous number of pilgrims needing health care, and nursing became a respected vocation. Although the early Middle Ages ended in chaos, nursing had developed purpose, direction, and leadership.

At the beginning of the 16th century, many Western societies shifted from a religious orientation to an emphasis on warfare, exploration, and expansion of knowledge. Many monasteries and convents closed, leading to a tremendous shortage of people to care for the sick. To meet this need, women who were convicted of crimes were recruited into nursing in lieu of serving jail sentences. In addition to having a poor reputation, nurses received low pay and worked long hours in unfavorable conditions.

Florence Nightingale and the Birth of Modern Nursing

From the middle of the 19th century to the 20th century, social reforms changed the roles of nurses and of women in general. It was during this time that nursing as we now know it began, based on many of the beliefs of Florence Nightingale. Born in 1820 to a wealthy family, she grew up in England, was well educated, and traveled extensively. Despite strong opposition from her family, Nightingale began training as a nurse at the age of 31. The outbreak of the Crimean War and a request by the British to organize nursing care for a military hospital in Turkey gave Nightingale an opportunity for achievement (Kalisch & Kalisch, 2004). As she successfully overcame enormous difficulties, Nightingale challenged prejudices against women and elevated the status of all nurses. After the war, she returned to England, where she established the first training school for nurses and wrote books about health care and nursing education. Florence Nightingale's contributions include:

- Identifying the personal needs of the patient and the role of the nurse in meeting those needs
- Establishing standards for hospital management
- Establishing a respected occupation for women
- Establishing nursing education
- Recognizing the two components of nursing: health and illness
- Believing that nursing is separate and distinct from medicine
- Recognizing that nutrition is important to health
- Instituting occupational and recreational therapy for sick people
- Stressing the need for continuing education for nurses
- Maintaining accurate records, recognized as the beginnings of nursing research

Florence Nightingale, other historically important nurses, and images of early nursing can be seen in Figure 1-1 (on page 8). People important to the development of nursing are listed in Table 1-1 (on page 9). A historical overview of the foundational documents for nursing is presented in Box 1-1 on page 10.

Development of Nursing from the 19th to 21st Centuries

Both the work of Florence Nightingale and the care provided for battle casualties during the Civil War focused attention on the need for educated nurses in the United States. Schools of nursing, founded in connection with hospitals, were established on the beliefs of Nightingale, but the training they provided was based more on apprenticeship than on educational principles. Hospitals saw an economic advantage in having their own schools, and most hospital schools were organized to provide more easily controlled and less expensive staff for the hospital. This resulted in a lack of clear guidelines separating nursing service and nursing education. As students and as graduates, female nurses were under the control of male hospital administrators and physicians. The lack of educational standards, the male dominance in health care, and the pervading Victorian belief that women were subordinate to men combined to contribute to several decades of slow progress toward professionalism in nursing (Kalisch & Kalisch, 2004).

World War II had an enormous effect on nursing. For the first time, large numbers of women worked outside the home. They became more independent and assertive. These changes in women and in society led to an increased emphasis on education. The war itself had created a need for more nurses and resulted in a knowledge explosion in medicine and technology, which broadened the role of nurses. After World War II, efforts were directed at upgrading nursing education. Schools of nursing were based on educational objectives and were increasingly developed in university and college settings, leading to degrees in nursing for men, women, and minorities.

Nursing has broadened in all areas, including practice in a wide variety of health care settings, the development of a specific body of knowledge, the conduct and publication of nursing research, and recognition of the role of nursing in promoting health. Increased emphasis on nursing knowledge as the base for evidence-based practice (EBP) has led to the growth of nursing as a professional discipline.

DEFINITIONS OF NURSING

The word *nurse* originated from the Latin word *nutrix*, meaning "to nourish." Most definitions of **nursing** describe the nurse as a person who nourishes, fosters, and protects and who is prepared to take care of sick, injured, and aged people. With the expanding roles and functions of the nurse in today's society, however, any one definition may be too limited.

Clara Barton, founder of the
American Red Cross in 1882

Florence Nightingale,
initiator of major reforms
in healthcare and nursing
training in England

Vassar training
camp classroom,
1918

Isabel Hampton Robb,
outstanding leader in
nursing and nursing
education

Mary Mahoney, America's
first African American nurse
to graduate from a school
of nursing

Philadelphia General Hospital
nurse, late 1800s

Post-WWII
nursing
school
poster

FIGURE 1-1. Images of nurses spanning more than 100 years of service. (Courtesy of the Center for the Study of the History of Nursing, University of Pennsylvania.)

The International Council of Nurses (2010) captures much of what nursing means in its definition:

> Nursing encompasses autonomous and collaborative care of individuals of all ages, families, groups, and communities, sick or well and in all settings. Nursing includes the promotion of health, prevention of illness, and the care of ill, disabled, and dying people. Advocacy, promotion of a safe environment, research, participation in shaping health policy and in patient and health systems management, and education are also key nursing roles.

The American Nurses Association (ANA) defines nursing as "the protection, promotion, and optimization of health and abilities, prevention of illness and injury, alleviation of suffering through the diagnosis and treatment of human response, and advocacy in the care of individuals, families, communities, and populations" (ANA, 2010). In addition to a definition of nursing, the ANA describes the social context of nursing, the knowledge base for nursing practice, the scope of nursing practice, standards of professional nursing practice, and the regulation of professional nursing in its *Nursing's Social Policy Statement* (2010). Within today's definitions of nursing we find all the elements of professional nursing. Nurses focus on human experiences and responses to birth, health, illness, and death within the context of individuals, families, groups, and communities. The knowledge base for nursing practice includes diagnosis, interventions, and evaluation of outcomes from an established plan of care. In addition, the nurse integrates objective data with knowledge gained from an understanding of the patient's or group's subjective experience, applies scientific knowledge in the nursing process, and provides a caring relationship that facilitates health and healing.

Table 1-1 PEOPLE IMPORTANT TO THE DEVELOPMENT OF NURSING IN NORTH AMERICA

PERSON	CONTRIBUTION
19th Century	
Florence Nightingale	Defined nursing as both an art and a science, differentiated nursing from medicine, created free-standing nursing education; published books about nursing and health care; is regarded as the founder of modern nursing (see text for further information)
Clara Barton	Volunteered to care for wounds and feed Union soldiers during the Civil War; served as the supervisor of nurses for the Army of the James, organizing hospitals and nurses; established the Red Cross in the United States in 1882
Dorothea Dix	Served as superintendent of the Female Nurses of the Army during the Civil War; was given the authority and the responsibility for recruiting and equipping a corps of army nurses; was a pioneering crusader for the reform of the treatment of the mentally ill
Mary Ann Bickerdyke	Organized diet kitchens, laundries, and an ambulance service, and supervised nursing staff during the Civil War
Louise Schuyler	A nurse during the Civil War; returned to New York and organized the New York Charities Aid Association to improve care of the sick in Bellevue Hospital; recommended standards for nursing education
Linda Richards	Graduated in 1873 from the New England Hospital for Women and Children in Boston, Massachusetts, as the first trained nurse in the United States; became the night superintendent of Bellevue Hospital in 1874 and began the practice of keeping records and writing orders
Jane Addams	Provided social services within a neighborhood setting; a leader for women's rights; recipient of the 1931 Nobel Peace prize
Lillian Wald	Established a neighborhood nursing service for the sick poor of the Lower East Side in New York City; the founder of public health nursing
Mary Elizabeth Mahoney	Graduated from the New England Hospital for Women and Children in 1879 as America's first African American nurse
Harriet Tubman	A nurse and an abolitionist; active in the underground railroad movement before joining the Union Army during the Civil War
Nora Gertrude Livingston	Established a training program for nurses at the Montreal General Hospital (the first 3-year program in North America)
Mary Agnes Snively	Director of the nursing school at Toronto General Hospital and one of the founders of the Canadian Nurses Association
Sojourner Truth	Provided nursing care to soldiers during the Civil War and worked for the women's movement
Isabel Hampton Robb	A leader in nursing and nursing education; organized the nursing school at Johns Hopkins Hospital; initiated policies that included limiting the number of hours in a day's work and wrote a textbook to help student learning; the first president of the Nurses Associated Alumnae of the United States and Canada (which later became the American Nurses Association)
20th Century	
Mary Adelaide Nutting	Became the first professor of nursing in the world as a faculty member of Teachers' College, Columbia University; with Lavinia Dock, published the four-volume *History of Nursing*
Elizabeth Smellie	A member of the original Victorian Order of Nurses for Canada (a group that provided public health nursing); organized the Canadian Women's Army Corps during World War II
Lavinia Dock	A nursing leader and women's rights activist; instrumental in the Constitutional amendment giving women the right to vote
Mary Breckenridge	Established the Frontier Nursing Service and one of the first midwifery schools in the United States
Margaret Sanger	Founder of Planned Parenthood

The central focus in all definitions of nursing is the patient (the person receiving care), which includes the physical, emotional, social, and spiritual dimensions of that person. Nursing is no longer considered to be concerned primarily with illness care. Nursing's concepts and definitions have expanded to include the prevention of illness and the promotion and maintenance of health for individuals, families, and communities.

BOX 1-1	TIMELINE OF THE DEVELOPMENT OF FOUNDATIONAL NURSING DOCUMENTS

1859	Florence Nightingale publishes *Notes on Nursing: What It Is and What It Is Not.*
1896	The Nurses' Associated Alumnae of the United States and Canada is founded. Later to become the American Nurses Association (ANA), its first purpose is to establish and maintain a code of ethics.
1940	A "Tentative Code" is published in the *American Journal of Nursing,* although never formally adopted.
1950	*Code for Professional Nurses,* in the form of 17 provisions that are a substantive revision of the "Tentative Code" of 1940, is unanimously accepted by the ANA House of Delegates.
1952	*Nursing Research* publishes its premiere issue.
1956	*Code for Professional Nurses* is amended.
1960	*Code for Professional Nurses* is revised.
1968	*Code for Professional Nurses* is substantively revised, condensing the 17 provisions of the code into 10 provisions.
1973	ANA publishes its first *Standards of Nursing Practice.*
1976	*Code for Nurses With Interpretive Statements,* a modification of the provision and interpretive statements, is published as 11 provisions.
1980	ANA publishes *Nursing: A Social Policy Statement.*
1985	The National Institutes of Health organizes the Center for Nursing Research.
	ANA publishes *Titling for Licensure.*
	Code for Nurses With Interpretive Statements retains the provisions of the 1976 version and includes revised interpretive statements.
	The ANA House of Delegates forms a task force to formally document the scope of practice for nursing.
1987	ANA publishes *The Scope of Nursing Practice.*
1990	The ANA House of Delegates forms a task force to revise the 1973 *Standards of Nursing Practice.*
1991	ANA publishes *Standards of Clinical Nursing Practice.*
1995	ANA publishes *Nursing's Social Policy Statement.*
	The Congress of Nursing Practice directs the Committee on Nursing Practice Standards and Guidelines to establish a process for periodic review and revision of nursing standards.
1996	ANA publishes *Scope and Standards of Advanced Practice Registered Nursing.*
1998	ANA publishes *Standards of Clinical Nursing Practice,* 2nd edition (also known as *Clinical Standards*).
2001	*Code of Ethics With Interpretive Statements* is accepted by the ANA House of Delegates.
	ANA publishes *Bill of Rights for Registered Nurses.*
2002	ANA publishes *Nursing's Agenda for the Future: A Call to the Nation.*
2003	ANA publishes *Nursing's Social Policy Statement,* 2nd edition.
2004	ANA publishes *Nursing: Scope and Standards of Practice.*
2008	*APRN Consensus Model* is published by the APRN Consensus Work Group and APRN Joint Dialogue Group.
	ANA publishes *Professional Role Competence Position Statement.*
	ANA publishes *Specialization and Credentialing in Nursing Revisited: Understanding the Issues, Advancing the Profession.*
2010	ANA publishes *Nursing's Social Policy Statement: The Essence of the Profession* ANA publishes *Nursing: Scope and Standards of Practice,* 2nd edition.

Source: American Nurses Association (ANA). (2010). *Nursing: Scope and standards of practice, 2nd ed.* Silver Spring, MD: Author. Reprinted with permission. All rights reserved.

NURSING'S AIMS AND COMPETENCIES

Four broad aims of nursing practice can be identified in the definitions of nursing:

1. To promote health
2. To prevent illness
3. To restore health
4. To facilitate coping with disability or death

To meet these aims, the nurse uses four blended competencies: *cognitive, technical, interpersonal,* and *ethical/legal.* More recently these have been further specified as the quality and safety education for nursing (QSEN, 2007) competencies: patient-centered care, teamwork

Table 1-2 — NURSING ROLES IN ALL SETTINGS

ROLE	FUNCTION
Caregiver	The provision of care to patients that combines both the art and the science of nursing in meeting physical, emotional, intellectual, sociocultural, and spiritual needs. As a caregiver, the nurse integrates the roles of communicator, teacher, counselor, leader, researcher, advocate, and collaborator to promote wellness through activities that prevent illness, restore health, and facilitate coping with disability or death. The role of caregiver is the primary role of the nurse.
Communicator	The use of effective interpersonal and therapeutic communication skills to establish and maintain helping relationships with patients of all ages in a wide variety of health care settings
Teacher/Educator	The use of communication skills to assess, implement, and evaluate individualized teaching plans to meet learning needs of patients and their families
Counselor	The use of therapeutic interpersonal communication skills to provide information, make appropriate referrals, and facilitate the patient's problem-solving and decision-making skills
Leader	The assertive, self-confident practice of nursing when providing care, effecting change, and functioning with groups
Researcher	The participation in or conduct of research to increase knowledge in nursing and improve patient care
Advocate	The protection of human or legal rights and the securing of care for all patients based on the belief that patients have the right to make informed decisions about their own health and lives
Collaborator	The effective use of skills in organization, communication, and advocacy to facilitate the functions of all members of the health care team as they provide patient care

and collaboration, quality improvement, safety, EBP, and informatics (Sherwood & Barnsteiner, 2012). These are described in Chapter 11. The Reflective Practice Boxes that begin each chapter of this book offer examples of practical challenges to these competencies that actual nursing students have encountered.

The primary role of the nurse as caregiver is given shape and substance by the interrelated roles of communicator, teacher, counselor, leader, researcher, advocate, and collaborator. These roles are described in Table 1-2 and are fully discussed in Unit V. The nurse carries out these roles in many different settings, with care increasingly provided in the home and in the community. Examples of settings for care are fully described in Unit II.

 RECALL Roberto Pecorini, the 38-year-old patient with metastatic cancer. When providing care for Mr. Pecorini, the nurse assumes the role of competent, caring, and responsible caregiver, creates a respectful partnership while identifying best practices, maintains the patient's safety throughout, and appropriately educates the patient and advocates for the patient's rights. ●

Promoting Health

Health is a state of optimal functioning or well-being. As defined by the World Health Organization (WHO), one's health includes physical, social, and mental components and is not merely the absence of disease or infirmity. Health is often a subjective state—a person may be medically diagnosed with an illness but still consider oneself healthy. Wellness, a term that is often associated with health, is an active state of being healthy by living a lifestyle that promotes good physical, mental, emotional, and spiritual health. Models of health and wellness are described in Chapter 3.

Health is an essential part of each of the other aims of nursing. Nurses promote health by identifying, analyzing, and maximizing each patient's own individual strengths as components of preventing illness, restoring health, and facilitating coping with disability or death.

 WHEN teaching Mr. Basshir, the patient described at the beginning of the chapter with risk factors for heart disease, the nurse would focus the teaching plan to rely on the patient's strengths. Although his statements reflect a reluctance to learn and change, emphasizing the patient's strengths would help the patient feel more in control of his health, and thus, hopefully, spur him to make the necessary changes. ●

Health promotion is motivated by the desire to increase a person's well-being and health potential. A person's level of health is affected by many different interrelated factors that either promote health or increase the risk for illness. These factors include genetic inheritance, cognitive abilities, educational level, race and ethnicity, culture, age and gender, developmental level, lifestyle, environment, and socioeconomic status. A level of health or wellness is also strongly influenced by what is termed "health literacy." Health literacy, defined by the U.S. Department of Health and Human Services in the document *Healthy People 2020,* is the ability of patients to obtain, process, and understand the basic information needed to make appropriate decisions about health. Examples of ways that nurses can promote health literacy are included throughout this text.

Healthy People 2020 also establishes health promotion guidelines for the nation as a whole. The guidelines are focused on meeting four overarching goals:

- Attain high-quality, longer lives free of preventable disease, disability, injury, and premature death.
- Achieve health equity, eliminate disparities, and improve the health of all groups.
- Create social and physical environments that promote good health for all.
- Promote quality of life, healthy development, and healthy behaviors across all life stages.

> (U.S. Department of Health and Human Services. Office of Disease Prevention and Health Promotion. *Healthy People 2020*. Washington, DC. Available at http://www.healthypeople.gov/2020/)

The guidelines also contain 12 Leading Health Indicators, which are used to measure the health of the nation over a 10-year period. The 2020 Leading Health Indicators, listed in Box 1-2 reflect the major health concerns in the United States at the beginning of the 21st century. They were selected on the basis of their ability to motivate action, availability to measure progress, and importance as public health issues.

Patient-centered health promotion is the framework for nursing activities. The nurse considers the patient's self-awareness, health awareness, and use of resources while providing care. Through knowledge and skill, the nurse accomplishes the following:

- Facilitates decisions about lifestyle that enhance quality of life and encourage acceptance of responsibility for one's own health
- Increases health awareness by assisting in the understanding that health is more than just not being ill, and by teaching that certain behaviors and factors can contribute to or diminish health
- Teaches self-care activities to maximize achievement of goals that are realistic and attainable; serves as a role model
- Encourages health promotion by providing information and referrals

 RECALL Michelle Fine, the young mother with a new baby who calls the nursery for help with breastfeeding. Making a referral for home care follow-up before Michelle's discharge from the hospital would have been an appropriate intervention to offer support, guidance, and additional teaching. ●

Preventing Illness

Prevention is "anticipatory action taken to prevent the occurrence of an event or to minimize its effects after it has occurred" (Turnock, 2009, p. 516). The objectives of illness-prevention activities are to reduce the risk for illness, to promote good health habits, and to maintain optimal functioning. Nurses prevent illness primarily by teaching and by personal example. Such activities include the following:

- Educational programs in areas such as prenatal care for pregnant women, smoking-cessation programs, and stress-reduction seminars
- Community programs and resources that encourage healthy lifestyles, such as aerobic exercise classes, "swim-nastics," and physical fitness programs
- Literature, television, radio, or Internet information on a healthy diet, regular exercise, and the importance of good health habits
- Health assessments in institutions, clinics, and community settings that identify areas of strength and risks for illness

 THINK back to Ahmad Basshir, the 62-year-old man at risk for heart disease who was described at the beginning of the chapter. The nurse participates in illness prevention, thus promoting healthier behavior by addressing his resistance to change and teaching him lifestyle modifications necessary to reduce his risk for developing heart disease. ●

Restoring Health

Activities to restore health encompass those traditionally considered to be the nurse's responsibility. These focus on the individual with an illness and range from early detection of a disease to rehabilitation and teaching during recovery. Such activities include the following:

- Performing assessments that detect an illness (e.g., taking blood pressure, measuring blood sugars)
- Referring questions and abnormal findings to other health care providers as appropriate

---

Box 1-2	HEALTHY PEOPLE 2020: LEADING HEALTH INDICATORS

- Access to health services
- Clinical preventive services
- Environmental quality
- Injury and violence
- Maternal, infant, and child health
- Mental Health
- Nutrition, physical activity and obesity
- Oral health
- Reproductive and sexual health
- Social determinants
- Substance abuse
- Tobacco

From U.S. Department of Health and Human Services. Office of Disease Prevention and Health Promotion. *Healthy People 2020*. Washington, DC. Available at http://www.healthypeople.gov/2020/. Accessed September 3, 2012.

- Providing direct care of the person who is ill by such measures as giving physical care, administering medications, and carrying out procedures and treatments
- Collaborating with other health care providers in providing care
- Planning, teaching, and carrying out rehabilitation for illnesses such as heart attacks, arthritis, and strokes
- Working in mental health and chemical-dependency programs

Facilitating Coping With Disability and Death

Although the major goals of health care are promoting, maintaining, and restoring health, these goals cannot always be met. Nurses also facilitate patient and family coping with altered function, life crisis, and death. Altered function decreases an individual's ability to carry out activities of daily living (ADLs) and expected roles. Nurses facilitate an optimal level of function through maximizing the person's strengths and potentials, through teaching, and through referral to community support systems. Nurses provide care to both patients and families during end-of-life care, and they do so in hospitals, long-term care facilities, hospices, and homes. Nurses are active in hospice programs, which assist patients and their families in multiple settings in preparing for death and in living as comfortably as possible until death occurs.

NURSING AS A PROFESSIONAL DISCIPLINE

As definitions of nursing have expanded to describe more clearly the roles and actions of nurses, increased attention has been given to nursing as a professional discipline. Nursing uses existing and new knowledge to solve problems creatively and meet human needs within ever-changing boundaries. Nursing is recognized increasingly as a **profession** based on the following defining criteria:

- Well-defined body of specific and unique knowledge
- Strong service orientation
- Recognized authority by a professional group
- Code of ethics
- Professional organization that sets standards
- Ongoing research
- Autonomy and self-regulation

Nursing involves specialized skills and application of knowledge based on an education that has both theoretical and clinical practice components. Nursing is guided by standards set by professional organizations and an established code of ethics. Nursing focuses on human responses to actual or potential health problems and is increasingly focused on wellness, an area of caring that encompasses nursing's unique knowledge and abilities. Nursing is increasingly recognized as scholarly, with academic qualifications, research, and publications specific to the profession that are widely accepted and respected. In addition, nursing interventions are focused on EBP, which is practice based on research and not intuition.

Nursing has evolved through history from a technical service to a person-centered process that maximizes potential in all human dimensions. This has been an active development process, using lessons from the past to gain knowledge for practice in the present and in the future.

EDUCATIONAL PREPARATION FOR NURSING PRACTICE

Educational preparation for nursing practice involves several different types of programs that lead to **licensure**, or the legal authority to practice as a nursing professional. Students may choose to enter a practical nursing program and become a licensed practical nurse (LPN) or they may enter a diploma, an associate degree, or a baccalaureate program to be licensed as a registered nurse (RN). State laws in the United States recognize both the LPN and the RN as credentials to practice nursing. Increasingly, various levels of nursing education are providing programs for educational advancement. For example, the LPN can complete an associate degree and become an RN, and the RN prepared at the diploma or associate degree level can attain a bachelor of science in nursing (BSN) degree. There are also programs that provide RN-to-master's degrees as well as BSN and master's degree-to-PhD. Graduate programs in nursing provide master's and doctoral degrees.

Educational preparation for the nurse has become a major issue in nursing; the multiple methods of preparation are confusing to employers, consumers of health care services, and nurses themselves. Nursing organizations are working hard to answer questions such as "What is technical nursing?" and "What is professional nursing?" as well as "Should graduates of different programs take the same licensing examination and have the same title?" These questions are likely to be resolved during your nursing career. The following sections discuss current education for LPNs and RNs, as well as graduate nursing education, continuing education for nurses, and in-service education.

Practical and Vocational Nursing Education

Practical (also labeled vocational) nursing programs were established to teach graduates to give bedside nursing care to patients. Schools for practical nursing programs are located in varied settings, such as high schools, technical or vocational schools, community colleges, and independent agencies. Most programs are 1 year in length, divided into one-third classroom hours and two-thirds clinical laboratory hours. On completion of the program, graduates can take the National Council Licensure Examination–Practical Nurse (NCLEX–PN) for licensure as an LPN. LPNs work under the direction of a physician or RN to give direct care to patients, focusing on meeting health care needs in hospitals, long-term care facilities, and home health agencies.

Table 1-3 SUMMARY OF TYPES OF EDUCATIONAL PROGRAMS FOR REGISTERED NURSES (RNs)

	DIPLOMA	ASSOCIATE DEGREE	BACCALAUREATE
Location	Hospital	Community college	Senior college or university
Study timeframe	24–36 months	2 academic or calendar years	4 academic years
Course work	Biologic science Physical science Nursing theory Nursing practice	Basic sciences Social sciences General education Nursing theory Nursing practice	Basic sciences General education Social sciences Nursing theory Nursing practice Nursing research Community health Management
Clinical component	Both hospital and community settings	Both hospital and community settings	A variety of settings in which health care and nursing care are provided
Further education opportunity	If affiliated with a college, may transfer some credit toward a bachelor of science in nursing (BSN) degree	Credits often apply toward a bachelor of science in nursing (BSN) degree	Base for advanced education at the master's and doctoral levels
Competencies on graduation	Plans and gives direct care to patients in structured settings Works with other members of the health care team to plan and provide care to mostly ill patients	Plans and gives direct care to patients in structured settings Works with other members of the health care team to plan and provide care to mostly ill patients	Plans and gives direct care to individual patients, groups, and communities Directs other members of the health care team in planning and providing care to ill and well patients in a variety of settings; assumes beginning leadership roles; provides comprehensive health care, including health promotion, illness prevention, and rehabilitative, educational, and health counseling

Registered Nursing Education

Three types of educational programs traditionally lead to licensure as an RN: (1) diploma, (2) associate degree, and (3) baccalaureate programs. Graduates of all three programs take the NCLEX–RN examination. Although it is a national examination, it is administered by—and the nurse is licensed in—the state in which the examination is taken and passed. *It is illegal to practice nursing unless one has a license verifying completion of an accredited (by state) program in nursing and has passed the licensing examination.* Nurses gain legal rights to practice nursing in another state by applying to that state's board of nursing and receiving reciprocal licensure. Table 1-3 summarizes the types of education for RNs. A more in-depth discussion of licensure is included later in this chapter under Nurse Practice Acts and Licensure.

The U.S. Department of Labor, Bureau of Labor Statistics (BLS) annually collects and publishes data on employment and earnings for more than 800 occupations. As of May 2011,

BLS estimates that there were 2,724,570 RNs employed in various settings in the United States (Figure 1-2).

Diploma in Nursing

Many nurses practicing in the United States today received their basic nursing education in a 3-year, hospital-based diploma school of nursing. The first schools of nursing established to educate nurses were diploma programs; until the 1960s, they were the major source of graduates. In recent years, the number of diploma programs has decreased greatly.

Graduates of diploma programs have a sound foundation in the biologic and social sciences, with a strong emphasis on clinical experience in direct patient care. Graduates work in acute, long-term, and ambulatory health care facilities.

Associate Degree in Nursing

Most associate degree in nursing (ADN) programs are offered by community or junior colleges. These 2-year educational

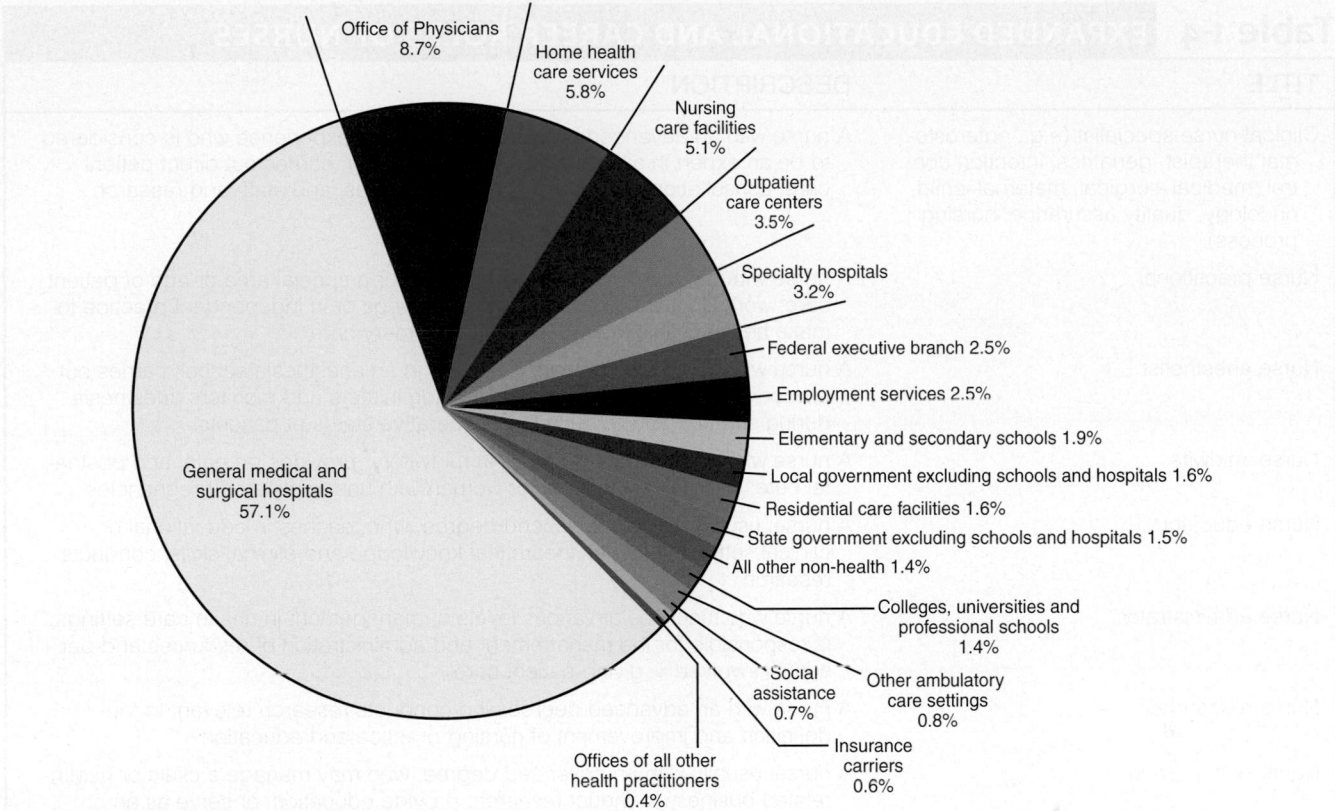

FIGURE 1-2. Employment settings of registered nurses in the United States, as of May 2011. (Source: McMenamin, P. [2012]. Compensation and employment of registered nurses: Part 1. One Strong Voice. American Nurses Association Blog. Available at: http://www.ananursespace.org/ANANURSESPACE/BlogsMain/BlogViewer/?BlogKey=e36976cc-ade3–480f-8fe0-ccbebdaf5506)

programs attract more men, more minorities, and more non-traditional students than do the other types of programs. Associate degree education prepares nurses to give care to patients in various settings, including hospitals, long-term care facilities, and home health care and other community settings. Graduates are technically skilled and well prepared to carry out nursing roles and functions. As defined by the National League for Nursing (NLN), competencies of the ADN on entry into practice encompass the roles of provider of care, manager of care, and member of the discipline of nursing.

Baccalaureate in Nursing

The first baccalaureate nursing programs were established in the United States in the early 1900s. The number of programs and the number of enrolling students, however, did not increase markedly until the 1960s. Most graduates receive a bachelor of science in nursing (BSN).

Recommendations by national nursing organizations that the entry level for professional practice be at the baccalaureate level have resulted in increased numbers of these programs. Although BSN nurses practice in a wide variety of settings, the 4-year degree is required for many administrative, managerial, and community health positions.

In BSN programs, the major in nursing is built on a general education base, with concentration on nursing at the upper level. Students acquire knowledge of theory and practice related to nursing and other disciplines, provide nursing care to individuals and groups, work with members of the health care team, use research to improve practice, and have a foundation for graduate study. Nurses who graduate from a diploma or associate degree program and wish to complete requirements for a BSN may choose to enroll in an on-campus, online, or external degree RN-to-BSN program. In addition, there are accelerated BSN programs for people who already have a degree in another area.

Emerging Entry Points

Beyond the traditional entry routes to a career as a registered nurse, a number of additional pathways are emerging and proving effective at attracting new audiences into the nursing profession. These alternative routes include entry-level master's programs, accelerated programs for graduates of nonnursing disciplines, community college–based baccalaureate programs, and RN completion programs for licensed practical nurses and other allied health providers (Raines & Taglaireni, 2008).

Table 1-4 EXPANDED EDUCATIONAL AND CAREER ROLES OF NURSES

TITLE	DESCRIPTION
Clinical nurse specialist (e.g., enterostomal therapist, geriatrics, infection control, medical–surgical, maternal–child, oncology, quality assurance, nursing process)	A nurse with an advanced degree, education, or experience who is considered to be an expert in a specialized area of nursing; carries out direct patient care; consultation; teaching of patients, families, and staff; and research
Nurse practitioner	A nurse with an advanced degree, certified for a special area or age of patient care; works in a variety of health care settings or in independent practice to make health assessments and deliver primary care
Nurse anesthetist	A nurse who completes a course of study in an anesthesia school; carries out preoperative visits and assessments; administers and monitors anesthesia during surgery; and evaluates postoperative status of patients
Nurse–midwife	A nurse who completes a program in midwifery; provides prenatal and postnatal care; and delivers babies for women with uncomplicated pregnancies
Nurse educator	A nurse, usually with an advanced degree, who teaches in educational or clinical settings; teaches theoretical knowledge and clinical skills; conducts research
Nurse administrator	A nurse who functions at various levels of management in health care settings; is responsible for the management and administration of resources and personnel involved in giving patient care
Nurse researcher	A nurse with an advanced degree who conducts research relevant to the definition and improvement of nursing practice and education
Nurse entrepreneur	A nurse, usually with an advanced degree, who may manage a clinic or health-related business, conduct research, provide education, or serve as an adviser or consultant to institutions, political agencies, or businesses

Graduate Education in Nursing

The two levels of graduate education in nursing are the master's and doctoral degrees. A master's degree prepares advanced practice nurses (APRNs) to function in educational settings, in managerial roles, as clinical specialists, and in various advanced practice areas, such as nurse–midwives and nurse practitioners (Table 1-4). Many master's graduates gain national certification in their specialty area, for example, as family nurse practitioners (FNPs) or nurse midwives. Nurses with doctoral degrees meet requirements for academic advancement and organizational management. They also are prepared to carry out research necessary to advance nursing theory and practice.

The newest graduate nursing degree is the doctor of nursing practice (DNP). In 2004, the American Association of Colleges of Nursing (AACN) in consultation with a variety of stakeholder groups, called for moving the current level of preparation necessary for advanced practice from the master's degree to the DNP by the year 2015. According to their position statement, the DNP is designed for nurses seeking a terminal degree in nursing practice and offers an alternative approach to research-focused doctoral programs. DNP-prepared nurses are well equipped to fully implement the science developed by nurse researchers prepared in PhD, DNSc, and other research-focused doctorates. For more information on the AACN's position, refer to the AACN Fact Sheet on the Doctor of Nursing Practice (2013; http://www.aacn.nche.edu/media-relations/fact-sheets/dnp).

Continuing Education

The ANA defines continuing education as those professional development experiences designed to enrich the nurse's contribution to health. Colleges, hospitals, voluntary agencies, and private groups offer formal continuing education through courses, seminars, and workshops. In many states, continuing education is required for an RN to maintain licensure.

In-Service Education

Many hospitals and health care agencies provide education and training for employees of their institution or organization, called in-service education. This is designed to increase the knowledge and skills of the nursing staff. Programs may involve learning, for example, a specific nursing skill or how to use new equipment.

PROFESSIONAL NURSING ORGANIZATIONS

One of the criteria of a profession is having a professional organization that sets standards for practice and education. Nursing's professional organizations are concerned with current issues in nursing and health care, and influence health care policy and legislation. The benefits of belonging to a professional nursing organization include networking with colleagues, having a voice in legislation affecting nursing, and keeping current with trends and issues in nursing.

International Nursing Organization

The International Council of Nurses (ICN), founded in 1899, was the first international organization of professional women. By sharing a commitment to maintaining high standards of nursing service and nursing education and by promoting ethics, the ICN provides a way for national nursing organizations to work together.

National Nursing Organizations

Professional nursing organizations in the United States include the American Nurses Association (ANA), the National League for Nursing (NLN), and the American Association of Colleges in Nursing (AACN). The National Student Nurses' Association (NSNA) prepares students to participate in professional nursing organizations.

American Nurses Association (ANA)

The ANA is the professional organization for RNs in the United States. Founded in the late 1800s, its membership is comprised of the state nurses' associations to which individual nurses belong. Its primary mission is to be involved in public education, clinical nursing standards, and lobbying state and federal lawmakers to advance the profession of nursing. The ANA addresses ethics, public policy, and the economic and general welfare of nurses. Publications of the ANA include *Code of Ethics, American Nurse Today, The American Nurse, OJIN: The Online Journal of Issues in Nursing,* and *NurseBooks.org.* ANA electronic newsletters include *ANA SmartBrief, Nursing Insider, ANA ImmuNews,* and *Capitol Update.*

National League for Nurses (NLN)

The NLN is an organization open to all people interested in nursing, including nurses, nonnurses, and agencies. Established in 1952, its objective is to foster the development and improvement of all nursing services and nursing education. The NLN conducts one of the largest professional testing services in the United States, including pre-entrance testing for potential students and achievement testing to measure student progress. It also serves as the primary source of research data about nursing education, conducting annual surveys of schools and new RNs. The organization also provides voluntary accreditation for educational programs in nursing.

American Association of Colleges of Nursing (AACN)

The AACN is the national voice for baccalaureate and higher-degree nursing education programs. The organization's goals focus on establishing quality educational standards,

---

BOX 1-3   EXAMPLES OF U.S. SPECIALTY PRACTICE AND SPECIAL INTEREST NURSING ORGANIZATIONS

- American Academy of Nurse Practitioners
- American Assembly for Men in Nursing
- American Association for the History of Nursing
- American Association of Nurse Attorneys
- American Holistic Nurses' Association
- Association of Nurses in AIDS Care
- American Association of Critical Care Nurses
- Dermatology Nurses Association
- Hospice Nurses Association
- Oncology Nurses Society
- Sigma Theta Tau International
- Transcultural Nursing Society

---

influencing the nursing profession to improve health care, and promoting public support of baccalaureate and graduate education, research, and nursing practice. National accreditation for collegiate nursing programs is provided (based on meeting standards) through the AACN by the Commission on Collegiate Nursing Education (CCNE).

National Student Nurses Association (NSNA)

Established in 1952 with the assistance of the ANA and the NLN, the NSNA is the national organization for students enrolled in nursing education programs. Through voluntary participation, students practice self-governance, advocate for student and patient rights, and take collective, responsible action on social and political issues.

Specialty Practice and Special Interest Nursing Organizations

A wide variety of specialty-practice and special-interest nursing organizations are available to nurses. These organizations provide information on specific areas of nursing, often have publications in the specialty area, and may be involved in certification activities. Examples of these organizations are listed in Box 1-3.

GUIDELINES FOR NURSING PRACTICE

Nursing controls and guarantees its practice through standards of practice, nurse practice acts and licensure, and the use of the nursing process. Each of these will guide your nursing education as a student and how you practice after graduation.

Standards of Nursing Practice

The ANA's 2010 *Nursing: Scope and Standards of Practice* defines activities that are specific and unique to nursing. **Standards** allow nurses to carry out professional roles, serving as protection for the nurse, the patient, and

BOX 1-4 ANA STANDARDS OF NURSING PRACTICE

Standards of Practice

- **Standard 1. Assessment**

  The registered nurse collects comprehensive data pertinent to the patient's health or the situation.

- **Standard 2. Diagnosis**

  The registered nurse analyzes the assessment data to determine the diagnoses or issues.

- **Standard 3. Outcomes Identification**

  The registered nurse identifies expected outcomes for a plan individualized to the patient or the situation.

- **Standard 4. Planning**

  The registered nurse develops a plan that prescribes strategies and alternatives to attain expected outcomes.

- **Standard 5. Implementation**

  The registered nurse implements the identified plan, coordinates care delivery, employs strategies to promote health and a safe environment (the advanced practice registered nurse [APRN] also provides consultation and uses prescriptive authority and treatment).

  Standard 5a. Coordination of Care
  The registered nurse coordinates care delivery.

  Standard 5b. Health Teaching and Promotion
  The registered nurse employs strategies to promote health and a safe environment.

  Standard 5c. Consultation
  The graduate-level prepared specialty nurse or APRN provides consultation to influence the identified plan, enhance the abilities of others, and effect change.

  Standard 5d. Prescriptive Authority and Treatment
  The APRN uses prescriptive authority, procedures, referrals, treatments, and therapies in accordance with state and federal laws and regulations.

- **Standard 6. Evaluation**

  The registered nurse evaluates progress toward attainment of outcomes.

Standards of Professional Performance

- **Standard 7. Ethics**

  The registered nurse practices ethically.

- **Standard 8. Education**

  The registered nurse attains knowledge and competence that reflects current nursing practice.

- **Standard 9. Evidence-Based Practice and Research**

  The registered nurse contributes to quality nursing practice.

- **Standard 10. Quality of Practice**

  The registered nurse contributes to quality nursing practice.

- **Standard 11. Communication**

  The registered nurse communicates effectively in all areas of practice.

- **Standard 12. Leadership**

  The registered nurse demonstrates leadership in the professional practice setting and the profession.

- **Standard 13. Collaboration**

  The registered nurse collaborates with the health care consumer, family, and others in the conduct of nursing practice.

- **Standard 14. Professional Practice Evaluation**

  The registered nurse evaluates her or his own nursing practice in relation to professional practice standards and guidelines, relevant statutes, rules, and regulations.

- **Standard 15. Resource Utilization**

  The registered nurse utilizes appropriate resources to plan and provide nursing services that are safe, effective, and financially responsible.

- **Standard 16. Environmental Health**

  The registered nurse practices in an environmentally safe and healthy manner.

- **Standard 17. Collegiality**

  The nurse interacts with and contributes to the professional development of peers and colleagues.

American Nurses Association. (2010). *Nursing: Scope and standards of practice, 2nd ed.* Silver Spring MD. Nursebooks.org; pp. 8–10. Reproduced with permission of the American Nurses Association.

the institution where health care is provided. Each nurse is accountable for his or her own quality of practice and is responsible for the use of these standards to ensure knowledgeable, safe, and comprehensive nursing care. The 2010 ANA standards outlined in Box 1-4 apply to the practice of professional nursing for all RNs, in all settings.

 Concept Mastery Alert

Standards of Practice address the key steps involved in caring for patients; Standards of Professional Performance address the key concepts that the nurse integrates into his or her role as a professional nurse.

Nurse Practice Acts and Licensure

Nurse practice acts are laws established in each state in the United States to regulate the practice of nursing. They are broadly worded and vary among states, but all of them have certain elements in common, such as the following:

- Protect the public by defining the legal scope of nursing practice, excluding untrained or unlicensed people from practicing nursing.
- Create a state board of nursing or regulatory body having the authority to make and enforce rules and regulations concerning the nursing profession.
- Define important terms and activities in nursing, including legal requirements and titles for RNs and LPNs.

• Establish criteria for the education and licensure of nurses.

The board of nursing for each state has the legal authority to allow graduates of approved schools of nursing to take the licensing examination. Those who successfully meet the requirements for licensure are then given a license to practice nursing in the state. The license, which must be renewed at specified intervals, is valid during the life of the holder and is registered in the state. Many states have a requirement for a specified number of continuing education units to renew and maintain licensure. There are two ways in which nurses can practice in a state other than in the one they were originally licensed. One is by **reciprocity**, which allows a nurse to apply for and be endorsed as a registered nurse by another state. There are also 24 states that are members of the Nurse Licensure Compact, allowing a nurse who is licensed and permanently lives in one of the member states to practice in the other member states without additional licensure (National Council of State Boards of Nursing, 2012). The license and the right to practice nursing can be denied, revoked, or suspended for professional misconduct (e.g., incompetence, negligence, chemical impairment, or criminal actions).

As nursing roles continue to expand and issues in nursing are resolved, revised nurse practice acts will reflect those changes. All nurses must be knowledgeable about the specific nurse practice act for the state in which they practice.

Nursing Process

The **nursing process** is another of the major guidelines for nursing practice. The essential activities involved in the nursing process are assessing, diagnosing, planning, implementing, and evaluating (see Unit III). Nurses implement their roles through the nursing process, which integrates both the art and the science of nursing—that is, the nursing process is nursing made visible.

The nursing process is used by the nurse to identify the patient's health care needs and strengths, to establish and carry out a plan of care to meet those needs, and to evaluate the effectiveness of the plan to meet established outcomes. The nursing process allows nurses to use critical thinking and clinical reasoning when providing care that is individualized and holistic, and to define those areas of care that are within the domain of nursing. Clinical reasoning and the nursing process are fully described in Unit III.

CURRENT TRENDS IN HEALTH CARE AND NURSING

The National Advisory Council on Nurse Education and Practice (NACNEP) identifies critical challenges to nursing practice in the 21st century: a growing population of hospitalized patients who are older and more acutely ill, increasing health care costs, and the need to stay current with rapid advances in medical knowledge and technology. You are sure to experience all of these as you begin your clinical experiences. Complicating these challenges are an existing shortage of nurses (Figure 1-3), an aging nurse workforce postponing retirement because of the country's recent economic downturn, and prospects of a worsening nurse shortage (NACNEP, 2010, p. 1).

According to the Association of American Medical Colleges (AAMC), many Americans are currently "medically homeless" and are finding it difficult to navigate the health care system when they need care or advice. In addition, this system financially rewards "patchwork" care provided by assorted clinicians instead of encouraging continuity and care coordination. These problems are compounded by a lack of shared health information systems that could make

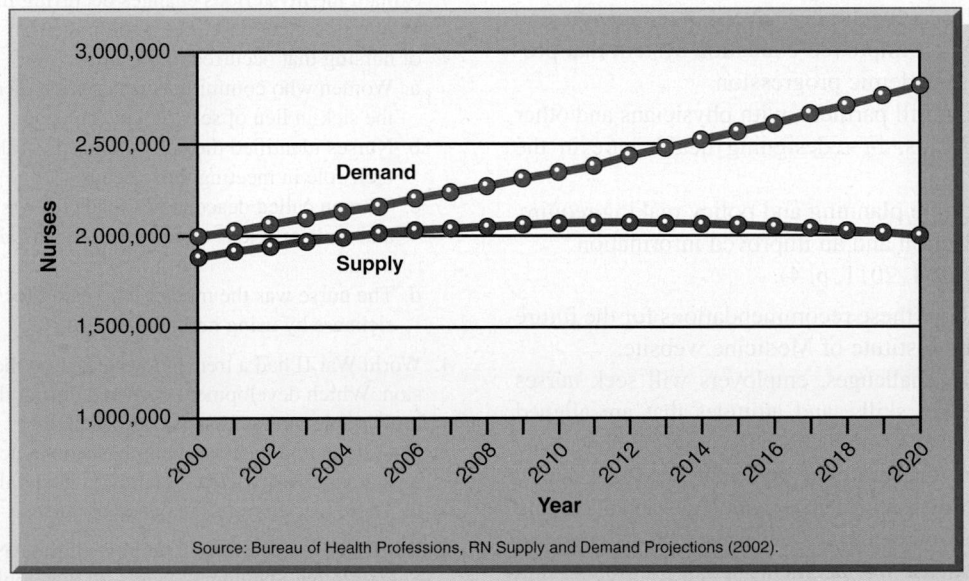

FIGURE 1-3. National supply and demand projection for full-time registered nurses: 2000 to 2020. (Source: U.S. Department of Health and Human Services Health Resources and Services Administration, Bureau of Health Professions [2002]. Projected supply, demand, and shortages of registered nurses: 2000–2020. Washington, DC. Author)

critical health information available to both patients and providers (AAMC, 2008, p. 2). You will learn more about these realities in Unit II. This much is clear: the public needs professional nurses who are "prepared to work when they are hired, willing to continue to learn, and ready to adapt their skills to the needs of the working environment" (NACNEP, 2010).

The NLN recently identified ten trends to watch for in nursing education (Heller, Oros, & Durneey-Crowley, 2011):

• Changing demographics and increasing diversity
• The technological explosion
• Globalization of the world's economy and society
• The era of the educated consumer, alternative therapies, and genomic and palliative care
• The shift to population-based care and the increasing complexity of patient care
• The cost of health care and the challenge of managed care
• The impact of health policy and regulation
• The growing need for interdisciplinary education and for collaborative practice
• The current nursing shortage/opportunities for lifelong learning and workforce development
• Significant advances in nursing science and research

To read more about how these trends are likely to influence your nursing education and practice, visit the National League for Nursing website (http://www.nln.org/nlnjournal/infotrends.htm).

Also in 2011, the Institute of Medicine (IOM) released the results of a groundbreaking study on the role of nurses in realizing a transformed health care system. The four key messages underlying their recommendations for transforming the nursing profession are:

1. Nurses should practice to the full extent of their education and training.
2. Nurses should achieve higher levels of education and training through an improved education system that promotes seamless academic progression.
3. Nurses should be full partners, with physicians and other health professionals, in redesigning health care in the United States.
4. Effective workforce planning and policy making require better data collection and an improved information infrastructure (IOM, 2011, p. 4).

To read more about these recommendations for the future of nursing, visit the Institute of Medicine website.

To address these challenges, employers will seek nurses who have knowledge, skills, and attitudes that are aligned with the requirements of their practice environments, can work effectively in interprofessional teams across a variety of health care settings, and can provide traditional nursing services, as well as other needed services such as case and practice leadership, case management, health promotion, and disease prevention.

Useful Web Resources for this chapter are available on thePoint website.

DEVELOPING CLINICAL REASONING

1. Consider the roles and functions of professional nursing (see Table 1-2, p. 11). Interview several nurses in different settings to see how much value they attach to these roles and how much time they are able to devote to them.

2. Describe how a nurse would meet the aims of nursing as described in this chapter (promoting health, preventing illness, restoring health, and facilitating coping with death or disability) when caring for the following patients:
   • A single mother who has just delivered her first child and is scheduled to be discharged 12 hours after delivery
   • An 82-year-old woman who wants to begin an exercise program
   • A 32-year-old man dying of AIDS at home

As you consider these situations, try to identify factors that either promote or inhibit the fulfilling of these aims.

PRACTICING FOR NCLEX

1. A nurse is caring for a patient in the ICU who is being monitored for a possible cerebral aneurysm following a loss of consciousness in the emergency room. The nurse anticipates preparing the patient for ordered diagnostic tests. This nurse's knowledge of the diagnostic procedures for this condition reflects which aspect of nursing?
   a. The art of nursing
   b. The science of nursing
   c. The caring aspect of nursing
   d. The holistic approach to nursing

2. Which nurse who was influential in the development of nursing in North America is regarded as the founder of American nursing?
   a. Clara Barton
   b. Lillian Wald
   c. Lavinia Dock
   d. Florence Nightingale

3. In early civilizations, the theory of animism attempted to explain the mysterious changes occurring in bodily functions. Which statement describes a component of the development of nursing that occurred in this era?
   a. Women who committed crimes were recruited into nursing the sick in lieu of serving jail sentences.
   b. Nurses identified the personal needs of the patient and their role in meeting those needs.
   c. Women called deaconesses made the first visits to the sick and male religious orders cared for the sick and buried the dead.
   d. The nurse was the mother who cared for her family during sickness by using herbal remedies.

4. World War II had a tremendous effect on the nursing profession. Which development occurred during this period?
   a. The role of the nurse was broadened.
   b. There was a decreased emphasis on education.
   c. Nursing was practiced mainly in hospital settings.
   d. There was an overabundance of nurses.

5. Which phrase describes a purpose of the ANA's Nursing's Social Policy Statement? Select all that apply.
   a. To describe the nurse as a dependent caregiver
   b. To provide standards for nursing educational programs
   c. To define the scope of nursing practice

d. To establish a knowledge base for nursing practice

e. To describe nursing's social responsibility

f. To regulate nursing research

6. One of the four broad aims of nursing practice is to restore health. Which examples of nursing interventions reflect this goal? Select all that apply.
   a. A nurse counsels adolescents in a drug rehabilitation program.
   b. A nurse performs range-of-motion exercises for a patient on bedrest.
   c. A nurse shows a diabetic patient how to inject insulin.
   d. A nurse recommends a yoga class for a busy executive.
   e. A nurse provides hospice care for a patient with end-stage cancer.
   f. A nurse teaches a nutrition class at a local high school.

7. Nursing is recognized increasingly as a profession based on which defining criteria? Select all that apply.
   a. Well defined body of general knowledge
   b. Interventions dependent upon the medical practice
   c. Recognized authority by a professional group
   d. Regulation by the medical industry
   e. Code of ethics
   f. Ongoing research

8. A nurse is practicing as a nurse-midwife in a busy OB-GYN office. Which degree in nursing is necessary to practice at this level?
   a. LPN
   b. ADN
   c. BSN
   d. MSN

9. Nurse practice acts are established in each state of the United States to regulate nursing practice. What is a common element of every state practice act?
   a. Defining the legal scope of nursing practice
   b. Providing continuing education programs
   c. Determining the content covered in the NCLEX examination
   d. Creating institutional policies for health care practices

10. The National Advisory Council on Nurse Education and Practice identifies critical challenges to nursing practice in the 21st century. What is a current health care trend contributing to these challenges?
    a. Decreased numbers of hospitalized patients
    b. Older and more acutely ill patients
    c. Decreasing health care costs due to managed care
    d. Slowed advances in medical knowledge and technology

ANSWERS WITH RATIONALES

1. *b.* The science of nursing is the knowledge base for care that is provided. In contrast, the skilled application of that knowledge is the art of nursing. Providing holistic care to patients based on the science of nursing is considered the art of nursing.

2. *d.* Florence Nightingale elevated the status of nursing to a respected occupation, improved the quality of nursing care, and founded modern nursing education. Clara Barton established the Red Cross in the United States in 1882. Lillian Wald is the founder of public health nursing. Lavinia Dock was a nursing leader and women's rights activist instrumental in womens' right to vote.

3. *d.* The theory of animism was based on the belief that everything in nature was alive with invisible forces and endowed with power. In this era, the nurse usually was the mother who cared for her family during sickness by providing physical care and herbal remedies. At the beginning of the 16th century the shortage of nurses led to the recruitment of women who had committed crimes to provide nursing care instead of going to jail. In the early Christian period, women called deaconesses made the first organized visits to sick people, and members of male religious orders gave nursing care and buried the dead. The influences of Florence Nightingale were apparent from the middle of the 19th century to the 20th century; one of her accomplishments was identifying the personal needs of the patient and the nurse's role in meeting those needs.

4. *a.* During World War II, large numbers of women worked outside the home. They became more independent and assertive, which led to an increased emphasis on education. The war itself created a need for more nurses and resulted in a knowledge explosion in medicine and technology. This trend broadened the role of nurses to include practicing in a wide variety of health care settings.

5. *c, d, e.* The ANA Social Policy Statement (2010) describes the social context of nursing, a definition of nursing, the knowledge base for nursing practice, the scope of nursing practice, standards of professional nursing practice, and the regulation of professional nursing.

6. *a, b, c.* Activities to restore health focus on the individual with an illness and range from early detection of a disease to rehabilitation and teaching during recovery. These activities include drug counseling, teaching patients how to administer their medications, and performing range-of-motion exercises for bedridden patients. Recommending a yoga class for stress reduction is a goal of preventing illness, and teaching a nutrition class is a goal of promoting health. A hospice care nurse helps to facilitate coping with disability and death.

7. *c, e, f.* Nursing is recognized increasingly as a profession based on the following defining criteria: well-defined body of specific and unique knowledge, strong service orientation, recognized authority by a professional group, code of ethics, professional organization that sets standards, ongoing research, and autonomy and self-regulation.

8. *d.* A master's degree (MSN) prepares advanced practice nurses. Many master's graduates gain national certification in their specialty area, for example, as family nurse practitioners (FNPs) or nurse midwives.

9. *a.* Nurse practice acts are established in each state to regulate the practice of nursing by defining the legal scope of nursing practice, creating a state board of nursing to make and enforce rules and regulations, define important terms and activities in nursing, and establish criteria for the education and licensure of nurses. The acts do not determine the content covered on the NCLEX, but they do have the legal authority to allow graduates of approved schools of nursing to take the licensing examination. The acts also may determine educational requirements for licensure, but do not provide the education. Institutional policies are created by the institutions themselves.

10. **b.** The National Advisory Council on Nurse Education and Practice identifies the following critical challenges to nursing practice in the 21st century: A growing population of hospitalized patients who are older and more acutely ill, increasing health care costs, and the need to stay current with rapid advances in medical knowledge and technology.

TAYLOR SUITE RESOURCES

Explore these additional resources to enhance learning for this chapter:

- NCLEX-Style Questions and other resources on thePoint, http://thePoint.lww.com/Taylor8e
- *Study Guide for Fundamentals of Nursing, 8th edition*
- Adaptive Learning | Powered by prepU, http://thepoint.lww.com/prepu

Bibliography

American Nurses Credentialing Center (ANCC). (2009). Available at http://www.nursecredentialing.org/

American Nurses Association (ANA). (2010). *Nursing's Social Policy Statement, 2010 edition.* Silver Spring, MD: Author.

American Nurses Association (ANA). (2010). *Nursing: Scope and standards of practice, 2nd ed.* Silver Spring, MD: Author.

American Nurses Association (ANA). (2005). *Core issues.* Washington, DC: Author.

American Nurses Association (ANA). (2009). *Considering nursing?* Available http://www.nursingworld.org/EspeciallyForYou/StudentNurses.aspx

American Association of Colleges of Nursing. (2013). AACN Fact Sheet on the Doctor of Nursing Practice. Available at http://www.aacn.nche.edu/media-relations/fact-sheets/dnp

Association of American Medical Colleges. (2008). The medical home: Position statement, p. 2. Available at https://www.aamc.org/download/60628/data/medicalhome.pdf

Benner, P., Sutphen, M., Leonard, V. & Day, L. (2010). *Educating nurses: A call for radical transformation.* San Francisco: Jossey-Bass.

Buerhaus, P. (2007). Dealing with reality: Confronting the global nursing shortage. *Reflections on Nursing Leadership, Fourth Quarter,* 6 p.

Buerhaus, P., Staiger, D., & Auerbach, D. (2009). *The future of the nursing workforce in the United States; Data, trends and implications,* p. 210. Studbury, MA: Jones & Bartlett.

D'Antonio, P. (2004). Women, nursing, and baccalaureate education in 20th century America. *Journal of Nursing Scholarship, 36*(4), 379–384.

D'Antonio, P. (2006). History for a practice profession. *Nursing Inquiry, 13*(4), 242–248.

Dolan, J. A., Fitzpatrick, M. L., & Herrmann, E. K. (1983). *Nursing in society: A historical perspective.* Philadelphia: W. B. Saunders.

Donley, R., Sr. (2005). Challenges for nursing in the 21st century. *Nursing Economics, 23*(6), 312–318.

Ellis, J., & Hartley, C. (2012). *Nursing in today's world: Challenges, issues, trends* (10th ed.). Philadelphia: Lippincott Williams & Wilkins.

Fairman, J. (2008). Context and contingency in the history of post World War II nursing scholarship in the United States. *Journal of Nursing Scholarship, 40*(1), 4–11.

Heller, B.R., Oros, M.T., & Durney-Crowley, J. The Future of Nursing Education: Ten Trends to Watch/National League for Nursing. Available at http://www.nln.org/nlnjournal/infotrends.htm

Hill, K. (2010) Improving quality and patient safety by retaining nursing expertise. *OJIN: The Online Journal of Issues in Nursing, 15*(3). DOI: 10.3912/OJIN.Vol15No03PPT03

International Council of Nurses. (2010). *The ICN definition of nursing.* Geneva: Imprimeries Populaires. Available at http://www.icn.ch/about-icn/icn-definition-of-nursing/

Kalisch, P. A., & Kalisch, B. J. (2004). *American nursing: A history.* Philadelphia: Lippincott Williams & Wilkins.

Lauridsen, B. (2005). Stepping stones on which today's nursing was built. *Nursing BC, 37*(2), 5.

McMenamin, P. (2012). Compensation and employment of registered nurses: Part 1. One Strong Voice. American Nurses Association Blog. Available at http://www.ananursespace.org/ANANURSESPACE/BlogsMain/BlogViewer/?BlogKey=e36976cc-ade3-480f-8fe0-ccbebdaf5506

National Advisory Council on Nurse Education and Practice. (2010). Addressing new challenges facing nursing education: Solutions for a Transforming Healthcare Environment. Eighth Annual Report to the Secretary of the U.S. Department of Health and Human Services and the U.S. Congress. Washington, DC.

National Council of State Boards of Nursing. (2012). Nurse licensure compact administration, Participating states in the NLC. Available at https://www.ncsbn.org/158.htm

National Research Council. The Future of Nursing: Leading Change, Advancing Health. Washington, DC: The National Academies Press, 2011.

Nightingale, F. (1992). *Notes on nursing: What it is and what it is not.* (Commemorative ed.). Philadelphia: J. B. Lippincott.

Price-Spratlen, L., & Mahoney, M. (2006). February, Black History Month: A time to review nursing's past, present, and future. *Washington Nurse, 36*(1), 12–13.

Quality and Safety Education for Nurses. (2007). Overview. Available at http://qsen.org/about/overview/

Raines. C. F., Taglaireni, M. E. (2008). Career Pathways in Nursing: Entry Points and Academic Progression. *OJIN: The Online Journal of Issues in Nursing, 13*(3).

Robert Wood Johnson Foundation. (2009). *The chronic care model.* Available at http://www.improvingchroniccare.org/index.php?p=The_Chronic_Care_Model&s=2.

Sherwood, G. & Barnsteiner, J. (2012)/ *Quality and safety in nursing: A competency approach to improving outcomes.* Hoboken, NJ: Wiley-Blackwell.

Smith, T. (2009). A policy perspective on the entry into practice issue. *OJIN: The Online Journal of Issues in Nursing, 15*(1).

Stanley, D. (2007). Lights in the shadows: Florence Nightingale and others who made their mark. *Contemporary Nurse, 24*(1), 45–51.

Turnock, B. J. (2009). *Public health: What it is and how it works.* Gaithersburg, MD: Aspen Publishers.

U.S. Department of Health and Human Services Health Resources and Services Administration. Research on the state of the healthcare workforce, tracking shortages, trends and issues as they develop. Health Workforce Analysis. Washington, DC: Author. Available at http://bhpr.hrsa.gov/healthworkforce/index.html

U.S. Department of Health and Human Services Health Resources and Services Administration. (2010). The Registered Nurse Population. Findings from the 2008 National Sample Survey of Registered Nurses. Washington, DC: Author. Available at http://bhpr.hrsa.gov/healthworkforce/rnsurveys/rnsurveyfinal.pdf

U.S. Department of Health and Human Services Health Resources and Services Administration, Bureau of Health Professions (2002). *Projected supply, demand, and shortages of registered nurses: 2000–2020.* Washington, DC: Author.

U.S. Department of Health and Human Services, Office of Disease Prevention and Health Promotion. (2010). *Healthy people 2010.* Washington, DC: Author.

U.S. Department of Health and Human Services, Office of Disease Prevention and Health Promotion. (2020). *Healthy people 2020.* Washington, DC: Author.

U.S. Department of Labor, Bureau of Labor Statistics. (2008). *Occupational Outlook Handbook, 2008–2009 Edition. Registered Nurses.* Washington, DC: Author. Available at http://www.bls.gov/oco/ocos083.htm

Wall, B. M. (2008). Celebrating nursing history. *American Journal of Nursing, 108*(6), 26–29.

West, R. A., Griffith, G. P., & Iphofen, R. (2007). A historical perspective on the nursing shortage. *MEDSURG Nursing, 16*(2), 124–130.

2 Theory, Research, and Evidence-Based Practice

JOE WIMMER

Joe, a first-time father of a healthy 8-lb baby girl delivered several hours ago, is visiting with his wife and new daughter. He asks, "Why is my daughter wearing that funny little cap on her head?"

CHARLOTTE HORN

Charlotte, the daughter of a 57-year-old patient being discharged with an order for intermittent nasogastric tube feedings, is being taught how to perform the procedure. During one of the teaching sessions, Charlotte asks, "How will I know that the tube is in the right place?"

MARIBELLA SANTOS

Maribella, who had just arrived back on the unit after undergoing abdominal surgery, is complaining of nausea. A while later she states, "My nausea is gone. The nurse did something with her hands and the feeling just went away."

Nursing is a unique health care discipline in which nurses provide a service based on knowledge and skill. Nursing has two essential elements: a body of knowledge and the application of that knowledge in nursing care interventions. The body of knowledge provides the rationale for nursing interventions. There is a growing knowledge base developed specifically for nursing through theory development and research (see the accompanying Reflective Practice display for an example). Rationales for nursing interventions also come from many different disciplines, including anatomy, physiology, chemistry, nutrition, psychology, and sociology. This chapter discusses the concepts of nursing knowledge, nursing theory, nursing research, and evidence-based practice as separate entities, but in fact, they are often intertwined in clinical practice.

NURSING KNOWLEDGE

Knowledge is an awareness of reality acquired through learning or investigation. Every individual collects, organizes, and arranges facts to build a knowledge base relevant to one's personal reality. The knowledge base for professional nursing practice includes nursing science, philosophy, and ethics; biology and psychology; and the social, physical, economic, organizational, and technological sciences. Nursing's Social Policy Statement (American Nurses Association [ANA], 2010, pp. 13–14) lists the following as issues that nurses address in partnership with individuals, families, communities, and populations:

- Promotion of health and wellness
- Promotion of safety and quality of care
- Care, self-care processes, and care coordination
- Physical, emotional, and spiritual comfort, discomfort, and pain
- Adaptation to physiologic and pathophysiologic processes
- Emotions related to the experience of birth, growth and development, health, illness, disease and death
- Meanings ascribed to health, illness, and other concepts
- Linguistic and cultural sensitivity
- Health literacy
- Decision making and the ability to make choices
- Relationships, role performance, and change processes within relationships
- Social policies and their effects on health
- Health care systems and their relationships to access, cost, and quality of health care
- The environment and the prevention of disease and injury

As you reflect on this list, you can see why your nursing education is so important and why professional nurses are lifelong learners.

Sources of Knowledge

Knowledge comes from a variety of sources and may be traditional, authoritative, or scientific.

Traditional Knowledge

Traditional knowledge is that part of nursing practice passed down from generation to generation. When questioned about the origin of such nursing practices, nurses might reply, "We've always done it this way." Changing bedclothes is an example of how traditional knowledge has affected nursing practice. It is customary in acute care settings to change a patient's bedclothes daily, whether soiled or not. There are no research data to support this, yet virtually millions of hospital beds are changed daily because this practice is accepted as a necessary component of quality patient care. Until this practice is challenged scientifically and its assumed value disproved, it will remain a traditional part of patient care.

Authoritative Knowledge

Authoritative knowledge comes from an expert and is accepted as truth based on the person's perceived expertise—

REFLECTIVE PRACTICE: CULTIVATING QSEN COMPETENCIES

CHALLENGE TO COGNITIVE SKILLS

One of the nurses, Danielle, on a surgical floor where I was assigned, took a course in therapeutic touch. When she returned to work, she was eager to use her new "intervention." My patient, Maribella Santos, had come back to the unit after undergoing abdominal surgery. Upon her return, she complained of nausea. Danielle used her "unruffling" technique to calm the patient, whose nausea then "disappeared." Excited, I reported this in postconference, only to learn from my instructor that therapeutic touch was "a lot of bunk" without scientific support.

Thinking Outside the Box: Possible Courses of Action

- Accept my instructor's dismissal of therapeutic touch.
- Learn more about therapeutic touch from my colleague Danielle and professional literature.
- Become an advocate for therapeutic touch if it *does* work!

Evaluating a Good Outcome: How Do I Define Success?

- Patient is not harmed by anyone using an unproven therapy.
- Patient benefits from my openness to new (potentially beneficial) therapies.
- I rely on research and evidence-based practice, not hearsay, as a basis for my clinical judgments and actions.

Personal Learning: Here's to the Future!

I was surprised to find the literature so inconclusive about the benefits of therapeutic touch. Obviously, its adherents claim that they can measure its efficacy. Others find these claims unsupported. Since this event happened at the beginning of my clinical rotation, I decided to observe Danielle throughout my rotation. What I saw made me a believer in this technique. Danielle was using therapeutic touch as an adjuvant to other therapies and it seemed to be working. I want to learn more about this technique. My goal is to attend a workshop on therapeutic touch to see if it is something I can incorporate into my practice.

Katherine Figliala, Georgetown University

REFLECTION ON QUALITY AND SAFETY COMPETENCIES

How do you think you would respond in a similar situation? Why? What does this tell you about yourself and about the adequacy of your competencies for professional practice? Can you think of other ways to respond? Do you agree with the criteria that the nursing student used to evaluate a successful outcome? Why or why not? What *knowledge, skills* and *attitudes* do you need to develop to continuously improve the quality and safety of care?

Patient-Centered Care: What information should be communicated to Maribella Santos and other patients about the use of therapeutic touch to involve them as partners in the use of this technique?

Teamwork and Collaboration/Quality Improvement: Other members of the professional caregiving team can have positive and negative effects on us. In what ways do you practice so as to remain open to learning new interventions from colleagues and not allow negativity to inhibit your creativity?

Safety/Evidence-Based Practice: What sources of knowledge did the nursing student use? Did the nursing student use theory and research? If so, please explain how. Would you consider therapeutic touch to be evidence-based practice? Why or why not? How might the patient's culture have affected the response? Might patients be harmed through the use of a new intervention such as therapeutic touch? What safeguards exist in practice sites to prevent reckless experimentation on patients? When a review of the literature proves inconclusive, on what should we base our judgment about the efficacy of therapeutic touch or other interventions?

Informatics: What research strategy is likely to yield the best evidence about the efficacy of therapeutic touch? Can you identify the essential information that must be available in a patient's record about the use of therapeutic touch?

for example, when a senior staff nurse teaches a new graduate nurse a more efficient method of doing a technical procedure, such as inserting an intravenous catheter. The senior nurse has gained knowledge through experience, and the new graduate nurse accepts it as truth based on the perceived authority of the experienced nurse. Authoritative knowledge generally remains unchallenged as long as presumed authorities maintain their perceived expertise.

Scientific Knowledge

Scientific knowledge is knowledge obtained through the scientific method (implying thorough research). New ideas are tested and measured systematically using objective criteria.

THINK back to Maribella Santos, the woman complaining of nausea after undergoing abdominal surgery. The nurse would integrate scientific knowledge about the effects of surgery and anesthesia on the body and the side effects of pain medication to develop the postoperative plan of care. ●

Significance of Knowledge Sources

All sources of knowledge are useful in the collective body of knowledge that constitutes the nursing profession. Although these three sources provide nursing with important contributions, each has inherent strengths and limitations. Both traditional and authoritative knowledge are practical to implement but are often based on subjective data, limiting their usefulness in a wide variety of practice settings. For this reason, nurses increasingly focus on scientific knowledge to provide care, commonly called evidence-based practice, a topic that will be thoroughly discussed later in this chapter.

Types of Knowledge

Some of the types of knowledge include science, philosophy, and process.

Science

Science is observing, identifying, describing, investigating, and explaining events and occurrences that are perceived in the world. It implies a body of knowledge. The science of nursing is the knowledge in and of nursing.

Philosophy

Philosophy is the study of wisdom, fundamental knowledge, and the processes used to develop and construct one's perceptions of life. Philosophy provides a viewpoint and implies a system of values and beliefs. Each individual develops a personal philosophy to give meaning to experiences and to guide behavior and attitudes. Personal philosophies are developed by learning from interpersonal relationships, through formal and informal educational experiences, through religion and culture, and from the environment.

Every nurse's philosophy, developed through education and practice, forms the basis for providing nursing care. Nurses demonstrate both a personal and professional philosophy through their values and beliefs about concepts such as goodness, health, illness, accountability, and ethics. In the same way, nursing education and nursing practice settings provide education or patient care based on philosophic beliefs about humans, health, teaching and learning, and quality patient care.

Process

A **process** is a series of actions, changes, or functions intended to bring about a desired result. During a process, one takes systematic and continuous steps to meet a goal and uses both assessments and feedback to direct actions to meet the goal. A particular theory or conceptual framework directs how these actions are carried out. The delivery of nursing care within the nursing process (described in Unit III) is directed by the way specific conceptual frameworks and theories define the person (patient), the environment, health, and nursing.

Historical Influences on Nursing Knowledge

The development of nursing knowledge has been influenced by the work of Florence Nightingale and by societal changes.

Nightingale's Contributions

Nightingale influenced nursing knowledge and practice by demonstrating efficient and knowledgeable nursing care, defining nursing practice as separate and distinct from medical practice, and differentiating between health nursing and illness nursing (see Chapter 1 for further information).

The training of nurses was initially carried out under the direction and control of the medical profession (Kalish & Kalish, 2004). Because the conceptual and theoretical basis for nursing practice came from outside the profession, nursing struggled for years to establish its own identity and to receive recognition for its significant contributions to health care.

Societal Influences on Nursing Knowledge

Most early schools of nursing established in the United States were adapted from Nightingale's model. There was no planned educational curriculum; instead, knowledge was acquired from lectures by physicians and through practical experience by caring for sick people in hospitals. This service orientation for nursing education remained the strongest influence on nursing practice until the 1950s. Nursing care was carried out under the control and direction of the hospital administration and physicians practicing in that hospital. Nursing care was based on traditional ideas about following orders, as well as on common wisdom about caring for others based on either "common sense" or widely accepted scientific principles (Chinn & Kramer, 2011). As a result, nursing knowledge remained undeveloped and fragmented.

During the first half of the 20th century, a change in the structure of society resulted in changed roles for women and, in turn, for nursing. As a result of World Wars I and II, women increasingly entered the workforce, became more independent, and sought higher education. At the same time, nursing education began to focus more on education than hands-on training, and nursing research was conducted and published. As women became more independent and assertive, nursing's need for a clearly defined identity based on unique contributions to the health care system emerged. In the mid-20th century, the idea of nursing as a science became more generally accepted, and philosophic beliefs and a knowledge base for nursing practice began to evolve. Today the proliferation of graduate nursing programs, including the PhD in nursing, demonstrate society's acceptance of nursing science.

In the 21st century, the Institute of Medicine (IOM) issued its seminal report, *The Future of Nursing* (IOM, 2011), which identifies research priorities for transforming nursing practice, nursing education, and nursing leadership. "Taken together, the recommendations are meant to provide a strong foundation for the development of a nursing workforce whose members are well educated and well prepared to practice to the full extent of their education, to meet the current and future health needs of patients, and to act as full partners in leading change and advancing health" (IOM, 2011, p. 271). The IOM report is available on their website: www.iom.edu.

NURSING THEORY

A **theory** is composed of a group of concepts that describe a pattern of reality. **Concepts**, like ideas, are abstract impressions organized into symbols of reality. Concepts describe objects, properties, and events and relationships among them. A group of concepts that follows an understandable pattern makes up a **conceptual framework or model**. Concepts can be thought of as the individual bricks and boards used to build a house, with the conceptual framework being the blueprint that specifies where each brick and board should go. Theories can be tested, changed, or used to guide research or to provide a base for evaluation. They are derived through two principal methods: **deductive reasoning**, in which one examines a general idea and then considers specific actions or ideas, and **inductive reasoning**, in which the reverse process is used—one builds from specific ideas or actions to conclusions about general ideas.

Nursing theory is developed to describe nursing. Nursing theory differentiates nursing from other disciplines and activities in that it serves the purposes of describing, explaining, predicting, and controlling desired outcomes of nursing care practices. Thus, theories provide a means of testing knowledge through research and for expanding nursing's knowledge base to meet the health care needs of patients in an ever-changing society.

Interdisciplinary Base for Nursing Theories

Nursing theories are often based on, and influenced by, other broadly applicable processes and theories. The ideas and principles of the theories described briefly in the following sections are basic to many nursing concepts and are a part of the nursing literature. Nurses need to understand these theories and terminologies as they develop their own knowledge base in nursing.

General Systems Theory

General systems theory has been used in a wide range of disciplines since it emerged in the 1920s. Its primary theorist, Ludwig von Bertalanffy, developed the theory for universal application. This theory describes how to break whole things into parts and then to learn how the parts work together in "systems." It emphasizes relationships between the whole and the parts and describes how parts function and behave. These concepts may be applied to different kinds of systems, for example, to molecules in chemistry, cultures in sociology, organs in anatomy, and health in nursing. The key points in general systems theory are outlined in Box 2-1.

 RECALL Maribella Santos, the woman described in the Reflective Practice box who received Therapeutic Touch? The nurse would need to integrate knowledge of systems theory, including system communication, open systems, and energy transfer to better understand the goal of this technique. ●

Adaptation Theory

Adaptation theory defines adaptation as the adjustment of living matter to other living things and to environmental conditions. Adaptation is a continuously occurring process that effects change and involves interaction and response. Human adaptation occurs on three levels: the internal (self), the social (others), and the physical (biochemical reactions). Chapter 41 describes adaptation in relation to stress.

Developmental Theory

Developmental theory outlines the process of growth and development of humans as orderly and predictable, beginning with conception and ending with death. Although the pattern has definite stages, the progress and behaviors of an individual within each stage are unique. Heredity, temperament, emotional and physical environment, life experiences, and health status influence the growth and development of an individual.

Several theorists have made important contributions to developmental theory, but only two are mentioned here because their work is often used to develop nursing theory and to organize nursing practice. Erik Erikson based his theory of psychosocial development on the process of socialization, emphasizing how individuals learn to interact with the world. Erikson recognized the role of social, biologic, and environmental factors in development, and defined specific tasks or conflicts that people accomplish or overcome during what he defined as the eight stages of life. Chapters 17 to 19 present more information on developmental theory.

Abraham Maslow developed his theory of human needs in terms of physical and psychosocial needs considered essential to human life, rather than by chronologic age as Erikson did. As described in Chapter 4, Maslow defined five levels of need in a hierarchy, with different needs existing simultaneously.

 THINK back to Joe Wimmer, the new father of a baby girl. When explaining about the use of the cap on the baby's head, the nurse would incorporate knowledge of Maslow's hierarchy of needs, specifically physiologic needs, and the need to minimize heat loss as a priority. ●

As you continue in your nursing education and practice, you will learn how systems, adaptation, and developmental theories are used in planning and giving holistic care to patients. The following sections on specific nursing theories will help you better understand the knowledge base used to develop the concepts unique to nursing.

Nursing Theories

Even though nurses have difficulty agreeing on precise definitions of nursing, theory-based nursing directs nurses toward a common goal, with the ultimate outcome being improved patient care. Nursing theory provides rational and knowledgeable reasons for nursing interventions, based on descriptions of what nursing is and what nurses do. Additionally, nursing theory gives nurses the knowledge base necessary for acting and responding appropriately in nursing care situations, provides a base for discussion, and, ideally, helps resolve current nursing issues. Theory gives nurses who know and practice theory better problem-solving skills, so that nursing interventions are better organized, considered, and purposeful. Nursing theory also prepares nurses to question assumptions and values in nursing, thus further defining nursing and increasing the knowledge base.

Nursing theories identify and define interrelated concepts important in nursing and clearly state the relationships between and among these concepts. Nursing theories should be simple and general; simple terminology and broadly applicable concepts ensure their usefulness in a wide variety of nursing practice situations. Nursing theories should also increase the nursing profession's body of knowledge by generating research to guide and improve practice. Overall, nursing theory guides nursing practice by providing a knowledge base, organizing concepts, providing guidelines for practice, and identifying nursing care goals.

Nursing theories may be descriptive or prescriptive (Meleis, 2012). Descriptive theories describe a phenomenon, an event, a situation, or a relationship. They further identify the properties and components of each of these as well as the circumstances in which it occurs. Prescriptive theories address nursing interventions and the consequences of those interventions; they are designed to control, promote, and change clinical nursing practice.

The aims of nursing, described in Chapter 1, are the same for all nursing theorists, but the values, assumptions, and beliefs individualize each theory when it is applied to nursing care. Theoretical frameworks of nursing provide a focus for nursing care activities. The person receiving care is the central theme, but the way each theorist defines that person, the environment, health, and nursing gives a unique focus specific to a particular theory. The ultimate goal of each framework is holistic patient care, individualized to meet needs, promote health, and prevent or treat illness. Selected theories of nursing are outlined in Table 2-1.

Common Concepts in Nursing Theories

Four concepts common in nursing theory that influence and determine nursing practice are (1) the person (patient), (2) the environment, (3) health, and (4) nursing. Each of these concepts is usually defined and described by a nursing theorist, and although these concepts are common to all nursing theories, both the definitions and the relations among them may differ from one theory to another. Of the four concepts, the most important is that of the person. The focus of nursing, regardless of definition or theory, is the person (Fig. 2-1).

Nursing Theory in Clinical Practice

As a discipline, nursing is increasingly defining its own independent functions and contributions to health care. The development and use of nursing theory provide autonomy (independence and self-governance) in the practice of nursing in many ways. As nurses demonstrate that nursing care does indeed make a difference and that nursing services are valuable, the discipline becomes more independent. Having a body of knowledge specific to the discipline allows members to be viewed by others as experts; this, in turn, gives nurses authority to carry out actions.

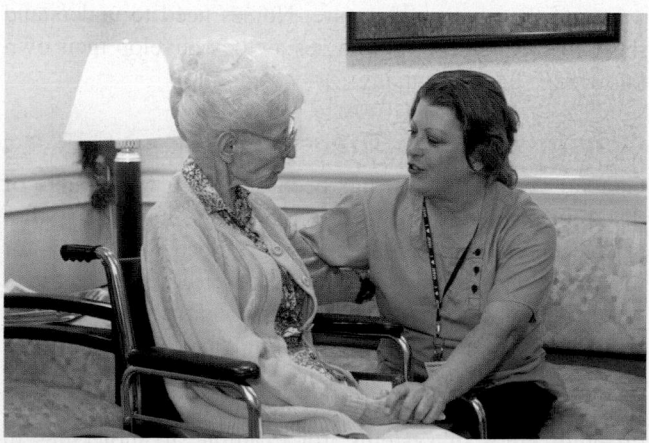

FIGURE 2-1. Four concepts common to all nursing theories are person, environment, health, and nursing. The most important concept, and the focus of nursing, is the person. (*Photo by Rick Brady.*)

Table 2-1	SELECTED THEORISTS AND THEORIES OF NURSING	
NURSING THEORIST AND DATE OF THEORY	**CENTRAL THEME**	**APPLICATION TO CLINICAL PRACTICE**
Florence Nightingale (1860)	Meeting the personal needs of the patient within the environment	Concern for the environment of the patient, including cleanliness, ventilation, temperature, light, diet, and noise
Hildegard Peplau (1952)	Nursing is a therapeutic, interpersonal, and goal-oriented process.	Nursing interventions are directed toward developing the patient's personality for productive personal and community living.
Virginia Henderson (1955)	The patient is an individual who requires help to reach independence.	Nursing practice is independent; autonomous nursing functions are identified, and self-help concepts are described.
Faye Abdullah (1960)	Nursing is a problem-solving art and science used to identify the nursing problems of patients as they move toward health and cope with illness-related health needs.	The 21 nursing-care problems identified were based on research and can be used to determine patient needs and formulate nursing-focused care.
Ida Jean Orlando (1961)	The nurse reacts to the patient's verbal and nonverbal expression of needs both to understand the meaning of the distress and to know what is needed to alleviate it.	Uses the nursing process to provide solutions to problems as well as to prevent problems.
Ernestine Wiedenbach (1964)	Nursing as an art; nursing is providing nurturing care to patients.	Clinical nursing includes a philosophy, a purpose, the practice, and the art. Care is directed toward a specific purpose to meet the patient's perceived health care needs.
Lydia E. Hall (1966)	A focus on rehabilitation, encompassing nursing's autonomy, is therapeutic use of self, treatment within the health care team (cure), and nurturing (care).	The major outcome of nursing care is rehabilitation and feelings of self-actualization by the patient.
Myra E. Levine (1967)	Emphasis is on the ill person in the health care setting; describes detailed nursing skills and actions.	The patient is the center of nursing activities, with nursing care provided based on four conservation principles to help patients adapt to their environment.
Martha Rogers (1970)	Emphasis on the science and art of nursing, with the unitary human being central to the discipline of nursing.	Nursing interventions are directed toward repatterning human environment fields or assisting in mobilizing inner resources.
Dorothea Orem (1971)	Self-care is a human need; self-care deficits require nursing actions.	Nursing is a human service, and nurses design interventions to provide or to manage self-care actions for sustaining health or recovering from illness or injury.
Imogene King (1971)	The patient is a personal system within a social system; the nurse and the patient experience each other and the situation, act and react, and transact.	Nursing is a process of human interactions as nurses and patients communicate to mutually set goals, and explore and agree on the means to reach those goals.
Betty Newman (1972)	Humans are in constant relationship with stressors in the environment.	The major concern for nursing is keeping the patient's system stable through accurately assessing the effects of environmental stressors and in assisting the patient with adjustments required for optimal wellness.
Sister Callista Roy (1974)	Humans are biopsychosocial beings existing within an environment. Needs are created within interrelated adaptive modes: physiologic self-concept, role function, and interdependence.	Nursing interventions are required when individuals demonstrate ineffective adaptive responses.
Madeline Leininger (1978)	Caring is the central theme of nursing care, knowledge, and practice.	Provides the foundation of transcultural nursing care. Caring improves human conditions and life processes.

(continued)

Table 2-1 SELECTED THEORISTS AND THEORIES OF NURSING *continued*

NURSING THEORIST AND DATE OF THEORY	CENTRAL THEME	APPLICATION TO CLINICAL PRACTICE
Jean Watson (1979)	Nursing is concerned with promoting and restoring health, preventing illness, and caring for the sick.	Clinical nursing care is holistic to promote humanism, health, and quality of living. Caring is universal and is practiced through interpersonal relationships.
Margaret A. Newman (1979)	Nursing interventions are purposeful, using a total-person approach to patient care to help individuals, families, and groups attain and maintain wellness.	Nursing care is directed toward reducing stress factors and adverse conditions that increase the risk for or actually affect optimal patient functions.
Dorothy E. Johnson (1980)	Nursing problems arise when there are disturbances in the system or subsystem, or the level of behavioral functioning is below an optimal level.	Nursing interventions are designed to support/maintain health, educate, counsel, and modify behavior.
Rosemarie Parse (1981)	The individual continually interacts with the environment and participates in maintaining health.	Health is a continual, open process (rather than an absence of illness), with nursing care planned based on the patient's perspective of health and care.
Nola Pender (1982)	The goal of nursing is the optimal health of the individual, with a focus on how individuals make health care decisions.	Factors significant to health-promoting behaviors include an individual's beliefs about the importance of health, the perceived benefits of, and perceived barriers to, those behaviors. Participation in health-promoting behaviors is modified by one's demographic and biologic characteristics, interpersonal influences, and situational and behavioral factors.
Patricia Benner & Judith Wrubel (1989)	Nursing practice within a context of caring and skill development. Caring is a common bond of persons situated in a state of being that is essential to nursing.	A systematic description of stages of nursing practice: novice, advanced beginner, competent, proficient, and expert.

In addition, interventions carried out and based on sound rationales are trusted and respected.

Today, it has become even more necessary and important for nurses to demonstrate efficient, cost-effective, high-quality care within organized health care delivery systems. By practicing theory-based nursing combined with clinical reasoning skills, nurses are able not only to deliver care that meets those criteria but also to describe and document what it is they do. Professional nurses use theories from nursing and from the behavioral sciences to collect, organize, and classify patient data and to understand, analyze, and interpret patients' health situations. Theoretical concepts and theories guide all phases of the nursing process, including planning, implementing, and evaluating nursing care, while also describing and explaining desired responses to and outcomes of care.

The major concepts of a chosen model or theory guide each step of the nursing process. The concepts serve as categories to guide the nurse in determining what information is relevant and should be collected to make assessments and to formulate nursing diagnoses. The concepts also suggest the appropriate types of nursing interventions and patient outcomes to be included in the care plan (see Table 2-1 for the purpose and clinical application of selected nursing theories). It is important to realize that as the focus of nursing changes, so does the applicability of the concepts within a specific theory.

NURSING RESEARCH

Research most simply defined means to examine carefully or to search again. Research as scientific inquiry is a process that uses observable and verifiable information (**data**), collected in a systematic manner, to describe, explain, or predict events. Research is conducted to validate and refine current knowledge or to develop new knowledge. The goals of research are to develop explanations (in theories) and to find solutions to problems.

 CONSIDER Charlotte Horn, the daughter who is being taught how to give tube feedings and is asking about ensuring proper tube placement. The nurse would recommend the best method to use based on scientific evidence from research. ●

Nursing research, broadly defined, encompasses research to improve the care of people in the clinical setting as well as the broader study of people and the nursing profession, including studies of education, policy development, ethics, and nursing history. Research is included as an essential component of nursing by the American Nurses

Used with permission. American Nurses Association (ANA). (2010a). *Nursing: Scope and standards of practice, 2nd ed.* Silver Spring, MD: Author, p. 51.

Box 2-2 ANA STANDARDS OF PROFESSIONAL NURSING PRACTICE

Standard 9. Evidence-Based Practice and Research
The registered nurse integrates evidence and research findings into practice.

Competencies

The registered nurse:

- Utilizes current evidence-based nursing knowledge, including research findings, to guide practice.
- Incorporates evidence when initiating changes in nursing practice.
- Participates as appropriate to education level and position, in the formulation of evidence-based practice through research.
- Shares personal or third-party research findings with colleagues and peers.

Association (ANA), by the International Council of Nurses, and by nursing specialty organizations (Box 2-2). One of the many ways to promote nursing's development of greater autonomy and strength is nursing research. Nurses, depending on their level of education, conduct or participate in research to improve their efforts to deliver high-quality, cost-efficient care. Nurses also increasingly use the findings of research to provide evidence-based nursing practice (discussed in the next section).

Nursing research is fundamental to the recognition of nursing as a profession. As an occupation, nursing has existed since the beginning of human history. One of the essential elements that differentiate a profession from an occupation is the existence of a unique and distinct knowledge base. The ultimate goal of expanding nursing's body of knowledge is to learn improved ways to promote and maintain health. As health care and illness patterns change, nursing interventions must change. Ongoing practice-based research reflects the nursing profession's commitment to meet the ever-changing demands of health care consumers.

 REMEMBER Joe Wimmer, the new father described at the beginning of the chapter. Before responding to Mr. Wimmer, the nurse would need knowledge of newborn heat loss and methods to minimize it. A review of the literature would provide theoretical information necessary to explain the scientific rationale for using caps on the heads of newborns to reduce heat loss. •

The Evolution of Nursing Research

While caring for victims of the Crimean War, Florence Nightingale kept careful and objective records. These records provided baseline data that she later used to deter-mine which nursing interventions were most effective in treating her patients.

Although nurses have always provided care through nursing interventions and have evaluated the response of the patient, for a long time those interventions were primarily based on a philosophy of "It's always been done that way." As advances were made in technology and medical research during the 20th century, nursing leaders realized that research about the practice of nursing was necessary to meet the health needs of modern society. Increasing numbers of nurses began to conduct research and publish articles telling other nurses how to conduct nursing research.

During the 1950s and 1960s, nursing research was increasingly recognized as important. Early studies provided the basis for the development of nursing practice standards and the most effective educational preparation for registered nurses. The ANA sponsored a series of nursing research conferences. A focus on clinical studies to examine quality of care and the development of outcomes of care grew out of the newly developed intensive care units (ICUs).

The 1970s and 1980s focused on clinical research, with published studies of clinical interventions, such as vital signs and treatment procedures. Primary patient care was a popular method of nursing care, with research investigating outcomes and quality of care. The nursing process also was studied, with research into assessment and effective nursing diagnosis of patient responses to the effects of illness. Studies of nursing education were concerned with student learning experiences and clinical evaluation methods, as well as differentiation of practice by educational preparation. In addition, models, conceptual frameworks, and theories were developed to guide nursing practice. More nurses were prepared at the master's and doctoral levels, and federal funding for nursing research increased. Journals specific to nursing research (both generally and in specialty areas) were published.

Of major importance was the ANA's 1985 creation of the National Center for Nursing Research, which was subsequently promoted to the National Institute of Nursing Research (NINR) in 1993, thereby gaining equal status with the other 27 National Institutes of Health. The NINR website funds research that establishes the scientific basis for quality patient care. According to the NINR, the goals of nursing research are to:

- Build the scientific foundation for clinical practice
- Prevent disease and disability
- Manage and eliminate symptoms caused by illness
- Enhance end-of-life and palliative care

The NINR website offers a series of "Featured Research Highlights," which summarize the recent work of NINR-supported researchers across the country. Box 2-3 (on page 32) is an example of one of these, concerning practices to decrease infection rates in the ICU.

Methods of Conducting Nursing Research

Nursing research is conducted by quantitative and qualitative methodology. Each method is summarized here to facilitate

Box 2-3 NINR FEATURED RESEARCH HIGHLIGHT

High compliance with "central line bundle" preventive practices can decrease infection rates in the ICU.

- Patients hospitalized in an intensive care unit (ICU) frequently need a central line—a special type of intravenous catheter surgically implanted into a major vein—for the delivery of fluids, nutrition, and medications.
- However, central lines are associated with a high risk of bloodstream infections (BSIs), which are very expensive to treat and can lead to disability or death. The Institute for Healthcare Improvement has promoted use of a "central line bundle" of clinical practices to reduce the incidence of BSIs associated with central lines.

For this study, the researchers focused on the use of three of the five elements of the bundle:

1. Maximal barrier precautions to maintain sterility when the line is inserted
2. Optimal selection of the insertion site to reduce chance of contamination
3. Daily review of the need for the central line, with prompt removal once no longer required

  - A survey of 415 ICUs in 250 hospitals across the United States found that about half had a written

central line bundle policy in place. However, only 45% of these units monitored compliance with this policy. Of these, 38% reported a high (>95%) compliance rate.
- Among the 312 ICUs that reported BSI rates, lower rates were achieved only for those that had a bundle policy in place, monitored compliance, and reported high compliance with at least one of the three central line bundle elements studied.
- The researchers estimate that an ICU moving from noncompliance to high compliance with at least one of these central line bundle elements could achieve a 38% reduction in BSIs. This result has the promise to reduce the risks associated with central lines, thereby lowering health care costs and improving health outcomes.

Citations

Furuya E. Y., Dick, A., Perencevich, E. N., Pogorzelska, M., Goldmann, D., Stone, P. W. (2011). Central line bundle implementation in US intensive care units and impact on bloodstream infections. *PLoS ONE*, 6, 1, e15452. DOI:10.1371/journal.pone.0015452
National Institute of Nursing Research: http://www.ninr.nih.gov/researchandfunding/researchhighlights/featuredarchive/stone-rh-archived#.UuF-8WQo5R4

---

understanding published research so that findings may be used in clinical practice.

Quantitative Research Methods

Quantitative research involves the concepts of basic and applied research. Box 2-4 provides definitions of important terms for quantitative research. **Basic research**, sometimes called pure or laboratory research, is designed to generate and refine theory, and the findings are often not directly useful in practice. **Applied research**, also called practical research, is designed to directly influence or improve clinical practice.

Box 2-4 IMPORTANT TERMS IN QUANTITATIVE RESEARCH

- *Variable:* Something that varies and has different values that can be measured
- *Dependent variable:* The variable being studied, determined as a result of a study
- *Independent variable:* Causes or conditions that are manipulated or identified to determine the effects on the dependent variable
- *Hypothesis:* Statement of relationships between the independent and dependent variables that the researcher expects to find
- *Data:* Information the researcher collects from subjects in the study (expressed in numbers)
- *Instruments:* Devices used to collect and record the data, such as rating scales, pencil-and-paper tests, and biologic measurements. Instruments should be both reliable (produce the same results [data] on repeated use) and valid (test what they are supposed to test).

The types of quantitative research depend on the level of current knowledge about a research problem (Table 2-2). The steps of quantitative research are followed carefully, although they may be designed in different ways. Table 2-3 presents an overview of the basic steps of the quantitative research process.

Qualitative Research Methods

Qualitative research is a method of research conducted to gain insight by discovering meanings. At its core is the idea that reality is based on perceptions, which differ for each person and change over time. The research design follows many of the same steps as quantitative research, but differs in that the researcher primarily analyzes words or narratives rather than numbers. Table 2-4 (on page 34) outlines and briefly describes the methods of qualitative research.

Protection of the Rights of Human Subjects

Many nurses work in health care institutions in which patients are invited to participate in clinical research. With their focus on the overall well-being of the patient, nurses play an important role in ensuring that patient interests are not sacrificed to research interests. Nursing priorities include determining that the studies have met appropriate scientific and ethical criteria before their implementation, and protecting patient rights. Specific patient rights include **informed consent**, the patient's right to consent knowledgeably to participate in a study without coercion (knowing that this consent may be withdrawn at any time) or to refuse to participate without jeopardizing the care that he or she will receive, the right to confidentiality, and the right to be

Table 2-2 TYPES OF QUANTITATIVE RESEARCH

TYPE	PURPOSE
Descriptive Research	To explore and describe events in real-life situations, describing concepts and identifying relationships between and among events. Often used to generate new knowledge about topics with little or no prior research.
Correlational Research	To examine the type and degree of relationships between two or more variables. The strength of the relationship varies from a −1 (perfect negative correlation, in which one increases as the other decreases) to a +1 (perfect positive correlation, with both variables increasing or decreasing together).
Quasi-experimental Research	To examine cause-and-effect relationships between selected variables. Often conducted in clinical settings to examine the effects of nursing interventions on patient outcomes.
Experimental Research	To examine cause-and-effect relationships between variables under highly controlled conditions. These are often conducted in a laboratory setting.

protected from harm. Nurse ethicist Christine Grady and her colleagues propose seven requirements that provide a coherent framework for evaluating the ethics of clinical research studies (Emmanuel, Wendler & Grady, 2000):

- Value: Enhancements of health or knowledge must be derived from the research.
- Scientific validity: The research must be methodologically rigorous.
- Fair subject selection: Scientific objectives, not vulnerability or privilege, and the potential for and distribution of risks and benefits, should determine communities selected

as study sites and the inclusion criteria for individual subjects.

- Favorable risk–benefit ratio: Within the context of standard clinical practice and the research protocol, risks must be minimized, potential benefits enhanced, and the potential benefits to individuals and knowledge gained for society must outweigh the risks.
- Independent review: Unaffiliated individuals must review the research and approve, amend, or terminate it.
- Informed consent: Individuals should be informed about the research and provide their voluntary consent.

Table 2-3 STEPS OF THE QUANTITATIVE RESEARCH PROCESS

STEP	DESCRIPTION
1. State the research problem.	Often stated as a question, which should be focused narrowly on the problem being studied. For example: "What is the optimal time for taking a rectal temperature with a digital thermometer?"
2. Define the purpose of the study.	The purpose explains "why" the problem is important and what use the findings will be.
3. Review-related literature.	The literature review provides information about what is already known, as well as providing information about concepts and how the concepts have been measured. It also identifies gaps in knowledge that will be studied.
4. Formulate hypotheses and variables.	Hypotheses are statements about two or more variables. Scientific hypotheses must be testable using variables that can be measured, manipulated, or controlled in a study.
5. Select the research design.	The design is a carefully determined, systematic, and controlled plan for finding answers to the question of the study. This provides a "road map" for all aspects of the study, including how to collect and analyze the data.
6. Select the population and sample.	The population is the group to be studied. The sample refers to specific people or events in the population from which data will be collected.
7. Collect the data.	Sources of data may include people, literature, documents, and findings (e.g., from sources such as laboratory data or measurements of vital signs). Data may be collected from interviews, questionnaires, direct measurement, or examinations (such as physical or psychological tests).
8. Analyze the data.	Statistical procedures are used to analyze the data and provide answers to the research question.
9. Communicate findings and conclusions.	Through publications and presentations, the researcher explains the results of the study and links them to the existing body of knowledge in the literature. The researcher also describes the implications of the study and suggests directions for further research.

Table 2-4 QUALITATIVE RESEARCH METHODS

METHOD	DESCRIPTION
Phenomenology	The purpose of phenomenology (both a philosophy and a research method) is to describe experiences as they are lived by the subjects being studied. Analysis of data provides information about the meaning of the experience within each person's own reality (e.g., the experience of health or of having a heart attack).
Grounded Theory	The basis of grounded theory methodology is the discovery of how people describe their own reality and how their beliefs are related to their actions in a social scene. The findings are grounded in the data from subjects and are used to formulate concepts and to generate a theory of the experience, supported by examples from the data (e.g., coping with a seriously ill child).
Ethnography	Developed by the discipline of anthropology, ethnographic research is used to examine issues of a culture that are of interest to nursing.
Historical	Historical research examines events of the past to increase understanding of the nursing profession today. Many historical studies focus on nursing leaders, but there is increasing interest in the historical patterns of nursing practice.

• Respect for enrolled subjects: Subjects should have their privacy protected, the opportunity to withdraw, and their well-being monitored.

Federal regulations require that institutions receiving federal funding or conducting studies of drugs or medical devices regulated by the Food and Drug Administration establish institutional review boards (IRBs). The IRBs review all studies conducted in the institution to determine the risk status of all studies and to ensure that ethical principles are followed (see Chapter 6 for full discussion of values and ethics in nursing).

Application of Research to Practice

The most common impediments to nursing research include restricted access to resources, limited time to participate in research-related activities, and lack of educational preparation needed by nurses for research. Research about nursing education, administration, and practice all affect patient care directly or indirectly. Too often, practicing nurses mistakenly think research is far removed from caring for patients at the bedside. This false impression has slowed the progress of practice-based nursing research. Yet much of what bedside nurses routinely do constitutes research. The nursing process (i.e., assessing, diagnosing, planning, implementing, and evaluating) represents the basic framework of the research process.

Unless the research findings of nurse researchers are used by practicing nurses to improve the quality of patient care, clinical nursing research is useless. Nursing students developing clinical skills must understand the scientific rationale that makes one course of action preferable to another (Fig. 2-2). Throughout this text, Research in Nursing boxes highlight current studies that have the potential to make a positive difference in nursing practice and patient outcomes.

EVIDENCE-BASED PRACTICE

Nurses make decisions about many different aspects of patient care each day. For example, questions for consideration range from "What route should I use to take an infant's temperature?" to "How can I move my patient in bed to decrease complications and promote safety?" Patient safety and health may be adversely affected unless the most current best evidence is used to answer questions and make clinical decisions.

Evidence-based practice (EBP) in nursing is a problem-solving approach to making clinical decisions, using the best evidence available (considered "best" because it is collected from sources such as published research, national standards and guidelines, and reviews of targeted literature). EBP blends both the science and the art of nursing so that the best patient outcomes are achieved. The information that is collected is analyzed and used to answer questions (the science of nursing), taking into consideration patient preferences and values, as well as the clinical experiences of the nurse (the art of nursing). EBP may consist of specific nursing interventions or may use guidelines established for the care of patients with certain illnesses, treatments, or surgical procedures.

FIGURE 2-2. A student questions her instructor about the discrepancy between what she sees staff nurses doing to treat a wound and what her text and literature search recommend.

Implementing EBP in clinical practice can present multiple challenges. Resistance to using EBP may arise in the current health care setting as a result of the nursing shortage, the acuity level of patients, nurses' skill in reading and evaluating published research, and an organizational culture that does not support change. However, to achieve desired outcomes for quality patient care and to demonstrate clinical nursing effectiveness, it is critical that nurses gain the necessary knowledge and skills to provide the best possible nursing care. The practice settings in which nurses work must support changes made based on EBP. The changes may be implemented by an individual nurse, by groups of nurses working together, or by interdisciplinary teams of health care providers.

The American Association of Critical Care Nurses (AACN) has developed useful EBP resources, which are shown in Box 2-5. The AACN website also offers a series of "Practice Alerts" that provide research-supported directives for specific clinical situations. Box 2-6 (on page 36) is an example of one AACN Practice Alert for catheter-associated urinary tract infections. Note that in all of these features you will find examples of (1) the scope and impact of the problem, (2) expected practice, (3) supporting evidence, (4) actions for nursing practice, (5) AACN levels of evidence (Armola et al., 2009), and (6) a section titled "Need more information or help?" with additional resources and pertinent references.

Box 2-5 | AACN EVIDENCE-BASED RESOURCES

- **Practice Alerts:** Practice alerts are succinct, dynamic directives from AACN that are supported by authoritative evidence to ensure excellence in practice and a safe and humane work environment.
- **AACN PEARL:** PEARL—an acronym for Practice, Evidence, Application, Resources, and Leadership—is an online collection of evidence-based tools and resources that simplify the process of sharing critical learning with peers, staff nurses, and hospital leadership.
- **Searching for Evidence Toolkit:** Tools to help you find and evaluate evidence.
- **Clinical Focus:** A knowledge portal for clinical topics of interest to acute care and critical care nurses.
- **Protocols for Practice:** *Protocols for Practice* provide bedside clinicians with the latest patient-care research findings. Available for purchase in the AACN Marketplace.
- **Procedure Manual:** The *AACN Procedure Manual for Critical Care* offers comprehensive coverage of procedures unique to the critical care environment.
- **Thunder Studies:** AACN's Thunder Project® was conceptualized and developed to provide critical care nurses with a research protocol ready for institutional review and implementation.

These resources are available at the American Association of Critical Care Nurses website. http://www.aacn.org/WD/Practice/Content/ebp.content?menu=Practice&lastmenu=

Rationale for Using EBP

The impetus for EBP is based in the Institute of Medicine report (2001) *Crossing the Quality Chasm: A New Health System for the 21st Century* that challenged health care professionals to provide care based on scientific evidence. In addition, those interested in quality and cost control want evidence that the services and interventions being funded or reimbursed are effective in securing valued goals.

Until the mid-1990s, many large hospitals had research utilization departments directed by doctorally prepared nurse scientists. These departments conducted research within the hospital to answer clinical practice questions, and used the research findings to dictate practice changes. Today, few hospitals use findings from their own research to direct clinical nursing practice. As a result of recent advances in information technology, findings from published literature can be found, analyzed, and applied to answer clinically relevant questions. Key databases and search engines may be easily accessed on most work computer stations as well as home computer systems. Many research articles in journals and guidelines developed by expert panels can be downloaded, read, evaluated, and shared with colleagues.

Therefore, the use of EBP mandates the analysis and systematic review of research findings. The first step for you as a student is to be able to read and understand a research article. To help you, the typical format of a research journal article with a description of each part is outlined in Table 2-5 (on page 37).

Steps in Implementing EBP

To practice EBP, nurses carry out the following 5 steps (Melnyk & Fineout-Overholt, 2005).

Step 1: Ask a question about a clinical area of interest or an intervention. There are several different methods that can be used to ask clinical questions. The most common method is the PICO format (Melnyk & Fineout-Overholt, 2002), described in Table 2-6 (on page 37). See the accompanying PICO in Practice (on page 38), for a sample of the development of a clinical question using PICO and the EBP decision-making process; additional samples are found in selected chapters of this book.

Step 2: Collect the most relevant and best evidence. It is important to collect information that is regarded as the strongest level of evidence. The level for strength of evidence is numerical, with level 1 being the strongest and level 7 the lowest. The strongest ("best") evidence is provided by findings from systematic reviews, EBP guidelines, and meta-analyses. **Systematic reviews** summarize findings from multiple studies of a specific clinical practice question or topic, and recommend practice changes and future directions for research. **Evidence-based practice guidelines** synthesize information from multiple studies and recommend best practices to treat patients with a disease (e.g., hypertension), a symptom (e.g., chronic pain), or a disability (e.g., cognitive impairment). These guidelines are typically

BOX 2-6	AACN PRACTICE ALERT: CATHETER-ASSOCIATED URINARY TRACT INFECTIONS

Scope and Impact of the Problem

Urinary tract infections (UTIs) are the most common nosocomial infection, accounting for up to 40% of infections reported by acute care hospitals.[1,2] Up to 80% of UTIs are associated with the presence of an indwelling urinary catheter.[3] A catheter-associated urinary tract infection (CAUTI) increases hospital cost and is associated with increased morbidity and mortality.[2,5,6] CAUTIs are considered by the Centers for Medicare and Medicaid Services to represent a reasonably preventable complication of hospitalization. As such, no additional payment is provided to hospitals for CAUTI treatment-related costs.[5]

Expected Practice

☑ Prior to placement of any indwelling urinary catheter, assess patient for accepted indications and alternatives. [Level C]

☑ Adhere to aseptic technique for placement, manipulation, and maintenance of indwelling urinary catheters. [Level E]

☑ Document all instances of indwelling urinary catheters, including insertion date, indication, and removal date. [Level C]

☑ Promptly discontinue indwelling urinary catheters as soon as indications expire. [Level C]

Supporting Evidence

- Prolonged catheterization is the major risk factor for CAUTIs.[7,8]
- Twenty-five percent of inpatients and up to 90% of patients in an ICU have a urinary catheter during hospitalization, often without an appropriate indication.[4] Indwelling urinary catheters are placed without sufficient rationale, and/or remain in place after indications expire.[9]
- CAUTIs can be decreased by interventions that facilitate removal of unnecessary catheters.[10,11]
- Most hospitals have not implemented effective strategies for preventing CAUTIs.[12,13]

Actions for Nursing Practice

- Develop written guidelines for urinary catheterization, include indications for indwelling urinary catheterization, and ensure that catheter placement is limited to patients who meet indications.
- Have available devices, supplies, and techniques that allow alternatives to indwelling catheters (eg, condom catheters, penis pouches, bladder scanners, incontinence products).
- Design and implement standards and training programs for catheter insertion and manipulation.
- Review the necessity of catheter continuation for all patients with urinary catheters on a daily basis.
- Develop systems to ensure prompt removal of catheters when no longer indicated.
- Implement infection surveillance programs that include unit-based urinary catheter days and rates of CAUTIs.
- Develop action plans to address needed improvements.

AACN Levels of Evidence

Level A   Meta-analysis of quantitative studies or metasynthesis of qualitative studies with results that consistently support a specific action, intervention, or treatment

Level B   Well-designed, controlled studies with results that consistently support a specific action, intervention, or treatment

Level C   Qualitative studies, descriptive or correlational studies, integrative reviews, systematic reviews, or randomized controlled trials with inconsistent results

Level D   Peer-reviewed professional organizational standards with clinical studies to support recommendations

Level E   Multiple case reports, theory-based evidence from expert opinions, or peer-reviewed professional organizational standards without clinical studies to support recommendations

Level M   Manufacturer's recommendations only

Need More Information or Help?

- Contact a clinical practice specialist for additional information (www.aacn.org); then select Practice Resource Network and Ask the Clinical Practice Team.
- Lo E, Lindsay N, Classen D, et al. Strategies to prevent catheter-associated urinary tract infections in acute care hospitals. *Infect Control Hosp Epidemiol.* 2008;29:S41–S50.
- HICPAC/Centers for Disease Control and Prevention. Guideline for Prevention of Catheter-Associated Urinary Tract Infections. 2009. http://www.cdc.gov/hicpac/cauti/001_cauti.html. Accessed October 5, 2011.

References

1. Edward JR, Peterson KD, Andrus ML, et al. National Health Safety Network (NHSN) report, data summary for 2006, issued June 2007. *Am J Infect Control.* 2007;35:290–301.
2. Klevans RM, Edwards JR, Richards CL, et al. Estimating health care-associated infections and deaths in US hospitals, 2002. *Pub Health Rep.* 2007;122:160–166.
3. Apisarnthanarak A, Rutjanawech S, Wichansawakun S, et al. Initial inappropriate urinary catheters use in a tertiary-care center. *Am J Infect Control.* 2007;35:594–599.
4. Laupland KB, Bagshaw SM, Gregson DB, Kirkpatrick AW, Ross T, Church DL. Intensive care unit-acquired urinary tract infections in a regional critical care system. *Crit Care.* 2005;9: R60–R65.
5. Wald HL, Kramer AM. Nonpayment for harms resulting from medical care. *JAMA.* 2007;298(23):2782–2784.
6. Platt R, Polk BF, Murdock B, et al. Mortality associated with nosocomial urinary-tract infections. *N Engl J Med.* 1982;307: 637–642.
7. Maki DG, Tambyah PA. Engineering out the risk of infection with urinary catheters. *Emerg Infect Dis.* 2001;7:1–6.
8. Tissot E, Limat S, Cornette C, Capellier G. Risk factors for catheter-associated bacteriuria in a medical intensive care unit. *Eur J Clin Microbiol Infect Dis.* 2001;20:260–262.
9. Saint S, Wiese J, Amory J, et al. Are physicians aware of which of their patients have indwelling urinary catheters? *Am J Med.* 2000;109:476–480.
10. Meddings J, Rogers MA, Macy M, Saint S. Systematic review and meta-analysis: reminder systems to reduce catheter-associated urinary tract infections and urinary catheter use in hospitalized patients. *Clin Infect Dis.* 2010; 51(5):550–560.
11. Elpern EH, Killeen K, Ketchem A, Wiley A, Patel G, Lateef O. Reducing use of urinary catheters and associated urinary tract infections. *Am J Crit Care.* 2009;18(6):535–541.
12. Saint S, Kowalski CP, Kaufman SR, et al. Preventing hospital-acquired urinary tract infections in the United States: a national study. *Clin Infect Dis.* 2008;46:243–250.
13. Saint S, Kowalski CP, Forman J, et al. A multicenter qualitative study on preventing hospital-acquired urinary tract infection in US hospitals. *Infect Control Hosp Epidemiol.* 2008;29: 333–341.

http://www.aacn.org/WD/practice/docs/practicealerts/catheter-associated-uti-practice-alert.pdf

Table 2-5	PARTS OF A RESEARCH JOURNAL ARTICLE
SECTIONS (IN USUAL ORDER)	**DESCRIPTION**
Abstract	The abstract is at the beginning of the article. It summarizes the entire article and usually provides the purpose of the study; a description of the subjects, data collection, and data analysis; and a summary of important findings.
Introduction • Review of the literature • Statement of the purpose	The literature review discusses relevant studies that have been conducted in the area of this study. A statement of the specific goals or purpose of the study often follows the review.
Method • Subjects • Design • Data collection • Data analysis	The methods section describes in detail how the study was conducted, including the type and number of subjects, the research design used, what data were collected and how, and the types of analysis done. There should be enough information so that the study could be replicated (repeated).
Results	The results (findings) are often presented both in words and in charts, tables, or graphs. It is important to understand what the results were and whether they are meaningful.
Discussion (Conclusions)	The discussion section reports what the results mean in regard to the purpose of the study and the literature review. It may also include suggestions for further research and application to nursing education or practice, as appropriate.
References	The references are at the end of the article and include a list of articles and books used by the researcher.

written by a panel of experts. A *meta-analysis* uses statistical analysis of the effect of a specific intervention across multiple studies, providing stronger evidence than results from a single study. If systematic reviews, EBP guidelines, and meta-analyses are not available, collect reviews of descriptive or qualitative studies or articles of original quantitative studies listed in databases such as MEDLINE and CINAHL (Cumulative Index to Nursing and Allied Health Literature). Box 2-7 (on page 38) provides a suggested list of resources for collecting evidence.

Step 3: Critically appraise the evidence. Ask three questions: (1) What were the results of the study? (2) Are the results valid (did the investigator measure what was intended to be measured) and reliable (were the measurements consistent across time)? (3) Will the results of the study improve patient care?

Step 4: Integrate the evidence with clinical expertise, patient preferences, and values in making a decision to change. Patients want to be involved in decision making about their care; if evidence is found to support

a change but the patient does not want it, the change should not occur. If the change that is proposed cannot be applied in a practical sense, or is too costly or too risky, then the change should also not occur. For example, the most reliable method to determine if a nasogastric tube is correctly placed is by x-ray examination. However, this method of verification is costlier and more risky to the patient (i.e., through exposure to radiation) than other methods; therefore, it is not considered the preferred method in many situations.

Step 5: Evaluate the practice decision or change. The evaluation step is essential to determining if the change is effective for a particular patient or setting and if the expected outcomes resulted from the change.

It is important for nurses and the patients they care for to implement EBP in their clinical practice. "In doing so, patients, healthcare professionals, and healthcare systems will be able to place more confidence in the care that is being delivered and know the best outcomes for patients and their families are being achieved" (Melnyk & Fineout-Overholt, 2005, p. 22).

Table 2-6	ASKING CLINICAL QUESTIONS IN PICO FORMAT	
COMPONENTS	**CONSIDERATIONS**	
P = Patient, population, or problem of interest	Need for explicit description; may include setting, limiting to subgroups (such as by age).	
I = Intervention of interest	The more defined, the more focused the search of the literature will be; may include exposure, treatment, patient perception, diagnostic test, or predicting factor.	
C = Comparison of interest	Usually the comparison is to another treatment or the usual standard of care.	
O = Outcome of interest	Specifically identifying the outcome to enable a literature search to find evidence that examined the same outcome, perhaps in different ways.	

ASKING CLINICAL QUESTIONS

Scenario: You are a staff nurse who works in a hospital-based long-term acute care facility (LTAC) that is associated with a level I trauma center. Most of your patients are adults who have had traumatic brain injuries, spinal cord injuries, and multiple-traumatic injuries. These patients are at risk for developing pressure ulcers. You serve as the chairperson of your unit-based council, which meets monthly. The nurse manager notes during a unit-based council meeting that the prevalence of pressure ulcers was higher this quarter than it had been the previous three quarters (i.e., three month timeframe) of this past year. She notes that a salesman has given her information on a new type of low air loss alternating pressure mattress that is reportedly "more effective in preventing pressure ulcers than the alternating pressure mattress overlays now in use." However, the low air loss alternating pressure mattress is more expensive. The nurse manager wonders if the new mattresses for the LTAC should be purchased. She asks you to charge the unit based council to form a task force that will perform a literature search and make an evidence-based recommendation to her whether or not to purchase the new mattress.

- POPULATION: Adult inpatients at risk for pressure ulcers
- INTERVENTION: Low air loss alternating pressure mattresses
- COMPARISON: Alternating pressure mattress overlays
- OUTCOME: Pressure ulcer rates

PICO Question: Is the use of low air loss alternating pressure mattresses associated with lesser rates of pressure ulcers than alternating pressure mattress overlays among adult inpatients at risk for pressure ulcers?

Finding: From a National Guidelines Clearinghouse search: National Pressure Ulcer Advisory Panel, European Pressure Ulcer Advisory Panel. (2009). *Pressure ulcer prevention recommendations.* Washington, DC: National Pressure Ulcer Advisory Panel.

Findings from multiple research studies on pressure ulcer prevention suggest that both alternating pressure mattresses and alternating pressure mattress overlays are effective in preventing pressure ulcers. However, there is no substantial evidence to suggest that one is superior to the other in preventing pressure ulcers.

Strength of Evidence: Level I—Systematic Review

Recommendation: You recommend that the nurse manager not purchase the more expensive low air loss alternating pressure mattresses.

BOX 2-7   AMERICAN ASSOCIATION OF CRITICAL CARE NURSES' RESOURCES FOR ONLINE SEARCHES

Systematic Reviews

A systematic review is a review of available research studies focusing on a single question. The systematic review summarizes, appraises, and synthesizes large bodies of evidence relevant to a focused research question.

- Cochrane Collaboration: www.cochrane.org
- Database of Abstracts of Reviews of Effectiveness (DARE): www.brad.ac.uk/library/elecinfo/dare.php
- Clinical Evidence: www.clinicalevidence.bmj.com
- The Joanna Briggs Institute (Library of Systematic Reviews): www.joannabriggs.edu.au/pubs/systematic_reviews.php
- PubMed: www.ncbi.nlm.nih.gov/entrez/query/static/clinical.shtml#reviews
- NHS Evidence Health Information Resources—Specialist Collections: www.library.nhs.uk/specialistlibraries/

Guideline Database

Guideline databases are searchable databases of evidence-based clinical practice guidelines.

- U.S. National Guideline Clearinghouse: www.guideline.gov
- U.S. Agency for Healthcare Research and Quality: www.ahrq.gov
- New Zealand Guidelines Group: www.nzgg.org.nz
- Trip Database: www.tripdatabase.com
- NHS Evidence National Library of Guidelines: www.library.nhs.uk/guidelinesfinder/
- Institute for Healthcare Improvement: www.ihi.org/IHI/topics/
- Centers for Disease Control: www.cdc.gov/hai/
- Australian National Health and Medical Research Council: www.nhmrc.gov.au/guidelines/index.htm
- Michigan Quality Improvement Consortium Guidelines: www.mqic.org/guidelines.htm

Professional Organizations

Professional organizations often offer position statements, guidelines, protocols and other documents to promote evidence-based practice.

- American Association of Critical Care Nurses: www.aacn.org
- Society of Critical Care Medicine: www.learnicu.org/Pages/Guidelines.aspx
- American College of Chest Physicians: www.chestnet.org

Online Clinical Databases

These databases allow literature searches for primary sources of evidence and research.

- The Cumulative Index of Nursing and Allied Health Literature (CINAHL) is a comprehensive resource for nursing and allied health literature. www.ebscohost.com/cinahl or access through www.aacn.org
- MEDLINE is the U.S. National Library of Medicine's® (NLM) database that references journal articles focused on biomedicine. Can be searched for free through PubMed: www.ncbi.nlm.nih.gov/pubmed

Journals

Professional journals may contain abstracts with expert commentaries. Here are some suggestions; others exist beyond this listing.

- *Evidence-Based Nursing:* www.ebn.bmj.com
- *Evidence-Based Medicine:* www.ebm.bmj.com
- BMJ's *Clinical Evidence:* www.clinicalevidence.com
- *American Journal of Critical Care,* Clinical Pearls Section: http://ajcc.aacnjournals.org/
- *American College of Physicians Journal Club:* www.annals.org/site/acpjc/

From AACN *Searching for Evidence Toolkit.* Resources for Online Search. Available at http://www.aacn.org/WD/Practice/Docs/Research/Resources%20for%20Online%20Search.pdf

DEVELOPING CLINICAL REASONING

1. Describe your own beliefs about the patient, the nurse, health, and what nursing is. Compare and contrast your answers with those of another student. How do they differ and how are they alike? How do you think such differences might influence nursing practice for each of you?

2. In preparation for your clinical assignment, you read three research articles about positioning and moving patients who are at risk for pressure ulcers (bedsores). The staff nurse responsible for the patient tells you, "Oh, I don't pay any attention to that stuff." How should you respond?

PRACTICING FOR NCLEX

1. When you ask an experienced nurse why it is necessary to change the patient's bed every day, the nurse says, "I guess we have just always done it that way." This answer is an example of what type of knowledge?
   a. Instinctive knowledge
   b. Scientific knowledge
   c. Authoritative knowledge
   d. Traditional knowledge

2. Which nursing actions reflect the use of philosophy as a knowledge base when delivering evidence-based care to patients? Select all that apply.
   a. A nurse interviews and examines a new patient diagnosed with prehypertension to formulate a care plan.
   b. A nurse draws from personal experiences of being a patient to establish a therapeutic relationship with a patient.
   c. A nurse searches the Internet to find the latest treatments for type 2 diabetes.
   d. A nurse uses spiritual training to draw strength when counseling a patient who is in hospice for an inoperable brain tumor.
   e. A nurse follows the protocol for assessing postoperative patients in the ICU.
   f. A nursing student studies anatomy and physiology of the body systems to understand the disease states of assigned patients.

3. A nurse is using general systems theory to describe the role of nursing to provide health promotion and patient teaching. Which statements reflect key points of this theory? Select all that apply.
   a. A system is a set of individual elements that rarely interact with each other.
   b. The whole system is always greater than its parts.
   c. Boundaries separate systems from each other and their environments.
   d. A change in one subsystem will not affect other subsystems.
   e. To survive, open systems maintain balance through feedback.
   f. A closed system allows input from and to the environment.

4. A charge nurse meets with staff to outline a plan to provide transcultural nursing care for patients in their health care facility. Which theorist promoted this type of

caring as the central theme of nursing care, knowledge, and practice?
   a. Madeline Leininger
   b. Jean Watson
   c. Dorothy E. Johnson
   d. Betty Newman

5. A student nurse interacting with patients on a cardiac unit recognizes the four concepts in nursing theory that determine nursing practice. Of these four, which is most important?
   a. Person
   b. Environment
   c. Health
   d. Nursing

6. A nurse manager schedules a clinic for the staff to address common nursing interventions used in the facility and to explore how they can be performed more efficiently and effectively. What is the term for this type of theory affecting change in clinical nursing practice?
   a. Prescriptive theory
   b. Descriptive theory
   c. Developmental theory
   d. General systems theory

7. When conducting quantitative research, the researcher collects information to support a hypothesis. This information would be identified as:
   a. The subject
   b. Variables
   c. Data
   d. The instrument

8. Which type of quantitative research is often conducted to examine the effects of nursing interventions on patient outcomes?
   a. Descriptive research
   b. Correlational research
   c. Quasi-experimental research
   d. Experimental research

9. Which method of qualitative research was developed by the discipline of anthropology?
   a. Historical
   b. Ethnography
   c. Grounded theory
   d. Phenomenology

10. A nurse is formulating a clinical question in PICO format. What does the letter *P* represent?
   a. Comparison to another similar treatment
   b. Clearly defined, focused literature review
   c. Specific identification of the desired outcome
   d. Explicit descriptions of the population of interest

ANSWERS WITH RATIONALES

1. ***d.*** Traditional knowledge is the part of nursing practice passed down from generation to generation, often without research data to support it. Scientific knowledge is that knowledge obtained through the scientific method (implying thorough research). Authoritative knowledge comes from an expert and is accepted as truth based on the person's perceived expertise. Instinct is not a source of knowledge.

2. **b, d.** Philosophy is the study of wisdom, fundamental knowledge, and the processes used to develop and construct one's perceptions of life. A philosophy is developed from personal experiences (such as the experience of being the patient), through formal and informal educational experiences, through religion and culture (such as using spiritual training as a source of strength), and from the environment. Interviewing and examining patients to formulate a care plan and using protocol for assessing patients in the ICU involve knowledge of processes. Researching the Internet and studying anatomy and physiology use scientific knowledge to deliver evidence-based care.

3. **b, c, e.** According to general systems theory, a system is a set of interacting elements contributing to the overall goal of the system. The whole system is always greater than its parts. Boundaries separate systems from each other and their environments. Systems are hierarchical in nature and are composed of interrelated subsystems that work together in such a way that a change in one element could affect other subsystems, as well as the whole. To survive, open systems maintain balance through feedback. An open system allows energy, matter, and information to move freely between systems and boundaries, whereas a closed system does not allow input from or output to the environment.

4. **a.** Madeline Leininger's theory provides the foundations of transcultural nursing care by making caring the central theme of nursing. Jean Watson stated that nursing is concerned with promoting and restoring health, preventing illness, and caring for the sick. The central theme of Dorothy E. Johnson's theory is that problems arise due to disturbances in the system or subsystem or functioning below optimal level. Betty Newman proposed that humans are in constant relationship with stressors in the environment and the major concern for nursing is keeping the patient system stable through accurate assessment of these stressors.

5. **a.** Of the four concepts, the most important is the person. The focus of nursing, regardless of definition or theory, is the person.

6. **a.** Prescriptive theories address nursing interventions and are designed to control, promote, and change clinical nursing practice. Descriptive theories describe a phenomenon, an event, a situation, or a relationship. Developmental theory outlines the process of growth and development of humans as orderly and predictable, beginning with conception and ending with death. General systems theory describes how to break whole things into parts and then to learn how the parts work together in "systems."

7. **c.** Data refers to information that the researcher collects from subjects in the study (expressed in numbers). A variable is something that varies and has different values that can be measured. Instruments are devices used to collect and record the data, such as rating scales, pencil-and-paper tests, and biologic measurements.

8. **c.** Quasi-experimental research is often conducted in clinical settings to examine the effects of nursing interventions on patient outcomes. Descriptive research is often used to generate new knowledge about topics with little or no prior research. Correlational research examines the type and degree of relationships between two or more variables. Experimental research examines cause-and-effect relationships between variables under highly controlled conditions.

9. **b.** Ethnographic research was developed by the discipline of anthropology and is used to examine issues of culture of interest to nursing. Historical research examines events of the past to increase understanding of the nursing profession today. The basis of grounded theory methodology is the discovery of how people describe their own reality and how their beliefs are related to their actions in a social scene. The purpose of phenomenology (both a philosophy and a research method) is to describe experiences as they are lived by the subjects being studied.

10. **d.** The *P* in the PICO format represents an explicit description of the patient population of interest. *I* represents the intervention, *C* represents the comparison, and *O* stands for the outcome.

TAYLOR SUITE RESOURCES

Explore these additional resources to enhance learning for this chapter:

- NCLEX-Style Questions and other resources on **thePoint,** http://thePoint.lww.com/Taylor8e
- *Study Guide for Fundamentals of Nursing, 8th edition*
- Adaptive Learning | Powered by prepU, http://thepoint.lww.com/prepu

Bibliography

Alligood, M., & Marriner-Tomey, A. (2010). *Nursing theory: Utilization and application* (4th ed.). Maryland Heights, MO: Elsevier Mosby.

Allyn, D. (2007). Primum non nocere (first, do no harm): Prayer, culture, and evidence-based practice. *Topics in Advanced Practice Nursing eJournal, 7*(2). Available at http://www.medscape.com/viewarticle/561760_print

American Nurses Association (ANA) (2010). *Nursing's Social Policy Statement,* 2010 ed. Silver Spring, MD: Author.

American Nurses Association (ANA). (2010). *Nursing: Scope and standards of practice, 2nd ed.* Silver Spring, MD: Author.

Armola, R. R., Bourgault, A. M., Halm, M. A., Board, R. M., Bucher, L., Harrington, L., ... Medina, J. (2009). Upgrading the American Association of Critical Care Nurses' evidence-leveling hierarchy. *American Journal of Critical Care, 18*(5), 405–409.

Burns, N., & Groves, S. (2011). *Understanding nursing research: Building an evidence-based practice* (5th ed.). Philadelphia: Elsevier Saunders.

Chinn, P., & Kramer, M. (2011). *Integrated knowledge development in nursing* (8th ed.). St. Louis: Mosby Elsevier.

Cronenwett, L., Sherwood, G., Barnsteiner, J., Disch, J., Johnson, J., Mitchell, P., Sullivan D.T., Warren, J. (2007). Quality and safety education for nurses. *Nursing Outlook, 55*(3), 122–131.

Dontje, K. (2007). Evidence-based practice: Understanding the process. *Topics in Advanced Practice Nursing eJournal, 7*(4). Available at http://medscape.com/viewarticle/567786_print

Emmanuel, E. J., Wendler, D., & Grady, C. (2000). What makes clinical research ethical? *Journal of the American Medical Association, 283*(20), 2701–2711.

Fawcett, J. (2005). Scholarly dialogue. Influences on advancement of nursing knowledge. *Nursing Science Quarterly, 18*(3), 227–232.

Fitne's Virtual Learning Resource Center. Nurse Theorists: Portraits of Excellence, Volumes I and II; Excellence in Action. Available at http://www.fitne.net/products.jsp

Furuya E. Y., Dick, A., Perencevich, E. N., Pogorzelska, M., Goldmann, D., & Stone, P. W. (2011). Central line bundle implementation in US intensive care units and impact on bloodstream infections. *PLoS ONE, 6*, 1, e15452. DOI:10.1371/journal.pone.0015452.

Grace, J., & Powers, B. (2009). Claiming our core: Appraising qualitative evidence for nursing questions about human response and meaning. *Nursing Outlook, 57*(1), 27–34.

Hood, L., & Leddy, S. (2010). *Leddy & Pepper's conceptual bases of professional nursing* (7th ed.). Philadelphia: Lippincott Williams & Wilkins.

Institute of Medicine (IOM). (2001). *Crossing the quality chasm: A new health system for the 21st century.* Washington, DC: National Academy of Sciences.

Institute of Medicine (IOM). (2011). The future of nursing: Leading change, advancing health. Washington, DC: The National Academies Press.

Kalish, P., & Kalish, B. (2004). American Nursing: A History (4th ed.). Philadelphia: Lippincott Williams & Wilkins.

Lamp, J., & Zadvinskis, I. (2008). Kangaroo care: Making the leap to an evidence-based practice. *American Nurse Today, 3*(3), 13–15.

Marriner-Tomey, A., & Alligood, M. (2010). *Nursing theorists and their work* (7th ed.). St. Louis, MO: Mosby.

McCutcheon, Z. (2005). Tradition, rituals, and standards: In a realm of evidence-based nursing care. *Contemporary Nurse, 18*(3), 300–308.

McEwen, M., & Wills, E. (2011). *Theoretical basis for nursing* (3rd ed.). Philadelphia: Lippincott Williams & Wilkins.

Meleis, A. I. (2012). *Theoretical nursing: Development and progress* (5th ed.). Philadelphia: Lippincott Williams & Wilkins.

Melnyk, B., & Fineout-Overholt, E. (2005). *Evidence-based practice in nursing: A guide to best practice.* Philadelphia: Lippincott Williams & Wilkins.

Melnyk, B., & Fineout-Overholt, E. (2002). Key steps in evidence-based practice. Asking compelling clinical questions and searching for the best evidence. *Pediatric Nursing, 28,* 262–263, 266.

National Institute of Nursing Research. (2011). Bringing science to life: Available at NINR strategic plan. Available at https://www.ninr.nih.gov/sites/www.ninr.nih.gov/files/ninr-strategic-plan-2011.pdf

National Institute of Nursing Research: http://www.ninr.nih.gov/

Pipe, T., Wellik, K., Buchda, V., Hansen, C., & Martyn, D. (2005). Implementing evidence-based nursing practice. *Urologic Nursing, 25*(5), 365–370.

Polit, D., & Beck, C. (2012). *Nursing research: Generating and assessing evidence for nursing practice* (9th ed.). Philadelphia: Lippincott Williams & Wilkins.

Rauen, C., Vollman, K., Arbour, R., & Chulary, M. (2008). Challenging nursing's sacred cows. *American Nurse Today, 3*(4), 23–26.

Remshardt, M., & Flowers, D. (2007). Understanding qualitative research. *American Nurse Today, 2*(9), 20–23.

Rycroft-Malone, J., Harvey, G., Seers, K., Kitson, A., McCormack, B., & Titchen, A. (2004). An exploration of the factors that influence the implementation of evidence into practice. *Journal of Clinical Nursing, 13*(8), 913–924.

Talsma, A., Grady P.A., Feetham, S., Heinrich, J., & Steinwachs, D. (2008). The perfect storm: Patient safety and nursing shortages within the context of health policy and evidence-based practice. *Nursing Research, 57*(1S): S15–S21.

Van Achterberg, T., Schoonhoven, L., & Grol, R. (2008). Nursing implementation science: How evidence-based nursing requires evidence-based implementation. *Journal of Nursing Scholarship, 40*(4), 302–310.

Winsett, R., & Cashion, A. (2007). The nursing research process. *Nephrology Nursing Journal, 34*(6), 635–643.

3 Health, Illness, and Disparities

RUTH JACOBI

Ruth is a 62-year-old woman who was hospitalized after a "mini-stroke." She has now returned to her pre-event level of functioning and is being prepared for discharge. She states, "I know that I have an increased risk for a major stroke, so I want to do everything possible to stay as active and as healthy as I possibly can."

SARA GELBART

Sara, a college freshman, is encouraged to visit the student health center by her roommate because she rarely visits the dining hall for meals, runs 5 to 8 miles a day, and has recently lost a significant amount of weight. She is very thin now and when she does eat a meal, she just seems to move the food around on her plate. Sara states, "I'm plenty healthy, just a bit 'nuts' about being fit!"

DANIEL STERNMAN

Daniel is a 27-year-old man with a history of schizophrenia. He comes to the mental health clinic, loudly demanding relief from the voices that are telling him to hurt himself. Mr. Sternman is well known by the clinic staff. His medical record reveals that he has had numerous visits to the clinic and that he has difficulty interacting and dealing with various staff members.

After completing the chapter, you will be able to accomplish the following:

1. Describe concepts and models of health, wellness, and illness.

2. Compare and contrast acute illness and chronic illness.

3. Discuss the factors that play a role in disparities in health care.

4. Explain how the human dimensions, basic human needs, and self-concept influence health and illness.

5. Summarize the role of the nurse in promoting health, preventing illness, and addressing disparities in health care.

6. Explain the levels of preventive care.

KEY TERMS

acute illness	health disparity	morbidity
chronic illness	health promotion	mortality
disease		remission
exacerbation	holistic care	risk factor
health	illness	wellness

The primary objectives of the nurse as caregiver are to promote health, to prevent illness, to restore health, and to facilitate coping with illness, disability, or death. These objectives focus care on maximizing the health of patients of all ages and in all populations, in all settings, and in both health and illness. Health is more than just the absence of illness; it is an active process in which a person moves toward one's maximum potential. It also has different definitions for different people. (See the accompanying Reflective Practice box (on page 44) for an example.) To give **holistic care**, care that addresses the many dimensions that comprise the whole person, the nurse must understand and respect each person's own definition of health and responses to illness and should be familiar with models of health and illness. The nurse's knowledge of health and illness is even more important because of today's focus on health promotion and advocacy, the continuing trend toward care being provided in the home and community, the increasing numbers of older adults, the growing incidence of chronic illnesses, and the ongoing efforts to maximize health care outcomes for all populations.

The recent 2013 report by the Institute of Medicine and the National Research Council provides additional impetus to foster positive health behaviors. Compared to sixteen other affluent countries, the United States has a serious health disadvantage despite the fact that the country spends twice as much per person on health care in comparison to the other nations in the survey. Americans fare worse in nine key health areas: infant mortality and low birth weight, injuries and homicides, teenage pregnancies and sexually transmitted infections, prevalence of human immunodeficiency virus (HIV) and acquired immunodeficiency syndrome (AIDS), drug-related deaths, obesity and diabetes, heart disease, chronic lung disease, and disability. There is agreement that the United States must vigorously investigate potential explanations for this health disadvantage. This includes intensifying efforts to strengthen systems responsible for health and social services, education and employment; promote healthy lifestyles; and design healthier environments. Some of these problems are long-standing concerns and many evidence-based strategies have been implemented to address these challenges. The United States can no longer afford to ignore these compelling issues. Better health must be an achievable outcome for all Americans (Woolf & Aron, 2013).

CONCEPTS OF HEALTH AND WELLNESS

Meguni Kuni, 4 years old, was born with cystic fibrosis. Although she requires ongoing treatment for this illness, she is now an active member of her preschool class, takes gymnastics lessons, and wants to be a doctor when she grows up. Shondra Cole, 34 years old, is married and has two school-aged children. She has chronic rheumatoid arthritis and is in a wheelchair. Shondra takes care of her house and family, using a specially designed car to get to her part-time job. Samuel Cohen is 67 years old. He was diagnosed with type 2 diabetes and high blood pressure last year and takes medications for both health problems. Samuel is retired but volunteers three days a week in a local hospital as a transport technician. Would Meguni, Shondra, and Samuel be described as healthy? Although they each have a physical condition that might lead them to define themselves as being ill, they are all productive members of their communities and would say they are healthy.

Health

A classic definition of **health** is that health is a state of complete physical, mental, and social well-being, not merely the absence of disease or infirmity (World Health Organization, 1974). The health of the public is measured globally by **morbidity**, how frequently a disease occurs, and **mortality**, the numbers of deaths resulting from a disease. On a personal level, however, most people define health according to how they feel ("I feel really sick"), the absence or presence of symptoms of illness ("I have a terrible pain in my stomach"), or their ability to carry out activities of daily living ("I felt so much better that I got up and cooked supper"). See the accompanying Through the Eyes of a Student (on page 45).

Each person defines health in terms of one's own values and beliefs. The person's family, culture, community, and society also influence this personal perception of health.

REFLECTIVE PRACTICE: CULTIVATING QSEN COMPETENCIES

CHALLENGE TO ETHICAL AND LEGAL SKILLS

My first college roommate, Sara Gelbart, seemed the ideal roommate when I first met her. A good student, she was thoughtful, outgoing, and fun. By October, however, I was really worried about her. I noticed that she rarely wanted to come to the dining hall with our group of friends. When she did come, she just seemed to pick at her food. She also spent a lot of time at the athletic center, running 5 to 8 miles almost daily. I wasn't surprised when she started losing significant amounts of weight. What worried me was her lack of willingness to talk about her nutritional habits and health. She told me that she was plenty healthy, just a bit "nuts" about being fit! She also kidded that I'd be healthier if I worked out more often with her. While she was certainly right about that, I was worried that she had a serious eating disorder and wasn't sure what I could do to help. She politely told me to "mind my own business" when I asked her if she had ever spoken with anyone about her health and eating.

Thinking Outside the Box: Possible Courses of Action

- Respect Sara's wishes and simply try to be a good friend without continuing to confront her about her nutritional status.
- Tell Sara I am concerned that she has a serious eating disorder, and then plan the next steps with her, fully respecting her right to seek or refuse professional help.
- Tell Sara that if she fails to get professional help, I will contact her parents or a counselor at school.

Evaluating a Good Outcome: How Do I Define Success?

- Sara gets whatever help she needs to address her eating problems and regain health.
- Sara's right to make her own decisions is respected.
- My obligations as a friend are fulfilled.
- My beginning ability to identify and correctly respond to health problems affirms my choice for nursing.

Personal Learning: Here's to the Future!

Unfortunately, I did not intervene because (1) I failed to recognize how serious a problem this would become, and (2) I wasn't sure what I could do after Sara refused my initial offers of help. Sara dropped out of school at the end of our freshman year and she has not returned my calls, so I'm not sure how she is doing. I've read more about eating disorders, and I now know how important it is to get professional help early. I learned too late that Sara had been in treatment for anorexia during high school and that the pressures of college life had led to a relapse. I think I valued her friendship more than I valued getting her the help that she needed to address a serious health problem.

REFLECTION ON QUALITY AND SAFETY COMPETENCIES

How do you think you would respond in a similar situation? Why? What does this tell you about yourself and about the adequacy of your skills for professional practice? Can you think of other ways to respond? Do you agree with the criteria that the nursing student used to evaluate a successful outcome? Why or why not? What *knowledge, skills,* and *attitudes* do you need to develop to continuously improve quality and safety when caring for patients like Sara?

Patient-Centered Care: What is the best approach when Sara denies that she has an eating problem? If Sara refuses any help, is it better to focus on her positive attributes and avoid conflict regarding her current situation? How might the student's and Sara's developmental level affected their responses? How should you, as her roommate and friend, proceed? What is the best way to communicate emotional support, concern, and caring to Sara?

Teamwork and Collaboration/Quality Improvement: What communication skills do you need in order to facilitate your role as a patient advocate for Sara? As a student nurse, what other skills do you need to respond appropriately in this situation? Should you offer to make an appointment for her with a professional (nutritionist, counselor, nurse) or offer to accompany her to an appointment?

Safety/Evidence-Based Practice: Can you secure any evidence in nursing literature that provides information related to eating disorders and the need for professional treatment? Should you share this information with Sara? What response best contributes to a safe environment for Sara?

Informatics: If you were completing a rotation in a clinical setting as a student nurse, what information should be electronically documented regarding your assessment of a patient like Sara and her response to any interventions?

THROUGH THE EYES OF A STUDENT

Carrie was a 17-year-old brunette who attended my high school, dated my best friend Ricky, and participated in many of the same clubs and activities as me. By looking at her, I never would have guessed anything was wrong. However, once I got to know her, I learned that she was diagnosed with cancer and that the disease had spread through her heart and lungs. The situation, as doctors continually told her, did not look promising. Yet, she never once let that slow her down, and she lived each day to the fullest. It was almost 1 year ago I watched this friend pass away from bone cancer. However, until the days before her last breath, in my eyes she was a happy and healthy girl. She never once let the disease get the best of her, and she fought for life every second of every day. Her constant optimism and determined smile touched and moved so many others. So you ask me, was Carrie healthy?

Health to me is a state of mind, not the physical condition of a person's body. Carrie, in my opinion, was the definition of healthy; she was happy, she lived her life to the fullest, and she continually inspired others to embrace life. The dictionary may state that health is the absence of a disease; however, for me it is the way a person thinks and reacts to life. A person's health consists of being able to work to the best of her capability, look out for herself, and her ability to respond to life enthusiastically. In my eyes, a person like Carrie can be physically unwell, but in terms of living, is healthy. Perhaps this is where health and wellness differ in that, to me, health means the person's entire state of being and is decided by the individual, whereas wellness refers more to the physical condition of a person and is determined more readily by society. The words *illness* and *disease* also correspond with these words. I believe that illness, like health, is a matter of thinking, while disease is a medical term that relates to physical condition and wellness. All of these states are constantly changing, and I have probably experienced the best and worst of all of them. However, as I embark on this new and exciting journey of college, I consider myself extremely healthy. I am living each day to the fullest, trying to impact other people's lives, and am filled with optimism. This all may change shortly, but as I look back on Carrie's life and the effect she has had on me, I will always try to live my life in a healthy and grateful way.

—*Molly Proskine, Georgetown University*

 THINK back to Sara Gelbart, the college freshman who rarely eats and runs several miles almost daily. According to her statement, she considers herself to be healthy. However, her roommate is concerned because of what she views as excessive exercise and Sara's poor nutrition. The nurse needs to investigate Sara's views further to determine exactly what Sara believes to be healthy. Doing so provides a foundation on which to develop an appropriate plan of care. ●

Health integrates all the human dimensions—the physical, intellectual, emotional, sociocultural, spiritual, and environmental aspects of the whole person. The nurse giving holistic nursing care must equally consider all these interrelated dimensions of the whole person (Fig. 3-1).

Wellness

Wellness—a term often used interchangeably with health—is an active state of being healthy, including living a lifestyle that promotes good physical, mental, and emotional health. Dunn (1980) described his model of high-level wellness as functioning to one's maximum potential while maintaining balance and a purposeful direction in the environment. Dunn differentiated "wellness" from "good health," believing that good health is a passive state simply denoting that the person is not ill at this time. Wellness is a more active state, regardless of one's level of health. Dunn also defined processes that help people know who and what they are. These processes, which are a part of each person's perception of one's own wellness state, are being (recognizing oneself as separate and individual), belonging (being part of a whole), becoming (growing and developing), and befitting (making personal choices to befit oneself for the future). Dunn's model encourages the nurse to care for the total person, with regard for all factors affecting the person's state of being while striving to reach maximum potential.

FIGURE 3-1. The human dimensions. All of these interdependent parts compose the whole person.

CONCEPTS OF ILLNESS AND DISEASE

Disease is a medical term, referring to pathologic changes in the structure or function of the body or mind. Box 3-1 lists examples of causes of disease. An **illness** is the response of the person to a disease; it is an abnormal process in which the person's level of functioning is changed when compared with a previous level. This response is unique for each person and is influenced by self-perceptions, others' perceptions, the effects of changes in body structure and function, the effects of those changes on roles and relationships, and cultural and spiritual values and beliefs. A disease is traditionally diagnosed and treatment is prescribed by a physician (although nurses with advanced educations are increasingly doing so), whereas nurses focus on the person with an illness. However, the two terms are often used interchangeably. It is important for nurses to remember that a person may have an illness or injury but still achieve maximum functioning and quality of life, and consider oneself to be healthy.

Classifications of Illness

Illnesses are classified as either acute or chronic. A person may have an acute illness, a chronic illness, or both at the same time; for example, an adult with diabetes (a chronic illness) may also have an acute episode of severely low blood sugar.

Acute Illness

An **acute illness** usually has a rapid onset of symptoms and lasts only a relatively short time. Although some acute illnesses are life threatening, with self-treatment and use of over-the-counter medications, simple acute illnesses such as the common cold or diarrhea do not usually require medical treatment. If medical care is required, a specific treatment with medication (e.g., an antibiotic for pneumonia), surgical procedures (e.g., an appendectomy for appendicitis), or another medical treatment usually return the person to normal functioning.

Chronic Illness

Chronic illness is a broad term that encompasses many different physical and mental alterations in health, with one or more of the following characteristics:

BOX 3-1   **COMMON CAUSES OF DISEASES**

- Inherited genetic defects
- Developmental defects resulting from exposure to such factors as virus or chemicals during pregnancy
- Biologic agents or toxins
- Physical agents such as temperature, chemicals, and radiation
- Generalized tissue responses to injury or irritation
- Physiologic and emotional reactions to stress
- Excessive or insufficient production of body secretions (hormones, enzymes, and so forth)

- It is a permanent change.
- It causes, or is caused by, irreversible alterations in normal anatomy and physiology.
- It requires special patient education for rehabilitation.
- It requires a long period of care or support.

Chronic illnesses usually have a slow onset and many have periods of **remission** (when the disease is present, but the person does not experience symptoms) and **exacerbation** (the symptoms of the disease reappear). Examples of common chronic illnesses are heart disease, diabetes mellitus, lung diseases, and arthritis.

 RECALL Daniel Sternman, the young man with schizophrenia. The nurse would integrate knowledge of this disorder, understanding that it is a chronic illness that can be treated. The patient's arrival at the clinic with reports of hearing voices would indicate to the nurse that symptoms of the disorder have reappeared, necessitating treatment. ●

Because chronic illnesses are the leading health problem in the world, the health promotion and illness prevention activities discussed later in this chapter are even more vital to nursing care. Current trends that result in an increase in chronic illnesses include growing numbers of older adults, lifestyle choices (such as smoking and drug use), environmental factors (increasing air and water pollution), the AIDS epidemic, and the effects of increasing obesity. Nurses will be caring for more patients with chronic illnesses in the future. Although not all people with a chronic illness require care, all who are chronically ill must accept certain conditions of life to be able to live with the illness on a day-to-day basis for the rest of their lives. Approximately 25% of people with chronic illnesses have one or more daily activity limitations (Centers for Disease Control and Prevention [CDC], 2012a). People with a chronic illness often grieve over losses or changes in physical structure and function; worry about their finances, status, roles, and dignity; and face the possibility of an earlier death. Of the 10 leading causes of death in the United States, seven are the result of chronic illnesses (heart disease, cancer, cerebrovascular disease, chronic lower respiratory disease, diabetes, Alzheimer disease, and kidney disease; National Center for Health Statistics, 2012).

To successfully adapt to a chronic illness, the person must learn to live as normally as possible and maintain a positive self-concept and sense of hope, despite symptoms and treatments that may make the person feel different from others. Activities of daily living, relationships, and self-care activities must often be modified, and it is important that the person maintain a feeling of being in control of one's own life and the prescribed treatments.

Nurses care for people of all ages with chronic illnesses, providing that care in all types of settings, including homes, hospitals, clinics, long-term care facilities, and other institutions. Regardless of the age of the patient or the effects and demands of the illness or the setting, the nurse must make every effort to promote health for patients with chronic

FIGURE 3-2. The nurse is assessing the patient as a basis for teaching healthy heart behaviors.

illness, with a focus of care that emphasizes what is possible rather than what can no longer be.

Illness Behaviors

When a person becomes ill, certain illness behaviors may occur in identifiable stages (Suchman, 1965). These behaviors are how people cope with altered functioning caused by the disease. They are unique to the person and are influenced by age, gender, family values, economic status, culture, educational level, and mental status.

There is no specific timetable for the stages-of-illness behaviors, which may occur rapidly or slowly. Nursing roles throughout the stages remain constant. In all stages, the nurse accepts the patient as an individual, gives nursing care based on prioritized needs, and facilitates recovery through physical care, emotional support, and health education (Fig. 3-2).

STAGE 1: EXPERIENCING SYMPTOMS

How do people define themselves as "sick"? The first indication of an illness usually is recognizing one or more symptoms that are incompatible with one's personal definition of health. Although pain is the most common symptom indicating illness, other common symptoms include a rash, fever, bleeding, or a cough. If the symptoms last for a short time or are relieved by self-care, the person usually takes no further action. If the symptoms continue, however, the person enters the next stage.

STAGE 2: ASSUMING THE SICK ROLE

The person now self-defines as being sick, seeks validation of this experience from others, gives up normal activities, and assumes a "sick role." At this stage, most people focus on their symptoms and bodily functions. Depending on individual health beliefs and practices, the person may choose to do nothing, may research symptoms on Internet sources, may buy over-the-counter medications, may try alternative remedies to relieve symptoms, or may seek out a health care provider for diagnosis and treatment. In our society, an illness becomes "legitimate" when a health care provider diagnoses it and prescribes treatment. After seeking help from the health care provider, the person becomes a patient and enters the next stage.

 RECALL Daniel Sternman, the young man with schizophrenia. His arrival at the mental health clinic indicates that he is seeking help from a health care provider. The nurse would interpret this behavior as signaling his assumption of the sick role. •

STAGE 3: ASSUMING A DEPENDENT ROLE

This stage is characterized by the patient's decision to accept the diagnosis and follow the prescribed treatment plan. The person may initially have difficulty conforming to the recommendations of the health care provider and may decide to seek a second opinion or deny the diagnosis. The lack of independence is more troubling for some people who, based on their diagnosis, often require assistance in carrying out activities of daily living, and need emotional support through acceptance, approval, physical closeness, and protection.

If the disease is serious (such as a heart attack or stroke), the patient may enter the hospital for treatment. If the symptoms can be managed by the patient or family alone or with the assistance of home care providers, the patient is cared for at home. To facilitate adherence to the treatment plan, the patient needs effective relationships with caregivers, knowledge about the illness, and an individualized plan of care. The patient's responses to care depend on a variety of factors, including the seriousness of the illness, the patient's degree of fear about the disease, the loss of roles, the support of others, and previous experiences with illness care. The optimal outcome expected by both caregivers and family is to get well and resume normal roles.

STAGE 4: ACHIEVING RECOVERY AND REHABILITATION

Recovery and rehabilitation might begin in the hospital and conclude at home, or may be totally concluded at a rehabilitation center or at home. Most patients complete this final stage of illness behavior at home. In this stage, the person gives up the dependent role and resumes normal activities and responsibilities. If the plan of care includes health education, the person may return to health at a higher level of functioning and health than before the illness.

 REMEMBER Ruth Jacobi, the woman being prepared for discharge after a mini-stroke. The patient's stated desire to be as active and as healthy as she possibly can reflects her desire to give up the dependent role. The nurse would use this knowledge as a basis for the patient's teaching plan, thereby fostering a return to health, possibly at a level higher than before the patient's mini-stroke. •

Effects of Illness on the Family

Most nursing care is given to patients with some form of support system, usually family members. When an illness occurs, daily life changes for both the patient and the family.

For example, a chronic illness creates stress for the patient and family because of possible lifelong alterations in roles or lifestyle, frequent hospitalizations, economic problems, and decreased social interactions among family members. The responses of family members to an illness are also individualized. Some family members want to be with the patient all the time, while others might avoid visiting. Parents of a sick child often react with blame, overprotection, and severe anxiety, and family members of patients requiring intensive care often feel alone and frightened. In both cases, they might also feel guilty and imagine the worst possible outcome. See Chapter 4 for more information.

DISPARITIES IN HEALTH CARE

Although health care increasingly focuses on the promotion of health and the prevention of illness, there continue to be disparities that lead to different health outcomes among different populations of people. A **health disparity** is defined by *Healthy People 2020* as a "particular type of health difference that is closely linked with social, economic, and/or environmental disadvantage" (Healthy People, 2010). Health disparities are influenced by many different factors, including racial and ethnic groups, poverty, gender, age, mental health, educational level, disabilities, sexual orientation, health insurance, and access to health care (U.S. Department of Health and Human Services [USDHHS], 2010).

Disparities in health outcomes are especially common in racial and ethnic minorities, in whom higher rates of obesity, cancer, diabetes mellitus, and AIDS are seen. For example, 13% of African Americans, 12% of Hispanics, and 12% of Native Americans develop adult-onset (type 2) diabetes, compared to the 8% rate in the White population (National Prevention Council, 2011). HIV rates demonstrate the most extreme chronic disease disparity, with African Americans experiencing HIV infections at 7.6 times the rate of Whites (The Office of Minority Health, 2012).

National trends in efforts to prevent health disparities focus on vulnerable populations, such as racial and ethnic minorities, those living in poverty, women, children, older adults, rural and inner-city residents, and people with disabilities and special health care needs. Emphasis is given to disparities in access to care, quality of care, health insurance status, specific sources of ongoing care, and quality and access to care for people with limited English proficiency. It is critical that nurses recognize that disparities exist and plan specific and individualized interventions for patients who are most at risk.

FACTORS AFFECTING HEALTH AND ILLNESS

Many factors influence a person's health status, health beliefs, and health practices. These factors may be internal or external and may or may not be under the person's conscious control. To plan and provide holistic care, the nurse must understand how these factors influence behavior in both healthy and ill patients.

Basic Human Needs

A basic human need is something essential that must be met for emotional and physiologic health and survival. A person whose needs are met may be considered to be healthy, and a person who has one or more unmet needs is at an increased risk for illness. (Basic human needs are discussed in detail in Chapter 4).

The Human Dimensions

The factors influencing a person's health–illness status, health beliefs, and health practices relate to the person's human dimensions (see Fig. 3-1, p. 45). Each dimension interrelates with each of the others and influences the person's behaviors in both health and illness. Nursing assessments of strengths and weaknesses in each dimension are used to develop a plan of care that is individualized and holistic. The nursing process, used to plan, implement, and evaluate plans of care, is discussed in Unit III.

Physical Dimension

The physical dimension includes genetic inheritance, age, developmental level, race, and gender. These components strongly influence the person's health status and health practices. For example, inherited genetic disorders include Down syndrome, hemophilia, cystic fibrosis, and color blindness. Toddlers are at greater risk for drowning, and adolescents and young adult males are at greater risk for automobile crashes from excessive speed. There are specific racial traits for disease, including sickle cell anemia, hypertension, and stroke. A young woman whose mother and grandmother had breast cancer is more likely to have an annual clinical breast examination and mammogram.

Emotional Dimension

How the mind affects body functions and responds to body conditions also influences health. Long-term stress affects body systems, and anxiety affects health habits; conversely, calm acceptance and relaxation can actually change the body's responses to illness. As examples of the negative effects of emotions, a student may always have diarrhea before examinations and an adolescent with poor self-esteem may begin to experiment with drugs. The positive effects of emotions include reducing surgical pain with relaxation techniques and reducing blood pressure with biofeedback skills.

 KNOWLEDGE of the emotional dimension would be important when planning care for Sara Gelbart, the college freshman described at the beginning of the chapter. The nurse needs to examine how she responds to stress and anxiety. ●

Intellectual Dimension

The intellectual dimension encompasses cognitive abilities, educational background, and past experiences. These influence the person's responses to teaching about health and reactions to nursing care during illness. They also play a major role in health behaviors. Examples involving this dimension include a young college student with diabetes who follows a diabetic diet but drinks beer and eats pizza with friends several times a week, and a middle-aged man who quits taking his high-blood-pressure medication after developing unpleasant side effects.

Environmental Dimension

The environment has many influences on health and illness. Housing, sanitation, climate, and pollution of air, food, and water are elements in the environmental dimension. Examples of environmental causes of illness include deaths in older adults from inadequate heating and cooling, an increased incidence of asthma and respiratory problems in large cities with smog, and an increased incidence of skin cancer in people who live in hot, sunny areas of the world.

Sociocultural Dimension

Health practices and beliefs are strongly influenced by a person's economic level, lifestyle, family, and culture. In general, low-income groups, racial and ethnic minorities, and other underserved populations are less likely to seek medical care to prevent illness and have fewer treatment options, while high-income groups are more prone to stress-related habits and illness. The family and the culture to which a person belongs influence the person's patterns of living and values about health and illness; such patterns are often unalterable. All of these factors are involved in personal care, patterns of eating, lifestyle habits, and emotional stability. Examples of other sociocultural situations that influence health and illness are an adolescent who sees nothing wrong with smoking or drinking because her parents smoke and drink, parents of a sick infant who do not seek medical care because they have no health insurance, a single parent (abused as a child) who in turn physically abuses her own small son, and a person of Asian descent who uses herbal remedies and acupuncture to treat an illness.

Spiritual Dimension

Spiritual beliefs and values are important components of a person's health and illness behaviors (see Chapter 45). It is important that nurses respect these values and understand their importance for the individual patient. Examples of the influences of the spiritual dimension on health care include the Roman Catholic requirement of baptism for both live births and stillborn babies; kosher dietary laws, prohibiting the intake of pork and shellfish, practiced by Orthodox and Conservative Jews; and opposition to blood transfusion, common to Jehovah's Witnesses.

Self-Concept

Another variable influencing health and illness is people's self-concept (see Chapter 40), which incorporates both how they feel about themselves (self-esteem) and the way they perceive their physical self (body image). Self-concept has both physical and emotional aspects and is an important

factor in the way a person reacts to stress and illness, follows self-care health practices, and relates to others.

 CONSIDER Sara Gelbart, the college freshman with a suspected eating disorder. Although she has lost a significant amount of weight, she states that she is healthy but just "nuts" about being fit. Her self-concept is most likely one of being overweight. Subsequently, she rarely eats. In contrast, people who are overweight may feel that nothing will change the way they look and refuse to follow a diet and exercise program. ●

A person's self-concept results from a variety of past experiences, interpersonal interactions, physical and cultural influences, and education. It includes perceptions of one's own strengths and weaknesses. Illness can alter a person's self-concept as it affects roles, independence, and relationships with important others.

Risk Factors for Illness or Injury

A **risk factor** is something that increases a person's chances for illness or injury. Like other components of health and illness, risk factors are often interrelated. Risk factors may be further defined as modifiable (things a person can change, such as quitting smoking) or nonmodifiable (things that cannot be changed, such as a family history of cancer). As a person's number of risk factors increases, so does the possibility of illness. For example, an overweight executive under pressure to increase sales may smoke and drink alcohol in excess. These factors, combined with a family history of heart disease, place this person at higher risk for illness. The six general types of risk factors are described in Table 3-1 (on page 50). Risk factors for each developmental level across the lifespan are included in Unit IV, and cultural influences on risk factors are discussed in Chapter 5.

HEALTH PROMOTION AND ILLNESS PREVENTION

Health promotion is the behavior of a person who is motivated by a personal desire to increase well-being and health potential. In contrast, illness/disease prevention, also called health protection, is behavior motivated by a desire to avoid or detect disease or to maintain functioning within the constraints of an illness or disability (Pender, Murdaugh, & Parsons, 2011). Health promotion and illness prevention activities are traditionally described as occurring on primary, secondary, and tertiary levels (Leavell & Clark, 1965). Definitions and examples of nursing activities for each level are discussed in the next section and are illustrated in Table 3-2 (on page 50).

Primary Health Promotion and Illness Prevention

Primary health promotion and illness prevention are directed toward promoting health and preventing the development of disease processes or injury. Nursing activities at the primary level may focus on people or groups. Examples of primary-level activities are immunization clinics, family planning

Table 3-1 MAJOR AREAS OF RISK FACTORS

RISK FACTOR	EXAMPLES
Age	School-aged children are at high risk for communicable diseases. After menopause, women are more likely to develop cardiovascular disease.
Genetic factors	A family history of cancer or diabetes predisposes a person to developing the disease.
Physiologic factors	Obesity increases the possibility of heart disease. Pregnancy places increased risk on both the mother and the developing fetus.
Health habits	Smoking increases the probability of lung cancer. Poor nutrition can lead to a variety of health problems.
Lifestyle	Multiple sexual relationships increase the risk for sexually transmitted infections (e.g., gonorrhea or AIDS). Events that increase stress (e.g., divorce, retirement, work-related pressure) may precipitate accidents or illness.
Environment	Working and living environments (such as hazardous materials and poor sanitation) may contribute to disease.

Table 3-2 EXAMPLES OF NURSING ACTIVITIES BY LEVEL OF HEALTH PROMOTION AND PREVENTIVE CARE

LEVEL	TOPIC
Primary	Weight loss Diet Exercise Smoking cessation Reduced alcohol consumption Avoidance of illicit drugs Farm safety Seat belts and child safety seats Immunizations Water treatment Safer sex practices Effective parenting
Secondary	Screenings (Blood pressure, cholesterol, glaucoma, HIV, skin cancer) Pap smears Mammograms Testicular examinations Family counseling
Tertiary	Medication Medical therapy Surgical treatment Rehabilitation Physical therapy Occupational therapy Job training

services, providing poison-control information, and accident-prevention education. Other nursing interventions include teaching about a healthy diet, the importance of regular exercise, safety in industry and farms, using seat belts, and safer sex practices.

Health-risk assessments are an important part of primary health promotion and preventive care. A health-risk assessment is an assessment of the total person. The resulting "picture" of the person indicates areas of risk for disease or injury as well as areas that support health. A variety of formats are used to perform this assessment, but all take a broad approach to health, focusing on lifestyle and behaviors. Box 3-2 contains an example of a health-style self-test the patient completes. As you work with patients to provide care, use this self-test to help your patients assess their state of health and health risks, and learn a new health style through recommended lifestyle practices that support health.

 Concept Mastery Alert

During primary prevention, teaching is an important activity. However, before teaching can be initiated, it is essential that the nurse engage the patient in a discussion about the health risks and the implications. Then once the risks are identified, the nurse can develop a patient-specific teaching strategy to help the patient address the risks.

Secondary Health Promotion and Illness Prevention

Secondary health promotion and illness prevention focus on screening for early detection of disease with prompt diagnosis and treatment of any found. The goals of secondary preventive care are to identify an illness, reverse or reduce its severity or provide a cure, and thereby return the person to maximum health as quickly as possible. The Patient Protection and Affordable Care Act of 2010, which broadens the scope of preventive care, also helps reduce health disparities so that underserved groups can reach their full health potential. Examples of nursing activities at this level are assessing children for normal growth and development and encouraging regular medical, dental, and vision examinations. Other activities include screenings (e.g., blood pressure, cholesterol, and skin cancer), recommending gynecologic examinations and mammograms for women at appropriate ages, and teaching testicular self-examination to men. Direct nursing care interventions at the secondary level include administering medications and caring for wounds.

 Concept Mastery Alert

Screenings are a major activity involved in secondary health promotion.

BOX 3-2   A HEALTH-STYLE SELF-TEST

All of us want good health, but many of us do not know how to be as healthy as possible. Health experts now describe *lifestyle* as one of the most important factors affecting health. In fact, it is estimated that as many as 7 of the 10 leading causes of death could be reduced through common-sense changes in lifestyle. That's what this brief test, developed by the Public Health Service, is all about. Its purpose is simply to tell you how well you are doing to stay healthy. The behaviors covered in the test are recommended for most Americans. Some of them may not apply to people with certain chronic diseases or disabilities, or to pregnant women. Such people may require special instructions from their physicians.

Cigarette Smoking

If you *never smoke,* enter a score of 10 for this section and go to the next section on Alcohol and Drugs.

almost always / sometimes / almost never

2 1 0   1. I avoid smoking cigarettes.
2 1 0   2. I smoke only low-tar and nicotine cigarettes *or* I smoke a pipe or cigars.

Smoking score: _____

Alcohol and Drugs

almost always / sometimes / almost never

4 1 0   1. I avoid drinking alcoholic beverages *or* I drink no more than one or two drinks a day.
2 1 0   2. I avoid using alcohol or other drugs (especially illegal drugs) as a way of handling stressful situations or the problems in my life.
2 1 0   3. I am careful not to drink alcohol when taking certain medicines (e.g., medicine for sleeping, pain, colds, and allergies), or when pregnant.
2 1 0   4. I read and follow the label directions when using prescribed and over-the-counter drugs.

Alcohol and drugs score: _____

Eating Habits

almost always / sometimes / almost never

4 1 0   1. I eat a variety of foods each day, such as fruits and vegetables, whole-grain breads and cereals, lean meats, dairy products, dry peas and beans, and nuts and seeds.
2 1 0   2. I limit the amount of fat, saturated fat, and cholesterol I eat (including fat on meats, eggs, butter, cream, shortenings, and organ meats such as liver).
2 1 0   3. I limit the amount of salt I eat by cooking with only small amounts, not adding salt at the table, and avoiding salty snacks.
2 1 0   4. I avoid eating too much sugar (especially frequent snacks of sticky candy or soft drinks).

Eating habits score: _____

Exercise and Fitness

almost always / sometimes / almost never

3 1 0   1. I maintain a desired weight, avoiding overweight and underweight.
3 1 0   2. I do vigorous exercises for 15 to 30 minutes at least three times a week (examples include running, swimming, brisk walking).
2 1 0   3. I do exercises that enhance my muscle tone for 15 to 30 minutes at least three times a week (examples include yoga and calisthenics).
2 1 0   4. I use part of my leisure time participating in individual, family, or team activities that increase my level of fitness (such as gardening, bowling, golf, and baseball).

Exercise/fitness score: _____

Stress Control

almost always / sometimes / almost never

2 1 0   1. I have a job or do other work that I enjoy.
2 1 0   2. I find it easy to relax and express my feelings freely.
2 1 0   3. I recognize early, and prepare for, events or situations likely to be stressful for me.
2 1 0   4. I have close friends, relatives, or others whom I can talk to about personal matters and call on for help when needed.
2 1 0   5. I participate in group activities (such as church and community organizations) or hobbies that I enjoy.

Stress control score: _____

Safety

almost always / sometimes / almost never

2 1 0   1. I wear a seat belt while riding in a car.
2 1 0   2. I avoid driving while under the influence of alcohol and other drugs.
2 1 0   3. I obey traffic rules and the speed limit when driving.
2 1 0   4. I am careful when using potentially harmful products or substances (such as household cleaners, poisons, and electrical devices).
2 1 0   5. I avoid smoking in bed.

Safety score: _____

What Your Scores Mean to You

Scores of 9 and 10

Excellent! Your answers show that you are aware of the importance of this area to your health. More important, you are putting your knowledge to work for you by practicing good health habits. As long as you continue to do so, this area should not pose a serious health risk. It's likely that you are setting an example for your family and friends to follow. Because you got a very high test score on this part of the test, you may want to consider other areas where your scores indicate room for improvement.

(continued)

BOX 3-2 A HEALTH-STYLE SELF-TEST *continued*

Scores of 6 to 8

Your health practices in this area are good, but there is room for improvement. Look again at the items you answered with "Sometimes" or "Almost never." What changes can you make to improve your score? Even a small change can often help you achieve better health.

Scores of 3 to 5

Your health risks are showing! Would you like more information about the risks you are facing and about why it is important for you to change these behaviors? Perhaps you need help in deciding how to make the changes you desire. In either case, help is available.

Scores of 0 to 2

Obviously, you were concerned enough about your health to take the test, but your answers show that you may be taking serious and unnecessary risks with your health. Perhaps you are unaware of the risks and what to do about them. You can easily get the information and help you need to improve, if you wish. The next step is up to you.

SUGGESTED SELF-CARE BEHAVIORS

Start by asking yourself a few frank questions: *Am I really doing all I can to be as healthy as possible? What steps can I take to feel better? Am I willing to begin now?* If you scored low in one or more sections of the test, decide what changes you want to make for improvement. You might pick that aspect of your lifestyle where you feel you have the best chance for success and tackle that one first. Once you have improved your score there, go on to other areas.

Lifestyle practices that promote health include:

- Sleeping regularly, 7 to 8 hours per night
- Eating regular meals, which include recommended food groups

- Maintaining ideal body weight
- Having a regular schedule of exercise
- Using alcohol in moderation, if at all
- Not smoking
- Maintaining positive mental health and self-concept
- Practicing safer sex
- Wearing seatbelts, using car seats for children, and wearing bicycle helmets
- Having recommended screenings and checkups by your medical and dental health care providers

If you already have tried to change your health habits (to stop smoking or exercise regularly, for example), don't be discouraged if you haven't yet succeeded. The difficulty you have encountered may be due to influences you've never really thought about—such as advertising—or to a lack of support and encouragement. Understanding these influences is an important step toward changing the way they affect you.

There's help available. In addition to personal actions you can take on your own, there are community programs and groups (such as the YMCA or the local chapter of the American Heart Association) that can assist you and your family to make the changes you want to make. If you want to know more about these groups or about health risks, contact your local health department or the National Health Information Clearinghouse. There's a lot you can do to stay healthy or to improve your health, and there are organizations that can help you. Start a new "health style" today!

For assistance in locating specific information on these and other health topics, write to the National Health Information Clearinghouse:

National Health Information Clearinghouse
P.O. Box 1133
Washington, DC 20013

(Adapted with permission of the National Health Information Clearinghouse.)

Tertiary Health Promotion and Illness Prevention

Tertiary health promotion and illness prevention begins after an illness is diagnosed and treated, with the goal of reducing disability and helping rehabilitate patients to a maximum level of functioning. Nursing activities on a tertiary level include teaching a patient with diabetes how to recognize and prevent complications, using physical therapy to prevent contractures in a patient who has had a stroke or spinal cord injury, and referring a woman to a support group after removal of a breast because of cancer. Nurses play an important role in monitoring the responses of the patient to the prescribed therapy and in providing services to facilitate the patient's recovery or improve quality of life while living with the effects of an illness or injury.

 THINK back to Sara Gelbart, the college freshman. If she is diagnosed with an eating disorder, the nurse would use tertiary preventive care by referring the patient to an eating disorders support group. For Ruth Jacobi, the woman being discharged

after a mini-stroke, tertiary preventive care would include educating her about the warning signs and symptoms of a major stroke and about measures to reduce her risk. ●

MODELS OF HEALTH PROMOTION AND ILLNESS PREVENTION

Models of why and how people behave in ways to promote health and prevent illness help health care providers understand health-related behaviors and adapt care to people from diverse economic and cultural backgrounds. This knowledge can be used to overcome barriers to health from disparities in care resulting from such factors as the increasing number of people without health insurance, a predicted increase in minority populations, and a lack of accessible and essential health care services for low-income and rural populations.

The Health Belief Model

Free or low-cost screens and health information are available in most areas to help detect disease early and to educate people about healthy living. Why, then, don't more people take advantage of these services or change their lifestyles?

This question can be answered with the widely used health belief model, which describes health behaviors.

The health belief model (Rosenstock, 1974) focuses on what people perceive or believe to be true about themselves in relation to their health. This model is based on three components of individual perceptions of threat of a disease: (1) perceived susceptibility to a disease, (2) perceived seriousness of a disease, and (3) perceived benefits of action.

Perceived susceptibility to a disease is the belief that one either will or will not contract a disease. It ranges from being afraid of developing a disease to completely denying that certain behaviors may cause illness. For example, one person who smokes cigarettes may believe he or she is at danger for lung cancer and may stop smoking, while another person may believe smoking poses no serious threat and continues to smoke.

Perceived seriousness of a disease concerns the person's perception of the threat disease poses to health and its effects on the person's lifestyle. Perceived seriousness depends on how much the person knows about the disease and can result in a change in health behavior. If a person who smokes knows that lung cancer can cause physical disability or death and therefore affect one's ability to work and care for the family, the person is more likely to stop smoking.

The perceived benefits of action are the person's beliefs about how effectively measures will prevent illness. This factor is influenced by the person's conviction that carrying out a recommended action will prevent or modify the disease and by the person's perception of the cost and unpleasant effects of performing the health behavior (compared with not taking any action). For example, the person may believe that stopping smoking will prevent future breathing problems and that the initial withdrawal symptoms can be overcome; therefore, the person may stop smoking.

In addition to these three components, a person's health beliefs are affected by modifying factors including demographic variables (such as age and gender), sociopsychological variables (such as personality and peer group pressure), and structural variables (such as knowledge and prior contact with the disease). These factors interact to influence the perceived benefits of preventive action minus the perceived barriers to preventive action. Another modifying factor is cues to action, including activities such as others' advice, mass-media campaigns, literature, appointment-reminder telephone calls or postcards, and the illness of a significant other. The likelihood of taking a recommended preventive health action is thus a composite of individual perceptions and modifying factors.

Recent research indicates that self-efficacy should be added as another component of the health belief model. Self-efficacy, one's own belief in the ability to reach goals and complete tasks, is a strong influence on a person's choices, particularly regarding health behaviors (Pender, Murdaugh, & Parsons, 2011).

The health belief model is useful when teaching about health and illness. You can assess the patient's related beliefs and together structure goals to help realistically meet health needs. Teaching and health promotion activities are ineffective, however, unless the patient believes that they are important and necessary.

 CONSIDER Ruth Jacobi, the woman being discharged after a mini-stroke. The patient indicates that she is positively motivated to achieve health, providing the nurse with valuable information about her health beliefs. Together, the nurse and patient can determine realistic goals. The nurse, then, could use this model to develop the patient's teaching plan, including information about the underlying disease process, risk factors for stroke, and ways to reduce the patient's risk for a major stroke. ●

The Health Promotion Model

The health promotion model (Pender, Murdaugh, & Parsons, 2006) was developed to illustrate how people interact with their environment as they pursue health. The model incorporates individual characteristics and experiences, as well as behavior-specific knowledge and beliefs, to motivate health-promoting behavior. Nurses can use the components of the model to design and provide interventions to promote health for people, families, and communities.

Individual characteristics and experiences can be useful to predict if a person will incorporate and use health-related behaviors. If a behavior has been used before and becomes a habit, it is more likely to be used again. Personal biologic, psychological, and sociocultural factors—including age, gender, strength, self-esteem, perceived health status, definition of health, acculturation, and socioeconomic status—all help predict a given health-related habit. For example, the person who has high self-esteem, defines self as healthy, and has an adequate income is less likely to use alcohol or tobacco and more likely to follow a healthy diet and take part in regular exercise. Conversely, a person with low self-esteem, a fatalistic attitude toward health, and low socioeconomic status is more likely to have poor nutrition, not exercise, and use addictive substances.

Behavior-specific knowledge, beliefs, and relationships are considered major motivators for health-promoting behaviors. These include the knowledge that that there will be a positive outcome from a specific health behavior, the belief that one has the skill and competence to engage in health behaviors, and the influences of others (especially family, peers, and health care providers). Situational influences, such as no-smoking policies, also influence health behaviors. Barriers to action, which include perceptions of unavailability, inconvenience, expense, difficulty, or time, usually result in avoidance of a behavior.

A revised health promotion model includes three additional variables: activity-related affect, a commitment to a plan of action, and immediate competing demands and preferences. Behaviors may induce either a positive or negative subjective response or affect. If the activity initiates a positive reaction, the behavior will likely be repeated; if the emotional reaction is negative, the person will likely avoid that behavior. A person initiates a health-related behavior by committing to a plan of action, accompanied by developing associated strategies to perform the valued behavior. Failure to sustain the behavior may result from competing demands. For example, a person may begin a low-fat diet but "give in" to the convenience of fast foods. Health-related behavior is the outcome of the model and is directed toward attaining positive health outcomes and experiences throughout the lifespan (Pender, Murdaugh, & Parsons, 2011).

The Health–Illness Continuum

The health–illness continuum is one way to conceptualize a person's level of health. This model views health as a constantly changing state, with high-level wellness and death at opposite ends of a graduated scale, or continuum (Fig. 3-3). This continuum illustrates the ever-changing state of health as a person adapts to changes in internal and external environments to maintain a state of well-being. For example, patients with cancer may view themselves at different points on the continuum at any given time, depending on how well they believe they are functioning with the illness.

 THINK back to Sara Gelbart, the college freshman described in the Reflective Practice display. The nurse could apply the health–illness continuum model when assessing this patient, recognizing that the stressors of college life have resulted in a shift along the continuum for this patient away from high-level wellness. ●

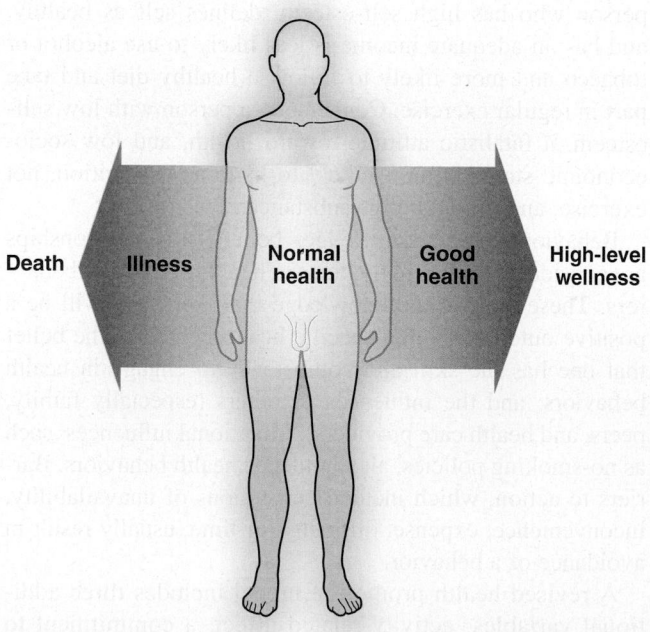

FIGURE 3-3. The health–illness continuum.

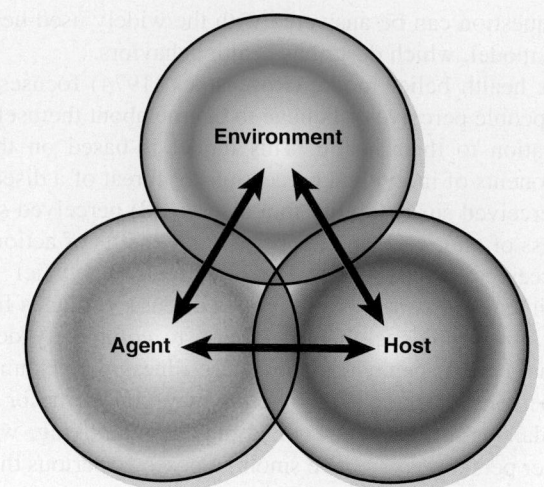

FIGURE 3-4. The agent–host–environment triangle.

The Agent–Host–Environment Model

The agent–host–environment model of health and illness, developed by Leavell and Clark (1965), views the interaction between an external agent, a susceptible host, and the environment as causes of disease in a person. It is a traditional model that explains how certain factors place some people at risk for an infectious disease. The triangle in Figure 3-4 illustrates how each of the agent–host–environment factors affects and is affected by the others. These factors are constantly interacting, and a combination of factors may increase the risk of illness. The use of this model is limited when dealing with noninfectious diseases, and other models have proved more useful (CDC, 2012b).

NURSING CARE TO PROMOTE HEALTH AND PREVENT ILLNESS

The current focus on health promotion and illness prevention at local, state, national, and global levels is important to nursing. Chapter 1 provides information about *Healthy People 2020,* a national agenda to promote health. Nursing interventions to promote health in the community are discussed in Chapters 4 and 9. Chapters 18 and 19 discuss recommended screenings, immunizations, and safety practices across the lifespan.

Nurses must take care of their own health to be able to give effective nursing care to others. Good personal health enables nurses not only to practice more efficiently but also to serve as role models for patients and families. Nurses can help patients acquire new health behaviors by modeling the very behaviors they are trying to promote. It is difficult for nurses to be sincerely attentive to the needs of patients when their own needs are not being met. Because no one is perfectly healthy all of the time, nurses who are preparing for professional practice should spend time getting to know themselves. From this self-knowledge should come a commitment to actively pursue holistic health. To help you increase your self-knowledge, complete the health-style self-test in Box 3-2, p. 51.

 Concept Mastery Alert

Primary role is not the same as primary prevention. Primary role is individually-directed; primary prevention focuses on activities that foster health for individuals, groups and communities.

The Promoting Health boxes highlighted throughout this text may also be useful to you, as well as to your patients. Use these guides to assess and identify both your strengths and risks for alterations in health. The guides can also serve as a basis for teaching self-care to patients.

As we move further into the 21st century, resources for health care practices for self and others, along with knowledge of health care trends, can help promote health and advocacy for patients and families of all ages and in all settings. Eliminating disparities in health care improves the quality of life for all people. Examples of nurse-led interventions that reduce disparities and provide access to quality health care include:

• A nurse-led clinic in an urban area in Milwaukee, Wisconsin, was established to treat low-income uninsured patients with hypertension and diabetes. Interventions include laboratory tests, low-cost medications, free patient education, and consultations as needed. This program was specifically designed "to reduce excessive wait times, inconvenient locations, and a lack of cultural awareness by healthcare providers" (Melville, 2011).

• A post-discharge, nurse-led clinic in San Francisco, California, helps patients transition from the inpatient to outpatient setting. This bridge clinic serves vulnerable populations including new immigrants, substance abusers, the homeless, and mentally ill patients. Outreach activities include review of medications, assessment of new symptoms, health promotion and education, and referrals as needed. Surveys of these patients have demonstrated significant improvement in self-management for this vulnerable population (Newbold, Schneidermann, & Horton, 2012).

• Residents of impoverished communities in Philadelphia, Pennsylvania, can receive a variety of services at one location. The Family Practice and Counseling Network (FPCN) includes three nurse-led health centers that provide immediate and long-term health care coordinated by a team of nurses including RNs and APRNs. This care coordination facilitates communication and produces quality patient outcomes (Trossman, 2012).

DEVELOPING CLINICAL REASONING

1. Identify a family in which someone has a chronic illness. Interview as many of the other family members as possible, and discuss the effect of the illness on them. What do you observe about the effects of the illness in relation to the patient's age, type of illness (e.g., AIDS versus cancer), gender, and family role?

2. List the six human dimensions described in this chapter, and identify your personal strengths and weaknesses in each area. For example, you may have inherited a genetic tendency toward being overweight (a weakness), but have controlled your weight through nutrition and exercise (a strength). After considering your strengths and weaknesses, develop a personal plan for health promotion.

3. In what ways can poverty, race or ethnic group, lack of education, and poor social support influence health outcomes? Does current information about the biologic and genetic characteristics of minority and underserved populations explain the health disparities experienced by these groups? Can you identify additional barriers that interfere with quality health care?

PRACTICING FOR NCLEX

1. A nurse assesses patients in a physician's office who are experiencing different levels of health and illness. Which statements best define the concepts of health and illness? Select all that apply.
   a. Health and illness are the same for all people.
   b. Health and illness are individually defined by each person.
   c. People with acute illnesses are actually healthy.
   d. People with chronic illnesses have poor health beliefs.
   e. Health is more than the absence of illness.
   f. Illness is the response of a person to a disease.

2. The student nurse learns that illnesses are classified as either acute or chronic. Which are examples of chronic illnesses? Select all that apply.
   a. Diabetes mellitus
   b. Bronchial pneumonia
   c. Rheumatoid arthritis
   d. Cystic fibrosis
   e. Fractured hip
   f. Otitis media

3. Despite a national focus on health promotion, nurses working with patients in inner-city clinics continue to see disparities in health care for vulnerable populations. Which patients would be considered vulnerable populations? Select all that apply.
   a. A White male diagnosed with HIV
   b. An African American teenager who is 6 months pregnant
   c. A Hispanic male who has type II diabetes
   d. A low-income family living in rural America
   e. A middle-class teacher living in a large city
   f. A White baby who was born with cerebral palsy

4. A nurse has volunteered to give influenza immunizations at a local clinic. What level of care is the nurse demonstrating?
   a. Tertiary
   b. Secondary
   c. Primary
   d. Promotive

5. A nurse's neighbor tells the nurse, "I have a high temperature, feel awful, and I am not going to work." What stage of illness behavior is the neighbor exhibiting?
   a. Experiencing symptoms
   b. Assuming the sick role
   c. Assuming a dependent role
   d. Achieving recovery and rehabilitation

6. Which clinic patient is most likely to have annual breast examinations and mammograms based on the physical human dimension?
   a. Jane, whose her best friend had a benign breast lump removed
   b. Sarah, who lives in a low-income neighborhood
   c. Tricia, who has a family history of breast cancer
   d. Nancy, whose family encourages regular physical examinations

7. Health promotion activities may occur on a primary, secondary, or tertiary level. Which activities are considered tertiary health promotion? Select all that apply.
   a. A nurse runs an immunization clinic in the inner city.
   b. A nurse teaches a patient with an amputation how to care for the residual limb.
   c. A nurse provides range-of-motion exercises for a paralyzed patient.
   d. A nurse teaches parents of toddlers how to childproof their homes.
   e. A school nurse provides screening for scoliosis for the students.
   f. A nurse teaches new parents how to choose and use an infant car seat.

8. The agent–host–environment model of health and illness is based on what concept?
   a. Risk factors
   b. Demographic variables
   c. Behaviors to promote health
   d. Stages of illness

9. When providing health promotion classes, a nurse uses concepts from models of health. What do both the health–illness continuum and the high-level wellness models demonstrate?
   a. Illness as a fixed point in time
   b. The importance of family
   c. Wellness as a passive state
   d. Health as a constantly changing state

10. A nurse follows accepted guidelines for a healthy lifestyle. How can this promote health in others?
    a. By being a role model for healthy behaviors
    b. By not requiring sick days from work
    c. By never exposing others to any type of illness
    d. By spending less money on food

ANSWERS WITH RATIONALES

1. **b, e, f.** Each person defines health and illness individually, based on a number of factors. Health is more than just the absence of illness; it is an active process in which a person moves toward one's maximum potential. An illness is the response of the person to a disease.

2. **a, c, d.** Diabetes, arthritis, and cystic fibrosis are chronic diseases because they are permanent changes caused by irreversible alterations in normal anatomy and physiology, and they require patient education along with a long period of care or support. Pneumonia, fractures, and otitis media are acute illnesses because they have a rapid onset of symptoms that last a relatively short time.

3. **b, c, d, f.** National trends in the prevention of health disparities are focused on vulnerable populations, such as racial and ethnic minorities, those living in poverty, women, children, older adults, rural and inner-city residents, and people with disabilities and special health care needs.

4. **c.** Giving influenza injections is an example of primary health promotion and illness prevention.

5. **b.** When people assume the sick role, they define themselves as ill, seek validation of this experience from others, and give up normal activities. In stage 1: experiencing symptoms, the first indication of an illness usually is recognizing one or more symptoms that are incompatible with one's personal definition of health. The stage of assuming a dependent role is characterized by the patient's decision to accept the diagnosis and follow the prescribed treatment plan. In the achieving recovery and rehabilitation role, the person gives up the dependent role and resumes normal activities and responsibilities.

6. **c.** The physical dimension includes genetic inheritance, age, developmental level, race, and gender. These components strongly influence the person's health status and health practices. A family history of breast cancer is a major risk factor.

7. **b, c.** Tertiary health promotion and disease prevention begins after an illness is diagnosed and treated to reduce disability and to help rehabilitate patients to a maximum level of functioning. These activities include providing ROM exercises and patient teaching for residual limb care. Providing immunizations and teaching parents how to childproof their homes and use an appropriate car seat are primary health promotion activities. Providing screenings is a secondary health promotion activity.

8. **a.** The interaction of the agent, host, and environment creates risk factors that increase the probability of disease.

9. **d.** Both these models view health as a dynamic (constantly changing state).

10. **a.** Good personal health enables the nurse to serve as a role model for patients and families.

TAYLOR SUITE RESOURCES

Explore these additional resources to enhance learning for this chapter:
- NCLEX-Style Questions and other resources on **thePoint**, http://thePoint.lww.com/Taylor8e
- *Study Guide for Fundamentals of Nursing, 8th edition*
- Adaptive Learning | Powered by prepU, http://thepoint.lww.com/prepu

Bibliography

Centers for Disease Control and Prevention (CDC). (2012a). *Chronic diseases and health promotion.* Available at http://www.cdc.gov/chronicdisease/overview/index.htm

Centers for Disease Control and Prevention (CDC). (2012b). *Lesson 1: Introduction to epidemiology.*

Available at http://cdc.gov/osels/scientific_edu/SS1978/Lesson1/Section8.html

Disparities in healthcare quality among racial and ethnic minority groups. Selected findings from the AHRQ 2010 NHQR and NHDR. (2011). Agency for Healthcare Research and Quality, Rockville, MD. Available at http://www.ahrq.gov/qual/nhqrdr10/nhqrdrminority10.htm

Dunn, H. (1980). *High-level wellness.* Thorofare, NJ: Slack, Inc.

Healthy People 2020. (2010). *Disparities.* Available at http://www.healthypeople.gov/2020/about/DisparitiesAbout.aspx

Leavell, H., & Clark, E. G. (1965). *Preventive medicine for the doctor in the community* (3rd ed.). New York: McGraw Hill.

Melville, N. (2011). *Nurse-led clinics show success in chronic disease management.* Available at http://www.medscape.com/viewarticle/753418_print

National Center for Health Statistics. (2012). Deaths: leading causes for 2009. Available at http://www.cdc.gov/nchs/data/nvsr/nvsr61/nvsr61_07.pdf

National Prevention Council. National Prevention Strategy, Washington, DC (2011). *Elimination of health disparities, p. 25.* Available at http://www.surgeon general.gov/initiatives/prevention/strategy/report.pdf

Newbold, E., Schneidermann, M. & Horton, C. (2012). The Bridge Clinic: A nurse-led postdischarge clinic improves care transitions in a public hospital. *American Journal of Nursing, 112*(7), 56–59.

The Office of Minority Health. (2012). *HIV/AIDS and African Americans.* Available at http://www.minorityhealth.hhs.gov/templates/content.aspx?ID=3019

Pender, N., Murdaugh, C., & Parsons, M. (2006). *Health promotion in nursing practice* (5th ed.). Upper Saddle River, NJ: Pearson Prentice Hall.

Pender, N., Murdaugh, C. & Parsons, M. (2011). *Health promotion in nursing practice* (6th ed.). Upper Saddle River, NJ: Pearson Education, Inc.

Rosenstock, I. (1974). Historical origin of the health belief model. *Health Education Monographs, 2*, 334.

Sherwood, G. & Barnsteiner, J. (2012). *Quality and Safety in Nursing: A competency approach to improving outcomes.* West Sussex, UK: Wiley-Blackwell.

Suchman, E. (1965). Stages of illness and medical care. *Journal of Health and Human Behavior, 6*, 114.

Trossman, S. (2012). Issues up close: Model of care coordination. *American Nurse, 7*(1), 38–39.

U.S. Department of Health and Human Services (USDHHS). (2010). Disparities. The Secretary's Advisory Committee on National Health Promotion and Disease Prevention Objectives for 2020. Phase 1 report recommendations for the framework and format of Health People 2020. Section IV. Advisory Committee findings and recommendations. Available at http://www.healthypeople.gov/hp2020/advisory/Phase1/sec4.html#_Toc211942917

Woolf, S. & Aron, S. Eds. (2013). *U.S. Health in International Perspective: Shorter Lives, Poorer Health.* National Research Council and Institute of Medicine. The National Academies Press. 2012 Patient-Centered Primary Care Collaborative/Millbank Memorial Fund.

World Health Organization. (1974). *Constitution of the World Health Organization: Chronicle of the World Health Organization.* Geneva: Author.

4 Health of the Individual, Family, and Community

ROLANDA SIMPKINS

Rolanda, a 16-year-old girl who is sexually active, comes to the clinic seeking information about contraception. She states, "My mother would 'kill me' if she knew I was asking about this."

SAMUEL KAPLAN

Samuel is the 80-year-old husband of a 76-year-old woman who was diagnosed with Alzheimer disease 1 year ago. Visibly tearful, he states, "I don't think that I can continue to care for my wife at home anymore. But how can I even consider putting her in a long-term care facility?"

CARLOTTA RIOS

Carlotta is a 17-year-old girl who was brought to the mental health–psychiatric unit because of attempted suicide. She does not speak English very well and lives with her sister because of the recent death of her mother. Further assessment reveals possible verbal abuse by her sister and a desire to "disappear" and not return to her sister's home.

LEARNING OBJECTIVES

After completing the chapter, you will be able to accomplish the following:

1. Describe each level of Maslow's hierarchy of basic human needs.

2. Explain nursing care necessary to meet needs in each level of Maslow's hierarchy.

3. Discuss family concepts, including family roles, structures, functions, developmental stages, tasks, and health risk factors.

4. Identify aspects of the community that affect individual and family health.

5. Describe nursing interventions to promote and maintain health of the individual as a member of a family and as a member of a community.

KEY TERMS

basic human needs	love and belonging needs	safety and security needs
blended family	nuclear family	self-actualization needs
community	physiologic needs	self-esteem needs
extended family		
family		

Humans are complex organisms, influenced by and responsive to both internal and external environments. Our behaviors, feelings about ourselves and others, values, and the priorities we set for ourselves all relate to our physiologic and psychosocial needs. These needs are common to all people, and meeting these needs is essential for the health and survival of all people; therefore, they are called **basic human needs**. Basic human needs can be met or unmet in a variety of ways. A person can meet some needs independently, but most needs require relationships and interactions with others for partial or complete fulfillment. Satisfying one's needs often depends on the physical and social environment, especially one's family and community.

Holistic nursing care, which is based on considering all human dimensions affecting how the patient's basic human needs are met in health and in illness, allows the nurse to provide individualized, health-oriented care. This chapter discusses how basic human needs, the family, and the community environment affect the health of every individual. (For an example, see the accompanying Reflective Practice box (on page 60)).

 Concept Mastery Alert

A holistic framework of care involves not just the individual patient but all those around the patient, most importantly the family and their active participation in promoting health.

THE INDIVIDUAL'S BASIC HUMAN NEEDS

In nursing, we consider both the physical and psychosocial needs of each individual patient. Abraham Maslow (1968) developed a hierarchy of basic human needs (Fig. 4-1 on page 61) that describes which needs of a person are the most important at any given time. Certain needs are more basic or essential than others and must be at least minimally met before other needs can be considered.

Maslow's hierarchy is useful for understanding relationships among basic human needs and for establishing priorities of care. The hierarchy is based on the theory that something is a basic need if it has the following characteristics:

• Its lack of fulfillment results in illness.
• Its fulfillment helps prevent illness or signals health.
• Meeting it restores health.
• It takes priority over other satisfactions when unmet.
• The person feels something is missing when the need is unmet.
• The person feels satisfaction when the need is met.

Maslow arranged the hierarchy to show that certain needs are more basic than others. Although all people experience all needs all the time, people generally strive to meet certain of the needs (at least to a minimal level) before attending to other needs. The five levels of needs, beginning with the most basic, are as follows:

Level 1: Physiologic needs
Level 2: Safety and security needs
Level 3: Love and belonging needs
Level 4: Self-esteem needs
Level 5: Self-actualization needs

Nursing care is often directed toward meeting unmet or threatened needs. Maslow's hierarchy provides a framework for nursing assessment and for understanding the needs of patients at all levels, so that interventions to meet priority needs become a part of the plan of care. Many nursing interventions are aimed at meeting patients' basic human needs. The following sections describe each level of need in more detail.

Physiologic Needs

Physiologic needs—for oxygen, water, food, elimination, temperature, sexuality, physical activity, and rest—must be met at least minimally to maintain life. These needs are the most basic in the hierarchy of needs, are the most essential to life and, therefore, have the highest priority. Most healthy children and adults meet their physiologic needs through self-care, but meeting physiologic needs is often a major part of the nursing care plan for young, old, disabled, and ill people who require assistance in meeting them.

Oxygen is the most essential of all needs because all body cells require oxygen for survival. Oxygenation of body cells is carried out primarily by the respiratory and cardiovascular systems, and any alteration in their structure or function

REFLECTIVE PRACTICE: CULTIVATING QSEN COMPETENCIES

CHALLENGE TO ETHICAL AND LEGAL SKILLS

Junior year was full of excitement and new experiences. I was both nervous and excited about our mental health clinical rotation. Although the staff was very helpful and cooperative to provide as great an experience as they could, I found this clinical rotation to be difficult. I was going to be speaking with patients who had mental-health problems and developing nurse–patient relationships that were different from the ones that I'd had in the past. To tell the truth, I was fearful. I was afraid I would say the wrong thing, causing the person to react, possibly injuring himself or others.

One patient really made an impression on me—Carlotta Rios, a 17-year-old girl who was brought to the unit because of attempted suicide. She did not speak English very well and lived with her sister because her mother had recently passed away. The nurses asked me to speak with her because I spoke Spanish.

When talking with her, I found out that Carlotta did not like living with her sister because the sister verbally abused her, always putting her down and constantly reminding Carlotta that the only reason she was here was because of her sister. Carlotta reported that her sister constantly told

her about all of the sacrifices that she was making just so that Carlotta could be with her. According to Carlotta, her sister said that Carlotta did not appreciate everything that her sister was doing. The sister constantly reminded Carlotta of everything she bought for her, keeping a record so that Carlotta would pay her back. Carlotta said that she was not happy and figured that the only way she would stop feeling bad and that her sister would be happy again would be if Carlotta disappeared. Carlotta no longer wanted to exist.

Talking with Carlotta further, I found out that she did not want to return to her sister's home. Unfortunately, this was a problem because legally she was not considered an adult. Therefore, Carlotta's sister would have to be contacted. Yet, it seemed that Carlotta's current family and living situation was not the safest. It also seemed to be the cause of Carlotta's desperate attempt to take her life. If she chose not to return to her sister's house, Carlotta would be taken to court in handcuffs and placed in a foster home. Although this placement would only be until she turned 18 years old, which was at the end of the month, it also meant that once she was 18 years old, she would be on her own. It was apparent that she was not ready for such a drastic change.

Thinking Outside the Box: Possible Courses of Action

- Call Carlotta's sister and have her pick Carlotta up, because she is legally responsible for the patient.
- Gain the trust of the patient by speaking to her as an adult and informing her of all the options, ultimately assisting her with carrying them out.

- Call someone with whom she felt comfortable to provide support and also to hear the options available; in this way, the patient would have the opinion of someone she knew and trusted before she made a decision on which course of action to take.

Evaluating a Good Outcome: How Do I Define Success?

- Patient's safety is ensured.
- Patient benefits from the course of action decided on.
- The patient's human dignity is respected.
- No violations of the American Nurses Association's Code of Ethics occur.

- Patient makes the most appropriate decision, resulting in the best outcome for her.
- The ethical and legal obligations for me and those of the hospital are met.

Personal Learning: Here's to the Future!

I figured the best way to approach this situation was to develop a trusting relationship. So, after getting Carlotta up, we went to a brighter, better-lit room, where we had breakfast. I started by asking simple questions, eventually progressing to those that pertained to why she was in the hospital. Throughout our talks, I reinforced that her sister was considered the person legally responsible for Carlotta, explaining that if Carlotta decided not to call home, she would be taken in handcuffs to court and then would be placed in a foster home. I told her that this would only be until she turned 18 years old; upon turning 18, she then would be on her own. After listening to all of her options,

she decided that she would call her sister to let her know where she was. She also told her sister that she would be staying with a best friend until she had figured things out. For Carlotta, this was the best decision to make because she felt safest. As a result of informing her sister, Carlotta would not have to go to court. Subsequently, any upset or disruption for her sister would be minimized, further adding to Carlotta's feelings of being safe. The priority for Carlotta was a safe environment. We were able to establish a trusting relationship and work together toward this end.

Stephanie Cuellar, Georgetown University

REFLECTION ON QUALITY AND SAFETY COMPETENCIES

How do you think you would respond in a similar situation? Why? What does this tell you about yourself and about the adequacy of your skills for professional practice? Can you think of other ways to respond? What *knowledge, skills,* and *attitudes* do you need to develop to continuously improve quality and safety when caring for patients like Carlotta?

Patient-Centered Care: What additional information would be important for the nursing student to obtain from Carlotta to provide a more complete picture of the family situation? What family risk factors were evident here? Have these factors been addressed? What is the best way to communicate emotional support to Carlotta?

REFLECTIVE PRACTICE: CULTIVATING QSEN COMPETENCIES *continued*

CHALLENGE TO ETHICAL AND LEGAL SKILLS

Teamwork and Collaboration/Quality Improvement:
What communication skills do you need to continue to function as a resource and advocate for Carlotta? Would collaboration with your instructor or her nurse have resulted in additional alternatives or another approach with Carlotta? Are there community resources that might prove helpful to Carlotta? Do you think some form of family therapy might prove helpful to Carlotta and her sister?

Safety/Evidence-Based Practice: Is there anything more you could have done to acknowledge that you understand Carlotta's concern about the future? How do you think your

response contributed to a safe environment for Carlotta? What evidence in nursing literature provides guidance for decision making regarding ensuring a safe environment and giving Carlotta the support that she needs?

Informatics: Can you identify essential information that must be documented in Carlotta's electronic record regarding communication that you had with her? Is it important to document your assessment of Carlotta's current mental status? Can you identify any additional information that supports safe patient care and coordination of care?

---

can result in an increased need for oxygen. This need may be acute (such as when cardiopulmonary resuscitation is needed) or chronic (requiring special positioning, treatments, and teaching). Nurses evaluate patients' oxygen needs by assessing skin color, vital signs, anxiety levels, responses to activity, restlessness, and mental responsiveness.

A balance between the intake and elimination of fluids is also essential to life. Healthy people drink fluids to satisfy thirst, and they maintain fluid balance through various physiologic processes. Disruption in the water balance of the body results in either dehydration or edema (the collec-

tion of fluid in body tissues). Dehydration results from conditions such as severe diarrhea or vomiting, whereas edema is caused by diseases of the cardiovascular or renal system, trauma, and other factors. Measuring intake and output, testing the resiliency of the skin, checking the condition of the skin and mucous membranes, and weighing the patient help assess a patient's water balance.

Food and elimination are related physiologic needs, with a balance maintained through digestive and metabolic processes. The need for food is manifested through hunger. Insufficient nutrient intake results in nutrient and electrolyte imbalances and weight loss. Waste products are eliminated from the body through the skin, lungs, kidneys, and intestines. A patient's nutritional status is assessed with a variety of indicators, including weight, muscle mass, strength, and laboratory values.

The human body functions best within a narrow temperature range, usually considered as plus or minus 98.6°F (37°C). Homeostatic mechanisms and adaptive responses, such as sweating or shivering, help maintain this temperature. Nurses assess body temperature as a vital sign (see Chapter 24).

Sexuality is an integral component of each person and may be affected by physical and emotional illnesses. Sexual practices depend on a variety of factors, such as a person's age, sociocultural background, self-esteem, and level of health. Health care practitioners are increasingly aware that consideration of sexuality is a vital part of holistic care.

 RECALL Rolanda Simpkins, the 16-year-old girl described at the beginning of the chapter requesting information about contraception. The nurse can use knowledge about Rolanda's sexuality and sexual practices to help determine the most appropriate method of contraception for her. ●

Physical activity and rest are also basic physiologic needs. Physical activity depends on intact and functioning neuromuscular and skeletal systems. Rest and sleep allow time for the body to rejuvenate and be free of stress. Individual

Self-actualization

Self-esteem

Higher-level needs

Safety and security

Lower-level needs

Physiologic

FIGURE 4-1. Maslow's hierarchy of basic human needs.

requirements for rest and sleep vary widely, but the adverse health effects of deprivation have been well documented. Factors that influence sleep include age, environment, exercise, stress, and drug use.

 THINK back to Samuel Kaplan, the older man caring for his wife with Alzheimer disease at home. The nurse assesses the effect of providing this care on his activity, rest, and sleep patterns, thereby developing an appropriate plan of care for Mr. Kaplan to ensure that his needs are met as well. •

Safety and Security Needs

Safety and security needs come next in priority and have both physical and emotional components. Physical safety and security means being protected from potential or actual harm. Nurses carry out a wide variety of activities to meet patients' physical safety needs, such as the following:

- Using proper hand hygiene and sterile techniques to prevent infection
- Using electrical equipment properly
- Administering medications knowledgeably
- Skillfully moving and ambulating patients
- Teaching parents about household chemicals that are dangerous to children

Specific safety interventions are discussed in Chapter 26.

Emotional safety and security involves trusting others and being free of fear, anxiety, and apprehension. Patients entering the health care system often fear the unknown and may have significant emotional security needs. Nurses can help meet such needs by encouraging spiritual practices that provide strength and support, by allowing as much independent decision making and control as possible, and by carefully explaining new and unfamiliar procedures and treatments.

 REMEMBER Carlotta Rios, the adolescent described in the Reflective Practice display. The nurse fosters the development of a trusting relationship to promote emotional safety and security. Doing so assists Carlotta in her decision-making process about going home. •

Love and Belonging Needs

All humans have a basic need for love and belonging. After physiologic and safety and security needs, this is the next priority and is often called a higher-level need. **Love and belonging needs** include the understanding and acceptance of others in both giving and receiving love, and the feeling of belonging to groups such as families, peers, friends, a neighborhood, and a community.

People who believe that their love and belonging needs are unmet often feel lonely and isolated. They may withdraw physically and emotionally, or they may become overly demanding and critical. Often, these behaviors signal that the person has unmet love and belonging needs. Nurses

FIGURE 4-2. By providing time for the mother and newborn to bond, the nurse is helping to fulfill the need for love and belonging of both mother and child.

should always consider love and belonging needs when developing a plan of care (Fig. 4-2), including nursing interventions such as:

- Including family and friends in the care of the patient
- Establishing a nurse–patient relationship based on mutual understanding and trust (by demonstrating caring, encouraging communication, and respecting privacy)
- Referring patients to specific support groups (such as a cancer support group or Alcoholics Anonymous)

 THINK back to Samuel Kaplan, the man caring for his wife with Alzheimer disease. The nurse could refer Mr. Kaplan to a support group for caregivers of patients with Alzheimer disease to help meet Mr. Kaplan's needs for love and belonging. •

Self-Esteem Needs

The next highest priority on the hierarchy is **self-esteem needs**, which include the need for a person to feel good about oneself, to feel pride and a sense of accomplishment, and to believe that others also respect and appreciate those accomplishments. Positive self-esteem facilitates the person's confidence and independence.

Many factors affect self-esteem. When a person's role changes (e.g., through illness or the death of a spouse), self-esteem can be seriously altered because the person's responsibilities and relationships also change. A change in body image, such as the loss of a breast, an injury, or a growth spurt during puberty, may also affect self-esteem. Nurses must remember that the person's perception of the change—rather than the actual change itself—is what affects that individual's self-esteem (see the Research in Nursing box).

Nurses can help meet patients' self-esteem needs by respecting their values and beliefs, encouraging patients to set attainable goals, and facilitating support from family or significant others. These actions promote a sense of worth and self-acceptance.

RESEARCH IN NURSING

BRIDGING THE GAP TO EVIDENCE-BASED PRACTICE

Understanding the Effect of Homelessness on the Health and Well-Being of Family Members

Families consisting of a single mother with children represent the fastest growing segment of the homeless population. From 2007 to 2009, there was a significant increase in the number of families who were homeless. Urban-dwelling minorities are the most likely group to lose affordable housing and become homeless. This negative life experience impacts the health and well-being of every member of the family and is particularly stressful for children. Both mothers and their children are more likely to suffer emotional problems or display depressive symptoms. Most of these women have also experienced physical and/or sexual assault at some time in their lives. People in this vulnerable group are at great risk for poor health and unsatisfactory health outcomes.

Related Research

Lee, R. (2012). Family homelessness viewed through the lens of health and human rights. *Advances in Nursing Science, 35*(2), E47–E59.

The purpose of this study was to document and interpret the effect of homelessness on the health and human rights of 12 Appalachian mothers and their children. Appalachian families are a unique cultural group; nursing care must recognize their values, beliefs, and practices in order to provide quality health care. The 12 mothers involved in this study resided in a homeless shelter in a large Midwestern city, were either African American or European American, and had one to five children ranging in age from 2 months to 15 years. The participants were interviewed two to four times for 1 to 2 hours. Three uni-versal themes were discovered during these interviews. First, each of the mothers described coping with challenging experiences that threatened their lives while attempting to support their children before coming to the shelter. These included job loss and/or a family illness. Second, all the mothers verbalized the struggle to earn the respect of self and others. The third universal theme dealt with the mothers remaining strong and supporting their children during this difficult time of living in a shelter and searching for stable housing. Each of the mothers also included having a place to live as part of their definition of health. They all verbalized experiences of discrimination and prejudice before and during their homelessness and expressed the feeling that they had been denied their inalienable human rights.

Relevance to Nursing Practice

The need for dignity and respect is a vital component of any definition of health and well-being. To provide individualized care for families who are homeless, nurses need to be aware of the cultural, ethnic, and religious orientations of their patients and understand the multiple factors that contribute to the homeless experience. Nurses must not impose their own interpretations on families that experience homelessness. This vulnerable population needs nurses to advocate on their behalf and identify available resources and plan interventions that will improve health outcomes for these families.

For additional research, visit thePoint.

Self-Actualization Needs

The highest level on the hierarchy of needs is **self-actualization needs**, which include the need for individuals to reach their full potential through development of their unique capabilities. In general, each lower level of need must be met to some degree before this need can be satisfied. The process of self-actualization continues throughout life. Maslow lists the following qualities that indicate achievement of one's potential:

* Acceptance of self and others as they are
* Focus of interest on problems outside oneself
* Ability to be objective
* Feelings of happiness and affection for others
* Respect for all people
* Ability to discriminate between good and evil
* Creativity as a guideline for solving problems and pursuing interests

To help meet patients' self-actualization needs, the nurse focuses on the person's strengths and possibilities rather than on problems. Following is an example of a nurse assisting a patient to meet self-actualization needs:

During a clinic visit, a diabetic patient expresses difficulty with his prescribed dietary recommendations but also rec-ognizes that he needs to be more careful or "I'll end up losing a leg or having trouble seeing because of this disease." A nurse coach recognizes that the patient is the best expert about his own health and listens carefully as he reviews his eating habits and discusses what he thinks he needs to do differently. Based on assessment data and the patient's desire to change his behavior, the nurse and patient together create an action plan to begin the process of change and move toward the optimal way for him to achieve his goals.

Nursing interventions are aimed at providing a sense of direction and hope and providing teaching that is aimed at maximizing potentials.

 RECALL Carlotta Rios, the 17-year-old who had attempted suicide. By focusing on her strengths as well as helping her explore alternatives to her current lifestyle, the nurse helps to meet Carlotta's self-actualization needs by fostering personal growth and assisting her to find meaning to her life. ●

Applying Maslow's Theory

Nurses can apply Maslow's hierarchy of basic needs in the assessment, planning, implementation, and evaluation of patient care. The hierarchy can be used with patients at any

Table 4-1   THE HUMAN DIMENSIONS AND BASIC HUMAN NEEDS

	BASIC HUMAN NEED	EXAMPLES
Physical dimension	Physiologic needs	Breathing Circulation Temperature Intake of food and fluids Elimination of wastes Movement
Environmental dimension	Safety and security needs	Housing Community/neighborhood Climate
Sociocultural dimension	Love and belonging needs	Relationships with others Communications with others Support systems Being part of a community Feeling loved by others
Emotional dimension	Self-esteem needs	Fear Sadness Loneliness Happiness Accepting self
Intellectual and spiritual dimensions	Self-actualization needs	Thinking Learning Decision making Values Beliefs Fulfillment Helping others

age, in all settings where care is provided, and in both health and illness. It helps the nurse identify unmet needs as they become health care needs. The hierarchy of basic needs allows the nurse to locate the patient on the health–illness continuum and to incorporate the human dimensions and health models into meeting needs (Table 4-1).

As the nurse identifies and carries out interventions to help meet patients' needs, it is important to remember that this is only a framework or guideline and that, in actuality, each person sets one's own priorities for needs. Additionally, basic human needs are interrelated and may require nursing actions at more than one level at a given time. For example, in caring for a person coming into the emergency department with a heart attack, the nurse's immediate concern is the patient's physiologic needs (e.g., oxygen and pain relief). At the same time, safety needs (e.g., for oxygen use precautions and for ensuring that the person does not fall off the examining table) and love and belonging needs (e.g., for having a family member nearby if possible) are

still major considerations. You will learn how nurses meet basic human needs throughout the rest of this book.

THE FAMILY

Almost every person is a member of a number of groups, such as friends, professional colleagues, a church congregation, or a school class. Each of these groups involves a specific part of the person's life and is important to the person. However, only one group—the family—is typically concerned with all parts of a person's life and with meeting the individual's basic human needs to promote health.

A **family** can be defined simply as any group of people who live together and depend on one another for physical, emotional, and financial support. Families are essential to the health and survival of the individual family members, as well as to society as a whole. The family is a buffer between the needs of the individual member and the demands and expectations of society. The role of the family is to help meet the basic human needs of its members while also meeting the needs of society (Pender, Murdaugh, & Parsons, 2011).

Family Structures

A family may consist of two or more people who may be related or unrelated either biologically or legally, may be of the same or different gender, and/or may span different generations. A family may include individuals with a meaningful commitment to each other outside of marriage (Pender, Murdaugh, & Parsons, 2011). Nurses must remember that there are no absolute "rights" or "wrongs" about what makes a family, and one person's values must not be imposed on another person. Respect for all kinds of family members and relationships is essential to holistic, individualized patient care.

Nuclear Family

The **nuclear family**, also called the traditional family, is composed of two parents and their children. Contemporary descriptions of a nuclear family vary. Pender, Murtaugh, & Parsons (2011) define a nuclear family as "two or more persons who depend on one another for emotional, physical, or financial support." The Centers for Disease Control and Prevention (CDC, 2010) summarizes a nuclear family as "one or more children living with two parents who are married to one another and are each biological or adoptive parents to all children in the family." One of the more contemporary definitions refers to the great variability in family structure as "postmodern families" (Williams, Sawyer, & Wahlstrom, 2008). The parents might be heterosexual or homosexual and are usually either married or in a committed relationship; family members live together until the children leave home as young adults. The nuclear family may be composed of biologic parents and children, adoptive parents and children, surrogate parents and children, or stepparents and children. Multiple research studies have concluded that family processes such as the quality of parenting and harmony between parents, rather than family structures, contribute to a child's well-being (American Academy of Pediatrics, 2012).

In contemporary nuclear families, one or both parents work, while the other or both share roles in providing physical and emotional safety and security. The two major causes of this change are increased education and career opportunities for women and changes in our economy resulting in a need for additional income to maintain a desired standard of living. This family group often lives in close geographic proximity to relatives, such as aunts, uncles, and grandparents, who are a part of the **extended family**. Couples without children and couples with grown children who no longer live at home are considered nuclear families as well. The **blended family** is another form of a nuclear family, formed when parents bring unrelated children from previous relationships together to form a new family.

Single-Parent Family

Single parents may be separated, divorced, widowed, or never married. Increasing numbers of never-married men and women are choosing to become parents. More than one fourth of all children in North America are now estimated to live in single-parent families (American Academy of Pediatrics, 2011). Many single-parent families are headed by women. Single parents often have special problems and needs, including financial concerns and role shifts (i.e., having the roles of both parents), becoming remarried or having new relationships. These problems are important considerations when planning and implementing nursing care.

Other Family Structures

In addition to traditional and single-parent families, cohabiting adults and single adults are other family structures. Cohabiting families are individuals who choose to live together for a variety of reasons, including relationships, financial need, or changing values. Cohabiting families include unmarried adults (of any age, including retired people who choose not to marry because it would impose financial hardship) living together, and communal or group marriages. Other family structures include binuclear (where divorced parents assume joint custody of children) and dyadic nuclear (in which the couple chooses not to have children).

Single adults may not be living with others, but they are part of a family of origin, usually have a social network with significant others, or may even regard a pet as family. Most single adults living alone are either young adults who achieve independence and enter the workforce or older adults who never married or are left alone after the death of a spouse.

With changes in family structure have come other influences on the basic human needs of family members. Considerations for the family, and for nursing care, include support systems (in our mobile society, family members may live hundreds or thousands of miles away), availability of childcare, time for leisure and recreation, struggles to meet financial commitments, and changing role models.

Family Functions

Families have important functions that affect how individual family members meet their basic human needs and maintain their health. The family provides the individual with an environment for development and social interactions. Families also are important to society as a whole because they provide new and socialized members for society.

Family functions occur in five major areas. Physically, the family provides a safe, comfortable environment necessary for growth, development, and rest or recuperation. Economically, the family provides financial aid to family members and also helps meet society's needs. The reproductive function of many families is to have and raise children. The affective and coping functions of the family provide emotional comfort to family members and help members establish their identity and maintain it in times of stress. Finally, through socialization, the family teaches; transmits beliefs, values, attitudes, and coping mechanisms; provides feedback; and guides problem solving (Friedman, Bowden, & Jones, 2003).

Developmental Tasks of Families

Duvall (1977) identified critical family developmental tasks and stages in a family life cycle. Duvall's theory, based on Erikson's theory of psychosocial development (described in Chapter 17), states that all families have certain basic tasks for survival and continuity as well as specific tasks related to developmental stages throughout the life of the family. These stages and developmental tasks are outlined in Table 4-2 (on page 66). If the family does not meet certain developmental tasks, societal disapproval may lead to intervention by children's services, social services, police departments, welfare agencies, or health departments (Edelman & Mandle, 2010). The successful mastery of each developmental stage is important to the family's adaptation and growth through successive stages.

The Family in Health and Illness

Individuals learn health care activities, health beliefs, and health values in the family. When patients enter the health care system, they bring their own personal behaviors and needs, but they also bring (in a sense) their family too.

Friedman and associates (2003) identified the importance of family-centered nursing care in four ways. First, the family is composed of interdependent members who affect one another. If some form of illness occurs in one member, all other members become involved in the illness. Second, because there is a strong relationship between the family and the health status of its members, the role of the family is essential in every level of nursing care. Third, the level of health of the family and in turn each of its members can be significantly improved through health promotion activities. Finally, illness of one family member may suggest the possibility of the same problem in other members. Through assessment and intervention, the nurse can assist in improving the health status of all family members.

Illness may precipitate a health crisis in a family. If an illness is relatively minor, such as a viral infection in a child, changes in family tasks may be minor and brief. But if a family

Table 4-2 FAMILY STAGES, TASKS, HEALTH RISK FACTORS, AND NURSING INTERVENTIONS TO PROMOTE HEALTH

FAMILY STAGE[a]	TASKS	STAGE-SPECIFIC RISK FACTORS	STAGE-SPECIFIC NURSING INTERVENTIONS/REFERRALS
Couple and family with young children	Establish a mutually satisfying marriage Plan to have or not to have children Have and adjust to infant Support needs of all family members Adjust to cost of family life Adapt to needs and activity of children Cope with loss of energy and privacy Encourage and support growth and development and educational achievements	Inadequate knowledge of contraception and family Inadequate knowledge of sexual and marital roles Lack of knowledge about child safety and health Child abuse and neglect First pregnancy before age 16	Family planning clinics Prenatal classes Well-child clinics Vision and hearing screenings Dental health information Parent support groups Safety in the home, daycare, school, neighborhood, and community
Family with adolescents and young adults	Maintain open communications Support moral and ethical family values Balance teenagers' freedom with responsibility Maintain supportive home base Strengthen marital relationships	Family of origin Family value of aggressiveness Inadequate problem-solving abilities Conflict between family members Physical or sexual abuse Sexually transmitted diseases	Accident prevention programs Sex education Mental health programs Screening for chronic illness
Family with middle-aged adults	Maintain ties with younger and older generations Prepare for retirement	Depression Exposure to environmental or work-related health risks, such as sunlight, asbestos, radiation, coal dust, and air or water pollution	Blood pressure screenings Screening for chronic illness
Family with older adults	Adjust to retirement Adjust to loss of spouse May move from family home	Increasing age with loss of physical function Chronic illness Depression Death of spouse	Screening for chronic illness Home safety information Retirement information Pharmacology information

Data from Duvall, E. (1977). *Marriage and family development* (5th ed.). Philadelphia: J. B. Lippincott; Aldous, J. (1975). *The developmental approach to family analysis*. Minneapolis: University of Minnesota Press.
[a]Family includes all forms: nuclear, extended, single-parent, etc.

member's injury or illness is serious, the roles and responsibilities, as well as functions, of other family members change. This is especially true if the illness is chronic and long term, results in disability, or decreases the person's time to live. Some families find it difficult to adapt to the stress of changes in financial, social, and caregiving resources, whereas other families experience renewed family closeness and stability. Regardless of how the family adapts, members of the family must constantly adjust roles and responsibilities to manage the needs of the ill family member and the family.

 REMEMBER Mr. Kaplan, the 80-year-old man caring for his wife with Alzheimer disease. Now the primary caregiver, Mr. Kaplan's role has changed. The disease and family role changes may affect the family's ability to function. The nurse would incorporate knowledge of this when developing the most appropriate plan for Mr. Kaplan and his wife. ●

Nursing interventions for a family in a health crisis include providing teaching that is honest, open, and respectful; using therapeutic communication skills; applying knowledge of family dynamics; and making referrals to community health care and financial resources to support realistic hope. In addition, it is important to involve family members in planning and implementing care.

Family Risk Factors

Family patterns of behavior, the environment in which the family lives, and genetic factors can all place family members at risk for health problems. Nurses should assess these factors before developing nursing care plans. Typical questions in a family assessment include the following (Pender, Murdaugh, & Parsons, 2011; Frampton & Wahl, 2012):

- What is the family's structure?
- What is the family's socioeconomic status?
- What are family members' cultural background and religious affiliation?
- Who cares for children if both parents work?
- What are the family's health practices (e.g., types of foods eaten, meal times, immunizations, bedtime, exercise)?
- How does the family define health?
- What habits are present in the family (e.g., do any family members smoke, drink to excess, or use drugs)?
- How does the family cope with stress?
- Is any family member the primary caregiver for another family member?
- Do close friends or family members live nearby and can they help if necessary?

 THESE questions are extremely important to ask when assessing Carlotta Rios, the adolescent described in the Reflective Practice display, and Samuel Kaplan, the older adult caring for his ill wife at home. Each person's answers provide the nurse with valuable information to help determine the best way to meet their needs. For Carlotta, this includes information about viable options for her living arrangements, including physical and emotional safety. For Mr. Kaplan, this assessment provides information about available sources of help so that he can continue to care for his wife at home, or if necessary, ease the transition and adjustment to moving his wife to a long-term care facility. ●

The health assessment for a family should also consider the risk factors for altered health described in Box 4-1.

Nursing Interventions to Promote Family Health

The nurse can help reduce risk factors with activities that promote health for all family members at any level of development. Recall that each person has one's own definition of health, based in part on family beliefs and values about health and illness. The nurse assists both the person and the family to meet their basic human needs. Examples of only stage-specific risk factors and nursing interventions to promote health in the family are shown in Table 4-2 (on page 66). Nurses may carry out such activities themselves or may refer the individual or family to other health care providers. Health promotion activities and nursing actions can reduce the risk for illness and facilitate healthy behaviors at any age within the family life cycle.

 CONSIDER Rolanda Simpkins, the adolescent seeking contraceptive information. The nurse needs to evaluate further her statement that her mother would "kill her," questioning Rolanda further to determine the family's health beliefs and practices. ●

BOX 4-1 RISK FACTORS FOR ALTERED FAMILY HEALTH

Lifestyle Risk Factors
- Lack of knowledge about sexual and marital roles, leading to teenage marriage and pregnancy; divorce; sexually transmitted infections; child, spouse, or elder abuse; and lack of prenatal or childcare
- Alterations in nutrition—either more or less than body requirements at any age
- Chemical dependency, including the use of alcohol, drugs, and nicotine
- Inadequate dental care and hygiene
- Unsafe or unstimulating home environment

Psychosocial Risk Factors
- Inadequate childcare resources, when both parents work, for preschool and school-aged children
- Inadequate income to provide safe housing, food, clothing, and health care
- Conflict between family members

Environmental Risk Factors
- Lack of knowledge or finances to provide safe and clean living conditions
- Work or social pressures that cause stress
- Air, water, or food pollution

Developmental Risk Factors
- Families who have new babies, especially if support systems are unavailable
- Older people, especially those living alone or on a fixed income
- Unmarried adolescent mothers who lack personal, economic, and educational resources

Biologic Risks
- Birth defects
- Mental retardation
- Genetic predisposition to certain diseases, including cardiovascular diseases and cancer

THE COMMUNITY

A person, as an individual and as a member of a family, is also a member of a community. The most basic definition of a **community** is a specific population or group of people living in the same geographic area under similar regulations and having common values, interests, and needs. A community may be a small neighborhood within a city or a large rural area, including a small town. Communities are based on shared characteristics of people, the area, social interaction, and familial, cultural, or ethnic heritage and ties. Within a community, people interact and share resources. The community environment affects the ability of the individual to meet basic human needs. This section discusses the relationship of the community to basic human needs, including influences on health and illness.

The physical and social environments of communities have been implicated by the Institute of Medicine and the National Research Council as possible contributing factors to health disadvantages in the United States as compared to other high-income countries (Woolf & Aron, 2013). Americans die younger and have a consistent pattern of poor health and death and suffering from illness and injuries compared to the other wealthiest nations in the world. Designing healthier community environments is one of the recommended strategies to promote more favorable health outcomes in the United States. See Chapter 3 for additional explanations of and implications for this U.S. health disadvantage.

Many community factors affect the health of residents. A healthy community enables people to maintain a high quality of life and productivity. For example, a healthy community:

- Offers access to health care services for all members of the community, which provide both treatment for illnesses and activities to promote health
- Has roads, schools, playgrounds, and other services to meet needs of the people in the community
- Maintains a safe and healthy environment

The health of a community's residents is affected by the social support systems, the community health structure, environmental factors, and agencies providing assistance for those in need of shelter, housing, and food. Examples of community factors affecting health are listed in Box 4-2 and are discussed further in the following sections.

Social Support Systems

A person's social support systems are made up of all the people who help meet financial, personal, physical, and emotional needs. In most instances, family, friends, and neighbors provide the best social support within a community. To understand the social support systems of a community, it is important to know who and what provide support (such as family, neighbors, friends, church, and organizations).

Community Health Care Structure

The health care structure of a community directly affects the health of the people living within it. The size and location of

BOX 4-2 EXAMPLES OF COMMUNITY FACTORS AFFECTING HEALTH

- Number and availability of health care institutions and services
- Housing codes
- Police and fire departments
- Nutritional services for low-income infants, mothers, school-aged children (e.g., lunch programs), and older people
- Zoning regulations separating residential and industrial areas
- Waste disposal services and locations
- Air and water pollution
- Food sanitation
- Health education services and dissemination
- Recreational opportunities
- Violent crimes or drug use

the community often determine what services are available. For example, urban residents may have public transportation to a variety of health care providers, whereas rural residents might need to travel long distances on their own for care. County and state funding for community health care services also determines the type and number of available health care institutions and agencies.

Economic Resources

Personal finances and health care insurance coverage affect a person's access to health care services within a community. As private health insurance costs continue to escalate, fewer citizens have it. Many part-time and unskilled jobs provide no insurance benefits at all, resulting in a substantial number of citizens without any financial assistance for health care screenings or care for illnesses.

Signed in March 2010, the Patient Protection and Affordable Care Act, often referred to simply as the Affordable Care Act (PPACA), aims to provide improved health security and access to health care for all Americans through comprehensive health insurance reforms being implemented in stages over several years. In addition to the major provisions that provide a right to coverage for Americans with pre-existing conditions, that allow young adults up to 26 years of age to continue to be covered under their parents' plan, and that end lifetime limits on coverage, this law expands Medicaid coverage to millions of low-income Americans and makes numerous improvements to the Children's Health Insurance Program (CHIP; Affordable Care Act, 2012). PPACA has many more provisions to facilitate health insurance coverage and help care for underserved populations and eliminate disparities in health care. Chapter 8 further discusses the costs of health care.

Environmental Factors

The community environment in which a person lives and works can have either helpful or harmful effects on health. The quality of air and water differs across communities. Large urban areas are often affected by air pollution, whereas many smaller communities are at risk for water pollution from run-off of chemical or livestock wastes. There is also increasing concern about how global warming and a growing potential for natural disasters affects health. Environmental barriers to accessing health care within a community may include lack of transportation, distance to services, and location of the services.

Effect on Individuals and Families

The community has a strong influence on health promotion and illness-prevention activities of individuals and families in the community (Fig. 4-3). Just as there are family risk factors for the health of individual members, so are there community risk factors involving resources, economics, and services. For nursing assessments and interventions to be comprehensive and individualized, the nurse must consider the community's influence.

Consider the following examples of how the community can affect the individual's and family's needs. Maria,

FIGURE 4-3. Many character-istics of a community influence the health of its members. This diagram shows six categories of characteristics that influence the health of a member of a community.

20 years old, lives in an inner-city, two-room apartment with her 6-month-old daughter. The apartment lacks adequate heat and plumbing. Maria has no family living nearby, and her husband has left her. Maria rarely leaves her apartment because she fears street gangs and drug addicts. She is on a public assistance program but has never taken her baby to a local clinic for checkups because of her concerns that the neighborhood is not safe.

Anne, 22 years old, lives in a small house in a rural area. Her 4-year-old son is in a community preschool program with afterschool care. She is a single mother and works as a secretary at an insurance agency. Anne often sees her family members, who live nearby. Anne and her son have regular health assessments.

These two different examples illustrate that the community plays a major role in the health of people who live there. Maria and her baby are at much greater risk for illness than are Anne and her son. Even if the two women had identical health care needs, their care plans would include different interventions because of their different community environments.

Nursing in the Community

In contrast to community health nursing, which focuses on whole populations within a community, community-based nursing is centered on the health care needs of individuals and families. Nurses practicing community-based nursing provide interventions to manage acute or chronic health problems, promote health, and facilitate self-care. Nursing care provided within a community must be culturally com-petent and family centered.

 Concept Mastery Alert

Community health nursing focuses on whole populations; community-based nursing focuses on the members of the population, specifically the individuals and families within the population.

Nurses providing community-based care must know about the location and specialty of health care providers, the availability and accessibility of services and supplies, and other public health services. Additional considerations include facilities (such as daycare or long-term care), hous-ing, and the number and type of agencies providing services.

The Future of Nursing, an Institute of Medicine report, emphasizes nursing as a vital component in all efforts to reform the health care system (Institute of Medicine, 2011). PPACA further reaffirms that nurse-managed centers in communities offer high-quality care to underserved popu-lations in a cost-effective manner (Domrose, 2012). More than 250 nurse-managed health centers in the United States are improving health outcomes in communities because they understand community needs (Collins, 2012).

Nurses in these centers carry out a variety of activities that focus on wellness and prevention, including immunizations,

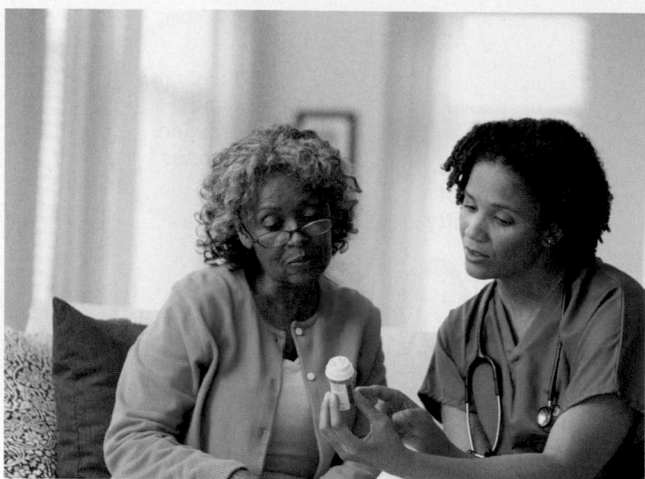

FIGURE 4-4. A nurse at work in a home health care setting.

prenatal care, health education, and medication supervision. Nurses promote health as individuals, as caregivers within institutional settings, and as community-based health care providers. Nurses also provide community services as volunteers in health-related activities (e.g., screenings, educational programs, and blood drives) and as role models for health practices and lifestyles. Nurses working in a variety of health care settings consider community influences when developing individualized nursing care plans and when making referrals to community agencies and support groups. Community-based nurses are employed in many different kinds of practice settings, including home care (Fig. 4-4), community health centers, school nursing, occupational nursing, and independent nursing practice. Community-based care is discussed in more detail in Chapter 9.

DEVELOPING CLINICAL REASONING

1. What do you believe to be the most important basic human need that is actually or potentially unmet in the following situations?
   - A toddler falls into a swimming pool.
   - An older woman falls at home and is not found for 3 days.
   - A preschooler is admitted to the hospital with multiple bruises and burn marks.
   - A teenager is constantly told "you are no good" by his parents.
   - A long-term care facility resident says, "I never did anything right in my life."

2. Our own family experiences often affect the way we relate to the families of our patients. Describe at least two possible responses to the families described below.
   - Suspecting child abuse, a nurse asks a mother about her child's bruises. The woman says, "In our family, we believe in 'spare the rod and spoil the child.'"
   - A single woman wants to have a child and comes to a fertility clinic for information on artificial insemination.
   - Several members of a patient's large extended family are in the patient's long-term care facility room and are trying to do everything for the patient.

PRACTICING FOR NCLEX

1. A nurse is providing care based on Maslow's hierarchy of basic human needs. For which nursing activities is this approach useful?
   a. Making accurate nursing diagnoses
   b. Establishing priorities of care
   c. Communicating concerns more concisely
   d. Integrating science into nursing care

2. The nurse is prioritizing nursing care for a patient in a long-term care facility. Which examples of nursing interventions help meet physiologic needs? Select all that apply.
   a. Preventing falls in the facility
   b. Changing a patient's oxygen tank
   c. Providing materials for a patient who likes to draw
   d. Helping a patient eat his dinner
   e. Facilitating a visit from a spouse
   f. Referring a patient to a cancer support group.

3. The nurse caring for patients postoperatively uses careful hand hygiene and sterile techniques when handling patients. Which of Maslow's basic human needs is being met by this nurse?
   a. Physiologic
   b. Safety and security
   c. Self-esteem
   d. Love and belonging

4. The nurse caring for patients in a long-term care facility knows that the highest level on Maslow's hierarchy of needs is self-actualization needs. Which statements accurately describe the achievement of self-actualization? Select all that apply.
   a. Humans are born with a fully developed sense of self-actualization.
   b. Self-actualization needs are met by depending on others for help.
   c. The self-actualization process continues throughout life.
   d. Loneliness and isolation occur when self-actualization needs are unmet.
   e. A person achieves self-actualization by focusing on problems outside self.
   f. Self-actualization needs may be met by creatively solving problems.

5. A nurse works with families in crisis at a community mental health care facility. What is the best broad definition of a family?
   a. A father, a mother, and children
   b. A group whose members are biologically related
   c. A unit that includes aunts, uncles, and cousins
   d. A group of people who live together and depend on each other for support

6. A nurse performs an assessment of a family consisting of a single mother, a grandmother, and two children. Which interview questions directed to the single mother could the nurse use to assess the affective and coping family function? Select all that apply.
   a. Who is the person you depend on for emotional support?
   b. Who is the breadwinner in your family?
   c. Do you plan on having any more children?
   d. Who keeps your family together in times of stress?
   e. What family traditions do you pass on to your children?
   f. Do you live in an environment that you consider safe?

7. The nurse caring for families in a free health care clinic identifies psychosocial risk factors for altered family health. Which example describes one of these risk factors?
   a. The family does not have dental care insurance or resources to pay for it.
   b. Both parents work and leave a 12-year old child to care for his younger brother.
   c. Both parents and their children are considerably overweight.
   d. The youngest member of the family has cerebral palsy and needs assistance from community services.

8. Shuba and Raul are a couple in their late seventies. According to Duvall, which developmental task is appropriate for this older adult family?
   a. Maintain a supportive home base
   b. Strengthen marital relationships
   c. Cope with loss of energy and privacy
   d. Adjust to retirement

9. A visiting nurse performs a community assessment in an area of the city in which the nurse will be working. What is one element of a healthy community?
   a. Meets all the needs of its inhabitants
   b. Has mixed residential and industrial areas
   c. Offers access to health care services
   d. Has modern housing and condominiums

10. A nurse is practicing community-based nursing in a mobile health clinic. What would be the central focus of this nurse's care?
    a. Individual and family health care needs
    b. Populations within the community
    c. Local health care facilities
    d. Families in crisis

ANSWERS WITH RATIONALES

1. *b.* Maslow's hierarchy of basic human needs is useful for establishing priorities of care.

2. *b, d.* Physiologic needs—oxygen, water, food, elimination, temperature, sexuality, physical activity, and rest—must be met at least minimally to maintain life. Providing food and oxygen are examples of interventions to meet these needs. Preventing falls helps meet safety and security needs, providing art supplies may help meet self-actualization needs, facilitating visits from loved ones helps meet self-esteem needs, and referring a patient to a support group helps meet love and belonging needs.

3. *b.* By carrying out careful hand hygiene and using sterile technique, nurses provide safety from infection. An example of a physiologic need is clearing a patient's airway. Self-esteem needs may be met by allowing an older adult to talk about a past career. An example of helping meet a love and belonging need is contacting a hospitalized patient's family to arrange a visit.

4. *c, e, f.* Self-actualization, or reaching one's full potential, is a process that continues throughout life. A person achieves self-actualization by focusing on problems outside oneself and using creativity as a guideline for solving problems and pursuing interests. Humans are not born with a fully developed sense of self-actualization, and self-actualization needs are not met specifically by depending on others for help. Loneliness and isolation are not always the result of unmet self-actualization needs.

5. *d.* Although all the responses may be true, the best definition is a group of people who live together and depend on each other for physical, emotional, or financial support.

6. *a, d.* The five major areas of family function are physical, economic, reproductive, affective and coping, and socialization. Asking who provides emotional support in times of stress assesses the affective and coping function. Assessing the breadwinner focuses on the economic function. Inquiring about having more children assesses the reproductive function, asking about family traditions assesses the socialization function, and checking the environment assesses the physical function.

7. *b.* Inadequate childcare resources is a psychosocial risk factor. Not having access to dental care and obese family members are lifestyle risk factors. Having a family member with birth defects is a biologic risk factor.

8. *d.* The developmental tasks of the family with older adults are to adjust to retirement and possibly to adjust to the loss of a spouse and loss of independent living. Maintaining a supportive home base and strengthening marital relationships are tasks of the family with adolescents and young adults. Coping with loss of energy and privacy is a task of the family with children.

9. *c.* A healthy community offers access to health care services to treat illness and to promote health. A healthy community does not usually meet all the needs of its residents, but should be able to help with health issues such as nutrition, education, recreation, safety, and zoning regulations to separate residential sections from industrial ones. The age of housing is irrelevant as long as residences are maintained properly according to code.

10. *a.* In contrast to community health nursing, which focuses on populations within a community, community-based nursing is centered on individual and family health care needs. Community-based nurses may help families in crisis and work in health care facilities, but these are not the focus of community-based nursing.

TAYLOR SUITE RESOURCES

Explore these additional resources to enhance learning for this chapter:
- NCLEX-Style Questions and other resources on the**Point**, http://thePoint.lww.com/Taylor8e
- *Study Guide for Fundamentals of Nursing, 8th edition*
- Adaptive Learning | Powered by prepU, http://thepoint.lww.com/prepu

Bibliography

Affordable Care Act (ACA). (2012). *Medicaid.gov.* Available at http://www.medicaid.gov/AffordableCare Act/Affordable-Care-Act.html

Aldous, J. (1975). *The developmental approach to family analysis.* Minneapolis: University of Minnesota Press.

American Academy of Pediatrics. (2011). *Family life: Single parent families.* Available at http://www.healthychildren.org/English/family-life/family-dynamics/types-of-families/pages/Single-Parent-Families.aspx

American Academy of Pediatrics. (2012). *Family life: Gay and lesbian parents.* Available at http://www.healthychildren.org/English/family-life/family-dynamics/types-of-families/Pages/Gay-and-Lesbian-Parents.aspx

Centers for Disease Control and Prevention (CDC). (2011). *Family Structure and Children's Health in the United States: Findings from the National Health Interview Survey, 2001–2007.* Vital and Health Statistics, Series 10, Number 246. Bethesda, MD.

Collins, A. (2012). Promoting community health: A nurse-managed health center bridges the gap to care. *American Journal of Nursing, 112*(6), 65–66.

Domrose, C. (2012). A healthy day in the neighborhood. *Nurse.com, 21*(8), 16–17.

Duvall, E. (1977). *Marriage and family development* (5th ed.). Philadelphia: J.B. Lippincott.

Edelman, C., & Mandle, C. (2010). *Health promotion throughout the lifespan* (7th ed.). St. Louis: Mosby Elsevier.

Ellis, J. & Hartley, C. (2012). *Nursing in today's world: Trends, issues, and management* (10th ed.). Philadelphia: Wolters Kluwer Health/Lippincott Williams & Wilkins.

Frampton, S. & Wahl, C. (2012). Partnering with families. *American Journal of Nursing, 112*(10), 11.

Friedman, M., Bowden, V., & Jones, E. (2003). *Family nursing: Research, theory, and practice* (5th ed.). Upper Saddle River, NJ: Prentice Hall.

Healthy People 2020. (2012). *Education and community-based programs.* Available at http://www.healthypeople.gov/2020/topicsobjectives2020/overview.aspx?topicid=11

Institute of Medicine. (2011). *The future of nursing: Focus on education.* Available at http://www.iom.edu/Reports/2010/The-Future-of-Nursing-Leading-Change-Advancing-Health/Report-Brief-Education.aspx

Lee, R. (2012). Family homelessness viewed through the lens of health and human rights. *Advances in Nursing Science, 35*(2), E47–E59.

Maklebust, J. (2011). Engaging the patient and family as partners in practice. *Nursing, 41*(6), 23–24.

Maslow, A. (1968). *Toward a psychology of being* (2nd ed.). New York: Van Nostrand–Reinhold.

NANDA International. (2012). *NANDA Nursing diagnoses: Definitions & classification, 2012–2014.* West Sussex, UK: Wiley-Blackwell.

Pender, N., Murdaugh, C., & Parsons, M. A. (2011). *Health promotion in nursing practice* (6th ed.). Upper Saddle River, NJ: Pearson Education, Inc.

Sherwood, G. & Barnsteiner, J. (2012). *Quality and safety in nursing.* West Sussex, UK: Wiley-Blackwell.

Stanhope, M., & Lancaster, J. (2010). *Foundations of community health nursing—community oriented practice* (3rd ed.). St. Louis: Mosby Elsevier.

Williams, B., Sawyer, S., & Wahlstrom, C. (2008). *Marriages, families & intimate relationships* (2nd ed.). Boston: Pearson.

Woolf, S. & Aron, L. Eds. (2013). *U.S. Health in international perspective: shorter lives, poorer health.* National Research Council and Institute of Medicine. Washington, DC: The National Academies Press. 2012 Patient-Centered Primary Care Collaborative/Millbank Memorial Fund. Available at http://www.iom.edu/Reports/2013/US-Health-in-International-Perspective-Shorter-Lives-Poorer-Health.aspx

5 Cultural Diversity

DANIELLE DORVALL

Danielle is an immigrant from Haiti who has been in the United States for approximately 8 months. She recently had surgical repair of a fractured femur and is now confined to a hospital bed in skeletal traction. She asks that a Haitian folk healer from her neighborhood be allowed to come to the hospital to help heal her broken leg.

KHALIFA ABDUL HAKIM

Khalifa, the husband of a Muslim patient, requests that only female health care practitioners care for his wife. In the Muslim culture, it is deemed immodest for the body of a married woman to be seen by any male other than her husband.

JANICE GOLDBERG

Janice, a 23-year-old woman of Jewish ancestry, comes to the women's health clinic for a routine examination. During the visit, she asks, "I've been dating this man who also is Jewish, and we're thinking about getting married and having children. But I've heard about a hereditary disorder called Tay-Sachs disease that occurs in Jews. Should I be concerned?"

LEARNING OBJECTIVES

After completing the chapter, you will be able to accomplish the following:

1. Explain concepts of cultural diversity.
2. Describe influences that affect culturally competent health care.
3. Discuss examples of how diversity affects health and illness care, including culturally based traditional care.
4. Identify factors commonly included in a transcultural assessment of health-related beliefs and practices.
5. Practice cultural competence when assessing and providing nursing care for patients from diverse cultural groups.
6. Discuss factors in the health care system and in nursing that facilitate or impede culturally competent nursing care.

KEY TERMS

cultural assimilation	cultural imposition	linguistic competence
cultural blindness	culture	personal space
	culture conflict	race
cultural competence	culture shock	stereotyping
	ethnicity	subculture
cultural diversity	ethnocentrism	transcultural nursing

Analysis of the 2010 U.S. census data reveals sweeping changes over the last 20 years. The U.S. population is bigger, older, more Hispanic and Asian, and less wedded to marriage and traditional families than in 1990. Other trends reveal that the U.S. is more embracing of several generations living under one roof, more inclusive of same-sex couples, more aware of multiracial identities, more suburban, and less rural. "The end of the first decade of the 21st century marks a turning point in the nation's social, cultural, geographic, racial and ethnic fabric. It's a shift so profound that it reveals an America that seemed unlikely a mere 20 years ago—one that will influence the nation for years to come in everything from who is elected to run the country, states and cities to what types of household will be built and where" (El Nassar & Overberg, 2011).

Our society is increasingly made up of people from many diverse backgrounds. The definition of **cultural diversity** includes, but is not limited to, people of varying cultural background, racial and ethnic origin, religion, language, physical size, gender, sexual orientation, age, disability, socioeconomic status, occupational status, and geographic location. The essential knowledge and skills for understanding cultural diversity and providing culturally competent care have become essential components of nursing practice. (For an example, see the accompanying Reflective Practice display). This chapter focuses on concepts of cultural diversity and discusses their influence on nursing care.

CONCEPTS OF CULTURAL DIVERSITY

Cultural diversity—including culture, ethnicity, and race—is an integral component of both health and illness because of the cultural values and beliefs that we learn in our families and communities, as well as the need for health care providers to understand physiologic characteristics common to certain populations that influence health. To be able to provide culturally competent care to people from diverse backgrounds, nurses must be sensitive to these factors. It is also vital to remember that each individual may be a member of multiple cultural, ethnic, and racial groups at one time. Therefore, different cultural values may guide an individual in different situations based on what is most important to that person at the time. In addition, any person should be viewed foremost as an individual, not as a representative of a cultural group.

Culture

Culture may be defined as a shared system of beliefs, values, and behavioral expectations that provides social structure for daily living. Culture influences roles and interactions with others as well as within families and communities, and is apparent in the attitudes and institutions unique to particular groups (Andrews & Boyle, 2012). The characteristics of culture include the following:

- Culture helps shape what is acceptable behavior for people in a specific group. It is shared by, and provides an identity for, members of the same cultural group.
- Culture is learned by each new generation through both formal and informal life experiences. Language is the primary means of transmitting culture.
- The practices of a particular culture often arise because of the group's social and physical environment.
- Cultural practices and beliefs may evolve over time, but they mainly remain constant as long as they satisfy a group's needs.
- Culture influences the way people of a group view themselves, have expectations, and behave in response to certain situations. Because a culture is made up of individuals, there are differences both within cultures and among cultures.

 RECALL Mr. Hakim, the Muslim man described in the Reflective Practice display. The nurse's knowledge of his culture and beliefs are important for ensuring culturally appropriate care as well as staffing needs. The nurse needs to understand actions and behaviors that would be acceptable to Mr. Hakim and his wife. ●

REFLECTIVE PRACTICE: CULTIVATING QSEN COMPETENCIES

CHALLENGE TO INTELLECTUAL SKILLS

I had thought that I was pretty much used to all sorts of questions from patients about why a guy like me would go into nursing. Today, however, I was surprised when Khalifa Abdul Hakim, the husband of a newly admitted patient, demanded that I leave his wife's room immediately. Stepping into the corridor with me, he explained that he and his family were Muslim and that in their culture it was deemed immodest for the body of a married woman to be seen by any male other than her husband. He asked me to make sure it was clear in his wife's chart that there should be no male nurses. He also asked about female physicians.

Since we were short-staffed and all trying to cover for one another to get through the day, I wasn't sure that I could make that promise, especially since our unit has three or four male nurses. I wasn't clear if this was just a personal preference or a religious or cultural matter or both, or if it really mattered at all. I had absolutely no clue how to respond. I understood the importance of culturally appropriate care, but couldn't remember learning how to respond to a request like this. I also wasn't sure if the hospital had a policy about something like this.

Thinking Outside the Box: Possible Courses of Action

- Find someone to swap patients with me and just not have to deal with the situation (probably the simplest response).
- Use the opportunity to research Muslim culture and talk with the patient's male family members about what is important to them. Since we are seeing more Muslim patients, suggest an in-service program on this topic for everyone.

- Explain to Mr. Hakim that his wife is in a U.S. hospital, and that while here, they should observe U.S. customs, meaning she may have male nurses or other male health care practitioners.
- Check the hospital's policy about this request and then follow it.

Evaluating a Good Outcome: How Do I Define Success?

- I know enough to do whatever is necessary to ensure the patient's health and well-being as well as respect the integrity of all participants involved.
- The patient and her family feel sufficiently comfortable in our environment (culturally appropriate care) for healing to be maximized.

- I know more at the end of the experience than when I started.

Personal Learning: Here's to the Future!

I was pretty surprised when two of the older, more experienced nurses said they had never encountered such a request and they didn't know if the hospital had a policy about it. Luckily, one of them referred me to our patient-advocate person, and she came right up to the unit. I had never met her before, but I was impressed with her knowledge and her strong commitment to patient advocacy. She showed me the hospital policy that obligates all workers to respect the beliefs and values of patients unless this entails

compromising their own integrity or the safety of other persons. She said that we will be seeing more Muslim patients in the future and recommended a website to get more information. I haven't checked it out yet, but I did talk some with the patient's family and have a better understanding why this matters to them. So now I'm trying to cultivate the attitude that each patient and family could be an important learning opportunity for me if I'm open to what they have to teach!

REFLECTION ON QUALITY AND SAFETY COMPETENCIES

How do you think you would respond in a similar situation? Why? Do you agree with the criteria this nursing student used to evaluate a successful outcome? Why or why not? What *knowledge, skills,* and *attitudes* do you need to develop to improve the quality and safety of care for families like the Hakims?

Patient-Centered Care: What role does the nurse's cultural sensitivity, respect, and accommodation play in creating a successful patient-centered partnership with the Hakims? What lessons did the student learn about the importance of cultural humility and competence?

Teamwork and Collaboration/Quality Improvement: What communication skills do you need to improve to ensure that you function as a valuable member of the

patient-care team and to obtain assistance when needed? What did you learn about the importance of a referral—in this case to the patient advocate? How could this experience be used to improve care for other Muslim families?

Safety/Evidence-Based Practice: What role should safety considerations play in evaluating whether or not there was adequate staff to meet Mr. Hakim's request? Are there research studies about how best to accommodate cultural beliefs and preferences?

Informatics: Can you identify the essential information that must be available in Ms. Hakim's electronic record to support safe patient care and coordination of care? Can you think of other ways to respond to or approach the situation?

Within most cultures are **subcultures**. A subculture is a large group of people who are members of the larger cultural group but who have certain ethnic, occupational, or physical characteristics that are not common to the larger culture. For example, nursing is a subculture of the larger health care system culture, and teenagers and older adults are often regarded as subcultures of the general population in the United States.

Most societies include both dominant culture groups and minority culture groups. The dominant group has the most ability to control the values and sanctions of the society. It usually is (but does not have to be) the largest group in the society. Minority groups usually have some physical or cultural characteristic (such as race, religious beliefs, or occupation) different from those of the dominant group.

When a minority group lives within a dominant group, many members may lose the cultural characteristics that once made them different, and they make take on the values of the dominant culture. This process is called **cultural assimilation** or acculturation. For example, when people immigrate and encounter a new dominant culture as they work, go to school, and learn the dominant language, they often move closer to the dominant culture. The process and the rate of assimilation are individualized.

Mutual cultural assimilation also occurs, with both groups taking on some characteristics of the other. For example, many Hispanic immigrants to the United States learn to speak English, and many Americans learn to cook and enjoy traditional Hispanic foods. We all gain from the many cultures with which we live. Although we seldom think about it, the clothes we wear, the foods we eat, the music we enjoy, many of the words we use, and the leisure activities we practice are all influenced by acculturation.

Another possibility is **culture shock**, the feelings a person may experience when placed in a different culture perceived as strange. Culture shock may result in psychological discomfort or disturbances, as the patterns of behavior a person found acceptable and effective in one's own culture may not be adequate or even acceptable in the new one. The person may then feel foolish, fearful, incompetent, inadequate, or humiliated. These feelings eventually can lead to frustration, anxiety, and loss of self-esteem.

Ethnicity

Ethnicity is a sense of identification with a collective cultural group, largely based on the group's common heritage. One belongs to a specific ethnic group or groups either through birth or through adoption of characteristics of that group. People within an ethnic group generally share unique cultural and social beliefs and behavior patterns, including language and dialect, religious practices, literature, folklore, music, political interests, food preferences, and employment patterns. Ethnicity largely develops through day-to-day life with family and friends within the community.

Race

Although the term *ethnicity* often is used interchangeably with **race**, these terms are not the same. Racial categories are typically based on specific physical characteristics such as skin pigmentation, body stature, facial features, and hair texture. Because of the significant blending of physical characteristics through the centuries, however, race is becoming harder to define using simple classifications, and physical characteristics are not considered a reliable way to determine an individual's race. Federal standards for race classification provide five categories including American Indian or Alaska Native, Asian, Black or African American, Native Hawaiian or Other Pacific Islander, and White, and provide the opportunity for individuals to identify themselves in multiple categories. Respondents are also asked about membership in one of two ethnic categories, "Hispanic or Latino" and "Not Hispanic or Latino." The American Anthropological Association recommends the elimination of the term "race" from the U.S. Census since "race" has been scientifically proven to not be a real, natural phenomenon. More specific social categories such as "ethnicity" or "ethnic group" are more salient for scientific purposes and have fewer of the negative, racist connotations for which the concept of race was developed.

Factors Inhibiting Sensitivity to Diversity

A variety of factors may affect a person's sensitivity to others. When one assumes that all members of a culture, ethnic group, or race act alike, **stereotyping** is at work. Stereotyping may be positive or negative. Negative stereotyping includes racism, ageism, and sexism. These are mistaken beliefs that certain races, an age group, or one gender is inherently superior to others, leading to discrimination against those considered inferior (Fig. 5-1).

Also affecting cultural sensitivity are **cultural imposition**, which is the belief that everyone else should conform to your own belief system, and **cultural blindness**, which occurs when one ignores differences and proceeds as though they do not exist. This has been true of the health care system, especially in regard to nontraditional methods of care. **Culture conflict** occurs when people become aware of cultural differences, feel threatened, and respond by ridiculing the beliefs and traditions of others to make themselves feel more secure about their own values (Andrews & Boyle, 2012).

CULTURAL INFLUENCES ON HEALTH CARE

The United States is multicultural, multiethnic, and multiracial. Therefore, nurses must be aware of, and sensitive to, the needs of a diverse patient population. Most people interpret the behaviors of others in terms of their own familiar culture. This process usually works both ways; for example, in a health care setting, the patient evaluates the attitudes and actions of the health care provider at the same time the health care provider interprets the behavior of the patient. What may seem reasonable and important to a patient may seem ridiculous and irrelevant to an insensitive nurse. The reverse is also true: practices a nurse perceives as logical and effective may seem senseless or even dangerous to a patient.

FIGURE 5-1. Identifying one's own prejudices is the first step toward eliminating them. Think about the assumptions you make regarding the people in these images.

 CONSIDER Danielle Dorvall, described at the beginning of the chapter. She might view skeletal traction as worthless, while the nurse may view her request for a folk healer in the same way. The nurse needs to be aware of these possible attitudes and beliefs to ensure maximum effective care while still meeting the patient's cultural needs. ●

The following sections describe general considerations in providing culturally competent care.

Physiologic Variations

Studies have shown that certain racial and ethnic groups are more prone to certain diseases and conditions. For example, a hereditary disorder, Tay-Sachs disease, is associated with individuals of Eastern European Jewish descent. Although the incidence of this disorder has declined over the years due to improved and earlier testing, it is still a concern. Use knowledge of such risk factors when interviewing a patient to complete a health history. Table 5-1 provides examples of diseases that are more often diagnosed in specific populations.

 RECALL Janice Goldberg, the young woman described at the beginning of the chapter. Knowledge of the Tay-Sachs disorder and screening and early detection methods would be important for the nurse to use as a foundation when counseling and teaching Janice. ●

Reactions to Pain

Health care researchers have discovered that many of the expressions and behaviors exhibited by people in pain are culturally prescribed. Some cultures allow or even encourage the open expression of emotions related to pain, whereas other cultures encourage suppression of such emotions.

The main issue for nurses in this area of cultural expression is their attitude toward patients who may be in pain. Nurses often assume that a patient who does not complain of pain is not having pain. Therefore, the pain-reduction needs of a patient who deals with pain quietly and stoically may be ignored. To avoid this, be sensitive to other signals of discomfort, such as holding or applying pressure to the painful area, avoiding activities that intensify the pain, and uncontrollable,

spontaneous expressions of discomfort, such as facial grimacing and moaning. You also should not consider patients who freely express their discomfort as constant complainers with excessive requests for pain relief. Pain is a warning from the body that something is wrong. Pain is what the patient says it is, and every complaint of pain should be assessed carefully.

Nursing care for a patient in pain is always individualized (see Chapter 34), but important culture-sensitive considerations include the following:

- Recognize that culture is an important component of individuality and that each person holds (and has the right to hold) various beliefs about pain.
- Respect patients' right to respond to pain in their own manner.
- Never stereotype a patient's perceptions of or responses to pain based on the person's culture.

Table 5-1	**EXAMPLES OF COMMON HEALTH PROBLEMS IN SPECIFIC POPULATIONS**
POPULATION	**COMMON HEALTH PROBLEMS**
Native Americans and Alaska Natives	Heart disease Cirrhosis of the liver Diabetes mellitus Fetal alcohol syndrome
African Americans	Hypertension Stroke Sickle cell anemia Lactose intolerance Keloids
Asians	Hypertension Cancer of the liver Lactose intolerance Thalassemia
Hispanics	Diabetes mellitus Lactose intolerance
Whites	Breast cancer Heart disease Hypertension Diabetes mellitus Obesity

Mental Health

Most mental health norms originate in research and observations made of White, middle-class people. But many ethnic groups have their own norms and acceptable patterns of behavior for psychological well-being, as well as different normal psychological reactions to certain situations. For example, many Hispanic people deal with problems within the family and consider it inappropriate to tell problems to a stranger. Traditional Chinese people often consider mental illness a stigma and seeking psychiatric help a disgrace to the family. In times of high stress or anxiety, some Puerto Ricans may demonstrate a hyperkinetic seizure-like activity known as *ataques*. This behavior is a culturally accepted reaction. Be aware of these variations and accept them as culturally appropriate.

Gender Roles

In many cultures, the man is the dominant figure and generally makes decisions for all family members. For example, if approval for medical care is needed, the man may give it regardless of which family member is involved. In male-dominant cultures, women are often passive. On the other hand, in many African American and White families, the woman is often dominant.

Knowing who is dominant in the family is important when planning nursing care. For example, if the dominant member is ill and can no longer make decisions, the whole family may be anxious and confused. If a nondominant family member is ill, the individual may need help in verbalizing needs, particularly if the needs differ from those the dominant member perceives as being important.

 THINK back to Mr. Hakim, the Muslim man concerned about his wife's care providers being male. Because Mr. Hakim, not his wife, made the request about no male care providers, the nurse would interpret this as indicating that Mr. Hakim is the dominant family member. •

Language (Linguistics) and Communication

When people from another part of the world move to the United States, they may speak their own language fluently but have difficulty speaking English. This is especially true for women or older adults in the family who do not work outside the home and for people who live in proximity to others who speak their primary language. Assimilation is likewise slower for people who stay at home, especially if they live in communities of their ethnic and cultural background. Children usually assimilate more rapidly and learn the language of the dominant culture quickly if they leave home each day to go to school and make new friends in the dominant culture. Wage earners also tend to learn a new language more quickly through the work setting. Language acquisition is thus tied to necessity and assimilation rather than to degree of difficulty.

Because the United States has such a diverse population, with many languages spoken, communication problems can arise during health care activities. This problem is not unique to non–English-speaking patients; even in different regions of the country, certain dialects or word meanings can cause differences in understanding. Consider how difficult it must be to describe symptoms or give a personal health history when you do not understand the questions being asked. In addition, patients may forget English words or revert to their more familiar language when experiencing the stress of an injury, illness, or pain. **Linguistic competence** refers to the ability of caregivers and organizations to understand and effectively respond to the linguistic needs of patients and their families in a health care encounter.

Nurses who work in a geographic area with a high population of residents who speak a language other than English should learn pertinent words and phrases in that language. See the accompanying Through the Eyes of a Student account. Many agencies also have a qualified interpreter, or one can be found in the community. To avoid misinterpretation of questions and answers, it is important to use an interpreter who understands the health care system. Sometimes a family member or friend can translate for the nurse, but such a person may be protective and not the most reliable means of transferring information, thus guidelines often discourage using family members or friends as translators. People sometimes talk more loudly to someone who does not understand what they are saying, but remember that this is a communication problem, not a hearing problem.

The U.S. Department of Health and Human Services Office of Minority Health created a health care language services implementation guide to help health care organizations implement effective language access services to meet the needs of their patients with limited English proficiency, thereby increasing their access to health care. Nurses will find many helpful resources at the website: https://hclsig.thinkculturalhealth.hhs.gov.

One of the most culturally variable forms of nonverbal communication is eye contact. Although the following examples are not true of all members of a group, they can provide some general guidelines. The American dominant culture emphasizes eye contact while speaking, but many other cultures regard this behavior in different ways. For example, direct eye contact may be considered impolite or aggressive by many Asians, Native Americans, Indochinese, Arabs, and Appalachians; these groups of people tend to avert their eyes while speaking. Hispanics may look downward in deference to age, gender, social position, economic status, or authority. Muslim–Arab women often indicate modesty by avoiding eye contact with men, and Hasidic Jewish men may avoid direct eye contact with women (Andrews & Boyle, 2012).

When caring for culturally and ethnically diverse patients, it is it important to perform a transcultural assessment of communication (adapted from Andrews & Boyle, 2012):

- What language does the patient speak during usual activities of daily living?
- How well does the patient speak and write in English?

THROUGH THE EYES OF A STUDENT

I was doing my maternity rotation and was assigned to labor and delivery. I was caring for a woman who spoke no English—she and her husband were from Central America and had been in the United States for only 2 months.

When I arrived at 7 AM, the night nurse was giving a report about my patient to the day nurse. The night nurse was frantic—no one understood the couple, all efforts to locate a translator had come up empty, and, quite frankly, she had no idea exactly what condition this woman was in.

I quickly began to think back on my 2 years of Spanish. Could I be of any help to this couple? I wondered. Would I remember enough to communicate with them about giving birth? Then I decided that any little bit of communication at this point was better than none, so I spoke up. I told both nurses that I spoke some Spanish and asked if I could be of any help. The night nurse literally hugged me!

I began by telling the expectant couple that I was a nursing student and that I spoke some Spanish. We exchanged introductions and then I asked the woman some assessment questions. Nothing I said was complicated—all of my sentences were short and simple, but who needed more than that?

Then the couple asked me some questions. They had heard about "cutting open the stomach" to deliver a baby. I naturally assumed that they meant a cesarean delivery. They looked so afraid but I had to be honest. They wanted to know how it was done and why. The words I could not remember or did not know I acted out. They looked so relieved when I was finished.

The man said that they thought all babies were born this way in our country. He said that they had never heard of this procedure until coming to the United States. No wonder they were so frightened!

The doctor came in, examined the woman, and said she was fully dilated. The doctor asked if I could teach a crash course in Lamaze breathing to the woman. She also asked me if I would stay throughout the delivery because she would need assistance in translating directions to the woman. Of course, I said yes.

The woman was terrified. I told her that it was normal to be afraid and that I would be with her during the delivery. She took my hand and whispered, "Muchas gracias." I never felt more useful than I did at that moment.

—*A. Kelly Gaylor, Holy Family College, Philadelphia*

- Does the patient need an interpreter? Are family members or friends available? Are there people the patient would not want to serve as an interpreter?
- How does the patient prefer to be addressed?
- What cultural values and beliefs of the patient may change your techniques of communication and care (such as eye contact, personal space, or social taboos)?
- How does the patient's nonverbal behavior affect the responses of members of the health care team?
- What are the cultural characteristics of the patient's communications with others?

Chapter 20 provides additional information on communicating with non–English-speaking patients.

Orientation to Space and Time

Personal space is the area around a person regarded as part of the person. This area, individualized to each person and to different cultures and ethnic groups, is the area into which others should not intrude during personal interactions. If others do not consider a person's personal space, that person may become uncomfortable or even angry. When providing nursing care that involves physical contact, you should know the patient's cultural personal space preferences. For example, people of Arabic and African origin commonly sit and stand close to one another when talking, whereas people of Asian and European descent are more comfortable with some distance between themselves and others.

Many people and almost all institutions in the United States value promptness and punctuality. When arriving for an appointment, doing a job, or carrying out an activity, being on time and getting the job done promptly are viewed as important. This is not true in some other cultures. For example, in some South Asian cultures, being late is con-

sidered a sign of respect. In addition, while some cultures are future oriented (including activities that promote future good health), other cultures are more concerned with the present or the past. Understanding the patient's orientation to time is important as you communicate, for example, the need to be on time for appointments for health care procedures and when taking medications.

Food and Nutrition

Food preferences and preparation methods often are culturally influenced. Certain food groups serve as staples of the diet based on culture and remain so even when members of that culture are living in a different country.

Patients in a hospital or long-term care setting often do not have much choice of foods. This means that people with cultural food preferences may not be able to select appealing foods and thus may be at risk for inadequate nutrition. When assessing the possible causes of a patient's decreased appetite, try to determine whether the problem may be related to culture. It may be possible for family or friends to bring in foods that satisfy the patient's nutritional needs while still meeting dietary restrictions. Dietary teaching must be individualized according to cultural values about the social significance and sharing of food.

Family Support

In many cultural and ethnic groups, people have large, extended families and consider the needs of any family member to be equal to or greater than their own. They may be unwilling to share private information about family members with those outside the family (including health care providers). Other cultural groups have great respect for the elders in the family and would never consider institutional care for them. Including the family in planning care for any patient is a major component in nursing care to meet individualized needs, especially if those needs can be met only through consideration of all members of the family.

Socioeconomic Factors

Low income is a major problem in the United States and is often described as having created a culture of poverty. A report from the U.S. Census Bureau (2012) noted that an estimated 15% of the U.S. population had an income below the poverty threshold. Of that population, the lowest income was found in African Americans, Native Americans, and Alaska Natives. The poverty rate in 2011 for children under age 18 was 21.9%.

There has been much debate about how to define poverty. In terms of economics, a person or family whose income falls below an established poverty line is considered poor. The U.S. Census Bureau defines poverty according to money/income guidelines that vary by family size and composition. If the family's total income is less than a set threshold, all members of the family are considered poor. Others have stated that poverty is a relative term that reflects a judgment based on community standards. Such standards vary at different times and in different places; what is judged to be poverty in one community might be regarded as wealth in another (Spector, 2009). No matter how poverty is defined, it is an increasingly devastating epidemic, fueled by real estate foreclosures and credit debt, that has evolved into a culture of its own. At highest risk are children, older people, families headed by single mothers, and the future generations of those now living in poverty. The amount of money a person or family has affects how they meet their basic needs and maintain their health. Poverty often leads to other problems such as lack of health insurance, inadequate care of infants and children, and homelessness. All these are of concern to nursing.

The feminization of poverty threatens to increase the number of people who are living at poverty level. The number of female-headed households is increasing as a result of divorce, abandonment, unmarried motherhood, and changes in abortion laws. Because it is now common that two incomes are required in a household for economic survival, a single woman supporting a household is at a financial disadvantage. The number of single-parent families headed by women is associated closely with the increasing number of children living in poverty and the number of homeless families with children.

The increasing population of older people has also raised problems associated with poverty. Many older people live on fixed incomes that often do not keep up with inflation, and many (particularly widows) are on the borderline of poverty or have already slipped below the poverty level. Socioeconomic status often differs by the cultural group of the older adult. For example, Pacific/Asian, African American, Native American, and Hispanic elders generally have lower incomes than elders in the majority population. The work history of the cultural group, especially those who have labored all their lives as agricultural workers, often means that an individual has no Social Security or Medicare benefits.

In some cases, the culture of poverty is passed from generation to generation. This appears to be especially true in such groups as migrant farm workers, families living on public assistance, and people who live in isolated areas of Appalachia. Poverty cultures often have the following characteristics:

- Feelings of despair, resignation, and fatalism
- Day-to-day attitude toward life, with no hope for the future
- Unemployment and need for financial or government aid
- Unstable family structure, possibly characterized by abusiveness and abandonment
- Decline in self-respect and retreat from community involvement

Poverty has long been a barrier to adequate health care. It prevents many people from consistently meeting their basic human needs. The lack of affordable or adequate housing is a problem experienced frequently by poor people. When low-income housing is available, it sometimes lacks such necessities as running water, heat, and electricity. To stretch their available money and to pool resources, many poor people live in crowded conditions, with several families living together in one household.

Research has demonstrated that crowded living conditions foster depersonalization, correlate with higher crime rates, and lead to psychological problems such as schizophrenia, alienation, and feelings of worthlessness (Spector, 2009). Such conditions also contribute to an increased incidence and severity of disease and illness because of the closer proximity of people, the sharing of utensils and belongings, poor sanitation, and poor health habits.

Accessing health care facilities frequently requires transportation, which often is neither affordable nor available to poor people. Their access to health insurance also is frequently limited, and they often must choose between purchasing food and obtaining health care. Those in upper-income groups tend to live longer and to experience less disability than those in lower-income groups. Other barriers to health care include isolation, language or communication difficulties, seasonal occupations, migration patterns, depersonalization, and institutional prejudice (Spector, 2009).

Health Disparities

Health disparities refer to health differences between groups of people; they can affect how frequently a disease affects a group, how many people get sick, or how often the disease causes death. You can read more about disparities in Chapter 3. Many different populations are affected by disparities, including racial and ethnic minorities; residents of rural areas; women, children, and the elderly; and persons with disabilities.

CULTURAL INFLUENCES ON HEALTH AND ILLNESS

People's values and beliefs about health, illness, and health care are influenced by cultural and ethnic groups. For example, in some groups, illnesses are classified as either natural or unnatural. "Natural illnesses" are caused by dangerous agents, such as cold air or impurities in the air, water, or food. "Unnatural illnesses" are punishments for failing to follow God's rules, resulting in evil forces or witchcraft causing physical or mental health problems.

In some cultures, the power to heal is thought to be a gift from God bestowed on certain people. People in these cultures believe that these folk or traditional healers know what is wrong with them through divine intervention and experience. A patient accustomed to traditional healers may think that health care providers are incompetent because they have to ask many questions before they can treat an illness. Traditional healers speak the patient's language, often are more accessible, and are usually more understanding of the patient's cultural and personal needs.

 THINK back to Danielle Dorvall, the immigrant from Haiti asking for a folk healer. Respecting her use of a folk healer, as appropriate, would demonstrate an understanding of her cultural beliefs. ●

People from different cultures may also have different beliefs about the best way to treat an illness or disease. For example, herbs are a common method of treatment in many cultures. In fact, many medications used today have a basis in herbs or other plant sources that have been used for centuries to cure illnesses. If a patient traditionally drinks an herbal tea to alleviate symptoms of an illness, there is no reason that both the herbal tea and prescribed medications cannot be used, as long as the tea is safe to drink and the ingredients do not interfere with or exaggerate the action of the medication.

Other traditional therapies include the use of cutaneous stimulation, therapeutic touch, acupuncture, and acupressure. Cutaneous stimulation by massage, vibration, heat, cold, or nerve stimulation reduces the intensity of the sensation of pain. Therapeutic touch is an intentional act that involves an energy transfer from the healer to the patient to stimulate the patient's own healing potential. Acupuncture, long used in China, is a method of preventing, diagnosing, and treating pain and disease by inserting special needles into the body at specified locations. Acupressure involves a deep-pressure massage of appropriate points of the body. Read more about these therapies in Chapter 27.

CULTURALLY COMPETENT NURSING CARE

Providing culturally competent nursing care means that care is planned and implemented in a way that is sensitive to the needs of individuals, families, and groups from diverse populations within society. Among the elements of **cultural competence** are (Purnell, 2009):

1. Developing an awareness of one's own existence, sensations, thoughts, and environment to prevent them from having an undue influence on those from other backgrounds
2. Demonstrating knowledge and understanding of the client's culture, health-related needs, and culturally specific meanings of health and illness
3. Accepting and respecting cultural differences in a manner that facilitates the client's and family's abilities to make decisions to meet their needs and beliefs
4. Not assuming that the health care provider's beliefs and values are the same as the client's
5. Resisting judgmental attitudes such as "different is not as good"
6. Being open to and comfortable with cultural encounters
7. Accepting responsibility for one's own education in cultural competence by attending conferences, reading professional literature, and observing cultural practices

These elements suggest that becoming culturally competent is a life-long challenge and that nurses should strive to be culturally humble—recognizing what we don't yet know about those entrusted to our care and being willing to learn what we need to know. The Office of Minority Health created "Think Cultural Health," an online service whose goal is to advance health equity at every point of contact through the development and promotion of culturally and linguistically appropriate services. Nurses who recognize and respect cultural diversity are better equipped to exhibit cultural sensitivity and provide nursing care that accepts the significance of cultural factors in health and illness. See Examples of NANDA-I Nursing Diagnoses.

The health care system is itself a culture with customs, rules, values, and a language of its own, with nursing as

EXAMPLES OF NANDA-I NURSING DIAGNOSES

CULTURAL DIVERSITY

The following nursing diagnoses are examples of those that might be appropriate for providing culturally competent care:

- Impaired Verbal Communication related to inability to speak English and interpreter unavailable
- Social Isolation related to recent move away from neighborhood and friends of same ethnic group
- Impaired Parenting related to use of culturally based discipline considered inappropriate or abusive by current country of residence
- Spiritual Distress related to inability to take part in significant culturally based rituals regularly

- Readiness for Enhanced Family Process related to request for information about childcare
- Ineffective Management of Therapeutic Regimen (Individual) related to mistrust of traditional health care personnel
- Situational Low Self-Esteem related to language difficulties and inability to secure employment
- Powerlessness related to inability to make health care providers understand the importance of dietary and social values and beliefs

BOX 5-1 CULTURAL NORMS OF THE HEALTH CARE SYSTEM

Beliefs
- Standardized definitions of health and illness
- Omnipotence of technology

Practices
- Maintenance of health and prevention of illness
- Annual physical examinations and diagnostic procedures

Habits
- Documentation
- Frequent use of jargon
- Use of a systematic approach and problem-solving methodology

Likes
- Promptness
- Neatness and organization
- Compliance

Dislikes
- Tardiness
- Disorderliness and disorganization

Customs
- Professional deference and adherence to the pecking order found in autocratic and bureaucratic systems
- Use of certain procedures attending birth and death

its largest subculture. As you progress through your education, you will be acculturated into the culture of the health care system and will develop values related to health and health care. Box 5-1 lists some common cultural norms of the health care system.

Although nursing as a whole is actively recruiting more diverse members, many nurses are members of, and have the same value systems as, the dominant U.S. middle-class culture. When a nurse with a particular set of cultural values about health interacts with a patient with a different set of cultural values about health, the following factors affect this interaction (Andrews & Boyle, 2012):

- The cultural background of each participant
- The expectations and beliefs of each about health care
- The cultural context of the encounter (e.g., hospital, clinic, home)
- The extent of agreement between the two persons' sets of beliefs and values

Nursing care can become complicated when the patient and the nurse have distinctly different cultural norms. Cultural imposition in health care is the tendency for health personnel to impose their beliefs, practices, and values on people of other cultures. Closely related to cultural imposition is **ethnocentrism**, the belief that the ideas, beliefs, and practices of one's own culture are superior to those of another's culture. When health professionals assume that they have the right to make choices and decisions for patients of another culture, patients may respond in the same way that minority cultures often respond to such an attitude by the dominant culture: by becoming passive, resistive, angry, or resistant to treatment.

Unless nurses are willing to examine carefully and clarify their own attitudes and values and to be sensitive to others who are "different," their use of cultural concepts when providing care will be unsuccessful. The nurse's role is to understand the patient's needs and to adapt care to meet those needs. A careful merging of modern and traditional cultural beliefs is a necessary prerequisite for safe, considerate, and successful nursing care of all patients.

National standards issued by the Office of Minority Health (2001) were developed to ensure that all people entering the health care system be provided equitable and effective treatment in a culturally and linguistically appropriate manner. Examples of these standards are provided in Box 5-2. In 2013, the Office of Minority Health released The National Standards for Culturally and Linguistically Appropriate Services in Health and Health Care.

BOX 5-2 ASSURING CULTURAL COMPETENCE IN HEALTH CARE

- Ensure that all patients/consumers receive from all staff members effective, understandable, and respectful care that is provided in a manner compatible with their cultural health beliefs and practices and preferred language.
- Implement strategies to recruit, retain, and promote at all levels of the organization a diverse staff and leadership that are representative of the demographic characteristics of the service area.
- Ensure that staff at all levels and across all disciplines receive ongoing education and training in culturally and linguistically appropriate service delivery.
- Offer and provide language assistance services, including bilingual staff and interpreter services, at no cost to each patient/consumer with limited English proficiency at

all points of contact, in a timely manner during all hours of operation.
- Make available easily understood patient-related materials and post signs in the language of the commonly encountered groups and/or groups represented in the service area.
- Ensure that data on the individual patient's/consumer's race, ethnicity, and spoken and written language are collected in health records, integrated into the organization's management information systems, and periodically updated.
- Maintain a current demographic, cultural, and epidemiologic profile of the community, as well as a needs assessment, to accurately plan for and implement services that respond to the cultural and linguistic characteristics of the service area.

Source: The Office of Minority Health, Public Health Service, U.S. Department of Health and Human Services. (2001). *Assuring cultural competence in health care: Recommendations for national standards and an outcomes-focused research agenda. Federal Register, 65*(247), 80865–80879.

BOX 5-3 TRANSCULTURAL ASSESSMENT: HEALTH-RELATED BELIEFS AND PRACTICES

1. To what cause(s) does the patient attribute illness and disease (e.g., divine wrath, imbalance in hot/cold or yin/yang, punishment for moral transgressions, hex, soul loss, pathogenic organism)?
2. What are the patient's cultural beliefs about the ideal body size and shape? What is the patient's self-image compared to the ideal?
3. What name does the patient give to his or her health-related condition?
4. What does the patient believe promotes health (e.g., eating certain foods; wearing amulets to bring good luck; sleep; rest; good nutrition; reducing stress; exercise; prayer; rituals to ancestors, saints, or intermediate deities)?
5. What is the patient's religious affiliation (e.g., Judaism, Islam, Pentecostalism, West African voodooism, Seventh-Day Adventism, Catholicism, Mormonism)? How actively involved in the practice of this religion is the patient?
6. Does the patient rely on cultural healers (e.g., curandero, shaman, spiritualist, priest, minister, monk)? Who determines when the patient is sick and when the patient is healthy? Who influences the choice/type of healer and treatment that should be sought?
7. In what types of cultural healing practices does the patient engage (e.g., use of herbal remedies, potions, massage; wearing of talismans, copper bracelets, or charms to discourage evil spirits; healing rituals, incantations, prayers)?
8. How are biomedical/scientific health care providers perceived? How does the patient and the patient's family perceive nurses? What are the expectations of nurses and nursing care?
9. What comprises appropriate "sick role" behavior? Who determines what symptoms constitute disease/illness? Who decides when the patient is no longer sick? Who cares for the patient at home?
10. How does the patient's cultural group view mental disorders? Are there differences in acceptable behaviors for physical versus psychological illnesses?

Adapted from Andrews, M., & Boyle, J. (2012). *Transcultural concepts in nursing care* (6th ed.). Philadelphia: Lippincott Williams & Wilkins.

Cultural Assessment

The National Center for Cultural Competence urges health care professionals who value cultural competence to enhance their understanding of the following:

- Beliefs, values, traditions and practices of a culture
- Culturally defined, health-related needs of individuals, families, and communities
- Culturally based belief systems of the etiology of illness and disease and those related to health and healing
- Attitudes toward seeking help from health care providers

When caring for patients from a different culture, it is important to first ask how they want to be treated based on their values and beliefs. An effective way to identify specific factors that influence a patient's behavior is to perform a cultural assessment. The primary informant should be the patient, if possible. If the patient is not able to respond to the questions, a family member or a friend can be consulted. A useful tool for this is the Andrews and Boyle Transcultural Nursing Assessment Guide (2012), part of which is included in Box 5-3. See also the Purnell model for cultural competence (Figure 5-2 on page 84). Similarly, the Giger and Davidhizar (2002) model takes into account six cultural phenomena: communication, space, social organization, time, environmental control, and biological variations. The Campinha-Bacote Model of Cultural Competence (2011) emphasizes becoming culturally competent and integrating cultural awareness, cultural knowledge, cultural skill, cultural encounters, and cultural desire.

You can also anticipate a patient's cultural needs by obtaining this information through research before initiating contact with the patient. Remember, however, that *information about any culture is general, and that it must be individualized for the specific patient once the actual interaction begins.*

Guidelines for Nursing Care

Transcultural nursing care, now both a specialty and a formal area of practice, resulted from work by Dr. Madeleine M. Leininger, a nurse–anthropologist. Her Theory of Cultural Care Diversity and Universality (1991) provides the foundation for providing culturally competent care for patients of all ages, as well as families, groups, and communities. A nurse who is culturally competent has the knowledge and skills to adapt nursing care to cultural similarities and differences. Cultural competence takes time. It involves developing awareness, acquiring knowledge, and practicing skills. Box 5-4 (on pages 85–87) lists information about selected diverse cultures to illustrate similarities and differences. Remember that these are only general guidelines and that each patient must be considered a unique individual. What is true of one person may not be true of another, even if they are from the same cultural background.

 Concept Mastery Alert

Regardless of the culture background of the patient, nurses need to assess each patient individually to provide culturally competent care. Asking open-ended questions provides an opportunity to obtain specific information from the patient about his or her beliefs related to health care.

When providing care to different people from different cultures, you may use past experiences as a guide but never as the answer to all cultural issues. Learn from your mistakes and do not repeat them. All nurses make mistakes at some time when caring for culturally different patients. Inadvertent mistakes are just that, but repeated mistakes are careless and disrespectful; they will adversely affect your interaction with patients and coworkers. The following

FIGURE 5-2. The Purnell Model for Cultural Competence. This schematic depicting the model is a circle with an outlying rim representing global society, a second rim representing community, a third rim representing family, and an inner rim representing the person. The interior of the concentric circles is divided into 12 pie-shaped wedges depicting cultural domains (constructs) and their concepts. The center of the model is empty, which represents unknown aspects about the cultural group. Along the bottom of the model is a saw-toothed line representing the concept of cultural consciousness. This line relates primarily to the health care provider, although organizations may also be represented on this nonlinear line according to their stage of cultural competence as an organization. (Reprinted by permission of SAGE Publications. From Purnell, L. [2002]. The Purnell model for cultural competence, *Journal of Transcultural Nursing 13*(3), 193–196.)

sections provide additional guidelines for providing culturally appropriate nursing care.

Develop Cultural Self-Awareness

Before you can provide culturally competent care to patients from diverse backgrounds, become aware of the role of cultural influences in your own life. Objectively examine your own beliefs, values, practices, and family experiences. As you become more sensitive to the importance of these factors, you will also become more sensitive to cultural influences in others' lives. Identify your biases. How do they affect your feelings about others? How could they affect your nursing care of others? Box 5-5 (on page 88) lists a cultural self-assessment that will help you gain the insight necessary to overcome ethnocentric tendencies and stereotypic behaviors.

Develop Cultural Knowledge

Learn as much as possible about the belief system and practices of people in your community and of patients in the area in which you work. Practice techniques of observation and listening to acquire knowledge of the beliefs and values of patients for whom you provide care. Some people, especially those of minority cultures, may have been belittled or ridiculed and may be hesitant to discuss their beliefs and practices. Approach this topic with patients carefully. If you are motivated by sincerity, respect, and concern, your attitude will convey this, and most patients will respond positively. On the other hand, if you are motivated by curiosity and have a condescending attitude, most patients will respond negatively.

| BOX 5-4 | CULTURAL FACTORS THAT AFFECT NURSING CARE |

White

Family
- Nuclear family is highly valued.
- Elderly family members may live in a long-term care facility when they can no longer care for themselves.

Folk and Traditional Health Care
- Self-diagnosis of illnesses
- Use of over-the-counter drugs (especially vitamins and analgesics)
- Dieting (especially fad diets)
- Extensive use of exercise and exercise facilities

Values and Beliefs
- Youth is valued over age
- Cleanliness
- Orderliness
- Attractiveness
- Individualism
- Achievement
- Punctuality

Nursing Considerations
- Careful assessment of client's use of over-the-counter medications (observe for signs and symptoms of toxic medication levels, especially fat-soluble vitamins)
- Nutritional assessments of dietary habits

African American

Family
- Close and supportive extended-family relationships
- Strong kinship ties with nonblood relatives from church or organizational and social groups
- Family unity, loyalty, and cooperation are important.
- Usually matriarchal

Folk and Traditional Health Care
- Varies extensively and may include spiritualists, herb doctors, root doctors, conjurers, skilled elder family members, voodoo, faith healing

Values and Beliefs
- Present oriented
- Members of the African American clergy are highly respected
- Frequently highly religious

Nursing Considerations
- Many African American families may still use various folk healing practices and home remedies for treating particular illnesses.
- Special care may be necessary for the hair and skin.
- Special consideration should be given to the sometimes extensive and frequently informal support networks of patients (e.g., religious and community group members who offer assistance in a time of need).

Asian
(Beliefs and practices vary, but most Asian cultures share some characteristics.)

Family
- Welfare of the family is valued above the person.
- Extended families are common.
- A person's lineage (ancestors) is respected.
- Sharing among family members is expected.

Folk and Traditional Health Care
- Theoretical basis is in Taoism, which seeks a balance in all things.
- Good health is achieved through the proper balance of yin (feminine, negative, dark, cold) and yang (masculine, positive, light, warm).
- An imbalance in energy is caused by an improper diet or strong emotions.
- Diseases and foods are classified as hot or cold, and a proper balance between them will promote wellness (e.g., treat a cold disease with hot foods).
- Many Asian health care systems use herbs, diet, and the application of hot or cold therapy. Also, many Asians believe that there are points on the body that are located on the meridians or energy pathways. If the energy flow is out of balance, treatment of the pathways may be necessary to restore the energy equilibrium.

  Acumassage—Technique of manipulating points along the energy pathways

  Acupressure—Technique for compressing the energy pathway points

  Acupuncture—Technique by which fine needles are inserted into the body at energy pathway points

Values and Beliefs
- Strong sense of self-respect and self-control
- High respect for age
- Respect for authority
- Respect for hard work
- Praise of self or others is considered poor manners
- Strong emphasis on harmony and the avoidance of conflict

Nursing Considerations
- Some members of Asian cultures may be upset by the drawing of blood for laboratory tests. They consider blood to be the body's life force, and some do not believe that it can be regenerated.
- Some members believe that it is best to die with the body intact, so they may refuse surgery except in dire circumstances.
- Members of many Asian cultures seldom complain about what is bothering them. Therefore, the nurse must carefully assess the patient for pain or discomfort by observing for nonverbal signs of discomfort, such as facial grimacing or wincing and holding of the painful area.
- Some Asians consider it polite to give a person the responses the person is expecting. Therefore, the client may transmit misinformation to the questioner in an effort to be respectful.
- Some members may change physicians in an attempt to be cured of an illness, but to avoid insulting or embarrassing a physician, they will not inform him or her that they are going to another practitioner. This can result in confusion, inaccuracies, and overmedication.
- Some Asians may refuse diagnostic studies because they believe that a skilled and competent physician can diagnose an illness solely through a physical examination.
- Some members may have a difficult time understanding the importance of a medication regimen because many folk treatments involve the ingestion of just one dose of herbal mixtures.
- Dietary counseling may be necessary if the patient is on a salt-restricted diet because many Asian foods have a high salt content related to the use of soy sauce.

(continued)

BOX 5-4 CULTURAL FACTORS THAT AFFECT NURSING CARE *continued*

Hispanic

Family
- Familial role is important.
- *Compadrazgo:* special bond between a child's parents and the child's grandparents
- Family is the primary unit of society.

Folk and Traditional Health Care
- *Curanderas(os):* folk healers who base treatments on humoral pathology—basic functions of the body are controlled by four body fluids or "humors":

  Blood—hot and wet

  Yellow bile—hot and dry

  Black bile—cold and dry

  Phlegm—cold and wet

- The secret of good health is to balance hot and cold within the body; therefore, most foods, beverages, herbs, and medications are classified as hot (*caliente*) or cold (*fresco, frio*) For example, a cold disease will be cured with a hot treatment).

Values and Beliefs
- Respect is given according to age (older) and sex (male).
- Roman Catholic Church may be very influential.
- God gives health and allows illness for a reason; therefore, many perceive illness as a punishment from God that can be cured through atonement and forgiveness.

Nursing Considerations
- It may be difficult to convince an asymptomatic patient that he or she is ill.
- Special diet considerations are necessary if the patient believes in the hot/cold theory of treating illnesses.
- Diet counseling may be necessary at times, because the usual diet of many members is high in starch.

Muslim

Family
- The family forms the basic building block of Muslim society. The man is considered the head of the family.
- Marriage forms the sole basis for sexual relations and parenthood.
- Islamic law generally discourages the use of contraception, extolling the virtues of large families, but there seems to be a trend toward smaller families.

Folk and Traditional Health Care
- Preventive health care strategies in Muslim experience include personal hygiene, dietary measures such as the restriction in eating specific ingredients (such as pork and its byproducts, and drinking alcohol), and the avoidance of addictive habits such as smoking tobacco or overconsumption of food.
- Some Muslims may perceive a sudden death or illness as a sign of punishment or a test from God.

Values and Beliefs
- Belief that there is no God but Allah and that Muhammad is his messenger.
- Belief that God created humans and gave them their bodies as gifts to be cared for through general hygiene, diet, and exercise.
- Belief that Allah will determine when they die; Death is an important part of the traditional Islamic life cycle. By tradition, family members wash the body of the deceased

and bury it as soon as possible. Cremation is not allowed under Islamic law, and embalming should be avoided unless it is required by civil law.

Nursing Considerations
- Respect the modesty needs of both men and women: special clothing or draping may be necessary, assign health care providers of the same sex, avoid touching patients of the opposite sex, and limit eye contact.
- Make accommodations for prayer needs.
- Maintain bodily purity by observing their cleansing and ablution rituals.
- Offer a halal diet free of alcohol and pork or pork products; make sure medications are alcohol- and pork-free.
- During Ramadan, Muslims must fast from sunrise to sunset. Fasting includes abstaining from all substances, including pharmaceuticals and IV drips. However, illness is an exception.

Native American
(Each tribe's beliefs and practices vary to some degree.)

Family
- Families are large and extended.
- Grandparents are official and symbolic leaders and decision makers.
- A child's namesake may become the equivalent to another parent to the child.

Folk and Traditional Health Care
- Medicine men (shaman) are heavily used.
- Heavy use of herbs and psychological treatments, ceremonies, fasting, meditation, heat, and massages

Values and Beliefs
- Present oriented. Taught to live in the present and not to be concerned about the future. This time consciousness emphasizes finishing current business before doing something else.
- High respect for age
- Great value is placed on working together and sharing resources.
- Failure to achieve a personal goal frequently is believed to be the result of competition.
- High respect is given to a person who gives to others. The accumulation of money and goods often is frowned on.
- Some Native Americans practice the Peyotist religion, in which the consumption of peyote, an intoxicating drug derived from mescal cacti, is part of the service. Peyote is legal if used for this purpose. It is classified as a hallucinogenic drug.

Nursing Considerations
- The family is expected to be part of the nursing care plan.
- Note taking often is taboo. It is considered an insult to the speaker because the listener is not paying full attention to the conversation. Good memory skills often are required by the nurse.
- Indirect eye contact is acceptable and sometimes preferred.
- It often is considered rude or impolite to indicate that you are not clearly hearing what they are saying.
- A low tone of voice often is considered respectful.
- A Native American patient may expect the caregiver to deduce the problem through instinct instead of asking many questions and history taking. If this is the case, it may help to use declarative sentences rather than direct questioning.

BOX 5-4 CULTURAL FACTORS THAT AFFECT NURSING CARE *continued*

Hawaiian

Family
- Familial role is important.
- *Ohana,* or extended families, are jointly involved in child-rearing.
- Hierarchy of family structure—each gender and age have specific duties.
- Closely knit families in small, isolated communities

Folk and Traditional Health Care
- *Kahuna La'au Lapa'au* is the ancient Hawaiian medical practitioner.
- View patient's illness as part of the whole.
- Relationships among the physical, psychological, and spiritual
- Emphasis on preventive medicine
- Treatment uses more than 300 medicinal plants and minerals

Values and Beliefs
- Aloha: a deep love, respect, and affection between people and the land
- Christian God replaced the myriad of Hawaiian gods.
- Lifestyle more revered than compliance with health care issues
- Present oriented, less initiative and drive rather than direction and achievement
- Death seen as part of life and not feared

Nursing Considerations
- Many Hawaiians may still use folk healing practices and home remedies.
- Special consideration given to the extensive family network during hospitalization

- Acceptance from health care practitioners of current health practices and lifestyle

Appalachian

Family
- Intense interpersonal relations
- Family is cohesive, and several generations often live close to each other.
- Elderly are respected as providers.
- Tend to live in rural, isolated areas

Folk and Traditional Health Care
- "Granny" woman, or folk healer, provides care and may be consulted even if receiving traditional care.
- Various herbs, such as foxglove and yellow root, are used for common illnesses such as malaise, chest discomfort, heart problems, and upper respiratory infections.
- Elderly may have had only limited contact with health care providers and may be skeptical of modern health care.

Values and Beliefs
- Independence and self-determination
- Isolation is accepted as a way of life.
- Person oriented
- May be fatalistic about losses and death
- Belief in a divine existence rather than attending a particular church

Nursing Considerations
- Treat each person with regard for personal dignity.
- Allow family members to remain with patient as support system.
- Accept the person's current health practices and lifestyle.
- Allow patients to make decisions about care.

Accommodate Cultural Practices in Health care

Incorporate factors from the patient's cultural background into health care whenever possible if the practices would not be harmful to the patient's health. To ignore or contradict the patient's background may result in the patient refusing care or failing to follow prescribed therapy. Modify care to include traditional practices and practitioners as much as possible, and be an advocate for patients from diverse cultural groups.

Accommodate the cultural dietary practices of patients as much as possible. Dietary departments in many hospitals and long-term care facilities can provide meals that are consistent with special dietary practices. Families may be encouraged to bring food from home for patients with particular preferences when this practice does not violate policy. Teaching patients and families about therapeutic diets may also be appropriate within the framework of particular cultural practices.

Respect Culturally Based Family Roles

Consider the cultural role of the family member who makes most of the important decisions. In some cultures it is the husband or father, whereas in others it may be a grandmother or another respected elder. To disregard this fact or to proceed

with nursing care that is not approved by this person can result in conflict or in disregard for the patient's and family's values. Be careful to involve this person in the nursing care planning.

Avoid Mandating Change

Keep in mind that health practices are part of the overall culture and that changing them may have widespread implications for the person. Provide support and reinforcement for the patient if it is necessary to change a health practice with a cultural basis.

Do not force patients to participate in care that conflicts with their values. If a patient is forced to accept such care, resulting feelings of guilt and alienation from a religious or cultural group are likely to threaten that patient's well-being.

Seek Cultural Assistance

Seek assistance from a respected family member, member of the clergy, or traditional healer, as appropriate, so that the patient is more likely to accept health care services. Acknowledging the role of the person's traditional healer can be an important way of building trust. Folk medicine practitioners can work closely with professional health practitioners in the interest of the patient and family. Such efforts promote mutual understanding, respect, and cooperation.

BOX 5-5 HOW DO YOU RELATE TO VARIOUS GROUPS OF PEOPLE IN SOCIETY?

Described below are different levels of response you might have toward a person. Reflect on which level of response best corresponds to how you believe you would respond.

Levels of Response

1. Greet: I can greet this person warmly and welcome the individual sincerely.
2. Accept: I can honestly accept this person as he or she is and be comfortable enough to listen to the individual's problems.
3. Help: I can genuinely try to help this person with his or her problems.

4. Background: I have the background of knowledge and/or experience to be able to help this person.
5. Advocate: I can honestly be an advocate for this person.

Instructions

The following is a list of individuals. Read down the list and place a checkmark next to anyone you could not greet, accept, help, use your background for, or advocate for. Try to respond honestly, not as you think would be socially or professionally desirable. Your answers are only for your personal use in clarifying your initial reactions to different people.

Individual	Level of Response				
	1	2	3	4	5
	Greet	Accept	Help	Background	Advocate
1. Haitian	☐	☐	☐	☐	☐
2. Child abuser	☐	☐	☐	☐	☐
3. Jewish person	☐	☐	☐	☐	☐
4. Person with hemophilia	☐	☐	☐	☐	☐
5. Neo-Nazi	☐	☐	☐	☐	☐
6. Mexican American	☐	☐	☐	☐	☐
7. IV drug user	☐	☐	☐	☐	☐
8. Senile, elderly person	☐	☐	☐	☐	☐
9. Prostitute	☐	☐	☐	☐	☐
10. Jehovah's Witness	☐	☐	☐	☐	☐
11. Gay/lesbian	☐	☐	☐	☐	☐
12. Person with AIDS	☐	☐	☐	☐	☐
13. African American	☐	☐	☐	☐	☐
14. Amputee	☐	☐	☐	☐	☐
15. Ku Klux Klansman	☐	☐	☐	☐	☐
16. Alcoholic	☐	☐	☐	☐	☐
17. Person with cancer	☐	☐	☐	☐	☐
18. Hispanic	☐	☐	☐	☐	☐
19. Amish person	☐	☐	☐	☐	☐
20. Atheist	☐	☐	☐	☐	☐
21. White American	☐	☐	☐	☐	☐

Adapted from the Association for the Care of Children's Health, 7910 Woodmont Avenue, Suite 300, Bethesda, MD 20814, from Randall-David, E. L. (1989). *Strategies for working with culturally diverse communities and clients*, pp. 7–9.

DEVELOPING CLINICAL REASONING

1. Analyze the following situations, identifying potential sources of cultural imposition:
   • A young Ethiopian woman with terminal breast cancer requests that all treatment decisions be made by her uncle, who is the family elder. Her primary nurse is an active feminist.
   • A Native American woman refuses a life-saving amputation of her leg because she believes it is essential to enter the next world "whole."

2. Interview family members or friends who have recently received health care, such as for a health screening, diagnostic testing, emergency care, routine checkup, office/clinic visit, or hospitalization. What aspects of the health care culture were most distressing to them? What factors were most helpful? Do their answers vary according to the setting for care or the attitudes of the health care practitioners involved? If so, why do you think they felt as they did?

3. College students have their own culture. What in your school's culture is influencing your health positively and negatively? If

you don't want to be the passive recipient of negative cultural forces, what choices do you have?

4. Visit the Georgetown University National Center for Cultural Competence website (http://nccc.georgetown.edu). Pay special attention to the self-assessment resources. Take the Self-Assessment Checklist test for personnel providing services and supports to LGBTQ Youth and Their Families. Share with your classmates what you learned about your own cultural competence/humility.

PRACTICING FOR NCLEX

1. Nurses caring for patients in health care facilities need to provide culturally competent care to an increasingly diverse population. Which statements accurately describe a characteristic of cultural diversity that exists in the United States? Select all that apply.
   a. The United States has become less inclusive of same-sex couples.

b. Cultural diversity is limited to people of varying cultures and races.

c. Cultural diversity is separate and distinct from health and illness.

d. Individuals may be members of multiple cultural groups at one time.

e. Culture guides what is acceptable behavior for people in a specific group.

f. Cultural practices may evolve over time but mainly remain constant.

2. In order to provide culturally competent care, nurses must be alert to factors inhibiting sensitivity to diversity in the health care system, including cultural imposition. Which examples exemplify cultural imposition? Select all that apply.

a. A hospital nurse tells a nurse's aide that patients should not be given a choice whether or not to shower or bathe daily.

b. A nurse treats all patients the same whether or not they come from a different culture.

c. A nurse tells another nurse that Jewish diet restrictions are just a way for them to get a special tray of their favorite foods.

d. A Catholic nurse insists that a patient diagnosed with terminal bladder cancer see the chaplain in residence.

e. A nurse directs interview questions to an elderly patient's daughter even though the patient is capable of answering them.

f. A nurse refuses to care for a married gay man who is HIV positive because she is against same-sex marriage.

3. A nurse caring for culturally diverse patients in a physician's office is aware that patients of certain cultures are more prone to specific disease states than the general population. Which patients would the nurse screen for diabetes mellitus based on the patient's race? Select all that apply.

a. A Native American patient

b. An African American patient

c. A Pacific Island patient

d. An Asian patient

e. A White patient

f. A Hispanic patient

4. A nurse is providing nutritional counseling to culturally diverse patients with dietary restrictions. Which statement accurately describes a dietary concern based on a specific culture?

a. Many Native Americans follow a diet that is alcohol- and pork-free.

b. Many White Americans have a diet that is high in starch.

c. Asians often eat a diet that is high in salt.

d. Muslims may have special diets based on the hot/cold theory of treating illness.

5. The nurse practitioner sees patients in a community clinic that is located in a predominately White neighborhood. After performing assessments on the majority of the patients visiting the clinic, the nurse notes that many of the minority groups living within the neighborhood have lost the cultural characteristics that made them different. What is the term for this process?

a. Cultural assimilation

b. Cultural imposition

c. Culture shock

d. Ethnocentrism

6. A nurse states, "That woman is 78 years old—too old to learn how to change a dressing." What is the nurse demonstrating?

a. Cultural imposition

b. Clustering

c. Cultural competency

d. Stereotyping

7. A young Hispanic mother comes to the local clinic because her baby is sick. She speaks only Spanish and the nurse speaks only English. What should the nurse do?

a. Use short words and talk more loudly

b. Ask an interpreter for help

c. Explain why care can't be provided

d. Provide instructions in writing

8. A nurse is interviewing a newly admitted patient. Which question would be considered culturally sensitive?

a. "Do you think you will be able to eat the food we have here?"

b. "Do you understand that we can't prepare special meals?"

c. "What types of food do you eat for meals?"

d. "Why can't you just eat our food while you are here?"

9. A nurse is telling a new mother from Africa that she shouldn't carry her baby in a sling created from a large rectangular cloth. The African woman tells the nurse that everyone in Mozambique carries babies this way. The nurse believes that bassinets are safer for infants. What term best describes what the nurse is doing?

a. Cultural imposition

b. Clustering

c. Cultural competency

d. Stereotyping

10. A nurse is teaching a novice nurse how to provide culturally competent care to patients in a culturally diverse community health clinic. Although all of the following are important to providing culturally competent nursing care, which one is most basic?

a. Learning the predominant language of the community

b. Obtaining significant information about the community

c. Treating each patient at the clinic as an individual

d. Recognizing the importance of the patient's family

ANSWERS WITH RATIONALES

1. *d, e, f.* Each individual may be a member of multiple cultural, ethnic, and racial groups at one time. Culture guides what is acceptable behavior for people in a specific group. Cultural practices and beliefs may evolve over time, but they mainly remain constant as long as they satisfy a group's needs. The United States has become more inclusive of same-sex couples. The definition of cultural diversity includes, but is not limited to, people of varying cultures, racial and ethnic origin, religion, language, physical size, gender, sexual orientation, age, disability, socioeconomic status, occupational status, and geographic location. Cultural diversity, including culture, ethnicity, and race, is an integral component of both health and illness.

2. *a, d.* Cultural imposition occurs when a hospital nurse tells a nurse's aide that patients should not be given a choice whether or not to shower or bathe daily and when a Catholic nurse insists that a patient diagnosed with terminal bladder cancer see the chaplain in residence. Cultural blindness occurs when a nurse treats all patients the same whether or not they come from a different culture. Cultural conflict occurs when a nurse

ridicules a patient by telling another nurse that Jewish diet restrictions are just a way for Jewish patients to get a special tray of their favorite foods. When a nurse refuses to respect an elderly person's ability to speak for oneself, or if the nurse refuses to treat a patient based on that patient's sexual orientation, the nurse is engaging in stereotyping.

3. *a, e, f.* Native Americans, Hispanics, and Whites are more prone to developing diabetes mellitus. African Americans are prone to hypertension, stroke, sickle cell anemia, lactose intolerance, and keloids. Asians and Pacific Islanders are prone to hypertension, liver cancer, thalassemia, and lactose intolerance.

4. *c.* The Asian diet is often high in salt due to cooking with soy sauce. Many Muslims follow a halal diet that is free of alcohol, pork, and pork products. Hispanics often have a diet that is high in starch. Hispanics also may practice the hot/cold theory of treating illness and require a special diet.

5. *a.* When minority groups live within a dominant group, many members lose the cultural characteristics that once made them different in a process called assimilation. Cultural imposition occurs when one person believes that everyone should conform to his or her own belief system. Culture shock occurs when a person is placed in a different culture perceived as strange, and ethnocentrism is the belief that the ideas, beliefs, and practices of one's own cultural group are best, superior, or most preferred to those of other groups.

6. *d.* Stereotyping is assuming that all members of a group are alike.

7. *b.* Many agencies have a qualified interpreter who understands the health care system and can reliably provide assistance.

8. *c.* Asking patients what types of foods they eat for meals is culturally sensitive.

9. *a.* The nurse is trying to impose her belief that bassinets are preferable to baby slings on the African mother—in spite of the fact that African women have safely carried babies in these slings for years.

10. *c.* In all aspects of nursing, it is important to treat each patient as an individual. This is also true in providing culturally competent care. This basic objective can be accomplished by learning the predominant language in the community, researching the patient's culture, and recognizing the influence of family on the patient's life.

TAYLOR SUITE RESOURCES

Explore these additional resources to enhance learning for this chapter:

- NCLEX-Style Questions and other resources on thePoint, http://thePoint.lww.com/Taylor8e
- *Study Guide for Fundamentals of Nursing, 8th edition*
- Adaptive Learning | Powered by prepU, http://thepoint.lww.com/prepu

Bibliography

American Anthropological Association. (1997). Response to OMB Directive 15: Race and Ethnic Standards for Federal Statistics and Administrative Reporting. Available at http://www.aaanet.org/gvt/ombdraft.htm.

Andrews, M. M., & Boyle, J. S. (2012). *Transcultural concepts in nursing care* (6th ed.). Philadelphia: Lippincott Williams & Wilkins.

Campinha-Bacote J. The process of cultural competence in the delivery of health care services. In: Douglas MK, Pacquiao DF, eds. *Core Curriculum for Transcultural Nursing and Health Care*. Thousand Oaks, CA: Sage Publications; 2011.

Douglas, M. K., Pierce, J. U., Rosenkoetter, M., Pacquiao, D., Callister, L. C., Hattar-Pollara, M., ... Purnell, L. Standards of practice for culturally competent nursing care: 2011 Update. *Journal of Transcultural Nursing*, 22:317. DOI: 10.1177/1043659611412965.

Eggenberger, S., Grassley, J., & Restrepo, E. (2006). Culturally competent nursing care for families listening to the voices of Mexican-American women. *The Online Journal of Issues in Nursing*, 11(3).

El Nassar, H. & Overberg, P. August 10, 2011. Census tracks 20 years of sweeping change. *USA Today*.

Engebretson, J., Mahoney, J., & Carlson, E. D. (2008). Cultural competence in the era of evidence-based practice. *Journal of Professional Nursing*, 24(3):172–178.

Expert Panel on Global Nursing and Health, American Academy of Nursing (2010). Standards of Practice for Culturally Competent Nursing Care Executive Summary. Available at http://www.tcns.org/files/Standards_of_Practice_for_Culturally_Compt_Nsg_Care-Revised_.pdf

Fadiman, A. (2012). *The spirit catches you and you fall down: A Hmong Child, Her American Doctors, and the Collision of Two Cultures*. New York: Farrar, Straus and Giroux.

Giger, J. N., & Davidhizar, R. (2002). The Giger and Davidhizar transcultural assessment model. *Journal of Transcultural Nursing*, 13(3), 185–188.

Giger, J. N., & Davidhizar, R. (2004). *Transcultural nursing: Assessment and intervention* (4th ed.). St. Louis: Mosby.

Hall, L., Callister, L. C., Berry, J. A., & Matsumura, G. (2007). Meanings of menopause: Cultural influences on perception and management of menopause. *Journal of Holistic Nursing*, 25(2), 106–118.

Kersey-Matusiak, G. (2012). Culturally competent care: Are we there yet? *Nursing Management*, 43(4), 34–39.

Leininger, M. M. (1991). *Culture care diversity and universality: A theory of nursing*. New York: John Wiley & Sons.

Limbo Sagar, P. (2012). Transcultural nursing theory and models. *Application in nursing education, practice and administration*. New York: Springer Publishing Company.

Muñoz, C., & Hilgenberg, C. (2005). Ethnopharmacology: Understanding how ethnicity can affect drug response is essential to providing culturally competent care. *American Journal of Nursing*, 105(8), 40–49.

Office of Minority Health, Public Health Service, U.S. Department of Health and Human Services. (2001). *National standards for culturally and linguistically appropriate services (CLAS) in health care*. Washington, DC: Office of Minority Health.

Pew Research Social and Demographic Trends. (2013). Race and ethnicity. Available at http://www.pewsocialtrends.org/topics/race-and-ethnicity/

Purnell, L. D. & Paulanka, B. J. (2009). *Guide to culturally competent health care* (2nd ed.). Philadelphia: F. A. Davis Company.

Purnell, L. (2000). A description of the Purnell model for cultural competence. *Journal of Transcultural Nursing*, 11(1), 40–46.

Pullen, R. L. (2007). Tips for communicating with a patient from another culture. *Nursing*, 37(10), 48–49.

Shrestha, L. B. & Heisler, E. J. (2011). The changing demographic profile of the United States. CRS Report for Congress: RL32701. Washington, DC: Congressional Research Service.

Spector, R. (2009). *Cultural diversity in health and illness* (7th ed.). Upper Saddle River, NJ: Prentice Hall.

Think Cultural Health. (2013). *The National Standards for Culturally and Linguistically Appropriate Services in Health and Health Care: A Blueprint for Advancing and Sustaining CLAS Policy and Practice (The Blueprint)*. Available at https://www.thinkculturalhealth.hhs.gov/Content/clas.asp

U.S. Census Bureau, (2012). Poverty. Social, Economic, and Housing Statistics Division: Poverty. http://www.census.gov/hhes/www/poverty/about/overview/

U.S. Department of Health and Human Services Office of Minority Health. (2013) Think Cultural Health. Available at: https://www.thinkculturalhealth.hhs.gov/Content/ContinuingEd.asp

U.S. Department of Health and Human Services. (2013). Transforming the face of health professions through cultural and linguistic competence education: the role of HRSA Centers of Excellence. Available at http://www.hopkinsmedicine.org/diversity_cultural_competence/resources/cultural_competency_resources.html

Yosef, A. R. O. (2008). Health beliefs, practice, and priorities for health care of Arab Muslims in the United States: Implications for care. *Journal of Transcultural Nursing*, 19(3), 284–291.

6 Values, Ethics, and Advocacy

CHENGYU ZHANG

Chengyu is an alert 32-year-old man in the intensive care unit who is begging to be removed from the ventilator. He understands that it is highly unlikely that he will be able to breathe on his own without the ventilator. He writes on the communication board, "If I die, I die. I can't keep living like this."

MARISSA SANDOVAL

Marissa, a 44-year-old woman who has just recently undergone extensive surgery to treat uterine cancer, is experiencing several serious postoperative complications. She states, "I don't know why all of these things are happening. I ask the doctors. So does my family. But we get no answers. We just want to know what is happening." The nurse is surprised to observe that the surgeon not only does not answer Marissa's questions but also dismisses her fears without any explanation.

WILLIAM RAINES

Mr. Raines, a homeless, 68-year-old indigent man diagnosed with schizophrenia, developmental delays, and uncontrolled hypertension, was admitted for control of moderately severe elevated blood pressure. A review of his medical record reveals that Mr. Raines was getting samples of medications for blood pressure treatment from the pharmaceutical representatives at the clinic, but recent policy changes stopped this practice approximately 4 weeks ago. Mr. Raines is about to be discharged with several prescriptions for medications but no way to fill them.

The unique nature of nursing places nurses both at the bedside and in groups of professionals where critical decisions are made about the best way to treat injury and illness and to solve health care problems. Often, the question confronting the nurse is not "How do I do this?" but, rather, "Should I do this?" The more that science and technology increase the options available to patients and health care professionals, the more frequently nurses will find themselves asking "We can do this, but should we, here and now, for this patient?" An example of this would be: "Should the professionals in the intensive care unit keep Mr. Zhang on ventilatory support?"

Nurses also are increasingly distressed by the failure of society to provide adequate care for its most vulnerable members. Nothing is more disturbing for professional nurses than seeing firsthand the consequences of unmet health care needs.

When nurses care for patients like Mr. Raines, who lack the financial resources to obtain the medications and treatment they need, they have special advocacy obligations. A shortage of nurses further complicates the nursing work environment, creating the necessity for nurses to be skilled advocates for safety and quality care as well as for their own needs. Never has it been more important for nurses to grasp the ethical dimensions of professional practice and to be confident in "doing the ethically right thing simply because it's the right thing to do!" With their moral integrity on the line every day, nurses understand the need to be as skilled ethically as they are intellectually, interpersonally, and technically. Nurses who understand how patients' values and their own values shape nurse–patient interactions, and who continually develop sensitivity to the ethical dimensions of nursing practice, are best able to provide quality care and advocate for their patients. (For an example, see the accompanying display, Reflective Practice: Challenge to Ethical and Legal Skills.)

VALUES

A **value** is a belief about the worth of something, about what matters, that acts as a standard to guide one's behavior. If you think back to how you spent your last weekend, you may observe something about your own values. The amount of time, passion, and money you devote to relationships, work, study, fitness activities, leisure, and other experiences reveals something about the importance (value) you attach to these endeavors.

A **value system** is an organization of values in which each is ranked along a continuum of importance, often leading to a personal code of conduct. A person's values influence beliefs about human needs, health, and illness; the practice of health behaviors; and human responses to illness. For example, individuals who place a high value on health and personal responsibility often work hard to reach their fitness goals. Individuals who value high-risk leisure activities may attach less value to life and health. Nurses who work effectively with patients are sensitive to how a patient's values and their own values influence their interactions.

Development of Values

An individual is not born with values; rather, values are formed during a lifetime involving influences from the environment, family, and culture.

 RECALL Chengyu Zhang, the 32-year-old man in the intensive care unit asking to be removed from the ventilator, even if it means that he will die. The nurse can integrate knowledge of the patient's culture and family and their influence on the patient's value of independence as a key aspect in planning his care. ●

As children observe the actions of others, they quickly learn what has high and low value for family members. If the parents spend a good portion of each day cooking, for example, and the family spends a long time eating and talking at the table, the children learn to value food and the good times

REFLECTIVE PRACTICE: CULTIVATING QSEN COMPETENCIES

CHALLENGE TO ETHICAL AND LEGAL SKILLS

I have faced a common ethical dilemma both as a student in the clinical area and as a summer nurse extern. My lack of confidence prevents me from being a patient advocate. My lack of status in the unit makes it very difficult for me to stand up to more senior, experienced staff to act as a patient advocate. However, patient advocacy is a crucial duty for any nurse. I feel that when I neglect this duty, I am being unethical because I am not fulfilling one of the most important nursing roles. An example of this dilemma occurred during one of my first weeks on the gynecologic surgical floor, where I was an extern this summer.

Mrs. Marissa Sandoval was a 44-year-old woman who had just recently undergone extensive surgery for treatment of newly diagnosed uterine cancer. She also developed several postoperative complications. Mrs. Sandoval and her family were unhappy about the lack of answers they were getting from the attending surgeon and the residents about the complications she was experiencing from the surgery. After observing the surgeon interacting with the patient and her family in her room, I could easily understand the patient's distress. In addition to the surgeon not answering any of the family's questions, he dismissed all of her legitimate fears without an explanation. I felt this was a terrible way to treat a patient and that as patient advocate, I had an ethical and professional duty to make sure the patient and her family received adequate answers.

Thinking Outside the Box: Possible Courses of Action

- Confront the surgeon, explaining the patient's anxiety and asking him to return to her room to answer the questions.
- Try to answer the patient's questions to the best of my ability.
- Pretend that the doctor was acting appropriately. Tell the patient that the doctor will return tomorrow during rounds, and that she will have the opportunity to ask questions then.
- Ask another, more experienced nurse to answer my patient's questions.
- Tell the patient not to worry so much because the doctors and nurses will take good care of her.

Evaluating a Good Outcome: How Do I Define Success?

- The patient receives satisfactory answers to her questions.
- The situation is handled in a respectful manner for all parties involved.
- The American Nurses Association's Bill of Rights for Registered Nurses is followed: "Nurses have the right to freely and openly advocate for themselves and their patients, without fear of retribution."
- No one involved in the situation suffers from a violation of integrity.
- The ANA Code of Ethics is followed: "The nurse promotes, advocates for, and strives to protect the health, safety, and rights of the patient."

Personal Learning: Here's to the Future!

In retrospect, when I examine the situation, I don't think that I handled the situation in the most ethical manner. Rather than dealing with the situation myself, I sought out the help of a more experienced nurse to answer the patient's questions to the best of her ability. Unfortunately, because of the complexity of the case, the more experienced nurse was not able to answer all of the questions adequately. I should have spoken with the surgeon and expressed my concern regarding the patient's questions going unanswered. However, I was greatly intimidated by this surgeon, and I did not want to confront him. My actions demonstrate that I was compromising my role as a patient advocate. I compromised this role because of personal anxiety and lack of confidence associated with confronting the surgeon.

I am trying to base my personal practice on a strong ethical foundation, and act accordingly, as I hold my own actions to a high ethical standard. However, I am not a very confrontational person. This, coupled with my great insecurities about working in the hospital, makes it difficult for me to confront other health care providers when I think they are acting in an unethical manner. Therefore, while I think my personal actions have a strong ethical foundation, I have a lot of room for growth when acting ethically to confront coworkers. I hope that as I grow more comfortable in the hospital, I will not compromise my role as a patient advocate because of my personal fears.

Elizabeth Nalli, Georgetown University

REFLECTION ON QUALITY AND SAFETY COMPETENCIES

How do you think you would respond in a similar situation? Why? What does this tell you about yourself and about the adequacy of your skills for professional practice? How was the nursing student's action ethical? Legal? Please explain. What other *knowledge, attitudes,* and *skills* do you need to develop to continuously improve the quality and safety of care for patients like Mrs. Sandoval?

Patient-Centered Care: What role did each member of the nursing team play in creating a partnership with Mrs. Sandoval to best coordinate her care? What special talents would you bring to this partnership?

Teamwork and Collaboration/Quality Improvement: What communication skills do you need to improve to ensure that you function as a competent, caring, and responsible member of the patient-care team and that you obtain assistance when needed? How would you have responded if experienced nurses, nursing leadership, and the patient's surgeon were not responsive to your concerns? What special talents would you bring to promoting a well-functioning interdisciplinary team?

Safety/Evidence-Based Practice: What priority did everyone involved in Mrs. Sandoval's care accord to her health, well-being, and safety? What evidence in the nursing literature supports practicing within the scope of practice and roles?

Informatics: Can you identify the essential information that must be available in Mrs. Sandoval's electronic record to support safe patient care and coordination of care? Can you think of other ways to respond to or approach the situation?

it represents. Similarly, children learn that helpfulness is a good and respected quality if praised when helping parents, grandparents, and siblings. Common modes of value transmission include modeling, moralizing, laissez-faire, rewarding and punishing, and responsible choice.

Through *modeling,* children learn what is of high or low value by observing parents, peers, and significant others. Thus, modeling may lead to socially acceptable or unacceptable behaviors. Children whose caregivers use the *moralizing* mode of value transmission are taught a complete value system by parents or an institution (e.g., church or school) that allows little opportunity for them to weigh different values.

Those who use the *laissez-faire* approach to value transmission leave children to explore values on their own (no single set of values is presented as best for all) and to develop a personal value system. This approach often involves little or no guidance and may lead to confusion and conflict.

Through *rewards* and *punishments,* children are rewarded for demonstrating values held by parents and punished for demonstrating unacceptable values. Finally, caregivers who follow the *responsible-choice* mode of value transmission encourage children to explore competing values and to weigh their consequences. Support and guidance are offered as children develop a personal value system. Reflect for a moment on values you hold and see if you can identify how you developed these values.

Values Essential to the Professional Nurse

Professional values provide the foundation for nursing practice and guide the nurse's interactions with patients, colleagues, and the public. In 1998, the American Association of Colleges of Nursing identified five values that epitomize the caring, professional nurse. Box 6-1 lists these values and sample behaviors illustrating each of them. Every nurse should critically examine one's personal values to see if they match these essential professional values. For example, if you value self-promotion to the extent that you won't make the sacrifices demanded by a genuine commitment to the welfare of the patients entrusted to your care, you will never be successful as a nurse. Similarly, if you attach low value to respecting people who are different from you, you may interact with patients and colleagues in a way that is demeaning and unprofessional. It is helpful to identify nurses in your practice setting who epitomize nursing's essential values and to learn from observing their behavior. It is never too late to develop the values that epitomize the caring, professional nurse.

To encourage health care professionals to respect and accept the individuality of patients, some educators have

---

| **Box 6-1** | **PROFESSIONAL VALUES** |

Altruism

Altruism is a concern for the welfare and well-being of others. In professional practice, altruism is reflected by the nurse's concern for the welfare of patients, other nurses, and other health care providers. Sample professional behaviors include the following:

- Demonstrates understanding of cultures, beliefs, and perspectives of others
- Advocates for patients, particularly the most vulnerable
- Takes risks on behalf of patients and colleagues
- Mentors other professionals

Autonomy

Autonomy is the right to self-determination. Professional practice reflects autonomy when the nurse respects patients' rights to make decisions about their health care. Sample professional behaviors include the following:

- Plans care in partnership with patients
- Honors the right of patients and families to make decisions about health care
- Provides information so that patients can make informed choices

Human Dignity

Human dignity is respect for the inherent worth and uniqueness of individuals and populations. In professional practice, human dignity is reflected when the nurse values and respects all patients and colleagues. Sample professional behaviors include the following:

- Provides culturally competent and sensitive care
- Protects the patient's privacy
- Preserves the confidentiality of patients and health care providers
- Designs care with sensitivity to individual patient needs

Integrity

Integrity is acting in accordance with an appropriate code of ethics and accepted standards of practice. Integrity is reflected in professional practice when the nurse is honest and provides care based on an ethical framework that is accepted within the profession. Sample professional behaviors include the following:

- Provides honest information to patients and the public
- Documents care accurately and honestly
- Seeks to remedy errors made by self or others
- Demonstrates accountability for own actions

Social Justice

Social justice is upholding moral, legal, and humanistic principles. This value is reflected in professional practice when the nurse works to assure equal treatment under the law and equal access to quality health care. Sample professional behaviors include the following:

- Supports fairness and nondiscrimination in the delivery of care
- Promotes universal access to health care
- Encourages legislation and policy consistent with the advancement of nursing care and health care

From American Association of Colleges of Nursing. (2008). *The essentials of baccalaureate education for professional nursing practice.* Washington, DC: Author.

advised that professionals be "value neutral" and "nonjudgmental" in their professional roles. Professional nurses do not assume that their personal values are more correct than those of their patients. This encourages effective care for patients with values different from the nurse's. For example, a nurse who strongly believes that any premarital or extramarital sex is wrong can still offer competent and compassionate nursing care to a young woman prostitute with active herpes lesions. On the other hand, when it comes to health, safety, and well-being, nurses do make judgments. If the same patient, after receiving education, indicates that she is unconcerned about whom she might infect in future sexual encounters, the nurse has an ethical obligation to try to protect the patient and others from the harm the patient's values may cause.

Values Clarification

Values clarification is a process by which people come to understand their own values and value system. It is a process of discovery, allowing the person to discover through feelings and analysis of behavior what choices to make when alternatives are presented. Values clarification is beneficial for nurses. When nurses understand the values that motivate patients' decisions and behaviors, they can tap these values when teaching and counseling patients. For example, a man who does not value his own health and well-being may be motivated by the value he attaches to being a good father for his children to make needed lifestyle changes.

Values theorists most often describe the process of valuing as focusing on three main activities (Raths, Simon, & Harmin, 1978):

1. Choosing
2. Prizing (treasuring)
3. Acting

When one decides to value something, one chooses freely from alternatives after careful consideration of the consequences of each alternative. Prizing something one values involves pride, happiness, and public affirmation. Finally, the person who values something acts by combining choice into one's behavior with consistency and regularity on the value.

Example of Values Clarification by the Nurse

If you value inherent human dignity in your nursing practice, you choose freely to believe in the worth and uniqueness of each individual, to realize that you have other options (e.g., you could treat with dignity only those people who are most like you), and to believe that respecting each person's human dignity yields the best consequences for you and for all of society.

You also will prize your choice. For example, you especially enjoy when patients let you know they appreciate your care and when nursing colleagues and supervisors compliment you on interpersonal skills. You also prize your ability to defend this value when someone's human dignity is being ignored.

Clarifying this value of respect for human dignity will motivate you to incorporate this value into your practice.

You strive to respect human dignity consistently in your personal as well as professional life.

As you become more conscious of this value, you will be sensitive to actions that are inconsistent with it. For example, you may feel uncomfortable hearing other nurses gossiping during break about a patient they do not like, realizing that this behavior contradicts a basic respect for human dignity.

Clinical Applications

Nurses who understand the valuing process can use this knowledge when counseling patients whose values fail to support healthy choices.

PATIENT PLACES LOW VALUE ON HEALTH AND HEALTH BEHAVIORS

You become frustrated when repeated attempts to teach or counsel a 26-year-old pharmaceutical salesperson meet with failure. Although hospitalized with a serious duodenal ulcer, all he can talk about is his job and meeting his sales quota.

To facilitate values clarification for this patient, first help him identify his basic values. Ask him, "What three things are most important to you in life?" or have him rank the following behaviors for how he would most likely spend an unexpected free day:

_____ Enjoy some quiet time alone (e.g., thinking, reading, listening to music)

_____ Spend time with family, friends

_____ Do something active (e.g., hiking, playing ball, swimming)

_____ Watch television

_____ Volunteer time and energy to help someone else

_____ Use time for my job

_____ Other

Discuss with the patient what his rankings suggest about his values. Ask whether his rankings would be different if asked how he *wished* he could spend the free day versus how he would *most likely* spend it.

VALUES OF PATIENT AND FAMILY MEMBERS CONFLICT

You sense a growing tension while counseling the young parents of a child with asthma. Questioning them ("You seem uncomfortable with what I'm saying now. Is there something wrong?") reveals that the wife smokes and has a pet cat and has told her husband that even if these behaviors are hurting their child, she is unwilling to give them up.

To facilitate values clarification, suggest that both parents complete the following exercise, then talk with them about their different responses:

Where do you stand on the following issues? (Mark each as SA, strongly agree; A, agree; D, disagree; SD, strongly disagree; U, undecided.)

_____ A parent's primary obligation is to meet the needs of his or her child.

_____ Each member of a family is entitled to pursue personal pleasures, even if these are not in the best interest of all.

_____ Pleasure is more important than health.

_____ The choices one family member makes can dramatically affect other family members (positively or negatively).

This exercise will help the parents to evaluate their basic values, explore areas of conflict, and perhaps move toward joint choosing, prizing, and acting on several health-promoting values.

ETHICS

Ethics is a systematic study of principles of right and wrong conduct, virtue and vice, and good and evil as they relate to conduct and human flourishing. The ability to be ethical, to make decisions and act in an ethical manner, begins in childhood and develops gradually. See Chapter 17 for two popular theories of moral development, Kohlberg's justice-based account and Gilligan's care-based account.

Many people use the term _ethics_ when describing the systematic ethics incorporated within a code of professional conduct, such as nursing codes of ethics. The term **morals**, although similar in meaning, usually refers to personal or communal standards of right and wrong. It is important to distinguish ethics from religion, law, custom, and institutional practices. For example, the fact that an action is legal or customary does not in itself make the action ethically or morally right.

Since our values reflect what we believe is important, they are intimately related to and direct our ethical conduct. If I place a high value on patient safety and well-being, I am more likely to inconvenience myself to secure the patient's safety and well-being—even when this entails sacrifice—than a nurse who places less value on securing the patient's interests.

 RECALL Mr. Raines, the 68-year-old indigent, homeless man who is being discharged with several medication prescriptions. Due to policy changes, this patient can no longer receive his medications at the clinic free of charge. Whether health care is a commodity that can be bought and sold in the marketplace ("Too bad, Mr. Raines, if you don't have insurance to cover your meds or money in your pocket...") or a social good owed everyone is a basic question in ethics. •

Nursing Ethics

The _Encyclopedia of Bioethics_ describes the scope of **bioethics** as a number of fields and disciplines grouped broadly under the rubric "the life sciences." At the heart of bioethics are three paramount human questions (Callahan, 1995):

• What kind of person should I be in order to live a moral life and make good ethical decisions?

• What are my duties and obligations to other individuals whose life and well-being may be affected by my actions?

• What do I owe the common good or the public interest in my life as a member of society?

Nursing ethics, which is a subset of bioethics, is the formal study of ethical issues that arise in the practice of nursing and of the analysis used by nurses to make ethical judgments.

As nurses assume increasing responsibility for managing care, we must be prepared to recognize the ethical dimensions of our practice and to participate competently in ethical decision making. Common ethical issues encountered by nurses in daily practice include cost-containment issues that jeopardize patient welfare, end-of-life decisions, breaches of patient confidentiality, and incompetent, unethical, or illegal practices of colleagues.

Theories of Ethics

Ethical theories or frameworks are systems of thought that attempt to explain how we ought to live and why. These theories may be broadly categorized as action-guiding theories that address the question "What should I do?" or character-guiding theories that address the question "What kind of person should I be?" Action-guiding theories fall into two main categories:

• **Utilitarian.** The rightness or wrongness of an action depends on the consequences of the action.

• **Deontologic.** An action is right or wrong based on a rule, independent of its consequences.

This distinction is important because it is involved in many ethical conflicts we experience in practice. For example, one nurse may believe that abortion is ethically justified in situations that result in the best consequences for the woman, child, and society (utilitarian argument). Another nurse may believe that abortion is wrong based on a rule that an innocent life should never be taken (deontologic argument).

 Concept Mastery Alert

The utilitarian focus is based on "usefulness," that is actions are right when they promote the greater good and wrong when they do not. The deontologic focus views actions as right or wrong, regardless of the ends.

Nurse ethicists frequently use two popular theoretical and practical approaches to "doing ethics"—the principle-based approach and the care-based approach.

Principle-Based Approach

The **principle-based approach** to ethics combines elements of both utilitarian and deontologic theories and offers specific action guides for practice. The Beauchamp and Childress principle-based approach to bioethics (2009) identifies four key principles: **autonomy, nonmaleficence, beneficence,** and **justice** (Table 6-1). Many nurses add **fidelity**, veracity, accountability, privacy, and confidentiality to this list because they play a central role in the tradition of nursing (and medical) ethics and guide the behavior of health care professionals toward patients and their families.

Table 6-1 PRINCIPLES OF BIOETHICS

PRINCIPLE	MORAL RULE	IMPLICATIONS FOR NURSING PRACTICE
Autonomy (self-determination)	Respect the rights of patients or their surrogates to make health care decisions.	Provide the information and support patients and families need to make the decision that is right for them, including collaborating with other members of the health care team to advocate for the patient.
Nonmaleficence	Avoid causing harm.	Seek not to inflict harm; seek to prevent harm or risk of harm whenever possible.
Beneficence	Benefit the patient, and balance benefits against risks and harms.	Commit yourself to actively promoting the patient's benefit (health and well-being or good dying). Be sensitive to the fact that individuals (patients, family members, and professional caregivers) may identify benefits and harms differently. A benefit to one may be a burden to another.
Justice	Give each his or her due; act fairly.	Always seek to distribute the benefits, risks, and costs of nursing care justly. This may involve recognizing subtle instances of bias and discrimination.
Fidelity	Keep promises.	Be faithful to the promise you made to the public to be competent and to be willing to use your competence to benefit the patients entrusted to your care. Never abandon a patient entrusted to your care without first providing for the patient's needs.

 RECALL Marissa Sandoval, the 44-year-old woman who developed complications following extensive surgery for uterine cancer. The nurse would likely feel that the surgeon and residents are not being faithful (principle of fidelity) to their responsibility to address the patient's questions and fears. Unless the nurse can effectively advocate for Marissa with the medical team, her own ability to be faithful to Marissa and accountable for her well-being will be compromised. ●

The principles offer general guides to action. All things being equal, we ought to act at all times in a manner that respects the autonomy of others, does not harm, does benefit others, treats others fairly, and is faithful to the promises we make to others. Rarely is this as simple as it sounds. Be sensitive to the fact that individuals (patients, family members, and professional caregivers) may identify benefits and harms differently. A benefit to one may be a burden to another.

 REVIEW the request by Mr. Zhang, the 32-year-old man described at the beginning of the chapter. Although the nurse may view the request for removal from the ventilator as harmful, most likely leading to the patient's death, the patient's view differs, that is, he does not want to be dependent on a ventilator to live. When conflict about how to apply these principles cannot be resolved, the nurse can request an ethics consult, which is described at the end of this chapter. ●

Ethical dilemmas arise when attempted adherence to basic ethical principles results in two conflicting courses of action. There is no foolproof method for identifying which principle is most important when there is conflict between competing principles. Popularized versions of the principle-based approach to bioethics have too frequently resulted in a type of "quandary ethics" that diminishes in importance the everyday ethical concerns of nurses (Taylor, 1997), and misleadingly suggests that how ethical dilemmas are resolved is unimportant, as long as one can justify one's recommendation with recourse to a principle. Thus, many health care professionals equate ethics with decisions about whether to "pull the plug," ignoring the ethical challenges involved in daily decisions about what constitutes an honest day's work, how respectful we are to others, how truthful, and how compassionate.

Care-Based Approach

Dissatisfaction with the principle-based approach to bioethics has led many nurses to look to care as the foundation for nursing's ethical obligations. The nurse–patient relationship is central to the **care-based approach**, which directs attention to the specific situations of individual patients viewed within the context of their life narrative. The care perspective directs that how you choose to "be" and act each time you encounter a patient or colleague is a matter of ethical significance. Ethics is not reduced to a decision to withhold or withdraw life-sustaining treatment. Characteristics of the care perspective include the following (Taylor, 1993):

- Centrality of the caring relationship
- Promotion of the dignity and respect of patients as people
- Attention to the particulars of individual patients
- Cultivation of responsiveness to others and professional responsibility
- A redefinition of fundamental moral skills to include virtues like kindness, attentiveness, empathy, compassion, reliability

Feminist Ethics

Feminist ethics is a particular type of ethical approach popular among nurses, both female and male. It critiques existing patterns of oppression and domination in society, especially as these affect women and the poor. The many forms of feminist ethics range in focus from gender-related inequities to concern for the least well off. Nurses working within a feminist framework promote social policy that reflects a fundamental trust in women and those on the margins. This trust is recognition that all persons deserve the opportunity to make legitimate choices about conditions that affect their lives and are deserving of respect whenever they exercise such agency. This approach reflects a full commitment to full personhood for marginalized persons and provides for basic human needs that are consistent with one's capacity to flourish and that honors human dignity and relationality (Holland, 2001, pp. 74–75).

An excellent example of feminist ethics is Holland's critique of human embryonic stem cell research:

> It is true that women, the poor, persons of color and marginals could benefit from the regenerative medical therapies and drug therapies heralded by hES (human embryonic stem) cell and EG (embryonic germ) cell research, but it is not at all likely that they will be the ones who do benefit. Such therapies, when they are perfected, are likely to be cost-prohibitive for all but the wealthy and the well-insured, assuming that insurance companies agree to such coverage, a big assumption in any case. The poor, who are primarily women and most persons of color, will simply be marginalized from these therapies, even as it is possible that their eggs are commercialized downstream for profit.
>
> (Holland, 2001, p. 83)

ETHICAL CONDUCT

Nurses committed to high-quality care base their practice on professional standards of ethical conduct as well as professional values. The study of professional ethical behavior begins in nursing school, continues in formal and informal discussions with colleagues and peers, and culminates when nurses "try on" and adopt the behaviors of role models who practice professional nursing consistent with high ethical standards. How do nurses learn the standards for professional ethical behavior? At the very least, nurses should cultivate the virtues of nursing, understand ethical theories that dictate and justify professional conduct, and be familiar with codes of ethics for nurses and standards for professional nursing conduct.

Ethical Agency

The fact that we want to be nurses does not automatically mean we have some natural ability to always do the ethically right thing because we know it is the right thing to do. This ability, **ethical agency** or ethical capacity, must be cultivated in the same way that nurses cultivate the ability to do the scientifically right thing when providing care.

The Virtues of Nurses

Virtues are human excellencies, cultivated dispositions of character and conduct that motivate and enable us to be good human beings. Clinical virtues enable nurses to provide good care to patients. While there is no official list of essential virtues of nurses, the following virtues are frequently named:

- Competence
- Compassionate caring
- Subordination of self-interest to patient interest
- Self-effacement
- Trustworthiness
- Conscientiousness
- Intelligence
- Practical wisdom
- Humility
- Courage
- Integrity

Since these human qualities cannot be "put on" the way one puts on a uniform or identity badge, it is important that they are part of the nurse's character, part of who the nurse is. Once again, nurses must work hard to cultivate the dispositions of character that invite the public's trust.

Nursing Codes of Ethics

According to the American Nurses Association (2000), individuals who become nurses are expected not only to adhere to the moral norms of the profession but also to embrace them as part of what it means to be a nurse. The ethical tradition of nursing is self-reflective, enduring, and distinctive. A **code of ethics** is a set of principles that reflect the primary goals, values, and obligations of the profession.

The Code of Ethics for Nurses serves the following purposes:

- It is a succinct statement of the ethical obligations and duties of every individual who enters the nursing profession.
- It is the profession's nonnegotiable ethical standard.
- It is an expression of nursing's own understanding of its commitment to society.

The International Council of Nurses writes that, to achieve its purpose, The Code of Ethics for Nurses must be available to students and nurses throughout their study and work lives. They recommend that nursing students:

- Study the standards under each element of the Code.
- Reflect on what each standard means to them. Think about how they can apply ethics in their own nursing domain: practice, education, research, and management.
- Discuss the Code with coworkers and others.
- Use a specific example from experience to identify ethical dilemmas and standards of conduct as outlined in the Code. Identify how they would resolve the dilemma.
- Work in groups to clarify ethical decision making and reach a consensus on standards or ethical conflict.
- Collaborate with their national nurses' association, coworkers, and others in continuous application of ethical standards in nursing practice, education, management, and research.

Codes help nurses accomplish these goals only to the extent that nurses uphold them. Code requirements may

BOX 6-2 THE INTERNATIONAL COUNCIL OF NURSES CODE OF ETHICS FOR NURSES

An international code of ethics for nurses was first adopted by the International Council of Nurses (ICN) in 1953. It has been revised and reaffirmed at various times since, most recently with this review and revision completed in 2012.

Preamble

Nurses have four fundamental responsibilities: to promote health, to prevent illness, to restore health and to alleviate suffering. The need for nursing is universal. Inherent in nursing is a respect for human rights, including cultural rights, the right to life and choice, to dignity, and to be treated with respect. Nursing care is respectful of and unrestricted by considerations of age, color, creed, culture, disability or illness, gender, sexual orientation, nationality, politics, race or social status. Nurses render health services to the individual, the family, and the community and coordinate their services with those of related groups.

The ICN Code

The *ICN Code of Ethics for Nurses* has four principal elements that outline the standards of ethical conduct.

1. Nurses and People

The nurse's primary professional responsibility is to people requiring nursing care. In providing care, the nurse promotes an environment in which the human rights, values, customs and spiritual beliefs of the individual, family, and community are respected.

The nurse ensures that the individual receives accurate, sufficient, and timely information in a culturally appropriate manner on which to base consent for care and related treatment.

The nurse holds in confidence personal information and uses judgement in sharing this information.

The nurse shares with society the responsibility for initiating and supporting action to meet the health and social needs of the public, in particular those of vulnerable populations.

The nurse advocates for equity and social justice in resource allocation, access to health care and other social and economic services.

The nurse demonstrates professional values such as respectfulness, responsiveness, compassion, trustworthiness, and integrity.

2. Nurses and Practice

The nurse carries personal responsibility and accountability for nursing practice, and for maintaining competence by continual learning.

The nurse maintains a standard of personal health such that the ability to provide care is not compromised.

The nurse uses judgement regarding individual competence when accepting and delegating responsibility.

The nurse at all times maintains standards of personal conduct which reflect well on the profession and enhance its image and public confidence.

The nurse, in providing care, ensures that use of technology and scientific advances are compatible with the safety, dignity, and rights of people.

The nurse strives to foster and maintain a practice culture promoting ethical behaviour and open dialogue.

3. Nurses and the Profession

The nurse assumes the major role in determining and implementing acceptable standards of clinical nursing practice, management, research, and education.

The nurse is active in developing a core of research-based professional knowledge that supports evidence-based practice.

The nurse is active in developing and sustaining a core of professional values.

The nurse, acting through the professional organisation, participates in creating a positive practice environment and maintaining safe, equitable social and economic working conditions in nursing.

The nurse practices to sustain and protect the natural environment and is aware of its consequences on health.

The nurse contributes to an ethical organisational environment and challenges unethical practices and settings.

4. Nurses and Co-Workers

The nurse sustains a collaborative and respectful relationship with co-workers in nursing and other fields.

The nurse takes appropriate action to safeguard individuals, families and communities when their health is endangered by a co-worker or any other person.

The nurse takes appropriate action to support and guide co-workers to advance ethical conduct.

Used with permission from the International Council of Nurses. © 2012 by ICN-3, place Jean-Marteau, 1201 Geneva (Switzerland).

exceed legal requirements. While violations of the law subject a nurse to civil or criminal liability (see Chapter 7), violations of the code of ethics may result in a reprimand, censure, suspension, or expulsion.

Codes of ethics for nursing include the International Council of Nurses (ICN) *ICN Code of Ethics for Nurses* (adopted in 1953 and revised in 1965, 1973, 2000, 2006, and 2012; Box 6-2); the *ANA Code for Nurses With Interpretive Statements* (adopted in 1950 and revised in 1968, 1976, 1985, and 2001; Box 6-3 (on page 100)); and the Canadian Nurses Association (CNA) *Code of Ethics for Registered Nurses* (adopted in 1980 and revised in 2002 and 2008; Box 6-4 on page 100). As we go to press the ANA is preparing to launch a new revision of the Code of Ethics in 2015. Check their website for the latest version. Students will also want to be familiar with the National

Student Nurses' Association Code of Academic and Clinical Conduct, which can be found on their website (www.nsna.org).

Nursing Standards of Practice

When the American Nurses Association revised its Standards of Clinical Nursing Practice in 1991, it developed standards of professional performance as well as standards of care. Standard 7 of professional performance, ethics, describes the nurse's ethical obligations; the registered nurse practices ethically. Measurement Criteria for Standard 7 (American Nurses Association, 2010, p. 47) follow.

The registered nurse:

• Uses *Code of Ethics for Nurses with Interpretive Statements* (ANA, 2001) to guide practice.

BOX 6-3 AMERICAN NURSES ASSOCIATION CODE FOR NURSES

1. The nurse, in all professional relationships, practices with compassion and respect for the inherent dignity, worth, and uniqueness of every individual, unrestricted by considerations of social or economic status, personal attributes, or the nature of health problems.
2. The nurse's primary commitment is to the patient, whether an individual, family, group, or community.
3. The nurse promotes, advocates for, and strives to protect the health, safety, and rights of the patient.
4. The nurse is responsible and accountable for individual nursing practice and determines the appropriate delegation of tasks consistent with the nurse's obligation to provide optimum patient care.
5. The nurse owes the same duties to self as to others, including the responsibility to preserve integrity, to maintain competence, and to continue personal and professional growth.

6. The nurse participates in establishing, maintaining, and improving health care environments and conditions of employment conducive to the provision of quality health care and consistent with the values of the profession through individual and collective action.
7. The nurse participates in the advancement of the profession through contributions to practice, education, administration, and knowledge development.
8. The nurse collaborates with other health professionals and with the public in promoting community, national, and international efforts to meet health needs.
9. The profession of nursing, as represented by associations and their members, is responsible for the articulating of nursing values, for maintaining the integrity of the profession and its practice, and for shaping social policy.

Reprinted with permission from *Code of Ethics for Nurses with Interpretive Statements.* © 2001 By American Nurses Association.

- Delivers care in a manner that preserves and protects health care consumer autonomy, dignity, rights, values, and beliefs.
- Recognizes the centrality of the health care consumer and family as core members of the health care team.
- Upholds health care consumer confidentiality within legal and regulatory parameters.
- Assists health care consumers in self-determination and informed decision making.
- Maintains a therapeutic and professional health care consumer–nurse relationship within appropriate professional role boundaries.

BOX 6-4 CANADIAN NURSES ASSOCIATION CODE OF ETHICS FOR REGISTERED NURSES[a]

A. Nurses provide safe, compassionate, competent, and ethical care.
B. Nurses work with people to enable them to attain their highest possible level of health and well-being.
C. Nurses recognize, respect, and promote a person's right to be informed and make decisions.
D. Nurses recognize and respect the intrinsic worth of each person.
E. Nurses recognize the importance of privacy and confidentiality and safeguard personal, family, and community information obtained in the context of a professional relationship.
F. Nurses uphold principles of justice by safeguarding human rights, equity, and fairness and by promoting the public good.
G. Nurses are accountable for their actions and answerable for their practice.

[a]This represents only one element of the code—values. Nurses in all domains of practice bear the ethical responsibilities identified under each of the seven primary nursing values. These are intended to help nurses apply the code.
Reprinted with permission from Canadian Nurses Association. (2008). *Code of ethics for registered nurses.* Ottawa, Ontario: Author.

- Contributes to resolving ethical issues involving health care consumers, colleagues, community groups, systems, and other stakeholders.
- Takes appropriate action regarding instances of illegal, unethical, or inappropriate behavior that can endanger or jeopardize the best interests of the health care consumer or situation.
- Speaks up when appropriate to question practice when necessary for safety and quality improvement.
- Advocates for equitable health care consumer care.

 REMEMBER Marissa Sandoval, the 44-year-old woman who wants answers but is not getting them? Integration of these standards would be essential for the nurse to act professionally and ethically when obtaining the needed answers. ●

Bill of Rights for Registered Nurses

Two of the chief reasons nurses cite for the declining quality of nursing care at their facilities are inadequate staffing and decreased nurse satisfaction. Advocacy on behalf of nurses and the profession has resulted in a tangible tool, the Bill of Rights for Registered Nurses, to aid in improving workplaces and ensuring nurses' ability to provide safe, quality patient care. The Bill of Rights is intended to empower nurses by making clear what is absolutely nonnegotiable in the workplace. "The ANA and its constituent member organizations will continue their longstanding work, through political and legislative activism, collective bargaining, workplace advocacy, and public education, to ensure that the basic tenets of this Bill of Rights are a reality for nurses across the country" (Wiseman, 2001).

The seven basic tenets of the Bill of Rights for Registered Nurses are (American Nurses Association, 2001, p. 1; used with permission):

1. Nurses have the right to practice in a manner that fulfills their obligations to society and to those who receive nursing care.

2. Nurses have the right to practice in environments that allow them to act in accordance with professional standards and legally authorized scopes of practice.
3. Nurses have the right to a work environment that supports and facilitates ethical practice, in accordance with the Code of Ethics for Nurses and its interpretive statements.
4. Nurses have the right to freely and openly advocate for themselves and their patients, without fear of retribution.
5. Nurses have the right to fair compensation for their work, consistent with their knowledge, experience, and professional responsibilities.
6. Nurses have the right to a work environment that is safe for themselves and their patients.
7. Nurses have the right to negotiate the conditions of their employment, either as individuals or collectively, in all practice settings.

ETHICAL EXPERIENCE AND DECISION MAKING

Ethical experience comes in many varieties for professional nurses. Two types of ethical problems commonly faced by nurses are ethical dilemmas and ethical distress. In an ethical dilemma, two (or more) clear moral principles apply but support mutually inconsistent courses of action. **Ethical distress** occurs when the nurse knows the right thing to do but either personal or institutional factors make it difficult to follow the correct course of action. When nurses are unable to translate their ethical judgments into action, their integrity is compromised. Nurses need sound analytic skills and the ability to engage in ethical reasoning to resolve ethical dilemmas and ethical distress. The American Association of Critical-Care Nurses has developed a helpful model to "rise above moral distress," which is illustrated in Figure 6-1.

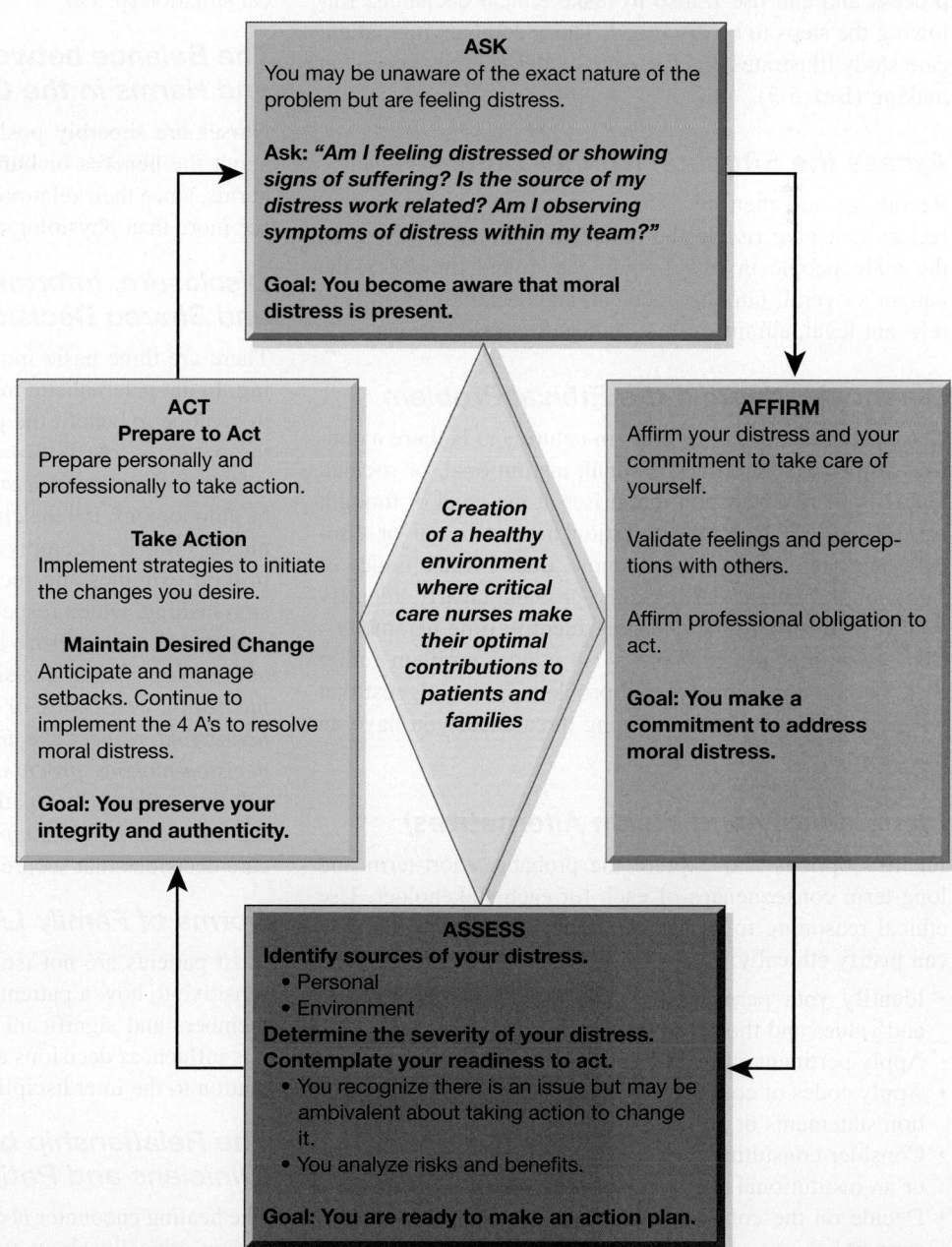

FIGURE 6-1. The 4 A's to Rise Above Moral Distress. (From American Association of Critical Care Nurses, available at http://www.aacn.org/WD/Practice/Docs/4As_to_Rise_Above_Moral_Distress.pdf.)

The Joint Commission mandates that all accredited agencies have a mechanism for addressing ethical problems. Nurses should be familiar with (and use) the resources within their institution. Most institutions have ethics committees (discussed later), and many employ staff ethicists. A few have nurse ethicists. Nurse will also find helpful resources for ethical decision making on the American Nurses Association (www.nursingworld.com) and American Association of Critical-Care Nurses (www.aacn.org) websites. Also see the section on creating and sustaining healthy work environments in Chapter 15.

Using the Nursing Process to Make Ethical Decisions

Every nurse needs to be confident in using a process of ethical decision making. Nurses are familiar with the nursing process and can use it also to make ethical decisions, following the steps to be discussed. The accompanying patient care study illustrates this five-step model of ethical decision making (Box 6-5).

Assess the Situation (Gather Data)

Recognize and then describe the situation and contextual factors that give rise to the ethical problem. This involves the main people involved (their views and interests); the patient's overall nursing, medical, and social situation; and relevant legal, administrative, and staff considerations.

Diagnose (Identify) the Ethical Problem

Clarify that the issue is ethical in nature: (1) Is there a conflict at the personal, interpersonal, institutional, or societal level? Is there a question that arises at the level of thought or feeling? (2) Does the question have a moral or ethical component? Why: for example, does it raise issues of rights, moral character? State the problem clearly. Identify your relationship to the decision. Identify time parameters. Make sure that the problem is an ethical problem rather than a communication or legal problem. Some suggest that whenever human dignity is being threatened, you have an ethical problem.

Plan (Identify and Weigh Alternatives)

Identify options and explore the probable short-term and long-term consequences of each for each stakeholder. Use ethical reasoning to decide on a course of action that you can justify ethically:

- Identify your personal and professional moral positions and values and those of other involved individuals.
- Apply pertinent ethical theories and principles.
- Apply codes of conduct and ethics, and professional position statements or guides, as applicable.
- Consider consulting with a respected and wise colleague or an institutional ethics committee.
- Decide on the course of action that you are best able to support.

Implement Your Decision

Implement your decision and begin to compare the outcome of your action with what you considered and hoped for in advance.

Evaluate Your Decision

What have you learned from this process that will help you in the future? How can you improve your reasoning and decision making in the future? In what ways does your institutional culture need to change to prevent similar conflicts in the future?

Ethically Relevant Considerations

Fletcher, Spencer, and Lombardo (2005) recommend attention to eight ethical considerations that have the greatest weight and relevance in the care of patients, which bridge between ethical principles, an ethics of caring, and the clinical situation (p. 12).

The Balance between Benefits and Harms in the Care of Patients

Nurses are superbly positioned to contribute to reasoning about the benefits or burdens of treatment and the related harms, since their relationships with patients enable them to see more than physiologic effects.

Disclosure, Informed Consent, and Shared Decision Making

There are three basic models of health care decision making. In the paternalistic model, clinicians decide what ought to be done to benefit the patient and inform the patient, and the patient's role is to comply. In the patient sovereignty model, patients or their surrogates, expressing their right to be autonomous, tell the clinician what they want, and the clinician's role is to comply. Most ethicists reject these models in their extremes and recommend a model of shared decision making, which respects and uses the preferences of the patient and the expertise and judgment of the clinician. *The object of all clinical decision making is decisions that secure the health, well-being, or good dying of the patient and that honor and respect the integrity of all participants in the decision-making process.* Nurses can play an important role in ensuring that patients and their surrogates receive the information *and support that they need* to make health care decisions that secure their interests.

Norms of Family Life

Most patients are not isolated individuals. Nurses who are sensitive to how a patient's injury or illness impacts family members and significant others can better appreciate how this influences decisions about care and can bring this information to the interdisciplinary team.

The Relationship between Clinicians and Patients

The healing encounter is central to nursing ethics. As nurses reason ethically about what should be done, it is always

Box 6-5 PATIENT CARE STUDY USING A FIVE-STEP PROCESS FOR RESOLVING ETHICAL CONFLICT

Jean Watts is a labor and delivery room nurse in a small community hospital that serves both private and clinic patients. Jean has always felt that certain members of the obstetrics–gynecology medical staff have treated these two groups of patients differently. On this particular morning, Jean is caring for a woman who is scheduled for an elective cesarean delivery. The woman (who is a clinic patient) has made it very clear that she wants to be awake for the delivery and has requested epidural or spinal anesthesia. Jean is dismayed when the anesthesiologist enters the delivery room because the anesthesiologist's success rate with epidural anesthesia is poor. The anesthesiologist unsuccessfully attempts to perform an epidural block. After waiting 20 minutes for results, the obstetrician is growing impatient and instructs the anesthesiologist to put the patient to sleep. Jean feels the rights of this patient are being violated but is unsure how she should respond.

Step 1: Assess the Situation (Gather Data)

The patient is in stable medical condition (elective cesarean delivery, not an emergency) and has made it very clear that she wishes to be awake for the delivery. The patient is not a private paying patient of the obstetrician. The nurse believes that her role is to promote and protect the patient's interests; she knows of no reason in this case why the patient's preferences should be disregarded.

The anesthesiologist has a poor success record with epidural anesthesia.

The obstetrician seems to want to complete the delivery quickly. In the past, he has seemed to give more weight to following wishes of private patients than those of clinic patients. He is the head of the obstetrics–gynecology department; he believes that nurses should obey physicians unquestioningly.

Nurses have in the past expressed dissatisfaction with the different levels of care being provided to private and clinic patients, but no one to date has formally addressed the concern.

Step 2: Diagnose (Identify) the Ethical Problem

Jean objects to the obstetrician's intent to disregard the patient's wish to be awake for her delivery; she is aware of no good reasons justifying this course of action.

The nurse will be a participant in carrying out the decision.

The decision for this case must be made immediately; it would also be helpful to plan to avoid situations like this in the future.

Step 3: Plan

a. Identify Options

The nurse can say nothing to the obstetrician and help with the delivery. If asked by the patient later why she needed to be put to sleep, the nurse can (1) tell the truth, (2) refer her to the obstetrician, (3) express sympathy that she could not be awake, or (4) say nothing. *Outcome:* The patient's wishes are disregarded; delivery occurs quickly, and the obstetrician is happy; the nurse fulfills obligation to the physician and hospital but feels she has betrayed the patient's trust. *Long-term outcome:* There is a good probability the same problem will happen again. *Or*

The nurse can remind the obstetrician that the patient was adamant about wanting to be awake and sug-

gest that a different anesthesiologist be called in. If the obstetrician agrees, the patient may get her wish and everyone is satisfied with the outcome (the nurse must still decide how to prevent recurrence of this dilemma). If the obstetrician refuses and insists that the patient be put to sleep, the nurse can (1) refuse to participate (but if another nurse is unavailable or unwilling to replace her, the nurse will have abandoned the patient and harm may ensue) or (2) participate and proceed as described or resolve to speak to the obstetrician in a "cool moment" after the delivery to see how to avoid this problem in the future. If the nurse is not satisfied with the obstetrician's response, then she must decide whether to move through the proper administrative channels. Depending on the institution and people involved, the nurse may be affirmed or censored for this move. *Long-term outcome:* Future patients may be helped by the nurse following through with her concerns.
Or
The nurse can say nothing and assist with this delivery, believing it to be the wisest course of action for the time being, but resolve to take the steps described to correct the perceived injustice. *Outcome:* There is no benefit for the present patient but there is potential benefit to future patients.

b. Think the Ethical Problem Through

Basic moral principles: The good of patients (beneficence) should be the nurse's primary concern (ANA Code of Ethics for Nurses); this strongly suggests that the nurse should act, but it does not address the nurse's obligation to do so if she feels it would jeopardize her own good (job security).

Respect for persons would suggest that the patient's autonomy (right to self-determination) should be respected unless there is strong justification for not doing so.

Justice would suggest that whether a patient pays the obstetrician privately should have no bearing on the quality of care received.

Care-based ethics would obligate Jean to serve as an effective advocate for her patient, respecting the nurse's commitment to be faithful to the nurse–patient relationship.

c. Make a Decision

Jean feels from past interactions with this obstetrician that her speaking up will not influence his decision to have the patient put to sleep. She decides to speak with the obstetrician after the delivery and follow up with whatever approach is necessary to avoid recurrence.

Steps 4–5: Implement and Evaluate Your Decision

Jean will never know if speaking up might have resulted in the patient's wishes being respected. Although she is dissatisfied with the outcome of this case, she hopes to prevent this from happening to other clinic patients in the future. In this instance, a hospital committee was formed to study the problem and make recommendations. If Jean had been told to "mind her own business" unless she wanted trouble, she would have had to make a decision weighing patient benefit on one hand with potential personal risk or harm on the other.

in the context of our relationships with patients and their families as well as with other professional caregivers. Much ethical distress for nurses results from the strong conviction that we owe individual patients more than our work environments allow us to deliver.

The Professional Integrity of Clinicians

While the 2001 ANA Code of Ethics for Nurses clearly states that the primary commitment of the nurse is the patient, it also states that the nurse owes the same duties to self as to others—including the responsibility to preserve integrity, to maintain competence, and to continue personal and professional growth. Nurses should think long and hard when they find themselves asked to sacrifice personal integrity to meet the needs of another.

Cost Effectiveness and Allocation

The increasing awareness of how difficult it is to make valued and scarce health resources available to all in need has resulted in new appreciation for the moral relevance of cost effectiveness. Nurses who are committed to patient advocacy bridge the sometimes overwhelming needs of patients and their families and the limited resources available to professional caregivers. Justice is the principle of bioethics that speaks to distributing the benefits and burdens of health care delivery fairly. Nurses are uniquely positioned within the interdisciplinary team to speak to what it means to give patients or patient cohorts "their due."

Issues of Cultural and/or Religious Variation

Since many conflicts about what should be done are rooted in different cultural or religious beliefs and values, nurses who are sensitive to the cultural and/or religious identity of patients and caregivers can help mediate these conflicts. Read more about culturally competent care in Chapter 3.

Considerations of Power

Differences in power underlie many of the ethical challenges encountered in clinical practice. Injury and illness make even sophisticated consumers of health care vulnerable. Nurses and other caregivers should be vigilant to challenge any abuses of power by clinicians. Clinicians who believe that they lack power to influence care settings and delivery may also experience ethical conflict and distress.

Examples of Ethical Problems

Ethical problems commonly arise between nurses and patients, nurses and physicians, nurses and other nurses, and nurses and their employing institutions. Moreover, nurses are often most conflicted when good practice seems to require acting against their personal moral convictions. As you read through the following mini-cases, try to determine how you would respond. The process of ethical decision making described previously should prove helpful. Note that many ethical challenges will be addressed in other chapters, especially Chapters 42 and 44.

Paternalism

An alert older resident who lives in a long-term care facility and who is now at high risk for falls refuses to call the nurse for assistance when getting out of bed. The nurse must decide whether to obtain an order to restrain the patient. Does preventing potential harm justify violating the patient's right to autonomy and make it acceptable for the nurse to act as a "parent," choosing an action the patient does not want because the nurse believes it to be in the patient's best interest?

Deception

A postoperative patient asks the student nurse, who is about to administer an intramuscular injection for pain, "Is this your first shot?" It does happen to be the student's first injection, and the student is anxious. Would the student's intent to decrease the patient's anxiety justify telling the patient, "No, I've given several before"?

Privacy

A nursing student in your class shows you her recent Facebook posting that includes a photo of a patient with a large sacral pressure ulcer. She says that since the patient is lying face down, this is not an invasion of privacy. What patient information can you post ethically on social media sites? How would you respond?

Confidentiality

A nurse asks a middle-aged woman who is crying quietly, "Would you like to share what's troubling you?" The woman tells the nurse that she has no idea how she will pay for this clinic visit because she entered the country illegally 2 months ago and is trying to earn enough money to help her family back home. She begs the nurse not to tell anyone. If the nurse believes that this anxiety is interfering with the patient's ability to obtain needed health care, would it be ethical to break the woman's confidence to obtain help for her?

Allocation of Scarce Nursing Resources

A nurse has just been pulled from your unit, leaving it understaffed. Among your patients is a 33-year-old man recovering from a heart attack who is being discharged in the morning (he tells you that he still has many questions), an older patient who is close to death, and a woman with cancer who has been vomiting all day and who is in severe pain. You know that you cannot meet everyone's needs well. How do you "distribute" your nursing care? (You really like the patient who is going home in the morning.)

Valid Consent or Refusal

A resident is attempting to perform a spinal tap on an adolescent who you know dislikes the resident. After one failed attempt, the adolescent tells the resident to stop. The resident asks you to administer an antianxiety medication to the patient to enable the resident to get the spinal tap done quickly. Should you administer the medication knowing that the patient no longer consents to the procedure?

Conflicts Concerning New Technologies

An infertile woman asks you what you think about in vitro fertilization. She tells you that she is "desperate to produce a child for her husband and in-laws" but also has grave reservations about the whole process. "I've read about couples who end up with seven frozen embryos, and I think that would kill me, thinking I've got seven potential kids 'on ice.'"

Unprofessional, Incompetent, Unethical, or Illegal Physician Practice

A nurse who works in the operating room notices that a pediatric surgeon who has been on the staff for several years and has done excellent work suddenly seems not to be concentrating during surgery and to be making more mistakes than usual. Rumors have been circulating about the surgeon having a problem with cocaine abuse after his recent divorce. The parents of one pediatric patient are dissatisfied with the progress the patient is making and ask the nurse for an opinion about the surgeon. Should the nurse voice personal concerns? Is the nurse ethically obligated to report the physician to the proper hospital authority for investigation?

Unprofessional, Incompetent, Unethical, or Illegal Nurse Practice

When you make your morning rounds, a patient tells you that one of the nurses fondled her body and made suggestive remarks during the previous night shift. You suspect that the patient may simply be trying to cause trouble, and because you like the nurse in question, you find it hard to believe the patient. What should you do?

Short Staffing and Whistle-Blowing

Restructuring has resulted in chronic understaffing on the unit where you work. You believe that patients are now at risk because there simply are not enough nurses to provide quality care. Some nurses are talking about forming a union and going on strike. Because yours is the only major hospital in a rural area, you are unsure whether striking is a morally legitimate option. Because efforts to get management to address the issues have repeatedly failed, you are also contemplating "going public" with your concerns. Your brother works for the local newspaper, and he would be willing to do a story about the situation at the hospital. What do you do?

Beginning-of-Life Issues

You are a psychiatric mental health nurse working in a Catholic hospital whose ethical and religious directives forbid abortion and abortion counseling. You are talking with a single woman recently hospitalized with bipolar disorder who is in the first trimester of an unplanned pregnancy and who is expressing great ambivalence about continuing the pregnancy. You personally believe that your ethical obli-gation is to assist this woman in exploring abortion as an option and to refer her to outside resources if she elects to abort. The charge nurse tells you that these are not appropriate options within this hospital.

End-of-Life Issues

You are the nurse case manager for a woman with a history of cancer whose cancer has recurred after many years and is now seriously advanced. She frequently tells you when you come to visit her at home that she is unwilling to fight anymore and wants to die with some dignity while she is still in control. She begs you to get her something that will "put me gently to sleep once and for all before my pain gets worse." You believe that this is her sincere wish, not just depression speaking, and you honestly believe that she would be better off spared the last stage of her fatal illness. According to your religious beliefs, however, assisted suicide is wrong under any circumstances. How do you reconcile your desire to help this woman with your profession's ethical code and your religious conviction that what she is asking for is wrong? For a fuller discussion of ethical issues at the end of life, see Chapter 42.

Nurses and Ethics Committees

An increasing number of health care institutions have developed ethics committees whose chief functions include education, policy making, case review, consultation, and in some cases research. Some committees focus on clinical ethics and some on organizational ethics. These committees are well equipped to deal with the complexities of modern health care because they are multidisciplinary and provide a forum for different views to be aired without fear of repercussion. Nurses bring an important voice to the ethics committee. When clinical issues are being reviewed, nurses can help to ensure that the technical facts are understood, that the appropriate decision makers have been identified, that the patient's medical and overall best interests have been identified, and that the course of action selected from the alternatives is justified by sound ethical principles. Nurses' strong backgrounds in interpersonal communications allow us to contribute unique knowledge about the patient and family to the discussion and to facilitate the ethics committee's group dynamics.

Nurses also play an important role in policy making. We are frequently able to identify what policies are needed to address recurring ethical concerns and to suggest needed modifications of existing policies.

ADVOCACY IN NURSING PRACTICE

Bridging vulnerable patients and the resources they need to secure health outcomes, nurses have always been strong patient advocates. **Advocacy** is the protection and support of another's rights. This role is increasingly important because of patients' changing expectations and demands, and because in our increasingly market-driven health care economy there are no guarantees that the health care system

NURSING ADVOCACY IN ACTION

Patient Scenario

Mrs. Abigail Winthur is repeatedly asking the staff in your nursing home *not* to encourage her husband to eat. Mr. Winthur, age 88, has advanced Alzheimer disease. He seems to enjoy eating and has no difficulty swallowing, but an aide has to sit by Mr. Winthur and lift the spoon to his mouth and place his cup in his hand. If you merely put the tray in front of him, he will most likely not eat.

Mrs. Winthur reports that her husband would never want to live the way he is now and she is sure that he would refuse to eat if capable of doing so. She also states that society is going to have to decide what to do about all the people we are currently "warehousing." She seems to love her husband, but she is very open about the horror of having been his caregiver for 3 years. He was always a gentle man, but then suddenly he became aggressive and would just as soon hit or punch you as take your hand.

Implications for Nursing Advocacy

How would you respond if you are Mr. Winthur's nurse? Talk with your classmates and experienced nurses about these questions:

- If you elect to advocate for Mr. and Mrs. Winthur, what practical steps can you take to ensure better health outcomes?
- What is it reasonable to expect of a student nurse, a graduate nurse, and an experienced nurse in this situation?
- What advocacy skills are needed to effectively respond to this challenge?

will work to secure their safety and health. See the Nursing Advocacy in Action box in this and other chapters.

Nurses who value patient advocacy:

- Make sure that their loyalty to their employing institution or colleagues does not compromise their primary commitment to the patient
- Give priority to the good of the individual patient rather than to the good of society in general
- Carefully evaluate the competing claims of the patient's autonomy (self-determination) and the patient's well-being

When respecting autonomy, the nurse supports the patient's right to make decisions with informed consent (Chapter 7). When promoting the patient's well-being, the nurse acts in the best interests of the patient. Ideally, both autonomy and patient well-being are promoted in every nurse–patient interaction; however, conflicts sometimes arise.

 FOR example, when Mr. Zhang, the 32-year-old man described at the beginning of the chapter, requests to be removed from the ventilator, the principle of autonomy demands respect for his treatment preferences at the same time that the principle of nonmaleficence obligates preventing the harm of his likely death. Nurses sensitive to the need to promote both patient autonomy and well-being may often experience conflict, but they are nonetheless more likely to succeed in securing the patient's genuine best interests. ●

Representing Patients

Most nurses would agree that much nursing time is spent representing patients' interests or guiding patients in protecting their own rights. The nurse is often involved as an intermediary between the patient and the family, especially when the patient and family have conflicting ideas about the management of health care situations (Fig. 6-2). For example, a patient with terminal cancer tells his nurse that he wants to go home to die. The patient's family, however, tells the nurse that they cannot care for him at home. As an advocate, the nurse recognizes the rights of both the patient

and his family. The nurse then works to help find a solution that benefits both the patient and the family. By informing the family of the availability of home care and hospice care, the nurse gives them information that may help satisfy the patient's desire for a dignified death. Working alone, most people could not get the financial help needed for such care. Nurses have the resources available to help them and can arrange referrals from other health care workers, such as social workers, to achieve the desired outcomes.

Nurses may also serve as intermediaries between patients and the medical profession. Nurse ethicist Patricia Murphy (1990) documented a moving account of how nurses interceded for a 43-year-old woman with amyotrophic lateral sclerosis who was on a ventilator but wished to die. The patient's primary physicians refused to help remove her from

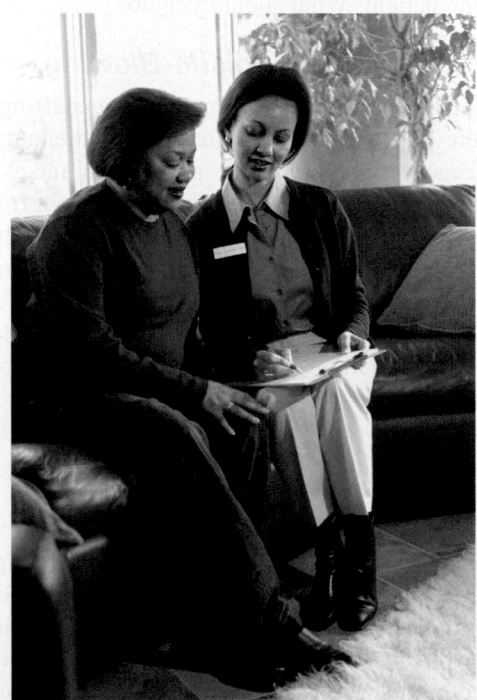

FIGURE 6-2. The nurse acts as a patient advocate in discussing all aspects of the patient's health care with family members.

the ventilator, and more than 20 other physicians declined to accept her as a patient when they learned what she wanted to do. After unsuccessful appeals for help to the county medical society and her own attorney, the patient's visiting nurse, working with a supportive social worker, contacted her state nurses association and finally secured the assistance needed to help the patient achieve her goal of a dignified death.

Patients with special advocacy needs include those who are uninformed about their rights and opportunities, those with sensory impairment, those who do not speak English well or at all, the very young and the elderly, those who are seriously ill, those who are mentally or emotionally impaired, those with physical disabilities, and those who lack adequate financial or human resources.

 CONSIDER Mr. Raines, the 68-year-old man described at the beginning of the chapter. Advocacy for his special needs would be critical in developing his discharge plan of care. ●

Promoting Self-Determination

Advocacy is linked to the belief that making choices about health is a fundamental human right that promotes the individual's dignity and well-being. Ethical dilemmas may arise when people are unable or unwilling to make choices or when they are not given the opportunity to do so. Faulty communication among patients, family members, and caregivers frequently contributes to these dilemmas. Nurses have an important advocacy role in educating the public about the value of written advance directives (described in Chapter 42).

Nurses as advocates must realize that they do not make ethical decisions for their patients. Instead, they facilitate their patients' own decision making. Nurses interpret findings for their patients, provide information to be considered, help them verbalize and organize their feelings, call in those people who should be involved in the decision making (e.g., family, primary nurse, physician, or clergy), and help patients assess all of their options. In this way, nurses advocate for the right of patients to make their own decisions concerning their health. Not all individuals want to make their own treatment decisions, however, and you should not violate the spirit of autonomy (self-determination) by forcing it on anyone. Nurses sometimes advocate for patients by helping them delegate decisions to a preferred decision maker whom they trust. In addition, when acting as a patient advocate, nurses must be careful to clarify exactly what it is that they mean by advocacy because, in most instances, this does not simply mean supporting patients in all of their preferences. For example, if a patient in the early stages of Alzheimer disease, with the support of her husband, asks a nurse for help in terminating her life, the nurse would have strong ethical grounds for refusing to advocate for that particular request.

 Concept Mastery Alert

Advocacy supports decision-making but it does not involve making the decision for the patient.

Whistle-Blowing

Every nurse who witnesses unsafe care has a duty to patients to report it. For too long, nurses have failed to speak up out of fear of retribution. In 2009, Anne Mitchell and Vicki Galle, two long-time registered nurses at Winkler County Memorial Hospital in Kermit, Texas, were charged with violating the law by sending an anonymous letter to the state medical board that expressed concern about Dr. Arafiles, who practiced at the hospital. After receiving a complaint of harassment from the physician, the Winkler County Sheriff's Department investigated and filed criminal charges against both nurses that carried potential penalties of 10 years imprisonment and a fine of up to $10,000. Mitchell and Galle, who had a combined 47 years of employment at the hospital, were also fired from their positions.

Charges of misuse of official information against Galle were dropped. Mitchell endured a 4-day jury trial and was found not guilty. The nurses then filed a federal civil suit against their accusers alleging violation of civil rights, among other violations, and won a $750,000 settlement. The Texas attorney general's office ultimately indicted the hospital and the government officials who had originally accused the nurses of wrongdoing. In 2011, Dr. Arafiles pleaded guilty and was sentenced to 60 days in jail and 5 years probation, a $5,000 fine, and surrendering his medical license. The Winkler County sheriff, county attorney, and hospital administrator received jail sentences for their roles in trying to silence the two nurses who complained to the Texas Medical Board about Arafiles. As expressed by the American Nurses Association, "The criminal convictions of all those involved in prosecuting the nurses sends a powerful message: Those who retaliate against nurses who speak up in the interests of patients will be held accountable" (ANA, 2011).

Being Politically Active

Nursing has also had a continuing voice in the political arena on behalf of those least well served by the health care system, including homeless people, minorities, women, and children. As the government becomes more involved in the delivery and funding of health care services, and as those designing rationing plans speak seriously of age and other variables as criteria for limiting care, nurses must continue to advocate for the health care needs of those least empowered to do so for themselves. Nurses are a powerful block of voters—three million strong—whose potential for influencing health care legislation is growing. See Chapter 7 for helpful guides to contacting your legislative representatives.

A Final Note About Trustworthiness

Common to all of the standards discussed previously is the obligation for nurses to be competent and willing to use their competence to secure the health and well-being or good dying of the patient. Who you choose to be on any day you arrive for practice literally has the power to influence how people are born, live, and die. When you become aware that something is interfering with patients getting the care that they need, you are responsible for responding within the scope of your power and responsibility. If you cannot independently resolve the problem, you are responsible for alerting the appropriate party, who may be the attending physician, a nursing supervisor, or a medical director. While some nurses believe that "the problem is out of my hands" once they notify the next person in the chain of command, the problem remains theirs until appropriate action is taken. Thus, you should know and use the chain of command and continue to refer a problem upwards until it is resolved and the patient's needs are met. Good professional nurses are competent, compassionate, collaborate advocates for patients and families. They are remembered for making the critical difference.

DEVELOPING CLINICAL REASONING

1. Students choose nursing as a career because of different values. A desire to help others, a desire for a steady income, wanting a career that allows you to work anywhere at any time, a commitment to provide for your children's well-being, a love of science and technology, and respect for your parents' wishes are all values that may lead to choosing nursing as a career.
   - Interview your classmates and identify the values that brought everyone to nursing. When a classmate lists more than one value, ask that classmate to rank them in order of their importance. Compare your lists.
   - Discuss which values, if any, provide the best motivation for professional nursing. Do you think that there are certain values that are incompatible with professional nursing and should be grounds for rejecting candidates for professional nursing?
   - Make a judgment about how well your personal values equip you for professional nursing. Would your patients affirm your values? Are any modifications needed?

2. Make a list of values that might positively or negatively influence someone's ability to lose weight. Think about how you could use this knowledge when counseling obese patients.

3. Another student tells you "Who I am outside of school is no one's business and has no effect on my nursing." Do you agree? Why or why not?

4. Using any current ethical issue (assisted suicide, human cloning, how to allocate scarce organs for transplantation, everyone's right to health care), poll your classmates to identify a range of opinions among them. Reflect on what it is that causes people to reach different conclusions about what is the ethically right thing to do. How might you use this knowledge as you experience ethical conflict in your professional practice?

5. During an observation experience in the operating room, you see the scrub nurse break the sterile field and continue as if nothing happened. Your clinical instructor is not in the hospital, and you don't know where your OR preceptor is at this moment. What should you do?

PRACTICING FOR NCLEX

1. A nurse caring for patients in the intensive care unit develops values from experience to form a personal code of ethics.

Which statements best describe a characteristic of the development of a personal value system? Select all that apply.
   a. People are born with values.
   b. Values act as standards to guide behavior.
   c. Values are ranked on a continuum of importance.
   d. Values influence beliefs about health and illness.
   e. Value systems are not related to personal codes of conduct.
   f. Nurses should not let their values influence patient care.

2. Five-year-old Bobby has dietary modifications related to his diabetes. His parents want him to value good nutritional habits and they decide to deprive him of a favorite TV program when he becomes angry after they deny him foods not on his diet. This is an example of what mode of value transmission?
   a. Modeling
   b. Moralizing
   c. Laissez-faire
   d. Rewarding and punishing

3. A nurse who is working in a hospital setting after graduation from a local college uses value clarification to help understand the values that motivate patient behavior. Which examples denote "prizing" in the process of values clarification? Select all that apply.
   a. A patient decides to quit smoking following a diagnosis of lung cancer.
   b. A patient shows off a new outfit that she is wearing after losing 20 pounds.
   c. A patient chooses to work fewer hours following a stress-related myocardial infarction.
   d. A patient incorporates a new low-cholesterol diet into his daily routine.
   e. A patient joins a gym and schedules classes throughout the year.
   f. A patient proudly displays his certificate for completing a marathon.

4. The American Association of Colleges of Nursing identified five values that epitomize the caring professional nurse. Which of these is best described as acting in accordance with an appropriate code of ethics and accepted standards of practice?
   a. Altruism
   b. Autonomy
   c. Human dignity
   d. Integrity

5. A professional nurse with a commitment to social justice is most apt to:
   a. Provide honest information to patients and the public
   b. Promote universal access to health care
   c. Plan care in partnership with patients
   d. Document care accurately and honestly

6. When an older nurse complains to a younger nurse that nurses just aren't ethical anymore, which reply reflects the best understanding of moral development?
   a. "Behaving ethically develops gradually from childhood; maybe my generation doesn't value this enough to develop an ethical code."
   b. "I don't agree that nurses were more ethical in the past. It's a new age and the ethics are new!"

c. "Ethics is genetically determined...it's like having blue or brown eyes. Maybe we're evolving out of the ethical sense your generation had."

d. "I agree! It's impossible to be ethical when working in a practice setting like this!"

7. A home health nurse who performs a careful safety assessment of the home of a frail elderly patient to prevent harm to the patient is acting in accordance with which of the principles of bioethics?
   a. Autonomy
   b. Beneficence
   c. Justice
   d. Fidelity
   e. Nonmaleficence

8. A professional nurse committed to the principle of autonomy would be careful to:
   a. Provide the information and support a patient needed to make decisions to advance one's own interests
   b. Treat each patient fairly, trying to give everyone his or her due
   c. Keep any promises made to a patient or another professional caregiver
   d. Avoid causing harm to a patient

9. Janie wants to call an ethics consult to clarify treatment goals for a patient no longer able to speak for himself. She believes his dying is being prolonged painfully. She is troubled when the patient's doctor tells her that she'll be fired if she raises questions about his care or calls the consult. This is a good example of:
   a. Ethical uncertainty
   b. Ethical distress
   c. Ethical dilemma
   d. Ethical residue

10. A student nurse begins a clinical rotation in a long-term care facility and quickly realizes that certain residents have unmet needs. The student wants to advocate for these residents. Which statements reflect a correct understanding of advocacy? Select all that apply.
    a. Advocacy is the protection and support of another's rights.
    b. Patient advocacy is primarily done by nurses.
    c. Patients with special advocacy needs include the very young and the elderly, those who are seriously ill, and those with disabilities.
    d. Nurse advocates make good health care decisions for patients and residents.
    e. Nurse advocates do whatever patients and residents want.
    f. Effective advocacy may entail becoming politically active.

ANSWERS WITH RATIONALES

1. **b, c, d.** A value is a belief about the worth of something, about what matters, which acts as a standard to guide one's behavior. A value system is an organization of values in which each is ranked along a continuum of importance, often leading to a personal code of conduct. A person's values influence beliefs about human needs, health, and illness; the practice of health behaviors; and human responses to illness. Values guide the practice of nursing care. An individual is not born with values; rather, values are formed during a lifetime from information from the environment, family, and culture.

2. **d.** When rewarding and punishing are used to transmit values, children are rewarded for demonstrating values held by parents and punished for demonstrating unacceptable values. Through modeling, children learn what is of high or low value by observing parents, peers, and significant others. Children whose caregivers use the moralizing mode of value transmission are taught a complete value system by parents or an institution (e.g., church or school) that allows little opportunity for them to weigh different values. Those who use the laissez-faire approach to value transmission leave children to explore values on their own (no single set of values is presented as best for all) and to develop a personal value system.

3. **b, f.** Prizing something one values involves pride, happiness, and public affirmation, such as losing weight or running a marathon. When choosing, one chooses freely from alternatives after careful consideration of the consequences of each alternative, such as quitting smoking and working fewer hours. Finally, the person who values something acts by combining choice into one's behavior with consistency and regularity on the value, such as joining a gym for the year and following a low-cholesterol diet faithfully.

4. **d.** The American Association of Colleges of Nursing defines integrity as acting in accordance with an appropriate code of ethics and accepted standards of practice. Altruism is a concern for the welfare and well-being of others. Autonomy is the right to self-determination, and human dignity is respect for the inherent worth and uniqueness of individuals and populations.

5. **b.** The American Association of Colleges of Nursing lists promoting universal access to health care as an example of social justice. Providing honest information and documenting care accurately and honestly are examples of integrity, and planning care in partnership with patients is an example of autonomy.

6. **a.** The ability to be ethical, to make decisions, and to act in an ethically justified manner begins in childhood and develops gradually.

7. **e.** Nonmaleficence is defined as the obligation to prevent harm. Autonomy is respect for another's right to make decisions, beneficence obligates us to benefit the patient, justice obligates us to act fairly, and fidelity obligates us to keep our promises.

8. **a.** The principle of autonomy obligates nurses to provide the information and support patients and their surrogates need to make decisions that advance their interests. Acting with justice means giving each person his or her due, acting with fidelity involves keeping promises to patients, and acting with nonmaleficence means avoiding doing harm to patients.

9. **b.** Ethical distress results from knowing the right thing to do but finding it almost impossible to execute because of institutional or other constraints (in this case, fear of losing her job). Ethical uncertainty results from feeling troubled by a situation but not knowing if it is an ethical problem. Ethical dilemmas occur when the principles of bioethics justify two or more conflicting courses of action. Ethical residue is what nurses experience when they seriously compromise themselves or allow themselves to be compromised.

10. *a, c, f.* Advocacy is the protection and support of another's rights. Among the patients with special advocacy needs are the very young and the elderly, those who are seriously ill, and those with disabilities; this is not a comprehensive list. Effective advocacy may entail becoming politically active. Patient advocacy is the responsibility of every member of the professional caregiving team—not just nurses. Nurse advocates do not make health care decisions for their patients and residents. Instead, they facilitate their decision making. Advocacy does not entail supporting patients in all their preferences.

TAYLOR SUITE RESOURCES

Explore these additional resources to enhance learning for this chapter:

- NCLEX-Style Questions and other resources on thePoint, http://thePoint.lww.com/Taylor8e
- *Study Guide for Fundamentals of Nursing, 8th edition*
- Adaptive Learning | Powered by prepU, http://thepoint.lww.com/prepu

Bibliography

American Association of Colleges of Nursing. (2008). *The essentials of baccalaureate education for professional nursing practice.* Washington, DC: Author.

American Association of Critical-Care Nurses. (n.d.). *4 A's to rise above moral distress.* Available at http://www.aacn.org/WD/Practice/Docs/4As_to_Rise_Above_Moral_Distress.pdf.

American Association of Critical-Care Nurses. (2005). *AACN standards for establishing and sustaining healthy work environments.* Available at http://www.aacn.org/WD/HWE/Content/hwehome.pcms?menu=Practice&lastmenu=

American Nurses Association. (2001). *Code for nurses with interpretive statements.* Washington, DC: Author.

American Nurses Association. (n.d.). Ethics and human rights. ANA policy statements. Available at http://www.nursingworld.org/MainMenuCategories/HealthcareandPolicyIssues/ANAPositionStatements/EthicsandHumanRights.aspx

American Nurses Association. (2010). *Nursing's social policy statement* (2010 ed.). Washington, DC: Author.

American Nurses Association. (2010). *Nursing: Scope and standards of practice* (2010 ed.). Washington, DC: Author.

American Nurses Association's Code of Ethics Task Force. (2000). A new code of ethics for nurses. *American Journal of Nursing, 100*(7), 69, 71–72.

Beauchamp, T. L., & Childress, J. F. (2009). *Principles of biomedical ethics* (6th ed.). New York: Oxford University Press.

Bishop, A. H., & Scudder, J. R. (1990). *The practical, moral, and personal sense of nursing.* Albany: State University of New York Press.

Burkhardt, M. A., & Nathaniel, A. K. (2008). *Ethical issues in contemporary nursing* (3rd ed.). Clifton Park, NY: Thomson Delmar Learning.

Callahan, D. (1995). Bioethics. In W. T. Reich (Ed.), *Encyclopedia of bioethics* (Rev. ed., pp. 247–256). New York: Macmillan.

Canadian Nurses Association. (2008). *Code of ethics for registered nurses.* Ottawa, Ontario: Author.

Corley, M. C., Elswick, R. K., Gorman, M., & Clor, T. (2001). Development and evaluation of a moral distress scale. *Journal of Advanced Nursing, 33*(2), 250–256.

Corley, M. C., Minick, P., Elswick, R. K., & Jacobs, M. (2005). Nurse moral distress and ethical work environment. *Nursing Ethics, 12*(4), 381–390.

DeWolf Bosek, M. S., & Savage, T. A. (2007). *The ethical component of nursing education.* Philadelphia: Lippincott Williams & Wilkins.

Fletcher, J. C., Spencer, E. M., & Lombardo, P. A. (Eds.). (2005). *Fletcher's introduction to clinical ethics* (3rd ed.). Hagerstown, MD: University Publishing Group.

Fowler, M. D. M. (Ed.). (2010 reissue). *Guide to the code of ethics for nurses: Interpretation and application.* Silver Spring, MD: American Nurses Association.

Fry, S. T., Veatch, R. M., & Taylor, C. (2011). *Case studies in nursing ethics* (4th ed.). Sudbury, MA: Jones and Bartlett Publishers.

Grace, P. J., & McLaughlin, M. (2005). Ethical issues. When consent isn't informed enough: What's the nurse's role when a patient has given consent but doesn't fully understand the risks? *American Journal of Nursing, 105*(4), 79, 81–84.

Grady, C., Danis, M., Soeken, K. L., O'Donnell, P., Taylor, C., Farrar, A., et al. (2008). Does ethics education influence the moral action of practicing nurses and social workers? *American Journal of Bioethics, 8*(4), 4–11.

Holland, S. (2001). Beyond the embryo: A feminist appraisal of the embryonic stem cell debate. In S. Holland, K. Lebacqz, & L. Zoloth (Eds.), *The human embryonic stem cell debate* (pp. 73–86). Cambridge, MA: A Bradford Book.

International Council of Nurses. (2012). *ICN code of ethics for nurses: Ethical concepts applied to nursing.* Geneva: Imprimeries Populaires.

Jensen, A., & Lidell, E. (2009). The influence of conscience in nursing. *Nursing Ethics, 16*(1), 31–42.

Lachman, V. D. (Ed.). (2006). *Applied ethics in nursing.* New York: Springer.

Lachman, V.D., Murray, J.S., Iseminger, K., & Ganske, K.M. (2012). Doing the right thing: Pathways to moral courage. *American Nurse Today, 7*(5):24.

McGowan, C. (2012). Patients' confidentiality. *Critical Care Nurse, 32*(5), 61–65.

Morris, P. E., & Dracup, K. (2008). Time for a tool to measure moral distress. *American Journal of Critical Care, 17*(5), 398–401.

Murphy, P. (1990). Helping Joanne die with dignity: A nursing profile in courage. *Nursing, 20*(9), 44–49.

National Student Nurses' Association. (2009). Code of Ethics: Part II. Code of Academic and Clinical Conduct and Interpretive Statements. Available at: www.nsna.org

Pavlish, C., & Hunt, R. (2012). An exploratory study about meaningful work in acute care nursing. *Nursing Forum, 47,* 113–122.

Pavlish, C., Brown-Saltzman, K., Hersh, M., Shirk, M., & Rounkle, A. M. (2011). Nursing priorities, actions, and regrets for ethical situations in clinical practice. *Journal of Nursing Scholarship, 43*(4), 385–395.

Pavlish, C., Brown-Saltzman, K., Hersh, M., Shirk, M., & Nudelman, O. (2011). Early indicators and risk factors for ethical issues in clinical practice. *Journal of Nursing Scholarship, 43*(1), 13–21.

Pinch, W. J. E., & Haddad, A. M. (2008). *Nursing and health care ethics: A legacy and a vision.* Silver Spring, MD: American Nurses Association.

Raths, L. E., Simon, S. B., & Harmin, M. (1978). *Values and teaching* (2nd ed.). Columbus, OH: Charles E. Merrill.

Schluter, J., Winch, S., Holzhauser, K., & Henderson, A. (2008). Nurses' moral sensitivity and hospital ethical climate: a literature review. *Nurse Ethics, 15*(3), 304–321.

Storch, J. L., Rodney, P., & Starzomski, R. (Eds.). (2013). *Toward a moral horizon: Nursing ethics for leadership and practice.* Toronto, Ontario: Pearson/Prentice Hall.

Storch, J. L., & Kenny, N. (2007). Shared moral work of nurses and physicians. *Nursing Ethics, 14*(4), 478–491.

Taylor, C. (1993). Nursing ethics: The role of caring. *AWHONN's Clinical Issues in Perinatal and Women's Health Nursing, 4*(4), 552–560.

Taylor, C. (1997). Everyday nursing concerns: Unique? Trivial? Or essential to healthcare ethics? *HEC Forum, 9*(1), 68–84.

The Patient Care Partnership. (2003). Available at http://www.aha.org/aha/issues/Communicating-With-Patients/pt-care-partnership.html

Ulrich, C.M. (2012). *Nursing Ethics in Everyday Practice.* Indianapolis: Sigmna Theta Tau.

Ulrich, C., Taylor, C., Soeken, K., O'Donnell, P., Farrar, A., Danis, M. & Grady, C. Everyday ethics: Ethical issues and stress in nursing practice. *Journal of Advanced Nursing, 66*(11):2510–2519. DOI: 10.1111/j.1365–2648.2010.05425.x

Wiseman, R. (2001). The ANA develops Bill of Rights for Registered Nurses. *American Journal of Nursing, 101*(11), 55, 57.

7 Legal Dimensions of Nursing Practice

RAMONE SCOTT

Ramone, a 66-year-old man, had surgery to repair a fractured hip earlier in the day. His nurse just administered a dose of an intravenous antibiotic that had been prescribed for a different patient.

MEREDITH BEDFORD

Meredith is the mother of a terminally ill child with a brain tumor who is admitted to a residential hospice for better pain and symptom management. One morning she tells the nurse, "I'm very unhappy with the care my son is receiving. I'm going to talk with my attorney as soon as possible to press charges against the hospice."

ELLA RODRIGUEZ

Ella, an 8-year-old girl, comes to the emergency department (ED) with a right forearm fracture. She requires diazepam (Valium) sedation for a closed reduction procedure. The ED's protocol for administration to a child states that a physician must be present throughout the entire sedation procedure. One of the physicians has been working his 14th hour, and the ED is overflowing. He orders the nurse to begin the sedation protocol, stating that he will be back in the room in 10 minutes.

LEARNING OBJECTIVES

After completing the chapter, you will be able to accomplish the following:

1. Define "law" and describe four sources of laws.
2. Describe the professional and legal regulation of nursing practice.
3. Identify the purpose of credentialing, using as examples accreditation, licensure or registration, and certification.
4. Identify grounds for suspending or revoking a license or registration.
5. Differentiate between intentional torts (assault and battery, defamation, invasion of privacy, false imprisonment, fraud) and unintentional torts (negligence).
6. Evaluate personal areas of potential liability in nursing.
7. Describe the legal procedure that occurs when a plaintiff files a complaint against a nurse for negligence.
8. Describe the roles of the nurse as defendant, fact witness, and expert witness.
9. Use appropriate legal safeguards in nursing practice.
10. Explain the purpose of incident reports.
11. Describe laws affecting nursing practice.

KEY TERMS

accreditation	defendant	malpractice
assault	expert witness	misdemeanor
battery	fact witness	negligence
certification	felony	plaintiff
common law	fraud	sentinel event
credentialing	liability	statutory law
crime	licensure	tort
defamation of character	litigation	whistle-blowing

As the roles and duties of nurses have expanded, so has our legal accountability. In the past, many nurses worked under the supervision of a physician, few carried liability insurance, and even if a nurse's actions directly caused harm to a patient, the primary liability for the nursing action fell on the employing agency or physician. In modern practice, nurses assess and diagnose patients and plan, implement, and evaluate nursing care. Full legal responsibility and accountability for these

nursing actions rest with the nurse. (See the accompanying Reflective Practice box for an example.) Nurses are increasingly the subjects of both civil and criminal negligence cases and are being brought to court to defend their practice. While nurses shouldn't practice in constant fear of being sued, it would be foolish not to learn how to be legally prudent.

Although many nurses continue to work in traditional settings like hospitals and long-term care facilities, more nurses are working in nontraditional community settings such as home care agencies, clinics, daycare centers, and nurse-managed health centers. Advanced practice nurses may have independent practices. It is critical for nurses to document their actions carefully and act in ways to prevent malpractice accusations. Nurses who wish to avoid legal conflicts need to develop trusting nurse–patient relationships (satisfied patients rarely sue), practice within the scope of their competence, and identify potential liabilities in their practice and work to prevent them. The most extensive malpractice study reviewed claims from 1991 to 2007 and found that there was one payment for every 2.7 active physicians (37%), one for every 32.5 active physician assistants (3.1%), and one for every 65.8 active and inactive advanced practice nurses (1.5%; Hooker, Nicholson, & Tuan, 2012). Nurses were less likely to be sued because they spent more time with patients and took time to answer their questions.

LEGAL CONCEPTS

As you begin professional practice, it is essential to understand how the law defines the nurse's legal responsibilities and duties.

Definition of Law

A law is a standard or rule of conduct established and enforced by the government that is intended chiefly to protect the rights of the public. Public law is law in which the government is involved directly. It regulates relationships between people and the government, for example, describing the powers of the government. Private law, also called civil law, regulates relationships among people. Civil law includes laws relating to contracts; ownership of property; and the practice of nursing, medicine, pharmacy, and dentistry. Criminal law, a type of public law, concerns state and federal criminal statutes, which define criminal actions such as murder, manslaughter, criminal negligence, theft, and illegal possession of drugs.

Sources of Laws

Four sources of laws exist at both the federal and state level: constitutions, statutory law, administrative law, and common law.

Constitutions

Federal and state constitutions indicate how the federal and state governments are created, and they give authority and state the principles and provisions for establishing specific laws. Although they contain relatively few laws (called

REFLECTIVE PRACTICE: CULTIVATING QSEN COMPETENCIES

CHALLENGE TO ETHICAL AND LEGAL SKILLS

This past summer, I worked in the emergency department of a very reputable hospital. Overall, I felt that the department was a desirable working environment and that the relationships between physicians and nurses were very open. However, one incident occurred that I felt put the patient's safety at risk.

Ella Rodriguez, an 8-year-old girl, had come to the emergency department with a right forearm fracture. She required diazepam (Valium) sedation for a closed reduction procedure. The ED's protocol for administration for a child states that a physician must be present throughout the entire sedation procedure. One of the physicians had been working for 14 hours, and the ED was overflowing. He ordered the nurse to begin the sedation protocol, stating that he would be back in the room in 10 minutes. The nurse taking care of the patient was a new graduate and did not feel comfortable giving the drug alone, but also did not feel comfortable speaking up to the doctor. She proceeded to go into the room and inject the first dose of diazepam (Valium), against protocol.

This nursing action completely undermined the patient's safety because the nurse not only stated previously that she did not feel comfortable with the sedation procedure, but she also went against protocol. Since both the physician and the nurse had a duty to follow the protocol, if harm resulted from their failure to do so, there would be grounds for negligence. Although the physician was also responsible for giving the nurse orders against protocol, her obligation to herself and the patient should have been the priority, and thus, she should have refused to give the drug until the physician was in the room.

Thinking Outside The Box: Possible Courses of Action

- Hope and pray that nothing happens to the patient until the physician comes back into the room.
- Get the physician back into the room; if he refuses an invitation to be present, report this to someone in a leadership position.
- Ask the nurse why she is violating protocol.
- Seek the help of my preceptor immediately.

Evaluating a Good Outcome: How Do I Define Success?

- Patient is benefited or at the very least not harmed.
- The physician, nurse, and unit leaders accept responsibility for safely implementing protocols.
- All health care team members demonstrate accountability for failures to adhere to protocols.
- Patient safety is put first, even when this means challenging other members of the team.

Personal Learning: Here's to the Future!

My preceptor, the charge nurse, realized that the nurse was in the room administering the medication. Once he realized this, he immediately got the physician to go into the patient's room. After the procedure was completed successfully, he discussed the implications of both the nurse's and the doctor's actions with each of them together and separately. I did not have time to respond to this incident because the charge nurse had acted so quickly and appropriately.

Obviously, I think that the nurse should have spoken to the physician and refused to give the medication, but I can understand her feelings, especially being a new graduate. The entire situation can be very intimidating, but as nurses, our responsibility is to the patient. By not standing up for the patient and herself, the nurse put the patient in danger and herself in danger, and did nothing to change the climate of the ED. The experienced and exceptionally capable charge nurse was not afraid to stand up to the doctor. Not only did his actions put the patient's safety first, but he also demonstrated to the nurse, myself, and other nurses that it is imperative that nurses stand up for themselves and patients.

I believe that no matter what the circumstance is, nurses need to stand up for themselves and their patients, especially now, when our health care climate yields to nurses' voices being heard. The only way that nurses' roles and reputations will change is if we, the nurses, speak up, and speak loudly. Right now, we have a unique opportunity to change the way medicine is practiced to benefit both patients and nurses. If all nurses grab this opportunity and make something of it, we can really make a difference, but it needs to be a collective effort to be successful. Regardless of how small the problem is, it must be addressed.

Julia Strobel, Georgetown University

REFLECTION ON QUALITY AND SAFETY COMPETENCIES

How do you think you would respond in a similar situation? Why? What does this tell you about yourself and about the adequacy of your skills for professional practice? How was the nurse's action ethical? Legal? Please explain. What other *knowledge, attitudes,* and *skills* do you need to develop to continuously improve the quality and safety of care for patients like Ella Rodriguez?

Patient-Centered Care: What role did each member of the nursing team play in creating a partnership with Ella's parents to best coordinate her care? What special talents do you bring to creating this partnership?

Teamwork and Collaboration/Quality Improvement: What communication skills do you need to improve to ensure that you function as a competent, caring, and responsible member of the patient-care team and that you obtain assistance when needed? How would you have responded if ordered by a physician to break protocol? What special talents do you bring to promoting a well-functioning interdisciplinary team?

Safety/Evidence-Based Practice: What priority did all involved in Ella's care accord to her health, well-being, and safety? What evidence in the nursing literature supports practicing as directed by this protocol? What in the safety literature dictates how nurses should respond in similar situations?

Informatics: Can you identify the essential information that must be available in Ella Rodriguez's electronic record to support safe patient care and coordination of care? Can you think of other ways to respond to or approach the situation?

constitutional laws), constitutions serve as guides to legislative bodies.

Statutory Law

A legislative body enacts **statutory law**. Statutory laws must be in keeping with both the federal constitution and the state constitution. Nurse Practice Acts are an example of statutory laws. These are discussed fully in the later section entitled "Professional and Legal Regulation of Nursing Practice."

Administrative Law

Executive officers (e.g., the President of the United States, state governors, or city mayors) administer agencies that, among other functions, are responsible for law enforcement. These agencies have the power to make administrative rules and regulations, in conformity with enacted law, that act as laws and are enforceable. Boards of nursing are administrative agencies at the state level. The rules and regulations that they adopt are administrative laws. An example of a municipal administrative agency is the city board of health.

Common Law

The government provides for a judiciary system, which is responsible for resolving controversies. It interprets legislation at the local, state, and national levels as it has been applied in specific instances and makes decisions concerning law enforcement. A body of law known as **common law** has evolved from these accumulated judiciary decisions. Common law is thus court-made law. Most law involving malpractice is common law.

Common law is based on the principle of *stare decisis,* or "let the decision stand." After a decision has been made in a court of law, the principle in that decision becomes the rule to follow in other similar cases. The case that first sets down the rule by decision is called a precedent. Court decisions can be changed, but only with strong justification. Common law helps prevent one set of rules from being used to judge one person and another set to judge another person in similar circumstances.

The Court System

A lawsuit is a civil action brought in a court of law. **Litigation** is the process of bringing and trying a lawsuit. The person or government who claims to have incurred losses as a result of an action by a **defendant** is called the **plaintiff**. The defendant is presumed innocent until proved guilty of a crime or tort. Criminal law is concerned with actions that are harmful to society as a whole. A prosecutor or district attorney brings charges against a person, persons, or corporate entity believed to have committed a crime.

 RECALL Meredith Bedford, the mother of the terminally ill child threatening to bring charges against the hospice. The mother would be considered the plaintiff, while those named in the lawsuit would be considered the defendants. ●

The two levels of courts in the United States are trial courts and appellate courts. The trial court, the first-level court, hears all the evidence in a case and makes decisions based on facts, usually through a jury. The appellate court hears only cases questioning a point of law decided by the trial court. No witnesses testify at the appellate court level. The opinions of appellate judges are published and become common law.

PROFESSIONAL AND LEGAL REGULATION OF NURSING PRACTICE

Nurses who practice safely respect both the voluntary and legal controls of nursing practice. Both of these controls are designed to ensure quality health care and to protect society from unsafe actions.

Nurse Practice Acts

Your state's Nurse Practice Act is the most important law affecting your nursing practice. Each state has a Nurse Practice Act that protects the public by broadly defining the legal scope of nursing practice. You should obtain a copy of this act from your state Board of Nursing and study it carefully. Visit the website of the National Council of State Boards of Nursing (NCSBN) for more information about nurse practice acts and how to contact your State Board of Nursing (https://www.ncsbn.org/about.htm). Each nurse is expected to care for patients within defined practice limits. Practicing beyond those limits (e.g., performing an appendectomy) makes you vulnerable to charges of violating the state Nurse Practice Act.

 CONSIDER Ella Rodriguez, the 8-year-old with the fractured arm requiring administration of sedation based on a protocol. The nurse should integrate knowledge of the state's Nurse Practice Act when administering the medication, understanding the need to adhere to the ED's protocol that requires a physician to be present throughout the administration. ●

Nurse Practice Acts list the violations that can result in disciplinary actions against a nurse and also intend to prevent untrained or unlicensed people from practicing nursing. Table 7-1 illustrates different sources of rules affecting nursing practice, examples of issues covered, where these rules are documented, and suggestions for initiating change. Sharp (2003, p. 12) claims that gaining legal power and influence for nurses is easier than we think: "Simple as it seems, the written word can get us exactly what we want and what our patients need—more nurses and improved working conditions.... To get what we want, we have to make sure our legislators hear us loud and clear. What easier way to do this than with a letter or e-mail?" An example of an e-mail to a member of Congress to support funding for the Nurse Reinvestment Act (NRA) is shown in Box 7-1, (on page 116) and a student describes a lobbying experience in Through the Eyes of a Student.

Table 7-1 WHO MAKES NURSING PRACTICE RULES?

SOURCE OF PRACTICE RULES	EXAMPLES OF ISSUES COVERED	WHERE RULES ARE DOCUMENTED	HOW TO INITIATE CHANGE
Federal legislation	• Medicare and Medicaid provisions related to reimbursement for nursing services	• Federal statutes	• Review documents. • Draft desired legislative changes. • Obtain support of colleagues, nursing organizations, other health care providers, and the public, if appropriate. • Obtain support and sponsorship from a U.S. congressperson or senator, who will introduce the bill. • Lobby for the bill's passage.
State legislation	• Scope of practice for RNs, LPNs, advanced practice nurses • Nursing educational requirements • Composition and disciplinary authority of board of nursing	• Nurse Practice Act • Medical Practice Act • Other statutes	• Review documents. • Draft desired legislative changes. • Obtain support of colleagues, nursing organizations, other health care providers, and the public, if appropriate. • Obtain support and sponsorship from a state legislator, who will introduce the bill. • Lobby for the bill's passage.
Board of nursing	• Delegation • Medication administration • Unprofessional conduct • Licensing	• Rules and regulations • Position statements • Declaratory rulings (as found in meeting minutes or newsletters), which may be specific to a particular setting or institution	• Review documents. • Initiate a formal query to the licensing board. • Obtain board support for change. • The board may issue a position statement or declaratory ruling or hold a formal public hearing before voting to promulgate new rules or change existing ones.
Health care institution	• Clinical procedures, such as wound dressing changes • Policies specific to the institution, specialty, or practice setting • Personnel and employment policies	• Unit-based policies • Institutional policies • Institutional credentialing policies	• Review institutional policies. • Follow institutional policies or the chain of command to make inquiries or propose change.

Reprinted with permission from Laskowshi-Jones, L. (1998). Reaching beyond the rules: Understanding—and influencing—your scope of practice. *Nursing, 28*(9), 45.

THROUGH THE EYES OF A STUDENT

I was extremely nervous to go to Capitol Hill and meet with my congressional representative; I had begun to feel so comfortable in my scrubs at the hospital that I felt out of place in a suit. I was very fortunate that Representative Christopher Shays agreed to meet with me to discuss my views on medical malpractice liability. Although the meeting was very short, Mr. Shays gave me his attention and respect and listened to my point of view and that of the ANA with political tact. He said that he appreciated my taking time to meet with him and share my views on the subject as a voter and student nurse. He found the issue to be especially important in Connecticut because our state is currently facing crises in regard to high medical malpractice insurance rates and a large number of physicians having to end their practice because of these rates. Mr. Shays shared his belief that it is critical to reform medical malpractice to provide quality, affordable health care. He explained his view that

excessive jury awards have driven the cost of health care up for everyone and that he believes a noneconomic damage cap of $250,000 will help in containing health care costs and make insurance more affordable to Americans. I was able to reiterate the ANA's view of postponing judgment on the institution of a medical malpractice cap until an impartial commission could complete and release a report on the effect of the controversial topic, helping him to make an informed decision. I thanked Mr. Shays for his time, and he thanked me for sharing my views on the subject and wished me luck in my study of such a "noble profession." It was thrilling to talk to Mr. Shays, if only briefly, and to feel like such an important part of the legislative process. Nurses definitely have the power to impact our nation's health care legislation.

—*Maureen McFadden, Georgetown University*

BOX 7-1 EXAMPLE OF AN E-MAIL TO CONGRESS TO SUPPORT FUNDING FOR THE NURSE REINVESTMENT ACT (NRA)

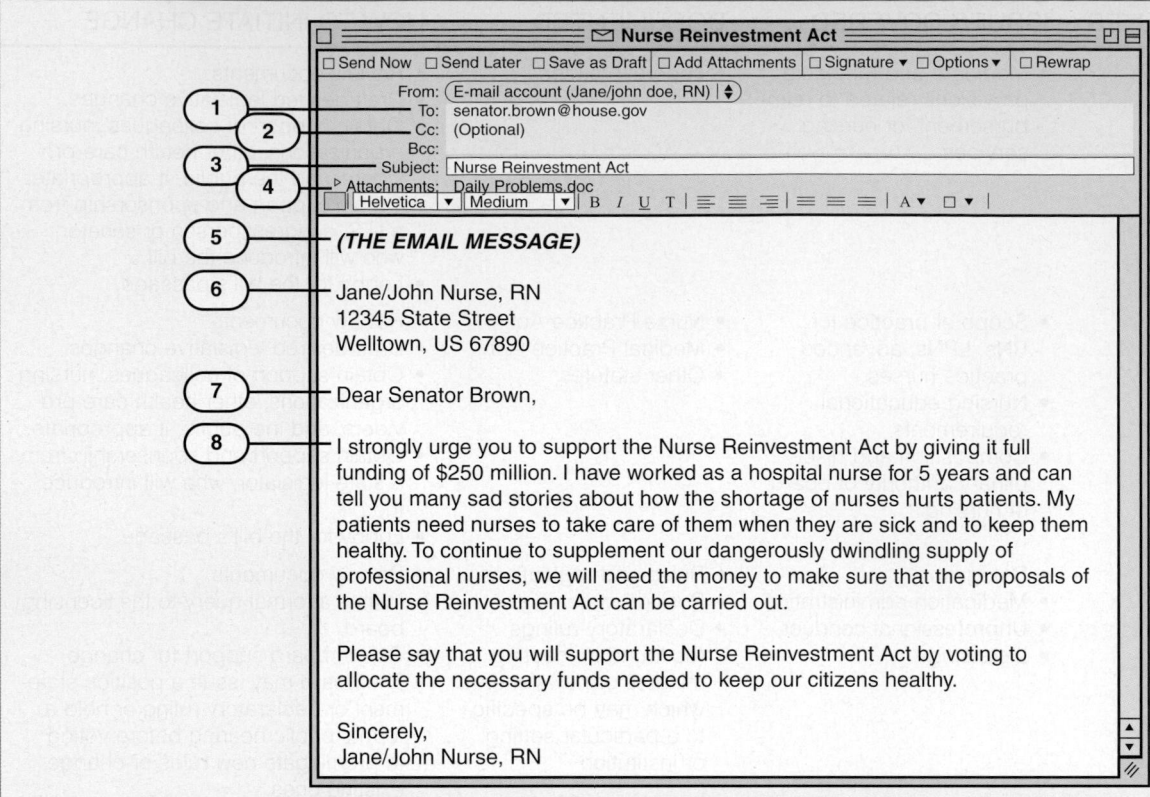

Explanation of Numbered Points

1. Use your Congress member's e-mail address, which can be found at http://www.house.gov and http://www.senate.gov. Send an individual e-mail to each member of Congress separately, with only one e-mail address in the "To:" line. You may want to send an e-mail to the member who represents voters from the place where you work, if you live in a different state or district from where you work. If you do this, be sure to write the e-mail to describe the impact that the legislation will have on your patients, who are the legislator's constituents.

2. You can copy this e-mail to a professional nursing organization or leave this blank. Do not copy it to another member of Congress.

3. State as clearly as possible the legislation you are addressing (e.g., nursing shortage). Although not necessary, you can use the bill number, if known.

4. If you want to attach a letter you have written that is longer and more fully explains your position, you may do so here.

5. An e-mail needs to be shorter and more succinct than a letter. The person reading it should be able to view your entire message on one screen without scrolling down. If you want to write more, attach a letter.

6. Put your name and address at the top to show the legislator that you are a voter in his or her district or state.

7. The legislator's title—either "Representative" or "Senator"—and last name make up the salutation.

8. Body of the e-mail:
   • State what you want the legislator to do in the first sentence.
   • Identify yourself as a concerned nurse.
   • Tell why the legislator should do what you are asking.
   • Ask the legislator to vote for/support what you are asking.

Finally, use spell-check and reread the e-mail to make sure the message you want to get across is clear and concise.

Used with permission. Sharp, N. (2003). The "write stuff." *Nursing Spectrum, 13*(2), 12–13.

Standards

Voluntary standards, developed and implemented by the nursing profession itself, are not mandatory but are used as guidelines for peer review. Professional nursing organizations continually reassess the functions, standards, and qualifications of their members. These organizations are guided by their own assessment of society's need for nursing and by the public's expectations of nursing. Examples of voluntary standards include the American Nurses Association (ANA) standards of practice (see Chapter 1), professional standards for the accreditation of education programs and service organizations, and standards for the certification of individual nurses in general and specialty areas of practice.

Legal standards, on the other hand, are developed by a legislature and are implemented by authority granted by the state to determine minimum standards for the education of nurses, to set requirements for licensure or registration, and to decide when a nurse's license may be suspended or revoked. Examples of legal standards include state Nurse Practice Acts and rules and regulations of nursing.

Credentialing

Nursing has taken several steps to ensure the competence of its practitioners, including the credentialing process. **Credentialing** refers to ways in which professional competence is ensured and maintained.

Three processes are used for credentialing in nursing. The first is **accreditation**, which is the process by which an educational program is evaluated and recognized as having met certain standards. The second is **licensure**, which is the process by which a state determines that a candidate meets certain minimum requirements to practice in the profession and grants a license to do so. The third is **certification**, which is the process by which a person who has met certain criteria established by a nongovernmental association is granted recognition in a specified practice area.

Accreditation

State constitutions give states a responsibility for the public welfare. State legislative bodies have used this principle to enact laws controlling occupational and professional groups. One function of these laws is to see that schools preparing practitioners maintain minimum standards of education. Nursing, like most other health care professions, operates under state laws that promote the general welfare by determining minimum standards of education through accreditation of schools of nursing. State-approved, or accredited, educational programs in nursing include practical or vocational, associate degree, diploma, baccalaureate, and graduate programs in nursing (see Chapter 1).

Legal accreditation of a school preparing nursing personnel by the state Board of Nursing is different from voluntary accreditation. The National League for Nursing Accrediting Commission (NLNAC) and the American Association of Colleges of Nursing (AACN) are voluntary agencies that accredit schools when they meet certain criteria. Most schools choose to seek this voluntary accreditation, and many prospective students prefer selecting accredited schools. Accreditation by NLNAC or AACN is not a legal requirement for a school to exist; state accreditation is a legal requirement.

Licensure

Licensure is a specialized form of credentialing based on laws passed by a state legislature. A license is a legal document that permits a person to offer to the public skills and knowledge in a particular jurisdiction, where such practice would otherwise be unlawful without a license. Licensure is discussed in Chapter 1. In addition to successfully completing an accredited nursing program of study and passing the National Council Licensure Examination (NCLEX), to maintain a license in good standing a nurse must meet other requirements as determined by the state or territory. These requirements typically include good moral character, continuing clinical competence or continuing education, the absence of a criminal record, English proficiency, and compliance with specific provisions of the state's nursing laws (Brous, 2012).

According to the National Council of State Boards of Nursing, a mutual recognition model of nurse licensure allows a nurse to have one license in his or her state of residency and to practice in other states (both physically and electronically) as well, subject to each state's practice law and regulation, unless otherwise restricted. This multistate nurse licensure model is governed by the Nurse Licensure Compact (NLC). All states that currently belong to the NLC also operate the single-state licensure model for those nurses who reside legally in an NLC state but do not qualify for multistate licensure. *You must legally reside in an NLC state to be eligible for a multistate license.* For questions related to the multistate license or privilege to practice, contact the Board of Nursing in your state of residence (https://www.ncsbn.org/nlc.htm).

Once earned, a license to practice is a property right and may not be revoked without due process. This includes notice of an investigation, a fair and impartial hearing, and a proper decision based on substantial evidence. Crucial to a nurse's successful defense are early legal counsel, character and expert witnesses, and thorough preparation for all proceedings.

State boards of nursing may revoke or suspend a nurse's license or registration for various reasons. Drug or alcohol abuse is currently the most frequent reason. Other reasons for revocation or suspension of a license or registration include fraud, deceptive practices, criminal acts, previous disciplinary action by other state boards, gross or ordinary negligence, and physical or mental impairments, including those resulting from aging.

Certification

Whereas licensure measures entry-level competence, certification validates specialty knowledge, experience, and clinical judgment. Nursing certification is offered by many U.S. professional organizations, including two primary organizations: the American Association of Critical-Care Nurses, which represents the specialty with the largest number of certified nurses, and the American Nurses Credentialing Center, a subsidiary of ANA, which began certifying nurses in 1974. The latter is the largest and most prestigious nurse credentialing organization in the United States and has certified more than a quarter million nurses since 1990 (http://www.nursecredentialing.org/Certification.aspx). Although certification, which involves special testing, is voluntary, nurse specialists are increasingly becoming certified.

Certification is one means to demonstrate advanced proficiency and a commitment to ensuring competence in the context of the current U.S. health care crisis, evidenced by daily reports of unsafe care, rising litigation, escalating costs, and a worsening nursing shortage.

 Concept Mastery Alert

Nursing deals with the public. Thus, the ultimate goal of all laws and professional regulations involved with nursing practice is public safety.

CRIMES AND TORTS

A wrong committed against a person or that person's property may be categorized as a crime or a tort, or sometimes both. A **crime** is a violation punishable by the state, whereas a **tort** is subject to action in a civil court with damages usually being settled with money. By its very nature, a wrong tried as a crime is considered a more serious offense, with more legal implications, than a tort.

Crime

Though there may only be one victim of a crime, criminal acts are considered to be against the public as well. In a criminal case, the government, called "the people," prosecutes the offender. When a crime is committed, the factor of intent to commit wrong is present in most cases. Nonetheless, people who break certain laws are guilty of a crime regardless of whether they intended it. For example, failure to observe the Federal Food, Drug, and Cosmetic Act may constitute a crime.

Criminal law is in most cases statutory law (e.g., Federal Controlled Substance Acts and kidnapping laws or state criminal codes that define murder, manslaughter, criminal negligence, rape, fraud, illegal possession of drugs, theft, assault and battery); only infrequently is it common law. Examples of common law are informed consent and the right to refuse treatment. Crimes are further classified as misdemeanors or felonies. A **misdemeanor** is a less serious crime, commonly punishable with a fine, imprisonment for less than 1 year, or both, or with parole. A **felony** (e.g., rape, murder) is punishable by imprisonment in a state or federal penitentiary for more than 1 year.

Torts

Torts may be intentional or unintentional acts of wrongdoing. Some of the intentional torts for which nurses may be held liable include assault and battery, defamation of character, invasion of privacy, false imprisonment, and fraud. A person committing an intentional tort is considered to have knowledge of the permitted legal limits of his or her words or acts. Violating these limits is grounds for prosecution. For example, although a policy specifies that a nurse may use restraints to protect an incompetent patient, restraining a competent patient to administer medications forcefully while the patient is refusing is assault and battery. Unintentional torts are referred to as negligence. A nurse who fails to initiate proper precautions to prevent patient harm (falls, skin breakdown) is subject to the charge of negligence. The nurse may not intend to cause harm, but harm results nevertheless.

An act that is a tort may also be a crime. For example, gross negligence demonstrating that the offender is guilty of complete disregard for another's life may be tried as both a civil and criminal action. It is then prosecuted under both civil and criminal law.

Intentional Torts

ASSAULT AND BATTERY

Assault is a threat or an attempt to make bodily contact with another person without that person's consent. **Battery** is an assault that is carried out and includes willful, angry, and violent or negligent touching of another person's body or clothes or anything attached to or held by that other person. Forcibly removing a patient's clothing, administering an injection after the patient has refused it, and pushing a patient into a chair are all examples of battery. Threatening to do any of these actions if the patient does not cooperate is assault. If an aggressive patient threatens harm, only actions necessary for self-protection or the aid of another are permitted.

Every individual has the right to be free from invasion of one's person, and adult patients who are alert and oriented have the right to refuse any treatment. The fact that treatment is desirable does not allow the nurse or physician to proceed without the consent of the patient or to go beyond the limits to which the patient has consented (see "Informed Consent or Refusal" within "Legal Safeguards for the Nurse").

DEFAMATION

Defamation of character is an intentional tort in which one party makes derogatory remarks about another that diminish the other party's reputation. Slander is spoken defamation of character; libel is written defamation. Defamation of character is grounds for an award of civil damages. Damages are awarded to the plaintiff based on the amount of harm done to the plaintiff. Nurses who make false or exaggerated statements about their patients or coworkers run the risk of being sued for slander or libel. A person charged with slander or libel may be found not liable if it can be proved that the statement was made not to injure another but was made for a nonmalicious, justifiable purpose. Social media have created new opportunities for defamation. Be familiar with guidelines for use of social media issued by the National Student Nurses' Association, American Nurses Association, and the National Council State Boards of Nursing. Read more about social media in Chapter 20.

INVASION OF PRIVACY

The U.S. Supreme Court has interpreted the right against invasion of privacy as a constitutional right. The Fourth Amendment gives citizens the right of privacy and the right to be left alone. State courts have also strongly protected a patient's right to have information kept confidential. What is confidential? All information about patients is considered private or confidential, whether written on paper, saved on a computer, or spoken aloud. This includes their name and all identifiers such as address, telephone and fax numbers, Social Security number, and any other personal information. It also includes the reason that the patient is sick or in the hospital, office, or clinic, the treatments the patient receives, and information about past health conditions. Protected health information may be found in the patient medical record, computer systems, telephone calls and voice mails, fax transmissions, e-mails that contain patient information, and conversations about patients between clinical staff.

The Health Insurance Portability and Accountability Act (HIPAA) was finalized in 2002. Most agencies now require workers to undergo HIPAA training and to review and sign a confidentiality agreement when hired and at each performance review. As a student in a health care setting, you should discuss privacy guidelines with your instructor and nurse mentors. HIPAA ensures that patients have a right:

- To see and copy their health record
- To update their health record
- To request correction of any mistakes
- To get a list of the disclosures a health care institution has made independent of disclosures made for the purposes of treatment, payment, and health care operations
- To request a restriction on certain uses or disclosures
- To choose how to receive health information

If a health institution wants to release a patient's health information for purposes other than treatment, payment, and routine health care operations, the patient must sign an authorization. Box 16-2 in Chapter 16 gives a list of permitted disclosures of patient health information and incidental disclosures. Other disclosure of confidential information, such as inappropriately discussing a patient's problem with a third party, may be construed as invasion of privacy and may subject the nurse to liability. The nurse's intimate knowledge of the patient increases legal risk in this regard.

The doctrine of privileged communication specifies that people in a protected relationship, such as a doctor and patient, cannot be forced, even during legal proceedings, to reveal communication between them unless the person who benefits from the protection agrees to it. State laws determine which relationships are protected by the privilege doctrine, and not all states privilege nurse–patient communication.

HIPAA includes punishments for anyone caught violating patient privacy: Those who do so for financial gain can be fined as much as $250,000 or be jailed for up to 10 years.

Even accidentally breaking the rules can result in penalties—and embarrassment—for you and your organization.

Certain acts by nurses could constitute invasion of privacy, as the following examples illustrate:

- Unnecessary exposure of patients while moving them through a corridor or while caring for them in rooms they share with others
- Talking with patients in rooms that are not soundproof
- Discussing patient information with people not entitled to the information (e.g., with the patient's employer or the press, or even the patient's family if not authorized to do so)
- Pressing the patient for information not necessary for care planning
- Interacting with the patient's family in ways not authorized by the patient
- Using tape recorders, dictating machines, computers, and the like without taking precautions to ensure the patient's confidentiality (see Chapter 16 and Box 7-2)
- Preparing written or oral class assignments about patients without concealing their identity
- Carrying out research without taking proper precautions to ensure the anonymity of patients

At times, a person's right to privacy may conflict with other rights, such as the public's right to information. When in doubt about disclosing confidential information, consult the nursing supervisor, ethics committee, or public relations department of the institution.

FALSE IMPRISONMENT

Unjustified retention or prevention of the movement of another person without proper consent can constitute false

BOX 7-2 PRIVACY AND CONFIDENTIALITY OF HEALTH CARE RECORDS

Security measures that a nurse should be aware of, particularly when using computerized health care records, include the following:

- Authorized users of an automated information system should have individual passwords and identification codes that are changed frequently. Nurses should never allow anyone else to use their log-on ID, nor should they perform any function using another person's log-on ID.
- Terminals, including those at the point of care, should have key locks as an additional measure to prevent unauthorized access to data.
- The computer system should "time out" when not in use for a specific period of time. The authorized user then needs to reenter the password and identification code to regain access.
- Nurses should log off the system when they leave a workstation and take other reasonable measures to ensure that unauthorized users cannot view or access confidential information.
  - Temporary employees, such as traveling nurses, should have temporary passwords assigned.
- Employees who leave the organization should have their passwords and IDs terminated.
- The system should be able to track which users viewed, deleted, or updated patient information.

- Some information, such as results of acquired immunodeficiency syndrome testing, should not be stored on a computer.
- Computer printouts must be discarded appropriately because they may contain sensitive data about a patient.
  - Nurses should not copy or provide data, either in printed or machine-readable form, for themselves or anyone else except as required to fulfill the responsibilities of their jobs.
  - Most nurses sign agreements that they will use Internet access only to perform the responsibilities of their job. Internet access is not to be used for non–job-related business.
- The organization should have a policy regarding the use of patient data in research. Patient identifiers should be removed before the data are analyzed.
- Every nurse must be aware of the laws and statutes that protect the confidentiality of medical records. Most states have guidelines on the sharing of medical information. Your State Board of Nursing may revoke your license for serious breaches of patient confidentiality.

Protecting the privacy and confidentiality of health care records is the duty of every nurse. Any nurse who is aware of an actual or suspected breach of confidentiality must report it.

imprisonment. For example, only a reasonable amount of restraint should be used in circumstances that warrant it. The indiscriminate and thoughtless use of restraints on a patient can constitute false imprisonment.

A person cannot be legally forced to remain in a health agency, such as a hospital, if that person is of sound mind, even when health practitioners believe that the individual should remain for additional care. Health agencies have special forms to use when a patient insists on being discharged against medical orders. The patient signs to indicate not holding the agency responsible for any harm that may result from leaving. People who are mentally ill may be committed to a psychiatric institution for treatment without their consent (involuntary commitment) only when it can be proved that they may be harmful to themselves or others.

FRAUD

Fraud is willful and purposeful misrepresentation that could cause, or has caused, loss or harm to a person or property. Misrepresentation of a product is a common fraudulent act. A person fraudulently misrepresenting oneself to obtain a license to practice nursing may be prosecuted under the state's Nurse Practice Act. Also, misrepresenting the outcome of a procedure or treatment may constitute fraud.

Unintentional Torts

NEGLIGENCE AND MALPRACTICE

Negligence is defined as performing an act that a reasonably prudent person under similar circumstances would not do or, conversely, failing to perform an act that a reasonably prudent person under similar circumstances would do. As the definition implies, an act of negligence may be an act of omission or commission. **Malpractice** is the term generally used to describe negligence by professional personnel. Reising (2012) identifies the following common categories of malpractice claims:

- Failure to follow standards of care: for example, you fail to follow the standards for administering insulin or other injectable medications
- Failure to use equipment in a responsible manner: for example, you attempt to use a bariatric patient lift for the first time without getting help and the patient falls
- Failure to assess and monitor: for example, you fail to follow your hospital's standards for postoperative assessments after receiving a patient from the operating room and response to a ruptured suture line is delayed
- Failure to communicate: for example, you fail to communicate your concerns about an elderly patient being discharged home; she lives alone and is soon rehospitalized because no provisions were made to secure the nursing care she needed after discharge
- Failure to document: for example, you work up the chain of command when your repeated calls to a physician to see a patient that you believe is in danger of arresting are ignored. Before any physician sees the patient, he arrests and, despite a code, dies. You document the arrest, code, and death but fail to document all the steps you took to

get the patient the medical attention he needed. Sixteen months later, the family sues and you try to remember what action you took that evening—most of which was never recorded.

- Failure to act as a patient advocate or to follow the chain of command: for example, you are in the operating room and watch a surgeon break the sterile field twice. No one else seems to notice. You are intimidated by this surgeon and fail to bring this to anyone's attention. You learn that the patient developed a serious infection postoperatively.

ELEMENTS OF LIABILITY

Liability involves four elements that must be established to prove that malpractice or negligence has occurred: duty, breach of duty, causation, and damages. Duty refers to an obligation to use due care (what a reasonably prudent nurse would do) and is defined by the standard of care appropriate for the nurse–patient relationship. Breach of duty is the failure to meet the standard of care. Causation, the most difficult element of liability to prove, shows that the failure to meet the standard of care (breach) actually caused the injury. Damages are the actual harm or injury resulting to the patient. Examples of these four elements are presented in Table 7-2.

STANDARDS OF CARE

Whether negligence has occurred depends on a standard of care—what a reasonably prudent person would or would not have done under similar circumstances. All nurses are responsible for following the standards of care for their particular

Table 7-2 | PROOF OF MALPRACTICE

An example of how a plaintiff (person bringing the lawsuit) proves that the nurse defendants are guilty of malpractice.

ELEMENT	EXAMPLE
Duty	Hospital staff nurses are responsible for: • Accurate assessment of patients assigned to their care • Alerting responsible health care professionals to changes in a patient's condition • Competent execution of safety measures for patients
Breach of duty	• Failure to note and report that an older adult patient assessed as alert on admission is exhibiting periods of confusion • Failure to execute and document use of appropriate safety measures (e.g., upper and lower bedside rails, use of restraints if necessary, assisted ambulation)
Causation	• Failure to use appropriate safety measures; this failure causes the patient to fall while attempting to get out of bed, resulting in a fractured left hip
Damages	• Fractured left hip, pain and suffering, lengthened hospital stay, and need for rehabilitation

areas of practice. For example, labor and delivery nurses must understand how standards for nursing practice differ from those for medical obstetric practice (according to the state's Nurse Practice Act), must be familiar with specific standards for obstetric nursing (e.g., Association of Women's Health, Obstetrics, and Neonatal Nursing [AWHONN]), and must carry out the nursing responsibilities detailed in the hospi-

tal's policies and procedures and in their job description. If hospital policy dictates an assessment of each woman in the early stages of labor every 30 minutes, for example, nurses must adhere to this standard unless they document a reason for doing otherwise.

Table 7-3 lists areas of potential liability associated with each of the ANA standards of clinical nursing practice.

Table 7-3 AREAS OF POTENTIAL LIABILITY FOR NURSES	
AREAS OF POTENTIAL LIABILITY	**EXAMPLES**
Standard I: Assessment The nurse collects patient health data. • Incomplete database obtained (occurs frequently when patient is too ill at admission to respond to questions) • Significant omissions or errors in recorded database • Failure to note in the patient's plan of care (and to execute) the need for more frequent nursing assessments • Failure to recognize and to report significant changes in the patient's condition	• Child too weak to be weighed on admission; chart contains no record of patient's weight; dosage of postoperative antibiotic therapy (which should be calculated on child's weight) too small to prevent infection; abscess develops • Nurse fails to detect and report observable signs that an older patient is at risk for abuse in her home from her granddaughter • Previously alert patient was exhibiting periods of confusion; found beating roommate with a hairbrush • Mother's labor is failing to progress, nurses unaware of signs of fetal distress; obstetrician not informed; irreversible cerebral damage to fetus • Healthy patient making slower than usual postanesthesia recovery; signs of developing cerebrovascular accident (slurred speech, difficulty moving extremities, falling to one side) present and unnoted
Standard II: Diagnosis The nurse analyzes the assessment data in determining diagnoses. • Failure to identify priority nursing diagnosis critical to the patient's care • Nursing diagnosis incorrectly developed and "labels" the patient negatively	• Nowhere in the resident's plan of care was it noted that the patient had a history of choking on food ("impaired swallowing") and that close supervision was indicated during meals; patient aspirated brussels sprout and died. • Homosexual male patient without acquired immunodeficiency syndrome (AIDS) admitted for gallbladder surgery questions the few interactions he has with staff; nursing diagnosis on Kardex reads "High Risk for Violence: Directed at Others (AIDS), related to homosexuality"
Standards III and IV: Outcome Identification and Planning The nurse identifies expected outcomes individualized to the patient and develops a plan of care that prescribes interventions to attain expected outcomes. • No indication in nursing care plan that nurses were aware of and sensitive to the patient's healthcare priorities	• Obese patient with a history of impaired circulation continually refuses to ambulate after major abdominal surgery; patient dies after a massive pulmonary embolism; plan of care showed no concern or attempt to compensate for patient's lack of mobility; family states that no nurse consulted them to encourage mobility
Standard V: Implementation The nurse implements the interventions identified in the plan of care. • Patient's record contains no documentation of attempts to teach appropriate self-care measures to patient and family • Nursing interventions deviate from usual standard of care (understaffing, indifference on part of nurse, inexperience of nurse, faulty or scarce equipment or resources)	• Male patient discharged from short-procedure unit on crutches; falls first day home, refracturing leg; alleges his not receiving instructions for crutch walking caused fall; patient record contains no documentation of client education • Skin breakdown on frail, older, homebound patient worsens with eventual muscle deterioration; sepsis; nurses seem confused about treatment regimen for pressure ulcers; treatment is inconsistent
Standard VI: Evaluation The nurse evaluates the patient's progress toward attainment of outcomes. • No evidence in plan of care and nursing notes that nurses evaluated whether the patient achieved target goals • Patient discharged before key goals are met and without follow-up instruction	• Male patient, newly started on insulin therapy, discharged after giving himself the insulin only once, and without understanding the relationship among food, exercise, and insulin. No referral made to visiting nurse; patient readmitted after 2 weeks with dangerously low blood sugar after overdose with insulin

American Nurses Association. (2010). *Nursing scope and standards of practice, 2010 edition.* Washington, DC: Author.

Nursing errors can result in serious outcomes for the patient, as these examples show. To read more about standards, see Chapters 13 and 15.

Malpractice Litigation

When a patient believes he or she has been injured because of the negligence of a nurse or other health care professional and pursues legal action, one of three outcomes usually occurs:

- All parties work toward a fair settlement.
- The case is presented to a malpractice arbitration panel (in the United States).
- The case is brought to trial court.

The steps involved in malpractice litigation are as follows:

1. The basis for the claim is determined to be appropriate and timely; all elements of liability are present (duty, breach of duty, causation, and serious damages).
2. All parties named as defendants (nurses, physicians, health care agency), as well as insurance companies and attorneys, work toward a fair settlement.
3. The case is presented to a malpractice arbitration panel. The panel's decision is either accepted or rejected, in which case a complaint is filed in trial court.
4. The defendants contest allegations (argue that there is no basis for alleging deviation from the appropriate standard of care or for proving causation and damages).
5. Pretrial discovery activities occur: review of medical records and depositions of plaintiff, defendants, and witnesses.
6. Trial takes place; both sides present their evidence and arguments.
7. Decision or verdict is reached by the judge and/or jury,
8. If the verdict is not accepted by both sides, it may be appealed to an appellate court.

The nurse may be involved in legal proceedings as a defendant, a fact witness, or an expert witness. For a tangible illustration of how the legal process operates, you and your class may want to implement the malpractice lawsuit simulation developed by Jenkins and Lemak (2009).

NURSE AS DEFENDANT

A nurse who is named a defendant should work closely with an attorney while preparing the defense. The attorney representing the nurse's interests is secured by either the nurse (if carrying personal liability insurance) or the employing agency. Recommendations for the nurse defendant include the following:

- Do not discuss the case with anyone at your agency (with the exception of the risk manager), with the plaintiff, with the plaintiff's lawyer, with anyone testifying for the plaintiff, or with reporters.
- Do not alter the patient's records. Tampering with a chart is the worst mistake you can make—you may well ruin your defense.
- Cooperate fully with your attorney. Do not hide any information from the attorney. Make sure you are fully prepared before you go on the witness stand.

- Be courteous on the witness stand. Do not volunteer any information.

NURSE AS FACT WITNESS

Either the defense or the prosecuting attorney may call a nurse who has knowledge of the actual incident prompting the legal case to testify as a **fact witness**. Fact witnesses, who are placed under oath, must base their testimony on only firsthand knowledge of the incident and not on assumptions. The nurse will be asked if the testimony is based on independent recollection of the incident or on documentation in the patient record. The nurse may testify, "I do not remember Ms. Jones, but I see from review of her record that I cared for her on the evenings of June 10, 13, 14, and 17." When in doubt about facts, the nurse should simply testify, "I do not remember that." New research into memory is showing that people often remember things differently from the way they were; this challenges the value of eyewitness memory. Thus, accurate documentation remains the nurse's best defense.

NURSE AS EXPERT WITNESS

A nurse may be called by either attorney to testify as an **expert witness** to explain to the judge and jury what happened based on the patient's record and to offer an opinion about whether the nursing care met acceptable standards. Nurse expert witnesses need a solid educational background and strong clinical experience comparable with those of the nurse defendant. The expert witness also needs an understanding of the legal aspects of nursing and malpractice liability as well as knowledge of the state Nurse Practice Act and the standard of nursing care where the incident occurred.

LEGAL SAFEGUARDS FOR THE NURSE

The U.S. health care system has a variety of safeguards to protect nurses from exposure to legal risks while performing the duties of their role and to ensure that the practice environment is geared towards enhancing patient and personal safety. As you read the following sections, consider the scenario featured in the Nursing Advocacy in Action display and the implications for nursing practice.

Competent Practice

Competent practice remains the nurse's most important and best legal safeguard (Fig. 7-1). Each nurse is responsible for making sure that one's educational background and clinical experience are adequate to fulfill the nursing responsibilities delineated in the job description. Legal safeguards include the following:

- Respecting legal boundaries of practice
- Following institutional procedures and policies
- "Owning" personal strengths and weaknesses; seeking means of growth, education, and supervised experience to ensure continued competence for new and evolving responsibilities
- Evaluating proposed assignments; refusing to accept responsibilities for which you are unprepared

NURSING ADVOCACY IN ACTION

Patient Scenario

Mr. Spahn is a 49-year-old attorney who suffered a cerebral bleed. After his brain surgery, his surgeon informed the family that Mr. Spahn has massive, irreversible neurologic damage. In short, barring an act of God or nature he will have no meaningful recovery. His wife is already suing the first hospital that treated her husband because they delayed performing the appropriate diagnostic tests. She and her daughter complain frequently about the nursing care Mr. Spahn is receiving now, and no one wants to take care of him because they are afraid of being named in a lawsuit. Mrs. Spahn keeps a notebook in which she writes down the name of every caregiver who helps her husband. She has placed numerous calls to complain to administration about everything from the cleanliness of the room to a torn sheet.

You believe that he is receiving less than optimal care because everyone is afraid of his family bringing a lawsuit.

Implications for Nursing Advocacy

How will you act if you are Mr. Spahn's nurse? Talk with your classmates and experienced nurses about the questions that follow.

- If you elect to advocate for Mr. Spahn, what practical steps can you take to ensure better health outcomes?
- What is it reasonable to expect of a student nurse, a graduate nurse, and an experienced nurse in this situation?
- What advocacy skills are needed to effectively respond to this challenge?

- Keeping current in nursing knowledge and skills
- Respecting patient rights and developing rapport with patients
- Keeping careful documentation
- Working within the agency to develop and support management policies

 THINK back to Ella Rodriguez, the girl with a fractured arm requiring the administration of sedation according to the agency's protocol. The nurse should incorporate knowledge of the legal safeguards for competent practice when preparing to administer the medication as well as knowledge of the unit's protocol. In addition, the nurse should identify personal limitations and confront the physician, stressing the need for his presence to ensure the patient's safety. ●

FIGURE 7-1. Competent practice is the nurse's most important legal safeguard. Careful documentation ensures a record of competent practice.

Competent practice includes developing sensitivity to common sources of patient injury, such as falls, restraints, and malfunctioning equipment, and then taking specific measures to prevent patient injury. Box 7-3 (on page 124) lists the most frequent allegations against nurses and related prevention tips.

The Impaired Nurse

About 1 in 10, or 10% to 15% of all nurses, may be impaired or in recovery from alcohol or drug addiction (Thomas & Siela, 2011). The stresses involved in nursing and health care combined with the availability of controlled substances makes nurses prime candidates for alcohol and drug addiction problems. Startlingly, more than half of all impaired nurses began abusing during their nursing education days. In the past, nurses with substance abuse problems usually were promptly punished by firing and license suspension. Today, substance abuse is recognized as a treatable disorder; the objective is to detect problems early and get nurses into treatment. The American Nurses Association strongly supports "alternative to discipline" or "peer assistance" programs and has an impaired nurse resource center. Students should recognize their level of risk and know to seek help promptly if they suspect a personal problem or a problem on the part of a classmate or colleague. Students can talk with a trusted faculty member. Practicing nurses should consult management. Box 7-4 describes signs and symptoms to watch for. The public's trust and well-being and the well-being of the nurse are both at stake.

Informed Consent or Refusal

Every person is granted freedom from bodily contact by another person unless consent is granted. In most states, you must be 18 to legally provide medical consent. States vary in the types of medical treatment they allow minors to authorize without their parents. Be sure to check your state law. In all health care agencies, informed and voluntary consent is needed for admission, for each specialized diagnostic or treatment procedure, and for any experimental treatments or procedures. The consent must be written, designated for the

BOX 7-3 NURSING MALPRACTICE PREVENTION

Most Frequent Allegations Against Nurses and Related Prevention Tips

1. **Failure to ensure patient safety**
   - Monitor patients in a timely manner consistent with agency policy and the changing needs of the patient. Assess and document potential for injury. Incorporate safety needs into the plan of care.
   - Clearly define criteria for use of restrictive devices. Ensure that the use of restrictive devices is consistent with agency policy. Use the least restrictive devices that will be effective in preventing injury.
   - Update your knowledge involving patient safety and new interventions to prevent and reduce injury.
   - Evaluate whether patients at high risk for injury are routinely identified before injury results.

2. **Improper treatment or performance of treatment**
   - Question treatments that you believe are improper. Know your agency's policy for questioning a problematic order.
   - Use proper techniques when performing procedures, and follow agency procedures.
   - Seek assistance when unsure of a new procedure. Never perform an intervention until you know what you are doing, why you are doing it, and your ongoing assessment and teaching responsibilities.
   - Update your clinical skills through continuing education classes, conferences, and workshops.

3. **Failure to monitor and report**
   - Follow physician orders regarding monitoring of patients unless changes in the patient's condition necessitate a change in the frequency of monitoring; report the need for change to the physician.
   - Report any requested information or significant changes in a patient's condition. If unsure of the significance of an observed change, consult with an experienced colleague.
   - Perform appropriate and timely nursing assessments.
   - Ensure that the nurse–patient ratio is adequate.

4. **Medication errors and reactions**
   - Verify any questionable medical orders.
   - Verify patient's name and date of birth before administering medication and use appropriate agency-specific identifiers such as bar coding.
   - Listen to any patient questions or objections regarding a medication, and investigate the patient's concerns before administering the medication.
   - Refer to a drug reference for any questions about appropriate dosages, side effects, and reactions.
   - Know your agency's policies on verbal and written medication orders and on medication administration.
   - Update your knowledge of medications and new medication administration protocols.

5. **Failure to follow agency procedure**
   - Know your agency's procedures. Ensure that your orientation to new responsibilities familiarizes you with pertinent policies and procedures.
   - If you must deviate from a procedure, discuss the incident with your supervisor and decide on appropriate action.
   - Advise the appropriate person of procedures that need to be revised.

6. **Documentation**
   - Document significant information about your patients objectively and factually.
   - Know and follow the agency's documentation policies.
   - Document specific times that you performed actions, made observations, or performed patient assessments.
   - Document legibly when writing, spell correctly, and use only agency-approved abbreviations.
   - Be sensitive to privacy considerations when documenting on a computer.
   - Routinely evaluate the quality of documentation and update your knowledge of new documentation methodologies.

7. **Equipment use**
   - Learn how to operate equipment in a safe and appropriate manner. Never operate equipment with which you are unfamiliar.
   - Use predetermined procedures when teaching patients how to use equipment, and ensure that all nurses involved in client education are teaching the same procedures.
   - Provide home care patients with the telephone number of a 24-hour backup hospital or home care service available in case of emergency.
   - Have patients demonstrate their competence with equipment before allowing them to use it.
   - Attend orientations and in-services on the use of new or modified equipment.

8. **Adverse incidents**
   - If an adverse incident occurs, complete the appropriate documentation and report the incident to the designated person following agency policy.
   - Do not assume, voice, or record any blame for the incident.
   - Know the institutional chain of command for reporting instances when patient care is at issue.
   - Support agency loss prevention programs that identify potential liabilities, guard against patient injuries, and maximize the defense of the agency and its employee nurses.

9. **Clients with human immunodeficiency virus (HIV)**
   - Be conscious of actions that could result in a lawsuit:
     - Discrimination in treatment
     - Nosocomial (in-hospital) transmission of virus
     - Breach of confidentiality
     - Participation in testing a patient for HIV without first obtaining informed consent
   - Know and follow agency policies and procedures for the care of patients with infectious diseases.
   - Update your knowledge of HIV infection; be familiar with national standards (such as those established by the Centers for Disease Control and Prevention) and pertinent state/province laws.

procedure to be performed, and signed by the patient or person legally responsible for the patient. A signed consent is not needed in an emergency if there is an immediate threat to life or health, if experts would agree that it is an emergency, and if the patient is unable to consent and a legally authorized person cannot be reached. While informed consent is a protection against lawsuits, the central values underlying informed consent include promoting the patient's well-being and respecting the patient's self-determination (President's Commission for the Study of Ethical Problems in Medicine

BOX 7-4	**SIGNS AND SYMPTOMS OF A SUBSTANCE-ABUSING NURSE**

As nurses we care for our patients, but we don't always care for our coworkers or ourselves. As you read the list below, you may discover that you are working with or have worked with a nurse who displays signs, symptoms, and behavioral changes that may indicate substance abuse.

Signs/Symptoms	Physical Signs	Behavior Changes
Brief, unexplained absences from the nursing unit	Shakiness and/or tremors	Frequent mood changes
Rounding at odd hours	Fatigue	Outburst of anger
		Defensiveness
Medication errors	Slurred speech	Inappropriate laughter
Isolation from peers	Frequent use of mouthwash or breath mints	Hyperactivity or hypoactivity
Mood changes after meals or breaks	Watery eyes	Lack of concentration
		Blackout periods
Frequent reports of lack of pain relief from assigned patients	Constricted/dilated pupils	Justify the addiction to "relax," "need to escape reality"
Narcotic or Pyxis obsession, offering to medicate coworkers, patients	Diaphoresis	Cold weather clothing in warm weather to hide track marks
Wasted narcotics attributed to a single nurse	Unsteady gait	Frequent accidents or emergencies
Increased narcotic sign-outs	Frequent runny nose	Personal relationship issues
Discrepancies with the narcotic record and/or the patient record	Frequent nausea, vomiting and diarrhea	Insomnia
		Frequent complaints of pain
Altered verbal or telephone medication orders	Weight gain or loss	Denial of problem
		Frequent lying
Decreased quality of care, documentation arriving late to work and requesting to leave early	Change in grooming	Decreased judgment in their own performance

Reprinted with permission from Thomas, C. M., & Siela, D. (2011). The impaired nurse: Would you know what to do if you suspected substance abuse? *American Nurse Today, 6*(8).

and Biomedical and Behavioral Research, 1982). For this reason, you should make sure that patients understand all the information they need to validly consent to or refuse what is being proposed. If patients do not speak English, they require the services of a translator. Be sure to check your agency's policies about translation and be familiar with resources. Using a family member to translate is rarely acceptable. Similarly, patients with low literacy may be unable to read what they are signing and require extra help. Elements of informed consent include disclosure, comprehension, competence, and voluntariness (Box 7-5).

Obtaining informed consent is the responsibility of the person who will perform the diagnostic or treatment procedure or the research study. Your role as a nurse is to confirm that a signed consent form is present in the patient's chart and to answer any patient questions about the consent. In some instances, you may be responsible for having a patient sign the consent form after a physician has explained the procedure, its risks and benefits, and alternative treatments to the patient. Increasingly, nurses are performing procedures requiring consent or are part of interdisciplinary teams that meet with the patient to obtain consent for complex interventions (e.g., bone marrow transplantation).

Documenting the consent process with a printed consent form should not be confused with the actual explanation given to the patient and the informed consent itself. When

BOX 7-5	**CHECKLIST TO ENSURE INFORMED CONSENT**

Disclosure

Patient/surrogate has been informed of the (1) nature of the procedure, (2) risks (nature of the risk, magnitude, probability that the risk will materialize) and benefits, (3) alternatives (including the option of nontreatment), and (4) fact that no outcomes can be guaranteed.

Comprehension

Patient/surrogate can correctly repeat in his or her own words that for which the patient/surrogate is giving consent.

Competence

The patient understands the information needed to make *this* decision, is able to reason in accord with a relatively consistent set of values, and can communicate a preference.

The surrogate (if needed) meets the above criteria, knows the patient's wishes to the extent that this is possible, and is free from undue emotional stress and conflict of interests.

Voluntariness

The patient is voluntarily consenting or refusing. Care has been taken to avoid manipulative and coercive influences.

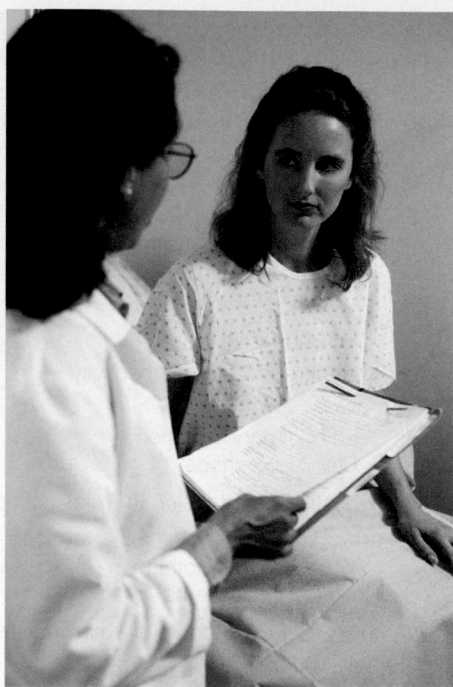

FIGURE 7-2. Informed consent is a process. A mere signature does not guarantee each of the elements of consent: disclosure, comprehension, competence, and voluntariness.

documenting consent, assess whether patients understand what they are signing and are acting voluntarily, and report any problems to the clinician doing the procedure. Having patients describe in their own words what they understand they are consenting to is the best way to make sure that they understand. Nurses often question the patient's understanding of the proposed procedure and its risks or the patient's ability to consent voluntarily to the procedure. Impediments include the effects of anxiety, pain, medication, depression, language barriers, and temporary or permanent states of disorientation and confusion. Unless you are obtaining consent for a nurse-prescribed and nurse-initiated intervention, as a nurse you sign the consent form as a witness to having seen the patient sign the form, not as having obtained the consent yourself (Fig. 7-2). Consequences of not obtaining a valid consent include the possibility of charges of battery against the nurse, the doctor, and the health care agency, which has a duty to protect patients and is responsible for its employees' actions.

 Concept Mastery Alert

Although there may be times when a nurse may be responsible for having a patient sign the consent form, in all instances, the nurse is responsible for answering any questions the patient may have and for making sure that the signed consent form is on the patient's chart. If the nurse determines that the patient is unsure or has questionable understanding, the nurse is responsible for notifying the person who had obtained the consent about the situation so that that person can clarify or re-explain the information.

A patient's refusal to sign a consent should be documented, and the patient should be informed of the possible consequences of the refusal. The patient should sign a release form indicating one's refusal to consent and releasing the nurse, physician, and agency from responsibility for outcomes of this act. This statement should be witnessed.

Contracts

A contract is an exchange of promises between two parties. The agreement may be in writing or oral, although oral contracts may be more difficult to prove. The law of contracts provides a remedy for a breach of contract so that the person who suffers from a broken contract may be compensated for any resulting loss. For a contract to be legally enforceable, it must involve real consent of the parties, a valid consideration, a lawful purpose, competent parties, and the format required by law.

Practicing nurses enter into legally valid and binding contracts with both their employers and their patients. Thus, it is important to understand and be able to fulfill the terms of a nursing agreement before agreeing to a contract. Your employment contract should specify what it is reasonable for you to expect of your employer and what the employer can expect of you. An employer that repeatedly expects you to assume supervisory responsibilities without benefit or who fires you without just cause is likely guilty of contract violations. Similarly, you may be guilty of contract violations if you refuse to accept reasonable assignments, repeatedly fail to arrive on time for work, or are habitually unable to complete reasonable work assignments. Any action by your employer that violates a federal or state law is the basis of a grievance, even if the employment contract permits the action. Examples include a female nurse receiving less pay for performing the same work as a male nurse, or a supervisor's failure to promote an employee based on race. When discrimination is suspected, complaints should be filed with the Equal Employment Opportunity Commission (EEOC).

Contracts with patients are often implied. There may not be a written contract specifying what is reasonable for patients to expect of nurses, but courts will uphold an implied contract obligating the nurse to be competent and to provide responsible care.

 REMEMBER Meredith Bedford, the mother of the terminally ill child threatening to sue the hospice. The nurse needs to understand the implied contract between the patient (and his family) and the health care team. ●

Collective Bargaining

The 2001 ANA Code of Ethics for Nurses states that the nurse "participates in establishing, maintaining and improving health care environments and conditions of employment conducive to the provision of quality health care and consistent with the values of the profession through individual and collective action."

Although individual contracts serve many nurses adequately, many nurses have joined other groups of workers whose interests are better protected when contracts are negotiated for them as a group. Collective bargaining is a legal process in which representatives of organized employees negotiate with employers about such matters as wages, hours, and conditions. Arbitration, strikes, and threats of strikes may be used to enhance the terms of employment and to enforce contracts. Many nurses choose their state nurses' association, rather than a trade organization, as their collective bargaining representative. Other nurses question whether collective bargaining is an appropriate role for a professional organization. When deciding whether to participate in collective bargaining, ask yourself:

* Will collective bargaining help my professional and economic status?
* Can I address my professional concerns through collective bargaining?
* Can I devote the time and effort that such organized activity demands?
* Can I change my working conditions as an individual, or do I need to organize with other nurses?

Patient Education

U.S. courts affirm the patients' right to know what is necessary to manage their health and view patient education as a legal duty of the nurse. Standards for patient education are derived from national professional standards and from state Nurse Practice Acts as well as the local standards described in agency policies, procedure manuals, and job descriptions. Special forms for documenting the nurse's assessment of the patient's learning needs and for subsequent teaching are available in some agencies. Failure to conduct or document an assessment of a patient's learning needs and teaching may later be construed as negligence.

Determine in your practice setting what specific aspects of patient education are the responsibility of nursing. Consult your job description, and be familiar with agency policies regarding patient education and its documentation. Remember that an important aim of nursing is to assist patients in managing their own care. Discuss the nursing plan of care with patients and family members, and identify their learning needs and learning readiness. Document the teaching plan as part of the nursing plan of care. Document all nursing efforts to educate the patient and family about health care management, and also document the patient's response. If a patient refuses health education or refers you to a family member (e.g., "Talk to my wife about my pills; she'll be giving them to me at home"), document this in the patient's record. If patient education greatly increases the patient's anxiety and the patient requests not to be given any more information, document the patient's initial response to teaching, the patient's request that it be stopped, and, if you complied, your reason for doing so.

Because a lack of time is frequently offered as the reason for failing to document patient education, assess what type of patient documentation is performed routinely in your setting. If possible, develop forms or checklists that will facilitate rapid documentation. For example, preoperative checklists make it easy to record preoperative teaching and are often introduced as evidence in court that preoperative teaching was done. Similarly, other forms have been developed for documenting diabetic patient teaching, teaching after a myocardial infarction, and teaching postpartum and baby care to mothers. The teaching role of the nurse is discussed in Chapter 21.

Executing Physician Orders

Nurses are legally responsible for carrying out the orders of the physician in charge of a patient unless a reasonable person would anticipate the order to lead to injury. Follow these guidelines:

1. Be familiar with the parties designated in your state's Nurse Practice Act who can legally write orders for the nurse to execute (in many states, a physician assistant cannot legally write orders for the nurse).
2. Be familiar with your institution's or agency's policy regarding physician orders.
3. Attempt to get all physicians' orders in writing. Verbal and telephone orders should be countersigned within 24 hours. Take the following steps to prevent errors caused by telephone orders:
   a. Limit telephone orders to true emergency situations when there is no alternative.
   b. Designate which nurses may take telephone orders (e.g., those who have more education and experience, such as primary nurses).
   c. Repeat the telephone order back to the physician for confirmation.
   d. Document the order, its time and date, the situation necessitating the order, the physician prescribing and reconfirming the order as it is read back, and your name; indicate if the order is a VO (verbal order) or TO (telephone order).
   e. When possible, have two nurses listen to a questionable telephone order, with both nurses countersigning the order. See Chapter 16 for additional guidelines on executing verbal, telephone, and fax orders.
4. Question any physician order that is:
   a. Ambiguous
   b. Contraindicated by normal practice (e.g., an abnormally high dose of medication)
   c. Contraindicated by the patient's present condition (e.g., as a patient's present condition improves, the patient may no longer need aggressive forms of treatment)

 REMEMBER Ella Rodriguez, the young girl requiring a sedation protocol for closed reduction of her fracture. The nurse should understand that the child is at risk for complications if the physician is not present during the drug administration. Therefore, the nurse should question the physician's order to "start without him" to ensure the patient's safety. ●

It is good practice to double-check any order that a patient questions. See Chapter 16 for another discussion of orders.

Delegating Nursing Care

Professional nurses are responsible for delegating nursing activities, but although RNs may delegate elements of care, they do not delegate the nursing process itself. As a nurse, you remain accountable for any actions you delegate. The ANA principles for delegation are described on the ANA site: www.nursingworld.com. Chapters 14 and 22 address nursing's delegation responsibilities.

Documentation

Documentation is discussed in detail in Chapter 16. Although most nurses prefer to spend their time interacting with patients rather than writing in a patient's record, careful documentation is a crucial legal safeguard for the nurse. Documentation must be factual, accurate, complete, and entered in a timely fashion. The law presumes that if something was not documented, it was not done. This includes even routine acts, such as taking vital signs, repositioning patients, and ensuring the patient's safety. In 2004, the Joint Commission created a list of "Do Not Use" abbreviations that should not be included in documentation. Be sure to check your agency's policies on what and how to document.

Be sure that the nursing plan of care is part of the patient's permanent record. Agencies should have flow sheets or a documentation form that enables you to check off routine aspects of care rapidly and completely. You should also write a comprehensive nursing note for each patient problem you address. This note should include the current nature of the problem, how you intervened, the patient's response, and, when appropriate, future priorities for care. After a problem is noted, nursing documentation should demonstrate continuity of care until the problem is resolved.

A common problem reported by nurses is not knowing how to document an incident, such as when you believe a patient needs medical attention but the responsible physicians are not responding to calls for assistance. In this case, the best legal safeguard is to document the facts of the incident, being careful not to make incriminatory statements, such as "Anyone could see we were losing this patient rapidly" or "Once again, Dr. Jones was unavailable when her patient needed her." The note should document the time the physician was called, the time of response or lack of response, and the subsequent nursing response (e.g., nursing supervisor notified). Such a note documents that you are carefully assessing the patient, recognizing significant cues, and reporting them appropriately. The nursing supervisor should write the next note after reviewing the case and choosing a course of action. Patient noncompliance with a treatment also should be documented, along with your attempts to increase compliance.

Adequate Staffing

Understaffing, sometimes called short staffing, is a problem that results in reduced quality of nursing care and may jeopardize patient safety. Temporary management solutions to understaffing, such as floating nurses from one unit to another or asking (or mandating) nurses to work overtime or double (back-to-back) shifts, are ineffective because they can further jeopardize patient safety. A nurse in an understaffed agency will be held to a professional standard of judgment for accepting responsibility for work and for delegating nursing responsibilities to others. Thus, if a patient claims negligent care, a nurse claiming to have been overworked that evening because of an unrealistic assignment does not have adequate grounds for a legal defense. If patient injury results, the agency and nurse employee will most likely be named as codefendants. Some state nursing associations are using "protest of assignment forms" to track employer practices of routine understaffing.

Whistle-blowing

Many nurses who are frustrated with unsafe practice environments are speaking up. **Whistle-blowing** is a warning from a present or past member of an organization to the public concerning a serious wrongdoing or danger created or masked by the organization (Lachman, 2008a). The decision to whistle-blow can be difficult since some nurses have been threatened with the loss of their jobs and licenses. Whistle-blower laws are intended to prevent employers from taking retaliatory action against nurses, such as suspension, demotion, harassment, or discharge, for reporting improper patient care or business practices. As part of the ANA Nationwide State Legislative Agenda, the ANA and State Nurses Associations are promoting strong whistle-blower laws on the state level that provide legal protections for nurses advocating for patients, without fear of reprisal. Many states now have protections in other legislation such as safe staffing and mandatory overtime prohibition. See information about whistle-blower protection at http://www.nursingworld.org to learn more, and see the whistle-blower section in Chapter 6.

Professional Liability Insurance

Although a nurse's best legal safeguard is always competent practice, the increasing number of malpractice claims naming nurses as defendants makes it wise for nurses to carry their own liability insurance. Nurses may obtain this insurance through the ANA and other nursing associations and other sources.

Reasons the ANA (1990) lists for purchasing a personal professional liability insurance policy are as follows:

• *Protection of the nurse's best interests.* If the nurse is named as a defendant in a malpractice action along with the agency, a conflict of interest could arise between the nurse and the agency. Nurses have no assurance that their best interest will be represented unless they have their own coverage, which provides their own attorney.

• *Limitations of employer's coverage.* Most health care facilities carry "claims made" insurance, which means that if the nurse is no longer working there or the facility closes, the nurse is not covered when a claim is filed.

• *Care or advice given outside of work.* An employer's policy covers the nurse only within the confines of the work setting.

Nurse attorney White (2011) explores the personal, professional, and historical influences on why nurses should or should not have their own malpractice insurance. As well, White urges nurses to regularly evaluate their circumstances and decide not only whether to carry their own malpractice insurance but what kind and how much.

Risk Management Programs

Hoping to reduce malpractice claims, many health care agencies have initiated risk management programs designed to identify, analyze, and treat risks. Elements of a comprehensive risk management program include the following:

• *Safety program.* The aim is to provide a safe environment in which the basic safety needs of patients, employees, and visitors are met.
• *Product safety program.* The aim is to ensure safe and adequate equipment; this involves ongoing equipment evaluation and maintenance.
• *Quality assurance program.* The aim is to provide quality health care to patients; this involves ongoing evaluation of all systems used in the care of patients.

Nurses with legal questions often find risk managers a helpful resource. Many risk managers encourage nurses and other clinicians to report "near misses" to better identify factors contributing to errors. A "near miss" is an error that would have happened except for someone's alertness and ability to identify and prevent the error.

Incident, Variance, or Occurrence Reports

An incident report, also called a variance or occurrence report, is used by health care agencies to document the occurrence of anything out of the ordinary that results in, or has the potential to result in, harm to a patient, employee, or visitor (Fig. 7-3). These reports are used for quality improvement and should not be used for disciplinary action against staff members. They are a means of identifying risks. More harm than good results from ignoring mistakes. Incident reports improve the management and treatment of patients by identifying high-risk patterns and initiating in-service programs to prevent future problems. These forms also make all the facts about an incident available to the agency in case of litigation. Increasingly, agencies use paperless computer-based reporting systems that are secure, timely, efficient, and effective. These may also offer online help and formal education and serve as a valuable tool for data analysis.

The nurse responsible for a potential or actual harmful incident or who witnesses an injury is the one who completes the incident form. This form should contain the complete name of the person or people involved and the names of all witnesses; a complete factual account of the incident; the date, time, and place of the incident; pertinent characteristics of the person or people involved (e.g., alert, ambulatory,

asleep) and of any equipment or resources being used; and any other variables believed to be important to the incident.

 THINK back to Ramone Scott, the patient who received the wrong medication. The nurse should document the incident, including the actions taken upon finding the error such as immediately stopping the medication, assessing the patient, and notifying the physician. In addition, the nurse should document continued follow-up assessments and interventions taken to ensure the patient's safety. ●

A physician completes one section of the incident form with documentation of the medical examination of the patient, employee, or visitor with an actual or potential injury.

In some states, incident reports may be used in court as evidence. When documenting a patient incident, be sure to include a complete account of what happened in the patient's record as well as in the incident report. *Documentation in the patient record, however, should not include the fact that an incident report was filed.*

Sentinel Events

The Joint Commission's Sentinel Event Policy defines a **sentinel event** as an unexpected occurrence involving death or serious physical or psychological injury, or the risk thereof. Serious injury specifically includes loss of limb or function. The phrase "or the risk thereof" includes any process variation for which a recurrence would carry a significant chance of a serious adverse outcome. Such events are called "sentinel" because they signal the need for immediate investigation and response. Common sentinel events have been wrong-side surgery, suicide, and operative and postoperative complications. Accredited organizations are expected to identify and respond appropriately to all sentinel events occurring in the organization or associated with services that the organization provides or provides for. Appropriate response includes a thorough and credible root cause analysis, implementation of improvements to reduce risk, and monitoring of the effectiveness of those improvements. Root cause analysis involves digging progressively deeper into the event, repeatedly asking why the event occurred, and exploring the circumstances that led to it to determine where improvements can be made. Nurses play a critical role in responding to sentinel events.

Never Events

In 2011, the National Quality Forum released a newly revised list of 29 events that they termed "serious reportable events," extremely rare medical errors that should never happen to a patient. Often termed "never events," these include errors such as surgery performed on the wrong body part or on the wrong patient, leaving a foreign object inside a patient after surgery, or discharging an infant to the wrong person. By reporting and following suggested guidelines when a never event occurs, the likelihood of such an error happening again is greatly decreased.

Medication Occurrence Information Report/PI
Send completed form to Risk Management
This document is part of a quality improvement process
CONFIDENTIAL: Do Not PHOTOCOPY
Do Not File in Patient Record
All Sections Must Be Completed

ADDRESSOGRAPH

Patient age:_____

Definition of occurrence: *Any preventable event that may cause or lead to inappropriate medication use or patient harm while the medication is in the control of the healthcare professional, patient, or consumer. Such events may be related to professional practice, healthcare products, procedures and systems, including prescribing, order communication, product labeling, packaging and nomenclature; compounding; dispensing; distribution; administration; education; monitoring; and use.*

Section A: Report filed by (please print): _____ Title: _____ Date/Time: _____
Location of event
Floor/Unit: _____ Date of event: _____ Time of event (24 hour): _____ ☐ Inpatient   ☐ Outpatient

Error discovered: ☐ Within same shift   ☐ Within 24 hours   ☐ Greater than 24 hours

Staff involved in initial error: ☐ Staff RN   ☐ Agency RN   ☐ Pharmacist   ☐ NP   ☐ House staff   ☐ Attending MD   Name: _____
Other staff also involved (i.e., perpetuated the error): ☐ Staff RN   ☐ Agency RN   ☐ Pharmacist   ☐ Physician

Staff that discovered error: ☐ Staff RN   ☐ Agency RN   ☐ Pharmacist   ☐ Physician

Physician notified? ☐ No   ☐ Yes   Date: _____ Time: _____ Attending: _____

Section B: Medication type: Medication(s) involved: Incident documented in medical record? ☐ Yes   ☐ No
         ☐ IV   A. _____   Patient/family aware of incident? ☐ Yes   ☐ No
         ☐ Non-IV   B. _____   *(If yes, please comment below)*

TYPE OF ERROR *(See reverse for definitions)*	**BREAKDOWN POINT** *(Where in process did the initial error occur?)*	**BREAKDOWN POINT** *(Where in process did the initial error occur?)* *(continued from the previous column)*

☐ Prescribing
☐ Omission—Total #
_____ Schedule: _____
☐ Monitoring error
☐ Wrong patient
☐ Wrong time
☐ Wrong route
☐ Wrong dose/quantity/extra dose
• dose ordered _____
• dose given _____
☐ Medication D/C'd, given
• extra doses:
_____
☐ Wrong drug
• med ordered _____
• med given _____
☐ Medication not ordered
• med given _____
• dose
☐ Wrong drug preparation
☐ Wrong rate of administration
☐ Given to patient with known allergy
☐ Investigational protocol not followed
☐ Other _____
	☐ Prescribing
	circle:
	• illegible handwriting
	• wrong chart/order sheet
	• incorrect order
	• incomplete order
	• other, please describe below
	☐ Order processing
	circle:
	• carbon not pulled/pulled late
	• order not transcribed
	• transcribed incorrectly
	• other, please describe below
	☐ Dispensing
	circle:
	• incorrectly entered into computer by pharmacist/not entered at all
	• wrong strength sent
	• wrong med sent
	• label incorrect/unclear
	• delay in delivery of medication
	• other, please describe below
	
	(continued next column)
		☐ Administration
		circle:
		• med given, but not charted
		• med charted, but not given
		• held med given
		• incorrect medication taken from floorstock/Pyxis and given
		• incorrect dose/rate calculation
		• pump error
		  –tubing clamped
		  –incorrect rate setting
		  –pump malfunction
		  –pump turned off
		☐ Other, please describe below
		ERROR SEVERITY/OUTCOME
		☐ **Category A:** Circumstances or events that have the capacity to cause error
		☐ **Category B:** Error occurred; medication not given
		☐ **Category C:** Medication given but did not cause patient harm
		☐ **Category D:** Resulted in the need for increased patient monitoring but no harm
		☐ **Category E:** Resulted in the need for treatment or intervention and caused temporary patient harm
		☐ **Category F:** Resulted in initial or prolonged hospitalization and caused temporary patient harm
		☐ **Category G:** Resulted in permanent patient harm
		☐ **Category H:** Resulted in a near-death event (e.g., anaphylaxis, cardiac arrest)
		☐ **Category I:** Resulted in patient death

COMMENTS/DESCRIBE EVENT (include any intervention/treatment given and outcome):
_____
_____
_____

Section C: ANALYSIS/RECOMMENDATIONS/ACTION PLAN *(Manager to complete):*
Possible causes: ☐ abbreviation ☐ calculation error ☐ communication confusing/intimidating/lacking
☐ computer order entry ☐ decimal point/leading zero missing/trailing zero ☐ equipment design ☐ facsimile order ☐ handwriting illegible ☐ inexperienced staff ☐ staffing level ☐ labeling (GUMC) confusing/incomplete/inaccurate ☐ labeling (manufacturer) confusing/incomplete/inaccurate ☐ similar name ☐ patient identification ☐ shift change ☐ floating staff ☐ poor lighting
☐ performance deficit ☐ preparation error ☐ procedure/protocol not followed ☐ reference manual confusing/inaccurate/unclear/outdated
☐ verbal order confusing/incomplete/misunderstood ☐ written order confusing/incomplete/misunderstood ☐ other _____
_____
_____

Signature of Manager: _____ Date: _____

FIGURE 7-3. Sample medication occurrence information report.

There is growing consensus that hospitals should not be reimbursed for the treatment of the consequences of never events. The Leapfrog Group, a voluntary program aimed at recognizing and rewarding big leaps in health care safety, quality, and customer value, gives public recognition to hospitals if they agree to the following if a never event occurs within their facility:

• We will apologize to the patient and/or family affected by the never event.
• We will report the event to at least one of the following agencies: The Joint Commission, as part of its Sentinel Events policy*; state reporting program for medical errors; or a Patient Safety Organization.
• We agree to perform a root cause analysis, consistent with instructions from the chosen reporting agency.
• We will waive all costs directly related to a serious reportable adverse event.
• We will make a copy of our policy available to patients and payers upon request.

See http://www.leapfroggroup.org/for_hospitals/leapfrog_ hospital_quality_ and_safety_survey_copy/never_events for more on the Leapfrog Group Position Statement on Never Events.

Patients' Rights

The American Hospital Association developed "A Patient's Bill of Rights" in 1972 (revised in 1992 and 2003; Box 7-6). Renamed "The Patient Care Partnership," it addresses the expectations, rights, and responsibilities of the patient while receiving care in the hospital, and ranges from "high-quality hospital care" to "helping prepare you and your family for when you leave the hospital." With care moving increasingly from the hospital to the community, legally prudent nurses must be familiar with how different institutions and professional groups define patient rights and responsibilities. Other bills of rights include the Pregnant Patient's Bill of Rights, the Indian Patient's Bill of Rights, a Nursing Home Bill of Rights, and the Veterans Administration Code of Patient Concern. Each emphasizes a specific aspect of patient rights within a particular health agency and implies a code of ethics that the nurse observes professionally.

Good Samaritan Laws

Good Samaritan laws are designed to protect health practitioners when they give aid to people in emergency situations. For example, a nurse at the scene of an automobile accident may give emergency care without fear of a legal suit if such care appears necessary, unless care is given in a grossly negligent manner.

Every state in the United States and the District of Columbia have Good Samaritan laws, although the laws vary considerably. Nurses are covered in some states but not in others; in some states, only certain acts are covered. While in many states no person has a legal obligation to help another (except in employment situations), and a health practitioner, like any other person, may choose to help or to leave the scene of an emergency, other states consider it mandatory for anyone to give help. Refer to the specific laws in your state. Regardless, in many situations, nurses may have an ethical responsibility to assist. In the event that health practitioners assist a person in an emergency situation when it is impossible to obtain consent for the care, they are expected to use good judgment to determine that an emergency exists and to give care that a reasonably prudent person with a similar background and in similar circumstances would provide.

STUDENT LIABILITY

As a student nurse, you are responsible for your own acts, including any negligence that may result in patient injury. Moreover, you are held to the same standard of care as a registered nurse. Your legal responsibilities include careful preparation for each new clinical experience and a duty to notify your clinical instructor if you feel in any way unprepared to carry out a nursing procedure. *For no reason should you attempt a clinical procedure if you are unsure of the correct steps involved.* You are also responsible for being familiar with agency policies and procedures.

A hospital may also be held liable for the negligence of a student nurse enrolled in a hospital-controlled program because the student is considered an employee of the hospital. The status of students enrolled in college and university programs is less clear, as is the liability of the educational institution in which they are enrolled and the health care agency offering a site for clinical practice.

Nursing instructors may share responsibility for damages in the event of patient injury if an assignment called for clinical skills beyond a student's competency or the instructor failed to provide reasonable and prudent clinical supervision. Because the status of patients can change rapidly, especially in an acute care setting, notify your instructor or a staff member of any significant changes in the patient's condition, even if you are unsure of the meaning of these changes.

Most nursing programs require students to carry personal professional liability insurance. *School policies provide coverage only for clinical nursing done for educational purposes at the direction of the school.* Moreover, student nurses who work as nursing assistants or in some other health care role are legally permitted to offer only those services included in their job description. Even if you feel confident with medication administration, catheter insertion, or another professional nursing act, you risk disciplinary action if you perform such a procedure outside the supervised clinical practice setting.

LAWS AFFECTING NURSING PRACTICE

Just as many safeguards help protect nurses from the risk of legal action, many laws govern the practice of nursing to protect both nurses and patients from harm.

*Reporting of sentinel events to the Joint Commission is voluntary for its accredited hospitals.

Box 7-6 THE PATIENT CARE PARTNERSHIP: UNDERSTANDING EXPECTATIONS, RIGHTS, AND RESPONSIBILITIES

When you need hospital care, your doctor and the nurses and other professionals at our hospital are committed to working with you and your family to meet your health care needs. Our dedicated doctors and staff serve the community in all its ethnic, religious, and economic diversity. Our goal is for you and your family to have the same care and attention we would want for our families and ourselves.

The sections below explain some of the basics about how you can expect to be treated during your hospital stay. They also cover what we will need from you to care for you better. If you have questions at any time, please ask them. Unasked or unanswered questions can add to the stress of being in the hospital. Your comfort and confidence in your care are very important to us.

What to Expect During Your Hospital Stay

- **High-quality hospital care.** Our first priority is to provide you the care you need, when you need it, with skill, compassion, and respect. Tell your caregivers if you have concerns about your care or if you have pain. You have the right to know the identity of doctors, nurses, and others involved in your care, as well as when they are students, residents, or other trainees.
- **A clean and safe environment.** Our hospital works hard to keep you safe. We use special policies and procedures to avoid mistakes in your care and keep you free from abuse or neglect. If anything unexpected and significant happens during your hospital stay, you will be told what happened and any resulting changes in your care will be discussed with you.
- **Involvement in your care.** You and your doctor often make decisions about your care before you go to the hospital. Other times, especially in emergencies, those decisions are made during your hospital stay. When they take place, making decisions should include:
  - *Discussing your medical condition and information about medically appropriate treatment choices.* To make informed decisions with your doctor, you need to understand several things:
    - The benefits and risks of each treatment
    - Whether it is experimental or part of a research study
    - What you can reasonably expect from your treatment and any long-term effects it might have on your quality of life
    - What you and your family will need to do after you leave the hospital
    - The financial consequences of using uncovered services or out-of-network providers

    Please tell your caregivers if you need more information about treatment choices.
  - *Discussing your treatment plan.* When you enter the hospital, you sign a general consent to treatment. In some cases, such as surgery or experimental treatment, you may be asked to confirm in writing that you understand what is planned and agree to it. This process protects your right to consent to or refuse a treatment. Your doctor will explain the medical consequences of refusing recommended treatment. It also protects your right to decide if you want to participate in a research study.
  - *Getting information from you.* Your caregivers need complete and correct information about your health and coverage so that they can make good decisions about your care. That includes:

- Past illnesses, surgeries, or hospital stays
- Past allergic reactions
- Any medicines or diet supplements (such as vitamins and herbs) that you are taking
- Any network or admission requirements under your health plan

- *Understanding your health care goals and values.* You may have health care goals and values or spiritual beliefs that are important to your well-being. They will be taken into account as much as possible throughout your hospital stay. Make sure your doctor, your family, and your care team know your wishes.
- *Understanding who should make decisions when you cannot.* If you have signed a health care power of attorney stating who should speak for you if you become unable to make health care decisions for yourself, or a "living will" or "advance directive" that states your wishes about end-of-life care, give copies to your doctor, your family, and your care team. If you or your family need help making difficult decisions, counselors, chaplains, and others are available to help.

- **Protection of your privacy.** We respect the confidentiality of your relationship with your doctor and other caregivers, and the sensitive information about your health and health care that are part of that relationship. State and federal laws and hospital operative policies protect the privacy of your medical information. You will receive a Notice of Privacy Practices that describes the ways that we use, disclose, and safeguard patient information and that explains how you can obtain a copy of information for our records about your care.

- **Help preparing you and your family for when you leave the hospital.** Your doctor works with hospital staff and professionals in your community. You and your family also play an important role. The success of your treatment often depends on your efforts to follow medication, diet, and therapy plans. Your family may need to help care for you at home.

  You can expect us to help you identify sources of follow-up care and to let you know if our hospital has a financial interest in any referrals. As long as you agree we can share information about your care with them, we will coordinate our activities with your caregivers outside the hospital. You can also expect to receive information and, where possible, training about the self-care you will need when you go home.

- **Help with your bill and filing insurance claims.** Our staff will file claims for you with health care insurers or other programs, such as Medicare and Medicaid. They will also help your doctor with needed documentation. Hospital bills and insurance coverage are often confusing. If you have questions about your bill, contact our business office. If you need help understanding your insurance coverage or health plan, start with your insurance company or health benefits manager. If you do not have health coverage, we will try to help you and your family find financial help or make other arrangements. We need your help with collecting needed information and other requirements to obtain coverage or assistance.

  While you are here, you will receive more detailed notices about some of the rights you have as a hospital patient and how to exercise them. We are always interested in improving. If you have questions, comments, or concerns, please contact _____.

Occupational Safety and Health

The Occupational Safety and Health Act of 1970 set legal standards in the United States in an effort to ensure safe and healthful working conditions for men and women. The act, intended to reduce work-related injuries and illnesses, has affected health care agencies and has increased certain responsibilities for many nurses. In 1991, the Occupational Safety and Health Administration (OSHA) established safety standards for workers who may be exposed to bloodborne pathogens in their employment. Following are examples of situations that could violate standards if care is not taken, because of the potential threat to worker safety:

- Use of electrical equipment
- Use of isolation techniques for patients with infectious diseases and the management of contaminated equipment and supplies
- Use of radiation, such as infrared or ultraviolet radiation, sound or radio waves, and laser beams
- Use of chemicals, such as those that are toxic or flammable

OSHA's regulations, frequently updated, have specific applications, and fines can be severe for infractions. Nurses can help implement this law by promoting health and safety precautions wherever they work. Nurses employed in industrial settings have a particularly important role. A new Office of Occupational Health Nursing was created at OSHA to underscore the major role that such nurses play in striving for safe and healthful workplaces.

National Practitioner Data Bank

The Health Care Quality Improvement Act of 1986 encourages identification and discipline of health care practitioners who engage in unprofessional conduct and to restrict their ability to move from state to state without a disclosure of their previous performance. When a state licenses, certifies, or registers practitioners, they become subject to the National Practitioner Data Bank requirements. The Act provides immunity from civil damages for peer review and establishes the National Practitioner Data Bank as an information clearinghouse. Nurses may be reported to the National Practitioner Data Bank for medical malpractice payments, adverse licensure actions, or adverse professional actions.

Reporting Obligations

Because of the unique nature of nurse–patient interactions, the nurse frequently has knowledge that a state requires to be reported, such as of child abuse, rape, or a communicable disease. Legislation varies, thus nurses must know what needs to be reported in their local area and to what authority.

Nurses are frequently the first members of the public to detect abuse. Abuse includes a physical, verbal, sexual, or emotional attack; neglect; and abandonment. Targets of abuse include infants, children, and adult men and women of all ages. Abusers are men and women of all ages, races, socioeconomic groups, and religious backgrounds. Nurses are obligated both ethically and legally to report abuse. In many states, the failure to report actual or suspected abuse is a crime in itself. Nurses are protected by law against suits from alleged abusers if they file a report of suspected abuse in good faith that turns out to be erroneous.

Controlled Substances

The United States has special laws governing the distribution and use of controlled substances (drugs with abuse potential) such as narcotics, depressants, stimulants, and hallucinogens. Drug abuse laws are specific, and violations are considered criminal acts. Nursing responsibilities for controlled substances include storing them in special locked compartments and adhering to specific documentation responsibilities.

Discrimination and Sexual Harassment

Title VII of the Civil Rights Act of 1964 protects employees from discrimination based on race, color, religion, sex, or national origin, and provides that pregnant women receive the same protection as other employees and applicants. The EEOC, which enforces Title VII, defines sexual harassment as "unwelcome sexual advances, requests for sexual favors, and other verbal or physical conduct of a sexual nature" occurring in the following circumstances:

- Submission to sexual advances is implicitly or explicitly considered a condition of employment.
- Submission to sexual advances is used as a basis for employment decisions.
- Sexual harassment interferes with job performance even if it only creates an intimidating, offensive, or hostile atmosphere. (EEOC, 1980, sections 3950.10 to 3950.11).

See Chapter 44 for a more detailed discussion of sexual harassment and hostile environment.

Health Insurance Portability and Accountability Act (HIPAA)

See the discussion of "Invasion of Privacy" on pages 118–119.

Restraints

The Nursing Home Reform Act of 1987 states that long-term care facility residents have the right to be free from physical or chemical restraints imposed for purposes of discipline or convenience and not required to treat medical symptoms. When caring for a patient who requires restraints, be sure that you are familiar with your institution's policies and the guidelines set forth by the Joint Commission. Safe use of restraints is discussed in Chapter 26.

People With Disabilities

At least 43 million Americans have physical or mental disabilities. Discrimination against such people persists in such crucial areas as employment, housing, public accommodations, education, transportation, communication, and health services. The 1990 Americans With Disabilities Act (ADA), amended in 2008, provides a broad definition of "disability" to cover any person who has a physical or mental impairment that substantially limits one or more major life activities or who has a record of such impairment. In addition to impairments that have traditionally been perceived as disabilities, the ADA also specifically protects people who have communicable diseases such as AIDS or HIV infection, people who are recovering from drug or alcohol addiction, and people who are regarded as being disabled, whether or not they are in fact disabled. The ADA imposes two requirements on businesses covered by the Act: it prohibits such entities from discriminating against people with disabilities and requires covered entities to "reasonably accommodate" people who are protected by the Act.

Wills

State and provincial laws regulate requirements for wills. The person who makes a will is called the testator. A will describes the intentions of a testator (for who will manage the estate and how property is to be disposed) to be carried out upon his or her death. A person who receives money or property from a will is called a beneficiary. Nurses are occasionally asked to witness a testator's signing of his or her will and should be familiar with the following guidelines:

- The witness should feel sure that the testator is of sound mind—that is, that the testator knows what he or she is doing and is free of the influence of drugs that could distort thinking.
- The witness should feel sure that the testator is acting voluntarily and is not being coerced in any way concerning the terms of his or her will.
- Witnesses should watch the testator sign the will, and they should sign in the presence of each other. State law indicates how many witnesses must acknowledge the testator's signature on a will; two or three witnesses are most commonly required.
- Witnesses to the signature on a will do not need to read it, but they should be sure that the document being signed is a will and not some other type of document.
- In most states, a person who is a beneficiary in a will is disqualified from being a witness to the testator's signature.

Legal Issues Related to Dying and Death

Legal responsibilities for the dying or deceased patient are discussed in Chapter 42. Legal issues include advance directives, do-not-resuscitate orders, assisted suicide, direct voluntary euthanasia, organ donation, autopsy, and inquest.

DEVELOPING CLINICAL REASONING

1. Nursing's collaborative responsibilities include helping other practitioners obtain informed and voluntary consent for treatment in difficult situations. How might a nurse facilitate the process of obtaining informed consent in the following situations?
   - A 15-year-old boy with cancer who is tired of therapy needs a new course of chemotherapy.
   - Vietnamese parents who speak little English are being asked to consent to surgery for their newborn.
   - An older adult who has had pain with eating for 6 months is being offered an exploratory laparotomy. She tells the surgeon, "I don't care what you do, just get rid of this pain."
   - Rehabilitation options are being considered for an older adult who is intermittently confused.

2. You are caring for a recently hospitalized patient who had been living in a retirement community. When his daughters, who tend to be critical, come to visit, they tell you that they hope their father's care here will be better than it was in the retirement community, which they are in the process of suing. How would you respond to the daughters, and what, if anything, would you share with other nurses about this incident?

3. The erratic behavior of a teenage patient on your unit is causing nurses to suspect that he is getting illegal drugs from his friends who visit. You are asked to keep a watchful eye. When changing his bed linens later in the day, you discover a cache of drugs. What are your next steps?

4. Recent layoffs have reduced the number of professional nurses on your unit, and you are increasingly concerned about patient safety as well as quality-of-care issues. What would you do about your concern for your personal liability for inadequate care?

5. When you bring an antipsychotic medication to your alert long-term care facility resident, she refuses to take it, saying, "I don't like the way it makes me feel." When you report this to one of the nurses, she tells you that they always crush the medication and administer it in food so that the resident doesn't know what she is getting. How do you respond?

PRACTICING FOR NCLEX

1. A state attorney decides to charge a nurse with manslaughter for allegedly administering a lethal medication. This is an example of what type of law?
   a. Public law
   b. Private law
   c. Civil law
   d. Criminal law

2. Newly hired nurses in a busy suburban hospital are required to read the state Nurse Practice Act as part of their training. Which topics are covered by this act? Select all that apply.
   a. Violations that may result in disciplinary action
   b. Clinical procedures
   c. Medication administration
   d. Scope of practice
   e. Delegation policies
   f. Medicare reimbursement

Questions 3 through 7 refer to the following scenario:

"Jean," a veteran nurse, pleaded guilty to a misdemeanor negligence charge in the case of a 75-year-old woman who died after slipping into a coma during routine outpatient eye surgery at an eye surgery center. Jean admitted that she failed to monitor the woman's vital signs during the procedure. The surgeon who performed the procedure called the nurse's action pure negligence, saying that the patient could have been saved. The patient was a vibrant grandmother of 10 who had walked three quarters of a mile the morning of her surgery and had sung in her church choir the day before. As part of her plea arrangement, the nurse agreed to serve

*6 months of probation—the first 2 months on house arrest—
and surrender her nursing license.*

3. Those bringing the charges against Jean are called:
   a. Appellates
   b. Defendants
   c. Plaintiffs
   d. Attorneys

4. Jean's attorney was careful to explain in her defense that Jean
   had specialty knowledge, experience, and clinical judgment
   and had met certain criteria established by a nongovernmental
   association, as a result of which she was granted recognition in
   a specified practice area. What is this sort of credential called?
   a. Accreditation
   b. Licensure
   c. Certification
   d. Board approval

5. If review of this patient's record revealed that she had never
   consented to the eye surgery, of which intentional tort might
   the surgeon have been guilty?
   a. Assault
   b. Battery
   c. Invasion of privacy
   d. False imprisonment

6. What must be established to prove that malpractice or negligence has occurred in this case?
   a. The surgeon who performed the procedure called the
      nurse's action pure negligence, saying that the patient
      could have been saved.
   b. The fact that this patient should not have died—she was a
      vibrant grandmother of 10 who had walked three quarters
      of a mile the morning of her surgery and had sung in her
      church choir the day before.
   c. The nurse intended to harm the patient and was willfully
      negligent.
   d. The nurse had a duty to monitor the patient's vital signs,
      failed to do so, the patient died, and it was Jean's failure to
      do her duty that caused the patient's death.

7. When the attorney representing the patient's family calls Jean
   and asks to talk with her about the case so that he can better
   understand her actions, how should Jean respond?
   a. "I'm sorry, but I can't talk with you. You'll have to contact
      my attorney."
   b. Answer the attorney's questions honestly and make sure
      that he understands her side of the story.
   c. Appeal to the attorney's sense of compassion and try to enlist
      his sympathy by telling him how busy it was that morning.
   d. "Why are you doing this to me? This could ruin me!"

8. A nurse administers the wrong medication to a patient and the
   patient is harmed. The physician who ordered the medication
   did not read the documentation that the patient was allergic
   to the drug. Which statement is true regarding liability for the
   administration of the wrong medication?
   a. The nurse is not responsible, because the nurse was merely
      following the doctor's orders.
   b. Only the nurse is responsible, because the nurse actually
      administered the medication.
   c. Only the physician is responsible, because the physician
      actually ordered the drug.
   d. Both the nurse and the physician are responsible for their
      respective actions.

9. A nurse answers a patient's call light and finds the patient
   on the floor by the bathroom door. After calling for assistance and examining the patient for injury, the nurse helps
   the patient back to bed and then fills out an incident report.
   Which statements accurately describe aspects of this procedure? Select all that apply.
   a. An incident report is used as disciplinary action against
      staff members.
   b. An incident report is used as a means of identifying
      risks.
   c. An incident report is used for quality control.
   d. The facility manager completes the incident report.
   e. An incident report makes facts available in case litigation
      occurs.
   f. Filing of an incident report should be documented in the
      patient record.

10. A nursing student asks the charge nurse about legal liability
    when performing clinical practice. Which statement regarding
    liability is true?
    a. Students are not responsible for their acts of negligence
       resulting in patient injury.
    b. Student nurses are held to the same standard of care
       that would be used to evaluate the actions of a registered
       nurse.
    c. Hospitals are exempt from liability for student negli-
       gence if the student nurse is properly supervised by an
       instructor.
    d. Most nursing programs carry group professional liability
       making student personal professional liability insurance
       unnecessary.

ANSWERS WITH RATIONALES

1. *d.* Criminal law concerns state and federal criminal statutes,
   which define criminal actions such as murder, manslaughter,
   criminal negligence, theft, and illegal possession of drugs.
   Public law regulates relationships between people and the
   government. Private or civil law includes laws relating to
   contracts, ownership of property, and the practice of nursing,
   medicine, pharmacy, and dentistry.

2. *a, d.* Each state has a Nurse Practice Act that protects the
   public by broadly defining the legal scope of nursing practice.
   Practicing beyond those limits makes nurses vulnerable to
   charges of violating the state Nurse Practice Act. Nurse Practice Acts also list the violations that can result in disciplinary
   actions against nurses. Clinical procedures are covered by the
   health care institutions themselves. Medication administration
   and delegation are topics covered by the board of nursing.
   Laws governing Medicare reimbursement are enacted through
   Federal legislation.

3. *c.* The person or government bringing suit against another
   is called the plaintiff. Appellates are courts of law, defendants are the ones being accused of a crime or tort, and
   attorneys are the lawyers representing both the plaintiff
   and defendant.

4. *c.* Certification is the process by which a person who has met
   certain criteria established by a nongovernmental association
   is granted recognition in a specified practice area. Nursing is
   one of the groups operating under state laws that promote the
   general welfare by determining minimum standards of education through accreditation of schools of nursing. Licensure is

a legal document that permits a person to offer to the public skills and knowledge in a particular jurisdiction, where such practice would otherwise be unlawful without a license. State board of approval ensures that nurses have received the proper training to practice nursing.

5. **b.** Assault is a threat or an attempt to make bodily contact with another person without that person's consent. Battery is an assault that is carried out. Every person is granted freedom from bodily contact by another person unless consent is granted. The Fourth Amendment gives citizens the right of privacy and the right to be left alone; a nurse who disregards these rights is guilty of invasion of privacy. Unjustified retention or prevention of the movement of another person without proper consent can constitute false imprisonment.

6. **d.** Liability involves four elements that must be established to prove that malpractice or negligence has occurred: duty, breach of duty, causation, and damages. Duty refers to an obligation to use due care (what a reasonably prudent nurse would do) and is defined by the standard of care appropriate for the nurse–patient relationship. Breach of duty is the failure to meet the standard of care. Causation, the most difficult element of liability to prove, shows that the failure to meet the standard of care (breach) actually caused the injury. Damages are the actual harm or injury resulting to the patient.

7. **a.** One of the cardinal rules for nurse defendants is: Do not discuss the case with anyone at your agency (with the exception of the risk manager), with the plaintiff, with the plaintiff's lawyer, with anyone testifying for the plaintiff, or with reporters.

8. **d.** Nurses are legally responsible for carrying out the orders of the physician in charge of a patient unless an order would lead a reasonable person to anticipate injury if it were carried out. If the nurse should have anticipated injury and did not,

both the prescribing physician and the administering nurse are responsible for the harms to which they contributed.

9. **b, c, e.** Incident reports are used for quality improvement and should not be used for disciplinary action against staff members. They are a means of identifying risks and are filled out by the nurse responsible for the injured party. An incident report makes facts available in case litigation occurs and in some states, incident reports may be used in court as evidence. A physician completes the incident form with documentation of the medical examination of the patient, employee, or visitor with an actual or potential injury. Documentation in the patient record should not include the fact that an incident report was filed.

10. **b.** Student nurses are held to the same standard of care that would be used to evaluate the actions of a registered nurse. Student nurses are responsible for their own acts of negligence if these result in patient injury. A hospital may also be held liable for the negligence of a student nurse enrolled in a hospital-controlled program because the student is considered an employee of the hospital. Nursing instructors may share responsibility for damages in the event of patient injury if an assignment called for clinical skills beyond a student's competency or the instructor failed to provide reasonable and prudent clinical supervision. Most nursing programs require students to carry personal professional liability insurance.

TAYLOR SUITE RESOURCES

Explore these additional resources to enhance learning for this chapter:

- NCLEX-Style Questions and other resources on thePoint, http://thePoint.lww.com/Taylor8e
- *Study Guide for Fundamentals of Nursing, 8th edition*
- Adaptive Learning | Powered by prepU, http://thepoint.lww.com/prepu

Bibliography

American Association of Critical-Care Nurses and AACN Certification Corporation. (2002). *Safeguarding the patient and the profession; Executive summary.* Aliso Viejo, CA: Author.

American Nurses Association. (1990). *Liability prevention and you: What nurses and employers need to know.* Washington, DC: Author.

American Nurses Association. (1994). *Guidelines on reporting incompetent, unethical or illegal practices.* Washington, DC: Author.

American Nurses Association. (2001). *Code for nurses with interpretive statements.* Washington, DC: Author.

American Nurses Association. (2010). *Nursing scope and standards of practice* (2nd ed.). Washington, DC: Author.

American Nurses Association. (2011). Navigating the World of Social Media. Available at http://www.nursingworld.org/Mobile/Nursing-Factsheets/navigating-the-world-of-social-media.html

American Nurses Association. (2011). 6 Tips for Nurses Using Social Media. http://bit.ly/HlvlVo

American Nurses Association (2011). Principles for Social Networking and the Nurse. Available at http://ana.nursingworld.org/MainMenuCategories/ThePracticeofProfessionalNursing/NursingStandards/ANAPrinciples.aspx

American Nurses Association. (2012). Frequently asked questions: Roles of State Boards of Nursing: Licensure, Regulation and Complaint Investigation. Available at http://www.nursingworld.org/MainMenu Categories/Tools/State-Boards-of-Nursing-FAQ.pdf

Ashley, R. C. (2004). Legal counsel. The first element of negligence. *Critical Care Nurse, 23*(6), 81.

Ashley, R. C. (2004). Legal counsel. The second element of negligence. *Critical Care Nurse, 24*(1), 68–69.

Ashley, R. C. (2004). Legal counsel. The third element of negligence. *Critical Care Nurse, 24*(3), 65–66.

Ashley, R. C. (2004). Legal counsel. The fourth element of negligence. *Critical Care Nurse, 24*(4), 78–79.

Brous, E. A. (2007). HIPAA vs. law enforcement: A nurse's guide to managing conflicting responsibilities. *American Journal of Nursing, 107*(8): 60–63.

Brous, E. (2012). Common misconceptions about professional licensure. *American Journal of Nursing, 112*(10):55–59.

Buppert, C. (2012). When does a nurse need a lawyer? MedScape News. Available at http://www.medscape.com/viewarticle/760437

CAN. Intervention: Risk Management Strategies for Impaired Nurses. CAN HealthPro VP07-1.

Cohen, M., Rosen, L. F., & Barbacci, M. (2008). Past, present, and future: The evolution of the nurse expert witness. *Journal of Legal Nurse Consulting, 19*(4), 3–8.

Croke, E. M. (2003). Nurses, negligence, and malpractice: An analysis based on more than 250 cases against nurses. *American Journal of Nursing, 103*(9), 54–64.

Equal Employment Opportunity Commission. (1980). Sex discrimination guidelines. In: *EEOC rules and regulations.* Chicago: Commerce Clearing House.

Glannon, J. W. *The Law of Torts: Examples and Explanations* (4th ed.). New York: Aspen Publishers; 2010.

Hooker, R., Nicholson, J., & Tuan, L. (2012). Does the employment of physician assistants and

nurse practitioners increase liability? *Journal of Medical Licensure and Discipline, 2009*(9):6–16. Available at http://www.paexperts.com/Nicholson%20-%20Hooker%20Article.pdf

Impaired Nurses Resource Center of the American Nurses Association: www.nursingworld.org/MainMenu Categories/WorkplaceSafety/Healthy-Work-Environment/Work-Environment/ImpairedNurse

Jenkins, R. C., & Lemak, C. H. (2009). A malpractice lawsuit simulation: Critical care providers learn as participants in a mock trial. *Critical care nurse, 29*(4), 52–60.

Joint Commission on Accreditation of Healthcare Organizations. (2012). Sentinel event policy and procedures. Available at http://www.jointcommission.org/Sentinel_Event_Policy_and_Procedures/

Karlsen, K. A., Hendrix, T. J., & O'Malley, M. (2009). Medical error reporting in America: A changing landscape. *Quality Management in Health Care, 18*(1), 59–70.

Kavalar, F., & Alexander, R. S. (2014). *Risk management in healthcare institutions* (3rd ed.). Burlington, MA: Jones & Bartlett Learning.

Lachman, V. D. (2008a). Whistleblowers: Troublemakers or virtuous nurses? *Dermatology Nursing, 20*(5), 394–396.

Lachman, V. D. (2008b). Whistleblowing: Role of Organizational Culture in Prevention and Management. *Dermatology Nursing, 20*(5), 390–393.

Laskowshi-Jones, L. (1998). Reaching beyond the rules: Understanding—and influencing—your scope of practice. *Nursing, 28*(9), 45.

McMullen, P. C., & Philipsen, N. C. (1996). Confidentiality: Computer security and data protection.

In B. R. Heller, M. E. Mills, & C. A. Romano (Eds.). *Information management in nursing and health care.* Springhouse, PA: Springhouse.

Midgley, M.S., Aumiller, L., Moskowitz, M., & Schultz, M. (2014). Every nurse is a risk manager. NURSE.com, 26–31.

Miller, L. A. (2011). The National Practitioner Data Bank: A Primer for Clinicians. *Journal of Perinatal and Neonatal Nursing, 25*(3), 224–225.

National Council of State Boards of Nursing (NCSBN). (2011). White Paper: A Nurses Guide to the Use of Social Media. Available at https://www.ncsbn.org/Social_Media.pdf

National Student Nurses' Association. Recommendations for Social Media Usage and Maintaining Privacy, Confidentiality and Professionalism. Available at http://www.nsna.org/Portals/0/Skins/NSNA/pdf/NSNA_Social_Media_Recommendations.pdf

Nurses Service Organization (NSO) and CAN HealthPro. (2011) Understanding Nurse Liability, 2006-2010: A three part approach. Available at: http://www.nso.com/pdfs/db/RN-2010-CNA-Claims-Study.pdf?fileName=RN-2010-CNA-Claims-Study.pdf&folder=pdfs/db&isLiveStr=Y

President's Commission for the Study of Ethical Problems in Medicine and Biomedical and Behavioral Research. (1982). *Making healthcare decisions: A report (Vol. 1).* Washington, DC: U.S. Government Printing Office.

Reising, D. L. (2012). Make your nursing care malpractice-proof. *American Nurse Today, 7*(1), 24–28.

Sharp, N. (2003). The "write stuff." *Nursing Spectrum, 13*(2), 12–13.

Smetzer, J. L. (1998). Lesson from Colorado: Beyond blaming individuals. *Nursing, 28*(5), 48–51.

Sorbello, B. (2008). Responding to a sentinel event. *American Nurse Today, 3*(10), 30–32.

Starr, K.T. (2014). Whistleblower liability: Are you ready to put your job on the line? *Nursing, 44*(2), 16–17.

Thede, L. (2010). Informatics: Electronic Health Records: A Boon or Privacy Nightmare? *OJIN: The Online Journal of Issues in Nursing, 15*(2).

Thomas, C. M., & Siela, D. (2011). The impaired nurse: Would you know what to do if you suspected substance abuse? *American Nurse Today, 6*(8).

Walker, R. (2011). Elements of negligence and malpractice. *The Nurse Practitioner, 36*(5), 9–11.

Weld, K. K., & Garmon, B. S. C. (2009). Concept analysis: Malpractice and modern-day nursing practice. *Nursing Forum, 44*(1), 2–10.

White, C. L. (2011). Do I need my own malpractice insurance? *Plastic Surgical Nursing, 31*(4), 185–187.

Health Care Delivery

Nurses care for patients in a wide variety of settings. As the health care environments change, nurses are increasingly providing care to promote wellness and restore health outside traditional hospital settings. Patients may receive health care services as inpatients or ambulatory outpatients in a hospital, through voluntary or public health agencies, in daycare centers and schools, in offices and clinics, in their home, or through crisis intervention centers. A health care team often provides care to meet a full range of physical, psychological, sociocultural, economic, and spiritual needs. Health care services may be financed through federal funding, health maintenance organizations, or private insurance. All these factors, combined with increasing concern about health care provision and costs, have raised questions about cost containment, consumer rights, fragmentation of care, vulnerable populations, and changing patient populations and needs.

As patients move among health care settings, the nurse is most often the member of the health care team responsible for coordinating care and teaching so that continuity of care is maintained. Unit II provides information about the various settings in which nursing care is provided and the resources for that care. Chapter 8 discusses the health care system as a whole, highlighting access, quality and safety, and affordability concerns. New models of organizing health care, such as patient-centered medical homes and accountable care organizations, are presented. Chapter 9 considers nursing care provided in the home and other community-based settings. Care coordination and continuity during handoffs are important as patients are admitted, transferred, and discharged from health care settings. Because health care is increasingly provided to patients in their own homes, Chapter 9 describes the characteristics and roles of the home health care nurse as well as the components of a home visit. The information in this unit enables the nurse to work within the health care system to meet individualized patient needs and provide holistic, person-centered care.

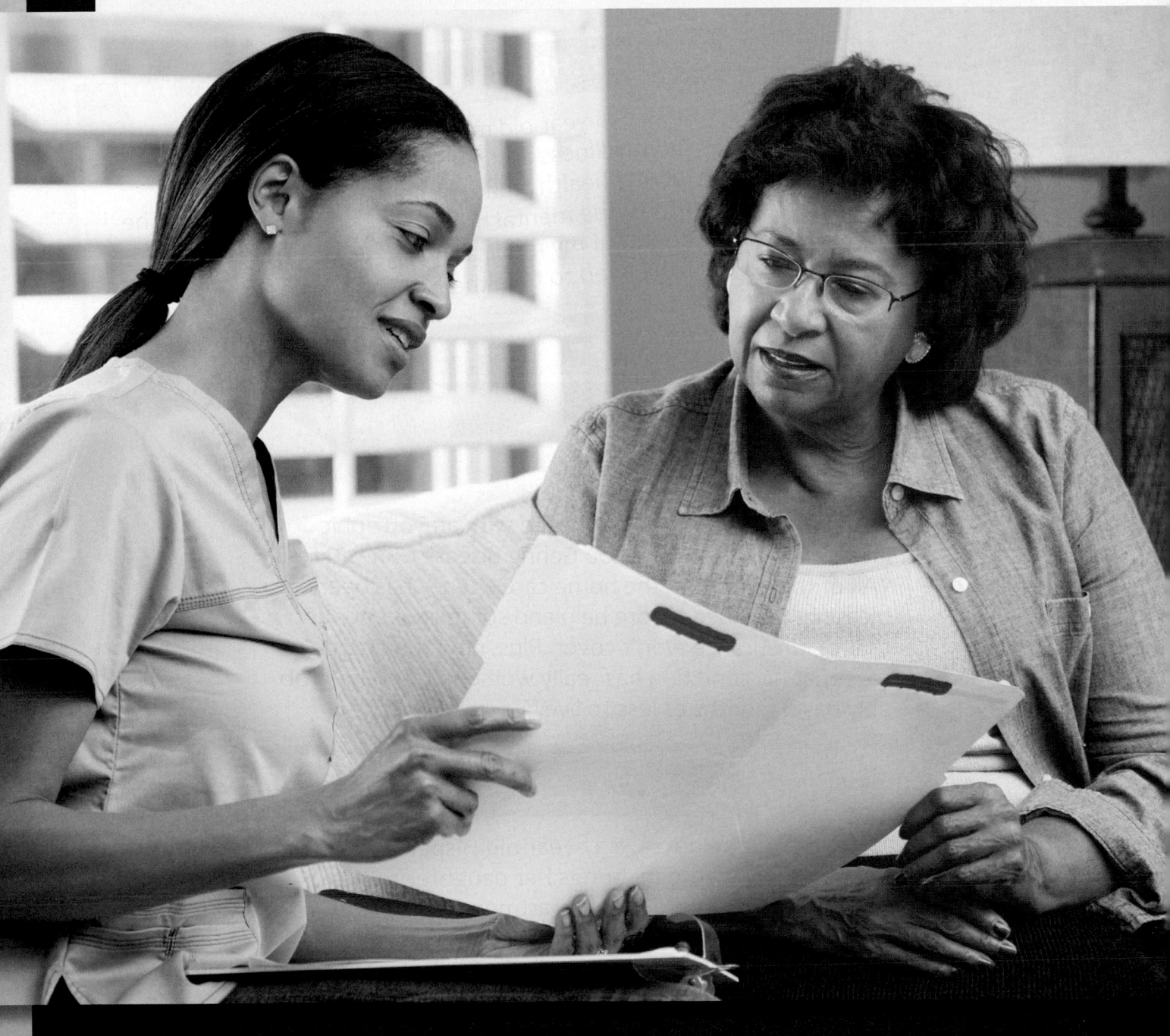

"… a realization that the call to the nurse is not only for the bedside care of the sick, but to help in seeking out the deep-lying basic causes of illness and misery, that in the future there may be less sickness to nurse and to cure."

Lillian Wald (1867–1940) a visionary humanitarian who initiated child-labor law revision, improved housing conditions in tenements, supported education for the mentally handicapped, originated public health nursing, and founded the Visiting Nurse Service at the Henry Street Settlement House, in New York City

8 The Health Care Delivery System

PAUL COCHRAN

Paul is a 38-year-old man with a history of mental illness and numerous visits to mental health inpatient and outpatient facilities; he comes to the mental health clinic for follow-up. He says, "I ran out of my medications last week, but I feel fine. Do I still need to take them?"

MARGARET RITCHIE

Margaret, a 63-year-old woman, is caring at home for her 67-year-old husband who has been diagnosed with amyotrophic lateral sclerosis (ALS, or Lou Gehrig disease). She states, "All of the help from the home care agency has been a blessing. But I need more help and some equipment now that our insurance won't cover. Plus, now the doctor says that his condition has really worsened, and he probably has 6 months or less to live."

MARITZA CORTES

Maritza, a 37-year-old Hispanic woman, brings her daughter to the emergency department. The child is diagnosed with a strep throat and is given a starting dose of penicillin. After receiving discharge instructions, including information about possible complications, and a prescription for additional doses of penicillin, she says, "I can't afford to get the prescription filled. Exactly what are these problems, and what are my son's chances for having them, too?"

LEARNING OBJECTIVES

After completing the chapter, you will be able to accomplish the following:

1. Identify elements of a well-functioning health care delivery system.

2. Describe strategies to increase access to affordable, high-quality care.

3. Compare and contrast these health care delivery systems: physicians and hospitals, multispecialty practice groups, community health centers, prepaid group practices, accountable care organizations, medical homes, and medical neighborhoods.

4. Evaluate four basic ways in which health care is paid for.

5. Compare and contrast settings and agencies that provide health care.

6. Describe the members of the interdisciplinary health care team.

7. Discuss selected trends and issues affecting health care delivery.

8. Describe the role of nursing in meeting the challenges of health care reform.

KEY TERMS

accountable care organization (ACO)	fee-for-service	multispecialty group practice
ambulatory care	Health Insurance Marketplace	outpatient
capitation	health maintenance organization (HMO)	palliative care
care coordination	hospice	Patient Protection and Affordable Care Act (PPACA)
community health center	inpatient	pay for performance
consumer	managed care	preferred provider organization (PPO)
diagnosis-related group (DRG)	Medicaid	respite care
entitlement reform	medical home	single-payer system
extended-care services	medical neighborhood	
	Medicare	
	multipayer system	

Designing a system for and delivering health care that adequately meets the needs of a diverse public is a complex challenge. Health care planners have always worried about access, quality, and cost. Who should get what quality of care at what cost? What you think about health care in the United States largely depends on your past experiences. If you are well insured or independently wealthy, you can access the best health care in the world. If you lack insurance and have limited financial resources, you may die of a disease that might have been prevented or treated in an early stage if you had access to quality care. The U.S. system has been criticized for providing too little care to some and too much of the wrong type of care to others. Many now believe that a moral society owes health care to its citizens—that health care is like clean water, sanitation, and basic education. Others, however, believe that health care is a commodity, like automobiles, to be sold and purchased in the marketplace—that if you lack the funds to buy a car, that may be sad, but society has no obligation to purchase a car for you. As you read this chapter, ask yourself what you believe about health care. Is it simply unfortunate if people cannot afford the health care that they and their families need? Learning about how health care works may not seem as exciting as learning how to administer medications safely, but your nursing practice every day will be affected by decisions made by governments, insurers, and health care institutions. Nursing's challenge as profits and politics increasingly dictate health priorities is to keep health care strongly focused on the needs of patients and the public. Health care in the United States is a business; revenues need to be generated to make care possible. But health care can never be *only* a business. First and primarily, it is a service a moral society provides for its vulnerable members. Nurses play a critical role in keeping health care centered on the patient and family. See the accompanying Reflective Practice display on page 142.

HEALTH CARE: THE BIG PICTURE

In 2001, describing a "new health system for the 21st century," the Institute of Medicine called for six outcomes envisioning a system that is safe, effective, efficient, patient-centered, timely, and equitable. More recently, the Institute of Medicine report *Best Care at Lower Cost* concluded that Americans would be better served by a more nimble health care system that is consistently reliable and that constantly, systematically, and seamlessly improves (Smith, Saunders, Stuckhardt, & McGinnis, 2012). It states its vision as follows: "…achieving a learning healthcare system—one in which science and informatics, patient–clinician partnerships, incentives, and culture are aligned to promote and enable continuous and real-time improvement, in both the effectiveness and efficiency of care—is both necessary and possible for the nation."

Access to Health Care

People have access to health care if they are able to obtain health care when they need it. Access depends on the ability to pay and the availability of services. Nearly 48 million nonelderly Americans were uninsured in 2011, a decline of 1.3 million since 2010. Decreasing the number of uninsured is a key goal of the 2010 **Patient Protection and Affordable Care Act (PPACA)**, which provides Medicaid or subsidized coverage to qualifying people with incomes up to 400% of

REFLECTIVE PRACTICE: CULTIVATING QSEN COMPETENCIES

CHALLENGE TO COGNITIVE SKILLS

Maritza Cortes, a 37-year-old Hispanic woman, came into the emergency department (ED) this summer with her daughter who was diagnosed with strep throat using a rapid strep test. The child was given an initial dose of penicillin and was getting ready for discharge. When I entered the patient's room to give her mother the discharge instructions and the prescription for 10 more doses of penicillin, Ms. Cortes said that she could not afford the medication and probably would not be able to have the prescription filled. I told her that it is essential to fill the medication because strep throat can lead to rheumatic fever and glomerulonephritis. She then asked me to elaborate, requesting exact information about the chances of her son also developing these complications. She wanted exact numbers and did not settle for my answer of "No matter what the percentage is, the medication is still necessary." She also wanted me to elaborate on the disease processes of rheumatic fever and glomerulonephritis. Although I do know basic information about these conditions, I did not feel comfortable being the primary and sole informer.

Thinking Outside the Box: Possible Courses of Action

- Make up a percentage to tell the mother and give a partial explanation of the diseases so that she would sign the discharge papers.
- Look up the answer in books available in the ED or search the Internet.
- Try to persuade her that numbers don't matter and that the possible diseases are very severe.
- Ask the nurse to inform me or explain the information to me while we are with the patient.
- Ask the physician to inform me or provide the information to me while we are with the patient.

Evaluating a Good Outcome: How Do I Define Success?

- Ms. Cortes receives adequate information regarding the medication and the conditions that may follow strep throat.
- Ms. Cortes obtains medication and gives it to her daughter, as prescribed.
- The standards of nursing care and protocols of the hospital are maintained.
- I am able to acknowledge that I need the help of others, seeking out their help; in return, those people help me.

Personal Learning: Here's to the Future!

Because I was working under my preceptor's license and he had to cosign my signature, I decided that he would be the best person to go to first. My preceptor said that this situation is a common occurrence in this ED because many people come in to get checked, even though they know that they cannot afford the medication, if necessary. As a justification to themselves, patients often want to know what are the exact chances for developing complications, which will likely influence whether or not they go ahead and fill the prescription.

My preceptor and I returned to the room, where he was able to explain rheumatic fever and glomerulonephritis in detail in Spanish. Because he was able to do this at the education level of the patient's mother and be very direct and persuasive, she was no longer concerned about exact numbers. She stated that she would try to get the medication filled, and then she signed the discharge document. Unfor-

tunately, there is no way to follow-up in these situations. I still wonder if the patient was able to get her medications.

Medical information is always changing, and what people held as standards of practice years ago differ from what we practice today. Similarly, what we hold today may be obsolete and even wrong in the years ahead. As a student, I find overwhelming the vast information that is necessary to be a competent nurse, especially in pharmacology. In this example, I should have probably been able to give the patient a comprehensive explanation of rheumatic fever and glomerulonephritis. However, I didn't feel comfortable. I do feel that I have learned a lot in the past years as a student, but I know that the knowledge I need to act as a professional nurse is much greater! While it is overwhelming and very challenging at times, I think continued learning is one reason why nursing is such a wonderful profession. I think it will never get boring.

Julia Strobel, Georgetown University

REFLECTION ON QUALITY AND SAFETY COMPETENCIES

How do you think you would respond in a similar situation? Why? What does this tell you about yourself and about the adequacy of your skills for professional practice? Can you think of other ways to respond? What other knowledge, attitudes and skills do you need to develop to continuously improve the quality and safety of care for patients like Ms. Cortes's daughter?

Patient-Centered Care: What made creating a partnership with Ms. Cortes and her daughter so challenging? What abilities did the student's preceptor possess and use to achieve a good outcome? What special talents do you bring to creating successful partnerships? Reread the preceptor's statement about this type of situation being common in the ED. Do such statements reflect culturally competent nursing? Or are such statements judgmental? Support your response.

Teamwork and Collaboration/Quality Improvement: What communication skills do you need to improve to ensure that you function as a competent, caring, and responsible member of the patient care team and that you obtain appropriate assistance when needed? What special talents do you bring to promoting a well-functioning team?

Safety/Evidence-Based Practice: What priority did all involved with Ms. Cortes accord to her daughter's health, well-being, and safety? What resources should be available to those who lack the financial resources to purchase prescribed medications or treatment? Were the team members successful advocates for this family? Did the nursing student seek out the most appropriate resources for information? Why or why not? What other resources could have been helpful? Do you agree with the criteria to evaluate a successful outcome? Did the nursing student meet the criteria? Explain your answers.

BOX 8-1 CHARACTERISTICS OF A CONTINUOUSLY LEARNING HEALTH CARE SYSTEM

Science and Informatics

Real-time access to knowledge: A learning health care system continuously and reliably captures, curates, and delivers the best available evidence to guide, support, tailor, and improve clinical decision making and care safety and quality.

Digital capture of the care experience: A learning health care system captures the care experience on digital platforms for real-time generation and application of knowledge for care improvement.

Patient-Clinician Partnerships

Engaged, empowered patients: A learning health care system is anchored on patient needs and perspectives, and promotes the inclusion of patients, families, and other caregivers as vital members of the continuously learning care team.

Incentives

Incentives aligned for value: A learning health care system has incentives actively aligned to encourage continuous improvement, identify and reduce waste, and reward high-value care.

Full transparency: A learning health care system systematically monitors the safety, quality, processes, prices, costs, and outcomes of care, and makes information available for care improvement and informed choices and decision making by clinicians, patients, and their families.

Continuous Learning Culture

Leadership-instilled culture of learning: A learning health care system is stewarded by leadership committed to a culture of teamwork, collaboration, and adaptability in support of continuous learning as a core aim.

Supportive system competencies: A learning health care system constantly refines complex care operations and processes through ongoing team training and skill building, systems analysis and information development, and creation of the feedback loops for continuous learning and system improvement.

Reprinted with permission from Smith, M., Saunders, R., Stuckhardt, L., & McGinnis, J. M., (Eds.). (2012). Best care at lower cost: The path to continuously learning healthcare in America. Washington, DC: The National Academies Press.

poverty, beginning in 2014. A key element of the health care law that took effect in 2014 provided a new way to get health insurance: the **Health Insurance Marketplace**. The Marketplace was designed to help people more easily find health insurance that fits their budget. Every health insurance plan in the new Marketplace must offer comprehensive coverage, from doctors to medications to hospital visits. People can compare all their insurance options in terms of price, benefits, quality, and other features that may be important to them, in plain language that makes sense. See HealthCare.gov for more information.

A Henry J. Kaiser Family Foundation brief, "Medicaid and the Uninsured" (2012), provides basic facts describing who the uninsured are and the effects of being uninsured:

1. Most of the nation's 47.9 million uninsured have low or moderate incomes.
2. More than three-quarters of the uninsured are in a working family.
3. Medicaid and the Children's Health Insurance Program (CHIP) provide a key source of coverage for many low-income families who lack access to other affordable coverage.
4. About one-quarter of uninsured adults go without needed care due to cost, compared to only 4% of those with private insurance.
5. Medical bills are a burden for the uninsured and frequently leave them with debt. When they receive care, the uninsured pay for more than one-third of their care out of pocket and are often charged higher amounts for their care than the insured pay.

A 2013 U.S. Subcommittee on Primary Health and Aging reported that nearly 57 million people in the United States—one in five Americans—live in areas without adequate access to primary health care due to a shortage of providers in their communities. The facts in this report are sobering:

- Fifty years ago, half of the doctors in the United States practiced primary care, but today fewer than one in three do.
- As many as 45,000 people die each year because they do not have health insurance and do not get to a doctor on time.
- The average primary care physician in the United States is 47 years old, and one-quarter are nearing retirement.
- In 2011, about 17,000 doctors graduated from American medical schools. Despite the fact that over half of patient visits are for primary care, only 7% of the nation's medical school graduates now choose a primary care career (Sanders, 2013).

The report cites nurse Linda Aiken noting that nurse practitioners are a good solution for the shortage of primary care predicted to worsen as millions of currently uninsured Americans get health insurance as a result of the Affordable Care Act. "Research shows that care by nurse practitioners is excellent, highly satisfactory to patients, accessible, and affordable."

Quality and Safety

The 1999 Institute of Medicine report, *To Err Is Human*, shocked the world when it claimed that at least 44,000 and perhaps as many as 98,000 people die in U.S. hospitals each year as a result of medical errors that could have been prevented. Even the lower number exceeds the combined annual deaths caused by automobile accidents, breast cancer, and AIDS. A common source of medical errors is the decentralized and fragmented nature of the health care delivery system—or "nonsystem." The report recommended a four-tiered strategy, which is now well underway:

- Establishing a national focus to create leadership, research, tools, and protocols to enhance our knowledge about safety
- Identifying and learning from errors by developing a nationwide public mandatory reporting system and by encouraging health care organizations and practitioners to develop and participate in voluntary reporting systems
- Raising performance standards and expectations for improvements in safety through the actions of oversight organizations, professional groups, and group purchasers of health care
- Implementing safety systems in health care organizations to ensure safe practices

In 2001, the Institute of Medicine defined quality as the degree to which health services for people and populations increase the likelihood of desired health outcomes and are consistent with professional knowledge. More simply, quality is the right care for the right person at the right time. Every year, the Agency for Health Care Research and Quality (AHRQ) issues national reports on quality and disparities. To learn more about health care quality, visit the websites listed in the Internet Resources for this chapter that can be found on thePoint.

Increasingly, quality of care is being measured and used to evaluate hospitals and other providers and to award reimbursement.

Pay for Performance

Pay for performance is a strategy using financial incentives to reward providers for the achievement of a range of payer objectives, including delivery efficiencies, submission of data and measures to the payer, and improved quality and patient safety. The National Committee for Quality Assurance (NCQA) developed the Healthcare Effectiveness Data and Information Set (HEDIS), a tool used by more than 90% of America's health plans to measure performance in important dimensions of care and service. Altogether, HEDIS consists of 80 measures across five domains of care. Because so many plans collect HEDIS data, and because the measures are so specifically defined, HEDIS makes it possible to compare the performance of health plans on an "apples-to-apples" basis. Health plans also use HEDIS results themselves to see where they need to focus their improvement efforts.

HEDIS measures address a broad range of important health issues. Among them are asthma medication use, persistence of beta-blocker treatment after a heart attack, controlling high blood pressure, comprehensive diabetes care, breast cancer screening, antidepressant medication management, childhood and adolescent immunization status, and childhood and adult weight/body mass index (BMI) assessment.

In 2011, Medicare finalized a plan to alter reimbursements based on the quality of care hospitals provide and patients' satisfaction during their stays. This was a dramatic step toward paying for better care, not just more care. Seventy percent of the bonuses initially were based on how often hos-

pitals followed guidelines on 12 clinical care measures. The other 30% were determined by how patients rated hospitals on their experiences (Rau, 2011). The Hospital Consumer Assessment of Healthcare Providers and Systems (HCAHPS) Survey is the first national, standardized, publicly reported survey of patients' perspectives of hospital care. HCAHPS (pronounced "H-caps"), also known as the CAHPS® Hospital Survey, is a 27-item survey instrument and data collection methodology for measuring patients' perceptions of their hospital experience. While many hospitals have collected information on patient satisfaction for their own internal use, until HCAHPS there were no common metrics and no national standards for collecting and publicly reporting information about patients' experience of care. Since 2008, HCAHPS has allowed valid comparisons to be made across hospitals locally, regionally, and nationally. The HCAHPS Survey asks recently discharged patients about aspects of their hospital experience that they are uniquely suited to address. The core survey items ask "how often" or whether patients experienced a critical aspect of hospital care, rather than whether they were "satisfied" with the care. Ten HCAHPS measures (six summary measures, two individual items, and two global items) are publicly reported on the Hospital Compare website (http://www.medicare.gov/hospitalcompare) for each participating hospital. The six composites summarize how well nurses and doctors communicate with patients, how responsive hospital staff are to patients' needs, how well hospital staff help patients manage pain, how well staff communicate with patients about medicines, and whether key information is provided at discharge. The two individual items address the cleanliness and quietness of patients' rooms, while the two global items report patients' overall rating of the hospital and whether they would recommend the hospital to family and friends (HCAHPS Fact Sheet, 2012).

Penalties for Excess Readmissions

In October 2012, more than 2,000 hospitals were penalized by the government because many of their patients were readmitted soon after discharge. These hospitals forfeited more than $280 million in Medicare funds because the government considers readmissions a prime symptom of an overly expensive and uncoordinated health system. Until now, hospitals had little financial incentive to ensure that patients get the care they need once they leave the hospital (Rau, 2012).

Affordability

Health care financing involves two streams of money: the collection of money for health care (money going in), and reimbursement of health care providers for health care (money going out). The United States is a **multipayer system** since its "payers" include both private insurance companies and the government. Distinctive to the United States is the dominance of the private element over the public (Chua, 2006). In 2012, the United States spent 17.9% of its gross domestic product (GDP) on health care—more than any other country in the world. The government estimates that an aging population, improving economy, and the health care overhaul will push spending on medical services to almost 20% of the U.S. gross domestic product by 2021 (Centers for Medicare and Medicaid, 2013). While some argue that nothing is more important than health and no price is too high to pay, the increasing percentage of the GDP being allocated to health care means less money for education, defense, public parks, the arts, and other priorities. See Table 8-1 for a description of strategies to reduce health care costs.

Many believe that the solution to rising U.S. health care costs is a **single-payer system**, that is, have one entity such as a government run the organization, collect all health care fees, and pay out all health care costs. In the current U.S. free market system, there are tens of thousands of different health care organizations and huge administrative waste. The Physicians for a National Health Program (PNHP) promote a single-payer system in which all hospitals, doctors, and other health care providers would bill one entity for their services. "This alone would reduce administrative waste greatly and save money, which could be used to provide care and insurance to those who currently don't have it" (PNHP, 2013). During President Obama's efforts to reform health care, the Senate did not allow discussion of a single-payer system.

How the U.S. Health Care Dollar Is Spent

Hospital care and physician/clinical services together account for 51% of the nation's health care expenditures. Figure 8-1 shows a breakdown of how the U.S. health care dollar is spent. The Institute of Medicine (IOM) Report *Best Care at Lower Cost* concluded that a substantial proportion of U.S. health care expenditures is wasted, leading to

little improvement in health or the quality of care. The IOM workshop summary, *The Health Care Imperative: Lowering Costs and Improving Outcomes,* estimates excess costs in six domains: unnecessary services, services inefficiently delivered, prices that are too high, excess administrative costs, missed prevention opportunities, and medical fraud (Yong, Saunders, & Olsen, 2010).

An International Comparison with the U.S. Health Care System

The 2010 Commonwealth Fund International comparison of the U.S. health care system concludes that despite having the most costly health system in the world, the United States consistently underperforms in most dimensions of performance relative to other countries. "Compared with six other nations—Australia, Canada, Germany, the Netherlands, New Zealand, and the United Kingdom—the U.S. healthcare system ranks last or next-to-last in five dimensions of a high-performance health system: quality, access, efficiency, equity, and healthy lives" (Davis, Schoen, & Stremikis, 2010). The report was hopeful that newly enacted health reform legislation in the United States would address these problems by extending coverage to those without and helping to close gaps in coverage—leading to improved disease management, care coordination, and better outcomes over time.

A discouraging 2013 Institute of Medicine report, *U.S. Health in International Perspective: Shorter Lives, Poorer Health,* concludes that while the United States is among the wealthiest nations in the world, it is far from the healthiest. Despite spending far more per person on health care than

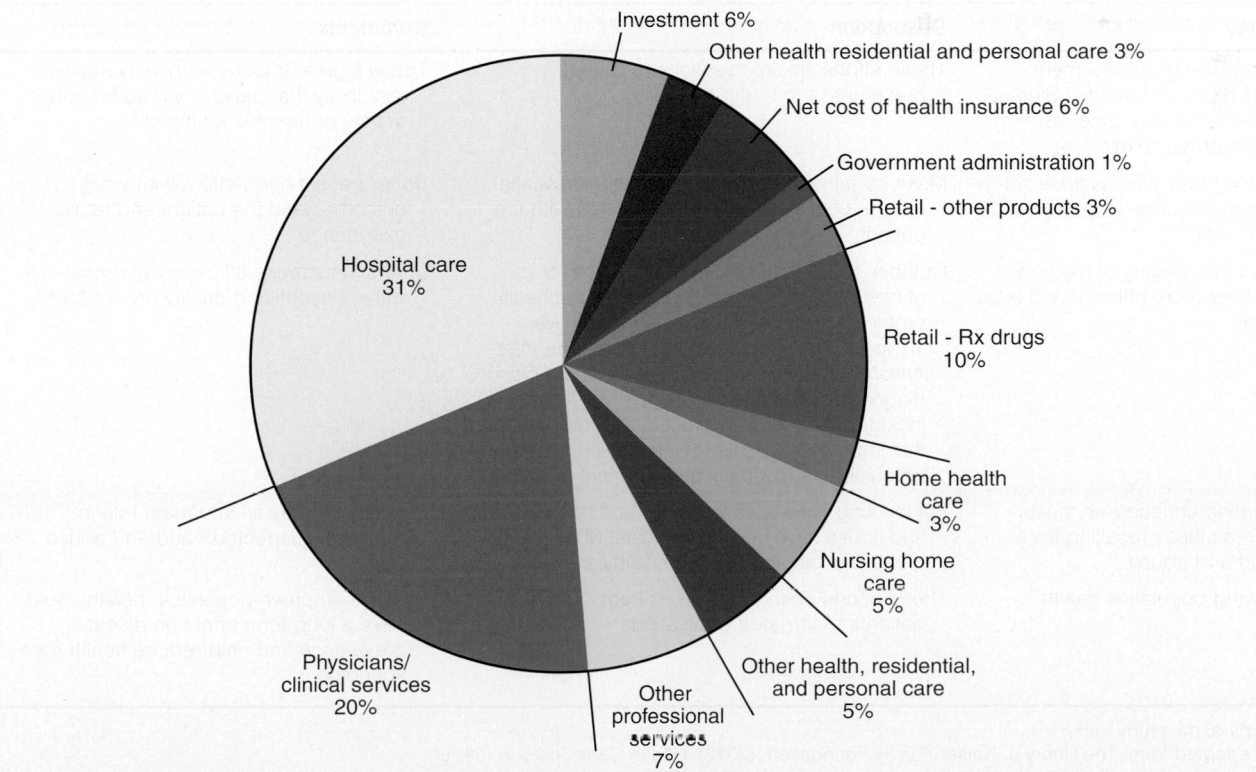

FIGURE 8-1. How the U.S. health care dollar is spent.

Table 8-1 STRATEGIES TO REDUCE HEALTH CARE COSTS

CHANGES IN REIMBURSEMENT AND REGULATORY ENVIRONMENT

Strategy	Description	Comments
Prospective Payment System: Diagnosis-Related Groups (DRGs) and Resource Utilization Groups (RUGs)	Grouped inpatient hospital services for Medicare patients into DRGs with a fixed reimbursement amount with adjustments based on case severity, rural/urban/regional costs, and teaching costs; RUGs in long-term care.	Changes the financial incentives linked to doing more in order to gain more reimbursement
Capitation and Managed Care	**Capitation** gives providers a fixed amount per enrollee of health plan. In managed care, the provider or system receives a capitated payment for each patient enrolled in the program and assumes financial risk.	Aims to build a payment plan for select diagnoses or procedures that consist of best standards of care at the lowest cost. Quality of care may suffer if there is too much emphasis on cost.
Bundled Payments	Provider receives a fixed sum of money to provide a range of services.	Again, the fixed sum aims to decrease costs of health care by changing the financial incentives.
Rate Setting	Government could set targets or caps for spending on health care services. Government could establish prices for services or even payment approaches that public and private payers would use.	Could equalize prices across payers and focus competition on health management and customer service. Diagnoses can be modified to game the system. Some see this as heavy-handed.
Comparative Effectiveness Analysis	Explicitly assess and weigh the benefits and costs of new technologies, and make decisions about whether a medical benefit is worth the cost and whether it should be covered by a public or private insurance program.	Forces providers to factor in costs when making decisions about new technologies; challenges the "more is always better" thinking
Increasing Patient Cost Sharing	Higher deductibles	Higher cost sharing reduces demand (and some people with few resources may not seek indicated services), which over the longer run will dampen incentives for research and investment. Can raise barriers to even necessary and appropriate care.

CHANGES IN CARE DELIVERY

Strategy	Description	Comments
Utilizing quality improvement tools (such as Lean Six Sigma, PDSA, etc.) to reduce waste and improve safety	These efforts link interventions to valued outcomes.	Today's greater focus on quality makes it less likely that patients will suffer unnecessary or harmful treatment.
Improving transitions across settings (to decrease 30-day readmissions)	Make sure that all the vital information essential to care coordination gets transferred with the patient.	Better patient hand-offs will improve outcomes and the patient and family experience.
Making the delivery of medical services more efficient and less costly	October 1, 2014, is the compliance date for use of new codes that classify diseases and health problems; estimated to save $6 billion over 10 years. These code sets, known as the *International Classification of Diseases, 10th Edition* diagnosis and procedure codes, or ICD-10, will include codes for new procedures and diagnoses that improve the quality of information available for quality improvement and payment purposes.	Efforts to increase efficiency and cost without sacrificing quality are welcome.
Eliminating unnecessary costs such as those resulting from fraud and abuse	For too long, measures to identify and address fraud and abuse have been inadequate, which have greatly contributed to rising health care costs.	Nurses can play an important role in reporting suspected fraud and abuse.
Improving population health	These efforts change the focus from individual patients to targeted populations.	Efforts to improve population health could have a long-term effect on disease prevalence and help reduce health care spending.

PDSA = plan, do, study, act
Partially adapted from: The Henry J. Kaiser Family Foundation. (2012). Health Care Costs: A Primer. Available at http://kff.org/health-costs/report/health-care-costs-a-primer/

any other nation, the United States has more people dying at younger ages than people in almost all other high-income countries. Among 16 peer nations, all affluent democracies, the United States is at or near the bottom in nine key areas of health: infant mortality and low birth weight, injuries and homicides, teenage pregnancies and sexually transmitted infections (STIs), prevalence of HIV and AIDS, drug-related deaths, obesity and diabetes, heart disease, chronic lung disease, and disability. Included as factors linked to the U.S. disadvantage are inadequate health care, unhealthy behaviors, and adverse economic and social conditions. "The tragedy is not that the U.S. is losing a contest with other countries, but that Americans are dying and suffering from illness and injury at rates that are demonstrably unnecessary" (Woolf & Aron, 2013).

HEALTH CARE REFORM

On March 23, 2010, President Obama signed comprehensive health reform legislation, the Patient Protection and Affordable Care Act (PPACA), into law. The intent of the law was to expand coverage, control health care costs, and improve the health care delivery system. While the law is complex, nurses should be familiar with how the law affects their practice, health care delivery, and the choices available to the public. Excellent information about the law can be found at www.heathcare.gov and www.nursingworld.org. The American Nurses Association website chronicles nurses' decades-long efforts to advocate for health care reforms that would guarantee access to high-quality health care for all. It acknowledges that with the passage of the PPACA, millions now have greater protection against losing or being denied health care coverage and better access

BOX 8-2	NURSES CAN MAKE A DIFFERENCE IN HEALTH CARE POLICY AND REFORM

- Stay informed about current issues and pending legislation.
- Write or e-mail members of Congress to support legislation to improve nursing and patient care. See Chapter 7.
- Belong to and participate in nursing organizations.
- Document the outcomes of nursing care and develop a database to influence health care costs and quality of care.
- Participate in efforts to design and implement innovative health care delivery models.
- Be a leader in local, state, and national nursing and consumer groups.
- Advocate for the rights of all people for equal, affordable, accessible, and knowledgeable health care.

to primary and preventive services. It also reminds us that the debate about health care is not over and offers practical strategies for nurses who choose to be politically active for continuing reform. See Box 8-2 for examples of ways that nurses can promote health care reform.

ORGANIZING HEALTH CARE: PRIMARY, SECONDARY AND TERTIARY CARE

Health care can be broken down into three levels: primary, secondary, and tertiary (Table 8-2). While these divisions seem simple, it is challenging to decide what resources should be allocated to each level. Many claim that the United

Table 8-2 PRIMARY, SECONDARY, AND TERTIARY HEALTH CARE

CARE LEVEL	GOAL	PRACTITIONER	PRACTICE SITE	ACTIVITIES
Primary Health Care	Common health problems (sore throats, diabetes, arthritis, depression, or hypertension) and preventive measures (vaccinations, mammograms) that account for 80% to 90% of visits to clinicians	Family practice physicians Nurse practitioners Midwives	Family planning centers Primary care centers Urgent care centers Employment health centers	Family planning Prenatal and well-baby care Immunization against specific diseases Health risk screenings Diagnostic tests Health education Medications
Secondary Health Care	Problems that require more specialized clinical expertise, such as hospital care for a patient with a myocardial infarction or stroke	Physicians in specialties such as internal medicine, pediatrics, neurology, psychiatry Advance practice nurses	Hospital-based clinics Emergency departments Hospitals Psychiatric institutes Same-day surgery units	Disease identification and management
Tertiary Health Care	Management of rare and complex disorders such as pituitary tumors and congenital malformations	Subspecialist physicians such as cardiovascular surgeons, pediatric hematologists Advance practice nurses	Tertiary care medical centers	Rare and complex disease management

Adapted from Bodenheimer, T., & Grumbach, K. (2012). Understanding health policy: A clinical approach (6th ed.). New York: McGraw Hill.

THROUGH THE EYES OF A NURSE

Asked to describe what keeps me up at night. I spoke about an upcoming summit ... one in which health care innovation would be featured prominently as part of a conversation about health care reform. I spoke about my concern, as the sole nurse leader in attendance, whether the space would be created in such an important forum for a larger conversation to take place—about how, in the face of emerging technologies and provider shortages, we can better utilize our health care workforce for potentially tens of millions who, under the Affordable Care Act, will likely soon find themselves with improved access to care.

...I believe the greatest challenge for nurse leaders is to influence the culture of care so that patients are able to optimally benefit from the knowledge, competencies, and skills of nurses. Nurses bring unique cost-saving value to health care and have the capacity to be system innovators. I believe nurses must be empowered to participate as leaders in care delivery redesign to assure changes will be meaningful for patients. And yet, nurses remain on the periphery of many policy and reform conversations.

• Care coordination managed by nurses decreases costs. One Institute of Medicine–commissioned study published in 2011 showed uncoordinated care raises costs by 75 percent, compared to similar cases with coordinated care.
• There is a strong link between patient satisfaction, nurse staffing, and revenue. Thirty percent of Medicare value-based performance scores are based on patient satisfaction scores (HCAHPS)—the single most important aspect of

which is patient perceptions of excellent nursing care. Additionally, increasing the proportion of RNs providing care within the team improves patient outcomes (decreased falls, reduced rates of complications, and lower mortality) and costs.
• Expanding access to advance practice registered nurses (APRNs) will provide additional primary coverage to individuals who otherwise find it difficult or impossible to have timely access to primary care.
• Women who deliver with midwives have fewer C-sections and higher breastfeeding rates, pointing to the cost effectiveness of midwifery services. A 2011 Agency for Healthcare Research and Quality brief found that the cost of a cesarean delivery was almost $2000 higher than for a vaginal delivery. Considering there are approximately four million births per year in this country and 32 percent are delivered by C-section, that is a total of $2.5 billion per year. Reducing this number by even 5 percent by increasing access to midwifery care for low-risk pregnancies would result in about $128 million in savings on hospitalizations alone.

These are just a few of the compelling arguments with respect to the value of nurses.

—Karen A. Daley, PhD, RN, FAAN, President,
American Nurses Association

Reprinted with permission from Daley, K. A. (2013). President's perspective: What keeps me up at night? *The American Nurse, 45*(1):3.

States has an illness care system rather than a health care system. As a result, a disproportionate percentage of our health care dollar goes to secondary and tertiary care at the expense of prevention and primary care. More attention is now being paid to prevention and primary care, and new opportunities are opening up for nurses at all levels of practice. If care coordination entails not only the right care for the right patient at the right time but also the right provider, decisions about how to organize care must also address which providers are best able to deliver affordable, safe, high-quality care. The Institute of Medicine Study Report, *The Future of Nursing, Leading Change, Advancing Health* (2011) calls on private and public funders, health care organizations, nursing education programs, and nursing associations to expand opportunities for nurses to lead and manage collective efforts with physicians and other members of the health care team to conduct research as well as redesign and improve practice environments and health systems. This is an exciting time to be a nurse. See the Through the Eyes of a Nurse display.

ORGANIZING HEALTH CARE: HEALTH CARE DELIVERY SYSTEMS AND CARE COORDINATION

For a long time, health care delivery in the United States has been characterized by fragmentation at the national, state, community, and practice levels. A 2008 Commonwealth

Fund study found that (Shih, Davis, Schoenbaum, Gauthier, Nuzum, & McCarthy, 2008):

• Patients and families navigate unassisted across different providers and care settings, fostering frustrating and dangerous patient experiences.
• Poor communication and lack of clear accountability for a patient among multiple providers lead to medical errors, waste, and duplication.
• The absence of peer accountability, quality improvement infrastructure, and clinical information systems foster poor overall quality of care.
• High-cost, intensive medical intervention is rewarded over higher-value primary care, including preventive medicine and the management of chronic illness.

As you read about the following delivery systems, note that great progress is being made to address this fragmentation, and nurses are playing ever more important roles in care coordination. See Chapter 9 for a discussion of the nurse navigator role. As noted in Chapter 1, The Institute of Medicine report on nursing states that "accessible, high quality care cannot be achieved without exceptional nursing care and leadership" (IOM, 2011, ix).

Physicians and Hospitals

Until recently, in the United States most medical care was delivered by fee-for-service private physicians in solo or small group practices. Most hospitals were not-for-profit community hospitals. Physicians, who were rarely employees of the hospital, wielded great power because hospitals depended on the patients whom physicians admitted or referred for treatment. Under a **fee-for-service** arrangement (in which everything a provider "does" for a patient leads to a bill generated and a fee paid), financial incentives reward doing more care, not necessarily better care.

Multispecialty Group Practice

As new drugs and technologies proliferated, it became increasingly difficult for general practitioners of medicine to provide all the services their patients needed. In the late 1800s, when the Mayo Clinic was founded in Rochester, Minnesota, physicians from different specialties united to share income, expenses, facilities, equipment, and support staff. The **multispecialty group practice** that resulted was better able to provide comprehensive care. While the Mayo Clinic generally served as a referral center, other multispecialty centers developed to serve specific communities.

Community Health Centers

Community health centers are regionalized services for vulnerable geographic populations with an emphasis on primary care and education. Their primary objective is to ensure that everyone who needs care has access regardless of ability to pay. Most of these services rely on nurses to provide primary care. Mary Breckinridge's Frontier Nursing Service, which successfully served a poor rural area in Kentucky that lacked basic medical and obstetric care, was a pioneer organization at its inception in the 1920s. Today the National Association of Community Health Centers (www.nachc.com) reports that community health centers serve the primary health care needs of more than 22 million patients in over 9,000 locations across the United States. According to NACHC, these health centers play a crucial role during tough economic times, providing affordable health services for millions of uninsured and newly jobless Americans. Community health centers save money every time an uninsured patient opts for an examination and treatment at the first sign of a health issue instead of waiting until a costly emergency room visit is the only option. These centers also save money for Americans looking for work whose families could otherwise face poor health without care or large medical debts.

Prepaid Group Practice

Health maintenance organizations (HMOs) are prepaid, group-managed care plans that allow subscribers to receive all the medical services they require through a group of affiliated providers. There may be no additional out-of-pocket costs, or subscribers may pay only a small fee, called a copayment. An HMO may employ all its providers (including physicians), or it may be a group of clinicians in alliance who provide care as independent practitioners. In most HMOs, the patient does not have a choice about health care providers but receives all services from clinicians who are associated with or part of the HMO. HMOs often have a goal of primary care to reduce costs by preventing illness. HMOs are popular with large employers who support the concept of **managed care**, and they are also associated with Medicare in some states.

Preferred provider organizations (PPOs) allow a third-party payer (agencies that pay health care providers for services provided to people, such as a health insurance company) to contract with a group of health care providers to provide services at a lower fee in return for prompt payment and a guaranteed volume of patients and services. Although patients are encouraged to use specific providers, they may also seek care outside the panel without referral by paying additional out-of-pocket expenses. One type of PPO is called a preferred provider arrangement, in which a contract is made with an individual health care provider rather than with a group of providers. Similarly, a point-of-service plan encourages the use of specified physicians and services but pays a portion of expenses for referrals made to physicians outside the organization by the patient's primary care physician.

Accountable Care Organizations

One of the more innovative models of care delivery to emerge from the Patient Protection and Affordable Care Act (PPACA) is the **accountable care organization (ACO)**. This new organizational structure is a departure from the traditional fee-for-service model of reimbursement. In the fee-for-service model, providers are incentivized to do more and more, but not necessarily in a coordinated manner. ACOs turn this model around by offering incentives to provide integrated, well-coordinated care to patients.

ACOs are made up of several types of organizations that deliver care: hospitals, primary care settings, and specialty care practices. Together, the organizations in an ACO come together to deliver the most efficient and high-quality care for the population served; only one bill is generated that covers *all* the care delivered across the various settings (e.g., before the hospitalization, during the inpatient stay, and after discharge from the hospital). In addition, when providers (hospitals and outpatient practice settings) deliver higher quality and more efficient care, they share in the savings from delivering well-integrated care.

Because nurses have the skill set to coordinate care across settings, they are especially well suited to make a real contribution to improved population health within ACOs.

Medical Homes to Medical Neighborhoods

A **medical home** is an enhanced model of primary care that provides whole-person, accessible, comprehensive, ongoing, and coordinated patient-centered care (Box 8-3). First advanced by the American Academy of Pediatrics in the 1960s, the concept gained momentum in 2007 when four major physician groups agreed to a common view of the patient-centered medical home (PCMH) model (AHRQ, 2012). As of January 2012, 41 states have adopted policies and programs to advance medical homes (National Academy

BOX 8-3 THE PATIENT-CENTERED MEDICAL HOME

Defining the Patient-Centered Medical Home (PCMH)

The medical home model holds promise as a way to improve health care in America by transforming how primary care is organized and delivered. Building on the work of a large and growing community, the Agency for Healthcare Research and Quality (AHRQ) defines a medical home not simply as a place but as a model of the organization of primary care that delivers the core functions of primary health care.

The medical home encompasses five functions and attributes:

1. Comprehensive Care

The primary care medical home is accountable for meeting the large majority of each patient's physical and mental health care needs, including prevention and wellness, acute care, and chronic care. Providing comprehensive care requires a team of care providers. This team might include physicians, advanced practice nurses, physician assistants, nurses, pharmacists, nutritionists, social workers, educators, and care coordinators. Although some medical home practices may bring together large and diverse teams of care providers to meet the needs of their patients, many others, including smaller practices, will build virtual teams linking themselves and their patients to providers and services in their communities.

2. Patient-Centered

The primary care medical home provides primary health care that is relationship-based with an orientation toward the whole person. Partnering with patients and their families requires understanding and respecting each patient's unique needs, culture, values, and preferences. The medical home practice actively supports patients in learning to manage and organize their own care at the level the patient chooses. Recognizing that patients and families are core members of the care team, medical home practices ensure that they are fully informed partners in establishing care plans.

3. Coordinated Care

The primary care medical home coordinates care across all elements of the broader health care system, including specialty care, hospitals, home health care, and community services and supports. Such coordination is particularly critical during transitions between sites of care, such as when patients are being discharged from the hospital. Medical home practices also excel at building clear and open communication among patients and families, the medical home, and members of the broader care team.

4. Accessible Services

The primary care medical home delivers accessible services with shorter waiting times for urgent needs, enhanced in-person hours, around-the-clock telephone or electronic access to a member of the care team, and alternative methods of communication such as email and telephone care. The medical home practice is responsive to patients' preferences regarding access.

5. Quality and Safety

The primary care medical home demonstrates a commitment to quality and quality improvement by ongoing engagement in activities such as using evidence-based medicine and clinical decision-support tools to guide shared decision making with patients and families, engaging in performance measurement and improvement, measuring and responding to patient experiences and patient satisfaction, and practicing population health management. Sharing robust quality and safety data and improvement activities publicly is also an important marker of a system-level commitment to quality.

AHRQ recognizes the central role of health IT in successfully operationalizing and implementing the key features of the medical home. Additionally, AHRQ notes that building a primary care delivery platform that the Nation can rely on for accessible, affordable, and high-quality health care will require significant workforce development and fundamental payment reform.

Without these critical elements, the potential of primary care will not be achieved.

Reprinted with permission from Agency for Healthcare Research and Quality (ARHQ). (2012). Defining the PCMH. Available at http://pcmh.ahrq.gov/page/defining-pcmh

for State Health Policy, 2013). The 2012 Patient-Centered Primary Care Collaborative research project demonstrated that the data about PCMHs are clear, consistent, and compelling: "The PCMH improves health outcomes, enhances the patient experience of care and reduces expensive, unnecessary hospital and ED care" (Nielsen, Langner, Zema, Hacker, & Grundy, 2012).

A 2011 Agency for Healthcare Research and Quality (AHRQ) white paper defines a **medical neighborhood** as a PCMH and the constellation of other clinicians providing health care services to patients within it, along with community and social service organizations as well as state and local public health agencies (Figure 8-2). Defined in this way, the PCMH and the surrounding medical neighborhood can focus on meeting the needs of the individual patient but also incorporate aspects of population health and overall community health needs in its objectives (Taylor, Lake, Nysenbaum, Peterson, & Meyers, p. 5). But despite

all our efforts to improve health care, the report starkly concludes:

The medical neighborhood in its current form is highly fragmented, with little coordination among the myriad clinicians and institutions.... primary care—and increasingly a PCMH as the provider of that primary care—should be at the core of the neighborhood, but for many patients it is not. Without a medical home, patients and their families often are left to navigate the system on their own. The current functioning of the neighborhood largely reflects the fee for service environment—in which few or no incentives exist for care coordination activities—and an historical emphasis on specialty-based medical practice in independent small groups or solo practice. Other factors, however, including existing professional norms and a lack of tools to share information across clinicians, also play a role in the way the medical neighborhood currently functions.

FIGURE 8-2. Medical neighborhood. (Reprinted with permission from Taylor, E.F., Lake, T., Nysenbaum, J., Peterson, G., & Meyers, D. [2011]. Coordinating care in the medical neighborhood: Critical components and available mechanisms. White Paper (prepared by Mathematica Policy Research under Contract No. HHSA290200900019I TO2). AHRQ Publication No. 11–0064. Rockville, MD: Agency for Healthcare Research and Quality).

Care Coordination

The AHRQ Care Coordination Measures Atlas acknowledges that there is no consensus definition for care coordination but offers the following (McDonald et al., 2010):

> **Care coordination** is the deliberate organization of patient care activities between two or more participants (including the patient) involved in a patient's care to facilitate the appropriate delivery of healthcare services. Organizing care involves the marshaling of personnel and other resources needed to carry out all required patient care activities and is often managed by the exchange of information among participants responsible for different aspects of care.

Nurses are critical to the success of any care coordination strategy. Chapter 9 explores this topic more fully.

PAYING FOR HEALTH CARE

Few citizens can afford to pay for health care from their own resources. The costs of most people's health care are covered by public or private health insurance. The four basic modes of paying for health care are out-of-pocket payment, individual private insurance, employer-based group private insurance, and government financing.

Out-of-Pocket Payment

During the first half of the twentieth century, most Americans paid for health care with cash payments. This simple method of financing is increasingly rare because today most families cannot afford the high costs of health care. Most Americans continue to believe that the basic health care needs of all should be met regardless of ability to pay.

Individual Private Insurance

Personal health care can be financed by private insurance through large, nonprofit, tax-exempt organizations or through smaller, private, for-profit insurance companies. To be insured, members pay monthly premiums either by themselves or in combination with employer payments. These plans are called third-party payers because the insurance company pays all or most of the cost of care. The premiums on private insurance plans tend to be higher than those for managed care plans, but members can choose their own physician and services desired.

Employer-Based Private Insurance

A majority of employers offer group health insurance policies to their employees and their families. In 2012, 61% of firms offered coverage to their employees. About half the people with employer-sponsored coverage are covered by their own employer (51%), and half are covered as an employee's dependent (49%). Health insurance rates vary among businesses, with large firms and those with more high-wage workers being more likely to offer coverage (Kaiser, 2012).

Government Financing

The largest federally funded health care programs are Medicare and Medicaid.

Medicare

The 1965 **Medicare** amendments to the Social Security Act established national and state health insurance programs for older adults under Title XVIII. Within a decade, almost all citizens over 65 years of age held Medicare insurance for hospital care, extended care, and home health care. Medicare coverage was increased in 1972 to include permanently disabled workers and their dependents, if they also qualified for Social Security benefits.

In 1983, Medicare converted to a prospective payment plan based on patient classification categories, called **diagnosis-related groups (DRGs)**. The federal government implemented DRGs in an effort to control rising health care costs. The plan pays the hospital a fixed amount that is predetermined by the medical diagnosis or specific procedure rather than by the actual cost of hospitalization and care. Medicare was expanded in 1988 to include catastrophic care costs and expensive medications. In 2007, based on changes in DRGs made by the Centers for Medicare and Medicaid Services (CMS), the reimbursement to hospitals became based on severity of illness and projected cost of care. The plan pays only the amount of money preassigned to a treatment for the diagnosis (e.g., an appendectomy); if the cost of hospitalization is greater than that assigned, the hospital must absorb the additional cost. If the cost is less than that assigned, the hospital makes a profit. In addition, Medicare no longer reimburses hospitals for conditions that result from preventable errors and lead to increased costs. Such conditions include pressure ulcers, injuries caused by falls, infections associated with indwelling urinary catheters, vascular catheter–associated infections, infections of the mediastinum after coronary artery bypass graft, air embolisms, adverse reactions to incompatible blood infusions, and sponges or instruments left inside a patient during surgery.

People who receive Medicare pay both a deductible cost and a monthly premium for full insurance coverage. Part A

of Medicare, which pays most inpatient hospital costs, is paid by the federal government. Part B of Medicare, which is voluntary, is paid by a monthly premium; it covers most outpatient costs for physician visits, medications, and home health services. Because the full cost of some services is not covered by Medicare, a supplemental insurance policy offered by a private insurance company is recommended. Also, because Medicare is federally funded, benefits may change annually according to Congressional decisions related to the federal budget. In the second decade of the twenty-first century there continues to be a national debate about whether the United States can continue to operate Medicare in the same form along with other government programs and still control spiraling health care costs. In the United States, as in other countries, **entitlement reform** is being considered for benefits paid by the government to citizens in order to improve the national budget and reduce debt.

 REMEMBER Margaret Ritchie, the older adult woman caring for her husband at home. Most likely, she and her husband have Medicare. Medicare does pay for home health care services if the patient meets specific criteria. However, Medicare does not cover all equipment that may be necessary. •

Medicaid

Medicaid was established in 1965 under Title XIX of the Social Security Act. Medicaid is a federally funded public assistance program for people of any age who have low incomes; for the blind, older adults, and disabled covered by supplemental security benefits; and for beneficiaries of Aid to Families With Dependent Children. This coverage depends on individual state regulations.

Current budgetary considerations are leading state and federal agencies to trim Medicaid expenditures. The rapid growth of an aging population and an increased number of poor people, many of whom are women and children, are draining the Medicaid budget. In an attempt to survive, Medicaid programs are implementing changes such as reduced benefits or placing patients into managed care programs.

Children's Health Insurance Program (CHIP)

The Children's Health Insurance Program (CHIP), formerly the State Children's Health Insurance Program (SCHIP), was created by the Balanced Budget Act of 1997, was enacted as Title XXI of the Social Security Act, and has allocated about $20 billion over 10 years to help states insure low-income children who are ineligible for Medicaid but cannot afford private insurance. States receive an enhanced federal match (greater than the state's Medicaid match) to provide this coverage. In 2007 the program was extended, and in 2009 was reauthorized by Congress and signed by President Obama. Together, Medicaid and CHIP serve more than 42 million children who would otherwise not have access to regular medical care. While Medicaid and CHIP have helped bring the rate of uninsured children to the lowest level in more than two decades, many more children are eligible but not covered as yet.

Veteran's Health Administration (VHA)

The Veterans Health Administration is home to the United States' largest integrated health care system, consisting of 152 medical centers, nearly 1,400 community-based outpatient clinics, community living centers, vet centers, and domiciliaries. Together these health care facilities and the more than 53,000 independent licensed health care practitioners who work within them provide comprehensive care to more than 8.3 million veterans each year. The VHA has an annual medical care appropriation of more than $47 billion.

HEALTH CARE SETTINGS AND SERVICES

Health care is provided within many different types of facilities to meet the varying needs of people. When one considers that only patients who require complex surgery, who are acutely ill or seriously injured, and some who are having babies are hospitalized—and then only for a minimum period of time—it is apparent that most health care services are provided in settings outside the hospital. These settings include clinics, homes, schools, prisons, daycare centers for children and older adults, crisis-intervention centers, mental health centers, drug and alcohol rehabilitation programs, storefront clinics, and churches.

Hospitals

There are approximately 5,000 community hospitals in the United States. Community hospitals are short-term, general, nonfederal, and special (e.g., orthopedic, cancer, and academic medical center) hospitals. Each year, community hospitals admit more than 35 million people, treat nearly 118 million people in their emergency departments, and deliver over 4 million babies (American Hospital Association, 2013). The average hospital stay in 2011 was 4.9 days, although longer stays occur in patients who have serious infections, major trauma, mental illnesses, and cardiovascular diseases (CDC, 2012). Shorter hospital stays have resulted from many factors, including improved treatment of diseases, an increased emphasis on preventive care, federal regulations, and other health care reimbursement policies. The shorter stay means that most hospital care is focused on the acute care needs of the patient.

Classification

Hospitals are classified as public or private, and as for profit or nonprofit. Public hospitals, which are nonprofit institutions, are financed and operated by local, state, or national agencies. Patients admitted to a public hospital may not have health insurance, and services are provided at little or no cost to the patient. Tax revenue or public funds cover the cost. Private hospitals may be for profit or nonprofit and are operated by communities, churches, corporations, and charitable organizations. Many patients cared for in private hospitals have some type of personal health insurance or health care plan.

Size and Services

Hospitals range in size from as few as 20 beds to large medical centers with hundreds of beds. Various services are provided, depending on the size and location of the hospital. Most hospitals provide emergency care, inpatient care, surgery, diagnostic tests, and patient education. Other hospital services might include intensive care, obstetric care, palliative care, social services, outpatient clinics and surgery, educational programs, and long-term skilled nursing care facilities. Hospitals may provide care for all types of illnesses and trauma or may specialize in the treatment of certain types of illness. Specialty hospitals, or special units in general hospitals, meet the varied needs of certain patient groups such as children and patients of all ages needing rehabilitation, cancer care, psychiatric or drug-dependency care, or patients with severe burns.

Inpatient and Outpatient Services

Hospitals provide both inpatient and outpatient services. An **inpatient** is a person who enters a hospital and stays overnight for an indeterminate time (from days to months). Hospitals also have many services for **outpatients**—those who are not hospitalized overnight but who require diagnosis or treatment. Patients who do not require inpatient care can receive treatment, care, and education on an outpatient basis. Examples of outpatient services include surgical procedures, diagnostic tests, medications, physical therapy, counseling, and health education. A form of hospital outpatient care occurs in short-stay units, where patients having diagnostic tests or surgery enter the hospital, have the procedure, and then return to the hospital room for a brief (1–6 hours) recovery period before going home. Patients may also be categorized as outpatients when they are admitted, treated, and discharged within 23 hours.

Nurses' Role in Hospitals

Although the trend is changing, hospitals still employ more nurses than any other type of facility. The percentage of RNs working in hospitals is declining, but about 58% of RNs are still employed in hospitals (U.S. Department of Labor, 2012). The U.S. Department of Labor projects that the number of RNs employed in hospitals will decrease while those employed in outpatient settings, home health, and long-term care will increase. Nurses employed in hospitals have many roles. Although many nurses are direct care providers, other roles include manager of other members of the health care team providing patient care, administrator, nurse practitioner, clinical nurse specialist, patient educator, in-service educator, and researcher.

The Magnet Recognition Program for Excellence in Nursing and the Pathway to Excellence Program are administered by the American Nurses Credentialing Center (ANCC), a subsidiary of the American Nurses Association. Magnet hospitals must meet strict requirements and standards that define the highest quality of nursing practice and patient care. A designation as a magnet hospital recognizes quality patient care, nursing excellence, and innovations in professional nursing practice (American Nurses Credentialing Center, 2013).

 THINK back to Maritza Cortes, the mother who brings her daughter to the emergency department for care. The nurse, in this situation, acts primarily in the caregiver role. However, the nurse also plays a major role as educator, using knowledge about the infection to teach the mother about possible complications and the need for continued antibiotic treatment. ●

Primary Care Centers

Physicians and advanced practice nurses provide primary health care services in offices and clinics. Services include the diagnosis and treatment of minor illnesses; performing minor surgical procedures; and providing obstetric care, well-child care, counseling, and referrals (Fig. 8-3). Federally qualified health centers (FQHCs) also known as community health centers, are nonprofit primary care clinics located in high-need areas across the country. Community health centers must serve everyone in the community, regardless of their health insurance and ability to pay, and often offer on-site mental health and dental services. An RN working in a health care provider's office makes health assessments, performs technical procedures, assists the physician, and provides health education and counseling.

Advanced practice registered nurses (APRNs), nurse practitioners, midwives, and clinical nurse specialists work independently or collaboratively with physicians to make assessments and care for patients who require health maintenance or health promotion activities. Depending on state regulations, APRNs may have their own offices and clinics to provide primary care and treatment to patients and refer only complex health problems to a physician.

FIGURE 8-3. A nurse assesses a patient during a well-child visit at a primary care center. (*Photo by Joe Mitchell.*)

 RECALL Maritza Cortes, the mother of the child with a strep throat. One might commonly think of primary health care services for typical childhood illnesses, but in this case, Ms. Cortes used the emergency department. Possibly, the mother thought that her child was too ill and needed to be seen immediately. In this case, the nurse would develop a teaching plan for Ms. Cortes about typical childhood illnesses. Maybe she did not know of anywhere else to obtain services. In this case, the nurse could contact social services to obtain information about community clinics for Ms. Cortes. Her finances may also have led to her decision to use the emergency department. In this case, the nurse also could contact social services to arrange for financial assistance. ●

Ambulatory Care Centers and Clinics

Ambulatory care centers and clinics (agencies that deliver outpatient medical care) may be located in hospitals, may be a freestanding service provided by a group of health care providers who work together, or may be managed by an APRN. Ambulatory care centers and clinics are often located in convenient areas such as shopping malls or other community agencies. Many ambulatory care centers and clinics offer walk-in services so that appointments are unnecessary, and many are also open at times other than traditional office hours. Small clinics staffed by APRNs are increasingly being established in nontraditional sites, such as drugstores and grocery stores. These clinics have dramatically improved access to care for the uninsured and those with other barriers to health care.

Nurses in ambulatory care centers and clinics provide technical services (e.g., administering medications), determine the priority of care needs, and provide teaching about all aspects of care. The urgent care center is a special type of ambulatory care center that provides walk-in care for illnesses and minor trauma. Outpatient or same-day surgical centers, discussed in Chapter 29, are another form of ambulatory care center.

Home Health Care

Home health care is one of the most rapidly growing areas of the health care system. Home health care may be provided through community health departments, visiting nurses' associations, hospital-based case managers, and home health agencies. These agencies provide many different health-related services, including skilled nursing assessment, teaching and support of patients and family members, and direct care for patients.

Home health care is important for many reasons. The prospective payment system of reimbursement encourages early discharge from the hospital, and has created a new, acutely ill population that needs skilled care at home. More older people are living longer and have multiple chronic illnesses, and with sophisticated technology people can live relatively comfortably in their own homes. Health care consumers demand that services be humane and that provisions be made for a dignified death at home. Read more about home care in Chapter 9.

Nurses who provide care in the home make assessments and provide physical care, administer medications, teach, and support family members. They also collaborate with other health care providers, such as physicians, physical therapists, occupational therapists, respiratory therapists, and social workers to plan and provide patient care.

Hospital At Home

In 1995, doctors at the John Hopkins School of Medicine developed a new program to provide safe and effective hospital-level care in the home (Box 8-4). Rather than being admitted to a hospital, persons who qualify are treated in their own homes by appropriate health care professionals. A National Demonstration and Evaluation Study tested the Hospital at Home program in three Medicare-managed care organizations and one Veterans Affairs medical center. Hospital at

BOX 8-4　THE HOSPITAL AT HOME

A Typical Hospital at Home Program Follows These Steps

- A patient requiring admission for one of the target illnesses is identified in the Emergency Department or ambulatory site. Staff assesses if the patient is a good candidate for the program using validated criteria.
- If the patient is eligible and consents to participate, the **Hospital at Home®** physician evaluates the patient and is then transported home, usually by ambulance.
- Once home, the patient receives extended nursing care for the initial portion of their admission, and then at least daily nursing visits according to clinical need. Nurses are available 24 hours a day/7 days a week for any urgent or emergent situation.
- The patient is evaluated daily by the **Hospital at Home** physician, who completes an assessment and continues to implement appropriate diagnostic and therapeutic measures. The physician makes one or more home visits per day and is available 24 hours a day/7 days a week for any urgent or emergent situation.
- The clinicians use care pathways, including illness-specific care maps, clinical outcome evaluations, and specific discharge criteria.
- The patient can receive diagnostic studies such as electrocardiograms, echocardiograms, and x-rays at home, as well as treatments, including oxygen therapy, intravenous fluids, intravenous antibiotics, and other medicines, respiratory therapy, pharmacy services, and skilled nursing services.
- Diagnostic studies and therapeutics that cannot be provided at home, such as computerized tomography, magnetic resonance imaging, or endoscopy, are available via brief visits to the acute hospital.
- The patient is treated until stable for discharge. When the patient is discharged by the **Hospital at Home** physician, care reverts to the patient's primary care physician.

Reprint with permission from Hospital at Home. Available at http://www.hospitalathome.org/about-us/how-it-works.php

Home met disease-specific quality standards at rates similar to the acute hospital. The average patient length of stay was shorter, and overall costs were a third lower than an inpatient stay. Patients also had a lower chance of developing delirium, requiring sedatives, or needing chemical restraints. In addition, both patients and family members were more satisfied with care compared to those treated in the hospital, and family member stress was lower. Patients also regained their ability to do usual tasks more quickly. In 2010, a public/private partnership tested a modified model of Hospital at Home in which home-based care is provided by nurses, with physician consult via biometrically enhanced, two-way telemedicine video. The new model is also managed by a physician group instead of a hospital (www.hospitalathome.org).

Extended Care

Extended-care services provide medical and nonmedical care for people with chronic illnesses or disabilities. Through a variety of services, family, and other caregivers, they assist with activities of daily living for people of any age who are physically or mentally unable to care for themselves independently. In 2012, about 9 million people over the age of 65 used long-term care services; that number is projected to increase to 12 million by 2020. Most extended care is provided to people by family or friends; for example, 70% of older adults requiring extended care are not in any type of facility (Medicare, 2013).

Extended care may last for periods ranging from days to years. Facilities that provide this care are often independent but may be associated with a hospital. Extended-care facilities include transitional subacute care, assisted-living facilities, intermediate and long-term care facilities, homes for medically fragile children, retirement centers, and residential institutions for mentally and developmentally or physically disabled patients of all ages. One of the newest concepts in extended care is called "aging in place." In this type of care, patients remain in their homes or move to a living space, such as an apartment, while they are still physically able to care for themselves, and then have access to services that are a part of the health care community as needed as long as they live. What is essential for this health care paradigm is a community committed to meeting one another's needs.

Extended-care facilities have proliferated in recent years for two reasons. First, as many patients are discharged from the hospital earlier in their recovery period, they require care that is beyond the scope of home care. These patients receive transitional, subacute care in an extended-care facility. Second, as the population ages, many older adults will not have caregivers available and would be unable to carry out activities of daily living independently. Although extended-care facilities, especially long-term care facilities, have had a negative image in the past, much has changed. Most long-term care facilities focus on maintaining residents' function and independence, with concern for the living environment as well as the health care provided. A focus on maximizing quality of life for residents has led to surroundings that include plants and animals as well as numerous intergenerational programs. Many of the overall improvements in long-term care resulted from the 1987 Omnibus Budget Reconciliation Act (OBRA), which included legislation to maintain standards of quality assurance in the long-term care industry.

Because patients entering extended-care facilities require so many different levels of care, it is difficult to generalize about the services provided. Those entering convalescent centers remain only until they have recovered. In some instances, an older adult may choose to move into a retirement or assisted-living facility that provides health care services only when needed. Other people who enter a long-term care facility may require complete care as long as they live. The nurse's roles in extended-care facilities may include being a provider of direct care, supervisor, administrator, or teacher. Because most patients are older, increasing numbers of gerontology nurse specialists are contributing their knowledge and expertise to the care of these patients. Almost all extended-care facilities require that skilled nursing care be available at all times. The care given to patients can be performed only by or under the direct supervision of a licensed nurse.

Specialized Care Centers and Settings

Specialized care centers and settings provide services for a specific population or group. They are usually located in easily accessible locations within a community.

Daycare Centers

Daycare centers have a variety of purposes. Some centers care for healthy infants and children whose parents work; some also care for children with minor illnesses. Eldercare centers and senior citizen centers provide a place for older adults to socialize and to receive care while family members work. Some daycare centers provide health-related services and care to people who do not need to be in a health care institution but cannot be at home alone. Such centers provide services to older people for physical rehabilitation, for people with special needs (e.g., cerebral palsy), and for chemical dependency and mental health.

Nurses who work in daycare centers administer medications and treatments, conduct health screenings, teach, and counsel.

Mental Health Centers

Mental health centers may be associated with a hospital or may provide services as an independent agency. The services provided may be crisis centered or may involve long-term counseling. Patients receive outpatient care through a variety of interventions, including individual and group counseling, medications, and assistance with independent living. Crisis intervention centers are also mental health centers. They typically provide 24-hour services and hotlines for people who are suicidal, abusing drugs or alcohol, or in abusive situations. These centers also provide information and services for victims of rape and abuse.

Nurses who work in mental health centers must have strong communication and counseling skills and must be thoroughly familiar with community resources specific to the needs of patients being served in order to make appropriate referrals.

 REMEMBER Paul Cochran, the patient with a mental illness who ran out of his medications. The nurse needs knowledge of local mental health centers to ensure continuity of care, including follow-up with medication regimen. ●

Rural Health Centers

Rural health centers are often located in geographically remote areas that have few health care providers. Many rural health centers are run by APRNs who serve as the patient's primary health provider for the care of minor acute illnesses as well as chronic illnesses. Patients who are seriously ill or injured are given emergency care and then transported to the nearest large hospital. Nurses who practice independently usually do so in collaboration with a physician who approves protocols for care. Many rural health care settings and providers now have immediate access to information about diagnosis and treatment of illness through telecommunication and computers.

Schools

School nurses are often the major source of health assessment, health education, and emergency care for the nation's children. The role of the school nurse reflects changes in society itself: children in schools today are from many different racial and ethnic groups, have varying socioeconomic backgrounds, and have more complex disabilities that require expert knowledge and skills for management during school hours. School nurses provide many different services, including maintaining immunization records, providing emergency care for physical and mental illnesses, administering prescribed medications, conducting routine health screenings (e.g., vision, hearing, scoliosis), and providing health information and education.

Industry

Many large industries have their own ambulatory care clinic, staffed primarily by nurses. Occupational health nurses in industrial clinics focus on preventing work-related injury and illness by conducting health assessments, teaching for health promotion (e.g., stopping smoking, eating sensibly, using safety equipment, exercising regularly), caring for minor accidents and illnesses, and making referrals for more serious health problems.

Homeless Shelters

Homeless shelters are usually living units, such as an apartment building or home, that provide housing for people who do not have regular shelter. The homeless are at increased risk for illness or injury because of factors such as exposure to the elements, exposure to violence, drug and alcohol addiction, poor nutrition, poor hygiene, and overcrowding. Services provided by nurses in homeless shelters include immunizing children, teaching pregnant women, treating infections and illnesses, referring for diagnosis and treatment of STIs, and providing information about maintaining health.

Rehabilitation Centers

Rehabilitation centers specialize in services for patients requiring physical or emotional rehabilitation and for treatment of chemical dependency. These centers may be freestanding or associated with a hospital. The goal is to return patients to optimal health and to the community as independent members of society. Rehabilitation centers often use a multidisciplinary team composed of physicians, nurses, physical therapists, occupational therapists, and counselors. The role of the nurse includes direct care, teaching, and counseling. The practice of rehabilitation nursing is based on a philosophy of encouraging independent self-care within the patient's capabilities.

Parish Nursing

Parish nursing is an expanding area of specialty nursing practice that emphasizes holistic health care, health promotion, and disease-prevention activities. It combines professional nursing practice with health ministry, emphasizing health and healing within a faith community. Parish nurses function as health educators, resource and referral aids, and facilitators of lay volunteer and support groups. Parish nurses reach out to those most vulnerable, such as older adults, those who have suffered a loss or change, single parents, and children. For more about parish nursing, see Chapter 45.

Health Care Services for the Seriously Ill and Dying

Health care services for the seriously ill and dying and for their families and caregivers include respite care, hospice, and palliative care. (End-of-life care is discussed further in Chapter 42.)

Respite Care

Respite care is a type of care provided for caregivers of homebound ill, disabled, or older patients. The main purpose is to give the primary caregiver some time away from the responsibilities of day-to-day care. Professionals or volunteers may provide care in an adult daycare center or in the patient's home. In most instances, the care is provided by trained nursing assistants or volunteers. Professional nurses provide information about how to access respite care and may make referrals. Medicaid and most insurance providers do not cover the costs of respite care.

Hospice Services

Hospice is a program of palliative and supportive care services providing physical, psychological, social, and spiritual care for dying people, their families, and other loved ones. The interdisciplinary hospice team:

- Manages the patient's pain and symptoms

- Assists the patient with emotional, psychosocial, and spiritual aspects of dying
- Provides needed drugs, medical supplies, and equipment
- Instructs the family on how to care for the patient
- Delivers special services like speech and physical therapy when needed
- Makes short-term inpatient care available when pain or symptoms become too difficult to treat at home, or the caregiver needs respite
- Provides bereavement care and counseling to surviving family and friends (National Hospice and Palliative Care Organization [NHPCO], 2013).

In 2011, an estimated 1.65 million patients received hospice services (NHPCO, 2013). Approximately 44.6% of all deaths in the United States in 2011 were under the care of a hospice program. The number of hospice programs nationwide has increased since the first program in 1974 to over 5,300 programs today. The Medicare hospice benefit, enacted by Congress in 1982, is the predominant source of payment for hospice care. To be eligible for hospice benefits from Medicare or Medicaid, the patient must have a serious, progressive illness with a life expectancy of 6 months or less.

 THINK back to Margaret Ritchie, who is caring for her husband at home. The physician recently informed her of her husband's prognosis. The nurse might anticipate that hospice care would be appropriate for Mrs. Ritchie and her husband. ●

The hospice nurse combines the skills of the home care nurse with the ability to provide daily emotional support to dying patients and their families. Hospice nurses are especially skilled in pain and symptom management. Their focus is on improving quality of life rather than merely prolonging its length, and on preserving dignity for the patient in death. After the death, the nurse continues to care for the patient's family during the bereavement period for up to 1 year. Nurses use this time to help families work through the grief process after their loss. (See Chapter 42 for more information).

Palliative Care

Palliative care evolved from the hospice experience but also exists outside of hospice programs. It is not restricted to the end of life and can be used from the point of initial diagnosis. Palliative care, which may be given in conjunction with medical treatment and in all types of health care settings, focuses on the relief of physical, mental, and spiritual distress. The goal of palliative care is to prevent and relieve suffering by early assessment and treatment of pain and other physical problems (such as difficulty breathing, nausea, fatigue, and problems with sleeping). Like hospice care, palliative care is provided by an interdisciplinary team.

HEALTH CARE AGENCIES

Many different types of agencies provide health care services. This section discusses voluntary agencies, religious agencies, and government agencies.

Voluntary Agencies

Community agencies are often nonprofit voluntary agencies. They are financed by private donations, grants, or fundraisers (although some may charge minimal fees). Examples of volunteer agencies are Meals on Wheels, which supplies meals to older and homebound people; transportation services for older and physically disabled people; and shopping or house-cleaning services. Other nonprofit voluntary community agencies include the American Heart Association and the American Lung Association. Physicians and nurses are often active members of these organizations, providing health screenings and educational programs.

Voluntary agencies may also provide a setting for support groups. These groups provide an education and support system for patients who are adjusting to their health problems. Members of these support groups have experienced the same type of problem. By sharing their experiences, members learn to solve problems when dealing with a stressful or crisis situation. Professional nurses most often provide information about and make referrals to these agencies to patients and family members. The following are examples of support groups:

- Alcoholics Anonymous—an international organization for recovering alcoholics. The purpose is to help people stop drinking and remain sober. Meetings are held in accessible community locations, such as churches and hospitals.
- Cancer support groups—focus on support and solving problems experienced by people diagnosed with cancer. Most cancer support group meetings are held at hospitals.
- Reach to Recovery—for women who have had a breast removed for cancer or have had breast reconstruction surgery. Among other activities, members visit women before surgery, teach exercises to prevent muscle atrophy, and provide information about prostheses and clothing.

Other Government Agencies

In addition to Medicare, Medicaid, and the Veteran's Association, described earlier, there are other government health agencies.

Public Health Service

The Public Health Service (PHS) is a federal health agency under the direction of the U.S. Department of Health and Human Services. The PHS is a multifaceted program with a wide range of services. It is the medical branch of the U.S. Coast Guard and the principal source of Native American health care through the Indian Health Services. The PHS supplies funds to health centers that provide care to migrant workers and to community agencies that supply health care to the poor and uninsured. The principal budget of the PHS goes to grant programs for poor and uninsured people.

The Centers for Disease Control and Prevention (CDC) in Atlanta and the National Institutes of Health (NIH) are both part of the PHS. The CDC focuses on the epidemiology, prevention, control, and treatment of communicable diseases, such as STIs. The NIH is engaged in both funding and conducting various health research activities.

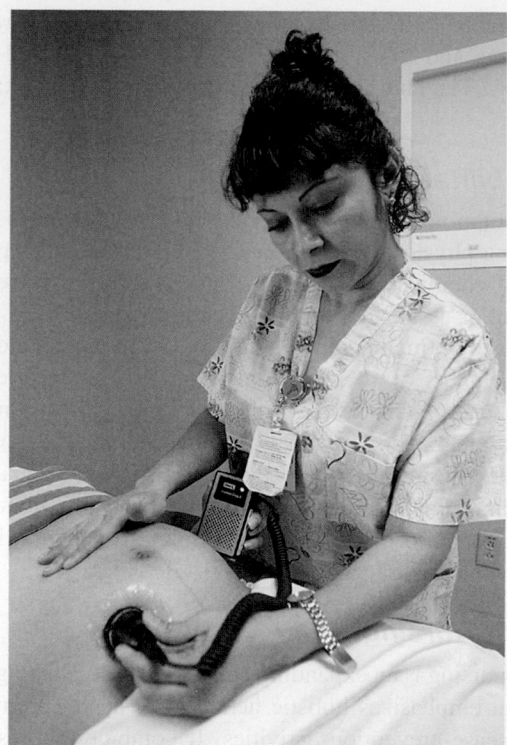

FIGURE 8-4. A nurse provides prenatal care at a public health clinic. (*Photo by Joe Mitchell.*)

The PHS also supplies health care professionals (e.g., nurses, physicians, dentists, pharmacists) to the U.S. Department of Justice to provide care in federal prisons. The service is also involved in some state-administered drug and alcohol abuse and mental health programs. PHS activities focus on community needs whenever possible. Nurses practicing in these settings provide direct care, provide information, and serve as patient advocates within the community.

Public Health Agencies

Public health agencies are local, state, and federal agencies that provide public health services at the local, county, state, or federal level. They are usually funded by taxes and run by elected or appointed administrators. Local agencies provide services and programs to promote health and prevent illness, such as providing immunizations and screening for tuberculosis and STIs. Public health agencies work with state and local departments to ensure public health through activities such as inspections of restaurants and water supplies. They also provide educational programs and may provide direct care services for low-income people or people living in rural, isolated areas. Nurses who practice in public health agencies focus on prenatal care, well-child care, screening programs, education, and outreach into the community (Fig. 8-4).

COLLABORATIVE CARE: THE HEALTH CARE TEAM

In any type of agency, setting, or framework, nurses work with other members of the interdisciplinary health care team to plan, provide, and evaluate patient care (Box 8-5). The

BOX 8-5 COLLABORATIVE ROLES OF MEMBERS OF THE HEALTH CARE TEAM

Physician

The physician is primarily responsible for the diagnosis of illness and the medical or surgical treatment of that illness. Physicians are granted the authority to admit patients to a health care agency by the health care agency or institution itself and to practice care within that setting through such actions as prescribing medications, interpreting the results of laboratory and diagnostic tests, and performing procedures and surgery. A person becomes a physician after extensive education and clinical practice and a licensing examination. Physicians may choose to be general practitioners or to specialize in the treatment of one type of illness or body system (such as a cardiologist) or a specific type of surgery (such as an orthopedic surgeon).

Hospitalists are physicians who provide care to patients when they visit the emergency department or are admitted to the hospital. They communicate with the patient's primary care physician but provide care while the patient is in the hospital. They also may take after-hour, weekend, and holiday calls and services for one or more physicians.

Physician Assistant

A physician assistant (PA) has completed a specific course of study and a licensing examination in preparation for providing support to the physician. The PA's responsibilities usually depend on the supervising physician and might include conducting physical examinations and suturing lacerations. In most states, nurses are not legally bound to follow a PA's orders unless a physician cosigns the orders. This is an important aspect to investigate if PAs are employed by hospitals in your area.

Nurse

Nurses supervise and coordinate direct care to patients and families. They teach the patient and family self-care and conduct research to ensure cost effectiveness and quality of care. Nurses coordinate the services of other health care providers. See Chapter 1 for a description of the many roles nurses play and their different levels of education.

Physical Therapist

A physical therapist (PT) seeks to restore function or to prevent further disability in a patient after an injury or illness. PTs use various techniques to treat patients, including massage, heat, cold, water, sonar waves, exercises, and electrical stimulation. Most PTs are also educated in the use of psychological strategies to motivate patients.

Occupational Therapist

Occupational therapists evaluate the patient's functional level and teaching activities to promote self-care in activities of daily living. They assess the home for safety and provide adaptive equipment as necessary.

Speech Therapist

A speech therapist is trained to help hearing-impaired patients speak more clearly, to assist patients who have had a stroke to relearn how to speak, and to correct or modify a variety of speech disturbances in children and adults. Speech therapists also diagnose and treat swallowing problems in patients who have had a head injury or a stroke.

Social Worker

Social workers assist patients and families in dealing with the social, emotional, and environmental factors that affect their well-being. They make referrals to appropriate community resources and provide assistance with securing equipment and supplies, as well as with health care finances. In recent years, their role in discharge planning has been highlighted.

Pharmacist

A pharmacist, prepared at the doctoral level, is licensed to formulate and dispense medications. The pharmacist is also responsible for keeping a file of all patient medications and for informing the physician when a potential or actual medication error in prescribing has occurred or when prescribed drugs may interact adversely. The pharmacist is an excellent resource for information related to medications for both patients and nurses.

Respiratory Therapist

A respiratory therapist (RT) is trained in techniques that improve pulmonary function and oxygenation. RTs may also be responsible for administering a variety of tests that measure lung function and for educating the patient about the use of various devices and machines prescribed by the physician.

Dietitian

A registered dietitian (RD) manages and plans for the dietary needs of patients, based on knowledge about all aspects of nutrition. RDs can adapt specialized diets for the individual needs of patients, counsel and educate individual patients, and supervise the dietary services of an entire facility.

Chaplain/Spiritual Care Provider

Spiritual care providers identify and respond to the spiritual needs of patients, families, and other members of the interdisciplinary team. They may be members of the clergy, pastoral care workers with graduate degrees, or lay volunteers.

Unlicensed Assistive Personnel

Unlicensed assistive personnel (UAPs) help nurses provide direct care to patients. As defined by individual state boards of nursing, UAPs may have the title of certified nursing assistants, orderlies, attendants, or technicians.

---

likelihood of achieving valued patient outcomes is greatly enhanced when nurses are skilled in collaborating with other members of the professional caregiving team. In 2012, The U.S. Department of Health and Human Services awarded $4 million over 5 years to fund a new coordinating center to promote interprofessional education and collaborative practice in health care at the University of Minnesota Academic Health Center. The goal is to foster efforts to create

a U.S. health care system that engages patients, families, and communities in collaborative, team-based care. Take advantage of every opportunity to get to know the members of the teams you will join as a student and learn what each member can contribute. Practice working collaboratively to make health care "work" for your patients and families. Read more about the care coordination role nurses play in Chapter 9.

THINK about Maritza Cortes, the woman who brought her daughter to the emergency department. Her statement about not having the money needed to have the prescription filled would alert the nurse to the need for consulting social service. The social worker could provide Ms. Cortes with information about available financial assistance and community resources. Which members of the health care team are best equipped to meet the health care needs of Maritza and her daughter, Margaret Ritchie and her husband, and Paul Cochran? How would you collaborate with these members of the team? ●

TRENDS AND ISSUES IN HEALTH CARE DELIVERY

This section discusses some current issues and trends in health care. In your career as a nurse, you may find that as some issues are resolved, other new challenges arise. It is important for you both personally and professionally to be knowledgeable about all health care trends affecting the health care delivery system (Box 8-6).

Focus on Preventive Care

People's health awareness and desire to be involved in their own health care have strongly influenced the delivery of health care services in our society. Stress management programs, nutritional awareness, exercise and fitness programs, and antismoking and antidrug campaigns are all examples of this trend. Equally important to health are measures such as legislating the use of seat belts, promoting automobile and airplane safety, controlling smog, controlling handguns, and eliminating hazardous wastes.

Knowledgeable and Engaged Consumers

A **consumer** is someone who uses a commodity or service. Health care consumers (patients) are increasingly knowledgeable about health, prefer to control and make decisions about their own health, and want to be active participants in planning and implementing their health care. It is therefore critical for nurses to develop skills for creating successful partnerships with patients and their families. Consumers of health care services are better educated about the services they require and the services that are available,

largely because so much health information is available on the Internet. They also are concerned about access to services, the cost of those services, and the quality of the care received. Consumers are questioning escalating costs and the proliferation and duplication of services. Consumers have become actively involved in the administration of health care agencies and have helped develop standards for care, patient rights, and cost-containment measures as protection for patients when they enter a health care setting.

The Centers for Medicare and Medicaid Services now requires providers to meet several patient engagement benchmarks. More than 50% of the patients that clinicians see must now get timely access to their health information, including diagnostic test results, medication lists, and a clinical summary of their office visit, within one business day. While this is an important effort by the U.S. government to engage the public in self-care, respectful, trusting, and compassionate health care professional–patient relationships remain the most effective strategy to achieve these goals.

Mobile Health

Paul Cerrato, editor of *InformationWeek Healthcare,* writes (Cerrato, 2013): "It's no exaggeration to describe consumers' and physicians' [and nurses'] embrace of mobile health apps, smartphones, and tablets as transformational." Tablets give access to electronic health record data, drug reference materials, and other valuable data that in the past was available only in the office or hospital. Patients, especially those with chronic illnesses, are similarly using apps and smartphone devices that let them measure blood pressure, blood glucose, and more. Many nurses are filming teachable moments, such as how to dress a port, and then e-mailing the video to the patient or family caregiver. This trend will only increase and provide more opportunities for nurses to provide effective, quality care.

HEALTH CARE: A RIGHT, A PRIVILEGE, OR AN OBLIGATION OF A MORAL SOCIETY?

Two major factors influencing the provision of health care in the United States are the ability to pay for care and the location of facilities. Poor or uninsured people, minorities, residents of rural areas, and older people often have inadequate access to health care services. In the United States, there are still too many who have inadequate health insurance or none at all. As this book goes to press, we are still waiting to see the effects of health reform as a result of the Affordable Care Act. Although many people assume that everyone has a right to health care, consider these questions that pose ethical dilemmas for nurses who provide care, as well as for consumers of health care services:

- Do people who engage in risky behaviors or who do not make necessary lifestyle changes deserve the same health care as people who live healthy lives?
- Who should pay for health care needed by the unemployed and homeless?
- Is someone who pays for national television coverage to ask for an organ donation for one's child any more deserving

---

BOX 8-6	**TRENDS TO WATCH IN HEALTH CARE DELIVERY**

- Changing demographics
- Increasing diversity
- Technology explosion
- Globalization of economy and society
- Educated and engaged consumers
- Increasing complexity of patient care
- Costs of health care
- Effect of health policy and regulation
- Shortages of key health care professionals and educators

than someone who has been waiting months for just such a transplant?

- Should citizens pay higher insurance premiums or taxes so that someone addicted to drugs who overdoses can have intensive care?
- Should undocumented workers in the United States have the same access to health care as U.S. citizens?
- If 20 people need a heart transplant and only one heart is available, who decides who gets another chance at life and how should these decisions be made?

These are only a few of the questions being raised, and there are no easy answers. Carefully review the *Code of Ethics for Nurses* (Chapter 6) and the American Nurses Association website resources on health care reform to guide your responses.

NURSES' ROLE IN HEALTH CARE REFORM

Since the delivery of health care continues to change rapidly, it is fitting to conclude with a note about nurses' continuing role in health care reform. Changes taking place in health care give nurses the opportunity to help shape health care for the future. Projections about competencies of future health care practitioners, coupled with the national health promotion and disease prevention objectives outlined in the *Healthy People 2020* project (www.healthypeople.gov), underscore the importance of nursing's role in improving access to care, quality of care, and cost of care.

The U.S. health care system is facing many challenges, including rapidly increasing numbers of older adults, changing expectations of health care consumers, rapidly expanding technologies, and an emphasis on improved quality and safety of care. The goals of health care reform focus on cost containment, improved access, and increased quality of services for all citizens. Where do nurses fit into the reform movement? First, nurses are becoming a stronger voice in protesting health-related problems in our nation and proposing solutions. Second, nurses in greater numbers are increasing their education and becoming APRNs. As such, more nurses now provide primary health care services in areas and to people long neglected: older adults, women, infants, the poor, and those living in rural areas. In addition, the focus of nursing care provided by all nurses is holistic care essential to promoting health and preventing illness. The issues of who gets health care and who pays the bills continue to have major importance for society in the 21st century. These issues will present both challenges and opportunities for nurses of the future.

DEVELOPING CLINICAL REASONING

1. How might prenatal and well-child care differ for two women—one without health insurance and the other with a good health insurance plan? Why do you think this happens? What can nurses do to ensure respectful, compassionate care of high quality for all?

2. Talk with your classmates about what should be in an essential health services package available for all. Would you include

dental care, mental health services, complementary and alternative treatment modalities, women's health services including birth control and abortion, long-term care? Why is it so difficult for health planners to agree on what services are essential?

3. Interview as many people as you can about what the government's role should be in providing health care. Why in the United States are so many distrustful of "big" government playing an expanded role in health care?

PRACTICING FOR NCLEX

1. Nursing students are reviewing information about health care delivery systems in preparation for a quiz the next day. Which statements describe current U.S. health care delivery practices? Select all that apply.
   a. Access to care depends only on the ability to pay, not the availability of services.
   b. The Patient Protection and Affordable Care Act provides private health care insurance to the underserved populations.
   c. Every health insurance plan in the Marketplace offers comprehensive coverage, from doctors to medications to hospital visits.
   d. The uninsured pay for more than one-third of their care out of pocket and are usually charged lower amounts for their care than the insured pay.
   e. Fifty years ago, half of the doctors in America practiced primary care, but today fewer than one in three do.
   f. Quality of care can be defined as the right care for the right person at the right time.

2. A nurse is providing secondary health care to patients in a health care facility. Which patients are receiving this level of care? Select all that apply.
   a. A patient enters a community clinic with signs of strep throat.
   b. A patient is admitted to the hospital following a myocardial infarction.
   c. A mother brings her son to the emergency department following a seizure.
   d. A patient with osteogenesis imperfecta is being treated in a medical center.
   e. A mother brings her son to a specialist to correct a congenital heart defect.
   f. A woman has a hernia repair in an ambulatory care center.

3. A nurse working in a physician's office prepares insurance forms in which the provider is given a fixed amount per enrollee of the health plan. What is the term for this type of reimbursement?
   a. Capitation
   b. Prospective payment system
   c. Bundled payment
   d. Rate setting

4. A nursing instructor is teaching students about the utilization of health care services and how the U.S. health care dollar is spent. Place the following care areas in order from the highest percentage of health care money spent to the lowest.
   a. Physician/clinical services
   b. Home health care
   c. Long-term care facility services
   d. Retail prescription drugs
   e. Government administration
   f. Hospital care

5. A nurse researcher keeps current on the trends to watch in health care delivery. What trends are likely included? Select all that apply.
   a. Globalization of economy and society
   b. Slowdown in technology development
   c. Decreasing diversity
   d. Increasing complexity of patient care
   e. Changing demographics
   f. Shortages of key health care professionals and educators

6. A nurse is caring for patients in a primary care center. What is the most likely role of this nurse based on the setting?
   a. Assisting with major surgery
   b. Performing a health assessment
   c. Maintaining patients' function and independence
   d. Keeping student immunization records up to date

7. A caregiver asks a nurse to explain respite care. How would the nurse respond?
   a. "A service that allows time away for caregivers"
   b. "A special service for the terminally ill and their family"
   c. "Direct care provided to individuals in a long-term care facility"
   d. "Living units for people without regular shelter"

8. A nurse caring for patients in a primary care setting submits paperwork for reimbursement from managed care plans for services performed. Which purpose best describes managed care as a framework for health care?
   a. A design to control the cost of care while maintaining the quality of care
   b. Care coordination to maximize positive outcomes to contain costs
   c. The delivery of services from initial contact through ongoing care
   d. Based on a philosophy of ensuring death in comfort and dignity

9. A nurse cares for dying patients by providing physical, psychological, social, and spiritual care for the patients, their families, and other loved ones. This service is known as:
   a. Respite care
   b. Palliative care
   c. Hospice care
   d. Extended care

10. A nurse is evaluating a patient diagnosed with renal disease for treatment in a Hospital at Home program. Which statement accurately describes a step in this program?
    a. The patient is evaluated upon hospital admission and is given daily nursing care in the home after discharge for as long as necessary.
    b. Any urgent or emergent situation requires an ambulance trip from the home to the hospital.
    c. Patients are transported to physicians' offices from the home for weekly evaluations.
    d. The clinicians use care pathways, clinical outcome evaluations, and specific discharge criteria.

ANSWERS WITH RATIONALES

1. *c, e, f.* The Marketplace is designed to help people more easily find health insurance that fits their budget. Every health insurance plan in the Marketplace offers comprehensive coverage, from doctors to medications to hospital visits. Fifty years ago, half of the doctors in America practiced primary care, but today fewer than one in three do. Quality is the right care for the right person at the right time. Access to care depends on both the ability to pay and the availability of services. The Patient Protection and Affordable Care Act provides Medicaid or subsidized coverage to qualifying people with incomes up to 400% of poverty. The uninsured pay for more than one-third of their care out of pocket and are often charged higher amounts for their care than the insured pay.

2. *b, c, f.* Secondary health care treats problems that require specialized clinical expertise, such as an MI, a seizure, and a hernia repair. Treating strep throat is primary health care. Tertiary health care involves management of rare and complex disorders, such as osteogenesis imperfecta and congenital heart malformations.

3. *a.* Capitation plans give providers a fixed amount per enrollee in the health plan in an effort to build a payment plan that consists of the best standards of care at the lowest cost. The prospective payment system groups inpatient hospital services for Medicare patients into DRGs. With bundled payments, providers receive a fixed sum of money to provide a range of services. Rate setting means that the government could set targets or caps for spending on health care services.

4. *f, a, d, c, b, e.* The national health expenditures in 2010 were hospital care 31%, physician/clinical services 20%, retail prescription drugs 10%, long-term care facility services 5%, home health care 3%, and government administration 1%.

5. *a, d, e, f.* Trends to watch in health care delivery include: globalization of the economy and society, increasing complexity of patient care, changing demographics, shortages of key health care professionals and educators, technology explosion, and increasing diversity.

6. *b.* Performing patient assessments is a common role of the nurse in a primary care center. Assisting with major surgery is a role of the nurse in the hospital setting. Maintaining patients' function and independence is a role of the nurse in an extended-care facility, and keeping student immunization records up to date is a role of the school nurse.

7. *a.* Respite care is provided to enable a primary caregiver time away from the day-to-day responsibilities of homebound patients.

8. *a.* Managed care is a way of providing care designed to control costs while maintaining the quality of care.

9. *c.* The hospice nurse combines the skills of the home care nurse with the ability to provide daily emotional support to dying patients and their families. Respite care is a type of care provided for caregivers of homebound ill, disabled, or older patients. Palliative care, which can be used in conjunction with medical treatment and in all types of health care settings, is focused on the relief of physical, mental, and spiritual distress. Extended-care facilities include transitional subacute care, assisted-living facilities, intermediate and long-term care, homes for medically fragile children, retirement centers, and residential institutions for mentally and developmentally or physically disabled patients of all ages.

10. *d.* In the Hospital at Home program, the clinicians use care pathways including illness-specific care maps, clinical outcome evaluations, and specific discharge criteria. A patient requiring admission for one of the target illnesses is identified in the emergency department or ambulatory site. Staff assess whether

the patient is a good candidate for the program using validated criteria. If the patient is eligible and consents to participate, the Hospital at Home physician evaluates the patient, who is then transported home, usually by ambulance. Nurses are available 24 hours a day/7 days a week for any urgent or emergent situations. The patient is evaluated daily in the home by the Hospital at Home physician, who completes an assessment and continues to implement appropriate diagnostic and therapeutic measures.

TAYLOR SUITE RESOURCES

Explore these additional resources to enhance learning for this chapter:

- NCLEX-Style Questions and other resources on thePoint, http://thePoint.lww.com/Taylor8e
- *Study Guide for Fundamentals of Nursing, 8th edition*
- Adaptive Learning | Powered by prepU, http://thepoint.lww.com/prepu

Bibliography

Agency for Healthcare Research and Quality (AHRQ). (2012). Defining the PCMH. Available at http://www.pcmh.ahrq.gov/portal/server.pt/community/pcmh__home/1483/pcmh_defining_the_pcmh_v2

American Association of Colleges of Osteopathic Medicine (AACOM). (2013). Primary care access: 30 million new patients and 11 months to go: Who will provide their care? Available at http://www.aacom.org/InfoFor/educators/naome/appprocess/Documents/AACOM%20Testimony%20Senate%20HELP%20Sub%20Primary%20Health%20and%20Aging%202-8-13.pdf

American Hospital Association (AHA). (2013). About the AHA. http://www.aha.org/about/index.shtml

American Nurses Association (ANA). (2013). Health care reform. Available at http://www.nursingworld.org/MainMenuCategories/Policy-Advocacy/HealthSystemReform

American Nurses Association (ANA). (2013). New care delivery models in health system reform: Opportunities for nurses and their patients. Available at http://www.nursingworld.org/MainMenuCategories/Policy-Advocacy/HealthSystemReform/HealthCareReformResources/Care-Delivery-Models.pdf

American Nurses Credentialing Center (ANCC). (2013). ANCC Magnet Recognition Program. ANCC Pathway to Excellence. Available at http://www.nursecredentialing.org/Magnet.aspx

Bodenheimer, T., & Grumbach, K. (2012). *Understanding health policy: A clinical approach* (6th ed.). New York: McGraw Hill.

Centers for Disease Control and Prevention (CDC). (2012). Hospital utilization (in non-Federal short stay hospitals). Available at http://www.cdc.gov/nchs/fastats/hospital.htm

Centers for Disease Control and Prevention (CDC). (April 2011). Rising health care costs are unsustainable. Available at http://www.cdc.gov/workplacehealthpromotion/businesscase/reasons/rising.html

Centers for Medicare and Medicaid Services, Office of the Actuary, National Health Statistics Group (2013). National health care expenditures data. Available at www.cms.gov/Research-Statistics-Data-and-Systems/Statistics-Trends-and-Reports/NationalHealthExpendData/index.html

Centers for Medicare and Medicaid Services. (2014). Medicare and you. Available at www.medicare.gov/Pubs/pdf/10050.pdf

Centers for Medicare and Medicaid Services (CMS) Press Office. (2011). Two year anniversary of children's health insurance law sees millions of newly insured children, families. Available at http://www.hhs.gov/news/press/2011pres/02/20110203b.html

Centers for Medicare and Medicaid Services (CMS) and Agency for Healthcare Research and Quality (AHRQ). (2012). HCAHPS Fact Sheet. Available at http://www.hcahpsonline.org/files/HCAHPS%20Fact%20Sheet%20May%202012.pdf

Cerrato, P. (2013). 5 Trends will reshape health IT in 2013. *Information Week* Health Care Digital Bundle. Available at http://www.informationweek.com/healthcare/leadership/5-trends-will-reshape-health-it-in-2013/240006254?pgno=1

Craig, C., Eby, D., & Whittington, J. (2011). Care coordination model: Better care at lower cost for people with multiple health and social needs. IHI Innovation Series white paper. Cambridge, Massachusetts: Institute for Healthcare Improvement. Available at http://www.ihi.org/knowledge/Pages/IHIWhitePapers/IHICareCoordinationModelWhitePaper.aspx

Chua, K-P. (2006). Overview of the U.S. health care system. Available at www.amsa.org/AMSA/Libraries/Committee_Docs/HealthCareSystemOverview.sflb.ashx

Daley, K. A. (2013). President's perspective: What keeps me up at night? *The American Nurse, 45*(1), 3.

Davis, K., Schoen, C., & Stremikis, K. (2010). Mirror, mirror on the wall: How the performance of the U.S. health care system compares internationally—2010 Update. The Commonwealth Fund. Available at http://www.commonwealthfund.org/Publications/Fund-Reports/2010/Jun/Mirror-Mirror-Update.aspx?page=all

Government Accountability Office (GAO). (2011). Use of Recovery Act and Patient Protection and Affordable Care Act funds for comparative effectiveness research. Available at http://www.gao.gov/products/GAO-11-712R

Healthcare.gov

Henry J. Kaiser Family Foundation. (2012). Kaiser Commission on Medicaid and the Uninsured. Available at http://kff.org/about-kaiser-commission-on-medicaid-and-the-uninsured/

Henry J. Kaiser Family Foundation. (2013). Health Policy Explained. U.S. health care costs. Available at: http://www.kaiseredu.org/issue-modules/us-health-care-costs/background-brief.aspx

Henry J. Kaiser Family Foundation. (2013). Health reform. Available at http://healthreform.kff.org

Henry J. Kaiser Family Foundation. (2013). The Uninsured: A Primer—Key Facts about health insurance on the eve of coverage expansions. Available at http://kff.org/uninsured/report/the-uninsured-a-primer-key-facts-about-health-insurance-on-the-eve-of-coverage-expansions/

HospitalatHome. (2013). www.hospitalathome.org

Institute for Healthcare Improvement (IHI). (2013). The IHI Triple Aim Initiative. Available at http://www.ihi.org/offerings/Initiatives/TripleAIM/Pages/default.aspx

Institute of Medicine (IOM). (1999). *To err is human: Building a safer health system.* Washington, DC: National Academy Press.

Institute of Medicine (IOM). (2001). *Crossing the quality chasm: A new health system for the 21st century.* Washington, DC: Author.

Institute of Medicine (IOM). (2011). *The future of nursing: Leading change, advancing health.* Washington, DC: The National Academies Press.

Institute of Medicine (IOM). (2012). *Best care at lower cost.* Washington, DC: The National Academies Press.

Kurtzman, E., & Buerhaus, P. (2008). New Medicare payment rules: Danger or opportunity for nursing? *American Journal of Nursing, 108*(6), 30–35.

Martin, A. B., Lassman, D., Washington, B., Catlin, A., & the National Health Expenditure Accounts Team. (2012). Growth in US health spending remained slow in 2010; Health share of gross domestic product was unchanged from 2009. *Health Affairs 31*(1):208–219.

McClellan, M., McKethan, A., Lewis, J., Roski, J., & Fisher, E. (2010). A national strategy to put accountable care into practice. *Health Affairs (Millwood), 29*(5):982–990. Available at http://content.healthaffairs.org/cgi/content/abstract/hlthaff.28.2.w219

McDonald, K. M., Schultz, E., Albin, L., Pineda, N., Lonhart, J., Sundaram, V.,... Malcolm, E. (2010). Care Coordination Atlas Version 3 (Prepared by Stanford University under subcontract to Battelle on Contract No. 290–04–0020). AHRQ Publication No. 11–0023-EF. Rockville, MD: Agency for Healthcare Research and Quality.

National Academy for State Health Policy. (2013). www.nashp.org

National Academy of Sciences. (2003). *Executive summary: Health professions education. A bridge to quality.* Available at http://www.nap.edu/openbook.php?record_id=10681&page=R1

National Association of Community Health Centers (NACHC). (2013). About our health centers. Available at www.nachc.com/about-our-health-centers.cfm

National Hospice and Palliative Care Organization (NHPCO). (2012). NHPCO Facts and Figures: Hospice Care in America, 2012 Edition. Available at http://www.nhpco.org/sites/default/files/public/Statistics_Research/2012_Facts_Figures.pdf

Nielson, M., Langner, B., Zema, C., Hacker, T. & Grundy, P. (2012). Benefits of Implementing the Primary Care Patient-Centered Medical Home: Cost and Quality Results, 2012. Patient-Centered Primary Care Collaborative. Available at www.pcpcc.org/sites/default/files/media/benefits_of_implementing_the_primary_care_pcmh.pdf

Physicians for a National Health Program. (2013). What is Single Payer? Available at http://www.pnhp.org/facts/what-is-single-payer.

Rau, J. (2011, April 29). Medicare announces rules for quality bonuses to hospitals. *Kaiser Health News.*

Rau, J. (2012, August 13). Medicare to penalize 2,217 hospitals for excess readmissions. *Kaiser Health News.*

Sanders, B. Subcommittee on Primary Health and Aging. (2013). Primary Care Access. Available at http://www.sanders.senate.gov/imo/media/doc/PrimaryCareAccessReport.pdf

Shih, A., Davis, K., Schoenbaum, S., Gauthier, A., Nuzum, R., & McCarthy, D. (2008). Organizing the U.S. Health Care Delivery System for High Performance. The Commonwealth Fund. Available at www.commonwealthfund.org/Publications/Fund-Reports/2008/Aug/Organizing-the-U-S–Health-Care-Delivery-System-for-High-Performance.aspx

Smith, M., Saunders, R., Stuckhardt, L. & McGinnis, J.M, Eds. (2012). Best care at lower cost: The path to continuously learning health care in America. Washington, DC: The National Academies Press.

Sofaer, S., & Schumann, M. J. (2013). Fostering successful patient and family engagement: Nursing's critical role. Available at http://www.naqc.org/WhitePaper-PatientEngagement

Taylor EF, Lake T, Nysenbaum J, Peterson G, Meyers D. Coordinating care in the medical neighborhood: critical components and available mechanisms. White Paper (Prepared by Mathematica Policy Research under Contract No. HHSA290200900019I TO2). AHRQ Publication No. 11-0064. Rockville, MD: Agency for Healthcare Research and Quality. June 2011. Available at http://pcmh.ahrq.gov/sites/default/files/attachments/Coordinating%20Care%20in%20the%20Medical%20Neighborhood.pdf

U.S. Department of Labor, Bureau of Labor Statistics. (2012). Occupational Outlook Handbook: Registered Nurses. Available at http://www.bls.gov/ooh/Healthcare/Registered-nurses.htm

Woolf, S. H. & Aron, L., Eds. (2013). *U.S. health in international perspective: Shorter lives, poorer health,* National Research Council and Institute of Medicine. The National Academies Press. 2012 Patient-Centered Primary Care Collaborative/Millbank Memorial Fund.

Yong, P. L., Saunders, R. S., & Olsen, L. (Eds.). (2010). The healthcare imperative: Lowering costs and improving outcomes. Workshop Series Summary. Washington, DC: The National Academies Press.

9

Care Coordination and Continuity in Health Care Settings and the Community

JEFF HART

Jeff is a 9-year-old with a genetic disease that includes severe mental retardation. He is transferred from the state home for children to the hospital for respiratory complications.

LAURA DEGAS

Laura, a 78-year-old woman, has been caring for her sister Ellen at home. She says, "She was diagnosed with Alzheimer disease 2 years ago. This surgery to fix her broken hip has really been tough. I want to take her home, but I'm not sure if I can give her the care that she needs now."

JOEY MARSHALL

Joey, an extremely low-birth-weight baby (1,100 g), spent 7 months in the hospital before being discharged home. His mother is caring for him, his twin (who is healthier), and their 3-year-old sister. Joey is still being fed artificially, is on a ventilator, and needs care round the clock.

After completing the chapter, you will be able to accomplish the following:

1. Describe the role of the nurse in ensuring continuity of care and coordinating care between and among health care settings and the home.

2. Describe the components of the home health care system, including agencies, patients, referrals, primary caregivers, reimbursement sources, and legal considerations.

3. Describe the qualities and roles of the home health nurse.

4. Explain the essential components of the pre-entry and entry phases of the home visit.

5. Explain the importance of documentation in home care.

6. Discuss considerations for establishing an effective nurse–patient relationship when admitting a patient to a health care setting.

7. Compare and contrast admission of a patient to an ambulatory care setting and a hospital setting.

8. Discuss transfer of patients within and among health care settings.

9. Explain how nurses use the components of discharge planning to provide continuity of care.

KEY TERMS

advocacy	community-based nursing	ISBARQ
care coordination	continuity of care	medication reconciliation
care coordinator	discharge planning	nurse navigator
care transition	handoffs	patient navigator
community-based care	home health care	SBAR

People enter health care settings and become consumers of health care services (patients) for many different reasons. Not all people have the same kinds of health care needs, nor are they alike as patients. Some are admitted to a treatment setting and discharged the same day, some remain in an acute care setting for months, and some require extended care at home or in another community setting. Increasingly, people are seeking health care services in the communities where they live, study, work, pray, and play.

Entering and leaving a health care setting, as well as receiving care at home, are experiences that produce anxiety for both patients and family members. The nurse is often the health care provider who helps the patient make a smooth transition from one care setting to another. (See the accompanying Reflective Practice display for an example on page 166). Three concepts essential to nursing care of patients within and across health care settings are **community-based nursing** care, continuity of care and care coordination. Planning for and providing individualized nursing interventions that promote health, prevent illness, and support coping with disability are critical in today's culturally diverse society. It is no longer enough only to consider the patient's needs within the hospital setting; nurses must also consider how those needs will be met as the patient makes the transition from the acute care setting to some type of long-term care or to care at home with support and services from the patient's community.

 CONSIDER Laura Degas, the sister of the woman with Alzheimer disease who has undergone a hip repair. Due to her sister's increased complexity of care, Ms. Degas is unsure if she can continue to care for her sister at home. The nurse would work with Ms. Degas to determine her needs and possibly enlist the aid of social services for assistance with a referral to home care and appropriate resources and community services. ●

COMMUNITY-BASED NURSING CARE

Community-based care is health care provided to people who live within a defined geographic area. That geographic area might be a small neighborhood within a large urban area or a large area of rural residents. Each community is unique and is defined by the people, area, social interactions, and common ties within that community. In contrast to community health and public health nursing (which are population based and focus on the health of the whole community), community-based care centers on individual and family health care needs. It emphasizes the provision of comprehensive, coordinated, and continuous services for patients with acute or chronic health problems. Within a framework of community-based care, nurses help people wherever they are, including where they live, work, play, worship, and go to school. Community-based practice sites can be as varied as neighborhood clinics, patients' homes, long-term care facilities, schools, churches, and prisons. Almost 30% of RNs work in such nonacute patient care settings, and this number is growing (Fig. 9-1). When health care is provided in the community, the nurse must adapt to the patient's environment and blend clinical skills with flexibility (Fig. 9-2).

 Concept Mastery Alert

Community-based care and community health care are different. A helpful way to remember the difference is to think that community is larger than community-based. So, community health care focuses on populations, whereas community-based care focuses on individuals and families.

REFLECTIVE PRACTICE: CULTIVATING QSEN COMPETENCIES

CHALLENGE TO TECHNICAL SKILLS

Joey Marshall, an extremely low-birth-weight baby (1,100 g) spent 7 months in the hospital before being discharged home. His mother is now at home full time caring for him, his twin (who is healthier), and their 3-year-old sister. Joey is still being fed via tube feedings, is on a ventilator, and needs care around the clock. When I first visited Joey on the day he was discharged home, I was frightened at the sight of such a small baby surrounded by beeping machines and tubes. While this was not a new sight for Joey's mom, she seemed very uncomfortable being his primary caregiver. She said she had lots of practice taking care of him in the hospital, but nothing had prepared her for the reality of his coming home and needing help around the clock.

Thinking Outside the Box: Possible Courses of Action

- Take a "pass" on this family and tell my instructor that this family's needs exceed my capacity to care; an adult with a lot of tubes is one thing, but a BABY!
- Ask for an experienced mentor to guide me through a comprehensive family assessment and planning to meet everyone's needs; use this as a challenge but ask for help until I feel competent and confident.
- Act like I know what I'm doing and pray I don't make mistakes!

Evaluating a Good Outcome: How Do I Define Success?

- Joey's mother develops the competence and confidence she needs to provide Joey's care at home.
- I am honest about my ability and seek help when I need it.
- I learn something from each situation that will prepare me to meet the next clinical challenge.
- I don't let my fear interfere with my learning.

Personal Learning: Here's to the Future!

I decided that options one (taking a pass) and three (acting like I knew what I was doing) weren't really options, although they seemed tempting. An experienced home health care nurse who once worked in the neonatal intensive care unit (NICU) agreed to visit this family with me, and she talked me through a comprehensive assessment. I was able to use my fear to identify with how Joey's mom was feeling, and I believe I was able to make her feel comfortable. I told her that we would learn how to do everything together! By the end of this rotation, we were both comfortable with Joey's care. I learned a valuable lesson: to seek help when I am in over my head and to relish a challenge. I hope I will remember this experience as I grow more confident so that I never forget how overwhelmed many families feel when they first bring a loved one home!

REFLECTION ON QUALITY AND SAFETY COMPETENCIES

How do you think you would respond in a similar situation? Why? What does this tell you about yourself and about the adequacy of your skills for professional practice? Can you think of other ways to respond? What other knowledge, attitudes, and skills do you need to develop to continuously improve the quality and safety of care for patients like Joey?

Patient-Centered Care: What made creating a partnership with Ms. Marshall so challenging? What abilities did the experienced home health care nurse and student use to achieve a good outcome? What special talents do you bring to creating successful partnerships?

Teamwork and Collaboration/Quality Improvement: What communication skills do you need to improve to ensure that you function as a competent, caring, and responsible member of the patient care team and that you obtain appropriate assistance when needed? How is teamwork different for home health care nurses? What special talents do you bring to promoting a well-functioning team? How did the student's commitment to quality care influence her response?

Safety/Evidence-Based Practice: What priority did the student give to Joey's health, well-being, and safety? What does research demonstrate about the safety of providing care in the home that once happened in the hospital? Did the nursing student seek out the most appropriate resources for help in responding to Joey and his mother's complex needs? What other resources could have been helpful? Do you agree with the criteria to evaluate a successful outcome? Did the nursing student meet the criteria? Explain your answer.

Nurses practicing community-based care consider the continuity of the care patients require when moving from one level or setting of care to another, providing interventions to promote health, manage acute or chronic illnesses, and promote self-care. Community-based care is designed to meet the needs of people as they move into, between, and among different health care settings within the overall health care system.

Until about 1990, community-based nurses were considered generalists, but recently many have gained advanced skills to meet the growing demands of acutely ill patients being cared for at home and in other community settings. These specialties include enterostomal therapy, cardiac care, mental health, maternal and child health, and palliative care. Specialized nursing knowledge and skills coupled with sophisticated technology increasingly allow many patients

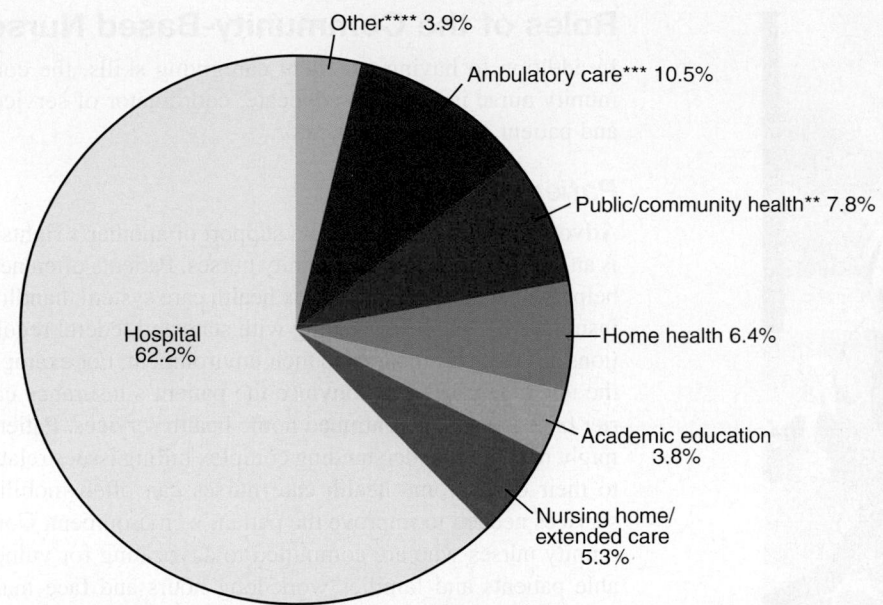

Other**** 3.9%

Ambulatory care*** 10.5%

Public/community health** 7.8%

Home health 6.4%

Academic education 3.8%

Nursing home/ extended care 5.3%

Hospital 62.2%

* Percents may not add to 100 due to the effect of rounding. Only RNs who provided setting information are included in the calculations used for this figure.

** Public/community health includes school and occupational health.

*** Ambulatory care includes medical/physician practices, health centers and clinics, and other types of non-hospital clinical settings.

**** Other includes insurance, benefits, and utilization review.

FIGURE 9-1. Employment sites of registered nurses (available at http://bhpr.hrsa.gov/healthworkforce/rnsurveys/rnsurveyfinal.pdf)

with acute and chronic health care needs to be treated safely and effectively in the home.

Qualities of the Community-Based Nurse

Nurses choose to practice community-based nursing in both urban and rural settings for various reasons. Many nurses

FIGURE 9-2. The nurse providing home health care must adapt to the patient's environment instead of the patient adapting to the hospital or clinic environment.

enjoy practicing in an autonomous setting where they can use their expertise in an expanded role. Others enjoy managing their time independently and like the satisfaction experienced when patients welcome them into their home and life. Community-based nurses find satisfaction in networking with community agencies to provide individualized care. Community settings also provide an opportunity for nurses to be creative in delivering care. Community-based nurses must possess several key qualities: they must be knowledgeable and skilled in their practice, able to make decisions independently, and must remain accountable. While these qualities hold true for all nurses, the fact that many nurses in the community work independently makes these qualities even more critical for community nurses. For example, if a home hospice nurse fails to appropriately assess a patient and report a developing complication to the team, the patient may never receive the needed proactive care.

Knowledgeable and Skilled

Nurses who provide care in the community must have the knowledge and skills needed to provide appropriate care. Both effective communication and clinical skills are essential (Fig. 9-3). In fact, many community-based agencies require a minimum of 1 year of clinical practice as a prerequisite for employment. Physical assessment skills are necessary to identify positive and negative changes in a patient's health status. Procedures such as administering intravenous fluids, changing complex wound dressings, caring for ostomies, and providing ventilator care are often required. Home health care nurses, for example, have identified the following areas of knowledge as most important in home care: legal

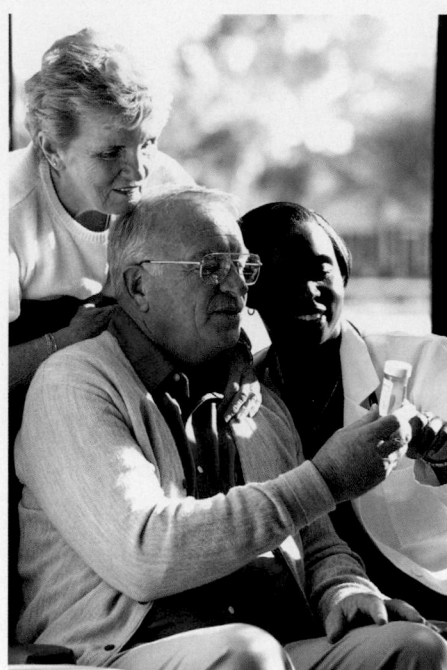

FIGURE 9-3. Home health care nurses combine effective communication skills with a sound clinical knowledge base when caring for patients and their families.

regulations, physical assessment, body mechanics, nursing diagnoses, and infection control.

Independent in Making Decisions

Nurses providing care in the community make independent decisions and assume responsibility for decision making. They are generally away from other health care providers when providing care and must be able to make patient care decisions independently. The combination of a sound theoretical foundation, proficiency in clinical skills, and ability to solve problems creatively enables the nurse to make appropriate patient care decisions.

Accountable

Accountability is another important characteristic of community-based nurses. In a hospital, the nurse generally works a shift and then reports to the next shift nurse, who continues to care for the patient. Nurses seeing patients in their homes generally are not followed by a next shift but instead rely on family or other caregivers to continue the care. If there is no caregiver in the home, the nurse returns to face the same issues at the next visit. The nurse is accountable to the patient, the family, and the primary health care provider. Community-based nurses must consider questions such as the following:

- Whom do I call if the patient's physician or nurse practitioner is not available?
- What should I do if a family member becomes acutely ill?
- How do I learn to perform advanced procedures?
- How do I document the patient's decisions about treatment?
- How do I ensure that other providers know about and document the plan of care?

Roles of the Community-Based Nurse

In addition to having excellent caregiving skills, the community nurse is a patient advocate, coordinator of services, and patient and family educator.

Patient Advocate

Advocacy—the protection and support of another's rights—is an important role of community nurses. Patients often need help understanding the complex health care system, handling insurance problems, or dealing with state and federal regulations affecting their care and their environment. For example, the nurse may have to convince the patient's insurance carrier of the need for continued home health services. Patients might need help understanding complex billing issues related to their care. Home health care nurses can often mobilize services needed to improve the patient's environment. Community nurses who are committed to advocating for vulnerable patients and families work long hours and face many challenges. It is sometimes difficult to establish and maintain professional boundaries and to sever ties when appropriate with families one has come to know and love. It is helpful to be aware of these challenges and to be able to discuss them with respected team leaders and colleagues.

Coordinator of Services

The community-based nurse generally coordinates all other health care providers visiting the patient and is the primary source of communication and coordination of the patient's care with the primary health care provider. The nurse uses effective communication skills with other health care providers while coordinating services for the patient.

A community-based nurse is also responsible for coordinating community resources needed by the patient. A sound knowledge of community resources enables the nurse to provide comprehensive services to the patient. For example, the nurse must understand the role of a social worker or physical therapist to determine a need for these services. The nurse should know about available community resources, such as Meals on Wheels, the American Cancer Society, services for patients who are visually or hearing impaired, and local services for the aging. As the coordinator of care, the nurse directs the various services toward a common goal of improving the patient's health and promoting independence.

Patient and Family Educator

Nurses providing community-based care in a clinic or home teach patients and families about all aspects of care, including disease processes and treatments, nutrition, medications, and treatment and care of wounds. The nurse identifies learning needs; then the nurse, patient, and family mutually develop goals for teaching information necessary to promote health. Family members or other caregivers may be taught any skill that they are able and willing to perform.

The nurse provides the information necessary to keep the patient safe until the next visit, using methods that work best in the home or other community setting. The goal is to increase the patient's ability to provide self-care and the caregiver's ability to care for the patient. The teaching and learning process is fully described in Chapter 21.

 REMEMBER Joey Marshall, the high-risk infant coming home after 7 months in the neonatal intensive care unit. In this situation, the home health care nurse fills many roles; one of the major roles will be that of educator, with the goal of teaching Joey's mother so that she can ultimately care for Joey independently. •

CONTINUITY OF CARE

Over their lifetimes, most people require many different health services offered in a variety of health care settings. Although a patient's health care may involve many different providers and settings (discussed in Chapter 8), the nurse is often the primary person responsible for communicating the patient's needs, teaching self-care, and, in many instances, providing care. As a result, one of the primary responsibilities of the nurse as caregiver is ensuring continuity of care. **Continuity of care** is a process by which health care providers give appropriate, uninterrupted care and facilitate the patient's transition between different settings and levels of care. Continuity of care ensures a smooth transition between ambulatory or acute care and **home health care** or other types of health care settings in the patient's community. Continuity depends on excellent communication as patients move from one caregiver or health care site to another. Too often communication breakdowns among caregivers result in medical errors or deficient plans of care. In recent years,

patient **handoffs**, transferring responsibility for a patient from one caregiver to another with the goal of providing timely, accurate information about a patient's plan of care, treatment, current condition and anticipated changes (Runy, 2013), have been carefully researched. In 2006, the Joint Commission National Patient Safety Goals required hospitals to implement a standardized approach to handoff communications that includes:

- The handoff situation
- Who is, or should be, involved in the handoff communication
- Opportunities for people involved in handoffs to ask and respond to questions
- An outline for when to use certain communication techniques, such as repeat-back or read-back or the Situation-Background-Assessment-Recommendation (SBAR) technique
- What print or electronic information should be available during the handoff (The Joint Commission, 2014)

One popular approach to handoffs is the **SBAR** (an acronym for situation, background, assessment, and recommendation) strategy described in Chapter 20. According to the Institute for Health Care Improvement, SBAR provides a framework for communication between members of the health care team about a patient's condition. It is an easy and focused way to set expectations for what will be communicated and how between members of the team, which is essential for developing teamwork and fostering a culture of patient safety. See Box 9-1 for examples of simple SBAR

BOX 9-1 | **SAMPLE SBAR (SITUATION-BACKGROUND-ASSESSMENT-RECOMMENDATION) COMMUNICATIONS**

SBAR Scenario #1

RN calling physician regarding patient's elevated temperature, breathing difficulties, and deteriorating condition

S—Jeff's temperature this evening shot up to 103 degrees and his respirations are labored; RR of 40, HR of 95 BPM, and O_2 Sat of 82% on room air. He is pale and also drooling.

B—Jeff was transferred two days ago from the state home for children with respiratory difficulties. Jeff is a 9-year-old with a genetic disease that includes severe mental retardation.

A—I am concerned about Jeff's deteriorating condition.

R—Another nurse is staying with Jeff, offering O_2 and positioning and suctioning, but I need you to come to the bedside and assess this patient.

SBAR Scenario #2

RN calling team manager regarding home hospice patient's inadequate pain management

S—Ms. Tadesse is grimacing and moaning—she appears uncomfortable.

B—She is in end-stage breast cancer and her family has been told that death is imminent—expected sometime this week.

A—Her daughter has been administering the PRN morphine sulfate as ordered, but it no longer seems to be keeping her mother comfortable.

R—Should we have the palliative care physician re-evaluate her analgesics and recommend a better pain management regimen?

SBAR Scenario #3

RN calling physician about inadequate social support services for a patient scheduled for a discharge from a hospital rehab unit to home

S—Mr. Ames is scheduled for discharge today. His wife appeared to "take him home" and arrived via taxi. She is a frail, 89-year-old woman who seems overwhelmed by the care she will need to provide in the home. She states that there are no family or friends capable of helping her care for her husband.

B—Mr. Ames has spent the last week in a hospital rehabilitation unit following a right-sided total knee replacement. He weighs 320 lbs. He has signed the discharge papers. There is no home care follow-up ordered.

A—I am concerned about the Ameses because Mr. Ames still needs help ambulating. Prior to his surgery, Mr. Ames, who is 75 years old, was the primary caretaker for the couple. Without good home care services I am concerned about their ability to manage.

R—Should we invite the social worker and the case manager to re-evaluate this family prior to his discharge and set up visiting nurses to assist?

communications. **ISBARQ** is a revised approach, adding introduction and question and answer components to SBAR (Runy, 2013):

- **I - Introduction:** People involved in the handoff identify themselves, their roles, and their jobs
- **S - Situation:** Complaint, diagnosis, treatment plan, and patient's wants and needs

- **B - Background:** Vital signs, mental and code status, list of medications, and lab results
- **A - Assessment:** Current provider's assessment of the situation
- **R - Recommendation:** Identify pending lab results and what needs to be done over the next few hours and other recommendations for care
- **Q - Question and answer:** An opportunity for questions and answers

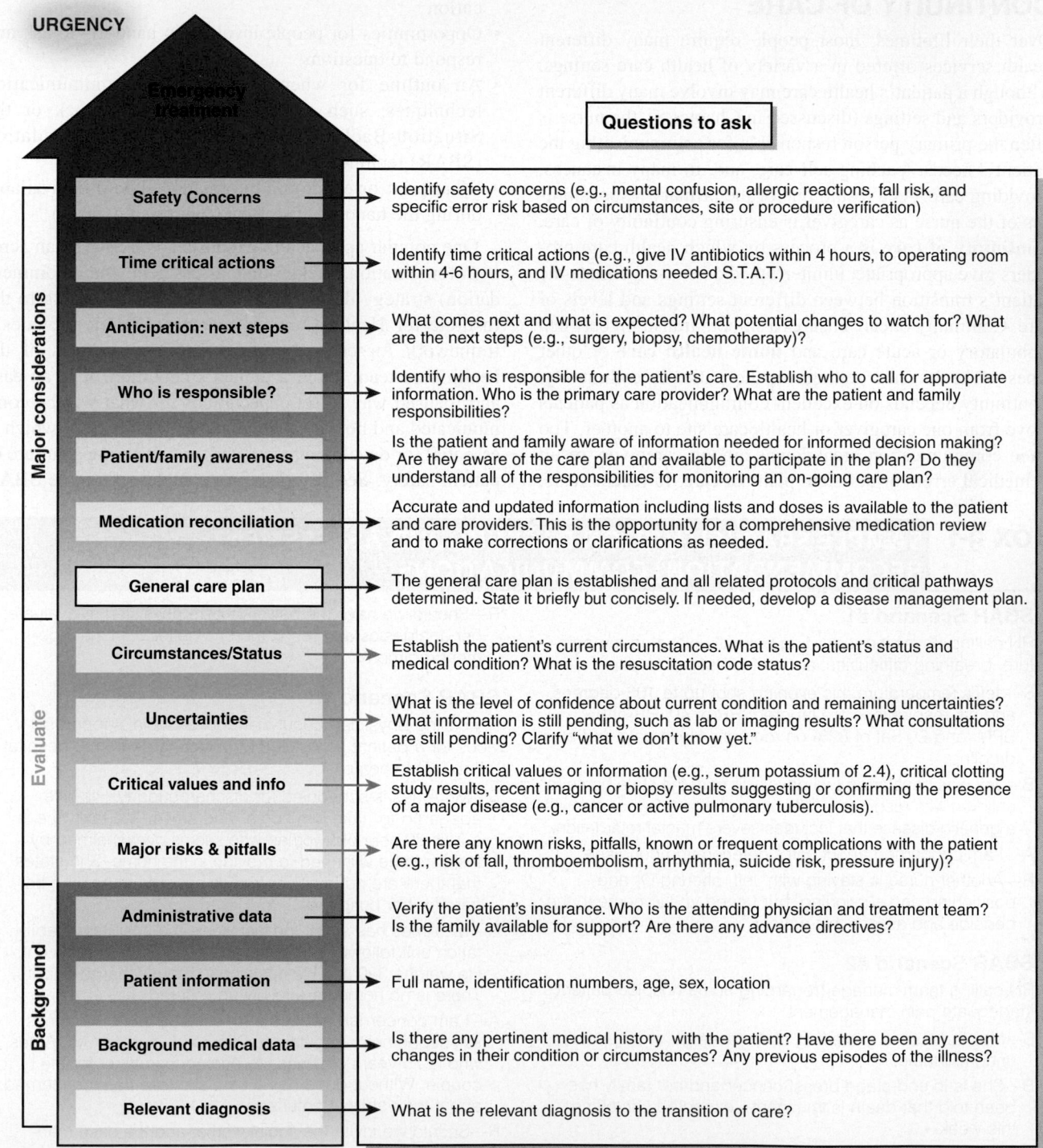

FIGURE 9-4. The U.S. Department of Defense Handoff Model. (Reprinted from Department of Defense Patient Safety Program. (2005). Healthcare Communications Toolkit to Improve Transitions in Care.)

Figure 9-4 illustrates a format for a more complex handoff. Following are ten tips for effective handoffs (Runy, 2013):

1. Allow for face-to-face handoffs whenever possible.
2. Ensure two-way communication during the handoff process.
3. Allow as much time as necessary for handoffs.
4. Use both verbal and written means of communication.
5. Conduct handoffs at the patient bedside whenever possible. Involve patients and families in the handoff process. Provide clear information at discharge.
6. Involve staff in the development of handoff standards.
7. Incorporate communication techniques, such as SBAR, in the handoff process. Require a verification process to ensure that information is both received and understood.
8. In addition to information exchange, handoffs should clearly outline the transfer of patient responsibility from one provider to another.
9. Use available technology, such as the electronic medical record, to streamline the exchange of timely, accurate information.
10. Monitor use and effectiveness of the handoff. Seek feedback from staff.

The Joint Commission Center for Transforming Healthcare describes targeted solutions for five specific causes of communication failures, as shown in Figure 9-5.

Targeting Solutions for Specific Causes of Communication Failure

Causes	**Solutions**
Culture does not promote successful hand-off, e.g., lack of teamwork and respect	• Make successful hand-offs an organization priority and performance expectation • Teach staff on what constitutes a successful hand-off • Standardize training on how to conduct a hand-off • Engage staff – real time performance feedback, just-in-time training
Ineffective communication method, e.g., verbal, recorded, bedside, written	• Sender uses standardized form, tool and method every time a hand-off occurs, e.g., checklists, SBAR tool • Identify new and existing technologies to assist in making the hand-off successful and complete, e.g., electronic medical records, PDAs • Develop and use standardized forms, tools and methods, e.g. checklists, SBAR tool
Inadequate amount of time provided for successful hand-off	• Sender identifies and stresses key information and critical elements about patient when talking to receiver • Sender synthesizes patient information from disparate sources prior to passing it on to the receiver
Sender provides inaccurate or incomplete information, e.g., medication list, DNR, concerns/issues, contact information	• Sender provides details of patient's history and status when speaking with receiver • Develop and use standardized forms, tools and methods, e.g., checklists, SBAR tool • Sender synthesizes patient information from disparate sources prior to passing it on to the receiver
Receiver has competing priorities and is unable to focus on transferred patient	• Establish workspace or setting that is conducive for sharing information about a patient; e.g., zone of silence • Hold staff managing patient's care responsible • Examine the work flow of healthcare workers to ensure a successful hand-off • Focus on the system, not just the people

FIGURE 9-5. Targeted solutions for specific causes of communication failures. (Reprinted with permission. Agency for Healthcare Research and Quality (AHRQ). (2012). Improving Transitions of Care: Hand-off Communications. Oakbrook Terrace, IL: Joint Commission for Transforming Healthcare, June 2012. Available at http://psnet.ahrq.gov/resource.aspx?resourceID=24737).

CARE COORDINATION

A recent Health Policy Brief describes **care transition** as a continuous process in which a patient's care shifts from being provided in one setting of care to another, such as from a hospital to a patient's home or to a skilled nursing facility and sometimes back to the hospital. It reports: "Poorly managed transitions can diminish health and increase costs. Researchers have estimated that inadequate care coordination, including inadequate management of care transitions, was responsible for $25 to $45 billion in wasteful spending in 2011 through avoidable complications and unnecessary hospital readmissions" (Health Policy Brief, 2012). Because of all the complexities in delivering safe and affordable health care of good quality (see Chapter 8), **care coordination** has emerged as a central responsibility of all health care professionals, and especially nurses. In simple terms, care coordination is a mechanism to make sure that patients get the right care at the right time in the most efficient and cost-effective manner, by the right person in the right setting. The aim is to link patients with resources in the community to enhance their well-being, improve information exchange, and reduce fragmentation and duplication of services.

A recent systematic review identified over 40 definitions for care coordination. The reviewers proposed the following broad definition: "Care coordination is the deliberate organization of patient care activities between two or more participants (including the patient) involved in a patient's care to facilitate the appropriate delivery of health care services. Organizing care involves the marshaling of personnel and other resources needed to carry out all required patient care activities and is often managed by the exchange of information among participants responsible for different aspects of care" (Agency for Healthcare Research and Quality [AHRQ], 2010). Figure 9-6 illustrates care coordination. Successes and failures in care coordination will be perceived in different ways depending on the perspective: patient/family, health care professional(s), or system representative(s). Patients and families are pleased when care coordination helps ensure that the patient's needs and preferences for health services and information sharing across people, functions, and sites are met over time. Patients are unhappy during transitions among different providers and settings when the effort to communicate their history and health care needs requires more effort. According to the AHRQ review, health care professionals notice failures in coordination particularly when the patient is directed to the wrong place in the health care system or has a poor health outcome as a result of poor handoffs or inadequate information exchanges. They also perceive failures in terms of an unreasonable effort needed by them to accomplish coordination during transitions among health care entities. System representatives focus more on coordination failures when patients experience a clinically significant mishap from fragmentation of care or when system finances are adversely affected, such as when a preventable hospital readmission occurs.

Why Care Coordination Now?

Changing demographics (increasing numbers of older adults), increasing chronic illness, and the increasing availability of costly medications and treatments have all led to a heavy

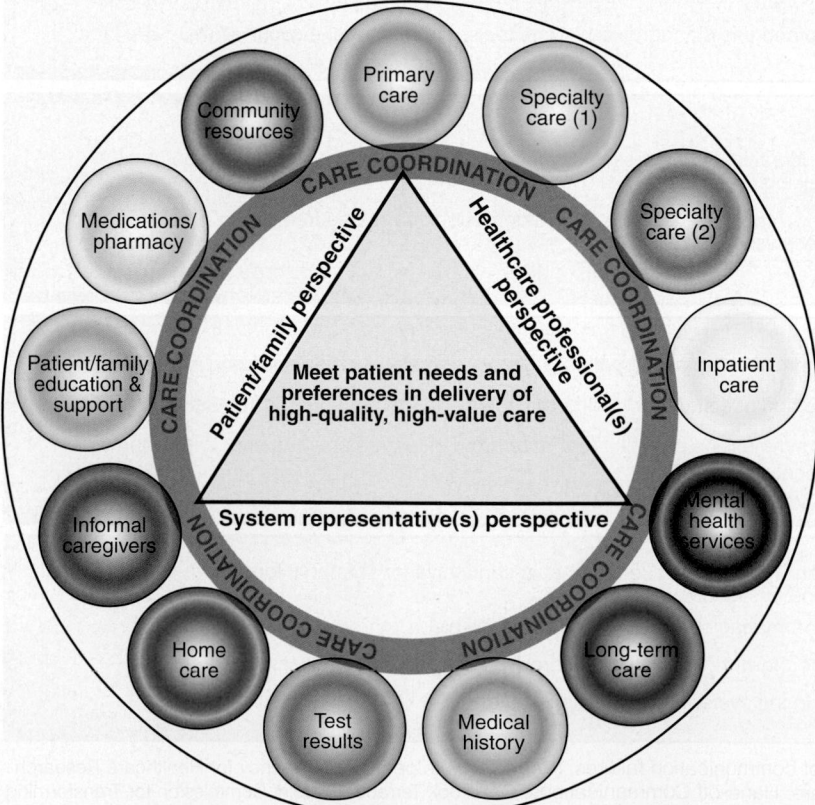

FIGURE 9-6. Care Coordination Ring. The central goal of care coordination is shown in the middle of the diagram. The colored circles represent some of the possible participants, settings, and information important to the care pathway and workflow. The blue ring connecting the colored circles is CARE COORDINATION—namely, anything that bridges gaps (*white spaces*) along the care pathway. (Reprinted with permission from McDonald, K. M., Schultz, E., Albin, L., Pineda, N., et al. [2010]. Care Coordination Atlas Version 3 (prepared by Stanford University under subcontract to Battelle on Contract No. 290–04–0020). AHRQ Publication No. 11–0023-EF. Rockville, MD: Agency for Healthcare Research and Quality.)

demand for care coordination. Care coordination is especially important following the passage of the Patient Protection and Affordable Care Act (PPACA). Financial incentives are shifting from giving more care (under the current fee-for-service model), to providing more integrated, less costly care. The move towards "bundled payment" with shared savings provides incentives for care coordination and avoiding fragmentation or duplication of services. Costs decrease when better information exchanges reduce the need for repeat procedures, which often happens when one provider doesn't know what others have ordered. Quality of care is enhanced when better handoffs result in treatment plans being aligned across settings. Chapter 8 describes some of the models of care coordination: physicians and hospitals, multispecialty group practice, community health centers, prepaid group practice, accountable care organizations, and medical homes/medical neighborhood. Care coordination in discharge planning is addressed later in this chapter.

The Care Coordinator

An Institute for Healthcare Improvement (IHI) white paper describes the **care coordinator** as the care provider (nurse case manager, social worker, community health worker, or lay person) who is responsible for identifying a person's health goals and coordinating services and providers to meet those goals. To be effective, care coordinators must have expertise in self-management and patient advocacy and be adept at navigating complex systems and communicating with a range of people, from family members to physicians and specialists. It is the responsibility of the care coordinator to identify life and health goals with the person and to coordinate services and community supports to work with the person toward better health outcomes. The care coordinator must also understand the strengths and gifts that the individual and family bring (their "assets").

This begins with conversations between the care coordinator and the person about life goals, health goals, and how they interact. These conversations must be nonjudgmental, as the care coordinator takes an open, learning stance to understand the person's life context, struggles, and gifts. The care coordinator has ultimate responsibility for ensuring that the care plan is delivered as described and for incorporating new knowledge to keep the care plan fresh and relevant. As the care coordinator and person learn more about what promotes and what gets in the way of improved health, they are able to modify the care plan to meet the person's emerging strengths and needs (Craig, Eby, and Whittington, 2011).

Patient navigation is just one of the new roles being developed to fill a void in care coordination. The Academy of Oncology Nurse Navigators clarifies the difference between a nurse navigator and a patient navigator:

• *Nurse navigator:* A clinically trained nurse responsible for the identification and removal of barriers to timely and appropriate cancer treatment. The nurse navigator guides the patient through the cancer care continuum from diag-

nosis through survivorship. More specifically, the nurse navigator acts as a central point of contact for a patient and coordinates all components involved in cancer care including surgical, medical, and radiation oncologists; social workers; patient education; community support; and financial and insurance assistance. This person has the clinical background and is a critical member of the multidisciplinary cancer team.

• *Patient navigator:* This term includes all models of navigation (nurse, social worker, lay person). The primary distinction is that this person does not have a clinical background and therefore focuses on the support aspects of care. Thus, this can be either a lay person or a social worker, and depending on background and training, the person's function can vary further. In general, the patient navigator provides assistance with scheduling, financial assistance, psychosocial support, and community support.

See Figure 9-7 for an example of an oncology nurse navigator.

Populations With Special Care Coordination Needs

The Urban Institute Health Policy Center describes vulnerable populations as groups that are not well integrated into the health care system because of ethnic, cultural, economic, geographic, or health characteristics. Their isolation can result in these groups not obtaining necessary health care. Examples of vulnerable populations include:

• People with disabilities or multiple chronic conditions (think of Jeff Hart or the Saxas discussed in Box 9-2)
• People with mental illnesses or substance abuse
• Cultural, racial, and ethnic minorities
• The rural and urban poor (poverty and homelessness)
• Undocumented immigrants

Nurses are often on the front lines of advocating for these groups, but this requires special knowledge, attitudes, and skills. We all have to ask ourselves, first, if we may have biases that interfere with our willingness to create respectful patient-centered partnerships with vulnerable people. Do we believe that chronic drug abusers, the homeless, "crazy old people," or people who do not speak English deserve the same respectful, compassionate person-centered care that we would want for those we love most? Are we moved by the plight of those most in need?

A *Washington Post* reporter recently wrote about the scandal that in a city like Washington, DC, with a $417 million budget, no one seemed to care about 600 kids crammed inside a scary, abandoned hospital serving as the city's makeshift family homeless shelter. "Stop and think about that. Six hundred kids with chubby cheeks and Spider-Man sneakers and Dora hats are beginning their journey in life on an army cot in a cafeteria or an old hospital bed in a city shelter. And that's an improvement from the time they spent sleeping in cars, bus shelters, Metro stations, apartment-house lobbies or on a different couch every night" (Dvorak, 2013).

One Patient's Story

Ellen McLoughlin, an oncology nurse navigator, helps Ms. Remos who is newly diagnosed with colon cancer.

Explanation

Ms. Remos has many questions about her ca zzncer after she gets home from her visit with her oncologist— questions she didn't think to ask. Her nurse navigator brings numerous resources and patience as she sits with Ms. Remos and answers Ms. Remos' questions. At this point she is building a trusting partnership with Ms. Remos and her husband.

Scheduling

The thought of scheduling surgery and follow up appointments that worked with the Remos' busy life was overwhelming Ms. Remos. The nurse navigator was able to schedule appointments for Ms. Remos that didn't interfere with when she needed to be home with her children or at work.

Information/Advice

Although Ms. Remos' surgeon talked with her about pre and post-operative care, Ms. Loughlin was able to explain how Ms. Remos could best prepare for surgery and what she could do afterwards to maximize her recovery. She was also able to help Mr. Remos plan to have family assist with childcare both during the hospitalization and after when Ms. Remos got home.

Support

The nurse navigator met with Ms. Remos the evening before her surgery and waited for her in the recovery room. Ms. Remos was grateful she could talk about her fears. The nurse navigator was also able to support Ms. Remos' husband and children.

FIGURE 9-7. An example of an oncology nurse navigator. (Adapted from Landro, L. (2011. August 16). When a doctor isn't enough. Nurse Navigators help patients through maze of cancer-treatment decisions, fears. *The Wall Street Journal*. Available a http://online.wsj.com/article/ SB10001424053111904253204576510472828240848.html).

Nurses have a proud tradition of seeking to meet the needs of the most vulnerable; will the next generation of nurses continue this?

Nurses also need specialized knowledge and skills to serve these people. It takes a special effort to "walk in the shoes" of a teenage single mother with three children under the age of four or a homeless man with a history of chronic drug and alcohol abuse to learn about who they are, what they need, and how best to help them. Think about a vulnerable population where you live, and try to interview some of its members. See if your class can devise a strategy to learn about and then begin to meet their needs. Think about how community-based care coordination efforts can improve the health and well-being of the most vulnerable in your region.

Admissions, Transfers, and Discharges

As a result of increasing costs and of health care cost reimbursement programs that are prospective rather than retrospective (meaning that costs are predetermined for specific illnesses or treatments, including severity of illness and costs of care), hospital admissions and lengths of hospital stay have decreased. More patients are having surgery, diagnostic tests, and emergency care in ambulatory care settings or on a hospital outpatient basis. Even patients who are admitted often stay for less than 24 hours, are admitted the morning of the surgery, or go home during an interim period between diagnosis and care. All this makes care coordination particularly challenging.

BOX 9-2 CARE COORDINATION AND CONTINUITY CASE STUDY

Read this scenario and discuss your answers to the questions that follow with your fellow students.

Mr. and Mrs. Saxa are an older couple (both in their mid-70s) who live independently. They live in the same house they raised their family in, and are active members of their church. They have two grown children who live across the country but who are attentive and visit regularly, and they have four young grandchildren. Mr. Saxa is still driving, but his children are increasingly concerned about his safety behind the wheel.

Mrs. Saxa has type 1 diabetes and hypertension but has been able to manage her diet well and maintains good control of her hypertension with her medications. She takes six medications.

Mr. Saxa is also hypertensive, and recently underwent hip replacement surgery. While hospitalized for this surgery he developed some difficulty urinating, and now sees a urologist. He also began anticoagulation therapy while hospitalized. Despite these issues, he has done quite well postoperatively, progressing from a walker to a cane that he now uses for stability. He currently takes seven medications.

The Saxas have a primary care provider (PCP) who has been their "family doctor" for decades. He is in a solo practice and does not have an electronic medical record system. In addition to their PCP, Mrs. Saxa sees an endocrinologist and a cardiologist, and Mr. Saxa sees a cardiologist, a urologist, and an orthopedic surgeon.

Mr. Saxa is a plumber. Mrs. Saxa did some secretarial work years ago but has primarily been a homemaker. Since Mr. Saxa retired and his employer does not offer retiree benefits, they rely on Medicare. They have a small nest egg of about $45,000.

In September, Mrs. Saxa has an episode of chest discomfort and shortness of breath, and is taken to the emergency department (ED) of the local hospital. A hospitalist evaluates her in the ED and sends her to the lab for blood work and to the radiology department for a chest film. He calls in a cardiology consult and subsequently admits her to the critical care unit with a diagnosis of congestive heart failure, ruling out myocardial infarction, renal insufficiency, and rheumatoid arthritis. The cardiologist on call orders a cardiac catheterization to rule out coronary artery disease. She is found to have significant occlusion of the left anterior descending artery and the right coronary artery. A cardiovascular surgeon is consulted and a coronary artery bypass graft (CABG) is scheduled and later performed.

Mrs. Saxa recovers from the surgery and is discharged to a rehabilitation facility. While she is in rehabilitation, there is an outbreak of seasonal flu, and although Mrs. Saxa doesn't actually get the flu, she is significantly impacted by staffing shortages. Meanwhile, Mr. Saxa is urged to get a flu shot by his daughter. Since his primary care provider is on vacation, he goes to an urgent care center in his local strip mall, where the nurse practitioner administers the flu shot. Mrs. Saxa receives physical and occupational therapy 3 times/week in rehab, and does quite well. She is discharged from rehab after 1 month, and is referred to home health care.

Two weeks after her discharge, she suffers a stroke and is readmitted to the hospital. Two weeks later she is again discharged to rehab, where she experiences another stroke, which leaves her with significant hemiparesis. Her progress is limited, and she is admitted to a long-term care facility. Mr. Saxa is now adamant about continuing to drive because he visits his wife daily. He is worried about how long they will be able to afford the long-term care facility, which is the only one close to their home.

Questions for Reflection and Discussion

1. What are the main health issues that would concern you with this family? What sort of nonphysical health care needs are the Saxas experiencing? Who is most likely to identify and respond to these needs?
2. What is it reasonable for the Saxas to expect of the nurses they encounter in each of the health care settings they experience?
3. How likely are the professional caregivers who encounter the Saxas in their multiple care settings to have complete histories of this couple, including both their medical and social histories? Would an electronic medical history that could be made available to new practitioners be helpful? Would an implantable microbiochip capable of being scanned and linked with medical records access be helpful? Could this information be misused?
4. How do the Saxas' various professional caregivers learn about new medications or treatments ordered by each other? Are there concerns with this?
5. How do you think the Saxas selected their professional caregivers and health care services? Do they have any way of knowing what quality to expect? If they are dissatisfied with the care they receive, what avenues are open to them to express their displeasure?
6. Make a list of all the different health care settings the Saxas are likely to experience. How well do you understand the services provided in each setting? What criteria would you use to select an excellent facility or service?
7. Make a list of all the different health care providers the Saxas are likely to experience. How well do you understand their respective roles? What criteria would you use to evaluate their care?
8. How will the Saxas' provider visits and hospitalizations be paid for? Will the Saxas bear any financial burden? What health care costs are they likely to incur? Medications? Medical supplies?
9. Think about how the Saxas' experience would differ if they were members of a vulnerable population, for example, urban poor, recent immigrants, non-English-speaking, rural, etc.
10. Who, if anyone, is best qualified to coordinate the care the Saxas are receiving? How likely are they to experience satisfactory care coordination and continuity?

(Adapted from Dr. Pat Cloonan, Georgetown University School of Nursing and Health Studies.)

All people who enter a health care setting take on a new role. They must add to their already established roles (e.g., spouse, parent, sibling, student) the role of patient. They also enter an environment in which strangers surround them and in which they encounter different sounds, sights, and smells. A competent, responsible, and caring nurse can make all the difference to an anxious, frightened, or confused patient and family.

To meet patients' health care needs during the admission process, nurses provide holistic care and establish the basis for how patients will respond to and evaluate the remainder of their stay. Box 9-3 describes guidelines for establishing

BOX 9-3 ESTABLISHING AN EFFECTIVE NURSE–PATIENT RELATIONSHIP ON ADMISSION

- Recognize and take steps to reduce the patient's anxiety. Anxiety is a natural reaction to the unknown, but it can be reduced by therapeutic communication, teaching, and acceptance. Some common concerns that cause anxiety are: *Will I have pain? Who will take care of my family if I die? Will strangers be looking at my body? How much will this cost? What if I can't keep my job?*
- Remember that the medical or surgical condition for which the patient is being treated is only one part of the patient's life. Other concerns include family needs, financial status, and the future.
- Communicate with patients as individuals so that they can maintain their own identity. Ask patients how you

should address them—some people prefer Mr., Mrs., Miss, or Ms. [last name]; others would rather be called by their first name. Do not call all older adults "Grandma" or "Grandpa." Do not refer to Mr. Jones, admitted to room 2218 for treatment of a ruptured appendix, as "the appendix in 2218."
- Take time to learn who the patient being admitted is, including that patient's cultural and religious background. Respect the patient's values and beliefs even though they may differ from yours.
- Encourage the patient's family to participate in and make decisions about all aspects of care.

an effective nurse–patient relationship to ensure that each patient is considered as an individual in any setting.

During admission, the nurse acts not only as a practitioner but also as an advocate concerned about the welfare of the patient and the family. The admission period corresponds to the orientation phase of the helping relationship described in Chapter 11. In addition, regulatory guidelines direct both the continuity and the quality of care. For example, the Joint Commission standards for admission to a hospital assert that each patient's need for nursing care should be assessed by a registered nurse. This assessment includes consideration of biophysical, psychosocial, environmental, self-care, educational, and discharge planning factors. In addition, nurses collaborate, as appropriate, with physicians and members of other clinical disciplines to make decisions regarding the patient's need for nursing care.

Admission to an Ambulatory Care Facility

In ambulatory care facilities, described in Chapter 8, the patient receives health care services but does not remain overnight. Ambulatory facilities include physician offices, clinics, hospital outpatient services, emergency departments, and same-day surgery centers. The goal of these facilities is to provide health care services to patients who are able to provide self-care at home. People go to ambulatory settings for health promotion, health maintenance, or medical or surgical treatment.

In most office and clinic facilities, patients enter a reception area, where they are asked to complete a short health history (unless they have already done so during a previous visit) and sign a statement acknowledging the HIPAA privacy rule (see Chapters 7 and 16). They then receive a physical assessment (often specific to the reason for the visit) in an examination room. Depending on their needs, patients may be given, for example, diagnostic tests, immunizations, or prescriptions for medications, or may undergo minor surgery. All patients require teaching, which should include written instructions about care at home, health promotion activities, and how to contact someone for further questions.

Referrals to community agencies, support groups, or other types of health care settings might also be necessary.

Admission to ambulatory or same-day surgery facilities is somewhat different. Screening tests, teaching, and admission procedures were usually completed previously. Patients arrive at the setting, have the procedure, and go home when recovery is satisfactory. If patients have outpatient or short-stay surgery in the hospital setting, the regular admission procedures are completed on arrival; in most instances, screening tests and teaching are done before the day of surgery. It is the nurse's responsibility to assess what has been done and tailor the care plan to the patient's needs.

 Concept Mastery Alert

Patients are admitted to all different types of ambulatory care facilities for many different reasons. Regardless of the setting or reason, teaching is a priority.

Admission to the Hospital

A scheduled admission to the hospital usually begins in the admitting office. Admitting office staff obtain information about the patient and input that information into the computer. The admission data become part of the patient's permanent record.

The identification number (often included as a barcode)—as well as the patient's name, physician's name, and any other information required by the particular institution—is printed on an identification wristband that is placed on the patient's wrist. This wristband is an important safety component during the patient's stay because it is one of two identifiers, required by The Joint Commission national safety standards (2014), used to identify accurately a patient during activities such as medication administration, blood and fluid administration, diagnostic tests, and surgery. A wristband is worn by all patients. The patient's date of birth is commonly used as the second identifier.

During the initial interview, the admitting staff provides other information about legal and ethical components of care. The patient is asked to sign forms that give consent to treatment and allow the hospital to contact health care insurance companies or public agencies (e.g., Medicare) for reimbursement of services. Patients are asked if they have established advance directives, such as a living will or durable power of attorney, to indicate their treatment preferences about prolonging life. If they have established advance directives, a copy becomes a part of their hospital record. If they have not, the purpose is explained and they are given a form to complete if they wish to do so. (Chapter 42 discusses advance directives and provides a sample form.) Providers must give patients a clear written explanation of how health information will be used and disclosed, and a privacy statement is signed. Patients may also be asked to provide the names of family or friends to whom health status information may be given. Finally, almost all hospitals give some form of a Patient Care Partnership (formerly titled a Patient Bill of Rights) to patients to inform them about what to expect while in the hospital. This document, usually available in several languages, includes the rights to high-quality hospital care, a clean and safe environment, involvement in care, protection of privacy, help when leaving the hospital, and help with insurance claims (American Hospital Association, 2008).

After the necessary forms have been completed in the admitting office, a nurse who works in that area might complete the admission health history and physical assessment, or patients may also be taken to an assigned room for these admission procedures. Laboratory studies and x-rays, as well as the admitting office procedures, are usually completed on an outpatient basis before the day of admission. If the patient has an unscheduled admission or will have only a limited stay (e.g., admitted the morning of a diagnostic examination

intending to return home later that day), admission procedures and assessments may be completed on the unit.

PREPARING THE ROOM FOR ADMISSION

The admitting office notifies the unit to which the patient is to be admitted before the patient arrives so that the room can be prepared. Although the nurse might delegate most of the activities in preparing the room for an admission, it is a nursing responsibility to ensure that other personnel do them. Guidelines for Nursing Care 9-1 outlines the activities carried out in anticipation of the patient's arrival.

ADMITTING THE PATIENT TO THE UNIT

Although other members of the health care team may assist in the admitting procedure, the nurse is responsible for ensuring the patient's safety, comfort, and well-being upon arrival in the unit. The admitting nursing history and assessment are described in Chapter 11. There you will find examples of paper and electronic assessment records. The admission assessment is used to develop the nursing care plan for the patient and also is used as a database for discharge planning and home care. In addition, an inventory of personal belongings and valuables is completed to ensure their return to the patient on discharge or their transfer with the patient to another unit or facility. A **medication reconciliation** form is completed on admission. The form is checked and filled out again with each transfer and on discharge to ensure that all medications have been correctly ordered or discontinued as the patient moves through the system.

Nurses should welcome the patient to the unit in the same courteous manner as when welcoming a guest into one's own home. In most instances, the patient is accompanied by family members who may either remain with the patient

GUIDELINES FOR NURSING CARE 9-1

PREPARING THE ROOM FOR PATIENT ADMISSION

- Position the bed. For ambulatory patients, the bed should be in its lowest position. Place the bed in its highest position if the patient will arrive on a stretcher. Ensure that the furniture in the room is arranged to allow easy access to the bed.
- Open the bed by folding back the top bed linens (see figure).
- Assemble routine equipment and supplies. A hospital admission pack (which contains such items as a bath basin, water pitcher, drinking glass, tissues, soap, and lotion) is placed in the room. A hospital gown or pajamas should be in the room, although the patient may choose to wear his or her own pajamas or gown. Equipment for taking vital signs (i.e., stethoscope, sphygmomanometer, thermometer) and height and weight should be in the room or readily available. If laboratory work has not been done previously, a container for a clean urine specimen should be available.
- Assemble special equipment and supplies. The patient may require oxygen therapy, cardiac monitoring, or suction

equipment. The nurse ensures that the equipment is functioning properly and is ready for the patient's use on arrival.
- Adjust the physical environment of the room. This may include turning on lights and setting the room temperature.

An "open" bed, ready for the patient's arrival.

to provide support and information or who may wait in the waiting room during the admission procedure. The nurse assesses the needs of the patient and family, and they should mutually agree about whether family should be present during admission.

Transferring Within and Between Health Care Settings

Patients often move within a setting as well as between settings, as in these examples:

- Within the hospital, such as from the emergency department to a hospital room, from an intensive care unit (ICU) to a hospital room (and vice versa), from one unit to another, or from one room to another room on the same unit
- To and from acute care settings and long-term settings
- From acute care settings to the patient's home
- From ambulatory care settings to acute care settings

When a transfer occurs, the patient must readjust to new surroundings, new roommates, new routines, and new people providing care. If the transfer is to a higher level of care, as in a move to the ICU, the patient and family often experience unfamiliar sights and sounds. A transfer to a long-term care facility may not be desired by the patient or family but may be necessary if family members cannot provide care at home or if no other support people are available. All of these factors cause stress and anxiety.

 RECALL Laura Degas, the woman who is not sure if she will be able to care for her sister at home. If it is determined that Ms. Degas cannot care for her sister at home, she may decide to have her sister transferred to a long-term care facility. In this case, the nurse must provide Ms. Degas with support and guidance to ease the transition and help minimize the stress and anxiety of this move. ●

The nurse may not be responsible for the actual physical move but is responsible for ensuring that the comfort, safety, and teaching needs of the patient and family are met. Although documentation and procedures differ depending on the institution and type of transfer, patient needs are always a priority in ensuring a smooth transition and continuity of care.

TRANSFER WITHIN THE HOSPITAL

When a patient is transferred within the hospital, personal belongings must be moved to the new room. Every effort must be made to ensure that belongings are not misplaced or lost. The patient's records are moved to the new unit or made available electronically. Other hospital departments (e.g., dietary, pharmacy, physical therapy) must be notified of the transfer.

When a patient is transferred to another unit, the nurse in the original area gives a verbal report about the patient to the nurse in the new area using the approved handoff technique. The report should include the patient's name, age, physicians, admitting diagnosis, surgical procedure (if applicable), current condition and manifestations, allergies, medications and

treatments, laboratory data, and any special equipment that will be needed to provide care. Nursing care priorities are identified, and the existence of advance directives is noted. Accurate, concise, and complete verbal communication is essential.

TRANSFER TO AN EXTENDED CARE FACILITY

When a patient is transferred from the hospital to an extended care facility or other community setting, the patient is discharged from the hospital and a copy of the medical record may be sent to the extended care facility (depending on the physician's preference and the agency's protocol). The original record, which is a legal document, remains at the hospital. All of the patient's belongings are sent to the facility with the patient. Prescriptions and appointment cards for return visits to the physician's office may also be sent.

In most instances, a detailed assessment and care plan is sent from the hospital to the extended care facility. In addition, the nurse at the hospital often provides a verbal report to the nurse at the new facility using the approved handoff technique.

 REMEMBER Jeff Hart, the 9-year-old boy transferred from the state facility to the hospital due to respiratory complications. Once the child's problems have been resolved, the nurse would prepare Jeff to be transferred back to the state facility. Information about the events of the hospitalization are documented and reported. In addition, communication between health care team members at the hospital and those at the state facility helps ensure continuity of care for Jeff. ●

Discharge From a Health Care Setting

Patients are discharged from a health care facility when the expected outcomes of care are met and the patient or caregiver has the necessary knowledge and skills to provide any additional care still needed. In meeting the needs of the patient being discharged from a health care setting, nurses consider that the person may be expecting a change from a dependent role to a more independent (self-care) role. Although discharge is almost always a welcome event, it also can be stressful.

DISCHARGE PLANNING

The purpose of planning for continuity of care, commonly referred to in hospitals and community agencies as **discharge planning**, is to ensure that patient and family needs are consistently met as the patient moves from a care setting to home. Essential components of discharge planning include assessing the strengths and limitations of the patient, the family or support person, and the environment; implementing and coordinating the plan of care; considering individual, family, and community resources; and evaluating the effectiveness of care.

Planning for discharge actually begins on admission, when information about the patient is collected and documented.

The key to successful discharge planning is an exchange of information among the patient, the caregivers, and those responsible for care while the patient is in a care setting and after the patient returns home. This coordination of care is usually the nurse's responsibility.

With earlier hospital discharges, patients often are still acutely ill when they go home, and many require complicated treatment and care by family members. It is no longer unusual for family members to change sterile dressings, administer tube feedings, monitor intravenous medications, manage high-technology equipment, give complete physical care, and prepare special diets. If they are unprepared or unable to carry out these interventions correctly, the patient may experience an exacerbation of the illness or complications that could require readmission or additional treatment. The nurse must ensure that family members are taught the necessary knowledge and skills and that referrals are made to agencies such as home health care or social services to provide support and assistance during the recovery period.

This process includes identifying which patients need which level of discharge planning. All patients need discharge planning in general, but certain patients have more comprehensive needs for specific services. The nurse who conducts the initial nursing assessment is in the best position to determine these special needs.

Patients who meet any of the following criteria need a formal discharge plan and referral to another agency:

- Lack of knowledge of the treatment plan
- Social isolation
- Recently diagnosed chronic disease
- Major surgery
- Prolonged recuperation from major surgery or illness
- Emotional or mental instability
- Complex home care regimen
- Financial difficulties
- Lack of available or appropriate referral sources
- Terminal illness

GUIDELINES FOR DISCHARGE PLANNING

For a patient hospitalized with a serious illness or injury, discharge planning may be done over time; for a patient treated in an ambulatory facility, it may be completed relatively quickly. A nursing case manager or discharge planner is often responsible for discharge planning for patients in acute care settings and may follow a plan of care or a critical path established for the patient. Regardless of the plan used, the nurse assesses the patient's needs and identifies problems, develops goals with the patient, carries out teaching, and makes referrals. An example of discharge planning is provided in Box 9-4.

BOX 9-4 A DISCHARGE PLANNING EXAMPLE

Scenario

Mr. Smith is a 55-year-old married man, admitted to the hospital with a diagnosis of stroke. He now has left-side weakness and difficulty communicating verbally. He has had a history of high blood pressure for 10 years. If his blood pressure remains stable, Mr. Smith is to be discharged from the hospital in 3 days. He will be going home with four new medications and an indwelling urinary catheter. A low-sodium diet is prescribed.

After reviewing the medical record, the nurse interviews Mr. and Mrs. Smith. The assessment reveals that Mr. Smith has a limited ability to transfer from bed to chair. Both Mr. and Mrs. Smith are fearful of discharge. Mr. Smith believes that he will be able to return to work as an accountant in 3 weeks and hates the thought of being an invalid at his age, but Mrs. Smith thinks he will never work again. They have never faced a life-threatening or disabling illness in the past. They have no strong cultural preferences for diet. They have two adult children who live out of state with their own families. Mrs. Smith has a younger sister who lives nearby. The Smiths are both college educated. They live in a suburban area in a two-story home with narrow stairs leading to the second floor's two baths and three bedrooms. They have adequate plumbing. Their doctor's office is about 1 mile away, and shopping is nearby.

Mrs. Smith is worried about managing care of the catheter and moving Mr. Smith in and out of bed. She needs instruction in the new medications and diet regimen. She is terrified that she may be unable to handle an emergency in the middle of the night. Financially, this two-income family has abruptly become a one-income family. Mr. Smith is not 65 years old and thus is not yet eligible for Medicare, although he does have disability insurance that will cover a portion of his salary.

Planning

How would the nurse coordinate this discharge plan? The physician must be consulted for diet, medication, other treatments, and home health care orders. The dietitian needs to counsel the Smiths on a low-sodium diet and on creative ways to prepare low-salt meals. Physical therapy has already been initiated at the hospital and will continue through home health care. An occupational therapist will visit to provide teaching about strengthening exercises and assistive devices, such as a walker. The social worker has been called for financial assessment to determine exactly what services the Smiths can expect to have reimbursed by their insurance plan and how they will manage their out-of-pocket expenses.

The nurse discusses Mr. and Mrs. Smith's health care needs with the home health care agency. A teaching plan for medications and care of the urinary catheter is implemented. Mrs. Smith demonstrates how to care for the catheter. The physical therapist teaches Mrs. Smith how to transfer Mr. Smith into and out of the bed and assures her that he will help her practice at home. Written information about high blood pressure, stroke, low-sodium diet, and prescribed medications is given to the Smiths, along with the telephone number of a local support group for people who have had strokes. Although Mrs. Smith still verbalizes concern about providing care at home, she says that she feels more in control now. Mr. Smith is beginning to realize that recovery may take longer than he anticipated. At the time of discharge, the nurse tells the Smiths that someone from the hospital will call them the next day and that the home health care nurse will visit them that afternoon.

FOCUSED ASSESSMENT GUIDE 9-1

DISCHARGE PLANNING

Factors to Assess	Questions and Approaches
Health data	Establish a database that includes age, gender, height and weight, medical diagnoses, past medical history, current health problems, surgery, and functional limitations (e.g., impaired sight or hearing, amputation, use of wheelchair or walker).
Personal data	Ask the patient: "What language do you prefer to use?" "How do you feel about being discharged?" "What are your expectations for recovery?" "What do you do to help you cope with stress? Are these things helpful?"
Caregivers	Establish the caregiver's age, gender, relationship to the patient, past experiences with this illness or treatment, values and beliefs, and cultural practices that might affect prescribed care. Ask the caregiver: "Do you live with the patient?" "What are your expectations about providing care at home?" "What are your fears about providing care at home?"
Environment	Assess the home, noting if there will be barriers to using prescribed assistive devices (e.g., wheelchairs or walkers); if the patient will be able to use bathroom facilities safely; and if hot water, heat, and room for supplies are available. Assess the community, noting location (such as rural or urban), whether health care is available and accessible, whether transportation is available, and any known environmental hazards.
Financial and support resources	Discuss expenses of prescribed care, including dressing supplies, medications, equipment, and special foods. Discuss available resources, including Medicare and Medicaid, parish nursing, and meal services to the home. Discuss, especially if the patient will be living alone, support services and resources and how they can be accessed. Include friends, church groups, and support groups specific to the patient's age and health care needs.

Assessing and Identifying Health Care Needs

The first step in discharge planning involves collecting and organizing data about the patient. When assessing the patient for discharge, the nurse includes the family, if possible, because both the patient and family must be actively involved for an effective transition from the health care setting to home. Factors to assess in discharge planning are listed in the accompanying Focused Assessment Guide 9-1. Other assessment formats may be used, depending on institutional procedures, to evaluate the patient's ability to carry out activities of daily living (e.g., bathing, dressing, toileting, transferring, continence, feeding) and instrumental activities of daily living (using the telephone, shopping, preparing food, doing housekeeping and laundry, taking medications, accessing transportation). The medical record and physician orders are also consulted for the exact medication and treatment plan before the nursing care plan is developed.

Nursing diagnoses, developed from the discharge planning assessment, identify the needs of both the patient and the family. Examples of nursing diagnoses for a patient being discharged are listed in the Examples of NANDA-I Nursing Diagnoses: Discharge From a Health Care Setting box. The nurse determines whether problems are present now or are potential problems. For example, a patient with chronic respiratory problems may have assistance from a member of the family who has come to stay for 1 month, but after that, the patient will be alone at home. In this case, the situation is not an actual problem now but could become one unless planning is done to meet needs when there is no longer a family caregiver.

Setting Goals With the Patient

The expected goals of the discharge plan are set mutually and must be realistic. If the patient is involved in establishing goals, the expected outcomes of the plan of care are more likely to be met. The patient may fail to follow the plan if the goals are not mutually agreed on or are not based on a complete assessment of the patient's needs. For example, the nurse or another health care provider may do a thorough job of teaching a patient about a special diet, but the patient may not actually follow the diet after discharge because of being unable to afford the special food, unable to get to the grocery store, or not having a refrigerator at home for food storage.

Teaching

Important teaching topics about self-care at home must be covered before discharge. These topics include medications, procedures and treatments, diet, referrals, and health status.

EXAMPLES OF NANDA-I NURSING DIAGNOSES

DISCHARGE FROM A HEALTH CARE SETTING

Nursing Diagnoses	Related Factors
Anxiety	Concern about uncertain future following radiation treatment for breast cancer
Risk for Caregiver Role Strain	Care of 75-year-old wife with dementia from Alzheimer disease
Readiness for Enhanced Coping	Attendance at support group meetings and verbally defining stressors as manageable
Delayed Surgical Recovery	Infection of large abdominal wound and needed help to complete self-care
Effective Enhanced Therapeutic Regimen Management	Demonstrates accurate dressing change and verbalizes confidence in managing recovery and preventing complications

The patient needs to understand the drug name, dosage, purpose, effects, times to be taken, and possible side effects. Information about medications should be given both verbally and in writing. Copies of the medication administration record are often given to the patient to use as a pattern for times and amounts of medications administered in the hospital. Patients often find it helpful when the nurse draws a clock face and writes the names of the medications in the correct time slots.

All steps of a procedure (e.g., dressing changes) should be demonstrated, practiced, and provided in writing. Some nurses make short videos to demonstrate complex procedures to patients that the patient takes home. The patient or caregiver should then perform the procedure or treatment in the presence of the nurse to demonstrate the ability to carry out the procedure. The caregiver should know the purpose of what is being done and how to get supplies.

Teaching should clearly describe the purpose of the diet and its expected outcomes. Patients find examples of written diet plans and meals helpful. If the patient has been in the hospital, it is helpful to save menu or meal forms to use as a reference at home.

Appointments for the first visit to a physician or agency are often made before discharge. In addition, the patient and family members should know how to contact the providers of follow-up care and should know whom to call if they have questions or problems. Nurses can help patients by making sure that they have the phone numbers of the primary care doctor and the names and phone numbers of community resources. Patients should also know the signs and symptoms of potential complications and know when to contact emergency care. This referral information takes into account the patient's economic situation, access to transportation, support systems, and home environment.

All aspects of the illness or effects of treatment should be clearly described, both verbally and in written materials. Many forms of written information are available for patients, ranging from printed literature (e.g., from the American Heart Association) to teaching materials developed by the health care facility. Written instructions are given to the patient. The patient should be able to talk about the anticipated physical and emotional effects of the illness and also describe what will be done to achieve the highest level of health possible. All teaching should be documented in the patient's record and the discharge summary. The patient's or family member's demonstrations of care procedures must be satisfactory, and the patient and caregiver must have exposure to and practice with the equipment that they will be using at home.

Meeting Eligibility Requirements for Community-based Settings

The physician must write an order for all home care services, and the patient must meet eligibility criteria for reimbursement for home health care visits. As much patient information as possible should be given to the home health agency, including the kind of surgery or injury, medications, the patient's physical and mental status, significant social factors (e.g., frail caregiver with health problems, or no caregiver), and the family's expected needs.

EVALUATING DISCHARGE PLANNING EFFECTIVENESS

Evaluating the discharge plan is crucial to ensure that the discharge planning works. Planning and referrals must be scrutinized to ensure the quality and appropriateness of services. Evaluation is ongoing, and care plans may need to be changed. A few weeks after the patient goes home, further evaluation of the discharge process is usually conducted by a telephone call, a questionnaire, or a home visit.

Leaving the Hospital Against Medical Advice

A patient sometimes decides to leave the hospital or other care setting against medical advice (AMA). Although the patient is legally free to do so, this choice carries a risk for increased illness or complications. A patient who decides to leave AMA must sign a form that releases the physician and health care institution from any legal responsibility for the patient's health status. The patient is informed of any possible risk before signing the form. The patient's signature must be witnessed, and the form becomes part of the patient's record.

Table 9-1 TYPES OF HOME HEALTH CARE AGENCIES

TYPE	DESCRIPTION
Official or public agencies	These agencies are operated by state or local governments and primarily financed by tax funds. Most offer home care and disease-prevention programs in the community.
Voluntary or private not-for-profit agencies	These agencies are supported by donations, endowments, charities (such as the United Way), and insurance reimbursements. They are governed by a board of directors, usually representing the community they serve.
Private, proprietary agencies	Most private, proprietary agencies are for-profit organizations governed by individual owners or national corporations. Their services are paid for through health care insurance or individual self-pay.
Institution-based agencies	These agencies operate under a parent organization, such as a hospital. The home care agency is governed by the institution, and most referrals for care come from within the institution.

HOME HEALTH CARE NURSING

This chapter would not be complete without addressing some of the particulars of home health care nursing, which is rapidly expanding for many reasons. The need for home health care services is increasing as the population ages. Because fewer people live in the same community as their parents, home health care providers may be needed to care for ill parents when children live far away. Because patients are discharged from hospitals earlier in their recovery, many need skilled professional care after they return home. As well, people are more often choosing to die with comfort and dignity in their own homes. In addition, third-party payers (such as insurance companies and managed care organizations) try to reduce the escalating costs of health care through the use of managed care programs that include home health care.

Nurses provide home health care within a system that includes home health agencies, patients, referral sources, physicians or other primary caregivers, reimbursement sources, and legal considerations. The system functions best when its members communicate, cooperate, and collaborate with each other.

Types of Home Health Care Agencies

There are several different kinds of public and private home health care agencies. All home health care agencies must meet uniform standards for licensing, certification, and accreditation by state agencies and/or federal programs (such as Medicare). Home care agencies differ in how they are organized and administered. Table 9-1 describes different types of home health care agencies.

Home health care agencies are either certified or not certified by Medicare. An agency must be certified by Medicare to receive reimbursement for services. Agencies may not be certified by Medicare for many reasons: for example, home care agencies that do not provide skilled nursing care (e.g., services provided by a registered nurse) cannot received Medicare reimbursement. Medicare is the largest single payer of home care services. It provides payment for services through a prospective payment plan based on an

Table 9-2 EXAMPLES OF HOME HEALTH CARE SERVICES

AREA OF SERVICE	TYPE OF SERVICE PROVIDED
High-technology pharmacy services	Intravenous therapy Home uterine monitoring Ventilator management Chemotherapy
Skilled professional/ paraprofessional services	Nursing care (provided by a licensed practical nurse, a registered nurse, a clinical nurse specialist, or a nurse practitioner) Home health care aides Personal care Physical therapy Occupational therapy Speech therapy Medical social work Respiratory therapy
Custodial services	Homemaking and house-keeping Hourly or shift coverage Live-in services Companionship
Home medical services	Providing durable medical equipment such as beds, braces, canes, crutches, wheelchairs, commodes, and oxygen
Hospice services	Pain management Physician services Spiritual support Respite care Bereavement counseling
Community support services	Meals on Wheels Transportation Friendly visitor Delivery services Emergency answering services

"episode of care" (usually considered a 60-day period). All patients receiving home health care services must have an order from their primary health care provider.

Home health care services include high-technology pharmacy services, skilled professional services, custodial care, medical equipment services, hospice and respite services (discussed in Chapter 8), and community support services. Table 9-2 lists examples of these services.

Depending on the agency and its geographic location, professional providers may include registered nurses, licensed practical/vocational nurses, nurse practitioners and clinical nurse specialists, home care aides, enterostomal therapists, mental health specialists, speech therapists, respiratory therapists, physical therapists, occupational therapists, social workers, dietitians, and a chaplain or spiritual care provider. Regardless of how many providers are involved, the responsibility for care coordination (also called case management) remains with the registered nurse.

Patients and Family Caregivers

The patient in home health care is both the person receiving care and the person's family, who often are also the caregivers. When a patient enters the hospital, the family most often plays a minor role in actual care. Families and friends visit with the patient and sometimes stay overnight, but they are generally not involved in direct patient care. Hospital staff provide personal care for the patient and administer medications and treatments. After the patient is discharged, the responsibility for care is shifted to family caregivers, who may or may not be physically or mentally able to handle this responsibility.

Today's emphasis on home health care means that family caregivers have increased responsibilities. Patients are discharged "quicker and sicker." Chronically ill patients may need long-term care at home that may not be covered by Medicare, and changes in Medicare funding may mean that fewer home visits are covered. The financial burden of care is more than many families can afford, and home health care nurses must be alert for signs of such financial problems (e.g., no food in the refrigerator or kitchen cupboards). A referral for services such as Meals on Wheels may be necessary to provide adequate nutrition for the patient.

In addition to the financial burden, family members face the challenges of handling equipment, providing new types of care to loved ones, and dealing with unfamiliar and often terrifying sounds, odors, and substances. Most caregivers are women, and many of them are over age 65. Older women may themselves have health problems or may not have the physical strength or energy to care for their husbands. Even family members who are themselves nurses may find that providing care at home is very different from providing care in the hospital. The accompanying Through the Eyes of the Family Caregiver display describes one such experience.

THROUGH THE EYES OF THE FAMILY CAREGIVER

"I'm so glad to have you home, but what do I do now?" (and this is just the first day....)

I am a nurse and have been a nurse for 30 years. I have a diploma in nursing, a baccalaureate in nursing, a master's in counseling, and a doctorate in nursing. I have taught others how to be nurses for more than 25 years. Nothing in all my educational and practice experiences prepared me to care for the complex needs of my husband, Jacque, when he had surgery 2 years ago. Following diagnosis of metastatic thyroid cancer, a large lower thoracic spinal cord tumor (which put pressure on the spinal nerves, causing leg weakness and bladder malfunction) and the thyroid gland were removed surgically, and steel rods were implanted almost the entire length of the spine. After 30 days in the hospital for diagnosis, surgery, and recovery, Jacque came home—unable to do more than move from the bed to a chair, and with a catheter in his bladder that was attached to a drainage bag.

Before he came home, I got a hospital bed with electric controls, a bedside commode, and a bedside table. I cleared out the family room furniture, got a friend to put the television up on a table (so it could be seen from the hospital bed), and thought I was all ready to give my husband expert care. The first challenge came when he got up in a chair to eat his dinner—we had no chairs with a high enough seat or a straight enough back to allow use of the bedside table. I ran up and down stairs to look at chairs, and finally decided the antique armchair in the living room would work, and it did. Now another problem—where to hang the catheter drainage bag? And how best to move so it didn't pull when he moved? And remember to empty the bag before he gets up!

I fixed a wonderful homecoming meal for this man I love, and he could only eat a few bites. Now back to bed and a new problem. He got out of the bed and into the chair just fine, but now he can't get out of the chair and into the bed because his legs are still so weak. What did I do wrong—it worked in the hospital. It took me 2 days to realize that I forgot to lower the bed height so Jacque wouldn't have to push up so hard to get his bottom on the bed.

Then, after finally literally hauling him back in bed, I realized that I did not know how to move him up in bed. The physical therapist had taught him how to get up in a chair, but not how to move himself up in bed (they always did it for him in the hospital). This is a 250-pound man we are talking about. I could turn him from side to side, but I couldn't physically move him up in bed and he couldn't stay where he was. After a lot of trials, we figured out that he could wiggle one side of his body at a time and slowly inch up in bed. Now, he was exhausted and in pain, and I felt totally incompetent. Thank goodness, the home health care nurse is coming to visit tomorrow.

If I felt this way, how must family members feel who know nothing about caring for someone who is sick or in pain? I have such respect for all those family members who provide such wonderful care and for the nurses who provide home care that calms the fears and answers the questions.

—Priscilla LeMone

BOX 9-5 DATA REQUIRED FOR AN EFFECTIVE HOME PLAN OF CARE

- Mental status
- Types of services and equipment required
- Prognosis and rehabilitation potential
- Functional limitations
- Activities permitted
- Nutritional requirements
- Medications and treatments
- Safety measures to protect against injury
- Instructions for timely discharge

The home health care nurse must identify the needs of the family and caregiver. The nurse assesses whether the patient and family understand and agree with the plan of care and determines if the caregivers understand the instructions provided and are capable of providing care. The nurse can help the patient and family identify and use community resources to meet their needs. If a caregiver feels overwhelmed, the nurse can provide resources to relieve the stress. The nurse also supports family decisions about complex treatments or end-of-life care. The following questions may be used for discussion:

- What is most important to you?
- What do you want for your life and your family's?
- How do you want to spend the rest of your life?
- How is this technology supporting or not supporting what you want?

Referrals for Home Care

A referral source is a person who recommends home care services and supplies the home health care agency with details about the patient's needs. The referral source may be a nurse, physician, social worker, therapist, or discharge planner. The referral may be to a home health agency, a hospice, or a community resource. Families sometimes generate their own referrals by contacting a home care agency. If the agency believes the patient qualifies for services, the agency contacts the patient's physician and requests a referral for the patient.

Orders for Home Care

Home health care cannot begin without an order from a primary caregiver (usually a physician, but may also be a nurse practitioner), nor can it proceed without the primary caregiver's approved treatment plan. This is a legal and reimbursement requirement. A nursing assessment visit to identify a patient's needs can be scheduled only after a referral is made and an initial set of primary caregiver's orders are received. At the nursing assessment visit, the nurse begins to formulate the plan of care and sends it to the primary caregiver for review and approval. Box 9-5 identifies the data needed to create an effective home plan of care. The primary caregiver's signature on the plan of care authorizes the home care agency to provide services. The plan is reviewed as necessary but at least once every 60 days.

Reimbursement Sources

A reimbursement source pays for home health care services. Although Medicare is the largest single source of reimbursement, services are also reimbursed by Medicaid, private insurance, patients or their families, and other public funding. The reimbursement source evaluates each plan of care, and only interventions identified on the plan are approved for reimbursement.

Medicare pays the cost of the first 100 home visits following a hospital stay (Centers for Medicare and Medicaid Services [CMS], 2009). Medicare does not reimburse visits to support general health, health promotion, or socioeconomic needs. To be approved for Medicare reimbursement, the patient must meet the criteria listed in Box 9-6.

In addition, Medicare provides reimbursement only if the nurse teaches about a new or acute situation, assesses an acute change in the patient's condition, or performs a skilled procedure requiring the professional skill, knowledge, ability, and judgment of a licensed nurse. It is imperative to thoroughly

BOX 9-6 ELIGIBILITY REQUIREMENTS FOR MEDICARE REIMBURSEMENT FOR HOME HEALTH CARE SERVICES

The home health care agency must be Medicare certified, and the patient must meet the following requirements:

- Be confined to the home
- Under the care of a physician
- Receiving services under a plan of care established and periodically reviewed by a physician
- Be in need of skilled nursing care on an intermittent basis (provided or needed on fewer than 7 days a week or less

than 8 hours of each day for periods of 21 days or less, although extensions may be possible)
- Have an intermittent need for physical therapy, speech–language therapy, or to continue occupational therapy

Although a patient may leave home for medical treatment or short infrequent trips for nonmedical reasons (such as to the barbershop or to attend religious services), leaving the home must require considerable and taxing effort.

(Source: U.S. Department of Health and Human Services, Centers for Medicare and Medicaid Services [USDHHS]. [2007]. *Medicare and home health. Section 1 Medicare coverage of home health care.* Available at http://www.medicare.gov/Publications/Pubs/pdf/10969.pdf)

Box 9-7 EXAMPLES OF RIGHTS AS A HOME HEALTH CARE PATIENT

Home health care patients have the right to:

- Be fully informed of all their rights and responsibilities by the home health care agency
- Choose care providers
- Receive reasonable continuity of care
- Receive information necessary to give informed consent before the start of any treatment or procedure
- Refuse treatment within the confines of the law and to be informed of the consequences of their action
- Have health care providers comply with advance directives in accordance with state law requirements
- Voice grievances and suggest changes in service or staff without fear of restraint or discrimination
- Be informed of what to do in the case of an emergency

(Source: These are part of a longer list of patient rights published by the National Association for Home Care & Hospice. [2014]. *Consumer information: What are my rights as a patient?* Available at http://www.nahch.org/what-are-my-rights-as-a-patient/)

document all nursing interventions with each home visit for reimbursement to occur.

Legal Considerations

Legal considerations in home care involve a variety of factors, including issues of privacy and confidentiality, the patient's access to health information, the patient's freedom from reasonable restraint, informed consent, and matters of negligence and malpractice. The same codes and standards that guide all other nurses also guide nurses providing care in the home. The American Nurses Association (ANA) *Home Health Nursing Scope and Standards of Practice* (2007) is the basis for practice in the home. The standards address the nursing process, interdisciplinary collaboration, quality assurance, professional development, and research. Another source of guidance is the National Association for Home Care (NAHC) Bill of Rights. Home care agencies are required by federal law to address the concepts in the Bill of Rights with all home care patients in the initial visit. Box 9-7 provides a few examples from the Bill of Rights. Nurses can best avoid lawsuits by knowing standards of practice, providing care that is consistent with agency policies, and documenting all care fully and accurately.

THE HOME VISIT

Home health care patients often feel frightened, in pain, and abandoned, and family members often feel nervous about their new roles as caregivers. The home health care nurse must keep these concerns and needs in mind when planning and carrying out care.

The Pre-entry Phase of the Home Visit

In the referral process, the physician or discharge planner of a hospital contacts the home care agency and provides a brief medical history, along with indications for home health services. During this pre-entry phase, the referral nurse at the home care agency collects as much information as possible about the patient's diagnoses, surgical experience, socioeconomic status, and treatments ordered. This is called the pre-entry phase. Once assigned the case, the nurse reviews the information and calls the patient to schedule a visit. During this phone conversation, the nurse can determine whether the patient's caregiver can answer questions related to the patient's and family's needs and can also learn about the patient's cognitive abilities, orientation, and caregiver status. This information is important to the nurse planning the first visit.

The nurse should evaluate safety issues before making the first home visit; this includes the safety of the neighborhood where the patient lives. The nurse may need to arrange the visit at a time when it is safe to be in that area and should always know the exact destination before arriving for the visit. In some unsafe areas, police or security officers may accompany the nurse. Other guidelines for safety include carrying a cell phone programmed with emergency numbers, making sure that someone from the agency knows the nurse's itinerary, and being continuously alert to the environment.

The Entry Phase of the Home Visit

The second phase of the visit is the entry phase. In the entry phase, the nurse develops rapport with the patient and family, makes assessments, determines nursing diagnoses, establishes desired outcomes (along with the patient and family), plans and implements prescribed care, and provides teaching. The nurse must remember that one is a guest in the patient's home and is offering services that the patient may accept or reject. Important considerations include negotiating and honoring visit times, establishing a rapport with the patient and family, defining what nursing care will be provided, and teaching to promote independence in self-care.

The nurse must gain the trust of the patient and family, and must recognize and respect their values. Accepting the patient's living conditions is necessary, even when they differ from those of the nurse. The nurse must ask permission before using the patient's home for activities such as handwashing. The nurse might believe that the furniture in the patient's home or sick room needs to be rearranged to allow the use of equipment and to remove safety hazards, but the patient should give permission before any changes are made.

Nurses who provide home health care interventions do so based on an individualized plan of care for each patient, based initially on identifying individualized health care needs. In identifying the patient's needs and determining the interventions, the nurse fulfills the roles discussed earlier in the chapter.

EXAMPLES OF NANDA-I NURSING DIAGNOSES

HOME HEALTH CARE

Nursing Diagnoses	Related Factors
Risk for Infection	Presence of large draining wound and unclean living environment
Impaired Home Maintenance	Fatigue and pain during recovery from injuries in automobile crash
Caregiver Role Strain	Requirement for 24-hour attention to needs and safety of husband with Alzheimer disease
Readiness for Enhanced Knowledge	Requests from family members for increased information about providing care and using community resources and support services
Readiness for Enhanced Parenting	Children express satisfaction with home environment

Identifying Needs and Determining Interventions

The ability to assess patients accurately is an important skill for home health care nurses. Most of the initial assessment takes place during the first home visit, although ongoing focused assessment occurs during subsequent visits. The nurse must be skilled not only in physical assessment but also in psychological, socioeconomic, environmental, spiritual, and cultural assessment. Skilled assessment allows the nurse to make appropriate diagnoses. (See Examples of NANDA-I Nursing Diagnoses: Home Health Care.) In addition, the nurse must determine and provide culturally sensitive care (see Chapter 5); although important for inpatients, this is even more important in the patient's home. Family caregivers must also be considered, taking into account the various roles that each family member plays and how they contribute to the patient's health status. Specific interventions are based on the patient's needs, but controlling infection and teaching the patient and caregiver are part of all home visits.

Teaching the Patient and Caregivers

Because home health care is meant to be short term and intermittent, the nurse includes the family and friends in the teaching process so that they can learn how to care for the patient after the nurse's home care is no longer needed. The nurse designs and implements the teaching plan based on the patient's and caregiver's readiness to learn. It must be adapted to the patient's and caregiver's physical and emotional status, and must be understandable and "doable."

 CONSIDER Joey Marshall, the infant discharged home after 7 months. Because of the complex technology associated with his care and because his mother feels anxious and afraid, the nurse needs to provide the necessary teaching about his care, but in small sessions to avoid overwhelming the mother. ●

Teaching should identify both the positive outcomes of following instruction and the serious consequences of failing to do so. The nurse points out the major problem areas specific to care in the home, focusing on the information needed to keep the patient safe until the nurse's next home visit.

Documenting Care Given in the Home

Documenting care given in the home is mandated by regulatory and federal agencies (see Chapter 16). The nurse may document the visit on preprinted forms or checklists or may use a computer.

The documented plan of care, the visit plan, and progress notes are routinely used by regulatory agencies and payer sources (e.g., private insurance or Medicare) to determine whether various state and federal regulations are being met and if payment is warranted. Figures 9-8 and 9-9 illustrate such documentation. The plan of care establishes specific measurable goals and specifies a time frame for reaching the goals. The plan of care accurately reflects the condition of the patient, the patient's functional limitations and safety needs, the need for skilled care, specific physician orders, anticipated progress, criteria for discharge, supplies needed, a visit schedule for all health care providers, and a list of support systems available.

The nurse writes (or types) progress notes to document each visit to the patient's home. These notes must accurately describe the patient's condition, the skilled care provided, the patient's response, the patient's progress toward discharge, and an ongoing plan for continued care. They also include the nurse's plan for the next visit. To meet reimbursement requirements, each progress note must indicate that the care provided requires the knowledge and skills of a professional nurse.

HOME HEALTH CERTIFICATION AND PLAN OF TREATMENT

1. Patient's HI Claim No.	2. Start Of Care Date	3. Certification Period		4. Medical Record No.	5. Provider No.
777-88-7788A	100311	From: 100311	To: 120311	S2521	78-9999

6. Patient's Name and Address	7. Provider's Name, Address and Telephone Number
Smythe, Samuel A. 25952 North Hawthorne Lane Sky City, WI 50000	BHC Home Care 2001 Oak Lane Sky City, WI 50000

8. Date of Birth 021730   9. Sex [X] M [ ] F

10. Medications: Dose/Frequency/Route (N)ew (C)hanged

11.ICD-9-CM	Principal Diagnosis	Date
890.1	Open wound, left hip	100115
12.ICD-9-CM	Surgical Procedure	Date
79.35	Open reduction, left femur	092715
13.ICD-9-CM	Other Pertinent Diagnoses	Date
820.9	Fracture, left femur	092615
428.0	Congestive heart failure	090515
715.09	Osteoarthritis	030015
250.00	NIDDM	010094

Cephradine 250 mg. Q 6 hrs. PO x 21 days
DC p̄ 10 AM dose 102400 (N)
Tolectin 400 mg. TID (C)
Furosemide 20 mg. Q AM PO (C)
KCl 10 mEq. Q AM PO (C)
Digoxin 0.125 mg. Q AM PO
Vitamin-mineral supplement 1 cap. QD PO
Acetaminophen tabs. 2 Q 4 hrs. PRN PO - pain

14. DME and Supplies   Wheelchair, walker

15. Safety Measures: Proper footwear, clear pathways when ambulating. O_2 precautions.

16. Nutritional Req.   1800 calorie ADA, 2 gm. Na

17. Allergies: No known allergies

18.A. Functional Limitations

1 [ ] Amputation	5 [ ] Paralysis	9 [ ] Legally Blind
2 [ ] Bowel /Bladder (Incontinence)	6 [X] Endurance	A [ ] Dyspnea With Minimal Exertion
3 [ ] Contracture	7 [X] Ambulation	B [X] Other (Specify)
4 [ ] Hearing	8 [ ] Speech	Occasional orthopnea

18.B. Activities Permitted

1 [ ] Complete Bedrest	6 [ ] Partial Weight Bearing	A [X] Wheelchair
2 [ ] Bedrest BRP	7 [ ] Independent At Home	B [X] Walker
3 [ ] Up As Tolerated	8 [ ] Crutches	C [ ] No Restrictions
4 [X] Transfer Bed/Chair	9 [ ] Cane	D [ ] Other (Specify)
5 [X] Exercises Prescribed		

19. Mental Status: 1 [X] Oriented   3 [ ] Forgetful   5 [ ] Disoriented   7 [ ] Agitated
2 [ ] Comatose   4 [ ] Depressed   6 [ ] Lethargic   8 [ ] Other

20. Prognosis: 1 [ ] Poor   2 [ ] Guarded   3 [X] Fair   4 [ ] Good   5 [ ] Excellent

21. Orders for Discipline and Treatments (Specify Amount/Frequency/Duration)

Wound care (L) hip daily: Irrigate with 1:1 H_2O_2/water, rinse with normal saline, pack with saline-soaked 4x4s, dress with gauze. O_2 2L PRN HS per cannula - orthopnea.

Skilled Nursing: Daily for 62 days. Assess wound, S/S fluid retention. Perform wound care. Teach diet, O_2 precautions; new/changed medications.

Physical Therapy: One visit first week, 3 times a week for 8 weeks. Evaluation, therapeutic exercises, gait training. Teach use of walker, transfer technique. Establish home program.

Home Health Aide: 3 times a week for 9 weeks. Personal care. Assist with transfers, home exercise program.

22. Goals/Rehabilitation Potential/Discharge Plans

Anticipate daily visits to end 010311. Rehab potential good for patient to ambulate independently with walker by 120311. Will be compliant with diet, medications, therapeutic regimen. Plan discharge to care of wife when wound complications resolved.

23. Nurse's Signature and Date of Verbal SOC Where Applicable: *Jane Jayes* RN 100311	25. Date HHA Received Signed POT OCT 13 2015
24. Physician's Name and Address Albert Richard, MD 1641 Pine Circle Sky City, WI 50000	26. I certify/recertify that this patient is confined to his/her home and needs intermittent skilled nursing care, physical therapy and/or speech therapy or continues to need occupational therapy. The patient is under my care, and I have authorized the services on this plan of care and will periodically review the plan.
27. Attending Physician's Signature and Date Signed *Albert Richard MD* 10/10/15	28. Anyone who misrepresents, falsifies, or conceals essential information required for payment of Federal funds may be subject to fine, imprisonment, or civil penalty under applicable Federal laws.

Form HCFA-485 (U-4) (02-94)

(Sample data © 1995 Beacon Health Corporation, Mequon WI. Used with permission.)

FIGURE 9-8. Example of home health plan of care.

SKILLED NURSING VISIT NOTE

Patient _____ Samuel Smythe _____

DATE 061315 TIME 11:00-11:45	No S/S fluid retention. Wound measures 9x5x3 cm. Small amount of purulent drainage. Wound bed 70% slough, 30% granulation tissue. Wound care performed: irrigated with normal saline, covered with ABD. Surrounding skin intact. Expresses discomfort during procedure Taught use of pain med 1 hr. before procedure. Reports occasional constipation. Observed aide transfer patient. Uses safe technique. Patient satisfied with care. Can demonstrate exercises but reluctant to do alone. Taught wife how to assist.

VISIT FREQUENCY **Daily**
☐ Change   ☐ Patient informed

BP 140/86 Standing (Sitting) Lying

TEMPERATURE   98.2°

PULSE 80, regular (Apical) Radial

RESPIRATIONS 26

LUNG SOUNDS Clear

DIET/APPETITE   1800 cal.   Taught fiber sources.

ACTIVITY LEVEL Weak. Transfers with 1.

AIDE SUPERVISION   Observed K. Jackson

PHYSICIAN CONTACT/APPT.   Appt. 061511

CARE COORDINATION   Reviewed PT program with aide.

CONFERENCE

☐ PROGRESS NOTE

SIGNATURE _Susan Jackson RN_

SKILLED NURSING VISIT NOTE

Patient _____ Samuel Smythe _____

DATE 091911 TIME 7:30-8:20	Venipuncture for FBS - (L) antecubital. Verbalizes routine for blood, urine testing. Still has difficulty performing finger stick. Does not get enough blood on strip for accurate reading. Demonstrated procedure for finger stick.

VISIT FREQUENCY **Weekly. Aide dc'd 0913**
☐ Change   ☒ Patient informed

BP 132/76 Standing (Sitting) Lying

TEMPERATURE   97.6°

PULSE 70, regular (Apical) Radial

RESPIRATIONS 22

LUNG SOUNDS Clear

DIET/APPETITE   1800 cal. ADA "Good appetite"

ACTIVITY LEVEL Ambulates 30' - walker No longer uses wheelchair.

AIDE SUPERVISION

PHYSICIAN CONTACT/APPT.   Appt. 092311

CARE COORDINATION

CONFERENCE

☒ PROGRESS NOTE   091915

Blood sugar 175-225.

Feeling more comfortable about performing care.

SIGNATURE _Susan Jackson RN_

FIGURE 9-9. Example of home health care nursing progress note.

DEVELOPING CLINICAL REASONING

1. Interview a nurse employed in a hospital and a nurse employed by a home health care agency. How are their roles and responsibilities alike? How do they differ? Ask both what they believe about the fragmentation of care in their setting. How well are nurses working with their colleagues to coordinate care?

2. Compare and contrast the needs of the following patients and their families:
   - A 2-year-old admitted to an ambulatory surgery center for minor surgery
   - A 34-year-old woman discharged home after treatment for a fractured arm in the emergency department
   - A 50-year-old woman returning to a clinic to learn the results of her mammogram
   - A 78-year-old man being transferred from the hospital to a long-term care facility

What care priorities are these patients and families likely to have? How can you best establish a partnership with these patients and families? How likely are today's health care providers to meet the holistic needs (physical, psychological, social, and spiritual) of these patients?

3. Discuss with your fellow students what you would do in the following home health care situations. What knowledge, attitudes, and skills are required to successfully address these needs?

   • An 85-year-old patient cannot move by himself and refuses to eat. His 83-year-old wife tries to care for him, but she is under a great deal of stress and begins to cry when you enter their apartment.

   • A 43-year-old woman is receiving home care after surgery to repair a herniated vertebral disc ("slipped disc"). When you arrive for the scheduled visit, you find that her speech is slurred and she does not remember how much pain medication she has taken.

   • A 2-year-old has a malignant brain tumor. He is not expected to live more than 1 week and is receiving hospice care.

   • A 55-year-old man with end-stage lung cancer is discharged home with a referral to a visiting nurse agency. He is receiving oxygen therapy. When the first visiting nurse enters his home, she finds the patient smoking, oblivious to the dangers with the oxygen in the room. When the nurse explains her safety concerns, he states that he might as well just die now if he isn't able to smoke because smoking is the only pleasure he has left.

4. How can continuity and care coordination be achieved for Jeff Hart, Laura Degas, and Joey Marshall?

PRACTICING FOR NCLEX

1. A nurse who is a discharge planner in a large metropolitan hospital is preparing a discharge plan for a patient after a kidney transplant. Which actions would this nurse typically perform to ensure continuity of care as the patient moves from acute care to home care? Select all that apply.
   a. Performing an admission health assessment
   b. Evaluating the nursing plan for effectiveness of care
   c. Participating in the transfer of the patient to the postoperative care unit
   d. Making referrals to appropriate agencies
   e. Maintaining records of patient satisfaction with services
   f. Assessing the strengths and limitations of the patient and family

2. A discharge nurse is evaluating patients and their families to determine the need for a formal discharge plan and/or referrals to another agency. Which patients would most likely be a candidate for these services? Select all that apply.
   a. An older patient who is diagnosed with dementia in the hospital
   b. A 45-year-old male who is diagnosed with Parkinson's disease
   c. A 35-year-old female who is receiving chemotherapy for breast cancer
   d. A 16-year-old who is being discharged with a cast on his leg
   e. A new mother who delivered a healthy infant via a cesarean birth
   f. A 59-year-old male who is diagnosed with end-stage bladder cancer

3. A home health care nurse is scheduled to visit a 38-year-old female client who has been discharged from the hospital with a new colostomy. Which duties would the nurse perform for this patient in the entry phase of the home visit? Select all that apply.
   a. Collect information about the patient's diagnosis, surgery, and treatments.
   b. Call the patient to make initial contact and schedule a visit.
   c. Develop rapport with the patient and her family.
   d. Assess the patient to identify her needs.
   e. Assess the physical environment of the home.
   f. Evaluate safety issues including the neighborhood in which she lives.

4. A hospital nurse is admitting a patient who sustained a head injury in a motor vehicle accident. Which activities could the nurse delegate to licensed assistive personnel?
   a. Collecting information for a health history
   b. Performing a physical assessment
   c. Contacting the physician for medical orders
   d. Preparing the bed and collecting needed supplies

5. A nurse is preparing an infant and his family for a hernia repair to be performed in an ambulatory care facility. What is the primary role of the nurse during the admission process?
   a. Assist with screening tests.
   b. Provide patient teaching.
   c. Assess what has been done and what still needs to be done.
   d. Assist with hernia repair.

6. A patient is being transferred from the ICU to a regular hospital room. What must the ICU nurse be prepared to do as part of this transfer?
   a. Provide a verbal report to the nurse on the new unit.
   b. Provide a detailed written report to the unit secretary.
   c. Delegate the responsibility for providing information.
   d. Make a copy of the patient's medical record.

7. Which statements or questions would be appropriate in establishing a discharge plan for a patient who has had major abdominal surgery?
   a. "I'll bet you will be so glad to be home in your own bed."
   b. "What are your expectations for recovery from your surgery?"
   c. "Be sure and take your pain medications and change your dressing."
   d. "You will just be fine! Please stop worrying."

8. A nurse is counseling an older female patient hospitalized for dehydration secondary to a urinary tract infection. The patient tells the nurse: "I don't like being in the hospital. There are too many bad bugs in here. I'll probably go home sicker than I came in." She also insists that she is going to get dressed and go home. She has the capacity to make these decisions. What is the legal responsibility of the nurse in this situation?
   a. To inform the patient that only the primary health care provider can authorize discharge from a hospital
   b. To collect the patient's belongings and prepare the paperwork for the patient's discharge
   c. To request a psych consult for the patient and inform her primary care provider of the results
   d. To explain that the choice carries a risk for increased complications and make sure that the patient has signed a release form

9. A nurse decides to become a home health care nurse. Which personal qualities are key to being successful as a community-based nurse? Select all that apply.
   a. Making accurate assessments
   b. Researching new treatments for chronic diseases
   c. Communicating effectively
   d. Delegating tasks appropriately
   e. Performing clinical skills effectively
   f. Making independent decisions

10. A nurse ensures that a hospital room prepared by an aide is ready for a new ambulatory patient. Which condition would the nurse ask the aide to correct?
    a. The bed linens are folded back.
    b. A hospital gown is on the bed.
    c. Equipment for taking vital signs is in the room.
    d. The bed is in the highest position.

ANSWERS WITH RATIONALES

1. *b, d, f.* The primary roles of the discharge planner as patients move from acute to home care are evaluating the nursing plan for effectiveness of care, making referrals for patients, and assessing the strengths of patients and their families. Although in smaller facilities a discharge planner may perform an admission health assessment and assist with patient transfers, it is not the usual job of the discharge planner. In most facilities, maintaining records of patient satisfaction is the role of the public relations manager or office manager.

2. *a, b, f.* The patients who are most likely to need a formal discharge plan and/or referral to another agency are those who are emotionally or mentally unstable (e.g., dementia), have recently diagnosed chronic disease (e.g., Parkinson disease), or have a terminal illness (e.g., end-stage cancer). Other candidates include patients who do not understand the treatment plan, are socially isolated, have had major surgery or illness, need a complex home care regimen, or lack financial services or referral sources.

3. *c, d, e.* In the entry phase of the home visit, the nurse develops rapport with the patient and family, makes assessments, determines nursing diagnoses, establishes desired outcomes, plans and implements prescribed care, and provides teaching. In the pre-entry phase of the home visit, the nurse collects information about the patient's diagnoses, surgical experience, socioeconomic status, and treatment orders. In the pre-

entry phase, the nurse also gathers supplies needed, makes an initial phone contact with the patient to arrange a visit, and assesses the patient's environment for safety issues.

4. *d.* The nurse may delegate preparation of the bed and collection of needed supplies to unlicensed personnel but would perform the other activities listed.

5. *c.* Although all the options may be performed by the ambulatory care nurse, it is the nurse's primary responsibility to assess what has been done and to tailor the plan of care to the patient's needs. Screening tests and teaching are usually completed prior to the patient entering an ambulatory care facility.

6. *a.* The ICU nurse gives a verbal report on the patient's condition and nursing care needs to the nurse on the new unit. This information is not given to a unit secretary, nor is it delegated to others. The medical record is transferred with the patient; a copy is not made.

7. *b.* It is important to assess the expectations of the patient (and family) when assessing health care needs for discharge planning.

8. *d.* The patient is legally free to leave the hospital against medical advice (AMA); however, patients who leave the hospital AMA must sign a form releasing the physician and hospital from legal responsibility for their health status. This signed form becomes part of the medical record.

9. *a, c, e, f.* Nurses working in the community must have the knowledge and skills to make accurate assessments, work independently, communicate effectively, and perform clinical skills accurately. Community-based nurses may be researchers and occasionally delegate care, but these are not key qualities for this type of nursing.

10. *d.* A properly prepared hospital room includes: a bed in the lowest position for an ambulatory patient, an open bed with top linens folded back, routine equipment and supplies and special equipment and supplies assembled, and the physical environment of the room adjusted.

TAYLOR SUITE RESOURCES

Explore these additional resources to enhance learning for this chapter:
- NCLEX-Style Questions and other resources on thePoint, http://thePoint.lww.com/Taylor8e
- *Study Guide for Fundamentals of Nursing, 8th edition*
- Adaptive Learning | Powered by prepU, http://thepoint.lww.com/prepu

Bibliography

Academy of Oncology Nurse Navigators. Frequently asked questions. http://www.aonnonline.org/about/faq

Agency for Healthcare Research and Quality (AHRQ). (2010). Care coordination measures atlas. AHRQ Publications No. 11-0023-EF. Available at http://www.ahrq.gov/professionals/systems/long-term-care/resources/coordination/atlas/atlas-coordination-measures-atlas.pdf

Agency for Healthcare Research and Quality (AHRQ). (2012). *Improving Transitions of Care: Hand-off Communications.* Oakbrook Terrace, IL: Joint Commission for Transforming Healthcare, June 2012. Available at http://psnet.ahrq.gov/resource.aspx?resourceID=24737)

American Hospital Association (AHA). (2008). *The patient care partnership.* Available at http://www.aha.

org/aha/issues/Communicating-With-Patients/pt-care-partnership.html

American Nurses Association (ANA). (2007). *Home health nursing scope and standards of practice.* Available at http://nursingworld.org

Arora, V. M., Greenstein, E. A., Woodruff, J. N., Staisiunas, P. G., & Farnan, J. M. (2014). Implementing peer evaluation of handoffs: associations with experience and workload. *Journal of Hospital Medicine, 8*:132–136.

Association of periOperative Registered Nurses. (2013). Patient Hand-Off Tool Kit. Available at www.aorn.org/PracticeResources/ToolKits/PatientHandOffToolKit

Buhler-Wilkerson, K. (2007). No place like home: A history of nursing and home care in the U.S. *Home Healthcare Nurse, 25*(4), 253–259.

Centers for Medicare & Medicaid Services (CMS). (2009). *Medicare & you.* Baltimore, MD: U.S. Department of Health and Human Services.

Centers for Medicare & Medicaid Services (CMS). (2008a). *Home health PPS.* Available at http://www.cms.hhs.gov/HomeHealthPPS/

Craig, C., Eby, D., & Whittington, J. (2011). Care Coordination Model: Better Care at Lower Cost for People with Multiple Health and Social Needs. IHI Innovation Series white paper. Cambridge, Massachusetts: Institute for Healthcare Improvement. Available at http://amlalliance.com.au/__data/assets/pdf_file/0003/46965/Care-Coordination-Model.pdf

Department of Defense Patient Safety Program. (2005). Healthcare Communications Toolkit to Improve Transitions in Care. Available at http://www.oumedicine.com/docs/ad-obgyn-workfiles/handofftoolkit.pdf?sfvrsn=2

Dvorak, P. (2013, February 8). 600 homeless children in DC, and no one seems to care. *The Washington Post.*

Health Affairs. (2012, September 13). Health Policy Brief: Improving Care Transitions. Available at http://www.healthaffairs.org/healthpolicybriefs/brief.php?brief_id=76

Johnson, M., Cowin, L. S. (2013). Nurses discuss bedside handover and using written handover sheets. *Journal of Nursing Management, 21*, 121–129.

The Joint Commission. (2014). Joint Commission Center for Transforming Healthcare Releases Tool to Tackle Miscommunication among Caregivers. Available at: http://www.jointcommission.org/center_transforming_healthcare_tst_hoc/

The Joint Commission. (2014). *National Patient Safety Goals.* Available at: http://www.jointcommission.org/standards_information/npsgs.aspx

Landro, L. (2011. August 16). When a doctor isn't enough. Nurse Navigators help patients through maze of cancer-treatment decisions, fears. *The Wall Street Journal.* Available at http://online.wsj.com/article/SB10001424053111904253204576510472828240848.html

McDonald, K. M., Schultz, E., Albin, L., Pineda, N., et al. (2010). Care Coordination Atlas Version 3 (prepared by Stanford University under subcontract to Battelle on Contract No. 290-04-0020). AHRQ Publication No. 11-0023-EF. Rockville, MD: Agency for Healthcare Research and Quality.

Middleton, B., Bloomrosen, M., Dente, M. A., et al. (2013). Enhancing patient safety and quality of care by improving the usability of electronic health record systems: recommendations from AMIA. *Journal of the American Medical Association,* 20:e2–e8.

NANDA International. (2012). *Nursing diagnoses: Definitions and classification 2012–2014.* West Sussex, UK: Wiley-Blackwell.

National Association for Home Care & Hospice. (2009). *Consumer information: What are my rights as a patient?* Available at http://www.nahch.org/consumer/rights.html.)

Peikes, D., Chen, A., Schore, J., & Brown, R. (2009). Effects of care coordination on hospitalization, quality of care, and health care expenditures among Medicare beneficiaries: 15 randomized trials. *Journal of the American Medical Association, 301*(6), 603–618. doi:10.1001/jama.2009.126

Rantz, M. J., Skubic, M., Alexander, G., Popescu, M., Aud, M. A., Wakefield, B. J., … Miller, S. J. (2010). Developing a comprehensive electronic health record to enhance nursing care coordination, use of technology, and research. *Journal of Gerontological Nursing, 36*(1), 13–17.

Runy, L. A. (2013). Patient Handoffs. Hospitals and Health Networks (H&HN). Available at http://www.hhnmag.com/hhnmag/jsp/articledisplay.jsp?dcrpath=HHNMAG/Article/data/05MAY2008/0805HHN_FEA_Gatefold&domain=HHNMAG

The National Transitions of Care Coalition. Care transition bundle: Seven Essential Intervention Categories. Available at http://www.tnpatientsafety.com/LinkClick.aspx?fileticket=uWHuqEalc28%3D&tabid=293

Urban Institute Health Policy Center. (2013). Vulnerable Populations. http://www.urban.org/health_policy/vulnerable_populations/index.cfm

U.S. Department of Health and Human Services (USDHHS). (2003). *Health information privacy: Guidance information for consumers.* Available at http://www.hhs.gov/ocr/privacy/hipaa/understanding/consumers//index.html

U.S. Department of Health and Human Services, Centers for Medicare and Medicaid Services (USDHHS). (2007). *Medicare and home health. Section 1 Medicare coverage of home health care.* Available at http://www.medicare.gov/Publications/Pubs/pdf/10969.pdf

Person-Centered Care and the Nursing Process

*T*he nursing process is a systematic, person-centered, goal-oriented method of caring *that provides a framework for nursing practice.* Unit III begins with an exploration of each element of thoughtful person-centered practice. Chapter 10 invites you to reflect on your readiness for practice. Is your motivation helping people who need nursing care? Do you have the personal attributes, knowledge base, and competencies to begin safe practice? Are you committed to learn how to reason clinically, to make judgments and decisions about treatment and care? This chapter introduces the five steps of the nursing process—assessing, diagnosing, outcome identification and planning, implementing, and evaluating. It also describes the blended and QSEN competencies nurses need to use the process for promoting patient well-being. Chapters 11 to 15 will explore each step of the nursing process. The unit concludes with Chapter 16, which focuses on documentation, reporting, conferring, and using informatics.

The steps of the nursing process are not separate items but rather parts of a whole, used to identify patient needs, establish priorities of care, maximize strengths, and resolve actual or potential alterations in human responses to health and illness, thereby promoting health to the highest level possible for each patient.

Assessment, the systematic and continuous collection and communication of data, allows analysis of data to identify problems and strengths of patients. During outcome identification and planning, the nurse and patient mutually identify expected outcomes and agree on nursing interventions necessary to meet these outcomes. The nurse implements the plan of care, adapting it to each person, documenting nursing actions and patient responses. After implementation, the nurse and patient evaluate the effectiveness of the plan based on achievement of outcomes, and determine if the plan should be continued, modified, or terminated.

The nursing process is nursing practice in action. Unit III provides the information necessary to begin to apply the nursing process. As blended competencies are learned and practiced (both by students and nurses), the process becomes an integral component of each nurse–patient interaction. The outcome is compassionate, comprehensive, and individualized nursing care.

"

... the nursing process is educative and therapeutic when nurse and patient can come to know and to respect each other, as persons who are alike, and yet different, as persons who share in the solution of problems."

Hildegard Peplau (1909–1999) was an active participant in ANA and NLN and a leader in recognizing the significance of interpersonal relationships in psychiatric nursing. Her landmark book integrated theory into her model at a time when nursing theory was in its infancy.

10

Blended Competencies, Clinical Reasoning, and Processes of Person-Centered Care

CHARLOTTE HORVATH

Charlotte is a single mother whose 5-year-old daughter will be discharged soon. Ms. Horvath is to learn how to perform wound care for her daughter at home. However, she has missed every planned teaching session thus far.

ADDIE WARNER

Addie is an African American woman who has suffered a cerebrovascular accident (CVA). She is currently being cared for in a neurologic step-down unit. The patient frequently uses her call light and is called "demanding" by some staff.

JERMAINE BYRD

Jermaine is a 58-year-old man who has just returned to the medical–surgical unit after undergoing vascular surgery on the femoral artery. Orders include assessing the distal pulses to ensure adequate blood flow. However, when the patient is assessed, the posterior tibial pulse is not palpable.

After completing the chapter, you will be able to accomplish the following:

1. Describe each element of thoughtful, person-centered practice: the nurse's personal attributes, knowledge base, and blended and QSEN competencies; clinical reasoning, judgment, and decision making; person-centered nursing process; and reflective practice leading to personal learning.

2. Assess one's capacity for competent, responsible, caring practice.

3. Contrast three approaches to problem solving.

4. Use the clinical reasoning model.

5. Describe the historic evolution of the nursing process.

6. Describe the nursing process and each of its five steps.

7. List five characteristics of the nursing process.

8. List three patient benefits and three nursing benefits of using the nursing process correctly.

9. Identify personal strengths and weaknesses in light of nursing's essential knowledge, attitudes, and skills.

10. Describe the steps in concept mapping care planning.

11. Value reflective practice as an aid to self-improvement.

KEY TERMS

assess	decision making	QSEN
blended competencies	evaluate	reflective practice
caring	expected outcomes	scientific problem solving
clinical judgment	implement	standards for critical thinking
clinical reasoning	intuitive problem solving	
concept mapping	nursing diagnoses	therapeutic relationship
creative thinking	nursing process	thoughtful practice
critical thinking	person-centered care	trial-and-error problem solving
critical thinking indicators	plan	

Traditionally, nurses prided themselves on comforting those who were ill and on executing with precision such tasks as dressing wounds, administering medications, and bathing, feeding, and ambulating patients. Physicians ordered many of these tasks, and few nurses in the past would have characterized their "work" as being independent, evidence-based, or creative.

But as society and the health care delivery system change, so does nursing. Nurses now work with healthy and ill patients in both private and institutional settings. In addition to their role as caregivers, nurses fill specialized roles as care managers/coordinators, teachers, counselors, advocates, and researchers. Nurses are responsible for a unique dimension of health care—"the diagnosis and treatment of human responses to actual or potential health problems" (American Nurses Association [ANA], 2010a) and, as such, are knowledgeable, competent, and independent professionals who work collaboratively with other health care professionals to design and deliver holistic care. As the role has changed, definitions of nursing have evolved to acknowledge essential features of professional nursing:

- Provision of a caring relationship that facilitates health and healing
- Attention to the range of human experiences and responses to health and illness within the patient's physical and social environments
- Integration of assessment data with knowledge gained from an appreciation of the patient's or group's subjective experience
- Application of scientific knowledge to the processes of diagnosis and treatment through the use of judgment and critical thinking
- Advancement of professional nursing knowledge through scholarly inquiry
- Influence on social and public policy to promote social justice
- Assurance of safe, quality, and evidence-based practice (ANA, 2010a).

Who nurses choose to be every time they show up for practice literally has the power to influence and in some cases to determine how people are born, live, suffer, and die. For this reason this text promotes thoughtful, person-centered practice. In this chapter you will learn what it takes to be a competent, responsible, and caring professional nurse. Committed nurses earn the public's trust every day.

THOUGHTFUL PRACTICE

A thoughtful nurse is a nurse who is considerate and compassionate, who always keeps the person at the center of caregiving in order to promote the humanity, dignity, and well-being of the patient. Thoughtful nurses value their own integrity and development, reflecting on each day's practice to better understand and learn from each day's challenges. Thoughtful nurses seek to establish powerful partnerships with patients and to deliver care through processes that are

REFLECTIVE PRACTICE: CULTIVATING QSEN COMPETENCIES

CHALLENGE TO ETHICAL AND LEGAL SKILLS

Recently, I spent time working as a pediatric nurse technician. My job was to provide basic care to patients, such as giving bed baths, assisting with meals, and changing linens. One of the nicest parts of my job was that I was able to spend more time than most nurses are able to, talking with my patients and getting to know them, and hopefully making a positive difference in their days. One day I was assigned to float to the neurologic step-down unit. Here, I met Addie Warner, an older African American woman who had suffered a cerebrovascular accident (CVA). Because of what happened

that day, I became responsible for her care for the rest of the day.

When I arrived on the unit that morning, a nurse told me what a "pain" Mrs. Warner was, describing how she kept demanding that the nurse come into her room and help her with this or that. They told me I should "ignore her," and they told me that I didn't need to listen to her. I was immediately appalled. I witnessed yet another nurse stand outside her door and condescendingly tell her in an annoyed voice, "I'll be with you when I have time." As I passed her room, Ms. Warner yelled out for attention.

Thinking Outside the Box: Possible Courses of Action

- Listen to all the nurses out of personal ignorance, out of fear for being reprimanded by them, or out of selfishness, and continue to ignore this patient and her needs just like everyone else was doing.
- Ask one of the nurses to go into the room with me to determine what the patient's needs were and to help me meet them, despite the nurses' obvious dislike of the patient and obvious lack of desire to help her.
- Go into the patient's room by myself, assess her needs for the simple purpose of relaying them to the nurse, and then not do anything to meet any of her needs myself.
- Enter the patient's room by myself, assess her needs, assure her that I would try to help her meet her needs

once the nurse became available, and then drop the ball in the end, not helping her much myself or with the nurse.
- Go into her room by myself, assess her needs, assure her that I would help her meet her needs, and take the steps to meet them later in the shift when I had more time.
- Proceed into her room by myself, assess her needs, assure her that I would help her meet them, and take the steps to meet them immediately and throughout the whole shift.
- Ignore the patient, stating that meeting her needs was not my job, but encourage the nurses to go into the room to assess and meet her needs.

Evaluating a Good Outcome: How Do I Define Success?

- The patient's needs are assessed and met by the most compassionate and most qualified professional possible.
- The patient feels heard and respected.
- I feel respected, feeling that I used my professional patient-care skills to the best of my ability to facilitate resolution of the patient's situation.
- The patient's inherent dignity, worth, and uniqueness is respected by everyone who comes into contact with her.

- The patient remains the primary commitment for me and the nurses.
- The patient feels that she is the primary commitment for the nurse and me.
- The health, safety, and rights of the patient are promoted, advocated for, and protected.
- The integrity of my patient, myself, and my fellow nurses is preserved.

Personal Learning: Here's to the Future!

Immediately upon starting my shift, I went into Ms. Warner's room to see what the problem was. She told me, in tears, that she's had to go to the bathroom for the past 2 hours, and that no one would help her. As a result, she ended up urinating on herself in bed. I immediately helped her out of bed into a chair, gave her soap and towels to start washing herself, and set about changing her linens. All the while, I listened to her talk about how humiliated and upset she was about having been forced to "wet the bed." She also was upset that she'd ruined the only pair of underwear she had with her in the hospital. So, I washed the underwear in the sink for her. I asked her questions about what had happened that morning and validated her feelings. I helped her finish bathing, set her up to be sitting comfortably in the chair, and got her lunch tray, which I then set up for her. Although, for the most part, she could feed herself, her CVA had left her with some residual weakness, necessitating some help with opening containers, cutting foods, and placing items within her reach on the tray. She also wanted me to bring her the phone and help her dial, which I did. I

let her eat and talk on the phone alone, promising I would come back to check on her soon.

Throughout the rest of the shift, I peeked my head into her room every half hour or so, eventually helping her back into her bed after she was comfortable, fed, and less upset. Probably the most important thing I did for her, besides resolving the wet bed situation, was to listen to her as she purged her feelings. I validated her feelings and did everything in my power to make sure that she experienced no further episodes of disrespect. Unfortunately, while the patient's needs were met by the most compassionate professional possible (me), they were not met by the most qualified professional possible (the nurse). I believe that the patient did feel heard and respected after our interactions. However, she stated that she felt ignored after her interactions with the nurses and physicians.

I felt that my actions were respected because none of the nurses gave me a difficult time or made fun of me for taking the extra time to soothe this patient. I did feel that I provided professional patient care to this patient in the best

(continued)

REFLECTIVE PRACTICE: CULTIVATING QSEN COMPETENCIES *continued*

CHALLENGE TO ETHICAL AND LEGAL SKILLS

manner I knew. I respected her inherent dignity, worth, and uniqueness, and I believe that the patient felt my primary commitment was to her. Unfortunately, this only highlighted the fact that no one else's primary commitment had been to her. I certainly promoted, advocated for, and strove to

protect this patient's health, safety, and rights. However, it seemed that the nurses went out of their way not to do that for this patient.

Tracey Sara Miller, Georgetown University

REFLECTION ON QUALITY AND SAFETY COMPETENCIES

How do you think you would respond in a similar situation? Why? What does this tell you about yourself and about the adequacy of your skills for professional practice? What *knowledge, attitudes,* and *skills* do you need to develop to continuously improve the quality and safety of care for patients like Ms. Warner?

Person-Centered Care: Why do you believe that the nursing staff was so critical of this patient? What was it about the student's attitudes and responses to Ms. Warner that created such a successful partnership?

Teamwork and Collaboration: Do you think that the nursing student should have approached the nursing staff about

what she found? How might a student or professional nurse effectively change negative staff behavior that is disrespectful of a patient's inherent dignity?

Safety/Evidence-Based Practice: What safety challenges resulted from the nursing staff's indifference and condescension, and how did the student correct these? What might the nursing research suggest as best practice in similar situations?

Informatics: Can you identify the essential information that must be available in Ms. Warner's electronic record to support safe patient care and coordination of care? Can you think of other ways to respond to or approach the situation?

holistic and tailored to meet the individual needs of patients. Care decisions are based on sound clinical reasoning and judgments that are evaluated and reviewed through reflective practice, so that there is continual learning in and from practice for the benefit of future patients (Dempsey, Hillege, & Hill, 2013, p. 239). Before reading further, take a minute to read the Reflective Practice display, review the concepts in Box 10-1 (p. 198), and the essential elements of thoughtful, person-centered care shown in Figure 10-1.

PERSON-CENTERED CARE

If you are new to health care, you probably can't imagine what health care would be like if it wasn't person centered. Sadly, U.S. health care in the twentieth century focused more on disease than on patients. Despite major efforts to refocus the delivery of health care based on the needs of the patient, we are in danger of failing again. Physician Abraham Verghese (2011) recently coined the term *iPatient:*

> I've gotten into some trouble in Silicon Valley for saying that the patient in the bed has almost become an icon for the real patient who is in the computer. I've actually coined a term for that entity in the computer. I call it the *iPatient.* The iPatient is getting wonderful care all across America. The real patient often wonders, where is everyone? When are they going to come by and explain things to me? Who's in charge? There's a real disjunction between the patient's perception and our own perceptions as physicians of the best medical care.

Nurses have always been on the frontlines of keeping care delivery focused on the needs of real patients in real time. But today's demanding work environments are forcing some nurses to focus more on accomplishing a set of

tasks than on helping patients. From the very beginning of your professional practice, remember that nursing is about creating therapeutic relationships with actual patients, about making health care work for all who need it. Being a good nurse isn't just a matter of being "busy" doing "tasks"—it is about being and making the critical difference for patients

Thoughtful Person-Centered Practice

FIGURE 10-1. The components of thoughtful practice are all interrelated and function together to create thoughtful, person-centered care. (Adapted from Dempsey, J., Hillege, S., & Hill, R. [2013]. *Fundamentals of Nursing and Midwifery: A Person-centered Approach to Care* (2nd ed.). Sydney: Wolters Kluwer/Lippincott Williams & Wilkins, p. 236.)

BOX 10-1 THOUGHTFUL PERSON-CENTERED PRACTICE

The Person

Each person is unique and has one's own set of beliefs, values, memories, hopes, and history. People are holistic beings with emotional, physical, social, and spiritual dimensions and needs that all meld together to create the whole individual person. The fact that a person has a disease is only one aspect of the whole in the same way as having red hair is only one aspect of the whole person. Therefore each person's health journey and personal care are individual. Clinical care is an interaction between the carer and the cared for. Each of the individuals within this relationship is unique, so the respect and valuing of the individual applies to both. Relationships based on this principle can become therapeutic.

The Professional Nurse

Professional nursing requires cultivated personal attributes, mastery of the science of nursing, and reflective clinical experience in which nurses develop the blended competencies and QSEN competencies that promote thoughtful and effective person-centered practice.

Reflective Practice Leading to Personal Learning

Reflective practice occurs when the carer has a profound awareness of self; awareness of one's own biases, prejudgments, prejudices, and assumptions; and understands how these may affect the therapeutic relationship. This awareness is developed through the process of reflection, thinking back on what has occurred for the purpose of learning in order to improve.

Clinical Reasoning, Judgment, and Decision Making

Clinical reasoning is the process for analyzing a situation, making a judgment, deciding on possible alternative reasons, and choosing an action to be taken. It is built on a foundation of knowledge, experience, and the personal attributes of the person doing the reasoning. Thinking is fundamental in the process of clinical reasoning. Care can become ritualistic and depersonalized when nurses fail in clinical reasoning.

Person-Centered Nursing Process

The nursing process describes the way in which care is organized through a series of actions undertaken in response to the individual needs of the patient. The components of the nursing process are assessing, diagnosing, planning, implementing, and evaluating.

The Nurse's Action in Response to Individual Clinical Need

The healing action that occurs in response to individual need completes the cycle of thoughtful practice when it is considered, personalized, appropriate, valued, and effective.

(Adapted from Dempsey, J., Hillege, S., & Hill, R. [2013]. *Fundamentals of nursing and midwifery: A person-centered approach to care* (2nd ed.). Sydney: Wolters Kluwer/Lippincott Williams & Wilkins, p. 237.)

and families with health care needs. Reflect for a moment on how you will respond when another nurse informs you that your patient is requesting medication for pain. How will your response differ if you have a person versus a task orientation? Hint: the nurse with a task orientation merely wants to safely administer and document the prescribed medication. The nurse with a person orientation uses every clinical encounter to assess how the person is doing and to communicate respect, compassion, and care.

The idea of **person-centered care** emerged about 30 years ago as a return to the holistic roots of health care. Promoters of this model of care included the Picker Institute, the Planetree membership network, and the 2001 Institute of Medicine's seminal report *Crossing the Quality Chasm*. With the introduction of the HCAHPS (Hospital Consumer Assessment of Healthcare Providers and Systems) patient experience of care survey, there now exists a standardized tool to evaluate the way care is provided from the patient's perspective (Frampton et al., 2008). While there are different definitions of person-centered care, the ten vital person-centered care principles listed in Box 10-2 offer a comprehensive illustration.

Theories of Caring

Nurses who practice person-centered care are committed to developing caring professional relationships based on respect and mutual trust. This approach is consistent with theories based on human caring, which use a holistic approach to promote humanism, health, and quality of living. Caring is viewed as universal and is practiced through interpersonal relationships. When the relationship between the carer and the cared for is used for promoting or restoring the health and well-being of people within the relationship, it becomes a **therapeutic relationship** (Dempsey et al., 2013). Dossey and Dossey (1998) write:

Our majestic predecessors in nursing, such as Florence Nightingale, spoke boldly about the need to honor the psychological and spiritual aspects of our patients. For her and many others, it was unthinkable to consider sick humans as mere bodies who could be treated in isolation from their minds and spirits. In Nightingale's holistic approach, the role of love and empathy was considered paramount.... But with the rise of scientific, materialistic medicine in the nineteenth and twentieth centuries, these lessons in love...were set aside and virtually lost.... In study after study, social contact, the richness of one's interactions with others, is correlated with positive health outcomes.... We're being asked to integrate a holistic approach and extend love, compassion, and empathy" (pp. 35–38).

Numerous nurse theorists have struggled to describe the caring central to the work of nursing. Travelbee (1971), an early nurse theorist, developed the Human-to-Human Relationship Model and defined nursing as an interpersonal

BOX 10-2	**REFLECTIVE PRACTICE: PERSON-CENTERED CARE**

Principles from: Rodak, S. (2012). 10 Guiding Principles for Patient-Centered Care. Available at: http://www.beckershospitalreview.com/quality/10-guiding-principles-for-patient-centered-care.html

1. All team members are considered caregivers.
   - Identify the team members you worked with while implementing the plan of care. Everyone in the workforce from housekeeping staff to the CEO is part of the patients' plan of care.
   - Next to each describe what they contributed to person-centered care for your patient.
   - Star or highlight those with whom you had meaningful conversations and briefly describe what you learned.

2. Care is based on continuous healing relationships.
   - Describe what you did to make your interactions with the patient/family qualify as a healing relationship versus a mere business transaction or provision of a service.
   - This principle reinforces a focus on the continuum of care. In what ways did your care anticipate and prepare your patient and family for the days ahead.

3. Care is customized and reflects patient needs, values, and choices.
   - Describe what you learned about this patient/family as unique individuals (strengths, needs, values, and preferences) that allowed you to creatively individualize the plan of care.
   - What strategies did you use to elicit the patient's needs, values, and choices?
   - In what specific ways is your plan of care different from any standardized plan of care?

4. Knowledge and information are freely shared between and among patients, care partners, physicians, and caregivers.
   - Describe one way you shared information with the patient/family and one way you shared information with the health care team that enhanced the partnership and the plan of care.
   - What did you learn from other members of the team that enhanced your ability to care for this patient/family?

5. Care is provided in a healing environment of comfort, peace, and support.
   - When we think healing environment we usually think of music, healing gardens, soothing colors. Assess your patient's healing environment and describe what you did to facilitate the creation of such an environment. How can you adapt these principles in critical care settings, emergency rooms, clinics, etc.?
   - In what ways are you able to address variables that negatively influence healing: Poverty, noise, time pressures, etc.
   - What percentage of the plan of care and *your* plan of care addresses patient needs other than physiological needs?
   - To what degree are the psycho-social-spiritual needs of the patients identified and addressed? To what degree do they appear in your plan of care?
   - Describe the measures you used to promote the patient's/family's comfort and peace and to provide support?

6. Families and friends of the patient are considered an essential part of the care team.
   - Has the patient identified family members or others he/she wishes to be part of the care team? If the patient is not able to articulate preferences, is there a legally valid surrogate making decisions? In what ways have you communicated with these individuals and provide the information and support they need to help the patient?

7. Patient safety is a visible priority.
   - What is the institutional commitment to safety measures like hand hygiene and other protocols to prevent hospital-acquired infections, medication and other errors, falls, etc.?
   - In what ways is this particular patient at risk for safety concerns, falls, infection, violence, etc. and what have you done to address these risks?

8. Transparency is the rule in the care of the patient.
   - True person-centered care requires transparency between providers and patients and among providers. Patients or their designees need information so they can make informed decisions. Does your patient have the information he/she needs to make informed decisions? If not, in what ways are you addressing this?

9. All caregivers cooperate with one another through a common focus on the best interests and personal goals of the patient.
   - In what ways are clinical decisions or institutional policies motivated by goals other than the best interests and personal goals of the patient and how is this constraining the plan of care? What have you done to address these variables?
   - What institutional resources exist to help you address these variables?

10. The patient is the source of control for their care.
    - Assess the degree to which your patient or her/his designee is the source of control for the plan of care.
    - What factors are constraining this and what are you doing to address these factors?

process whereby the professional nurse practitioner assists an individual, family, or community to prevent or cope with the experience of illness and suffering and, if necessary, to find meaning in these experiences. Benner and Wrubel (1989) write that caring is a basic way of being in the world and that caring is central to human expertise, curing, and healing. "Nursing is viewed as a caring practice whose science is guided by the moral art and ethics of care and responsibility.... Nurses provide care for people in the midst of health, pain, loss, fear, disfigurement, death, grieving, challenge, growth, birth, and transition on an intimate front-line basis. Expert nurses call this the *privileged place of nursing*" (p. xi). Watson's

(2008) theory of transpersonal caring begins with the conviction that humans are to be valued, cared for, respected, nurtured, understood, and assisted. She believes that caring can be demonstrated and practiced, and that nurses should create caring environments in which patients are accepted as they are and are invited to grow and realize their full potential. She reminds nurses that this model is transformative in that the nurse–patient relationship influences both the nurse and the patient for better or for worse. Finally, Swanson (1991) identifies five caring processes and defines caring as "a nurturing way of relating to a valued other toward whom one feels a personal sense of commitment and responsibility" (p. 165). There is no universally accepted definition of caring. You should become familiar with the care models described in Table 10-1 and see if you agree with the convictions held by nurse members of the International Association of Human Caring (IAHC). Members of the IAHC believe:

- **Caring** is the human mode of being.
- Caring is the essence of nursing and the moral imperative that guides nursing praxis (education, practice and research).
- Caring is both spiritual and human consciousness that connects and transforms everything in the universe.
- Caring in nursing is action and competencies that aim toward the good and welfare of others.
- Caring in nursing is a special way of being, knowing, and doing with the goal of protection, enhancement, and preservation of human dignity.
- Care is culturally diverse and universal, and provides the broadest and most important means to study and explain nursing knowledge and nursing care practices (www. humancaring.org)

Before reading further, reflect on how these convictions will influence your future practice. If you agree that caring is essential to being human and is the way nurses promote healing, what are your personal strengths and growth opportunities for caring? How can you plan to focus your attention on human caring as you struggle to master tasks like safely transferring patients, assisting with bathing, or administering medications? How likely are the recipients of your care to describe you as a competent, compassionate, caring nurse? In what ways might nurses relate to patients who may evoke negative feelings? How will you prevent this in your practice? You can read more about care ethics in Chapter 6 and about how to become a healing presence in Chapter 45.

THE PROFESSIONAL NURSE

Nurses committed to person-centered care are careful to assess whether or not they possess the prerequisite personal attributes along with learned knowledge, blended competencies, and QSEN competencies.

Personal Attributes

Not everyone "has what it takes" to be a professional nurse. As you read the following list of attributes, reflect on how well they characterize you at this stage of your human development.

Openmindedness. This might also be termed humility. Are you open to learn what your patients, families, and colleagues have to teach you?

Profound sense of the value of the person. Do you believe that everyone, literally everyone, matters? Can you think of anyone who deserves less than your best care

Table 10-1	**COMPARISON OF BENNER'S THE HELPING ROLE OF THE NURSE WITH SWANSON'S CARING PROCESS AND WATSON'S CARATIVE FACTORS**	
BENNER: THE HELPING ROLE OF THE NURSE	**SWANSON'S CARING PROCESS**	**WATSON'S CARATIVE FACTORS**
• Creating a climate for establishing a commitment to healing • Providing comfort measures and preserving personhood in the face of pain and extreme breakdown • Presencing • Maximizing the patient's participation and control in the patient's recovery • Interpreting kinds of pain and selecting appropriate strategies for pain management and control • Providing comfort and communication through touch • Providing emotional and informational support to patients and families • Guiding patients through emotional and developmental changes	• Knowing: avoiding assumptions, centering on the one cared for, assessing thoroughly, seeking cues, engaging the self of both • Being with: being there, conveying ability, sharing feelings, not burdening • Doing for: comforting, anticipating, performing competently/skillfully, protecting, preserving dignity • Enabling: informing/explaining, supporting/allowing, focusing, generating alternatives/thinking it through, validating/giving feedback • Maintaining belief: believing in/holding in esteem, maintaining a hope-filled attitude, offering realistic optimism, "going the distance"	• Humanistic altruistic system of values • Instillation of faith/hope • Sensitivity to self and others • Helping/trusting human care relationship • Expressing positive and negative feelings • Creating problem-solving caring process • Transpersonal teaching/learning • Supportive, protective, and/or corrective mental, physical, societal, and spiritual environment • Human needs assistance • Existential–phenomenological–spiritual forces

(Adapted from Benner, P., & Wrubel, J. (1989). *The primacy of caring in health and illness* (p. 50). Menlo Park, CA: Addison-Wesley; Swanson, K. M. (1991). Empirical development of a middle range theory of caring. *Nursing Research, 49* (3), 161–166; and Watson, J. (2008). Nursing: The Philosophy and Science of Caring (rev. ed.), Boulder: University Press of Colorado.)

effort? Are you willing to go to bat for the most vulnerable in our midst? Are you committed to learning how to advocate for those not well served by today's health care system?

Self-awareness and knowledge of own beliefs and values. Do you know what you believe, why you believe it, and the consequences of your beliefs? Are you sensitive to how your beliefs and values influence your professional relationships?

Sense of personal responsibility for actions. At the end of the day, will people (your patients and team) be better because of their experiences with you? Are you committed to using your personal expertise, time, and power to coordinate all the care patients and families need?

Motivation to do what you do to the best of your ability because you care about the well-being of those entrusted to your care. Does love get you up and motivate your study and practice? Do you want to be your personal best for those who will count on you?

Leadership skills. Have you tried to use your influence to help others attain valued goals? Are you committed to using your leadership strengths with patients, families, and colleagues to achieve valued health goals?

Bravery to question the "system." When the plan of care isn't working for a patient or your work environment is interfering with your ability to give good care, are you willing to challenge the status quo, and can you do this effectively? Denise Thornby, previous president of the American Association of Critical Care Nurses, was famous for challenging nurses to "make waves" when change was needed—even when this demanded personal courage. She reminded all of us that the day we don't wake up we will have already created our legacy: "Every day, every moment, you make choices on how to act or respond. Through these acts, you have the power to positively influence. As John Quincy Adams sagely said, 'The influence of each human being on others in this life is a kind of immortality.' So I ask you: What will be your act of courage? How will you influence your environment? What will be your legacy?" When the day arrives that you are no longer able to show up for practice, what do you want colleagues to say about you? What will be *your* legacy?

Knowledge Base

In order to reason through a clinical situation, you must be able to draw upon a body of nursing knowledge that comes from the sources of knowledge described in Chapter 2. Added to this must be research evidence. Box 10-4 on page 205, outlines the knowledge required for competent clinical reasoning in nursing. The specific knowledge in a given care interaction depends on the actual clinical situation. For example, if the situation calls for reasoning about the manifestation of a clinical problem, the nurse will need to understand the disease or condition, its epidemiology, the mechanisms of its pathophysiology, its physical and psychological mani-

festations, signs and symptoms, and the probabilities of its progression or outcome.

 THINK back to the nurse who could not locate Jermaine's tibial pulse. The nurse needs to know the complications of vascular surgery on the femoral artery and the significance of not being able to palpate the tibial pulse. ●

If the clinical situation involves a problematic hospital discharge of a patient with disabilities, for example, the nurse's knowledge base must include knowledge of support services available in the local community or knowledge of how and when to contact other team members with this expertise (Dempsey et al., 2013, pp. 257–258). These knowledge requirements are essential for the development of clinical reasoning and judgment, discussed later in this chapter.

Blended Competencies

Nurses aim to design and manage each patient's care scientifically, holistically, and creatively. To do this successfully, nurses need many cognitive, technical, interpersonal, and ethical/legal competencies, along with the willingness to use them creatively and critically when working with patients to promote or restore health, to prevent disease or illness, and to facilitate coping with altered functioning. Understanding the importance of these competencies helps you work consciously to develop them while beginning to master the nursing process. Cognitive and technical competencies equip nurses to manage clinical problems stemming from the patient's changing health or illness state. Interpersonal and ethical skills are essential, moreover, for nurses concerned about the patient's broader well-being. This text uses the term "blended competencies" because in most instances, nursing actions require all four competencies. A nurse who sets out to suction a patient, for example, must understand the evidence that supports this action, be skilled in handling the required equipment, use the encounter to promote the patient's sense of well-being, and practice in an ethically and legally defensible manner. Few nurses excel naturally in all four of these competencies, and even experienced nurses continue working on becoming more proficient in the knowledge, attitudes, and skills that lead to excellence. These competencies were first introduced and defined in Chapter 1. Box 10-3 (on page 202) will help you to assess your proficiency in these competencies.

Developing Cognitive Competencies

Cognitively skilled nurses are critical thinkers. **Critical thinking** is defined as "a systematic way to form and shape one's thinking. It functions purposefully and exactingly. It is thought that is disciplined, comprehensive, based on intellectual standards, and, as a result, well-reasoned" (Paul, 1993, p. 20). Alfaro (2014) defines critical thinking as "your ability to focus your thinking to get the results you need in various situations" and claims that "critical thinking makes the difference between whether you succeed or fail" (p. 2).

Box 10-3 TAKE THE CHALLENGE

Read the following professional behaviors, and circle the number that best reflects the proficiency you now have in each of these essential nursing competencies.

1 = no skills   3 = moderately skilled   5 = excellent skills
2 = somewhat skilled 4 = well skilled

Cognitive Competencies

1 2 3 4 5   • Offer a scientific rationale for the plan of care.
1 2 3 4 5   • Select those nursing interventions that are most likely to yield desired outcomes.
1 2 3 4 5   • Use critical thinking to problem solve creatively.

Technical Competencies

1 2 3 4 5   • Use technical equipment with sufficient competence and ease to achieve goal with a minimum of distress to involved participants.
1 2 3 4 5   • Creatively adapt equipment and technical procedures to the needs of particular patients in diverse circumstances.

Interpersonal Competencies

1 2 3 4 5   • Creative use of looks, speech, and touch to communicate respect and to enhance sense of worth
1 2 3 4 5   • Skilled use of presence and conversation to demonstrate empathy and to obtain sufficient knowledge about the patient to personalize care and serve as an effective advocate
1 2 3 4 5   • Responsible, competent attentiveness to the holistic needs of patients such that trust is built and patients experience comfort of security
1 2 3 4 5   • Value mutual enrichment of both participants in the nurse–patient relationship

Ethical/Legal Competencies

1 2 3 4 5   • Self-motivated to act in ways that advance the interests of patients (consistently trustworthy)
1 2 3 4 5   • Accountable for practice to self, patients served, the caregiving team, and society
1 2 3 4 5   • Consistently serve as effective patient advocate
1 2 3 4 5   • Skilled in mediating ethical conflict among the patient, significant others, health care team, and other interested parties
1 2 3 4 5   • Practice nursing faithful to the tenets of professional codes of ethics
1 2 3 4 5   • Use legal safeguards that reduce the risk of litigation

DEVELOPING THE METHOD OF CRITICAL THINKING

To develop the critical thinking skills essential to quality nursing practice, nurses find it helpful when posed with a challenge to work methodically through a set of five types of considerations: the purpose of thinking, adequacy of knowledge, potential problems, helpful resources, and critique of judgment/decision.

Purpose of Thinking

The first step when thinking critically about a situation is to identify the purpose or goal of your thinking. This helps to discipline your thinking by directing your thoughts toward the goal. The purpose of critical thinking might be to make a judgment about a particular patient or situation or to make a decision about how best to intervene.

Adequacy of Knowledge

At the outset of critical thinking, you need to judge whether the knowledge you have is accurate, complete, factual, timely, and relevant. If you reason with false information or a lack of important data, it is impossible to draw a sound conclusion. You also want to be sure that you understand all the details relevant to the issue. What is at stake? How much

time do you have to make a decision? How much room is there for error?

 CONSIDER Addie Warner, the patient described as "demanding" by some staff. Rather than accept that description, the nurse answers the patient's call light, thereby obtaining information from which to make an informed decision. ●

Potential Problems

As you become skilled in critical thinking, you will learn to "flag" and remedy pitfalls to sound reasoning. Common problems include working with untested or faulty assumptions, accepting an unproven claim or line of argument, allowing bias to color your thinking, and reasoning illogically, such as making a generalization on the basis of a single experience or case or allowing emotion to rule reason. The more familiar you are with these common blocks to critical thinking, the easier it is to detect them in your own thinking.

Helpful Resources

Wise professionals are quick to recognize their limits and seek help to remedy their deficiencies. Experienced clinicians know that learning is continuous and expect their practice to involve challenges that demand new knowledge. Critical thinkers know what help they need to assist their reasoning and what resources to tap. Key resources include experienced clinicians, texts and journals, institutional policies and procedures, and professional groups and writings.

Critique of Judgment/Decision

Ultimately, you must identify alternative judgments or decisions, weigh the merits of each, and reach a conclusion. It helps to try to predict the consequences of your major options before concluding your reasoning. You will also want to evaluate the alternative you selected as your decision begins to influence your actions.

After using this method to work through an intellectually challenging situation, critique your use of the method in light of the **standards for critical thinking**: clear, precise, specific, accurate, relevant, plausible, consistent, logical, deep, broad, complete, significant, adequate (for the purpose), and fair.

Focused Critical Thinking Guides

The display box Focused Critical Thinking Guide 10-1 (on page 204) illustrates the use of these five considerations to facilitate critical thinking about a care dilemma experienced by a nursing student. The merits of thinking critically about which of the options is most likely to meet that patient's needs are easily seen. Because nurses are accountable for the well-being of their patients, sloppy reasoning is both dangerous and inexcusable—even for someone new to nursing and clinical practice. Other examples of this method are found throughout the book.

DEVELOPING THE PERSONAL ATTRIBUTES TO THINK CRITICALLY

Reasoning has a logical or cognitive (thinking) component as well as an emotional or affective (feeling) component, both of which are affected by the personal attributes of the thinker. Critical thinking is also affected by one's beliefs and values. For example, nurses must be independent thinkers. Nurses who are independent thinkers are careful not to allow the status quo or a persuasive person to control their thinking.

 REMEMBER Addie Warner, the older woman who was considered to be demanding by some staff. The student demonstrated independent thinking by not accepting that emotional description of the patient. Rather, the student confronted the situation, obtained information, and then acted based on this information. ●

When confronted with an intellectual challenge, such as "Why does this patient resist change?" the nurse should proceed cautiously, consulting with the patient and respected colleagues and reviewing the literature. Only then can the nurse reach a true clinical judgment. Compare this with a nurse who makes a snap judgment that a patient is "unreasonable" based only on hearing the comments of another nurse—even if this nurse is the nurse manager.

 RECALL Charlotte Horvath, the single mother needing wound care teaching. A nurse who is not an independent thinker might quickly assume that Ms. Horvath just wasn't interested in caring for her child at home. But a nurse who is an independent thinker would investigate the situation further before making a decision. ●

Alfaro-LeFevre (2011) has carefully developed a list of **critical thinking indicators** (CTIs™), which are evidence-based descriptions of behaviors that demonstrate the knowledge, characteristics, and skills that promote critical thinking in clinical practice (Boxes 10-4 and 10-5 on pages 205 and 206). If you are serious about developing the critical thinking skills needed for professional practice, now would be a good time to sit down with someone who knows you well to see which critical thinking characteristics you possess and which need work. One way to do this is to ask these questions about each characteristic in Box 10-5:

1. On a scale of 1 to 7 (with 1 being almost never and 7 always), to what degree do I demonstrate this characteristic that promotes critical thinking?
2. Think of examples of times when you demonstrated and failed to demonstrate these characteristics. What were the consequences in these situations?

It can be helpful to see if you and others you invite to evaluate your characteristics reach the same conclusions about your strengths and areas for improvement.

Another way to use this list is to try to determine as a class which characteristics in Box 10-5 accurately describe your class! Alternatively, you can compare groups. For example, as a rule, which characteristics do nurses as a group and physicians as a group demonstrate?

As you begin clinical practice, you can also use the lists in Box 10-4 to critique your competence for professional practice.

Developing Technical Competencies

Some people are naturally "good with their hands" and quickly master intricate procedures that involve working with technical equipment. Others have to practice procedures many times before they feel competent handling the equipment and performing clinical activities independently. Whatever your natural level of technical skill, developing the following habits can help you master the manual skills essential in the nursing process:

- When a procedure demands manual dexterity and/or a complex series of steps, practice the necessary skill until you feel confident in your ability before attempting to perform it with a patient.
- Take time to familiarize yourself with new equipment before using it in a clinical procedure. Understand how it works and what supplies are needed to ensure optimal functioning. If possible, anticipate problems and know how to remedy them.

FOCUSED CRITICAL THINKING GUIDE 10-1

WESTERN VS. ALTERNATIVE MEDICINE

You are a nursing student. Your friend, Amy Chang, confides to you that she is very worried about her grandmother. When you meet Mrs. Chang, she demonstrates many of the assessment findings related to heart failure. Although her family has entreated her to seek medical attention, Mrs. Chang insists on relying on herbal teas and traditional Chinese remedies. Now 88 years old, Mrs. Chang came to America from mainland China when she was 14. Although she raised a family that is now thoroughly "Americanized," Mrs. Chang has resisted embracing her new culture and now wants nothing to do with "American medicine." Amy, who is also a nursing student, loves her grandmother dearly and is frustrated by her stubborn refusal to see an internist. Both of you have reason to believe that she could be helped by medical attention. What do you do?

1. Identify goal of thinking

Clarify your thinking about alternative medicine so that you can decide how you ought to respond to Mrs. Chang's worsening physical condition.

2. Assess adequacy of knowledge

Pertinent circumstances: Although you have strong reason to believe that Mrs. Chang is suffering from congestive heart failure, she has not been medically diagnosed, and you lack definitive knowledge about her medical condition and the likelihood that she would respond to treatment. You do know that she places a high value on traditional Chinese culture and strongly believes that if she is to be healed, the healing will result from herbal teas and traditional Chinese remedies. She has no confidence in American medicine. Her family describes her as being extremely strong willed and very lovable. You do not know if she has the benefit of seeing a competent practitioner of Chinese medicine.

Prerequisite knowledge: To decide how you should respond in this situation, you need to know that traditional Western medicine is not the only beneficial system of medicine. It would be helpful for you and Mrs. Chang's family to learn more about Chinese medicine and the probability of its benefiting her (as well as the possibility of its harming her) in her present condition. You will also need to learn more about what is essential to Mrs. Chang's well-being. How much value does she place on physical health? How important is it for her to live (and possibly die) within the familiar and comforting boundaries of her culture? You will want to assess what teaching, counseling, and support Mrs. Chang needs to reach an informed and voluntary decision that is right for her.

Room for error: Because Mrs. Chang's life may literally be at stake, there is not much room for error in the manner you and her family choose to respond. Even if her condition is not life threatening, her sense of well-being may be severely threatened if she feels forced to pursue treatment that is alien and frightening.

Time constraints: Although you are uncertain about the seriousness of her condition, you understand that the sooner Mrs. Chang receives effective therapy, the better. Unless her condition suddenly deteriorates, this is not a decision that needs to be made within the next 24 hours.

3. Address potential problems

The most serious obstacle to critical thinking in this situation would be an inability to weigh the respective merits of alternative healing systems. Cultural bias may result in the untested assumption that American medicine is necessarily superior to all other systems of healing and that it would be morally wrong to support a choice of anything else. The love of Mrs. Chang's family and their desire to do everything possible to keep her well may interfere with their ability to allow her the freedom to make the choice that is right for her.

4. Consult helpful resources

Your first challenge will be to learn more about traditional Chinese medicine by consulting with local authorities and available literature. The National Institutes of Health have now established an Office of Alternative Medicine, which may provide helpful information and which is easily accessed through their website. Your most important resource may be Mrs. Chang herself; it will be important to try to learn from her as much as you can about what she values and what her goals are at this point in her life. You will also want to be sure that Mrs. Chang has the benefits of a competent practitioner of Chinese medicine.

5. Critique judgment/decision

After getting to know Mrs. Chang better, you realize that she is firmly committed to her ways and adamant about not going to an American doctor or into a hospital at this point of her life. Thus, you (with her family) have several options: to force her to see an internist against her will, possibly deceiving her to get her to the internist's office, or to support her choice to rely on familiar remedies, which may or may not successfully resolve her problems. The first alternative may save her life, and her family can see no other choice. You realize that by making this choice, the family is imposing its values on Mrs. Chang and violating her autonomy, her right to determine the course of her life. You decide to support her and to try to explain to her family the importance of doing this. You understand that if her condition is serious and her traditional remedies prove ineffective, her death may be hastened, but she accepts this consequence and prefers it to embracing an alien and frightening culture. An alternative strategy that might result in a win–win result would be to find an American Chinese physician who practices both Chinese and Western medicine. If Mrs. Chang could be persuaded to visit this practitioner, she would experience the best of both medical traditions.

BOX 10-4 KNOWLEDGE AND INTELLECTUAL SKILLS CTIs

Knowledge

Requirements vary, depending on context (e.g. specialty practice):

Relates Knowledge of:
❏ Nursing and medical terminology
❏ Nursing vs. medical and other models, roles, and responsibilities.
❏ Scope of nursing practice (qualifications; applicable standards, laws, and rules and regulations).
❏ Related anatomy, physiology, and pathophysiology
❏ Spiritual, social, and cultural concepts
❏ Normal and abnormal growth and development (pediatric, adult, and gerontologic implications).
❏ Normal and abnormal function (bio-psycho-social-cultural-spiritual)
❏ Factors affecting normal function (bio-psycho-social-cultural-spiritual)
❏ Nutrition and pharmacology principles
❏ Behavioral health and disease management
❏ Signs and symptoms of common problems and complications.
❏ Nursing process, nursing theories, research, and evidence-based practice.
❏ Reasons behind policies, procedures and interventions; diagnostic studies implications
❏ Ethical and legal principles
❏ Risk management and infection control
❏ Safety standards, healthy workplace standards, and principles of learning and safety cultures
❏ Inter-relationship of health care disciplines and systems.
❏ Reliable information resources

Demonstrates:
❏ Focused nursing assessment skills (e.g., breath sounds or IV site assessment)
❏ Mathematical problem solving for drug calculations
❏ Related technical skills (e.g., n/g tube or other equipment management)

Clarifies:
❏ Personal biases, values, beliefs, needs
❏ How own culture, thinking, personality, and learning style preferences differ from others'
❏ Level of commitment to organizational mission and values

Intellectual Skills/Competencies

Demonstrates Nursing Process and Decision-Making Skills:
❏ Communicates effectively orally and in writing
❏ Identifies practice scope: applies standards, principles, laws, and ethics codes
❏ Makes safety and infection control a priority; prevents and deals with mistakes constructively
❏ Includes patient, family, and key stakeholders in decisionmaking; teaches patient, self and others
❏ Identifies purpose and focus of assessment
❏ Assesses systematically and comprehensively.
❏ Distinguishes normal from abnormal; identifies risks for abnormal
❏ Distinguishes relevant from irrelevant; clusters relevant data together
❏ Identifies assumptions and inconsistencies; checks accuracy and reliability (validates data)
❏ Recognizes missing information; gains more data as needed.
❏ Concludes what's known and unknown; draws reasonable conclusions—gives evidence to support them
❏ Identifies both problems and their underlying cause(s) and related factors; includes patient and family perspectives
❏ Recognizes changes in patient status; takes appropriate action
❏ Considers multiple ideas, explanations, and solutions
❏ Determines individualized outcomes and uses them to plan and give care
❏ Manages risks, predicts complications
❏ Weighs risks and benefits; anticipates consequences and implications—individualizes interventions accordingly
❏ Sets priorities and makes decisions in a timely way
❏ Reassesses to monitor outcomes (responses)
❏ Promotes health, function, comfort, and well-being
❏ Identifies ethical issues and takes appropriate action
❏ Uses human and information resources; detects bias

Additional Related Skills:
❏ Advocates for patients, self, and others
❏ Engages and empowers patients, families, peers, and coworkers
❏ Fosters positive interpersonal relationships; addresses conflicts fairly; promotes healthy workplace and learning cultures
❏ Promotes teamwork (focuses on common goals, respects diversity; encourages others to contribute in their own way)
❏ Facilitates and navigates change
❏ Organizes and manages time and environment
❏ Gives and takes constructive criticism
❏ Delegates appropriately (matches patient needs with worker competencies; determines worker learning needs, supervises and teaches as indicated; monitors results personally)
❏ Leads, inspires, and helps others move toward common goals.
❏ Demonstrates systems thinking (shows awareness of relationships existing within and across healthcare systems).

Reprinted with permission from Alfaro-LeFevre, R. (2014). Critical Thinking Indicators (CTIs). Available at www.AlfaroTeachSmart.com

• Identify nurses who are technical experts, and ask them to share their secrets. Many experienced clinicians have developed quality, time-saving techniques they are willing to share.

• Never be ashamed to ask for help when feeling unsure of how to perform a procedure or manage equipment. Don't overlook the patient or family caregiver as a source of helpful hints for care they routinely provide. Never forget that the patient's well-being and sometimes the patient's life depend on your technical competence.

Many nursing procedures are described in the clinical chapters in this text. Performance checklists break each procedure down into its component parts, allowing you to

BOX 10-5 PERSONAL CRITICAL THINKING INDICATORS (CTIs)

PERSONAL CTIs are brief descriptions of behaviors, attitudes and characteristics often seen in critical thinkers. These are the behaviors that promote development of critical thinking habits. The below is the ideal—no one's perfect. Characteristics vary depending on circumstances such as comfort and familiarity with the people and situations at hand. What matters is *patterns* of behavior over time (is the behavior usually evident?). If you're a critical thinker, you probably can pick some characteristics you'd like to improve (critical thinkers are inately focused on improvement).

❑ **SELF-AWARE:** Identifies own learning, personality, and communication style preferences; clarifies biases, strengths, and limitations; acknowledges when thinking may be influenced by emotions or self-interest.

❑ **GENUINE/AUTHENTIC:** Shows true self; demonstrates behaviors that indicate stated values.

❑ **EFFECTIVE COMMUNICATOR:** Listens well (shows deep understanding of others' thoughts, feelings and circumstances); speaks and writes with clarity (gets key points across to others).

❑ **CURIOUS AND INQUISITIVE:** Asks questions; looks for reasons, explanations, and meaning; seeks new information to broaden understanding.

❑ **ALERT TO CONTEXT:** Looks for changes in circumstances that warrant a need to modify approaches; investigates thoroughly when situations warrant precise, in depth thinking.

❑ **REFLECTIVE AND SELF-CORRECTIVE:** Carefully considers meaning of data and interpersonal interactions, asks for feedback; corrects own thinking, alert to potential errors by self and others, finds ways to avoid future mistakes.

❑ **ANALYTICAL AND INSIGHTFUL:** Identifies relationships; expresses deep understanding.

❑ **LOGICAL AND INTUITIVE:** Draws reasonable conclusions (if this is so, then it follows that because...); uses intuition as a guide; acts on intuition only with knowledge of risks involved.

❑ **CONFIDENT AND RESILIENT:** Expresses faith in ability to reason and learn; overcomes problems and disappointments.

❑ **HONEST AND UPRIGHT:** Looks for the truth, even if it sheds unwanted light; demonstrates integrity (adheres to moral and ethical standards; admits flaws in thinking).

❑ **AUTONOMOUS / RESPONSIBLE:** Self-directed, self-disciplined, and accepts accountability.

❑ **CAREFUL AND PRUDENT:** Seeks help as needed; suspends or revises judgment as indicated by new or incomplete data.

❑ **OPEN AND FAIR-MINDED:** Shows tolerance for different viewpoints; questions how own viewpoints are influencing thinking.

❑ **SENSITIVE TO DIVERSITY:** Expresses appreciation of human differences related to values, culture, personality, or learning style preferences; adapts to preferences when feasible.

❑ **CREATIVE:** Offers alternative solutions and approaches; comes up with useful ideas.

❑ **REALISTIC AND PRACTICAL:** Admits when things aren't feasible; looks for useful solutions.

❑ **PROACTIVE:** Anticipates consequences, plans ahead, acts on opportunities.

❑ **COURAGEOUS:** Stands up for beliefs, advocates for others, doesn't hide from challenges

❑ **PATIENT AND PERSISTENT:** Waits for right moment; perseveres to achieve best results.

❑ **FLEXIBLE:** Changes approaches as needed to get the best results.

❑ **HEALTH-ORIENTED:** Promotes a healthy lifestyle; uses healthy behaviors to manage stress.

❑ **IMPROVEMENT- ORIENTED (SELF, PATIENTS, SYSTEMS): Self**—Identifies learning needs; finds ways to overcome limitations, seeks out new knowledge. **Patients**—Promotes health; maximizes function, comfort, and convenience. **Systems**—Identifies risks and problems with health care systems; promotes safety, quality, satisfaction, and cost containment.

Reprinted with permission from Alfaro-LeFevre, R. (2014). Critical Thinking Indicators (CTIs). Available at www.AlfaroTeachSmart.com.

evaluate your performance of each step of the procedure. This type of self-knowledge enables you to identify quickly and remedy any deficiencies in technical skills.

Developing Interpersonal Competencies

Interpersonal skills are essential to the practice of thoughtful person-centered practice. Interpersonal caring involves promoting the dignity and respect of patients as people and establishing a caring relationship. As a result, both the nurse and patient experience mutual enrichment.

PROMOTING HUMAN DIGNITY AND RESPECT

Nurses committed to respecting the human dignity of patients find it helpful to reflect on these questions:

• What obligates me to respect patients' human dignity? Why should I respect all patients equally? Are some patients more deserving of respect than others? Can a patient ever forfeit the right to be respected?

• What does it mean to respect the dignity of patients? What are five concrete ways I can demonstrate respect?

• What are my strengths and deficiencies when it comes to respecting patients?

• In what ways (if any) must I change to be faithful to the duty of respecting the dignity of patients?

• What patients most challenge my ability to give care respectfully? How do I respond to this challenge? What does this teach me for the future?

Nurses often underestimate their power to help a patient heal simply through their respectful and caring presence. Each time a nurse walks into a room, the nurse communicates one of two messages: (1) "You are a job to be done—you mean nothing to me" or (2) "You are a person of worth, and I care about you." Even a 60-second nurse–patient interaction can enhance or jeopardize human well-being. Therefore nurses must be sensitive about what their looks, speech, and touch communicate to patients and colleagues. The more vulnerable the patient and the more threatened the patient's sense of self, the more powerful effect the nurse's message has on the person's sense of worth and well-being.

 CONSIDER Addie Warner, the patient described in the Reflective Practice display. Imagine the message that she received from staff who consider her difficult when she used her call light to ask for help. Most likely, the message conveyed was negative. Compare this to the message communicated by the nursing student who helped get her out of bed and get washed: a more positive message supporting the patient's self-worth. •

The learning activity in Box 10-6 was developed for nurses caring for older patients in a long-term care facility. To help develop interpersonal skills, try these activities with a friend. Take turns being both the nurse and the older adult, and talk about how different types of nursing presence makes you feel.

ESTABLISHING CARING RELATIONSHIPS

Increasingly, nurses report that new systems of care and the demand to work "harder, faster, and smarter" to keep up in today's competitive health care arena are making traditional nurse–patient relationships difficult to attain. As you begin your nursing practice, ask yourself what priority you assign to caring. Nurses who accept that there can be no excellence in nursing in the absence of this relationship commit themselves to finding creative means to establish caring relationships. Obviously, many variables influence the quality of relationships that are possible, not the least of which is how sick the patient is and the patient's length of stay. Helpful reflection questions include the following:

- Do I know my patients well enough to promote anything more than their physical well-being?
- If asked to describe a patient, would I be able to report on anything other than the patient's physical condition?
- Is the care I routinely provide really holistic, individualized, prioritized according to medical need and the

---

BOX 10-6 DEVELOPING INTERPERSONAL SKILLS

Human Dignity: How Who I Am as a Caregiver Affects Others

Description
The purpose of this exercise is to explore the notion of "therapeutic use of self." You will be challenged to reflect on the effect your looks, speech, and touch have on other people. Role play and guided discovery will be used to enable you to experience the affirming and negating influences of different means of human relating.

Objectives
Upon conclusion of this exercise, you will be able to:
1. Demonstrate how looks, words, and touch can be used to harm or benefit others
2. Describe how the way you approach others enhances or diminishes their well-being
3. Identify one care behavior you plan to modify to improve your nursing practice

Learning Activities
Invite an experienced nurse to demonstrate how looks, words, and touch can be used to communicate two different messages to others: "You are a job to be done—you mean nothing to me" and "You are precious, and I care about you." After the demonstration, team up with another student, and experience giving and receiving these messages. Share the feelings that you both experienced. After these preliminary exercises, role play the following suggested nursing situations (or others of your choosing), and once again process the experience. Talk about the relevance of this experience to human interaction in general, and conclude the exercise by writing a goal for your practice.

Worksheet
A. Practice looking at a colleague two different ways:
   1. "You are a job to be done—you mean nothing to me."
   2. "You are precious, and I care about you."

B. Practice speaking to a colleague in two different ways:
   1. Indifferent: "Your patient, your light."
   2. Helpful: "I think Mrs. Jones's light is on again. Do you need help?"
C. Practice touching a colleague in two different ways:
   1. Indifferent: Pick up your colleague's wrist and feel for a pulse.
   2. Using warm lotion, massage your colleague's hands.
D. Talk about how each of these looks, words, and touches made you feel. Talk about how you think they make patients feel.
E. Role play each of the following situations in two different ways, trying to incorporate looks, words, and touches that communicate:

   First time: You are a job to be done—you mean nothing to me.

   Second time: You are precious, and I care about you.

   1. Student feels overwhelmed by patient care assignment and approaches clinical instructor to discuss her options.
   2. Student walks into patient's room to begin morning care.
   3. Student assists older patient to stand and ambulate around room.
   4. Student brings medication to patient.
   5. Student approaches another student and asks for help changing the bed linens of an obese patient who is on complete bed rest.
F. Name one thing you have decided to try to do differently when you take care of your patients as a result of this session.
G. Does what you experienced today have any implications for who you are when you are not nursing?

THROUGH THE EYES OF A PATIENT

I recently spent 2 months in a university teaching hospital while doctors tried to find a way to regulate my heartbeats. Many of the days were filled with tests, some of which were frightening. I was given many drugs—most of which turned out not to be helpful. I was a 2-hour car ride away from my home, family, and friends—which meant there wasn't always a familiar face at my bedside.

I quickly learned I could judge what kind of day I was going to have as soon as I saw my nurse each morning. All of them brought my medicines and helped with the treatment plan. With some nurses, however, I also experienced the comfort and security of knowing that my expressed needs would be promptly and respectfully tended to. If I needed help getting up to the bathroom or asked for something for

pain, I could count on help coming quickly. And finally there were those few with whom I knew I was going to have a great day because they would "make it happen" no matter how sick I was feeling. These were the nurses who offered a hug with their medicines, who had a moment to sit and listen, who teased about the "fashion statements" I was making with my nightgowns, and who "walked me through" new tests so that at least I felt better prepared to face the unknown. Most often, it wasn't what they did but how they did it.

I wish all nurses understood the power they have to influence a patient's basic sense of well-being. A hospital can be a pretty scary, lonely place. Nurses can make all the difference!

—Mildred Taylor, Pottsville, PA

patient's interests, and continuous? Do my care plans reflect this?
- What does the content of the patient report and nursing documentation communicate about nursing priorities in my practice setting?
- What are my strengths and deficiencies in creating caring relationships?
- In what ways (if any) must I change to establish better caring relationships?

Nurses committed to caring relationships routinely use opportunities for conversation to communicate genuine interest in who the patient is and what the patient is experiencing to provide meaningful nursing assistance. For example, rather than just chatting aimlessly with a talkative patient, a nurse skilled in developing caring relationships will direct the conversation. Leading statements or questions that are often successful in eliciting useful information from older patients include the following:

- "Tell me something about your life at home. What do you miss most now that you are here?"
- "What family members and friends do you see most often? Who do you think knows you best and would you trust to speak for you if you were ever unable to speak for yourself?"
- "Most of us have some goal or dream that keeps us going. It might be owning our own home, seeing some relationship patched up, or being able to celebrate the birth of a grandchild. What is your dream?"
- "When you've had troubles in the past, what did you draw on for strength? What keeps you going?"
- "Looks like you've got a lot of time for thinking these days...would you like to share what's been on your mind?"
- "Looks like we'll be spending some time together...what would you like to do with this time? How may I help you?"
- "What would you like us to know that will help us to better meet your needs?"
- "Hospitals can be scary places...how can I help you?"

Nurses who are sensitive to the well-being of their patients can find many ways to communicate caring. Happily, most caring is mutually enriching, and nurses who care find themselves re-energized for the more demanding aspects of their practice. Read one patient's account of the importance to her of nurse caring in the accompanying Through the Eyes of a Patient display.

ENJOYING THE REWARDS OF MUTUAL EXCHANGE

In any helping profession, but especially in nursing, countless opportunities exist to interact with others. Those committed to interpersonal caring enrich everyday interactions by investing them with something of themselves and, in return, receiving something from the other (Fig. 10-2). Think of your last encounter with a patient. Whether you were administering a medication, checking vital signs, or preparing the patient for discharge, you had the choice of merely accomplishing the given task or accomplishing the task while simultaneously communicating a personal gift of support, caring, strength, and peacefulness. Frequently overlooked, these interpersonal gifts might contribute to a patient's healing as significantly as medical interventions. Rather than deplete their giver, these

FIGURE 10-2. Interpersonal caring enriches the lives of everyone participating, providing a mutual exchange of giving and receiving.

interpersonal gifts invite similar gifts from the recipient, which in return enrich the caregiver. Nothing causes burnout faster than a practice that is reduced to the performance of multiple tasks stripped of their human significance. When a patient is given care in a way that "makes a difference" in terms of his or her well-being, the patient's gratitude, even when unspoken, helps renew the nurse's energy. Too seldom do we stop our busy practices long enough to reflect on how who we are that day is influencing the well-being of those receiving our care. It is helpful to question:

- How conscious am I of how my mood influences the well-being of others?
- Have I ever consciously tried to transmit strength, peace, support, or joy to another? What were the results?
- Am I aware of any situation in which my fatigue, anxiety, frustration, or negativity was communicated to a patient in a manner that negatively influenced the patient's well-being?
- Am I conscious of ways in which patients enrich me personally or enrich my practice?
- In what ways is my practice different when I am attuned to the interpersonal dimensions of nurse–patient interactions?
- In what ways must my practice change if I am to facilitate healing in every patient encounter?

Developing Ethical/Legal Competencies

Nurses who prize their role in securing patient well-being are sensitive to the ethical and legal implications of nursing practice. Chapters 6 and 7 describe essential components of ethical and legal competence for nurses. Although it can take years to master effective patient advocacy skills and to become proficient in mediating ethical conflict, even beginning nurses are responsible for certain basic ethical skills. For example, one of the greatest challenges nursing students face is balancing the competing demands of home life, school, and the hospital or practice setting. Learning to be true to oneself, to the patients for whom one is responsible, to the caregiving team, and to the profession and society is an ongoing struggle. Examining one's sense of accountability is crucial as one assumes professional responsibilities. Nurses committed to interpersonal caring hold themselves accountable for the human well-being of patients entrusted to their care. Being accountable means being attentive and responsive to the health care needs of individual patients. It means that your concern for the patient transcends whatever happens during your shift, and that you ensure continuity of care when you leave a patient. In today's system of increasingly fragmented care, patients often find themselves unable to point to any single caregiver who knows their overall situation and is capable and willing to coordinate the efforts of the health care team. Being responsive and responsible earns a patient's trust that "all will be well" as health care needs are addressed. Nurses committed to responsible caring reflect on the following:

- To what extent does my commitment to securing the human well-being of those in my care dictate my work priorities?

- How comfortable am I voicing unmet patient needs to other members of the health care team? Is meeting the patient's needs more important to me than remaining in my comfort zone?
- Do other caregivers listen when I present patient concerns because of my successful record of patient advocacy?
- What system variables (e.g., nurse–patient ratios, skill mix, availability of resources) need to change for us to better meet the human needs of our patients?
- In what ways must I change for my patients to be able to count on me to respond in a responsible way to their needs?

Nurses who are sensitive to the legal dimensions of practice are careful to develop a strong sense of both ethical and legal accountability. Competent practice is a nurse's best legal safeguard. Nurses seeking to develop legal competence might find it helpful to ask the following questions:

- Do I know the legal boundaries of my practice?
- Am I familiar with pertinent institutional procedures and policies?
- Do I "own" my personal strengths and weaknesses and seek assistance as needed?
- Am I careful never to accept responsibility for an assignment for which I am unprepared?
- Am I knowledgeable about, and respectful of, patient rights?
- Does my documentation provide a legally defensible account of my practice?

When working to develop ethical and legal accountability, nurses must recognize that both deficiencies and excesses of responsible caring are problematic. Although it is reasonable to hold oneself accountable for promoting the human well-being of patients, nurses can err by setting unrealistic standards of responsiveness and responsibility for themselves. Prudence is always necessary to balance responsible self-care with care of others. Inexperienced nurses might feel totally responsible for effecting patient outcomes beyond their control and become frustrated and sad when unable to produce the desired outcome. Conversations with other nurses about what is reasonable to hold ourselves and others accountable for are always helpful.

QSEN Competencies

The overall goal of the **Quality and Safety Education for Nurses (QSEN)** project is to meet the challenge of preparing future nurses who will have the knowledge, skills, and attitudes (KSAs) necessary to continuously improve the quality and safety of the health care systems within which they work.

Using the Institute of Medicine competencies, QSEN faculty and a National Advisory Board defined quality and safety competencies for nursing and proposed targets for the knowledge, skills, and attitudes to be developed in nursing pre-licensure programs for each competency. See the QSEN website (www.qsen.org) and Box 10-7 for a description of these competencies. To highlight the importance of these competencies, each chapter in this text has a feature entitled *Reflective Practice: Developing QSEN Competencies*. These

BOX 10-7 THE NEW FUNDAMENTALS IN NURSING: INTRODUCING BEGINNING QUALITY AND SAFETY EDUCATION FOR NURSES (QSEN) COMPETENCIES

Patient-Centered Care

The traditional concept involves listening to the patient and demonstrating respect and compassion. The QSEN competency emphasizes recognition of the patient or designee as the source of control and full partner in providing compassionate and coordinated care based on respect for patient's preferences, values, and needs. The KSAs include:

- K—Integrate understanding of multiple dimensions of person-centered care: patient, family, and community preferences and values; coordination and integration of care; information, communication, and education; physical comfort and emotional support; involvement of family and friends; and transition and continuity.
- S—Elicit patient values, preferences, and expressed needs as part of the clinical interview, implementation of care plan, and evaluation of care.
- A—Value seeing healthcare situations "through patients' eyes."

Teamwork and Collaboration

The traditional view of teamwork may involve working side by side with other healthcare professionals while forming nursing skills. The updated QSEN definition calls for functioning effectively within nursing and interprofessional teams, fostering open communication, mutual respect, and shared decision making to achieve quality patient care. Important beginning KSAs include:

- K—Describe scope of practice and roles of healthcare team members.
- S—Follow communication practices that minimize risk associated with handoff among providers and across transition in care.
- A—Acknowledge own potential to contribute to effective team functioning.

Evidence-Based Practice

Traditional practices involve adhering to internal policies to standardize skills execution. The QSEN definition specifies the integration of best current evidence with clinical expertise and patient and family preferences and values for delivery of optimal healthcare. Important, beginning KSAs reveal significant changes in fundamentals of nursing:

- K—Describe evidence-based practice to include components of research evidence, clinical expertise, and patient and family values.
- S—Base individualized care plan on patient values, clinical expertise, and evidence.
- A—Value the concept of evidence-based practice as integral to determining best clinical practice.

Quality Improvement

A long-standing approach to quality involves routinely updating nursing policies and procedures. The QSEN updated concept of quality improvement recommends use of data to monitor the outcomes of care processes and use of improvement methods to design and test changes to continuously improve the quality and safety of healthcare systems. The KSAs recommended for early introduction include:

- K—Recognition that nursing and other health professions students are parts of systems of care and care processes that affect outcomes for patients and families.
- S—The delphi ratings did not identify a beginning skill in quality improvement but rather recommended introduction and emphasis in intermediate or advanced experiences.
- A—Appreciate continuous quality improvement as essential in the daily work of all healthcare professionals.

Safety

A simplistic, traditional definition of safety is to use bed rails properly to ensure "that my patient does not fall during my shift." The QSEN update assures recognition of a culture of safety and minimization of risk of harm to patients through both system effectiveness and individual performance. Safety KSAs rated as important to introduce early include:

- K—Examine human factors and other basic safety design principles as well as commonly used unsafe practices (e.g., workarounds, dangerous abbreviations).
- S—Demonstrate effective use of strategies to reduce risk of harm to self or others.
- A—Value the contributions of standardization and reliability to safety.

Informatics

Traditionally, documentation consists of timely and accurate charting. However, the QSEN updated definition is expanded and calls for using information and technology to communicate, manage knowledge, mitigate error, and support decision making. The KSAs identified as important for early introduction include:

- K—Explain why information and technology skills are essential for safe patient care.
- S—Apply technology and information management tools to support safe processes of care.
- A—Value technologies supporting decision making, error prevention, and care coordination.

(Reprinted with permission from Preheim, G., Armstrong, G. E., & Barton, A. (2009). The NEW fundamentals in nursing: Introducing beginning quality and safety education for nurses (QSEN) competencies. *Journal of Nursing Education, 48*(12), 694–698.)

displays are written by nursing students and will help you to assess your developing mastery of these competencies.

Clinical Reasoning, Judgments, and Decision Making

Many use the terms *critical thinking, clinical reasoning,* and *clinical judgment* interchangeably. Alfaro-LeFevre (2014, p. 8) offers these helpful distinctions:

- Critical thinking—a broad term—includes reasoning both outside and inside of the clinical setting. Clinical reasoning and clinical judgment are key pieces of critical thinking in nursing.
- Clinical reasoning—a specific term—usually refers to ways of thinking about patient care issues (determining, preventing, and managing patient problems). For reasoning about other clinical issues (e.g., teamwork, collaboration,

and streamlining work flow), nurses usually use critical thinking.

- **Clinical judgment** refers to the result (outcome) of critical thinking or clinical reasoning—the conclusion, decision, or opinion you make.

People use critical thinking skills whenever they want to use clear, focused thinking to achieve a result. You can think critically about how to survive the day's challenges, to find a partner for life, to pass a licensing exam, or to become president! Critical thinking applied to clinical reasoning and judgment in nursing practice (Alfaro-LeFevre, 2014, p. 8):

- Is guided by standards, policies, and procedures, ethics codes, and laws (individual state practice acts)
- Is based on principles of nursing process, problem solving, and the scientific method (requires forming opinions and making decisions based on evidence)
- Carefully identifies the key problems, issues, and risks involved, including patients, families, and major care providers in decision making

- Is driven by patient, family, and community needs, as well as nurses' needs to give competent, efficient care (e.g., streamlining paperwork to free nurses for patient care)
- Calls for strategies that make the most of human potential and compensate for problems created by human nature (e.g., finding ways to prevent errors, using information technology, and overcoming the powerful influence of personal views)
- Is constantly re-evaluating, self-correcting, and striving to improve

Levett-Jones et al. (2010) prepared the clinical reasoning (CR) model depicted in Figure 10-3 after studying the work of Hoffman (2007), Alfaro-LeFevre (2013) and Andersen (1991). They describe eight main steps or phases in the clinical reasoning cycle. However, in reality, the distinctions between these phases are not so clear. While clinical reasoning can be broken down into steps—look, collect, process, decide, plan, act, evaluate, and reflect—these phases often merge and the boundaries between them become blurred.

Describe or list facts, context, objects or people.

Review current information (e.g. handover reports, patient history, patient charts, results of investigations and nursing/medical assessments previously undertaken).
Gather new information (e.g. undertake patient assessment)
Recall knowledge (e.g. physiology, pathophysiology, pharmacology, epidemiology, therapeutics, culture, context of care, ethics, law etc)

Contemplate what you have learned from this process and what you could have done differently.

Consider the patient situation

Collect cues & information

Reflect on process and new learning

Interpret: analyze data to come to an understanding of signs or symptoms. Compare normal v/s abnormal.
Discriminate: distinguish relevant from irrelevant information; recognize inconsistencies, narrow down the information to what is most important and recognize gaps in cues collected.
Relate: discover new relationships or patterns; cluster cues together to identify relationships between them.
Infer: make deductions or form opinions that follow logically by interpreting subjective and objective cues; consider alternatives and consequences.
Match current situation to past situations or current patient to past patients (usually an expert thought process).
Predict an outcome (usually an expert thought process).

Clinical reasoning cycle

Evaluate the effectiveness of and actions outcomes. Ask: "has the situation improved now?"

Evaluate outcomes

Process information

Take action

Select a course of action between different alternatives available.

Establish goal(s)

Identify problems/ issues

Describe what you want to happen, a desired outcome, a time frame...

Synthesize facts and inferences to make a definitive diagnosis of the patient's problem.

FIGURE 10-3. The clinical reasoning cycle. (Reprinted with permission from Levett-Jones, T., Hoffman, K., Dempsey, J., Jeong, S. Y-S, Noble, D., Norton, C.A., ... Hickey, N. [2010]. The 'five rights' of clinical reasoning: An educational model to enhance nursing students' ability to identify and manage clinically 'at risk' patients. *Nurse Education Today, 30*(6), 515–520, DOI: 10.1016/j.nedt.2009.10.020.)

Remember to learn to recognize, understand, and work through each phase, rather than making assumptions about patient problems and initiating interventions that have not been adequately considered. Effective use of the CR model by nursing students and its application in practice by novice nurses are directly linked to the five rights of clinical reasoning: the ability to collect the right cues and take the right action for the right patient at the right time and for the right reason (Levett-Jones et al., 2010). The demand on nurses to execute higher-order reasoning skills is increasing as clinical environments become more complex. This complexity requires nurses to be capable of clear, ordered thinking, identifying problems accurately, and effective decision making that demonstrates good clinical judgment (Dempsey, Hillege and Hill, 2013, p. 258). Clinical reasoning includes the ability to recognize clinical problems and to solve them using the cognitive skills of critical thinking, creative thinking, and intuitive thinking. Using all of these skills, the clinician in the nursing context is capable of "thinking like a nurse" (Tanner, 2006, p. 204) in order to make a clinical judgment and come to a decision that results in a nursing action. Each of the nursing process chapters that follow has a section highlighting the type of clinical reasoning necessary to successfully implement that step of the nursing process.

Problem Solving

One of the strengths of clinical reasoning is that it is based on a methodology that is familiar to most nursing students—problem solving. Problem solving is a basic life skill; identifying a problem and then taking steps to resolve it are a matter of common sense. However, different approaches to problem solving yield different results, some of which are more successful than others.

TRIAL-AND-ERROR PROBLEM SOLVING

Trial-and-error problem solving involves testing any number of solutions until one is found that works for that particular problem. This method is not efficient for the nurse and can be dangerous to the patient; it is therefore not recommended as a guide for nursing practice. For example, although you might enjoy experimenting with different types of ethnic food as you discover and develop personal food preferences, you would not want to use the trial-and-error method of determining food preferences for a dehydrated and malnourished patient. You want to know, based on clinical research, exactly what food and fluid supplements are most likely to reverse the patient's deficiencies.

 CONSIDER Jermaine Byrd, the patient who has returned from vascular surgery and whose posterior tibial pulse cannot be palpated. The nurse might use trial-and-error to determine if the pulse is indeed absent or just difficult to palpate or locate. For example, the nurse might try to reposition the fingers for palpation or apply less pressure during palpation to determine if the pulse can be palpated. ●

SCIENTIFIC PROBLEM SOLVING

Scientific problem solving is a systematic, seven-step, problem-solving process that involves (1) problem identification, (2) data collection, (3) hypothesis formulation, (4) plan of action, (5) hypothesis testing, (6) interpretation of results, and (7) evaluation, resulting in conclusion or revision of the hypothesis. This method is used most correctly in a controlled laboratory setting but is closely related to the more general problem-solving processes commonly used by health care professionals as they work with patients, such as the nursing process.

 AGAIN, think back to Jermaine Byrd, the postoperative patient with a nonpalpable pulse. The nurse uses scientific problem solving to investigate the situation. For example, after attempts at repositioning yield no change, the nurse would collect more data, such as the temperature and the color of the patient's extremity when compared with the opposite leg, existence of pulses above and below the posterior tibial pulse, complaints of pain, numbness, or tingling in the extremity, and the patient's overall condition. These findings would lead the nurse to identify if the patient is experiencing vascular compromise, if the pulse was difficult to palpate, or if the nurse needs more skill in palpation. In addition, the nurse could summon the assistance of another nurse to negate or validate the findings. Once the problem is identified, the nurse can then plan care appropriately to meet the patient's need. ●

INTUITIVE PROBLEM SOLVING

For years, nurse theorists and educators argued that clinical judgments should be based on data alone (the logical, scientific, evidence-based method) in an attempt to establish nursing as a science, worthy of the respect of other professions. Today, nurses acknowledge the role of intuitive thinking in making clinical decisions. Many veteran nurses can describe situations in which an "inner prompting" led to a quick nursing intervention that saved a patient's life. When they directly apprehend a situation based on its similarity or dissimilarity to other situations they have experienced, they use intuitive problem solving. **Intuitive problem solving** is thus a direct understanding of a situation based on a background of experience, knowledge, and skill that makes expert decision making possible. A recovery room nurse who realizes that a postoperative patient is deteriorating before there are measurable signs to suggest trouble is using intuitive problem solving, as is an oncology nurse who somehow senses the right moment to teach, offer encouragement, affirm, or simply listen.

Advocates of intuition recommend the following:

- Welcoming flashes of intuition as additions to logical reasoning, rather than as disruptions.
- Validating intuitions: When an intuition cannot be validated (e.g., when the nurse senses that something is wrong with the patient, although there are no clinical signs), careful monitoring of the patient should be initiated.

• Furthering nursing research to help find ways to (1) cultivate intuition and its typical results (accurate and early diagnosis, vigilant monitoring, better patient care) and (2) document the information that intuition supplies (Rew, 1987).

Beginning nurses must use nursing knowledge and scientific problem solving as the basis of care they give; intuitive problem solving comes with years of practice and observation. If the beginning nurse has an intuition about a patient, that information should be discussed with the faculty member, preceptor, or supervisor.

CRITICAL THINKING: INTUITIVE, LOGICAL, OR BOTH?

While this text makes a strong case for clinical reasoning that is logical, scientific, and evidence-based, it also promotes clinical reasoning that is creative and intuitive. Alfaro-LeFevre, an expert in critical thinking, is quick to note that critical thinking is contextual and changes depending on the circumstances. As examples, she cites brainstorming sessions as a good method for nurturing intuition because logical thinking might constrain and block ideas. On the other hand, developing policies, procedures, and plans of care requires more logical, evidence-based thought. In summary, when intuition is used alone, there are increased risks and fewer benefits. Intuition often moves problem solving forward quickly, but it might result in a lot of trial-and-error approaches. Logic is the safest approach, but it doesn't foster out-of-the-box ideas and might inhibit right-brain thinkers from getting started. Pairing intuitive and logical thinkers who have learned specific strategies to promote reasoning (e.g., mind mapping) can bring great results (Alfaro-LeFevre, 2009).

 Concept Mastery Alert

Critical thinking often involves scientific problem solving but it also involves intuition, logic, and creative thinking. A person integrates and adapts the use of all these strategies to address the situation.

Creative Thinking

Critical thinking and clinical reasoning also involve reflection and creative thinking. **Creative thinking** involves imagination, intuition, and spontaneity, factors that underpin the art of nursing. Creative thinking is brought into play when you ask "why" or "what if" questions and is most useful when conventional solutions have not resolved a situation. Creative nurse thinkers are able to "think outside the box" and imagine possible consequences, generate original approaches, and identify alternative perspectives. The solution to a challenge might involve resources as yet untapped, effective, and cost saving and lead to interventions as yet undiscovered and untried. The process of brainstorming might bring out, along with unworkable options, one or two realistic suggestions that would not have surfaced otherwise. Each Reflective Practice box that opens a chapter

invites readers to think outside the box as they contemplate possible courses of action.

Decision Making and Clinical Reasoning

Nurses make decisions every day. We decide what to eat, where to work, whether or not to exercise. While some use the phrases *problem solving* and *decision making* synonymously, not all decisions result from problems. Decision making is about choosing from options. Lipe and Beasley (2004) define **decision making** as "purposeful, goal directed effort applied in a systematic way to make a choice among alternatives," and they explain that even choosing not to act in a certain situation is a decision (p. 37). They also emphasize that all decisions have consequences. Since the nurse's decisions about patient care have the power to literally determine how people are born, live, suffer, and die, it is critical for nurses to be skilled in making decisions.

Potential errors in decision making include (Lipe & Beasley, 2004, p. 46):

• *Bias*
  • Placing excess emphasis on first data received
  • Avoiding information contrary to one's opinion
  • Selecting alternatives to maintain status quo
  • Being predisposed to a single solution
  • Stating the problem in a way to support one's choices
  • Making decisions to support past choices
• *Failure to consider the total situation*
  • Using inaccurate data
  • Not clearly identifying the problem
  • Failing to prioritize or rank the problems in order of importance
  • Using unrealistic goals
• *Impatience*
  • Failing to identify multiple solutions
  • Incorrectly implementing the decision
  • Failing to use appropriate resources

THE NURSING PROCESS

As the practice of nursing became more complex in the second half of the twentieth century, nurses began to study the process of nursing to both understand and improve the means that nurses use to accomplish their aims.

Historical Perspective

Since Hall first used the term "nursing process" in 1955, many nurses have struggled to define exactly what constitutes the "work of nursing" and what makes nurses successful. In the 1960s, nursing theorists began to describe nursing as a distinct entity among the health care professions and also delineated specific steps in a process approach to nursing practice. In 1967, Yura and Walsh published the first comprehensive book on nursing process, in which they described four steps in the nursing process: assessment, planning, intervention, and evaluation. They viewed the nursing diagnosis as the logical conclusion of the assessment phase, whereas Gebbie and Lavin (1974) later made nursing diagnosis a separate step in the process. These and other studies led to the development of the five-step nursing process commonly used today: assessment, diagnosis, outcome identification and planning, implementation, and evaluation.

The steps of the nursing process were legitimized in 1973, when the ANA Congress for Nursing Practice developed standards of practice to guide nursing performance. The following definition serves as the foundation for the scope and standards of nursing practice: "Nursing is the protection, promotion, and optimization of health and abilities, prevention of illness and injury, alleviation of suffering through the diagnosis and treatment of human response, and advocacy in the care of individuals, families, communities, and populations" (ANA, 2010a, p. 6). The scope defines the range and boundaries of nursing practice (see Chapter 1 for more information). The standards are authoritative statements by which the nursing profession describes responsibilities for which its practitioners are accountable. These standards were revised in 1991, 1998, 2004, and 2010. The six *standards of practice* (assessment, diagnosis, outcome identification, planning, implementation, and evaluation) describe a competent level of nursing care as demonstrated by the critical thinking model of the nursing process. The nursing process encompasses all significant actions taken by registered nurses and forms the foundation of the nurse's decision making (ANA, 2010).

Although the ANA refers to a six-step nursing process, many practitioners still commonly refer to a five-step nursing process that combines outcome identification and planning into one step. The five-step nursing process is presented throughout this textbook.

The Joint Commission requires that care be documented according to the nursing process, and the National League for Nursing has recommended that educational programs incorporate the nursing process as their intellectual process. In 1982, the state board examinations for professional nursing practice underwent major revisions and began to use the nursing process as an organizing concept. The revised examinations are structured to test the practitioner's ability to assess patients, to diagnose health problems amenable to nursing therapy, and to plan, implement, and evaluate nursing care. The examinations had previously organized content on a medical model, structured according to medical specialties—medicine, surgery, maternity, pediatrics, and psychiatry.

Description of the Nursing Process

The **nursing process** is a systematic method that directs the nurse and patient, as together they accomplish the

Nurses and patients work together as partners to
• promote health
• prevent disease/illness
• restore health
• facilitate coping with altered functioning

Assessing

Diagnosing

Outcome identification and planning

Implementing

Evaluating

Termination of nursing care OR Revision of plan of care

FIGURE 10-4. The steps in the thoughtful, person-centered, outcome-oriented nursing process are dynamic and interrelated. Each of the five steps depends on the accuracy of the preceding step.

following: (1) **assess** the patient to determine the need for nursing care, (2) determine **nursing diagnoses** for actual and potential health problems, (3) identify **expected outcomes** and **plan** care, (4) **implement** the care, and (5) **evaluate** the results. The steps in this person-centered, outcome-oriented process are interrelated; each step depends on the accuracy of the steps preceding it. The process provides a framework that enables the nurse and patient to accomplish the following:

- Systematically collect patient data (assessing)
- Clearly identify patient strengths and actual and potential problems (diagnosing)
- Develop a holistic plan of individualized care that specifies the desired patient goals and related outcomes and the nursing interventions most likely to assist the patient to meet those expected outcomes (planning)
- Execute the plan of care (implementing)

- Evaluate the effectiveness of the plan of care in terms of patient goal achievement (evaluating)

 CONSIDER Addie Warner, the older patient who had suffered a CVA and is considered "demanding" by some staff. The nurse uses this framework to determine the patient's presenting problem, that is, the reason for using the call light. By systematically collecting information, determining the patient's strengths and needs, quickly developing a plan for these needs, executing it, and then determining the effectiveness of the plan, the nurse provides the patient with safe, quality, effective care. ●

The five steps of the nursing process are shown in Figure 10-4 and described in Table 10-2. In each step of the process, the nurse and patient work together as partners

Table 10-2	OVERVIEW OF THE NURSING PROCESS		
COMPONENT	**DESCRIPTION**	**PURPOSE**	**ACTIVITIES**
Assessing	Collection, validation, and communication of patient data	Make a judgment about the patient's health status, ability to manage his or her own health care, and need for nursing. Plan individualized holistic care that draws on patient strengths and is responsive to changes in the patient's conditions.	1. Establish the database: • Nursing history • Physical assessment • Review of patient record and nursing literature • Consultation with the patient's support people and health care professionals 2. Continuously update the database. 3. Validate data. 4. Communicate data.
Diagnosing	Analysis of patient data to identify patient strengths and health problems that independent nursing intervention can prevent or resolve	Develop a prioritized list of nursing diagnoses.	1. Interpret and analyze patient data. 2. Identify patient strengths and health problems. 3. Formulate and validate nursing diagnoses. 4. Develop prioritized list of nursing diagnoses.
Outcome identification and planning	Specification of (1) patient outcomes to prevent, reduce, or resolve the problems identified in the nursing diagnoses; and (2) related nursing interventions	Develop an individualized plan of nursing care. Identify patient strengths that can be tapped to facilitate achievement of desired outcomes.	1. Establish priorities. 2. Write outcomes and develop an evaluative strategy. 3. Select nursing interventions. 4. Communicate plan of nursing care.
Implementing	Carrying out the plan of care	Assist patients to achieve desired outcomes—promote wellness, prevent disease and illness, restore health, and facilitate coping with altered functioning.	1. Carry out the plan of care. 2. Continue data collection, and modify the plan of care as needed. 3. Document care.
Evaluating	Measuring the extent to which the patient has achieved the outcomes specified in the plan of care; identifying factors that positively or negatively influenced outcome achievement; revising the plan of care if necessary	Continue, modify, or terminate nursing care.	1. Measure how well the patient has achieved desired outcomes. 2. Identify factors that contribute to the patient's success or failure. 3. Modify the plan of care (if indicated).

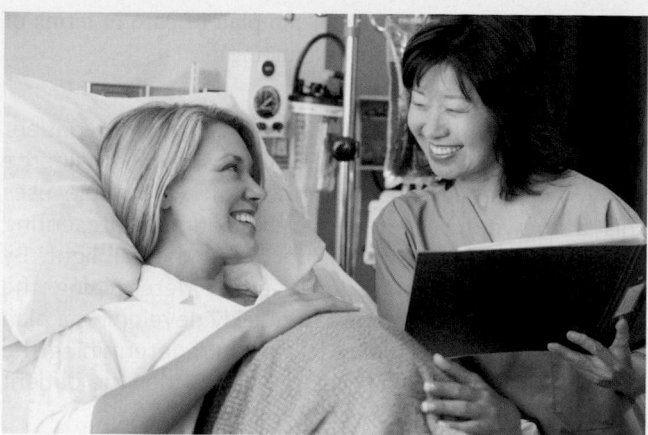

FIGURE 10-5. Nurses work collaboratively with patients when using the nursing process to plan and deliver care.

(Fig. 10-5); the patient's health state and resources influence the patient's level of participation. When the patient is an infant or is unconscious or uncooperative, the nurse works through the steps of the process with the help of a family member or support person whenever possible.

 Concept Mastery Alert

Assessment is the first step in the nursing process and always involves gathering data. Data can be obtained from the patient, family, or other sources as well as from the physical examination.

Nursing Process Trends

Although experienced nurses might tell stories about lengthy handwritten plans of individualized care, the trend today is toward standardization and computerization. Nurses at centralized or bedside computer terminals have access to databases that allow them to plan and document care easily. Critical pathways (see Chapter 13)—which target desired outcomes for particular illnesses, procedures, or conditions—and accompanying multidisciplinary staff actions along a timeline provide the standard guidelines for care in many institutions. Facilitating this work are national efforts to develop the state of nursing knowledge and science and a standard nursing language (Table 10-3). This work is described in subsequent chapters on diagnosis, planning, and implementation. Two recent milestone

Table 10-3	**EXAMPLES OF GROUPS DEVELOPING STANDARD LANGUAGES (VOCABULARIES)**	
GROUP NAME	**FOCUS**	**PURPOSE**
North American Nursing Diagnosis Association (NANDA) International	Diagnoses	Increase the visibility of nursing's contribution to patient care by continuing to develop, refine, and classify phenomena of concern to nurses (see Nursing Diagnosis Quick Reference section). **Web site:** http://www.nanda.org
Nursing Interventions Classification (NIC)	Interventions	Identify, label, validate, and classify actions nurses perform, including direct and indirect care interventions (interventions done directly with patients, e.g., teaching; those done indirectly, e.g., obtaining laboratory studies). **Web site:** http://www.nursing.uiowa.edu/excellence/nursing_knowledge/clinical_effectiveness/index.htm
Nursing-Sensitive Outcomes Classification (NOC)	Outcomes	Identify, label, validate, and classify nursing-sensitive patient outcomes and indicators to evaluate the validity and usefulness of the classification, and define and test measurement procedures for the outcomes and indicators. **Web site:** http://www.nursing.uiowa.edu/excellence/nursing_knowledge/clinical_effectiveness/index.htm
Home Health Care Classification (HHCC)	Diagnoses, Interventions, and Outcomes	Provide a structure for documenting and classifying home health and ambulatory care. Consists of two interrelated taxonomies: HHCC of Nursing Diagnoses and HHCC of Nursing Interventions. **Web site:** http://www.sabacare.com
International Classification for Nursing Practice (ICNP®)	Diagnoses, Interventions, and Outcomes	Capture nursing's contributions to health and provide a framework into which existing vocabularies and classifications can be cross-mapped, enabling comparison of nursing data from various countries throughout the world. **Web site:** http://www.icn.ch/icnp.htm
SNOMED CT (Systematized Nomenclature of Medicine—Clinical Terms)	Comprehensive clinical terminology	Integrate, link, and map terms from various disciplines such as medicine, nursing, and occupational therapy. **Web site:** http://www.nlm.nih.gov/research/umls/Snomed/snomed_main.html

(Reprinted with permission from Alfaro-LeFevre, R. [2010]. *Applying nursing process: A tool for critical thinking* (7th ed., p. 100). Philadelphia: Lippincott Williams & Wilkins.)

monographs in nursing science are *Unifying Nursing Languages: The Harmonization of NANDA, NIC, and NOC* (Dochterman & Jones, 2003) and *Clinical Information Systems: A Framework for Reaching the Vision* (Androwich, 2002).

Characteristics of the Nursing Process

Various words and phrases have been used to describe the nursing process. Key descriptors include systematic, dynamic, interpersonal, outcome oriented, and universally applicable.

Systematic

Each nursing activity is part of an ordered sequence of activities. Moreover, each activity depends on the accuracy of the activity that precedes it and influences the actions that follow it. Without a complete and accurate database, the nurse cannot identify patient strengths and problems. Lacking knowledge of these, the nurse and patient cannot develop a plan of care based on realistic and valued patient goals. Unless the goals and outcomes are well written, nursing actions and evaluation lack focus and might be ineffective. The nursing process directs each step of nursing care in a sequential, ordered manner.

Dynamic

Although the nursing process is presented as an orderly progression of steps, in reality, there is great interaction and overlapping among the five steps. No single step in the nursing process is a one-time phenomenon; each step flows into the next step. In some nursing situations, all five stages occur almost simultaneously.

Interpersonal

Always at the heart of nursing is the human being. Read one student's account of this truth in the accompanying Through the Eyes of a Student display. The nursing process ensures that nurses are person centered rather than task centered (Fig. 10-6). Rather than simply approaching a patient to take vital signs, the nurse might ask, "How are you today,

FIGURE 10-6. Nurses focus on people, not problems or tasks. The nursing process is person centered, not task centered.

Mr. Byrd? Are our nursing actions helping you to achieve your goals? What are the most important things you'd like me to do?" The nurse might also consider any new data that indicate a need to modify the patient's plan of care.

 CONSIDER Charlotte Horvath, the single mother who requires wound care teaching but has failed to attend any scheduled teaching sessions. A nurse who values the interpersonal dimensions of nursing would investigate with Ms. Horvath the reasons underlying her inability to make the teaching sessions. This investigation may reveal many reasons, such as an inability to get away from work, fear, feelings of being overwhelmed, or lack of awareness about the importance of the wound care. ●

The nursing process encourages nurses to work together to help patients use their strengths to meet all their human health needs. This is different from viewing the patient as a "problem to be solved" and interacting mechanically to provide the solution. Working intimately with patients helps nurses to explore their own strengths and limitations and to develop themselves personally and professionally.

THROUGH THE EYES OF A STUDENT

My first experience with an open wound was with a woman who had a stage IV sacral decubitus. I needed to do a dressing change with packing. I was fearful of what the wound would look like. I thought for sure I was going to be "grossed out," and I was—not by the appearance of the wound, but by the odor. The stench was awful! I started to feel queasy and began to sweat, and I thought I was going to pass out and fall right over on the patient. While I was packing the wound, I kept thinking that I was never going to get out of that room. I looked over at my clinical instructor and searched her face for approval of my technique, and I wondered if she also smelled anything and if it was making her feel sick too!

After the procedure was over and I left the room, I asked my instructor if all wounds smell that awful and would the

smell always make me feel sick. Her response was that sometimes an odor will be really bad, and it might make me feel sick. With this kind of reassurance, I thought this is it—I never want to smell that again, and no way do I want to be a nurse.

Later, I realized that I had forgotten there was someone else in that room: the patient. She had to stay in there with that wound and its odor. It was for this reason I changed my mind about leaving nursing. I remembered that it was wanting to help patients to deal with their wounds that made me decide to be a nurse in the first place.

—Barbara L. Dlugosz
Holy Family College, Philadelphia, PA

Outcome Oriented

The nursing process offers a means for nurses and patients to work together to identify specific outcomes related to health promotion, disease and illness prevention, health restoration, and coping with altered functioning; to determine which outcomes are most important to the patient; and to match them with the appropriate nursing actions. When these outcomes are recorded in the plan of care and prioritized, each nurse can quickly determine the patient's priorities and begin nursing with a clear sense of how to proceed. The patient benefits from continuity of care, and each nurse's care moves the patient closer to outcome achievement.

Universally Applicable in Nursing Situations

The one constant in health care is change. When nurses have a working knowledge of the nursing process, they find that they can practice nursing with well or ill people, young or old, in any type of practice setting. Mastering the nursing process gives you a valuable tool you can use with ease in any nursing situation.

It should be clear from this discussion that the nursing process provides a framework for all the nurse's activities. In each nurse–patient interaction, it is important to assess the patient, note any significant alterations in health status, determine whether the nursing action is helping the patient achieve his or her goals, and modify the plan of care as necessary. Thus, the nurse who feeds a child through a special tube as ordered by a physician continually assesses how the child is responding to the feeding and whether the child or family will be able to manage the feedings independently when the child is discharged. Depending on the results of the nursing assessment, new nursing diagnoses might be

needed, along with related additions to the plan of care. The nursing process offers direction for all the activities carried out by the nurse when caring for patients.

Documenting the Nursing Process

The ability to communicate clearly is a critical nursing skill. Accurate, concise, timely, and relevant documentation provides all the members of the caregiving team with a picture of the patient. The patient record is the chief means of communication among members of the interdisciplinary team. Legally speaking, a nursing action that was not documented was not performed. If accused of negligent care, a nurse might tell the court of having faithfully assessed the patient's needs, diagnosed problems, and implemented and evaluated an effective plan of care. However, unless the patient's health records contain documentation supporting these claims, the court has no reason to accept the nurse's word rather than that of the patient or family who are claiming that such care was not given.

Each chapter in this unit offers specific documentation guidelines for nursing process activities; Chapter 16 discusses documentation in general. It is helpful to practice documentation while learning any given nursing activity; like any other nursing skill, documentation improves with practice. Examples of nursing documentation, nursing assessments, plans of care, and notes are provided throughout this text.

Benefits of the Nursing Process

When used well, the nursing process achieves for the patient scientifically based, holistic, individualized care; the opportunity to work collaboratively with nurses; and continuity of care. Nurses who use the nursing process in a thoughtful and systematic way achieve a clear, efficient,

---

BOX 10-8 | EXAMPLE OF THE NURSING PROCESS IN ACTION

Assessing

You are checking on a patient who had abdominal surgery yesterday and hear that the patient has considerable pain: "It kept me up all night." The patient has been reluctant to ask for any pain medication, fearing effects of the drug. "I don't want to become a junkie." The patient's blood pressure and pulse rate are slightly elevated.

Diagnosing

You analyze the data just described and write the nursing diagnosis: *Unrelieved pain related to a fear of taking pain-relieving medications.* The patient agrees that this is becoming a problem.

Outcome Identification and Planning

You decide to work with the patient to achieve the outcome: *By 3:00 PM, patient reports sufficient relief of pain to enable him to rest and to get out of bed to go to the bathroom.* The patient wants to accomplish the outcome. You identify teaching as the primary nursing intervention.

Implementing

After asking the patient about his experiences with pain-relieving medications, you explain that although many of these drugs are addictive when abused, there is no harm if they are taken as prescribed postoperatively. You also explain that it is important for him to experience enough pain relief to be able to cough and deep breathe, ambulate, and do other things important to his recovery. You suggest that the medication will be most effective if taken before his pain peaks and becomes intense. You administer the prescribed medication for pain when the patient indicates that he is willing to give it a try.

Evaluating

After enough time has elapsed for the medication to take effect, you check back with the patient to evaluate whether he has obtained relief and met his outcome. If the patient is satisfied and you both feel that comfort is no longer a problem, you terminate the plan of care for this diagnosis. If the patient still feels pain or is dissatisfied with the medication, each of the preceding steps of the nursing process is re-evaluated, and necessary changes are made in the plan of care.

PROMOTING HEALTH LITERACY

IN PATIENTS AND FAMILIES WITH ASTHMA

Patient Scenario

Your mom calls to tell you that your neighbor back home spent the night in the emergency department with her 3-year-old son Bobby, whom you used to baby-sit. When Bobby experienced chest tightness and shortness of breath, his pediatrician recommended a quick trip to the local emergency department. For the present, Bobby's parents are comforted that he was able to be discharged and is now breathing easier. They were terrified, however, to learn that he may have asthma and wanted your opinion on what they should do. They have an appointment scheduled with their pediatrician.

Nursing Considerations: *Tips for Improving Health Literacy*

Call Bobby's mom and give her an information sheet about childhood asthma and tips on finding out more information

about the disease online from a credible source. Explain that it is a potentially serious disorder if not treated properly, but with good management children are able to sleep, learn, and play. Encourage her to follow the pediatrician's recommendations and to be prepared to ask her pediatrician three questions:

- What is Bobby's main problem?
- What do they need to do?
- Why is it important for them to do this?

What additional measures can you take to help increase health literacy in this patient/family? What other measures would be helpful if Bobby's parents do not speak English, cannot read, or have other learning deficits?

and cost-effective plan of action by which the entire nursing team can achieve the best results for patients; the satisfaction that they are making an important "difference" in the lives of their patients; and the opportunity to grow professionally as they evaluate the effectiveness of interventions and variables that contribute positively or negatively to the patient's achievement of valued outcomes. See Box 10-8 for an example of the nursing process in action. The accompanying Promoting Health Literacy box is another example of how nurses can make a difference.

Evaluating the Use of the Nursing Process

The primary purpose of the nursing process is to help nurses committed to thoughtful person-centered practice manage each patient's care scientifically, holistically, and creatively. To do this successfully, the nurse needs the correct personal attributes, a sound knowledge base, and many competencies, along with the willingness to use them creatively and critically when working with patients to promote or restore health, prevent disease or illness, and facilitate coping with altered functioning.

The chapters that follow in this unit describe each step of the nursing process in detail. Student nurses beginning to use the nursing process should evaluate their growing skill in using the nursing process correctly. The assessment tool in Box 10-9 helps you assess your proficiency in the skills essential for competent use of the nursing process. After completing the exercise, share your self-evaluation with a trusted colleague or clinical instructor and see whether your assessments of your abilities agree. Celebrate your natural and developed strengths. Begin now to plan a strategy to boost those skills in which you are deficient. It may sound trite but it is true: Your patients will be grateful you cared enough to be your best. Nurses sensitive to mastering both the art and the science

of thoughtful, person-centered care evaluate whether they have the prerequisite skills for each nurse–patient encounter, as well as the skills needed to perceive, respond to, and appreciate the uniqueness of each patient. Quality care is each nurse's responsibility.

Concept Mapping

Concept mapping is an instructional strategy in which learners identify, graphically display, and link key concepts. Concept maps, also called cognitive maps, mind maps, and meta cognitive tools for learning, are a proven means to promote critical thinking and self-directed learning. McHugh Schuster (2002) recommends concept mapping as a "critical-thinking approach to care planning":

The important ideas that must be linked together during clinical care planning are the medical and nursing diagnoses, along with all pertinent clinical data. Concept map care planning can be used to promote critical thinking about patient problems and treatment of problems. Through concept mapping of diagnoses and clinical data, you can evaluate what you know about the care of a patient and what further information you need to provide safe and effective nursing care. The visual map of relationships among diagnoses allows you and your clinical faculty to exchange views on why relationships exist among diagnoses. It also allows you to recognize missing diagnoses and linkages, thus suggesting further learning. (p. 3)

Steps in concept map care planning are:

1. Develop a basic skeleton diagram.
2. Analyze and categorize data.
3. Analyze nursing diagnoses relationships.
4. Identify goals, outcomes, and interventions.
5. Evaluate patient's responses.

BOX 10-9 CHECKLIST FOR EVALUATING YOUR USE OF THE NURSING PROCESS

Assessing
- ❑ The initial database is obtained by means of a nursing history and nursing examination.
- ❑ Assessment data are documented:
  - ❑ Accurately—Questionable data are validated.
  - ❑ Completely—Use of a systematic guide ensures that recorded data describe (1) the patient's functional ability to meet each basic human need, and (2) responses to health and illness.
  - ❑ Concisely—Irrelevant data and meaningless generalizations are avoided.
  - ❑ Factually—Patient behaviors are recorded rather than the nurse's interpretation of these behaviors.
  - ❑ Timely—Current data are recorded for the team.
- ❑ The initial database communicates a "real sense" of the patient that makes possible individualized care.
- ❑ Focused assessment data are recorded for each patient problem.
- ❑ Data collection and documentation are ongoing and responsive to changes in the patient's condition.

Diagnosing
- ❑ A prioritized list of nursing diagnoses is in the plan of care.
- ❑ Each nursing diagnosis describes an actual or potential patient health problem that independent nursing intervention can prevent or resolve. Each nursing diagnosis:
  - ❑ Is derived from an accurate and validated interpretation of a cluster of significant patient data or "cues"
  - ❑ Contains a precise problem statement describing what is unhealthy about the patient and what needs to change—suggests patient goals
  - ❑ Identifies factors that contribute to the problem (etiology)—these suggest nursing interventions
  - ❑ Uses nonjudgmental language and is written using legally advisable terms
- ❑ Old nursing diagnoses are deleted from the plan of care once resolved, and new diagnoses are added as soon as identified.

Outcome Identification and Planning
- ❑ A comprehensive, individualized, and up-to-date plan of care that specifies patient outcomes and nursing orders for each nursing diagnosis is developed with the assistance of the patient and family.

- ❑ Planning is comprehensive:
  - ❑ Initial
  - ❑ Ongoing
  - ❑ Discharge
- ❑ Long-term goals alert the entire nursing team to realistic patient expectations after discharge.
- ❑ Short-term outcomes:
  - ❑ When achieved, demonstrate a resolution of the problem specified in the nursing diagnosis
  - ❑ Describe a single, observable, and measurable patient behavior
  - ❑ Are valued by the patient and family
  - ❑ Are realistic in terms of the resources of the patient and the nurse
- ❑ Nursing orders:
  - ❑ Clearly and concisely describe the nursing intervention to be performed (ongoing assessment; nursing treatments and procedures; teaching, counseling, advocacy)
  - ❑ Are individualized to the patient
  - ❑ Are consistent with standards of care and supportive of other therapies
  - ❑ Are effective in accomplishing the desired patient outcomes
- ❑ The plan of care encourages patient and family participation.

Implementing
- ❑ The patient record contains daily documentation of the nursing measures used to (1) assist the patient to meet basic human needs, (2) resolve health problems, and (3) implement select aspects of the medical plan of care.
- ❑ The plan of care is implemented:
  - ❑ Competently
  - ❑ Confidently
  - ❑ Caringly
  - ❑ Creatively

Evaluating
- ❑ Evaluative statements are recorded on the plan of care to document the patient's level of outcome achievement at targeted times.
- ❑ Ongoing evaluation of the patient's responses to the plan of care is used to make decisions about terminating, continuing, or modifying nursing care.

Examples of concept maps prepared by a student at Delaware County Community College with the related patient database problem list forms are illustrated in Figure 10-7. Simple concept maps demonstrating the nursing process for featured patients can be found in selected chapters in Units VI, VII, and VIII.

REFLECTIVE PRACTICE

Reflection is a normal human activity. We frequently think about what has just happened and how it has affected us, but often this reflection is superficial. **Reflective practice** is a purposeful activity that leads to action, improvement of practice, and better patient outcomes. It is about looking at an event, understanding it, and learning from it. Learning

from reflection is not automatic and requires a deeper understanding of how and why reflection contributes to the competence of the effective nurse. Schon (1983) has identified three types of reflection.

- *Reflection in action* happens in the here and now of the activity and is also known as "thinking on your feet."
- *Reflection on action* occurs after the fact and involves thinking through a situation that has occurred in the past. It is used as a means of evaluating the experience and deciding what could have been done differently.
- *Reflection for action* is the desired outcome of the first two types of reflection, and helps the person to think about how future actions might change as a result of the reflection.

(text continues on page 226)

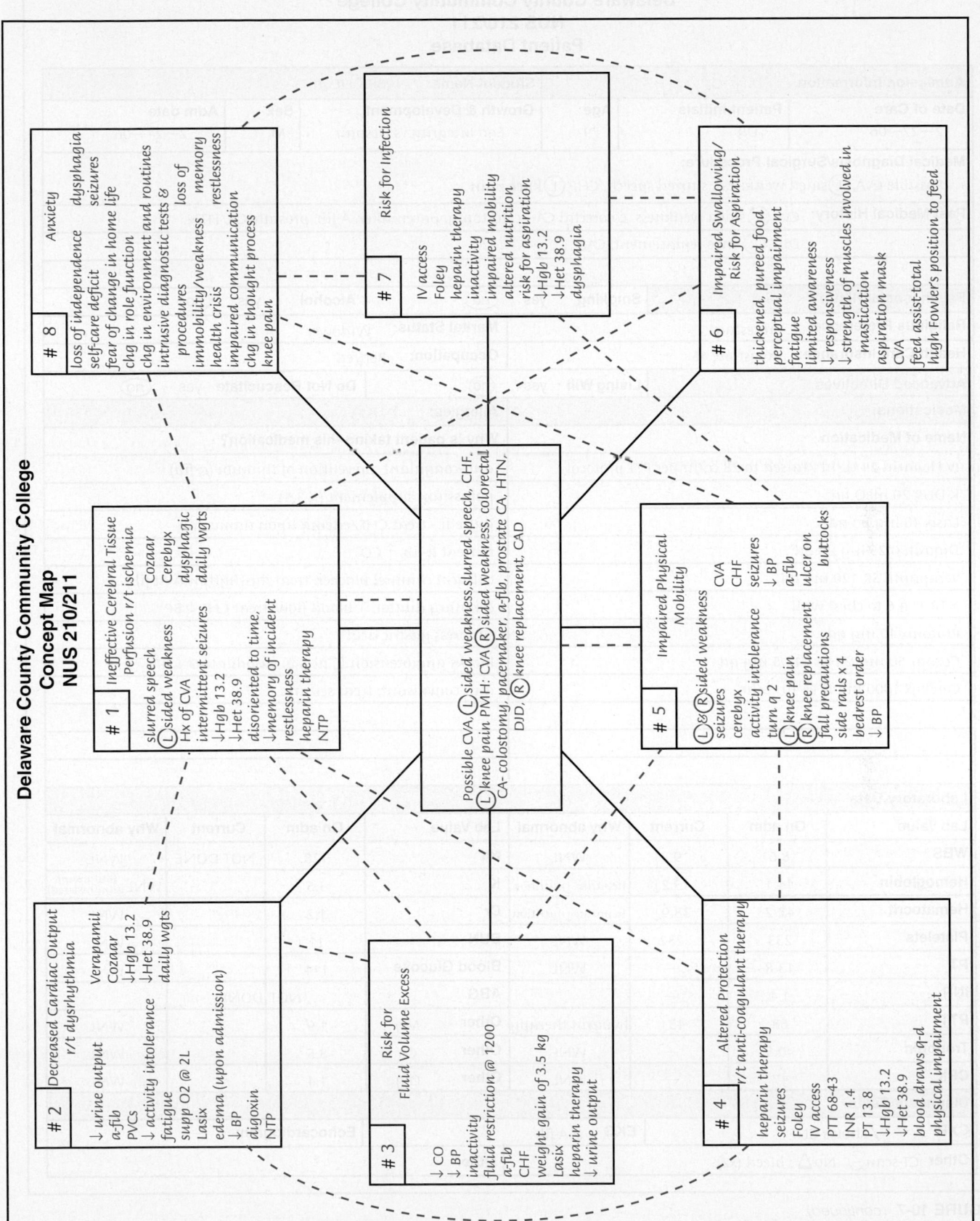

Delaware County Community College Concept Map NUS 210/211

 # 1 Ineffective Cerebral Tissue Perfusion r/t ischemia

slurred speech   Cozaar
Ⓛ sided weakness   Cerebyx
Hx of CVA   dysphagia
intermittent seizures daily wgts
↓Hgb 13.2
↓Hct 38.9
disoriented to time,
↓ memory of incident
restlessness
heparin therapy
NTP

 # 2 Decreased Cardiac Output r/t dysrhythmia

↓ urine output   Verapamil
a-fib   Cozaar
PVCs   ↓Hgb 13.2
↓ activity intolerance ↓Hct 38.9
fatigue   daily wgts
supp O2 @ 2L
Lasix
edema (upon admission)
↓ BP
digoxin
NTP

 # 3 Risk for Fluid Volume Excess

↓ CO
↓ BP
inactivity
fluid restriction @ 1200
a-fib
CHF
weight gain of 3.5 kg
Lasix
heparin therapy
↓ urine output

 # 4 Altered Protection r/t anti-coagulant therapy

heparin therapy
seizures
Foley
IV access
PTT 68-43
INR 1.4
PT 13.8
↓Hgb 13.2
↓Hct 38.9
blood draws q-d
physical impairment

(Center box)

Possible CVA, Ⓛ sided weakness, slurred speech, CHF, Ⓛ knee pain PMH: CVA Ⓡ sided weakness, colorectal CA- colostomy, pacemaker, a-fib, prostate CA, HTN, DJD, Ⓡ knee replacement, CAD

 # 8 Anxiety

loss of independence   dysphagia
self-care deficit   seizures
fear of change in home life
chg in role function
chg in environment and routines
intrusive diagnostic tests &
procedures   loss of
immobility/weakness   memory
health crisis   restlessness
impaired communication
chg in thought process
knee pain

 # 7 Risk for Infection

IV access
Foley
heparin therapy
inactivity
impaired mobility
altered nutrition
risk for aspiration
↓Hgb 13.2
↓Hct 38.9
dysphagia

 # 6 Impaired Swallowing/ Risk for Aspiration

thickened, pureed food
perceptual impairment
fatigue
limited awareness
↓ responsiveness
↓ strength of muscles involved in
mastication
aspiration mask
CVA
feed assist-total
high Fowler's position to feed

 # 5 Impaired Physical Mobility

Ⓛ & Ⓡ sided weakness   CVA
seizures   CHF
cerebyx   seizures
activity intolerance   ↓ BP
turn q 2   a-fib
Ⓛ knee pain   ulcer on
Ⓡ knee replacement   buttocks
fall precautions
side rails x 4
bedrest order
↓ BP

FIGURE 10-7. Sample concept map and supporting data. (Adapted from Schuster, P. M. [2002]. *Concept mapping: A critical-thinking approach to care planning.* Philadelphia: F. A. Davis. Completed forms used with permission from Janet Heck, Delaware County Community College.) *(continued)*

221

Delaware County Community College
NUS 210/211
Patient Database

Admission Information

			Student Name:	JANET HECK		

Date of Care	Patient Initials	Age	Growth & Development	Sex	Adm date
2—27—06	DR	79	Ego Integrity vs Despair	M	2—24—06

Medical Diagnosis/Surgical Procedure:

Possible CVA, (L)sided weakness, slurred speech, CHF, (L)knee pain

Past Medical History: CVA (R) sided weakness, colorectal CA—colostomy, pacemaker, A-fib, prostate CA, HTN, DJD, (R) knee replacement, CAD

Psychosocial History	**Smoking** yes (no)	**Alcohol** yes (no)
Religious Preference: Protestant		**Marital Status:** Widower
Health Care Insurance: Keystone 65		**Occupation:** Retired

Advanced Directives	**Living Will** yes (no)	**Do Not Rescucitate** yes (no)

Medications:	**Allergies:** NKA

Name of Medication	Why is patient taking this medication?
IV Heparin 24 cc/hr /raised to 28 cc/hr per PTT protocol	anti-coagulant -prevention of thrombi (a-fib)
K-DUR 20 meQ qd	potassium supplement (K 3.5)
Lasix 40 mg po qd	diuretic - treat CHF/edema upon admission
Digoxin 0.25 mg po qd	to treat a-fib, ↑ CO
Verapamil SR 120 mg qd	calcium channel blocker, treat dysrhythmia (a-fib)
NTP 1" q 6 to chest wall	coronary dilator, ↑ blood flow, treat CHF ↓ BP
Protonix 40 mg qd	suppress gastric acid
Cozaar 50 mg & Het 212.5 mg qd	blocks angiotension II, acts to vasodilate & ↓ BP
Cerebyx 1000 mg IV @ 10 cc/hr	anti-convulsant; treat seizures

Laboratory Data

Lab Value	On adm	Current	Why abnormal	Lab Value	On adm	Current	Why abnormal
WBS	8.6	9.2	WNL	Na	128	NOT DONE	WNL
Hemoglobin	14.1	13.2↓	heparin; ↓nutrition	K	3.5	"	WNL (but K supp administered)
Hematocrit	42.2	38.9↓	heparin; ↓nutrition	Cr	1.2	"	WNL
Platelets	233	232	WNL	BUN	11	"	WNL
PT	13.8	—	WNL	Blood Glucose	114	"	WNL
INR	1.4	—		ABG		NOT DONE	
PTT	68	43↓	heparin therapy	Other Mg	1.9	"	WNL
Troponin	<0.5	—	WNL	Other CA	8.5	"	WNL
CPK	47	—	WNL	Other Dig	1.4	"	WNL

Diagnostic Tests

CXR ✓shows CHF	EKG ✓A-fib	Echocardiogram —
Other CT-scan⊖ No △; bleed (x2)	**Other**	

FIGURE 10-7. *(continued)*

Treatments:	Daily wgts
	Pulse Ox q shift – > 90% (on 2L NC)
	No neuro checks ordered
	Turn q 2●

Diet

Type: Pureed, ↓NA 2 gm	Restrictions: thickened only 1200 cc po fluid	Appetite: Good
Difficulty Swallowing: (yes) no		Assist with Feeds: (yes) no

Fluid Status

IV solution & rate: Heparin 28 cc/hr	Type of IV access: Peri	Site condition: Ø swelling, Ø redness
24 hr intake: 1460	24 hr output: 1000	Balance: +460
5 hr intake: 480	5 hr output: 250	Balance: +230
Weight: 86.2 kg admin; 89.7 kg		Amount of gain or loss: +3.5 kg

Elimination

Continent:	Bladder: (yes) no	Bowel: (yes) no
Foley: (yes) no	Urine color: dark amber	Last BM: 2/27/06

Activity

Activity Order:	Gait:	Use of Assistive Devices:
Bedrest	N/A	N/A
Risk for Falls: (yes) no	Weakness: (yes) no	Restraints: yes (no)

Vital Signs 8 am	BP 112/60	P 66	R 16	T 97 SAO2 99%
Any additional vs 1200	94/60	70	18	97 (AX) SAO2 99%

Narrative Assessment Notes for Clinical Day:

2/27/06 0800. Rec'd pt sleeping– responsive to verbal stimuli. Pt is oriented to person, place only. Responds slowly c̄ one word answers or head motion. Heparin infusion running at 24 cc/hr s̄ incident IV site #11 shows ↓ swelling and ↓ redness. Pt denies pain. VS BP 112/60, T 97+(0); P66, R16, Pt on 2L O_2 via nc, SAO2 @ 99%. Pt has colostomy bag - no BM present. Foley draining c̄ dark amber urine. Pt's lungs are clear but decreased in bases. BS⊕, Radial and DI pulses palpable +2. Skin warm and dry. Rash evident on face– pt picks and scratches at face especially nose and mouth frequently. Inspected nose and mouth, both clear c̄ no evidence of inflammation or sores. Pt weak in both LE and upper extremities, limited mvmt. Pt grimaces upon manipulation or mvmt of (L) knee. (R) arm spasms frequently– subsides c̄ touch. Pt dozes on & off but responsive to verbal stimuli. Pt has duoderm on (L) buttock - unable to inspect wound. Complete bed bath given c̄ mouthcare, pt tolerated well. Capillary refill brisk. ↓ edema present. PEARL; heart sounds S, S_2 c̄ murmur ————————————— JM DCCCSN

FIGURE 10-7. *(continued)*

Delaware County Community College Concept Map Care Plan

Problem #1 *Ineffective Cerebral Tissue Perfusion r/t ischemia (thrombosis)*
Short-term Goal: *Cerebral perfusion pressure will be maintained during hospital stay.*
Long-term Goal: *Pt will participate in rehabilitation exercises to regain optimal strength in (L) extremities.*

Nursing Interventions:	Patient's Response:
1. *Monitor VS q 4, check pupils*	1. *BP 112/60, T97, P66, RR16, PEARL @ 0800*
2. *Monitor I & O strict q shift.*	2. *BP 94/60, T97, P70, RR18, PEARL @ 1200*
3. *Monitor pulse Ox q shift*	3. *Pt on restricted 1200 cc fluids po, 5 hr intake=480, SAO$_2$ 99% on 2L NC.*
4. *Keep head of bed 30 or lower (except when feeding)*	4. *Pt responsive to verbal stimuli, oriented to person & place.*
5. *Cluster activities to ↓ ICP.*	5. *Pt tolerated assessment, bath and feeding before tiring.*
6. *Administer heparin infusion.*	6. *Pts PTT 68 to 43.*

Summarize your impressions of patient progress towards goals *Pt displays Ø worsening of symptoms of reduced of cerebral perfusion. Continue interventions.*

Problem #2 *Decreased Cardiac Output r/t dysrhythmia*
Short-term Goal: *Pt will maintain optimally compensated cardiac output evidenced by clear lung sounds, Ø SOB, increased urine output on ↑ activity tolerance while hospitalized.*
Long-term Goal: *Pt will comply c̄ medication regimen to maintain optimal cardiac output after discharge.*

Nursing Interventions:	Patient's Response:
1. *Assess rate & quality of apical & peripheral pulses.*	1. *Pulses palpable +2, apical rate S$_1$S$_2$ c murmur; Ø pulse deficit.*
2. *Assess BP q 4*	2. *BP 112/60 @ 0800, 94/80 @ 1200.*
3. *Assess lung sounds q 2*	3. *Lungs clear but decreased in bases bilaterally.*
4. *Assess urine output.*	4. *Urine output 50 cc/hr (250 in 5 hrs)*
5. *Assess SAO$_2$.*	5. *Pt SAO$_2$ 99% c 2L O$_2$ via nc.*
6. *Weigh pt daily.*	6. *Pt has gained 3.5 kg from 2/24 to 2/27.*

Summarize your impressions of patient progress towards goals *Pt is maintaining good cardiac output as evidenced by ↑ urine output, clear lung sounds and ↓ edema. Continue interventions.*

Problem #3 *Risk for Fluid Volume Excess*
Short-term Goal: *Pt will maintain optimal fluid balance as evidenced by stable wgt, clear lung sounds, Ø edema and adequate urine output.*
Long-term Goal: *Pt will maintain fluid balance upon discharge by compliance c̄ medication regimen and fluid intake.*

Nursing Interventions:	Patient's Response:
1. *Weigh pt daily.*	1. *Pt gained 3.5 kg since admission.*
2. *Monitor strict I & O (1200 cc/24 hr)*	2. *Pt's intake was 480, output 250 in 5 hrs.*
3. *Evaluate urine output.*	3. *Urine output is 50 cc/hr for 5 hrs (0800—1300)*
4. *Administer Lasix as ordered.*	4. *Lasix given @ 1000 40 mg po.*
5. *Monitor electrolytes (side effect of diuretic)*	5. *All electrolytes WNL.*
6. *Assess for edema.*	6. *Ø edema present.*

Summarize your impressions of patient progress towards goals *Pt is maintaining optimum fluid balance presently c̄ exception of wgt gain. Continue interventions.*

Problem #4 *Altered Protection r/t anticoagulant therapy*
Short-term Goal: *Pt will maintain therapeutic blood level of anticoagulant as evidenced by PTT, PT and INR WNL.*
Long-term Goal: *Pt will set up schedule for bloodwork to be drawn after discharge to maintain therapeutic levels.*

Nursing Interventions:	Patient's Response:
1. *Monitor pt for adverse effects to anti-coagulant.*	1. *Pt shows Ø signs of unexplained bleeding– Ø bruising, Ø petechic.*
2. *Monitor vs q 4.*	2. *Pts BP 112/60, T978, P66, RR16 @ 0800, 94/60, T974, P20, RR18@1200.*
3. *Ensure IV infusion & site is uninterrupted.*	3. *Heparin infusing s̄ incident, IV site shows Ø signs of inflammation or bleeding.*
4. *Monitor lab results of PTT, PT, INR and intact.*	4. *Pts PTT 68 to 43, PT 13.8, INR 1.4.*
5. *Monitor Hgb & Hct for internal bleeding.*	5. *Hgb ↓ 13.2, Hct 38.9 ↓*

Summarize your impressions of patient progress towards goals *Pt currently shows Ø signs of bleeding caused by anti-coagulant therapy. Continue to monitor –check H&H to see if continues downward trend. Continue interventions.*

FIGURE 10-7. *(continued)*

Delaware County Community College Concept Map Care Plan

Problem #5 *Impaired Physical Mobility*
Short-term Goal: *Pt will maintain maximum level of function and risk of complications will be reduced while hospitalized.*
Long-term Goal: *Pt will regain optimal level of functioning as dictated by severity of CVA.*

Nursing Interventions:	Patient's Response:
1. *Assess pt's degree of weakness in both upper & lower extremities.*	1. *Pt's ⓁL side shows ↑ weakness to ⓇR side.*
2. *Determine active & passive ROM capabilities.*	2. *Pt can move ⓇR arm independently, other extremities require passive ROM.*
3. *Monitor skin integrity for potential breakdown.*	3. *Pt's skin intact c̄ exception of ⓁL buttock -opaque dsg- cannot assess.*
4. *Change pt's position q 2.*	4. *Pt appears comfortable, Ø breakdown present.*
5. *Use pressure relieving devices to ↓ stress.*	5. *Placed pillows under legs to elevate heels, pillow under ⓇR or ⓁL side to ↓ pressure on sacrum.*
6. *Implement fall precautions for pt safety.*	6. *Side rails x 4, bed in low, locked position.*

Summarize your impressions of patient progress towards goals   *Pt has Ø falls. Pt shows Ø skin breakdown and passive ROM performed on lower extremities & ⓁL arm. Continue interventions.*

Problem #6 *Impaired Swallowing/Risk for Aspiration*
Short-term Goal: *Pt will not experience aspiration while hospitalized.*
Long-term Goal: *Pt will maintain adequate nutrition, as evidenced by stable wgt and albumin WNL.*

Nursing Interventions:	Patient's Response:
1. *Before mealtime, provide adequate rest periods.*	1. *Pt was able to stay alert through meal.*
2. *Provide oral care before feeding.*	2. *Pt's mouth moistened, displayed good appetite.*
3. *Place pt in high Fowler's position for feeding.*	3. *Pt swallowed and chewed well.*
4. *Prompt pt to chew/swallow.*	4. *Pt responsive to prompts.*
5. *Identity food given to pt before each mouthful.*	5. *Pt nodded recognition- frowned to display distaste.*
6. *Crush pills and place in pureed food.*	6. *Pt took all medications s̄ incident*

Summarize your impressions of patient progress towards goals   *Pt did not aspirate and completed 75% of meals. Continue interventions.*

Problem #7 *Risk for Infection*
Short-term Goal: *Pt will remain free of infection as evidenced by VS WNL, Ø purulent drainage from tubes.*
Long-term Goal: *Pt will remain free of infection post discharge.*

Nursing Interventions:	Patient's Response:
1. *Monitor VS q 4.*	1. *VS WNL: Temp 97, HR66.*
2. *Monitor WBC.*	2. *WBC WNL - 9.2.*
3. *Monitor pt for S & S of infection.*	3. *Pt shows Ø S & S of inflammation, swelling, drainage at any IV site.*
4. *Practice aseptic technique at all times.*	4. *Pt remains free of infection.*
5. *Monitor appearance of urine.*	5. *Pt's urine is dark, amber color. MD notified. Culture ordered.*
6. *Encourage intake of protein & calorie rich foods.*	6. *Pt completes app. 75% of food offered.*

Summarize your impressions of patient progress towards goals   *Pt has remained free of S/S of infection—awaiting results of urine culture. Continue interventions.*

Problem #8 *Anxiety*
Short-term Goal: *Pt will demonstrate a reduced level of anxiety evidenced by ↓ seizures, ↓ restlessness.*
Long-term Goal: *Pt will demonstrate positive coping mechanisms.*

Nursing Interventions:	Patient's Response:
1. *Acknowledge awareness of pt's anxiety.*	1. *Pt appeared grateful, nodded affirmatively.*
2. *Maintain a calm manner c̄ pt.*	2. *Pt appears calm and responsive.*
3. *Maintain frequent contact c̄ pt.*	3. *Pt demonstrates recognition when I appear.*
4. *Use simple language & brief statements to explain procedures & tasks.*	4. *Pt followed commands appropriately.*
5. *Reduce sensory stimuli.*	5. *Pt appears calm and resting comfortably.*

Summarize your impressions of patient progress towards goals   *Pt is experiencing less restlessness and appears more comfortable c̄ environment. Continue interventions.*

FIGURE 10-7. *(continued)*

Table 10-4 GIBBS'S MODEL OF REFLECTION

Description	What happened? Don't make judgments yet or try to draw conclusions; simply describe.
Feelings	What were your reactions and feelings? Again, don't move to analyzing these yet.
Evaluation	What was bad or good about the experience? Make value judgments.
Analysis	What sense can you make of the situation? Bring in ideas from outside the experience to help you. What was really going on? Were different people's experiences similar or different in important ways?
Conclusions (general)	What can be concluded, in a general sense, from these experiences and the analyses you have undertaken?
Conclusions (specific)	What can be concluded about your own specific, unique, personal situation or way of working?
Personal Action Plan	What are you going to do differently in this type of situation next time? What steps are you going to take on the basis of what you have learned?

Reprinted with permission from Gibbs, G. (1988). Learning by doing: A guide to teaching and learning methods. Further Education Unit, Oxford, UK: Polytechnic. Available at http://www.brookes.ac.uk/services/upgrade/study-skills/reflective-gibbs.html

Gibbs's model of reflective practice is used by many nurses to learn from and improve their practice (Table 10-4).

SUPPOSE the nursing student caring for Addie Warner mistakenly gives her the medications she was supposed to give to another patient. She can use the critical reflection in action through the critical incident analysis described in Table 10-5 to learn from this experience.

Try to identify a recent situation that left you feeling disappointed in yourself. Then use Gibbs's reflective cycle questions to analyze what happened so that you can use what you learned about yourself to guide future experiences.

Table 10-5 CRITICAL REFLECTION IN ACTION THROUGH CRITICAL INCIDENT ANALYSIS

REFLECTIVE PRACTICE	REFLECTIVE QUESTIONS	LEARNING
Self-awareness These questions are aimed at helping the nursing student to become more aware of self.	What was my role in the incident?	I gave the drug to the wrong patient. The drug was meant for my second patient—not Addie Warner. I was in a rush and did not check the eleven rights of drug administration.
	What did I learn about myself?	When I am in a rush I take shortcuts.
Reflection These questions are aimed at helping the student to identify deficits in knowledge and the actions or inactions that contributed to the situation.	What circumstances may have contributed to my error?	The unit was very busy and I was already behind on my work and trying to do three things at once. I asked someone to check the drug with me, but I knew they were also busy and not focused on the task at hand.
	Were there any knowledge deficits that contributed to my error? If so, how might I overcome these?	I already knew the eleven rights but did not check them, so the deficit relates to acting on my knowledge rather than a lack of knowledge.
	Were there any environmental issues that may have contributed to the error occurring?	This patient had been so demanding all morning that she certainly had me "on edge" and worried about finishing all I had to do before needing to leave the floor for post-conference.
	What did I learn from the incident?	This reinforced the importance of checking and also of my role in safe administration of medication. I also learned why I can't let demanding patients "rattle" me. Luckily the patient did not suffer an adverse reaction, but it did make me stop and think about my practice.
	How might I act differently in the future?	I will think about the patient first and ensure I am not rushed during drug administration. I will ask for help.

(Reprinted with permission from Dempsey, J., Hillege, S., & Hill, R. (2013). *Fundamentals of nursing and midwifery: A person-centered approach to care* (2nd ed.) (p. 248). Sydney: Wolters Kluwer/Lippincott Williams & Wilkins.)

Nurses who are sincerely committed to quality person-centered care learn early to make reflection and self-evaluation an integral part of their nursing practice. Self-evaluation skills promote professional development, enhance self-esteem, and help one develop self-awareness. The Reflective Practice exercises in each chapter illustrate this practice. Each exercise describes a particular challenge to the student's competence, a range of possible responses, the criteria the student used to evaluate a good response, and a brief statement about what the student learned from this experience. A nurse who is just beginning to develop in the caregiver role might find it helpful to conclude each caregiving experience with a brief moment of reflection that identifies and celebrates the nursing skills used and targets skills that still need to be developed. This practice can keep you from feeling overwhelmed by everything that remains to be mastered and yet strongly motivated to learn new skills.

DEVELOPING CLINICAL REASONING

1. A nursing student realizes that her college roommate's behavior has changed dramatically during the past month. Once outgoing and funny, she is now withdrawn and moody, rebuffing efforts to discuss her change. Compare and contrast the processes and likely outcomes of using different methods of problem solving (trial-and-error, scientific, intuitive) and the nursing process to address the roommate's needs.

2. The nursing process is an interpersonal process that is always person centered rather than task centered. Discuss with other students the meaning of this claim. Think through (and discuss) the implications of approaching patients as "problems to be solved" rather than as unique human beings with inherent dignity.

3. Describe how you would structure an assessment of the following situation, using critical thinking considerations: purpose of thinking, adequacy of knowledge, potential problems, helpful resources, and critique of judgment/decision.
   - A 28-year-old woman is admitted to a hospital for multiple contusions and a hairline fracture of the skull. She claims that she "fell down the steps," but on examination, several of the injuries seem inconsistent with a fall. The woman sticks to her story that her fall was an accident. You are her nurse.
   - Assess whether your attitudes and dispositions would help or hinder the task of critical thinking if you were the nurse in this situation. Share your self-evaluation with another student and compare your responses.

4. Using the just described scenario, identify the cognitive, technical, interpersonal, and ethical/legal skills you would need to meet the nursing needs of this woman. If possible, compare your list with that of an experienced nurse and discuss differences.

PRACTICING FOR NCLEX

1. Read the following patient scenario and identify the step of the nursing process represented by each numbered and bold-faced nursing activity.

   Annie seeks the help of the nurse in the student health clinic because she suspects that her roommate, Angela, suffered date rape. She is concerned because Angela chose not to report the rape and does not seem to be coping well. (1) ***After talking with Annie, the nurse learns that although Angela blurted out that she had been raped when she first came home, since then she has refused verbalization about the rape ("I don't want to think or talk about it"), has stopped attending all college social activities (a marked change in behavior), and seems to be having nightmares.*** *After analyzing the data, the nurse believes that Angela might be experiencing* (2) ***rape-trauma syndrome: silent reaction.*** *Fortunately, Angela trusts Annie and is willing to come to the student health center for help. A conversation with Angela confirms the nurse's suspicions, and problem identification begins. The nurse talks further with Angela* (3) ***to develop some treatment goals and formulate outcomes.*** *The nurse also begins to think about the types of nursing interventions most likely to yield the desired outcomes. In the initial meeting with Angela,* (4) ***the nurse encourages her expression of feelings and helps her to identify personal coping strategies and strengths.*** *The nurse and Angela decide to meet in 1 week* (5) ***to assess her progress toward achieving targeted outcomes.*** *If she is not making progress, the plan of care might need to be modified.*

   (1) _____

   (2) _____

   (3) _____

   (4) _____

   (5) _____

2. A female patient who is receiving chemotherapy for breast cancer tells the nurse, "The treatment for this cancer is worse than the disease itself. I'm not going to come for my therapy anymore." The nurse responds by using critical thinking skills to address this patient problem. Which action is the first step the nurse would take in this process?
   a. The nurse judges whether the patient database is adequate to address the problem.
   b. The nurse considers whether or not to suggest a counseling session for the patient.
   c. The nurse reassesses the patient and decides how best to intervene in her care.
   d. The nurse identifies several options for intervening in the patient's care and critiques the merit of each option.

3. The nursing process ensures that nurses are person centered rather than task centered. Rather than simply approaching a patient to take vital signs, the nurse thinks, "How is Mrs. Barclay today? Are our nursing actions helping her to achieve her goals? How can we better help her?" This demonstrates which characteristic of the nursing process?
   a. Systematic
   b. Interpersonal
   c. Dynamic
   d. Universally applicable in nursing situations

4. An experienced nurse tells a beginning nurse not to bother studying too hard, since most clinical reasoning becomes "second nature" and "intuitive" once you start practicing. What thinking below should underlie the beginning nurse's response?
   a. Intuitive problem solving comes with years of practice and observation, and novice nurses should base their care on scientific problem solving.
   b. For nursing to remain a science, nurses must continue to be vigilant about stamping out intuitive reasoning.

c. The emphasis on logical, scientific, evidence-based reasoning has held nursing back for years; it's time to champion intuitive, creative thinking!

d. It's simply a matter of preference; some nurses are logical, scientific thinkers, and some are intuitive, creative thinkers.

5. The nurse uses blended competencies when caring for patients in a rehabilitation facility. Which examples of interventions involve cognitive skills? Select all that apply.

a. The nurse uses critical thinking skills to plan care for a patient.

b. The nurse correctly administers IV saline to a patient who is dehydrated.

c. The nurse assists a patient to fill out an informed consent form.

d. The nurse learns the correct dosages for patient pain medications.

e. The nurse comforts a mother whose baby was born with Down syndrome.

f. The nurse uses the proper procedure to catheterize a female patient.

6. A nurse uses critical thinking skills to focus on the care plan of an elderly patient who has dementia and needs placement in a long-term care facility. Which statements describe characteristics of this type of critical thinking applied to clinical reasoning? Select all that apply.

a. It functions independently of nursing standards, ethics, and state practice acts.

b. It is based on the principles of the nursing process, problem solving, and the scientific method.

c. It is driven by patient, family, and community needs as well as nurses' needs to give competent, efficient care.

d. It is not designed to compensate for problems created by human nature, such as medication errors.

e. It is constantly re-evaluating, self-correcting, and striving for improvement.

f. It focuses on the big picture rather than identifying the key problems, issues, and risks involved with patient care.

7. A nurse is caring for a patient who has complications related to type 2 diabetes mellitus. The nurse researches new procedures to care for foot ulcers when developing a plan of care for this patient. Which QSEN competency does this action represent?

a. Patient-centered care

b. Evidence-based practice

c. Quality improvement

d. Informatics

8. A nurse is assessing a 15-year-old female patient who is diagnosed with anorexia. Following the assessment, the nurse recommends that the patient meet with a nutritionist. This action best exemplifies the use of:

a. Clinical judgment

b. Clinical reasoning

c. Critical thinking

d. Blended competencies

9. A nurse working in a long-term care facility bases patient care on five caring processes: knowing, being with, doing for, enabling, and maintaining belief. This approach to patient care best describes the theory of which theorist?

a. Travelbee

b. Watson

c. Benner

d. Swanson

10. The nurse practices using critical thinking indicators (CTIs) when caring for patients in the hospital setting. The best description of CTIs is:

a. Evidence-based descriptions of behaviors that demonstrate the knowledge that promotes critical thinking in clinical practice

b. Evidence-based descriptions of behaviors that demonstrate the knowledge and skills that promote critical thinking in clinical practice

c. Evidence-based descriptions of behaviors that demonstrate the knowledge, characteristics, and skills that promote critical thinking in clinical practice

d. Evidence-based descriptions of behaviors that demonstrate the knowledge, characteristics, standards, and skills that promote critical thinking in clinical practice

ANSWERS WITH RATIONALES

1. (1) is an illustration of assessing: the collection of patient data. (2) is an illustration of the identification of a nursing diagnosis: a health problem that independent nursing intervention can resolve. (3) is an illustration of planning: outcome identification and related nursing interventions. (4) is an illustration of implementing: carrying out the plan of care. (5) is an illustration of evaluating: measuring the extent to which Angela has achieved targeted outcomes.

2. *c.* The first step when thinking critically about a situation is to identify the purpose or goal of your thinking. Reassessing the patient helps to discipline thinking by directing all thoughts toward the goal. Once the problem is addressed, it is important for the nurse to judge the adequacy of the knowledge, identify potential problems, use helpful resources, and critique the decision.

3. *b,* interpersonal. All of the other options are characteristics of the nursing process, but the conversation and thinking quoted best illustrates the interpersonal dimension of the nursing process.

4. *a.* Beginning nurses must use nursing knowledge and scientific problem solving as the basis of care they give; intuitive problem solving comes with years of practice and observation. If the beginning nurse has an intuition about a patient, that information should be discussed with the faculty member, preceptor, or supervisor. Answer *b* is incorrect because there is a place for intuitive reasoning in nursing, but it will never replace logical, scientific reasoning. Critical thinking is contextual and changes depending on the circumstances, not on personal preference.

5. *a, d.* Using critical thinking and learning medication dosages are cognitive competencies. Performing procedures correctly is a technical skill, helping a patient with an informed consent form is a legal/ethical issue, and comforting a patient is an interpersonal skill.

6. *b, c, e.* Critical thinking applied to clinical reasoning and judgment in nursing practice is guided by standards, policies and procedures, and ethics codes. It is based on principles of nursing process, problem solving, and the scientific method. It carefully identifies the key problems, issues, and risks involved, and is driven by patient, family, and community

needs, as well as nurses' needs to give competent, efficient care. It also calls for strategies that make the most of human potential and compensate for problems created by human nature. It is constantly re-evaluating, self-correcting, and striving to improve (Alfaro-LeFevre, 2014).

7. *c.* Quality improvement involves routinely updating nursing policies and procedures. Providing patient-centered care involves listening to the patient and demonstrating respect and compassion. Evidence-based practice is used when adhering to internal policies and standardized skills. The nurse is employing informatics by using information and technology to communicate, manage knowledge, and support decision making.

8. *a.* Although all the options refer to the skills used by nurses in practice, the best choice is clinical judgment as it refers to the result or outcome of critical thinking or clinical reasoning—in this case the recommendation to meet with a nutritionist. Clinical reasoning usually refers to ways of thinking about patient care issues (determining, preventing, and managing patient problems). Critical thinking is a broad term that includes reasoning both outside and inside of the clinical setting. Blended competencies are the cognitive, technical, interpersonal, and ethical/legal skills combined with the willingness to use them creatively and critically when working with patients.

9. *d.* Swanson (1991) identifies five caring processes and defines caring as "a nurturing way of relating to a valued other toward whom one feels a personal sense of commitment and responsibility. Travelbee (1971), an early nurse theorist, developed the Human-to-Human Relationship Model and defined nursing as an interpersonal process whereby the professional nurse practitioner assists an individual, family, or community to prevent or cope with the experience of illness and suffering, and if necessary to find meaning in these experiences. Benner and Wrubel (1989) write that caring is a basic way of being in the world and that caring is central to human expertise, curing, and healing. Watson's theory is based on the belief that all humans are to be valued, cared for, respected, nurtured, understood, and assisted.

10. *c,* evidence-based descriptions of behaviors that demonstrate the knowledge, characteristics, and skills that promote critical thinking in clinical practice.

TAYLOR SUITE RESOURCES

Explore these additional resources to enhance learning for this chapter:
- NCLEX-Style Questions and other resources on thePoint, http://thePoint.lww.com/Taylor8e
- *Study Guide for Fundamentals of Nursing, 8th edition*
- Adaptive Learning | Powered by prepU, http://thepoint.lww.com/prepu

Bibliography

Alfaro-LeFevre, R. (2013). *Critical thinking, clinical reasoning, and clinical judgment* (5th ed.). St. Louis: Elsevier/Saunders.

Alfaro-LeFevre, R. (2009). *Critical thinking and clinical judgment: A practical approach* (4th ed.). St. Louis: Elsevier/Saunders.

Alfaro-LeFevre, R. (2012). Teaching Smart/Learning Easy. Available at http://www.AlfaroTeachSmart.com

Alfaro-LeFevre, R. (2014). *Applying nursing process: The Foundation for Clinical Reasoning* (8th ed.). Philadelphia: Wolters Kluwer/Lippincott Williams & Wilkins.

American Association of Colleges of Nursing (AACN). (2008). The essentials of baccalaureate education for professional nursing practice. Washington, DC: Author.

American Nurses Association (ANA). (2001). *Code for nurses with interpretive statements.* Washington, DC: Author.

American Nurses Association (ANA). (2010a). Nursing's Social Policy Statement, 2010 edition. Silver Spring, MD: Author.

American Nurses Association (ANA). (2010b). *Nursing: Scope and standards of practice,* 2nd ed. Silver Spring, MD: Author.

Andersen, B. (1991). Mapping the terrain of the discipline. In G. Gray and R. Pratt (eds.) *Towards a discipline of nursing* (pp. 95–124). Melbourne: Churchill Livingstone.

Androwich, I. (Ed.), American Medical Informatics Association, American Nurses Association, American Nurses Pub. (2002). *Clinical information systems: A framework for reaching the vision.* Washington, DC: American Nurses Association.

Baxter, P. E., & Boblin, S. (2008). Decision making by baccalaureate nursing students in the clinical setting. *Journal of Nursing Education, 47*(8), 345–350.

Benner, P. (2001). *From novice to expert.* Menlo Park, CA: Addison-Wesley.

Benner, P. (2005). Extending the dialogue about classification systems and the work of professional nurses. *American Journal of Critical Care, 14*(3), 242–243, 272.

Benner, P., & Wrubel, J. (1989). *The primacy of caring in health and illness.* Menlo Park, CA: Addison-Wesley.

Bulechek, G. M., Butcher, H. K., & Dochterman, J. (Eds.). (2013). *Nursing interventions classification [NIC]* (6th ed.). St. Louis, MO: Elsevier.

Craft-Rosenberg, M., & Delaney M. (1997). Nursing diagnosis extension and classification (NDEC). In M. J. Rantz & D. LeMone (Eds.), *Classification of nursing diagnoses: Proceedings of the Twelfth Conference North American Nursing Diagnosis* (pp. 26–31). Glendale, CA: CINAHL Information Services.

Cronenwett, L., Sherwood, G., Barnsteiner J., Disch, J., Johnson, J., Mitchell, P.,.... Warren, J. (2007). Quality and safety education for nurses. *Nursing Outlook, 55*(3)122–131.

Daley, B. J. (1996). Concept maps: Linking nursing theory to clinical nursing practice. *Journal of Continuing Education in Nursing, 27*(1), 17–27.

Davies, E. (1995). Reflective practice: A focus for caring. *Journal of Nursing Education, 34*(4), 167–174.

Dempsey, J., Hillege, S., & Hill, R. (2013). *Fundamentals of nursing and midwifery: A person-centered approach to care* (2nd ed.). Sydney: Wolters Kluwer/ Lippincott Williams & Wilkins.

Diers, D. (2004). *Speaking of nursing...Narratives of practice, research, policy and the profession.* Sudbury, MA: Jones and Bartlett Publishers.

DiVito-Thomas, P. (2000). Identifying critical thinking behaviors in clinical judgments. *Journal of Nursing Staff Development, 16*(3), 174–180.

DiVito-Thomas, P. (2005). Nursing student stories on learning how to think like a nurse. *Nurse Educator, 30*(3), 133.

Dochterman, J. M., & Jones, D. A. (2003). *Unifying nursing languages: The harmonization of NANDA, NIC, NOC.* Washington, DC: American Nurses Association.

Dossey, B. M., & Dossey, L. (1998). Body, mind, spirit. Attending to holistic care. *American Journal of Nursing, 98*(8), 35–38.

Ferrario, C. G. (2003). Experienced and less-experienced nurses' diagnostic reasoning: Implications for fostering students' critical thinking. *International Journal of Nursing Terminologies and Classifications, 14*(2), 41–52.

Ferrario, C. G. (2004). Developing nurses' critical thinking skills with concept mapping. *Journal for Nurses in Staff Development, 20*(6), 261–267.

Frampton, S., Guastello, S., Brady, C., Hale, M., Horowitz, S., Smith, S.B. & Stone, S. (2008). Person-centered care improvement guide. Available at http://planetree.org/wp-content/uploads/2012/01/Person-centered-Care-Improvement-Guide-10-28-09-Final.pdf

Gebbie, K., & Lavin, M. A. (1974). Classification of nursing diagnosis. *American Journal of Nursing, 74,* 250–253.

Glaze, J. E. (2002). Stages in coming to terms with reflection: Student advanced nurse practitioners' perceptions of their reflective journeys. *Journal of Advanced Nursing, 37*(3), 265–272.

Hall, L. E. (1955). Quality of nursing care. Address given at the Department of Baccalaureate and Higher Degree Programs of the New Jersey League for Nursing. *Public Health News (June).* Trenton, NJ: New Jersey State Department of Health.

Hansten, R., & Washburn, M. (2001). Intuition in professional practice: Executive and staff perceptions. *Journal of Nursing Administration, 30*(4), 185–188.

Hill, C. (2006). Integrating clinical experiences into the concept mapping process. *Nurse Educator, 31*(1), 36.

Hinck, S. M., Webb, P., Sims-Giddens, S., Helton, C., Hope, K. L., Utley, R.,...Yarbrough, S. (2006). Student learning with concept mapping of care plans in community-based education. *Journal of Professional Nursing, 22*(1), 23.

Hoffman, K. (2007). Unpublished PhD thesis, A comparison of decision-making by "expert" and "novice" nurses in the clinical setting, monitoring patient haemodynamic status post abdominal aortic aneurysm surgery. University of Technology, Sydney.

Institute of Medicine (IOM). (2003). Health professions education: A bridge to quality. Washington DC: National Academies Press.

Iowa Intervention Project. (1997). Nursing interventions classification (NIC): An overview. In M. J. Rantz & P. LeMone (Eds.), *Classification of nursing diagnoses: Proceedings of the Twelfth Conference, North American Nursing Diagnosis* (pp. 32–39). Glendale, CA: CINAHL Information Systems.

Irvine, L. (1995). Can concept mapping be used to promote meaningful learning in nurse education. *Journal of Advanced Nursing, 21,* 1175–1179.

Jackson, M., Ignatavicius, D., & Case, B. (Eds.). (2004). *Conversations in critical thinking and clinical judgment.* Pensacola, FL: Pohl Publishing.

Joint Commission on Accreditation of Healthcare Organizations (JCAHO). (2005). *Accreditation manual for hospitals.* Oakbrook Terrace, IL: Author.

King, M., & Shell, R. (2002). Teaching and evaluating critical thinking with concept maps. *Nurse Educator, 27*(5), 214.

Lamond, D., & Thompson, C. (2000). Intuition and analysis in decision making and choice. *Journal of Nursing Scholarship, 32*(3), 411–414.

Levett-Jones, T., Hoffman, K., Dempsey, J., Jeong, S. Y-S, Noble, D., Norton, C.A., ... Hickey, N. (2010). The 'five rights' of clinical reasoning: An educational model to enhance nursing students' ability to identify and manage clinically 'at risk' patients. *Nurse Education Today, 30*(6), 515–520, DOI: 10.1016/j.nedt.2009.10.020

Lewenson, S. B., & Truglio-Londrigan, M. (2008). *Decision-making in nursing: Thoughtful approaches for practice.* Boston: Jones and Bartlett.

Lipe, S. K., & Beasley, S. (2004). *Critical thinking in nursing: A cognitive skills workbook.* Philadelphia: Lippincott Williams & Wilkins.

Locsin, R. C. (1995). Machine technologies and caring in nursing. *Image—The Journal of Nursing Scholarship, 27*(3), 201–203.

Moorhead, S., Johnson, M., Maas, M. L., & Swanson, E. (2013). *Nursing outcomes classification (NOC)* (5th ed.). St. Louis: Elsevier.

Mueller, A., Johnston, M., & Bligh, D. (2002). Joining mind and mapping care planning to enhance student critical thinking and achieve holistic nursing care. *Nursing Diagnosis, 13*(1), 24–27.

Myrick, R., & Yonge, O. (2004). Enhancing critical thinking in the preceptorship experience in nursing education. *Journal of Advanced Nursing, 45*(4), 371–380.

NANDA International. (2009). *Nursing diagnoses: Definitions & classification, 2012–2014.* West Sussex, UK: Wiley-Blackwell.

Paul, R. W. (1993). *Critical thinking: How to prepare students for a rapidly changing world.* Santa Rosa, CA: Foundation for Critical Thinking.

Preheim, G., Armstrong, G. E., & Barton, A. (2009). The NEW fundamentals in nursing: Introducing beginning quality and safety education for nurses (QSEN) competencies. *Journal of Nursing Education, 48*(12), 694–698.

Profetto-McGrath, J. (2003). The relationship of critical thinking skills and critical thinking dispositions of baccalaureate nursing students. *Journal of Advanced Nursing, 43*(6), 569–577.

Rew, L. (1987). Nursing intuition: Too powerful— and too valuable—to ignore. *Nursing, 17*(7), 43–45.

Rodak, S., (2012). 10 Guiding Principles for Patient-Centered Care. Available at http://www.beckershospitalreview.com/quality/10-guiding-principles-for-person-centered-care.html

Scheffer, B., & Rubenfeld, M. (2000). A consensus statement on critical thinking in nursing. *Journal of Nursing Education, 39*(8), 352–359.

Schuster, P. M. (2002). *Concept mapping: A critical-thinking approach to care planning.* Philadelphia: F. A. Davis.

Schön, D. (1983). *The Reflective Practitioner, How Professionals Think In Action, Basic Books.*

Swanson, E. (2008). *Nursing Outcomes Classification (NOC)* (4th ed.). St. Louis: Elsevier/Mosby.

Swanson, K. M. (1991). Empirical development of a middle range theory of caring. *Nursing Research, 49*(3), 161–166.

Tanner, C. (2006). Thinking like a nurse: A research-based model of clinical judgment in nursing. *Journal of Nursing Education, 45*(6), 204–211.

Taylor, C. (1995). Rethinking nursing's basic competencies. *Journal of Nursing Care Quality, 9*(4), 1–13.

Travelbee, J. (1971). *Interpersonal aspects of nursing* (2nd ed.). Philadelphia: F.A. Davis.

Verghese, A. (2011). A doctor's touch. TED talk. Available at: http://www.ted.com/talks/abraham_verghese_a_doctor_s_touch.html

Watson, J. (2008). Nursing: The Philosophy and Science of Caring (rev. ed.), Boulder: University Press of Colorado.

Yura, H., & Walsh, M. B. (1988). *The nursing process: Assessing, planning, implementing, evaluating* (5th ed.). Norwalk, CT: Appleton-Century-Crofts.

11 | Assessing

SUSAN MORGAN

Susan is a 34-year-old woman newly diagnosed with multiple sclerosis (MS). She says, "How am I going to tell my husband? We were just married last year and planned to do lots of hiking and outdoor sports. It's not fair for him to be tied down to me if I can't be the wife and partner that he thought he had married."

SYLVIA WU

Sylvia, a 17-year-old woman, has just arrived back in the United States after a visit to her family in mainland China. She comes to the emergency department because she woke up that morning with flu-like symptoms (cough, sore throat, fever, muscle aches, fatigue). "I'm scared because of everything I've seen on television and read in the newspapers about that new virus."

JAMES FARREN

James is a college junior who comes to the student health center complaining of difficulty sleeping, eating, and studying. He reveals that his mother died when he was 8 years old, and last semester his father died suddenly in a car crash. "Ever since my dad died, nothing seems to mean anything anymore. All I see is gray."

LEARNING OBJECTIVES

After completing the chapter, you will be able to accomplish the following:

1. Define and describe the purpose of four types of nursing assessments.

2. Explain the relationship between nursing assessment and medical assessment.

3. Differentiate between objective and subjective data.

4. Identify five sources of patient data useful to the nurse.

5. Describe the purpose of nursing observation, interview, and physical assessment.

6. Obtain a nursing history using effective interviewing techniques.

7. Plan patient assessments by identifying assessment priorities and structuring the data to be collected systematically.

8. Identify common problems encountered in data collection, noting their possible causes.

9. Explain when data need to be validated and several ways to accomplish this.

10. Describe the importance of knowing when to report significant patient data and of proper documentation.

11. Obtain and document purposeful, prioritized, complete, systematic, accurate, and relevant patient data in a standard format.

KEY TERMS

assessing	initial assessment	physical assessment
cue	interview	review of systems (ROS)
data	minimum data set	subjective data
database	nursing history	time-lapsed assessment
emergency assessment	objective data	validation
focused assessment	observation	
inference		

Assessing is the systematic and continuous collection, analysis, validation, and communication of patient **data**, or information. These data reflect how health functioning is enhanced by health promotion or compromised by illness and injury. A **database** includes all the pertinent patient information collected by the nurse and other health care professionals. The database enables you to partner with patients to develop a comprehensive and effective plan of care. Assessment is the first of six nursing standards (Box 11-1); collecting patient data is a vital step in the nursing process because the remaining steps depend on purposeful, prioritized, complete, systematic, accurate, and relevant data. Assessment is critical for safety, accuracy, and efficiency (Alfaro, 2014, p. 46).

 REFER to the Reflective Practice box regarding Sylvia Wu, a patient who fears that she has a virus. The nurse's assessment would reveal possible risk factors. Additionally, the patient's statements about her fears provide further data on which to develop a plan of care. ●

BOX 11-1 AMERICAN NURSES ASSOCIATION (ANA) STANDARDS OF PRACTICE: STANDARD 1, ASSESSMENT

The registered nurse collects comprehensive data pertinent to the healthcare consumer's health and/or the situation.

Measurement Criteria

The registered nurse:

Collects comprehensive data including but not limited to physical, functional, psychosocial, emotional, cognitive, sexual, cultural, age-related, environmental, spiritual/transpersonal, and economic assessments in a systematic and ongoing process while honoring the uniqueness of the person.

Elicits the healthcare consumer's values, preferences, expressed needs, and knowledge of the healthcare situation.

Involves the healthcare consumer, family, and other healthcare providers, as appropriate, in holistic data collection.

Identifies barriers (e.g., psychosocial, literacy, financial, cultural) to effective communication and makes appropriate adaptations.

Recognizes the impact of personal attitudes, values, and beliefs.

Assesses family dynamics and impact on healthcare consumer health and wellness.

Prioritizes data collection activities based on the healthcare consumer's immediate condition, or the anticipated needs of the patient or situation.

Uses appropriate evidence-based assessment techniques, instruments, and tools.

Uses analytical models and problem-solving tools.

Synthesizes available data, information, and knowledge relevant to the situation to identify patterns and variances.

Applies ethical, legal, and privacy guidelines and policies to the collection, maintenance, use, and dissemination of data and information.

Recognizes the healthcare consumer as the authority on her or his own health by honoring their care preferences.

Documents relevant data in a retrievable format.

Reprinted with permission from American Nurses Association (ANA). (2010). *Scope and standards of practice* (2nd ed., p. 39–40). Silver Spring, MD: Author.

REFLECTIVE PRACTICE: CULTIVATING QSEN COMPETENCIES

CHALLENGE TO INTELLECTUAL SKILLS

While on a clinical rotation in the emergency department, I met Sylvia Wu, a 17-year-old woman who had just arrived back in the United States after a visit to her family in mainland China. She came to the emergency department because she woke up that morning with flu-like symptoms (cough, sore throat, fever, muscle aches, fatigue) and was terrified because of everything she had seen on television and read in the newspapers about the latest virus. Of the 64 people who have died already, she knows that most of the cases are in Asia. She came to the emergency department begging to be told that she doesn't have the virus but just fatigue or a cold. I want to calm her, but I honestly don't know what she has. Besides, I am starting to feel a bit anxious myself because the one thing everyone knows about this virus is the fact that it is extremely "contagious." I could feel myself recoil when Sylvia sneezed.

Thinking Outside the Box: Possible Courses of Action

- Reassure Sylvia and tell her not to worry because the overwhelming probability is that her symptoms aren't anything serious.
- Quickly get someone with more experience to care for Sylvia because I don't want to be anywhere near her if she does have this virus.
- Document and report her concerns, trying to keep her isolated and away from other patients, while trying to find more information about this new virus quickly, since I'm not sure about its signs and symptoms.

Evaluating a Good Outcome: How Do I Define Success?

- Sylvia gets the medical treatment she needs, and her fears are appropriately addressed.
- In the event that Sylvia does have a highly communicable disease, the risk for disease transmission to others is reduced.
- I manage to control my fears, being able to respond to Sylvia's concerns appropriately.
- I learn something about my immediate response to feeling at risk and my commitment to professionalism.

Personal Learning: Here's to the Future!

Although I am not proud of my response, I falsely reassured Sylvia that this was probably nothing. As a result, I did not report or document her fears. Unfortunately, Sylvia was diagnosed with the virus, and several others in our emergency department at that time became infected. For some reason, I escaped. In the future, I hope I'll never be so insensitive to a patient's concerns or insights again.

REFLECTION ON QUALITY AND SAFETY COMPETENCIES

How do you think you would respond in a similar situation? Why? What does this tell you about yourself and about the adequacy of your skills for professional practice? What factors might have influenced this nursing student's actions? What types of data could have led the nursing student to a different course of action? How might the nursing student have assessed the patient differently? Do you agree with the criteria that the nursing student used to evaluate a successful outcome? Why or why not? What *knowledge, skills,* and *attitudes* do you need to develop to continuously improve the quality and safety of care for patients like Ms. Wu?

Patient-Centered Care: How would you develop a partnership with Ms. Wu, knowing her fears? If steps are needed to keep others safe, how can you communicate to Ms. Wu that she is your care priority?

Teamwork and Collaboration/Quality Improvement: What communication skills do you need to improve to ensure that you function as a member of the patient care team and to obtain assistance when needed? How might the transmission of this infection have been prevented?

Safety/Evidence-Based Practice: What does the evidence point to as "best practice" in situations like this to keep everyone safe and to treat Ms. Wu effectively?

Informatics: Can you identify the essential information that must be available in Ms. Wu's electronic record to support safe patient care and coordination of care? Can you think of other ways to respond to or approach the situation? What else might the nursing student have done to ensure a successful outcome?

The initial comprehensive nursing assessment results in baseline data that enable the nurse to:

- Make a judgment about an individual's health status, ability to manage his or her own need for self-care and need for nursing care.
- Plan and deliver thoughtful, person-centered nursing care that draws on the individual's strengths and promotes optimum functioning, independence, and well-being

- Refer the patient to a physician or other health care professional, if indicated.

In addition to an initial assessment of the patient, the nurse makes ongoing assessments. These assessments alert the nurse to changes in the patient's responses to health and illness and suggest necessary changes in the plan of nursing care or care offered by other health care professionals.

Assessing
- Preparing for data collection
- Collecting data
- Indentifying cues and making inferences
- Validating data
- Clustering related data and indentifying patterns
- Reporting and recording data

Diagnosing

Outcome identification and planning

Evaluating

Implementing

FIGURE 11-1. Assessing. The primary source of patient information is the patient. Resources include the patient's support people, the patient record, information from other health care professionals, and information from nursing and health care literature.

During the assessment step of the nursing process, the nurse establishes the database by interviewing the patient to obtain a nursing history. The **nursing history** identifies the patient's health status, strengths, health problems, health risks, and need for nursing care. The nurse may also perform a nursing physical examination to collect data. Other sources of patient information used by the nurse include the patient's family and significant others, the patient record, other health care professionals, and nursing and other health care literature.

After the nurse has established the database, data about the patient are collected continuously because the patient's health status can change quickly. Questionable data are verified (validated) as part of the assessment step of the nursing process. All pertinent data are recorded and communicated to other health care professionals so that the data can best benefit the patient (Fig. 11-1). In addition to collecting data, nurses might use intuition to assess patients (see Chapter 10).

UNIQUE FOCUS OF NURSING ASSESSMENT

When nurses make nursing assessments, they do not duplicate medical assessments. Medical assessments target data pointing to pathologic conditions, whereas nursing assessments focus on the patient's responses to health problems. For example, is there interference with the patient's ability to meet basic human needs? Can the patient perform the activities of daily living? Although the findings from a nursing assessment may contribute to the identification of a medical diagnosis, the unique focus of nursing assessments is on the patient's responses to actual or potential health problems.

 REMEMBER Susan Morgan, a patient recently diagnosed with MS? By looking at the data supplied by the patient, the nurse would be able to determine that the patient's new diagnosis of MS is affecting her body image and self-esteem. The nurse then would use this information to focus assessment questions to obtain additional information to be included in the database, from which a plan of care specific to Susan's needs can be developed. ●

ASSESSMENT AND CLINICAL REASONING

Since the entire nursing process rests on the initial and ongoing assessment of the patient, it is imperative to use excellent critical thinking and clinical reasoning skills when gathering, analyzing, validating, and communicating data. Among the critical thinking activities linked to assessment are (Alfaro, 2010, p. 49):

- Assessing systematically and comprehensively, using a nursing framework to identify nursing concerns and a body systems framework to identify medical concerns

- Detecting bias and determining the credibility of information sources
- Distinguishing normal from abnormal findings and identifying the risks for abnormal findings
- Making judgments about the significance of data, distinguishing relevant from irrelevant
- Identifying assumptions and inconsistencies, checking accuracy and reliability, and recognizing missing information

To promote sound clinical reasoning, your nursing assessments should have the following characteristics:

Purposeful. When preparing for data collection, identify the purpose of the nursing assessment (comprehensive, focused, emergency, time-lapsed) and then gather the appropriate data. The circumstances of the patient's situation may also dictate the nature and amount of data collected.

Prioritized. It is essential to get the most important information first. We address how to do this later in this chapter.

Complete. As much as possible, identify all the patient data needed to understand a patient health problem and develop a plan of care to maximize the patient's health and well-being. For example, knowing that a patient has lost weight is not fully meaningful until you discover (1) if the weight loss was intentional or unintentional, (2) if it was related to a change in eating or exercise patterns or to some underlying pathologic condition, and (3) how the patient views and is responding to the weight loss.

Systematic. Using a systematic way to gather data, you will always know if you've missed something important.

Factual and accurate. Both the patient and the nurse may intentionally or unintentionally misrepresent or distort patient information. For example, a patient who values being thin may describe a weight gain of several pounds as the onset of obesity. Nurses concerned with accuracy and factual reality continually verify what they hear with what they observe, using other senses and validating all questionable data. At the outset of data collection, it is crucial to determine whether the patient or caregiver who is supplying the data is reliable. If nurses suspect that their own personal bias or stereotyping may be influencing their data collection, they should consult with another nurse. It is also best to describe observed behavior rather than to interpret the behavior. Such a description may read: "Patient frequently is observed lying with his face to the wall. Attempts to engage him in conversation fail. He refused lunch today and ate only soup for dinner." In contrast, the statement "Patient is depressed" is an interpretation of the patient's behavior, not a factual statement. Recording the patient's behaviors factually allows other health care professionals to explore causes of the behavior with the patient.

Relevant. Because recording comprehensive data can be very time consuming, one challenge facing nurses is to determine what types of and how much data to collect for each patient. As described throughout this chapter, the aim is to record concisely all pertinent data. Often, only experience teaches nurses what data are needed in specific cases.

Recorded in a standard manner. Data cannot be efficiently used unless the information is recorded according to agency policy so that all caregivers can easily access what you learned.

Learning how to collect, validate, and communicate data that are purposeful, prioritized, complete, systematic, accurate, and relevant is the focus of the remainder of this chapter. Many assessment activities are challenging for those new to nursing, who often lack the sorts of clinical experience that facilitate expert clinical reasoning. Thus, students are urged to ask questions frequently about data and to test their inferences and judgments.

ASSESSMENT AND INTERPERSONAL COMPETENCE

The nurse's interpersonal competence is critical beginning with the very first assessment by the nurse. The patient's initial impression of the nurse is crucial, especially with patients who are new to the health care environment. *The patient may judge all nurses encountered in the future in light of this first impression.* When the nurse communicates respect and genuine concern for the patient, the patient is encouraged to discuss health concerns and problems freely. The nurse's competence and professionalism as well as the interpersonal qualities of being respectful and caring invite the patient's confidence and assure the patient that help is available. Successful assessments begin with the trust and confidence an interpersonally competent nurse inspires. See the Guidelines for Nursing Care: Promoting a Caring Interview on page 245.

TYPES OF NURSING ASSESSMENTS

Nursing assessments include the comprehensive initial assessment, the focused assessment, the emergency assessment, and the time-lapsed assessment. This chapter focuses on assessing the health status of an individual patient, but as you develop expertise in nursing assessments you will also be able to assess communities and special populations, such as schoolchildren or people with AIDS or other infectious diseases.

Initial Assessment

The **initial assessment** is performed shortly after the patient is admitted to a health care agency or service. Most institutions have policies specifying the time interval within which this assessment must be completed. The purpose of this assessment is to establish a complete database for problem identification and care planning. The nurse collects data concerning all aspects of the patient's health, establishing priorities for ongoing focused assessments and creating a

Esposito, Tomas Gender: Male , DOB: 1/16/1967 (46y)   Height: **72 in** Weight: **185 lb**   MRN: **984521**   Allergies: Penicillin
Primary Adm Dx: Pneumonia   Location: Mercy Hospital Rm: 412   Contact Precaution: Standard
Adm Provider: Tom Rankle, Admitting   Adm On: 11/29/2013 14:45 (3 day(s))   Adv Directive: Full Code

| Patient Information | Assessment | ADLs | Notes | Nursing Dx | Orders | MAR | I/O | Vital Signs | Diagnostics | Flowsheet | Monday, December 2, 2013 15:56:35 |

Back To Current Assessment

Charted at 12/2/2013 14:45 By: Tom Rankle, Admitting

ADL Assessment
✓ Bed mobility
Description of assessment activity: Limited assistance
✓ Transfer
Description of assessment activity: Limited assistance
✓ Walking
Description of assessment activity: Supervision needed
✓ Dressing
Description of assessment activity: Extensive assistance
✓ Eating
Description of assessment activity: Limited assistance
✓ Toilet use
Description of assessment activity: Extensive assistance
✓ Personal hygiene
Description of assessment activity: Limited assistance
✓ Bathing
Description of assessment activity: Total dependence

Diet Consumption
○ 25%
○ 50%
✓ 75%
○ 100%

Diet Assessment
☐ Increased appetite
✓ Decreased appetite
☐ Aspiration risk
☐ Difficulty chewing
☐ Dysphagia
☐ Weight gain
☐ Weight loss

Communication
✓ Short-term memory intact
✓ Long-term memory intact
✓ Has ability to understand
✓ Has ability to make self-understood

Speech Assessment
☐ Rate
☐ Rhythm
✓ Content
Speech clear and appropriate.

☐ Loudness
☐ Fluency
☐ Quantity
☐ Articulation
☐ Pattern

Mood and Behavior
☐ Verbal expression of distress
☐ Loss of interest
☐ Sleep pattern disturbance
☐ Apathetic
☐ Anxious
☐ Sad appearance
✓ Appropriate for patient

Notes:

How does the resident make decisions about ADLs
Patient requires direction to complete personal hygiene ADLs.

FIGURE 11-2. Section of sample electronic nursing admission assessment form. (© Cerner Corporation. All rights reserved. Reprinted with permission.)

reference baseline for future comparison. See Figure 11-2 for a sample of an initial assessment in an electronic medical record. For an example of a handwritten admission database, see Figure 11-3.

Focused Assessment

In a **focused assessment**, the nurse gathers data about a specific problem that has already been identified. Helpful questions include:

- What are your signs and symptoms?
- When did they start?
- Were you doing anything different than usual when they started?
- What makes your symptoms better? Worse?
- Are you taking any remedies (medical or natural) for your symptoms?

A focused assessment may be done during the initial assessment if the patient's health problems surface, but it is routinely part of ongoing data collection. Another purpose of the focused assessment is to identify new or overlooked problems. Quick priority assessments (QPA) are short, focused, prioritized assessments you do to gain the most important information you need to have first. They are

important because they can "flag" existing problems and risks (Alfaro, 2014, 50).

 RECALL Sylvia Wu, the 17-year-old who comes to the emergency department because she thinks that she might have a virus. The nurse would use a focused assessment to evaluate her complaints that relate specifically to her respiratory status. If you suspect a communicable disease, you also need to consider what precautions to take before continuing with your assessment. This information would be supplemented by additional data about the patient's recent travel to mainland China. ●

Emergency Assessment

When a physiologic or psychological crisis presents, the nurse performs an **emergency assessment** to identify life-threatening problems. A long-term care facility resident who begins choking in the dining room, a bleeding patient brought to the emergency department with a stab wound, an unresponsive patient in the rehabilitation unit, and a factory worker threatening violence are all candidates for an emergency assessment. In the first example, the source of the choking

Jefferson University Hospitals

* 001504 . 1009 *

MR# 56923

Acct# 06947328

Name Martha Rosenfeld

DOB 04/17/1948

Nursing Admission History

COMPLETE OR IMPRINT WITH ADDRESS-O-PLATE

Admission Data

Date 8/19/2015 Time 2100

T 38.5 P 92 R 18

BP 108/76 Ht Wt

☒ ID Bracelet ON Patient

Allergies
☐ No Known Allergies ☐ Allergy Bracelet On
☒ Medication   Reaction
Morphine   Rash
Penicillin   Rash

☐ Food
☐ Latex   ☐ IV Contrast (Dye)/Iodine
☐ Uncertain
☐ Other _____

Advance Directives

1. Advance Directive Information was provided to the patient.
☒ Yes ☐ No

2. Does the patient have an Advance Directive?
☒ Yes ☐ No

3. If patient has an Advance Directive, is it on the chart?
☒ Yes ☐ No

4. If patient has an Advance Directive and it is not on chart, was a request made to provide a copy of Advance Directive for chart?
☐ Yes ☐ No N/A

5. If patient has an Advance Directive, do they want to review or revise it?
☐ Yes ☒ No

6. If patient does not have an Advance Directive, would they like assistance in developing one?
☐ Yes ☐ No N/A

7. If patient does not have an Advance Directive and would like assistance in developing or if patient would like assistance in revising an Advance Directive, was Social Work consulted?
☐ Yes ☐ No ☒ N/A

Non-RN Signature

Orientation to Room/Unit
☒ Light/Emerg Call   ☒ Patient Handbook
☒ Bed Controls/Siderails ☒ Safety
☒ Visiting Hours   ☒ TV/Pt Ed Channels
☒ Oriented to JDU   ☒ Hourly Rounds
☐ Inability to Understand Instructions
   Explained to: ☐ Family ☒ Patient

Health History (see review of systems on back)
Information Source
☒ Patient ☐ Other (name/relationship):

Stated Reason for Hospitalization
uncontrolled pain & nausea r/t cancer
☐ Unable to Obtain Hx at Present
   Reason:

☒ History of falls at home/prior hospitalizations
   ☒ Yes ☐ No

☒ Patient is afraid of falling?
   ☒ Yes ☐ No

☒ Chemotherapy ☐ Radiation Therapy
☐ Transplant (type) _____
☒ Cancer (type) Stomach
☒ Past Surgeries J-tube placement, Mediport

☐ Isolation Care Precaution Other than Standard
   Type _____
   Other Pertinent Info _____

Medications ☐ None
Current medications being taken:
(include over-the-counter medications, herbals, and non-traditional medications)

Name/Dose/Frequency	Last Taken
Oxycontin 60mg BID	0800
Reglan 10mg TID	0800
Protonix 40mg daily	0800
Peri-colace 2 tabs BID	0800

Are you taking investigational study drugs? ☐ Yes ☒ No
(specify) _____

Are you currently using any mode of alternative therapy? ☒ Yes ☐ No
(specify) Medical Cannabis

Unit Date/Time

Spiritual/Cultural/Social Information
Are there any religious traditions, ethnic practices or cultural practices that need to be part of your care
☒ No ☐ Yes (explain):

☐ Unable to Obtain Social/Discharge info due to:

Lives: ☐ Alone ☒ Spouse ☐ Children ☐ Parents
   ☐ Other (specify) _____
☐ Smokes
   How Long? _____ Packs/Day _____
   Time of first cigarette. _____
   ☐ Informed of Hospital Smoking Policy
   ☐ Interested in Smoking Cessation Education
   Would you like to have nicotine replacement therapy while here in the hospital?
   ☐ Yes ☐ No
☐ Alcohol
   How Long? _____ Amount? _____
   ☐ Last Drink
      (time/amount) _____
   ☐ Previous treatment and response.

☒ Recreational Drugs (type/amount/last used)
   Medical Cannabis daily 8/18
   ☐ Previous treatment and response.

Contact/Support Person Present: ☒ Yes ☐ No
Name David Rosenfeld
Relationship Spouse
Home Phone _____
Work Phone _____

Valuable/Personal Property
Prosthetic Devices ☐ None
                          With Pt: Yes No
☐ Dentures   ☐   ☐
   ☐ Type: _____
☒ Glasses   ☒   ☐
☐ Contact Lenses   ☐   ☐
☒ Hearing Aid (R/L)   ☒   ☐
☐ Limb Prosthesis   ☐   ☐
☐ Glass Eye   ☐   ☐

Assistive Devices ☐ None
                          With Pt: Yes No
☐ _____   ☐   ☐

Valuable/Personal Items/Medications
Item   Home W/Pt Secured
_____   ☐   ☐   ☐
_____   ☐   ☐   ☐
☒ Sent Home with (relationship) Spouse
☐ Secured Location

FIGURE 11-3. Nursing admission database. (Used with permission, Jefferson University Hospitals.) *(continued)*

Nursing Admission History

Patient Name: Rosenfeld, Martha   DOB: 04/17/1948   MR#: SC923

Social Work/Case Management Screen
Enter consult in **Jeff Chart** or call SW/CM Consult line at 5-2587 if any condition is present.
- ☐ Trauma or New SCI
- ☐ Difficulty Coping with Diagnosis/Traumatic Incident
- ☐ Mental Health Impairment (eating disorder/suicide)
- ☐ Unknown Identity/Unknown Next of Kin
- ☐ No Parent on Admission for a Minor Under 18
- ☐ Boarding Home/Nursing Home Return
- ☐ Unable to Return Home
- ☐ Financial Difficulties (lack of gas, electric, water, medication coverage, etc.)
- ☐ Lack of Transportation for Discharge
- ☐ Assistance with Advance Directive
- ☐ Abuse/Neglect (child/older adult/domestic violence)
- ☐ Drug/Alcohol/Substance Abuse
- ☐ Positive Drug Screen of Newborn/Parent of Newborn/Child
- ☐ No Prenatal Care
- ☐ Pregnant Woman Under 16
- ☐ Fetal Demise
- ☐ Adoption/Foster Care Placement
- ☐ Other Concerns that would impede Discharge
- ☐ Other Concerns Impeding Psychosocial Functioning (non-compliance, end of life issues)
- ☐ Other ____
- ☒ **No Conditions Identified**

Screening Criteria for Nutrition
Enter consult in **Jeff Chart** or contact Department of Nutrition and Dietetics at ext. 5-7144 if any condition is present.
- ☐ Food Allergy
- ☒ Unintentional Weight Loss > 15lbs in past 3 months
- ☒ On Tube Feeding or anticipate Tube Feeding
- ☐ On TPN or anticipate TPN
- ☐ Stage 2 or greater Decubitus Ulcer or Non-healing Wound
- ☐ Jaw/Mandibular Fx/Wired Jaw
- ☐ Anorexia Nervosa or Bulimia
- ☐ Difficulty swallowing or other problems that prevent eating
- ☐ Continuous vomiting > 5 days
- ☐ Esophagectomy
- ☐ Enterocutaneous Fistula or Repair
- ☐ Radical Neck Surgery
- ☐ Whipple Procedure
- ☐ Other ____
- ☐ **No Conditions Identified**

Pregnant Woman (above criteria plus the following)
- ☐ Gestational Diabetic
- ☐ Hyperemesis
- ☐ Lactating (assessment by RN/Lactation specialist at Center City)
- ☐ Other ____
- ☒ **No Conditions Identified**

Rehab Screen
Physician order in Jeff Chart for new onset of deficits in:
Occupational Therapy
- ☐ Bathing   ☐ Dressing/Grooming
- ☐ Feeding   ☐ Toileting
- ☐ Range of Motion   ☐ Home Management
- ☐ Judgement/Safety   ☐ Vision
- ☐ Cognition and Perception
- ☒ **No Conditions Identified**

Physical Therapy
- ☐ Strength, Balance Coordination, Range of Motion
- ☐ Transfers   ☐ Stairs   ☐ Bed Mobility
- ☐ Wheel Chair Mobility   ☐ Ambulation
- ☐ Other ____
- ☒ **No Conditions Identified**

Speech Language Pathology
- ☐ Communication   ☐ Speech/Language
- ☐ Swallowing
- ☐ Other ____
- ☒ **No Conditions Identified**

RN Signature: *Katherine Blalock, RN*   Unit: C53   Date/Time: 8/19/2015

MRSA Screen
Has patient been diagnosed with MRSA?   ☐ Yes ☒ No
If yes, document facility and date and order MDRO Precautions.

____

Were you admitted from an outside facility?
If yes, order MRSA screen.
Were you hospitalized within the past 30 days?
If yes, order MRSA screen.

EENT   ☒ No Hx/Conditions Identified
- ☐ Glaucoma/ Cataracts   ☐ Sinus Problems
- ☐ Loose Teeth   ☐ Difficulty Hearing   ☐ TMJ
- ☐ Airway Device ____
- ☐ Hoarseness   ☐ Mouth Sores
- ☐ Dental Problems   ☐ Stiff Neck
- ☐ Bleeding Gums   ☐ Epistaxis
- Hearing Deficit: ☐ Right   ☒ Left   *wears hearing aid*
- Vision Deficit: ☐ Right   ☐ Left
- Comments:

Resp   ☐ No Hx/Conditions Identified
- ☐ Tuberculosis   ☒ Asthma   ☐ Pneumonia
- ☐ COPD   ☐ Emphysema   ☐ Home O₂
- Cough: ☐ Productive   ☐ Non-Productive
- Dyspnea: ☐ At Rest   ☐ With Exertion
  - ☐ Sleep Apnea (at home use of):
    - ☐ BiPap   ☐ CPAP
- Comments: *No exacerbation >5 years, no meds*

Cardiac   ☒ No Hx/Conditions Identified
- ☐ High Blood Pressure   ☐ Irregular Heartbeat
- ☐ Palpitations   ☐ Murmur   ☐ Chest Pain/Angina
- ☐ Heart Attack   ☐ Phlebitis/Varicose Veins
- ☐ Bleeding Disorder   ☐ Angioplasty/Stents
- ☐ Pacemaker   ☐ Implanted Defibrillator/AICD
- ☐ Venous Access Device (e.g. PICC, Infusaport)
- Comments:

GI   ☐ No Hx/Conditions Identified
- ☒ Nausea   ☐ Vomiting   ☐ Diarrhea
- ☐ Ulcers   ☐ Blood in Stool   ☒ Constipation
- ☐ Liver Disease   ☐ Jaundice
- ☐ Gallbladder Prob.   ☐ Hepatitis
- ☐ Inflammatory Bowel Disease   ☐ Pancreatitis
- ☒ Hiatal Hernia ☐ Heartburn/Acid Reflux
- ☐ Incontinence   ☐ GI Diversion
- Weight: ☐ Recent Gain   ☒ Recent Loss
- Last BM: *8/16*
- Comments: *Diagnosed stomach cancer 5/2015*

GU/Repro   ☒ No Hx/Conditions Identified
- ☐ Kidney Disease   ☐ Kidney Stones
- ☐ Blood in Urine   ☐ Difficulty Urinating
- ☐ Prostate Problems   ☐ Hesitancy   ☐ Urgency
- ☐ Dribbling   ☐ Incontinence   ☐ Frequency
- ☐ Nocturia
- Urinary Diversion ____
- Indwelling Foley ____
- When/Where inserted? ____
- ☐ Dialysis Access Location ____
- ☐ Vaginal/Penile Discharge
- ☐ Breast Problems   ☐ Hysterectomy
- ☐ Vaginal Bleeding
- ☐ LMP ____   ☐ Pregnant (____ weeks)
- Comments: *post-menopause*
- (Call pharmacy at 5-7147 if pregnant or lactating)
- ☐ Pharmacy called

Neuromuscular   ☒ No Hx/Conditions Identified
- ☐ Back Pain   ☐ Arthritis/Gout
- ☐ Joint Pain/Swelling
- ☐ Amputation ____
- ☐ Contracture ____
- ☐ Fractures ____
- ☐ Unsteady Gait
- ☐ Requires Assistance to Ambulate
- ☐ Limited ROM
- ☐ Unable to Bear Weight (RLE / LLE)
- ☐ Blurred Vision   ☐ Migraines   ☐ Headaches
- ☐ Seizures   ☐ Dizziness   ☐ Stroke
- ☐ Numbness/Tingling
- ☐ Paralysis: location
- ☐ Inappropriate Behavior
- ☐ Slurred Speech   ☐ Aphasia   ☐ Dysphagia
- Muscle: ☐ Weakness   ☐ Flaccid   ☐ Spastic
- Location ____
- Comments:

Endocrine   ☐ No Hx/Conditions Identified
- ☐ Thyroid Disease/Goiter
- ☐ Heat or Cold Intolerance
- ☐ Long Term Steroids
- ☐ Fever   ☐ Night Sweats
- ☐ Diabetes Type 1   ☒ Diabetes Type 2
- ☐ Diabetes Other
- Comments: *Diet Controlled*

Comfort   ☐ No Hx/Conditions Identified
- Patient Goal *improve pain & nausea*
- Where is Pain Now?

- Describe the pain *Aching, dull*
- How long have you had this pain? *4 months*
- What relieves the pain? *nothing*
- What makes it worse? *nothing*
- List pain meds *Oxycontin*
- Are they effective? *No*
- Does pain interfere with daily activities? *Yes*
- With sleep? *yes*
- Which number best describes your pain?
- (no pain) 0 1 2 3 4 5 6 7 ⑧ 9 10 (worst pain)

Psych   ☐ No Hx/Conditions Identified
- ☐ Alcohol/Drug Abuse   ☐ Other Addictions
- ☐ Psychiatric Disorder   ☐ Suicidal Ideations
- ☐ Grieving   ☐ Chronic Anxiety
- ☒ Depressed Affect   ☐ Hallucinations
- ☐ Confusion   ☐ Aggressive behavior
- ☐ Restraint use ____
- Comments: *has appointment with psychiatrist*

Skin   ☒ No Hx/Conditions Identified
- ☐ Skin Problems   ☐ Rashes   ☐ Ulcers
- ☐ Infection: site ____
- Comments:

Updated By ____   Unit ____   Date/Time ____

IMPORTANT: DO NOT WRITE IN MARGINS

PAGE 2 OF 2

FIGURE 11-3. *(continued)*

is assessed; in the second, the blood loss and wound characteristics; and in the third, the potential for immediate harm.

Time-Lapsed Assessment

The **time-lapsed assessment** is scheduled to compare a patient's current status to the baseline data obtained earlier. Most patients in residential settings and those receiving nursing care over longer periods of time, such as homebound patients with visiting nurses, are scheduled for periodic time-lapsed assessments to reassess their health status and to make necessary revisions in the plan of care. This assessment can be comprehensive or focused.

PREPARING FOR DATA COLLECTION

When preparing for data collection, establishing assessment priorities and systematically structuring data collection are two important considerations.

Establishing Assessment Priorities

Before beginning to collect data on any patient, think carefully about the type of data needed to develop a satisfactory plan of care. This also includes identifying data of a lower priority that you may not repeatedly collect. For example, data already collected from the patient and in the patient record should not be repeatedly sought unless there is a need for validation. Repetitious questioning can be annoying to a patient and may cause the patient to wonder about a lack of communication among health care professionals. A careful review of the patient record before interviewing the patient helps prevent this problem.

Nurses spend more or less time on different assessment components depending on the patient's reason for needing nursing care. For example, pediatric nurses are careful to establish the developmental age and milestones obtained by children admitted to a pediatric unit so that they can respect and promote these achievements. A school nurse who suspects child abuse pays careful attention to the child's statements about living conditions at home and relationships with family members and caregivers. A nurse preparing to discharge a patient from same-day surgery makes sure that the patient has the human and physical resources needed for appropriate postoperative care.

The purpose for which the assessment is being performed offers the best guidance for what type and how much data to collect. Assessment priorities are influenced by the patient's health orientation, developmental stage, culture, and need for nursing. Following the comprehensive nursing assessment, the patient's health problems dictate assessment priorities for future nurse–patient interactions.

Health Orientation

Nurses may use health assessments, such as the Health-Style Self-Test in Chapter 3 and the Promoting Health displays in each clinical chapter, to help patients identify potential and actual health risks and to explore their habits, behaviors, beliefs, attitudes, and values that influence their wellness.

The literature abounds in specialized assessment tools that focus on relationships; psychological, environmental, and physical self-care; relaxation; spirituality; humor and play; movement and exercise; sleep and dreams; nutrition; and sexuality. These assessments generally gather a different type of patient data compared to the assessments of patients being hospitalized for disease-related treatment.

Developmental Stage

Nursing assessments vary according to the patient's developmental needs. For example, when assessing an infant, special attention is given to weight gain and physical growth, feeding and elimination problems, sleep–activity cycles, and the parenting skills of caregivers. When children are hospitalized, it is important to note how independent the child is with basic care measures (toileting, hygiene, dressing, eating), what words the child uses to indicate the need to void and defecate, play preferences, and so on.

Culture

When assessing patients from different cultural backgrounds (e.g., racial, ethnic, religious, socioeconomic), remember all the influences of cultural factors. Consideration of the patient's culture begins with how you approach the patient and whether or not you make direct eye contact or shake the person's hand. Chapter 5 offers practical guidelines for incorporating cultural considerations into nursing assessments. Also assess the need for an interpreter. In what language does the patient wish to communicate? If an interpreter is necessary, be sure to follow your agency's policy about using a professional interpreter, since it is inappropriate to rely on the patient's family members for this service.

Need for Nursing

The likely duration of the nurse's interaction with the patient (e.g., same-day surgery versus surgery requiring a long recovery in an intensive care unit) and the nature of nursing care needed by the patient (e.g., assistance with the birth of a baby versus support and home care throughout a terminal illness)—both of these factors powerfully influence the type of data the nurse collects. A general assessment guideline is to gather only data that are helpful when planning and delivering care. It would be inappropriate, for example, to collect a detailed sexual history of a patient admitted to the hospital overnight after a slight concussion. Conversely, a nurse should not fail to ask a pregnant woman admitted to the hospital for observation because of bleeding during her first trimester whether she has any questions about resuming sexual activity after she gets home.

 THINK back to James Farren, the college junior described at the beginning of the chapter. The nurse would assess his sleeping, eating, and activity habits as well as his emotional status to gain further insight into his possible problems. However, a detailed assessment of his elimination habits would probably be inappropriate at the present time. ●

Structuring the Assessment

Because many different types of data are collected about patients, data collection must be structured systematically. Systematic guidelines specifically developed for a nursing assessment help ensure that comprehensive, holistic data are collected for each patient and lead easily to formulating nursing diagnoses. When the nurse internalizes such assessment guidelines, it is easier to focus on the patient during the assessment rather than worrying about what to assess next.

Most schools of nursing and health care institutions have a **minimum data set** that specifies the information that must be collected from every patient and uses a structured assessment form to organize or cluster this data. Many nursing assessment guides are based on holistic models rather than medical models. Gordon's (1994) framework identifies 11 functional health patterns and organizes patient data within these patterns. Maslow's hierarchy of five levels of human needs may also be used to organize data. A medical model often organizes data collection according to body systems.

BOX 11-2   MODELS FOR ORGANIZING OR CLUSTERING DATA

Holistic			Medical
Human Needs (Maslow)	**Functional Health Patterns (Gordon)**	**Human Response Patterns (Unitary Person)**	**Body System Model**
Physiologic (Survival) Needs: Food, fluids, oxygen, elimination, warmth, physical comfort	*Health Perception/Health Management:* Perception of general health status and well-being; adherence to preventive health practices	*Exchanging:* Nutritional status, temperature, elimination, oxygenation, circulation, fluid balance, skin, and mucous membranes, risk for injury	Neurologic Cardiovascular Respiratory Gastrointestinal Musculoskeletal Genitourinary Psychosocial
Safety and Security Needs: Things necessary for physical safety (e.g., a cane) and psychological security (e.g., a child's favorite toy)	*Nutritional–Metabolic:* Patterns of food and fluid intake, fluid and electrolyte balance, general ability to heal	*Communicating:* Ability to express thoughts verbally; orientation, speech impairments, language barriers	
Love and Belonging Needs: Family and significant others	*Elimination:* Patterns of excretory function (bowel, bladder, skin) and client's perception	*Relating:* Establishing bonds, social interaction, support systems, role performance (including parenting, occupation, and sexual role)	
Self-Esteem Needs: Things that make people feel good about themselves and confident in their abilities (e.g., being well groomed, having accomplishments recognized)	*Activity/Exercise:* Pattern of exercise, activity, leisure, recreation, and ADLs; factors that interfere with desired to expected individual pattern	*Valuing:* Religious and cultural preference and practices, relationship with deity, perception of suffering; acceptance of illness	
Self-Actualization Needs: Need to grow, change, and accomplish goals	*Cognitive–Perceptual:* Adequacy of sensory modes such as vision, hearing, taste, touch, smell, pain perception, cognitive functional abilities	*Choosing:* Ability to accept help and make decisions, adjustment to health status, desire for independence/dependence, denial of problem, adherence to therapies	
	Sleep/Rest: Patterns of sleep and rest–relaxation periods during a 24-hour day, as well as quality and quantity	*Moving:* Activity tolerance, ability for self-care, sleep patterns, diversional activities, disability history, safety needs, breastfeeding	
	Self-Perception/Self-Concept: Attitudes about self, perception of abilities, body image, identity, general sense of worth, and emotional patterns	*Perceiving:* Body image, self-esteem, ability to use all five senses, amount of hopefulness, perception of ability to control current situation	
	Role/Relationship: Perception of major roles and responsibilities in current life situation	*Knowing:* Knowledge about current illness or therapies; previous illnesses; risk factors, expectations of therapy, cognitive abilities; readiness to learn, orientation, memory	
	Sexuality and Reproductive: Perceived satisfaction or dissatisfaction with sexuality; reproductive state and pattern	*Feeling:* Pain, grieving, risk for violence, anxiety level, emotional integrity	
	Coping/Stress Tolerance: General coping pattern, stress tolerance, support systems, perceived ability to control and manage situations		
	Value-Belief: Values, goals, or beliefs that guide choices or decisions		

Adapted from Alfaro-LeFevre, R. (2014). *Applying nursing process. The foundation for clinical reasoning* (8th ed.). Philadelphia: Wolters Kluwer Health/Lippincott Williams & Wilkins.

Although the medical model is helpful for formulating diagnoses related to physiologic problems, it neglects patient problems and strengths in psychosocial and spiritual dimensions of health and well-being. Box 11-2 describes models for organizing assessment data.

COLLECTING DATA

There are two types of data: subjective and objective. **Subjective data** are information perceived only by the affected person; these data cannot be perceived or verified by another person. Examples of subjective data are feeling nervous, nauseated, or chilly, and experiencing pain. Subjective data also are called symptoms or covert data.

Objective data are observable and measurable data that can be seen, heard, felt, or measured by someone other than the person experiencing them. Objective data observed by one person can be verified by another person observing the same patient. Examples of objective data are an elevated temperature reading (e.g., 101°F), skin that is moist, and refusal to look at or eat food. Objective data also are called signs or overt data. Table 11-1 compares subjective and objective data.

Paying attention to both subjective and objective data promotes clinical reasoning because often the two types of data complement and clarify one another.

REVIEW the data provided in the scenario for Sylvia Wu in the Reflective Practice display. Her complaints of flu-like symptoms provide the nurse with subjective data. Hearing her cough, noting any sputum produced, inspecting her throat for redness and irritation, and checking her temperature would provide the nurse with objective data that help to clarify and substantiate the patient's complaints. •

Table 11-1	COMPARISON OF OBJECTIVE AND SUBJECTIVE DATA
OBJECTIVE DATA	SUBJECTIVE DATA

32-year-old man
Height: 5'8"
Weight:
  9/18/14—224 lb
  2/4/15—202 lb
	"I'm beginning to feel better about myself now that I'm losing weight and I seem to have more energy."

Posterior, left midcalf is warm and red.	"My leg hurts when I walk."
Patient observed fidgeting with bed covers; facial features are tightly drawn.	"I'm so afraid of what they might find when they cut me open tomorrow."

Sources of Data
Patient

The patient is the primary and usually the best source of information. Unless specified otherwise, the data recorded in the nursing history are assumed to have been collected from the patient. Most patients are willing to share information when they know it is helpful for planning their care. See the Through the Eyes of a Student display. Although subjective data collected from the patient are usually accurate, the nurse should be alert for certain difficulties. For example, a patient who is acutely ill may not be able to communicate adequately if the pain is severe or if consciousness is altered. An emotionally upset patient may distort information; for example, patients who are fearful because they think their illness may threaten their work or life may deny certain

THROUGH THE EYES OF A STUDENT

During my chronic medical–surgical rotation, my clinical group was placed on an oncology floor. My first thought was "Oh no, not the cancer floor!" The word *fear* didn't even begin to describe how I felt. These patients had enough problems without some "green" nursing student aggravating them all day. I kept thinking these people are extremely ill and won't want to be bothered by my intruding questions.

Nonetheless, I knew I had to do it. Not only did I have to take care of this patient all day, but I also had to develop a database and plan of care. I knew I would have to do a lot more than give him his morning care and leave him alone. I would have to carry on an extended conversation with this patient to get all the information I needed.

As if all of this wasn't enough to make me throw in the white flag, when my patient assignment was given, I discovered my patient was a man only 1 year older than me. A 28-year-old man with terminal cancer—this was too scary!

Clinical day came, as I knew it would, and I was shaking. I walked in that room and together the patient and I planned his care. I explained to him the things I needed to talk about with him and I couldn't believe it—he didn't tell me to go

away! We talked at length about his disease process and how it had affected his plans and goals. He opened up to me about his spirituality, his relationships with friends and family, and other personal subjects. Periodically, he would cringe, and I could tell it was time for a break. He was hurting too badly to go on at that time.

At the end of that day, my viewpoint was totally different than it had been that morning. I walked away from that room and off that floor feeling like I had made a difference for this person. We had shared a lot and he seemed so appreciative for the time I took to talk with him. The information he shared helped me to develop a better plan of care that was more responsive to his particular needs. The amazing part was that all I had to do was just be myself and allow him to do the same and our day flowed smoothly. The lesson I learned here was important for me: Keep calm and hold on to compassion, and nursing offers many rewards!

—Nancy E. Driskill, Southeast Missouri State University
Cape Girardeau, Missouri

symptoms or deliberately give misleading facts. If the nurse becomes aware that a patient's report of symptoms differs from physical findings or data obtained from other sources, note this and explore the cause of the discrepancy.

Data from patients with limited mental or communication capacity, such as young children and older adults with dementia, cannot be relied on as accurate. Children and people with decreased mental capacity or impaired verbal ability should, however, be encouraged to respond to interview questions as best as they can. Automatically turning to a family member, friend, or caregiver for information instead communicates powerfully that the nurse either has no time for the patient to express his or her needs or mistakenly doubts the patient's ability to communicate these needs.

Family and Significant Others

Family members, friends, and caregivers are especially helpful sources of data when the patient is a child or has limited capacity to share information with the nurse. Partners can supply information concerning their spouses. Friends often accompany a patient to a health agency and can supply useful information. Take care to determine that the patient does not object to you gathering data from family and friends and that they want to participate. Also, everyone involved should clearly understand the confidentiality of this data. Whenever data are gathered from support people, indicate this in the nursing history.

Patient Record

Records prepared by different members of the health care team provide information essential to comprehensive nursing care. The nurse should review records early when gathering data—in some instances, before the first contact with the patient. This review helps to focus the nursing assessment and to confirm and amplify information obtained from other sources.

The patient's health record or chart, which lists such information as age, sex, occupation, religious preference, next of kin, and financial status, is one type of record. The health record includes information entered by various health care professionals such as physicians, social workers, dietitians, physiotherapists, and laboratory technicians.

 FOR Susan Morgan, the 34-year-old patient recently diagnosed with MS, the nurse would review her medical record for information related to her diagnosis and treatment plans, including specialized consultations and therapy, as well as her current home situation. This information would help the nurse determine the approach to performing the nursing history and physical examination, as well as planning the patient's care. •

Nurses who want their care to be supportive of the patient while responding to changes in health status must be familiar with the many sections of the patient record in addition to the documentation of the nursing plan of care and nursing notes. The following parts of the patient record are important sources of data for the nurse.

MEDICAL HISTORY, PHYSICAL EXAMINATION, AND PROGRESS NOTES

These parts of the record include the findings of physicians as they assess and treat the patient; they focus on identifying pathologic conditions and their causes and on determining the medical regimen for treatment.

CONSULTATIONS

The patient's physicians may invite specialists to assess and treat the patient. The focus of these parts of the record is additional findings related to the patient's medical diagnosis and treatment.

REPORTS OF LABORATORY AND OTHER DIAGNOSTIC STUDIES

Reports of laboratory studies and other diagnostic tests, such as radiographs, include objective data that can either confirm or conflict with data collected during the nursing history or examination. Diagnostic studies help physicians establish a diagnosis and monitor the patient's response to treatment. The results of these studies may also help nurses evaluate the success of nursing interventions.

REPORTS OF THERAPIES BY OTHER HEALTH CARE PROFESSIONALS

Other health care professionals who interact with the patient also record their findings and note what progress the patient is making in their specific areas—for example, nutrition, physical therapy, or speech therapy. These reports also help the nurse assess the patient's progress and help determine the patient's ability to return home and manage care independently. For example, a nurse would carefully check a speech therapist's evaluation of a patient's ability to swallow while working with a dietitian to develop and administer the plan of care for nutrition via a feeding tube.

Records of previous admissions for health care and records from other health agencies, such as a social service agency or a home health care agency, are also valuable sources of data. They contain information about the patient's previous medical or surgical problems and response patterns, which may be important determinants of the current plan of care. See Chapters 16 and 20 for a description of the critical information that should be shared when patients are "handed off" or transitioned from one caregiver or team to another.

Assessment Technology

Nurses can also gain valuable data about patients from technologies such as cardiac and respiratory monitors. For example, a patient's bedside monitoring can provide round-the-clock information on blood pressure, heart rate, respirations, and cardiac activity.

Other Health Care Professionals

Nurses can learn a great deal about a patient's normal health habits and patterns and response to illness by talking with other nurses, physicians, social workers, and others on the

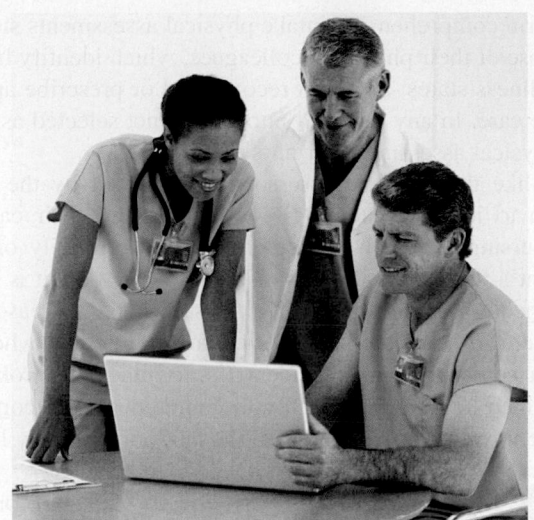

FIGURE 11-4. Nurses can learn a great deal about a patient's health habits, patterns, and responses to illness by talking with other nurses, physicians, social workers, and other members of the health care team. This exchange of information is particularly important when patients transfer from one health care setting to another, or to home.

health care team (Fig. 11-4). Although such communication is always important, it is especially critical when patients are transferred from home to an institution or from one hospital or institution to another. The only way to ensure continuity of care is to make special efforts to share pertinent information.

Nursing and Other Health Care Literature

To obtain a comprehensive patient database, it may be necessary to consult the nursing and related literature on specific health problems. For example, a nurse who has not cared for a patient with Paget disease before should read about the clinical manifestations of the disease and its usual progression to know what to look for when assessing the patient. In addition to information about medical diagnoses, treatment, and prognosis, a literature review offers nurses important information about nursing diagnoses, developmental norms, and psychosocial and spiritual practices that is helpful when assessing and caring for patients.

 FOR Sylvia Wu, the possible diagnosis of a virus that is potentially lethal is very frightening. To provide the most appropriate care, the nurse would need to know as much as possible about the disease. Then the nurse would be better able to act as an advocate for the patient. ●

Methods of Data Collection

The nursing history and physical assessment are primary components of data collection (see Chapter 25). These data may be documented on separate assessment tools or incorporated into a combined database assessment form, as shown in Figure 11-2 on page 236.

Observation is a key nursing skill when performing both the nursing history and the physical examination. **Observation** is the conscious and deliberate use of the five senses to gather data. Skilled nurses observe and interpret meaningful stimuli (data) in each nurse–patient interaction. You can develop such observation skills by training yourself to carefully observe the following each time you encounter a patient:

- What are the patient's current responses (physical and emotional) to his or her situation? Be alert to signs of distress—difficulty breathing, bleeding, pain, heightened anxiety—as well as anything out of the ordinary, such as sudden eruption of rash or a change in level of consciousness.
- What is the patient's current ability to manage his or her care (need for additional information or nursing assistance)?
- What factors are relevant in the immediate environment? Consider the safety of the environment as well as the functioning of equipment (e.g., intravenous therapy, oxygen, drains). Who are the people in the room and at home? What are the temperature and odor of the room?
- What other factors are relevant in the larger environment (hospital or community)?

Nursing History

Ideally, the nursing history captures and records the uniqueness of the patient so that care may be planned to meet the patient's individual needs. The nursing history should be obtained as soon as possible after a patient presents for care and should be followed by the nursing physical assessment. The nursing history should clearly identify the patient's strengths and weaknesses; health risks, such as hereditary and environmental factors; and potential and existing health problems. The nursing history focuses on getting to know the person.

 WHEN obtaining the nursing history from Sylvia Wu, the nurse would ascertain when the patient had traveled in China, how long she had been there, how long she had been home, with whom she may have been in contact, and whether these individuals exhibited any signs and symptoms. This information is important for determining the patient's actual risk for developing a particular virus. ●

COMPONENTS OF A NURSING HISTORY
Components of a nursing history include:

- Profile: name, age, sex, race/ethnicity, marital status, religion, occupation, education
- Reason for seeking health care
- Usual health habits and patterns and related needs for nursing assistance
- Cultural considerations in relation to diet, decision making, and activities
- Current state of health, functioning of body systems, degree of pain, and past medical and surgical history

- Current medications, allergies, and record of immunizations and exposure to communicable diseases
- Perception of health status and what health and illness mean to the patient, as well as usual responses or coping patterns
- Developmental history, family history, environmental history, and psychosocial history
- Patient's and family's expectations of nursing and of the health care team
- Patient's and family's educational needs and ability and willingness to learn
- Patient's and family's ability and willingness to participate in the plan of care
- Whether an advance directive exists or if the patient wants help to prepare an advance directive
- Patient's personal resources (strengths) and deficits
- Patient's potential for injury

PATIENT INTERVIEW

The nurse obtains the nursing history by interviewing the patient. An **interview** is a planned communication. Strong interviewing skills are needed to establish a successful working partnership with the patient, to communicate care and concern for the patient, and to obtain the necessary patient data. See the accompanying Guidelines for Nursing Care for promoting a caring and effective interview. See Figure 11-5 for seating and distance tips. The interview occurs in four phases: the preparatory phase, introduction, working phase, and termination. More detailed information on interviewing techniques is provided in Chapter 20.

Physical Assessment

Physical assessment is the examination of the patient for objective data that may better define the patient's condition and help the nurse plan care. The physical assessment normally follows the nursing history and interview and may verify data gathered during the history or yield new data. Physicians traditionally have performed the intake physical assessment, which commonly is the mechanism of entry into the health care delivery system as well as the basis for medical treatment. Some nurses in advanced practice roles

perform comprehensive intake physical assessments similar to those of their physician colleagues, which identify health and illness states, and then recommend or prescribe appropriate care. In any case, all nurses conduct selected aspects of physical assessment for nursing purposes.

Unlike the physical assessment performed by the physician to identify pathologic conditions and their causes, the nursing physical assessment focuses primarily on the patient's functional abilities. If a neurologic deficit is present, the nurse identifies how it affects the patient's reasoning and sensorimotor abilities. For example, a patient who has had a cerebrovascular accident (brain attack or stroke) is examined to determine ability to comprehend and communicate information and perform the tasks of everyday life.

 THE physical assessment for Susan Morgan, the young woman newly diagnosed with MS described at the beginning of the chapter, would include investigation of the patient's muscle strength and endurance level and the effects of MS on the patient's ability to perform daily activities. In the physical examination the nurse would be alert for indications of fatigue or inability to complete specific activities. This information would help the nurse to respond appropriately to the patient's concerns about her marriage. •

The purposes of the nursing physical assessment include the appraisal of health status, the identification of health problems, and the establishment of a database for nursing interventions (Figure 11-6).

Nurses practicing in different settings may use different physical assessment techniques for different purposes. Nurses in the coronary care unit use sophisticated, high-technology assessment techniques, whereas nurses in a rehabilitation center use a wide range of physical assessment skills that focus on identifying functional and nonfunctional response patterns to disabilities.

FIGURE 11-5. In the interview, both the seating arrangement and the distance from the patient are important in establishing a relaxed and comfortable environment for data collection. *(Photo B. Proud)*

FIGURE 11-6. The nurse conducts a physical examination. No matter what the setting or the age of the patient, the physical examination should include appraisal of health status, identification of health problems, and establishment of a database for nursing intervention. *(Photo by B. Proud.)*

PROMOTING A CARING INTERVIEW

These guidelines can help you to establish trust, create a positive attitude, and reduce anxiety—both yours and the patient's!

How to Establish Rapport

Before you go into the interview

- Get organized. Be sure that you have everything you need to have with you.
- Prepare for the interview by reading current and past records and reports.
- Don't rely on memory: Have a printed or electronic assessment tool to guide the questions you will ask.
- Plan enough time: The admission interview usually takes 30 to 60 minutes.
- Ensure privacy: Make sure that you have a quiet, private setting, free from interruptions or distractions.
- Get focused: Clear your mind of other concerns. Say to yourself, "Getting to know this person is the most important thing I have to do right now."
- Visualize yourself as being confident, warm, and helpful: This helps you to be confident, warm, and helpful—your genuine interest comes through.
- Approach the patient with an open mind and be aware of any stereotypes or prejudices that might affect this encounter.

When you begin the interview

- Begin by sitting at eye level with the patient (Fig. 11-5). Chairs placed at right angles to each other and about 3 to 4 feet (0.9–1.2 m) apart facilitate an easy exchange of information. If the patient is in bed, placing the chair at a 45-degree angle to the bed is helpful.
- Introduce yourself and give your name and position. This sends the message that you accept responsibility and are willing to be accountable for your actions. This is especially important if you are a student.
- Verify the person's name and ask what he or she would like to be called. This communicates your respect for the patient and that you recognize the patient as an individual with likes and dislikes.
- In unusual situations in which a contractual agreement that clearly identifies the responsibilities of both patient and nurse is indicated (e.g., a gerontologic nurse entrepreneur), terms are discussed at this time.

During the interview

- Give the person—not your notes or computer—your full attention. This will take practice.
- Avoid rushing. Become comfortable with the patient's silence.

How to Listen

- Listen actively—listen for feelings as well as words.
- Let the person know in a diplomatic manner when you see body language that sends a message that conflicts with what is being said, for example, "You say that you aren't having pain, but you look uncomfortable to me."
- Use short, supplemental phrases that let the person know you understand and encourage the person to continue, for example, "I see," Mmhm," and "Then what?"
- Be patient if the person has a memory block.
- Avoid the impulse to interrupt.

- Allow for pauses in conversation. Silence gives both you and the person time to gather thoughts, and allows you to reflect on the accuracy of the information the patient has provided.

How to Ask Questions

- Ask questions about the person's main problems first, for example, "What are the main reasons you are here today?" and "What do you hope happens today (or during your visit/time here)?"
- Focus your questions to gain specific information about signs and symptoms, for example, "Show me where the problem is" and "Can you describe how this feels more specifically?"
- Don't use leading questions, for example, "You don't smoke, do you?"
- Do use exploratory statements, for example, "Tell me more about your sleeping patterns."
- Use communication techniques that enhance your ability to think critically and get the facts:
  1. Use phrases that help you see the other person's perspective, for example, "What are the problems as you see them?"
  2. Restate the person's own words, for example, "Let me repeat what you said to make sure I understand."
  3. Ask open-ended questions, for example, "How are you feeling?" rather than "Are you feeling well?"
  4. Avoid close-ended questions—those requiring a one word answer—unless the person is too ill to elaborate or you are trying to clarify a response by getting a yes or no.

What to Observe

- Carefully assess areas connected to verbal complaints.
- Use your senses.
- Note general appearance.
- Observe body language. Does the person appear comfortable? Nervous? Withdrawn? Apprehensive? What behaviors do you see?
- Notice interaction patterns. Be aware of the person's responses to your interviewing style (e.g., sometimes cultural and personal differences create communication barriers).

How to Terminate the Interview

- Give a warning, for example, "We have 5 minutes to finish up…let's be sure we have covered the most important things you want us to know."
- Ask people to summarize their most important concerns and then summarize the most important concerns as you see them.
- Ask, "What else?," for example, "Is there anything else you want us to know to better plan your care?"
- Offer yourself as a resource, for example, "Let me know if anything changes or you have any questions."
- Explain care routines and provide information about who is accountable for nursing care decisions. Patients are often confused about who is responsible for what.
- Explain where the data being recorded are stored, how they will be used, and who has access to them.
- End on a positive note and encourage the person to become an active participant, for example, "We have a good start here. We want you to be actively involved in making decisions about your care."

(Adapted from Alfaro, R. (2014). *Applying nursing process. The foundation for clinical reasoning* (8th ed.). Philadelphia: Wolters Kluwer Health/Lippincott Williams & Wilkins, pp. 62–65.)

The nursing physical assessment involves the examination of all body systems, called the **review of systems (ROS)**, in a systematic manner, commonly using a head-to-toe format. Four methods are used to collect data during the physical assessment: inspection, palpation, percussion, and auscultation. Nurses may also use physical assessment skills to evaluate selected body systems. These techniques and the basic skills for physical assessment are described in Chapter 25.

Problems Related to Data Collection

Common problems encountered during data collection include inappropriate organization of the database, omission of pertinent data, inclusion of irrelevant or duplicate data, erroneous or misinterpreted data, failure to establish rapport and partnership with the patient, recording an interpretation of data rather than observed behavior, and failure to update the database. Table 11-2 and Table 11-3 describe possible causes and remedies for such problems.

IDENTIFYING CUES AND MAKING INFERENCES

Nurses now use the language of cues and inferences to describe the early analysis of data. The subjective and objective data you identify ("the patient does not respond when I speak to him on his left side") is a **cue** that something may be wrong. The judgment you reach about the cue (the patient's hearing may be impaired on his left side) is an **inference**. Until you check the patient's hearing, you cannot be sure that your inference is correct. Inferences may be validated in multiple ways:

- Physical examination, using the proper equipment and procedure (you may need to have an expert confirm your findings)
- Clarifying statements ("You said this is not a problem, but I sense you may still be worried.")
- Sharing your inferences with other respected members of the team and seeking consensus
- Checking your findings with research reports, textbooks, or journals
- Comparing cues to your knowledge base of normal function
- Checking consistency of cues

Figure 11-7 (on page 248) illustrates the process for validating inferences.

The nurse may validate data during collection or at the end of the data-gathering process. When it is clear that the

Table 11-2	PATIENT VARIABLES THAT CAN NEGATIVELY INFLUENCE AN INTERVIEW AND SUGGESTED NURSING RESPONSES	
PATIENT VARIABLES	EFFECT ON INTERVIEW	NURSING RESPONSE
High anxiety	Patient may speak rapidly or incoherently and may jump from one topic to another; patient may deny or misrepresent what he or she is experiencing.	Normalize anxiety: "Many people find it difficult to talk about their health and become anxious"; approach patient gently, speak slowly and softly; underscore importance of the patient sharing what he or she is experiencing so that nurses can help.
Pain	Patient offers clipped responses and "yes" or "no" answers whenever possible; overriding concern is pain relief.	Do everything possible to make patient comfortable before the interview, including obtaining an order for and administering pain medication; if pain persists, obtain only vital data and defer remainder of interview until patient is more comfortable.
Language difficulty (patient not fluent in nurse's language because patient speaks a different language, has a limited education, or fears saying the "wrong thing")	Vital patient data will not be communicated; patient may mistakenly be labeled "indifferent" or "noncommunicative."	Speak clearly (do not raise voice) using simple language; whenever possible, obtain the assistance of an interpreter and follow agency guidelines.
Previous negative experience with nurses or health care delivery system	Patient is aloof, unwilling to participate in interview; general attitude: "Why should I waste my time telling you anything...it won't do me any good."	"I know other people who have had a tough time with nurses or the system...life isn't perfect...but how about giving us a chance this time to show you what nurses can do?" Communicate respect for the patient and competence.
Unrealistic expectations of health care professionals	Patient expects nurses and other health care professionals magically to know everything about the patient and to "take care" of the patient; "surrenders" self to the system—"you know best" attitude.	Communicate clearly that no one knows or understands the patient like the patient does, and invite the patient to become involved in his or her care; "No two people are alike, and unless you tell me a little more about yourself and how you are feeling, there is no way we'll be able to plan good care."

Table 11-3 COMMON PROBLEMS OF DATA COLLECTION, POSSIBLE CAUSES, AND SUGGESTED REMEDIES

PROBLEM	POSSIBLE CAUSES	SUGGESTED REMEDIES
Database inappropriately organized	Failure to plan for the assessment by identifying needed data; use of inappropriate tools for data collection	Review the guidelines for specifying pertinent data. Consider modifying tool for data collection or select an alternative tool.
Pertinent data omitted	Not following up on cues during data collection; inappropriate guidelines	Identify potentially relevant factors in advance of collection. Practice interview strategies.
Irrelevant or duplicate data collected	Failure to identify specific purpose of data collection; failure to review available patient records; use of inappropriate tools for data collection	Determine specific purpose of data collection for each patient. Consider existing data before initiating collection. Consider modifying data collection tool or selecting alternative.
Erroneous or misinterpreted data collection	Failure to observe carefully or validate during data collection; interviewer prejudices or stereotypes	Sharpen observation skills by independently observing the same situation with a peer and comparing notes afterward. Role play several validation techniques.
Failure to establish rapport	Failure to establish sufficient rapport or use appropriate communication techniques with patient; failure to know what information is wanted	Review and practice communication techniques discussed in Chapter 20. Role play several explanations of purpose of data collection. Identify general data desired before collection.
Interpretation of data is recorded rather than the observed behavior	Nurse jumps to hasty conclusion about patient's behavior and deprives others of exploring with patient possible causes of the behavior; deficient validation	Review the distinction between data and interpretation of data. Practice documenting observed patient behavior concisely.
Failure to update the database	Erroneous belief that assessment is concluded after the initial database is recorded; low priority attached to ongoing data collection	Recollect that it is impossible to give quality, individualized care without knowledge of changes in the patient's status. Ongoing data collection is critical to the deletion or modification of old problems and the identification of new problems.

data are correct, the nurse is ready to analyze the data and formulate nursing diagnoses—the next step of the nursing process. Figure 11-8 (on page 249) illustrates the role clinical reasoning plays in moving from assessment to diagnosis.

VALIDATING DATA

Validation is the act of confirming or verifying. The purpose of validating is to keep data as free from error, bias, and misinterpretation as possible. Validation is an important part of assessment because invalid information can lead to inappropriate nursing care. Because it is neither possible nor necessary to validate all data, nurses need to decide which items need verification. For example, data need to be verified when there are discrepancies: a patient tells you he is fine and has no concerns, but you note that he demonstrates tense body musculature and seems curt in his responses. When there is a discrepancy between what the person is saying and what you are observing, validation is necessary to determine accuracy. Validation in this instance may take the form of your saying, "You tell me you feel fine, but right now your body and behaviors are telling me something else. Tell me more about this."

Data also need verification when they lack objectivity. For example, you suspect that the patient hears in one ear but does not seem to hear well in the other. You should validate the data before proceeding and should determine whether the

patient does indeed have a hearing problem. Suspicions are not objective. In this instance, you need to test the patient's hearing in both ears. Speaking toward the suspected better ear, you explain, "It seems to me that you hear better out of one ear than the other. I would like to test this. I'll bring a watch slowly toward your right ear first and then toward your left. Please look straight ahead and tell me when you first hear the watch ticking." You can then record how far the watch was from each ear when the patient first heard it ticking.

 Concept Mastery Alert

Whenever there is any data discrepancy or conflict, the nurse must investigate further, gathering focused information to support, confirm, or negate the suspicions.

CLUSTERING RELATED DATA AND IDENTIFYING PATTERNS

As described earlier, as you prepare to collect your data you also decide how to organize or cluster the data. Box 11-2 on page 240 illustrates three holistic models (Maslow's human needs, Gordon's functional health patterns, and human response patterns) along with the body system medical model. Once you have organized your data according to the

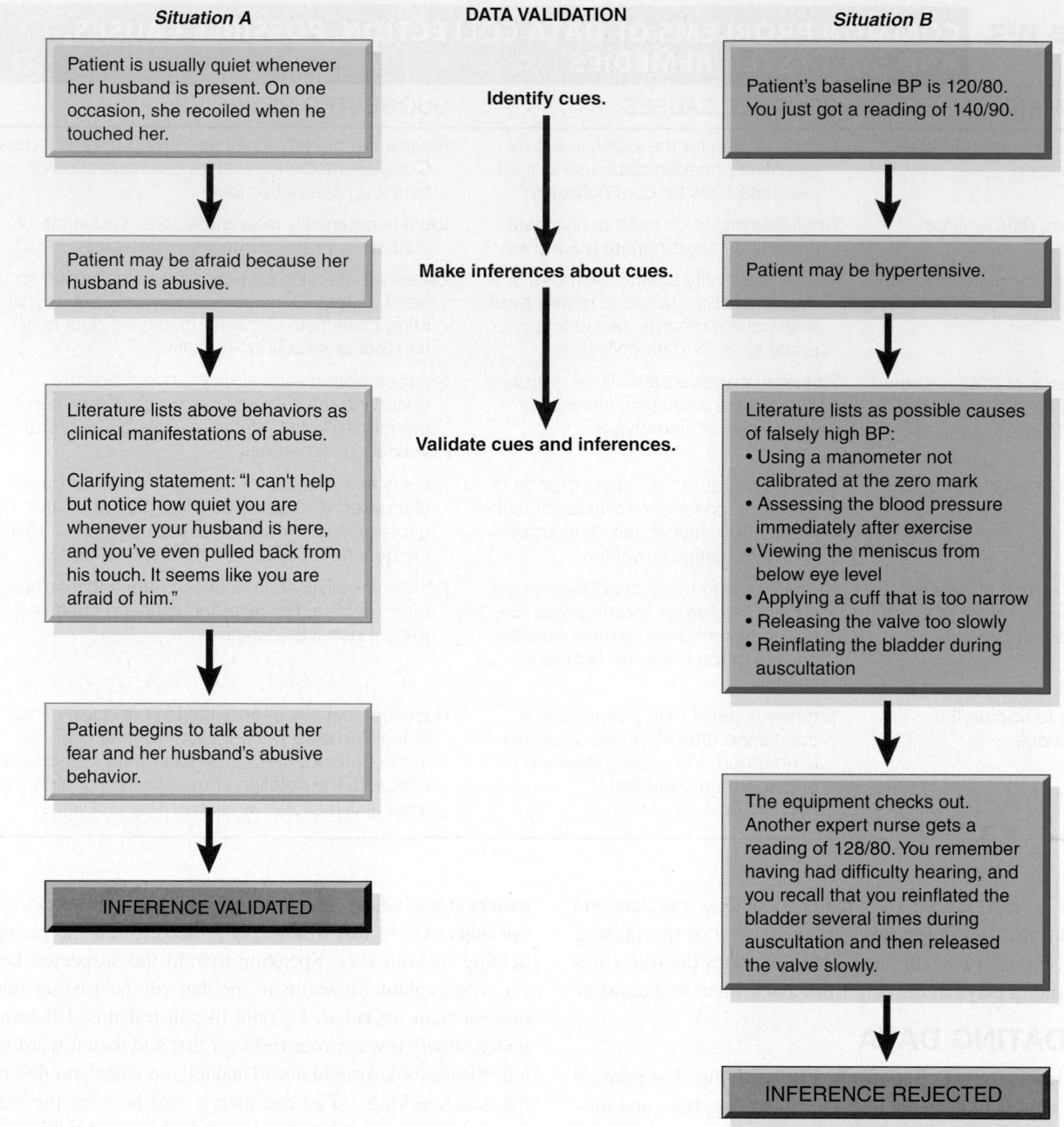

FIGURE 11-7. The process used to validate cues and inferences.

purpose of your assessment, you begin to look for and test your initial impressions about patterns of human functioning. Alfaro (2014) recommends testing your first impressions to decide what's relevant, making tentative decisions about what the data suggest, and focusing your assessment to gain more in-depth information to better understand the patient's situation. She stresses the importance of trying to learn why the pattern came to be, remembering that there is usually more than one contributing factor because health problems are complex.

REPORTING AND RECORDING DATA

The patient data the nurse collects, both initially and as patient contact continues, are of no benefit to the patient

and the health care team unless they are appropriately communicated. See the legal alert in Box 11-3. Appropriate communication involves correct timing and proper documentation.

Timing

Data should be reported verbally immediately whenever assessment findings reveal a critical change in the patient's health status that necessitates the involvement of other nurses or health care professionals. A nurse who observes an elevated temperature of 103.2°F (39.5°C) in a patient scheduled for surgery that morning must report this to the charge nurse and to the surgeon, who might then cancel surgery. Failure to communicate this finding could result in

ASSESSMENT

- ☐ Collecting Data
- ☐ Identifying Cues and Making Inferences
- ☐ Validating Data
- ☐ Clustering Related Data and Indentifying Patterns
- ☐ Reporting and Recording Data

⬇

Clinical Reasoning
(analyzing, synthesizing, reflecting, making judgments and drawing conclusions)

⬇

DIAGNOSIS

FIGURE 11-8. How the phases of assessment set the stage for diagnosis. (Reprinted with permission from Alfaro, R. (2014). *Applying nursing process. The foundation for clinical reasoning* (8th ed.). Philadelphia: Wolters Kluwer Health/Lippincott, Williams & Wilkins, p. 49.)

the patient's receiving preoperative sedation, being taken to the operating room, and even having the surgery performed under less than optimal conditions. Similarly, a nurse who hears a patient making suicidal remarks must communicate this information to the health care team so that all are alerted to the danger and so that suicide precautions may be taken immediately.

A nurse who is unsure of the significance of a particular finding should consult with another nurse. In some situations, years of experience are needed to distinguish significant from insignificant findings. Neither ignorance nor the fear of appearing less than competent justifies failure to report critical data.

 THE nurse would need to report Sylvia Wu's complaints along with the underlying history of travel to China immediately to the appropriate health care personnel. Doing so ensures that the necessary precautions are taken to reduce the risk of infection transmission with highly communicable viruses. •

Documentation

The patient's initial database is entered into the computer or recorded in ink, using the designated agency protocol or forms, the same day the patient is admitted to the agency. If,

Box 11-3 | LEGAL ALERT

Nurses are responsible for alerting the appropriate health care professional whenever assessment data differ significantly from the patient's baseline, indicating a potentially serious problem. Interventions for which the nurse may be legally responsible include increasing the frequency of assessments and initiating necessary changes in the treatment regimen.

for any reason, important data cannot be obtained during the initial assessment, this should be documented so that they are obtained as soon as possible. Objective and subjective patient data should be summarized and written so that the data communicate a unique sense of the patient and are comprehensive, concise, and easily retrievable. The data should be written legibly, using good grammar and only standard medical abbreviations. To facilitate quick data retrieval, data should be presented under clearly marked headings.

Whenever possible, subjective data should be recorded using the patient's own words within quotation marks: "I feel tired from the moment I first get up in the morning. It seems I have no energy at all." Patient reports may also be paraphrased: Patient reports feeling dyspneic, has difficulty catching breath when walking one flight of stairs.

Avoid the tendency to record data using nonspecific terms with different meanings or interpretations—words like *adequate, good, average, normal, poor, small, large*. One nurse's idea of what "average" fluid intake is may be very different from that of another nurse. Always be specific. Chapter 16 offers general documentation guidelines.

REFLECTIVE PRACTICE LEADING TO PERSONAL LEARNING

Remember that the goal of reflective practice is to look at an experience, understand it, and learn from it. As you begin to develop expertise in assessing patients' health status and well-being, reflect on your experiences—successes and failures—in order to improve your practice. How can you do it better next time? What did you learn today that can help you tomorrow? Begin your reflection by paying close attention to the following during the assessing phase of the nursing process:

- Did your preparation for the assessing experience bring you to the interview and physical examination feeling confident in your ability to gather reliable, accurate, and complete data while inspiring the patient's confidence and trust?
- How confident are you that the data you reported and recorded accurately communicates the health problems, issues, risks, and strengths of the patient? How successfully have you communicated who this patient/family are to your interdisciplinary colleagues?
- Were you aware of any stereotypes or prejudices that might have negatively influenced the clinical encounter? If yes, how did you address these?
- Was patient/family participation in the process at an optimal level? How might you have better engaged the patient and family? As you concluded your assessment, did the patient know your name, know what to expect of you and of nursing, sense that you are competent, respectful, and caring, and know what is expected in terms of developing the plan of care and participating in its execution?

Perhaps the most important question to reflect on is: Are your patients and families better for having had you share in the critical responsibility of assessing their health problems and identifying and tapping their strengths? Will your patients now receive individualized, prioritized, holistic, evidence-based treatment and care because of your efforts?

DEVELOPING CLINICAL REASONING

1. Working with another student, interview patients in both their home and institutional settings, and record your findings separately. Make a list of the objective and subjective data you gather about each patient interviewed and the inferences you make from these cues. Compare your data lists and inferences. Describe to each other how you plan to validate your inferences. Explore possible reasons for the differences you discover.

2. Allow another student to perform a comprehensive nursing assessment (interview and physical assessment) on you. Reflect on what you experienced. Offer the student feedback about which of her or his behaviors were helpful, comforting, or distressing. Change roles and talk about what you learned from this experience.

3. Collect several different forms for recording the initial comprehensive nursing assessment (hospital, long-term care facility, home care, school of nursing forms). Identify differences and explain them. Experiment with using the different forms, and make a list of features that help you get all the data you need in the easiest way possible. Review Table 11-2 on page 246. What other patient variables might negatively influence an interview? Nursing variables? How should you address these?

PRACTICING FOR NCLEX

1. Read the following scenario and identify the term for the characteristics of patient data that are numbered below. Place your answers on the lines provided.

   The nurse is conducting an initial assessment of a 79-year old female patient admitted to the hospital with a diagnosis of dehydration. The nurse: (1) uses clinical reasoning to identify the need to perform a comprehensive assessment and gather the appropriate patient data, (2) first asks the patient about the most important details leading up to her diagnosis, (3) collects as much information as possible to understand the patient's health problems, (4) collects the patient data in an organized manner, (5) verifies that the data obtained is pertinent to the patient care plan, and (6) records the data according to agency policy.

   (1) _____
   (2) _____
   (3) _____
   (4) _____
   (5) _____
   (6) _____

2. The nurse practitioner is performing a short assessment of a newborn who is displaying signs of jaundice. The nurse observes the infant's skin color and orders a test for bilirubin levels to report to the primary care provider. What type of assessment has this nurse performed?
   a. Comprehensive
   b. Initial
   c. Time-lapsed
   d. Quick priority

3. The nurse is admitting a 35-year-old pregnant woman to the hospital for treatment of preeclampsia. The patient asks the nurse: "Why are you doing a history and physical exam when the doctor just did one?" Which statements best explain the primary reasons a nursing assessment is performed? Select all that apply.
   a. "The nursing assessment will allow us to plan and deliver individualized, holistic nursing care that draws on your strengths."
   b. "It's hospital policy. I know it must be tiresome, but I will try to make this quick!"
   c. "I'm a student nurse and need to develop the skill of assessing your health status and need for nursing care."
   d. "We want to make sure that your responses to the medical exam are consistent and that all our data are accurate."
   e. "We need to check your health status and see what kind of nursing care you may need."
   f. "We need to see if you require a referral to a physician or other health care professional."

4. When you receive the shift report, you learn that your patient has no special skin care needs. You are surprised during the bath to observe reddened areas over bony prominences. What action is appropriate?
   a. Correct the initial assessment form.
   b. Redo the initial assessment and document current findings.
   c. Conduct and document an emergency assessment.
   d. Perform and document a focused assessment of skin integrity.

5. A student nurse attempts to perform a nursing history for the first time. The student nurse asks the instructor how anyone ever learns all the questions the nurse must ask to get good baseline data. What would be the instructor's best reply?
   a. "There's a lot to learn at first, but once it becomes part of you, you just keep asking the same questions over and over in each situation until you can do it in your sleep!"
   b. "You make the basic questions a part of you and then learn to modify them for each unique situation, asking yourself how much you need to know to plan good care."
   c. "No one ever really learns how to do this well because each history is different! I often feel like I'm starting afresh with each new patient."
   d. "Don't worry about learning all of the questions to ask. Every agency has its own assessment form you must use."

6. The nurse collects objective and subjective data when conducting patient assessments. Which patient conditions are examples of subjective data? Select all that apply.
   a. A patient tells the nurse that she is feeling nauseous.
   b. A patient's ankles are swollen.
   c. A patient tells the nurse that she is nervous about her test results.
   d. A patient complains of having a rash on her arm that is itchy.
   e. A patient rates his pain as a 7 on a scale of 1 to 10.
   f. A patient vomits after eating supper.

7. When a nurse enters the patient's room to begin a nursing history, the patient's wife is there. What should the nurse do?
   a. Introduce oneself and thank the wife for being present.
   b. Introduce oneself and ask the wife if she wants to remain.
   c. Introduce oneself and ask the wife to leave.
   d. Introduce oneself and ask the patient if he would like the wife to stay.

8. A nurse is performing an initial comprehensive assessment of an 84-year-old male patient admitted to a long-term care facility from home. The nurse begins the assessment by asking the patient, "How would you describe your health status and well-being?" The nurse also asks the patient, "What do you do to keep yourself healthy?" Which model for organizing data is this nurse following?
   a. Maslow's human needs
   b. Gordon's functional health patterns
   c. Human response patterns
   d. Body system model

9. The nurse is surprised to detect an elevated temperature (102°F) in a patient scheduled for surgery. The patient has been afebrile and shows no other signs of being febrile. What is the first thing the nurse should do?
   a. Inform the charge nurse.
   b. Inform the surgeon.
   c. Validate the finding.
   d. Document the finding.

10. A student nurse tells the instructor that a patient is fine and has "no complaints." What would be the instructor's best response?
   a. "You made an inference that she is fine because she has no complaints. How did you validate this?"
   b. "She probably just doesn't trust you enough to share what she is feeling. I'd work on developing a trusting relationship."
   c. "Sometimes everyone gets lucky. Why don't you try to help another patient?"
   d. "Maybe you should reassess the patient. She has to have a problem—why else would she be here?"

ANSWERS WITH RATIONALES

1. (1) Purposeful: The nurse identifies the purpose of the nursing assessment (comprehensive) and gathers the appropriate data.
   (2) Prioritized: The nurse gets the most important information first.
   (3) Complete: The nurse gathers as much data as possible to understand the patient health problem and develop a plan of care.
   (4) Systematic: The nurse gathers the information in an organized manner.
   (5) Factual and accurate: The nurse verifies that the information is reliable.
   (6) Recorded in a standard manner: The nurse records the data according to agency policy so that all caregivers can easily access what is learned.

2. *d.* Quick priority assessments (QPA) are short, focused, prioritized assessments nurses do to gain the most important information they need to have first. The comprehensive initial assessment is performed shortly after the patient is admitted to a health care agency or service. The time-lapsed assessment is scheduled to compare a patient's current status to baseline data obtained earlier.

3. *a, e, f.* Medical assessments target data pointing to pathologic conditions, whereas nursing assessments focus on

the patient's responses to health problems. The initial comprehensive nursing assessment results in baseline data that enable the nurse to make a judgment about a patient's health status, the ability to manage his or her own health care and the need for nursing. It also helps nurses plan and deliver individualized, holistic nursing care that draws on the patient's strengths and promotes optimum functioning, independence, and well-being, and enables the nurse to refer the patient to a physician or other health care professional, if indicated. The fact that this is hospital policy is a secondary reason, and although it may be true that a nurse may need to develop assessment skills, it is not the chief reason the nurse performs a nursing history and exam. The assessment is not performed to check the accuracy of the medical examination.

4. *d.* Perform and document a focused assessment on skin integrity since this is a newly identified problem. The initial assessment stands as is and cannot be redone or corrected. This is not a life-threatening event; therefore, there is no need for an emergency assessment.

5. *b.* Once you learn what constitutes the minimum data set, you can adapt this to any patient situation. It is not true that each assessment is the same even when you are using the same minimum data set, nor is it true that each assessment is uniquely different. Nurses committed to thoughtful, person-centered practice tailor their questions to the uniqueness of each patient and situation. Answer *d* is incorrect because relying solely on standard agency assessment tools does not allow for individualized patient care or critical thinking.

6. *a, c, d, e.* Subjective data are information perceived only by the affected person; these data cannot be perceived or verified by another person. Examples of subjective data are feeling nervous, nauseated, itchy, or chilly and experiencing pain. Objective data are observable and measurable data that can be seen, heard, or felt by someone other than the person experiencing them. Examples of objective data are an elevated temperature reading (e.g., 101°F), edema, and vomiting.

7. *d.* The patient has the right to indicate whom he would like to be present for the nursing history and exam. You should neither presume that he wants his wife there nor that he does not want her there. Similarly, the choice belongs to the patient, not the wife.

8. *b.* Gordon's functional health patterns begin with the patient's perception of health and well-being and progress to data about nutritional–metabolic patterns, elimination patterns, activity, sleep/rest, self-perception, role relationship, sexuality, coping, and values/beliefs. Maslow's model is based on the human needs hierarchy. Human responses include exchanging, communicating, relating, valuing, choosing, moving, perceiving, knowing, and feeling. The body system model is based on the functioning of the major body systems.

9. *c.* The nurse should first validate the finding if it is unusual, deviates from normal, and is unsupported by other data. Should the initial recording prove to be in error, it would have been premature to notify the charge nurse or the surgeon. The nurse should be sure that all data recorded are accurate, thus all data should be validated before documentation if there are any doubts about accuracy.

10. *a.* The instructor is most likely to challenge the inference that the patient is "fine" simply because she is telling you

that she has no problems. It is appropriate for the instructor to ask how the student nurse validated this inference. Jumping to the conclusion that the patient does not trust the student nurse is premature and is an invalidated inference. Answer c is wrong because it accepts the invalidated inference. Answer d is wrong because it is possible that the condition is resolving.

Bibliography

Alfaro-LeFevre, R. (2010). *Applying nursing process: A tool for critical thinking* (7th ed.). Philadelphia: Wolters Kluwer Health/Lippincott Williams & Wilkins.

Alfaro, R. (2014). *Applying nursing process. The foundation for clinical reasoning* (8th ed.). Philadelphia: Wolters Kluwer Health/Lippincott Williams & Wilkins.

American Nurses Association (ANA). (2010). *Standards of clinical nursing practice* (2nd ed.). Silver Spring, MD: Author.

American Nurses Association (ANA). (2010). *Nursing's social policy statement* (2010 ed.). Silver Spring, MD: Author.

Armstrong, J., & Mitchell, E. (2008). Comprehensive nursing assessment in the care of older people. *Nursing Older People, 20*(10), 36–40.

Bickley, L. (2013). *Bates' guide to physical examination and history taking* (11th ed.). Philadelphia: Wolters Kluwer Health/Lippincott Williams & Wilkins.

Dykes, P. C., Kim, H. E., Goldsmith, D. M., Choic, J., Esumi, K., & Goldberg, H. S. (2009). The adequacy of ICNP Version 1.0 as a representational model for electronic nursing assessment documentation. *Journal of the American Medical Informatics Association, 16*(2), 238–246.

Fawcett, T., & Rhynas, S. (2012). Taking a patient history: The role of the nurse. *Nursing Standard, 26*(24), 41–46.

Gordon, M. (1994). *Nursing diagnosis: Process and application* (3rd ed.). St. Louis, MO: Mosby - Year Book.

Johnson, M., Jefferies, D., & Nicholls, D. (2012). Developing a minimum data set for electronic nursing handover. *Journal of Clinical Nursing, 21*(3–4), 331–343.

Kumekawa, J. K. (2001, September 30). Health information privacy protection: Crisis or common sense? *Online Journal of Issues in Nursing, 6*(3), manuscript 2. Available at http://www.nursingworld.org/MainMenuCategories/ANAMarketplace/ANA-Periodicals/OJIN/TableofContents/Volume62001/No3Sept01/PrivacyProtectionCrisis.asp

Maxson, P. M., Derby, K. M., Wrobleski, D. M., & Foss, D. M. (2012). Bedside nurse-to-nurse handoff promotes patient safety. *Medsurg Nursing, 21*(3), 140–145.

U.S. Department of Health and Human Services (USDHHS), Office for Civil Rights. (2003). HIPAA: Summary of the HIPAA security rule. Available at http://www.hhs.gov/ocr/privacy/hipaa/understanding/srsummary.html

TAYLOR SUITE RESOURCES

Explore these additional resources to enhance learning for this chapter:
- NCLEX-Style Questions and other resources on **the Point**, http://thePoint.lww.com/Taylor8e
- *Study Guide for Fundamentals of Nursing, 8th edition*
- Adaptive Learning | Powered by prepU, http://thepoint.lww.com/prepu

12 Diagnosing

MARTIN PRESCOTT

Martin, a 46-year-old man, comes to the health clinic for a routine physical examination. During the assessment, he states, "I've had problems with constipation and have seen some blood when I wipe myself after a bowel movement. It's just hemorrhoids, right? Nothing to worry about?"

ANTONIA ZUCCARELLI

Antonia is a middle-aged woman newly diagnosed with cancer that is treatable. However, she continually fails to show up for follow-up appointments for both diagnosis and treatment.

ANGIE CLARKSON

Angie, a college sophomore, tearfully reports to her student nurse colleague that she believes she was a victim of date rape. She had too much to drink at a party and can only remember waking up in a strange room with a guy she just met, unsure if she passed out because of the alcohol or date-rape drugs. A virgin, Angie was sure there was penetration because of blood and semen stains she discovered upon waking. It is now a month later and she has not been able to "get her life together" and move on.

LEARNING OBJECTIVES

After completing the chapter, you will be able to accomplish the following:

1. Describe the term *nursing diagnosis,* distinguishing it from a collaborative problem and a medical diagnosis.
2. Describe the four steps involved in data interpretation and analysis.
3. Use the guidelines for writing nursing diagnoses when developing diagnostic statements.
4. Identify five types of nursing diagnoses.
5. Describe means to validate nursing diagnoses.
6. Describe the benefits and limitations of nursing diagnoses.

KEY TERMS

actual nursing diagnoses	health problem	risk nursing diagnoses
collaborative problems	medical diagnoses	standard
cue	nursing diagnoses	syndrome nursing diagnoses
data cluster		
diagnosing	possible nursing diagnoses	wellness diagnoses
diagnostic error		

Assessment

- ☐ Collecting Data
- ☐ Identifying Cues and Making Inferences
- ☐ Validating (Verifying) Data
- ☐ Clustering Related Data
- ☐ Identifying Patterns/Testing First Impressions
- ☐ Reporting and Recording Data

Clinical reasoning
(analyzing, synthesizing, reflecting, drawing conclusions)

Diagnosis

- ☐ Creating a list of suspected problems/diagnoses
- ☐ Ruling out similar problems/diagnoses
- ☐ Naming actual and potential problems/diagnoses and clarifying what's causing or contributing to them
- ☐ Determining risk factors that must be managed
- ☐ Identifying resources, strengths, and areas for health promotion

FIGURE 12-1. This diagram shows how the activities of *assessment* lead to a *pivotal* point in the nursing process: *diagnosis.* Diagnosis is a pivotal point for the following reasons:

1. **The purpose of diagnosis is to clarify the exact nature of the problems and risks that must be addressed to achieve the overall expected outcomes of care.** If you do not completely understand the problems and what factors are contributing to them, how do you know what to do about them? If you don't pay attention to risks, how are you going to prevent problems?
2. **The conclusions you make during this phase affect the entire plan of care.** If your conclusions are correct, your plan is likely to be on target. If they are not—for example, if you are operating on *assumptions* rather than sound reasoning that is based on evidence—your plan is likely to be flawed, maybe even dangerous.

(Used with permission from Alfaro-LeFevre, R. (2014). *Applying nursing process: The Foundation for Clinical Reasoning* (8th ed.). Philadelphia: Wolters Kluwer Health/Lippincott Williams & Wilkins, p. 91.)

Diagnosing—the second step in the nursing process—begins after the nurse has collected and recorded the patient data. The purposes of **diagnosing** are to (1) identify how a person, group, or community responds to actual or potential health and life processes; (2) identify factors that contribute to or cause health problems (etiologies); and (3) identify resources or strengths that the person, group, or community can draw on to prevent or resolve problems. See the accompanying Reflective Practice display for an example.

In the diagnosing step of the nursing process, the nurse interprets and analyzes data gathered from the nursing assessment (Fig. 12-1). The data help the nurse identify patient strengths and health problems. A **health problem** is a condition that necessitates intervention to prevent or resolve disease or illness or to promote coping and wellness.

Alfaro-LeFevre (2014) counsels nurses to understand the types of problems they should focus on to better understand their responsibilities relating to the diagnosis and management of health problems. She lists the following as concerns that are central to your role as a nurse (Alfaro-LeFevre, 2014, p. 92):

- Recognizing safety and infection–transmission risks and addressing these immediately.

- Identifying human responses—how problems, signs and symptoms, and treatment regimens *impact on patients' lives*—and promoting optimum function, independence, and quality of life
- Anticipating possible complications and taking steps to prevent them
- Initiating urgent interventions—you do not want to wait to make a final diagnosis if there are signs and symptoms indicating the need for immediate treatment.

When a health problem is identified, the nurse must decide which health care professional can best address the problem. Actual or potential health problems that can be prevented or resolved by independent nursing intervention are termed **nursing diagnoses**. The nurse formulates, validates, and lists nursing diagnoses for each patient

REFLECTIVE PRACTICE: CULTIVATING QSEN COMPETENCIES

CHALLENGE TO COGNITIVE AND INTERPERSONAL SKILLS

Angie Clarkson, a college sophomore, told me, her college friend, tearfully that she believes she was a victim of daterape her first week in school. She knows she had too much to drink at a party and can only remember waking up in a strange room with a guy she met at the party. She is not sure if she passed out because of the alcohol or if one of the date-rape drugs was involved. A virgin, Angie was sure there had been penetration because of the blood and semen stains she discovered upon waking. It is now a month later and she has not been able to "get her life together" and move on. Angie told me that I am the first person she has told because she feels "so ashamed" and can't believe she let this happen to her. This is my first encounter with an experience like this. I don't do drugs or alcohol and am not sexually active.

Thinking Outside the Box: Possible Courses of Action

- Try to be a good friend and simply suggest she get professional help.
- Advocate for Angie by finding out what resources exist on campus.

- Inform Angie that everything she is describing sounds like the defining characteristics of rape-trauma syndrome and explain how to get professional help and why getting help is so important.

Evaluating a Good Outcome: How Do I Define Success?

- Angie gets the professional help she needs to survive this well.
- I prove worthy of her trust in me.

- I use this experience to learn more about a common problem on campus and the adequacy of existing resources.
- I learn something about my ability to diagnose a health problem and plan accordingly.

Personal Learning: Here's to the Future!

Responding to Angie's clear cry for help certainly moved me out of my comfort zone and made me aware of how my newly developing clinical skills will at times complicate something as simple as being a friend. I felt somewhat responsible for helping Angie cope with being raped and believed that I had to do more than simply provide a listening ear. I was pleasantly surprised to discover all the resources that exist on campus. I guess I wasn't surprised that it took quite a bit of coaxing to get Angie to seek professional help. When I showed her some of what is written about the diagnosis of rape-trauma syndrome, she seemed to find her experience validated and finally agreed to try the student health service counseling center. I felt positive about my role in helping to make this happen.

REFLECTION ON QUALITY AND SAFETY COMPETENCIES

How do you think you would respond in a similar situation? Why? What does this tell you about yourself and about the adequacy of your personal attributes and competencies for professional practice? Do you agree with the criteria that the nursing student used to evaluate a successful outcome? Why or why not? What *knowledge, skills,* and *attitudes* do you need to develop to continuously improve the quality and safety of care for patients like Ms. Clarkson?

Patient-Centered Care: How would you develop a partnership with Ms. Clarkson, knowing her fears? How can you communicate to her that she is your care priority and that she can trust you?

Teamwork and Collaboration/Quality Improvement: In this case, your teamwork will involve campus resources.

What communication skills do you need to improve to ensure that you can access these resources and make them work for Ms. Clarkson? If your research revealed inadequate campus resources, what could you do to advocate for improved quality?

Safety/Evidence-Based Practice: What does the evidence point to as "best practice" in a situation like this? Can you think of campus activities that would promote enhanced safety for all students?

Informatics: Can you identify electronic resources that might help Ms. Clarkson or you? Can you think of other ways to respond to or approach the situation? What else might the nursing student have done to ensure a successful outcome?

(Fig. 12-2 on page 256). Nursing diagnoses provide the basis for selecting nursing interventions that will achieve valued patient outcomes for which the nurse is responsible (Fig. 12-3 on page 256). See Box 12-1 (on page 257) for Alfaro's rule about the legal implications of diagnoses.

Alfaro recommends using both a nursing model and a body systems approach (see Chapter 11) to organize assessment data to detect both nursing and medical problems.

EVOLUTION OF NURSING DIAGNOSES

The term *nursing diagnosis* first appeared in the literature in the 1950s. As early as 1966, Hammond wrote that nurses need to be competent in information-seeking strategies and should have a good background of theoretical knowledge to search for cues and evaluate evidence. These skills and

FIGURE 12-2. Diagnosing is the interpretation and analysis of patient data to identify patient strengths and health problems that nursing intervention can prevent or resolve. Nursing diagnoses may change from day to day as the patient's responses to health and illness change. *(Photo by B. Proud.)*

knowledge result in accurate diagnosing. Key elements in the evolution of nursing diagnosis as an integral component of the nursing process include the following:

- In 1953, the term *nursing diagnosis* was introduced by V. Fry (1953) to describe a step necessary in developing a care plan.
- In 1972, the New York State Nurse Practice Act identified diagnosing as part of the legal domain of professional nursing; practice acts in many other states have been revised similarly since then.
- In 1973, the American Nurses Association's Standards of Practice included diagnosing as a function of professional nursing.
- Also in 1973, Gebbie and Lavin, of St. Louis University, called the First National Conference on Classification of Nursing Diagnoses, beginning a national effort to identify, standardize, and classify health problems treated by

nurses. At this first meeting, the National Group, since renamed the North American Nursing Diagnosis Association (NANDA) and subsequently renamed NANDA International (NANDA-I), appointed a task force to accomplish the following goals:
- Gather information and disseminate it through the Clearinghouse for Nursing Diagnosis.
- Encourage educational activities at regional and state levels to promote the implementation of nursing diagnoses. These activities include conferences to organize nurses to identify additional diagnostic labels and workshops to teach nurses about nursing diagnoses.
- Promote and organize activities to continue the development, classification, and scientific testing of nursing diagnoses. These activities include planning national conferences, identifying criteria for accepting diagnoses, surveying current research activities, and exploring varied methods for classification.

FIGURE 12-3. The relationship of nursing diagnosis to accountability and autonomy. (Used with permission from Carpenito-Moyet, L. J. [2008]. *Nursing diagnosis: Application to clinical practice* [12th ed.]. Philadelphia: Lippincott Williams & Wilkins.)

BOX 12-1 LEGAL ALERT: ALFARO'S RULE

Legal Implications of Using the Word *Diagnosis*

The term *diagnosis* implies that there's a situation or problem requiring appropriate, qualified treatment. This means that if you identify a problem, you must decide if you are *qualified* to treat it and willing to *accept responsibility* for treating it. If you are not, you are responsible for getting help.

Source: Alfaro-LeFevre, R. (2014). *Applying nursing process: The Foundation for Clinical Reasoning* (8th ed.). Philadelphia: Wolters Kluwer Health/Lippincott Williams & Wilkins, p. 92.

- In 1980, the American Nurses Association (ANA) Social Policy Statement defined nursing as "the diagnosis and treatment of human response to actual or potential health problems" (ANA, 1980).
- In March 1990, at the Ninth Conference of NANDA, the General Assembly approved an official definition of nursing diagnosis:

    Nursing diagnosis is a clinical judgment about individual, family, or community responses to actual or potential health problems/life processes. Nursing diagnosis provides the basis for selection of nursing interventions to achieve outcomes for which the nurse is accountable. (NANDA, 1990)

- In March 1990, the first issue of *Nursing Diagnosis,* NANDA's official journal, was published.
- In 2004, the ANA Standards of Nursing Practice revised the Standard 2 Diagnosis, to include the word *issues:* The registered nurse analyzes the assessment data to determine the diagnoses or issues (ANA, 2010) (Box 12-2). Alfaro-LeFevre (2014) believes that adding "issues" to the standard reflects the realities of today's health care setting. Today's nurses deal with specific problems (diagnoses) and ill-defined problems (issues).
- NANDA-I conferences are held every 2 years, during which much progress continues to be made in defining, classifying, and describing nursing diagnoses—internationally.

Now an accepted and essential step in the nursing process, nursing diagnosis was initially confused with medical diagnosis, sparking controversy. Although this confusion has been resolved, many nurses have been slow to understand and to accept the "work" of diagnosing.

UNIQUE FOCUS OF NURSING DIAGNOSIS

In the diagnosing step of the nursing process, the nurse expresses nursing's unique concern for a patient (i.e., what it is about the patient that gives rise to the need for nursing, as opposed to the need for medicine or for physical therapy). Nursing diagnoses are written to describe patient problems or issues that nurses can treat independently, such as activity, pain and comfort, and tissue integrity and perfusion problems.

BOX 12-2 ANA STANDARDS OF PRACTICE: STANDARD 2, DIAGNOSIS

The registered nurse analyzes the assessment data to determine the diagnoses or issues.

Competencies

The registered nurse:

Derives the diagnoses or issues based from assessment data.

Validates the diagnoses or issues with the healthcare consumer, family, and other healthcare providers when possible and appropriate.

Identifies actual or potential risks to the healthcare consumer's health and safety or barriers to health, which may include but are not limited to interpersonal, systematic, or environmental circumstances.

Uses standardized classification systems and clinical decision support tools, when available, in identifying diagnoses.

Documents diagnoses or issues in a manner that facilitates the determination of the expected outcomes and plan.

Reprinted with permission from American Nurses Association (ANA). (2010). *Scope and standards of practice* (p. 34). Silver Spring, MD: Author.

 CONSIDER Antonia Zuccarelli, the middle-aged woman recently diagnosed with cancer but failing to maintain follow-up. Although the patient's diagnosis of cancer is important, the nurse would focus on the patient's lack of follow-up and the possible underlying reasons. For example, the patient may not realize the importance of the follow-up, thereby indicating a lack of knowledge. Or the patient may be too overwhelmed with the diagnosis, possibly denying its existence and being unable to cope. ●

In her latest book on the nursing process, Alfaro-LeFevre (2014, pp. 93–94) describes the shift from diagnose and treat (DT) to predict, prevent, manage, and promote (PPMP). The latter approach focuses on early evidence-based intervention to prevent and manage problems and their potential complications. It requires three activities for nurses:

1. In the presence of known problems, predict the most common and most dangerous complications and take immediate action to (a) prevent them, and (b) manage them in case they cannot be prevented.
2. Whether problems are present or not, look for evidence of risk factors (things that evidence suggests contribute to health problems). If you identify risk factors, you aim to reduce or control them, thereby preventing the problems themselves.
3. In all situations, ensure that safety and learning needs are met, and promote optimum function and independence.

As nurses interpret and analyze patient data, they may identify health problems that are better treated by physicians (medical diagnoses) or by nurses working with other health care professionals (collaborative problems). In such a case, the nurse reports the findings to the physician or other appropriate health care professionals and works collaboratively with them to resolve the problem.

Nursing Diagnosis Versus Medical Diagnosis

Medical diagnoses identify diseases, whereas nursing diagnoses focus on unhealthy responses to health and illness. Medical diagnoses describe problems for which the physician directs the primary treatment, whereas nursing diagnoses describe problems treated by nurses within the scope of independent nursing practice. A medical diagnosis remains the same for as long as the disease is present, whereas a nursing diagnosis may change from day to day as the patient's responses change. These distinctions reflect key differences in medical and nursing practices.

Myocardial infarction (heart attack) is a medical diagnosis. Examples of nursing diagnoses for a person with myocardial infarction may include Fear, Altered Health Maintenance, Deficient Knowledge, Pain, and Altered Tissue Perfusion.

 THINK back to Angie Clarkson, the college sophomore who was a victim of daterape. Possible nursing diagnoses might include Ineffective Coping, RapeTrauma Syndrome, Post-Trauma Syndrome, Risk for Situational Low Self-Esteem, and Risk for Infection. ●

Nursing Diagnosis Versus Collaborative Problem

Nursing diagnoses are also different from collaborative problems. Together, nursing diagnoses and collaborative problems constitute the range of responses that nurses treat; as such, they define the unique nature of nursing. Carpenito defines **collaborative problems** as "certain physiologic complications that nurses monitor to detect onset or changes in status. Nurses manage collaborative problems using physician-prescribed and nurse interventions to minimize the complications of the event" (Carpenito, 2013, p. 23).

Unlike medical diagnoses, collaborative problems are the primary responsibility of nurses. Unlike nursing diagnoses, with collaborative problems, the prescription for treatment comes from nursing, medicine, and other disciplines. When the nurse writes patient outcomes that require delegated medical orders for goal achievement, the situation is not a nursing diagnosis, but a collaborative problem. Because collaborative problems involve potential complications, they must be identified early so that preventive nursing care can be instituted early. Figure 12-4 shows collaborative problems identified by a nurse caring for a patient with ovarian cancer. These problems are related to a medical disease, a medical treatment, and a diagnostic study.

 Concept Mastery Alert

A helpful way to remember the difference between nursing diagnoses and collaborative problems is to connect the "C's," that is, collaborative equals complications.

To write a diagnostic statement for a collaborative problem, focus on the potential complications of the problem. Use "PC" (for potential complication), followed by a colon, and list the complications that might occur. For clarity, link the potential complications and the collaborative problem by using "related to." Example: "PC: Paralytic ileus related to anesthesia."

Table 12-1 shows how health care professionals successfully interpret different clusters of data to identify a nursing diagnosis, collaborative problem, and medical diagnosis. In the first example, a nursing diagnosis is identified and successfully treated. In the next example, the nurse identifies a collaborative problem and initiates intervention within the scope of nursing practice. When this fails to resolve the problem, a physician is contacted to order medication or a catheterization. In this example, the nurse's early detection

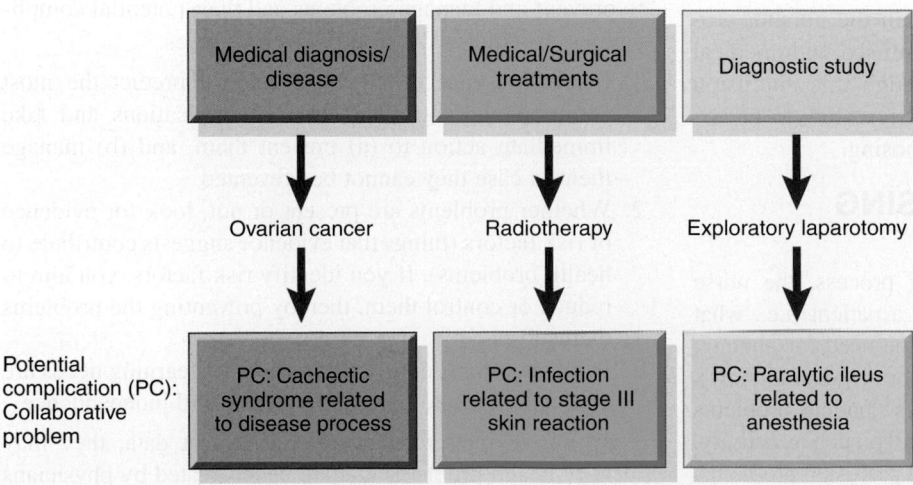

FIGURE 12-4. Collaborative problems.

Table 12-1 A COMPARISON: NURSING DIAGNOSIS, COLLABORATIVE PROBLEM, MEDICAL DIAGNOSIS

	NURSING DIAGNOSIS	COLLABORATIVE PROBLEM	MEDICAL DIAGNOSIS
Definition	A nursing diagnosis is a clinical judgment about individual, family, or community responses to actual or potential health problems or life processes. Nursing diagnosis provides the basis for selection of nursing interventions to achieve outcomes for which the nurse is accountable (NANDA-I).	Certain physiologic complications that nurses monitor to detect onset of changes in status (Carpenito-Moyet, 2010)	Traumatic or disease condition or syndrome validated by medical diagnostic studies
Focus	Monitoring human responses to actual and potential health problems	Monitoring pathophysiologic responses of body organs or systems	Correcting or preventing pathology of specific organs or body systems
Sample data cluster	56-year-old mother of seven; 5'4", 167 lb; "Whenever I sneeze lately, I dribble urine. This is embarrassing."	42-year-old woman; 1 hour after delivery; spinal anesthesia; 1,500 mL fluid infused in past 4 hours without patient voiding; unable to void	"Whenever I have to urinate, it burns terribly. I also feel like I have to go all the time—real bad." Small, frequent voidings, cloudy urine; T—100.8°F
Diagnostic statement	Stress Urinary Incontinence related to degenerative changes in pelvic muscles and structural supports associated with advanced age, obesity, gravid uterus	Potential complication: Urinary Retention related to fluid overload and effects of anesthesia	Cystitis
Select nursing responses	Teach Kegel exercises to increase muscle tone; explore patient's willingness and motivation to pursue weight reduction and exercise program; evaluate need for bladder-training program.	Monitor for signs of increasing urine retention; offer bedpan, and encourage voiding with running water, warm water dripped over perineum, and so forth; if no result, administer physician-prescribed medication; if no result, perform physician-prescribed catheterization.	Report signs and symptoms to physician; obtain urine culture; report results to physician; administer appropriate physician-prescribed antibiotic.

and reporting of the problem to the physician lead to the physician's prompt medical diagnosis of cystitis and successful antibiotic therapy.

DIAGNOSTIC REASONING AND CLINICAL REASONING

Successful implementation of each step of the nursing process requires high-level skills in clinical reasoning. To correctly diagnose health problems:

- Be familiar with nursing diagnoses and other health problems; read professional literature and keep reference guides handy.
- Trust clinical experience and judgment, but be willing to ask for help when the situation demands more than your qualifications and experience can provide.
- Respect your clinical intuition, but before writing a diagnosis without evidence, increase the frequency of your observations and continue to search for cues to verify your intuition.
- Recognize personal biases and keep an open mind.

Questions to facilitate critical thinking during diagnostic reasoning include:

- Are my data accurate and complete? Do the objective data support the subjective data? How do I know that this information is reliable?
- Have I correctly distinguished normal from abnormal findings and decided if abnormal data may be signs and symptoms of a specific health problem?
- Have I made and validated deductions or opinions that follow logically from patient cues?
- Has the patient or the patient's surrogates validated (if able to do so) that these are important problems?
- Have I given the patient or the patient's surrogate an opportunity to identify problems that I may have missed?
- Is each diagnosis supported by evidence? Might these cues signify a different problem or diagnosis?
- Have I tried to identify what is causing the actual or potential problem, and what strengths/resources the patient might use to avoid or resolve the problem?
- Have I followed agency guidelines to correctly document diagnostic statements in a way that clearly communicates patient problems to other health care professionals?
- Is this a problem that falls within nursing's independent domain or does it signify a medical diagnosis or collaborative problem?

DIAGNOSTIC REASONING AND INTERPERSONAL COMPETENCE

NANDA-I is quick to point out that nursing diagnoses are best used by nurses who have strong interpersonal and communication skills. These skills translate into patients being able to trust nurses sufficiently to talk about their responses to health problems and life processes. You must be able to demonstrate your desire to listen to the patient's narrative to gain trust.

> The best use of nursing diagnosis is in partnership with patients, families, groups and communities.... To work in partnership, nurses need to speak to people with respect and care, listen effectively, respect the opinions and views of others, and know how to validate perceptions with patients and families. Learning these skills is a challenge, so the interpersonal aspects of nursing need to be an integral part of learning to use nursing diagnoses (NANDA-I, 2012, p. 74).

DATA INTERPRETATION AND ANALYSIS

Most experienced nurses begin the work of interpreting and analyzing data while they are still collecting (assessing) it. The term **cue** is often used to denote significant data or data that influence this analysis. Significant data should "raise a red flag" for the nurse, who then looks for patterns or clusters of data that signal an actual or possible nursing diagnosis.

 RECALL Martin Prescott, the 46-year-old man with bleeding associated with bowel movements. The report of bleeding accompanied by the patient's complaint of constipation should alert the nurse to a potential problem involving the patient's bowel elimination. ●

Recognizing Significant Data

Sorting out healthy patient responses from those that are not healthy is not as clear-cut as it may seem. To avoid erroneously labeling selected patient health patterns as unhealthy (**diagnostic error**) while failing to detect an actual unhealthy behavior, nurses must be familiar with comparative standards to be used in data interpretation and analysis.

A **standard**, or a norm, is a generally accepted rule, measure, pattern, or model to which data can be compared in the same class or category. For example, when determining the significance of a patient's blood pressure reading, appropriate standards include normative values for the patient's age group, race, and illness category. The patient's own normal range, if known, is an important standard. A pressure of 150/90 mm Hg may be high for someone whose pressure normally is 120/70 mm Hg, but it may be normal for a person with hypertension. Examples of how standards can be used to identify significant cues include the following (Gordon, 1994):

1. Changes in a patient's usual health patterns that are unexplained by expected norms for growth and development:

Example—An infant who took to breastfeeding easily as a newborn suddenly stops sucking when put to the breast and begins to lose weight.
2. Deviation from an appropriate population norm: *Example*—A first-year college student begins to accelerate her exercise habits dramatically and starts inducing vomiting after binge eating. She rapidly loses weight.
3. Behavior that is nonproductive in the whole-person context: *Example*—A college student breaks up with her boyfriend and begins to believe that she is "unfit" for any other relationship, withdrawing from her friends and social activities.
4. Behavior that indicates a developmental lag or evolving dysfunctional pattern: *Example*—A 16-year-old single mother with a 6-month-old infant continues to "party hard" with her friends, hangs out at the mall, and shows no interest in caring for her son, who is repeatedly left with concerned family members.

Recognizing Patterns or Clusters

A **data cluster** is a grouping of patient data or cues that points to the existence of a health problem. Nursing diagnoses should always be derived from clusters of significant data rather than from a single cue. The danger of deriving a nursing diagnosis from a single cue is illustrated in the following example. Diagnosing a woman recovering from gallbladder surgery with Ineffective Coping solely on the basis of tears may misinterpret the patient's crying, which may be a healthy release of emotion. If the same patient begins to exhibit a cluster of significant cues, such as refusing to eat, preferring bed rest to scheduled ambulation, and reporting increasing discomfort, an unhealthy pattern is emerging.

 THINK back to Angie Clarkson, the college sophomore. Her verbalization of the rape trauma is significant. However, even more significant is Angie's report that the event happened more than 1 month ago and she is having difficulty "getting her life together" and moving on. ●

Table 12-2 offers examples of how clusters of significant data lead to formulation of accurate nursing diagnoses.

Identifying Strengths and Problems

The next step in analyzing data is to determine the patient's strengths and problems. It also helps to determine whether the patient agrees with the nurse's identification of strengths and problems and is motivated to work toward problem resolution.

Determining Patient and Family Strengths

If a patient appears to meet a standard, the nurse concludes that the patient has strength in that particular area, and that this strength contributes to the patient's level of wellness. For example, a person with a history of maintaining a well-balanced diet is usually better able to cope with illness than a person who has a history of eating poorly.

Table 12-2 FORMULATING ACCURATE NURSING DIAGNOSIS BASED ON DATA CLUSTERS

DATA INTERPRETATION AND ANALYSIS		FORMULATION OF TENTATIVE NURSING DIAGNOSIS	VALIDATION OF NURSING DIAGNOSIS
Significant Cues	*Sample Data Clusters*		
Patient 1 Change in a patient's usual health patterns that is unexplained by expected norms for growth and development	• "I guess I lost about 20 to 30 pounds over the last 6 months—I think I've just been too busy to eat." • Height: 5'8" • Weight: 102 lb • 35-year-old mother of twin boys; returned to work (executive secretary) for first time since delivery of twins 7 months ago	Imbalanced Nutrition: Less Than Body Requirements, related to stress of new job; role conflict and demands	Accurate diagnosis: Patient validates this diagnosis, agreeing with contributing factors
Patient 2 Deviation from an appropriate population norm	• Teacher notices and reports frequency of bruises on third-grade boy who is repeatedly observed alone during recess periods and who is withdrawn in classroom. • In conversation with the school nurse, one parent remarks: "That boy brings out the worst in me! I don't know why, but I often have to smack him hard to make him listen."	Risk for Other-Directed Violence (Child Abuse) related to? Etiology (deficient parenting skills?)	Incomplete diagnosis: Additional data collection yields new information: • Father out of work for past 18 months • Father was abused as a child Diagnosis restated: Risk For Other-Directed Violence (Child Abuse) related to increased family stress and father's history of being abused
Patient 3 Behavior that is nonproductive in the whole-person context	• Fiancé abruptly terminated relationship 3 months before established wedding date • Noticeable change in physical appearance; frequently wears same clothes; makeup, jewelry, hair-styling are absent; strong body odors present • No desire to be with others; goes home (lives alone) immediately after work • Stopped attending aerobics classes	Risk for Situational Low Self-Esteem related to feeling rejected by fiancé	Premature diagnosis resulting from incomplete data collection. Patient has a long history of major depressive states, one of which may have resulted in the breakup of this relationship. Medical diagnosis and treatment indicated. Changes in appearance are indicative of depressive state. Need to explore related nursing diagnoses.
Patient 4 Behavior indicating developmental lags or evolving dysfunctional patterns	• Admitted to long-term care facility 2 months ago • "I have nothing to live for anymore…why don't I die?" • Wishes to remain in room seated in chair—will only ambulate with great urging • Anything requiring movement has become "too much bother." • Decreased muscle mass, tone, and strength, reduced joint mobility	Impaired Physical Mobility related to difficult transition to long-term care facility	Accurate but routinized diagnosis that may result in staff's acceptance of status quo unless a more specific cause is identified

Patient strengths might include healthy physiologic functioning, emotional health, cognitive abilities, coping skills, interpersonal strengths, and spiritual strengths. Resources such as the presence of support people, adequate finances, and a healthy environment may all contribute to patient strengths. Many people take their strengths for granted and might not know how to use them effectively when responding to illness. Discussing observed strengths with patients and counseling patients about ways to develop and use their strengths are important nursing measures.

Determining the Patient's Problem Areas

A person who does not meet a certain health standard probably has a limitation in that area and may benefit from professional care. For example, a person with a long history of constipation probably needs care to help overcome this problem. As stated previously, the nurse decides whether the data represent a nursing diagnosis or a collaborative problem, or whether the data should be reported to the physician because they might lead to a medical diagnosis.

Determining Problems the Patient Is Likely to Experience

Nurses also identify potential health problems. For example, a nurse notes that a patient has signs of a wound infection, but laboratory test results show that the patient's white blood cell count has not increased, as is usual when such an infection is present. The nurse concludes that the body apparently is not building up normal defenses to combat the infection. The nurse then predicts the problems this patient is likely to encounter, such as a longer-than-normal healing period. Potential nursing diagnoses alert other caregivers to problems the patient may experience if certain trends in the patient's condition continue unreversed. This prediction has implications for nursing care such as measures related to the patient's diet, fluid intake, urine output, and mobility.

Identifying Potential Complications

Patients may experience many complications related to their diagnoses, medications or treatment regimens, or invasive diagnostic studies. While new to nursing, you can more easily prevent potential complications or at least make sure that they are detected early and managed well if you research the potential complications associated with your patient's diagnoses, diagnostics, and treatment, and if you report all abnormal data. For example, slurred speech, changes in skin color or moistness, inability to move an extremity or abnormal movement, and changes in levels of consciousness may all be indications of serious and life-threatening complications (Alfaro-LeFevre, 2014).

Reaching Conclusions

The nurse reaches one of four basic conclusions after interpreting and analyzing the patient data. Different nursing responses result from each conclusion:

No Problem
- No nursing response is indicated.
- Reinforce the patient's health habits and patterns.
- Initiate health-promotion activities to prevent disease or illness or to promote a higher level of wellness.
- Wellness diagnosis might be indicated.

Possible Problem
- Collect more data to confirm or disprove a suspected problem.

Actual or Potential Nursing Diagnosis
- Begin planning, implementing, and evaluating care designed to prevent, reduce, or resolve the problem.
- If unable to treat the problem because the patient denies the problem and refuses treatment, make sure that the patient understands the possible outcomes of this stance.

Clinical Problem Other Than Nursing Diagnosis
- Consult with the appropriate health care professional and work collaboratively on the problem.
- Refer to medical or other services, as indicated.

Partnering with the Patient and Family

Remember that your best source of information usually is an aware patient. While some patients still enter the health care system expecting physicians and nurses to tell them what is "wrong" and to "fix it," increasingly patients want to play a leading role in identifying and treating their health problems. Be sure to ask patients what they believe their most important problems or issues are and have them confirm what your assessment reveals and help you prioritize the resulting list of diagnoses.

FORMULATING AND VALIDATING NURSING DIAGNOSES
Terminology for Writing Nursing Diagnoses

When the nurse recognizes a cluster of significant patient data indicating a health problem that can be treated by independent nursing interventions, a nursing diagnosis should be written. If you are just beginning to understand and write nursing diagnoses, consult the list of health problems accepted by NANDA-I for testing and study (Box 12-3). The NANDA-I list is a beginning list of suggested terms for health problems that might be identified and treated by nurses. Each of the diagnoses in *NANDA International Nursing Diagnoses: Definitions and Classification, 2012–2014* is presented in taxonomic order and includes the basic components of a nursing diagnosis: definition, defining characteristics, and related factors or risk factors (Box 12-4 on page 266).

There are distinct advantages to nurses' use of common terminology when formulating nursing diagnoses. These range from communication advantages (everyone uses the same words to describe common problems) to promoting the development of nursing science by facilitating research

(text continues on page 265)

BOX 12-3 NANDA-I NURSING DIAGNOSES 2012–2014

This list represents the nursing diagnoses approved by NANDA-I for clinical use and testing.

Domain 1: Health Promotion

Definition

The awareness of well-being or normality of function and the strategies used to maintain control of and enhance that well-being or normality of function

Approved Diagnoses

Deficient Diversional Activity
Sedentary Lifestyle
Deficient Community Health
Risk-Prone Health Behavior
Ineffective Health Maintenance
Readiness for Enhanced Immunization Status
Ineffective Protection
Ineffective Self-Health Management
Readiness for Enhanced Self-Health Management
Ineffective Family Therapeutic Regimen Management

Domain 2: Nutrition

Definition

The activities of taking in, assimilating, and using nutrients for the purpose of tissue maintenance, tissue repair, and the production of energy

Approved Diagnoses

Insufficient Breast Milk
Ineffective Infant Feeding Pattern
Imbalanced Nutrition: Less Than Body Requirements
Imbalanced Nutrition: More Than Body Requirements
Readiness for Enhanced Nutrition
Risk for Imbalanced Nutrition: More Than Body Requirements
Impaired Swallowing
Risk for Unstable Blood Glucose Level
Neonatal Jaundice
Risk for Neonatal Jaundice
Risk for Impaired Liver Function
Risk for Electrolyte Imbalance
Readiness for Enhanced Fluid Balance
Deficient Fluid Volume
Excess Fluid Volume
Risk for Deficient Fluid Volume
Risk for Imbalanced Fluid Volume

Domain 3: Elimination and Exchange

Definition

Secretion and excretion of waste products from the body

Approved Diagnoses

Functional Urinary Incontinence
Overflow Urinary Incontinence
Reflex Urinary Incontinence
Stress Urinary Incontinence
Urge Urinary Incontinence
Risk for Urge Urinary Incontinence
Impaired Urinary Elimination
Readiness for Enhanced Urinary Elimination
Urinary Retention
Constipation
Perceived Constipation
Risk for Constipation
Diarrhea
Dysfunctional Gastrointestinal Motility
Risk for Dysfunctional Gastrointestinal Motility
Bowel Incontinence
Impaired Gas Exchange

Domain 4: Activity/Rest

Definition

The production, conservation, expenditure, or balance of energy resources

Approved Diagnoses

Insomnia
Sleep Deprivation
Readiness for Enhanced Sleep
Disturbed Sleep Pattern
Risk for Disuse Syndrome
Impaired Bed Mobility
Impaired Physical Mobility
Impaired Wheelchair Mobility
Impaired Transfer Ability
Impaired Walking
Disturbed Energy Field
Fatigue
Wandering
Activity Intolerance
Risk for Activity Intolerance
Ineffective Breathing Pattern
Decreased Cardiac Output
Risk for Ineffective Gastrointestinal Perfusion
Risk for Ineffective Renal Perfusion
Impaired Spontaneous Ventilation
Ineffective Peripheral Tissue Perfusion
Risk for Decreased Cardiac Tissue Perfusion
Risk for Ineffective Cerebral Tissue Perfusion
Risk for Ineffective Peripheral Tissue Perfusion
Dysfunctional Ventilatory Weaning Response
Impaired Home Maintenance
Readiness for Enhanced Self-Care
Bathing Self-Care Deficit
Dressing Self-Care Deficit
Feeding Self-Care Deficit
Toileting Self-Care Deficit
Self-Neglect

Domain 5: Perception/Cognition

Definition

The human information-processing system, including attention, orientation, sensation, perception, cognition, and communication

Approved Diagnoses

Unilateral Neglect
Impaired Environmental Interpretation Syndrome

(continued)

BOX 12-3 | NANDA-I NURSING DIAGNOSES 2012–2014 *continued*

Acute Confusion
Chronic Confusion
Risk for Acute Confusion
Ineffective Impulse Control
Deficient Knowledge
Readiness for Enhanced Knowledge
Impaired Memory
Readiness for Enhanced Communication
Impaired Verbal Communication

Domain 6: Self-Perception
Definition
Awareness about the self

Approved Diagnoses
Hopelessness
Risk for Compromised Human Dignity
Risk for Loneliness
Disturbed Personal Identity
Risk for Disturbed Personal Identity
Readiness for Enhanced Self-Concept
Chronic Low Self-Esteem
Situational Low Self-Esteem
Risk for Chronic Low Self-Esteem
Risk for Situational Low Self-Esteem
Disturbed Body Image

Domain 7: Role Relationships
Definition
The positive and negative connections or associations between people or groups of people and the means by which those connections are demonstrated

Approved Diagnoses
Ineffective Breastfeeding
Interrupted Breastfeeding
Readiness for Enhanced Breastfeeding
Caregiver Role Strain
Risk for Caregiver Role Strain
Impaired Parenting
Readiness for Enhanced Parenting
Risk for Impaired Parenting
Risk for Impaired Attachment
Dysfunctional Family Processes
Interrupted Family Processes
Readiness for Enhanced Family Processes
Ineffective Relationship
Readiness for Enhanced Relationship
Risk for Ineffective Relationship
Parental Role Conflict
Ineffective Role Performance
Impaired Social Interaction

Domain 8: Sexuality
Definition
Sexual identity, sexual function, and reproduction

Approved Diagnoses
Sexual Dysfunction
Ineffective Sexuality Pattern

Ineffective Childbearing Process
Readiness for Enhanced Childbearing Process
Risk for Ineffective Childbearing Process
Risk for Disturbed Maternal–Fetal Dyad

Domain 9: Coping/Stress Tolerance
Definition
Contending with life events/life processes

Approved Diagnoses
Post-Trauma Syndrome
Risk for Post-Trauma Syndrome
Rape-Trauma Syndrome
Relocation Stress Syndrome
Risk for Relocation Stress Syndrome
Ineffective Activity Planning
Risk for Ineffective Activity Planning
Anxiety
Defensive Coping
Ineffective Coping
Readiness for Enhanced Coping
Ineffective Community Coping
Readiness for Enhanced Community Coping
Compromised Family Coping
Disabled Family Coping
Readiness for Enhanced Family Coping
Death Anxiety
Ineffective Denial
Adult Failure to Thrive
Fear
Grieving
Complicated Grieving
Risk for Complicated Grieving
Readiness for Enhanced Power
Powerlessness
Risk for Powerlessness
Impaired Individual Resilience
Readiness for Enhanced Resilience
Risk for Compromised Resilience
Chronic Sorrow
Stress Overload
Autonomic Dysreflexia
Risk for Autonomic Dysreflexia
Disorganized Infant Behavior
Readiness for Enhanced Organized Infant Behavior
Risk for Disorganized Infant Behavior
Decreased Intracranial Adaptive Capacity

Domain 10: Life Principles
Definition
Principles underlying conduct, thought, and behavior about acts, customs, or institutions viewed as being true or having intrinsic worth

Approved Diagnoses
Readiness for Enhanced Hope
Readiness for Enhanced Spiritual Well-Being
Readiness for Enhanced Decision-Making

BOX 12-3 NANDA-I NURSING DIAGNOSES 2012–2014 *continued*

Decisional Conflict
Moral Distress
Noncompliance
Impaired Religiosity
Readiness for Enhanced Religiosity
Risk for Impaired Religiosity
Spiritual Distress
Risk for Spiritual Distress

Domain 11: Safety/Protection

Definition
Freedom from danger, physical injury, or immune-system damage; preservation from loss; and protection of safety and security

Approved Diagnoses
Risk for Infection
Ineffective Airway Clearance
Risk for Aspiration
Risk for Bleeding
Impaired Dentition
Risk for Dry Eye
Risk for Falls
Risk for Injury
Impaired Oral Mucous Membrane
Risk for Perioperative Positioning Injury
Risk for Peripheral Neurovascular Dysfunction
Risk for Shock
Impaired Skin Integrity
Risk for Impaired Skin Integrity
Risk for Sudden Infant Death Syndrome
Risk for Suffocation
Delayed Surgical Recovery
Risk for Thermal Injury
Impaired Tissue Integrity
Risk for Trauma
Risk for Vascular Trauma

Risk for Other-Directed Violence
Risk for Self-Directed Violence
Self-Mutilation
Risk for Self-Mutilation
Risk for Suicide
Contamination
Risk for Contamination
Risk for Poisoning
Risk for Adverse Reaction to Iodinated Contrast Media
Latex Allergy Response
Risk for Allergy Response
Risk for Latex Allergy Response
Risk for Imbalanced Body Temperature
Hyperthermia
Hypothermia
Ineffective Thermoregulation

Domain 12: Comfort

Definition
Sense of mental, physical, or social well-being or ease

Approved Diagnoses
Impaired Comfort
Readiness for Enhanced Comfort
Nausea
Acute Pain
Chronic Pain
Social Isolation

Domain 13: Growth/Development

Definition
Age-appropriate increase in physical dimensions, maturation of organ systems, and/or progression through the developmental milestones

Approved Diagnoses
Risk for Disproportionate Growth
Delayed Growth and Development
Risk for Delayed Development

Reprinted with permission from North American Nursing Diagnosis Association International (NANDA-I). (2012). *Nursing Diagnoses: Definitions and Classification 2012–2014*. Oxford, UK: Wiley-Blackwell.
In order to make safe and effective judgments using NANDA-I nursing diagnoses, it is essential that nurses refer to the definitions and defining characteristics of the diagnoses listed in this work.

and the dissemination of research findings to establishing the foundation for any cost/benefit analysis for nursing practice.

The NANDA-I structure has been simplified to facilitate the parallel development of an electronic database for nursing diagnoses. The five-digit code structure provides for the growth and development of the classification structure without having to change codes when new diagnoses, refinements, and revisions are added. The code structure is compliant with recommendations from the National Library of Medicine concerning health care terminology codes.

Pocket-sized handbooks of NANDA-I–approved nursing diagnoses are available and help students unfamiliar with this grouping of health problems. Nurses who encounter different health problems within the scope of their practice that

they believe to be nursing diagnoses may submit these to the NANDA-I Diagnosis Review Committee.

Types of Nursing Diagnoses

NANDA-I describes five types of nursing diagnoses: actual, risk, possible, wellness, and syndrome.

Actual Nursing Diagnoses

Actual nursing diagnoses represent problems that have been validated by the presence of major defining characteristics. This type of nursing diagnosis has four components: label, definition, defining characteristics, and related factor.

BOX 12-4 COMPONENTS OF A NANDA-I NURSING DIAGNOSIS

Label
Imbalanced Nutrition: More Than Body Requirements (1975, 2000).

Definition
Intake of nutrients that exceeds metabolic needs.

Defining Characteristics
- Concentrating food intake at the end of the day
- Dysfunctional eating pattern (e.g., pairing food with other activities)
- Eating in response to external cues (e.g., time of day, social situation)
- Eating in response to internal cues other than hunger (e.g., anxiety)
- Sedentary activity level
- Triceps skin fold greater than 25 mm in women, greater than 15 mm in men
- Weight 20% over ideal for height and frame

Related Factors
- Excessive intake in relation to metabolic need.
- Excessive intake in relation to physical activity (caloric expenditure)

Reprinted with permission from North American Nursing Diagnosis Association International (NANDA-I). (2012). *NANDA International nursing diagnoses: Definitions and classification, 2012–2014* (p. 174). Oxford, UK: Wiley-Blackwell.

Risk Nursing Diagnoses

Risk nursing diagnoses are clinical judgments that a person, family, or community is more vulnerable to develop the problem than others in the same or similar situation.

Possible Nursing Diagnoses

Possible nursing diagnoses are statements describing a suspected problem for which additional data are needed. Additional data are used to confirm or rule out the suspected problem.

An actual nursing diagnosis for a patient who has experienced vomiting, diarrhea, and excessive diaphoresis for 3 days is Deficient Fluid Volume related to abnormal fluid loss. If the diarrhea persists and weakness interferes with the patient's normal perineal hygiene, the patient might be at risk for skin breakdown. This is written as the risk diagnosis, Risk for Impaired Skin Integrity. If the nurse suspects that a disturbance of self-concept is also present but lacks the necessary data (defining characteristics) to confirm this, it can be written as a possible diagnosis: Possible Chronic Low Self-Esteem. This alerts other nurses to the need to collect more data about the patient's self-esteem.

Wellness Diagnoses

Wellness diagnoses are clinical judgments about a person, group, or community in transition from a specific level of wellness to a higher level of wellness. Wellness diagnoses are often more applicable in nursing settings that deal primarily with healthy patients. Two cues must be present for a valid wellness diagnosis:

- A desire for a higher level of wellness
- An effective present status or function (Carpenito-Moyet, 2010, p. 17)

The diagnostic statement for wellness diagnoses is a one-part statement that contains the label Readiness for Enhanced, followed by the desired higher-level wellness. Related factors are not included. Examples include Readiness for Enhanced Family Coping, Readiness for Enhanced Health Maintenance, Readiness for Enhanced Parenting, and Readiness for Enhanced Self-Esteem.

Syndrome Nursing Diagnoses

Syndrome nursing diagnoses comprise a cluster of actual or risk nursing diagnoses that are predicted to be present because of a certain event or situation; for example, Rape-Trauma Syndrome or Post-Trauma Syndrome.

Parts of Nursing Diagnosis Statements

Most nursing diagnoses are written either as two-part statements listing the patient's problem and its cause or as three-part statements that also include the problem's defining characteristics (Table 12-3).

 Concept Mastery Alert

The acronyms, PE and PED, can be helpful in remembering how to write a nursing diagnosis. PE stands for "problem" and "etiology"; PED stands for "problem," "etiology," and "defining characteristics."

Problem

The purpose of the problem statement is to describe the health state or health problem of the patient as clearly and concisely as possible. Because this section of the nursing diagnosis identifies what is unhealthy about the patient and what the patient would like to change in his or her health status, it suggests patient outcomes. NANDA-I recommends the use of quantifiers or descriptors to limit or specify the meaning of a problem statement. For example, the descriptor "anticipatory" placed before the concept "grieving" clarifies the nursing diagnosis for a pregnant couple informed prenatally that their child will most likely be stillborn and who are already grieving the death of their child. Some common descriptors are listed in Table 12-4.

Etiology

The etiology identifies the physiologic, psychological, sociologic, spiritual, and environmental factors believed to be related to the problem as either a cause or a contributing factor. Because the etiology identifies the factors that maintain the unhealthy patient state and prevent the desired change, the etiology directs nursing intervention. Unless the

Table 12-3 FORMULATION OF NURSING DIAGNOSIS STATEMENTS

	DEFINITION	PURPOSE	EXAMPLE
Problem	Identifies what is unhealthy about the patient, indicating the need for change (clear, concise statement of the patient's health problem)	Suggests the patient outcomes (expectations for change)	Bathing/Hygiene Self-Care Deficit ↓ related to ↓
Etiology	Identifies the factors that are maintaining the unhealthy state or response (contributing or causative factors)	Suggests the appropriate nursing measures	Fear of falling in the tub and obesity ↓ as manifested by ↓
Defining characteristics	Identify the subjective and objective data that signal the existence of the problem (cues that reflect the existence of a problem)	Suggest evaluative criteria	Strong body and urine odor, unclean hair: "I'm afraid I'll fall in the tub and break something." (5′4″, 170 lb)

Examples:

Two-part diagnostic statement: Bathing/Hygiene Self-Care Deficit related to fear of falling in tub and obesity

Three-part diagnostic statement: Bathing/Hygiene Self-Care Deficit related to fear of falling in tub and obesity, as manifested by strong body and urine odor, unclean hair, statement of fearing fall in tub, and height and weight: 5′4″, 170 lb

Table 12-4 COMMON JUDGMENTS USED TO CLARIFY A DIAGNOSTIC FOCUS

DESCRIPTOR	MEANING
Complicated	Intricately involved, complex
Compromised	Damaged, made vulnerable
Decreased	Lessened (in size, amount, or degree)
Deficient	Insufficient, inadequate
Delayed	Late, slow or postponed
Disabled	Limited, handicapped
Disorganized	Not properly arranged or controlled
Disproportionate	Too large or too small in comparison with a norm
Disturbed	Agitated, interrupted, interfered with
Dysfunctional	Not operating normally
Effective	Producing the intended or desired result
Excessive	Greater than necessary or desirable
Imbalanced	Out of proportion or balance
Impaired	Damaged, weakened
Ineffective	Not producing the intended or desired effect
Interrupted	Having its continuity broken
Low	Below the norm
Organized	Properly arranged or controlled
Perceived	Observed through the senses
Readiness for	In a suitable state for an activity or situation
Situational	Related to a particular circumstance

Reprinted with permission from North American Nursing Diagnosis Association International (NANDA-I). (2012). *NANDA International nursing diagnoses: Definitions and classification, 2012–2014* (p. 60). Oxford, UK: Wiley-Blackwell.

etiology is correctly identified, nursing actions might be inefficient and ineffective. For example, a diabetic patient who is frequently admitted to the hospital with hyperglycemia and who has a poor history of dietary and pharmacologic management is diagnosed to be noncompliant. Mistakenly assuming that the noncompliance is related to a knowledge deficit, channeling all nursing activities and energies into teaching the patient how to manage the diabetes would be useless if the noncompliance was actually a result of the patient's decreased will to live, which would necessitate a different group of nursing interventions.

 RECALL Antonia Zuccarelli, the middle-aged woman recently diagnosed with cancer who fails to maintain follow-up. A nursing diagnosis that might be appropriate would be "Noncompliance related to repeated failure to maintain appointments for follow-up treatment and diagnostic testing." ●

Defining Characteristics

The subjective and objective data that signal the existence of the actual or possible health problem are the third component of the nursing diagnosis. NANDA-I has identified defining characteristics for each accepted nursing diagnosis; familiarity with these characteristics helps nurses recognize clusters of significant data. Table 12-3 defines the three components of a nursing diagnosis statement and shows how they affect patient outcomes, nursing measures, and evaluation. Other examples of nursing diagnosis statements are found throughout the book.

Guidelines for Writing Nursing Diagnoses

Remember the following to ensure that your diagnostic statements are correctly written.

1. Phrase the nursing diagnosis as a patient problem or alteration in health state rather than as a patient need.

Table 12-5 COMMON ERRORS IN WRITING NURSING DIAGNOSES AND RECOMMENDED CORRECTIONS

ERROR	EXAMPLE	CORRECTION	EXAMPLE
Writing the diagnosis in terms of needs and not response	Needs assistance with bathing related to bed rest	Write the diagnosis in terms of response rather than need.	Bathing/Hygiene Self-Care Deficit related to immobility
Making legally inadvisable statements	Noncompliance due to hostility toward nursing staff (the words *due to* imply a direct cause-and-effect relationship) Spouse Abuse related to husband's immaturity and violent temper Impaired Skin Integrity related to patient's lying on back all night	Use "related to" rather than "due to" or "caused by" to link the etiology to the problem statement. Write diagnosis in legally advisable terms: statements that may be interpreted as libel or that imply nursing negligence are legally hazardous to all the nurses caring for the patient.	Noncompliance related to hostility toward nursing staff (denotes a relation between the problem and etiology but not necessarily a causal relation) High Risk for Violence: Spouse Abuse related to husband's reported inability to control behavior Impaired Skin Integrity related to mobility deficit
Identifying as a problem a patient response that is not necessarily unhealthy	Mild Anxiety related to impending surgery	Include in the problem statement of the nursing diagnosis only patient responses that are unhealthy or that the patient wants to change.	No need for nursing diagnosis: mild anxiety before surgery is a healthy response that motivates preoperative self-care behavior
Identifying as a problem signs and symptoms of illness	Cough related to long history of smoking	Avoid including signs and symptoms of illness in the problem statement of the nursing diagnosis.	Ineffective Airway Clearance related to 20-year history of smoking
Identifying as a patient problem or etiology what cannot be changed	Alterations in Bowel Elimination: Permanent Colostomy related to cancer of bowel Grieving related to death of spouse	Express the problem statement and etiologic factors in terms that can be changed; otherwise, nursing energies are being directed to a hopeless task.	Self-Care Deficit: Care of Colostomy, related to severe anxiety about cancer and feelings of powerlessness Dysfunctional Grieving related to inability to accept death of spouse
Identifying environmental factors rather than patient factors as a problem	Cluttered Home related to inability to discard anything	Express the problem statement in terms of unhealthy patient responses rather than environmental conditions.	Risk for Injury related to cluttered home (inability to discard anything)
Reversing clauses	Deficient Knowledge related to alteration in parenting	Avoid reversing the problem statement and etiologic statement.	Impaired Parenting related to knowledge deficit: child growth and development, discipline
Having both clauses say the same thing	Impaired Comfort related to pain (pain is the comfort alteration—what is contributing to the pain?)	Be sure that the two parts of the diagnosis do not mean the same thing.	Unrelieved Incisional Pain related to fear of addiction
Including value judgments in the nursing diagnosis	Poor Home Maintenance related to laziness	Write the diagnosis without value judgments; avoid words such as *poor, inadequate, abnormal, unhealthy.*	Impaired Home Maintenance related to low value ascribed to home safety and cleanliness
Including the medical diagnosis in the diagnostic statement	Impaired Home Maintenance related to arthritis	Do not include the medical diagnosis in the nursing diagnosis statement	Impaired Home Maintenance related to mobility, endurance, and comfort alterations

Common errors adapted from Mundinger, M. O., & Jauron, G. D. (1975). Developing a nursing diagnosis. *Nursing Outlook, 23*(2), 94–98. Guidelines for writing nursing diagnoses adapted from Iyer, P., Taptich, B., & Bernocchi-Losey, D. (1991). *Nursing process and nursing diagnoses* (2nd ed.). Philadelphia: W. B. Saunders.

2. Check to make sure that the patient problem precedes the etiology and that the two are linked by the phrase "related to."
3. Defining characteristics, when included in the nursing diagnosis, should follow the etiology and be linked by the phrase "as manifested by" or "as evidenced by."
4. Write in legally advisable terms.
5. Use nonjudgmental language.
6. Be sure the problem statement indicates what is unhealthy about the patient or what the patient wants to change (enhance).
7. Avoid using defining characteristics, medical diagnoses, or something that cannot be changed in the problem statement.
8. Reread the diagnosis to make sure that the problem statement suggests patient outcomes and that the etiology will direct the selection of nursing measures.

 RECALL Angie Clarkson, the college sophomore who was a victim of daterape. An appropriate nursing diagnosis could be "Rape-Trauma Syndrome related to feelings of embarrassment and shame as manifested by the patient's reporting of event 1 month after it happened, and by patient's statements of inability to get life together and move on." ●

Common errors in writing nursing diagnoses are shown in Table 12-5, along with suggestions for correcting them.

When recording nursing diagnoses in electronic health records (EHRs), remember that different EHRs organize data differently and that the documentation for nursing assessments and for risk nursing diagnoses, health promotion diagnoses, and actual nursing diagnoses may vary. Be sure to check your agency's policies. You should be able to select your nursing diagnoses within the system's problem lists, and the problem list may trigger a message to place an order for an intervention or care set of orders for the patient if this is not already present (NANDA-I, 2012).

What Is Not a Nursing Diagnosis

The nursing diagnosis statement is written in terms of a patient problem, alteration in health state, or patient strength for which nursing provides the primary therapy. Table 12-6 uses a patient with diabetes mellitus to illustrate what nursing

Table 12-6 WHAT A NURSING DIAGNOSIS IS NOT, AND WHY

WHAT A NURSING DIAGNOSIS IS NOT	EXAMPLE	RATIONALE
Medical diagnosis	Diabetes mellitus	Although there is nursing care associated with medical illnesses, the illness is not primarily amenable to nursing intervention. Nursing's concern is the *person* who has the illness and the effect of the illness on human functioning.
Medical pathology	Hypoglycemia	Nurses need to understand the pathology underlying disease states to plan appropriate nursing care, but once again, nursing's focus is the person, not the pathology. The person's response to hypoglycemia, how hypoglycemia affects human functioning—these are the domain of *nursing* diagnoses.
Diagnostic tests, treatments, equipment	Fasting blood glucose, Insulin therapy, Insulin syringe, Infusion pump	Nursing's concern is the person's response to the diagnostic study, treatment, or equipment. If the need for insulin therapy reveals a deficient knowledge or self-care deficit, this becomes the nursing diagnosis, not insulin therapy in and of itself.
Therapeutic patient needs	Needs to learn the relation among diet, exercise, and insulin	The diagnosis should be written as a patient health problem rather than a patient need. *Example:* Impaired Health Maintenance (Diabetic Care) related to lack of knowledge of relation among diet, exercise, and insulin.
Therapeutic nursing goals	To develop therapeutic diabetic self-care behaviors	The diagnosis should be written from the patient perspective rather than the nursing perspective and phrased as a patient health problem. *Example:* Self-Care Deficit: Diabetic Self-Care Behaviors, related to decreased value on life and decreased motivation to learn.
A single sign or symptom	After successfully administering own insulin for 3 days, patient tells nurse, "You give me my shot today."	A nursing diagnosis is not developed until a pattern or cluster of significant cues is detected. The signs and symptoms lead to the identification of the problem statement but are not the problem statement. In this situation, no nursing diagnosis is indicated until further data collection, interpretation, and analysis take place.
An *unvalidated* nursing inference	Above incident leads to the nursing inference: Noncompliance related to depression	This is a premature nursing diagnosis that may not accurately reflect a patient problem. More data and the validation of the tentative nursing diagnosis (nursing inference) are needed before the diagnosis can be recorded.

diagnoses are not. For example, nursing diagnoses are not medical diagnoses or statements of patient need.

Validating Nursing Diagnoses

After a tentative nursing diagnosis is formulated, it should be validated. An affirmative response to each of the following questions validates a tentative diagnosis:

- Is my patient database (assessment data) sufficient, accurate, and supported by nursing research?
- Does my synthesis of data (significant cues) demonstrate the existence of a pattern?
- Are the subjective and objective data I used to determine the existence of a pattern characteristic of the health problem I defined?
- Is my tentative nursing diagnosis based on scientific nursing knowledge and clinical expertise?
- Is my tentative nursing diagnosis able to be prevented, reduced, or resolved by independent nursing action?
- Is my degree of confidence above 50% that other qualified practitioners would formulate the same nursing diagnosis based on my data?

Remember that you are responsible for validating the diagnoses you write, even when using computer-assisted diagnosis. The use of standardized language and electronic health records may make diagnosis writing easier by suggesting possible diagnoses to match your recorded assessment findings. However, computers cannot replace humans and critical thinking, especially when it comes to complex diagnostic reasoning. While the computer can process data faster than you can, it will not be aware of what is happening to your patient at this moment in time. You need to validate diagnoses and recognize when your computer is making an obvious error.

In addition, patients who are able to participate in decision making should be encouraged to validate the diagnosis. "It seems to me that bathing has become a problem now that you are afraid of falling in the tub. What's your sense of this?" Table 12-2 on page 261 lists possible outcomes of validating tentative nursing diagnoses.

DOCUMENTING NURSING DIAGNOSES

The nurse documents validated nursing diagnoses in the patient record. Depending on the documentation system in use, nursing diagnoses might be recorded in the nursing plan of care and on the multidisciplinary problem list at the front of the patient record. Table 12-3 on page 267 illustrates how to document nursing diagnoses using both two- and three-part diagnostic statements.

At one time, nurses were urged to only use NANDA-I accepted terms to state nursing diagnoses. Today, accepted terms vary. Nurses should use the terms recommended by their school, employer, or specialty organization (e.g., Association of Perioperative Nurses [AORN] or Association of Rehabilitation Nurses [ARN]). The terms most commonly used will be the terms chosen for standard plans and computerized systems.

Importance of Nursing Diagnoses in Electronic Health Records (EHRs)

The goal of the EHR is to enable the interdisciplinary team caring for the patient to more easily view the patient's risks, health promotion possibilities, and actual long-term care problems. NANDA-I (2012, p. 100) writes that the documentation of nursing diagnoses is important for the patient and others providing care, and recommends that students use the EHR to:

- View the patient's ongoing risks (Risk for Aspiration, Risk for Falls, etc.) and problems (Impaired Gas Exchange, Bowel Incontinence, etc.) that others have identified and documented
- Decide on and document new nursing diagnoses based on the patient assessment findings
- Facilitate communication of the patient's actual problems (Urinary Retention, Impaired Skin Integrity, etc.) with nurses and others on the care team
- Use nursing diagnosis to make decisions about what mutual goals the patient desires (patient outcomes) and what can be done (nursing interventions)
- Determine and document when the nursing diagnoses (risk, health promotion, or actual problem) are resolved

NURSING DIAGNOSIS: A CRITIQUE

Current nursing diagnosis literature contains many examples of nurses writing about how using nursing diagnoses has improved their clinical practice; articles also detail the many benefits nursing diagnosis brings to the profession. Conversely, other articles point out the limitations of nursing diagnosis and urge nurses to be cautious so that an uncritical use of nursing diagnosis does not restrict their practices.

The primary benefit of nursing diagnosis for the patient is the individualization of patient care. For example, nurses might be caring simultaneously for three women who have had a modified radical mastectomy because of breast cancer. Although the postoperative nursing management of these women is similar, priorities of care may differ. A prioritized list of nursing diagnoses enables nurses to direct their energies toward these differing patient priorities. Different examples of nursing diagnoses for women with modified radical mastectomy follow.

Patient A
- Disturbed Body Image
- Ineffective Coping

Patient B
- Pain
- Bathing/Hygiene Self-Care Deficit

Patient C
- Sexual Dysfunction
- Powerlessness

The use of nursing diagnoses also allows patients to be informed and willing participants in their care, as they validate their diagnoses and assist in prioritizing them. The process of prioritizing nursing diagnoses is the first step in planning care, addressed in Chapter 13.

Improved communication among nurses and other health care professionals is probably the most important benefit of accurate, up-to-date diagnoses—expressed in well-defined and standardized terminology—for nurses. This communication aids in planning, charting, patient data retrieval, health team conferences, change-of-shift reports, and health care follow-up. It also promotes nursing accountability for the problems that nurses diagnose.

Among the other benefits of nursing diagnoses for the profession is help in defining the domain of nursing for health care administrators, legislators, and other health care providers. This is important when seeking funding for nursing and reimbursement for nursing services. Nursing diagnoses are also used to define curriculum content and to direct specialization and advancement in nursing and nursing research.

If the diagnostic process is used incorrectly, however, a patient might be "misdiagnosed." Common sources of error include:

- *Premature diagnoses based on an incomplete database:* For example—A diagnosis of Defensive Coping is made after the patient verbally attacks one nurse who was attempting to teach him self-care for his wound.
- *Erroneous diagnoses resulting from an inaccurate database or a faulty data analysis:* For example—A diagnosis of Dysfunctional Grieving is made in a patient observed crying after learning that her cancer had returned, before anyone had time to evaluate whether this was simply an appropriate response to bad news.
- *Routine diagnoses resulting from the nurse's failure to tailor data collection and analysis to the unique needs of the patient:* For example—A diagnosis of Deficient Knowledge is made in a diabetic patient who is frequently hospitalized with diabetes-related complications, when she actually has excellent knowledge of diabetes and related self-care demands, but has lacked the motivation to care for herself appropriately.
- *Errors of omission:* Failure to modify diagnoses and to identify new diagnoses as the patient's status changes may also be problematic. Failures in diagnosis lead to failures in nursing care.

 RECALL Martin Prescott, the 46-year-old man with rectal bleeding and constipation. Although an initial nursing diagnosis may involve Deficient Knowledge related to possible causes of rectal bleeding, further assessment may reveal that the patient's constipation resulting from a diet inadequate in fiber and fluids is the underlying cause of the bleeding. Thus, the nurse would need to revise the nursing diagnosis to focus on Constipation related to inadequate intake of high-fiber foods and fluids as manifested by hard stool and rectal bleeding, and Deficient Knowledge related to foods high in fiber. ●

These are not so much limitations of nursing diagnosis as they are problems of nurses diagnosing incorrectly. More serious criticisms of nursing diagnoses are raised by nurses who claim that a classification of standardized nursing diagnoses limits nursing, curbing nurses' originality and ability to think things through.

Although some nurses believe that diagnosis offers a valued shortcut to practice, critics find this attitude offensive and respond that rather than invest nursing's energies in perfecting a shortcut, nurses need to change working conditions that interfere with in-depth problem solving and thoughtful nursing care.

Critics of diagnostic labeling point out that instead of identifying what is unique and positive about nursing, nursing diagnoses make a clear statement that nurses are concerned about what is deviant, wrong, or pathologic (Hagey & McDonough, 1984). The ever-changing and dynamic human person with a need for nursing care becomes objectified (Gebbie, 1984). The practice of many experienced nurses who find nursing diagnoses helpful in targeting care for patients with diverse needs counters these concerns.

Nurses who are sensitive to transcultural issues raise important concerns about the cultural limitations of the NANDA-I diagnoses. Foremost among these concerns is that NANDA-I diagnoses and behaviors assume that the patient is "wrong" and the provider is "right," and deny the validity of cultural and health care beliefs and practices that are different from those of the nurse (Geissler, 1991). Examples of nursing diagnoses that often are misused in labeling such cultural deviations as abnormal include Impaired Verbal Communication, Impaired Social Interaction, and Noncompliance. Nurses who provide culturally sensitive care (see Chapter 5) and who work collaboratively with the patient as a partner avoid these problems.

In conclusion, nursing diagnosis has become a valued and essential step in the nursing process. Used correctly, it is a powerful tool for individualizing patient care and ensures that nurses' energies are being used in the most efficient way to meet prioritized and holistic patients' needs. Nurses who are as concerned about the art and spirit of nursing as they are about its science are careful to avoid labeling patients in a way that objectifies them or limits the potential range of nurse–patient interactions.

REFLECTIVE PRACTICE LEADING TO PERSONAL LEARNING

Remember that the object of reflective practice is to look at an experience, understand it, and learn from it. As you begin to develop your expertise in diagnosing health problems and identifying patient strengths, reflect on your experiences—successes and failures—in order to improve your practice. How can you do it better next time? What did you learn today that can help you tomorrow? Alfaro (2014) recommends paying close attention to the following during the diagnosing phase of the nursing process:

- Has patient/family participation in the process been at an optimal level? How might you have better engaged the patient and family?
- Are your data reliable, accurate, and complete? How do you know this?

- Have you identified the assumptions you made about patient cues?
- Are your conclusions based on facts (evidence) rather than guesswork?
- Have you considered alternate conclusions, ideas and solutions?

Perhaps the most important question to reflect on is: Are your patients and families better for having had you share in the critical responsibility of diagnosing their health problems and identifying and tapping their strengths? Are your patients now receiving individualized, prioritized, holistic, evidence-based treatment and care because of your efforts?

DEVELOPING CRITICAL REASONING

1. Find a patient with a well-established medical condition. List potential medical and nursing diagnoses and collaborative problems. Explain the differing purposes of medical and nursing diagnoses and collaborative problems. What is nursing's diagnostic contribution to the interdisciplinary team's effort to care for this patient?

2. Interview several experienced nurses. Find at least one nurse who is strongly committed to using nursing diagnoses and another who believes they are a waste of time. Interview both until you can explain their different experiences with nursing diagnoses. Try to identify different patient outcomes related to their use or nonuse of nursing diagnoses. List the benefits and limitations of using nursing diagnoses.

3. Interview two patients with the same medical diagnosis. Develop a prioritized list of nursing diagnoses for both, and reflect on the differences. Compare and contrast the strengths of both patients. If you can do this exercise with another student, it would be helpful to explore why there are differences in your lists of nursing diagnoses and patient strengths.

4. Reflective nurses realize that they bring their personal attributes, knowledge, and competencies to the process of diagnosing. What personal strengths and limitations do you expect to influence your ability to diagnose health problems and identify and tap strengths?

PRACTICING FOR NCLEX

1. A registered nurse is writing a diagnosis for a 28-year-old male patient who is in traction due to multiple fractures from a motor vehicle accident. Which nursing actions are related to this step in the nursing process? Select all that apply.
   a. The nurse uses the nursing interview to collect patient data.
   b. The nurse analyzes data collected in the nursing assessment.
   c. The nurse develops a care plan for the patient.
   d. The nurse points out the patient's strengths.
   e. The nurse assesses the patient's mental status.
   f. The nurse identifies community resources to help his family cope.

2. A nurse is caring for an older adult patient who presents with labored respirations, productive cough, and fever. What would be appropriate nursing diagnoses for this patient? Select all that apply.
   a. Bronchial pneumonia
   b. Impaired gas exchange
   c. Ineffective airway clearance

   d. Potential complication: sepsis
   e. Infection related to pneumonia
   f. Risk for septic shock

3. After assessing a patient who is recovering from a stroke in a rehabilitation facility, a nurse interprets and analyzes the patient data. Which of the four basic conclusions has the nurse reached when identifying the need to collect more data to confirm a diagnosis of situational low self-esteem?
   a. No problem
   b. Possible problem
   c. Actual nursing diagnosis
   d. Clinical problem other than nursing diagnosis

4. A nurse assesses a patient and formulates the following nursing diagnosis: Risk for Impaired Skin Integrity related to prescribed bedrest as evidenced by reddened areas of skin on the heels and back. Which phrase represents the etiology of this diagnostic statement?
   a. Risk for Impaired Skin Integrity
   b. Related to prescribed bedrest
   c. As evidenced by
   d. As evidenced by reddened areas of skin on the heels and back

5. A nurse is counseling a 60-year-old female patient who refuses to look at or care for a new colostomy. She tells the nurse, "I don't care what I look like anymore, I don't even feel like washing my hair, let alone changing this bag." The nurse diagnoses Altered Health Maintenance. This is an example of what type of problem?
   a. Collaborative problem
   b. Interdisciplinary problem
   c. Medical problem
   d. Nursing problem

6. To determine the significance of a blood pressure reading of 148/100, it is first necessary for the nurse to:
   a. Compare this reading to standards.
   b. Check the taxonomy of nursing diagnoses for a pertinent label.
   c. Check a medical text for the signs and symptoms of high blood pressure.
   d. Consult with colleagues.

7. When the initial nursing assessment revealed that a patient had not had a bowel movement for 2 days, the student nurse wrote the diagnostic label "constipation." Which of the following comments is the nurse most likely to hear from the instructor?
   a. "Hold on a minute…Nursing diagnoses should always be derived from clusters of significant data rather than from a single cue."
   b. "Job well done…you've identified this problem early and we can manage it before it becomes more acute."
   c. "Is this an actual or a possible diagnosis?"
   d. "This is a medical, not a nursing problem."

8. A nurse makes a clinical judgment that an African American male patient in a stressful job is more vulnerable to developing hypertension than White male patients in the same or similar situation. The nurse has formulated what type of nursing diagnosis?
   a. Actual
   b. Risk
   c. Possible
   d. Wellness

9. A nurse is writing nursing diagnoses for patients in a psychiatrist's office. Which nursing diagnoses are correctly written as two-part nursing diagnoses?
    (1) Ineffective Coping related to inability to maintain marriage
    (2) Defensive Coping related to loss of job and economic security
    (3) Altered Thought Processes related to panic state
    (4) Decisional Conflict related to placement of parent in a long-term care facility
        a. (1) and (2)
        b. (3) and (4)
        c. (1), (2), and (3)
        d. All of the above

10. A nurse writes nursing diagnoses for patients and their families visiting a community health clinic. Which nursing diagnoses are correctly written as three-part nursing diagnoses?
    (1) Disabled Family Coping related to lack of knowledge about home care of child on ventilator
    (2) Imbalanced Nutrition: Less Than Body Requirements related to inadequate caloric intake while striving to excel in gymnastics as evidenced by 20-pound weight loss since beginning the gymnastic program, and greatly less than ideal body weight when compared to standard height weight charts
    (3) Need to learn how to care for child on ventilator at home related to unexpected discharge of daughter after 3-month hospital stay as evidenced by repeated comments "I cannot do this," "I know I'll harm her because I'm not a nurse," and "I can't do medical things"
    (4) Spiritual Distress related to inability to accept diagnosis of terminal illness as evidenced by multiple comments such as "How could God do this to me?," "I don't deserve this," "I don't understand. I've tried to live my life well," and "How could God make me suffer this way?"
    (5) Caregiver Role Strain related to failure of home health aides to appropriately diagnose needs of family caregivers and initiate a plan to facilitate coping as evidenced by caregiver's loss of weight and clinical depression
        a. (1) and (3)
        b. (2) and (4)
        c. (1), (2), and (3)
        d. All of the above

ANSWERS WITH RATIONALES

1. *b, d, f.* The purposes of diagnosing are to identify how an individual, group, or community responds to actual or potential health and life processes; identify factors that contribute to or cause health problems (etiologies); and identify resources or strengths the individual, group, or community can draw on to prevent or resolve problems. In the diagnosing step of the nursing process, the nurse interprets and analyzes data gathered from the nursing assessment, identifies patient strengths, and identifies resources the patient can use to resolve problems. The nurse assesses and collects patient data in the assessment step and develops a care plan in the planning step of the nursing process.

2. *b, c, f.* Nursing diagnoses are actual or potential health problems that can be prevented or resolved by independent nursing interventions, such as impaired gas exchange, ineffective airway clearance, or risk for septic shock. Bronchial pneumonia and infection are medical diagnoses, and "potential complication: sepsis" is a collaborative problem.

3. *b.* When a possible problem exists, such as situational low self-esteem related to effects of stroke, the nurse must collect more data to confirm or disprove the suspected problem. The conclusion "no problem" means no nursing response is indicated. When an actual problem exists, the nurse begins planning, implementing, and evaluating care to prevent, reduce, or resolve the problem. A clinical problem other than nursing diagnosis requires that the nurse consult with the appropriate health care professional to work collaboratively on the problem.

4. *b.* "Related to prescribed bedrest" is the etiology of the statement. The etiology identifies the contributing or causative factors of the problem. "Risk for Impaired Skin Integrity" is the problem, and "as evidenced by reddened areas of skin on the heels and back" are the defining characteristics of the problem.

5. *d.* Nursing Problem, because it describes a problem that can be treated by nurses within the scope of independent nursing practice. Collaborative and interdisciplinary problems require a teamwork approach with other health care professionals to resolve the problem. A medical problem is a traumatic or disease condition validated by medical diagnostic studies.

6. *a.* A standard, or a norm, is a generally accepted rule, measure, pattern, or model to which data can be compared in the same class or category. For example, when determining the significance of a patient's blood pressure reading, appropriate standards include normative values for the patient's age group, race, and illness category. Deviation from an appropriate norm may be the basis for writing a diagnosis.

7. *a.* A data cluster is a grouping of patient data or cues that points to the existence of a patient health problem. Nursing diagnoses should always be derived from clusters of significant data rather than from a single cue. There may be a reason for the lack of a bowel movement for 2 days, or it might be this individual's normal pattern.

8. *b.* A clinical judgment that an individual, family, or community is more vulnerable to develop the problem than others in the same or similar situation is a Risk nursing diagnosis.

9. *d.* Each of the four diagnoses is a correctly written two-part diagnostic statement that includes the problem or diagnostic label and the etiology or cause.

10. *b.* (1) is a two-part diagnosis, (3) is written in terms of needs and not an unhealthy response, and (5) is a legally inadvisable statement.

TAYLOR SUITE RESOURCES

Explore these additional resources to enhance learning for this chapter:
* NCLEX-Style Questions and other resources on thePoint, http://thePoint.lww.com/Taylor8e
* *Study Guide for Fundamentals of Nursing, 8th edition*
* Adaptive Learning | Powered by prepU, http://thepoint.lww.com/prepu

Bibliography

Alfaro-LeFevre, R. (2009). *Critical thinking and clinical judgment: A practical approach* (4th ed.). St. Louis: Elsevier/Saunders.

Alfaro-LeFevre, R. (2013). *Critical thinking, clinical reasoning, and clinical judgment* (5th ed.). St. Louis: Elsevier/Saunders.

Alfaro-LeFevre, R. (2014). *Applying nursing process: The Foundation for Clinical Reasoning* (8th ed.). Philadelphia: Wolters Kluwer Health/Lippincott Williams & Wilkins.

American Association of Colleges of Nursing (AACN). (2008). *The essentials of baccalaureate education for professional nursing practice*. Washington, DC: Author.

American Nurses Association (ANA). (2001). *Code for nurses with interpretive statements*. Washington, DC: Author.

American Nurses Association (ANA) (1980, 2010). *Nursing's social policy statement*. Silver Spring, MD: Author.

American Nurses Association (ANA). (2004, 2010). *Nursing: Scope and standards of practice* (2nd ed.). Silver Spring, MD: Author.

Aspinall, M. J. (1976). Nursing diagnosis: The weak link. *Nursing Outlook, 24*(7), 433–436.

Benner, P. (2005). Extending the dialogue about classification systems and the work of professional nurses. *American Journal of Critical Care, 14*(3), 242–243, 272.

Carpenito, L.J. (2013). *Nursing Diagnosis: Application to Clinical Practice* (14th ed.). Philadelphia: Wolters Kluwer Health/Lippincott Williams & Wilkins.

Carpenito-Moyet, L. J. (2010). *Nursing care plans and documentation: Nursing diagnoses and collaborative problems* (5th ed.). Philadelphia: Wolters Kluwer Health/Lippincott Williams & Wilkins.

Carroll-Johnson, R. M. (Ed.). (1991). *Classification in nursing diagnosis: Proceedings of the ninth national conference*. Philadelphia: J. B. Lippincott.

Dochterman, J. M., & Jones, D. A. (2003). *Unifying nursing languages: The harmonization of NANDA, NIC, NOC*. Washington, DC: The American Nurses Association.

Dossey, B., & Guzzetta, C. E. (1981). Nursing diagnosis. *Nursing, 11*(6), 34–38.

Dougherty, C. M., Jankin, J. J., Lunney, M. R., & Whitley, G. G. (1993). Conceptual and research-based validation of nursing diagnoses: 1950–1993. *Nursing Diagnosis, 4*(4), 156–165.

Fry, V. S. (1953). The creative approach to nursing. *American Journal of Nursing, 53*, 301–302.

Gebbie, K. M. (Ed.). (1975). *Summary of the second national conference*. St. Louis: Clearinghouse for Nursing Diagnoses.

Gebbie, K. M. (1984). Nursing diagnosis: What is it and why does it exist? *Topics in Clinical Nursing, 5*(4), 1–9.

Gebbie, K. M., & Lavin, M. A. (1973). *Summary of the first national conference*. St. Louis: C. V. Mosby.

Geissler, E. M. (1991). Transcultural nursing and diagnosis. *Nursing and Health Care, 12*(4), 190–192, 203.

Gordon, M. (1976). Nursing diagnosis and the diagnostic process. *American Journal of Nursing, 76*(8), 1298–1300.

Gordon, M. (1994). *Nursing diagnosis: Process and application* (3rd ed.). St. Louis: C. V. Mosby.

Hagey, R. S., & McDonough, P. (1984). The problem of professional labeling. *Nursing Outlook, 32*(3), 151–157.

Hammond, K. R. (1966). Clinical inference in nursing: A psychologist's viewpoint. *Nursing Research, 15*(1), 27–38.

Herdman, T. H. (2008). Nursing diagnosis: Is it time for a new definition? *International Journal of Nursing Terminologies & Classifications, 19*(1), 2–13.

Hurley, M. (Ed.). (1986). *Classification of nursing diagnoses: Proceedings of the sixth conference*. St. Louis: C. V. Mosby.

Iyer, P., Taptich, B., & Bernocchi-Losey, D. (1991). *Nursing process and nursing diagnoses* (2nd ed.). Philadelphia: W. B. Saunders.

Kerr, M., Hoskins, L. M., Fitzpatrick, J. J., Warren, J. J., Avant, K. C., & Hurley, M., et al. (1993). Taxonomic validation: An overview. *Nursing Diagnosis, 4*(1), 6–14.

Kim, M. J., McFarland, G. K., & McLane, A. M. (Eds.). (1984). *Classification of nursing diagnosis: Proceedings of the fifth national conference*. St. Louis: C. V. Mosby.

Kim, M. J., & Moritz, D. A. (1982). *Classification of the third and fourth national conferences*. Hightstown, NJ: McGraw-Hill.

Kritek, P. B. (1985). Nursing diagnosis in perspective: Response to a critique. *Image—The Journal of Nursing Scholarship, 16*(1), 3–8.

Kurashima, S., Kobayaski, K., Toyabe, S., & Akazawa, K. (2008). Accuracy and efficiency of computer-aided nursing diagnosis. *International Journal of Nursing Terminologies and Classifications, 19*(3), 95–101.

Lindsey, A. M. (1990). Identification and labeling of human responses. *Journal of Professional Nursing, 6*(3), 143–150.

Lipe, S. L., & Beasley, S. (2004). *Critical thinking in nursing*. Philadelphia: Lippincott Williams & Wilkins.

Lunney, M. (1982). Nursing diagnosis: Refining the system. *American Journal of Nursing, 82*(3), 456–459.

Lunney, M. (2008). The need for international nursing diagnosis research and a theoretical framework.

International Journal of Nursing Terminologies and Classifications, 19(1), 28–34.

Lunney, M. (2010). Use of critical thinking in the diagnostic process. *International Journal of Nursing Terminologies and Classifications, 21*(2), 82–88.

McLane, A. M. (Ed.). (1987). *Classification of nursing diagnoses: Proceedings of the seventh conference*. St. Louis: C. V. Mosby.

Mitchell, G. J. (1991). Nursing diagnosis: An ethical analysis. *Image—The Journal of Nursing Scholarship, 23*(2), 99–103.

Mueller, A., Johnston, M., & Bligh, D. (2002). Joining mind mapping and care planning to enhance student critical thinking and achieve holistic nursing care. *Nursing Diagnosis, 13*(1), 24.

Muller-Staub, M., Lavin, M. A., Needham, I., & van Achterberg, T. (2007). Meeting the criteria of a nursing diagnosis classification: Evaluation of ICNP, ICF, NANDA and ZEFP. *International Journal of Nursing Studies, 44*(5), 702–713.

Mundinger, M. O., & Jauron, G. D. (1975). Developing a nursing diagnosis. *Nursing Outlook, 23*, 94–98.

North American Nursing Diagnosis Association (NANDA). (1990). *Taxonomy I revised with official diagnostic categories*. St. Louis: Author.

North American Nursing Diagnosis Association International (NANDA-I). (2012). *NANDA international nursing diagnoses: Definitions and classification, 2012–2014*. Oxford, UK: Wiley-Blackwell.

Popkess, S. (1981). Diagnosing your patient's strengths. *Nursing, 11*(7), 34–37.

Popkess, S., &Vawter, S. (1991). Wellness nursing diagnosis: To be or not to be? *Nursing Diagnosis, 2*(1), 19–25.

Porter, E. J. (1986). Critical analysis of NANDA nursing diagnosis taxonomy I. *Image—The Journal of Nursing Scholarship, 18*(4), 136–139.

Rasch, R. F. R. (1987). The nature of taxonomy. *Image— The Journal of Nursing Scholarship, 19*(3), 147–149.

Shamansky, S. L., & Yanni, C. R. (1983). In opposition to nursing diagnosis: A minority opinion. *Image— The Journal of Nursing Scholarship, 15*(2), 47–50.

Tanner, C.A. (2006). Thinking like a nurse. A research-based model of clinical judgment in nursing. *Journal of Nursing Education, 45*(6), 204–211.

Vincent, K. G., & Coler, M. S. (1990). A unified nursing diagnostic model. *Image—The Journal of Nursing Scholarship, 22*(2), 93–95.

Warren, J., & Hoskins, L. (1990). The development of NANDA's nursing diagnosis taxonomy. *Nursing Diagnosis, 1*(4), 162–168.

Wilkinson, J. M. (2000). *Nursing diagnosis handbook with NIC interventions and NOC outcomes* (7th ed.). Upper Saddle River, NJ: Prentice Hall Health.

Wong, E. (2008). Coining and defining novel nursing technology. Part 1: Critical incident nursing diagnosis. *International Journal of Nursing Technologies and Classifications, 19*(3), 89–94.

13 | Outcome Identification and Planning

GLENDA KRONK

Glenda, a 35-year-old woman, comes to the health center for a routine checkup. During the visit, she expresses a strong motivation and desire to become physically fit, lose weight, increase her muscle tone, and improve her cardiorespiratory capacity. "I know it will involve some major lifestyle changes, including diet. What's with all these diets and diet supplements now?" she asks.

DARLA JEFFERSON

Darla, a 29-year-old single woman, is about 14 weeks pregnant. She describes herself as a "hopeless addict" who has tried to stop "more times than I can remember." Although currently drug-free, she is not hopeful of preventing relapse. She does not know the baby's father and has mixed feelings about keeping the baby, saying, "On the one hand I want someone to love me, but I'm not sure I'd want me for a mother."

ELIJAH WOLINSKI

Elijah is a thin, frail, 85-year-old man who is bed-bound due to severe degenerative joint disease. He is being cared for by his 56-year-old nephew at his home. Assessment on a home visit reveals Elijah lying on soiled linens with a large pressure ulcer on his sacrum, approximately 3" in diameter and about 1" deep with purulent drainage.

After the nurse collects and interprets patient data, identifying patient strengths and health problems, it is time to plan for nursing actions (see the accompanying Reflective Practice box for an example). During the **outcome identification** and **planning** steps of the nursing process, the nurse works in partnership with the patient and family to:

- Establish priorities
- Identify and write expected patient outcomes
- Select evidence-based nursing interventions
- Communicate the plan of nursing care (Fig. 13-1 on page 278)

A **goal** is an aim or an end. A **patient outcome** is an expected conclusion to a patient health problem, or in the event of a wellness diagnosis, an expected conclusion to a patient's health expectation. The words *goal, objective,* and *outcome* are often used interchangeably. In some practice settings, the term *goal* or *objective* is used to describe what is wanted, and the term *outcome* is used to describe the results achieved. In nursing, the phrase **expected outcomes** is used to refer to the more specific, measurable **criteria** used to evaluate the extent to which a goal has been met. This chapter uses *outcome* to refer to expected patient outcomes.

The nurse, patient, and family should work together as much as possible in the outcome identification and planning stage. If the outcomes specified in the plan of care are not valued by the patient or do not contribute to the prevention, resolution, or reduction of the patient's problems or the achievement of the patient's health expectations, the plan of care may be ineffective. Outcome determination is, therefore, a critical skill for successfully intervening with patients.

This chapter describes outcome identification and planning as a formal process, a deliberate step in the nursing process. A formal plan of care allows nurses to:

- Individualize care that maximizes outcome achievement
- Set priorities
- Facilitate communication among nursing personnel and their colleagues
- Promote continuity of high-quality, cost-effective care
- Coordinate care
- Evaluate the patient's responses to nursing care
- Create a record that can be used for evaluation, research, reimbursement, and legal purposes
- Promote the nurse's professional development

Nurses also engage in informal planning in practice. This is the link between identifying a patient's strength or problem and providing an appropriate nursing response. When a nurse on a busy surgical unit learns that a postoperative patient is complaining of incisional pain and quickly reshuffles priorities to allow time to assess the course and qualities of the pain and determine nursing measures to reduce discomfort, planning has occurred. When a postpartum nurse on the 3-to-11 shift realizes the evening before the mother's discharge that he or she has not seen a particular father hold his new daughter and makes a mental note to observe the father–daughter interactions that evening and facilitate their bonding, planning has occurred. When a nurse in a geriatric daycare center hears a patient choking and rushes to his side to perform the Heimlich maneuver if necessary, planning

REFLECTIVE PRACTICE: CULTIVATING QSEN COMPETENCIES

CHALLENGE TO ETHICAL AND LEGAL SKILLS

While working in a women's shelter, I met Darla Jefferson, a 29-year-old single woman who was about 14 weeks pregnant. Darla described herself as a "hopeless addict" who had tried to stop "more times than I can remember." She was drug-free at the moment but not hopeful of preventing relapse. She did not know her baby's father and had mixed feelings about keeping the baby. She said, "On the one hand I want someone to love me, but I'm not sure I'd want me for a mother." I knew I needed to explore her commitment to this pregnancy, but I am strongly opposed to abortion and did not think I could talk with her objectively about her decision. I needed to develop a plan for dealing with this issue.

Thinking Outside the Box: Possible Courses of Action

- Tell Darla that I believe it is her responsibility to have this baby and to then make a decision about whether to offer the baby for adoption based on her assessment of her parenting readiness.

- Help Darla assess her readiness to become a parent and, in light of this, explore all her options regarding continuing or terminating the pregnancy.
- Get someone else to talk with Darla so that she gets the counseling she needs and I am not morally compromised.

Evaluating a Good Outcome: How Do I Define Success?

- Darla gets the help she needs to make the decision that is right for her and her unborn baby.

- I am faithful to both my nursing responsibilities to counsel this patient and my duty to maintain my moral integrity.

Personal Learning: Here's to the Future!

Unfortunately, I overestimated my ability to counsel Darla without compromising myself, and as a result, I don't think I was as helpful to her as I should have been. Ideally, I planned to objectively explore her readiness to be a mother and then have an open and unbiased discussion about her options. When she began to talk about getting an abortion, I found myself urging her to have the baby and then place the baby up for adoption if she still felt she couldn't care for the infant after delivery. Regrettably, I let my personal opinions come through in the discussion. Through my actions, I think she lost trust in me. I'm going to talk with other nurses to see how they handle this challenge.

REFLECTION ON QUALITY AND SAFETY COMPETENCIES

How would you respond in a similar situation? Why? What does this tell you about yourself and about the adequacy of your competencies for professional practice? Can you think of other ways to respond? What actions might have proved more effective? What actions might be helpful for the nursing student so that when faced with similar situations in the future, the outcome would be more positive? Do you agree with the criteria that the nursing student used to evaluate a successful outcome? Why or why not? What *knowledge, skills,* and *attitudes* do you need to develop to continuously improve the quality and safety of care for patients like Ms. Jefferson?

Patient-Centered Care: How would you develop a successful partnership with Ms. Jefferson, knowing that she may choose an alternative that is unethical for you? Are nurses obligated to be ethically neutral when issues like this come up? How can you best communicate empathy and that you respect her even when you disagree with choices she makes?

Teamwork and Collaboration/Quality Improvement: What communication and interpersonal skills do you need to improve to ensure that you function as a member of the patient-care team and to obtain assistance when needed? What does quality care for Ms. Jefferson "look like"?

Safety/Evidence-Based Practice: What does the evidence point to as "best practice" for Ms. Jefferson? What safety needs does she and her unborn baby have and how can you meet them?

Informatics: Can you identify the essential information that must be available in Ms. Jefferson's electronic record to support safe patient care and coordination of care? Can you think of other ways to respond to or approach the situation? What else might the nursing student have done to ensure a successful outcome?

has occurred. Informal planning on a more deliberate level is illustrated by a hospice nurse who drives home pondering how best to support a patient with terminal cancer who is gradually relinquishing her hold on life. The hospice nurse may elect to initiate a more formal process of planning the next day when consulting with colleagues who have cared for patients with similar health needs. In each of these examples, the process of informal planning allowed an individual nurse to think about how best to help a particular patient—

ideally, with good results. What is lacking is a coordinated plan known by everyone caring for the patient.

UNIQUE FOCUS OF NURSING OUTCOME IDENTIFICATION AND PLANNING

The primary purpose of the outcome identification and planning step of the nursing process is to design a plan of care

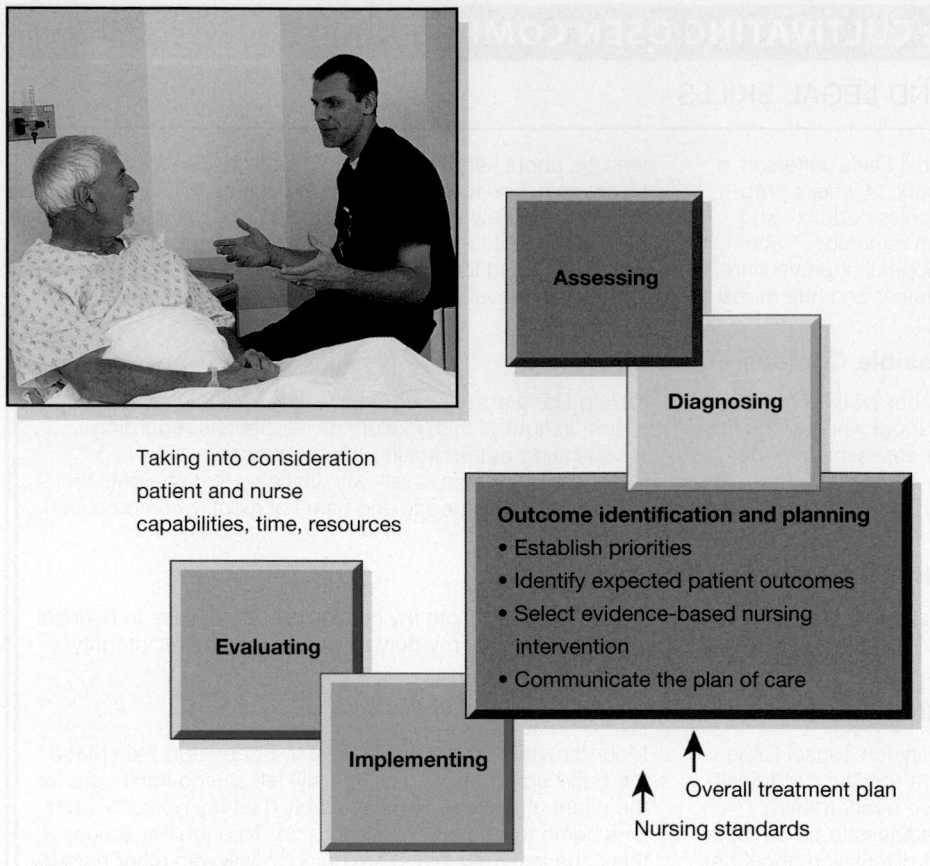

Taking into consideration patient and nurse capabilities, time, resources

Assessing

Diagnosing

Outcome identification and planning
- Establish priorities
- Identify expected patient outcomes
- Select evidence-based nursing intervention
- Communicate the plan of care

Evaluating

Implementing

↑ Overall treatment plan
Nursing standards

FIGURE 13-1. Outcome identification and planning. The nurse and patient work together to establish priorities, identify expected patient outcomes, and select evidence-based nursing interventions. The plan of care should be consistent with nursing standards, congruent with other planned therapies, and realistic in terms of the patient's and nurse's abilities or resources. Ensuring that the plan of care is recorded is also an important nursing responsibility. *(Photo by B. Proud.)*

with and for the patient that, once implemented, results in the prevention, reduction, or resolution of patient health problems and the attainment of the patient's health expectations, as identified in the patient outcomes (Box 13-1).

 THINK back to Glenda Kronk, the woman verbalizing a need to improve her fitness level. Based on a comprehensive patient assessment, together the nurse and patient would develop an appropriate plan to achieve this improved level of health, such as planning for 20-minute walks three times a week, eating a nutritious diet, and making routine follow-ups to determine the patient's progress toward the ultimate outcome. ●

A comprehensive plan of care additionally specifies any routine nursing assistance the patient needs to meet basic human needs (e.g., assistance with hygiene or nutrition) and describes appropriate nursing responsibilities for fulfilling the collaborative and medical plan of care. For example, physicians may delegate to nurses caring for a surgical patient the redressing of the surgical incision, the administration of prescribed medications and intravenous therapy, and the responsibility for scheduling laboratory studies. Nurses design plans of care that incorporate their independent, dependent, and collaborative responsibilities. See the clinical decision-making process illustrated in Figure 13-2 (on page 280) to help determine when you can act independently. Because nursing is concerned with the patient's responses to health and illness,

the plan of care is supportive of nursing's broad aims: to promote wellness, prevent disease and illness, promote recovery, and facilitate coping with altered functioning.

OUTCOME IDENTIFICATION, PLANNING, AND CLINICAL REASONING

Successful implementation of each step of the nursing process requires high-level skills in clinical reasoning. To plan health care correctly, in your role as nurse you must:

- Be familiar with standards and agency policies for setting priorities, identifying and recording expected patient outcomes, selecting evidence-based nursing interventions, and recording the plan of care (Box 13-2).
- Remember that the goal of person-centered care is to keep the patient and the patient's interests and preferences central in every aspect of planning and outcome identification
- Keep the "big picture" in focus: What are the discharge goals for this patient, and how should this direct each shift's interventions?
- Trust clinical experience and judgment but be willing to ask for help when the situation demands more than your qualifications and experience can provide; value collaborative practice
- Respect your clinical intuitions, but before establishing priorities, identifying outcomes, and selecting nursing interventions, be sure that research supports your plan
- Recognize your personal biases and keep an open mind

BOX 13-1 AMERICAN NURSES ASSOCIATION (ANA) STANDARDS OF PRACTICE: STANDARDS THREE AND FOUR, OUTCOME IDENTIFICATION AND PLANNING

Outcome Identification

Competencies

The registered nurse:

Involves the patient, family, healthcare providers, and others in formulating expected outcomes when possible and appropriate

Derives culturally appropriate expected outcomes from the diagnoses

Considers associated risks, benefits, costs, current scientific evidence, expected trajectory of the condition, and clinical expertise when formulating expected outcomes

Defines expected outcomes in terms of the healthcare consumer, healthcare consumer culture, values, ethical considerations

Includes a time estimate for attainment of expected outcomes

Develops expected outcomes that provide direction for continuity of care

Modifies expected outcomes based on changes in the status of the patient or evaluation of the situation

Documents expected outcomes as measurable

Planning

The registered nurse develops a plan that prescribes strategies and alternatives to attain expected outcomes.

Competencies

The registered nurse:

Develops an individualized plan in partnership with the person, family, and others considering the person's characteristics or the situation including but not limited to values, beliefs, spiritual and health practices, preferences, devel-

opmental level, coping style, culture and environment, and available technology

Establishes the plan priorities with the healthcare consumer, family, and others, as appropriate

Includes strategies within the plan that address each of the identified diagnoses or issues. These may include but are not limited to strategies for:

- Promotion and restoration of health
- Prevention of illness, injury, and disease
- The alleviation of suffering
- Supportive care for those who are dying

Includes strategies for health and wholeness across the lifespan

Provides for continuity in the plan

Incorporates an implementation pathway or timeline within the plan

Considers the economic impact of the plan on the healthcare consumer, family, caregivers, or other affected parties

Integrates current scientific evidence, trends, and research

Utilizes the plan to provide direction to other members of the healthcare team

Explores practice setting and safe space and time for the nurse and the healthcare consumer to explore suggested, potential, and alternative options

Defines the plan to reflect current statutes, rules and regulations, and standards

Modifies the plan according to the ongoing assessment of the healthcare consumer's response and other outcome indicators

Documents the plan in a manner that uses standardized language or recognized terminology

Reprinted with permission from American Nurses Association (ANA). (2010 edition). *Scope and standards of practice* (2nd ed.). Silver Spring, MD: Author.

 REMEMBER Darla Jefferson, the pregnant woman with a history of drug abuse described in the Reflective Practice box. Although the nursing student planned to engage the patient in an unbiased discussion of her alternatives, the student was unable to adhere to the plan, inserting personal opinions in the discussion. As a result, the plan of care was thwarted and the patient lost trust in the student. •

BOX 13-2 APPLYING STANDARDS TO PLAN NURSING CARE

The standards you must apply when identifying outcomes and related nursing interventions are determined by:

- *The law.* Your state's nurse practice act outlines the scope of nursing practice. Your state board of nursing also outlines what you are and are not allowed to do.
- *National practice standards,* such as those of the American Nurses Association.
- *Specialty professional organizations,* such as the American Association of Critical Care Nurses or Emergency Nurses Association, which develop standards for specialty practice.

- *The Joint Commission.* This powerful accrediting body has developed detailed standards that must be followed to keep accreditation.
- *The Agency for Healthcare Research and Quality (AHRQ).* This organization develops, reviews, and updates clinical guidelines to aid health care providers to prevent, diagnose, and manage clinical conditions.
- *Your employer.* Each facility usually develops its own unique set of standards (standards of care, guidelines, policies, procedures, critical pathways, standard care plans, and so forth) that reflect how nursing care should be given in specific situations.

Reprinted with permission from Alfaro-LeFevre, R. (2010). *Applying nursing process: A tool for critical thinking* (7th ed., pp. 144–145). Philadelphia: Wolters Kluwer Health/Lippincott Williams & Wilkins.

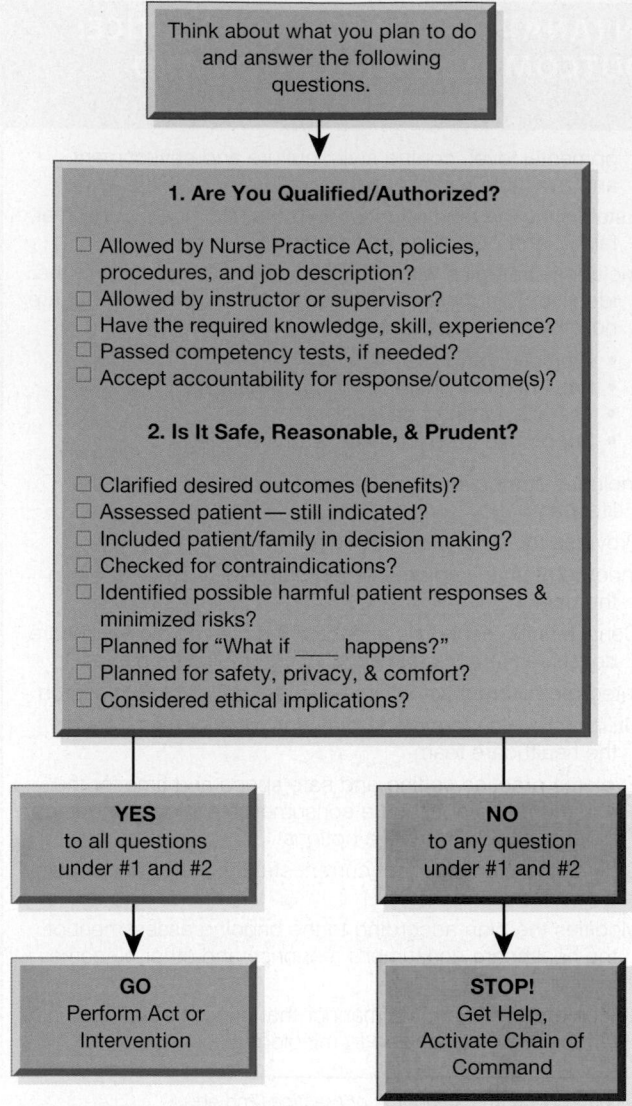

Think about what you plan to do and answer the following questions.

1. Are You Qualified/Authorized?

☐ Allowed by Nurse Practice Act, policies, procedures, and job description?
☐ Allowed by instructor or supervisor?
☐ Have the required knowledge, skill, experience?
☐ Passed competency tests, if needed?
☐ Accept accountability for response/outcome(s)?

2. Is It Safe, Reasonable, & Prudent?

☐ Clarified desired outcomes (benefits)?
☐ Assessed patient—still indicated?
☐ Included patient/family in decision making?
☐ Checked for contraindications?
☐ Identified possible harmful patient responses & minimized risks?
☐ Planned for "What if ____ happens?"
☐ Planned for safety, privacy, & comfort?
☐ Considered ethical implications?

YES
to all questions
under #1 and #2

NO
to any question
under #1 and #2

GO
Perform Act or
Intervention

STOP!
Get Help,
Activate Chain of
Command

FIGURE 13-2. Clinical decision-making process for determining your ability to act independently. (© 2009 R. Alfaro-LeFevre. Reprinted with permission from www.AlfaroTeachSmart.com.)

Questions to facilitate clinical reasoning during planning and outcome identification include:

- *Setting priorities:* Which problems require my immediate attention or that of the team? Which problems are my responsibility, and which should I refer to someone else? Which problems are most important to the patient?
- *Identifying outcomes:* What must I observe in the patient to demonstrate the resolution of the problems identified by the nursing diagnoses and general problem list? What is the time frame for accomplishing these outcomes? Do the outcomes need to be modified in light of the patient's response (or lack of response) to the planned interventions?
- *Selecting evidence-based nursing interventions:* What do nursing science and my clinical experience suggest is the likelihood that this particular nursing intervention will help the patient realize his or her expected outcomes? How can I tailor my interventions to increase the likelihood of patient benefit? What is the worst thing that might happen

with this intervention, how likely is it to happen, and what can I do to minimize the possibility of this harm?
- *Communicating the plan of care:* Does the plan of care adequately address the patient's priorities today? If the plan of care is computerized or standardized, does it adequately address the specific needs of this particular patient? Can anyone reading the plan of care know how to intervene effectively with this patient?

OUTCOME IDENTIFICATION, PLANNING, AND INTER-PERSONAL COMPETENCE

As in every phase of the nursing process, your interpersonal competence influences your success in planning. It is nurses' unique ability to understand the patient's and family's needs, expectations, hopes, and fears that allows nurses to develop effective plans of care. Unless patients believe that you are committed to meeting their health and well-being needs, they have little incentive for partnering with you. The more active that patients and families are in the planning process, the more motivated they will be to achieve valued goals. While standardized care plans predominate in care settings today, your challenge is to individualize such plans to the unique needs of your patients.

COMPREHENSIVE PLANNING

In acute care settings, three basic stages of planning are critical to comprehensive nursing care: initial, ongoing, and discharge. In other settings such as long-term care, hospice care, or a community clinic, initial and ongoing planning may be the primary types of planning. If a nurse develops a comprehensive plan of care on the patient's first day but fails to update the plan, the plan will not be effective or efficient. Failure to update the plan of care as needed is a common problem in all health care settings.

Initial Planning

Initial planning is performed by the nurse with the admission nursing history and the physical assessment. This comprehensive plan addresses each problem listed in the prioritized nursing diagnoses and identifies appropriate patient goals and the related nursing care. **Standardized care plans** are prepared plans of care that identify the nursing diagnoses, outcomes, and related nursing interventions common to a specific population or health problem. (An example of a standardized care plan is shown later in the chapter.) They can provide an excellent basis for the initial plan if the nurse individualizes them. Resources for standardized plans include computerized plans, textbooks with prepared care plans, and agency-developed plans/maps/critical pathways. By using such standardized plans, the nurse is free to direct time and expertise to individualizing the plan.

Ongoing Planning

Ongoing planning is carried out by any nurse who interacts with the patient. Its chief purpose is to keep the plan up to date to facilitate the resolution of health problems, manage risk factors, and promote function. The nurse caring for the patient uses new data as they are collected and analyzed to make the plan more specific and accurate and, therefore, more effective. The work of ongoing planning includes stating nursing diagnoses more clearly (both the problem statement and the cause), developing new diagnoses, adjusting patient outcomes to be more realistic, developing new outcomes as needed, and identifying nursing interventions that will best accomplish the patient goals.

 CONSIDER Elijah Wolinski, the frail, older adult who developed a pressure ulcer. Ongoing planning is necessary because the patient's pressure ulcer would most likely take some time to heal or improve. In addition, other needs might become apparent during subsequent home visits, requiring the nurse to update the plan of care. ●

At this stage of planning, standardized plans based on medical conditions or procedures might be useful in developing new nursing diagnoses and related nursing interventions, but individualizing the plan is necessary to meet unique patient needs. For example, the standard nursing order "force fluids" might be rewritten as "offer 60 mL cranberry or orange juice between meals, and keep fresh water at bedside." A preliminary order such as "explore with the patient existing supports" might be replaced with "keep daughter Barbara informed of mother's progress and coach her in effective support strategies: Barbara Clems, (h) 448-3211, (w) 654-8999."

Discharge Planning

Discharge planning is best carried out by the nurse who has worked most closely with the patient and family, possibly in conjunction with a nurse or social worker with a broad knowledge of existing community resources. In acute care settings, comprehensive discharge planning begins when the patient is admitted for treatment—or even before admission. Careful planning ensures that the nurse uses teaching and counseling skills effectively to help the patient and family develop sufficient knowledge of the health problem and the therapeutic regimen to carry out necessary self-care behaviors at home competently. Discharge planning is further discussed in Chapter 9.

ESTABLISHING PRIORITIES

To develop a prioritized list of nursing diagnoses, the nurse needs guidelines for ranking diagnoses as high, medium, or low priority. High-priority diagnoses pose the greatest threat to the patient's health and well-being. Diagnoses that are not life threatening are ranked as medium priorities, and diagnoses that are not specifically related to the current level of health or well-being are of low priority. In all levels, psychosocial needs must be considered as well as physiologic needs.

In addition to developing a prioritized list of nursing diagnoses, nurses working within an interdisciplinary team need to set priorities for nursing care that take account of all the patient's health needs, as recorded on the general problem list. This involves looking at all problems to determine the relationships among the problems (what's causing or contributing to what). Thus, it generally makes sense to deal with medical (or suspected medical) problems first. If these can be resolved, many human response problems are gone. If a nurse sees the classic signs and symptoms of appendicitis and tries to identify and manage a nursing diagnosis of pain without consulting a physician or nurse practitioner, the patient's appendix might rupture before a nursing plan to relieve pain is even developed!

Three helpful guides to facilitate clinical reasoning when prioritizing patient problems include Maslow's hierarchy of human needs, patient preference, and anticipation of future problems.

Maslow's Hierarchy of Human Needs

Because basic needs must be met before a person can focus on higher ones, patient needs may be prioritized according to the following hierarchy:

1. Physiologic needs
2. Safety needs
3. Love and belonging needs
4. Self-esteem needs
5. Self-actualization needs

For example, a geriatric patient who is incontinent of urine and sitting in a wet disposable brief (physiologic need) will be unable to participate fully in a music therapy diversional activity (self-esteem need) until the more basic need is met. (Chapter 4 more fully discusses basic human needs.)

Patient Preference

Thoughtful, person-centered nursing directs you to first meet the needs that the patient thinks are most important, as long as this order does not interfere with other vital therapies. For example, a woman is admitted to an orthopedic unit with a fractured pelvis and multiple lacerations after an automobile accident. The morning after the accident, she complains of pain and needs assistance with bathing and attention to her lacerations, but she refuses to do anything until she calls home to find out who is caring for her 15-month-old twins. The nurse should help her to call home before beginning other care as long as it does not interfere with life-saving emergency care.

Anticipation of Future Problems

Nurses must tap their knowledge base to consider the potential effects of different nursing actions. Assigning low priority to a diagnosis that the patient wants to ignore but can result in harmful future consequences for the patient might be nursing negligence. For example, an obese patient with multiple sclerosis and greatly decreased limb strength who spends most of her day in bed may see no value in diet modification and position changes. A nurse who is alert to the potentially serious problem of pressure ulcers would assign high priority to this diagnosis, nonetheless, and incorporate weight management and position changes into the plan of care despite the patient's reluctance.

Clinical Reasoning and Establishing Priorities

The work of setting priorities demands careful clinical reasoning. Alfaro-LeFevre (2010, p. 148) suggests that nurses ask:

1. What problems need immediate attention and which ones can wait?
2. Which problems are your responsibility and which do you need to refer to someone else?
3. Which problems can be dealt with by using standard plans (e.g., critical paths, standards of care)?
4. Which problems aren't covered by protocols or standard plans but must be addressed to ensure a safe hospital stay and timely discharge (or simply safe care of high quality)?

 THINK back to Darla Jefferson, the pregnant woman with a history of drug abuse. The nurse would incorporate clinical reasoning by asking these four questions, thereby ultimately arriving at the patient problems requiring the most immediate attention. •

When planning nursing care for each day, consider the following:

- Have changes in the patient's health status influenced the priority of nursing diagnoses? For example, when a routine home visit to an older adult reveals evidence of possible elder abuse, a new diagnosis may result in a new set of care priorities.
- Have changes in the way the patient is responding to health and illness or the plan of care affected those nursing diagnoses that can be realistically addressed? For example, a nurse might have identified Ineffective Coping as a high-priority diagnosis for the patient after the patient learned the medical diagnosis and planned to initiate counseling. If the patient adamantly requests to be left alone for a day to think things through, however, the nurse has to modify priorities of care for that day.
- Are there relationships among diagnoses that require that one be worked on before another can be resolved?
- Can several patient problems be dealt with together?

After answering these questions, the nurse ranks the diagnoses in the order in which they should be addressed. Setting priorities enables the nurse to make sure that time and energy are being directed first to the patient's most important problems.

IDENTIFYING AND WRITING OUTCOMES

Learning to identify and write appropriate outcomes takes practice. The following sections and the guidelines in Box 13-1 on page 279 will help you to identify outcomes that will maximize your effectiveness when working with patients.

Table 13-1	EXAMPLES OF GOALS/OUTCOMES TO RELIEVE PROBLEMS
PROBLEM STATEMENT OF THE NURSING DIAGNOSIS	**RELATED PATIENT GOAL/OUTCOME**
Pain	Within 8 hours, patient will report pain is absent or diminished
Imbalanced Nutrition: More Than Body Requirements	By 12/6/15, patient will reach target weight of 122 lb
Impaired Physical Mobility	Before discharge, patient will ambulate length of hallway independently

Deriving Outcomes from Nursing Diagnoses

Outcomes are derived from the problem statement of the nursing diagnosis. For each nursing diagnosis in the plan of care, at least one outcome should be written that, if achieved, demonstrates a direct resolution of the problem statement (Table 13-1).

Other outcomes that contribute to the resolution of the problem may be written. For example, for the nursing diagnosis Imbalanced Nutrition: More Than Body Requirements related to excessive snacking and inactivity, in addition to the outcome "within 12 weeks (12/6/15), the patient will lose 20 pounds and reach target weight (122 lb)," the following goals are appropriate: "within 3 days of teaching: the patient will identify 10 low-calorie snack foods he is willing to try; the patient will have 3-day diet recall consistent with nutritionally balanced 1,500-calorie diet; the patient will report incorporating three half-hour periods of walking at 5 miles per hour into each week." If the patient can identify low-calorie snack foods and adopt a more active lifestyle, there is a greater likelihood that he will reach his target weight, but it is entirely possible for a patient to achieve these secondary outcomes without resolving the chief problem. Remember, at least one outcome per nursing diagnosis must directly resolve the problem statement in the nursing diagnosis.

The **Nursing Outcomes Classification (NOC)** developed by the Iowa Outcomes Project presents the first comprehensive standardized language used to describe the patient outcomes that are responsive to nursing intervention (Moorhead, Johnson, Maas, & Swanson, 2013). The current classification lists 490 outcomes with definitions, indicators, measurement scales, and supporting references. The outcomes may be used for individuals, families, or communities. Examples of NOC outcomes are found in each clinical chapter. Explicit linkages between the North American Nursing Diagnosis Association International (NANDA-I) diagnoses and the NOC facilitate a comprehensive approach to care planning. Remember whenever you use standardized language to ensure that it adequately captures the uniqueness of your patients and families.

Establishing Long-Term Versus Short-Term Outcomes

Outcomes might be either long term or short term. Long-term outcomes require a longer period (usually more than a week) to be achieved than do short-term outcomes. They also may be used as discharge goals, in which case they are more broadly written and communicate to the entire nursing team the desired end results of nursing care for a particular patient. For example, two women, both 77 years of age, are on a nursing unit after undergoing similar operations for fractured left hips. One woman has spent the past 2 years in bed in a long-term care facility; the other woman fractured her hip at the YMCA, where she swims daily. Their nursing care should not be the same because it is directed toward different long-term goals, even though their short-term goals might be similar (see Box 13-3).

Box 13-3 EXAMPLES OF LONG-TERM AND SHORT-TERM OUTCOMES

Patient on Bedrest From Long-Term Care Facility
Long-Term Outcome
Mrs. Goldstein returns to the long-term care facility pain free with her incision healed and her left leg in good alignment.

Short-Term Outcomes
• Whenever observed, patient will be lying in bed with legs in correct alignment (abductor pillow in place, if ordered).
• Before discharge, Mrs. Goldstein's hip incision will show signs of healing (skin surfaces approximate, free from signs of infection—redness, swelling, heat, purulent drainage).
• Whenever observed, patient will report that comfort measures and medication are satisfactorily managing pain.

Active Patient from Private Home
Long-Term Outcome
Mrs. Silverstein returns home to her husband pain free with incision healed, fully mobile (full weight bearing on left leg), and capable of independent activities of daily living.

Short-Term Outcomes
• By 1/28/15, the patient will verbalize willingness to participate in physical therapy program.
• By 2/4/15, the patient will ambulate (with nursing assistance and walker) to bathroom (full weight bearing).
• By 2/11/15, the patient will ambulate with nursing assistance only (no walker) in her room.
• Goals for incision and pain relief same as for Mrs. Goldstein.

 CONSIDER Elijah Wolinski, the frail, older adult with a pressure ulcer. The nurse might establish a long-term outcome such as, "The patient's sacral area will exhibit no evidence of a pressure ulcer." Short-term outcomes might include, "The patient's sacral pressure ulcer demonstrates an absence of purulent drainage within 1 week of initiating wound care. By week 2, the patient's pressure ulcer has decreased in size by a quarter-inch. By week 2, the patient's caregiver demonstrates measures to relieve pressure on the skin while the patient is in bed." ●

Determining Patient-Centered Outcomes

Alfaro-LeFevre (2014, p. 136) recommends that nurses first ask patients to describe two or three major goals they would like to achieve. Nurses then should be realistic and consider:

• Patient's health state, overall prognosis
• Expected length of stay
• Growth and development
• Patient values and cultural considerations
• Other planned therapies for the patient
• Available human, material, and financial resources
• Risks, benefits, and current scientific evidence
• Changes in status that indicate you need to modify usual expected outcomes

Moorhead et al. (2013, p. 32) recommend considering the following factors when selecting outcomes: (1) the type of health concern, (2) the nursing or medical diagnoses, (3) patient characteristics, (4) available resources, (5) patient preferences, and (6) treatment potential.

One of the most important considerations in writing outcomes is to encourage the patient and family to be as involved in goal development as their abilities and interest permit. When developing patient outcomes, the nurse and patient look at the problem statement of the nursing diagnosis and ask, "What patient changes or outcomes will result in the prevention or resolution of this problem?" The answer, when carefully worded, becomes the patient outcome.

Ensuring Quality Outcomes

The Committee on Quality Health Care in America of the Institute of Medicine (2001), in its report *Crossing the Quality Chasm*, highlights six aims to be met by health care systems with regard to the quality of care:

• Safe: avoiding injury
• Effective: avoiding overuse and underuse
• Patient-centered: responding to patient preferences, needs, and values
• Timely: reducing waits and delays
• Efficient: avoiding waste
• Equitable: providing care that does not vary in quality to all recipients

Institutions measuring their achievement of these aims will welcome nursing's efforts to determine its effectiveness (Moorhead et al., 2013, p. 32).

The Joint Commission publishes standards and requirements for Joint Commission accreditation and certification programs. Be sure to check their website and pay special attention to the National Patient Safety Goals, which became effective in January, 2013 (available at www.jointcommission.org).

Using Cognitive, Psychomotor, and Affective Outcomes

Outcomes may be categorized according to the type of change needed by a patient. Cognitive outcomes describe increases in patient knowledge or intellectual behaviors—for example: "Within 1 day after teaching, the patient will list three benefits of continuing to apply moist compresses to leg ulcer after discharge." Psychomotor outcomes describe the patient's achievement of new skills—for example, "By 6/12/15, the patient will correctly demonstrate application of wet-to-dry dressing on leg ulcer." Affective outcomes describe changes in patient values, beliefs, and attitudes. Difficult both to write and to evaluate, affective outcomes could be critical to the resolution of a complex patient problem—for example, "By 6/12/15, the patient will verbalize valuing health sufficiently to practice new health behaviors to prevent recurrence of leg ulcer." In this example, even if the patient intellectually grasps the reasons for taking care of her leg and can competently redress her ulcer, unless she is motivated to take care of herself, her knowledge and skills will not result in healthy outcomes. See Chapter 15 for other examples of these outcomes.

Identifying Clinical, Functional, and Quality-of-Life Outcomes

Another way to think about the types of outcomes to identify is to categorize them as clinical, functional, or quality of life. Alfaro-LeFevre (2014) presents them as follows:

Clinical outcomes describe the expected status of health issues at certain points in time, after treatment is complete. They address whether the problems are resolved or to what degree they are improved.

Functional outcomes describe the person's ability to function in relation to the desired usual activities.

Quality-of-life outcomes focus on key factors that affect someone's ability to enjoy life and achieve personal goals (p. 137).

Identifying Culturally Appropriate Outcomes

The American Nurses Association (ANA) Standards of Practice (see Box 13-1, p. 279) direct the nurse to derive *culturally appropriate expected outcomes* from the diagnoses. See Chapter 5 for a discussion of culturally appropriate care.

Identifying Outcomes Supportive of the Total Treatment Plan

When identifying outcomes, always remember that nurses nurse people, not problems. This means that every outcome

you write should support the overall treatment plan and "make sense" in terms of the overall goals for the patient. For example, identifying nutritional outcomes may be appropriate for a patient who is losing weight, but if this patient is in a hospice and dying, this may not be an appropriate outcome if it is incompatible with the overall goal of a peaceful death with dignity.

Writing Patient-Centered Measurable Outcomes

To be measurable, outcomes should have the following:

- *Subject:* the patient or some part of the patient
- *Verb:* indicates the action the patient will perform

  Verbs helpful in writing measurable outcomes include:

Define	List	Explain
Prepare	Verbalize	Select
Identify	Describe	Apply
Design	Choose	Demonstrate

- *Conditions:* specifies the particular circumstances in or by which the outcome is to be achieved. Not every outcome specifies conditions.
- *Performance criteria:* describe in observable, measurable terms the expected patient behavior or other manifestation
- *Target time:* specifies when the patient is expected to be able to achieve the outcome. The target time or time criterion may be a realistic, actual date or other statement indicating time, such as before discharge, after viewing film, whenever observed.

Following are examples of properly constructed measurable outcomes:

- During the next 24-hour period, the patient's fluid intake will total at least 2,000 mL.
- At the next visit, 12/23/15, the patient will correctly demonstrate relaxation exercises.

It often helps to include special conditions when writing an outcome if this information is important for other nurses (e.g., "Before discharge, the patient will ambulate independently the length of hallway and back, using a Philadelphia collar to support cervical vertebrae").

A memory jog for writing goals and outcomes is the word SMART (Doran, 1981):

S – specific
M – measurable
A – attainable
R – realistic
T – timebound

Avoiding Common Errors in Outcomes

Common errors when writing patient outcomes include the following:

- *Expressing the patient outcome as a nursing intervention.*
  Incorrect: "Offer Mr. Myer 60 mL fluid every 2 hours

while awake." Correct: "Mr. Myer will drink 60 mL fluid every 2 hours while awake, beginning 2/24/15."

- *Using verbs that are not observable and measurable.* Incorrect: "Mrs. Gaston will know how to bathe her newborn." Correct: "After attending the infant care class, Mrs. Gaston will correctly demonstrate the procedure for bathing her newborn." Verbs to be avoided when writing goals include "know," "understand," "learn," and "become aware." These verbs are too general and cannot be measured. Verbs for writing outcomes should be observable and measurable (as listed previously).
- *Including more than one patient behavior/manifestation in short-term outcomes.* Incorrect: "Patient will list dangers of smoking and stop smoking." Correct: "By next meeting, 3/11/15, the patient will (1) identify three dangers of smoking and (2) describe a plan he is willing to try to stop smoking. By 6/20/15, the patient will report that he no longer smokes."
- *Writing outcomes that are so vague that other nurses are unsure of the goal of nursing care.* Incorrect: "Patient will cope better." Correct: "After teaching, 10/20/15, the patient will (1) describe two new coping strategies he is willing to try and (2) demonstrate decreased incidence of previously observed ineffective coping behaviors (chain smoking, withdrawal behavior, heavy alcohol consumption)."

IDENTIFYING NURSING INTERVENTIONS

The Nursing Interventions Classification (NIC) project defines a **nursing intervention** as "any treatment based upon clinical judgment and knowledge that a nurse performs to enhance patient/client outcomes" (Bulechek, Butcher, Dochterman, & Wagner, 2013, p. 2). The NIC project further goes on to describe the types of interventions:

> The Classification includes interventions that nurses do on behalf of patients, both independent and collaborative interventions, both direct and indirect care. NIC interventions include both the physiological (e.g., Acid–Base Management) and the psychosocial (e.g., Anxiety Reduction).... Interventions are included for illness treatment (e.g., Hyperglycemia Management), illness prevention (e.g., Fall Prevention), and health promotion (e.g., Exercise Promotion). Most of the interventions are for use with individuals, but many are for use with families (e.g., Family Integrity Promotion) and some for entire communities (e.g., Environmental Management: Community). Indirect care interventions (e.g., Supply Management), are also included.

Carpenito-Moyet (2010, p. 42) describes how the major focus of intervention differs according to the type of nursing diagnoses or collaborative problem being addressed. For actual nursing diagnoses, interventions seek to:

- Reduce or eliminate contributing factors of the diagnosis
- Promote higher-level wellness
- Monitor and evaluate status

For risk nursing diagnoses, interventions seek to:
- Reduce or eliminate risk factors
- Prevent the problem
- Monitor and evaluate status

For possible nursing diagnoses, interventions seek to:
- Collect additional data to rule out or confirm the diagnosis.

For collaborative problems, interventions seek to:
- Monitor for changes in status
- Manage changes in status with nurse-prescribed and physician-prescribed interventions
- Evaluate response

Your challenge in the planning phase of the nursing process is to identify the nursing interventions most likely to achieve the outcomes. There are nurse-initiated, physician-initiated, and collaborative interventions.

Nurse-Initiated Interventions

A **nurse-initiated intervention** is an autonomous action based on scientific rationale that a nurse executes to benefit the patient in a predictable way related to the nursing diagnosis and projected outcomes. Nursing interventions are actions performed by the nurse to (Alfaro-LeFevre, 2014, p. 142–143):

1. Monitor patient health status and response to treatment
2. Reduce risks
3. Resolve, prevent, or manage a problem
4. Promote independence with activities of daily living
5. Promote optimum sense of physical, psychological, and spiritual well-being
6. Give patients the information they need to make informed decisions and be independent

Nurse-initiated interventions do not require a physician's (or other team member's) order. Nurse-initiated interventions, like patient goals, are derived from the nursing diagnosis. But whereas the problem statement of the diagnosis suggests the patient goals, it is the cause of the problem (etiology) that suggests the nursing interventions (Fig. 13-3 on page 288). Effective nurses select nursing interventions that specifically address factors that cause or contribute to the patient's problems. For example, many factors may contribute to obesity, such as deficient nutritional knowledge, convenience of high-calorie fast foods, lifetime snacking habits, limited food budget, little exercise, and low self-esteem. The nurse working with a patient who wants to lose weight could attempt to deal with all these factors, but this approach would be inefficient. When a carefully developed nursing diagnosis identifies the specific factors that contribute to a particular patient's weight problem, nursing interventions can be selected to deal directly with these factors.

 REMEMBER Glenda Kronk, the woman desiring to improve her fitness. Based on assessment, the nurse determines the factors that have played a role in the patient's current status, developing appropriate nursing diagnoses and outcomes from which to establish appropriate interventions. For example, if the patient has been sedentary over the past several years, interventions should focus on measures to increase the patient's activity level, thereby promoting improvement in her overall health and fitness. ●

Similarly, nursing interventions for a patient with the diagnosis Imbalanced Nutrition: More Than Body Requirements related to lifetime snacking habits and heavy reliance on high-calorie fast foods might include education about the fat content and calories in fast foods and exploration of ways the patient could change eating habits to eat more nutritionally balanced meals with fewer calories. Thus, the nursing approach is not the same for every patient with a weight problem. The art of nursing involves the careful identification of the specific nursing interventions needed by particular patients to meet their individual needs.

Identifying and Selecting Appropriate Nurse-Initiated Interventions

After writing the patient outcomes, the nurse identifies various nursing interventions to help the patient achieve the outcomes. The **Nursing Intervention Classification (NIC)**, the first comprehensive, validated list of nursing interventions applicable to all settings that can be used by nurses in multiple specialties, greatly facilitates the work of identifying appropriate interventions. Table 13-2 illustrates the NIC taxonomy structure designed to help clinicians locate and select interventions most helpful for patients. Bulechek et al. (2013) write that the selection of a nursing intervention for a particular patient is part of the clinical judgment of the nurse. They identify six factors that should be considered when choosing an intervention: (1) desired patient outcomes, (2) characteristics of the nursing diagnosis, (3) research base for the intervention, (4), feasibility for doing the intervention, (5) acceptability to the patient, and (6) capability of the nurse (p. 13). Examples of using NIC to facilitate care planning for specific patient health problems may be found in each clinical chapter of this text.

The effectiveness of the nurse is directly proportional to the nurse's knowledge of varied nursing strategies. Consider the following different nursing care options identified by three nurses when they are asked to describe nursing care

Table 13-2 NURSING INTERVENTIONS CLASSIFICATION (NIC) TAXONOMY

DOMAIN I	DOMAIN II	DOMAIN III
Level 1 Domains		
1. Physiologic: Basic Care that supports physical functioning	**2. Physiologic: Complex** Care that supports homeostatic regulation	**3. Behavioral** Care that supports psychosocial functioning and facilitates lifestyle changes
Level 2 Classes		
A **Activity and Exercise Management:** Interventions to organize or assist with physical activity and energy expenditure	G **Electrolyte and Acid–Base Management:** Interventions to regulate electrolyte/acid–base balance and prevent complications	O **Behavior Therapy:** Interventions to reinforce or promote desirable behaviors or alter undesirable behaviors
B **Elimination Management:** Interventions to establish and maintain regular bowel and urinary elimination patterns and manage complications due to altered patterns	H **Drug Management:** Interventions to facilitate desired effects of pharmacologic agents	P **Cognitive Therapy:** Interventions to reinforce or promote desirable cognitive functioning or alter undesirable cognitive functioning
C **Immobility Management:** Interventions to manage restricted body movement and the sequelae	I **Neurologic Management:** Interventions to optimize neurologic function	Q **Communication Enhancement:** Interventions to facilitate delivering and receiving verbal or nonverbal messages
D **Nutrition Support:** Interventions to modify or maintain nutritional status	J **Perioperative Care:** Interventions to provide care before, during, and immediately after surgery	R **Coping Assistance:** Interventions to assist another to build on own strengths, to adapt to a change in function, or to achieve a higher level of function
E **Physical Comfort Promotion:** Interventions to promote comfort using physical techniques	K **Respiratory Management:** Interventions to promote airway patency and gas exchange	S **Patient Education:** Interventions to facilitate learning
F **Self-Care Facilitation:** Interventions to provide or assist with routine activities of daily living	L **Skin/Wound Management:** Interventions to maintain or restore tissue integrity	T **Psychological Comfort Promotion:** Interventions to promote comfort using psychological techniques
	M **Thermoregulation:** Interventions to maintain body temperature within a normal range	
	N **Tissue Perfusion Management:** Interventions to optimize circulation of blood and fluids to the tissue	

Reprinted with permission from Bulechek, G. M., Butcher, H. K., & Dochterman, J. (Eds.). (2008). *Nursing interventions classification (NIC)* (5th ed., pp. 74–75). St. Louis: Elsevier/Mosby.

for a woman 2 days after cesarean delivery who is complaining of pain in the incisional area.

Nurse A

- Check to see what type of pain medication is ordered, and give it if the time interval is sufficient.

Nurse B

- Assess the quality of the pain, and use this time to communicate support by means of expression and squeeze of hand.
- Administer analgesic if indicated.
- Assess effectiveness of the analgesic ordered.

Nurse C

- Assess quality of the pain, and explore the possibility of contributing factors such as the effects of increased gas in the abdominal area or concern about the newborn, herself, or other family members.
- Use empathic listening (possibly touch) to communicate support and to encourage the mother to share her concerns.
- Change the patient's position in bed.
- Offer a backrub.

- If appropriate, suggest activity that will distract attention from the pain (e.g., watching a film about newborn care or listening to music).
- Give the prescribed medication for pain and observe its effect.
- When administering the medication, use the power of positive suggestion to enhance its effectiveness: "This will start taking the pain away in about 10 minutes and will help you relax."

It is possible that the patient simply needs her prescribed analgesic to achieve the outcome: "Patient will report minimal to no pain at assessment every 2 hours." In that case, all three nurses would be effective in meeting the patient's need for nursing care. It is highly possible, however, that the prescribed medication is not sufficient or the pain is compounded by the mother's fears about caring for her new baby or by her worries that the baby will ruin her relationship with her husband. Therefore, nurse C, whose knowledge level is more comprehensive, is likely to be most effective in resolving the patient's problem.

The more varied the options available to the nurse, the more effective the nursing response. In different situations,

DOMAIN IV	DOMAIN V	DOMAIN VI	DOMAIN VII
4. Safety Care that supports protection against harm	**5. Family** Care that supports the family unit	**6. Health System** Care that supports effective use of the health care delivery system	**7. Community** Care that supports the health of the community
U **Crisis Management:** Interventions to provide immediate short-term help in both psychological and physiologic crises V **Risk Management:** Interventions to initiate risk reduction activities and continue monitoring risk over time	W **Childbearing Care:** Interventions to assist in understanding and coping with the psychological and physiologic changes during the childbearing period X **Lifespan Care:** Interventions to facilitate family unit functioning and promote the health and welfare of family members throughout the lifespan	Y **Health System Mediation:** Interventions to facilitate the interface between patient/family and the health care system Z **Childrearing Care:** Interventions to assist in raising children a. **Health System Management:** Interventions to provide and enhance support services for the delivery of care b. **Information Management:** Interventions to facilitate communication among health care workers	c. **Community Health Promotion:** Interventions that promote the health of the whole community d. **Community Risk Management:** Interventions that assist in detecting or preventing health risks to the whole community

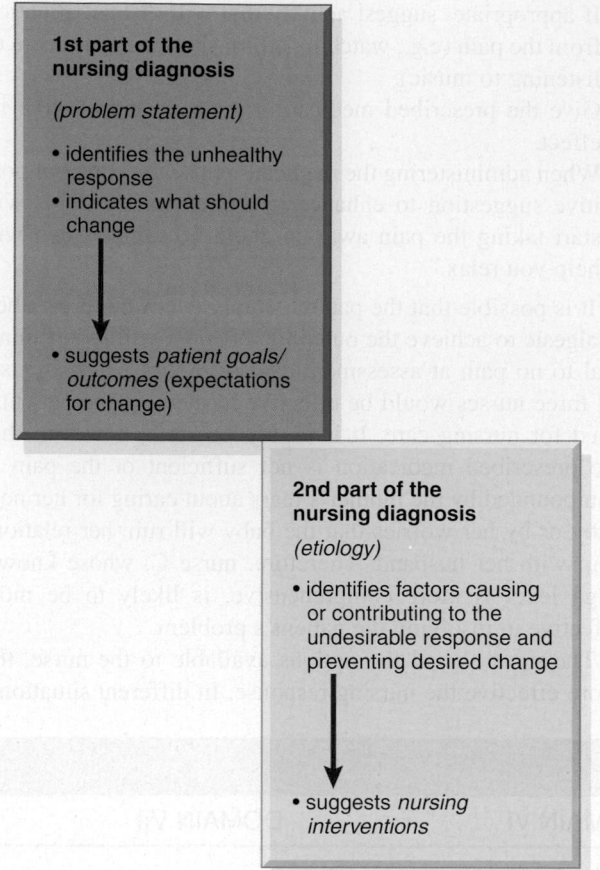

FIGURE 13-3. Deriving patient goals/outcomes and nursing orders from nursing diagnoses.

a skilled nursing procedure, the appropriate use of silence, respectful listening, humor, teaching, counseling, and touch can all be effective nursing strategies. Nurses who are merely task oriented and satisfied to meet every patient problem with a mechanical procedure are limiting their effectiveness.

When selecting nursing interventions for individual patients, use the guidelines in Box 13-4. These guidelines help ensure that the patient will achieve the outcome. Ongoing evaluation enables the nurse to determine the effectiveness of the selected interventions.

BOX 13-4 | **GUIDELINES FOR SELECTING NURSING INTERVENTIONS**

Nursing interventions should be:

- Appropriate in terms of the nursing diagnosis and related patient outcomes, safe, and efficient
- Consistent with research findings and standards of care
- Realistic in terms of the abilities, time, and resources available to the nurse and patient
- Compatible with the patient's values, beliefs, and cultural and psychosocial background
- Valued, whenever possible, by the patient and family
- Compatible with other planned therapies

Individualizing Evidence-Based Interventions

Nurse researchers are attempting to establish a statistical pattern for predicting the probability of success for select nursing interventions. Using the student plan of care at the end of this chapter, review the scientific rationale for the selected nursing orders. You should always be prepared to explain why you are doing intervention "a" as opposed to intervention "b" or "c." You should know how likely it is that the proposed intervention will achieve the desired outcomes and what the associated risks are. Alfaro-LeFevre (2010, p. 163) recommends that nurses answer four key questions when determining individualized evidence-based interventions:

1. What can be done to prevent or minimize the risks or causes of this problem?
2. What can be done to manage the problem?
3. How can I tailor interventions to meet expected outcomes?
4. How likely are we to get desired versus adverse responses to the interventions, and what can we do to reduce the risks and increase the likelihood of beneficial responses?

You can learn more about evidence-based practice in Chapter 2 and in the Research in Nursing and PICO in Practice recurring displays in the clinical chapters (Units VI and VII). Competent nurses use research findings (science of nursing), experience, and knowledge of the patient (art of nursing) to help select effective nursing interventions. Consultation with nurse colleagues and continuing education also assist nurses to develop effective nursing approaches to patients' problems.

Recording Nurse-Initiated Interventions in the Patient Record

Nursing interventions describe, and thus communicate to the entire nursing staff and health care team, the specific nursing care to be implemented for the patient. Each nursing intervention should include:

- *Date*
- *Verb:* Action to be performed
- *Subject:* Who is to do it
- *Descriptive phrase:* How, when, where, how often, how long, or how much

Well-written nursing interventions accomplish the following:

- Assist the patient to meet specific outcomes that are related directly to one outcome
- Clearly and concisely describe the nursing action to be performed (answer the questions who, what, where, when, and how)
- Are dated when written and when the plan of care is reviewed
- Are signed by the nurse prescribing the order or intervention
- Use only those abbreviations accepted in the institution (these are usually found in the agency's policy manual; a list of commonly accepted abbreviations appears in Chapter 16)
- Refer the nurse to the agency's procedure manual or other literature for the steps of routine, lengthy procedures

Following are examples of well-stated nursing interventions:

- Offer patient 60 mL water or juice (prefers orange or cranberry juice) every 2 hours while awake for a total minimum PO intake of 500 mL.
- Teach patient the necessity of carefully monitoring fluid intake and output; remind patient each shift to mark off fluid intake on record at bedside.
- Walk with patient to bathroom for toileting every 2 hours (on even hours) while patient is awake.

 Concept Mastery Alert

Outcome statements reflect the result or what to achieve; interventions state how the nurse will go about trying to achieve the result.

The set of nursing interventions written to assist a patient to meet an outcome must be comprehensive. Comprehensive nursing interventions specify what *observations* (assessments) need to be made and how often, what nursing *interventions* need to be done and when they must be done, and what *teaching, counseling,* and *advocacy* needs patients and families have.

Many sets of nursing interventions are inadequate because they fail to indicate the ongoing assessment priority needs for a specific problem or goal. Clearly stating assessment priorities helps all nurses to be more sensitive to important patient data.

 REVIEW the scenario at the beginning of the chapter for Glenda Kronk. The nurse would need to establish assessment priorities. For example, when assisting Glenda, who wants to lose weight to reach her target weight, appropriate nursing interventions might include the following: "6/17/15: Continue to assess (1) patient's motivation to participate in weight-loss program and (2) factors that positively or negatively influence weight loss." ●

Similarly, it is often assumed that all patients have the same teaching needs. Nothing is farther from the truth. In fact, many patients have an excellent knowledge base (which might be greater than that of the nurse for a particular disease). Their need for nursing might be a need for counseling, instead of teaching, as they learn to live with a chronic illness. However, it is important to obtain proof of the patient's knowledge or competency before proceeding with the plan of care. For example, a diabetic patient would need to state the signs and symptoms of hypo- and hyperglycemia or to give a return demonstration of doing a fingerstick blood glucose test. In summary, comprehensive nursing interventions relate to individual patient needs.

Physician-Initiated and Collaborative Interventions

An intervention is initiated by a physician in response to a medical diagnosis but is carried out by a nurse in response to a doctor's order. For example, a physician examining a patient brought into the emergency department after a motor vehicle accident might ask the nurse to administer a medication to relieve pain and to schedule the patient for radiographs and other diagnostic tests. The nurse who performs these interventions is implementing **physician-initiated interventions**. Both the physician and nurse are legally responsible for these interventions, and nurses are expected to be knowledgeable about how to execute these interventions safely and effectively. Nurses who question the appropriateness of physician-initiated interventions are legally responsible to seek clarification of the order with responsible parties. Under no circumstances should a nurse implement a questionable intervention, even at the urging of a physician or other professional. Chapter 7 addresses nurses' legal responsibility for their actions. Nurses also carry out treatments initiated by other providers such as pharmacists, respiratory therapists, or physician assistants, which are **collaborative interventions**. For example, nurses caring for a patient after a motor vehicle accident might eventually implement interventions written by a physical therapist, occupational therapist, or other member of the health care team.

Structured Care Methodologies

Efforts to standardize nursing care have taken different forms. Popular past approaches have included procedures (1960s), standards of care (1970s), algorithms (1980s), and clinical practice guidelines (1990s). Each of these approaches aims to help the nurse identify and select interventions that produce optimal care, reduce legal risks, and lower health care costs.

- *Procedure:* A set of how-to action steps for performing a clinical activity or task
- *Standard of care:* A description of an acceptable level of patient care or professional practice
- *Algorithm:* A set of steps that approximates the decision process of an expert clinician and is used to make a decision; these clinical rules are typically embedded in a branching flow chart
- *Clinical practice guideline:* A statement or series of statements outlining appropriate practice for a clinical condition or procedure

National guidelines such as those published by the U.S. Agency for Health Care Research and Quality (AHRQ; http://www.ahrq.gov) and the Cochrane Library (http://www.cochrane.org/cochrane/cc-broch.htm#CC and http://www.cochrane.org/reviews/clibintro.htm) are generally based on the latest, most comprehensive scientific evidence and expert analysis. They provide standards for delivering and evaluating care for patients with the same diagnosis. Box 13-5 compares structured care methodologies. Additional examples are provided in Chapter 15.

Consulting

A nurse designing the plan of care might discover that more information is needed about the nature of the problems

BOX 13-5 STRUCTURED CARE METHODOLOGIES

Algorithm

- Useful in management of high-risk subgroups within the cohort; may be "layered" on top of a pathway to control care practices that are used to manage a specific problem
- Binary decision trees that guide stepwise assessment and intervention
- Intense specificity; no provider flexibility
- May use analytical research methods to ensure cause and effect

Critical Pathway

- Represents a sequential, interdisciplinary, minimal practice standard for a specific patient population
- Provides flexibility to alter care to meet individualized patient needs
- Abbreviated format, broad perspective
- Phase or episode driven
- Ability to measure cause-and-effect relationship between pathway and patient outcomes prohibited by lack of control; changes in patient outcomes directly attributable to the efforts of the collaborative practice team

Guideline

- Broad, research-based practice recommendations
- May or may not have been tested in clinical practice
- Practice resources helpful in construction of structured care methodologies
- No mechanism for ensuring practice implementation

Order Set

- Preprinted provider orders used to expedite the order process after a practice standard has been validated through analytical research
- Complements and increases compliance with existing practice standards
- Can be used to represent the algorithm or protocol in order format

Protocol

- Prescribes specific therapeutic interventions for a clinical problem unique to a subgroup of patients within the cohort
- Multifaceted; may be used to drive practice for more than one discipline
- Broader specificity than an algorithm; allows for minimal provider flexibility by way of treatment options
- May be "layered" on top of a pathway

Agency for Health Care Policy and Research's (now Agency for Healthcare Research and Quality) Clinical Practice Guideline Development, AHCPR program note in Publication 93-0023, 1993.

underlying the need for nursing or about specific interventions. **Consultation,** a process in which two or more people with varying degrees of experience and expertise discuss a problem and its solution, often proves helpful. Nurses might consult with nurse specialists and other members of the health care team, including physicians, nutritionists, social workers, therapists, pastoral caregivers, and ethicists (Fig. 13-4). Consultations are a valuable means for nurses to expand their nursing knowledge and repertoire of effective strategies.

 REVIEW the Reflective Practice box describing Darla Jefferson. The nurse would consult other health care team members for assistance. For

example, the nurse might consult social services for assistance with drug treatment and rehabilitation. Should the patient decide to keep her baby, social services also would be helpful, such as with obtaining food stamps and infant formula through government programs, appropriate housing, and follow-up in the community. A consultation with a nutritionist would be helpful prenatally to help Darla meet the requirements for herself and her fetus, and also postpartum to ensure that the infant is receiving adequate nutrition to grow and develop. ●

DEVELOPING EVALUATIVE STRATEGIES

Well-written outcomes define evaluative strategies to be used by the nurse. Patient outcomes are meaningless unless nurses evaluate the patient's progress toward their achievement. The nurse records the date the outcome was written and the date it is achieved. Evaluative statements (Box 13-6) include a statement about achievement of the desired outcome (met, partially met, not met) and list actual patient behavior as evidence supporting the statement. If the plan is not achieved, recommendations for revising the plan of care are included in the evaluative statement. Chapter 15 deals specifically with the evaluative component of the nursing process.

COMMUNICATING AND RECORDING THE PLAN OF NURSING CARE

The **plan of nursing care** (patient care plan) is the written guide that directs the efforts of the nursing team working

FIGURE 13-4. Consulting with a nursing colleague or other member of the health care team can help the nurse develop an effective nursing plan of care. *(Photo © B. Proud.)*

BOX 13-6 EVALUATIVE STATEMENT

Documents that patient has met, partially met, or not met the goal/outcome

Goal/Outcome Statement

Beginning 6/8/15, the patient will ambulate half the length of hallway with assistance three times daily.

Evaluative Statement

6/8/15—Goal partially met; patient refused to ambulate in the morning but did walk to the bathroom once in the afternoon with the assistance of one nurse.

Recommendation: Review reason for progressive ambulation with patient; assess motivation to increase independence.

—*M. Stenulis, RN*

with patients to meet their health goals. It specifies nursing diagnoses, outcomes, and associated nursing interventions. Well-written plans of care offer many benefits to the patient, nurse, nursing unit, nursing administration, and nursing profession. Primarily, plans of nursing care ensure that the nursing team works efficiently to deliver holistic, goal-oriented, individualized care to patients. A well-written plan of nursing care accomplishes the following:

- Represents an effective philosophy of nursing and advances nursing's four aims: promotes health, prevents disease and illness, promotes recovery, facilitates coping with altered functioning
- Is prepared by the nurse who best knows the patient and is recorded on the day the patient presents for treatment and care according to agency policy; modifications to the initial plan are signed and dated
- Is responsive to the individual characteristics and needs of the patient; is culturally appropriate
- Clearly identifies the nursing assistance the patient needs and nursing's collaborative responsibilities for fulfilling the medical and interdisciplinary plan of care (clearly specifies nursing diagnoses, patient outcomes, nursing interventions, and evaluative strategies)
- Directs the nurse's assessment priorities, caregiving behaviors, and teaching, counseling, and advocacy behaviors
- Is based on scientific principles and incorporates findings of nursing research
- Meets the developmental, psychosocial, and spiritual needs of the patient, as well as the patient's physiologic needs
- Is updated to reflect changes in the patient's status and related needs for nursing care
- Addresses the discharge needs of the patient and family
- Provides for as much patient and family participation as possible
- When appropriate, is compatible with the medical plan of care and that of the interdisciplinary team
- Creates a record that can be used for evaluation, research, reimbursement, and legal purposes

Many suggestions for plans of care appear in the nursing literature. Each school of nursing and each health care institution and agency has its own format, which may reflect a particular nursing theory. Common to all formats is a minimum of three columns for documenting nursing diagnoses, patient outcomes, and nursing interventions. Formats vary in the ways assessment data and the nursing evaluation are addressed.

Institutional and Agency Plans of Care

The Joint Commission requires health care institutions and agencies to formulate, maintain, and support a patient-specific plan for care, treatment, and rehabilitation.

Types of Nursing Care

In most institutions and agencies, the plans of care, regardless of their format, communicate directions for three different types of nursing care: nursing care related to basic human needs, nursing care related to nursing diagnoses, and nursing care related to the medical and interdisciplinary plan of care.

NURSING CARE RELATED TO BASIC HUMAN NEEDS

The plan should concisely communicate to caregivers the data about the patient's usual health habits and patterns, obtained during the nursing history, that are needed to direct daily care. For example, it is important to know whether a toddler is toilet-trained and what words the child uses to indicate the need to void or defecate. Directives about the patient's usual health habits and patterns might be modified by current treatment orders, such as an order to fast for a diagnostic procedure or to limit or increase activity. This information is useful to caregivers only if it is kept current as the patient's condition changes. Any nurse should be able to find in the plan of care the instructions needed to provide competent care.

NURSING CARE RELATED TO NURSING DIAGNOSES

The plan contains outcomes and nursing interventions for every nursing diagnosis, as well as a place to note the patient's responses to care. This section is the heart of the nursing care plan because it represents the independent component of nursing practice. When well developed, it demonstrates the nurse's clinical competence (knowledge of the science of nursing), sensitivity to the individual needs of the patient, and creativity in mobilizing the resources of the patient and the caregiving team to meet the patient's health needs.

NURSING CARE RELATED TO THE MEDICAL AND INTERDISCIPLINARY PLAN OF CARE

The plan of care also records current medical orders for diagnostic studies and treatment and specified related nursing care.

Formats for Plans of Care

A great variety of formats are used to communicate the plan of care. In addition to traditional written plans of care, you should be familiar with the following.

COMPUTERIZED PLANS OF CARE

Nurses now often use **computerized plans of nursing care** as part of the electronic medical record. The benefits of computerized plans include ready access to a large knowledge base, improved record keeping and a resulting improvement in audits and quality assurance, documentation by all members of the health care team with printouts for the patient's

record and for change-of-shift reports, and less time spent on paperwork. One nurse researcher, however, has studied a potential negative impact of computerized plans on the professionalization of staff nurses. Harris (1990) cautions that computerized systems for patient care planning and the larger systems in which they are embedded contribute to the loss of autonomy, loss of individualization of care, and loss of nursing expertise. Individual nurses, as well as researchers, need to respond to this challenge from Harris: "Does a lot of nursing time spent in procedural, rule-governed, step-by-step thinking processes destroy part of the nurse's ability to care, to empathize, to intuit, to gain insight, to function in the expert mode?" (1990, p. 73).

Concept Mapping

FIGURE 13-5. This map identifies and prioritizes key problems/nursing diagnoses and uses lines to illustrate the relationships between problems. (Reprinted with permission from Schuster, D. M. [2012]. *Concept mapping: A critical thinking approach to care planning* [3rd ed.]. Philadelphia: F. A. Davis, p. 10.)

CONCEPT MAP PLANS OF CARE

A concept map care plan is a diagram of patient problems and interventions. Your ideas about patient problems and treatments are the "concepts" that are diagrammed. These maps are used to organize patient data, analyze relationships in the data, and enable you to take a holistic view of the patient's situation (Schuster, 2012). Examples of concept map care plans are shown in Chapter 10 and throughout the text. Figure 13-5 illustrates a concept map that identifies and prioritizes key problems/nursing diagnoses and uses lines to illustrate the relationships between problems. Figure 13-6 illustrates how one diagnosis, Risk for Falls, is worked up in the plan of care.

CHANGES OF SHIFT REPORTS

Chapter 9 describes the importance of critical patient information being communicated with each patient transfer or "hand-off." This includes what happens each time nurses finish their shift and "hand off" patients to other nurses. Many agencies have developed forms to facilitate this exchange of information, including the SBAR/ISBARQ (Situation-Background-Assessment-Recommendation/Introduction-Situation-Background-Assessment-Recommendation-Question and Answer) formats described in Chapters 9 and 16. Alfaro-LeFevre (2014) describes three advantages of using a standardized hand-off tool:

1. Helps you get organized
2. Prevents omissions of key information that must be communicated
3. Promotes dialogue and critical thinking between caregivers

See Figure 13-7 (on page 294) for a standardized hand-off tool different from the SBAR. As you rotate through different clinical agencies, pay attention to their policies and procedures for hand-offs, and follow them carefully.

MULTIDISCIPLINARY (COLLABORATIVE) PLANS OF CARE

Clinical pathways (critical pathways, CareMaps) are tools used in case management to communicate the standardized, interdisciplinary plan of care for patients. Case management is a health care delivery system intended to provide high-quality, cost-effective care for individuals, families, and groups. The emphasis is on clearly stating expected patient outcomes and the specific times within which it is reasonable to achieve these outcomes. Chapter 16 provides examples of how critical pathways are used with select documentation tools in a computerized system. Figure 13-8 (on page 295) illustrates a standardized plan of care for patients with a total knee replacement. Care guidelines and outcomes are specified for each day of the patient's stay. In this case, patients receive a version of their plan of care on admission, based on the rationale that knowing what to expect will result in less stress, quicker recovery, and earlier discharge.

Student Plans of Care

The care plans that students are required to develop are often more detailed than those used in practice settings. The aim is to assist students to assimilate each of the five steps of the nursing process. Although care plan formats vary among different nursing programs, most are designed so that the student systematically proceeds through the interrelated steps of the nursing process. Many use a five-column format.

Problem #_____2_____ : Risk for Falls
General Goal: Patient does not fall

Predicted Behavioral Outcome Objective(s): The patient will . . . remain free from falling on day of care.

Nursing Strategies	Patient Responses (Evaluation)
1. Assess risk for falls	1. Patient at risk due to age, confusion, insomnia, edema & leg brace
2. Assist with ambulation Wear brace	2. Ambulated to PT and lunch Wears brace all day
3. Make sure glasses are clean & in place	3. Wore glasses all day except while shaving
4. Keep one side rail up	4. Side rail remained up
5. Dangle before standing	5. Always sat up with feet on ground before rising to standing postion
6. Use wheelchair if weak or tired	6. Did not have to use wheelchair, ambulated safely
7. Room clear of hazards	7. Room with obstructing furniture, no small items on floor
8. Shoes, slippers, socks, nonskid	8. Nonskid shoes worn

Summarize patient progress toward outcomes objectives: The patient ambulated safely and remained free of falls, protective environment was maintained.

FIGURE 13-6. Identification of goals, outcomes, and strategies, and patient responses for one nursing diagnosis in the concept map. (Reprinted with permission from Schuster, D. M. [2012]. *Concept mapping: A critical thinking approach to care planning* [3rd ed.]. Philadelphia: F. A. Davis, p. 12.)

Date/Time:

ISHAPED Patient Centered Bedside Report Tool

I Introduction

Patient Label:

Room #: _____ Code Status _____ Do Not Announce? _____

Attending: _____ Consults: _____

Primary/Family Contact Information:

S Story

CC: _____ Diagnosis: _____

Communication Issues: Interpreter Needed?: □ Yes □ No Language: _____ Deaf □ HOH □ Auxiliary Aids: _____ □ Blind

Admission Process: □ Admission HX □ Med Rec □ Vaccine Screening □ MRSA Screening □ Pt Belongings List □ Fall Safety Contract

H History

Past Medical History: _____

Allergies: Home O2 □ Yes □ No Smoker □ Yes □ No □ Other: _____

A Assessment

Last Vital Signs: Time: _____ BP: _____ HR: _____ R: _____ Temp: _____ O2 Sat: _____ Freq: _____

Pain: □ Yes □ No Location: _____ Level/Scale: _____ Last Pain Med/Time: _____ Type: _____

IV access: Type: PIV/CVL/PICC Site: _____ Fluid: _____

PIV/CVL/PICC Site: _____ Fluid: _____

Drips: _____

Abnormal Labs: _____

AccuChecks: Schedule and Coverage: _____

Neurological Status: A & O x _____ □ Other: _____

Musculoskel./Activity: □ OOB Ad Lib □ OOB assist □ Total Care □ Bed Rest □ PT/OT Consult (date): _____ □ Other: _____

Cardiovascular: □ Regular □ Irregular □ Edema □ Pacemaker □ Remote Telemetry □ Dialysis: schedule _____

Respiratory Status: □ WNL □ Exceptions: _____ SpO2 _____% on _____L/min _____(mode) □ Chest Tube

Oxygen: O2 order verified □ Yes □ NA Weaning O2 □ Yes □ No Bipap/ Cpap Pulse-ox Monitoring Cont □ Other _____

GI: Diet: _____ □ Feeder □ Assist □ Independent □ Tube Feed via _____ (mode)

Last BM: _____ NGT: Suction _____ □ Ostomy: _____ □ Other: _____

GU: □ Voids □ Foley: Insertion Date: _____ Indication: _____ □ D/C'd: _____ Due to Void: _____

Skin: Pressure Ulcer: □ Yes □ No □ at risk Location(s) _____ □ Documented Pt Last Turned: _____

□ WOCN Consult (date): _____ Incisions/Drains: □ Yes □ No Location(s) _____

Wound Care/Dressings Changes: □ Yes □ No Site(s): _____ □ Frequency: _____ last changed _____

Psychosocial/Family:

P Plan

Today's Goal(s): _____

Oxygen wean goal: _____

Tests/Procedures/Labs: _____

PRN Meds/Last Dose: _____

Discharge Plan/teaching: _____

CM / SW needs: _____

Core Measures: □ Checklist

□ CHF

□ Pneumonia

□ AMI

□ SCIP

E Error-Prevention

Isolation: □ No □ Yes Type: _____ Organism/Site: _____

Fall Risk: □ Low □ Moderate □ High Score: _____ Bed Alarm On: □ No □ Yes □ Interventions/Orders Initiated _____ □ Safety Plan

High Risk Medications:

RISKS:	Sepsis	Aspiration	Elopement	Suicide	Restraints	Seizure	ETOH Withdraw
	□ Yes □ No	□ Yes □ No	□ Yes □ No	□ Yes □ No	□ Yes □ No	□ Yes □ No	□ Yes □ No
		Precautions Initiated:			□ Behavior □ Medical	□ Bed Padded	CIWA: _____
		□ Yes □ No					

D Dialogue

Question and answer occurred: □ Yes □ No   Patient/family had opportunity to participate: □ Yes □ No If no, why:

Not part of the Permanent Medical Record: 2012-2013

FIGURE 13-7. Nurse-to-nurse shift reports are essential elements of care coordination. (Used with permission, Inova Health System Foundation, Falls Church, VA.)

TOTAL KNEE REPLACEMENT PATIENT CARE PLAN

Care	Day of Surgery	Day 1 Post-Op	Day 2 Post-Op	Days 2-4 Post-Op	Discharge Goals
Nutrition	⇨ Intravenous (IV) started for fluids & medications ⇨ Catheter inserted in bladder & urine output monitored for 24 hours ⇨ Diet as tolerated	⇨ Fluids taken as tolerated ⇨ Sit up for meals as able ⇨ IV as needed ⇨ Catheter removed ⇨ Start bowel routine ⇨ Go to bathroom by commode chair/walker with help	⇨ Diet as tolerated ⇨ Sit up in chair for all meals ⇨ Discontinue IV if no nausea and no IV medications	⇨ Sit up in chair for all meals ⇨ Enema or suppository given if no bowel movement	⇨ Eating and bowel movements returning to normal
Hygiene	⇨ Assisted mouth & skin care as needed	⇨ Wash at sink or basin		⇨ Shower if able & if wound drainage device removed	⇨ Patient manages independently
Wound Care	⇨ Dressing checked & reinforced as needed ⇨ Fluid from surgery wound drained by device as needed	⇨ Wound checked daily ⇨ Removed dressing & redress if draining ⇨ Wound drainage device removed at 24 hours	⇨ Remove dressing & redress if draining	⇨ Expose incision when wound is dry	⇨ Surgical wound is clean & dry, or wound care management arranged for home ⇨ Staple/suture removal arranged
Pain Control/ Medication	⇨ IV or Oral medications for pain control once spinal wears off ⇨ May have epidural	⇨ Continue IV or oral pain medication ⇨ Patient to ask for pain medication when needed	⇨ Pain medication as needed & coordinated with activity or rehabilitation schedule	⇨ Pain control medication prior to exercise ⇨ Review home instructions for self-administering anti-coagulant to help prevent blood clotting	⇨ Pain management discussed with & understood by patient ⇨ Required prescriptions provided to patient
Activity/ Rehab	⇨ Patient does the following post-operative exercises every hour when awake: • Deep breathing & coughing • Foot & ankle exercises ⇨ Avoid resting knee in bent position on pillow ⇨ Sit up on side of bed & stand with help ⇨ Walk if able & as requested by doctor ⇨ Apply ice	⇨ Deep breathing & coughing ⇨ Transfer to/from bed & chair with help ⇨ Sit up in chair for short periods ⇨ Apply ice, elevate leg ⇨ Walk using walker/ crutches with help (not exceeding doctor-ordered weight limit on operated leg) ⇨ Begin daily rehab to increase range of motion & exercises to strengthen operated leg	⇨ Deep breathing & coughing ⇨ Increase frequency of transfers to/from bed & chair, & increase independence of transfers ⇨ Apply ice, elevate leg ⇨ Increase distance & frequency of walks Progress to crutches as able ⇨ Continue exercises (with therapist & independently) ⇨ Occupational therapy initiated as needed	⇨ Deep breathing & coughing ⇨ Progress to crutches as appropriate ⇨ Review procedure for going up & down stairs ⇨ Review home exercises ⇨ Apply ice, elevate leg ⇨ Continue to increase independent transfers to/from bed & chair, & walking to bathroom & in hallway as able ⇨ Attend physiotherapy session ⇨ Attent occupational therapy session to review tub transfers & dressing if needed	⇨ Patient is able to: • Achieve minimum 70° flexion in operated leg • Transfer to/from bed & chair, & stand independently & safely • Walk 30 metres using walking aid without exceeding doctor-ordered weight limit on operated leg • Go up & down stairs safely • Perform home exercises & daily living activities safely (or has support in place at home for required activities) • Patients requiring more rehab will be transferred to sub-acute facility
Discharge Planning	⇨ Expected length of stay is 3–4 days ⇨ Planned day of discharge is written on bedside communication board	⇨ Discharge needs discussed with patient's care provider(s) (i.e. equipment, services)	⇨ Nurse, physio and occupational therapists confirm discharge plan & equipment in place ⇨ Resources contacted as needed (i.e. sub-acute facility, Home Care, mobile lab)	⇨ Arrange out-patient physiotherapy if requested by surgeon (when new knee has less than 70° of flexion and/or thigh muscles significantly weak)	⇨ Patient is given & understands: • Discharge instructions • Required exercise routine • Follow-up appointment dates

FIGURE 13-8. Standardized plan of care for a patient with a total knee replacement. (Available at http://www.palomarhealth.org/media/File/Joint/PtCarePathTKR.pdf)

The sample student plan of care shown in Box 13-7 (on pages 296–297) demonstrates a plan developed for a 72-year-old woman admitted to the hospital after experiencing a mini-stroke/brain attack (transient ischemic attack) at home. Her condition is stable, and the three prioritized diagnoses written in the plan address her inability to deal with this new medical diagnosis and to prevent a major stroke (high priority), ineffective coping (medium priority), and constipation (low priority).

Assessing

The student records the assessment data that led to the determination of each diagnosis in the assessment/diagnosis column. Recording these data helps to link specific defining characteristics with diagnostic problem statements.

Diagnosing

Nursing diagnoses are recorded in the assessment/diagnosis column in a prioritized list beginning with the top-priority diagnosis. For each diagnosis, a clear and concise problem statement is followed by an etiology statement that identifies specific contributing factors.

Outcome Identification and Planning

The outcome identification and planning column contains the expected changes in patient health status or in patient

behaviors (i.e., patient outcomes). If achieved, these resolve the problem statement in the nursing diagnosis.

Implementing

Sets of nursing orders that describe specific nursing interventions are written for each patient outcome. These specify what nursing interventions are to be performed, how they are to be performed, when they are to be performed, and who is to perform them. In many nursing programs, students are asked to document the source of their proposed nursing interventions. Although students might be able to "pull from their head" some nursing strategies, developing the practice of consulting the nursing literature is a sure means to increase nursing knowledge. Some programs also require students to provide a scientific rationale for the interventions they propose. A succinct rationale statement demonstrates that the student is deliberately choosing the nursing intervention because of its high probability to effect the desired change.

Evaluating

Incorporating evaluative statements in the plan of care clearly communicates the message that nursing care is never complete until achievement of patient outcomes is evaluated. Just as some say that teaching does not occur if learning does

(text continues on page 298)

Box 13-7 SAMPLE STUDENT PLAN OF CARE

Assessment/Diagnosis	Goal/Outcome	Nursing Orders

Subjective data: "Will I get a stroke now? I don't think I could handle that." "How can I help myself prevent it?"
Objective data: Admitting diagnosis: TIA
BP: 184/120
Strengths: Past pattern of adhering to prescribed health behaviors.
 	
Nursing diagnosis: Ineffective Health Maintenance Response to TIA and Stroke Prevention related to knowledge deficit
	Before discharge, the patient will:
	• Describe the terms *TIA* and *stroke,* identifying the underlying disease process, causes, symptoms, and treatment
	
	After discussion with the physician and nurse, the patient will:
	• Correctly describe the treatment plan:
	  • Medications (drugs, intended effect, dose, time, route)
	  • Dietary modifications
	  • Exercise prescription
	  • Signs and symptoms to report
	• Follow-up appointment date
		Assess what the patient knows about TIA and stroke (correct any misinformation). Assess learning needs, readiness to learn, and factors that will influence learning.
		Plan teaching and learning sessions to involve family members designated by patient.
		Include in the teaching plan a description of TIA and stroke and the underlying disease process, causes, symptoms, and treatment plan.
		After the treatment plan has been developed, make sure the patient and family can restate it (teaching) and value the prescribed lifestyle modification (counseling).

Subjective data: Husband died 8 months ago; moved in with daughter 6 months ago after selling family home. Daughter reports mother had been a very independent, strong woman in the past—seemed to "crumple" after husband's death. History of headaches *Objective data:* Clutches daughter's hand *Strengths:* History of handling life stressors well *Limitations:* In the past, her husband was her primary support **Nursing diagnosis:** Ineffective Coping related to illness, recent death of husband, and relocation with daughter	Beginning 9/7/15, the patient will: • Verbalize her feelings related to the loss of her husband, loss of family home, loss of health • Identify coping patterns that have helped her in the past • Identify three personal strengths and three outside supports that will help her now Before discharge, the patient will: • Verbalize that she feels "okay" (sufficiently in charge of her life) about returning home	Once during each shift, primary nurse should sit at patient's bedside for at least several minutes to communicate caring and to explore with the patient her current stressors and the adequacy of her coping response. • Assess factors compounding her losses. • Reinforce her personal strengths and support systems; counsel her to tap into these now. • Suggest local support groups, if indicated. Primary nurse to explore with daughter, Lisa, how her mother's moving in with her has affected the family. Recommend support systems.

Subjective data: "I move my bowels every 2 or 3 days; get constipated at least once a week. Often Metamucil helps."
"I drink plenty of fluids and eat fruits and vegetables."
History of hemorrhoids secondary to straining
Objective data: No bowel movement in past 4 days
On bedrest since hospitalized
Nursing diagnosis: Constipation related to decreased physical activity and long-term laxative use (Metamucil)
	Beginning 9/7/15, the patient will:
	• Pass soft, formed stool every 1 to 3 days without use of laxatives
	By 9/10/15, the patient will:
	• Verbalize the importance of the following natural aids to bowel elimination:
	  • Daily intake of foods high in bulk
	  • Daily fluid intake of 8 to 10 glasses
	  • Regular time for elimination
	  • Daily physical exercise: walking
		Monitor bowel elimination patterns; identify causative factors of constipation and successful corrective measures.
		Explain the importance of adhering to a regular time for defecation (patient suggests after breakfast)—adhere to this in the hospital.
		When given medical clearance, assist patient with progressive ambulation.
		Recommend that she include brisk walking into daily health habits (build strength to 20- to 30-minute brisk walk daily).
		Explain the long-term effects of laxative abuse on the bowel, and discourage use of laxatives.
		Reinforce the patient's fluid intake and ingestion of high-bulk foods, such as fresh fruits and salad.

Scientific Rationale	Evaluation
Each person's learning needs are different; each person learns in one's own unique way; learning is dependent on readiness.	9/10/15—Outcome not met. Patient says her head is "too old" to learn all this stuff. Equates stroke with death. *Revision:* Reteach content in simpler terms. Reassess learning readiness. —*M. Foley, SN*
The more support people knowledgeably committed to the plan of care, the greater the probability the patient will achieve goals. New self-care behaviors are dependent on knowledge.	
New self-care behaviors are dependent on motivation. Unless the patient is committed to stroke prevention and values this outcome, she will not follow the treatment plan.	9/10/15 Too early to evaluate. —*M. Foley, SN*
The nurse's unhurried, attentive, and caring presence communicates to the patient that she is important to the nurse and that the nurse values her well-being. It is an invitation to the patient to become actively involved in recovery. Also, it is logical to explore adequacy of past and current coping mechanisms before suggesting new approaches.	9/10/15 Outcome partially met. Patient speaks freely about how much she misses her husband and how fearful this hospitalization makes her. When asked about living with her daughter, she becomes uncharacteristically quiet. —*M. Foley, SN* 9/10/15 Outcome met. Patient talks about how everything seemed better in the past after she talked it over with her husband and God. —*M. Foley, SN* 9/10/15 Outcome not met. Patient couldn't think of anything about herself that is healthy or strong. Says "maybe" her family can help her now.
Adult children of aging parents frequently experience overwhelming stress as they try to deal with their own and their parents' problems. Supporting this family is supporting the patient indirectly.	*Revision:* Counsel regarding personal strengths. Help her to experience them. —*M. Foley, SN* 9/11/15 Too early to evaluate. —*M. Foley, SN*
This patient's elimination problems will not be resolved until all the specific causes of her constipation and successful corrective measures are identified. Needs to be an ongoing assessment priority. This encourages positive use of circadian rhythms. Peristalsis is stimulated by physical exercise.	9/10/15 Outcome partially met. Soft, formed stool passed every 2 to 3 days with aid of Colace. —*M. Foley, SN* 9/10/15 Outcome met. Patient correctly related value of four natural aids to elimination. Questions whether she will be strong enough to walk. *Revision:* Encourage assisted ambulation. —*M. Foley, SN*
Laxative abuse leads to decreased peristaltic response to food and loss of intestinal tone. Commenting on these positive self-care behaviors reinforces them.	

not take place, so nursing care is incomplete if the desired patient goals are not achieved.

PROBLEMS RELATED TO OUTCOME IDENTIFICATION AND PLANNING

Problems commonly encountered while developing plans of nursing care include failure to involve the patient in the planning process, insufficient data collection, use of inaccurate or insufficient data to develop nursing diagnoses, outcomes that are stated too broadly, outcomes that are derived from poorly developed nursing diagnoses, failure to write nursing orders clearly, written nursing orders that do not resolve the problem, and failure to update the plan of care.

 RECALL Elijah Wolinski, the frail, older adult with a pressure ulcer. Since the nurse is providing care in the patient's home, a written plan of care is extremely important because more than one caregiver may be involved in the patient's care. In addition, the nurse must update the plan regularly to ensure that regardless of who is providing the care, the correct care is given consistently. ●

A FINAL WORD ABOUT NIC/NOC AND STANDARDIZED LANGUAGES

Moorhead, Johnson, Maas, and Swanson (2013) lament that while nurses' clinical-reasoning and decision-making skills are integral to quality health care and account for much of the health care system "safety net," little attention has been focused on the outcomes of nursing interventions. They write that, as part of improving health care quality and safety, "it is imperative that nursing define its interventions and outcomes and that these standardized nomenclatures be included in clinical nursing information systems and in large data sets used for systematic analysis" (p. 3).

The use of Nursing Interventions Classification (NIC; Bulechek, Butcher, & Dochterman, 2013, p. vi):

* Helps demonstrate the impact that nurses have on the system of health care delivery
* Standardizes and defines the knowledge base for nursing curricula and practice
* Facilitates the appropriate selection of a nursing intervention
* Facilitates communication of nursing treatments to other nurses and other providers
* Enables researchers to examine the effectiveness and cost of nursing care
* Assists educators to develop curricula that better articulate with clinical practice
* Facilitates the teaching of clinical decision making to novice nurses
* Assists administrators in planning more effectively for staff and equipment needs
* Promotes the development of a reimbursement system for nursing services

* Promotes the development and use of nursing information systems
* Communicates the nature of nursing to the public

REFLECTIVE PRACTICE LEADING TO PERSONAL LEARNING

Remember that the object of reflective practice is to look at an experience, understand it, and learn from it. As you begin to develop your expertise in outcome identification and planning, reflect on your experiences—both successes and failures—in order to improve your practice. How can you do it better next time? What did you learn today that can help you tomorrow? Begin your reflection by paying close attention to the following during the planning phase of the nursing process:

* Did your preparation for your partnering with the patient and family to identify outcomes and plan bring you to this experience feeling confident in your ability to identify pertinent outcomes, select evidence-based interventions, and communicate the plan of care? Did you inspire the patient's confidence and trust?
* How confident are you that once implemented, this plan will address the clinical, functional, and quality-of-life concerns of the patient? How can you become more familiar with the many outcomes and interventions that may be applicable for future patients?
* Were you aware of any personal stereotypes or prejudices that might have negatively influenced this clinical encounter? If yes, how did you address them?
* Was the patient's/family's participation in the process at an optimal level? How might you have better engaged the patient and family? Does the plan of care accurately reflect patient priorities and preferences? To what degree do you think the patient's participation in planning will influence the achievement of outcomes?

Perhaps the most important question to reflect on is: Are your patients and families better for having had *you* share in the critical responsibility of partnering with them to identify outcomes and plan the care that will result in them achieving these outcomes? Will your patients now receive individualized, prioritized, holistic, evidence-based treatment and care because of your efforts?

DEVELOPING CLINICAL REASONING

1. Write nursing diagnoses for three obese patients, and make sure that the etiologies for the problem statement (Imbalanced Nutrition: More Than Body Requirements) differ. Describe how these different etiologies result in different plans of care.

2. Use one of the nursing diagnoses from Exercise 1 and write related cognitive, psychomotor, and affective goals for this patient. Explain the different purposes of each type of goal and why it may be necessary to include all three to resolve a patient problem successfully.

3. An alert 82-year-old widow, who has a history of unsafe behaviors, has recently been discharged from the hospital to

her home. Caregivers attempted to secure her consent to be transferred to a long-term care facility, but she flatly refused. Responsible for her home care, you list Risk for Injury as a priority nursing diagnosis. First, list the nursing measures that you believe are most likely to achieve the outcome of preventing injury. Then talk with several other students to compare your lists of interventions and the evidence that supports each; then discuss how practicing nurses can be sure they select the best nursing interventions for each expected patient outcome.

PRACTICING FOR NCLEX

1. A nurse is planning care for a male adolescent patient who is admitted to the hospital for treatment of a drug overdose. Which nursing actions are related to the outcome identification and planning step of the nursing process? Select all that apply.
   a. The nurse formulates nursing diagnoses.
   b. The nurse identifies expected patient outcomes.
   c. The nurse selects evidence-based nursing interventions.
   d. The nurse explains the nursing care plan to the patient.
   e. The nurse assesses the patient's mental status.
   f. The nurse evaluates the patient's outcome achievement.

2. A nurse on a busy surgical unit relies on informal planning to provide appropriate nursing responses to patients in a timely manner. What are examples of this type of planning? Select all that apply.
   a. A nurse sits down with a patient and prioritizes existing diagnoses.
   b. A nurse assesses a woman for postpartum depression during routine care.
   c. A nurse plans interventions for a patient who is diagnosed with epilepsy.
   d. A busy nurse takes time to speak to a patient who received bad news.
   e. A nurse reassesses a patient whose PRN pain medication is not working.
   f. A nurse coordinates the home care of a patient being discharged.

3. When helping a patient turn in bed, the nurse notices that his heels are reddened and plans to place him on precautions for skin breakdown. This is an example of what type of planning?
   a. Initial planning
   b. Standardized planning
   c. Ongoing planning
   d. Discharge planning

4. A nurse is prioritizing the following patient diagnoses according to Maslow's hierarchy of human needs:
   (1) Disturbed Body Image
   (2) Ineffective Airway Clearance
   (3) Spiritual Distress
   (4) Impaired Social Interaction

   Which answer choice below lists the problems in order of highest priority to lowest priority based on Maslow's model?
   a. 2, 4, 1, 3
   b. 3, 1, 4, 2
   c. 2, 4, 3, 1
   d. 3, 2, 4, 1

5. A nurse is using critical pathway methodology for choosing interventions for a patient who is receiving chemotherapy for breast cancer. Which nursing actions are characteristics of this system being used when planning care? Select all that apply.
   a. The nurse uses a minimal practice standard and is able to alter care to meet the patient's individual needs.
   b. The nurse uses a binary decision tree for stepwise assessment and intervention.
   c. The nurse is able to measure the cause-and-effect relationship between pathway and patient outcomes.
   d. The nurse uses broad, research-based practice recommendations that may or may not have been tested in clinical practice.
   e. The nurse uses preprinted provider orders used to expedite the order process after a practice standard has been validated through research.
   f. The nurse uses a decision tree that provides intense specificity and no provider flexibility.

6. A nurse is identifying outcomes for a patient who has a leg ulcer related to diabetes. An example of an affective outcome for this patient is:
   a. Within 1 day after teaching, the patient will list three benefits of continuing to apply moist compresses to leg ulcer after discharge.
   b. By 6/12/15, the patient will correctly demonstrate application of wet-to-dry dressing on leg ulcer.
   c. By 6/19/15, the patient's ulcer will begin to show signs of healing (e.g., size shrinks from 3″ to 2.5″).
   d. By 6/12/15, the patient will verbalize valuing health sufficiently to practice new health behaviors to prevent recurrence of leg ulcer.

7. A nurse is preparing a clinical outcome for a 32-year-old female runner who is recovering from a stroke that caused right-sided paresis. An example of this type of outcome is:
   a. After receiving 3 weeks of physical therapy, patient will demonstrate improved movement on the right side of her body.
   b. By 8/15/15, patient will be able to use right arm to dress, comb hair, and feed herself.
   c. Following physical therapy, patient will begin to gradually participate in walking/running events.
   d. By 8/15/15, patient will verbalize feeling sufficiently prepared to participate in running events.

8. A nurse is caring for an elderly male patient who is receiving fluids for dehydration. Which outcome for this patient is correctly written?
   a. Offer the patient 60 mL fluid every 2 hours while awake.
   b. During the next 24-hour period, the patient's fluid intake will total at least 2,000 mL.
   c. Teach the patient the importance of drinking enough fluids to prevent dehydration by 1/15/15
   d. At the next visit, 12/23/15, the patient will know that he should drink at least 3 liters of water per day.

9. A nurse is collecting more patient data to confirm a diagnosis of emphysema for a 68-year-old male patient. What type of diagnosis does this intervention seek to confirm?
   a. Actual
   b. Possible
   c. Risk
   d. Collaborative

10. A nurse is caring for a patient who is diagnosed with conges-tive heart failure. Which statement below is *not* an example of a well-stated nursing intervention?
    a. Offer patient 60 mL water or juice (prefers orange or cranberry juice) every 2 hours while awake for a total minimum PO intake of 500 mL.
    b. Teach patient the necessity of carefully monitoring fluid intake and output; remind patient each shift to mark off fluid intake on record at bedside.
    c. Walk with patient to bathroom for toileting every 2 hours (on even hours) while patient is awake.
    d. Manage patient's pain.

ANSWERS WITH RATIONALES

1. *b, c, d.* During the outcome identification and planning step of the nursing process, the nurse works in partnership with the patient and family to establish priorities, identify and write expected patient outcomes, select evidence-based nursing interventions, and communicate the plan of nursing care. Although all these steps may overlap, formulating and validating nursing diagnoses occurs most frequently during the diagnosing step of the nursing process. Assessing mental status is part of the assessment step, and evaluating patient outcomes occurs during the evaluation step of the nursing process.

2. *b, d, e.* Informal planning is a link between identifying a patient's strength or problem and providing an appropriate nursing response. This occurs, for example, when a busy nurse first recognizes postpartum depression in a patient, takes time to assess a patient who received bad news about tests, or reassesses a patient for pain. Formal planning involves prioritizing diagnoses, formally planning interven-tions, and coordinating the home care of a patient being discharged.

3. *c.* Ongoing planning is problem oriented and has as its pur-pose keeping the plan up to date as new actual or potential problems are identified. Initial planning addresses each problem listed in the prioritized nursing diagnoses and identifies appropriate patient goals and the related nursing care. Standardized care plans are prepared plans of care that identify the nursing diagnoses, outcomes, and related nurs-ing interventions common to a specific population or health problem. During discharge planning, the nurse uses teaching and counseling skills effectively to help the patient and family develop sufficient knowledge of the health problem and the therapeutic regimen to carry out necessary self-care behaviors competently at home.

4. *a.* 2, 4, 1, 3. Because basic needs must be met before a person can focus on higher ones, patient needs may be prioritized according to Maslow's hierarchy: (1) physiologic needs, (2) safety needs, (3) love and belonging needs, (4) self-esteem needs, and (5) self-actualization needs. #2 is an example of a physiologic need, #4 is an example of a love and belonging need, #1 is an example of a self-esteem need, and #3 is an example of a self-actualization need.

5. *a, c.* A critical pathway represents a sequential, interdis-ciplinary, minimal practice standard for a specific patient population that provides flexibility to alter care to meet individualized patient needs. It also offers the ability to measure a cause-and-effect relationship between pathway and patient outcomes. An algorithm is a binary decision tree that guides stepwise assessment and intervention with intense specificity and no provider flexibility. Guidelines are broad, research-based practice recommendations that may or may not have been tested in clinical practice, and an order set is a preprinted provider order used to expedite the order process after a practice standard has been validated through analytical research.

6. *d.* Affective outcomes describe changes in patient values, beliefs, and attitudes. Cognitive outcomes (*a*) describe increases in patient knowledge or intellectual behaviors; psychomotor outcomes (*b*) describe the patient's achievement of new skills. *c* is an outcome describing a physical change in the patient.

7. *a.* Clinical outcomes describe the expected status of health issues at certain points in time, after treatment is complete. Functional outcomes (*b*) describe the person's ability to function in relation to the desired usual activities. Quality-of-life outcomes (*c*) focus on key factors that affect someone's ability to enjoy life and achieve personal goals. Affective outcomes (*d*) describe changes in patient values, beliefs, and attitudes.

8. *b.* The outcomes in *a* and *c* make the error of expressing the patient goal as a nursing intervention. Incorrect: "Offer the patient 60 mL fluid every 2 hours while awake." Correct: "The patient will drink 60 mL fluid every 2 hours while awake, beginning 1/3/15." The outcome in *d* makes the error of using verbs that are not observable and measurable. Verbs to be avoided when writing goals include "know," "under-stand," "learn," and "become aware."

9. *b.* An intervention for a possible diagnosis is to collect more patient data to confirm or rule out the problem. An inter-vention for an actual diagnosis is to reduce or eliminate contributing factors to the diagnosis. Interventions for a risk diagnosis focus on reducing or eliminating risk factors, and interventions for collaborative problems focus on monitoring for changes in status and managing these changes with nurse- and physician-prescribed interventions.

10. *d.* This statement lacks sufficient detail to effectively guide nursing intervention. The set of nursing interventions written to assist a patient to meet an outcome must be comprehen-sive. Comprehensive nursing interventions specify what observations (assessments) need to be made and how often, what nursing interventions need to be done and when they must be done, and what teaching, counseling, and advocacy needs patients and families may have.

TAYLOR SUITE RESOURCES

Explore these additional resources to enhance learning for this chapter:
- NCLEX-Style Questions and other resources on thePoint, http://thePoint.lww.com/Taylor8e
- *Study Guide for Fundamentals of Nursing, 8th edition*
- Adaptive Learning | Powered by prepU, http://thepoint.lww.com/prepu

Bibliography

Alfaro-LeFevre, R. (2010). *Applying nursing process: A tool for critical thinking* (7th ed.). Philadelphia: Wolters Kluwer Health/Lippincott Williams & Wilkins.

Alfaro-LeFevre, R. (2013). *Critical thinking, clinical reasoning, and clinical judgment: A practical approach* (5th ed.). St. Louis: Elsevier.

Alfaro, R. (2014). *Applying nursing process. The foundation for clinical reasoning* (8th ed.). Philadelphia: Wolters Kluwer Health/Lippincott Williams & Wilkins.

American Nurses Association (ANA). (2010). *Standards of clinical nursing practice* (2nd ed.). Silver Spring, MD: Author.

American Nurses Association (ANA). (2010). *Nursing's social policy statement* (2010 ed.). Silver Spring, MD: Author.

Atay, S., & Karabacak, U. (2012). Care plans using concept maps and their effects on critical thinking dispositions of nursing students. *International Journal of Nursing Practice, 18*, 233–239.

Bulechek, G. M., Butcher, H. K., Dochterman, J., & Wagner, C.M. (Eds.). (2013). *Nursing interventions classification (NIC)* (6th ed.). St. Louis: Elsevier.

Carpenito, L. J. (2013). *Nursing diagnosis: Application to clinical practice* (14th ed.). Philadelphia: Wolters Kluwer Health/Lippincott Williams & Wilkins.

Carpenito-Moyet, L. J. (2010). *Nursing care plans and documentation: Nursing diagnoses and collaborative problems* (5th ed.). Philadelphia: Wolters Kluwer Health/Lippincott Williams & Wilkins.

Committee on Quality Health Care in America, Institute of Medicine (IOM). (2001). *Crossing the qual-ity chasm: A new health system for the 21st century.* Washington, DC: National Academy Press.

Concept Mapping. www.nursingconceptmapping.com

Daley, B. J. (1999). Concept maps: A strategy to teach and evaluate critical thinking. *Journal of Nursing Education, 38*(1), 42.

Doran, G. T. (1981). There's a S.M.A.R.T. way to write management's goals and objectives. *Management Review, 70*(11), (AMA FORUM), 35–36.

Ferrario, C. G. (2003). Experienced and less-experienced nurses' diagnostic reasoning: Implications for fostering students' critical thinking. *International Journal of Nursing Terminologies and Classifications, 14*(2), 41–52.

Ferrario, C. G. (2004). Developing nurses' critical thinking skills with concept mapping. *Journal for Nurses in Staff Development, 20*(6), 261–267.

Fowler, M. D. M. (Ed.) (2010 reissue). *Guide to the Code of Ethics for Nurses.* Silver Spring, MD: American Nurses Association.

Harris, B. L. (1990). Becoming deprofessionalized: One aspect of the staff nurse's perspective on computer-mediated nursing care plans. *Advances in Nursing Science, 13*(2), 63–74.

Hendry, C., & Walker, A. (2004). Priority setting in clinical nursing practice: Literature review. *Journal of Advanced Nursing, 47*(4), 427.

Iowa Intervention Project. (1997). Nursing interventions classification (NIC): An overview. In M. J. Rantz & P. LeMone (Eds.), *Classification of Nursing Diagnoses: Proceedings of the Twelfth Conference, North American Nursing Diagnosis* (pp. 32–39). Glendale, CA: CINAHL Information Systems.

Johnson, M., Bulechek, G., McCloskey Dochterman, J., Maas, M., & Moorhead, S. (Eds.). (2001). *Nursing diagnoses, outcomes and interventions: NANDA, NIC, NOC, linkages.* St. Louis: Mosby.

The Joint Commission. (2012). National Patient Safety Goal. Available at http://www.jointcommission.org/assets/1/18/NPSG_Chapter_Jan2013_HAP.pdf

King, M., & Shell, R. (2002). Teaching and evaluating critical thinking with concept maps. *Nurse Educator, 27*(5), 214.

LaDuke, S. (2008). Viewpoint: Death to nursing care plans! *American Journal of Nursing, 108*(6), 13.

Lunney, M. (2006). Helping nurses use NANDA, NOC and MC: Novice to expert. *Nurse Educator, 31*(1), 40–46.

Moorhead, S., Johnson, M., Maas, M. L., & Swanson, E. (Eds.). (2013). *Nursing outcomes classification (NOC)* (5th ed.). St. Louis, MO: Elsevier.

Mueller, A., Johnston, M., & Bigh, D. (2002). Joining mind mapping and care mapping to enhance student critical thinking and achieve holistic nursing care. *Nursing Diagnosis, 13*(1), 24–27.

Schnehl, P. (2014). *Introduction to concept mapping in nursing.* Burlington, MA: Jones & Bartlett.

Schuster, D. M. (2012). *Concept mapping: A critical thinking approach to care planning* (3rd ed.). Philadelphia: F. A. Davis.

St. Cyr, S., & All, A. (2009). Concept mapping: A road to critical thinking. *Journal for Nurses in Staff Development, 25*(2), 70–74.

Swanson, F. (2008). *Nursing Outcomes Classification (NOC)* (4th ed.). St Louis: Elsevier/Mosby.

14 Implementing

ANTOINETTE BROWNE

Antoinette, a toddler, is brought to the well-child community clinic by her grandmother. The health history reveals recurrent nausea, vomiting, and diarrhea. Her physical examination reveals a negligible gain in height and weight, lethargy, and a delay in achieving developmental milestones.

ESTELLE MORRISSEY

Estelle is an 86-year-old woman who is in a long-term care facility because of multiple chronic health problems. She is alert and oriented to person, place, and time. She states, "I'm all alone. There's no one left and I want to die. Can you help me?"

JAMES MCMAHON

James, a 62-year-old man, is admitted to the intensive care unit in hepatic failure. He is critically ill, being monitored continuously, and receiving intravenous fluids and medications via central and peripheral IV catheters.

LEARNING OBJECTIVES

After completing this chapter, you will be able to accomplish the following:

1. List advantages of using a standard classification of nursing interventions and outcomes.

2. Use cognitive, interpersonal, technical, ethical/legal, and QSEN competencies to implement a plan of nursing care.

3. Use eight guidelines for implementation.

4. Describe six variables that influence the way a plan of care is implemented.

5. Use ongoing data collection to determine how to safely and effectively implement a plan of care.

6. Explain why reassessment after nursing intervention is important.

7. Describe the risks and responsibilities of delegating nursing interventions.

KEY TERMS

delegation	implementing	protocols
direct care intervention	indirect care intervention	standing orders
evidence-based practice	nursing intervention	unlicensed assistive personnel (UAP)

During the **implementing** step of the nursing process, nursing actions planned in the previous step are carried out. The purposes of implementation are to help the patient achieve valued health outcomes: promote health, prevent disease and illness, restore health, and facilitate coping with altered functioning. For an example, see the accompanying Reflective Practice box on page 304. The plan of care is best implemented when patients who are able and willing to participate have maximum opportunities to engage in self-care. Family members and other support people, as well as other health care professionals, may also be involved in successfully implementing the plan of care (Table 14-1 on page 305). During the implementation step, the nurse continues to collect data and to modify the plan of care as needed (Fig. 14-1 on page 306). All activities are documented in the format used by the nurse's institution or agency.

UNIQUE FOCUS OF NURSING IMPLEMENTATION

In all nurse–patient interactions, the nurse is concerned with the patient's response to health and illness and the patient's ability to meet basic human needs. Whereas other health care professionals focus on selected aspects of the patient's treatment regimen, nurses are concerned with how the patient is responding to the plan of care in general. Standards of practice for implementation are described in Box 14-1.

The Nursing Interventions Taxonomy Structure

In 1992, McCloskey Dochterman and Bulechek published *Nursing Interventions Classification (NIC),* a report of research to construct a taxonomy of nursing interventions.

BOX 14-1 THE REGISTERED NURSE IMPLEMENTS THE IDENTIFIED PLAN

Standard 5. Implementation
The registered nurse implements the identified plan.
Competencies
The registered nurse:

Partners with the person, family, significant others, and caregivers as appropriate to implement the plan in a safe, realistic, and timely manner.

Demonstrates caring behaviors toward health care consumers, significant others, and groups of people receiving care.

Utilizes technology to measure, record, and retrieve health care consumer data, implement the nursing process, and enhance nursing practice.

Utilizes evidence-based interventions and treatments specific to the diagnosis or problem.

Provides holistic care that addresses the needs of diverse populations across the lifespan.

Advocates for health care that is sensitive to the needs of health care consumers with particular emphasis on the needs of diverse populations.

Applies appropriate knowledge of major health problems and cultural diversity in implementing the plan of care.

Collaborates with health care providers from diverse backgrounds to implement and integrate the plan.

Accommodates for different styles of communication by health care consumers, families, and health care providers.

Integrates traditional and complementary health care practices as appropriate.

Implements the plan in a timely manner in accordance with patient safety goals.

Promotes the health care consumer's capacity for the optimal level of participation and problem-solving.

Documents implementation and any modifications, including changes or omissions, of the identified plan.

Standard 5A. Coordinator of Care
The registered nurse coordinates care delivery.

Standard 5B. Health Teaching and Health Promotion
The registered nurse employs strategies to promote health and a safe environment.

Reprinted with permission from American Nurses Association (ANA). (2010). *Scope and Standards of Practice.* Silver Spring, MD: Author.

REFLECTIVE PRACTICE: CULTIVATING QSEN COMPETENCIES

CHALLENGE TO TECHNICAL SKILLS

James McMahon, a 62-year-old man, is admitted to the intensive care unit (ICU) in hepatic failure. He is critically ill, being monitored continuously, and receiving intravenous (IV) fluids and medications via central and peripheral IV catheters. During a recent clinical rotation in the ICU, I followed an extremely busy nurse who was caring for Mr. McMahon. He had several IV infusion lines and required numerous technologic devices for monitoring and care. The nurse asked me to hang a new bag of IV medication. I found myself completely overwhelmed and confused by the myriad tangle of IV lines and knew that I wouldn't be able to determine how to run the medication without the guidance of the nurse. I became frustrated because I should have been able to perform this task quickly and correctly if I had been working independently. I didn't want to risk hanging the IV medication and infusing it into a line with another fluid that was possibly incompatible. Nor did I want to risk running the medication through the incorrect port. The nurse was extremely busy, and I felt pressured to perform this task immediately.

Thinking Outside the Box: Possible Courses of Action

- Request that the nurse hang the medication once she was through with her other tasks.
- Hang the medication, hoping that it was compatible with the other fluids that were already infusing.
- Ask another nurse on the unit to hang the medication.
- Wait until the nurse was through with what she had to do, admit to her that I felt uncomfortable hanging the medication on my own, and then ask that she walk me through the process.

Evaluating a Successful Outcome: How Do I Define Success?

- The patient remains free from harm while receiving the necessary medication.
- The nurse recognizes the need to provide me with more guidance.
- I feel comfortable and competent in my skills.
- The patient receives efficient, safe care.

Personal Learning: Here's to the Future!

Luckily, there was a positive ending to this situation. I explained to the nurse that I was confused by the maze of IV lines and that I was uncomfortable administering the IV medication on my own. The nurse immediately recognized that the patient's lines were tangled and disorganized and some were unlabeled. With me at her side, she took the time to reorganize and label all of the lines, making it easier to visualize all of the medications and fluids the patient was receiving. We referenced a drug book to ensure that the medication was compatible with the other fluids that were running. She also walked me through the process of hanging the medication and connecting it to the appropriate port. The nurse appreciated the fact that I waited to ask her for help. As a result, the patient remained safe from injury. In addition, she realized that she shouldn't have asked me to perform this task independently. I benefited from the experience because I became more familiar with this particular skill. As of now, I still find myself feeling somewhat anxious and uncomfortable with certain technical skills. However, I am finding that with each new clinical experience, I become more comfortable and more independent in my practice.

Colleen Kilcullen, Georgetown University

REFLECTION ON QUALITY AND SAFETY COMPETENCIES

How do you think you would respond in a similar situation? Why? What does this tell you about yourself and about the adequacy of your competencies for professional practice? Do you agree with the criteria that the nursing student used to evaluate a successful outcome? Why or why not? What *knowledge, skills,* and *attitudes* do you need to develop to continuously improve the quality and safety of care for patients like Mr. McMahon? What factors might have influenced the nurse in assigning this task to the student? Did the nurse effectively delegate this intervention? Why or why not? Did the student adhere to ethical and legal guidelines with the response? If so, explain how. If not, what issues were present?

Patient-Centered Care: How can you keep your focus on providing respectful and compassionate care for Mr. McMahon—even when feeling overwhelmed?

Teamwork and Collaboration/Quality Improvement: What communication and interpersonal skills do you need to be able to approach other nurses and team members when you need help? What does quality care for Mr. McMahon "look like"? What did the experienced nurse teach the student by taking the time to label the lines and medications?

Safety/Evidence-Based Practice: What does the evidence point to as "best practice" for administering Mr. McMahon's medications? What safety needs does he have and how can you meet them? What have you learned about the dangers of "busyness"?

Informatics: Can you identify the essential information that must be available in Mr. McMahon's drug record to support safe patient care and coordination of care? Can you think of other ways to respond to or approach the situation? What else might the nursing student have done to ensure a successful outcome?

Table 14-1 PROFESSIONAL NURSING RELATIONSHIPS: ROLE RESPONSIBILITIES AND RELATED COMPETENCIES

RELATIONSHIP	ROLE RESPONSIBILITIES	RELATED COMPETENCIES
Nurse–patient	• Communicate to patients that someone is concerned about them (as well as the disease) and is interested in how change in health state will affect their overall well-being. • Create an environment in which patients can commit their energies to health promotion or restoration or peaceful dying, confident that basic human needs are being addressed. • Challenge patients to develop self-care abilities that promote holistic health.	• Repertoire of therapeutic interpersonal behaviors: attending, listening, interviewing, nonverbal communication, touching, facilitating, coaching • Ability to establish trusting nurse–patient–family relationships • Demonstrated competence in the nursing roles of caregiver, teacher, counselor, advocate
Nurse–patient–family	• Develop in the patient and family the knowledge, attitude, and skills that will enable them to respond to the self-care challenges of their health or illness state. • Intervene as appropriate to promote healthy family functioning. • Educate the family to be wise and assertive health care consumers.	
Nurse–nurse	• Support one another's efforts to deliver quality nursing care; work collaboratively with nursing administration to improve quality care. • Provide creative leadership—formally or informally—to make the nursing unit a satisfying and challenging place to work. • Supervise the nursing care given by other nursing personnel; affirm the nursing strengths of others, and constructively address the nursing deficiencies encountered. • Enhance the professional development of self and other nurses through active participation in professional organizations.	Communication Teaching/counseling/advocacy Assertiveness Collaboration Coordination Group process Organization Leadership Delegation Change strategies Problem solving Decision making Conflict resolution
Nurse–health care team	• Communicate clearly nursing's perspective regarding the patient and family to the health care team. • Coordinate the inputs of the multidisciplinary team into a comprehensive plan of care. • Serve as a liaison between the patient and family and the health care team, as necessary.	

New editions appeared in 1996, 2000, 2004, 2008, and 2013. Each of the interventions listed has a label, a definition, a set of activities that a nurse performs to carry out the intervention, and a short list of background readings. Advantages of having a standard classification of nursing interventions are discussed in Chapter 13. Table 13-2 on page 286 illustrates the NIC taxonomy structure designed to help clinicians locate and select the interventions most helpful for patients.

The researchers involved in the development of NICs are also committed to developing a classification of patient outcomes for nursing interventions, called Nursing Outcomes Classifications (NOCs). This research aims to:

1. Identify, label, validate, and classify nursing-sensitive patient outcomes and indicators
2. Evaluate the validity and usefulness of the classification in clinical field testing
3. Define and test measurement procedures for the outcomes and indicators

This research continues in an effort to develop a common nursing language to optimize the design and delivery of safe, high-quality, and cost-effective care.

For examples of how NIC and NOC can be used to plan and implement care, see the box "Examples of Nursing Interventions and Nursing Outcomes Classifications (NIC/NOC)" (on page 306) in this chapter and in each clinical chapter. The examples in this chapter illustrate how NIC and NOC can be used to implement care for a patient and family who require assistance to maintain the home as a clean, safe, and pleasant place. The box lists representative nursing activities for the intervention Home Maintenance Assistance and suggested outcomes for Impaired Home Maintenance.

Care Coordination, Continuity, and the Nurse

One of nursing's major contributions to the health care team is the role of coordinator (discussed in Chapter 9). Care can easily become fragmented when patients are seen by numerous specialists—each interested in a different aspect of the patient—and in different settings. At best, patients complain that no single one person really knows them and can talk with them about what is going on and how it all may affect them in the future. At worst, the orders of different specialists may

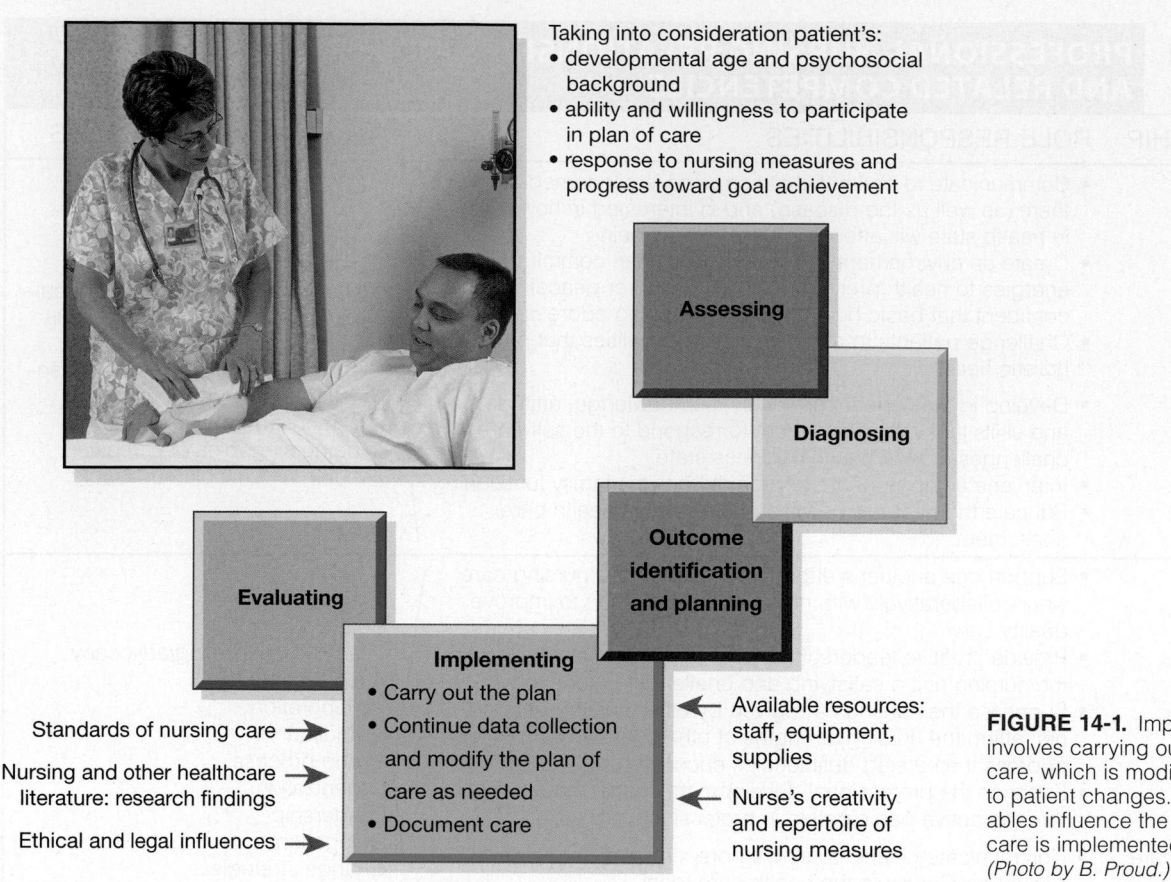

Taking into consideration patient's:
- developmental age and psychosocial background
- ability and willingness to participate in plan of care
- response to nursing measures and progress toward goal achievement

Assessing

Diagnosing

Outcome identification and planning

Evaluating

Implementing
- Carry out the plan
- Continue data collection and modify the plan of care as needed
- Document care

Standards of nursing care →

Nursing and other healthcare literature: research findings →

Ethical and legal influences →

← Available resources: staff, equipment, supplies

← Nurse's creativity and repertoire of nursing measures

FIGURE 14-1. Implementing involves carrying out the plan of care, which is modified in response to patient changes. Numerous variables influence the way the plan of care is implemented (see arrows). *(Photo by B. Proud.)*

conflict with one another and be counterproductive. Therefore, it is important for you as the nurse to make rounds with other health care professionals and to read the results of consultations that patients have had with specialists. You can then interpret the specialists' findings for patients and

family members, prepare patients to participate maximally in the plan of care before and after discharge, and serve as a liaison among the members of the health care team. Nurse case managers and navigators are specialists in the role of care coordinator.

EXAMPLES OF NURSING INTERVENTIONS AND NURSING OUTCOMES CLASSIFICATIONS (NIC/NOC)

HOME MAINTENANCE ASSISTANCE

Nursing Interventions	Nursing Outcomes
• Determine patient's home maintenance requirements. • Involve patient and family in deciding home maintenance requirements. • Suggest necessary structural alterations to make the home accessible. • Provide information on how to make the home environment safe and clean. • Advise for the alleviation of all offensive odors. • Suggest services for pest control, as needed. • Offer solutions to financial difficulties. • Order homemaker services, as appropriate. • Provide information on respite care, as needed.	• Family Social Climate • Family Functioning • Caregiver Emotional Health • Self-Care Status • Role Performance • Safe Home Environment • Self-Care: Instrumental Activities of Daily Living (IADL)

Adapted from Bulechek, G. M., Butcher, H. K., Dochterman, J., & Wagner, C. M. (Eds.). (2013). *Nursing interventions classification (NIC)* (6th ed.). St. Louis: Elsevier/Mosby, p. 218; and Moorhead, S., Johnson, M., Maas, M. L., & Swanson, E. (Eds.). (2013). *Nursing outcomes classification (NOC)* (5th ed.). St. Louis: Elsevier, p. 601.
    (A full listing of nursing activities for each nursing intervention and indicators for each nursing outcome can be found in these books.)

THINK back to Antoinette Browne, the toddler described at the beginning of the chapter. As a result of the child's delays, multiple disciplines would likely be involved in caring for her. The nurse would play a major role as coordinator for the child's care, ensuring communication among all team members. Additionally, the nurse would act as the liaison between the other members of the team to ensure that the child's grandmother understands the plan of care. ●

CLINICAL REASONING AND IMPLEMENTING

As you implement the plan of care, you are constantly engaging in clinical reasoning about what you are doing. Since patient conditions can change dramatically in minutes, you must reassess the patient for changes in status that might dictate a different set of interventions. You also want to be sure that research supports the interventions you have selected and be open to better ways of addressing patient problems and issues. In every clinical setting, we should hear nurses and other members of the team actively questioning whether there are better ways to achieve desired patient outcomes. Finally, you are always monitoring the patient's responses to your interventions so that you can modify the plan of care if needed. Remember Alfaro's Rule: "assess, re-assess, revise, record: *Assess* patients before performing nursing actions. *Re-assess* them to determine their responses after you perform nursing actions. *Revise* your approach as indicated. *Record* patient responses and any changes you made in the plan of care" (Alfaro-LeFevre, 2014, p, 161).

As a student, you should always ask if you are competent to implement the plan of care. If you doubt that your cognitive, interpersonal, or technical competencies are adequate to successfully implement the plan of care, it is your responsibility to ask for help. Getting help when you need it demonstrates your primary commitment to the patient. Expert nurses understand that learning is a lifelong practice and that we need one another to continue to master clinical skills.

IMPLEMENTING AND INTERPERSONAL COMPETENCE

Nursing is rarely a solo activity. Nurses are always working with patients, families, communities, and other nurses and health care professionals. While nurses need knowledge of best practice interventions and technical skills to implement the plan of care, it is also true that the nurse's interpersonal competence to a large degree determines how successfully the plan is implemented. If your patients and team do not trust you, it will be difficult to motivate everyone's best effort toward achieving goals. Alfaro-LeFevre (2014) writes that "your ability to communicate (listen, speak, and write effectively) with patients, families, unlicensed workers, and other professionals makes the difference between competent, efficient care and care that is sloppy, unprofessional, and prone to errors" (p. 161). You may want to talk with patients about what qualities and attributes they value in a nurse. You are sure to discover

that your respect, empathy, compassion, accountability, and trustworthiness are highly valued.

TYPES OF NURSING INTERVENTIONS

The Nursing Interventions Classification (NIC) project defines a **nursing intervention** as "any treatment based upon clinical judgment and knowledge that a nurse performs to enhance patient/client outcomes" (Bulechek, Butcher, & Dochterman, 2008, p. xxi). The NIC project further goes on to describe the types of interventions:

Nursing interventions include both direct and indirect care; those aimed at individuals, families and community; and those for nurse-initiated and other provider-initiated treatments.

A **direct care intervention** is a treatment performed through interaction with the patient(s). Direct care interventions include both physiological and psychosocial nursing actions and include both the 'laying of hands' actions and those that are more supportive and counseling in nature.

An **indirect care intervention** is a treatment performed away from the patient but on behalf of a patient or group of patients. Indirect care interventions include nursing actions aimed at management of the patient care environment and interdisciplinary collaboration. These actions support the effectiveness of direct care interventions.

A community (or public health) intervention is targeted to promote and preserve the health of populations. Community interventions emphasize the health promotion, health maintenance, and disease prevention of populations and include strategies to address the social and political climate in which the population resides. (Bulechek, Butcher, & Dochterman, 2008, p. xxi)

When you carry out the interventions identified in the plan of care, you are implementing the plan of care. When implementing the plan of care, you function independently and collaboratively. See Chapter 13 for descriptions of nurse-initiated, physician-initiated, and collaborative interventions.

 THE three types of nursing interventions can be illustrated by the example of Antoinette Browne, the toddler with gastrointestinal symptoms and delayed growth and development. If the physician orders a series of gastrointestinal studies, it is the nurse's responsibility to prepare the patient by executing the physician's order for cleansing the bowel. This nursing action is a physician-initiated intervention. When the nurse senses that the grandmother seems unusually fearful of the outcome of the studies, and explores the grandmother's fears and then follows up with appropriate teaching and counseling, the nurse is using nurse-initiated interventions. When a multidisciplinary team conference is held to discuss the patient's failure to progress, the nurse works collaboratively with the psychiatrist, gastroenterologist, social worker, and child development specialist to develop a comprehensive plan of care; this involves collaborative nursing interventions. ●

Carpenito-Moyet (2010, p. 42) describes how the major focus of intervention differs according to the type of nursing diagnoses or collaborative problem being addressed. For actual nursing diagnoses, interventions seek to:

- Reduce or eliminate contributing factors of the diagnosis
- Promote higher-level wellness
- Monitor and evaluate status

For risk nursing diagnoses, interventions seek to:

- Reduce or eliminate risk factors
- Prevent the problem
- Monitor and evaluate status

For possible nursing diagnoses, interventions seek to:

- Collect additional data to rule out or confirm the diagnosis

For collaborative problems, interventions seek to:

- Monitor for changes in status
- Manage changes in status with nurse-prescribed and physician-prescribed interventions
- Evaluate response

Protocols and standing orders expand the scope of nursing practice in certain clearly defined situations. **Protocols** are written plans that detail the nursing activities to be executed in specific situations. Although some protocols specify routine aspects of nursing care (e.g., protocols that describe nursing responsibilities when a patient is admitted to or discharged from the institution), other protocols include **standing orders** that empower the nurse to initiate actions that ordinarily require the order or supervision of a physician. Examples include admission protocols for obstetric and gynecology patients, protocols for bowel programs that allow the nurse to select and administer necessary bowel interventions, standard orders for narcotic overdoses that specify the agents the nurse is to administer to reverse respiratory depression in an emergency, and standard orders for pain management that enable the nurse to select the strength of the medication to be given within preset ranges.

IMPLEMENTING THE PLAN OF CARE

When carrying out the plan of care, nurses use specialized abilities to (1) determine the patient's new or continuing need for nursing assistance, (2) promote self-care, and (3) assist the patient to achieve valued health outcomes.

Reassessing the Patient and Reviewing the Plan of Care

A patient's condition can change dramatically in a matter of minutes. Therefore, it is critical to assess the patient carefully before initiating any nursing intervention to make sure that the plan of care is still responsive to the patient's needs and prioritized to the most pressing of those needs. Each nurse implementing the plan should:

- Be sure that each nursing intervention is supported by a sound scientific rationale, as demanded by an **evidence-based practice** (see Chapter 2)

- Be sure that each nursing intervention is consistent with professional standards of care and consistent with the protocols, policies, and procedures of the institution or agency
- Be sure that the nursing actions are safe for this particular patient and individualized to his or her preferences
- Clarify any questionable orders

Clarifying Prerequisite Nursing Competencies

To implement the plan of nursing care, nurses need blended intellectual, interpersonal, technical, and ethical/legal competencies as well as mastery of the Quality and Safety Education for Nurses Competencies that are described in Chapter 10 and illustrated in the Reflective Practice displays that introduce each chapter. Each nurse has a unique blend of these competencies and can act effectively to the extent that her or his abilities match the patient's need for nursing care.

 REMEMBER James McMahon, the critically ill patient in the intensive care unit. Although technological skills are key in this area, the nurse also needs to implement care that integrates intellectual, interpersonal, and ethical and legal competencies because of the patient's complex needs. The Quality and Safety Education for Nursing (QSEN) competencies also promote a good outcome: patient-centered care, teamwork and collaboration, evidence-based practice, quality improvement, safety, and informatics. ●

Always notify your nursing instructor or nurse mentor if you believe that you lack any competencies needed to safely implement the plan of care.

Organizing Resources

Successful implementation of the plan of care requires a high degree of organization and efficiency in today's hectic health care environments.

Patient and Patient Visitors

Make sure that patients are physically and psychologically prepared for what you are going to do. Give nursing interventions the best chance for success by ensuring that patients are not in too much pain to cooperate, understand what is being attempted and why they should cooperate, and are not distracted (e.g., by wanting to talk with visitors or watch TV). If visitors are in the room, check with patients to see if they want the visitor(s) to stay during the procedure. If a family caregiver needs to learn new caregiving skills, try to schedule your interventions at a time both appropriate for the patient and convenient for the family caregiver.

Equipment

Anticipate all the equipment you will need to successfully carry out the intervention, and arrange it so that it is easily accessible. Be sure to order sufficient supplies at the beginning of the shift for the care you expect to provide, and be thoughtful of the nurse who will follow you by leaving adequate supplies. Follow agency policy when ordering supplies to ensure proper charges. To avoid injury on the job, take the time to use proper assistive devices, such as lifts for heavy patients or transfer boards for patients with limited mobility.

Environment

Think through the proper environment for each intervention. Thoughtful, person-centered practice means paying special attention to respecting the patient's dignity, privacy, and safety needs. Remember routine measures as simple as closing a door or pulling drapes. These considerations are of special importance when patients or residents share rooms. For example, administering an enema can be embarrassing for the patient and unpleasant for the patient's roommate. With some planning, the intervention can be scheduled in a private bathroom or at a time when the roommate is absent.

Personnel

Identify whether you can carry out the planned intervention alone or if you need assistance. To avoid injury to both patients and professional caregivers, be sure that interventions are attempted by the right person or by a sufficient number of people. Because it is easy to underestimate the strength it takes to lift or support a large patient, it is always safer to err on the side of having too much help rather than not enough. Teams of student nurses can begin each rotation by asking, "Who thinks they might need help today?" The team can then plan to coordinate care so that help is available when needed.

Anticipating Unexpected Outcomes/Situations

When you learn about new nursing procedures and interventions, you often see a list of possible adverse effects. While everyone hopes never to encounter these complications, they do occur with some frequency. The skilled nurse knows what might happen if an intervention "goes wrong" and is prepared to deal with the new challenge. This may be as simple as accurately assessing how much support a patient may need to avoid a fall when ambulating for the first time after surgery or being prepared to respond to complaints of burning at a new IV site. For further consideration of unexpected outcomes and situations, refer to *Taylor's Clinical Nursing Skills* by Pamela Lynn and *Taylor's Video Guide to Clinical Nursing Skills* by Lippincott Williams & Wilkins.

Preventing Errors and Omissions

Alfaro-LeFevre (2014) counsels nurses to keep patients safe during implementation by preventing errors and omissions and building safety nets (Fig. 14-2). Starting with your first clinical experience, develop the habit of monitoring closely for error-prone situations. The goal is to "catch" possible

Potential Dangerous Situations

TECHNICAL ISSUES
Examples: alarms not working, broken equipment, computer issues

HUMAN ISSUES
Examples: poor attention, knowledge, or skill; fatigue; failure to follow policies and procedures

SYSTEM FAILURE ISSUES
Examples: poor staffing; poor training; room design that makes it difficult for nurses to maintain infection control; poorly designed workflow. Technical and human issues on left may also be the result of system failure issues.

NURSING SURVEILLANCE AND SAFETY NETS
Monitoring for the above dangerous situations; interrupting and correcting error-prone situations; building safety nets to catch mistakes before they happen.

☐ Early detection, prevention, and correction of errors.
☐ Reporting of organizational failure issues.

RESULTS
☐ **No adverse patient outcome** (or reduction in severity of adverse patient outcome)
☐ **Correction of system failure issues**—improved organization safety measures

FIGURE 14-2. How monitoring for dangerous situations promotes early correction of problems and keeps patients safe (© 2010 www.Alfaro TeachSmart.com. Used with permission.)

Box 14-2   IMPROVE SAFETY: URGE YOUR PATIENTS TO SPEAK UP®

The Joint Commission (TJC) encourages patients to become active, involved, and informed participants on the health care team. The following simple steps are based on research showing that patients who take part in decisions about their health care are more likely to have better outcomes.

- Speak up if you have questions or concerns, and if you don't understand, ask again. It's your body and you have a right to know.
- Pay attention to the care you are receiving. Make sure you're getting the right treatments and medications by the right health care professionals. Don't assume anything.

- Educate yourself about your diagnosis, the medical tests you are undergoing, and your treatment plan.
- Ask a trusted family member or friend to be your advocate.
- Know your medications and why you take them. Medication errors are the most common health care errors.
- Use a hospital, clinic, surgery center, or other type of health care organization that has undergone a rigorous on-site evaluation against established state-of-the-art quality and safety standards, such as that provided by TJC.
- Participate in all decisions about your treatment. You are the center of the health care team.

(Courtesy of The Joint Commission (TJC). Complete Speak Up® document available at: http://www.jointcommission.org/assets/1/6/Facts_Speak_Up.pdf

errors and omissions early. Remember that anyone can make a mistake and everyone needs surveillance.

 REMEMBER James McMahon, the critically ill patient in the intensive care unit. When the nurses caring for Mr. McMahon spent times relabeling and organizing his lines they were preventing a possible error. •

Henneman et al. (2010) recommends the following strategies to identify, interrupt, and correct errors:

- *Error identification strategies:* knowing the patient, knowing the "players," knowing the plan of care, surveillance, knowing policy/procedure, double-checking, using systematic processes, and questioning
- *Error interruption strategies:* offering help, clarifying, and verbally interrupting
- *Error correction strategies:* persevering, being physically present, reviewing or confirming the plan of care, offering options, referencing standards or experts, and involving another nurse or physician

Box 14-2 describes the Joint Commission's initiative to get patients more actively participating in their care by speaking up.

Promoting Self-Care: Teaching, Counseling, and Advocacy

Although most people can meet their basic human needs independently, illness and the stress of diagnostic and therapeutic measures may interfere with a person's usual practice of self-care. The nurse assesses patients' abilities to meet their human needs independently. Nurses can fail patients by doing too much for them and by encouraging negative, sick-role behaviors, such as inappropriate dependence. Conversely, there is a time and a place for the "tender loving care" that says to a patient "I know you may be able to do this for yourself, but just this once, how about if I do it and we'll talk!" Balancing the need to encourage a patient's best self-care effort with the effort to make each patient feel cared for is an important component of the art of nursing.

If patients and their families want to participate actively in seeking wellness, preventing disease and illness, recovering health, and learning to cope with altered functioning, they need effective self-care behaviors. Nurses sensitive to the importance of patients learning to direct and manage their own care use nurse–patient interactions for both planned and spontaneous teaching, counseling, and advocacy. These nursing roles are described in Chapter 6 and Chapter 21.

NURSING ADVOCACY IN ACTION

Patient Scenario

The emergency department is very rushed and overcrowded. Mrs. Penuela, who speaks little English, grabs you when you walk into the waiting area and begs someone to look at her husband, who is holding his head and moaning. When you finally get him in the unit to be assessed, he has a blood pressure of 240/150 mm Hg. He speaks a little more English than his wife, but is not fluent. However, you are able to learn that he stopped taking his blood pressure medication because he couldn't afford the prescription. He also lost his job and the family lost their house because of an inability to make mortgage payments. They are now living with her brother. Mr. Penuela is in the emergency department for several hours while intravenous medications are administered. You are shocked to discover that the only discharge orders

for Mr. Penuela are a prescription for the same medication he was on previously, which he couldn't afford. His doctor tells you that the ED isn't a charity or social service—"our job is to fix medical problems."

Implications for Nursing Advocacy

How will you respond if you are Mr. Penuela's nurse? Talk with your classmates and experienced nurses about the questions that follow.

- If you elect to advocate for the Penuelas, what practical steps can you take to ensure better health outcomes?
- What is it reasonable to expect of a student nurse, a graduate nurse, and an experienced nurse in this situation?
- What advocacy skills are needed to effectively respond to this challenge?

THROUGH THE EYES OF A FAMILY CAREGIVER

"The nurses never told me there'd be days like this."

I wasn't prepared for a roller coaster ride when my husband became ill. My husband was admitted to the hospital in an emergency condition, became confused when his electrolytes were off balance, went into cardiac arrest and had CPR, was placed on a ventilator, and was sedated because he was too apprehensive about the ventilator. I had reached the lowest point as I sat by his bedside for days, talking to him and wondering if he heard me.

My spirits soared the day they brought him out of his sleep state and he recognized me and was hungry for real food. The next day when I went to the hospital, I plummeted to the low point again when he was crumpled in bed like a confused rag doll with his hospital gown up to his chest and the sheet to his ankles. I started to cry, and the nurse came and put her arm around me. She said, "Don't think he's taken a turn for the worse. There will be good days and bad days as he recovers." No one had prepared me for that—and her arm around me and her words were so consoling.

When I brought him home after 6 weeks in the hospital, I was not prepared for his anger at being confined to the house (in a heat wave) and not being allowed to drive. His reasoning that he had to get a haircut because he hadn't had one in 2 months made sense to him. My saying that no one would care about the length of his hair did not soothe his anger.

He couldn't accept the fact that he was too weak to go up and down the steps more than once a day, so he insisted on going to the basement. Going down was simple; coming up wasn't. We forgot there was no railing (which he needed to haul himself up) on the last four steps. He solved the problem by sitting on the steps and lifting himself up a step at a time. Then he got to the floor at the top and couldn't stand up. I couldn't lift him. We were stuck. Again, I took a nose dive.

I thought I understood how difficult it would be for him to readjust. I knew he would be depressed and expected him to lean on me. But I was not prepared for his frustration to come out as anger at me. It would have been helpful to have someone prepare me. Or, it would be nice to have a nurse put her arm around me now when my roller coaster plummets.

—*Eleanor Faven, Philadelphia, Pennsylvania*

(See also the accompanying Nursing Advocacy in Action box.) Referring families to a community support group or other resources further enhances the self-care behaviors being developed. See Through the Eyes of a Family Caregiver for a description of one wife's experiences when her husband was discharged home.

Assisting Patients to Meet Health Outcomes

In this phase of the implementation process, the nursing team carries out the nursing orders detailed in the nursing plan of care. If the plan of care is well constructed, carrying out its orders is the nurse's most important task and should receive top priority. The nursing actions planned to promote patient goal/outcome achievement and the resolution of health problems should be carefully executed. Implementation guidelines are listed in Box 14-3.

Because understaffing is a problem in many practice settings, nurses must learn to use their time wisely and to maximize each patient encounter. A patient bath can be simply that, or it can be an opportunity to gather additional focused data, to communicate concern for what the patient is experiencing and offer support, and to teach and counsel as appropriate. How the nurse uses the 30 minutes for the bath determines how effective the nurse is in helping the patient to achieve the patient's goals/outcomes. See the accompanying Through the Eyes of a Student display (on page 312) for one student's account of an important bath.

Variables That Influence Outcome Achievement

When working with patients to achieve the outcomes specified in the plan of care, remember that nothing about the

plan of care is fixed. Some of the most important variables that influence how the plan of care is implemented follow.

PATIENT VARIABLES

Ideally, the patient is primary in determining how nursing interventions are implemented. Successful nurses modify their

BOX 14-3 | IMPLEMENTING GUIDELINES

- When implementing nursing care, remember to act in partnership with the patient/family.
- Before implementing any nursing action, reassess the patient to determine whether the action is still needed.
- Approach the patient competently. Know how to perform the nursing action, why the action is being performed, and potential adverse responses. Have all equipment and supplies ready.
- Approach the patient caringly. Explain the nursing action using language the patient understands. Communicate genuine concern for what the patient is experiencing.
- Modify nursing interventions according to the patient's (1) developmental and psychosocial background, (2) ability and willingness to participate in the plan of care, and (3) responses to previous nursing measures and progress toward goal/outcome achievement.
- Check to make sure that the nursing interventions selected are consistent with standards of care and within legal and ethical guides to practice.
- Always question that the nursing intervention selected is the best of all possible alternatives. Consult colleagues and the nursing and related literature to see if other approaches might be more successful. Evaluate the effectiveness of the intervention selected, noting any factors that positively or negatively influenced the outcome.
- Develop a repertoire of skilled nursing interventions. The more options one can choose from, the greater the likelihood of success.

THROUGH THE EYES OF A STUDENT

One of my first patients was a woman with a history of Alzheimer disease. When I was assigned this patient, I knew that I was not going to have a good day. I had been introduced to her the week before, when I had orientation. She was sitting in a geriatric chair in the hallway, where she sang at the top of her lungs and threw tissues on the floor. Occasionally, she would curse at a person passing by.

I took a deep breath and entered her room. At her bedside, I introduced myself. With a few choice words, she told me to get out of her room. I tried to ignore her response and prepared her breakfast tray. She proceeded to throw her scrambled eggs around the room. After I took the tray away from her and finished cleaning up the mess, it was time for preconference. At preconference, my instructor told me that we were going to "tub" my patient. I had visions of a grand fiasco in the tub room, and I dreaded giving her the bath.

My instructor and I took her to the tub room by wheelchair. Once we convinced her to get in the tub, she did nothing but yell that it was cold. We started the water and she yelled even louder. I knew everyone could hear her in the hallway as she cursed and yelled, but as the bath proceeded,

she quieted down and stopped fighting me. We completed the bath and wheeled her back down the hall to her room. I bundled her up in blankets and put her in the gerry chair in the hallway. She was so relaxed from the bath that she let me brush her hair and put it in a ponytail. While I was brushing her hair, she fell asleep. I did my chart until her lunch arrived. When I set her up for her lunch and told her I would be leaving, she thanked me, and it made my day. All the struggling I went through all day with her and she thanked me. When I went home, I felt really good about helping her. During all my worrying about the day being a fiasco and the embarrassment of having a patient yell at me, I had lost sight of the patient herself and what she needed me to do for her. By her thanking me at the end of the day, I realized that when my clinical instructor forced me to do something for my patient that the regular staff of the hospital wouldn't do, I was meeting her basic needs, and my patient recognized that.

—*Jeanene C. Smith*
Delaware County Community College, Media, Pennsylvania

nursing actions according to the patient's (1) changing ability and willingness to participate in the plan of care and (2) previous responses to nursing interventions and progress toward achieving goals/outcomes. Other important variables are the patient's developmental stage and psychosocial background.

Developmental Stage

Addressing the developmental needs of a patient involves identifying the patient's developmental stage, as well as the developmental tasks related to this stage and their relationship to nursing care. Be careful not to let stereotypes about developmental stages and tasks influence patient care. To implement a comprehensive and holistic plan of care, nurses must find creative ways to meet developmental needs. This is of greatest importance when patients are separated from their families and home environments for long periods.

THINK back to Antoinette Browne, the toddler with physical and developmental delays. The nurse would creatively adapt interventions to meet the needs of this toddler. •

Psychosocial Background

The same is true of the psychosocial needs of patients. When choosing nursing interventions, the nurse should consider and respect the patient's socioeconomic background and culture. Confronted with a malnourished patient on a limited income who rents a single room in a boarding home, a nurse cannot simply teach the importance of including more protein in the diet. To be effective, the nurse must explore the realistic issue of whether the patient can afford and obtain foods rich in protein. Moreover, the nurse needs to assess whether the patient values this intervention and is willing to make the necessary changes.

NURSE VARIABLES

Nurse variables that influence the implementation of the plan of care include levels of expertise, creativity (ability to match patient needs with specific nursing strategies), willingness to provide care, and available time. Focused Critical Thinking Guide 14-1 illustrates the importance of a nurse's ability to think critically about intervention strategies.

RESOURCES

The most elaborately designed plan of care cannot be fully effective without adequate staff, equipment, and supplies. These resources are all important determinants of patient care. The patient's financial resources and the adequacy of community-based resources also influence the plan of care.

CURRENT STANDARDS OF CARE

All nursing actions for implementing the plan of care must be consistent with standards of practice. See Chapter 15 for a discussion of these standards. All nurses are responsible for learning the standards that dictate practice in their specialty. Failure to practice according to these standards may result in a charge of negligence.

RESEARCH FINDINGS

Nurses concerned about improving the quality of nursing care use research findings to enhance their nursing practice. Reading professional nursing journals and attending continuing education workshops and conferences are excellent ways to learn about new nursing strategies that have proved effective. Evidence-based practice resources include:

- Agency for Healthcare Research and Quality (AHRQ) (http://ahrq.gov)
- Reviews on effective quality improvement and implementation (http://epoc.cochrane.org)

FOCUSED CRITICAL THINKING GUIDE 14-1

INTERVENTION STRATEGIES

One of the nurses on the oncology unit where you have been working for 6 months since graduation wants to develop a "humor room" where patients, their families, and staff can "take a break" from the serious business of illness. Designed to lift the spirits, amuse, distract, and thus speed the healing process, humor rooms are gaining popularity as new therapeutic tools. Funny books, comic movies on a large-screen TV, games and puzzles—and ideally, even clowns, magicians, musicians, and stand-up comedians—are being envisaged. Several nurses have vocally expressed their lack of support for the project and think the idea is "stupid" at best, and potentially a great waste of money, time, and energy that could be devoted to "tried and true" methods of healing. You have been asked to support the project and must decide how to respond.

1. Identify goal of thinking

Clarify your thinking about humor as a therapeutic measure so that you can decide whether to support this project.

2. Assess adequacy of knowledge

Pertinent circumstances: The nurse who wants to develop the humor room is more popular with patients than she is with her colleagues. Her nurse friends are quick to point out that while it's true that she is "a bit flaky" and unorthodox, she is an efficient nurse who is well loved by her patients and their families. The hospital is in the midst of cutting expenses and has laid off both professional and nonprofessional employees.

Prerequisite knowledge: To decide how you should respond in this situation, you need to research the healing benefits of humor. Are there clinical studies demonstrating its effectiveness as a therapeutic measure? If studies point to humor's effectiveness, you will need to determine (1) what priority it should have among other treatment modalities and (2) the feasibility of creating a humor room in the current climate of cutting expenses. Is there a creative way to finance this venture?

Room for error: Since life and death do not hinge on how you elect to respond to this plea for support, there is a relatively wide margin for error. Because personal energy

and finances are limited, however, you do not want to involve your unit in a futile project.

Time constraints: There is no rush for an immediate decision on your part, which gives you adequate time to develop the knowledge base you need to make an informed decision.

3. Address potential problems

The most serious obstacle to critical thinking in this situation would be the lack of an open mind and refusal to weigh the merits of a new treatment modality. Complicating factors include divided loyalties among the nurses and the tendency to support or refuse support for the project on the basis of whether one likes the nurse advocating the project, rather than on the merits of the project. Finally, the lowered morale caused by layoffs may squash all creativity and willingness to "dream new dreams."

4. Consult helpful resources

Your first challenge will be to learn more about humor as a healing measure. Ideally, you may be able to consult a local expert and invite the expert to meet with the staff. Alternately, you can research the literature, looking for clinical studies and reports of the first-person experiences of others.

5. Critical judgment/decision

After a search of the literature convinced you and some of the other nurses of the clinical benefits of humor, you decide to explore the feasibility of developing a humor room. Your options are to "play it safe" and not rock the boat during a difficult period in the hospital by trying something new, or to become an advocate for the project and commit your energies to making it happen. You decide that a creative project may be exactly what the staff needs to rediscover the "joy of nursing" and begin to explore means to fund the project. You plan to "start small" and to reassess the project every 6 months. Since your research educated you about the potential benefits *and harms* humor can create, you decide that your first objective must be to educate the staff.

- Toolkit: Implementation of clinical practice guidelines (http://www.rnao.org)
- Intervention mapping step 5: Adoption and implementation. (http://interventionmapping.com)
- AACN Practice alerts (http://www.aacn.org/WD/Practice/Content/practicealerts.content?menu=Practice&lastmenu=)

Research in Nursing boxes throughout this text demonstrate the difference nursing research can make in improving patient outcomes. Proponents of nursing implementation science are beginning to address the challenges of imple-

menting research findings into practice (van Achterberg, Schoonhoven, & Grol, 2008).

ETHICAL AND LEGAL GUIDES TO PRACTICE

To practice good nursing, you need to be knowledgeable about the laws and regulations that affect health care and the ethical dimensions of clinical practice. Without this understanding, a sincere motivation to benefit the patient and a conscientious attempt to implement nursing orders will not be sufficient. Each nurse is responsible for becoming sensitive to the ethical and legal dimensions of practice, and moral and legal accountability are inherent in the practice of professional nursing.

 LOOK back on the scenario presented at the beginning of the chapter for Estelle Morrissey. Ethical and legal guidelines are crucial in determining how the nurse intervenes. Additionally, the nurse needs to evaluate the ethical and legal ramifications of one's actions in light of the patient's request to die. •

Chapters 6 and 7 discuss the ethical and legal dimensions of practice. Hospital risk managers and ethics committees are increasingly available as institutional resources for nurses.

CONTINUING DATA COLLECTION AND RISK MANAGEMENT

An important nursing intervention is ongoing data collection. In every patient encounter, it is important to be sensitive to both subtle and dramatic changes in the patient's condition. Skilled nurses monitor the patient's responses to planned interventions to determine if the plan of care is working. These assessment findings are used to update and revise the plan of care. Sensitivity to how the patient is responding to nursing interventions and to the patient's progress toward outcome achievement allows the nurse to modify nursing interventions appropriately.

Another vital nursing intervention is ongoing risk management. While monitoring the patient's responses to the plan of care, nurses are also alert to the development of new problems that may result in the identification of new diagnoses or collaborative problems. As nurses get to know patients and recognize clusters of significant data, they can identify problems for which the patient is at risk and intervene appropriately to promote health and to prevent disease.

DOCUMENTING NURSING CARE

Remembering the legal truth, "It wasn't done if it wasn't documented," each nurse carefully documents all nursing interventions. See Chapter 16 for guidelines for written documentation, and see the plans of nursing care at the end of each clinical chapter for samples of documented nursing interventions.

WHEN A PATIENT DOES NOT COOPERATE WITH THE PLAN OF CARE

When a patient does not follow the plan of care despite your best efforts, it is time to reassess strategy. The first objective is to identify why the patient is not following the therapy. One possibility is that the plan of care may not be right for this patient. In this event, what is needed is not a change in the patient but rather a change in the plan of care. If you determine, however, that the plan of care is adequate, you must identify and remedy the factors contributing to the patient's noncompliance. Common reasons for noncompliance include:

• Lack of family support
• Lack of understanding about the benefits of compliance

• Low value attached to outcomes or related interventions
• Adverse physical or emotional effects of treatment (such as pain and fatigue)
• Inability to afford treatment
• Limited access to treatment

DELEGATING NURSING CARE

Because of the pressure to reduce health care costs and the increasing demand for nursing services in the midst of a critical shortage of professional nurses, many employers of nurses have increased their use of unlicensed assistive personnel (UAP) or "nurse extenders." **Unlicensed assistive personnel** are people who are trained to function in an assistive role to the licensed registered nurse (RN) in the provision of patient activities as delegated by and under the supervision of the registered professional nurse. **Delegation** is the transfer of responsibility for the performance of an activity to another person while retaining accountability for the outcome. In some cases, the new mix of professional and nonprofessional staff is threatening patient safety. Never has it been more important for nurses to critically identify which nursing interventions require professional nurses and which can be safely delegated. This can be especially challenging for new nurses. See Box 14-4 for Boucher's list of "Essentials of Effective Delegation." Chapter 22 includes additional discussion of delegation, including the American Nurses Association's new *Principles for Delegation*.

BOX 14-4 | **ESSENTIALS OF EFFECTIVE DELEGATION**

The following will help you with the essential responsibilities and techniques of delegating care tasks:

• Know your state and institutional policies on delegation (the policy and procedure manual is available on each unit; for state policies, contact the state nurse association).
• Be clear on the difference between nursing process and nursing tasks.
• Know the training and background of the unlicensed assistive personnel (UAP). (Administration must have a standard and process to validate the UAP's preparation.)
• Know the patient's needs and what he or she is at risk for.
• Know what clinical cues the UAP should be alert for and why.
• Assess which tasks can be safely delegated.
• Have the UAP repeat your instructions to be sure you have communicated them clearly.
• Make frequent walking rounds to assess patients.
• When talking with the patient, members of the patient's family, or UAPs, listen for cues that indicate changes in the patient's condition.
• Take frequent mini-reports from the UAP.
• Evaluate the UAP's performance and the patient's response.

Reprinted with permission from Boucher, M. A. (1998). Delegation alert! *American Journal of Nursing, 98*(2), 26–32.

REVIEW the patient scenario for James McMahon, the critically ill patient described at the beginning of the chapter and in "Reflective Practice: Challenge to Technical Skills." The nurse's ability to delegate effectively is important for providing safe, efficient care. •

Delegation and the Student Nurse

Student nurses may find themselves the recipient of delegated care that they cannot safely perform. Whenever you are asked by a staff nurse to perform an intervention for which you lack training, consult with your instructor to see if you can safely perform it with supervision. Never attempt to perform interventions beyond your capacity without supervision, even if instructed to do so by a staff nurse. Students who work as nursing assistants while enrolled in professional programs are especially likely to be asked to perform interventions beyond their mastery. You may be able to turn these requests into learning opportunities. For example, you might say, "I've never practiced that procedure but I'd love the opportunity to observe one of the experienced nurses do this."

GUIDE FOR STUDENTS
Organizing Care

Student nurses organizing their nursing care in advance for a particular clinical day can use the guidelines for student clinical responsibilities in Box 14-5 to help identify nursing measures for which they will be responsible. After this, working out a time schedule may provide clear direction for the clinical day and ensure that the patient's needs are met. Some faculty require students to prepare clinical logs, which are also an excellent guide to organization. Figure 14-3 (on page 316) illustrates guidelines for a clinical log.

Nursing Oneself

It is difficult for nurses to be sincerely attentive to patient needs if their own human needs are not met. Make sure you come to clinical well rested and having had a nutritious meal. Because no one is perfectly healthy or "whole" all the time, nurses preparing for professional practice should spend time getting to know themselves. Activities that promote psychological health when practiced regularly include self-awareness, communication, time management, preparation for crisis and loss, developing and maintaining support systems, and practicing self-care in all areas. The characteristics of emotional health include self-esteem, self-knowledge, satisfying interpersonal relationships, environmental mastery, stress management, a positive body image, a sense of humor, and the ability to experience pleasure.

Nurses who want to be competent practitioners learn early to nurse themselves and other nurses before attempting to nurse patients. Good personal health enables nurses not only to practice more efficiently, but also to be a health model for patients and their families. Nurses can help patients to imitate good health behaviors and eventually integrate them into their daily life through the process of identification. Use the Promoting Health displays in each clinical chapter (Units VI and VII) for yourself as well as for your patients.

REFLECTIVE PRACTICE LEADING TO PERSONAL LEARNING

Remember that the object of reflective practice is to look at an experience, understand it, and learn from it. As you begin to develop your expertise in implementing the plan of care, reflect on your experiences—successes and failures—in order to improve your practice. How can you do it better next time? What did you learn today that can help you tomorrow? Begin your reflection by paying close attention to the following during the implementing phase of the nursing process:

- Did your commitment to engage your patients and families and to collaborate with your fellow students, instructor, and other members of the team as you implemented the plan of care result in successful partnerships?
- Did your preparation result in your feeling confident about the nursing interventions you performed? Did your competence and confidence inspire the patient's and team's trust?
- Did your patients make real progress toward realizing expected outcomes as a result of your interventions?

Box 14-5 | ORGANIZING STUDENT CLINICAL RESPONSIBILITIES

To organize clinical responsibilities, check:
1. Patient profile
2. Name by which patient wishes to be addressed
3. Patient's chief complaint and reason for admission
4. Patient's current health status: Note any physical or emotional changes indicating the need to modify the plan of care.
5. Routine assistance patient needs to meet basic human needs
6. Priorities for nursing care:
   - Priorities identified by the patient as "most important." The nurse might state, "I'll be your nurse until 3 PM, and I'm interested in learning what you would most like to accomplish today."

- Prioritized nursing diagnoses, patient outcomes, and related nursing interventions
- Medical orders that need to be implemented
- Interdependent or collaborative nursing responsibilities
7. Special "events" of the day that may require special observation of the patient, teaching, preparation, or aftercare:
   - Diagnostic tests
   - Consultations with specialists
   - New therapies (physical therapy, medications, surgery, radiotherapy, and the like)
8. Special safety or risk management needs
9. Special teaching, counseling, or advocacy needs
10. Special needs of the family

Student		Date		

Element/Criteria	Points possible	Score
Epidemiology of Primary Diagnosis • Incidence • Prevalence • Risk Factors • Case-Fatality Rate	10	
Pathophysiology • presented in understandable patient education terms • brief explanation is congruent with actual physiologic processes of disease	10	
Tests/Procedures • brief explanation of why indicated • analysis of findings accurate • pre-post patient education developmentally appropriate • pre-post nursing interventions appropriate	10	
Medications • provide a list of all medications that the patient is receiving • brief explanation of the indication in terms that a patient would understand	10	
Physiologic/Psychosocial Assessment Summary • assessment findings accurate • includes physiologic, psychosocial and spiritual findings (as identified)	10	
Nursing Diagnosis • 5 appropriate nursing diagnoses identified • diagnoses presented in appropriate format (alt...r/t...aeb...) • priority nursing diagnosis selected is appropriate	10	
Nursing Process: Interventions/Rationale/Evaluation. (Determined by clinical faculty weekly) • Measurable goals established/Short-term goal supports achievement of long-term goal but are not the same goal • Interventions are clear and concise and include frequency of action • 3 appropriate interventions provided for each LT and ST goal • Rationales clearly support intervention in plan of care and are referenced • Evaluation statements for short-term goal are clear, and concise (LTG not evaluated) • Unmet goals include action plan	20	
Self-identified strengths and opportunities for self improvement • congruent with strengths identified by instructor	2	
National Patient Safety Goals: Indentify one of the National Patient Safety Goals and how you addressed it during your shift (use a different one for each log).	4	
Cultural Considerations appropriately incorporated in your care with an example	2	
Values: Describe an example of how your nursing care emulates the principles of Social Justice, Human Flourishing, OR Commitment to the Common Good that we stand for in the Department of Nursing at Georgetown University	4	
Professional Roles • self-identities roles utilized in providing care	2	
Reflective Practice: Thought question of the week • Question posed by student upon reflecting on the day of care. May be based on patient care or condition, nursing, staff issues, etc.	2	
Format: typed, spelling, grammar, APA for references	4	
Note: Papers are due within 48 hours. Please submit to your clinical faculty member via e-mail or Blackboard as per their preference. Rules for grading apply as with all NHS papers.	100	

FIGURE 14-3. Evaluation tool for clinical logs. (Used with permission. Georgetown University School of Nursing and Health Studies.)

• Did you need to modify the plan of care as a result of ongoing assessments? Did you think of better interventions to produce the expected outcomes?

• Did your vigilance and awareness of potential error and omissions prevent error?

Perhaps the most important question to reflect on is: Are your patients and families better for having had *you* share in the critical responsibility of partnering with them to implement the plan of care?

DEVELOPING CLINICAL REASONING

1. Team up with another student and take turns role-playing a nurse visiting a homebound older man who needs his vital signs and nutritional status assessed. Discuss with each other the truth or falsity of this claim: "Who the nurse is, is as important as, and sometimes more important than, what the nurse does."

2. Receive the same clinical assignment as another student and independently outline your care priorities, specifying what you plan to accomplish during each of your clinical hours. Talk with the other student about the differences in what you both hope to accomplish and how you would do this. Try to imagine what these differences would mean to the patient.

3. You are the only RN on a 50-bed wing in a long-term care facility. You have one LPN working with you and two personal care assistants. Each of the 50 residents requires assistance with activities of daily living, all take at least some medications, and most require monitoring for multiple chronic (and sometimes acute) illnesses. How will you decide which interventions to delegate? When the home is short-staffed, you are sometimes the only RN covering two 50-bed units.

4. Describe how you would probably respond, and how you would like to respond (if these are different), to hearing another nurse in the shift report say that one of the patients you are assigned to was a real "PIB" ("pain in the butt") all day and "just impossible" to care for. Reflect on the importance of the language we use to report on a patient to one another.

PRACTICING FOR NCLEX

1. A school nurse notices that a female adolescent student is losing weight and decides to perform a focused assessment of her nutritional status to determine if she has an eating disorder. How should the nurse proceed?
   a. Perform the focused assessment. This is an independent nurse-initiated intervention.
   b. Request an order from Jill's physician since this is a physician-initiated intervention.
   c. Request an order from Jill's physician since this is a collaborative intervention.
   d. Request an order from the nutritionist since this is a collaborative intervention.

2. A nurse is using the implementation step of the nursing process to provide care for patients in a busy hospital setting. Which nursing actions best represent this step? Select all that apply.
   a. The nurse carefully removes the bandages from a burn victim's arm.
   b. The nurse assesses a patient to check nutritional status.
   c. The nurse formulates a nursing diagnosis for a patient with epilepsy.
   d. The nurse turns a patient in bed every 2 hours to prevent pressure ulcers.
   e. The nurse checks a patient's insurance coverage at the initial interview.
   f. The nurse checks for community resources for a patient with dementia.

3. Nurses use the Nursing Interventions Classification Taxonomy structure as a resource when planning nursing care for patients. What information would be found in this structure?
   a. Case studies illustrating a complete set of activities that a nurse performs to carry out nursing interventions
   b. Nursing interventions, each with a label, a definition, and a set of activities that a nurse performs to carry it out, with a short list of background readings
   c. A complete list of nursing diagnoses, outcomes, and related nursing activities for each nursing intervention
   d. A complete list of reimbursable charges for each nursing intervention

4. A new RN is being oriented to a nursing unit that is currently understaffed and is told that the UAPs have been trained to obtain the initial nursing assessment. What is the best response of the RN?
   a. Allow the UAPs to do the admission assessment and report the findings to the RN.
   b. Do his or her own admission assessments but don't interfere with the practice if other professional RNs seem comfortable with the practice.
   c. Tell the charge nurse that he or she chooses not to delegate the admission assessment until further clarification is received from administration.
   d. Contact his or her labor representative and complain about this practice.

5. A nurse performs nurse-initiated nursing actions when caring for patients in a skilled nursing facility. Which are examples of these types of interventions? Select all that apply.
   a. A nurse administers 500 mg of ciprofloxacin to a patient with pneumonia.
   b. A nurse consults with a psychiatrist for a patient who abuses pain killers.
   c. A nurse checks the skin of bedridden patients for skin breakdown.
   d. A nurse orders a kosher meal for an orthodox Jewish patient.
   e. A nurse records the I&O of a patient as prescribed by his physician.
   f. A nurse prepares a patient for minor surgery according to facility protocol.

6. A nurse is about to perform pin site care for a patient who has a halo traction device installed. What is the first nursing action that should be taken prior to performing this care?
   a. Administer pain medication.
   b. Reassess the patient.
   c. Prepare the equipment.
   d. Explain the procedure to the patient.

7. A student nurse is on a clinical rotation at a busy hospital unit. The RN in charge tells the student to change a surgical

dressing on a patient while she takes care of other patients. The student has not changed dressings before and does not feel confident with the procedure. What would be the student's best response?

a. Tell the RN that he or she lacks the technical competencies to change the dressing independently.

b. Assemble the equipment for the procedure and follow the steps in the procedure manual.

c. Ask another student nurse to work collaboratively with him or her to change the dressing.

d. Report the RN to his or her instructor for delegating a task that should not be assigned to student nurses.

8. A nurse develops a detailed plan of care for a 16-year-old female who is a new single mother of a premature infant. The plan includes collaborative care measures and home health care visits. When presented with the plan, the patient states, "We will be fine on our own. I don't need any more care." What would be the nurse's best response?

a. "You know your personal situation better than I do, so I will respect your wishes."

b. "If you don't accept these services, your baby's health will suffer."

c. "Let's take a look at the plan again and see if we can adjust it to fit your needs."

d. "I'm going to assign your case to a social worker who can explain the services better."

9. An RN working on a busy hospital unit delegates patient care to unlicensed assistive personnel (UAPs). Which patient care could the nurse most likely delegate to a UAP safely? Select all that apply.

a. Performing the initial patient assessments

b. Making patient beds

c. Giving patients bed baths

d. Administering patient medications

e. Ambulating patients

f. Assisting patients with meals

10. A student nurse is organizing clinical responsibilities for an 84-year-old female patient who is diabetic and is being treated for foot ulcers. The patient tells the student, "I need to have my hair washed before I can do anything else today; I'm ashamed of the way I look." The patient's needs include diagnostic testing, dressing changes, meal planning and counseling, and assistance with hygiene. How would the nurse best prioritize this patient's care?

a. Explain to the patient that there is not enough time to wash her hair today because of her busy schedule.

b. Schedule the testing and meal planning first and complete hygiene as time permits.

c. Perform the dressing changes first, schedule the testing and counseling, and complete hygiene last.

d. Arrange to wash the patient's hair first, perform hygiene, and schedule diagnostic testing and counseling.

ANSWERS WITH RATIONALES

1. *a.* Performing a focused assessment is an independent nurse-initiated intervention, thus the nurse does not need an order from the physician or the nutritionist.

2. *a, d, f.* During the implementing step of the nursing process, nursing actions planned in the previous step are carried out.

The purpose of implementation is to assist the patient in achieving valued health outcomes: promote health, prevent disease and illness, restore health, and facilitate coping with altered functioning. Assessing a patient for nutritional status or insurance coverage occurs in the assessment step, and formulating nursing diagnoses occurs in the diagnosing step.

3. *b.* The Nursing Interventions Classification Taxonomy lists nursing interventions, each with a label, a definition, a set of activities that a nurse performs to carry it out, and a short list of background readings. It does not contain case studies, diagnoses, or charges.

4. *c.* The nurse should not delegate this nursing admission assessment because only nurses can perform this intervention. The nurse should seek clarification for this policy from the nursing administration.

5. *c, d, f.* Nurse-initiated interventions, or independent nursing actions, involve carrying out nurse-prescribed interventions resulting from their assessment of patient needs written on the nursing plan of care, as well as any other actions that nurses initiate without the direction or supervision of another health care professional. Protocols and standard orders empower the nurse to initiate actions that ordinarily require the order or supervision of a physician. Consulting with a psychiatrist is a collaborative intervention.

6. *b.* Before implementing any nursing action, the nurse should reassess the patient to determine whether the action is still needed. Then the nurse may collect the equipment, explain the procedure, and if necessary administer pain medications.

7. *a.* Student nurses should notify their nursing instructor or nurse mentor if they believe they lack any competencies needed to safely implement the plan of care. It is within the realm of a student nurse to change a dressing if he or she is technically prepared to do so.

8. *c.* When a patient does not follow the plan of care despite your best efforts, it is time to reassess strategy. The first objective is to identify why the patient is not following the therapy. If the nurse determines, however, that the plan of care is adequate, the nurse must identify and remedy the factors contributing to the patient's noncompliance.

9. *b, c, e, f.* Performing the initial patient assessment and administering medications are the responsibility of the registered nurse. In most cases, patient hygiene, bed-making, ambulating patients, and helping to feed patients can be delegated to a UAP.

10. *d.* As long as time constraints permit, the most important priorities when scheduling nursing care are priorities identified by the patient as being most important. In this case, washing the patient's hair and assisting with hygiene puts the patient first and sets the tone for an effective nurse–patient partnership.

TAYLOR SUITE RESOURCES

Explore these additional resources to enhance learning for this chapter:

- NCLEX-Style Questions and other resources on thePoint, http://thePoint.lww.com/Taylor8e
- *Study Guide for Fundamentals of Nursing, 8th edition*
- Adaptive Learning | Powered by prepU, http://thepoint.lww.com/prepu

Bibliography

Alfaro, R. (2014). *Applying nursing process. The foundation for clinical reasoning* (8th ed.). Philadelphia: Wolters Kluwer Health/Lippincott Williams & Wilkins.

Alfaro-LeFevre, R. (2010). *Applying nursing process: A tool for critical thinking* (7th ed.). Philadelphia: Wolters Kluwer Health/Lippincott Williams & Wilkins.

Alfaro-LeFevre, R. (2013). *Critical thinking, clinical reasoning, and clinical judgment: A practical approach* (5th ed.). St. Louis: Elsevier.

American Nurses Association (ANA). (2007). *ANA's principles of environmental health for nursing practice with implementation strategies.* Washington, DC: Author.

American Nurses Association (ANA). (2010). *Nursing's social policy statement* (2010 ed.). Silver Spring, MD: Author.

American Nurses Association (ANA). (2010). *Standards of clinical nursing practice* (2nd ed.). Silver Spring, MD: Author.

American Nurses Association (ANA). (2012). *Principles for Delegation.* Silver Spring, MD: Author.

Benner, P. (1984). *From novice to expert: Excellence and power in clinical nursing practice.* Menlo Park, CA: Addison-Wesley.

Benner, P., & Wrubel, J. (1989). *The primacy of caring: Stress and coping in health and illness.* Menlo Park, CA: Addison-Wesley.

Bulechek, G. M., Butcher, H. K., & Dochterman, J. C. (Eds.). (2008). *Nursing Interventions Classification (NIC)* (5th ed.). St. Louis, MO. Elsevier/Mosby.

Bulechek, G. M., Butcher, H. K., Dochterman, J. C., & Wagner, C. M. (Eds.). (2013). *Nursing interventions classification (NIC)* (6th ed.). St. Louis: Elsevier.

Boucher, M. A. (1998). Delegation alert! *American Journal of Nursing, 98*(2), 26–32.

Carpenito, L. J. (2013). *Nursing diagnosis: Application to clinical practice* (14th ed.). Philadelphia: Wolters Kluwer Health/Lippincott Williams & Wilkins.

Carpenito-Moyet, L. J. (2010). *Nursing care plans and documentation: Nursing diagnoses and collaborative problems* (5th ed.). Philadelphia: Wolters Kluwer Health/Lippincott Williams & Wilkins.

Dall, T. M., Chen, Y. J., Seifert, R. F., Maddox, T. J., & Hogan, T. F. (2009). The economic value of professional nursing. *Medical Care, 47*(1), 1–8.

Eisenhauer, L. A. (1994). A typology of nursing therapeutics. *Image—The Journal of Nursing Scholarship, 26*(4), 261–264.

Fowler, M. D. M. (Ed.). (2010 reissue). *Guide to the Code of Ethics for Nurses.* Silver Spring, MD: American Nurses Association.

Henneman, E., Gaawlinski, A, Blank, F., Henneman, P., Jordan, D., & McKenzie, J. (2010). Strategies to identify, interrupt, and correct medical errors: Theoretical framework. *American Journal of Critical Care, 19*(6), 500–509.

Holleman, G., Eliens, A., Van Vliet, M., & van Achterberg, T. (2006). Promotion of evidence-based practice by professional nursing associations: Literature review. *Journal of Advanced Nursing, 53,* 702–709.

Iowa Intervention Project. (1993). The NIC taxonomy structure. *Image—The Journal of Nursing Scholarship, 25*(3), 187–192.

Iowa Intervention Project. (1997). Nursing interventions classification (NIC): An overview. In M. J. Rantz & P. LeMone (Eds.), *Classification of nursing diagnoses: Proceedings of the Twelfth Conference, North American Nursing Diagnosis* (pp. 32–39). Glendale, CA: CINAHL Information Systems.

Joint Commission on Accreditation of Healthcare Organizations. (2013). Standards. Available at http://www.jointcommission.org/

Maxfield, D., Grenny, J., Patterson, K., McMillan, R., & Switzler, A. (2005). Silence kills: The seven crucial conversations in healthcare. Available at http://www.aacn.org/WD/Practice/Docs/PublicPolicy/SilenceKillsExecSum.pdf

McCauley, K. M. (2005). A message from the American Association of Critical Care Nurses. *American Journal of Critical Care, 14*(3), 186–197.

McCloskey Dochterman, J. C., & Bulechek, G. M. (Eds.). (1992). *Nursing interventions classification (NIC).* St. Louis: Mosby–Year Book.

McCloskey Dochterman, J. C., & Bulechek, G. M. (1995). Validating and coding of the NIC taxonomy structure. *Image—The Journal of Nursing Scholarship, 27*(1), 43–49.

McCloskey Dochterman, J. C., & Bulechek, G. M. (Eds.). (1996). *Nursing interventions classification (NIC)* (2nd ed.). St. Louis: Mosby–Year Book.

McCloskey Dochterman, J. C., & Bulechek, G. M. (Eds.). (2000). *Nursing interventions classification (NIC)* (3rd ed.). St. Louis: Mosby–Year Book.

McCloskey Dochterman, J., & Bulechek, G. M. (Eds.). (2004). *Nursing interventions classification (NIC)* (4th ed.). St. Louis: Mosby.

Moorhead, S., Johnson, M., Maas, M. L., & Swanson, E. (Eds.). (2008). *Nursing outcomes classification (NOC)* (4th ed.). St. Louis: Elsevier/Mosby.

Moorhead, S., Johnson, M., Maas, M. L., & Swanson, E. (Eds.). (2013). *Nursing outcomes classification (NOC)* (5th ed.). St. Louis, MO: Elsevier.

NANDA International (NANDA-I). (2012). *Nursing Diagnoses: Definitions & classification, 2012–2014.* Oxford, UK: Wiley-Blackwell.

Titler, M. G., Kleiber, C., Steelman, V., Rakel, B., Budreau, G., Everett, L. Q., et al. (2001). The Iowa Model of evidence-based practice to promote quality care. *Critical Care Nursing Clinics of North America, 13,* 497–509.

van Achterberg, T., Schoonhoven, L., & Grol, R. (2008). Nursing implementation science: How evidence-based nursing required evidence-based implementation. *Journal of Nursing Scholarship, 40*(4), 302–310.

15

Evaluating

TYLER JAMESON

Tyler, a term neonate born 30 hours ago, has yet to pass stool. Follow-up assessment reveals that he does not have a patent anus, a finding that was not detected in the neonate's initial assessment.

MIOSHI OTSUKI

Mioshi, an older adult woman with a history of heart failure being treated with diuretics, is receiving home care. Questioned about her prescribed drug-therapy regimen, the patient states, "I take this one labeled 'furosemide' every day in the morning along with this other one labeled 'Lasix.'"

NICHOLAS SOROS

Nicholas is a 68-year-old patient newly diagnosed with diabetes. His initial assessment revealed that he was about 50 pounds overweight due to poor diet and lack of exercise. A plan was developed to help Mr. Soros better manage his diabetes through planned weight reduction and regular exercise. At a follow-up visit, assessment reveals a weight gain of 5 pounds. He stated, "I'm too old to worry about diet and exercise. You can control my diabetes with medication, right?"

LEARNING OBJECTIVES

After completing the chapter, you will be able to accomplish the following:

1. Describe evaluation, its purpose, and its relation to the other steps in the nursing process.

2. Evaluate the patient's achievement of four types of outcomes specified in the plan of care.

3. Manipulate factors that contribute to success or failure in outcome achievement.

4. Use the patient's response to the plan of care to modify the plan as needed.

5. Explain the relation between quality-assurance/quality-improvement programs and excellence in health care.

6. Describe the AACN standards for establishing and sustaining healthy work environments and describe the seven crucial conversations in health care.

7. Value self-evaluation as a critical element in developing the ability to deliver quality, person-centered nursing care.

KEY TERMS

concurrent evaluation

criteria

evaluating

evaluative statement

evidence-based practice

National Database of Nursing Quality Indicators (NDNQI)

nursing-sensitive quality indicators

outcome evaluation

peer review

performance improvement

process evaluation

quality-assurance program

quality improvement (QI)

retrospective evaluation

standards

structure evaluation

In the fifth step of the nursing process, **evaluating**, the nurse and patient together measure how well the patient has achieved the outcomes specified in the plan of care. When evaluating patient outcome achievement, the nurse identifies factors that contribute to the patient's ability to achieve expected outcomes and, when necessary, modifies the plan of care (Fig. 15-1 on page 323). The purpose of evaluation is to allow the patient's achievement of expected outcomes to direct future nurse–patient interactions. Based on the patient's responses to the plan of care, the nurse decides to:

• Terminate the plan of care when each expected outcome is achieved

• Modify the plan of care if there are difficulties achieving the outcomes

• Continue the plan of care if more time is needed to achieve the outcomes

When evaluation points to the need to modify nursing care, the nurse reviews each preceding step of the nursing process (assessing, diagnosing, planning, and implementing). Successful evaluation helps ensure that valued patient outcomes are attained. It also enhances the public's image of nursing and promotes continued selection and funding of nursing services in the competitive health care market.

UNIQUE FOCUS OF NURSING EVALUATION

As members of the health care team, nurses are involved in many types of evaluation. Nurses measure patient outcome achievement, how effectively nurses help targeted groups of patients to achieve their specific outcomes, the competence of individual nurses, and the degree to which external factors—such as different types of health care services, specialized equipment or procedures, or socioeconomic factors—influence health and wellness. *The patient, however, is always the nurse's primary concern.* A nurse may perform a nursing procedure competently, creatively, and with care, but if this nursing intervention does not help the patient reach desired outcomes, it is not fully meaningful. Either directly or indirectly, the aim of all nursing evaluation is quality nursing care that aids patient outcome achievement. Therefore, the most important act of evaluation performed by nurses is evaluating outcome achievement with the patient (see the accompanying Reflective Practice box for an example on page 322).

The Institute of Medicine's Committee on Quality of Health Care in America is educating the public about what patients can reasonably expect from their health care (Box 15-1 on page 323). Even beginning nurses can use these guidelines to evaluate the care they are providing.

CLINICAL REASONING AND EVALUATING

The five classic elements of evaluation are (1) identifying evaluative criteria and standards (what you are looking for when you evaluate, e.g., expected patient outcomes), (2) collecting data to determine whether these criteria and standards are met, (3) interpreting and summarizing findings, (4) documenting your judgment, and (5) terminating, continuing, or modifying the plan. Each element requires the nurse to use clinical reasoning about how best to evaluate the patient's progress toward valued health outcomes. In the nursing process, evaluative criteria are the patient outcomes developed during the planning step. Because these reflect desired changes in patient status and because nursing actions are directed toward these outcomes, they are the core of evaluation in thoughtful, person-centered nursing practice. Determining whether these outcomes have been or are being met and then identifying the appropriate nursing response are the functions of evaluation.

REFLECTIVE PRACTICE

CHALLENGE TO INTERPERSONAL SKILLS: CULTIVATING QSEN COMPETENCIES

I first met Mr. Nicholas Soros, a 68-year-old patient newly diagnosed with diabetes, in the clinic. He was about 50 pounds overweight, and his health history revealed the need for major dietary changes and an exercise program. The interdisciplinary team devised a plan to help Mr. Soros better manage his diabetes through planned weight reduction and regular exercise, for which I did much of the initial teaching. Unfortunately, when Mr. Soros returned for his next check-up, he had gained 5 additional pounds and reported being "too old" to worry about diet and exercise. "You can control my diabetes with medication, right?" When I reported this to the nurse practitioner, he told me that Mr. Soros knows what to do and now it is his responsibility. I wasn't perfectly comfortable with this response and thought that Mr. Soros needed more than someone wagging a finger in his face.

Thinking Outside the Box: Alternate Courses of Action

- Remind Mr. Soros of what he needs to do and tell him that responsibility for this is his!
- After I make sure that he does indeed know what to do, spend time making sure that he values his health sufficiently to try these new behaviors.
- Make sure that Mr. Soros trusts us sufficiently to value working with us to achieve his health goals.

Evaluating a Good Outcome: How Do I Define Success?

- Mr. Soros achieves his target weight and is faithful to a program of regular exercise.
- Mr. Soros feels that his independence and ability to determine his own life plan are respected, at the same time feeling that we care about his health status.
- I learn more about developing a trusting nurse–patient relationship, exploring the relationship's role in helping patients to achieve valued health outcomes.

Personal Learning: Here's to the Future!

I learned something about myself and an important distinction between teaching and counseling. Clearly, just teaching Mr. Soros about diet and exercise wasn't sufficient. Mr. Soros was in no way going to change his lifestyle until he valued his health enough to make needed changes, including understanding why these changes were important. I also learned how important nurse–patient relationships are. When Mr. Soros came for his third visit, he asked the nurse who greeted him where I was, telling her "I want to see that nurse who cared about me!"—positive reinforcement for the relationship's importance.

Megan Kyle, Georgetown University

REFLECTION ON QUALITY AND SAFETY COMPETENCIES

How do you think you would respond in a similar situation? Why? What does this tell you about yourself and about the adequacy of your competencies for professional practice? Do you agree with the criteria that the nursing student used to evaluate a successful outcome? Describe the type of teaching plan that the nursing student may have used at the initial teaching session. How might that teaching plan have changed based on the patient's response at the next visit? Would the outcomes identified initially need to be revised based on any changes in the teaching plan? Explain why or why not. What *knowledge, skills,* and *attitudes* do you need to develop to continuously improve the quality and safety of care for patients like Mr. Soros?

Patient-Centered Care: How can you establish a successful partnership with a patient who lacks the motivation to make critical lifestyle changes?

Teamwork and Collaboration/Quality Improvement: When colleagues aren't willing to go that "extra mile" to work with vulnerable patients, how can you intervene successfully? What needs to change to improve quality in this setting? What does quality care for Mr. Soros "look like"?

Safety/Evidence-Based Practice: What does the evidence point to as "best practice" for Mr. Soros? What safety needs does he have and how can you meet them?

Informatics: Can you identify the essential information that must be available in Mr. Soros's record to support safe patient care and coordination of care? Are there any apps that might be useful in coaching Mr. Soros? Can you think of other ways to respond to or approach the situation? What else might the nursing student have done to ensure a successful outcome?

THINK back to Nicholas Soros, the 68-year-old man diagnosed with diabetes who needs to lose weight and to exercise. The outcomes identified initially most likely focused on weight loss and adherence to an exercise program. Teaching at this initial visit also focused on ways to achieve these outcomes. However, the patient's statements and weight gain on his next clinic visit would lead the nurse to the conclusion that the outcomes identified were not being achieved. Therefore, some changes in the patient's plan of care are necessary. ●

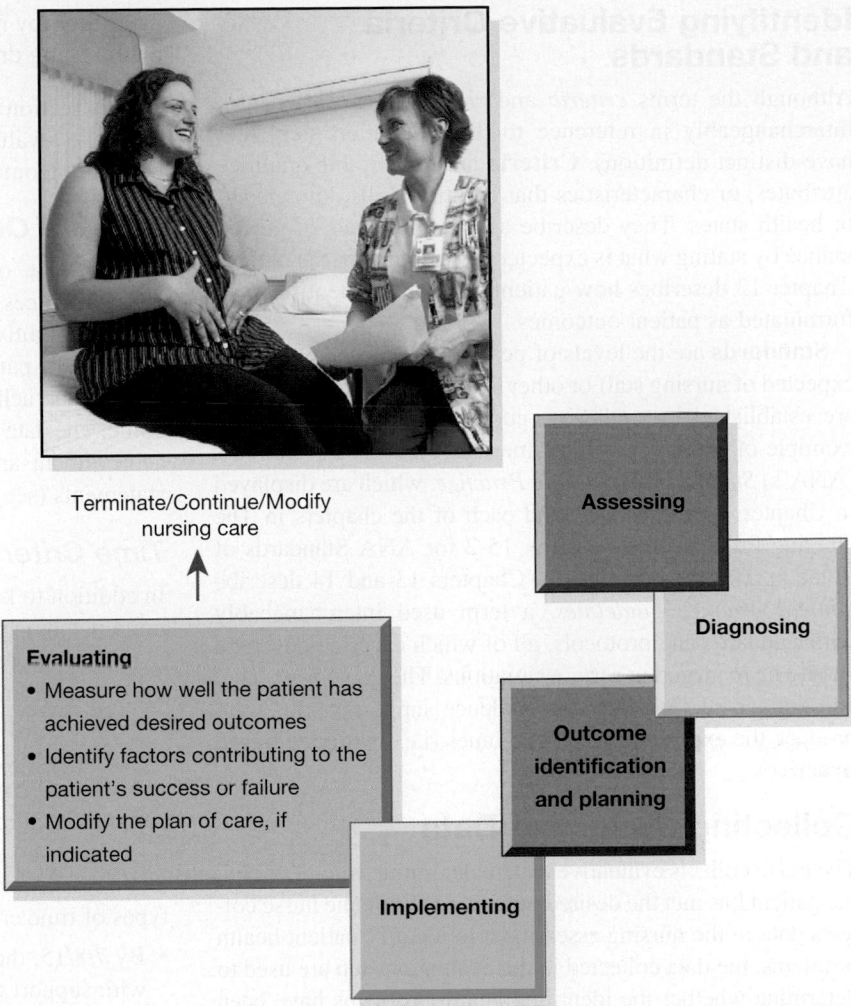

Terminate/Continue/Modify
nursing care

Evaluating
- Measure how well the patient has achieved desired outcomes
- Identify factors contributing to the patient's success or failure
- Modify the plan of care, if indicated

Assessing

Diagnosing

Outcome identification and planning

Implementing

FIGURE 15-1. Evaluating. The nurse and patient together measure how well the patient has achieved the outcomes specified in the plan of care. Factors that contribute to the patient's success or failure are identified, and the plan of care is modified if necessary. Patient responses to the plan of care determine whether nursing care is to be continued as is, modified, or terminated. *(Photo by Joe Mitchell.)*

BOX 15-1 WHAT PATIENTS SHOULD EXPECT FROM THEIR HEALTH CARE

1. **Beyond patient visits:** You will have the care you need when you need it . . . *whenever* you need it. You will find help in many forms, not just in face-to-face visits. You will find help on the Internet, on the telephone, from many sources, by many routes, in the form you want it.
2. **Individualization:** You will be known and respected as an individual. Your choices and preferences will be sought and honored. The usual system of care will meet most of your needs. When your needs are special, the care will adapt to meet you on your own terms.
3. **Control:** The care system will take control only if and when you freely give permission.
4. **Information:** You can know what you wish to know, when you wish to know it. Your medical record is yours to keep, to read, and to understand. The rule is: "Nothing about you without you."
5. **Science:** You will have care based on the best available scientific knowledge. The system promises you excellence as its standard. Your care will not vary illogically from doctor to doctor or from place to place. The sys-

tem will promise you all the care that can help you, and will help you avoid care that cannot help you.
6. **Safety:** Errors in care will not harm you. You will be safe in the care system.
7. **Transparency:** Your care will be confidential, but the care system will not keep secrets from you. You can know whatever you wish to know about the care that affects you and your loved ones.
8. **Anticipation:** Your care will anticipate your needs and will help you find the help you need. You will experience proactive help, not just reactions, to help you restore and maintain your health.
9. **Value:** Your care will not waste your time or money. You will benefit from constant innovations, which will increase the value of care to you.
10. **Cooperation:** Those who provide care will cooperate and coordinate their work fully with each other and with you. The walls between professions and institutions will crumble, so that your experiences will become seamless. You will never feel lost.

Identifying Evaluative Criteria and Standards

Although the terms *criteria* and *standards* are often used interchangeably in reference to the evaluation step, they have distinct definitions. **Criteria** are measurable qualities, attributes, or characteristics that identify skills, knowledge, or health states. They describe acceptable levels of performance by stating what is expected of the nurse or the patient. Chapter 13 describes how patient criteria are identified and formulated as patient outcomes.

Standards are the levels of performance accepted by and expected of nursing staff or other health team members. They are established by authority, custom, or consent. A good example of standards is the American Nurses Association's (ANA's) *Standards of Nursing Practice,* which are displayed in Chapter 1, this chapter, and each of the chapters in The Nursing Process unit. See Box 15-2 for ANA Standards of Practice related to evaluation. Chapters 13 and 14 describe *clinical practice guidelines,* a term used interchangeably with standards and protocols, all of which describe how care should be managed in certain situations. The goal is to design and deliver nursing care that evidence supports as likely to produce the expected patient outcomes (i.e., **evidence-based practice**).

Collecting Evaluative Data

The nurse collects evaluative data to determine whether or not the patient has met the desired outcomes. While the nurse collects data in the nursing assessment to identify patient health problems, the data collected in the evaluation step are used to determine whether the identified health problems have been or are being resolved through outcome achievement.

 CONSIDER Mrs. Otsuki, the older adult who is inadvertently taking double the dose of prescribed diuretic. This initial assessment indicates a need for teaching. Thus, when evaluating outcome achievement for this patient, the nurse would determine whether the patient demonstrates understanding of her drug therapy regimen and is no longer taking two doses of the same drug. ●

This section discusses (1) the different types of data collected to evaluate the achievement of different types of patient outcomes and (2) time criteria for data collection.

Types of Outcomes

Nurses write outcomes during the planning phase of the nursing process. Chapter 13 describes four types of outcomes: cognitive, psychomotor, affective, and physiologic. The type of patient data collected to support the evaluation of outcome achievement depends on the nature of the outcome. The data collected to determine the degree of outcome achievement are recorded in the corresponding evaluative statements (see Box 15-3).

Time Criteria

In addition to knowing what type of data to collect to determine outcome achievement, the nurse needs to know when to collect the data. When the patient outcomes were developed, a time frame was established for determining whether the specified changes have been achieved. At the designated time, the nurse, in collaboration with the patient, the family, and other members of the nursing team, evaluates the patient's attainment of the outcome. If outcomes are developed in observable and measurable terms, the task of collecting data for evaluation is clear-cut. Examples of three types of time criteria follow:

- By 7/8/15, the patient will walk the length of the hallway with support of a walker.
- Beginning 7/8/15, the patient will demonstrate a weight loss of 3 lb per month until target weight (135 lb) is achieved (6/8/15, weight: 151 lb).
- Before discharge, parents will correctly demonstrate chest physiotherapy procedures for patient.

Nurses should evaluate patient outcome achievement as early as possible. Celebrating outcome attainment with the patient usually helps encourage the patient and leads to

---

BOX 15-2 **AMERICAN NURSES ASSOCIATION (ANA) STANDARDS OF PRACTICE: STANDARD 6, EVALUATION**

The registered nurse evaluates progress toward attainment of outcomes.

Competencies

The registered nurse:

Conducts a systematic, ongoing, criterion-based evaluation of the outcomes in relation to the structures and processes prescribed by the plan of care and the indicated timeline.

Collaborates with the healthcare consumer and others involved in the care or situation in the evaluative process.

Evaluates, in partnership with the healthcare consumer, the effectiveness of the planned strategies in relation to the healthcare consumer's responses and the attainment of the expected outcomes.

Uses ongoing assessment data to revise the diagnoses, outcomes, the plan, and the implementation as needed.

Disseminates the results to the healthcare consumer, family and others involved, in accordance with the state and federal laws and regulations.

Participates in assessing and assuring the responsible and appropriate use of interventions in order to minimize unwarranted or unwanted treatment and healthcare consumer suffering.

Documents the results of the evaluation.

Used with permission from American Nurses Association (ANA). (2010). *Scope and standards of practice.* Silver Spring, MD: Author.

BOX 15-3 EVALUATING FOUR TYPES OF OUTCOMES IN THE PLAN OF NURSING CARE

Nursing Diagnosis

High Risk for Altered Parenting related to no previous experience in childrearing (fear)

Assessment Data

Subjective: "My husband and I are both afraid we won't know what to do when we get the baby home."

Objective: Both parents are single children, report no childrearing experience; healthy newborn son delivered 2/4/15; first born

Strengths

VIB (very important baby): parents are both 38; history of infertility with one miscarriage; strong motivation to learn and use good parenting skills; strong support network

Expected Outcomes	Nursing Interventions	Evaluative Statement (Actual Outcomes)
Psychomotor Outcomes Before discharge, parents will demonstrate confidence in: • Holding baby • Diapering, dressing baby • Bathing baby • Feeding baby	Assess both parents' knowledge of childrearing practices; identify and reinforce motivation to learn; correct any misinformation. Develop and implement at a time convenient for both parents a teaching plan to include: • The primary nurse role-modeling techniques for comfortably and safely holding, talking to, and dressing baby • Parents independently viewing videos on: baby care, baby bath, and breastfeeding, followed by one-on-one discussion • Class for new parents: nurse to demonstrate baby bath and discuss general principles of care • Primary nurse observing mother and infant during initial feeding sessions and offering teaching and support as necessary	2/6/15 Outcome partially met. Both parents have correctly demonstrated safe techniques for holding, dressing, and bathing baby. Mother is still concerned baby is not getting enough milk. *Revision:* Continue to spend time with mother and infant during feeding—provide positive reinforcement. *F. Morales, RN*
Cognitive Outcomes By 2/6/15, parents will report appropriate action to be taken if questions or problems arise after discharge: • Name and number of primary nurse • Name and number of pediatrician • La Leche League contact and number	Answer parents' questions and address related concerns. Assess parents' knowledge of infant problems frequently encountered by new parents. Inform parents of available community resources and describe appropriate action to take if questions or problems arise.	2/6/15 Outcome met. Parents discussed some infant problems related to feeding, elimination, and illness and reported appropriate community resource to contact. *F. Morales, RN*
Affective Outcome Before discharge, parents will verbalize decreased anxiety in regard to caring for son.	Assess parents' level of anxiety and potential negative effects on childrearing. Discuss this with parents. Explore adequacy of parents' coping strategies—increased knowledge, practice in supportive environment, community resources. Counsel as necessary. Compliment parents on new parenting skills. Allow for ventilation of anxiety or specific fears. Respond with teaching or emotional support, as necessary.	2/6/15 Outcome partially met. Except for concern about breastfeeding, *both* parents expressed feeling comfortable and eager to care for their son at home. *F. Morales, RN*
Physiologic Outcomes At 1-month postpartal telephone interview, 3/4/15 (by parents' report), the baby will demonstrate adequate: • Weight gain (birth weight, 7 lb 6 oz) • Sleep–wakefulness patterns • Comfort level indicating adequate parenting	Use a 1-month postdelivery telephone interview to assess the adequacy of parenting skills. With positive report of growth and development, compliment (reinforce) the parents. With negative report, teach or counsel and refer as appropriate.	3/4/15 Outcome met. Parents' report of baby's weight gain and behavior indicates good parenting skills. *F. Morales, RN*

further outcome achievement. When failure to meet designated outcomes is detected early, the plan of care can be modified to remedy the failure.

 THINK back to Nicholas Soros, the 68-year-old patient with diabetes. By recognizing the lack of outcome achievement on the next visit, the nurse can gather additional data to revise the plan of care. For example, perhaps Mr. Soros did not completely understand the nurse's teaching. Or, he may have had difficulty accepting his diagnosis, thereby interfering with his ability to comply with the plan, ultimately leading to weight gain instead of a weight loss. •

The most common mistake nurses make when evaluating in acute care settings is waiting until the day the patient is to be discharged before evaluating outcome achievement. At that point, it is too late to revise the plan of care.

Interpreting and Summarizing Findings

Before the nurse can make a judgment about the patient's achievement of outcomes, it is necessary to study and interpret the data collected. Just as clusters of data are interpreted before the nurse identifies and validates a nursing diagnosis, so too do evaluative data need to be interpreted. For example, a patient who is expected to walk the length of the hallway with support of a walker asks to be taken back to her room because she feels weak. The nurse must gather more data to determine if this is a one-time incident linked to medications or a temporary metabolic imbalance, or whether it signals a consistent inability to achieve this behavior. Interpreting evaluative data requires clinical reasoning and is a skill that must be practiced.

When interpreting and summarizing findings, consider factors that influence outcome achievement. Numerous patient, nurse, and health care system variables contribute positively or negatively to patient outcome achievement. Identifying these variables allows the nurse to reinforce positive factors by drawing on them in the future, as well as to deal with other variables that are creating problems. The more sensitive and responsive nurses are to these variables, the more rewarding their practices will be.

Examples of positive factors include a patient's strong motivation to learn new health behaviors, a nurse who comes to work well rested and with a new care idea learned from a nursing journal, and a health care institution or agency that offers incentives for quality nursing and has an optimal nurse-to-patient ratio.

A nurse who understands what factors are helpful to the patient who is trying to reach desired outcomes can often manipulate these factors. For example, if a patient is learning to ambulate independently after hip surgery and you notice that he seems to make his best effort when his wife is present, mention this to her and plan to ambulate the patient at least once a day when she is present. Conversely, if a patient seems more fearful when his wife is present, note in the plan

of care that ambulation is best attempted when the patient's wife is not on the unit. Ideally, this fear would be explored with the patient before discharge so that he can continue to make progress when he is discharged home with his wife.

Table 15-1 presents variables that commonly negatively influence patient outcome achievement. Tentative nursing approaches are suggested. Nurses need to think critically about the effects of these variables and respond creatively to them.

Documenting Your Judgment

After the data have been collected and interpreted to determine patient outcome achievement, the nurse makes and documents a judgment summarizing the findings. This is termed the **evaluative statement**. The two-part evaluative statement includes a decision about how well the outcome was met, along with patient data or behaviors that support this decision. Outcomes may have been met, partially met, or not met:

- 1/21/15—Outcome met. Patient reports 1 week of no tobacco use. C. Taylor, RN
- 1/21/15—Outcome partially met. Patient reports decreasing tobacco use from one pack per day to 4 to 6 cigarettes per day. Continue to implement and monitor plan. C. Taylor, RN
- 1/21/15—Outcome not met. Patient reports no change in tobacco use. Revision: Re-explore patient's commitment to try tobacco-use control strategies and adequacy of personal support systems to eliminate tobacco use. C. Taylor, RN

The nurse signs and dates the evaluative statement (see Box 15-3) or follows the documentation guidelines specified in the institution's computerized documentation systems.

Modifying the Plan of Care

When evaluation reveals that the patient has made little or no progress toward outcome achievement, the nurse needs to re-evaluate each preceding step of the nursing process to try to identify the contributing factors causing problems with the plan of care. New assessment data might need to be collected, diagnoses may be added or altered, outcomes might need to be modified or rewritten, nursing orders may be changed, or evaluation may be targeted more frequently.

 REMEMBER Tyler Jameson, the neonate who has not passed any stool after 30 hours. The initial outcome may have stated that the neonate would pass stool within 18 to 24 hours after birth. However, this outcome was developed based on data that was inaccurate. Therefore, the nurse, learning of the new data, would revise the outcome to correlate with the neonate's condition, dependent on the treatment to correct the anomaly. •

Review the checklist in Box 10-9 on page 220 for help in evaluating your use of the nursing process. Table 15-2 (on pages 328–329) suggests appropriate nursing responses to common problems encountered during evaluation of each step in the nursing process.

Table 15-1 PATIENT, NURSE, AND HEALTH CARE SYSTEM VARIABLES THAT MAY DETRACT FROM QUALITY NURSING CARE

VARIABLES	POSSIBLE SOLUTION
Patient Variables Patient who is physically and cognitively capable of self-care gives up—refuses to cooperate with therapeutic regimen or thwarts the regimen	Identify one nurse who is able to develop a trusting relationship with the patient and determine the reason underlying the observed behavior: • No longer finds meaning and purpose in life • Overwhelming sense of powerlessness • Previous history of being "hurt," "exploited," "cheated" by the health care system • Inability to accept illness and related lifestyle changes Counsel appropriately. Use a team conference to develop a consistent plan of nursing care.
Patient who quietly accepts whatever is done or not done for him or her; seldom communicates needs or dissatisfaction	Note on the plan of care the need to assess this patient thoroughly because the patient will probably not advocate for self. Educate the patient to become a more assertive health care consumer.
Nurse Variables Nurse who sincerely desires to give 150% all the time and who becomes quickly frustrated when observing substandard care; may feel alienated from other staff; excellent candidate for burnout	Learn to give quality care during designated work period; leave on time; avoid the temptation to do the work of others; leave work concerns at work. After establishing a reputation for delivering quality nursing care, seek creative solutions for nursing problems (strategies to increase nursing resources, motivation, morale) and try them—hopefully with a support network. View concerns as challenges rather than overwhelming obstacles. Develop a realistic sense of how much nursing care and of what quality can be delivered with existing resources. If resources do not permit quality care, explore change strategies within the institution. If administration is not supportive, explore other practice settings.
Nurse with overwhelming outside concerns: • Preparation for marriage, childbirth, divorce • Illness (self or family members) • Role conflict (familial roles, school, work, and the like) • New apartment, house	During periods of peak demand, may need to accept less than optimal performance at work. If this becomes the norm rather than the exception, carefully evaluate priorities. May need to cut work hours rather than "cheat" patients.
Nurse who is bored	After reflection, write down *personal* objectives related to work. Explore avenues within work setting for professional growth and development: initiate changes in nursing unit to improve patient care and to stimulate peer development; join institutional committees; participate actively in staff development programs; develop patient and family support groups. Look for new position that offers new challenges within or outside the institution. Join professional organizations and participate actively. Evaluate educational goals and explore possibilities—continuing education programs and degree work.
Health Care System Variables Inadequate staffing	Develop and use a patient classification system that incorporates an identification of the kind and amount of nursing services required. Record staffing patterns and relate to needs for nursing care and patient outcomes. Clearly demonstrate and document that adequate staffing makes a difference. Present these data to nursing administration with the request for additional staff. If necessary, use professional bargaining unit.
Nursing administration has sold out nursing; insensitivity to nursing demands within the institution	It may be impossible to practice quality, progressive nursing in this environment. If there seems to be no hope for change after appropriate channels have been explored, look for a new practice setting. Evaluate the new setting on the basis of what experience has taught you.

After identifying the factors contributing to the outcomes not being achieved, use the evaluative statement to suggest necessary revisions in the plan of care: (1) delete or modify the nursing diagnosis, (2) make the outcome statement more realistic, (3) increase the complexity of the outcome statement, (4) adjust time criteria in outcome statement, or (5) change the nursing intervention. Increasing the complexity of an outcome after it has been achieved facilitates optimal function. For example, the initial outcome for a patient with the diagnosis "Impaired Physical Mobility"

Table 15-2 COMMON PROBLEMS NOTED DURING EVALUATION OF THE NURSING PROCESS

PROBLEM	NURSING RESPONSE
Assessing	
1. Inaccurate database → inaccurate nursing diagnoses and a distorted plan of care	1. a. Identify the patient or nurse variables responsible for inaccuracy. b. Revise the recorded database.
2. Database does not reflect changes in patient condition.	2. Review with the *entire* nursing staff the importance of making assessment a priority in every patient interaction as well as the recording of the new data obtained.

3. Database is superficial:
• Fails to communicate uniqueness of patient
• Lacks sufficient detail on major problems or developments
	3. a. Rethink the critical relation between an adequate database and quality care.
	   b. Develop interviewing and physical assessment skills.
	   c. Begin to identify the key data that need to be collected for specific nursing diagnosis and medical diagnosis and to assess patient response to therapeutic regimen (use of a nursing diagnosis handbook may be helpful).

Diagnosing	
1. General sense that nursing diagnoses are "common sense" and, therefore, do not need to be put in writing → failure to address patient's real problems	1. Carefully develop and record priority nursing diagnoses for several patients and fairly evaluate whether this makes a difference in terms of the continuity of quality care.
2. General sense that nurses are too busy doing treatments, "passing meds," and doing paperwork to develop nursing diagnoses carefully → independent dimension of nursing remains underdeveloped	2. Examine practice and see whether *independent* nursing has a place; what percentage of every day is devoted to independent nursing functions? If this percentage is nonexistent or small, there understandably may be *no felt need* for nursing diagnoses—but a desperate need to revise practice priorities.

3. Nursing diagnoses are too vague to be helpful → routinized patient care	3. a. Revise the problem statement to describe more accurately what is *unhealthy* about the patient (the behavior that needs to be changed).
	   b. Revise the etiology to more accurately identify what is making the problem a problem—this should be a guide to nursing intervention.
	   c. Check NANDA-I lists.

4. Nursing diagnoses are not up to date → no one uses the plan of care	4. Have a process for periodically reviewing the plan of care to delete nursing diagnoses when problems have been resolved and to add a new diagnosis as needed.
Planning	
1. The plan of care contains only the standard knowledge most nurses would know without a written plan.	1. Make use of standardized (computerized) plans as a basis for care planning. Devote nursing energies to *individualizing* this plan.
2. The long-term goal is vague, standard; fails to make clear the discharge goal for this patient.	2. Practice writing specific long-term goals that clarify for all nurses the aim toward which all nursing care is directed (e.g., patient returns home ambulatory with walker, right hip incision healing, able to manage activities of daily living with minimal assistance from spouse).
3. The nursing outcomes, even if met, do not necessarily guarantee a resolution of the patient problem.	3. When writing goals, it often helps to develop outcomes related to etiologic factors. Because the stated etiology may be incomplete or inaccurate, at least *one outcome* must be written so that if it is achieved, the problem in the nursing diagnosis is resolved.
4. The outcomes are incorrectly developed; progress toward goal achievement is difficult to evaluate.	4. After writing outcomes, check them against the following criteria: • Subject is the patient or some part of the patient. • The patient behavior is stated in observable, measurable terms. • Criteria of acceptable performance are specified. • Time criteria are included in notes.
5. Nursing orders are superficial → patient receives routinized care.	5. Review nursing orders to ensure that they indicate the *specific* nursing strategies or interventions most likely to result in successful outcome achievement *for this patient* (e.g., particular comfort measures that are successful adjuncts to analgesic administration for a particular patient). In specifying the "who, what, when, where, how, and how much" of nursing interventions, be sure to list the type of equipment and supplies needed in various treatments. As new patient data are obtained, update nursing orders. Delete inappropriate or unnecessary orders.

Table 15-2 **COMMON PROBLEMS NOTED DURING EVALUATION OF THE NURSING PROCESS** *continued*

PROBLEM	NURSING RESPONSE
6. The initial plan of care fails to be updated → plan of care will not be consulted by nurses—if used, it will be to patient's detriment.	6. If personal accountability for updating plan fails, develop a process on the nursing unit to ensure care plan review and revision.
7. The plan of care addresses the immediate needs of the patient but fails to anticipate discharge needs → patient returns home unable to manage self-care activities.	7. Work hard at developing the ability to project yourself into the patient's home after discharge. Learn to anticipate problems and concerns and prepare the patient and family for these. Use all discharge resources in the institution. Learn from patients what their needs were after previous discharge.
Implementing	
1. Nurses are not aware of patient priorities and the plan of care; lack of continuity; inefficient use of nursing resources → patient fails to achieve goals/outcomes.	1. a. Use shift report to update staff on status of priority nursing diagnosis and concomitant nursing care. b. Review plan of care and nursing notes before beginning care.
2. Nursing care becomes routine and mechanized → patient never has the sense of being personally known by nurses.	2. Explore creative strategies to make quality nursing care on this particular unit a *challenge* rather than a *burden;* use ongoing education, problem-solving strategies by the nursing team, gaming, and other incentives.
3. Documentation is inadequate → because there is no complete written record of nursing care, *legally* this care was never provided.	3. a. Develop the philosophy that quality nursing care *deserves* to be documented. Review legal reasons for careful documentation. b. Become familiar with the flow sheets and note format used within the work setting so that charting can be done quickly and comprehensively.
Evaluating	
1. It is not done → mastery of nursing process is stunted; severely limits accomplishment of nursing aims.	1. Develop the belief that quality nursing care does not happen automatically and that only ongoing evaluation will identify needed areas of revision. Devise an evaluative strategy and carry it out. Study its effect on quality of care after 6 months' implementation.

might be "patient transfers from the bed to the chair." After this is achieved, however, the outcome needs to be stepped up in complexity to "patient walks around room with support of walker."

Following is an example of a specified outcome for a resident in long-term care: "Resident will participate in a minimum of two planned social activities per week beginning 9/16/15." If the resident did not meet that outcome, this evaluative statement may be written: "9/27/15—Outcome not met. Resident chose not to participate in any group activities this week." Many courses of action are then available to the nurse. Possible revisions to any plan of care include the following:

- *Delete or modify the nursing diagnosis.* This might not be a problem or concern for the resident. Evaluate and validate data pointing to the nursing diagnosis.
- *Make the outcome statement more realistic.* Carefully determine the resident's need for activities and ability or desire to participate in activities.
- *Adjust time criteria in outcome statement.* Re-evaluate after 3 weeks; resident may need more time to adjust to being institutionalized and more encouragement.
- *Change nursing interventions.* Make a special effort to familiarize yourself with the resident's interests, and match these with available programs and activities.

Once the nurse, in partnership with the patient if possible, makes a decision about how to respond, this must be com-

municated to the patient or the patient's surrogate and to other members of the professional caregiving team, via the patient's record.

 THINK back to Mioshi Otsuki, the older adult taking too much diuretic medication. The home care nurse would work with the patient to develop a teaching plan about her heart failure, specifically related to her drug-therapy regimen. This plan then would be documented in the patient's record and communicated to all people involved in the patient's care, such as other home care agency nurses who may be on call or filling in to visit the patient or home health aides involved in providing personal care and hygiene for the patient. ●

EVALUATING QUALITY CARE

In addition to each nurse's evaluation of patient outcome achievement and subsequent modifications to the plan of care, many informal and formal mechanisms are used to ensure quality nursing care.

Performance Improvement in Everyday Clinical Practice

Nurses sometimes discover problems with the delivery of nursing care in their practice setting. The Institute of Medicine's Committee on Quality of Health Care in America

(Kohn, Corrigan, & Donaldson, 2000) suggests 10 rules to redesign and improve care:

1. Care based on continuous healing relationships
2. Customization based on patient needs and values
3. The patient as the source of control
4. Shared knowledge and the free flow of information
5. Evidence-based decision making
6. Safety as a system priority
7. The need for transparency
8. Anticipation of patient's needs
9. Continuous decrease in waste
10. Cooperation among clinicians

Each nurse must decide how to respond when compromised patient care has been identified. Nurses committed to healthier patients, quality care, reduced costs, and the personal satisfaction of knowing that they *are actually making a difference* versus merely *wishing things were different* value **performance improvement**. The following four steps are crucial in improving performance (Haase & Miller, 1999):

1. Discover a problem.
2. Plan a strategy using indicators.
3. Implement a change.
4. Assess the change; if the outcome is not met, plan a new strategy.

See Box 15-4 for an example of a performance-improvement strategy. Remember, the central focus of these efforts is always improving the patient's experience and outcomes. In this example, oncology nurses believe that advance directives are not being used optimally to improve end-of-life care for the seriously ill and dying.

An important resource for nurses committed to performance improvement is *Quality and Safety Education for Nurses* (QSEN). The overall goal of QSEN Institute initiatives is to prepare nurses with the knowledge, skills, and attitudes (KSAs) necessary to continuously improve the quality and safety of their health care systems. Visit the website (www.qsen.org) to view a variety of educational materials.

Peer review, the evaluation of one staff member by another staff member on the same level in the hierarchy of the organization, is an important mechanism nurses can use to improve their professional performance. This can be done formally or informally by inviting a peer you respect to give you feedback on nursing skills you are trying to develop. "How do you think that session went with the patient's daughter? She's been so critical of us and I'm trying to understand the situation from her point of view and respond appropriately."

Establishing and Sustaining Healthy Work Environments

According to the study Silence Kills: The Seven Crucial Conversations for Healthcare (Maxfield, Grenny, McMillan, Patterson, & Switzler, 2005), the prevalent culture of poor communication and collaboration among health professionals is significantly related to continued medical errors and staff turnover. Additionally, a lack of adequate support systems, skills, and personal accountability results in communication gaps that can cause harm to patients. Results of the national study conducted by the American Association of Critical-Care Nurses (AACN) and VitalSmarts of more than 1,700 health professionals include these facts:

- 84% of physicians and 62% of nurses and other clinical-care providers have seen coworkers taking shortcuts that could be dangerous to patients.
- 88% of physicians and 48% of nurses and other providers work with people who show poor clinical judgment.
- Fewer than 10% of physicians, nurses, and other clinical staff directly confront their colleagues about their concerns, and one in five physicians said they have seen harm come to patients as a result.

BOX 15-4 **EXAMPLE OF STEPS IN PERFORMANCE IMPROVEMENT**

The following four steps are crucial in improving performance:

- **Discover a problem**
  Advance directives are a powerful legal tool for people to indicate their end-of-life care preferences. Nurses on an oncology unit are becoming frustrated because many of the patients on their unit lack advance directives. By the time decisions need to be made about ventilators, coding, dialysis, and so forth, patients are often no longer able to communicate their preferences. The hospital has a policy about advance directives, but no one seems to be taking responsibility for initiating discussions with patients when they are first admitted–or in the outpatient setting.

- **Plan a strategy using indicators**
  The nurses call an interdisciplinary meeting with the oncologists, social workers, and spiritual caregivers, who decide that the nurse case manager will be responsible for working with patients on admission to see if they want help in

preparing an advance directive. Each case manager will be responsible for documenting within 48 hours of admission the patient's decision regarding an advance directive. Staff nurses will be able to direct patient and family requests to do advance planning to the case manager and appropriate team members. The ethics committee was asked to do an in-service on advance directives for the team.

- **Implement a change**
  Case managers begin assuming this responsibility, and one nurse volunteers to monitor progress at 3-month intervals by checking charts for advance directive content and by speaking with the staff nurses who voiced the initial frustration about decision making.

- **Assess the change**
  If the goal is not met, plan a new strategy. At the end of 6 months, everyone seems satisfied that the new plan is working, but a decision is made to schedule a 6-month follow-up evaluation to prevent backsliding.

Reprinted with permission from Haase, R., & Miller, K. (1999). Performance improvement in everyday clinical practice. *American Journal of Nursing,* 99(5), 52, 54.

- The 10% of health care workers who raise these crucial concerns observe better patient outcomes, work harder, and are more satisfied and more committed to staying in their jobs (Executive Summary).

The study pinpoints seven categories of common communication problems that are rarely addressed. See Table 15-3 for examples of the seven crucial conversations in health care that nurses and other professionals must learn to master. If you find yourself in one of these situations, ask an experienced and trusted colleague how best to respond and don't accept an answer such as "Spare yourself some grief and do nothing." A follow-up to this study conducted by VitalSmarts, AACN, and the Association of periOperative Registered Nurses (AORN) revealed that safety tools fail to address a second category of communication breakdowns: "undiscussables." These are risks that are widely known but not discussed: (1) dangerous shortcuts, (2) incompetence, and (3) disrespect (Maxfield, Grenny, Lavandero & Groah, 2010). This study revealed that too many nurses are in situations in which they feel unsafe to speak up about problems or are unable to get others to listen.

AACN's commitment *to actively promote the creation of healthy work environments that support and foster excellence in patient care* is a superb example of nursing leadership. See Box 15-5 for AACN's six essential standards for establishing and sustaining healthy work environments. The standards represent *evidence-based* and *relationship-centered* principles of professional performance. Each standard is

Table 15-3 THE SEVEN CRUCIAL CONVERSATIONS IN HEALTH CARE

CATEGORY OF CONVERSATION	EXAMPLES	RECOMMENDATIONS
1. Broken rules	Colleague fails to wash hands.	Confront your colleague and tell her that you noticed that she failed to wash her hands and that this could be harmful to herself, the patient, or other patients. If the behavior continues, report your concerns to the nurse manager and work up the chain of command.
2. Mistakes	Nurse administers medication to the wrong patient and asks you to keep an eye on the patient for adverse reactions. She does not plan to report the error.	Tell your colleague that you'll be happy to help watch the patient but that a full report needs to be made. If appropriate, help your colleague identify what contributed to her giving the medication to the wrong patient.
3. Lack of support	Nurse refuses to help a colleague move an obese patient although she has time to do so.	Explain to this nurse that teamwork is essential to good outcomes and that her behavior is simply unacceptable. "When we have patients with special needs and need all hands on deck, everyone who's free is obligated to help out!" Develop and enforce zero tolerance for selfish behavior.
4. Incompetence	Nurse fails to correctly administer dialysis. She wasn't finished with her orientation to the unit and attempted a procedure before she was prepared to do it solo.	In addition to reporting the error, help the nurse identify that overconfidence in one's abilities can have deadly results for patients. The nurse manager will need to address the incompetence.
5. Poor teamwork	A particularly difficult family is splitting the team by choosing (and rewarding) favorites among the staff and complaining to them about other workers. The staff is encouraging this behavior.	Someone needs to call the team together and name the divisive behavior and get everyone working together again. If there is staff who are problematic, appropriate channels need to be used to address these behaviors.
6. Disrespect	When a student nurse asks a physician if she has time to answer a few questions for her patient, the physician screams at her and tells her that she has more important things to do than babysit her patient and tells the student to find someone else to answer the questions.	The student should calmly tell the physician that her response is inappropriate and that she is entitled to respectful conversation, then seek the counsel of an experienced nurse. The physician's behavior should be reported.
7. Micromanagement	A student asks her clinical preceptor, "Will you walk me through this procedure before I do it, since it's my first time?" The preceptor then takes over, doing the procedure for the student, and starts watching her every move.	The student should inform her preceptor that she merely wanted to review the steps of the procedure to make sure that she would perform it correctly and that it is essential for the student to gain experience by trying new procedures. If the preceptor's behavior does not change, the student should seek the counsel of her instructor.

Adapted from Maxfield, D., Grenny, J., Patterson, K., McMillan, R., & Switzler, A. (2005). Silence Kills. Available at http://www.aacn.org/WD/Practice/Docs/PublicPolicy/SilenceKillsExecSum.pdf

BOX 15-5 THE AMERICAN ASSOCIATION OF CRITICAL-CARE NURSES STANDARDS FOR ESTABLISHING AND SUSTAINING HEALTHY WORK ENVIRONMENTS

- **Skilled Communication.** Nurses must be as proficient in communication skills as they are in clinical skills.
- **True Collaboration.** Nurses must be relentless in pursuing and fostering true collaboration.
- **Effective Decision Making.** Nurses must be valued and committed partners in making policy, directing and evaluating clinical care, and leading organizational operations.

- **Appropriate Staffing.** Staffing must ensure the effective match between patient needs and nurse competencies.
- **Meaningful Recognition.** Nurses must be recognized and must recognize others for the value each brings to the work of the organization.
- **Authentic Leadership.** Nurse leaders must fully embrace the imperativeness of a healthy work environment, authentically live it, and engage others in its achievement.

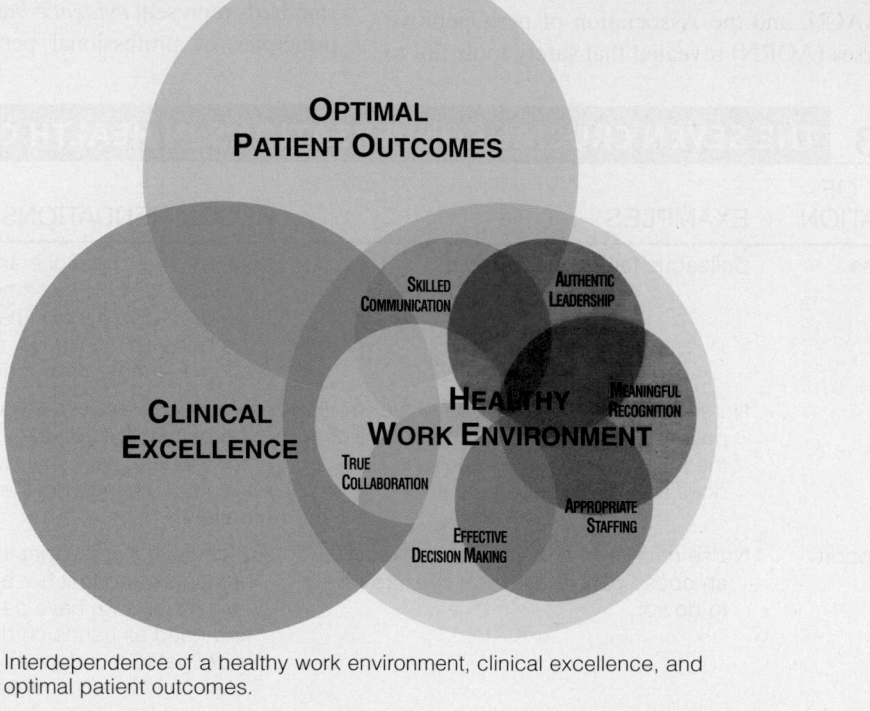

Interdependence of a healthy work environment, clinical excellence, and optimal patient outcomes.

Used with permission from American Association of Critical-Care Nurses (AACN). (2005). *AACN standards for establishing and sustaining healthy work environments: A journey to excellence* (pp. 13–14). Aliso Viejo, CA: Author.

considered essential because studies show that effective and sustainable outcomes do not emerge when any standard is considered optional. For copies of the Silence Kills report and the AACN Standards for Establishing and Sustaining Healthy Work Environments, visit www.aacn.org or www.silenttreatmentstudy.com.

Evaluative Programs

In the United States, regulatory agencies, such as state boards of nursing, the Joint Commission, the Professional Standards Review Organization, and the National Health Planning and Resources Development Act of 1975, require nurses to document that nursing standards are being implemented and maintained. Each of these agencies is concerned with quality care and quality control. The decreased availability of resources to treat patients in hospitals and the unavailability of sufficient alternative treatment settings pose a strong challenge to the nursing profession to find ways to avoid compromising quality of care. Numerous professional organizations are working to meet this challenge

(see Table 15-4). Selected Web resources for patients and families can be found on thePoint website.

Quality Assurance

Quality-assurance programs are special programs that promote excellence in nursing. These range from small programs conducted by nurses on a small nursing unit to those developed for an entire institution, state, province, or country.

Quality-assurance programs enable nursing to be accountable to society for the quality of nursing care. Such programs also respond to the public mandate for professional accountability. They help ensure survival of the profession, encourage nursing's fidelity to its moral and ethical responsibilities, and assist nursing to comply with other external pressures.

There are two different approaches to ensuring quality. *Quality by inspection* focuses on finding deficient workers and removing them. Nurses and others working in a setting using this approach may be afraid to admit a mistake or error and wrongly attempt to hide a problem. Such behavior is never

Table 15-4 NATIONAL QUALITY INITIATIVES

ORGANIZATION	INITIATIVE	DESCRIPTION
The Joint Commission http://www.jointcommission.org/assets/1/6/ORYX_for_Hospitals.pdf	ORYX	Integrates use of outcomes and performance measures into accreditation process; requires accredited general medical/surgical hospitals to collect and transmit data on a minimum of six core measures.
NCQA (National Committee for Quality Assurance) Accrediting body for managed care http://www.ncqa.org	HEDIS (Health Plan Employer Data and Information Set)	HEDIS targets these areas: effectiveness of care, access and availability of care, patient satisfaction, health plan stability, use of services, costs, and health plan descriptive information. Quality Compass reports (available on CD-ROM/electronic data file) include performance data on managed care plans.
ANA (American Nurses Association) https://www.nursingquality.org/	The National Database of Nursing Quality Indicators (NDNQI®)	NDNQI is the only national nursing quality measurement program that provides hospitals with unit-level performance reports with comparisons to national averages, percentile rankings, and other important data. All indicator data are collected and reported at the nursing-unit level. NDNQI's nursing-sensitive indicators reflect the structure, process, and outcomes of nursing care. NDNQI's mission is to aid the nursing provider in patient safety and quality improvement efforts by providing research-based national comparative data on nursing care and the relationship to patient outcomes. The database collects and evaluates unit-specific nurse-sensitive data from hospitals in the United States.
Centers for Medicare and Medicaid Services http://www.cms.hhs.gov/oasis/default.asp	OASIS (Outcome and Assessment Information Set)	Set of assessment questions to collect clinical, financial, and administrative data in home health care agencies. Goals of OASIS: to improve quality of care delivered to home health care patients and to provide data to HCFA.
National Quality Forum (NQF) http://www.qualityforum.org/Home.aspx	Manages a portfolio of more than 700 best-in-class quality measures	NQF operates under a three-part mission to improve the quality of American health care by: • Building consensus on national priorities and goals for performance improvement and working in partnership to achieve them • Endorsing national consensus standards for measuring and publicly reporting on performance • Promoting the attainment of national goals through education and outreach programs To ensure that all patients are protected from injury while receiving care, NQF has developed and endorsed a set of Serious Reportable Events (SREs). This set is a compilation of serious, largely preventable, and harmful clinical events, designed to help the health care field assess, measure, and report performance in providing safe care.
Institute for Healthcare Improvement (IHI) http://www.ihi.org/Pages/default.aspx	5 Million Lives Campaign, Triple Aim	An independent, not-for-profit organization founded in the 1980s to redesign health care into a system without errors, waste, delay, and unsustainable costs. IHI is a leading innovator in health and health care improvement worldwide. To accelerate the path to the health and care we need, IHI created the Triple Aim, a framework for optimizing health system performance by simultaneously focusing on the health of a population, the experience of care for people within that population, and the per capita cost of providing that care.

acceptable and may result in serious harm to patients. *Quality as opportunity,* on the other hand, focuses on finding opportunities for improvement and fosters an environment that thrives on teamwork, with people sharing the skills and lessons they have learned. Mistakes are viewed not as being caused by a lack of motivation or lack of effort by a worker but rather as a result of a problem in the system. In work environments using

this approach, nurses respond with openness and a desire to learn because their integrity and self-worth are not threatened. Our outcome should be to work in an environment in which quality measurements encourage our best efforts.

The American Nurses Association (ANA) in 1975 developed a model quality-assurance program consisting of seven steps: (1) identify values; (2) identify structure, process, and outcome standards and criteria; (3) measure the degree of attainment of criteria and standards; (4) make interpretations about strengths and weaknesses based on such measurements; (5) identify possible courses of action; (6) choose a course of action; and (7) take action. The ANA hoped the model would be used to develop and implement quality-assurance programs within institutions.

The ANA model directs attention to three essential components of quality care: structure, process, and outcome. Other types of quality-assurance programs may focus only on one of these components or on a mixture of components.

A **structure evaluation** or audit focuses on the environment in which care is provided. Standards describe physical facilities and equipment; organizational characteristics, policies, and procedures; fiscal resources; and personnel resources.

The focus of a **process evaluation** is the nature and sequence of activities carried out by nurses implementing the nursing process. Criteria make explicit acceptable levels of performance for nursing actions related to patient assessment, diagnosis, planning, implementation, and evaluation.

Outcome evaluation focuses on measurable changes in the health status of the patient or the end results of nursing care. While the proper environment for care and the right nursing actions are important aspects of quality care, the critical element in evaluating care is demonstrable changes in patient health status.

 Concept Mastery Alert

It is important to distinguish the different types of evaluation in quality assurance. A helpful way to remember the different types is to focus on the meaning of the word. For example, structure implies buildings or facilities; process implies action or activities; outcome implies changes in health.

From Quality Assurance to Quality Improvement

Concerns about the spiraling costs of health care, coupled with the success of industrial models for quality improvement, led to a strong commitment to quality improvement in the 1990s. **Quality improvement (QI)** (also known as continuous quality improvement [CQI] or total quality management [TQM]) is "the commitment and approach used to continuously improve every process in every part of an organization, with the intent of meeting and exceeding customer expectations and outcomes" (Schroeder, 1994, p. 3). Unlike quality assurance, quality improvement is internally driven, focuses on patient care rather than organizational structure, focuses on processes rather than people, and has no end points. Its goal is *improving* quality rather than *assuring* quality. The major premises of quality improvement are as follows (Schroeder, 1994, pp. 5–8):

• Focus on organizational mission
• Continuous improvement

• Customer orientation
• Leadership commitment
• Empowerment
• Collaboration/crossing boundaries
• Focus on process
• Focus on data and statistical thinking

From the patient's point of view, one of the most important outcomes of quality improvement is the recognition that patient satisfaction in health care is as important as customer satisfaction in retail business. With increased competition for the health care dollar, providers are learning that it is important to offer services that patients value and to offer them in a way that is valued by patients. By re-emphasizing the critical nature of nursing's *person* versus *task* orientation, quality improvement underscores the need for nurses to blend cognitive, technical, interpersonal, and ethical/legal competencies successfully.

Patient Satisfaction

An evaluative program that focuses on patient satisfaction is a powerful tool for patients and families who want to know what care will be like before choosing a health care facility. Hospital Consumer Assessment of Healthcare Providers and Systems (HCAHPS), the Centers for Medicare and Medicaid Services patient satisfaction program, is the first national, standardized, publicly reported survey of patients' perspectives of hospital care. The program provides consumers with information about a hospital's performance in key areas of communication, pain control, timeliness of care, discharge instructions, hospital cleanliness, and treatment with courtesy and respect. The survey was designed to produce data about patients' perspectives of care that allow objective and meaningful comparisons of hospitals on topics that are important to consumers. Public reporting of the survey results creates new incentives for hospitals to improve quality of care. Public reporting also serves to enhance public accountability in health care by increasing the transparency of the quality of hospital care provided in return for the public investment.

Are you helping or hurting your hospital? With your first clinical rotation, you can ask yourself how you think your patients would respond if asked the following questions: During this hospital stay, how often did nurses (1) treat you with courtesy and respect? (2) listen carefully to you? (3) explain things in a way you could understand? (Never, Sometimes, Usually, or Always?) And (4) During this hospital stay, after you pressed the call button, how often did you get help as soon as you wanted it? (Never, Sometimes, Usually, Always, or I never pressed the call button?) You can see how your local hospitals compare by searching the website www. hospitalcompare.hhs.gov. To learn more about HCAHPS visit www.cms.hhs.gov/HospitalQualityInits/.

Nursing's Safety and Quality Initiative

In March of 1994, the ANA Board of Directors launched a major multiphase initiative to investigate the impact of health care restructuring on the safety and quality of patient care as well as on nursing. Through Nursing's Safety & Quality Initiative, the ANA highlights the strong linkages between nursing actions and patient outcomes. **Nursing-sensitive quality indicators** are those indicators that capture care or its outcomes most affected by nursing care. Examples of nursing-sensitive quality indicators for acute care settings are the mix of RNs, LPNs, and unlicensed staff caring for patients in acute care settings, the total number of nursing care hours provided per patient day, pressure ulcers, and patient falls. In 1998, the ANA funded the development of a national database to house nursing-sensitive quality indicators. The goals of the National Database of Nursing Quality Indicators (NDNQI) are to promote and facilitate the standardization of information submitted by hospitals across the United States on nursing quality and patient outcomes (www.nursingworld.org).

The ANA Safety & Quality Initiative has focused on educating RNs about quality measurement; informing the public and purchasing/regulating constituencies about safe, quality health care; and investigating research methods and data sources to empirically evaluate the safety and quality of patient care.

Concurrent Versus Retrospective Evaluation

Nursing care and patient outcomes may be evaluated while the patient is receiving care (i.e., a concurrent evaluation) or after the patient has been discharged (i.e., a retrospective evaluation). **Concurrent evaluation** is conducted by using direct observation of nursing care, patient interviews, and chart review to determine whether the specified evaluative criteria are met.

Retrospective evaluation may use postdischarge questionnaires, patient interviews (by telephone or face to face), or chart review (nursing audit) to collect data. The type of retrospective audit most familiar to nurses working in hospitals is the Joint Commission retrospective chart review. This accrediting body initially required hospitals to conduct a certain number of audits per year.

REFLECTIVE PRACTICE LEADING TO PERSONAL LEARNING

Remember that the object of reflective practice is to look at an experience, understand it, and learn from it. As you begin to develop your expertise in evaluating the plan of care, reflect on your experiences—successes and failures—in order to improve your practice. How can you do it better next time? What did you learn today that can help you tomorrow? Begin your reflection by paying close attention to the following:

- How effectively did you engage your patients and families in evaluating the plan of care? To what degree does patient/family satisfaction motivate your efforts to provide high quality, safe care?
- What value do you attach to monitoring the patient's achievement of expected outcomes? In what ways did this monitoring result in valuable changes to the plan of care?

- Did your experience with evaluation reveal the need for changes in yourself or in your practice setting? How might these be accomplished?

The cultivation of evaluation as a critical component of the nursing process helps ensure nursing's continued success in achieving desired changes in patient health status. Nursing actions are far too valuable and costly to be haphazardly implemented. Evaluation that is carefully planned and executed can direct and redirect these actions to maximize the patient's benefit. This is the outcome and challenge of nursing evaluation.

Perhaps the most important question to reflect on is: Are your patients and families better for having had *you* share in the critical responsibility of partnering with them to evaluate the development and implementation of the plan of care?

DEVELOPING CLINICAL REASONING

1. Interview five students who have personal fitness goals. Ask them to describe what personal factors have helped or hindered achieving their goals. Note commonalities and differences. Reflect on how you can help patients tap their own personal strengths to achieve their outcomes more successfully.

2. Interview several patients and ask them what qualities in a nurse are most helpful as they try to achieve their health outcomes. Similarly, ask what nurse qualities are most problematic. Reflect on how you measure up in terms of both positive and negative nurse qualities.

3. Interview three or more experienced nurses in the same practice setting. Ask them what system variables (such as philosophy of care, nurse-to-patient ratio, professional and nonprofessional staff mix, nursing management, adequacy of resources) most influence their ability to deliver quality care. Identify variables you want to look for when you interview for a job.

4. Specify how nurses might use the AACN standards and crucial conversation recommendations to change the outcomes in the following situations:
   - A nurse knows that a patient's pain medication isn't working but decides not to call his attending physician because the physician was verbally abusive to her in the past and believes his patients "don't need analgesics."
   - A new policy was developed to make sure that obese patients are transferred safely without harm to themselves or staff. The nurse manager places the new policy in the policy manual but fails to educate staff in the new bariatric unit. Moreover, some nurses have been quite vocal about not putting themselves at risk with these patients and have refused to participate in collaborative efforts to move these patients safely.
   - Two nurses call in sick and staffing is at an all-time low. Additional patients are added to each nurse's assignment, increasing the probability that errors will be made. The nurses are frustrated and angry.

PRACTICING FOR NCLEX

1. A student health nurse is counseling a female college student who wants to lose 20 pounds. The nurse develops a plan to increase the student's activity level and decrease the consumption of the wrong types of foods and excess calories.

The nurse plans to evaluate the student's weight loss monthly. When the student arrives for her first "weigh-in," the nurse discovers that instead of the projected weight loss of 5 pounds, the student has lost only 1 pound. Which is the best nursing response?
a. Congratulate the student and continue the plan of care.
b. Terminate the plan of care since it is not working.
c. Try giving the student more time to reach the targeted outcome.
d. Modify the plan of care after discussing possible reasons for the student's partial success.

2. A nurse uses the following classic elements of evaluation when caring for patients. Which item below places them in their correct sequence?
(1) Interpreting and summarizing findings
(2) Collecting data to determine whether evaluative criteria and standards are met
(3) Documenting one's judgment
(4) Terminating, continuing, or modifying the plan
(5) Identifying evaluative criteria and standards (what one is looking for when evaluating, e.g., expected patient outcomes)
   a. 1, 2, 3, 4, 5
   b. 3, 2, 1, 4, 5
   c. 5, 2, 1, 3, 4
   d. 2, 3, 1, 4, 5

3. A new nurse who is being oriented to the subacute care unit is expected to follow existing standards when providing patient care. Which nursing actions are examples of these standards? Select all that apply.
a. Monitoring patient status every hour
b. Using intuition to troubleshoot patient problems
c. Turning a patient on bed rest every 2 hours
d. Becoming a nurse mentor to a student nurse
e. Administering pain medication ordered by the physician
f. Becoming involved in community nursing events

4. A nurse is collecting evaluative data for a patient who is finished receiving chemotherapy for an osteosarcoma. Which nursing action represents this step of the nursing process?
a. The nurse collects data to identify health problems.
b. The nurse collects data to identify patient strengths.
c. The nurse collects data to justify terminating the plan of care.
d. The nurse collects data to measure outcome achievement.

5. A nurse writes the following outcome for a patient who is trying to stop smoking: "The patient appreciates or values a healthy body sufficiently to stop smoking." This is an example of what type of outcome?
a. Cognitive
b. Psychomotor
c. Affective
d. Physical changes

6. A nurse writes the following outcome for a patient who is trying to lose weight: "The patient can explain the relationship between weight loss, increased exercise, and decreased calorie intake." This is an example of what type of outcome?
a. Cognitive
b. Psychomotor

c. Affective
d. Physical changes

7. A nurse is writing an evaluative statement for a patient who is trying to lower her cholesterol through diet and exercise. Which evaluative statement is written correctly?
a. "Outcome not met."
b. "1/21/15—Patient reports no change in diet."
c. "Outcome not met. Patient reports no change in diet or activity level."
d. "1/21/15—Outcome not met. Patient reports no change in diet or activity level."

8. A nurse is attempting to improve care on the pediatric ward of a hospital. Which nursing improvements might the nurse employ when following the recommendations of the Institute of Medicine's Committee on Quality of Health Care in America? Select all that apply.
a. Basing patient care on continuous healing relationships
b. Customizing care to reflect the competencies of the staff
c. Using evidence-based decision making
d. Having a charge nurse as the source of control
e. Using safety as a system priority
f. Recognizing the need for secrecy to protect patient privacy

9. A quality-assurance program reveals a higher incidence of falls and other safety violations on a particular unit. A nurse manager states, "We'd better find the folks responsible for these errors and see if we can replace them." This is an example of:
a. Quality by inspection
b. Quality by punishment
c. Quality by surveillance
d. Quality by opportunity

10. After one nursing unit with an excellent safety record meets to review the findings of the audit, the nurse manager states, "We're doing well, but we can do better! Who's got an idea to foster increased patient well-being and satisfaction?" This is an example of leadership that values:
a. Quality assurance
b. Quality improvement
c. Process evaluation
d. Outcome evaluation

ANSWERS WITH RATIONALES

1. *d.* Since the student has only partially met her outcome, the nurse should first explore the factors making it difficult for her to reach her outcome and then modify the plan of care. It would not be appropriate to continue the plan as it is since it is not working, and it is premature to terminate the plan of care since the student has not met her targeted outcome. The student may need more than time to reach her outcome, which makes (c) the wrong response.

2. *c.* The five classic elements of evaluation in order are (1) identifying evaluative criteria and standards (what you are looking for when you evaluate, e.g., expected patient outcomes), (2) collecting data to determine whether these criteria and standards are met, (3) interpreting and summarizing findings, (4) documenting your judgment, and (5) terminating, continuing, or modifying the plan.

3. *a, c, e.* Standards are the levels of performance accepted and expected by the nursing staff or other health care team members. They are established by authority, custom, or consent.

4. *d,* The nurse collects evaluative data to measure outcome achievement. While this may justify terminating the plan of care, that is not necessarily so. Data to assess health problems and patient variables are collected during the first step of the nursing process.

5. *c.* Affective outcomes pertain to changes in patient values, beliefs, and attitudes. Cognitive outcomes involve increases in patient knowledge; psychomotor outcomes describe the patient's achievement of new skills; physical changes are actual bodily changes in the patient (e.g., weight loss, increased muscle tone).

6. *a.* Cognitive outcomes involve increases in patient knowledge; psychomotor outcomes describe the patient's achievement of new skills; affective outcomes pertain to changes in patient values, beliefs, and attitudes; and physical changes are actual bodily changes in the patient (e.g., weight loss, increased muscle tone).

7. *d.* The evaluative statement must contain a date; the words "outcome met," "outcome partially met," or "outcome not met"; and the patient data or behaviors that support this decision. Answers *a, b,* and *c* are incomplete statements.

8. *a, c, e.* Care should be based on continuous healing relationships and evidence-based decision making. Customization should be based on patient needs and values with the patient as the source of control. Safety should be used as a system priority, and the need for transparency should be recognized.

9. *a.* Quality by inspection focuses on finding deficient workers and removing them. Quality as opportunity (*d*) focuses on finding opportunities for improvement and fosters an environment that thrives on teamwork, with people sharing the skills and lessons they have learned. Answers *b* and *c* are distractors.

10. *b.* Unlike quality assurance, quality improvement is internally driven, focuses on patient care rather than organizational structure, focuses on processes rather than individuals, and has no end points. Its goal is improving quality rather than assuring quality. Answers *c* and *d* are types of quality-assurance programs.

TAYLOR SUITE RESOURCES

Explore these additional resources to enhance learning for this chapter:

- NCLEX-Style Questions and other resources on thePoint, http://thePoint.lww.com/Taylor8e
- *Study Guide for Fundamentals of Nursing, 8th edition*
- Adaptive Learning | Powered by prepU, http://thepoint.lww.com/prepu

Bibliography

Albanese, M. P., Evans, D. A., Schantz, C. A., Bowen, M., Disbot, M., Moffa, J. S., … Polomano, R. C. (2010). Engaging clinical nurses in quality and performance improvement activities. *Nursing Administration Quarterly, 34*(3), 226–245. doi: 10.1097/NAQ.0b013e3181e702ca.

Alfaro, R. (2014). *Applying nursing process. The foundation for clinical reasoning* (8th ed.) Philadelphia: Wolters Kluwer Health/Lippincott Williams & Wilkins.

Alfaro-LeFevre, R. (2013). *Critical thinking, clinical reasoning, and clinical judgment: A practical approach* (5th ed.). St. Louis: Elsevier.

American Association of Critical-Care Nurses (AACN). (2005). *AACN standards for establishing and sustaining healthy work environments: A journey to excellence.* Aliso Viejo, CA: Author.

American Nurses Association (ANA). (1975). *A plan for implementation of the standards of nursing practice.* Kansas City, MO: Author.

American Nurses Association (ANA). (1976). *ANA quality assurance workbook.* Kansas City, MO: Author.

American Nurses Association (ANA). (1999). *Nursing quality indicators: Guide for implementation* (2nd ed.). Washington, DC: Author.

American Nurses Association (ANA). (2001). *Code for nurses with interpretive statements.* Washington, DC: Author.

American Nurses Association (ANA). (2010). *Nursing's social policy statement* (2010 ed.). Silver Spring, MD: Author.

American Nurses Association (ANA). (2010). *Standards of clinical nursing practice* (2nd ed.). Silver Spring, MD: Author.

Bloch, D. (1975). Evaluation of nursing care in terms of process and outcome: Issues in research and quality assurance. *Nursing Research, 24,* 256–263.

Bulechek, G. M., Butcher, H. K., Dochterman, J., & Wagner, C. M. (Eds.). (2013). *Nursing interventions classification (NIC)* (6th ed.). St. Louis: Elsevier.

Carpenito, L. J. (2013). *Nursing diagnosis: Application to clinical practice* (14th ed.). Philadelphia: Wolters Kluwer Health/Lippincott Williams & Wilkins.

Carpenito-Moyet, L. J. (2009). *Nursing care plans and documentation: Nursing diagnoses and collaborative problems* (5th ed.). Philadelphia: Wolters Kluwer Health/Lippincott Williams & Wilkins.

Donabedian, A. (1980). *The definition of quality and its approaches.* Ann Arbor, MI: Health Administration Press.

Donabedian, A. (1982). *The criteria and standards of quality: Explorations in quality assessment and monitoring.* Ann Arbor, MI: Health Administration Press.

Fowler, M. D. M. (Ed.) (2010 reissue). *Guide to the Code of Ethics for Nurses.* Silver Spring, MD: American Nurses Association.

Haase, R., & Miller, K. (1999). Performance improvement in everyday clinical practice. *American Journal of Nursing, 99*(5), 52, 54.

HealthGrades, Inc. (2004). *HealthGrades Quality Study: Patient safety in American hospitals.* Golden, CO: Author.

Institute of Medicine (IOM). (1999). *Measuring the quality of health care.* Washington, DC: National Academy Press.

Institute of Medicine (IOM). (2001). *Crossing the quality chasm: A new health system for the 21st century.* Washington, DC: National Academy Press.

Institute of Medicine (IOM). (2007). *Advancing QI research: Challenges and opportunities.* Washington, DC: National Academies Press.

Institute of Medicine (IOM). (2008). *Knowing what works in healthcare: A roadmap for the nation.* Washington, DC: National Academies Press.

The Joint Commission. (2010). Implementation guide for the NQF endorsed nursing-sensitive care measure set, 2009. Available at http:// http://www.jointcommission.org/assets/1/6/NSC%20Manual.pdf

The Joint Commission. (2013). Sentinel event policy and procedures. Available at http://www.jointcommission.org/Sentinel_Event_Policy_and_Procedures/

Kohn, L. T., Corrigan, J. M., & Donaldson, M. S. (Eds.), Committee on Quality of Health Care in America, Institute of Medicine (IOM). (2000). *To err is human: Building a safer health system.* Washington, DC: National Academy Press.

Manojlovich, M., & DeCicco, B. (2007). Healthy work environments, nurse–physician communication, and patients' outcomes. *American Journal of Critical Care, 16*(6), 536–543.

Maxfield, D., Grenny, J., Lavandero, R., & Groah, L. (2010). The silent treatment: Why safety tools and checklists aren't enough to save lives. Available at www.silenttreatmentstudy.com

Maxfield, D., Grenny, J., McMillan, R., Patterson, K., & Switzler, A. (2005). *Silence kills: The seven crucial conversations for healthcare.* Available at http://www.aacn.org/WD/Practice/Docs/PublicPolicy/SilenceKillsExecSum.pdf

Moorhead, S., Johnson, M., Maas, M. L., & Swanson, E. (Eds). (2013). *Nursing outcomes classification (NOC)* (5th ed.). St. Louis, MO: Elsevier.

Phaneuf, M. (1976a). *The nursing audit: Self-regulation in nursing practice.* New York: Appleton-Century-Crofts.

Phaneuf, M. (1976b). Quality assurance: A nursing view. *New Zealand Nursing Journal, 69*(2), 9–11.

Ratz, M., Bostick, J., & Riggs, C. J. (2002). *Nursing quality measurement: A review of nursing studies 1995–2000.* Washington, DC: American Nurses Association.

Salmon, M. (2007). Care, quality and safety: Same old? *Nursing Outlook, 55*(3), 117–119.

Schroeder, P. (1994). *Improving quality and performance: Concepts, programs, and techniques.* St. Louis, MO: C. V. Mosby.

Wright, D. (1984). An introduction to the evaluation of nursing care: A review of literature. *Journal of Advanced Nursing, 9*(5), 457–467.

16

Documenting, Reporting, Conferring, and Using Informatics

PHILLIPPE BARON

Phillippe is a 52-year-old man being discharged from the outpatient surgery department after undergoing a colonoscopy for removal of three polyps. He will be going home with his wife, who is a nurse, and they both require discharge teaching.

MILLIE DELONG

Millie, a 44-year-old woman, develops a wound infection following abdominal surgery. Wound care with normal saline irrigations is ordered 4 times a day.

JASON CHANDLER

Jason, 15 years old and in police custody, is brought to the emergency department for treatment because he allegedly consumed a handful of individually wrapped crack rocks (estimated to be about 30 rocks) to avoid arrest. Treatment with insertion of nasogastric tube and bowel preparation solution is ordered. Jason is refusing treatment because he denies possession of drugs entirely.

LEARNING OBJECTIVES

After completing the chapter, you will be able to accomplish the following:

1. List guidelines for effective documentation, including those of the American Nurses Association.

2. Identify measures to protect confidential patient information.

3. Identify approved abbreviations and symbols used for documentation and distinguish these from error-prone abbreviations and symbols.

4. Describe the purposes of patient records.

5. Compare and contrast different methods of documentation: electronic health record, source-oriented record; problem-oriented record; PIE—problem, intervention, evaluation; focus charting; charting by exception; and case management model.

6. Describe the purpose and correct use of each of the following formats for nursing documentation: nursing assessment, nursing care plan, critical/collaborative pathways, progress notes, flow sheets, discharge summary, and home care documentation.

7. Document nursing interventions completely, accurately, currently, concisely, and factually—avoiding legal problems.

8. Describe the nurse's role in communicating with other health care professionals by reporting and conferring.

9. Describe nursing informatics and its contributions to nursing and health care.

KEY TERMS

change-of-shift report

charting by exception (CBE)

collaborative pathway

confer

consultation

critical pathway

discharge summary

documentation

electronic health record (EHR)

flow sheet

focus charting

graphic record

hand-off

health information exchange (HIE)

incident/variance report

ISBAR communication

meaningful use

minimum data set

narrative notes

nursing informatics

OASIS

occurrence/variance charting

patient record

personal health record (PHR)

PIE charting

problem-oriented medical record (POMR)

progress notes

read back

referral

SOAP format

source-oriented record

variance report

Effective communication among health care professionals is essential to the coordination and continuity of person-centered care. Communicating effectively enables personnel to support and to complement one another's services and to avoid duplications and omissions in care. This chapter describes three methods of communication central to nurses' professional role: documenting, reporting, and conferring, as well as some of the newer informatics technologies that assist communication. The first day you care for patients, you will find yourself conferring with colleagues, recording your interventions, and reporting on your patient's progress toward valued goals and outcomes. As you develop these skills, you will quickly see a link between communicating information and clinical reasoning and judgment. As you document data, you are looking for relationships and patterns—things that might otherwise be overlooked. As you confer with the patient and the patient's family and professional caregivers, you might learn something about the patient or situation that enhances your data set and clarifies the patient's health problem and related need for care (see the accompanying Reflective Practice box for an example on page 340). This chapter will help you assume these responsibilities with greater confidence and skill. The communication process itself and specific communication techniques are discussed in Chapter 20.

DOCUMENTING CARE

Documentation is the written or electronic legal record of all pertinent interactions with the patient—assessing, diagnosing, planning, implementing, and evaluating. Increasingly sophisticated management information systems help manage patient-specific data and information. These records contain data used to facilitate quality, evidence-based patient care, serve as financial and legal records, help in clinical research, and support decision analysis. Information specialists aim to create an environment that supports timely, accurate, secure, and confidential recording and use of patient-specific information.

The **patient record** is a compilation of a patient's health information. Each health care institution or agency has policies that specify the nurse's documentation responsibilities. The Joint Commission specifies that nursing care data related to patient assessments, nursing diagnoses or patient needs, nursing interventions, and patient outcomes are permanently integrated into the patient record. Each nurse is expected to practice according to local policies and professional standards.

Guidelines for Effective Documentation

The patient record is the only permanent legal document that details the nurse's interactions with the patient and is the nurse's best defense if a patient or patient surrogate alleges nursing negligence. Unfortunately, there are often crucial omissions in the nursing documentation, along with meaningless repetitious or inaccurate entries. Although these errors might go undetected and have no effect on the patient, they might also seriously affect the care the patient receives,

REFLECTIVE PRACTICE: CULTIVATING QSEN COMPETENCIES

CHALLENGE TO ETHICAL AND LEGAL SKILLS

Working in the emergency department (ED) this summer never ceased to amaze me. Police brought Jason Chandler to the ED, a 15-year-old male who was in custody for drug charges. Apparently, as police approached Jason, he consumed a handful of individually wrapped crack rocks (estimated to be about 30 rocks) to avoid arrest. He was brought to the ED as a precaution. If this bag broke inside his gastrointestinal tract, it would obviously have serious consequences. Jason was refusing treatment because he denied the possession of drugs entirely. The ED attending physician was unsure of his legal rights for treating the boy and called the hospital attorney. The attorney said the doctor could force treatment if there were probable signs that ingestion had occurred. However, the boy was not showing any clinical manifestations of chemical ingestion. This was a dilemma because if the bag of drugs burst open inside the boy, the

physician stated that he most likely would not survive. The legal issue was whether or not the officer's statement of witnessing the ingestion was enough to constitute the need for treatment. The doctor was about to begin treating the patient when his mother arrived, threatening to sue anyone and everyone who "touched her little boy."

My preceptor and I were assigned to this patient and were given orders to insert a nasogastric (NG) tube so that a bowel preparation solution (GoLYTELY) could be used to flush out the drugs. The hospital attorney concluded that there was probable cause to justify forced treatment. However, the mother was furious and said she would sue under these circumstances, despite what the doctor or attorney said. As we entered the room to insert the NG tube and begin treatment, the boy, who was handcuffed to the bed, was screaming at us not to touch him.

Thinking Outside the Box: Possible Courses of Action

- Go with my preceptor and assist with the NG tube insertion.
- Refuse to treat the patient for fear of becoming part of a lawsuit.
- Allow my preceptor to sedate the patient against his will, to make the NG tube insertion easier.

- Inform the physician that I do not feel comfortable proceeding with treatment on a patient who refuses it and shows no clinical manifestations of drug toxicity.

Evaluating a Good Outcome: How Do I Define Success?

- The patient is benefited or, at the very least, not harmed by our actions.
- The hospital and its employees act in a legally defensible manner and (hopefully!) are not sued by the patient's family.

- The patient accepts treatment.
- The mother is able to realize the need for medical intervention.
- Hospital policy is maintained.
- I learn more about my legal and ethical responsibilities.

Personal Learning: Here's to the Future!

My preceptor and I went into the room and explained to the patient and his mother the procedure of NG tube insertion and what the bowel preparation solution was expected to do. I think the mother appreciated that we were not talking to them in a condescending fashion and, therefore, began to see us as trying to help her son, not harm him. She asked a couple of questions about side effects of the medication and how the NG tube worked. She began to show signs of calming down until the physician walked into the room. Then she started to show her frustration again. Therefore, my preceptor politely asked the doctor to leave. Subsequently, we were able to insert the NG tube, despite some resistance from the patient. Several hours later, the patient passed a bag of crack rocks intact.

Obviously, this situation was very new to me. I had never dealt with a patient who was threatening to sue and who was clearly upset by what was happening. I was able to see the

collaboration between the attending physician, the toxicologist, the hospital attorney, and the nurses and myself. This was an interesting case because the treatments were clearly necessary for the patient's well-being, but everyone wanted to make sure they were legally able to impose treatment. I learned that a hospital attorney is a good resource when legal questions or ambiguous situations arise.

I think that my professional legal skills need a fair amount of work. Unfortunately, I also believe that nurses violate the law more often than is recognized—for example, subtle breaches of the law such as failure to ensure patient safety and failure to follow agency policy. Although I feel that I understand many of the obvious legal violations, I think I have a lot to learn regarding legal issues in the nursing practice.

Julia Strobel, Georgetown University

REFLECTION ON QUALITY AND SAFETY COMPETENCIES

How do you think you would respond in a similar situation? Why? What does this tell you about yourself and about the adequacy of your competencies for professional practice? Can you think of other ways to respond? What legal and ethical principles were involved in this situation? Which ones had the potential to be violated? Did the preceptor and nursing student ensure the patient's rights? How might this situation have been different if the patient were over 18 years of age? What *knowledge, skills,* and *attitudes* do you need to develop to continuously improve the quality and safety of care for patients like Jason?

Patient-Centered Care: How can you establish a successful partnership with a patient and family refusing treatment?

Teamwork and Collaboration/Quality Improvement: What role did the hospital attorney play? What other team members would be helpful? What needs to change to improve quality in this setting?

Safety/Evidence-Based Practice: What does the evidence point to as "best practice" for Jason? What safety needs does he have and how can you meet them?

Informatics: Can you identify the essential information that must be available in Jason's record to support safe patient care and coordination of care? Can you think of other ways to respond to or approach the situation? What else might the nursing student have done to ensure a successful outcome?

undermine nursing's credibility as a professional discipline, and cause legal problems for the nurses responsible. Adherence to the documentation guidelines shown in Box 16-1 (on page 342) helps to prevent errors. Be sure to also check the guidelines later in this chapter for electronic documentation.

Responding to the widespread nursing concern that the time spent documenting nursing care comes at the expense of providing safe, quality patient care, the American Nurses Association (ANA) introduced a tool to streamline the nursing documentation process in 2003 and revised this in 2010. Available as a brochure titled *Principles for Documentation,* this guide includes policy statements, principles, and recommendations to assist nurses with documentation and to comply with institutional and regulatory requirements.

The policy statements and principles outlined in the guide are based on the ANA *Code of Ethics for Nurses With Interpretive Statements* (ANA, 2001) and *Scope and Standards of Practice,* 2010 edition (ANA, 2010). In addition, the formulated principles in many instances are based on standards set forth by state and federal regulatory agencies, the Centers for Medicare and Medicaid Services (CMS), and through accrediting organizations, such as the Joint Commission and the National Committee for Quality Assurance (NCQA). The ANA standards identify the following characteristics of effective documentation: accessible; accurate, relevant, and consistent; auditable; clear, concise, and complete; legible/readable (particularly in terms of the resolution and related qualities of EHR content as it is displayed on the screens of various devices); thoughtful; timely, contemporaneous, and sequential; reflective of the nursing process; and retrievable on a permanent basis in a nursing-specific manner (ANA, 2010, p. 12).

Privacy and Confidentiality

Nurses and other professional caregivers learn and communicate private information about patients and their families every day.

What Information Is Confidential?

All information about patients is considered private or confidential, whether written on paper, saved on a computer, or spoken aloud. This includes their names and all identifiers such as address, telephone and fax number, Social Security number, and any other personal information. It also includes the reason the patient is sick or in the hospital, office, or clinic, the assessments and treatments the patient receives, and information about past health conditions. Protected health information might be found in the patient medical record, computer systems, telephone calls, voice mails, fax transmissions, e-mails that contain patient information, and conversations about patients among clinical staff.

While most nurses are staunch advocates of a patient's right to privacy and confidentiality, it is possible to violate these rights thoughtlessly. For example, one nurse gives patient information over the phone to a patient's alleged spouse without knowing whether or not the patient wants his wife to know, another talks about a difficult patient in the eleva-

tor on the way to dinner, and another gives patient information to a professional caregiver who "knows" the patient but is not involved in the patient's care. Additional examples of breaches of confidentiality and security include the following:

- Discussing patient information in any public area where those who have no need to know the information can overhear
- Leaving patient medical information in a public area
- Leaving a computer unattended in an accessible area with medical record information unsecured
- Failing to log off a computer terminal
- Sharing or exposing passwords
- Copying or providing data, either in paper or machine-readable form, for one's self, coworkers, or any other party, except as required to fulfill job responsibilities
- Improperly accessing, reviewing, and/or releasing birth dates and addresses of friends or relatives, or requesting another person to do so
- Improperly accessing, reviewing, and/or releasing the record of a patient out of concern or curiosity, or requesting another person to do so
- Improperly accessing, reviewing, and/or releasing a patient record to use information in a personal relationship
- Improperly accessing, reviewing, and/or releasing the patient record of a public personality for the intent of giving or selling information to the media
- Improperly accessing, reviewing, and/or releasing confidential information of another member of the workforce who is also a patient
- Improperly accessing, reviewing, and/or releasing confidential information that may bring harm to the organization or people associated with it

Table 16-1 (on page 343) provides specific measures to use to ensure that information about your patients remains confidential.

Professional codes of ethics, agency policies, and state and federal privacy legislation dictate how patient information can be communicated (spoken verbally and in writing), where and how it can be stored, the appropriate people and entities to whom it may be divulged, and the purposes for which it may be divulged. Nurses must be familiar with these guidelines.

Take note! There have been reports of school suspensions for nursing and medical students who unprofessionally share patient experiences on Facebook, MySpace, blogs, and YouTube. What may start as a prank may lead to your suspension or dismissal. Take the time to review the social media guidelines for nurses developed by the American Nurses Association (www.nursingworld.org), National Student Nurses Association (www.nsna.org), and the National Council of State Boards of Nursing (www.ncsbn.org).

Health Information Privacy

The U.S. Office for Civil Rights enforces the Health Insurance Portability and Accountability Act (HIPAA) Privacy Rule, which protects the privacy of individually identifiable health information; the HIPAA Security Rule, which sets

BOX 16-1 DOCUMENTATION GUIDELINES

Aim: Complete, accurate, concise, current, factual, and organized data communicated in a timely and confidential manner to facilitate care coordination and serve as a legal document.

Content

- Enter information in a *complete, accurate, concise, current,* and *factual* manner.
- Make sure your documentation reflects the nursing process and your professional responsibilities.
- Record patient findings (observations of behavior) rather than your interpretation of these findings.
- Avoid words such as "good," "average," "normal," or "sufficient," which may mean different things to different readers.
- Avoid generalizations such as "seems comfortable today." A better entry would be "on a scale of 1 to 10, patient rates back pain 2 to 3 today as compared with 7 to 9 yesterday; vital signs returned to baseline."
- Note problems as they occur in an *orderly, sequential manner;* record the nursing intervention and the patient's response; update problems or delete as appropriate.
- Record precautions or preventive measures used.
- Document in a *legally prudent manner.* Know and adhere to professional standards and agency/institutional policy for documentation.
- Document the nursing response to questionable medical orders or treatment (or failure to treat). Factually record the date and time the physician was notified of the concern and the exact physician response. If this occurs by phone, have a second nurse listen to the conversation and cosign the note. If a nurse administrator was contacted, document this. Documentation should give legal protection to the nurse, other caregivers, the health care agency or institution, and the patient.
- Avoid stereotypes or derogatory terms when charting.

Timing

- Document in a *timely* manner. Follow agency policy regarding the frequency of documentation and *modify this if changes in the patient's status warrant more frequent documentation.*
- Indicate in each entry the date and both the time the entry was written and the time of pertinent observations and interventions. This is crucial when a case is being reconstructed for legal purposes.
- Most agencies use military time, one 24-hour time cycle, to avoid confusion between AM and PM times (see accompanying figure).
- Document nursing interventions as closely as possible to the time of their execution. The more seriously ill the patient, the greater the need to keep documentation current. Never leave the unit for a break when caring for a seriously ill patient until all significant data are recorded.
- *Never document interventions before carrying them out.*
- Write a progress note for each of these instances:
  - Upon admission, transfer to another unit, and discharge
  - When a procedure is performed
  - Upon receiving a patient postoperatively or post-procedure
  - Upon communicating with physicians regarding critical patient information (e.g., abnormal lab value result)
  - For any change in patient status

Format

- Check to make sure you have the correct chart before writing.
- Record on the proper form or screen as designated by agency policy.
- With paper charts, print or write legibly in *dark* ink to ensure permanence. Use correct grammar and spelling. Use **standard terminology**, only commonly accepted terms and abbreviations and symbols (see Box 16-3 on page 345). Alternately, follow computer documentation guidelines.
- Date and time each entry.
- Record nursing interventions chronologically on consecutive lines. Never skip lines. Draw a single line through blank spaces.

Accountability

- Sign your first initial, last name, and title to each entry. Do not sign notes describing interventions not performed by you that you have no way of verifying.
- Do not use dittos, erasures, or correcting fluids. Draw a single line through an incorrect entry, and write the words "mistaken entry" or "error in charting" above or beside the entry and sign. Then rewrite the entry correctly.
- Identify each page of the record with the patient's name and identification number.
- Recognize that the patient record is *permanent.* Follow agency policy pertaining to the color of ink and the type of pen or ink to be used. Ensure that the patient record is complete before sending it to medical records.

Confidentiality

- Patients have a moral and legal right to expect that the information contained in their patient health record will be kept private. Students should be familiar with agency policy and pertinent legislation about who has access to patient records other than the immediate caregiving team, and the process used to obtain access (see HIPAA guidelines).
- Most agencies allow students access to patient records for educational reasons. Students using patient records are bound professionally and ethically to keep in strict confidence all the information they learn by reading patient records. Actual patient names and other identifiers should not be used in written or oral student reports.

The military clock uses one 24-hour time cycle instead of two 12-hour cycles (e.g., 9:00 AM is 0900 and 9:00 PM is 2100).

Table 16-1 TIPS FOR PREVENTING BREACHES IN PATIENT CONFIDENTIALITY

TYPE OF BREACH	HOW TO PREVENT IT
Computers Displaying information on a screen (especially handheld computers) that is viewed by unauthorized users	Make sure display screens do not face public areas. For portable devices, install encryption software that makes information unreadable or inaccessible.
Sending confidential e-mail messages via public networks such as the Internet, where they can be read by unauthorized users	Use encryption software when sending e-mail over public networks.
Sharing printers among units with differing functions and information (unauthorized users can read printouts)	Request that your unit have a separate printer not shared with another unit.
Copiers Discarded copies of patient health information in trash cans adjacent to copiers	Use secure disposal containers (similar to mailboxes) adjacent to copiers.
Cordless and Cellular Phones Holding conversations vulnerable to eavesdropping outsiders with scanning equipment	Use phones with built-in encryption technology.
Fax Machines Faxing confidential information to unauthorized persons	Before transmission, verify the fax number and that the recipient is authorized to receive confidential information.
Voice Pagers Sending confidential messages that can be overheard on the pager	Restrict use of voice pagers to nonconfidential messages.

Reprinted with permission from Holmes, H. N. (Ed.). (2006). *Documentation in action*. Philadelphia: Wolters Kluwer Health/Lippincott Williams & Wilkins.

national standards for the security of electronic protected health information; the HIPAA Breach Notification Rule, which requires covered entities and business associates to provide notification following a breach of unsecured protected health information; and the confidentiality provisions of the Patient Safety Rule, which protect identifiable information being used to analyze patient safety events and improve patient safety (www.HHS.gov). Congress passed HIPAA in 1996. The final regulations were released in August 2002. Most agencies now require workers to undergo HIPAA training and to review and sign a confidentiality agreement both when hired and at each performance review. As a student in a health care setting, you should discuss privacy guidelines with your instructor and nurse mentors. According to HIPAA, patients have a right to:

• See and copy their health record
• Update their health record
• Get a list of the disclosures that a health care institution has made independent of disclosures made for the purposes of treatment, payment, and health care operations
• Request a restriction on certain uses or disclosures
• Choose how to receive health information

 CONSIDER Jason Chandler, the adolescent brought to the emergency department by the police. The nurse needs to be knowledgeable about HIPAA regulations to ensure that Jason's confidentiality is maintained. In addition, the nurse should keep in mind that Jason is a minor, and any authorizations would probably require a parent's consent. •

If a health institution wants to release a patient's health information for purposes other than treatment, payment, or routine health care operations, the patient must be asked to sign an authorization (see Box 16-2 (on page 344) for a list of permitted disclosures of patient health information and incidental disclosures).

Take note! HIPAA legislation includes punishments for anyone caught violating patient privacy. Those who do so for financial gain can be fined as much as $250,000 or go to jail as long as 10 years! Even accidentally breaking the rules can result in penalties—and embarrassment—for you and your organization.

Agency Policies

Most agencies have specific policies regarding patient records. Everyone with access to the record (direct caregivers) is expected to maintain its confidentiality (see the earlier discussion about privacy). Most agencies grant student nurses access to patient records for education purposes. In this instance, *the student assumes responsibility to hold patient information in confidence.* Never use a patient's name when preparing written or oral reports for school.

Agency policies also indicate which personnel are responsible for recording on each form in the record; such policies might also describe the order in which the forms are to appear in the record. Additional policies might concern the frequency with which entries are to be made, whether routine care is recorded, how health personnel identify themselves after making an entry, which abbreviations are acceptable, and the manner in which recording errors

BOX 16-2 THE HEALTH INSURANCE PORTABILITY AND ACCOUNTABILITY ACT OF 1996 AUTHORIZATION RULE

If a health institution wants to release a patient's health information (PHI) for purposes other than treatment, payment, and routine health care operations, the patient must be asked to sign an authorization.

Permitted Disclosure of PHI

While the authorization rule covers most situations in which patient information is released for purposes other than treatment, payment, and routine health care operations, there are some exceptions to the authorization rule for the good of the general population.

These three exceptions show situations in which authorization is *not* required prior to releasing the patient's information:

Public health activities	• Tracking and notification of disease outbreaks • Infection control • Statistics related to dangerous problems with drugs or medical equipment
Law enforcement and judicial proceedings	• Medical records crucial to the investigation and prosecution of a crime • Medical records to identify victims of crime or disasters • Medical personnel reporting incidents of child abuse, neglect, or domestic violence • Medical records released according to a valid subpoena
Deceased people	• PHI needed by coroners, medical examiners, and funeral directors • PHI needed to facilitate organ donations • PHI provided to law enforcement in the case of a death from a potential crime

Incidental Disclosure of PHI

Incidental disclosure of PHI is defined as a secondary disclosure that cannot reasonably be prevented, is limited in nature, and occurs as a byproduct of an otherwise permitted use or disclosure of PHI.

Examples of incidental disclosures that are permitted:

Permitted Disclosure	Necessary Conditions
• Use of sign-in sheets	• Provided that the sign-in sheet does not contain information on the reason for the patient's visit
• The possibility of a confidential conversation being overheard	• Provided that the surroundings are appropriate for a confidential conversation and voices are kept down
• Placing patient charts outside exam rooms	• Provided that unauthorized public traffic is not permitted in the area of the exam rooms and face sheets are turned toward the wall
• Use of white boards	• Provided that only the minimum information needed for the purpose of the white board is used
• X-ray light boards that can be seen by passers-by	• Provided that patient x-rays are not left unattended on the light board
• Calling out names in the waiting room	• Provided that the reason for the patient's visit is not mentioned
• Leaving appointment reminder voicemail messages	• Provided that the minimum amount of information is disclosed

---

are handled. Box 16-3 provides a list of commonly used abbreviations. Table 16-2 (on pages 346–348) identifies the Institute for Safe Medication Practices (ISMP) list of error-prone abbreviations, symbols, and dose designations. One of the strategies the Joint Commission is using to achieve National Patient Safety Goals is a list of "do not use" abbreviations, acronyms, and symbols (Table 16-3 on page 349). Be sure to know the latest Joint Commission and agency policies regarding the use of abbreviations, acronyms, and symbols in your practice setting. It is now recommended that students minimize the use of abbreviations and instead write or type out the full terms and other words to create a clear record for the caregivers who follow. An issue of growing importance concerns documentation made by unlicensed personnel. Because professional nurses frequently supervise the care that unlicensed personnel give, it must be clear which assessments and interventions may be charted by unlicensed personnel and which require documentation by a professional nurse.

The storage of patient records after treatment is a function of the health agency's record department. Many patient records are microfilmed for compact storage or are entered into a computer to expedite accessibility of information.

You should also know your agency's policies regarding the patient's right to access records. Be sure to check the policy where you work to find out answers to the following common questions from patients:

• Can I take my chart home?
• Can I take my discharge instructions or medical record home electronically?
• How long do you retain records?
• How long will it take to get a copy of my record?
• How much does it cost?
• I do not want some parts of my record (e.g., psychiatric information) released to anyone. What do I do?
• May I look at my family's medical record?
• Who can look at my record?
• Who do I tell if my name has changed?

Your agency should have an information officer or clinical informaticist who can help you answer these questions.

Box 16-3 ABBREVIATIONS AND SYMBOLS COMMONLY USED BY HEALTH PRACTITIONERS*

Activities
AMB — ambulatory
BRP — bathroom privileges
CBR — complete bed rest
OOB — out of bed
up ad lib — up as desired

Assessment Data
abd — abdomen
BP — blood pressure
bx — biopsy
C — Celsius (centigrade)
c/o — complains of
CTA — clear to auscultation
dx — diagnosis
F — Fahrenheit
FUO — fever of unknown origin
GI — gastrointestinal
GU — genitourinary
H/A — headache
h/o — history of
HPI — history of present illness
Imp — impressions
lt or Ⓛ — left
MAE — moves all extremities
NAD — no apparent distress
NKA — no known allergies
N/V — nausea and vomiting
neg — negative
P — pulse
PE — physical examination
PMH — past medical history
R — respirations
R/O — rule out
ROS — review of systems
rt or Ⓡ — right
SOB — short of breath
Sx — symptoms
T — temperature
⊕ — positive
⊖ — negative

Diseases
ASCVD — arteriosclerotic cardio-vascular disease
ASHD — arteriosclerotic heart disease
BPH — benign prostatic hypertrophy
CA — cancer

CAD — coronary artery disease
CHF — congestive heart failure
COPD — chronic obstructive pulmonary disease
CVA — cerebrovascular accident
DM — diabetes mellitus
HTN (↑BP) — hypertension
MI — myocardial infarction
PE — pulmonary emboli
PVD — peripheral vascular disease
STD — sexually transmitted disease
STI — sexually transmitted infection
URI — upper respiratory infection

Diagnostic Studies
ABG — arterial blood gases
BE — barium enema
CBC — complete blood count
CO_2 — carbon dioxide
C&S — culture and sensitivity
CXR — chest x-ray
ECG (EKG) — cardiogram
lytes — electrolytes
RBC — red blood cells
UA — urinalysis
UGI — upper GI
WBC — white blood cells

Symbols
↑ — increase
↗ — increasing
↓ — decrease
↙ — decreasing
2° — secondary to
= — equal to
≠ — unequal
♀ — female
♂ — male
° — degree
▲ — change
x̄ — except

Miscellaneous
ā — before
ad lib — as desired

AMA — against medical advice
ASAP — as soon as possible
BM — bowel movement
BSD — bedside drainage
c̄(C) — with
CABG — coronary artery bypass graft
CPR — cardiopulmonary resuscitation
DNR (no code) — do not resuscitate
Dsg — dressing
dx — diagnosis
FOB — foot of bed
Fx — fracture
GHWT — good handwashing technique
HOB — head of bed
Hx — history
I&O — intake and output
IV — intravenous
KVO — keep vein open
NG — nasogastric
noc — night
NPO (npo) — nothing by mouth
NS (NIS) (N/S) — normal saline
O_2 — oxygen
OT — occupational therapy
p̄ — after
postop — postoperative
preop — preoperative
prep — preparation
PRN (p.r.n.) — as needed
PT — physical therapy
pt — patient
ROM — range of motion
RX — treatment
s̄ (S) — without
SOB — side of bed
S/P — status post
STAT — immediately
TF — tube feeding
TPR — temperature, pulse, respirations
TX — treatment
VS — vital signs
WA — while awake
× — times

*Use only those abbreviations and symbols accepted by your institution.

Purposes of Patient Records

Patient records serve many purposes. The ANA states that the most important of these is "communicating within the health care team and providing information for other professionals, primarily for individuals and groups involved with accreditation, credentialing, legal, regulatory and legislative, reimbursement, research, and quality activities" (ANA, 2010, p. 5).

Communication

The primary purpose of the patient record is to help health care professionals from different disciplines (who interact with the patient at different times) communicate with one another. Communication fosters continuity of care. For example, a critically ill patient in an academic health center may be seen by an attending physician, several consulting

(text continues on page 349)

Table 16-2 ISMP ERROR PRONE ABBREVIATIONS

The abbreviations, symbols, and dose designations found in this table have been reported to ISMP through the ISMP National Medication Errors Reporting Program (ISMP MERP) as being frequently misinterpreted and involved in harmful medication errors. They should **NEVER** be used when communicating medical information. This includes internal communications, telephone/verbal prescriptions, computer-generated labels, labels for drug storage bins, medication administration records, as well as pharmacy and prescriber computer order entry screens.

ABBREVIATIONS	INTENDED MEANING	MISINTERPRETATION	CORRECTION
μg	Microgram	Mistaken as "mg"	Use "mcg"
AD, AS, AU	Right ear, left ear, each ear	Mistaken as OD, OS, OU (right eye, left eye, each eye)	Use "right ear," "left ear," or "each ear"
OD, OS, OU	Right eye, left eye, each eye	Mistaken as AD, AS, AU (right ear, left ear, each ear)	Use "right eye," "left eye," or "each eye"
BT	Bedtime	Mistaken as "BID" (twice daily)	Use "bedtime"
cc	Cubic centimeters	Mistaken as "u" (units)	Use "mL"
D/C	Discharge or discontinue	Premature discontinuation of medications if D/C (intended to mean "discharge") has been misinterpreted as "discontinued" when followed by a list of discharge medications	Use "discharge" and "discontinue"
IJ	Injection	Mistaken as "IV" or "intrajugular"	Use "injection"
IN	Intranasal	Mistaken as "IM" or "IV"	Use "intranasal" or "NAS"
HS hs	Half-strength At bedtime, hours of sleep	Mistaken as bedtime Mistaken as half-strength	Use "half-strength" or "bedtime"
IU**	International unit	Mistaken as IV (intravenous) or 10 (ten)	Use "units"
o.d. or OD	Once daily	Mistaken as "right eye" (OD-oculus dexter), leading to oral liquid medications administered in the eye	Use "daily"
OJ	Orange juice	Mistaken as OD or OS (right or left eye); drugs meant to be diluted in orange juice may be given in the eye	Use "orange juice"
Per os	By mouth, orally	The "os" can be mistaken as "left eye" (OS-oculus sinister)	Use "PO," "by mouth," or "orally"
q.d. or QD**	Every day	Mistaken as q.i.d., especially if the period after the "q" or the tail of the "q" is misunderstood as an "i"	Use "daily"
qhs	Nightly at bedtime	Mistaken as "qhr" or every hour	Use "nightly"
qn	Nightly or at bedtime	Mistaken as "qh" (every hour)	Use "nightly" or "at bedtime"
q.o.d. or QOD**	Every other day	Mistaken as "q.d." (daily) or "q.i.d. (four times daily) if the "o" is poorly written	Use "every other day"
q1d	Daily	Mistaken as q.i.d. (four times daily)	Use "daily"
q6PM, etc.	Every evening at 6 PM	Mistaken as every 6 hours	Use "daily at 6 PM" or "6 PM daily"
SC, SQ, sub q	Subcutaneous	SC mistaken as SL (sublingual); SQ mistaken as "5 every;" the "q" in "sub q" has been mistaken as "every" (e.g., a heparin dose ordered "sub q 2 hours before surgery" misunderstood as every 2 hours before surgery)	Use "subcut" or "subcutaneously"
ss	Sliding scale (insulin) or ½ (apothecary)	Mistaken as "55"	Spell out "sliding scale;" use "one-half" or "½"

Table 16-2 | ISMP ERROR PRONE ABBREVIATIONS *continued*

ABBREVIATIONS	INTENDED MEANING	MISINTERPRETATION	CORRECTION
SSRI	Sliding scale regular insulin	Mistaken as selective-serotonin reuptake inhibitor	Spell out "sliding scale (insulin)"
SSI	Sliding scale insulin	Mistaken as Strong Solution of Iodine (Lugol's)	
i/d	One daily	Mistaken as "tid"	Use "1 daily"
TIW or tiw	3 times a week	Mistaken as "3 times a day" or "twice in a week"	Use "3 times weekly"
U or u**	Unit	Mistaken as the number 0 or 4, causing a 10-fold overdose or greater (e.g., 4U seen as "40" or 4u seen as "44"); mistaken as "cc" so dose given in volume instead of units (e.g., 4u seen as 4cc)	Use "unit"
UD	As directed ("ut dictum")	Mistaken as unit dose (e.g., diltiazem 125 mg IV infusion "UD" misinterpreted as meaning to give the entire infusion as a unit [bolus] dose)	Use "as directed"

DOSE DESIGNATIONS AND OTHER INFORMATION	INTENDED MEANING	MISINTERPRETATION	CORRECTION
Trailing zero after decimal point (e.g., 1.0 mg)**	1 mg	Mistaken as 10 mg if the decimal point is not seen	Do not use trailing zeros for doses expressed in whole numbers
"Naked" decimal point (e.g., .5 mg)**	0.5 mg	Mistaken as 5 mg if the decimal point is not seen	Use zero before a decimal point when the dose is less than a whole unit
Abbreviations such as mg. or mL. with a period following the abbreviation	mg mL	The period is unnecessary and could be mistaken as the number 1 if written poorly	Use mg, mL, etc. without a terminal period
Drug name and dose run together (especially problematic for drug names that end in "l" such as Inderal40 mg; Tegretol300 mg)	Inderal 40 mg Tegretol 300 mg	Mistaken as Inderal 140 mg Mistaken as Tegretol 1300 mg	Place adequate space between the drug name, dose, and unit of measure
Numerical dose and unit of measure run together (e.g., 10mg, 100mL)	10 mg 100 mL	The "m" is sometimes mistaken as a zero or two zeros, risking a 10- to 100-fold overdose	Place adequate space between the dose and unit of measure
Large doses without properly placed commas (e.g., 100000 units; 1000000 units)	100,000 units 1,000,000 units	100000 has been mistaken as 10,000 or 1,000,000; 1000000 has been mistaken as 100,000	Use commas for dosing units at or above 1,000, or use words such as 100 "thousand" or 1 "million" to improve readability

DRUG NAME ABBREVIATIONS	INTENDED MEANING	MISINTERPRETATION	CORRECTION
To avoid confusion, do not abbreviate drug names when communicating medical information. Examples of drug name abbreviations involved in medication errors include:			
APAP	acetaminophen	Not recognized as acetaminophen	Use complete drug name
ARA A	vidarabine	Mistaken as cytarabine (ARA C)	Use complete drug name
AZT	zidovudine (Retrovir)	Mistaken as azathioprine or aztreonam	Use complete drug name
CPZ	Compazine (prochlorperazine)	Mistaken as chlorpromazine	Use complete drug name

(continued)

Table 16-2 ISMP ERROR PRONE ABBREVIATIONS *continued*

DRUG NAME ABBREVIATIONS	INTENDED MEANING	MISINTERPRETATION	CORRECTION
DPT	Demerol-Phenergan-Thorazine	Mistaken as diphtheria-pertussis-tetanus (vaccine)	Use complete drug name
DTO	Diluted tincture of opium, or deodorized tincture of opium (Paregoric)	Mistaken as tincture of opium	Use complete drug name
HCl	hydrochloric acid or hydrochloride	Mistaken as potassium chloride (The "H" is misinterpreted as "K")	Use complete drug name unless expressed as a salt of a drug
HCT	hydrocortisone	Mistaken as hydrochlorothiazide	Use complete drug name
HCTZ	hydrochlorothiazide	Mistaken as hydrocortisone (seen as HCT250 mg)	Use complete drug name
MgSO4**	magnesium sulfate	Mistaken as morphine sulfate	Use complete drug name
MS, MSO4**	morphine sulfate	Mistaken as magnesium sulfate	Use complete drug name
MTX	methotrexate	Mistaken as mitoxantrone	Use complete drug name
PCA	procainamide	Mistaken as patient controlled analgesia	Use complete drug name
PTU	propylthiouracil	Mistaken as mercaptopurine	Use complete drug name
T3	Tylenol with codeine No. 3	Mistaken as liothyronine	Use complete drug name
TAC	triamcinolone	Mistaken as tetracaine, Adrenalin, cocaine	Use complete drug name
TNK	TNKase	Mistaken as "TPA"	Use complete drug name
ZnSO4	zinc sulfate	Mistaken as morphine sulfate	Use complete drug name

STEMMED DRUG NAMES	INTENDED MEANING	MISINTERPRETATION	CORRECTION
"Nitro" drip	nitroglycerin infusion	Mistaken as sodium nitroprusside infusion	Use complete drug name
"Norflox"	norfloxacin	Mistaken as Norflex	Use complete drug name
"IV Vanc"	intravenous vancomycin	Mistaken as Invanz	Use complete drug name

SYMBOLS	INTENDED MEANING	MISINTERPRETATION	CORRECTION
ℨ	Dram	Symbol for dram mistaken as "3"	Use the metric system
ℳ	Minim	Symbol for minim mistaken as "mL"	
x3d	For three days	Mistaken as "3 doses"	Use "for three days"
> and <	Greater than and less than	Mistaken as opposite of intended; mistakenly use incorrect symbol; "< 10" mistaken as "40"	Use "greater than" or "less than"
/ (slash mark)	Separates two doses or indicates "per"	Mistaken as the number 1 (e.g., "25 units/10 units" misread as "25 units and 110" units)	Use "per" rather than a slash mark to separate doses
@	At	Mistaken as "2"	Use "at"
&	And	Mistaken as "2"	Use "and"
+	Plus or and	Mistaken as "4"	Use "and"
°	Hour	Mistaken as a zero (e.g., q2° seen as q 20)	Use "hr," "h," or "hour"
Φ or ⌀	zero, null sign	Mistaken as numerals 4, 6, 8, and 9	Use 0 or zero, or describe intent using whole words

**These abbreviations are included on The Joint Commission's "minimum list" of dangerous abbreviations, acronyms, and symbols that must be included on an organization's "Do Not Use" list, effective January 1, 2004. Visit www.jointcommission.org for more information about this Joint Commission requirement.

Table 16-3   JOINT COMMISSION OFFICIAL "DO NOT USE" LIST[a]

DO NOT USE	POTENTIAL PROBLEM	USE INSTEAD
U, u (for unit)	Mistaken for "0" (zero), the number "4" (four), or "cc"	Write "unit"
IU (International Unit)	Mistaken for IV (intravenous) or the number 10 (ten)	Write "International Unit"
Q.D., QD, q.d., qd (daily)	Mistaken for each other.	Write "daily"
Q.O.D., QOD, q.o.d, qod (every other day)	Period after the Q mistaken for "I" and the "O" mistaken for "I"	Write "every other day"
Trailing zero (X.0 mg)[b]	Decimal point is missed.	Write X mg
Lack of leading zero (.X mg)		Write 0.X mg
MS	Can mean morphine sulfate or magnesium sulfate	Write "morphine sulfate" Write "magnesium sulfate"
MSO₄ and MgSO₄	Confused for one another.	

[a]Applies to all orders and all medication-related documentation that is handwritten (including free-text computer entry) or on preprinted forms.
[b]Exception: A "trailing zero" may be used only when required to demonstrate the level of precision of the value being reported, such as for laboratory results, imaging studies that report the size of lesions, or catheter/tube sizes. It may not be used in medication orders or other medication-related documentation.

©The Joint Commission, 2013 Reprinted with permission. Available at http://www.jointcommission.org/assets/1/18/Do_Not_Use_List.pdf

physicians, different teams of residents, an assigned social worker or case manager, assorted therapists, a hospital chaplain, and many nurses. Because these people are never all in the same room at the same time, the patient record is the primary means of communication. A nurse may check the patient record to see if the physician has spoken with the patient or the patient's surrogate about a do-not-resuscitate order. The physician may read the nurse's note to see how the family is responding to the recommendation to withhold or withdraw life-sustaining treatment.

Note also that other health care professionals make judgments about nurses and nursing's contributions to the health care team partially on the basis of what is documented in the patient record.

Diagnostic and Therapeutic Orders

Patient records also include diagnostic and therapeutic orders. Anyone reviewing the chart can find all the diagnostic studies ordered for the patient since admission, the results of these studies, and related orders for care. Illegible handwritten notes and typos have been the source of many errors. Whenever you are unsure of what has been written or entered in an electronic record, check the order. Never guess about what is written. A patient's life and your license are literally at risk if you incorrectly transcribe or execute an order.

VERBAL ORDERS

In most agencies, the only circumstance in which an attending physician, nurse practitioner, or house officer may issue orders verbally is in a medical emergency when the physician/nurse practitioner is present but finds it impossible, due to the emergency situation, to write the order. The order must be given directly by the physician or nurse practitioner to a registered professional nurse or registered professional pharmacist, who receives, reads back, documents, and executes

the order. In "**read back**," the recipient reads back the message as he or she heard and interpreted it. The person giving the order then confirms that such recording and interpretation of the order is correct. Verbal orders may not be given, received, or executed under any other circumstances. A sample policy for verbal orders follows:

A. The registered professional nurse or registered professional pharmacist who receives the verbal order will:
   1. Record the orders in the patient's medical record.
   2. Read back the order to verify accuracy of the order.
   3. Date and note the time the orders were issued during the emergency.
   4. Record VOs (verbal orders), the name of the physician or nurse practitioner who issued the orders, followed by the nurse's own name and title.
B. Immediately after the conclusion of the emergency, the physician or nurse practitioner who issued the verbal orders must:
   1. Review the orders to ascertain whether they are correct
   2. Sign the orders with name, title, and pager number
   3. Date and note the time he or she signs the orders
C. The registered professional nurse must see that the orders are transcribed according to procedure.

"Recommendations to ameliorate potential dangers associated with verbally communicated orders include 'read-backs' and other strategies to improve the safety of verbal orders and/or limit their use, and to ensure that the verbal communication was understood and accurately transcribed into the hospitals' ordering systems" (Wakefield et al., 2012, p. 11).

Care Planning

Each health care professional working with the patient has access to the patient's baseline and ongoing data and can see how the patient is responding to the treatment plan from day to day. For example, if recorded data indicate that a patient is gradually becoming weaker and cannot now tolerate ambulation, orders for physical therapy and other nurse-initiated ambulation need to be modified. Modifications of the plan of care are based on these data.

 THINK back to Phillippe Baron, the patient who had undergone a colonoscopy. The nurse uses the patient's chart to obtain information about the patient, including events of the colonoscopy and how the patient responded, to develop an individualized discharge teaching plan. ●

Quality Process and Performance Improvement

"Documentation is the primary source of evidence used to continuously measure performance outcomes against predetermined standards" (ANA, 2010, p. 7). Records might be reviewed to evaluate the quality of care patients have received and the competence of the nurses providing that care. For example, in a nursing audit, a committee decides in advance the standards of care it wants to evaluate (e.g., pertaining to nursing assessment, nursing documentation, or safety measures). A number of records are then randomly selected and reviewed for evidence that the nurses met the selected standards of care. If deficiencies are found, in-service training can be used to remedy the problem and improve the quality of care. Accrediting agencies, such as the Joint Commission, might also use record review to determine whether a particular agency or health care institution is meeting its standards.

Research

Researchers might study patient records, hoping to learn how best to recognize or treat identified health problems from the study of similar cases. The aim is to promote evidence-based practice in nursing and quality health care.

Decision Analysis

Information from record review often provides the data needed by administrative strategic planners to identify needs as well as the means and strategies most likely to address these needs. Record review might reveal both underused and overused services, patients with prolonged stays who require special assistance, and financial information about which services generate revenue compared with those that cost the institution or agency money.

Education

Health care professionals and students reading a patient's record can learn a great deal about the clinical manifestations of particular health problems, effective treatment modalities, and factors that affect patient goal achievement.

Credentialing, Regulation, and Legislation

Documentation allows reviewers to monitor health care practitioners' and the health care facility's compliance with standards governing the profession and provision of care.

Legal Documentation

Patient records are legal documents that might be used as evidence in court proceedings. One in four malpractice suits are decided on the basis of the patient's record. Documentation plays an important role in implicating or absolving health care practitioners charged with improper care. The record can also be used in accident or injury claims made by the patient. No nurse can afford to be ignorant of or careless about agency policies and professional standards for documentation.

Reimbursement

Patient records are used to demonstrate to payers (e.g., insurance companies) that patients received the intensity and quality of care for which reimbursement is being sought.

Historical Documentation

Because all entries on records are dated, the record has value as a historical document. Years later, information concerning a patient's past health care might be pertinent.

Methods of Documentation

While the different methods of documentation might initially seem confusing, each is designed to achieve certain aims. Understanding a variety of systems helps nurses adapt quickly in new practice settings.

Computerized Documentation and Electronic Health Records (EHRs)

Increasingly, computer systems are used for nursing documentation in the patient record. In such systems the nurse may:

1. Call up the admission assessment tool on the computer screen and key in patient data (see Chapter 11 for illustrations)
2. Develop the plan of care using computerized care plans available for each North American Nursing Diagnosis Association (NANDA)–approved diagnosis or approved problem list
3. Add to the patient database as new data are identified and modify the plan of care accordingly
4. Receive a work list showing the treatments, procedures, and medications necessary for each patient throughout the shift
5. Document care immediately using the computer terminal at the patient's bedside

According to the Office of the National Coordinator for Health Information Technology (ONC), once fully functional and exchangeable, the benefits of electronic health records (EHRs) offer far more than a paper record can do ("Benefits of electronic health records," n.d.). EHRs:

• Improve quality and convenience of patient care
• Increase patient participation in their care (see Figure 16-1)
• Improve accuracy of diagnoses and health outcomes
• Improve care coordination

FIGURE 16-1. Computerized bedside charting allows the nurse to remain in contact with the patient while electronically documenting patient information. *(Photo by B. Proud.)*

- Increase practice efficiencies and cost savings. For this reason the Medicare and Medicaid EHR incentive programs provide a financial incentive for achieving **meaningful use**, which is the use of certified EHR technology to achieve health and efficiency goals. The ultimate goal is to bring about health care that is patient centered, evidence based, prevention- oriented, efficient, and equitable.
- Service elements (such as admission and discharge dates and expected payer for services)

With computer-based records, or **electronic health records (EHRs)**, data can be distributed among many caregivers in a standardized format, allowing them to compare and uniformly evaluate patient progress easily. Besides tracking the progress of individual patients, computerized outcome information can compare the progress of groups of patients with similar diagnoses. These results will contribute to research, education, and, ultimately, better and more efficient nursing practice. Table 16-4 describes terms used to discuss electronic records in health care.

The Agency for Healthcare Research and Quality (AHRQ, 2012) reports the following:

- Nurses from hospitals with fully implemented EHRs were significantly less likely to report unfavorable outcomes compared to nurses working in hospitals without fully implemented EHRs.
- Fewer nurses in the fully implemented hospitals reported frequent medication errors, poor quality of care, and poor confidence in a patient being ready for discharge. These nurses also had a 14% decrease in the odds of reporting that "things fell between the cracks" when patients were transferred between units. They were also less likely to report that patient safety is a low priority for hospital management.

With the increasing use of computerized patient information systems to store and analyze patient data have come policies and procedures to ensure the privacy and confidentiality of patient information. Policies should specify what types of patient information can be retrieved, by whom, and for what purpose. Patient consent is necessary for the use and release of any stored information that can be linked to the patient.

The American Nurses Association, the American Medical Record Association, and the Canadian Nurses Association offer the following guidelines and strategies for safe computer charting:

- Never give your personal password or computer signature to anyone, including another nurse in the unit, a float nurse, or a doctor.

Table 16-4	DESCRIPTIONS OF TERMS USED TO DISCUSS ELECTRONIC RECORDS IN HEALTH CARE	

ENTITY	DESCRIPTION
Health care smart card	The health care smart card is similar to a credit card, with a magnetic strip that either contains vital emergency health care information or creates a link to information in another location. Using the cardholder's personal identification number (PIN) and entering the card into a reader enables emergency providers to retrieve designated health-related information about a given patient. People should always carry their PIN with them to permit access in an emergency.
Electronic Health Record (EHR)	The EHR is the patient care record created when agencies under different ownership share their data. The goal is for this sharing to be nationwide, creating a situation in which a person's health care record is accessible by designated health care providers anywhere in the nation. The patient will decide which portions of a record will be available to whom.
Electronic Medical Record (EMR)	An EMR is an electronic patient care record created by an agency or agencies having common ownership. Although these EMRs today are often called EHRs, they are not true EHRs because the data is not shared between providers in agencies under different ownership.
Health Information Exchange (HIE)	An HIE is an organization that provides services to enable the electronic sharing of health-related information.
Electronic database	An electronic database is a collection of data that allows easy searching and easy retrieval of similar pieces of data from many records.

Adapted from Thede, L. (2008). The electronic health record: Will nursing be on board when the ship leaves? *OJIN: The Online Journal of Issues in Nursing, 13*(3). Available at www.nursingworld.org/MainMenuCategories/ANAMarketplace/ANAPeriodicals/OJIN/Columns/Informatics/Electronic HealthRecord.aspx

- Don't leave a computer terminal unattended after you have logged on.
- Follow the correct protocol for correcting errors. To correct an error after it has been entered, mark the entry "mistaken entry," add the correct information, and date and initial the entry. If you record information in the wrong chart, write "mistaken entry—wrong chart" and sign off. Follow similar guidelines in electronic records.
- Never create, change, or delete records unless you have specific authority to do so.
- If you inadvertently delete part of the permanent record, type an explanation into the computer file with the date, time, and your initials, and submit an explanation in writing to your manager.
- Don't leave information about a patient displayed on a monitor where others may see it. Keep a log that accounts for every printout of a computerized file that you've generated from the system.
- Never use e-mail to send protected health information unless it has been encrypted to protect it from unauthorized access.
- Follow the agency's confidentiality procedures for documenting sensitive material, such as a diagnosis of acquired immunodeficiency syndrome (AIDS) or human immunodeficiency virus (HIV) infection.

Remember, each time you log in to an electronic medical record with your password you create a trail that can be traced.

PERSONAL HEALTH RECORDS (PHRs)

Many people today are preparing online **personal health records (PHRs)** to manage their health care via computer. These records contain the person's medical history, including diagnoses, symptoms, and medications. Some patients scan in doctors' notes, test results, CT images, and insurance information. They may give health care professionals their password so that they can log on, and may give permission to share the record with other family members. The chief reason for a personal health record is to provide easy access to up-to-date, complete health information to assist in self-care and communication with providers. Patients with chronic illnesses and caregivers who care for children or aging adults with complex medical histories and needs are most likely to benefit from comprehensive digital medical records. ONC differentiates two types of PHRs ("Are there different types," n.d.):

- *Standalone Personal Health Records:* With a standalone PHR, patients fill in information from their own records, and the information is stored on patients' computers or the Internet. In some cases, a standalone PHR can also accept data from external sources, including providers and laboratories. With a standalone PHR, patients could add diet or exercise information to track progress over time. Patients can decide whether to share the information with providers, family members, or anyone else involved in their care.
- *Tethered/Connected Personal Health Records:* A tethered, or connected, PHR is linked to a specific health care organization's electronic health record (EHR) system or to a health plan's information system. With a tethered PHR, patients can access their own records through a secure portal and see, for example, the trend of their lab results over the last year, their immunization history, or due dates for screenings.

When talking with patients who are considering using a personal health record, advise them to check the service's privacy policy carefully to see how much control they will have over their information and whether the service can share or exchange their data, and ask their health care providers if they are willing to read their PHR.

An informational website, www.myPHR.com, offers a guide to creating a personal health care record, how-to information on obtaining medical records, privacy rights, and downloadable health record forms. Other suggestions for online and password-protected PHR products that let users upload and input a wide variety of personal health information include:

- http://www.medicare.gov/manage-your-health/personal-health-records/personal-health-records.html
- www.thesmartphr.com

HEALTH INFORMATION EXCHANGE (HIE)

An electronic **health information exchange (HIE)** allows doctors, nurses, pharmacists, other health care providers, and patients to appropriately access and securely share a patient's vital medical information electronically—improving the speed, quality, safety, and cost of patient care. Appropriate, timely sharing of vital patient information can better inform decision making at the point of care and allows providers to avoid readmission and medication errors, improve diagnoses, and decrease duplicate testing ("Health information exchange," n.d.). Benefits of an HIE include:

- Provides a vehicle for improving quality and safety of patient care
- Provides a basic level of interoperability among EHRs maintained by individual physicians and organizations
- Stimulates consumer education and patients' involvement in their own health care
- Helps public health officials meet their commitment to the community
- Creates a potential loop for feedback between health-related research and actual practice
- Facilitates efficient deployment of emerging technology and health care services
- Provides the backbone of technical infrastructure for leverage by national and state-level initiatives ("Health information exchange," n.d.).

The following resources provide more information about electronic health and medical records and health information exchange:

- American Nursing Informatics Association (www.ania.org)
- HealthIT.gov (www.healthit.gov/)

- HealthcareITNews (www.healthcareitnews.com)
- HIMSS—Transforming health through IT (www.himss.org)

Source-Oriented Records

Many nurses, especially in rural and underserved areas, continue to practice in settings not using electronic medical records. Traditional paper records are still used in such settings, including a variety of different formats. A **source-oriented record** is a paper format in which each health care group keeps data on its own separate form. Sections of the record are designated for nurses, physicians, laboratory, x-ray personnel, and so on. Notations are entered chronologically, with the most recent entry being nearest the front of the record. An advantage of the source-oriented record is that each discipline can easily find and chart pertinent data. The main disadvantage is that data are fragmented, making it difficult to track problems chronologically with input from different groups of professionals.

Although the specifics vary among health agencies, the general characteristics of source-oriented records are essentially the same. Types of forms typically used in a source-oriented patient record are shown in Table 16-5 (on page 354). Notes written to inform caregivers of the progress a patient is making toward achieving expected outcomes are called **progress notes**. Progress notes written by nurses in a source-oriented record are **narrative notes** and address routine care, normal findings (findings that do not call for changes in the plan of care), and patient problems identified in the plan of care. They include a description of the status of the problem, related nursing interventions, patient responses, and needed revisions to the plan of care.

Problem-Oriented Medical Records

Another type of paper record used in some health agencies is the **problem-oriented medical record (POMR)**, or problem-oriented record, originated by Dr. Lawrence Weed in the 1960s (See a sample POMR on thePoint). The POMR is organized around a patient's problems rather than around sources of information. With POMRs, all health care professionals record information on the same forms. The advantages of this type of record are that the entire health care team works together in identifying a master list of patient problems and contributes collaboratively to the plan of care. Progress notes clearly focus on patient problems. The POMR includes the defined database, problem list, care plans, and progress notes.

The **SOAP format** (**S**ubjective data, **O**bjective data, **A**ssessment [the caregiver's judgment about the situation], **P**lan) is used to organize entries in the progress notes of the POMR. Caregivers select numbered problems from the master list on the front of the patient record and then work up the problem or "SOAP it" on the progress sheet. Some nurses believe that the SOAP method of charting focuses too narrowly on problems and advocate instead a return to the traditional narrative format. Variants of the SOAP format include SOAPE, SOAPIE, and SOAPIER (**I**ntervention, **E**valuation, and **R**esponse).

PIE—Problem, Intervention, Evaluation

The **PIE charting** system is unique in that it does not develop a separate plan of care. The plan of care is incorporated into the progress notes, which identify problems by number (in the order they are identified). In this documentation system, a patient assessment is performed and documented at the beginning of each shift using preprinted fill-in-the-blank assessment forms (flow sheets). Patient problems identified in these assessments are numbered, documented in the progress notes, worked up using the **P**roblem, **I**ntervention, **E**valuation (PIE) format, and evaluated each shift. Resolved problems are dropped from daily documentation following the nurse's review. Continuing problems are documented and numbered each day. One advantage of this system is that it promotes continuity of care. It also saves time because there is no separate plan of care. The disadvantage of not having a formal care plan is that nurses need to read all the nursing notes to determine problems and planned interventions before initiating care. Unlike the SOAP method, which originated from the medical record, the PIE format has a nursing origin (See a sample PIE patient care note on thePoint).

Focus Charting

The purpose of **focus charting** is to bring the focus of care back to the patient and the patient's concerns. Instead of a problem list or list of nursing or medical diagnoses, a focus column is used that incorporates many aspects of a patient and patient care. The focus might be a patient strength, problem, or need. Topics that may appear in the focus column include patient concerns and behaviors, therapies and responses, changes of condition, and significant events such as teaching, consultations, monitoring, management of activities of daily living, or assessment of functional health patterns. The narrative portion of focus charting uses the **D**ata, **A**ction, **R**esponse (DAR) format (Fig. 16-2 on page 355). The principal advantage of focus charting is the holistic emphasis on the patient and the patient's priorities. Ease of charting is also cited as an advantage of focus charting because each note does not need to incorporate data, action, and response. Some nurses report, however, that the DAR categories are artificial and not helpful when documenting care.

 FOR Mr. Baron, the nurse may use focus charting to document specific aspects of teaching related to the colonoscopy and postprocedural care. In addition, due to the effects of anesthesia from the colonoscopy procedure, Mr. Baron might not completely remember all that is taught. Therefore, the nurse documents to include the patient's wife in the discharge teaching to ensure that the information taught was indeed understood. Remember that Mrs. Baron is a nurse. Her clinical knowledge and any necessary reinforcement of information would also be documented. ●

Charting by Exception

Charting by exception (CBE) is a shorthand documentation method that makes use of well-defined standards of

Table 16-5 EXAMPLES OF FORMS AND INFORMATION IN SOURCE-ORIENTED PATIENT RECORDS

FORM	TYPICAL CLIENT INFORMATION
Admission sheet	Legal name, identification number Age, birth date, sex Marital status Occupation and employer Religious preference Next of kin and person to notify in case of emergency Date, time, reason for admission Name of the attending physician Insurance information Discharge data
Admission nursing assessment (See Chapter 11)	Results of nursing history and physical assessment
Graphic sheet	Daily temperatures, pulse and respiratory rates, blood pressure (vital signs), pain level Daily weight Special measurements, such as the patient's fluid intake and output
Flow sheet to record routine care (see Fig. 16-5, p. 358)	Respiratory Hygiene Cardiac Activity Pain Sleep Nutrition Safety Elimination Equipment IV therapy Teaching Wound Progress sheet Tubes
Narrative nurse's notes	Descriptions of pertinent observations of patient Statements that specify the nursing care, including teaching, received by patient and patient's responses to nursing care Statements that describe patient's condition and progress, or lack of progress, toward recovery and goal achievement Descriptions of patient's complaints and how patient is coping or failing to cope with them, and nursing's response
Medication sheet (see Chapter 28)	Name of prescribed medications administered on a regular or PRN basis Dosage of medication administered Route by which medication was administered, unless given orally Time medication was administered Name or initials of person administering the medication
Medical history and examination sheet	Results of physical examination performed by physician Current medical condition Health history, including previous illnesses Family medical history Confirmed or tentative diagnosis Plan of medical therapy
Physician's order sheet	Orders for medications Orders for treatments Other directives pertinent to a particular patient's care
Physician's progress notes	Interpretations of patient's pathology Responses of patient to medical therapy
Miscellaneous forms	Laboratory reports X-ray film reports Consultation reports Dietary requirements Results of social service consultations Types and results of physical, respiratory, and x-ray therapy

Date/Time	Focus	Patient Care Notes
7/11/15 9:15 am	High risk for trauma	**DATA:** *Patient crying when I entered room; confided that she is afraid to go home because her injuries are the result of husband's battery* **ACTION:** *Attending notified and discharge cancelled; Abuse network called with patient's permission and they are sending a counselor this afternoon to talk with her.* ————————————————————————— — *C. Taylor, RN*
10:00 am	Pain	**DATA:** *Patient complaining of pain in right rib area* **ACTION:** *Tylenol 3 administered as ordered.*————————— ————————————————————————— — *C. Taylor, RN*
10:30 am	Pain	**RESPONSE:** *Patient reports relief from rib pain, still anxious about aftermath of discharge.*———————————— ————————————————————————— — *C. Taylor, RN*

FIGURE 16-2. Sample focus patient care notes.

practice; only significant findings or "exceptions" to these standards are documented in narrative notes. Benefits of this approach include less time needed for charting (freeing more time for direct patient care), a greater emphasis on significant data, easy retrieval of significant data, timely bedside charting, standardized assessment, greater interdisciplinary communication, better tracking of important patient responses, and lower costs.

A significant drawback to charting by exception is its limited usefulness when trying to prove that high-quality safe care was given if a negligence claim is made against nursing. As more facilities move to a totally electronic medical record, even facilities not previously using a CBE system are considering doing so.

Case Management Model

Managed care's emphasis on quality, cost-effective care delivered within a limited time frame has led to the development of interdisciplinary documentation tools that clearly identify those outcomes that select groups of patients are expected to achieve on each day of care. The case management model promotes collaboration, communication, and teamwork among caregivers; makes efficient use of time; and increases quality by focusing care on carefully developed outcomes. One limitation of this model, however, is that it works best for "typical" patients with few individualized needs. At present, there is little consensus about which documentation tools are best for recording routine aspects of care and avoiding repetition.

COLLABORATIVE PATHWAYS

Collaborative pathways (may also be called **critical pathways** or **care maps**) are used in the case management model. The collaborative pathway specifies the plan of care linked to expected outcomes along a timeline (see the example in Chapter 13). In some documentation systems, the collaborative pathway is part of a computerized documentation system that integrates the collaborative pathway and documentation flow sheets designed to match each day's

expected outcomes. Charting by exception is frequently used with collaborative pathway documentation systems.

OCCURRENCE CHARTING

When a patient fails to meet an expected outcome or a planned intervention is not implemented in the case management model, this variance from the plan is documented. The usual format for **occurrence** or **variance charting** is the unexpected event, the cause of the event, actions taken in response to the event, and discharge planning, when appropriate. The variances most likely to be documented are those that affect quality, cost, or length of stay.

 CONSIDER Millie Delong, the woman who developed a wound infection. Typically, after abdominal surgery, infection is a complication, not a normal or expected occurrence. Therefore, using the case management model, the nurse needs to document this unexpected outcome with variance charting. ●

Formats for Nursing Documentation

When the nursing process is fully implemented, nursing documentation in the patient's permanent record includes the following formats.

Initial Nursing Assessment

A typical electronic form used to record the initial database obtained from the nursing history and physical assessment is illustrated in Chapter 11. Accurate documentation of these data is important to provide a baseline for later comparisons as the patient's condition changes.

 THINK back to Jason Chandler, the adolescent brought to the emergency department in police custody. Due to the nature of the admission, a complete nursing assessment would be inappropriate. However, the nurse needs to thoroughly assess the patient for signs and symptoms indicating problems associated with swallowing the bag of drugs. Later on,

FIGURE 16-3. Electronic patient care summary. (© Cerner Corporation. All rights reserved. Used with permission.)

once the initial situation is resolved, an initial history and physical examination would be performed. ●

Care Plan

Patient records must communicate the patient's problems or diagnoses; related goals, outcomes, and interventions; and progress or resolution of the problems. The nursing plan of care may be written separately or incorporated into a multidisciplinary plan. In a traditional plan of nursing care, nursing diagnoses, goals and expected outcomes, and nursing interventions are written for each patient (see the sample student plan in Chapter 13 and the plans of care at the end of each clinical chapter). Standardized plans of care may also be used that identify common problems and related care for select patient groups. These generally incorporate standards of high-quality care, but unless such care plans are individualized, they might not sufficiently address individual patient needs. Formats for plans of care vary greatly.

Patient Care Summary

The patient care summary contains an overview of valuable patient information such as documentation, lab and test results, orders, and medications. Figure 16-3 shows one such example.

Critical/Collaborative Pathways

The case management plan is a detailed, standardized plan of care that is developed for a patient population with a designated diagnosis or procedure. It includes expected outcomes, a list of interventions to be performed, and the sequence and timing of those interventions. The critical/collaborative pathway, illustrated in Chapter 13, is an abbreviated summary of key information taken from the more detailed case management plan.

Progress Notes

The purpose of progress notes is to inform caregivers of the progress a patient is making toward achieving expected outcomes. The method used to record the patient's progress depends on the documentation system being used. Common examples include narrative nursing notes, SOAP notes, PIE notes, focus charting, charting by exception, and the case management model. Figure 16-4 shows an example of a home hospice nurse's charting following a home visit.

FIGURE 16-4. Electronic nursing documentation following a home hospice visit. (© Cerner Corporation. All rights reserved. Used with permission.)

Flow Sheets and Graphic Records

Flow sheets are documentation tools used to efficiently record routine aspects of nursing care (see Fig. 16-5 on page 358). Well-designed flow sheets enable nurses to quickly document the routine aspects of care that promote patient goal achievement, safety, and well-being. The **graphic record** is a form used to record specific patient variables such as pulse, respiratory rate, blood pressure readings, body temperature, weight, fluid intake and output, bowel movements, and other patient characteristics.

A graphic record would be used for both Millie Delong and Phillippe Baron, described at the beginning of the chapter. Specifically for Ms. Delong, documentation of vital signs is significant because she has wound infection. Because Mr. Baron is postcolonoscopy, his vital signs also need to be assessed frequently. In addition, fluid intake and output are key postoperative assessment findings to be documented. ●

Medication Record

The patient's medication record must include documentation of all the medications administered to the patient (drug, dose, route, time), the nurse administering the drug, and for some medications (e.g., analgesics), the reason the drug was administered and its effectiveness. Sample medication records are shown in Chapter 28.

Acuity Records

Twenty-four-hour reports are increasingly used in conjunction with acuity reports, with which nurses rank patients as high-to-low acuity in relation to both the patient's condition and need for nursing assistance or intervention. A trauma patient whose condition is changing rapidly and who requires intensive nurse monitoring and intervention merits a higher acuity rank than a patient whose condition is stable. Acuity rankings are often used to determine staffing requirements. A nursing unit with patients with higher acuity rankings requires more professional nurses than a unit with the same number of patients who have lower acuity ranks.

Discharge and Transfer Summary

When a patient is discharged from care or transferred from one unit, institution, or agency to another, a **discharge summary** should be written that concisely summarizes the reason for treatment, significant findings, the procedures performed and treatment rendered, the patient's condition on discharge or transfer, and any specific pertinent instructions given to the patient and family. You can imagine how frustrating it would be for patients and their family caregivers to arrive in a new treatment setting and have to inform

08 March 2015 00:00 EST - 10 March 2015 23:59 EDT						
Today's Intake: 100 Output: 0 Balance: 100		Yesterday's Intake: Output: Balance:				
	C3/09/15					
	11:00 EDT - 11:59 EDT	12:00 EDT - 12:59 EDT	1300 EDT - 13:59 EDT	14:00 EDT - 14:59 EDT	15:00 EDT - 15:59 EDT	Evening Shift Total
− Intake Total	100					100
− Continuous Infusions	100	☑	☑			100
Sodium Chloride 0.9%, Intravenous 1000 mL mL	100	100	100			100
− Medications						
− Transfusions						
− Output Total						
− Urine Output						
Urine Voided mL						
− Emesis Output						
− Gastric Tube Outputs						
Balance	100					100

FIGURE 16-5. Intake and output flow sheet. (© Cerner Corporation. All rights reserved. Used with permission.)

professional caregivers about their needs because the plan of care didn't accompany them. Review the discharge instructions in Chapter 9.

 CONSIDER Phillippe Baron, the man who had undergone a colonoscopy. The nurse is responsible for completing the discharge summary, making sure to include specific aspects of self-care teaching and both the patient's and wife's understanding of the teaching. ●

Home Health Care Documentation

Documentation of home health care visits that reports the patient's progress serves multiple purposes. Sent to the attending physician with a request for signed medical orders to continue treatment, these records ensure continuity of care. Sent to third-party payers, they establish the need for continuing home care with continued reimbursement for necessary services. Medicare, for example, reviews progress summaries to determine whether a patient meets one of these Medicare requirements:

- The patient is homebound and still needs skilled nursing care.
- Rehabilitation potential is good (or the patient is dying).
- The patient's status is not stabilized.
- The patient is making progress in expected outcomes of care.

The Outcome and Assessment Information Set, or **OASIS**, is a group of data elements that:

- Represent core items of a comprehensive assessment for an adult home care patient

- Form the basis for measuring patient outcomes for purposes of outcome-based quality improvement (OBQI)

The OASIS is a key component of Medicare's partnership with the home care industry to foster and monitor improved home health care outcomes. Overall, the OASIS items are useful for outcome monitoring, clinical assessment, care planning, and other internal agency-level applications. OASIS data items encompass sociodemographic, environmental, support system, health status, and functional status attributes of adult (nonmaternity) patients. In addition, selected attributes of health service use are included (see http://cms.hhs.gov/oasis). Chapter 9 contains a sample home health certification and a skilled nursing note.

Long-Term Care Documentation

Documentation in long-term care settings is specified by the Resident Assessment Instrument (RAI), which helps staff gather definitive information on a resident's strengths and needs and addresses these in an individualized plan of care. The RAI helps staff track changes in a resident's status by evaluating resident goal achievement and making appropriate revisions in the plan of care. The goal is to coordinate the efforts of the multidisciplinary team to ensure that residents achieve the highest level of functioning possible (quality of care) and maintain their sense of individuality (quality of life).

The RAI consists of four basic components:

- *Minimum data set:* A core set of screening, clinical, and functional status elements that forms the foundation of the comprehensive assessment of all residents in long-term care facilities certified to participate in Medicare or Medicaid. The items in the minimum data set standardize communication about resident problems and condition.

- *Triggers:* Specific resident responses for one or a combination of minimum data set elements that identify residents who either have or are at risk for developing specific functional problems and who require further evaluation using resident assessment protocols.
- *Resident assessment protocols:* Structured, problem-oriented frameworks for organizing minimum data set information and examining additional clinically relevant information about a resident. Resident assessment protocols help identify social, medical, nursing, and psychological problems and form the basis for individualized care planning.
- *Utilization guidelines:* Specified in state operation manuals that direct when and how to use the RAI.

Statutory law, federal regulations, and the Health Care Financing Administration specify how the RAI is implemented. An RAI must be completed for residents of Medicare skilled nursing facilities or Medicaid nursing facilities, hospice residents, and short-term stay or respite residents who reside in a facility for longer than 14 days.

Benefits of using the RAI process include the following:

- Residents respond to individualized care.
- Staff communication becomes more effective.
- Resident and family involvement increases.
- Documentation becomes clearer.

REPORTING CARE

To report is to give an account of something that has been seen, heard, done, or considered. Reporting is the oral, written, or computer-based communication of patient data to others. A laboratory report, for example, might communicate to the health care team that a patient's cardiac enzymes are normal or that a biopsy of breast tissue revealed malignant or atypical cells. A nurse's shift or hand-off report or nursing note might communicate the progress a patient is making toward goal achievement. Common methods for reporting among health practitioners, in addition to the patient record, include face-to-face meetings, telephone conversations, messengers, written messages, audiotaped messages, and computer messages. Each of these methods has certain benefits and limitations, as detailed in Table 16-6.

The Joint Commission included "managing hand-off communications" among its 2009 national patient-safety goals. The Institute for Health Care Improvement (www.ihi.org) is promoting the **ISBAR communication** (Identity/Introduction, Situation, Background, Assessment, Recommendation) technique as a framework for communication between members of the health care team about a patient's condition.

- *Identity/Introduction:* Communicate who you are, where you are, and why you are communicating.
- *Situation:* Communicate what is occurring and why the patient is being handed off to another department or unit.

Table 16-6 COMMON METHODS OF COMMUNICATION AMONG HEALTH CARE PROFESSIONALS

METHOD	ADVANTAGES	DISADVANTAGES
Face-to-face meeting	• Message can be delivered immediately. • Nonverbal messages are readily conveyed. • Message can be clarified; receiver's questions can be raised and answered.	• Both the communicating and the receiving people must be available at the same time, in the same place. • Ordinarily, there is no permanent record for later use.
Telephone conversation	• Message can be delivered immediately. • Message can be clarified; receiver's questions can be raised and answered. • Two parties need not be present in same place.	• Only the tone of voice and voice inflections can be communicated—no nonverbal messages unless skype or some other synchronous means are used. • Ordinarily, there is no permanent record.
Written message	• Message can be exchanged at times convenient for the people involved. • Record is available. • Time efficient if message is understood	• Message usually cannot be validated with the sender.
Audiotaped message	• Message can be exchanged at times convenient for the people involved. • Record is available. • Time efficient if information communicated is complete.	• Message usually cannot be validated with the sender.
Computer message	• Message can be delivered immediately—even to those at a great distance. • Parties need not be present in same place. • Two-way communication is possible by e-mail. • Record is available. • Many people can participate in exchange.	• No nonverbal messages can be communicated. • Privacy concerns remain an issue.

- *Background:* Explain what led up to the current situation and put in context if necessary.
- *Assessment:* Give your impression of the problem.
- *Recommendation:* Explain what you would do to correct the problem.

Note that there are different ISBAR formats: earlier versions used simply SBAR, and some newer versions use ISBARR, with the last R being a read-back of orders/response. See Chapters 9 and 20 for more on ISBAR and other frameworks for patient hand-offs. ISBAR is an easy-to-remember, concrete mechanism useful for framing any conversation, especially critical ones, requiring a clinician's immediate attention and action. It allows for an easy and focused way to set expectations for what will be communicated and how between members of the team, which is essential for developing teamwork and fostering a culture

of patient safety. Many students find calling their physician colleagues about changes in a patient's condition challenging. See Box 16-4 for suggestions about how to do this well.

Be professional whenever making a report about care. Ensure that you have all the pertinent data, and be concise. Most importantly, keep the report focused on the patient and avoid gossip, floor politics, and social plans. It is never professional to speak disrespectfully about a patient or family; such comments may negatively dispose a colleague to patients and the coming shift.

Change-of-Shift/Hand-off Reports

A **change-of-shift report** or **hand-off** is given by a primary nurse to the nurse replacing him or her or by the charge nurse to the nurse who assumes responsibility for continuing care of the patient. The change-of-shift report might be

BOX 16-4 ISBARR REPORT TO A PHYSICIAN

Before calling the physician:
1. Assess the patient.
2. Review the record for the appropriate physician to call.
3. Know the admitting diagnosis.
4. Read the most recent physician and nursing notes.

5. Have the record at hand and be ready to report allergies, medications, IV fluids, and lab and test results.
6. Every ISBARR report is different. Focus on the problem. Be concise. Not everything in the following outline needs to be reported—just what is needed for the situation.

I Identity/Introduction	State **NAME, TITLE**, and **UNIT**	I am Ellen McLoughlin, a Georgetown University nursing student, working on 3 Main.
S Situation	I am calling about: (**Patient Name and Room Number**) The **PROBLEM** I am calling about is:	I am calling about Ms. Miriam Klein, room 9. She is scheduled this morning for a prophylactic bilateral mastectomy to prevent breast cancer but she is now having second thoughts.
B Background	State **Admission Diagnosis and Admission Date** State Pertinent **Medical History** Brief Synopsis of **Treatment** if pertinent **Most recent Vital Signs** **Changes in VS** or **Assessment from Prior assessment**	Ms. Klein was admitted yesterday. She has a strong family history of breast and ovarian cancer. She tested positive earlier this year for *BRCA1* (breast cancer gene). She signed the informed consent for the mastectomy in your office and had all her preop testing done, but she has been up all night expressing second thoughts.
A Assessment	Give your conclusions about the present situation. Words like "might be" or "could be" are helpful. A diagnosis is not necessary. If the situation is unclear, at least try to indicate what **body system** might be involved. State how severe the problem seems to be. If appropriate, state that the problem could be **life threatening**.	This seems to be more than the usual presurgery jitters. She has clearly stated that she regrets signing the informed consent and wishes to withdraw her consent.
R Recommendation	Say what you think would be helpful or needs to be done (medications, treatment, tests, X-rays, EKG, CT, transfer to critical care, physician evaluation, consultant evaluation) Ask about any **Changes in Orders**	Shall I hold the preop orders and notify the OR that we need to place the surgery on hold until you can see her and determine if she wants this done? Is there anything else I can do at this time?
R Read Back	Restate orders you have been given. Clarify how often to do vital signs. Under what circumstances to call back.	I understand you want me to hold the preop medications and call the OR to place the surgery on hold. Thank you. I will tell her that you should be here within the hour.

Note: Be sure to document the change in condition and the physician notification.
Adapted from ISBARR (Critical Situation) Report, © Joint Commission Resources; and Enlow, M., Shanks, L., Guhde, J. & Perkins, M. (2010). Incorporating interprofessional communication skills (ISBARR) into an undergraduate nursing curriculum. *Nurse Educator, 35*(4), 176–180.

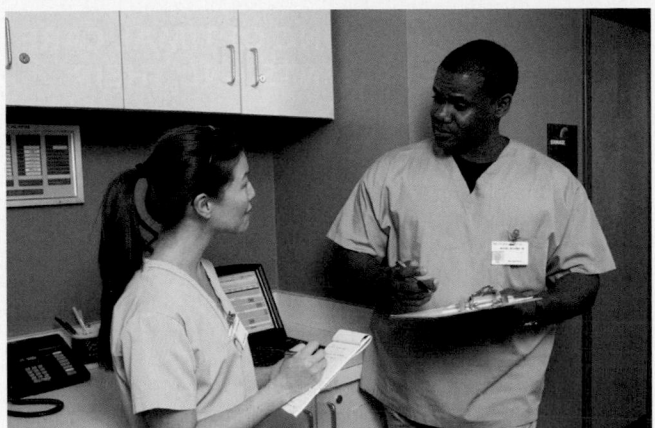

FIGURE 16-6. During a change-of-shift report, a nurse from the ending shift provides a summary of the patient's condition and current status of care to the nurse coming on duty. *(Photo by B. Proud.)*

given in written form or orally in a meeting (Fig. 16-6), or it may be audio- or videotaped. The trend today is toward a standardized, streamlined shift report system at the bedside (see Chapters 9 and 20), which is driven by patient safety and enhanced patient/family participation. Vital elements of the bedside report include the oncoming and outgoing nurse seeing the patient together, reviewing medication records and the physician's and nursing orders, and establishing patient goals for the shift.

Typical information shared among nurses, patients, and families in a change-of-shift report includes the following:

- Basic identifying information about each patient—name, room number, bed designation, diagnosis, and attending and consulting physicians
- Current appraisal of each patient's health status:
  - Changes in patient's status during your shift and the patient's response to medical therapy
  - Pertinent monitoring, lab, and/or radiology data; data that are irregular or data that have been noted to be irregular in the past and have now been resolved
  - Abnormal findings in your physical/head-to-toe assessment
  - Where the patient stands in relation to identified nursing diagnoses and goal achievement
  - Pain level and pain management needs
- Current orders (especially any newly changed orders):
  - Changes in medications, intravenous fluids, diet, toileting, and activity level
  - Upcoming or ongoing tests and procedures, and specific instructions for these such as NPO after midnight
- Abnormal occurrences during your shift
- Any unfilled orders that need to be continued onto the next shift
- Patient/family questions, concerns, needs
- Reports on patients who have been transferred or discharged

Telephone/Telemedicine Reports

Telephones and telemedicine equipment can link health care professionals immediately and enable nurses to receive and give critical information about patients in a timely fashion. For example, the hematology lab might call to report a dangerously low platelet count, and the nurse might in turn call the attending physician to obtain new medical orders. When reporting significant changes in a patient's condition to physicians and other health care professionals, be prepared to do the following:

- Identify yourself and the patient, and state your relationship to the patient. ("Dr. Gomez-Lobo, this is Ellen McLouglin, and I'm calling about Mr. Clouser, a patient of yours who was just discharged home following a work-up for recurrent chest pain. I'm his new nurse case manager.")
- Report concisely and accurately the change in the patient's condition that is of concern and what has already been done in response to this condition. ("When I first arrived in his home, he was complaining of feeling dizzy, and his blood pressure was 190/110. Yesterday morning in the hospital, it was 150/90. His wife appears very flustered and says she doesn't know how she is going to take care of him. I had him rest for 30 minutes, and when I checked his pressure at that time, it was still 186/110.")
- Report the patient's current vital signs and clinical manifestations.
- Have the patient's record at hand to make knowledgeable responses to any physician's inquiries. In this example, the physician will probably want to know all the vital signs and may ask questions about the treatment regimen, both in the hospital and upon discharge.
- Concisely record the time and date of the call, what was communicated to the physician, and the physician's response. Read back any changes to the orders.

Transfer and Discharge Reports

Nurses report a summary of a patient's condition and care when transferring patients from one unit, institution, or agency to another (e.g., from the postanesthesia care unit to a surgical floor) and when discharging patients. The nurse making the report should concisely summarize all the patient data that caregivers need to provide immediate care. See Chapter 9 for transfer and discharge reporting guidelines.

Reports to Family Members and Significant Others

Nurses play a crucial role in keeping the patient's family and significant others updated about the patient's condition and progress toward goal achievement. Always clarify with the patient which visitors, if any, are entitled to progress reports. "Mrs. Neale, do you object to our disclosing your health information to family or friends?" Similarly, clarify what types of information may be communicated, and be familiar with agency policy about such communications. Some agencies provide family members approved by the patient a "code" to use when calling the agency to ask about the patient's condition. If the patient objects to disclosure, nurses are not permitted to discuss the patient's health condition with family or friends. If a patient is not able to communicate objections, such as in an emergency situation or when a patient is unconscious, professional caregivers must use their best professional judgment to decide whether to talk to family and friends.

For example, the nurse is generally not the caregiver who informs family members that a patient's biopsy has revealed a malignancy. The nurse does, however, often explain what this will mean for the patient after the family has this information. Information should be shared in a manner that is honest, compassionate, and respectful of the person's ability to understand medical concepts.

Incident Reports

An **incident report**, also termed a **variance report** or occurrence report, is a tool used by health care agencies to document the occurrence of anything out of the ordinary that results in or has the potential to result in harm to a patient, employee, or visitor. These reports are used for quality improvement and should not be used for disciplinary action against staff members. They are a means of identifying risks. More harm than good results from ignoring mistakes. Incident reports improve the management and treatment of patients by identifying high-risk patterns so that in-service programs can be initiated to prevent future problems. These forms also make all the facts about an incident available to the agency in case of litigation. You should be familiar with agency policy about your responsibilities and obligations if involved personally in an incident that results in or has the potential to result in harm to a patient, employee, or visitor, or if you witness such an incident. An example of an incident report form and a fuller discussion of this topic appear in Chapter 7.

CONFERRING ABOUT CARE

To **confer** is to consult with someone to exchange ideas or to seek information, advice, or instructions. A nurse might consult with another nurse, such as when a primary care nurse consults with a nurse clinical specialist about a particular patient's care. A school nurse might confer with a child's teacher or a psychologist about a behavior problem. A community health nurse and a physician might confer about a patient's activity regimen. Health practitioners also confer with each other to validate information. Health care professionals increasingly use electronic support groups to consult with clinicians who share similar interests or who have expertise in other specialty areas. See Box 16-5 for an illustration of how one health care system is using creative conferrals to motivate change in contemporary nursing practice and nursing care delivery.

 THINK back to Jason Chandler, the adolescent who was brought into the emergency department by the police. He was refusing treatment. To determine the legal implications of administering treatment to the patient, the physician consulted the hospital's attorney for legal guidance. Doing so helped to clarify what actions were and were not acceptable. ●

BOX 16-5 DELIVERING OPTIMAL CARE TO PATIENTS AND THEIR FAMILIES

Nursing leadership at MedStar Health is committed to leading the organization along a path to a clearly defined goal: the delivery of optimal care to patients and their families. To guide these efforts, the *MedStar Way*, a set of 14 activities, has been devised to motivate change in contemporary nursing practice and nursing care delivery.

1. Senior Leader Rounding—to promote communication and access within the nursing team
2. Multidisciplinary Team Rounding—to ensure consistent documentation and timely communication, and discuss the care plan
3. Nurse Leader Rounding—to support a culture of service, assess patient and staff needs, and promote the patient/family experience
4. Nursing Staff Hourly Rounds—to anticipate and evaluate patient needs, and improve safety and satisfaction
5. Nurse-to-Nurse Bedside Shift Reports—to ensure safe handoffs, and keep the patient and family involved in the care plan
6. Huddles at the Beginning of Each Shift—to improve teamwork and communication, and ensure timely response to issues and concerns
7. White Boards in Patient Rooms—to encourage communication, teamwork and efficiency, and to assure the patient that the team is working together to provide optimal care
8. Post-Visit Phone Calls—to ensure quality clinical outcomes and increase patient satisfaction

Reprinted with permission. (June 2013). The MedStar Way: Delivering Optimal Care to Patients and Their Families. *MedStar Nursing, Insights and Innovations, 1*(2), 7.

Consultations and Referrals

When nurses detect problems they cannot resolve because they are outside the scope of independent nursing practice or their expertise, they make consultations or referrals to other professionals. The process of inviting another professional to evaluate the patient and make recommendations to you about the patient's treatment is called a **consultation**. The electronic medical record may be designed to automatically make nursing consults to selected services based on what the nurse documents. For example, if you click on the "yes" box when answering the question, "Does the patient have financial concerns regarding hospitalization?" a nursing consult is automatically sent to the social work department.

The process of sending or guiding the patient to another source for assistance is called a **referral**. A patient might be referred by a hospital to a community health nursing service for assistance with home care. A school nurse might refer a student to a hospital emergency department. A community health nurse who learns that a patient with multiple sexual contacts is HIV positive will refer to the Department of Health for tracking of these contacts.

Most health agencies have policies for referrals. An agency may use a special form for making referrals. Referral policies usually indicate who may initiate a referral, how it is to be done, and so on. Referrals are especially important for providing continuity of care for people who need a variety of services. The health practitioners to whom a patient is referred must receive the information that is most useful to the continuity of care. The key question is "What would I want to know about this patient if I were the person who will continue his or her care?" The patient must know and approve of a referral to another agency or to other health personnel.

Before requesting a consultation or making a referral, determine which profession has the needed expertise and which of its practitioners are appropriate for consultation or referral. A great disservice is done to patients when referrals are poorly made. Patients and family members also appreciate a phone number and practical tips about how to easily reach the referred practitioner.

 RECALL Millie Delong, the woman with the wound infection. Obtaining a consultation from a wound, ostomy, and continence nurse might be appropriate to assist with measures for wound care. Additionally, consultation with an infection-control nurse may be necessary if the patient's wound remains infected or fails to heal. ●

Nursing and Interdisciplinary Team Care Conferences

Nurses and other health care professionals frequently confer in groups to plan and coordinate patient care. Such conferences are also used for instructing students and practitioners. A nursing care conference is a meeting of nurses to discuss some aspect of a patient's care. For example, several nurses who are caring for a generally uncooperative patient might initiate a conference. This would allow each nurse an opportunity to offer one's opinion about the patient's problem and its cause, and then together they could discuss possible solutions to the problem.

Nurses might invite other health care practitioners to a nursing care conference concerning a patient's care. For example, a clinical psychologist might be invited in the preceding example to address the possibility that a mental disorder is influencing this patient's behavior.

Nursing Care Rounds

Nursing care rounds are procedures in which a group of nurses visit selected patients individually, at each patient's bedside. The primary purposes of nursing care rounds are to gather information to help plan nursing care, to evaluate the nursing care patients have received, and to provide them with an opportunity to discuss their care with those administering it. As each patient is visited, the nurse assigned provides a short summary of the patient's nursing diagnoses and goals and the care being given. Nursing care rounds have two principal advantages over discussions in a meeting room: Nursing personnel can actually see the patient as a

report of care is given, and the patient and family can participate in discussions of patient-centered care.

Nurses should use language the patient can understand when holding discussions at the bedside. Otherwise, the patient is likely to feel excluded and cannot intelligently participate in the discussion. Nurses might also make rounds with physicians to share nursing's perspective with them.

USING NURSING INFORMATICS

According to the ANA Scope and Standards of Nursing Informatics Practice, **nursing informatics** is a specialty that integrates nursing science, computer science, and information science to manage and communicate data, information, and knowledge in nursing practice. Nursing informatics facilitates the integration of data, information, and knowledge to support patients, nurses, and other providers in their decision making in all roles and settings. This approach uses information structures, information processes, and information technology (ANA, 2008). As more nurses have become informaticists, the tangible benefits of their efforts become clear:

• Increases in the accuracy and completeness of nursing documentation
• Improvement in the nurse's workflow and an elimination of redundant documentation
• Automation of the collection and reuse of nursing data
• Facilitation of the analysis of clinical data (Joint Commission indicators, core measures, federal- or state-mandated data and facility-specific data; Barthold, Duecker, Guinn, & MacCallum, 2009).

Increasingly, nurses are "involved with developing and implementing cutting-edge technologies and tools that are revolutionizing the way they work while improving safety and quality of care for patients" (Spader, 2009). Nurses' identification badges can now be used for hands-free, instant, two-way voice communication. This allows nurses to answer calls without stopping what they are doing or breaking a sterile field. It also can provide institutions with a record of where nurses are during every minute of their shifts. Smart devices are making an amazing amount of information readily available to nurses. For example, Wolters Kluwer Health offers a Nursing Drug Handbook app, which provides fast access to nursing-specific drug information, allowing nurses to find drug facts anytime, anywhere in seconds. This app features drug monographs addressing more than 900 generic and nearly 3,000 brand-name drugs. It currently has the most comprehensive collection of pill images—more than 400—to help nurses confidently identify their patients' medications. The app allows nurses to search for desired drugs alphabetically, by pharmacologic class, or by therapeutic class. It includes a dosage calculator, customizable notes, a favorites list, and detailed monographs, all in a user-friendly program.

As nursing apps are constantly changing, we recommend that you consult with your faculty about what apps will be most helpful for your clinical experiences and NCLEX

BOX 16-6 **NURSING INFORMATICS AND TECHNOLOGY: PREPARING WORK ENVIRONMENTS ORGANIZED AROUND ACCOUNTABLE CARE**

The health care environment is changing. The industry is moving from volume to value, provider-centric to patient-centric, fee-for-service to bundled payment, and delivery of extreme care to accountable care and population health management. Nurses will play a growing and vital role if they can master, adopt, use, and promote technologies related to patient engagement, telemedicine and mobile health, population health management, clinical integration, and performance management.

Nurses can play important roles as coordinators, communicators, and quality managers. They can also add value as communicators, explaining treatment options to patients and families and sharing insights related to disease and condition risk factors, causes, diagnoses, discharge instructions, and prevention of complications and readmissions. Finally, they can improve quality through evidence-based nursing practice, data analysis, and evaluation of cost and quality measures.

To fulfill these vital roles, nurses must master a variety of technologies, among them:

Patient engagement technologies: Patient engagement occurs when patients and families become actively involved in their own care. Nurses can support engagement through the adoption, use, and further development of patient portals. Engagement happens when portals deliver access to an electronic medical record (EMR) system and personal health information, online appointment scheduling, and personalized, condition-focused alerts and reminders in the form of e-mails, automated telephone calls, or text messages.

Telemedicine and mobile technologies: Accountable care organizations (ACOs) need to extend the boundaries of care beyond the confines of the traditional hospital or primary care practice. Telemedicine and mobile health facilitate patient engagement, while helping providers deliver more cost-effective care. While telemedicine embraces applications and services that include two-way video communications, e-mail, and wireless phones, mobile health features multiple technologies integrated into the increasingly wireless and mobile health care delivery system. The *New York Times* has already reported on the growing significance of mobile devices in nurse education, while Apple developed a list of top apps for nurses now available in the iTunes Store. Meanwhile, the market

for remote patient monitoring topped $204 million in 2012, according to GBI Research.

Data aggregation technologies: Nurses will play a growing role in data aggregation, a process that involves data collection, analysis, use, reporting, and delivery of feedback throughout the organization. ACOs will use process and outcomes data to measure what they achieve for patients and population-based communities. This means offering information to influence care decision making at the point of care through clinical decision support (CDS) and integrating responses from patient experience and satisfaction surveys. Even ACOs that aren't associated with the Medicare program will need to achieve accountability on measures like patient safety, patient/provider experience, care coordination, and preventive health. The best data aggregation technologies will support advanced practice nurses (APRNs) with easy access, user-friendly search, and training in data collection, analysis, use, and reporting.

Population health management technologies: ACOs are designed to improve outcomes, which should improve population health management. ACOs must know a population's health status and utilization patterns to develop targeted wellness and prevention programs. That, in turn calls for technologies that perform data mining, risk stratification, and analysis. Nurses will engage with longitudinal tracking mechanisms that integrate with CDS systems for real-time patient management, while also conducting searches for disease trends, diagnoses, procedures, and missed appointments.

Other technologies will be equally vital to nurses within ACOs. Among them are clinical integration technologies that offer integration of patient medical records, clinician/physician patient care portals, and notifications and reminders; performance management technologies that provide quality measures, best practices, evidence-based data, regulatory compliance, real-time reporting, and benchmarking; and reporting technologies that feature patient health record integration, standardized reporting measures, e-distribution of outcomes, information access for clinical decision making, and statistical summaries and compilations. APRNs may also interface with financial technologies involving medical necessity, authorization, scheduling, billing, and image retrieval.

Reprinted with permission from Sportsman, S. (2013). Nursing informatics & technology: A blog for all levels of users. Prepare for a work environment organized around accountable care. Available at http://community.advanceweb.com/blogs/nurses_18/archive/2013/08/28/prepare-for-a-work-environment-organized-around-accountable-care.aspx

preparation. If you use the search phrase "apps for nurses," you will find multiple recommendations for helpful apps.

See Box 16-6 for a description of the new technologies nurses must master to play important roles as care coordinators, communicators, and quality managers in the new health care environment.

DEVELOPING CLINICAL REASONING

1. Interview three practicing nurses and ask them to describe the documentation methods they have used in their practice. Which methods did they prefer? Which method was more effective, time efficient, and easiest to use?

2. A nurse overhears you complaining about writing narrative nursing notes and says to you, "Don't sweat it. I never worry about documentation—it's a waste of time. I'd rather spend my time doing things for patients than writing up what I did." Think about what you would like to say to this nurse and your rationale for this. Ask other students for their response, and compare your answers.

3. Imagine that you are a nurse in a long-term care facility and that you and the facility are being sued for negligence by the family of an older resident who fell and fractured her hip last year. You know the resident but do not remember much about the day she fell. What data do you hope to find recorded in her health record? Which documentation system would most likely

provide the type of information you think you need to reconstruct the events surrounding her fall?

4. How would you respond to each of the following requests for patient information? Compare your responses with those of another student and talk about any differences.
   - The mayor of your town, who is up for re-election, was just admitted to your unit after an acute myocardial infarction. You receive a phone call from his office requesting information about his condition.
   - A woman you have never seen approaches you in the hallway, identifies herself as a close friend of a married male patient on your unit, and requests information about his condition.
   - A case manager from a managed care organization calls you to ask about the progress an older surgical patient is making postoperatively. You have heard that the organization is eager to discharge her quickly, and you feel uncomfortable reporting any information over the phone.
   - A family member asks your advice about developing a personal health record. She says she has heard that there are privacy concerns. How do you respond?

PRACTICING FOR NCLEX

1. A nurse is documenting patient data in the medical record of a patient admitted to the hospital with a diagnosis of appendicitis. The physician has ordered 10 mg morphine IV every 3 to 4 hours. Which examples of documentation of care for this patient follows recommended guidelines? Select all that apply.
   a. 6/12/15 0945 Morphine 10 mg administered IV. Patient's response to pain appears to be exaggerated. M. Patrick, RN
   b. 6/12/15 0945 Morphine 10 mg administered IV. Patient seems to be comfortable. M. Patrick, RN
   c. 6/12/15 0945 30 minutes following administration of morphine 10 mg IV patient reports pain as 2 on a scale of 1 to 10. M. Patrick, RN
   d. 6/12/15 0945 Patient reports severe pain in right lower quadrant. M. Patrick, RN
   e. 6/12/15 0945 Morphine IV 10 mg will be administered to patient every 3 to 4 hours. M. Patrick, RN
   f. 6/12/15 0945 Patient states she does not want pain medication despite return of pain. After discussing situation, patient agrees to medication administration.

2. A nurse is documenting the care given to a 56-year-old patient diagnosed with an osteosarcoma, whose right leg was amputated. The nurse accidentally documents that a dressing changed was performed on the left leg. What would be the best action of the nurse to correct this documentation?
   a. Erase or use correcting fluid to completely delete the error.
   b. Draw a single line through the entry and rewrite it above or beside it.
   c. Use a permanent marker to block out the mistaken entry and rewrite it.
   d. Remove the page with the error and rewrite the data on that page correctly.

3. A nurse is discharging a patient from the hospital following a heart stent procedure. The patient asks to see and copy his medical record. What is the nurse's best response?
   a. "I'm sorry, but patients are not allowed to copy their medical records."
   b. "I can make a copy of your record for you right now."

c. "You can read your record while you are still a patient, but copying records is not permitted according to HIPAA rules."
   d. "I will need to check with our records department to get you a copy."

4. According to the Health Insurance Portability and Accountability Act of 1996, if a health institution wants to release a patient's health information (PHI) for purposes other than treatment, payment, and routine health care operations, the patient must be asked to sign an authorization. The nurse is aware that there are exceptions to this requirement. In which of the following cases is an authorization form not needed? Select all that apply.
   a. News media are preparing a report on the condition of a public figure.
   b. Data are needed for the tracking and notification of disease outbreaks.
   c. Protected health information is needed by a coroner.
   d. Child abuse and neglect are suspected.
   e. Protected health information is needed to facilitate organ donation.
   f. The sister of a patient with Alzheimer's wants to help provide care.

5. A friend of a nurse calls and asks if she is still working at Memorial Hospital. The nurse replies, "Yes." The friend tells the nurse that his girlfriend's father was just admitted as a patient and he wants the nurse to find out how he is. The friend states, "Sue seems unusually worried about her dad, but she won't talk to me and I want to be able to help her." What is the best initial response the nurse should make?
   a. "You shouldn't be asking me to do this. I could be fined or even lose my job for disclosing this information."
   b. "Sorry, but I'm not able to give information about patients to the public—even when my best friend or a family member asks."
   c. "Because of the Health Insurance Portability and Accountability Act, you shouldn't be asking for this information unless the patient has authorized you to receive it! This could get you in trouble!"
   d. "Why do you think Sue isn't talking about her worries?"

6. A patient has an order for an analgesic medication to be given PRN. When would the nurse administer this medication?
   a. Every three hours
   b. Every four hours
   c. Daily
   d. As needed

7. A resident who is called to see a patient in the middle of the night is leaving the unit but then remembers that he forgot to write a new order for a pain medication a nurse had requested for another patient. Tired and already being paged to another unit, he verbally tells the nurse the order and asks the nurse to document it on the physician's order sheet. The nurse's best response is:
   a. "Thank you for taking care of this!"
   b. Get a second nurse to listen to the order, and after writing the order on the physician order sheet, have both nurses sign it.
   c. "I am sorry, but verbal orders can only be given in an emergency situation that prevents us from writing them out. I'll bring the chart and we can do this quickly."
   d. Try calling another resident for the order or wait until the next shift.

8. A nurse is looking for trends in a postoperative patient's vital signs. Which documents would the nurse consult first?
   a. Admission sheet
   b. Admission nursing assessment
   c. Activity flow sheet
   d. Graphic record

9. A nurse is using the SOAP format of documentation to document care of a patient who is diagnosed with type 2 diabetes. Which source of information would be the nurse's focus when completing this documentation?
   a. A patient problem list
   b. Notes describing the patient's condition
   c. Overall trends in patient status
   d. Planned interventions and patient outcomes

10. A nurse is using the ISBARR physician reporting system to report the deteriorating mental status of Mr. Sanchez, a male patient who has been prescribed morphine via a patient-controlled analgesia pump (PCA) for pain related to pancreatic cancer. Place the following nursing statements related to this call in the order in which they should be performed.
    a. "I am calling about Mr. Sanchez in Room 202 who is receiving morphine via a PCA pump for pancreatic cancer."
    b. "Mr. Sanchez has been difficult to arouse and his mental status has changed over the past 12 hours since using the pump."
    c. "You want me to discontinue the PCA pump until you see him tonight at patient rounds."
    d. "I am Rosa Clark, an RN working on the second floor of South Street Hospital."
    e. "Mr. Sanchez was admitted two days ago following a diagnosis of pancreatic cancer."
    f. "I think the dosage of morphine in Mr. Sanchez's PCA pump needs to be lowered."

ANSWERS WITH RATIONALES

1. **c, d, f.** The nurse should enter information in a *complete, accurate, concise, current,* and *factual* manner and indicate in each entry the date and both the time the entry was written and the time of pertinent observations and interventions. When charting, the nurse should avoid the use of stereotypes or derogatory terms as well as generalizations such as "seems comfortable today." The nurse should never document an intervention before carrying it out.

2. **b.** The nurse should not use dittos, erasures, or correcting fluids. A single line should be drawn through an incorrect entry, and the words "mistaken entry" or "error in charting" should be printed above or beside the entry and signed. The entry should then be rewritten correctly.

3. **d.** According to HIPAA, patients have a right to see and copy their health record; update their health record; get a list of the disclosures a health care institution has made independent of disclosures made for the purposes of treatment, payment, and health care operations; request a restriction on certain uses or disclosures; and choose how to receive health information. The nurse should be aware of agency policies regarding the patient's right to access and copy records.

4. **b, c, d, e.** Authorization is not required for tracking disease outbreaks, providing PHI to a coroner, reporting incidents of child abuse, or facilitating organ donations. Under no circumstance can a nurse provide information to a news reporter without the patient's express authorization. An authorization form is still needed to provide PHI for a patient who has Alzheimer's disease.

5. **b.** The nurse should immediately clarify what he or she can and cannot do. Since the primary reason for refusing to help is linked to the responsibility to protect patient privacy and confidentiality, the nurse should not begin by mentioning the real penalties linked to abuses of privacy. Finally, it is appropriate to ask about Sue and her worries, but this should be done after the nurse clarifies what he or she is able to do.

6. **d.** PRN means "as needed."

7. **c.** In most agencies, the only circumstance in which an attending physician, nurse practitioner, or house officer may issue orders verbally is in a medical emergency, when the physician/nurse practitioner is present but finds it impossible, due to the emergency situation, to write the order.

8. **d.** While one recording of vital signs should appear on the admission nursing assessment, the best place to find sequential recordings that show a pattern or trend is the graphic record. The admission sheet does not include vital sign documentation, and neither does the activity flow sheet.

9. **a.** When using the SOAP format, the problem list at the front of the chart alerts all caregivers to patient priorities. Narrative notes allow nurses to describe a condition, situation, or response in their own terms. Abnormal status can be seen immediately when using charting by exception, and planned interventions and patient expected outcomes are the focus of the case management model.

10. **d, a, e, b, f, c.** The order for ISBARR is: identity/introduction, situation, background, assessment, recommendation, and read-back.

TAYLOR SUITE RESOURCES

Explore these additional resources to enhance learning for this chapter:
- NCLEX-Style Questions and other resources on thePoint, http://thePoint.lww.com/Taylor8e
- *Study Guide for Fundamentals of Nursing, 8th edition*
- Adaptive Learning | Powered by prepU, http://thepoint.lww.com/prepu

Bibliography

Agency for Healthcare Research and Quality. (May 2012). Electronic health records improve nursing care, coordination, and patient safety: Research Activities, No. 381. Rockville, MD: Author. Available at http://www.ahrq.gov/news/newsletters/research-activities/may12/0512RA11.html

Are there different types of personal health records (PHRs)? (n.d.) Retrieved from http://www.healthit.gov/providers-professionals/faqs/are-there-different-types-personal-health-records-phrs

American Nurses Association (ANA). (2001). *Code of ethics for nurses with interpretive statements.* Washington, DC: Author.

American Nurses Association (ANA). (2010). *Principles for documentation.* Silver Spring, MD: Author.

American Nurses Association (ANA). (2008). *Nursing informatics: Scope and standards of practice.* Silver Spring, MD: Author.

American Nurses Association (ANA). (2010). *Scope and Standards of Practice* (2nd ed.). Silver Spring, MD: Author.

Barthold, M. F., Duecker, T., Guinn, P., & MacCallum, R. (2009). Nursing Informatics 101. Available at http://www.himss.org/handouts/NI101.pdf

Benefits of electronic health records (EHRs). (n.d.) Retrieved from http://www.healthit.gov/providers-professionals/benefits-electronic-health-records-ehrs

Brusco, J. M. (2011). Electronic health records: what nurses need to know. *AORN Journal, 93*(3), 371–379.

Buckley-Womack, C., & Gidney, B. (1987). A new dimension in documentation: The PIE method. *Journal of Neuroscience Nursing, 19*(5), 256–260.

Burke, L., & Murphy, J. (1988). *Charting by exception: A cost-effective quality approach.* Albany, NY: Delmar.

Centers for Medicare and Medicaid Services. (n.d.) Nursing Home Quality Initiative. Available at: http://www.cms.gov/Medicare/Quality-Initiatives-Patient-Assessment-Instruments/NursingHomeQualityInits/index.html?redirect=/NursingHomeQualityInits/45_NHQIMDS30TrainingMaterials.asp

Cibulka, N. J., & Crane-Wider, L. (2011). Introducing personal digital assistants to enhance nursing education in undergraduate and graduate nursing programs. *The Journal of Nursing Education, 50*(2), 115–118.

Courtney, K. L., Goodwin, L. K., & Aubrecht, J. (2011). Database management systems–their place in nursing informatics education. *Computers, Informatics, Nursing : CIN, 29*(1), 7–12.

Enlow, M., Shanks, L., Guhde, J., & Perkins, M. (2010). Incorporating interprofessional communication skills (ISBARR) into an undergraduate nursing curriculum. *Nurse Educator, 35*(4), 176–180.

Gendreau-Webb, R. (2007). Put PDAs to work in your practice. *Nursing, 37*(10), 62–63.

George, L., & Davidson, L. (2005). PDA use in nursing education: Prepared for today, poised for tomorrow. *Online Journal Nursing Informatics, 9*(2). Available at http://ojni.org/9_2/george.htm

Healthcare Information and Management Systems Society (HIMSS). Available at: http://www.himss.org/AboutHIMSS/index.aspx?navItemNumber=17402

Health Information Exchange (HIE). (n.d.) Retrieved from http://www.healthit.gov/providers-professionals/health-information-exchange/what-hie

The Health Insurance Portability and Accountability Act (HIPAA). (1996). Public Law, 104–191. http://www.hhs.gov/ocr/hipaa.

Holmes, H. N. (Ed.). (2006). *Documentation in action.* Philadelphia: Wolters Kluwer Health/Lippincott Williams & Wilkins.

Institute for Healthcare Improvement. SBAR technique for communication: a situational briefing model.

Available at http://www.ihi.org/IHI/Topics/Patient-Safety/SafetyGeneral/Tools/SBARTechniquefor CommunicationASituationalBriefingModel.htm

The Joint Commission. (2012). *2013 Hospital Accreditation Standards.* Washington, DC: Author.

The Joint Commission. (n.d.) Facts About the Official "Do Not Use" List. Available at http://www.joint-commission.org/assets/1/18/Do_Not_Use_List.pdf

Kahn, J., Aulak, V., & Bosworth, A. (2009). What it takes: Characteristics of the ideal personal health record. *Health Affairs, 28*(2), 369–376.

Keys to successful adoption of electronic medical record systems. (2009, August). *AACN Bold Voices, 1*(2), 11.

Kunz, M. K. (2010). Embracing the electronic medical record: helping nurses overcome possible barriers. *Nursing for women's health, 14*(4), 290–300.

Kutney-Lee, A., & Kelly, D. (2011). The effect of hospital electronic health record adoption on nurse-assessed quality of care and patient safety. *Journal of Nursing Administration, 41*(11), 466–472.

Liaw, S. T., & Gray, K. (2010). Clinical health informatics education for a 21st Century World. *Studies in health technology and informatics, 151*, 479–491.

McGraw, D., Dempsey, J. X., Harris, L., & Goldman, J. (2009). Privacy as an enabler, not an impediment: Building trust into health information exchange. *Health Affairs, 28*(2), 416–427.

Muller-Staub, M., Lunney, M., Odenbreit, M., Needham, I., Lavin, M. A., & van Achterberg, T. (2009). Development of an instrument to measure the quality of documented nursing diagnoses, interventions and outcomes: The Q-DIO. *Journal of Clinical Nursing, 18*(7), 1027–1037.

Murphy, E. K. (2003). Charting by exception—OR nursing law. *AORN Journal.* Available at http://www.findarticles.com/p/articles/mi_m0FSL/is_5_78/ai_111011830.

National Alliance for Health Information Technology. (2008). Health IT terms established. Available at www.endonurse.com/hotnews/health-it-terms-set-alliance.html.

Saranto, K., & Kinnunen, U. (2009). Evaluation nursing documentation—Research designs and methods: Systematic review. *Journal of Advanced Nursing, 65*(3), 464–476.

Siegrist, L., Stocks, B., & Dettor, R. (1985). The PIE system: Complete planning and documentation of nursing care. *QRB, 11*(6), 186–189.

Simpson, R. L. (2011). Nurse informaticians critical to proving meaningful use. *Nursing administration quarterly, 35*(1), 82–84.

Spader, C. (2009). Cool tools. Cutting-edge gadgets sharpen nurses' efficiency. *Nursing Spectrum (Washington, DC/MD/VA edition), 19*(11), 20–21.

Sportsman, S. (2013). Nursing informatics & technology: A blog for all levels of users. Prepare for a work environment organized around accountable care. Available at http://community.advanceweb.com/blogs/nurses_18/archive/2013/08/28/prepare-for-a-work-environment-organized-around-accountable-care.aspx

Thede, L. Q. (2010). *Informatics and nursing: Competencies and applications* (3rd ed.). Philadelphia: Wolters Kluwer Health/Lippincott Williams & Wilkins.

Thompson, P., & Bell, P. (2007) Potential student abuse of technology in the clinical setting. *Nurse Educator, 32*(4), 145–146.

von Krogh, G., & Naden, D. (2008). A nursing-specific model of EPR documentation: Organizational and professional requirements. *Journal of Nursing Scholarship, 40*(1), 68–75.

U.S. Department of Health and Human Services. (n.d.) Health Information Privacy. Available at http://www.hhs.gov/ocr/privacy/hipaa/understanding/

Wakefield, D. S., Wakefield, B. J., Despins, L., Brandt, J., Davis, W., Clements, K., & Steinman, W. (2012). A review of verbal order policies in acute care hospitals. *The Joint Commission Journal on Quality and Patient Safety, 38*(1), 11–22.

Weaver, C. A., Delaney, C. W., Weber, P., & Carr, R. (Eds.). (2006). *Nursing and informatics for the 21st Century: An international look at practice, trends and the future.* Chicago: HIMSS.

Williams, C., Mostashari, E., Mertz, K., Hogin, E., & Atwal, P. (2012). From the office of the national coordinator: The strategy for advancing the exchange of health information. *Health Affairs, 31*(3), 527–536.

Windle, P. E. (1994). Critical pathways: An integrated documentation tool. *Nursing Management, 25*(9), 80F–L, 80P.

Promoting Health
Across the Lifespan

*T*he chapters in Unit IV focus on growth and development through the life cycle. By considering all aspects of the person, nurses provide health care oriented toward wellness and maximize each patient's strengths to reach his or her potential. (The influences of the family on growth and development are discussed fully in Chapter 4.)

Chapter 17 gives an overview of developmental concepts and theories necessary to understanding growth and development across the lifespan. Major theorists and their contributions to the understanding of psychosocial, physical, cognitive, moral, and faith development are described.

Chapter 18 considers the individual from conception through young adulthood. Influences on growth and development, as well as physiologic, cognitive, psychosocial, moral, and spiritual development, are discussed. Common health problems of each age group and the role of the nurse in health promotion and illness prevention for each age group are considered.

Chapter 19 discusses the adult years in early, middle, and older-adult stages. Common health problems and the nurse's role in health care for the adult continue to be important through older adulthood. The chapter ends with a look at the paradigm of aging and stereotypes of older adults. Gerontology and the health care system related to this field are discussed.

> *Basic to any philosophy of nursing seems to be these three concepts: (1) reverence for the gift of life; (2) respect for the dignity, worth, autonomy, and individuality of each human being; (3) resolution to act dynamically in relation to one's beliefs."*

Ernestine Wiedenbach (1900–1996) a faculty member at Yale University School of Nursing, where she developed her model of nursing from years of experience in various nursing positions

> *"The concern of nursing is with man in his entirety, his wholeness. Nursing's body of scientific knowledge seeks to describe, explain, and predict about human beings."*

Martha Rogers (1914–1994) a nationally renowned nurse theoretician, author, lecturer, and consultant, whose "theory of man" inspired tremendous creativity, research activity, and intellectual growth in the nursing profession

17 Developmental Concepts

MELANIE KIMBER

Melanie, a 24-year-old single mother, voices concerns about rearing her 12-month-old son by herself. "He is just so active, putting toys in his mouth, and getting into everything. I'm afraid to look away for even a second because he might get hurt. I don't know how other parents do it."

JUAN ALVAREZ

Juan, an 8-year-old boy with encephalitis, becomes violent and combative at times, throwing himself against the bed and muttering words. He immediately calms down when an interpreter visits with him who speaks to him in Spanish and when some of the nurses use Spanish words with him.

JOSEPH LOGAN

Joseph, a 70-year-old man who fell and fractured his hip while repairing the exterior of his home, states, "Go away and leave me alone. I'm a grown man, I can take care of myself. . . and get rid of this tray. I'm not hungry." Further investigation reveals that Mr. Logan has been the traditional head of his household and is now troubled by needing others, including his wife, to care for him.

After completing the chapter, you will be able to accomplish the following:

1. Summarize basic principles of growth and development.
2. Discuss the theories of Freud, Erikson, Havighurst, Gould, Levinson, Piaget, Kohlberg, Gilligan, and Fowler.
3. Describe the importance of incorporating theories of growth and development in assessing and planning nursing care for individuals.
4. Explain implications for nursing practice based on an understanding of growth and development.

KEY TERMS

accommodation	developmental task	growth
assimilation		moral development
cognitive development	faith	
development	genome	pharmaco-genetics
	genomics	

Humans grow and develop throughout life. **Growth** is an increase in body size or changes in body cell structure, function, and complexity. **Development** is an orderly pattern of changes in structure, thoughts, feelings, or behaviors resulting from maturation, experiences, and learning. Development is a dynamic and continuous process as one proceeds through life, characterized by a series of ascents, plateaus, and declines. The human processes of growth and development result from the interrelated effects of heredity and environment. Humans simultaneously grow and develop in physical, cognitive, psychosocial, moral, and spiritual dimensions, with each dimension being an essential part of the whole person.

Nurses promote health in people from birth to death. All people, regardless of age, have unique health care needs that result from their physical, intellectual, emotional, sociocultural, spiritual, and environmental dimensions at their developmental level. To plan and give holistic and individualized care, the nurse must understand typical growth and development characteristics, tasks, and needs of patients of all ages. (See the accompanying Reflective Practice box on page 372.)

This chapter presents theories and principles of growth and development across the lifespan that help us understand both healthy and ill people at various life stages. The major theories examining cognitive, psychosocial, spiritual, and moral development are discussed.

PRINCIPLES OF GROWTH AND DEVELOPMENT

Everyone's physical development has a predetermined genetic base because of inheritance patterns carried on the chromosomes. Thus, an unborn child begins life with specific physical attributes. Environmental factors from birth through the early years of growth provide initial psychological and social contact through positive or negative experiences with caregivers. As environmental influences expand beyond the immediate caregivers or family, development is influenced by a wide variety of psychosocial experiences as well as circumstances in the physical environment. Cognitive, moral, and spiritual development are fostered through interactions within the family, school, and community. The nurse can better understand these interrelated variables at specific life stages through theories of human growth and development.

Growth and development are orderly and sequential as well as continuous and complex. All humans experience the same general growth patterns and developmental levels, but because these patterns and levels are individualized, a wide variation in biologic and behavioral changes is normal. Within each developmental level, certain milestones can be identified, such as the first time the infant rolls over, crawls, walks, or says his or her first words. Although growth and development occur in individual ways for different people, certain generalizations can be made about the nature of human development for everyone. These generalizations, outlined in Box 17-1 (on page 373), form the principles that help us understand growth and development.

FACTORS INFLUENCING GROWTH AND DEVELOPMENT

Many different factors influence both growth and development. One's growth and development might be facilitated or delayed by genetic heredity; prenatal, individual, and caregiver factors; and environment and nutrition. Other factors influencing growth and development are health–illness state (discussed in Chapters 3, 4, 18, and 19) and culture (discussed in Chapter 5).

 THINK back to Juan, the 8-year-old boy with encephalitis described at the beginning of the chapter. Although his behavior could be attributed to his infection, culture also may be a contributory factor for his behavior. ●

Because of these often interrelated and interdependent factors, each person's growth and development is individualized. Scientists also continue to debate the relative importance of the combined genes and environment that affect the development of a person ("nature versus nurture").

Genetic Heredity

At conception, every human receives an equal number of chromosomes from each parent. The characteristics inherited from each parent are carried in gene pairs on the 23 pairs of chromosomes, which carry the genetic information that

REFLECTIVE PRACTICE: CULTIVATING QSEN COMPETENCIES

CHALLENGE TO ETHICAL AND LEGAL SKILLS

Two summers ago, while working in a nurse externship program, I worked with Juan, a Spanish-speaking 8-year-old boy diagnosed with encephalitis. The boy would become violent and combative at times, throwing himself against the bed and muttering words. Although his underlying disease was a likely cause of this behavior, he became calm when an interpreter was with him. The interpreter would speak to him in Spanish and he seemed to calm down. He also would appear calmer when nurses spoke Spanish words to him. Unfortunately, most nurses and physicians would ignore his screams in a language they did not understand, complaining about his behavior, and relying on medication to calm him.

On one particular day, I was in the room with a physician who was writing an assessment note for Juan while I was getting his bath water ready for morning care. As usual, Juan was muttering words and thrashing in the bed. I knew some measures to calm him; for example, speaking the few Spanish words I knew. The physician remained in her chair, looking at me and complaining about Juan's behavior, not making any effort to calm him. She said that she could not do anything to calm him down except prescribe sedative medications. I felt bad for the patient and knew he was frustrated. I knew that I could possibly help in this situation, but did not want to show disrespect to the physician.

Thinking Outside the Box: Possible Courses of Action

- I could nod in agreement with the physician. After all, I was only a nursing student and "didn't know better" than she did.

- I could tell her what measures I had used to help calm Juan.
- I could refrain from saying anything at all, wait until the physician had left, and then try to calm Juan.

Evaluating a Good Outcome: How Do I Define Success?

- Patient benefited from my actions.
- I did not disrespect the physician.
- I was able to use my intuition, authority, and common sense to the best of my ability.

- Did I have the authority to jump in and give the physician advice on how to care for the patient?
- In this situation, my intuition and common sense told me to jump up and take action to calm down poor Juan, who was frustrated and upset.

Personal Learning: Here's to the Future!

Unfortunately, in this situation, I did not respond as I would have liked to. I did not say anything, but watched Juan become upset and mutter Spanish words. During this whole time, the physician shook her head, looked down on him, and told me she just "couldn't do anything about him" except to give him medications. I waited until the physician left, and then tried to calm Juan myself. In this situation, I should have let the physician know about the methods used to calm Juan previously, not just the simple use of drugs to

sedate him. However, as a junior level nursing student, I did not feel comfortable enough to use this type of authority. I now see how important it is for nurses and all staff members to communicate their opinions, beliefs, and observations about patients for the benefit of the patient. These suggestions and opinions need to be heard so that patients receive the best possible care. In the future, as a practicing nurse, I will respect my fellow staff members, but always make sure that my voice is heard concerning a patient's needs.

REFLECTION ON QUALITY AND SAFETY COMPETENCIES

How do you think you would respond in a similar situation? Why? What does this tell you about yourself and about the adequacy of your skills for professional practice? Can you think of other ways to respond or approach the situation? What *knowledge, skills,* and *attitudes* do you need to develop to continuously improve quality and safety when caring for patients like Juan?

Patient-Centered Care: What do you think Juan might have been experiencing and why? What if the nursing student had approached the physician about using other methods to calm Juan? Would you consider that action to be disrespectful? How do you think the physician would have responded to the nursing student's feedback about the use of the Spanish language to calm Juan?

Teamwork and Collaboration/Quality Improvement: Do you think that you would act differently if the physician were male or older? What communication skills do you need to improve to ensure that you function as a member of the patient care team and minimize risk of harm to Juan? Would collaboration with your instructor or Juan's nurse

have resulted in additional alternatives or another approach to communicate calmly and safely with Juan?

Safety/Evidence-Based Practice: Would Juan's stage of growth and development influence your nursing care? Do you think that the nursing student's stage of growth and development may have played a role in the student's response? Why or why not? Would an effort to identify common Spanish words and phrases and have them available to all caregivers help Juan to remain calm and less frustrated and not require the use of sedatives? What evidence in nursing literature provides guidance for decision making about methods to ensure a safe environment for a young child who does not understand English?

Informatics: Can you identify the essential information that needs to be included and documented in Juan's electronic record regarding efforts to communicate with him and give nursing care? Is it important to document your assessments and interventions? Can you identify any additional information that supports safe patient care and coordination of care?

BOX 17-1 PRINCIPLES OF GROWTH AND DEVELOPMENT

Growth and development are orderly and sequential, as well as continuous and complex. All humans experience the same growth patterns and developmental levels. Because these patterns and levels are individualized, a wide variation in biologic and behavioral changes is considered normal. Within each developmental level, certain milestones can be identified; for example, the time the infant rolls over, crawls, walks, and says his or her first words.

Growth and development follow regular and predictable trends. Cephalocaudal (proceeding from head to tail) development is the first trend, with the head and brain developing first, followed by the trunk, legs, and feet. The second trend is proximodistal development, which means that growth progresses from gross motor movements (such as learning to lift one's head) to fine motor movements (such as learning to pick up a toy with the fingers). The last trend is symmetric development of the body, with both sides of the body developing equally.

Growth and development are both differentiated and integrated. As nerve pathways develop, they become more specialized, allowing the growing child to respond to different stimuli. Throughout the lifespan, each new learned ability builds on previously learned abilities so that increasingly complex tasks can be accomplished. For example, the toddler learning to use a spoon combines motor skills, hand–eye coordination, cognitive patterning, and social imitation from watching others. As children grow and develop, the task of learning to use a spoon becomes basic, forming the foundation for learning skills requiring more manual dexterity.

Different aspects of growth and development occur at different stages and at different rates, and can be modified. For example, muscles and bones both grow most rapidly during the first year of life. During the toddler and preschool years, bone growth slows, but muscle fibers increase in size and strength. The most intense period of speech development is between 3 and 5 years of age. Sexual maturity begins during the preadolescent years and progresses into the adult years, but is based on gender and sex role identity established from birth. Many factors can modify growth and development, including nutrition, environment, love and affection from caregivers, and illnesses.

The pace of growth and development is specific for each person. Both physical and psychological skills and maturation vary among people. For example, while learning to walk, a child may concentrate energies on the task and temporarily slow down in language development. Racial variations may also be seen; Asian children tend to be smaller than White children of the same age. In addition, one's genetic heredity places restrictions on the upper limits that can be achieved in growth and development.

---

determines the person's cellular differentiation, growth, and function. As a result, physical characteristics such as height, bone size, and eye and hair color are inherited from our family of origin. Other characteristics, such as personality, are not as clearly identified with genetic heredity, but research is ongoing in this area. Genetic heredity also influences the development of many diseases, such as cancer and diabetes.

The Human Genome Project, completed in 2003, was a national and international 13-year research project to map the estimated 20,000 to 25,000 genes in human DNA (Human Genome Project Information, 2011a). All the DNA in an organism, including its genes, is referred to as a **genome**. The challenging complexity of this project is recognized when one understands that human DNA developed from four different chemical building blocks called bases involves approximately 3 billion bases arranged along the chromosomes in a particular order that is unique for each person (Human Genome Project Information, 2011b). The Human Genome Project has already identified more than 1,800 disease genes, but the genetic factors of complex diseases such as heart disease and cancer remain elusive. The Cancer Genome Atlas, a new initiative, is attempting to identify the genetic abnormalities seen in 50 major types of cancer (Human Genome Project, 2011). Currently, more than 2,000 genetic tests are available for human conditions.

Genomics is the study of the structure and interactions of all the genes in the human body, including their interactions with each other as well as the environment. In the very near future, all health care providers will be challenged to integrate genomics into their research, education, and practice (*Healthy People 2020,* 2012). Genetic tests plus family history tools have the potential to identify people at risk for diseases. Two emerging challenges related to genomic discoveries include the following:

- Evidence-based review panels are needed to thoroughly evaluate the possible benefits and harms related to the expanding number of genetic tests and family health history tools.
- Valid and reliable national data are needed to establish baseline measures and track progress toward targets (*Healthy People 2020,* 2012).

Research is also focusing on **pharmacogenetics**, the study of how genetic variation affects a person's response to drugs. Pharmacogenetic tests can determine if a patient is likely to have a strong therapeutic response to a drug or suffer adverse reactions from the medication. Genetic variation can either accelerate or slow the metabolism of many drugs (Lehne, 2013; Human Genome Project, 2011).

Nurses must be prepared to answer questions and discuss the impact of genetic findings on health and illness. Patient assessments, nursing care, and health teaching will all depend on this knowledge base. Therefore, nurses need to know how to find information about genetics and genomics and how to use this data (Goldberg, Jenkins, & Spahis, 2010). Resources for genetic technology and information are included in Table 17-1 (on page 374).

Prenatal, Individual, and Caregiver Factors

Prenatal, individual, and caregiver factors influence development. Fetal development can be affected by maternal

Table 17-1	GENETIC TECHNOLOGY AND INFORMATION RESOURCES	
ORGANIZATION	**ACTIVITIES**	
National Human Genome Research Institute www.genome.gov	Helps health care practitioners understand concepts and issues related to genetic services	
My Family Health Portrait https://familyhistory.hhs.gov	Aids in construction of a family pattern of diseases	
Gene Tests http://www.ncbi.nlm.nih.gov/gtr/	Provides information on breast cancer screening and government-related labs	
National Society of Genetic Counselors www.nsgc.org	Locates genetic nurse counseling services according to zip code location	

age (with greater risk in mothers younger than 15 years of age or older than 35 years of age), inadequate prenatal care, inadequate maternal nutrition, and maternal substance abuse. Individual factors that can affect development from birth through adolescence include congenital or genetic disorders, brain damage from accidents or abuse, vision and hearing impairments, chronic illness, inadequate nutrition, chemotherapy or radiation therapy, lead poisoning, poverty, and substance abuse. Caregiver factors that negatively affect development include neglect and abuse, mental illness, mental retardation, or a severe learning disability.

Environment and Nutrition

Environment and nutrition influence all stages of development. Environmental factors that might alter development include poverty, violence, unsafe living conditions, the presence of lead or mold in the home, and the quality of air and water in the surrounding environment. The effect of each can occur independently, but they are more likely to be interrelated, as seen in these examples:

- Infants who are malnourished in utero develop fewer brain cells than infants who have had adequate prenatal nutrition.
- Substance abuse by a pregnant woman increases the risk for congenital anomalies, low birth weight, and prematurity in her developing fetus.
- Federally sponsored school meal programs support enhanced learning with adequate nutrition.
- Failure to thrive, a condition of early infancy, has been linked to both nutritional and emotional deprivation.
- Environmental challenges, such as substandard housing and inadequate medical care, can further compound the effects of poor nutrition.

- Child abuse is an extreme example of physical and emotional harm or deprivation, leading to deficits in physical or psychosocial development, or both.
- Substance abuse by adolescents and young adults is associated with an increased incidence of teenage pregnancy, violence, accidents, and suicide. Abuse of alcohol and drugs is more prevalent in teenagers who have poor family relationships, low self-esteem, and poor social skills.
- Nutritional influences such as overeating and inactivity as well as genetic factors are directly related to obesity.

OVERVIEW OF DEVELOPMENTAL THEORIES

Human development and behavior have been studied since the beginning of the 20th century, and many theories have been developed to explain human responses normally occurring at certain ages during life. Although a psychological approach is common to most developmental theories, each theory has a different focus. The theories discussed in the following sections examine cognitive, social, and instinctual influences on human growth and development, and key points are summarized in Table 17-2.

Theory of Psychoanalytic Development: Sigmund Freud

Freud's theory emphasizes the effect of instinctual human drives on behavior. Freud identified the underlying stimulus for human behavior as sexuality, which he called *libido*. Libido is defined as general pleasure-seeking instincts rather than purely genital gratification.

The four major components of the mind according to Freud's theory are:

- the unconscious mind
- the id
- the ego
- the superego

The unconscious mind contains memories, motives, fantasies, and fears that are not easily recalled but that directly affect behavior. The id is the part of the mind concerned with self-gratification by the easiest and quickest available means. Defense mechanisms are a means of unconscious coping to reduce stress in the conscious mind when the id's impulses cannot be satisfied. (Defense mechanisms are discussed in Chapter 41.)

The ego is the conscious part of the mind that serves as a mediator between the desires of the id and the constraints of reality so that one can live effectively within one's social, physical, and psychological environment. The ego includes intelligence, memory, problem solving, separation of reality from fantasy, and incorporation of experiences and learning into future behavior. Freud noted that the death of a loved one can result in the loss of one's sense of identity, but once the loss is accepted, the ego is able to reconcile the loss and search for new attachments. Development of the ego allows the infant, by 6 months of age, to view self as separate from

Table 17-2 KEY POINTS OF DEVELOPMENTAL THEORIES

	FREUD	ERIKSON	HAVIGHURST	PIAGET	FOWLER	KOHLBERG
Theme	Psychosexual	Psychosocial	Developmental	Cognitive	Faith	Moral
Infancy to toddler-hood	Oral stage; anal stage	Trust versus mistrust; autonomy versus shame and doubt	Learning to walk; learning to talk; learning to control body waste elimination	Basic reflexes; coordinates more than one thought at a time; begins to reason and anticipate events	Centers on relation-ship with primary caregiver	Oriented to obedience and punish-ment
Preschool to early school years	Phallic stage	Initiative versus guilt	Learning sex differ-ences; forming concepts; getting ready to read	Increased language; increased under-standing of life events and rela-tionships	Imitates religious behaviors of others	Defines acts satisfying to self and some satisfying to others as right
School years	Latent stage	Industry versus inferiority	Learning physical skills; learning to get along with others; develop-ing conscience and morality	Develops logical thinking; incor-porates others' perspectives; uses abstract thinking and deductive rea-soning; tests beliefs to estab-lish values	Accepts exis-tence of deity; sto-ries define religious and moral beliefs	Morality of maintaining good rela-tions and approval of others; aware of need to respect authority
Adoles-cent to adult years	Genital stage	Intimacy versus generation	Achieving gender-specific social role; achieving independence; acquiring a set of values and an ethical system to guide behavior	Adopts life-guiding values or reli-gious practices	Selects prin-ciples to follow; con-cern for the rights and needs of others	
Middle adult years		Generativ-ity versus stagnation	Achieving social and civic respon-sibility; accepting and adjusting to physical changes			
Later adult years		Ego integrity versus despair	Adjusting to decreasing phys-ical status and health; adjusting to retirement			

others and to begin to alter behaviors in response to cues. Ego development continues throughout life.

The superego is the part of the mind commonly called the conscience. It develops from the ego during the first year of life, as the child learns praise versus punishment for actions. The superego represents the internalization of rules and val-ues so that socially acceptable behavior is practiced.

Each of the following stages typically involves certain issues; any unresolved issues can persist into adulthood.

Oral Stage (Ages 0 to 18 Months)

During the oral stage, the infant uses the mouth as the major source of gratification and exploration. Pleasure is experienced from eating, biting, chewing, and sucking. The infant's primary need is for security. A major conflict occurs with weaning.

 RECALL Ms. Kimber, the young, single, frus-trated mother of a 12-month-old child. The nurse might apply the concepts of Freud's the-ory in the nursing care of Ms. Kimber and her child by explaining the oral behaviors typical of the stage of her child's development. ●

Anal Stage (Ages 8 Months to 4 Years)

This stage begins with the development of neuromuscular control to allow control of the anal sphincter. Toilet train-ing is a crucial issue, requiring delayed gratification as the

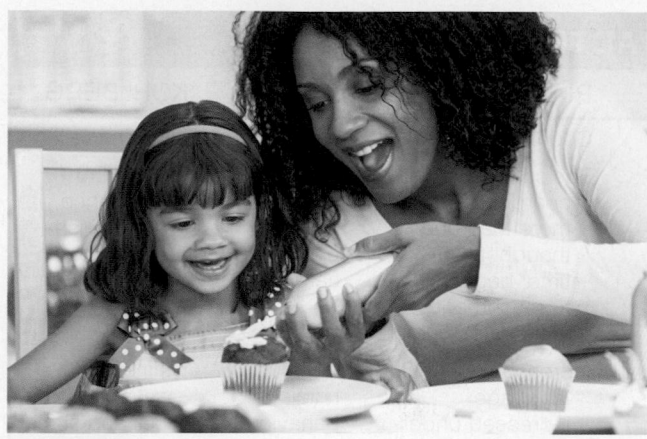

FIGURE 17-1. Sharing baking experiences allows this preschool girl to imitate activities that she often sees her mother enjoy.

child compromises between enjoyment of bowel function and limits set by social expectations.

Phallic Stage (Ages 3 to 7 Years)

The child has increased interest in gender differences and his or her own gender (Fig. 17-1). The child experiences conflict and resolution of that conflict with the parent of the same sex (named the Oedipus complex in boys and the Electra complex in girls, based on feelings of intimate sexual possessiveness for the opposite-sex parent). Curiosity about the genitals and masturbation increase during this stage.

Latency Stage (Ages 7 to 12 Years)

This stage marks the transition to the genital stage during adolescence. Increasing sex-role identification with the parent of the same sex prepares the child for adult roles and relationships.

Genital Stage (Ages 12 to 20 Years)

At this stage, sexual interest can be expressed in overt sexual relationships. Sexual pressures and conflicts typically cause turmoil as the adolescent makes adjustments in relationships.

Theory of Cognitive Development: Jean Piaget

Piaget and Inhelder (1969) developed a theory of **cognitive development** from infancy through adolescence. Piaget believed that learning occurs as a result of the internal organization of an event, forming a mental schema (plan) and serving as a base for further schemata as one grows and develops. Intellectual growth is a continual restructuring of knowledge to progress to higher levels of problem solving and critical thinking. Two continual processes of restructuring knowledge, assimilation and accommodation, stimulate intellectual growth in the child. **Assimilation** is the process of integrating new experiences into existing schemata. **Accommodation** is an alteration of existing thought processes to manage more complex information. Piaget described four stages of cognitive development.

Sensorimotor Stage (Birth to 24 Months)

This stage is marked by progression through a series of developmental tasks, for example:

- 0 to 1 month—Demonstrates basic reflexes, such as sucking
- 1 to 4 months—Discovers enjoyment of random behaviors (such as smiling or sucking thumb) and repeats them
- 4 to 8 months—Relates own behavior to a change in environment, such as shaking a rattle to hear the sound or manipulating a spoon to eat
- 8 to 12 months—Coordinates more than one thought pattern at a time to reach a goal, such as repeatedly throwing an object on the floor; only objects in sight are considered permanent
- 12 to 18 months—Recognizes the permanence of objects, even if out of sight; can understand simple commands
- 18 to 24 months—Begins to develop reasoning and can anticipate events

 RECALL Ms. Kimber, the single mother of a 12-month-old infant. Applying Piaget's theory, the nurse could develop a teaching plan for the mother that addresses appropriate anticipatory guidance to prevent injury while fostering the child's cognitive development. ●

Preoperational Stage (Ages 2 to 7 Years)

This stage is characterized by the beginning use of symbols, through increased language skills and pictures, to represent the preschooler's world (Fig. 17-2). This stage is divided into two parts: the preconceptual stage (ages 2–4 years) and the intuitive stage (ages 4–7 years). Play activities during this time help the child to understand life events and relationships.

Concrete Operational Stage (Ages 7 to 11 Years)

During this stage, children learn by manipulating concrete or tangible objects and can classify articles according to two or more characteristics. Logical thinking is developing, with

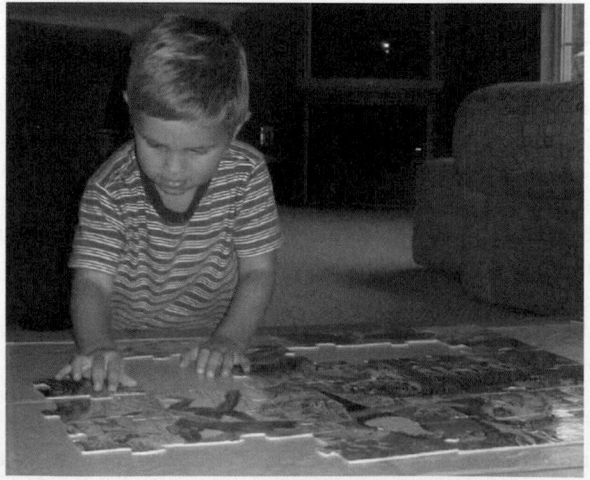

FIGURE 17-2. This child's cognitive development is characterized by the ability to learn simple sequences and relationships.

an understanding of reversibility, relations between numbers, and loss of egocentricity, in addition to the ability to incorporate another's perspective. Children become increasingly aware of external events and realize that their feelings and thoughts are unique and may not be the same as those of other children their age. They have the ability to focus on multiple parts of a problem at the same time.

Formal Operational Stage (Age 11 Years or Older)

This stage is characterized by the use of abstract thinking and deductive reasoning. General concepts are related to specific situations and alternatives are considered. The world is evaluated by testing beliefs in an attempt to establish values and meaning in life.

Theories of Psychosocial Development

Erik Erikson

Erikson's (1963) developmental theory expanded from Freud's work to include cultural and social influences in addition to biologic processes. His psychosocial theory is based on four major organizing concepts:

- Stages of development
- Developmental goals or tasks
- Psychosocial crises
- The process of coping

Erikson believed that development is a continuous process made up of distinct stages, characterized by the achievement of developmental goals that are affected by the social environment and significant others. He identified eight stages that progress from birth to old age and death. Each stage is characterized by a developmental crisis to be mastered, with possible successful or unsuccessful resolution of the crisis. Unsuccessful resolution at any one stage might delay progress through the next stage, but mastery can occur later.

TRUST VERSUS MISTRUST (INFANCY)
The infant learns to rely on caregivers to meet basic needs of warmth, food, and comfort, forming trust in others. Mistrust can result from inconsistent, inadequate, or unsafe care (Fig. 17-3).

AUTONOMY VERSUS SHAME AND DOUBT (TODDLER)
As motor and language skills develop, the toddler (ages 1 to 3 years) learns from the environment and gains independence through encouragement from caregivers to feed, dress, and toilet self. If the caregivers are overprotective or have expectations that are too high, shame and doubt, as well as feelings of inadequacy, might develop in the child.

 THINK back to Ms. Kimber, the single mother. The nurse could apply Erikson's theory to explain the child's "getting into everything" as his need for learning about the environment and gaining independence. Additionally, the mother's anxiety level

FIGURE 17-3. This caregiver provides comfort and affection to his daughter, teaching her to trust in others. (*Photo by Joe Mitchell.*)

and the child's attempts to investigate the environment through locomotion and oral exploration place the child at risk for injury from a fall or aspiration of a small object. With astute observation and knowledge of child development, the nurse plays a primary role in prevention by educating the mother. ●

INITIATIVE VERSUS GUILT (PRESCHOOL)
Confidence gained as a toddler allows the preschooler (ages 4 to 6 years) to take the initiative in learning so that the child actively seeks out new experiences and explores the how and why of activities. If the child experiences restrictions or reprimands for seeking new experiences and learning, guilt results, and the child hesitates to attempt more challenging skills in motor or language development.

INDUSTRY VERSUS INFERIORITY (SCHOOL-AGED CHILDREN)
Focusing on the end result of achievements, the school-aged child gains pleasure from finishing projects and receiving recognition for accomplishments (Fig. 17-4 on page 378). If the child is not accepted by peers or cannot meet parental expectations, a feeling of inferiority and lack of self-worth might develop.

 THINK back to Juan, the 8-year-old boy described at the beginning of the chapter. The nurse could help to foster Juan's industry by offering positive reinforcement for his ability to calm down when spoken to in Spanish. The nurse also could incorporate activities into Juan's plan of care that would provide him with opportunities to succeed. ●

IDENTITY VERSUS ROLE CONFUSION (ADOLESCENCE)
With many physical changes occurring, the adolescent is in transition from childhood to adulthood. Hormonal changes

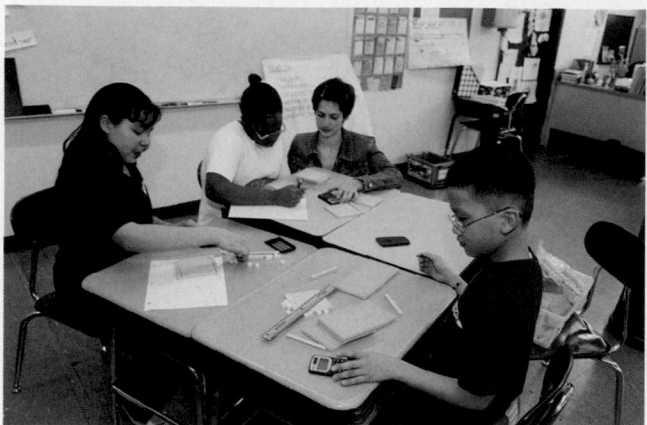

FIGURE 17-4. School-aged children focus on the end results of accomplishments—recognition and praise from family, teachers, and peers—in their development of a sense of competition and industry.

produce secondary sex characteristics and mood swings. Trying on roles and even rebellion can be normal behaviors as the adolescent acquires a sense of self and decides what direction to take in life. Role confusion occurs if the adolescent is unable to establish identity and a sense of direction.

INTIMACY VERSUS ISOLATION (YOUNG ADULTHOOD)

The tasks for the young adult are to unite self-identity with identities of friends and to make commitments to others. Fear of such commitments results in isolation and loneliness.

 REMEMBER Ms. Kimber, the single mother described at the beginning of the chapter. She appears to have a limited support system. Recognizing this, the nurse can assess further to identify the mother's potential problems with intimacy and subsequently, her progression toward generativity. ●

GENERATIVITY VERSUS STAGNATION (MIDDLE ADULTHOOD)

The middle adult years are marked by involvement with family, friends, and community. This is also a time for becoming concerned for the next generation and desiring to make a contribution to the world. If this task is not met, stagnation results, and the person becomes self-absorbed and obsessed with one's own needs or regresses to an earlier level of coping.

EGO INTEGRITY VERSUS DESPAIR (LATER ADULTHOOD)

As one enters the older years, reminiscence about life events provides a sense of fulfillment and purpose. Some older adults may not be fearful of dying if they feel they have achieved integrity. If one believes that one's life has been a series of failures or missed directions, a sense of despair might prevail.

 THINK back to Mr. Logan, the 70-year-old man who broke his hip. Applying Erikson's theory, the nurse could assess Mr. Logan for indications of despair due to his feelings of dependency on others, and plan appropriate interventions to foster a sense of fulfillment and purpose. ●

Robert J. Havighurst

Havighurst (1972) believed that living and growing are based on learning, and that a person must continuously learn to adjust to changing conditions. He described learned behaviors as **developmental tasks** that occur at certain periods in life. Successful achievement leads to happiness and success in later tasks, whereas unsuccessful achievement leads to unhappiness, societal disapproval, and difficulty in later tasks. The developmental tasks arise from maturation, personal motives, and values that determine occupational and family choices and civic responsibility.

INFANCY AND EARLY CHILDHOOD

Developmental tasks for infancy and early childhood include:

- Achieving physiologic stability
- Learning to eat solid foods
- Learning to walk and talk
- Forming simple concepts of social and physical reality
- Learning to relate emotionally to parents, siblings, and other people
- Learning to control the elimination of body wastes
- Learning to distinguish between right and wrong
- Learning sex differences and sexual modesty

MIDDLE CHILDHOOD

Developmental tasks for middle childhood include:

- Learning physical skills necessary for games
- Learning to get along with age-mates
- Developing fundamental skills in reading, writing, and mathematics
- Developing a conscience, morality, and a scale of values
- Achieving personal independence

ADOLESCENCE

Developmental tasks for adolescence include:

- Accepting one's body and using it effectively
- Achieving a masculine or feminine gender role
- Achieving emotional independence from parents and other adults
- Preparing for a career
- Preparing for marriage and family life
- Desiring and achieving socially responsible behavior
- Acquiring an ethical system as a guide to behavior (see the accompanying Research in Nursing box)

YOUNG ADULTHOOD

Developmental tasks for young adulthood include:

- Selecting a mate (Fig. 17-5)
- Learning to live with a marriage partner
- Starting a family and rearing children
- Managing a home
- Getting started in an occupation
- Taking on civic responsibility
- Finding a congenial social group

RESEARCH IN NURSING

BRIDGING THE GAP TO EVIDENCE-BASED PRACTICE

Comparison of Adolescent Concerns Between the First and Fourth Year of High School

Adolescence can be a tumultuous period of change, including the transition into high school and accompanying concerns about relationships, expectations, and personal identity. Adolescents experience changes in biologic, cognitive, and psychosocial development. Accelerated growth and hormonal changes lead to changes in body image. Adolescents develop increased competence in cognitive skills and begin to develop the ability to respond to new and demanding social situations. Peers become a growing influence, and adolescents continue the transition toward independence from their parents. As adolescents continue to move through the high school years, they develop their own personal identity, values, and interests.

Related Research

Rew, L., Tyler, D., Fredland, N., & Hannah, D. (2012). Adolescents' concerns as they transition through high school. *Advances in Nursing Science, 35*(3), 205–221.

In this study, the concerns of 216 adolescents were analyzed as they transitioned from entry into public high school and graduation from high school. The purpose was to analyze self-reported concerns that express the unique perspective of adolescents and to discern interventions that promote optimal health for most

high school students at all levels through this time period. This group of participants completed written surveys during each of the four years they attended high school. The sample included 142 females and 72 males (two others did not include gender data in their information). Twenty-one categories of concerns were identified, with education, relationships, expectations, and the future most commonly mentioned during the first year of high school. Three of these concerns differed considerably by the fourth year of high school. In the fourth year there was more concern about education, less concern about relationships, and more concern about the future. There was no significant difference in concerns about expectations.

Relevance to Nursing Practice

The findings of this study support nursing interventions that are developmentally appropriate for nurses who work with adolescents. During the high school years, nurses have the opportunity to interact and develop relationships with high school students and maintain positive support systems. Nurses can help students adopt life-long healthy behaviors. Understanding the concerns of adolescents during this transitional phase of their lives provides a basis for nursing interventions.

For additional research, visit thePoint.

MIDDLE ADULTHOOD

Developmental tasks for middle adulthood include:

- Accepting and adjusting to physical changes
- Attaining and maintaining a satisfactory occupational performance

- Assisting children to become responsible adults
- Relating to one's spouse as a person
- Adjusting to aging parents
- Achieving adult social and civic responsibility

LATER MATURITY

Developmental tasks for later maturity include:

- Adjusting to decreasing physical strength and health
- Adjusting to retirement and reduced income
- Adjusting to death of a spouse
- Establishing an explicit affiliation with one's age group
- Adjusting and adapting social roles in a flexible way
- Establishing satisfactory physical living arrangements

FIGURE 17-5. Choosing a life partner is often an important developmental task for young adults.

 RECALL Mr. Logan, the older adult male with the fractured hip described at the beginning of the chapter. Based on his comments, the nurse could apply Havighurst's theory to conclude that Mr. Logan might be fluctuating between feelings of nonadjustment and feelings of acceptance of his declining health. ●

Roger Gould

Gould (1978) studied men and women between the ages of 16 and 60 years, labeling the central theme for the adult years as "transformation," with specific beliefs and developmental phases.

AGES 18 TO 22

During the young adult years, individuals typically struggle with leaving their parents' world and challenging false assumptions from their child-like consciousness (e.g., "Only my parents can guarantee my safety"). However, these assumptions may be replaced with new false assumptions, such as "Rewards will come automatically if we do what we are supposed to do."

AGES 22 TO 28

Individuals in their 20s feel established as adults and separate from their families, but believe they must still demonstrate their competence as independent adults to their parents. They want to enjoy the present but build for the future.

AGES 29 TO 34

Self-acceptance increases as the need to prove oneself disappears. Marriage and careers are generally well established, and young parents want to accept their own children for what they are becoming without imposing rules. Questions about life in general are still present.

AGES 35 TO 43

Adults in this age group tend to continually look inward and question themselves, their values, and life. They see time as having an end and believe they have little time left to shape the behavior of their adolescent children (Fig. 17-6). They may be critical of their own parents, blaming them for many of their own problems.

AGES 43 TO 50

At this phase, adults accept the reality of boundaries for the lifespan and believe that personalities are set. They are interested in an active social life, church activities, community service, friends, and spouse. Life is viewed as neither simple nor controllable, which might result in periods of passivity, rage, depression, and despair.

AGES 50 TO 60

Previous patterns of reflection and contemplation generally result in increased self-approval and self-acceptance.

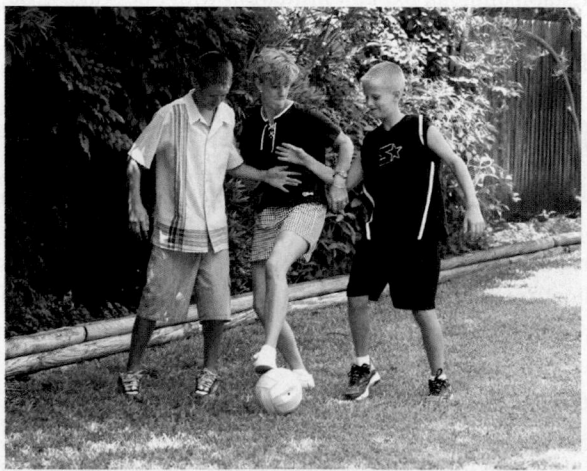

FIGURE 17-6. As her sons grow into young adults, this mom adapts to remain a positive influence in their lives. *(Photo by Joe Mitchell.)*

Increased marital happiness and contentment are associated with seeing one's spouse as a valued companion.

Daniel Levinson and Associates

Levinson, Darrow, Klein, Levinson, and McKee (1978) based their theory on the organizing concept of "individual life structure." The theory centered on the belief that the pattern of life at any point in time is formed by the interaction of three components: the self (values, motives), the social and cultural aspects of one's life (family, career, religion, ethnic background), and the particular set of roles in which one participates (husband, father, friend, student). When anything changes in one component, the whole life structure must then reorganize. According to Levinson and associates, there are five major phases in young and middle adult life.

EARLY ADULT TRANSITION

The major concerns of the young adult (age 18–22) are to break away from one's parents, make initial career choices, and establish intimate relationships. Many separations, losses, and transformations are necessary to terminate old relationships. This is also a time to begin to select personal values and establish goals, as one's life structure begins to be more integrated.

ENTERING THE ADULT WORLD

The years of the middle to late 20s (age 22–28) are a time to build on previous decisions and choices, and to try different careers and lifestyles. By the late 20s, the young adult enters the age-30 transition period. The person often feels uneasy that something is missing. During this transition, decisions are made either to find a new direction in life or to make a stronger commitment to previous choices.

SETTLING DOWN

In the settling-down phase (age 30–40), the adult invests energy into the areas of life that are most personally important. The areas of investment are primarily family, work, and community. The person strives to gain respect, status, and a sense of authority.

MIDLIFE TRANSITION

Midlife transition (age 40–45) involves a reappraisal of one's goals and values. The established lifestyle may continue, or the person may choose to reorganize and change careers. This is an unsettled time, with the person often anxious and fearful.

THE PAY-OFF YEARS

The years from 45 to 65 are a time of maximum self-direction and self-approval. Physical and mental changes increase one's awareness of aging and mortality.

Theories of Moral Development

Lawrence Kohlberg

Kohlberg (1969) developed a theory of **moral development** in levels that closely follow Piaget's theory of cognitive development. Kohlberg recognized that a person's moral development is influenced by cultural effects on one's perceptions

FIGURE 17-7. This grandfather reads traditional stories to his young granddaughter, teaching her important cultural values and beliefs, thereby influencing her moral development. *(Photo by Joe Mitchell.)*

of justice in interpersonal relationships. A child's beginnings of moral development result from caregiver–child communications during the early childhood years, as the young child tries to please his or her parents (Fig. 17-7). The concept of morality emerges as a subset of a person's beliefs or values and governs choices made throughout life. Kohlberg's stages of moral development begin in childhood but may develop well into adolescence and adulthood. Rules and regulations established by society are eventually challenged and evaluated as a person either accepts societal rules into one's own internal set of values or rejects them.

 REMEMBER Juan, the 8-year-old with encephalitis. Juan's language barrier and cultural heritage may be adding to the child's already heightened fears and anxieties due to hospitalization. The nurse's astute observation and application of Kohlberg's theory can further an understanding of the child's perceptions, beliefs, and, ultimately, choices and actions. •

PRECONVENTIONAL LEVEL

The preconventional level is based on external control, as the child learns to conform to rules imposed by authority figures. At stage 1, punishment and obedience orientation, the motivation for choices of action is the fear of physical consequences of authority's disapproval. As a result of the consequences, a perception of goodness or badness develops. At stage 2, instrumental relativist orientation, the thought of receiving a reward overcomes fear of punishment, thus actions that satisfy this desire are selected.

CONVENTIONAL LEVEL

The conventional level involves identifying with significant others and conforming to their expectations. The person respects the values and ideals of family and friends, regardless of consequences. In stage 3, "good boy–good girl" orientation, the person strives for approval in an attempt to be viewed as "good." At stage 4, "law and order" orientation, behavior follows social or religious rules from a respect for authority. In his later work, Kohlberg maintained that many adults are at this stage because they think abstractly and view themselves as members of society.

POSTCONVENTIONAL LEVEL

The postconventional level involves moral judgment that is rational and internalized into one's standards or values. At stage 5, social contract and utilitarian orientation, correct behavior is defined in terms of society's laws. Laws can be changed, however, to meet society's needs, while maintaining respect for self and others. Stage 6, universal ethical principle orientation, represents the person's concern for equality for all human beings, guided by personal values and standards, regardless of those set by society or laws. Justice might be internalized at an even higher level than society's level. Few adults ever reach this stage of development.

Carol Gilligan

Gilligan (1977; 1982) originally worked with Kohlberg. As she listened to women discuss their own real-life moral conflicts, she recognized that there was a conception of morality from the female viewpoint that was not represented in Kohlberg's work. Gilligan's theory views females as developing a morality of response and care, and males as developing a morality of justice.

In Gilligan's theory, males and females have different ways of looking at the world. Males are more likely to associate morality with obligations, rights, and justice. Females are more likely to see moral requirements emerging from the needs of others within the context of a relationship. This moral orientation of females is called the ethic of care, which develops through three levels. Each level ends with a transitional period—a time when the female considers new approaches to moral considerations and moves to a new level.

LEVEL 1—SELFISHNESS

In level 1, the focus is on one's own needs. "Should" and "would" are the same. Morality is seen in terms of sanctions by society. Relationships are often disappointing, and as a result, a woman might isolate herself to avoid getting hurt. The transition that follows this level is characterized by the move from selfishness to responsibility—a move that integrates the responsibility to care for oneself with the desire to care for others.

LEVEL 2—GOODNESS

In level 2, moral judgment is based on shared norms and expectations, and societal values are adopted. Acceptance by others becomes critical, and the ability to protect and care for others becomes the defining characteristic of female goodness. This characteristic is upheld through beliefs that one is responsible for the actions of others but that others are responsible for the choices they make. As a woman examines her self-sacrifice, the second transition occurs, with the woman asking if her own needs are not also important. A shift from goodness to truth (as well as a new conception of goodness) takes place.

 THINK back to Ms. Kimber, the single mother. The nurse could apply Gilligan's theory to assist Ms. Kimber in adjusting to her role as both a single parent caring for a child and as a woman with her own set of needs. •

LEVEL 3—NONVIOLENCE

In level 3, a changed understanding of self and a redefinition of morality allow reconciliation of selfishness and responsibility. Nonviolence (the injunction against hurting) governs all moral judgments and actions. Care becomes a universal obligation toward self and others. Moral problems are usually considered within the contexts of maintaining relationships and of promoting the welfare or preventing the harm of others.

Theory of Faith Development: James Fowler

Fowler (1981) postulated a developmental theory of the spiritual identity of humans, based on work by Piaget, Kohlberg, and Erikson. Fowler describes **faith** as follows:

> Faith is not always religious in its content or context.... Faith is a person's or group's way of moving into the force field of life. It is our way of finding coherence in and giving meaning to the multiple forces and relations that make up our lives. Faith is a person's way of seeing him or herself in relation to others against a background of shared meaning and purpose. Faith, therefore, is not necessarily religious, but it comprises the reasons one finds life worth living. (p. 4)

Fowler's theory is composed of a prestage and six stages of faith development. The age when a certain stage occurs varies, but the sequence does not. Fowler explained that a relationship among self, shared causes or values, and others is the unifying factor in all stages and is based on trust. Equilibrium, or a plateau in faith development, can occur at any stage from stage 2 and beyond.

Prestage: Undifferentiated Faith

During the prestage, trust, courage, hope, and love compete with threats of abandonment and inconsistencies in the infant's environment. The strength of faith in this stage is based on the infant's relationship with the primary caregiver.

Stage 1: Intuitive–Projective Faith

Intuitive–projective faith is most typical of the 3- to 7-year-old child. Children imitate religious gestures and behaviors of others, primarily their parents. They take on their parents' attitudes toward religious or moral beliefs without a thorough understanding of them. Imagination in this stage leads to long-lived images and feelings that they must question and reintegrate in later stages.

Stage 2: Mythical–Literal Faith

Mythical–literal faith predominates in the school-aged child, who is having more social interaction. Stories represent religious and moral beliefs, and the child accepts the existence of a deity. The child can appreciate the perspectives of others as well as the concept of reciprocal fairness.

Stage 3: Synthetic–Conventional Faith

Synthetic–conventional faith is the characteristic stage of many adolescents. As the person experiences increasing demands from work, school, family, and peers, the basis for identity becomes more complex. The person has an emerging ideology but has not closely examined it until now. The person begins to question life-guiding values or religious practices in an attempt to stabilize one's own identity.

FIGURE 17-8. (**A**) To provide holistic and individualized care, the nurse applies theories of growth and development when she communicates caring and provides emotional support to a young hospitalized child. (**B**) The nurse caring for an older adult includes the daughter, with whom the patient now lives, in discharge teaching. (B: Photo by B. Proud.)

BOX 17-2 INCORPORATING PRINCIPLES AND THEORIES OF GROWTH AND DEVELOPMENT

General guidelines for incorporating principles and theories of growth and development and family dynamics into daily practice of nursing care are listed here. They are provided as suggestions for working with patients of all ages.

- Be knowledgeable about the various stages of cognitive, psychosocial, moral, and spiritual development and prepared to support developmental stages typical of certain ages.
- Maintain flexibility in assessing patients, and respect the uniqueness of each person. Although the literature describes development typical of a particular age, not everyone fits into an exact mold.
- Anticipate possible regression during difficult periods or times of crisis, then accepting and supporting a person's return to a forward progression in development.
- Understand that environmental and cultural influences have a strong effect on development, especially psychosocial development. A deprived environment can be detrimental, whereas an enriched environment enhances development.

- Assess each person with an awareness that within each stage of development, a person may retain some behaviors of a previous stage, attain goals of the current stage, and begin to exhibit behaviors of the next stage. There is a time of transition to the next stage with no definite beginning or ending to the particular stage of development.
- Remember that patients are members of families and that the family can have both positive and negative influences on the development of individual members. Attempt to support good family relationships and healthy environments that assist members to reach their greatest potential for growth. Provide patient teaching to individuals and their families to aid in their understanding of periods of development.
- Be ready to provide health care to patients who are ill or who fail to meet developmental goals. Collaborate with other members of the health care team in providing care to prevent or minimize disruption of development and to promote optimal health throughout life.
- Provide environments and experiences that are developmentally challenging.

Stage 4: Individuative–Reflective Faith

Individuative–reflective faith is crucial for older adolescents and young adults because they become responsible for their own commitments, beliefs, and attitudes. Many adults do not develop to this stage, and for some people, it does not emerge until they are in their 30s or 40s. Searching for self-identity no longer defined by the faith compositions of significant others is a primary concern.

Stage 5: Conjunctive Faith

Conjunctive faith integrates other viewpoints about faith into one's understanding of truth. One can see the real nature of one's own beliefs. Along with this realization, one observes the divisions of faith development among people.

Stage 6: Universalizing Faith

Universalizing faith involves making tangible the values of absolute love and justice for humankind. The faith relationship is characterized by total trust in the principle of actively "being in relation" to others in whom we invest commitment, belief, love, risk, and hope, and in the existence of the future, regardless of what religion or image of faith is involved.

APPLYING THEORIES OF GROWTH AND DEVELOPMENT TO NURSING CARE

The complex and interrelated elements that contribute to human growth and development involve not only biophysical factors, but also factors of personality development. The theories summarized in this chapter help us understand cognitive, psychosocial, moral, and spiritual development. To understand the whole person, nurses need to evaluate all the components of growth and development to understand certain life events or concerns (Fig. 17-8).

Although these theories offer a great deal of insight into the processes of human growth and development, they do have some limitations. When planning holistic nursing care for patients with diverse needs, backgrounds, and ages, nurses should assess the patient as an individual and use interventions based on rationales from multiple developmental theories to provide comprehensive health care. Guidelines for incorporating the principles and theories of growth and development in nursing care are listed in Box 17-2.

Health care needs change quickly as a person grows and passes through life. These needs are unique for each person but have certain similarities in specific developmental stages. The nurse must plan care based on the patient's general and unique health needs and must continually revise aspects of care as the growth process evolves or alterations in health status occur.

The nurse is also uniquely positioned to address the sensitive emotional, psychological, and educational issues related to genomic discoveries. This focus on health, rather than disease, has the potential to result in significantly positive outcomes for the growth and development of all people.

DEVELOPING CLINICAL REASONING

1. Identify developmental challenges for five of your family members or friends at different ages across the lifespan. Explain why meeting developmental needs is an essential role of nursing.

2. Compare and contrast the psychosocial theories of Erikson and Gould. Are the concepts in these theories relevant today? If yes, explain why. If no, what would you delete and what would you add?

3. Using Piaget's theory of cognitive development, describe how you would explain the death of a parent to children 4, 9, and 13 years of age.

PRACTICING FOR NCLEX

1. A nurse examining a toddler in a pediatric office documents that the child is in the 90th percentile for height and weight and has blue eyes. These physical characteristics are primarily determined by:
   a. Socialization with caregivers
   b. Maternal nutrition during pregnancy
   c. Genetic information on chromosomes
   d. Meeting developmental tasks

2. The nurse caring for infants in a hospital nursery knows that newborns continue to grow and develop according to individual growth patterns and developmental levels. Which terms describe these patterns? Select all that apply.
   a. Orderly
   b. Simple
   c. Sequential
   d. Unpredictable
   e. Differentiated
   f. Integrated

3. A 2-year-old grabs a handful of cake from the table and stuffs it in his mouth. According to Freud, what part of the mind is the child satisfying?
   a. Id
   b. Superego
   c. Ego
   d. Unconscious mind

4. A nurse is teaching parents of preschoolers what type of behavior to expect from their children based on developmental theories. Which statements describe this stage of development? Select all that apply.
   a. According to Freud, the child is in the phallic stage.
   b. According to Erikson, the child is in the trust versus mistrust stage.
   c. According to Havighurst, the child is learning to get along with others.
   d. According to Fowler, the child imitates religious behavior of others.
   e. According to Kohlberg, the child defines satisfying acts as right.
   f. According to Havighurst, the child is achieving gender-specific roles.

5. A nurse caring for elderly patients in a long-term care facility encourages an older adult to reminisce about her past life events. This life review, according to Erikson, is demonstrating what developmental stage of the later adult years?
   a. Ego integrity
   b. Generativity
   c. Intimacy
   d. Initiative

6. A nurse researcher studies the effects of genomics on current nursing practice. Which statements identify genetic principles that will challenge nurses to integrate genomics in their research, education, and practice? Select all that apply.
   a. Genetic tests plus family history tools have the potential to identify people at risk for diseases.
   b. Pharmacogenetic tests can determine if a patient is likely to have a strong therapeutic response to a drug or suffer adverse reactions from the medication.
   c. Evidence-based review panels are in place to evaluate the possible risks and benefits related to genetic testing.
   d. Valid and reliable national data are available to establish baseline measures and track progress toward targets.
   e. Genetic variation can either accelerate or slow the metabolism of many drugs.
   f. It is beyond the role of the nurse to answer questions and discuss the impact of genetic findings on health and illness.

7. A nurse who is working with women in a drop-in shelter studies Carol Gilligan's theory of morality in women to use when planning care. According to Gilligan, what is the motivation for female morality?
   a. Law and justice
   b. Obligations and rights
   c. Response and care
   d. Order and selfishness

8. Which factor initially influences moral development as described in Kohlberg's theory?
   a. Parent–child communications
   b. Societal rules and regulations
   c. Social and religious rules
   d. One's beliefs and values

9. The school nurse uses the principles and theories of growth and development when planning programs for high school students. According to Havighurst, what is a developmental task for this age group?
   a. Finding a congenial social group
   b. Developing a conscience, morality, and a scale of values
   c. Achieving personal independence
   d. Achieving a masculine or feminine gender role

10. A nurse is interviewing Anthony, a 42-year-old patient who visits his internist for a blood pressure screening. Anthony tells the nurse that he is currently a sales associate but is considering a different career. He states that he is "a little anxious about the process." According to Levinson, what phase of adult life is Anthony experiencing?
    a. Entering the adult world
    b. Settling down
    c. Midlife transition
    d. The pay-off years

ANSWERS WITH RATIONALES

1. **c.** Physical appearance and growth have a predetermined genetic base in inheritance patterns carried on the chromosomes.

2. **a, c, e, f.** Growth and development are orderly and sequential, as well as continuous and complex. Growth and development follow regular and predictable trends, and are both differentiated and integrated.

3. **a.** Freud defined the id as the part of the mind concerned with self-gratification by the easiest and quickest available means.

4. **a, d, e.** According to Freud, the child is in the phallic stage. According to Fowler, the child imitates religious behavior of others. According to Kohlberg, the child defines satisfying acts as right. According to Erikson, the child is in the initiative versus guilt stage. According to Havighurst, the child is learning sex differences, forming concepts, and getting ready

to read. According to Havighurst, the adolescent, not the preschooler, is achieving gender-specific social roles.

5. *a.* Reminiscence during the older years of one's life provides a sense of fulfillment and purpose (ego integrity). Generativity is a developmental stage of the middle adult years. Intimacy is a developmental task of the adolescent to adult years, and initiative is a task of the preschooler to early school-age years.

6. *a, b, e.* In the very near future, all health care providers will be challenged to integrate genomics into their research, education, and practice (*Healthy People 2020,* 2012). Genetic tests plus family history tools have the potential to identify people at risk for diseases. Pharmacogenetics is the study of how genetic variation affects an individual's response to drugs. Pharmacogenetic tests can determine if a patient is likely to have a strong therapeutic response to a drug or suffer adverse reactions from the medication. Genetic variation can either accelerate or slow the metabolism of many drugs (Lehne, 2013; Human Genome Project, 2011). Two emerging challenges related to genomic discoveries are (1) the need for evidence-based review panels to thoroughly evaluate the possible benefits and harms related to the expanding number of genetic tests and family health history tools, and (2) valid and reliable national data are needed to establish baseline measures and track progress toward targets (*Healthy People 2020,* 2012). Nurses must be prepared to answer questions and discuss the impact of genetic findings on health and illness.

7. *c.* In Gilligan's theory, males and females have different ways of looking at the world. Males are more likely to associate

morality with obligations, rights, and justice. Females are more likely to see moral requirements emerging from the needs of others within the context of a relationship.

8. *a.* Moral development in the young child results from communications as the child tries to please his or her parents.

9. *d.* According to Havighurst, it is the role of the adolescent to achieve a masculine or feminine gender role. Developing a conscience, morality, and a scale of values and achieving personal independence are roles of middle childhood. Finding a congenial social group is a role of young adulthood.

10. *c.* Midlife transition (age 40–45) involves a reappraisal of one's goals and values. The established lifestyle may continue, or the individual may choose to reorganize and change careers. This is an unsettled time, with the individual often anxious and fearful. The years of the middle to late 20s (age 22–28) are a time to build on previous decisions and choices and to try different careers and lifestyles. In the settling-down phase (age 30–40), the adult invests energy into the areas of life that are most personally important. The years from 45 to 65 are a time of maximum self-direction and self-approval.

TAYLOR SUITE RESOURCES

Explore these additional resources to enhance learning for this chapter:

- NCLEX-Style Questions and other resources on thePoint, http://thePoint.lww.com/Taylor8e
- *Study Guide for Fundamentals of Nursing, 8th edition*
- Adaptive Learning | Powered by prepU, http://thepoint.lww.com/prepu

Bibliography

Calendra, J. (2011). Effective parenting: Innate or learned? *Nurse.com, (20)*13, 34–39.

Erikson, E. H. (1963). *Childhood and society* (2nd ed.). New York: Norton.

Fowler, J. W. (1981). *Stages of faith: The psychology of human development and the quest for meaning.* New York: Harper & Row.

Fowler, J. W. (1991). *Weaving the new creation: Stages of faith and the public church.* San Francisco: HarperCollins.

Freud, S., & Strachey, J. (1960). *The ego and the id: The standard edition of the complete psychological works of Sigmund Freud.* New York: Norton.

Gilligan, C. (1977). In a different voice: Women's conceptions of the self and of morality. *Harvard Educational Review, 47,* 481–517.

Gilligan, C. (1982). *In a different voice.* Cambridge, MA: Harvard University Press.

Goldberg, P., Jenkins, S., & Spahis, J. (2010). Genetics: Soon to be a part of nursing practice. *Nursing Spectrum, 19*(15), 26–31.

Gould, R. (1978).*Transformations.* New York: Simon & Schuster.

Havighurst, R. J. (1972). *Developmental tasks and education.* New York: David McKay.

Healthy People 2020 (2012). Genomics. Available at http://www.healthypeople.gov/2020/topicsobjectives2020/overview.aspx?topicid=15

Human Genome Project. (2011). NIH Fact Sheet. Available at http://report.nih.gov/NIHfactsheets/ViewFactSheet.aspx?csid=45

Human Genome Project Information. (2011a). *About the human genome project.* Available at http://ornl.gov/sci/techresources/Human_Genome/project/about.shtml

Human Genome Project Information. (2011b). *Frequently asked questions.* Available at http://www.ornl.gov/sci/techresources/Human_Genome/faq/faqs1.shtml

Kohlberg, L. (1969). Stage and sequence: The cognitive–developmental approach to socialization. In D. Gaslin (Ed.), *Handbook of socialization: Theory and research* (pp. 347–380). Chicago: Rand McNally.

Lehne, R. (2013). *Pharmacology for Nursing Care* (8th ed.). St. Louis, Missouri: Elsevier.

Levinson, D., Darrow, C., Klein, E., Levinson, M., & McKee, B. (1978). *The seasons of a man's life.* New York: Knopf.

NANDA International (NANDA-I). (2012). *Nursing diagnoses: Definitions & classification 2012–2014.* West Sussex, UK: Wiley-Blackwell.

Pender, N., Murdaugh, C., & Parsons, M. (2011). *Health Promotion in Nursing Practice* (6th ed.). Upper Saddle River, NJ: Pearson Education, Inc.

Piaget, J., & Inhelder, B. (1969). *The psychology of the child.* New York: Basic Books.

Rew, L., Tyler, D., Fredland, N., & Hannah, D. (2012). Adolescents' concerns as they transition through high school. *Advances in Nursing Science, 35*(3), 205–221.

Sherwood, G., & Barnsteiner, J. (2012). *Quality and Safety in Nursing: A Competency Approach to Improving Outcomes.* West Sussex, UK: Wiley-Blackwell.

18 | Conception Through Young Adult

NATE PELTON

Nate, who is 11 years old, collided with another player while running in the outfield during a Little League baseball game. He was removed from the game after the collision because he complained of a headache and, according to his coaches, appeared slightly dazed. His parents took him to the emergency department (ED) at the local hospital where Nate told the ED nurse, "I felt a little dizzy after the collision but I feel fine now."

DARLENE JENKINS

Darlene, a pregnant 14-year-old in her third trimester, comes to the prenatal clinic for the first time. Her history reveals sexual activity with multiple partners, smoking two packs of cigarettes per day, beer "4 or 5 nights a week," and eating mostly "fast foods." She has had no prenatal care and hasn't been taking any prenatal vitamins. She is homeless but occasionally stays with an older girlfriend since her parents "threw me out of the house."

HILLARIE BROWNING

Hillarie, who is 2 years old, is brought to the ED by her father, James Browning. She is unresponsive. Mr. Browning says that she "took a tumble" down the stairs, but assessment reveals that her injuries are inconsistent with this type of fall.

LEARNING OBJECTIVES

After completing the chapter, you will be able to accomplish the following:

1. Summarize major physiologic, cognitive, psychosocial, moral, and spiritual developments from conception through young adulthood.
2. List common health problems of each age period from conception through young adulthood.
3. Describe nursing interventions to promote health in patients from conception through young adulthood.

KEY TERMS

adolescence	neonate	sudden infant death syndrome (SIDS)
attachment	preschooler	
bonding	puberty	
child maltreatment	regression	sudden unexplained infant death (SUID)
colic	school-aged child	
failure to thrive (FTT)	separation anxiety	temperament
infant	sexually transmitted infection (STI)	toddler
negativism		young adult

Growth and development occur throughout the lifespan. The nurse's knowledge of growth and developmental milestones provides a base for planning and implementing holistic, individualized nursing care. This chapter continues the discussion of developmental theories introduced in Chapter 17, with specific information related to the sequential stages of growth and development from conception through young adulthood.

Although divided into different stages, childhood encompasses the entire period before young adulthood. Included within this time span are the fetus, neonate, infant, toddler, preschooler, school-aged child, and adolescent. This chapter's discussion of each of these stages includes, as appropriate, physiologic, cognitive, psychosocial, and moral and spiritual development; health; and the nurse's role in promoting health. For an example addressing the adolescent, see the accompanying Reflective Practice box on page 388.

CONCEPTION AND PRENATAL DEVELOPMENT

Human growth and development begin at the moment the ovum is fertilized by the sperm. The fertilized ovum (zygote) contains the full complement of genetic information provided by each parent that determines gender and influences personality, intellect, and physical and psychological traits. The growth and development stages of the fetus are orderly and continuous, and proceed as follows.

Pre-embryonic Stage

The pre-embryonic stage lasts for about 3 weeks. The zygote, which implants in the uterine wall, has three distinct cell layers. The endoderm (inner layer) becomes the respiratory system, the digestive system, the liver, and the pancreas. The mesoderm (middle layer) becomes the skeleton; connective tissue; cartilage; muscles; and the circulatory, lymphoid, reproductive, and urinary systems. The ectoderm (outer layer) becomes the brain, spinal cord, nervous system, and outer body parts (skin, hair, and nails).

Embryonic Stage

The embryonic stage occurs from the 4th through the 8th week. Rapid growth and differentiation of the cell layers take place. By the end of this stage, all basic organs have been established, the bones have begun to ossify, and some human features are recognizable. Because this is a period of such rapid growth and change, the embryo is especially vulnerable to any factor that might cause congenital anomalies (such as maternal use of alcohol, nicotine, over-the-counter medications, or drugs).

Fetal Stage

The fetal stage lasts from 9 weeks to birth. All body organs and systems continue to grow and develop. At the end of the first trimester (12 weeks' gestation), some reflexes are present, kidney secretion begins, the heartbeat can be heard by Doppler, and the sex of the fetus is distinguishable by outward appearance. At the end of the second trimester (24 weeks' gestation), fetal heart tones are audible by stethoscope, the liver and pancreas are functioning, hair forms, sleep–wake patterns are established, lung surfactant is produced, and the eyelids open. At the end of the third trimester (40 weeks' gestation), the testes have descended, lung alveoli are formed, subcutaneous fat is deposited, and the fetus actively kicks. By birth, the average neonate weighs 7.5 lb (3.4 kg) and is 20 inches (50.8 cm) long.

During pregnancy, adequate maternal nutrition is essential for normal growth and development of the embryo and fetus. A fetus not receiving adequate nutrition might be small for gestational age, fail to have normal brain development, have learning disabilities as a child, and be at increased risk for chronic illnesses as an adult. Vitamin and mineral deficiencies can result in fetal megaloblastic anemia and neural tube defects (folic acid deficiency), inadequate bone calcification (vitamin D and calcium deficits), and hypothyroidism (iodine deficiency).

During the past decade, the number of premature births (those occurring before 37 weeks' gestation) has decreased. Approximately 12% of the births in the United States in 2011 were premature, but this rate is still higher than levels reported during the 1980s and most of the 1990s (Hamilton,

REFLECTIVE PRACTICE: CULTIVATING QSEN COMPETENCIES

CHALLENGE TO ETHICAL AND LEGAL SKILLS

I was admitting Darlene Jenkins, a pregnant, unmarried, 14-year-old to the prenatal clinic. This was her first visit and she was already in her third trimester. A quick history revealed multiple factors putting both her and her fetus at risk for health problems: lack of family (or other) support (homeless, occasionally staying with an older girlfriend), father of the baby unknown, multiple sexual partners, diet consisting mainly of fast food, no prenatal vitamins, little to no exercise, and history of smoking (2 packs of cigarettes per day) and alcohol consumption ("beer 4 to 5 times a week"). When she was seen by the medical resident, he asked her quite curtly if she was trying to "kill your baby," telling her that it was probably too late for her to get the care she needed. "Why should we waste our time on you when other women here really want to be helped?" Although Darlene was acting "tough," I could tell from her expression that she was both angry and hurt. While I was upset by the choices that she had made so far and shared some of the resident's frustration, I knew we had to give her a reason to trust us if we wanted her to start taking better care of herself and her baby. I was also upset by the resident's lack of professionalism and wondered if I should say something to him.

Thinking Outside the Box: Possible Courses of Action

- Play the "good cop–bad cop" routine; after the resident finished his visit, I could try to be especially caring and explain why we were all concerned about her and her baby. Then I could talk to her about what she needed to do to maximize good outcomes.
- Challenge the resident in the patient's presence, thereby showing her that at least I honestly cared about her.

- Confront the resident later in a "cooler moment," hoping that this behavior doesn't repeat itself, while being prepared to report my concerns to a "higher authority" should this behavior occur again.
- Approach the resident outside the patient's presence and explain my concerns. Persuade the resident to apologize to Darlene in the interests of winning the patient's trust and compliance with the prenatal care program.

Evaluating a Good Outcome: How Do I Define Success?

- The respect for each person's human dignity (Darlene, the resident, myself) is affirmed.
- Each person feels empowered to make personal decisions that advance one's interests and goals.

- The patient makes the needed lifestyle changes, with good outcomes for herself and her baby.
- Personal integrity is maintained; no one has to sacrifice beliefs and values.
- Professional integrity is maintained.

Personal Learning: Here's to the Future!

In this situation, I don't think that I chose the best alternative because I tried to comfort Darlene and make "excuses" for the resident's behavior. I tried to explain that the resident was very busy and simply "out of sorts." I have to admit that, initially, I was probably just as shocked by the resident's response as Darlene. Personally, I knew that I'd die if someone said something like that to me. After I spoke with the resident, I realized there might be some value in shocking a patient into seeing the harm of her ways. However, in this encounter, Darlene had no way of knowing whether this response was well-intended (if indeed it was!) or not. While talking further with Darlene, I became convinced that she wouldn't start listening to us until she could trust us. I wish I had the courage to ask the resident to apologize to Darlene. His apology might have been exactly what was needed to get her to trust us. I'm learning that when patient welfare is at stake, I might have to sacrifice my own comfort level to challenge other professional caregivers. Hopefully, I'll learn how to do this in a way that promotes respectful, collaborative relationships.

REFLECTION ON QUALITY AND SAFETY COMPETENCIES

How do you think you would respond in a similar situation? Why? What does this tell you about yourself and the adequacy of your skills for professional practice? Can you think of other ways to respond? What *knowledge, skills,* and *attitudes* do you need to develop to continuously improve quality and safety when caring for patients like Darlene?

Patient-Centered Care: What information should be communicated to Darlene regarding concerns about her pregnancy and the developing fetus? How could you involve the patient as a partner in coordinating her care to promote trust? How might you talk with Darlene about the various risk factors contributing to her health and that of her baby? What is the best way to communicate emotional support to Darlene?

Teamwork and Collaboration/Quality Improvement: What communication skills do you need to continue to function as a resource and advocate for Darlene? What if the nurse confronted the resident in front of the patient? Would you consider this professional behavior? Do you feel that the resident functioned in a professional manner? Do you agree with the nurse in her thinking that an apology from the resident would help encourage Darlene to trust health care professionals? Why or why not? Are there other community resources that might help Darlene in the care of her baby following the baby's birth?

Safety/Evidence-Based Practice: Is there anything more you could have done to acknowledge you understand Darlene's reasons for lack of trust and possible unwillingness to make changes to promote a positive outcome? How might a nurse's developmental stage have affected the actions taken toward the resident and the patient? What evidence in nursing literature provides guidance for decision-making regarding ensuring a safe environment and giving Darlene the support that she needs?

Informatics: Can you identify essential information that must be documented in Darlene's electronic record about efforts to communicate with her and the specific concerns that she expressed? What other information must be available to support safe care for Darlene and her fetus and coordination of her care? Can you think of other ways to respond or approach the situation?

Martin & Ventura, 2012). Low birth weight is one of the leading causes of infant mortality and the leading cause of infant death during the first month of life. Infants born prematurely are at increased risk for disorders such as cerebral palsy, mental retardation, and chronic respiratory problems (Centers for Disease Control and Prevention [CDC], 2013e). Many people, including health care workers, are unaware of the magnitude of this problem.

Other health risks for the developing fetus are discussed later in this chapter.

NEONATE: BIRTH TO 28 DAYS

At birth, the **neonate** must adapt to extrauterine life through several significant physiologic adjustments. The most important occur in the respiratory and circulatory systems as the neonate begins breathing and becomes independent of the umbilical cord. The neonate is assessed immediately after birth. Of several existing measurement scales, the Apgar rating scale is the most commonly used. This scale is used to assess neonates 1 minute and 5 minutes after birth (Table 18-1).

Physiologic Development

The physical characteristics and behaviors of normal neonates are as follows:

- Reflexes include the Moro reflex, the stepping reflex, grasp reflex, hand-to-mouth activity, sucking, swallowing, blinking, sneezing, and yawning (Fig. 18-1 on page 390).
- Body temperature responds quickly to the environmental temperature.
- Senses are used to respond to the environment; see color and form; hear and turn toward sound, smell, and taste; and feel touch and pain.
- Stool and urine are eliminated.
- Both an active crying state and a quiet alert state are exhibited (see Fig. 18-1).

The neonate inherits a transient immunity from infections as a result of maternal immunoglobulins that cross the placenta. Breastfeeding provides further protection against bacterial and viral infections through antibodies, immunoglobulins, and leukocytes in breast milk. The high lactose content in breast milk, combined with limited protein, promotes an acid environment that is unsuitable for bacterial growth.

Health of the Neonate

Difficulties related to the birth process, the transition to extrauterine life, or congenital anomalies might require intervention by health care personnel.

Respiratory difficulties might occur, especially if drugs given to the mother during labor and delivery have sedated the neonate. Premature neonates are vulnerable to respiratory distress syndrome because of the relatively immature lung function. Neonates delivered by cesarean birth are at risk for respiratory difficulties because of excess mucus in the lungs and might require frequent suctioning.

Incompatibility between the neonate's and mother's blood groups requires prompt care at birth. Congenital malformations, such as cleft palate and cleft lip or neural tube defects (such as spina bifida) and hydrocephalus, might result in long-term health problems. Birth traumas that cause temporary symptoms are of concern because the parents need to be reassured that the symptoms will disappear. Examples include caput succedaneum (localized edema of the scalp), molding (elongation of the skull as the baby passes through the birth canal), and subconjunctival hemorrhage. The nonthreatening nature of physiologic jaundice, which commonly occurs in the neonate's first days, should also be explained to the parents.

Neonates born to mothers who smoke cigarettes, drink alcohol, or use drugs are at risk for developmental deficits as well as complications during birth. Smoking during pregnancy might cause low birth weight. Fetal alcohol syndrome caused by maternal drinking is believed to be a leading cause of birth defects, including growth retardation, developmental delay, and impaired intellectual ability.

A woman who uses drugs during pregnancy puts herself as well as her baby at risk. For example, maternal use of methamphetamine increases the probability of congenital anomalies, prematurity, low birth weight, and drug withdrawal symptoms. Methamphetamine use can result in abrupt changes in the mother's blood pressure, resulting in decreased fetal blood flow and oxygenation. Babies born to meth-addicted mothers may grow more slowly in utero and can be jittery, irritable, intolerant of cuddling, and feed

Table 18-1 APGAR SCORING CHART

CATEGORY[a]	0	1	2
Heart rate	Absent	Slow (less than 100 beats/min)	More than 100 beats/min
Respiratory effort	Absent	Slow, irregular	Good, crying
Muscle tone	Flaccid	Some flexion of extremities	Active motion
Reflex irritability	No response	Weak cry or grimace	Vigorous cry
Color	Blue, pale	Body pink, extremities blue	Completely pink

[a]Each category is rated as 0, 1, or 2. The rating for each category is then totaled to a maximum score of 10. Normal neonates score between 7 and 10. Neonates who score between 4 and 6 require special assistance; those who score below 4 are in need of immediate life-saving support.

Grasp reflex *(Photo by Joe Mitchell.)*

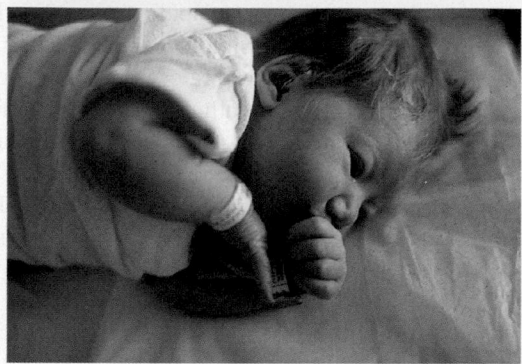

Hand to mouth and sucking activity

Moro reflex *(Photo by Joe Mitchell.)*   Stepping reflex *(Photo by Joe Mitchell.)*

FIGURE 18-1. Reflexes and behaviors of the neonate.   Quiet alert state   Active crying state *(Photo by Joe Mitchell.)*

poorly (American College of Obstetricians and Gynecologists (ACOG), 2011).

INFANT: 1 MONTH TO 1 YEAR

The neonate becomes an **infant** at 1 month, a period lasting until the first birthday (Fig. 18-2).

Physiologic Development

The physical characteristics of the infant include the following:

- Brain grows to about half the adult size.
- Body temperature stabilizes.
- Motor abilities develop, allowing use of building blocks, attempting to feed self, crawling, and walking.
- Eyes begin to focus and fixate.
- Heart doubles in weight, heart rate slows, and blood pressure rises.

- Deciduous teeth begin to erupt at 4 to 6 months.
- Birth weight usually triples by 1 year, when the average male infant weighs 22 lb (10 kg) and the average female infant weighs 21 lb (9.5 kg). Length increases by 50%.

Cognitive Development

Infants from birth to 1 year are in the sensorimotor stage of development described by Piaget. Language development is in the prelinguistic phase. Babies begin to coo and make sounds soon after birth, and by 12 months of age, they can convey their wishes through a few key words. Language development in infants has several consistent characteristics that occur with all languages:

- Use of syllable repetition (such as ma-ma, da-da, bye-bye)
- Universal early phonetic expressions (babbling sounds)
- Imitation of sounds and intonations spoken by caregivers

Bonding might occur in the first few hours after birth or later in the first few months and is necessary for later attachment. *(Photo by Joe Mitchell.)*

Developmental tasks of the first year include taking solid food.

As the infant enters the second half of her first year, play will begin to involve manipulation of objects and the environment.

Later infancy is characterized by the ability to pull-to-stand, cruise, and often walk.

FIGURE 18-2. Development in the infant.

Psychosocial Development

Developmental Theories

In terms of the developmental theories discussed in Chapter 17, the infant has the following characteristics:

- Is in the oral stage (Freud), striving for immediate gratification of needs and having a strong sucking need
- Develops trust (Erikson) if the caregiver can be counted on to provide food when the infant is hungry; trust is also facilitated by diaper changing, warmth, and comforting
- Meets developmental tasks (Havighurst) by learning to take solid food, walk, and talk

Special Considerations

Other components of psychosocial development in the neonate and infant include attachment, bonding, play, and temperament.

ATTACHMENT AND BONDING

Attachment is an active, affectionate, reciprocal relationship between two people, which is somewhat different from bonding. **Bonding**, described by Klaus and Kennell (1982), occurs during a sensitive period in the first few hours after birth (although bonding also might occur later in the first few months) and is necessary for later attachment. Bonding might be considered the emotional linkage of two people, and attachment the long-term maintenance and strengthening of the linked state.

PLAY

Infants and children discover their environment and begin to learn how to control it through play. Beginning as soon as the baby is aware of sensations and the pleasure they produce, play progresses from self-pleasure to interaction with others. The two dimensions of play are social play and cognitive play.

Social play, such as rolling a ball back and forth between two children, is motivated by a desire for fun, pleasure, and relationships with others. Cognitive play, as when a child puts a puzzle together, is motivated by the desire to learn.

TEMPERAMENT

Temperament is primarily inborn, although it is influenced by environment. A baby or child might be said to be "easy," "slow to warm," or "difficult" (Thomas, Chess, & Birch, 1968). The "easy" infant sleeps, eats, and eliminates easily; smiles spontaneously; and cries in response to significant needs. The "slow-to-warm" infant is more passive and distant. The "difficult" infant has volatile and labile responses, often is a restless sleeper, is highly sensitive to noises, and eats poorly. These traits often remain fairly consistent throughout the person's life. The behavior of caregivers as they care for the baby can positively or negatively influence the degree to which temperament dictates behavioral style.

Health of the Infant

Various health problems in infancy might require the intervention of health care personnel. Gastroenteritis and food allergies are common. Skin disorders, such as diaper dermatitis (diaper rash), seborrheic dermatitis (infant dandruff), prickly heat rash, acute infantile eczema, and thrush (infection of the oral mucous membrane by the fungus *Candida albicans*), also are common. Infant colic, failure to thrive, accidents, sudden infant death syndrome, and child maltreatment are of particular concern during infancy.

Infant Colic

Colic is uncontrollable, extended crying in an otherwise healthy and well-fed baby. Colic generally occurs during the first 3 months of life and has been referred to as the "100-day syndrome." This continuous crying can occur at any time but usually worsens in the evening. The infant cries loudly and draws the legs up to the abdomen. Despite the symptoms, the infant gains weight. Parents and other family members might experience stress and anxiety due to the constant crying (see Through the Eyes of a Caregiver).

The exact cause of colic is not known. One common belief is that an immature digestive system might be the cause. Swallowing excess air, feeding too rapidly or too much, improper feeding techniques, or allergies might lead to spasmodic contractions of the intestines, with acute abdominal pain. Another belief is that an immature nervous system might be the cause. Normal external stimulation might cause the baby to tense up.

Failure to Thrive

Failure to thrive (FTT) is a condition of inadequate growth in height and weight resulting from the infant's inability to obtain or use calories needed for growth. Infants with FTT have signs of malnutrition and delayed development. Causes and contributing factors might include physiologic causes, inadequate funds to buy sufficient food, the use of a fad diet, inadequate nutritional knowledge, insufficient breast milk, and disturbances in maternal–child attachment. In most cases of FTT not caused by a physiologic problem, a team of health care providers is needed to meet the complex needs of the infant and caregivers.

Accidental Injuries

Safety issues must be addressed during infancy. The swallowing reflex matures progressively from birth, but until it is fully developed, aspiration is a risk. Because infants often put small objects in their mouths, choking is a risk.

THROUGH THE EYES OF A CAREGIVER

When my son Luke was first born, he was an easy-going, pleasant baby. Then, when he was about 3 weeks old, it started. He cried inconsolably every night from 5 PM until 12 AM. We could do nothing to comfort him. We took him to the pediatrician. The doctor said the word we already expected to hear: "colic." He gave us a prescription for an antacid and a muscle relaxant. He gave us some advice on how to comfort him...wrap him snugly, hold him like a football, eliminate milk and dairy from my diet (I was breast-feeding), and put pressure on his belly. None of these things worked. Eventually, we discovered that rocking him in our arms as we ran the shower seemed to calm him. Pink Floyd and *Dark Side of the Moon* also comforted him. We found this out quite accidentally when we played the CD in an attempt to drown out his crying. These methods somewhat helped with the crying, but little helped my anxiety. I was concerned for my little son, who was clearly upset or in pain. At the same time, I found it very difficult to bond with him. I'd find myself dreading the evening; dreading being with my baby. When I'd come home from work, I'd take a deep breath and stand paralyzed at the front door, wondering if I had to go in. I could hear his crying from the doorstep. I felt horrible about these feelings. I questioned my parenting skills. At one point, I spoke with a nurse whose daughter had colic. She said, "My daughter's colic lasted 100 days, but it has taken me 14 years to forgive her!" This made me laugh for the first time in weeks. Then she asked how I was doing and if I wanted to talk about how I was feeling. I hadn't told anyone how I was feeling toward my son. How could I? I confided in her, though. I knew she wouldn't judge me. I knew she'd understand. After speaking with the nurse, I felt a lot better knowing that it was OK to feel the way I did. As time went on, Luke's crying spells got shorter and shorter, until the 99th day; then, miraculously, it ended. We had a party the next day, with a cake that said "Day 100. We made it." Today, he is a sweet, healthy child. He is no fussier than any other 3-year-old child. We have bonded exceptionally well. My husband and family were supportive and helped care for Luke when he had colic, but it was the nurse who helped care for me!

—*Dana Jameson, Philadelphia, PA*

EXAMPLES OF NANDA-I NURSING DIAGNOSES

INFANCY THROUGH SCHOOL AGE

Nursing Diagnoses	Possible Related Factor
Risk for Infection	Exposure to other children in childcare and at school
Deficient Fluid Volume	Severe case of vomiting and diarrhea
Risk for Suffocation	Caregiver's lack of knowledge of safety precautions
Risk for Poisoning	Caregiver's lack of knowledge of proper storage of hazardous liquids
Risk for Injury	Lack of knowledge about proper use of skates, bicycles, roller blades, and trampolines
Risk for Situational Low Self-Esteem	History of physical abuse by caregiver

Choking might also result from small pieces of food, nuts, and popcorn. If the airway is obstructed and the child is not coughing forcefully or does not have a strong cry, parents and caregivers need instruction to use five quick back blows between the infant's shoulders while holding the infant prone over one arm. If this does not dislodge the object, the infant should be placed in a supine position over the rescuer's thighs with the infant's head supported. Five downward chest thrusts to the lower third of the sternum should be given quickly. If this technique is ineffective and the infant becomes unresponsive, CPR needs to be initiated (U.S. National Library of Medicine, 2013).

As the infant becomes more mobile, the risk for falls or for being caught in a dangling cord (such as in mini-blinds) increases. Preventive measures against such safety hazards must be taught to new parents. In addition, the law requires using special car safety seats and restraints for infants. See Examples of NANDA-I Nursing Diagnoses: Infancy Through School Age.

Sudden Infant Death Syndrome (SIDS)

Sudden infant death syndrome (SIDS) refers to the sudden death of an infant under the age of 1 year when consideration of the infant's history, a postmortem examination, and investigation of the scene where the death occurred fails to reveal a cause of death. **Sudden unexplained infant death (SUID)** is an all-encompassing term used for sudden, unexplained infant deaths that occur suddenly and unexpectedly and the cause of death cannot readily be identified prior to an investigation. More than 4,500 infants between 1 month and 1 year of age die suddenly and unexpectedly each year in the United States (Matthews & Moore, 2013). In an effort to improve diagnostic and reporting practices, the CDC began the SUID initiative to monitor national trends, identify risk factors, and focus on interventions to prevent these infant deaths (CDC, 2011). In addition to SIDS, other SUIDs can be caused by metabolic disorders such as hypothermia or hyperthermia, neglect, poisoning, homicide, and accidental suffocation. SIDS accounts for at least 50% of all these SUID cases,

and most incidences of SIDS occur between 2 and 3 months of age (Matthews & Moore, 2013). The exact cause is still unknown but researchers are determining the importance of various risk factors for SIDS. The rate of infant deaths attributed to SIDS has declined significantly since the early 1990s when the Back to Sleep campaign promoted placing infants on their back to sleep rather than in the prone position. In 2011, the American Academy of Pediatrics (AAP) issued updated safe sleep guidelines for infants that further emphasize the importance of all caregivers placing the child in the supine position for every sleep period, including those occurring in childcare settings. These guidelines also encourage removing bumper pads and avoiding loose bedding, soft objects, and pillows in the infant's sleep environment.

Suffocation

Nearly 1,000 children under the age of one year die annually from unintentional suffocation (CDC, 2012d). Suffocation deaths have occurred when infants co-sleep with adults, other children, or animals (AAP, 2013). These accidental deaths occur most commonly when infants share a bed with parents (co-sleeping) and are inadvertently wedged beneath another person, trapped in a dangerous position, such as between the bed and the wall, and suffocated by bedding or being placed in an unapproved infant sleep positioner (ISP). Such devices are intended to keep an infant in a specific position while sleeping, but most infant deaths associated with ISPs occurred because the infant was placed in a side position and later discovered in the prone position unresponsive. In the past, some of these deaths may also have been classified as of unknown cause. Nurses should speak to parents to promote a safe sleeping environment by placing infants on their backs in a safety-approved crib, encouraging co-sleeping with the infant in a three-sided bassinet placed next to the bed rather than in the same bed as the parent, and recommending against use of pillows, comforters, other soft bedding and toys in the crib. The CDC encourages parents and caregivers to remember the ABCs of safe sleeping for infants: place infants *alone,* on their *back,* and in a bare *crib* (CDC, 2012c).

Child Maltreatment

Although **child maltreatment** may occur at any age, most victims are from birth to age 4 years. The CDC defines child maltreatment as "an act or series of acts of commission or omission by a parent or other caregiver that results in harm, potential for harm, or threat of harm to a child" (CDC, 2012a). Forms of child maltreatment include child abuse (acts of commission) and child neglect (acts of omission). In the United States in 2010, over 695,000 children were victims of maltreatment, and approximately 1,560 children died from abuse and neglect (CDC, 2012b).

Neglect, the most common form of maltreatment, is the failure of a caregiver to provide for the child's basic needs with an adequate level of care or the failure to supervise and protect a child from harm or potential harm (CDC, 2012a). Child abuse can be physical, sexual, or psychological in nature. Physical abuse, often referred to as *battered child syndrome,* refers to deliberate physical abuse and is typically inflicted by a parent or caregiver. Sexual abuse includes incest, molestation, exhibitionism, child pornography, child prostitution, and pedophilia. When committed by a caregiver such as a parent or babysitter, these acts are considered sexual abuse. When a stranger commits such an act, it is considered sexual assault. Psychological or emotional abuse includes belittling behavior on the part of the parent or caregiver that harms a child's self-worth or emotional well-being, placing a child in a dangerous situation, unreasonable confinement, exploiting or corrupting a child, and failing to express any emotion toward a child (CDC, 2010). Other forms of child maltreatment include violent shaking, called *shaken baby syndrome,* especially in infants younger than 6 months of age (resulting in brain trauma), and Munchausen syndrome by proxy, which is an illness fabricated or induced in another person. It is most often the mother who fabricates or causes an illness in a child to gain attention from health care providers.

Childhood sexual abuse has long-term consequences for health. When it occurs early in a child's life and is severe, it can affect the structure and function of the brain, causing an imbalanced stress reaction and a negative effect on the immune response. Adults who experienced childhood sex-ual abuse are more likely to report serious health problems (Wilson & Severson, 2012). Such problems include inflammatory disorders and autoimmune diseases such as irritable bowel syndrome, fibromyalgia, rheumatoid arthritis, and type 1 diabetes. Cardiovascular diseases are also more common when immune function and the inflammatory response have been compromised, such as in adults who survived childhood sexual abuse (Wilson & Severson, 2012).

Although child abuse occurs in all ethnic groups and at all levels of society, certain factors increase the risk, including the following:

- Parents experiencing stress from unemployment, depression, poor social and marital relationships, substance abuse, or health problems
- Children who cry frequently; have sleep difficulties; wet the bed; are hyperactive or aggressive; have difficult temperaments; or have physical, emotional, or cognitive disabilities
- Caregivers' lack of knowledge about parenting and the normal behaviors of children
- Lack of family and social support for caregivers

The fact that many cases of child abuse are not reported to police or social services is a national concern. Health care providers and facilities, teachers, daycare providers, and social workers are in an excellent position to recognize families at risk and offer interventions. In all 50 states, these professionals have a legal obligation to report suspected maltreatment (see Chapter 7). Organizations that serve as resources for child abuse concerns are listed in Table 18-2. The long-term treatment of abused children and their families is complex and multidisciplinary.

Role of the Nurse in Promoting Health and Preventing Illness

The most essential role of the nurse in promoting health of the infant is teaching family members and caregivers. Teaching ranges from providing basic information about prevention of diaper rash to facilitating grieving in parents who have lost a baby to SIDS. Examples of specific areas of preventive teaching for parents of infants are given in Teaching Tips 18-1.

Table 18-2 CHILD ABUSE RESOURCES

ORGANIZATION	ACTIVITIES
U.S. Department of Health and Human Services Children's Bureau http://www.acf.hhs.gov/programs/cb/index.htm	Assists states in the delivery of child welfare services.
Childhelp National Child Abuse Hotline http://www.childhelp.org Phone: 1-800-4-A-CHILD (1-800-422-4453)	Hotline counselors are available and can provide phone numbers for reporting abuse situations.
Prevent Child Abuse America http://www.preventchildabuse.org Phone: 1-800-244-5373 or 312-663-3520	National organization that provides access to hotlines, self-help groups, publications, and volunteer opportunities.
Child Welfare Information Gateway http://www.childwelfare.gov/ Phone: 1-800-394-3366	Provides access to information and resources to help protect children and strengthen families.

TEACHING TIPS 18-1

INFANTS

Health Topic	Teaching Tip	Why Is This Important?
Safety	• Feed the baby slowly and "burp" often. • Do not prop bottles and leave the baby unattended. • If choking occurs, follow appropriate procedure to give back blows and chest thrusts or CPR. • Place infants on their back in safe cribs with no crib bumpers, loose bedding, or toys. Keep the crib rails up at all times. • Avoid co-sleeping with parents, other children, and animals. • Never leave the baby unattended in or near water. • Use approved car seat. • Keep small objects out of reach. • Never leave the baby unattended on a table, chair, or regular bed. • Place the baby on his or her back for sleeping. • Keep plastic bags and mini-blind cords out of reach. • Block stairs with gates. • Cover electrical outlets.	The leading causes of death in infants are drowning, suffocation, and falls. Infants wiggle, roll, creep, crawl, walk, and reach for objects. Propping bottles, even in later infancy, might increase the risk of aspiration and tooth decay. Placing babies on their back to sleep has significantly reduced the incidence of SIDS.
Nutrition	• How to breastfeed, if chosen. • Preparing formula, information about positioning for feeding, and the importance of holding the baby for feeding, if this method is chosen. • Introducing solid foods, as prescribed by the health care provider. Do not add sugar, salt, or honey to foods. • Weaning is usually completed by the end of the first year.	Feeding is a time for the caregiver and baby to strengthen attachment and bonding. There is no one best time to introduce solid foods, but they should be started one at a time. Overfeeding or adding extra calories might cause obesity in the infant or in later life.
Hygiene	• Bathing the baby and caring for the umbilical cord. • Provide skin care for boys if circumcision is chosen. • Keep the diaper area clean and dry.	Skin care, as well as care for the umbilical cord and circumcision site, are necessary for preventing infections and excoriations.
Elimination	• By 2 months, babies usually have 2 stools a day. • Breastfed babies vary more in bowel consistency, color, and times than do babies fed formula.	Renal and intestinal physiology develop throughout the first year of life.
Growth and Development	• Provide consistent care and love. • Growth and development differ for each infant, but there are some predictable milestones. • Provide educational toys appropriate to the age of the infant. • Talk and read to the baby. • Allow the baby to explore different shapes, sizes, tastes, and experiences.	The infant must be consistently loved and cared for in order to thrive, learn to trust, and achieve developmental tasks. Stimulation with age-appropriate toys and the freedom to explore influence intellectual development.
Promoting Health and Preventing Illness	• If a danger of lead ingestion exists, take appropriate measures and have the baby screened. • Maintain schedule of immunizations. • Contact health care provider for care of respiratory infections. • Wean baby off pacifier in the second 6 months of life. • Stress importance of supplemental fluoride if water is not fluoridated. • Continue well-baby checkups as recommended. • Do not smoke in the house or car with the baby. • Keep infants younger than 6 months out of direct sunlight and covered with protective clothing and hats.	Infants who ingest lead, such as from eating peeling lead-based paint, are at risk for brain damage, behavioral problems, and mental deficiency. Immunizations are an essential part of health care. Upper respiratory infections may spread to involve the middle ear or lungs. Fluoride is necessary for tooth structure. Cigarette smoke of any type (active or passive) is dangerous and might increase the risk of respiratory illnesses, asthma, and ear infections. Infants in daycare have increased exposure to respiratory and skin infections and infestations.

2013 Recommended Immunizations for Children from Birth Through 6 Years Old

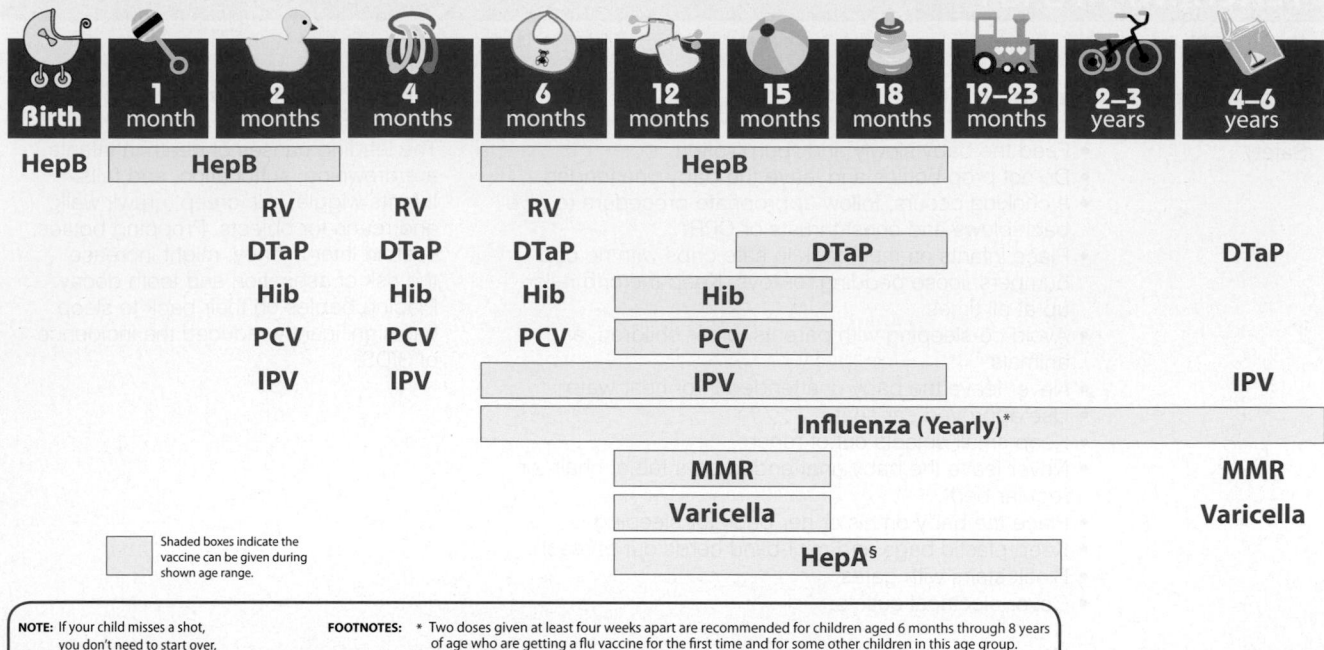

Birth	1 month	2 months	4 months	6 months	12 months	15 months	18 months	19–23 months	2–3 years	4–6 years

HepB	HepB				HepB					
		RV	RV	RV						
		DTaP	DTaP	DTaP		DTaP				DTaP
		Hib	Hib	Hib	Hib					
		PCV	PCV	PCV	PCV					
		IPV	IPV		IPV					IPV
					Influenza (Yearly)*					
					MMR					MMR
					Varicella					Varicella
					HepA§					

Shaded boxes indicate the vaccine can be given during shown age range.

NOTE: If your child misses a shot, you don't need to start over, just go back to your child's doctor for the next shot. Talk with your child's doctor if you have questions about vaccines.

FOOTNOTES: * Two doses given at least four weeks apart are recommended for children aged 6 months through 8 years of age who are getting a flu vaccine for the first time and for some other children in this age group.

§ Two doses of HepA vaccine are needed for lasting protection. The first dose of HepA vaccine should be given between 12 months and 23 months of age. The second dose should be given 6 to 18 months later. HepA vaccination may be given to any child 12 months and older to protect against HepA. Children and adolescents who did not receive the HepA vaccine and are at high-risk, should be vaccinated against HepA.

If your child has any medical conditions that put him at risk for infection or is traveling outside the United States, talk to your child's doctor about additional vaccines that he may need.

2013 Recommended Immunizations for Children from 7 Through 18 Years Old

7–10 YEARS	11–12 YEARS	13–18 YEARS
Tdap [1]	Tetanus, Diphtheria, Pertussis (Tdap) Vaccine	Tdap
	Human Papillomavirus (HPV) Vaccine (3 Doses) [2]	HPV
MCV4	Meningococcal Conjugate Vaccine (MCV4) Dose 1 [3]	MCV4 Dose 1 [3] / Booster at age 16 years
Influenza (Yearly) [4]		
Pneumococcal Vaccine [5]		
Hepatitis A (HepA) Vaccine Series [6]		
Hepatitis B (HepB) Vaccine Series		
Inactivated Polio Vaccine (IPV) Series		
Measles, Mumps, Rubella (MMR) Vaccine Series		
Varicella Vaccine Series		

These shaded boxes indicate when the vaccine is recommended for all children unless your doctor tells you that your child cannot safely receive the vaccine.

These shaded boxes indicate the vaccine should be given if a child is catching-up on missed vaccines.

These shaded boxes indicate the vaccine is recommended for children with certain health conditions that put them at high risk for serious diseases. Note that healthy children **can** get the HepA series[6]. See vaccine-specific recommendations at www.cdc.gov/vaccines/pubs/ACIP-list.htm.

FOOTNOTES

[1] Tdap vaccine is combination vaccine that is recommended at age 11 or 12 to protect against tetanus, diphtheria and pertussis. If your child has not received any or all of the DTaP vaccine series, or if you don't know if your child has received these shots, your child needs a single dose of Tdap when they are 7-10 years old. Talk to your child's health care provider to find out if they need additional catch-up vaccines.

[2] All 11 or 12 year olds – both girls *and* boys – should receive 3 doses of HPV vaccine to protect against HPV-related disease. Either HPV vaccine (Cervarix® or Gardasil®) can be given to girls and young women; only one HPV vaccine (Gardasil®) can be given to boys and young men.

[3] Meningococcal conjugate vaccine (MCV) is recommended at age 11 or 12. A booster shot is recommended at age 16. Teens who received MCV for the first time at age 13 through 15 years will need a one-time booster dose between the ages of 16 and 18 years. If your teenager missed getting the vaccine altogether, ask their health care provider about getting it now, especially if your teenager is about to move into a college dorm or military barracks.

[4] Everyone 6 months of age and older—including preteens and teens—should get a flu vaccine every year. Children under the age of 9 years may require more than one dose. Talk to your child's health care provider to find out if they need more than one dose.

[5] A single dose of Pneumococcal Conjugate Vaccine (PCV13) is recommended for children who are 6 - 18 years old with certain medical conditions that place them at high risk. Talk to your healthcare provider about pneumococcal vaccine and what factors may place your child at high risk for pneumococcal disease.

[6] Hepatitis A vaccination is recommended for older children with certain medical conditions that place them at high risk. HepA vaccine is licensed, safe, and effective for all children of all ages. Even if your child is not at high risk, you may decide you want your child protected against HepA. Talk to your healthcare provider about HepA vaccine and what factors may place your child at high risk for HepA.

FIGURE 18-3. Recommended childhood and adolescent immunization schedules—United States, 2013. Footnote information available online. (Reprinted from Centers for Disease Control and Prevention; available at www.cdc.gov/vaccines/schedules/index.html)

Immunization against contagious diseases begins during the first year of life and should follow a regular schedule, as outlined in Figure 18-3. In recent years, controversy has arisen regarding a possible relationship of immunization vaccines to the development of autism disorders. Some parents were concerned with a vaccine preservative, thimerosal, which contains mercury. Research by both the Food and Drug Administration (FDA) and the Institute of Medicine (IOM), however, demonstrated that thimerosal-containing vaccines do not place children at risk for autism or result in any indications of mercury toxicity (Offit, 2012). As a precaution, recommended childhood vaccines today in the United States no longer use thimerosal as a preservative. Some formulations of flu vaccine in multidose vials still use thimerosal for its preservative effect (CDC, 2012f). Health care providers need to listen to parents' concerns about immunization and guide them to resources with current immunization information and schedules. Vaccine information is available from CDC at http://www.cdc.gov/vaccines/programs/vfc/index.html.

It is also important to assess the infant's growth and development. Growth rate is assessed in comparison with standardized growth charts developed for boys and girls, whose growth rates differ. Be careful when comparing an individual child's growth to standards on a chart for the following reasons:

- Every child has individual variations and short-term spurts and lags in growth.
- Atypical infants, such as those who are premature or have low birth weight, are not taken into account in such charts.
- Growth charts might be ethically and socioeconomically weighted in favor of White, middle-class children.

The inexpensive Denver Developmental Screening Test (DDST) is commonly used to quickly assess for atypical developmental patterns in infants and children. The crucial areas of development assessed in the DDST are gross motor behavior and skills, fine motor behavior and skills, language acquisition, and personal and social interaction. The test identifies problem areas that require more precise assessments. The DDST is described in more detail in most pediatric nursing texts.

When an infant in late infancy is hospitalized, separation anxiety behaviors are common. **Separation anxiety** occurs when a child is separated from loved ones who offer security. It usually begins at about 6 months of age and continues through the preschool period. At a later age, the young child is able to predict this happening and feels anxiety even before the separation occurs. The infant might initially cry and scream in the phase of protest but then stop crying and appear depressed, which is the despair phase (Hockenberry & Wilson, 2013). Nurses should encourage parents to stay with the hospitalized infant and provide care, and when that is not possible, consistent health care providers are important to maintain the infant's trust in others.

TODDLER: 1 TO 3 YEARS

From 1 to 3 years of age, the child is considered a **toddler** (Fig. 18-4 on page 398).

Physiologic Development

Physiologic development continues steadily through the toddler years, but the pace is considerably slower than that in infancy. Growth and development highlights include the following:

- Has rapid brain growth; increase in length of long bones of the arms and legs; growth of muscles
- Uses fingers to pick up small objects
- Walks forward and backward, runs, kicks, climbs stairs, and rides a tricycle
- Drinks from a cup and uses a spoon
- At 2 years of age, the toddler is typically four times the birth weight, averaging 30 to 35 lb (13.6–15.9 kg) and 23 to 37 inches (58.4–94 cm) in height.
- Has bladder control during the day and sometimes during the night (2.5–3 years of age)
- Turns pages in a book, and by 3 years of age, draws stick people

Cognitive Development

Toddlers are in Piaget's last two stages of sensorimotor development: beginning to understand object permanence, following simple commands, and anticipating events. Toddlers can understand self as separate from others and have a beginning perception of body image. Toddlers can identify and name several body parts, and have a sense of gender identity. Language begins at about 1 year of age, with the use of single or bisyllable sounds. At about 2 years of age, children begin to use short sentences.

Psychosocial Development

Freud's Theory

The toddler is in Freud's anal stage. Increased muscle development and sphincter control encourage the child to focus on the pleasure of sphincter contraction and relaxation. Toilet training becomes a major focus during this period.

Erikson's Theory

The toddler enters Erikson's stage of autonomy versus shame and doubt. Autonomy is developing from independence in feeding, walking, dressing, and toileting, as well as the ability to express wishes verbally. Children who do not feel autonomous might be reluctant to explore and might be fearful of activities and people.

Negativism (characteristically expressed by saying no) and outbursts of temper result from the toddler's efforts at control over the environment. **Regression**, behavior that is more characteristic of a younger age, can occur at any time in response to stressful circumstances. The most common regressive behaviors are excessive clinging to caregivers, loss of control over elimination, and the use of more infantile speech patterns.

Separation anxiety in response to separation from the mother figure intensifies at about 18 to 24 months and can be as intense for the toddler as it was for the infant. The child

Toddlers enter a stage of autonomy, promoting exploration.

The curious and independent toddler often has a desire to do things by himself.

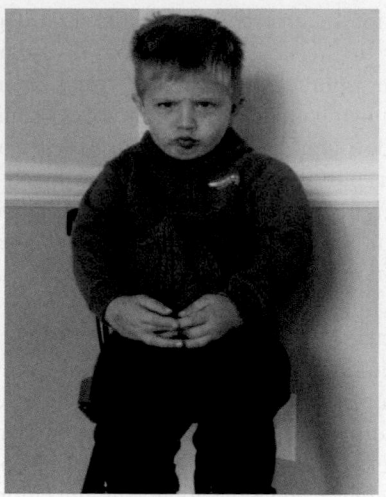

Discipline helps toddlers learn inner control and understand limits.

Cognitive development can be promoted by allowing the toddler the opportunity to observe and imitate. Younger siblings particularly enjoy mimicking older siblings.

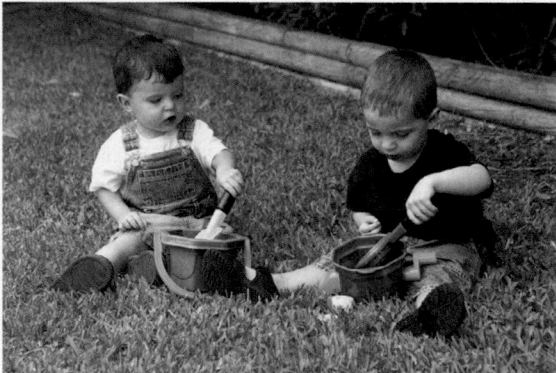

Play in toddlerhood might be solitary or parallel. *(Photo by Joe Mitchell.)*

FIGURE 18-4. Development in the toddler.

might have feelings of anger, fear, grief, and revenge during this period, but by 24 months the toddler begins to demonstrate increased independence from the mother (Pillitteri, 2010).

Havighurst's Theory

The toddler has the developmental task of learning to control the elimination of urine and feces and begins to learn sex differences, form concepts, learn language, and distinguish right from wrong.

Health of the Toddler

Accidents—such as motor vehicle crashes, poisonings, burns, drowning, choking and aspirations, and falls—are the major cause of death in toddlers. The number of young children visiting the ED due to ingestion of small button batteries has significantly increased. Of these children, 75% are younger than 5 years of age. These batteries are commonly found in toys and games and some household objects (Potera, 2013). Most batteries pass through the body, but some can lodge in the esophagus and cause serious injury requiring surgery or other treatment. Dental problems are also common, espe-

cially if the toddler is allowed to go to sleep while sucking on a bottle of milk or sweetened liquid. Respiratory tract and middle-ear infections are common. Some surgeries, such as repair of a cleft lip and palate, might be done in the toddler years. Autistic disorder—with abnormal behavior, social interactions, and communication—is usually diagnosed by the time the child is 3 years old.

Over-the-counter (OTC) cold medications can have serious adverse effects in infants and toddlers. Both the Consumer Healthcare Products Association (CHPA) and the FDA support product labels on OTC cough and cold medicines that state "do not use" in children under the age of 4 years (FDA, 2012). In addition to the concerns about misuse of the drugs, data indicate that they have minimal therapeutic value for this age group.

Role of the Nurse in Promoting Health and Preventing Illness

The role of the nurse in promoting health in the toddler continues to be primarily teaching, as shown by the examples in Teaching Tips 18-2. An important part of teaching is helping

TEACHING TIPS 18-2

TODDLERS

Health Topic	Teaching Tip	Why Is This Important?
Safety	• Lock medicines, cleaning supplies, and yard-care products out of reach. • Use safety plugs in electrical outlets. • Block stairs with gates. • Use approved car seat. • Never leave toddler unattended near water. Have toddler wear Coast Guard–approved life jackets around pools. • Do not give toddler small hard foods, small toys or toy parts, or balloons. • Keep plastic bags and mini-blind cords out of reach. • Teach danger in simple terms ("stove hot"). • Do not toss toddler in the air or swing by the arms.	Accidents are a leading cause of injuries and death in toddlers. It is necessary to childproof the home to prevent injury, as the toddler moves quickly, lacks judgment, and explores the world by seeing, touching, and tasting. Small objects or balloons might be aspirated and cause suffocation. Joints might be dislocated by swinging the child.
Nutrition	• Do not scold for messiness while eating. • Provide finger foods. • Short periods of loss of appetite are normal. • Avoid foods that are high in fat, sugar, and salt (often found in fast foods). • Watch for signs of food allergies. Reactions to milk, egg, peanuts, tree nuts, fish, shellfish, soy, and wheat are the most common.	The toddler is growing less rapidly than the infant and does not require as many calories. Feeding self, even if messy, promotes independence. Giving too much food or food that is high in calories might result in obesity. In recent years, food allergies have increased almost 20% in children under 18 months. Children with food allergies are more likely to develop asthma or other allergies.
Hygiene	• Teach hand washing after eating and toileting. • Teach how to brush teeth. • Schedule dentist visit.	It is important to establish good hygiene and to serve as a role model. The first dentist visit might be just to become familiar with the office and provider.
Elimination	• Physical development is necessary for toilet training. • Begin training with bowel elimination. • Watch for signs of readiness (realizing wetness, staying dry for 2 or more hours). • Night dryness occurs later than day dryness.	The neuromuscular control necessary for elimination occurs between 1 and 3 years. Bowel training is a less complex task than bladder training.
Growth and Development	• Encourage independence in eating, dressing, and toileting. • Provide toys that emphasize gross motor skills and creativity. • Parallel play with other children is normal. • The concept of sharing is not yet developed. • Saying "no" to almost everything is normal.	The toddler gains a sense of security and control by being able to eat, dress, toilet self, and say "no."
Promoting Health and Preventing Illness	• If a danger of lead ingestion exists, take appropriate measures and have the toddler screened. • Complete immunizations. • See health care professionals for treatment of respiratory infections. • Do not smoke in the house or car with the child. • Limit sun exposure or use sun protection practices. • Learn CPR for emergencies.	Toddlers who ingest lead, such as from eating peeling lead-based paint, are at risk for brain damage, behavioral problems, and mental deficiency. Immunizations are an essential part of health care. Respiratory infections might lead to ear infections. Avoid smoking to reduce risk of respiratory illness, asthma, and ear infections. Passive smoke is dangerous. Infants in daycare have increased exposure to respiratory and skin infections and infestations. Children at high risk for development of skin cancer include those with light skin, freckling, or a family history.

caregivers encourage their toddler's independence while setting firm limits.

Toddlers who require hospital care experience stress and separation anxiety when parents are not present. To decrease stress from unfamiliar surroundings and caregivers, parents should be encouraged to provide care and remain with the toddler as much as possible. Every effort should be made to have consistency of health care providers and to maintain familiar routines and rituals. When ill or in pain, toddlers often regress to earlier behaviors, such as wanting a bottle to drink from.

 RECALL 2-year-old Hillarie Browning, who is unresponsive. The nurse could apply knowledge about the feelings of stress and separation for a hospitalized toddler when developing the plan of care for this child, especially in light of possible child abuse. Consistency in staff members caring for the child and maintaining rituals would help foster trust and minimize upset. ●

PRESCHOOLER: 3 TO 6 YEARS

At around age 3, toddlers begin to move into the next stage: **preschooler**. Although growth and development are slower than in infancy and toddlerhood, they are still steady (Fig. 18-5).

Physiologic Development

The physical characteristics of the preschooler include the following:

- Head is close to adult size by 6 years of age.
- The body is less chubby and becomes leaner and more coordinated.

Preschooler play is associative and cooperative in its social dimension, and cognitive development is demonstrated in constructive and pretend play.

Motor abilities include throwing and catching a ball.

Safety is a common concern for caregivers.

Preschoolers enjoy imitative play.

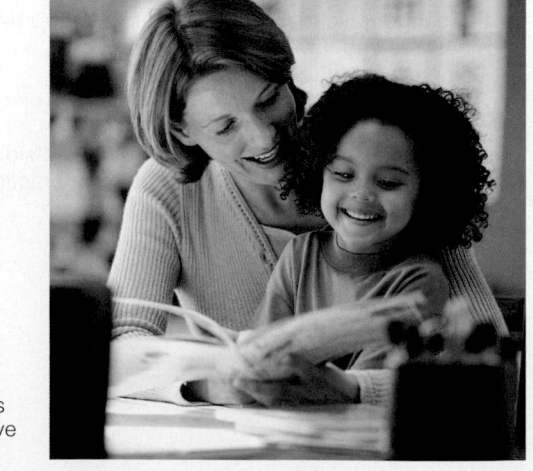

Cognitive development produces improved reasoning ability and readiness to read.

FIGURE 18-5. Development in the preschooler.

- Motor abilities include skipping, throwing and catching a ball, copying figures, and printing letters and numbers.
- Full set of 20 deciduous teeth is present; baby teeth begin to fall out and are replaced by permanent teeth.
- Average weight at 5 to 6 years of age is 45 lb (20.4 kg), with boys being slightly heavier than girls.

Cognitive Development

Preschoolers are in Piaget's preoperational stage of development. Passing through the preconceptual and intuitive phases, preschoolers demonstrate the following transitional changes:

- Egocentrism decreases as socialization with other children increases, and the ability to express self verbally improves.
- Play is more related to real-life events (rather than fantasy).
- Basic curiosity results in constant questions and improved reasoning ability.

Language development is seen in more elaborate and grammatically correct sentences, with 6- to 18-word sentences becoming common by 6 years of age. Incessantly asking "Why?" increases the child's knowledge, encourages further conversations, and helps develop language abilities.

Preschoolers clearly identify themselves as male or female, can understand basic body functions, and have a curiosity about sex differences. This curiosity often leads to "playing doctor," which is normal behavior at this stage. Many children in this age group want to look special or dressed up and gain increased self-esteem from compliments about their appearance.

Psychosocial Development

Freud's Theory

The preschooler is in Freud's phallic stage, with the biologic focus primarily genital. The child has a sexual desire for the opposite-sex parent but, as a means of defense, strongly identifies with the same-sex parent; as a result of this conflict resolution, the superego and conscience begin to develop.

Erikson's Theory

The preschooler is in Erikson's stage of initiative versus guilt. Inner turmoil occurs when natural curiosity is pitted against a constant examination of the propriety of one's actions by a rigid conscience. Realistic self-limits are learned through social interactions.

Havighurst's Theory

According to Havighurst, the preschooler has four developmental tasks to accomplish: to learn sex differences and modesty, to describe social and physical reality through concept formation and language development, to get ready to read, and to learn to distinguish right from wrong.

Special Considerations

Preschoolers often have fears—most commonly fear of new places, fear of the dark, and fear during nightmares. These fears are often made worse by the child's own fertile imagination and ability to fantasize. Support and validation of the preschooler's feelings by caregivers are essential.

Moral and Spiritual Development

Kohlberg's preconventional phase of moral reasoning dominates at this age. The focus of this stage is obeying rules to avoid punishment or receive a reward. The cognitive, psychosocial, and moral developments of the preschooler provide a base for spiritual development, as described by Fowler. The preschooler might attend activities at church or synagogue with the family, but does not understand religious concepts. The concept of a deity is literal, with God usually being viewed as a male human. Concepts such as heaven, hell, and holy spirits are incomprehensible and often frightening.

Health of the Preschooler

Preschoolers continue to have the health problems that are common in toddlerhood. Communicable diseases and respiratory tract infections are common, especially with increased interaction with other children at nursery schools and daycare. Preschoolers are prone to accidents because of their increased curiosity about the world. Some congenital disorders—such as hypospadias, inguinal hernias, and cardiac anomalies—require surgery at this time. Dental caries become common if teeth are neglected. As language becomes more sophisticated, speech disorders might become apparent.

In the United States as well as worldwide, obesity is a significant threat to the health of children. Over the past 30 years, the incidence of obesity has doubled in children and tripled in adolescents (CDC, 2013b). Currently, more than one-third of children and adolescents are overweight or obese; young children who are obese are more likely to become obese adults. Obese children are at risk for developing immediate and long-term medical problems in addition to suffering self-esteem issues from being teased or bullied by other children (Kids Health, 2012). The alarming rise in type 2 diabetes and cardiovascular disease, in addition to other conditions seen typically during the adult years, is further evidence of the devastating toll of obesity. Body mass index (BMI) is now recommended for basic screening and identification of obesity at routine physical examinations at 2 years of age and all subsequent examinations (Himes, 2013). BMI measurement is discussed in detail in Chapter 35.

Role of the Nurse in Promoting Health and Preventing Illness

Teaching Tips 18-3 (on page 402) provides examples of teaching to promote health in preschoolers. Nurses play a vital role in identifying children at risk for obesity, teaching families about the health consequences, providing information and health teaching, and promoting wellness in this vulnerable population. (See the accompanying PICO in Practice display on page 403.) Assessments of dietary patterns and physical activity level of family members guide nursing interventions. The CDC provides weight management

TEACHING TIPS 18-3

PRESCHOOLERS

Health Topic	Teaching Tip	Why Is This Important?
Safety	• Lock medicines and cleaning and gardening supplies out of reach. • Use safety plugs in electrical outlets. • Teach child how to go up and down stairs. • Do not give small hard foods, small toys, or balloons. • Tape shut battery compartments of toys and household objects to limit access to button batteries. • Use approved car seat and bicycle helmets. • Teach simple traffic safety. • Teach to never talk to or get in the car with a stranger. Include information about inappropriate touching. • Never leave the child alone in public or unattended in a car. • Begin swimming lessons and teach water safety. • Teach danger of fire and have a home fire safety plan. • Limit use of bouncers or moonwalks and trampolines. Limit the number of children using them at one time. Always have a parent present.	Accidents are the leading cause of injury and death in preschoolers, most often from motor vehicles, drowning, burns, and poisoning. Even minor head trauma may cause hematoma formation. Children are at risk for harm from physical and sexual abuse and must be taught how to avoid situations that might increase that risk. Broken bones and sprains are the most common type of bounce-related injuries. The number of U.S. children with this type of injury is 15 times higher now than 15 years ago.
Nutrition	• A gradual increase in calories, with nutritious snacks, is necessary. • Children who follow their own appetite patterns are less likely to be overweight. • Avoid foods that are high in fat, sugar, and salt (found in most fast foods). • Preschoolers like to eat one food at a time and prefer those that are mildly flavored and lukewarm.	The preschool child needs the same food group nutrition as the adult, but in lesser amounts.
Hygiene	• Stress importance of hand washing before meals and after toileting. • Assist with brushing and flossing teeth after eating. • Teach disposal of used tissues. • Maintain regular dental checkups and care.	Preschoolers are able to carry out basic hygiene but continue to need assistance and reminders. Dental caries often begins during this age.
Elimination	• Toilet training is completed, but night wetting may persist.	Recognizing the need to empty the bladder during sleep takes a longer time in some children. They should not be punished for wetting the bed.
Growth and Development	• Night fears and bad dreams are common. • Make-believe play and imaginary friends are normal. • Although each child grows and develops differently, there are ranges of normal. • Play occupies most of the child's time; the child can play with others for periods of time. • Provide play materials that encourage physical activity, dramatic play, quiet play, and creativity. • Provide consistent, fair, and kind limits for behavior. • Masturbation is normal, although the child should learn that it is not acceptable in public.	Sleep problems usually resolve on their own; calm reassurance by parents is appropriate when they occur. Play is the work of the child; adults should provide time, space, equipment, and safety, but should not structure the child's play.
Promoting Health and Preventing Illness	• If a danger of lead ingestion or poisoning exists, take appropriate measures and have the child screened. • Maintain immunizations. • Have vision tested. • Have hearing tested if necessary (e.g., child does not seem to listen). • Maintain regular well-child checkups. • Preschoolers often fear dental and medical treatments. Avoid hospitalization if possible, but if necessary, prepare the child before the procedure.	Lead poisoning in preschoolers causes brain dysfunction. Immunizations and health-related checkups are essential in promoting health. Preschoolers often see dental or medical procedures as a punishment and fear damage to their bodies. Parents should set a good example and be honest with the child. Preparation for procedures and hospitalization can help decrease fear and separation anxiety.

PICO IN PRACTICE

ASKING CLINICAL QUESTIONS

Scenario: Your cousin Kara is a first-time parent of a 4-year-old named Kermit. One Saturday afternoon, you pay a visit to your cousin in her home. Kermit had been taking his daily afternoon nap when you arrived and woke after you rang the doorbell. Kara meets you at the door, and the two of you walk to Kermit's bedroom. He says, "Mommy, I am sorry but I wet myself again." He is wearing a pull-up diaper. After Kara cleans and changes him, she tells you that she doesn't know why Kermit still wets himself during sleep once or twice weekly after he has been toilet-trained during waking hours for the past 10 months. She asks you, "Is this normal for Kermie to bed -wet? Should I ask his pediatrician to prescribe some medicine for him to treat this?"

- POPULATION: Four-year-old boy
- INTERVENTION: Pharmacologic agent
- COMPARISON: None
- OUTCOME: Cessation of bed-wetting

PICO Question: Are pharmacologic agents indicated in 4-year-old boys who bed-wet once or twice weekly?

Finding: From the National Guideline Clearinghouse: National Clinical Guideline Centre. (2010). *Nocturnal enuresis: The management of bedwetting in children and young people.* London, UK: National Institute for Health and Clinical Excellence (NICE).

This guideline notes that one in five children under 5 years of age wets the bed at least once a week. The authors of this guideline recommend that clinicians reassure parents and caregivers of children that many children under 5 years of age wet the bed. Therefore, pharmacologic agents to treat this are not indicated. Parents and caregivers should be advised to try not using pull-up diapers at least two nights or naptimes in a row to see if that may result in less frequent bed-wetting. The child of this age that bed-wets should also be assessed for constipation, since this frequently is associated with bed-wetting.

Strength of Evidence: Level I

Recommendation: You share these recommendations with Kara. You tell her that Kermit's bed-wetting is not a cause for concern, given his age. You assess Kermit's bowel habits with Kara to see if Kermit may be constipated, and note to Kara that constipation may be associated with bed-wetting in children of Kermit's age. You recommend to Kara that she try not giving Kermit pull-up diapers for a couple of sequential nights or naptimes to see if that results in improved urinary continence.

---

guidelines and tips at http://www.cdc.gov/nccdphp/dnpa/obesity/childhood/tips_for_parents.htm.

When caring for a preschool-aged child who is scheduled for surgery or requires hospitalization, nurses must recognize the importance of the child's fear of pain as well as separation anxiety. The nurse can help decrease fears by explaining procedures in language the child can understand and by being honest about how much pain a procedure will cause. Many health care institutions and agencies have preprocedure visits so that the child having surgery becomes familiar with the setting and the activities that will be done. Allowing the child to practice procedures on a doll and encouraging the child to express his or her feelings openly are also beneficial (Fig. 18-6). Encouraging caregivers to take an active role in the child's care helps to reduce fear and separation anxiety.

SCHOOL-AGED CHILD: 6 TO 12 YEARS

School-aged children, from 6 to 12 years of age, are typically sturdy and strong. Physical growth during this time is relatively slow but continues steadily, with both refinement and subtle changes taking place (Fig. 18-7 on page 404).

Physiologic Development

Physiologic development of school-aged children includes the following:

- The brain reaches 90% to 95% of adult size; by 12 years of age, the nervous system is almost completely matured, resulting in coordinated body movements.

- Motor abilities progress from the ability to hold a pencil and print words at 6 years of age to the ability to write in script and in sentences at 12 years of age.
- Sexual organs grow but are dormant until late in this period, when hormonal changes begin.

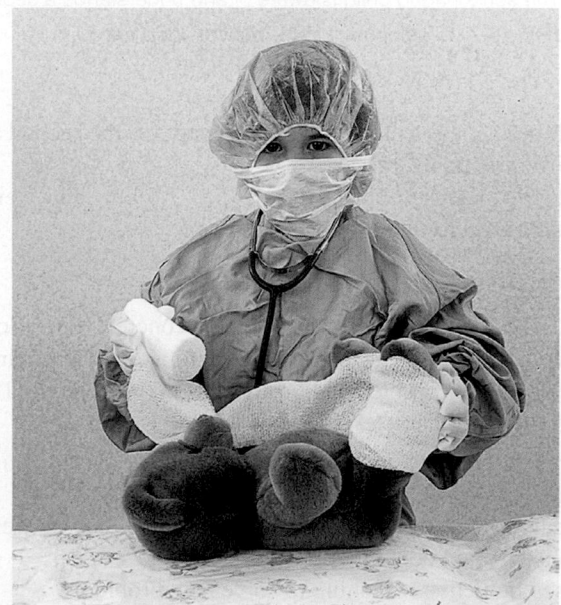

FIGURE 18-6. Abstract reasoning is necessary for children to understand that painful medical treatments given now will make them feel better later. Dramatic play may help the preschool child, who is not old enough to have developed abstract reasoning, to understand the uncomfortable experiences of the hospital stay. *(Photo by B. Proud.)*

Play involves development of skill, games with rules, and competitive activities.

The school-aged child is aware of and understands a sequence of events.

Making friends is important to the school-aged child.

FIGURE 18-7. Development in the school-aged child.

- All permanent teeth are present, except for the second and third molars, by 12 years of age.
- Height increases 2 to 3 inches (5.1–7.6 cm) and weight increases 3 to 6 lb (1.4–2.7 kg) a year.

Cognitive Development

The school-aged child is in Piaget's concrete operational stage of development, organizing facts about the environment to use for problem solving. In this period, the child has the following characteristics:

- Thinks logically and develops concepts of mass, volume, weight, and measurement
- Deals best with actual objects and people, but can relate concepts and compare events
- Uses inductive reasoning to solve new problems
- Generalizes about people, places, and things
- Develops classification systems
- Develops an awareness and understanding of other people's feelings and points of view
- Understands reversal of events

School-aged children have well-developed language skills, using language in a more sophisticated manner. Their ability to store information in long-term memory and retrieve it in the remembering (recall) process is more efficient.

Psychosocial Development

Freud's Theory

The school-aged child is in the latency stage of Freud's theory, with psychosocial energies being channeled toward strong identification with one's own sex and creative activities. Privacy and understanding one's body are important at this age.

Erikson's Theory

The school-aged child is in the industry-versus-inferiority stage of Erikson's theory, with the child focused on learning useful skills and thereby developing positive self-esteem. A sense of identity begins to emerge, and values are integrated. The emphasis is on doing, succeeding, and accomplishing.

THINK back to Nate Pelton, the 11-year-old baseball player. The nurse could apply Erikson's theory to understand that joining a sports team offers Nate the opportunity to develop physical skills, to learn to play as a member of a team, and to improve self-esteem. When children participate in sports, their parents need to be actively involved to ensure safety while understanding that support and positive reinforcement help to promote a positive experience that will shape values and behaviors for adult life. ●

Havighurst's Theory

According to Havighurst, the school-aged child has the following developmental tasks:

- Learning physical game skills
- Learning appropriate social roles
- Developing fundamental skills in reading, writing, and calculating
- Developing concepts necessary for everyday living
- Achieving personal independence
- Developing conscience, morality, and a scale of values

Special Considerations

Peer relationships become the major gauge for determining status, skill, and ability to be personable. Peer groups in middle childhood help prepare the child for getting along in the larger world and may begin to introduce messages regarding sexual orientation. They also act as transition modes for the child as the child leaves the total caregiver influence and heads toward adult independence. Unfortunately, as children become members of social groups, they may experience some form of bullying. Data indicate that bullying behavior becomes more common at school during unstructured moments such as recess and may be related to gender, physical appearance, disability or ability, and intellect. Bullying behavior intends to embarrass or harm the victim, and creates a perceived imbalance of power between the aggressor(s) and the victim (Hockenberry & Wilson, 2013).

Body image, self-concept, and sexuality are interrelated. Sexual development results in a strong need to understand body function and to have accurate information about sexuality.

Moral Development

Most of middle childhood is spent in the conventional phase of moral development. Behavior is based on familial and peer group beliefs, and conformity to the norm is common. Following school regulations, respecting teachers, and viewing justice as a means of fair play are all important.

Spiritual Development

In Fowler's theory, school-aged children view religious faith as a relationship that involves reciprocal fairness. They take part in rituals of their faith, with a basic understanding of the ritual's significance. The importance of spiritual beliefs and the possibility of life after death is accepted, even if not totally understood.

Health of the School-Aged Child

Accidents continue to be common in school-aged children. With increased interactions with other children in school, communicable conditions such as scabies, impetigo, and head lice are more prevalent. The CDC recommends the vaccination of 11- and 12-year-old girls with three doses of human papilloma virus (HPV) vaccine to prevent the types of HPV that can cause cervical cancer and genital warts (CDC, 2012g). Other common health-related problems of the school-aged child include obesity, attention deficit hyperactivity disorder (ADHD) and learning disability (LD), and enuresis (bed wetting). In addition, chronic conditions such as sickle cell anemia, hyperactivity, seizure disorders, hypertension, diabetes mellitus, and obesity might affect the school-aged child. Scoliosis, an abnormal curvature of the spine, occurs most often in girls between the ages of 10 and 13 years.

Obesity

Over the past 20 years, obesity among school-aged children has more than doubled (CDC, 2013b). A sedentary lifestyle is a contributing factor as children spend many hours using electronic devices, playing video games, and watching TV rather than actively playing. Many obese school-aged children also have diets that are high in saturated fats, do not meet fruit and vegetable daily requirements, are low in fiber, and are low in calcium. As with adults, obesity in children results from consuming more calories than are expended. Genetics and health factors may be a contributing factor. (See Research in Nursing box on page 406.)

In response to the increasing numbers of obese children, revised standards for national school breakfast and lunch programs will be phased in over a 3-year period beginning with the 2012 to 2013 school year. The changes created by the U.S. Department of Agriculture include an increased emphasis on fruits and vegetables; fat-free or low-fat milk options; more whole-grain offerings; and less calories, sodium, and saturated and trans fat in the meals (Wallis, 2013).

ADHD and Learning Disabilities

ADHD is a developmentally inappropriate degree of inattention, impulsiveness, and hyperactivity. To be diagnosed with this disorder, the child must have manifested symptoms before 7 years of age, and symptoms must be present in at least two settings. Recently, some physicians have expressed concern that the diagnosis of ADHD and the medications prescribed to treat it are overused in American children. The commonly used medications have also been associated with addiction and anxiety, and their misuse appears to be rising (Schwarz & Cohen, 2013). Learning disabilities (LD) is a group of disorders in which the child has significant difficulty in listening, speaking, reading, writing, reasoning, mathematic abilities, or social skills

RESEARCH IN NURSING

BRIDGING THE GAP TO EVIDENCE-BASED PRACTICE

Exploring the Daily Lifestyles of Obese Children to Determine Factors that Affect Their Weight Status

Most people are aware that obesity has become an epidemic. In the United States, by 2030 approximately 40% of Americans are projected to be obese. Child obesity has also reached epidemic levels and is a concern as a predictor of future adult obesity and overall poor health. Increasing the level of physical activity and moderating a child's diet do not seem to dramatically reduce obesity. Experts contend that it is a much more complicated situation. Behavioral aspects should also be considered because they provide a clearer understanding of the risk factors for child obesity and possibly more effective interventions.

Related Research

Okely, A., Pearson, P., Puglisi, L., & Vialle, W. (2013). Understanding the day-to-day lives of obese children and their families. *Family & Community Health, 36*(1), 42–50.

The goal of this inquiry was to understand the complexity of child obesity and determine factors involved in this problem. Investigators observed the daily lives of these obese children and factors that influenced their weight-related behaviors. This research process involved a naturalistic approach with which the researcher observed families in their day-to-day environments. Six obese children and their families participated in the study and were observed 3 days in summer and 3 days in winter from awakening to bedtime. There were approximately 95 hours of observation for each family. Every action and behavior of the children was observed and recorded, including recording all conversations. Both casual conversations and digital photographs contributed to the explanation of their daily activities.

After data was analyzed, common themes became evident among the six families. It was determined there was a lack of parenting skills and role modeling. Parents had unhealthy behaviors and poor eating patterns that their children observed on a regular basis. Energy-dense and nutrient-poor foods were readily available in all the homes, and the school cafeteria provided similar foods. In all the families, physical activities were limited. These children also had poor self-images and often perceived themselves as incompetent in many situations. This study provided further confirmation that parental practices are major influences on the occurrence of obesity in their children. It also contributed additional information to the literature on child obesity risk factors and associated behaviors. Nonetheless, child obesity still has a very complex nature.

Relevance to Nursing Practice

The results of this study give some direction to nurses and health care providers in their efforts to devise intervention strategies that address the health problem of child obesity. In addition to parents, school and community environments must be considered as influences on the behaviors of obese children. Childhood is a critical period, and it is important to determine the factors that affect a child's weight status.

For additional research, visit thePoint.

(Hockenberry & Wilson, 2013). Both of these conditions affect all areas of the life of the child, but they are most noticeable in the classroom. Multiple approaches are used in management, including medication, environmental strategies, and classroom education. Based on the Education for All Handicapped Children's Act, children with ADHD and LD must receive free public education in the least restrictive environment.

Enuresis

Enuresis is diagnosed when a child is at least 5 years of age and is still having involuntary urination, usually at night. Although this problem is significant to the child and his or her parents, it is a benign and self-limiting disorder, usually ending between 6 and 8 years of age.

Role of the Nurse in Promoting Health and Preventing Illness

The nurse's role in promoting health for the school-aged child involves individual and family teaching, often conducted by school nurses. Multiple strategies can be implemented in schools to address the obesity epidemic. Parents, teachers, administrators, and the school nurse can collaborate to assess the current programs available in the school and take action. Recommended approaches include increasing opportunities for students to become involved in physical activities and ensuring that students have healthy food and beverage choices while at school. Because school violence has become more common, school nurses must be prepared for a potential crisis. They need to be alert for warning signs of bullying and other dangerous behaviors and be involved in efforts to promote a safe environment in playgrounds, buses, and schools. This often includes collaboration between the school nurse, parents, and educators to determine creative strategies that promote healthier lifestyles and environments for school-aged children. Teaching Tips 18-4 provides examples of nursing activities specific for this age group. In addition, nurses often function as advocates for vulnerable populations (see the Nursing Advocacy in Action display on page 408).

Because school-aged children are striving for independence and control, hospitalization might mean a loss of freedom of choice (e.g., types of food, clothing, activities). Children of this age should be allowed to have some measure of control over allowable activities and should be

TEACHING TIPS 18-4

SCHOOL-AGED CHILDREN

Health Topic	Teaching Tip	Why Is This Important?
Safety	• Teach and require pedestrian traffic safety. • Wear seat belts and bicycle helmets. • Emphasize bicycle, scooter, skate, and skateboard safety. • Provide swimming lessons and water safety rules. • Rural children should be taught farm safety. • Teach how to "stop, drop, and roll" to extinguish clothing fire. • Teach the dangers of dangerous products and chemicals. • Keep guns locked up. Teach gun safety rules. • Teach use of proper equipment for contact sports. • Be alert for concussion sports injuries, use proper equipment, and follow treatment recommendations for concussions.	Accidents are the leading cause of death in school-aged children, most often caused by motor vehicle crashes, fires, falls, drowning, and poisonings. Gun accidents to themselves and others occur in school-aged children. Accident prevention and safety education should be taught and reinforced both at home and at school. Concussions that are not treated properly increase the risk for long-term problems.
Nutrition	• School-aged children need adequate calories and might also require increased amounts of vitamin D and calcium. • Provide foods that meet nutritional needs and do not supply empty calories (as found in junk food and fast food). • Do not overemphasize table manners to keep meal times more pleasant.	Increased vitamin D and calcium are needed as bones enlarge and for girls to prevent later osteoporosis. American children eat too much salt, sugar, and fats; nearly 1/4 of all school-aged children have an elevated cholesterol level. Eating patterns for school-aged children will improve over time. Both undernutrition and overnutrition are seen in this age group.
Hygiene	• Teach girls how to wipe from front to back after urination. • Teach children not to share hats or combs.	Girls are prone to urinary infections because of their short urethra. Head lice and ringworm are common in school-aged children and are easily spread to others.
Sexual Development	• Both girls and boys have characteristics of sexual maturity, including a growth spurt, growth of body hair, changes in body proportion, and the beginning of secondary physical sex changes. • Provide accurate information and answer questions honestly about sex, including anatomy, physiology, birth control, and STIs (including AIDS). • Monitor TV watching and computer use.	Girls have breast development, grow axillary and pubic hair, and may begin to menstruate. Boys have testicular growth and grow axillary and pubic hair, and the penis enlarges. Boys may also have temporary breast enlargement. School-aged children are curious, and if unsupervised, may watch pornographic television or computer material. In addition, the violence in television shows or video games may lead to aggressive behavior.
Growth and Development	• Best friends and groups of peer friends are important to the school-aged child. • Rules are rigidly followed during games with peers. • Encourage both quiet and active play activities. • Provide guidance and set limits for behavior, focusing on only one incident at a time. • Encourage feelings of industry by having realistic expectations and recognizing unique abilities and talents. • Provide positive statements demonstrating that the child is valued, loved, and important.	From ages 7 to 9, close friends are usually the same gender and age. This is not as important from ages 10 to 12. Unrealistic expectations or excessive discipline might result in stress and feelings of inferiority.

(continued)

TEACHING TIPS 18-4

SCHOOL-AGED CHILDREN   *continued*

Health Topic	Teaching Tip	Why Is This Important?
Promoting Health and Preventing Illness	• Maintain records of immunizations, and have boosters as recommended. CDC recommends 3 doses of HPV vaccine for 11- and 12-year-old girls. Gardasil (one of the FDA-approved HPV vaccines) is also recommended for males starting at 9 years of age to protect against genital warts. • Promote regular physical activity and exercise. • Teach how to "just say no" to smoking, alcohol, and drugs. • Maintain dental examinations. • Maintain well-child checkups, and have screenings (if at risk or indicated by symptoms) and treatment for chronic conditions such as asthma, diabetes mellitus, sickle cell anemia, hypertension, seizure disorder, hyperactivity, and obesity. • Have vision tested if school problems with reading, coordination, or inability to see screen or monitor in front of the room occur.	Maintaining immunizations is essential to health; records are required for enrollment in school. Children need to know how to handle peer pressure to smoke, drink, and take drugs. Many school-aged children are at risk for and exhibit symptoms of chronic illnesses.

encouraged to do what they can, such as playing competitive games and making their own bed (Fig. 18-8).

 RECALL 11-year-old Nate Pelton, who suffered a possible concussion during a baseball game as a result of a blow to his head in a collision with another teammate. Nurses working in the ED, schools, and public health settings should use the nursing process to provide education about the recognition and treatment of concussions and to collaborate with parents, young athletes, coaches, and school faculty to prevent and treat these injuries. ●

THE ADOLESCENT AND YOUNG ADULT

The adolescent and young adult years are a time of both change and stability. **Adolescence** begins with puberty and extends from 12 to 20 years of age; the **young adult** period is considered to be the 20s and 30s. However, these time periods are highly individualized. A person is defined as an adult when that person is "physically and psychologically mature, ready to assume adult responsibilities and be self-sufficient" (Murray & Zentner, 2001, p. 525).

After experiencing rapid growth and development during adolescence, the young adult completes physical growth and develops internal and external controls and values acceptable to society. There are no specific measurements of maturity; each person is an individual and a wide range of normal values and behaviors are considered healthy (Fig. 18-9).

Physiologic Development

Changes in the adolescent's body transform the adolescent from a child to an adult in appearance. Physiologic development includes the following:

• The feet, hands, and long bones grow rapidly, accompanied by an increase in muscle mass (especially in boys).
• Primary and secondary sexual development occurs, with maturation of the genitalia; presence of body hair; breast

NURSING ADVOCACY IN ACTION

Patient Scenario

You are working as a school nurse in a district where there are many poor families who have come to the United States (many illegally) to find work. At present, there is a lively debate in the country about whether these families should be identified and "shipped home" or supported. Many of the parents are afraid of being deported, and you learn that some have taken their children out of school. You know that the children benefit from being in school. In addition to the education, the free school lunch program is for many children the one meal of the day they can count on.

Implications for Nursing Advocacy

How will you respond if you are the school nurse approached by faculty who want to help the children? Talk with your classmates and experienced nurses about these questions:

• If you elect to advocate for these children, what practical steps can you take to ensure better health outcomes?
• What is it reasonable to expect of a student nurse, a graduate nurse, and an experienced nurse in this situation?
• What advocacy skills are needed to effectively respond to this challenge?

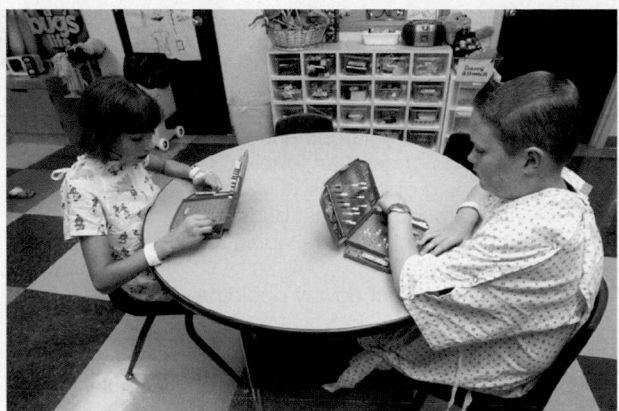

FIGURE 18-8. Allowing school-aged children to play competitive games promotes a positive hospital experience. *(Photo by Joe Mitchell.)*

development and menstruation in girls; facial hair growth, voice changes, and spermatogenesis in boys.

- **Puberty** (the time when the ability to reproduce begins) starts at 9 to 13 years of age in girls (with menstruation usually beginning between 10 and 14 years of age) and at 11 to 14 years of age in boys.
- Sebaceous and axillary sweat glands become active.
- Full adult size is reached, although some young men might continue to grow in their 20s. Puberty can be divided into the following three stages (Table 18-3 on page 410):
  - *Prepubescence:* Secondary sex characteristics begin to develop, but the reproductive organs do not yet function.
  - *Pubescence:* Secondary sex characteristics continue to develop, and ova and sperm begin to be produced by the reproductive organs.
  - *Postpubescence:* Reproductive functioning and the development of secondary sex characteristics reach adult maturity.

Cognitive Development

According to Piaget, adolescence is the stage when the cognitive development of formal operations is developed. Deductive, reflective, and hypothetical reasoning are possible, and abstract concepts can be used. Long-term goals can be set as

Peer relationships are particularly influential during adolescence.

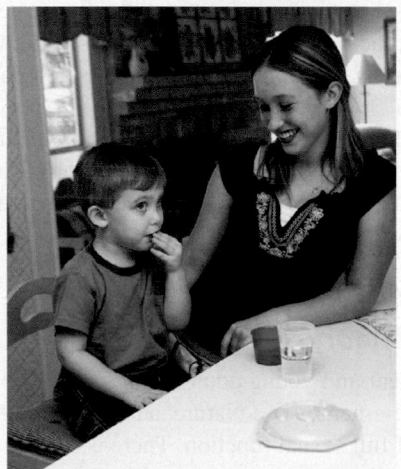

Babysitting offers an opportunity to practice formal adult skills. *(Photo by Joe Mitchell.)*

The development of self-identity in adolescence involves discovering talents and becoming emotionally independent.

FIGURE 18-9. Development in the adolescent.

A primary developmental task of adolescence is to achieve new and more mature relationships.

Table 18-3 ADOLESCENT SEXUAL DEVELOPMENT

STAGE	MALES	FEMALES
Prepubescence	• Progressive enlargement of testicles, seminal ducts, prostate gland • Enlargement and reddening of the scrotal sac • Increase in length and circumference of penis • Appearance of downy pubic hair	• Progressive enlargement of the ovaries • Ripening of graafian follicles • Rounding of the hips • Appearance of breast buds • Enlargement of the fallopian tubes, vagina, and uterus • Appearance of downy pubic hair
Pubescence	• Increase in amount, pigmentation, and curling of pubic hair • Growth spurt involving height and weight increase • Deepening of the voice due to growth of larynx • Enlargement of testicles • Increased pigmentation and growth of scrotum • Growth of penis in length and circumference • Beginning of spermatogenesis	• Increase in amount, pigmentation, and curling of pubic hair • Growth spurt involving height and weight increase • Menarche • Appearance of axillary hair • Enlargement of vulva and clitoris • Development of breast tissue • Ovulation
Postpubescence	• Completion of sexual growth and development • Fertility	• Completion of sexual growth and development • Fertility

the concept of time, its passage, and the future become real. Challenging the decision making of adults is common. Egocentrism returns, and imaginary audiences and daydreaming are common.

Young adults, in comparison to the adolescent, are more creative in thought, are objective and realistic, and are less self-centered. Their learning is enhanced through educational and life experiences.

Psychosocial Development

Freud's Theory

The adolescent and young adult are in Freud's genital stage. The libido re-emerges in a mature, adult form, and the person is capable of full sexual function. There is a sense of self and others, extending to other adults and peers of the opposite gender. Creativity and pleasure are found in love and in work.

Erikson's Theory

According to Erikson's theory, the adolescent tries out different roles, personal choices, and beliefs in the stage called identity versus role confusion. Self-concept is being stabilized, with the peer group acting as the greatest influence.

 THINK back to Darlene Jenkins, the 14-year-old pregnant teenager. The nurse could apply knowledge of Erikson's theory to foster a sense of identity in Darlene by explaining about important self-care measures and encouraging her participation in her pregnancy. In addition, establishing a trusting relationship with Darlene and subsequently between her and other members of the health care staff would help to further promote her identity. ●

The young adult, in the intimacy-versus-isolation stage, needs to complete tasks such as achieving independence

from parents, establishing intimate relationships, and choosing an occupation or career. If such developmental tasks are not accomplished, the young adult may become isolated and self-absorbed.

Havighurst's Theory

According to Havighurst, more mature relationships with both boys and girls of the same age are achieved, a masculine or feminine social role is developed, one's personal appearance is accepted, and a set of values and ethical system as a guide to behavior are internalized.

Levinson's Theory

In Levinson's theory of individual life structure, the years from 18 to 22 are characterized by early adult transition (Levinson, Darrow, Klein, Levinson, & McKee, 1978). This is a time of making initial career choices, establishing personal relationships, and selecting personal values and lifestyles. During the years from 22 to 28, the young adult builds on previous choices, but there might be a transient quality to occupational choices and friendships.

Gould's Theory

Gould's (1972) theory of transformation views young adults as having established their own control as adults separate from the family. They want to enjoy the present but also build for the future.

Special Considerations

CHOOSING AN OCCUPATION OR CAREER

A major psychosocial developmental requirement for the young adult is choosing a vocation. The decision to enter the world of work is strongly influenced initially by the need to become independent of one's family and to be self-sufficient. The choice of an occupation or a career is also

Graduating college or trade school is an important developmental milestone.

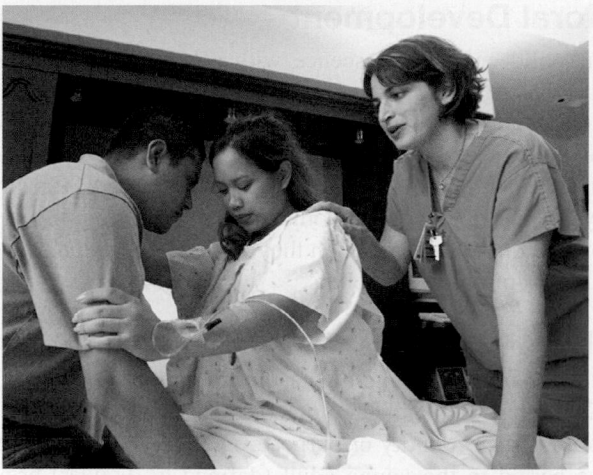

Choosing an occupation and starting a career are also important developmental milestones.

Developmental tasks of the young adult center on establishing intimate relationships, a home, and a family.

FIGURE 18-10. Development in the young adult.

guided by factors such as the desire to get married, raise a family, and become part of the community (Fig. 18-10).

Occupational and career choices are largely tied to educational choices. Many careers require a college education. Adults learn from both informal and formal experiences and are largely goal-directed learners. If the person's identified goals are to increase career opportunities, maintain financial stability, and pursue upward mobility, the adult will be motivated to learn and change. The major factor in achieving satisfaction with one's vocational choice is the belief that one is functioning to capacity and making a contribution to society.

ESTABLISHING A FAMILY

As discussed in Chapter 4, there are many different types and configurations of families. Families provide a safe zone and a buffer between the needs of individuals and the expectations of society. Each has the potential to provide a caring, supportive environment. Establishing a family involves both parents, even though the physiologic changes of pregnancy

take place in the woman. Pregnancy is a period of adjustment requiring family members to be flexible enough to adapt to the changes that pregnancy and a new family member will bring. The cognitive, psychosocial, cultural, and educational dimensions of the prospective parents influence completion of the tasks.

The verification of pregnancy might raise conflicting emotions in the woman, influenced by such factors as whether the pregnancy was planned or unplanned and how the baby may affect career goals. As body changes occur and fetal movement is felt, the woman begins to visualize herself as a mother and normally assumes responsibility for the health of the growing baby. As the time for delivery becomes closer, the woman centers on maternal tasks (such as preparing the baby's room and having clothing ready) and prepares herself for labor and delivery. During the pregnancy, the expectant father needs to learn the normal physiologic and psychological changes of pregnancy, accept his supportive role in meeting maternal needs, and explore his feelings about the developing infant and the birth.

Moral Development

The child enters adolescence with a law-and-order orientation and might never progress beyond that point. Young adults who have mastered previous levels of moral development reach the conventional level and are concerned with maintaining expectations. They also value conformity, loyalty, and social order. Some people might enter the postconventional stage, in which they make moral judgments on the basis of universal beliefs.

Spiritual Development

Adolescents and young adults can think in the abstract and might question beliefs and practices that no longer serve to stabilize their identity or purpose. The individuating-reflective period in the young adult (defined by Fowler) brings discovery of the meaning of values as they relate to the achievement of social purposes and the acceptance of the value systems of others. Often, adolescents or young adults temporarily abandon traditional religious practices.

Health of the Adolescent and Young Adult

Although adolescence and young adulthood are times of maximum physiologic development and health, a wide variety of health problems can occur. Health promotion focuses on nutrition, relationships with self and others, and safety. The Advisory Committee on Immunization Practices now recommends routine vaccination with one dose of meningococcal conjugate vaccine for all people 11 to 18 years of age (CDC, 2013a). College freshmen living in dormitories and young adults living in military barracks are at risk for meningococcal disease and require the vaccine for protection from it. Young adults should have a tetanus and diphtheria booster every 10 years. Since 2000, there has been a recurrence of pertussis (whooping cough), and a tetanus, diphtheria, and acellular pertussis vaccine (Tdap) has been developed to provide immunity against pertussis. Tdap should replace one dose of Td when it is recommended for this age group (Fryhofer, 2013). The CDC also recommends the vaccination of girls and women ages 13 through 26 who did not receive the three doses of the HPV vaccine when they were younger. The HPV vaccine prevents the types of HPV that most commonly cause cervical cancer and genital warts (CDC, 2012g). See Examples of NANDA-I Nursing Diagnoses: Adolescence for health issues in adolescents.

Injuries

Injuries are the leading cause of death for adolescents and young adults. Motor vehicle crashes are the most common cause of mortality, often associated with the use of alcohol or other drugs. Drivers 16 to 19 years of age are more likely to be involved in a fatal crash than drivers 20 and older (CDC, 2013d). According to the CDC (2012h), homicide is the second leading cause of death in the 10- to 24-year age group. In 2011, more than 707,000 youths in this age group were treated in emergency departments for injuries related to a physical assault (CDC, 2012h). Among adolescents 10 to 17 years of age, more than one million serious sports-related injuries occur each year (*Healthy People 2020*, 2012).

Substance Abuse

Smoking and the use of illegal drugs pose serious health risks, and the use of alcohol is significantly related to risk-taking behavior for adolescents and young adults. According to a 2012 survey of adolescent substance abuse, prescription medications, most often obtained from family and friends, and over-the-counter (OTC) medications were among the most common drugs abused by high school seniors (National Institute on Drug Abuse, 2013). OTC drugs most commonly misused by this age group include dextromethorphan (found

EXAMPLES OF NANDA-I NURSING DIAGNOSES

ADOLESCENCE

Nursing Diagnoses	Possible Related Factor
Imbalanced Nutrition: More Than Body Requirements	Sedentary lifestyle
Imbalanced Nutrition: Less Than Body Requirements	Self-imposed dieting
Risk for Injury	Risk-taking behavior while driving
Social Isolation	Perceived inability to be popular
Risk for Impaired Parenting	Teenage pregnancy
Disturbed Personal Identity	Discrimination due to sexual orientation
Anxiety	Fear of failure in school
Ineffective Health Maintenance	Frequent use of alcohol and drugs
Risk-Prone Health Behavior	Smoking

in common cold and cough medicines), caffeine medicines and energy drinks, and diet pills. Opioid analgesics and amphetamine-dexamphetamine (Adderall), a stimulant prescribed to treat attention deficit hyperactivity disorder (ADHD), are among the more commonly abused prescription medications in this age group. Inhaling the vapors of toxic substances with the intent of causing a mind-altering effect (or "high") can damage the kidneys, brain, and liver and lead to cardiopulmonary arrest. Types of products abused include solvents such as glue and paint thinners, aerosols such as spray paint and hair spray, gas inhalants found in whipped cream containers, and nitrites (also referred to as "poppers"). Marijuana use has increased, and fewer adolescents perceive this drug as harmful. Researchers are increasingly concerned that regular use of marijuana during the high school years increases the risk of addiction; as well, marijuana is believed to lower IQ and impair mental abilities (National Institute on Drug Abuse, 2012). Substance abuse, including tobacco and alcohol, is further discussed in Chapter 26.

Suicide

The suicide rate of adolescents has increased drastically, with suicide being more prevalent in adolescents than in any other age group. Suicide is the third leading cause of death of 15- to 24-year-olds and the second leading cause of death for adults 25 to 34 years of age (CDC, 2012e). Although females attempt suicide more often than males, males are more likely to succeed. A history of previous suicide attempts and depression are possible risk factors. Verbal or nonverbal indicators of suicide should not be ignored; rather, an immediate referral should be made to a professional trained in suicide intervention.

Pregnancy

The United States leads the developed countries in the number of pregnancies among adolescents 15 to 19 years old. These pregnancies are physically, psychologically, and economically costly for the adolescent mother, the infant, the family, and society. Many adolescent mothers are poor, do not complete high school, and are at high risk for complications involving the pregnancy and the infant.

Nutritional Problems

Fad dieting and habitually eating fast foods are common among adolescents and young adults. For those obsessed with body image (particularly girls and young women), severe eating disorders can result. The most common are anorexia nervosa (compulsive dieting to the point of self-starvation) and bulimia (a destructive cycle of binge eating followed by self-induced vomiting in an effort to prevent weight gain). The psychodynamics of these conditions are complex but almost always involve a negative self-concept. Although these disorders were once considered uncommon, 5% of adolescent girls report symptoms of anorexia; approximately 5% to 10% of cases of anorexia are male (Hockenberry & Wilson, 2013). Bulimia occurs more frequently in older adolescent girls who are either average or slightly above average weight and is more rare in males.

Adolescents and young adults are consuming energy drinks with increasing frequency. These drinks have high levels of caffeine, which is not always disclosed on the label, and are advertised to boost energy and improve mental and physical performance. There has been a 50% increase in ED visits due to adverse reactions from consuming these beverages. Excessive caffeine levels can result in anxiety, rapid pulse, abnormal cardiac rhythms, nervousness, and panic disorders (McGraw, 2013).

Sexually Transmitted Infections

Adolescents and young adults who engage in unprotected sexual intercourse are at a higher risk for contracting **sexually transmitted infections (STIs)** and their complications than are adults, and account for more than the 20 million new STIs that occur each year in the United States (Wisnieski & Matzo, 2013). Lack of knowledge, lack of psychosocial maturity, embarrassment, and a lack of planning ahead and not using condoms are the most common reasons for this increased risk. Trichomonal and monilial infections, as well as human papillomavirus, are common.

Chlamydia, an infection of the genital tract, is the most common STI in the United States (CDC, 2013c). Chlamydial infections occur in both genders, as do syphilis and herpes simplex type II (genital herpes). These STIs pose serious health threats.

Acquired immunodeficiency syndrome (AIDS) poses the greatest single threat to people and society as a whole. Although AIDS can be transmitted through means other than sexual contact, transmission is primarily through genital, oral, or anal sexual activities. AIDS is a major cause of death in the world, and its incidence is predicted to increase still further.

Developmental and Situational Stressors

Adolescents and young adults have to deal with many stressors as a result of their choices about lifestyle, occupation, and relationships. Adolescence is usually the time when peer pressure and fear of being different can result in young people questioning their sexual orientation. Sexual orientation defines a person's physical and emotional attraction to a person of the same and/or opposite gender. This attraction is an evolving process but typically emerges between middle childhood and early adolescence. Sexual orientation does not appear to be related to genetic, hormonal, developmental, social, or cultural influences, but there is agreement that a person has little or no choice regarding it. There is also consensus that sexual orientation cannot be changed by medicine or therapy. Common terms used to describe sexual orientation include *heterosexual* (attraction to members of the opposite sex), *homosexual* (attraction to someone of the same sex), and *bisexual* (attracted to both sexes). Homosexual persons may also be labeled *lesbian* (women attracted to women) or *gay* (men attracted to men). When a person's internal feelings of being male or female differ from his or

TEACHING TIPS 18-5

ADOLESCENTS AND YOUNG ADULTS

Health Topic	Teaching Tip	Why Is This Important?
Safety	<ul><li>Encourage drivers' education classes for adolescents, if available.</li><li>Discuss the relationship of alcohol and drug consumption to motor vehicle crashes.</li><li>Provide information about water safety, gun safety, and sports safety.</li></ul>	Most deaths in people between the ages of 15 and 24 are the result of motor vehicle crashes, homicide, and suicide.
Nutrition	<ul><li>Encourage a diet based on the food groups, with added calories during the adolescent growth spurt.</li><li>Refer for counseling for extremes in either underweight or overweight.</li><li>Discuss nutritional problems that may result from too much fast food and too many soft drinks.</li><li>A balance of food intake, exercise, and rest is important.</li></ul>	Nutritional needs increase to meet the accelerated physical growth and development during adolescence. Underweight may result from an inadequate intake of calories, or in extreme cases from anorexia nervosa or bulimia. Overweight results from an intake of calories in excess of metabolic needs.
Sexual Development	<ul><li>Secondary sex characteristics are fully developed.</li><li>Both males and females are physically capable of reproduction.</li><li>Discuss sexual behavior openly and honestly with adolescents.</li></ul>	The development of secondary sex characteristics that began in the school-aged child is completed during adolescence. Sexual behavior in adolescents and young adults might result in disease or pregnancy, as well as decreased self-esteem.
Growth and Development	<ul><li>The adolescent is primarily influenced by the peer group.</li><li>Risk-taking behavior, especially in males, is common.</li><li>Maintaining open communications with teens is important.</li><li>Encourage increasing independence in the adolescent and young adult, but continue to provide love and support.</li><li>Assist with clarifying values and goals for future occupation.</li></ul>	Peer groups may have positive or negative effects. The rapid physical and emotional changes of adolescence require revising self-concept and body image. These should stabilize by late adolescence. The young adult is usually living independently and has an occupation of choice.
Promoting Health and Preventing Illness	<ul><li>Have immunizations and boosters as recommended. CDC recommends a series of three HPV vaccinations for women ages 13–26 who did not receive them when they were younger. Gardasil, one of the FDA-approved HPV vaccines, is also recommended for men through 26 years of age to protect against genital warts.</li><li>Have regular physical, vision, and dental examinations.</li><li>Always have a physical examination before participating in sports activities.</li><li>Do a breast self-exam (females) and a testicular self-exam (males) each month.</li><li>Learn to say "no" to pressures to have sexual activity.</li><li>Engage in safe-sex practices if sexually active.</li><li>Have an annual Pap test and pelvic examination if sexually active.</li><li>Know the dangers of STIs (from genital, oral, and anal sex) and have HIV testing if safe sex is not practiced.</li></ul>	Immunizations and regular health-related examinations are essential to maintaining health. Chronic illnesses such as hypertension, cardiovascular disease, and diabetes mellitus might appear during adolescence and young adulthood. Sexual desires are high, and sexual activity is common. STIs and AIDS are a major health problem, with more than two-thirds of those infected younger than 25. Untreated STIs may result in sterility in females and males or infection of an unborn baby.

her physical anatomy, the term *transgender* is used to refer to gender identity. The term *questioning* defines a person unsure of sexual orientation. The acronym LGBTQ is commonly used in the United States to refer to all these alternatives collectively. People who identify themselves as gay, lesbian, bisexual, or transgender may experience prejudice and discrimination that can cause negative psychological outcomes. Adolescents may be reluctant to reveal their sexual orientation or gender identity for fear of ridicule, rejection, or harassment from family and friends, or they may receive unconditional support and love from both groups.

Family-centered stressors include both positive and negative factors, such as marriage, divorce, parenthood, and death of a parent. Stress might precipitate mental or physical health problems, aggravated by ineffective coping mechanisms such as substance abuse, child abuse, spousal abuse, decreased nutrition and rest, and risk-taking behavior.

 CONSIDER Darlene Jenkins, the 14-year-old pregnant adolescent described in the case file at the beginning of the chapter. Analysis of this patient's assessment reveals multiple developmental and situational stressors affecting Darlene that place her and her fetus at high risk for problems. Using this information, the nurse could develop a highly individualized plan of care that focuses on these stressors (e.g., her lack of adequate supports, multiple sexual partners, poor nutritional habits), ultimately to the benefit of Darlene and her baby. ●

An increasing number of men and women are remaining single, either by choice or situation. Singlehood status has advantages and disadvantages. Being single gives one the freedom to come and go as one chooses, to have more autonomy, to pursue or create one's own career vision, and to spend money and time as one wishes. On the other hand, external pressures to marry and the desire for love, to belong, and to raise a family might make a young adult question the decision to remain single.

Couples might encounter difficulties conceiving, delay childbearing until their careers are established, or choose not to have children. If they want to have children, infertility (defined as the inability to conceive after 1 year of coitus without contraception) might add even more stress. Women who have postponed having children might realize in their middle to late 30s that their so-called biologic clock is winding down; an increasing number of women in this age group are having their first child.

Divorce is common in our society, with rates being highest among those marrying young, having low income, and having low educational levels. It separates children from their families, has long-term emotional costs, and increases the number of single-parent families headed by women.

Role of the Nurse in Promoting Health and Preventing Illness

A true assessment of adolescent development must include the profound changes in reproductive functioning. Teaching

FIGURE 18-11. Adolescents with chronic illnesses can avoid feelings of isolation by using social networking sites to communicate with their peers.

activities to promote health for adolescents and young adults are listed in Teaching Tips 18-5. Perhaps one of the more significant nursing activities for people in this stage is facilitating healthy family relationships. Mutual respect, open communications, and accurate information exchange among family members pave the road for a healthy transition from adolescence to adulthood.

Acute illness is often more of an annoyance than of serious consequence. If hospitalized, an adolescent's and young adult's motivation to recover and to resume normal activities is strong. Because independence and self-sufficiency are important to adolescents and young adults, they will not easily accept the dependent sick role.

Although chronic illnesses are less common, their occurrence can lead to delayed development, loss of independence, and permanent changes in personal and career goals. Prolonged hospitalization, long-term care, or home care increases the adolescent's feelings of isolation and may disrupt normal development. Educational and recreational activities should be provided, if at all possible (Fig. 18-11).

DEVELOPING CLINICAL REASONING

1. Based on the information presented in Chapters 17 and 18, describe nursing interventions to meet developmental needs for the following:
   - An infant hospitalized for treatment of a serious birth defect involving the heart and lungs
   - A toddler with a fracture of the left leg, treated in the emergency department and then sent home
   - A school-aged child, now in rehabilitation, with burns on both arms
   - A 20-year-old hospitalized for injuries resulting from an automobile accident after drinking alcohol
2. During your home visit for a 16-year-old with cancer, she says, "I don't believe in God." What would you reply? Why would you respond this way?

3. During a clinic visit, a 2-month-old appears listless and constantly cries. The mother tells you that he has colic, so she has been diluting his formula with water. What would you do now?

PRACTICING FOR NCLEX

1. A nurse performing an assessment of a newborn in the neonatal unit records these findings: heart rate 85 bpm, irregular respiratory rate, normal muscle tone, weak crying, and bluish tint to skin. Using the APGAR scoring chart (see Table 18-1, p. 389) what would be the score for this newborn?
   a. 5
   b. 7
   c. 8
   d. 10

2. The nurse records an APGAR score of 4 for a newborn. What would be the priority intervention for this newborn?
   a. No interventions are necessary; this is a normal score.
   b. Provide respiratory assistance.
   c. Perform CPR.
   d. Wait 5 minutes and repeat the scoring process.

3. A school nurse is preparing a talk on safety issues for parents of school-aged children to present at a parent–teacher meeting. Which topics should the nurse include based on the age of the children? Select all that apply.
   a. Child-proofing the home
   b. Choosing a car seat
   c. Teaching pedestrian traffic safety
   d. Providing swimming lessons and water safety rules
   e. Discussing alcohol and drug consumption related to motor vehicle safety
   f. Teaching child how to "stop, drop, and roll"

4. The nurse encourages parents of hospitalized infants and toddlers to stay with their child to help decrease what potential problem?
   a. Problems with attachment
   b. Separation anxiety
   c. Risk for injury
   d. Failure to thrive

5. A nurse is teaching parents of toddlers how to spend quality time with their children. Which activity would be developmentally appropriate for this age group?
   a. Playing video games
   b. Playing peek-a-boo
   c. Playing in a sand box
   d. Playing board games

6. A mother tells the nurse that she is worried about her 4-year-old daughter because she is "overly attached to her father and won't listen to anything I tell her to do." What would be the nurse's best response to this parental concern?
   a. Tell the mother that this is normal behavior for a preschooler.
   b. Tell the mother that she and her family should see a counselor.
   c. Tell the mother that she should try to spend more time with her daughter.
   d. Tell the mother that her child should be tested for autism.

7. A high school nurse is counseling parents of teenagers who are beginning high school. Which issues would be priority topics of discussion for this age group? Select all that apply.
   a. The influence of peer groups
   b. Bullying
   c. Water safety
   d. Eating disorders
   e. Risk taking behavior
   f. Immunizations

8. A nurse working with adolescents in a group home discusses the developmental tasks appropriate for adolescents with the staff. What is an example of a primary developmental task of the adolescent?
   a. Working hard to succeed in school
   b. Spending time developing relationships with peers
   c. Developing athletic activities and skills
   d. Accepting the decisions of parents

9. Following assessment of an obese adolescent, a nurse considers nursing diagnoses for the patient. Which diagnosis would be most appropriate?
   a. Risk for injury
   b. Risk for delayed development
   c. Social isolation
   d. Disturbed body image

10. A nurse is teaching new mothers about infant care and safety. What would the nurse accurately include as a teaching point?
    a. Keep infants younger than 6 months out of direct sunlight.
    b. Use honey instead of sugar in homemade baby food.
    c. Place the baby on his or her stomach for sleeping.
    d. Keep crib rails down at all times.

ANSWERS WITH RATIONALES

1. *a.* A newborn with a heart rate less than 100 bpm, irregular respiratory effort, normal muscle tone, weak cry, and bluish tint to the skin scores a 5 on the APGAR chart.

2. *b.* A newborn who scores a 4 on the APGAR chart requires special assistance such as respiratory assistance. Normal APGAR scores are 7 to 10. Neonates who score between 4 and 6 require special assistance, and those who score below 4 are in need of life-saving support.

3. *c, d, f.* Important safety topics for school-aged children include pedestrian traffic safety, water safety, and fire safety. Childproofing a home would be appropriate for parents of a toddler, choosing a car seat would be an appropriate topic for parents of an infant or toddler, and teaching drug and alcohol as it relates to motor vehicle safety would be a more appropriate topic for parents of adolescents.

4. *b.* Separation anxiety, with crying initially and then appearing depressed, is common during late infancy in infants who are hospitalized.

5. *c.* Playing in a sand box with toys that emphasize gross motor skills and creativity is a developmentally appropriate activity for a toddler. Video games are appropriate for school-aged children and adolescents, but should be monitored. Playing peek-a-boo is developmentally appropriate for an infant, and playing board games usually begins with preschool and older children.

6. *a.* Preschoolers, according to Freud, are in the phallic stage, with the biologic focus primarily genital. The child has a sexual desire for the opposite-sex parent, but as means of defense strongly identifies with the same-sex parent. This is normal behavior for a preschooler, and the family does not need counseling or autism testing. Spending more time with the child is always a good idea, but is not the solution to this concern.

7. *a, b, d, e.* Appropriate topics of discussion for parents of adolescents include peer groups, bullying, eating disorders, and risk-taking behaviors. Immunizations would be appropriate for parents of children from infants to school-age, and water safety should be taught in the preschool years.

8. *b.* Adolescence is a time to establish more mature relationships with both boys and girls of the same age.

9. *d.* Adolescents who are obese are at high risk for a disturbed body image. Risk for injury would be appropriate for a risk taker, a risk factor for delayed development may be ADHD, and social isolation may occur with low self-esteem.

10. *a.* Nurses should teach parents to keep infants younger than 6 months out of direct sunlight and cover them with protective clothing and hats. The nurse should also teach parents not to add honey or sugar to homemade baby food, to place the baby on the back for sleeping to prevent SIDS, and to keep the crib rails up at all times.

TAYLOR SUITE RESOURCES

Explore these additional resources to enhance learning for this chapter:

- NCLEX-Style Questions and other resources on thePoint, http://thePoint.lww.com/Taylor8e
- *Study Guide for Fundamentals of Nursing, 8th edition*
- Adaptive Learning | Powered by prepU, http://thepoint.lww.com/prepu

Bibliography

American Academy of Pediatrics. (2013). Reduce the risk of SIDS. Available at http://www.healthychildren.org/English/ages-stages/baby/sleep/Pages/Preventing-SIDS.aspx

American College of Obstetricians and Gynecologists (ACOG). (2011). *Tobacco, alcohol, drugs, and pregnancy.* Available at http://www.acog.org/~/media/For%20Patients/faq170.pdf?dmc=1&ts=20140125T1801364339

Centers for Disease Control and Prevention (CDC). (2010). Understanding child maltreatment. Available at http://www.cdc.gov/violenceprevention/pdf/CM-FactSheet-a.pdf

Centers for Disease Control and Prevention (CDC). (2011). CDC's sudden unexpected infant death initiative. Available at http://www.cdc.gov/sids/suidabout.htm

Centers for Disease Control and Prevention (CDC). (2012a). Child maltreatment: Definitions. Available at http://www.cdc.gov/violenceprevention/childmaltreatment/definitions.html

Centers for Disease Control and Prevention (CDC). (2012b). Child maltreatment: Facts at a glance. Available at http://www.cdc.gov/violenceprevention/pdf/cm_datasheet2012-a.pdf

Centers for Disease Control and Prevention (CDC). (2012c). Sleep safely and soundly. Available at http://www2c.cdc.gov/podcasts/media/pdf/mmwr5_112912_transcript.pdf

Centers for Disease Control and Prevention (CDC). (2012d). Suffocation deaths associated with use of infant sleep positions—United States, 1997–2011. *Morbidity and Mortality Weekly Report (MMWR)* 2012;61(46), 933–937.

Centers for Disease Control and Prevention (CDC). (2012e). *Suicide: Facts at a glance.* Available at http://www.cdc.gov/ViolencePrevention/pdf/suicide_DataSheet-a.pdf

Centers for Disease Control and Prevention (CDC). (2012f). Understanding thimerosal, mercury, and vaccine safety. Available at http://www.cdc.gov/vaccines/hcp/patient-ed/conversations/downloads/vacsafe-thimerosal-bw-office.pdf

Centers for Disease Control and Prevention (CDC). (2012g). Vaccine safety: Frequently asked questions about HPV vaccine safety. Available at http://www.cdc.gov/vaccinesafety/Vaccines/HPV/hpv_faqs.html

Centers for Disease Control and Prevention (CDC). (2012h). Youth violence: Facts at a glance. Available at http://cdc.gov/violenceprevention/pdf/YV-DataSheet-a.pdf

Centers for Disease Control and Prevention (CDC). (2013a). 2013 Recommended immunizations for children from 7 through 18 years old. Available at http://www.cdc.gov/vaccines/who/teens/downloads/parent-version-schedule-7–18yrs.pdf

Centers for Disease Control and Prevention (CDC). (2013b). Childhood obesity facts. Available at http://www.cdc.gov/healthyyouth/obesity/facts.htm

Centers for Disease Control and Prevention (CDC). (2013c). Chlamydia—CDC fact sheet. Available at http://www.cdc.gov/std/chlamydia/STDFact-Chlamydia.htm

Centers for Disease Control and Prevention (CDC). (2013d). Teen drivers. Available at http://www.cdc.gov/Motorvehiclesafety/Teen_Drivers/index.html

Centers for Disease Control and Prevention (CDC). (2013e). What is premature birth? Available at http://www.cdc.gov/features/prematurebirth/

Fryhofer, S. (2013). New adult immunization schedule: A quick overview. Available at http://www.medscape.com/viewarticle/778046

Gould, R. (1972). The phases of adult life: A study in developmental psychology. *American Psychiatry,* 129, 33–43.

Hamilton, B., Martin, J., & Ventura, S. (2012). Births: Preliminary data for 2011. *National Vital Statistics Reports, 61*(5), 1–5.

Healthy People 2020. (2012). Injury and violence. Available at http://healthypeople.gov/2020/LHI/injuryViolence.aspx?source=govdelivery&tab=determinants

Himes, J. (2013). Challenges of accurately measuring and using BMI and other indicators of obesity in children. *Pediatrics, 124*(Suppl 1), S3–22. Available at http://pediatrics.aappublications.org/content/124/Supplement_1/S3.full

Hockenberry, M., & Wilson, D. (2013). *Wong's Essentials of Pediatric Nursing* (9th ed.). St. Louis: Elsevier.

KidsHealth. (2012). Overweight and obesity. Available at http://kidshealth.org/parent/general/body/overweight_obesity.html

Klaus, M. H., & Kennell, J. H. (1982). *Parent–infant bonding.* St. Louis: C. V. Mosby.

Levinson, D., Darrow, C., Klein, E., Levinson, M., & McKee, B. (1978). *The seasons of a man's life.* New York: Knopf.

McGraw, M. (2013). Are energy drinks safe? *Nursing, 43*(3), 68.

Matthews, R., & Moore, A. (2013). Babies are still dying of SIDS. *American Journal of Nursing, 113*(2), 59–64.

Murray, R., & Zentner, J. (2001). *Health promotion strategies through the life span* (7th ed.). Upper Saddle River, NJ: Prentice Hall.

NANDA International. (2012). *Nursing diagnoses: Definitions & classification 2012–2014.* West Sussex, UK: Wiley-Blackwell.

National Institute on Drug Abuse. (2012). Regular marijuana use by teens continues to be a concern. Available at http://www.drugabuse.gov/news-events/news-releases/2012/12/regular-marijuana-use-by-teens-continues-to-be-concern

National Institute on Drug Abuse. (2013). Prevention efforts focused on youth reduce prescription abuse into adulthood. Available at http://www.drugabuse.gov/news-events/news-releases/2013/02/prevention-efforts-focused-youth-reduce-prescription-abuse-adulthood

Norton, C., Feltz, S., Brocker, A., & Granitto, M. (2013). Tackling long-term consequences of concussion. *Nursing, 43*(1), 50–55.

Offit, P. (2012). Thimerosal in vaccines: What are the facts? Available at http://www.medscape.com/viewarticle/776762

Okely, A., Pearson, P., Puglisi, L., & Vialle, W. (2013). Understanding the day-to-day lives of obese children and their families. *Family & Community Health, 36*(1), 42–50.

Pillitteri, A. (2010). *Maternal & child health nursing: Care of the childbearing & childrearing family* (6th ed.). Philadelphia: Wolters Kluwer Health/Lippincott Williams & Wilkins.

Potera, C. (2012). ED visits from battery injuries on the rise in children. *American Journal of Nursing, 112*(8), 16.

Schwarz, A., & Cohen, S. (2013). A.D.H.D. seen in 11% of U.S. children as diagnoses rise. Available at http://www.nytimes.com/2013/04/01/health/more-diagnoses-of-hyperactivity-causing-concern.html?_r=0

Sherwood, G., & Barnsteiner, J. (2012). *Quality and Safety in Nursing.* West Sussex, UK: Wiley-Blackwell.

Thomas, A., Chess, S., & Birch, H. G. (1968). *Temperament and behavior discussed in children.* New York: New York University Press.

U.S. Food and Drug Administration (FDA) (2012). Using over-the-counter cough and cold products. Available at http://www.fda.gov/ForConsumers/ConsumerUpdates/ucm048515.htm

U.S. National Library of Medicine. (2013). Choking—infant under 1 year. Medline Plus. Available at http://www.nlm.nih.gov/medlineplus/ency/article/000048.htm

Wallis, L. (2013). School lunch standards. *American Journal of Nursing, 113*(1), 17.

Wilson, D., & Severson, M. (2012). Long-term health outcomes of childhood sexual abuse. *American Nurse today.* Available at http://www.americannursetoday.com/Popups/ArticlePrint.aspx?id=11782

Wisnieski, D., & Matzo, M. (2013). Promoting healthy sexual behavior in adolescents. *American Journal of Nursing, 113*(6), 67–70.

19 The Aging Adult

ETHEL PEABODY

Ethel, an 88-year-old single woman with beginning dementia who was treated for cardiac problems, is being discharged. She has no family and lives in a small, two-story house with her three cats. There is some concern about her safety at home. She depends on a neighbor for some help and refuses to consider moving to a retirement community or extended-care facility.

LARRY JENKINS

Larry, a 67-year-old man with diabetes, states, "Everything's gone downhill since I retired 5 months ago. He reports being "bored out of my mind" and drinking more alcohol simply because "there's nothing else to do!"

ROSEMARY MASON

Rosemary, a 59-year-old woman who comes to the clinic with her 64-year-old husband, confides that she wishes that Viagra had never been discovered. "I was happier when we just cuddled at night. Now he wants to try all sorts of things, and I'm just not ready for this!"

After completing the chapter, you will be able to accomplish the following:

1. Summarize the theories that describe how and why aging occurs.

2. Describe major physiologic, cognitive, psychosocial, moral, and spiritual developments and tasks of middle and older adulthood.

3. Describe common health problems of middle and older adults.

4. Discuss physiologic and functional changes that occur with aging.

5. Describe common myths and stereotypes that perpetuate ageism.

6. Describe nursing interventions to promote health for middle and older adults.

7. Identify the health care needs of older adults in terms of chronic illnesses, accidental injuries, and acute care needs.

KEY TERMS

ageism	gerontologic nursing	reality orientation
Alzheimer disease	gerontology	reminiscence
cascade iatrogenesis	life review	social isolation
delirium	middle adult	sundowning syndrome
dementia	older adult	
functional health	polypharmacy	

Aging is a gradual process, characterized by continued development and maturation. The changes of aging begin as one enters middle adulthood. The onset and effects of those changes throughout the middle and older adult years are influenced by numerous biologic, psychosocial, and environmental factors (described in the Theories of Aging section). The physiologic changes of aging, first experienced in middle adulthood, become more obvious in older adults. Continued development throughout one's adult life depends to a great extent on a person's sense of self-concept and prior ability to adapt. This chapter continues the discussion of growth and development from previous chapters, focusing on the aging years. For an example addressing the older adult, see the accompanying Reflective Practice box on page 420.

THEORIES OF AGING

As one ages, changes in cells, tissues, organs, and organ systems occur. Scientists do not fully understand why some people, even within the same family or environment, age much more rapidly than others. Although internal processes may in part determine aging, other factors, such as nutrition and the environment, may also play a role. Numerous theories describe how and why aging occurs, but none is universally accepted. These theories focus on a variety of factors, including genetic inheritance, cell metabolism and function, and the immune system.

Genetic Theory of Aging

The genetic theory of aging holds that lifespan depends to a great extent on genetic factors. Genes within the organism control "genetic clocks," which determine the occurrence and rate of metabolic processes, including cell division. According to the wear-and-tear theory, organisms wear out from increased metabolic functioning, and cells become exhausted from continual energy depletion from adapting to stressors (Eliopoulos, 2010).

Immunity Theory of Aging

The immunity theory of aging focuses on the functions of the immune system. This system—composed primarily of the bone marrow, thymus, spleen, and lymph nodes—seeks out and destroys foreign agents (such as viruses, bacteria, and perhaps cells undergoing neoplastic changes). The immune response declines steadily after younger adulthood as the thymus loses size and function. Age-associated changes in the immune system, also known as *immunosenescence,* are thought to be responsible for the increase in infections such as pneumonia and septicemia, immune disorders, and cancer as adults age (Chettle, 2009). Some authorities believe that nutrition plays an important role in maintaining the immune response; therefore, there is much interest in vitamin supplements (such as vitamin E) that are believed by some to improve immune function.

Cross-Linkage Theory

Cross-linkage is a chemical reaction that produces damage to the DNA and cell death. As one ages, cross-links accumulate, leading to essential molecules in the cell binding together and interfering with normal cell function.

Free Radical Theory

Free radicals, formed during cellular metabolism, are molecules with separated high-energy electrons, which can have adverse effects on adjacent molecules. Lipids, found in cell membranes, as well as proteins and cell organelles, are affected. Over time, irreversible damage results from the accumulated effects of this damage.

THE MIDDLE ADULT

The **middle adult** years are generally considered to be ages 40 to 65. This is a period of gradual, individualized changes in both physical and psychosocial dimensions. As the average lifespan has increased, most people at this age still consider themselves young compared with the older population. Visible signs of aging and a heightened awareness of the time left

REFLECTIVE PRACTICE: CULTIVATING QSEN COMPETENCIES

CHALLENGE TO ETHICAL AND LEGAL SKILLS

Mrs. Ethel Peabody is an 88-year-old single woman with beginning dementia hospitalized for cardiac problems. She has no family and her only visitor is a neighbor. She lives alone in a small, two-story home with her three cats.

When the doctor ordered her discharge, I had grave worries about her ability to live safely on her own. When I asked her if she had ever thought about moving to a long-term care facility or retirement community, she said, "I'd rather die than go to one of those places!" When I told her I was worried about her safety, she told me her cats would take care of her! When I repeated this conversation to the charge nurse, she said, "There is nothing we can do if the patient isn't willing to explore other options."

Thinking Outside the Box: Possible Courses of Action

- Feel satisfied that I had reported my concerns to the charge nurse and let whatever happens happen.
- Explore hospital and other resources to determine realistic options for someone like Mrs. Peabody and the obligations of caregivers and the hospital.

- Find my instructor and seek her counsel.
- Seek out the unit's social worker, confide my worries, and see if she has other recommendations.

Evaluating a Good Outcome: How Do I Define Success?

- Both Mrs. Peabody's safety and ability to make decisions (autonomy) are respected.
- I feel at peace with the decision that was made for the patient and the role I played in this decision.

- My personal and professional integrity are intact.
- My legal responsibilities and those of the institution are met.

Personal Learning: Here's to the Future!

Sadly, I must confess that I was invited to accompany another patient for a diagnostic study off the unit, so I never followed through on my concerns. Mrs. Peabody was discharged to her home, and I never learned what happened to her. However, I was troubled by my inaction and discussed this situation with my instructor. As a result, I am now aware of more options available that I can use when faced with similar situations in the future. The number of older adults will continue to grow, presenting many similar challenges in the future. I want to make sure I'm prepared for my next "Mrs. Peabody." Meanwhile, I will be talking with our patient-relations person, the social worker, hospital risk manager, and our office on aging to increase my knowledge of support services for older adults.

REFLECTION ON QUALITY AND SAFETY COMPETENCIES

How do you think you would respond in a similar situation? Why? What does this tell you about yourself and about the adequacy of your skills for professional practice? Can you think of other ways to respond? What could the nursing student have done differently? What *knowledge, skills,* and *attitudes* do you need to develop to continuously improve quality and safety when caring for patients like Mrs. Peabody?

Patient-Centered Care: How might the student have interacted with the charge nurse and the social worker and other pertinent hospital personnel to promote a safe, structured home environment for Mrs. Peabody while respecting her preferences? What alternatives are available to allow this patient to remain in her home while ensuring her safety? If available options to assist Mrs. Peabody had been explored during her hospitalization, what nursing actions might be helpful as this information is shared with the patient?

Teamwork and Collaboration/Quality Improvement: What communication skills do you need to develop in order to facilitate your role as a patient advocate? What skills would be of particular importance when dealing with the charge nurse? What strategies might be appropriate to ensure that you function as a valued member of the health care team?

Safety/Evidence-Based Practice: How might the lack of any home care interventions affect the outcome for Mrs. Peabody? What safety measures could be enacted that would allow Mrs. Peabody the opportunity to request assistance when needed? What evidence in nursing literature provides guidance for decision-making regarding patients living alone with impaired cognition?

Informatics: Can you identify essential information that must be documented in Mrs. Peabody's electronic record regarding her cardiac condition and treatment? Why is it important to document an assessment of the patient's current mental health status? Can you identify any other essential information that supports safe patient care and that should be included in the electronic record?

to live, however, lead middle adults to evaluate their achievement of goals and influence their adaptation to older age.

Physiologic Development

In the early years of this period of life, physical functions are usually still effective. As time passes, gradual internal and external physiologic changes occur. These are not pathologic changes, but normal changes that result from aging. The person must modify self-image and self-concept to adapt successfully to and to accept these normal changes. Physical changes of the middle adult are outlined in Box 19-1.

BOX 19-1   PHYSICAL CHANGES IN THE MIDDLE ADULT

- Fatty tissue is redistributed; men tend to develop abdominal fat, women thicken through the middle.
- The skin is drier.
- Wrinkle lines appear on the face.
- Gray hair appears, and men may lose hair on the head.
- Cardiac output begins to decrease.
- Muscle mass, strength, and agility gradually decrease.
- There is a loss of calcium from bones, especially in perimenopausal women.
- Fatigue increases.
- Visual acuity diminishes, especially for near vision (presbyopia).
- Hearing acuity diminishes, especially for high-pitched sounds.
- Hormone production decreases, resulting in menopause or andropause.

The hormonal changes that take place in midlife affect men and women differently. Women undergo menopause, a gradual decrease in ovarian function, with subsequent depletion of estrogen and progesterone. This change usually occurs between 40 and 55 years of age. With the cessation of ovulation, menstrual periods stop either gradually or abruptly, causing many women to experience hot flashes, mood swings, and fatigue. The loss of estrogen also increases the risk for osteoporosis and heart disease. The process can last for several years; afterward, the woman can no longer become pregnant. Men do not experience physical symptoms from the decreased levels of hormones, called andropause. Androgen levels diminish slowly; the man may have some loss of sexual potency but is still capable of reproduction.

 REMEMBER Rosemary Mason, the 59-year-old woman described at the beginning of the chapter. The nurse could incorporate information about the differences in hormonal changes for men and women into a teaching plan to help Rosemary understand and adjust to the changes that are occurring. ●

Cognitive Development

Cognitive and intellectual abilities of middle adults change little from young adulthood. There often is increased motivation to learn, especially if the knowledge gained can be applied immediately and has personal relevance. Problem-solving abilities remain throughout adulthood, although response time may be slightly longer. This is due not to any decreased ability but, rather, to a longer search through more memories and to a desire to think a problem through before responding.

Psychosocial Development

The middle adult years often are a time of increased personal freedom, economic stability, and social relationships (Fig. 19-1 on page 422). This is also a time of increased responsibility and an awareness of one's own mortality. One realizes that one's life may be half or more past and may feel many things are still undone. This realization can lead to a developmental crisis and situational stressors. Several theorists describe developmental tasks of middle adulthood, as follows.

Erikson's Theory

According to Erikson's theory (1963), the middle adult is in a period of generativity versus stagnation. The tasks are to establish and guide the next generation, accept middle-age changes, adjust to the needs of aging parents, and reevaluate one's goals and accomplishments. Adults who do not achieve these tasks tend to focus on themselves, becoming overly concerned with their own physical and emotional health needs.

Havighurst's Theory

The developmental tasks of the middle adult described by Havighurst (1972) are learned behaviors arising from maturation, personal motives and values, and civic responsibility. To successfully master this developmental stage, the middle adult must accept and adjust to physical changes, maintain a satisfactory occupation, assist children to become responsible adults, adjust to aging parents, and relate to one's spouse or partner as a person.

Levinson's Theory

Levinson (Levinson, Darrow, Klein, Levinson, & McKee, 1978) theorized that the middle adult may choose either to continue an established lifestyle or to reorganize one's life in a period of midlife transition.

Gould's Theory

Gould (1972) viewed the middle years as a time when adults look inward (ages 35 to 43); accept their lifespan as having definite boundaries, and have a special interest in spouse, friends, and community (ages 43 to 50); and increase their feelings of self-satisfaction, value spouse as a companion, and become more concerned with health (ages 50 to 60).

Adjusting to the Changes of Middle Adulthood

Various changes can take place during the middle years. These include changes in employment, relationships with a spouse or partner, relationships with children who are becoming adults, and relationships with aging parents. Midlife transition might occur in both men and women in their 40s. Although one does not feel that one is aging, realizing that others consider you older can be stressful.

Employment

Middle-aged adults might experience changes in employment. They may opt for a career change and return to school to obtain new knowledge and skills. These changes often result from a need for increased job satisfaction, satisfying a life-long goal, or economic conditions. Many employees

FIGURE 19-1. The middle adult years are characterized by greater expendable wealth, renewed relationship with one's spouse or partner, and expanded social relationships and family roles.

in this age group have lost their jobs due to company downsizing during the recent economic turmoil and have had to acquire new skills and additional education to find employment in other areas. Women who have been immersed in a career may decide to have children and either become "stay at home moms" or reduce their workload. Increasing numbers of middle-aged adults are self-employed, often working from home.

As the 50s approach, questions about retirement and economic security become more prevalent, with an increased interest in the benefits of financial and retirement plans. These concerns can be heightened by overall economic conditions. For example, many people who had planned on an early retirement decide to continue their active employment status. The security of retirement investments and income is critical to ensure that people remain financially stable and that workers receive the pensions they are working toward or have already achieved.

Spousal Relationships

Relationships with one's spouse or partner may change. Although for many this is a time of greater security and stability, with stronger emotional commitment and sharing, for some it is a time of disenchantment. Either partner may develop negative or critical feelings and attitudes as a result of changes in physical appearance, energy levels, or sexual needs and abilities.

 RECALL Rosemary Mason, the 59-year-old woman, voicing displeasure with her husband's desire to "try all sorts of things" sexually. The nurse could use this information about spousal relationships to gather additional assessment data about the couple's relationship before her husband started Viagra. This would help develop an appropriate plan of care that addresses Rosemary's current displeasure. ●

Dissatisfaction with not achieving career or family goals contributes to the stresses placed on the marriage. Extramarital affairs and divorce may result.

Loss of a spouse or partner is more likely in the middle adult years. The loss is a major crisis and a threat to one's self-concept, as well as a major role change. Many changes may occur, including a reduced income, changes in lifestyle and social relationships, and the need for help to work through the loss and grief (see Chapter 42).

Relationships With Children and Aging Family Members

Middle-aged adults may be caught in a "generation sandwich." Their children may be independent and married, with children of their own, or may be recent college graduates who have returned home to live. Difficulty finding employment coupled with the burden of student loans often necessitates the postponement of independent living.

Although much has been written about the "empty-nest syndrome" that occurs when the last child leaves home, most middle-aged parents welcome the increased space, time, and independence they have when active parenting ceases. As their involvement with and responsibility for children decrease, they may have an increased need to help care for aging parents and other family members. The physical aging or death of a parent makes one's own aging and inevitable death a reality.

Moral Development

According to Kohlberg (1969), a middle adult may either remain at the conventional level or move to the postconventional level of moral development, especially if the individual has had sustained responsibility for the welfare of others and has consistently applied ethical principles developed in adolescence. At this level, the adult believes that the rights of others take precedence and takes steps to support those rights.

Spiritual Development

As with moral development, not all adults progress to Fowler's (1991) paradoxical–consolidative state of spiritual development. Fowler believed that only some people reach this stage and only after 30 years of age. Most middle adults are less rigid in their beliefs and have increased faith in a supreme being as well as trust in spiritual strength.

Health of the Middle Adult

Middle adults are subject to physical and emotional health problems associated with lifestyle behaviors, developmental or situational crises, family history, and the environment. Both acute and chronic illnesses are more likely to occur, and recovery takes longer. This is a result of slower and more prolonged responses to stressors, more pronounced reactions to an illness, and the possibility of more than one illness being present at a time.

The leading causes of death in the middle adult years, according to 2009 statistics, are malignant neoplasms; cardiovascular disease; unintentional injury including poisoning, motor vehicle accidents, and falls; diabetes mellitus; chronic lower respiratory disease; and cerebrovascular causes (Heron, 2012). Other major health problems include rheumatoid arthritis, obesity, alcoholism, and depression.

The risk for these common health problems often depends on a combination of lifestyle factors and aging. As one gets older, energy requirements decrease. Middle adults tend to maintain previous eating patterns and caloric intake while being less physically active. This trend can result in obesity and atherosclerosis, with an increased risk for high blood pressure, coronary artery disease, renal failure, and diabetes. Additionally, smoking and alcohol consumption put the person at greater risk for cancer, chronic respiratory diseases, and liver disease.

Chronic illness in middle adults has a major effect on self-concept and may precipitate changes in life structure. For example, after a serious heart attack, a man may face changes in his family role, his earning capacity, and his social relationships. Such changes usually cause great stress.

Middle age does not automatically result in physical or emotional health problems. Many men and women remain healthy throughout their lives, but knowing preventive health care practices and their special needs at this age can help middle adults have improved quality and quantity of life.

Role of the Nurse in Promoting Health and Preventing Illness

The nurse has a major role in promoting health and preventing illness in middle adults by teaching, serving as a role model, and encouraging self-care responsibilities. See Examples of NANDA-I Nursing Diagnoses: The Middle Adult on page 424.

Health-related screenings, examinations, and immunizations for adults are outlined in Table 19-1 on page 424. Additionally, the following health-promotion activities are recommended:

- Eat a diet low in fat and cholesterol, including fruits, vegetables, and fiber; use sugar, salt, and sodium in moderation.
- Make regular exercise a part of life.
- Drink alcohol in moderation, if at all.
- Do not smoke.

The middle adult needs to know the dangers of substance abuse. Referrals to support groups and individual counseling may be necessary to strengthen a middle adult's coping mechanisms and promote acceptance of personal and family changes. Having successfully met developmental tasks, the healthy middle adult is ready to enjoy the rest of life. A sense of continuity and adaptability from the early 20s through the 50s is essential to meeting the developmental tasks of aging satisfactorily and to enjoying one's remaining years.

EXAMPLES OF NANDA-I NURSING DIAGNOSES

THE MIDDLE ADULT

Nursing Diagnoses	Possible Related Factor
Risk for Imbalanced Nutrition: More Than Body Requirements	High-calorie diet and sedentary lifestyle
Risk for Impaired Skin Integrity	Lifetime of sun exposure
Caregiver Role Strain	Long-term care of aging parents
Sedentary Lifestyle	Lack of resources (time, money, facilities)
Stress Overload	Chronic illness
Risk-Prone Health Behavior	Inadequate comprehension
Ineffective Relationship	Stressful life events

Table 19-1 GUIDELINES FOR HEALTH-RELATED SCREENINGS, EXAMINATIONS, AND IMMUNIZATIONS FOR THE AGING ADULT

HEALTH-RELATED AREA	RECOMMENDATIONS
Physical examination	• Every 3 years to age 40 • Every year from age 40 • The Affordable Care Act provides free annual wellness visits for people enrolled in Medicare.
Breast cancer (women)	• Breast self-examination each month • Breast clinical examination every 3 years to age 40, then every year • Mammogram every year beginning age 40
Cervical cancer (women)	• Pelvic examination with Papanicolaou (Pap) exam at least every 3 years • Women who have had a total hysterectomy (removal of the uterus and cervix) do not need cervical cancer screening, unless the surgery was for cervical precancer or cancer. • Women over age 65 to 70 with at least 3 normal Pap tests and no abnormal Pap tests in the last 10 years should consult with their health care provider about continuing cervical cancer screening.
Prostate (men, beginning age 50)	• Prostate-specific antigen (PSA) test every year (some advisory groups now do not recommend an annual PSA because results may be misleading; schedule should be discussed with physician) • Digital rectal examination (DRE) every year • Begin at age 45 if African American or a family history of prostate cancer. • Screening is individualized based on health care provider and the person's concerns.
Testicular cancer (men)	• Testicular self-examination every month
Colorectal cancer (men and women, beginning age 50)	• Fecal occult blood test every year • Digital rectal examination (DRE) every year • Flexible sigmoidoscopy every 3–5 years, or • Colonoscopy with follow-up every 3–5 years depending on size of polyps
Skin cancer (men and women)	• Self-examination every month • Clinical skin examination every year
Oral cancer (men and women)	• Every year as part of medical or dental checkups
Bone density	• Those at risk: postmenopausal women, maternal history of hip fracture, fracture after age 50, tall height at age 25
Vision	• Eye examination, with a test for glaucoma, every year
Immunizations	• Tetanus, diphtheria (Td) or Tdap: 1-dose booster every 10 years of either Td or Tdap; Tdap recommended for adults 65 and older if in contact with a child <12 months of age • Influenza: 1 dose every year • Pneumococcal polysaccharide vaccine (PPV): 1 dose every year up to age 64 for those with medical indications; 1 dose for those unvaccinated by age 65, or who received the first dose more than 5 years previously (before age 65) • Zoster vaccine, live (Zostavax): Recommended for adults 60 years and older to prevent herpes zoster (shingles) (CDC, 2012b).

THE OLDER ADULT

Society has arbitrarily labeled the **older adult** as a person older than 65 years of age. The older adult period is often further divided into the young-old (ages 60 to 74 years), the middle-old (ages 75 to 84 years), and the old-old (ages 85 years and older).

American society is aging—dramatically, rapidly, and largely well. With birthrates down and some baby boomers already reaching retirement age, we are on the threshold of the first-ever "mass geriatric society." In the years since 1975, life expectancy for men has increased from 67 years to 76.2 years and for women from just below 75 to 81 years (National Center for Health Statistics, 2013). Older women outnumber older men. In 2010, women age 65 and older accounted for 57% of this population, a number increasing to 67% by 85 years of age (Federal Interagency Forum on Aging Related Statistics, 2012). Between 1990 and 2010, the life expectancy at birth increased 6 years for the African American population compared to 2.8 years for the White population, thus narrowing the gap between the two groups (National Center for Health Statistics, 2013). By 2030, approximately 20% of the population will be 65 years or older. For the first time in history, by 2030, the population of Americans over 65 years old will be larger than the population of children 0 to 14 years of age. Medical advances, including control of infectious diseases, improvements in food handling and sanitation, and safer drinking water, along with an increased emphasis on health hazards such as tobacco use, are largely responsible for this population shift (Van Leuven, 2012).

A Unique Population

The older adult population is the most unique group in society today because its members have lived the longest and have participated in and adapted to complex societal changes. Within the lifespan of many older adults, society developed from a rural agricultural culture through industrialization to a service-oriented, high-technology culture. In the early 1900s, a 20-mile trip meant an all-day undertaking in a horse-drawn wagon; today, a person can fly across the continent in less time and with considerably less effort. Lighting has progressed from kerosene and gas lamps to electricity. Information that once took weeks or months to be received now is instantaneous. Most older adults have lived through the trauma of world wars. Many had parents with strong ethnic ties to another country, and many were immigrants themselves. Older adults have lived through the Great Depression of the 1930s and developed self-sufficiency.

Further adaptations become necessary with advancing age because of physical or cognitive limitations, retirement, loss of a spouse or family members, or changing income. Older adults face numerous role changes related to their age or health status. Lost roles must be replaced with new roles and activities that are acceptable and satisfying to the person.

RECALL Larry Jenkins, the 67-year-old complaining of his life going downhill since he retired. The nurse could incorporate knowledge of role changes to develop an appropriate plan of care for the patient that fosters adjustment to his role changes. ●

Older people are thus living in a world that requires them to change and to adapt. Senior years are a time to reach one's potential and to satisfy long-range goals that may have been delayed because of other responsibilities. It can also be a time for older adults to turn over to others certain tasks, such as career or community leadership. Due to recent economic challenges, some older adults have chosen to remain in the work force out of necessity while others enjoy the socialization and intellectual stimulation that continues with employment. Research has shown that most older adults do adjust and adapt to new roles, and most are satisfied with their lives and with what they have. Depending on the older adult's adaptability and supportive resources, older adulthood may be a time of happiness, peace, and understanding or of sorrow, conflict, and confusion.

Ageism and Common Stereotypes

Sometimes, older adults are a victim of ageism. **Ageism** is a form of prejudice, like racism, in which older adults are stereotyped by characteristics found in only a few members of their group. Fundamental to ageism is the view that older people are different and will remain different; therefore, they do not experience the same desires, needs, and concerns as other adults. Our industrial technological world places a high priority on productivity, and some may think that retired people have "outlived their usefulness."

THINK back to Larry Jenkins, the 67-year-old retiree. The nurse could incorporate knowledge of ageism as a basis for obtaining additional assessment data, examining possible factors contributing to the patient's feelings of boredom and uselessness. ●

As well, younger generations often have lost ties to the older generation because of increased mobility of the family; thus many young adults lack experiences with older relatives and their friends.

Older people may be incorrectly viewed as being rigid or narrow-minded, unable to learn, unreliable because of memory loss, too old to enjoy sexual pleasure, or child-like and dependent. Many people fear advancing age because of pervasive views that older people are poor, lonely, in frail health, and headed for institutionalization in a long-term care facility. These descriptors are not true for most older adults (Fig. 19-2 on page 426). Common myths are compared with the realities in Table 19-2 on page 426.

Most older adults are satisfied with their lives, finding retirement and old age more enjoyable than they had anticipated. Three-fourths live in their own homes, and one third

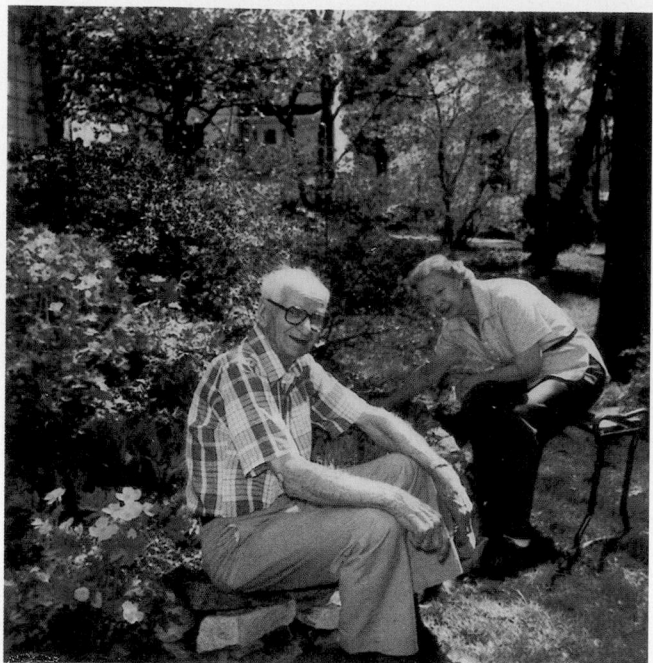

FIGURE 19-2. This couple, married 61 years, enjoys gardening together. They've found that they can continue most activities with only minor adjustments.

of these live alone. Most older adults maintain close ties with their families and have incomes above the poverty level (Eliopoulos, 2010).

Physiologic Development

In older adults, all organ systems undergo some degree of decline in overall functioning, and the body becomes less efficient. Normal physiologic changes in structure and func-

tion of the body with aging are outlined in Box 19-2. Body functions that require integrated activity of several organ systems are affected the most. For example, aging of the cardiac muscles causes fluid retention in both peripheral tissues and the lungs, causing swelling of the legs and making breathing more difficult. The most commonly encountered chronic disorders are hypertension, arthritis, heart disease, cancer, diabetes, and sinusitis (Gray-Vickrey, 2010).

 RECALL Ethel Peabody, the 88-year-old woman with dementia and cardiac problems. Knowledge of physiologic changes associated with aging could help with developing an appropriate plan of care for this patient after discharge. ●

Most older adults regard themselves as healthy and say they do not experience severe limitations in activities. Most are never institutionalized, nor do they suffer the effects of senility. Being healthy, however, does not necessarily mean without disease. The term *sarcopenia* refers to the loss of muscle mass that frequently occurs in older adults; *sarcopenic obesity* describes the muscle loss combined with an increase in body fat as people age (Benton, Whyte, & Dyal, 2012). This condition can result in loss of strength and function and a reduced quality of life that is significant for older adults. Resistance training and adequate dietary protein are management strategies that can prevent or reverse this process. More than four of five older adults suffer from at least one chronic illness. Like younger adults, they define their health in relation to how well they function. Functional health includes a person's ability to remain self-reliant, to "make do," and to maintain a sense of independence and control over oneself and one's environment. There is a trend in health care today toward fostering increasing independence

Table 19-2 MYTHS AND REALITIES ABOUT OLDER ADULTS

MYTH	REALITY
Old age begins at 65 years of age.	Defining 65 years of age as "old age" happened arbitrarily when 65 years of age was set for Social Security payments in the 1930s, based on the labor market and the economy of that time.
Most older adults live in long-term care facilities.	Only about 4% of older adults live in long-term care facilities. Most older adults own their own homes; 29% live alone, 55% live with spouses, and the rest live with family or friends.
Most older adults are sick.	Fully 76% of all older adults rate their health as good or excellent.
Old age means mental deterioration.	Although response time may be prolonged from a longer processing time, neither intelligence nor personality normally decreases because of aging.
Older adults are not interested in sex.	Although sexual activity may be less frequent, the ability to perform and enjoy sexual activity lasts well into the 90s in healthy older adults.
Older adults don't care how they look.	Older adults want to be attractive to others.
Most older adults are isolated and lonely.	Loneliness results from death of loved ones or other losses, just as it does for people of all ages. Many older adults are active in social and community activities.
Bladder problems are a problem of aging.	Incontinence is not a part of aging; it requires medical attention.
Older adults do not deserve aggressive treatment for serious illnesses.	Older adults deserve aggressive treatment if they want it.

BOX 19-2   NORMAL PHYSIOLOGIC CHANGES OF OLDER ADULTS

General Status
- Progressively decreasing efficiency of physiologic processes results in a fragile balance and hinders the body's ability to maintain homeostasis.
- Physical or emotional stressors cause the older adult to be more vulnerable because of decreased physiologic reserves.
- The older adult may continue to engage in all activities of middle age but intuitively adjusts to a modified pace and more frequent rest periods.

Integument
- Wrinkling and sagging of skin occur with decreased skin elasticity; dryness and scaling are common.
- Balding becomes common in men, and women also experience thinning of hair; hair loses pigmentation.
- Skin pigmentation and moles are common, although the skin may become pale because of loss of melanocytes.
- Nails typically thicken, becoming brittle and yellowed.
- The blood vessels in the dermis become more fragile, causing increased bruising and purpura (hemorrhaging into the skin).

Musculoskeletal
- Decreases in subcutaneous tissue and weight commonly are found in the old-old.
- Muscle mass and strength decrease.
- Bone demineralization occurs; bones become porous and brittle. Fracture is more common.
- Joints tend to stiffen and lose flexibility, and range of motion may decrease.
- Overall mobility commonly slows, and posture tends to stoop. Height may decrease 1 to 3 inches.

Neurologic
- The central nervous system responds more slowly to multiple stimuli. Hence, the cognitive and behavioral response of the older adult may be delayed.
- Rate of reflex response decreases.
- Temperature regulation and pain/pressure perception become less efficient.
- There may be a loss of sensation in the extremities.
- The older adult may also experience difficulty with balance, coordination, fine movements, and spatial orientation, resulting in an increased risk for falls.
- Sleep at night typically shortens, and the older adult may awaken more easily. Catnaps become common.

Special Senses
- Diminished visual acuity (presbyopia) occurs, with increased sensitivity to glare, decreased ability to adjust to darkness, decreased accommodation, decreased depth perception, and decreased color discrimination. Cataracts may further obscure vision. Difficulty reading small print might result. Daytime or night driving might be compromised.
- Diminished hearing acuity (presbycusis) occurs, particularly diminished pitch discrimination in the presence of environmental noises. Cerumen buildup is common. As a result of hearing problems, the older adult may withdraw from social events.
- The senses of taste and smell are decreased. Sweet and salty tastes diminish first. Sensitivity to odors might be reduced. Problems with nutrition may result.

Cardiopulmonary
- Blood vessels become less elastic and often rigid and tortuous. Venous return becomes less efficient. Fatty plaque deposits continue to occur in the linings of the blood vessels. Lower-extremity edema and cooling may occur, particularly with decreased mobility. Peripheral pulses are not always palpable. Orthostatic hypotension can occur.
- The body is less able to increase heart rate and cardiac output with activity.
- Pulmonary elasticity and ciliary action decrease, so that clearing of the lungs becomes less efficient. Respiratory rate may increase, accompanied by diminished depth.

Gastrointestinal
- Digestive juices continue to diminish, and nutrient absorption decreases.
- Malnutrition and anemia become more common.
- With reduced muscle tone and decreased peristalsis, constipation and indigestion are common complaints.
- Diminished saliva production leads to dry mouth problems.

Dentition
- Tooth decay and loss continue for most older adults.
- Eating habits may change, particularly if the older adult lacks teeth or has ill-fitting dentures.

Genitourinary
- Blood flow to the kidneys decreases with diminished cardiac output.
- The number of functioning nephron units decreases by 50%; waste products may be filtered and excreted more slowly.
- Fluids and electrolytes remain within normal ranges, but the balance is fragile.
- Bladder capacity decreases by 50%. Voiding becomes more frequent; two or three times a night is usual. A decrease in bladder and sphincter muscle control may result in stress incontinence or incomplete bladder emptying.
- About 75% of men over 65 years of age experience hypertrophy of the prostate gland; surgery may be required if urinary retention occurs.
- The older woman's genital tract experiences atrophy, decrease of secretions, and thinning.

---

and self-care in older adults. Those who live alone are at greatest risk for loss of independence and increased need for assisted living or long-term care.

 REMEMBER Ethel Peabody, the woman described in the Reflective Practice box. The nurse can apply knowledge about functional health to determine the patient's needs for safety and independence while, at the same time, fostering the patient's view of herself. ●

There is growing evidence that aging is not synonymous with loss of function and disability. At least 80% of older adults have at least one chronic disorder, and most have at least two; yet their ability to adapt determines whether they are ill or healthy (Eliopoulos, 2010). Most continue their activities from middle age and adapt intuitively to the gradual limitations of aging, although it may take longer to complete an activity or the activity may need to be modified. For example, an older adult with arthritis may need to use an electric can opener rather than a manual one, or a person with heart disease may need 3 hours to garden, resting several times, rather than the former 1 hour.

 Concept Mastery Alert

As people age, their ability to adapt, not the time it takes for them to adapt, is the key determinant for whether they will be ill or healthy.

The greatest threat to the health of older adults is loss of the physiologic reserve of the various organ systems. When illness occurs, increased physical and emotional stress places an older adult at risk for complex reactions. An older adult is more likely to develop complications and to recover more slowly (Fig. 19-3). For instance, an older patient with a hip fracture is at high risk for pneumonia and skin breakdown because of immobility, a decreased ability to expel pulmonary secretions, and thinner, more fragile skin.

Cognitive Development

The term *cognition* indicates cerebral functioning, including the ability to perceive and understand one's world. Cognition does not change appreciably with aging. In fact, intelligence increases into the 60s, and learning continues through life. It is normal for an older adult to take longer to respond and react, however, particularly in new or unfamiliar surroundings. Knowing this, the nurse should slow the pace of care and allow older patients extra time to ask questions or complete activities. Mild short-term (recent) memory loss is common but can be remedied by an older adult using notes, schedules, and calendars. Long-term memory usually remains intact. Dementia, Alzheimer disease, depression, and delirium might occur and cause cognitive impairment.

FIGURE 19-3. The hospitalized older adult requires nursing interventions to prevent complications. *(Photo by Kathy Sloane.)*

These conditions are discussed later in relation to the health of the older adult.

Psychosocial Development

Most theorists agree that a person's self-concept is relatively stable throughout adult life. An older adult who has a strong sense of self-identity and has successfully met challenges earlier in life will probably continue to do so. This person substitutes new roles for old roles and perhaps continues former roles in a new context. For example, business managers after retirement may continue to use their leadership talents in community or volunteer organizations. Older adults with a strong self-concept typically describe themselves as being healthier than others or "young for my years." Maslow, in his hierarchy of human needs, describes the level of self-actualization as the desire to become the most that one can be. A self-actualized person has realistic perceptions of self, is a problem solver, is usually spontaneous, needs time to focus on one's own individual potential, and views the world with a sense of appreciation. On the other hand, events that may accompany aging can threaten a person's self-concept. Depending on the person's outlook on life and past ability to cope, events such as retirement, loss of health or income, loss of ability to operate a motor vehicle, and isolation can be devastating. For example, a retired teacher whose sense of identity was closely tied to career may suddenly be in the position of having lost friends, income, and sense of accomplishment, and may consequently feel a great loss of control and self-identity.

The loss of the privilege of driving has serious repercussions for older adults. Aging results in slower reaction times and changes in vision such as increased sensitivity to the glare from approaching headlights as well as alterations in peripheral vision. Certain adjustments can prolong an older person's ability to drive safely. These include driving only during daylight hours and avoiding travel at stressful times such as morning and evening rush hours. Keeping a safe distance from the car ahead and a watchful eye on unsafe weather conditions are also helpful. When it becomes obvious for safety reasons that an older driver should stop driving altogether, it is best if family members address their concerns with their older adult in an honest, forthright manner. Losing driving privileges is disheartening and can cause older adults to feel anxious and lonely, which may be viewed as another negative consequence of aging. This lack of independence may also result in less opportunity for activities or interactions with friends and family. Alternative means of transportation are always a concern, and their availability should be explored. The state Department of Transportation is an additional resource and may request that an older driver be retested based on identification of a concern from a health care provider, a police or accident report, or written expressed concern from a family member. As the number of older drivers increases, so do the challenges to promote safe driving and find alternatives to driving (Talking with Older Drivers, 2011; Bartley & Shiflett, 2010).

Disengagement Theory

An early psychosocial theory, called the disengagement theory, maintained that older adults often withdraw from usual roles and become more introspective and self-focused. This withdrawal was theorized as intrinsic and inevitable, necessary for successful aging, and beneficial for both the person and for society.

Later studies showed that isolation is not desired or acceptable and that as societal interactions decrease, healthy older adults increase their close relationships with family and friends. According to the activity theory, successful aging includes the ability to maintain high levels of activity and functioning. An older adult may substitute activities but does not slow down or disengage from society. The identity-continuity theory assumes that healthy aging is related to the older adult's ability to continue similar patterns of behavior from young and middle adulthood.

Erikson's Theory

Erikson (1963) identified ego integrity versus despair and disgust as the last stage of human development, which begins at about 60 years of age. Older adults continue to look forward but now also look back and begin to reflect on their life. It is a time for realization of a "wholeness" perspective, with an inner search for meaning and order in the life cycle. Older adults search for emotional integration and acceptance of the past and present, as well as acceptance of physiologic decline without fear of death. Older adults often like to tell stories of past events. This phenomenon, called **life review** or **reminiscence**, has been identified worldwide. In a sense, this is a way for an older adult to relive and restructure life experiences and is part of achieving ego integrity (Klever, 2013; Fig. 19-4). Nurses can also use reminiscence as a therapy to facilitate adaptation to present circumstances.

 THINK back to Larry Jenkins, the 67-year-old male described at the beginning of the chapter. The nurse could use life review to foster the patient's ego integrity. ●

Ego integrity is facilitated when an older adult has successfully accomplished tasks earlier in life. Older adulthood can be a time for the person to look backward with pride and without regrets and forward with optimism and enthusiasm. A person who regrets the past and sees current problems as insurmountable, however, may despair. This person may view life as a series of unresolved problems and missed opportunities and feel worthless or hopeless. A despairing person may want to do things over but fears the lack of time before death.

The tasks of midlife continue or may resurface. Older adults still strive to guide the coming generations and to leave something behind (generativity versus stagnation). Their need for love and closeness continues (intimacy versus isolation), as does a strong sense of who one is in relation to family and community (identity versus role diffusion).

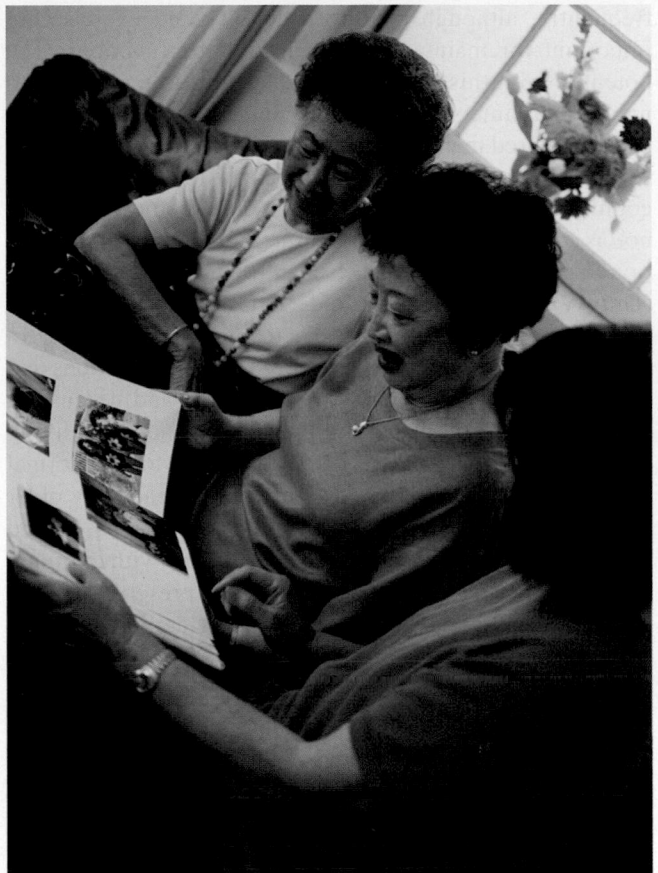

FIGURE 19-4. Reminiscing is a culturally universal phenomenon of aging. It is a way for the older adult to reassess life experiences and further develop a sense of accomplishment, fulfillment, and reward in life.

Because of physical and social changes associated with aging, older adults are repeatedly faced with the need to adapt and to again face already completed tasks.

Havighurst's Theory

According to Havighurst (1972), the major tasks of old age are primarily concerned with the maintenance of social contacts and relationships. Successful aging depends on a person's ability to be flexible and adapt to new age-related roles. The person must find new and meaningful roles in old age while being reasonably comfortable with the social customs of the times.

Adjusting to the Changes of Older Adulthood

Older adults use their years of experience as a guide to adjusting to the changes that come with increasing age. These changes, based on Havighurst's tasks for later life, involve many areas of life, as described in the following sections.

Physical Strength and Health

Most older adults gradually modify their lifestyle to accommodate for declining strength and health. They rest more frequently, although continued activity and exercise are important for maintaining all physiologic functions. The potential with this age group for sleep disorders accompanied by daytime sleepiness contributes to slower response time, impaired memory, and behavior that may be mistaken for some form of cognitive impairment. Confusion and cognitive impairment in an older adult should be viewed not as a normal consequence of aging but instead in relation to an acute problem such as infection or polypharmacy (Gray-Vickrey, 2010). An older adult is at high risk for accidents and falls and may need to curtail driving or use a cane or other aid to remain mobile. Diet modifications and prescribed medications may be necessary, and because of chronic illness, an older adult may need to adjust to living with some pain. Pain should not be assumed to be a normal consequence of aging, but it is often experienced by older adults and frequently is undertreated. Attitudes toward treating pain in this population may interfere with optimum pain relief. Older adults are frequently prescribed lower doses of opioid analgesics than younger adults, and poor clinical outcomes can result (Sullivan, 2011). Delirium, sleep disturbances, cognitive changes, and diminished functional abilities may result when pain is not managed adequately. Additional information about pain management for older adults can be found in Chapter 34. With severe illness, loss of independence can occur. The loss of health is difficult to adjust to because it affects every aspect of life.

Retirement and Reduced Income

Retirement brings a change in a person's concept of time. Many older adults must learn to occupy their leisure time in ways that maintain their self-esteem while being personally satisfying. Satisfaction with retirement is closely tied to income and the relationships one has outside of work. While many older adults have adequate retirement income, for others a lack of adequate income can affect their ability to meet their needs, such as for medical care and housing or social and creative interests.

The Health of One's Spouse or Partner

When one's spouse or partner becomes ill, numerous and difficult adjustments must be made. An older adult may face new roles for the first time, such as cooking meals or handling family finances. These role changes come at a time when stress is already high. Giving physical care can be an overwhelming task if the other spouse or partner is also frail or in poor health. Adaptations may be needed in living conditions and lifestyle, and one spouse may need to plan social and recreational events alone.

The need for love and belonging does not diminish with age and may become acute with the loss of one's spouse or partner through illness or institutionalization. Humans are sexual beings, and sexual behavior does not necessarily stop in old age. Sexuality is part of who we are, and older adults are no exception. Like younger adults, older adults need to express their intimacy physically by touching and

FIGURE 19-5. Stereotypical images of the older adult as narrow-minded, forgetful, sexless, and dependent are untrue of most older adults. This couple exhibits the vitality, sensuality, joy, and playfulness of a young couple.

sexual activity and emotionally by sharing joys, sorrows, ideas, and values (Fig. 19-5).

Relating to One's Age Group

With an aging population, social organizations for older adults are becoming more numerous. For example, most communities have senior citizens' centers that offer meals, social and informational programs, and other activities for a nominal fee. Other organizations offer opportunities for travel, cultural events, and political involvement. Affiliation with others of the same age allows older adults to share common interests and concerns and to find status among their peers. Some adults reside in retirement communities that provide a multitude of opportunities for social engagement. It should not be assumed, however, that older adults want to associate only with others their age (Fig. 19-6).

Social Roles

Social roles change with the developmental tasks and adjustments of older adulthood, but the need to feel valued, useful, and productive continues. Older adults may develop

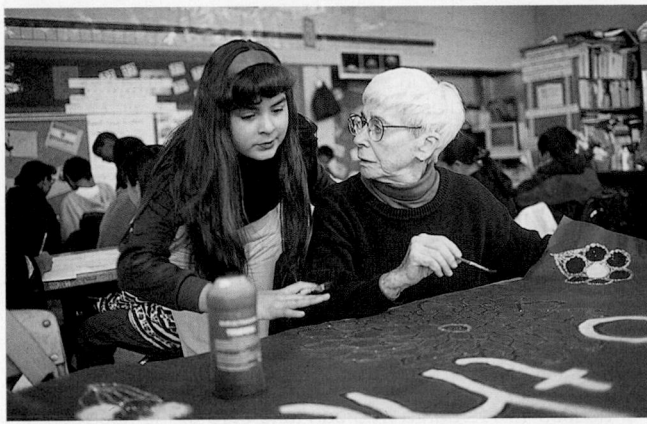

FIGURE 19-6. Social relationships and satisfying leisure activities remain important throughout life. This older adult volunteers in art class with 6th-grade Asian and Latina girls. *(Photo by Kathy Sloane.)*

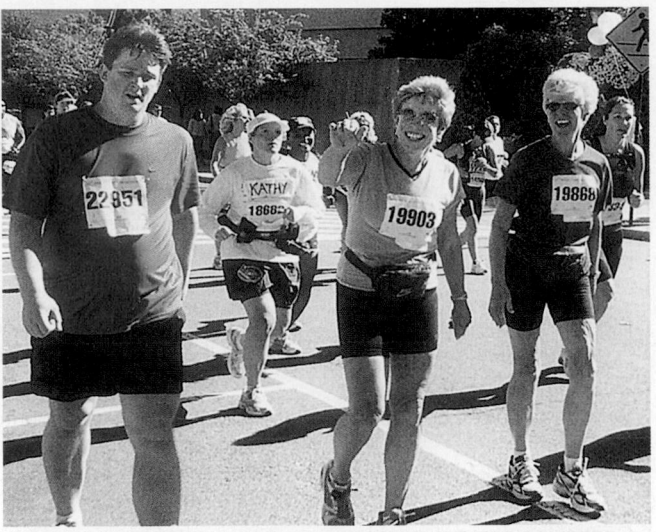

new hobbies or increase their involvement in community, church, or family affairs (Fig. 19-7). They may do volunteer work or even begin a new career. If an older adult cannot adjust and form new relationships, social isolation can become a problem. **Social isolation** is a sense of being alone and lonely as a result of having fewer meaningful relationships. It may occur because of declining health or income, transportation problems, or ageism. Whatever the cause, prolonged social isolation has been associated with declining health and higher mortality rates.

 Concept Mastery Alert

Social isolation is different from ineffective coping. Social isolation is the feeling of being alone; ineffective coping refers to difficulty in adapting or responding to the changes associated with the situation. Ineffective coping can lead to social isolation.

Living Arrangements

Various types of housing options for older adults are outlined in Table 19-3 on page 432. The ability to function safely and independently at home depends a great deal on one's functional health, transportation, income, and family. An older adult, for example, may need assistance with home repairs, house cleaning, or grocery shopping. Architectural barriers, such as steps, may need to be modified. Easy access to medical and recreational facilities and churches may become more important. Many older adults in poor health can continue living at home with some assistance from visiting nurses or with the aid of other services, such as home-delivered meals and senior transportation. Assisted-living housing is becoming more common, providing such requirements as meals, health care services, and housekeeping services.

Most older adults prefer to live in their own home and find it difficult to move. Over half of this population lives with a spouse or partner, but this number decreases with increasing age and the death of the significant other (Administration on Aging, 2011). Moving in with adult children

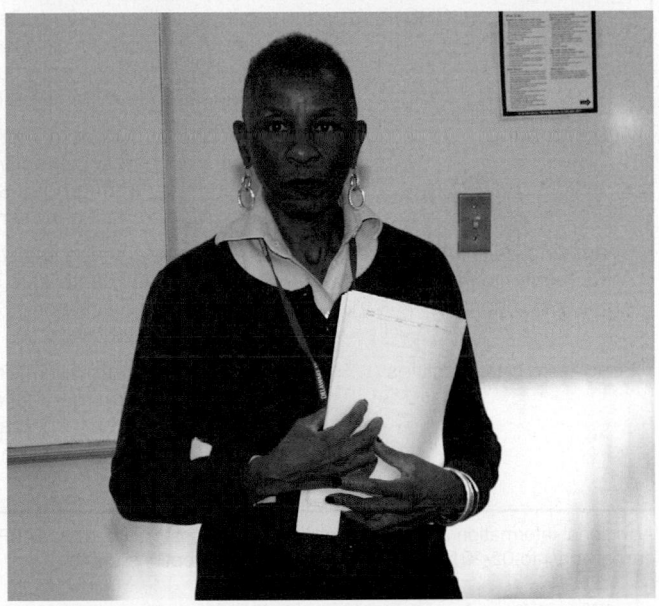

FIGURE 19-7. Older adults who exercise regularly improve their physical strength as well as overall stamina, mood, and mental health. Opportunities for involvement outside the home give an older adult a sense of personal control and engagement.

creates changes in roles and authority. In 2010, approximately 1.94 million grandparents over the age of 65 lived in a home with a grandchild (Administration on Aging, 2011). If the older adult is chronically ill or cognitively impaired, the family caregivers face the need for daily caregiving, lack of freedom, and emotional stress. When a person moves to a long-term care facility, the loss of one's home and possessions and the need to conform to the routines of institutional living can be traumatic for the person and family. Approximately 4.1% of older adults live in an institutional setting, but this number increases dramatically with more advanced age (Administration on Aging, 2011). Some people, however, choose to move for convenience, social relationships, or needed health care.

Additional options for older adults include quality patient-centered programs with a focus on providing long-term care

Table 19-3 HOUSING OPTIONS FOR OLDER ADULTS

Home modification	By making changes, older adults may be able to stay in their own homes. Examples of modifications are replacing doorknobs with handles, replacing faucet handles with levers, and installing grab bars in bathtubs.
Homesharing	Two or more people may share an apartment or house. Each person usually has a private bedroom and shares the other living spaces. These homes may be sponsored by faith-based groups or community agencies.
Accessory apartments	A separate apartment is constructed in part of an existing house, such as a basement or attic. This allows older adults to live independently and privately while not being alone.
Elderly cottage housing opportunities (ECHO)	ECHO homes are small portable cottages that are placed (most often) in the yard of an adult child's home. These units typically cost $28,000 or more, but do allow living independently but close to support.
Senior retirement communities	A grouping of rental apartments or houses for residents who can take care of themselves and are mobile. Meals may be available in a central dining room, and housekeeping services may be offered (at additional cost). Social and recreational activities are usually offered.
Continuing care retirement communities (CCRC)	This type of housing community offers several options and services, depending on the needs of the resident. Residents usually begin by living independently in apartments, and then move to an assisted-living facility on the same grounds. A skilled nursing center is also part of the community and available when needed. Sometimes called "aging-in-place" models, this type of housing tends to be expensive.
Assisted living	These facilities generally provide housing, group meals, personal care and support services, and social activities in a social setting. Some health care may be provided. Costs vary from around $29,000 to $66,000 annually depending on location. Some states pay for personal care services for those with limited incomes.
Board and care homes Adult family home Adult group homes	Smaller in scale than assisted-living facilities, these services provide a room, meals, and help with daily activities. They may be licensed or unlicensed. Costs average $33,000 per year for a private room; Supplemental Security Income (SSI) will help pay for those with very limited incomes.
Long-term care facilities	These facilities provide skilled nursing care and/or long-term care, including meals, personal care, and medical care. Bedrooms and bathrooms may be shared. Costs average $66,000 per year, but many are more expensive. Medicare provides only short-term coverage following a hospitalization. Medicaid provides coverage for low-income, low-asset people.

Additional information about these housing options is provided by AARP at http://www.aarp.org/relationships/caregiving/info-02-2012/caregiving-assisted-living-options-tool.html

to older adults who want to remain in the community. Several examples include:

- PACE, the Program of All-Inclusive Care for the Elderly, in which adults age 55 years or older who meet specific criteria can receive comprehensive interdisciplinary care. They also receive support to live in the community as long as possible. Approximately 80 PACE programs are active around the country (Gibbons, 2010).
- A growing senior population in one community formed a new association called Naturally Occurring Retirement Communities (NORCs). This collaboration necessitated the hiring of a geriatric care manager who helped the residents negotiate the health care system and enabled them to remain in their homes. In this setting, tasks are shared based on the abilities of their members (Guteri, 2012).
- REACH programs (Racial and Ethnic Approaches to Community Health) represent an effort by the CDC to establish community-based, culturally appropriate programs and eliminate health disparities among racial and ethnic groups. African Americans, American Indians, Hispanics/Latinos, Asian Americans, Alaska Natives, and

Pacific Islanders all benefit from these programs. Currently REACH funds 50 communities and six minority-serving national organizations (CDC, 2012d).

Retirement centers and senior citizens' housing have become common. For the family members of older adults who need health care, alternative methods of care have become available. Examples include respite care facilities, which allow the family a needed rest by temporarily housing and caring for an ailing older family member, and day-care centers, which provide a safe, stimulating environment during the day when family caregivers must work. Nurses should be knowledgeable about what health care and social services are available in the patient's community so that the patient and family can be referred.

The old-old have special significance for nursing care because they are more likely to need help with mobility and basic activities of daily living. They may need increasing assistance to maintain a safe and comfortable living environment. The older the person, the more likely that the individual needs family and community support to maintain functional health. Additional resources for community

Table 19-4 RESOURCES FOR OLDER ADULTS

ORGANIZATION	ACTIVITIES
U.S. Department of Health and Human Services (DHHS) http://www.hhs.gov	Government agency charged with protecting health through the delivery of human services
Administration on Aging (AoA) http://www.aoa.gov	Provides home- and community-based services to older adults through programs funded under the Older Americans Act.
Centers for Medicare and Medicaid Services (CMS) http://www.cms.gov	DHHS agency assigned to maintain health care security for its beneficiaries.
Eldercare Locator http://www.eldercare.gov/Eldercare.NET/Public/ Index.aspx	Connects older adults and families by zip code, city, state or county to eldercare resources in the community.
National Association for Area Agencies on Aging (n4a) http://www.n4a.org	Helps older people and those with disabilities to live with dignity and choices in their homes and communities for as long as possible.
Meals on Wheels Association of America (MOWAA) http://www.mowaa.org	Provides lunch and dinner to older adults and people with disabilities.
NIH Senior Health http://www.nihseniorhealth.gov	Includes health and wellness information for older adults.
Senior Housing Finder http://www.communityresourcefinder.org	The Alzheimer's Association Senior Housing Finder searches a current list of licensed assisted-living residences, long-term care facilities, and other types of senior housing.
Lotsa Helping Hands http://www.lotsahelpinghands.com	Provides communication resources to support family caregivers, including help from volunteers and community.

support services that help older adults live independently are located in Table 19-4.

 REMEMBER Ethel Peabody, the 88-year-old woman with beginning dementia who lives alone. The nurse could work with social services to investigate possible community support resources available for the patient so that she can safely maintain her independence as much as possible. ●

Family and Role Reversal

An older adult's spouse and other family members are natural support systems that help the person maintain functional health and independence and meet the developmental tasks of old age. Supportive assistance may include providing transportation, food, shelter, social interactions, and even complex medical and nursing treatments. Significant others, such as close friends and neighbors, may also take on tasks formerly assumed to be the responsibilities of the traditional family.

Not all families can assist an aged member satisfactorily because of geographic distance, low income, poor health, strained marital relationships, or infringement on career or lifestyle. Adult children may feel "sandwiched" between responsibilities for their own children and careers and the needs of older parents. It can be a guilt-ridden and emotionally draining time for all involved when an older adult's physical or emotional illness reverses roles (with the child now assuming the role of parent, while the parent becomes dependent as the "child") and strains family resources.

The nurse must view the whole family as the recipient of care and assess the family for capabilities and limitations for assisting the aged member. The nurse can help ease the strain by listening to the patient's and family's concerns and by validating the importance of family needs. The nurse assists the patient and family to find workable solutions and may refer the family to community support services.

Moral and Spiritual Development

Older adults, according to Kohlberg (1969), have completed their moral development. Most are at the conventional level, following society's rules in response to others' expectations. Spiritually, an older adult may remain at an earlier level, often at the individuative-reflective level. Many older adults, however, demonstrate conjunctive faith, integrating faith and truth to see the reality of their own beliefs, or universalizing faith, in which they trust a greater power and believe in the future.

Self-transcendence is a characteristic of later life that helps one expand beyond personal limits to reach out to others and the environment and a greater awareness of others' beliefs and values. Integration of the past and future in the present facilitates acceptance of where one is in life without regretting past mistakes or fearing the future (Reed, 1996). As a person ages, spirituality and transcendence are a resource and a source of strength when faced with inevitable change and loss.

Health of the Older Adult

As the number of older adults increases, nurses will spend more time providing care for this population. Older adults who require care are in all types of health care settings, including hospitals, long-term care facilities, emergency departments, outpatient surgeries, and homes. Nursing care for older adults should be based on two principles:

- Most older people are not impaired but are functional in the community, thereby benefiting from health-oriented interventions.
- Older people are more vulnerable to physical, emotional, and socioeconomic problems than people in other age groups and may require special attention to health promotion and maintenance.

This section provides a broad introduction to the health care needs of the older adult in terms of chronic illness, accidental injuries, and acute illness.

Chronic Illness

The probability of a person becoming ill increases with age. Chronic health problems or disability also may result from acute illnesses or accidents such as fractures, pneumonia, motor vehicle accidents, and falls. The leading causes of death in older adults are heart disease, cancer, and stroke (Federal Interagency Forum on Aging Related Statistics, 2012).

Although illness affects all dimensions of a person regardless of age, older adults have to contend with a variety of problems as they live with chronic illness. Aging is a normal process, and chronic illness is a pathologic process, but both often occur at the same time. The interrelated changes of aging and the needs imposed by chronic illness increase the risk for problems in all areas of life, including—but not limited to—self-care, lifestyle, economics, social factors, and living arrangements. Chronic health conditions can negatively affect an older adult's functioning and quality of life, but many of these can be prevented or modified with behavioral interventions.

 THINK back to Ethel Peabody, the 88-year-old woman with beginning dementia and cardiac disease. The nurse could use the knowledge of chronic illness as a basis for a teaching plan that addresses the patient's increased needs for safety. •

IMPLICATIONS FOR HEALTH CARE

Consider the following:

- Older adults use more health care than any other age group. The health care costs for those older adults with no chronic conditions averaged $5500 yearly but rise to $24,500 per year for older adults with five or more conditions (Federal Interagency Forum on Aging Related Statistics, 2012).
- Meeting the expenses of health care is often difficult for older adults and their families.
- Medication costs related to chronic illness typically continue for the rest of a person's life, with multiple medications being the rule rather than the exception. **Polypharmacy**, the use of many medications at the same time, can pose many hazards for older adults. Complicated

regimens need careful review to minimize risks and complications and maximize benefits (see Research in Nursing: Bridging the Gap to Evidence-Based Practice). Alternative therapies such as herbal remedies have the potential to interact with prescribed drugs and cause dangerous effects (Bilyeu, Gumm, Fitzgerald, Fox, & Selig, 2011; Lynn 2012). Nurses must be able to recognize adverse drug reactions in this population instead of mistaking them for age-related changes. Refer to Chapter 28 for additional information regarding altered drug response in older adults.

- Hospitalization costs continue to rise, and the price of high-quality, long-term care may well be beyond the patient's or family members' ability to pay.
- Special diets, special equipment, and medical supplies increase economic difficulties.
- Family members must learn how to cope with the needs of the ill person. Included are personal hygiene, medication administration, special diets, elimination, activities of daily living, and recognition of symptoms that necessitate medical attention.
- Family members must also adapt to psychological stressors such as changes in communications, changes in roles (e.g., an older mother becomes dependent), and changes in their own lifestyle as they become the caregivers.

DIVERSITY AND CHRONIC ILLNESS

As the U.S. population ages dramatically and becomes more diverse, it is important to consider how cultural differences can affect future patterns of disease, disability, and health care use. Minority populations continue to grow; by 2020, 24% of older adults will be minorities compared to 20% in 2010. Between 2010 and 2030, the White population 65 years and older is expected to increase by 59%, in contrast to a 160% increase in all older minorities; Hispanics are projected to have the most growth (202%; Administration on Aging, 2011).

The prevalence of certain diseases varies among racial and ethnic groups; research has not yet proven definitively what effect early health behaviors and practices have on the disease patterns of older adults in these various groups. Health disparities that exist between nonminority populations and racial and ethnic minorities are recognized and are particularly prevalent in the older populations. Poverty, the presence of chronic illnesses, and difficulty accessing the health care system make older adults much more vulnerable to a diminished quality of life caused by disease.

Profiles of various racial and ethnic groups indicate the following patterns of diseases:

- African American men are 30% more likely to die from heart disease than non-Hispanic White men. African American adults are diagnosed with diabetes and die from diabetes almost twice as often as White adults. African Americans have the highest mortality rate of any minority for most major cancers. Lung, prostate, and gastric cancer are also more prevalent in this group, who account for 43% of HIV/AIDS cases (Office of Minority Health, 2012a).

RESEARCH IN NURSING

BRIDGING THE GAP TO EVIDENCE-BASED PRACTICE

Medication Compliance and Health Literacy in Older Adults

By 2050, older adults will comprise an estimated 25% of the population. Medication regimens for this population are often complex due to the presence of multiple chronic diseases. The ability to read, understand, and translate information promotes adherence to multiple medication schedules. These medications may be prescribed for varying times of the day, and medication errors often occur. The patient's limited health literacy can result in confusion, lack of self-confidence for managing medications, and even serious consequences, including death.

Related Research

Martin, D., Kripalani, S., & Durapau, VJ. (2012). Improving medication management among at-risk older adults. *Journal of Gerontological Nursing, 38*(6), 24–34.

The goal of this study was to foster older adults' adherence to their medication regimen while addressing low health literacy. This quality improvement project involved 20 older adults (ages 59–89) enrolled at an inner-city adult daycare center in New Orleans. All participants were enrolled in Medicare and, at their medical appointments at this facility, expressed difficulty understanding their medication regimens. Approximately 40% of Medicare recipients read at less than a sixth-grade level, making it difficult for them to understand instructions for administration of multiple medications. In the initial face-to-face meeting, participants consented to join the study, baseline data were collected, and health literacy was assessed. The interventions in this study involved distribution of personalized, illustrated medication instructions. The educational aid, PictureRx™, uses simple language and very specific instructions about the timing and reason for each medication. The researchers conducted an educational session with each participant that terminated with a teach-back to confirm that all participants evaluated PictureRx™ as helpful and used it regularly. Participants had improved adherence to their medication schedule and improved confidence in their ability to manage their prescriptions. The Joint Commission recommends using both illustrated aids and the teach-back method to communicate health instructions.

Relevance to Nursing Practice

Given the growth of the older adult population, nurses must design interventions that improve medication compliance in all settings. Consideration of health literacy level is essential in designing health teaching and education to promote understanding and improve adherence and self-confidence. This particular study demonstrated the efficacy of using pictorial aids and the teach-back approach to confirm that medication schedules and directions are understood.

For additional research, visit thePoint.

- The leading causes of illness and death for Hispanic Americans are heart disease, cancer, unintentional injuries (accidents), stroke, and diabetes. Hispanics have higher rates of obesity than non-Hispanic Whites. Asthma, chronic obstructive pulmonary disease (COPD), HIV/AIDS, suicide, and liver disease also are more common in this population (Office of Minority Health, 2012d).
- Asian Americans are most at risk for cancer, heart disease, stroke, accidents, and diabetes. Tuberculosis is 11 times more common in this group than the White population. Asian American women have the highest life expectancy (85.8 years) of any ethnic group in the United States (Office of Minority Health, 2012c).
- American Indian/Alaska Natives have an infant mortality rate 60% higher than that of Whites. Leading causes of death and illness are heart disease, cancer, accidents, diabetes, and stroke. They also have a higher risk for mental health issues including suicide, as well as obesity, substance abuse, and SIDS. (Office of Minority Health, 2012b).

Refer to Chapter 5 for additional discussion of cultural variations and influences on health care.

Accidental Injuries

The older adult is at increased risk for accidental injury because of changes in vision and hearing, loss of mass and strength of muscles, slower reflexes and reaction time, and decreased sensory ability. Many older adults limit their activities because of fear of a fall that might result in serious health consequences. Falls are the most common cause of injuries and hospital admission in older adults. Approximately 30% to 40% of adults over 65 years of age living in the community fall at least once per year (Edelman & Ficorelli, 2012). Falls may result in a traumatic brain injury (TBI), which accounts for 46% of fatal falls among older adults (CDC, 2012a). Approximately 95% of hip fractures are caused by a fall (CDC, 2012a). Recommendations for prevention of falls in older adults now include an exercise component and vitamin D supplementation. The U.S. Preventive Services Task Force recently reviewed the evidence and identified those interventions as effective in helping prevent falls in community-dwelling older adults (Scudder, 2012). Chapters 26 and 32 have expanded information regarding the risk for falls and developmental considerations related to ambulation. The CDC (2012c) has compiled a collection of fall prevention guides, available at: http://www.cdc.gov/HomeandRecreationalSafety/Falls/pubs.html.   See Examples of Nursing Interventions and Nursing Outcomes Classifications (NIC/NOC): Fall Prevention on page 436.

In addition, the combined effects of chronic illness and medications may make an older adult more prone to accidents. Older adults with reduced income may live in

EXAMPLES OF NURSING INTERVENTIONS AND NURSING OUTCOMES CLASSIFICATIONS (NIC/NOC)

FALL PREVENTION

Nursing Interventions	Nursing Outcomes
• Identify behaviors and factors that affect risk of falls. • Monitor gait, balance, and fatigue level with ambulation. • Assist unsteady individual with ambulation. • Post signs to alert staff that patient is at high risk for falls. • Instruct patient to wear prescription glasses, as appropriate, when out of bed. • Avoid clutter on floor surfaces. • Educate family members about risk factors that contribute to falls and how they can decrease these risks.	• Balance • Fall Prevention Behavior • Knowledge: Fall Prevention • Mobility • Risk Control • Safe Home Environment • Sensory Function: Vision • Ambulation

Bulechek, G., Butcher, H., & Dochterman, J., & Wagner, C. (2013). *Nursing interventions classification (NIC)* (6th ed., p. 188). St. Louis: Elsevier/Mosby. *A full listing of nursing activities for each nursing intervention can be found in this book.*

Moorhead, S., Johnson, M., Maas, M., & Swanson, E. (2013). *Nursing outcomes classification (NOC)* (5th ed., p. 654). St. Louis: C.V. Mosby. *A full listing of nursing outcomes for each nursing diagnosis can be found in this book.*

inadequate housing in neighborhoods with heavy traffic or high crime rates. They may be isolated from family members, and many live alone. Combined with the normal changes of aging and the effects of any illness, older people not only are at increased risk but also have a more difficult time regaining health after an injury. Refer to Chapter 26 for additional information related to risk for accidental injuries in older adults.

Dementia, Depression, and Delirium

When a serious mental impairment occurs, the effect on the patient and family can be devastating. **Dementia** refers to various organic disorders that progressively affect cognitive functioning. Dementia is chronic and usually develops gradually. Of the dementias that affect older adults, **Alzheimer disease** (AD) is the most common degenerative neurologic illness and the most common cause of cognitive impairment (CDC, 2011). It is irreversible and progresses from deficits in memory and thinking skills to an eventual inability to perform even the simplest of tasks (National Institute on Aging, 2012). The first indications of AD usually occur after 60 years of age, and nearly half of 85-year-old adults have the disease (CDC, 2011). Scientists estimate that at least 5 million people have Alzheimer disease (National Institute on Aging, 2012).

Alzheimer disease affects brain cells and is characterized by patchy areas of the brain that degenerate. It is a progressively serious and ultimately fatal disorder. At first, forgetfulness and impaired judgment may be evident. Over a period of several years, the person becomes progressively more confused, forgetting family and becoming disoriented in familiar surroundings. A common problem in patients with dementia is **sundowning syndrome**, in which an older adult habitually becomes confused, restless, and agitated after dark. When the ability to perform simple activities of daily living is lost, the person requires constant supervision

and care, often in a long-term care facility. There is no effective medical treatment for AD at this time.

People with dementia are hospitalized more frequently than other older adults. The precipitating factor may be a medical–surgical problem or behavioral or psychiatric symptoms that occur with dementia. Often, a medical or nursing intervention can trigger a sequence of adverse events in a frail older adult. This downward spiral and decline is referred to as **cascade iatrogenesis**. An episode of confusion and wandering at night may lead to a fall that results in a hip fracture. During the resulting hospitalization, the insertion of an indwelling catheter can precipitate a urinary tract infection that requires use of an antibiotic and possibly the development of antibiotic-resistant organisms.

Recognizing patients at risk for cascade iatrogenesis may help avoid its occurrence. Communication with family members and a systematic approach to assessment is required. The Fulmer SPICES tool has proved effective in identifying common problems experienced in older adults that can lead to negative outcomes. The acronym SPICES facilitates assessment and information gathering about the following:

- **S** – Sleep disorders
- **P** – Problems with eating or feeding
- **I** – Incontinence
- **C** – Confusion
- **E** – Evidence of falls
- **S** – Skin breakdown (Fulmer & Wallace, 2012)

This instrument can be used in all settings and alerts nurses to quickly identify interventions to individualize an older patient's care.

Comprehensive and empathetic nursing care is important. Both the patient and family caregivers need emotional support and teaching, and may benefit from community resources that can ease the family's burden.

Table 19-5 ONLINE TOOLS FOR ASSESSMENT OF DELIRIUM AND DEMENTIA

ASSESSMENT TOOL	DESCRIPTION
CAM (Confusion Assessment Method) http://www.consultgerirn.org/uploads/File/trythis/ try_this_13.pdf	Identifies delirium quickly. Long and short version are available.
NEECHAM Confusion Scale http://www.unc.edu/courses/2005fall/nurs/213/001/ neuropsychiatric/neecham.html	Consists of nine items and is used to detect early stages of delirium. Does not differentiate between dementia and delirium.
Mini-Cog http://www.bami.us/Neuro/MiniCog.html	Two-part test to determine if dementia or cognitive impairment is present (even in early stages). Takes 3–5 minutes to administer.

Sometimes delirium and depression in an older adult are mistaken for true dementia. **Delirium**, a temporary state of confusion, is an acute illness that can last from hours to weeks and resolves with treatment. Drug interactions, circulatory or metabolic problems, nutritional deficiencies, or a worsening illness are likely the real cause. An older adult may also become confused when too many changes or losses occur at one time or when moved to a different environment. As many as 87% of critically ill older patients in an intensive care unit (ICU) setting experience an episode of delirium during a hospitalization (Brooks, 2012). Incidences of postoperative delirium are more likely to occur with extended ICU stays and increased use of ventilators, increasing the risk of death (American Nurse, 2012). Treatment of delirium may include stopping unnecessary medications, as well as interventions to resolve infection and metabolic alterations. Medications that reduce agitation may be prescribed in certain circumstances. The benzodiazepines are usually avoided because they may increase confusion and cause oversedation. Delirium may be managed by incorporating a bundle of evidence-based strategies into routine care. The acronym ABCDE is used for these interventions and assessments that focus on *A*wakening and *B*reathing coordination, choice of *C*areful sedation, monitoring *D*elirium, and *E*arly progressive mobility (American Nurse, 2012).

The nurse can help other members of the health team determine the cause of a patient's confusion and help reorient the patient. The nurse can use **reality orientation**, which involves interventions to redirect the patient's attention to what is real in the environment. See Table 19-5 for online resources for assessing for dementia and delirium. When assessing behavioral changes, remember that an older adult with dementia may also develop delirium or depression.

Extreme or prolonged sadness in an older adult may be a warning sign of depression. Death of a spouse or friends and changes in living environment and financial resources can precipitate feelings of depression. There is usually a distinct change of behavior accompanied by other specific signs and symptoms of depression, such as sleep disturbances, weight loss, difficulty with concentration, and suicidal thoughts or preoccupation with death (Naegle, 2011; Cahoon, 2012). Depression usually does not resolve without treatment and is frequently underdiagnosed. About 14% of people over

the age of 65 experience significant periods of depression (Dang, 2010). The Geriatric Depression Scale (short form), a 15-question screening tool, can be used effectively in older adults in any setting. When combined with a mental health assessment by a professional, it can facilitate a diagnosis of depression (Naegle, 2011). The Geriatric Depression Scale: Short Form is available at http://www.healthcare.uiowa.edu/igec/tools/depression/GDS.pdf.

Treatment of depression usually involves psychotherapy or counseling along with antidepressant medication. In an older adult, hopelessness rather than sadness is more often associated with suicidal intent. Alcohol or prescription drug abuse is most often associated with suicides in this age group (Naegle, 2011).

Elder Maltreatment

The increase in the number of older adults coupled with increasing lifespan has resulted in greater awareness about the problem of elder maltreatment, including abuse and neglect. Some estimate that as many as two million people older than 65 years of age suffer from abuse, neglect, or exploitation that is inflicted by family members in 90% of cases (Stark, 2012). It is difficult to determine an accurate number of elder maltreatment incidents because 84% of elder abuse cases are never reported (Stark, 2012). Elder abuse most commonly occurs in women over 80 years of age. Physical abuse, sexual abuse, emotional or psychological abuse, neglect, abandonment, and financial or material exploitation are all types of elder maltreatment (National Center on Elder Abuse, 2011).

Neglect accounts for more than half of all elder maltreatment reports made to adult protective service agencies. It can be active or passive and occurs when a caregiver fails to adequately meet the physical, social, or emotional needs of an older adult, resulting in harm to that person. Poor hygiene, inadequate nutrition, untreated injuries, and lack of assistance with care needs are indicators of neglect. Physical abuse causes pain, impairment, or deliberate physical injury to an older adult. Hitting, assault of any kind, slapping, and restraining are all examples of forms of physical abuse. Older adults who have been physically abused present with injuries that are incompatible with the older adult or caregiver's version of how the injury occurred. Evidence of

Table 19-6 ELDER ABUSE RESOURCES

ORGANIZATION	ACTIVITIES
National Center on Elder Abuse http://www.ncea.aoa.gov Phone: 1-800-677-1116	This site is a gateway to resources on elder abuse, neglect, and exploitation.
U.S. Administration on Aging, Eldercare Locator http:www.aoa.gov/naic/elderloc. html Phone: 1-800-677-1116	Connects older adults and caregivers with sources of information on senior services.
Law Enforcement Agencies Dial 911	For use when an older adult is in immediate, life-threatening danger or when reporting suspected abuse is mandatory.

previously untreated injuries or suspicious cuts and bruises should alert health care providers to the possibility of physical abuse. Sexual abuse involves nonconsensual sexual contact of any kind with an elderly person (Stark, 2012). Emotional abuse occurs when threats, intimidation, or isolation result in anguish for the elder person, while financial abuse involves exploitation or misuse of another's property.

Identification of elder abuse requires an alert health care provider. Indications of abuse are often misinterpreted as normal signs of aging. Careful observation of the relationship between the older adult and the caregiver may be the first evidence that the older adult is a victim of abuse. Pay attention to interactions involving voice tone, caring behaviors, and personal touch. If you suspect abuse, attempt to speak to the older adult in a private setting away from the caregiver. A victim may deny abuse or choose not to report it because of shame, fear of abandonment, worry about retaliation, or dementia. All assessment data should be objectively documented, including direct quotes from both parties. The Elder Assessment Instrument (EAI) is appropriate for all clinical settings and allows practicing nurses to screen for maltreatment in suspected cases (Fulmer, 2012). It requires an interview and physical assessment for data collection and is available at http://consultgerirn.org/uploads/File/trythis/try_this_15.pdf. Most states require that health care professionals report any suspected cases of elder abuse to designated official agencies. Table 19-6 lists various organizations that provide additional information and support about elder abuse.

Older Adults and the Health Care System

Our knowledge of aging has increased dramatically in the past 40 years. **Gerontology** is the scientific and behavioral study of all aspects of aging and its consequences. Normal changes that occur with aging result from complex interactions among genetics, biologic systems, and physical and social environments. Disease complicates a person's ability to adapt and maintain **functional health** (the ability to carry out usual and desired daily activities). Mental or physical decline in older adults often may not be directly related to the aging process but may result from the absence of supportive care and services that could prevent disease and help maintain the older adult's ability to function.

The increasing aging population has greatly strained a health care system that has traditionally focused on cures and acute disease processes. For an older patient with chronic disorders, the focus of care should include the patient's and family's goals and promote functional health and independent living to the greatest extent possible. **Gerontologic nursing** combines the basic knowledge and skills of nursing with a specialized knowledge of aging in both illness and health. The terms *geriatrics* and *gerontology* are sometimes used interchangeably. *Geriatrics* is a branch of medicine that focuses on the study of health and disease later in life, while *gerontology* represents the scientific study of the effects of aging and age-related diseases on humans. As of 2011, only 1% of RNs were certified in gerontology, and only one third of BSN programs included a geriatrics course in their curriculum (Cutugno, 2011). Given the increasing numbers of older adults, it is imperative for nurses to address the challenges of an aging population, be competent in geriatric care, and be prepared to make a difference in outcomes for this vulnerable population.

Role of the Nurse in Promoting Health and Preventing Illness

The nurse should teach the patient and family general health-promotion activities. This is important because older people often believe themselves "too old" to worry about nutrition, exercise, health screenings, and immunizations. In addition to the recommended screenings, examinations, and immunizations outlined in Table 19-1 on page 424, the following should be emphasized:

- Eat a diet that includes all food groups; is low in fat, saturated fat, and cholesterol; balances calories with physical activity; has recommended amounts of fruits, vegetables, and grains; and uses sugar and salt in moderation.
- Make exercise a part of daily activities. Multiple studies have demonstrated that regular aerobic exercise can reduce the risk for dementia and that resistance training may improve cognition (Brauser, 2012).
- Discuss with your primary physician whether to include a vitamin D supplement as part of your daily routine. Vitamin D is considered moderately beneficial for helping prevent hip fractures and other broken bones in older adults (CDC, 2012a; Lehne, 2013).
- Drink alcohol in moderation.
- Do not smoke.

An older adult who requires surgery or medical treatment for chronic or acute illness has special, age-related needs regardless of the setting for care. Nursing care to meet age-related needs in any setting is outlined in Table 19-7.

Table 19-7   PROMOTING HEALTH IN OLDER ADULTS

AREA OF CONCERN	NURSING ACTIONS
Physiologic function	• Maintain physiologic reserves. Maintain ongoing assessments for early detection of problems. • Review perceptions of current health status, health problems, and prescribed or over-the-counter medications. • Include nursing care that maintains physical status, such as skin care and planned rest and activity.
Cognitive function	• Slow pace of activity and wait for responses. • Be sure eyeglasses and hearing aids are used; ensure that lenses are clean and batteries are strong.
Psychosocial needs	• Be aware that illness, hospitalization, or changes in living arrangements are major stressors. • Assess and support sources of strength, including cultural and spiritual values and rituals. • Encourage use of support systems: family, friends, community resources, and pets. • Set mutual goals and encourage the patient's role in making decisions about care. • Encourage life review and reminiscence. • Encourage self-care. • Consider the patient's background, interests, capabilities, values, culture, and lifestyle when planning care.
Nutrition	• Assess for lost or damaged teeth; ensure that dentures fit properly. Provide foods appropriate to the patient's ability to chew. • Assess height, weight, eating patterns, and food choices. If weight is being lost, assess income, storage, and transportation. • Assess swallowing ability. • Consider using supplements.
Sleep and rest	• Discourage excessive napping. • Assess normal bedtime, time for rising, bedtime rituals, effects of pain, medications, anxiety, and depression.
Elimination	• Assess frequency of bladder elimination as well as problems with incontinence. • Assess normal times for bowel movements, changes in activity, privacy, and medications. • Ensure that the floor is not cluttered, the toilet is easily accessible, lighting is adequate, and privacy is provided. • Suggest having safety bars installed in the bathroom. • Review diet for necessary fluid and fiber content.
Activity and exercise	• Assess ability to walk; ensure that assistive devices (such as a walker or cane) are available. • Consider effects of illness, surgery, medications, and changes in diet and fluid intake on strength and motor function. • Ensure an uncluttered environment with good lighting; suggest using a night light and removing throw rugs. • Slow the pace of care, allowing extra time to carry out activities.
Sexuality	• Assist as necessary with hygiene, hair care, oral care, clean clothing and bedding, makeup, and shaving. • Maintain a clean, odor-free environment. • Demonstrate genuine caring: ask preferred name, listen carefully, and respect belongings. • Discuss safer sex if appropriate. • Discuss water-soluble lubricants with women; refer men for evaluation if erectile dysfunction is a concern.
Meeting developmental tasks	• Promote continued development and maintenance of functional health by identifying unmet tasks, feelings of isolation, and physical or sensory limitations. • Assist in finding creative solutions to developmental tasks. • Collaborate with other health care providers to provide information and referral to community resources for the patient and family.

EXAMPLES OF NANDA-I NURSING DIAGNOSES

THE OLDER ADULT

Nursing Diagnoses	Possible Related Factor
Disturbed Personal Identity	Social role change and depression
Risk for Injury	Unstable gait and decreased vision from cataracts
Risk for Loneliness	Death of spouse
Ineffective Coping	Diagnosis of chronic illness
Impaired Physical Mobility	Severe arthritic changes in legs
Impaired Memory	Cognitive impairment from onset of Alzheimer disease
Powerlessness	Institutional environment
Risk for Acute Confusion	Dementia

Although nursing care adapted to the needs of older patients is described throughout this text, general principles for care are included here. Nurses must recognize physiologic and psychosocial interrelationships and view older patients holistically. See Examples of NANDA-I Nursing Diagnoses: The Older Adult.

Illness can severely disrupt an older adult's ability to function independently. The ill patient is under increased physical and emotional stress, which increases the risk for complications because of the lack of physiologic reserves. When a patient is hospitalized or institutionalized, family and community interactions are severely inhibited. The acute care environment itself adds new stressors such as diagnostic tests, treatments, and surgery. In the face of new and unfamiliar routines and sensory stimulation, prior coping skills may not work, and an older patient may feel less able to understand and control the new environment. An older patient is more likely than a younger patient to suffer multisystem dysfunctions, iatrogenic complications (caused by medications or treatments), accidents such as falls, and increasing dependence and confusion. Hospitalization of an older patient can also substantially accelerate cognitive decline.

The focus of nursing care is to assist older patients to function as independently as possible and to support their individual strengths. The nurse collaborates with the family and other disciplines to prevent complications of illness, to secure a safe and comfortable environment, and to promote the patient's return to health.

CARING FOR AN AGING POPULATION

Medical advances have enabled elderly and frail patients with serious and chronic illnesses and disabilities to survive much longer than they could in the past. American society faces the dilemma of how to care for this population. Already, millions of American families are struggling nobly to provide steady and demanding long-term care for their incapacitated loved ones, often with little respite or communal support and usually for many years. It seems unlikely that increasing paid caregiving will be able to alleviate the growing strains on family caregivers. The pool of workers available for paid home health care is shrinking. Factors reducing the number of home health aides and nurses include the strenuousness of the work involved, inadequate financial compensation, difficult relationships with patients, language barriers, an aging nursing workforce, and the lack of health insurance and other benefits. Caring for older adults is complicated but rewarding, and challenges nurses to remember that the patient and family are an integral part of the team, which together must strive to find strategies to promote health and diminish or postpone frailty in this older population.

DEVELOPING CLINICAL REASONING

1. Complete the following sentences, then analyze the reasons for your answers:
   - When my parents can no longer care for themselves, I will _____.
   - If my parents were living in a long-term care facility, I would want the nurses to _____.
   - When I am old, I want my family to _____.

2. Consider your own family. Can you identify developmental tasks for family members who are middle adults and older adults? What factors in your family facilitate or impede meeting these tasks?

PRACTICING FOR NCLEX

1. A nurse caring for adults in a physician's office notes that some patients age more rapidly that other patients of the same age. The nurse researches aging theories that attempt to

describe how and why aging occurs. Which statements apply to the immunity theory of aging? Select all that apply.
a. Chemical reactions in the body produce damage to the DNA.
b. Free radicals have adverse effects on adjacent molecules.
c. Decrease in size and function of the thymus causes infections.
d. There is much interest in the role of vitamin supplementation.
e. Lifespan depends on a great extent to genetic factors.
f. Organisms wear out from increased metabolic functioning.

2. A nurse caring for older adults in a long-term care facility knows that several physical changes occur in the aging adult. Which characteristics best describe these changes? Select all that apply.
a. Fatty tissue is redistributed.
b. The skin is drier and wrinkles appear.
c. Cardiac output increases.
d. Muscle mass increases.
e. Hormone production increases.
f. Visual and hearing acuity diminishes.

3. Based on Erikson's theory, middle adults who do not achieve their developmental tasks may be considered to be in stagnation. Which statement is one example of this finding?
a. "I am helping my parents move into an assisted-living facility."
b. "I spend all of my time going to the doctor to be sure I am not sick."
c. "I have enough money to help my son and his wife when they need it."
d. "I earned this gray hair and I like it!"

4. Which of the following nursing diagnoses would be appropriate for many middle adults?
a. Risk for Imbalanced Nutrition: Less Than Body Requirements
b. Delayed Growth and Development
c. Self-Care Deficit
d. Caregiver Role Strain

5. An experienced nurse tells a younger nurse who is working in a retirement home that older adults are different and do not have the same desires, needs, and concerns as other age groups. The nurse also comments that most older adults have "outlived their usefulness." What is the term for this type of prejudice?
a. Harassment
b. Whistle blowing
c. Racism
d. Ageism

6. A nurse who is caring for older adults in a senior daycare center documents findings as related to which normal aging process? Select all that apply.
a. A patient's increased skin elasticity causes wrinkles on the face and arms.
b. Exposure to sun over the years causes a patient's skin to be pigmented.
c. A patient's toenails have become thinner with a bluish tint to the nail beds.
d. A patient experiences a hip fracture due to porous and brittle bones.
e. Fragile blood vessels in the dermis allow for more easy bruising of a patient's forearm.
f. Increased bladder capacity causes decreased voiding in an older patient.

7. A nursing instructor teaching classes in gerontology to nursing students discusses myths related to the aging of adults. Which statement is a myth about older adults?
a. Most older adults live in their own homes.
b. Healthy older adults enjoy sexual activity.
c. Old age means mental deterioration.
d. Older adults want to be attractive to others.

8. What is the leading cause of cognitive impairment in old age?
a. Stroke
b. Malnutrition
c. Alzheimer disease
d. Loss of cardiac reserve

9. A nurse is caring for an 80-year-old female patient who is living in a long-term care facility. To help this patient adapt to her present circumstances, the nurse is using reminiscence as therapy. Which question would encourage reminiscence?
a. "Tell me about how you celebrated Christmas when you were young."
b. "Tell me how you plan to spend your time this weekend."
c. "Did you enjoy the choral group that performed here yesterday?
d. "Why don't you want to talk about your feelings?"

10. Following a fall that left an elderly male patient temporarily bedridden, the nurse is using the SPICES assessment tool to evaluate him for cascade iatrogenesis. Which are correct aspects of this tool? Select all that apply.
a. S – Senility
b. P – Problems with feeding
c. I – Irritableness
d. C – Confusion
e. E – Edema of the legs
f. S – Skin breakdown

ANSWERS WITH RATIONALES

1. *c, d.* The immunity theory of aging focuses on the functions of the immune system and states that the immune response declines steadily after younger adulthood as the thymus loses size and function, causing more infections. There is much interest in vitamin supplements (such as vitamin E) to improve immune function. In the cross-linkage theory, cross-linkage is a chemical reaction that produces damage to the DNA and cell death. The free radical theory states that free radicals, formed during cellular metabolism, are molecules with separated high-energy electrons, which can have adverse effects on adjacent molecules. The genetic theory of aging holds that lifespan depends to a great extent on genetic factors. According to the wear-and-tear theory, organisms wear out from increased metabolic functioning, and cells become exhausted from continual energy depletion from adapting to stressors (Eliopoulos, 2010).

2. *a, b, f.* Physical changes occurring with aging include these: fatty tissue is redistributed, the skin is drier and wrinkles appear, and visual and hearing acuity diminishes. Cardiac output decreases, muscle mass decreases, and hormone production decreases, causing menopause or andropause.

3. *b.* Middle adults who do not reach generativity tend to become overly concerned about their own physical and emotional health needs.

4. *d.* Many middle adults help care for aging parents and have concerns about their own health and ability to continue to care for an older family member. Caregivers often face 24-hour care responsibilities for extended periods of time, which creates physical and emotional problems for the caregiver.

5. *d.* Ageism is a form of prejudice in which older adults are stereotyped by characteristics found in only a few members of their age group. Harassment occurs when a dominant person takes advantage of or overpowers a less dominant person (may involve sexual harassment or power struggles). Whistle blowing involves reporting illegal or unethical behavior in the workplace. Racism is prejudice against other races and ethnic groups.

6. *b, d, e.* Exposure to sun over the years can cause a patient's skin to be pigmented. Bone demineralization occurs with aging, causing bones to become porous and brittle, making fractures more common. The blood vessels in the dermis become more fragile, causing an increase in bruising and purpura. Wrinkling and sagging of skin occur with decreased skin elasticity. A patient's toenails may become thicker, with a yellowish tint to the nail beds. Bladder capacity decreases by 50%, making voiding more frequent; two or three times a night is usual.

7. *c.* Although response time may be longer, intelligence does not normally decrease because of aging. Most older adults own their own homes, and although sexual activity may be less frequent, the ability to perform and enjoy sexual activity lasts well into the 90s in healthy older adults. Older adults want to be attractive to others.

8. *c.* Alzheimer disease is the most common degenerative neurologic illness and the most common cause of cognitive impairment. It is irreversible, progressing from deficits in memory and thinking skills to an inability to perform even the simplest of tasks.

9. *a.* Asking questions about events in the past can encourage the older adult to relive and restructure life experiences.

10. *b, d, f.* The SPICES acronym is used to identify common problems in older adults and stands for:

   S – Sleep disorders

   P – Problems with eating or feeding

   I – Incontinence

   C – Confusion

   E – Evidence of falls

   S – Skin breakdown (Fulmer & Wallace, 2012).

TAYLOR SUITE RESOURCES

Explore these additional resources to enhance learning for this chapter:

- NCLEX-Style Questions and other resources on thePoint, http://thePoint.lww.com/Taylor8e
- *Study Guide for Fundamentals of Nursing, 8th edition*
- Adaptive Learning | Powered by prepU, http://thepoint.lww.com/prepu

Bibliography

Administration on Aging. (2011). A profile of older Americans: 2011. Available at http://www.aoa.gov/aoaroot/aging_statistics/Profile/2011/docs/2011profile.pdf

American Nurse. (2012). *Delirium affects 80 percent of critically ill, 44*(2), 15.

Bartley, M., & Shiflett, L. (2010). Handle older trauma patients with care. *Nursing, 40*(8), 24–29.

Benton, M., Whyte, M., & Dyal, B. (2011). Sarcopenic obesity: Strategies for management. *American Journal of Nursing, 111*(12), 38–44.

Bilyeu, K., Gumm, C., Fitzgerald, J., Fox, S., & Selig, P. (2011). Reducing the use of potentially inappropriate medications in older adults. *American Journal of Nursing, 111*(1), 47–52.

Brauser, D. (2012). Weight training, walking improve cognition in the elderly. Available at http://www.medscape.com/viewarticle/767452

Brooks, P. (2012). Postoperative delirium in elderly patients. *American Journal of Nursing, 112*(9), 38–49.

Cahoon, C. (2012). Depression in older adults. *American Journal of Nursing, 112*(11), 22–29.

Centers for Disease Control and Prevention (CDC). (2011). Alzheimer's disease. Available at http://www.cdc.gov/aging/aginginfo/alzheimers.htm

Centers for Disease Control and Prevention (CDC). (2012a). Falls among older adults: An overview. Available at http://www.cdc.gov/HomeandRecreational Safety/Falls/adultfalls.html

Centers for Disease Control and Prevention (CDC). (2012b). Recommended adult immunization schedule—United States, 2012. *Morbidity and Mortality Weekly Report, 61*(4), 1–7.

Centers for Disease Control and Prevention (CDC). (2012c). Older adult falls publications. Available at http://www.cdc.gov/HomeandRecreationalSafety/Falls/pubs.html

Centers for Disease Control and Prevention. (CDC). (2012d). REACH. Available at http://www.cdc.gov/healthycommunitiesprogram/communities/reach/

Chettle, C. (2009). Aging immune systems more vulnerable to attack. *Nursing Spectrum, 18*(6), 20–25.

Cutugno, C. (2011). The "graying" of trauma care: Addressing traumatic injury in older adults. *American Journal of Nursing, 111*(11), 40–48.

Dang, M. (2010). Walking away the blues: Exercise for depression in older adults. *Nursing, 40*(11), 33–36.

Edelman, M., & Ficorelli, C. (2012). Keeping older adults safe at home. *Nursing, 42*(1), 65–66.

Eliopoulos, C. (2010). *Gerontological nursing* (7th ed.). Philadelphia: Wolters Kluwer Health/Lippincott Williams & Wilkins.

Erikson, E. (1963). *Childhood and society* (2nd ed.). New York: Norton.

Federal Interagency Forum on Aging Related Statistics. (2012). Older Americans 2012: Key indicators of well-being. Available at http://www.agingstats.gov/agingstatsdotnet/main_site/default.aspx

Fowler, J. W. (1991). *Weaving the new creation: Stages of faith and the public church.* San Francisco: HarperCollins.

Fulmer, T. (2012). Elder mistreatment assessment. *Hartford Institute for Geriatric Nursing, College of Nursing, 15,* 1–2.

Fulmer, T., & Wallace, M. (2012). Fulmer SPICES: An overall assessment tool for older adults. *Hartford Institute for Geriatric Nursing, College of Nursing, 1,* 1–2.

Gibbons, M. (2010). It takes a community. *Advance for Nurses, 12*(20), 10–11.

Gould, R. (1972). The phases of adult life: A study in developmental psychology. *American Psychiatry, 129,* 33–43.

Gray-Vickrey, P. (2010). Gathering "pearls" of knowledge for assessing older adults. *Nursing, 40*(3), 34–43.

Guteri, G. (2012). The graying of healthcare. *Advance for Nurses, 14*(11), 16–21.

Havighurst, R. J. (1972). *Developmental tasks and education* (3rd ed.). New York: David McKay.

Heron, M. (2012). Deaths: Leading causes for 2009. *National Vital Statistics Reports, 61*(7), 8–18.

Klever, S. (2013). Reminiscence therapy: Finding meaning in memories. *Nursing, 43*(4), 36–37.

Kohlberg, L. (1969). Stage and sequence: The cognitive–developmental approach to socialization. In D. Gaslin (Ed.), *Handbook of socialization: Theory and research* (pp. 347–380). Chicago: Rand McNally.

Lehne, R. (2013). *Pharmacology for Nursing Care* (8th ed.). St. Louis: Elsevier/Saunders.

Levinson, D., Darrow, C., Klein, E., Levinson, M., & McKee, B. (1978). *The seasons of a man's life.* New York: Knopf.

Lynn, S. (2012). Adverse drug reactions in the elderly. Available at http://www.medscape.com/viewarticle/758855

Martin, D., Kripalani, S., & DuRapau, V. (2012). Improving medication management among at-risk older adults. *Journal of Gerontological Nursing, 38*(6), 24–34.

McCloskey Dochterman, J., & Bulechek, G. (Eds.). (2004). *Nursing interventions classification (NIC)* (4th ed.). St. Louis: Mosby.

Moorhead, S., Johnson, M., Maas, M., & Swanson, E. (Eds.). (2008). *Nursing outcomes classification (NOC)* (4th ed.). St. Louis: Mosby.

Naegle, M. (2011). Detecting and screening for depression in older adults. *American Nurse Today, 6*(11), 18–20.

NANDA International (NANDA-I). (2012). *NANDA nursing diagnoses: Definitions & classification 2012–2014.* West Sussex, UK: Wiley-Blackwell.

National Center on Elder Abuse (NCEA). (2011). Major types of elder abuse. Available at http://www.ncea.aoa.gov/FAQ/Type_Abuse/index.aspx

National Center for Health Statistics. (2013). *Health, United States 2012: With Special Feature on Emergency Care.* Hyattsville, MD.

National Institute on Aging. (2012). *Alzheimer's disease fact sheet.* Available at http://www.nia.nih.gov/sites/default/files/alzheimers_disease_fact_sheet_0.pdf

Office of Minority Health. (2012a). African American Profile. Available at http://minorityhealth.hhs.gov/templates/browse.aspx?lvl=2&lvlid=51

Office of Minority Health. (2012b). American Indian/ Alaska Native Profile. Available at http://minorityhealth. hhs.gov/templates/browse.aspx?lvl=2&lvlid=52

Office of Minority Health. (2012c). Asian American/Pacific Islander Profile. Available at http://minorityhealth.hhs.gov/templates/browse. aspx?lvl=2&lvlid=53

Office of Minority Health. (2012d). Hispanic/Latino Profile. Available at http://minorityhealth.hhs.gov/ templates/browse.aspx?lvl=2&lvlid=54

Pennsylvania Department of Transportation. (n.d.) Talking with older drivers: A guide for family and friends. Available at http://www.dmv.state.pa.us/ pdotforms/misc/Pub_345.pdf

Reed, P. (1996). Transcendence: Formulating nursing perspectives. *Nursing Science Quarterly, 9*(1), 2–4.

Scudder, L. (2012). New USPSTF recommendations for prevention of falls in elderly patients. Available at http://www.medscape.org/viewarticle/765310

Sherwood, G., & Barnsteiner, J. (2012). *Quality and Safety in Nursing.* West Sussex, UK: Wiley-Blackwell.

Stark, S. (2012). Elder abuse: Screening, intervention, and prevention. *Nursing, 42*(10), 24–29.

Sullivan, J. (2011). Caring for older adults after surgery. *Nursing, 41*(4), 48–51.

Van Leuven, K. (2012). Population aging: Implications for nurse practitioners. Available at http://www. medscape.com/viewarticle/767243_print

Roles Basic to Nursing Care

Unit V discusses the nurse's professional roles of communicator, teacher, counselor, leader, and manager. These roles are interdependent, and each is an integral part of the broad nursing role of caregiver. The nurse in these roles helps patients of all ages to meet needs along the health continuum.

To be effective as a caregiver, the nurse must be proficient in both the art and the science of nursing. Communication is essential to each professional nursing role and is the heart of caring. Nursing is a person-centered service, based on relationships with patients, peers, and other members of the health care team. By developing effective interpersonal skills and using therapeutic communication skills, nurses can establish and maintain helping relationships.

As teacher, the nurse uses communication skills to teach individuals and families. Teaching is used throughout the nursing process to meet learning needs. As counselor, the nurse provides information, makes appropriate referrals, and assists the patient in developing a systematic approach to problem solving and decision making. The nurse as a leader and/or manager practices assertive, self-directed nursing. Abilities to lead and to bring about change begin with the student nurse and progress as the nurse develops self-confidence and skill in interpersonal relationships and experience in health care settings. Unit V, therefore, enables beginning nurse caregivers to enrich their professional practice by integrating the professional nursing roles of communicator, teacher, counselor, leader, and manager. Nursing practice, as a specialized and unique service to others, is based on the application of knowledge and skills presented in this unit.

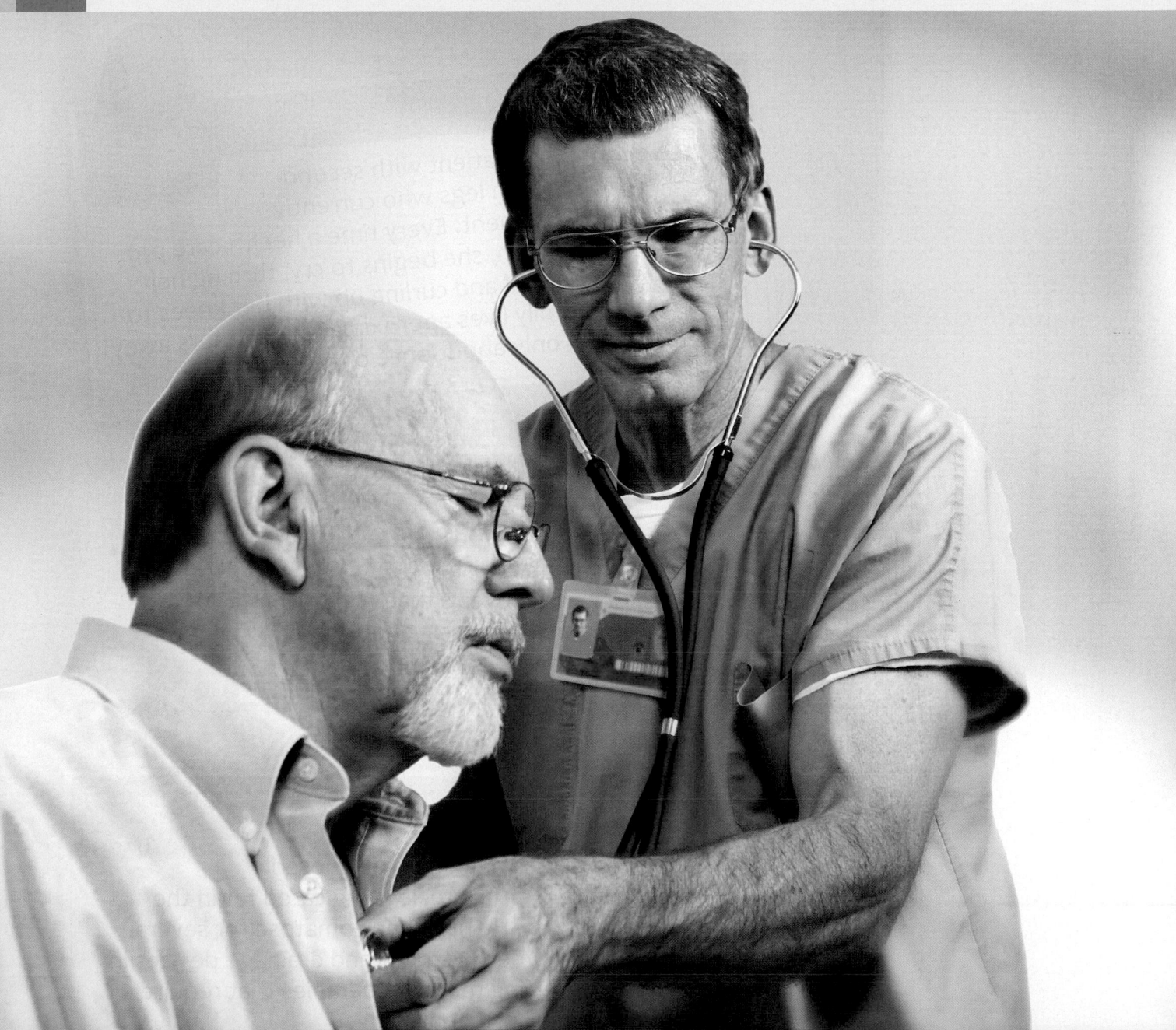

“Clinical competence . . . has three dimensions. . . . Care is the fundamental things we do to make a patient comfortable . . . . curative nursing, . . . the broader group of restorative and rehabilitative activities . . . and counseling, . . . [providing] emotional, intellectual, and psychological support . . . ”

Frances Reiter (1904–1977) the first chairperson of the American Nurses Association Committee on Education, she coined the term “nurse clinician” and advocated advanced preparation of nurse clinicians.

Communicator

SUSIE MUSASHI

Susie is a 3-year-old patient with second-degree burns on both legs who currently is receiving débridement. Every time a health care provider enters her room, she begins to cry, turning her body toward the wall and curling up with her knees to her chest. Her family lives approximately 1½ hours away and can visit her only about once or twice a week.

IRWINA RUSSELLINSKI

Irwina, a 75-year-old woman transferred from the emergency department, is diagnosed with pneumonia. Her chart reveals that she is hard of hearing, "pleasantly confused" at times, and speaks "broken English." A nursing assessment is needed.

RANDOLPH GORDON

Randolph, a middle-aged man diagnosed with end-stage liver failure, is being cared for in the intensive care unit. He has been comatose for several weeks. He has numerous tubes and drainage devices in place and is receiving multiple therapies that require continuous electronic monitoring.

LEARNING OBJECTIVES

After completing the chapter, you will be able to accomplish the following:

1. Describe the communication process, identifying factors that influence communication.

2. List at least eight ways in which people communicate nonverbally.

3. Discuss professional responsibilities when using electronic communication.

4. Describe the interrelation between communication and the nursing process.

5. Identify patient goals for each phase of the helping relationship.

6. Use effective communication techniques when interacting with patients from different cultures.

7. Use a standardized communication technique (SBAR) to communicate with physicians and transfer patient information to other nurses.

8. Evaluate yourself in terms of the interpersonal competencies needed in nursing.

9. Describe how each type of ineffective communication hinders communication.

10. Describe strategies that counteract disruptive professional behaviors.

11. Establish therapeutic relationships with patients assigned to your care, and describe effective interventions for patients with impaired verbal communication.

KEY TERMS

aggressive behavior	horizontal violence	professionalism
assertive behavior	incivility	rapport
body language	interpersonal communication	receiver (decoder)
bullying	interviewing techniques	SBAR
channel	intrapersonal communication	semantics
cliché	language	small-group communication
communication	message	social media
empathy	noise	source (encoder)
feedback	nonverbal communication	stimulus
group dynamics	organizational communication	verbal communication
helping relationship		

Any nurse who wishes to be an effective caregiver must first learn how to be an effective communicator. Good communication skills enable nurses to get to know their patients and, ultimately, to diagnose and meet their needs for nursing care. Nursing students who sit face to face with patients to obtain a comprehensive nursing history intuitively grasp the importance of the nurse's communicator role. To adequately document the patient's health history, the nursing student must understand and implement proper communication techniques. Communication skills are the building blocks of professional relationships between nurse and patient, nurse and nurse, and nurse and other health-team members. (See the accompanying Reflective Practice box for an example on page 448.)

Many experienced nurses identify the quality of their interpersonal relationships as the single most significant element in determining their helper effectiveness. Studies have shown that on nursing units where nurses freely exchange ideas and information, solve problems together when something goes wrong rather than assigning blame, compliment one another, and use humor creatively, staff morale is high, and there is a higher level of attainment of patient outcomes. On the other hand, when harassment or disruptive communication behaviors occur in the workplace between health care professionals, the consequences can affect the emotional and physical well-being of those involved in the abusive behavior, the functioning of the organization, and the safety of patient care.

THE PROCESS OF COMMUNICATION

Communication is the process of exchanging information and generating and transmitting meanings between two or more people. It is the foundation of society and the most primary aspect of a nurse–patient interaction. Without communication, it would be impossible to share family experiences, gain knowledge, establish and maintain practice protocols, and enhance caregiving. By nature, humans are social beings, and human needs are met in collaboration with other humans. Human relationships enable us to meet our physical and safety needs. Communication also assists in meeting our psychosocial needs of love, belonging, and self-esteem. The ability to communicate is basic to human functioning and well-being.

David K. Berlo (1960) is credited with the classic description of the communication process, which involves a source (encoder), message, channel, and receiver (decoder). This communication process is initiated based on a **stimulus**, in this case a patient need that must be addressed. The need might be due to a patient's discomfort or desire for information or to address any uncertainty the patient might be experiencing. The sender or **source (encoder)** of the message is a person or group who initiates or begins the communication process.

The **message** is the actual communication product from the source. It might be a speech, interview, conversation, chart, gesture, memorandum, or nursing note. The **channel** of communication is the medium the sender has selected

REFLECTIVE PRACTICE: CULTIVATING QSEN COMPETENCIES

CHALLENGE TO ETHICAL AND LEGAL SKILLS

Recently, I was accompanying a nurse in the intensive care unit (ICU) when I encountered some behaviors that I found to be unprofessional and lacking in interpersonal skills. We were caring for Mr. Randolph Gordon, a middle-aged patient who was in end-stage liver failure and had been comatose for several weeks. The extent of drains, tubes, and technologies being used to care for Mr. Gordon was overwhelming. It was almost difficult to recognize him as a human being. I was taken aback when the nurse and some residents entered the patient's room and immediately began to assess the technological equipment, without any regard for or recognition of the patient. They proceeded to have a conversation about the patient's poor condition, unsightly appearance, and foul smell at the bedside, in the direct presence of the patient. They did not speak to the patient and they made no attempt to interact with the patient, not even the slightest touch of a hand.

Thinking Outside the Box: Possible Courses of Action

- Ignore the conversation between the nurse and residents and acknowledge the patient through words or touch.
- Calmly ask the nurse and residents to leave the room before discussing the patient's condition.
- Confront the nurse and residents, stating that they need to pay attention to the patient and his psychosocial and emotional well-being.

Evaluating a Good Outcome: How Do I Define Success?

- The patient's health care team will act with professionalism.
- Health care team will demonstrate respect for the patient's human dignity.
- We will have regard for the whole patient, with attention to spiritual, emotional, and social issues.
- We will set a good example for others in our expression of caring.

Personal Learning: Here's to the Future!

I was somewhat disappointed by my actions in this situation because I did not confront the nurse and the residents when they were acting unethically and unprofessionally. I did, however, ask the nurse if this was common behavior in the ICU, that is, demonstrating little regard for the patient's holistic well-being. The nurse stated that unfortunately this was the case. The patients in the ICU are critically ill, and many health care professionals become extremely focused on the physical and technological aspects of care. I was hesitant to interrupt the nurse and the residents because of my status as a nursing student. I feared that my opinion would not be respected. I know that I will not be able to change the actions of everyone. However, in the future, I will demonstrate my concern for the patient, hoping that those around me will follow my example. I think that I should have immediately gone to the patient and said hello or touched his hand, even if he was comatose. Maybe my actions would have reminded the nurse and residents that there was a person in that bed. Then, possibly, they might have followed my lead.

Colleen Kilcullen, Georgetown University

REFLECTION ON QUALITY AND SAFETY COMPETENCIES

How do you think you would respond in a similar situation? Why? What does this tell you about yourself and about the adequacy of your skills for professional practice? What knowledge, skills, and attitudes do you need to develop to continuously improve quality and safety in a situation like the one experienced by this student nurse?

Patient-Centered Care: How could the nursing student's communication skills have demonstrated empathy and emotional support for this patient? Did her handling of this situation facilitate her ability to deliver effective care and treatment in other environments? What reasons can you propose to suggest the rationale for the nurse's and residents' behavior?

Teamwork and Collaboration/Quality Improvement: How do you think that the residents would have reacted if the nursing student had approached them about their behavior? Can you think of other ways to respond? Describe a plan that the nursing student could use to go about changing the staff's behavior. What communication skills might effectively communicate empathy and caring by all the professional staff caring for this patient?

Safety/Evidence-Based Practice: Do you agree with the criteria to evaluate a positive outcome in this situation? Did the nursing student meet the criteria? Please explain why or why not. Should one of the priorities of care for Mr. Gordon have included a review at the bedside of his current condition and treatment therapies with respect to the possibility that the patient might be able to hear the discussion even though he is not able to communicate with the staff? What evidence in nursing literature provides guidance for the student when caring for an unresponsive patient?

Informatics: Can you identify essential information that should be documented in Mr. Gordon's electronic record regarding physical assessments and electronic monitoring in addition to efforts to communicate with this patient? Do you think the understanding you gained from this situation improves your ability to care effectively for other comatose patients and communicate respect and emotional support?

to send the message. The channel might target any of the receiver's senses. The message can be sent to the receiver through the following channels:

- Auditory—spoken words and cues
- Visual—sight, observations, and perception
- Kinesthetic—touch

Nurses use all three of these channels to communicate with patients.

The **receiver (decoder)** must translate and interpret the message sent and received. Through the translation of the message, the receiver must then make a decision about an accurate response. To be an effective communicator, the nurse needs to be considerate of the receiver, and select a message that appeals to the patient's interests and that requires minimal effort and time to decode.

 RECALL Randolph Gordon, the middle-aged man who was comatose. When planning Mr. Gordon's care, the nurse would need to incorporate knowledge about changes in mental status and their effect on communication. The patient's current mental status mandates that the messages sent by the nurse and other health care providers be simple, clear, and easy to understand. ●

Confirmation of the message provides **feedback** (i.e., evidence) that the receiver has understood the intended message. **Noise**—factors that distort the quality of a message—can interfere with communication at any point in the process. These distractors might be from the television, or from pain or discomfort experienced by the patient.

Communication is a reciprocal process in which both the sender and the receiver of messages participate simultaneously. The communication process is illustrated in Figure 20-1. Messages might be influenced on either end by the person's previous knowledge, past experiences, feelings, or sociocultural level.

Test your knowledge of communication by reading the situation in Box 20-1 (on page 450).

FORMS OF COMMUNICATION

The sending and receiving of messages is accomplished through verbal and nonverbal communication techniques. These can occur separately or simultaneously.

Verbal Communication

Verbal communication is an exchange of information using words, including both the spoken and written word. Verbal communication depends on **language**, or a prescribed way of using words so that people can share information effectively. Language includes a common definition of words and a method of arranging the words in a certain order.

A person's use of written and spoken language forms reveals aspects of the person's intellectual development, educational level, and geographic and cultural origin. Nurses must also consider whether English is a second language for the patient. Language helps nurses assess what the

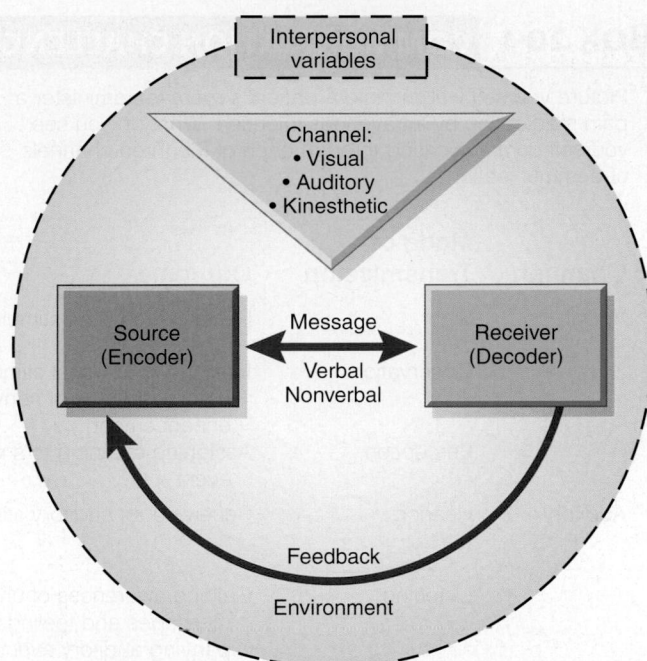

FIGURE 20-1. The various components in the process of communication.

patient knows and feels. In turn, nurses must develop their own language skills to assist in reciprocal responses in the communication process.

 THINK back to Irwina Russellinski, the older adult woman admitted with pneumonia. According to her medical record, the patient speaks "broken English." Therefore, the nurse must incorporate knowledge of this when attempting to communicate verbally with the patient, making adaptations during the interaction to ensure that messages are clear. ●

Nurses use verbal communication extensively when providing patient care, including verbal interactions with patients and family, giving oral reports to other nurses, writing care plans, and recording progress in the patient's chart. Other examples of verbal communication include public speaking, writing for publication, and composing signs and posters. Words and language in the previous examples communicate messages to others.

Nonverbal Communication

The transmission of information without the use of words is termed **nonverbal communication**, also known as **body language**. It often helps nurses to understand subtle and hidden meanings in what the patient is saying verbally. For example, a nurse asks the patient, "How do you feel today?" The patient responds, "I feel all right." However, the nurse notes that the patient does not maintain eye contact and his facial expression is tense. This would indicate that the nurse should investigate further because of the incongruence of the patient's verbal and nonverbal communication (Fig. 20-2 on page 450).

BOX 20-1 | COMMUNICATION CHALLENGES

Picture yourself walking into a patient's room to administer a pain medication by intravenous injection. What do you see yourself communicating through each of the three channels of communication?

Then read the following scenario and think about all the ways nurses might unintentionally communicate that they are not concerned about the patient or his pain. Use this exercise to guide both your verbal and nonverbal messages to patients.

Channel	Mode of Transmission	Outcome	Nursing Behavior
Visual	Sight	Receiving a visual stimulus	Patient sees nurse walking into the room holding desired medication.
	Observation	Interpreting a visual stimulation by making note of nonverbal enhancement	Patient makes note of the nurse's sense of competence, confidence, and sympathetic expression.
	Perception	Assigning meaning to a visual event	Patient concludes that the nurse is willing and able to help him and feels comforted.
Auditory	Hearing	Receiving an auditory stimulus	Patient hears the nurse say, "I understand your hip is hurting. This injection should help you to start feeling better within minutes."
	Listening	Gaining awareness of underlying messages and feelings accompanying auditory events	Patient senses that the nurse said he should start feeling better soon and really wants this to happen because she cares about him.
Kinesthetic	Procedural touch	Performing nursing procedures and techniques	Patient feels the nurse touching him while preparing to inject the medication into the IV access.
	Caring touch	Conveying emotional support	Patient feels that the nurse cares about him as a person when she touches his shoulder upon first entering the room while asking about his pain.

FIGURE 20-2. Eye contact, the lack of it, facial expression, posture, gesture, and silence send nonverbal messages to the receiver. What messages do you receive from each of these photographs?

CONSIDER Susie Musashi, the 3-year-old described at the beginning of the chapter. Interpretation of her nonverbal behavior is essential to implementing an effective plan of care. For example, the nurse needs to interpret what her crying indicates, such as fear, pain, or loneliness. In addition, the nurse needs to examine the meaning of the child's turning away from the door. Does she want to be left alone? Is she frightened? Once this information is obtained and analyzed, the nurse is better equipped to develop a plan of care to meet the child's needs. ●

Information is exchanged through nonverbal communication in various ways. It is generally accepted that nonverbal communication expresses more of the true meaning of a message than verbal communication. Therefore, nurses must be aware of both the nonverbal messages they send and the nonverbal messages they receive from patients. Nurses working with patients from diverse cultural backgrounds should attempt to understand cultural variations to avoid misunderstanding nonverbal communication. The various forms of nonverbal communication follow.

Touch

Tactile sense has been studied seriously as a form of nonverbal communication only since the 1960s. Touch is a personal behavior and means different things to different people. Familial, regional, class, and cultural influences largely shape tactile experiences. Factors such as age and sex also play a key role in meanings associated with touch. Despite its individuality, touch is viewed as one of the most effective nonverbal ways to express feelings of comfort, love, affection, security, anger, frustration, aggression, excitement, and many others.

RECALL Mr. Gordon, the patient with end-stage liver disease who is in a coma. Although the patient may not respond verbally or be able to comprehend, the nurse could use touch to indicate concern and respect for the patient, thus sending a message that someone is there for him. ●

Eye Contact

Communication often begins with eye contact. A glance, for example, is often an attention-getting method to open conversation. In many cultures, eye contact suggests respect and a willingness to listen and to keep communication open. Its absence often indicates anxiety or defenselessness, or avoidance of communication. Some view eye contact as the nonverbal communication that reveals a person's true nature. However, some Asian and Native American cultures view eye contact as an invasion of a person's privacy. In other cultures, people are taught to avoid eye contact or, out of respect, not to make eye contact with a superior.

In addition to the messages sent by eye contact, the eyes carry other nonverbal messages. For example, the eyes fix in a stare during anger, tend to narrow in disgust, and ordinarily open wide in fear. Some people who experience fear might be unable to speak and only their eyes will send the message of anxiety. A blank stare can indicate daydreaming or inattentiveness.

Facial Expressions

The face is the most expressive part of the body. Examples of the various messages facial expressions convey are anger, joy, suspicion, sadness, fear, and contempt. Some people have extremely expressive faces, whereas others mask their feelings, making it more difficult to determine what the person is really thinking. Nurses need to learn to control their own facial expressions.

TAKE, for example, Susie Musashi, the 3-year-old with burns. Preschoolers are naturally curious. So, she might watch the nurse's reaction when the nurse changes the burn dressings for the first time. Any sign of repulsion or disgust could greatly impact the child's self-image and recovery. ●

Posture

The way a person holds the body carries nonverbal messages. People in good health and with a positive attitude usually hold their bodies in good alignment. Depressed or tired people are more likely to slouch. Posture also often provides nonverbal clues concerning pain and physical limitations, for instance, a rigid, stiff appearance might be a good indicator of tension and pain.

Gait

A bouncy, purposeful walk usually carries a message of well-being. A less purposeful, shuffling gait often means the person is sad or discouraged. Certain gaits are associated with illness. For example, patients recovering from recent abdominal surgery usually walk slightly bent over and slowly and might need the assistance of handrails or a helping person.

Gestures

Gestures using various parts of the body can carry numerous messages—for example, thumbs up means victory, kicking an object often expresses anger, wringing the hands or tapping a foot usually indicates anxiety or anger, and a waving hand serves to beckon someone to come on, or if waved in another way, signifies that someone should leave. Gestures are often used extensively when two people speaking in different languages attempt to communicate with each other.

REMEMBER Mrs. Russellinski, the 75-year-old with pneumonia. Gestures would be very helpful in communicating with the patient, especially in light of the patient's hearing and language deficits. ●

General Physical Appearance

Most illnesses cause at least some alterations in general physical appearance. Observing for changes in appearance is an important nursing responsibility for detecting illness or evaluating the effectiveness of care and therapy. For example, a person with an insufficient intake of fluids has dry skin that wrinkles easily, eyes that might be sunken and dull in appearance, and poor muscle tone. On the other hand, the person in good health tends to radiate a healthy status through general appearance.

Mode of Dress and Grooming

A person's clothing and grooming practices carry significant nonverbal messages. For example, healthy people tend to pay attention to details of dress and grooming, whereas people feeling ill often demonstrate little interest in personal appearance. It is often a sign of returning health when interest in their physical appearance and mode of dress returns.

Sounds

Crying, moaning, gasping, and sighing are oral but nonverbal forms of communication. Such sounds can be interpreted in numerous ways. For example, a person might cry because of sadness or joy. Gasping often indicates fear, pain, or surprise. A sigh might be a sign of reluctant agreement to do something or of relief.

Silence

Periods of silence during a conversation often carry important nonverbal messages. A silence between two people might indicate complete understanding of each other, that both of the two people are thinking, or that they are angry with each other. Silence and its possible uses and meanings are discussed later in this chapter.

Electronic Communication

The Internet and a variety of social websites provide new and challenging opportunities for nurses to communicate and collaborate with other health care providers. The challenges of using social media include protecting patient privacy and confidentiality and preventing unintended consequences for the employer or the nurse. Protocols for using e-mail, sending text messages, and accessing the social media sites are vital for wise use of these forms of electronic communication. Student nurses also must know these guidelines for use of electronic communication venues. Educational institutions should orient students to their social networking policies as well as those of health care facilities where students have clinical experiences (Spector & Kappel, 2012).

Social Media

Social media are web-based technologies that allow users to create, share, and participate in dialogue in virtual communities and networks. The availability of social media sites has dramatically changed communications among people, communities, and organizations. Social media networks allow nurses to share ideas, develop professional connections, access educational offerings and forums, receive support, and investigate evidence-based practices. Facebook, Twitter, and LinkedIn are common websites used by nurses (Duffy, 2011a). Concerns about social media occur when nurses inadvertently reveal information about patients that compromise the patients' privacy. Nurses must adhere to Health Insurance Portability and Accountability Act (HIPAA) regulations that protect patient confidentiality and privacy and be aware of their employer's policies about using social media. Health care facilities may specifically address personal use of computers in the facility and types of websites that may be accessed during working hours from employer computers. Health care facility policies often do not address employee use of social media when not at work, but disclosing information that violates the privacy and confidentiality of patients or professional standards, and posting defamatory remarks about an employer, supervisor, co-worker or patient has serious consequences for nurses (National Council of State Boards of Nursing [NCSBN], 2011). Derogatory comments can also lead to civil lawsuits against the nurse (Prinz, 2011).

Both the American Nurses Association (ANA) and the NCSBN have issued guidelines for RNs regarding use of social media. They agree that professional boundaries must be followed in the social media environment. In a 2010 NCSBN survey of Boards of Nursing (BON), a majority stated that they had received complaints regarding nurses who violated patient privacy by providing information or photos of patients on social media websites (NCSBN, 2011). The response from the BON varied from a letter of concern to suspension of the nurse's license. See Box 20-2 for the six principles for social networking endorsed by the ANA.

In most cases, inappropriate disclosures of information are unintentional. Nurses may expect that information they post is private, but in reality it can be shared with multiple

---

BOX 20-2 AMERICAN NURSES ASSOCIATION'S PRINCIPLES FOR SOCIAL NETWORKING

1. Nurses must not transmit or place online individually identifiable patient information.
2. Nurses must observe ethically prescribed professional patient–nurse boundaries.
3. Nurses should understand that patients, colleagues, institutions, and employers may view postings.
4. Nurses should take advantage of privacy settings and seek to separate personal and professional information online.
5. Nurses should bring content that could harm a patient's privacy, rights, or welfare to the attention of appropriate authorities.
6. Nurses should participate in developing institutional policies governing online conduct.

Reprinted with permission from American Nurses Association (ANA). (2011). *ANA's Principles for Social Networking and the Nurse.* Silver Springs, MD: Nursesbooks.org.

other recipients. As well, it is also incorrect to assume that once information has been deleted from a site, it is no longer available. Describing a patient by using a room number or diagnosis rather than a name is still considered a breach of confidentiality and a violation of patient privacy. When your relationship with a health care institution is apparent, use a disclaimer to verify that any views expressed are yours alone and not your employer's (Pagana, 2011a). Employers also may use social media to screen potential employees as long as they do not violate discrimination laws. Any information you have provided about yourself on a social media website may influence a hiring decision. The ease with which information can be posted on a social media site allows minimal time to consider the implications and the effect a posting can have on a nurse's personal and professional life (NCSBN, 2011).

E-Mail and Text Messages

E-mail and text messages are efficient means to communicate with staff members and, in some cases, patients. The risk for violating patient privacy and confidentiality exists any time a message is sent electronically. Health care agencies usually have security measures in place to safeguard e-mail and text communications. E-mail and text messages should be concise and avoid text abbreviations (Pagana, 2012). Nurses should be aware of agency policies and guidelines regarding the use of electronic communication with patients. The patient may have to sign an authorization permitting e-mail communication from the health care agency. Any e-mails sent to a patient must be duplicated and become part of the medical record for that patient. While e-mail and text messages are additional communication tools, it is always necessary to follow agency policies and adhere to your professional code of conduct. Individualizing patient care requires nurses to determine which form of communication is most beneficial for each patient.

LEVELS OF COMMUNICATION

Throughout our lives and the lives of our patients, communication occurs at varying levels. Nurses engage in four levels of communication during practice: intrapersonal communication, interpersonal communication, small-group communication, and organizational communication.

Intrapersonal Communication

Intrapersonal communication, or self-talk, is communication within a person. This communication is crucial because it affects the nurse's behavior and can enhance or detract from positive interactions with the patient and family. Imagine two different nursing students preparing for the first experience with a critically ill patient. Both are frightened. One tells herself, "Calm down, you've been in challenging situations before and always survived. You can handle this." The other repeatedly tells himself, "There's no way you can survive this experience. The instructor will be all over you, and you might as well admit defeat before you start."

Obviously, the first student's positive self-talk is more helpful than that of the second student.

 CONSIDER Susie Musashi, the 3-year-old receiving treatment for her burns. The nurse may use self-talk when preparing to interact with the child, thereby helping her to focus on the child and her behaviors. In doing so, the nurse may be better able to interpret the child's messages. The nurse might say to herself, "I will use broad opening statements to help the patient and family express their feelings. I will talk to the patient on her level. I must maintain eye contact with the patient and family and answer their questions. I will not make light of the situation or appear unconcerned." ●

Understanding the importance of intrapersonal communication can also help you to work with patients and families whose negative self-talk affects their health and self-care abilities.

Interpersonal Communication

Interpersonal communication occurs between two or more people with a goal to exchange messages. Most of the nurse's day is spent communicating with patients, family members, and members of the health care team. The ability to communicate effectively at this level influences your sharing, problem solving, goal attainment, team building, and effectiveness in critical nursing roles (e.g., caregiver, teacher, counselor, leader, manager, patient advocate).

Group Communication

Group communication includes small-group and organizational group communication. To determine the effectiveness or ineffectiveness of a group, one studies the group dynamics.

Small-Group Communication

Small-group communication occurs when nurses interact with two or more people. To be functional, members of the small group must communicate to achieve their goal. Examples of small-group communication include staff meetings, patient care conferences, teaching sessions, and support groups. The more people involved in the communication process, the more complex it becomes.

Organizational Communication

Organizational communication occurs when people and groups within an organization communicate to achieve established goals. Nurses on a practice council meeting to review unit policies, or nurses working with interdisciplinary groups on strategic planning or quality assurance, use organizational communication to achieve their aims.

Group Dynamics

When determining the effectiveness or ineffectiveness of a group, one studies the group dynamics. **Group dynamics** involve how individual group members relate to one another during the process of working toward group goals.

Table 20-1	CHARACTERISTICS OF EFFECTIVE AND INEFFECTIVE GROUPS	
VARIABLE	EFFECTIVE GROUP	INEFFECTIVE GROUP
Group identity	Members value and "own" the aims of the group; aims are clearly articulated.	Group's aims are not of major importance to members.
Cohesiveness	Members generally trust and like one another and are loyal to the group; high commitment; high degree of cooperation.	Members often feel alienated from the group and from one another; low commitment; members tend to work better alone than with the group.
Patterns of interaction	Honest, direct communication flows freely; members support, praise, and critique one another.	Communication is sparing; little self-disclosure; self-serving roles (i.e., dominator, blocker, or aggressor) may be unchecked.
Decision making	Problems are identified, appropriate method of decision making is used (i.e., individual, minority, majority, consensus, or unanimous); decision is implemented and followed through; group commitment to decision is high.	Problems are allowed to build without resolution; little responsibility is shown for problem solving; group commitment to decision is low.
Responsibility	Members feel strong sense of responsibility for group outcomes.	Little responsibility for group felt by group members.
Leadership	Effective style of leadership to meet desired aims	Ineffective leadership styles
Power	Sources of power are recognized and used appropriately; needs or interests of those with little power are considered.	Power is used and abused to "fix" immediate problems; little attention to needs of powerless.

Although effective leadership facilitates a group's achievement of its goals, success or failure largely results from members' behavior. Ideally, all group members use their talents and interpersonal strengths to help the group to accomplish its goals. The group's ability to function at a high level depends on each member's sensitivity to the needs of the group and its individual members. Effective groups have members who are mutually respectful. If a group member dominates or thwarts the group process, then the leader or other group members must confront that member to promote the needed collegial relationship. Effective and ineffective groups are contrasted in Table 20-1.

FACTORS INFLUENCING COMMUNICATION

Factors influencing communication include level of development; gender; sociocultural differences; roles and responsibilities; space and territoriality; physical, mental, and emotional state; and environment.

Developmental Level

The rate of language development is directly correlated with the patient's neurologic competence and cognitive development. Thus, it is helpful to understand the process of language development and the stages of intellectual and psychosocial development. This helps you communicate effectively with patients and family of all age ranges.

 REMEMBER Susie Musashi, the 3-year-old child with burns. The nurse would incorporate knowledge of the typical preschooler fears (such as fear of new places and fear of the dark) when developing the child's plan of care. Preschoolers gain self-esteem by receiving compliments about their appearance. The presence of the burns directly affects the child's appearance, possibly threatening self-esteem. Therefore, the nurse also needs to consider the child's current fears related to her burns and burn treatment and their effect on the child's self-esteem. ●

The stages of development are presented in Chapters 17, 18, and 19. Knowing how each age group commonly perceives health, illness, and body functions should guide your interactions with patients. For instance, a 10-year-old child has limited understanding of what an infection is; therefore, explain things in simple terms so that the child cooperates with the treatment without being frightened. Because adolescents are developing abstract thinking, more detailed and accurate explanations can be given to them. Being familiar with commonly used slang usually helps when communicating with adolescents. Communicating with adults can be affected by their past positive or negative health-related experiences and by inaccurate information. When communicating with older patients, assess for any problems with hearing or sight (discussed later in this chapter), confusion, or depression, any of which could affect nurse–patient interaction.

Gender

Men and women have differing communication styles and might give different interpretations to the same conversation. Tannen (1990) believes that this is because girls and boys grow up communicating differently. Whereas girls generally play with "best friends" and use language to seek confirmation, minimize differences, and establish or reinforce intimacy, boys use language to establish their independence and to negotiate status activities in large groups. In contrast, Townsend (2009) states that gender roles are changing in American society because sexual roles are becoming less distinct. Factors contributing to this change are the growing use of the term "unisex" and the fact that women and men enter professions previously dominated by the other sex. It is necessary to be sensitive to the fact that men and women might communicate differently. As such, when working with patients of the opposite gender, you'll need to validate that both you and your patient are accurately receiving the message the other is trying to communicate.

Sociocultural Differences

Nurses need to recognize ways in which culture, economic condition, and overall lifestyle influence a patient's preferred mode of communicating. This helps one understand what the patient understands. Currently, approximately one in five U.S. residents speaks a language other than English (Ashton, 2012).

Culture refers to the common lifestyles, languages, behavior patterns, traditions, and beliefs that are learned and passed from one generation to the next. The first step toward cultural competence requires becoming aware of your own personal cultural beliefs and identifying "prejudices or attitudes that could be a barrier to good communication" (Gerace & Salimbene, 2010). Likewise, understanding a patient's culture helps you understand nonverbal communication and deliver accurate nursing care to the patient and family. For example, women in some cultures might speak of personal things only to their spouses. For this reason, a maternal care nurse might talk with the patient's husband about the woman's postdelivery care.

The health care system is a culture with its own customs, values, and language. Patients with limited proficiency in English have difficulty understanding medical instructions and understanding test results and diagnoses. Try to remain aware of these cultural variations and be careful to use lay terminology when speaking with patients, unless you know that the patient is a health care professional. Use of medical terminology (e.g., myocardial infarction for heart attack, cerebrovascular accident for stroke [brain attack], or cholecystectomy for gallbladder operation) usually alienates patients and can inhibit further communication. A patient's language proficiency should be evaluated upon admission to a health care facility, and medical interpreters should be available to facilitate any communication and improve the quality of care (Ashton, 2012). The recent Joint Commission Standards for Patient-Centered Communication and criteria for accreditation are discussed in detail in Chapter 21.

Roles and Responsibilities

A person's occupation might give the nurse a general supposition of that individual's abilities, talents, interests, and economic status. Stereotyping a person according to occupation, however, can be misleading and should be avoided.

This can be particularly dangerous when nurses assume that patients who are health care professionals know everything about their condition and need little nursing assistance, teaching, and counseling. The challenge in the provision of care is to respect the patient's roles and responsibilities, especially because these influence their preferred manner of communicating, without denying the patient needed care. For example, a successful attorney might have a "take-charge" demeanor and seem utterly self-sufficient; a skilled nurse will note this but still provide an opening for the patient to verbalize his or her needs. "You seem well prepared for this procedure and in control, but I know that patients often have questions that never get answered or fears that remain unvoiced. Is there anything I can help you with while I'm here?" Similarly, be careful not to ignore an uncomplaining patient who never asks for anything, because the power differences in the health care professional–patient relationship may make communication intimidating.

Space and Territoriality

People are most comfortable in areas they consider their own. We generally feel relief when we come home, take our shoes and professional clothes off, and relax. This urge to maintain an exclusive right to certain space is termed territoriality. You might have already noticed that patients behave differently when being interviewed in their homes, at a health fair in the mall, or in an institutional setting. Similarly, health care professionals might behave differently when they are "on their own turf" in a health care setting compared to when they enter a patient's home as a guest caregiver. It is important to understand how territoriality influences the nurse–patient relationship.

The actual physical difference between the nurse and patient during interaction is also important. *Proxemics* is the study of distance zones between people during communication (Videbeck, 2011). Each person has a sense of how much personal or private space is needed and what distance between people is optimum. Figure 20-3 (on page 456) demonstrates the four communication zones. Activities that are likely to occur during each of these zones include:

- Intimate zone: interaction between parents and children or people who desire close personal contact
- Personal zone: distance when interacting with close friends
- Social zone: space when interacting with acquaintances such as in a work or social setting
- Public zone: communication when speaking to an audience or small groups

Some aspects of communication zones are dictated through culture, and some are idiosyncratic. Anywhere from 18 inches to 4 feet might be optimal distance to sit from a patient during an intake interview. For example, European Americans and African Americans require more personal space between two people who are speaking than other cultures (Mediterranean, Hispanic, Asian, Middle Eastern, East Indian) who are comfortable at a closer distance when speaking (Videbeck, 2011). People in the United States usually

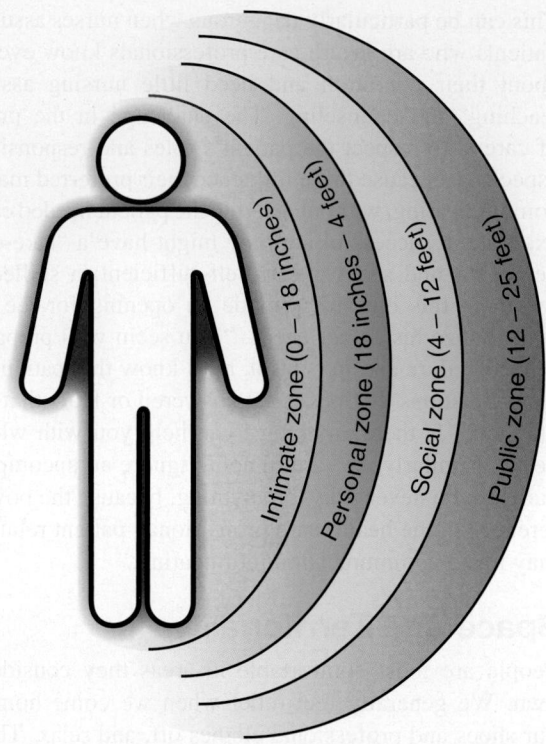

Intimate zone (0 – 18 inches)

Personal zone (18 inches – 4 feet)

Social zone (4 – 12 feet)

Public zone (12 – 25 feet)

FIGURE 20-3. These four distance zones around the body are recognized as personal territories.

are comfortable standing about 3 feet away from each other when speaking (Pagana, 2011b). It is best to take cues from patients, noting whether they are moving backward from you if you are too near or leaning forward to get closer to you. Because many nursing interventions place one in proximity to a patient and entail forced intimacy, be sensitive to how offensive this might be to certain patients who are accustomed to large areas of private space. Develop the habit of seeking the patient's permission before touching areas within

a patient's private zones. Although most people consider their hands, arms, shoulders, and back within a social zone, increasing levels of privacy are according to (1) mouth and feet; (2) face, neck, and front of body; and (3) genitalia.

Physical, Mental, and Emotional State

The degree to which people are physically comfortable and mentally and emotionally free to engage in interactions also influences communication. A full bladder, a dull headache, crushing chest pain, anxiety about a pending diagnosis or concern about what is happening at home or at work, and fear can all negatively influence communication. For example, patients who think that a nurse wants to hurt them will be difficult to interview. Be sensitive to the patient's physical, mental, and emotional barriers to effective communication.

Cognitively impaired patients present special communication challenges. For example, an older patient who has aphasia and is agitated due to pain from an abscessed tooth might be unable to communicate with the nurse.

The accompanying box, Examples of Nursing Interventions and Nursing Outcomes Classifications (NIC/NOC), suggests helpful cognitive stimulation activities and expected outcomes when communicating with these patients.

 REMEMBER Irwina Russellinski, the 75-year-old woman who was described as "being pleasantly confused" at times and requiring a nursing assessment. The patient's level of confusion presents challenges for the nurse when eliciting information for the nursing history. This challenge could be further complicated by the patient's difficulty speaking English. The nurse needs to speak clearly, distinctly, and in terms that the patient understands. In addition, the nurse needs to allow ample time for the patient to respond and explore other sources for needed information. ●

EXAMPLES OF NURSING INTERVENTIONS AND NURSING OUTCOMES CLASSIFICATIONS (NIC/NOC)

COGNITIVE STIMULATION AND COGNITIVE ORIENTATION

Nursing Interventions	**Nursing Outcomes**

• Consult with family to establish patient's cognitive baseline.
• Inform patient of recent nonthreatening news events.
• Offer environmental stimulation through contact with varied personnel.
• Provide a calendar.
• Orient to time, place, and person.
• Provide planned sensory stimulation.
• Use television, radio, or music as part of planned stimuli program.
• Reinforce or repeat information.
• Present change gradually.
• Talk to patient.
	• Cognitive Orientation
	  • Identifies significant current events.
	  • Identifies self.
	  • Identifies significant other.
	  • Identifies current place.
	  • Identifies correct day.
	  • Identifies correct month.
	  • Identifies correct year.

Bulechek, G., Butcher, H., Dochterman, J., & Wagner, C. (2013). *Nursing interventions classification (NIC)* (6th ed., p. 125). St. Louis: Elsevier/Mosby. A full listing of nursing activities for each nursing intervention can be found in this book.
Moorhead, S., Johnson, M., Maas, M., & Swanson, E. (2013). *Nursing outcomes classification (NOC)* (5th ed., p. 157). St. Louis: Elsevier/Mosby. A full listing of indicators for each nursing outcome can be found in this book.

Values

Communication is influenced by the way people value themselves, one another, and the purpose of any human interaction. Nurses who believe that teaching is an important aspect of nursing and who value empowering patients will communicate this to patients. Conversely, a nurse who believes teaching is an unimportant chore is unlikely to be an effective teacher. Similarly, the patient's motivation (or lack of motivation) to develop new self-care behaviors cannot help but influence nurse–patient communication.

Environment

Communication happens best when the environment facilitates an easy exchange of needed information. The environment most conducive to communication is one that is calm and nonthreatening. The goal is to minimize distractions and ensure privacy. The use of music, art, and interior decorations might help put the patient at ease. A patient with newly diagnosed human immunodeficiency virus (HIV) infection will find it difficult to discuss sexual history or genital warts in an area that lacks privacy. A toddler might find it easier to communicate if a parent, favorite stuffed animal, or blanket is nearby.

USING THERAPEUTIC COMMUNICATION IN THE NURSING PROCESS

The ability to communicate with patients and other nurses is essential for effective use of the nursing process. Knowledge of the communication process and effective communication techniques is fundamental to all steps of the nursing process. At the same time, the nursing process provides the guidance and direction needed to communicate with patients clearly, effectively, and compassionately.

Assessing

The major focus of assessment is to gather information in both verbal and nonverbal communication forms. Before the assessment, the nurse should determine if the patient needs any assistive devices in order to communicate effectively and understand conversations (e.g., hearing aid, glasses, etc.). Identify the patient's preferred language and secure an interpreter if one is needed. Assessment is also the appropriate time to ascertain from the patient if there are any additional challenges such as understanding health care information and participating in treatment (Bombard, 2012).

The written word is used to obtain patient data and when reading patients' records or charts before meeting them. The spoken word is used to give and to receive reports to and from other health personnel. This is commonplace when admitting a patient to a hospital unit or before visiting the patient at home. One-to-one communication is used with patients to obtain thorough nursing histories and physical examinations. Effective communication techniques, as well as observational skills, are used extensively during this phase. The data collected verbally and nonverbally are analyzed and then passed on to the appropriate people through oral and written communication.

Diagnosing

Following the formulation of the nursing diagnoses, the nurse communicates findings to other nursing professionals through the use of the written and spoken word. The written diagnosis becomes a permanent part of the patient's record.

Outcome Identification and Planning

The planning step requires communication among the patient, nurse, and other team members as mutually agreed-upon outcomes are developed and interventions are determined. Because a nurse is rarely able to implement all parts of a plan alone, oral and written communication is needed to inform others of what needs to be done to meet the set objectives or goals. The formal written plan of care is a form of communication. Without communication, the nursing plan could not be implemented.

Implementing

Nurses assume many roles when they implement the plan of care. Verbal and nonverbal communication enhance basic caregiving measures and are used to teach, counsel, and support patients and their families during the implementation phase. Even a simple nursing order, such as "encourage patient to drink 100 mL of fluid every hour while awake," requires countless messages to be sent and received between the nurse and the patient. The nurse explains the importance of an adequate fluid intake, along with the amount and frequency of intake. The patient, in turn, speaks of his or her ability or inability to meet targeted objectives. The patient's verbal and nonverbal messages are assessed during each nurse–patient interaction. The implementation of the plan of care is then documented in the patient's record.

Evaluating

Nurses often rely on verbal and nonverbal cues from patients to verify whether patient objectives or goals have been achieved. Communication, through the exchange of positive and negative messages between the nurse and the patient, also facilitates the revision of parts of the care plan.

Documenting Communication

Continual assessment of the patient's needs and conditions requires accurate documentation in the appropriate place. This documentation helps promote the continuity of care given by nurses and other health care providers. Because one nurse cannot provide 24-hour coverage for patients, significant information must be passed on to others through nursing progress notes and care plans. Documentation and the use of electronic communication are discussed in detail in Chapter 16.

Using Hand-off Communication: SBAR Technique

Hand-off communication involves the process of accurate presentation and acceptance of patient-related information from one caregiver or team to another caregiver or team using effective communication. It is estimated that 80% of serious medical errors occur due to miscommunication between caregivers when patients are handed off or transferred, and at least one-third of all patient hand-offs are problematic (Joint Commission Center for Transforming Healthcare, 2012; Jukkala, James, Autrey, Azuero, & Millner, 2012). Hand-off communication can occur with other hospital departments, nurse-to-nurse report, or nurse-to-physician discussions. In an effort to eliminate breakdowns in communication and potential adverse events, the Joint Commission (TJC) includes a goal to improve the effectiveness of communication among caregivers as a National Patient Safety Goal. Both TJC and the Institute for Healthcare Improvement (IHI) have recommended using SBAR reports to improve hand-off communication. **SBAR**, which stands for **S**ituation, **B**ackground, **A**ssessment, and **R**ecommendations, provides a consistent method for hand-off communication that is clear, structured, and easy to use. This technique was originally developed by the U.S. Navy to accurately transmit critical information and initially adapted by Kaiser Permanente of Colorado to facilitate nurse and physician communication. The S (Situation) and B (Background) provide objective data, whereas the A (Assessment) and R (Recommendations) allow for presentation of subjective information. The SBAR format is widely used in health care and can be modified to meet the specific situations related to shift reports, conversations with physicians, and transfers of patients. Wentworth et al. (2012) concluded in their research that an electronic SBAR tool was effective for hand-off communication for noncomplicated routine patients. Figure 20-4 provides an example of a basic SBAR communication tool used between a nurse and physician. SBAR is also discussed in Chapters 9, 13, and 16.

The QSEN Institute revised the standard SBAR form to include an initial identification of yourself and the patient (I) and the opportunity to ask and respond to questions or readback (R) at the close of the communication (QSEN Institute, 2008). This reformulated I-SBAR-R allows a nurse to clearly introduce oneself and the patient when communicating with a caregiver during patient hand-offs or conversations with physicians. Many health care institutions are using this revised I-SBAR-R format.

The Joint Commission Center for Transforming Healthcare has developed a Targeted Solutions Tool™ (TST) that measures the effectiveness of hand-off communication in Joint Commission–accredited institutions and suggests

proven effective solutions (Joint Commission for Transforming Healthcare, 2013). This application involves an accurate measurement of an organization's hand-off communication, identification of any barriers occurring during communication, and solutions that are targeted to the specific institution. Using SBAR or another hand-off tool enables nurses to communicate in a collegial, collaborative manner with the focus on patient safety.

USING THERAPEUTIC COMMUNICATION IN THE HELPING RELATIONSHIP

Nurses and other health care personnel enter health care in order to help people. Relationships between health care providers and patients do not develop but occur through purposeful communication. A **helping relationship** exists among people who provide and receive assistance in meeting human needs. It sets the climate for the participants to move towards common goals. Therefore, the patient's needs are met as the result of a successful helping relationship. In this book, the term *helping relationship* is used to refer to such relationships between nurses and patients (Fig. 20-5).

When a nurse and patient are involved in a helping relationship, sometimes called the nurse–patient relationship, the nurse is the helper and the patient is the person being helped. The quality of the relationship between these individuals is the most significant element in determining helping effectiveness. "Of all the problems that can arise in nursing care, perhaps the most common is failure to establish rapport and a helping–trust relationship with the other person" (Watson, 1985, p. 24). Communication is the means used to establish rapport and helping–trust relationships.

A Helping Relationship Versus a Social Relationship

The difference between a helping relationship and a friendship is important. Helping relationships contain many of the

FIGURE 20-5. A helping relationship between the nurse and patient sets the climate for participants to move toward common goals.

S

SITUATION

I am calling about _____

The patient's Code status is: _____

The problem I am calling about is: _____

(e.g. I AM CONCERNED THE PATIENT IS GOING TO ARREST)

I have just assessed the patient personally:

Vital signs are: Blood Pressure_____/_____, Pulse_____,

Respiration_____, and temperature_____

I am concerned about the:

Blood pressure because it is	over 200 or	less than 100 or	30 mmHg below usual
Pulse because it is	over 130 or	less than 40 and smptomatic	
Respiration because it is	less than 8 or	over 30	
Temperature because it is	less than 96 or	over 104	
Urine output because it is	less than 25ml/hr or 200 ml/8hrs		
O_2 saturation because it is	less than 88% on 6/liters nasal cannula		
Other: _____			

B

BACKGROUND

The patient's mental status is:

Alert and oriented to person, place, and time

Confused and cooperative or non-cooperative

Agitated or combative

Lethargic but conversant and able to swallow

Stuporous and not talking clearly and possibly not able to swallow

Comatose Eyes closed Not responding to stimulation.

The skin is:

Warm and dry

Pale

Mottled

Diaphoretic

Extremities are cold

Extremities are warm

The patient is not or is on oxygen.

The patient has been on _____ (l/min) or (5) oxygen for _____ minutes (hours)

The oximeter is reading _____ %

The oximeter does not detect a good pulse and is giving erratic readings.

A

ASSESSMENT

This is what I think the problem is: _____

"SAY WHAT YOU THINK IS THE PROBLEM"

The problem seems to be cardiac infection neurologic respiratory

I am not sure what the problem is but the patient is deteriorating.

The patient seems to be unstable and may get worse, we need to do something.

R

RECOMMENDATION

From Physician _____

Transfer the patient to Critical Care

Come to see the patient at this time

Talk to the patient or family about Code status

Ask a consultant to see patient now.

Are any tests needed:

Do you need any tests like CXR ABG EKG CBC BMP

Others:_____

If a change in treatment is ordered then ask:

How often do you want vital signs?

How long do you expect this problem will last?

If the patient does not get better when would you want us to call again?

FIGURE 20-4. Sample SBAR Communication Tool. (Reprinted with permission from the Institute for Healthcare Improvement. Available at http://www.ihi.org/knowledge/Pages/Tools/SampleSBARCommunicationTool.aspx)

qualities of a social relationship—they have in common the components of care, concern, trust, and growth. They are also very different:

- The helping relationship does not occur spontaneously, as do most social relationships. It occurs for a specific purpose with a specific person.
- The helping relationship is characterized by an unequal sharing of information. The patient shares information related to personal health problems, whereas the nurse shares information in terms of a professional role. In a friendship, information sharing is more likely to be similar in quantity and type.
- The helping relationship is built on the patient's needs, not on those of the helping person. In a friendship, needs of both participants are generally considered. A friendship might grow out of a helping relationship, but this is separate from the purposeful, time-limited interaction described as a helping relationship.

It is of great importance to remember that helping relations are professional relationships. It can be helpful to identify nurse models who, through their appearance, demeanor, and behavior, communicate a clear sense of **professionalism** or confidence and expertise in their practice. Patients and the public are more likely to trust and value nurses who appear competent and confident and who are focused on the patients entrusted to their care. Rudeness, sloppiness, inattention to person, sexually inappropriate behavior, and other breaches of professionalism undermine nursing's professional image and the effectiveness of individual nurses.

 THINK back to Mr. Gordon, the patient described in the Reflective Practice display, and consider the behavior of the nurse and residents caring for the patient. Unfortunately, their focus was not on the patient as a whole but rather on the patient's devices and technologic equipment. The nurse needs to keep in mind the highly technical nature of the intensive care unit and work to implement a plan of care that focuses on the "whole" patient. ●

Characteristics of the Helping Relationship

The helping relationship is intangible and, therefore, difficult to describe. Most authorities agree, however, that it has at least the following three basic characteristics:

- It is dynamic. Both the person providing the assistance and the person being helped are active participants to the extent each is able.
- It is purposeful and time limited. This means there are specific goals that are intended to be met within a certain period.
- Although both parties in the helping relationship have responsibilities, the person providing the assistance is professionally accountable for the outcomes of the relationship and the means used to attain them. Helping persons should present their helping abilities as honestly as possible and not promise to provide more assistance than they can offer.

Goals of the Helping Relationship

The goals of a helping relationship between a nurse and a patient are determined cooperatively and are defined in terms of the patient's needs. Broadly speaking, common goals might include increased independence for the patient, greater feelings of worth, and improved health and well-being. Selected nursing interventions will help the person move toward the goal. As the patient's needs and goals change, so do the nursing care interventions implemented to attain the patient's goals. You might also have many needs to be met, but in the helping relationship between the nurse and the patient, those are temporarily set aside—the focus is on the patient's needs.

Phases of the Helping Relationship

The helping relationship is ordinarily described as having three phases: (1) the orientation phase, (2) the working phase, and (3) the termination phase. In the helping relationship, the communication process follows the sequence of the nursing process. Both processes are continuous and reciprocal. Box 20-3 summarizes goals for patients during the three phases of an effective helping relationship. In some situations, one nurse initiates the helping relationship and works with the patient and family through to termination. More often (e.g., in hospital settings), different nurses at different times are implementing different phases of the relationship. In preparation for the orientation phase, you might use interpersonal communication to prepare for the data-gathering phase of the interaction with the patient.

BOX 20-3 | **SUMMARY OF PATIENT GOALS FOR THE THREE PHASES OF THE HELPING RELATIONSHIP**

Orientation Phase
- The patient will call the nurse by name.
- The patient will accurately describe the roles of the participants in the relationship.
- The patient and nurse will establish an agreement about:
  - Goals of the relationship
  - Location, frequency, and length of the contacts
  - Duration of the relationship

Working Phase
- The patient will actively participate in the relationship.
- The patient will cooperate in activities that work toward achieving mutually acceptable goals.
- The patient will express feelings and concerns to the nurse.

Termination
- The patient will participate in identifying the goals accomplished or the progress made toward goals.
- The patient will verbalize feelings about the termination of the relationship.

Orientation Phase

The helping relationship ideally begins between the nurse and patient during the data-gathering part of the nursing process. It can also be initiated at other times during the nurse–patient relationship. In the orientation phase, the tone and guidelines for the relationship are established. You and the patient meet and learn to identify each other by name. It is especially important to introduce yourself to the patient; it might even be helpful to write your name for the patient. Failure to do so might result in the patient becoming confused and mistrustful because of the number of caregivers with whom most patients come in contact.

The following activities generally occur during the orientation phase of the helping relationship:

- The roles of both people in the relationship are clarified.
- An agreement or contract about the relationship is established. The agreement is usually a simple verbal exchange related to goals and the means of achieving them or occasionally a written document, especially if the relationship extends over a long period of time.
- The patient is provided with an orientation to the health care facility, its services, admission routines, and any pertinent information the patient requires to decrease anxiety. This orientation should be identified as one of the goals in the nurse–patient helping relationship.

The development of a trusting relationship is critical to the development of the nurse–patient relationship. Exhibiting openness and interest in the concerns of the patient paves the way for developing trust and communicating care and respect.

Working Phase

The working phase is usually the longest phase of the helping relationship. During this phase, the nurse works together with the patient to meet the patient's physical and psychosocial needs. Interaction is the essence of the working phase. Nurse–patient interactions that occur at this time are purposeful in that they are designed to ensure achievement of health goals or objectives that were mutually agreed upon.

In addition, the nurse as caregiver provides the patient with whatever assistance might be needed to perform activities of daily living. For example, if a patient with impaired mobility is unable to get out of bed except to use a bedside commode, the nurse or caregiver needs to help with daily hygiene.

The nursing roles of teacher and counselor (see Chapter 21) are performed primarily during this phase. These roles involve motivating the patient to learn and to implement health-promotion activities, to facilitate the patient's ability to execute the plan of care, and to express feelings about health problems, nursing care, any progress or setbacks, and any other areas of concern. This is where your interpersonal skills are used to their fullest (see the discussions of interpersonal skills and effective communication techniques later in this chapter). A breakdown of the helping relationship on one of these levels could result in serious consequences.

Satisfactory interaction preserves people's integrity while promoting an atmosphere characterized by minimal fear, anxiety, distrust, and tension. People feel harmonious and contented with each other as they work cooperatively to reach common goals.

Termination Phase

The termination phase occurs when the conclusion of the initial agreement is acknowledged. This might happen at change-of-shift time, when the patient is discharged, or when a nurse leaves on vacation or for employment elsewhere. At this point, you'll examine with the patient the goals of the helping relationship for indications of their attainment or for evidence of progress toward them. If the goals/outcomes have been reached, this fact should be acknowledged. Such acknowledgment generally results in a feeling of satisfaction for the patient and nurse. If the goals/outcomes have not been reached, the progress can be acknowledged and either the patient or you might make suggestions for future efforts.

Ordinarily, emotions are associated with the termination of a helping relationship. If the goals have been met, there is often regret about ending a satisfying relationship, even though a sense of accomplishment persists. If the goals have not been achieved, the patient might experience anxiety and fear about the future. Whatever the feelings, patients should be encouraged to express their emotions about the termination.

You can prepare for the termination of the helping relationship in various ways. It is thoughtful to set the stage for the patient to establish a helping relationship with another nurse, if appropriate. You can also assist the patient transferring from one agency to another or from one unit in an agency to another by offering explanations concerning the transfer. In some instances, you might introduce the patient to personnel who will be giving care.

Interpersonal relations are discussed in greater detail in the classic works of nursing theorists Orlando (1961), Paterson and Zderad (1976), Peplau (1952), Travelbee (1971), and Watson (1985).

Factors Promoting Effective Communication Within the Helping Relationship

Despite the fact that patient stays in health care facilities are shorter than in the past and there is now an increased reliance on technology, therapeutic communication with patients and their families is essential and remains a vital part of a helping relationship. Nurses who are competent, honest, skilled communicators are viewed as effective and compassionate caregivers. This focus on helping relationships is a critical component of what nurses do and plays a vital role in promoting healing, enhancing safety, and improving clinical outcomes.

Dispositional Traits

A dispositional trait is a characteristic or customary way of behaving. Nurses who consistently demonstrate warmth and friendliness; openness and rapport; empathy, honesty, authenticity and trust; caring; and competence are well disposed to communicate effectively.

WARMTH AND FRIENDLINESS

The helping relationship depends on the nurse's ability to begin the orientation phase successfully. A pleasant greeting and friendly smile can facilitate this phase and place the patient at ease. By maintaining qualities of warmth and friendliness throughout the helping relationship, you will convey continuous acceptance of the patient and interest in discussing the patient's feelings and concern.

OPENNESS AND RESPECT

One key factor to effective communication is to be open, accepting, frank, respectful, and without prejudice. Patients who feel that a nurse is being judgmental might withhold

significant information. You need to develop sensitivity to the unique challenges presented by each patient. Attention to patient variables that might influence the process of communicating (e.g., gender, developmental level, culture, life experience) can make the difference between effective and ineffective interactions. Box 20-4 highlights guidelines for relating to patients from different cultures (see also Chapter 5).

EMPATHY

Empathy is identifying with the way another person feels. An empathic nurse is sensitive to the patient's feelings and problems, but remains objective enough to help the patient work to attain positive outcomes. By retaining this quality, you can establish successful helping relationships without appearing cold or stern. Sympathy differs from empathy because it shifts the emphasis from the patient to the nurse

---

BOX 20-4   RELATING TO PATIENTS FROM DIFFERENT CULTURES

Assess your personal beliefs surrounding people from different cultures.

- Review your personal beliefs and past experiences.
- Set aside any values, biases, ideas, and attitudes that are judgmental and may negatively affect care.

Assess communication variables from a cultural perspective.

- Determine the ethnic identity of the patient, including generation in America.
- Use the patient as a source of information when possible.
- Assess cultural factors that may affect your relationship with the patient and respond appropriately.

Plan care based on the communicated needs and cultural background.

- Learn as much as possible about the patient's cultural customs and beliefs.
- Encourage the patient to reveal cultural interpretation of health, illness, and health care.
- Be sensitive to the uniqueness of the patient.
- Identify sources of discrepancy between the patient's and your own concepts of health and illness.
- Communicate at the patient's personal level of functioning.
- Evaluate effectiveness of nursing actions and modify nursing care plan when necessary.

Modify communication approaches to meet cultural needs.

- Be attentive to signs of fear, anxiety, and confusion in the patient.
- Respond in a reassuring manner in keeping with the patient's cultural orientation.
- Be aware that in some cultural groups, discussion concerning the patient with others may be offensive and may impede the nursing process.

Understand that respect for the patient and communicated needs is central to the therapeutic relationship.

- Communicate respect by using a kind and attentive approach.
- Learn how listening is communicated in the patient's culture.

- Use appropriate active listening techniques.
- Adopt an attitude of flexibility, respect, and interest to help bridge barriers imposed by culture.

Communicate in a nonthreatening manner.

- Conduct the interview in an unhurried manner.
- Follow acceptable social and cultural amenities.
- Ask general questions during the information-gathering stage.
- Be patient with a respondent who gives information that may seem unrelated to the patient's health problem.
- Develop a trusting relationship by listening carefully, allowing time, and giving the patient your full attention.

Use validating techniques in communication.

- Be alert for feedback that the patient is not understanding.
- Do not assume meaning is interpreted without distortion.

Be considerate of reluctance to talk when the subject involves sexual matters.

- Be aware that in some cultures, sexual matters are not discussed freely with members of the opposite sex.

Adopt special approaches when the patient speaks a different language.

- Use a caring tone of voice and facial expression to help alleviate the patient's fears.
- Speak slowly and distinctly, but not loudly.
- Use gestures, pictures, and play acting to help the patient understand.
- Repeat the message in different ways if necessary.
- Be alert to words the patient seems to understand and use them frequently.
- Keep messages simple and repeat them frequently.
- Avoid using medical terms and abbreviations that the patient may not understand.
- Use an appropriate language dictionary.

Use interpreters to improve communication.

- Ask the interpreter to translate the message, not just the individual words.
- Obtain feedback to confirm understanding.
- Use an interpreter who is culturally sensitive.

Used with permission from Gieger, J. N., & Davidhizar, R. E. (2008). *Transcultural nursing: Assessment and intervention* (5th ed.). St. Louis: Elsevier/Mosby.

as the nurse shares feelings and personal concerns and projects them onto the patient, limiting ability to focus objectively on the patient's needs (Videbeck, 2011). For example, although it is understandable for team members to become impatient with family members who never seem satisfied with the care their loved one is receiving, it helps to empathize with the family who might be feeling frightened and helpless. "This must be a hard time for you...how are you coping?" "Is there any way I can be of help?" When the patient and family sense that you have some idea of what they are experiencing and that you are committed to helping, the basis is set for a trusting therapeutic relationship.

HONESTY, AUTHENTICITY, AND TRUST

Patients should be able to trust that nurses are who they say they are (professional helpers), and that they can be trusted to do everything within their level of expertise to secure the resources and to help meet the patient needs.

CARING

Patients quickly sense whether they are merely a "task to be performed" (task-centered caring), or a person of worth who is both cared about and cared for (relation-centered caring). Expert nurses know how to communicate genuine caring the minute they step into a patient's space by how they look at and touch the patient and what they say and do. Patients who feel cared for will feel accepted.

 THINK back to Susie Musashi, the 3-year-old child with burns. How the nurse approaches the child will set the stage for the interaction. Consider how the child would respond to a nurse who enters the room and scolds the child for crying as compared to the nurse who enters the room and approaches the child's bed, touching the child's shoulder or hand gently and softly. The message conveyed by the second action would be much more caring. ●

COMPETENCE

Competent nurses are skilled in all aspects of basic nursing and can meet their patients' health care needs through their technical, cognitive, interpersonal, and ethical/legal skills. Take responsibility for evaluating your own strengths and weaknesses so that your patients will receive optimal care. Consequently, your patients will develop trust in and respect for you as their nurse, facilitating helping relationships and good communication.

Rapport Builders

Rapport, a feeling of mutual trust experienced by people in a satisfactory relationship (Fig. 20-6), facilitates open communication. Good rapport can be achieved by paying attention to the following variables.

SPECIFIC OBJECTIVES

Having a purpose for an interaction provides guidance toward achieving a meaningful encounter with the patient. One objective might be to perform a head-to-toe physical

FIGURE 20-6. Rapport between the nurse and the patient/family is a necessary first step in planning care.

assessment when greeting the patient and at the beginning of each shift. Another objective might be the discussion of a patient's feelings about being newly diagnosed with diabetes. The shortest encounter with a patient can have an objective, even if it is as simple as conveying a feeling of friendliness. Be flexible at all times, and follow the patient's cues to work toward meeting all needs.

COMFORTABLE ENVIRONMENT

A comfortable environment, in which both the patient and the nurse are at ease, helps to promote interactions. Suitable furniture, proper lighting, and a moderate temperature are important. Also, effective relationships are enhanced when the atmosphere is relaxed and unhurried. If you seem preoccupied and on the run, or if the patient is ill at ease for fear of missing visitors or because of another commitment, communication is impaired.

PRIVACY

It might not always be possible to carry on conversations alone with the patient in a room, but every effort should be made to provide privacy and to prevent conversations from being overheard by others. Sometimes merely drawing the curtains around the bed in a hospital or long-term care facility or sitting in a corner of the waiting room or lounge can provide the sense of privacy that is so important in most interactions. Home visits might need to be timed to ensure the privacy the patient desires and needs.

CONFIDENTIALITY

The confidentiality with which patient information is to be treated should be established with the patient. Indicate with whom the information that the patient gives will be shared. The patient should know about the right to specify who might have access to the information. Failure to consider this factor can be considered a breach of the patient's right to privacy. See Chapter 16 for guidelines concerning patient confidentiality.

PATIENT VERSUS TASK FOCUS

Communication in the nurse–patient relationship should focus on the patient and patient needs, not on the nurse or an activity in which the nurse is engaged (see the accompanying box: Through the Eyes of a Patient). Consider the following example, in which the nurse's comment focuses on the patient and the patient needs:

Patient: I don't know why these injections scare me, but they do.

Nurse: You are afraid of these injections?

In contrast, consider this example, in which the nurse's comment focuses instead on the nursing activity:

Patient: I don't know why these injections scare me, but they do.

Nurse: I give hundreds of injections. Don't be so immature.

USING NURSING OBSERVATIONS

Observations, which involve both seeing and interpreting, are especially useful for validating information. For example, a nurse suspects that a patient is afraid to hear the results of certain blood tests, but the patient insists that the results are unimportant. The nurse then observes the patient pacing in the corridor, apparently deep in thought. Observing the patient's behavior helps validate the nurse's suspicion that the patient is fearful and the patient's assertion of being unconcerned appears to be a cover-up for truer feelings.

Observation serves several important purposes:

* It helps increase awareness of a patient's nonverbal messages.
* It is the primary source of information when a patient is unwilling or unable to communicate verbally.
* It demonstrates caring and interest in the patient. (Patients often recognize when a nurse is unobservant and, rightly or wrongly, usually conclude that the nurse does not care about them.)

OPTIMAL PACING

Consider the pace of any conversation or encounter with a patient. For instance, it would be ineffective to rush through a list of questions when obtaining a nursing history; it is more effective to let the patient set the pace. Let the patient

know at the beginning of the interaction if time is limited so that the patient does not feel that you are rushing because of a lack of concern or personal interest.

DEVELOPING THERAPEUTIC COMMUNICATION SKILLS

Although humans communicate during virtually all waking moments, the therapeutic use of communication requires training and practice. Box 20-5 contrasts therapeutic and nontherapeutic communication. Nursing students might feel awkward when first trying to develop therapeutic relationships. Practice makes perfect, however, and you will soon feel at ease if you work on developing the following communication skills.

Conversation Skills

Conversation, or the exchange of verbal communication, is a social interaction. As social beings, humans learn as children how to converse with others; nursing students, therefore, have already had years of experience communicating verbally. However, you can improve your communications with patients and achieve a more effective helping relationship in the following ways:

* Control the tone of your voice so that you are conveying exactly what you mean to say and not a hidden message. Your tone should indicate interest rather than boredom, patience rather than anger, acceptance rather than hostility, and so forth.
* Be knowledgeable about the topic of conversation and have accurate information. When possible, be familiar with the subject of conversation before discussing it with the patient. If the topic is unfamiliar to you (e.g., the availability of community resources for family caregivers of patients with special needs), admit that to the patient and family and direct them to other resources. Convey confidence and honesty to the patient.
* Be flexible. You might want to discuss a certain subject but learn that the patient wishes to discuss something else.

THROUGH THE EYES OF A PATIENT

I know you come to clinical every day with your head full of all the important things you need to do for me. Probably you worry about whether or not you will remember the steps to both simple and complex procedures and fear that you will never get everything done in the time allotted. I'm sure that there are many things that your clinical instructor will use as a basis for your evaluation and perhaps other things that are important to you for your self-evaluation. But I thought you might like to know what's important to me. Most of what I've listed are simple things that you can communicate each time you walk into my home or room.*

* Really listen to me.
* Ask me what I think.
* Don't dismiss my concerns.
* Don't treat me like a disease, treat me like a person.

* Talk *to* me, not *at* me.
* Respect my privacy.
* Don't keep me waiting.
* Don't tell me what to do without telling me how to do it.
* Keep me informed.
* Remember who I used to be.
* Let me know you care.

Thanks for giving me this chance to share with you what matters to me.

---

*The list of nursing interventions that are valued highly by patients was compiled by Roberta Messner after a review of many patient satisfaction studies. These are cited in Messner, R. L. (1993). What patients really want from their nurses. *American Journal of Nursing, 93*(8), 38–41.

BOX 20-5 | THERAPEUTIC VERSUS NONTHERAPEUTIC COMMUNICATION

Patient Scenario

Mr. Commens is a 65-year-old divorced man who lives alone. His grown children are married and live out of town. He was recently diagnosed with cancer of the colon and underwent a colon resection. He is now home recuperating and has received a new diagnosis. The home health care nurse is scheduled to visit Mr. Commens.

Nontherapeutic Communication

Nurse: Hello, Mr. Commens! I'm glad you're home. I only have 30 minutes to visit with you. It's been a very busy day.

Mr. Commens: I'm sorry you are having a bad day. I have been to the doctor and I'm very concerned about the report I received.

Nurse: Yes, I've had a busy day but not a bad day. I guess your day has been busy too. What report are you talking about?

Mr. Commens: Well, I need more tests because they think the cancer has spread.

Nurse: Now, who told you that? Maybe the test was wrong or you misunderstood the physician. Mr. Commens, I'll call your physician. Is there anything else bothering you?

Mr. Commens: No.

Nurse: I'll call your doctor and then call you tomorrow.

In this scenario, the nurse seems unconcerned about Mr. Commens' test results and gives him the idea the nurse does not believe the information he has relayed. The nurse is more concerned about his or her own busy day and less concerned about the patient.

Therapeutic Communication

Nurse: Hello, Mr. Commens! I'm sorry I am running a little behind schedule. Now that I'm here, we will have as much time as we need to discuss how you're feeling and your visit to the physician. How are you feeling?

Mr. Commens: (His eyes are cast down to the floor and he is wringing his hands.) Well, I feel all right. I've had some pain in my right side.

Nurse: Mr. Commens, how would you rate your pain on a scale of 1 to 10?

Mr. Commens: About an 8.

Nurse: Mr. Commens, you seem concerned and a little preoccupied. Is there something bothering you?

Mr. Commens: Yes, I suppose there is. My doctor said my cancer has spread to my hip. I guess that's why I have pain in my right side. I have so many decisions to make and I'm very confused. The doctor said I need to start chemotherapy. I don't even know how I'll get there. My family is out of town.

Nurse: Mr. Commens, would it help if I spoke to your physician to obtain specific details about your treatment plan? This would then assist me in obtaining some help when you begin your chemotherapy.

Mr. Commens: That would be wonderful! If you call the doctor, then you can explain everything to me, and maybe it will help me to understand what I'll be going through. Also, it might help me in making decisions about my treatments.

Nurse: Mr. Commens, would you then like me to be here when you call your children about your diagnosis and treatment plan? I might be able to answer some of the questions they might have about your treatments.

Mr. Commens: That would be wonderful. I feel so much more relaxed knowing you are going to help me. Thank you so much.

Nurse: Mr. Commens, I'll call your physician and clarify the information you have received, and I'll be back at 5 PM. Maybe at that time, we can call your family.

Mr. Commens: That sounds like a good plan, but we might need to call my children at 6 PM.

Nurse: That's just fine. I will be back at 5 PM to discuss the information I have, and we will call your children at 6 PM.

Interpretation

The first example of communication focuses on the nurse's needs, not the patient's needs. Most of the interaction in the first scenario blocks the communication process. The second example allows the patient to verbalize his concerns and his lack of decision making. The nurse provides the patient with broad opening statements and patient goals to assist in his planning and decision making.

It is better to follow the patient's lead whenever possible; in due time, you can return to the subject. For example, you arrive at the patient's bedside to administer a medication, but the patient begins to talk about diet issues. It is better to take a little time to talk about the patient's interest than to insist on talking about only the procedure at hand, as long as there is enough time for the conversation.

• Be clear and concise, and make statements as simple as possible. Patients are often anxious and fail to understand the message unless the patient understands the language used. Stay on one subject at a time. This helps prevent confusion.

• Avoid words that might have different interpretations. The study of the meaning of words is called **semantics**. Even when two people speak the same language, some words—such as love, hate, freedom, and health—might have different meanings to different people.

• Be truthful. A patient who is given false information will soon distrust the nurse. If you're not sure about something, admit you don't know and seek an answer rather than make a comment that may be an error.

• Keep an open mind. An attitude of "I know better than the patient" is quickly discerned by the patient. Patients can make valuable contributions to their own health care.

• Take advantage of available opportunities. During most caregiving situations, you can facilitate conversation that makes even the most routine task meaningful. For instance, when giving a bed bath to a patient, ask about the patient's employment. This would allow the patient to verbalize any positive or negative feelings about the job and being temporarily absent from it, reducing the anxiety that often occurs with the loss of work. It is often comforting to know that someone understands and cares.

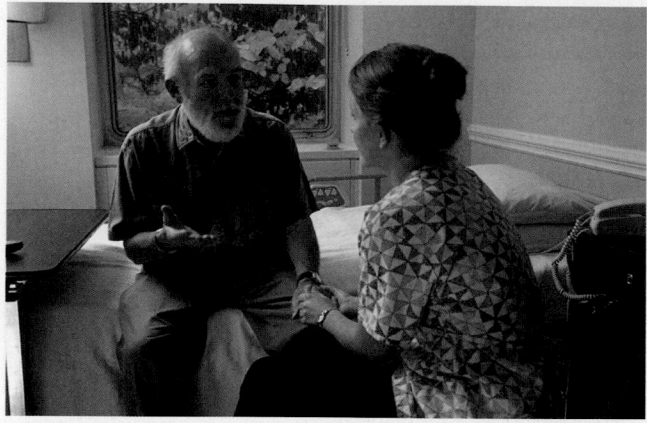

FIGURE 20-7. Listening attentively, with concentration and genuine concern, is key to productive communication.

Listening Skills

Listening is a skill that involves both hearing and interpreting what the other says. It requires attention and concentration to sort out, evaluate, and validate clues to better understand the true meaning of what is being said (Fig. 20-7). The accompanying box, Through the Eyes of a Student, relates one student's experience with attentive listening. The following techniques are recommended to improve listening skills:

- When possible, sit when communicating with a patient. Do not cross your arms or legs because that body language conveys a message of being closed to the patient's comments.
- Be alert and relaxed and take sufficient time so that the patient feels at ease during the conversation.

- Keep the conversation as natural as possible, and avoid sounding overly eager.
- If culturally appropriate, maintain eye contact with the patient, without staring, in a face-to-face pose. This technique conveys interest in the conversation and willingness to listen.
- Indicate that you are paying attention to what the patient is saying by using appropriate facial expressions and body gestures. Be attentive to both your own and the patient's verbal and nonverbal communication.
- Think before responding to the patient. Responding impulsively tends to disrupt communication and listening.
- Do not pretend to listen. Most patients are sensitive to an attitude of feigned attention or to boredom and apathy.
- Listen for themes in the patient's comments. What are the repeated themes in the person's speech and behavior? What topics does the patient tend to avoid? What subjects tend to make the patient shift the conversation to other subjects? What inconsistencies and gaps appear in the patient's conversations?

Silence

The nurse can use silence appropriately to wait for the patient to initiate or to continue speaking (Videbeck, 2011). During periods of silence, reflect on what has already been shared and observe the patient without having to concentrate simultaneously on the spoken word. Periods of silence during communication can carry a variety of meanings, including the following:

- The patient might be comfortable and content in the nurse–patient relationship. Continuous talking is unnecessary.

THROUGH THE EYES OF A STUDENT

It was my first day of clinical rotation and I was assigned to Mr. Anderson, who was in his early 90s. He was in the hospital because he had a second heart attack. Mr. Anderson had lived alone for 5 years after the death of his wife. He wanted to remain independent, but his daughter, who was herself in her late 60s, and his doctor believed that he would not be able to function well on his own any longer. Mr. Anderson was distressed about this belief.

Because it was my first day and, unlike some of my classmates, I had never worked in a hospital before, I felt insecure and nervous. There really wasn't a lot of work for us to do. We weren't allowed to give medication yet, and my patient was pretty self-sufficient. Because my skills were shaky, I took my time taking vital signs, assisted Mr. Anderson with his bath and toileting, and made his bed. After checking his chart, I began my nursing interview with him. I was overjoyed to discover that he was a real talker! His memory was tremendous—either that or he was a great improviser! He recalled stories about his childhood and his wife with great detail and emotion. He smiled and laughed when he spoke of his daughter and grandchildren. He told me about his daughter's childhood illnesses, as well as his own. We talked

about the Depression and world wars and about music, art, and education. He asked me about my family, and I felt like I had made a friend.

The next day, Mr. Anderson told me about his fears. He talked about losing his wife, about his health and body deteriorating, and about losing his independence and home. He despised having to be sent to a long-term care facility and having to depend on others. It hurt him a lot and made me sad. Mr. Anderson left on my second day, and as I said goodbye I wished I could do something for him.

I thought about him a lot since then, and I've come to realize that in those 2 days that I knew Mr. Anderson, I did do something for him besides washing him and changing his sheets. I listened to him. Although his family had little time for him and the doctors quickly flew in and out of the room, I let him talk and heard all he said, both in words and in his eyes. He will always be a good memory for me—and I think I'll be a good memory for him.

—Kristina Hofmeister
Holy Family College, Philadelphia, PA

- The patient might be trying to demonstrate stoicism and the ability to cope without help.
- The patient might be exploring inner thoughts or feelings, and conversation would disrupt this. In effect, the patient is really saying, "I need some time to think."
- The patient might be fearful and use silence as an escape from a threat.
- The patient might be angry and use silence to display this emotion.
- The patient's culture may require longer pauses between verbal communication.

In due time, you might discuss the silence with the patient, especially if you wish to understand its meaning. Fear of silence sometimes leads to too much talking by the nurse. Also, excessive talking tends to place the focus on the nurse rather than on the patient.

Touch

Touch is a powerful means of communication with multiple meanings. It can connect people; provide affirmation, reassurance, and stimulation; decrease loneliness; increase self-esteem; and share warmth, intimacy, approval, and emotional support. It can also communicate frustration, anger, aggression, and punishment, and invade personal space and privacy (Videback, 2011). Because of the personal nature of touching, be sure to weigh the benefit of touch against the detrimental use of touch for each patient. Touch can be a powerful therapeutic tool when used at the right time. Anxiety or discomfort might result, however, when a patient does not understand the meaning of a tactile gesture or when the patient simply dislikes being touched.

Touch is the most highly developed sense at birth. Tactile experiences of infants and young children appear to be essential for the normal development of self and awareness of others. It has also been found that many older people long for touch, especially when isolated from loved ones because of hospitalization or being in a long-term care facility. Many older people have no living family to provide them with the caring touch so necessary for the sense of well-being. In such an instance, you can provide some special care by holding the patient's hand (Fig. 20-8).

Many situations require touching the patient while implementing nursing care. Physical closeness between the patient and the nurse is essential and inevitable. Therefore, every nurse needs to become comfortable with the judicious use of this nonverbal communication technique so that a sense of security, rather than anxiety, results. As well, dexterity and sureness in the use of the hands help to assure the patient of your expertise when measuring blood pressure or giving an injection.

Interest has continued to grow in the phenomenon known as therapeutic touch. Therapeutic touch involves "unruffling," or clearing, congested areas of energy in the body and redirecting this energy. After assessing a patient's "energy field," the nurse uses therapeutic touch to promote comfort, relaxation, healing, and a sense of well-being. Many

FIGURE 20-8. A reassuring handclasp uses touch to convey a message. Sometimes touch can be a more effective way of expressing concern and interest than verbal communication. *(Photo by B. Proud.)*

nurses are studying therapeutic touch in nursing educational programs and through special courses or workshops. It is becoming a widely accepted form of therapy, as well as a subject for nursing research. Many patients testify to the benefits of therapeutic touch. Refer to Chapters 27 and 34 for additional discussion of therapeutic touch.

Humor

Humor is increasingly valued as both an interpersonal skill for the nurse and a healing strategy for patients. Nurses can use humor effectively to maintain a balanced perspective in their work and to encourage patients to do the same. Nurses with a sense of humor are able to laugh at themselves and accept their failures, confront the absurdities of everyday practice without falling apart, and challenge patients to situate their current dilemma within the context of their larger life experiences. Laughter releases excess physical and psychological energy and reduces stress, anxiety, worry, and frustration. Humor, like other interpersonal competencies, is a learned skill. When used inappropriately, however, it can be destructive. You'll need an awareness of how various cultures perceive the use of humor in the presence of an illness. You might also find it helpful to identify nurses who use humor well and to "try on" observed behaviors. The use of humor is also discussed in Chapters 27 and 34.

Interviewing Techniques

The purpose of the patient interview is to obtain accurate and thorough information. In nursing, the interview is a major tool for collecting data during the assessment step of the nursing process (see Chapter 11). Consequently, every nurse needs to become proficient in the use of the communication techniques described previously as well as interviewing techniques designed to gather and validate information.

All interviews should begin with an explanation of the purpose of the interview. During the interview, you'll use **interviewing techniques** to obtain needed information while remaining flexible in approach. The interview itself is a therapeutic interaction and might be an essential part of the orientation phase of the helping relationship. At the end of the interview, plans for further interactions can be made. The following interviewing techniques are useful in nearly all nurse–patient interactions, especially the interview.

Open-Ended Question or Comment

When obtaining a nursing history, use the open-ended question technique to allow the patient a wide range of possible responses. It allows patients to express what they understand to be true, yet is specific enough to prevent digressing from the issue at hand. It encourages free verbalization. The greatest advantage of this technique is that it prevents the patient from giving a simple yes or no answer that has the effect of limiting the patient's response. The following is an example of an open-ended question and the response:

> *Nurse:* What did your physician tell you about your need for this hospitalization?
>
> *Patient:* He told me that my blood pressure is dangerously high and that I need some special tests done while I am here.

Closed Question or Comment

The closed question provides the receiver with limited choices of possible responses and might often be answered by one or two words, "yes" or "no." Closed questions are used to gather specific information from a patient and to allow the nurse and patient to focus on a particular area. Closed questions are often a barrier to effective communication. The following is an example of an appropriate use of a closed question:

> *Nurse:* What medicines have you been taking at home?
>
> *Patient:* Let me see, my doctor gave me a water pill and a blood pressure pill to take every day.

Validating Question or Comment

This type of question or comment serves to validate what the nurse believes he or she has heard or observed. Overusing validating questions and comments might lead the patient to think the nurse is not listening, however. To continue the example used in the previous technique, the nurse could validate the patient's reply as follows:

> *Nurse:* At home, you have been taking both a water pill and a blood pressure pill every day. Did you take them today?
>
> *Patient:* Yes, I took one of each with my breakfast.

Clarifying Question or Comment

The use of the clarifying question or comment allows the nurse to gain an understanding of a patient's comment. When used properly, this technique can prevent possible misconceptions that could lead to an inappropriate nursing diagnosis. However, overuse of clarifying questions or comments can lead the patient to believe that the nurse is not listening or lacks appropriate knowledge. The following is an example of effective use of this technique:

> *Patient:* I have never needed to take medicine before in my life.
>
> *Nurse:* Is this the first health problem you have had?
>
> *Patient:* Yes, I've always been healthy.

Reflective Question or Comment

The reflective question technique involves repeating what the person has said or describing the person's feelings. It encourages patients to elaborate on their thoughts and feelings. An example of this technique follows:

> *Patient:* I've been really upset about my blood pressure and have to take these pills.
>
> *Nurse:* You've been upset...
>
> *Patient:* I guess I'm worried about what could happen if my blood pressure gets too bad.

Sequencing Question or Comment

Sequencing is used to place events in a chronologic order or to investigate a possible cause-and-effect relationship between events. Nursing assessment is facilitated when events leading to a problem are placed in sequence. This technique is evident in the following example:

> *Patient:* I don't feel like myself anymore since I've been taking my blood pressure medicine. I'm tired and don't have any energy.
>
> *Nurse:* Your tiredness began after you started taking your medicine?

Directing Question or Comment

It might become necessary at times to obtain more information about a topic brought up earlier in the interview or to introduce a new aspect of the current topic. In this way, the nurse can gain additional valuable information to consider in assessing the patient's health status and educational or counseling needs. The following is an example of this technique:

> *Nurse:* You mentioned your dad earlier. Did he develop complications related to high blood pressure?
>
> *Patient:* Yes.
>
> *Nurse:* What sort of complications?
>
> *Patient:* Kidney failure. He was on dialysis for years before getting a transplant.
>
> *Nurse:* Are you afraid this might happen to you?

Assertive Versus Aggressive Behavior

When interacting with patients, family members, other nurses, physicians, and other members of the health care team, nurses should communicate in a way that demonstrates respect for all parties. **Assertive behavior** is the ability to stand up for oneself and others using open, honest, and direct communication. The focus is on the issue and not the person. Assertive behaviors, which are one hallmark of professional nursing relationships, are very different from aggressive (i.e., harsh, injurious, or destructive) behaviors. They also differ greatly from avoidance or acquiescent behaviors. The key to assertiveness is expressing feelings and beliefs in a nondefensive manner. "I" statements—"I feel…" and "I think…"—play an important role in assertive statements. They communicate personal feelings and preferences without expressing a judgment or blaming another person (Hodgetts, 2011). Table 20-2 gives examples of assertive, nonassertive, and aggressive speech.

Characteristics of the assertive nurse's self-presentation include a confident, open body posture; eye contact; use of clear, concise "I" statements; and the ability to share effectively one's thoughts, feelings, and emotions. The assertive nurse's attitude toward work is characterized by working to capacity with or without supervision, the ability to remain calm under supervision, the freedom to ask for help when necessary, the ability to give and accept compliments, and honesty in admitting mistakes and taking responsibility for them.

Aggressive behavior, on the other hand, involves asserting one's rights in a negative manner that violates the rights of others. Aggression can be verbal or physical. It is communication that is marked by tension and anger, and inhibits the formation of good relationships and collaboration.

Characteristics of aggressive verbal behavior include using an angry tone of voice, making accusations, and demonstrating belligerence and intolerance (Zeiler, 2010). Aggressive behavior is rude and threatening. The focus is usually on "winning at all costs" and/or demonstrating personal excellence (Marquis & Huston, 2012). Comments such as "do it my way" or "that's just enough out of you" are examples of aggressive verbal statements. People speaking in an aggressive manner may invade another's personal space, speak loudly, and use gestures that are very emphatic or threatening. Aggressive people enhance their self-esteem and prove their superiority through destructive comments directed at others.

BLOCKS TO COMMUNICATION

Nurses who have a good understanding of their own feelings and responses are better able to communicate and respond to others. The failure to verbalize clearly and compassionately, however, blocks effective communication. Recognition of the patient as a human being, listening carefully, and avoiding nontherapeutic statements help the nurse to provide optimal, compassionate patient care. Respectful behavior and communication between nurses and other members of the health care team promotes a safer patient environment with positive outcomes and improved job satisfaction.

Table 20-2	EXAMPLES OF ASSERTIVE, NONASSERTIVE, AND AGGRESSIVE SPEECH		
	ASSERTIVE	**NONASSERTIVE**	**AGGRESSIVE**
Nurse to Nurse	"I know we all lose track of time occasionally, but I'm finding it harder and harder to cover for you when you take extra time for lunch. I don't think it's fair for your patient and me to have to wait an extra 30 minutes every day for you to come back from lunch. Can we talk about this?"	"Huh? No, I didn't really mind. Luckily I wasn't too busy today." Thought: "What a sucker I am. Now I'll have to grab a quick bite so that I can get back to the unit in time to do 2 PM treatments."	"I'm sick and tired of covering for you. You are lazy and unreliable and I'm going to talk to the unit leader about you and let her know how irresponsible you are! What kind of nurse are you! I hope you lose your job!"
Nurse to Physician	"I know we talked about Mr. Esposito's pain medication before, but I've collected some new data. Even with the change in dosage, he is only getting 1 to 1½ hours of relief. I believe a different analgesic agent might work better for him."	"Um…yes I know you already changed the dosage. It's just that I thought it still wasn't working. Maybe I didn't give it enough time. Thanks for listening to me anyway. I'm sorry to bother you with this."	"What is it going to take to convince you that Mr. Esposito is not exaggerating his pain level so he can get more meds? I thought nurses and doctors were going to be more respectful of each other and collaborate, but this whole attempt to talk to you is a disaster. I need to report you to someone and maybe none of us will have to deal with you anymore. You give doctors a bad name."
Student Nurse to Preceptor	"Miss Cheng has a new order to be straight cathed. I reviewed the procedure, but I'd sure appreciate your talking me through this because I've never done it before and I'm terrified."	"Uh…I'm sorry to be such a pain again. I have to do this cath and don't know where to begin. I know you must be busy, but, uh, is there any way you might have time for me?"	"If this is an example of how helpful experienced nurses on this unit are to student nurses, then the profession is in a lot of trouble. Are you one of the believers in that saying that 'nurses eat their young'? Remind me to try and avoid you in the future."

Failure to Perceive the Patient as a Human Being

Nurses must focus on the whole patient and not merely the patient's diagnosis. Patients report that nothing is more discomforting than to be treated as merely an object of care rather than a patient. Patients should be addressed by a formal name such as Mr., Mrs., Ms., or Dr. rather than slang terminology such as "honey" or "sweetie." What distinguishes nursing from other health professions is its focus on the whole person, not simply the illness or dysfunction.

 THINK back to Mr. Gordon, the patient with end-stage liver disease. In the scenario, the nursing student voiced concerns about the staff nurse and residents focusing only on the technical aspects of the patient's care. To effectively communicate this concern to these individuals, the nurse would use open, honest, and direct communication when speaking with them, stressing the need for providing care to the whole patient. •

Failure to Listen

Patients might or might not feel able to speak freely to the nurse. Often, the signals indicating their readiness to talk are subtle. Don't miss valuable opportunities for important communication by approaching patients with a closed mind or focusing on your own needs rather than on the patient's needs. Nurses who lack confidence in their own ability to meet the challenges a patient presents might become defensive in response to a patient's comments. Nurse defensiveness is a huge barrier to open and trusting communication.

Nontherapeutic Comments and Questions

Certain types of comments and questions should be avoided in most situations because they tend to impede effective communications. A description of each type follows.

Using Clichés

A **cliché** is a stereotyped, trite, or pat answer. Most health care clichés suggest that there is no cause for anxiety or concern, or they offer false assurance. Patients tend to interpret them as a lack of real interest in what they have said. For example, even though the common question "How are you?" could start a conversation, it can cause a problem if patients hearing this suspect that the nurse is not sincerely interested in how they feel. Avoid the following common clichés because they tend to impede effective communication:

"Everything will be all right."

"Don't worry. You will be just fine in another day or two."

"Your doctor knows best."

"Cheer up. Tomorrow is another day."

Another type of cliché makes a sweeping generalization that does not necessarily apply to a specific patient. It also tends to

cut off communications and makes people feel as though they are insignificant. Consider the following examples:

"Men tolerate pain poorly. That must be why you are complaining of severe pain."

"Everybody is afraid of surgery. Why should you be any different?"

"You teenagers are all alike. You aren't cooperative because you deny authority."

Such comments rarely promote communication with the patient to whom they are addressed.

Using Questions Requiring Only a Yes or No Answer

Questions that can be answered by simply saying yes or no tend to cut off discussion, even when the person might wish to continue. Consider the following question:

Nurse: Did you have a good day?

The question begs for a noncommittal answer, which tells the nurse little. This is a better question:

Nurse: Tell me about your sessions in therapy. How did you feel they went today?

Another pitfall is to pose a question to which the patient can say no when that answer could present a problem. Consider the following question that a nurse asks a postoperative patient:

Nurse: Are you ready to get out of bed?

By offering the patient the chance to say no, the nurse might have created difficulties if the patient should be getting out of bed.

At times, of course, questions that can be answered with yes or no are appropriate, such as in these examples:

Nurse: Did you take your insulin before breakfast this morning?

Nurse: Do you have pain when I move your arm this way?

The problem with yes or no questions arises when seeking more detailed information or when the question might create difficulty.

Using Questions Containing the Words Why and How

Questions using the words *why* and *how* are intimidating to many patients. Consider the following questions:

Nurse: Why were you not tired enough to sleep?

Nurse: How did you ever decide to go on a crash diet?

These two questions would be better stated as follows:

Nurse: What were you doing while you were unable to sleep?

Nurse: What things prompted you to decide to go on a crash diet?

Using Questions That Probe for Information

Questions that too obviously probe for information might cut off communication. Patients who are made to feel as though they are receiving the "third degree" become resentful, usually stop talking, and try to avoid further conversation. Although more information might be needed, it is better to follow the patient's lead. Letting the patient take the initiative allows you to delve more deeply at a time when the patient is ready. A nurse who says, "Let's get to the bottom of this" is likely to destroy conversation, unless the patient is ready to face the real cause of the problem.

Using Leading Questions

A leading question suggests what response the speaker wishes to hear. Leading questions tend to produce answers that might please the nurse but are unlikely to encourage the patient to respond honestly without feeling intimidated. Consider the following examples:

Nurse: You aren't going to smoke that cigarette, are you?

Nurse: You have been well cared for by your nurses, haven't you?

These questions direct patients to give an answer that pleases the nurse rather than to express their own thoughts.

Using Comments That Give Advice

Giving advice often implies that the nurse knows what is best for patients and denies them the right to make decisions and have feelings. It also tends to increase the patient's dependence on caregivers. However, advice does have a rightful place when it is requested and when the person giving the advice has expert knowledge that the patient does not.

Using Judgmental Comments

Judgmental comments tend to impose the nurse's standards on the patient. Consider the comment of a nurse who notes that a young woman is crying:

Nurse: You aren't acting very grown up. How do you think your husband would feel if he saw you crying like this?

The nurse judges the patient as being immature, and the nurse's apparent hostility could end effective communication. A better comment in this situation might be as follows:

Nurse: I would like to help. Tell me, what is making you cry?

Consider the following exchange between a nurse and a patient about to have surgery:

Patient: I think I have a right to be afraid of this operation.
Nurse: Tell me what makes you feel afraid.

This patient is likely to feel safe when allowed to express feelings without being judged.

 REMEMBER Susie Musashi, the 3-year-old with burns who is crying. A response such as "You're acting like a baby. You're a big girl now" would be intimidating, especially to a young child who is striving for acceptance. Instead, a response such as "Can you tell me what is making you cry or feel so sad?" would allow the child to verbalize her concerns without feeling intimidated or scolded. This response also would help in establishing a trusting nurse–patient relationship. ●

Changing the Subject

A quick way to stop conversation is to change the subject. The patient might be at a point of readiness to discuss something and will likely feel frustrated if put off by a change in the topic of conversation, as in this following example:

Patient: When can I expect to be told about my insulin?

Nurse: Let's discuss your diet now so that you will know what to eat when you get home. We can discuss your insulin some other time.

A nurse might also change the subject when feeling uncomfortable about the topic of conversation. For example, the patient's needs are being met when the nurse allows the patient to speak of impending death, thoughts of suicide, or contemplated abortion. The nurse is ignoring the patient, however, if the nurse changes the subject because of feeling uncomfortable talking about it.

Giving False Assurance

Because it is easier and more pleasant to deal with positive outcomes than negative outcomes, nurses might try to convince the patient that things are going to turn out well even when knowing the chances are not good. False assurance might give patients the impression that the nurse is not interested in their problems. The use of clichés gives a patient false assurance. Communication might be impeded when providing the patient and family with false assurance. If you inadvertently do use false assurance, then you should explain with an apology and implement effective communication techniques.

Gossip and Rumor

Gossip and rumor are common forms of communication, particularly in health care settings, sometimes referred to as "the grapevine." Gossip and rumor can produce detrimental effects on relationships and group building. Gossiping might be used to inform, influence others, entertain, or ventilate. It can be harmless but could also damage the reputation of others. Rumors serve similar functions but become more widespread. Both rumors and gossip might cause blocks to team building and damage the reputations of the people who are the subject of the information.

Disruptive Interpersonal Behavior

Disruptive behavior has a negative effect on clinical outcomes and interpersonal relationships. Adverse events occur when communication between health care professionals is ineffective, abusive, or negative. The Joint Commission (TJC), in an effort to eliminate disruptive behavior in hospitals, issued a leadership standard that requires hospitals to establish a code of conduct defining acceptable and unacceptable behavior. Hospitals are also required to have policies in place to address these incidents when they occur. Additionally, TJC advises hospitals to educate all staff about the code of conduct, develop reporting systems, use mediators when necessary, and document all efforts to address unacceptable behavior (TJC, 2008). Disruptive interpersonal behavior compromises patient safety, influences satisfaction with care, and contributes to medical errors.

Incivility is rude, intimidating, and undesirable behavior directed at another person. This behavior is recognized as a major concern among health care workers (Stokowski, 2011). Incivility is considered by some as a precursor to bullying behavior or lateral violence and by others as a form of bullying (Lower, 2012).

Bullying

Anger and aggressive behavior between nurses, or nurse-to-nurse hostility, has been labeled **horizontal violence**. This negative behavior is also referred to as **bullying**, lateral violence, and professional incivility. Bullying often occurs repetitively, whereas horizontal or lateral violence can occur as a single event (Stokowski, 2010). All are forms of psychological and social harassment and involve covert or overt behaviors (Flateau-Lux & Gravel, 2013). Covert bullying includes withholding information from a colleague, gossiping and spreading rumors, nonverbal communication such as eye rolling and other body language, and social isolation. Overt bullying behaviors include accusing a nurse of errors made by someone else (scapegoating) or humiliating a person in the presence of others.

NURSE BULLYING

Bullying behaviors occur in all health care environments and affect nurses at all levels of practice, including new graduates and nursing students (see the accompanying Research in Nursing box). According to recent surveys, the occurrence in the United States of nurses reporting being bullied ranges from 18% to 31% (ANA, 2012). The potential source of the disruptive behavior, the bully, may be a co-worker, supervisor, or physician. Medical–surgical units have the highest frequency, but incidents of bullying are also more common in critical care units, emergency departments, perioperative areas, and obstetric departments (Stokowski, 2010). According to a recent survey of new RNs in the United States, 60% quit a job after 6 months of employment as a result of being bullied (Flateau-Lux & Gravel, 2013; Townsend, 2012). Bullying also affects patient safety because teamwork is negatively influenced, resulting in deterioration in the quality of care and a greater potential for error. The physical and emotional toll on those employed in a toxic work environment can be significant. Commonly reported physical consequences include frequent headaches, sleep disturbances, gastrointestinal symptoms, and decreased energy. Psychological manifestations such an increased level of stress, anxiety, fear, frustration, and loss of self-esteem can result in burnout and emotional exhaustion (ANA, 2012).

RESEARCH IN NURSING

BRIDGING THE GAP TO EVIDENCE-BASED PRACTICE

Recognizing the Effects of Workplace Mistreatment on New Graduates

Given the increasing numbers of older adults and the expected shortage of RNs due to retirements, new graduates are a valuable resource. It is predicted that, in the United States, there will be a shortage of almost one million nurses by 2030; in Canada, it is projected that 60,000 more RNs will be needed by 2022. Incivility and bullying behaviors in the workplace negatively impact new RNs and are responsible for decreased retention of this vulnerable population. As many as one-third of graduate nurses admitted to experiencing workplace mistreatment during the first year of their employment as an RN. Research had not clearly indicated what factors are correlated with experiences of incivility and bullying and the related outcomes of these behaviors for these new graduates. This study explored both types of disruptive behavior and their impact on these new professionals.

Related Research

Read, E., & Laschinger, H. (2013). Correlates of new graduate nurses' experiences of workplace mistreatment. *Journal of Nursing Administration, 43*(4), 221–228.

A total of 342 RNs in Ontario, Canada, participated in this study by completing a survey consisting of standardized questions. The majority of the respondents were women with an undergraduate degree in nursing and one year of nursing experience in either medical–surgical or critical care nursing. Many new graduate nurses recounted experiencing humiliating comments, a lack of support, limited opportunities for new learning experiences, and sometimes even verbal threats while

practicing nursing. The researchers proposed that a supportive work environment, including respectful leaders who do not tolerate bullying and incivility and an empowering workplace, played a key role in the development of a positive work environment and job satisfaction. Personal resources such as resiliency, a positive outlook, and the ability to accept challenges and respond positively to adversity appear to help RNs address negative work experiences. Results of this research indicated that bullying, co-worker incivility, and supervisor incivility in the workplace are correlated with decreased job and career satisfaction and poor mental health accompanied by physical and emotional exhaustion. New graduate nurses who are subjected to this type of toxic behavior are more likely to leave their nursing position and possibly even leave the profession.

Relevance to Nursing Practice

Nursing is considered a caring profession. Given the effects of bullying and incivility on new and seasoned practitioners, professionals are calling for zero tolerance of these behaviors. They negatively impact teamwork, collaboration, and communication with co-workers and may ultimately pose a safety threat to patients. A strong sense of community coupled with an empowering work environment may be an important step to address bullying and incivility in the workplace and eradicate it. A proactive approach has the potential to increase job satisfaction, foster personal growth, and positively impact the retention of registered nurses.

For additional research, visit thePoint.

Nurses who refuse to be a victim can help break this cycle of violence. Once bullying is recognized as a problem, the need for a culture change is evident. Education is crucial; nurses need to learn effective communication strategies to combat bullying. Proactive behavior includes learning how to react professionally and protectively "in the moment," documenting and reporting the incident, welcoming new nurses, using conflict-management strategies when responding to a bully, and insisting that this abuse is addressed. Nurses who have always cared for others need to also care for themselves and their peers.

NEGATIVE COMMUNICATION BETWEEN THE NURSE AND PHYSICIAN

Nurses continue to report the occurrence of negative communication with physicians. In a 2012 survey, 42% of nurse leaders reported that physician abuse or disrespect of nurses is still common (Gessler, Rosenstein, & Ferron, 2012). This factor is often cited as a contributor to poor job satisfaction and jeopardizes nurse retention. Nurses describe this disruptive behavior by physicians as rude, intimidating, and belittling, and state that it occurs more frequently with older physicians than among younger ones. In settings where teamwork is essential, such as operating rooms and intensive care areas, the relationship between nurse and physician is more positive. Nurses who remain current in their field of expertise, become involved in informal collaborative work groups, and participate in interdisciplinary hospital committees feel more empowered in their encounters with physicians. It is a mistake to permit negative behavior by a physician to discourage any future communication. When disruptive physician behavior occurs, it is best to respond assertively and confront the physician directly. If this is not possible, ask to speak to the physician in private and address any disrespectful remarks or behaviors. Nurses should factually document the occurrence of any bullying behaviors and speak to a nurse-manager if the behavior continues (Gessler, Rosenstein, & Ferron, 2012). Nurses who stay focused and professional and approach physicians in a collegial manner will be better prepared to avoid negative communication. If it occurs, the hospital administration policies and procedures should be implemented to deal with individual situations in a constructive manner.

Organizational Response to Disruptive Behaviors

Addressing disruptive behaviors requires the determination that bullying will no longer be tolerated in order to promote a healthy work environment. The Joint Commission standard regarding preventing disruptive behaviors in health care facilities includes the following key recommendations:

- Education must be provided for all staff regarding respectful, professional behavior.
- All staff members must be held accountable for their behavior.
- Zero-tolerance policies must be implemented regarding disruptive behaviors and protection must be provided for those who report these behaviors.
- Those in leadership positions must attend training regarding professional standards of behavior and function as a positive role model.
- Surveillance and reporting systems must be available to identify unprofessional behaviors.
- Emphasis must be placed on the importance of documenting bullying behaviors (TJC, 2008).

An organizational response coupled with individual nurses' efforts to address disruptive behaviors at all levels can create a healthy work environment, positively impact job satisfaction, improve the retention of nurses, and result in more positive patient outcomes.

IMPAIRED VERBAL COMMUNICATION

The ability to communicate is our most human characteristic. Human communication is essential for learning, working, and social interaction. Impaired communication can affect every aspect of a person's life. Impaired Verbal Communication is an approved North American Nursing Diagnosis Association International (NANDA-I) nursing diagnosis. According to NANDA-I, Impaired Verbal Communication is defined as decreased, delayed, or absent ability to receive, process, transmit, and/or use a system of symbols. (See Examples of NANDA-I Nursing Diagnoses: Communication.)

EXAMPLES OF NANDA-I NURSING DIAGNOSES

COMMUNICATION

Nursing Diagnoses	Related Factors	Sample Defining Characteristics
Impaired Verbal Communication	Decrease in circulation to the brain; brain tumor; physical barrier (tracheostomy, intubation); anatomic defect, cleft palate; psychological barriers (psychosis, lack of stimuli); cultural differences; developmental or age related	Individual is able to speak dominant language; speaks or verbalizes with difficulty; does not or cannot speak; stutters; slurs; has difficulty forming words or sentences; has difficulty expressing thoughts verbally; uses inappropriate verbalization; has dyspnea; is disoriented
Disturbed Energy Field	Slowing or blocking of energy flows secondary to illness, injury, immobility, pain, anxiety, or age-related developmental crises	Perceptions of changes in patterns of energy flow such as movement, sounds, temperature, visual change, and disruption of the field

BOX 20-6 COMMUNICATING WITH PATIENTS WHO HAVE SPECIAL NEEDS

Patients Who Are Visually Impaired
- Acknowledge your presence in the patient's room.
- Identify yourself by name.
- Remember that the visually impaired patient will be unable to pick up most nonverbal cues during communication. Speak in a normal tone of voice.
- Explain the reason for touching the patient before doing so.
- Indicate to the patient when the conversation has ended and when you are leaving the room.
- Keep a call light or bell within easy reach of the patient.
- Orient the patient to the sounds in the environment and to the arrangement of the room and its furnishings.
- Be sure the patient's eyeglasses are clean and intact or that contacts are in place.

Patients Who Are Hearing Impaired
- Orient the patient to your presence before initiating conversation. This may be done by gently touching the patient or moving so that you can be seen.
- Talk directly to the patient while facing him or her. If the patient is able to lip read, use simple sentences and speak in a quiet, natural manner and pace. Be aware of nonverbal communication.
- Do not chew gum or cover your mouth when talking with the patient.
- Demonstrate or pantomime ideas you wish to express, as appropriate.
- Use sign language or finger spelling, as appropriate.
- Write any ideas that you cannot convey to the patient in another manner.
- Be sure that hearing aids are clean, functioning, and inserted properly.

Patients With a Physical Barrier (Laryngectomy or Endotracheal Tube)
- Select one or more simple means of communication that the patient is physically able to use. Options include eye blinks or hand squeezes to communicate yes or no; writing pads or magic slates; communication boards with words, letters, or pictures; flash cards; sign language.
- Be sure that everyone communicating with the patient— family, friends, and caregivers—understands and is able to use the communication devices selected.

- Demonstrate patience with the time needed to communicate effectively, and reinforce the patient's efforts.
- Ensure that the patient has an effective means of signaling need for assistance, such as a call bell or alarm.

Patients Who Are Cognitively Impaired
- Establish and maintain eye contact with the patient to hold attention.
- Communicate important information in a quiet environment where there is little to distract the patient's attention.
- Keep communication simple and concrete. Break down instructions into simple tasks and avoid lengthy explanations. Do not use pronouns or abstract terms. Use pictures or drawings when appropriate.
- Whenever possible, avoid open-ended questions. Ask "Would you like to wear the brown pants or the gray pants?" instead of "What would you like to wear?"
- Be patient and give the patient time to respond. If the patient does not respond after 2 minutes, repeat what you said. If there is still no response, take a break before continuing the conversation so that neither you nor the patient becomes frustrated.

Patients Who Are Unconscious
- Be careful of what is said in the patient's presence. Hearing is believed to be the last sense lost; therefore, the unconscious patient is often likely to hear even though there is no apparent response.
- Assume that the patient can hear you. Talk in a normal tone of voice about things you would ordinarily discuss.
- Speak with the patient before touching. Remember that touch can be an effective means of communication with the unconscious patient.
- Keep environment noises at as low a level as possible. This helps the patient focus on the communication.

Patients Who Do Not Speak English
- Use an interpreter whenever possible.
- Use a dictionary that translates words from one language to another so that you can speak at least some words in the patient's language.
- Speak in simple sentences and in a normal tone of voice.
- Demonstrate or pantomime ideas you wish to convey, as appropriate.
- Be aware of nonverbal communication. Remember that many nonverbal communication cues are universal.

Specific communication strategies may be necessary for older adults who have speech, language, and hearing disorders. Nurses and other caregivers should avoid "elderspeak" when communicating with older adults. Elderspeak involves using speaking patterns and words mimicking "baby talk" that imply that the older person is not competent. It is actually a form of ageism and used more commonly with frail older adults in long-term care facilities. Communication adjustments may be necessary but must be respectful, positive, and individualized. Chapter 19 also addresses communication with older adults.

Box 20-6 offers guidelines for communicating with patients with special needs. The causes of hearing loss include chronic ear infections, heredity, birth defects, health problems at home, certain drugs, head injury, viral or bacterial infection, exposure to loud noise, aging, and tumors.

Causes of speech and language disorders are related to hearing loss, cerebral palsy, and other nerve and muscle disorders; severe head injury; stroke (brain attack); viral diseases; mental retardation; certain drugs; physical impairments, such as cleft lip or palate; vocal abuse or misuse; and inadequate speech and language.

 FOR Irwina Russellinski, the older adult woman admitted with pneumonia, the nurse needs to investigate the cause and degree of the patient's hearing loss and what, if any, treatments or measures have been used to manage the problem. The nurse also needs to gather additional data about the patient's confusion and her cultural background. Based on this information, the nurse would be able to develop a plan of care that addresses Mrs. Russellinski's needs. ●

A nurse who suspects a speech, language, or hearing problem should refer the patient to a speech–language pathologist or audiologist. A speech–language pathologist is a professional educated in the study of human communication, its development, and its disorders. An audiologist is a professional educated in the study of normal and impaired hearing.

DEVELOPING CLINICAL REASONING

1. Working with another student, attempt to express the following using nonverbal communication only:
   - I am in pain.
   - I am genuinely concerned about your well-being.
   - I couldn't care less that you are my patient, and I wish I were anywhere else but here caring for you.
   - I am afraid that you will hurt me.

   Describe what this exercise can teach you about the importance of nonverbal communication. Explain how this understanding will influence your nursing practice.

2. Conversation is both an art and an essential nursing tool. If you had 30 minutes to spend with each of the following patients while doing a procedure that allows you to communicate, what would you talk about (communicate) and why? Compare your answers with another student's, and explore what your conversations would communicate to the patients involved.
   - An older adult recently admitted to a long-term care facility
   - A 6-year-old boy newly admitted to a hospital for asthma
   - An HIV-positive, 33-year-old man who has just been given the news that he has acquired immunodeficiency syndrome (AIDS)
   - A 45-year-old amputee who has been in a rehabilitation hospital for 3 weeks after a motorcycle accident
   - A 19-year-old woman who has just had an elective abortion and is in the recovery unit
   - An unconscious patient in a critical care unit

3. An experienced nurse observes your distress after leaving the room of a patient who has just told her family that her cancer has recurred and is in an advanced state. She tells you that you better "toughen up" if you want to survive in nursing. She counsels not getting emotionally involved with patients and families: "Become a rock." How do you respond to this nurse and why? Of what value, if any, is empathy?

PRACTICING FOR NCLEX

1. During rounds, a charge nurse hears the patient care technician yelling loudly to a patient regarding a transfer from the bed to chair. When entering the room, what is the nurse's best response?
   a. "You need to speak to the patient quietly. You are disturbing the patient."
   b. "Let me help you with your transfer technique."
   c. "When you are finished, be sure to apologize for your rough demeanor."
   d. "When your patient is safe and comfortable, meet me at the desk."

2. A public health nurse is leaving the home of a young mother who has a special needs baby. The neighbor states, "How is she doing, since the baby's father is no help?" What is the nurse's best response to the neighbor?
   a. "New mothers need support."
   b. "The lack of a father is difficult."
   c. "How are you today?"
   d. "It is a very sad situation."

3. A 3-year-old child is being admitted to a medical division for vomiting, diarrhea, and dehydration. During the admission interview, the nurse should implement which communication techniques to elicit the most information from the parents?
   a. The use of reflective questions
   b. The use of closed questions
   c. The use of assertive questions
   d. The use of clarifying questions

4. A nurse enters a patient's room and examines the patient's IV fluids and cardiac monitor. The patient states, "Well, I haven't seen you before. Who are you?" What is the nurse's best response?
   a. "I'm just the IV therapist checking your IV."
   b. "I've been transferred to this division and will be caring for you."
   c. "I'm sorry, my name is John Smith and I am your nurse."
   d. "My name is John Smith, I am your nurse and I'll be caring for you until 11 p.m."

5. A nurse enters the room of a patient with cancer. The patient is crying and states, "I feel so alone." Which statement is the most therapeutic?
   a. The nurse stands at the patient's bedside and states, "I understand how you feel. My mother said the same thing when she was ill."
   b. The nurse places a hand on the patient's arm and states, "You feel so alone."
   c. The nurse stands in the patient's room and asks, "Why do you feel so alone? Your wife has been here every day."
   d. The nurse holds the patient's hand and asks, "What makes you feel so alone?"

6. A nurse caring for a patient who is hospitalized following a double mastectomy is preparing a discharge plan for the patient. Which action should be the focus of this termination phase of the helping relationship?
   a. Determining the progress made in achieving established goals
   b. Clarifying when the patient should take medications
   c. Reporting the progress made in teaching to the staff
   d. Including all family members in the teaching session

7. A nursing student is nervous and concerned about the work she is about to do at the clinical facility. To allay anxiety and be successful in her provision of care, it is most important for her to:
   a. Determine the established goals of the institution
   b. Be sure her verbal and nonverbal communication is congruent
   c. Engage in self-talk to plan her day and decrease her fear
   d. Speak with her fellow colleagues about how they feel

8. A nurse in the rehabilitation division states to her head nurse, Mr. Tyler, "I need the day off and you didn't give it to me!" The head nurse replies, "Well, I wasn't aware you needed the day off, and it isn't possible since staffing is so inadequate." Instead of this exchange, what communication by the nurse would have been more effective?

a. "Mr. Tyler, I placed a request to have August 8th off, but I'm working and I have a doctor's appointment."

b. "Mr. Tyler, I would like to discuss my schedule with you. I requested the 8th of August off for a doctor's appointment. Could I make an appointment?"

c. "Mr. Tyler, I will need to call in on the 8th of August because I have a doctor's appointment."

d. "Mr. Tyler, since you didn't give me the 8th of August off, will I need to find someone to work for me?"

9. During a nursing staff meeting, the nurses resolve a problem of delayed documentation by agreeing unanimously that they will make sure all vital signs are reported and charted within 15 minutes following assessment. This is an example of which characteristics of effective communication? Select all that apply.

a. Group decision making

b. Group leadership

c. Group power

d. Group identity

e. Group patterns of interaction

f. Group cohesiveness

10. A nurse sees a patient walking to the bathroom with a stooped gait, facial grimacing, and gasping sounds. It is important that the nurse assess the patient for:

a. Pain

b. Anxiety

c. Depression

d. Fluid volume deficit

11. A nursing student is preparing to administer morning care to a patient. What is the most important question that the nursing student should ask the patient about personal hygiene?

a. "Would you prefer a bath or a shower?"

b. "May I help you with a bed bath now or later this morning?"

c. "I will be giving you your bath. Do you use soap or shower gel?"

d. "I prefer a shower in the evening. When would you like your bath?"

12. A nurse is providing instruction to a patient regarding the procedure to change his colostomy bag. During the teaching session, he asks, "What type of foods should I avoid to prevent gas?" The patient's question allows for what type of communication?

a. A closed-ended answer

b. Information clarification

c. The nurse to give advice

d. Assertive behavior

13. When interacting with a patient, the nurse answers, "I am sure everything will be fine. You have nothing to worry about." This is an example of what type of inappropriate communication technique?

a. Cliché

b. Giving advice

c. Being judgmental

d. Changing the subject

14. A 76-year-old patient states, "I have been experiencing complications of diabetes." The nurse needs to direct the patient to gain more information. What is the most appropriate comment or question to elicit additional information?

a. "Do you take two injections of insulin to decrease the complications?"

b. "Most physicians recommend diet and exercise to regulate blood sugar."

c. "Most complications of diabetes are related to neuropathy."

d. "What specific complications have you experienced?"

15. During an interaction with a patient diagnosed with epilepsy, a nurse notes that the patient is silent after she communicates the plan of care. What would be appropriate nurse responses in this situation? Select all that apply.

a. Fill the silence with lighter conversation directed at the patient.

b. Use the time to perform the care that is needed uninterrupted.

c. Discuss the silence with the patient to ascertain its meaning.

d. Allow the patient time to think and explore inner thoughts.

e. Determine if the patient's culture requires pauses between conversation.

f. Arrange for a counselor to help the patient cope with emotional issues.

ANSWERS WITH RATIONALES

1. *d.* The charge nurse should direct the patient care technician to determine the patient's safety. Then the nurse should address any concerns regarding the patient care technician's communication techniques privately. The nurse should direct the patient care technician on aspects of therapeutic communication.

2. *a.* The nurse must maintain confidentiality when providing care. The statement "New mothers need support" is a general statement that all new parents need help. The statement is not judgmental of the family's roles.

3. *d.* The use of the clarifying question or comment allows the nurse to gain an understanding of a patient's comment. When used properly, this technique can avert possible misconceptions that could lead to an inappropriate nursing diagnosis. The reflective question technique involves repeating what the person has said or describing the person's feelings. Open-ended questions encourage free verbalization and expression of what the parents believe to be true. Assertive behavior is the ability to stand up for oneself and others using open, honest, and direct communication.

4. *d.* The nurse should identify himself, be sure the patient knows what will be happening, and the time period he will be with his patient.

5. *d.* The use of touch conveys acceptance, and the implementation of an open-ended question allows the patient time to verbalize freely.

6. *a.* The termination phase occurs when the conclusion of the initial agreement is acknowledged. Discharge planning coordinates with the termination phase of a helping relationship. The nurse should determine the progress made in achieving the goals related to the patient's care.

7. *c.* By engaging in self-talk, or intrapersonal communication, the nursing student can plan her day and enhance her clinical performance to decrease fear and anxiety.

8. *b.* Effective communication by the sender involves the implementation of nonthreatening information by showing respect to the receiver. The nurse should identify the subject of the meeting and be sure it occurs at a mutually agreed upon time.

9. *a, d, e, f.* Solving problems involves group decision making; ascertaining that the staff completes a task on time and that all members agree the task is important is a characteristic of group identity; group patterns of interaction involve honest communication and member support; and cohesiveness occurs when members generally trust each other, have a high commitment to the group, and a high degree of cooperation. Group leadership occurs when groups use effective styles of leadership to meet goals; with group power, sources of power are recognized and used appropriately to accomplish group outcomes.

10. *a.* A patient who presents with nonverbal communication of a stooped gait, facial grimacing, and gasping sounds is most likely experiencing pain. The nurse should clarify this nonverbal behavior.

11. *b.* The nurse should ask permission to assist the patient with a bath. This allows for consent to assist the patient with care that invades the patient's private zones.

12. *b.* The patient's question allows the nurse to clarify information that is new to the patient or that requires further explanation.

13. *a.* Telling a patient that everything is going to be all right is a cliché. This statement gives false assurance and gives the patient the impression that the nurse is not interested in the patient's condition.

14. *d.* Requesting specific information regarding complications of diabetes will elicit specific information to guide the nurse in further interview questions and specific assessment techniques.

15. *c, d, e.* The nurse can use silence appropriately by taking the time to wait for the patient to initiate or to continue speaking. During periods of silence, the nurse should reflect on what has already been shared and observe the patient without having to concentrate simultaneously on the spoken word. In due time, the nurse might discuss the silence with the patient in order to understand its meaning. Also, the patient's culture may require longer pauses between verbal communication. Fear of silence sometimes leads to too much talking by the nurse, and excessive talking tends to place the focus on the nurse rather than on the patient. The nurse should not assume silence requires a consult with a counselor.

TAYLOR SUITE RESOURCES

Explore these additional resources to enhance learning for this chapter:

* NCLEX-Style Questions and other resources on **thePoint**, http://thePoint.lww.com/Taylor8e
* *Study Guide for Fundamentals of Nursing, 8th edition*
* Adaptive Learning | Powered by prepU, http://thepoint.lww.com/prepu

Bibliography

American Nurses Association (ANA). (2012). *Bullying in the workplace: Reversing a culture.* Silver Springs, MD: Author.

American Nurses Association (ANA). (2011). *Principles for social networking and the nurse.* Silver Springs, MD: Author.

Ashton, L. (2012). Caring for patients in any language: Does it matter? *Nursing, 42*(6), 65–66.

Berlo, D. (1960). *The process of communication: An introduction to theory and practice.* New York: Holt, Rinehart & Winston.

Bombard, C. (2012). Effective communication with patients. *Nurse.com, 21*(16), 21–25.

Bulechek, G., Butcher, H., Dochterman, J., & Wagner, C. (2013). *Nursing interventions classification (NIC)* (6th ed., p. 125). St. Louis: Elsevier/Mosby.

Duffy, M. (2011a). Facebook, Twitter, and LinkedIn, Oh My! *American Journal of Nursing, 111*(4), 56–59.

Duffy, M. (2011b). Patient privacy and company policy in online life. *American Journal of Nursing, 111*(9), 65–69.

Eliopoulos, C. (2010). *Gerontological nursing* (7th ed.). Philadelphia: Wolters Kluwer Health/Lippincott Williams & Wilkins.

Flateau-Lux, L., & Gravel, T. (2013). Put a stop to bullying new nurses. *Nursing, 43*(6), 24–28.

Gerace, L., & Salimbene, S. (2010). Culturally diverse nursing staff: Working together. *Nurse.com, 19*(20), 26–31.

Gessler, R., Rosenstein, A., & Ferron, L. (2012). How to handle disruptive physician behaviors. *American Nurse Today, 7*(11), 8–10.

Gieger, J. N., & Davidhizar, R. E. (2008). *Transcultural nursing: Assessment and intervention* (5th ed.). St. Louis: Elsevier/Mosby.

Hodgetts, S. (2011). Being assertive benefits everyone. Available at http://www.nursingtimes.net/nursing-practice/clinical-zones/management/being-assertive-benefits-everyone/5038545.article

The Joint Commission (TJC). (2008). *Sentinel Event Alert.* Available at http://www.jointcommission.org/assets/1/18/SEA_40.PDF

Joint Commission Center for Transforming Healthcare. (2012). Facts about the hand-off communications project. Available at http://www.centerfortransforminghealthcare.org/assets/4/6/CTH_HOC_Fact_Sheet.pdf

Joint Commission for Transforming Healthcare. (2013). Targeted solutions tool. Available at http://www.centerfortransforminghealthcare.org/tst_hoc.aspx

Jukkala, A., James, D., Autrey, P., Azuero, A., & Millner, R. (2012). Develop a standardized tool to improve nurse communication during shift report. *Journal of Nursing Care Quality, 27*(3), 240–246.

Lower, J. (2012). Civility starts with you. *American Nurse Today, 7*(5), 21–22.

Marquis, B., & Huston, C. (2012). *Leadership roles and management functions* (7th ed.). Philadelphia: Wolters Kluwer Health/Lippincott Williams & Wilkins.

Messner, R. L. (1993). What patients really want from their nurses. *American Journal of Nursing, 93*(8), 38–41.

Moorhead, S., Johnson, M., Maas, M., & Swanson, E. (2013). *Nursing outcomes classification (NOC)* (5th ed., p. 157). St. Louis: Elsevier/Mosby.

NANDA International (NANDA-I). (2012). *NANDA Nursing diagnoses: Definitions and classification, 2012–2014.* West Sussex, UK: Wiley-Blackwell.

National Council of State Boards of Nursing (NCSBN). (2011). White Paper: A Nurse's Guide to the Use of Social Media. Available at https://www.ncsbn.org/Social_media_guidelines.pdf

Orlando, I. J. (1961). *The dynamic nurse–patient relationship.* New York: G. P. Putnam's Sons.

Pagana, K. (2011a). After shock: Nurses respond to episodes of violence by writing new policies. *Nurse.com, 20*(14), 21–25.

Pagana, K. (2011b). Mind your manners…Multiculturally. *Nurse.com, 20*(11), 38–43.

Pagana, K. (2012). How to keep your communications professional. *American Nurse Today, 7*(9), 56–58.

Paterson, J., & Zderad, L. (1976). *Humanistic nursing.* New York: Wiley.

Peplau, H. (1952). *Interpersonal relations in nursing.* New York: Putnam.

Prinz, A. (2011). Professional social networking for nurses. *American Nurse Today, 6*(7), 30–32.

QSEN Institute. (2008). *Reformulating SBAR to "I-SBAR-R."* Available at http://qsen.org/reformulating-sbar-to-i-sbar-r/

Read, E., & Laschinger, H. (2013). Correlates of new graduate nurses' experiences of workplace mistreatment. *Journal of Nursing Administration, 43*(4), 221–228.

Sherwood, G., & Barnsteiner, J. (2013). *Quality and Safety in Nursing.* West Sussex, UK: Wiley-Blackwell.

Spector, N., & Kappel, D. (2012). Guidelines for using electronic and social media. Available at http://www.medscape.com/viewarticle/780050

Stokowski, L. (2010). A matter of respect and dignity: Bullying in the nursing profession. Available at http://www.medscape.com/viewarticle/729474

Stowkowski, L. (2011). The downward spiral of incivility in nursing. Available at http://www.medscape.com/viewarticle/739328

Tannen, D. (1990). *You just don't understand: Women and men in conversation.* New York: Morrow.

Townsend, M. (2009). *Psychiatric mental health nursing: Concepts of care* (6th ed.). Philadelphia: F. A. Davis.

Townsend, T. (2012). Break the bullying cycle. *American Nurse Today, 7*(1), 12–15.

Travelbee, J. (1971). *Interpersonal aspects of nursing* (2nd ed.). Philadelphia: F. A. Davis.

Videbeck, S. (2011). *Psychiatric mental health nursing* (5th ed.). Philadelphia: Wolters Kluwer Health/Lippincott Williams & Wilkins.

Watson, J. (1985). *Nursing: The philosophy and science of caring.* Boulder, CO: Colorado Associated University Press.

Wentworth, L., Diggins, J., Bartel, D., Johnson, M., Hale, J., & Gaines, K. (2012). SBAR: Electronic handoff tool for noncomplicated procedural patients. *Journal of Nursing Care Quality, 27*(2), 125–131.

Zeiler, K. (2010). Assertive versus aggressive. *Advance for Nurses, 9*(26), 4–8.

21

Teacher and Counselor

MARCO GARCÍA RAMÍREZ

Marco accompanies his wife, Claudia, to the antepartal clinic for a routine visit. They are expecting their first child in 5 months. He reports that they are happy and excited but also scared and very nervous. They are planning for a home birth, asking lots of questions about childbirth and their new responsibilities as parents: "We're both wondering if we'll be good parents."

RACHEL BLUMENTHAL

Rachel, age 40, is the second wife of a 57-year-old man who has suffered a serious myocardial infarction. They have been married for only 1 year. She says, "I'm a little embarrassed to talk with the cardiologist, but I have lots of questions about what my husband will be able to do after he gets home. I'm also wondering about resuming sexual activity."

ALICIA BONET

Alicia is the young mother of a baby boy; the baby's physician is recommending that he start long-term aspirin therapy. Ms. Bonet is quite concerned about agreeing to long-term aspirin therapy and asks, "I've heard so much about Reye syndrome and aspirin. What should I do? What would you recommend?"

LEARNING OBJECTIVES

After completing the chapter, you will be able to accomplish the following:

1. Describe the teaching–learning process, including domains, developmental concerns, and specific principles.
2. Describe the factors that should be assessed in the learning process.
3. Discuss strategies that improve health literacy and promote patient safety.
4. Describe the factors that influence patient compliance with the therapeutic plan.
5. Formulate diagnoses for identified learning needs.
6. Explain how to create and implement a culturally competent, age-specific teaching plan for a patient.
7. Discuss the role of a nurse coach in promoting behavior change.
8. Name three methods for evaluating learning.
9. Explain what should be included in the documentation of the teaching–learning process.
10. Discuss the nurse's role as a counselor.
11. Summarize how the nursing process is used to help patients solve problems.
12. Describe how to use the counseling role to motivate a patient toward health promotion.

KEY TERMS

affective learning	health literacy	patient education
andragogy	informal teaching	pedagogy
cognitive learning	learning	positive reinforcement
contractual agreement	learning readiness	psychomotor learning
counseling	literacy	situational crisis
developmental crisis	negative reinforcement	teaching– learning process
formal teaching	nurse coach	

Helping patients and their families learn how to respond to their health care problems and how to protect their health is one of the most important nursing functions. Many patients lack the knowledge and self-care abilities they need to achieve their health goals. To work effectively with these patients, nurses must be skilled teachers and counselors. Both roles require strong communication skills. Current trends toward shorter hospital stays and decreased time for interactions between health care professionals and patients, dependence on complex technologies, health promotion/consumer empowerment, cost containment, and increased chronic illnesses have increased the need for effective teaching and counseling. Nurses are challenged with the task of teaching large amounts of information, with limited time and resources, to patients who might or might not be ready, willing, or able to learn. (See the accompanying Reflective Practice box for an example on page 480–481.)

Never has the demand for quality education and counseling been greater. Nurses who are skilled educators and counselors can improve patients' health and well-being and reduce the demand for professional services. The Joint Commission (TJC) has identified goals and standards for patient and family teaching and included them throughout its accreditation manual. These standards help ensure that the patient and family receive the information they need to maintain optimal health. They address an understanding of health status including disease and its treatment, informed decision making, and the promotion of healthy lifestyles. In 2002, TJC began sponsoring the "Speak Up" initiative. This is an effort to educate patients how to get involved in their care and prevent health care errors. The Speak Up campaign now includes 20 brochures and 8 videos that address topics such as things you can do to prevent infection, pain management recommendations, and how patients can avoid mistakes with their medications (TJC, 2012b). All these are available in English and Spanish. The complete list of "Speak Up" informational brochures and videos is available at http://www.jointcommission.org/speakup.aspx.

AIMS OF TEACHING AND COUNSELING

Patient education is the process of influencing the patient's behavior to effect changes in knowledge, attitudes, and skills needed to maintain and improve health. Research supports the fact that educated patients experience better health and have fewer complications. This results in fewer hospitalizations and emergency department, clinic, and physician visits. To be successful, patient education must be ongoing and interactive. It must also take into account the patient's plan of care, educational level, and need for care across the continuum from the hospital to home care to long-term care. Patient education plans should be developed in collaboration with the entire health care team, including members of the hospital team (e.g., dietitians, respiratory therapists, social workers, pharmacists) as well as home care agencies, wellness facilities, and long-term care agencies.

The basic purpose of teaching and counseling is to help patients and families develop the self-care abilities (knowledge, attitude, skills) they need to maximize their functioning and quality of life (or to have a dignified death). For example, a patient newly diagnosed with diabetes must (1) acquire knowledge about diabetes as a disease process and related medical management and self-care; (2) value health sufficiently to make certain lifestyle modifications (attitude);

REFLECTIVE PRACTICE: CULTIVATING QSEN COMPETENCIES

CHALLENGE TO ETHICAL AND LEGAL SKILLS

It was during my senior practicum in pediatrics last spring that I met Alicia Bonet, the young mother of a baby boy for whom I was caring. The baby's physician was recommending long-term aspirin therapy (unfortunately, I cannot remember what condition the child had for which long-term aspirin therapy was being recommended). Ms. Bonet was quite concerned about agreeing to aspirin therapy, asking me if I knew much about Reye syndrome. Then she asked me what I would recommend about whether or not to agree to long-term aspirin therapy. Not really understanding the risks versus the benefits of aspirin therapy or how it actually ties into Reye syndrome, I did not feel competent to answer Ms. Bonet's questions, let alone make an educated recommendation to her.

Thinking Outside the Box: Possible Courses of Action

- Tell the mother that I could not be of help to her in making this decision because of my lack of knowledge about either topic.
- Inform her that I would have to ask other nurses and physicians to explain both topics to me (due to my lack of knowledge) before I could give her my opinion.
- Tell her that because I didn't know very much about either aspirin therapy or Reye syndrome, I would research the topics in books and on the Internet when I had time and would get back to her with a recommendation based on my research.
- Be honest with the mother about my lack of knowledge about either aspirin therapy or Reye syndrome and offer to gather information from reputable sources for both of us so that we could discuss the topics.
- Provide her with information from the hospital library or the Internet so that she could educate herself (but not for my education so that I could assist her in making her decision).
- Lie to the mother (or withhold the fact that I did not know much about aspirin therapy or Reye syndrome) and make an uneducated recommendation simply because I had the "authority" to do so.
- Ignore the mother's request, pretending not to have time to discuss her questions, rather than admitting my own ignorance or taking the time to educate myself.

Evaluating a Good Outcome: How Do I Define Success?

- The mother's needs are met. Not only does she receive a professional, educated, and competent recommendation, but she also is given the opportunity to make her own educated decisions by being given the information she needs.
- My intellectual competence is challenged and improved. I am able to admit a deficit in my knowledge and embrace the opportunity to improve it.
- The mother and patient benefit from my actions (or at least are not harmed) by the mother's informed choice.
- The mother's autonomy is encouraged—by providing her with all the necessary information, I enable her to make a healthy, educated decision.
- Quality care is provided to the patient and his family by competent professionals.
- The mother expresses an understanding of the information presented to her, feels comfortable asking additional questions, and makes an educated decision with which she is comfortable.

Personal Learning: Here's to the Future!

After explaining to the mother that I was not very familiar with aspirin therapy or Reye syndrome, I first attempted to gather research information off the Internet for her. However, because I did not have a password to access the Internet from the nurse's station, I could not obtain the research I needed on my own. My next step was to ask my preceptor how to gather data for the mother if I could not get it off the Internet. She suggested calling down to the hospital library and asking them to put together an information packet that could be easily understood by a patient. I did this, and several hours later, the packet arrived on the floor. After flipping through it briefly, I was satisfied with its contents and delivered it to Ms. Bonet. While I wished I had had the time to read all the information myself so that I could sit down with the mother and discuss it in detail, the day had been particularly busy. The best I could do was to pass the information on to the mother and hope she would read it herself. She was very grateful that I went to the trouble of gathering so much information for her, and she did not seem at all annoyed or disappointed that I did not have time to sit down with her to review the material. I did let her know that she could feel free to ask me any questions after she read the material, but she never got a chance to read the packet before my shift ended (because her son had visitors). As a result, we never got around to discussing her concerns.

One of the things that I learned from this experience is that it is okay to admit to a patient that you do not have all the answers. Moreover, admitting this helps to allay any doubt that he or she may have about my intellect or abilities as a nurse. Admitting a lack of knowledge is not a weakness, but a strength, for half the battle is knowing what you do not know. If anything, my willingness to admit my lack of knowledge and eagerness to educate both myself and my patient (by doing research) helped inspire trust and faith in me by my patient. I also learned that sometimes doing the best we can is better than doing nothing at all, even if the best we can do is not very much. Although I really needed to be able to sit down with Ms. Bonet and review the research with her, simply providing her with the material was enough to enable her to make an informed decision on her own. That simple act most likely empowered her to be much more comfortable with her decision in the end.

Although this occurred only a few months ago, I feel safe saying that my professional intellectual skills are quite adequate now—actually, they were quite adequate back

REFLECTIVE PRACTICE: CULTIVATING QSEN COMPETENCIES *continued*

CHALLENGE TO ETHICAL AND LEGAL SKILLS

then, too. Not knowing everything in nursing is not a reflection of inadequate professional intellectual skills, because it is impossible to know everything in this field. The fact that I knew that my knowledge was lacking, but that I knew where to go to find an answer, tells me my professional intellectual skills are more than adequate.

Tracey Sara Miller, Georgetown University

REFLECTION ON QUALITY AND SAFETY COMPETENCIES

How do you think you would respond in a similar situation? Why? What does this tell you about yourself and about the adequacy of your skills for professional practice? What *knowledge, skills,* and *attitudes* do you need to develop to continuously improve quality and safety in a situation like the one experienced by this student nurse?

Patient-Centered Care: How did the nursing student's communication skills improve the nurse–patient relationship? Did her handling of this situation facilitate her ability to deliver effective care and treatment in other environments? What, if any, teaching and learning principles did the nursing student use?

Teamwork and Collaboration/Quality Improvement: How important are effective communication skills when collaborating with other team members and hospital staff? Are there other referrals or community resources that might prove helpful to Ms. Bonet regarding her questions about long-term aspirin use for her child?

Safety/Evidence-Based Practice: Is there anything else the nursing student could have done to facilitate a positive outcome? Do you agree with the criteria to evaluate a successful outcome? Did the nursing student meet the criteria? What evidence in nursing literature provides guidance to assist Ms. Bonet with effective decision-making in this situation? If time had not been a factor and you were able to discuss the materials in the packet with the baby's mother, would that have been an opportunity to assess Ms. Bonet's understanding of the information provided?

Informatics: Can you identify essential information that should be documented in the child's electronic record regarding your efforts to communicate with the mother about the specific concerns she expressed? Do you think the self-confidence gained from dealing effectively with this situation improves your ability to respond to patient's questions and accurately document their concerns?

---

and (3) master certain skills, such as insulin injection. When done effectively, teaching and counseling are powerful tools for helping patients achieve health goals. Teaching provides the knowledge that patients need to make informed health care decisions and to implement a plan of care.

 RECALL Alicia Bonet, the young mother worried about long-term aspirin therapy and Reye syndrome. By providing Ms. Bonet with information, the nurse enables her to reach a decision that is based on sound knowledge and one with which she is comfortable. •

Counseling provides the resources and support that patients need to participate actively in self-care and to facilitate their coping with what cannot be changed.

Maintaining and Promoting Health

Nurses can help patients to value health and develop specific health practices that promote wellness. Health teaching is varied and ranges from teaching passive exercises to a patient with left-sided paralysis to designing a safe exercise program for a young athlete.

Preventing Illness

Illness prevention, a major theme in health teaching and counseling, takes many forms. You can counsel women of childbearing age about health practices that promote optimal fetal development, teach parents how to make their home safe for a toddler, or counsel people at high risk for heart disease, cancer, or communicable diseases.

Restoring Health

Once a patient is ill, teaching and counseling focus on developing self-care practices that promote recovery. Preoperative and postoperative teaching, sexual counseling for a patient recovering from a myocardial infarction, and lifestyle counseling for a patient with an ostomy are all examples of teaching and counseling directed at restoring health.

 CONSIDER Rachel Blumenthal, the wife of the patient who had suffered a myocardial infarction. She is concerned about his activity level. When developing an appropriate teaching plan, the nurse would need to assess Mrs. Blumenthal's knowledge base before determining her actual teaching needs. In addition, the nurse would need to consult with the patient's cardiologist to determine the patient's status and what he will be allowed to do. These actions help to ensure that the teaching plan includes accurate information and is individualized to Mrs. Blumenthal's needs. •

Facilitating Coping

Developmental lifestyle changes and acute, chronic, and terminal illness all place demands on patients and families that may become overwhelming. As a nurse, you will work not only with patients but also with their families and friends to help them to come to terms with illness and whatever lifestyle modifications may be required. Not all patients fully recover from their illness or injury; many patients will need to learn to cope with permanent health alterations.

Outcomes

Nurse caregivers who are skilled teachers and counselors can promote the following outcomes:

- High-level wellness and related self-care practices
- Disease prevention or early detection
- Quick recovery from trauma or illness with minimal or no complications
- Enhanced ability to adjust to developmental lifestyle changes and acute, chronic, and terminal illness
- Family acceptance of the lifestyle changes necessitated by illness or disability

 REMEMBER Marco García Ramírez, the father-to-be described in the beginning of the chapter. Pregnancy and childbirth are considered developmental lifestyle changes. The nurse needs to incorporate knowledge of these changes when preparing an appropriate teaching plan for Mr. García Ramírez and his wife. The goal of teaching would be a positive adaptation to their new role as parents. ●

General topics for health teaching are listed in Box 21-1.

THE NURSE AS TEACHER

Teaching is a planned method or series of methods used to help someone learn. The person using these methods is the teacher. **Learning** is the process by which a person acquires or increases knowledge or changes behavior in a measurable way as a result of the experience. You assume the role of teacher and your patient assumes the role of learner when there are identifiable learning needs. This teacher–learner relationship is enhanced by the helping relationship (see Chapter 20), in which mutual respect and trust are established. You build on this trust by sharing information that you and your patient mutually identify as important.

 THINK back to Alicia Bonet, the young mother with questions about long-term aspirin therapy. The nurse developed trust with Ms. Bonet by honestly admitting that she lacked the necessary knowledge about the therapy. The nurse promoted an ongoing therapeutic relationship by seeking the information, thereby solidifying the trust. ●

The patient may ask for this information, or you may initiate teaching after assessing and diagnosing a learning need. Much patient education focuses on three critical areas:

- Preparation for receiving care
- Preparation before discharge from a health care facility
- Documentation of patient education activity

BOX 21-1 | **TOPICS FOR HEALTH TEACHING AND COUNSELING**

Promoting Health
- Developmental and maturational issues
- Normal childbearing
- Hygiene
- Nutrition
- Exercise
- Mental health
- Spiritual health

Preventing Illness
- First aid
- Safety
- Immunizations
- Screening
- Identification and management of risk factors

Restoring Health
- Orientation to treatment center and staff
- Patients' and nurses' expectations of one another
- The illness and physical condition: anatomy and physiology, etiology of problem, significance of symptoms, prognosis
- The medical and nursing regimens and how the patient can participate in care
- Self-care practices the patient and family need to manage the patient's condition independently

Facilitating Coping
- How the patient's physical and mental condition affects other areas of functioning; lifestyle counseling
- Measures that maximize independence and enhance self-concept
- Stress management
- Environmental alterations
- Community resources
- Appropriate referrals (e.g., physical therapy, occupational therapy, self-help groups, psychiatric–mental health counselor)
- Grief and bereavement counseling

Like other clinical interventions, effective patient teaching demands analytic and problem-solving skills. To maximize the effectiveness of patient teaching, remember the acronym TEACH:

T: Tune into the patient.

E: Edit patient information.

A: Act on every teaching moment.

C: Clarify often.

H: Honor the patient as a partner in the education process.

Learning to be an effective teacher is a critical component of professional development. A basic understanding of the **teaching–learning process** helps you develop your own teaching and learning skills. The process of patient teaching, which resembles the nursing process, consists of several steps that are necessary to provide teaching and to measure learning (Box 21-2). This process is often condensed because of limited time or resources, but the basic principles apply each time teaching–learning occurs.

BOX 21-2   STEPS OF THE TEACHING–LEARNING PROCESS

Assess Learning Needs and Learning Readiness

1. Use all appropriate sources of information.
2. Identify the knowledge, attitudes, or skills needed by the patient and family.
3. Assess the patient's emotional and experiential readiness to learn.
4. Assess factors affecting the patient's ability to learn, including age and development level, family support networks and financial resources, cultural influences, literacy, and language barriers.
5. Develop critical pathways or teaching plans that span care delivery settings from hospital to home to take advantage of optimal learning readiness.
6. Identify the patient's strengths.
7. Use anticipatory guidance.

Diagnose the Patient's Learning Needs

1. Be realistic.
2. Validate with patient or family through conversations, questionnaires, and checklists.

Develop Learning Outcomes

1. Identify specific, attainable, measurable, and short-term outcomes for patient learning.
2. Make sure that proposed behavioral changes are realistic and explored in the context of the patient's resources and lifestyle.
3. Decide which domain of learning is involved (cognitive, psychomotor, affective).
4. Prioritize.
5. Include the patient and family. Unless the patient values these outcomes, little learning is likely to occur.

Develop a Teaching Plan

1. Select content, content sequencing, and appropriate teaching strategies/activities.
2. Relate the teaching content to the patient's learning style, interests, resources, and patterns of everyday living.
3. Pay careful attention to time constraints, scheduling, and the physical environment.
4. Decide on group versus individual teaching and formal versus informal methodologies.
5. Formulate a verbal or written contract with the patient.

Implement Teaching Plan and Strategies

1. Prepare the physical environment, with attention to comfort and privacy.
2. Communicate effectively with individuals, small groups, and, in some instances, large groups.
3. Gather all audiovisual materials and equipment.
4. Deliver the content in an organized manner using the selected teaching strategies.
5. Be flexible.
6. Keep teaching sessions short.
7. Vary strategies for sensory stimulation, which promotes learning.
8. Relate the material to the patients' life experiences, which will help them assimilate new knowledge.
9. Plan how you will evaluate learning.
10. Assess verbal and nonverbal feedback.

Evaluate Learning

1. Evaluate whether the learner outcomes were met:
   - Observe a return demonstration.
   - Ask the patient to restate the instructions.
   - Ask the patient questions to determine whether teaching reinforcement is needed.
   - Use written test or questionnaires.
   - Consult with the patient's family.
   - Consider patient feedback and comments.
2. Reinforce and celebrate learning.
3. Evaluate teaching:
   - Self-evaluation
   - Patient questionnaires
4. Revise the plan if the learner outcome is not met:
   - Alter content and teaching strategies.
   - Use motivational counseling.
   - Reschedule teaching sessions.
5. Document the teaching–learning process:
   - Patient and family learning needs and identified barriers to learning
   - Mechanisms used to overcome learning barriers
   - Patient and family readiness to learn
   - Current knowledge regarding the patient's condition and health status
   - Learning outcomes agreed on by the nurse, patient, and family
   - Identification of learning outcomes
   - Information and skills taught
   - Teaching methods used
   - Patient and family response
   - Evaluation of what patient and family learned and need for follow-up

Being a successful teacher requires excellent communication skills and sensitivity to all the factors that affect the patient's ability to learn (Fig. 21-1).

Factors Affecting Patient Learning

By taking into consideration the patient's age and developmental level, family support networks and financial resources, cultural influences and language deficits, and health literacy level, you can individualize the teaching plan and maximize learning. This will support the nursing goal of helping the patient to manage one's own health care needs.

FIGURE 21-1. Effective communication is essential in the teaching–learning process.

Age and Developmental Level

People learn throughout life, although what they learn and how learning occurs change according to developmental stages. Three critical developmental areas to consider when developing a teaching plan are the patient's physical maturation and abilities, psychosocial development, and cognitive capacity. Other concerns related to the teaching–learning process include the patient's emotional maturity and moral and spiritual development.

CHILD AND ADOLESCENT LEARNERS

Piaget's theory of intellectual development is a major learning theory (see Chapter 17). By understanding how children and adolescents develop learning abilities, you can use this knowledge when teaching patients. When the patient is an infant, teaching is directed toward the parents. Toddlers and preschoolers may have some degree of understanding about medical tests or procedures, but health teaching continues to be directed toward the parents. For patients in this age range, it helps for one nurse to establish a relationship with the patient and family and to be consistently involved in patient-teaching activities. An example of teaching considerations for young children would be the case of a 4-year-old girl diagnosed with diabetes: the child must begin to take insulin every day, and the nurse should recognize the child's limitations in understanding diabetes. Information should be simplified to include only the most basic facts, with concrete examples or demonstrations; a detailed discussion of the pathophysiology of diabetes would not be appropriate. The girl could be told that she needs a shot every day to keep her from getting sick or feeling "funny." She could be allowed to play with the syringes and to give shots to a doll. Children today, even at very young ages, have likely been exposed to online games with colorful animations that teach basic information. Their manual dexterity skills may be more advanced, and they may be more comfortable with tasks previously viewed as challenging for them. Preschool children are often eager to demonstrate a skill they have been taught and may ask many questions. Explanations should be short and composed of simple words. Compared to adults, children have shorter attention spans and a greater need for nurturing, support, and creative participation in learning activities.

School-aged children are capable of logical reasoning and should be included in the teaching–learning process whenever possible. Teaching strategies that include clear explanations and reasons for procedures, stated in a simple and logical manner, are most successful. These children are open to new learning experiences but need learning to be reinforced by either a parent or health care personnel as they become more involved with their friends and school activities.

The cognitive processes of adolescents are similar to those of adults, thus the content and strategies of patient teaching resemble those used for teaching adults. There are some important considerations to keep in mind, however. For example, when teaching a sexually active 16-year-old girl about contraceptive methods, you would assess whether the young patient has reached the stage Piaget refers to as formal operations (the ability to use logical reasoning to solve hypothetical problems). If the patient's intellectual development is delayed and she is still in the period of concrete operations (use of logical reasoning to solve concrete problems), she may be less skilled in thinking abstractly—that is, she may not perceive pregnancy as a real possibility and, therefore, may not fully understand the need for contraception. If so, you can alter the teaching plan to include online teaching aids that are easily accessible and explain the topic in concrete terms. Peer group acceptance is critical for most adolescents. Teaching strategies designed for an adolescent patient should recognize the adolescent's need for independence and the need to establish a trusting relationship that demonstrates respect for the adolescent's opinions.

Motor development is also a concern in the teaching–learning process. A 4-year-old girl diagnosed with diabetes may not be able to administer her own insulin shots if she lacks the fine motor skills needed to manipulate the equipment, but a 13-year-old patient could probably master the technique quickly.

ADULT LEARNERS

As people age, their personalities and learning abilities change. Most psychologists who have studied the teaching–learning process base their work on children and adolescents because a large amount of learning occurs early in life. The science of teaching (**pedagogy**) generally refers to the teaching of children and adolescents. In recent years, however, the study of teaching adults (**andragogy**) has gained more attention.

Adults need to be taught differently than children. Knowles (1990) listed the following four assumptions about adult learners:

1. As people mature, their self-concept is likely to move from dependence to independence.
2. The previous experience of the adult is a rich resource for learning.
3. An adult's readiness to learn is often related to a developmental task or a social role.
4. Most adults' orientation to learning is that material should be useful immediately, rather than at some time in the future.

Thus, andragogy focuses on a specific problem or need and on the immediate application of new material. In general, adult learners must believe that they need to learn before they become willing to learn. Nurses often must use their counseling skills (discussed later) to motivate patients to participate in the teaching–learning process. Adults may need to be shown the importance of learning new information, health practices, or skills.

Because health promotion and injury avoidance are important activities throughout the lifespan, teaching methods need to be further modified when working with older patients. When developing a teaching plan for older adults, first identify any learning barriers such as sensory loss, limited physical mobility, or inability to comply with the recommended therapeutic regimen. Sensory deficits that can affect learning in older adults include the presence of cataracts that can cloud vision, a decrease in lens accommodation that necessitates adequate lighting, a decrease in peripheral vision that requires that teaching materials be kept immediately in front of the learner, or a hearing loss that make it imperative for the teacher to speak slowly and clearly (Nigolian & Miller, 2011). Successful teaching plans for older adults incorporate extra time, short teaching sessions, accommodation for sensory deficits, and reduction of environmental distractions. Older adults also benefit from instruction that relates new information to familiar activities or information.

Family Support Networks and Financial Resources

No matter what the patient's age, working with the patient's family can be a great help in patient teaching. Assess the family's function and style by talking with them and observing how the patient and family interact. This assessment will yield information about family function, stress, transitions, and expectations. Informal conversations with both the patient and family can provide data that will help in developing the teaching plan. The COPE model described in Box 21-3 is one method of helping family members to become effective problem solvers and support your teaching efforts.

Almost one third of American families have a caregiver who provides unpaid assistance for an older adult family member (Nigolian & Miller, 2011). This family caregiver also provides support when the patient is hospitalized and needs to be involved in collaboration with hospital staff regarding discharge planning. When teaching long-term family caregivers, include information about the disease process and resources available in the community that can help them with disease management and education, with a focus on planning, caregiving, decision making, and problem solving. Always view the family caregiver as a partner in providing care and view yourself as a health educator

---

BOX 21-3   THE COPE MODEL

C: Creativity

Help the family overcome obstacles to carrying out health care management and learning how to generate alternatives.

O: Optimism

Help the family caregivers learn how to view the caregiving situation with confidence.

P: Planning

Help the family learn how to plan for future problems and how to develop contingency plans that reduce uncertainty.

E: Expert Information

Help the family learn how to obtain expert information from health care providers about what to do in specific situations. This information empowers caregivers by encouraging them to develop plans for solving caregiving problems.

BOX 21-4   CULTURALLY COMPETENT PATIENT TEACHING

- Develop an understanding of the patient's culture.
- Work with a multicultural team in developing educational programs.
- Be aware of personal assumptions, biases, and prejudices.
- Understand the core cultural values of the patient or group.
- Develop written materials in the patient's native language.
- Use testimonials of people with the same cultural background as the patient.

---

who teaches families how to solve problems, rather than as an expert meant to solve problems for them.

In addition, evaluate the family's financial resources, because the patient may be unable to afford to follow a new treatment regimen. If needed, refer patients and families to community-based support groups and funding sources.

Cultural Influences and Language Deficits

As our society becomes more ethnically diverse, nurses are continuously faced with the challenge of providing care and education to patients from many different cultural and ethnic backgrounds. To do so successfully, you may need to seek information from a variety of sources, such as the nursing literature and textbooks that describe the health practices and values of other cultures. Box 21-4 outlines strategies for providing patient education in a culturally competent manner.

In addition, be sure to identify language deficits or barriers and develop strategies to address them, clearly communicating this in the plan of care. Do not assume that a family member is adequately translating information critical to the patient's learning. In July, 2012, TJC initiated a new accreditation requirement that hospitals must accommodate the oral and written communication needs of all patients (TJC, 2012a). This includes translated, clearly stated patient education information. To help deal with a culturally and ethnically diverse population, patient education specialists from four health systems in central Ohio offer free, easy-to-read, copyrighted health information in multiple languages on the website HealthInfoTranslations.org. More than 300 education topics are available. TJC has identified this website as a "best practice resource" (Moyer, Guthrie, & Wingert, 2012). The National Library of Medicine on Medline Plus also has patient education materials in multiple languages that include tutorials with animated graphic materials and accompanying handouts (Lorenz, 2011). This site links many interactive health tutorials with HealthInfoTranslations.org (Moyer, Guthrie, & Wingert, 2012).

Health Literacy

According to a report by TJC (2012), approximately 90 million Americans lack the basic **literacy** skills (the ability to read and write) needed to function successfully in our society.

Health literacy is the ability to read, understand, and act on health information. The National Center for Education Statistics identifies the lack of health literacy skills, reporting that only approximately 12% of Americans are proficient in health literacy (Robert Wood Johnson Foundation, 2011). Even though this is true of all populations, minority and groups of lower socioeconomic status more commonly lack health literacy skills (U.S. Department of Health and Human Services [DHHS], 2010). Given the complexity of health care, it is clear that many people are unable to understand basic health information, search for health information, adopt healthy behaviors, and make appropriate health care decisions. This population is more likely to avoid medical screenings and require emergency department attention.

Federal initiatives such as the Affordable Care Act of 2010 and the National Action Plan to Improve Health Literacy from DHHS have made health literacy a national priority to improve the health of all Americans (Koh et al., 2012). The scope of the problem is challenging, in part because health care information and directions have traditionally been written at a 10th-grade level or higher, while educational material is generally more easily understood when written at a 5th-grade level. Low health literacy affects all segments of our population and threatens the quality and safety of our health care.

The National Patient Safety Foundation collaborated with the Partnership for Clear Health Communication to promote awareness of the need for improved health literacy and to seek solutions that result in more positive patient outcomes. The Ask Me 3 brief tool is intended to promote understanding and improve communication between patients and their providers. It involves three simple questions that patients should ask their health care providers during every encounter. Providers are encouraged to answer these questions in a clear, forthright manner. The Ask Me 3 questions are:

- What is my main problem?
- What do I need to do?
- Why is it important for me to do this?

The health care provider's response should include plain language without medical jargon, may incorporate the use of visual models to explain a disease or procedure, and may involve patients in a "teach back" demonstration that verifies their understanding of the information presented (National Patient Safety Foundation, 2013). See the accompanying Promoting Health Literacy display in this and other chapters throughout this book for an example in action.

The teach-back tool assesses health literacy, seeking to confirm that the learner understands the health information received from the health professional. It is important when

PROMOTING HEALTH LITERACY

IN PATIENTS WHO SMOKE

Patient Scenario

Jack Boyer is 37 years old and has been smoking since he was 17 years of age. During a routine physical, he admits to a one pack per day habit. In response to a question from his physician, Jack admits that several previous attempts to stop smoking failed after a day or two. He states on his history form that he is married and has two sons, 7 and 3 years of age, and also lists that his father died following a heart attack at the age of 60. Jack tells his physician that he is essentially healthy but is under a lot of stress. Because of the downturn in the economy, his job in automotive sales is at risk. His wife works full-time as an administrative assistant. The physician expresses concern to Jack about the effects of second-hand smoke on his family. Jack states, "I know all about that and when I smoke in the car, I keep the window down and blow the smoke outside. At home, I try to smoke outside most of the time except when the weather is bad." The physical examination reveals that Jack has hypertension (BP 164/92), is 15 pounds overweight, and is currently having difficulty sleeping. The physician explains that he would like to monitor Jack's blood pressure for 1 month before prescribing antihypertensive medication. He recommends that Jack make a serious effort to stop smoking and reviews the harmful effects of nicotine use and the long-term benefits for Jack as well as his family if he stops smoking. The physician explains that the nurse will give Jack information about quitting smoking when he makes an appointment for his next visit. As Jack is speaking with the nurse, he comments that maybe he'll switch to chewing tobacco since there's no smoke involved with that.

Nursing Considerations: *Tips for Improving Health Literacy*

Provide Jack with information about ways to help him quit smoking. Mention that counseling and behavior cessation therapies have proven effective and that often it takes repeated attempts to quit. Jack needs to understand the harmful effects of second-hand smoke on his family, as well as the fact that people who stop smoking greatly reduce their risk of lung cancer, heart disease, and respiratory symptoms. Explain to him that smokeless tobacco is also a significant health risk and not a safe substitute for smoking cigarettes. Give him information about nicotine replacement products (gum, inhalers, patches) found effective in treating tobacco dependence. Several nonnicotine medications are also available but need to be prescribed by his physician. For extra help, tell him to call 1-800-QUIT-NOW. When Jack returns for his follow-up appointment, he needs to be prepared to ask his physician the following questions to help him understand that tobacco addiction is a chronic condition and what the positive outcomes of quitting will be:

- What is my main problem?
- What do I need to do?
- Why is it important for me to do this?

What additional measures can you take to help increase health literacy in this patient? What other measures would be helpful if Jack did not speak English, could not read, or had other learning deficits?

a person has difficulty reading and comprehending written materials or has limited English proficiency. Patients and caregivers have the opportunity to repeat back to the health care provider the key points they understand from a teaching session. The health care provider should speak slowly and clearly and focus on the most important concepts. The health care provider should ask any questions in a shame-free manner, using open-ended questions. An interpreter may be required in some instances (Nigolian & Miller, 2011). Dickens and Piano (2013) report that even though the teach-back method has been proven to be effective, it is not used consistently.

An additional tool has recently been developed to assess the level of a patient's understanding of new health information. The Understanding Personal Perception (UPP) tool is an attempt to determine if additional education is necessary. The nurse asks the patient to look at the images on the tool and decide which of the figures most accurately indicates the patient's understanding of the new health education materials. This tool has images ranging from either a bright sun (signifying that the patient completely understands the material) to gray clouds (confusions exists) to dark clouds blocking the sun (new information is not understood; Murdock & Griffin, 2013).

The Newest Vital Sign (NVS) is an additional reliable screening tool to assess health literacy. It was developed by Pfizer to improve communications between patients and providers and can be administered during initial assessments to assess the patient's literacy skills involving both numbers and words (Pfizer Clear Health Communication, 2012). The Newest Vital Sign tool consists of a nutrition label from an ice cream container (Fig. 21-2) and a score sheet for recording the patient's answers to six oral questions referring to the label (Fig. 21-3 on page 488). Literacy is interpreted according to the number of correct responses on the score sheet. The time spent administering this tool more than compensates for the time providers might need clarifying a diagnosis, treatment, or medications if they had not recognized a patient's limited literacy.

Learning Domains

Patients learn in three domains: cognitive, psychomotor, and affective (Bloom, 1956). The ability of patients to manage their daily life and resume their former roles depends on the extent to which their cognitive, psychomotor, and affective learning results in behavioral changes. These domains influence the nurse's selection of teaching and evaluation strategies. Effective teaching often involves the promotion of behaviors in all three domains.

Cognitive learning involves the storing and recalling of new knowledge in the brain (e.g., the patient describes how salt intake affects blood pressure). Cognitive learning includes intellectual behaviors such as the acquisition of knowledge, comprehension, application (using abstract ideas in concrete situations), analysis (relating ideas in an organized way), synthesis (assimilating parts of information as a whole), and evaluation (judging the worth of a body of information).

Nutrition Facts		
Serving Size		½ cup
Servings per container		4
Amount per serving		
Calories 250	Fat Cal	120
		%DV
Total Fat 13g		20%
Sat Fat 9g		40%
Cholesterol 28mg		12%
Sodium 55mg		2%
Total Carbohydrate 30g		12%
Dietary Fiber 2g		
Sugars 23g		
Protein 4g		8%

*Percentage Daily Values (DV) are based on a 2,000 calorie diet. Your daily values may be higher or lower depending on your calorie needs.

Ingredients: Cream, Skim Milk, Liquid Sugar, Water, Egg Yolks, Brown Sugar, Milkfat, Peanut Oil, Sugar, Butter, Salt, Carrageenan, Vanilla Extract.

FIGURE 21-2. The Newest Vital Sign (NVS) Health Literacy Assessment Tool. Available at http://www.pfizerhealthliteracy.com/asset/pdf/NVS_Eng/files/nvs_flipbook_english_final.pdf (Reprinted with permission.)

Learning a physical skill involving the integration of mental and muscular activity is called **psychomotor learning** (e.g., the patient demonstrates how to change dressings using clean technique).

Affective learning includes changes in attitudes, values, and feelings (e.g., the patient expresses renewed self-confidence after physical therapy).

 RECALL Marco García Ramírez, the father-to-be with concerns about his new role. The nurse would develop a teaching plan that focuses on the three domains of learning. The nurse would address the cognitive domain by teaching Mr. García Ramírez and his wife about labor and delivery, including the labor process and what events will occur. Teaching the couple about newborn care and breathing techniques to use during labor would address the psychomotor domain. Learning in the affective domain would be demonstrated if Mr. García Ramírez reports that the he and his wife do not fear labor and feel comfortable handling a newborn. ●

Effective Communication Techniques

A critical component of effective patient education is the nurse's ability to be an effective communicator. Key points

Score Sheet for the Newest Vital Sign
Questions and Answers

READ TO SUBJECT:
This information is on the back of a container of a point of ice cream.

	ANSWER CORRECT?	
	yes	no

1. If you eat the entire container, how many calories will you eat?
   Answer: 1,000 is the only correct answer

2. If you are allowed to eat 60 grams of carbohydrates as a snack, how much ice cream could you have?
   Answer: Any of the following is correct: 1 cup (or any amount up to 1 cup), half the container. Note: If patient answers "two servings," ask "How much ice cream would that be if you were to measure it into a bowl?"

3. Your doctor advises you to reduce the amount of saturated fat in your diet. You usually have 42 g of saturated fat each day, which includes one serving of ice cream. If you stop eating ice cream, how many grams of saturated fat would you be consuming each day?
   Answer: 33 is the only correct answer

4. If you usually eat 2,500 calories in a day, what percentage of your daily value of calories will you be eating if you eat one serving?
   Answer: 10% is the only correct answer

READ TO SUBJECT:
Pretend that you are allergic to the following substances: penicillin, peanuts, latex gloves, and bee stings.

5. Is it safe for you to eat this ice cream?
   Answer: No

6. (Ask only if the patient responds "no" to question 5): Why not?
   Answer: Because it has peanut oil.

Number of correct answers:

Interpretation
Score of 0-1 suggests high likelihood (50% or more) of limited literacy.
Score of 2-3 indicates the possibility of limited literacy.
Score of 4-6 almost always indicates adequate literacy.

Working together for a healthier world™

February 2011

FIGURE 21-3. The Score Sheet for The Newest Vital Sign (NVS) includes questions and answers that refer to the label. Available at http://www.pfizerhealthliteracy.com/asset/pdf/NVS_Eng/files/nvs_flipbook_english_final.pdf (Reprinted with permission.)

of effective communication associated with patient teaching include the following:

- Be sincere and honest; show genuine interest and respect.
- Avoid giving too much detail; stick to the basics.
- Ask if the patient has any questions.
- Be a "cheerleader" for the patient. Avoid lecturing.
- Use simple words.
- Vary your tone of voice.
- Keep the content clear and concise.
- Listen and do not interrupt when the patient speaks.
- Ensure that the environment is conducive to learning and free of interruptions.
- Be sensitive to the timing of teaching sessions. A shorter session is best for a younger child, and an adult may need to choose an opportune time to learn new information.

NURSING PROCESS FOR PATIENT AND CAREGIVER TEACHING

Patient teaching is approached most effectively using the steps of the nursing process. The teaching–learning process and the nursing process are interdependent.

Assessing

Usually, patients themselves are the best source of assessment information. Patients are considered primary sources of information. By using effective interviewing techniques (see Chapter 20), you can obtain the data needed to identify learning needs. In addition, relevant information can be obtained before actually meeting the patient by reviewing the patient's past and current medical records. These records are considered secondary sources of information; they can provide a history of medical problems as well as documentation of the nursing assessments, nursing diagnoses, nursing physical examinations, and nursing interventions that have been performed.

The patient's family and significant others are also valuable sources of assessment data. They are sometimes needed to provide assessment data when the patient cannot communicate because of health problems, language barriers, or impaired sensory functions. At other times, family members or significant others might be the most appropriate source of certain information; for example, if seeking information about how much salt is used in the family's cooking, you could speak with the person who prepares the meals at home and include that person in any teaching about food preparation. The patient's permission is needed before family members are involved in the teaching–learning process.

Assessment Parameters

Four elements should be considered in each assessment of patient learning needs (Box 21-5). First, identify what new knowledge, attitudes, or skills are necessary for patients and families to learn in order to manage their health care. Second, focus on **learning readiness**, the

---

BOX 21-5 ASSESSMENT PARAMETERS: FACTORS THAT AFFECT LEARNING

1. **Knowledge, attitudes, and skills needed for the patient and family to manage health care independently**
2. **Readiness to learn**
   - Emotional readiness
     Emotional health
     Motivation for learning
     Self-concept and body image
     Sense of responsibility for self
   - Experiential readiness
     Social and economic stability
     Past experiences with learning
     Attitude toward learning
     Culture
3. **Ability to learn**
   - Physical condition
   - Cognitive ability to learn
   - Acuity of senses
   - Developmental considerations
   - Level of education
   - Literacy
   - Communication skills
   - Primary language
4. **Learning strengths**
   - Successful learning in the past
   - Above-average comprehension, reasoning, memory, or psychomotor skills
   - High motivation
   - Strong network
   - Adequate financing

---

patient's willingness to engage in the teaching–learning process (emotional readiness) and to begin the challenge of learning. Barriers to learning readiness include a patient's denial of being ill, lack of physical endurance, lack of human or financial resources, a perceived benefit of continuing in the sick role, and a disparity of values between the patient and the health care provider. Readiness is distinguished from the patient's actual ability to learn, which is the third element. The fourth element of assessment is the patient's strengths, which are the personal resources that you can help the patient to tap.

MOTIVATION

When assessing a patient's learning readiness, consider the patient's motivation. Patients who are ready to learn are able and motivated to process new information, develop new skills, and explore new attitudes and behaviors. Motivation is an internal impulse (such as emotion or physical pain) that encourages the patient to take action or change behavior.

 THINK back to Rachel Blumenthal, the wife of the patient who had a myocardial infarction. Although further assessment is necessary, analysis of Mrs. Blumenthal's questions would lead the nurse to suspect that she is interested in finding out information, showing motivation and a beginning readiness to learn. ●

A patient's health beliefs can have great influence on motivation. The health belief model identifies several health beliefs as critical for patient motivation (Rosenstock, 1974). Motivation is enhanced when:

- Patients view themselves as susceptible to the disease in question
- Patients view the disease as a serious threat
- Patients believe there are actions they can take to reduce the probability of contracting the disease
- Patients believe the threat of taking these actions is not as great as the disease itself

The health belief model was designed to explain why people are willing to take actions to support their health, but it evolved into a strategy for predicting the likelihood that patients would comply with therapies. Motivation plays a key role in the health belief model because it spurs the patient to behave in ways for health promotion and disease protection. Examples of motivational triggers include personal crisis and loss of social role due to disease symptoms. You can use the health belief model when developing teaching plans, evaluating the ideas or beliefs that motivate a patient, and applying these to the teaching plan. For example, if you are able to modify a patient's perception of disease susceptibility, the patient might become more receptive to learning.

COMPLIANCE

Nursing assessment of the patient's learning needs is vital to developing a plan of care with which the patient can comply. Patients are considered compliant when they follow the treatment plan and use the information they have been taught. When patients understand their diagnosis, treatment rationale, medication regimen, and the benefits of compliance, they are more likely to comply. Noncompliance occurs when patients ignore instructions or do not follow them appropriately. Noncompliance can be associated with a lack of learning readiness and motivation, confusion, disappointment, misunderstanding, fear, inability to learn, or inadequate finances. Noncompliance can hurt the patient's health.

Patients control the choices they make about following the plan of care and using what they have been taught, but it is your responsibility as a nurse to help patients improve their health by sharing knowledge, solving problems, and providing support while the patient integrates the new knowledge and practices the new skills. Increased patient compliance results directly from effective patient teaching. Box 21-6 lists ways to help patients and families become compliant with the plan of care.

BOX 21-6 **PROMOTING PATIENT AND FAMILY COMPLIANCE**

- Be certain that health care instructions are understandable and designed to support patient goals.
- Include the patient and family as partners in the teaching–learning process.
- Use interactive teaching strategies.
- Remember that teaching and learning are processes that rely on strong interpersonal relationships with patients and their families.

Diagnosing

If the patient lacks the required knowledge, attitudes, or skills to support health promotion, you should diagnose the deficit. Use diagnoses or problem statements approved by the North American Nursing Diagnosis Association-International (NANDA-I) as a guide when diagnosing learning needs (see Chapter 12). If you believe that a patient's knowledge deficit is the primary problem, write a diagnosis identifying a specific knowledge deficit as the problem, followed by its etiology and the related signs and symptoms. For example, Deficient Knowledge: Breastfeeding related to inexperience, as manifested by anxiety and multiple questions.

A knowledge deficit usually results in an actual or potential problem; therefore, the knowledge deficit is written as the etiology (second part of the diagnostic statement): for example, Imbalanced Nutrition: Less Than Body Requirements related to mother's lack of knowledge about infant feeding and deficient learning readiness (as manifested by mother's quick frustration when breastfeeding, refusal to engage in learning process, infant's weight loss).

If you learn that a pregnant woman plans to breastfeed but knows nothing about breastfeeding, "Deficient Knowledge: Breastfeeding" is the problem statement. The goal is to increase the mother's knowledge. If, on the other hand, you observe a newborn failing to gain weight appropriately, and it is reasonable to suspect that the mother's lack of knowledge about how to breastfeed is interfering with the infant's nutritional intake, "Deficient Knowledge: Breastfeeding" is the etiology. The goal is to ensure the infant's proper nutrition.

Related nursing diagnoses include the following:

- Ineffective Health Maintenance
- Ineffective Therapeutic Regimen Management
- Noncompliance
- Self-Care Deficit (specify)

In addition to identifying the patient's learning needs, you should assess your own knowledge base and teaching skills. Nurses cannot teach information and skills to patients if they themselves lack the information and skills

BOX 21-7 SAMPLE TEACHING PLAN

Diagnosis: Ineffective breastfeeding related to deficient knowledge (nipple care)
Signs and Symptoms: complaints of sore nipples, redness, cracking

Long-term Outcome: Woman will be able to breastfeed as long as desired without nipple problems

Learner Outcome	Met	Content	Teaching Strategy	Learner Activity
Woman describes measures to prevent nipple cracking (cognitive)	8/10/14 L.I.	Protective measures: • Avoid soap. • Avoid exposure to air and sunlight.	Discussion Audiovisual: flip chart on breastfeeding	Read handout: Nipple care View "Breastfeeding—skin and nipple changes"; available at http://www.nlm.nih.gov/medlineplus/ency/patientinstructions/000632.htm
Woman begins protective measures immediately (psychomotor)	8/10/14 L.I.	• Apply lanolin or vegetable oil. • Avoid plastic liners in bra or bra pads.		
Woman describes the correct procedure for breastfeeding (cognitive)	8/10/14 L.I.	Preparation for breastfeeding • Nipple roll before the feeding.	Discussion Audiovisual: flip chart on breastfeeding	Read handout: Sore nipples
Woman explains why feedings should be shorter and more frequent (cognitive)	8/10/14 L.I.	Breastfeeding the baby • Feed baby every 2 hours during the day. • Start baby on less sore side.	Discovery: guide through each step; assist as necessary Return demonstration	Read handout: Positioning baby for breastfeeding View "Breastfeeding Tips"; available at http://www.nichd.nih.gov/health/topics/breastfeeding/conditioninfo/Pages/how-is-it-done.aspx
Woman demonstrates correct procedure for breastfeeding (psychomotor)	8/10/14 L.I.	• Get baby onto areola area. • Position properly. • Change position for each feeding. • Remove baby from breast.		
Display increasing confidence in breastfeeding skills and self-care (affective)	8/10/14 L.I.	After feeding • Air dry the nipples. • Inspect for open or cracked areas. • Apply lanolin or vegetable oil.	Discovery	
Value good nutrition and rest at home (affective)	8/10/14 L.I.	Home considerations • Maintain "demand feedings." • Ensure good nutrition. • Get adequate rest. • Know the signs and symptoms of thrush.	Lecture with discussion Audiovisual: poster	Refer to handouts at home as needed; call maternity department's information number for any questions.
List the signs of thrush (cognitive)	8/10/14 L.I.			

to be taught. Often, knowing where to find information or an appropriate resource person is the first step in correcting one's own knowledge deficits.

Outcome Identification and Planning

Planning for learning involves the development of a teaching plan. Teaching plans are similar to nursing care plans—both follow the steps of the nursing process. One type of teaching plan is presented in Box 21-7. It is directed toward teaching appropriate nipple care to reduce the likelihood of nipple cracking and redness in breastfeeding women.

Standardized teaching plans are available for major topics of health teaching. Such plans must be tailored to the patient's learning needs and abilities. Remember that factors such as age, developmental level, family support networks, financial resources, cultural influences, language deficits, and health literacy affect the patient's ability to learn; consider them when individualizing the teaching plan. Examples of teaching plans that are incorporated into critical path documentation systems are featured in Chapters 13 and 16.

Thoughtful planning of patient teaching maximizes the patient's learning while ensuring the most efficient use of your time and skills. Learner outcomes are developed for each diagnosis of a learning need. The nursing orders become the content, teaching strategy, and learner activity columns of the written plan. This phase requires thought and creativity. Your efforts are rewarded when the patient meets the outcomes at the end of the implementation phase.

When planning for learning, decide together with the patient who should be included in the learning sessions. When the patient is a young child, one or both parents may be the primary learners. For an adult patient, a spouse or close friend who will be giving the care that is to be learned may be included. For instance, the person who does the household's cooking is usually asked to be present for nutritional teaching. Teaching plans are developed according to the needs of the people being taught.

One or several nurses can prepare and use a teaching plan. When two or more nurses plan and coordinate the implementation of the plan, this is called team teaching. An advantage of team teaching is that it takes advantage of the talents of more than one nurse.

Duplicating teaching that has already been completed by other members of the health care team wastes time and causes frustration. Accurate and thorough documentation of all patient teaching, along with review of the medical record before teaching sessions and effective communication with members of the interdisciplinary team, can prevent this problem.

Several factors should be considered while formulating any teaching plan, as discussed in the next sections.

Patient Learning Outcomes

Learner outcomes are written in the same manner as the patient outcomes in the nursing process (see Chapter 13). When planning for the patient's learning, first determine which of the three learning domains (cognitive, psychomotor, or affective) is the focus of teaching. Then write learning outcomes that reflect what learning is to occur. Learning outcomes should be stated as desired or expected patient behaviors, rather than as nursing interventions. For a patient having difficulty sleeping, for example, an appropriate learning outcome is "Avoid foods, beverages, and OTC medications in the evening that contain caffeine" rather than "Teach the patient about foods and beverages that contain caffeine," which states a nursing behavior. A well-constructed learning outcome is measurable and serves as a guide for planning evaluation methods.

Choosing the verb for a learning outcome is probably the most difficult part of writing outcomes (Box 21-8). But a careful choice makes it easier to plan the content, teaching strategies, learner activities, and evaluation.

 Concept Mastery Alert

The domains of learning guide the learning outcomes. It is helpful to remember the following: "cognitive" is "knowledge"; "psychomotor" is "action"; "affective" is "feelings."

BOX 21-8 **VERBS THAT CAN BE USED WHEN WRITING LEARNER OUTCOMES**

Cognitive Domain		Psychomotor Domain	
compares	identifies	adapts	manipulates
defines	names	arranges	moves
describes	prepares	assembles	organizes
designs	plans	begins	rearranges
differentiates	solves	changes	shows
explains	states	constructs	starts
gives	summarizes	creates	works
examples		demonstrates	

Affective Domain	
chooses	justifies
defends	relates
displays	revises
forms	selects
gives	shares
helps	uses
initiates	values

The number of outcomes needed for each diagnosis varies. It is better to have several specific outcomes than to try to cover everything with only one or two broad outcomes. Many nurses write one long-term, general outcome for each diagnosis, followed by several short-term, specific outcomes. For example, a long-term outcome for the sample teaching plan could be: "The patient will be able to breastfeed her infant as long as desired without sore nipples." This outcome could be met in 2 weeks or 2 years, depending on how long the woman decides to breastfeed. Long-term outcomes are general statements. On the other hand, the outcomes written in the learner outcome column of the sample teaching plan are short-term, specific behaviors to be accomplished within a specified time (e.g., "The patient immediately begins protective measures to prevent nipple cracking").

Patients and appropriate family members or significant others should be included in planning the outcomes. When patients value the learning outcomes, their readiness to learn is enhanced, increasing the likelihood that they will achieve the goals.

Teaching Content

After writing the learner outcomes, decide what information the patient needs to complete them. This is the content of the teaching plan. The most effective teaching plans address the most important topics relevant to the patient's care. New nurses usually need to research the subject to be taught to determine what information exists about the topic. Extensive information is easily accessible online, along with handouts, books, and journal articles available in many nursing units. Content supported by nursing research is called evidence-based and reflects the most accurate and clinically supported information (see Chapter 2).

Nurses are often concerned about just how much patients should learn about topics such as illness, procedures, medications, and surgeries. Patients benefit, for example, from explanations of the physical sensations they will experience during a procedure. They appreciate knowing in advance what they will feel, taste, hear, see, and smell.

Content explaining why certain treatments and medications are needed is included in the teaching plan. Information on the prevention of illness or its complications should also be covered. Again, patients are more likely to implement a plan that they understand and value.

Teaching Strategies

The techniques used by a teacher to promote learning are called teaching strategies. Plan teaching strategies before the actual teaching sessions so that every content area and learner outcome can be matched with an effective teaching technique. Choose strategies depending on your familiarity with the method, the availability of educational resources and teaching aids, and other factors affecting the patient's learning, such as educational level and cultural background. Also use age-appropriate methods; for example, a 10-year-old will be more receptive to a comic book on personal safety, whereas an adult could learn similar material by discussing safety measures with you.

Education experts generally agree that using a variety of teaching strategies enhances learning. In addition, some methods are better suited for certain learning outcomes. Box 21-9 gives suggested teaching strategies for the three learning domains. The sample teaching plan shows how teaching strategies vary according to the learner outcomes

BOX 21-9 SUGGESTED TEACHING STRATEGIES FOR THE THREE LEARNING DOMAINS

Cognitive Domain

Lecture or discussion
Panel discussion
Discovery
Audiovisual materials
Printed materials
Programmed instruction
Computer-assisted instruction programs

Affective Domain

Role modeling
Discussion
Panel discussion
Audiovisual materials
Role playing
Printed materials

Psychomotor Domain

Demonstration
Discovery
Audiovisual materials
Printed materials

and content of that particular plan. Again, be creative in choosing your methods. Try to stimulate as many of the patient's senses as possible when teaching. Seeing, hearing, and touching are superior to reading or hearing alone. It is often said that we remember 10% of what we read, 20% of what we hear, 30% of what we see, 50% of what we see and hear, and 80% of what we say and do. Descriptions of common teaching strategies follow.

ROLE MODELING

The old saying "actions speak louder than words" explains why role modeling is effective. Patients watch their nurses closely; use this as an opportunity to improve a patient's behavior. For example, nurses who formerly smoked can be role models for patients who are trying to quit smoking. Nurses who diligently wash their hands before any patient encounter or procedure demonstrate the value and importance of hand washing.

 CONSIDER Marco García Ramírez, the father-to-be concerned about his role as a parent. The nurse acts as a role model to the couple when demonstrating newborn care. ●

LECTURE

The term "lecture" means a presentation of information by a teacher to a learner. To be more effective, lectures can include question-and-answer periods and collaboration with the learner. This strategy can be used to deliver information to a large group of patients but is more effective when the session is interactive; it is rarely used for individual instruction, except in combination with other strategies.

DISCUSSION

Discussion involves a two-way exchange of information, ideas, and feelings between the teacher and learners. It is an effective method when used by a nurse who is comfortable with leading a group and knowledgeable about group processes (see Chapter 20). It can also be an effective method for one-on-one instruction.

 REMEMBER Alicia Bonet, the young mother who had to make a decision about long-term aspirin therapy for her baby. The nurse could use a discussion to present information to Ms. Bonet about aspirin therapy, its risks and benefits, and Reye syndrome. The nurse would also provide time for Ms. Bonet to ask questions and think about the information presented. ●

PANEL DISCUSSION

A panel discussion involves a presentation of information by two or more people. Panel discussions can be used to impart factual material but are also effective for sharing experiences and emotions. Debates are a form of panel discussion that includes multiple sides of a controversial topic.

DEMONSTRATION

Demonstration of techniques, procedures, exercises, and the use of special equipment, combined with a lecture and discussion, is an effective strategy. You can evaluate the patient's learning using a return demonstration, as with the teach-back technique described earlier. Practice sessions are often included for the learner. Models of body parts or practice models, such as a resuscitation model, are frequently used. When teaching breast self-examinations, you can use a breast model to let the learner feel different types of lumps commonly found in breast tissue. Childbirth educators usually demonstrate the birth of a baby by using a pelvic model, knitted uterus, and baby doll.

DISCOVERY

In discovery learning, a problem or situation is presented to the patient or group of patients, who are then guided to discover the solution or approach. Discussion of other possible approaches and solutions can follow the patient's own solutions. This is a good method for teaching problem-solving techniques and independent thinking. For instance, you could give a group of diabetic patients a short description of a situation that includes signs and symptoms, asking them to decide whether they indicate hypoglycemia (low blood sugar) or hyperglycemia (high blood sugar) and what measures to take. Then discuss the group's decision as a further learning experience. Even if the patients choose a poor solution, it can be turned into an effective learning experience.

 RECALL Rachel Blumenthal, the wife of the patient who had a myocardial infarction. The nurse could present Mrs. Blumenthal with a "what-if" situation, such as "What if your husband started to have chest pain while you were cuddling and kissing? How would you handle the situation?" From her answer, the nurse would be able to tell how well she understands her husband's condition. The nurse would also have an opportunity for reinstruction, reinforcement, and validation of learning. •

ROLE PLAYING

Role playing gives the learner a chance to experience, relive, or anticipate an event. You explain a scenario and allow the patient to play out the scene with you or with one or more other learners. Role playing can be used to work through emotional traumas or to plan for possible traumas. For example, role playing could help a teenage girl prepare to tell her parent about her pregnancy by letting the girl play herself while you play the girl's parent. This would help the patient rehearse what she wanted to say and anticipate the emotional atmosphere that she will experience. Role playing is a good strategy for children as well as adults. Puppets and dolls can be used as part of the process to help young children express negative feelings about hospitalization and traumatic procedures (Fig. 21-4).

FIGURE 21-4. Role playing can help children learn and express negative feelings resulting from hospitalization and traumatic procedures. *(Photo by Joe Mitchell.)*

AUDIOVISUAL MATERIALS

Audiovisual (AV) materials such as computer programs, online courses, PowerPoint presentations, films, television programs, DVDs, overhead transparencies, flip charts, posters, and diagrams are popular and effective teaching strategies when combined with a lecture or discussion. As discussed earlier, never assume that the patient is literate. As well, never use AV materials as the sole source of learning for a patient. The patient may view the AV material alone, but it should be preceded and followed with a discussion of the material.

PRINTED MATERIAL

The first consideration with printed material is availability. Many brochures, fact sheets, and pamphlets are available at no cost from online sources. Many nurses have also written materials for distribution to patients. Writing instruction sheets, books, and comic books for health teaching can be rewarding as well as useful. Like AV materials, printed materials are generally used in conjunction with other strategies. It is also relatively easy to make games, which are a popular and fun way for patients to learn. For instance, cards with pictures of foods can be used to create a nutritional instruction game.

Select printed materials carefully based on how well they present the needed content in a format that is attractive, understandable, and helpful. A sample of patient education material appears in Box 21-10.

 CONSIDER how the nurse handled the situation of Alicia Bonet, the young mother described in the Reflective Practice box. The nurse provided Ms. Bonet with written materials that were at a level she could understand, thereby helping her make her decision. •

PROGRAMMED INSTRUCTION

Most programmed instruction books or booklets are prepared so that learners can use them independently of a

BOX 21-10 HEART ATTACK: KNOW THE SYMPTOMS. TAKE ACTION

Important Information
Fill out the next two sections and put this card in your wallet with your ID.
It will help emergency medical staff treat you after you call 9-1-1.

Medicines you are taking:

_____
_____
_____

Medicines you are allergic to:

_____
_____
_____

Health Care Provider
Name: _____
Office phone: _____
After-hours phone: _____

Person You Would Like Contacted If You Go to the Hospital
Name: _____
Home phone: _____
Work phone: _____

- **Chest Pain or Discomfort**
  Discomfort in the center or left side of the chest that lasts more than a few minutes or goes away and comes back. May feel like pressure, squeezing, fullness, or pain. May also feel like heartburn or indigestion.

- **Other Upper Body Pain or Discomfort**
  May be felt in one or both arms, the back, shoulders, neck, jaw, or upper part of the stomach (above the belly button).

- **Shortness of Breath**
  May be the only symptom, or it may occur before or along with chest pain or discomfort. May occur when resting or during easy activities.

- **Other Possible Symptoms**
  May include breaking out in a cold sweat, feeling unusually tired, nausea, or light-headedness. Any sudden new symptom or change in usual symptoms also should be a concern.

If you think you might be having heart attack symptoms or a heart attack, call 9-1-1 immediately. Don't ignore your pain or discomfort. Every minute matters when it comes to getting treatment for heart attacks.

Never delay calling 9-1-1 to take espirin or do anything else you think might help.

If you are unable to reach 9-1-1, have someone else drive you to the hospital right away. Don't drive yourself to the hospital. You may cause a car accident.

Available @http://www.nhlbi.nih.gov/health/public/heart/mi/heart_attack_wallet_card.pdf

teacher. However, educators generally agree on the need to spend time with the learner before and after the program to clarify the information, answer questions, and provide the personal touch necessary for a learner's motivation. Because this is a self-paced strategy, it can be beneficial for many learners.

WEB-BASED INSTRUCTION AND TECHNOLOGY
Websites appropriate to the patient's disease process, wellness interests, or health promotion focus can be valuable teaching and learning resources. Access to the Internet is common, and many websites can support instruction. These sites provide consumer information that is formatted for easy reading and access. Programmed instruction or web-based instruction can be particularly useful for patients in isolated areas, especially when it is interspersed with opportunities to see the nurse or health care provider in person. Be sure to evaluate the website chosen by the patient and advise the patient on its suitability and accuracy because some information found on the Internet is not grounded in scientific, medical, or nursing research. Holt, Flint, and Bowers (2011) cite the use of mobile phone technology to supplement discharge instructions and facilitate demonstration of procedures necessary to manage wound care in the home. The patient's mobile phone with camera and voice memo capabilities was used

to track the steps required for a complicated dressing change. Both the patient and the nurse were familiar with this technology, which suited this patient's learning style.

Contractual Agreements
A **contractual agreement** is a pact between two people setting out mutually agreed-on goals. Contracts between nurses and patients are common in many health care settings. The contracts are usually informal and not legally binding. When teaching a patient, such an agreement can serve to motivate both the patient and you as the teacher to do what is necessary to meet the patient's learning outcomes. The agreement notes the responsibilities of both the teacher and the learner, emphasizing the importance of the mutual commitment (Box 21-11 on page 496). If the contracted outcomes are achieved, you can boost the patient's self-esteem with rewards; if the outcomes are not achieved, you can try different teaching techniques.

Learning Activities
While planning teaching strategies, also decide what learning activities the patient should do independently. There are many ways that the patient can preview new material or reinforce what has already been taught. Printed materials, AV materials, and programmed instruction materials are often assigned in the learning activity column of

BOX 21-11 EXAMPLE OF A CONTRACTUAL AGREEMENT BETWEEN A NURSE AND A CLIENT

I will participate in the learning activities needed to help me learn about my low-salt diet. During my hospital stay, I will attend the class on low-salt diets, read the materials given to me, and ask questions as I need to. I will work with S. Moore, RN, to plan my meals and food preparation at home. If I need help when I get home, I will contact S. Moore.

Jim Mall

I will provide Jim Mall with the experiences needed for him to follow his low-salt diet accurately.

S. Moore, RN

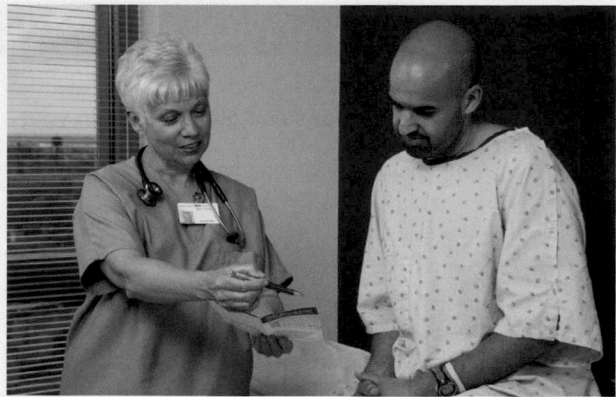

FIGURE 21-5. One-to-one teaching is used in many nurse–patient situations. The nurse must be able to assess whether individual teaching is needed or whether learning can occur in a group. *(Photo by B. Proud.)*

the teaching plan. Use this column to guide the patient in learning activities before, between, and after planned learning sessions. Practical considerations for planning learning activities follow.

TIME CONSTRAINTS

Consider time constraints when planning the patient's learning, as nurses often have a problem finding time to meet patients' needs. Set priorities in order to teach essential content thoroughly. Teach less important content last so that the more important learner outcomes can be met within the time available. If time permits, the remaining content can be addressed.

To meet time constraints, nurses often plan together. Teamwork and cooperation allow nurses to meet deadlines. If teaching must continue beyond the hospitalization, home visit, or clinic visit, schedule additional learning opportunities through outpatient programs or referrals to community-based programs. Home health care nurses often receive referrals from hospital nurses to continue the teaching begun during a patient's hospitalization. Discharge planning must be started early to ensure continuity of teaching.

SCHEDULING

It is better to plan shorter, more frequent teaching sessions than one or two longer sessions. Short sessions allow patients to digest the new material and prevent them from becoming too tired or uncomfortable because of a health problem. Sessions of 15 to 30 minutes are generally well tolerated. Usually, more formal classroom programs last for more than 1 hour. In such cases, provide a break after every 50 minutes of class time. Include the patient when planning the time and frequency of lessons. Scheduling teaching sessions when the patient is least stressed will enhance teaching.

GROUP VERSUS INDIVIDUAL TEACHING

Several factors are important when choosing the teaching setting. Some learner outcomes are met more readily in a one-to-one encounter (Fig. 21-5), whereas others are achieved more easily in a group. For example, the out-

come "The patient will change the dressing using sterile technique" is best taught and evaluated in a private session. The outcome "The patient will discuss feelings about diabetes self-management" might be met more easily in a group discussion with other patients (see the accompanying Research in Nursing box).

FORMAL VERSUS INFORMAL TEACHING

Most nurse–patient interactions can include **informal teaching**. These unplanned teaching sessions are often effective because they deal with the patient's immediate learning needs and concerns. Something as simple as responding to a question about the timing of a medication or verifying information about a scheduled procedure is actually teaching. Informal teaching might also lead to additional planned, formal sessions. **Formal teaching** is the planned teaching done to fulfill learner outcomes. Both forms are effective when used appropriately.

Implementing

Implementing the teaching plan requires interpersonal skills and effective communication techniques. Teaching the patient can be a major part of the working phase of the helping relationship (see Chapter 20). You must continually observe the patient for additional assessment data that could alter the original teaching plan. This requires skill in adapting and reorganizing the teaching plan. Following are important considerations when implementing a teaching plan:

- Promote patient learning by using a warm and accepting approach. Your attitude has more effect on the patient than any other factor (Fig. 21-6). Avoid taking a condescending attitude and using technical and medical terms (unless the patient has a background in this area). A nonthreatening teaching–learning atmosphere allows learning to occur.
- Consider the physical environment when implementing the teaching plan. Some planning may be needed to ensure adequate space and lighting, comfortable chairs, and good ventilation. Privacy is also important, as is freedom from distractions and interruptions.

RESEARCH IN NURSING

BRIDGING THE GAP TO EVIDENCE-BASED PRACTICE

Measuring the Effectiveness of a Group Teaching Intervention To Manage Diabetes Care

It is estimated that due to increasing levels of obesity coupled with a sedentary lifestyle and the growing population of older adults, there is an increasing incidence of type 2 diabetes. During the next 15 years, approximately 333 million people in the United States will be diagnosed with type 2 diabetes. Most health care educators agree that diabetes education is most effective when a patient-centered, interactive approach is used. A variety of teaching strategies have been attempted including individual appointments prior to a group session, group sessions without individual sessions, or some type of one-time-only program. Diabetes occurs more frequently in minority populations and those with lower incomes; these underserved people may experience poor health status, poor health outcomes, and a lesser quality of care.

Related Research

Esden, J., & Nichols, M. (2013). Patient-centered group diabetes care: A practice innovation. *The Nurse Practitioner: The American Journal of Primary Health Care, 38*(4), 42–48.

The purpose of this study was to deliver a group approach for a patient-centered model of care that involved interactive self-management education for diabetic patients at a clinic in Central Florida. The options for diabetic education for this underserved population in Central Florida were limited. Participants in this study were recruited at office visits and via phone calls from office staff, and were required to speak, read, and write in English. The study used three measurement tools pre- and postintervention to assess patients' knowledge of diabetes, their perceived self-efficacy and attitudes toward diabetes, and barriers to diabetes self-care. The group sessions were held once a month for 3 months; each session lasted about 2.5 hours not including an additional hour for session one and three to complete pre- and postassessment tools. Topics at the sessions included the pathophysiology of the disease, dietary implications and choices, the various types of medications available and their administration, and the implications of laboratory results and risk-factor reduction. Group bonding activities were used throughout the sessions. The total number of participants who attended all the sessions was eight. All had been diagnosed with type 2 diabetes and were considered obese using body mass index (BMI) calculations. Most participants were Hispanic, and most were taking oral medication for their diabetes.

The results of this study indicated that there was improved knowledge and understanding of diabetes and its treatment, particularly with self-efficacy, for this group of participants. They expressed satisfaction with the group activity, enjoyed the social support of the group, and indicated that they wished the group activity could continue.

Relevance to Nursing Practice

This group approach involving self-management education for an underserved diabetic population was viewed positively by the participants. It is a supplement but not a replacement for regular office visits at the clinic. This type of interaction has potential for replication in various other settings where knowledge deficits and issues with self-efficacy can interfere with positive self-care behaviors regarding other chronic conditions. Nurses have many opportunities to influence patient education about chronic disease conditions and also foster a safer care environment.

For additional research, visit thePoint.

• Review the patient's expectations and role functions as a learner. To avoid any misunderstandings, review the contractual agreement before implementing the teaching plan. The patient is expected to listen, observe, and attempt to understand what is being taught.

FIGURE 21-6. The nurse's warm approach is an important factor in interpersonal relationships.

• Assess the patient's comfort level. Some people are uncomfortable in the role of learner, and you need to recognize this problem in order to assist the patient to assume the role more easily. If the patient must learn special techniques or procedures (e.g., colostomy care, self-injections, or eye medication instillation), assure the patient that it takes time and practice before anyone can perform new skills confidently.

• Be prepared and organized before implementing the teaching plan. Gather and organize all teaching aids (e.g., posters, films, or printed materials) before the teaching session. A disorganized teacher distracts the learner and hinders learning. Also, a procedure or skill must be taught in the correct sequence so that the patient does not become confused.

• Make each learning session interesting and enjoyable for the patient. Have an enthusiastic and positive attitude, and make learning fun by creative use of planned teaching strategies. When you approach teaching positively, the patient is more likely to approach learning in a similar way.

The Role of the Nurse as Coach

With the implementation of the 2010 Affordable Care Act and the goals outlined in the *Healthy People 2020* initiative, there is a clear need to address the direction of health care in the future. Health challenges are more complex these days, and nurses need to be prepared to move from a disease-based model of care toward a health and wellness promotion model. The Institute of Medicine Report (2010) also emphasizes the need for nurses to assume a leadership role that includes collaborating and coordinating care across teams of health professionals. The nurse coach role is an integral component of this partnership and assists patients and families to make changes that promote healthier lifestyles.

Nurses who incorporate coaching into their professional practice can improve the quality and effectiveness of care A **nurse coach** is a "registered nurse who integrates coaching competencies into any setting or specialty area of practice to facilitate a process of change or development that assists individuals or groups to realize their potential" (Hess et al, 2013). A nurse coach establishes a partnership with a patient and uses discovery to identify the patient's personal goals and agenda in a way that will result in change rather than using teaching and education strategies directed by the nurse as the expert. Nurse coaches may practice in a specialty area, such as diabetes education or cardiac rehabilitation, and may be staff nurses, advanced practice nurses, educators, and administrators. The nurse coach role is supported by coaching education, training, and experience and is influenced by the population served.

The nurse coaching process includes the following:

- Establishing relationships and identifying readiness for change
- Identifying opportunities, issues, and concerns
- Establishing patient-centered goals
- Creating the structure of the coaching interaction
- Empowering and motivating patients to reach goals
- Assisting the patient to determine progress toward goals (Hess et al., 2013)

The role of nurse coach is evolving and should not be confused with that of a preceptor or mentor. A nurse coach explores the patient's readiness for coaching, designs the structure of a coaching session, supports the achievement of the patient's desired goals, and with the patient determines how to evaluate the attainment of patient goals (Hess et al., 2013). Health maintenance organizations and various health and wellness programs have nurse coaches to assist patients to improve health outcomes. Professional nursing organizations recognize the need to further define the definition of a nurse coach and develop a nurse coach certification program and process.

Evaluating

The nurse and the patient together measure how well the patient has achieved the outcomes specified in the plan of care.

Evaluating Learning

Nurses cannot be sure that patients have actually learned the content without some type of proof or feedback. The key to evaluation is the learner outcomes in the teaching plan that describe what behaviors to measure. Methods for obtaining feedback about learning are discussed in the following section.

METHODS OF EVALUATION

There are several methods of evaluation. For instance, cognitive domain learning may be evaluated through oral questioning, affective domain learning through the patient's response, and psychomotor domain learning by a return demonstration. Consider this learner outcome in the cognitive domain: "The patient will be able to describe what a blood pressure reading represents." To evaluate this, you could ask the patient, "Tell me what this blood pressure reading means to you." The patient then has a chance to talk about the reading while you evaluate the patient's understanding of it.

Asking direct questions is often an efficient method of evaluating learner outcomes. Simply ask the patient a question, and the answer reflects the patient's level of knowledge about a topic. Direct questions can also be used to evaluate the patient's affective learning.

Another way to decide whether learner outcomes have been met is to analyze the patient's own comments. Patients may state that they understand the information while avoiding further discussion of the topic. In such instances, using effective communication techniques when reintroducing the topic at a later time might provide the evaluation data needed.

Sometimes observational skills can help determine whether the patient is using the material learned. For example, observing what the patient has ordered for lunch shows whether dietary lessons are being put into practice. A nurse also uses observation when evaluating the patient's psychomotor skills. A return demonstration is an excellent way of evaluating psychomotor domain learning (Fig. 21-7). Letting patients change their own dressing, for example, provides concrete evidence of satisfactory or unsatisfactory performance of the procedure. However, you must take care to promote a nonstressful environment when the time comes for the patient's return demonstration.

TIMING OF EVALUATION

Evaluation of learning is ongoing. If learning is only evaluated as soon as teaching is completed, the results may be misleading. Home health care nurses may evaluate what the patient learned in the hospital, as well as what is being taught during home visits. Hospital nurses often check with family members or significant others after discharge to evaluate whether learner outcomes have been met.

Reinforcing and Celebrating Learning

Most people feel encouraged and supported when their efforts are acknowledged by another person, especially

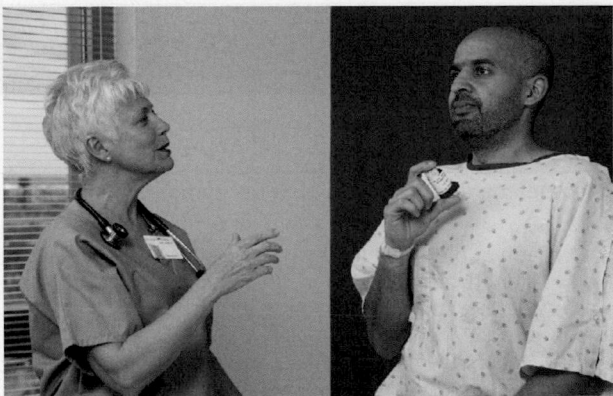

FIGURE 21-7. If the patient can correctly demonstrate what you've taught, you know learning has occurred. *(Photo by B. Proud.)*

BOX 21-12 | **COMMON TEACHING MISTAKES**

- Ignoring the restrictions of the patient's environment
- Failing to accept that patients have the right to change their mind
- Using medical jargon
- Failing to negotiate goals
- Duplicating teaching that other team members have done
- Overloading the patient with information
- Choosing the wrong time for teaching
- Not evaluating what the patient has learned
- Not reviewing educational media, or relying exclusively on media
- Failing to document patient teaching and plan for follow-up or teaching reinforcement

---

when they trust and value the other person. This is especially true in health care, where patients often feel overwhelmed by their illness. To make the most of this dynamic, use **positive reinforcement** to affirm the efforts of patients who have mastered new knowledge, attitudes, or skills. Reinforcement may be as simple as a few words of acknowledgment ("You've mastered this diet quickly"), as spontaneous as a warm hug, or as planned as the entire staff joining to celebrate a patient's independent ambulation. **Negative reinforcement**—criticism or punishment—is generally ineffective; undesirable behavior is usually best ignored. Behavior modification programs that reward desired behaviors and ignore undesired behaviors can be designed for some patients.

Evaluating Teaching

Evaluation of teaching must occur so that you can capitalize on your strengths and work on improving weaknesses. Like all nursing roles, effective teaching requires practice and experience. Even nurse educators agree that they are always discovering better ways to promote learning. It is important not to feel discouraged when evaluations of one's teaching are less than perfect.

It is best to evaluate one's own teaching effectiveness immediately after a teaching session. This involves a quick review of how well you feel you implemented the plan. Mentally noting both the strengths and weaknesses of the teaching session helps you plan better for subsequent sessions.

You can also seek feedback from patients. You can use a simple questionnaire at the end of a teaching session or after discharge to gain the patient's perception of your teaching effectiveness. Use a standardized questionnaire in the hospital or agency or prepare your own. When using an outcome format that requires only circles or checkmarks as answers, provide space for comments.

Revising the Plan

During evaluation, you or your patient might decide that revisions are needed in the teaching plan. When revis-

ing the plan, you should identify teaching factors that might have reduced teaching effectiveness (Box 21-12). A reassessment might indicate that some patient factors were not considered in the original plan, and adjustments might be made accordingly to meet the patient's needs. Often, the use of a different teaching strategy is all that is needed for a patient to achieve the learner outcomes.

Revision is a natural part of the teaching–learning process and should not be viewed negatively. Neither you nor the patient has "failed" when an outcome is not met. Most outcomes can be met with a change in approach, although sometimes the learner outcomes are unrealistic. Further assessment might reveal that the content might be too complex or the time too short for successful achievement.

Documenting

The nurse is legally responsible for documenting teaching in the patient's record. Documentation of the teaching–learning process includes a summary of the learning need, the plan, the implementation of the plan, and the evaluation results. The evaluative statement is crucial and must show concrete evidence that demonstrates that learning has occurred. If the desired learning has not occurred, your notes or the electronic record should indicate how the problem was resolved. It is not enough to document only what you taught; your charting must show evidence that the patient or significant other has actually learned the material taught.

THE NURSE AS COUNSELOR

Counseling is the interpersonal process of helping patients make decisions that promote their overall well-being. Family members or significant others are often included in counseling sessions. Everyone participating must feel comfortable

Table 21-1 ANALYSIS OF NURSING RESPONSES IN COMMON COUNSELING SITUATIONS

INEFFECTIVE RESPONSE	ANALYSIS	EFFECTIVE RESPONSE	ANALYSIS
Situation A: You walk into the room of Ms. Goldstein, who learned earlier in the day that her tumor is malignant. She is crying.			
"Oh cheer up! Tomorrow's got to be a brighter day."	Provides false reassurance; communicates insensitivity to patient's feelings.	Touch forearm and sit next to her quietly. After several minutes, say, "I can't even begin to imagine how difficult this must be for you. Please let me know if there is anything I can do to help."	Uses touch, silence, and caring appropriately.
Situation B: You have been teaching 60-year-old Mr. Hyong diabetic self-care for 4 days, and he is still asking the same questions and refusing to administer his own insulin or check his blood sugar.			
"Well, I guess we are getting nowhere here. Is there anyone else who might be able to do this for you?"	Rejects patient without first evaluating the teaching plan and exploring patient variables that might be hindering learning.	"We may have a bit of a problem here.... I hear you asking the same questions every day. Let's see if together we can figure out why this isn't making sense to you."	Enlists patient in problem solving.
Situation C: One morning, you walk into the room of an older resident who had withdrawn and become totally dependent on the nurses for basic care on her transfer into the long-term care facility. You are surprised to discover that she has washed and dressed herself—for the first time.			
"Well, I'm happy to see that you have rejoined the ranks of the living. Did you wash off your glasses?"	Misses opportunity to celebrate the resident's achievement of an important goal.	Hugs resident warmly, looks her in the eye, and exclaims, "Don't you look wonderful today? What are you celebrating?" Defers an assessment of how thorough the morning care has been until later.	Rejoices spontaneously in the resident's achievement and reinforces this behavior. Gives the resident a reason to continue to make progress. Uses touch appropriately.
Situation D: You are helping Mr. Stein out of bed; he has been on bed rest for 2 weeks because of a painful and debilitating illness. A fiercely independent man, he is embarrassed to need your support and looks disgusted with himself when he steps on your foot.			
"What's the problem, Honey? Haven't been eating your Wheaties?"	Uses terms of endearment, which often denote disrespect and condescension to patients, no matter in what spirit they are uttered.	"No problem, Mr. Stein, my husband steps on my toes all the time when we go dancing!" After a few minutes... "It must be hard when you are used to doing everything for yourself to all of a sudden find yourself needing others for simple things...."	Uses humor and empathy appropriately; invites the patient to share his feelings.
Situation E: Ms. Berretta recently underwent surgery resulting in a urinary diversion. She should be able to change her own ostomy bag by this time, but she is still unwilling to look at the stoma, and participate alone in her care. The nurses are getting impatient with her "childish" refusals to learn.			
"Really Helen, I'll do it myself but you'll be the loser once you get home with this thing and there's no one around to help."	Uses a threat in an attempt to coerce learning (negative reinforcement). Displays unwillingness to explore what is blocking Ms. Berretta's readiness to learn.	Before beginning Ms. Berretta's care: "I think we need to talk before your treatment today. You will be discharged soon, and I want you to feel confident about caring for your stoma. I understand that until you can accept it, you don't want to learn anything about it. Would you like to talk about this with me, or would you prefer me to make a referral to someone else?"	Communicates respect for patient and sensitivity to her needs, without ignoring what is a real problem. Offers the possibility of a referral to another health care professional if the patient so wishes.

in the situation and surroundings. Like teaching, counseling may be formal or informal.

The interpersonal skills of warmth, friendliness, openness, and empathy are necessary for successful counseling. An effective counselor needs to be a caring person. Caring is based on a humanistic philosophy (Watson, 1985), which is the core of nursing practice. A humanistic approach to counseling rooted in professional caring helps the patient strive toward the greatest health potential. Caring is important in all nursing roles but is fundamental in the counseling role.

Some advanced-practice psychiatric mental health nurses specialize in counseling, and this form of counseling has an important professional role. The focus in this chapter, however, is on the everyday counseling that is a basic component of all nurses' practice. This counseling involves listening carefully to the patient's or family's questions, concerns, demands, and complaints and then responding in an effective manner.

 CONSIDER Rachel Blumenthal, the wife of the patient who had a myocardial infarction. By carefully listening to Mrs. Blumenthal's concerns, including her comment about being embarrassed to talk with her husband's cardiologist, the nurse helps to establish a trusting relationship that forms the basis for counseling. •

Knowing appropriate responses to what a patient says might be difficult at first, but practice helps develop this skill.

Each nurse–patient (or nurse–family) interaction is unique; a nurse's response that works well with one patient might intimidate or anger another. Sensitivity to the unique needs of each patient and a willingness to get involved and make a difference are essential for effective counseling. Because counseling skills take time to cultivate, nursing students and new nurses should be aware of their limits and not rush to counsel without first considering consultation with more experienced nurses. Table 21-1 presents typical counseling situations you might experience in your first year of nursing and analyzes both effective and ineffective nursing responses. You might want to role play these situations with a friend. Nurses who wish to succeed as caregivers and counselors need to master the communication techniques described in Chapter 20.

In counseling situations, you do not tell patients what to do to solve the problem but instead assist and guide them to solve problems and make decisions. If the patient lacks the knowledge and skills to approach a problem systematically, you can combine the teaching and counseling roles to help the patient solve the dilemma successfully.

The nursing process is an essential tool when guiding and teaching patients. Nurses are educated to approach all nursing situations in a logical, systematic way. In a situation that needs counseling, whether minor problem or major crisis, share your problem-solving abilities with patients. The nursing process is used to organize the nurse–patient counseling situation described in Box 21-13. For

BOX 21-13 AN EXAMPLE OF PROBLEM SOLVING THAT FOLLOWS THE NURSING PROCESS

Situation
Monday, 7:30 PM, Amy Purcell has been admitted to the children's unit with dehydration resulting from diarrhea. Amy is responding well to intravenous (IV) fluids. Her mother is visibly distraught.

Assessing
Amy is doing well but will need 24 hours of IV therapy.

Amy and her twin sister Susan have never been separated from their parents or each other. They are 2 years old.

Ms. Purcell has no idea who will care for Susan when Mr. Purcell goes to work in the morning.

The Purcells have no regular childcare arrangements and have no family members in the area.

Ms. Purcell wants to stay with Amy during her hospitalization.

The Purcells' neighbor is home during the day. Sometimes Amy and Susan play at her house.

There is a daycare center near their home, but Susan might be upset about going there. It's also expensive.

Mr. Purcell cannot afford to take Tuesday off but will take Wednesday morning off.

Insurance does not cover a private room, which would allow Susan to come to stay in the hospital too.

Diagnosing
Anxiety related to stress of daughter's hospitalization, need for childcare for Susan, and uncertain resources.

Planning Goal
Ms. Purcell will demonstrate decreased anxiety over the care of Susan during Amy's hospitalization.

Together, Ms. Purcell and the nurse have planned the following:

- The neighbor will come to the Purcell home to care for Susan when Mr. Purcell leaves for work on Tuesday morning.
- The neighbor will bring Susan to the hospital for the afternoon visiting hours to be with Ms. Purcell and Amy.
- Mr. Purcell will come to the hospital after work to have dinner with the family.
- Mr. Purcell will take Susan home for bedtime.
- On Wednesday morning, Mr. Purcell will take off work in the morning. He and Susan will go to the hospital to pick up Ms. Purcell and Amy.

Implementing
Plan implemented by the Purcells with support of the nursing staff.

Evaluating
Ms. Purcell told the nurse that she feels that both Amy and Susan did well with the care they received from their parents. The family's stress was minimized, and she is relieved that everything went so well. The nurse decides that the goals were met.

EXAMPLES OF NANDA-I NURSING DIAGNOSES

COUNSELING NEEDS

Nursing Diagnoses	Related Factors
Decisional Conflict	Inability to authorize withdrawal of life-sustaining treatment despite believing this to be in the patient's best interests
Hopelessness	Progression of debilitating symptoms and belief that "even God has abandoned me"
Impaired Social Interaction	Communication barriers
Situational Low Self-Esteem	Recent lay-off and divorce

the type of counseling that may be indicated, see Examples of NANDA-I Nursing Diagnoses: Counseling Needs for diagnoses.

Types of Counseling

Counseling may be situational, developmental, or motivational, as well as short- or long-term.

Short-Term Counseling

Short-term counseling focuses on the immediate problem or concern of the patient or family. It can be a relatively minor concern or a major crisis, but in any case, it needs immediate attention (Fig. 21-8). Short-term counseling might be used during a **situational crisis**, which occurs when a patient faces an event or situation that causes a disruption in life. For example, a male patient in the hospital finds out that his wife has been involved in a car accident; she received only a few scratches, but their only car was demolished. As a nurse, you are in an excellent position to help the patient decide what can be done to solve this situational crisis. You can guide the patient to resources to help solve the travel, financial, and emotional difficulties that arise as a result of the accident. This holistic approach is especially important because the crisis could hinder the patient's recovery.

FIGURE 21-8 Counseling may involve a concern that needs immediate attention. *(Photo by Rick Brady.)*

Long-Term Counseling

Long-term counseling extends over a prolonged period. A patient might need the counsel of the nurse at daily, weekly, or monthly intervals. A patient experiencing a developmental crisis, for example, might need long-term counseling. A **developmental crisis** can occur when a person is going through a developmental stage or passage. For example, many women going through menopause need help adjusting to the changes they experience. Long-term counseling may occur in nurse-led support groups.

Motivational Interviewing

Motivational interviewing is an evidence-based counseling approach that involves discussing feelings and incentives with the patient. Nurses often become frustrated because their patients do not seem to want to get better or to learn how to care for themselves. Perhaps some patients do not have the inner drive or motivation to cooperate in their own health care. Some patients say, "I have nothing to live for." By establishing a helping relationship with the patient early on, you can help the patient work through these feelings of despair. You might be able to get the patient to talk about what is generating the lack of interest in recovery. If a problem is identified, you can use the problem-solving technique with the patient to work toward an acceptable solution. Gance-Cleveland (2013) proposes that the traditional model of counseling may not prove effective for an issue such as the childhood obesity epidemic. Instead, a collaborative, family-centered model that includes motivational interviewing may help the family identify health goals. Instead of focusing on solutions to the obesity issue, the nurse attempts to gain a better understanding of the barriers that exist to changing family behaviors. With this technique, families gain the self-confidence needed to promote better health outcomes. This is not the traditional approach, and it requires time to establish relationships and explore family perspectives, but many experts recommend motivational interviewing as an effective alternative to deal with a severe health problem.

When assessing a motivational problem, always consider the patient's cultural values. Often the way a person feels about something is strongly influenced by that individual's cultural background. For instance, if a person has grown up in a family in which illness is perceived as an inevitable result of aging, it will be difficult to motivate that person to practice preventive measures for health (see Chapter 5). Such a problem may seem insurmountable, yet a caring nurse can work toward helping patients with this mindset become interested in promoting their own health. When discouraged, confer with a colleague to help solve patient-centered problems.

Referrals

Sometimes a patient needs specialized counseling from a nurse with advanced training or from other health care professionals. In these cases, offer to refer the patient to the appropriate professional (e.g., psychiatric or mental health nurse, psychologist or psychiatrist, social worker, clergy, financial counselor, sex therapist, or occupational therapist). In other cases, a simple referral to a community resource, such as a neighborhood support group, may be all the patient needs. When making a referral, be sure to address any barriers that might prevent the patient from acting on the referral. Patients might fail to follow up with a referral for financial reasons, because they do not understand the reason for or value the referral, because they lack transportation, or because the agency is not open at times convenient for them.

DEVELOPING CLINICAL REASONING

1. Explain what the following statement means: "It is as important for patients to understand and value the proposed treatment regimen as it is for them to understand how to implement the proposed regimen." What are the implications of this for teaching and counseling?

2. A patient your age has just learned that she has tested positive for the human immunodeficiency virus (HIV). Make a list of some of the learning (cognitive, psychomotor, affective) that you think should take place. What sorts of things might affect her readiness to learn? How would you tailor your nursing in response to these variables?

3. Mrs. Riley is being readmitted to your hospital unit with complications related to her diabetes. A coworker voices her frustrations and says, "We've taught her everything she needs to know to do a better job of managing her diabetes. I don't know what more we can do." How do you respond?

PRACTICING FOR NCLEX

1. A nurse is teaching first aid to counselors of a summer camp for children with asthma. This is an example of what aim of health teaching?
   a. Promoting health
   b. Preventing illness
   c. Restoring health
   d. Facilitating coping

2. A nurse is teaching patients of all ages in a hospital setting. Which examples demonstrate teaching that is appropriately based on the patient's developmental level? Select all that apply.
   a. The nurse plans long teaching sessions to discuss diet modifications for an older adult diagnosed with type 2 diabetes.

   b. The nurse recognizes that a female adolescent diagnosed with anorexia is still dependent on her parents and includes them in all teaching sessions.
   c. The nurse designs an exercise program for a sedentary older adult male patient based on the activities he prefers.
   d. The nurse includes an 8-year-old patient in the teaching plan for managing cystic fibrosis.
   e. The nurse demonstrates how to use an inhaler to an 11-year-old male patient and includes his mother in the session to reinforce the teaching.
   f. The nurse continues a teaching session on STIs for a sexually active male adolescent despite his protest that "I've heard enough already!"

3. A nurse is teaching a 50-year-old male patient how to care for his new ostomy appliance. Which teaching aid would be most appropriate to confirm that the patient has learned the information?
   a. Ask Me 3
   b. Newest Vital Sign
   c. Teach-back tool
   d. TEACH acronym

4. A nurse is planning teaching strategies for patients addicted to alcohol, in the affective domain of learning. What are examples of strategies promoting behaviors in this domain? Select all that apply.
   a. The nurse prepares a lecture on the harmful long-term effects of alcohol on the body.
   b. The nurse explores the reasons alcoholics drink and promotes other methods of coping with problems.
   c. The nurse asks patients for a return demonstration for using relaxation exercises to relieve stress.
   d. The nurse helps patients to reaffirm their feelings of self-worth and relate this to their addiction problem.
   e. The nurse uses a pamphlet to discuss the tenants of the Alcoholics Anonymous program to patients.
   f. The nurse reinforces the mental benefits of gaining self-control over an addiction.

5. A nurse is preparing to teach a 45-year-old male patient with asthma how to use his inhaler. Which teaching tool is one of the best methods to teach the patient this skill?
   a. Demonstration
   b. Lecture
   c. Discovery
   d. Panel session

6. A nurse has taught a diabetic patient how to administer his daily insulin. The nurse should evaluate the teaching–learning process by:
   a. Determining the patient's motivation to learn
   b. Deciding if the learning outcomes have been achieved
   c. Allowing the patient to practice the skill he has just learned
   d. Documenting the teaching session in the patient's medical record

7. A registered nurse assumes the role of nurse coach to provide teaching to patients who are recovering from strokes. One example of an intervention the nurse may provide related to this role is:
   a. The nurse uses discovery to identify the patients' personal goals and create an agenda that will result in change.
   b. The nurse is the expert in providing teaching and education strategies to provide dietary and activity modifications.

c. The nurse becomes a mentor to the patients and encourages them to create their own fitness programs.

d. The nurse assumes an authoritative role to design the structure of the coaching session and support the achievement of patient goals.

8. A nurse is counseling a 19-year-old male athlete who had his right leg amputated below the knee following a motorcycle accident. During the rehabilitation process, the patient refuses to eat or get up to ambulate on his own. He says to the nurse, "What's the point. My life is over now and I'll never be the football player I dreamed of becoming." What is the nurse counselor's best response to this patient?

a. "You're young and have your whole life ahead of you. You should focus on your rehabilitation and make something of your life."

b. "I understand how you must feel. I wanted to be a famous singer, but I wasn't born with the talent to be successful at it."

c. "You should concentrate on other sports that you could play even with a prosthesis."

d. "I understand this is difficult for you. Would you like to talk about it now or would you prefer me to make a referral to someone else?"

9. A nurse is caring for a 42-year-old male patient who is admitted to the hospital with injuries sustained in a motor vehicle accident. While he is in the hospital, his wife tells him that the bottom level of their house flooded, damaging their belongings. When the nurse enters his room, she notes that the patient is visibly upset. The nurse is aware that the patient will most likely be in need of which type of counseling?

a. Long-term developmental

b. Short-term situational

c. Short-term motivational

d. Long-term motivational

10. A nurse who is caring for a morbidly obese male teenager forms a contractual agreement with him to achieve his weight goals. Which statement best describes the nature of this agreement?

a. "This agreement forms a legal bond between the two of us to achieve your weight goals."

b. "This agreement will motivate the two of us to do what is necessary to meet your weight goals."

c. "This agreement will help us determine what learning outcomes are necessary to achieve your weight goals."

d. "This agreement will limit the scope of the teaching session and make stated weight goals more attainable."

ANSWERS WITH RATIONALES

1. *b.* Teaching first aid is a function of the goal to prevent illness. Promoting health involves helping patients to value health and develop specific health practices that promote wellness. Restoring health occurs once a patient is ill, and teaching focuses on developing self-care practices that promote recovery. When facilitating coping, nurses help patients come to terms with whatever lifestyle modification is needed for their recovery or to enable them to cope with permanent health alterations.

2. *c, d, e.* Successful teaching plans for older adults incorporate extra time, short teaching sessions, accommodation for

sensory deficits, and reduction of environmental distractions. Older adults also benefit from instruction that relates new information to familiar activities or information. School-aged children are capable of logical reasoning and should be included in the teaching–learning process whenever possible; they are also open to new learning experiences but need learning to be reinforced by either a parent or health care provider as they become more involved with their friends and school activities. Teaching strategies designed for an adolescent patient should recognize the adolescent's need for independence, as well as the need to establish a trusting relationship that demonstrates respect for the adolescent's opinions.

3. *c.* The teach-back tool is a method of assessing literacy and confirming that the learner understands health information received from a health professional. The Ask Me 3 is a brief tool intended to promote understanding and improve communication between patients and their providers. The Newest Vital Sign (NVS) is a reliable screening tool to assess low health literacy, developed to improve communications between patients and providers. The TEACH acronym is used to maximize the effectiveness of patient teaching by *t*uning into the patient, *e*diting patient information, *a*cting on every teaching moment, *c*larifying often, and *h*onoring the patient as a partner in the process.

4. *b, d, f.* Affective learning includes changes in attitudes, values, and feelings (e.g., the patient expresses renewed self-confidence to be able to give up drinking). Cognitive learning involves the storing and recalling of new knowledge in the brain, such as the learning that occurs during a lecture or by using a pamphlet for teaching. Learning a physical skill involving the integration of mental and muscular activity is called psychomotor learning, which may involve a return demonstration of a skill.

5. *a.* Demonstration of techniques, procedures, exercises, and the use of special equipment is an effective patient teaching strategy for a skill. Lecture can be used to deliver information to a large group of patients but is more effective when the session is interactive; it is rarely used for individual instruction, except in combination with other strategies. Discovery is a good method for teaching problem-solving techniques and independent thinking. Panel discussions can be used to impart factual material but are also effective for sharing experiences and emotions.

6. *b.* The nurse cannot assume that the patient has actually learned the content unless there is some type of proof of learning. The key to evaluation is meeting the learner outcomes stated in the teaching plan.

7. *a.* A nurse coach establishes a partnership with a patient and, using discovery, facilitates the identification of the patient's personal goals and agenda to lead to change rather than using teaching and education strategies with the nurse as the expert. A nurse coach explores the patient's readiness for coaching, designs the structure of a coaching session, supports the achievement of the patient's desired goals, and with the patient determines how to evaluate the attainment of patient goals.

8. *d.* This answer communicates respect and sensitivity to the patient's needs and offers an opportunity to discuss his feelings with the nurse or another health care professional. The other answers do not allow the patient to express his feelings and receive the counseling he needs.

9. **b.** Short-term counseling might be used during a situational crisis, which occurs when a patient faces an event or situation that causes a disruption in life, such as a flood. Long-term counseling extends over a prolonged period; a patient experiencing a developmental crisis, for example, might need long-term counseling. Motivational interviewing is an evidence-based counseling approach that involves discussing feelings and incentives with the patient. A caring nurse can motivate patients to become interested in promoting their own health.

10. **b.** A contractual agreement is a pact two people make setting out mutually agreed-on goals. Contracts are usually informal and not legally binding. When teaching a patient, such an agreement can help motivate both the patient and the teacher to do what is necessary to meet the patient's learning outcomes. The agreement notes the responsibilities of both the teacher and the learner, emphasizing the importance of the mutual commitment.

TAYLOR SUITE RESOURCES

Explore these additional resources to enhance learning for this chapter:

- NCLEX-Style Questions and other resources on thePoint, http://thePoint.lww.com/Taylor8e
- *Study Guide for Fundamentals of Nursing, 8th edition*
- Adaptive Learning | Powered by prepU, http://thepoint.lww.com/prepu

Bibliography

Bloom, B. S. (1956). *Taxonomy of educational objectives: The classification of educational goals.* New York: David McKay.

Dickens, C., & Piano, M. (2013). Health literacy and nursing: An update. *American Journal of Nursing, 113*(6), 52–57.

Esden, J., & Nichols, M. (2013). Patient-centered group diabetes care: A practice innovation. *The Nurse Practitioner: The American Journal of Primary Health Care, 38*(4), 42–48.

Gance-Cleveland, B. (2013). Motivational interviewing for adolescent obesity. *American Journal of Nursing, 113*(1), 11–12.

Hess, D., Dossey, B., Southard, M., Luck, S., Gulino-Schaub, B., & Bark, L. (2013). *The art and science of nurse coaching: The provider's guide to coaching scope and competencies.* Silver Spring, MD: American Nurses Association.

Holt. J., Flint, E., & Bowers, M. (2011). Got the picture? Using mobile phone technology to reinforce discharge instructions. *American Journal of Nursing, 111*(8), 47–51.

Institute of Medicine (IOM). (2010). *The future of nursing: Leading change, advancing health.* Washington, DC: National Academies Press. Available at http://www.iom.edu/Reports/2010/The-Future-of-Nursing-Leading-Change-Advancing-Health.aspx

The Joint Commission (TJC). (2012a). Facts about patient-centered communications. Available at http://www.jointcommission.org/assets/1/18/Patient_Centered_Communications_7_3_12.pdf

The Joint Commission (TJC). (2012b). The Joint Commission releases Speak Up: What you need to know about your serious illness and palliative care. Available at http://www.jointcommission.org/the_joint_commission_releases_speak_up_what_you_need_to_know_about_your_serious_illness_and_palliative_care_/

Knowles, M. S. (1990). *The adult learner: A neglected species* (4th ed.). Houston: Gulf Publishing.

Koh, H., Berwick, D., Clancy, C., Baur, C., Brach, C., Harris, L., & Zerhusen, E. (2012). New Federal Policy initiatives to boost health literacy can help the nation move beyond the cycle of costly "crisis care." Available at http://content.healthaffairs.org/content/31/2/434.full?ijkey=HfkOgU2splhhQ&keytype=ref&siteid+healthaff

Lorenz, J. (2011). Health education and promotion. *Advance for Nurses, 13*(15), 20–23.

Mauk, K. (2006). Reaching and teaching older adults. *Nursing, 36*(2), 17.

Moyer, D., Guthrie, K., & Wingert, B. (2012). It's all in the translation. *American Nurse Today, 7*(5), 50–51.

Murdock, A., & Griffin, B. (2013). How is patient education linked to patient satisfaction? *Nursing, 43*(6), 43–45.

National Patient Safety Foundation. (2014). Ask Me 3. Available at http://www.npsf.org/for-healthcare-professionals/programs/ask-me-3/

Nigolian, C., & Miller, K. (2011). Teaching essential skills to family caregivers. *American Journal of Nursing, 111*(11), 52–58.

North American Nursing Diagnosis Association–International (NANDA-I) (2012). *Nursing diagnoses: Definitions & classification 2012–2014.* West Sussex, UK: Wiley-Blackwell.

Pfizer Clear Health Communication. (2012). The Newest Vital Sign: A health literacy assessment tool for patient care and research. Available at http://www.pfizerhealthliteracy.com/public-policy-researchers/NewestVitalSign.aspx

Robert Wood Johnson Foundation. (2011). Health Literacy: Reducing the burden of a complex healthcare system. Available at http://www.rwjf.org/en/blogs/new-public-health/2011/10/health-literacy-reducing-the-burden-of-a-complex-healthcare-system.html

Rosenstock, I. (1974). Historical origins of the health belief model. *Health Education Monograph, 2*, 354.

Sherwood, G., & Barnsteiner, J. (2012). *Quality and Safety in Nursing.* West Sussex, UK: Wiley-Blackwell.

Simonson, M., Smaldini, S., Albright, M., & Zvacek, S. (2012). *Teaching and Learning at a Distance: Foundations of Distance Education* (5th ed.). Boston, MA: Pearson.

U.S. Department of Health and Human Services (DHHS), Office of Disease Prevention and Health Promotion (2010). *National Action Plan to Improve Health Literacy.* Wshington, DC: Author.

Watson, J. (1985). *Nursing: The philosophy and science of caring.* Denver: Colorado University Press.

22 Nurse Leader, Manager, and Care Coordinator

REHEMA KOHLS

Rehema is a college sophomore who comes to the health care center requesting information about sexually transmitted infections (STIs). During the visit, she says, "So many of my friends are concerned about STIs. They all say we should start a group on campus to discuss this problem, and they want me to set it up and be the leader. But I wouldn't know where to start or what to do!"

STEPHEN WALL

Stephen, a 65-year-old widower who lives alone, is admitted to the intensive care unit after an automobile accident in which he sustained trauma to the head, chest, abdomen, and lower extremities. He is being monitored continuously via numerous invasive devices and requires complex care. His closest family member, a 40-year-old son, lives approximately 75 miles away.

JACK CAMP

Jack, a middle-aged single man with a history of diabetes mellitus, is receiving care for a compound fracture of his left lower extremity being treated with an external fixator. Compliance with his diabetic therapy regimen is questionable; he states, "I really love my sweets!" The patient frequently voices loud complaints about his room, the food, and the hospital routine. He also uses his call light very frequently, stating, "I just want to see if it's working and if the nurses will come check on me."

LEARNING OBJECTIVES

After completing the chapter, you will be able to accomplish the following:

1. Identify the qualities, four skills, and differing styles of leaders.

2. List the four managerial functions.

3. Discuss the difference between leadership and management.

4. Discuss the significance of Magnet recognition for a health care organization.

5. Summarize the steps in the process of change.

6. Describe areas in which beginning nurses can develop leadership skills.

7. Recognize the responsibilities associated with the delegation of nursing care.

8. Describe the role of a mentor.

KEY TERMS

autocratic leadership

change

decentralized decision-making process

delegation

democratic leadership

explicit power

implied power

just culture

laissez-faire leadership

leadership

management

planned change

power

quantum leadership

self-governance

transactional leadership

transformational leadership

Today, health care providers are experiencing changes such as fiscal constraints, workforce shortages, sophisticated health care consumers, and technological/pharmacologic advances. Never before has there been such a need for nurses to work competently and collaboratively with other health care professionals to deliver cost-effective, high-quality health care to all. Although nurses might assume leadership roles by virtue of their positions, they only become effective leaders over time by understanding the complexities of coordinating care, remaining open to differing points of view, and understanding the interdependency of the entire health care team (see the accompanying Reflective Practice box on page 508). Leadership and management are intertwined, but leadership roles differ from management tasks or functions. In *The Seven Habits of Highly Effective People,* Stephen Covey (1999) clarified the difference, citing a quote from Peter Drucker: "Management is doing things right; leadership is doing the right things." This suggests that leadership involves philosophy, perception, and judgment, whereas management tasks are the core of the

management role (Stachowiak & Bugel, 2013). A supportive leader uses strategies that facilitate the delivery of safe, high-quality patient care in a positive environment.

Now, more than ever, it is important for nursing as a profession to be self-directed as it charts its future. The American Nurses Association (ANA) currently recommends recognition and reimbursement for the role that nurses play in providing effective care coordination. This core competency for RNs positively impacts patient outcomes and the quality of care and reduces health care costs through more efficient use of resources (ANA, 2013). Nurses' efforts to effectively influence health care reform require familiarity with the health care organization in which they are employed as well as the health care system at large.

LEADERSHIP

The concept of leadership is one of the most researched, studied, and debated fields of inquiry. Paradoxically, it is at the same time clear and vivid, as well as elusive and subtle. **Leadership** has been described as the ability to direct or motivate a person or group to achieve set goals. Effective leaders in groups or systems do this by encouraging others to be their best selves as they work collaboratively in the pursuit of common organizational or unit goals. Leaders have power, whether explicit or implied. For example, elected class leaders have **explicit power** by virtue of their position. However, students in the class with no designated leadership position might, by force of their personality, have more power to influence the class than designated leaders; this is **implied power**.

 CONSIDER Jack Camp, the patient described in the Reflective Practice scenario. The patient assumed a position of "running things in his business," thus having the explicit power of his position. In addition, the patient used "implied power" while hospitalized to exert control over his situation. The nurse's understanding of power would be important in developing a plan to deal with the patient's behavior. ●

Power to influence a group depends on the person's leadership style and how the person fulfills leadership responsibilities. The dynamics of leadership involve applying that power for personal or organizational growth or change. Nurses who use leadership skills can become proficient in effecting desired changes in many areas, including their patients' health patterns, the health care agency, the community, the nursing profession, and the health care system in general.

Leadership Qualities

Most people admire a charismatic, dynamic, enthusiastic, visionary leader who is poised, confident, and self-directed. These characteristics define leaders such as Mother Teresa, John Kennedy, Martin Luther King, Gandhi, and others. Not everyone can be as dynamic and inspirational as these individuals, however. Yet leaders do need to be comfortable with themselves (i.e., have a positive self-image) and present

REFLECTIVE PRACTICE: CULTIVATING QSEN COMPETENCIES

CHALLENGE TO ETHICAL AND LEGAL SKILLS

While in a clinical rotation my junior year, I was assigned the dreaded Jack Camp (I still remember his name). He was a middle-aged single man receiving care for a compound fracture of his left lower extremity being treated with an external fixator. He had a bad case of diabetes, and an even worse sweet tooth. Before I even met him, the nurses on the floor were saying things like "good luck," which made this junior nursing student extra paranoid (although I was grateful for the warning). The patient was known

for voicing loud complaints about his room, the food, and the hospital routine. He also was using his call light very frequently. The nurses called him names and discussed their dislike of him in the nurses' station, which was in the center of the unit.

As the day progressed, I found out that all this patient wanted was some attention, because he was used to running things in his business. I actually found him entertaining.

Thinking Outside the Box: Possible Courses of Action

- Ignore the comments of the other nurses on the floor, hoping that no one else hears them.
- Report the nurses to my clinical instructor, possibly causing tension on the floor.

- Politely tell the nurses to keep it down and refrain from talking about the patient, risking my own comfort level; after all, I am only a visiting student—what do I know?

Evaluating a Good Outcome: How Do I Define Success?

- Act as a patient advocate despite my limited power, which means correcting unethical behaviors as cordially as possible.

- Have the courage to go to the next level if the nurses' behavior is not corrected.
- Inform the patient politely to modify his behavior.

Personal Learning: Here's to the Future!

My response was to ignore the nurses' comments and hope no one else heard them either. I was not courageous enough to be the patient advocate that we had been taught to be. I knew my response should have been to ask them to keep it down, which would allow them to maintain their personal opinions while at the same time keeping the comments from jeopardizing patient confidentiality. From this experience, I learned that you have to be a leader, speak up, and take the risk. Part of that means being able to go

against the group, risking being ostracized. In doing so, others may follow your lead, but if they choose not to follow, at least you know you advocated for your patient. Since this experience, I have not been in a situation that has challenged my personal ethics, but I have the self-confidence to believe that I can be the leader that I spoke so passionately about.

Kim Gray, Georgetown University

REFLECTION ON QUALITY AND SAFETY COMPETENCIES

How do you think you would respond in a similar situation? Why? What does this tell you about yourself and about the adequacy of your skills for professional practice? What *knowledge, skills,* and attitudes do you need to develop to continuously improve quality and safety in a situation like the one experienced by this student nurse?

Patient-Centered Care: How could the nursing student initiate improved communication between Mr. Camp and the nurses working on his unit? Did her handling of this situation facilitate her ability to advocate for patients in similar situations? Would it be helpful to elicit Mr. Camp's preferences and expressed needs and ensure that they are included as part of the plan of care?

Teamwork and Collaboration/Quality Improvement: How do you think the nursing staff would have reacted had the nursing student approached them regarding their comments about Mr. Camp? Can you think of other ways

to respond? Describe a plan the nursing student could use to go about changing the staff's behavior. Which type of leadership style might have been most effective with this group?

Safety/Evidence-Based Practice: Is there anything more the nursing student could have done to contribute to a safe patient care environment, confront her fears, and promote a positive outcome in this situation? What evidence in nursing literature provides guidance for the leadership qualities necessary to enlist support and cooperation with the nursing staff in this environment?

Informatics: What information should be included in the patient handoff at the close of the student nurse's shift? Can you identify the essential information that must be available in Mr. Camp's electronic record to support safe patient care, coordination of care, and communication with staff?

BOX 22-1	ANA STANDARDS OF NURSING PRACTICE

Standard 12. Leadership

The registered nurse demonstrates leadership in the professional practice setting and the profession.

Competencies

The registered nurse:

- Oversees the nursing care given by others while retaining accountability for the quality of care given to the healthcare consumer.
- Abides by the vision, the associated goals, and the plans to implement and measure progress of an individual healthcare consumer or progress within the context of the healthcare organization.

- Demonstrates a commitment to continuous, lifelong learning and education for self and others.
- Mentors colleagues for the advancement of nursing practice, the profession, and quality healthcare.
- Treats colleagues with respect, trust, and dignity.
- Develops communication and conflict resolution skills.
- Participates in professional organizations.
- Communicates effectively with the healthcare consumer and colleagues.
- Seeks ways to advance nursing autonomy and accountability.
- Participates in efforts to influence healthcare policy involving healthcare consumers and the profession.

American Nurses Association. (2010). *Nursing scope and standards of practice* (2nd ed.). Washington, DC: Author.

themselves as role models for followers. Ideally, they also have a vision that energizes the group and brings forth the best efforts of members. Critical thinkers and responsible decision makers commit high energy to achieving goals and are skilled in enlisting support and cooperation.

Leaders value learning and must be knowledgeable. Nurse leaders and managers cannot be knowledgeable about all aspects of the profession, but they must be creative in the development and use of scarce resources. For example, nurse leaders can use one another and other health care workers as resources, respecting each other's expertise. Contemporary nurse managers draw upon their own staff for clinical and organizational knowledge.

Political awareness is also important for nurse leaders. Knowing how to map the political terrain of the workplace is just as valuable as knowing how legislation at the local, state, and national levels affects the health care delivery system.

Flexibility is a must for all nursing leaders. All nursing functions and roles require flexibility. The needs of patients, families, and the nursing team can change from minute to minute. For example, a nurse coordinator might plan to involve staff in a discussion about how best to distribute new work responsibilities, but if there are three unexpected new admissions to the unit, the discussion may need to be postponed to a quieter time.

Leadership potential is present in all nurses. With education and practice, these qualities can be developed to the point at which a nurse is skilled in the many behaviors necessary for leadership. In 2010, the American Nurses Association (ANA) in *Nursing: Scope and Standards of Nursing Practice,* 2nd edition, defined specific professional performance guidelines for leadership (see Box 22-1). Professional nurses are accountable for these standards.

A full discussion of all these qualities is beyond the scope of this text, but Box 22-2 (on page 510) summarizes how one might approach the role of leader. Beginning nurses can monitor their progress by periodically reviewing the checklist provided in Box 22-2.

 RECALL Rehema Kohls, the college sophomore considering starting a campus group on STIs. The nurse would apply knowledge of leadership qualities when helping Rehema to decide about leading the group. In addition, the nurse would demonstrate these qualities when interacting with Rehema. ●

Personal Leadership Skills

Nurses recognize key qualities that are vital for a successful leader. The following list includes basic skills needed for nursing leadership and is not meant to be all inclusive, but instead to serve as a basis for development:

- Commitment to excellence
- Problem-solving skills including a clear vision and strategic focus that allow movement forward toward a creative solution (see the accompanying Nursing Advocacy in Action display on page 511)
- Commitment to and passion for one's work
- Trustworthiness and integrity
- Respectfulness
- Accessibility
- Empathy and caring
- Responsibility to enhance the personal growth of all staff (Sherman, 2012b)

The ability to know oneself is the cornerstone of success in either implicit or explicit leadership roles. In a *Harvard Business Review* article, Peter Drucker (1999), a scholar of leadership, wrote that to be successful in our current knowledge culture (of which nursing is a part), one must possess self-knowledge; with self-knowledge, we can place ourselves in positions in which we can make the greatest contribution. In terms of nursing leadership roles, this translates into formal authority of position, such as a unit coordinator or director or a clinical leader without a formal title (see Box 22-3 on page 511).

BOX 22-2 CHECKLIST FOR THE BEGINNING NURSE WHO WISHES TO DEVELOP LEADERSHIP SKILLS

Basic Attitudes and Skills

Read the statements on the right and circle the appropriate response: (1) rarely characterizes me, (2) sometimes characterizes me, and (3) often characterizes me.

1 2 3   1. I am self-directed. I know what I want and take the necessary steps to get it.

1 2 3   2. I know my strengths and limitations and feel confident with who I am and who I am becoming.

1 2 3   3. I get an idea ("vision") and energize others to help me "make it happen."

1 2 3   4. I coordinate or direct the activities of others, matching their abilities to the necessary task.

1 2 3   5. I think critically about a situation without letting my feelings or those of others bias my analysis.

1 2 3   6. Once I have identified a problem, I work at it until I resolve it—to the extent that this is within my power.

1 2 3   7. When I need help, I know where to find it and ask for it.

1 2 3   8. I recognize and encourage the talents of others and offer sincere compliments.

1 2 3   9. I accept responsibility for my decisions and behavior.

1 2 3   10. I accept compliments and enjoy my success.

1 2 3   11. I confront individuals who are abusing my rights or those of others in my group.

1 2 3   12. I use assertiveness techniques when defending rights.

1 2 3   13. I am flexible and can change direction once I see the value of another course of action.

1 2 3   14. I follow an appropriate chain of command when problem solving.

1 2 3   15. I question how nursing interventions might be improved.

The higher your score the better. Reread the statements where you checked "1" and see how you might plan to improve in these areas.

Beginning Execution of Leadership Role Responsibilities

Read the list of behaviors on the right and check the appropriate box—met or not met.

Met	Not Met	
☐	☐	1. Recognize some personal need you have been ignoring and take steps to ensure that it is met.
☐	☐	2. Think of some group you belong to (e.g., school, work, church, or social) whose members' needs are not being met, and plan with other members to tackle the problem.
☐	☐	3. Recognize the special advocacy needs of a patient you believe is being underserved by the health care system. Become an advocate for this patient.
☐	☐	4. Find a nursing research study that recommends a specific type of care for one of your patients. Implement the recommendation and compare your findings with those of the researchers. Work collaboratively with the interdisciplinary team to implement needed changes.
☐	☐	5. Join a professional nursing organization and become an active member.
☐	☐	6. Analyze the media's portrayal of nurses in a specific television program, film, or book. Talk with a friend about how this portrayal of nursing influences your profession. Share your comments with the producer or author.
☐	☐	7. Contact your legislator to share your views about pending legislation.
☐	☐	8. Think about leaders you admire and respect; interview current nursing leaders; develop a plan for personal professional growth and development.
☐	☐	9. Develop a mentoring relationship with a nursing leader.

 THINK back to Rehema Kohls, the college sophomore who is thinking about starting a campus discussion group on STIs. The nurse would incorporate knowledge of Drucker's identified need for self-knowledge and personal inquiries when helping Rehema decide about starting and leading the group. ●

Leadership Styles

Many different styles of leadership are present in contemporary health care settings. The complexity and persistent, rapid change in health care drive many of the leadership styles that you will observe. It is helpful to think of leadership as a behavior, as something one person does to influence another. This influence takes many forms and requires much creativity, intellect, and savvy. Different styles are applicable in different contexts and with different levels of employees. Some of those styles are explained in the next section. New graduates should carefully choose organizations that match their preferred leadership style.

Autocratic Leadership

Autocratic leadership, also called directive leadership or authoritarian leadership, involves the leader assuming control over the decisions and activities of the group. It is often an efficient process, yet many people may resent this leadership approach when used regularly. Staff and team

NURSING ADVOCACY IN ACTION

Patient Scenario

Everybody loves Sarah. Mature for her 9 years, Sarah has advanced leukemia, and her only medical hope now is to transfer to a hospital 3,000 miles from home that has the bone marrow that she needs. There are, however, several problems.

1. Sarah's family is homeless and visits rarely. She makes excuses for them—saying how hard it is to be on the street and always trying to find shelter—but she couldn't hide her disappointment when no one visited on Christmas and her birthday. You have met the parents and were struck by their immaturity.
2. Sarah's physician is working passionately to get Sarah to the transplant center; the latest hurdle is ensuring that they will accept her given the fact that the family has no insurance or finances.
3. Many of Sarah's professional caregivers aren't sure that the bone marrow transplant is a good idea. It is doubt-

ful the funds would be found to send any of her family with her, and the possibility exists that, if unsuccessful, she could die at the transplant center surrounded by strangers.

You mention these concerns to Sarah's doctor, who replies, "But this is her only hope for cure!"

Implications for Nursing Advocacy

How will you respond if you are Sarah's nurse? Talk with your classmates and experienced nurses about the questions that follow.

- If you elect to advocate for Sarah, what practical steps can you take to ensure better health outcomes?
- What is it reasonable to expect of a student nurse, a graduate nurse, and an experienced nurse in this situation?
- What advocacy skills are needed to effectively respond to this challenge?

---

members have limited opportunity to contribute suggestions and participate in organizational decisions. High staff turnover and burnout are more common with this style of leadership.

 CONSIDER Stephen Wall, the 65-year-old patient in the intensive care unit. The nurse would demonstrate autocratic leadership to perform specific care activities and to delegate responsibilities to appropriate personnel. •

Many experienced nurses are used to working under autocratic leaders because this approach was used in most hospitals in earlier years. It might have evolved from nursing's historical military and religious past, or from the industrial model of command and control prevalent in many organizations. This style of leadership is gradually being replaced by the democratic style of leadership as nurses demand and receive more say in decision making. Some health care workers still respond best to the directive approach.

In addition, some situations may require an autocratic leadership style. For example, Nurse A discovers that one of her patients is bleeding excessively from his surgical incision. She knows that he needs immediate attention, so she gives specific orders to another team member to attend to the other patients. She tells the registered nurse on her team to call the surgical resident to come as soon as possible. She implements a nursing plan of care to prevent further blood loss or complications. Nurse A assumed the autocratic style of leadership in this situation so that all necessary tasks would be accomplished immediately. Although she rarely uses this style, she implemented it effectively in this emergency situation. This example illustrates that leadership is context dependent.

Democratic Leadership

Democratic leadership, also called participative leadership, is characterized by a sense of equality among the leader and other participants. Decisions and activities are shared.

BOX 22-3 PERSONAL INQUIRIES FOR DETERMINING COMPLEMENTARY LEADERSHIP ROLES AND WORKING ENVIRONMENTS

- *Identify your strengths:* Continually improve the things you do best; discover your "intellectual arrogance" (being bright is no substitute for knowledge); work on acquiring the skills and knowledge you need to fully realize your strengths; remedy your bad habits.
- *Evaluate how you accomplish work:* We all work in ways that yield the best results for us. Are you a visual or auditory learner? Do you learn best by reading or writing? Do you work more productively in teams or alone? Are you more productive as a decision maker or as an advisor?
- *Clarify your values:* Working in an organization or on a unit whose value system is unacceptable or incompatible

with yours will lead to frustration and poor performance. Identify your values and seek a work environment that is complementary, not adversarial.
- *Determine where you belong and what you can contribute:* In small or large organizations, as a decision maker or as an advisor, prepare for opportunities that emerge in response to these queries. In this dynamic industry, set reasonable short- to medium-range goals.
- *Assume responsibility for relationships:* Cultivate relationships and analyze the differences you may have with others. Know and understand the strengths, performance modes, and values of your coworkers and managers.

Participants are encouraged to develop their skills and strengths within the group. The group and leader work together to accomplish mutually set goals and outcomes. As professionals, nurses generally respond well to this style of leadership when they are the followers and feel more comfortable when they are the leaders of democratic groups. Group satisfaction and motivation are excellent benefits of this style. In situations in which a rapid response is essential, however, a democratic approach to leadership that requires gathering the input of team members may slow decision making.

 RECALL Stephen Wall, the patient in the intensive care unit. The nurse would use democratic leadership to work collaboratively with other health care disciplines to plan the most effective care for the patient. For example, the nurse might need to work with the surgical and neurologic staff, respiratory therapy, physical therapy, and social services in developing the patient's plan of care. ●

An example of democratic leadership follows. Nurse B, a head nurse, observes that staff members have not been documenting patient teaching and learning in their progress notes. Nurse B is not sure why this is occurring but believes that this problem must be solved. He calls a staff meeting and leads a discussion to seek information on possible causes and solutions. Nurse B decides that staff members need to be included in the problem-solving approach. He thinks the staff will be more motivated to document their teaching and the patients' learning if they have a say in what changes in practice are necessary and how they will be implemented. Nurse B has used the democratic style of leadership and **decentralized decision-making process** to resolve this issue.

Laissez-Faire Leadership

In **laissez-faire leadership**, also called nondirective leadership, the leader relinquishes power to the group, such that an outsider could not identify the leader in the group. This approach encourages independent activity by group members. This style depends on the strengths of followers to direct the group activities. It is most effective when all staff are clinical experts with a deep understanding of both clinical and administrative processes. This style is rarely useful because task achievement is difficult when each nurse is working independently, and the staff on most units and departments have varying levels of clinical maturity. However, it can be used effectively when the leader wants a problem to be solved completely by expert staff group members.

 CONSIDER Stephen Wall, the patient with multiple trauma who is in the intensive care unit. The patient has multiple priority needs, requiring interdependent actions of many individuals. Use of laissez-faire leadership would not be effective in this situation. ●

Quantum Leadership

Porter-O'Grady and Malloch (2003), in *Quantum Leadership: A Textbook of New Leadership,* argued that leaders must move beyond the traditional modes used by all levels of workers. They, like Drucker (1999) and others, focused on the impact of the information age, identified at the turn of the century, on work and workers. The vertical command and control structures that generated the leadership styles previously mentioned are no longer useful for managers and workers, nor do they yield productivity for organizations. The explosion of information and technology in health care, as in other industries, has spawned, by necessity, the "knowledge worker." This social transformation is affecting aspects of all of our lives including, perhaps most importantly, how we lead and manage our organizations.

We are in a difficult transition period between the old and the new. In the old, change was viewed as an entity to be planned, carefully managed, and accepted. In the new "quantum age," change is conceived as dynamic, ever present, and continually unfolding. We are forced to experience change at the same time we perceive it, with little or no opportunity to definitively and laboriously plan and manage it. **Quantum leadership** theory views an organization and its members as interconnected and collaborative—a helpful approach when unpredictable events and changing environments present themselves (Curtin, 2013). Nursing leaders can model these new behaviors by combining these new attributes with the requisite technical skills.

Transactional Leadership

Transactional leadership style is based on a task-and-reward orientation. Team members agree to a satisfactory salary and working conditions in exchange for commitment and compliance to their leader. Health care organizations have often used transactional leadership strategies to provide direction and recognize employees' progress in meeting pre-established goals and work deadlines. Transactional leaders maintain control by rewarding good behavior and punishing behavior they perceive as detrimental or negative. Employees have minimal opportunities for creative thinking and involvement in organizational decisions, and employer and employee may not share a common vision. Transactional leaders provide little inspiration for nurses to participate in reforming health care, problem solving, or engaging in practices and research that promote nursing excellence (Habel & Sherman, 2012).

Transformational Leadership

Transformational leadership can create revolutionary change. Often described as charismatic, transformational leaders are unique in their ability to inspire and motivate others. They create intellectually stimulating practice environments and challenge themselves and others to grow personally and professionally, and to learn. Gifted in creating a common vision, they demonstrate passion for their vision and keep others similarly focused. One of the unique qualities of transformational leaders is their vulnerability. They communicate honestly and openly and can express emotions as well as ideas as they share themselves with others. They show concern and care for others and are willing to take risks. They pay attention to process as well as outcomes.

An example of transformational leadership is as follows. Nurse C is troubled by the plight of women and children in the inner city where she lives. She unites with other nurses and health care professionals to design and implement strategies to meet their needs. Within 18 months, a nursing center is funded and running, improving maternal–child outcomes in the area. The founding group of health care professionals continues to meet monthly to dream about future strategies and to support each other in their work. They are proudest of the improved self-esteem and independence in many of the women they serve.

Transformational leaders have a positive and compelling vision, fostering a new culture for nursing practice and patient care (Habel & Sherman, 2012). This style of leadership is a key component of organizations that achieve Magnet® status.

DEVELOPMENT OF THE MAGNET® RECOGNITION PROGRAM

More than two decades ago, Task Force on Nursing Practice in Hospitals of the American Academy of Nursing (AAN) conducted a study of 41 hospitals to identify and describe variables that created an environment that attracted and retained well-qualified nurses who promoted quality patient care through providing excellence in nursing services. These institutions were called "magnet" hospitals because they attracted and retained professional nurses who experienced a high degree of professional and personal satisfaction through their practice. These institutions used a decentralized decision-making process, **self-governance** at the unit level, and respect for and acknowledgment of professional autonomy. In

1990, the American Nurses Credentialing Center (ANCC), a subsidiary of ANA, developed a formal process to recognize excellence in nursing service and to confer "magnet" status. Magnet status is awarded for 4 years, after which organizations must reapply. Originally, 14 characteristics, called the Forces of Magnetism, were recognized that identified quality patient care, excellent nursing care, and innovations in professional nursing practice. A statistical analysis and review of evaluators' reports has resulted in the configuration of the original 14 attributes into 5 model components, effective in 2009 (Table 22-1). This new model includes the original 14 forces but reflects a greater focus on measuring outcomes and eliminates redundancy in documentation.

SIGNIFICANCE OF MAGNET® RECOGNITION

Research and surveys support that magnet hospitals have better patient outcomes, shorter lengths of stay, higher patient satisfaction, and higher nurse job satisfaction and nurse retention than hospitals without this governance style of leadership (ANCC, 2013; Habel & Sherman, 2012; Hawkins & Shell, 2012). The achievement of magnet status has a profound impact on the quality of patient care and nursing practice. According to Bashaw (2011), magnet recognition has become the "apex of achievement for nursing professionals and health care organizations." Almost 400 hospitals have achieved magnet status. Additional information regarding the Magnet® Recognition Program is available at the American Nurses Credentialing Center at http://www.nursecredentialing.org.

IMPLEMENTATION OF A "JUST CULTURE"

Health care organizations that achieve magnet status have created a focus on positive patient care outcomes, collaboration, shared decision making, and a climate in which patient safety is a priority. Creation of a **"just culture"** indicates an organizational commitment to accountability

Table 22-1	QUALITY STANDARDS AND INDICATORS FOR THE MAGNET® RECOGNITION PROGRAM

14 FORCES OF MAGNETISM	MAGNET® RECOGNITION PROGRAM COMPONENTS
1. Quality of Nursing Leadership 2. Organizational Structure 3. Management Style 4. Personnel Policies and Programs 5. Professional Models of Care 6. Quality of Care 7. Quality Improvement 8. Consultation and Resources 9. Autonomy 10. Community and Health 11. Nurses as Teachers 12. Image of Nursing 13. Interdisciplinary Relationships 14. Professional Development	1. Transformational Leadership 2. Structural Empowerment 3. Exemplary Professional Practice 4. New Knowledge, Innovation, and Improvements 5. Empirical Quality Results

©2013 American Nurses Credentialing Center. All Rights Reserved. Reproduced with the permission of the American Nurses Credentialing Center. Available at http://www.nursecredentialing.org/Magnet/ProgramOverview/New-Magnet-Model

and universal safety in health care. Nurses are encouraged to disclose clinical errors and potential error situations without the fear of punitive actions. This accountability then allows other nurses to learn from this experience. The open communication resulting from development of a just culture allows health care workers to discuss concerns and challenges related to patient care and turn them into opportunities for improvement. The combination of magnet principles and a just culture can produce a health care vision focused on transparency, accountability, communication, collaboration, and the pursuit of health care excellence (Bashaw, 2011; Shepard, 2011; Bashaw, Rosentein, & Lounsbury, 2012).

MANAGEMENT

All nurses, to the extent that they work with others and influence others to be their best, can become leaders. However, some nurses hold positions in the health care system that also make them managers. The role of **management** is to plan, organize, direct, and control available human, material, and financial resources to deliver quality care to patients and families. The managerial role is frequently conceptualized as the technical dimension of formal leadership roles. These technical areas of expertise, particularly in the financial or clinical resource management dimension, are mandatory for contemporary nurse managers. A few of their direct responsibilities, identified in a previous section, can be viewed in these traditionally broad areas:

- *Planning:* identifying problems and developing goals, objectives, and related strategies to meet the demands of the clinical arena
- *Organizing:* acquiring, managing, and mobilizing resources to meet both clinical and financial objectives
- *Staffing:* hiring, orienting, scheduling to facilitate team building; also includes staff development
- *Directing:* leading others in achieving goals within the constraints of the current fiscal and workforce shortage scenarios, a demanding task for managers and staff alike
- *Controlling:* implementing mechanisms for ongoing evaluation, particularly in areas of clinical quality and financial accountability (Marquis & Huston, 2012)

 REMEMBER Jack Camp, the patient with diabetes and an external fixator. The nurse manager for this unit could address the problem of the staff's overt criticism of the patient. Using planning, organizing, directing, and controlling, the nurse manager could ultimately create an environment that is conducive to the patient's recovery and health and satisfying to staff caring for this patient. ●

It is increasingly challenging for the nurse manager to be both a clinical and a managerial expert; the explosion of clinical knowledge and expectations for managerial expertise place unrealistic demands on this role. Typical nurse managers are expected to manage their unit budget within prescribed constraints, deliver a high level of quality care to patients on the unit, develop and serve as mentors for junior staff, comply with regulatory requirements, and be experts at human resource management. Although the role might seem overwhelming, it can also be quite satisfying to the manager, the staff, and the organization. Collaboration and appropriate support from both superiors and subordinates can empower and motivate staff, facilitating a highly functioning team and best-practice clinical environment.

Marquis and Huston (2012) caution that management and leadership should be intertwined for each to be effective. Some view leadership as an expected function of management, while others consider leadership as more complex with an emphasis on improving productivity and empowering the workforce rather than just controlling specific organizational details. However, a leader without management skills can cause chaos in an organization, while a manager who fails to lead is equally ineffective. Nurse managers must be effective leaders to be successful. Nurse managers who cannot create a healthy group environment; who fail to resolve interpersonal issues that lower morale and result in numerous complaints from patients, nurses, and physicians; and who cannot develop a plan to resolve detrimental interpersonal issues lack leadership skills.

Centralized and Decentralized Management Structures

In a centralized management structure, senior managers generally make decisions. Those further down in the hierarchy of the organization are often responsible for implementing decisions into which they had little input. In a decentralized management structure, on the other hand, decisions are made by those who are most knowledgeable about the issues being decided. Nurses are thus intimately involved in decisions concerning patient care. Nurse managers are accountable for what happens on their nursing unit, including patient census, staffing, supplies, and budget. A decentralized system invites greater accountability and responsibility because most nurses feel more responsible for decisions they have made themselves. However, you will most likely experience both modes of decision making, centralization and decentralization, in nursing units. Financial targets and other broad strategic directions are frequently established at executive levels of the organization. Clinical issues, processes of care delivery, clinical outcomes, and unit governance are usually resolved at the unit or department level.

Conflict Management

Nurse managers frequently encounter conflict between employees and between themselves and employees. Unresolved conflict can lower morale and threaten quality care. Marquis and Huston (2012) described six styles for dealing with conflict—avoiding, accommodating, competing, compromising, collaborating, and smoothing—and noted that "the situation itself, the urgency of the decision, the power and status of the players, the importance of the issue, and

Table 22-2 CONFLICT RESOLUTION STRATEGIES

STRATEGY	DEFINITION
Avoiding	There is awareness of the conflict situation, but the parties involved decide to either ignore the conflict or avoid/postpone its resolution. The conflict has not been resolved and may resurface later in an exaggerated form.
Collaborating	This is a joint effort to resolve the conflict with a win–win solution. All parties set aside previously determined goals, determine a priority common goal, and accept mutual responsibility for achieving this goal. This focus on problem solving is based on mutual respect, honest communication, and shared decision making.
Competing	This approach results in a win for one party at the expense of the other group. This win–lose confrontation can leave the loser frustrated, with a desire to get even in the future. This strategy may be utilized when one party has more knowledge regarding the situation or when resistance is appropriate because of ethical concerns or unsafe patient care practices.
Compromising	For this technique to be effective, both parties must be willing to relinquish something of equal value. If that does not occur, either or both parties may feel that they have lost the conflict and given up more than the other group.
Cooperating/Accommodating	One party makes a conscious decision to let the other group win and frequently collects an "IOU" for use in the future. This party's original loss may result in a more positive outcome in the future.
Smoothing	Smoothing is an effort to compliment the other party and focus on agreement rather than disagreement, thus reducing the emotion in the conflict. The original conflict is rarely resolved with this technique.

Adapted from Marquis, B., & Huston, C. (2012). *Leadership roles and management functions in nursing* (7th ed., pp. 474–475). Philadelphia: Wolters Kluwer Health/Lippincott Williams & Wilkins.

the maturity of the people involved in the conflict" determine which strategy is most appropriate. Table 22-2 further defines these conflict resolution strategies.

Johansen (2012) describes a nursing management situation that demonstrates these conflict resolution strategies. Nurse C, who works in an emergency department, receives her assignment and notices that Nurse J has a much lighter assignment. Nurse J has a reputation for being difficult and always getting her way. Because of the number of her assigned patients and the severity of their conditions, Nurse C approaches the charge nurse, Nurse S, and asks her to modify her assignment. Nurse S declines to change it, does not want to address this with Nurse J, and reminds Nurse C how difficult Nurse J can be if confronted with an unpleasant situation. Nurse C decides to discuss this situation with Nurse P, the nurse manager. To manage this conflict, Nurse P can use one of the following strategies:

- *Avoid* the situation, with the result that both Nurse C and Nurse P feel frustrated and powerless.
- Respond in a dominating or *competing* manner and tell Nurse S that the assignments are unacceptable. She intimidates Nurse S and also is upset because the nurses on the unit are not resolving their own problems.
- Ask Nurse C to accept the assignment in order to *accommodate* the charge nurse. Nurse P understands the inequity of this assignment but lets Nurse C know that she appreciates her team commitment and will remember this in the future.
- Attempt a *compromise* by providing Nurse S with a rationale for modifying the assignment. Both Nurse C and

Nurse S should discuss the assignment with Nurse J and see if they can find a mutually agreeable solution.

- *Collaborate* with all parties to resolve the assignment issue and promote a safer work situation.
- Use a *smoothing* approach that involves complimenting all parties in an attempt to prevent emotional outbursts and focus on agreement.

A problem can occur if one habitually uses one style of conflict resolution, which might not always be best for particular situations. The best outcome is to create a win–win situation for all those involved. While this is not always possible, conflict resolution strategies may lessen existing differences and prevent all parties from feeling overwhelmed. Effective nurses try out each style and learn to use the style best suited for each situation. This ability to determine the appropriate response to conflict and create a win–win solution for all parties is critical for a nurse to be an effective manager.

Managing Change

Change is the process of transforming or modifying something. It might be planned, unplanned, developmental, or, as Porter-O'Grady and Malloch suggested, quantum and ever-present. Nursing and the health care system are continually changing and evolving—that momentum will only escalate in the years to come. Factors such as the increasing number of chronically ill and older people, the increasing role of government and industry in health care, the rising cost of health care, and the changing patterns of health care delivery have produced a need for innovation and change in health care. Patient care safety and quality issues play a vital role in the transformation occurring in the health care system. Nurse managers, once they have assessed the need for change, function as visionary, assertive, and supportive role models in the implementation of the planned change.

Change Theory

There are many theories of change, most based on the classic theory of change proposed by Kurt Lewin (1951). Lewin identified three stages of change:

* *Unfreezing:* The need for change is recognized.
* *Moving:* Change is initiated after a careful process of planning.
* *Refreezing:* Change becomes operational.

These three rather simplistic stages do not fully reveal the very dynamic and personal nature of change of any kind. In health care, we can find numerous examples of using change theory to transform practice. Not so long ago, childbirth in the United States was routinely "medicalized." Women came to the hospital to deliver their babies; pain medications that interfered with the natural process of labor were routinely administered, necessitating forceps and assisted deliveries; and husbands, partners, and siblings were banished from the delivery room. Nurse midwives and others recognized the need for change (*unfreezing*) and set about researching childbirth and ways to improve infant and family outcomes. After a careful process of planning (*moving*), multiple natural childbirth options in health care facilities and in the home were made available to women and couples; today they represent mainstream care (*refreezing*).

Similarly, someone who takes good health for granted might fail to develop healthy lifestyle practices until illness results in recognition of the need for change (*unfreezing*).

A careful process of consultation and study might lead to the development of a well-developed fitness plan (*moving*), which ideally becomes part of the person's everyday life (*refreezing*). Effective nurses pay attention to their ability to influence the person's thinking and behavior in each stage of change.

Planned Change

Planned change is a purposeful, systematic effort to bring about change. Nurse managers most often implement planned change. The eight steps in the process of change, which are somewhat similar to the steps of the nursing process, are shown in Box 22-4. Kotter (1996) emphasized that for change to be successful, it is important to progress in sequence through each of the eight stages. Skipping any of the steps can result in the vision being sabotaged, momentum faltering, and frustration increasing for all involved in the process.

Before planning to make a change, a nurse manager should consider the following:

* What is amenable to change? Considering this question might reveal a behavior not amenable to change.
* How does the group function as a unit? Certain forces within a group may favor change, whereas other forces may resist it.
* Is the person or group ready for change and, if so, at what rate can that change be expected to be accepted? The pace of change must be consistent with the person's or group's readiness to assimilate change. Readiness involves both the ability and willingness to change. In contemporary health care organizations, change is dynamic, persistent, and very challenging. The concept of flexibility previously mentioned is put to a real test in any clinical or managerial arena.

BOX 22-4 PLANNED CHANGE: AN EIGHT-STEP PROCESS

Planned change is a purposeful, systematic effort to alter or bring about change through the intervention of a change agent. The same steps apply whether dealing with individuals or groups.

1. *Recognize symptoms that indicate a change is needed and collect data.*
2. *Identify a problem to be solved through change.* Analyze the symptoms and reach a conclusion. Note resistance or barriers to change and factors that promote the desired change.
3. *Determine and analyze alternative solutions to the problem.* Consider the advantages, disadvantages, and consequences of each alternative. An analysis of various proposed solutions to a problem may result in using a combination of alternatives.
4. *Select a course of action from possible alternatives.* Avoid initiating too many courses of action and thereby dissipating resources and energy.
5. *Plan for making the change.* This step is crucial to effect change successfully. Start by stating specific

objectives, designing a plan for change, developing timetables, selecting people to assist with making the change, and anticipating how to stabilize change and deal with resistance to change. Unless a plan is clearly designed, effecting change is likely to be a chaotic experience.

6. *Implement the selected course of action to effect change.* Put the plan for change into effect. During this period, flexibility is important to adapt to unforeseen problems.
7. *Evaluate the effects of change by comparing them with objectives stated in the plan for change.* Adjustments can be made in the plan as necessary after evaluation. If the results of evaluation indicate that the course of action selected to solve a problem has been unsuccessful, an adjustment should be made or another course of action selected.
8. *Stabilize the change.* When a solution has been found, take measures to make the change permanent. Continue follow-up until the change is firmly established.

- Are the changes major or minor? A series of small changes might be more easily accomplished than one large, dramatic change. The nursing leader/manager must support the staff during the difficult task of acquiring new skills and frequently new professional identities.

In today's dynamic health care environment, nurses play a pivotal role in the change process. They must be prepared to initiate and implement quality change projects. The Robert Wood Johnson Foundation and the Institute for Healthcare Improvement originated a program called Transforming Care at the Bedside (TCAB) that focuses on instituting changes to improve patient care on medical–surgical units. Nurses are empowered to address inefficiencies and changes in work flow in an effort to improve the quality of patient care. An additional change effort, the Care Innovation and Transformation (CIT) initiative, was developed by the American Organization of Nurse Executives (AONE). This program supports nurse managers and provides training and tools to ensure a successful change environment. As of 2013, both of these programs have been adopted in more than 150 hospitals (Burke & McLaughlin, 2013).

Resistance to Change

People might resist change for various reasons. The nurse manager/leader must identify whether any resistance is present, which would determine which techniques are needed to overcome it. Change alters the balance of a group and resistance is an expected accompaniment to change.

THREAT TO SELF

People generally view change in terms of how they are affected personally. Personal threats might include a loss of self-esteem, a belief that more work will be required, or a belief that social relationships will be disrupted. For example, when hospitals began to use more unlicensed assistive personnel (UAP) for routine nursing care, many nurses resisted not only because of quality concerns but also because they found themselves legally and professionally responsible for supervising the care given by these aides. There was also concern that some professional nurses would be replaced by unlicensed assistive personnel.

LACK OF UNDERSTANDING

Someone who does not understand the nature of change is likely to resist. The people who will be affected by the change must become involved and educated if their resistance is to be overcome. For example, nurses who do not realize the effectiveness of using plans of care tend to resist preparing them because they believe they are not beneficial for providing patient care.

LIMITED TOLERANCE FOR CHANGE

Some people simply do not like to function in a state of flux or disequilibrium. A person might understand the need for change but might be unable to cope emotionally with it. For example, a nurse might resist change because of the temporary confusion the change is likely to cause.

DISAGREEMENTS ABOUT THE BENEFITS OF CHANGE

Resistance might occur when the change agent and those resisting change have different information. If the information known by the people resisting change is more accurate and relevant than the change agent's information, their resistance might be beneficial. For example, the supervisor of community health services proposes to implement, in a low-income neighborhood, a home health care plan that has been effective in a middle-class section of the city. The nurse in charge of the health program in the low-income area resists, believing that the same plan would not be successful in a financially and educationally disadvantaged neighborhood.

FEAR OF INCREASED RESPONSIBILITY

Many people are worried about having to take on more complex responsibilities, especially if they feel unprepared for the planned changes. The changes might seem overwhelming, so they naturally resist them.

Overcoming Resistance to Change

Resistance can be subtle or distinct, gentle or aggressive. Responding to resistance is both a leadership responsibility and a challenge in which the leader uses leadership qualities, leadership style, and knowledge of group dynamics to influence others toward a desired outcome. Nurses acting as change agents find the following guidelines helpful for overcoming resistance to change:

- Explain the proposed change to all affected people in simple, concise language.
- List the advantages of the proposed change, both for the individual and for members of the group.
- Relate the proposed change to the person's or group's existing beliefs and values.
- Help overcome resistance by providing opportunities for open communication and feedback.
- Indicate clearly how the change will be evaluated.
- If possible, introduce change gradually. Involve everyone affected by the change in the design and implementation of the process.
- Provide incentives for commitment to change, such as money, status, time off, or a better working environment.

 THINK back to Jack Camp, the patient described in the Reflective Practice display. The nurse could apply these guidelines when attempting to change staff behavior and the patient's behavior. Ultimately, a positive outcome for both could be achieved. ●

Power

Nurses in leadership and managerial roles who wish to be effective change agents are sensitive to both the uses and abuses of power. **Power**, the ability to influence others to achieve a desired effect, has many sources. Nurses in management positions within an institution (e.g., director of

Table 22-3 TYPES OF POWER

TYPE	DEFINITION
Reward power	Rewarding employees with something they deem valuable. May take the form of a raise, a promotion, comp time, or simply a compliment.
Coercive power	The opposite of reward power: utilizing threat of punishment to force someone to comply or do something the individual does not want to do. May be conveyed via threats of losing one's job, demotion, or receiving a poor performance review or evaluation.
Legitimate power	Accompanies a position of power or authority in an organization. Creates feelings of obligation or responsibility. Once the position or title is lost, the power is lessened or disappears.
Expert power	The perception of expertise based on knowledge, skills, or experience. Expert power leaders are able to influence and convince subordinates to trust them and work toward meeting goals.
Referent power	Occurs when one person receives approval or personal acceptance from another person. The leader is often viewed as a role model and trusted and respected by other people. However, this type of power is easily lost.
Informational power	Occurs when one has information or facts that others need to accomplish tasks or meet goals. Includes using information to persuade others or providing rational arguments for the acceptance of information.

Adapted from Marquis, B., & Huston, C. (2012). *Leadership roles and management functions in nursing* (7th ed.). Philadelphia: Wolters Kluwer Health/Lippincott Williams & Wilkins.

nursing or nursing coordinator) have ascribed power associated with the role. A group might attribute power to different individuals because of their expertise, leadership, or charisma. When introducing change, it is helpful to recognize and enlist the support of key power players who can then encourage others to become involved. You can probably think of people in the groups to which you belong (school, church, civic groups) who are "natural leaders" because of their demonstrated ability to influence others. These are the "key power players" whose support is essential to effecting change. Various types of power are outlined in Table 22-3.

All nurses should recognize the inherent power they have to ensure safe, quality, person-centered care and to cause change. Various nursing leaders have repeatedly emphasized that nurses need to utilize this power and be proactive rather than reactive to have a significant impact on a new vision for nursing. The following factors can have a role in increasing the power base of nursing:

- *Right timing:* Consumers and legislators are frustrated with errors reported in the health care system, the number of uninsured people, and overall problems with the health care system in the United States. Nurses, as the most respected health care providers, are poised to help improve health care and implement health care reform.
- *Size of the nursing profession:* This is one of nursing's greatest assets, with at least 3 million RNs in the United States. Nurses are an impressive voting bloc.
- *Nursing's referent power:* The public has expressed a high degree of trust and credibility in the nursing profession.
- *Increasing knowledge base and education for nurses:* More nurses are assuming advanced practice roles, and nursing graduates are strongly encouraged to achieve higher levels of education.

- *Nursing's unique perspective:* The caring component of nursing coupled with evidence-based practice and critical thinking has positioned nurses to deliver complex care to a variety of patients and positively impact quality of care.
- *Desire of consumers and providers for change:* Consumers are increasingly aware of the need for accessible, affordable, and safe quality care (Marquis & Huston, 2012).

Transformational leaders empower their staff by communicating and encouraging learning as well as promoting and verifying a sense of value about the powerful, life-saving work that nurses perform. Nurses who feel they have no control over their environment are more likely to express frustration toward a coworker and to leave their position or even the profession (Stringer, 2012).

 RECALL Rehema Kohls, the college sophomore considering starting a campus discussion group about STIs. The nurse at the health care center sees that Rehema is considered by her peers to have power and to be a leader. The nurse would integrate this information in helping Rehema develop the group. ●

Although power and gender issues are still present in our society, this situation has been changing over the last few decades. Women are accomplished professionals and occupy powerful leadership positions in corporations, health care organizations, and political arenas. The proverbial "glass ceiling" barrier has been broached—communication skills that promote group and team initiatives, long thought to be skills associated with females, are now valued by all. People are realizing that techniques for achieving and managing power vary and that gender differences create unique approaches to increase effectiveness and promote positive outcomes (Marquis & Huston, 2012).

IMPLEMENTING LEADERSHIP AND MANAGEMENT SKILLS IN NURSING CARE

No one is born a leader. People develop leadership qualities through observation, knowledge, and experience. Nurses develop their leadership qualities in the same way, although they might enter nursing with some leadership experience. Nursing students and beginning practicing nurses have some leadership responsibilities but are usually still working at developing leadership skills and learning where and how to apply them. Fortunately, they have support systems for guidance.

Approach leadership like any other new role or skill: slowly and carefully. Nursing students and beginning nurses should be prepared with all of the necessary tools or skills before attempting a new leadership role. Initially, nurses develop leadership skills in well-defined clinical situations. With each experience, growth occurs and leadership is strengthened. Remember that all nurse managers, nurse administrators, and nursing leaders began as inexperienced nurses. The accompanying Research in Nursing display discusses the need to cultivate and nurture nursing leaders.

Evidence-Based Strategies to Improve Leadership Skills

Nurses are familiar with the use of evidence-based practices in their clinical care but are less familiar with evidence-based strategies that support leadership development. Research has identified strategies and guidelines that can assist nurses to be more effective leaders. They include the following:

- *Strive to become an authentic leader:* Clearly communicate factual information while maintaining your core values and tolerance for those with differing viewpoints.
- *Develop leadership skills:* A Nurse Manager Leadership Collaborative model has been developed that identifies competencies and skills needed to lead in today's complex health care environment.

RESEARCH IN NURSING

BRIDGING THE GAP TO EVIDENCE-BASED PRACTICE

Identifying Predictors Indicating RN Interest in Leadership Roles

Today's nurses face many challenges. Nurse leaders and managers have considerable responsibility for patient outcomes and function in complex, high-stress environments. The path to a leadership role requires resilience, commitment, and a belief that leaders can make a difference and have a positive impact on the health care environment. Given the increasing responsibility that nurses will assume with health care reforms, it is imperative that efforts be made to identify and develop nurse leaders. Ultimately, an effective nurse leader shapes and influences nursing practice.

Related Research

Bulmer, J. (2013). Leadership aspirations of registered nurses: Who wants to follow us? *Journal of Nursing Administration, 43*(3), 130–134.

Currently, fewer than 12% of RNs have expressed an interest in leadership roles. They cite lack of support, life and job stresses, and fear of failure as reasons for avoiding leadership responsibility. This descriptive correlational study reviewed perceived support, career stage, educational preparation, and leadership aspirations in registered nurses to determine characteristics of nurses who have interest and potential for development of leadership skills. The sample consisted of RNs who were not currently in leadership positions in an urban hospital in Pennsylvania. Thirteen (13) men and 190 women responded to the 21-question survey; close to a majority (n = 98, 48%) had a bachelor's degree in nursing. Educational preparation for the remainder of the participants ranged from diploma graduates to one RN with a doctorate in nursing. Experience as an RN was divided into five career stages ranging from less than 2 years (exploration stage) to 25 years or more experience (late career). Results of the survey indicated that there was limited aspiration on the part of all the RNs surveyed to attain a leadership position (14%) and, unexpectedly, those RNs with the least amount of experience (less than 2 years) expressed the most interest in a leadership role. Economic and childcare challenges as well as a focus on the quality of life and planning for retirement may contribute to less leadership interest in those RNs with more experience. Respondents to the survey reported that colleagues consistently provided the most support, while supervisors' support ranked the lowest, although reassurance in abilities and acknowledgement of efforts from supervisors did contribute to leadership aspirations. There was no correlation between the support of colleagues and leadership aspirations. RNs with graduate degrees were more likely to be interested in a leadership role than those with other educational preparation. Overall, the years of experience (less than 2 years), educational preparation (highest nursing degree completed), and informational support provided by a nonwork individual or mentor were associated with the greatest measure of interest in leadership roles.

Relevance to Nursing Practice

This study is one example of how nursing research can provide insight into those characteristics recognized as critical to encouraging nurses to aspire to leadership positions. A nurse manager or mentor acting as a coach and nurse leader residency programs have been mentioned in the literature as supportive of cultivating nursing leaders. Finding and encouraging RNs with interest and potential leadership qualities is a serious issue in nursing that needs to be addressed. Nurses can use these leadership skills to become proficient in effecting change in many areas of health care.

For additional research, visit thePoint.

- *Promote a healthy work environment:* Staff satisfaction, retention, and improved patient outcomes depend on a healthy work environment in which nurses have a role in necessary improvements and can achieve personal satisfaction in their job.
- *Engage staff to commit to their best effort at work:* When the environment is healthy and staff feel they have control over their practice, they are more likely to be engaged and committed to their work.
- *Assist new graduates to transition into the RN role:* Evidence suggests that new graduates need preceptors and mentors who support them during their first 12 months of practice (Sherman, 2012a).

Nurses who become effective leaders can play a major role in influencing future changes in the health care system.

Clinical Nurse Leader Role

To have a positive effect on fragmented health care and promote improved collaboration within the entire health care team, the American Association of Colleges of Nursing (AACN) created the nursing professional role of clinical nurse leader (CNL). This master's-prepared nurse has earned the certified CNL credential. The CNL works collaboratively with the health care team to facilitate, coordinate, and oversee care provided to patients (Stachowiak & Bugel, 2013: Sheets et al., 2012). This role is not considered an administrative or management role but rather one of leadership in all health care settings. The CNL should be able to clearly communicate with other health care professionals, integrate evidence-based practices into patient care, and evaluate risks and outcomes that may require change in care plans for patients (AACN, 2012). The person-centered focus of the CNL role includes functioning as a patient advocate, educator, and provider of patient care in complex situations.

Questions have arisen about a perceived overlap or duplication between the roles of the CNL and those of the clinical nurse specialist and case manager. Some nursing professionals also question the need for the CNL at this time. Clinical nurse specialists are advanced practice nurses with specialist education in a defined area of practice, however, whereas case managers are closely involved with discharge plans, length-of-stay issues, and insurance constraints (Stachowiak & Bugel, 2013). Refer to Chapters 8 and 9 for additional discussion regarding case management.

Guidelines for Delegating Nursing Care

New graduate nurses use leadership techniques when they direct the work of nonprofessional staff and volunteers and when they delegate tasks to nonprofessional staff. These individuals who are unlicensed and function in an assistive role to RNs are referred to as unlicensed assistive personnel (UAP) by the American Nurses Association (ANA), replacing the former term, nursing assistive personnel (NAP). UAP may include nurses' aides, certified nursing assistants,

or other unlicensed caregivers within the health care environment. The ANA in 2012 released a revised position statement that supported the safe and effective use of delegation. The *Principles for Delegation by Registered Nurses to Unlicensed Assistive Personnel (UAP)* guides RNs practicing in all settings across the continuum of care (ANA, 2012c). **Delegation** involves the transfer of responsibility for the performance of an activity to another person while retaining accountability for the outcome. It is a critical competency and essential skill for a registered nurse in today's health care environment. RNs may never delegate any elements of the nursing process itself.

The ANA, which is committed to monitoring the regulation, education, and use of UAPs, recommends adherence to eleven broad principles guiding RNs prior to delegating care (ANA, 2012c). In addition to the RN's responsibility, several principles focus on the accountability of the health care organization. Initially, the RN must be fully aware of the parameters for delegation as outlined in their state's Nurse Practice Act as well as the employing organization's policies and procedures regarding delegation (Daley, 2013). Facilities are responsible for ensuring that UAPs are qualified and capable of performing nursing tasks that RNs may delegate to them. Registered nurses should have involvement in the development of agency policies regarding delegation and also have access to any information regarding competency of the UAPs on their team. Before the RN delegates any nursing intervention, a number of additional factors, including the qualifications and capabilities of the UAP, should be considered: (1) the stability of the patient's condition, (2) the complexity of the activity to be delegated, (3) the potential for harm, (4) the predictability of the outcome, and (5) the overall context of other patient needs (ANA, 2012c). The RN remains accountable for any delegated nursing care or outcomes and is responsible for the supervision of the UAP to whom tasks are delegated. UAPs need an awareness of any patient precautions, when to seek assistance, and what should immediately be reported to the RN. Inappropriate delegation decisions can jeopardize the safety of patients and endanger a nurse's professional practice.

Delegation skills must be developed, practiced, and strengthened. Nurse educators are encouraged by the ANA to integrate principles for delegation into the curriculum and ensure that nursing students have opportunities to practice delegation skills (Chapter 14 has additional information on delegation and the student nurse). Professional development offerings assist RNs to develop critical thinking skills that promote good judgment and provide strategies to delegate effectively. Experienced and reliable UAPs who perform delegated skills competently allow RNs to focus more on assessment and development or revision of the nursing care plan and learn skills that improve their nursing practice (Trossman, 2012). The Decision Tree for Delegation by Registered Nurses distributed by the ANA is a helpful guide for nurses who are learning to delegate (Fig. 22-1). Refer to Chapter 14 for additional information on nursing delegation.

FIGURE 22-1. Sample decision tree for delegation by registered nurses. (Reprinted with permission from the American Nurses Association, © 2012 American Nurses Association.)

Gradually, new nurses assume increased leadership responsibilities as they become primary nurses, case managers, or unit coordinators. An understanding of the function and organization of both the nursing department and health care organization is required to be an effective leader.

Nursing Department

The nursing team can also be viewed in the broader context of the entire nursing department of a health care institution or agency. Nurses should have an interest in the functioning of the department. Using this knowledge, nurses can seek information or change through appropriate channels. The more nurses understand how the nursing department runs, the better able they are to work constructively to meet the department's objectives.

Employing Institution or Agency

Nurses at all levels need to be knowledgeable about the administrative structure and functions of their employing institution or agency. When problems arise concerning professional, unit, departmental, or institutional or agency objectives, nurses must be able to use the proper channels of communication. For example, if a nurse believes that work assignments are routinely incompatible with basic patient safety and quality but gets no response after discussing this with an immediate nursing supervisor, the nurse should take those complaints to the director of nursing. If the director of nursing fails to respond adequately, the nurse should determine to whom the director of nursing reports and should approach that person. Similarly, a nurse concerned about medical care should first approach the medical attending. If the medical attending fails to respond, the nurse must then contact the nursing coordinator and, in consult with the nursing coordinator, approach the medical director. The structure of these channels is shown in the agency's organization chart, which details the relationships among the various administrative positions, departments, and job titles. Sometimes, the nurse is referred to committees that deal with specific issues.

Support for Leadership Training

Nurses intent on developing their leadership ability have multiple resources available to them—mentorship, preceptorship, participation in professional organizations, and continuing education.

Mentorship

Mentorship is a relationship in which an experienced person (the mentor) advises and assists a less experienced person (protégé). This is an effective way of easing a new nurse into leadership responsibilities. Mentors link with protégés by common interest and provide support, information, and network links. The relationship does not include financial reward. The advantages of having an effective mentor are highlighted in Box 22-5.

Mentorship is valuable in all types of nursing positions. As a nurse climbs the ladder of leadership responsibility, a mentor who is experienced in management and administrative functions might be of great assistance. A mentor can be key in helping a less experienced nurse assume added responsibilities and position changes. Many mentorship relationships also become lasting friendships.

Preceptorship

An alternative model is preceptorship. The preceptor (experienced nurse) is selected (and generally paid) to introduce an employee to new responsibilities through teaching and guidance. This orientation ensures that the new RN gains the appropriate knowledge, skills, and support to care for patients safely and efficiently. Preceptors also assist new RNs to learn the policies and procedures of a new facility, and can serve as a mentor by modeling excellent nursing practice (Keasler, 2013). The relationship is limited by the new employee's needs (Fig. 22-2).

Participation in Nursing and Other Professional Organizations

The many nursing organizations at the international, national, state, district, and local levels are discussed in Chapter 1.

FIGURE 22-2. The nurse preceptor advises and teaches nursing students by example. *(Photo by Joe Mitchell.)*

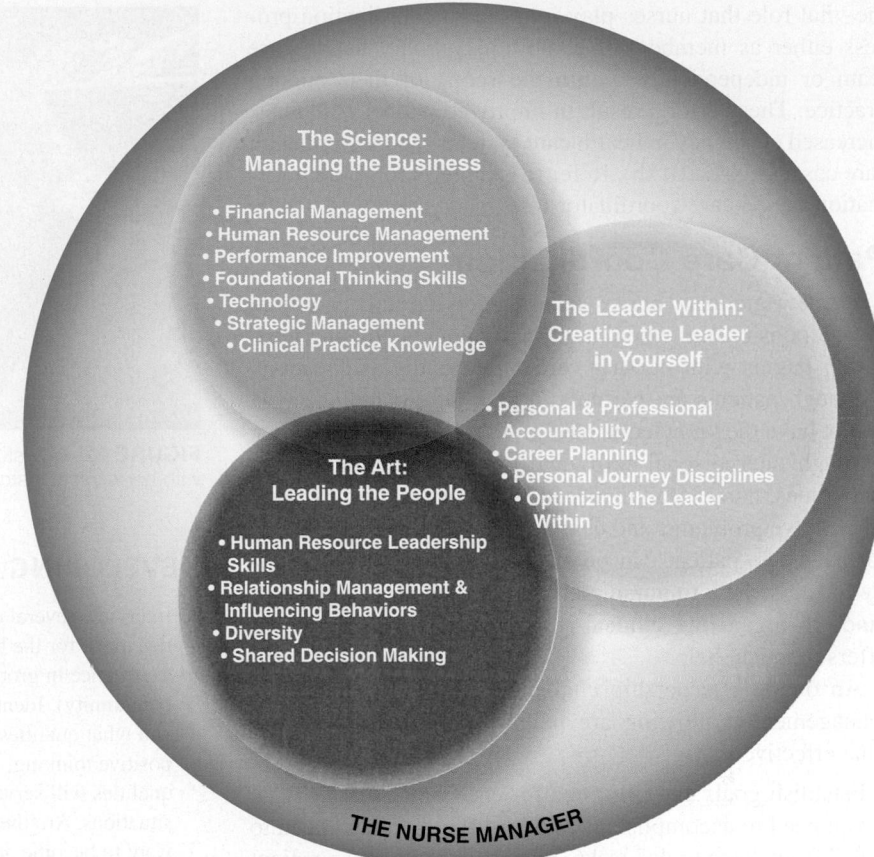

The Science:
Managing the Business

• Financial Management
• Human Resource Management
• Performance Improvement
• Foundational Thinking Skills
• Technology
• Strategic Management
• Clinical Practice Knowledge

The Leader Within:
Creating the Leader
in Yourself

• Personal & Professional
  Accountability
• Career Planning
• Personal Journey Disciplines
• Optimizing the Leader
  Within

The Art:
Leading the People

• Human Resource Leadership
  Skills
• Relationship Management &
  Influencing Behaviors
• Diversity
• Shared Decision Making

THE NURSE MANAGER

FIGURE 22-3. Nurse manager learning domain framework. (©2006 Nurse Manager Leadership Partnership. Reprinted with permission from American Organization of Nurse Executives (AONE). (2012). Available at http://www.aone.org/resources/leadership%20tools/NMLPframework.shtml)

They are major forces for nursing leadership and have active groups throughout the United States and abroad. The more than 100 professional organizations address specialty interests, goals, and purposes, as well as advocate for nurses and nursing (Matthews, 2012). Representatives of these nursing organizations also work with ANA lobbyists in Congress and state legislatures regarding nursing concerns, health care issues, and quality care. The American Organization of Nurse Executives (AONE), recognizing the need for leadership development for nurse managers, united with the American Association of Critical-Care Nurses (AACN) and the Association of PeriOperative Registered Nurses (AORN) to develop a model that includes content on the science, art, and creation of the leader within oneself (AONE, 2012) (see Figure 22-3). These are intended to engage nurses in exploring potential solutions to achieve their management goals. Nursing leadership can define what the future should look like and help make it happen. Participation in nursing and other professional organizations provides important opportunities for nurses to develop and exhibit leadership.

Continuing Education

Many programs for developing leadership, managerial, and administrative skills are available to nurses. Courses can also be taken by correspondence or over the Internet. Periodicals and books also provide continuing education for emerging leaders. Many continuing education programs are available to prepare nurses before they assume higher levels of leadership; some are geared to nurses already in such positions. Nurses should choose a program that matches their learning needs. Many State Boards of Nursing require evidence of continuing education credits prior to renewal of RN licenses.

CARE COORDINATION AND THE ROLE OF NURSING

Nurses have long been involved in care coordination activities, but only recently have these efforts been recognized as an integral contribution to effective and efficient use of health care resources and quality patient outcomes. Care coordination is defined as the organization of patient care activities to facilitate the delivery of quality health care services in an efficient person-centered manner (ANA, 2013). Nurses have developed care plans that account for patients' needs and preferences, conducted health teaching for patients and their families prior to discharge, and coordinated care across a variety of settings following discharge from a health care facility (ANA, 2012a).

Validation of Care Coordination Activities

The ANA has launched an effort to validate the care coordination activities of RNs and seek funding for these essential components of patient care. Its position statement affirms the vital role that nurses play in the care coordination process either as members of a multidisciplinary health care team or independently within the scope of their nursing practice. These efforts result in improved patient outcomes, increased efficiency in health care systems, and lower health care costs (ANA, 2012b). Refer to Chapter 9 for more information on the care coordinator role.

Patient Care Coordination

Even new graduate nurses have leadership and coordination responsibilities when they begin nursing. Nursing leadership begins with nursing care of the individual patient. Although patients are partners in their care planning, most do not have the knowledge base and skills to direct the plan. Through interpersonal skills and effective communication techniques, nurses lead their patients to acquire new knowledge, solve problems, and change behaviors. Managing care for even one patient can be an overwhelming responsibility for those new to nursing and its challenges. The student guide to organizing clinical responsibilities in Chapter 14 offers practical help.

An ongoing leadership challenge for all nurses is time management. Following are helpful steps for using your time effectively:

- Establish goals and priorities for each day. Identify what you need to accomplish each day, differentiating "need to do" from "nice to do" tasks. Be sure to include the patient and/or the patient's family in establishing these priorities. Ask, "What is it important for you to accomplish today?"
- Evaluate your goals in terms of their ability to meet the needs of the patients entrusted to your care as well as your duties to yourself and your colleagues (other students and members of the team). If one student has a patient whose care requires assistance, other students can plan their day to be able to help at a particular time. This sort of teamwork is an important element of care coordination.
- Establish a time line. Allocate priorities to hours in your workday so that you will recognize when you are falling behind schedule in time to correct it before the day is lost.
- Evaluate your success or failure in managing time. If you fail to accomplish your goals in the time available, determine whether your goals were overambitious, whether things happened beyond your control (e.g., your patient's condition worsened, requiring more care, or another student required your assistance), or whether you wasted time that could have been better spent (Fig. 22-4).
- Use the results of this evaluation to direct your next day's priorities and time line.

 REMEMBER Stephen Wall, the 65-year-old patient in the intensive care unit with multiple injuries. Due to his multiple and complex needs, time management for the nurse is crucial. Applying the steps just identified in this situation would be very helpful when planning and providing care. ●

FIGURE 22-4. A student reviews her success in managing time with her clinical instructor. *(Photo by Joe Mitchell.)*

DEVELOPING CLINICAL REASONING

1. Interview several experienced nurses and ask them what qualities make for the best nursing leaders. Reflect on your personal experience in groups (e.g., within your family, church, school, community). Identify the roles you characteristically assume and what qualities you bring to the group (e.g., enthusiasm, positive thinking, vision, self-direction). Consider whether those qualities will serve you well in professional nursing groups and situations. Are there new qualities you need to develop if you want to become an effective nurse leader? Why?

2. Identify a situation in your class or school that "cried out for change." Discuss with your classmates which students emerged as leaders to address the need for change. Review and critique the steps they engaged in to bring about change. See if your group can reach consensus about the adequacy of their leadership behaviors.

PRACTICING FOR NCLEX

1. A charge nurse in a busy hospital manages a skilled nursing unit using an autocratic style of leadership. Which leadership tasks best represent this style of leadership? Select all that apply.
   a. The charge nurse polls the other nurses for input on nursing protocols.
   b. The charge nurse dictates break schedules for the other nurses.
   c. The charge nurse schedules a mandatory in-service on new equipment.
   d. The charge nurse allows the other nurses to divide up nursing tasks.
   e. The charge nurse delegates nursing responsibilities to the staff.
   f. The charge nurse encourages the nurses to work independently.

2. A nurse who is newly hired to manage a busy pediatric office is encouraged to use a transactional leadership style when dealing with subordinates. Which activities best exemplify the use of this type of leadership? Select all that apply.
   a. The manager institutes a reward program for employees meeting goals and work deadlines.

b. The manager encourages the other nurses to participate in health care reform by joining nursing organizations.

c. The manager promotes compliance by reminding subordinates that they have a good salary and working conditions.

d. The manager makes sure all the employees are kept abreast of new developments in pediatric nursing.

e. The manager works with subordinates to accomplish all the nursing tasks and goals for the day.

f. The manager allows the other nurses to set their own schedules and perform nursing care as they see fit.

3. A nurse manager of a busy cardiac unit observes disagreements between the RNs and the LPNs related to schedules and nursing responsibilities. At a staff meeting, the manager compliments all the nurses on a job well done and points out that expected goals and outcomes for the month have been met. The nurse concludes the meeting without addressing the disagreements between the two groups of nurses. Which of the following conflict resolution strategies is being employed by this manager?
   a. Collaborating
   b. Competing
   c. Compromising
   d. Smoothing

4. A nurse manager in a long-term care facility threatens to fire subordinates who refuse to work overtime when needed. This manager is displaying what type of power?
   a. Expert power
   b. Referent power
   c. Coercive power
   d. Informational power

5. A nurse manager is attempting to update a physician's office from paper to electronic health records (EHR) by using the eight-step process for planned change. Place the following actions in the order in which they should be initiated:
   a. The nurse devises a plan to switch to electronic health records.
   b. The nurse records the time spent on written records vs. electronic health records.
   c. The nurse seeks approval from management for new computers
   d. The nurse analyzes all options for converting to electronic health records.
   e. The nurse installs new computers and provides an in-service for the staff.
   f. The nurse explores possible barriers to changing to electronic health records.
   g. The nurse follows up with the staff to check compliance with the new system.
   h. The nurse evaluates the effects of changing to electronic health records.

6. A nurse manager who is attempting to institute the SBAR process to communicate with physicians and transfer patient information to other nurses is meeting staff resistance to the change. Which action would be most effective in approaching this resistance?
   a. Containing the anxiety in a small group and moving forward with the initiative
   b. Explaining the change and listing the advantages to the individual and the organization

c. Reprimanding those who oppose the new initiative and praising those who willingly accept the change

d. Introducing the change quickly and involving the staff in the implementation of the change

7. A nurse is asked to act as a mentor to a new nurse. Which nursing action is related to this process?
   a. The nurse mentor accepts payment to introduce the new nurse to his or her responsibilities.
   b. The nurse mentor hires the new nurse and assigns duties related to the position.
   c. The nurse mentor makes it possible for the new nurse to participate in professional organizations.
   d. The nurse mentor advises and assists the new nurse to adjust to the work environment of a busy emergency department.

8. An RN on a surgical unit is behind schedule administering medications. Which of the RN's other tasks can be safely delegated to a UAP?
   a. The assessment of a patient who has just arrived on the unit
   b. Teaching a patient with newly diagnosed diabetes about foot care
   c. Documentation of a patient's I & O on the flow chart
   d. Helping a patient who has recently undergone surgery out of bed for the first time

9. A nurse is using time management techniques when planning activities for patients. Which nursing action reflects effective time management?
   a. The nurse asks patients what is their priority to accomplish each day.
   b. The nurse includes a "nice to do" for every "need to do" task on the list.
   c. The nurse "front loads" the schedule with "must do" priorities.
   d. The nurse avoids helping other nurses if scheduling does not permit it.

10. A new nurse manager at a small hospital is interested in achieving Magnet® status. Which action would best help the hospital to achieve this goal?
    a. Centralizing the decision-making process
    b. Promoting self-governance at the unit level
    c. Deterring professional autonomy to promote teamwork
    d. Promoting evidence-based practice over innovative nursing practice

ANSWERS WITH RATIONALES

1. *b, c, e.* Autocratic leadership involves the leader assuming control over the decisions and activities of the group, such as dictating schedules and work responsibilities, and scheduling mandatory in-services. Democratic leadership is characterized by a sense of equality among the leader and other participants, with decisions and activities being shared—polling the other nurses is an example. In laissez-faire leadership, the leader relinquishes power to the group and encourages independent activity by group members. Examples of laissez-faire leadership style are allowing the nurses to divide up the tasks and encouraging them to work independently.

2. *a, c.* Transactional leadership style is based on a task-and-reward orientation. Team members agree to a satisfactory salary and working conditions in exchange for commitment and compliance to their leader. Leaders using transformational leadership style encourage nurses to participate in health care reform. Keeping abreast of new developments in nursing care is a characteristic of quantum leadership. The group and leader work together to accomplish mutually set goals and outcomes with the democratic leadership style, and the laissez-faire style encourages independent activity by group members, such as setting their own schedules and work activities.

3. *d.* The manager who resolves conflict by smoothing compliments the other party and focuses on agreement rather than disagreement, thus reducing the emotion in the conflict. The original conflict is rarely resolved with this technique. Collaborating is a joint effort to resolve the conflict with a win–win solution. All parties set aside previously determined goals, determine a priority common goal, and accept mutual responsibility for achieving this goal. Competing results in a win for one party at the expense of the other group. Compromising occurs when both parties relinquish something of equal value.

4. *c.* Managers exerting coercive power use punishment to force someone to comply or do something that individual does not want to do. Leaders using expert power are able to influence and convince subordinates to trust them and work toward meeting goals. Referent power occurs when one person receives approval or personal acceptance from another person. Informational power uses information to persuade others or provides rational arguments for the acceptance of information.

5. *b, f, d, c, a, e, h, g.* Planned change involves the following steps: (1) recognize symptoms that indicate a change is needed and collect data, (2) identify a problem to be solved through change, (3) determine and analyze alternative solutions, (4) select a course of action from possible solutions, (5) plan for making the change, (6) implement the change, (7) evaluate the change, and (8) stabilize the change.

6. *b.* Change is ubiquitous, as is resistance to change. The manager should explain the proposed change to all affected, list the advantages of the proposed change for all parties, introduce the change gradually, and involve everyone affected by the change in the design and implementation of the process. The manager should not use the reward/punishment style to overcome resistance to change.

7. *d.* Mentorship is a relationship in which an experienced person (the mentor) advises and assists a less experienced person (protégé). This is an effective way of easing a new nurse into leadership responsibilities. The preceptor (experienced nurse) is selected (and generally paid) to introduce an employee to new responsibilities through teaching and guidance. The nurse mentor does not hire or schedule new nurses. Nurses do not need mentors to join professional organizations.

8. *c.* Nursing care that should never be delegated to a UAP includes the initial nursing assessment for a patient, patient teaching that requires an assessment, and any nursing intervention that requires professional nursing knowledge and judgment.

9. *a.* In order to manage time, the nurse should establish goals and priorities for each day and include the patient in prioritizing tasks, identify what needs to be accomplished each day, differentiating "need to do" from "nice to do" tasks, establish a time line and allocate priorities to hours in the workday to recognize any falling behind and correct the problem before the day is lost, and use teamwork appropriately to enhance the schedule.

10. *b.* Magnet hospitals use a decentralized decision-making process, self-governance at the unit level, and respect for and acknowledgment of professional autonomy. In magnet hospitals, 14 characteristics, the Forces of Magnetism, have been recognized that identify quality patient care, excellent nursing care, and innovations in professional nursing practice.

TAYLOR SUITE RESOURCES

Explore these additional resources to enhance learning for this chapter:

- NCLEX-Style Questions and other resources on thePoint, http://thePoint.lww.com/Taylor8e
- *Study Guide for Fundamentals of Nursing, 8th edition*
- Adaptive Learning | Powered by prepU, http://thepoint.lww.com/prepu

Bibliography

American Association of Colleges of Nursing (AACN). (2012). Leading initiatives: Frequently asked questions. Available at http://www.aacn.nche.edu/cnl/frequently-asked-questions

American Nurses Association (ANA). (2010). *Scope and Standards of Practice: Nursing* (2nd ed.). Silver Spring, MD: Author.

American Nurses Association (ANA). (2012a). American Nurses Association urges recognition and funding for nurses' essential role in patient care coordination. Available at http://www.nursingworld.org/MainMenu Categories/Policy-Advocacy/Positions-and-Resolutions/Issue-Briefs/Care-Coordination/Recognition-for-Nurses-Essential-Role-in-Patient-Care-Coordination.pdf

American Nurses Association (ANA). (2012b). Care coordination should be reimbursed. Available at http://news.nurse.com/article/20120612/NATIONAL02/106250001

American Nurses Association (ANA). (2012c). *Principles for Delegation by Registered Nurses to Unlicensed Assistive Personnel (UAP)*. Silver Springs, MD: Author.

American Nurses Association (ANA). (2013). Care coordination and the essential role of nurses. Available at http://www.nursingworld.org/care-coordination

American Nurses Credentialing Center (ANCC). (2013). *Magnet recognition program model*. Available at http://www.nursecredentialing.org/Magnet/ProgramOverview/New-Magnet-Model

American Organization of Nurse Executives (AONE). (2012). NMLP Learning Domain Framework. Available at http://www.aone.org/resources/leadership%20tools/NMLPframework.shtml

Bashaw, E. (2011). Fusing Magnet and just culture. *American Nurse Today, 6*(9), 42–45.

Bashaw, E., Rosenstein, A., & Lounsbury, K. (2012). Culture trifecta: Building the infrastructure for Magnet and just culture. *American Nurse Today, 7*(9), 36–41.

Bulmer, J. (2013). Leadership aspirations of registered nurses: Who wants to follow us? *Journal of Nursing Administration, 43*(3), 130–134.

Burke, W., & McLaughlin, D. (2013). Partnering for change. *American Journal of Nursing, 113*(2), 47–51.

Covey, S. (1999). *The seven habits of highly effective people*. London: Simon and Schuster.

Curtin, L. (2013). Quantum leadership: Upside down. *American Nurse Today, 8*(3), 56.

Daley, K. (2013). Helping nurses strengthen their delegation skills. *American Nurse Today, 8*(3), 18.

Douglass, L. M. (1995). *The effective nurse: Leader and manager* (5th ed.). St. Louis: Elsevier/Mosby–Year Book.

Drucker, P. (1999). Managing oneself. *Harvard Business Review*, March–April, 65–74.

Habel, M., & Sherman, R. (2012). Transformational leadership: A growing promise for nursing. *Nurse.com, 21*(15), 24–29.

Hawkins, J., & Shell, A. (2012). Magnet hospitals are attracted to the BSN but what's in it for nurses? *Nursing, 42*(3), 50–52.

Institute of Medicine (IOM). (2010). The future of nursing leading change, advancing health. Available at http://www.iom.edu/Reports/2010/The-Future-of-Nursing-Leading-Change-Advancing-Health/Report-Brief.aspx

Johansen, M. (2012). Keeping the peace: Conflict management strategies for nurse managers. *Nursing Management, 43*(2), 50–54.

Keasler, T. (2013). Nurse residency program empowers new grads. *The American Nurse, 45*(4), 13.

Kotter, J. (1996). *Leading change.* Boston: Harvard Business School Press.

Lewin, K. (1951). *Field theory in social science.* New York: Harper & Row.

Manion, J. (1995). Understanding the seven stages of change. *American Journal of Nursing, 95*(4), 41–43.

Marquis, B., & Huston, C. (2012). *Leadership roles and management functions in nursing* (7th ed.). Philadelphia: Wolters Kluwer Health/Lippincott Williams & Wilkins.

Matthews, J. (2012). Role of professional organizations in advocating for the nursing profession. Available at http://www.medscape.com/viewarticle/766817

Porter-O'Grady, T., & Malloch, K. (2003). *Quantum leadership: A textbook of new leadership.* Boston: Jones & Bartlett.

Sheets, M., Bonnah, B., Kareivis, J., Abraham, P., Sweeney, M., & Strauss, J. (2012). CNLs make a difference. *Nursing, 42*(8), 54–58.

Shepard, L. (2011). Creating a foundation for a just culture workplace. *Nursing, 41*(8), 46–48.

Sherman, R. (2012a). Evidence-based effective nursing leadership. *Nurse.Com, 21*(9), 50–55.

Sherman, R. (2012b). What followers want in their nurse leaders. *American Nurse Today, 7*(9), 62–64.

Sherwood, G., & Barnsteiner, J. (2012). *Quality and Safety in Nursing.* West Sussex, UK: Wiley-Blackwell.

Stachowiak, M., & Bugel, M. (2013). The clinical nurse leader and the case manager: Are both roles needed? *American Journal of Nursing, 113*(1), 59–63.

Stringer, H. (2012). Powerful nurses can create change. *Nurse.com, 21*(2), 16–17.

Trossman, S. (2012). Nurse leadership: Is it OK to delegate? *The American Nurse, 44*(6), 1, 6.

Actions Basic to Nursing Care

Unit VI focuses on the actions basic to practice—the nursing interventions planned, implemented, and evaluated to meet the health care needs of patients at any age, at any point along the health–illness continuum, and in all settings. The nursing interventions discussed in this unit are assessing vital signs, conducting a health history and physical assessment, maintaining safety, administering medications, and providing perioperative care.

Chapter 23 explains medical and surgical aseptic techniques necessary to prevent and control the spread of microorganisms. Chapter 24 describes assessing vital signs, and Chapter 25 discusses conducting a health history and physical assessment. Nursing assessment is both an art and a science. The art of performing a skill is integrated into the science of nursing so that variations from normal are identified and evaluated and necessary nursing interventions are implemented. The findings from assessments provide a database necessary to maintain or restore health and promote wellness.

Nurses are responsible for meeting basic human needs for physical safety and security. Chapter 26 discusses promoting environmental safety (including threats from bioterrorism), identifying risk factors for patients at any age, and implementing teaching and other nursing actions to prevent accidents. Chapter 27 discusses complementary and alternative therapies, an ever-increasing component of health care.

Chapters 28 and 29 focus on collaborative and independent nursing interventions used to accurately and safely administer medications and provide perioperative care. In most instances, the physician prescribes the medications and performs the surgery while the nurse orders and implements nursing interventions to promote patient safety and knowledge and to facilitate optimal function or recovery in both hospital and home settings. Although institutional procedures and protocols are often used in these situations, nursing interventions are individualized to the unique needs of each person requiring care.

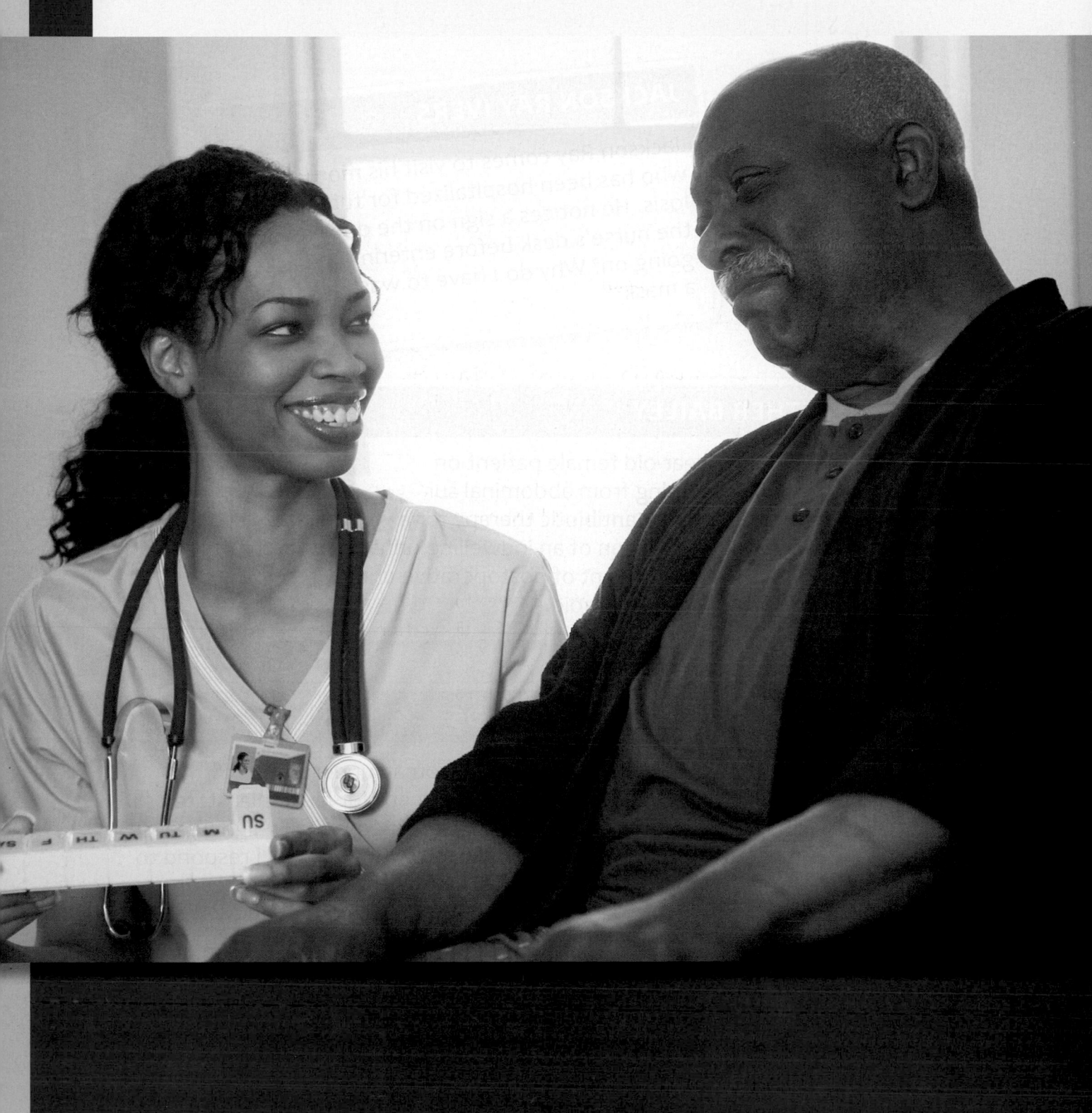

"*Our intent when we lay hands on the patient in bodily care is to comfort.*"

Lydia Hall (1906–1969) an innovator in nursing practice, she developed the theory that the direct nurse-to-patient relationship is itself therapeutic and that nursing care is the chief therapy for critically ill patients.

23

Asepsis and Infection Control

JACKSON RAY IVERS

Jackson Ray comes to visit his mother, who has been hospitalized for tuberculosis. He notices a sign on the door to check at the nurse's desk before entering. He asks, "What's going on? Why do I have to wash my hands and wear a mask?"

ESTHER BAILEY

Esther, a 72-year-old female patient on the unit recovering from abdominal surgery and receiving antibiotic therapy for a wound infection, requires insertion of an indwelling urinary catheter due to the development of postoperative urinary retention and an inability to void.

GISELLE TURHEIS

Giselle, a 38-year-old woman undergoing chemotherapy treatment for leukemia, states: "I know that my risk for infection is really high because of my poor immune status. But how do I respond to my Sunday school class, who are used to greeting me with a big hug? I want to be safe, but I know that I need these hugs too!"

LEARNING OBJECTIVES

After completing the chapter, you will be able to accomplish the following:

1. Explain the infection cycle.
2. List the stages of an infection.
3. Identify patients at risk for developing an infection.
4. Describe nursing interventions used to break the chain of infection.
5. Identify situations in which hand hygiene is indicated.
6. Identify multidrug-resistant organisms that are prevalent in hospitalized patients and community settings.
7. List nursing diagnoses for a patient who has or is at risk for infection.
8. Describe strategies for implementing CDC guidelines for standard and transmission-based precautions when caring for patients.
9. Implement recommended techniques for medical and surgical asepsis.

KEY TERMS

aerobic	health care–associated infection (HAI)	reservoir
anaerobic		standard precautions
antibody	host	
antigen	iatrogenic infection	sterilization
antimicrobial		surgical asepsis
asepsis	isolation	
bacteria	medical asepsis	transmission-based precautions
bundles	nosocomial	
colonization	parasites	vector
disinfection	pathogens	virulence
endemic	personal protective equipment (PPE)	virus
endogenous		
exogenous		
fungi		

A major concern for health practitioners is the danger of spreading microorganisms from person to person and from place to place. Microorganisms are naturally present in almost all environments. Some are beneficial; some are not. Some are harmless to most people, and others are harmful to many people. Still others are harmless except in certain circumstances.

Government agencies at the international, national, state, and local levels, health personnel, and laypeople recognize the need for an organized, systematic approach to the control of infections. For example, the Centers for Disease Prevention and Control (CDC) is the U.S. government agency responsible for investigating, preventing, and controlling disease. Efforts by these agencies and people include mass immunization programs, laws concerning safe sewage disposal, regulations for the control of communicable diseases, and hospital infection–surveillance programs. Medical science continues to grapple with problems caused by increasingly virulent organisms that have become drug resistant and problems related to patients who are immunologically compromised.

Prevention of infection is a major focus for nurses. The Quality and Safety Education for Nurses (QSEN) initiative has identified safety as one of the leading issues in health care. The focus on safety includes effective infection control practices. As primary caregivers, nurses are involved in identifying, preventing, controlling, and teaching the patient about infection (see the accompanying Reflective Practice box on page 532). Use of the nursing process can prove critical in breaking the cycle of infection.

INFECTION
Infection Cycle

An **infection** is a disease state that results from the presence of **pathogens** (disease-producing microorganisms) in or on the body. An infection occurs as a result of a cyclic process, consisting of six components, as shown in Figure 23-1 (on page 533). These components are:

- Infectious agent
- Reservoir
- Portal of exit
- Means of transmission
- Portals of entry
- Susceptible host

Infectious Agent

Some of the more prevalent agents that cause infection are bacteria, viruses, and fungi. **Bacteria**, the most significant and most commonly observed infection-causing agents in health care institutions, can be categorized in various ways. They are categorized by shape as spherical (cocci), rod shaped (bacilli), or corkscrew shaped (spirochetes). Bacteria can be categorized as either gram positive or gram negative, based on their reaction to the Gram stain. For example, gram-positive bacteria have a thick cell wall that resists decolorization (loss of color) and are stained violet. However, gram-negative bacteria have chemically more complex cell walls and can be decolorized by alcohol. Thus, gram-negative bacteria do not stain. This information is crucial for physicians when prescribing the most appropriate antibiotic therapy because antibiotics are classified as specifically effective against only gram-positive organisms or as broad spectrum and effective against several groups of microorganisms. Another distinguishing characteristic of (or way of categorizing) bacteria is their need for oxygen. Most

REFLECTIVE PRACTICE: CULTIVATING QSEN COMPETENCIES

CHALLENGE TO ETHICAL AND LEGAL SKILLS

This is my last clinical rotation before graduation and it has been a difficult year. My focus has been somewhat off for a while, and I haven't been as prepared as I should have been for my clinical and classroom experiences. My clinical instructor has been on my case for the last few weeks. I'm also realizing that in no time at all I will be out of school and on my own when it comes to patient care. So, all of a sudden, I'm eager for as many clinical experiences as I can get. To make a long story short, I'm thrilled when offered the opportunity to catheterize Esther Bailey, a 72-year-old female patient on my unit. I quickly review the procedure and go to the patient's room, with the catheterization supplies in hand, feeling semi-confident. After introducing my clinical instructor and myself and explaining what I'm about to do, I open the sterile package, prepare the sterile field,

and cleanse the meatus. In one quick moment, as the patient asks a question and diverts my instructor's gaze, I realize to my horror that I've contaminated the catheter. I've got a split second to decide what to do. I can tell my instructor what happened, obtain a new kit, and proceed anew, or pretend nothing happened and continue. I don't like that I'm even considering not admitting the mistake, after everything that has been drilled into us about the importance of sterility and the consequences of nosocomial infections. But I'm also prudent enough to realize that it is time to leave the unit because the rest of the group is waiting for postconference. Plus, after all, there are financial costs to ordering another tray. But what if I do not admit the error and by chance the instructor did see me contaminate the catheter? Then my goose is really cooked!

Thinking Outside the Box: Possible Courses of Action

- Obviously the simplest solution: admit my error and accept the consequences.
- Request a new catheter and inform my instructor later that the patient moved just as I was preparing to enter the meatus (a bit of deception but this makes the error not my fault).

- Alternatively, pretend that nothing happened and pray that no harm comes to the patient. (After all, how much bacteria do you need to contaminate a catheter?… and the patient is receiving antibiotic therapy anyway.)
- Continue and not even be bothered by the contamination. (Life is one big risk for everyone, right? All that matters is that you take care of #1.)

Evaluating a Good Outcome: How Do I Define Success?

- Patient benefited from my actions or, at the very least, was not harmed.
- No one's integrity is compromised or sacrificed.

- No violations of the standards of practice or the American Nurses Association's Code of Ethics occurred.

Personal Learning: Here's to the Future!

At least I can say there was a happy ending to this story. I did stop, explain what happened, and waited while someone ran for a new catheterization tray. Amazingly, my instructor told me later that she valued my maturity and honesty and ability to put the needs of the patient

ahead of my own needs, stating that I "might just have what it takes after all!" I'm not sure how often I'll be called upon to put the needs of a patient ahead of my own needs but hopefully I'll be ready to respond selflessly each time.

REFLECTION ON QUALITY AND SAFETY COMPETENCIES

How do you think you would respond in a similar situation? Why? Do you agree with the criteria that the nursing student used to evaluate a successful outcome? Why or why not? What *knowledge, skills,* and *attitudes* do you need to develop to continuously improve quality and safety when caring for patients like Mrs. Bailey?

Patient-Centered Care: What information regarding this procedure needs to be communicated to the patient? Does Mrs. Bailey understand why the Foley catheter is being inserted and the preferred target time for its removal?

Teamwork and Collaboration/Quality Improvement: What communication skills do you need to provide clear, comprehensive information to Mrs. Bailey? Did you explain

to Mrs. Bailey why there was a pause in the procedure? Was your request for the additional supplies clearly and respectfully communicated to a team member?

Safety/Evidence-Based Practice: Is there anything you could have done to anticipate the unexpected? How do you think your response affected the situation? What evidence in nursing literature provides guidance for decision-making regarding infection control?

Informatics: Can you identify the essential information that must be available in Mrs. Bailey's electronic record to support safe patient care? Is it important to electronically document daily the reasons why the Foley is still in place?

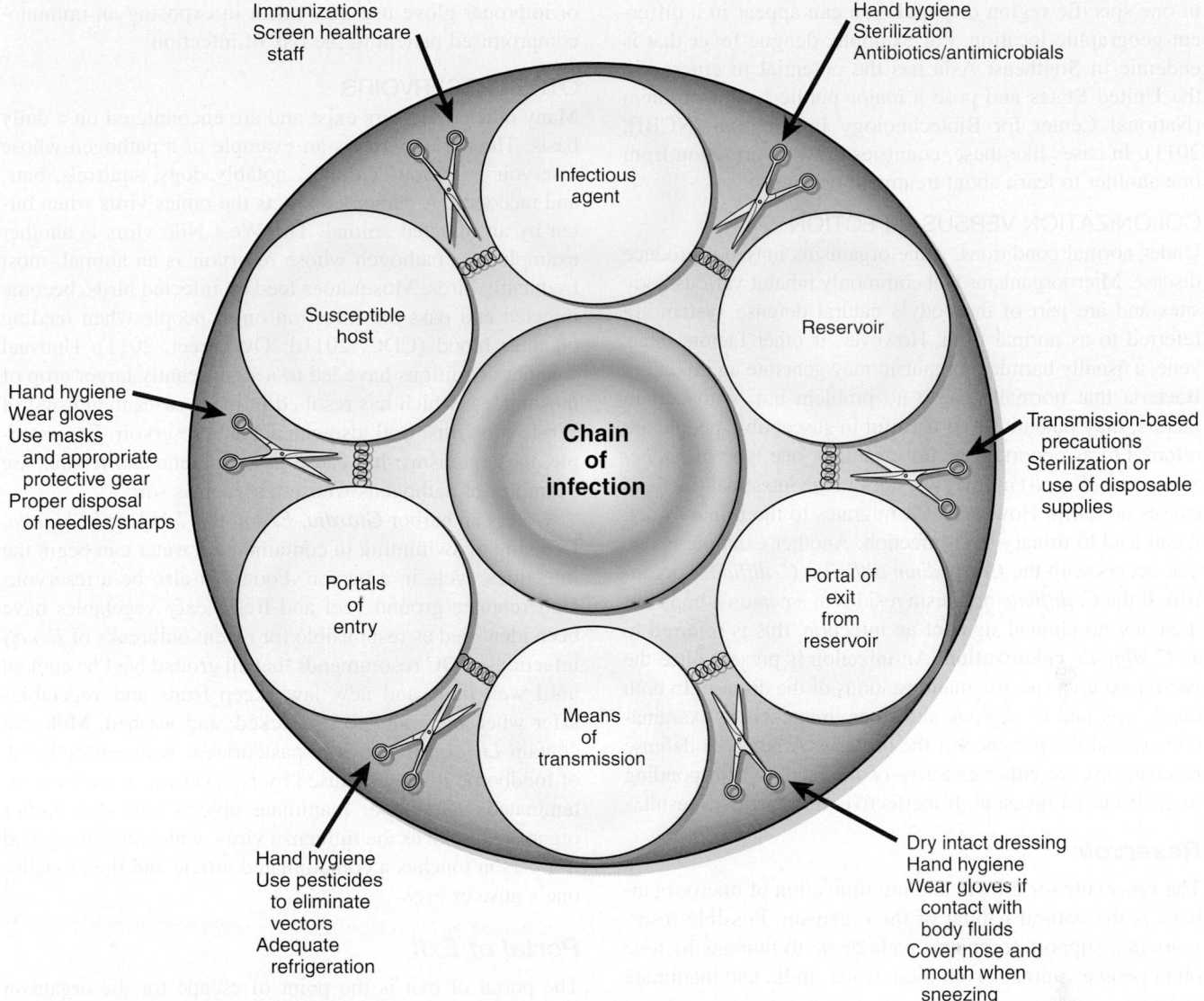

Immunizations
Screen healthcare staff

Hand hygiene
Sterilization
Antibiotics/antimicrobials

Infectious agent

Reservoir

Susceptible host

Chain of infection

Hand hygiene
Wear gloves
Use masks and appropriate protective gear
Proper disposal of needles/sharps

Transmission-based precautions
Sterilization or use of disposable supplies

Portals of entry

Portal of exit from reservoir

Means of transmission

Hand hygiene
Use pesticides to eliminate vectors
Adequate refrigeration

Dry intact dressing
Hand hygiene
Wear gloves if contact with body fluids
Cover nose and mouth when sneezing

FIGURE 23-1. The infection cycle is demonstrated as a chain. The goal is to break the links of the chain to end the cycle. (Adapted from Murphy, D. [1998]. Infectious microbes and disease: General principles. *Nursing Spectrum,* 7[2], 12–14.)

bacteria require oxygen to live and grow and are, therefore, referred to as **aerobic**. Those that can live without oxygen are **anaerobic** bacteria.

A **virus** is the smallest of all microorganisms, visible only with an electron microscope. Viruses cause many infections, including the common cold, hepatitis B and C, and acquired immunodeficiency syndrome (AIDS). Antibiotics have no effect on viruses. However, there are some antiviral medications available that are effective with some viral infections. When given in the prodromal stage of certain viruses, these medications can shorten the full stage of the illness.

Fungi, plant-like organisms (molds and yeasts) that also can cause infection, are present in the air, soil, and water. Some examples of infections caused by fungi include athlete's foot, ringworm, and yeast infections. These infections are treated with antifungal medications; however, many infections due to fungi are resistant to treatment. **Parasites** are organisms that live on or in a host and rely on it for nourish-

ment. Malaria is a serious disease that occurs when a parasite infects a certain type of mosquito that then feeds on humans.

Not all organisms to which a person is exposed cause disease. An organism's potential to produce disease in a person depends on a variety of factors, including:

- Number of organisms
- **Virulence** of the organism, or its ability to cause disease
- Competence of the person's immune system
- Length and intimacy of the contact between the person and the microorganism

IDENTIFICATION OF INFECTIOUS AGENTS

Identifying the type of infection and infectious agent is not always an easy process. Sometimes new diseases appear and health care workers race to identify them so that treatment can begin. This is the process that occurred with AIDS and with severe acute respiratory syndrome (SARS). Other times, a disease that is **endemic** or occurs with predictability in one specific region or population can appear in a different geographic location. For example, dengue fever that is endemic in Southeast Asia has the potential to emerge in the United States and pose a major public health problem (National Center for Biotechnology Information [NCBI], 2011). In cases like these, countries draw information from one another to learn about treatment options.

COLONIZATION VERSUS INFECTION

Under normal conditions, some organisms may not produce disease. Microorganisms that commonly inhabit various body sites and are part of the body's natural defense system are referred to as normal flora. However, if other factors intervene, a usually harmless organism may generate an infection. Bacteria that normally cause no problem but, with certain factors, may potentially be harmful in susceptible people are referred to as opportunists. For example, one type of *Escherichia coli* (*E. coli*) normally resides in the intestinal tract and causes no harm. However, if it migrates to the urinary tract, it can lead to urinary tract infection. Another example is one that occurs with the *Clostridium difficile* (*C. difficile*) organism. If the *C. difficile* organism resides in a person's body but there are no clinical signs of an infection, this is referred to as *C. difficile* **colonization**. An infection is present once the person exhibits specific manifestations of the disease. In both the *E. coli* and *C. difficile* situations, microscopic examinations reveal the presence of the bacteria. A person's defense mechanisms are either effective or ineffective in responding to the bacterial invasion. If ineffective, infection will result.

Reservoir

The **reservoir** for growth and multiplication of microorganisms is the natural habitat of the organism. Possible reservoirs that support organisms pathogenic to humans include other people, animals, soil, food, water, milk, and inanimate objects.

OTHER PEOPLE

Some people act as reservoirs for the infectious agent and demonstrate signs and symptoms of the disease, while other people act as reservoirs for the infectious agent but do not exhibit any manifestations of the disease. These people are considered carriers. Carriers, although asymptomatic, can transmit the disease. For example, a person who has tested positive for the human immunodeficiency virus (HIV) antibody is probably infected with HIV. However, this person may not exhibit any signs and symptoms of the disease at the time of testing. Moreover, the signs and symptoms of AIDS may not occur for years. However, the person may transmit the virus to others, for example, by intimate sexual contact or by sharing a contaminated needle and syringe. An infected pregnant woman may transmit the virus to her child during pregnancy, birth, or breastfeeding. Children in daycare centers can spread *E. coli* from one child to another child. Nurses can also serve as reservoirs and inadvertently transfer pathogenic organisms to patients. For example, a nurse with artificial nails may harbor a large number and variety of microbes under the nails. Ineffective handwashing or improper glove use may result in exposing an immunocompromised patient to the risk of infection.

OTHER RESERVOIRS

Many other reservoirs exist and are encountered on a daily basis. The rabies virus is an example of a pathogen whose reservoir is various animals, notably dogs, squirrels, bats, and raccoons. A person contracts the rabies virus when bitten by an infected animal. The West Nile virus is another example of a pathogen whose reservoir is an animal, most frequently birds. Mosquitoes feed on infected birds, become infected and pass the infection on to people when feeding on their blood (CDC, 2011d; Overstreet, 2011). Unusual weather conditions have led to a significantly larger crop of mosquitoes, which has resulted in more cases than usual of West Nile virus. Soil also can act as a reservoir. For example, the organisms that cause gas gangrene and tetanus are examples of pathogens whose reservoir is soil.

Water can harbor *Giardia, E. coli* 0157-H7, and *Shigella*. Drinking or swimming in contaminated water can begin the infectious cycle in a person. Food can also be a reservoir. Undercooked ground beef and fresh leafy vegetables have been identified as responsible for recent outbreaks of *E. coli* infections. CDC recommends that all ground beef be cooked until well done and new laws keep fruits and vegetables safer when they are grown, picked, and washed. Milk can contain *Listeria* unless it is pasteurized. A recent outbreak of foodborne illnesses caused by *Listeria* was traced to contaminated cantaloupe. Inanimate objects can also harbor organisms, such as the influenza virus, which may be spread if a person touches a contaminated article and then touches one's nose or eyes.

Portal of Exit

The portal of exit is the point of escape for the organism from the reservoir. The organism cannot extend its influence unless it moves away from its original reservoir. Usually, each type of microorganism has a primary exit route. In humans, common portals of exit or escape routes include the respiratory, gastrointestinal, and genitourinary tracts, as well as breaks in the skin. Blood and tissue can also be portals of exit for pathogens.

Means of Transmission

An organism may be transmitted from its reservoir by various means or routes. Some organisms can be transmitted by more than one route. Organisms can enter the body by way of the contact route, either directly or indirectly. Direct contact involves proximity between the susceptible host and an infected person or a carrier, such as through touching, kissing, or sexual intercourse. Health care workers have the potential to directly transmit organisms to susceptible people through touching. The indirect contact route involves personal contact with an inanimate object, such as touching a contaminated instrument. Recent research indicated that pathogenic bacteria were found on more than 60% of nurses' scrubs (Guolette, 2012). Proper hand hygiene and glove use can interrupt the transmission of dangerous bacteria from nurses to patients. Paper has also been identified as a surface where bacteria can survive; pathogens can possibly be transferred from a paper document to a health care worker's hands to the patient (Hubner, Hubner, Kramer, & Assadian, 2011).

 RECALL Esther Bailey, the woman described at the beginning of the chapter in the Reflective Practice box, who was catheterized. In this situation, the catheter becomes contaminated. Indirect contact occurs if this catheter is inserted, predisposing her to an infection. ●

Contaminated blood, food, water, or inanimate objects (fomites) are vehicles of transmission. **Vectors**, such as mosquitoes, ticks, and lice, are nonhuman carriers that transmit organisms from one host to another by injecting salivary fluid when a human bite occurs.

Microorganisms can also be spread through the airborne route when an infected host coughs, sneezes, or talks, or when the organism becomes attached to dust particles. Another means of transmission is through droplets. Droplet transmission is similar to airborne transmission. However, airborne particles are less than 5 mcm, and droplet particles are greater than 5 mcm. Table 23-1 summarizes the means of transmission for several organisms, their reservoirs, and examples of diseases they transmit.

Portal of Entry

The portal of entry is the point at which organisms enter a new host. The organism must find a portal of entry to a host or it may die. The entry route into the new host often is the same as the exit route from the prior reservoir. The urinary, respiratory, and gastrointestinal tracts and the skin are common portals of entry.

 Concept Mastery Alert

The respiratory, gastrointestinal, genitourinary tracks, and skin are common portals for organism entry and exit.

Susceptible Host

Microorganisms can continue to exist only in a source that is acceptable (a **host**) and only if they overcome any resistance mounted by the host's defenses. Susceptibility is the degree of resistance the potential host has to the pathogen. Hospital patients are often in a weakened state of health because of illness and have less resistance. Thus, they are more susceptible for infection. Many factors influence a host's susceptibility; these are discussed later in the chapter.

 REMEMBER Giselle Turheis, the woman with leukemia and a compromised immune status. Her susceptibility to infection is increased because of the lack of an adequate functioning immune system. ●

Stages of Infection

An understanding of the stages in the development of an infection is necessary to intervene and disrupt the infection cycle. An infection progresses through the following phases:

* Incubation period
* Prodromal stage

Table 23-1	ORGANISMS CAPABLE OF CAUSING DISEASE		
ORGANISM	**RESERVOIR**	**MEANS OF TRANSMISSION**	**DISEASE TRANSMITTED**
Staphylococcus aureus	Skin surface Mouth Nose Throat	Contact (direct)	Wound infection Abscess Carbuncle Boil
Hepatitis B virus	Blood Feces Body fluids and excretions	Contact (indirect)	Hepatitis B
Human immunodeficiency virus	Blood Semen Vaginal secretions Breast milk	Contact (direct) Contact (ingestion)	Acquired immunodeficiency syndrome
Mycobacterium tuberculosis	Sputum (respiratory tract)	Airborne	Tuberculosis
Borrelia burgdorferi	Ticks (sheep, cattle, deer, mice) Contact (direct)	Vectors	Lyme disease
Escherichia coli	Feces Undercooked meat (beef) Unpasteurized apple juice Tomatoes, peppers, spinach	Contact (ingestion)	*E. coli* infection
Salmonella	Intestinal tracts of humans and other animals, including birds	Contact (ingestion)	Diarrheal illness

- Full stage of illness
- Convalescent period

The course and severity of the infection, as well as the patient's response, influence the type and extent of nursing care provided.

Incubation Period

The incubation period is the interval between the pathogen's invasion of the body and the appearance of symptoms of infection. During this stage, the organisms are growing and multiplying. The length of incubation may vary. For example, the common cold has an incubation period of 1 to 2 days, whereas tetanus has an incubation period ranging from 2 to 21 days.

Prodromal Stage

A person is most infectious during the prodromal stage. Early signs and symptoms of disease are present, but these are often vague and nonspecific, ranging from fatigue and malaise to a low-grade fever. This period lasts from several hours to several days. During this phase, the patient often is unaware of being contagious. As a result, the infection spreads.

Full Stage of Illness

The presence of specific signs and symptoms indicates the full stage of illness. The type of infection determines the length of the illness and the severity of the manifestations. Symptoms that are limited or occur in only one body area are referred to as localized symptoms, whereas symptoms manifested throughout the entire body are referred to as systemic symptoms.

Convalescent Period

The convalescent period is the recovery period from the infection. Convalescence may vary according to the severity of the infection and the patient's general condition. The signs and symptoms disappear, and the person returns to a healthy state. However, depending on the type of infection, there may be a temporary or permanent change in the patient's previous health state even after the convalescent period.

A person may continually pass through the four phases with the same infectious process, such as with herpes simplex. Although there may have been only one infectious exposure, the infection may continue to cycle through the phases.

The Body's Defense Against Infection

One of the first lines of defense against infection is the body's normal flora. Flora helps to keep potentially harmful bacteria from invading the body. In addition to the normal flora that inhabit various body sites, other defense systems help a person combat infection. These include the inflammatory response and immune response.

Inflammatory Response

The inflammatory response is a protective mechanism that eliminates the invading pathogen and allows for tissue repair to occur. Inflammation helps the body to neutralize, control, or eliminate the offending agent and to prepare the site for repair (Smeltzer, Bare, Hinkle, & Cheever, 2010). In addition to infection, the inflammatory response also occurs in response to injury. It is either an acute or chronic process.

The cardinal signs of acute infection are redness, heat, swelling, pain, and loss of function, usually appearing at the site of the injury or inflammation. The vascular and cellular stages are the main components of the inflammatory process; these physiologic processes are responsible for the appearance of the cardinal signs. Initially, in the vascular stage, small blood vessels constrict in the area followed by vasodilatation of arterioles and venules that supply the area. This increase in blood flow results in redness and heat in the area. Histamine also is released, leading to an increased permeability of vessels, which allows protein-rich fluid to pour into the area. At this point, swelling, pain, and loss of function can occur.

During the cellular stage, white blood cells (leukocytes) move quickly into the area. Neutrophils, the primary phagocytes, engulf the organism and consume cell debris and foreign material. Exudate composed of fluid, cells, and inflammatory byproducts is released from the wound. The exudate may be clear (serous), contain red blood cells (sanguinous), or contain pus (purulent). The amount of exudate depends on the size and location of the wound. The damaged cells then are repaired by either regeneration (replacement with identical cells) or the formation of scar tissue (Porth, 2011). Refer to Chapters 31 and 41 for additional discussion of the inflammatory response.

Immune Response

Another defense system is the immune response. The immune response involves specific body responses to an invading foreign protein, such as bacteria, or in some cases, to the body's own proteins. The complex mechanisms that constitute the immune response occur as the body attempts to protect and defend itself. The foreign material is called an **antigen**, and the body commonly responds to the antigen by producing an **antibody**. This antigen–antibody reaction, also known as humoral immunity, is one component of the overall immune response. The other component that also helps the body defend against invaders is a cell-mediated defense, or cellular immunity. It involves an increase in the number of lymphocytes (white blood cells) that destroy or react with cells the body recognizes as harmful. Although these complicated chemical and mechanical responses are not completely understood, it is known that they help to defend the body specifically against bacterial, viral, and fungal infections, as well as malignant cells.

Factors Affecting the Risk for Infection

The susceptibility of the host depends on various factors:

- Integrity of skin and mucous membranes, which protect the body against microbial invasion

FOCUS ON THE OLDER ADULT

AGE-RELATED CHANGES PREDISPOSING TO INFECTION

Infection Risk	Age-Related Changes	Nursing Strategies
Pulmonary infections	• Decreased cough reflex • Decreased elastic recoil of lungs • Decreased activity of cilia • Abnormal swallowing reflexes	• Place patient in sitting position to eat and drink. • Encourage patient to drink plenty of fluids unless contraindicated. • Encourage patient to cough and deep breathe or use incentive spirometer as ordered. • Recommend pneumococcal vaccination once in a lifetime and influenza vaccination annually.
Urinary tract infections	• Incomplete emptying of bladder • Decreased sphincter control • Bladder-outlet obstruction due to enlarged prostate gland • Pelvic floor relaxation due estrogen depletion • Reduced renal blood flow	• Discuss with patient need to void at regular intervals. • Encourage patient to drink plenty of fluids unless contraindicated. • Administer medications for enlarged prostate (benign prostate hypertrophy) and estrogen depletion as ordered. • If patient wears absorbent product such as incontinence pad, instruct patient to change pad frequently and perform good "pericare." • Assess for UTIs (may be atypical in elderly patient). • Discuss the need for patient to void immediately after sexual intercourse.
Skin infections	• Loss of elasticity • Increased dryness • Thinning of epidermis • Slowing of cell replacement • Decreased vascular supply	• Encourage patient to drink plenty of fluids, unless contraindicated. • Help patient to perform good hygiene practices daily. • Apply lotion to skin as needed. • Assess frequently for any breaks in skin integrity, rashes, or changes in skin.

Note: Atypical clinical manifestations of infection in an older adult include confusion, disorientation, lethargy, anorexia, delayed fever response, falls, incontinence, and failure to thrive.

• pH levels of the gastrointestinal and genitourinary tracts, as well as the skin, which help to ward off microbial invasion
• Integrity and number of the body's white blood cells, which provide resistance to certain pathogens
• Age, sex, race, and hereditary, which influence susceptibility. Neonates and older adults appear to be more vulnerable to infection. (See the accompanying box, Focus on the Older Adult.)
• Immunizations, natural or acquired, which act to resist infection
• Level of fatigue, nutritional and general health status, the presence of preexisting illnesses, previous or current treatments, and certain medications, which play a part in the susceptibility of a potential host
• Stress level, which if increased, may adversely affect the body's normal defense mechanisms
• Use of invasive or indwelling medical devices, which provide exposure to and entry for more potential sources of disease-producing organisms, particularly in a patient whose defenses are already weakened by disease

 THINK back to Esther Bailey, the woman being catheterized who also has developed a postoperative wound infection. Undergoing abdominal surgery disrupts the integrity of the skin and mucous membranes, thereby increasing her risk for a wound infection. ●

Health habits that promote wellness can reduce potential risk factors, thus decreasing the susceptibility of a host. Sensible nutrition, adequate rest and exercise, stress-reduction techniques, and good personal hygiene habits can help maintain optimum bodily function and immune response. Unsafe sex practices and sharing intravenous (IV) needles are potentially dangerous, providing an opportunity for pathogens to enter a host and cause an infection.

THE NURSING PROCESS FOR INFECTION PREVENTION AND CONTROL

It is imperative that health care practitioners safeguard the people entrusted to their care by controlling diseases and preventing the spread of infection. Vigilant preventive care can limit exposure to potentially harmful infectious organisms and reduce the occurrence of infection.

Assessing

The nurse plays a critical role in preventing and controlling infection. This role begins with early detection

BOX 23-1 LABORATORY DATA INDICATING AN INFECTION

- Elevated white blood cell (leukocyte) count—normal value is 5,000 to 10,000/mm^3
- Increase in specific types of white blood cells (differential count or percentage of each cell type)

Neutrophils	Normal = 60%–70%	Increased in acute infections that produce pus; increased risk for acute bacterial infection if decreased; may also be increased in response to stress
Lymphocytes	Normal = 20%–40%	Increased in chronic bacterial and viral infections
Monocytes	Normal = 2%–8%	Increased in severe infections and function as a scavenger or phagocyte
Eosinophil	Normal = 1%–4%	May be increased in allergic reaction and parasitic infection
Basophil	Normal = 0.5%–1%	Usually unaffected by infections

- Elevated erythrocyte sedimentation rate—red blood cells settle more rapidly to the bottom of a tube of whole blood when an inflammation is present
- Presence of pathogen in urine, blood, sputum, or other draining cultures

and surveillance techniques. The extent of nursing interventions depends on the susceptibility of the host, the virulence of the organism, and the patient's signs and symptoms.

Inquire about the patient's immunization status and previous or recurring infections. Observe nonverbal cues and gather information about the history of the current disease. Nursing assessments include observing for signs and symptoms of a local or systemic infection. A localized infection can result in redness, swelling, warmth in the involved area, pain or tenderness, and loss of function of the affected part. Manifestations of a systemic infection include fever, often accompanied by an increase in pulse and respiratory rate, lethargy, anorexia, and tenderness and enlargement of lymph nodes that drain the area when an infection is present. Laboratory data can provide further insight into the presence of an infectious process. Any of the laboratory test results outlined in Box 23-1 may indicate the presence of an infection.

Compilation of this assessment data constitutes a unique nursing database that suggests nursing interventions for patients at risk for infection or those in whom an infection is already present.

Diagnosing

The potential for infection or the presence of an infection in a patient suggests possible nursing diagnoses. The focus of nursing care depends on a nursing diagnosis that accurately reflects the patient's condition. The following are examples of nursing diagnoses related to an infectious process:

- Risk for Infection related to presence of chronic disease; altered immune response; effects of medication; altered skin integrity; malnutrition; presence of invasive or indwelling medical device; lack of proper immunization
- Social Isolation related to presence of communicable disease (AIDS)
- Impaired Oral Mucous Membrane related to ineffective dental hygiene; trauma; side effect of medication; presence of invasive medical device

- Deficient Diversional Activity related to lack of visitors; restrictions imposed by airborne precautions
- Risk for Imbalanced Body Temperature related to infectious process; dehydration
- Anxiety related to high risk for infection; social isolation

See additional examples of nursing diagnoses with defining characteristics in the accompanying NANDA-I box.

Outcome Identification and Planning

The nurse develops appropriate patient outcomes after reviewing the assessment data, considering the cycle of events resulting in an infection, and incorporating the principles of infection control. Planning outcomes that prevent infection or interfere with the infection cycle is an exciting challenge, providing an opportunity to see the positive results from one's efforts, that is, effective nursing interventions aimed at controlling or preventing infection. The following examples of expected patient outcomes are appropriate for preventing infection and using infection control techniques. The patient will:

- Demonstrate effective hand hygiene and good personal hygiene practices
- Identify the signs of an infection
- Maintain adequate nutritional intake
- Demonstrate proper disposal of soiled articles
- Use appropriate cleansing and disinfecting techniques
- Demonstrate an awareness of the necessity of proper immunizations
- Demonstrate stress-reduction techniques
- Verbalize an understanding of health risks associated with a latex allergy

Implementing

The practice of **asepsis** includes all activities to prevent infection or break the chain of infection. The nurse uses aseptic techniques to halt the spread of microorganisms and minimize the threat of infection. There are two asepsis categories: medical asepsis and surgical asepsis. **Medical asepsis**, or clean technique, involves procedures

EXAMPLES OF NANDA-I NURSING DIAGNOSES

ASEPSIS AND INFECTION CONTROL

Nursing Diagnoses	Related Factors	Sample Defining Characteristics
Anxiety	Social isolation High risk for infection	"I'm afraid I won't see the nurses very much because they have to put on all this equipment whenever they come into my room." "You don't get many visitors when you're isolated like this. Everyone's afraid they'll get what I have." "In class, I sit next to the girl who was rushed to the hospital with meningitis. I'm so nervous that I'll get it, too. She's really sick!"
Activity Intolerance	Effects of infectious process Generalized weakness	"I knew I should have gotten the flu shot. I've been so sick with it and feel so weak that I can hardly get out of bed." Patient admitted with probable diagnosis of tuberculosis. Awaiting results of AFB smears. He is acutely ill, has extreme fatigue, productive cough, low-grade fever, and chills and sweats at night. Isolation is standard precaution with additional airborne precautions. Required assistance with all ADLs.

and practices that reduce the number and transfer of pathogens. Medical asepsis procedures include performing hand hygiene and wearing gloves. **Surgical asepsis**, or sterile technique, includes practices used to render and keep objects and areas free from microorganisms. Surgical asepsis procedures include inserting an indwelling urinary catheter or inserting an IV catheter.

Using Medical Asepsis

Medical asepsis techniques are used continuously both within and outside health agencies, based on the assumption that pathogens are likely to be present. For example, shared drinking cups are considered unsanitary because a person harboring pathogens may transfer them to the cup when used. In a health care facility, if a specific pathogen is known to be present, special methods of medical asepsis are used to prevent further spread of the organism. Nearly every nursing activity includes practices of medical asepsis. Therefore, the nurse assumes a major responsibility for breaking the cycle of infection by providing safe patient care and protecting the patient, as well as the nurse, from microorganisms that may cause disease. Box 23-2 highlights the basic practices of medical asepsis for nurses to use when giving care to patients.

Limiting the dissemination of pathogens will decrease the transfer of pathogens from person to person. The most practical way to accomplish this is through the use of barriers that prevent common vehicles from transmitting the pathogens. Barriers are ways to decrease the spread of pathogens and include hand hygiene, personal protective

BOX 23-2 PRACTICING BASIC PRINCIPLES OF MEDICAL ASEPSIS IN PATIENT CARE

- Practice good hand hygiene.
- Keep soiled items and equipment from touching the clothing. Carry soiled linens or other used articles so that they do not touch your clothing.
- Do not place soiled bed linen or any other items on the floor, which is grossly contaminated. It increases contamination of both surfaces.
- Avoid allowing patients to cough, sneeze, or breathe directly on others. Provide them with disposable tissues, and instruct them, as indicated, to cover their mouth and nose to prevent spread by airborne droplets.
- Move equipment away from you when brushing, dusting, or scrubbing articles. This helps prevent contaminated particles from settling on the hair, face, and clothing.
- Avoid raising dust. Use a specially treated cloth or a dampened cloth. Do not shake linens. Dust and lint particles constitute a vehicle by which organisms may be transported from one area to another.
- Clean the least soiled areas first and then the more soiled ones. This helps prevent having the cleaner areas soiled by the dirtier areas.

- Dispose of soiled or used items directly into appropriate containers. Wrap items that are moist from body discharge or drainage in waterproof containers, such as plastic bags, before discarding into the refuse holder so that handlers will not come in contact with them.
- Pour liquids that are to be discarded, such as bath water, mouth rinse, and the like, directly into the drain to avoid splattering in the sink and onto you.
- Sterilize items that are suspected of containing pathogens. After sterilization, they can be managed as clean items, if appropriate.
- Use practices of personal grooming that help prevent spreading microorganisms. Examples include shampooing the hair regularly, keeping it short or pinned up to limit the possibility of carrying microorganisms on hair shafts, keeping the fingernails short and free of broken cuticles and ragged nail edges, and avoiding wearing rings with grooves and stones that may harbor microorganisms.
- Follow guidelines conscientiously for standard and transmission-based precautions as prescribed by your agency.

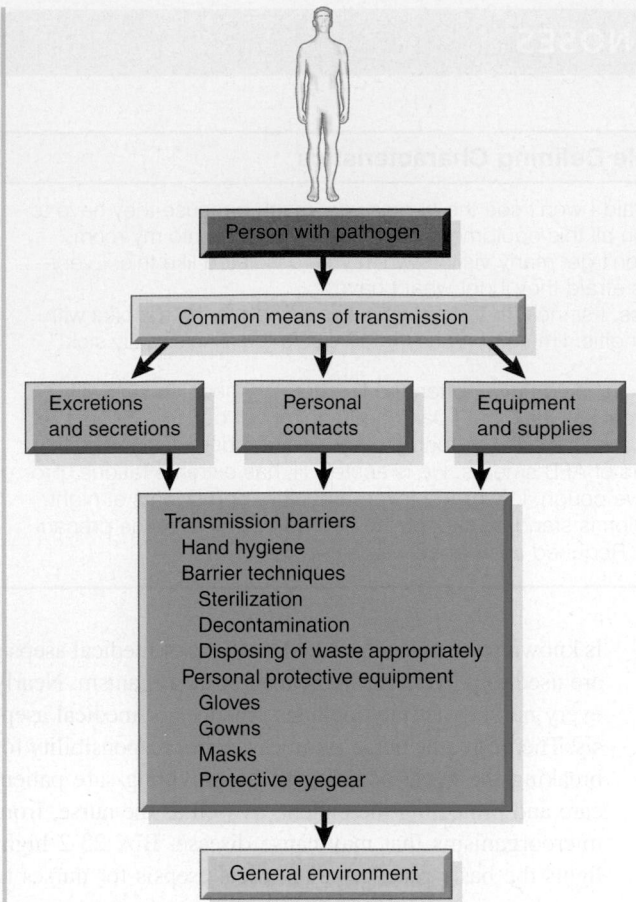

Person with pathogen

Common means of transmission

Excretions and secretions

Personal contacts

Equipment and supplies

Transmission barriers
Hand hygiene
Barrier techniques
Sterilization
Decontamination
Disposing of waste appropriately
Personal protective equipment
Gloves
Gowns
Masks
Protective eyegear

General environment

FIGURE 23-2. Transmission barriers help prevent the transporting of pathogens from the infected person to the general environment.

equipment (discussed later), and other barrier techniques. Figure 23-2 shows how barriers break the infection cycle. Nurses must understand the various precautions or barrier techniques if they are to use them correctly and minimize infection risks to patients as well as to themselves (see Promoting Health 23-1).

PERFORMING HAND HYGIENE

Hand hygiene is the most effective way to help prevent the spread of infectious agents. There is general consensus that most health care–associated pathogens are transmitted via the contaminated hands of health care workers. According to the CDC, each year approximately 2 million patients or nearly 1 in 20 people get a hospital-acquired infection (CDC, 2011a). The CDC issued the initial guidelines for hand hygiene in health care settings in 2002. The term *hand hygiene* applies to either handwashing with plain soap and water, use of antiseptic handrubs including waterless alcohol-based products, or surgical hand antisepsis. Although there is agreement that hand hygiene is the most important procedure for preventing infections, this procedure is still not performed consistently in health care

settings. Compliance rates are generally below 50% and less than 41% when gloves are used (Fuller et al., 2011). The Joint Commission Center for Transforming Healthcare (2012a) cites some of the factors that contribute to poor compliance with hand hygiene practices:

- Dispensers or sinks are placed in inappropriate locations.
- Hand hygiene compliance data is collected or reported inaccurately.
- There is a lack of accountability.
- There is a failure to stress the importance of hand hygiene for all staff.
- Education regarding hand hygiene is ineffective or insufficient.
- Hands are full with equipment or supplies.
- The belief may exist that hand hygiene is not required when gloves are worn.
- Inattentiveness or other factors can distract health care workers.

The World Health Organization (WHO) clearly defined the "Five Moments for Hand Hygiene." These include:

- Moment 1 – Before touching a patient
- Moment 2 – Before a clean or aseptic procedure
- Moment 3 – After a body fluid exposure risk
- Moment 4 – After touching a patient
- Moment 5 – After touching patient surroundings

Johnson, Kaehler, Siska, Lecy, and O'Neil (2011) express the need to focus attention on a cultural change generated by an institution-wide commitment to compliance with hand hygiene recommendations. The Joint Commission Center for Transforming Healthcare (2012b) has initiated a campaign inviting all Joint Commission accredited organizations to improve patient safety and lower the cost of health care. The Hand Hygiene Project takes advantage of their Targeted Solutions Tool™ (TST) that facilitates a "step-by-step process to accurately measure an organization's actual performance, identify their barriers to excellent performance, and direct them to proven solutions that are customized to address their particular barriers." The initial group of eight major health care organizations who participated in this project demonstrated significant gains in performance of hand hygiene. Compliance rates that initially were less than 50% have improved to 82%; this level has been maintained over an 8-month period.

The CDC also encourages consumers to help prevent infections by a personal commitment to practicing hand hygiene and a reminder to insist on hand hygiene measures from all health care staff involved in their care. (Refer to the accompanying Research in Nursing box for a discussion of hand hygiene in the community setting on page 542.)

Bacteria. Two types of bacterial flora are normally found on the hands: transient bacteria and resident bacteria (Table 23-2). Transient bacteria, although usually easily

PROMOTING HEALTH 23-1

INFECTION CONTROL PRECAUTIONS AND BARRIER TECHNIQUES

Use the assessment checklist to determine how well you are observing infection control or barrier precautions as you care for patients in a health care facility or in a community setting. Then develop a prescription for self-care by choosing appropriate behaviors from the list of suggestions.

Assessment Checklist

❑ almost always   ❑ sometimes   ❑ almost never

❑ ❑ ❑   1. Perform hand hygiene before and after contact with a patient.

❑ ❑ ❑   2. I wear PPE if contact with blood or body fluids is a possibility.

❑ ❑ ❑   3. I cover my nose and mouth when coughing and sneezing and properly dispose of tissues.

❑ ❑ ❑   4. I use additional protective equipment (gowns, masks, goggles, face shields) when necessary.

❑ ❑ ❑   5. I avoid recapping any needles.

❑ ❑ ❑   6. I place needles or other sharp objects in a puncture-proof disposable container.

❑ ❑ ❑   7. I dispose of used or contaminated objects and equipment in a leak-resistant plastic trash bag.

Self-Care Behaviors

1. Read infection control standards published by OSHA and CDC.
2. Attend programs that provide updates on current CDC/OSHA policies and survey literature regularly to determine best practices.
3. Maintain strict personal hygiene habits.
4. Obtain immunizations when available.
5. Assess for any signs and symptoms of an infection.
6. Perform hand hygiene frequently.
7. Perform hand hygiene immediately after removing gloves.
8. Practice cough etiquette to prevent transmission of respiratory infections.
9. Protect myself with the barriers necessary to prevent exposure to blood, body fluids, or secretions.
10. Follow agency policy if any exposure to blood or body substance occurs.
11. Never eat, drink, smoke, apply cosmetics or lip moistener, or handle contact lenses in an area where occupational exposure is possible.

removed by thorough handwashing, have the potential to adjust to the environment of the skin when they are present in large numbers over a long period and become resident bacteria. If pathogenic organisms become resident bacteria on the skin, the hands then become carriers of the particular organism. Therefore, to help prevent transient bacteria from becoming resident bacteria, it is important to clean the hands promptly when they are visibly soiled, after each contact with contaminated materials, and after removing gloves. (See the accompanying PICO in Practice box on page 543.) In addition, the CDC Guideline for Hand Hygiene in Health-Care Settings (2002) specifies

that health care personnel involved in patient care should not wear artificial nails because they are more likely to be associated with higher bacterial counts. In fact, wearing artificial nails in the operating room (OR) is a citable offense during The Joint Commission accreditation process. Natural nails should be less than one quarter (1/4) of an inch long.

Cleansing Agents. Various hand hygiene products are available. Soaps and detergents, also referred to as non-antimicrobial agents, are considered adequate for routine mechanical cleansing of the hands and removal of most

Table 23-2   BACTERIAL FLORA ON THE HANDS

TYPES OF BACTERIAL FLORA	CHARACTERISTICS	EFFECTIVE HAND HYGIENE MEASURES
Transient	• Occur on hands with activities of daily living • Relatively few in number on clean and exposed areas of the skin • Attached loosely on skin usually in grease, fats, and dirt • Found in greatest number under the fingernails • Can be pathogenic or nonpathogenic	Can be removed relatively easily by frequent and thorough handwashing.
Resident	• Normally found in creases in the skin • Usually stable in number and type • Cling tenaciously to skin by adhesion and absorption	Considerable friction with a brush is required to remove them. Less susceptible to antiseptics than are transient bacteria.

RESEARCH IN NURSING

BRIDGING THE GAP TO EVIDENCE-BASED PRACTICE

Hand Hygiene Practices of Nurses in A Community Environment

Hand hygiene is recognized as one of the most effective measures to prevent the spread of infection yet adherence on the part of health care workers is poor. Multiple studies have observed hand hygiene practices in health care facilities, but compliance with recommended hand hygiene practices has rarely been verified in a community setting. It is not uncommon for patients to be discharged to home requiring intravenous medication or care of nasogastric tubes, central lines, and catheters. These more complicated care routines coupled with an increase in community-acquired infections make hand hygiene safety in this setting a major challenge and concern. Little is also known regarding how aware home care nurses are of the WHO's "Five Moments for Hand Hygiene," which is considered a standard for hand hygiene. The WHO guidelines represent specific recommendations that should be implemented in any situation or setting where health care is provided.

Related Research

Felembam, O, St. John, W., & Shaban, R. Z. (2012). Hand hygiene practices of home visiting community nurses: perceptions, compliance, techniques, and contextual factors of practice using the World Health Organization's "five moments for hand hygiene." *Home Healthcare Nurse*, 30(3), 152–160.

The goal of this observational study included investigation of the current hand hygiene practices of community nurses related to contemporary WHO standards. Additional aims of this study involved exploration of the nurses' perceptions regarding hand hygiene practices and identification of contextual factors that influence hand hygiene in community settings. The two home care agencies involved in the study were located in Queensland, Australia. Direct observation methods were used to review current hand hygiene practices and to assess barriers that influenced compliance. Participants in this study also completed a brief questionnaire that included

demographic information and explored their perspective on hand hygiene. Eight nurses performed hand hygiene 61 of the 103 opportunities. They preferred soap and water 75% of the time rather than alcohol rubs even though both agencies supplied alcohol rubs to the nurses. Two tools were used for data collection. One was based on the WHO guidelines, while the other tool gathered information about physical surroundings and availability of equipment and hand hygiene facilities in patients' homes. Most participants practiced appropriate hand hygiene techniques the majority of time, but the most common violation of correct technique was failure to vigorously rub or lather hands with soap and water and alcohol rubs. Findings also indicated that 60% of the participants had not attended any recent continuing education on hand hygiene. The conclusion of this study was that this group of community health nurses did not consistently use best practices for hand hygiene.

Relevance to Nursing Practice

This study verified the need for community nurses to attend regular in-service offerings on best practices for hand hygiene and thus gain familiarity with contemporary standards. It also indicated the importance of nursing input into decisions that impact actual practice. In this study, the agencies provided alcohol rubs to all their nurses since this is considered the global standard for routine hand hygiene. These participants rarely used this method. Easy access is usually a positive indicator for improved hand hygiene technique. Nurses' preferences and convenience are factors that need to be considered if the use of alcohol rubs is promoted as standard practice. A strong commitment by health care agencies and nurses is an effective approach to increase knowledge and improve hand hygiene practices.

For additional research, visit thePoint.

---

transient microorganisms. They help remove soil because they lower surface tension and act as emulsifying agents. Bar, liquid, leaflet, and powdered soaps are all effective. Use of a particular type in a health care agency often depends on personnel or agency preference.

Using handwashing products that contain an **antimicrobial** or antibacterial ingredient is recommended in any setting where the risk for infection is high. When present in certain concentrations, these agents can kill bacteria or suppress their growth. Numerous studies have documented that alcohol-based handrubs, in most situations, more effectively reduce bacterial and viral counts on the hands of health care personnel than antimicrobial soap does (Institute for Healthcare Improvement [IHI], 2011). Alcohol-based handrubs have an alcohol concentration between 60% and 95% and are available as foam, gel, or lotions.

Techniques. If the health care worker's hands are not visibly soiled, alcohol-based handrubs are recommended because they save time, are more accessible and easy to use, and reduce bacterial count on the hands. The following are clinical situations when an alcohol-based handrub can be used to decontaminate hands:

- Before direct contact with patients
- After direct contact with patient's skin
- After contact with body fluids, mucous membranes, nonintact skin, and wound dressings, if hands are not visibly soiled
- After removing gloves
- Before inserting urinary catheters, peripheral vascular catheters, or invasive devices that do not require surgical placement
- Before donning sterile gloves prior to an invasive procedure (e.g., inserting a central intravascular catheter)

PICO IN PRACTICE

ASKING CLINICAL QUESTIONS

Scenario: You are a staff nurse newly hired to a general medicine unit. Your assigned preceptor calls in sick one day. Another seasoned nurse assigned to the unit, Donna, agrees to serve as your substitute preceptor for that shift. One of your assigned patients must have a nasogastric tube placed. You ask Donna to observe you perform this procedure; you do so without incident, following the hospital's nursing policies and procedures for inserting nasogastric tubes. You washed your hands and donned nonsterile gloves to prepare for the procedure, and Donna had done the same, anticipating that you might require some assistance. However, when you both take off your gloves, only you wash your hands. After you leave the patient's room, you ask Donna why she hadn't washed her hands when she removed her gloves. She shrugs at you, visibly annoyed, and retorts: "Well, my hands were clean when I put my gloves on and the gloves weren't dirty, so why should I?" You wonder whether or not this is appropriate hand hygiene policy to follow on your unit, and whether washing nonsoiled hands after removing gloves could reduce rates of hospital-associated infections. The next day, your preceptor Lisa returns to work. You have developed excellent rapport with Lisa, and discretely ask her about the appropriateness of Donna's actions. Lisa notes that the current hospital hand hygiene policy does not specify whether or not nonsoiled hands should be washed after gloves are removed. She tasks you with developing an evidence-based recommendation that you and she will then take to your unit-based council and nurse manager.

- POPULATION: Direct-care gloved nurses without soiled hands
- INTERVENTION: Handwashing after removal of gloves
- COMPARISON: Removal of gloves only without handwashing
- OUTCOME: Lower rates of hospital-associated infections on the unit

PICO Question: Among direct-care gloved nurses who have not soiled their hands, is handwashing after removal of gloves associated with lower rates of hospital-associated infections on the unit than removal of gloves without handwashing?

Finding: From the National Guidelines Clearinghouse:

Betsy Lehman Center for Patient Safety and Medical Error Reduction, JSI Research and Training Institute, Inc. (2008). Prevention and control of healthcare-associated infections in Massachusetts. Executive Summary: Part 1. Final recommendations of the Expert Panel. Boston, MA: Massachusetts Department of Public Health, pp. 36–41.

This expert panel strongly recommends that all health care providers that come in contact with patients wash their hands after gloves are removed.

Level of Evidence: Level I

Recommendation: You and Lisa propose to your nurse manager and your unit-based council that steps be taken to revise the existing hand hygiene policy so that nurses are advised to wash their hands after removal of gloves, regardless of whether or not their hands are soiled.

- If moving from a contaminated body site to a clean body site during patient care
- After contact with objects (including equipment) located in the patient's environment (IHI, 2011).

When used repeatedly, alcohol-based handrubs cause less dryness and skin irritation than soap products do. Those who have sensitive skin may benefit from use of an alcohol-based product that contains lotion. See Guidelines for Nursing Care 23-1 for directions on how to use an alcohol-based handrub.

 Concept Mastery Alert

Alcohol-based handrubs are a quick way to remove germs when hands are not visibly soiled.

Controversy does exist regarding the use of alcohol-based handrubs when *C. difficile* organisms have been identified. *C. difficile* is a gram-positive, anaerobic, spore-forming bacterium that is a common cause of diarrhea affecting children, adults, and older adults. The morbidity and mortality associated with *C. difficile* infections (CDI) has motivated health care providers to improve prevention strategies. Alcohol does not kill *C. difficile* spores. In fact, soap and water is considered more effective at removing *C. difficile* spores from the hands of health care providers when an outbreak of *C. difficile* occurs (Jabbar et al., 2010). Therefore, soap and water is the preferred hand hygiene method. However, additional information seems to confirm that glove use is the best preventative measure to control this infection

GUIDELINES FOR NURSING CARE 23-1

HAND HYGIENE: USING AN ALCOHOL-BASED HANDRUB

- Apply product to the palm of one hand, using the amount of product recommended on the package (it will vary according to the manufacturer but usually is 1 to 3 mL).

- Rub hands together, making sure to cover all surfaces of the hands, fingers, and in between the fingers. Also, clean the fingertips and the area beneath the fingernails.
- Continue rubbing until the hands are dry (at least 15 seconds).

(CDC, 2012c). *C. difficile* infection is discussed later in this chapter.

If a health care worker's hands are visibly soiled or contaminated with blood or body fluids, washing the hands with either antimicrobial soap or nonantimicrobial soap and water is required. Handwashing is also required before eating and after using the restroom. Effective handwashing requires at least a 20-second scrub with plain soap or disinfectant and warm water. Hands that are visibly soiled need a longer scrub. Recommended handwashing techniques for medical asepsis are listed in Skill 23-1 on pages 558–560.

Hand antisepsis before assisting with a surgical procedure involves a more lengthy scrub, reducing resident and transient flora from the forearms and hands. This procedure, known as surgical hand scrub, incorporates surgical asepsis and is described in texts that deal with operating and delivery room procedures. The CDC guideline recommends using an antimicrobial soap or alcohol-based surgical hand scrub product with persistent activity for surgical hand antisepsis. Scrub time is also reduced significantly when alcohol-based scrub agents are used.

Preventing Health Care–Associated Infections

For various reasons and sometimes despite best efforts, certain patients in health care agencies develop **health care–associated infections (HAIs)** during the course of treatment for other conditions that were not present in this patient on admission. The term **nosocomial** is used specifically to indicate something originating or taking place in a hospital. The source of infection may be either exogenous or endogenous. An infection is referred to as **exogenous** when the causative organism is acquired from other people. An **endogenous** infection occurs when the causative organism comes from microbial life harbored in the person. An infection is referred to as **iatrogenic** when it results from a treatment or diagnostic procedure. Not all nosocomial infections are iatrogenic.

Prevention of HAIs is a major challenge for health care providers. In the United States, HAIs account for tens of thousands of deaths and $28 billion to $33 billion dollars of additional health care costs annually (Agency for Healthcare Research and Quality [AHRQ], 2010). A patient who is hospitalized for a medical or surgical condition and acquires an HAI requires, on average, a 19-day longer hospital stay (Keefe, 2011). The cost of the additional hospital care days necessary to treat an HAI is staggering, particularly in light of the efforts to control spiraling health care expenses. With its focus on patient safety, The Joint Commission mandated that death or serious injury caused by an infection-related event must be reported as a sentinel event (see Chapter 26 for a discussion of sentinel events; Joint Commission, 2012). Effective October 1, 2008, the Centers for Medicare and Medicaid Services (CMS) no longer reimburses

hospitals for preventable hospital-acquired conditions in ten categories. Urinary tract infections from improper use of catheters, vascular catheter–associated infections, and certain surgical site infections are included in the list. In order to comply with this ruling, hospitals must report whether these conditions existed when the patients were admitted to their facility (CMS, 2012). Though this is an evolving process, there is potential that the critical impact that nurses have on decreasing the number of HAIs will be recognized and more easily verified.

Healthy People 2020 (2012) has included a "disproportionate nurse-to-patient ratio" as an issue that may have an impact on HAIs. Staffing takes into account registered nurse-to-patient ratios, level of RN education and experience, and the use of temporary workers. Failure to perform appropriate hand hygiene can occur when a nurse has a heavy patient load or when an inexperienced nurse is overwhelmed with her assignment.

Based on the premise that most HAIs are preventable, the U.S. Department of Health and Human Services (USDHHS), in conjunction with multiple other federal agencies, has formed a Steering Committee that is committed to coordinating strategies to reduce the transmission of HAIs. Nine targets have been identified and goals have been established for each target. Progress is measured annually, moving toward a 5-year completion date for the current action plan. Included in the targeted infections are four categories that are responsible for a majority of HAIs in the acute care hospital setting. These include:

• Urinary tract infections
• Surgical site infections
• Bloodstream infections
• Pneumonia (USDHHS, 2012b)

Coinciding with the imperative to address these infections, HHS has also implemented a national awards program to recognize sustained progress toward eliminating HAIs. The initial group of hospitals and health care agencies were honored for their efforts to reduce ventilator-associated pneumonia and bloodstream infections related to central intravenous lines in critical care areas (USDHHS, 2011).

Mandatory public reporting of HAI rates is required in a large number of states (Zastrow, 2011). Advocates of mandatory reporting believe that all agencies should report HAI rates. This public disclosure will allow consumers to make more informed choices regarding the selection of a health care facility based on an institution's efforts to prevent HAIs. However, a recent report confirmed that only 1% of adverse events, including HAIs, were actually reported to the various states. Researchers believe that this failure to report is likely due to staff ignorance of regulations and what they need to report rather than a cover-up effort. In the future, electronic records may serve as a surveillance system for tracking these events (USDHHS, 2012a).

USING INVASIVE MEDICAL DEVICES

Most HAIs are caused by bacteria, such as *E. coli, Staphylococcus aureus, Streptococcus faecalis, Pseudomonas aeruginosa,* and *Klebsiella* species. Many HAIs can be traced to an invasive device, such as a urinary catheter or venous access catheter. For example, catheter-associated urinary tract infections (CAUTIs) are the most common type of HAIs, accounting for more than 30% of HAIs in acute care hospitals (CMS, 2012). Infection control measures include adherence to recommended best practices, or **bundles**. Bundles are evidence-based best practices that have proven positive outcomes when implemented together to prevent infection (Dumont & Nesselrodt, 2012; Puliti, 2011). This has resulted in progress toward the 5-year 25% reduction of urinary tract infections according to the action plan goals monitored by the HHS Steering Committee (USDHHS, 2012c). The same reduction is on track for surgical site infections.

 CONSIDER Esther Bailey, the 72-year-old woman who has had abdominal surgery and developed a wound infection. The patient already has one infection. However, insertion of the catheter increases her risk for an additional infection, directly related to the use of the catheter. ●

Patients receiving mechanical ventilation are especially at risk for ventilator-associated pneumonia (VAP). This infection occurs when pathogens gain access to a patient's lungs via either an endotracheal tube or a tracheostomy tube. Central line–associated bloodstream infections (CLABSIs) have a high mortality rate and are very costly. There has been a significant reduction in the incidence of CLABSI because CDC central-line insertion guidelines require health care practitioners to perform proper hand hygiene beforehand, don sterile apparel, prepare the patient's skin with the recommended antiseptic, and allow the antiseptic to dry before insertion of the central line. The 5-year target goal for CLABSI is a 50% reduction in the number of cases; latest figures show a 33% reduction to date. Some ICUs report zero CLABSIs following these efforts (Dumont & Nesselrodt, 2012).

DEALING WITH MULTIDRUG-RESISTANT ORGANISMS

A significant and disturbing trend continues to be the development of microorganisms, primarily bacteria, resistant to one or more classes of antibiotics. The indiscriminate use of broad-spectrum antibiotics has allowed once-susceptible bacteria to develop defenses against antibiotics. As a result, resistant organisms, such as methicillin-resistant *Staphylococcus aureus* (MRSA), vancomycin-resistant *Staphylococcus aureus* (VRSA), and carbapenem-resistant Enterobacteriaceae (CRE) have emerged. According to the World Health Organization (WHO), a concerted effort is needed to limit the impact of drug-resistant bacteria (WHO, 2011).

MRSA. *Staphylococcus aureus* bacteria are normally found in the nasal mucous membranes, on the skin, and in the respiratory and gastrointestinal tracts. Approximately one-third of the people in the United States are colonized with "staph," meaning that the organism is present in these locations but the person does not have symptoms, and remains healthy and uninfected. They can, however, pass the organism on to others. In the 1960s, a strain of this bacteria emerged that was resistant to the broad-spectrum antibiotic (methicillin), normally the drug of choice used to treat these infections. The very powerful antibiotic, vancomycin, had to be used to treat the MRSA infections that primarily occurred in health care settings. In the late 1990s, a type of MRSA appeared in the wider community. Community-associated MRSA (CA-MRSA), a common cause of skin and soft-tissue infections in the United States, has been increasing rapidly (CDC, 2011b). Those most at risk are young children, older adults, and people in close physical proximity, including athletes and military personnel (Neville-Swensen & Clayton, 2011).

Treatment options for CA-MRSA include incision and drainage of abscesses in patients who are afebrile and healthy with mild, uncomplicated abscesses. Antimicrobial therapy may not be required. If incision and drainage are not effective and systemic or serious infection results, antimicrobial therapy may be necessary. Prior to antibiotic therapy, wound drainage should be sent for culture and sensitivity testing (Neville-Swensen & Clayton, 2011).

The health care–associated MRSA strain, on the other hand, has more serious implications. However, CDC research indicates that life-threatening MRSA infections in health care settings are declining. Patients who have surgery or other invasive procedures, have invasive devices, or are immunocompromised are at risk for developing a MRSA infection. It can be responsible for bloodstream infections, wound infections, ventilator-associated pneumonia, and multidrug resistance. Intravenous vancomycin is the drug of choice for health care–associated MRSA, but if the bacteria develop resistance to vancomycin, then the infection can be treated with a synthetic antibiotic, such as linezolid (Zyvox). In a health care setting, the main mode of transmission is through contact with the contaminated hands of health care personnel or contact with equipment (CDC, 2011c). Basic infection control practices are the key to the prevention and control of MRSA.

VISA, VRSA and VRE. Vancomycin intermediate-resistant *Staphylococcus aureus* (VISA) emerged in 2002 in the United States closely followed by vancomycin-resistant *Staphylococcus aureus* (VRSA) that was totally resistant to vancomycin. Once bacteria develop drug resistance, they progress from being sensitive to an antibiotic to an intermediate resistance followed by complete resistance to the antibiotic. Since October 2010, all cases of VISA and VRSA have been successfully treated with other drugs approved by the Food and Drug Administration agency. Patients at risk of developing VISA and

VRSA are those with a history of kidney disease or diabetes, a previous MRSA infection, presence of an invasive catheter, or recent exposure to vancomycin. Effective infection control measures are imperative to control the spread of VISA and VRSA; prudent use of vancomycin is an important preventive measure.

Vancomycin-resistant enterococci (VRE) are another serious pathogen in hospitals. Enterococci, a species of *Streptococcus* often found in normal intestinal and female genital tracts, can cause HAIs with a high mortality rate if the organism is vancomycin resistant. Originally treated with penicillin, ampicillin, and then gentamicin, the enterococci became resistant to each drug. Subsequently, physicians again prescribed vancomycin as the drug of choice. However, resistance has developed to this and VRE must be treated with antibiotics other than vancomycin. Risk factors for VRE include:

- Compromised immune systems
- Recent abdominal or chest surgery
- Presence of urinary or central IV catheter
- Prolonged antibiotic use, especially with vancomycin
- Lengthy hospital stay, especially in an ICU (Riley, 2012; CDC, 2010c).

VRE is spread via contact with the feces, urine, or blood of an infected or colonized person. Health care providers have the potential to spread VRE on their hands from one patient to another. Medical equipment and environmental surfaces can also harbor this organism. Appropriate hand hygiene and contact precautions can halt the spread of VRE. Careful assessment, intervention, and evaluation of high-risk patients and situations by nurses helps to minimize infection and reduce the unnecessary suffering imposed on patients.

CRE. Carbapenem-resistant Enterobacteriaceae (CRE) are very difficult to treat and represent a public health threat. This disease was first reported in 2001 in the United States and is associated with a 40% to 50% mortality rate. *Klebsiella* species and *Escherichia coli* are examples of Enterobacteriaceae normally found in the human intestine. These bacteria are carbapenem resistant (CDC, 2012d). Carbapenem antimicrobial drugs are broad-spectrum antimicrobials and the agents of choice for serious infections when an organism is resistant to other primary antibiotics (CDC, 2010b). Resistance to carbapenems leaves few other treatment options. These organisms are readily passed from patient to patient. People who have bladder or venous catheters in place, require ventilator assistance to breathe, those taking antibiotics for a lengthy period of time, or people who have frequent hospitalizations or long-term care facility stays are at risk for developing CRE (Kelly, 2011). The plan of care requires laboratory testing to detect resistance to carbapenems; decisions on treatment of infections with CRE are based on these results. The CDC recommends that the patient be placed on contact precautions. A focus on hand hygiene and education regarding prevention of CRE transmission are vital to prevent transmission of the deadly infection.

Acinetobacter baumannii. *Acinetobacter baumannii* is a gram-negative bacterium that is frequently isolated from war wounds. Soldiers who were injured in Iraq and Afghanistan acquired the organisms in emergency departments and ICUs of combat zone hospitals prior to their return home to the United States with *A. baumannii* infections. It has spread through health care facilities and continues to develop resistance to many antibiotic regimens. The extensive use of antibiotics in hospitals has facilitated drug resistance—*A. baumannii* is resistant to three of the four classes of antimicrobial agents and is very difficult to eradicate. The fear is that at some point there may not be another treatment option (Chettle, 2011). Patients who have compromised immune systems—such as older adults, those with invasive devices or open wounds, and chronically hospitalized people—are at greater risk. When people repeatedly transfer between hospital and long-term care facilities, they can introduce this organism into the hospital environment if infection control policies are not stringent. Because *A. baumannii* can also sustain itself in the environment, the patient's room and all mechanical equipment must be cleaned and disinfected. The infected person is placed on contact precautions and health care workers need to carefully follow all infection control guidelines (Patton, 2012; Delahanty & Myers, 2010).

Clostridium difficile. While rates of some HAIs have declined in recent years, *C. difficile* infection (CDI) rates and associated deaths have risen. It is considered responsible for about 14,000 deaths annually in the United States; this infection costs the health care system billions of dollars each year (CDC, 2012b). Health care experts are concerned that the number of deaths caused by *C. difficile* may actually be considerably higher since the CDC data is based on death certificates. Often, one of the complications of *C. difficile* may be listed as the cause of death and the infection is not listed. Those most at risk are older adults who are receiving medical care and taking antibiotics. Hospital-acquired CDI rates have also increased significantly in children, but the severity of those cases has remained constant. Both symptomatic and asymptomatic people serve as reservoirs for *C. difficile,* as do any surfaces or objects contaminated with feces. This organism normally resides in the intestinal tract. When antibiotics are prescribed or taken for a prolonged period of time, particularly broad-spectrum ones, helpful bacteria are destroyed and *C. difficile* bacteria can grow out of control, creating a bacterial imbalance. Watery diarrhea, fever, and mild abdominal cramping are some of the more common signs and symptoms (Snow, 2011). When antibiotics are discontinued, 20% of the cases of CDI resolve but 80% of those diagnosed with this infection require further antibiotic therapy. The CDC recommends the following to prevent CDI:

- Prescribe antibiotics cautiously.
- Use contact precautions for patients confirmed or suspected of having CDI. This includes a private room,

as well as use of gown and gloves when entering the room and during patient care.

- Use effective hand hygiene (discussed earlier in this chapter on pages 540–544).
- Have room and nondisposable equipment cleaned with bleach or other appropriate disinfectant.
- Upon transfer out of the facility, notify the new facility about the *C. difficile* infection (Splete, 2012).

The CDC emphasizes that following these guidelines can eradicate *C. difficile* infection. In England and some European countries, the government requires that all hospitals report cases of CDI. In addition, antibiotic use is carefully monitored. These measures have resulted in a 50% drop in CDI cases since 2008. A new requirement to report CDI was scheduled to take effect in 2013 in the United States.

STERILIZING AND DISINFECTING

Cleansing, disinfection, and sterilization help to break the cycle of infection and prevent disease. Several processes are used to destroy microorganisms. **Disinfection** destroys all pathogenic organisms except spores; **sterilization** destroys all microorganisms, including spores. Disinfection can be used when preparing the skin for a procedure or cleaning a piece of equipment that does not enter a sterile body part. Sterilization is usually performed on equipment that is entering a sterile portion of the body. Disinfection and sterilization of contaminated or infected objects and good hand hygiene diminish and often eliminate microorganisms as potential sources of infection.

Method Selection. Various factors influence the choice of sterilization and disinfection methods, including the following:

- Nature of organisms present: The CDC recommends that all supplies, linens, and equipment in a health care setting should be treated as if the patient were infectious. Some organisms are easily destroyed, whereas others can withstand certain common sterilization and disinfection methods.
- Number of organisms present: The more organisms present on an item, the longer it takes to destroy them.
- Type of equipment: Equipment with small lumens, crevices, or joints requires special care. Certain articles that may be damaged by various sterilization and disinfection methods require special handling.
- Intended use of equipment: The need for medical or surgical asepsis influences the preparation and cleaning of equipment. In the home, it may be safe to use equipment and supplies that are clean, but most health care agencies use sterilized articles for patient care.
- Available means for sterilization and disinfection: The choice of chemical or physical means of sterilization and disinfection depends on the nature and number of organisms, the type and intended use of the equipment, and the availability and practicality of the means. (Table 23-3 lists the types of methods for sterilization and disinfection.)
- Time: Time is a key factor when sterilizing or disinfecting articles. Failure to follow the recommended time periods is grossly negligent.

Table 23-3 METHODS OF STERILIZATION AND DISINFECTION

METHOD	DISCUSSION	CAUTION
Physical		
Steam	Higher temperature caused by higher pressure destroys organisms (e.g., autoclaving)	Most plastic and rubber devices are damaged by autoclaving.
Boiling water	Frequently used in the home—simple and inexpensive; boil item for at least 10 minutes	Spores and some viruses are not destroyed by boiling.
Dry heat	Alternative sterilization method for home Used for metal items. Heat oven to 350°F for 2 or more hours.	Insufficient to destroy all microorganisms. Not used in health care agencies.
Radiation	Used for pharmaceuticals, foods, plastics, and other heat-sensitive items	Object must be directly exposed to ultra-violet radiation on all surfaces. Poses risk to personnel.
Chemical		
Ethylene oxide gas	Destroys microorganisms and spores by interfering with metabolic processes in cells. Gas is released while items (oxygen and suction gauges, blood pressure equipment) are contained in autoclave.	Precautions necessary because gas is toxic to humans.
Chemical solutions	Generally used for instrument and equipment disinfection and for housekeeping disinfection. Chlorines are useful for disinfecting water and for housekeeping purposes. A solution of sodium hypochlorite (household bleach) in a 1:100 dilution effectively inactivates human immu-nodeficiency virus. Betadine and alcohol are also used as disinfectants.	Method does not destroy all spores and may cause corrosion on metal surfaces.

USING PERSONAL PROTECTIVE EQUIPMENT AND SUPPLIES

According to the 1992 Occupational Safety and Health Administration (OSHA) ruling, health care agencies must provide employees with the equipment and supplies necessary to minimize or prevent exposure to infectious material. This **personal protective equipment (PPE)** includes gloves, gowns, masks, and protective eye gear. Skill 23-2 on pages 561–564 illustrates the proper use of this equipment.

Gloves. Gloves, not a substitute for good hand hygiene, are worn only once and discarded appropriately according to agency policy. Then hands are thoroughly decontaminated with meticulous hand hygiene. When nursing care activities do not involve the possibility of soiling the hands with body fluids, gloves are not necessary. Activities such as turning a patient, feeding a patient, taking vital signs, and changing IV fluid bags do not require the use of gloves as long as the potential contact with body fluids is not present.

However, when there is a possibility of soiling the hands with body fluids, gloves must be worn. Each patient interaction requires a clean pair of gloves. Some care activities for an individual patient may necessitate changing gloves more than once. Gloves should always be changed prior to moving from a contaminated task to a clean one.

While wearing gloves, never leave the patient's room (unless transporting a contaminated item or a patient requiring transmission-based precautions), never write in the patient's chart, and never use the computer keyboard or telephone in the nurses' station. Also, health care workers should not touch their pagers or cell phones without performing good hand hygiene first.

Wearing gloves does not eliminate the need for proper hand hygiene. In reality, the warmth and moisture inside gloves create an ideal environment for bacteria to multiply, making it even more important to perform good hand hygiene before and after using gloves. Research also indicates that gloving does not guarantee complete protection from infectious organisms. Gloves provide a barrier but are not impenetrable. It has been shown that many times glove-barrier failure goes undetected by the health care worker. Double gloving (putting on two gloves on one hand) is recommended if the health care worker is involved in a procedure during which exposure to blood or body fluids is expected, such as in an OR setting.

Approximately 2% to 17% of health care workers and less than 1% of the general population are sensitized to traditional latex, with reactions ranging from local skin reactions to urticaria (hives) to systemic anaphylaxis, an exaggerated allergic reaction that can result in death (Behrman & Schraga, 2011; Altrich, 2012). The cornstarch powder or talc used to make gloves easier to put on is a major causative factor in any latex allergy. The powder binds with the latex protein and becomes airborne, where it can remain for 5 to 12 hours after health care workers don or remove gloves. Powder particles may be inhaled or absorbed into skin or mucous membranes or enter the bloodstream. Repeated exposures have been shown to lead to a latex sensitivity. If the person continues to be exposed to latex after a sensitivity has developed, the person may demonstrate signs of a latex allergy. At present, there is no cure for a latex allergy.

The National Institute for Occupational Safety and Health (NIOSH) recommends that nonlatex gloves or powder-free, low-allergen latex gloves (if latex gloves are used) be available for use. Research has indicated that using powder-free latex gloves resulted in a significant reduction in latex sensitivity and there was also a 25% reduction in latex sensitivity when latex gloves were replaced with nonlatex gloves (Kelly et al., 2011). Also, according to the OSHA Bloodborne Pathogens Standard, employers must provide alternative gloves if necessary. Because a totally "latex-free" environment is considered unattainable given the ubiquitous nature of latex, a "latex-safe" health care environment is essential for patients and health care providers with a latex allergy. All health care facilities are required to have a written policy that identifies how to deal with latex-sensitive employees and patients. Awareness of an allergy to latex is also important for safe home care. Nurses need to ask whether patients have experienced any unusual signs or symptoms when blowing up balloons, using latex condoms, or wearing rubber gloves for dishwashing or cleaning. Box 23-3 summarizes information on latex allergy for health care personnel and patients.

Gowns. Gowns are usually worn to prevent soiling of the health care worker's clothing by the patient's blood and body fluids. They provide barrier protection and are donned immediately before entering the patient's room. Individual gown technique is recommended. This technique involves wearing a gown only one time and then discarding it appropriately according to agency policy. A waterproof or impervious gown is used if there is an increased likelihood of contact with the patient's blood or body fluids. If a gown becomes heavily soiled or moistened with blood or body fluids when caring for a patient, remove it, perform thorough hand hygiene, and put on a clean gown. There is no single special technique for applying a gown used as a barrier, but recommended practices for removing a soiled gown are described in Skill 23-2 on page 561–564.

Masks. Masks help prevent the wearer from inhaling large-particle aerosols, which usually travel short distances (about 3 feet), and small-particle droplet nuclei, which can remain suspended in the air and travel longer distances. They also protect the patient from the respiratory secretions of the health care worker. Masks discourage the wearer from touching the eyes, nose, and mouth, thus limiting contact of organisms with mucous membranes.

Various mask practices are used. In some instances, all personnel and all the patient's visitors wear masks; in other situations, a patient requiring specific precautions wears the mask when transported outside his or her room

BOX 23-3 LATEX ALLERGY SUMMARY

Risk Factors

- Health care workers who wear latex gloves
- People with allergic tendencies
- People with food allergies, specifically banana, papaya, avocado, potatoes, kiwi fruit, chestnuts, and pineapples
- Latex-industry workers
- People with asthma, spina bifida, or a history of multiple surgical procedures or exposures to latex

Frequently Used Products That Contain Latex

- Gloves
- Blood pressure cuffs
- Electrode pads
- Stethoscopes
- IV tubing
- Foley catheters
- Tourniquets
- Syringes
- Surgical masks
- Baby bottle nipples and pacifiers

Types of Reactions

- *Irritant contact dermatitis:* most common reaction usually restricted to hands that have made contact with the latex; symptoms include dry, irritated skin associated with pruritus.
- *Allergic contact dermatitis or delayed hypersensitivity:* allergic contact dermatitis, displayed as dry, crusty bumps, erythema, pruritus, scaling vesicles, papular lesions at site of contact, including the palms; symptoms usually appear in 24–96 hours.
- *Latex allergy or immediate hypersensitivity:* systemic reactions usually happen within minutes of exposure; displayed as rhinitis, conjunctivitis, angioedema,

bronchospasm, shock, and/or systemic anaphylactic reactions; this is a life-threatening sensitivity that is rarely the first reaction to latex exposure.

Diagnosis

- RAST (radioallergosorbent test): blood test for IgE antibodies to latex
- Skin prick: small amount of serum derived from latex placed on small prick in skin

Treatment

- Prevention: avoidance of latex-containing products
- Localized reaction: treat with oral diphenhydramine, cool compresses, and hydrocortisone 1% cream
- Systemic reaction: possibly treated with epinephrine subcutaneously, systemic steroids, antihistamines, with transport to the emergency department
  - Remove all latex-containing articles from the room
  - Place three-way stopcocks in IV lines for medication administration; place tape over any injection ports on IV tubing

Patient Teaching (If Diagnosed with Latex Allergy)

- Avoid all latex-containing products and avoid inhaling powder used in latex gloves.
- Inform employer and other health professionals of latex allergy.
- Wear medical alert bracelet.
- Follow doctor's recommendations.
- Inform physician/nurse of allergy prior to any injections/immunizations; a latex-free vile stopper should be used.
- Ensure that physician is aware of allergy prior to any medical procedure or surgery.

Adapted from: *NIOSH Fast Facts—Home healthcare workers: How to prevent latex allergy.* (2012). Available at http://www.cdc.gov/niosh/docs/2012-119/pdfs/2012-119.pdf

---

to protect health care personnel and other patients from any exposure to pathogens.

A mask is worn only once and never lowered around the neck and then brought back over the mouth and nose for reuse. How long one can wear one mask while caring for one patient is the subject of debate. Regardless of the time worn, a mask must be changed before it becomes damp from the wearer's exhalations. (See Skill 23-2, pp. 561–564 for the recommended practice for applying and removing a mask.)

The serious increase in the number of multidrug-resistant tuberculosis cases prompted new guidelines to prevent the transmission of this disease. According to CDC guidelines, either a high-efficiency particulate air (HEPA) filter respirator or N95 respirator certified by NIOSH must be worn when entering the room of a patient with known or suspected tuberculosis, SARS, or influenza.

The respirators filter inspired air, whereas surgical masks filter only expired air. Caregivers have expressed difficulty wearing the HEPA-style respirator for extended periods of time, but the N95 respirator, which is designed to filter out particles as small as 1 mcm with 95% efficiency, fits more comfortably against the face (Fig. 23-3 on page 550). The elastic straps on these respirators pro-

vide more protection and a better fit than the ties on regular surgical masks.

 THINK back to Jackson Ray Ivers, the son coming to visit his mother who is hospitalized with tuberculosis. The nurse would incorporate knowledge of tuberculosis transmission and appropriate barriers to explain to Mr. Ivers about the need for wearing a mask, or, in this case, a respirator. ●

Protective Eyewear. Protective eyewear, such as goggles or a face shield, must be available whenever there is a risk of contaminating the mucous membranes of the eyes. For example, suctioning a tracheostomy or assisting with an invasive procedure that may result in splattering of blood or other body fluids requires protection for the caregiver. Plain glasses are unacceptable because side shields are required.

HANDLING AND DISPOSING OF SUPPLIES

Used equipment may be disposed of after use or, if reusable, bagged according to agency policy, sent to a central cleaning area, and sterilized or disinfected. Double bagging may be required if the single bag is not secure or is

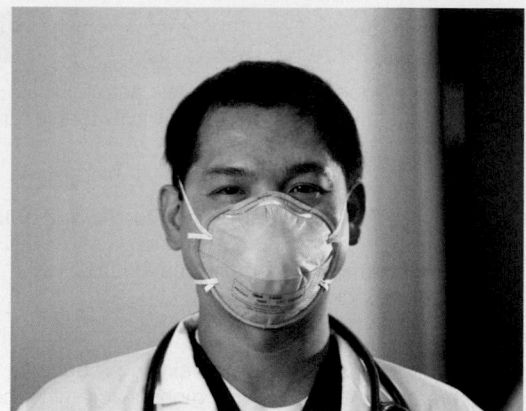

FIGURE 23-3. The Type N95 health care particulate respirator is NIOSH approved. It meets CDC guidelines for tuberculosis exposure control and is designed specifically for use in a health care setting. *(Courtesy of 3M Health Care.)*

soiled on the outside. A contaminated item must never be used for another patient.

Double bagging of trash and linen is usually needed only if the outside of the bag is visibly soiled. Some linen bags are water soluble and dissolve in hot water, making it unnecessary for workers to handle the contaminated linen. The use of paper trays and plastic eating utensils does not prevent transmission of organisms and is no longer recommended. The combined hot water and detergent used in commercial dishwashers sufficiently decontaminates dishes, glasses, and utensils. All spills of body fluids or substances must be immediately cleaned with the appropriate chemical germicide or disinfectant.

When collecting a specimen, take care to prevent the outside of the container from becoming contaminated with any secretions or body fluids. Place all laboratory specimens in plastic bags and seal the bags to prevent leakage during transportation. A bag marked "BIOHAZARDS" is used to dispose of trash that contains liquid or semiliquid blood or other potentially infective material (OPIM), trash contaminated with blood or OPIM that would release these substances if compressed, and trash that is caked with dried blood or OPIM and is capable of releasing these materials during handling.

USING STANDARD AND TRANSMISSION-BASED ISOLATION PRECAUTIONS

In addition to barriers, specific precautions have been established to prevent the transmission of infection. Historically, the term **isolation**, a protective procedure that limits the spread of infectious diseases among hospitalized patients, hospital personnel, and visitors, has been used. In 2007, the CDC updated its specific guidelines for transmission-based precautions, which are currently in use.

Current CDC Guidelines. The 2007 CDC guidelines update previous recommendations from the 1996 Guidelines for Isolation Precautions in Hospitals. These guidelines recognize that health care delivery occurs in other settings beside acute care hospitals. They reflect the emergence of new pathogens (e.g., SARS, *C. difficile,* MRSA), methods to prevent transmission of multidrug-resistant organisms, and the CDC's concern regarding biological terrorism. In these recent guidelines, the term "nosocomial infection" has been replaced with "health care–associated infection." Nurses must understand the various precautions or barrier techniques if they are to use them correctly and minimize infection risks to patients as well as to themselves (see Promoting Health 23-1: Infection Control Precautions and Barrier Techniques, p. 541).

The revised guidelines continue the designation of two tiers of precautions:

- **Standard precautions:** precautions used in the care of all hospitalized patients regardless of their diagnosis or possible infection status. These precautions apply to blood, all body fluids, secretions, and excretions except sweat (whether or not blood is present or visible), nonintact skin, and mucous membranes. Additions are respiratory hygiene/cough etiquette, safe injection practices, and directions to use a mask when performing high-risk prolonged procedures involving spinal canal punctures.
- **Transmission-based precautions:** precautions used in addition to standard precautions for patients in hospitals with suspected infection with pathogens that can be transmitted by airborne, droplet, or contact routes. The 2007 guidelines include a directive to don personal protective equipment (PPE) when entering the room of a patient on contact or droplet precautions. Previously, PPE was only required when the nurse was delivering care within 3 feet of the patient. These categories recognize that a disease may have multiple routes of transmission.

 RECALL Jackson Ray Ivers, the son of a patient with tuberculosis. Based on the nurse's knowledge of disease transmission, the nurse institutes airborne precautions for the patient and instructs Mr. Ivers in the need for proper hand hygiene and the use of a mask. ●

The three types of transmission-based precautions (airborne, droplet, or contact) may be used alone or in combination, but always in addition to standard precautions. Box 23-4 summarizes the current CDC guidelines along with a listing of specific recommendations for both tiers of precautions. Hospitals are encouraged to modify these recommendations as needed for implementation of their infection control strategy.

Controversy does exist concerning the use of contact precautions for prevention of transmission in a patient colonized with multidrug-resistant organisms. According to the Association for Professionals in Infection Control and Epidemiology (APIC), as many as 40% of states require active surveillance or testing for colonization of multidrug-resistant organisms in patients in certain settings (APIC, 2010). If these organisms are present, contact precautions are ordered. APIC does not support legislation providing for routine surveillance for colonization. The

BOX 23-4	SUMMARY OF CDC GUIDELINES FOR ISOLATION PRECAUTIONS IN HEALTH CARE SETTINGS 2007

Standard Precautions (Tier 1)

- Follow hand hygiene techniques.
- *Wear clean nonsterile gloves* when touching blood, body fluids, excretions or secretions, contaminated items, mucous membranes, and nonintact skin. Change gloves between tasks on the same patient as necessary and remove gloves promptly after use.
- *Wear personal protective equipment* such as mask, eye protection, face shield, or fluid-repellent gown during procedures and care activities that are likely to generate splashes or sprays of blood or body fluids. Use gown to protect skin and prevent soiling of clothing.
- *Follow respiratory hygiene/cough etiquette.* Any patients, family members, and visitors with undiagnosed, transmissible respiratory infections require education to cover their mouth and nose with a tissue when coughing and promptly dispose of the tissue. During periods of increased occurrence of respiratory infections, offer a surgical mask to coughing patients and other symptomatic people upon entry to the health care facility or office. Encourage the coughing patient to maintain more than a 3-foot separation from other people in the health care facility or office.
- *Avoid recapping used needles.* If you must recap, never use two hands. Use a needle-recapping device or the one-handed scoop technique. Place needles, sharps, and scalpels in appropriate puncture-resistant containers after use.
- *Use safe injection practices* including single-dose vials when possible; use disposable needles and syringes for each injection, and prevent contamination of injection equipment and medication.
- *Wear face mask* if placing a catheter or injecting material into the spinal or epidural space.
- *Handle used patient care equipment that is soiled with blood or identified body fluids, secretions, and excretions carefully* to prevent transfer of microorganisms. Clean and reprocess items appropriately if used for another patient.
- *Use adequate environmental controls* to ensure that routine care, cleaning, and disinfection procedures are followed.
- *Review room assignments carefully.* Place patients who may contaminate the environment in private rooms (such as an incontinent patient).

Transmission-Based Precautions (Tier 2)

The following precautions are recommended in addition to standard precautions:

Airborne Precautions

Use these for patients who have infections that spread through the air such as tuberculosis, varicella (chicken pox), rubeola (measles), and possibly SARS (severe acute respiratory syndrome).

- Place patient in a private room that has monitored negative air pressure in relation to surrounding areas, 6 to 12 air changes per hour, and appropriate discharge of air outside or monitored filtration if air is recirculated. Keep door closed and patient in room.
- Wear a mask or respirator when entering room of patient with known or suspected tuberculosis. If patient has known or suspected rubeola (measles) or varicella (chicken pox), respiratory protection should be worn unless the person entering room is immune to these diseases.
- Transport patient out of room only when necessary and place a surgical mask on the patient if possible.
- Consult CDC Guidelines for additional prevention strategies for tuberculosis.

Droplet Precautions

Use these for patients with an infection that is spread by large-particle droplets such as rubella, mumps, diphtheria, and the adenovirus infection in infants and young children.

- Use a private room, if available. Door may remain open.
- Wear PPE upon entry into the room for all interactions that may involve contact with the patient and potentially contaminated areas in the patient's environment.
- Transport patient out of room only when necessary and place a surgical mask on the patient if possible.
- Keep visitors 3 feet from the infected person.

Contact Precautions

Use these for patients who are infected or colonized by a multidrug-resistant organism (MDRO).

- Place the patient in a private room, if available.
- Wear PPE whenever you enter the room for all interactions that may involve contact with the patient and potentially contaminated areas in the patient's environment. Change gloves after having contact with infective material. Remove PPE before leaving the patient environment, and wash hands with an antimicrobial or waterless antiseptic agent.
- Limit movement of the patient out of the room.
- Avoid sharing patient-care equipment.

Adapted from Siegel, J. D., Rhinehart, E., Jackson, M., Chiarello, L., & the Healthcare Infection Control Practices Advisory Committee. (2007). 2007 Guideline for Isolation Precautions: Preventing Transmission of Infectious Agents in Healthcare Settings. Available at http://www.cdc.gov/hicpac/pdf/isolation/Isolation2007.pdf

CDC prefers that institutions make their decision based on available data and risk assessments rather than a mandate ordering them to do so. The CDC and other infection control agencies do support use of contact precautions in patients colonized with these organisms (Zastrow, 2011).

Due to the recent appearance of individuals in the United States who are positive for the Ebola virus, the CDC has issued revised guidelines for healthcare workers caring for these patients. The revised guidelines focus on repeated hands-on training with PPE before treating patients, avoidance of skin exposure when PPE is worn, and supervision by a trained monitor of the application and removal of PPE. The complete guideline is available at: http://www.cdc.gov/vhf/ebola/hcp/procedures-for-ppe.html.

PREVENTING OCCUPATIONAL EXPOSURES

OSHA, the Occupational Safety and Health Administration, developed the Bloodborne Pathogens Standard in 1991 to protect health care workers from exposure or risk of exposure to pathogens such as HIV and hepatitis B virus (HBV). This was revised in 2000 by the passage of The Needlestick Safety and Prevention Act that had more specifications for employers and more detail about how health care practitioners should participate in decisions and ensure safe practice regarding needlestick injuries and bloodborne exposures. The Needlestick Safety and Prevention Act requires health care providers to:

- Identify and provide safer medical devices that reduce or eliminate injuries from sharps
- Involve health care workers in the selection process of these safer devices
- Provide engineering controls for sharps disposal containers, self-sheathing needles, and other safety devices to reduce or eliminate sharps injuries
- Educate employees regarding how to safely use these devices
- Keep a sharps injury log (Delisio, 2012)

Since the law went into effect, there has been a significant decrease in sharps injuries in health care workers except for those staff who work in the operating room. Approximately 385,000 needlestick injuries occur every year in U.S. hospitals, but risks also exist in other settings (Delisio, 2012). Needlestick injuries are also a significant occupational hazard for health care workers visiting private homes (see Box 23-5). It is not always the nurse or original person using the device who sustains the injury. Other clinicians, housekeeping, or laundry staff could also come in contact with these devices and sustain an injury. Nurses suffer the largest proportion of these needlestick injuries when administering injections.

The most serious risk associated with needlestick injuries or mucous membrane exposure is the possible risk of infection with pathogens such as HBV, hepatitis C virus (HCV), and HIV. Health care facilities now purchase needles with built-in safety features and needleless, protected, or recessed IV systems. Although this equipment is more expensive, the higher costs may almost be totally offset due to fewer needlestick injuries. Knowledge of safety devices and prevention of bloodborne pathogen exposures creates a safer workplace environment and protects nurses from potentially life-threatening injuries.

REPORTING ACCIDENTAL EXPOSURES

Nurses are accountable for their own safety. Any needlestick injury or accidental exposure to blood or body fluids must be reported immediately so that appropriate interventions can be used. Underreporting of exposures is believed to be widespread, ranging anywhere from 29% to 98% (Delisio, 2012). Reasons for not reporting exposures include belief that the injury is insignificant, reporting it requires too much time, concern about negative consequences if the injury is reported, and belief that these types of injuries are to be expected. It is imperative that nurses and other health care workers report these injuries promptly so that they receive any appropriate postexposure treatment and prophylaxis. An agency's plan for this type of exposure typically includes the following:

- Washing the exposed area immediately with warm water and soap
- Reporting the incident to the appropriate person and completing an incident or injury report if required by the agency
- Informing the agency of the source (patient's name) and nature of the exposure
- Consenting to an initial baseline blood test, if agreeable, to determine personal HIV and HBV status, with repeat blood testing 6 weeks after exposure and at 3-month, 6-month, and 1-year intervals
- Consenting to postexposure prophylaxis, if recommended, at the appropriate time
- Awaiting blood test results of the involved patient (with the patient's consent) to determine HIV, HBV, and HCV status. State laws may vary concerning this practice
- Attending counseling session regarding safe practices to protect self and others

PROVIDING CARE IN SPECIAL SITUATIONS

Occasionally, nurses need to use neutropenic precautions for a patient whose immune system is compromised (e.g., recovering from transplantation surgery or receiving chemotherapy). Those who are immunosuppressed more

---

Box 23-5 | **PREVENTING NEEDLESTICK INJURIES TO HOME HEALTH CARE WORKERS**

Nurses working in private homes need to be aware of the factors that contribute to risks in these settings. They include:

- Avoid using needles whenever safe and effective alternatives are available.
- Avoid recapping or bending needles that might be contaminated.
- Bring standard-labeled, leak-proof, puncture-resistant sharps containers to the patients' homes and promptly dispose of used needles and sharps in this container.
- Plan for safe handling and disposal of needles before use.
- Keep sharps container out of the reach of children, pets, and anyone not needing access to it.

- Ensure that sharps container is secure to prevent spilling before transporting it.
- Follow standard precautions, infection prevention, and general hygiene practices consistently.
- Participate in your employer's bloodborne pathogens training program.
- Help your employer elect and evaluate safety devices and equipment.
- Use devices with safety features provided by your employer.
- Report any needlestick or other sharps injury immediately to your employer.

Adapted from: NIOSH Fast Facts—Home healthcare workers: How to prevent needlestick and sharps injuries. (2012). DHHS (NIOSH) Publication No. 2012-123. Available at http://www.cdc.gov/niosh/docs/2012-123/pdfs/2012-123.pdf

often than not become infected by organisms harbored in their own bodies, rather than by pathogens present in the environment or transmitted from other people. As with all patients, standard precautions are required, but some additional measures are helpful when a patient's ability to withstand any bacterial invasion is compromised.

Recommendations in this situation include the following:

- Ensure that caregiver is healthy.
- Restrict visits from friends and family members who have colds or contagious illnesses.
- Avoid collection of standing water in the room (e.g., with flowers or in humidifiers) to prevent bacteria typically found in this water.

The latest CDC isolation guidelines also address environmental controls that foster a "protective environment" to decrease the risk of infection in the most severely immunocompromised patients.

The increasing number of people who are ill or immunocompromised, coupled with increasingly virulent organisms, poses sterilization and disinfection concerns for home environments. Common measures that reduce the risk of infection at home include the following:

- Wash hands frequently—before preparing food, before eating, and after using the restroom.
- Keep immunizations up to date.
- Clean and disinfect kitchen surfaces, especially when preparing meat, chicken, and fish.
- Avoid sharing personal items.
- Cook food to the proper internal temperature.
- Promptly refrigerate or freeze perishables, prepared foods, and leftovers.

After thorough cleaning, some contaminated items may be disinfected by placing them in boiling water or using common household disinfectants such as bleach, isopropyl alcohol (70%), or acetic acid (white vinegar).

Controlling disease and preventing infections from spreading is a vital home care consideration for everyone.

Using Surgical Asepsis

Surgical asepsis techniques, used regularly in the operating room, labor and delivery areas, and certain diagnostic testing areas, are also used by the nurse at the patient's bedside. Procedures that involve the insertion of a urinary catheter, sterile dressing changes, or preparing an injectable medication are examples of surgical asepsis techniques. An object is considered sterile when all microorganisms, including pathogens and spores, have been destroyed. For example, the needle for an injection must be handled so that it is sterile when inserted into a patient. Sterile forceps or gloves are used to handle sterile dressings to protect against contamination. The basic principles of surgical asepsis are listed in Box 23-6.

When observing *medical asepsis,* areas are considered contaminated if they bear or are suspected of bearing pathogens; whereas when following *surgical asepsis,* areas are considered contaminated if they are touched by any object that is not also sterile. One of the most important aspects of surgical and medical asepsis is that the effectiveness of both depends on faithful and conscientious practice by those carrying them out. It is far better to err on the side of safety when using surgical asepsis than to take the slightest chance of possible contamination. Being a patient advocate requires vigilant aseptic technique and a willingness to speak up if the patient's safety has been compromised by improper procedures.

 THINK back to Esther Bailey, the woman described in the Reflective Practice box. The nurse acted appropriately by speaking up about the possible contamination of the catheter. Had this catheter been used, the patient's safety would have been compromised. •

BOX 23-6 PRACTICING BASIC PRINCIPLES OF SURGICAL ASEPSIS

- Allow only a sterile object to touch another sterile object. Unsterile touching sterile means contamination has occurred.
- Open sterile packages so that the first edge of the wrapper is directed away from the worker to avoid the possibility of a sterile surface touching unsterile clothing. The outside of the sterile package is considered contaminated. Opening a sterile package is shown and described in Skill 23-3.
- Avoid spilling any solution on a cloth or paper used as a field for a sterile setup. The moisture penetrates through the sterile cloth or paper and carries organisms by capillary action to contaminate the field. A wet field is considered contaminated if the surface immediately below it is not sterile.
- Hold sterile objects above the level of the waist. This will ensure keeping the object within sight and preventing accidental contamination.
- Avoid talking, coughing, sneezing, or reaching over a sterile field or object. This helps to prevent contamination

by droplets from the nose and the mouth or by particles dropping from the worker's arm.
- Never walk away from or turn your back on a sterile field. This prevents possible contamination while the field is out of the worker's view.
- Keep all items sterile that are brought into contact with broken skin, or used to penetrate the skin to inject substances into the body, or to enter normally sterile body cavities. These items include dressings used to cover wounds and incisions, needles for injection, and tubes (catheters) used to drain urine from the bladder.
- Use dry, sterile forceps when necessary. Forceps soaked in disinfectant are not considered sterile.
- Consider the edge (outer 1 inch) of a sterile field to be contaminated.
- Consider an object contaminated if you have any doubt as to its sterility.

Explaining the surgical asepsis procedure to patients facilitates their cooperation. Inform the patient about which objects and areas may not be touched, and direct the patient to avoid sudden movements that might contaminate the equipment. This helps the patient assist in maintaining the sterility of the procedure.

OPENING A STERILE PACKAGE AND PREPARING A STERILE FIELD

Commercially prepared sterile items may be sealed in paper or packaged in plastic containers. Sterile packages may be opened on a flat surface or while held in the hands. Skill 23-3 on pages 564–569 illustrates how to open a sterile package and prepare a sterile field. A sterile item should be covered if it is not used immediately. Reapply the cover by touching only the outside of the wrapper and reversing the opening order.

POURING STERILE SOLUTIONS

Care is necessary when pouring sterile liquids onto a sterile dressing or into a sterile basin. The outer surfaces of the bottle and cap are considered unsterile, whereas the inside areas and the solution are considered sterile. After a solution has been opened, the outer bottle should be labeled with date and time if it is to be reused. Most solutions are considered sterile for 24 hours after they are opened. When pouring from a bottle, grasp the bottle so that the label is in the palm of your hand. This action prevents any of the liquid from running over the label and making it illegible. Avoid splashing the liquid since this would contaminate the sterile field (see Skill 23-3, p. 564–569).

ADDING STERILE SUPPLIES TO A STERILE FIELD

After establishing a sterile field, it may be necessary to add items such as instruments or additional supplies to the sterile field. Item 6 in Skill 23-3 on page 567 demonstrates this technique. Once a sterile field is established, objects on a field may be handled only by using sterile forceps or with hands wearing sterile gloves.

PUTTING ON STERILE GLOVES

Sterile gloves are donned in a way that allows only the inside of the gloves to come in contact with the hands.

Skill 23-4 on pages 570–573 describes the proper technique for putting on sterile gloves.

After the gloves are on, only sterile items may be handled with the sterile-gloved hands. Careful removal of the gloves reduces any hand contact with contaminated materials. Good hand hygiene technique before and after putting on sterile gloves is imperative.

POSITIONING A STERILE DRAPE

The sterile drape, which ideally is waterproof, may be used to extend the sterile working area. Using sterile gloves allows the nurse to handle the entire drape surface. For protection when positioning, fold the upper edges of the drape over the sterile-gloved hands (Fig. 23-4). When sterile gloves are not worn, the nurse can touch only the outer 1 inch (2.5 cm) of the drape. Use caution when gently shaking the drape open so as not to touch one's clothing or an unsterile object. Hold the drape by the 1-inch upper edge and position the drape over the desired area. Do not reach over the drape because this would contaminate a sterile area.

Meeting Needs of Patients Requiring Infection Control Precautions

The psychological implications of infection control precautions are usually great, whether the patient is strictly separated from others or needs only to observe relatively simple precautions (see the accompanying box, Through the Eyes of a Student).

The current CDC standard precautions treat all people in a similar manner and greatly minimize the psychological trauma of feeling unclean and undesirable, which often occurred with earlier measures. However, sensory deprivation and loss of self-esteem may occur with transmission-based precautions. Friends and relatives, as well as health care personnel, may be inclined to spend less time with the patient because they are afraid that they will contract the disease or because of the inconvenience of coping with specific transmission precaution procedures. This may lead to inconsistent recording of vital signs, irregular documentation, and less patient monitoring on the part of caregivers. Research has also verified that patients placed in isolation because of the presence of a communicable disease may suffer unintended consequences such as an

FIGURE 23-4. Techniques of cuffing a sterile drape over gloved hands.

THROUGH THE EYES OF A STUDENT

She was the cutest little girl I have ever known. She was infected with HIV from birth. Her mother was an IV drug user and engaged in unprotected sex with multiple partners. This little girl, who came into the world with an innocent, fresh, new face full of unconditional love, could not walk, could not talk, could not chew, could not control her urine or bowel movements—but boy, could she smile! In the beginning, I was so terrified of contracting AIDS that I couldn't walk into her room without a mask, gown, gloves, protective eyewear, and basically a full protective body spacesuit. At the end, I wanted to take her into my home and give her all the love, support, and care she needed. I am not saying that I didn't wear gloves when I changed her diapers or when I flushed her heparin lock because I did… I was very careful. But I realized that she is a person, a person full of feelings, a person who needed me, and from whom I could learn. People with the AIDS virus are just that—people. We need to learn to treat them as such.

I also learned not to fear the person who is diagnosed with HIV infection or AIDS. I know that I will take the proper safety precautions with this person. The person I need to fear is the cute little old man who would never have AIDS because "he's not the type." If I don't use precautions, it is possible that one day I'll become infected through contact with someone who is "not the type." If that should ever happen, I hope everyone who cares for me will treat me as a real person and not be afraid.

—*Karmi N. Soder*
Georgetown University, Washington, DC

increase in incidents of depression, anxiety, fewer visits from health care staff, and an increase in the number of adverse events (Zastrow, 2011). Nursing measures to help prevent the sensory deprivation and loss of self-esteem associated with isolation precautions are discussed in Chapters 40 and 43.

Health teaching about transmission-based precautions can ease the fears of patients and family members. Both must understand the pertinent epidemiologic facts and how to carry out the specific precautions. It is helpful to emphasize the following:

- Precautions are temporary.
- The precautions and protective equipment worn by the staff protect the patient, the caregiver, and other patients.
- Proper hand hygiene before and after visiting the patient is the most effective measure to prevent spread of the disease.
- Continued explanations about procedures and continued updates on progress help to minimize anxiety.

Nurses must document their health teaching about barrier precautions in the patient's plan of care. A well-informed nurse who understands how to protect both self and patients and a well-informed patient who is cooperating in one's own care represent superior communicable disease precautions.

Raising Ethical Concerns About Infection Risks

Infection control and precautions minimize infection risks for patients as well as health care workers. However, the increasing numbers of people infected with HIV, HBV, and HCV have led to serious ethical concerns and controversy related to the risk for transmitting these diseases. At issue are the rights of the patient versus the rights of the health care worker and the health care agency. Refer to the accompanying box, Nursing Advocacy in Action, for an example of a situation in which the nurse must reconcile the patient's right to make choices versus the well-being of family members.

Questions such as the following are being debated:

- Should all hospital patients be routinely tested for HCV infection?
- Should HBV testing be mandatory for all foreign born residents of the United States?
- Should health care workers infected with HIV be permitted to perform exposure-prone invasive procedures?
- Should you address hand hygiene with another RN whom you have observed never washes her hands after removing gloves?
- Should pregnant health care providers be expected to care for patients with infectious diseases?

The CDC and various medical and nursing groups are seeking consensus on these issues, based on scientific information and valid statistical evidence. Although the CDC has issued guidelines related to these topics, not all states have adopted the guidelines. Additionally, some states have revised them. All agree, however, that health care workers who conscientiously adhere to appropriate infection-control precautions seriously reduce the risk for infection for patients and themselves.

Working With the Infection Preventionist

In the hospital, the nurse is responsible for educating patients and staff about effective infection control techniques and for collecting statistics about infections. Many hospitals rely on this specialized practitioner, referred to as the infection preventionist, to survey laboratory reports and review records for patients at risk, as well as suggest approaches to potentially dangerous situations. Other responsibilities include:

- Developing a plan to reduce the occurrence of HAIs
- Collaborating with state and local health departments regarding recommended or mandatory reporting of HAIs
- Developing a plan to respond to an act of bioterrorism
- Evaluating new products
- Providing routine consultations to staff and patients regarding infection control issues

NURSING ADVOCACY IN ACTION

Patient Scenario

Ms. Samol is a 38-year-old patient in the medical intensive care unit who is dying of AIDS-related complications. Since being diagnosed with AIDS, she has refused to inform her husband and family of her AIDS status. She even has an advance directive, which forbids the disclosure of her diagnosis when she can no longer advocate for herself. Her husband and mother cannot understand why the doctors and nurses cannot treat her "pneumonia"—the only diagnosis she gave them. The doctors and nurses caring for Ms. Samol believe that her husband has the right to know his wife's diagnosis so that he can make decisions in his own best interest about being tested, having their children tested, etc.

Implications for Nursing Advocacy

What would you do if you were Ms. Samol's nurse? Talk with your classmates and experienced nurses about the questions that follow.

- If you elect to advocate for the Samols, what practical steps can you take to ensure better health outcomes? Are there any legal guidelines for what you can and cannot do?
- What is reasonable to expect of a student nurse, a graduate nurse, and an experienced nurse in this situation?
- What advocacy skills are needed to effectively respond to this challenge?

Intensive investigative strategies create a positive environment that significantly reduces the incidence of HAIs in health care facilities. The infection preventionist knows the devastating effects of infection, and is intent on promoting a safe environment and fostering a systematic approach to infection control.

In the home, the infection preventionist's duties include surveillance for agency-associated infections, education, consultation, epidemiologic investigation, quality-improvement activities, and policy and procedure development. OSHA regulations state that home care agencies must have an infection control program and that OSHA infection control standards and policies must be available to all staff for reference.

Teaching About Infection Control

Teaching about medical asepsis and infection control is a challenging nursing responsibility. Patients need to be aware of techniques that prevent the spread of infection. Use of the nursing process in infection control protects both the patient and the nurse.

Medical asepsis techniques are appropriate for most procedures in the home, except for self-injection technique and venous catheter care, which require surgical asepsis. The patient frequently must make adjustments and improvise with the resources and supplies available for his or her use. In addition, the nurse emphasizes effective hand hygiene and other hygiene practices that interrupt the infection cycle. To satisfy OSHA requirements, many home care agencies have either a full-time or part-time infection preventionist.

Teach patients to use basic principles of asepsis at home and in public facilities. These involve the activities of daily living (see Chapter 30 for a discussion of personal hygiene). Following are examples of medical asepsis practices recommended in the home:

- Washing hands before preparing food and before eating
- Preparing foods at temperatures high enough to ensure that they are safe to eat (e.g., preparation of fresh meat)
- Washing hands, cutting boards, and utensils with hot, soapy water before and after handling raw poultry and meat

- Keeping foods refrigerated, especially those containing mayonnaise
- Washing raw fruits and vegetables before serving them
- Using pasteurized milk and fruit juices
- Washing hands after using the bathroom
- Using individual personal care items, such as washcloths, towels, and toothbrushes, rather than sharing

 THINK back to Giselle Turheis, the woman with leukemia and a compromised immune system. When teaching the patient about measures to prevent infection, the nurse would stress the use of proper practices in the home to reduce the patient's risk for infection. •

Teach patients about ways to prevent infection in public facilities, such as the following:

- Wash hands after using any public bathroom.
- Use paper towels or hot-air dryers in restrooms.
- Use individually wrapped drinking straws.
- Use tongs to lift food from common service trays in cafeterias, food stores, and salad bars.

The community reinforces medical asepsis practices in various ways, including the following:

- Using sterilized combs and brushes in barber and beauty shops
- Performing examination of food handlers for evidence of disease
- Encouraging food handlers to receive the hepatitis A vaccination
- Enforcing frequent handwashing by food handlers

Evaluating

Nurses as primary caregivers can intervene in and positively affect a patient's outcome. By assessing the person at risk, selecting appropriate nursing diagnoses, planning, and intervening to maintain a safe environment, the nurse can reduce a patient's potential for developing an infection (see the accompanying concept map for an example).

Esther Bailey, age 72, is 4 days postoperative abdominal surgery and has a wound infection. She is receiving continuous intravenous (IV) fluids of 5% dextrose and 0.45% normal saline with 20 mEq potassium chloride at 75 mL/hour and an IV antibiotic once a day. She has a nasogastric tube connected to suction. Upon assessment, you find bowel sounds are absent and the abdomen is slightly distended. The midline incision is draining small amount of tan purulent material and has a gauze dressing in place. During the dressing change, you note the skin edges are reddened and edematous. Wound cultures reveal heavy growth of *S. aureus*. Her temperature has been as high as 101°F in the past 24 hours. Lab work is significant for an elevated white blood cell count (WBC) . Esther has been using the incentive spirometer but has poor inspiratory effort due to incisional pain. You find her lung sounds are clear but diminished in the bases. Her urinary catheter was removed 8 hours ago. Since then, she has been unable to void, so the catheter is going to be reinserted.

Priority 1

Risk for Infection, actual and potential, related to documented wound infection and an increased risk of infection due to invasive therapy
Supporting Data:
- Abdominal incision reddened and edematous with tan purulent drainage
- Wound culture shows *S. aureus*
- Receiving IV antibiotics
- Temperature max 101°F
- Elevated WBC
- IV catheter and parenteral therapy
- Indwelling urinary catheter insertion

Priority 2

Ineffective Breathing Pattern related to postoperative incisional pain, increasing risk of atelectasis
Supporting Data:
- Poor effort with use of incentive spirometer
- Experiencing incisional pain
- Elevated WBC
- Temperature max 101°F
- Lung sounds clear but diminished in bases

Priority 3

Imbalanced Body Temperature related to an infectious process
Supporting Data:
- Temperature max 101°F
- Wound culture shows *S. aureus*
- Elevated WBC
- Abdominal incision reddened and edematous with tan purulent drainage

Outcome:
Patient will demonstrate signs of wound healing and no further signs of infection; WBC and temperature will return to normal.

Outcome:
Patient will perform coughing and deep breathing exercises; inspiratory effort will improve; and patient will remain free from a pulmonary infection.

Outcome:
Patient will maintain body temperature within normal limits.

Nursing Interventions:
- Assess temperature every 4 hours
- Monitor WBC count
- Administer antibiotics as prescribed
- Maintain aseptic technique with indwelling urinary catheter insertion and parenteral therapy
- Change abdominal dressing using sterile technique once a day and prn
- Dispose of soiled dressings appropriately
- Utilize proper handwashing technique
- Note appearance of incision
- Monitor characteristics of urine

Nursing Interventions:
- Encourage coughing and deep breathing exercises every 2 hours; assist to splint incision
- Assess pain level (scale of 0–10)
- Administer pain medication as prescribed
- Encourage use of incentive spirometer every hour as prescribed
- Auscultate lungs for presence of abnormal sounds
- Note characteristics of any sputum produced
- OOB to chair/reposition every 2 hours

Nursing Interventions:
- Assess temperature every 4 hours
- Administer antibiotics as prescribed
- Administer antipyretics as prescribed
- Remove excessive blankets when febrile
- If diaphoretic with fever, bathe and change linens as needed

Evaluation: Catheter was inserted using aseptic technique. Catheter draining clear yellow urine. Temperature returned to normal. WBC count remains elevated. No significant change noted in incision. Continue interventions.

Evaluation: Patient is performing coughing and deep breathing exercises effectively after adequate pain control. Occasional cough is nonproductive. Lungs are now clear with equal bilateral breath sounds. Continue interventions.

Evaluation: Esther's temperature has returned to normal. Continue to monitor.

- - - - - **Relationship**   ■ **Assessment**   ■ **Nursing Diagnosis**   ■ **Outcome Identification**   ■ **Interventions**   ■ **Evaluation**

Concept map displaying the nursing process for Esther Bailey.

Evaluation of the plan of care determines whether the person's need for safety is being met effectively. Ongoing systematic evaluation is crucial for nurses who strive to maintain a secure environment for their patients as well as themselves. If patient goals have been met and evaluative criteria have been satisfied, the patient will accomplish the following:

- Correctly use techniques of medical asepsis
- Identify health habits and lifestyle patterns that promote health
- State the signs and symptoms of an infection
- Identify unsafe situations in the home environment

 SKILL 23-1 PERFORMING HAND HYGIENE USING SOAP AND WATER (HANDWASHING)

DELEGATION CONSIDERATIONS

The application and use of hand hygiene is appropriate for all health care providers.

EQUIPMENT

- Antimicrobial or nonantimicrobial soap (if in bar form, soap must be placed on a soap rack)
- Paper towels
- Oil-free lotion (optional)

IMPLEMENTATION

ACTION	RATIONALE
1. Gather the necessary supplies. Stand in front of the sink. Do not allow your clothing to touch the sink during the washing procedure (Figure 1).	The sink is considered contaminated. Clothing may carry organisms from place to place.
2. Remove jewelry, if possible, and secure in a safe place. A plain wedding band may remain in place.	Removal of jewelry facilitates proper cleansing. Microorganisms may accumulate in settings of jewelry. If jewelry was worn during care, it should be left on during handwashing.
3. Turn on water and adjust force (Figure 2). Regulate the temperature until the water is warm.	Water splashed from the contaminated sink will contaminate clothing. Warm water is more comfortable and is less likely to open pores and remove oils from the skin. Organisms can lodge in roughened and broken areas of chapped skin.

FIGURE 1. Standing in front of sink.

FIGURE 2. Turning on the water at the sink.

ACTION	RATIONALE

ACTION

4. Wet the hands and wrist area. Keep hands lower than elbows to allow water to flow toward fingertips (Figure 3).

5. Use about 1 teaspoon liquid soap from dispenser or rinse bar of soap and lather thoroughly (Figure 4). Cover all areas of hands with the soap product. Rinse soap bar again and return to soap rack without touching the rack.

RATIONALE

Water should flow from the cleaner area toward the more contaminated area. Hands are more contaminated than forearms.

Rinsing the soap before and after use removes the lather, which may contain microorganisms.

FIGURE 3. Wetting hands to the wrist.

FIGURE 4. Lathering hands with soap and rubbing with firm circular motion.

6. With firm rubbing and circular motions, wash the palms and backs of the hands, each finger, the areas between the fingers (Figure 5), and the knuckles, wrists, and forearms. **Wash at least 1 inch above area of contamination.** If hands are not visibly soiled, wash to 1 inch above the wrists (Figure 6).

Friction caused by firm rubbing and circular motions helps to loosen dirt and organisms that can lodge between the fingers, in skin crevices of knuckles, on the palms and backs of the hands, and on the wrists and forearms. Cleaning less contaminated areas (forearms and wrists) after hands are clean prevents spreading microorganisms from the hands to the forearms and wrists.

FIGURE 5. Washing areas between fingers.

FIGURE 6. Washing to 1 inch above the wrist.

7. Continue this friction motion for at least 20 seconds.

Length of handwashing is determined by degree of contamination. Hands that are visibly soiled need a longer scrub.

(continued)

SKILL 23-1 PERFORMING HAND HYGIENE USING SOAP AND WATER (HANDWASHING) *continued*

ACTION	RATIONALE

8. Use fingernails of the opposite hand or a clean orangewood stick to clean under fingernails (Figure 7).

Area under nails has a high microorganism count, and organisms may remain under the nails, where they can grow and be spread to other persons.

9. Rinse thoroughly with water flowing toward fingertips (Figure 8).

Running water rinses microorganisms and dirt into the sink.

FIGURE 7. Using fingernails to clean under nails of opposite hand.

FIGURE 8. Rinsing hands under running water with water flowing toward fingertips.

10. Pat hands dry with a paper towel, beginning with the fingers and moving upward toward forearms, and discard it immediately. Use another clean towel to turn off the faucet. Discard towel immediately without touching other clean hand.

Patting the skin dry prevents chapping. Dry hands first because they are considered the cleanest and least contaminated area. Turning the faucet off with a clean paper towel protects the clean hands from contact with a soiled surface.

11. Use oil-free lotion on hands if desired.

Oil-free lotion helps to keep the skin soft and prevents chapping. It is best to apply after patient care is complete and from a small, personal container. Oil-based lotions should be avoided because they can cause deterioration of gloves.

DOCUMENTATION

The performance of handwashing is not generally documented.

SPECIAL CONSIDERATIONS

General Considerations

- An antimicrobial soap product is recommended with handwashing before participating in an invasive procedure and after exposure to blood or body fluids. The length of the scrub will vary based on need.
- Liquid or bar soap, granules, or leaflets are all acceptable forms of nonantimicrobial soap.

Home Care Considerations

- Home care providers should consider bringing their own liquid soap and disposable paper towels into the home for washing and drying their hands instead of using potentially contaminated bar soap and towels in the patient's home (Grossman & DeBartolomeo, 2008).
- Proper hand hygiene before leaving a home and immediately upon entering another home is imperative (Kenneley, 2010; McGoldrick & Rhinehart, 2007).

SKILL 23-2 | USING PERSONAL PROTECTIVE EQUIPMENT (PPE)

DELEGATION CONSIDERATIONS

The application and use of PPE is appropriate for all health care providers.

EQUIPMENT

- Gloves
- Mask (surgical or particulate respirator)
- Impervious gown

- Protective eyewear (does not include eyeglasses)

Note: Equipment for PPE may vary depending on facility policy.

IMPLEMENTATION

ACTION	RATIONALE
1. Check medical record and nursing plan of care for type of precautions and review precautions in infection control manual.	Mode of transmission of organism determines type of precautions required.
2. Plan nursing activities before entering patient's room.	Organization facilitates performance of task and adherence to precautions.
3. Perform hand hygiene.	Hand hygiene prevents the spread of microorganisms.
4. Provide instruction about precautions to patient, family members, and visitors.	Explanation encourages cooperation of patient and family, and reduces apprehension about precaution procedures.
5. Put on gown, mask, protective eyewear, and gloves based on the type of exposure anticipated and category of isolation precautions.	Use of PPE interrupts chain of infection and protects patient and nurse. Gown should protect entire uniform. Gloves protect hands and wrists from microorganisms. Masks protect nurse or patient from droplet nuclei and large-particle aerosols. Eyewear protects mucous membranes in the eye from splashes.
a. Put on the gown, with the opening in the back. Tie gown securely at neck and waist (Figure 1).	Gown should fully cover the torso from the neck to knees, arms to the end of wrists, and wrap around the back.
b. Put on the mask or respirator over your nose, mouth, and chin (Figure 2). Secure ties or elastic bands at the middle of the head and neck. If respirator is used, perform a fit check. Inhale; the respirator should collapse. Exhale; air should not leak out.	Masks protect nurse or patient from droplet nuclei and large-particle aerosols. A mask must fit securely to provide protection.

FIGURE 1. Tying gown at neck and waist.

FIGURE 2. Applying mask over nose, mouth, and chin.

(continued)

SKILL 23-2 USING PERSONAL PROTECTIVE EQUIPMENT (PPE) *continued*

ACTION

c. Put on goggles (Figure 3). Place over eyes and adjust to fit. Alternately, a face shield could be used to take the place of the mask and goggles (Figure 4).

d. Put on clean disposable gloves. Extend gloves to cover the cuffs of the gown (Figure 5).

RATIONALE

Eyewear protects mucous membranes in the eye from splashes. Must fit securely to provide protection.

Gloves protect hands and wrists from microorganisms.

FIGURE 3. Putting on goggles.

FIGURE 4. Putting on face shield.

FIGURE 5. Putting on gloves, ensuring gloves cover gown cuffs.

6. Identify the patient. Explain the procedure to the patient. Continue with patient care as appropriate.

Patient identification validates the correct patient and correct procedure. Discussion and explanation help allay anxiety and prepare the patient for what to expect.

Remove PPE

7. Remove PPE: Except for respirator, remove PPE at the doorway or in an anteroom. **Remove respirator after leaving the patient's room and closing the door.**

a. If impervious gown has been tied in front of the body at the waistline, untie waist strings before removing gloves.

Proper removal prevents contact with and the spread of microorganisms. Removing respirator outside of the patient's room prevents contact with airborne microorganisms.

Outside front of equipment is considered contaminated. The inside, outside back, ties on head and back, are considered clean, which are areas of PPE that are not likely to have been in contact with infectious organisms. Front of gown, including waist strings, are contaminated. If tied in front of body, the ties must be untied before removing gloves.

ACTION

b. Grasp the outside of one glove with the opposite gloved hand and peel off, turning the glove inside out as you pull it off (Figure 6). Hold the removed glove in the remaining gloved hand.

c. Slide fingers of ungloved hand under the remaining glove at the wrist, **taking care not to touch the outer surface of the glove** (Figure 7).

d. Peel off the glove over the first glove, containing the one glove inside the other (Figure 8). Discard in appropriate container.

e. To remove the goggles or face shield: Handle by the head-band or earpieces (Figure 9). Lift away from the face. Place in designated receptacle for reprocessing or in an appropriate waste container.

RATIONALE

Outside of gloves are contaminated.

Ungloved hand is clean and should not touch contaminated areas.

Proper disposal prevents transmission of microorganisms.

Outside of goggles or face shield is contaminated; **Do not touch.** Handling by headband or earpieces and lifting away from face prevents transmission of microorganisms. Proper disposal prevents transmission of microorganisms.

FIGURE 6. Grasping the outside of one glove and peeling off.

FIGURE 7. Sliding fingers of ungloved hand under the remaining glove at the wrist.

FIGURE 8. Pulling glove off the hand and over the other glove.

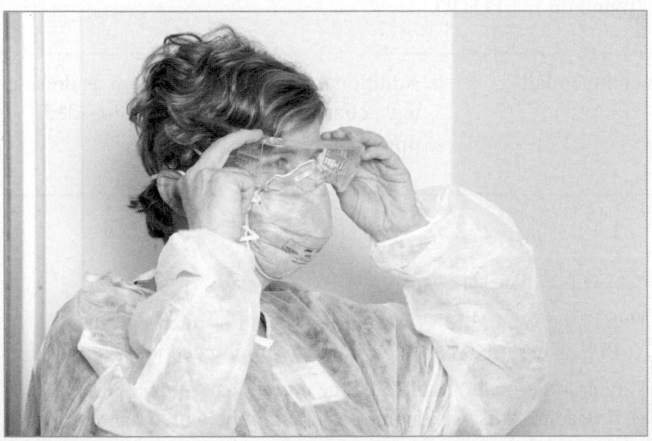

FIGURE 9. Removing goggles by grasping earpieces.

(continued)

SKILL 23-2 USING PERSONAL PROTECTIVE EQUIPMENT (PPE) *continued*

ACTION	RATIONALE
f. To remove gown: Unfasten ties, if at the neck and back. Allow the gown to fall away from shoulders. **Touching only the inside of the gown**, pull away from the torso. Keeping hands on the inner surface of the gown, pull gown from arms. Turn gown inside out. Fold or roll into a bundle and discard.	Gown front and sleeves are contaminated. Touching only the inside of the gown and pulling it away from the torso prevents transmission of microorganisms. Proper disposal prevents transmission of microorganisms.
g. To remove mask or respirator: Grasp the neck ties or elastic, then top ties or elastic and remove. **Take care to avoid touching front of mask or respirator.** Discard in waste container. If using a respirator, save for future use in the designated area.	Front of mask or respirator is contaminated; **Do not touch.** Not touching the front and proper disposal prevent transmission of microorganisms.
8. Perform hand hygiene immediately after removing all PPE.	Hand hygiene prevents spread of microorganisms.

DOCUMENTATION	It is not usually necessary to document the use of specific articles of PPE or each application of PPE. However, document the implementation and continuation of specific transmission-based precautions as part of the patient's care.

UNEXPECTED SITUATIONS AND ASSOCIATED INTERVENTIONS	• *You did not realize the need for protective equipment at beginning of task:* Stop task and obtain appropriate protective wear. • *You are accidentally exposed to blood and body fluids:* Stop task and immediately follow agency protocol for exposure, including reporting the exposure.

SKILL 23-3 PREPARING A STERILE FIELD AND ADDING STERILE ITEMS TO A STERILE FIELD

DELEGATION CONSIDERATIONS	Procedures requiring the use of a sterile field and other sterile items are not delegated to nursing assistive personnel (NAP) or unlicensed assistive personnel (UAP). Depending on the state's nurse practice act and the organization's policies and procedures, these procedures may be delegated to licensed practical/vocational nurses (LPN/LVN). The decision to delegate must be based on careful analysis of the patient's needs and circumstances, as well as the qualifications of the person to whom the task is being delegated. Refer to the Delegation Guidelines in Appendix A (found on thePoint).

EQUIPMENT	• Sterile wrapped drape or commercially prepared sterile package	• Additional sterile supplies, such as dressings, containers, or solution, as needed • PPE, as indicated

IMPLEMENTATION

ACTION	RATIONALE
1. Perform hand hygiene and put on PPE, if indicated.	Hand hygiene and PPE prevent the spread of microorganisms. PPE is required, based on transmission precautions.
2. Identify the patient. Explain the procedure to the patient.	Patient identification validates the correct patient and correct procedure. Discussion and explanation help allay anxiety and prepare the patient for what to expect.

ACTION

Preparing a Sterile Field

3. Check that packaged sterile drape is dry and unopened. Also, note expiration date, making sure that the date is still valid.

4. Select a work area that is waist level or higher.

5. Open sterile wrapped drape or commercially prepared kit following the directions below.

For a Prepackaged Sterile Drape

a. Open the outer covering of the drape. Remove sterile drape, lifting it carefully by its corners. Hold away from body and above the waist and work surface.

b. Continue to hold only by the corners. Allow the drape to unfold, away from your body and any other surface (Figure 1).

c. Position the drape on the work surface with the moisture-proof side down (Figure 2). This would be the shiny or blue side. Avoid touching any other surface or object with the drape. If any portion of the drape hangs off the work surface, that part of the drape is considered contaminated. Do not touch or reach over the sterile field.

RATIONALE

Moisture contaminates a sterile package. Expiration date indicates period that package remains sterile.

Work area is within sight. Bacteria tend to settle, so there is less contamination above the waist.

Outer 1 inch (2.5 cm) of drape is considered contaminated. Any item touching this area is also considered contaminated.

Touching outer side of wrapper maintains the sterile field. Contact with any surface would contaminate the field.

Moisture-proof side prevents contamination of the field if it becomes wet. The moisture penetrates the sterile cloth or paper and carries organisms by capillary action to contaminate the field. A wet field is considered contaminated if the surface immediately below it is not sterile.

FIGURE 1. Holding drape by corners and allowing it to unfold away from body and surfaces.

FIGURE 2. Positioning drape on work surface with the moisture-proof side down.

For a Commercially Prepared Kit or Tray

a. Open the outside cover of the package and remove the kit or tray (Figure 3). Place in the center of the work surface, with the topmost flap positioned on the far side of the package. Discard outside cover.

b. Reach around the package and grasp the outer surface of the end of the topmost flap, holding no more than 1 inch from the border of the flap. Pull open away from the body, keeping the arm outstretched and away from the inside of the wrapper (Figure 4). Allow the wrapper to lie flat on the work surface.

This allows sufficient room for sterile field.

This maintains sterility of inside of wrapper, which is to become the sterile field. Outer surface of the wrapper is considered unsterile. Outer 1-inch border of the wrapper is considered contaminated.

(continued)

SKILL 23-3

PREPARING A STERILE FIELD AND ADDING STERILE ITEMS TO A STERILE FIELD *continued*

ACTION	RATIONALE

FIGURE 3. Opening outside cover of package.

FIGURE 4. Pulling top flap open, away from body.

c. Reach around the package and grasp the outer surface of the first side flap, holding no more than 1 inch from the border of the flap. Pull open to the side of the package, keeping the arm outstretched and away from the inside of the wrapper (Figure 5). Allow the wrapper to lie flat on the work surface.

This maintains sterility of inside of wrapper, which is to become the sterile field. Outer surface of the wrapper is considered unsterile. Outer 1-inch border of the wrapper is considered contaminated.

d. Reach around the package and grasp the outer surface of the remaining side flap, holding no more than 1 inch from the border of the flap. Pull open to the side of the package, keeping the arm outstretched and away from the inside of the wrapper (Figure 6). Allow the wrapper to lie flat on the work surface.

This maintains sterility of inside of wrapper, which is to become the sterile field. Outer surface of the wrapper is considered unsterile. Outer 1-inch of border of the wrapper is considered contaminated.

FIGURE 5. Pulling open the first side flap.

FIGURE 6. Pulling open the remaining side flap.

e. Stand away from the package and work surface. Grasp the outer surface of the remaining flap closest to the body, holding not more than 1 inch from the border of the flap. Pull the flap back toward the body, keeping arm outstretched and away from the inside of the wrapper (Figure 7). Keep this hand in place. Use other hand to grasp the wrapper on the underside (the side that is down to the work surface). Position the wrapper so that when flat, edges are on the work surface, and do not hang down over sides of work surface (Figure 8). Allow the wrapper to lie flat on the work surface.

f. The outer wrapper of the package has become a sterile field with the packaged supplies in the center (Figure 9). Do not touch or reach over the sterile field.

This maintains sterility of inside of wrapper, which is to become the sterile field. Outer surface of the wrapper is considered unsterile. Outer 1-inch border of the wrapper is considered contaminated.

Sterility of the field and contents are maintained.

FIGURE 7. Pulling open flap closest to body.

FIGURE 8. Positioning wrapper on work surface.

FIGURE 9. Outside wrapper of package is now sterile field.

Adding Items to a Sterile Field

6. Place additional sterile items on field as needed.

Sterility of the field is maintained.

To Add an Agency-Wrapped and Sterilized Item

a. Hold agency-wrapped item in the dominant hand, with top flap opening away from the body. With other hand, reach around the package and unfold top flap and both sides.

Only sterile surface and item are exposed before dropping onto sterile field.

(continued)

SKILL 23-3 PREPARING A STERILE FIELD AND ADDING STERILE ITEMS TO A STERILE FIELD *continued*

ACTION	RATIONALE
b. Keep a secure hold on item through the wrapper with the dominant hand. Grasp the remaining flap of the wrapper closest to the body, taking care not to touch the inner surface of the wrapper or the item. Pull the flap back toward the wrist, so the wrapper covers the hand and wrist.	Only sterile surface and item are exposed before dropping onto sterile field.
c. Grasp all the corners of the wrapper together with the non-dominant hand and pull back toward wrist, covering hand and wrist. Hold in place.	Only sterile surface and item are exposed before dropping onto sterile field.
d. Hold the item 6 inches above the surface of the sterile field and drop onto the field. Be careful to avoid touching the surface or other items or dropping onto the 1-inch border.	This prevents contamination of the field and inadvertent dropping of the sterile item too close to the edge or off the field. Any items landing on the 1-inch border are considered contaminated.

To Add a Commercially Wrapped and Sterilized Item

ACTION	RATIONALE
a. Hold package in one hand. Pull back top cover with other hand. Alternately, carefully peel the edges apart using both hands (Figure 10).	Contents remain uncontaminated by hands.
b. After top cover or edges are partially separated, hold the item 6 inches above the surface of the sterile field. Continue opening the package and drop the item onto the field (Figure 11). **Be careful to avoid touching the surface or other items or dropping onto the 1-inch border.**	This prevents contamination of the field and inadvertent dropping of the sterile item too close to the edge or off the field. Any items landing on 1-inch border are considered contaminated.
c. Discard wrapper.	A neat work area promotes proper technique and avoids inadvertent contamination of the field.

FIGURE 10. Carefully peeling edges apart.

FIGURE 11. Dropping sterile item onto sterile field.

To Add a Sterile Solution

ACTION	RATIONALE
a. Obtain appropriate solution and check expiration date.	Once opened, label any bottles with date and time. Solution remains sterile for 24 hours once opened.
b. Open solution container according to directions and **place cap on table away from the field with edges up (Figure 12).**	Sterility of inside cap is maintained.
c. Hold bottle outside the edge of the sterile field with the label side facing the palm of your hand and prepare to pour from a height of 4 to 6 inches (10 to 15 cm). **Never touch the tip of the bottle to the sterile container or field.**	Label remains dry, and solution may be poured without reaching across sterile field. Minimal splashing occurs from that height. Accidentally touching the tip of the bottle to a container or dressing contaminates them both.

d. Pour required amount of solution steadily into sterile container previously added to sterile field and positioned at side of sterile field or onto dressings (Figure 13). **Avoid splashing any liquid.**

e. Touch only the outside of the lid when recapping. Label solution with date and time of opening.

A steady stream minimizes the risk of splashing; moisture contaminates sterile field.

Solution remains uncontaminated and available for future use.

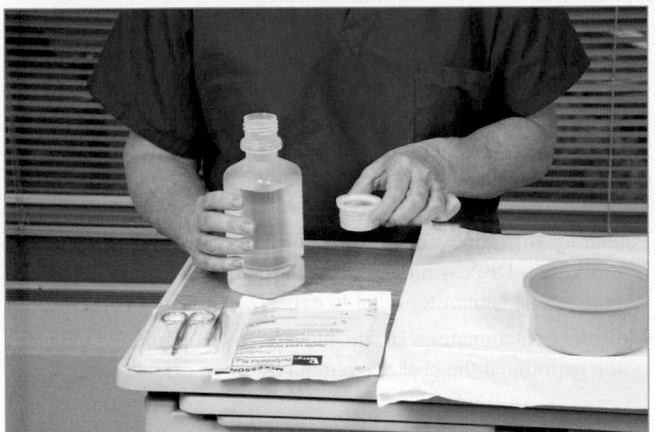

FIGURE 12. Opening bottle of sterile solution and placing cap on table with edges up.

FIGURE 13. Pouring solution into sterile container.

7. Continue with the procedure as indicated.

8. When procedure is completed, remove PPE, if used. Perform hand hygiene.

Removing PPE properly reduces the risk for infection transmission and contamination of other items. Hand hygiene prevents the spread of microorganisms.

DOCUMENTATION

It is not usually necessary to document the preparation of a sterile field. However, documentation should be recorded regarding the use of sterile technique for any procedure performed using sterile technique.

UNEXPECTED SITUATIONS AND ASSOCIATED INTERVENTIONS

- *The item being added falls close to or on the edge of the field:* Consider the outer 1-inch edge of a sterile field to be contaminated. Any item within the outer 1-inch is considered contaminated.

- *A part of the sterile field becomes contaminated:* When any portion of the sterile field becomes contaminated, discard all portions of the sterile field and start over.

- *The nurse realizes a supply is missing after setting up the sterile field:* Call for help. Do not leave the sterile field unattended. If the nurse is not able to visualize the sterile field at all times, it is considered contaminated.

- *The patient touches the sterile field:* If the patient touches the sterile field, discard the supplies and prepare a new sterile field. If the patient is confused, have someone assist by holding the patient's hands and/or reinforcing what is happening.

SKILL 23-4 PUTTING ON STERILE GLOVES AND REMOVING SOILED GLOVES

DELEGATION CONSIDERATIONS	Procedures requiring the use of sterile gloves and other sterile items are not delegated to nursing assistive personnel (NAP) or unlicensed assistive personnel (UAP). Depending on the state's nurse practice act and the organization's policies and procedures, these procedures may be delegated to licensed practical/vocational nurses (LPNs/LVNs). The decision to delegate must be based on careful analysis of the patient's needs and circumstances, as well as the qualifications of the person to whom the task is being delegated. Refer to the Delegation Guidelines in Appendix A (found on thePoint).
EQUIPMENT	• Sterile gloves of the appropriate size • PPE, as indicated

IMPLEMENTATION

ACTION	RATIONALE
1. Perform hand hygiene and put on PPE, if indicated.	Hand hygiene and PPE prevent the spread of microorganisms. PPE is required based on transmission precautions.
2. Identify the patient. Explain the procedure to the patient.	Patient identification validates the correct patient and correct procedure. Discussion and explanation help allay anxiety and prepare the patient for what to expect.
3. Check that the sterile glove package is dry and unopened. Also note expiration date, making sure that the date is still valid.	Moisture contaminates a sterile package. Expiration date indicates the period that the package remains sterile.
4. Place sterile glove package on clean, dry surface at or above your waist.	Moisture could contaminate the sterile gloves. Any sterile object held below the waist is considered contaminated.
5. Open the outside wrapper by carefully peeling the top layer back (Figure 1). Remove inner package, handling only the outside of it.	This maintains sterility of gloves in inner packet.
6. Place the inner package on the work surface with the side labeled "cuff end" closest to the body.	Allows for ease of glove application.
7. Carefully open the inner package. Fold open the top flap, then the bottom and sides (Figure 2). **Take care not to touch the inner surface of the package or the gloves.**	The inner surface of the package is considered sterile. The outer 1-inch border of the inner package is considered contaminated. The sterile gloves are exposed with the cuff end closest to the nurse.

FIGURE 1. Pulling top layer of outside wrapper back.

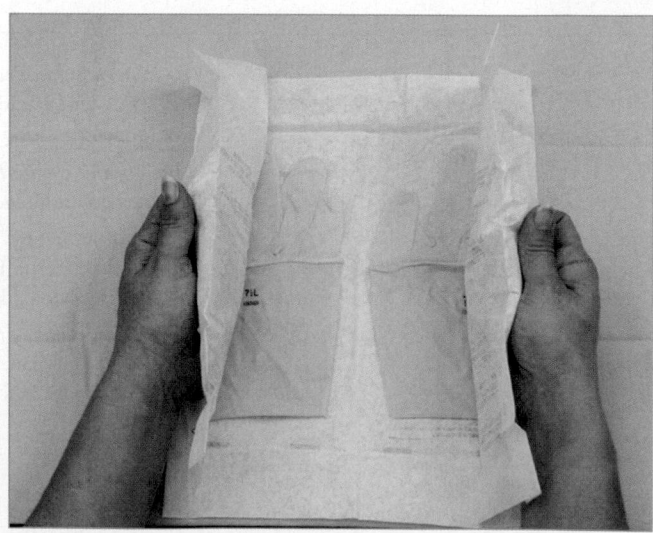

FIGURE 2. Folding back side flaps.

ACTION

8. With the thumb and forefinger of the nondominant hand, grasp the folded cuff of the glove for the dominant hand, touching only the exposed inside of the glove (Figure 3).

9. Keeping the hands above the waistline, lift and hold the glove up and off the inner package with fingers down (Figure 4). **Be careful that it does not touch any unsterile object.**

10. Carefully insert dominant hand palm up into glove (Figure 5) and pull glove on. Leave the cuff folded until the opposite hand is gloved.

11. Hold the thumb of the gloved hand outward. Place the fingers of the gloved hand inside the cuff of the remaining glove (Figure 6). Lift it from the wrapper, taking care not to touch anything with the gloves or hands.

RATIONALE

Unsterile hand touches only inside of glove. Outside remains sterile.

Glove is contaminated if it touches any unsterile objects.

Attempting to turn upward with unsterile hand may result in contamination of sterile glove.

Thumb is less likely to become contaminated if held outward. Sterile surface touching sterile surface prevents contamination.

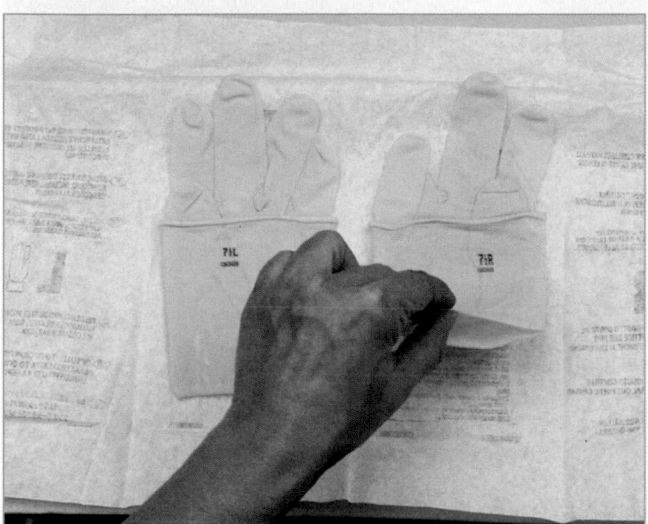

FIGURE 3. Grasping cuff of glove for dominant hand.

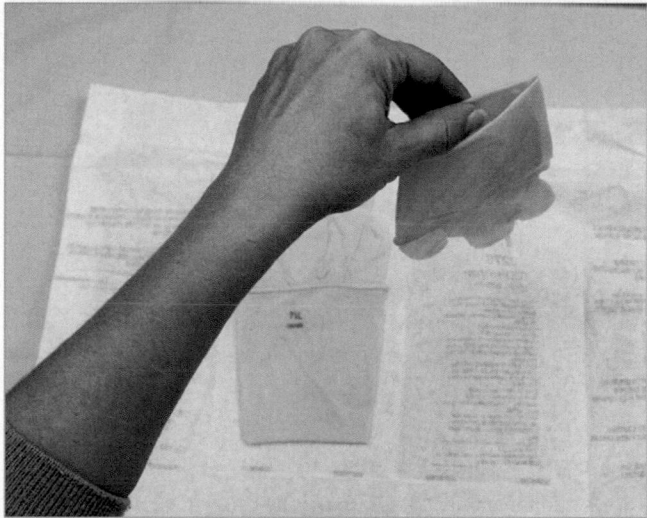

FIGURE 4. Lifting glove from package.

FIGURE 5. Inserting dominant hand into glove.

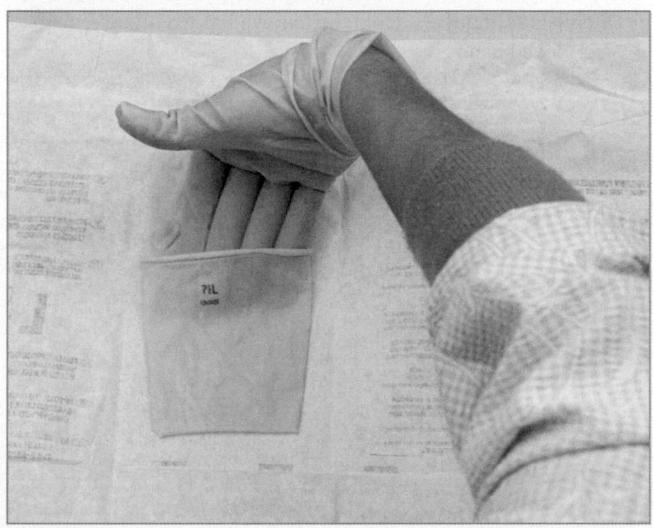

FIGURE 6. Sliding fingers under cuff of glove for nondominant hand.

(continued)

SKILL 23-4 | PUTTING ON STERILE GLOVES AND REMOVING SOILED GLOVES *continued*

ACTION	**RATIONALE**
12. Carefully insert nondominant hand into glove. Pull the glove on, taking care that the skin does not touch any of the outer surfaces of the gloves.	Sterile surface touching sterile surface prevents contamination.
13. **Slide the fingers of one hand under the cuff of the other and fully extend the cuff down the arm, touching only the sterile outside of the glove (Figure 7). Repeat for the remaining hand.**	Sterile surface touching sterile surface prevents contamination.
14. Adjust gloves on both hands if necessary, **touching only sterile areas with other sterile areas** (Figure 8).	Sterile surface touching sterile surface prevents contamination.
15. Continue with procedure as indicated.	

FIGURE 7. Sliding fingers of one hand under cuff of other hand and extending cuff down the arm.

FIGURE 8. Adjusting gloves as necessary.

Removing Soiled Gloves

16. Use dominant hand to grasp the opposite glove **near cuff end on the outside exposed area.** Remove it by pulling it off, inverting it as it is pulled, keeping the contaminated area on the inside (Figure 9). Hold the removed glove in the remaining gloved hand.

Contaminated area does not come in contact with hands or wrists.

FIGURE 9. Inverting glove as it is removed.

ACTION	RATIONALE
17. Slide fingers of ungloved hand between the remaining glove and the wrist (Figure 10). **Take care to avoid touching the outside surface of the glove.** Remove it by pulling it off, inverting it as it is pulled, keeping the contaminated area on the inside, and securing the first glove inside the second (Figure 11).	Contaminated area does not come in contact with hands or wrists.

FIGURE 10. Sliding fingers of ungloved hand inside remaining glove.

FIGURE 11. Inverting glove as it is removed, securing first glove inside it.

ACTION	RATIONALE
18. Discard gloves in appropriate container. Remove additional PPE, if used. Perform hand hygiene.	Proper disposal and removal of PPE reduces the risk for infection transmission and contamination of other items. Hand hygiene prevents the spread of microorganisms.

DOCUMENTATION

It is not usually necessary to document the addition of sterile items to a sterile field. However, document the use of sterile technique for any procedure performed using sterile technique.

UNEXPECTED SITUATIONS AND ASSOCIATED INTERVENTIONS

- *Contamination occurs during application of the sterile gloves:* Discard gloves and open new package of sterile gloves.

- *A hole or tear is noticed in one of the gloves:* Discard gloves and open a new package of sterile gloves.

- *A hole or tear is noticed in one of the gloves during the procedure:* Stop procedure. Remove damaged gloves. Wash hands or perform hand hygiene (depending on whether soiled or not) and put on new sterile gloves.

- *The patient touches the nurse's hands or the sterile field:* If the patient touches your hands and nothing else, you may remove the contaminated gloves and put on new, sterile gloves. It is always a good idea to bring two pairs of sterile gloves into the room, depending on facility policy. If the patient touches the sterile field, discard the supplies and prepare a new sterile field. If the patient is confused, have someone assist you by holding the patient's hands or reinforcing what is happening.

- *Patient has a latex allergy:* Obtain latex-free sterile gloves.

DEVELOPING CLINICAL REASONING

1. A nurse cannot help but notice that whenever a particular surgeon makes rounds, he ignores basic principles of asepsis. He moves from one patient to another, touching dressings without washing his hands between patients. He is also inconsistent in his practice of sterile technique. You suspect that there is a higher rate of postoperative infection among his patients. What do you do?

2. A friend who is a nursing student always wears gloves when doing anything for ill patients. You are more selective in your use of gloves. She tells you that you are a fool for "taking chances" because you never know what you may pick up and bring home. Is this a matter of personal preference? Is one position more consistent with good nursing? Are your instructors consistent in how they respond to these questions?

PRACTICING FOR NCLEX

1. A nurse is following the principles of medical asepsis when performing patient care in a hospital setting. Which nursing action performed by the nurse follows these recommended guidelines?
   a. The nurse carries the patients' soiled bed linens close to the body to prevent spreading microorganisms into the air.
   b. The nurse places soiled bed linens and hospital gowns on the floor when making the bed.
   c. The nurse moves the patient table away from the nurse's body when wiping it off after a meal.
   d. The nurse cleans the most soiled items in the patient's bathroom first and follows with the cleaner items.

2. A school nurse is performing an assessment of a student who states: "I'm too tired to keep my head up in class." The student has a low-grade fever. The nurse would interpret these findings as indicating which stage of infection?
   a. Incubation period
   b. Prodromal stage
   c. Full stage of illness
   d. Convalescent period

3. A nurse is caring for patients in an isolation ward. In which situations would the nurse appropriately use an alcohol-based handrub to decontaminate the hands? Select all that apply.
   a. The nurse is providing a bed bath for a patient.
   b. The nurse has visibly soiled hands after changing the bedding of a patient.
   c. The nurse removes gloves when patient care is completed.
   d. The nurse is inserting a urinary catheter for a female patient.
   e. The nurse is assisting with a surgical placement of a cardiac stent.
   f. The nurse removes old magazines from a patient's table.

4. A nurse is performing hand hygiene after providing patient care. The nurse's hands are not visibly soiled. Which steps in this procedure are performed correctly? Select all that apply.
   a. The nurse removes all jewelry including a platinum wedding band.
   b. The nurse washes hands to one inch above the wrists.
   c. The nurse uses approximately two teaspoons of liquid soap.
   d. The nurse keeps hands higher than elbows when placing under faucet.
   e. The nurse uses friction motion when washing for at least 15 seconds.
   f. The nurse rinses thoroughly with water flowing toward fingertips.

5. The nurse has opened the sterile supplies and put on two sterile gloves to complete a sterile dressing change, a procedure that requires surgical asepsis. The nurse must:
   a. Keep splashes on the sterile field to a minimum.
   b. Cover the nose and mouth with gloved hands if a sneeze is imminent.
   c. Use forceps soaked in a disinfectant.
   d. Consider the outer 1 inch of the sterile field as contaminated.

6. The nurse caring for patients in a hospital setting institutes CDC standard precaution recommendations for which category of patients?
   a. Only patients with diagnosed infections
   b. Only patients with visible blood, body fluids, or sweat
   c. Only patients with nonintact skin
   d. All patients receiving care in hospitals

7. In addition to standard precautions, the nurse would initiate droplet precautions for which patients? Select all that apply.
   a. A patient diagnosed with rubella
   b. A patient diagnosed with diptheria
   c. A patient diagnosed with varicella
   d. A patient diagnosed with tuberculosis
   e. A patient diagnosed with MRSA
   f. An infant diagnosed with adenovirus infection

8. A nurse is preparing a sterile field using a packaged sterile drape for a confused patient who is scheduled for a surgical procedure. When setting up the field, the patient accidentally touches an instrument in the sterile field. What is the appropriate nursing action in this situation?
   a. Ask another nurse to hold the hand of the patient and continue setting up the field.
   b. Remove the instrument that was touched by the patient and continue setting up the sterile field.
   c. Discard the supplies and prepare a new sterile field with another person holding the patient's hand.
   d. No action is necessary since the patient has touched his or her own sterile field.

9. A nurse who created a sterile field for a patient is adding a sterile solution to the field. What is an appropriate action when performing this task?
   a. Place the bottle cap on the table with the edges down.
   b. Hold the bottle inside the edge of the sterile field.
   c. Hold the bottle with the label side opposite the palm of the hand.
   d. Pour the solution from a height of 4 to 6 inches (10 to 15 cm).

10. A nurse is finished with patient care. How would the nurse remove PPE when leaving the room?
    a. Remove gown, goggles, mask, gloves, and exit the room.
    b. Remove gloves, perform hand hygiene, then remove gown, mask, and goggles.
    c. Untie gown waiststrings, remove gloves, goggles, gown, mask; perform hand hygiene.
    d. Remove goggles, mask, gloves, gown, and perform hand hygiene.

11. A nurse who is caring for a patient diagnosed with HIV/AIDS incurs a needlestick injury when administering the patient's medications. What would be the priority action of the nurse following the exposure?
    a. Report the incident to the appropriate person and file an incident report.
    b. Wash the exposed area with warm water and soap.
    c. Consent to postexposure prophylaxis at appropriate time.
    d. Set up counseling sessions regarding safe practice to protect self.

12. The nurse assesses patients to determine their risk for health care–associated infections. Which hospitalized patient is most at risk for developing this type of infection?
    a. A 60-year-old patient who smokes two packs of cigarettes daily
    b. A 40-year-old patient who has a white blood cell count of 6,000/mm³
    c. A 65-year-old patient who has an indwelling urinary catheter in place
    d. A 60-year-old patient who is a vegetarian and slightly underweight

13. A nurse is caring for an obese 62-year-old patient with arthritis who has developed an open reddened area over his sacrum. What is a priority nursing diagnosis for this patient?
    a. Imbalanced Nutrition: More Than Body Requirements related to immobility
    b. Impaired Physical Mobility related to pain and discomfort
    c. Chronic Pain related to immobility
    d. Risk for Infection related to altered skin integrity

14. A nurse teaches a patient at home to use clean technique when changing a wound dressing. This practice is considered:
    a. The nurse's preference
    b. Safe for the home setting
    c. Unethical behavior
    d. Grossly negligent

15. A nurse is using personal protective equipment (PPE) when bathing a patient diagnosed with *C. difficile* infection. Which nursing action related to this activity promotes safe, effective patient care?
    a. The nurse puts on PPE after entering the patient room.
    b. The nurse works from "clean" areas to "dirty" areas during bath.
    c. The nurse personalizes the care by substituting glasses for goggles.
    d. The nurse removes PPE prior to leaving the patient room.

ANSWERS WITH RATIONALES

1. *c.* According to the principles of medical asepsis, the nurse should move equipment away from the body when brushing, scrubbing, or dusting articles to prevent contaminated particles from settling on the hair, face, or uniform. The nurse should carry soiled items away from the body to prevent them from touching the clothing. The nurse should not put soiled items on the floor, as it is highly contaminated. The nurse should also clean the least soiled areas first and then move to the more soiled ones to prevent having the cleaner areas soiled by the dirtier areas.

2. *b.* During the prodromal stage, the person has vague signs and symptoms, such as fatigue and a low-grade fever. There

are no obvious symptoms of infection during the incubation period, and they are more specific during the full stage of illness, before disappearing by the convalescent period.

3. *a, c, d, f.* It is recommended to use an alcohol-based handrub in the following situations: before direct contact with patients; after direct contact with patient skin; after contact with body fluids *if hands are not visibly soiled;* after removing gloves; before inserting urinary catheters, peripheral vascular catheters, or invasive devices that *do not require surgical placement;* before donning sterile gloves prior to an invasive procedure; if moving from a contaminated body site to a clean body site; and after contact with objects contaminated by the patient.

4. *b, e, f.* Proper hand hygiene includes removing jewelry with the exception of a plain wedding band, wetting the hands and wrist area with the hands lower than the elbows, using about one teaspoon of liquid soap, using friction motion for at least 15 seconds, washing to one inch above the wrists with a friction motion for at least 15 seconds, and rinsing thoroughly with water flowing toward fingertips.

5. *d.* Considering the outer inch of a sterile field as contaminated is a principle of surgical asepsis. Moisture such as from splashes contaminates the sterile field, and sneezing would contaminate the sterile gloves. Forceps soaked in disinfectant are not considered sterile.

6. *d.* Standard precautions apply to all patients receiving care in hospitals, regardless of their diagnosis or possible infection status. These recommendations include blood; all body fluids, secretions, and excretions except sweat; nonintact skin; and mucous membranes.

7. *a, b, f.* Rubella, diphtheria, and adenovirus infection are illnesses transmitted by large-particle droplets and require droplet precautions in addition to standard precautions. Airborne precautions are used for patients who have infections spread through the air with small particles, for example, tuberculosis, varicella, and rubeola. Contact precautions are used for patients who are infected or colonized by a multidrug-resistant organism (MDRO), such as MRSA.

8. *c.* If the patient touches a sterile field, the nurse should discard the supplies and prepare a new sterile field. If the patient is confused, the nurse should have someone assist by holding the patient's hand and reinforcing what is happening.

9. *d.* To add a sterile solution to a sterile field, the nurse would open the solution container according to directions and place the cap on the table away from the field with the edges up. The nurse would then hold the bottle outside the edge of the sterile field with the label side facing the palm of the hand and prepare to pour from a height of 4 to 6 inches (10 to 15 cm).

10. *c.* If an impervious gown has been tied in front of the body at the waist, the nurse should untie the waist strings before removing gloves. Gloves are always removed first because they are most likely to be contaminated, followed by the goggles, gown, and mask, and hands should be washed thoroughly after the equipment has been removed and before leaving the room.

11. *b.* When a needlestick injury occurs, the nurse should wash the exposed area immediately with warm water and soap, report the incident to the appropriate person and complete an incident injury report, consent to and await the results of

blood tests, consent to postexposure prophylaxis, and attend counseling sessions regarding safe practice to protect self and others.

12. *c.* Indwelling urinary catheters have been implicated in most health care–associated infections. Cigarette smoking, a normal white blood cell count, and a vegetarian diet have not been implicated as risk factors for HAIs.

13. *d.* The priority diagnosis in this situation is the possibility of an infection developing in the open skin area. The others may be potential or probable diagnoses for this patient and may also require nursing interventions after the first diagnosis is addressed.

14. *b.* In the home setting, where the patient's environment is more controlled, medical asepsis is usually recommended, with the exception of self-injection. This is the appropriate procedure for the home and is neither unethical nor grossly negligent.

15. *b.* When using PPE, the nurse should work from "clean" areas to "dirty" ones, put on PPE before entering the patient room, always use goggles instead of personal glasses, and remove PPE in the doorway or anteroom.

TAYLOR SUITE RESOURCES

Explore these additional resources to enhance learning for this chapter:

- NCLEX-Style Questions and other resources on thePoint, http://thePoint.lww.com/Taylor8e
- *Study Guide for Fundamentals of Nursing, 8th edition*
- Adaptive Learning | Powered by prepU, http://thepoint.lww.com/prepu
- *Skill Checklists for Fundamentals of Nursing, 8th edition*
- *Taylor's Clinical Nursing Skills:* Chapter 1, Asepsis and Infection Control
- *Taylor's Video Guide to Clinical Nursing Skills:* Asepsis

Bibliography

Agency for Healthcare Research and Quality (AHRQ). (2010). *AHRQ's efforts to prevent and reduce healthcare-associated infections.* Available at http://www.ahrq.gov/qual/haiflyer.pdf.

Altrich, M. (2012). Diagnosis of latex allergy. *The Alert Newsletter,* pp. 1–6. Slinger, WI: American Latex Allergy Association.

Association for Professionals in Infection Control and Epidemiology (APIC). (2010). *Guide to the elimination of methicillin-resistant Staphylococcus aureus (MRSA) transmission in hospital settings* (2nd ed.). Washington, DC: Author.

Behrman, A., & Schraga, E. (2011). *Latex allergy.* Available at http://emedicine.medscape.com/article/756632-overview

Betsy Lehman Center for Patient Safety and Medical Error Reduction, JSI Research and Training Institute, Inc. (2008). Prevention and control of healthcare-associated infections in Massachusetts. Executive Summary: Part 1. Final recommendations of the Expert Panel. Boston, MA: Massachusetts Department of Public Health, pp. 36–41.

Bulechek, G., Butcher, H., Dochterman, J. & Wagner, C. (2013). *Nursing Interventions Classification (NIC),* (6th ed.). St. Louis: Elsevier/Mosby.

Chettle, C. (2011). *Acinetobacter baumannii:* Winning the battle against antibiotics. *Nursing Spectrum, 20*(8), 20–25.

Centers for Disease Control and Prevention (CDC). (2002). Guideline for hand hygiene in health-care settings. *Morbidity and Mortality Weekly Report 2002, 51*(RR16), 1–45.

Centers for Disease Control and Prevention (CDC). (2010a). CAUTI guideline fast facts. Available at http://www.cdc.gov/hicpac/CAUTI_fastFacts.html#1.

Centers for Disease Control and Prevention (CDC). (2010b). Laboratory detection of imipenem or meropenem resistance in gram-negative organisms. Available at http://www.cdc.gov/HAI/settings/lab/lab_imipenem.html.

Centers for Disease Control and Prevention (CDC). (2010c). Vancomycin-resistant enterococci (VRE) in healthcare settings. Available at http://www.cdc.gov/HAI/organisms/vre/vre.html.

Centers for Disease Control and Prevention (CDC). (2011a). Hand hygiene basics. Available at http://www.cdc.gov/handhygiene/Basics.html.

Centers for Disease Control and Prevention (CDC). (2011b). MRSA statistics. Available at http://cdc.gov/mrsa/statistics/index.html.

Centers for Disease Control and Prevention (CDC). (2011c). Protect yourself from MRSA. Available at http://www.cdc.gov/Features/MRSAinHealthcare/

Centers for Disease Control and Prevention (CDC). (2011d). West Nile virus: What you need to know. Available at http://www.cdc.gov/ncidod/dvbid/westnile/wnv_factsheet.htm.

Centers for Disease Control and Prevention (CDC). (2012a). Carbapenem-resistant enterobacteriaceae (CRE). Available at http://www.cdc.gov/hai/organisms/cre/index.html

Centers for Disease Control and Prevention (CDC). (2012b) *Clostridium difficile* infection. Available at http://www.cdc.gov/HAI/organisms/cdiff/Cdiff_infect.html

Centers for Disease Control and Prevention (CDC). (2012c). Frequently asked questions about *Clostridium difficile* for healthcare providers. Available at http://www.cdc.gov/HAI/organisms/cdiff/Cdiff_faqs_HCP.html.

Centers for Disease Control and Prevention (CDC). (2012d). General information about CRE. Available at http://www.cdc.gov/hai/organisms/cre/cre-patientgeneral.html.

Centers for Medicare and Medicaid Services (CMS). (2012). Hospital-acquired conditions. Available at http://www.cms.gov/Medicare/Medicare-Fee-for-Service-Payment/HospitalAcqCond/Hospital-Acquired_Conditions.html.

Centers for Disease Prevention and Control (CDC). (2014). Guidance on personal protective equipment to be used by healthcare workers during management of patients with ebola virus disease in U.S. hospitals, including procedures for putting on (donning) and removing (doffing). Available at http://www.cdc.gov/vhf/ebola/hcp/procedures-for-ppe.html.

Delahanty, K., & Myers, F. (2010). 3 Bad bugs. *Nursing, 40*(3), 24–30.

Delisio, N. (2012). Bloodborne infection from sharps and mucocutaneous exposure: A continuing problem. *Nursing, (7)*5, 35–38.

Drug–resistant bacteria growing challenge, WHO says. (2011). *Nurse.com, 20*(10), 18.

Dumont, C., & Nesselrodt, D. (2012). Preventing CLABSI (central line-associated bloodstream infections). *Nursing, 42*(6), 41–47.

Felembam, O, St. John, W., & Shaban, R. Z. (2012). Hand hygiene practices of home visiting community nurses: perceptions, compliance, techniques, and contextual factors of practice using the World Health Organization's "five moments for hand hygiene." *Home Healthcare Nurse, 30*(3), 152–160.

Fuller, C., Savage, J., Besser, S., Hayward, S., Cookson, B., Cooper, B., & Stone, S. (2011). The dirty hand in the latex glove: a study of hand hygiene compliance when gloves are worn. *Infection Control & Hospital Epidemiology, 32*(12), 1194–1199.

Grossman, S. & DeBartolomeo Mager, D. (2008). Managing the threat of methicillin-resistant Staphylococcus aureus in home care. *Home Healthcare Nurse, 26*(6), 356–366.

Guolette, C. (2012). Should nurses be required to wear hospital-laundered scrubs to help prevent the spread of pathogens. *Advance for Nurses,* Available at http://nursing.advanceweb.com/Editorial/Content/PrinterFriendly.aspx?CC=249728

Healthy People 2020. (2012). Healthcare-associated infections. Available at http:www.healthypeople.gov/2020/topicsobjectives2020/overview.aspx?topicid=17

Hubner, N., Hubner, C., Kramer, A., & Assadian, O. (2011). Survival of bacterial pathogens on paper and bacterial retrieval from paper to hands: Preliminary results. *American Journal of Nursing, 111*(12), 30–34.

Institute for Healthcare Improvement (IHI). (2011). *How-to guide: Improving hand hygiene.* Available at http://www.ihi.org/knowledge/Pages/Tools/HowtoGuideImprovingHandHygiene.aspx

Jabbar, U., Leischner, J., Kasper, D., Gerber, R., Sambol, S., Parada, J., Johnson, S., & Gerding, D. (2010). Effectiveness of alcohol-based hand rubs for removal of *Clostridium difficile. Infection Control & Hospital Epidemiology, 30*(10), 565–570.

Johnson, M., Kaehler, B., Siska, M., Lecy, B., & O'Neil, M. (2011). Healing touch: Tips for successful hand hygiene. *Nursing, 41*(11), 18.

The Joint Commission. (2012). Sentinel Event Alert, Issue 28: Infection control related sentinel events. Available at http://www.jointcommission.org/sentinel_event_alert_issue_28_infection_control_related_sentinel_events/

The Joint Commission. Center for Transforming Healthcare. (2012a). Facts about the hand hygiene project. Available at http://www.centerfortransforminghealthcare.org/assets/4/6/CTH_HH_Fact_Sheet.pdf

Joint Commission Center for Transforming Healthcare. (2012b). Facts about Targeted Solutions Tool™. Available at http://www.centerfortransforminghealthcare.org/news/detail.aspx?Articleid=293998

Keefe, S. (2011). Prioritizing infection prevention. *Advance for Nurses, 13*(3), 13–14.

Kelly, K., Wang, M., Klancnik, M., & Peterson, E. (2011). Prevention of IgE sensitization to latex in health care workers after reduction of antigen exposures. *Journal of Occupational and Environmental Medicine, 53*(8), 934–940.

Kelly, M. (2011). Battling super bugs. *Nursing Spectrum, 20*(10), 13.

Kenneley, I.L. (2010). Infection control and the home care environment, *Home Health Care Management & Practice, 22*(3), 195–201.

Lowes, R. (2011). Hospitals make progress toward reducing some infections: CDC. Available at http://www.medscape.com/viewarticle/751877_print

McGoldrick, M. & Rhinehart, E. (2007). Managing multi-drug-resistant organisms in home care and hospice: Surveillance, prevention, and control. *Home Healthcare Nurse, 25*(9), 580–588.

Meyers, F. (2011). Making the case for fecal bacteriotherapy. *Nursing, 41*(12), 50–53.

Moorhead, S., Johnson, M., Maas, M., & Swanson, E. (2013). *Nursing Outcomes Classification (NOC).* (5th ed.). St. Louis: Elsevier/Mosby.

National Center for Biotechnology Information (NCBI). (2011). Dengue fever. Available at http://www.ncbi.nlm.nih.gov/pubmedhealth/PMH0002350/.

National Institute for Occupational Safety and Health (NIOSH). (2012). NIOSH fast facts—Home healthcare workers: How to prevent latex allergies. Available at http://www.cdc.gov/niosh/docs/2012-119/pdfs/2012-119.pdf

Neville-Swensen, M., & Clayton, M. (2011). Outpatient management of community-associated methicillin-resistant *Staphylococcus aureus* skin and soft tissue infection. Available at http://www.medscape.com/viewarticle/748722_print

North American Diagnosis Association (NANDA) International. (2012). *Nursing diagnoses: Definitions and classifications 2012–2014.* West Sussex, UK: Wiley-Blackwell.

Occupational Safety and Health Administration (OSHA). (2011). Most frequently asked questions concerning the bloodborne pathogens standard. Available at http://www.osha.gov/pls/oshaweb/owadisp.show_document?p_table=INTERPRETATIONS&p_id=21010&p_text_version=FALSE

Overstreet, M. (2011). West Nile virus. *Nursing, 41*(6).

Patton, M. (2012). Combating an emerging bacterium. *Advance for Nurses, 14*(10), 12–20.

Phillips, E., & Dawson, J. (2012). Environment, health, and safety: Sharps safety is as important as ever. *American Nurse Today, 7*(3), 34.

Porth, C. (2011). *Essentials of pathophysiology: Concepts of altered health states* (3rd ed.). Philadelphia: Lippincott Williams & Wilkins.

Puliti, B. (2011). Infection prevention. *Advance for Nurses, 13*(14), 10–11.

Riley, M. (2012). Vancomycin-resistant enterococci. *Nursing.com, 21*(2), 20–25.

Sherwood, G., & Barnsteiner, J. (2012). *Quality and safety in nursing: a competency approach to improving outcomes.* West Sussex, UK: Wiley-Blackwell.

Siegel, J. D., Rhinehart, E., Jackson, M., Chiarello, L., & the Healthcare Infection Control Practices Advisory Committee. (2007). 2007 Guideline for Isolation Precautions: Preventing Transmission of Infectious Agents in Healthcare Settings. Available at http://www.cdc.gov/hicpac/pdf/isolation/Isolation2007.pdf

Simko, L. (2012). Breaking sterility: Dealing with procedural violations in healthcare. *Nursing, 42*(8), 22–26.

Smeltzer, S., Bare, B., Hinkle, J. H., & Cheever, K. H. (2010). *Brunner & Suddarth's textbook of medical–surgical nursing* (12th ed.). Philadelphia: Lippincott Williams & Wilkins.

Snow, M. (2011). *Clostridium difficile:* Trouble for adult and children. *Nursing, 41*(8), 67–68.

Splete, H. (2012). *C. difficile* infections hit all-time high. *Family Practice News.* Available at http://www.familypracticenews.com/news/more-top-news/single-view/ic-difficilei-infections-hit-all-time-high/dfae3e52c5.html.

U.S. Department of Health & Human Services (USDHHS). (2011). HHS recognizes progress toward eliminating healthcare-associated infections. Available at http://www.hhs.gov/ash/news/20110502a.html

U.S. Department of Health & Human Services (USDHHS). (2012a). Few adverse events in hospitals were reported to state adverse event reporting systems.

Available at https://oig.hhs.gov/oei/reports/oei-06-09-00092.asp

U.S. Department of Health & Human Services (USDHHS). (2012b). Healthcare-associated infection (HAI). Available at http://www.hhs.gov/ash/iniatives/hai/index.html

U.S. Department of Health & Human Services (USDHHS). (2012c). National targets and metrics: Monitoring progress toward action plan goals. Available at http://www.hhs.gov/ash/initiatives/hai/nationaltargets/index.html

U.S. Department of Health & Human Services (USDHHS). (2012d). NIOSH Fast Facts—Home healthcare workers: How to prevent needlestick and sharps injuries. DHHS (NIOSH) Publication No. 2012-123. Available at http://www.cdc.gov/niosh/docs/2012-123/pdfs/2012-123.pdf

U.S. Department of Health & Human Services (USDHHS). (2012e). NIOSH Fast Facts—Home healthcare workers: How to prevent latex allergy. Available at http://www.cdc.gov/niosh/docs/2012-119/pdfs/2012-119.pdf

World Health Organization. (2009). WHO guidelines on hand hygiene in health care. Available at http://whqlibdoc.who.int/publications/2009/9789241597906_eng.pdf

World Health Organization (2011). Race against time to develop new antibiotics. *Bulletin of the World Health Organization. 89*(2), 81-160.

Zastrow, R. (2011). The contact precautions controversy. *American Journal of Nursing, 111*(3), 47–52.

24 Vital Signs

NOAH SHOOLIN

Noah is a 2-year-old who is brought to the emergency department by his mother. When the nurse attempts to obtain a tympanic temperature, the child begins to scream uncontrollably, crying and pushing the device away from his ear.

TOMAS ESPOSITO

Tomas is a middle-aged man admitted to the hospital. He is placed in a private room with transmission-based infection control precautions, requiring staff to put on a gown and gloves when entering the room each time. A morning assessment, including vital signs, is needed.

DORETHA RENFROW

Doretha brings her 65-year-old husband with high blood pressure to the clinic for evaluation. He is 5'10" and overweight. Mrs. Renfrow states, "I really would like to learn how to take my husband's blood pressure so that I can keep track of his progress. Can you teach me how to do it?"

LEARNING OBJECTIVES

After completing the chapter, you will be able to accomplish the following:

1. Explain the physiologic processes involved in homeostatic regulation of temperature, pulse, respirations, and blood pressure.
2. Compare and contrast factors that increase or decrease body temperature, pulse, respirations, and blood pressure.
3. Identify sites for assessing temperature, pulse, and blood pressure.
4. Assess temperature, pulse, respirations, and blood pressure accurately.
5. Demonstrate knowledge of the normal ranges for temperature, pulse, respirations, and blood pressure across the lifespan.
6. Provide information to patients about measuring pulse and blood pressure at home.

KEY TERMS

afebrile	febrile	pulse
apnea	fever	pulse deficit
blood pressure	hypertension	pulse pressure
bradycardia	hyperthermia	respiration
bradypnea	hypotension	systolic pressure
diastolic pressure	hypothermia	tachycardia
dyspnea	Korotkoff sounds	tachypnea
dysrhythmia	orthopnea	temperature
eupnea	orthostatic hypotension	vital signs

Vital **signs** are a person's temperature, pulse, respiration, and blood pressure (abbreviated as T, P, R, BP). Pain, often included as the fifth vital sign, is discussed in Chapter 34. Pulse oximetry, the noninvasive measurement of arterial oxyhemoglobin saturation, is also often included with the measurement of vital signs in hospitalized patients and is discussed in Chapter 38. The health status of a person is reflected in these indicators of body functions, regulated through homeostatic mechanisms, and falling within certain normal ranges. A change in vital signs might indicate a change in health.

Assessing vital signs as part of a nursing assessment is an important component of care in all health care settings. Nurses assess vital signs and compare findings with accepted normal values and the patient's usual patterns in a wide variety of instances. Examples of appropriate times to measure

vital signs include, but are not limited to, screenings at health fairs and clinics, in the home, upon admission to a health care setting, when medications are given that affect cardiac rate and rhythm, before and after invasive diagnostic and surgical procedures, and in emergency situations. Nurses obtain vital signs as often as a patient's condition requires such assessment, prioritizing and adapting assessment of vital signs to address the patient's unique situation (Box 24-1). Frequency of assessment should be based on the patient's medical diagnosis, co-morbidities, types of treatments received, and the patient's level of acuity. Patients who are at greatest risk for an adverse outcome should receive more frequent assessments (Schulman, 2010).

In addition, institutional and agency policies govern when and how frequently vital signs are assessed. For example, vital signs are assessed at least every 4 hours in hospitalized patients with elevated temperatures, with high or low blood pressures, with changes in pulse rate or rhythm, or with respiratory difficulty. In critical care settings, technologically advanced devices are used to continually monitor patients' vital signs. Regulations require monthly vital sign measurements in long-term care residents, but for residents classified as Medicare A (meaning they have been discharged from the hospital and now Medicare is paying for their stay to receive skilled nursing care) vital signs are taken daily. In the home and in some self-care and psychiatric units, assessments are made only as frequently as the nurse judges necessary.

Although vital sign assessment may be delegated to other health care personnel when the condition of the patient is stable, it is the nurse's responsibility to ensure the accuracy of the data, interpret vital sign findings, and report abnormal findings. Principles of delegation should be followed. (Delegation is discussed in Chapters 14 and 22). If a patient has abnormal or unusual physical signs or symptoms (e.g., chest pain or dizziness) or has unexpected changes in vital signs, the nurse should validate the findings and further assess the patient. (See the accompanying Reflective Practice box for an example on page 580.) The nurse should know the normal variations in vital signs that occur at various ages as listed in Table 24-1 on page 581.

BOX 24-1 WHEN TO ASSESS VITAL SIGNS

- On admission to any health care agency or institution
- Based on agency or institutional policy and procedures
- Any time there is a change in the patient's condition
- Any time there is a loss of consciousness
- Before and after any surgical or invasive diagnostic procedure
- Before and after activity that may increase risk, such as ambulation after surgery
- Before administering medications that affect cardiovascular and respiratory function

REFLECTIVE PRACTICE: CULTIVATING QSEN COMPETENCIES

CHALLENGE TO ETHICAL AND LEGAL SKILLS

At clinical 2 weeks ago, I had four patients for the first time and I was very busy. One of my patients, Tomas Esposito, required transmission-based infection control precautions. So, every time I entered his room, I had to put on a gown and gloves. It was getting to be late in the morning and I still had not completed this patient's full assessment, including his vital signs. Upon entering the patient's room, I discovered that the separate stethoscope usually found in isolation rooms was not there. As a result, I had to remove my gown and gloves and go find the nurse to help me locate the stethoscope. Ultimately, the nurse had to get me a new isolation stethoscope set and put it together for me. Unfortunately, these stethoscopes are poor in quality.

I went back to the patient's room and put on a new gown and gloves. By this time, Mr. Esposito was very irritable, and just wanted me to do the assessment quickly and leave him alone. I attempted to listen to measure his blood pressure, but I couldn't hear any sound after opening the valve on the blood pressure cuff. I played with the stethoscope for a few minutes and tried again, but I still couldn't hear anything. My patient kept telling me to leave him alone. Being a 4th-year nursing student and self-sufficient in doing the basic patient assessment, I felt stupid going to get the nurse or my instructor and telling her I couldn't obtain a blood pressure. I was really pressed for time and now was faced with a critical decision.

Thinking Outside the Box: Possible Courses of Action

- Remove my gown and gloves, get my instructor and the nurse and tell them that I was unable to hear any sounds to obtain a blood pressure measurement, and request their assistance.
- Leave the patient alone as he requested, saving precious time, pretending that I completed vital signs and his assessment, and charting the same findings as the previous shift's assessment.

- Explain to the nurse that the patient wasn't cooperating and ask her to do the blood pressure and assessment without my instructor knowing about it.
- Try to complete the vital signs and assessment using my own stethoscope and risk transmission of potentially infectious microorganisms to other patients on the unit.

Evaluating a Good Outcome: How Do I Define Success?

- Patient receives the highest quality of care.
- Professional integrity of all health care team members involved is maintained.

- All documented information is accurate.
- Professional, ethical, and legal principles are maintained.

Personal Learning: Here's to the Future!

Luckily, my conscience and my desire to always give the best care to my patients pushed me to the right decision. I took the time to remove my gown and gloves and went to find my instructor and the nurse. I told the nurse that I was having trouble hearing the patient's blood pressure. She was very understanding and came to the room with me and tried herself. Upon further investigation, we found that the problem was a broken stethoscope, not my incompetence to complete an assessment. After assessing the patient with a properly functioning stethoscope, I obtained his blood pres-

sure, and also found expiratory wheezing and documented it. This finding provided a clue that I should probably keep a very close eye on this patient. Mr. Esposito ended up experiencing increasing difficulty breathing and his oxygen saturation levels began to drop into the 80% range. As a result, I realized just how important the initial assessment is when caring for a patient throughout the day. Hopefully, the lesson about how important it is to do the "right" thing for the patient will stick with me forever.

Catherine Barrell, Georgetown University

REFLECTION ON QUALITY AND SAFETY COMPETENCIES

How do you think you would respond in a similar situation? Why? Do you agree with the criteria that the nursing student used to evaluate a successful outcome? Why or why not? What *knowledge, skills, and attitudes* do you need to develop to continuously improve the quality and safety of care for patients like Mr. Esposito?

Patient-Centered Care: What information should be communicated to the patient about the care provided? How could you involve Mr. Esposito as a partner in coordinating his care to minimize frustration on the part of the patient and student? What might you have done to prevent the numerous trips in and out of the patient's room?

Teamwork and Collaboration/Quality Improvement: What communication skills do you need to improve to

ensure that you function as a member of the patient-care team and to obtain assistance when needed? How should you follow up regarding the defective equipment?

Safety/Evidence-Based Practice: What might you have done to determine whether the stethoscope was functioning properly? How do you think your time management and organizational skills affect the situation? What evidence in nursing literature provides guidance for decision making regarding infection control?

Informatics: Can you identify the essential information that must be available in Mr. Esposito's electronic record to support safe patient care and coordination of care? Can you think of other ways to respond to or approach the situation?

Table 24-1 · AGE-RELATED VARIATIONS IN NORMAL VITAL SIGNS

AGE	TEMPERATURE °C °F	PULSE BEATS/MIN	RESPIRATIONS BREATHS/MIN	BLOOD PRESSURE MM HG
Newborn[a]	35.9–36.9 96.7–98.5	70–190	30–55	73/55
Infants[b]	37.1–38.1 98.7–100.5	80–150	20–40	85/37
Toddler[b]	37.1–38.1 98.7–100.5	70–120	20–30	89/46
Child[c]	36.8–37.8 98.2–100	70–115	20–25	95/57
Preteen[d]	35.8–37.5 96.4–99.5	65–110	18–26	102/61
Teen[d]	35.8–37.5 96.4–99.5	55–105	12–22	112/64
Adult[d]	35.8–37.5 96.4–99.5	60–100	12–20	120/80
Aged Adult[d] (65+ years)	35.8–36.8 96.4–98.3	40–100	16–24	120/80

[a]Temperature is axillary measurement.
[b]Temperature is temporal measurement.
[c]Temperature is tympanic measurement.
[d]Temperature is oral measurement.

Adapted from Boltz, M., Capezuti, E., Fulmer, T., & Zwicker, D. (eds.) (2012). *Evidence-based geriatric nursing protocols for best practice* (4th ed.). New York: Springer Publishing Company; Jensen, S. (2011). *Nursing Health Assessment. A best practice approach.* Philadelphia. Wolters Kluwer Health/Lippincott Williams & Wilkins; and Kyle, T., & Carman, S. (2013). *Essentials of pediatric nursing.* (2nd ed.). Philadelphia: Wolters Kluwer Health/Lippincott Williams & Wilkins.

RECALL Tomas Esposito, the patient requiring initial assessment described in the Reflective Practice display. The nurse's inability to auscultate heart and lung sounds would be an important finding that requires additional assessment. The nurse would need to evaluate these findings in conjunction with the patient's other vital signs and symptoms. ●

The skills of assessing each of the vital signs, with rationale for each action, and a discussion of normal and abnormal findings are presented in this chapter. See Chapter 25 for additional information about health assessment.

TEMPERATURE

Body **temperature** is the difference between the amount of heat produced by the body and the amount of heat lost to the environment measured in degrees. Heat is generated by metabolic processes in the core tissues of the body, transferred to the skin surface by the circulating blood, and then dissipated to the environment. Core body temperature (intracranial, intrathoracic, and intra-abdominal) is higher than surface body temperature. Normal body temperature ranges from 35.9°C to 38°C (96.7°F to 100.5°F), depending on the route used for measurement (Jensen, 2011).

There are individual variations of these temperatures as well as variations related to age, gender, physical activity, state of health, and environmental temperatures. Body temperature also varies during the day, with temperatures being

lowest in the early morning and highest in the late afternoon (Grossman, 2014).

Physiology of Body Temperature

The core body temperature of a healthy person is maintained within a fairly constant range by the thermoregulatory set point of the thermoregulatory center in the hypothalamus. This center receives messages from cold and warm thermal receptors located throughout the body, compares that information with its temperature set point, and initiates responses to either produce or conserve body heat or to increase heat loss.

Heat Production

The primary source of heat in the body is metabolism, with heat produced as a byproduct of metabolic activities that generate energy for cellular functions. Various mechanisms increase body metabolism, including hormones and exercise. When additional heat is required to maintain balance, epinephrine and norepinephrine (sympathetic neurotransmitters) are released to rapidly alter metabolism so that energy production decreases and heat production increases. Thyroid hormone, produced by the thyroid gland, also increases metabolism and heat production, but over a much longer time period. Shivering, a response that increases the production of heat, is initiated by the hypothalamus and results in muscle tremors, causing the production of heat. In addition, the contraction of pilomotor muscles of the skin, as occurs with shivering, causes piloerection, or "goose bumps," and reduces the surface area of skin available for heat loss. Physical exertion increases heat production through muscle movements.

Heat Loss

The skin is the primary site of heat loss. The circulating blood brings heat to the skin's surface, where small connections between the arterioles and the venules lie directly below the skin surface. These connections, called arteriovenous shunts, may remain open to allow heat to dissipate (e.g., during exercise in hot environmental temperatures) to the skin and then to the external environment, or they may close and retain heat in the body (e.g., when the body is exposed to cold environmental temperatures). The sympathetic nervous system controls the opening and closing of the shunts in response to changes in core body temperature and in environmental temperature (Grossman, 2014). Heat is transferred to the external environment through the physical processes of radiation, convection, evaporation, and conduction. These processes are defined and illustrated in Table 24-2. Other heat losses occur through evaporation of sweat, through warming and humidifying of inspired air, and through elimination of urine and feces.

Factors Affecting Body Temperature

A variety of factors affect body temperature. These factors include time of day (circadian rhythms), age, gender, physical activity, state of health, and environmental temperatures.

Circadian Rhythms

Many environmental and physiologic processes occur in repeated cycles of time. Some events in humans recur at 24-hour intervals, referred to as circadian (meaning nearly every 24 hours) rhythm. Predictable fluctuations in measurements of body temperature and blood pressure are examples of functions that have a circadian rhythm. For instance, body temperature is usually about 0.6°C (1° to 2°F) lower in the early morning than in the late afternoon and early evening. This variation tends to be somewhat greater in infants and children. The peak elevation of a person's temperature occurs in late afternoon and early evening, between 4 and 8 PM.

Age and Gender

Older adults lose some thermoregulatory control with aging; body temperatures in older adults may be lower than the average adult temperature (Lu, Leasure, & Dai, 2009). Both the very old and the very young are more sensitive to changes in environmental temperature. Older adults are at risk for harm from extremes of temperature due to impaired thermoregulatory responses. The body temperature of infants and children changes more rapidly in response to both hot and cold air temperatures.

Table 24-2 MECHANISMS OF HEAT TRANSFER

	RADIATION	CONVECTION	EVAPORATION	CONDUCTION
Definition	The diffusion or dissemination of heat by electromagnetic waves	The dissemination of heat by motion between areas of unequal density	The conversion of a liquid to a vapor	The transfer of heat to another object during direct contact
Example	The body gives off waves of heat from uncovered surfaces.	An oscillating fan blows currents of cool air across the surface of a warm body.	Body fluid in the form of perspiration and insensible loss is vaporized from the skin.	The body transfers heat to an ice pack, causing the ice to melt.

Radiation   Convection   Evaporation   Conduction

CONSIDER Noah Shoolin, the 2-year-old brought to the emergency department by his mother. The nurse assessing the child's temperature would need to keep in mind the effect of environmental temperature changes on a child of this age. Efforts to prevent chilling and overheating would be incorporated into the child's plan of care. ●

Women tend to experience more fluctuations in body temperature than do men, probably the result of changes in hormones. The increase in progesterone secretion at ovulation increases body temperature as much as 0.3° to 0.6°C (0.5°–1°F).

Physical Activity

Physical exertion increases body temperature. Increased metabolism resulting from muscle activity results in the production of heat. The nurse should consider whether the patient has participated in physical activity when evaluating temperature measurements.

State of Health

Alterations in a person's health can contribute to variations in body temperature. The presence of certain disease conditions and other health problems may result in alterations in body temperature. Refer to the Increased Body Temperature and Decreased Body Temperature discussions later in this section.

Environmental Temperature

Most of us respond to changes in environmental temperature by wearing clothing that either allows increased heat loss when it is hot or retains heat when it is cold. When one is exposed to extreme cold without adequate protective clothing, heat loss may be increased to the point of **hypothermia** (low body temperature). Similarly, if one is exposed to extremes of heat for long periods of time, **hyperthermia** (high body temperature) may result. Both hypothermia and hyperthermia may cause serious illness or death.

Normal Body Temperature

Body temperature varies among individuals, with a range of 0.3° to 0.6°C (0.5°–1.0°F) from the average temperature considered to be within normal limits. However, wider variations from the average temperature may be normal for some people. A person with a normal body temperature is referred to as **afebrile** ("without fever"). Table 24-3 shows the average normal temperature standards for healthy adults at various body sites.

Increased Body Temperature

Fever (pyrexia) is an increase above normal in body temperature. A person with a fever is said to be **febrile**. Fever occurs in response to an upward displacement of the thermoregulatory set point in the hypothalamus, caused by pyrogens (substances that cause fever). Substances that can trigger this increase in temperature include bacteria, bacterial products, and whole microorganisms, such as viruses. Fever may also occur as a result of chemicals produced in the body in response to tissue injury, such as from myocardial infarction (MI), pulmonary emboli, cancer, trauma, and surgery. Although the purpose of fever is not fully understood, it signals increased immune function and inflammation, and is a valuable indicator of health status.

Most fevers, unless extremely high (above 40°C/104°F), are not harmful (Grossman, 2014). In fact, there are many beneficial effects of fever, including destruction of disease-causing microorganisms, increased susceptibility of disease-causing microorganisms to anti-infective agents, and enhanced response by the immune system (Cunha, 2011). However, when fever is equal to or greater than 41°C (106°F), it is referred to as hyperpyrexia and is a medical emergency. The body must be cooled rapidly to prevent brain damage (Hinkle & Cheever, 2014).

When the thermostatic set point of the hypothalamus is increased in response to a pyrogen, the hypothalamus initiates temperature-rising mechanisms: shivering, piloerection, vasoconstriction, and increased metabolism. After the body temperature rises to the new set point, heat-loss mechanisms (sweating, vasodilation, increased respirations) keep the body temperature from rising to dangerous levels. Most fevers are self-limiting, and the temperature returns to normal after the factors causing it are controlled. Box 24-2 (on page 584) lists terms used to describe types of fever.

The onset and significance of a fever from an illness differs according to age. The onset of a fever, which can be sudden or gradual, typically is more rapid in children than in adults. A mild elevation in temperature might indicate a serious infection in infants younger than 3 months of age who do not have well-developed temperature-control mechanisms. Older adults often have a lower baseline body temperature. Therefore, fever may be one of the later signs

Table 24-3 AVERAGE NORMAL TEMPERATURES FOR HEALTHY ADULTS AT VARIOUS SITES

ORAL	RECTAL	AXILLARY	TYMPANIC	TEMPORAL ARTERY
37.0°C	37.5°C	36.5°C	37.5°C*	37°C
98.6°F	99.5°F	97.7°F	99.5°F	98.6°F

*The average normal tympanic temperature depends on the calibration and mode setting of the tympanic membrane thermometer.

BOX 24-2 TERMS AND DEFINITIONS FOR TYPES OF FEVER

Intermittent: The body temperature returns to normal at least once every 24 hours.

Remittent: The body temperature does not return to normal and fluctuates a few degrees up or down.

Sustained or Continuous: The body temperature remains above normal with minimal variations.

Relapsing or Recurrent: The body temperature returns to normal for one or more days with one or more episodes of fever, each as long as several days.

(Adapted from Grossman, S. (2014). Porth's pathophysiology: concepts of altered health states. (9th ed.). Philadelphia: Wolters Kluwer Health/Lippincott Williams & Wilkins.

of illness with temperature elevations of only slightly above normal, even in a serious infection.

Other types of increased body temperature are hyperthermia, neurogenic fever, and fever of unknown origin (FUO). Hyperthermia differs from fever in that the hypothalamic set point is not changed, but in situations of extreme heat exposure or excessive heat production (e.g., during strenuous exercise), the mechanisms that control body temperature are ineffective. Neurogenic fever is the result of damage to the hypothalamus from pathologies such as intracranial trauma, intracranial bleeding, or increased intracranial pressure. This type of fever does not respond to antipyretic medications (Grossman, 2014). A fever of 38.3°C (101°F) or higher that lasts for 3 weeks or longer without an identified cause is diagnosed as an FUO.

Physical Effects of Fever

Patients with fever may experience loss of appetite; headache; hot, dry skin; flushed face; thirst; muscle aches; and fatigue. Respirations and pulse rate increase. Young children with high fevers may experience seizures and older adults may have periods of confusion and delirium. Fever blisters may develop in some people as the fever activates the type I herpes simplex virus. Fluid, electrolyte, and acid–base imbalances are potentially dangerous complications of fever.

Treatment of Fever

Fever is an important part of a person's defense mechanisms against infection. Determining the cause of the fever and treating its underlying cause is an important part of patient care. Nursing care related to fever focuses on increasing patient comfort and preventing complications.

If the fever is the result of a bacterial or other type of microbial infection, the appropriate antibiotic or anti-infective may be prescribed. Antipyretic (fever-reducing) drugs, such as aspirin, ibuprofen, or acetaminophen, may be administered in certain circumstances. These drugs reset the elevated set point regulated by the hypothalamus.

The National Reye's Syndrome Foundation, the U.S. Surgeon General, the Food and Drug Administration (FDA), the Centers for Disease Control and Prevention (CDC), the American Academy of Pediatrics (AAP), and the World Health Organization (WHO) recommend that aspirin and combination products containing aspirin not be taken by anyone younger than 19 years during fever-causing or flu-like illnesses (National Reye's Syndrome Foundation, 2012).

Modifications of the external environment may be implemented to increase heat transfer from the internal to the external environment, including the use of cool sponge baths, cool packs, and hypothermia (cooling) blankets. Guidelines for Nursing Care 24-1 outlines the procedure for using a hypothermia blanket. Oral fluids are increased to maintain cellular and intravascular status and prevent dehydration. Simple carbohydrates are included in the diet to prevent tissue breakdown from the hypermetabolic state.

Nursing interventions and expected outcomes for the patient with a fever are outlined in the Examples of Nursing Interventions and Nursing Outcomes Classifications (NIC/NOC) box.

Decreased Body Temperature

Hypothermia is a body temperature below the lower limit of normal. Hypothermia occurs when the compensatory physiologic responses meant to produce and retain heat are overwhelmed by unprotected exposure to cold environments. This may be a result of accidental exposure or impaired perception of cold, which occurs particularly in older adults or the disabled. Chronic conditions—such as alcoholism, malnutrition, and hypothyroidism—increase the risk of hypothermia. Patients in the perioperative period and newborn infants are also at increased risk. Death may occur when body temperature falls below 35°C (95°F), but survival has been reported in isolated cases (such as in drowning in very cold water or burial in snow) when body temperatures have fallen in the range of severe hypothermia (28°C, or 82.4°F). Survival is possible because rates of chemical reactions in the body are slowed, thereby decreasing the metabolic demands for oxygen.

Physical Effects of Hypothermia

Patients with hypothermia may experience poor coordination, slurred speech, poor judgment, amnesia, hallucinations, and stupor. Respirations increase, and the pulse becomes weak and irregular, with lowering blood pressure.

Treatment of Hypothermia

Treatment of hypothermia includes rewarming the patient. Rewarming can be accomplished by covering with additional clothing and blankets, the use of heating blankets and pads, and radiant warmers. Warm fluids are administered either orally or through the intravenous route.

Assessing Temperature

To accurately assess body temperature, the nurse must know what equipment to use, which site to choose, and what method is appropriate. Although the measurement of temperature may be delegated to unlicensed assistive personnel, the nurse is responsible for assessing the findings, assessing the effect of changes in body temperature, and for

GUIDELINES FOR NURSING CARE 24-1

USING A HYPOTHERMIA BLANKET TO REGULATE BODY TEMPERATURE

A hypothermia blanket, or cooling pad, is a blanket-sized aquathermia pad that conducts a cooled solution, usually distilled water, through coils in a plastic blanket or pad. It operates much like an aquathermia pad (discussed in Chapter 32), except that the liquid is cooled instead of heated. Placing a patient on a hypothermia blanket or pad helps to lower body temperature. The nurse monitors the patient's body temperature and can reset the blanket setting accordingly. The blanket also can be preset to maintain a specific body temperature; the device continually monitors the patient's body temperature using a temperature probe (which is inserted rectally or in the esophagus, or placed on the skin) and adjusts the temperature of the circulating liquid accordingly. When applying a hypothermia blanket, follow these steps:

- Apply lanolin or a mixture of lanolin and cold cream to the patient's skin where it will be in contact with the blanket.
- Turn on the blanket and make sure the cooling light is on. Verify that the temperature limits are set within the desired safety range.
- Place the hypothermia blanket on the bed and cover it with a sheet so that the patient's skin does not come in direct contact with the cold blanket. Position the patient on the blanket so that the top edge of the pad is aligned with the patient's neck.

- Lubricate the rectal probe and insert it into the patient's rectum unless contraindicated. Or tuck the skin probe deep into the patient's axilla and tape it in place. For patients who are comatose or anesthetized, use an esophageal probe. Attach the probe to the control panel for the blanket.
- Recheck the thermometer and settings on the control panel.
- Turn and position the patient regularly (every 30 minutes to 1 hour). Keep linens free from condensation. Reapply cream, as needed. Observe the patient's skin for change in color, changes in lips and nail beds, edema, pain, and sensory impairment.
- Monitor vital signs and perform a neurologic assessment, per facility policy, usually every 15 minutes, until the body temperature is stable. In addition, monitor the patient's fluid and electrolyte status.
- Observe for signs of shivering, including verbalized sensations, facial muscle twitching, hyperventilation, or twitching of extremities.
- Turn off the blanket according to facility policy, usually when the patient's body temperature reaches 1 degree above the desired temperature. Continue to monitor the patient's temperature until it stabilizes.

implementing appropriate interventions. The nurse is also responsible for teaching the patient and caregivers about methods of temperature measurement, normal values, and the need to report abnormal findings.

Equipment

Body temperature, measured in degrees, may be assessed with a variety of devices—electronic and digital thermometers, tympanic membrane thermometers, disposable single-use thermometers, temporal artery thermometers, and

automated monitoring devices. Figure 24-1 (on page 586) illustrates several different types of thermometers. No matter which type of thermometer is used, it is very important to follow the manufacturer's instructions to ensure an accurate measurement. Body temperature is documented in either Celsius or Fahrenheit degrees. Table 24-4 (on page 586) provides equivalent Celsius and Fahrenheit values as well as a method for conversion.

Glass thermometers with mercury-filled bulbs have been used in the past for measuring body temperature. They are

EXAMPLES OF NURSING INTERVENTIONS AND NURSING OUTCOMES CLASSIFICATIONS (NIC/NOC)

FEVER/HYPERTHERMIA

Nursing Interventions	Nursing Outcomes
• Monitor temperature as frequently as appropriate. • Monitor blood pressure, pulse, and respirations as appropriate. • Monitor intake and output. • Monitor for fever-related complications. • Administer antipyretic medication as appropriate.	• Vital Signs • Hydration • Thermoregulation • Risk Control: Hyperthermia

From: Bulechek, G. M., Butcher, H. K., Dochterman, J. M., & Wagner, C. M. (Eds.). (2013). *Nursing interventions classification (NIC)*. (6th ed., p. 196). St. Louis: Mosby Elsevier; and Moorhead, S., Johnson, M., Maas, M. L., & Swanson, E. (Eds.). (2013). *Nursing outcomes classification (NOC)*. (5th ed., p. 602). St. Louis: Mosby Elsevier. A full listing of nursing activities for each nursing intervention and outcomes can be found in these books.

FIGURE 24-1. Types of thermometers used to assess body temperature. (**A**) Electronic thermometer. (**B**) Tympanic membrane thermometer. (**C**) Disposable thermometer for measuring oral temperature; the dots change color to indicate temperature. (**D**) Temporal artery thermometer.

not used in health care institutions, based on federal safety recommendations (U.S. Environmental Protection Agency [EPA], 2012). However, patients may still have mercury thermometers at home and may be continuing to use them. Nurses should encourage patients to use alternative devices

Table 24-4 EQUIVALENT CELSIUS AND FAHRENHEIT TEMPERATURES*

CELSIUS	FAHRENHEIT
35.0	95.0
36.0	96.8
36.5	97.6
37.0	98.6
37.5	99.5
38.0	100.4
38.5	101.3
39.0	102.2
40.0	104.0
41.0	105.8

*To convert Celsius to Fahrenheit, multiply by 9/5 and add 32. To convert Fahrenheit to Celsius, subtract 32 and multiply by 5/9.

to measure body temperature and include patient teaching as part of nursing care. Bulb-type glass thermometers containing liquids other than mercury are available. This type of thermometer is prone to breakage and should never be used to take a temperature for a person who is unconscious or irrational, or for infants and young children.

ELECTRONIC AND DIGITAL THERMOMETERS
Electronic and digital thermometers measure oral, rectal, or axillary body temperature over a time period from 1 to 60 seconds, depending on the site and product used. These battery-operated devices provide a numerical temperature display. The devices also have disposable probe covers to reduce the risk of infection transmission. Some models also provide the last measurement, a full 60-second pulse timer, and automatic conversion from the Fahrenheit to the Celsius scale.

TYMPANIC MEMBRANE THERMOMETERS
Tympanic membrane thermometers use infrared sensors to detect heat given off by the tympanic membrane. The probe is covered with a probe cover and inserted into the ear canal tightly enough to seal the opening. The reading takes from 1 to 3 seconds, depending on the product. Studies conflict regarding the accuracy of this method (Davie & Amoore, 2010; Jensen, 2011; Lawson et al., 2007). As such, it is

important to use proper technique and adhere to manufacturer's guidelines for use.

 REMEMBER Noah Shoolin, the toddler described at the beginning of the chapter? Although a tympanic thermometer yields a quick reading, the nurse would need to verify the accuracy of the reading, especially in light of the child's current upset state, possibly by asking the mother if she had taken the child's temperature before coming to the emergency department or by using an alternative method. ●

DISPOSABLE SINGLE-USE THERMOMETERS

Disposable single-use thermometers are nonbreakable and register the temperature within seconds. Because they are used only once, they eliminate the danger of cross-infection and are sometimes used for patients requiring transmission-based precautions.

Temperature-sensitive patches or tape, commonly applied to the abdomen or forehead, change color at different temperature ranges. These devices may be used to screen the temperature of a toddler or young child. A thermometer should be used to reassess the temperature if the color on the tape or patch indicates that the temperature is out of the normal average range.

TEMPORAL ARTERY THERMOMETERS

Temporal artery thermometers measure body temperature by capturing the heat emitted by the skin over the temporal artery. These devices are battery operated and have a temperature display. Lawson et al. (2007) found oral and temporal artery measurements more accurate and precise than those taken by the axillary and tympanic routes.

AUTOMATED MONITORING DEVICES

Automated monitoring devices are used in various health care settings to measure body temperature, pulse, respirations, and blood pressure simultaneously. They require less of the nurse's time, especially when these assessments are required frequently.

Sites and Methods of Assessing Body Temperature

Health agency policies and procedures often specify the site to be used for assessing patients' temperatures. However, the nurse is expected to choose an alternate, appropriate site, and the correct equipment, based on the patient's condition, facility policy and medical orders. Factors affecting site selection include the patient's age, state of consciousness, amount of pain, and other care or treatments (such as oxygen administration) being provided. If a temperature reading is obtained from a site other than the oral route, it is important to document the site of the measurement along with the result to ensure accurate comparison of data. If no site is listed with the documentation, it is generally assumed to be the oral route.

The sites most commonly used to assess body temperature are oral (sublingual), tympanic, temporal artery, rectal, and axillary. An electronic probe is placed under the tongue (sublingual area) of a person's mouth to assess an oral temperature, in the anal canal to assess a rectal temperature, or in an axilla (armpit) to assess an axillary temperature. A probe is placed in the ear to assess a tympanic temperature. Temporal artery thermometers are swiped over the skin covering the temporal artery. Single-use thermometers are placed over the skin, usually the forehead. For most clinical purposes, it is satisfactory to assess an oral, tympanic, temporal artery, axillary, or rectal temperature, provided proper technique is used, the site of the temperature is documented, and normal variations among the methods are considered. Comparing the recordings using two different sites is a method for double-checking the validity of an unusual measurement. The procedures for assessing body temperature at each site, with rationale for each step, are outlined in Skill 24-1 on pages 604–612.

ASSESSING AN ORAL TEMPERATURE

When selecting the oral site, the patient must be able to close his or her mouth around the probe. The probe must remain in the sublingual pocket for the full period of measurement (Davie & Amoore, 2010). If a patient has had either hot or cold food or fluids or has been smoking or chewing gum, the general recommendation is to wait 15 to 30 minutes to allow the oral tissues to return to normal temperature. Oral temperatures should not be taken in people with diseases of the oral cavity and in those who have had surgery of the nose or mouth. In addition, oral temperatures should not be assessed in patients receiving oxygen by mask, because the time it takes to assess a reading is likely to result in a serious drop in the patient's blood oxygen level. Oral temperature readings range from 35.8°C to 37.5°C (96.4°F–99.5°F; Jensen, 2011).

ASSESSING A TYMPANIC MEMBRANE TEMPERATURE

Infrared sensors in the thermometer sense heat from the body given off by the tympanic membrane. The thermometer does not touch the tympanic membrane. This site allows easy and safe measurement of temperature and is readily accessible. However, it should not be used for patients who have drainage from the ear, ear pain, ear infection, or scars on the tympanic membrane. Temperature readings are not significantly altered by the presence of cerumen (earwax) or otitis media (infection of the middle ear). Tympanic temperature readings are approximately equal to oral (Jensen, 2011).

 Concept Mastery Alert

If a patient has drainage from the ear, ear pain, ear infection or scarring on the tympanic membrane on one side, then the opposite ear may be used to measure the tympanic temperature.

ASSESSING A TEMPORAL ARTERY TEMPERATURE

Measurement on the right or left side of the forehead is equally effective. When taking a temporal artery temperature, assess for head coverings. Anything covering the area—such as a hat, hair, wigs, or bandages—would insulate the area, resulting in falsely high readings. If a patient is lying on the side, measure only the side of the head exposed to the environment. Do not measure temporal artery temperature over scar tissue, open lesions, or abrasions. Move the thermometer across the forehead slowly and remain in contact with the skin to ensure accurate results. Temporal artery temperature readings are approximately equal to oral (Jensen, 2011).

ASSESSING AN AXILLARY TEMPERATURE

The axillary site may be used when both oral and rectal sites are contraindicated or when these sites are inaccessible. Place the probe in the center of the axilla; hold the patient's arm by the patient's side until the measurement is complete (Garner & Fendius, 2010). Axillary temperature readings are approximately 1 degree lower than oral (Jensen, 2011).

ASSESSING A RECTAL TEMPERATURE

The rectal temperature, a core temperature, is considered to be one of the most accurate routes. However, many patients are embarrassed at having their temperature taken rectally. The rectal site should not be used in newborns, children with diarrhea, and in patients who have undergone rectal surgery or have a disease of the rectum. Because the insertion of the thermometer into the rectum can slow the heart rate by stimulating the vagus nerve, assessing a rectal temperature for patients with heart disease or after cardiac surgery may not be allowed in some institutions. In addition, assessing a rectal temperature is contraindicated in patients who are neutropenic (have low white blood cell counts, such as in leukemia) and in patients who have certain neurologic disorders (e.g., spinal cord injuries). Do not insert a rectal thermometer into a patient who has a low platelet count. The rectum is very vascular, and a thermometer could cause rectal bleeding. Rectal temperature readings are approximately 1 degree higher than oral (Jensen, 2011).

PULSE

The peripheral **pulse** is a throbbing sensation that can be palpated over a peripheral artery, such as the radial artery or the carotid artery. Peripheral pulses are palpable when blood is ejected as the left ventricle contracts and pumps blood into the vascular system. As the heart contracts to eject blood into an already full aorta, smooth muscle in the arteries expands to compensate for the increase in pressure of the blood. This rhythmic distention of the arterial walls is the result of surges of blood as the heart beats. The distention of the arteries moves along the arterial system until it reaches the capillaries, where vessel walls lack elasticity and peripheral resistance to blood flow. The peripheral pulses may be felt wherever an artery passes over a solid structure, such as bone or cartilage.

Characteristics of the peripheral pulse, including rate, quality (strong or weak), rhythm, and volume of blood ejected with each heartbeat (also referred to as stroke volume), are indicators of the effectiveness of the heart as a pump and the adequacy of peripheral blood flow. The heart rate affects the amount of blood ejected by the heart with each beat by determining the frequency with which the ventricle contracts. The quality and rhythm affect how much blood is ejected and whether the beat is regular in rhythm. Further information about the control and mechanisms involved with blood flow and stroke volume is provided later with the discussion of blood pressure.

An apical pulse may also be auscultated (listened to) over the apex of the heart as the heart beats. Heart sounds, which are produced by closure of the valves of the heart, are characterized as "lub-dub." The apical pulse is the result of closure of the mitral and tricuspid valves ("lub") and aortic and pulmonic valves ("dub"). The combination of the two sounds is counted as one beat.

Further information related to the characteristics of pulses is discussed later in this chapter.

Physiology of the Pulse

The pulse is regulated by the autonomic nervous system through the sinoatrial (SA) node (the pacemaker) of the heart. Parasympathetic stimulation of the SA node via the vagus nerve decreases the heart rate, and sympathetic stimulation of the SA node increases the heart rate and force of contraction. Additional information about the conduction system and function of the heart is discussed in Chapter 38. The pulse rate is the number of pulsations felt over a peripheral artery or heard over the apex of the heart in 1 minute. This rate normally corresponds to the same rate at which the heart is beating.

Factors Affecting the Pulse

Many factors can affect both the heart rate and volume; however, compensatory mechanisms attempt to maintain a sufficient supply of blood to the cells at all times. For example, when the stroke volume decreases, such as when the blood volume is decreased because of hemorrhage, the heart rate increases to try to maintain the same cardiac output. Conversely, in a physically fit athlete whose heart pumps a maximum volume of blood per stroke, the heart rate may be at the low range or below the range of normal, yet the body cells remain adequately supplied. When assessing a patient's pulse, consider factors that could influence the pulse rate, including age, gender, physical activity, fever, stress, medication use, and the presence of disease.

Age and Gender

Women on average have slightly higher pulse rates than men. Pulse rate decreases as a person ages due to decreased metabolic rate.

Physical Activity

The pulse rate increases with exercise. However, well-conditioned athletes may have a significantly decreased pulse rate. This is due to greater efficiency and strength of the heart muscle from regular cardiovascular exercise.

Fever and Stress

An elevated body temperature causes increased pulse rate due to increased metabolic demands and compensatory mechanisms to increase heat loss. Increased levels of stress cause an increased pulse rate. Common sources of stress associated with increased pulse rate include pain, fear, and anxiety.

Medications

There are many medications that can cause alterations in pulse rate. Some medications increase a patient's pulse rate and others decrease a patient's pulse rate. Changes in pulse related to medication use can be an intended effect or an unintended adverse effect.

Disease

Many acute and chronic health conditions affect a patient's pulse rate. Some diseases, such as chronic obstructive pulmonary disease and pneumonia, impair oxygenation and alter the pulse rate. Other health problems, such as sepsis, alter the pulse rate as a result of the body's response to infection.

Normal Pulse Rate

The normal pulse rate for adolescents and adults ranges from 60 to 100 beats/min. The pulse rate increases and decreases in response to a variety of physiologic mechanisms. It might also be altered by any of the factors discussed previously. Normal pulse rates change across the lifespan, gradually diminishing from birth to adulthood (see Table 24-1, p. 581).

Increased Pulse Rate

As the heart rate increases, cardiac output usually also increases. However, **tachycardia**, a rapid heart rate, decreases cardiac filling time, which, in turn, decreases stroke volume and cardiac output. An adult has tachycardia when the pulse rate is 100 to 180 beats/min. Box 24-3 lists factors that may contribute to tachycardia.

Box 24-3   FACTORS CONTRIBUTING TO TACHYCARDIA

- A decrease in blood pressure, such as occurs with blood loss, when the heart's compensatory mechanisms attempt to meet the need for increased cardiac output
- An elevated temperature, which usually causes an increase of about 7 to 10 beats/min for each 0.6°C (1°F) of elevation above normal
- Any condition resulting in poor oxygenation of blood, for example, chronic pulmonary disease or anemia
- Exercise, when the heart's compensatory ability attempts to meet the need for increased blood circulation
- Prolonged application of heat
- Pain
- Strong emotions, such as fear, anger, anxiety, and surprise
- Some medications (e.g., epinephrine [Adrenalin®])

Decreased Pulse Rate

Bradycardia is a pulse rate below 60 beats/min in an adult. The pulse rate is normally slower during sleep in men and in people who are thin. It slows during hypothermia as metabolic processes decrease. The pulse also tends to become slower with aging. Some medications, whose action is specific to the work of the heart, slow the heart rate while also strengthening the force of contraction to increase cardiac output.

Sinus bradycardia results when the SA node generates a slower-than-normal impulse rate. This type of bradycardia occurs at times when metabolic needs are decreased (e.g., during sleep, in hypothermia, in trained athletes at rest); from certain medications, such as beta blockers; from vagal stimulation (e.g., from bearing down to have a bowel movement), during suctioning of respiratory secretions, with severe pain, and in increased intracranial pressure and MI. The nurse should immediately report bradycardia associated with difficult breathing, changes in level of consciousness, decreased blood pressure, ECG changes, and angina (heart pain). Emergency treatment consists of administering atropine intravenously to block vagal stimulation and to restore normal heart rate.

Pulse Amplitude and Quality

The pulse amplitude describes the quality of the pulse in terms of its fullness and reflects the strength of left ventricular contraction. It is assessed by the feel of the blood flow through the vessel. The amplitude of each pulse beat is normally strong at all areas where an artery can be palpated. There are several systems for grading the amplitude of arterial pulses. Nurses should be familiar with the system in use at their facility or institution. Table 24-5 presents a scale often used to describe and document pulse amplitude. In addition, the peripheral pulse may be described and documented as full and bounding when it is forceful or weak and thready when it is feeble.

Pulse Rhythm

Pulse rhythm is the pattern of the beats and the pauses between them. Pulse rhythm is normally regular; the beats

Table 24-5   PULSE AMPLITUDE

GRADE	DESCRIPTION
0	Absent, unable to palpate
+1	Diminished, weaker than expected
+2	Brisk, expected (normal)
+3	Bounding

Adapted from Hirsch, A. T., et al. (2006). ACC/AHA 2005 guidelines for the management of patients with peripheral arterial disease (lower extremity, renal, mesenteric, and abdominal aortic): executive summary a collaborative report from the American Association for Vascular Surgery/Society for Vascular Surgery, Society for Cardiovascular Angiography and Interventions, Society for Vascular Medicine and Biology, Society of Interventional Radiology, and the ACC/AHA Task Force on Practice Guidelines (Writing Committee to Develop Guidelines for the Management of Patients With Peripheral Arterial Disease). *Circulation, 113*(11), e463–e654.

and the pauses between occur at regular intervals. An irregular pulse rhythm occurs when the beats and pauses between beats occur at unequal intervals. An irregular pattern of heartbeats is called a **dysrhythmia**. Report any irregularity in the heartbeat immediately.

Assessing the Pulse

The pulse may be assessed by palpating peripheral arteries or by auscultating the apical pulse with a stethoscope. It is important to know how to use a stethoscope and which site and method are appropriate.

 REMEMBER Tomas Esposito, the middle-aged man requiring transmission-based infection-control measures and assessment? Although the nurse had difficulty auscultating his heart and lung sounds, the nurse would need to assess both his radial and apical pulse. It is possible that by palpating his radial pulse and then attempting to auscultate his apical pulse and not hearing anything, the nurse might have a clue leading her to suspect that the stethoscope was not functioning properly. ●

Equipment

Nurses most often assess the pulse by using their fingers to palpate (feel) the radial artery. However, various types of equipment may be used to assess the pulse. For example, the stethoscope is typically used to auscultate the apical pulse. In critical or emergency care, a cardiac monitor may be used to assess the apical pulse. The monitor produces a graph or digital reading of the pulse rate and amplitude.

STETHOSCOPE

The acoustical stethoscope, the most common type used, has an amplifying mechanism connected to earpieces by tubing (Fig. 24-2). The most common amplifying mechanisms of a stethoscope are the *diaphragm,* which is a large, flat disk, and the *bell,* which has a hollowed, upright, curved appearance. The diaphragm is more useful for hearing high-frequency sounds, such as respiratory sounds, because it screens out low-frequency sounds. The bell screens out high-frequency sounds and is more useful for hearing low-frequency sounds, such as those commonly made by the heart and the blood within the vessels.

FIGURE 24-2. A stethoscope. The two sides of the stethoscope amplifier are used for different purposes: the diaphragm is more useful for hearing high-frequency sounds; the bell is more useful for hearing low-frequency sounds.

The earpieces of the stethoscope should be selected to fit one's ear canals comfortably and snugly for the most effective auscultation. The tips should be directed into the ear canal, not against the ear itself. They should be large enough to block out extraneous noises in the environment when the stethoscope is being used.

DOPPLER ULTRASOUND

A Doppler ultrasound device may be used to assess pulses that are difficult to palpate or auscultate. The device has an audio unit with an ultrasound transducer. Techniques for assessing pulses with a Doppler ultrasound device are outlined in Guidelines for Nursing Care 24-2.

Sites and Methods of Assessing the Pulse

Nurses must know the correct site and method for assessing the pulse for individual patients. Although peripheral pulses are most commonly assessed, an apical pulse or an apical-radial pulse should be assessed in certain situations, described later.

ASSESSING PERIPHERAL ARTERIAL PULSES

Many peripheral artery sites might be used to assess the pulse by palpation. Figure 24-3 illustrates the most commonly used

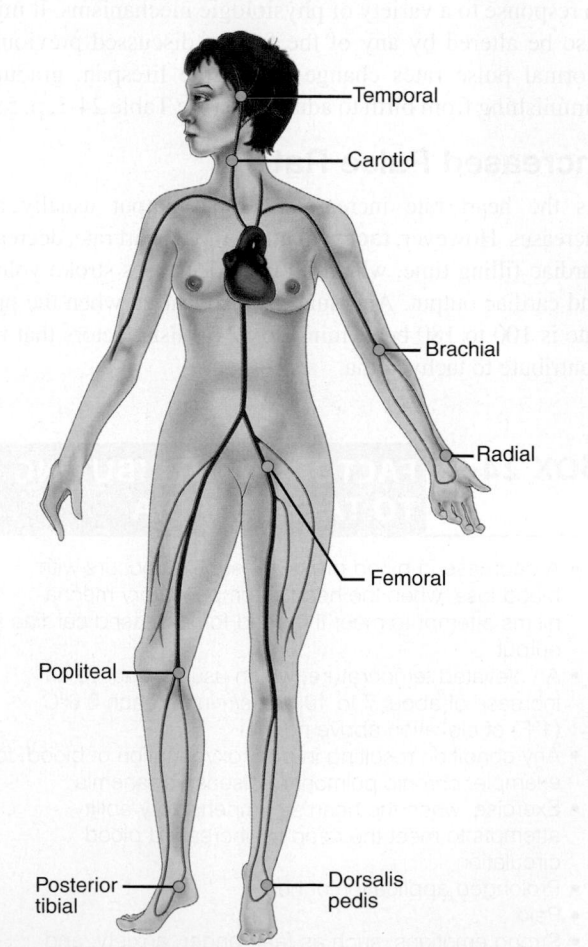

FIGURE 24-3. These arteries are located near the surface of the body. The pulse can be detected in any of these sites by light palpation.

GUIDELINES FOR NURSING CARE 24-2

ASSESSING PERIPHERAL PULSE USING A PORTABLE DOPPLER ULTRASOUND DEVICE

- Determine the need to use a Doppler ultrasound device for pulse assessment.
- Select the appropriate peripheral site based on assessment data.
- Move the patient's clothing to expose only the site chosen.
- Remove the Doppler from the charger and turn it on. Make sure that the volume is set at low.
- Apply conducting gel to the site where you are auscultating the pulse.
- Hold the Doppler base in your nondominant hand. With your dominant hand, place the Doppler probe tip in the gel. Adjust the volume as needed. Move the Doppler tip around until the pulse is heard (see Figure).
- Using a watch with a second hand, count the heartbeat for 1 minute.
- Remove the Doppler tip and turn the Doppler off. Wipe excess gel off of the patient's skin with a tissue.
- Place a small × over the spot where the pulse is located with an indelible pen, depending on facility policy. Marking the site allows for easier future assessment. It can also make palpating the pulse easier since the exact location of the pulse is known.
- Cover the patient and help the patient to a position of comfort.

- Wipe off any gel remaining on the Doppler probe with a tissue. Clean the Doppler probe per facility policy or manufacturer's recommendations.
- Return the Doppler to the charge base.
- Record pulse rate, rhythm, and site, and the fact that it was obtained with a Doppler ultrasound device.

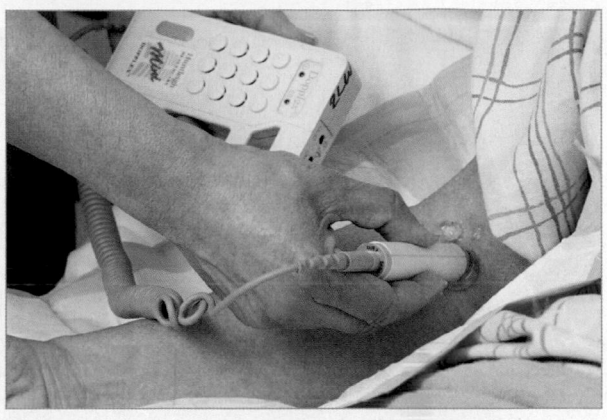

sites. Of these sites, the radial pulse site is assessed most often in children and adults. Skill 24-2 on pages 612–614 describes the steps for assessing a peripheral pulse via palpation.

Circulation to the legs and feet may be assessed at the femoral, popliteal, posterior tibial, or dorsalis pedis sites. The carotid pulse site is used during emergency assessments, such as for patients who are in shock or have had a cardiac arrest. When taking a carotid pulse, lightly palpate only one side at a time to prevent any decrease in cerebrovascular circulation. The brachial pulse site is used most often for infants in these situations.

ASSESSING THE APICAL PULSE

If a peripheral pulse is difficult to assess accurately because it is irregular, weak, or very rapid, the apical rate should be assessed using a stethoscope. An apical pulse is also assessed when giving medications that alter heart rate and rhythm. Apical pulse measurement is also the preferred method of pulse assessment for infants and children less than 2 years of age (Jarvis, 2012). The contraction of the heart can be heard in the space between the fifth and the sixth ribs, about 8 cm (3 inches) to the left of the median line and slightly below the nipple (Guidelines for Nursing Care 24-3 on page 592). The apical rate of an infant can also be easily palpated with the fingertips as well as being auscultated.

ASSESSING THE APICAL-RADIAL PULSE

Counting of the pulse at the apex of the heart and at the radial artery simultaneously is used to assess the apical-radial pulse rate. A difference between the apical and radial pulse rates is called the **pulse deficit** and indicates that all of the heartbeats are not reaching the peripheral arteries or are too weak to be palpated. Guidelines for Nursing Care 24-4 (on page 592) outlines the technique for taking an apical-radial pulse.

RESPIRATIONS

Respiration involves ventilation, diffusion, and perfusion. Ventilation (or breathing) is movement of gases in and out of the lungs; inspiration (or inhalation) is the act of breathing in, and expiration (or exhalation) is the act of breathing out. Unlike heart rate, which is controlled by the autonomic nervous system, ventilation has both autonomic and voluntary control. Diffusion is the exchange of oxygen and carbon dioxide between the alveoli of the lungs and the circulating blood. Perfusion is the exchange of oxygen and carbon dioxide between the circulating blood and tissue cells.

Although nurses assess the manifestations of changes in all of these respiratory events, the component that is measured as a vital sign is ventilation, more commonly called **respirations**. Respiratory system assessment is described further in Chapter 25. Measuring respirations allows for baseline assessment of respiratory function. Respiratory rate can give early indications of physiologic deterioration (Parkes, 2011).

Physiology of Respirations

The rate and depth of breathing can change in response to tissue demands. These changes are brought about by the inhibition or stimulation of the respiratory muscles by the

GUIDELINES FOR NURSING CARE 24-3

ASSESSING THE APICAL PULSE

- Use an alcohol swab to clean the diaphragm of the stethoscope. Use another swab to clean the earpieces if necessary.
- Assist the patient to a sitting or reclining position and expose the chest area; move the patient's clothing to expose only the apical site.
- Hold the stethoscope diaphragm against the palm of your hand for a few seconds (to warm it).

- Palpate the space between the fifth and sixth ribs (fifth intercostal space), and move to the left midclavicular line. Place the diaphragm over the apex of the heart (see Figure).
- Listen for heart sounds ("lub-dub"). Each "lub-dub" counts as one beat.
- Using a watch with a second hand, count the heartbeat for 1 minute.
- Clean the diaphragm of the stethoscope with an alcohol swab.

The apical pulse is usually found at (**A**) the fifth intercostal space just inside the midclavicular line and can be heard (**B**) over the apex of the heart.

---

respiratory centers in the brain. Activation of the respiratory centers occurs via impulses from chemoreceptors located in the aortic arch and carotid arteries, via stretch and irritant receptors in the lungs, and via receptors in muscles and joints. An increase in carbon dioxide is the most powerful respiratory stimulant, causing an increase in respiratory depth and rate. The cerebral cortex of the brain allows voluntary control of breathing, such as when singing or playing a musical instrument. See Chapter 38 for a further discussion of respiratory physiology.

The rate and depth of inhalation and exhalation are normally smooth, effortless, and without conscious effort. However, factors such as environmental changes and patho-

physiologic alterations in various body systems may result in increases or decreases in respiratory rate and depth.

Factors Affecting Respirations

Many different factors affect respiratory rate and depth. These factors include exercise; respiratory and cardiovascular disease; alterations in fluid, electrolyte, and acid–base balances; medications; trauma; infection; pain; and emotions. Box 24-4 outlines the factors that affect respiratory rate, depth, and movements. Refer to the accompanying Research in Nursing display regarding the effects of music on the respiratory rate, heart rate, and blood pressure of postoperative abdominal surgery patients.

GUIDELINES FOR NURSING CARE 24-4

TAKING AN APICAL-RADIAL PULSE

The following techniques are recommended to assess an apical-radial pulse rate:

- Two nurses are needed; one listens with a stethoscope over the apex of the heart for the heartbeat, and the other counts the rate at the radial artery.
- The patient's chest wall is exposed so that the stethoscope can be placed directly on the skin of the chest wall.

- One watch with a sweep second hand is placed, so that both nurses can read it simultaneously.
- The nurses determine where they can best hear and feel the pulse and decide on a time to start counting, such as when the second hand on the watch is at a specified place (e.g., the number 12).
- Both nurses count for 1 full minute and record their counts.

BOX 24-4 FACTORS AFFECTING RESPIRATORY RATE, DEPTH, AND MOVEMENTS

- **Age:** The respiratory rate decreases with age, ranging from a normal range of 30 to 55 breaths/min in a newborn to 12 to 20 breaths/min in an adult.
- **Exercise:** Exercise increases respiratory rate and depth.
- **Acid–base balance:** Alterations in acid–base balance (especially acidosis) commonly result in increased rate and depth of respirations (hyperventilation).
- **Brain lesions:** Lesions of the brain (such as hemorrhage or tumors) or brainstem can cause a change in both the depth and rate of respirations, most commonly manifested as Cheyne-Stokes respirations.
- **Increased altitude:** As an adaptation to higher altitudes, healthy people may exhibit Cheyne-Stokes respirations, especially when asleep. Higher altitudes also increase respiratory rate and depth prior to adaptation by increasing hemoglobin levels.

- **Respiratory diseases:** Any alterations in the normal respiratory structures may result in changes in respiratory rate, depth, and patterns, most often manifested as difficult breathing, using accessory muscles of respiration (such as the intercostal muscles), and increased rate. The depth may be shallower. Smoking can alter the pulmonary airways, resulting in an increase in respiratory rate at rest.
- **Anemia:** Anemia, a decrease in oxygen-carrying hemoglobin, may result in an increased rate of respirations.
- **Anxiety:** Anxiety can cause sighing type respirations (increased depth) and increased rate.
- **Medications:** Medications—such as narcotics, sedatives, and general anesthetics—slow respiratory rate and depth. Other drugs, including amphetamines and cocaine, may increase rate and depth.
- **Acute pain:** Acute pain increases respiratory rate but may decrease respiratory depth.

Normal Respiratory Rate

Under normal conditions, healthy adults breathe about 12 to 20 times each minute; infants and young children breathe more rapidly (see Table 24-1, p. 581). Normal, unlabored respiration is called **eupnea**. The relationship of one respiration to four heartbeats is fairly consistent in healthy people.

 THINK back to Noah Shoolin, the 2-year-old brought to the emergency department. The nurse would anticipate that the child's respiratory rate would be increased most likely as a result of his screaming and emotional upset. ●

Increased Respiratory Rate

Tachypnea, an increased respiratory rate, may occur in response to an increased metabolic rate, such as when a person has a fever. Cells require more oxygen at this time and produce more carbon dioxide that must be removed. The rate increases as much as 4 breaths/min with every 0.6°C (1°F) that the temperature rises above normal. Any condition

RESEARCH IN NURSING

BRIDGING THE GAP TO EVIDENCE-BASED PRACTICE

Music and Postoperative Recovery

Surgery and postoperative pain cause increased heart rate and blood pressure. Postoperative pain can alter respiratory function, and interfere with deep breathing, coughing, and moving. An important part of nursing care in the postoperative period includes nursing interventions to prevent complications from surgery. Listening to music can focus attention, facilitate breathing, and stimulate the relaxation response, aiding in pain control. Decreased pain allows patients to participate in important activities to prevent postoperative complications.

Related Research

Vaajoki, A., Kankkunen, P., Pietilä, A.M., & Vehviläinen-Julkunen, K. (2011). Music as a nursing intervention: Effects of music listening on blood pressure, heart rate, and respiratory rate in abdominal surgery patients. *Nursing and Health Sciences, 13*(4), 412–418.

The aim of this study was to evaluate the effects of music listening on blood pressure, heart rate, and respiratory rate on operation day, and on the first, second, and third postoperative days in abdominal surgery patients. Abdominal surgery patients were assigned every second week to the music group (n = 83) or to the control group (n = 85) for 25 months. Patients in the music group chose their favorite music. In

the music group, the respiratory rate was significantly lower after intervention on both the first and second postoperative days compared with the control group. A significant reduction in systolic blood pressure was demonstrated in the group that received music compared with the control group on both the first and second postoperative days. There were no differences between the two groups in diastolic blood pressure or heart rate.

Evaluation of the long-term effects of music on physiologic factors showed that the respiratory rate in the music group was significantly lower compared with the control group.

Relevance to Nursing Practice

Listening to music can significantly lower systolic blood pressure and respiratory rate in the postoperative period and was identified as a positive experience for patients. Nurses should strengthen their knowledge of the benefits of music listening as a nonpharmacologic intervention. Music can be used as part of the healing environment to support surgical patients during their recovery period, and can positively influence patient's experiences while in the hospital.

For additional research, visit thePoint.

causing an increase in carbon dioxide and a decrease in oxygen in the blood increases the rate and depth of respirations, **hyperventilation**. Respiratory diseases such as acute pneumonia or may cause tachypnea or hyperventilation.

Decreased Respiratory Rate

Bradypnea, a decrease in respiratory rate, occurs in some pathologic conditions. An increase in intracranial pressure depresses the respiratory center, resulting in irregular or shallow breathing, slow breathing, or both. Certain drugs, such as opioids (e.g., morphine, hydromorphone), can depress the respiratory rate.

Respiratory Depth and Rhythm

The depth of respirations normally varies from shallow to deep. The depth of each respiration is about the same when resting or sleeping. Periodically, each person automatically inhales deeply (sighs), filling the lungs with more air than with the usual depth of respiration.

Certain terms are used to describe the nature and depth of respirations. **Apnea** refers to periods during which there is no breathing. If apnea lasts longer than 4 to 6 minutes, brain damage and death might occur. **Dyspnea** is difficult or labored breathing. A dyspneic patient usually has rapid, shallow respirations and appears anxious. Dyspneic people can often breathe more easily in an upright position, a condition known as **orthopnea**. While sitting or standing, gravity lowers organs in the abdominal cavity away from the diaphragm. This gives the lungs more room for expansion within the chest, allowing the intake of more air with each breath. Table 24-6 describes and illustrates various respiratory patterns.

 ## Assessing Respirations

The nurse assesses respiratory rate (breaths per minute), depth (deep or shallow), and rhythm (regular or irregular) by inspection (observing and listening) or by listening with the stethoscope. Other methods of assessing respiratory effectiveness include monitoring arterial blood gas results and using a pulse oximeter to determine oxygenation of blood. A description of a pulse oximeter and a procedure for using it are found in Chapter 38. Skill 24-3 on pages 614–615 describes how to assess the respiratory rate. Further assessments of respirations are described in Chapter 25.

BLOOD PRESSURE

Blood pressure refers to the force of the moving blood against arterial walls. Maximum blood pressure is exerted on the walls of arteries when the left ventricle of the heart contracts and pushes blood through the aortic valve into the aorta at the beginning of systole. The pressure rises as the ventricle contracts (systole) and falls as the heart relaxes (diastole). This continuous contraction and relaxation of the left ventricle creates a pressure wave that is transmitted through the arterial system (Grossman, 2014). The highest pressure, created during ventricular contraction, is the **systolic pressure**. When the heart rests between beats during ventricular diastole, the pressure drops. The lowest pressure present on arterial walls at this time is the **diastolic pressure**. The difference between the systolic and diastolic pressures is called the **pulse pressure**. Additional information about the function of the heart is discussed in Chapter 38.

Stroke volume and heart rate determine cardiac output (discussed in Chapter 38). Cardiac output and peripheral resistance determine both systolic and diastolic pressures. Peripheral resistance reflects the viscosity (thickness of the blood) and the changes in the radius of the arterioles.

Blood pressure is measured in millimeters of mercury (mm Hg) and is recorded as a fraction. The numerator is the systolic pressure; the denominator is the diastolic pressure. For example, if the blood pressure is 120/80 mm Hg,

Table 24-6 PATTERNS OF RESPIRATIONS

	DESCRIPTION	PATTERN	ASSOCIATED FEATURES
Normal	12–20 breaths/min Regular		Normal pattern
Tachypnea	>24 breaths/min Shallow		Fever, anxiety, exercise, respiratory disorders
Bradypnea	<10 breaths/min Regular		Depression of the respiratory center by medications, brain damage
Hyperventilation	Increased rate and depth		Extreme exercise, fear, diabetic ketoacidosis (Kussmaul's respirations)
Hypoventilation	Decreased rate and depth; irregular		Overdose of narcotics or anesthetics
Cheyne-Stokes respirations	Alternating periods of deep, rapid breathing followed by periods of apnea; regular		Drug overdose, heart failure, increased intracranial pressure, renal failure
Biot's respirations	Varying depth and rate of breathing, followed by periods of apnea; irregular		Meningitis, severe brain damage

120 represents the systolic pressure, and 80 represents the diastolic pressure. The pulse pressure, in this case, is 40 mm Hg.

Physiology of Blood Pressure

Arterial walls contain elastic tissue that allows them to stretch and distend (called compliance) as blood enters with each ventricular contraction. When the heart rests between each beat, the walls of the arteries return to their original position, although pressure in them does not drop to zero. The arterioles offer resistance to the pressure of the blood and keep the blood entering the capillaries in a continuous flow rather than in spurts. Therefore, the elasticity of the arterial walls, in addition to the resistance of the arterioles, helps to maintain normal blood pressure. With increased age, the walls of arterioles become less elastic, which interferes with their ability to stretch and dilate. This can subsequently limit adequate blood flow and contribute to rising pressure within the vascular system.

Although blood moves through the circulatory system from areas of higher pressure to areas of lower pressure, blood pressure is controlled by various short-term and long-term mechanisms. These mechanisms regulate the blood pressure so that blood flow (and pressure) remains relatively constant.

Short-term Regulation of Blood Pressure

The mechanisms for short-term blood pressure regulation (occurring over minutes or hours) are primarily neural (nerve) and humoral (pertaining to body fluids). These mechanisms correct temporary changes in pressure that occur during activities such as changing position or exercising, and are also responsible for maintaining blood pressure during life-threatening situations. In addition, increased cardiac output (from a stronger contraction and increased stroke volume) results in an increased blood pressure while a weak contraction of the heart with decreased cardiac output causes a decrease in blood pressure.

The neural centers for blood pressure regulation are located in the brain in an area called the cardiovascular center. The cardiovascular center transmits parasympathetic impulses to the heart via the vagus nerve and sympathetic impulses to the heart and blood vessels via the spinal cord and peripheral sympathetic nerves. Stimulating the vagus nerve slows the heart rate; sympathetic stimulation increases the heart rate.

 Concept Mastery Alert

The vagus nerve and parasympathetic stimulation go hand-in-hand. So parasympathetic slows while sympathetic speeds.

Pressure-sensitive receptors, called baroreceptors, are located in the heart and walls of arteries (such as the aortic arch and carotid). They are stimulated by changes in stretch of the blood vessel as blood pressure changes and send impulses to the cardiovascular center to initiate the appropriate changes in heart rate and vascular smooth muscle. For example, blood pressure normally decreases when rising from a lying to an upright position, resulting in decreased stretch of baroreceptors. In response, heart rate and peripheral vascular resistance increase in turn to increase blood pressure. During life-threatening situations, such as a serious hemorrhage, the same mechanisms are activated.

Many different humoral mechanisms, along with hormones, also help regulate blood pressure. Epinephrine, a sympathetic neurotransmitter, is released by the adrenal gland to increase heart rate and contractility, thereby increasing cardiac output. The renin-angiotensin-aldosterone system, through angiotensinogen II, causes vasoconstriction in the arterioles. This leads to increased peripheral vascular resistance as a short-term mechanism, and also increases sodium and water retention by the kidneys to increase circulatory fluid volume, thus increasing blood pressure as a long-term mechanism (see discussion in the next section). Vasopressin (antidiuretic hormone [ADH]) is released from the posterior pituitary when stimulated by decreased blood volume and blood pressure, or by an increased osmolality of body fluids. It has a direct vasoconstricting effect on blood vessels, increasing peripheral resistance.

Long-term Regulation of Blood Pressure

Long-term mechanisms are responsible for the ongoing regulation of blood pressure. These mechanisms regulate extracellular fluid volume through the kidneys. They function by regulating blood pressure for an individual person's equilibrium point. Arterial pressure rises when the body contains too much extracellular fluid. In response, increased amounts of sodium and fluid are excreted by the kidneys to return the blood pressure to the person's equilibrium point. When blood pressure decreases due to decreased extracellular fluid, the opposite effect occurs. Extracellular fluid volume regulates blood pressure directly by increasing cardiac output and renal blood flow and indirectly by autoregulation of blood flow, in which autoregulatory mechanisms redirect blood flow to various blood tissues.

Factors Affecting Blood Pressure

Because of the many factors that influence blood pressure, a single blood pressure measurement is not necessarily significant. Box 24-5 (on page 596) lists factors that commonly cause variations in blood pressure.

Normal Blood Pressure

Studies of healthy people indicate that blood pressure can be within a wide range and still be normal. Because of individual differences, it is important to know the normal blood pressure of a particular person. A rise or fall of 20 to 30 mm Hg in a person's blood pressure is significant, even if it is within the generally accepted normal range. Although blood pressure varies constantly, sustained long-term changes are not considered normal. Table 24-7 (on page 596) lists the categories for blood pressure levels in adults.

Box 24-5 FACTORS CONTRIBUTING TO BLOOD PRESSURE VARIATIONS IN HEALTHY PEOPLE

- **Age:** The older adult has decreased elasticity of the arteries, which increases peripheral resistance and, therefore, increases blood pressure.
- **Circadian rhythm:** Normal fluctuations occur during the day. The blood pressure is usually lowest on arising in the morning. Blood pressure has been noted to rise as much as 5 to 10 mm Hg by late afternoon, and gradually falls again during sleep.
- **Gender:** Women usually have lower blood pressure than men of the same age until menopause.
- **Food intake:** Blood pressure increases after eating food.
- **Exercise:** Systolic blood pressure rises during periods of exercise and strenuous activity.

- **Weight:** Blood pressure is usually higher in people who are obese than in those who are thin.
- **Emotional state:** Emotions, such as anger, fear, excitement, and pain, generally cause the blood pressure to rise, but the pressure falls to normal when the situation passes.
- **Body position:** Blood pressure tends to be lower in a prone or supine position than when sitting or standing.
- **Race:** Race is a factor in increased blood pressure (hypertension), which is more prevalent and more severe in African American men and women.
- **Drugs/Medications:** Oral contraceptives cause a mild increase in blood pressure in many women.

The American Heart Association (AHA) recommends that blood pressure readings be measured on two or more subsequent occasions before determining if the blood pressure is outside acceptable parameters (AHA, 2012). Measurements should be taken after the patient rests for at least 5 minutes and has not consumed caffeine or smoked for 30 minutes before the measurement.

Increased Blood Pressure

Hypertension, one of the most common health problems, is blood pressure that is above normal for a sustained period. A diagnosis of hypertension is made when the systolic pressure is 140 mm Hg or higher or the diastolic pressure is 90 mm Hg or higher. The AHA (2012) estimates that 76.4 million adults in the United States have been diagnosed with hypertension. Of this number, the prevalence of hypertension is greater in African American adults than in White or Hispanic American adults. Its prevalence is also greater in older adults. This trend can be expected to continue with the aging of the "baby boomers," as the number of people with hypertension increases with aging. In addition, overweight and obesity is on the rise in youth younger than 18 years old. As a result, prehypertension and high blood pressure are also becoming more common in this age group. African American and Mexican American youth are more likely to have high blood pressure and prehypertension than White youth. Also, boys are at higher risk for high blood pressure than girls (National Heart Blood and Lung Institute [NHBLI], 2011). Hypertension is a major risk factor for heart disease and is the most important risk factor associated with stroke. It is often called "the silent killer" because there are few symptoms beyond increased blood pressure. The NHBLI has outlined standards for diagnosing hypertension (see Table 24-7).

The two major classifications of hypertension are primary hypertension and secondary hypertension. Primary hypertension (also called essential hypertension) has no known cause. It is characterized by an increase above normal in both the systolic and diastolic pressures. Secondary hypertension, which is much less common than primary hypertension, is caused by another disease condition. Some of the common causes of secondary hypertension are kidney disease, disorders of the adrenal cortex, and disorders of the aorta.

The basis for hypertension is thought to be dysfunction of the neurohormonal system. Overactivation of both angiotensin and aldosterone result in an increase in blood pressure. Over time, this sustained increase results in a permanent remodeling and thickening of the blood vessels. As a result, there is increased peripheral resistance and a backup of pressure to organs affected by the vascular system, such as the brain, heart, and kidneys. Disorders resulting from hypertension include thickening of the myocardium, enlargement of the ventricles, congestive heart failure, MI, stroke, and kidney damage.

There are many risk factors for the development of hypertension. Significant risks are a family history of hypertension, race, aging, and metabolic disorders such as type 2 diabetes

Table 24-7 CATEGORIES FOR BLOOD PRESSURE LEVELS IN ADULTS (AGES 18 AND OLDER)

CATEGORY	BLOOD PRESSURE LEVEL (MM HG)		
	Systolic		Diastolic
Normal*	<120	and	<80
Prehypertension	120–139	or	80–89
High Blood Pressure			
Stage 1	140–159	or	90–99
Stage 2	≥160	or	≥100

*In regard to risk of heart disease, optimal is defined as less than 120/80 mm Hg.

Source: National Heart, Lung, and Blood Institute (NHLBI). National Institutes of Health (NIH). (2011). What is high blood pressure? Available at http://www.nhlbi.nih.gov/health/health-topics/topics/hbp/printall-index.html.

mellitus, obesity, and high cholesterol. Lifestyle risk factors include a sedentary lifestyle; high dietary intake of salt, fats, and calories; use of oral contraceptives in women; and sleep apnea. Other high-risk factors include cigarette smoking and regular alcohol consumption.

 REMEMBER Mrs. Renfrow, the wife of a man who is overweight and diagnosed with hypertension? The nurse would need to incorporate information about various risk factors for developing hypertension as well as information about risk related to hypertension in the teaching plan for Mrs. Renfrow. ●

Hypertension can be controlled by medications and lifestyle changes. The categories of antihypertensive medications include diuretics (to decrease fluid volume), beta-adrenergic blockers (to block sympathetic stimulation and decrease cardiac output), vasodilators and calcium channel blockers (to relax smooth muscles of arterioles and decrease peripheral vascular resistance), and angiotensin-converting enzyme (ACE) inhibitors (to prevent vasoconstriction by angiotensin II and decrease circulatory fluid volume by reducing aldosterone production). Lifestyle changes include following a low-calorie, low-fat diet; losing excess weight and maintaining weight loss; limiting alcohol intake; eliminating smoking; reducing salt intake; and engaging in regular physical activity. Nurses can influence the health of the public through screenings, education, and referrals. See Promoting Health Literacy in Patients With Hypertension for more information.

Decreased Blood Pressure

Hypotension is below-normal blood pressure. A consistently low blood pressure (e.g., a systolic reading of 90–115 mm Hg) is normal in some adults, such as trained athletes. However, most cases of hypotension are the result of pathology. Pathologic hypotension might result from vasodilation of the arterioles, failure of the heart to function as an effective pump, or loss of blood volume (such as with a hemorrhage). The nurse should immediately report assessments of hypotension, tachycardia, pallor, increased sweating, and confusion.

Orthostatic hypotension (postural hypotension) is a decrease in systolic blood pressure of 20 mm Hg or a decrease in diastolic blood pressure of 10 mm Hg within 3 minutes of standing when compared with blood pressure from the sitting or supine position (Lanier, Mote, & Clay, 2011). It results from an inadequate physiologic response to postural (positional) changes in blood pressure. Orthostatic hypotension may be acute or chronic, as well as symptomatic or asymptomatic (Lanier et al., 2011, p. 527). It is associated with dizziness, lightheadedness, blurred vision, weakness, fatigue, nausea, palpitations, and headache. Older adults may experience orthostatic hypotension without associated symptoms, leading to falls (Gray-Miceli, Ratcliffe, Liu, Wantland, & Johnson, 2012). Orthostatic hypotension occurs when one rises to an erect position, either supine to sitting, supine to standing, or sitting to standing. It is caused by dehydration or blood loss; problems of the neurologic, cardiovascular or endocrine systems; and/or use of certain classes of medications.

There are many nonpharmacologic interventions that may be used to control or prevent orthostatic hypotension. Arising and moving about slowly, especially after a period of bed rest, might prevent orthostatic hypotension. When ambulating patients after surgery or prolonged bed rest, first raise the head of the bed, then assist the patient to a sitting

PROMOTING HEALTH LITERACY

IN PATIENTS WITH HYPERTENSION

Patient Scenario

Harry Miller, 66 years old, went to his primary health care provider for his annual health assessment. He had gained 15 pounds in the past year. When the office nurse took his blood pressure, it was 166/92 mm Hg. The nurse took Mr. Miller's blood pressure again and then repeated it later after his health assessment was completed. Although the reading varied by a few points, it remained consistently high. Mr. Miller was obviously surprised at having hypertension, because he said, "It has never been this high before. There must be something wrong with your machine." His health care provider tried to discuss the need for changes in his lifestyle as well as the need to take the medication prescribed for his blood pressure, but Mr. Miller said he had no questions and rushed out of the examining room.

Nursing Considerations: *Tips for Improving Health Literacy*

Provide Mr. Miller with printed literature about high blood pressure, including causes and risks. Explain that it is important

to control his high blood pressure to prevent serious risks, such as heart attack and stroke. Urge Mr. Miller and his wife to talk to a dietitian about a nutritious diet that would help him lose weight; contains recommended servings of fiber, fruits, and vegetables; and contains less salt. Explain the action of the prescribed medication and the importance of taking the medication to reduce and control his blood pressure. Encourage Mr. Miller to make an appointment to return to the office on a regular basis and to be prepared to ask his provider the following three questions:

- What is my main problem?
- What do I need to do?
- Why is it important for me to do this?

What additional measures can you take to help maintain health literacy in this patient and his wife? What other measures would be helpful for Mr. Miller if he did not speak English, could not read, or had other learning deficits?

GUIDELINES FOR NURSING CARE 24-5

ASSESSING ORTHOSTATIC HYPOTENSION

If orthostatic blood pressure measurements are ordered, use the following guidelines:

Throughout the procedure, assess for signs and symptoms of hypotension, such as dizziness, lightheadedness, pallor, diaphoresis, or syncope. If the patient is attached to a cardiac monitor, assess for arrhythmias. Immediately return the patient to a supine position if symptoms appear during the procedure. Do not have the patient stand if symptoms of hypotension occur when the patient is sitting.

- Lower the head of the bed. Place the bed in a low position.
- Ask the patient to lie in a supine position for 3 to 10 minutes. At the end of this time, take initial blood pressure and pulse measurements.
- Assist the patient to sit on the side of the bed with legs dangling. After 1 to 3 minutes, take the blood pressure and pulse measurements.

- Assist the patient to stand (unless contraindicated). Wait 2 to 3 minutes and then take blood pressure and pulse measurements.
- Record the measurements for each position. A decrease in systolic blood pressure of ≥20 mm Hg or a decrease in diastolic blood pressure of ≥10 mm Hg within 3 minutes of standing when compared with blood pressure from the sitting or supine position (Lanier, et al., 2011).

Adapted from Lanier, J. B., Mote, M. B., & Clay, E. C. (2011). Evaluation and management of orthostatic hypotension. *American Family Physician, 84*(5), 527–536; and Pickering, T., Hall, J., Appel, L., et al. (2004). American Heart Association Scientific Statement. Recommendations for blood pressure measurement in humans and experimental animals. Part 1: Blood pressure measurement in humans: A statement for professionals from the subcommittee of professional and public education of the American Heart Association Council on High Blood Pressure Research. Available at http://hyper.ahajournals.org/cgi/content/full/45/1/142.

position on the side of bed (often called "dangling") for a few minutes to assess for dizziness or faintness, and then assist to a standing position. If the patient becomes dizzy or feels faint, return the patient to bed and place in a supine position, which restores blood flow to the brain. Administer contributing medications at bedtime if possible, especially antihypertensives. Patients should ensure adequate hydration. Exercise programs to improve conditioning and exercises involving the arms, legs, and abdominal muscles during positional changes or prolonged standing may also help (Lanier et al., 2011). Guidelines for Nursing Care 24-5 describes how to assess orthostatic hypotension.

Assessing Blood Pressure

To accurately assess blood pressure, the nurse must know the appropriate equipment to use, how to describe the sounds that are heard, and which site to choose.

Equipment

Blood pressure may be assessed with different types of devices. Most commonly, nurses assess blood pressure by

using a stethoscope and sphygmomanometer. Auscultation is the preferred method of obtaining blood pressure readings in children older than one year (NHLBI, 2005; Ogedegbe & Pickering, 2010). Blood pressure may also be estimated with a Doppler ultrasound stethoscope (described in the discussion of the pulse), estimated by palpation, and assessed with electronic or automated devices.

SPHYGMOMANOMETER

A sphygmomanometer is used to assess blood pressure. The sphygmomanometer consists of a cuff and the manometer (Fig. 24-4). The cuff contains an airtight, flat, rubber bladder covered with cloth. Selecting a cuff of the proper width (ranging from neonate to adult thigh) is essential to obtain an accurate blood pressure reading. The correct cuff should have a bladder length that is 80% of the arm circumference and a width that is at least 40% of the arm circumference, with a length-to-width ratio of 2:1. The bladder inside the cuff should enclose a child's entire limb. If the cuff is too narrow, the reading could be erroneously high because the pressure is not evenly transmitted to the artery. This occurs, for example, when an average-sized cuff is used on an obese

FIGURE 24-4. Sphygmomanometer. (**A**) Three cuff sizes: a small cuff for a child or a small or frail adult, a normal-sized cuff, and a large adult cuff. A cuff sized for use on the thigh is also available. (**B**) An aneroid manometer.

Table 24-8 RECOMMENDED BLOOD PRESSURE CUFF SIZES

CUFF SIZE	CUFF MEASUREMENTS	ARM CIRCUMFERENCE*
Newborn–premature infants	4 × 8 cm	
Infants	6 × 12 cm	
Older children	9 × 18 cm	
Small adult size	12 × 22 cm	22–26 cm
Adult size	16 × 30 cm	27–34 cm
Large adult size	16 × 36 cm	35–44 cm
Adult thigh size	16 × 42 cm	45–52 cm

*Select a blood pressure cuff that has a bladder width that is at least 40% of the arm circumference midway between the olecranon and the acromion.
  Adapted from Pickering, T., Hall, J., Appel, L., et al. (2004). American Heart Association Scientific Statement. Recommendations for blood pressure measurement in humans and experimental animals. Part 1: Blood pressure measurement in humans: A statement for professionals from the subcommittee of professional and public education of the American Heart Association Council on High Blood Pressure Research. Available at http://hyper.ahajournals.org/cgi/content/full/45/1/142.

person. If a cuff is too wide (e.g., using an adult cuff on the arm of a child), the reading may be erroneously low because pressure is dispersed over a disproportionately large surface area. Recommendations by the AHA for the selection of an appropriately sized cuff are given in Table 24-8.

 THINK back to Mrs. Renfrow, the wife of a patient with hypertension who is overweight. The nurse would need to caution Mrs. Renfrow to make sure that the device she uses to measure her husband's blood pressure is sized adequately. Otherwise, the readings may be erroneous, possibly leading to inappropriate management based on inaccurate readings or a false sense of security that the hypertension is being controlled. ●

Depending on the product, cuffs may be disposable or reusable. They are closed around the limb with contact closures, such as nylon fabric that can be fastened to itself with Velcro® or hooks. Some long cuffs are applied by encircling the arm several times. Two tubes are attached to the bladder within the cuff. One is connected to a manometer and the other is attached to a bulb used to inflate the bladder. The bladder is inflated enough to obstruct the flow of blood through the artery. A needle valve on the bulb allows the cuff to be deflated while the pressure is being read.

AUTOMATED BLOOD PRESSURE MONITORS

Automated, electronic blood pressure monitors determine blood pressure by analyzing the sounds of blood flow or measuring oscillations (fluctuations) in blood flow (Fig. 24-5). The machine can be set to take and record blood pressure readings at preset intervals. Irregular heart rates, excessive patient movement, and environmental noise can interfere with the readings. Because electronic equipment is more sensitive to outside interference, and the monitors require routine validation of accuracy, these readings are susceptible to error. There is some evidence to suggest that these devices should not be used in some specific circumstances, such as in management of hypertension, with patients who have experienced trauma, or where there is

significant potential for deterioration in the patient's condition. Blood pressure should be measured using an auscultatory device in these situations (Skirton, Chamberlain, Lawson, Ryan, & Young, 2011). When using an automatic blood pressure monitor for serial readings, check the cuffed limb frequently. Incomplete deflation of the cuff between measurements can lead to inadequate arterial perfusion and venous drainage, compromised the circulation in the limb (Bern et al., 2007; Pickering, Hall, & Appel, 2004). These devices may also provide measurements of pulse rate, pulse oximetry, and/or temperature.

DOPPLER ULTRASOUND

Blood pressure may be taken with a Doppler ultrasound device, which amplifies sounds. This device is especially useful if the sounds are indistinct or are inaudible with a regular stethoscope. This method only provides an estimate of systolic blood pressure. See Guidelines for Nursing Care 24-6 (on page 600) for assessment technique.

DIRECT ELECTRONIC MEASUREMENT

It is possible to measure blood pressure directly through the insertion of a thin catheter into an artery (an arterial line). The tip of the catheter senses the pressure and transmits this information to a machine that displays the systolic and

FIGURE 24-5. The automatic blood pressure monitor reports systolic, diastolic, and mean blood pressure. (*Photo by B. Proud*)

GUIDELINES FOR NURSING CARE 24-6

ASSESSING BLOOD PRESSURE USING A DOPPLER ULTRASOUND

- Select the appropriate limb for application of cuff.
- Have the patient assume a comfortable lying or sitting position with the appropriate limb exposed.
- Center the bladder of the cuff over the artery, lining the artery marker on the cuff up with the artery.
- Wrap the cuff around the limb smoothly and snugly, and fasten it. Do not allow any clothing to interfere with the proper placement of the cuff.
- Check that the needle on the aneroid gauge is within the zero mark. If using a mercury manometer, check to see that the manometer is in the vertical position and that the mercury is within the zero level with the gauge at eye level.
- Place a small amount of conducting gel over the artery.
- Hold the Doppler in your nondominant hand. Using your dominant hand, place the Doppler tip in the gel. Adjust the volume as needed. Move the Doppler tip around until you hear the pulse.
- Once the pulse is found using the Doppler, close the valve to the sphygmomanometer. Tighten the screw valve on the air pump.

- Inflate the cuff while continuing to use the Doppler on the artery. Note the point on the gauge where the pulse disappears.
- Open the valve on the manometer and allow air to escape quickly. Repeat any suspicious reading, but wait at least 1 minute between readings to allow normal circulation to return in the limb. Deflate the cuff completely between attempts to check the blood pressure.
- Remove the Doppler tip and turn the Doppler off. Wipe excess gel off of the patient's skin with tissue. Remove the cuff.
- Wipe off any gel remaining on the Doppler probe with a tissue. Clean the Doppler according to facility policy or manufacturer's recommendations.
- Return the Doppler to the charge base.
- Remove PPE, if used. Perform hand hygiene.
- Record the findings on paper, flow sheet, or computerized record. Identify arm used and site of assessment if other than brachial, and the fact that it was obtained with a Doppler.

---

diastolic pressure in a waveform. This technique is used primarily in intensive care areas.

Korotkoff Sounds

The series of sounds for which the nurse listens when assessing the blood pressure are called **Korotkoff sounds**, described and illustrated in Table 24-9. These sounds are only heard when using a stethoscope to assess blood pressure.

In some adults, each of these sounds is distinct, whereas in others only the beginning and ending sounds are heard. It is important to determine agency policy for recording blood pressure sounds and to be consistent in taking and documenting the readings.

The blood pressure is most commonly recorded with two numbers, written as a fraction. The first sound heard through the stethoscope, which is the onset of phase I, represents the systolic pressure. It is recorded as the first number in the fraction—for example, if the blood pressure reading is 120/80 mm Hg, 120 is the systolic pressure. The second number, which represents the diastolic pressure (in this case, 80), notes the level at which the sounds disappear completely. There has been discussion in the past as to using phase IV or V of the Korotkoff sounds for recording diastolic pressure, but there is now a general consensus that phase V should be used (Jarvis, 2012; Pickering et al., 2004). In situations in which sounds were heard all the way down to zero—for example, in pregnant women and patients with arteriovenous fistulas—the blood pressure recording would include phase IV (112/62/0). Blood pressure readings for children are recorded in the same manner (Kyle, 2012).

  ### Sites and Methods of Assessing the Blood Pressure

Although various sites may be used to assess the blood pressure, the brachial artery and the popliteal artery are most commonly used. Equipment has been developed to measure blood pressure at the forearm also.

ASSESSING BLOOD PRESSURE AT THE BRACHIAL ARTERY

It is recommended that blood pressure should be checked in both arms at the first examination. It has been shown that most individuals have differences in blood pressure readings between arms. When there is a consistent inter-arm difference, the arm with the higher pressure should be used (Pickering et al., 2004). A brachial artery blood pressure assessment should not be taken on an arm with an intravenous line or with an arteriovenous fistula or shunt. Blood pressure assessment should also be avoided in the arm on the side of an axillary node dissection or mastectomy because the pressure may increase the risk of lymphedema developing in the affected arm.

Skill 24-4 on pages 616–620 describes how to assess the blood pressure using the brachial artery. Table 24-10 describes the common causes associated with blood pressure assessment errors.

ASSESSING BLOOD PRESSURE AT THE RADIAL ARTERY

The radial artery is used to auscultate the Korotkoff sounds when assessing blood pressure in the forearm. This site is becoming commonly used. Forearm measurements tend

Table 24-9 · KOROTKOFF SOUNDS

PHASE	DESCRIPTION	ILLUSTRATION
Phase I	Characterized by the first appearance of faint but clear tapping sounds that gradually increase in intensity; the first tapping sound is the systolic pressure	

FIGURE A. Blood flow interrupted by inflated cuff.

Phase II	Characterized by muffled or swishing sounds; these sounds may temporarily disappear, especially in hypertensive people; the disappearance of the sound during the latter part of phase I and during phase II is called the *auscultatory gap* and may cover a range of as much as 40 mm Hg; failing to recognize this gap may cause serious errors of underestimating systolic pressure or overestimating diastolic pressure

FIGURE B. As the pressure in the cuff is released, blood starts flowing again and Korotkoff sounds are audible.

Phase III	Characterized by distinct, loud sounds as the blood flows relatively freely through an increasingly open artery
Phase IV	Characterized by a distinct, abrupt, muffling sound with a soft, blowing quality; in adults, the onset of this phase is considered to be the first diastolic pressure
Phase V	The last sound heard before a period of continuous silence; the pressure at which the last sound is heard is the second diastolic pressure

FIGURE C. Cuff is completely deflated after Phase V, restoring complete blood flow.

to be higher than the upper arm measurements (Domiano, et al., 2008; Frese et al., 2011). The accuracy of readings with forearm monitors is affected by the position of the wrist relative to the heart. This can be avoided if the wrist is always at heart level when the reading is taken (Pickering et al., 2004).

The site has been suggested as an alternative for obtaining blood pressure readings for obese individuals, as it is often difficult to obtain the appropriately sized cuff for the upper arm, given arm circumference and conical-shaped upper arms common in obesity. The conical shape of the upper arm makes it difficult to fit the cuff to the arm, increasing

Table 24-10 · BLOOD PRESSURE ASSESSMENT ERRORS AND CONTRIBUTING CAUSES

ERROR	CONTRIBUTING CAUSES
Falsely low assessments	• Hearing deficit • Noise in the environment • Viewing the meniscus from above eye level • Applying too wide a cuff • Inserting earpieces of stethoscope incorrectly • Using cracked or kinked tubing • Releasing the valve rapidly • Misplacing the bell beyond the direct area of the artery • Failing to pump the cuff 20–30 mm Hg above the disappearance of the pulse
Falsely high assessments	• Using a manometer not calibrated at the zero mark • Assessing the blood pressure immediately after exercise • Viewing the meniscus from below eye level • Applying a cuff that is too narrow • Releasing the valve too slowly • Reinflating the bladder during auscultation

GUIDELINES FOR NURSING CARE 24-7

ASSESSING BLOOD PRESSURE AT THE POPLITEAL ARTERY

- Place the patient in the prone position, if possible. If that position is not possible, place the patient in the supine position, with the knee slightly flexed.
- Use a cuff that is specifically made for this assessment, or one that is large enough to make an accurate assessment.
- Place the cuff 2.5 cm (1 inch) above the popliteal artery, with the bladder over the posterior of the midthigh (see Figure).
- Follow the same procedure for auscultation as for the brachial artery.

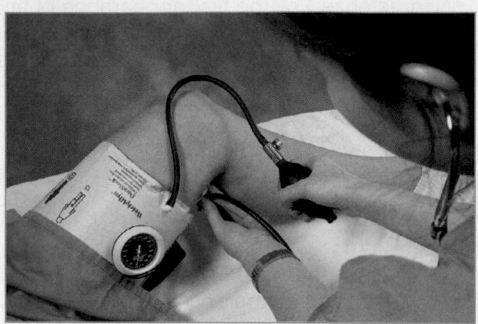

Thigh blood pressure. (From Jensen, S. (2011). *Nursing Health Assessment. A best practice approach.* Philadelphia: Wolters Kluwer Health/Lippincott Williams & Wilkins.)

the likelihood of inaccurate blood pressure measurement (Palatini & Parati, 2011). Measurement in the forearm is a possible solution to this problem.

ASSESSING BLOOD PRESSURE AT THE POPLITEAL ARTERY

When the patient's brachial artery is inaccessible and/or the use of the upper arm is contraindicated, the nurse can assess the blood pressure using the popliteal artery in the leg. The systolic pressure is normally 10 to 40 mm Hg higher at this site, although the diastolic pressure is the same. The technique for assessment is outlined in Guidelines for Nursing Care 24-7.

PALPATING THE BLOOD PRESSURE

Assessing the blood pressure through palpation is sometimes referred to as the sensory detection method. It requires only the use of the sphygmomanometer. The cuff is inflated

30 mm Hg above the point at which the pulsation in the artery disappears. As the air in the cuff is released, the nurse feels for the return of the pulse. Usually, no diastolic pressure is recorded because the artery continues to pulsate as long as blood flows through it.

NURSING DIAGNOSES

The data collected about the patient's vital signs may lead to the development of one or more nursing diagnoses related to alterations in vital signs. The etiology of the problem directs nursing interventions. Data collected during the nursing assessment may also lead to the identification of a collaborative problem.

Examples of diagnoses, etiologic factors, and defining characteristics appear in Examples of NANDA-I Nursing Diagnoses: Altered Vital Signs.

EXAMPLES OF NANDA-I NURSING DIAGNOSES

ALTERED VITAL SIGNS

Nursing Diagnosis	Related Factors	Sample Defining Characteristics
Hyperthermia	Dehydration Illness Trauma Vigorous activity	Flushed skin, tachycardia, tachypnea, increase in body temperature above normal range
Ineffective Peripheral Tissue Perfusion	Hypertension, smoking, diabetes mellitus	Absent or diminished pulses, blood pressure changes in extremities, capillary refill time >3 seconds, altered skin characteristics
Ineffective Breathing Pattern	Anxiety, hyperventilation, pain, neurologic damage	Alterations in depth of breathing, dyspnea, tachypnea, use of accessory muscles to breathe
Decreased Cardiac Output	Altered heart rate, altered rhythm, altered contractility, altered afterload	Arrhythmias, palpitations, orthopnea, variations in blood pressure readings, decreased peripheral pulses

From NANDA International. (2012). *Nursing diagnoses: Definitions & classification 2012–2014.* West Sussex, UK: Wiley-Blackwell.

TEACHING VITAL SIGNS FOR SELF-CARE AT HOME

Patients and/or their family members often need to check their own temperature, pulse, and/or blood pressure at home. Guidelines for teaching self-assessment are presented in Teaching Tips 24-1. Home blood pressure monitoring (HBPM) is being increasingly recommended (Parati, Krakoff, & Verdecchia, 2010; Pickering et al., 2008). Research has shown that readings at home are reliable, are often lower than those taken in a health care provider setting, contribute to better adherence treatment, and provide multiple readings taken over prolonged periods, giving a better picture of the patient's status and response to treatment (Leblanc, Cloutier, & Veiga,

2011; Ogedegbe & Pickering, 2010). Recommended guidelines for HBPM include:

- Advise patients to buy oscillometric BP monitors that measure BP on the upper arm with an appropriate cuff size.
- Explain that home monitoring devices should be checked for accuracy every one to two years. Readings should be compared with auscultated measurement by a health care practitioner to ensure accuracy.
- Explain that 3 readings, at least one minute apart, should be taken while in a sitting position, both in the morning and at night. Measurement should occur after resting quietly in a chair for 3 to 5 minutes, with the upper arm at heart level. The readings should be recorded to show to the health care provider.

TEACHING TIPS 24-1

SELF-CARE: MEASURING TEMPERATURE, PULSE, AND BLOOD PRESSURE

Health Topic	Teaching Tips	Why Is This Important?
Measuring Temperature	• Body temperature varies during the day. It is lower in the morning and higher in the evening. It may vary somewhat based on the method used to take the temperature, the person's condition, and the time of day. • Measure temperature the same way every time. • Read the thermometer and write the numbers down on paper. • Clean the thermometer with soap and water, or alcohol. • When reporting temperature measurements to a health care provider, be sure to say which method was used.	If the temperature is very high or low, or if you have any concerns, contact your health care provider. Ensures accuracy and provides accurate information.
Using a thermometer in the mouth	• Wait 20–30 minutes after drinking or eating to measure oral temperature. • Turn the thermometer on. • Put the thermometer in the mouth and under the tongue in the back. Close the lips around the thermometer. Do not bite down with the teeth. • Listen for the signal or beep. • Remove the thermometer.	Consuming hot or cold foods can affect the reading.
Using a tympanic membrane thermometer	• Turn the thermometer on. • Insert the ear probe snugly into the ear canal using gentle but firm pressure, angling toward the jaw. If the person is younger than 3 years, pull the ear lobe back and down. • Push the button to take the temperature and hold until reading is obtained. • Remove the thermometer.	Using equipment properly ensures accurate measurements.
Using a temporal artery thermometer	• Turn the thermometer on. • Place it firmly against the center of the forehead. • Push the "on" button. Keep the button depressed while taking the temperature. • Slowly slide the thermometer straight across the forehead to the hairline. • Lift the thermometer from the forehead and touch it to the neck just behind the ear lobe. • Release the button.	
Using a thermometer under the arm	• Turn the thermometer on. • Put the thermometer under the arm. • Fold the arm down and across the chest to hold it in place. • Listen for the signal or beep. • Remove the thermometer.	
Measuring the Pulse	• The pulse is often taken before taking certain medications, such as those to make the heartbeat slower or stronger. People who exercise and want to monitor the effect of the exercise on heart function may also take their pulse. • It is necessary to be able to see a watch or a clock with a second hand when taking the pulse.	If the pulse is very fast, very slow, or irregular, or if you have any concerns, contact your health care provider.

(continued)

TEACHING TIPS 24-1 *continued*

SELF-CARE: MEASURING TEMPERATURE, PULSE, AND BLOOD PRESSURE

Health Topic	Teaching Tips	Why Is This Important?
Measuring the Pulse (continued)	• Place one arm on a firm surface so that the palm is upward. Using the middle three fingers of the other hand, gently feel the outside of the arm just below the wrist with the fingertips. Do not press hard. When pulsations are felt, observe the second hand of the watch or clock and begin to count when the second hand reaches 12 (any number is fine, but it is often easier to remember to always begin counting when the second hand is on 12). Count each pulsation (beat) for 1 minute (when the second hand again reaches 12), and write the number down.	
Measuring Blood Pressure	• The blood pressure is often taken to determine how well medications are working to control high blood pressure. The blood pressure is usually checked once a week, or as instructed. Readings may be taken in the morning and evening. A record of blood pressure readings over time is more important than one reading. • Use a validated monitor with an automatic inflation cuff. • Avoid food, caffeine, tobacco and alcohol for 30 minutes before taking a measurement. • Take your blood pressure before (not after) you eat. • Rest 3–5 minutes before taking your blood pressure. • Sit comfortably with your back supported and both feet on the floor (don't cross your legs). • Elevate your arm to heart level on a table or a desk. • Use the proper sized cuff. It should fit smoothly and snugly around your bare upper arm. There should be enough room to slip a fingertip under the cuff. The bottom edge of the cuff should be 1 inch above the crease of the elbow. • Ideally, take 3 measurements at one sitting and record the average. • Follow instructions that come with the home device.	Home blood pressure monitoring is the ideal method for monitoring the response to treatment for high blood pressure. If the blood pressure numbers increase or decrease by more than 10, or if you have any concerns, contact your health care provider. Ensures accuracy of readings.

SKILL 24-1 ASSESSING BODY TEMPERATURE

DELEGATION CONSIDERATIONS

Assessment of body temperature may be delegated to nursing assistive personnel (NAP) or to unlicensed assistive personnel (UAP), as well as to licensed practical/vocational nurses (LPN/LVNs). The decision to delegate must be based on careful analysis of the patient's needs and circumstances, as well as the qualifications of the person to whom the task is being delegated. Refer to the Delegation Guidelines in Appendix A (found on thePoint).

EQUIPMENT

- Digital, glass, or electronic thermometer, appropriate for site to be used
- Disposable probe covers
- Water-soluble lubricant for rectal temperature measurement
- Nonsterile gloves, if appropriate
- Additional personal protective equipment (PPE), as indicated
- Toilet tissue, if needed
- Pencil or pen, paper or flow sheet, computerized record

IMPLEMENTATION

ACTION

1. Check the medical order or nursing care plan for frequency of measurement and route. More frequent temperature measurement may be appropriate based on nursing judgment.

RATIONALE

Assessment and measurement of vital signs at appropriate intervals provide important data about the patient's health status. Bringing everything to the bedside conserves time and energy. Arranging items nearby is convenient, saves time, and avoids unnecessary stretching and twisting of muscles on the part of the nurse.

ACTION

RATIONALE

2. Perform hand hygiene and put on PPE, if indicated.

Hand hygiene and PPE prevent the spread of microorganisms. PPE is required based on transmission precautions.

3. Identify the patient.

Identifying the patient ensures that the right patient receives the intervention and helps prevent errors.

4. Close the curtains around the bed and close the door to the room, if possible. Discuss the procedure with the patient and assess the patient's ability to assist with the procedure.

This ensures the patient's privacy. Explanation relieves anxiety and facilitates cooperation. Dialogue encourages patient participation and allows for individualized nursing care.

5. Assemble equipment on the overbed table within reach.

Organization facilitates performance of task.

6. Ensure that the electronic or digital thermometer is in working condition.

Improperly functioning thermometer may not give an accurate reading.

7. Put on gloves, if indicated.

Gloves prevent contact with blood and body fluids. Gloves are usually not required for an oral, axillary, or tympanic temperature measurement, unless contact with blood or body fluids is anticipated. Gloves should be worn for rectal temperature measurement.

8. Select the appropriate site based on previous assessment data.

This ensures safety and accuracy of measurement.

9. Follow the steps as outlined below for the appropriate type of thermometer.

10. When measurement is completed, remove gloves, if worn. Remove additional PPE, if used. Perform hand hygiene.

Removing PPE properly reduces the risk for infection transmission and contamination of other items. Hand hygiene prevents the spread of microorganisms.

Measuring an Oral Temperature

11. Remove the electronic unit from the charging unit, and remove the probe from within the recording unit.

Electronic unit must be taken into the patient's room to assess the patient's temperature. On some models, by removing the probe the machine is already turned on.

12. Cover thermometer probe with disposable probe cover and slide it on until it snaps into place (Figure 1).

Using a cover prevents contamination of the thermometer probe.

13. **Place the probe beneath the patient's tongue in the posterior sublingual pocket (Figure 2). Ask the patient to close his or her lips around the probe.**

When the probe rests deep in the posterior sublingual pocket, it is in contact with blood vessels lying close to the surface.

FIGURE 1. Putting probe cover on the thermometer.

FIGURE 2. Inserting thermometer under the tongue in the posterior sublingual pocket.

(continued)

SKILL 24-1 | ASSESSING BODY TEMPERATURE *continued*

ACTION	RATIONALE
14. Continue to hold the probe until you hear a beep (Figure 3). Note the temperature reading.	If left unsupported, the weight of the probe tends to pull it away from the correct location. The signal indicates that the measurement is completed. The electronic thermometer provides a digital display of the measured temperature.
15. Remove the probe from the patient's mouth. Dispose of the probe cover by holding the probe over an appropriate receptacle and pressing the probe release button (Figure 4).	Disposing of the probe cover ensures that it will not be reused accidentally on another patient. Proper disposal prevents spread of microorganisms.

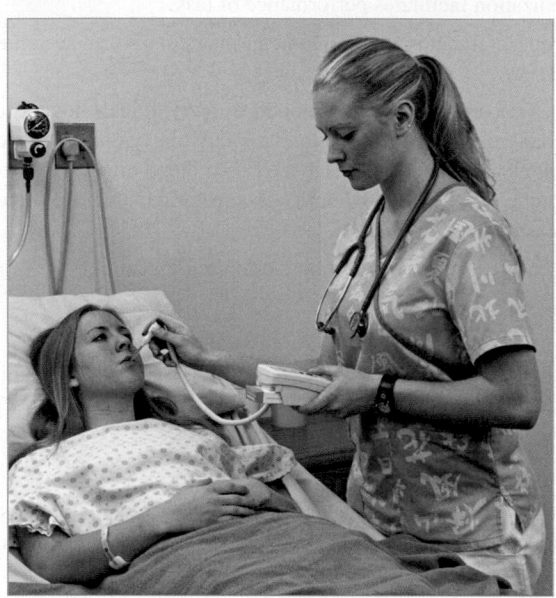

FIGURE 3. Holding probe in the patient's mouth.

FIGURE 4. Pushing button to dispose of cover.

16. Return the thermometer probe to the storage place within the unit. Return the electronic unit to the charging unit, if appropriate.	The thermometer needs to be recharged for future use. If necessary, the thermometer should stay on the charger so that it is ready to use at all times.

Measuring a Tympanic Membrane Temperature

17. If necessary, push the "ON" button and wait for the "ready" signal on the unit (Figure 5).	For proper function, the thermometer must be turned on and warmed up.

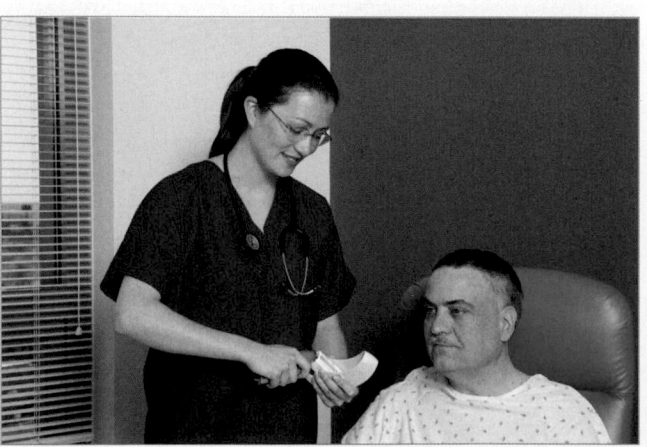

FIGURE 5. Turning unit on and awaiting the ready signal.

ACTION

18. Slide the disposable cover onto the tympanic probe.

19. **Insert the probe snugly into the external ear using gentle but firm pressure, angling the thermometer toward the patient's jaw line (Figure 6). Pull the pinna up and back to straighten the ear canal in an adult.**

20. Activate the unit by pushing the trigger button. The reading is immediate (usually within 2 seconds). Note the reading.

21. Discard the probe cover in an appropriate receptacle by pushing the probe-release button or use the rim of cover to remove it from the probe (Figure 7). Replace the thermometer in its charger, if necessary.

RATIONALE

Use of a disposable cover deters the spread of microorganisms.

If the probe is not inserted correctly, the patient's temperature may be noted as lower than normal.

The digital thermometer must be activated to record the temperature.

Discarding the probe cover ensures that it will not be reused accidentally on another patient. Proper disposal prevents the spread of microorganisms. If necessary, the thermometer should stay on the charger so that it is ready to use at all times.

FIGURE 6. Thermometer in patient's ear canal with pinna pulled up and back.

FIGURE 7. Disposing of probe cover.

Measuring Temporal Artery Temperature

22. Brush the patient's hair aside if it is covering the temporal artery area.

Anything covering the area—such as a hat, hair, wigs, or bandages—would insulate the area, resulting in falsely high readings. Measure only the side of the head exposed to the environment.

23. Apply a probe cover.

Using a cover prevents contamination of the thermometer probe.

24. Hold the thermometer like a remote control device, with your thumb on the red "ON" button. Place the probe flush on the center of the forehead, with the body of the instrument sideways (not straight up and down), so that it is not in the patient's face (Figure 8).

Allows for easy use of the device and reading of the display. Holding the instrument straight up and down could be intimidating for the patient, particularly young patients and/or those with alterations in mental status.

FIGURE 8. Placing the thermometer probe on the center of the forehead.

(continued)

SKILL 24-1 | ASSESSING BODY TEMPERATURE *continued*

ACTION	RATIONALE

ACTION

25. Depress the "ON" button. Keep the button depressed throughout the measurement.

26. Slowly slide the probe straight across the forehead, midline, to the hairline (Figure 9). The thermometer will click; fast clicking indicates a rise to a higher temperature, slow clicking indicates that the instrument is still scanning, but not finding any higher temperature.

27. Brush hair aside if it is covering the ear, exposing the area of the neck under the ear lobe. Lift the probe from the forehead and touch on the neck just behind the ear lobe, in the depression just below the mastoid (Figure 10).

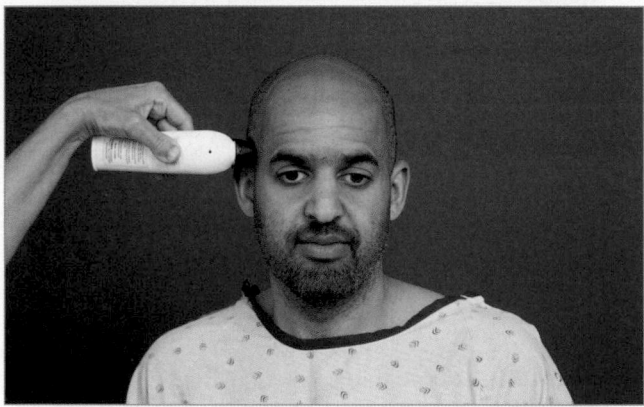

FIGURE 9. Sliding the probe across the forehead to the hairline.

28. Release the button and read the thermometer measurement.

29. Hold the thermometer over a waste receptacle. Gently push the probe cover with your thumb against the proximal edge to dispose of the probe cover.

30. The instrument will automatically turn off in 30 seconds, or press and release the power button.

Measuring Axillary Temperature

31. Move the patient's clothing to expose only the axilla (Figure 11).

RATIONALE

Midline on the forehead, the temporal artery is less than 2 mm below the skin; whereas at the side of the face, the temporal artery is much deeper. Measuring there would result in falsely low readings.

Sweat causes evaporative cooling of the skin on the forehead, possibly leading to a falsely low reading. During diaphoresis, the area on the head behind the ear lobe exhibits high blood flow necessary for the arterial measurement; it is a double check for the thermometer (Exergen, 2007).

FIGURE 10. Touching the probe behind the ear.

Discarding the probe cover ensures that it will not be reused accidentally on another patient.

Turns thermometer off.

The axilla must be exposed for placement of the thermometer. Exposing only the axilla keeps the patient warm and maintains his or her dignity.

FIGURE 11. Exposing axilla to assess temperature.

ACTION

32. Remove the probe from the recording unit of the electronic thermometer. Place a disposable probe cover on by sliding it on and snapping it securely.

33. **Place the end of the probe in the center of the axilla (Figure 12). Have the patient bring the arm down and close to the body.**

34. Hold the probe in place until you hear a beep, and then carefully remove the probe. Note the temperature reading.

35. Cover the patient and help the patient to a position of comfort.

36. Dispose of the probe cover by holding the probe over an appropriate waste receptacle and pushing the release button.

37. Place the bed in the lowest position and elevate rails, as needed. Leave the patient clean and comfortable.

38. Return the electronic thermometer to the charging unit.

RATIONALE

Using a cover prevents contamination of the thermometer probe.

The deepest area of the axilla provides the most accurate measurement; surrounding the bulb with skin surface provides a more reliable measurement.

Axillary thermometers must be held in place to obtain an accurate temperature.

Ensures patient comfort.

Discarding the probe cover ensures that it will not be reused accidentally on another patient.

Low bed position and elevated side rails provide for patient safety.

Thermometer needs to be recharged for future use.

FIGURE 12. Placing thermometer in center of axilla.

FIGURE 13. Removing appropriate probe and attaching disposable probe cover.

Measuring Rectal Temperature

39. Adjust the bed to a comfortable working height, usually elbow height of the care giver (VISN 8 Patient Safety Center, 2009). Put on nonsterile gloves.

40. Assist the patient to a side-lying position. Pull back the covers sufficiently to expose only the buttocks.

41. Remove the rectal probe from within the recording unit of the electronic thermometer. Cover the probe with a disposable probe cover and slide it into place until it snaps in place (Figure 13).

Having the bed at the proper height prevents back and muscle strain. Gloves prevent contact with contaminants and body fluids.

The side-lying position allows the nurse to visualize the buttocks. Exposing only the buttocks keeps the patient warm and maintains his or her dignity.

Using a cover prevents contamination of the thermometer.

(continued)

SKILL 24-1 ASSESSING BODY TEMPERATURE *continued*

ACTION

42. **Lubricate about 1 inch of the probe with a water-soluble lubricant (Figure 14).**

43. Reassure the patient. Separate the buttocks until the anal sphincter is clearly visible.

44. **Insert the thermometer probe into the anus about 1.5 inches in an adult or no more than 1 inch in a child (Figure 15).**

RATIONALE

Lubrication reduces friction and facilitates insertion, minimizing the risk of irritation or injury to the rectal mucous membranes.

If not placed directly into the anal opening, the thermometer probe may injure adjacent tissue or cause discomfort.

Depth of insertion must be adjusted based on the patient's age. Rectal temperatures are not normally taken in an infant, but may be indicated. Refer to the Special Considerations section at the end of the skill.

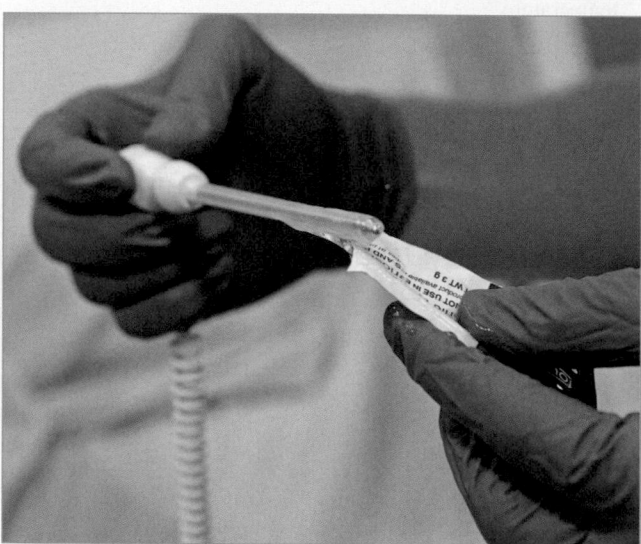

FIGURE 14. Lubricating thermometer tip.

FIGURE 15. Inserting thermometer into the anus.

45. Hold the probe in place until you hear a beep, then carefully remove the probe. Note the temperature reading on the display.

46. Dispose of the probe cover by holding the probe over an appropriate waste receptacle and pressing the release button.

47. Using toilet tissue, wipe the anus of any feces or excess lubricant. Dispose of the toilet tissue. Remove gloves and discard them.

48. Cover the patient and help the patient to a position of comfort.

49. Place the bed in the lowest position; elevate rails as needed.

50. Return the thermometer to the charging unit.

If left unsupported, movement of the probe in the rectum could cause injury and/or discomfort. The signal indicates that the measurement is completed. The electronic thermometer provides a digital display of the measured temperature.

Proper probe cover disposal reduces risk of microorganism transmission.

Wiping promotes cleanliness. Disposing of the toilet tissue avoids transmission of microorganisms.

Ensures patient comfort.

These actions provide for the patient's safety.

The thermometer needs to be recharged for future use.

DOCUMENTATION

Guidelines

Record temperature on paper, flow sheet, or computerized record. Report abnormal findings to the appropriate person. Identify the site of assessment if other than oral.

Sample Documentation

Lippincott DocuCare Practice documenting body temperature and other vital signs in Lippincott DocuCare.

10/20/15 Tympanic temperature assessed. Temperature 102.5°F. Patient states she has "a pounding" headache; denies chills, malaise. Physician notified. Received order to give 650 mg PO acetaminophen now. Incentive spirometer × 10 q 2 hours.

—*M. Evans, RN*

UNEXPECTED SITUATIONS AND ASSOCIATED INTERVENTIONS

- *Temperature reading is higher or lower than expected based on your assessment:* Reassess temperature with a different thermometer. The thermometer may not be calibrated correctly. If using a tympanic thermometer, you will get lower readings if the probe is not inserted far enough into the ear.
- *During rectal temperature assessment, the patient reports feeling lightheaded or passes out:* Remove the thermometer immediately. Quickly assess the patient's blood pressure and heart rate. Notify the physician. Do not attempt to take another rectal temperature on this patient.

SPECIAL CONSIDERATIONS

General Considerations

- Nonmercury glass thermometers used for oral readings commonly have long, thin bulbs. Those for rectal readings have a blunt bulb to prevent injury.
- If the patient smoked, chewed gum, or consumed hot or cold food or fluids recently, wait 30 minutes before taking an oral temperature to allow the oral tissues to return to baseline temperature.
- Nasal oxygen is not thought to affect oral temperature readings. Do not assess oral temperatures in patients receiving oxygen by mask. Removal of the mask for the time period required for assessment could result in a serious drop in the patient's blood oxygen level.
- When using a tympanic thermometer, make sure to insert the probe into the ear canal sufficiently tightly to seal the opening to ensure an accurate reading.
- A dirty probe lens and cone on the temporal artery thermometer can cause a falsely low reading. If the lens is not shiny in appearance, clean the lens and cone with an alcohol preparation or swab moistened in alcohol.
- If the patient's axilla has been washed recently, wait 15 to 30 minutes before taking an axillary temperature to allow the skin to return to baseline temperature.
- Axillary temperatures are generally about one degree less than oral temperatures; rectal temperatures are generally about one degree higher.

Infant and Child Considerations

- Pull the pinna back and down when measuring tympanic temperature on a child younger than 3 years of age. For children older than 3 years of age, there is no need to manipulate the pinna (Kyle & Carman, 2013).
- Small children have a limited attention span and difficulty keeping their lips closed sufficiently long to obtain an accurate oral temperature reading. Based on an assessment of the child's ability to cooperate, it may be more appropriate to use the temporal or tympanic site.
- Chemical dot thermometers (liquid crystal skin contact thermometers) are sometimes used as alternatives in pediatric settings. These single-use, disposable, flexible thermometers have specific chemical mixtures in circles on the thermometer that change color to measure temperature increments of two tenths of a degree. Place the thermometer in the mouth with the dot side (sensor) down, into the posterior sublingual pocket. Keep this type of thermometer in the mouth for 1 minute, in the axilla 3 minutes, and in the rectum 3 minutes. Read the color change 10 to 15 seconds after removing the thermometer. Read away from any heat source. Wearable, continuous-use chemical dot thermometers are available. These are placed under the axilla and must remain in place at least 2 to 3 minutes before taking the first reading; continuously thereafter. Replace thermometer and assess the underlying skin every 48 hours (Higgins, 2008; Perry et al., 2010).
- The Society of Pediatric Nurses (SPN) recognizes that temporal artery thermometry is accurate for infants less than 90 days old without fever, as well as for all patients more than 90 days of age with or without fever, ill or well. The SPN recommends that the temporal artery method should not be used in infants 90 days or younger who are ill, have a fever, or have an ill diagnosis (Asher & Northington, 2008, p. 235). The rectal method should be used for these infants unless contraindicated by diagnosis, in which case the axillary method should be used. In addition, in children 6 months of age or older, the tympanic or oral methods may be used with correct positioning of the ear (tympanic) and if the patient can cooperate (oral) (Asher & Northington, 2008).

(continued)

SKILL 24-1 ASSESSING BODY TEMPERATURE *continued*

Home Care Considerations

- Teach patients who use electronic or digital thermometers to clean the probe after use to prevent transmission of microorganisms between family members. Clean according to manufacturer's directions.
- Teach patients using nonmercury glass thermometers to clean the thermometer after use in lukewarm soapy water and rinse in cool water. Store it in an appropriate place to prevent breakage and injury from the glass.
- Pacifier thermometers, which use the supralingual area, are available to screen for fever. These thermometers give an approximation to rectal temperature measurement in the home setting (Braun, 2006). Leave this thermometer in place for 3 to 6 minutes, based on the manufacturer's recommendations.

SKILL 24-2 ASSESSING A PERIPHERAL PULSE BY PALPATION

DELEGATION CONSIDERATIONS

The assessment of the radial and brachial peripheral pulses may be delegated to nursing assistive personnel (NAP) or unlicensed assistive personnel (UAP). The assessment of peripheral pulses may be delegated to licensed practical/vocational nurses (LPN/LVN). The decision to delegate must be based on careful analysis of the patient's needs and circumstances, as well as the qualifications of the person to whom the task is being delegated. Refer to the Delegation Guidelines in Appendix A (found on thePoint).

EQUIPMENT

- Watch with second hand or digital readout
- Pencil or pen, paper or flow sheet, computerized record
- Nonsterile gloves, if appropriate; additional PPE, as indicated

IMPLEMENTATION

ACTION	RATIONALE
1. Check medical order or nursing care plan for frequency of pulse assessment. More frequent pulse measurement may be appropriate based on nursing judgment.	Assessment and measurement of vital signs at appropriate intervals provide important data about the patient's health status.
2. Perform hand hygiene and put on PPE, if indicated.	Hand hygiene and PPE prevent the spread of microorganisms. PPE is required based on transmission precautions.
3. Identify the patient.	Identifying the patient ensures that the right patient receives the intervention and helps prevent errors.
4. Close the curtains around the bed and close the door to the room, if possible. Discuss the procedure with the patient and assess the patient's ability to assist with the procedure.	This ensures the patient's privacy. Explanation relieves anxiety and facilitates cooperation.
5. Put on gloves, if indicated.	Gloves are not usually worn to obtain a pulse measurement unless contact with blood or body fluids is anticipated. Gloves prevent contact with blood and body fluids.
6. Select the appropriate peripheral site based on assessment data.	Ensures safety and accuracy of measurement.
7. Move the patient's clothing to expose only the site chosen.	The site must be exposed for pulse assessment. Exposing only the site keeps the patient warm and maintains his or her dignity.

ACTION	RATIONALE
8. Place your first, second, and third fingers over the artery (Figure 1). **Lightly compress the artery so pulsations can be felt and counted.**	The sensitive fingertips can feel the pulsation of the artery.
9. Using a watch with a second hand; count the number of pulsations felt for 30 seconds (Figure 2). Multiply this number by 2 to calculate the rate for 1 minute. **If the rate, rhythm, or amplitude of the pulse is abnormal in any way, palpate and count the pulse for 1 minute.**	Ensures accuracy of measurement and assessment.

FIGURE 1. Palpating the radial pulse.

FIGURE 2. Counting the pulse.

ACTION	RATIONALE
10. Note the rhythm and amplitude of the pulse.	Provides additional assessment data regarding the patient's cardiovascular status.
11. When measurement is completed, remove gloves, if worn. Cover the patient and help the patient to a position of comfort.	Removing PPE properly reduces the risk for infection transmission and contamination of other items. Ensures patient comfort.
12. Remove additional PPE, if used. Perform hand hygiene.	Removing PPE properly reduces the risk for infection transmission and contamination of other items. Hand hygiene prevents the spread of microorganisms.

DOCUMENTATION

Guidelines

Record pulse rate, amplitude, and rhythm on paper, flow sheet, or computerized record. Identify site of assessment. Report abnormal findings to the primary care provider.

Sample Documentation

DocuCare **Practice documenting pulse and other vital signs in Lippincott DocuCare.**

> <u>2/6/15</u> 1000 Pulses 84, regular, 2+ and equal in radial, popliteal, and dorsalis pedis sites.
>
> —M. Evans, RN

UNEXPECTED SITUATIONS AND ASSOCIATED INTERVENTIONS

- *The pulse is irregular:* Monitor the pulse for a full minute. If the pulse is difficult to assess, validate pulse measurement by taking the apical pulse for 1 minute. If this is a change for the patient, notify the primary care provider.

- *The pulse is palpated easily, but then disappears:* Apply only moderate pressure to the pulse. Applying too much pressure may obliterate the pulse.

- *You cannot palpate a pulse:* Use a portable Doppler ultrasound to assess the pulse. If this is a change in assessment or if you cannot find the pulse using a Doppler ultrasound, notify the primary care provider. If you can find the pulse using a Doppler ultrasound, place a small X over the spot where the pulse is located. This can make palpating the pulse easier because the exact location of the pulse is known.

(continued)

SKILL 24-2 ASSESSING A PERIPHERAL PULSE BY PALPATION *continued*

SPECIAL CONSIDERATIONS

General Considerations

- The normal heart rate varies by age.
- When palpating a carotid pulse, lightly press only one side of the neck at a time. Never attempt to palpate both carotid arteries at the same time. Bilateral palpation could result in reduced cerebral blood flow (Hogan-Quigley, Palm, & Bickley, 2012).
- If a peripheral pulse is difficult to assess accurately because it is irregular, feeble, or extremely rapid, assess the apical rate.

Infant and Child Considerations

- For children younger than 10 years of age, the apical pulse measurement is the preferred method of pulse assessment (Jarvis, 2012) (see Guidelines for Nursing Care 24-3 on page 592). Do not measure the radial pulse in children younger than 2 years of age, because it is difficult to palpate accurately in this age group (Kyle & Carman, 2013). In older children, measure the radial pulse for a full minute.
- Measure the apical rate if the child has a cardiac problem or congenital heart defect (see Guidelines for Nursing Care 24-3 on page 592).

Home Care Considerations

- Teach the patient and family members how to take the patient's pulse, if appropriate.
- Inform the patient and family about digital pulse monitoring devices.
- Teach family members how to locate and monitor peripheral pulse sites, if appropriate.

 # SKILL 24-3 ASSESSING RESPIRATION

DELEGATION CONSIDERATIONS

The assessment of respiration may be delegated to nursing assistive personnel (NAP) or unlicensed assistive personnel (UAP), as well as to licensed practical/vocational nurses (LPN/LVN). The decision to delegate must be based on careful analysis of the patient's needs and circumstances, as well as the qualifications of the person to whom the task is being delegated. Refer to the Delegation Guidelines in Appendix A (found on thePoint).

EQUIPMENT

- Watch with second hand or digital readout
- Pencil or pen, paper or flow sheet, computerized record
- PPE, as indicated

IMPLEMENTATION

ACTION	RATIONALE
1. While your fingers are still in place for the pulse measurement, after counting the pulse rate, observe the patient's respirations (Figure 1).	The patient may alter the rate of respirations if the patient is aware they are being counted.

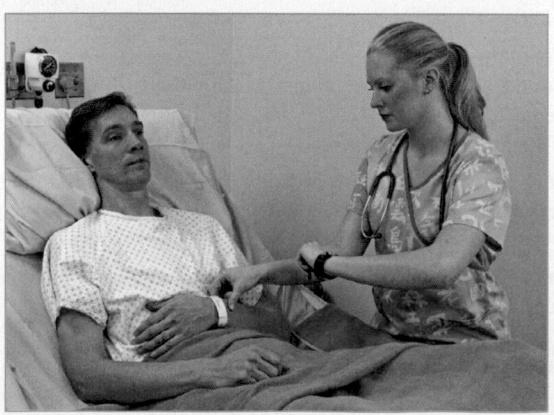

FIGURE 1. Assessing respirations.

ACTION	RATIONALE
2. Note the rise and fall of the patient's chest.	A complete cycle of an inspiration and an expiration composes one respiration.
3. Using a watch with a second hand, count the number of respirations for 30 seconds. Multiply this number by 2 to calculate the respiratory rate per minute.	Sufficient time is necessary to observe the rate, depth, and other characteristics.
4. **If respirations are abnormal in any way, count the respirations for at least 1 full minute.**	Increased time allows the detection of unequal timing between respirations.
5. Note the depth and rhythm of the respirations.	Provides additional assessment data regarding the patient's respiratory status.
6. When measurement is completed, remove gloves, if worn. Cover the patient and help the patient to a position of comfort.	Removing gloves properly reduces the risk for infection transmission and contamination of other items. Ensures patient comfort.
7. Remove additional PPE, if used. Perform hand hygiene.	Removing PPE properly reduces the risk for infection transmission and contamination of other items. Hand hygiene deters the spread of microorganisms.

DOCUMENTATION

Guidelines

Document respiratory rate, depth, and rhythm on paper, flow sheet, or computerized record. Report any abnormal findings to the appropriate person.

Sample Documentation

DocuCare Practice documenting respiration and other vital signs in *Lippincott DocuCare*.

<u>10/23/15</u> 0830 Patient breathing at a rate of 16 respirations per minute. Respirations regular and unlabored.

—M. Evans, RN

UNEXPECTED SITUATIONS AND ASSOCIATED INTERVENTIONS

- *The patient is breathing with such shallow respirations that you cannot count the rate:* Sometimes it is easier to count respirations by auscultating the lung sounds. Auscultate lung sounds and count respirations for 30 seconds. Multiply by 2 to calculate the respiratory rate per minute. If the respiratory rate is irregular, count for a full minute. Notify the physician of the respiratory rate and the shallowness of the respirations.

SPECIAL CONSIDERATIONS

General Considerations

- If respiratory rate is irregular, count respirations for 1 minute.

Infant and Child Considerations

- For infants, count respirations for 1 full minute due to a normally irregular rhythm.
- Assess respirations in infants and children when the child is resting or sitting quietly, because respiratory rate often changes when infants or young children cry, feed, or become more active. The most accurate respiratory rate is obtained before disturbing the infant or child (Kyle & Carman, 2013).
- Infants' respirations are primarily diaphragmatic; count abdominal movements to measure respiratory rate. After 1 year of age, count thoracic movements (Kyle & Carman, 2013).

SKILL 24-4 ASSESSING BLOOD PRESSURE BY AUSCULTATION

DELEGATION CONSIDERATIONS

The assessment of brachial artery blood pressure may be delegated to nursing assistive personnel (NAP) or unlicensed assistive personnel (UAP), as well as to licensed practical/vocational nurses (LPN/LVN). The decision to delegate must be based on careful analysis of the patient's needs and circumstances, as well as the qualifications of the person to whom the task is being delegated. Refer to the Delegation Guidelines in Appendix A (found on thePoint).

EQUIPMENT

- Stethoscope
- Sphygmomanometer
- Blood pressure cuff of appropriate size
- Pencil or pen, paper, flow sheet, or computerized record
- Alcohol swab
- PPE, as indicated

IMPLEMENTATION

ACTION	RATIONALE
1. Check the medical order or nursing care plan for frequency of blood pressure measurement. More frequent measurement may be appropriate based on nursing judgment.	Provides for patient safety.
2. Perform hand hygiene and put on PPE, if indicated.	Hand hygiene and PPE prevent the spread of microorganisms. PPE is required based on transmission precautions.
3. Identify the patient.	Identifying the patient ensures the right patient receives the intervention and helps prevent errors.
4. Close the curtains around the bed and close the door to the room, if possible. Discuss procedure with the patient and assess the patient's ability to assist with the procedure. Validate that the patient has relaxed for several minutes.	This ensures the patient's privacy. Explanation relieves anxiety and facilitates cooperation. Activity immediately before measurement can result in inaccurate results.
5. Put on gloves, if indicated.	Gloves prevent contact with blood and body fluids. Gloves are usually not required for measurement of blood pressure, unless contact with blood or body fluids is anticipated.
6. Select the appropriate arm for application of the cuff.	Measurement of blood pressure may temporarily impede circulation to the extremity.
7. Have the patient assume a comfortable lying or sitting position with the forearm supported at the level of the heart and the palm of the hand upward (Figure 1). If the measurement is taken in the supine position, support the arm with a pillow. In the sitting position, support the arm yourself or by using the bedside table. If the patient is sitting, have the patient sit back in the chair so that the chair supports the patient's back. In addition, make sure the patient keeps the legs uncrossed.	The position of the arm can have a major influence when the blood pressure is measured; if the upper arm is below the level of the right atrium, the readings will be too high. If the arm is above the level of the heart, the readings will be too low (Pickering, et al., 2004). If the back is not supported, the diastolic pressure may be elevated falsely; if the legs are crossed, the systolic pressure may be elevated falsely (Pickering et al., 2004). This position places the brachial artery on the inner aspect of the elbow so that the bell or diaphragm of the stethoscope can rest on it easily. This sitting position ensures accuracy.

FIGURE 1. Proper positioning for blood pressure assessment using brachial artery. (*Photo by B. Proud*)

ACTION

8. Expose the brachial artery by removing garments or move a sleeve, if it is not too tight, above the area where the cuff will be placed.

9. Palpate the location of the brachial artery. **Center the bladder of the cuff over the brachial artery, about midway on the arm, so that the lower edge of the cuff is about 2.5 to 5 cm (1 to 2 inches) above the inner aspect of the elbow. Line up the artery marking on the cuff with the patient's brachial artery.** The tubing should extend from the edge of the cuff nearer the patient's elbow (Figure 2).

10. Wrap the cuff around the arm smoothly and snugly, and fasten it. Do not allow any clothing to interfere with the proper placement of the cuff.

11. Check that the needle on the aneroid gauge is within the zero mark (Figure 3). If using a mercury manometer, check to see that the manometer is in the vertical position and that the mercury is within the zero level with the gauge at eye level.

RATIONALE

Clothing over the artery interferes with the ability to hear sounds and can cause inaccurate blood pressure readings. A tight sleeve would cause congestion of blood and possibly inaccurate readings.

Pressure in the cuff applied directly to the artery provides the most accurate readings. If the cuff gets in the way of the stethoscope, readings are likely to be inaccurate. A cuff placed upside down with the tubing toward the patient's head may give a false reading.

A smooth cuff and snug wrapping produce equal pressure and help promote an accurate measurement. A cuff wrapped too loosely results in an inaccurate reading.

If the needle is not in the zero area, the blood pressure reading may not be accurate. Tilting a mercury manometer, inaccurate calibration, or improper height for reading the gauge can lead to errors in determining the pressure measurements.

FIGURE 2. Placing the blood pressure cuff. (*Photo by B. Proud*)

FIGURE 3. Ensuring gauge starts at zero. (*Photo by B. Proud*)

Estimating Systolic Pressure

12. Palpate the pulse at the brachial or radial artery by pressing gently with the fingertips (Figure 4).

Palpation allows for measurement of the approximate systolic reading.

FIGURE 4. Palpating the brachial pulse. (*Photo by B. Proud*)

(continued)

SKILL 24-4 ASSESSING BLOOD PRESSURE BY AUSCULTATION *continued*

ACTION	**RATIONALE**
13. Tighten the screw valve on the air pump.	The bladder within the cuff will not inflate with the valve open.
14. **Inflate the cuff while continuing to palpate the artery. Note the point on the gauge where the pulse disappears.**	The point where the pulse disappears provides an estimate of the systolic pressure. To identify the first Korotkoff sound accurately, the cuff must be inflated to a pressure above the point at which the pulse can no longer be felt.
15. Deflate the cuff and wait 1 minute.	Allowing a brief pause before continuing permits the blood to refill and circulate through the arm.

Obtaining Blood Pressure Measurement

ACTION	**RATIONALE**
16. Assume a position that is no more than 3 feet away from the gauge.	A distance of more than about 3 feet can interfere with accurate readings of the numbers on the gauge.
17. Place the stethoscope earpieces in your ears. Direct the earpieces forward into the canal and not against the ear itself.	Proper placement blocks extraneous noise and allows sound to travel more clearly.
18. Place the bell or diaphragm of the stethoscope firmly but with as little pressure as possible over the brachial artery (Figure 5). Do not allow the stethoscope to touch clothing or the cuff.	Having the bell or diaphragm directly over the artery allows more accurate readings. Heavy pressure on the brachial artery distorts the shape of the artery and the sound. Placing the bell or diaphragm away from clothing and the cuff prevents noise, which would distract from the sounds made by blood flowing through the artery.
19. Pump the pressure 30 mm Hg above the point at which the systolic pressure was palpated and estimated. Open the valve on the manometer and allow air to escape slowly (allowing the gauge to drop 2 to 3 mm per second).	Increasing the pressure above the point where the pulse disappeared ensures a period before hearing the first sound that corresponds with the systolic pressure. It prevents misinterpreting phase II sounds as phase I sounds.
20. **Note the point on the gauge at which the first faint, but clear, sound appears that slowly increases in intensity. Note this number as the systolic pressure (Figure 6). Read the pressure to the closest 2 mm Hg.**	Systolic pressure is the point at which the blood in the artery is first able to force its way through the vessel at a similar pressure exerted by the air bladder in the cuff. The first sound is phase I of Korotkoff sounds.

FIGURE 5. Proper placement of diaphragm of stethoscope. (*Photo by B. Proud*)

FIGURE 6. Measuring systolic blood pressure. (*Photo by B. Proud*)

ACTION	**RATIONALE**
21. Do not reinflate the cuff once the air is being released to recheck the systolic pressure reading.	Reinflating the cuff while obtaining the blood pressure is uncomfortable for the patient and can cause an inaccurate reading. Reinflating the cuff causes congestion of blood in the lower arm, which lessens the loudness of Korotkoff sounds.

ACTION	RATIONALE
22. **Note the point at which the sound completely disappears. Note this number as the diastolic pressure (Figure 7). Read the pressure to the closest 2 mm Hg.**	The point at which the sound disappears corresponds to the beginning of phase V Korotkoff sounds and is generally considered the diastolic pressure reading (Pickering et al., 2004).

FIGURE 7. Measuring diastolic blood pressure. (*Photo by B. Proud*)

ACTION	RATIONALE
23. Allow the remaining air to escape quickly. Repeat any suspicious reading, but wait at least 1 minute. Deflate the cuff completely between attempts to check the blood pressure.	False readings are likely to occur if there is congestion of blood in the limb while obtaining repeated readings.
24. When measurement is completed, remove the cuff. Remove gloves, if worn. Cover the patient and help the patient to a position of comfort.	Removing gloves properly reduces the risk for infection transmission and contamination of other items. Ensures patient comfort.
25. Clean the bell or diaphragm of the stethoscope with the alcohol wipe. Clean and store the sphygmomanometer, according to facility policy.	Appropriate cleaning deters the spread of microorganisms. Equipment should be left ready for use.
26. Remove additional PPE, if used. Perform hand hygiene.	Removing PPE properly reduces the risk for infection transmission and contamination of other items. Hand hygiene deters the spread of microorganisms.

DOCUMENTATION

Guidelines

Record the findings on paper, flow sheet, or computerized record. Report abnormal findings to the appropriate person. Identify arm used and site of assessment if other than brachial.

Sample Documentation

Lippincott **DocuCare** Practice documenting blood pressure and other vital signs in *Lippincott DocuCare*.

10/18/15 0945 Blood pressure taken in right arm 180/88. Physician notified. Ordered captopril 25 po mg b.i.d. Blood pressure to be repeated 30 minutes after administering medication.

—*M. Evans, RN*

SPECIAL CONSIDERATIONS

General Considerations

• It is recommended that blood pressure measurements should be checked in both arms at the first examination. Most people have differences in blood pressure readings between arms. It is normal to have a 5- to 10-mm Hg difference in the systolic reading between arms. When there is a consistent interarm difference, use the arm with the higher pressure (Pickering et al., 2004).

• If you have difficulty hearing the blood pressure sounds, raise the patient's arm, with cuff in place, over the patient's head for 30 seconds before rechecking the blood pressure. Inflate the cuff while the arm is elevated, and then gently lower the arm while continuing to support it. Position the stethoscope and deflate the cuff at the usual rate while listening for Korotkoff sounds. Raising the arm over the head reduces vascular volume in the limb and improves blood flow to enhance the Korotkoff sounds (Pickering et al., 2004).

(continued)

SKILL 24-4 | ASSESSING BLOOD PRESSURE BY AUSCULTATION *continued*

- Blood pressure can be assessed using an automatic electronic blood pressure monitor or Doppler ultrasound.

- Many versions of automatic electronic blood pressure monitors are not recommended for patients with irregular heart rates, tremors, or the inability to hold the extremity still. The presence of these conditions may cause the monitor to incorrectly overinflate the cuff, causing pain for the patient. Check the manufacturer's guidelines when considering use with these patients.

- Diastolic pressure measured while the patient is sitting is approximately 5 mm Hg higher than when measured while the patient is supine; systolic pressure measured while the patient is supine is approximately 8 mm Hg higher than when measured in the patient who is sitting (Pickering et al., 2004).

- Measuring blood pressure in the forearm by auscultating the radial artery for the Korotkoff sounds is becoming more common. Forearm measurements tend to be higher than the upper arm measurements (Domiano et al., 2008; Frese et al., 2011). The accuracy of readings with forearm monitors is affected by the position of the wrist relative to the heart. This can be avoided if the wrist is always at heart level when the reading is taken (Pickering et al., 2004). This site for measurement has been suggested as an alternative for obtaining blood pressure readings in people who are obese. It is often difficult to obtain the appropriately sized cuff for the upper arm, given arm circumference and conical-shaped upper arms common in obesity. The conical shape of the upper arm makes it difficult to fit the cuff to the arm, increasing the likelihood of inaccurate blood pressure measurement (Palatini & Parati, 2011). Thus, measurement in the forearm can be a possible solution to this problem.

- When the patient's brachial artery is inaccessible and/or the use of the upper arm is contraindicated, the nurse can assess the blood pressure using the popliteal artery in the leg. The systolic pressure is normally 10 to 40 mm Hg higher at this site, although the diastolic pressure is the same.

Infant and Child Considerations

- In infants and small children, the lower extremities are commonly used for blood pressure monitoring. The more common sites are the popliteal, dorsalis pedis, and posterior tibial. Blood pressures obtained in the lower extremities are generally higher than if taken in the upper extremities. In children over 1 year of age, the systolic pressure in the thigh tends to be 10 to 40 mm Hg higher than in the arm; the diastolic pressure remains the same (Kyle & Carman, 2013).

- Infants and children presenting with cardiac complaints may have blood pressures assessed in all four extremities. Large differences among blood pressure readings can indicate heart defects.

- The fifth Korotkoff sound corresponds to diastolic blood pressure in children. In some children, the Korotkoff sounds continue to 0 mm Hg. In this situation, document the reading as systolic pressure over "P" for pulse (Kyle & Carman, 2013).

Home Care Considerations

- Automated blood pressure devices in public locations are generally inaccurate and inconsistent. In addition, the cuffs on these devices are inadequate for persons with large arms (Pickering et al., 2004).

- Explain to the patient that it is important to use a cuff size appropriate for limb circumference. Inform the patient that cuff sizes range from a pediatric cuff to a large thigh cuff and that a poorly fitting cuff can result in an inaccurate measurement.

- Inform the patient about digital blood pressure monitoring equipment. Although more costly than manual cuffs, most provide an easy-to-read recording of systolic and diastolic measurements.

- Explain that three readings, at least 1 minute apart, should be taken while in a sitting position, both in the morning and at night. Measurement should occur after resting quietly in a chair for 3 to 5 minutes, with the upper arm at heart level. The readings should be recorded to show to the health care provider.

- Explain that home monitoring devices should be checked for accuracy every 1 to 2 years. Readings should be compared with auscultated measurement by a health care practitioner to ensure accuracy.

DEVELOPING CLINICAL REASONING

1. Take your own pulse several times a day, such as when you first get up, before and after meals, and before and after exercise. Write down the rate, rhythm, and quality of the pulse. What changes did you see? What are the physiologic rationales for these changes?

2. Describe differences you might expect to find in the vital signs of the following individuals, and include the physiologic reasons for these differences:
   • A teenager who has his first football practice in 95°F heat
   • An infant with a bacterial ear infection
   • A young woman arriving at the emergency department after an attempted assault
   • A middle-aged man who sustained serious trauma and bleeding in an automobile crash
   • A 92-year-old woman with a chronic respiratory disease

PRACTICING FOR NCLEX

1. A nurse assesses an oral temperature for an adult patient. The patient's temperature is 37.5°C (99.5°F). What term would the nurse use to report this temperature?
   a. Febrile
   b. Hypothermia
   c. Hypertension
   d. Afebrile

2. A nurse is assessing the vital signs of patients who presented at the emergency department. Based on the knowledge of age-related variations in normal vital signs, which patients would the nurse document as having a normal vital sign? Select all that apply.
   a. A 4-month old infant whose temperature is 38.1°C (100.5°F)
   b. A 3-year old whose blood pressure is 118/80
   c. A 9-year old whose temperature is 39°C (102.2°F)
   d. An adolescent whose pulse rate is 70 bpm
   e. An adult whose respiratory rate is 20 bpm
   f. A 72-year old whose pulse rate is 42 bpm

3. A patient who is febrile may lose body heat through perspiration. The nurse recognizes that this is an example of what mechanism of heat loss?
   a. Evaporation
   b. Convection
   c. Radiation
   d. Conduction

4. The rectal temperature, a core temperature, is considered to be one of the most accurate routes. In which cases would taking a rectal temperature be contraindicated? Select all that apply.
   a. A newborn who has hypothermia
   b. A child who has pneumonia
   c. An older patient who is post myocardial infarction (heart attack)
   d. A teenager who has leukemia
   e. A patient receiving erythropoietin to replace red blood cells
   f. An adult patient who is newly diagnosed with pancreatitis

5. While taking an adult patient's pulse, a nurse finds the rate to be 140 beats/min. What should the nurse do next?
   a. Check the pulse again in 2 hours.
   b. Check the blood pressure.
   c. Record the information.
   d. Report the rate to the primary care provider.

6. A patient complains of severe abdominal pain. When assessing the vital signs, the nurse would not be surprised to find what assessments? Select all that apply.
   a. An increase in the pulse rate
   b. A decrease in body temperature
   c. A decrease in blood pressure
   d. An increase in respiratory depth
   e. An increase in respiratory rate
   f. An increase in body temperature

7. Two nurses are taking an apical-radial pulse and note a difference in pulse rate of 8 beats per minute. The nurse would document this difference as which of the following?
   a. Pulse deficit
   b. Pulse amplitude
   c. Ventricular rhythm
   d. Heart arrhythmia

8. The nurse instructor is teaching student nurses about the factors that may affect a patient's blood pressure. Which statements accurately describe these factors? Select all that apply.
   a. Blood pressure decreases with age.
   b. Blood pressure is usually lowest on arising in the morning.
   c. Women usually have lower blood pressure than men until menopause.
   d. Blood pressure decreases after eating food.
   e. Blood pressure tends to be lower in the prone or supine position.
   f. Increased blood pressure is more prevalent in African Americans.

9. A patient is having dyspnea. What would the nurse do first?
   a. Remove pillows from under the head
   b. Elevate the head of the bed
   c. Elevate the foot of the bed
   d. Take the blood pressure

10. A student nurse is learning to assess blood pressure. What does the blood pressure measure?
    a. Flow of blood through the circulation
    b. Force of blood against arterial walls
    c. Force of blood against venous walls
    d. Flow of blood through the heart

11. Prioritization: Place the following descriptions of the phases of Korotkoff sounds in order from Phase I to Phase V.
    a. Characterized by muffled or swishing sounds that may temporarily disappear; also known as the auscultatory gap
    b. Characterized by distinct, loud sounds as the blood flows relatively freely through an increasingly open artery
    c. The last sound heard before a period of continuous silence, known as the second diastolic pressure
    d. Characterized by the first appearance of faint but clear tapping sounds that gradually increase in intensity; known as the systolic pressure
    e. Characterized by a distinct, abrupt, muffling sound with a soft, blowing quality; considered to be the first diastolic pressure

12. A patient has a blood pressure reading of 130/90 mm Hg when visiting a clinic. What would the nurse recommend to the patient?
    a. Follow-up measurements of blood pressure
    b. Immediate treatment by a physician
    c. No action, because the nurse considers this reading is due to anxiety
    d. A change in dietary intake

13. A nurse is documenting a blood pressure of 120/80 mm Hg. The nurse interprets the 120 to represent:
    a. The rhythmic distention of the arterial walls as a result of increased pressure due to surges of blood with ventricular contraction
    b. The lowest pressure present on arterial walls while the ventricles relax
    c. The highest pressure present on arterial walls while the ventricles contract
    d. The difference between the pressure on arterial walls with ventricular contraction and relaxation

14. It is important to have the appropriate cuff size when taking the blood pressure. What error may result from a cuff that is too large or too small?
    a. An incorrect reading
    b. Injury to the patient
    c. Prolonged pressure on the arm
    d. Loss of Korotkoff sounds

15. A patient has intravenous fluids infusing in the right arm. When taking a blood pressure on this patient, what would the nurse do in this situation?
    a. Take the blood pressure in the right arm
    b. Take the blood pressure in the left arm
    c. Use the smallest possible cuff
    d. Report inability to take the blood pressure

ANSWERS WITH RATIONALES

1. *d.* Afebrile means without fever. This temperature is within the normal range for an adult. Fever (pyrexia) is an elevation of body temperature; a person with fever is said to be febrile. Hypothermia is a low body temperature and hyperthermia is a high body temperature.

2. *a, d, e, f.* The normal temperature range for infants is 37.1°C to 38.1°C (98.7°F–100.5°F). The normal pulse rate for an adolescent is 55 to 105. The normal respiratory rate for an adult is 12 to 20 bpm and the normal pulse for an older adult is 40 to 100 bpm. The normal blood pressure for a toddler is 89/46 and the normal temperature for a child is 36.8°C to 37.8°C (98.2°F–100°F; refer to Table 24-1, Age-Related Variations in Normal Vital Signs).

3. *a.* Evaporation is the conversion of a liquid to a vapor as occurs when body fluid in the form of perspiration is vaporized from the skin. With convection, the heat is disseminated by motion between areas of unequal density, for example, the action of a fan blowing cool air over the body. An example of radiation (diffusion of heat by electromagnetic waves) is the body giving off heat from uncovered areas. In conduction, the heat is transferred to another object during direct contact, for example, body heat melting an ice pack.

4. *a, c, d, e.* The rectal site should not be used in newborns, children with diarrhea, and in patients who have undergone rectal surgery. The insertion of the thermometer can slow the heart rate by stimulating the vagus nerve, thus patients post–MI should not have a rectal temperature taken. Assessing a rectal temperature is also contraindicated in patients who are neutropenic (have low white blood cell counts, such as in leukemia), in patients who have certain neurologic disorders, and in patients with low platelet counts.

5. *d.* A rate of 140 beats/min in an adult is an abnormal pulse and should be reported to the primary care provider or the nurse in charge of the patient.

6. *a, e.* The pulse often increases when a person is experiencing pain. Pain does not affect body temperature and may increase (not decrease) blood pressure. Acute pain may increase respiratory rate but decrease respiratory depth.

7. *a.* The difference between the apical and radial pulse rate is called the pulse deficit.

8. *b, c, e, f.* Blood pressure increases with age due to a decreased elasticity of the arteries, increasing peripheral resistance. Blood pressure is usually lowest on arising in the morning. Women usually have lower blood pressure than men until menopause occurs. Blood pressure increases after eating food. Blood pressure tends to be lower in the prone or supine position. Increased blood pressure is more prevalent and severe in African American men and women.

9. *b.* Elevating the head of the bed allows the abdominal organs to descend, giving the diaphragm greater room for expansion and facilitating lung expansion.

10. *b.* Blood pressure is the measurement of the force of blood against arterial walls.

11. *d, a, b, e, c.* Phase I is characterized by the first appearance of faint but clear tapping sounds that gradually increase in intensity; the first tapping sound is the systolic pressure. Phase II is characterized by muffled or swishing sounds, which may temporarily disappear, especially in hypertensive people; the disappearance of the sound during the latter part of phase I and during phase II is called the *auscultatory gap*. Phase III is characterized by distinct, loud sounds as the blood flows relatively freely through an increasingly open artery. Phase IV is characterized by a distinct, abrupt, muffling sound with a soft, blowing quality; in adults, the onset of this phase is considered to be the first diastolic pressure. Phase V is the last sound heard before a period of continuous silence; the pressure at which the last sound is heard is the second diastolic pressure.

12. *a.* A single blood pressure reading that is mildly elevated is not significant, but the measurement should be taken again over time to determine if hypertension is a problem. The nurse would recommend a return visit to the clinic for a recheck.

13. *c.* The systolic pressure is 120 mm Hg. The diastolic pressure is 80 mm Hg, the lowest pressure present on arterial walls when the heart rests between beats. The difference between the systolic and diastolic pressures is called the pulse pressure. The rhythmic distention of the arterial walls as a result of increased pressure due to surges of blood with ventricular contraction is the pulse.

14. *a.* A blood pressure cuff that is not the right size may cause an incorrect reading.

15. *b.* The blood pressure should be taken in the arm opposite the one with the infusion.

TAYLOR SUITE RESOURCES

Explore these additional resources to enhance learning for this chapter:

- NCLEX-Style Questions and other resources on thePoint, http://thePoint.lww.com/Taylor8e
- *Study Guide for Fundamentals of Nursing, 8th edition*

- Adaptive Learning | Powered by prepU, http://thepoint.lww. com/prepu
- *Skill Checklists for Fundamentals of Nursing, 8th edition*

- *Taylor's Clinical Nursing Skills:* Chapter 2, Vital Signs
- *Taylor's Video Guide to Clinical Nursing Skills:* Vital Signs
- *Lippincott DocuCare* Fundamentals cases

Bibliography

Ackley, B. J., & Ladwig, G. B. (2011). *Nursing Diagnosis Handbook* (9th ed.). St. Louis: Mosby/Elsevier.

Alexis, O. (2009). Providing best practice in manual blood pressure measurement. *British Journal of Nursing, 18*(7), 410–415.

Alexis, O. (2010). Providing best practice in manual pulse measurement. *British Journal of Nursing, 19*(4), 228–234.

American Heart Association. (2012). About high blood pressure. Available at http://www.heart. org/HEARTORG/Conditions/HighBloodPressure/ AboutHighBloodPressure/About-High-Blood-Pressure_ UCM_002050_Article.jsp.

Asher, C., & Northington, L. (2008). Society of Pediatric Nurses. Position statement for measurement of temperature/fever in children. *Journal of Pediatric Nursing, 23*(3), 234–236.

Beard, R., & Day, M. (2008). Fever and hyperthermia: Learn to beat the heat. *Nursing, 38*(6), 28–31.

Bern, L., Brandt, M., Mbelu, N., Asonye, U., Fisher, T., Shever, Y., & Serrill, C. (2007). Differences in blood pressure values obtained with automated and manual methods in medical inpatients. *MEDSURG Nursing, 16*(6), 356–362.

Boltz, M., Capezuti, E., Fulmer, T., & Zwicker, D. (eds.) (2012). *Evidence-based geriatric nursing protocols for best practice* (4th ed.). New York: Springer Publishing Company.

Braun, C. (2006). Accuracy of pacifier thermometers in young children. *Pediatric Nursing, 32*(5), 413–418.

Bulechek, G. M, Butcher, H. K., Dochterman, J. M., & Wagner, C. M. (Eds.). (2013). *Nursing interventions classification (NIC)* (6th ed.). St. Louis: Mosby Elsevier.

Carr, M. A., Wilmoth, M. L., Eliades, A. B., Baker, P. J., Shelestak, D., Heisroth, K. L., & Stoner, K. H. (2011). Comparison of temporal artery to rectal temperature measurements in children up to 24 months. *Journal of Pediatric Nursing, 26*(3), 179–185.

Cunha, B. A. (2011). Fever myths and misconceptions: The beneficial effects of fever as a critical component of host defenses against infection. *Heart & Lung, 41*(1), 99–101.

Davie, A., & Amoore, J. (2010). Best practice in the measurement of body temperature. *Nursing Standard, 24*(42), 42–49.

Domiano, K. L., Hinck, S. M., Savinske, D. L., & Hope, K. L. (2008). Comparison of upper arm and forearm blood pressure. *Clinical Nursing Research, 17*(4), 241–250.

Exergen. (2007). Temporal scanner reference manual. Watertown, MA: Author. Available at http://www. exergen.com/medical/PDFs/tat2000instrev6.pdf

Frese, E. M., Fick, A., & Sadowsky, H. S. (2011). Blood pressure measurement guidelines for physical therapists. *Cardiopulmonary Physical Therapy Journal, 22*(2), 5–12.

Gangavati, A., Hajjar, I., Quach, L., Jones, R. N., Kiely, D. K., Gagnon, P., & Lipsitz, L. A. Hypertension, orthostatic hypotension, and the risk of falls in a community-dwelling elderly population: The maintenance of balance, independent living, intellect, and zest in the elderly of Boston study. *Journal of the American Geriatric Society, 59*(3), 383–389.

Garner, A., & Fendius, A. (2010). Temperature physiology, assessment, and control. *British Journal of Neuroscience Nursing, 6*(8), 397–400.

Gillespie, C., Kuklina, E. V., Briss, P. A., Blair, N. A., & Hong, Y. (2011) Vital Signs: Prevalence, treatment, and control of hypertension—United States, 1999–2002 and 2005–2008. *Morbidity and Mortality Weekly Report, 60*(4), 103–108.

Gray-Miceli, D., Ratcliffe, S. J., Liu, S., Wantland, D., & Johnson, J. (2012). Orthostatic hypotension in older nursing home residents who fall: Are they dizzy? *Clinical Nursing Research, 21*(1), 64–78.

Grossman, S., & Porth, C. M. (2014). Porth's pathophysiology: concepts of altered health states. (9th ed.). Philadelphia: Wolters Kluwer Health/Lippincott Williams & Wilkins.

Higgins, D. (2008). Patient assessment Part 2: Measuring oral temperature. *Nursing Times, 104*(8), 24–25.

Hinkle, J. L. & Cheever, K. H. (2014). *Brunner & Suddarth's Textbook of Medical-Surgical Nursing* (13th ed.). Philadelphia: Wolters Kluwer Health | Lippincott Williams & Wilkins.

Hirsch, A. T., Haskal, Z. J., Hertzer, N. R., Bakal, C. W., Creager, M. A., et al. (2006). ACC/AHA 2005 guidelines for the management of patients with peripheral arterial disease (lower extremity, renal, mesenteric, and abdominal aortic): executive summary a collaborative report from the American Association for Vascular Surgery/Society for Vascular Surgery, Society for Cardiovascular Angiography and Interventions, Society for Vascular Medicine and Biology, Society of Interventional Radiology, and the ACC/AHA Task Force on Practice Guidelines (Writing Committee to Develop Guidelines for the Management of Patients With Peripheral Arterial Disease). *Circulation, 113*(11), e463–e654.

Hogan-Quigley, B., Palm, M. L., & Bickley, L. (2012). *Bates' Nursing Guide to Physical Examination and History Taking.* Philadelphia: Wolters Kluwer Health/Lippincott Williams & Wilkins.

Huether, S. E., & McCance, K. L. (2012.) *Understanding Pathophysiology* (5th ed.). St. Louis: Elsevier.

Jarvis, C. (2012). *Physical examination & health assessment* (6th ed.). St. Louis: Saunders/Elsevier.

Jensen, S. (2011). *Nursing Health Assessment. A best practice approach.* Philadelphia: Wolters Kluwer Health/Lippincott Williams & Wilkins.

Kyle, T., & Carman, S. (2012). *Essentials of pediatric nursing.* (2nd ed.). Philadelphia: Wolters Kluwer Health/Lippincott Williams & Wilkins.

Lanier, J. B., Mote, M. B., & Clay, E. C. (2011). Evaluation and management of orthostatic hypotension. *American Family Physician, 84*(5), 527–536.

Lawson, L., Bridges, E., Ballou, I., Eraker, R., Greco, S., Shively, J., & Sochulak, V. (2007). Accuracy and precision of noninvasive temperature measurement in adult intensive care patients. *American Journal of Critical Care, 16*, 485–496.

Leblanc, M. E., Cloutier, L., & Veiga, E. V. (2011). Knowledge and practice outcomes after home blood pressure measurement education programs. *Blood Pressure Monitoring, 16*(6), 265–269.

Lee, G., Flannery-Bergey, D., Randall-Rollins, K., Curry, D., Rowe, S., Teague, M., Tuininga, C., & Schroeder, S. (2011). Accuracy of temporal artery thermometry. *Advances in Neonatal Care, 11*(1), 62–70.

Lu, S. H., Leasure, A. R., & Dai, Y. T. (2009). A systematic review of body temperature variations in older people. *Journal of Clinical Nursing, 19*(1–2), 4–16.

Massey, D. (2010). Respiratory assessment 1: Why do it and how to do it? *British Journal of Cardiac Nursing, 5*(11), 537–541.

Mayo Clinic. (2011). High blood pressure (hypertension). Get the most out of home blood pressure monitoring. Available at http://www.mayoclinic.com/health/ high-blood-pressure/HI00016

Moorhead, S., Johnson, M., Maas, M. L., & Swanson, E. (Eds.). (2013). *Nursing Outcomes Classification (NOC).* (5th ed.). St. Louis: Mosby Elsevier.

NANDA International. (2012). *Nursing diagnoses: Definitions & classification 2012–2014.* West Sussex, UK: Wiley-Blackwell.

National Heart, Lung, and Blood Institute (NHLBI). National Institutes of Health (NIH). (2011). What is high blood pressure? Available at http://www.nhlbi.nih. gov/health/health-topics/topics/hbp/printall-index.html.

National Heart, Lung, and Blood Institute (NHLBI). National Institutes of Health (NIH). (2005). *The fourth report on the diagnosis, evaluation, and treatment of high blood pressure in children and adolescents.* (NIH Publication No. 05-5267). Washington, D.C.: U.S. Department of Health and Human Services.

National Reye's Syndrome Foundation. (2012). *The aspirin link.* Available at http://www.reyessyndrome. org/aspirin.html.

Ogedegbe, G., & Pickering, T. (2010). Principles and techniques of blood pressure measurement. *Cardiology Clinics, 28*(4), 571–586.

Palatini, P., & Parati, G. (2011). Blood pressure measurement in very obese patients: a challenging problem. *Journal of Hypertension, 29*(3), 425–429.

Parati, G., Krakoff, L. R., & Verdecchia, P. (2010). Methods of measurements: home and ambulatory blood pressure monitoring. *Blood Pressure Monitoring, 15*(2), 100–105.

Parkes, R. (2011). Rate of respiration: The forgotten vital sign. *Emergency Nurse, 19*(2), 12–17.

Paul, S. P., Mayhew, J., & Mee, A. (2011). Safe management and prescribing for fever in children. *Nurse Prescribing, 9*(11), 539–544.

Perry, S. E., Hockenberry, M. J., Lowdermilk, D. L., & Wilson, D. (2010). *Maternal child nursing care.* (4th ed.). Maryland Heights, MI: Mosby Elsevier.

Pickering, T., Miller, N., Ogedegbe, G., et al. (2004). American Heart Association Scientific Statement. Recommendations for blood pressure measurement in humans and experimental animals. Part 1: Blood pressure measurement in humans: A statement for professionals from the subcommittee of professional and public education of the American Heart Association Council on High Blood Pressure Research. Available at http://hyper.ahajournals.org/cgi/content/full/45/1/142

Pickering, T., Miller, N., Ogedegbe, G., Krakoff, L., Artinian, N., & Goff, D. (2008). Call to action on use and reimbursement for home health pressure monitoring: Executive summary. *Journal of Clinical Hypertension, 10*(6), 467–476.

Prosad Paul, S., Jayhew, J., & Mee, A. (2011). Safe management and prescribing for fever in children. *Nurse Prescribing, 9*(11), 539–544.

Pursell, E., While, A., & Coomber, B. (2009). Tympanic thermometry—normal temperature and reliability. *Paediatric Nursing 21*(6), 40–43.

Quatrara, B., Coffman, J., Jenkins, T., Mann, K., McGough, K., Conaway, M., & Burns, S. (2007). The effects of respiratory rate and ingestion of hot and cold beverages on the accuracy of oral temperatures measured by electronic thermometers. *MEDSURG Nursing, 16*(2), 105–108, 100.

Schulman, C. S. (2010). Ask the experts. Standards for frequency of measurement and documentation of vital signs and physical assessments. *Critical Care Nurse, 30*(3), 74–76.

Skirton, H., Chamberlain, W., Lawson, C., Ryan, H., & Young, E. (2011). A systematic review of variability and reliability of manual and automated blood pressure readings. *Journal of Clinical Nursing, 20*(5/6), 602–613.

Smitz, S., Van de Winckel, A., & Smitz, M. F. (2009). Reliability of infrared ear thermometry in the prediction of rectal temperature in older inpatients. *Journal of Clinical Nursing, 18*(3), 451–456.

Sund-Levander, M., & Grodzinsky, E. (2009). Time for a change to assess and evaluate body temperature in clinical practice. *International Journal of Nursing Practice, 15*(4), 241–249.

Tabloski, P. (2010). *Gerontological nursing* (2nd ed.). Upper Saddle River, NJ: Pearson.

Taylor, J. J., & Cohen, B. J. (2013). *Memmler's structure and function of the human body* (10th ed.). Philadelphia: Wolters Kluwer Health/Lippincott Williams & Wilkins.

U.S. Environmental Protection Agency (EPA). (2012). Mercury. Thermometers. Available at http:// epa.gov/hg/thermometer-main.html

Vaajoki, A., Kankkunen, P., Pietilä, A. M., & Vehviläinen-Julkunen, K. (2011). Music as a nursing intervention: Effects of music listening on blood pressure, heart rate, and respiratory rate in abdominal surgery patients. *Nursing and Health Sciences, 13*(4), 412–418.

VISN 8 Patient Safety Center (2009). *Safe patient handling and movement algorithms.* Tampa, FL: Author. Available http://www.visn8.va.gov/visn8/ patientsafetycenter/safePtHandling/default.asp

25

Health Assessment

BILLY COLLINS

Billy, a 9-year-old boy with a history of allergies, including an allergy to insect stings, is spending a week at summer camp. He reports to the camp counselor that he was just stung by a bee.

TAMMY BROWNING

Tammy, who is expecting her first child, is about to be moved to the delivery room. She and her partner, both in their late 20s, have a history of substance abuse, primarily alcohol and marijuana. A urine specimen is to be collected for routine evaluation and a drug screen. Tammy is unaware that drug testing will be done.

RAMONA LEWIS

Ramona, a 22-year-old college student, was recently discharged from the inpatient unit with a diagnosis of anorexia nervosa. She is living with her partner, Karen, and her mother, in her mother's home. A home health nurse is visiting Ramona for follow-up services.

LEARNING OBJECTIVES

After completing the chapter, you will be able to accomplish the following:

1. Explain the purposes and types of health assessment.
2. Prepare the patient and the environment for a health assessment.
3. Follow guidelines for conducting a health history.
4. Use the techniques of inspection, palpation, and auscultation appropriately during a physical assessment.
5. Conduct a physical assessment in a systematic manner.
6. Document health assessment findings in a concise, descriptive, and legally appropriate manner.
7. Describe nursing responsibilities before, during, and after diagnostic procedures.

KEY TERMS

activities of daily living (ADLs)
adventitious breath sounds
auscultation
body mass index (BMI)
bronchial sounds
bronchovesicular sounds
bruits
comprehensive assessment
cyanosis
diaphoresis
ecchymosis
edema
emergency assessment
erythema
focused assessment
health history
inspection
instrumental activities of daily living (IADLs)
jaundice
ongoing partial assessment
pallor
palpation
percussion
petechiae
physical assessment
precordium
review of systems
turgor
vesicular breath sounds
waist circumference

Conducting a health assessment involves collecting, validating, and analyzing subjective data (also called symptoms) and objective data (also called signs) to determine the overall level of physical, psychological, sociocultural, developmental, and spiritual health of a patient. Subjective data are experienced or known only by the patient (e.g., pain and nausea) and are gathered by verbal report during the health history. Objective data are directly observed or elicited through physical examination techniques.

Although most components of a health assessment are described in this chapter, some of the assessments included in a comprehensive or focused examination (such as an internal eye examination, a vaginal examination, or a rectal examination) are usually carried out by advanced practice professionals, health care providers with advanced education. Refer to information on thePoint or a health assessment text for details of these advanced assessment skills.

HEALTH ASSESSMENT

Health assessment involves gathering information about the health status of the patient. The nurse then evaluates and synthesizes the information (data). The nurse plans appropriate nursing interventions based on this data and evaluates patient care outcomes to deliver the best possible care for each patient. A health assessment includes a health history and a physical assessment. A **health history** is a collection of subjective information that provides information about the patient's health status. **Physical assessment** is a collection of objective data that provides information about changes in the patient's body systems.

A health assessment may be comprehensive, ongoing partial, focused, or emergency. A **comprehensive assessment** with a health history and complete physical examination is usually conducted when a patient first enters a health care setting, with information providing a baseline for comparing later assessments. An **ongoing partial assessment**, or follow-up assessment, is one that is conducted at regular intervals (e.g., at the beginning of each home health visit or each hospital shift) during care of the patient. This type of assessment concentrates on identified health problems to monitor positive or negative changes and evaluate the effectiveness of interventions. A **focused assessment** is conducted to assess a specific problem. For example, if a woman is having abdominal pain, the nurse asks questions about urinary problems, bowel problems, allergies, and menstrual history during the health history and then assesses vital signs and abdominal structures during the physical assessment. An **emergency assessment** is a type of rapid focused assessment conducted when addressing a life-threatening or unstable situation. Assessment of the airway, breathing, and circulation when encountering a patient with traumatic injury as a result of a motor vehicle accident is an example of an emergency assessment.

 CONSIDER Billy Collins, the 9-year-old who was stung by a bee. In this situation, the nurse would conduct an emergency assessment to determine the immediate effects of the bee sting, assessing for indications of an allergic reaction such as respiratory difficulty. Once this emergency assessment is completed and any immediate treatments initiated, the nurse would complete a health history to identify the boy's history of allergies and other relevant health issues. ●

Health assessment is an integral component of preventive health care. A preventive health assessment includes the patient's health history, risk for depression, functional ability, level of safety, a physical examination, and patient education and counseling. Annual wellness visits include the patient's health history, blood pressure, height, weight, screening for cognitive impairment and potential risk factors related to depression, functional ability, and safety, as well as health education and preventive counseling. These services are part of the benefits offered for patients covered by Medicare, for example, as part of health promotion and disease prevention and detection (Centers for Medicare and Medicaid Services [CMS], 2012).

A nursing health assessment differs from other types of health assessments (e.g., one performed by a physician) in that it is a holistic collection of information about factors that affect or are affected by one's level of health. Health assessment is an integral component of nursing care and is the foundation of the nursing process. The information from the nursing health assessment is used to formulate nursing diagnoses that require nursing care. Assessments are used to plan, implement, and evaluate teaching and care to promote an optimal level of health through interventions to prevent illness, restore health, and facilitate coping with disabilities or death. The information is also used to identify health problems that require interdisciplinary care or immediate referral to other health care providers. This chapter provides information necessary to identify risks for or actual alterations in health, perform the skills of physical examination, and identify normal age-related variations in physical structures and functions. Health assessments are a part of nursing care for patients across the lifespan and may be conducted in any setting. Refer to the accompanying Reflective Practice box for an example. Additional information about assessment is found in Chapter 11.

Lifespan Considerations

A comprehensive assessment includes cognitive, psychosocial, and emotional development in addition to physical growth (Jensen, 2011). The nurse should identify growth and development patterns from infancy through adolescence, adulthood, and into older age. Refer to Chapters 17, 18, and 19 for more information related to these assessments.

Cultural Considerations and Sensitivity

Each person is a unique individual. Nurses must consider patients within the context of family, culture, and community. Nurses and other health care professionals need to provide health care services in a sensitive, knowledgeable, and nonjudgmental manner with respect for people's health beliefs and practices when they are different than those of the care provider (Ritter & Hoffman, 2010). Nurse should be familiar with the general health beliefs and variances of various groups to improve the effectiveness of health care services and provide care within a cultural context (Ritter & Hoffman, 2010). Nurses should know risk factors for alterations in health that are based on racial inheritance and ethnic

backgrounds, as well as normal variations that occur within races. In addition, it is important to consider how religion and spirituality may impact health. Chapter 5 provides information about cultural diversity and the importance of providing culturally sensitive nursing care.

 Concept Mastery Alert

All patients, regardless of their race or culture, have the same basic human needs. However, the nurse needs to keep in mind any cultural influences or factors affecting anatomy and physiology, health beliefs, and alterations in health.

Patient Preparation

When conducting a nursing health assessment, it is important to consider and remain sensitive to the patient's physiologic needs (e.g., pain or decreased stamina because of age or illness) and psychological needs (e.g., anxiety about having the examination). Explain that the first part of the assessment will involve questions about the patient's health concerns, health habits, and lifestyle and that the information will only be shared with the patient's other health care providers. Inform the patient that after the health history is completed, body structures will be examined.

The patient may be anxious for various reasons. Reassure the patient by explaining that the assessments should not be painful. Explaining the assessment in general terms can help decrease the patient's embarrassment, fear of possible abnormal physical findings, or fear of "failing" a test. Be sure to then explain each assessment in greater detail as it is performed. Explain that drapes (covers) will be used during the examination, and only the area being assessed will be exposed. Answer the patient's questions directly and honestly.

 THINK back to Ramona Lewis, the college student who was recently discharged after treatment for anorexia nervosa. The nurse would need to incorporate knowledge of the emotional and physical effects of eating disorders when communicating with Ms. Lewis. In addition, the patient's anxiety is likely to be high; thus, using empathy, taking the time to explain things slowly, and establishing a trusting nurse–patient relationship are important. ●

Environmental Preparation

Privacy and respect for the patient are primary concerns when conducting a health assessment. In an outpatient setting, such as a clinic or primary care provider office, separate examination rooms provide a quiet, private space for assessment. Prepare the examination room before the health assessment is conducted by preparing the examination table, providing a gown and drape for the patient, and gathering instruments and special supplies needed for the assessment. In a hospital or community-based facility, the health assessment usually takes place in the patient's room. If the area

REFLECTIVE PRACTICE: CULTIVATING QSEN COMPETENCIES

CHALLENGE TO ETHICAL AND LEGAL SKILLS

I have always been interested in labor and delivery, so I was very excited to have the opportunity to follow a nurse in labor and delivery, and assist and witness the beginning of life. I had no idea that the whole process could be so complicated.

It was here that I met Tammy Browning, who was expecting her first child. She and her partner were in their late 20s or early 30s. She was going to be moved to the delivery room shortly. Before entering the room, the nurse gave me a brief rundown of what we were expected to do throughout the morning.

On entering the patient's room for the first time, I was shocked at what I saw. The room was dark and extremely cluttered with food, candy wrappers, and trash overflowing onto the floor. The patient's partner had been sleeping in the room and both of their belongings were all over the place. I could not believe it! When we left the room, the nurse told me that both the patient and her partner had a history of drug use, mainly alcohol and marijuana. We had to get a urine sample from her to do a dipstick test. The specimen was also going to be used for a drug screen, but the patient was not going to be told about this. I was shocked and confused by this action. I thought that we had to tell the patient everything we were going to do—right?

Thinking Outside the Box: Possible Courses of Action

- Go along with what the nurse decided to do, and when we got out of the patient's room, ask why she decided to take this course of action.
- Inform myself of the legality of taking this route of action.

- Inform my instructor and head nurse about the case, asking if this was a usual occurrence and requesting that they tell or educate me on what basis they were allowed to do this.

Evaluating a Good Outcome: How Do I Define Success?

- Safety of patient and neonate is ensured.
- Patient and baby benefit from the decided-on course of action.
- No breach of duty or harm is done.

- Patient receives proper care and treatment regardless of her past drug use and results of the drug tests.
- Respect for patient is maintained.

Personal Learning: Here's to the Future!

I really had no idea what to do. Because I did not feel legally competent to challenge the nurse and suggest a different course of action, I followed her and went along with her story. Afterward, I asked her if we were allowed to do this. Her answer was that she was doing it because the patient had a history of drug use and she suspected that she had been smoking marijuana throughout her stay. The test was not going to harm the baby or the mother; if anything, the test was going to be beneficial in providing the most adequate care for her and her baby. It was also going to assist in preparing for any complications that may arise during the delivery.

When she gave me this explanation, I figured that her reasons were valid and it was all right to do this since no one was going to get hurt and it would be beneficial. However, I was left with the thought that we were violating the patient's privacy. I also spoke with my clinical instructor about the situation. Through this experience, I realized that I need to educate myself more on the legal aspects of nursing. I had never paid much attention to the fact that I am exposed to many legal situations every day as a health care provider. Therefore, I must be prepared to confront them. I think that it is vital to be skilled as well as to be competent medically and legally. By having this knowledge, many difficult situations may be avoided and/or resolved. With this knowledge, I will also be a better advocate for my patients.

Stephanie Cuellar, Georgetown University

REFLECTION ON QUALITY AND SAFETY COMPETENCIES

How do you think you would respond in a similar situation? Why? What does this tell you about yourself and about the adequacy of your skills for professional practice? Do you agree with the criteria that the nursing student used to evaluate a successful outcome? Are there any other criteria that would be appropriate to use? Did the nursing student meet the criteria? Why or why not? What *knowledge*, *skills*, and *attitudes* do you need to develop to continuously improve the quality and safety of care for patients like Ms. Browning?

Patient-Centered Care: What do you think might have happened if the patient were told about the drug testing? Do you feel that the nurse's action of not telling the patient was based on appropriate ethical and legal principles? Why or why not? If so, what ethical and legal principles formed the basis for the action? If not, what ethical and legal principles were violated?

Teamwork and Collaboration/Quality Improvement: What communication skills do you need to improve to ensure that you function as a member of the patient-care team? What skills do you need to implement effective strategies for communicating and resolving conflict? What skills do you need to assert your own position/perspective in discussions about patient care?

Safety/Evidence-Based Practice: What evidence in nursing literature provides guidance for decision making regarding care of this patient?

Informatics: Can you identify the essential information that must be available in Ms. Browning's electronic health record to support safe patient care and coordination of care? Can you identify the appropriate process to protect confidentiality of protected health information in the patient's health records? Can you think of other ways to respond to or approach the situation?

is open to others, an enclosure with a curtain or screen is essential. The room should be warm enough to prevent chilling, and the area or room should be adequately lighted, either by sunlight or overhead lighting.

When patients are seen in their home, an assessment may be performed in the patient's bedroom or another private area. Direct the patient to a private dressing area or to a comfortable area in the home and ask the patient to change into a gown, if possible.

For all settings, if necessary, assist the patient with undressing. Ask the patient to empty the bladder before the examination to promote patient comfort during the assessment and to facilitate assessment of the abdomen by the nurse.

THE HEALTH HISTORY

A health history is a collection of data that provides a detailed profile of the patient's health status. Nurses use therapeutic communication skills and interviewing techniques during the health history to establish an effective nurse–patient relationship and to gather data to identify actual and potential health problems as well as health-promotion activities and sources of strength. Effective interviewing skills are described in Chapters 11 and 20.

Information is collected during an interview with the patient, who is the primary source of data. The patient's family members and/or caregivers may also be an important source of data. They can sometimes offer insight that cannot be gained from patients who may be acutely ill, in pain, or cognitively impaired. Fawcett and Rhynas (2012) suggest, "Nurses need to balance the benefits of obtaining information from family members with the potentially conflicting motivations of patients and their families." The health records of the patient, if available, can also be used to collect additional information. Nurses should know and be sensitive to cultural differences that influence how both verbal and nonverbal communications are interpreted.

Components of the health history include biographical data, the reason the patient is seeking health care, present health or history of present health concern, past health history, family history, functional health, psychosocial and lifestyle factors, and a review of systems. The nurse should adapt questions to the individual patient, omitting questions that do not apply and adding questions that seem pertinent, based on the setting, situation, the individual patient, and ongoing information as the health assessment proceeds. Be sure to use language the patient can understand; avoid using medical terms and jargon. Refer to Focused Assessment Guide 25-1 for examples of appropriate questions related to health history, family history, functional health, and psychosocial and lifestyle factors. Examples of health history questions related to each body system (review of systems) are included in the discussion of each region of the physical examination later in the chapter.

Biographical Data

Depending on the health care setting, some biographical data may be collected by people other than the nurse. For example, someone in the admissions department or a receptionist in a medical office may obtain demographic data, including the patient's name, address, billing and insurance information. Additional biographical information includes gender, age and birth date, marital status, occupation, race, ethnic origin, religious preference, and the patient's primary health care provider. The source of the information is also recorded. Differences in language and culture may have an effect on the quality and safety of health care. Language barriers appear to increase the risks to patient safety (Divi, Koss, Schmaltz, & Loeb, 2007). It is important to note the patient's preferred language for discussing health care, as well as any sensory or communication needs. This is a requirement for hospitals, based on the Joint Commission Standards (Joint Commission, 2010).

Reason for Seeking Health Care

The reason for requesting care is a statement in the patient's own words that describes the patient's reason for seeking care. This can help to focus the rest of the assessment. Ask an open-ended question, such as, "Tell me why you are here today." Try to record whatever the person has to say in the individual's exact words. Avoid paraphrasing or interpreting. For example, if Nina Dunning comes into the clinic and tells you "I am having trouble sleeping. At night, I can't seem to stop my thoughts. All I do is worry," it is important to document the patient's own words. It would be incorrect to document the following: "Patient complains of insomnia and anxiety." Correct documentation may include the following: "Patient states, 'I am having trouble sleeping. At night, I can't seem to stop my thoughts. All I do is worry.'"

History of Present Health Concern

When taking the patient's history of present health concern, be sure to explore the symptoms thoroughly. Encourage the patient to describe and explain any symptoms. The description should include information regarding the onset of the problem, location, duration, intensity, quality/description, relieving/exacerbating factors, associated factors, past occurrences, any treatments, and how the problem has affected the patient. Refer to Focused Assessment Guide 25-1 for examples of appropriate questions related to this component.

Past Health History

A patient's past health history may provide insight into causes of current symptoms. It also alerts the nurse to certain risk factors. A past health history includes childhood and adult illnesses, chronic health problems and treatment, and previous surgeries or hospitalizations. This history should also include accidents or injuries, obstetric history, allergies, and the date of most recent immunizations. Vaccine recommendations are updated each year by the Centers for Disease Control and Prevention (CDC). Current guidelines for different age groups can be found on the CDC's website at www.cdc.gov (CDC, 2012). Ask the patient about health maintenance screenings, including dates and results, as well as the use of safety measures. Ask the patient about prescribed and

FOCUSED ASSESSMENT GUIDE 25-1

HEALTH HISTORY

Factors to Assess	Questions and Approaches
Present Health History	• "When did you first begin having this problem?" • "Did it happen suddenly or slowly?" • "Show me exactly where you are having this problem." • "What other symptoms have you had with this problem?" • "How have you treated this problem?"
Past Health History	• "Tell me about the childhood illnesses, such as measles or mumps, that you had." • "What are you allergic to?" • "Describe any accidents, injuries, and surgeries you have had." • "What prescribed or over-the-counter medications do you use?" • "Do you take any herbal or dietary supplements?" • "What is the date of your most recent immunization for tetanus; pertussis; polio; measles; rubella; mumps; influenza; hepatitis A, B, and C; and pneumococcus?"
Family History	• "How old are the members of your family?" • "If any members of your family are not living, what caused their death?" • "Is there any history of this health problem you have in other family members?" • "Do any family members have long-term illnesses?"
Functional Health	• "Do you have difficulty or require assistance with bathing or dressing?" • "Do you have difficulty or require assistance with toileting or moving around?" • "Do you have difficulty or require assistance with eating or preparing meals?" • "Do you have difficulty or require assistance with shopping or administering your own medications?" • "Tell me about your driving. Who provides transportation?" • "Do you have difficulty or require assistance with housekeeping, finances, or laundry?"
Psychosocial/Lifestyle Factors	• "Do you smoke, drink, or use drugs? If so, what kind, for how long and how much?" • "Describe the foods you eat during a typical day." • "Tell me about how well you sleep." • "How much exercise do you get each day?" • "Who in your family or community is available to help you with health problems if you need it?" • "Does your religious faith or spirituality play an important part in your life?" • "Tell me about how you deal with stress." • "Describe any changes that you have had in your mood or feelings." • "Have you ever been treated for any problems with your mood or behavior?" • "Tell me about your use of seat belts in cars." • "Tell me about your family's use of sports helmets, padding, or other protective equipment."

over-the-counter medications, including vitamins, supplements, and any home or herbal remedies. Include the name, dose, route, frequency, and purpose for each medication. Refer to Focused Assessment Guide 25-1 for examples of appropriate questions related to this component.

Family History

Information about a person's family history will provide information about diseases and conditions for which an individual patient may be at increased risk. Certain disorders have genetic links. For example, a family history of cancer is a risk factor for cancer. Information regarding contact with family members with communicable diseases or environmental hazards can provide clues to the patient's current health or risk factors for health issues. It would be important to note that a family member had recently recovered from pertussis (whooping cough), especially if the patient

presented with respiratory symptoms. This information can also identify important topics for health teaching and counseling. For example, if a child with asthma is living in a household with family members who smoke, the child is at great risk for exacerbations of the disease. Family counseling regarding asthma and smoking would be an important health care intervention. Refer to Focused Assessment Guide 25-1 for examples of appropriate questions related to this component.

Functional Health Assessment

A functional health assessment focuses on the effects of health or illness on a patient's quality of life, including the strengths of the patient and areas that need to improve. Assess the patient's ability to perform **activities of daily living (ADLs)** or self-care activities. Eating, bathing, dressing, and toileting are examples of ADLs. Assess the patient's ability to perform **instrumental activities of daily living (IADLs)** or those needed for independent living. Housekeeping, meal preparation, management of finances, and transportation are examples of IADLs. Functional health may be further assessed using a formal tool, such as the Katz Index of Independence in Activities of Daily Living, which is used with older adults. This tool can be found in Chapter 32 on page 1057. Refer to Focused Assessment Guide 25-1 for examples of appropriate questions related to this component.

Psychosocial and Lifestyle Factors

A patient's lifestyle contributes to his or her overall health and well-being. For example, smoking is related to many health problems. Discussion of one or more of these topics may cause strong personal reactions by a patient. It is very important to be nonjudgmental and explain why you need to know certain information (Hogan-Quigley, Palm, & Bickley, 2012). Consider assessing these factors at the end of the interview, because these issues may naturally arise during the review of systems. Also, a trusting relationship has been established, making the discussion of personal issues easier (Jensen, 2011).

Ask about the patient's social support and network of available assistance. Ask about confidants, skillful supporters, and individuals that are able to help the patient to cope with any health alteration, illness, or other change. Support provided by caregivers, family, friends, and social organizations can ensure that a patient's recovery is more successful and prevent complications in the future (Price, 2011).

Ask about the patient's level of activity and exercise, sleep and rest, and nutrition. Obtain information related to the patient's interpersonal relationships and resources; values, beliefs, and spiritual resources; self-esteem and self-concept (Chapter 40); and coping and stress management. Question the patient regarding personal habits, including use of alcohol, illicit drugs, and/or tobacco; exposure to environmental and occupational hazards; intimate partner and family violence; sexual history and orientation; and mental health.

"Mental health is an integral part of a patient's well-being; thus, the assessment of mental health status is essential" (Jensen, 2011, p. 198). Regular screenings in primary care and other health care settings enables earlier identification of mental health and substance use disorders, leading to earlier treatment and care. Screenings should be provided to people of all ages, even the young and the elderly (Substance Abuse and Mental Health Services Administration [SAMHSA] and the Health Resources and Services Administration [HRSA] Center for Integrated Health Solutions, 2012). There are many assessment tools available to assist with screening for mental health disorders. Specific tools are available to screen for depression or suicide, for example, and to be used with specific populations, such as adolescents or the elderly. The Patient Health Questionnaire-9 (PHQ-9), the most common screening tool to identify depression, is one example of a mental health assessment tool (Box 25-1).

 REMEMBER Tammy Browning, the young mother who is having her first child. The nurse would include an assessment of current and past use of alcohol and drugs as part of Tammy's admission to the obstetric unit. This assessment would include questions regarding the type and amount of drugs and alcohol she has used or is using, as well as the frequency of use. ●

Refer to Focused Assessment Guide 25-1 for examples of appropriate questions related to this component.

Review of Systems

The **review of systems** is a series of questions about all body systems that helps to reveal concerns or problems as part of the health history. Many times, these questions can be incorporated into the physical examination of each region, such as asking about bowel habits when listening to bowel sounds in the abdomen. In addition, many questions relate to one or more body systems, thus the information obtained may pertain to more than one area. For example, asking about recent changes in weight is part of the overall health state, but it also provides information about fluid balance and edema (Jensen, 2011), and may offer information about appetite and functional ability. Examples of health history questions related to each body system are included in the discussion of each region of the physical examination later in the chapter.

PHYSICAL ASSESSMENT

A physical assessment is the systematic collection of objective information. The physical assessment is usually conducted in a head-to-toe sequence or a system sequence but can be adapted to meet the needs of the patient. It is often necessary to modify the sequence, positions, and specific assessments based on the patient's age, energy level, and cognitive and physical state, as well as time constraints. Even when modified, it is important to conduct the physical assessment in an organized and knowledgeable manner. Conducting an accurate physical assessment takes time and practice. Note that not all assessments included in a comprehensive physical assessment are covered in this chapter. The information reviewed here addresses the assessments that may be used by beginning practitioners. Consult an assessment textbook for additional information related to more advanced assessment procedures.

Preparing for a Physical Examination

Prior to beginning a physical examination, think about how to make the patient comfortable and relaxed. Be sure to use appropriate verbal and nonverbal communication techniques. Refer to the discussion earlier in this chapter. Think about the sequence of the examination—what order will be used to assess the areas required by the examination. Adjust the lighting and the environment; good lighting and a quiet environment are important, but not always possible. Do the best you can to make the conditions as favorable as possible (Hogan-Quigley et al., 2012). Refer also to the discussion of environmental preparation earlier in the chapter. Gather and

BOX 25-1 THE PATIENT HEALTH QUESTIONNAIRE-9 (PHQ-9)

Over the last 2 weeks, how often have you been bothered by any of the following problems? *(Use "✓" to indicate your answer)*	Not At All	Several Days	More Than Half the Days	Nearly Every Day
1. Little interest or pleasure in doing things	0	1	2	3
2. Feeling down, depressed, or hopeless	0	1	2	3
3. Trouble falling or staying asleep, or sleeping too much	0	1	2	3
4. Feeling tired or having little energy	0	1	2	3
5. Poor appetite or overeating	0	1	2	3
6. Feeling bad about yourself—or that you are a failure or have let yourself or your family down	0	1	2	3
7. Trouble concentrating on things, such as reading the newspaper or watching television	0	1	2	3
8. Moving or speaking so slowly that other people could have noticed. Or the opposite—being so fidgety or restless that you have been moving around a lot more than usual.	0	1	2	3
9. Thoughts that you would be better off dead or of hurting yourself in some way	0	1	2	3

FOR OFFICE CODING 0 + _____ + _____ + _____

= Total Score: _____

If you checked off any problems, how difficult have these problems made it for you to do your work, take care of things at home, or get along with other people?

Not difficult at all ☐	Somewhat difficult ☐	Very difficult ☐	Extremely difficult ☐

How to Score PHQ-9

Major Depressive Syndrome is suggested if:

- Of the 9 items, 5 or more are checked as at least "More than half the days"
- Either item #1 or #2 is positive, that is, at least "More than half the days"

Other Depressive Syndrome is suggested if:

- Of the 9 items, 2, 3, or 4 are checked as at least "More than half the days"
- Either item #1 or #2 is positive, that is, at least "More than half the days"

From Patient Health Questionnaire (PHQ) Screeners. Developed by Drs. Robert L. Spitzer, Janet B. W. Williams, Kurt Kroenke and colleagues, with an educational grant from Pfizer Inc. No permission required to reproduce, translate, display or distribute. Available at http://www.phqscreeners.com/

check the equipment needed for the examination. Assist the patient to the appropriate position to start the examination. Use proper hand hygiene techniques and standard precautions when performing physical examinations. Transmission-based precautions are implemented in addition as needed. Refer to Chapter 23 for information about hand hygiene, standard precautions, and transmission-based precautions.

Equipment

The equipment used in a physical assessment should be readily accessible, clean, and in proper working order. Equipment that will touch the patient should be warmed (by the examiner's hands or warm water) before use. Following are details about the equipment most likely used by beginning practitioners. However, beginning practitioners may observe or assist with more advanced assessments. Refer to Figure 25-1 (on page 632) for equipment that may be used by more advanced practitioners. Nurses will need a watch with a second hand in addition to the materials to follow.

Clean equipment after use with each patient, based on facility policies, to prevent transmission of organisms between patients or between the patient and the nurse.

THERMOMETER AND SPHYGMOMANOMETER

The thermometer is used to measure the patient's body temperature. A sphygmomanometer is used to measure blood pressure. Manual measurement with a sphygmomanometer is preferred over an electronic device. Refer to Chapter 24 for a more detailed discussion of equipment to measure vital signs.

SCALE

A scale (Fig. 25-2 on page 632) with height attachment is used to weigh the patient and measure height. Chair scales are available for patients who are unable to stand. Infants and children less than 2 or 3 years of age are weighed on a platform-type balance scale (Jarvis, 2012). Beds for use in hospitals and other facilities may have a scale built into the bed. Height may also be measured using a stadiometer, a device for measuring height that consists of a vertical ruler

FIGURE 25-1. Equipment used in advanced assessment. (**A**) Ophthalmoscope. (**B**) Otoscope. (**C**) Percussion hammer. (**D**) Nasal speculum. (**E**) Vaginal speculum and water-soluble lubricant.

with a sliding horizontal rod or paddle, which is adjusted to rest on the top of the head. It is often wall mounted, but is used horizontally on a tabletop for infants and young children to measure length.

FLASHLIGHT OR PENLIGHT

A light source is used to assist in viewing inside the mouth and nose. It is also used to determine the reactions of the pupils of the eyes.

STETHOSCOPE

The stethoscope, illustrated and described in Chapter 24, is used to measure blood pressure. It is also used to auscultate (listen to) heart, lung, abdomen, and cardiovascular sounds (Fig. 25-3). The bell of the stethoscope is used to listen to low-pitched sounds (such as heart murmurs). Use gentle pressure against the body part being examined when assessing low-pitched sounds. The diaphragm of the stethoscope is used to listen to high-pitched sounds such as normal heart sounds, breath sounds, and bowel sounds. Use firm pressure against the body part being examined when assessing high-pitched sounds. When using the stethoscope, expose the body part to be auscultated and try to minimize environmental noises.

METRIC TAPE MEASURE AND RULER

A tape measure is used to measure waist circumference in adults. It is also used to measure head circumference in infants and children up to 2 to 3 years of age, as well as chest circumference in infants. A ruler is used to measure abnormal findings on the skin, such as wounds, incisions, or lesions.

FIGURE 25-2. A scale with height attachment is used to weigh the patient and measure height. (Jensen, S. (2011). *Nursing health assessment: A best practice approach.* Philadelphia: Wolters Kluwer Health/Lippincott Williams & Wilkins.)

Bell side   **Diaphragm side**

FIGURE 25-3. Stethoscope bell and diaphragm. Use the *bell* of the stethoscope to detect low-pitched sounds. The bell should be at least 1 inch wide. Hold the bell lightly against the body part being auscultated. Use the *diaphragm* of the stethoscope to detect high-pitched sounds. The diaphragm should be at least 1.5 inches wide for adults and smaller for children. Hold the diaphragm firmly against the body part being auscultated.

FIGURE 25-4. Snellen chart.

FIGURE 25-5. Tuning forks.

EYE CHART

A Snellen eye chart (Fig. 25-4), or other vision assessment tool, is used to screen for distant vision. The Snellen chart consists of characters arranged in lines of different-sized type; the line of largest characters is at the top of the chart and the line of smallest characters is at the bottom. Scores ranging from 20/10 (the smallest line of characters) to 20/200 (the largest line of characters) indicate visual acuity.

A handheld vision screener, such as a Jaeger card, can be used to test near vision. The Jaeger card also consists of characters arranged in lines of different-sized type, like the Snellen chart. A distance equivalent based on the Snellen chart is shown on the side of the card.

TUNING FORK

A tuning fork (Fig. 25-5) is a two-pronged metal instrument used to test vibratory perception. The fork is activated to vibrate by holding the base and gently tapping the prongs against the palm of the examiner's hand. Once vibrating, the fork is held at the base to avoid diminishing the vibration.

Positioning and Draping

A variety of positions may be used during a physical assessment (Box 25-2 on page 634). During positioning, it is important to consider the patient's age, culture, health status, mobility, physical condition, energy level, and privacy.

Positioning patients who are weak or have physical limitations may require assistance. Positioning should be adjusted to accommodate patient limitations, such as arthritis, confusion, pain, or respiratory problems. Uncomfortable or embarrassing positions should not be maintained for long periods. The assessment should be organized so that several body systems can be assessed with the patient in one position, thus minimizing unneeded and possibly tiring movements.

Draping prevents unnecessary exposure, provides privacy, and keeps the patient warm during the physical assessment. Drapes may be paper, cloth, or bed linens. When conducting an assessment, expose only the body parts being assessed to maintain the patient's modesty and comfort.

Techniques of Physical Assessment

The four primary assessment techniques are inspection, palpation, percussion, and auscultation. These techniques are most often used in the sequence listed; variations are noted in the discussion of specific body areas later in the chapter. Bilateral body parts are always compared; for example, the assessment findings of one leg are compared with those of the other leg. Bilateral body parts are normally symmetric; that is, they have the same size and shape as well as the same characteristics, such as movement or pulses. Assess any areas that are likely to be painful or cause the patient extreme discomfort at the end of the examination.

Inspection

Inspection is the process of performing deliberate, purposeful observations in a systematic manner. Closely observe visually but also use hearing and smell to gather data throughout the assessment. Assess details of the patient's appearance, behavior, and movement. Inspection begins with the initial patient contact and continues through the entire assessment. Adequate natural or artificial lighting is essential for distinguishing the color, texture, and moisture of body surfaces.

Inspect each area of the body for size, color, shape, position, movement, and symmetry, noting normal findings and any deviations from normal. Inspection, followed by palpation, may sequentially be used during the assessment of each body part.

Palpation

Palpation uses the sense of touch. The hands and fingers are sensitive tools that can assess skin temperature, turgor,

BOX 25-2   POSITIONS USED DURING PHYSICAL ASSESSMENT

Standing

The patient stands erect. This position should not be used for patients who are weak, dizzy, or prone to fall. It is used to assess posture, balance, and gait (while walking upright).

Standing

Sitting

The patient may sit in a chair or on the side of the bed or examining table, or remain in bed with the head elevated. It allows visualization of the upper body, facilitates full lung expansion, and is used to assess vital signs and the head, neck, anterior and posterior thorax, lungs, heart, breasts, and upper extremities.

Sitting

Supine

The patient lies flat on the back with legs extended and knees slightly flexed. It facilitates abdominal muscle relaxation and is used to assess vital signs and the head, neck, anterior thorax, lungs, heart, breasts, abdomen, extremities, and peripheral pulses.

Supine

Dorsal Recumbent

The patient lies on the back with legs separated, knees flexed, and soles of the feet on the bed. It is used to assess the head, neck, anterior thorax, lungs, heart, breasts, extremities, and peripheral pulses. It should not be used for abdominal assessment because it causes contraction of the abdominal muscles.

Dorsal recumbent

Sims Position

The patient lies on either side with the lower arm below the body and the upper arm flexed at the shoulder and elbow. Both knees are flexed, with the upper leg more acutely flexed. It is used to assess the rectum or vagina.

Sims position

Prone

The patient lies flat on the abdomen with the head turned to one side. It is used to assess the hip joint and the posterior thorax.

Prone

Lithotomy

The patient is in the dorsal recumbent position with the buttocks at the edge of the examining table and the heels in stirrups. It is used to assess female genitalia and rectum.

Lithotomy

Knee–chest

The patient kneels, with the body at a 90-degree angle to the hips, back straight, arms above the head. It is used to assess the anus and rectum.

Knee-chest

FIGURE 25-6. (Left) Palmar surfaces of the examiner's fingertips and fingerpads are used for discriminatory sensation such as texture, vibration, presence of fluid, or size and consistency of a mass. **(Right)** The dorsum, or back of the hand, is used to assess surface temperature.

texture, and moisture, as well as vibrations within the body (such as the heart) and shape or structures within the body (e.g., the bones). Specific parts of the hand are more effective at assessing different qualities (Fig. 25-6). The dorsum (back) surfaces of the hand and fingers are used for gross measure of temperature. The palmar (front) surfaces of the fingers and fingerpads are used to assess firmness, contour, shape, tenderness, and consistency. The fingerpads are best at fine discrimination. Use fingerpads to locate pulses, lymph nodes, and other small lumps, and to assess skin texture and edema. Vibration is palpated best with the ulnar, or outside, surface of the hand.

The nurse's hands should be warm and the fingernails short. Inform the patient about the areas to be palpated and ask for permission to use touch. When conducting palpation, any area of tenderness is palpated last. Light (gentle), moderate, or deep palpation may be used, controlling the depth by the amount of pressure applied. For light palpation, apply pressure with the fingers together and depressing the skin and underlying structures less than 1 cm (0.5″; Fig. 25-7). Moderate palpation is conducted by depressing

FIGURE 25-7. In light palpation, light pressure is applied by placing the fingers together and depressing the skin and underlying structures about 1 cm (½″). *(Photo by B. Proud.)*

Table 25-1 | **CHARACTERISTICS OF MASSES DETERMINED BY PALPATION**

QUALITY	CHARACTERISTICS TO DETERMINE
Shape	Round Ovoid Tubular Irregular
Size	Measured in cm
Consistency	Firm Edematous Spongy Cystic
Surface	Smooth Nodular Granular
Mobility	Fixed or nonmobile Mobile
Tenderness	Amount of tenderness to touch
Pulsatile	Pulsation can or cannot be felt in the mass

the skin surface 1 to 2 cm (0.5″ to 0.75″). Deep palpation, which carries a risk of internal injury, should be used cautiously and only by experienced advanced practitioners. Characteristics of masses, as determined by palpation, are described in Table 25-1.

Percussion

Percussion is the act of striking one object against another to produce sound. The fingertips are used to tap the body over body tissues to produce vibrations and sound waves. The characteristics of the sounds produced are used to assess the location, shape, size, and density of tissues. Abnormal sounds suggest alteration of tissues, such as an emphysematous lung, or the presence of a mass, such as an abdominal tumor. A quiet environment allows sounds to be heard. Refer to information on thePoint or a health assessment text for details.

Auscultation

Auscultation is the act of listening with a stethoscope to sounds produced within the body. Auscultation is performed by placing the stethoscope diaphragm or bell against the body part being assessed. When auscultating, expose the part listened to, use the proper part of the stethoscope (diaphragm or bell) for specific sounds (see previous discussion of a stethoscope), and listen in a quiet environment.

Four characteristics of sound are assessed by auscultation: (1) pitch (ranging from high to low), (2) loudness (ranging from soft to loud), (3) quality (e.g., gurgling or swishing), and (4) duration (short, medium, or long).

Conducting a Physical Assessment

Although there are various organizing structures for conducting a physical assessment, one often used proceeds from head to toe. Although each body system is discussed individually here, in reality, nurses usually combine several systems (e.g., while assessing the head and neck they also assess the cranial nerves, which are part of the neurologic system). The accompanying head-to-toe assessment video demonstrates proper technique.

Performing a General Survey

The general survey is the first component of the physical assessment, beginning with the first moment of patient contact and continuing throughout the nurse–patient relationship. The general survey contributes to the overall impression of the patient. It includes observing the patient's overall appearance and behavior, taking vital signs, measuring height, weight, and waist circumference, and calculating the body mass index (BMI). Information from the general survey provides clues to the patient's overall health.

HEALTH HISTORY

Identify risk factors for altered health during the health history by asking about the following:

- History of changes in weight
- History of pain or discomfort
- Sleeping patterns, difficulty sleeping

APPEARANCE AND BEHAVIOR

Observations of the patient's appearance and behavior provides information about various aspects of the patient's health. While collecting information during the health history, inspect the patient's body build, posture, and gait. Note proportion of height to weight, which provides insight into nutritional status. Observe whether the patient has an erect or slumped posture, and evaluate movements and gait pattern for coordination. Uncoordinated or spontaneous movements may suggest neurologic problems. Note signs of illness and/or distress, such as changes in posture, skin color, and respirations; nonverbal communication of pain; and short attention span.

Observe hygiene and grooming (cleanliness, body odors) and note any deficits, which may indicate other problems. For example, patients with inappropriate dress (e.g., wrong for the season) or worn or dirty clothing may be experiencing feelings of depression or have inadequate financial resources. Assess cognitive processes (speech content and patterns; orientation to person, place, and time; appropriate verbal responses). As cognitive processes are controlled by the neurologic system, these are discussed later in the chapter.

Clues to mood and mental health are provided by speech, facial expressions, ability to relax, eye contact, and behavior. If depression, anxiety, or other mental health disorders are suspected, use appropriate screening tools and refer the patient to the appropriate health care professionals as necessary. Box 25-3 presents the Geriatric Depression Scale, a useful tool in screening older adults for depression. This tool is completed by the patient and reviewed by the practitioner.

HEIGHT AND WEIGHT

The ratio of height to weight is an assessment of overall health and overnutrition or undernutrition. Measure height and weight using accurate scales and measuring devices. Ask the patient to remove shoes and heavy clothing if the measurements are taken before undressing (Guidelines for Nursing Care 25-1). If the patient cannot stand erect, obtain

---

Box 25-3 GERIATRIC DEPRESSION SCALE (GDS)

Instructions: Circle the answer that best describes how you felt over the <u>past week</u>.

	yes	no
1. Are you basically satisfied with your life?	yes	no
2. Have you dropped many of your activities and interests?	yes	no
3. Do you feel that your life is empty?	yes	no
4. Do you often get bored?	yes	no
5. Are you in good spirits most of the time?	yes	no
6. Are you afraid that something bad is going to happen to you?	yes	no
7. Do you feel happy most of the time?	yes	no
8. Do you often feel helpless?	yes	no
9. Do you prefer to stay at home, rather than going out and doing things?	yes	no
10. Do you feel that you have more problems with memory than most?	yes	no
11. Do you think it is wonderful to be alive now?	yes	no
12. Do you feel worthless the way you are now?	yes	no
13. Do you feel full of energy?	yes	no
14. Do you feel that your situation is hopeless?	yes	no
15. Do you think that most people are better off than you are?	yes	no

Total Score _____

Scoring Instructions: Score 1 point for "no" to questions 1, 5, 7, 11, and 13. Score 1 point for "yes" to other questions. A total score of 5 or more suggests depression.

Reprinted with permission from Yesavage, J. A. (1986). The use of Rating Depression Series in the Elderly. In L. W. Poon (Ed.). *Clinical memory assessment of older adults.* Washington, DC: American Psychological Association.

GUIDELINES FOR NURSING CARE 25-1

OBTAINING HEIGHT AND WEIGHT WITH AN UPRIGHT BALANCE SCALE

Obtaining Height
- Ask the patient to remove shoes.
- Raise L-shaped sliding arm on the measuring device attached to the scale somewhat higher than the patient's approximate height.
- Ask the patient to step on the platform of the scale and stand erect with the back to the measuring device and the heels together.
- Lower the L-shaped sliding arm until it rests on top of the patient's head.
- Read the height in inches and record.
- Ask the patient to step down from the platform.

Obtaining Weight
- Balance the scale on zero.
- Ask the patient to remove shoes (and coat, if appropriate) and step onto the platform.
- Move the sliding indicator to the left until the scale balances.
- Read the weight in pounds and record.
- Ask the patient to step down from the platform.
- Return the scale weight indicator to zero.
- Considerations: Daily weights should be obtained at the same time each day (usually early morning), with the patient wearing the same clothing, and using the same scale.

Photo by B. Proud.

weight using a chair or bed scale. Refer to Skill 25-1 on pages 672–674 for instructions to obtain a patient's weight using a bed scale.

Make sure to measure the height of children 2 years of age and younger in the recumbent position with the legs fully extended. Weigh infants without any clothing, and weigh children in their underwear.

 REMEMBER Ramona Lewis, the young woman with anorexia nervosa. The nurse would use baseline data, including Ramona's height and weight, to monitor Ramona's health status. ●

BODY MASS INDEX AND WAIST CIRCUMFERENCE
Body mass index (adults and children) and waist circumference (adults) are the preferred methods to establish ideal body weight. **Body mass index (BMI)** is a ratio of weight to height. BMI is used as an initial assessment of nutritional status, and is an indicator of obesity or malnutrition. BMI also provides an estimation of relative risk for some diseases. Calculate the BMI after obtaining the patient's height and weight. Refer to the discussion of BMI, including method for calculation, in Chapter 35.

Waist circumference is the measurement around a patient at the level of the umbilicus and is a good indicator of abdominal fat. The location of excess body fat is thought to be an important and reliable indicator of risk for

diseases. Refer to the discussion of waist circumference in Chapter 35.

VITAL SIGNS
Vital signs are measured to establish a baseline for the database and to detect actual or potential health problems. Some facilities, particularly hospitals, may include measurement of oxygen saturation as part of the vital signs. Vital signs are discussed in detail in Chapter 24. Oxygen saturation is discussed in Chapter 38.

PAIN
Pain assessment is often considered the fifth vital sign. Assessment of pain is part of the initial assessment of a patient, and continues throughout the nurse–patient relationship. Assessment of pain is discussed in Chapter 34.

Assessing the Integument
The integument is comprised of the skin, nails, hair, and scalp. Assessing the integumentary structures provides information about the patient's overall health status, as well as clues to local or systemic health problems. It also provides data about self-care activities to maintain health, hygiene, and nutrition. Assessing for skin cancer is essential and provides the base for teaching skin cancer prevention. Refer to Box 25-4 (on page 638) for guidelines on assessing for melanoma. Additional information related to assessment of the integument is discussed in Chapter 31.

BOX 25-4 ASSESSING FOR MELANOMA

Warning Signs: The ABCDEs of Melanoma

A: Asymmetry

If a line is drawn through a mole, the two halves will not match.

B: Border

The borders of an early melanoma tend to be uneven. The edges may be scalloped or notched.

C: Color

Having a variety of colors is another warning signal. A number of different shades of brown, tan, or black could appear. A melanoma may also become red, blue, or some other color.

D: Diameter

Melanomas usually are larger in diameter than the size of the eraser on your pencil (1/4 inch or 6 mm), but they may sometimes be smaller when first detected.

E: Evolving

Any change—in size, shape, color, elevation, or another trait, or any new symptom such as bleeding, itching or crusting—points to danger.

Source: Skin Cancer Foundation. (2012). Melanoma. Available at http://www.skincancer.org/skin-cancer-information/melanoma

FIGURE 25-8. The skin is inspected for color, vascularity, and lesions. (*Photo by B. Proud.*)

HEALTH HISTORY

Identify risk factors for altered health during the health history by asking about the following:

- History of rashes, lesions, change in color, or itching
- History of bruising or bleeding in the skin
- History of allergies to medications, plants, foods, or other substances
- Exposure to the sun and sunburn history
- History of bathing routines and products
- Presence of lesions (wounds, bruises, abrasions, or burns)
- Presence of body piercings and/or tattoos
- Change in the color, size, or shape of a mole
- Recent chemotherapy or radiation therapy
- Exposure to chemicals that may be harmful to the skin, hair, or nails
- Degree of mobility
- Types of food eaten and liquids consumed each day
- Cultural practices related to skin

PHYSICAL ASSESSMENT

The skin, hair, and nails are assessed by inspection and palpation. Assessment of the skin should begin with the general survey and continue throughout the physical examination. Protect the patient's privacy by exposing only the body part being examined. If the patient has lesions of the skin (including the scalp) or an infestation of the hair with lice, wear gloves during palpation.

The skin is a general indicator of the patient's health status and provides information that might indicate an underlying disease. Begin the assessment with an overall inspection of the skin's condition. Assess specific areas of the skin during other body system assessments (e.g., you may assess the skin on the abdomen while performing other abdominal assessments). Ensure adequate lighting, which is essential for accurate assessments. Inspect the skin for color, vascularity, and lesions (Fig. 25-8), and palpate for temperature, moisture, turgor, and texture.

Inspecting Skin Color

Skin color varies among races and among individuals, ranging from a pinkish white to various shades of brown. Skin areas that are normally exposed, such as the face and hands, may have a somewhat different color from areas that are usually covered by clothing, but otherwise skin color is relatively constant. Take special care to detect color changes in patients with dark skin tones. Some body areas of people with darker skin tones, such as the palms of the hands and the soles of the feet, normally have less pigmentation than other body areas.

Changes in skin color include erythema, cyanosis, jaundice, and pallor (Table 25-2). These color changes are often easier to assess in people with light skin tones. **Erythema**, redness of the skin, is caused by dilation of superficial blood vessels. It is associated with sunburn, inflammation, fever, trauma, and allergic reactions. When assessing for erythema in people with darker skin tones, it is important to assess skin temperature; areas of erythema will feel warm compared with surrounding skin.

 THINK back to Billy Collins, the child who was stung by a bee. The nurse would use inspection skills to observe for erythema in the area of the sting. ●

Cyanosis is a bluish or grayish discoloration of the skin in response to inadequate oxygenation. Cyanosis is assessed as a blue tinge in patients with white skin and as dullness in patients with dark skin tones. **Jaundice** is a yellow color of the skin resulting from elevated amounts of bilirubin in

Table 25-2 SKIN COLOR ASSESSMENT

COLOR VARIATIONS	ASSESSMENT AREAS	POSSIBLE CAUSES
Redness (erythema, flushing)	Facial area, localized area of skin on the body	Blushing, alcohol intake, fever, injury trauma, infection
Bluish (cyanosis)	Exposed areas, particularly the ears, lips, inside of the mouth, hands and feet, and nail beds	Cold environment, cardiac or respiratory disease (decreased oxygenation)
Yellowish (jaundice)	Overall skin areas, mucous membranes, and sclera	Liver disease (increase in bilirubin levels)
Paleness (pallor)	Exposed areas, particularly the face and lips, conjunctivae, and mucous membranes	Anemia (decreased hemoglobin) Shock (decreased blood volume)
Vitiligo (whitish patchy areas on the skin)	Overall skin areas, lips, nail beds, and conjunctivae	Depigmentation (congenital or autoimmune conditions)
Tanned or brown	Sun-exposed areas	Overexposure (increased melanin production), pregnancy (brown spots)

the blood. It is associated with liver and gallbladder disease, some types of anemia, and excessive hemolysis (breakdown of red blood cells). It usually develops first in the sclera of the eyes and then in the skin and mucous membranes. It is more difficult to observe jaundice on the trunk of the body in patients with darker skin tones but the sclera, oral mucous membranes, palms, and soles appear yellow to yellow-orange. **Pallor**, or paleness of the skin, often results from a decrease in the amount of circulating blood or hemoglobin, causing inadequate oxygenation of the body tissues. Depending on severity, pallor may be visible over the entire skin surface or only in the lips, nail beds, mucous membranes, and conjunctiva. Pallor in patients with dark skin tones is seen as an ashen gray or yellow tinge.

Inspecting Skin Vascularity and Lesions

Inspect the skin for vascularity, bleeding, or bruising; these signs might relate to a cardiovascular, hematologic, or liver dysfunction. **Ecchymosis** is a collection of blood in the subcutaneous tissues, causing purplish discoloration. **Petechiae** are small hemorrhagic spots caused by capillary bleeding. If they are present, assess their location, color, and size.

Lesions are areas of diseased or injured tissue such as bruises, scratches, cuts, burns, insect bites, and wounds (breaks in the continuity of the skin). Lesions are categorized as primary or secondary. Primary lesions are those that may arise from previously normal skin (Table 25-3 on page 640). Secondary lesions result from changes in primary lesions (Table 25-4 on page 641). Assess lesions and wounds for size, shape, depth, location, and presence of drainage or odor. Wounds are discussed in Chapter 31. Scars are healed wounds. Describe rashes (skin eruptions) in terms of their type, size, elevation, coloring, and presence of drainage or itching. Assess the location and condition of body piercings and/or tattoos. Document the exact body surface areas involved.

Palpating Skin Temperature, Texture, Moisture, and Turgor

The skin is normally warm and dry. An increase in skin temperature and moisture can indicate an elevated body temperature. The texture of the skin varies from smooth and soft to rough and dry. In the dehydrated patient, the texture is dry, loose, and wrinkled, and the mucous membranes are cracked and dry. An excessive amount of perspiration, such as when the entire skin is moist, is called **diaphoresis**.

Turgor is the fullness or elasticity of the skin. It is usually assessed on the sternum or under the clavicle by lifting a fold of skin with the thumb and first finger (Fig. 25-9). Skin turgor is normal when the fold returns to its usual shape when released. When the patient is dehydrated, the skin's elasticity is decreased, and the skin fold returns slowly. Decreased skin turgor may be a normal finding in older patients, as a result of decreased elasticity and thinning of the dermis as a person ages.

Difficulty in lifting a skin fold may indicate **edema** (excess fluid in the tissues). Edema is characterized by swelling, with taut and shiny skin over the edematous area. If the area of edema is palpated with the fingers, an indentation (measured in mm for depth of the indentation) may remain after the pressure is released; if the indentation is very deep, it is called pitting edema. Edema may be graded; refer to Chapter 39 for a visual representation of a grading system.

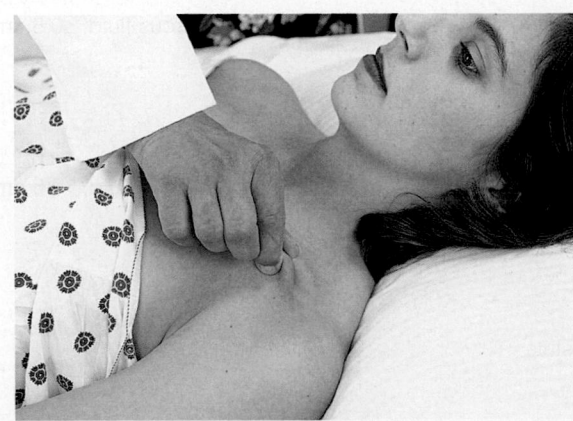

FIGURE 25-9. To assess skin turgor, a small fold of skin is picked up and then released to return to its normal shape. Difficulty in lifting a skin fold may indicate presence of edema. *(Photo by B. Proud.)*

Table 25-3   PRIMARY SKIN LESIONS

LESION NAME	DESCRIPTION	EXAMPLE	ILLUSTRATION
Circumscribed, Flat, Nonpalpable Change in Skin Color			
Macule	Lesion ≤1 cm	Petechiae, freckle	Macule
Patch	Lesion >1 cm	Vitiligo	Patch
Palpable, Elevated Solid Masses			
Papule	Mass ≤0.5 cm	Mole	Papule
Plaque	Mass >0.5 cm	Coalesced papules	Plaque
Nodule	Mass 0.5–2 cm; firmer than a papule	Nevus (wart)	Nodule
Tumor	Mass >2 cm	Lipoma	Tumor
Wheal	Irregular, superficial area of localized skin edema	Hives, mosquito bite	Wheal
Circumscribed, Superficial Skin Elevations Formed by Free Fluid in a Cavity Within the Skin Layers			
Vesicle	Filled with serous fluid, ≤0.5 cm	Herpes simplex	Vesicle
Bulla	Filled with serous fluid, >0.5 cm	2nd-degree burn	Bulla
Pustule	Filled with pus	Acne, impetigo	Pustule

Table 25-4 SECONDARY AND MISCELLANEOUS SKIN LESIONS

LESION NAME	DESCRIPTION	EXAMPLE
Secondary Lesions		
Loss of Skin Surface		
Erosion	Loss of superficial epidermis, moist, nonbleeding surface	Moist area after rupture of a vesicle, as in chickenpox
Ulcer	Loss of epidermis and dermis, may bleed and scar	Stasis ulcer
Fissure	Deep linear crack, extends into dermis	Athlete's foot
Material on the Skin Surface		
Crust	Dried residue of serum, pus, or blood	Impetigo
Scale	Thin flake of exfoliated dermis	Dandruff, dry skin
Miscellaneous Lesions		
Lichenification	Thickened and roughened epidermis, with increased visibility of skin furrows	Atrophic dermatitis
Atrophy	Thinning of the skin, loss of skin furrows, shiny appearance	Peripheral vascular disease
Excoriation	Scratch of the epidermis	
Scar	Fibrous tissue replaces tissue in the dermis or subcutaneous layer	
Keloid	Hypertrophied scar	
Other Common Skin Lesions, Not Technically Primary or Secondary		
Comedo	Plugged opening of a sebaceous gland, a hallmark of acne	Common blackhead
Telangiectasia	Small, dilated, red or bluish surface vessels, may be part of a basal cell carcinoma or skin injury from radiation	
Nevus	Flat to slightly elevated, round, evenly pigmented	Common mole

Edema may be the result of overhydration, heart failure, kidney failure, trauma, or peripheral vascular disease.

Inspecting the Nails

Inspect the nails for shape, angle, texture, and color. The nails should be somewhat convex and should follow the natural curve of the finger. The angle between the nail and its base should be about 160 degrees. The nails should be smooth, and the nail base, when palpated, should be firm and nontender. Abnormal findings include indentations called Beau's lines (from acute illness), infection, painless separation of the nail plate from the nail bed (onycholysis) due to infection or trauma, increased brittleness or thickness and angulation (from anemia or iron deficiency anemia), and clubbing (from long-term lack of oxygenation). Figure 25-10 (on page 642) illustrates nail abnormalities.

Inspecting the Hair and Scalp

Hair is found on all body surfaces except the palms of the hands, the soles of the feet, and parts of the genitalia. Assess the hair for color, texture, and distribution. The hair is normally resilient, evenly distributed, and neither excessively dry nor oily. Abnormal findings include unusual balding (alopecia) and excessive amounts of hair on the face and body (hirsutism). Hair loss may be normal or may be the result of chemotherapy, radiation therapy, infection, hormonal disorders, or inadequate nutrition. Decreased oxygenation of peripheral tissues, especially of the lower extremities, may cause loss of hair. Excessive hair growth may occur in persons with hormonal disorders.

Separate the hair to inspect the scalp for color, dryness, scaliness, lumps, lesions, or lice. Nits, which are the white eggs of lice, can be differentiated from dandruff or lint because they are attached to the hair shaft. If any lumps or masses are palpated, note their location, size, tenderness, and mobility.

NORMAL AGE-RELATED VARIATIONS

Infant/Child

Common skin variations in newborns and children include:

- Jaundice and milia (whiteheads) in newborns
- Fine downy hair (lanugo) for the first 2 weeks of life
- Smooth, thin skin at birth
- Pubic hair development at the onset of puberty

Older Adult

Common skin variations in the older adult include:

- Wrinkles, dryness, scaling, decreased turgor
- Raised dark areas (senile keratosis)
- Flat, brown age spots (senile lentigines)
- Small, round red spots (cherry angioma)
- Fine, brittle gray or white hair
- Hair loss
- Coarse facial hair in women, decreased body hair in men and women
- Thick, yellow toenails

Assessing the Head and Neck

Assessment of the head and neck includes the skull, face, eyes, ears, nose and sinuses, mouth and pharynx, trachea, thyroid gland, and lymph nodes. During the health history, note any health problems such as headaches or dizziness. If the patient smokes, include a discussion about ways to

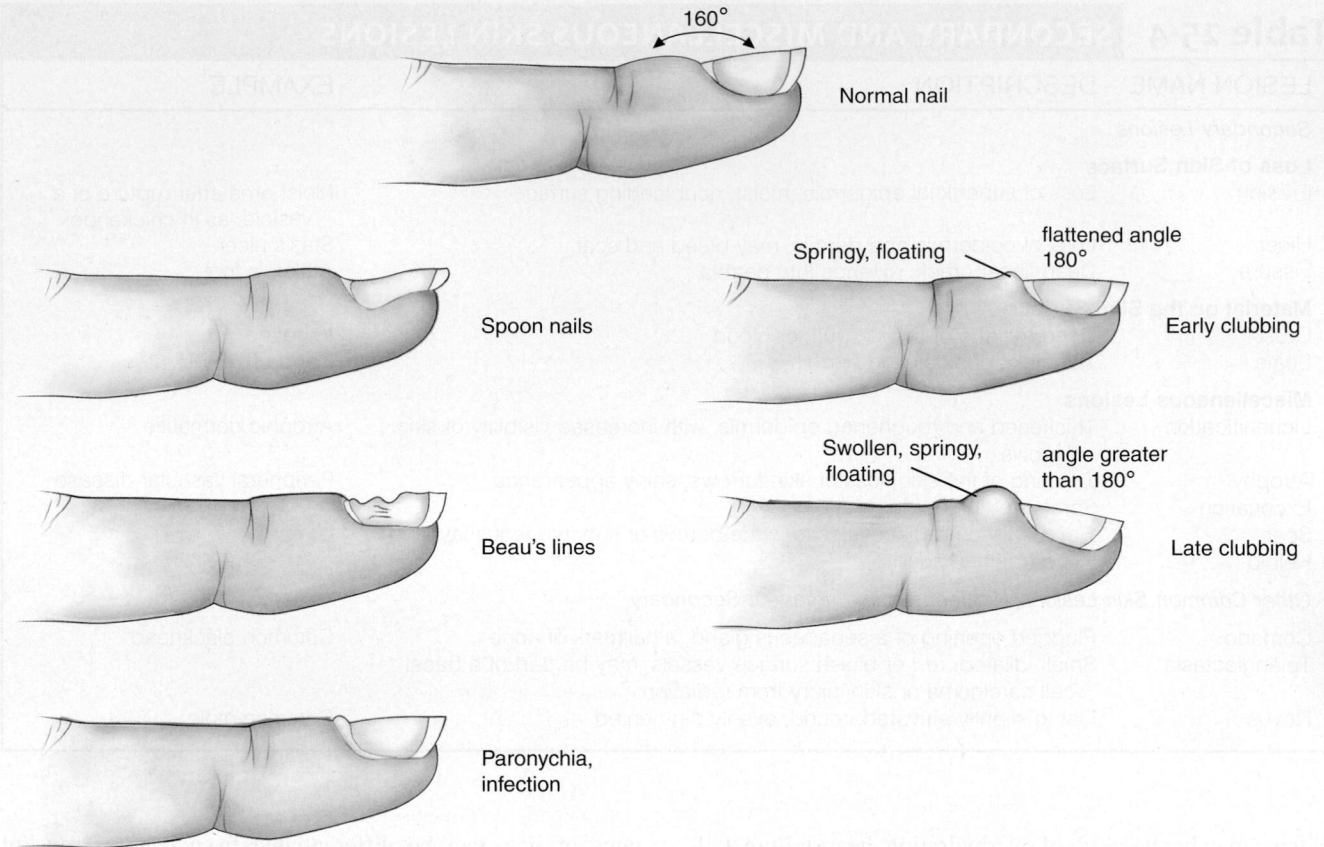

FIGURE 25-10. Examples of nail abnormalities.

stop smoking in the plan of care. Physical examination of the structures of the head and neck provides data about the shape and structure of cranial bones, function of special senses (sight, hearing, taste, smell), nasal and oral structures, and any swelling or pain in the lymph nodes in the neck. Assessment of the size and consistency of the thyroid gland is performed by advance practice professionals. Refer to a health assessment text for details.

HEALTH HISTORY

Identify risk factors for altered health during the health history by asking about the following:

- Changes in vision or hearing with aging
- History of use of corrective lenses or hearing aids
- Loss of an eye (use of artificial eye)
- History of allergies
- History of disturbances in vision or hearing
- History of chronic illnesses such as hypertension, diabetes mellitus, or thyroid disease
- Exposure to harmful substances or loud noises
- Exposure to ultraviolet light
- History of smoking (how long, how many packs/day), chewing tobacco, or cocaine use
- Presence of body piercings and/or tattoos
- History of eye or ear infections
- History of head trauma
- History of persistent hoarseness
- Oral and dental care practices

PHYSICAL ASSESSMENT

Inspecting and Palpating the Head and Face

Inspect and palpate the head for size and shape. The parts of the head and face should be in proportion to each other and symmetric. Although the shape of the normal skull varies considerably, generally the shape is gently curved with prominences at the frontal and parietal bones. Abnormal findings include lack of symmetry or unusual size or contour of the skull (either may be the result of trauma or diseases affecting the growth of bone) and tenderness. If the skull of a child or an adult appears disproportionately large or small, measure the circumference. Measuring head circumference is a normal part of infant assessment to the age of 2 to 3 years and should be conducted at each health-related visit.

Inspect the face for color, symmetry, and distribution of facial hair. Edema of the face, especially around the eye (periorbital edema), and involuntary facial movements (e.g., tics, fasciculations, tremors) are abnormal findings. If abnormalities are noted, document the location, amount, duration, and timing.

Inspecting the Eyes

Assess the structures and functions of the eyes by using a penlight and an eye chart. Inspection is the primary assessment technique used. Assessment includes the external eye structures, visual acuity, extraocular movements, and peripheral vision. Advanced practitioners usually perform assessment of the internal eye structures with an ophthalmoscope,

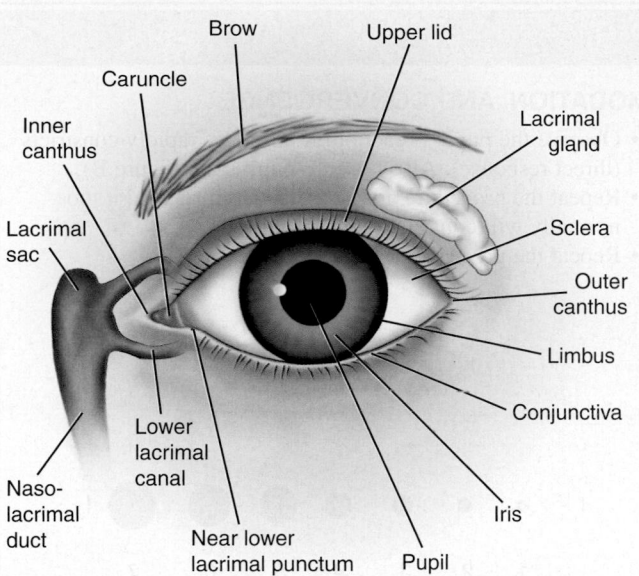

FIGURE 25-11. The eye and surrounding structures.

[Figure labels: Brow, Upper lid, Caruncle, Inner canthus, Lacrimal gland, Lacrimal sac, Sclera, Outer canthus, Limbus, Conjunctiva, Lower lacrimal canal, Naso-lacrimal duct, Near lower lacrimal punctum, Pupil, Iris]

which is an advanced assessment skill. Refer to information on thePoint or a health assessment text for details.

Inspecting External Eye Structures. Inspect the eyes, eyebrows, eyelids, eyelashes, lacrimal glands, pupils, and iris for position and alignment (Fig. 25-11). Asymmetry of position and alignment of the eyes may be caused by muscle weakness or a congenital abnormality. The eyebrows should be equally distributed; the eyelashes should curl outward.

Inspect the eyelids for color, edema, and equal coverage of the eyeball. Abnormal findings include drooping of the upper lids (ptosis), which may be attributable to damage to the oculomotor nerve, myasthenia gravis, or a congenital disorder; inward turning of the lower lid and lashes (entropion); outward turning of the lower lid and lashes (ectropion); and redness or drainage (from infection of the lid margins, conjunctivae, or hair follicles). Inspect and palpate the lacrimal glands for edema and pain.

The pupils are normally black, equal in size, round, and smooth. The pupils may be pale and cloudy if the patient has cataracts (loss of opacity of the lens). Injury to the eye, glaucoma, and certain medications may cause the pupil to dilate (mydriasis); certain drugs can cause constriction (miosis), and unequal pupils may result from central nervous system injury or illness.

Assess the pupils for reaction to light and accommodation and for convergence (Guidelines for Nursing Care 25-2 on page 644). Decreased or absent pupillary response indicates blindness or serious brain damage. Inability of the eyes to accommodate or converge is abnormal.

Assessing Visual Acuity, Extraocular Movements, and Peripheral Vision. Assess visual acuity with the Snellen chart. Have the patient stand 20 feet from the chart and ask the patient to read the smallest line of letters possible, first with both eyes

and then with one eye at a time (with the opposite eye covered). Note whether the patient's vision is being tested with or without corrective lenses.

Visual acuity is measured by using the standardized numbers listed on the side of the chart. The numerator is 20, representing the distance in feet the patient was from the test. The denominator represents the smallest line read accurately by the patient. Visual acuity is recorded as a fraction and is written as 20 over the smallest line read by the patient with no more than two inaccurate readings (such as "20/30–2 with glasses"). Thus, the larger the denominator, the poorer the vision (Jensen, 2011). Use a Snellen picture chart or Snellen E chart to test vision in patients who are unable to read English and in young children. The E chart uses the capital letter E in varying sizes pointing in different directions. The patient points his or her fingers in the direction the legs of the E are pointing.

Test near vision with a handheld vision screen with varying sizes of print. A Jaeger card can be used for this measurement. The patient holds the card 14 inches from the eyes. Ask the patient to read the smallest line of letters possible, with one eye at a time (with the opposite eye covered), and corrective lenses in place, if used. The results are recorded as a fraction and written as 14 over the smallest line read by the patient. A normal result is 14/14.

Test extraocular movements by assessing the cardinal fields of vision for coordination and alignment. Normally both eyes move together, are coordinated, and are parallel. Tests for peripheral vision (or visual fields) are used to assess retinal function and optic nerve function. Full peripheral vision is normal. Guidelines for Nursing Care 25-3 (on page 645) describe how to assess extraocular movements and peripheral vision.

Inspecting Internal Eye Structures. The internal eye is examined with the ophthalmoscope to assess the fundus, including the retina, optic nerve disc, macula, fovea centralis, and retinal vessels. Abnormal findings include cloudiness of the lens (from cataracts), changes in the size and shape of blood vessels (from hypertension or arteriosclerosis), and changes in color and surface characteristics (from such health problems as diabetes mellitus, hypertension, trauma, inflammation, or a detached retina).

Using the ophthalmoscope to inspect the internal eye structures is an advanced assessment skill and usually performed by advanced practitioners. Refer to information on thePoint or a health assessment text for details.

Inspecting and Palpating the Ears

Assess the external ear by inspection and palpation. An otoscope is used to inspect the ear canal and tympanic membrane, which is usually performed by advanced practitioners, being an advanced assessment skill. Refer to information on thePoint or a health assessment text for details.

Inspecting and Palpating the External Ear. Inspect the external ear (Fig. 25-12 on page 645) for shape, size, and lesions. The external surfaces of the ear should be smooth, and the

GUIDELINES FOR NURSING CARE 25-2

MEASURING PUPILLARY REACTION, SIZE, ACCOMMODATION, AND CONVERGENCE

Pupillary Reaction

- Darken the room.
- Ask the patient to look straight ahead.
- Bring the penlight from the side of the patient's face and briefly shine the light on the pupil (Figure A).

FIGURE A. Assessing papillary reaction.

Accommodation

- Hold the forefinger, a pencil, or other straight object about 10 to 15 cm (4″ to 6″) from the bridge of the patient's nose.

- Observe the pupil's reaction; it normally rapidly constricts (direct response). Also observe pupil size (Figure B).
- Repeat the procedure and observe the other eye; it too normally will constrict (consensual reflex).
- Repeat the procedure with the other eye.

1 2 3 4 5 6 7

FIGURE B. Pupillary gauge measures pupils (dilation or constriction) in millimeters (mm).

- Ask the patient to first look at the object, then at a distant object, then back to the object being held. The pupil normally constricts when looking at a near object and dilates when looking at a distant object (Figure C).

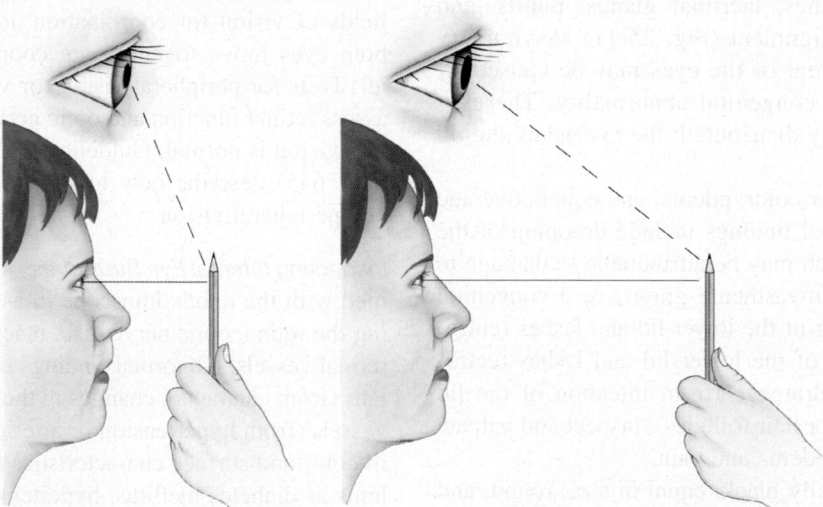

FIGURE C. Assessing accommodation.

Convergence

- Hold your finger about 6″ to 8″ from the bridge of the patient's nose.
- Move your finger toward the patient's nose to assess convergence (Figure D). The patient's eyes should normally converge (assume a cross-eyed appearance).

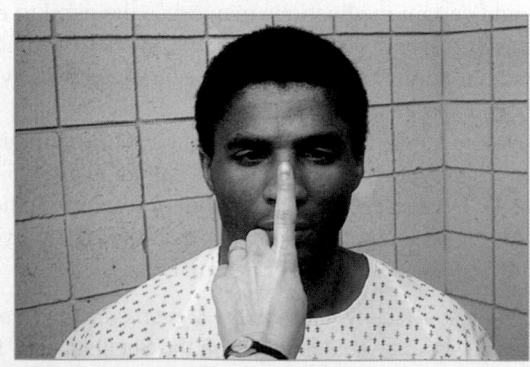

FIGURE D. Assessing convergence.

GUIDELINES FOR NURSING CARE 25-3

ASSESSING EXTRAOCULAR MOVEMENTS AND PERIPHERAL VISION

Extraocular Movements

- Ask the patient to sit or stand about 2 feet away, facing you sitting or standing at eye level with the patient.
- Ask the patient to hold the head still and follow the movement of your forefinger or a penlight with the eyes.
- Keeping your finger or light about 1 foot from the patient's face, move it slowly through the cardinal positions: up and down, left and right, diagonally up and down to the left, diagonally up and down to the right (see Figure).

Peripheral Vision

- Have the patient stand or sit about 2 feet away, facing you at eye level.
- Ask the patient to cover one eye with a hand or an index card.
- Ask the patient to look directly at your nose and fix the eyes on that spot.
- Cover your own eye opposite the patient's closed eye.
- Hold one arm outstretched to one side (right or left) equidistant from you and the patient, and move your fingers into the visual fields from various peripheral points.
- Ask the patient to tell you when the fingers are first seen (both you and the patient should see the fingers at the same time).
- Repeat the procedure for the other eye.

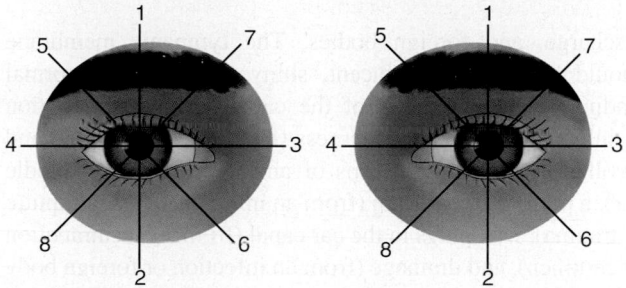

Testing extraocular movement of the eye.

---

shape and size of the ears should be symmetric and proportional to the head. Abnormal findings include unequal height and size, uneven color, and lesions. Gently palpate the external ear for pain, edema, or presence of lesions. Pain when manipulating the pinna is a symptom of an infection of the external ear.

FIGURE 25-12. External structures of the ear.

Assessing Hearing and Sound Conduction. Assess hearing in one ear at a time by determining whether the patient can hear a whispered voice. Assess hearing acuity out of the patient's line of vision (to prevent lip reading), with the opposite ear covered. Determine whether the patient can hear a whispered sentence or group of numbers from a distance of 1 to 2 feet. Ask the patient to repeat what you said.

Tuning fork tests, such as the Weber and Rinne tests, measure hearing by air conduction or by bone conduction, in which sound vibrates through the cranial bones to the inner ear. Traditionally, these tests have been included in physical assessment content. However, there is evidence to show that these tests are inaccurate and do not provide accurate or reliable information. The Weber and Rinne tests should not be used for general screening (Jarvis, 2012; Bagai, Thavendiranathan, & Detsky, 2006). Screening tests that are proven to be useful include the whisper test, audiometer (formal evaluation of hearing that measures hearing at frequencies varying from low pitches to high pitches), and self-report questionnaires. These are good tests to use initially in the evaluation of hearing loss (American Hearing Research Foundation, 2008).

Inspecting the Ear Canal and Tympanic Membrane. The otoscope is used to examine the ear canal and the tympanic membrane (Fig. 25-13 on page 646). The ear canal should be smooth and pink. The canal is examined for wax,

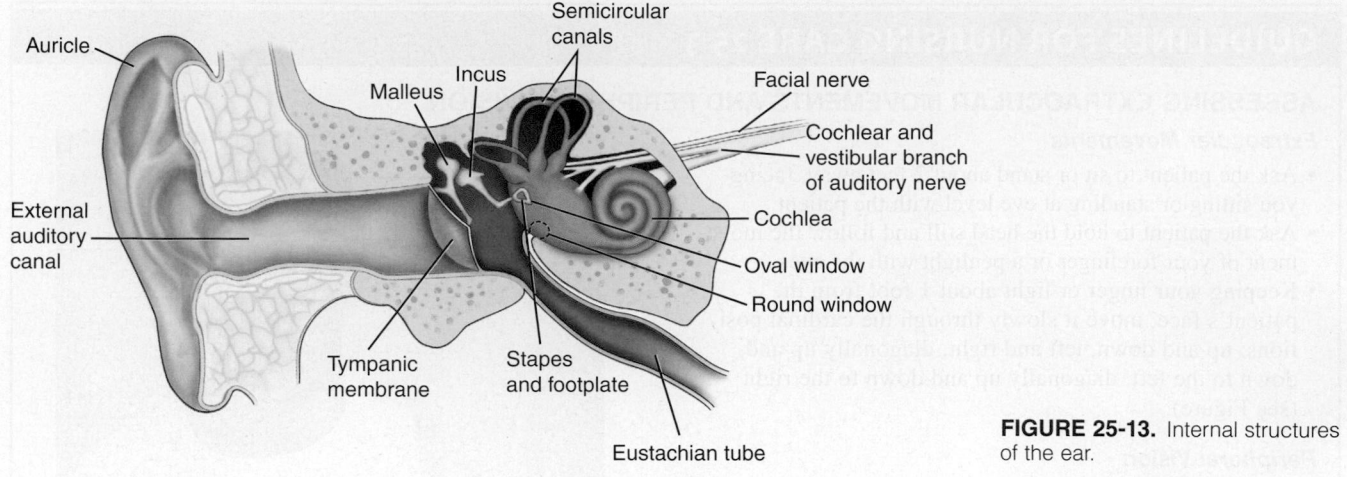

FIGURE 25-13. Internal structures of the ear.

discharge, and foreign bodies. The tympanic membrane should be intact, translucent, shiny, and gray. Abnormal findings include redness of the canal (from inflammation or infection), mastoid tenderness (from infection), a red and swollen eardrum (symptoms of an infection in the middle ear), a perforated eardrum (from an infection causing rupture or trauma), wax plugs in the ear canal (from an accumulation of cerumen), and drainage (from an infection or foreign body in the ear canal). Using the otoscope to inspect the ear canal and tympanic membrane is an advanced assessment skill, usually performed by advanced practitioners. Refer to information on the**Point** or a health assessment text for details.

Inspecting the Nose
Assessment of the nose involves examining the external nose, the nares, and the turbinates (Fig. 25-14). Inspect the nose and inspect and palpate the sinuses with the patient sitting and his or her head slightly tilted back, if possible.

Assess the nose for patency by occluding one nostril at a time and asking the patient to inhale and exhale through the nose. Inspect each anterior nares and turbinates by tipping the patient's head back slightly and shining a light into the nares. Examine the mucous membranes for color and the presence of lesions, exudate, or growths. Also, inspect the nasal septum for intactness and deviation.

Normally, the nasal mucosa is moist and darker red than the oral mucosa. Abnormal findings are swelling of the mucosa, bleeding or discharge (indicating allergies with inflammation or infection), perforation or deviation of the nasal septum (cocaine use may cause perforation; a deviated septum may be congenital or from trauma), and polyps (often seen with chronic allergies).

Palpating the Sinuses
The frontal and maxillary sinuses, located in the frontal and maxillary bones, respectively, are palpated for pain and edema. The frontal sinuses are palpated by gently pressing upward on the bony prominences located above each eye. The maxillary sinuses are palpated by gentle pressure on the bony prominences of the upper cheek (Fig. 25-15). Normally, the

sinuses are not painful when palpated. Pain may be a finding if the sinuses are infected or obstructed.

Inspecting the Mouth and Pharynx
The mouth and pharynx include the lips, tongue, teeth, gums, hard and soft palate, salivary gland, tonsillar pillars, and tonsils (Fig. 25-16). Equipment used to assess the mouth, pharynx, and neck includes a penlight, a tongue blade, a 4″ × 4″ gauze sponge, and gloves.

Assess the mouth and pharynx by inspecting the lips, gums and teeth, tongue, and hard and soft palates. Have the patient sit with the head tilted backward, if possible, and the mouth opened wide. Use palpation if any abnormalities

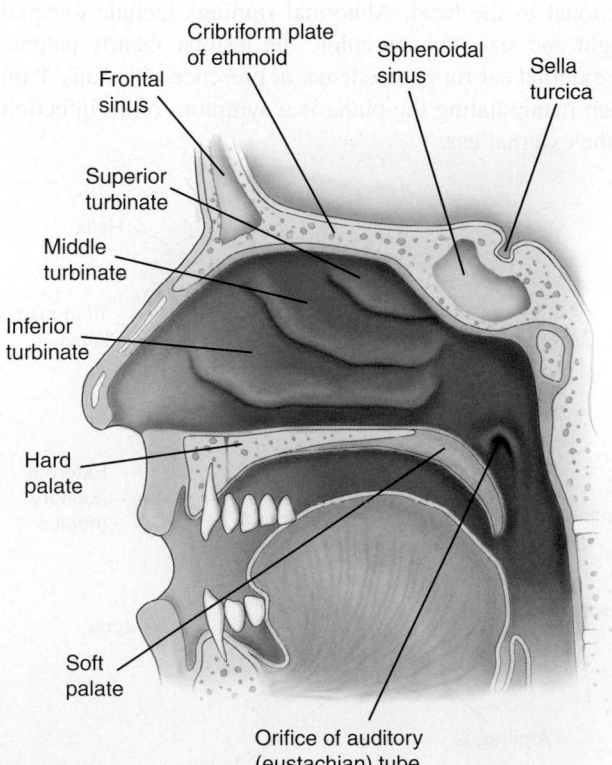

FIGURE 25-14. Cross-section of the nasal cavity.

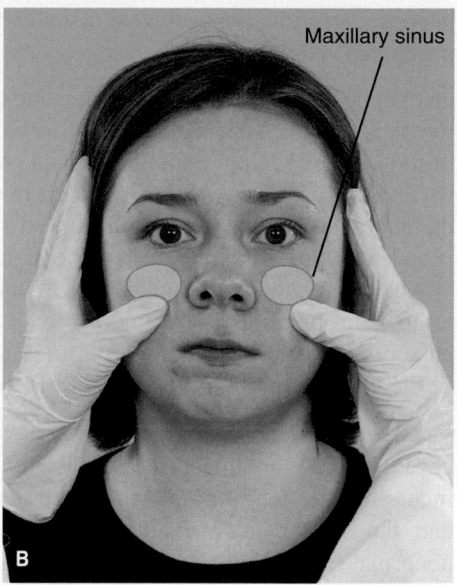

Frontal sinus

Maxillary sinus

FIGURE 25-15. (**A**) The frontal sinuses are palpated by gently pressing upward on the bony prominences above each eye. (**B**) The maxillary sinuses are palpated by applying gentle pressure on the bony prominences of the upper cheek. *(Photos by B. Proud.)*

are noted during inspection. Wear gloves when assessing a patient's mouth and use 4″ × 4″ gauze to hold the tongue for palpation.

The lips should be pink, moist, and smooth. The tongue and mucous membranes are normally pink, moist, and free of swelling or lesions. If the patient wears dentures, ask the patient to remove them for inspection of the gums and roof of the mouth. The gums should be pink and smooth. With the patient's tongue relaxed on the floor of the mouth, examine the mucous membrane of the oropharynx while depressing the base of the tongue with a tongue depressor. The uvula is normally centered and freely movable. The tonsils, if present, are small, pink, and symmetric in size. The teeth should be regular and free of cavities or have dental restoration.

Abnormal findings are pallor, cyanosis, or redness and swelling of the mucous membranes; lesions of the mucosa and lips; swollen, red tonsils (indicating infection); swollen, red, and bleeding gums (from nutritional deficits, inflammation or infection, poorly fitted dentures, or poor oral hygiene); poorly aligned, missing, or carious teeth; a white coating on the tongue (from poor oral hygiene, irritation, or smoking); a fissured tongue (from dehydration); a bright-red tongue (seen in deficiencies of iron, vitamin B$_{12}$, or niacin); or a black, hairy tongue (from antibiotic use).

Inspecting the Neck

Assessments of the neck include the trachea, lymph nodes, and thyroid gland (Fig. 25-17). Assess the neck with the patient sitting and the neck slightly hyperextended, if possible. Ask the patient to tilt the head backward, forward, and side to side to assess range of motion (ROM). The neck should be symmetric, with ROM. Also assess the neck for

Frenulum of upper lip

Buccinator muscle

Uvula

Palatine tonsil

Frenulum of lower lip

Hard palate

Soft palate

Posterior wall of oropharynx

Dorsum of tongue

Gingiva

Vestibule of mouth

FIGURE 25-16. Structures of the mouth.

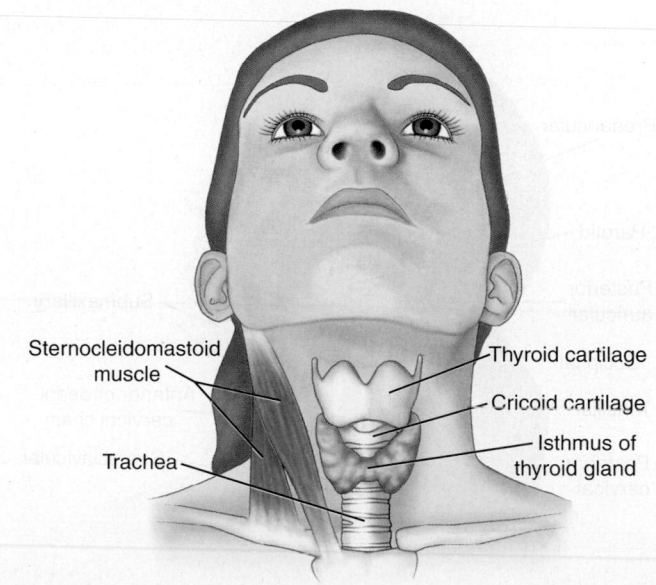

Sternocleidomastoid muscle

Trachea

Thyroid cartilage

Cricoid cartilage

Isthmus of thyroid gland

FIGURE 25-17. Structures of the neck.

venous distention. No neck vein distention (indicating heart problems) should be visible.

Inspecting the Thyroid Gland. Assess the thyroid gland with the neck slightly hyperextended. Observe the lower portion of the neck overlying the thyroid gland. Assess for symmetry and visible masses. Ask the patient to swallow. Observe the area while the patient swallows. Offer a glass of water, if necessary, to make it easier for the patient to swallow.

Abnormal findings include asymmetry, enlargement, lumps, and bulging. These findings may indicate the presence of enlargement of the thyroid (a goiter), inflammation of the thyroid (thyroiditis), or cancer of the thyroid.

Palpating the Trachea and Lymph Nodes. Palpate the trachea, normally midline at the suprasternal notch, for alignment and position. An unequal space between the trachea and the sternocleidomastoid muscle on each side is an abnormal finding indicating tracheal displacement.

Palpate the lymph nodes (Fig. 25-18) with the pads of the fingers for enlargement, tenderness, and mobility. The nodes are generally not palpable; if palpable, they should be small, mobile, smooth, and nontender. If lymph nodes are palpable, assess location, size, consistency, mobility, and tenderness. Enlarged lymph nodes (lymphadenopathy) may indicate infection, autoimmune disorders, or metastasis of cancer.

Palpating the Thyroid Gland

Palpate the thyroid for size, shape, symmetry, tenderness, and presence of any nodules. If palpable, the thyroid gland should feel soft but elastic. It should be nontender and should have no enlargement, masses, or nodules (which may indicate thyroid gland disease, infection of the thyroid, or cancer). Palpation of the thyroid is an advanced assessment skill, usually performed by advanced practitioners. Refer to information on thePoint or a health assessment text for details.

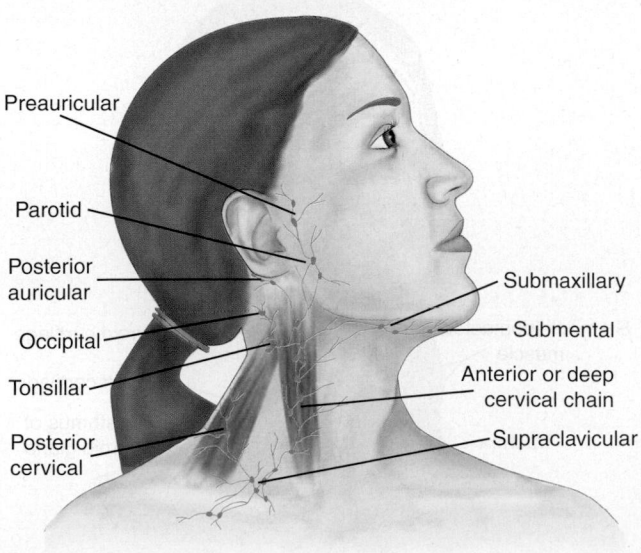

FIGURE 25-18. Location of the lymph nodes of the neck.

NORMAL AGE-RELATED VARIATIONS
Infant/Child

Common head and neck variations in newborns and children include:

- Closing of posterior fontanel at 8 weeks of age; soft anterior fontanel at about 18 months of age
- Gazing at and following bright objects by 1 month of age
- Focusing with both eyes by 6 months of age
- Pupils at the inner folds (pseudostrabismus)
- Startle reflex in newborns

Older Adult

Common head and neck variations in the older adult include:

- Impaired near vision (presbyopia)
- Decreased color vision and peripheral vision
- Decreased adaptation to light and dark
- A white ring around the cornea (arcus senilis)
- Entropion and ectropion
- Hearing loss (presbycusis)
- Impaired conductive hearing
- Elongated ear lobes
- Prominent ear landmarks
- Decreased neck ROM
- Nodular thyroid gland
- Smaller, more easily palpated lymph glands

Assessing the Thorax and Lungs

The thorax (Fig. 25-19) comprises the lungs, rib cage, cartilage, and intercostal muscles. Data from the health history may elicit a health problem, such as dyspnea or chest pain, as well as information about sleep patterns, cough, and sputum. A history of smoking indicates the need to include ways to stop smoking in the plan of care. Environmental exposure to certain inhalants (such as secondhand smoke, paint, air pollution, or asbestos fibers) in the home or workplace may increase the risk of respiratory diseases and cancer. Physical examination provides data about the bony structures of the thorax, respiratory effort, chest expansion, and breath sounds. Additional information related to assessment of the thorax and lungs is discussed in Chapters 25 and 38.

HEALTH HISTORY

Identify risk factors for altered health during the health history by asking about the following:

- History of trauma to the ribs or lung surgery
- Number of pillows used when sleeping
- History of chest pain with deep breathing
- History of persistent cough with or without producing sputum
- History of allergies
- Environmental exposure to chemicals, asbestos, or smoke
- History of smoking (how long, how many packs/day)
- History of lung disease in family members or self
- History of frequent or chronic respiratory infections

PHYSICAL ASSESSMENT

Physical assessment of the thorax and lungs requires a stethoscope and a tape measure. Make sure that the environment is

FIGURE 25-19. Thoracic landmarks. (**A**) Anterior. (**B**) Posterior.

warm and adequately lit. The techniques for this assessment include inspection, palpation, percussion, and auscultation. The patient sits during the assessment. Percussion of the thorax is an advanced assessment technique, usually performed by advanced practitioners. Refer to information on thePoint or a health assessment text for details.

Inspecting the Thorax

Begin inspection by observing the patient's chest for color, shape or contour, breathing patterns, and muscle development. The color should be even and consistent with the color of the patient's face. The shape or contour should have a downward equal slope at the rib cage. The chest should be symmetric, with the transverse diameter greater than the anteroposterior diameter. An increased anteroposterior diameter, as seen in chronic lung diseases, is described as barrel chest (Fig. 25-20). Respirations should be smooth and even, ranging from 12 to 20 breaths/min (adults).

Abnormal findings include an increase in chest size and contour, abnormal breathing patterns with use of accessory muscles (symptoms of respiratory disease, such as chronic obstructive pulmonary disease or asthma), unequal chest expansion (may occur in chest trauma or pneumonia), and abnormal respirations.

Palpating the Thorax

Palpation is used to detect areas of sensitivity, chest expansion during respirations, and vibrations (fremitus). Use the palmar surface of the hands to palpate the anterior and posterior thoracic landmarks (Fig. 25-21 on page 650) in

Normal adult chest   Barrel chest

FIGURE 25-20. Profile and anteroposterior diameter of normal adult chest and barrel chest.

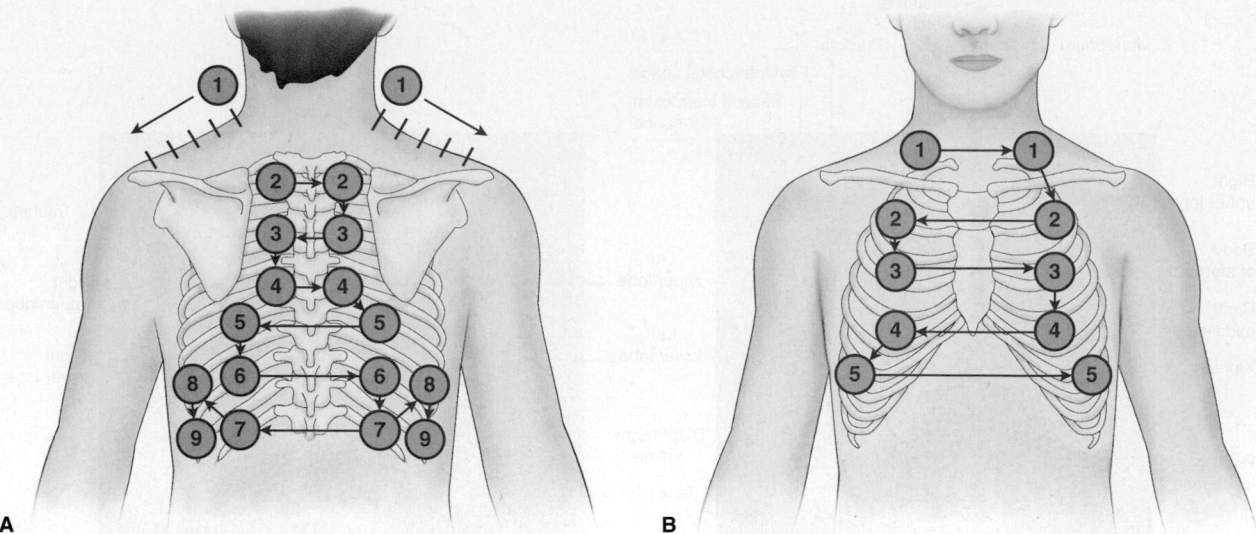

FIGURE 25-21. Posterior (**A**) and anterior (**B**) chest—landmarks and systematic sequence of assessment. The pattern is used for palpation, percussion, and auscultation of the chest.

a sequential pattern for temperature, moisture, muscular development, and any tenderness or masses. The skin should be warm and dry, with symmetric muscular development, and no tenderness, masses, or vibrations. Abnormal findings may be cool or excessively dry or moist skin, muscle asymmetry, tenderness, masses, and vibrations.

Chest expansion is determined by placing the hands over the posterior chest wall, with the fingers at the level of T9 or T10. Ask the patient to take a deep breath, and observe the movement of your thumbs. The thorax should expand symmetrically (Fig. 25-22).

Auscultating Breath Sounds

Auscultation is used to detect airflow within the respiratory tract. Ask the patient to breathe slowly and deeply through the mouth. Place the warmed diaphragm of the stethoscope over the thoracic landmarks and auscultate breath sounds in the same sequential pattern as used for palpation (see Fig. 25-21). Normally, breath sounds result from the free movement of air into and out of all parts of the bronchial tree. Listen for the duration, pitch, and intensity of the sounds.

Normal breath sounds (Table 25-5) vary over different parts of the lungs. **Bronchial sounds** heard over the larynx and trachea are high-pitched, harsh "blowing" sounds, with sound on expiration being longer than inspiration. **Bronchovesicular sounds** are heard over the mainstem bronchus and are moderate blowing sounds, with inspiration equal to expiration. **Vesicular breath sounds** are soft, low-pitched, whispering sounds, heard over most of the lung fields, with sound on inspiration being longer than expiration.

FIGURE 25-22. Palpating the posterior thorax excursion. The examiner's hands are placed symmetrically on the patient's back (**A**). As the patient inhales, the examiner's hands should move apart symmetrically (**B**). (*Photos by B. Proud.*)

Table 25-5   NORMAL BREATH SOUNDS

TYPE, DESCRIPTION, AND LOCATION	RATIO OF INSPIRATION TO EXPIRATION
Bronchial or Tubular	
Blowing, hollow sounds; auscultated over the larynx and trachea	Sound on expiration is longer, lower, and higher-pitched than inspiration.
Bronchovesicular	
First and second interspaces	
Medium-pitched, medium intensity, blowing sounds; auscultated over the first and second interspaces anteriorly and the scapula posteriorly	Inspiration and expiration sounds have similar pitch and duration.
Vesicular	
Soft, low-pitched, whispering sounds; heard over most of the lung fields	Sound on inspiration is longer, louder, and higher-pitched than expiration.

Adventitious breath sounds (added, abnormal sounds) are not normally heard in the lungs but, if present, may be auscultated. These adventitious sounds result from air moving through moisture, mucus, or narrowed airways. These abnormal sounds also result from sudden opening of collapsed alveoli. Refer to Table 25-6 (on page 652) for an explanation of these abnormal sounds. If any of these sounds are heard, listen for the loudness, pitch, duration, timing in the respiratory cycle (inspiration versus expiration), location on the chest wall, variations with breathing, and any change after a cough or deep breath (Jensen, 2011). If a productive cough occurs during assessment of the thorax and lungs, the sputum should be assessed for color, consistency, and amount.

THINK back to Billy Collins, the 9-year-old who was stung by a bee. Incorporating knowledge of the signs and symptoms of an allergic reaction, the nurse would inspect Billy's chest for accessory muscle use and auscultate his lungs, noting any evidence of wheezing, which is commonly observed with allergic reactions. ●

NORMAL AGE-RELATED VARIATIONS
Infant/Child
Common thorax and lung variations in newborns and children include:

- Louder breath sounds on auscultation
- More rapid respiratory rate (until 8 to 10 years of age)
- Use of abdominal muscles during respiration

Older Adult
Common thorax and lung variations in older adults include:

- Increased anteroposterior chest diameter
- Increase in the dorsal spinal curve (kyphosis)
- Decreased thoracic expansion
- Use of accessory muscles to exhale

Table 25-6 ADVENTITIOUS BREATH SOUNDS

TYPE AND CHARACTERISTICS	ILLUSTRATION
Wheeze (Sibilant) • Musical or squeaking • High-pitched, continuous sounds • Auscultated during inspiration and expiration • Air passing through narrowed airways	
Rhonchi (Sonorous Wheeze) • Sonorous or coarse; snoring quality • Low-pitched, continuous sounds • Auscultated during inspiration and expiration • Coughing may clear the sound somewhat • Air passing through or around secretions	
Crackles • Bubbling, crackling, popping • Low- to high-pitched, discontinuous sounds • Auscultated during inspiration and expiration • Opening of deflated small airways and alveoli; air passing through fluid in the airways	
Stridor • Harsh, loud, high-pitched • Auscultated on inspiration • Narrowing of upper airway (larynx or trachea); presence of foreign body in airway	
Friction Rub • Rubbing or grating • Loudest over lower lateral anterior surface • Auscultated during inspiration and expiration • Inflamed pleura rubbing against chest wall	

Assessing the Cardiovascular and Peripheral Vascular Systems

Cardiovascular and peripheral vascular assessment includes assessment of the heart and the extremities. Questions in the health history can identify supporting subjective data such as leg pain, chest pain, or dyspnea on exertion. Data can also be used to identify activities of daily living and health behaviors that increase the risk of cardiovascular disease, including smoking, lack of exercise, and a diet high in calories, fats, and salt. If these risks are identified, the plan of care should include referral for additional diagnostic testing and teaching about health promotion activities. The physical examination is used to identify signs and symptoms of heart disease and peripheral vascular disease (most often found in the lower extremities). Additional information related to assessment of the cardiovascular and peripheral vascular systems is discussed in Chapters 24 and 38.

HEALTH HISTORY

Identify risk factors for altered health during the health history by asking about the following:

- History of chest pain, palpitations, or dizziness
- Swelling in the ankles and feet
- Number of pillows used to sleep
- Type and amount of medications taken daily
- History of heart defect, rheumatic fever, or chest or heart surgery
- Personal and family history of hypertension (high blood pressure), myocardial infarction (heart attack), coronary artery disease, high blood cholesterol levels, or diabetes mellitus
- History of smoking (how long, how many packs/day)
- History of alcohol use
- Type and amount of exercise
- Usual foods eaten each day
- Changes in color or temperature of the extremities
- History of pain in the legs when sleeping or pain that is worsened by walking
- History of blood clots or sores on the legs that do not heal

PHYSICAL ASSESSMENT

The techniques used for cardiovascular assessment are inspection, palpation, and auscultation. Necessary equipment includes a stethoscope with a bell and diaphragm and a sphygmomanometer. The patient may be in a sitting position or in a supine position with the head raised about 30 degrees, if possible. Adequate lighting is essential for inspection of color and for pulsations. A quiet environment is necessary for accurate auscultation of heart sounds. The nurse is usually positioned at the right side of the patient. Figure 25-23 provides a view of the heart, including the heart valves responsible for heart sounds.

Peripheral vascular assessment includes measuring the blood pressure and assessing the skin and perfusion of the extremities and the peripheral pulses. Assessments are made by inspection and palpation, with the patient sitting or supine. Peripheral vascular assessments may be combined with assessment of other body areas. Many practitioners assess the neuromuscular, musculoskeletal, and peripheral vascular systems as an integrated assessment. Refer to Skill 25-2 on pages 674–681 for an example of a systematic, integrated assessment of these systems.

Inspecting the Neck and Precordium

Observe the neck and **precordium** (the portion of the body over the heart and lower thorax, encompassing the aortic, pulmonic, tricuspid, and apical areas, and Erb's point) (Fig. 25-24) for visible pulsations. Pulsations usually are absent except for the apical impulse, located at about the fourth or fifth intercostal space at the left midclavicular line. Inspect the epigastric area at the tip of the sternum for pulsation of the abdominal aorta. Findings of neck vein distention (indicating heart disease) or visible pulsations in precordial areas

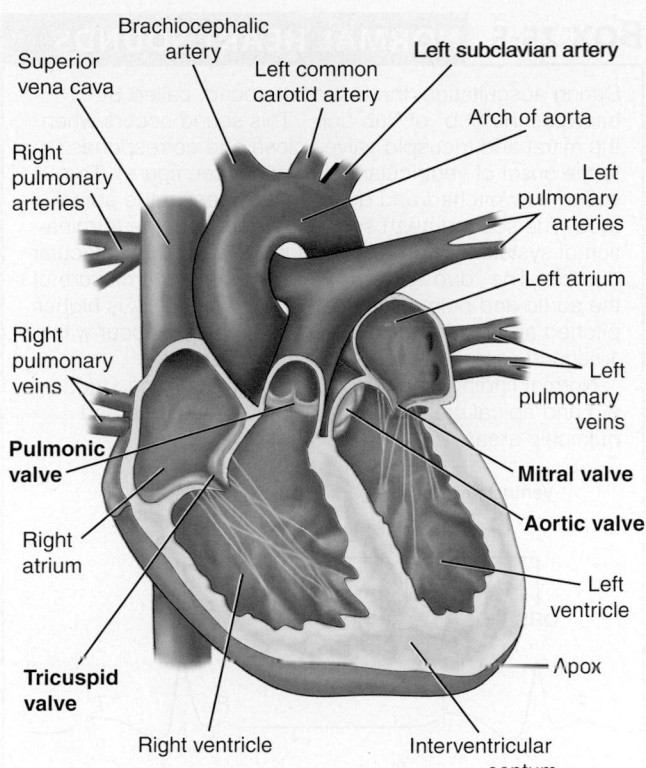

Brachiocephalic artery
Superior vena cava
Right pulmonary arteries
Right pulmonary veins
Pulmonic valve
Right atrium
Tricuspid valve
Right ventricle
Left common carotid artery
Left subclavian artery
Arch of aorta
Left pulmonary arteries
Left atrium
Left pulmonary veins
Mitral valve
Aortic valve
Left ventricle
Apex
Interventricular septum

FIGURE 25-23. View of the interior of the heart showing the atrioventricular and semilunar valves responsible for normal heart sounds.

FIGURE 25-25. Palpate the carotid artery medial to the sternomastoid muscle in the neck between the jaw and the clavicle. (Jensen, S. (2011). *Nursing health assessment*. Philadelphia, PA: Lippincott Williams & Wilkins.)

other than the apical impulse (which may result from abnormalities of the ventricle) are considered abnormal.

Palpating the Neck and Precordium

Warm your hands, if necessary. Palpate the carotid artery medial to the sternomastoid muscle in the neck between the jaw and the clavicle (Fig. 25-25). Palpate the carotid arteries one at a time to avoid obstructing both arteries simultaneously, reducing blood flow to the brain and potentially

Aortic area
Pulmonic area
Erb's point
Tricuspid area
Mitral (apical) area

Midsternum   Midclavicular line

FIGURE 25-24. The precordium with the traditional cardiac landmarks and areas for auscultation.

causing dizziness or loss of consciousness (Jensen, 2011). Note the strength of the pulse and grade it as with peripheral pulses (refer to discussion later in this section). Normal findings include equal pulses bilaterally, with a strength of +2/3. Abnormal findings include an absent, weak, thready pulse (which may indicate a decreased cardiac output), a forceful or bounding pulse (seen in hypertension and circulatory fluid overload), and an asymmetric pulse (related to impaired circulation).

Using the palmar surface of the hand with the four fingers held together, gently palpate the precordium for pulsations (Fig. 25-26 on page 654). Palpate in a systematic manner, assessing specific cardiac landmarks—the aortic, pulmonic, tricuspid, and mitral areas, as well as Erb's point. Palpate the apical impulse in the mitral area. Note size, duration, force, and location in relationship to the midclavicular line. Normal findings include no pulsation palpable over the aortic and pulmonic areas, with a palpable apical impulse. Abnormal findings include precordial thrills, which are fine, palpable, rushing vibrations over the right or left second intercostal space, and lifts or heaves, which involve a rise along the border of the sternum with each heartbeat.

Auscultating Heart Sounds

Auscultation is used to determine the heart sounds caused by closure of the heart valves. Ask the patient to breathe normally. Use systematic auscultation, beginning at the aortic area, moving to the pulmonic area, then to Erb's point, then to the tricuspid area, and finally to the mitral area (see Fig. 25-24). Use the diaphragm of the stethoscope first to listen to high-pitched sounds. Then use the bell to listen to low-pitched sounds. Focus on the overall rate and rhythm of the heart and the normal heart sounds (Box 25-5 on page 654).

Abnormal findings include extra heart sounds at any of the cardiac landmarks and abnormal rate or rhythm. Extra heart sounds are often heard when the patient has anemia or heart disease. A wide variety of conditions may alter the normal heart rate or rhythm, including serious infections, diseases of the heart muscle or conducting system, dehydration or

FIGURE 25-26. Palpating areas of the precordium: (**A**) aortic area, (**B**) pulmonic area, and (**C**) apical (mitral) and tricuspid area. (*Photos by Ken Kasper.*)

BOX 25-5 NORMAL HEART SOUNDS

During auscultation, the first heart sound, called S_1, is heard as the "lub" of "lub-dub." This sound occurs when the mitral and tricuspid valves close and corresponds to the onset of ventricular contraction (see figure). The sound, low pitched and dull, is heard best at the apical area. The second heart sound, S_2, occurs at the termination of systole and corresponds to the onset of ventricular diastole. The "dub" of "lub-dub" represents the closure of the aortic and pulmonic valves. The sound of S_2 is higher pitched and shorter than S_1. The two sounds occur within 1 second or less, depending on the heart rate.

Normal findings include S_1, that is louder at the tricuspid and apical areas, with S_2 louder at the aortic and pulmonic areas.

Heart sounds in relation to the cardiac cycle and an electrocardiogram.

---

grading depend on the adequacy of valve function, rate of blood flow, and size of the valve opening. Usually, nurses are more concerned with recognizing changes in murmurs rather than in diagnosing and labeling them (Jensen, 2011). Refer to a health assessment text for grading details.

Inspecting the Extremities

Inspect the skin of the extremities for color, temperature, continuity, lesions (as described previously for assessment of the integument), venous patterns, and edema. Normally, venous patterns, varicosities, rashes, ulcers, or edema are absent on the lower extremities. However, if the patient has peripheral vascular disease (resulting in decreased blood flow and oxygenation of tissues), the skin of the lower extremities is typically pale and cool, shiny with brown discolorations, and hairless. The toenails are thickened. Phlebitis (inflammation of a vein) of the lower extremity is indicated by pain, redness, and swelling of the affected calf or thigh.

Palpating Peripheral Pulses and Capillary Refill

Use the pads of the index and middle fingers to palpate peripheral pulses for amplitude and symmetry. Palpate,

overhydration, endocrine disorders, respiratory disorders, and head trauma. Extra heart sounds may be S_3, S_4, murmurs, or bruits.

S_3, known as the third heart sound, follows S_2 and is often represented by a "lub-dub-dee" pattern ("dee" being S_3). This sound is best heard with the stethoscope bell at the mitral area, with the patient lying on the left side. S_3 is considered normal in children and young adults and abnormal in middle-aged and older adults. S_4 is the fourth heart sound, occurring right before S_1, and is often represented by a "dee-lub-dub" pattern ("dee" being S_4). S_4 is considered normal in older adults but abnormal in children and adults. Heart murmurs are extra heart sounds caused by some disruption of blood flow through the heart. The characteristics of a murmur and

FIGURE 25-27. Assessing capillary refill. (Reprinted with permission from Jensen, S. [2011]. *Nursing health assessment.* Philadelphia: Wolters Kluwer Health/Lippincott Williams & Wilkins.)

carefully and one at a time, the carotid, brachial, radial, femoral, popliteal, dorsalis pedis, and posterior tibial pulses (see Fig. 24-3 on page 590). These should be strong and equal bilaterally. The amplitude of the pulses, with a scale that may be used for documentation, is described in Table 24-5 on page 589. Using your thumb and forefinger, squeeze the patient's fingernail or toenail until it blanches (turns white). Release the pressure and observe the time it takes for normal color to return (Fig. 25-27). Normal capillary refill is <3 seconds (Jensen, 2011).

Abnormal findings include an absent, weak, thready pulse (which may indicate a decreased cardiac output), a forceful or bounding pulse (seen in hypertension and circulatory fluid overload), and an asymmetric pulse (related to impaired circulation). Prolonged capillary refill is associated with alterations in peripheral perfusion and cardiac output.

Other assessments to determine arterial blood flow include Allen's test and Buerger's test, usually performed by advanced practice professionals thus are not discussed here. Refer to an assessment text for details.

Assessing Neurovascular Status

Musculoskeletal trauma, crush injuries, orthopedic surgery, and external pressure from a cast or tight-fitting bandage can cause damage to blood vessels and nerves. This damage causes localized inflammation and tissue edema, which can lead to significantly diminished perfusion and severe ischemia, with resulting severe and permanent dysfunction of the affected area and/or loss of a limb. Assessment of neurovascular status is an important nursing intervention leading to early identification of neurovascular impairment and timely intervention (Johnston-Walker & Hardcastle, 2011). A neurovascular assessment includes assessing for changes in circulation, oxygenation, and nerve function. Box 25-6 outlines the components of a neurovascular assessment.

NORMAL AGE-RELATED VARIATIONS
Infant/Child

Common cardiovascular and peripheral vascular variations in newborns and children include:

- Visible cardiac pulsation if the chest wall is thin
- Sinus dysrhythmia (the rate increases with inspiration and decreases with expiration)
- Presence of S_3 (in about one-third of all children)
- More rapid heart rate (until about 8 years of age)

Older Adult

Common cardiovascular and peripheral vascular variations in older adults include:

- Difficult-to-palpate apical pulse
- Difficult-to-palpate distal arteries
- Dilated proximal arteries
- More prominent and tortuous blood vessels; varicosities common
- Increased systolic and diastolic blood pressure
- Widening pulse pressure

Box 25-6 COMPONENTS OF A NEUROVASCULAR ASSESSMENT

- **Pain:** Extreme pain, especially on passive motion, is a significant sign of probable neurovascular impairment in an extremity. Subjective and objective assessments should be included. Opioid analgesia is unlikely to relieve the pain.
- **Pallor (perfusion):** Comparison between affected and unaffected limb is important. Assess color and temperature of the extremity. Pale skin, decreased tone, or white color may indicate poor arterial perfusion. Cyanosis may indicate venous stasis. Coolness or decreased temperature may indicate decreased arterial supply. Compare distal to proximal temperature variation in affected limb. Assess capillary refill.
- **Peripheral Pulses:** Comparison between affected and unaffected limb is important. Assess the consistency of arterial blood flow (pulse presence, rate, quality) to and

past the affected area. Assess capillary refill, especially in patients whose pulses cannot be palpated due to casts or bandages (Judge, 2007; Johnston-Walker & Hardcastle, 2011) and in non-verbal patients.
- **Paresthesia (sensation):** May be first symptom of changes in sensory nerves to appear. Numbness, tingling, or "pins and needles" sensations may be reported. Evaluate the areas above and below the affected area.
- **Paralysis (movement):** The ability of the patient to move the extremity distal to the injury. Paralysis of an extremity may be the result of prolonged nerve compression or irreversible muscle damage.
- **Pressure:** Comparison between affected and unaffected limb is important. Affected area may become taut and firm to the touch, with surrounding skin appearing shiny. The feeling of tightness or pressure may be present.

Adapted from Hinkle, J. L., & Cheever, K. H. (2014). *Brunner & Suddarth's Textbook of Medical–Surgical Nursing* (13th ed.). Philadelphia: Wolters Kluwer Health/Lippincott Williams & Wilkins; and Johnston-Walker, E. & Hardcastle, J. (2011). Neurovascular assessment in the critically ill patient. *Nursing in Critical Care, 16*(4), 170–177.

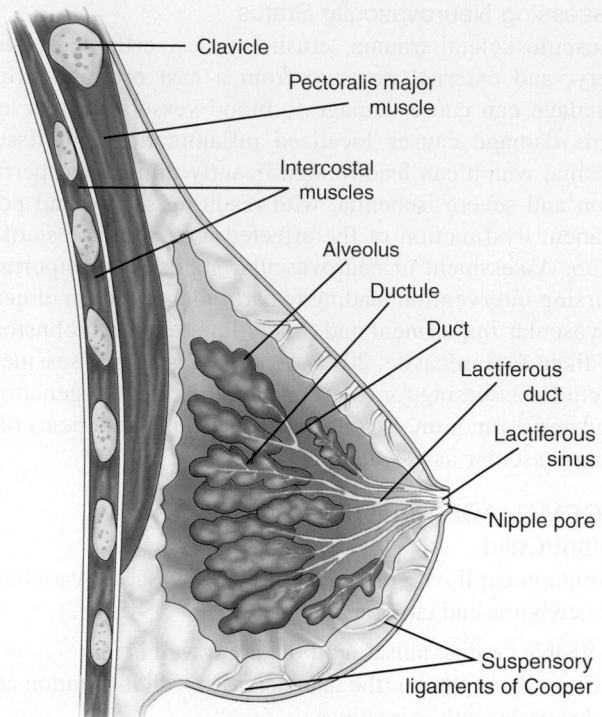

FIGURE 25-28. Lateral view of the female breast.

Assessing the Breasts and Axillae

Each breast has a lymphatic network that drains into the underlying axilla (Fig. 25-28). Although the assessments and disorders described here focus on the female breast, men also are at risk for breast disease. The health history elicits risk factors for cancer of the breast, especially in females. Physical assessment of the breasts and axilla are primarily conducted to identify any lumps in the breasts and/or enlargement or pain in axillary lymph nodes; if assessed, the patient should have further diagnostic tests. Review or teach the procedure for self breast examination after completion of the physical exam.

HEALTH HISTORY

Identify risk factors for altered health during the health history by asking about the following:

- History of pain in one or both breasts, including relationship to menstrual period
- History of lumps or swelling, redness, change in size, or dimpling in the breasts
- History of discharge from the breast
- Family history of ovarian or breast cancer
- History of breast disease, biopsy, or surgery
- Menstrual and pregnancy history
- Use of hormones, oral contraceptives
- Exposure to radiation, benzene, or asbestos
- Usual dietary intake and alcohol consumption
- Knowledge and practice of breast self-examination
- Most recent clinical breast examination and mammogram

PHYSICAL ASSESSMENT

Assess the breasts and axilla in both men and women using inspection and palpation. The patient can be sitting or lying supine. When sitting, the patient should sit erect, with arms at sides or raised overhead, if possible. When supine, the patient's hand on the side being examined is placed under the head, if possible. Examination of the breast and axilla are often performed sequentially with the assessment of the thorax, lungs, and heart.

Inspecting the Breasts

Inspect the breasts for size, shape, symmetry, color, texture, and skin lesions. The breasts should be relatively symmetric, although variations are normal. The size varies among individuals. The shape of the breasts is round and smooth, and there should be no skin depressions (retraction) or puckering (dimpling). The color should be consistent with the rest of the skin, and the texture of the skin should be soft.

Inspect the areola and nipples for size and shape and the nipples for discharge, crusting, and inversion. The areolar and nipple areas should be equal in size, round or oval, with a smooth surface. Montgomery's tubercles (sebaceous glands on the areolae of the breasts) are a normal component of the areola. The nipples are normally everted. Discharge from the nipples is an abnormal finding except in pregnancy (leaking is normal during pregnancy and breastfeeding). Other abnormal findings include dimpling, lesions, and asymmetry.

Palpating the Breasts and Axillae

Palpate the breasts in each of the four quadrants (the upper outer quadrant, the lower outer quadrant, the upper inner quadrant, and the lower inner quadrant) to detect any abnormal lumps (Fig. 25-29). Guidelines for Nursing Care 25-4 provides instructions for palpation.

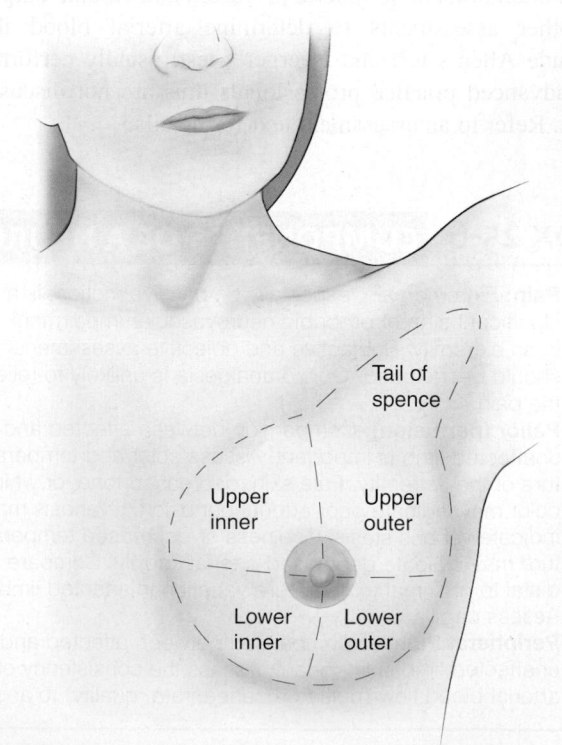

FIGURE 25-29. Location of assessment findings of the breast are identified by quadrant.

GUIDELINES FOR NURSING CARE 25-4

PALPATING THE BREASTS

Palpate each quadrant of each breast in a systematic method, either the circular, wedge, or vertical strip technique. The patient should be supine with a small pillow or towel beneath her back and the arm on the side of the breast to be examined raised above her head.

Circular

- Start at the tail of Spence and move in increasing smaller circles (Figure A).
- Use the pads of the first three fingers to gently compress the breast tissue against the chest wall.

FIGURE B. Wedge technique.

Vertical Strip

- Start at the outer edge of the breast and palpate up and down the breast (Figure C).
- Use the pads of the first three fingers to gently compress the breast tissue against the chest wall.

FIGURE A. Circular technique.

Wedge

- Work in a clockwise direction and palpate from the periphery toward the areola (Figure B).
- Use the pads of the first three fingers to gently compress the breast tissue against the chest wall.

FIGURE C. Vertical strip technique.

Palpate the nipple and areola, and gently compress the nipple between the thumb and forefinger to assess for discharge. The breast tissue should be smooth and firm, with a granular consistency. If a mass is detected, carefully assess its location, size, shape, consistency, and tenderness. The breasts are normally tender during the week before menstruation.

An increase in the nodularity and tenderness of the breasts may be associated with the menstrual period or may indicate fibrocystic disease. Discharge, lumps, lesions, dimpling, asymmetry, and palpable lymph nodes may be indicative of breast cancer.

Palpate the axillary areas for lymph nodes (Fig. 25-30), which normally are nonpalpable and nontender. If any nodes are palpable, assess their location, size, shape, consistency, tenderness, and mobility. Palpable lymph nodes are an abnormal finding.

NORMAL AGE-RELATED VARIATIONS
Infant/Child
Common breast and axillae variations in newborns and children include:

- Breast enlargement and a white discharge from the nipples (up to 2 weeks of age)

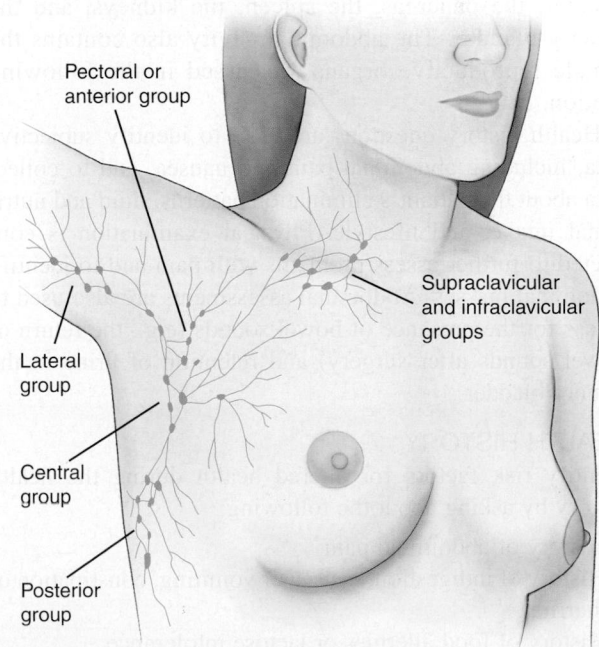

FIGURE 25-30. Location of the cervical, axillary, and mammary lymph nodes.

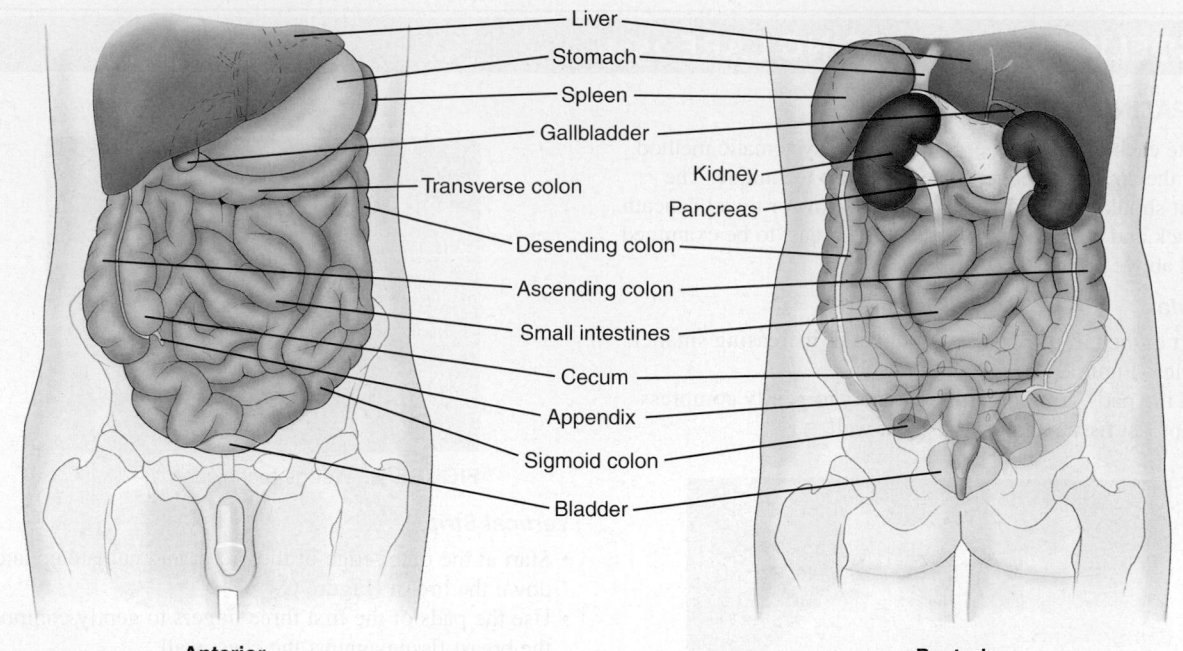

Anterior

Posterior

FIGURE 25-31. Organs of the abdominal cavity.

- Female breast growth beginning at 10 or 11 years of age
- Temporary enlargement of one or both breasts (gynecomastia) in pubescent boys

Older Adult

Common breast and axillae variations in older adults include:

- Granular, pendulous breasts in women

Assessing the Abdomen

The abdominal cavity (Fig. 25-31) contains the stomach, the small intestine, the large intestine, the liver, the gallbladder, the pancreas, the spleen, the kidneys, and the urinary bladder. The abdominal cavity also contains the female reproductive organs, discussed in the following section.

Health history questions are used to identify subjective data, including abdominal pain and nausea, and to collect data about the patient's elimination patterns, fluid and nutritional intake, and lifestyle. Physical examination is conducted to further assess problems with pain and to identify abdominal masses. Abdominal assessments are also used to assess for the presence of bowel sounds (e.g., the return of bowel sounds after surgery) and retention of urine in the urinary bladder.

HEALTH HISTORY

Identify risk factors for altered health during the health history by asking about the following:

- History of abdominal pain
- History of indigestion, nausea or vomiting, constipation or diarrhea
- History of food allergies or lactose intolerance
- Appetite and usual food and fluid intake
- Usual bowel and bladder elimination patterns

- History of gastrointestinal disorders, such as peptic ulcer disease, bowel disease, gallbladder disease, liver disease, or appendicitis
- History of urinary tract disorders such as infections, kidney stones, or kidney disease
- History of abdominal surgery or trauma
- Type and amount of prescribed and over-the-counter medications used
- Amount and type of alcohol ingestion
- For women, menstrual history

PHYSICAL ASSESSMENT

Use a warm stethoscope (it can be warmed with your hand) and ensure that lighting is adequate when assessing the abdomen. Also, make sure that your hands are warm and your fingernails are trimmed short. Ask the patient to empty the bladder. Place the patient in the supine position with the head slightly elevated and arms at the sides, if possible. Place small pillows under the head and knees for comfort. Make sure that the patient is warm and comfortable to help prevent contraction of the abdominal muscles, which makes palpation difficult.

To locate organs more easily and to make documentation more specific, the abdomen can be divided into four quadrants: right upper, right lower, left upper, and left lower (Fig. 25-32). The sequence of techniques used to assess the abdomen is inspection, auscultation, percussion, and palpation. Percussion and palpation are done *after* auscultation because they stimulate bowel sounds. Ask the patient to breathe slowly and deeply through the mouth during the examination to promote relaxation. Ask the patient to identify painful areas of the abdomen and explain that you will assess these at the end of the examination. Percussion of the abdomen is an advanced assessment technique, usually

Midline

Right Upper Quadrant
- Pylorous
- Duodenum
- Liver
- Right kidney and adrenal gland
- Hepatic flexure of colon
- Head of pancreas

Left Upper Quadrant
- Stomach
- Spleen
- Left kidney and adrenal gland
- Splenic flexure of colon
- Body of pancreas

Right Lower Quadrant
- Cecum
- Appendix
- Right ovary and fallopian tube (female)
- Right ureter and lower kidney pole
- Right spermatic cord (male)

Left Lower Quadrant
- Sigmoid colon
- Left ovary and fallopian tube (female)
- Left ureter and lower kidney pole
- Left spermatic cord (male)

Midline
- Urinary bladder
  Urethra (female)

FIGURE 25-32. Diagram of abdominal quadrants and outline of underlying organs.

performed by advanced practitioners. Refer to information on thePoint or a health assessment text for details.

Inspecting the Abdomen
Sit at the side of the patient and look across the abdomen. A tangential view enhances shadows and contours. Inspect skin color and surface characteristics, including the umbilicus, contour, symmetry, peristalsis, pulsations, and visible masses. The skin color may be slightly lighter than exposed areas. Fine white or silver lines (striae) may be visible, often the result of skin stretching from weight gain or pregnancy. The umbilicus should be centrally located and may be flat, rounded, or concave. The abdomen should be evenly rounded or symmetric, without visible peristalsis. In thin people, an upper midline pulsation may normally be visible. Abnormal findings include asymmetry (possibly from an enlarged organ or mass), distension (possibly indicating retained gas or air; obesity), swelling of the abdomen (possibly indicating fluid retention called ascites), and abdominal masses or unusual pulsations.

Auscultating Bowel Sounds and Vascular Sounds
Auscultation is used to assess bowel sounds and vascular sounds. Warm the stethoscope and using light pressure, place the flat diaphragm on the right lower quadrant of the abdomen, then move to right upper quadrant, left upper quadrant, and finally to the left lower quadrant. Listen carefully for bowel sounds (gurgles and clicks), and note their frequency and character (usually occur every 5 to 34 seconds). Before documenting bowel sounds as absent, the nurse must listen for 2 minutes or longer in each abdominal quadrant. Abnormal findings include increased bowel sounds (often heard with diarrhea or in early bowel obstruction), decreased bowel sounds (heard after abdominal surgery or late bowel obstruction), or absent bowel sounds (indicating peritonitis or paralytic ileus). Bowel sounds of high-pitched tinkling or rushes of high-pitched sounds indicate a bowel obstruction.

Using the bell of the stethoscope, auscultate over the abdominal aorta, femoral arteries, and iliac arteries for **bruits**. Bruits are abnormal "swooshing or blowing" sounds heard over a blood vessel, caused by blood that is swirling in the vessel, rather than normal smooth flow. A bruit may be heard in the presence of stenosis (narrowing) or occlusion of an artery. Bruits may also be caused by abnormal dilation of a vessel. Report and document changes in or absence of bowel and vascular sounds.

Palpating the Abdomen
The pads of the fingers are used to palpate with a light, gentle, dipping motion approximately 1 to 2 cm (Jensen, 2011). Watch the patient's face for nonverbal signs of pain during palpation. Palpate each quadrant in a systematic manner, noting muscular resistance, tenderness, enlargement of the organs, or masses. If the patient complains of abdominal pain, palpate the area of pain last. The abdomen should normally be soft, relaxed, and free of tenderness. Abnormal findings include involuntary rigidity, spasm, and pain (which may indicate trauma, peritonitis, infection, tumors, or enlarged or diseased abdominal organs).

NORMAL AGE-RELATED VARIATIONS
Infant/Child
Common abdominal variations in newborns and children include:

- Umbilical cord in newborns; dries and falls off within the first few weeks of life
- A "pot-belly" (under 5 years of age)
- Visible peristaltic waves

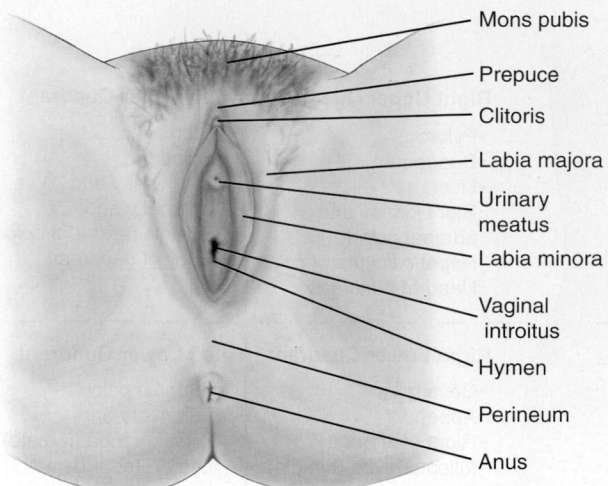

Mons pubis
Prepuce
Clitoris
Labia majora
Urinary meatus
Labia minora
Vaginal introitus
Hymen
Perineum
Anus

FIGURE 25-33. External female genitalia.

Older Adult

Common abdominal variations in older adults include:

- Decreased bowel sounds
- Decreased abdominal tone
- Fat accumulation on the abdomen and hips

Assessing Female Genitalia

The external female genitalia consist of the mons pubis, labia majora and minora, clitoris, vestibular glands, vaginal vestibule, vaginal orifice, and urethral opening (Fig. 25-33). Information collected during the health history is especially helpful in identifying risk factors for cancer and health-related behaviors that may lead to sexually transmitted infections. During the physical assessment, the external genitalia may be examined. The female genitalia are assessed for lesions, discharge, masses, and enlargement of internal organs. The rectum and anus may be assessed during part of this examination if a complete health assessment is being performed. Information about rectal examination is provided later in this chapter. The internal pelvic examination is an advanced skill, usually performed by an advanced practice professional. Refer to information on thePoint or a health assessment text for details of this advanced assessment skill.

HEALTH HISTORY

Identify risk factors for altered female health during the health history by asking about the following:

- Menstrual history (age of first and last period, length of flow, type of flow, pain)
- Sexual history (age at which sexual activity began, number and gender of partners)
- Pain with intercourse, difficulty achieving orgasm
- Number of pregnancies and live births
- History of sexually transmitted infection
- Use of contraceptives
- Frequency of pelvic examinations and Pap smears
- History of vaginal discharge, itching, or pain on urination
- Family history of reproductive or genital cancer

- Use of hormones and tobacco (how long, how much, how many packs/day)

PHYSICAL ASSESSMENT

Assess the genitalia by inspection and palpation. A description of an internal pelvic assessment of women is included in this chapter. This is an advanced assessment technique, but nurses often assist in performing vaginal examinations and need to be familiar with the procedure. In many instances, male health care providers will ask that a female be present in the room during the examination. Women from some cultures or who practice certain religions (e.g., Islam) may agree to a physical examination of the genitalia only by a female nurse or female practitioner. Equipment required includes a good light source and disposable gloves.

Inspecting and Palpating the External Genitalia

Ask the patient to empty her bladder before the examination. Explain the procedure to her and help her to relax as it is performed. The patient should be supine or lying on her side.

Inspect the external genitalia for color, size of the labia majora and vaginal opening, lesions, and discharge. The vulva normally has more pigmentation than other skin areas, and the mucous membranes are dark pink and moist. The skin and mucosa should be smooth, without lesions or swelling. The labia should be symmetric without lesions or swelling. Lesions may be the result of infections (such as herpes or syphilis). There may normally be a small amount of clear or whitish vaginal discharge. The vaginal orifice varies in size, depending on the woman's age, sexual history, and having vaginal delivery. In children, loss of hymenal tissue between the 3 o'clock and 9 o'clock position indicates trauma (from digits, penis, or foreign objects). Palpate the labia for masses.

Inspecting Internal Genitalia

Examination of the internal genitalia is an advanced assessment technique and usually performed by advanced practitioners. The patient is placed in the lithotomy position on the examination table, with the legs in stirrups, and draped so that only the genitalia are exposed. Explain the procedure and help the patient to relax as it is performed. The examination is outlined here to provide the student with an understanding of the examination if asked to assist. A speculum, consisting of two blades and an adjustment device, is lubricated and inserted into the vagina. This allows inspection of the cervix and other internal genitalia for abnormalities. Specimens for a Papanicolaou (Pap) test for cervical and vaginal cancer can be obtained, as well as specimens for gonorrhea and chlamydia cultures, and to test for human papillomavirus (HPV). The vaginal wall is inspected as the speculum is removed. With lubricated fingers, the advanced practice professional palpates the internal genitalia for location, size, mobility, tenderness, and masses. Refer to a health assessment text for additional details of this advanced assessment skill. The examination of the rectum is often included at this time. This examination is discussed later in the chapter on page 662.

Abnormal findings include redness, swelling of glands, discharge, lesions, and pain, which may indicate infection,

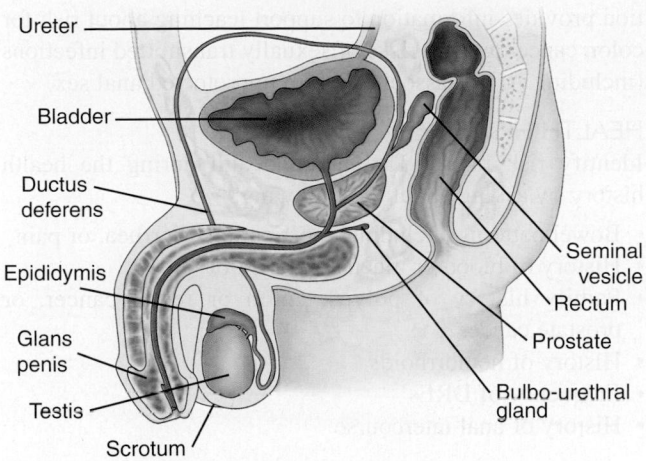

FIGURE 25-34. Organs of the male genital system.

an abscess, a polyp, or cancer. For related assessments of the urinary tract and sexually transmitted infections, see Chapters 36 and 44.

NORMAL AGE-RELATED VARIATIONS
Infant/Child

Common genitalia variations in newborns (resulting from exposure to maternal hormones in utero, normally seen in the first week after birth and subsiding by the second week after birth) and children include:

- Enlarged labia and clitoris
- Breast enlargement in both boys and girls
- Vaginal discharge in girls, called pseudomenstruation
- Pubic hair and breast development occur at puberty and follow a regular sequence of development.
- Menstruation begins about 2.5 years after puberty begins.
- Irregular menstrual cycle for first 2 years

Older Adult

Common genitalia variations in older women include:

- Decreased size of labia and clitoris
- Decreased amount of pubic hair
- Decreased vaginal secretions
- Pale, thin, and dry vaginal mucosa

Assessing Male Genitalia

The male genitalia (Fig. 25-34) include the penis, testicles, epididymis, scrotum, prostate gland, and seminal vesicles. In addition, the inguinal area may be assessed as part of this assessment. Information from the health history is helpful in identifying self-care and lifestyle factors that increase the risk of illnesses, such as testicular cancer or sexually transmitted infections. The physical examination is focused on detecting abnormal findings so that early diagnosis and treatment can be initiated. Review or teach the procedure for testicular self-examination after completion of the physical exam. Figure 25-35 reviews the procedure for testicular self-examination.

HEALTH HISTORY

Identify risk factors for altered male health during the health history by asking about the following:

- Frequency of digital rectal examinations
- Frequency of testicular self-examination
- Use of contraceptives
- Occupational exposure to chemicals (tire and rubber manufacturing, farming, mechanics)
- History of sexually transmitted infection
- History of discharge from the penis
- Difficulty with urination (incontinence, hesitancy, frequency, voiding at night)
- History of erectile dysfunction

PHYSICAL ASSESSMENT

The patient may be standing or supine. Gloves are worn during this assessment.

Inspecting and Palpating the External Genitalia

The external genitalia are inspected for size, placement, contour, appearance of the skin, redness, edema, and discharge. If the patient is uncircumcised, retract the foreskin

FIGURE 25-35. Testicular self-examination is to be performed once a month. A convenient time is after a warm bath or shower when the scrotum is relaxed. Both hands are used to palpate the testis; the normal testicle is smooth and uniform in consistency. (**A**) With the index and middle finger under the testis and the thumb on tip, roll the testis gently in a horizontal plane between the thumb and fingers, feeling for any evidence of a small lump or abnormality. (**B**) Follow the same procedure for palpation in a vertical plane. (**C**) Locate the epididymis (cord-like structure on the top and back of the testicle that stores and transports sperm). Repeat the examination for the other testis; it is normal to find one testis larger than the other. Any evidence of a small pea-sized lump should be checked by an advance practice professional. It may be due to an infection or a tumor growth.

for inspection of the glans penis. Assess the location of the urinary meatus. Inspect the scrotum for symmetry; it is not unusual for the left testicle to lie lower in the scrotal sac than the right testicle. Palpate the testes. The size, shape, and consistency of the scrotal contents (i.e., testes) should be similar bilaterally. Normal findings include skin that is free of lesions, and a foreskin (if present) that is intact, uniform in color, and easily retracted. The urinary meatus is normally located in the center of the glans penis and is free of discharge. The scrotum and testes should be free of masses and nontender.

Abnormal findings include lesions, redness, edema, pain, discharge, fluid-filled masses in the scrotum (symptoms of a hydrocele or varicocele), and displacement of the urinary meatus or difficulties with voiding. Edema, redness, discharge, or pain may indicate an infection. Voiding difficulties may result from scarring caused by infections or prostate enlargement. (See Chapters 36 and 44 for additional discussion of the male urinary tract and sexually transmitted infections.)

Inspecting and Palpating the Inguinal Area

The inguinal area may be inspected at this time by asking the patient to bear down. Normally, the inguinal area is free of bulges. Further assessment for inguinal hernia, inguinal lymph nodes, and femoral hernia are usually performed by an advanced practice professional. Refer to a health assessment text for details.

NORMAL AGE-RELATED VARIATIONS
Infant/Child

Common genitalia variations in newborns (resulting from exposure to maternal hormones in utero, normally seen in the first week after birth and subsiding by the second week after birth) and children include:

- Breast enlargement
- Development of pubic hair and enlargement of the scrotum, testes, and penis occurs at puberty and follows a regular sequence to adult configuration.
- Spontaneous nocturnal emission of seminal fluid occurs at puberty.

Older Adult

Common genitalia variations in older adults include:

- Decreased penis size
- Decreased pubic hair
- Decreased size and firmness of testes

Assessing the Rectum and Anus

Although the rectum and anus are not assessed in all patients, this assessment is a part of a total health assessment for both men and women. Assessments of the rectum and anus are usually performed by advanced practice professionals. Information from the health history provides information about normal patterns of bowel elimination and identifies risks for illness (such as colon cancer) and health behaviors (such as frequency of digital rectal examinations [DRE] to assess for cancer or engaging in anal intercourse). Physical examina-

tion provides information to support teaching about risk for colon cancer and the risks of sexually transmitted infections (including AIDS) associated with unprotected anal sex.

HEALTH HISTORY

Identify risk factors for altered health during the health history by asking about the following:

- Bowel patterns, including constipation, diarrhea, or pain
- History of blood or mucus in the stool
- Family history of polyps, colon or rectal cancer, or prostate cancer
- History of hemorrhoids
- Frequency of DREs
- History of anal intercourse

PHYSICAL ASSESSMENT

Techniques used to assess the rectum and anus include inspection and palpation. Gloves and good lighting are necessary equipment. The patient may be in the knee–chest or side-lying position.

Inspection is used to assess the anal area, which normally has increased pigmentation and some hair growth. Assess for lesions, ulcers, fissures, inflammation, and external hemorrhoids (dilated veins appearing as reddened protrusions). Ask the patient to bear down as though having a bowel movement. Assess for the appearance of internal hemorrhoids or fissures. Normally, there is no protrusion of tissue. Abnormal findings include relaxed sphincter tone; skin cracks, nodules, or hemorrhoids at the anal sphincter; and bleeding (which may indicate hemorrhoids or colorectal cancer). Advanced practice professionals usually perform palpation of the anal canal and sphincter and the prostate gland in men. Refer to a health assessment text for details.

NORMAL AGE-RELATED VARIATIONS
Infant/Child

Normally physical examination of the rectum and anus is not performed in young children or adolescents.

Older Adult

Common variations in older men include:

- Anus is darker in color.
- Hemorrhoids are often present.

Assessing the Musculoskeletal System

The primary structures of the musculoskeletal system are the bones, muscles, cartilage, ligaments, tendons, and joints. Health history information is used to evaluate the patient's ability to carry out activities of daily living and to collect data about areas such as pain, stiffness, and ability to move. Physical examination provides information about posture, gait, bone size and structure, joint ROM, and muscle strength. Normally, the joints are bilaterally equal in size, shape, and color; are free of swelling, pain, nodules, or crepitus (grating sounds on movement); and can move through full ROM. Abnormal findings include deformity, crepitus, and limited ROM (indicating injury, inflammation and/or arthritis of the affected joints or bones, and muscle pain and/or weakness caused by injury or disease). Many practitioners assess the neuromuscular, musculoskeletal, and peripheral vascular systems as an integrated assessment. Refer to Skill 25-2 on pages 674–681 for an example of a systematic, integrated assessment of these systems.

HEALTH HISTORY

Identify risk factors for altered health during the health history by asking about the following:

- History of trauma, arthritis, or neurologic disorder
- History of pain or swelling in the muscles and/or joints
- Frequency and type of usual exercise
- Dietary intake of calcium
- History of any surgery on muscles or joints
- History of smoking (how long, how many packs/day)
- History of alcohol intake

PHYSICAL ASSESSMENT

The patient assumes a variety of positions, including standing, sitting, and supine, if possible. Assessments of the musculoskeletal system can be integrated into assessment of other body systems.

Inspecting and Palpating the Muscles

Examine the muscles by inspection and palpation of muscle groups and by testing muscle tone and strength. Muscle groups are observed for bilateral symmetry and palpated for tenderness. Normally, they are symmetric and nontender. Evaluate muscle tone (the normal condition of a muscle at rest) by putting each joint and extremity through passive ROM. Assess muscle strength. Guidelines for Nursing Care 25-5 (on pages 664–665) describes testing muscle strength.

Abnormal findings include atrophy (a decrease in size), tremors (involuntary movements), and flaccidity (without tone) of muscles. Other abnormal findings are loss of strength and tone, decreased ROM, uncoordinated movements, swelling, and pain. Abnormal findings may indicate a musculoskeletal disease, trauma, or a neurologic disease.

Palpating the Bones

Palpate the bones for normal contour and prominence and for bilateral symmetry. Abnormal findings include pain, enlargement, asymmetry, and changes in contour. Abnormal findings may indicate trauma, degenerative joint disease, musculoskeletal disease, or a neurologic disease.

Inspecting and Palpating the Joints

Each joint is put through its full ROM to assess the degree of movement. Joint movements include flexion, extension, hyperextension, abduction, adduction, supination, and pronation. Normally, each joint has full ROM, is nontender, and moves smoothly. Palpate joints for the abnormal findings of pain, swelling, nodules, and crepitation (a grating sound heard or felt on movement).

Inspecting Spinal Curves

With the patient standing, inspect the spine from the back and from the side. The spine normally has concave curves at the cervical and lumbar spine and convex curves at the thoracic and sacrococcygeal spine. The lumbar curve may be flattened with a herniated disc. Kyphosis (an increased thoracic spinal curve) is more often seen in older adults. An exaggerated lumbar curve (lordosis) is often seen during pregnancy or in obesity. Scoliosis is a lateral curvature of the spine with increased convexity on the side that is curved. School nurses often first identify scoliosis during screenings, which are recommended for girls in grades 5 and 7 and for boys in grades 8 or 9. Findings indicating scoliosis are illustrated in Figure 25-36.

A

| Is the head level and centered over the trunk? | Are the shoulders the same height? |

B

| Are the hips at the same level? | When bent forward with arms dropping toward feet, is rib cage level on both sides? |

FIGURE 25-36. Screening for scoliosis. (**A**) Normal position and spinal curves. (**B**) Scoliosis indicators.

GUIDELINES FOR NURSING CARE 25-5

ASSESSING MUSCLE STRENGTH

Assess muscle strength by asking the patient to move against resistance. Bilateral equal resistance should be present. Observe muscle contraction and determine muscle strength exerted. Muscle strength should be bilaterally equal, with a slight increase on the dominant side. Techniques for assessing the muscles include:

Shoulder Flexion

The patient flexes shoulder muscle against resistance of the examiner's hand (Figure A).

FIGURE A

Elbow Extension and Flexion

• The patient first extends the elbow against resistance by the examiner (Figure B).

FIGURE B

• Then the patient flexes the elbow against resistance (Figure C).

FIGURE C

Wrist Extension

The patient makes a fist and resists examiner's attempts to pull down wrist (Figure D).

FIGURE D

Grip

The patient squeezes the examiner's index and middle fingers (Figure E).

FIGURE E

Hip Flexion

The patient attempts to raise the thigh against examiner's resistance (Figure F).

FIGURE F

GUIDELINES FOR NURSING CARE 25-5 *continued*

ASSESSING MUSCLE STRENGTH

Knee Flexion and Extension

- With the patient's knee bent and foot on the examining table, the patient attempts to keep foot down while the examiner attempts to straighten the patient's leg to test flexion (Figure G).

FIGURE G

- To test extension, the examiner supports the patient's knee and the patient attempts to straighten the leg against resistance at the ankle (Figure H).

FIGURE H

(Photos by Ken Casper.)

Ankle Plantar Flexion and Dorsiflexion

- The patient first pushes the balls of the feet against resistance of the examiner's hands (Figure I).

FIGURE I

- Then, the patient attempts to pull against examiner's resistance (Figure J).

FIGURE J

NORMAL AGE-RELATED VARIATIONS
Infant/Child

Common musculoskeletal variations in newborns and children include:

- C-shaped curve of spine at birth; the anterior cervical curve develops at about 3 to 4 months of age, and the anterior lumbar curve develops between 12 and 18 months of age
- Lordosis (an exaggerated lumbar curve)
- Pronation of the feet in children between 12 and 30 months of age
- Genu varum (bowleg) for 1 year after learning to walk

Older Adult

Common musculoskeletal variations seen in older adults include:

- Loss of muscle mass and strength
- Decreased ROM
- Kyphosis
- Decreased height
- Osteoarthritic changes in joints

Assessing the Neurologic System

Neurologic assessment includes cerebral function, cranial nerve function, cerebellar function, motor and sensory function, and reflexes. The health history is useful in obtaining information about activities of daily living and other pertinent data, such as dizziness, loss of sensation, headaches, and ability to see, hear, taste, and detect sensations. Physical examination is conducted to identify mental status and level of consciousness, cranial nerve function, muscle strength and coordination, and reflexes. Normally, the patient is alert and responsive, has full sensory function, and all muscle groups are bilaterally strong. Abnormal findings are discussed with specific parts of the examination that follow. Many practitioners assess the neuromuscular, musculoskeletal, and peripheral vascular systems as an integrated assessment. Refer to Skill 25-2 on pages 674–681 for an example of a systematic, integrated assessment of these systems.

HEALTH HISTORY

Identify risk factors for altered health during the health history by asking about the following:

- History of numbness, tingling, or tremors
- History of seizures
- History of headaches
- History of dizziness
- History of trauma to the head or spine
- History of infections of the brain
- History of stroke
- Changes in the ability to hear, see, taste, or smell
- Loss of ability to control bladder and bowel
- History of high blood pressure
- History of smoking (how long, how many packs/day)
- History of chronic alcohol use
- History of diabetes mellitus or heart disease
- Use of prescription and over-the-counter medications
- Family history of high blood pressure, Alzheimer's disease, epilepsy, cancer, or Huntington's chorea
- Frequency of blood cholesterol tests and results
- Exposure to environmental hazards (e.g., lead, insecticides)

PHYSICAL ASSESSMENT

Evaluate cerebral function by observing the patient's behavior throughout the health history interview and physical assessment. Assess the patient's mental status, memory, emotional status, cognitive abilities, and behavior. Evaluate cerebellar function by assessing fine motor skills, coordination, and balance. Assess the sensory system by having the patient identify various sensory stimuli, and evaluate the reflexes by contraction of specific muscles.

Equipment for a neurologic assessment includes vials of aromatic substances (e.g., peppermint and vanilla), a visual acuity chart, a penlight, a sharp object (e.g., a large safety pin), cotton balls, vials of solution to test taste (e.g., salt or sugar), a tuning fork, a tongue depressor, and familiar objects, such as a key or coin. The patient should be sitting, if possible, and the environment should be quiet. Advanced practice professionals typically perform assessment of deep tendon reflexes to determine the functional ability of specific spinal segment levels. Refer to a health assessment text for details.

Assessing Mental Status

Mental status assessment includes level of awareness, level of consciousness, behavior and appearance, memory, abstract reasoning, and language. On initial contact, begin to evaluate the patient's orientation to person, place, and time, as well as cognitive abilities and affect (whether the patient knows who he or she is, where he or she is, and the day or month or year). Observe the patient's appearance, general behavior, ability to speak clearly, and respond to questions. Note any variation in responses.

Assess the patient's overall appearance. The patient should have a clean, neat appearance with erect posture; should be oriented to person, place, and time; should have memory recall (both short-term and long-term memory); and should be able to demonstrate coherent and logical thought processes. Abnormal findings include poor hygiene, inappropriate dress, disorientation, absent memory recall, and incoherent or illogical thought processes. These abnormal findings may indicate a mental health disorder, developmental delay, brain disease, cerebrovascular disorder, alcohol or drug intoxication, or a tumor.

 THINK back to Tammy Browning, the pregnant woman with a history of substance abuse. The nurse would assess the patient's mental status for clues suggesting recent drug use, incorporating knowledge of abnormal findings into the assessment. ●

The following discussion of each of the mental status components includes sample questions or specific assessments to use during the assessment.

Assessing Level of Awareness. Assess awareness by evaluating orientation to time, place, and person. The following questions may be used:

- *Time:* What is today's date? What day of the week is it? What season of the year is this? What was the last holiday?
- *Place:* Where are you now? What is the name of this city? What state are we in?
- *Person:* What is your name? How old are you? Who came to visit you this morning?

Although exceptions may occur, people who have impaired awareness first lose time orientation, followed by place orientation, and then person orientation. Remember that it is often difficult to know the exact date when one is ill, in pain, or in unfamiliar surroundings.

Assessing Level of Consciousness. Consciousness is the degree of wakefulness or the ability of a person to be aroused. This is not the same as orientation; a patient may be conscious but not oriented. Level of consciousness is described as follows:

- Awake and alert: fully awake; oriented to person, place, and time; responds to all stimuli, including verbal commands
- Lethargic: appears drowsy or asleep most of the time but makes spontaneous movements; can be aroused by gentle shaking and saying patient's name

Table 25-7 GLASGOW COMA SCALE

The Glasgow Coma Scale (GCS) evaluates three key categories of behavior that most closely reflect activity in the higher centers of the brain: eye opening, verbal response, and motor response (Waterhouse, 2005). Within each category, each level of response is given a numerical value. The maximal score is 15, indicating a fully awake, alert, and oriented patient; the lowest score is 3, indicating deep coma (Hickey, 2009). The GCS is used in conjunction with other neurologic assessments, including pupillary reaction and vital sign measurement, to evaluate a patient's status (Waterhouse, 2005).

COMPONENT	SCORE	RESPONSE
Eye opening	4	Opens eyes spontaneously when someone approaches
	3	Opens eyes in response to speech (normal tone or shouting)
	2	Opens eyes only to painful stimuli (apply pressure with a pen to the lateral outer aspect of the second or third finger, up to 10 seconds, then release)
	1	No response to painful stimuli
Motor response	6	Accurately responds to instructions; obeys a simple command, such as "Lift your left hand off the bed"
	5	Localizes (moves hand to point of stimulation) to painful stimuli and attempts to remove source
	4	Flexion reflex action, but unable to locate the source of pain; purposeless movement in response to pain
	3	Flexes elbows and wrists while extending lower legs to pain; decorticate posturing
	2	Extends upper and lower extremities to pain; decerebrate posturing
	1	No motor response to pain on any limb
Verbal response	5	Converses; oriented to time, place, and person
	4	Converses; disoriented to time, place, or person; any one or all indicators
	3	Converses only in words or phrases that make little sense in the context of the questions
	2	Responds with incomprehensible sounds; no understandable words and/or moaning, groaning, or crying in response to painful stimuli
	1	No response

Adapted from Hickey, J. V. (2009). *The clinical practice of neurological and neurosurgical nursing* (6th ed.). Philadelphia, PA: Wolters Kluwer Health/Lippincott Williams & Wilkins; Caton-Richards, M. (2010). Assessing the neurological status of patients with head injuries. *Emergency Nurse, 17*(10), 28–31; and Teasdale, G. & Jennett, B. (1974). Assessment of coma and impaired consciousness. A practical scale. *Lancet, 2*(7872), 81–84.

- Stuporous: unconscious most of the time; has no spontaneous movement; must be shaken or shouted at to arouse; can make verbal responses, but these are less likely to be appropriate; responds to painful stimuli with purposeful movements
- Comatose: cannot be aroused, even with use of painful stimuli; may have some reflex activity (such as gag reflex); if no reflexes present, is in a deep coma

The Glasgow Coma Scale (GCS) (Table 25-7) is a standardized assessment tool that assesses level of consciousness. Three parameters are evaluated: eye opening, motor response, and verbal response. Scores are given in each category, and a total score is recorded, with higher scores indicating a more normal level of functioning. A score of 7 or less defines coma. This is a more accurate evaluation of mental status over time. Some limitations to using the GCS include the inability to assess the verbal score after the patient has been intubated; a lack of assessment of respiration and brainstem reflexes; inability to assess a possible developing vegetative state; and inability to recognize pseudocoma.

The newer FOUR (Full Outline of Un-Responsiveness) score coma scale (Table 25-8 on page 668) can be used to assess for signs of decreasing consciousness, increasing intracranial pressure, and brain herniation, as well as to predict patient outcome (Sadaka, Patel, & Lakshmanan, 2012; Barker, 2008). It includes important information not assessed by the GCS, including measurement of brainstem reflexes; determination of eye opening, blinking, and tracking; a broad spectrum of motor responses; and the presence of abnormal breath rhythms and a respiratory drive. Because the FOUR score, unlike the GCS, does not include an assessment of verbal response, it is more useful for assessing critically ill patients who have undergone intubation (Sadaka et al., 2012; Iyer et al., 2009). The components of the scale are not totaled or summed, but a FOUR score of 0 would likely indicate that the patient could fulfill the criteria of brain death (Barker, 2008). Refer to the accompanying Research in Nursing box on page 668.

Assessing Memory. Assess memory by asking questions that require answers demonstrating immediate recall and recall for past events. To assess immediate memory, ask the patient to repeat a series of numbers forward or backward (e.g., 3, 6, 9). Start with three numbers and gradually increase the digits until the patient cannot respond correctly. Most adults can repeat a series of five to eight numbers forward and four to six digits backward. You might also ask, "What did you eat for breakfast this morning?" To assess past memory, ask, "When is your birthday?" or "When is your wedding anniversary?"

Table 25-8 FULL OUTLINE OF UN-RESPONSIVENESS (FOUR) COMA SCALE

The FOUR score coma scale combines the most important neurologic signs into an easy-to-use scale with four components. The maximum score in each of these components is 4. The components are not totaled or summed and can be used to detect decreasing consciousness, increasing intracranial pressure and brain herniation, as well as predict patient outcome (Sadaka et al., 2012; Iyer et al., 2009; Barker, 2008).

	0	1	2	3	4
Eye Response	E0: Eyelids remain closed with pain	E1: Eyelids closed but open to pain	E2: Eyelids closed but open to loud voices	E3: Eyelids open but not tracking	E4: Eyelids open or opened, tracking or blinking to command
Motor Response *Note: Ask patients to make a peace sign, a fist, and show thumbs up*	M0: No response to pain	M1: Extension response to pain	M2: Flexion response to pain	M3: Localizing to pain	M4: Thumbs-up, fist, or peace sign
Brainstem Reflexes	B0: Absent pupil, corneal, and cough reflex	B1: Pupil and corneal reflexes absent	B2: Pupil or corneal reflexes absent	B3: One pupil wide and fixed	B4: Pupil and corneal reflexes present
Respiration	R0: Breathes at ventilator rate or apnea	R1: Breathes above ventilatory rate	R2: Not intubated, irregular breathing	R3: Not intubated, Cheyne-Stokes breathing pattern	R4: Not intubated, regular breathing pattern

Adapted from Barker, E. (2008). *Neuroscience nursing* (3rd ed.). St. Louis: Elsevier/Mosby; Iyer, V. N., Mandrekar, J. N., Danielson, R. D., Zubkov, A. Y., Elmer, J. L., & Wijdicks, E. F. (2009). Validity of the FOUR score coma scale in the medical intensive care unit. *Mayo Clinic Proceedings*, *84*(8), 694–701; and Sadaka, F., Patel, D., & Lakshmanan, R. (2012). The FOUR score predicts outcome in patients after traumatic brain injury. *Neurocritical Care*, *16*(1), 95–101.

Assessing Abstract Reasoning. Ask the patient to explain a proverb such as "the early bird catches the worm." If intellectual ability is impaired, the patient usually gives a literal explanation or repeats the phrase. Be sure that the phrase is not culture specific.

Assessing Language

The cerebral cortex controls the ability to express self through writing, words, or gestures and to understand the spoken and written word. Some simple methods of assessing language capabilities include asking the patient to name

RESEARCH IN NURSING

BRIDGING THE GAP TO EVIDENCE-BASED PRACTICE

Coma and the FOUR (Full Outline of Un-Responsiveness) Score

The newer FOUR (Full Outline of Un-Responsiveness) score coma scale can be used to assess for signs of decreasing consciousness, increasing intracranial pressure, and brain herniation, as well as predict patient outcome. It includes important information not assessed by the Glasgow Coma Scale.

Related Research

Sadaka, F., Patel, D., & Lakshmanan, R. (2012). The FOUR score predicts outcome in patients after traumatic brain injury. *Neurocritical Care*, 16(1), 95–101.

This study's goal was to determine whether the Full Outline of Un-Responsiveness (FOUR) score is an accurate predictor of outcome in traumatic brain injury patients and to compare its performance to the Glasgow Coma Scale (GCS), the most widely used and studied coma score to date. Fifty-one patients admitted to a neurologic intensive care unit over the course of 7 months were evaluated using the FOUR score and GCS. Outcomes were evaluated at 3 and 6 months, including in-hospital mortality, and poor neurologic outcomes. The

researchers concluded that the FOUR score is an accurate predictor of outcome in traumatic brain injury patients and it offers some advantages over the GCS. Advantages of the FOUR score include the ability to identify subtle changes in alteration of consciousness and relative ease of use. In addition, the FOUR score can be used to assess an intubated patient (unlike the GCS), and is faster to use.

Relevance to Nursing Practice

Nurses should continually search for interventions to improve patient care. Assessment and monitoring of a patient's neurologic status is an important nursing intervention. Nurses spend the greatest amount of time with patients, providing direct care, allowing for early detection of changes in a patient's condition. Nurses should consider discussing possible evaluation of the FOUR score for use by a facility when caring for neurologically compromised patients.

For additional research, visit thePoint.

items in the room (e.g., bed, flowers, gown, pajamas), to follow simple commands (such as "Point to your head"), to read a short sentence aloud, or to match printed and spoken words with appropriate pictures. Injury to the cortex can cause aphasia, which is a disorder of language ability. Aphasia may be expressive (the individual understands written and spoken words but cannot write or speak to communicate effectively) or receptive (the individual cannot understand written or spoken words). These aphasias may also be combined.

Assessing Cranial Nerve Function

The function of the 12 cranial nerves is assessed primarily during the neurologic assessment, although parts of cranial nerve function are assessed with other body systems (e.g., capillary response during assessment of the face). Each nerve has a specific function and is evaluated individually. Table 25-9 outlines the cranial nerves, with their function and assessment methods.

Assessing Motor and Sensory Function

Motor ability is evaluated by assessing balance, gait, and coordination. Sensory function is assessed by testing sensory discrimination of pain, light touch, and vibrations.

Inspecting Balance and Gait. Evaluate balance and gait by having the patient walk across the room on the toes, on the heels, and heel to toe. Observe posture, balance, and arm and leg movements. The posture should be erect, with slight swaying in the standing position. Walking (gait) should be smooth and rhythmic, with arms swinging at the sides.

Assessing Motor Function and Coordination. Evaluate motor function and coordination by having the patient rapidly touch each finger with the thumb, rapidly pat the hand on the thigh, and tap the foot on the floor (or against your hand, if the patient is supine). Repeat the sequence on the opposite limb. Normally, the movements are coordinated. If the patient is unable to perform these movements, it may indicate disease of the upper motor neurons or cerebellum.

Assessing Sensory Perception. Test sensory perception by evaluating the patient's response to pain, light touch, normal shapes, and vibration. With the patient's eyes closed, randomly touch the skin on the upper and lower extremities and the trunk with a sharp object and a soft object. The assessment proceeds from distal (hands, arms, feet, or legs) to proximal (the trunk). The patient should be able to distinguish between

Table 25-9	**SUMMARY OF CRANIAL NERVES**		
NERVE (NUMBER)	**TYPE**	**FUNCTIONS**	**METHODS FOR EXAMINING NERVE**
Olfactory (I)	Sensory	Sense of smell	Test each nostril for smell reception with various agents and interpretation.
Optic (II)	Sensory	Sense of vision	Test vision for acuity and visual fields.
Oculomotor (III)	Motor	Pupil constriction Raise eyelids	Test pupillary reaction to light and ability to open and close eyelids.
Trochlear (IV)	Motor/ Proprioceptor	Downward, inward eye movement	Test for downward and inward movement of the eye.
Trigeminal (V)	Motor	Jaw movements—chewing and mastication	Ask patient to open and clench jaws while you palpate the jaw muscles.
	Sensory	Sensation on the face and neck	Test face and neck for pain sensations, light touch, and temperature.
Abducens (VI)	Motor	Lateral movement of the eyes	Test ocular movement in all directions.
Facial (VII)	Motor	Muscles of the face	Ask the patient to raise eyebrows, smile, show teeth, and puff out cheeks.
	Sensory	Sense of taste on the anterior two thirds of the tongue	Test for the taste sensation with various agents.
Acoustic (VIII)	Sensory	Sense of hearing	Test hearing ability.
Glossopharyngeal (IX)	Motor	Pharyngeal movement and swallowing	Ask the patient to say "ah," and have patient yawn to observe upward movement of the soft palate; elicit gag response; note ability to swallow.
	Sensory	Sense of taste on the posterior one third of the tongue	Test for taste with various agents.
Vagus (X)	Motor/Sensory	Swallowing and speaking	Ask the patient to swallow and speak; note hoarseness.
Accessory (XI)	Motor/Sensory	Movement of shoulder muscles	Ask the patient to shrug shoulders against your resistance.
Hypoglossal (XII)	Motor	Movement of the tongue; strength of the tongue	Ask the patient to protrude tongue; ask patient to push tongue against cheek.

sharp (painful) and soft or dull touch. The same process is repeated by using the tuning fork to test for vibratory sensation by placing the activated fork on bony prominences. Sensory perception may also be assessed by asking the patient to close the eyes and identify familiar objects (such as a coin or key) by touching them. Abnormal findings include inability to perceive pain or light touch, inability to identify the location of touch, inability to identify familiar objects, and absence of vibratory sensation.

Neurovascular Assessment. Assessment of neurovascular status is an important nursing intervention leading to early identification of neurovascular impairment and timely intervention (Johnston-Walker & Hardcastle, 2011). Refer to the discussion of neurovascular assessment earlier in the chapter. See Box 25-6 on page 655 for an outline of the components of a neurovascular assessment.

NORMAL AGE-RELATED VARIATIONS
Infant/Child
Common neurologic variations for newborns and children include:

- Positive Babinski's reflex (normal in children between 12 and 24 months)
- Grasp reflex (present at birth)
- Motor control develops in head, neck, trunk, and extremities sequence

Older Adult
Common neurologic variations for older adults include:

- Slower thought processes and verbal responses
- Decreased sensory ability (hearing, sight, smell, taste, temperature, pain)
- Slower coordination and voluntary movements

BOX 25-7 DOCUMENTING A HEALTH ASSESSMENT

Mrs. D. comes to a local community outpatient agency for intolerance of eating fatty foods. She says, "I just started having a lot of gas and was sick to my stomach after eating fried foods." The nurse in charge of the agency makes the following assessments.

Health History

Mrs. D. is a 52-year-old woman who lives with her 54-year-old husband on a farm in a rural midwestern area. She graduated from high school and is employed as a secretary for a local insurance agency. Mrs. D. is well groomed, alert, and oriented. She occasionally takes over-the-counter medications for constipation and colds. She takes a prescription medication twice a day for "high blood pressure." She says she has about two mixed drinks a week and does not smoke. She has had five pregnancies, resulting in five living children.

Mrs. D. had her tonsils removed at 5 years of age, had an appendectomy at 22 years of age, and is allergic to penicillin (causes rash and difficulty breathing). She has had all her immunizations, but her last tetanus shot was 10 years ago. Her family history of illness is as follows:

Maternal grandfather died of heart problems at 77 years of age.

Maternal grandmother died of diabetes complications at 69 years of age.

Paternal grandfather died of stroke at 82 years of age.

Paternal grandmother died of unknown causes at 56 years of age.

Sister, 49 years of age, healthy

Brother died at 22 years of age in a car accident.

Physical Assessment

Vital signs: T = 98.8°F (orally), P = 82 beats/min, R = 16 breaths/min, BP = 150/88 mm Hg

Height/weight: 5 feet, 4 inches tall, 178 pounds

Integument: Skin warm and dry, normal turgor. Numerous freckles over face and arms. Old scar, RLQ (appendectomy). Nails convex and smooth. Hair dark brown, shiny, normal distribution.

Head and neck: Skull size and shape normal. Facial features symmetric. Can raise eyebrows, close eyes, smile, and puff out cheeks. External eye structures symmetric. Sclera white, conjunctiva pink. Wears glasses to correct near-sightedness. Vision with glasses 20/30-2 on Snellen chart. Pupils equal, round, and react to light bilaterally. Demonstrates accommodation, convergence, and peripheral vision. Lens clear. External ears symmetric. Canals smooth and pink without excess cerumen. Tympanic membranes intact, without redness or drainage. Right nostril clear, left nostril occluded with mucus. Left maxillary sinus slightly tender on palpation. Teeth in good repair with six fillings. Oral mucous membranes pink. Tonsils absent. Trachea midline, thyroid nonpalpable. No lymph nodes palpable.

Thorax/lungs/heart: Thorax symmetric with equal expansion. Respirations even and unlabored. Lung sounds clear. No visible pulsations noted in neck or precordium. S_1 and S_2 heard at pulmonic, aortic, tricuspid, and mitral areas. No extra heart sounds, murmurs, or bruits heard. Apical pulse 84 beats/min and regular.

Breasts and axilla: Skin pink. No dimpling or retraction noted. Areolae and nipples dark brown, no crusting or drainage. No masses palpated in breasts. Axillary lymph nodes are not palpable. To have mammogram at next visit.

Abdomen: Obese, rounded. Umbilicus midline. No pain on light palpation. Bowel sounds heard in all four quadrants. No bruits heard on auscultation.

Peripheral vascular: Pulses equal in both arms. Pulses equal in both legs. No edema present. Superficial varicose veins present on both lower extremities between ankle and knee. Toenails thick and yellow.

Genitalia: Will be assessed at next visit with pelvic and Papanicolaou's smear.

Rectum and anus: Inspected only. Small external hemorrhoids noted.

Musculoskeletal: Stands erect. Normal spinal curves. No joint deformities, tenderness, or crepitation. Full active ROM in all joints. Muscle strength equal bilaterally, slightly stronger on the right (dominant side).

Neurologic: Alert and oriented to time, place, and person. Facial expressions appropriate. Speech clear and appropriate. Demonstrates long-term and short-term memory. All cranial nerves tests were intact. Fine motor movements intact. Gait even. Perceives pain or light touch appropriately.

- Decreased reflex responses
- Appearance of confusion in unfamiliar surroundings
- Slower gait, with a wider base and flexed hips and knees
- Diminished deep tendon reflexes

DOCUMENTATION OF DATA

After completing the health history and physical assessment, organize all health assessment data to identify actual and potential health problems, identify nursing diagnoses, plan appropriate care, and evaluate the patient's responses to interventions. A pattern is often established that begins during the history and is confirmed during the physical assessment. For example, a health history of a woman diagnosed with multiple sclerosis (a neurologic disorder) might include data about fatigue and increased weakness and muscle spasms in the legs. Physical examination findings would include decreased muscle strength in the lower extremities. These data are used to support the nursing diagnosis of Activity Intolerance related to fatigue and lower extremity weakness. Document the data, with each system recorded individually. Box 25-7 illustrates an example of documentation.

THE NURSE'S ROLE IN DIAGNOSTIC PROCEDURES

Diagnostic procedures and tests provide crucial information about a patient's health; their results become a part of the total health assessment. Nurses assist before, during, and after diagnostic tests. The nurse is also responsible for other activities associated with diagnostic tests, such as witnessing the patient's consent, scheduling the test, preparing the patient physically and emotionally for the test, providing care, and teaching the patient and/or caregivers about the ordered procedures or tests. Table 25-10 presents an overview of different types of diagnostic procedures.

 THINK back to Tammy Browning, the pregnant woman with a history of substance abuse. A urine specimen was to be obtained for routine testing. In addition, the specimen was to be used for drug testing without the patient's knowledge. Typically, a signed consent form is not necessary for urine specimens. However, the nurse would need to know the facility's policy and legal statutes of the area regarding consent for drug testing before obtaining the specimen. ●

Table 25-10 A GUIDE TO COMMON LABORATORY AND DIAGNOSTIC PROCEDURES

PROCEDURE	DESCRIPTION	EXAMPLES
Aspiration procedures	Studies in which a needle or similar instrument is inserted into a body organ or cavity. Fluid or tissue is aspirated, prepared, labeled, and sent to the laboratory for examination.	Liver biopsy Lumbar puncture Paracentesis Thoracentesis
Electrical impulse procedures	Studies that use a machine with electrodes attached to the body to monitor electric activity. Electric impulses are recorded on a graph and displayed on paper or an oscilloscope screen.	Electrocardiogram (ECG) Electroencephalogram (EEG)
Endoscopic procedures	Studies that allow for direct visual examination of various body cavities and organs by means of a hollow, lighted tube called an endoscope. The tube may be flexible or rigid. May be used to obtain tissue specimens for biopsy or microscopic examination.	Bronchoscopy Colonoscopy Gastroscopy Sigmoidoscopy Laparoscopy
Laboratory procedures	Studies in which body fluids, secretions, or tissues are sent to the laboratory for analysis.	Blood studies Urine studies Sputum studies Fecal studies Biopsies
Radiography procedures	Because of the ability of x-rays to penetrate human tissues, x-ray studies provide a picture of body structures that looks like a negative of a photograph.	Chest x-ray Dye-enhanced cardiac catheterization
Magnetic resonance imaging (MRI)	The computer-based procedure provides physiologic information and detailed views of fluid-filled soft tissues.	MRI of the brain, spine, extremities, joints, heart, pelvis, and abdomen
Nuclear scanning	Studies that use the administration of a radionuclide and subsequent measurement of radiation from an organ to detect functional abnormalities	Brain scan Heart scan Lung scan Bone scan
Ultrasonography	Studies in which a harmless, high-frequency sound wave is emitted that penetrates the organ being studied. The sound waves bounce back to the sensor and are electronically converted into a picture of the organ or the contents of the organ.	Ultrasound of the pelvis, abdomen, heart, uterus

SKILL 25-1 USING A BED SCALE

DELEGATION CONSIDERATIONS

The measurement of body weight may be delegated to nursing assistive personnel (NAP) or unlicensed assistive personnel (UAP), as well as to licensed practical/vocational nurses (LPN/LVNs). The decision to delegate must be based on careful analysis of the patient's needs and circumstances, as well as the qualifications of the person to whom the task is being delegated. Refer to the Delegation Guidelines in Appendix A (found on thePoint).

EQUIPMENT

- Bed scale with sling
- Cover for sling
- Sheet or bath blanket
- PPE, as indicated

IMPLEMENTATION

ACTION	RATIONALE
1. Check the medical order or nursing plan of care for frequency of weight measurement. More frequent measurement of the patient's weight may be appropriate based on nursing judgment. Obtain the assistance of a second caregiver, based on the patient's mobility and ability to cooperate with the procedure.	This provides for patient safety and appropriate care.
2. Perform hand hygiene and put on PPE, if indicated.	Hand hygiene and PPE prevent the spread of microorganisms. PPE is required based on transmission precautions.
3. Identify the patient.	Identifying the patient ensures that the right patient receives the intervention and helps prevent errors.
4. Close curtains around the bed and close the door to the room if possible. Discuss the procedure with the patient and assess the patient's ability to assist with the procedure.	This ensures the patient's privacy. Explanation relieves anxiety and facilitates cooperation.
5. Place a cover over the sling of the bed scale.	Using a cover deters the spread of microorganisms.
6. Attach the sling to the bed scale. Lay the sheet or bath blanket in the sling. Turn the scale on. **Balance the scale so that weight reads 0.0.**	Scale will add the sling into the weight unless it is zeroed with the sling, blanket, and cover.
7. Adjust the bed to a comfortable working position, usually elbow height of the caregiver (VISN 8, 2009). Position one caregiver on each side of the bed if two caregivers are present. Raise side rail on the opposite side of the bed from where the scale is located, if not already in place. Cover the patient with the sheet or bath blanket. Remove other covers and any pillows.	Having the bed at the proper height prevents back and muscle strain. Having one caregiver on each side of the bed provides for patient safety and appropriate care. The side rail assists patient with movement. The blanket maintains the patient's dignity and provides warmth.
8. Turn the patient onto his or her side facing the side rail, keeping the patient's body covered with the sheet or blanket. Remove the sling from the scale. Place the cover on the sling. Roll the cover and sling lengthwise. Place the rolled sling under the patient, making sure the patient is centered in the sling.	Rolling the patient onto his or her side facilitates placing the patient onto the sling. The blanket maintains the patient's dignity and provides warmth.
9. Roll the patient back over the sling and onto the other side. Pull the sling through, as if placing the sheet under the patient, unrolling the sling as it is pulled through.	This facilitates placing the patient onto the sling.
10. Roll the scale over the bed so that the arms of the scale are directly over the patient. **Spread the base of the scale.** Lower the arms of the scale and place the arm hooks into the holes on the sling.	By spreading the base, you are giving the scale a wider base, thus preventing the scale from toppling over with the patient. Hooking the sling to the scale provides secure attachment to the scale and prevents injury.

ACTION	RATIONALE
11. Once the scale arms are hooked onto the sling, gradually elevate the sling so that the patient is lifted up off of the bed (Figure 1). **Assess all tubes and drains, making sure that none have tension placed on them as the scale is lifted. Once the sling is no longer touching the bed, ensure that nothing else is hanging onto the sling (e.g., ventilator or IV tubing). If any tubing is connected to the patient, raise it up so that it is not adding any weight to the patient.**	The scale must be hanging free to obtain an accurate weight. Any tubing that is hanging off the scale will add weight to the patient.

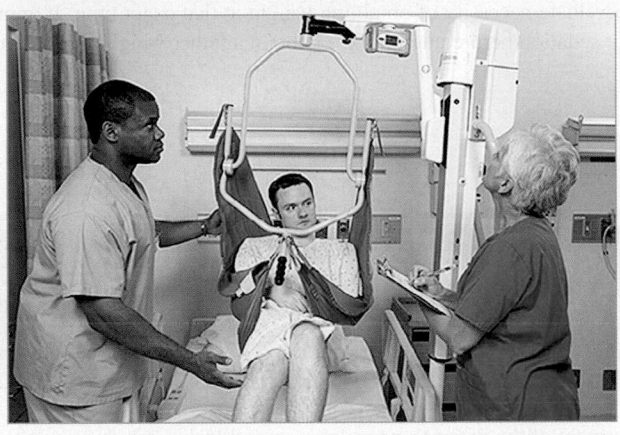

FIGURE 1. Using a bed scale.

ACTION	RATIONALE
12. Note the weight reading on the scale. Slowly and gently, lower the patient back onto the bed. Disconnect the scale arms from the sling. Close the base of the scale and pull it away from the bed.	Lowering the patient slowly does not alarm the patient. Closing the base of the scale facilitates moving the scale.
13. Raise the side rail. Turn the patient to the side rail. Roll the sling up against the patient's backside.	Raising the side rail is a safety measure.
14. Raise the other side rail. Roll the patient back over the sling and up, facing the other side rail. Remove the sling from the bed. Remove gloves, if used. Raise the remaining side rail.	The patient needs to be removed from the sling before it can be removed from the bed.
15. Cover the patient and help him or her to a position of comfort. Place the bed in the lowest position.	Ensures patient comfort and safety.
16. Remove the disposable cover from the sling and discard in the appropriate receptacle.	Using a cover deters the spread of microorganisms.
17. Remove additional PPE, if used. Clean equipment based on facility policy. Perform hand hygiene.	Removing PPE properly reduces the risk for infection transmission and contamination of other items. Cleaning equipment prevents transmission of microorganisms. Hand hygiene deters the spread of microorganisms.
18. Replace the scale and sling in the appropriate spot. Plug the scale into the electrical outlet.	Scale should be ready for use at any time.

DOCUMENTATION

Guidelines Document weight, unit of measurement, and scale used.

Sample Documentation

> 10/15/15 0230 Patient reports pain in legs 5/10. Premedicated with Percocet 2 tabs po before obtaining weight per order. Patient weighed using bed scale, 75.2 kg.
>
> —M. Evans, RN

(continued)

SKILL 25-1 USING A BED SCALE *continued*

UNEXPECTED SITUATIONS AND ASSOCIATED INTERVENTIONS

- *As the patient is being lifted, the scale begins to tip over:* Stop lifting the patient. Slowly lower the patient back to the bed. Ensure that the base of the scale is spread wide enough before attempting to weigh the patient.

- *Weight differs from the previous day's weight by more than 1 kg:* Weigh the patient using the same scale at the same time each day. Check calibration of the scale. Make sure that the patient is wearing the same clothing. Make sure that no tubes or containers are hanging on the scale. If the patient is incontinent, make sure undergarments are clean and dry.

- *The patient becomes agitated as the sling is raised into the air:* Stop lifting the patient and reassure him or her. If the patient continues to be agitated, lower the patient back to the bed. Reevaluate necessity of obtaining weight at that exact time. If appropriate, obtain an order for sedation before attempting to obtain another weight measurement.

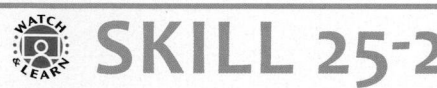

SKILL 25-2 ASSESSING THE NEUROLOGIC, MUSCULOSKELETAL, AND PERIPHERAL VASCULAR SYSTEMS

DELEGATION CONSIDERATIONS

The assessment of the patient's neurologic, musculoskeletal, and peripheral vascular systems should not be delegated to nursing assistive personnel (NAP) or unlicensed assistive personnel (UAP). Some items may be noticed while providing care and noted by the NAP or UAP. The nurse must then validate, analyze, document, communicate, and act on these findings, as appropriate. Depending on the state's nurse practice act and the organization's policies and procedures, the licensed practical/vocational nurses (LPN/LVNs) may perform some or all of the parts of assessment of the patient's neurologic, musculoskeletal, and peripheral vascular systems. The decision to delegate must be based on careful analysis of the patient's needs and circumstances, as well as the qualifications of the person to whom the task is being delegated. Refer to the Delegation Guidelines in Appendix A (found on thePoint).

EQUIPMENT

- PPE, as indicated
- Bath blanket or other drape
- Tongue depressor
- Examination gown
- Gloves

- Containers of odorous materials (e.g., coffee or chocolate) and substances for taste assessment (e.g., sugar, salt, vinegar)
- Miscellaneous items (e.g., coin, pin, cotton, key, and paper clip)
- Cotton-tipped applicators

IMPLEMENTATION

ACTION	RATIONALE
1. Perform hand hygiene and put on PPE, if indicated.	Hand hygiene and PPE prevent the spread of microorganisms. PPE is required based on transmission precautions.
2. Identify the patient.	Identifying the patient ensures that the right patient receives the intervention and helps prevent errors.
3. Close the curtains around the bed and close the door to the room, if possible. Explain the purpose of the neurologic, musculoskeletal, and peripheral vascular examinations and what you are going to do. Answer any questions.	This ensures the patient's privacy. Explanation relieves anxiety and facilitates cooperation.

ACTION	RATIONALE
4. Help the patient undress, if needed, and provide a patient gown. Assist the patient to a supine position, if possible. Use the bath blanket to cover any exposed area other than the one being assessed.	Having the patient wear a gown facilitates examination of the neurologic, musculoskeletal, and peripheral vascular systems. Use of a bath blanket provides for comfort and warmth.
5. Begin with a survey of the patient's overall hygiene and physical appearance.	This provides initial impressions of the patient. Hygiene and appearance can provide clues about the patient's mental state and comfort level.
6. Assess the patient's mental status.	
a. Evaluate the patient's orientation to person, place, and time.	This helps identify the patient's level of awareness.
b. Evaluate level of consciousness.	The patient should be awake and alert. Patients with an altered level of consciousness may be lethargic, stuporous, or comatose.
c. Assess memory (immediate recall and past memory).	Memory problems may indicate neurologic impairment.
d. Assess abstract reasoning by asking the patient to explain a proverb, such as "The early bird catches the worm."	If intellectual ability is impaired, the patient usually gives a literal interpretation or repeats the phrase.
e. Evaluate the patient's ability to understand the spoken and written word.	This helps assess for aphasia.
7. Test cranial nerve (CN) function.	
a. Ask the patient to close the eyes, occlude one nostril, and then identify the smell of different substances, such as coffee, chocolate, or alcohol. Repeat with the other nostril.	This action tests the function of CN I (olfactory nerve).
b. Test visual acuity and pupillary constriction. Refer to the previous discussion in the assessment of the head and neck.	This tests function of CN II and CN III (optic and oculomotor nerves).
c. Move the patient's eyes through the six cardinal positions of gaze. Refer to previous discussion in the assessment of the head and neck.	This testing evaluates the functions of CN III, CN IV, and CN VI (oculomotor, trochlear, and abducens nerves).
d. Ask the patient to smile, frown, wrinkle the forehead, and puff out cheeks (Figure 1).	This maneuver evaluates the motor function of CN VII (facial nerve).
e. Ask the patient to protrude the tongue and push against the cheek with the tongue.	This evaluates the function of CN XII (hypoglossal nerve).

FIGURE 1. Puffing out cheeks. (Weber, J.R., & Kelley, J.H. (2014). *Health assessment in nursing* (5th ed.). Philadelphia: Wolters Kluwer Health | Lippincott Williams & Wilkins.)

(continued)

SKILL 25-2 ASSESSING THE NEUROLOGIC, MUSCULOSKELETAL, AND PERIPHERAL VASCULAR SYSTEMS *continued*

ACTION	RATIONALE
f. Palpate the jaw muscles. Ask the patient to open and clench jaws. Stroke the patients face with a cotton ball.	This evaluates the function of CN V (trigeminal nerve).
g. Test hearing with the whispered voice test. Refer to previous discussion in the assessment of the head and neck.	This evaluates the function of CN VIII (acoustic nerve).
h. Put on gloves. Ask the patient to open the mouth. While observing the soft palate, ask the patient to say "ah"; observe upward movement of the soft palate. Test the gag reflex by touching the posterior pharynx with the tongue depressor. Explain to patient that this may be uncomfortable. Ask the patient to swallow. Remove gloves.	Gloves prevent contact with blood and body fluids. An intact gag reflex and swallowing indicates normal functioning of CN IX and CN X (glossopharyngeal and vagus nerves).
i. Place your hands on the patient's shoulders (Figure 2) while he or she shrugs against resistance. Then place your hand on the patient's left cheek, then the right cheek, and have the patient push against it.	These actions check CN XI (spinal accessory nerve) function and trapezius and sternocleidomastoid muscle strength.
8. Check the patient's ability to move his or her neck. Ask the patient to touch the chin to the chest and to each shoulder, then move each ear to the corresponding shoulder (Figure 3), and then tip the head back as far as possible.	These actions assess neck ROM, which is normally smooth and controlled.

FIGURE 2. Assessing strength of the trapezius muscle. (Weber, J.R., & Kelley, J.H. (2014). *Health assessment in nursing* (5th ed.). Philadelphia: Wolters Kluwer Health | Lippincott Williams & Wilkins.)

FIGURE 3. Moving each ear to the corresponding shoulder. (From Jensen, S. (2011.) *Nursing health assessment. A best practice approach.* Philadelphia: Wolters Kluwer Health/Lippincott Williams & Wilkins, p. 654, Figure 23.16B.)

9. Inspect the upper extremities. Observe for skin color, presence of lesions, rashes, and muscle mass. Palpate for skin temperature, texture, and presence of masses.	Examination of the upper extremities provides information about the circulatory, integumentary, and musculoskeletal systems.
10. Ask the patient to extend the arms forward and then rapidly turn the palms up and down.	This maneuver tests proprioception and cerebellar function.
11. Ask the patient to flex the upper arm and to resist the examiner's opposing force (Figure 4).	This technique assesses the muscle strength of the upper extremities.
12. Inspect and palpate the hands, fingers, wrists (Figure 5), and elbow joints.	Inspection and palpation provide information about abnormalities, tenderness, and ROM.
13. Ask the patient to bend and straighten the elbow, and flex and extend the wrists and hands.	Tests ROM of the elbow joint and wrists.

ACTION

FIGURE 4. Assessing elbow muscle strength. (From Jensen, S. (2011). *Nursing health assessment. A best practice approach.* Philadelphia: Wolters Kluwer Health/Lippincott Williams & Wilkins, p. 658, Figure 23.20.)

14. Palpate the skin and the radial and brachial pulses. Assess the pulse rate, quality or amplitude, and rhythm. Test capillary refill.

15. Have the patient squeeze two of your fingers (Figure 6).

16. Ask the patient to close the eyes. Using your finger or applicator, trace a one-digit number on the patient's palm and ask the patient to identify the number. Repeat on the other hand with a different number (Figure 7).

FIGURE 6. Testing grip. Patient squeezes nurse's index and middle fingers. *(Photo by B. Proud.)*

17. Ask the patient to close the eyes. Place a familiar object, such as a key, in the patient's hand and ask the patient to identify the object. Repeat using another object for the other hand.

RATIONALE

FIGURE 5. Palpating the wrist. *(Photo by B. Proud.)*

Pulse palpation and capillary refill evaluates the peripheral vascular status of the upper extremities.

This maneuver tests the muscle strength of the hands.

This test evaluates tactile discrimination, specifically graphesthesia.

FIGURE 7. Testing tactile discrimination (graphesthesia). *(Photo by B. Proud.)*

This test evaluates tactile discrimination, specifically stereognosis.

(continued)

SKILL 25-2

ASSESSING THE NEUROLOGIC, MUSCULOSKELETAL, AND PERIPHERAL VASCULAR SYSTEMS *continued*

ACTION	RATIONALE
18. Assist the patient to a supine position. Palpate (Figure 8-A) and then use the bell of the stethoscope to auscultate the femoral pulses in the groin (Figure 8-B), if not done during assessment of the abdomen. Note the strength of the pulse and grade it as with peripheral pulses.	This technique assesses flow of blood through the arteries. Auscultation can detect a bruit.

 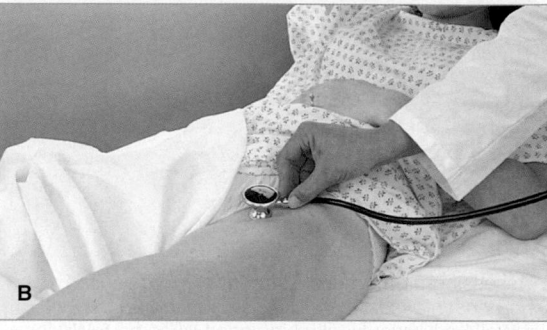

FIGURE 8. Palpating (**A**) and auscultating (**B**) the femoral pulses. *(Photos by B. Proud.)*

19. Examine the lower extremities. Inspect the legs and feet for color, lesions, varicosities, hair growth, nail growth, edema, and muscle mass.	Inspection provides information about peripheral vascular function.
20. Assess for pitting edema in the lower extremities by pressing fingers into the skin at the pretibial area and dorsum of the foot (Figure 9-A). If an indentation remains in the skin after the fingers have been lifted, pitting edema is present (Figure 9-B).	This technique reveals information about excess interstitial fluid. Refer to an edema scale in assessing the amount of edema: 1+ about 2 mm deep to 4+ about 8 mm deep.

FIGURE 9. Assessing for pitting edema in lower extremities. (From Hogan-Quigley, B., Palm, M.L., & Bickley, L. (2012). *Bates' nursing guide to physical examination and history taking.* Philadelphia: Wolters Kluwer Health/ Lippincott Williams & Wilkins, p. 412.)

ACTION

21. Palpate for pulses and skin temperature at the posterior tibial, dorsalis pedis, and popliteal areas. Assess the pulse rate, quality or amplitude, and rhythm. Test capillary refill.

22. Have the patient perform the straight leg test with one leg at a time (Figure 10).

23. Ask the patient to move one leg laterally with the knee straight to test abduction and medially to test adduction of the hips.

24. Ask the patient to raise the thigh against the resistance of your hand (Figure 11); next have the patient push outward against the resistance of your hand; then have the patient pull backward against the resistance of your hand. Repeat on the opposite side.

RATIONALE

Pulses, skin temperature, and capillary refill provide information about the patient's peripheral vascular status.

This test checks for vertebral disc problems.

This maneuver assesses ROM and provides information about joint problems.

These measures assess motor strength of the upper and lower legs.

FIGURE 10. Performing straight leg test. *(Photo by B. Proud.)*

FIGURE 11. Testing motor strength of upper leg. Patient attempts to raise thigh against nurse's resistance. *(Photo by B. Proud.)*

25. Test plantar reflex. Stroke the sole of the patient's foot with the end of a hard object such as the edge of a tongue depressor or a key. Begin at the heel and apply firm but gentle pressure to the lateral aspect of the foot. Continue to the base of the toes (Figure 12). Repeat on the other side.

Flexion of all the toes is considered a normal finding in an individual 18 months of age and older: a negative Babinski reflex.

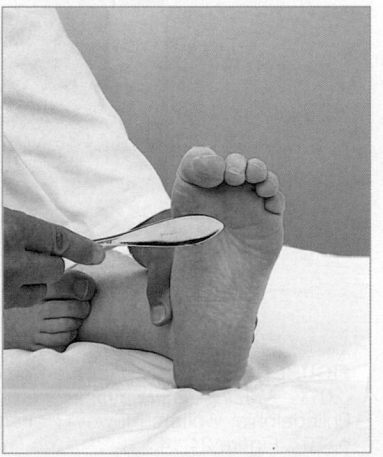

FIGURE 12. Eliciting plantar reflex.

(continued)

SKILL 25-2 ASSESSING THE NEUROLOGIC, MUSCULOSKELETAL, AND PERIPHERAL VASCULAR SYSTEMS *continued*

ACTION	RATIONALE
26. Ask patient to dorsiflex and then plantarflex both feet against opposing resistance (Figure 13).	These measures test foot strength and ROM.

FIGURE 13. (**A**) Testing ankle flexion and dorsiflexion. The patient first pushes the balls of the feet against resistance of the nurse's hands. (**B**) Then attempts to pull against nurse's resistance. *(Photos by B. Proud.)*

27. As needed, assist the patient to a standing position. Observe the patient as he or she walks with a regular gait, on the toes, on the heels, and then heel to toe (Figure 14).	This procedure evaluates cerebellar and motor function.
28. Perform the Romberg test; ask the patient to stand straight with feet together, both eyes closed with arms at side (Figure 15). Wait 20 seconds and observe for patient swaying and ability to maintain balance. Be alert to prevent patient fall or injury related to losing balance during this assessment.	This test checks cerebellar functioning and evaluates balance, equilibrium, and coordination. Slight swaying is normal, but the patient should be able to maintain balance.

FIGURE 14. Testing heel to toe walking. (From Jensen, S. (2011). Nursing health assessment. A best practice approach. Philadelphia: Wolters Kluwer Health/Lippincott Williams & Wilkins, p. 707, Figure 24.13.)

FIGURE 15. Positioning for the Romberg test. (From Jensen, S. (2011). *Nursing health assessment. A best practice approach.* Philadelphia: Wolters Kluwer Health/Lippincott Williams & Wilkins, p. 707, Figure 24.14.)

ACTION

29. Assist the patient to a comfortable position.

30. Remove PPE, if used. Perform hand hygiene. Continue with assessments of specific body systems, as appropriate, or indicated. Initiate appropriate referral to other health care practitioners for further evaluation, as indicated.

RATIONALE

This ensures the patient's comfort.

Removing PPE properly reduces the risk for infection transmission and contamination of other items. Hand hygiene prevents the spread of microorganisms. Additional assessments should be completed, as indicated, to evaluate the patient's health status. Intervention by other health care providers may be indicated to evaluate and treat the patient's health status.

DOCUMENTATION

Guidelines

Document assessment techniques performed, along with specific findings. Note the cognitive responses of the patient, the tested cranial nerves, and sensation and motor responses. Document any patient statements of pain, muscle weakness, or joint abnormality. Record findings, including color, turgor, temperature, pulses, and capillary refill.

Sample Documentation

DocuCare Practice documenting assessment techniques and findings in *Lippincott DocuCare.*

4/4/15 Patient alert, oriented, cognitively appropriate. Cranial nerves intact. Sensation intact. Full ROM of all joints. Muscles soft, firm, nontender, no atrophy. Patient states pain in right calf. Right calf skin paler tone and slightly cooler compared to left calf. Peripheral pulses 72, +2, regular rhythm, equal bilaterally; exception—right posterior tibial and dorsalis pedis pulses +1. Capillary refill right lower extremity sluggish, >3 seconds.

—S. Moses, RN

SPECIAL CONSIDERATIONS

General Considerations

- Before asking questions related to the mental status examination, inform the patient that some of the questions may seem unusual, but that you are attempting to evaluate overall cognitive function.

Infant and Child Considerations

- In an infant, jerky and brief twitching of the extremities may be noted and is considered a normal finding.
- The Babinski sign is typically elicited in children age 18 months and younger.
- The infant's extremities move symmetrically through ROM but lack full extension.
- The Barlow-Ortolani maneuver is used to assess hip abduction and adduction in an infant. (Refer to a pediatrics text for more information.)
- Before age 5 years, sensory function is normally not tested.
- Coordination of movement varies according to the developmental level of the young child.

Older Adult Considerations

- Be aware that short-term memory, such as recall of recent events, may diminish with age, as well as slowed reaction time.
- In the older adult patient, expect to find decreased musculoskeletal function, such as loss of muscle strength.
- Keep in mind that older adults may take longer to perform certain actions, such as completing activities for testing coordination.

DEVELOPING CLINICAL REASONING

1. Describe how you would explain a cardiovascular assessment to the following patients:
   - A healthy 5-year-old
   - A college student who has never been ill
   - A 50-year-old man who has never had a physical assessment
   - An 85-year-old woman with heart problems

2. When you are conducting a health history, your patient gives you strange answers. Later, during the mental status assessment, she gives you the wrong answers for the date and place. She also cannot remember what medications she takes. How would you document this information? What would you do next?

3. When you make a home visit to conduct an initial health history and physical assessment, the patient refuses to let you do more than assess vital signs. What would you do?

PRACTICING FOR NCLEX

1. A home health care nurse takes the vital signs of a patient who is receiving supplemental oxygen at home for chronic obstructive pulmonary disease (COPD). This is the nurse's fourth visit to the patient's home. The nurse records the data collected on the patient's chart. What type of assessment has this nurse performed?
   a. Comprehensive
   b. Ongoing partial assessment
   c. Focused assessment
   d. Emergency assessment

2. A nurse caring for patients in a long-term care facility is performing a functional assessment of a new patient. Which questions would the nurse ask? Select all that apply.
   a. Are you able to dress yourself?
   b. Do you have a history of smoking?
   c. What is the problem for which you are seeking care?
   d. Do you prepare your own meals?
   e. Do you manage your own finances?
   f. Whom do you rely on for support?

3. A nurse is assessing a patient's eyes for extraocular movements. Which action correctly describes a step the nurse would take when performing this test?
   a. Ask the patient to sit about 3 feet away facing the nurse.
   b. Keep a penlight about 1 foot from the patient's face and move it slowly through the cardinal positions.
   c. Move a penlight in a circular motion in front of the patient's eyes.
   d. Ask the patient to cover one eye with a hand or index card.

4. Which actions would the nurse perform when using the technique of palpation during the physical assessment of a patient? Select all that apply.
   a. The nurse compares the patient's bilateral body parts for symmetry.
   b. The nurse takes a patient's pulse.
   c. The nurse touches a patient's skin to test for turgor.
   d. The nurse checks a patient's lymph nodes for swelling.
   e. The nurse taps a patient's body to check the organs.
   f. The nurse uses a stethoscope to listen to a patient's heart sounds.

5. When inspecting the skin of a patient who has cirrhosis of the liver, the nurse notes that the skin has a yellow tint. What would the nurse document related to this finding?
   a. Jaundice
   b. Cyanosis
   c. Erythema
   d. Pallor

6. After inspecting the skin of a patient, the nurse documents the presence of a skin lesion as a palpable solid mass measured at 1 cm. What types of skin lesions might this describe? Select all that apply.
   a. Macule
   b. Patch
   c. Plaque
   d. Nodule
   e. Bulla
   f. Pustule

7. A patient's visual acuity is assessed as 20/40 in both eyes using the Snellen chart. The nurse interprets this finding as:
   a. The patient can see twice as well as normal.
   b. The patient has double vision.
   c. The patient has less than normal vision.
   d. The patient has normal vision.

8. When assessing a patient's breath sounds, the nurse hears a high-pitched continuous sound. What type of breath sound would the nurse document?
   a. Rhonchi
   b. Crackles
   c. Stridor
   d. Wheezes

9. A nurse is using the FOUR Coma Scale to assess the neurologic status of a patient following surgery to remove a brain tumor. The nurse rates the patient as M2 for motor response. What condition does this number represent?
   a. Localizing to pain
   b. Flexion response to pain
   c. Extension response to pain
   d. No response to pain

10. A nurse auscultates the thorax and lungs and hears coarse, low-pitched, continuous sounds on expiration. When the patient coughs, the sounds clear up somewhat. The nurse would document these sounds as:
    a. Adventitious breath sounds
    b. Bronchovesicular breath sounds
    c. Vesicular breath sounds
    d. Bronchial sounds

11. A nurse is assessing a patient's eyes for accommodation. What actions would the nurse perform during this test? Select all that apply.
    a. Bring a penlight from the side of the patient's face and briefly shine the light on the pupil.
    b. Hold a forefinger, a pencil, or other straight object about 10 to 15 cm (4″ to 6″) from the bridge of the patient's nose.
    c. Hold a finger about 6″ to 8″ from the bridge of the patient's nose.
    d. Darken the room.
    e. Ask the patient to look straight ahead.
    f. Ask the patient to first look at a close object, then at a distant object, then back to the close object.

12. A nurse is palpating the breast of a woman during an assessment. Which technique is performed correctly?
    a. The nurse starts at the tail of Spence and moves in increasing smaller circles.
    b. The nurse uses the palms of the hands to gently compress the breast tissue against the chest wall.
    c. The nurse works in a counterclockwise direction and palpates from the periphery toward the areola.
    d. The nurse starts at the inner edge of the breast and palpates up and down the breast.

13. During a physical assessment, a nurse inspects a patient's abdomen. What assessment technique would the nurse perform next?
    a. Percussion
    b. Palpation
    c. Auscultation
    d. Whichever is more comfortable for the patient

14. A nurse is assessing the level of consciousness of a patient who sustained a head injury in a motor vehicle accident. The nurse notes that the patient appears drowsy most of the time but makes spontaneous movements. The nurse is able to wake the patient by gently shaking him and calling his name. What level of consciousness would the nurse document?
    a. Awake and alert
    b. Lethargic
    c. Stuporous
    d. Comatose

15. A nurse is conducting an assessment of a patient's cranial nerves. The nurse asks the patient to raise the eyebrows, smile, and show the teeth to assess which cranial nerve?
    a. Olfactory
    b. Optic
    c. Facial
    d. Vagus

ANSWERS WITH RATIONALES

1. *b.* An ongoing partial assessment, or follow-up assessment, is conducted at regular intervals (e.g., at the beginning of each home health visit or each hospital shift) during care of the patient. This type of assessment concentrates on identified health problems to monitor positive or negative changes and evaluate the effectiveness of interventions. A comprehensive assessment with a health history and complete physical examination is usually conducted when a patient first enters a health care setting, with information providing a baseline for comparing later assessments. A focused assessment is conducted to assess a specific problem. An emergency assessment is a type of rapid focused assessment conducted when addressing a life-threatening or unstable situation.

2. *a, d, e.* A functional health assessment focuses on the effects of health or illness on a patient's quality of life, including the strengths of the patient and areas that need to improve. The nurse would assess the patient's ability to perform ADLs and IADLs such as dressing, grooming, preparing meals, and managing finances. A history of smoking is a lifestyle factor and the chief complaint is the reason for seeking health care, both assessed during the health history. Social networks and support persons are assessed as psychosocial factors related to the health history.

3. *b.* The steps in testing for extraocular movement are: (1) Ask the patient to sit or stand about 2 feet away, facing the nurse, who is sitting or standing at eye level with the patient; (2) ask the patient to hold the head still and follow the movement of a forefinger or a penlight with the eyes; (3) keeping the finger or light about 1 foot from the patient's face, move it slowly through the cardinal position—up and down, left and right, diagonally up and down to the left, diagonally up and down to the right.

4. *b, c, d.* During palpation, the nurse uses the sense of touch to take a pulse, test for skin turgor, and check lymph nodes. With inspection, a comparison of bilateral body parts is necessary for recognizing abnormal findings. During percussion, the fingertips are used to tap the body over body tissues to produce vibrations and sound waves. The characteristics of the sounds produced are used to assess the location, shape, size, and density of tissues. Auscultation is the act of listening with a stethoscope to sounds produced within the body.

5. *a.* Jaundice is a yellowish skin color caused by liver disease. Cyanosis is a bluish skin color caused by a cold environment or decreased oxygenation. Erythema is a reddish color caused by blushing, alcohol intake, fever, injury trauma, or infection. Pallor is a paleness caused by anemia or shock.

6. *c, d.* Plaque and nodules are palpable, elevated, solid masses that may measure 1 cm. Macules and patches are circumscribed, flat, nonpalpable changes in skin color. Macules are less than or equal to 1 cm and patches are greater than 1 cm. Bulla and pustules are circumscribed, superficial skin elevations formed by free fluids in a cavity with skin layers. Bulla are greater than 0.5 cm and pustules are filled with pus.

7. *c.* Normal vision is 20/20. A finding of 20/40 would mean that a patient has less than normal vision.

8. *d.* Wheezes are musical or squeaking high-pitched, continuous sounds heard as air passes through narrowed airways. Rhonchi are low-pitched, continuous sounds with a snoring quality that occur when air passes through secretions. Crackles are bubbling, cracking or popping, low- to high-pitched, discontinuous sounds that occur when air passes through fluid in the airways. Stridor is a harsh, loud, high-pitched sound due to narrowing of the upper airway.

9. *b.* To assess motor response, patients are asked to make a peace sign, a fist, and show thumbs up. Patients are scored as follows:
    M4 Thumbs-up, fist, or peace sign
    M3 Localizing to pain
    M2 Flexion response to pain
    M1 Extension response to pain
    M0 No response to pain

10. *a.* Adventitious breath sounds are sounds not normally heard in the lungs.
    Bronchovesicular breath sounds are normal sounds heard on inspiration and expiration. Vesicular breath sounds are soft, low-pitched, whispering sounds; heard over most of the lung fields. Bronchial sounds are blowing, hollow sounds, auscultated over the larynx and trachea.

11. *b, f.* To test accommodation the nurse would hold the forefinger, a pencil, or other straight object about 10 to 15 cm (4″ to 6″) from the bridge of the patient's nose. Then the

nurse would ask the patient to first look at the object, then at a distant object, then back to the object being held. The pupil normally constricts when looking at a near object and dilates when looking at a distant object. To test for convergence, the nurse would darken the room and ask the patient to look straight ahead. The nurse would then bring the penlight from the side of the patient's face and briefly shine the light on the pupil, observing the reaction. When testing convergence the nurse would hold a finger about 6″ to 8″ from the bridge of the patient's nose and move it toward the patient's nose.

12. *a.* When palpating the breast, the nurse would palpate each quadrant of each breast in a systematic method using either the circular, wedge, or vertical strip technique and then use the pads of the first three fingers to gently compress the breast tissue against the chest wall. In the circular method, the nurse would start at the tail of Spence and move in increasing smaller circles. In the wedge method, the nurse would work in a clockwise direction and palpate from the periphery toward the areola. In the vertical strip method, the nurse would start at the outer edge of the breast and palpate up and down the breast.

13. *c.* When assessing the abdomen, the sequence is inspection, auscultation, percussion, and palpation. Auscultation follows inspection because percussion and palpation stimulate bowel sounds.

14. *b.* The stages of consciousness are:
Awake and alert: fully awake; oriented to person, place, and time; responds to all stimuli, including verbal commands.

Lethargic: appears drowsy or asleep most of the time but makes spontaneous movements; can be aroused by gentle shaking and saying patient's name.
Stuporous: unconscious most of the time; has no spontaneous movement; must be shaken or shouted at to arouse; can make verbal responses, but these are less likely to be appropriate; responds to painful stimuli with purposeful movements.
Comatose: cannot be aroused, even with use of painful stimuli; may have some reflex activity (such as gag reflex); if no reflexes present, is in a deep coma

15. *c.* Motor function of the facial nerve (cranial nerve VII) is assessed by asking the patient to raise the eyebrow, smile, and show the teeth. The olfactory nerve (cranial nerve I) is tested by testing smell reception with various agents. The nurse tests the optic nerve (cranial nerve II) for acuity and visual fields and the vagus nerve (cranial nerve X) by asking the patient to swallow and speak, noting hoarseness.

TAYLOR SUITE RESOURCES

Explore these additional resources to enhance learning for this chapter:

- NCLEX-Style Questions and other resources on thePoint, http://thePoint.lww.com/Taylor8e
- *Study Guide for Fundamentals of Nursing, 8th edition*
- Adaptive Learning | Powered by prepU, http://thepoint.lww.com/prepu
- *Skill Checklists for Fundamentals of Nursing, 8th edition*
- *Taylor's Clinical Nursing Skills:* Chapter 3, Health Assessment
- *Taylor's Video Guide to Clinical Nursing Skills:* Physical Assessment
- *Lippincott DocuCare* Fundamentals cases

Bibliography

American Hearing Research Foundation. (2008). Hearing testing. Available at http://american-hearing.org/disorders/hearing-testing/

Armstrong, J., & Mitchell, E. (2008). Comprehensive nursing assessment in the care of older people. *Nursing Older People, 1*(20), 36–40.

Bagai, A., Thavendiranathan, P., & Detsky, A.S. (2006). Does this patient have hearing impairment? *Journal of the American Medical Association, 295*(4), 416–428.

Barker, E. (2008). *Neuroscience nursing* (3rd ed.). St. Louis: Elsevier/Mosby.

Boltz, M., Capezuti, E., Fulmer, T., & Zwicker, D. (eds.) (2012). *Evidence-based geriatric nursing protocols for best practice* (4th ed.). New York: Springer Publishing Company.

Centers for Disease Control and Prevention (CDC). (2012). *Immunization schedules.* Available at http://www.cdc.gov/vaccines/schedules/index.html

Centers for Medicare and Medicaid Services. (2012). Quick reference information: The ABCs of providing the initial preventive physical examination. Available at http://www.cms.gov/Outreach-and-Education/Medicare-Learning-Network-MLN/MLNProducts/downloads/MPS_QRI_IPPE001a.pdf

Divi, C., Koss, R. G., Schmaltz, S. P., & Loeb, J. M. (2007). Language proficiency and adverse events in U.S. hospitals: A pilot study. *International Journal for Quality in Health Care, 19*(2), 60–67.

Dudek, S. (2014). *Nutrition essentials for nursing practice* (7th ed.). Philadelphia: Wolters Kluwer Health/Lippincott Williams & Wilkins.

Fawcett, T., & Rhynas, S. (2012). Taking a patient history: the role of the nurse. *Nursing Standard, 15*(26), 41–46.

Fennessey, A., & Wittmann-Price, R. A. (2011). Physical assessment: A continuing need for clarification. *Nursing Forum, 46*(1), 45–50.

Fletcher, J. (2009). Identifying patients at risk of malnutrition: Nutrition screening and assessment. *Gastrointestinal Nursing, 7*(5), 12–17.

Foret Giddens, J., & Eddy, L. (2007). A survey of physical examination skills taught in undergraduate nursing programs: Are we teaching too much? *Journal of Nursing Education, 48*(1), 24–29.

Giddens, J. (2007). A survey of physical assessment techniques performed by RNs: Lessons for nursing education. *Journal of Nursing Education, 46*(2), 83–87.

Harkin, H., & Kelleher, C. (2011). Caring for older adults with hearing loss. *Nursing Older People, 23*(9), 22–28.

Hassall, S., & Butler-Williams, C. (2010). Assessment of airway and breathing in adults. *British Journal of Neuroscience Nursing, 6*(6), 288–291.

Hickey, J. V. (2009). *The clinical practice of neurological and neurosurgical nursing.* (6th ed.). Philadelphia: Wolters Kluwer Health/Lippincott Williams & Wilkins.

Hinkle, J. L., & Cheever, K. H. (2014). *Brunner & Suddarth's Textbook of Medical-Surgical Nursing* (13th ed.). Philadelphia: Wolters Kluwer Health/Lippincott Williams & Wilkins.

Hogan-Quigley, B., Palm, M. L., & Bickley, L. (2012). *Bates' Nursing Guide to Physical Examination and History Taking.* Philadelphia: Wolters Kluwer Health/Lippincott Williams & Wilkins.

Hotta, T. (2011). The basics of a health assessment. *Plastic Surgical Nursing, 31*(3), 100–104.

Husky, M. M., Miller, K., McGuire, L., Flynn, L., & Olfson, M. (2011). Mental health screening of adolescents in pediatric practice. *Mental Health Screening, 38*(2), 159–169.

Iyer, V. N., Mandrekar, J. N., Danielson, R. D., Zubkov, A. Y., Elmer, J. L., & Wijdicks, E. F. (2009). Validity of the FOUR score coma scale in the medical intensive care unit. *Mayo Clinic Proceedings, 84*(8), 694–701.

Jarvis, C. (2012). *Physical examination and health assessment* (6th ed.). St. Louis: Elsevier/Saunders.

Jensen, S. (2011). *Nursing Health Assessment: A best practice approach.* Philadelphia: Wolters Kluwer Health/Lippincott Williams & Wilkins.

Johnston-Walker, E., & Hardcastle, J. (2011). Neurovascular assessment in the critically ill patient. *Nursing in Critical Care, 16*(4), 170–177.

Judge, N. L. (2007). Neurovascular assessment. *Nursing Standard, 21*(45), 39–44.

The Joint Commission. (2010). Advancing effective communication, cultural competence, and patient- and family-centered care: A roadmap for hospitals. Available at http://www.jointcommission.org/assets/1/6/ARoadmapforHospitalsfinalversion727.pdf

Kee, J. L., Hayes, E. R., McCuistion, L. E. (2012). *Pharmacology: A Nursing Process Approach* (7th ed.). St. Louis: Elsevier/Saunders.

Keveric, J., Jelinek, G. A., Knott, J., & Weiland, T. J. (2011). Validation of the Full Outline of Unresponsiveness (FOUR) Scale for conscious state in the emergency department: comparison against the Glasgow Coma Scale. *Emergency Medicine Journal, 28*(6), 486–490.

Kyle, T., & Carman, S. (2013). *Essentials of pediatric nursing* (2nd ed.). Philadelphia: Wolters Kluwer Health/Lippincott Williams & Wilkins.

Lloyd, H., & Craig, S. (2007). A guide to taking a patient's history. *Nursing Standard, 22*(13), 42–48.

Lynn, P. (2015). *Taylor's clinical nursing skills: A nursing process approach* (4th ed.). Philadelphia: Lippincott Williams & Wilkins.

Massey, D. (2010). Respiratory assessment 1: Why do it and how to do it? *British Journal of Cardiac Nursing, 6*(11), 537–541.

Meredith, T., & Massey, D. (2011). Respiratory assessment 2: More key skills to improve care. *British Journal of Cardiac Nursing, 6*(2), 63–68.

National Institutes of Health (NIH), National Heart, Lung and Blood Institute (NHLBI). (2012a). How are overweight and obesity diagnosed? Available at http://www.nhlbi.nih.gov/health/health-topics/topics/obe/diagnosis.html

National Institutes of Health (NIH), National Heart, Lung and Blood Institute (NHLBI). (2012b). What are overweight and obesity? Available at http://www.nhlbi.nih.gov/health/health-topics/topics/obe/

Parkes, R. (2011). Rate of respiration: The forgotten vital sign. *Emergency Nurse, 19*(2), 12–17.

Perry, S. E., Hockenberry, M. J., Lowdermilk, D. L., & Wilson, D. (2010). *Maternal child nursing care* (4th ed.). Maryland Heights, MO: Elsevier/Mosby.

Price, B. (2011). How to map a patient's social support network. *Nursing Older People, 23*(2), 28–35.

Ritter, L. A., & Hoffman, N. A. (2010). *Multicultural health.* Boston: Jones and Bartlett.

Romanelli, L., Landsverk, J., Levitt, J. M., Leslie, L. K., Hurley, M. M., Bellonci, C., Gries, L. T., ... the Child Welfare–Mental Health Best Practices Group. (2009). Best practices for mental health in child welfare: Screening, assessment and treatment guidelines. *Child Welfare, 88*(1), 163–188.

Sadaka, F., Patel, D., & Lakshmanan, R. (2012). The FOUR score predicts outcome in patients after traumatic brain injury. *Neurocritical Care, 16*(1), 95–101.

Skin Cancer Foundation. (2012). Melanoma. Available at http://www.skincancer.org/skin-cancer-information/melanoma

Spector, R. E. (2009). *Cultural diversity in health and illness* (7th ed.). Upper Saddle River, NJ: Pearson/Prentice Hall.

Substance Abuse and Mental Health Services Administration (SAMHSA) and the Health Resources and Services Administration (HRSA), SAMHSA-HRSA Center for Integrated Health Solutions (CIHS). (2012). Screening tools. Available at http://www.integration.samhsa.gov/clinical-practice/screening-tools

Tabloski, P. (2010). *Gerontological nursing* (2nd ed.). Upper Saddle River, NJ: Pearson/Prentice Hall.

Taylor, J. J., & Cohen, B. J. (2013). *Memmler's structure and function of the human body* (10th ed.). Philadelphia: Wolters Kluwer Health/Lippincott Williams & Wilkins.

Waterhouse, C. (2005). The Glasgow Coma Scale and other neurological observations. *Nursing Standard, 19*(33), 56–64c.

VISN 8 Patient Safety Center. (2009). *Safe patient handling and movement algorithms.* Tampa, FL: Author. Available http://www.visn8.va.gov/visn8/patientsafetycenter/safePtHandling/default.asp.

Yesavage, J. A. (1986). The use of Rating Depression Series in the Elderly. In L. W. Poon (Ed.): *Clinical memory assessment of older adults.* Washington, DC: American Psychological Association.

26

Safety, Security, and Emergency Preparedness

KARA GREENWOOD

Kara, a high school junior class representative and peer counselor, comes to the local community health center for a routine examination. During the interview, she says, "My guidance counselor has asked me and a few of my friends to develop a talk for our classmates on the dangers we face as adolescents. I know everybody is worried about terrorism, but I want to make sure that we talk about other safety issues, too."

BESSIE WASHINGTON

Bessie, a 77-year-old woman, was recently discharged to her home after suffering a cerebrovascular accident (stroke). She lives alone in a small, one-bedroom apartment and uses a walker to ambulate. She says, "I have so much stuff crammed into this small apartment! I almost fell this morning going from my bedroom to the kitchen."

JUANITA AND INEZ FLORES

Juanita is a young mother of a 1-year-old girl, Inez. Today they are at the clinic for a well-child visit. While sitting on a cot with her daughter, whose legs are dangling at the edge of the cot about a foot above ground level, Juanita turns to get something out of her purse and the child falls to the floor and begins to cry loudly.

After completing the chapter, you will be able to accomplish the following:

1. Identify factors that affect safety in a person's environment.
2. Identify patients at risk for injury.
3. Describe specific safety risk factors for each developmental stage.
4. Select nursing diagnoses for patients in unsafe situations.
5. Describe health-teaching interventions to promote safety for each developmental stage.
6. Describe strategies to decrease the risk for injury in the home.
7. Describe nursing interventions to prevent injury to patients in health care settings.
8. Identify alternatives to using restraints.
9. Explore resources for developing and evaluating an emergency management plan.
10. Evaluate the effectiveness of safety interventions.

KEY TERMS

asphyxiation	ground	poison control center
bioterrorism	intimate	
chemical terrorism	partner violence (IPV)	restraint
cyber terror	nuclear terrorism	safety event report
disaster		sentinel event

Safety and security are basic human needs. Safety—or freedom from danger, harm, or risk—is a paramount concern that underlies all nursing care. In addition, patient safety is a responsibility of all health care providers. The Institute of Medicine (IOM) report "To Err is Human," which was introduced in 2000, recognized the need for a renewed focus on a culture of safety that promotes safe, effective, person-centered delivery of care. The IOM identified safety as an organizational priority and emphasized that medical errors are more frequently due to system problems rather than human error. Evidence-based research has identified tools and techniques that have eliminated errors and promoted a safer health care environment (ANA, 2014). However, individual performance is paramount in a culture of safety. Communication, leadership, teamwork, and staff empowerment not only improve the work environment but are effective strategies that focus on safe high-quality care (Domrose, 2010). Since nurses comprise the largest number of health care workers, their role is prominent and they have an unparalleled opportunity to influence the lives of their patients. Safety is a focus in all health care facilities as well as in the home, workplace, and community. Many safety and security concerns are universal for all age groups, but there are unique considerations for each developmental stage.

Since the mass casualties that occurred in the terrorist attacks of September 11, 2001, as well as terrorist attacks in other parts of the world, the health care community has become increasingly aware of the need to be prepared should future incidents occur. Nurses are a vital part of any emergency response team and need knowledge about biological, chemical, and radioactive agents as well as the skills and competencies required to respond safely and effectively.

This chapter provides practical information on safety and security, and introduces concepts of emergency preparedness. The nursing process facilitates the nurse's ability to recognize, assess, diagnose, and plan nursing interventions to ensure safety for all ages in all environments. (See the accompanying Reflective Practice box on page 688.)

FACTORS AFFECTING SAFETY

Promoting safety and preventing injury are dual responsibilities of the nurse. Being aware of factors that affect safety, such as developmental level, lifestyle, mobility, sensory perception, knowledge level, communication ability, physical health state, and psychosocial state allows nurses to identify potential hazards and promote wellness. Injuries and deaths from motor vehicle accidents, falls, fire, suffocation, and poisoning occur with alarming regularity across the lifespan. Many of these injuries and deaths can be prevented with appropriate safety awareness and precautions. Violent behavior and its aftermath has also become a significant factor that affects public safety.

Ideally, the nurse and the patient or family should work together to eliminate or reduce accident risks in the home, community, or health care setting. Nationally, community-based nurses and emergency nurses are establishing partnerships and venturing into the community to offer injury prevention activities to children and families. Nurses who role model good health behaviors are more effective teachers.

Developmental Considerations

Each developmental level carries its own particular risks. Health care needs and safety risks change as people progress from infancy to the older adult stage. In addition, safety risks exist from conception. Studies have confirmed, for example, that pregnant women who use drugs, consume alcohol, or smoke expose their unborn children to substances that may adversely affect their normal growth and development.

Physical and cognitive changes reflect the sequential developmental stages of infancy through older adult. Ensuring that the environment is safe and secure requires an awareness of potential hazards for each developmental level. Prompt recognition of the potential or actual threat to safety is crucial; the nursing assessment may play a vital role in identifying a harmful environment.

REFLECTIVE PRACTICE: CULTIVATING QSEN COMPETENCIES

CHALLENGE TO ETHICAL AND LEGAL SKILLS

I first met Juanita Flores while working at a children's hospital two summers ago in a nurse externship program. Juanita was the mother of a 1-year-old girl diagnosed with failure to thrive who had been on the rehabilitation unit for some time. The child was very small and had a feeding program prescribed. One day while I was in the room, Juanita was sitting on the cot with her daughter, whose legs were dangling at the edge of the cot, about 1 foot above ground level. I was taking the child's vital signs. As the mother turned her back for a minute to grab something from her bag, I turned away to wash my hands in the sink. All of a sudden, I heard

a thud and crying as the child fell to the floor. Juanita tried to comfort her, picking her up and rocking and singing to her. Although I knew it was not completely my fault, I felt horrible about turning my back on the child for only the few seconds to wash my hands, the seconds that it took for the child to fall. Although Juanita was in the room, the child had been unsupervised for only a few seconds. However, I was not watching her at the moment the child fell. I wanted to tell my preceptor right away and knew I should in case anything had happened to the child, but I was nervous and afraid that I would get into trouble.

Thinking Outside the Box: Possible Courses of Action

- Tell my preceptor immediately that the child had fallen, and risk being asked why I had turned my back on the child.
- Report later that morning that the child had fallen earlier, and not make a big deal of it.
- Not mention it at all.

Evaluating a Good Outcome: How Do I Define Success?

- Patient is benefited by my actions, or at least is not harmed.
- My professional integrity is not compromised, nor is the personal integrity of the patient.
- A level of respect is maintained between the preceptor and student.
- Institutional policy for incident reporting is not violated.

Personal Learning: Here's to the Future!

Although I did tell my preceptor what had happened, I was not pleased by the way I handled the situation. Instead of reporting the incident right away, I waited until my preceptor was in the room with me, a half-hour or so later. I casually mentioned that the child had fallen earlier that morning but seemed to be fine. When my preceptor asked why I did not inform her earlier, I said that I couldn't find her and assumed that she was busy—plus, the child seemed fine and her mother was with her.

I was disappointed in how I dealt with this situation. Although I did not get reprimanded for the situation, an incident report was written documenting that the child

had fallen. The physician also came to examine the child to ensure that the child was indeed okay. My preceptor stressed the importance of reporting incidents as soon as they happen, rather than delaying or ignoring them. This time the child was uninjured, but I learned that in the future I will report any problem immediately. A patient's fall could be detrimental. It is also very important to follow the institution's policy for reporting incidents to ensure both your professional integrity and the well-being of the patient.

Anne Hrynko, Georgetown University

REFLECTION ON QUALITY AND SAFETY COMPETENCIES

How do you think you would respond in a similar situation? Why? What does this tell you about yourself and about the adequacy of your skills for professional practice? Is the nurse extern's fear justification for the action? Please explain. What ethical and legal principles, if any, were violated in this situation? What liability would the nurse extern be required to assume? Can you think of other ways to respond? What knowledge, skills, and attitudes do you need to develop to continuously improve quality and safety when caring for patients like Juanita and Inez Flores?

Patient-Centered Care: How might the nurse extern have interacted with the mother to promote the child's safety? What information should the nurse extern discuss with Juanita Flores concerning providing a safe environment for her child at various developmental stages? How could the nurse extern further involve the mother as a partner in maintaining safety through all hospital encounters?

Teamwork and Collaboration/Quality Improvement: What communication skills do you need to improve to

ensure that you function as a member of the patient care team and minimize risk of harm to patients? How do you think this incident affected the relationship between the nurse extern and the preceptor?

Safety/Evidence-Based Practice: How might the delay in reporting the child's fall have affected the outcome of this situation? Should the extern initiate a discussion with her preceptor to review personal accountability and reporting procedures in a timely manner for any safety violations or incidents? What evidence in nursing literature provides guidance for decision making regarding ensuring a safe patient care environment? Given the focus on a culture of safety, should the health care team review what went wrong to allow this incident to occur, rather than who let it happen?

Informatics: Can you identify essential information that must be documented in the child's electronic record regarding the fall she experienced? What other actions should be documented regarding the institution's response to the incident?

For children, potential hazards multiply as their motor skills develop and their environment expands. Nurses promote safe sleeping practices for infants when they advise parents to avoid stuffed animals and crib bumpers that increase the risk for suffocation. The risk of falling is noticeably higher for children. Toddlers are increasingly active and need appropriate safeguards to prevent falls in the home. Attentive supervision and age-appropriate playground equipment protect children from injuries when playing outside. Adolescents face great dangers when they abuse drugs or alcohol or engage in high-risk sexual activity. Devastating outcomes of these unsafe behaviors include alcohol-related motor vehicle accidents, pregnancy, sexually transmitted infections (STIs), and suicide. Drug and/or alcohol abuse are concerns for young and middle-aged adults employed in stressful work environments. Older adults experiencing altered balance or decline in cognitive abilities are increasingly vulnerable to falls and episodes of confusion. Nurses have firsthand experience with the specific hazards confronting each age group and situation.

Education to promote awareness of potentially dangerous situations must begin as early as possible and continue throughout the lifespan. Assessment of specific risks for each developmental level and appropriate nursing interventions are discussed later in this chapter.

Lifestyle

Certain occupations and recreational activities place people in more hazardous situations. For example, health care staff who suffer sleep deprivation due to extended work hours and variable shift assignments are more likely to commit errors and be a factor in adverse events (see further discussion in Chapter 33).

Occupation

Occupation and work environment often contribute to a person's safety. People who work in certain occupations may experience exposure to health hazards, such as excessive noise, pollution, toxic chemicals or vapors, or infectious agents. For example, a worker who operates industrial machinery or works with chemicals has a greater risk for accidental injury. Nurses working in the operating room are regularly exposed to surgical smoke, a byproduct of laser and electrocautery procedures. Surgical smoke contains chemicals that cause upper respiratory tract irritation and inflammation (Waddell, 2010). Reproductive hazards may exist for women with long-term exposure to certain anesthetic agents. An antiviral preparation (ribavirin) used for respiratory infections in hospitalized infants and children and treatment of chronic hepatitis C may be harmful to a developing fetus (Pillitteri, 2010). Exposure to excessive noise (e.g., a construction site, extremely loud music) may lead to hearing loss.

Certain occupations are also associated with increased risks of specific injuries. Nurses remain at serious risk for needlestick injuries and blood-borne infections despite safer needle devices that are available widely (Foley, 2012). The Occupational Safety and Health Administration (OSHA) identifies risks and develops standards to prevent serious injuries and illnesses caused by work-related musculoskeletal disorders resulting from repetitive motions. Back pain and carpal tunnel syndrome may occur from work-related repetitive motion. Nurses need to be proactive about their own safety in the workplace and share in the responsibility to eliminate any hazards. Injuries should not be considered "part of the job" because most are preventable. Involvement in safety committees helps to ensure that procedures and personal safety equipment are available, and that incidents and accidents are reviewed and remedied (Garcia, 2012).

Social Behavior

Some people by nature are more inclined to take risks and place themselves at jeopardy for injury. For example, failure to wear seat belts or to follow safety precautions is common behavior for some people. Others do not use appropriate protective equipment, such as wearing a helmet when riding a motorcycle. Such behaviors increase the risk for injury.

Stress may precipitate an unhealthful lifestyle that involves drug or alcohol abuse. For example, a high school student involved in multiple school activities and intent on maintaining excellent grades may turn to an addictive substance such as methamphetamine as a stimulant. This drug temporarily allows the student to remain alert for more hours each day and complete required class assignments.

Vulnerable populations, such as people who have made poor lifestyle choices, also need support and attention. Nurses have always been strong patient advocates regarding safety concerns for this population group. See Nursing Advocacy in Action (see page 690) for an example of a nurse supporting a vulnerable patient's safety and health.

Environment

Although much has been done to identify and control environmental pollutants, many U.S. residents still remain at risk for exposure to potentially unhealthy substances in the environment. In addition, certain environmental areas, like high-crime neighborhoods, have proven to be more hazardous.

Living in an area where crime is prevalent can pose a threat to physical security and emotional well-being. Violence, acts of aggression, and terrorism are components of 21st-century life. Security measures such as locks, security systems, and exterior lighting can promote safety.

It is imperative that community nurses are aware of risks or hazards in certain settings that have the potential to result in violence and cause personal injury. In high-crime areas, a personal escort may be required to ensure a safe nurse visit. Each home care agency must have a policy in place that recognizes violent behavior and has a strategy to deal with it. Agency risk assessment takes into account crime patterns in the area, the willingness and availability of law enforcement to assist with dangerous situations, and staff impressions about previous visits, including the type of

NURSING ADVOCACY IN ACTION

Patient Scenario

Ms. Jackson was admitted to the labor and delivery unit in active labor. She is in prison for killing her husband and is accompanied to the hospital by two armed guards. She is in shackles in the labor room "to prevent her escape." When you begin your shift, you find a woman in hysterics who has been in labor for 12 hours because of the position of the baby. You want to get her shackles off to try to make her more comfortable, but the guards aren't willing to help. They explain that it is policy to keep them on for felons like Ms. Jackson. You are horrified.

Implications for Nursing Advocacy

How will you respond if you are Ms. Jackson's nurse? Talk with your classmates and experienced nurses about the questions that follow.

- If you elect to advocate for Ms. Jackson and other women like her, what practical steps can you take to ensure better labor and delivery care?
- What is reasonable to expect of a student nurse, a graduate nurse, and an experienced nurse in this situation?
- What advocacy skills are needed to effectively respond to this challenge?

environment that was encountered. Examples of high-risk situations and behaviors include weapons that are visible in the home, history of past violent behavior in this setting, high-crime buildings or neighborhoods, substance abuse by either the patient or a family member, and a situation in which a child is being considered for removal from an abusive environment (McPhaul, 2011). Programs that monitor staff and dangerous situations protect nurses on their visits to patients' homes. Use Promoting Health 26-1 as a tool for self-evaluation of safety behaviors in the community setting before using it with others.

Mobility

Any limitation in mobility is potentially unsafe. An older patient with an unsteady gait is more prone to falling. Furthermore, if the patient is in an unfamiliar setting, such as a health care facility, the problem may be aggravated. Someone with paralysis or a spinal cord injury may require assistance with even simple movements. Supportive devices—such as canes, walkers, and wheelchairs—may facilitate movement, but they require careful patient instruction and preparation for safe use. Recent surgery or a prolonged illness can temporarily affect a patient's mobility and necessitate special precautions to prevent falls or injuries. Nurses must assess a patient's risk for injury with a view toward maintaining independence and fostering self-esteem while providing a safe and predictable environment.

 THINK back to Bessie Washington, the 77-year-old woman with a cerebrovascular accident (stroke) who lives alone in a small apartment and requires a walker to ambulate. To ensure that the patient remains safe, the nurse needs to assess the patient's home environment closely for hazards. This is especially important for Bessie based on her statement that she almost fell recently. ●

PROMOTING HEALTH 26-1

SAFETY IN THE COMMUNITY

Use the assessment checklist to determine how well you are meeting your needs for maintaining personal safety as you assist with health care delivery in the community. Then develop a prescription for self-care by choosing appropriate behaviors from the list of suggestions.

Assessment Checklist

☐ almost always ☐ sometimes ☐ almost never

☐ ☐ ☐   1. I wear a badge or clothing that identifies me as a health care worker.

☐ ☐ ☐   2. I dress in an unobtrusive, professional manner.

☐ ☐ ☐   3. I keep my car in good working order.

☐ ☐ ☐   4. I am aware of neighborhoods where personal safety and security may be a problem.

☐ ☐ ☐   5. I confirm directions to the patient's residence before the visit.

☐ ☐ ☐   6. I enter patients' homes only when invited in by a responsible adult.

Self-Care Behaviors

1. Call patients to schedule visits for an agreeable time.
2. Carry a map of the communities you plan to visit.
3. Avoid isolated areas.
4. Request that pets be secured before your visit.
5. Do not carry money, credit cards, or handbag on your person. If necessary, lock them in your trunk.
6. Avoid wearing expensive jewelry.
7. Carry a cell phone.
8. Request escort services as appropriate or make joint visits.
9. Keep your car locked when driving and when parked.
10. Make sure agency is aware of time/location of scheduled visits.

Sensory Perception

Alterations in sensory perception can have a devastating effect on safety. Any impairment in sight, hearing, smell, taste, or touch can reduce a person's sensitivity to the environment. Visual changes may cause a person to stumble, lose one's balance, and fall. A patient with a hearing deficit may not be able to hear safety alarms, automobile horns, or sirens and may not hear health care instructions. A patient with a reduced ability to distinguish odors may fail to detect leaking gas or smoke. A patient with a loss of taste may have unsafe eating habits or may eat tainted food. A patient whose tactile sense is impaired may not perceive temperature extremes that are a threat to safety.

Knowledge

An awareness of safety and security precautions is crucial for promoting and maintaining wellness throughout the lifespan. Patients need instructions, for example, to adhere to a medical regimen or to follow safety precautions when oxygen is in use. They require a certain amount of knowledge to manage new equipment and unfamiliar procedures. Nursing assessment includes identifying and recognizing potentially threatening circumstances caused by a lack of knowledge regarding safety and security precautions. Patient teaching about safety is crucial. Recommendations for specific safety and security precautions are included throughout this chapter.

 RECALL Juanita Flores, the young mother of a 1-year-old who fell from a cot. The nurse's knowledge of potential threats to safety for infants, in conjunction with providing anticipatory guidance to the mother about safety issues for infants, would be essential to prevent future potential injury. ●

Ability to Communicate

The ability to communicate is basic to many safety practices. The nurse must assess any factor that influences the patient's ability to receive and send messages. Fatigue, stress, medication, aphasia, and language barriers are examples of factors that can affect personal communication and prevent the patient from accurately perceiving events. For example, a medication side effect of drowsiness may interfere with a health teaching session between the nurse and the patient taking this drug. A valid assessment by the nurse not only identifies the patient's level of understanding, but also facilitates a positive communication experience.

Physical Health State

Anything that affects the patient's health state potentially can affect the safety of the environment. When a person is chronically ill or in a weakened state, the focus of health care includes preventing accidents as well as promoting wellness and restoring the person to a healthy state. The nurse caring for a patient who is recovering from a stroke (also referred to as brain attack), for example, identifies the patient's neuromuscular impairment, pays particular attention to health teaching concerning the person's ability to maintain a sense of balance, and carefully assists the patient with ambulation to prevent falls. Many patients who fall have a primary or secondary diagnosis of cardiovascular disease, such as a stroke. Prevention of complications and return to the optimal level of functioning require attention to safety and become primary concerns in a rehabilitation program. The nurse strives to maximize the patient's potential by considering safety factors in all phases of the illness and recovery experience.

 CONSIDER Bessie Washington, the woman who is now at home after having a stroke. The nurse would incorporate knowledge of safety factors along with knowledge of Bessie's mobility limitations to develop a plan of care that maximizes her potential while maintaining her safety. ●

Psychosocial Health State

Stressful situations tend to narrow a person's attention span and make the individual more prone to accidents. Stress may occur over a long period, but the effects tend to be more devastating in the person's later years, when there is typically less adaptive and coping capacity. Depression may result in confusion and disorientation, accompanied by reduced awareness or concern about environmental hazards. Social isolation or lack of social contact may lead to a reduced level of concentration, errors in judgment, and a diminished awareness of external stimuli.

THE NURSING PROCESS FOR MAINTAINING SAFETY

Assessing

When performing a safety assessment, the nurse focuses on three categories: the person, the environment, and specific risk factors.

Assessing the Person

Assessment of the person consists of a nursing history and a physical examination.

NURSING HISTORY

Be alert to any history of falls or accidents, because a person with a history of falling is likely to fall again. Note any assistive devices that the patient uses (e.g., a cane or walker). Be alert to any history of drug or alcohol abuse. Family members and significant others are often valuable resources. Knowledge of family support systems and the home environment is crucial for the nurse to plan protective health measures. The initial assessment performed by the nurse upon admission to a health care facility summarizes all of this information (refer to Nursing History in Chapter 11).

Some people seem more likely than others to have accidents. Some children, for example, are involved in multiple mishaps resulting in fractured bones or minor injuries requiring surgical repair. Adults at any age may also have this tendency. Experts disagree about the cause of accident-prone behavior, but most agree that a patient with a history of accidents is likely to have another one.

PHYSICAL EXAMINATION

Assess the patient's mobility status, ability to communicate, level of awareness or orientation, and sensory perception in the physical examination. Early identification of any potential safety hazards is essential. Recognize any manifestations that suggest domestic violence or neglect. Chapters 3 and 18 discuss families experiencing violence, neglect, or abuse.

Assessing the Environment

Assessment of the environment requires the same attention to safety. Risks in the home, community, and health care agency may cause injury.

Environmental safety hazards can result in falls, fires, poisoning, suffocation, and accidents involving motor vehicles, equipment, and procedures. Nursing assessment includes identifying people at risk and recognizing unsafe situations. This requires knowledge of the factors that influence safety and predispose people to accidents. Recognizing these factors helps the nurse develop an individualized plan of care and nursing interventions for protecting the patient. Assessment includes an awareness of risk factors in both the home and the health care agency, with the focus on the patient's developmental level and health status.

As student nurses become increasingly involved in community and home care settings, they need also to assess their own environmental safety when visiting unfamiliar areas.

Performing a Specific Risk Factor Assessment

Be aware of those patients who are most at risk for injury as well as specific hazards. The following are common safety risks that nurses should assess.

FALLS

Falls can occur at any age, but they are the leading cause of injury fatality among adults older than 65 years of age (Jorgensen, 2011). Falls are the most common reason for admissions to hospitals for injuries in older adults. A large portion of health care for the older adult is used to care for fall-related injuries. Medicare costs for the treatment of falls in this population continue to climb and are expected to rise to $54.9 billion by 2020 (Centers for Disease Control and Prevention [CDC], 2012c). Falls occur in community settings, as well as in acute and long-term care facilities. Nearly one-third of older adults fall at home each year, and the most common injuries that result from a fall include hip or other fractures, head trauma, or soft-tissue injury (Ponce, 2012). Many falls at home go unreported because they do not cause injuries

requiring medical attention. However, injuries from falls may also go unreported because older adults fear activity restrictions, loss of independence, or placement in a long-term care facility. The fear of falling can also cause anxiety and panic, which may make an older adult more vulnerable to a fall.

Assessment of the risk for falling includes the use of nursing history and physical examination. The nursing history and physical examination include inquiring about, and inspecting for, factors that contribute to falls and an understanding of the types of or reasons for falls. Falls can be categorized as either *accidental* (clutter or a spill cause a person to trip), *an anticipated physiologic fall* (a direct consequence of gait imbalances, effects of medication, or dementia), *unanticipated physiologic falls* (caused by unknown or unexpected medical issues such as a stroke or seizure), or *intentional falls* (occur when patients act out behaviorally with intent to fall; Quigley & Goff, 2011). Some of these falls are preventable and nursing assessment can determine the optimal interventions to promote patient safety.

A person is considered at high risk for a fall if he or she has any of the following characteristics:

- Age older than 65 years
- Documented history of falls
- Impaired vision or sense of balance
- Altered gait or posture
- A medication regimen that includes diuretics, tranquilizers, sedatives, hypnotics, or analgesics
- Postural hypotension
- Slowed reaction time
- Confusion or disorientation
- Impaired mobility
- Weakness and physical frailty
- Unfamiliar environment

Falls in the older adult can be prevented if they can be predicted. Therefore, continuous surveillance for environmental hazards is crucial in the health care facility and the home environment and of patients who are at risk for falls. Family members are an invaluable resource in assessing a patient's risk for a fall. They can provide information regarding periods of weakness, confusion/disorientation, and a history of unreported falls.

 RECALL Bessie Washington, the older adult woman described at the beginning of the chapter. Based on the assessment of the patient, the nurse would identify Bessie's risk for falls as high. It would be crucial to incorporate this information into her plan of care to ensure her safety. ●

Most health care agencies have fall-prevention programs. One research study used a fall prevention "tool kit" to significantly reduce the rate of falls in four urban hospitals (Dykes et al., 2010). For this research intervention, nurses provided the risk-assessment data and an electronic program provided patient-specific fall prevention interventions, educational handouts, and alerts for placement over the patient's bed. Nurses are responsible for identifying patients who are at high risk for falls, documenting pertinent assessments on the chart, and planning appropriate interventions to ensure their safety. Just as pain is now regarded as the fifth vital sign, some health care experts suggest that fall risk assessment should be considered the sixth vital sign (Younce, Hinton, Haynes, & Berg, 2011). A nurse whose behavior is reasonable and prudent and similar to the behavior that would be expected of another nurse in similar circumstances is unlikely to be found liable if a patient falls, even if an injury results. Checklists for preventing falls at home and in health care facilities appear in Box 26-1 on page 694. See the accompanying PICO in Practice box.

Older adults are not the only population at high risk for falling; in the United States, many children visit hospital emergency departments as a result of falls. More than 200,000 children ages 14 and younger suffer fall injuries; almost half of these injuries are severe, resulting in fractures, concussions, or internal injuries (CDC, 2012e). Climbing equipment on public playgrounds and swings on home playgrounds are responsible for the majority of pediatric fall injuries. Specific interventions to diminish this fall risk for children are discussed later in this chapter.

FIRES

Of all fire deaths in the United States, 85% occur in the home (CDC, 2011a). Many home fires are started because someone was smoking in bed or fell asleep while smoking on a sofa or chair. Kitchen stoves, candles, and electric heaters are other causes of home fires. Faulty wiring and unsafe electrical equipment cause fires in homes and health care facilities. Most fatal home fires occur while people are sleeping, and most people who die in house fires die of smoke inhalation rather than burns.

The risk for home fires can be determined by assessing the knowledge of family members and the presence of functioning smoke detectors. More than one-third of home fire deaths occur in a home without a smoke detector (CDC, 2011a).

Ask people with limited financial resources about how they heat their house because the electricity or gas may have been turned off and space or kerosene heaters, wood stoves, or a fireplace may be the sole source of heat. Box 26-1 (on page 694) lists important fire safety issues as well as other safety issues that should be addressed when assessing for risk factors in the home.

Fire prevention and emergency response programs in health care facilities are sometimes viewed by staff as time-consuming or unnecessary exercises, but nurses must be prepared at all times to protect patients from injury. Hospitals are required by law to establish safety boards and to inspect the facility regularly for possible hazards. Equipment must be checked periodically, and escape routes must be kept open. Nurses, as part of their daily care procedures, must be aware of their agency's policies, review equipment and its proper functioning, and assess when and how often drills are performed.

PICO IN PRACTICE

ASKING CLINICAL QUESTIONS

Scenario: You are a faith community nurse employed by a rural Christian parish. Many members of your congregation are retired, older adults living in the homes where they had raised their children. You have noted over the past several months that several older adult parishioners fell at home, necessitating hospitalization. Some of these parishioners had significant injuries, including hip fractures. You decide to implement an intervention aimed at reducing the risk of falls among your older adult parishioners. A member of your congregation is a tai chi instructor, and offers to run classes in the parish hall three times weekly for a nominal charge. Your pastor wonders whether developing and distributing an educational brochure that highlights methods aimed at preventing falls might be a more effective use of limited parish funds.

- POPULATION: Community-dwelling older adults
- INTERVENTION: Group tai chi classes
- COMPARISON: Educational brochures
- OUTCOME: Rate of falls at home

PICO Question: Are group tai chi classes more effective at reducing the rate of falls than distributing educational brochures about fall prevention among community-dwelling older adults?

Finding: From the Cochrane Collaboration: Gillespie, L. D., Robertson, M. C., Gillespie, W. J., Sherrington, C., Gates, S., Clemson, L. M., et al. (2013). Interventions for preventing falls in older people living in the community. *Cochrane Database of Systematic Reviews*, 9, CD007146.

Group tai chi exercise programs effectively reduce the rate of falls among community dwelling older adults. It is uncertain whether or not providing older adults living in the community only educational materials on fall prevention reduces the rate of falls.

Strength of Evidence: Level I

Recommendation: You recommend to your pastor that the limited funds available to institute a fall-prevention program for older adult parishioners be spent on tai chi classes. If additional funds become available, then developing and distributing educational brochures on fall prevention may be a reasonable supplemental intervention.

BOX 26-1 **HOME SAFETY CHECKLIST**

Fire and Burn Safety

❑ Have a list of emergency phone numbers posted near the phone.

❑ Install smoke detectors in each room (or at a minimum, on each floor).

❑ Replace smoke detector batteries when you reset your clock.

❑ Have a fire extinguisher available on each floor, and know how to use it.

❑ Practice a fire escape plan with your family.

❑ Teach all family members to stop, drop, and roll if clothing catches on fire.

❑ Keep matches and lighters out of reach of children.

❑ Keep lighted candles out of children's reach.

❑ Buy flame-resistant children's clothing, particularly sleepwear.

❑ Keep bedroom doors closed while sleeping (use monitor to listen for a child).

❑ Have ashtrays readily available if there is a smoker in the house.

❑ Enforce a strict "no smoking in bed" policy.

❑ After a party, check wastebaskets, ashtrays, furniture, and carpets for carelessly discarded cigarettes.

❑ Turn off a kerosene heater when no one is in the room and at bedtime.

❑ Operate your fireplace or wood-burning stove safely (flue open, fire screen covering the opening, annual chimney cleaning, proper disposal of ashes).

❑ Prevent trash or paint-saturated rags from accumulating in your garage.

❑ Store oily rags, gasoline, or other flammables away from heating sources or open flames, such as the pilot light of the water heater.

❑ Cook on back burners, and turn pot handles toward the back of the stove.

❑ Keep hot dishes away from the edges of tables and counters.

❑ Set water heater at a safe temperature (below 120°F).

❑ Check bath water temperature with the back of your wrist before placing a child in bath.

❑ Use sunscreen and protective clothing to minimize exposure to the sun and prevent sunburn.

Electrical Safety

❑ Maintain electrical cords in good condition.

❑ Protect unused electric outlets with safety covers.

❑ Use the proper replacement for a blown fuse.

❑ Keep an electric space heater away from curtains and flammable material.

❑ Turn off appliances before going to bed or leaving the house.

❑ Hire a professional to do electrical repairs.

❑ Never overload wall outlets or extension cords.

❑ Unplug appliances that are not in use.

❑ Do not permit children to use the microwave.

Preventing Poisoning

❑ Keep the phone number for the local poison control center next to the phone.

❑ Color-code medication bottles for those who are visually impaired.

❑ Syrup of ipecac is no longer recommended if poisoning should occur. Immediately contact the Poison Control Center (1-800-222-1222).

❑ Store all medicines in child-resistant containers in a locked medicine cabinet.

❑ Destroy old medicines (flush down the toilet).

❑ Keep all poisonous plants out of a child's reach.

❑ Avoid eating any fresh or prepared foods that look or smell spoiled.

❑ Store cleaning products, insecticides, and corrosives safely out of a child's reach.

❑ Avoid mixing caustic products with any other household product (dangerous chemical reactions may occur).

❑ Keep shampoos and cosmetics in a safe place.

❑ Use safety latches on cabinets.

❑ Store alcoholic beverages out of a child's reach.

❑ Check that paint or finish on furniture and toys is nontoxic.

❑ Install a carbon monoxide detector in your home.

❑ Have your furnace professionally inspected each year.

❑ Keep vents and chimneys clear of debris, and have them checked seasonally.

❑ Don't operate cars, motorized equipment, or charcoal or gas grills in enclosed spaces.

Preventing Falls and Other Injuries

❑ Keep stairways clear and uncluttered.

❑ Maintain walkways, stairs, and railings in good repair.

❑ Keep stairs, hallways, outside walkways, and working areas well lit.

❑ Install safety gates at tops and bottoms of stairways.

❑ Paint the bottom step of the stairs a different color.

❑ Apply nonslip adhesive strips to the bottom surface of the tub or shower.

❑ Have a raised toilet seat with support arms available if necessary.

❑ Provide grab bars next to the toilet and in the tub or shower area.

❑ Use sturdy chairs that have armrests.

❑ Eliminate scatter rugs, or secure them with adhesive strips on the underside.

❑ Use a handheld device, such as pincers, when reaching for inaccessible items.

❑ Buckle a child into an approved automobile safety seat even when making short trips.

Firearm Safety

❑ Keep guns and ammunition stored separately and locked up.

❑ Install trigger locks on all guns.

❑ Make certain that the key to the locked gun storage area is not available to a child or young person.

❑ Discuss the risk for injury from guns with your children.

❑ Instruct your child never to touch a gun or remain in a friend's house where a gun is accessible.

Preventing Asphyxiation or Choking

❑ Keep plastic bags out of a child's reach.

❑ Check that crib slats are no more than 2⅜ inches apart.

❑ Ensure that the mattress fits the sides of the crib snugly.

❑ Remove soft pillows or thick blankets from your infant's crib.

❑ Never place an infant on a waterbed to sleep.

❑ Cut food into small pieces before giving it to a young child.

❑ Supervise young children when eating and drinking.

❑ Avoid giving peanuts, hard candy, or other small treats to a young child.

❑ Keep small objects, such as jewelry, buttons, and safety pins, out of a child's reach.

❑ Use toys appropriate for the child's age.

❑ Always watch a child who is in the tub.

❑ Cover wading pools and sandboxes when not in use.

❑ Check that nearby swimming pools are enclosed with a fence that your child cannot easily climb over.

❑ Keep pool rescue equipment nearby.

❑ Supervise your child closely when near water.

❑ Know how to perform cardiopulmonary resuscitation and the Heimlich maneuver.

Table 26-1   COMMON AGENTS IN CHILDHOOD POISONING

POISONOUS AGENT	SOURCE	COMMON CLINICAL MANIFESTATIONS	TREATMENT
Acetaminophen	Products containing acet-aminophen (Tylenol)	Anorexia, nausea, vomiting, and liver toxicity	In the emergency department (ED), activated charcoal or acetylcyste-ine either orally or via NG tube
Hydrocarbons	Gasoline Kerosene Furniture polish Lamp oil	Gagging, coughing, choking, dys-pnea, grunting, nausea, chills, fever, lethargy	*Never induce vomiting!* Contact physician or poison control center (PCC)
Caustics	Oven cleaner Drain openers Toilet bowl cleaners Battery contents Rust removers Hair perms	Burning pain in mouth and throat, drooling, edema of lips; oral, esophageal, gastric burns; vom-iting, hemoptysis	*Never induce vomiting!* Never attempt to neutralize the caustic. Dilute with milk or water. Contact physician or PCC
Iron	Vitamin preparations (partic-ularly pregnancy vitamins)	Nausea, vomiting, diarrhea, abdominal pain, melena, hematemesis, lethargy, coma	Contact PCC. In ED, stomach lavage (may remove unabsorbed pills); possible use of cathartic. If dose is toxic, use chelating agent.
Lead	Paint chips Paint dust Fumes from burning or swal-lowed batteries	May be asymptomatic, anorexia, abdominal pain, anemia, lead encephalitis, neurobehavioral deficits	Chelation therapy and monitoring of lead levels
Insecticides	Insecticide sprays	Nausea, vomiting, diarrhea, excessive salivation, confusion, depressed reflexes, seizures	Activated charcoal if swallowed. If clothing is contaminated, wash skin and hair. IV atropine and a cholinesterase reactivator possible to ease symptoms.

Adapted from Pillitteri, A. (2010). *Maternal and child health nursing* (6th ed.). Philadelphia: Wolters Kluwer Health/Lippincott Williams & Wilkins.

POISONING

Although the death rate from childhood poisoning has fallen drastically in the past 30 years, accidental poisoning from ingestion of medications is now responsible for more than half of the childhood poisoning deaths (Safe Kids Worldwide, 2012). According to the latest government statistics, over 300 children in the United States are treated daily in an emergency department due to poisonings (CDC, 2012g). Causes of unintentional poisoning in children are listed in Table 26-1. Analgesics, antihistamines, and sedatives are the drugs most often implicated in poisoning deaths in young children (Safe Kids Worldwide, 2012). Factors that put children most at risk for exposure to toxic substances include unsafe storage in the home, spending time in environments other than the home, lack of attention on the part of the caregiver, the rise in multigenerational families that give children an opportunity to access grandparents' medications, and the presence of multiple pharmaceuticals and vitamins and dietary supplements in the home (Safe Kids Worldwide, 2012). In 2011, U.S. poison control centers reported approximately 2.3 million calls related to poisons or possible poisons. Nearly 76% of these incident reports involved unintentional poison exposure (National Capital Poison Center, 2014).

Consider the person's developmental stage when making a safety assessment. Younger children are more apt to ingest household chemicals, whereas older children may swallow medicines in a suicide attempt. Preschoolers are also at risk for ingestion of lead-containing substances in the home. Adolescents and young adults who experiment with drugs may experience accidental poisoning and death. The ready availability of inhalants on store shelves and in the home may provide the opportunity for children to sniff or "huff" these dangerous substances. An older person may inadvertently take an overdose of a medication because of confusion or forgetfulness. Poor vision is also a factor in accidental poisoning in older adults.

 RECALL Kara Greenwood, the adolescent asking for information about adolescent dangers. An important area to include in the discussion would be drug experimentation. ●

Most exposures to toxic fumes occur in the home. Poisoning may result from improper mixing of household substances, prolonged use of strong cleaning products, or malfunctioning household appliances (gas, oil, and kerosene heaters) that can release carbon monoxide. Carbon monoxide (CO) is a colorless, odorless, tasteless, and nonirritating gas, which makes it especially dangerous. Exposure can result in mild symptoms or progress to a life-threatening problem or long-term effects. Carbon monoxide toxicity can cause severe organ damage in a very short period of time and is the third most common cause of death from toxicity in the United States (Laing, 2010).

Poison control centers provide checklists for "poison-proofing" a home and provide lists of toxic household items. Such lists are helpful when assessing and teaching the family about poisonous materials (see Box 26-1, p. 694).

SUFFOCATION AND CHOKING

Suffocation, or **asphyxiation**, may occur at any age, but the incidence is greater in children. In suffocation, air does not reach the lungs and breathing stops. Common causes of suffocation are drowning, choking on a foreign substance inhaled into the trachea, and gas or smoke poisoning. An infant may suffocate when a pillow or a piece of plastic inadvertently covers the nose and mouth. Infants are most at risk of suffocation when they are sleeping (CDC, 2012h). A young child may be strangled accidentally by the shoulder harness of a seat belt or become trapped while playing in a discarded refrigerator and suffocate.

Drowning is a form of suffocation. It is the leading cause of injury death for children ages 1 to 4 (CDC, 2012f). Most drowning deaths in young children occur because of inadequate adult supervision of a child in or near a bathtub or pool, even a small wading pool. Older children are more likely to drown while swimming or boating.

Educating the public about the causes of suffocation can save many lives. Assessing the knowledge level of people, especially parents, is vital. Nurses need to be alert to hazards that might cause a child to asphyxiate or choke (see Box 26-1, p. 694).

FIREARM INJURIES

Preventing injuries caused by firearms has become a major concern for health care professionals. Intentional injuries caused by firearms are a leading cause of mortality in children. Some people believe that keeping a gun in the home provides protection for family and property. However, when a gun is available it is more likely that the owner or a family member, rather than an intruder, will suffer a fatal injury. The presence of a gun in the home is a huge risk factor. If not stored properly, guns can be extremely dangerous. Young children are curious and like to explore their surroundings—when they encounter a loaded gun, the outcome is often tragic. Also, having a gun in the house increases the risk for domestic homicide threefold.

Emergency medical care for gunshot victims has a huge impact on health care systems, with treatment costs averaging up to $4 billion annually (Narang et al., 2010). Recent mass shootings, gang violence incidents, activities related to drug procurement, interpersonal disagreements, and activities associated with law enforcement are examples of potential risks for injuries and fatalities associated with firearms. Gun ownership is a sensitive issue, thus nurses need to approach this topic in a nonjudgmental manner with the focus on injury prevention. The intent is to inform families about the risks of firearm injury and discuss appropriate safety measures (see Box 26-1, p. 694).

Diagnosing

Unsafe situations and patients at risk are reflected in the nursing diagnosis and plan of care. The statement of the patient's actual or potential health status must be followed by the appropriate contributing factors or risk factors to individualize the nursing plan of care. Nursing diagnoses involving safety risks may include the following:

- Risk for Injury related to lack of awareness of environmental hazards; visual or auditory sensory deficits; history of falling; unsteady gait; substance abuse; refusal to use seat belt or child safety seat; effects of medication; age greater than 65 years; generalized weakness; biological, chemical, or nuclear exposure
- Risk for Poisoning related to impaired vision; medications stored in unlocked medicine cabinet that is accessible to a child; presence of poisonous plants; excess alcohol intake; use of illicit drugs; knowledge deficit; chemical contamination of food and water
- Risk for Suffocation related to a plastic bag that is accessible to a young child; child left unattended in bathtub; smoking in bed; placing an infant prone in a water bed; lack of safety precautions (door left on discarded refrigerator); unfamiliarity with fire prevention guidelines; household gas leaks
- Risk for Disuse Syndrome related to use of physical restraints
- Risk for Contamination related to chemical contamination of food or water, exposure to bioterrorism, exposure to radiation, flaking or peeling paint in presence of young children, playing in outdoor areas where environmental contaminants are used, smoking

Outcome Identification and Planning

Many accidental injuries and deaths are preventable. Consider the various factors and the environment that affect the patient's safety and formulate expected outcomes uniquely suited to each situation and circumstance. Nursing interventions focus on meeting these safety needs. Some expected outcomes for patients that promote safety and prevent injury are as follows.

The patient will:

- Identify unsafe situations in his or her environment
- Identify potential hazards in his or her environment
- Demonstrate safety measures to prevent falls and other accidents
- Establish safety priorities with family members or significant others
- Demonstrate familiarity with his or her environment
- Identify resources for safety information
- Remain free of injury during hospitalization

EXAMPLES OF NURSING INTERVENTIONS AND NURSING OUTCOMES CLASSIFICATIONS (NIC/NOC)

ENVIRONMENTAL MANAGEMENT: SAFETY

Nursing Interventions	Nursing Outcomes

• Identify safety hazards in the environment (i.e., physical, biological, and chemical).
• Modify the environment to minimize hazards and risks.
• Provide patient with emergency phone numbers (e.g., police, local health department, poison control center).
• Initiate and/or conduct screening programs for environmental hazards (e.g., lead and radon).
• Educate high-risk individuals and groups about environmental hazards.
	• Safe Home Environment
	  • Space to move safely in dwelling
	  • Carbon monoxide detector maintenance
	  • Smoke detector maintenance
	  • Safe storage of medications
	  • Safe storage of firearms
	  • Correction of lead hazard risks
	  • Arrangement of furniture to reduce fall risks

Adapted from Bulechek, G., Butcher, H. Dochterman, J., & Wagner, C. (2013). *Nursing interventions classification (NIC)* (6th ed., p. 179). St. Louis: Elsevier/Mosby. A full listing of nursing activities for each nursing intervention can be found in this book; and Moorhead, S., Johnson, M., Maas, M., & Swanson, E. (2013). *Nursing outcomes classification (NOC)* (5th ed., pp. 460–461). St. Louis: Elsevier/Mosby. A full listing of indicators for each nursing outcome can be found in this book.

See additional examples of nursing outcomes and interventions in the Examples of Nursing Interventions and Nursing Outcomes Classifications (NIC/NOC) display.

Implementing

Patient safety is integral to the nursing plan of care. It is important to intervene in order to control or modify the patient's environment. Safety recommendations in the following sections apply to health agency settings, the home, and the community. Nursing interventions are designed for each developmental level as well as for specific hazards in the environment. Adults who are developmentally disabled or who are experiencing dementia or delirium frequently need the same safety measures as those for children. Injury control includes preventing injuries, providing acute care for injured patients, and rehabilitation services. Most importantly, injury prevention allows for the reduction of injuries through eliminating risky events, measuring the consequences of these events, and reducing the severity of injuries. There are many strategies for preventing injury. Interventions that include modification of the environment and education for individuals at risk have proved effective. Laws or regulations, such as those imposed by OSHA, also help to modify at-risk behavior.

Teaching to Promote Safety

PREVENTING ACCIDENTS

Teaching is an important intervention for accident prevention and health promotion. Many teaching opportunities concerning safety measures arise while the nurse performs regular patient care, and many resources are available to supplement health teaching (Fig. 26-1 on page 698). Careful assessment, diagnosis, and planning prepare nurses to use these opportunities wisely.

Assessment data and statistical information often prove helpful to health care personnel who are developing a safety program for patients at risk. Safety education classes, in addition to situational health teaching, can be worthwhile for hospitalized patients and their family members. Studies have demonstrated that early assessment of vulnerable patients and preventive education programs can decrease the incidence of falls.

A school nurse has many opportunities and a ready audience for health teaching about safety, including screening programs (e.g., vision and hearing), fire prevention sessions, drug and alcohol prevention programs, firearm safety, and classes on various accident prevention techniques. Managing minor accidents at school often provides an opportunity for additional preventive teaching. School nurses also interact with parents. In this setting, formal or informal health teaching can occur, which should include encouragement to do the following:

• Monitor the child's use of the Internet.
• Get involved in school activities and ask pertinent questions.
• Volunteer for safety committees that include staff and parents.
• Ensure that the school's emergency preparedness plan is current.

ADDRESSING DEVELOPMENTAL CONSIDERATIONS

Teaching Tips 26-1 (on page 699) lists common types of safety risks according to developmental age, along with sample teaching tips to discuss with parents and in the school. The following discussions of developmental stages are also applicable to teaching.

Neonate and Infant. Safety considerations begin with an awareness of behaviors that may harm the developing fetus. Newborns of mothers who smoke have a lower birth weight. Excessive alcohol consumption and use of

All-purpose fire
extinguishers
for the home

Toddler gates at
stairs and doors

Outlet covers
protect curious
tots from
electrical shock

Carbon monoxide detectors for the home
(Photo courtesy of First Alert.)

Car seats for infants
and children

FIGURE 26-1. The nurse's responsibilities in home safety are primarily that of education and counseling, including providing information about home safety devices and sources for additional information.

drugs may cause adverse effects that are readily apparent at birth. Reinforce a pregnant woman's knowledge of the risks associated with excess alcohol consumption, smoking, drug use, and exposure to other dangers in the environment (see Teaching Tips 26-1). It is also important to stress the importance of regular doctor visits and the use of prenatal vitamins.

The nurse has many opportunities to educate parents about safety and accident prevention for infants. Young infants' lack of mobility limits opportunities for hazardous activity, but minimal safeguards are vital to prevent accidents. Safe care includes never leaving the infant

unattended, using crib rails, and monitoring the setting for objects that the infant could place in the mouth and swallow. As the child becomes more active, parents and caregivers must be alert to hazards that a curious, mobile child may encounter. All items within reach must be carefully inspected and, if dangerous, kept in a safe place, out of the child's reach. Because infants frequently climb or pull up on objects, hot liquids and sharp instruments must be placed out of their reach. Also, remind parents that items that are small enough to fit through a standard toilet paper tube represent a potential choking hazard for young children.

TEACHING TIPS 26-1

PREVENTING ACCIDENTS AND PROMOTING SAFETY AT VARYING DEVELOPMENTAL STAGES

Developmental Stage/ Safety Risks	Teaching Tip	Why This Is Important
Fetus Abnormal growth and development	• Abstain from alcohol and caffeine while pregnant. • Stop smoking or reduce the number of cigarettes smoked per day. • Avoid all drugs, including OTC drugs, unless prescribed by a physician, midwife, or other licensed independent practitioner. • Avoid exposure to pesticides and certain environmental chemicals. • Avoid exposure to radiation.	Any factors, chemical or physical, can adversely affect the fertilized ovum, embryo, and developing fetus. A fetus is extremely vulnerable to environmental hazards.
Neonate (first 28 days of life) Infection Falls SIDS	• Wash hands frequently. • Never leave infant unsupervised on a raised surface without side rails. • Use appropriate infant car seat that is secured in the back seat facing the rear of the car. • Handle infant securely while supporting the head. • Place infant on back to sleep.	Physical care for the newborn includes maintaining a patent airway, protecting the baby from infection and injury, and providing optimal nutrition.
Infant Falls Injuries from toys Burns Suffocation or drowning Inhalation or ingestion of foreign bodies	• Supervise child closely to prevent injury. • Select toys appropriate for developmental level. • Use appropriate safety equipment in the home (e.g., locks for cabinets, gates, electrical outlet covers). • Never leave child alone in the bathtub. • Childproof the entire house.	Infants progress from rolling over to sitting, crawling, and pulling up to stand. They are very curious and will explore everything in their environment that they can.
Toddler Falls Cuts from sharp objects Burns Suffocation or drowning Inhalation or ingestion of foreign bodies/poisons	• Have poison control center phone number in readily accessible location. • Use appropriate car seat for toddler. • Supervise child closely to prevent injury. • Childproof house to ensure that poisonous products, drugs, and small objects are out of toddler's reach. • Never leave child alone and unsupervised outside. • Keep all hot items on stove out of child's reach.	Toddlers accomplish a wide variety of developmental tasks and progress to walking and talking. They become more independent and continue to explore their environment.
Preschooler Falls Cuts Burns Drowning Inhalation or ingestion Guns and weapons	• Teach child to wear proper safety equipment when riding bicycles or scooters. • Ensure that playing areas are safe. • Begin to teach safety measures to child. • Do not leave child alone in the bathtub or near water. • Practice emergency evacuation measures. • Teach about fire safety.	Though more independent, preschoolers still have an immature understanding of dangerous behavior. They may strive to imitate adults and thus attempt dangerous behavior.
School-aged child Burns Drowning Broken bones Concussions (TBI) Inhalation or ingestion Guns and weapons Substance abuse	• Teach accident prevention at school and home. • Teach child to wear safety equipment when playing sports. • Reinforce teaching about symptoms that require immediate medical attention. • Continue immunizations as scheduled. • Provide drug, alcohol, and sexuality education. • Reinforce use of seat belts and pedestrian safety.	School-aged children have developed more refined muscular coordination, but increasing involvement in sports and play activities increases their risk for injury. TBI can cause disruption in brain function and death. Cognitive maturity improves their ability to understand safety instructions.

(continued)

TEACHING TIPS 26-1 *continued*

PREVENTING ACCIDENTS AND PROMOTING SAFETY AT VARYING DEVELOPMENTAL STAGES

Developmental Stage/ Safety Risks	Teaching Tip	Why This Is Important
Adolescent Motor vehicle accidents Drowning Guns and weapons Inhalation and ingestion	• Teach responsibilities of new freedoms that accompany being a teenager. • Enroll teen in safety courses (driver education, water safety, emergency care measures). • Emphasize gun safety. • Get physical examination before participating in sports. • Make time to listen to and talk with your adolescent (helps with stress reduction). • Follow healthy lifestyle (nutrition, rest, etc.). • Teach about sexuality, sexually transmitted infections, and birth control. • Encourage child to report any sexual harassment or abuse of any kind.	Adolescence is a critical period in growth and development. The adolescent needs increasing freedom and responsibility to prepare for adulthood. During this time, the mind has a great ability to acquire and use knowledge. The teen's peer group is a greater influence than parents during this stage.
Adult Stress Domestic violence Motor vehicle accidents Industrial accidents Drug and alcohol abuse	• Practice stress reduction techniques (e.g., meditation, exercise). • Enroll in a defensive driving course. • Evaluate the workplace for safety hazards and utilize safety equipment as prescribed. • Practice moderation when consuming alcohol. • Avoid use of illegal drugs. • Provide options and referrals to domestic violence victims.	As people progress through the adult years, visible signs of aging become apparent. Lifestyle behaviors and situational or family crises can also impact an adult's overall health and cause stress. Preventive health practices help adults improve the quality and duration of life.
Older Adult Falls Motor vehicle accidents Elder abuse Sensorimotor changes Fires	• Identify safety hazards in the environment. • Modify the environment as necessary. • Attend defensive driving courses or courses designed for elderly drivers. • Encourage regular vision and hearing tests. • If prescribed, ensure that eyeglasses and hearing aids are available and functioning. • Wear appropriate footwear. • Have operational smoke detectors in place. • Objectively document and report any signs of neglect and abuse.	Accidental injuries occur more frequently in older adults because of decreased sensory abilities, slower reflexes and reaction times, changes in hearing and vision, and loss of strength and mobility. Collaboration between family and health care providers can ensure a safe, comfortable environment and promote healthy aging.

All 50 states mandate the use of infant car seats and carriers when transporting a child in a motor vehicle. According to the CDC, nearly 40% of all children who ride with an unbelted driver are not secured with child safety seats or seat belts (CDC, 2012b). The American Academy of Pediatrics (AAP) now recommends that infants and toddlers up to 2 years of age (or up to the maximum height and weight for the seat) remain in a rear-facing safety seat. This position provides more support for the head, neck, and spine should a crash occur (AAP, 2012). The high force of sudden air bag inflation can cause injury to an infant in a safety seat or a child in the front seat. One recent study found that 72% of parents in the 3,500 instances in which car and booster seats were observed used car seats incorrectly, increasing a child's risk of injury should a crash occur (CDC, 2012b). Most parents do not secure the car seat tightly enough with the seat belt or fail to tighten the car seat's harness straps. These seemingly simple omissions can lead to tragic consequences. (See Teaching Tips 26-1 for additional safety counseling measures that focus on health teaching for this developmental level.)

Toddler and Preschooler. To prevent accidental injury and death in toddlers and preschoolers, parents need to childproof the home environment. Play areas should allow for exploration but still provide for safety. Vigilant supervision by parents and guardians should anticipate hazards in the environment and protect the child with precautionary devices. Childproofing products are available that help parents and children recognize dangerous items in the home and prevent injury.

RECALL Juanita Flores, the mother of the child who fell off a cot. As part of the plan of care, review safe infant care with Juanita and provide anticipatory guidance related to toddler safety in preparation for the child's discharge home. ●

Ingestion of poisons or medications is a major threat for preschoolers. Their overconfidence and initiative also make them more likely to dart into the street while chasing a ball, climb into a discarded refrigerator, or play with matches. In addition, any child who is older than 2 years or more than the maximum height and weight listed on the safety seat should be placed in a forward-facing safety seat in the back seat of the vehicle. A safety concern exists regarding overweight children fitting properly into a safety seat. Several manufacturers of car seats have introduced car safety seats with higher weight and height limits in response to this challenge (AAP, 2011).

Protecting a child also includes being alert to manifestations that indicate child maltreatment or abuse (Box 26-2). Each year, in the United States, 3.3 million reports of child abuse are filed and five children die every day from child abuse. Of these children, 80% are under the age of four (Childhelp, 2012). Abuse can be physical, sexual, or emotional and may also be a result of neglect. All 50 states have laws that require health care personnel to report suspected child abuse. Contact The National Child Abuse Hotline at 1-800-422-4453. (See Teaching Tips 26-1 for health teaching topics that help safeguard toddlers and preschoolers.)

School-Aged Child. Although school-aged children are increasingly independent, they still need help avoiding activities that are potentially dangerous. Accidents continue to be a leading cause of death. The nurse should counsel parents of school-aged children about specific interventions for safety at home, at school, and in the neighborhood.

All school-aged children need to be secured in safety seats, belt-positioning booster seats, or shoulder lap belts for their size. The National Highway Traffic Safety Administration recommends booster seats for children until they are 4′9″ tall and weigh between 80 and 100 pounds. Use the Safety Belt Fit Test to determine when a child may safely use a seat belt without a booster (Box 26-3). All children 12 years of age and younger should ride in the back seat, whenever possible, to eliminate the risk of injury from airbag deployment (National Highway Traffic Safety Administration [NHTSA], 2010). If no other arrangement is possible and an older child must ride in the front seat, move the vehicle seat as far back as possible away from the air bag and restrain the child properly based on the child's size.

Each year, a significant number of children younger than 10 years are injured in *bicycle accidents.* Many of these injuries involve the head or face. The protective effect of bicycle helmets among children is well documented. Studies indicate that legislation and injury prevention strategies have had a positive impact on increasing helmet use and decreasing the number and severity of bicycle

---

BOX 26-2   MANIFESTATIONS OF CHILD MALTREATMENT

The four common types of child abuse or maltreatment include:

Physical Abuse

Unexplained or repeated injuries resulting from physical force.

Manifestations include bruises, fractures (arms, legs, facial, ribs), burns, bite marks, head injuries and any other indications of force.

Sexual Abuse

Engaging a child in sexual acts including fondling, rape, and exposing a child to other sexual activities.

Can be manifested by vaginal discharge, urinary tract infection, difficulty walking or sitting, sexually transmitted infections, and genital pain.

Emotional Abuse

Behaviors that harm a child's self-worth or emotional well-being.

Manifestations can include extremes in behavior, sleep problems, headaches or stomachaches, avoiding activities.

Neglect

Failure to meet a child's basic needs including housing, food, clothing, education, and access to medical care.

Adapted from Centers for Disease Control and Prevention (CDC). (2010). *Understanding child maltreatment: Fact sheet.* Available at http://www.cdc.gov/violenceprevention/pdf/CM-FactSheet-a.pdf

---

BOX 26-3   SAFETY BELT FIT TEST

If a child meets all of the following criteria, the child may sit in the back seat of a vehicle with a lap and shoulder belt in place:

- Have the child sit in the back seat with the entire back against the vehicle's seat back. If the child's knees bend at the edge of the seat, go on with the test.
- Buckle the seat belt. If it stays low on the hips and is not resting on the soft part of the stomach, go on with the test.
- Check the shoulder belt. If it lays on the collarbone and shoulder, go on with the test.
- If the child is able to maintain the correct seating position with the shoulder belt on the shoulder and the lap belt low across the hips, then the child has passed the seat belt fit test.

Failure to meet these criteria at any point requires that the child continue using a booster seat. Retest once each month.

Adapted from Safe Kids Worldwide. (2014). Seat belt safety for big kids. Available at http://www.safekids.org/tip/seat-belt-safety-big-kids

accidents that result in a head injury in this very vulnerable population. However, their use is far from universal. Because of their multiple experiences with children and parents, nurses—whether in the emergency department or a well-child setting—have many opportunities for health teaching related to bicycle safety and helmet use. Points to include in any teaching session include the following:

- Children should wear helmets at all times when riding a bicycle.
- Young children who are secured in a child seat as a passenger on a bicycle should also wear a properly sized helmet.
- The helmet should rest flat on the top of the child's head (approximately 1″ above the eyebrows) and fit snugly.
- The chinstrap on the helmet should be adjusted so that it fits securely. If you can slide two fingers under the strap, the helmet is too loose.
- Any helmet that is involved or damaged in a crash should be discarded and replaced.
- Parents are effective role models for their children when they also wear helmets while riding a bicycle.

Sports or recreation-related activities can result in traumatic brain injury (TBI). A TBI usually results from a blow, bump, or jolt to the head that causes disruption in brain function (Tavernero & Solheim, 2012). *Concussion* is a milder form of TBI that is usually sports related. The direct blow to the head causes the brain to accelerate into the skull and then return and bounce off the opposite side of the skull. The brain can also rotate inside the skull, resulting in further damage. In the United States, approximately 3.8 million concussions are reported each year, but this number does not take into account whether loss of consciousness (LOC) occurs. Given the criteria of LOC, 300,000 concussions are reported annually but LOC occurs less than 10% of the time (Goldsmith, 2011). Nurses in a variety of settings need to be alert for indications of concussion. The common manifestations can be subtle, but parents, teachers, and nurses need to be aware of the following descriptions of symptoms by category that may require a 911 call and immediate emergency department attention:

- Physical: headache, vomiting, problems with balance, fatigue, dazed or stunned appearance
- Cognitive: mentally foggy, difficulty concentrating and remembering, confusion, forgets recent activities
- Emotional: irritability, nervousness, very emotional behavior
- Sleep: drowsiness, difficulty falling asleep, sleeping more or less than usual

Evaluation immediately following a concussion includes assessment of airway, breathing, and circulation (ABCs) and any indication of a cervical spine injury (Goldsmith, 2011). Some assessment tools are available for use and can be administered quickly. Treatment for an uncomplicated concussion includes physical and cognitive rest

until a licensed physician medically clears the athlete to return to activity. Cognitive rest entails avoidance of reading, watching TV, and playing games of any kind. A Sports Concussion Assessment Tool (SCAT) is available on thePoint.

The possibility of *child abduction* also needs to be addressed with parents and kids for this age group. Abduction occurs for a number of reasons and is a tragedy that devastates parents, families, and communities. Strangers, family members, friends, or neighbors may kidnap children. Some children suffer sexual assault or are murdered by their captors. Adults who prey on children often take advantage of the innocent and trusting nature of children to persuade the child to accompany them.

Children, even the very young, need basic instructions on how to recognize and respond to a potentially dangerous situation. Health teaching should also emphasize the need for parents to be alert and vigilant at all times regarding the whereabouts of their children.

Teach parents and caregivers about the Amber Alert System, which can be activated when a child is missing and believed to be kidnapped. This critical response program uses the resources of law enforcement and the media to notify the public about an abduction. Identifying information is broadcast via radio, television, and highway bulletin boards. The Amber Alert is a powerful tool that helps recover kidnapped children and return them to their families.

Adolescent. Much of the adolescent's time is spent away from home, with his or her peer group. Adolescents are particularly at risk for *motor vehicle accidents* because they spend so much time in automobiles and are prone to distracted driving and driving under the influence of substances. The CDC (2012j) lists motor vehicle accidents as the number-one cause of death for adolescents. Although the number of teenagers who drink and drive decreased by 54% between 1991 and 2011, 85% of teenagers who reported drinking and driving admitted to binge drinking before driving (CDC, 2012i). The definition of binge drinking is having five or more alcoholic drinks within a short period of time.

Alcohol use among teenagers is more common than that of tobacco or illicit drugs; each year, underage drinking claims the lives of approximately 5,000 people under the age of 21 (USDHHS, 2011). Almost 2,000 of these deaths occur from motor vehicle accidents. When young people drink alcohol, they are more likely to consume alcoholic drinks in significant number (i.e., binge drinking). Enforcement of zero tolerance laws regarding drinking age and driving while under the influence of alcohol, prevention programs in schools, and family efforts to influence whether their children consume alcohol are all significant factors aimed at preventing underage drinking.

Distracted driving is a troubling trend for all age groups, but particularly for adolescents who comprise the largest percentage of distracted drivers. In addition to talking on a cell phone or texting while driving, talking to other passengers, eating, performing grooming activities, changing music, or reading directions all cause drivers to take their eyes off the road and lose concentration on driving. According to Tumolo (2012), texting while driving "takes your eyes off the road an average of 4.6 seconds—at 55 mph, that is equivalent to driving the length of an entire football field blind." In their various roles, nurses have the potential to educate teenagers about this very dangerous risk to themselves and others.

Nurses and parents should collaborate to reinforce safety behaviors in adolescents. Minimum legal drinking ages, zero tolerance laws, the increased involvement of parents, and graduated driver licensing systems are all considered factors in keeping adolescents from the perils of driving and drinking. Education to prevent motor vehicle accidents should focus on safe driving skills, the importance of wearing a seat belt, limited nighttime driving, obeying speed limits, never using a cell phone or texting while driving, and limiting the number of other teenagers in the car (CDC, 2012i). In addition, teaching should include discussions about drug and alcohol use.

Substance abuse is a significant concern in the adolescent population. Teenagers abuse legally available drugs such as prescription medications and over-the-counter (OTC) cough, cold, sleep, and diet medications. They also abuse illegal substances such as marijuana, stimulants including cocaine and methamphetamine, heroin, opiates, and designer drugs (Ecstasy). Synthetic marijuana is an emerging public health concern because it is widely available and difficult to detect with current drug screens. The concern is that this substance is wrongly viewed as a safe alternative to marijuana and is growing in popularity in the teenage population. The synthetic stimulant known as "bath salts" has recently been declared a controlled substance. It is a powder that can be smoked, snorted, injected, or ingested and has an effect similar to amphetamines or cocaine (Lowry, 2011). Users of bath salts present to the emergency department with severe anxiety and agitation, bizarre behavior, and hallucinations (McGraw, 2012). Presently, there is no antidote available for this substance and treatment is supportive. The National Institute on Drug Abuse (NIDA) reports that marijuana use among teenagers has been on the increase and the abuse of prescription medication and OTC drugs has remained at a high level (NIDA, 2012). Abuse of these legal drugs can also have serious consequences, progressing from mild effects on health to addiction and death. Warning signs of alcohol and drug abuse during adolescence include physical fatigue, personality change, poor judgment, sudden mood changes, withdrawal from the family, a variety of school-related issues (negative attitude, drop in grades, failure), and social problems. Parents need to focus on open communication with their teenagers, role model–appropriate behavior, and seek appropriate help and guidance once a problem with alcohol or drug abuse is recognized.

Tobacco is an additional health problem for teenagers. Approximately one in five (20%) high school students reported using some type of tobacco product and electronic cigarette use doubled among middle and high school students from 2011 to 2012 (CDC, 2012l; CDC, 2014). Federal law mandates a minimum age of 18 years to purchase tobacco products and bans billboard advertising within 1,000 feet of schools and playgrounds. Teenagers and younger children are influenced to use tobacco products via advertisements, TV, and movies.

Educational programs and information can play a role in delaying or preventing smoking among young adults but concerned, involved parents have significant influence on their child's decision to smoke. Conversations regarding the risks of smoking can begin as early as 5 to 6 years of age because many children start using tobacco products at 11 years of age and may be addicted by age 14 (American Cancer Society [ACS], 2010).

Body piercing has become increasingly popular with adolescents and young adults. Common sites for piercing include the ears, nose, eyebrows, lips, tongue, nipples, navel, and genitals. It is a quick procedure that does not require anesthesia, but the risk for infection, tissue trauma, and transmission of hepatitis B, hepatitis C, and HIV is real.

Tattoos have also become increasingly popular. Tattoos are permanent markings on skin surfaces viewed as a form of body art. They carry similar risks as body piercings do. To prevent the spread of viruses and bacteria from one surface to another, the tattooist should wear disposable gloves and change them when necessary, wash hands often, disinfect surfaces between procedures, clean reusable tools before sterilization, and use disposable supplies when possible (Mayo Clinic, 2012). Meticulous post-piercing and tattoo care reduce the risk for developing an infection. Nurses need to be informed about the health risks in order to be effective and well-informed health educators.

There are significant security issues related to adolescents and the *use of guns*. Homicide rates for youths using firearms are higher than any other age group. The most recent statistics indicate that youths between 10 and 19 years of age committed almost 1,500 suicides using firearms (Kegler, Annest, Kresnow, & Mercy, 2011). Adolescents need encouragement and education about ways to solve arguments without guns and violence, and guidance and direction for developing a healthful lifestyle while coping with the stresses of daily living.

 THINK back to Kara Greenwood, the adolescent who is to present a discussion on adolescent dangers. Numerous issues face adolescents today; providing safety information is crucial to help adolescents make mature decisions about health hazards they are likely to encounter. ●

The use of the *Internet* has grown, particularly among teenagers. This has prompted legitimate safety concerns by parents. Certain people take advantage of the vulnerability of young children and teenagers by stalking them online and exploiting them sexually. Most research confirms that the Internet provides easy access for offenders to meet a teenager or younger child to engage in sexual abuse, pornography, or prostitution (Dowdell, Burgess, & Flores, 2011). Meeting someone with whom the person has communicated online poses the greatest safety risk for children. Safety guidelines for parents include addressing the following with their children:

- Discuss the dangers associated with the Internet with children. Review the family rules for online activity.
- Keep identifying information private (e.g., full name, address, telephone number). Children need to be reminded that anything posted on the Internet is available to the public at large. Use a screen name that does not contain any identifying information. Parents have the right to have an online site delete any personal information it has about their child.
- Investigate filtering software or methods of blocking out objectionable information.
- Be aware of the sites and services that your children access when online. Parents should be aware of their children's user names and passwords and maintain access to their e-mails. Also maintain "friend" status on your child's Facebook account.
- Avoid public chat rooms and forums. Computer sex offenders often use chat rooms to contact potential victims.
- Never allow a child to arrange a meeting alone with someone the child has met online. Parents should be involved if a meeting is planned and accompany their child.
- Never respond to e-mails or messages that are suggestive, obscene, threatening, or inappropriate in any way. If a parent becomes aware of the transmission or viewing of child pornography while online, the parent should report this immediately to the local FBI office and the CyberTipline at the National Center for Missing and Exploited Children (1-800-843-5678).
- Emphasize that a good amount of what is said or read online may not be true.
- Monitor and set rules regarding the amount of time that children spend on the computer. Children are at the greatest risk when they are online in evening hours. Hours spent online late at night may indicate a potential problem.
- Be alert for downloaded files with suffixes that indicate images or pictures (e.g., .jpg, .gif, .bmp, .tif, or .pcx).
- Consider setting up the computer in a central location in the house, rather than in a child's bedroom.

According to the American Academy of Child and Adolescent Psychiatry, as many as 50% of children are bullied during their school years. Some experts believe that cyber bullying is more dangerous and damaging to children than bullying that occurs in the schoolyard (Puliti, 2011). Children who are bullied have a greater risk for depression and anxiety and are more likely to consider thoughts about suicide. Often, academic efforts decline and bullied children are more likely to have assorted health complaints. People who bully may have a history of abusive behavior as well as substance abuse issues. Cyber bullying can take the form of cruel text messages, using Internet chat rooms, and sending rumors via e-mails or social websites with the purpose of causing embarrassment (Puliti, 2011).

Unfortunately, there are real dangers associated with online communication. Parents need to have serious discussions about them with their children. (See Teaching Tips 26-1, pp. 699–700 for additional safety topics.)

Adult. Young and middle-aged adults need to be reminded about the effects of stress on their lifestyle and health. Coping with the demands of raising a family and succeeding in a career may lead to unsafe health habits and a reliance on drugs or alcohol.

Domestic violence is widespread in the United States. Studies indicate that each year, more than 12 million adult men and women in the United States are victims of **intimate partner violence (IPV)**, which is domestic violence or battering between two people in a close relationship (CDC, 2012k). These statistics include incidents of rape, physical violence, and stalking by an intimate partner. According to the National Center for Injury Prevention and Control, IPV includes physical violence, sexual violence, threats of physical or sexual violence, and emotional abuse (CDC, 2012k). Many men who batter their spouses also batter their children. Recent evidence suggests a relationship between childhood sexual abuse and certain physical symptoms in adulthood, such as gastrointestinal symptoms, eating disorders, and substance abuse. The nurse is often the initial health care provider in contact with an abused child or a battered woman or man. Prompt recognition of the potential or actual threat to safety is crucial, and the nursing assessment may play a vital role in identifying a harmful environment. The nurse may be involved directly in health education and counseling measures or may suggest other resources to the family as additional support for safety and well-being and to interrupt the cycle of violence.

It is not always easy to confirm that a person has sustained injuries as a result of domestic abuse. Most victims of IPV are reluctant to admit any abuse and may even deny that it has occurred (Gerlock, Grimesey, Pisciotta, & Harel, 2011). Some studies have suggested that routine screening can prove to be effective, but most experts agree that asking simple, specific questions in a private setting can also prove to be helpful. Box 26-4 is an example of an assessment tool that the nurse can use to identify victims of domestic violence.

It is vital that the caregiver follow the facility's protocol for addressing IPV. This will most likely include careful assessment of the victim's situation, the opportunity to

Box 26-4   ABUSE ASSESSMENT SCREEN

1. WITHIN THE LAST YEAR, have you been hit, slapped, kicked, or otherwise physically   YES   NO
   hurt by someone?
   If YES, by whom? _____
   Total number of times _____

2. SINCE YOU'VE BEEN PREGNANT, have you been hit, slapped, kicked, or otherwise   YES   NO
   physically hurt by someone?
   If YES, by whom? _____
   Total number of times _____

MARK THE AREA OF INJURY ON THE BODY MAP. SCORE EACH INCIDENT   SCORE
ACCORDING TO THE FOLLOWING SCALE:

1 = Threats of abuse including use of a weapon.
2 = Slapping, pushing: no injuries and/or lasting pain
3 = Punching, kicking, bruises, cuts and/or continuing pain
4 = Beating up, severe contusions, burns, broken bones
5 = Head injury, internal injury, permanent injury
6 = Use of weapon; wound from weapon

If any of the descriptions for the higher number apply, use the higher number.

3. WITHIN THE LAST YEAR, has anyone forced you to have sexual activities?   YES   NO

   If YES, who? _____
   Total number of times _____

Developed by the Nursing Research Consortium on Violence and Abuse. Readers are encouraged to reproduce and use this assessment tool.

speak with a trained victim advocate, information about safety options, and respect for the victim's right to self-determination without judging (Gerlock et al., 2011).

Even if an abuse victim is not able or willing to take action when the question of domestic violence is addressed, information about making a safety plan is vital. These are critical steps that will provide a safety lifeline once the decision is made to break the cycle of violence. If in immediate danger, the abuse victim should call the police. Additional resources include the National Domestic Violence Hotline (1-800-799-SAFE), which will provide contact information regarding local domestic violence shelters and other resources.

A safety plan should include arrangements for a sudden departure and a list of actions and items the abuse victim will need to take during the escape. A safety plan is an initial step in the right direction toward a healthier, violence-free life. The following is a sample list:

- A place to stay if a sudden departure from home is necessary
- An escape route
- A person you can call in a crisis
- A signal to a neighbor that indicates you need immediate help
- Keys for the house and car
- Secure copies of important papers (e.g., birth certificates, Social Security cards, marriage and driver's licenses, passports, car title, insurance information, school and health records, bank account information)
- A packed bag with clothes, money, medications and prescriptions, credit cards

- Additional addresses and phone numbers for family, friends, a victim advocate, community resources, and legal assistance (U.S. Department of Veteran Affairs, 2011).

Older Adult. Most accidents that involve older adults are preventable. Falls and motor vehicle accidents are significant hazards for this age group. Visual changes, slowed reaction time, and impaired thinking due to mental illness are realistic concerns that affect the older driver. Some become overly cautious, whereas others are prone to careless behavior. Teach the following interventions to help older adults drive safely: maintain the automobile in optimal driving condition, schedule regular eye examinations, wear corrective lenses when necessary, and keep noise from the radio and other equipment to a minimum. Some states require additional testing for older adults before they can renew their driver's license.

Fires also are a significant hazard for older adults. Factors such as confusion, forgetfulness, and diminished visual and olfactory senses place them at greater risk for burn injuries. Health teaching should include safety precautions if the older adult smokes in the home. Because it may be difficult to distinguish the intensity of temperatures, heating devices often used by older adults need to be carefully monitored and regulated. Smoke detectors indicate the presence of a fire that may not be recognized by an older person with a diminished sense of smell.

Accidental overdosing on medications is also a safety risk, possibly related to poor eyesight or confusion. Special devices such as medication trays can be prefilled to help prevent older patients from taking additional doses. (See Teaching Tips 26-1, pp. 699–700 for additional health teaching interventions directed at helping to promote a safe environment for older patients at home.)

In the United States, 5 million older Americans are abused yearly; almost 40% of elder abuse occurs with people over the age of 80 (Richards, 2011). Given the expanding number of people over 65 years of age, the incidence of maltreatment in this vulnerable population is expected to escalate. In 90% of the reported cases, a family member is the one who abused the older adult (Stark, 2012). Sadly, the majority of abuse situations are never reported. Nurses must be alert to any indications of elder abuse, document any injuries or behaviors that suggest elder abuse, and report suspected incidents to appropriate agencies in states where it is required. It is important to observe and objectively document voice tone, interactions, and personal touch between the older adult and a caregiver, and, if abuse is suspected, speak to the older adult in a private setting away from the caregiver.

Orienting the Person to Surroundings

A person who is familiar with one's surroundings is less likely to experience an accidental injury. As part of the hospital admission routine, orient the patient to the safety features and equipment in the room. An explanation and demonstration of the adjustable bed and side rails, call system, telephone, television, and bathroom help the patient adjust to the new environment. The patient identification bracelet and a discussion of agency routine further ensure safety and assist the patient to adapt to the unfamiliar setting. Similarly, teach the importance of orienting an older person to new surroundings when the older person moves in with a family member or other caregiver.

Preventing Falls

PREVENTING FALLS IN THE HOME

Major causes of falls in the home include slippery surfaces, poor lighting, clutter, and improperly fitting clothing or slippers. Common traffic pathways in the home, the bathroom, and access areas to and from the home are hazardous areas for older adults. Measures as simple as installing hand rails in bathrooms and on stairs, ensuring good lighting, and discarding or repairing broken equipment around the home help prevent accidents (see Box 26-1, p. 694). Assessments by the nurse can play a vital role in promoting safety in the home. Home health care nurses frequently use the acronym DAME to assess the risk for falling in older adults at home. The assessment, as summarized by Kulik (2011), includes consideration of:

- **D** – Drug and alcohol use
- **A** – Age-related physiologic status
- **M** – Medical problems
- **E** – Environment

 CONSIDER Bessie Washington, the older woman who ambulates with a walker after suffering a stroke. Key to the patient's plan of care would be a thorough home safety assessment by the home care nurse. This assessment would be valuable in identifying areas that promote patient safety and hazards that need to be addressed. ●

Research appears to support the positive role that calcium supplementation and vitamin D play in promoting skeletal health and reducing fall risk for this population. Regular exercise has a positive effect on bone and muscle strength, balance, and flexibility of joints. Women who participate in a regular walking regimen plus other leisure activities are 55% less likely to suffer a hip fracture than sedentary women (Ponce, 2012). The martial art of tai chi is another exercise routine that has proved particularly effective. It involves slow, deliberate movements that can be practiced almost anywhere. Tai chi helps to prevent falls by developing balance control and stability in older adults.

PREVENTING FALLS IN THE HEALTH CARE FACILITY

As mentioned earlier, falls among older adults are the most common cause of hospital admissions for trauma. The Joint Commission requires that hospitals implement fall prevention assessments and programs. The Centers for Medicare and Medicaid Services (CMS) have identified falls as a "never event" because they are preventable and should never occur. Falls and trauma are also on the CMS list of Hospital-Acquired Conditions that result in limited reimbursement, especially those falls that result in injuries (The Joint Commission Center for Transforming Healthcare, 2012). Safety measures recommended to reduce the number of falls in acute and extended-care facilities are given in Box 26-5.

One simple evaluation tool can help identify hospitalized patients at risk for falling. According to accreditation standards, The Hendrich II Fall Risk Model, which can be administered quickly, evaluates eight independent risk factors. This tool also includes the Get Up and Go Test that measures a person's ability to rise from a seated position. Performance on each physiologic factor merits a specific score and identifies individuals most at risk for falls. View the Hendrich II Fall Risk Model on thePoint.

In response to the The Joint Commission's mandate that accredited health care organizations must reduce the risk of harm to patients resulting from falls, hospitals have implemented effective programs to safeguard their patients from falls. Examples of these improvement strategies include:

- *Fall Scene Investigations (FSI):* A collaborative effort to examine the scene where the fall occurred and explore possible causes using a documentation tool that addresses safety hazards, future prevention strategies, and lessons learned (Boothe & Harris, 2010).

BOX 26-5 NURSING INTERVENTIONS TO PREVENT FALLS IN A HEALTH CARE FACILITY

- Complete a risk assessment.
- Indicate risk for falling on patient's door and chart.
- Keep bed in low position.
- Keep wheels on bed and wheelchair locked.
- Leave call bell within patient's reach.
- Instruct patient regarding use of call bell.
- Answer call bells promptly.
- Leave a night light on.
- Eliminate all physical hazards in the room (clutter, wet areas on the floor).
- Provide nonskid footwear.

- Leave water, tissues, bedpan/urinal within patient's reach.
- Document and report any changes in patient's cognitive status to the physician and other nurses at the change of shift.
- Use alternative strategies when necessary instead of restraints.
- As a last resort, use the least restrictive restraint according to agency policy.
- If restraint is applied, assess patient at the required intervals.

- *Hourly Patient Rounding:* A proactive approach that involves hourly visits to patients during day and evening hours and 2-hour visits during the night to address patient concerns that may result in a fall (need for pain medication, position change, or a visit to the bathroom). These regularly scheduled visits reassure patients that their needs will be met in a timely manner. Some hospitals use managers or specially assigned nursing staff to conduct the rounding (Davies, 2010).
- *Root Cause Analysis (RCA):* Involves an investigation of the environment, collection of evidence regarding the contributing factors that caused the fall, and an actual drawing of the fall scene that details the patient's location, the position of the bed, and presence of any assistive devices. An interdisciplinary team then revisits the incident, looks for patterns and relationships, and reviews systems and processes with the goal of identifying patients at risk and system changes that are needed to ensure that the revised safety plan is effective (Shell, 2011).

Polypharmacy has long been listed as a risk factor but research has indicated that adverse effects related to the specific medication categories of antiepileptics and benzodiazepine drugs are more predictive of falling. A history of a previous fall has consistently been identified as a predictor of another fall. If a fall occurred as a direct result of a risk factor that has been resolved, one fall may not necessarily indicate that another fall is likely. Some

common safety devices used in health care facilities are shown in Figure 26-2.

Using Restraints in Health Care Facilities

Restraints are physical devices used to limit a patient's movement. Side rails, geriatric chairs with attached trays, and appliances tied at the wrist, ankle, or waist are types of physical restraints. Figure 26-3 (on page 708) shows examples of physical restraints that can be used for adults and children. Drugs that are used to control behavior and are not included in the person's normal medical regimen can be considered chemical restraints.

In the past, it was considered acceptable bedside care to restrain patients to protect them from harm, but recent studies have indicated that the use of restraints for this purpose is potentially dangerous. Physical restraints increase the possibility of serious injury due to a fall— they do not prevent falls. The adverse health consequences associated with restraint use actually result in the need for additional staff because the condition of residents in long-term care facilities can deteriorate when restraints are employed. Additional negative outcomes of restraint use include skin breakdown and contractures, incontinence, depression, delirium, anxiety, aspiration and respiratory difficulties, and even death.

In the late 1970s, more than 25% of U.S. residents in long-term care facilities were restrained compared to a current average of 5% (Restraint use cut in half, 2010). Older adults with dementia are most at risk of being

FIGURE 26-2. Some of the safety devices used in health care agencies and in the home to prevent falls. (**A**) Side rails on bed raised at the patient's request; the patient must be able to raise and lower the side rail without help. (**B**) Locking devices on wheeled equipment. (**C**) Nonskid slippers. *(Photos by B. Proud.)*

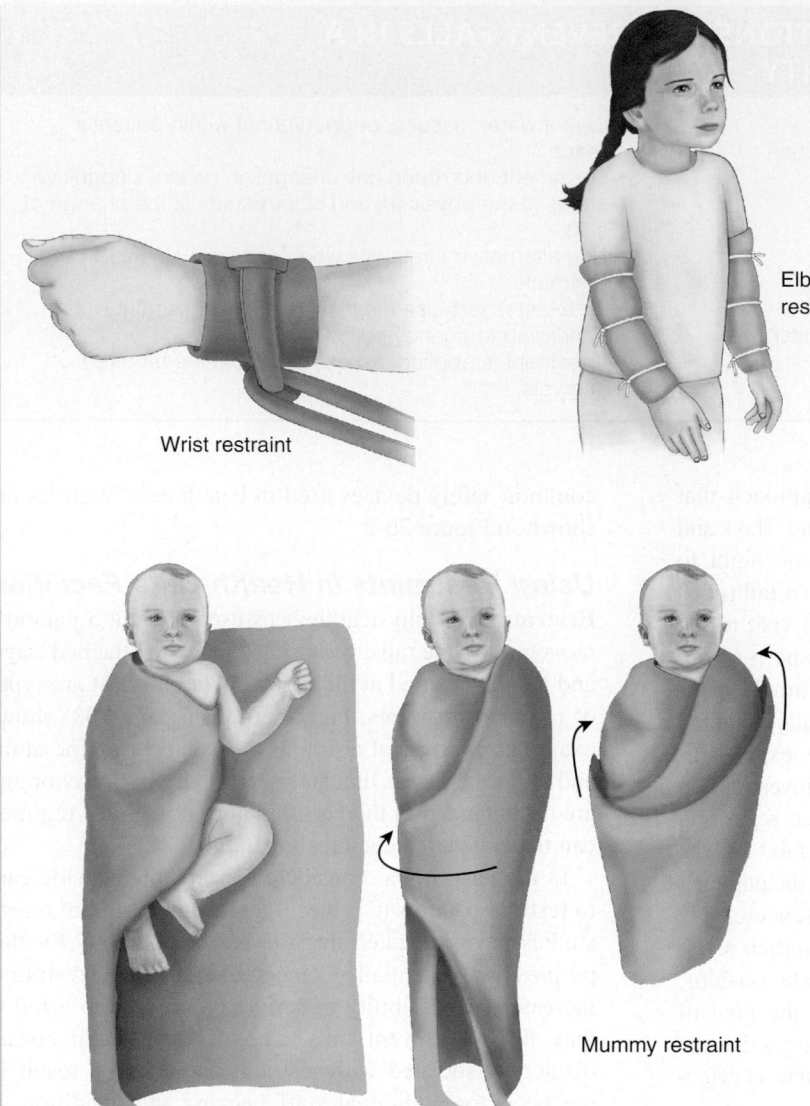

Wrist restraint

Elbow restraint

Mummy restraint

FIGURE 26-3. A variety of restraints used for adults and children. The purpose of restraints is to help prevent the patient from being harmed. Restraints should not interfere with physiologic functioning such as impairing circulation, limiting muscular activity to the point of immobilization, or interfering with respiration. Restraints that can be adjusted to the desired activity limitation are most likely to be accepted by the patient and family.

restrained except for the ICU setting, in which younger adults are restrained at approximately the same percentage as older adults. The use of restraints is definitely declining as health care providers become more educated about the risks associated with their use.

Since 1987, the federal government and accrediting agencies have worked to reduce or eliminate the use of restraints. Initial guidelines formulated by the Health Care Financing Administration as part of the 1987 Omnibus Budget Reconciliation Act encouraged the limited use of restraints in long-term settings. The current standard for long-term care facilities is to provide safe care without the use of physical or chemical restraints. Federal and state mandates, as well as The Joint Commission (TJC), recommend that acute-care agencies use restraints only as a last resort.

Federal guidelines reinforce that in all settings the primary responsibility is to protect and promote patient's rights and that restraints may only be used to protect the patient, staff, or others. They must be discontinued at the earliest possible time. Any health care facility that accepts Medicare and Medicaid reimbursement must abide by the federal guidelines for the use of restraints. In 2002, the Sentinel Event Advisory Group was formed within TJC to develop patient safety goals. These help accredited agencies address specific areas of concern related to patient safety. According to TJC, a **sentinel event** is an unexpected occurrence involving death or serious physical or psychological injury, or the risk of death or injury (TJC, 2011). These signal the need for an immediate investigation and response. The American Nurses Association (ANA) has approved a position statement defining the nurses' role in reducing restraint use in health care. Their recommendations are included in Box 26-6.

USING SIDE RAILS AS RESTRAINTS

In the past, side rails were used to provide support and aid equilibrium, but it is now recognized that they can pose serious risks for a confused or agitated patient. A 1995 FDA Safety Alert informed health care agencies

BOX 26-6 AMERICAN NURSES ASSOCIATION (ANA) BOARD OF DIRECTORS POSITION STATEMENT: REDUCTION OF PATIENT RESTRAINT AND SECLUSION IN HEALTH CARE SETTINGS

Recommendations: To ensure safe, quality care for all patients in the least restrictive environment, ANA supports nursing efforts to:

1. Educate nurses, nursing students, unlicensed personnel, other members of the interdisciplinary team, and family caregivers on the appropriate use of restraint and seclusion, and on the alternatives to these restrictive interventions;
2. Ensure sufficient nursing staff to monitor and individualize care with the goal of only using restraint when no other viable option is available;
3. Ensure policies and environment support services are in place to provide feasible alternatives to physical and chemical restraints;

4. Move progressively toward a restraint-free environment while providing a therapeutic sanctuary for all;
5. Enforce documentation requirements and education about what should be documented;
6. Explore the ethical implications of restraining patients with nursing students and discuss the need for institutional policy that clarifies when, where, and how clients are to be restrained and monitored while restrained;
7. Be aware of all implications of allowing the application of restraints in health care settings. The nurse administrator should make consultation available to nurses, including ethical consultation about decisions to restrain; and
8. Develop clear policies based on accepted national standards to guide decision-making regarding restraints.

American Nurses Association (ANA). (2011). ANA Position Statement: Reduction of Patient Restraint and Seclusion in Health Care Settings. Available at http://www.nursingworld.org/restraintposition

---

of the hazards associated with side rail use. A person of small stature has a greater risk for entrapment or injury. Death from asphyxiation has occurred when patients have become wedged between the mattress and the bed frame or side rail. Although patient entrapment is uncommon, it can be fatal. Most of the victims of side rail fatalities are frail, elderly, or confused, many with uncontrolled body movement. Most incidents of entrapment occur in a long-term care setting.

A side rail is not considered a restraint if the patient requests that it be raised to aid in getting in or out of bed. Some patients may request that side rails be used at night while they sleep so that they may feel more secure (see Fig. 26-2A). Patients requesting side rails must be able to raise and lower the side rails themselves. If a family member requests the use of side rails for a patient, it is the nurse's responsibility to review benefits and risks associated with their use and periodically evaluate the reason for their use. Side rails are not routinely recommended for all situations. It is the responsibility of health care facilities to evaluate existing bed systems for entrapment risks and investigate corrective actions that may be necessary to provide a safe environment for patients.

USING ALTERNATIVES TO RESTRAINTS

Careful nursing assessment is the key to identifying appropriate alternatives to restraint use and finding an individualized solution (Box 26-7 on page 710). Nursing interventions may be used to reduce confusion or agitation and provide a safe environment. Using a restraint on an older patient who tends to wander is unjustified because a variety of alternative options can be used to keep such patients safe. Figure 26-4 shows an example of a position-sensitive electronic device (Ambularm) that is an alternative to using restraints. A variety of electronic alarms and monitors are available for chairs, beds, and doors.

USING RESTRAINTS AS A LAST RESORT

Despite all efforts, restraints may be the only solution in some situations. The least restrictive restraint should be the first option. Restraints must never be applied for the convenience of the staff. The patient's family must be consulted and involved in the plan of care before applying restraints in a long-term care setting. They must be informed of the agency's policy regarding applying and removing restraints and may be asked to sign a release form to protect the agency from liability. Agency policy, TJC, and state and federal guidelines require an order from a physician or a licensed independent practitioner (LIP). The order should include the type of restraint, justification for the restraint, and criteria for removal. The order must never be written for PRN use.

In an emergency, the physical restraint can be applied, but an order from a physician or LIP must be obtained immediately or within a few minutes according to Joint Commission Standards. The order must state the

FIGURE 26-4. Ambularm device. *(Photo courtesy of AlertCare, Inc.)*

BOX 26-7 CHOOSING ALTERNATIVES TO RESTRAINTS

- Determine whether behavior pattern exists.
- Assess for pain and treat appropriately.
- Rule out causes for agitation. Assess respiratory status, vital signs, blood glucose level, fluid and electrolyte issues, and medications. Use standardized screening tools to evaluate change in function.
- Involve the family in patient's care.
- Ask family members or significant other to stay with the patient.
- Reduce stimulation, noise, and light.
- Distract and redirect, using a calming voice.
- Use simple, clear explanations and directions.
- Check environment for hazards.
- Use night light.
- Identify door of room (e.g., use of balloon, sign, patient's picture, ribbon).
- Use an electronic alarm system on a temporary basis (e.g., bed or position-sensitive alarms) to warn of unassisted activity.
- Allow restless patient to walk after ensuring that environment is safe.
- Use a large plant or piece of furniture as a barrier to limit wandering from designated area.
- Use low-height beds.
- Place floor mats on each side of the bed.
- Ensure the use of glasses and hearing aids, if necessary.
- Use pillows wedged against the side of the chair to keep patient positioned safely.
- Use full-length body pillows, a swimming pool noodle, or a rolled blanket to indicate the edge of the bed.
- Assist with toileting at frequent intervals.
- Arrange for a bedside commode.
- Make the environment as home-like as possible; provide familiar objects.
- Provide a warm beverage.
- Provide comfortable rocking chairs.
- Use therapeutic touch.
- Play music or video selections of the patient's choice.
- Offer diversional activities, such as games and books.
- Encourage daily exercise/provide exercise and activities or relaxation techniques.
- Consider relocation of the patient to a room closer to the nursing station.
- Conceal tubing necessary for care. Anchor tubing securely. Conceal tubing with gauze wrap; unwrap regularly to assess site for complications.
- Investigate possibility of discontinuing bothersome treatment devices (e.g., intravenous line, catheter, feeding tube).

intended duration of use. The patient must be monitored and assessed at least every hour or according to agency policy. An inpatient psychiatric patient in restraints requires continual observation, including specific assessments every 15 minutes. Documentation must reflect the date and time the restraint is applied, the type of restraint, alternatives that were attempted (including their results), and notification of the patient's family and physician. Include the frequency of assessment, your findings, regular intervals when the restraint is removed, and nursing interventions. Constant re-evaluation of the need for the restraint is vital. Chapter 7 discusses the legal issues involved when restraints are used. Student nurses, from their earliest clinical experiences, need help to identify and assess the cause of a patient's behavior and not just the behavior itself. Careful patient assessment is needed to develop creative alternative strategies. Skill 26-1 on pages 719–722 demonstrates the proper method for applying restraints should they be necessary.

 Concept Mastery Alert

Restraints may be applied without a physician's order if the situation is an emergency and the threat to safety is imminent. However, an order must be obtained immediately afterward.

Preventing Fires and Maintaining Fire Safety

Careless smoking, faulty electrical equipment, and combustion of anesthetic agents are the most common causes of hospital fires. Orientations in health care agencies emphasize fire prevention information and the agency's smoking policy. Nurses are responsible for patients' safety and need to be familiar with the agency's fire safety plan, exits, the location and operation of fire extinguishers, and any special instructions for reporting a fire.

Most hospital procedures emphasize the following priorities and recommend that staff members remember the acronym RACE as a guide:

- **R**escue anyone in immediate danger.
- **A**ctivate the fire code system and notify the appropriate person.
- **C**onfine the fire by closing doors and windows.
- **E**vacuate patients and other people to a safe area.

Type ABC fire extinguishers are the most common kind used in health care agencies. In the home setting, cigarettes, grease, and electrical problems are most often responsible for fires. Educating parents about home fire safety includes having a plan of action similar to that used in health care settings. (See Box 26-1, p. 694 for priorities and practical suggestions for fire and burn safety.)

Preventing Poisoning

Concerted efforts by people, communities, state governments, and the federal government have reduced the number of accidental deaths by poisoning. Childproof containers are primarily responsible for this reduction.

Nursing interventions involve health education aimed at preventing accidental poisoning in the home. Every household must have the telephone number of the nearest poison control center (PCC) readily available. Emphasize that parents should call the poison control center immediately, before attempting any home remedy. Parents may be instructed to bring the child immediately to an emergency facility for treatment. The focus of emergency treatment of poisoning is to stabilize vital body functions, prevent the absorption of the poison, and encourage excretion of the toxic substance.

Activated charcoal is considered the most effective agent for preventing absorption of the ingested toxin. It is not recommended for storage or use at home. Activated charcoal can be administered through a nasogastric tube in the emergency department for serious poisonings after the risks and benefits have been determined (National Capital Poison Center, 2012). Syrup of ipecac is no longer recommended because vomiting may be dangerous. A toxic substance may prove more hazardous coming up rather than when it was swallowed. Gastric lavage is no longer prescribed routinely for treatment of ingestion of a toxic substance because it may propel the poison into the small intestine, where absorption will occur. The amount of toxin removed by gastric lavage is relatively small.

Nursing education efforts can also change behaviors that place older adults at risk for medication-related poisoning. Although poisonings happen more frequently in children, poison control centers receive many calls from adults, particularly older adults, regarding accidental poisonings. Suggestions for preventing poisoning in older adults are included in the accompanying box, Focus on the Older Adult.

All health care providers should recommend that a carbon monoxide detector be installed to alert family members to toxic levels of the gas. Gas or oil companies and the local health authority can help identify and remove sources of contamination. Many states and communities now require installation of carbon monoxide detectors in residences. (See Box 26-1, p. 694 for additional tips for preventing poisoning.)

Preventing Suffocation

As a result of suffocation, unconsciousness, respiratory failure, and cardiac arrest can occur. Emergency measures must start without delay, beginning with the removal of any obstruction and administration of cardiopulmonary resuscitation. When teaching parents, the nurse should emphasize careful supervision of children and should outline specific situations that place children at risk for suffocation. Health education is a valuable preventive force (see Box 26-1, p. 694 for specific interventions.)

Preventing Injury From Firearms

Nurses are in a unique position to raise awareness and to help reduce high-risk behavior that may lead to firearm injuries and deaths. In homes, schools, and other health care settings, nurses can provide information on how parents can keep guns out of the hands of children. Parents may be unaware of how common gunshot injuries are or the dangers that can occur when a gun is accessible to children and young adults. As a prevention partner, the nurse can begin to have an impact on the epidemic of gun-related injuries and death (see Box 26-1, p. 694 for measures to prevent injury from firearms).

Preventing Equipment-Related Accidents

With the marked increase in the use of highly sophisticated electronic equipment in health care settings, health care practitioners must learn to use the equipment properly and must recognize signs of malfunctioning equipment. Suction devices with inadequate vacuum and rate regulators or infusion equipment that delivers erratic amounts of solution have resulted in equipment-related accidents. Failure to use protective belts or side rails on stretchers and to lock wheelchair wheels can result in patient injury.

FOCUS ON THE OLDER ADULT

TEACHING TIPS TO PREVENT MEDICATION-RELATED POISONING

Age Related Changes	Nursing Strategies
Confusion	• Do not hesitate to call the physician, nurse, or pharmacist with any questions. • Develop good communication with your physician, nurse, and pharmacist. • Use a medication calendar or diary to keep track of your dosing schedule. • Use a pill dispenser as a reminder tool.
Reduced vision	• Request large-print labels from your pharmacist.
Polypharmacy	• Report side effects from medications to your health care provider. • Do not share medications with others or take their pills. • When a drug is discontinued, throw away any remaining medication.
Effect of drugs in the aging body	• Keep the telephone numbers for your health care providers and the poison control center in a readily accessible place. • Do not stop taking any prescription drug or change the dose without first consulting the physician or nurse. • Avoid doubling a dose if you forget a medication. Check with the physician or nurse first. • Avoid mixing alcohol with medicines without first checking with the pharmacist.

Box 26-8 DECREASING EQUIPMENT-RELATED ACCIDENTS

- Use equipment only for the use for which it was intended.
- Do not operate equipment with which you are unfamiliar.
- Handle equipment with care to prevent damaging it.
- Use three-prong electric plugs whenever possible.
- Do not twist or bend electric cords. The wires inside the cord may break.
- Be alert to signs that indicate equipment is faulty such as breaks in electric cords, sparks, smoke, electric shocks, loose or missing parts, and unusual noises or odors. Report signs of trouble immediately.
- Make certain that electric cords are not in a position to be trapped as beds are raised or lowered. This can strip insulation covering the electric wires.
- Be alert for wet surfaces on areas where electric cords or connections are present.
- Make certain when charging defibrillator batteries that "charging" indicator light is on.
- Implement a process for reporting and addressing problems with equipment.

FIGURE 26-5. An essential nursing responsibility is checking the patient's identification bracelet before any procedure. Here, the nurse checks the patient's identification before administering medications.

Electrical equipment can present a safety hazard to both the patient and health care practitioner when safety measures are ignored. Most electrical equipment used in hospitals is equipped with three-prong plugs. The third prong, when inserted into a properly wired wall outlet, provides a ground for the piece of equipment. A **ground** is a connection from an electricity source to the earth through which electric current leakage can be harmlessly conducted. Box 26-8 lists guidelines to help reduce the number of equipment-related accidents. Hospitals and long-term care facilities are required by federal law and Food and Drug Administration (FDA) regulations to report to the FDA and the manufacturer of a device any suspected deaths or serious injuries related to use of the device (FDA, 2012).

Accidents in the home frequently result from careless use of equipment or from malfunctioning or poorly maintained equipment. Many injuries and deaths from electric shock can be prevented. Overloaded electrical circuits, faulty appliances, frayed wires, careless use of electrical equipment, and handling of electrical devices and cords with wet hands or while wearing wet shoes can result in injury or death. (See Box 26-1, p. 694 for specific guidelines to prevent electrical injury.)

Preventing Procedure-Related Accidents

The nurse must always be cautious and alert to prevent procedure-related accidents. Errors are possible when administering medications or intravenous solutions, transferring a patient, changing a dressing, or applying external heat to a patient's extremity. Therefore, nurses must follow correct procedures when administering care (see the Research in Nursing box that describes the development of a tool to simplify and standardize procedures). Safeguards to prevent errors include making sure

that the patient is identified correctly (Fig. 26-5). The nurse should use all available resources to answer any questions about correct procedure.

In an effort to promote a culture of safety, The Joint Commission publishes an annual list of National Patient Safety Goals. These are established based on sentinel events that have been reported and include the corrective actions recommended as a response to these sentinel events. Some goals are ongoing while others may get removed from the annual list once the hospitals have incorporated the recommended practices to meet a particular safety goal into their standards of operation (TJC, 2012). The goals and related requirements are specific to each accreditation program (e.g., ambulatory care, assisted living, long-term care). Accreditation by TJC requires that a health care organization provide evidence that these goals have been addressed and requirements have been met. Effective alternatives may be acceptable, depending on the services provided by the particular health care organization. National Patient Safety Goals are available on The Joint Commission Web site at http://www.jointcommission.org/standards_information/npsgs.aspx

Filing a Safety Event Report

An accident or incident that compromises safety in a health care agency requires the completion of a **safety event report**. This is a confidential document, formerly referred to as an incident report, which objectively describes the circumstances of the accident or incident. The report also details the patient's response and the examination and treatment of the patient after the incident. The nurse completes the event report immediately after the incident and is responsible for recording the circumstances and the effect on the patient in the medical record. The safety event report is not a part of the medical record and should not be mentioned in the documentation. Because laws vary in different states, nurses must know their own state law regarding safety event reports.

RESEARCH IN NURSING

BRIDGING THE GAP TO EVIDENCE-BASED PRACTICE

Developing a Tool to Reduce Errors of Omission in Pediatric Intensive Care Units

Children admitted to pediatric intensive care units (PICUs) require complex interventions and administration of multiple medications. Because of their complicated and often unstable condition, they are also particularly vulnerable to iatrogenic injuries. Research studies have indicated that, on average, patients receive approximately half of the care that is recommended for their condition. The reported international incidence of adverse events in PICUs is 2.7 to 33.4 complications or adverse events per 100 PICU days. The steps that health care providers may omit when caring for critically ill patients increase the risk for errors.

Related Research

Ullman, A., Long, D., Horn, D., Woosley, J., & Coulthard, M. (2013). The KIDS SAFE checklist for pediatric intensive care units. *American Journal of Critical Care, 22*(1), 61–69.

Checklists are often used as a valuable tool to prevent omission of vital steps in a procedure. The objective of this study was to develop an evidence-based checklist as a tool to prevent the occurrence of adverse events and improve the quality of clinical care in a pediatric intensive care environment. Mnemonic checklists are easy to remember and help simplify standard procedures or behaviors that are complex. A previous mnemonic, FASTHUG, has improved outcomes for adult ICU patients. In order to develop this checklist, researchers at Royal Children's Hospital in Brisbane,

Australia reviewed the literature to determine adverse events (preventable and nonpreventable) that occurred when children were admitted to PICUs. Following this, a multidisciplinary group of health care representatives established a list of items that were prone to errors of omission and that should be included in a PICU checklist. The resultant KIDS SAFE checklist includes 8 areas of care for PICU patients: *k*ids' developmental needs, *i*nfection, *p*rophylaxis for deep vein thrombosis, *s*edation, *s*kin integrity, *a*nalgesia, *f*amily, and *e*nteral needs. This checklist does not include all preventable adverse events in a PICU but does focus on delivering holistic care to children and quick recall of steps and events via this mnemonic device.

Relevance to Nursing Practice

Nurses are instrumental in improving patient outcomes. The QSEN initiative focuses on the development of a patient safety culture. Standardizing and simplifying procedures through the use of checklists reduces reliance on memory and minimizes the risk of harm to patients. The KIDS SAFE checklist is simple and addresses the needs of children who are critically ill. Future studies are needed to demonstrate its effectiveness in reducing errors of omission and preventable adverse events.

For additional research, visit thePoint.

All safety event reports are reviewed carefully to detect any potentially threatening situation or pattern. These reports are discussed in more detail in Chapter 7.

 RECALL Juanita Flores, the young mother whose child fell off the cot. As a result of the fall, a safety event report was completed. ●

When an incident results in a patient injury, the nurse has a responsibility to speak openly and honestly with the patient and family. The National Patient Safety Foundation (2011), in an effort to focus on safe delivery of high-quality care, has developed a framework outlining a true partnership between patients and providers. The Universal Patient Compact: Principles for Partnership (Box 26-9 on page 714) describes a patient-/family-centered process that "creates an understanding between the parties about how they will work together." The National Patient Safety Foundation's Principles for Partnership represent a concerted effort to demonstrate a health care organization's commitment to respect the rights of patients and incorporate these beliefs into their mission.

Maintaining Emergency Preparedness

Emergency preparedness has always been a concern for health care workers. Nurses, as members of emergency

response teams, need to be aware of their role when an emergency or disaster occurs. Existing community resources are usually sufficient to respond to an emergency situation, such as a multiple vehicle collision, a fire in an apartment complex involving a significant number of burn injuries, or an explosion or plane crash. Since the September 11, 2001, terrorist attacks in New York, Washington, D.C., and Pennsylvania and the subsequent anthrax attacks, attention has been focused on national security and strategies for sustaining emergency preparedness levels, as well as the need for communities to step up the level of their involvement in emergency preparedness for any disaster.

A **disaster** is broadly defined as a tragic event of great magnitude that requires the response of people outside the involved community. Disasters can be categorized as natural (e.g., massive flooding following a hurricane or an earthquake) or man-made (e.g., a toxic spill, war, or a terrorist event). In any disaster, the lives of the victims, their families, and the community and nation are affected in incalculable ways.

 THINK back to Kara Greenwood, the adolescent described in the beginning of the chapter. Her statement revealed her peer group's

BOX 26-9	THE UNIVERSAL PATIENT COMPACT™: PRINCIPLES FOR PARTNERSHIP

As your healthcare partner, we pledge to:

- Include you as a member of the team
- Treat you with respect, honesty, and compassion
- Always tell you the truth
- Include your family or advocate when you would like us to
- Hold ourselves to the highest quality and safety standards
- Be responsive and timely with our care and information to you
- Help you to set goals for your healthcare and treatment plans
- Listen to you and answer your questions
- Provide information to you in a way you can understand
- Respect your right to your own medical information
- Respect your privacy and the privacy of your medical information
- Communicate openly about benefits and risks associated with any treatments
- Provide you with information to help you make informed decisions about your care and treatment options
- Work with you, and other partners who treat you, in the coordination of your care

As a patient, I pledge to:

- Be a responsible and active member of my healthcare team
- Treat you with respect, honesty, and consideration
- Always tell you the truth
- Respect the commitment you have made to healthcare and healing
- Give you the information that you need to treat me
- Learn all that I can about my condition
- Participate in decisions about my care
- Understand my care plan to the best of my ability
- Tell you what medications I am taking
- Ask questions when I do not understand and until I do understand
- Communicate any problems I have with the plan for my care
- Tell you if something about my health changes
- Tell you if I have trouble reading
- Let you know if I have family, friends, or an advocate to help me with my healthcare

awareness of terrorism. Kara would need to obtain additional information about terrorism from community sources when preparing the discussion. ●

Based on national and world events, the efforts of government agencies, nongovernmental agencies, the private sector, communities, and people are all vital components of health and emergency response systems when a disaster occurs. In addition, accreditation bodies such as The Joint Commission have contributed to the considerable progress that hospitals have made in disaster preparedness (*Healthy People 2020,* 2012). Disaster training is more rigorous and standardized, and encompasses the entire community and its resources. These health care coalitions provide the foundation for improved response capacity.

The National Disaster Medical System (NDMS) has responsibility for the coordination of health care practitioners who supplement local disaster responses in large-scale disasters. In collaboration with USDHHS, Homeland Security, Veterans Affairs, and the Defense Department, they supply funds, equipment, training and medical and support personnel (Murray, 2012), Nurses have a critical role in caring for victims of a disaster.

The CDC is also committed to responding rapidly to mass trauma events and chemical, biological, radiologic, and nuclear agents. The CDC's Health Alert Network has upgraded the capacity of state and local health agencies to detect and communicate varying health threats (CDC, 2012d). The CDC has also collaborated with pharmaceutical companies and other partners to create quickly regional stockpiles of the drugs that would be needed to treat man-made outbreaks of disease, such as anthrax,

plague, and other diseases. It is a prescription for great danger if the United States does not continue to develop the optimal emergency preparedness capabilities that it needs to protect its communities. As we have seen with previous disasters, older Americans are particularly vulnerable. The 85-and-older population is the fastest growing segment of older adults and they are at high risk during a disaster. Deficits in strength and mobility, vision and hearing loss, multiple chronic illnesses, and possible dependence on life-saving equipment make it challenging to meet their many needs (Habel, 2012).

ADDRESSING BIOLOGICAL THREATS

Bioterrorism involves the deliberate spread of pathogenic organisms into a community to cause widespread illness, fear, and panic (CDC, 2007). The organisms used in a mass attack may not be routine, and the clinical manifestations may be vague and nonspecific. Table 26-2 outlines some of the more common biological agents, including symptoms and interventions. If an unusual number of people suddenly experience similar signs and symptoms, health care personnel should consider whether they may have been exposed to a biological agent.

Health care personnel must adhere to the Standard Precautions recommended by the CDC. For certain diseases, additional safeguards may be necessary. If a contagious disease is suspected, the patient should be isolated accordingly. Although not usually required with biological agents, decontamination may be necessary if a patient's exposure status is uncertain. The patient may need to bathe or shower with soap and place his or her clothing in sealed plastic bags.

Table 26-2 BIOLOGICAL AGENTS OF CONCERN

AGENTS	CLINICAL MANIFESTATIONS	TREATMENT/PROTECTION
Anthrax (*Bacillus anthrax*)	Symptoms variable based on form of anthrax: • Cutaneous: skin lesion with local edema that progresses, enlarges, ulcerates, and becomes necrotic • Gastrointestinal: nausea, vomiting, fever, abdominal pain, hematemesis, severe diarrhea • Inhalational: fever, fatigue, cough, dyspnea, pain; may progress to meningitis, septicemia, shock, and death	Standard precautions Decontamination possibly required for recent exposure Rapid administration of antimicrobial therapy Supportive therapy for shock, fluid volume deficit, and airway management Vaccine available; currently recommended only for high-risk populations
Plague or "black death" (*Yersinia pestis*)	Expected attack most likely airborne (inhalation of bacilli) with sudden appearance in ED of multiple patients with respiratory symptoms Symptoms similar to a severe respiratory infection Progresses rapidly to severe pneumonia, sepsis, and death	Standard precautions with droplet precautions until 48 hours after initiation of antibiotic therapy Antibiotic of choice: streptomycin (IM) or gentamicin sulfate (IM or IV). Possible use of oral antibiotics (effective when mass numbers of people are ill). Fatality rate of 100% for those not receiving treatment within 24 hours of onset of symptoms
Smallpox (*Variola major*, viral agent)	Spread via direct contact or inhalation of respiratory droplets; most likely to be spread via aerosol route Flu-like symptoms Characteristic rash that progresses to crusted scabs in 5 days, most prominent on face and extremities	Strict contact and airborne precautions for duration of illness—vaccination for those exposed No proven treatment Supportive care including possible antibiotics if secondary infections develop Use of antiviral agents under investigation Vaccine available; currently recommended only for high-risk populations
Botulism (*Clostridium botulinum*)	Possible release via airborne method, or contaminated food supplies Ocular symptoms such as blurred vision Skeletal muscle paralysis that progresses symmetrically and in a descending manner Muscle weakness that can result abruptly in respiratory failure	Standard precautions Passive immunization with botulinum antitoxin Supportive respiratory care
Tularemia (*Francisella tularensis*)	Transmission via contaminated water, food, and soil; most likely aerosolization of bacteria for use as a biological weapon Fever Nonproductive or productive cough Possible progression to respiratory failure	Standard precautions Drug therapy such as streptomycin or gentamicin sulfate Fluid and respiratory support measures Vaccine under investigation
Viral hemorrhagic fevers (e.g., Lassa, Ebola, Marburg, yellow, and dengue fevers)	Possible spread via aerosol infection Fever Myalgias Conjunctival symptoms Mild hypotension Petechial hemorrhages Progresses to shock and hemorrhage	Standard, droplet, and contact precautions for the duration of illness; additional precautions, including use of negative-pressure room, N95 or higher respirator Use of personal protective equipment (PPE) (see Chap. 26) No proven treatment other than supportive care Avoidance of aspirin or other anticlotting drugs

Adapted from: Centers for Disease Control and Prevention (CDC). (2006). General fact sheets on specific bioterrorism agents. Available at http://emergency.cdc.gov/bioterrorism/factsheets.asp

ADDRESSING CHEMICAL THREATS

The use of chemical agents as a terrorist weapon is a growing concern. **Chemical terrorism** involves the deliberate release of a chemical compound that has the potential for harming people's health (CDC, 2006). The chemical would probably be dispersed in an enclosed space, such as a subway or a closed sports arena, to cause the maximum effect. Chemical agents act rapidly, and immediate decontamination is crucial before patients are transported to a hospital. Emergency preparedness requires the swift transfer of portable decontamination units, equipment, and trained personnel to the site of the chemical attack.

Several categories of chemicals can be used as weapons of mass destruction:

- Choking/lung/pulmonary agents
- Blood agents
- Vesicants/blister Agents
- Nerve agents
- Incapacitating agents

Box 26-10 summarizes the effects of the various chemical agents.

ADDRESSING RADIATION THREATS

Nuclear terrorism involves intentional introduction of radioactive materials into the environment for the purpose of causing injury and death (CDC, 2011b). The attack might involve use of a radiation dispersion device ("dirty bomb"), a planned assault at a nuclear power station or weapons facility, or dispersal of radioactive material into the food or water supply. Even a small amount of radioactive material can have devastating effects.

Radiation burns occur as a result of exposure to a radioactive source. The severity of injury depends on a variety of factors, including the duration of the exposure and the distance between the source and the person. A higher dose increases the likelihood of developing later effects such as bone marrow depression and cancer. Lymph tissue and bone marrow are the tissues most sensitive to radiation while the skin, kidneys, intestines, and gonads are the most radiation-sensitive organs (Slepski, 2011). Although the likelihood of a nuclear attack may be small, nurses need to be well informed, familiar with their agency's emergency response plan, and prepared to deal with a nuclear emergency.

Nurses serving on a radiologic emergency response team must protect themselves and wear the necessary equipment, including a radiation detection device. They will assess patients in a radiation emergency area (REA) designated by the hospital's emergency response plan. If patients have not been decontaminated at the scene of the attack, decontamination will occur at the medical facility.

ADDRESSING CYBER TERROR

Cyber terror involves the use of high technology to disable or delete critical infrastructure data or information (Tafoya, 2011). It is a serious threat to national security and very difficult to identify a perpetrator who resides in cyberspace. The federal agencies responsible for investigating cyber terror must remain vigilant because it is difficult to predict such attacks. Authorities agree that it is not a question of if a cyber terror attack will occur, but rather when it will occur. These criminals are constantly searching for vulnerabilities and looking for opportunities to launch an attack. Intruders can break into supposedly secure systems to alter files and steal confidential information. An attack on a hospital network could potentially compromise physicians' and nurses' ability to care for patients and respond to health care emergencies. The resulting chaos could be devastating to patient safety (UC Davis Health System, 2010).

PREPARING FOR MASS TRAUMA TERRORISM

Terrorists have used bombs and other explosives in a variety of ways (e.g., roadside devices, on public transportation) to inflict mass trauma injuries and cause multiple fatalities. Proximity to the detonation determines the severity of injuries and mortality rates. Blast lung injury (BLI) has recently been recognized as a direct consequence of the blast wave from a high explosive detonation (CDC, 2012a). Once the condition is diagnosed, the patient may require complex care and should be admitted to an intensive care unit. Few emergency health care

---

BOX 26-10 CATEGORIES OF CHEMICAL AGENTS

Choking Lung/Pulmonary Agents
Examples: phosgene (CG), diphosgene (DP), chlorine (CL)
Effects: dyspnea, cough, pulmonary edema

Blood Agents
Examples: hydrogen cyanide (AC), cyanogen chloride (CK)
Effects: loss of consciousness, convulsions, respiratory arrest

Vesicants/Blister Agents
Examples: sulfur mustard (H or HD), lewisite (L)
Effects: skin erythema and blisters, eye irritation, progressively severe respiratory symptoms, damage to bone marrow

Nerve Agents
Examples: tabun (GA), sarin (GB), soman (GD)
Effects: constricted pupils, reddened eyes, loss of consciousness, convulsions, respiratory arrest

Incapacitating Agents
Examples: glycolate anticholinergic compound (BZ), Agent 15
Effects: hyperthermia, bizarre behavior, delirium

Adapted from Centers for Disease Control and Prevention (CDC). (2006). *Emergency preparedness: Chemical categories.* Available at http://emergency.cdc.gov/agent/agentlistchem-category.asp

Table 26-3 EMERGENCY PREPAREDNESS RESOURCES

ORGANIZATION	ACTIVITIES
National Disaster Medical System (NDMS) http://www.hhs.gov/aspr/opeo/ndms/index.html	Has responsibility for managing and coordinating the federal medical response to major emergencies and federally declared disasters
Federal Emergency Management Agency (FEMA) http://www.fema.gov	Works to build and support the national emergency management system
Centers for Disease Control and Prevention (CDC) http://www.cdc.gov	Acts as the lead federal agency for disease prevention and control activities; provides backup support to state and local health departments
The Joint Commission (TJC) http://www.jointcommission.org	Accredits facilities according to established safety and quality standards; revises the emergency management standards for health care facilities
American Red Cross http://www.redcross.org	Acts as the lead nongovernmental agency that provides safety information and disaster response
Department of Homeland Security http://www.dhs.gov/index.shtm	Protects the nation against further terrorist attacks and coordinates the response for future emergencies

providers in the United States have experience treating patients with explosion-related injuries.

IDENTIFYING DISASTER RESOURCES

Each health care facility should determine in advance how to deliver care should an emergency or disaster occur. This involves collaboration with internal committees and external agencies. Organizations that serve as resources for recommendations and updated information are listed in Table 26-3.

In any disaster, nurses will have multiple roles. In addition to clinical expertise, nurses may be responsible for triage, various treatments, counseling, and assistance with distribution of resources. There are many unresolved issues regarding the legal, ethical, and personal responsibilities of a nurse when a disaster occurs. There may be concerns about personal safety, legal implications, and the ethical decisions they may be called on to make in a disaster. Nurses may be less willing to respond to a crisis if their own personal disaster plan is not in place and there are concerns about family members, pets, and personal responsibilities (Smith, 2010). The ANA is partnering with government agencies, employers, and individual nurses to resolve these issues and allow nurses to respond confidently with their usual compassionate response and attitude (ANA, 2010).

Disaster preparedness is imperative at all levels. In order to reduce confusion and lessen the impact of a disaster, people need to take responsibility, include the family in all discussions, and develop a personal disaster plan. Emergency food, supplies, and medications should be assembled; a communication routine should be established, and sources for reliable information should be monitored when disaster strikes (Brewer, 2011). Multiple resources are available to assist in this preparation. They include FEMA (http://www.ready.gov/are-you-ready-guide) and the CDC (http://emergency.cdc.gov/preparedness/).

ADDRESSING PSYCHOLOGICAL ASPECTS OF DISASTERS

Disasters affect the lives of victims, family members, and health care personnel in many ways. Fear and panic can be expected, as well as anger, horror, and real and exaggerated concerns about possible future events. Nurses and other health care providers, as first responders, rescue and recovery workers, or staff at a medical facility, can help to minimize panic by addressing risks and providing careful explanations. Anxiety can be treated with reassurance. The impact of a disaster on each person varies, and it can have lingering effects. Most disaster survivors experience normal stress reactions, but some may exhibit acute stress disorder or posttraumatic stress disorders that require treatment. Emergency preparedness education and planning must also address mental health issues.

Evaluating

Evaluation is the final step of the nursing process. The accompanying concept map on page 718 illustrates the nursing process for the care of Bessie Washington. Nurses must evaluate the effectiveness of their interventions to promote environmental safety, prevent injury, and promote emergency preparedness. If the expected patient outcomes have been met and evaluative criteria have been satisfied, the patient should be able to accomplish the following:

- Correctly identify real and potential unsafe environmental situations
- Implement safety measures in the environment
- Use available resources to obtain safety information
- Incorporate accident prevention practices into activities of daily living
- Remain free of injury

Bessie Washington, age 77, has been discharged to home after sustaining a cerebral vascular accident (CVA). She is experiencing residual weakness in her right arm and leg and she has a right visual field cut that affects her ability to see things in her right field of vision. She is taking metoprolol for hypertension and an anticoagulant to prevent further CVAs. In the hospital, Ms. Washington's blood pressure was 110/60mm Hg and her heart rate was 62 beats per minute and irregular. She was discharged with a referral to visiting nurse and home physical therapy. The visiting nurse finds that she lives alone in a first floor apartment and uses a walker to ambulate. She tells the visiting nurse, "I have so much stuff crammed into this small apartment. I almost fell going from my bedroom to the kitchen." The nurse notes that Ms. Washington drags her right leg when ambulating and drifts to her weak side when sitting. When asked about activities of daily living, Ms. Washington says that she has been unable to perform chores.

Priority 1

Nursing Diagnosis: Risk for Fall related to physical disability and environmental conditions.
Supporting Data:
• Experiencing right-sided weakness
• Uses walker to ambulate
• Experiencing right visual field cut
• Takes multiple medications
• BP 110/60mm Hg; HR 62 bpm, irregular
• Lives in a cluttered environment

Priority 2

Nursing Diagnosis: Impaired Mobility related to recent CVA.
Supporting Data:
• Experiencing right-sided weakness
• Drags rt. leg when ambulating
• Uses walker to ambulate
• Drifts to weak side when sitting or ambulating

Priority 3

Nursing Diagnosis: Impaired Home Maintenance related to acute illness.
Supporting Data:
• "I almost fell going from my bedroom to the kitchen."
• Unable to perform house chores
• Lives alone in first-floor apartment
• Recent CVA

Outcome:
Patient will demonstrate safety measures to prevent falls.

Outcome:
Patient will demonstrate safe ambulation techniques, participate in physical therapy and prescribed treatment, and increase strength.

Outcome:
Patient will maintain her environment, utilize resources to assist with house chores, and incorporate adaptive strategies to assist with activities of daily living.

Nursing Interventions:
• Encourage patient to turn head from side to side to see all of environment.
• Teach patient to sit upright at first and then rise slowly to prevent orthostatic hypotension.
• Remove any throw rugs or obstacles.
• Obtain assistive equipment such as raised toilet seat, grab bars, shower chair, etc.
• Reinforce importance of having prescribed lab work to maintain therapeutic anticoagulant levels.
• Identify resources to assist in clearing cluttered environment.

Nursing Interventions:
• Assess level of mobility and strength.
• Assess patient's insight into own motor deficit.
• Reinforce proper techniques for use of walker as taught by physical therapy.
• Encourage patient to perform prescribed exercises throughout the day
• Encourage frequent rest periods.

Nursing Interventions:
• Perform home evaluation.
• Request referral to occupational therapy to assist with adaptive strategies to perform activities of daily living.
• Identify family and community resources to assist with chores around house within financial constraints.

Evaluation: Ms. Washington demonstrated proper techniques while ambulating. Her children have offered to straighten up her apartment. Throw rugs were removed. She has had her lab work drawn and her anticoagulant medication was adjusted. Continue home visits for reinforcement.

Evaluation: Ms. Washington is performing exercises as prescribed. Her strength is rated a +2 on the right side and a +4 on the left side. She does more than the prescribed exercise and needs to be reminded to rest. She is attempting to ambulate too quickly. Instructed to slow down.

Evaluation: OT is working with Ms. Washington. Adaptive strategies were devised and she has demonstrated these strategies. Church resources were identified to assist with chores during the recovery period. Continue visiting nurse to monitor home maintenance.

- - - - - **Relationship**   **Assessment**   **Nursing Diagnosis**   **Outcome Identification**   **Interventions**   **Evaluation**

Concept map displaying the nursing process for Bessie Washington.

SKILL 26-1 APPLYING AN EXTREMITY RESTRAINT

DELEGATION CONSIDERATIONS	After assessment of the patient by the RN, the application of an extremity restraint may be delegated to nursing assistive personnel (NAP) or unlicensed assistive personnel (UAP), as well as to licensed practical/vocational nurses (LPN/LVN). The decision to delegate must be based on careful analysis of the patient's needs and circumstances, as well as the qualifications of the person to whom the task is being delegated. Refer to the Delegation Guidelines in Appendix A (found on thePoint).
EQUIPMENT	• Appropriate cloth restraint for the extremity that is to be immobilized • Padding, if necessary, for bony prominences • PPE, as indicated

IMPLEMENTATION

ACTION	RATIONALE
1. Determine need for restraints. Assess the patient's physical condition, behavior, and mental status.	Restraints should be used only as a last resort when alternative measures have failed and the patient is at increased risk for harming self or others.
2. Confirm agency policy for application of restraints. **Secure an order from the primary care provider, or validate that the order has been obtained within the required time frame.**	Policy protects the patient and the nurse and specifies guidelines for application as well as type of restraint and duration. **Each order for restraint or seclusion used for the management of violent or self-destructive behavior that jeopardizes the immediate physical safety of the patient, a staff member, or others may only be renewed in accordance with the following limits for up to a total of 24 hours: (A) 4 hours for adults 18 years of age or older; (B) 2 hours for children and adolescents 9 to 17 years of age; or (C) 1 hour for children under 9 years of age. After 24 hours, before writing a new order for the use of restraint or seclusion for the management of violent or self-destructive behavior, a physician or other licensed independent practitioner who is responsible for the care of the patient must see and assess the patient (CMS, 2006).**
3. Perform hand hygiene and put on PPE, if indicated.	Hand hygiene and PPE prevent the spread of microorganisms. PPE is required based on transmission precautions.
4. Identify the patient.	Identifying the patient ensures that the right patient receives the intervention and helps prevent errors.
5. Explain the reason for restraint use to the patient and family. Clarify how care will be given and how needs will be met. Explain that restraint is a temporary measure.	Explanation to the patient and family may lessen confusion and anger and provide reassurance. A clearly stated agency policy on application of restraints should be available for the patient and family to read. In a long-term care facility, the family must give consent before a restraint is applied.
6. Include the patient's family and/or significant others in the plan of care.	This promotes continuity of care and cooperation.
7. Apply restraint according to manufacturer's directions:	Proper application prevents injury.
a. Choose the least restrictive type of device that allows the greatest possible degree of mobility.	This provides minimal restriction.
b. Pad bony prominences.	Padding helps prevent skin injury.

(continued)

SKILL 26-1 | APPLYING AN EXTREMITY RESTRAINT *continued*

ACTION	RATIONALE
c. Wrap the restraint around the extremity with the soft part in contact with the skin (Figure 1). If a hand mitt is being used, pull over the hand with the cushion to the palmar aspect of the hand (Figure 2).	This prevents excess pressure on extremity.

FIGURE 1. Wrapping the restraint around the extremity with the soft part in contact with the skin. (From Craven, C. F. & Hirnle, C. J. (2013). *Fundamentals of nursing (7th ed.)* Philadelphia: Wolters Kluwer Health/Lippincott Williams & Wilkins, p. 596, Figure 1.)

FIGURE 2. Using a hand mitt. (From Craven C. F. & Hirnle, C. J. (2013). *Fundamentals of nursing (7th ed)*. Philadelphia: Wolters Kluwer Health/Lippincott Williams & Wilkins, p. 597, Figure 4.)

ACTION	RATIONALE
8. Secure in place with the Velcro straps or other mechanism, depending on specific restraint device (Figure 3). Depending on characteristics of specific restraint, it may be necessary to tie a knot in the restraint ties, to ensure that the restraint remains secure on the extremity.	Proper application secures restraint and ensures that there is no interference with patient's circulation and potential alteration in neurovascular status.
9. **Ensure that two fingers can be inserted between the restraint and patient's extremity (Figure 4).**	Proper application ensures that nothing interferes with patient's circulation and potential alteration in neurovascular status.

FIGURE 3. Securing restraint on extremity. (From Craven, C. F., & Hirnle, C. J. (2013). *Fundamentals of nursing (7th ed.)*. Philadelphia: Wolters Kluwer Health/Lippincott Williams & Wilkins, p. 597, Figure 2.)

FIGURE 4. Ensuring that two fingers can be inserted between the restraint and the patient's wrist. (From Craven, C. F., & Hirnle, C. J. (2013). *Fundamentals of nursing (7th ed.)*. Philadelphia: Wolters Kluwer Health/Lippincott Williams & Wilkins, p. 597, Figure 3.)

ACTION

10. Maintain restrained extremity in normal anatomic position. **Use a quick-release knot to tie the restraint to the bed frame, not side rail (Figure 5).** The restraint may also be attached to a chair frame. The site should not be readily accessible to the patient.

FIGURE 5. Securing restraint to bed frame. (Reprinted with permission from Craven, C.F., & Hirnle, C. J. (2009). *Fundamentals of nursing (6th ed.).* Philadelphia: Wolters Kluwer Health/Lippincott Williams & Wilkins.)

11. Remove PPE, if used. Perform hand hygiene.

12. Assess the patient at least every hour or according to facility policy. Assessment should include the placement of the restraint, neurovascular assessment of the affected extremity, and skin integrity. In addition, assess for signs of sensory deprivation, such as increased sleeping, daydreaming, anxiety, panic, and hallucinations.

13. **Remove the restraint at least every 2 hours, or according to agency policy and patient need.** Perform range-of-motion exercises.

14. Evaluate the patient for continued need of restraint. Reapply restraint only if continued need is evident and the order is still valid.

15. Reassure the patient at regular intervals. Provide continued explanation of rationale for interventions, reorientation if necessary, and plan of care. **Keep the call bell within the patient's easy reach.**

RATIONALE

Maintaining a normal position lessens possibility of injury. A quick-release knot ensures that the restraint will not tighten when pulled and can be removed quickly in an emergency. Securing the restraint to a side rail may injure the patient when the side rail is lowered. Tying the restraint out of the patient's reach promotes security.

Removing PPE properly reduces the risk for infection transmission and contamination of other items. Hand hygiene prevents transmission of microorganisms.

Improperly applied restraints may cause skin tears, abrasions, or bruises. Decreased circulation may result in paleness, coolness, decreased sensation, tingling, numbness, or pain in extremity. Use of restraints may decrease environmental stimulation and result in sensory deprivation.

Removal allows you to assess the patient and re-evaluate need for restraint. It also allows interventions for toileting, provision of nutrition and liquids, exercise, and change of position. Exercise increases circulation in the restrained extremity.

Continued need must be documented for reapplication.

Reassurance demonstrates caring and provides an opportunity for sensory stimulation as well as ongoing assessment and evaluation. The patient can use the call bell to summon assistance quickly.

DOCUMENTATION

Guidelines

Document alternative measures attempted before applying restraint. Document patient assessment before application. Record patient and family education and understanding regarding restraint use. Document family consent, if necessary, according to facility policy. Document the reason for restraining the patient, date and time of application, type of restraint, times when removed, and result and frequency of nursing assessment.

(continued)

SKILL 26-1 APPLYING AN EXTREMITY RESTRAINT *continued*

Sample Documentation

7/10/15 0830 Patient disoriented and combative. Attempting to remove trache-ostomy and indwelling urinary catheter. Sitting at bedside, patient continued to tug at catheter and pull on tracheostomy. Family unwilling to sit with patient. Wrist restraints applied bilaterally as ordered.

—*K. Urhahn, RN*

7/10/15 1030 Patient continues to be disoriented and combative. Wrist restraints removed for 30 minutes during patient's bath; skin intact, hands warm, even skin tone, + radial pulses, + movement; passive and active range of motion completed. Wrist restraints reapplied.

—*K. Urhahn, RN*

UNEXPECTED SITUATIONS AND ASSOCIATED INTERVENTIONS	• *Patient has an IV catheter in the right wrist and is trying to remove drain from wound:* The left wrist may have a cloth restraint applied. Due to the IV in the right wrist, alternative forms of restraints should be tried, such as a cloth mitt or an elbow restraint. • *Patient cannot move left arm:* Do not apply restraint to an extremity that is immobile. If the patient cannot move the extremity, there is no need to apply a restraint. Restraint may be applied to the right arm after obtaining an order from the primary care provider.
SPECIAL CONSIDERATIONS	• Do not position the patient flat in a supine position with wrist restraints. If the patient vomits, aspiration may occur. • Check the restraint for correct size before applying. Extremity restraints are available in different sizes. If the restraint is too large, the patient may free the extremity. If the restraint is too small, circulation may be affected. • Consider keeping a pair of scissors with emergency supplies in case the restraints cannot be untied quickly.

DEVELOPING CLINICAL REASONING

1. You are the visiting nurse for a frail older patient who lives alone in her own home and prizes her independence. You assess her to be at high risk for falls because of her general weakness, the medication she takes, and a long history of indifference to safety counseling. What nursing interventions are likely to be most effective in ensuring her safety?

2. Identify the safety hazards and threats to security for which you and family members of different ages are most at risk. What anticipatory planning and teaching could be done to prevent these hazards? Note your willingness and that of your family to make the necessary changes, and identify the nursing strategies that would be most likely to secure patient cooperation in making the needed changes.

PRACTICING FOR NCLEX

1. The nurse caring for patients in a long-term care facility knows that there are factors that place certain patients at a higher risk for falls. Which patients would the nurse consider to be in this category? Select all that apply.
   a. A patient who is older than 60 years
   b. A patient who has already fallen twice
   c. A patient who is taking antibiotics
   d. A patient who experiences postural hypotension
   e. A patient who is experiencing nausea from chemotherapy
   f. A 70-year old patient who is transferred to long-term care

2. A school nurse is teaching parents about home safety and fires. What information would be accurate to include in the teaching plan? Select all that apply.
   a. 60% of U.S. fire deaths occur in the home.
   b. Most fatal fires occur when people are cooking.
   c. Most people who die in fires die of smoke inhalation.
   d. Over 1/3 of fire deaths occur in a home without a smoke detector.
   e. Fires are more likely to occur in homes without electricity or gas.
   f. More fires occur in homes occupied by single parents.

3. A nurse is assessing the following children. Which child would the nurse identify as having the greatest risk for choking and suffocating?
   a. A toddler playing with his 9-year-old brother's construction set
   b. A 4-year-old eating yogurt for lunch
   c. An infant covered with a small blanket and asleep in the crib
   d. A 3-year-old drinking a glass of juice

4. While discussing home safety with the nurse, a patient admits that she always smokes a cigarette in bed before falling asleep at night. Which nursing diagnosis would be the priority for this patient?
   a. Impaired Gas Exchange related to cigarette smoking
   b. Anxiety related to inability to stop smoking
   c. Risk for Suffocation related to unfamiliarity with fire prevention guidelines
   d. Deficient Knowledge related to lack of follow-through of recommendation to stop smoking

5. A nurse working in a busy emergency department is caring for a teenage patient who presents with a burning pain in his mouth, edema of the lips, vomiting, and hemoptysis. The teen admits that he was playing a dare game with friends and was forced to swallow a drain opener preparation. What would be the nurse's priority intervention?
   a. Induce vomiting and call the primary care provider.
   b. Perform stomach lavage and call the poison control center.
   c. Give activated charcoal orally and call the physician.
   d. Dilute the poison with milk and call the primary care provider.

6. A nurse is teaching parents in a parenting class about the use of car seats and restraints for infants and children. Which information is accurate and should be included in the teaching plan?
   a. Booster seats should be used for children until they are 4′9″ tall and weigh between 80 and 100 pounds.
   b. Most U.S. states mandate the use of infant car seats and carriers when transporting a child in a motor vehicle.
   c. Infants and toddlers up to 2 years of age (or up to the maximum height and weight for the seat) should be in a front-facing safety seat.
   d. Children older than 6 years may be restrained using a car seat belt in the back seat.

7. A nurse working with adolescents in a juvenile detention center teaches parents about behaviors that place adolescents at high risk for injury. Which statements accurately describe these risks? Select all that apply.
   a. Each year, underage drinking claims the lives of approximately 5,000 individuals under the age of 21.
   b. Approximately one in three high school students reported using some type of tobacco product.
   c. The CDC (2012i) lists motor vehicle accidents as the number-one cause of death for adolescents.
   d. Marijuana use among teenagers has been on the increase and the abuse of prescription medication and OTC drugs has remained at a high level.
   e. Homicide rates for adolescents are high, and youths aged 10–19 years committed almost 500 suicides using firearms.
   f. As many as 30% of children are bullied during their school years and cyber bullying is even more damaging to children.

8. When describing safety issues and related mortality to a local senior citizens group, what would the nurse identify as the leading cause of hospital admissions for trauma in older adults?
   a. Fires
   b. Exposure to temperature extremes
   c. Intimate partner violence
   d. Falls

9. What consideration should the nurse keep in mind regarding the use of side rails for a confused patient?
   a. They prevent confused patients from wandering.
   b. A history of a previous fall from a bed with raised side rails is insignificant.
   c. Alternative measures are ineffective to prevent wandering.
   d. A person of small stature is at increased risk for injury from entrapment.

10. When a fire occurs in a patient's room, what would be the nurse's priority?
    a. Rescue the patient.
    b. Extinguish the fire.
    c. Sound the alarm.
    d. Run for help.

11. When completing a safety event report, the nurse should:
    a. Include suggestions on how to prevent the incident from recurring.
    b. Provide minimal information about the incident.
    c. Discuss the details with the patient before documenting them.
    d. Objectively describe the incident in detail.

12. When discussing emergency preparedness with a group of first responders, what information would be important to include about preparation for a terrorist attack?
    a. Posttraumatic stress disorders can be expected in most survivors of a terrorist attack.
    b. The FDA has collaborated with drug companies to create stockpiles of emergency drugs.
    c. Even small doses of radiation result in bone marrow depression and cancer.
    d. Blast lung injury is a serious consequence following detonation of an explosive device.

13. An older resident who is disoriented likes to wander the halls of his long-term care facility. Which action would be most appropriate for the nurse to use as an alternative to restraints?
    a. Sitting him in a geriatric chair near the nurses' station
    b. Using the sheets to secure him snugly in his bed
    c. Keeping the bed in the high position
    d. Identifying his door with his picture and a balloon

14. The Joint Commission issues guidelines regarding the use of restraints. In which case is a restraint properly used?
    a. The nurse positions a patient in a supine position prior to applying wrist restraints.
    b. The nurse ensures that two fingers can be inserted between the restraint and patient's ankle.
    c. The nurse applies a cloth restraint to the left hand of a patient with an IV catheter in the right wrist.
    d. The nurse ties an elbow restraint to the raised side rail of a patient's bed.

15. A nurse orients an older patient to the safety features in her hospital room. What is a priority component of this admission routine?
    a. Explain how to use the telephone.
    b. Introduce the patient to her roommate.
    c. Review the hospital policy on visiting hours.
    d. Explain how to operate the call bell.

ANSWERS WITH RATIONALES

1. *b, d, f.* Risk factors for falls include age over 65 years, documented history of falls, postural hypotension, and unfamiliar environment. A medication regimen that includes diuretics, tranquilizers, sedatives, hypnotics, or analgesics is also a risk factor, not chemotherapy or antibiotics.

2. *c, d, e.* Of all fire deaths in the United States, 85% occur in the home (CDC, 2011a). Most fatal home fires occur while people are sleeping, and most people who die in house fires die of smoke inhalation rather than burns. More than one-third of home fire deaths occur in a home without a smoke detector (CDC, 2011a). People with limited financial resources should be asked about how they heat their house because the electricity or gas may have been turned off and space or kerosene heaters, wood stoves, or a fireplace may be the sole source of heat. Being a single parent is not a risk factor for fire occurrences.

3. *a.* A young child may place small or loose parts in the mouth; a toy that is safe for a 9-year-old could kill a toddler. An infant sleeping in a crib without a pillow or large blanket and a 3-year-old and a 4-year-old drinking juice and eating yogurt are not particular safety risks.

4. *c.* Because Mrs. Fuller is not aware that smoking in bed is extremely dangerous, she is at risk for suffocation from fire. The other three nursing diagnoses are correctly stated but are not a priority in this situation.

5. *d.* For the ingestion of drain opener, the nurse should never induce vomiting; instead, the poison should be diluted with milk or water and the primary care provider should be called. For vitamin preparations, stomach lavage is used to remove undigested pills and for acetaminophen poisoning, activated charcoal may be used.

6. *a.* Booster seats should be used for children until they are 4'9" tall and weigh between 80 and 100 pounds. All 50 U.S. states mandate the use of infant car seats and carriers when transporting a child in a motor vehicle. Infants and toddlers up to 2 years of age (or up to the maximum height and weight for the seat) should be in a rear-facing safety seat. Many children older than 6 years should still be in a booster seat.

7. *a, c, d.* Each year, underage drinking claims the lives of approximately 5,000 people under the age of 21. The CDC (2012j) lists motor vehicle accidents as the number one cause of death for adolescents. Marijuana use among teenagers has been on the increase and the abuse of prescription medication and OTC drugs has remained at a high level. Approximately one in five (20%) high school students reported using some type of tobacco product. Homicide rates for youths using firearms are higher than any other age group and the most recent statistics indicate that youths aged 10–19 years committed almost 1,500 suicides using firearms (Kagler, Annest, Kresnow & Mercy, 2011). According to the American Academy of Child & Adolescent Psychiatry, as many as 50% of children are bullied during their school years and some experts believe that cyber bullying is more dangerous and damaging to children than bullying that occurs in the schoolyard.

8. *d.* Falls among older adults are the most common cause of hospital admissions for trauma. Fires and temperature extremes are also significant hazard for older adults but are not the most common cause of trauma admissions. Intimate partner violence occurs more frequently in adults as opposed to older adults.

9. *d.* Studies of restraint-related deaths have shown that people of small stature are more likely to slip through or between the side rails. The desire to prevent a patient from wandering is not sufficient reason for the use of side rails. Creative use of alternative measures indicates respect for the patient's dignity and may in fact prevent more serious fall-related injuries. A history of falls from a bed with raised side rails carries a significant risk for a future serious incident.

10. *a.* The patient's safety is always the priority. Sounding the alarm and extinguishing the fire are important after the patient is safe. Calling for help, if possible, rather than running for assistance, allows you to remain with your patient and is more appropriate.

11. *d.* A safety event report is a legal document, which must be as objective and complete as possible. It is not a collaborative effort with the patient, and any suggestions to prevent the occurrence from happening again should be discussed at a postincident conference.

12. *d.* Blast lung injury is a recognized consequence following exposure to an explosive device. The CDC is the federal agency that has collaborated with the pharmaceutical companies to stockpile drugs for an emergency. A high dose of radiation exposure can result in bone marrow depression and cancer. Most survivors of a terrorist event will experience stress and some (possibly one-third of survivors) may exhibit posttraumatic stress disorder.

13. *d.* This allows the resident to be on the move and be more likely to find his room when he wants to return. The alternative would be to not allow him to wander. Many facilities use this kind of approach. Identifying his door with his picture and a balloon may work as an alternative to restraints. Using the geriatric chair and sheets are forms of physical restraint. Leaving the bed in the high position is a safety risk and would probably result in a fall.

14. *b.* The nurse should be able to place two fingers between the restraint and a patient's wrist or ankle. The patient should not be put in a supine position with restraints due to risk of aspiration. Due to the IV in the right wrist, alternative forms of restraints should be tried, such as a cloth mitt or an elbow restraint. Securing the restraint to a side rail may injure the patient when the side rail is lowered.

15. *d.* Knowing how to use the call bell is a safety priority; knowing how to use the phone, meeting the roommate, and knowledge of visiting hours will not necessarily prevent an accidental injury.

TAYLOR SUITE RESOURCES

Explore these additional resources to enhance learning for this chapter:

- NCLEX-Style Questions and other resources on thePoint, http://thePoint.lww.com/Taylor8e
- *Study Guide for Fundamentals of Nursing, 8th edition*
- Adaptive Learning | Powered by prepU, http://thepoint.lww.com/prepu
- *Skill Checklists for Fundamentals of Nursing, 8th edition*
- *Taylor's Clinical Nursing Skills:* Chapter 4, Safety

Bibliography

American Academy of Pediatrics (AAP). (2011). Child passenger safety. Available at http://pediatrics. aappublications.org/content/127/4/e1050.full

American Academy of Pediatrics (AAP). (2012). AAP updates recommendation on car seats. Available at http://www.aap.org/en-us/about-the-aap/aap-press-room/Pages/AAP-Updates-Recommendation-on-Car-Seats.aspx

American Cancer Society (ACS). (2010). Child and teen tobacco use. Available at http://www.cancer.org/acs/groups/cid/documents/webcontent/002963-pdf.pdf

American Cancer Society (ACS). (2011). *Child and teen tobacco use.* Available at http://www.cancer.org/Cancer/CancerCauses/TobaccoCancer/ChildandTeen TobaccoUse/child-and-teen-tobacco-use-what-to-do

American Nurses Association (ANA). (2010). Who will be there? Ethics, the law, and a nurse's duty to respond in a disaster. Available at http://www.nursing world.org/MainMenuCategories/Policy-Advocacy/Positions-and-Resolutions/Issue-Briefs/Disaster-Preparedness.pdf

American Nurses Association (ANA). (2012). Reduction of patient restraint and seclusion in health care settings. Available at http://www.nursingworld.org/restraintposition

American Nurses Association. (2014). OSHA releases new resources to protect hospital workers and enhance patient safety. Available at http://nursing-world.org/HomepageCategory/NursingInsider/OSHA-Releases-Resources-to-Protect-Hospital-Workers.html

Barnsteiner, J. (2012). Teaching the culture of safety. Available at http://www.medscape.com/view-article/758853

Boothe, D., & Harris, S. (2010). Fall scene investigation: A proactive approach to fall prevention. *Nursing, 40*(8), 67.

Brewer, K. (2011). Issues up close: Preparing for the worst is the key to surviving disasters. *American Nurse Today, 6*(9), 33–34.

Bulechek, G., Butcher, H., Dochterman, J. & Wagner, C. (2013). *Nursing interventions classification (NIC)* (6th ed., p. 179). St. Louis: Elsevier/Mosby.

Cahill, K., Nickles, D., & Fonder, P. (2012). Okay to play? A discussion about sports-related concussion. Available at http://www.americannursetoday.com/Popups/ArticlePrint.aspx?id=10514

Centers for Disease Control and Prevention (CDC). (2006). Chemical emergencies overview. Available at http://emergency.cdc.gov/chemical/overview.asp

Centers for Disease Control and Prevention (CDC). (2007). Bioterrorism overview. Available at http://www.bt.cdc.gov/bioterrorism/overview.asp

Centers for Disease Control and Prevention (CDC). (2011a). Fire deaths and injuries: Fact sheet. Available at http://www.cdc.gov/HomeandRecreationalSafety/Fire-Prevention/fires-factsheet.html

Centers for Disease Control and Prevention (CDC). (2011b). Types of radiation emergencies. Available at http://emergency.cdc.gov/radiation/typesofemergencies.asp

Centers for Disease Control and Prevention (CDC). (2012a). Blast injuries: Blast lung injury. Available at http://emergency.cdc.gov/masscasualties/blastlung injury.asp

Centers for Disease Control and Prevention (CDC). (2012b). Child passenger safety: Fact sheet. Available at http://www.cdc.gov/MotorVehicleSafety/Child_Passenger_Safety/CPS-Factsheet.html

Centers for Disease Control and Prevention (CDC). (2012c). Costs of falls among older adults. Available at http://www.cdc.gov/HomeandRecreationalSafety/Falls/fallcost.html

Centers for Disease Control and Prevention (CDC). (2012d). Health alert network (HAN). Available at http://www.bt.cdc.gov/HAN/

Centers for Disease Control and Prevention (CDC). (2012e). Playground injuries: Fact Sheet. Available at http://www.cdc.gov/homeandrecreationalsafety/Playground-Injuries/playgroundinjuries-factsheet.htm

Centers for Disease Control and Prevention (CDC). (2012f). Protect the ones you love: Drowning. Available at http://www.cdc.gov/safechild/Drowning/index.html

Centers for Disease Control and Prevention (CDC). (2012g). Protect the ones you love: Poisonings. Available at http://www.cdc.gov/safechild/Poisoning/index.html

Centers for Disease Control and Prevention (CDC). (2012h). Protect the ones you love: Suffocation. Available at http://www.cdc.gov/safechild/Suffocation/index.html

Centers for Disease Control and Prevention (CDC). (2012i). Teen drinking and driving. Available at http://www.cdc.gov/vitalsigns/TeenDrinking AndDriving/

Centers for Disease Control and Prevention (CDC). (2012j). Teen drivers. Available at http://www.cdc.gov/Motorvehiclesafety/Teen_Drivers/index.html

Centers for Disease Control and Prevention (CDC). (2012k). Understanding intimate partner violence: Fact sheet. Available at http://www.cdc.gov/violence prevention/pdf/IPV_Factsheet2012-a.pdf

Centers for Disease Control and Prevention (CDC). (2012l). Youth and tobacco use. Available at http://www.cdc.gov/tobacco/data_statistics/fact_sheets/youth_data/tobacco_use/index.htm

Centers for Disease Control and Prevention (CDC). (2014). Youth and tobacco use. Available at http://www.cdc.gov/tobacco/data_statistics/fact_sheets/youth_data/tobacco_use/

Centers for Medicare & Medicaid Services (CMS). (2006). Department of Health and Human Services. Federal Register. 42 CFR Part 482. Conditions of Participation: Patients' Rights. Final Rule. Available at http://www.cms.gov/Regulations-and-Guidance/Legislation/CFCsAndCoPs/downloads/finalpatient rightsrule.pdf.

Childhelp. (2012). National child abuse statistics: Child abuse in America. Available at http://www.child-help.org/pages/statistics

Davies, K. (2010). Hourly patient rounding. *Advance for Nurses, 12*(13), 13–15.

Domrose, C. (2010). The time is now. *Nurse.com, 19*(14), 12–13.

Dowdell, E., Burgess, A., & Flores, J. R. (2011). Online social networking patterns among adolescents, young adults, and sexual offenders. *American Journal of Nursing, 111*(7), 28–36.

Dykes, P., Carroll, D., Hurley, A., Lipsitz, S., Benoit, A., Chang, F., Meltzer, S., … Middleton, B. (2010). Fall prevention in acute care hospitals. *Journal of the American Medical Association, 304*(17):1912–1918. Available at http://www.ncbi.nlm.nih.gov/pmc/articles/PMC3107709/

Foley, M. (2012). Essential elements of a comprehensive sharps injury-prevention program. *The American Nurse Today, 7*(9), 2–4.

Garcia, A. (2011). Healthy nurse: Nine strategies to keep you safe at work. *American Nurse Today, 7*(1), 18.

Gerlock, A., Grimsey, J. Pisciotta, A. & Harel, O. (2011). Ask a few more questions: Identifying and responding to perpetrators of intimate partner violence in the clinical setting. *American Journal of Nursing, 111*(11), 35–39.

Goldsmith, C. (2011). Sports-related concussions: Tackling a growing trend. *Nursing Spectrum, 20*(5), 30–34.

Habel, M. (2012). Protecting seniors in disasters. *Nurse.com, 21*(4), 20–25.

Healthy People 2020. (2012). *Preparedness.* Available at http://www.healthypeople.gov/2020/topics objectives2020/overview.aspx?topicid=34

Hooven, C., Walsh, E., Pike, K., & Herting, J. (2012). Promoting care: Including parents in youth suicide prevention. *Community Health, 35*(3), 225–235.

The Joint Commission (TJC). (2011). Sentinel Events (SE). Available at http://www.jointcommission.org/assets/1/6/2011_CAMBHC_SE.pdf

The Joint Commission (TJC). (2012). National patient safety goals. Available at http://www.joint commission.org/standards_information/npsgs.aspx

The Joint Commission Center for Transforming Healthcare. (2012). Facts about the preventing falls with injury project. Available at http://www.center fortransforminghealthcare.org/assets/4/6/CTH_PFWI_Fact_Sheet.pdf

Jorgensen, J. (2011). Reducing patient falls: A call to action. *The American Nurse Today, 6*(2), 2–5.

Kegler, S., Annest, J. L., Kresnow, M. & Mercy, J. A. (2011). Violence-related firearm deaths among residents of metropolitan areas and cities: United States, 2006–2007. Available at http://www.medscape.com/viewarticle/742893

Kulik, C. (2011). Components of a comprehensive fall-risk assessment. *The American Nurse Today, 6*(2), 6–7.

Laing, C. (2010). Acute carbon monoxide toxicity. *Nursing, 40*(11), 39–44.

Lowry, F. (2011). DEA moves to make "bath salts" illegal as overdoses rise. Available at http://www.medscape.com/viewarticle/749304

Mayo Clinic. (2012). Tatoos: Understand risks and precautions. Available at http://www.mayoclinic.com/health/tattoos-and-piercings/MC00020/

McGraw, M. (2012). Bath salts. *Nursing, 42*(1), 26–33.

McPhaul, K. (2011). Safe at home. *Advance for Nurses, 13*(12), 17–18.

Moorhead, S., Johnson, M., Maas, M., & Swanson, E. (2013). *Nursing outcomes classification (NOC)* (5th ed., pp. 460–461). St. Louis: Elsevier/Mosby.

Murray, J. (2012). National disaster medical system. *American Journal of Nursing, 112*(2), 58–63.

NANDA International. (2012). *NANDA nursing diagnoses: Definitions & classification: 2012–2014.* West Sussex, UK: Wiley-Blackwell.

Narang, P., Paladugu, A., Manda, S., Smock, W., Gosnay, C., & Lippmann, S. (2011). Do guns provide safety? At what cost? Available at http://www.medscape.com/viewarticle/717278

National Capital Poison Center (2012). What is ipecac syrup? Available at http://www.poison.org/prepared/ipecac.asp

National Capital Poison Center (2014). Poisonings: The national picture. Available at http://www.poison.org/stats/

National Highway Traffic Safety Administration (NHTSA). 2010. Securing our most precious cargo. Available at http://www.nhtsa.dot.gov/staticfiles/DOT/NHTSA/Traffic%20Injury%20Control/Articles/Associated20Files/LATCH-factsheet.pdf

National Institute on Drug Abuse (NIDA). (2012). Drug facts: High school and youth trends. Available at http://www.drugabuse.gov/publications/drugfacts/high-school-youth-trends

National Patient Safety Foundation (NPSF). (2011). The universal patient compact: Principles for partnership. Available at http://www.npsf.org/wp-content/uploads/2011/10/UniversalPatientCompact.pdf

Phillips, J. (2010). The ABCs of safety and quality. *Nursing, 40*(3), 55.

Pillitteri, A. (2010). *Maternal & child nursing: Care of the childbearing and childrearing family* (6th ed.). Philadelphia: Wolters Kluwer Health/Lippincott Williams & Wilkins.

Ponce, M. (2012). How to prevent falls among older adults in outpatient settings. Available at http://www.americannursetoday.com/Popups/ArticlePrint.aspx?id=10854

Puliti, B. (2011). Bullying in school: Nurses educate students on the negative effects. Available at http://nursing.advanceweb.com/Editorial/Content/Print Friendly.aspx?CC=241315

Quigley, P., & Goff, L. (2011). Current and emerging innovations to keep patients safe. *The American Nurse Today, 6*(2), 14–17.

(2010). Restraint use cut in half. *Nursing, 40*(10), 20.

Richards, E. (2011). Stop the silence of elder abuse. Available at http://www.americannursetoday.com/article.aspx?id=8112&fid=8078

Safe Kids Worldwide. (2014). Seat belt safety for big kids. Available at http://www.safekids.org/tip/seat-belt-safety-big-kids

Safe Kids Worldwide. (2012). *Safe storage, safe dosing, safe kids.* Available at http://www.safekids.

org/assets/docs/safety-basics/safety-tips-by-risk-area/medicine-safety-study-2012.pdf

Shell, L. (2011). Preventing falls: Root cause analysis can help you see what you're not looking for. *Advance for Nurses, 13*(18), 14.

Sherwood, S., & Barnsteiner, J. (2012). *Quality and Safety in Nursing.* West Sussex, UK: Wiley-Blackwell.

Slepski, L. (2011). Radiation: Incidents and emergency preparedness. *Nursing Spectrum, 20*(6), 20–25.

Smith, J. (2010). Mass casualty events: Are you prepared? *Nursing, 40*(4), 40–45.

Stark, S. (2012). Elder abuse: Screening, intervention, and prevention. *Nursing, 42*(10), 24–30.

Tafoya, W. (2011). Cyber terror. Available at http://www.fbi.gov/stats-services/publications/law-enforcement-bulletin/november-2011/cyber-terror

Taverno, T., & Solheim, J. (2012). Traumatic brain injury. Available at http://ce.nurse.com/course/ICE07/traumatic-brain-injury/

Tumulo, J. (2012). Fatal distractions. *Advance for Nurses, 14*(4), 11.

UC Davis Health System. (2010). Experts: Cyberattacks threaten hospitals. Available at http://www.ucdmc.ucdavis.edu/welcome/features/2010–2011/08/20100811_cyberterrorism.html

Ullman, A., Long, D., Horn, D., Woosley, J., & Coulthard, M. (2013). The KIDS SAFE checklist for pediatric intensive care units. *American Journal of Critical Care, 22*(1), 61–69.

U.S. Department of Health and Human Services (USDHHS). (2009). Violence against women: Domestic and intimate partner violence. Available at http://www.womenshealth.gov/violence-against-women/types-of-violence/domestic-intimate-partner-violence.html

U.S. Department of Health and Human Services (USDHHS). (2011). Underage drinking. Available at http://report.nih.gov/nihfactsheets/ViewFactSheet.aspx?csid=21&key=U

U.S. Department of Veteran Affairs (VA). (2011). Intimate partner violence. Available at http://www.ptsd.va.gov/public/types/violence/domestic-violence.asp

U.S. Food and Drug Administration (FDA). (2012). Medical device reporting. Available at http://www.fda.gov/MedicalDevices/Safety/ReportaProblem/default.htm

Waddell, A. (2010). Implementing surgical smoke evacuation in the operating room. *American Journal of Nursing, 110*(1), 54–58.

Younce, A., Hinton, D., Haynes, D., & Berg, J. (2011). Make fall risk the sixth vital sign. *Nursing, 41*(4), 62–64.

27 Complementary and Alternative Therapies

BRIAN LEGETT

Brian, a 30-year-old man with a long history of back problems due to a work injury, comes to the clinic for evaluation. He states, "I've had so many kinds of treatment, and nothing seems to work. Maybe I should see a chiropractor?"

SYLVIA PUENTES

Sylvia, a middle-aged woman, is scheduled for abdominal surgery next week. She comes to the outpatient clinic for preoperative evaluation and laboratory testing and says, "I'm really anxious about the surgery, but I don't want to take any medicines. Is there anything I can do to help me relax?"

LEE CHEN

Lee, a 65-year-old man dying of lung cancer, was brought to the United States from China by his two daughters, who believed that U.S. medicine would cure him. Mr. Chen did not respond to any of the therapies that were attempted, and the team wants to transition to palliative care. The daughters are unwilling to authorize removal of ventilatory support or sign a do-not-resuscitate order. They request an acupuncturist, but the physician refuses their request.

LEARNING OBJECTIVES

After completing the chapter, you will be able to accomplish the following:

1. Differentiate complementary and alternative therapies from allopathic medicine.

2. Compare and contrast the beliefs about the origin of disease and ways to promote health of each of the five main categories of CAT.

3. Describe ways in which nurses can use knowledge of complementary and alternative therapies in providing patient care.

4. Identify the knowledge the public should possess about CAT if they wish to be informed consumers.

5. Describe ways in which nurses can use selected complementary and alternative therapies for self-care and health promotion.

KEY TERMS

acupuncture	dosha	nurse healer
allopathic medicine	healing touch (HT)	qi
alternative modalities	holism	qi gong
aromatherapy	holistic nursing	relaxation response
aura	homeopathy	shamanism
Ayurveda	imagery	therapeutic touch (TT)
chakra	integrative care	traditional Chinese medicine (TCM)
chiropractic medicine	intercessory prayer	yin-yang theory
complementary therapies	meridian	
	naturopathic medicine	

Many people in the United States are using complementary and alternative therapies (CAT) to promote health and assist with healing from illness. The term *complementary and alternative therapies* refers to interventions that are **complementary therapies** (they can be used with traditional medical interventions and thus complement them) as well as **alternative modalities** (not included in the scope of conventional medical care). However, CAT are neither standardized nor part of an existing system, as is conventional medical care. The term *complementary and alternative medicine* (CAM) is widely used; however, many nurses use CAT instead, because people without medical degrees practice CAM/CAT. This chapter discusses basic CAT that a practicing nurse needs to understand to provide safe nursing care.

Nurses need to be knowledgeable about CAT primarily for three reasons. First, patients, families, physicians, and institutions increasingly expect practicing nurses to be knowledgeable about CAT. Many patients use these types of therapies as outpatients and want to continue their use as inpatients. They or family members may expect nurses to administer herbal preparations or nutritional supplements. Also, it is not uncommon for people to retain health care practices brought from other countries although they reside in the United States. In these situations, nurses can assist patients by accommodating special CAT healing practices as much as possible. In addition, as evidence grows demonstrating the effectiveness of selected CAT, many institutions now provide complementary therapies to inpatients as part of total patient care. See the accompanying Reflective Practice display.

Second, many nurses are expanding their clinical practice by incorporating CAT. Many state Boards of Nursing recognize select alternative/complementary modalities as part of nursing practice and have provisions for the safe practice of these modalities by registered nurses.

Finally, although CAT may seem totally safe, some therapies have led to harmful and, at times, lethal outcomes. Nurses play an important role in educating the public about how these therapies can be used safely and effectively. This chapter will provide helpful resources for education.

INTRODUCTION TO COMPLEMENTARY AND ALTERNATIVE THERAPIES

Although the use of most complementary and alternative therapies predates modern medicine, it was not until recently that nursing and medical schools began to teach about their use. The sharp divide between traditional medicine and CAT has now softened, and successful practitioners know how to combine the two successfully.

Traditional Medicine and CAT

Allopathic medicine (or biomedicine) has been dominant for about 100 years and has spearheaded remarkable advances in biotechnology, surgical interventions, pharmaceutical approaches, and diagnostic tools. Allopathic medical care is particularly effective when aggressive treatment is needed in emergency or acute situations.

However, allopathic medical care has not been totally effective in dealing with chronic illness, a persistent problem. Increasingly, CAT are being used as an "answer" to the problem of chronic illness. The CAT and allopathic systems differ fundamentally in several ways (Table 27-1 on page 730). Until recently, the majority of decision making in CAT has been based on observation, experience, and traditional healing manuscripts in contrast to allopathic medicine, which has moved away from these methodologies to evidence-based practice.

Many CAT are based on a theory and philosophy of holism upon which holistic nursing also is based. Many practitioners and consumers of health care choose to combine allopathic

REFLECTIVE PRACTICE: CULTIVATING QSEN COMPETENCIES

CHALLENGE TO COGNITIVE SKILLS

This spring, while working on an oncology floor, I was caring for Lee Chen, a 65-year-old man dying of lung cancer. His two daughters, who were living in the United States, had brought him from China to the United States, believing that U.S. medicine would cure him. Unfortunately, Mr. Chen's cancer had not responded to any of the therapies that were attempted. All of his professional caregivers believed that the goal of treatment should now be preparation for a comfortable and dignified death using compassionate palliative care. His daughters, however, were unwilling to accept this goal and would not authorize removing him from ventilatory support or issuing a do-not-resuscitate order. Mr. Chen could no longer speak on his own behalf. One afternoon, one of his daughters informed Mr. Chen's physician that she was going to bring an acupuncturist in to work on her father. The physician told her in no uncertain terms that he would not allow "voodoo medicine" on his unit. I wasn't sure what to do, because both daughters were growing more and more upset, and this answer seemed like the "last straw."

Thinking Outside the Box: Possible Courses of Action

- Accept the status quo and try to comfort the daughters.
- Support the physician's judgment and try to get the daughters to see things his way.
- Learn more about acupuncture and related benefits and harms (I have never seen it done and know very little about what to expect).
- Find out if the physician really had the authority to forbid acupuncture on this patient.
- Advocate for the patient and his family if there is a possibility that acupuncture will benefit him.

Evaluating a Good Outcome: How Do I Define Success?

- Patient receives culturally appropriate, person-centered care consistent with the goals of compassionate palliative care.
- The patient is not harmed.
- Mr. Chen's daughters feel supported as they struggle with decisions and anticipatory grieving.
- All health care team members (including Mr. Chen's physician) learn about acupuncture and other complementary and alternative therapies, as well as about the hospital's policies regarding their use.
- The physician is confronted in a professional manner about the behavior as increasing the stress on the family caregivers.
- I grow in my knowledge of how to incorporate CAM into my care.

Personal Learning: Here's to the Future!

I was so upset by the daughters' distress that I decided to learn more about acupuncture. After searching the Internet and talking with a nurse who was receiving acupuncture treatments, I decided that acupuncture treatments were unlikely to harm the patient; in fact, the treatments just might help to increase his comfort level. At the very least, Mr. Chen's daughters would believe that we respected and supported their efforts to help their father. I was also hopeful that the professional caregiving team would learn more about culturally competent care. When I spoke with the head nurse, she was understanding about my goals and actually confronted Mr. Chen's doctor and secured his approval for having the acupuncturist visit. I learned that the acupuncturist had to be credentialed by our hospital. While Mr. Chen's cancer did not respond to the acupuncture treatment, he did seem more comfortable, and his daughters couldn't thank me enough. I talked with them about how impressive their devotion to their father was and also mentioned that they may need to give him one last gift, the gift of "letting go." Unfortunately, I never saw this family again because this was my last week on this unit.

Melinda Ventura, Georgetown University

REFLECTION ON QUALITY AND SAFETY COMPETENCIES

How do you think you would respond in a similar situation? Why? What does this tell you about yourself and about the adequacy of your competencies for professional practice? Can you think of other ways to respond?

What *knowledge, skills,* and *attitudes* do you need to develop to continuously improve the quality and safety of care for patients like Mr. Chen?

Patient-Centered Care: How can you establish a successful partnership with family members discouraged by a patient's worsening condition who want to try complementary and alternative therapies? How did the nursing student promote respectful, patient-centered, culturally competent care?

Teamwork and Collaboration/Quality Improvement: What factors do you think may have played a role in the physician's answer? Imagine if the nursing student (rather than the head nurse) had approached the physician to allow the acupuncturist to visit. Do you think that the physician's answer would have been the same as it was when the head nurse confronted him? Please explain why or why not. What competencies do you need to develop to get the team to work well together? What needs to change to improve quality in this setting?

Safety/Evidence-Based Practice: What does the evidence point to as "best practice" in a situation like this? What safety needs does Mr. Chen have and how can you meet them?

Informatics: Can you identify the essential information that must be available in Mr. Chen's record to support safe patient care and coordination of care? Can you think of other ways to respond to or approach the situation? What else might the nursing student have done to ensure a successful outcome?

| **Table 27-1** | BELIEFS UNDERLYING COMPLEMENTARY AND ALTERNATIVE THERAPIES AND THE ALLOPATHIC THERAPIES |

COMPLEMENTARY AND ALTERNATIVE THERAPIES	ALLOPATHIC THERAPIES
Mind, body, and spirit are integrated and together influence health and illness.	Illness occurs in either the mind or the body, which are separate entities.
Health is a balance of body systems: mental, social, and spiritual, as well as physical.	Health is the absence of disease.
Illness is a manifestation of imbalance or disharmony.	The main causes of illness are considered to be pathogens (bacteria or viruses) or biochemical imbalances.
Symptoms are a sign or reflection of a deeper instability within the person; restoring physical and mental harmony will alleviate the symptoms. Healing is a slow process that involves the whole person.	Curing seeks to destroy the invading organism or repair the affected part.
Emphasis is on health. Healing is done by the patient; care is individualized.	Emphasis is on disease and high technology. Drugs, surgery, and radiation are among the key tools for dealing with medical problems.

modalities and CAT using an integrative approach. These concepts are discussed in the following sections.

Holism

Holism is a theory and philosophy that focuses on connections and interactions between parts of the whole. In contrast, the prevailing scientific approach has focused on reductionism, the goal of which is to reduce all phenomena to the smallest possible atom, particle, or interaction. Using a holistic perspective, all living organisms, including humans, are continuously connecting and interacting with their environment. Further, parts of the organism, whether they are systems, subsystems, or cells, are also continuously interacting and changing. This continual interaction and change means that the body is not the sum of its parts (as in reductionism), but that it is a unified, dynamic whole.

Although one might view holism as a recently developed belief system, holism in fact was the predominant belief throughout history until sometime before René Descartes, a French philosopher who lived in the early part of the 17th century. He and other influential thinkers asserted that the mind and body were separate from each other. That belief lasted until the early 20th century, when researchers began to prove that there was a connection between the mind and the body.

One of the 20th-century researchers, Hans Selye, developed the term *general adaptation syndrome* (GAS) to describe the general holistic pattern that emerges when people experience stress/illness. The GAS reflects a general response that occurs in various parts of the body. This theory holds that when someone is sick, that person is "sick all over," not just where symptoms manifest. Selye also demonstrated that adrenal exhaustion can be caused by emotional tension, such as suppressed rage or frustration. (For more on the GAS, see Chapter 41.)

A holistic philosophy underlies many CAT. People have a mind, body, emotions, and spirit that are connected and function as a unified whole. A change in any part of the organism will be reflected in other parts. When someone feels the emotion of sadness, that individual may have a physical response of crying. In addition, when a person feels stressed and overwhelmed, the face and body language frequently reflect these conditions.

Holistic nursing is nursing practice built on a holistic philosophy. Healing the whole person is its goal. Since holism is a philosophy and not a specific nursing role, holistic nurses can be found in all varieties of health care settings as well as in independent practice settings. In addition, holistic nurses frequently add CAT to their practice. Most holistic nurses use CAT for self-care, an essential component of holistic practice. The American Holistic Nurse Association (AHNA) promotes the education of nurses, other health care professionals, and the public in all aspects of holistic caring and healing. AHNA authors Dossey and Keegan (2013, p. xxvii) challenge nurses to explore three questions:

1. What do you know about the meaning of healing?
2. What do you do each day to facilitate healing in yourself?
3. How can you be an instrument of healing and a nurse healer?

Read through the accompanying Through the Eyes of a Nurse and reflect on your commitment to holistic person-centered nursing and healing. The efforts of AHNA recently resulted in the recognition of holistic nursing as an "official nursing specialty" by the American Nurses Association. In 2000, the American Holistic Nursing Association published standards for holistic nursing practice (Frisch, Dossey, Guzzetta, & Quinn, 2000). Registered nurses can become certified in basic and advanced holistic nursing through the American Holistic Nurses' Certification Corporation (AHNCC).

Integrative Care

A person who uses **integrative care** uses some combination of allopathic medicine and CAT (Table 27-2). There are

THROUGH THE EYES OF A NURSE

Healing is a lifelong journey into understanding the wholeness of human existence. Along this journey, our lives mesh with those of clients, families, and colleagues, where moments of new meaning and insight emerge in the midst of crisis. Healing occurs when we help clients, families, others, and ourselves embrace what is feared most. It occurs when we seek harmony and balance. Healing is learning how to open what has been closed so that we can expand our inner potentials. It is the fullest expression of oneself that is demonstrated by the light and shadow, and the male and female principles that reside in each of us. It is accessing what we have forgotten about connections, unity, and interdependence. With a new awareness of these interrelationships, heal-ing becomes possible, and the experience of the nurse as an instrument of healing and as a nurse healer becomes actualized. A **nurse healer** is one who facilitates another person's growth toward wholeness (body–mind–spirit) or who assists another with recovery from illness or transition to peaceful death. Healing is not just curing symptoms. Rather, it is the exquisite blending of technology with caring, love, compassion, and creativity.

—Barbara Montgomery Dossey, Lynn Keegan

Used with permission. (2013). *Holistic Nursing: A handbook for practice* (6th ed.). Burlington, MA: Jones & Bartlett Learning.

---

several types of integrative care models used throughout the United States, which can be housed in virtually all health care delivery structures. Optimally, these models include sensitive and knowledgeable health care providers who work with patients to design a plan of care that is responsive to the patient's preferences and combines the best of allopathic medicine and CAT while avoiding harmful interactions.

CAT and Nursing

CAT consists of a large variety of therapies that are based on a set of beliefs different from those of allopathic medicine. Some of these modalities have developed fairly recently (e.g., guided imagery), while others have been used for thousands of years as components of ancient healing systems (e.g., Ayurveda or traditional Chinese medicine). Some therapies can be used effectively without assistance (e.g., nutritional approaches, deep breathing exercises), while others (e.g., naturopathy, acupuncture) are more effective when used with guidance from practitioners who have particular knowledge and expertise.

Many people use CAT for stress management/reduction. Techniques such as relaxation with focused breathing, meditation, imagery, biofeedback, and massage are used in all stages of health and illness to promote healing and/or

manage symptoms. Because stress can contribute to illness, CAT can sometimes be effective in reducing symptoms and enhancing quality of life. Nurses can assist clients—and themselves—with these therapies.

 RECALL Sylvia Puentes, the anxious patient scheduled for surgery. The nurse's knowledge of CAT would be important in helping this patient to reduce her preoperative anxiety. The nurse could discuss various methods available, allowing the patient to select the one that seems best for her. Such actions help develop a trusting nurse–patient relationship and foster a sense of self-esteem in the patient by allowing her to participate in the plan of care and decision making. •

Use of CAT in the United States

The most comprehensive and reliable findings to date on Americans' use of CAT are released by the National Center for Complementary and Alternative Medicine (NCCAM) and the National Center for Health Statistics (NCHS), part of the Centers for Disease Control and Prevention (CDC). The following findings are based on the 2008 edition of the NCHS's National Health Interview Survey (NHIS), an annual study in which tens of thousands of Americans are interviewed about their health- and illness-related experiences (Barnes, Bloom, & Nahin, 2008). The report is available, along with a press release and graphics, at nccam.nih. gov/news/camstats/.

Prevalence of CAT

The 2007 survey found that in the United States, approximately 38% of adults (about 4 in 10) and approximately 12% of children (about 1 in 9) were using some form of CAT in the 12 months before the survey. Consistent with results from the 2002 NHIS, in 2007, CAT use was more prevalent among women, adults aged 30 to 69, adults with higher levels of education, adults who were not poor, adults living in the West, former smokers, and adults who were hospitalized in the last year. In both the 2002 and 2007

Table 27-2	INTEGRATIVE CARE OF THE COMMON COLD*
COMPLEMENTARY AND ALTERNATIVE THERAPIES	**ALLOPATHIC APPROACHES**
Acupuncture to appropriate areas to reduce sinus congestion	Decongestant over-the-counter medications
Rest and fluids	Rest and fluids
Herbs, vitamin C to stimulate immune system	Vitamin C to stimulate immune system

*In this example, adding herbs and/or acupuncture to a typical allo-pathic approach would represent integrative care.

surveys, adults younger than 65 years of age and those with private health insurance were more likely than those with public health insurance or uninsured adults to use CAT. There also are cultural variations. The breakdown of CAT use by race or ethnicity among adults is as follows: American Indian/Alaska Native, 50.3%; White, 43.1%; Asian, 39.9%; African American, 25.5%; and Hispanic, 23.7%.

The American Association of Retired Persons (AARP) and NCCAM partnered on a telephone survey of over 1,000 people aged 50 and older. Just over half of those surveyed reported using complementary and alternative medicine and over a third take some type of herbal product or dietary supplement. Yet only a third of all respondents and a little over half of CAM users said they have ever discussed CAM with their health care providers. These findings highlight the need for nurses to ask about CAM use at every patient visit and the need for people aged 50 and older to know that CAM use is something that is important to discuss with their conventional health care providers (AARP & NCCAM, 2010). The National Cancer Institute's Office of Cancer Complementary and Alternative Medicine makes *Talking about Complementary and Alternative Medicine with Health Care Providers: A Workbook and Tips* available for patients and professionals on their website: http://cam.cancer.gov/ attachments/workbook/talking_about_cam_workbook.pdf. You will find it to be a valuable teaching resource.

Reasons for Using CAT

People use CAT for an array of diseases and conditions. Generally, people who choose CAT approaches are seeking ways to improve their health and well-being or to relieve symptoms associated with chronic, even terminal, illnesses or the side effects of conventional treatments for them. Other reasons for choosing to use CAT include having a holistic health philosophy or a transformational experience that changes one's worldview and wanting greater control over one's own health. For example, American adults are most likely to use CAT for musculoskeletal problems such as back, neck, or joint pain. However, the use of CAT for head or chest colds decreased from 2002 to 2007.

Most Frequently Used CAT

In 2007, the CAT most commonly used by U.S. adults in the past 12 months were nonvitamin, nonmineral, natural products (17.7%); deep breathing exercises (12.7%); meditation (9.4%); chiropractic or osteopathic manipulation (8.6%); massage (8.3%); and yoga (6.1%). Among U.S. adults, the use of some mind–body therapies, specifically deep breathing exercises, meditation, and yoga, increased between 2002 and 2007. Between 2002 and 2007, increased use was also seen for acupuncture, massage therapy, and naturopathy. Between 2002 and 2007, there was a significant decrease in the use of the Atkins diet.

Use of CAT With Children

In 2007, the CAT most commonly used by U.S. children in the past 12 months included nonvitamin, nonmineral, natu-

ral products (3.9%); chiropractic or osteopathic manipulation (2.8%); deep breathing exercises (2.2%); yoga (2.1%); and homeopathic treatment (1.3%). Children whose parents used CAT were about twice as likely as all U.S. children to have used nonvitamin, nonmineral, natural products (9.2% vs. 3.9%); chiropractic or osteopathic manipulation (5.7% vs. 2.8%); deep breathing exercises (5.4% vs. 2.2%); yoga (4.7% vs. 2.1%); and homeopathic treatment (2.8% vs. 1.3%) in the past 12 months.

Growth of the CAT Industry

Americans spent $33.9 billion out-of-pocket on CAT over the previous 12 months according to the 2007 government survey. Of schools of nursing responding to a survey, 85% reported that CAT was included in their curricula (Fenton & Morris, 2003). Approximately two thirds of medical schools in the United States offer courses in CAT, either as elective or required courses. Insurers increasingly pay for selected CAT for particular identified conditions. Scores of private organizations provide classes and workshops for consumers as well as education and practical experience for health care providers.

Many private and governmental organizations have been developed to deal with CAT. The National Center for Complementary and Alternative Medicine (NCCAM) in the National Institutes of Health (NIH) funds research on CAT and is a great first resource for professionals and the pubic seeking information about CAT. See Box 27-1 for NCCAM's advice to the public about being an informed consumer. The special White House Commission on Complementary and Alternative Medicine Policy (WHCCAMP) issued an extensive report in March 2002, addressing policy issues specific to CAT. The following are the 10 guiding principles they used before issuing recommendations (www. whccamp.hhs.gov/es.html):

1. A wholeness orientation in health care delivery
2. Evidence of safety and efficacy
3. The healing capacity of the person
4. Respect for individuality
5. The right to choose treatment
6. An emphasis on health promotion and self-care
7. Partnerships as essential to integrated health care
8. Education as a fundamental health care service
9. Dissemination of comprehensive and timely information
10. Integral public involvement

Health care professionals and consumers can find valuable information about the safety and efficacy of CAT on the NCCAM website.

The U.S. Food and Drug Administration (FDA) is seeking to increase regulations for dietary supplements. In 2013, the FDA offered six "tip-offs" to help consumers identify "rip-offs" (FDA, 2013):

• *One product does it all.* Be suspicious of products that claim to cure a wide range of diseases. A New York firm claimed that its products marketed as dietary supplements could treat or cure senile dementia; brain atrophy;

| BOX 27-1 | COMPLEMENTARY AND ALTERNATIVE MEDICINE (CAM): BE AN INFORMED CONSUMER |

- Take charge of your health by being an informed consumer.
- Talk with your health care providers when making any decisions about using complementary and alternative medicine (CAM). Your health care providers can give you advice based on your medical needs.
- If you are thinking about using a CAM therapy, learn the facts. Is it safe? Does it work?
- Find out what scientific studies have been done. It is not a good idea to use a CAM therapy simply because you have seen it in an advertisement or on a Web site or because people have told you that it worked for them.
- Keep in mind that the number of Web sites offering health-related resources grows every day. Many sites provide valuable information, while others may have information that is unreliable or misleading. To evaluate the

quality of a Web site, take a look at who runs the site, who pays for it, and the purpose of the site. Also, check out where the information comes from, how it is selected, and how current it is.
- Scientific research on many CAM therapies is relatively new, so information about safety and effectiveness may not be available for every therapy. However, many studies of CAM treatments are underway, and researchers are always learning more about CAM.
- You can find reliable information on CAM through the National Institutes of Health's National Center for Complementary and Alternative Medicine (NCCAM). The NCCAM Web site (http://nccam.nih.gov/) provides a variety of useful information as well as links to other trustworthy sources. You can also contact the NCCAM Clearinghouse staff (call toll-free at: 1-888-644-6226 or e-mail info@nccam.nih.gov for help).

Adapted from National Institutes of Health. http://nihseniorhealth.gov/complementaryhealthapproaches/informedconsumer/01.html

atherosclerosis; kidney dysfunction; gangrene; depression; osteoarthritis; dysuria; and lung, cervical, and prostate cancer. In October 2012, at FDA's request, U.S. marshals seized these products.

- *Personal testimonials.* Success stories, such as, "It cured my diabetes" or "My tumors are gone," are easy to make up and are not a substitute for scientific evidence.
- *Quick fixes.* Few diseases or conditions can be treated quickly, even with legitimate products. Beware of language such as, "lose 30 pounds in 30 days" or "eliminates skin cancer in days."
- *"All natural."* Some plants found in nature (such as poisonous mushrooms) can kill when consumed. Moreover, FDA has found numerous products promoted as "all natural" that contain hidden and dangerously high doses of prescription drug ingredients or even untested active artificial ingredients.
- *"Miracle cure."* Alarms should go off when you see this claim or others like it such as, "new discovery," "scientific breakthrough," or "secret ingredient." If a real cure for a serious disease were discovered, it would be widely reported through the media and prescribed by health professionals—not buried in print ads, TV infomercials, or on Internet sites.
- *Conspiracy theories.* Claims like "The pharmaceutical industry and the government are working together to hide information about a miracle cure" are always untrue and unfounded. These statements are used to distract consumers from the obvious, common-sense questions about the so-called miracle cure.

Even with these tips, fraudulent health products are not always easy to spot. FDA recommends that if you're tempted to buy an unproven product or one with questionable claims, check with your doctor or other health care professional first.

Consumers can subscribe to the FDA RSS feed (http://www.fda.gov/AboutFDA/ContactFDA/StayInformed/RSSFeeds/default.htm) that will send information on fraudulent products to your smart phone or computer and help keep you from being duped or hurt by these products. Lastly, the Foundation for Alternative Medicine (NFAM) is engaged in international research to determine "best practices" for cancer treatment.

CAT CATEGORIES

NCCAM classifies the major CAT into five categories (or domains): whole medical systems, mind–body therapies, energy medicine, biologically based practices, and manipulative and body-based practices. Each category contains several therapies. For example, meditation is a therapy included in the mind–body category. Box 27-2 (on page 735) describes each of the categories. Table 27-3 (on page 734) lists examples of alternative treatments from these categories that work on pain, describing what they help and how they work. This chapter includes information on some of the most widely used CAT of interest to practicing nurses.

Whole Medical Systems

A whole medical system (or alternative medical system) consists of a philosophy and theory about health and illness along with specific types of treatment. These systems have developed independently from allopathic medicine and are generally culturally based. Ayurveda, traditional Chinese medicine, shamanism (which includes native traditions), homeopathy, naturopathy, and chiropractic medicine are examples of whole medical systems.

Ayurveda

Ayurveda originated in the Vedic civilization of India about 4,000 years ago and is one of the world's oldest medical

Table 27-3 ALTERNATIVE TREATMENTS THAT WORK ON PAIN

TYPE	WHAT THEY HELP	HOW THEY HELP	EXAMPLES
Movement-Based Therapies: Physical exercises and practices	Musculoskeletal pain, joint pain, and lower-back pain	By strengthening muscles supporting joints, improving alignment, and releasing endorphins	• *Physical therapy:* Specialized movements to strengthen weak areas of the body, often through resistance training • *Yoga:* An Indian practice of meditative stretching and posing • *Pilates:* A resistance regimen that strengthens core muscles • *Tai chi:* A slow, flowing Chinese practice that improves balance • *Feldenkrais:* A therapy that builds efficiency of movement
Nutritional and Herbal Remedies: Food choices and dietary supplements (ask your doctor before using supplements)	All chronic pain but especially abdominal discomfort, headaches, and inflammatory conditions, such as rheumatoid arthritis	By boosting the body's natural immunity, reducing pain-causing inflammation, soothing pain, and decreasing insomnia	• *Anti-inflammatory diet:* A Mediterranean eating pattern high in whole grains, fresh fruits, leafy vegetables, fish, and olive oil • *Omega-3 fatty acids:* Nutrients abundant in fish oil and flaxseed that reduce inflammation in the body • *Ginger:* A root that inhibits pain-causing molecules • *Turmeric:* A spice that reduces inflammation • *MSM:* Methylsulfonylmethane, a naturally occurring nutrient that helps build bone and cartilage
Mind–Body Medicine: Using the powers of the mind to produce changes in the body	All types of chronic pain	By reducing stressful (and, hence, pain-inducing) emotions such as panic and fear, and by refocusing attention on subjects other than pain	• *Meditation:* Focusing the mind on something specific (such as breathing or repeating a word or phrase) to quiet it • *Guided imagery:* Visualizing a particular outcome or scenario with the goal of mentally changing one's physical reality • *Biofeedback:* With a special machine, becoming alert to body processes, such as muscle tightening, to learn to control them • *Relaxation:* Releasing tension in the body through exercises such as controlled breathing
Energy Healing: Manipulating the electrical energy—called chi in Chinese medicine—emitted by the body's nervous system	Pain that lingers after an injury heals, as well as pain complicated by trauma, anxiety, or depression	By relaxing the body and the mind, distracting the nervous system, producing natural painkillers, activating natural pleasure centers, and manipulating chi	• *Acupuncture:* The insertion of hair-thin needles into points along the body's meridians, or energetic pathways, to stimulate the flow of energy throughout the body; proven helpful for postsurgical pain and dental pain, among other types • *Acupressure:* Finger pressure applied to points along the meridians, to balance and increase the flow of energy • *Chi gong:* Very slow, gentle physical movements, similar to tai chi, that cleanse the body and circulate chi • *Reiki:* Moving a practitioner's hands over the energy fields of the client's body to increase energy flow and restore balance
Physical Manipulation: Hands-on massage or movement of painful areas	Musculoskeletal pain, especially lower-back and neck pain; pain from muscle underuse or overuse; and pain from adhesions or scars	By restoring mobility, improving circulation, decreasing blood pressure, and relieving stress	• *Massage:* The manipulation of tissue to relax clumps of knotted muscle fiber, increase circulation, and release patterns of chronic tension • *Chiropractic:* Physically moving vertebrae or other joints into proper alignment, to relieve stress • *Osteopathy:* Realigning vertebrae, ribs, and other joints, as with chiropractic; osteopaths have training equivalent to that of medical doctors

Table 27-3 ALTERNATIVE TREATMENTS THAT WORK ON PAIN *continued*

TYPE	WHAT THEY HELP	HOW THEY HELP	EXAMPLES
Lifestyle Changes: Developing healthy habits at home and work	All types of chronic pain	By strengthening the immune system and enhancing well-being, and by reframing one's relationship to (and, thus, experience of) chronic pain	• *Sleep hygiene:* Creating an optimal sleep environment to get deep, restorative rest; strategies include establishing a regular sleep–wake schedule and minimizing light and noise. • *Positive work environment:* Having a comfortable workspace and control over one's activities to reduce stress and contribute to the sense of mastery over pain. • *Healthy relationships:* Nurturing honest and supportive friendships and family ties to ease anxiety that exacerbates pain. • *Exercise:* Regular activity to build strength and lower stress

Research shows these therapies can ease discomfort. For more information, visit the website of the National Center for Complementary and Alternative Medicine (www.nccam.nih.gov).

systems. The aim of Ayurvedic medicine is to integrate and balance the body, mind, and spirit. This is believed to prevent illness and promote wellness (NCCAM, 2009a).

Central to Ayurvedic medicine is an understanding of the patient's basic constitution, or **dosha**. The three doshas in Ayurvedic medicine are *vata* (changeable), *pitta* (intense), and *kapha* (relaxed). People can display one dosha predominately or a combination of two or three doshas. One's dosha can be equated with one's genetic make-up. A person whose doshas are balanced experiences health and well-being in mind, body, and spirit. Since each dosha has particular characteristics, when a dosha is out of balance, a person typically displays signs and symptoms (including disease) characteristic of the imbalance. Imbalance in the doshas can be caused by a number of factors, including stress, lifestyle, and improper diet.

Diagnosis is made by information obtained in a detailed holistic history, review of symptoms, and selected physical observations. Ayurveda includes mind–body medicine and biologically based practices. Many treatment modalities are specific for each dosha and may include nutrition, exercise, herbs, breathing, meditation, massage, aromatherapy, yoga, and purification. The quality of care received from an Ayurvedic practitioner can vary considerably based on the practitioner's educational preparation. A person can be certified as an Ayurvedic practitioner after attending a qualified 2-year program. In addition, there are prerequisites for background preparation.

Special considerations may be necessary for patients who want to continue their Ayurvedic program while hospitalized. For example, some people may have special dietary (e.g., vegetarian) needs, some may need time set aside for self-care such as meditation, and some may desire to continue taking an herbal supplement. All precautions related to herbal and pharmaceutical interactions should be followed when using Ayurvedic herbal preparations.

BOX 27-2 CAT DOMAINS

Whole (or alternative) medical systems are similar to the Western, allopathic model in that they are complete systems of theory and practice. They consist of a set of beliefs about the origin of diseases, ways to promote health, and types of treatment.

Mind–body medicine uses a variety of techniques designed to enhance the mind's ability to affect bodily function and symptoms.

Energy medicine involves the use of energy fields, such as magnetic fields or biofields (energy fields that some believe surround and penetrate the human body).

Manipulative and body-based practices work with the structures and systems of the body, including bones and joints, soft tissues, and circulatory and lymphatic systems.

Biologically based practices include the use of botanicals (herbs), animal-derived extracts, vitamins, minerals, fatty acids, amino acids, proteins, prebiotics and probiotics, whole diets, and functional foods.

Source: National Center for Complementary and Alternative Medicine, http://www.nccam.nih.gov.

YOGA

Yoga, one practice used in Ayurvedic medicine, is a mind and body practice with historical origins in ancient Indian philosophy. In the United States, yoga is practiced independently or paired with other health-promoting activities that assist people to achieve unity and wholeness. Generally, yoga consists of various physical postures that are practiced to promote strength and flexibility, increase endurance, promote relaxation, and reduce one's response to stress. Breathing exercises, posture awareness, spiritual practices, and mind–body centering can be added to the basic postures. Basic yoga postures are illustrated in Figure 27-1. Common types of yoga include:

- Ashtanga, which focuses on synchronizing breathing with a fast-paced series of postures
- Bikram, which is done in a studio heated to 105°F and involves 26 set postures

- Iyengar, which focuses on proper alignment and holding poses for a relatively longer time
- Kripaula, or "gentle yoga," which focuses on relaxation and coming into balance

Yoga can be used throughout the lifespan. Some postures are contraindicated during menstruation, after surgery, and in the presence of disease. Consumers can buy yoga videos or attend yoga classes. Yoga instructors come from a variety of backgrounds and usually are happy to discuss their preparation and knowledge with potential students. Encourage patients to find a type of yoga that is compatible with their physical condition and goals.

Traditional Chinese Medicine (TCM)

Underlying the practice of **traditional Chinese medicine (TCM)** is a unique view of the world and the human body

FIGURE 27-1. Sample yoga poses.

Gate pose

Down dog pose

Tree pose

Virabhadrasana I pose
(Warrior I pose)

Parivrtta trikonasana
(Revolved triangle pose)

that is different from Western medicine concepts. This view is based on the ancient Chinese perception of humans as microcosms of the larger surrounding universe—interconnected with nature and subject to its forces. The human body is regarded as an organic entity in which the various organs, tissues, and other parts have distinct functions but are all interdependent. In this view, health and disease relate to balance of the functions.

The theoretical framework of TCM has a number of key components:

- **Yin-yang theory**—the concept of two opposing, yet complementary, forces that shape the world and all life—is central to TCM.
- In the TCM view, a vital energy or life force called **qi** circulates in the body through a system of pathways called **meridians**. Health is an ongoing process of maintaining balance and harmony in the circulation of qi.
- The TCM approach uses eight principles to analyze symptoms and categorize conditions: cold/heat, interior/exterior, excess/deficiency, and yin/yang (the chief principles). TCM also uses the theory of five elements—fire, earth, metal, water, and wood—to explain how the body works; these elements correspond to particular organs and tissues in the body (NCCAM, 2010c).

The goal of the TCM diagnostic process is to arrive at the pattern of disharmony that is being manifested by the person. TCM practitioners obtain a holistic history; observe particular parts of the body, such as the tongue; and palpate pulses. TCM includes energy medicine and biology-based practices; treatment may consist of acupuncture, with or without moxibustion (burning an herb above the acupuncture needle), dietary prescriptions, herbs, massage, and energy exercises, such as qi gong. Accredited schools that provide TCM education require extensive college-level coursework followed by an educational program of about 4 years.

ACUPUNCTURE

Although records document the existence of traditional acupuncture treatments in China dating back 5,000 years, **acupuncture** has been prevalent in the United States only since the 1970s. Acupuncture gained national media attention in 1971 when James Reston, a correspondent for the *New York Times,* had an appendectomy in Beijing using acupuncture instead of general anesthesia and postoperative analgesia. Reston's reports of his experience stimulated significant interest in acupuncture and TCM.

 REMEMBER Lee Chen, the terminally ill patient whose daughters asked for an acupuncturist. When developing the plan of care, the nurse would need to investigate Mr. Chen's culture and examine the beliefs associated with acupuncture. Based on an understanding of this information, the nurse would be better prepared to advocate for the patient and daughters. •

FIGURE 27-2. Acupuncture meridians.

Acupuncture addresses a person's qi. Qi (chi in Japanese) is believed to flow vertically in the body through an intricate structure of 12 primary meridians, energy circuits that nourish and support all cells and organs of the body (Fig. 27-2). Acupuncture consists of placing very thin, short, sterile needles at particular acupoints, believed to be centers of nerve and vascular tissue, along a meridian (Fig. 27-3). Acupuncture either increases or decreases the flow of qi along the meridian, restoring the balance of yin and yang. This change in the flow of energy contributes to healing.

FIGURE 27-3. Placement of acupuncture needles.

CONSIDER Mr. Chen, the terminally ill patient whose daughters requested that he receive acupuncture. Applying the theory underlying acupuncture's mechanism of action, the nurse would understand that the daughters' request is based on their belief and desire for their father's condition to improve. The nurse would incorporate this understanding in discussions with the daughters about their father's condition. In addition, the nurse would also begin assisting the daughters to "let go" and begin the grieving process should the patient's condition remain unchanged, even after the acupuncture. ●

Acupuncture is used for a variety of reasons, including reducing pain, promoting adherence to substance abuse programs, and minimizing nausea and vomiting due to chemotherapy and pregnancy. Licensed acupuncturists have graduated from an accredited acupuncture school after significant college-level coursework. In addition, they have passed a licensure examination.

Acupuncture is generally provided in clinics or private offices, although it is possible for acupuncturists to provide acupuncture on inpatients. In this situation, patients may need up to 1 hour of uninterrupted time in bed while the needles are in place.

QI GONG AND TAI CHI

Qi gong is a system of postures, exercises (both gentle and dynamic), breathing techniques, and visualization that regulates the qi. The majority of qi gong exercises or meditations enhance systemic health. They are designed to restore the healing system, the body's innate intelligence, so it knows how to correct and heal itself. Qi gong postures are illustrated in Figure 27-4. For techniques specific to particular diseases, a patient can consult a qi gong teacher. Tai chi, a martial art, mind–body practice, which many say developed from qi gong, has been used successfully in patients in long-term care facilities to promote balance and coordination. A

review of scientific literature suggests that there is strong evidence of beneficial health effects of tai chi and qi gong, including for bone health, cardiopulmonary fitness, balance, and quality of life. Both tai chi and qi gong (also known as qigong) have origins in China and involve physical movement, mental focus, and deep breathing (NCCAM, 2010b). As with yoga, qi gong and tai chi can be learned through the use of videos or in a class. Encourage those interested to ask potential instructors about their background and knowledge.

Shamanism

Shamanism has been the most widely practiced medical system on our planet. Shamanism originated with indigenous people in many geographic areas of the world, including Hawaii, Ecuador, Tibet, West Africa, Israel, Peru, Colombia, and East Asia. In shamanism, illness and other forms of distress are thought to originate in the spirit world. The shaman or medicine man/woman possesses the ability to access the spirit world, which is done on behalf of people or the community, and return to "ordinary reality" with information on the proper treatment. Particular emphasis is on the classic shamanic journey, one of the most remarkable visionary methods used by humankind to explore the hidden universe otherwise known mainly through myth and dream. Treatment may consist of retrieving lost soul energy, restoring the person to the right relationship with the spirit world, and treating symptoms. General healing techniques involve native plants and herbs, animals, rituals, ceremonies, and purification techniques.

In the United States, many ethnic cultures commonly practice some form of shamanism, so the nurse needs to have an awareness of and tolerance for shamanic practice. For example, in the United States, traditional Hmong and Native American populations may have particular beliefs related to health and illness, and may practice specific ceremonies and rituals to properly care for the spirit of the deceased.

The American Cancer Society has a website that includes information about how different groups of people make treatment decisions. The website reports that the most common aspects of Native American healing include the use of herbal remedies, purifying rituals, shamanism, healing myths, and spiritual healing to treat illnesses of both the body and spirit. Traditional healers aim to "make whole" by restoring well-being and harmonious relationships with the community and the spirit of nature.

Nurses need to be aware of the beliefs of various ethnic groups. For example, Native American beliefs about healing include the following:

- Illness stems from spiritual problems.
- Diseases are more likely to invade the body of a person who is imbalanced, has negative thinking, and lives an unhealthy lifestyle.
- Spirit is an inseparable element of healing, and medicine is part of spirit.
- Healing takes time.
- The distractions of modern life interfere with potential healing agents.

FIGURE 27-4. Qi gong postures.

- Modern culture encourages us to maintain a low level of emotional awareness.
- Ceremony is important to receive guidance and assistance from the spiritual dimension.

Homeopathy

Samuel Hahnemann, a German physician, developed **homeopathy** approximately 200 years ago.

The allopathic approach to dealing with illness is frequently to suppress symptoms; for example, acetaminophen can be given to reduce a fever. In contrast, homeopaths believe that when symptoms are suppressed in this manner, the condition "goes deeper" into the body, making it ultimately more difficult to cure. Supporters of homeopathy point to two unconventional theories:

- "Like cures like": the notion that a disease can be cured by a substance that produces similar symptoms in healthy people
- "Law of minimum dose": the notion that the *lower* the dose of the medication, the *greater* its effectiveness. Many homeopathic remedies are so diluted that no molecules of the original substance remain.

Homeopathic remedies are derived from substances that come from plants, minerals, or animals, such as red onion, arnica (mountain herb), crushed whole bees, white arsenic, poison ivy, belladonna (deadly nightshade), and stinging nettle. Homeopathic remedies are often formulated as sugar pellets to be placed under the tongue; they may also be in other forms, such as ointments, gels, drops, creams, and tablets. Treatments are "individualized" or tailored to each person—it is not uncommon for different people with the same condition to receive different treatments. According to NCCAM, there is little evidence to support homeopathy as an effective treatment for any specific condition. Although people sometimes assume that all homeopathic remedies are highly diluted and therefore unlikely to cause harm, some products labeled as homeopathic can contain substantial amounts of active ingredients, thus could cause side effects and drug interactions (NCCAM, 2013a).

Naturopathy

Naturopathy is a relatively new system of medicine that began in the early 1900s in the United States. It evolved from a combination of traditional practices and health care approaches popular in Europe during the 19th century. "**Naturopathic medicine** is not only a system of medicine but also a way of life, with emphasis on client responsibility, client education, health maintenance, and disease prevention. It may be the model health system of the future with the movement toward healthy lifestyles, healthy diets, and preventive health care" (Fontaine, 2005, p. 173).

Naturopaths believe that health is a dynamic state of being that provides abundant energy for people to deal with life in our complex society. Much of illness can be attributed, at least in part, to ignoring "natural laws," such as engaging in a sedentary lifestyle without adequate time for exercise; exposing oneself to environmental toxins; eating processed, overcooked foods; engaging in negativity or harboring negative thoughts; and not getting adequate rest or relaxation.

The principles underlying the practice of naturopathy include (NCCAM, 2012b):

- *First do no harm.* Try to minimize harmful side effects and avoid suppression of symptoms.
- *Physician as teacher.* Educate patients and encourage them to take responsibility for their own health.
- *Treat the whole person.* Consider all factors (e.g., physical, mental, emotional, spiritual, genetic, environmental, social) when tailoring treatment to each patient.
- *Prevention.* Assess risk factors and, in partnership with patients, make appropriate interventions to prevent illness.
- *Healing power of nature.* Seek to identify and remove obstacles to the body's natural processes for maintaining and restoring health.
- *Treat the cause.* Focus on the causes of a disease or condition, rather than its symptoms.

NCCAM is careful to note, however, that "natural" does not necessarily mean "safe." Some therapies used in naturopathy, such as herbal supplements and restrictive or unconventional diets, have the potential to be harmful if not used under the direction of a well-trained practitioner.

Naturopathic physicians may have responsibility for their patients while they receive inpatient care in a hospital or other health care institution. Patients who are being treated by a naturopathic physician will probably have a different plan of care than those being treated by allopathic physicians.

Chiropractic Medicine

Chiropractic medicine is a health care profession that focuses on the relationship between the body's structure—mainly the spine—and its functioning. Although practitioners may use a variety of treatment approaches, they primarily perform adjustments (manipulations) to the spine or other parts of the body with the goal of correcting alignment problems, alleviating pain, improving function, and supporting the body's natural ability to heal itself. NCCAM reports that most research on chiropractic has focused on spinal manipulation. Spinal manipulation appears to benefit some people with low-back pain and may also be helpful for headaches, neck pain, upper- and lower-extremity joint conditions, and whiplash-associated disorders. Chiropractors may combine the use of spinal adjustments and other manual therapies with several other treatments and approaches such as (NCCAM, 2012a):

- Heat and ice
- Electrical stimulation
- Relaxation techniques
- Rehabilitative and general exercise
- Counseling about diet, weight loss, and other lifestyle factors
- Dietary supplements

Doctors of chiropractic medicine (DC) are licensed and attend 4 years of chiropractic school after prerequisite coursework. At this time, most chiropractic treatment is conducted on outpatients. A good understanding of chiropractic medicine will allow you to answer patients' questions and ask questions about a patient's current treatments. This knowledge also helps you to be able to refer patients asking questions about chiropractic medicine to reliable sources of information.

 RECALL Brian Legett, the patient with chronic back problems who has experienced little relief and is asking about seeing a chiropractor. When responding to Mr. Legett, the nurse would need to explain the underlying principles of chiropractic science. In addition, the nurse, in conjunction with other health care team members involved in the patient's plan of care, would need to review the patient's history thoroughly to identify (if possible) the underlying cause of his back problems and the various treatments attempted. This review would be important in determining if a referral to a chiropractor would be appropriate. •

Mind–Body Modalities

Most people acknowledge that there is a strong mind–body connection. Common everyday occurrences indicate that some connection does indeed exist. For example, students may experience insomnia related to anxiety the night before a major examination or suffer a migraine headache triggered by a fight with a spouse or good friend. Recent research has expanded our knowledge of how the mind and body communicate with each other.

Knowing how this communication between the mind and body occurs assists in the understanding of the mind–body modalities of relaxation, meditation, and imagery. These three therapies can be useful for patients as well as self-care for nurses.

 THINK back to Sylvia Puentes, the anxious preoperative patient. The nurse would need to incorporate an understanding of the mind–body connection when discussing possible suggestions for anxiety relief. •

The scientific field of psychoneuroimmunology (PNI) studies neurochemicals such as neuropeptides that are now believed to be the messenger molecules that connect the body and mind. Neuropeptides have properties that allow them to affect neurologic and physiologic tissue receptors. Many neuropeptide receptor sites lie along the gastrointestinal tract; this explains why people can experience a large variety of gastrointestinal symptoms in response to emotional situations. Neuropeptides are produced as needed and travel through all spaces of the body in blood as well as other body fluids. Because they frequently travel and act quickly and are produced only as needed, there is as yet no way to measure them in the body.

Benson (1975) studied the **relaxation response** extensively. Dossey and Keegan (2013) described this response as "an alert, hypokinetic process of decreased sympathetic

nervous system arousal that may be achieved in a number of ways, including through breathing exercises, relaxation and imagery exercises, biofeedback, and prayer. A degree of discipline is required to evoke this response, which includes mental and physical well-being" (p. 328).

Relaxation

Relaxation techniques promote parasympathetic activity, helping to reduce sympathetic activity and restore the balance of the two systems.

Sympathetic system dominance, characterized by increased epinephrine levels in the body, can contribute to symptoms such as hypertension, cool hands and feet, tight muscles, increased heart rate, and increased respiratory rate (Dossey & Keegan, 2013). The ultimate goal is to increase the parasympathetic system influence in the mind–body and thus reduce the effect of stress and stress-related illness on the body.

Relaxation can be useful whether a patient is experiencing a single stressful event, such as surgery, or chronic stress. Patient benefits include reduced anxiety, reduced muscle tension and pain, improved functioning of the immune system, enhanced sleep and rest, and an improved overall sense of well-being.

Dossey and Keegan (2013) discussed several relaxation techniques, including meditation and modern relations methods such as progressive muscle relaxation, autogenic training, biofeedback, body scanning, and hypnosis. Because these modalities are quite different, the type of relaxation modality chosen needs to be individually suited to the patient.

 RECALL Mr. Chen, the terminally ill patient described in the Reflective Practice display. When developing the plan of care, the nurse needs to include the patient's daughters. Therefore, when interacting with the patient's daughters, the nurse would also assess their stress level as they cope with their father's deteriorating condition. This assessment could provide valuable information about the cultural beliefs and values of each daughter, leading the nurse to suggest possible culturally appropriate methods for relaxation. •

Nurses can assist patients to begin to achieve a relaxation response by focusing on their breathing. Patients can breathe into a stressful or painful area, lengthen their breathing, or focus on abdominal or diaphragmatic breathing. Benson (1975) found it helpful to use a mental device such as a repetitive phrase to remind the body to relax.

Nurses can also practice relaxation as part of their self-care, enabling them to better deal with personal and work-related stress. Relaxation exercises can be done anywhere, at any time, and without cost. Numerous relaxation guides and CDs are available online. Some of the benefits of relaxation for the nurse and holistic nursing practice follow. Relaxation (Dossey and Keegan, 2013, p. 331):

• Cultivates a centered, calm practice
• As a self-care practice offers insights into challenges and benefits patients will experience

- Offers a vehicle to modulate and self-regulate the nurse's own stress response in stress-filled work settings
- Supports a therapeutic energetic bond and connectedness when practicing with patients or colleagues
- Creates opportunity for intuitive exploration, insight, and understanding of self and others, issues, and problems—an essential dimension of reflective practice
- Can be a spiritual practice for opening ourselves to deeper ways of being

Meditation

Meditation has been part of many spiritual and healing traditions for hundreds of years. Meditation refers to a group of techniques, such as mantra meditation, relaxation response, mindfulness meditation, and Zen Buddhist meditation. In meditation, a person learns to focus attention. Some forms of meditation instruct the practitioner to become mindful of thoughts, feelings, and sensations and to observe them in a nonjudgmental way. This practice is believed to result in a state of greater calmness and physical relaxation, as well as psychological balance. Practicing meditation can change how a person relates to the flow of emotions and thoughts.

Most types of meditation have four elements in common (NCCAM, 2010a):

- *A quiet location:* Meditation is usually practiced in a quiet place with as few distractions as possible. This can be particularly helpful for beginners.
- *A specific, comfortable posture:* Depending on the type being practiced, meditation can be done while sitting, lying down, standing, walking, or in other positions.
- *A focus of attention:* Focusing one's attention is usually a part of meditation. For example, the meditator may focus on a mantra (a specially chosen word or set of words), an object, or the sensations of the breath. Some forms of meditation involve paying attention to whatever is the dominant content of consciousness.
- *An open attitude:* Having an open attitude during meditation means letting distractions come and go naturally without judging them. When the attention goes to distracting or wandering thoughts, they are not suppressed; instead, the meditator gently brings attention back to the focus. In some types of meditation, the meditator learns to "observe" thoughts and emotions while meditating.

Patients seeking inpatient care might have a meditation practice they want to continue. Nurses can provide the time necessary for this. Nurses could benefit from a meditation practice as well, and could experience a brief meditation during breaks from patient care activities.

Guided Imagery

Guided imagery focuses on evoking pleasant images to replace negative or stressful feelings and to promote relaxation. Children with leukemia first used guided imagery in the 1970s as an adjunct to chemotherapy. These children imagined their white blood cells "gobbling up" the cancer cells.

Imagery involves using all five senses to imagine an event or body process unfolding according to a plan. When all senses are involved in the experience, the imaginary situation is more fully encoded in the body and more likely to take place. A relaxation technique is frequently used to prepare the mind and body before beginning an imagery session. Research studies have demonstrated that imagery assists patients with AIDS and cancer to extend their lives, as well as enhance their quality of life. You can assist clients with imagery in several ways:

- Many kinds of imagery recorded material with scripts are available that patients can use independently. If some of these are available on the nursing unit, patients can determine what types of recorded material they would like to use or purchase. Patients can also be assisted to write a script and record it for their own use.
- Nurses can work with patients using "outcome imagery," which might consist of using a picture or photograph to visualize the desired outcome in a body part or in a situation. Patients can add to the visual cue and develop a total image.
- During a painful or stressful event, such as an intravenous line being started, the patient can "go to a favorite place" and imagine being there with all the pleasant experiences related to that space.

 THINK back to Sylvia Puentes, the anxious patient scheduled for surgery. Any of these types of imagery techniques would be appropriate suggestions for the patient. However, the nurse needs to assess the patient's preferences, beliefs, and ability to participate in these techniques to determine the best recommendation. ●

The American Holistic Nurses Association (AHNA) endorses the Nurses Certificate Program in Imagery. Visit the Internet Resources on thePoint website for information.

Prayer

According to the NCCAM, when prayer is included in the definition of CAT, the domain of mind–body medicine is the most commonly used domain (53%). **Intercessory prayer** involves praying for the benefit of another person to the Judeo-Christian God. Dossey (1993) thoroughly explored this subject, exploring areas such as beliefs about prayer, the process of praying, and whether a physician's beliefs are important in the healing relationship. This area can be controversial and needs to be explored with patients using sensitivity and cultural knowledge. Additional information and nursing considerations are covered in Chapter 45, Spirituality.

Aromatherapy

Aromatherapy using essential oils was practiced in ancient Egypt and India more than 6,000 years ago. Oils were used in religious ceremonies, for medicinal purposes, and in perfumes and cosmetics. Today, one cannot go to a shopping mall without seeing scented candles and various other "aromatherapy" products.

Medicinally, aromatherapy is the use of essential oils of plants as a therapy to improve physical, emotional, and spiritual well-being. The fragrance of these oils is believed to ultimately affect the very sensitive amygdala of the limbic system in the brain, where emotional memories are stored and released. Laboratory and animal studies have shown that certain oils have antibacterial, antiviral, antifungal, calming, and energizing effects. Commonly used essential oils in a health care setting are ginger or peppermint for nausea and lavender or chamomile for insomnia. Essential oils vary in quality and potency depending on the manufacturing processes. If specific essential oils are approved for use in an inpatient setting, provide education on these oils. Some people are highly sensitive to strong fragrances, particularly concentrated essential oils. This might preclude their use in some patient settings.

Certification in Aromatherapy for Health Professionals is available. This course is endorsed by AHNA, and information is available in the Internet Resources found on thePoint website.

Energy Medicine Modalities

Without realizing it, you may have heard a person talk about energy. The terms "resonance" ("I really resonate with you") and "wavelength" ("We are on the same wavelength") were used in Einstein's theory of physics. Today, Einstein's theory of physics, or energy theory, has been added to the sciences of biology and chemistry to express ideas about health and illness as well as to explain the human organism (Gerber, 2001).

All organisms are dependent on a subtle vital force that creates order in the system (Gerber, 2001). This vital force has been known to healing systems and people in various cultures for centuries and has been called a variety of names throughout history, such as vital life force (general usage), *pneuma* (ancient Greece), *qi* or *chi* (China and Japan), and *pran* (India). Many traditions consider this subtle energy to reflect the spiritual nature of people and to refer to individuals as mind, body, and spirit.

This life force feeds and nourishes the organism and is carried via two energetic structures that interact with each other: chakras and the etheric body. **Chakras** are concentrated areas of energy aligned vertically in the body that relate to each other as well as to specific areas of the body, mind, and spirit. Different traditions present different numbers of chakras. An **aura** (Fig. 27-5) is a vague, luminous glow surrounding something that may be an information-containing electromagnetic field, which can be likened to the data contained within a computer (Dossey and Keegan, 2013, p. 751). There is scientific evidence that following conception, energetic structures are the first to develop and, in some cases, serve as templates for cellular and organ development (Gerber, 2001). This finding supports the expression, "We are energy first." Energy therapies used for healing are based on the belief that they can affect this primary life force and thus contribute to physiologic healing.

FIGURE 27-5. First four layers of the human aura.

— Etheric or vital layer
— Emotional layer
— Mental layer
— Intuitive or spiritual layer (also called the astral body)

The North American Nursing Diagnosis Association (NANDA) recognizes disturbed energy field as a nursing diagnosis. Defining characteristics of the disturbed field relate to movement, sounds, temperature change, visual changes, and disruption. There are many forms of energy work that seek to reduce disturbance in the energy field. Qi gong and acupuncture were discussed earlier in the chapter; additional therapies are discussed in the next section.

Therapeutic Touch

Therapeutic touch (TT), founded by Delores Krieger in the 1970s, is the use of the hands on or near the body with the intent to help or heal. The TT process consists of centering, assessing the energy field, and rebalancing the field using modulation, "unruffling," and other techniques (Krieger, 1993).

TT uses four primary scientific premises (Krieger, 1993, pp. 12–13):

1. All the life sciences agree that, physically, a human being is an open energy system.
2. Anatomically, a human being is bilaterally symmetrical.
3. Illness is an imbalance in a person's energy field.
4. Human beings have natural abilities to transform and transcend their conditions of living.

Workshops and other learning opportunities are available for nurses to learn energy healing techniques. Energy work can assist patients in virtually all settings and all age groups, although advanced knowledge is necessary to work with babies and other vulnerable populations.

Registered nurses can become credentialed in TT. Details are available on the Nurse Healers Web site (see Internet Resources on thePoint website).

Healing Touch

Healing Touch (HT), founded by Janet Mengten in the 1980s, uses a collection of energy techniques to assess and treat the human energy system, thus effecting physical, emotional, mental, and spiritual health and healing. The current HT textbook contains about 20 specific energy techniques to be used in particular patient situations. The goal of HT is to restore wholeness through harmony and balance (Hover-Kramer, 2011). The Healing Touch Program lists the following benefits of HT:

- *Non-Invasive.* Healing touch is done without the use of invasive procedures such as injections, inserting tubes, medication, or surgery.
- *Effective.* Research has shown that healing touch facilitates the relaxation response and enhances the healing process.
- *Non-Toxic.* Medications can cause side effects and must be monitored. Healing touch restores balance and harmony to our natural biofield without the use of pharmaceuticals.
- *Economical.* Healing touch does not require the use of equipment or substances and can be done in any setting. An open heart, a set of hands, and a willing spirit is all that is needed (http://www.healingtouchprogram.com)

HT energy techniques have been collected from well-known healers as well as shamanic and aborigine traditions. Instructors certified by Healing Touch International teach these techniques in three or more leveled workshops.

Box 27-3 describes when HT can be used. Certification in HT for people from various backgrounds is available through Healing Touch International after completion of a series of classes and experiences. The program is endorsed by AHNA, and class information is available on the AHNA website.

Sound Healing

Sound is an ancient form of healing. Examples include the central importance of drum and flutes for American Indians and Tibetan bowls, which are used to simulate chakras (Dossey and Keegan, 2013). Music helps many to relax and is increasingly used in hospice to comfort the dying.

Music can be used to promote healing in several ways. Patients can listen to their favorite music prior to surgery or other stressful events, during imagery, and while relaxing. Music is frequently played in operating rooms and harp or piano music is played in patient lounges and lobbies.

BOX 27-3 WHEN HEALING TOUCH CAN BE USED

- To stimulate wound healing
- To relieve pain
- To reduce anxiety and stress
- To energize the auric field
- To promote health
- To assist patients before and after medical treatments and procedures such as surgery
- To support the dying process

 REMEMBER Sylvia Puentes, the anxious preoperative patient described at the beginning of the chapter. Based on an assessment of the patient's likes and dislikes, the nurse might suggest music therapy as a means to reduce the patient's preoperative anxiety. •

Biologically Based Practices

Botanical agents (herbs) and nutritional supplements are chemical compounds that are ingested with the hope of achieving a therapeutic goal. They are becoming increasingly popular with consumers, who can buy many of these preparations over the counter or from company distributors. Currently, dietary supplements (which include herbs and nutritional supplements) are considered foods, thus manufacturers need to follow FDA labeling requirements. Some product sample analyses have revealed inconsistencies in the amount of active ingredients. Because of these inconsistencies as well as for other reasons, in 2004 the Institute of Medicine issued a report (IOM, 2005) recommending a framework for cost-effective and science-based evaluation of dietary supplements by the FDA.

Botanicals (Herbal Products) and Nutritional Supplements

Some consumers and practitioners are attracted to herbs because they are "natural" plant products, which are perceived as more compatible with the body than manufactured pharmaceutical agents. In fact, some pharmaceutical agents (e.g., Digitalis) were first produced as natural products derived from plants and now are produced chemically.

In many countries, herbal products are regulated and available through the primary health care system. In Germany, for example, "Commission E" reviews scientific data and establishes prescriptive standards for pharmaceuticals, including conventional drugs and plant products used for healing. In the United States, FDA classifies herbs as a food and not a drug. This is important because herbs are not regulated for quality and potency as drugs are, and herbal formulas can be sold without being studied to see if they are helpful or harmful.

Many whole medical systems use herbs in their system. Alternatively, herbs can be used for treatment of disease and reduction of symptoms. Echinacea and goldenseal (separately or in combination) are frequently used for respiratory infections, and ginkgo biloba is frequently used to dilate cerebral blood vessels and reduce symptoms of memory loss and mental confusion.

Nutritional supplements are chemical compounds that contain ingredients (vitamins, minerals, enzymes, amino acids, essential fatty acids) believed to promote health. These products have a wide range of safety and effectiveness.

Increasing numbers of patients are using herbs and supplements. Nurses need to be aware of the various products available and provide education to patients to ensure safety with their use (Teaching Tips 27-1 on page 744).

TEACHING TIPS 27-1

USING HERBS AND SUPPLEMENTS

Teaching Tip	Why Is This Important?
Get information from knowledgeable and reliable sources.	Advertising media and many sources on the Internet frequently seek primarily to sell the product, not educate the consumer.
Buy name-brand products that are produced by reputable companies to increase your chances of getting a high-quality product.	Since this industry is not regulated, contamination and inconsistency in the amount of product sometimes occur.
The word "standardized" on an herbal product means that it consistently contains the percentage of the herb stated on the label.	A standardized product means that it contains a certain amount of active ingredient.
Whenever possible, buy single products.	If the product contains several ingredients and you have a reaction or positive response, you won't know which ingredient was the causative agent.
Take the proper dose and monitor side effects.	Herbal remedies are natural medicines and can be toxic in higher-than-recommended doses.
Give the product adequate time to work.	Herbs frequently take longer to produce a therapeutic effect than allopathic preparations.
Become knowledgeable about the product and your reason for using it.	Consumers who initiate any type of self-care tend to make better decisions if they are well informed.

Modified from Fontaine, K. L. (2005). *Healing practices* (2nd ed., pp. 136–137). Upper Saddle River, NJ: Prentice-Hall.

Extensive specialized education is required before a nurse can be competent to advise patients on the use of herbs and supplements. However, nurses are finding that information about certain herbs adds an aspect of safety to their practice. For example, some herbs and/or supplements may interact with prescribed medications patients are taking. Ginkgo biloba, the most widely sold herb in Europe and used by many to improve memory, affects platelet function, thus should not be used concurrently with warfarin or aspirin. Some nursing pharmacology courses include information on commonly used herbs. Women who are pregnant or nursing and children should be especially cautious about using herbal supplements either alone or in mixtures, since these products can act like drugs.

"Natural" does not mean safe. For example, the herbs kava and comfrey have been linked to serious liver damage.

Nutritional Therapy

The eating habits of people in the United States are being scrutinized because of the alarming increase in obesity, particularly in children, and chronic illnesses in all age groups. The so-called typical American diet—consisting of prepared and processed foods and large amounts of meat, dairy products, and sugar—is highly suspect.

People with a variety of credentials have endorsed many popular eating plans that purport to address these health problems. The diversity of these approaches is understandably very confusing to the consumer. Although an examination of these popular diets is beyond the scope of this book, it does appear that people have individual needs and preferences with respect to foods. In fact, this belief has been a cornerstone of holistic nutritional approaches for centuries in the TCM and Ayurvedic systems (see also Chapter 35). Teaching Tips 27-2 provides guidelines for teaching about holistic approaches to food choices. It is common to find many of these approaches endorsed by naturopathic practitioners.

Manipulative and Body-Based Practices

This group of therapies includes therapeutic massage—an assortment of techniques that involve manipulation of soft tissues of the body through pressure and movement, as well as a variety of techniques such as Rolfing, shiatsu, Feldenkrais, Alexander, myofascial release, and others. The goal is to break up tension held in body structures, promote communication between mind–body structures, promote detoxification, and generally improve body functioning. Some of these therapies can be painful while they work to oxygenate tissues, break up lymphatic congestion, release muscle tightness, and promote circulation. These therapies require specialized preparation and are typically useful in rehabilitation or health-promotion types of settings.

NURSING IMPLICATIONS OF CAT

The development of CAT continues to be a market-driven and, in some respects, a patient-driven phenomenon. Many

TEACHING TIPS 27-2

HOLISTIC APPROACHES TO FOOD CHOICES

Teaching Tip	Why Is This Important?
Reduce amounts of processed foods.	Processing frequently reduces the nutrients available for absorption. For example, canned foods frequently have lower nutritional values than frozen foods.
Reduce/eliminate soft drinks (carbonated/sugar-sweetened beverages).	They are "fake food" and have no nutritional value.
Avoid eating foods with preservatives.	Preservatives are artificial substances that the body ultimately needs to excrete, usually through the urine or feces. This excretion process diverts energy the body could use for other processes.
Reduce intake of refined and natural sugars.	The "average" individual in the United States consumes an unhealthy amount of glucose. Among other things, excess glucose places an increased demand on the pancreas, kills the natural bacterial flora found in the gastrointestinal tract that is necessary for absorption, and interferes with cellular absorption of nutrients.
Reduce intake of artificial sweeteners, including aspartame.	Since aspartame is not a food, it needs to be excreted, and there is some evidence that it is toxic to humans. In some countries (Japan), aspartame is extensively regulated. Replace aspartame with stevia, a natural sweetener available in liquid or granulated form.
Eat organically grown foods.	If grown according to rigorous organic regulations, these foods contain no pesticides or chemical byproducts, which are toxins in the body.
Reduce intake of dairy products.	Many dairy cows are regularly given antibiotics and, in some cases, hormones. Breakdown products from these substances may be found in milk.
Consider adopting a vegetarian diet.	Animals are increasingly fed antibiotics and potentially contaminated foods. Increasingly, fish are being contaminated with mercury and other pollutants.
Eat foods in season.	Foods produced "out of season" are treated with chemicals to ripen them since they are picked before ripening.
Be aware of genetically engineered, radiated food.	Become informed about these processes before you make a decision as to whether you want to eat these foods.

patients/consumers are unsatisfied with allopathic treatments and are turning to CAT for relief of symptoms and healing. Since health care currently operates on a business model, it is probable that more CAT will become available to deal with real or perceived market needs. Third-party payers do not cover many of these therapies, which means that consumers must pay out of pocket for them. In addition, government and professional groups do not regulate most of the therapies. Because of this lack of regulation, there can be inconsistencies among the preparation and care provided by practitioners.

There is a great opportunity here for nurses to expand their practice to meet existing patient needs, as well as to promote health. See Focused Assessment Guide 27-1: Holistic Care (on page 746) for an identification of areas in which a holistic nurse can improve patient care. As new therapies demonstrate their effectiveness, they can be added to the assessment.

Nursing is expanding its knowledge base to include information that explains selected CAT. For example, pharmacology courses in schools of nursing frequently include information on herbs. Certifications in basic holistic nursing for nurses with a baccalaureate degree and in advanced holistic nursing for nurses with a master's degree are available through the American Holistic Nurses' Certification Corporation (AHNCC). It is expected that CAT will become a larger part of practice for some nurses. See the accompanying Research in Nursing (on page 746) and PICO in Practice boxes (on page 747).

Patient education about CAT is essential. Patients and the public need to know about the safe and effective use of CAT. Numerous resources exist to educate health care professionals and the public. The NCCAM health topics page is always a good place to start. For information about how to evaluate web-based health resources, check out the websites found in the Internet Resources on thePoint website.

FOCUSED ASSESSMENT GUIDE 27-1

HOLISTIC CARE

Factors to Assess	Questions and Approaches
Stress	What measures does the patient use to reduce stress? If the patient wants to continue a meditation, relaxation, or imagery practice while receiving care, explore ways in which that can be accomplished.
Music/sound preferences	What preferences does the patient have for music or environmental sounds (e.g., ocean waves, birds) either while meditating or relaxing? Music could be provided by the patient if preferred music is not available.
Diet	What dietary preferences does the patient have (e.g., vegetarian, no processed foods)? Communicate these preferences to nutritional services.
Environmental sensitivity	Is the patient sensitive to environmental odors or fragrances? If so, can an air purifier be brought to the room?
Use of herbs and supplements	Is the patient taking any herbs or supplements as directed by a CAT practitioner or purchased over the counter? If so, obtain the names of the herbs/supplements, dosages, and reasons for their use. If these substances are in the patient's possession, follow applicable institutional policies.
Use of CAT health care provider	Is the patient planning to use a primary CAT provider while receiving allopathic care? If so, convey appropriate information to the primary allopathic provider.

RESEARCH IN NURSING

BRIDGING THE GAP TO EVIDENCE-BASED PRACTICE

Hatha Yoga and Zen Meditation

Stress is considered a crucial trigger for physical and mental illness. Many therapies are helpful in reducing stress but we still need research to demonstrate best practices.

Hatha Yoga: Related Research

Huang, F.-J., Chien, D.-K., & Chung, U.-L. (2013). Effects of Hatha yoga on stress in middle-aged women. *Journal of Nursing Research*, *21*(1), 59–66.

This study investigated the comparative effectiveness of a single 90-minute Hatha yoga class and an 8-week, 90-minute-class-per-week course on stress reduction. Subjects were 63 female community residents, randomly divided into an experimental and control group. The experimental group received the Hatha yoga class. After a single 90-minute class of Hatha yoga, experimental group perceived stress scale scores were significantly less than those of the control group ($p = .001$) and heart rate variability was significant. These findings support the position that regular, long-term practice of Hatha yoga provides clear and significant health benefits. Participation in a single 90-minute Hatha yoga class can significantly reduce perceived stress. Doing Hatha yoga regularly can reduce perceived stress even more significantly.

Zen Meditation: Related Research

Lu, C.-F., Smith, L. N., & Gau, C.-H. (2012). Exploring the Zen meditation experiences of patients with generalized anxiety disorder: A focus group approach. *Journal of Nursing Research*, *20*(1), 43–52. doi: 10.1097/JNR.0b013e3182466e83

Most of the many studies on the efficacy of meditation on anxiety disorders over the past half century have been quantitatively studied and lacked consensus. Studies into the experiences of meditation practitioners are lacking. Taiwan has a high prevalence of generalized anxiety disorders (GAD), and Zen meditation is popular there. The study site was a psychiatric outpatient department in a general hospital in Taiwan. Two groups of adult patients with GAD ($n = 9$) and without any kind of meditation experience ($n = 12$) enrolled in and attended a Zen meditation program. Results: A major theme, "The process of Zen meditation," emerged. It was underpinned by the three categories: "struggling to reach a state of calm," "signs of improvement," and "an individual process." Signs of improvement included "finding a personal way to enter a state of calm," "changing the sense of time," and "adjusting Zen meditation practice goals." Findings provide a better understanding of essential elements of Zen meditation complementing quantitative studies and may be used by professionals who intend to apply Zen meditation as an alternative therapy for patients with GAD.

Implications for Nursing

Both of these studies are significant in that they demonstrate culturally sensitive effective therapies for reducing stress among the Taiwanese. Since both Hatha yoga and Zen medication are popular practices in Taiwan, nurses can now confidently employ these therapies in their practice. U.S. nurses will want to replicate the studies to see if these therapies prove as effective in reducing stress and anxiety in the United States.

PICO IN PRACTICE

ASKING CLINICAL QUESTIONS

Scenario: You are a staff nurse who works in an outpatient oncology clinic, a position that you have held for the past 8 months. You are also a licensed massage therapist, and practiced massage therapy at a health spa for several years before going back to school to study nursing. Over the course of the past several months, you note that many of the patients who come to the clinic for chemotherapy complain of stress and sleep disorders. You believe that implementing massage techniques with some of these patients could help improve their sleep patterns.

- POPULATION: Patients with cancer who receive chemotherapy in a clinic
- INTERVENTION: Therapeutic massage
- COMPARISON: None
- OUTCOME: Improved sleep patterns

PICO Question: Can therapeutic massage result in improved sleep patterns in patients with cancer who receive chemotherapy in an oncology clinic?

From the Oncology Nursing Society (ONS): Oncology Nursing Society Putting Evidence into Practice (PEP) (2013). ONS PEP research evidence table: Sleep-wake disturbance. Available at www.ons.org/Research/PEP/media/ons/docs/research/outcomes/sleep/table-of-evidence.pdf

Evidence from this table notes multiple limitations of four studies conducted with patients with cancer who received therapeutic massage. Results from these studies do not clearly advocate that therapeutic massage improves sleep in patients with cancer, though it apparently does not cause any undue effects or harm to them.

Level of Evidence: Level III

Recommendation: You make an appointment to meet with your facility's nurse researcher to ask if it is advisable to conduct a pilot study with a small group of patients treated at your clinic to determine whether therapeutic massage improves their sleep patterns.

DEVELOPING CLINICAL REASONING

1. You are caring for a culturally diverse population. How would you appropriately assess for and implement CAT into your nursing care, simultaneously demonstrating respect for your patients' beliefs and preferences while honoring your commitment to evidence-based nursing/medicine?

2. The family of a woman dying of cancer approaches you with a brown paper bag of ground herbs and asks you to mix them with the patient's next tube feeding. They are very upset that she isn't healing and believe the herbs might help. How do you respond and what is the basis for your response? Talk with other students about what they would do and compare your responses.

3. A nurse who practices therapeutic touch tells you that she finds it very helpful for all sorts of patients. When you press her for details, you learn that she even practices this technique on patients without their consent while they are sleeping. Are you troubled by this? Is patient consent needed for CAT in the same way it is needed for allopathic treatments?

4. A patient brings you a clipping from the December 11, 2011 *Chicago Times* with an article by Trine Tsouderos. "Thanks to a $374,000 taxpayer-funded grant, we now know that inhaling lemon and lavender scents doesn't do a lot for our ability to heal a wound. With $666,000 in federal research money, scientists examined whether distant prayer could heal AIDS. It could not. The National Center for Complementary and Alternative Medicine also helped pay scientists to study whether squirting brewed coffee into someone's intestines can help treat pancreatic cancer (a $406,000 grant) and whether massage makes people with advanced cancer feel better ($1.25 million). The coffee enemas did not help. The massage did." He asks you how he can know "what works?" How do you reply?

PREPARING FOR NCLEX

1. At a follow-up visit, a patient recovering from a myocardial infarction tells the nurse: "I feel like my life is out of control ever since I had the heart attack. I would like to sign up for yoga, but I don't think I'm strong enough to hold poses for long." What would be the nurse's best response?
   a. "Right now you should concentrate on relaxing and taking your blood pressure medicine regularly, instead of worrying about doing yoga."
   b. "There is a slower-paced yoga called Kripaula that focuses on coming into balance and relaxation that you could look into."
   c. "Ashtanga yoga is a gentlepaced yoga that would help with your breathing and blood pressure."
   d. "Yoga is contraindicated for patients who have had a heart attack."

2. A nurse is providing a lecture on CAT to a group of patients in a rehabilitation facility. Which teaching point should the nurse include?
   a. CAT is a safe intervention used to supplement traditional care.
   b. Many patients use CAT as outpatients, but do not wish to continue as inpatients.
   c. Many nurses are expanding their clinical practice by incorporating CAT to meet the demands of patients.
   d. Most complementary and alternative therapies are relatively new and their efficacy has not been established.

3. A nurse mentor is teaching a new nurse about the underlying beliefs of CAT vs. allopathic therapies. Which statements by the new nurse indicate that teaching was effective? Select all that apply.
   a. "CAT proponents believe the mind, body, and spirit are integrated and together influence health and illness."

b. "CAT proponents believe that health is a balance of body systems: mental, social and spiritual, as well as physical."

c. "Allopathy proponents believe that the main cause of illness is an imbalance or disharmony in the body systems."

d. "Curing according to CAT proponents seeks to destroy the invading organism or repair the affected part."

e. "The emphasis is on disease for allopathic proponents and drugs, surgery, and radiation are key tools for curing."

f. "According to CAT proponents, health is the absence of disease."

4. A nurse is caring for a patient who has crippling rheumatoid arthritis. Which nursing intervention best represents the use of integrative care?

a. The nurse administers Naproxen (Aleve) and uses guided imagery to take the patient's mind off the pain.

b. The nurse prepares the patient's physician-approved herbal tea and uses meditation to relax the patient prior to bed.

c. The nurse administers Naproxen (Aleve) and performs prescribed range-of-motion exercises.

d. The nurse arranges for acupuncture for the patient and designs a menu high in Omega-3 fatty acids.

5. A nurse works for a physician who practices the naturopathic system of medicine. What is the focus of nursing actions based on this type of medical practice? Select all that apply.

a. Treating the symptoms of the disease

b. Providing patient education

c. Focusing on treating individual body systems

d. Making appropriate interventions to prevent illness

e. Believing in the healing power of nature

f. Encouraging patients to take responsibility for their own health

6. A nurse cares for patients in a chiropractic office. What patient education might this nurse perform? Select all that apply.

a. Applying heat or ice to an extremity

b. Explaining the use of electrical stimulation

c. Teaching a patient relaxation techniques

d. Teaching a patient about a prescription

e. Explaining an invasive procedure to a patient

f. Teaching about dietary supplements

7. A nurse is caring for a postoperative patient who is experiencing pain. Which CAT involves active participation by the patient and is effective for pre- or postoperative pain control?

a. Acupuncture

b. Therapeutic touch

c. Botanical supplements

d. Guided imagery

8. A nurse is guiding a patient in the practice of meditation. Which teaching point is most useful in helping the patient to achieve a state of calmness, physical relaxation, and psychological balance?

a. Teach the patient to always lie down in a comfortable position during meditation.

b. Teach the patient to focus on multiple problems that the patient feels demand attention.

c. Teach the patient to let distractions come and go naturally without judging them.

d. Teach the patient to suppress distracting or wandering thoughts to maintain focus.

9. A nurse working in a long-term care facility incorporates aromatherapy into her practice. For which patient would this nurse use the herb ginger?

a. A patient who has insomnia

b. A patient who has nausea

c. A patient who has dementia

d. A patient who has migraine headaches

10. A nurse manager who works in a hospital setting is researching the use of energy healing to use as an integrative care practice. Which patient would be the best candidate for this type of CAT?

a. A patient who is anxious about residual pain from cervical spinal surgery

b. A patient who is experiencing abdominal discomfort

c. A patient who has chronic pain from diabetes

d. A patient who has frequent cluster headaches

ANSWERS WITH RATIONALES

1. *b.* Kripaula, or "gentle yoga," focuses on relaxation and coming into balance. Ashtanga focuses on synchronizing breath with a fast-paced series of postures. The nurse should not discourage the use of yoga in patients who are healthy enough to participate. Yoga is not contraindicated in patients with controlled high blood pressure.

2. *c.* Many nurses are expanding their clinical practice by incorporating CAT. Although CAT may seem totally safe, some therapies have led to harmful and at times lethal outcomes. Many patients use these types of therapies as outpatients and want to continue their use as inpatients. Although the use of most complementary and alternative therapies predates modern medicine, it was not until recently that nursing and medical schools began to teach about their use.

3. *a, b, e.* With CAT, mind, body, and spirit are integrated and together influence health and illness, and illness is a manifestation of imbalance or disharmony. Allopathic beliefs include: the main causes of illness are considered to be pathogens (bacteria or viruses) or biochemical imbalances, curing seeks to destroy the invading organism or repair the affected part, and emphasis is on disease and high technology. Drugs, surgery, and radiation are among the key tools for dealing with medical problems. According to allopathic beliefs, health is the absence of disease.

4. *a.* Adding guided imagery (CAT) to the administration of pain medications (allopathy) is an example of integrative care. A person who uses integrative care uses some combination of allopathic medicine and CAT.

5. *b, d, e, f.* Naturopathic medicine is not only a system of medicine, but also a way of life, with emphasis on client responsibility, client education, health maintenance, and disease prevention. Its principles include minimizing harmful side effects and avoiding suppression of symptoms, educating patients and encouraging them to take responsibility for their own health, treating the whole person, preventing illness, believing in the healing power of nature, and treating the cause of a disease or condition rather than its symptoms.

6. *a, b, c, f.* Chiropractors may combine the use of spinal adjustments and other manual therapies with several other

treatments and approaches including heat and ice, electrical stimulation, relaxation techniques, rehabilitative and general exercise, counseling about weight and diet, and using dietary supplements. Chiropractors do not prescribe medication or perform invasive procedures.

7. **d.** Imagery involves using all five senses to imagine an event or body process unfolding according to a plan. A patient can be encouraged to "go to a favorite place." With the other modalities, the patient is more passive.

8. **c.** Meditators should have an open attitude by letting distractions come and go naturally without judging them. They should also maintain a specific, comfortable posture lying down, sitting, standing, walking, etc.; focus attention on a mantra, object, or breathing; and not suppress distracting or wandering thoughts, instead they should gently bring attention back to focus.

9. **b.** Commonly used essential oils in a health care setting are ginger or peppermint for nausea and lavender or chamomile for insomnia.

10. **a.** Energy healing is focused on pain that lingers after an injury heals, as well as pain complicated by trauma, anxiety, or depression. Nutritional and herbal remedies treat all chronic pain, but especially abdominal discomfort, headaches, and inflammatory conditions, such as rheumatoid arthritis.

TAYLOR SUITE RESOURCES

Explore these additional resources to enhance learning for this chapter:

- NCLEX-Style Questions and other resources on thePoint, http://thePoint.lww.com/Taylor8e
- *Study Guide for Fundamentals of Nursing, 8th edition*
- Adaptive Learning | Powered by prepU, http://thepoint.lww.com/prepu

Bibliography

Achterberg, J. (1985). *Imagery in healing: Shamanism and modern medicine.* Boston: Shambhala.

Adams, I., & Tovey, P. (2007). *Complementary and alternative medicine in nursing and midwifery: Towards a critical social science.* New York: Routledge.

American Association of Retired Persons (AARP), National Center for Complementary and Alternative Medicine (NCCAM). (2011). Complementary and Alternative Medicine: What People Aged 50 and Older Discuss With Their Health Care Providers. Available at http://assets.aarp.org/rgcenter/health/complementary-alternative-medicine-nccam.pdf

American Cancer Society (ACS). Native American Healing. (2008) Available at http://www.cancer.org/docroot/ETO/content/ETO_5_3X_Native_American_Healing.asp?sitearea=ETO

Barnes, P. M., Powell-Griner, E., McFann, K., & Nahin, R. L. (2004). Complementary and alternative medicine use among adults: United States, 2002. Advance data from vital and health statistics; no. 343. Hyattsville, MD: National Center for Health Statistics.

Barnes, P. M., Bloom, B., & Nahin, R. (2008). CDC National Health Statistics Report #12. Complementary and Alternative Medicine Use Among Adults and Children: United States, 2007. Available at nccam.nih.gov/news/camstats/.

Benson, H. (1975). *The relaxation response.* New York: William Morrow & Co.

Benson, H. (1984). *Beyond the relaxation response.* New York: Times Books.

Denner, S. S. (2008). The evolving doctrine of informed consent for complementary and integrative therapy. *Holistic Nursing Practice, 22*(1), 37–43.

Dossey, B. M., & Keegan, L. (2013). *Holistic nursing. A handbook for practice* (6th ed.). Burlington, MA: Jones & Bartlett Learning.

Dossey, L. (1993). *Healing words.* New York: HarperCollins.

Eisenberg, D. M., Davis, R. B., Ettner, S. L., Appel, S., Wilkey, S., Van Rompay, M., et al. (1998). Trends in alternative medicine use in the United States, 1990–1997. *New England Journal of Medicine, 280*(18), 1569–1575.

Eisenberg, D. M., Kessler, R. C., Foster, C., Norlock, F. E., Calkins, D. R., & Delbanco, T. L. (1993). Unconventional medicine in the United States. *New England Journal of Medicine, 328*(4), 246–252.

Ernst, E. (2006). Acupuncture—a critical analysis. *Journal of Internal Medicine, 259*(2), 125–137.

Fenton, M.V. & Morris, D.L. (2003). The integration of holistic nursing practices and complementary and alternative modalities into curricula of schools of nursing. *Alternative Therapies in Health and Medicine, 9*(4), 62–67.

Fontaine, K. L. (2005). *Healing practices* (2nd ed.). Upper Saddle River, NJ: Pearson Education.

Fontaine, K.L. (2010). *Complementary & alternative therapies for nursing practice* (3rd ed.). Upper Saddle River, NJ: Prentice Hall.

Freeman, L. (2004). *Mosby's complementary & alternative medicine.* St. Louis: Elsevier/Mosby.

Frisch, N., Dossey, B., Guzzetta, C., & Quinn, J. (2000). *AHNA standards of holistic nursing practice: Guidelines for caring and healing.* Gaithersburg, MD: Aspen Publishers.

Frisch, N. (2001). Standards for holistic nursing practice: A way to think about our care that includes complementary and alternative modalities. *Online Journal of Issues in Nursing, 6*(2), Manuscript 4.

Gerber, R. (2000). *Vibrational medicine for the 21st century.* New York: HarperCollins.

Gerber, R. (2001). *Vibrational medicine* (3rd ed.). Rochester, VT: Bear & Company.

Horrigan, B. (1996). Janet Quinn, RN, PhD: Therapeutic Touch and a healing way. *Alternative Therapies in Health and Medicine, 2*(4), 69–75.

Horrigan, B. (1999). Michael Murray, ND: A natural approach to health. *Alternative Therapies in Health and Medicine, 5*(2), 77–84.

Horrigan, B. (2003). Ken Cohen, MA, MSTH: Healing through ancient traditions: Qigong and Native American medicine. *Alternative Therapies in Health and Medicine, 9*(3), 83–91.

Hover-Kramer, D. (2002). *Healing Touch. A guidebook for practitioners.* Albany, NY: Delmar.

Hover-Kramer, D. (2011). Healing Touch. Essential energy medicine for yourself and others. Boulder, CO: Sounds True, Inc.

Institute of Medicine, Committee on the Use of Complementary and Alternative Medicine by the American Public. (2005). Complementary and alternative medicine (CAM) in the United States. Washington, DC: National Academy Press.

Krieger, D. (1993). *Accepting your power to heal.* Santa Fe, NM: Bear & Company.

National Cancer Institute (NCI). (2010). Acupuncture (PDQ). Available at http://www.cancer.gov/cancertopics/pdq/cam/acupuncture.

National Cancer Institute (NCI) Office of Cancer Complementary and Alternative Medicine. (n.d.) Talking about Complementary and Alternative Medicine with Health Care Providers: A Workbook and Tips. Available at http://cam.cancer.gov/attachments/workbook/talking_about_cam_workbook.pdf

National Center for Health Statistics. (2007). National health interview survey (NHIS): 2007 data release. Available at http://www.cdc.gov/nchs/about/major/nhis/nhis_2007_data_release.htm.

National Center for Complementary and Alternative Medicine (NCCAM). (2005). Expanding horizons of health care: Strategic plan 2005–2009. Available at http://nccam.nih.gov/about/plans/2005

National Center for Complementary and Alternative Medicine (NCCAM). (2009a). Ayurvedic medicine.

NCCAM Pub No. D287. Available at http://nccam.nih.gov/health/ayurveda/introduction.htm

National Center for Complementary and Alternative Medicine (NCCAM). (2009b). Time to talk. Available at http://nccam.nih.gov/timetotalk/

National Center for Complementary and Alternative Medicine (NCCAM). (2010a). Meditation: an introduction. NCCAM. Pub No: D308. Available at http://nccam.nih.gov/health/meditation/overview.htm

National Center for Complementary and Alternative Medicine (NCCAM). (2010b). Research Spotlight: tai chi and qi gong show some beneficial health effects. Available at http://nccam.nih.gov/research/results/spotlight/071910.htm

National Center for Complementary and Alternative Medicine (NCCAM). (2010c). Traditional Chinese medicine. NCCAM Pub No. D428. Available at http://nccam.nih.gov/health/whatiscam/chinesemed.htm

National Center for Complementary and Alternative Medicine (NCCAM). (2012a). Chiropractic: An Introduction. NCCAM Pub No. D403. Avialable at http://nccam.nih.gov/health/chiropractic/introduction.htm

National Center for Complementary and Alternative Medicine (NCCAM). (2012b). Naturopathy: An Introduction. NCCAM Pub No. D372. Available at: http://nccam.nih.gov/health/naturopathy/naturopathyintro.htm

National Center for Complementary and Alternative Medicine (NCCAM). (2013a). Homeopathy: An Introduction. NCCAM Pub No. D439. Available at: http://nccam.nih.gov/health/homeopathy

National Center for Complementary and Alternative Medicine (NCCAM). (June 2013b). Yoga for health. NCCAM Pub No. D472. Available at: http://nccam.nih.gov/health/yoga/introduction.htm

National Center for Health Statistics. (2008). National Health Interview Survey (NHIS): Public-use data release. NHIS survey description. Available at ftp://ftp.cdc.gov/pub/Health_Statistics/NCHS/Dataset_Documentation/NHIS/2007/srvydesc.pdf

Pert, C. (1999). *Molecules of emotion: The science behind mind–body medicine.* New York: Simon & Schuster.

Rossman, M. L. (2000). *Guided imagery for self-healing.* Tiburon, CA: H. J. Kramer.

Seskevich, J. E., Crater, S. W., Lane, J. D., & Krucof, M. W. (2004). Beneficial effects of noetic therapies on mood before percutaneous intervention for unstable coronary syndromes. *Nursing Research, 53*(2), 116–121.

Sparber, A. (2001). State boards of nursing and scope of practice of registered nurses performing complementary therapies. *Online Journal of Issues in Nursing, 6*(2), 6–7.

U.S. Food and Drug Administration (FDA). (2013). 6 tip-offs to rip-offs: Don't fall for health fraud scams. Available at http://www.fda.gov/ForConsumers/ConsumerUpdates/ucm341344.htm.

Weil, A. (1988). *Health and healing.* Boston: Houghton Mifflin.

28 Medications

REGINA SAUDER

Regina, a 73-year-old woman with a history of lymphoma, has presented to the emergency department with pain, swelling, and erythema (redness and inflammation) of her left calf. She has been diagnosed with a left leg deep vein thrombosis (DVT). She is receiving intravenous heparin and oral warfarin. When she is discharged, she will need to have weekly blood testing to ensure therapeutic levels of the warfarin.

MILDRED CAMPBELL

Mildred, a 65-year-old woman with a history of arthritis and hypertension (high blood pressure), comes to the clinic for evaluation of her painful joints. She states, "I just saw this new medicine advertised on television that is supposed to be really helpful in relieving joint pain. What do you think? Is it something I should try?"

FRANÇOIS BAPTISTE

François is an elderly man with a wound infection requiring intravenous antibiotic therapy. He is scheduled to receive his next dose at 10 AM. The medication delivered by the pharmacy is labeled with the correct drug and dose, but with a different patient's name.

After completing the chapter, you will be able to accomplish the following:

1. Discuss drug legislation in the United States.

2. Describe basic principles of pharmacology, including drug nomenclature and types of drug preparations.

3. Develop an understanding of basic principles of pharmacology, including mechanisms of drug action, adverse drug effects, and factors affecting drug action.

4. Discuss principles of medication administration, including an understanding of medication orders, dosage calculations, and medication safety measures.

5. Obtain patient information necessary to establish a medication history.

6. Describe principles used to prepare and administer medications safely by the oral, parenteral, topical, and inhalation routes.

7. Use the Nursing Process to safely administer medications.

8. Develop teaching plans to meet patient needs specific to medication administration.

KEY TERMS

absorption	intradermal injection	placebo
adverse drug effect	intramuscular injection	PRN order
allergic effect	intravenous route	stat order
ampule	medication reconciliation	subcutaneous injection
anaphylactic reaction	metabolism	synergistic effect
anaphylaxis	mini-infusion pump	teratogenic
antagonist effect	official name	therapeutic range
cumulative effect	parenteral	topical application
distribution	peak level	toxic effect
drug tolerance	pharmaco-dynamic	trade name
ethnopharma-cology	pharmaco-kinetics	trough level
excretion	pharmacology	vial
generic name	pharmaco-therapeutics	volume-control administration set
half-life		
idiosyncratic effect	piggyback delivery system	Z-track technique
inhalation		

A drug or medication is any substance that modifies body functions when taken into the body. The study of drugs and their effect on the body's functioning is called **pharmacology**. A pharmacist is a person licensed to prepare and dispense drugs. Physicians, dentists, psychiatrists, podiatrists, physician assistants, and advance practice nurses have prescriptive authority. Prescriptive authority for advance practice nurses (clinical nurse specialists, nurse practitioners, certified nurse anesthetists, nurse midwives) and physician assistants varies in the degree of independence and the medications that may be prescribed from state to state. Nurses must be familiar with the laws relative to prescriptive authority in their state of practice. The prescriber conveys medication plans to others by an order called a prescription. In a hospital or other health care facility, after the pharmacist prepares the medication, the nurse administers the medication to the patient. This chain provides a check-and-balance system for medication administration. If an error is made when the order is written, the pharmacist or nurse administering the medication has the opportunity to note the discrepancy. If an error occurs when the pharmacy dispenses the medication, the administering nurse has the opportunity to note this discrepancy. See the accompanying Reflective Practice box on pages 752–753 for an example.

Medication administration is a basic nursing function that involves skillful technique and consideration of the patient's development, health status, and safety. The nurse administering medications needs to have a knowledge base about drugs, including drug names, preparations, classifications, adverse effects, and physiologic factors that affect drug action. Information about specific drugs is available in pharmacology texts and drug reference books. Computer programs and electronic databases are available for up-to-date medication information. Nurses must have sufficient knowledge about the drugs being administered to safely care for their patients. The Joint Commission (TJC) has made several recommendations regarding safe practice when administering medications. Up-to-date information about these recommendations can be found at www.jointcommission.org/PatientSafety/NationalPatientSafetyGoals/.

The nursing process can be applied to medication administration. Assessment includes a comprehensive medication history, awareness of the patient's allergies, and patient assessment, as well as ongoing assessments of the patient's response during and after medication administration. Nursing diagnoses are developed from the assessment data. Patient-centered outcomes are evaluated after implementation of the plan of care and are tailored to the patient's needs.

PRINCIPLES OF PHARMACOLOGY

An overview of basic pharmacology includes drug nomenclature, types of drug preparations, drug classification, drug indication, mechanisms of drug action, adverse drug effects, and factors affecting drug action, as well as drug blood level monitoring and pertinent U.S. drug legislation.

REFLECTIVE PRACTICE: CULTIVATING QSEN COMPETENCIES

CHALLENGE TO ETHICAL AND LEGAL SKILLS

During my clinical rotation for complex care a few weeks ago, I met François Baptiste, an elderly man with a wound infection requiring intravenous antibiotic therapy. He was due for a certain IV antibiotic to be hung at 1000. When I checked his drawer at 0800 and 0900, the antibiotic was not there. However, the nurse I was working with told me not to call pharmacy about it yet since the pharmacy staff often comes and replaces the drawers in the medication carts before 1000 anyway. So, I didn't call pharmacy. Sure enough, a pharmacy representative came up that hour and changed the medication drawers. At 1000, I went to look in my patient's drawer. What I found confused me a great deal! Yes, the bag of medication was in there. Yes, it was the right drug and the right dose. However, it was the wrong patient! The label on the bag in my patient's drawer had another patient's name on it. I looked up information on that other patient, and it turned out he was also a patient on the unit. This patient was also receiving the same drug at the same dose but at a different time. I wondered if I should hang this bag for my patient because he was due for it, even though it had someone else's name and medical record number on the label. It was, after all, the same drug and the same dose.

Thinking Outside the Box: Possible Courses of Action

- Change the patient's name on the label and hang the bag.
- Call pharmacy to ask about the mix-up. If the bag did, indeed, contain the same medication at the same dose, then change the patient's name on the label and hang it for my patient.
- Check the other patient's medication administration record (MAR) to confirm that he is, indeed, receiving the same drug at the same dose as my patient, and if so, use this bag for my patient (since it is in my patient's drawer and my patient is due for it).
- Ask my nurse and/or preceptor what to do. Is it okay, safe, and legal to use this bag if someone else's name is on the label? If they say yes, check with the nurse caring for the patient whose name is on the label to make sure she does not need the medication right now.
- Send the bag back to pharmacy, requesting they send up a new one with an accurate label.
- Call pharmacy, ask them to send up a new bag with an accurate label, and tell them I am giving the other bag to the other patient's nurse.

Evaluating a Good Outcome: How Do I Define Success?

- The right patient receives the right drug, at the right dose, at the right time, via the right route, with the right documentation, understanding the right rationale.
- The patient feels comfortable and safe with the drug being administered to him.
- The needs of my patient and those of the patient whose name was on the bag are assessed and met. Both patients have the medication available to them when they need it and are due for it.
- My education and my license, along with that of my nurse and preceptor, are not put at risk by an avoidable medication error.
- My legal skills are sharpened by thinking through and working through the situation.

Personal Learning: Here's to the Future!

Ultimately, I addressed the situation step by step to make sure all the bases were covered. First, I checked the other patient's drawer to see if he had a bag of this IV antibiotic. He did not, which led me to believe that either his bag was placed in my drawer by accident, or his bag had not been made yet (that the bag in my patient's drawer was intended for my patient but had the wrong label on it). Then I checked my patient's MAR and that of the other patient. Indeed, both were ordered to receive the same drug at the same dose via the same route. However, my patient was due for it at 1000, the other patient was due for it at 1400. Next, I brought the medication bag, the MARs, and my other paperwork to my clinical preceptor and to the nurses caring for my patient and the other patient. They all agreed that the bag that was in my drawer was the right drug at the right dose, even though it had the wrong name on the label. However, it is not the nurse's responsibility or legal right to dispense medication. For this reason, the bag of medication needs to be returned to the pharmacy because it was labeled with the wrong name. The pharmacist must re-label the medication, preparing and dispensing a correctly labeled dose for each patient. I called the pharmacy, explained what I had found, and told them I would be returning the dose that had been delivered to my patient. I requested a correct dose for 1000 for my patient.

The pharmacy delivered a new bag of medication, correctly labeled, in time for the patient's 1000 dose. After checking everything again, I administered the medication to my patient. My patient did not have an adverse reaction, the other patient got his medication when it was due, and no mistakes were made by any of the nurses. The only mistake that was made was by pharmacy, which put the wrong label on the bag and then put the bag in the drawer.

I learned that checking and double-checking medication labels is extremely important. After a while, we all have a tendency to get into the habit of glancing at things when we are in a hurry, especially when it involves labels we look at all the time, feeling confident that we would recognize a problem. This is not the first time I could have missed a change on the label—there have been several times when I did not think to check every single thing on a label. That's because after giving it so many times, I felt it had become routine. But every time I am tempted not to double-check a label, I am reminded of this situation. As a result, I triple-check things, because those are the times when I may not be paying as close attention as I need to be. I do not think my professional legal skills are quite as adequate as they need to be. Because I do not have my license yet, I am not quite as driven to protect it by knowing all the laws pertinent to nurses as I should or

REFLECTIVE PRACTICE: CULTIVATING QSEN COMPETENCIES *continued*

CHALLENGE TO ETHICAL AND LEGAL SKILLS

will be. However, as a student nurse, I am careful to avoid any mistakes that could place me in jeopardy legally for areas of which I *am* aware. In addition, I am always careful to protect my education and my future as a nurse by not doing things about which I am uncertain. I always ask my preceptor or my nurse for help or advice when I need it. Moreover, I have carried professional liability malpractice insurance since the day I started nursing school, fearing for the financial viability of my life and my future. Therefore, while my legal skills probably need some work, they are certainly not terrible, and my skills and I are moving in the right direction.

Tracey Sara Miller, Georgetown University

REFLECTION ON QUALITY AND SAFETY COMPETENCIES

How do you think you would respond in a similar situation? Why? What does this tell you about yourself and about the adequacy of your skills for professional practice? Do you agree with the criteria to evaluate a successful outcome? Did the nursing student validate the rationale for the outcome? What *knowledge, skills, and attitudes* do you need to develop to continuously improve the quality and safety of care for patients like Mr. Baptiste?

Patient-Centered Care: Would it have been appropriate for the nursing student to change the name on the label? Why or why not? How did the nursing student's actions adhere to ethical and legal principles? Did the nursing student act as an advocate for Mr. Baptiste?

Teamwork and Collaboration/Quality Improvement: What communication skills do you need to improve to ensure that you communicate appropriately in situations like this? What communication skills do you need to improve to ensure that you could address this issue as a member of the patient-care team? How can you ensure that this event

is used to prevent similar issues in the future to improve the patient's quality of care?

Safety/Evidence-Based Practice: How can you communicate observations or concerns related to hazards and errors to patients, families, and the health care team? What is your role in preventing errors? What legal principles did the nursing student adhere to with the described actions? Suppose the nursing student had given the medication without double checking all of the information. What legal principles might have been violated? What evidence in nursing literature provides guidance for decision making regarding care of this patient? What does this tell you about yourself and about the adequacy of your skills for professional practice?

Informatics: Can you identify the essential information that must be available in Mr. Baptiste's electronic health record to support safe patient care and coordination of care? What information should be documented in the electronic health record regarding the student's assessment and interventions? Can you think of other ways to respond to or approach the situation?

Drug Nomenclature

Drugs have several names, including chemical, generic, official, and trade names. The chemical name is a precise description of the drug's chemical composition. The chemical name identifies the drug's atomic and molecular structure using exact chemical language and terminology. The **generic name**, which identifies the drug's active ingredient, is the name assigned by the manufacturer that first develops the drug. Often, the generic name is derived from the chemical name. The generic name is not owned by any drug company and is universally accepted. The **official name** is the name by which the drug is identified in the official publications, United States Pharmacopeia and National Formulary (USP and NF). The official name is often the generic name. The **trade name**, also referred to as the brand name or proprietary name, is selected by the pharmaceutical company that sells the drug and is protected by trademark. A drug can have several trade names when produced by different manufacturers.

Nurses should be familiar with a drug's generic and trade names. For example, acetaminophen (generic name) has trade names such as Tylenol, Tempra, and Liquiprin. Recognizing a drug's name is an important part of the nurse's

responsibilities when transcribing orders and administering medication therapies.

Types of Drug Preparations

Drugs are available in many forms, or preparations. The form in which the drug is prepared may determine the route of administration. Drug preparations are available for oral, topical, and parenteral administration. Some drugs may be prepared in only one form to be administered by a certain route. Others may be supplied in several preparations, allowing them to be given through various routes. One type of preparation may be desirable in a given situation. For example, a liquid preparation of a medication would be indicated for a young child who cannot swallow solid preparations, such as tablets. A suppository may be indicated to deliver a medication for a patient who cannot take anything by mouth. Table 28-1 (on page 754) describes drug preparations commonly used by nurses.

Drug Classifications

Drug classifications, or drug classes, are groups of drugs that share similar characteristics. Drugs are classified in several ways. For example, drugs may be classified by effect on

Table 28-1 COMMON TYPES OF DRUG PREPARATIONS

PREPARATION	DESCRIPTION
Capsule	Powder or gel form of an active drug enclosed in a gelatinous container; may also be called liquigel
Elixir	Medication in a clear liquid containing water, alcohol, sweeteners, and flavor
Enteric coated	A tablet or pill coated to prevent stomach irritation
Extended release	Preparation of a medication that allows for slow and continuous release over a predetermined period; may also be referred to as CR or CRT (controlled release), SR (sustained or slow release), SA (sustained action), LA (long acting), or TR (timed release)
Liniment	Medication mixed with alcohol, oil, or soap, which is rubbed on the skin
Lotion	Drug particles in a solution for topical use
Lozenge	Small oval, round, or oblong preparation containing a drug in a flavored or sweetened base, which dissolves in the mouth and releases the medication; also called *troche*
Ointment	Semisolid preparation containing a drug to be applied externally; also called an *unction*
Pill	Mixture of a powdered drug with a cohesive material; may be round or oval
Powder	Single or mixture of finely ground drugs
Solution	A drug dissolved in another substance (e.g., in an aqueous solution)
Suppository	An easily melted medication preparation in a firm base such as gelatin that is inserted into the body (rectum, vagina, urethra)
Suspension	Finely divided, undissolved particles in a liquid medium; should be shaken before use
Syrup	Medication combined in a water and sugar solution
Tablet	Small, solid dose of medication, compressed or molded; may be any color, size, or shape; *enteric-coated tablets* are coated with a substance that is insoluble in gastric acids to reduce gastric irritation by the drug
Transdermal patch	Unit dose of medication applied directly to skin for diffusion through skin and absorption into the bloodstream

body systems (e.g., drugs that affect the respiratory system, drugs that affect the cardiovascular system), by chemical composition, or by the clinical indication for the drug or therapeutic action (e.g., analgesic, antibiotic). Knowledge related to the class of drug can be applied to individual drugs in that class.

Drug Indication

Pharmacotherapeutics is the achievement of the desired therapeutic goal from drug therapy. It is the clinical purpose (the indication) for administering a drug (Aschenbrenner & Venable, 2012). Understanding the desired outcome of administering a drug is an important part of nursing responsibilities related to medication administration. Nurses are legally responsible for understanding the pharmacotherapeutics of all drugs they administer (Aschenbrenner & Venable, 2012). This knowledge is required to enable the nurse to assess the appropriateness of the medication, as well as provide appropriate and accurate patient education.

Mechanisms of Drug Action

Pharmacokinetics

Pharmacokinetics is the effect of the body on the drug, once the drug enters the body. It is the movement of drug molecules in the body in relation to the drug's absorption, distribution, metabolism, and excretion.

ABSORPTION

Absorption is the process by which a drug is transferred from its site of entry into the body to the bloodstream. Absorption of a drug is influenced by the following factors.

Route of Administration

The rate of absorption depends on the route of administration. Drugs given orally usually take the longest to be absorbed. Injected medications are usually absorbed more rapidly than oral medications. Drugs administered intravenously are placed directly into the bloodstream, thus technically are not absorbed and take effect quickly (Aschenbrenner & Venable, 2012). Many drugs, such as eye drops, eardrops, nasal sprays, respiratory inhalations, and transdermal drugs, have little absorption; the action of these drugs is mostly local, at the site of administration (Kee, Hayes, & McCuistion, 2012).

Lipid Solubility

Cell membranes have a fatty acid layer. A drug that is more lipid soluble can be absorbed more readily and pass more easily through the cell membrane.

pH

Acidic drugs are well absorbed in the stomach. Drugs that are basic remain ionized or insoluble in an acid environment. These drugs are not absorbed before reaching the small intestine. The concept of acid–base balance is further discussed in Chapter 39.

Blood Flow

Absorption is increased with increased blood flow. Patients with impaired circulatory function absorb drugs less rapidly than do patients with normal circulatory function.

Local Conditions at the Site of Administration

The more extensive the absorbing surface, the greater the absorption of the drug and the more rapid the effect. For example, a patient with burns would have poor absorption from an intramuscular injection. Food in the stomach can delay the absorption of some medications or enhance the rate of absorption of other drugs. Drug absorption can be manipulated with sustained-release preparations or enteric-coated preparations. Enteric-coated preparations are resistant to the digestive action of the stomach. Contact time also affects absorption. If a drug is not in contact with the absorption site for a specific period of time, the drug will not be completely absorbed. Patients with alterations in intestinal function, such as those with diarrhea, may experience decreased absorption from a drug due to increased peristalsis, resulting in a decreased amount of time the drug is in contact with intestinal mucosa (Janda & Fagan, 2010).

Drug Dosage

A loading dose, or a larger than normal dose, is usually given when a patient is in acute distress and the maximum therapeutic effect is desired as quickly as possible. If drug toxicity occurs, it can be detected quickly and treated in the controlled hospital environment. A maintenance dose is a lower dosage that becomes the usual or daily dosage. Patients who receive digoxin or phenobarbital, for example, may receive loading doses when therapy is initiated. The goal of drug dosing is to give a dose that achieves the desired therapeutic effect of the drug (pharmacotherapeutics) without causing other undesirable effects (*adverse effects,* discussed later; Aschenbrenner & Venable, 2012).

DISTRIBUTION

Distribution occurs after a drug has been absorbed into the bloodstream and the drug is distributed throughout the body, becoming available to body fluids and body tissues. Distribution depends on blood flow to the tissues, the drug's ability to leave the bloodstream, and the drug's ability to enter the cells (Aschenbrenner & Venable, 2012). Certain other factors may also influence distribution. The drug may bind to plasma proteins, which causes unequal distribution and prevents the drug from reaching its intended site of action. Another factor affecting distribution is the blood–brain barrier. The blood–brain barrier is a structure made up of tightly packed capillary walls that supply blood to the brain. It prevents toxins and poisons from reaching the brain. Unfortunately, many drugs cannot penetrate the barrier, obviously influencing distribution. Some drugs fail to penetrate the tissues of the central nervous system as readily as others. The placenta, on the other hand, is an ineffective barrier. Drugs readily move across the placenta, and many drugs produce harmful effects in the fetus. These factors must be considered when planning and implementing drug therapies. Any concern about the safe use of a medication during pregnancy can be identified in a pharmacology text, through consultation with a pharmacist, or from trusted comptuer programs and electronic databases.

METABOLISM

Metabolism, or biotransformation, is the change of a drug from its original form to a new form. The liver is the primary site for drug metabolism. Various processes and enzymes are involved in metabolism. Most drugs are inactivated by the liver and transformed to inactive substances for excretion (discussed in the next section). Physiologic changes associated with aging, the presence of liver disease, or other factors that impair the functioning of the liver decrease its ability to metabolize drugs. Other tissues, such as those of the gastrointestinal tract, lungs, kidney, and skin, also have a role in drug metabolism (Aschenbrenner & Venable, 2012).

Some drugs move from the intestinal lumen to the liver by way of the portal vein and do not go directly into the systemic circulation following oral absorption. This is called the first-pass effect, or hepatic first pass. Some drugs are metabolized by the liver to an inactive form, reducing the amount of active drug left in the body. Other drugs do not undergo metabolism at all in the liver, and others may be metabolized to an active drug metabolite (another form), and may be more active than the original drug. Warfarin (Coumadin) is an example of a drug with first-pass metabolism. Some drugs with extensive first-pass effect, like lidocaine, are not given orally because most of the drug would be destroyed, with little or no drug left to work in the body (Kee et al., 2012, p. 4). Pharmacology texts provide more detailed explanations of the metabolism of drugs.

EXCRETION

After the drug is broken down to an inactive form, **excretion** of the drug occurs. Excretion is the process of removing a drug, or its metabolites (products of metabolism), from the body. The kidneys excrete most drugs. The lungs are the primary route for the excretion of gaseous substances, such as inhalation anesthetics. Many drugs are excreted through bile in the gastrointestinal tract. The sweat, salivary, and mammary glands are also routes of drug excretion.

Some medications may be contraindicated, or dosages may need to be adjusted, if renal excretion is impaired. Changes associated with aging, disease, or the presence of other factors that impair the functioning of the kidneys can decrease their ability to excrete drugs. Manufacturers are required by law to include specific information regarding implications for geriatric patients on the package inserts of certain drugs. Of particular concern are details concerning the excretion of these drugs in older adults whose renal function has declined. This law affects psychotropic drugs, nonsteroidal anti-inflammatory agents (NSAIDs), oral hypoglycemic agents, anticoagulants, certain broad-spectrum antibiotics, and cardiac drugs.

Pharmacodynamics

Drugs act at the cellular level to achieve the desired effects. The process by which drugs alter cell physiology and affect the body is called **pharmacodynamics** (Aschenbrenner & Venable, 2012). Drugs turn on, turn off, promote, or block responses that are part of the body's processes. One mechanism of drug action is a drug–receptor interaction, in which the drug interacts with one or more cellular structures to alter cell function. These specialized structures are called receptor sites. The drug fits the receptor as a key fits a lock. Drugs may also combine with other molecules in the body to achieve their effect. For example, a drug may combine with an enzyme to achieve the desired effect, which is referred to as a drug–enzyme interaction. Other drugs act on the cell membrane or alter the cellular environment to achieve their effect.

Adverse Drug Effects

Although therapeutic effect is the desired outcome in medication administration, sometimes secondary undesirable effects occur. Undesirable effects other than the intended therapeutic effect of a drug are known as **adverse drug effects** (Tabloski, 2010; Aschenbrenner & Venable, 2012).

Some adverse effects are predictable and may be tolerated as part of the therapy. For example, morphine, an opioid agonist, is used to treat moderate to severe and chronic pain. A known adverse effect with morphine use is constipation. However, the benefit of pain relief usually outweighs the adverse effect of constipation, so that the adverse effect is often accepted and managed with stool softeners and laxatives. On the other hand, adverse effects can be severe and may require discontinuation of the drug, depending on whether the benefit of the drug outweighs the harm from the adverse effect. For example, a common adverse effect of morphine is nausea and vomiting. If uncontrollable and severe, persistent nausea and vomiting will result in discontinuation of the morphine and a switch to another type of pain medication.

Another example of an adverse drug effect is the development of an iatrogenic disorder caused unintentionally by drug therapy. Neutropenia caused by chemotherapy is an example of this. Other types of adverse effects to be discussed include allergic effects, drug tolerance, toxic effects, idiosyncratic effects, and drug interactions.

It is important for nurses and other health care professionals to monitor for adverse effects from drug therapy. Serious adverse reactions must be documented according to agency policy and should be reported to a national database, such as MedWatch. MedWatch is a safety information and voluntary adverse events reporting program, sponsored by the U.S. Food and Drug Administration (FDA). This program provides nationwide tracking of all serious adverse drug reactions, along with up-to-date information about medication errors and potential or actual medical-product problems and errors (Aschenbrenner & Venable, 2012). According to FDA criteria, a serious adverse drug event is defined as an action that is life threatening, requires intervention to prevent death or permanent impairment, and/or leads to death, hospitalization, disability, or congenital anomaly. Reporting of serious adverse effects is necessary for corrective action

to take place to protect patients. This information is used to revise drug labels, add warnings for health care providers, create patient medication guides, or withdraw a drug from the market (U.S. FDA, 2012c). Additional information regarding reporting adverse events is discussed at the end of the chapter, in the section on Preventing and Responding to Medication Errors.

Allergic Effect

An **allergic effect** is an immune system response that occurs when the body interprets the administered drug as a foreign substance and forms antibodies against the drug. Drug allergies can be manifested in a variety of symptoms ranging from minor to serious. The reaction can occur immediately after the patient receives the medication or be delayed for hours to days. Symptoms may become more severe each time the drug is introduced into the body. Some of the signs and symptoms of a drug allergy are rash, urticaria, fever, diarrhea, nausea, and vomiting. The most serious allergic effect is called an **anaphylactic reaction** (**anaphylaxis**). Anaphylaxis is life threatening and results in respiratory distress, sudden severe bronchospasm, and cardiovascular collapse. This reaction is treated with vasopressors, bronchodilators, corticosteroids, oxygen therapy, intravenous fluids, and antihistamines.

Drug Tolerance

Drug tolerance occurs when the body becomes accustomed to the effects of a particular drug over a period of time. Larger doses of the drug must be taken to produce the desired effect. For example, patients using morphine for an extended period of time become tolerant to the drug's therapeutic effects and eventually need higher and higher doses to control their pain.

Toxic Effect

Toxic effects (toxicities) are specific groups of symptoms related to drug therapy that carry risk for permanent damage or death (Aschenbrenner & Venable, 2012). The organ or system affected by the toxicity is used to name the toxicity, as in hepatotoxicity, or damage to the liver. Toxicities can occur from a **cumulative effect**. A cumulative effect occurs when the body cannot metabolize one dose of a drug before another dose is administered. The drug is taken in more frequently than it is excreted, and each new dose increases the total quantity in the body. Older patients are at risk for experiencing a cumulative effect, related to altered drug metabolism and elimination due to impaired hepatic metabolism and renal clearance related to normal changes with aging.

Idiosyncratic Effect

An **idiosyncratic effect** (sometimes called paradoxical effect) is any unusual or peculiar response to a drug that may manifest itself by overresponse, underresponse, or even the opposite of the expected response. Idiosyncratic effects are related to a patient's unique response to a drug and are thought to be the result of genetic enzyme deficiencies that lead to an abnormal mechanism of drug breakdown. Older patients often have unpredictable or erratic responses to medications.

Drug Interactions

Drug interactions occur when one drug is affected in some way by another drug, a food, or another substance that is taken at the same time. Drug interactions may be advantageous when, for example, a medication is given to decrease the adverse effects of a drug or increase its therapeutic effects. Other drug interactions are not beneficial: for example, interactions that decrease the therapeutic effect and/or increase the adverse effects. In a drug–drug interaction, the combined effect of two or more drugs acting simultaneously produces an effect either less than that of each drug alone (**antagonist effect**) or greater than that of each drug alone (**synergistic effect**). Alcohol and barbiturates, for example, when taken together create an unbeneficial synergistic effect with the potential for significantly increased central nervous system depression. It is important to be knowledgeable about, and alert for, drug interactions and the effects of drug therapy.

Drug interactions in older adults are a very real and dangerous problem because older adults are more likely to take more than one drug (Lorenz, 2010; Tabloski, 2010). Older patients often see more than one physician and do not always remember to bring the medications that they are taking to each physician they see. This leads to polypharmacy (the taking of more than two medications at a time), which can result in serious drug interactions.

 THINK back to Mildred Campbell, the 65-year-old woman with arthritis and hypertension (high blood pressure) asking about a recently advertised medication for joint pain relief. The nurse should assess the patient's medication history to determine her current medication regimen. This information is crucial to obtain so that the nurse can evaluate for possible polypharmacy and potential risks for drug interactions, even before discussing whether the advertised medication would be appropriate. ●

Dietary supplements and herbal and "natural" remedies are another potential problem area for drug interactions. Many patients do not consider dietary supplements and herbal and natural remedies to be medications because they can purchase these items at a store selling nutritional products, thus consider them safe to use. However, many of these products have recognized pharmacologic effects, unexpected allergic reactions, and problematic drug–supplement interactions (Marik & Flemmer, 2012; Dudek, 2010). When asking patients if they are taking any medications, specifically ask if they are taking any herbal or natural supplements. Health care providers need to be aware of the intended benefits, possible adverse effects, potential drug interactions, and perioperative implications related to these types of supplements. Further information related to dietary supplements and natural and herbal products can be found at the U.S.

Food and Drug Administration's website (www.fda.gov/AboutFDA/Transparency/Basics/ucm193949.htm) and the National Center for Complementary and Alternative Medicine (NCCAM) website (http://nccam.nih.gov/).

Factors Affecting Drug Action

Certain variables can influence the action or effect of a medication. These variables include developmental considerations, patient's body weight, patient's gender, genetic and cultural factors, psychological factors, pathology, environment, and timing of medication administration.

Developmental Considerations

During pregnancy, many drugs are contraindicated because of their possible adverse effects on the fetus. Certain drugs, referred to as **teratogenic**, are known to have the potential to cause developmental defects in the embryo or fetus and are definitely contraindicated. Examples of teratogenic drugs include cocaine, alcohol, phenytoin (Dilantin, an anticonvulsant), and isotretinoin (Accutane, a medication used to treat severe acne). Some drugs cross into breast milk, putting breastfed infants at risk for adverse effects from drugs in the mother's circulation. Small body size, reduced weight, and reduced body water also alter distribution, as do decreases in cardiac output and organ perfusion. Therefore, a child's medication dose is smaller than an adult's dose. Infants are especially sensitive to medications because of the immaturity of their organs and immaturity of the blood–brain barrier. Older people are sensitive to medications because their bodies have experienced physiologic changes associated with the aging process, including decreased gastric motility, muscle mass, acid production, and blood flow, which affect drug absorption. They may also be more susceptible to certain adverse effects. Liver function declines with advancing age, and changes occur in the hepatic enzymes involved in drug metabolism. Blood flow to the liver decreases secondary to a decrease in cardiac output. Drugs are excreted more slowly from the body as a result of changes in kidney function. Receptor sensitivity is altered in older people, and their sensitivity to certain drugs increases. The physiologic changes in older people that increase drug susceptibility are summarized in the accompanying display, Focus on the Older Adult (on page 758).

 RECALL Mr. Baptiste, the elderly patient receiving intravenous antibiotics for a wound infection. The nurse would need to consider age-related changes that might interfere with the drug action, being especially alert for signs and symptoms of drug toxicity. ●

Weight

Expected responses to drugs are based largely on the reactions that occur when the drugs are given to healthy adults (18 to 65 years of age, 150 lb [68 kg]). It is important to know the usual dose for a medication before administering

FOCUS ON THE OLDER ADULT

NURSING STRATEGIES TO ADDRESS AGE-RELATED CHANGES IN DRUG RESPONSE

Age-Related Changes	Implication or Response	Nursing Strategies
Decreased gastric motility; increased gastric pH	Stomach irritation; nausea; vomiting; gastric ulceration	• Assess for symptoms of gastrointestinal discomfort. • Assess stools for blood.
Decreased lean body mass; decreased total body water	Decreased distribution of water-soluble drugs and higher plasma concentrations, leading to increased possibility of drug toxicity	• Assess for signs of drug interactions or toxicity. • Monitor blood levels of drugs. • Monitor fluid balance—intake and output.
Increased adipose tissue	Accumulation of fat-soluble drugs; delay in elimination from and accumulation of drug in the body, leading to prolonged action and increased possibility of toxicity	• Assess for signs of drug interactions or toxicity. • Monitor blood levels of drugs.
Decreased number of protein-binding sites	Higher drug plasma concentrations, leading to increased possibility of drug toxicity	• Assess for signs of drug interactions or toxicity. • Monitor blood levels of drugs. • Monitor laboratory values—albumin and prealbumin.
Decreased liver function; decreased enzyme production for drug metabolism; decreased hepatic perfusion	Decreased rate of drug metabolism; higher drug plasma concentrations, leading to prolonged action and increased possibility of drug toxicity	• Assess for signs of drug interactions or toxicity. • Monitor blood levels of drugs. • Monitor laboratory values—hepatic enzymes.
Decreased kidney function, renal mass, and blood flow	Decreased excretion of drugs, leading to possible increased serum levels/toxicity	• Assess for signs of drug interactions or toxicity. • Particularly monitor NSAID use; may decrease renal blood flow and function. • Monitor blood levels of drugs. • Monitor laboratory values—creatinine clearance, blood urea nitrogen, serum creatinine.
Alterations in normal homeostatic responses; altered peripheral venous tone	Exacerbated response to cardiovascular drugs; more pronounced hypotensive effects from medications	• Assess for signs of drug interactions or toxicity. • Monitor blood levels of drugs. • Monitor vital signs. • Orthostatic hypotension precautions
Alterations in blood–brain barrier	Enhanced central nervous system penetration of fat-soluble drugs; increased possibility for alterations in mental status, dizziness, gait disturbances	• Assess for signs of drug interactions or toxicity. • Assess for dizziness and light-headedness. • Fall safety precautions
Decreased central nervous system efficiency	Prolonged effect of drugs on the central nervous system; exacerbated response to analgesics and sedatives	• Assess for signs of drug interactions or toxicity. • Assess for alterations in neurologic status. • Monitor vital signs and pulse oximetry.
Decreased production of oral secretions; dry mouth	Difficulty swallowing oral medications	• Monitor ability to swallow medications, especially tablets and capsules. • Discuss changing medications to forms that can be crushed and/or liquid forms with prescribing practitioner.
Decreased lipid content in skin	Possible decrease in absorption of transdermal medications	• Monitor effectiveness of transdermal preparations.

Adapted from Aschenbrenner, D., & Venable, S. (2012). *Drug therapy in nursing* (4th ed.). Philadelphia: Wolters Kluwer Health/Lippincott Williams & Wilkins; Hinkle, J. L., & Cheever, K. H. (2014). *Brunner & Suddarth's Textbook of Medical-Surgical Nursing* (13th ed.). Philadelphia: Wolters Kluwer Health/Lippincott Williams & Wilkins; Tabloski, P. (2010). *Gerontological nursing* (2nd ed.). Upper Saddle River, NJ: Pearson/Prentice Hall; and Grossman, S., & Porth, C.M. (2014). *Porth's pathophysiology: concepts of altered health states.* (9th ed.). Philadelphia: Wolters Kluwer Health/Lippincott Williams & Wilkins.

it. Body surface area (BSA) is the area of the external surface of the body, expressed in square meters (m²). BSA method is considered the most accurate way to calculate the drug dose for infants, children, older adults, patients receiving oncologic medications, and patients with low body weight (Kee et al., 2012). Drug doses for children are calculated by weight in kilograms or BSA.

Gender

The difference in the distribution of body fat and fluids in men and women is a minor factor affecting the action of some drugs. To date, most research on drugs and their actions and effects has been conducted on men. Future clinical drug trials are expected to include more women to document the effects of hormonal fluctuations.

Cultural and Genetic Factors

Religious restrictions and beliefs or cultural practices may affect the patient's acceptance of, response to, and compliance with certain drug therapies. Health care providers need an understanding of a patient's cultural values, beliefs, and practices to provide culturally acceptable care (Ritter & Hoffman, 2010). For example, Christian Scientists place their faith in spiritual healing; therefore, they do not take medicine. A Christian Scientist would not participate in a childhood vaccination program or pharmaceutical therapy to manage disease (Ward, 1988). Herbal treatments that are popular in some cultures may interfere with or counteract the action of prescribed medication.

Ethnopharmacology is the study of the effect of ethnicity on responses to prescribed medication, especially drug absorption, metabolism, distribution, and excretion. It includes pharmacogenetics, the study of genetic varia-

tions in response to drugs. Differences in the responses of patients receiving the same medication may result from genetic differences, such as genetic variations in certain enzymes that may cause differing drug response. Ethnicity influences response to certain medications. Certain ethnic groups have more of these variations than do others (Ward-Smith, 2010; Muñoz & Hilgenberg, 2005). Nurses need to know about medications that may produce varied responses in patients from different ethnic groups. Specifically, there may be important variations in the therapeutic dose and/or incidence of adverse effects. Some patients in certain ethnic groups obtain therapeutic responses at lower doses than those usually prescribed, while other patient groups experience less effect or more effect from prescribed medications than expected. For example, certain angiotensin-converting enzyme (ACE) inhibitors have been found to be less effective in members of the African American population. Alternately, certain thiazide diuretics appear to be better for controlling hypertension in African Americans. African American, Japanese, and Taiwanese patients may experience elevated serum drug levels when lithium is prescribed in the usual dosages, thus experiencing symptoms of drug toxicity. Care must be taken, however, to avoid making sweeping generalizations and assumptions. Ethnicity influences responses to certain medications, but no two people are alike.

General and specific cultural knowledge allows the health care provider to ask the right questions when interacting with patients of varying backgrounds. Nurses who are aware of the specific needs and beliefs of culturally diverse patient populations are better able to communicate effectively and provide optimal care. Box 28-1 gives guidelines for effective communication about medication with culturally diverse patients.

BOX 28-1 | **TIPS FOR COMMUNICATING EFFECTIVELY ABOUT MEDICATION WITH CULTURALLY DIVERSE PATIENTS**

- Acquire basic information about health beliefs and practices of various cultural groups in your health care setting. This provides a basis for assessing patient's beliefs and practices. Recognize, however, that within all cultures and ethnic groups, there are members who do not hold all the values of the group.
- Be alert to atypical drug responses or unexpected adverse effects that may occur in certain ethnic groups. This knowledge helps you direct assessment questions as appropriate.
- Ask specifically about the use of folk or home remedies prescribed by a nontraditional healer.
- Ask specific questions about possible adverse effects, rather than asking general questions or waiting for the patient to voice concerns. For example, do not ask, "Are you having any problems with your medicine?" Instead, ask, "Have you noticed any unusual, involuntary movements?"
- Consider culture when teaching patients and families. Ask, "What do you think caused your health problem?"

and "What treatment do you think will help?" Include culturally sensitive information in all basic health teaching.
- Determine the patient's language preferences for spoken and written communication.
- Use printed or audiovisual information that is in the language spoken by your patients.
- Encourage cultural sensitivity in health care workers in your particular setting.
- Recognize that diversity exists within cultural groups. For example, the Hispanic population includes Mexicans, Cubans, Puerto Ricans, and other Latino groups.
- Emphasize threads or messages in health teaching that are common to all cultures (e.g., concern about family, faith, and home).
- Help culturally diverse patients to value and understand the importance of communicating concerns and asking questions about prescribed medications. Patients and families need to know how to identify major adverse effects of the medications they are taking and the appropriate person(s) to contact if these effects are noted.

Adapted from Ritter, L. A., & Hoffman, N. A. (2010). *Multicultural health*. Boston: Jones and Bartlett; and Muñoz, C., & Hilgenberg, C. (2005). Ethnopharmacology. *American Journal of Nursing, 105*(8), 40–47.

Psychological Factors

The patient's expectations of the medication may affect the response to the medication, as, for instance, in studies of drug effects in which some patients receive a placebo. A **placebo** is a pharmacologically inactive substance. In clinical drug trials, one group of patients receives the active drug, whereas another group receives a placebo to study the drug's effects. Some patients appear to have the same response with the placebo as with the active drug.

Pathology

The presence of disease can affect drug action. For example, the liver is the primary organ for drug breakdown, so pathologic conditions that involve the liver may slow metabolism and alter the dosage of the drug needed to reach a therapeutic level. The kidneys excrete most drugs and their byproducts from the body. Pathologic conditions that involve the kidneys would change excretion and alter the dosage of the drug required to obtain a therapeutic serum level. These types of conditions also influence the presence of adverse effects, such as toxicities.

Environment

A patient's environment may influence that individual's response to medications. Sensory deprivation and overload may affect drug responses. The patient who receives pain medication or a sedative in an active, noisy environment may not be able to benefit fully from the medication's effects, whereas those receiving pain medication in a quiet environment and using an additional relaxation method, such as guided imagery, may have a longer benefit from the pain medication. The relative oxygen deprivation at high altitudes may increase sensitivity to some drugs.

In addition, nutritional state can also affect the body's reaction to certain drugs. When dietary factors are altered, drug therapy may produce different effects in the body than would normally occur. For example, many drugs normally bind to proteins in the plasma. Lowered protein levels in the body means less drug bound to plasma proteins, leading to a higher concentration of free drug in the body. A higher drug concentration increases the drug's effect in the body and the risk for adverse effects (Aschenbrenner & Venable, 2012).

Timing of Administration

The presence of food in the stomach can delay the absorption of orally administered medications. Alternately, some medications should be given with food to prevent gastric irritation; the nurse should consider this when establishing a patient's medication schedule. Other medications may have enhanced absorption if taken with certain foods. Circadian rhythms and cycles may also influence drug action.

Drug Dose and Serum Drug Levels

Blood levels of a drug are often measured to help evaluate whether a drug's dose is at a level to achieve the desired effect and below the level at which adverse effects occur (Aschenbrenner & Venable, 2012).

After a drug has been absorbed, its serum level can be monitored by drawing a blood specimen and measuring the level of the drug in the serum. This is recommended for certain medications (e.g., aminoglycoside antibiotics, digoxin, warfarin) to ensure that a therapeutic range is maintained. A drug's **therapeutic range** is the concentration of drug in the blood serum that produces the desired effect without causing toxicity. The **peak level**, or highest plasma concentration, of the drug should be measured when absorption is complete. The peak level may be affected by factors that affect drug absorption as well as the route of administration. The **trough level** is the point when the drug is at its lowest concentration, indicating the rate of elimination. This specimen is usually drawn in the 30-minute interval before the next dose. The dosage schedule, as well as the half-life of the drug, can modify the trough level. A drug's **half-life** is the amount of time it takes for 50% of the blood concentration of a drug to be eliminated from the body. Monitoring these levels ensures that therapeutic ranges are obtained without reaching toxic levels.

 CONSIDER Regina Sauder, the woman admitted to the hospital with a deep vein thrombosis. She is receiving intravenous heparin and oral warfarin, both of which are monitored using blood tests. Her dose of each drug is adjusted based on the results to ensure the appropriate therapeutic effect. ●

Drug Legislation

In 1906, the Pure Food and Drug Act designated the United States Pharmacopeia and the National Formulary as the official drug standards in the United States, which set national standards for drug quality. This act also empowered the federal government to enforce these standards. This legislation was updated in 1938 by the Federal Food, Drug and Cosmetic Act, prohibiting adulterated or mislabeled drugs from being made available. The Food and Drug Administration (FDA) enforces this law. Extensive testing of new drugs is required before they may be marketed for use. The Durham-Humphrey amendment to the Federal Food, Drug and Cosmetic Act in 1952 distinguished prescription drugs from nonprescription (over-the-counter) drugs and provided directions for dispensing prescription drugs.

The Kefauver-Harris Amendment of 1962 increased controls on drug safety, requiring tighter testing of drugs and written inclusion in the drug literature of adverse reactions and contraindications for approved drugs. The Comprehensive Drug Abuse Prevention and Control Act, also known as the Controlled Substances Act, was passed in 1970. This law regulates the distribution of narcotics and other drugs of abuse. Such drugs have been categorized according to their therapeutic usefulness and potential for abuse. Government programs for the prevention and treatment of drug abuse were established. In 1983, the Drug Enforcement Administration (DEA), a part of the Department of Justice, was identified as the nation's sole legal drug enforcement agency.

More current drug-related legislation includes the Food and Drug Administration Modernization Act of 1997. This act provides for accelerated review and use of new drugs and approves drug testing in children before marketing. In addition, it necessitates the inclusion of clinical trial data for experimental drug use for serious or life-threatening health conditions and requires drug companies to provide information related to "off-label" drugs (drugs not approved by the FDA), including their uses and costs. The act provides that drug companies planning to discontinue drugs must inform health professionals and patients at least six months before stopping drug production (Kee et al., 2012).

In 2003, the Pediatric Research Equity Act was signed into legislation. This act authorizes the FDA to require testing by drug manufacturers of drugs and biologic products for their safety and effectiveness in children. Drug manufacturers must not assume that children are small adults (Kee et al., 2012). Also in 2003, Congress approved the Medicare Prescription Drug Improvement and Modernization Act (MMA). This legislation provides financial assistance to seniors to purchase needed prescription medications.

PRINCIPLES OF MEDICATION ADMINISTRATION
Medication Orders

No medication may be given to a patient without a medication order from a licensed practitioner. Each health agency has a policy specifying the manner in which the practitioner writes an order. In some instances, orders are written on a form designed specifically for a primary care provider's order. This becomes part of a patient's permanent record. Prescribers are able to make use of electronic prescribing systems, sending medication prescriptions electronically to outpatient pharmacies. Most health care facilities are beginning to use computer prescriber order-entry systems (CPOE). CPOE systems allow the prescriber to enter medication orders in a standard format. CPOEs guide the prescriber in complete, accurate, and appropriate ordering. The computer sends the order directly to the pharmacy and enters the order into the patient's permanent record. This prevents any guessing when handwriting is illegible or drug names are similar. Some of the information this system provides includes recommended dosing of medications, drug-specific information, current patient information, laboratory tests that monitor the action of the drug, and potential interactions that may occur with other medications or food. A computerized order-entry system can make medication administration safer and reduce adverse drug events.

Safe practice dictates that a nurse follows only a written or typed order, or an order entered into a computer order-entry system because these types of orders are less likely to result in error or misunderstanding. Under certain circumstances, such as in an emergency, a verbal order from the physician may be given to a registered nurse or a pharmacist. In most settings, a student nurse is not permitted to accept a verbal order from a physician. The legal implications for dispensing and administering an agent without a written order vary, and nurses must be familiar with the exact agency policy whenever called on to administer therapeutic agents. The legal implications of verbal orders are discussed in Chapter 7.

Usual hospital policy dictates that when a patient is admitted, unless specific orders to the contrary are written, all drugs that may have been ordered while the patient was at home are discontinued. This can be a problem when a patient brings medications from home to the hospital. To avoid the possibility of having the patient continue to take the home medications while receiving the same ones or others under new orders, all medications should be sent home with the family or removed from the patient's unit and placed in safekeeping. This requires an explanation to the patient and the family of how the patient's drug plan is to be implemented.

However, in some inpatient facilities, patients keep their medications at their bedside and learn, or continue, to administer them as they would at home. It is believed that this approach helps to promote patients' independence. Be aware when patients are allowed to take their own medications while hospitalized and know each medication's purpose and possible adverse effects. Also, make a notation on the patient's plan of care so that everyone knows the patient has medications at the bedside.

When a patient has had surgery, is transferred to another clinical service, or is transferred to another health agency, it is general practice that all orders related to drugs are discontinued and new orders are written in the new setting. It is important to carefully check that all appropriate medications are reordered. **Medication reconciliation**, the process of specifying medications and maintaining a current, accurate list of medications the patient is receiving, has been shown to decrease the incidence of medication errors that occur during care at points of transition (Barnsteiner, 2005). The accuracy of the list is validated, reviewed, and amended. Verification of admission medication lists with outpatient provider lists may improve accuracy (Balon & Thomas, 2011). Medication reconciliation should occur at the time the patient enters a facility or agency, continuing across the continuum of care (Dinescu et al., 2012), and at the time of patient discharge from a facility, with the primary care provider identifying those drugs to be continued and those to be discontinued (Barnsteiner, 2005). The Joint Commission includes medication reconciliation as part of the 2014 National Patient Safety Goals. Goal 3 identifies the collection of a patient's current medication list, informing patients of the importance of maintaining an accurate medication list, and comparison of medications taken with the newly prescribed medications, to prevent duplications, omission, or interactions (TJC, 2014).

Types of Orders

There are several types of orders that a prescriber may write. A standing order (or routine order) is carried out as specified until it is canceled by another order. Many practitioners whose practices are limited to a particular clinical area have a specified set of written orders for all their hospitalized patients. These are also referred to as standing orders. A practitioner may write a standing order with specified limitations; that is, the prescriber specifies that a certain order is to be carried out for a stated number of days or times. After the stated period has passed, the order is canceled automatically.

The prescriber may write a **PRN order** ("as needed") for medication. The patient receives medication when it is requested or required. PRN orders are commonly written for treatment of symptoms. For example, medications used for pain relief, to relieve nausea, and for sleep aids are often written as a PRN or as-needed order.

Another type of order is the single, or one-time, order. With this type of order, the directive is carried out only once, at a time specified by the prescriber. Medication to be administered immediately before surgery is an example of a single order. A **stat order** also is a single order, but it is carried out immediately. A stat order for a bronchodilator or an antihistamine would be carried out immediately for a patient who is experiencing an anaphylactic drug reaction.

Parts of the Medication Order

The medication order consists of seven parts:

1. Patient's name
2. Date and time the order is written
3. Name of drug to be administered
4. Dosage of the drug
5. Route by which the drug is to be administered
6. Frequency of administration of the drug
7. Signature of person writing the order

Medication orders require the drug, dose, rate, route, frequency, and, when appropriate, duration to be explicit and specific to the needs of the patient in order to achieve the desired outcome (Shane, 2009). In effect, medication orders are sentences where an error or lack of precision in any of the elements of the order can result in unintended consequences (Shane).

PATIENT'S NAME
The patient's full name is used. The middle name or initial should be included to avoid confusion with other patients. In agencies using paper records, the patient's full name and identification number and the primary care provider's name are labeled on all sheets on the patient's chart, including the medical order sheet. Be extremely careful when administering medications when there is more than one patient on the unit with the same last name. Not only can the nurse give the wrong patient the wrong medication, but also a prescriber may enter an order in the wrong patient's medical record.

DATE AND TIME THE ORDER IS WRITTEN
The date the order is written is given, sometimes including the time as well. Because the nursing staff in inpatient agencies changes several times during each 24-hour period, the date and time help to prevent errors of oversight as different nurses take charge of the patient's care. When an order

is to be followed for a specified number of days, the date and time are important so that the discontinuation date and time can be determined accurately. State law determines the length of time an order for a narcotic remains valid. Therefore, the date and time the order is written are essential for determining when the order for a narcotic becomes invalid. Hospitals are utilizing many computer applications in patient care. Examples of such technology include a computer-generated database, computer-generated medication administration orders, and computer-generated flow sheets, as well as electronic medical records. This technology is helping to improve patient safety, but it also requires that nurses check patient information frequently for changes in the patient's status as well as implementation of new medication orders.

NAME OF DRUG TO BE ADMINISTERED
The name of the drug is stated in the order, either by the brand name or by the generic name. Certain brand names are well known, but the practice of using the generic name is considered safest and is required by some health care agencies.

A nurse unfamiliar with a drug can use several sources to obtain information. The United States Pharmacopeia-National Formulary (USP-NF) is the official source in the United States. Most other countries have similar references that describe official therapeutic agents. Most facilities also provide their own formulary, listing the drugs stocked by the facility. Health care agencies also provide access to online medication information sites. The *Physicians' Desk Reference* (PDR) is another source of information that is supplied by pharmaceutical companies. In addition, information about drugs can be obtained from the hospital pharmacist, the prescriber, and any of several texts written specifically for the nursing role in the management of drug therapy. Many of these nursing-specific texts are available as software and can be loaded onto handheld devices such as tablets and smartphones.

DOSAGE OF THE DRUG
The dosage of a drug can be stated in either the metric or the household system. These systems are described in the section Dosage Calculations. The metric system has been adopted internationally, is the most widely used, and is the safest measurement system for drug dosages. Self-administered drugs are commonly labeled in household measurements to facilitate administration for the patient. The household system of measurement may also be used in community settings, such as a person's home (Kee et al., 2012). It is important to be familiar with common equivalent measurements when using household equipment, such as teaspoons and tablespoons, because the home is usually not equipped with special measuring devices. However, instruct patients to use measuring spoons and *not* silverware if administration equipment is not available due to the variability of the amount silverware can hold. The most common equivalents are in Appendix B (found on thePoint).

Certain standard abbreviations are used to indicate drug amounts; it is important to know the common abbreviations before administering drugs. Refer to Box 16-3 in Chapter 16 for common abbreviations used in drug orders. Several abbreviations used in the past have been identified as having the potential to cause errors. The Joint Commission (TJC) has identified an official "do not use" list of abbreviations. See Table 16-3 on page 349 for this list. The use of ambiguous medical abbreviations has been identified by The Institute for Safe Medication Practices (ISMP) and the U.S. Food and Drug Administration (FDA) as one of the most common but preventable sources of medication errors (ISMP, 2012). Refer to the website for the ISMP at www.ismp.org/tools/abbreviations/ for more information about their campaign to eliminate the use of error-prone abbreviations. In addition, the ISMP has identified a list of error-prone abbreviations, symbols, and dose designations that should never be used when communicating medical information (ISMP, 2013). See Table 16-2 on pages 346–348 for this list.

ROUTE BY WHICH THE DRUG IS TO BE ADMINISTERED

The route to be used when administering a medication is stated clearly because some drugs can be given in more than one way and others may be used safely through only one route. Table 28-2 describes common routes by which medications are administered. Refer to "The Nursing Process for Administering Medications" beginning on page 769 for guidelines on administering drugs by these routes.

Table 28-2 ROUTES FOR ADMINISTERING DRUGS

TERMS USED TO DESCRIBE ROUTE	HOW DRUG IS ADMINISTERED
Oral route	Having patient swallow drug
Enteral route	Administering drug through an enteral tube
Sublingual administration	Placing drug under tongue
Buccal administration	Placing drug between cheek and gum
Parenteral route	Injecting drug into
Subcutaneous injection	Subcutaneous tissue
Intramuscular injection	Muscle tissue
Intradermal injection	Corium (under epidermis)
Intravenous injection	Vein
Intra-arterial injection	Artery
Intracardial injection	Heart tissue
Intraperitoneal injection	Peritoneal cavity
Intraspinal injection	Spinal canal
Intraosseous injection	Bone
Topical route	Applying drug onto skin or mucous membrane
Vaginal administration	Vagina
Rectal administration	Rectum
Inunction	Rubbing drug into skin
Instillation	Placing drug into direct contact with mucous membrane
Irrigation	Flushing mucous membrane with drug in solution
Skin application	Applying transdermal patch
Pulmonary route	Having patient inhale drug

FREQUENCY OF ADMINISTRATION OF THE DRUG

The time and frequency with which a drug is to be administered are usually stated in standard abbreviations in the medication order, although many abbreviations used in the past have been phased out due to error and safety concerns (See Table 16-3). The use of ambiguous medical abbreviations has been identified by The Institute for Safe Medication Practices (ISMP) and the U.S. Food and Drug Administration (FDA) as one of the most common but preventable sources of medication errors (ISMP, 2012). Refer to the website for the ISMP at www.ismp.org/tools/abbreviations/ for more information about their campaign to eliminate the use of error-prone abbreviations. Common abbreviations used in writing prescriptions, including time and frequency, are listed in Box 16-3 on page 345.

The nursing service, facility policy, and pharmacy departments of inpatient facilities usually determine the hours at which routine drugs are given. For example, an every–4-hour drug administration may be at the times of noon, 4 PM, 8 PM, midnight, 4 AM, and 8 AM. Another agency may use the hours 1 PM, 5 PM, 9 PM, 1 AM, 5 AM, and 9 AM. To lessen the risk for error, many health care facilities use the 24-hour clock (or military time), which designates midnight as 0000 hours and runs until 2400 hours. If an administration order states that the drug is to be given before or after meals, the time of administration depends on the hours at which meals are served. It is a nursing and pharmacy responsibility to check that times for medication administration correspond to safe practice for that drug.

If a drug is to be given only once or twice a day, the decision about which hours to use depends on the nature of the drug and the patient's plan of care, as well as the standard facility administration times. Whenever possible, consider the patient's choice of time.

Administer drugs punctually, as ordered. A nurse administering drugs to several patients, however, cannot give all of the drugs exactly on the hour indicated. Facility policies vary, but a common one is that drugs should be administered within a half-hour before or after the indicated hour. Thus, a drug to be administered at 9 AM can be administered any time between 8:30 AM and 9:30 AM using this policy. However, it is important to note that this policy does not apply to all drugs. A preoperative medication ordered to be given at 7:30 AM should be administered at that hour because the time was planned in relation to the time that surgery is to begin. Preoperative medications may also be given when the nursing unit receives a call from the operating room to premedicate the surgical patient. This also holds true when patients are given drugs before certain diagnostic procedures and with stat orders.

SIGNATURE OF PERSON WRITING THE ORDER

Prescribers using a computer prescriber order-entry system (CPOE) access the system using a unique username and password. The identifying information of the prescriber, such as name and title, is automatically recorded when the system is accessed, and a handwritten signature is not necessary. When it is necessary to handwrite an order, the signature, with title, of the person writing the order follows the order. Many facilities require prescribers to also print their name with the signature, to facilitate reading of the prescriber's name.

This identifying information is important for legal reasons because the authority to prescribe drugs is defined by state laws. Also, if there is a question about the order, the identifying information indicates who should be contacted.

Checking the Medication Order

Facility or agency policy specifies the manner in which the medication order is checked. Various systems are used; nurses should be familiar with the system used in the agency where they work and should implement it correctly to minimize errors.

The patient's medication record, often called an MAR (medication administration record) is a complete list of all medications prescribed for the patient. Increasing numbers of health care facilities are computerizing patient records, including medication records (CMAR [computerized medication administration record]). The nurse is responsible for checking that the medication order was transcribed correctly by comparing it with the original order, depending on the type of system in use. The nurse is also responsible for double-checking the dosage and appropriateness of the medication.

Questioning the Medication Order

Nurses are legally responsible for the drugs they administer. Therefore, it is important to question any drug order suspected to be in error. The suspected error may be in any part of the order. When preparing to administer a medication, ask (Hughes & Ortiz, 2005): Do the patient's condition, symptoms, and health status warrant receiving this medication? Does it make sense for the patient to have this medication? Is the correct dose and preparation ordered? The legal implications are serious in a situation in which there is an error in a drug order and the nurse could be expected, based on knowledge and experience, to have noted and reported the error.

On occasion, the nurse may not think that there is an error in the order but may not understand why the medication has been prescribed. In such instances, ask the prescriber how the order relates to the patient's plan of care. This may prevent a medication error if the wrong medication has been ordered.

Confusion over the placement of a decimal point can lead to a medication error. A zero should always precede a decimal point (e.g., 0.1 mg) for clarity. The use of a trailing zero (e.g., 1.0) is not considered good practice and has been included in the Joint Commission's "Do not use" list. See Table 16-3 on page 349 for additional abbreviations included in this list.

A drug to which the patient is allergic may be prescribed inadvertently. Best practice is to question the patient about ever having received the medication and ask whether the patient is aware of any reaction to the medication. The patient may describe past adverse reactions with the drug. It is general practice to indicate clearly on the patient's chart any drug allergies. The drug should not be given and the order should be questioned when, in the nurse's judgment, the patient is allergic to a drug. In many health care facilities, the patient may also wear a wristband that indicates specific allergies. An allergic reaction can be life threatening to the patient.

In addition, a drug may be ordered that would potentially interact with another medication the patient is taking. It is important that nurses verify all medications that they are unfamiliar with before administration to avoid possible drug interactions. If a nurse has difficulty reading an order, guessing is gross carelessness; checking with the person who wrote the order is the only safe procedure.

Nurses have the right to refuse to administer any medication that, based on their knowledge and experience, may be harmful to the patient. Although this situation seldom occurs, it is important to understand that the patient's safety is a primary objective in the administration of medications. Always notify the primary care provider of the refusal to administer any medication. Document any concerns regarding medication orders in the patient's medical record, and note having contacted the primary care provider, the response of the primary care provider, and any related interventions.

Medication Supply Systems

Medications are supplied in a number of ways. Many facilities make use of one or more systems in conjunction with each other, or variations of systems. Unit dose dispensing on a patient-specific basis is now the standard of practice for most hospitals. Pharmaceutical manufacturers should also provide all medications in health systems in unit dose packages (American Society of Health-System Pharmacists [ASHP], 2009). Computerized automated dispensing cabinets (ADCs) are a technology based on stock supply of unit dose medications. A large cabinet containing stock medications for the unit is used. The nurse accesses the system with a user name and password, calling up a medication list for a specific patient or a list of available medications. In many systems, only medications entered for a specific patient are available for withdrawal at any one time. A computerized medication dispensing system is shown in Figure 28-1. With an individual unit dose supply system, each patient is supplied with the medication needed for a period of time. The nurse is responsible for accurately obtaining the prescribed medications from the patient's supply. In the unit dose system, the pharmacist simplifies medication preparation by packaging and labeling each dosage for a 24-hour period.

Some nursing units use a medication cart for the administration of medications. The standard cart contains individual drawers into which the medications for each patient are placed. The drawer is labeled with the patient's name. The nurse moves the cart from room to room when dispensing medications.

Another medication delivery system uses bar-code–enabled medication administration (BCMA). BCMA prevents one "wrong-patient" error and almost five "wrong-time" errors each day (Shane, 2009). Just as a CPOE has improved the

FIGURE 28-1. Computerized medication dispensing system.

safe prescribing of medications, the use of BCMA technology can improve patient safety and the accuracy of medication administration and documentation (ASHP, 2009). When using a computerized bar-coded administration system, each patient and each nurse wear identification with a unique bar code to identify the person. Each drug is packaged with a bar code that includes its unique National Drug Code number to identify the form and dosage. The nurse scans his or her own ID, the patient's ID, and each package of medication to be administered. The system confirms the nurse's dispensing authority and the patient's ID, matching the patient with his medication profile. If any of the information is incorrect or does not match, an alert message will appear on the screen notifying the nurse of the discrepancy. The system also records the medication administration and stores the information (ASHP).

Dosage Calculations

Systems of Measurement

Nurses need to be proficient in the use of weights and measures as well as systems of measurement to calculate drug dosages and prepare medications for administration. Two systems of measurement are used in the United States for administering medications: the metric system and the household system. The apothecary system was used infrequently in the past and is no longer used for measurement of medications (Kee et al., 2012). The nurse may be called on to convert dosages from metric to household and household to metric. It is extremely important to be able to calculate commonly used equivalents, as listed in Appendix B (found on thePoint). Practice the Medication Calculation Problems at the end of this chapter to develop your dose calculation skills.

METRIC SYSTEM

The metric system is the most widely accepted and convenient system of measurement. The basic units of measurement are the meter (linear), the liter (volume), and the gram (weight). The metric system is a decimal system, in which each unit can be divided into multiples of 10 (10, 100, 1,000). Calculations in the metric system often involve moving the decimal point to the right or left. In the preparation of medications, the following metric units are typically used:

Weight
- 1 kilogram = 1,000 grams
- 1 gram = 1,000 milligrams
- 1 milligram = 1,000 micrograms

Volume
- 1 liter = 1,000 milliliters or cubic centimeters

It may be necessary to convert drug dosages to a different unit in the metric system. To convert a larger unit into a smaller unit, move the decimal point to the right (the new number is larger than the original). To convert a smaller unit into a larger unit, move the decimal point to the left (the new number is smaller than the original). *Example 1:* 0.5 g equals how many milligrams? Move the decimal point three places to right; the answer is 500 mg. *Example 2:* 900 mg equals how many grams? Move the decimal point three places to the left; the answer is 0.9 g.

HOUSEHOLD SYSTEM

The household system is not widely used except in some community settings, such as a person's home. Teaspoon, tablespoon, and glass are commonly used household measures. The household system is not as accurate as the metric system because of the lack of standardization of spoons, cups and glasses. The measurements are approximate. A teaspoon is considered to be equivalent to 5 mL. Three teaspoons equal one tablespoon. One ounce is considered to be equivalent to 30 mL. As discussed previously, teaspoon and tablespoon refer to measuring spoons, not silverware.

Methods for Computing Drug Dosages

Drugs are sometimes prepared and supplied in the amount ordered by the prescriber, and the nurse can see when checking the medication label that no calculation is necessary. At other times, drugs are not prepared and supplied in the exact quantities called for in the medication order, and the nurse must do a dosage calculation to determine what quantity of medication the patient is to receive.

FORMULA METHODS

Several formulas can be used to calculate drug dosages. One such formula consists of ratios to set up a proportion and can be used to calculate dosages for both solid and liquid preparations. A ratio shows the relation between numbers. A proportion contains two ratios. The nurse is usually seeking the quantity of on-hand medication that is equal to the desired dosage (the dosage ordered). The formula is as follows:

$$\frac{\text{dose on hand}}{\text{quantity on hand}} = \frac{\text{dose desired}}{X \text{ (quantity desired)}}$$

The dosage must be in the same unit of measurement. This applies to the quantity as well. Dosages are on the top line of the proportion, quantities on the bottom line. After the numbers are placed in the proportion, cross-multiply to find the desired quantity.

Example: Amoxicillin, 625 mg PO, is ordered. It is supplied as a liquid preparation containing 250 mg in 5 mL. How much does the nurse administer?

$$\frac{250 \text{ mg}}{5 \text{ mL}} = \frac{625 \text{ mg}}{X \text{ mL}}$$

Cross-multiply:

$$3,125 = 250X$$

$$X = 12.5 \text{ mL}$$

Example: Digoxin (Lanoxin) 0.125 mg PO daily is ordered. It is available as a liquid in a unit dose container labeled 500 mcg/10 mL. How many mL does the nurse the nurse administer? There are two systems of measurement in this problem. The nurse knows that 1 mg is equal to 1,000 mcg; therefore, 0.125 mg equals 125 mcg.

$$\frac{10 \text{ mL}}{500 \text{ mcg}} = \frac{X \text{ mL}}{125 \text{ mcg}}$$

Cross-multiply:

$$500X = 1250$$

$$X = 2.5 \text{ mL}$$

Another formula that can be used to calculate drug dosages is as follows:

$$\frac{\text{dose desired}}{\text{dose on hand}} \times \text{quantity on hand} = \text{desired quantity}$$

Using this formula, the previous example would be solved as

$$\frac{125 \text{ mcg}}{500 \text{ mcg}} \times 10 \text{ mL} = 2.5 \text{ mL}$$

This formula can be used for both liquid dosages and fractions of tablets.

DIMENSIONAL ANALYSIS

Another method that is used to compute medication dosages is dimensional analysis. Dimensional analysis, also known as factor-labeled method, is a systematic, straightforward approach to setting up and solving problems that require conversions. It is a way of thinking about problems that can be used when two quantities are directly proportional to each other, but one needs to be converted using a conversion factor in order for the problem to be solved (Craig, 2009). When using dimensional analysis, the first numerator must be what you are solving for. For instance, in the amoxicillin example, you would set up the equation like this:

$$\text{mL} = (5 \text{ mL}/250 \text{ mg}) \times 625 \text{ mg} = 12.5 \text{ mL}$$

Dimensional analysis can also encompass conversion factors all in the same formula. For instance, the nurse is

to administer 50 mcg fentanyl. The pharmacy supplies the nurse with an ampule of fentanyl 0.1 mg/2 mL. How much should the nurse administer? To solve the problem, the mg needs to be converted to mcg. This can all be done in the same calculation.

$$\text{mL} = (2 \text{ mL}/0.1 \text{ mg}) \times (1 \text{ mg}/1,000 \text{ mcg}) \times 50 \text{ mcg}$$
$$= 1 \text{ mL}$$

Pediatric Calculations

According to Kyle (2013), the most common method for calculating pediatric medication doses is based on body weight, due to the wide range of size differences from infants to toddlers to school-aged children. The recommended dosage is usually expressed as the amount of drug to be given over a 24-hour period (mg/kg/day) or as a single dose (mg/kg/dose). When calculating pediatric drug dosages, check whether the prescribed amount is per dose or per 24-hour period. A medication overdose can occur if the nurse does not note that the calculation is per 24 hours and gives the total amount of medication in one dose. Weigh the child and, if necessary, convert the weight into kilograms by dividing the child's weight in pounds by 2.2 to compute the equivalent kilograms of weight. Then multiply the child's weight in kilograms by the prescribed dose to obtain the appropriate dose for the child. A drug reference book will identify the safe dose range for pediatric drug dosages based on weight.

Using Safety Measures While Preparing Drugs

Medication errors are defined as the preventable inappropriate use of medications. These errors occur when medications are ordered, transcribed, dispensed, administered, and monitored. Medication errors may or may not have serious consequences (Hughes & Ortiz, 2005). Medication errors can occur with almost any type of drug. Errors are more common with certain classes of medications, such as analgesics, antibiotics, anticoagulants, chemotherapeutic agents, diabetic medications, and cardiovascular agents. This is thought to possibly be due to the pharmacologic properties of the drugs that result in more adverse effects, toxicities, and interactions. Medication errors are also common in drugs with narrow therapeutic levels and in drugs prescribed frequently (Hughes & Ortiz). Safety is of the utmost importance in preparing and implementing drug administration. There are many interventions that can minimize the risk for medication errors. The following is a discussion of nursing interventions to reduce this risk.

Three Checks and the Rights of Medication Administration

Use of the three checks and the rights of medication administration when administering medications can assist with safe administration of medications. The use of the previously discussed technology, such as bar-code labeling and medication administration, does not relieve the nurse of responsibility for assuring safe medication administration. Check the label on the medication package or container

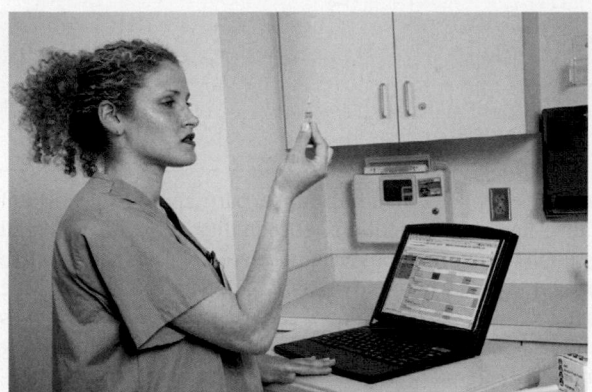

FIGURE 28-2. Comparing medication label with CMAR.

three times during medication preparation and administration. The label should be read:

1. **When the nurse reaches for the unit dose package or container**
2. **After retrieval from the drawer and compared with the CMAR/MAR, or compared with the CMAR/MAR immediately before pouring from a multi-dose container**
3. **Before giving the unit dose medication to the patient, or when replacing the multi-dose container in the drawer or shelf**

Figure 28-2 illustrates the comparison of a medication label with the CMAR (second label check) to ensure accuracy.

The rights of medication administration can help to ensure accuracy when administering medications. However, the Institute for Safe Medication Practices (2007) states "They (rights of medication administration) are merely broadly stated goals or desired outcomes of safe medication practices." The rights themselves do not ensure medication safety. The nurse assumes individual accountability for safe drug administration by engaging in behavior that follows standards of practice and behaviors prescribed by the institution to achieve the goals of the rights (Aschenbrenner & Venable, 2012). Suggested rights of administration vary slightly between references. However, in general, eight to ten rights of medication administration seem to be common in the literature (Elliott & Liu, 2010; Macdonald, 2010; Kee et al., 2012). Ensure that the (1) **right medication** is given to the (2) **right patient** in the (3) **right dosage** (in the right form) through the (4) **right route** at the (5) **right time** for the (6) **right reason** based on the (7) **right (appropriate) assessment data** using the (8) **right documentation** and monitoring for the (9) **right response** by the patient. Additional rights have been suggested to include (10) the **right to education**, ensuring that patients receive accurate and thorough information about the medication, and (11) the **right to refuse**, acknowledging that patients can and do refuse to take a medication. Validating the right reason requires the nurse to understand the rationale for administration and answer the questions, "Does it make sense?" and "Is it appropriate for this person?" The right documentation refers to accurate and timely documentation of administration. The right response

refers to the evaluation by the nurse related to the effectiveness of the medication's intended purpose, monitoring the patient for the desired response. When a patient refuses to take a medication, the nurse should try to determine the reason for the refusal and take reasonable measures to convince the patient to take the medication (Kee et al., 2012). In addition, the nurse should explain the risk of refusing to take the medication and reinforce the reason for the medication (Kee et al., 2012). Documentation of the refusal is necessary, as well as any education and/or explanation provided related to trying to facilitate administration. The primary care provider should be informed of the refusal when the omission poses a specific threat to the patient (Kee et al., 2012).

In addition, it is important to acknowledge that nurses are not the only professionals responsible for the medication administration process. Medication administration is a process with many interconnected players, including nurses, physicians, advanced practice professionals, pharmacists, and patients. All involved in the process share the responsibility for a safe medication system (Macdonald, 2010).

 THINK back to Mr. Baptiste, the patient described in the beginning of the chapter and the Reflective Practice display. By adhering to the rights of medication administration, the nurse would be able to determine that the medication delivered by the pharmacy was labeled incorrectly. ●

Maintaining a Safe Environment

An environment that promotes safety and good working habits contributes to accuracy in the preparation of drugs for administration. Refer to the Research in Nursing display (on page 768) "Practice Environments and Medication Errors." Simmons et al. (2009) discuss physical working conditions that can influence the nurse's ability to perform safely. Good lighting must be present when preparing drugs. Increased noise and noise disruptions decrease the ability to concentrate. Nurses should be aware of the higher risk of making an error when their work flow is disrupted from either a distraction or interruption (Unver, Tastan, & Akbayrak, 2012; Popescu, Cjrrey, & Botti, 2011). Therefore, it is important to prepare drugs in a relatively quiet location. The nurse who is preparing drugs should work alone. This practice helps to avoid distractions and interruptions, which may lead to errors (Klejka, 2012; Unver et al.; Popescu et al.).

After beginning to prepare drugs for administration, do not leave them unattended. If it is imperative to leave for a short time, place the prepared drugs in a locked area, such as in the medication cart. The nurse who prepares the medication also administers the drug and records the drug administration. When not working at the medication dispensing system or medication cart, keep it locked. This is a requirement of the certifying bodies of hospitals.

Handling Controlled Substances Safely

Medication dispensing systems should be locked; this includes securement of controlled substances. Depending

RESEARCH IN NURSING

BRIDGING THE GAP TO EVIDENCE-BASED PRACTICE

Practice Environments and Medication Errors

Medication errors occur frequently and are a serious problem in health care. Medication errors may have serious consequences. What factors affect nurses' ability to identify and intercept medication errors?

Related Research

Flynn, L., Liang, Y., Dickson, G. L., Xie, M., & Suh, D. C. (2012). Nurses' practice environments, error interception practices, and inpatient medication errors. *Journal of Nursing Scholarship, 44*(2), 180–186.

This study explored the relationships among characteristics of the nursing practice environment, nurse staffing levels, nurses' error interception practices, and rate of nonintercepted medication errors in acute care hospitals. A total of 686 registered nurses on 82 units from 14 hospitals were surveyed. Data included the number of medication errors per 1,000 patient days and the number of RN hours per patient day. Nurse survey data included a measure of environmental characteristics and a measure of nurses' interception practices. A supportive practice environment was measured with items consistent with the five domains of the practice environment as characterized by the Nursing Organization and

Outcomes Model, including nurse participation in hospital affairs, nursing foundations for quality of care, collegial nurse–physician relations, a supportive and competent nurse manager, and staffing and resource adequacy. Results of the survey showed that a supportive practice environment was positively associated with error interception practices among nurses in the study. Importantly, nurses' interception practices were inversely associated with medication error rates. The authors concluded that a supportive practice environment enhances nurses' error interception practices. These interception practices play a role in reducing medication errors.

Relevance to Nursing Practice

Nurses should advocate for interventions by institutions to provide and support the best environment possible. Nurses should be actively involved in the environment of the institution. When supported by their practice environments, nurses employ practices that can assist in interrupting medication errors before they reach the patients.

For additional research, visit thePoint.

---

on the system used, controlled substances may be kept in a locked drawer or container as an added safety measure, providing for a "double locked" system. Opioids or other controlled substances may be ordered only by physicians; in some states, nurse practitioners and physician assistants who are registered with the Department of Justice, Bureau of Narcotics, and Dangerous Drugs may order them as well. According to federal law, a record must be kept for each narcotic that is administered. Although methods of recording may differ, the following information usually is required:

- Name of the patient receiving the controlled substance
- Amount of the substance used
- Hour the controlled substance was given
- Name of the physician or advanced practice practitioner who prescribed the substance
- Name of the nurse who administered the substance

It is common practice to check controlled substances daily at specified intervals. In hospitals, checking is usually performed at each shift change. The amount of controlled substances on hand is counted and must be accounted for in the administration records. Many facilities use various computerized systems for dispensing narcotics. This is often a component of the computerized automated dispensing cabinets (ADCs) that supply stock unit dose medications for the unit. The nurse has a secure identification code that provides access into the system, identifies the patient by name or identification number, and verifies the count for each drug as it is removed. Because this secure identification code is equivalent to the nurse's signature, it should never be given

out to other staff members. Unless the controlled substance count is incorrect, this eliminates the need to check the narcotic count at specific intervals each day. A controlled substance count that does not check properly must be reported immediately. The law requires these special precautions to aid in the control of drug abuse by patients and health care workers.

The nurse administering controlled substances has an important responsibility to see that the federal law is observed. If for any reason a controlled substance prepared for administration has to be discarded, a second nurse should act as a witness. This validation by two nurses is recorded, based on the requirements of the medication system in use. Document with a witness any time a full dosage is not given and some of the controlled substance needs to be disposed of. For instance, if 3 mg of an opioid has been ordered and the nurse uses a 4-mg syringe, the remaining 1 mg should be disposed of while a witness is watching, and both nurses should record the transaction, according to facility policy and medication system in use.

Identifying the Patient

Positive identification of the patient is essential to safe drug administration. Before administering the drug, check carefully to see that the right drug is being given to the right patient. Patients in inpatient health care agencies usually wear identification bracelets. Identify the patient by checking the identification bracelet, as shown in Figure 28-3. Validate the patient's name (first identifier) and identification

FIGURE 28-3. Checking patient's identity.

number, medical record number, and/or birth date (second identifier), comparing with the CMAR or MAR. Specific identifiers used depend on facility policy. Also, ask the patient to state his or her name if possible. It is considered unsafe to call the patient by name because the patient may respond even if the nurse uses the wrong name. If using a bar-code system, the nurse will also scan the patient's bracelet. The computer system will validate the patient's identification. In some long-term care facilities a current

photograph of the resident, displayed above the resident's bed, can also be used for identification. The 2013 National Patient Safety Goals established by The Joint Commission state that whenever administering patient medications, at least two patient identifiers should be used (TJC, 2013). The patient's room number or physical location may not be used to validate patient identification (TJC).

THE NURSING PROCESS FOR ADMINISTERING MEDICATIONS
Assessing

Assessment of the patient receiving medications begins during a nursing history. One component of this is the medication history. During the interview, the nurse can adapt questions to meet the patient's needs and level of understanding. Avoid using medical jargon that the patient may not understand; instead, use familiar terms. For instance, the patient may refer to a diuretic as the "water pill" or to an anticoagulant as a "blood thinner." Areas to be included in the medication history are listed in the accompanying Focused Assessment Guide.

FOCUSED ASSESSMENT GUIDE 28-1

MEDICATIONS

Factors to Assess	Questions and Approaches
Previous and current drug use	What medications are you taking that the primary care provider prescribed for you? What over-the-counter medications, natural, or herbal supplements are you taking on a regular basis? Do you use nonmedicinal drugs (e.g., alcohol, caffeine, home remedies)? How often do you use them? What is the reason for taking the medication? What medications have you taken during the past year and for what reasons? Is there anything else you have tried to alleviate your symptoms?
Medication schedule	At what times do you take your medications? Is there any special way your medication has to be prepared (e.g., crushing and mixing with applesauce)? Do you have any special method for remembering to take your medications?
Response to medications	Have the medications had the expected effects? Have you ever experienced any adverse or unexpected reactions to the medications? Is there a family history of this type of reaction to medication? Do you have any allergies to medications? What happens when you take this medication?
Attitude toward drugs and use of drugs	How do you feel about taking medications? Why do you take the medications?
Compliance with regimen	Can you tell me your understanding of the reason for taking the medications? Can you describe how you follow the medication schedule? Are there any problems that prevent you from following the medication regimen?
Storage	Where are your medications stored at home? How long do you keep medications in the home? Can you show me any medications you have on hand?

THE nurse caring for Mildred Campbell would need to incorporate the information the patient shared regarding her interest in an advertised medication when assessing the patient. This information is extremely important to prevent possible drug interactions should the patient decide to use the medication advertised on television. ●

Additional information to be assessed includes the patient's health status, current and past illnesses, laboratory test results, known drug allergies, and religious beliefs and/or ethnic practices. Assess the patient with regard to medications during the nursing history and continue the assessment during and after medication administration.

Diagnosing

Data that the nurse collects may lead to the development of several nursing diagnoses related to medication administration. Each nursing diagnosis statement identifies a patient problem and suggests expected patient outcomes. The etiology of the problem directs nursing interventions. The following are examples of appropriate nursing diagnoses:

- Ineffective Health Maintenance related to lack of knowledge about anticoagulant medication regimen
- Anxiety related to daily self-injection of insulin
- Disturbed Body Image related to effects of chemotherapy
- Constipation related to use of an opioid
- Risk for Aspiration related to impaired swallowing of oral medications
- Deficient Knowledge related to interactions between herbal remedies and prescribed medications

- Noncompliance with Medication Regimen related to adverse drug effects, cost of medications, confusion, lack of motivation, visual impairment, complexity of regimen

Additional examples of diagnoses with related etiologic factors and defining characteristics appear in Examples of NANDA-I Nursing Diagnoses: Medications.

Outcome Identification and Planning

Nursing measures for patients receiving medication are directed toward the patient's achievement of the following goals:

- Expected therapeutic effects will be demonstrated within a specified time frame
- Expected change in symptoms: for example, the patient's pain will be relieved, or vital signs will return to baseline
- Maintenance of therapeutic blood levels of medication
- The patient will demonstrate knowledge regarding his or her medications

Implementing

Remain with the patient and make sure that the medication is taken. If the patient receives several drugs, offer them separately so that if one is refused or dropped, positive identification can be made and the drug can be recorded or replaced. Never leave medications at the bedside for the patient to take later. This is an unsafe practice because the patient may forget to take the medication, or someone else may take the medication. Record medication administration immediately, or as soon as possible, after the patient takes the medication. Some agencies allow patients to self-administer certain drugs to promote

---

EXAMPLES OF NANDA-I NURSING DIAGNOSES

MEDICATIONS

Nursing Diagnoses	Related Factors	Sample Defining Characteristics
Constipation	Dehydration, opiate use, irregular defecation habits, anesthesia, decreased physical activity	*"I feel bloated."* Seventy-year-old man 5 days after a left thoracotomy. Abdomen slightly distended, with hypoactive bowel sounds. Severe flatus. Last bowel movement day of surgery.
Deficient Knowledge	Lack of interest in learning, information misinterpretation, lack of recall	Fifty-year-old woman with recently diagnosed diabetes. "I don't see why all this is necessary. I don't have time for all this!" Asking friends and family to provide snacks and food from home in addition to her meal trays. Unable to verbalize information regarding new oral hypoglycemic agent she is taking, unable to demonstrate fingerstick blood sugar procedure.
Sexual Dysfunction related to adverse effects of antihypertensive drug	New medication regimen, including antihypertensive agent	"I hate the way I feel. My wife doesn't understand. I think I should stop taking that blood pressure pill." Patient and wife verbalize dissatisfaction with sexual function and inability to achieve desired satisfaction since beginning oral antihypertensive therapy.

Table 28-3 ENSURING CORRECT ADMINISTRATION OF MEDICATIONS

"RIGHT" TO ENSURE	QUESTIONS TO ASK	ACTIONS TO TAKE
When Preparing to Give Medication		
Right drug	• Has the patient been given this medication before? • Given the patient's symptoms and diagnosis, does it make sense for the patient to have this medication?	• Determine if the patient has any known drug allergies or sensitivities. • Assess the patient's other medications to detect possible contraindications. • Make sure it is the right medication; packaging, labeling, and spelling of some drugs look alike. • Have another person double-check all medications and mathematical calculations.
Right reason	• Do the patient's condition, symptoms, and health status warrant receiving this medication?	• Determine if the patient has the condition the medication is used for.
Right dose, route, and preparation	• Is the correct dose being administered? • How is the medication administered?	• Ensure that labeling is legible and clearly understood.
Immediately before Administering the Medication		
Right patient	• Is this the right patient to receive this medication?	• Verify the identity of the patient using at least two identifiers: name and date of birth (check wristband, ask patient to state name).
Right time	• Is this the correct time for the medication to be administered?	• Check when the medication was last administered. If the drug is new, document when it is first given.
Right assessment data	• Is it appropriate to administer the medication, based on the specific data collected?	• Collect appropriate assessment data related to mechanism of action and/or therapeutic effect.
Right route	• Is it appropriate to administer the medication orally, intravenously, by injection, or other route?	• Check the original orders to verify the route of administration.
Right education	• Is the patient familiar with the medication? Does the patient understand the purpose, dosing, and administration information, as well as other information specific to medication?	• Assess patient's level of knowledge. Provide patient education as necessary.
After the Medication has been Administered		
Right documentation	• Has the correct documentation been completed according to facility policy?	• Complete documentation according to facility policy immediately after administering any medication. • Document and communicate to the appropriate health care provider any signs and symptoms indicative of any adverse effects.

Right response	• How is the patient responding to the medication?	• Monitor the patient to:
		  • determine the efficacy of the drug
		  • detect and prevent complication
		  • evaluate and document changes in health status
		• When applicable, assess the patient's laboratory values to detect changes.
		• Provide patient education, when possible, so patient is alert to adverse effects and changes in how he feels.

Modified from Aschenbrenner, D., & Venable, S. (2013). *Drug therapy in nursing* (4th ed.). Philadelphia: Wolters Kluwer Health|Lippincott Williams & Wilkins; Kee, J. L., Hayes, E. R., & McCuistion, L. E. (2012). *Pharmacology. A Nursing Process Approach* (7th ed.). St. Louis: Elsevier/Saunders; and Hughes, R., & Ortiz, E. (2005). Medication errors. *American Journal of Nursing, 105*(Suppl 35), 14–24.

the patient's independence. Be familiar with agency policy on this matter.

Table 28-3 summarizes questions to ask and actions to take when administering drugs by any route to ensure the correct administration of medications, as well as examples of nursing interventions to promote safe medication

administration and appropriate outcomes. The accompanying Examples of Nursing Interventions and Nursing Outcomes Classifications (NIC/NOC) box (on page 772) lists standardized nursing interventions and corresponding outcomes related to promoting safe and effective medication administration.

EXAMPLES OF NURSING INTERVENTIONS AND NURSING OUTCOMES CLASSIFICATIONS (NIC/NOC)

MEDICATION

Nursing Interventions	Nursing Outcomes
• Medication Administration • Teaching: Prescribed Medication • Medication Reconciliation • Medication Management • Analgesic Administration	• Knowledge: Medication • Medication Response • Client Satisfaction: Teaching • Pain Control

From: Bulechek, G. M., Butcher, H. K., Dochterman, J. M., & Wagner, C. M. (Eds.). (2013). *Nursing interventions classification (NIC)*. (6th ed., pp. 79, 255, 264, 266, 512). St. Louis: Elsevier/Mosby; and Moorhead, S., Johnson, M., Maas, M. L., & Swanson, E. (Eds.). (2013). *Nursing outcomes classification (NOC)*. (5th ed., pp. 154, 328, 363, 390). St. Louis: Elsevier/Mosby. A full listing of nursing activities for each nursing intervention and outcomes can be found in these books.

Administering Oral Medications

Drugs given orally are intended for absorption in the stomach and small intestine. The oral route is the most commonly used route of administration. It is usually the most convenient and comfortable for the patient. Drug action has a slower onset and a more prolonged, but less potent, effect with oral administration of drugs compared to administration via other routes. There are certain situations in which oral medications should not be administered, such as when the patient has difficulty swallowing, is unconscious, is to receive nothing by mouth, or is vomiting. Occasionally, a patient may unintentionally or intentionally hide a medication in the mouth, or "cheek" it. Check that the medication was actually swallowed before recording that it has been taken.

Oral medications are available in solid and liquid form. Solid preparations include tablets, capsules, and pills. Some tablets are scored for easy breaking if a partial quantity is needed. Unless a tablet is scored, do not break it because doing so could result in an inaccurate dose. Enteric-coated tablets are covered with a hard surface that impedes absorption until the tablet has left the stomach; thus, the medication is released in the small intestine. Enteric-coated tablets are used when the active ingredient of the drug is irritating to the stomach mucosa. As a result, less gastrointestinal irritation occurs, and the medication is protected from destruction by gastric acid. Enteric-coated tablets should not be chewed or crushed because crushing the medication destroys the action of the coating. Other forms of oral medications that should not be chewed or crushed without checking with the prescriber include any of the extended-release forms, such as SR (sustained release), XL (extended release), CR or CRT (controlled release), SA (sustained action), or LA (long acting). Chewing and/or crushing these medications destroys their extended-release delivery mechanism and may result in potentially toxic peaks and low troughs.

Liquid preparations include elixirs, spirits, suspensions, and syrups. Some are water-based solutions, and others are alcohol-based solutions. If the patient has had a previous drug or alcohol addiction, it is important to avoid medications containing alcohol. Disposable, calibrated cups are available for the administration of liquid medications. For patients who find it difficult to take liquids from a cup, the medication can be placed in the mouth directly using a plastic oral syringe. A needle is not used with this type of syringe. Place the syringe between the gum and cheek and give the liquid to the patient slowly. This technique, in addition to having the patient in an upright or side-lying position, helps prevent the patient from choking and aspirating the medication. Shake emulsions and suspensions well and administer them promptly to ensure accurate dosage.

Liquids are available in multidose bottles and single-dose containers. If a label becomes difficult to read or accidentally comes off the container, return the container to the pharmacy. Never give a medication from a bottle without a label or with a label that cannot be read with accuracy. Because of the danger of error, do not return unused medications to their bottles. Exercise care in pouring to prevent unnecessary loss. Do not transfer medications from one pharmacy container to another. Many medication bottles now have an identification code number on them. If similar medications were mixed and a patient had a reaction, it would be difficult to identify which drug was responsible. Do not use a medication with an unexpected precipitate, or one that has changed color. Skill 28-1 on pages 802–808 describes the techniques for preparing and administering oral medications.

SPECIAL TECHNIQUES

Certain drugs that are given orally can discolor the teeth or damage the enamel. The administration technique for this medication is to mix it well with water or some other liquid, have the patient take the medication mixed with liquid through a drinking straw, and encourage the patient to drink water after administration. This practice reduces the strength of the drug that comes in contact with the teeth.

Some patients object to the taste of certain medications. The following techniques help disguise or mask an objectionable taste:

- Crush the medication (if appropriate for type of medication) and add it to food or a drink so that the patient can swallow it. Many times the food or drink will mask the flavor of the medication. However, as previously discussed, some drugs cannot be crushed (e.g., enteric-coated and sustained-release capsules). Check with the pharmacist or a pharmacology reference if you are uncertain about crushing a medication.
- Allow the patient to suck on a small piece of ice for a few minutes before taking the medication. The ice numbs the taste buds, and the objectionable taste is less discernible.
- Store oily medications in the refrigerator. Cold oil is less aromatic than oil at room temperature.
- Place the medication in a syringe, and place the syringe well back on the tongue, being careful not to trigger the patient's gag reflex. This places the medication on the part of the tongue with few taste buds.
- Offer oral hygiene immediately after giving the medication.
- Give the medication with generous amounts of water or other liquids, if permitted, to dilute the taste.

Children. It can be challenging and frustrating to administer medications to infants and children. Children younger than 5 years have difficulty swallowing tablets and capsules. Therefore, most medications are available in liquid form. Nursing responsibility includes teaching and preparing family members to administer medications to a child at home. In addition to understanding the medication order and the reason for the medication, the caregiver should be able to demonstrate any special techniques involved in administering the prescribed drugs. Actions to take to prevent errors when parents or other caregivers need to administer medications include asking, demonstrating, and planning. Question caregivers about their experiences giving medications to their children, about access to proper dosing devices, and previous use of the devices. Demonstrate how to use the appropriate dosing device that will be used at home. Ensure that the caregivers give a correct return demonstration. Help caregivers plan for the times of the day to give the medication. In addition, provide written instructions that clearly state the dose and times of the day for administration. Helpful strategies for administering oral medications to children include the following:

- Use a dropper to give infants or very young children liquid medications while holding them in a sitting or semi-sitting position. Place the medication between the gum and cheek to prevent aspiration.
- Crush uncoated tablets or empty a soft capsule (if appropriate for form of medication) and mix the medication with soft foods—such as potatoes, pudding, ice cream, or cooked or hot cereal—for children who are

likely to aspirate liquids. However, as previously discussed, some drugs cannot be crushed (e.g., enteric-coated and sustained-release capsules). Check with the pharmacist or a pharmacology reference if you are uncertain about crushing a medication.

- Take care when selecting the food to be mixed with the medication. The item should not be an essential part of the child's diet, such as formula or the child's favorite food. The child may refuse to eat a food associated with medications.
- If a medication has an objectionable taste, warn the child if he or she is old enough to understand. Failing to warn the child is likely to decrease the child's trust in the nurse.
- Offer the child a flavored ice pop or frozen fruit bar immediately before taking the medication. It numbs the tongue, making the taste of the medication less evident.
- Praise the child for a job well done after the child swallows the medication.

Older Adults. Techniques for administering medications to older people include the following:

- Allow extra time to administer medications to older patients because their reflexes may be slowed and their understanding of the treatment decreased.
- Older patients may have difficulty swallowing medications and may find it easier to take their medications when crushed or given in liquid form. Initiate swallowing by gently massaging the laryngeal prominence or the area just below the chin prominence. The pressure from the gentle massage creates the desire to swallow. A speech therapist may offer additional suggestions for patients who have difficulty swallowing.
- Reevaluation of the drug dosage is necessary with the older patient. Weight and age should be used as criteria for determining the dosage.
- Assist the older patient to set up a schedule as a reminder to take medications as scheduled at home.
- Monitor the patient carefully for adverse effects that may result from the drug regimen. These may be magnified in older adults.
- Teach patients the names of drugs, rather than distinguishing them by color. Manufacturers may vary the colors of generic drugs, and the visual changes associated with aging may make it more difficult to identify medications by their color.

In older adults, successful self-management of medication may be promoted by establishing habits, adjusting routines, tracking medications, simplifying medication practices, and improving patient education regarding the relationship of medications to maintaining health (Swanlund, Scherck, Metcalfe, & Jesek-Hale, 2008).

ADMINISTERING MEDICATIONS THROUGH AN ENTERAL FEEDING TUBE

Patients with a gastrointestinal tube (nasogastric, nasointestinal, percutaneous endoscopic gastrostomy [PEG], or jejunostomy [J] tube) often receive medication through the tube. The insertion of the tube and care of the patient with an enteral feeding tube are described in Chapter 35. The following are suggestions for giving medications through the tube:

- Use liquid medications when possible because they are absorbed readily and less likely to cause tube occlusions (Toedter Williams, 2008).
- Certain solid dosage medications can be crushed and combined with liquid. (Refer to previous discussion regarding crushing of medications.) Crush medication to a fine powder and mix it with 15 to 30 mL of water before delivery through the tube (Best & Wilson, 2011).
- Certain capsules may be opened, emptied into liquid, and administered through the tube (Toedter Williams, 2008). Check manufacturer recommendations and/or with a pharmacist to verify.
- Bring the liquid medication to room temperature. Cold liquids may cause patient discomfort.
- Elevate the head of the bed to prevent reflux.
- Remove the clamp from the tube and use the recommended procedure for checking tube placement in the stomach or intestine before administering the drug.
- Flush the tube with 15 to 30 mL water (5 to 10 mL for children) before giving the medication and immediately after giving the medication. Flushing helps to maintain tube patency.
- Give medications separately and flush with water between each drug (Best & Wilson). Some medications may interact with each other or become less effective if mixed with other drugs.
- If the tube is connected to suction, keep it disconnected from the suction and clamped for 20 to 30 minutes after administration of the medication to allow absorption.
- If the patient is receiving tube feedings, review information about the drugs to be administered. Absorption of some drugs, such as phenytoin (Dilantin), is affected by tube-feeding formulas. Discontinue a continuous tube feeding and leave the tube clamped for the required period of time before and after the medication has been given, according to the reference and facility protocol.
- Document the water intake and liquid medication by tube on the intake and output record. Adjust the amount of water used if the patient's fluid intake is restricted.

 Concept Mastery Alert

When administering medications via an enteral tube, the same amount of fluid—15 to 30 mL—is used to mix the medication and to flush the tube afterward.

ADMINISTERING SUBLINGUAL AND BUCCAL MEDICATIONS

Certain drugs, such as nitroglycerin, are administered sublingually; that is, a tablet is placed under the patient's tongue. Another method is to administer the medication between the cheek and gum, known as buccal administration. These areas are rich in superficial blood vessels, which allow the drug to be absorbed relatively rapidly into the bloodstream for quick systemic effects. Sublingual and buccal medications should not be swallowed, but rather held in place so that complete absorption can occur. Before administering a sublingual or buccal drug, offer the patient a drink of water (if the patient is permitted to have fluids) or oral care (if the patient is NPO). This ensures that the tablet will dissolve appropriately. Certain opioids that were previously available for parenteral administration only can now also be administered in a lollipop or oral-transmucosal form.

Administering Parenteral Medications

The word **parenteral** means outside the intestines or alimentary canal. Several methods to administer a medication by the parenteral route involve injecting the medication into those body tissues outside of the intestines or alimentary canal and into the circulatory system. Table 28-2 on page 763 defines terms used to describe various types of parenteral injections. Advanced injection techniques consist of injecting medications into an artery, the peritoneum, heart tissues, the spinal canal, and bones. Techniques for injecting medications into these areas are discussed in clinical texts. In most instances, physicians or specialized advanced practitioners are responsible for these procedures.

EQUIPMENT

Needles and Syringes. Needles are available in various lengths and gauges, with different sizes of bevels. The needle length used depends on the route of administration. The gauge refers to the diameter of the needle. Needle gauges are numbered 18 through 30. As the diameter of the needle increases, the gauge number decreases. For example, an 18-gauge needle is larger in diameter than a 30-gauge needle. The bevel of the needle is its sloped edge, designed to make a narrow, slit-like opening that closes quickly.

 Concept Mastery Alert

Opposites rule. The larger the gauge of a needle, the smaller the diameter.

Syringes are supplied in various sizes. Most syringes are plastic and disposable. Some syringes are supplied with the needle attached; others are not, in which case you should select an appropriate needle. Figure 28-4 shows the parts of a needle and the parts of a syringe.

Choose the equipment needed for an injection based on the following criteria:

- *Route of administration:* A longer needle is required for an intramuscular injection than for an intradermal or a subcutaneous injection. See the discussion related

FIGURE 28-4. Parts of a needle and syringe.

to each individual route for specific guidelines regarding needle length and gauge.

- *Viscosity of the solution:* Some medications are more viscous than others and require a large-lumen needle to inject the drug.
- *Quantity to be administered:* The larger the amount of medication to be injected, the greater the capacity of the syringe.
- *Body size:* An obese person requires a longer needle to reach muscle tissue than does a thin person. A thin person or an older adult with decreased muscle mass requires a shorter needle.
- *Type of medication:* There are special syringes for certain uses. An example is the insulin syringe used to inject insulin.

Once used, do not recap needles. After use, place needles and syringes in puncture-resistant containers without being recapped because most needlestick injuries occur during recapping. Health care facilities are required to provide needles with needle guards to prevent accidental injury. After the injection is given, push the needle guard into place, preventing injury. Other needle and syringe combinations have a retractable needle that locks and seals inside the syringe barrel. Prefilled syringes are manufactured with retractable needle sheath covers. With these syringes, once the needle is contaminated, the top

slides forward and over the needle to prevent a needlestick injury. If recapping is absolutely unavoidable, use the one-handed technique. This technique and additional measures to protect health care workers from accidental transmission of infectious diseases are discussed in Chapter 23.

When administering parenteral injections, maintain surgical asepsis and use strict sterile technique to avoid introducing organisms into the body. The parts of the syringe and needle that must be kept sterile during the procedure of preparing and administering an injection include the inside of the barrel, the part of the plunger that enters the barrel, the tip of the barrel, and the needle, except for the exterior of the needle hub. Surgical asepsis also applies to cleaning the skin for an injection. Cleanse the skin with alcohol or another antimicrobial in a circular motion, working from the center of the designated site outward.

Needleless Systems. The risk for accidental needlesticks and exposure to blood-borne pathogens is reduced significantly with the use of needleless devices or protected needles. Chapter 23 describes the rationale for these systems of protection for health care workers. Needleless systems are available for intravenous use, including recessed and shielded intravenous needle connectors, as well as blunt cannulas that are inserted into special receptor sites on tubing or lock setups. Discard all needleless devices or blunt cannulas in special containers that are puncture-proof, leak-proof, and labeled clearly. Figure 28-5 (on page 776) shows an example of a needleless administration device.

PREPARING MEDICATIONS FOR ADMINISTRATION BY INJECTION

Drugs that are administered by injection are packaged in several ways. Those that deteriorate in solution are usually dispensed as powders and are reconstituted immediately before injection. Drugs that remain stable in solution are usually dispensed in ampules, bottles, prefilled cartridges, or vials in an aqueous or oily solution or suspension. Drugs may be dispensed in single-dose glass ampules, single-dose rubber-capped vials, multidose rubber-capped vials, and prefilled cartridges.

Removing Medication from an Ampule. An **ampule** is a glass flask that contains a single dose of medication for parenteral administration. Figure 28-6 (on page 776) shows an example of an ampule. There is no way to prevent airborne contamination of any unused portion of medication after the ampule is opened; if not all the medication is used, discard the remainder. Medication is removed from an ampule after its thin neck is broken. Take special care when breaking the ampule so that you do not get cut. If you cut yourself on the ampule, discard the ampule and medication. Because of the risk of small glass shards falling into the ampule, use a filter needle to remove the medication from the vial and then discard it

FIGURE 28-5. (**A**) Needleless administration devices. (**B**) Syringe attached to needleless administration device. *(Photos by B. Proud.)*

appropriately. Place an unfiltered needle of appropriate size on the syringe before administering the medication. Invert the ampule or place it on a flat surface to draw the solution into the syringe. Care must be taken not to contaminate the needle by touching the rim of the ampule. Skill 28-2 on pages 808–811 shows how to remove medication from an ampule.

Removing Medication from a Vial. A **vial** is a plastic or glass bottle with a self-sealing stopper through which the medication is removed (Fig. 28-7). For safety in transporting and storing, the vial is usually covered with a soft metal cap that can be removed easily. The rubber stopper that is then exposed is the means of entrance into the vial.

Some drugs are dispensed in vials that contain several doses. This means that the nurse can remove several doses from the same container. To prevent microbial growth in the vial, each multidose vial is usually good for only 24 hours. Label the vial with the time and date when first used. After the initial use of the multidose vial, wipe the rubber stopper with alcohol each time the medication is removed from the vial. To facilitate removal of medication, inject air into the vial. The amount of air injected into the vial is the same amount as the desired quantity of solution. The Centers for Disease Control and Prevention (CDC)

recommends that medications packaged as multiuse vials be assigned to a single patient whenever possible (CDC, 2011). In addition, it is recommended that the top of the vial be cleaned prior to each entry and that a new sterile needle and syringe is used with each entry. Skill 28-3 on pages 811–813 details how to remove medication from a vial.

Using a Prefilled Cartridge or Syringe. Prefilled cartridges provide a single dose of medication. Insert the cartridge into a reusable holder or injection device. Before giving the injection, check the dosage in the cartridge and clear the cartridge of excess air. Most prefilled cartridges are overfilled; therefore, eject any excess medication to give an exact dose and avoid a medication error. Tubex® and Carpuject® are two types of prefilled cartridges. Figure 28-8 shows examples of prefilled cartridges and injector devices.

Similar to prefilled cartridges are prefilled syringes. These are syringes that are already filled with a medication and usually have their own needle attached. Like prefilled cartridges, these syringes also come with excess air. In some cases, this air should *not* be expelled before administering the medication. Enoxaparin (Lovenox) is an example of a syringe for which the air should not be expelled before administering (Sanofi Aventis, 2012).

FIGURE 28-6. Ampule. *(Photo by B. Proud.)*

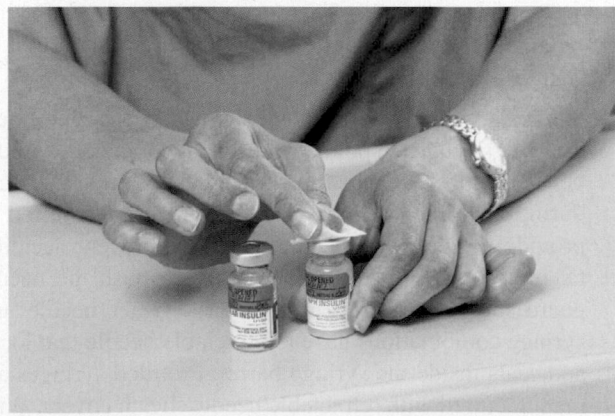

FIGURE 28-7. Vials. *(Photo by B. Proud.)*

FIGURE 28-8. Prefilled cartridge and injector device. *(Photo by B. Proud.)*

Mixing Medications in One Syringe. When considering mixing two medications in one syringe, first ensure that the two drugs are compatible. Certain medications, such as diazepam (Valium), are incompatible with other drugs in the same syringe. Other drugs have limited compatibility and should be administered within 15 minutes of preparation. Incompatible drugs may become cloudy or form a precipitate in the syringe. Discard these medications and re-prepare the drugs in separate syringes. Mixing more than two drugs in one syringe is not recommended. If it must be done, contact the pharmacist to determine the compatibility of the three drugs, as well as the compatibility of their pH values and the preservatives that may be present in each drug. A drug compatibility table should be available to nurses who are preparing medications.

Preparation of medications in one syringe depends on how the medication is supplied. When using a single-dose vial and a multidose vial, inject air into both vials and draw the medication in the multidose vial into the syringe first. This prevents the contents of the multidose vial from being contaminated with the medication in the single-dose vial. The steps to follow when preparing medications from two multidose vials in one syringe are illustrated in Figure 28-9. When preparing medications from an ampule and a vial, prepare the medication in the vial first. Draw up the medication in the ampule after the medication in the vial.

Mixing Insulins in One Syringe. Insulin, a naturally occurring hormone produced by the pancreas, enables cells to use carbohydrates. Two of the issues relative to insulin in patients with diabetes mellitus include no insulin production or insufficient insulin production. Many types of insulin are available for use by patients with diabetes mellitus. Insulins vary in their onset and duration of action and are classified as rapid acting, short acting, intermediate acting, and long acting (Aschenbrenner & Venable, 2012). A patient may receive more than one type of insulin. A patient may be treated with a basal insulin, such as insulin glargine (Lantus), insulin detemir (Levemir), or NPH insulin to cover the body's basal

FIGURE 28-9. Mixing medications (insulin) in one syringe.

metabolic needs. In addition, the patient will probably also be treated with a prandial (with a meal) or preprandial (before a meal) insulin, such as insulin lispro (Humalog) or insulin aspart (NovoLog), to prevent postprandial (after meal) hyperglycemia (high blood glucose). Lantus and Levemir cannot be mixed with other insulins. Patients treated with other insulins may require the mixing of the two insulins in one syringe. Before administering any insulin, be aware of the onset time, peak, and duration of effects and ensure that proper food is available. Refer to a drug reference for a listing of the different types of insulin and action specific to each type.

Insulin dosages are calculated in units. The scale commonly used is U100, which is based on 100 units of insulin contained in 1 mL of solution. An insulin syringe is also calibrated in units. Insulin is also available in injection pens. Before administering insulin, check the dosage with the medical orders. Skill 28-4 on pages 814–817 gives the steps for mixing two types of insulin in the same syringe. Insulin administration is discussed later in the chapter in the section Administering Medications Subcutaneously.

Reconstituting Powdered Medications. Occasionally, a drug is supplied as a powder in a vial. A liquid, or diluent, must be added to the powder before it is administered as a solution. The technique of adding a diluent to a powdered drug is called reconstitution. Information needed for reconstitution, such as the specific solution to use for the diluent and dosage calculation, is usually found on the vial label. Additional sources of information about reconstitution of medications are package inserts and the pharmacist.

Another form that powdered medications may come in is an Act-O-Vial® (Pfizer). Act-O-Vials have the diluent and powder in the same vial but separated by a rubber stopper. When the nurse is ready to administer the medication, the rubber stopper is deployed, and the Act-O-Vial is agitated gently to mix the diluent and powder.

ADMINISTERING MEDICATIONS INTRADERMALLY

Intradermal injections are administered into the dermis, just below the epidermis. The intradermal route has the longest absorption time of all the parenteral routes. For this reason, intradermal injections are used for sensitivity tests, such as tuberculin and allergy tests, and local anesthesia. The advantage of the intradermal route for these tests is that the body's reaction to substances is easily visible, and degrees of reaction are discernible by comparative study.

Sites commonly used are the inner surface of the forearm and the upper back, under the scapula. Equipment used for an intradermal injection includes a tuberculin syringe calibrated in tenths and hundredths of a milliliter. A 1/4″ to 1/2″, 25- or 27-gauge needle is used. The dosage given intradermally is small, usually less than 0.5 mL. The angle of administration for an intradermal injection is 5 to 15 degrees. Skill 28-5 on pages 818–822 demonstrates how to administer an intradermal injection.

ADMINISTERING MEDICATIONS SUBCUTANEOUSLY

Subcutaneous injections are administered into the adipose tissue layer just below the epidermis and dermis. This tissue has few blood vessels, thus drugs administered here have a slow, sustained rate of absorption into the capillaries. This route is used to administer drugs such as insulin and heparin.

Subcutaneous Injection Sites. Various sites may be used for subcutaneous injections, including the outer

FIGURE 28-10. Sites on the body where subcutaneous injections can be given.

aspect of the upper arm, the abdomen (from below the costal margin to the iliac crests), the anterior aspects of the thigh, the upper back, and the upper ventral or dorsogluteal area (Fig. 28-10). Avoid sites that are bruised, tender, hard, swollen, inflamed, or scarred. These conditions could affect absorption or cause discomfort and injury (Hunter, 2008). Absorption rates differ among the various sites. Injections in the abdomen are absorbed most rapidly; ones in the arms are absorbed somewhat more slowly; those in the thighs, even more slowly; and those in the upper ventral or dorsogluteal areas have the slowest absorption (American Diabetes Association [ADA], 2004).

Equipment. It is important to choose the right equipment to ensure depositing the medication into the intended tissue layer and not the underlying muscle. Equipment used for a subcutaneous injection includes a syringe of appropriate volume for the amount of drug being administered. A 25- to 30-gauge, 3/8″ to 1″ needle can be used. The 3/8″ and 5/8″ needles are most commonly used. Choose the needle length based on the amount of subcutaneous tissue present, which is based on the patient's body weight and build (Annersten & Willman, 2005). Usually, no more than 1 mL of solution is given subcutaneously. Giving larger amounts adds to the patient's discomfort and may predispose to poor absorption. Some medications are packaged in prefilled cartridges with a needle attached. Enoxaparin (Lovenox), for example, is provided this way. Confirm that the provided needle is appropriate for the patient before use. If not, the medication will have to be transferred to another syringe and the appropriate needle attached.

Procedure. Subcutaneous injections are administered at a 45- to 90-degree angle. Choose the angle of needle insertion based on the amount of subcutaneous tissue present and the length of the needle. Generally, the shorter, 3/8″ needle should be inserted at a 90-degree angle, and the longer, 5/8″ needle is inserted at a 45-degree angle. Recommendations differ regarding pinching or bunching of a skin fold for administration. Pinching is advised for thinner patients and when a longer needle is used to lift the adipose tissue away from underlying muscle and tissue. If pinching is used, once the needle is inserted, release the skin to avoid injecting into compressed tissue.

Aspiration, or pulling back on the plunger to check that a blood vessel has been entered, is not necessary and has not proved to be a reliable indicator of needle placement. The likelihood of injecting into a blood vessel is small (Crawford & Johnson, 2012). Aspiration is definitely contraindicated with administration of heparin because this action can result in hematoma formation. The American Diabetes Association (ADA, 2004) has stated that routine aspiration is not necessary when injecting insulin.

If blood or clear fluid appears at the site after withdrawing the needle, apply gentle pressure. Massaging the site is not necessary and can damage underlying tissue as well as increase the absorption of the medication. Massaging after heparin administration can contribute to hematoma formation.

It is necessary to rotate sites or areas for injection if the patient is to receive frequent injections. This helps to prevent buildup of fibrous tissue and permits complete absorption of the medication. Because absorption rates vary from site to site, it is recommended that patients administering their own insulin use the same area of the body at the same time every day to ensure more consistent absorption and prevent tissue changes from repeated use of the same site (Aschenbrenner & Venable, 2012; ADA, 2004). For instance, every morning the patient may use the abdomen for insulin injection, and every evening before dinner, the patient may inject the insulin into the arms or thighs. In each case, the injections should be given an inch away from the previous injection site so that the same area will not be used again in the same month. A small spot bandage or piece of tape can be used to mark the first injection site, with subsequent injections rotated in a circle around that site. After this area has been used, an adjacent site, an inch away, can be selected, using the same rotation format. A marked diagram incorporated into the patient's plan of care is also helpful for noting alternative sites. Do not rely on memory. The patient cannot always recall the site of the previous injection, thus the site of administration must be recorded in the patient's record.

Skill 28-6 on pages 822–827 shows the procedure for administering medications subcutaneously. Techniques for reducing discomfort in subcutaneous administrations are listed in Box 28-2.

Drug-Specific Equipment and Techniques. Various drugs require very specific equipment and/or techniques. Insulin is prepared using an insulin syringe. Other drugs are never administered with an insulin syringe. Insulin syringes are available with 28- to 30-gauge, 5/16″ and 1/2″ length needles, and in 3/10-mL to 1-mL sizes. The shorter needles (5/16″) are becoming the more common length used. Shorter needles are less painful, and there is less risk for inadvertent injection into muscle tissue.

BOX 28-2 REDUCING DISCOMFORT IN SUBCUTANEOUS AND INTRAMUSCULAR ADMINISTRATIONS

The following are recommended techniques for reducing discomfort when injecting medications subcutaneously or intramuscularly:

- Select a needle of the smallest gauge that is appropriate for the site and solution to be injected, and select the correct needle length.
- Be sure the needle is free of medication that may irritate superficial tissues as the needle is inserted. The recommended procedure is to use two needles—one to remove the medication from the vial or ampule and a second one to inject the medication. If medication is in a prefilled syringe with a nonremovable needle and has dripped back on the needle during preparation, gently tap the barrel to remove the excess solution.
- Use the Z-track technique for intramuscular injections to prevent leakage of medication into the needle track, thus minimizing discomfort.
- Inject the medication into relaxed muscles. There is more pressure and discomfort when the medication is injected into a contracted muscle.

- Do not inject areas that feel hard on palpation or tender to the patient.
- Insert the needle with a dart-like motion without hesitation, and remove it quickly at the same angle at which it was inserted. These techniques reduce discomfort and tissue irritation.
- Do not administer more solution in one injection than is recommended for the site. Injecting more solution creates excess pressure in the area and increases discomfort.
- Inject the solution slowly so that it may be dispersed more easily into the surrounding tissue (10 seconds per 1 mL).
- Apply gentle pressure after injection, unless this technique is contraindicated.
- Allow patients who are fearful of injections to talk about their fears. Answer patients' questions truthfully, and explain the nature and purpose of the injection. Taking the time to offer support often allays fears and decreases discomfort.
- Rotate sites when the patient is to receive repeated injections. Injections in the same site may cause undue discomfort, irritation, or abscesses in tissues.

GUIDELINES FOR NURSING CARE 28-1

USING AN INSULIN PEN

- Perform hand hygiene and put on PPE, as indicated.
- **Identify the patient. Compare the information with the CMAR/MAR. The patient should be identified using at least two methods (TJC, 2013).**
- Explain procedure to the patient.
- Close the door to the room or pull the bedside curtain.
- **Complete necessary assessments before administering medications. Check the patient's allergy bracelet or ask the patient about allergies. Explain the purpose and action of the medication to the patient.**
- Scan the patient's bar code on the identification band, if required.
- **Based on facility policy, the third check of the label may occur at this point. If so, recheck the labels with the CMAR/MAR before administering the medications to the patient.**
- Select an appropriate administration site.
- Assist the patient to the appropriate position for the site chosen. Drape, as needed, to expose only area of site to be used.
- Identify the appropriate landmarks for the site chosen.
- Remove the pen cap.
- Insert an insulin cartridge into the pen, if necessary, following the manufacturer's directions.
- Clean the tip of the reservoir with alcohol.
- Invert the pen 20 times to mix if using an insulin suspension.
- Remove the protective tab from the needle.
- Screw the needle onto the reservoir.
- Remove the outer and inner needle caps.
- Hold the pen upright and tap to force any air bubbles to the top.
- Dial the dose selector to 2 units to perform an "air shot" to get rid of bubbles.
- Hold the pen upright and press the plunger firmly. Watch for a drop of insulin at the needle tip.

- Check the drug reservoir to make sure enough insulin is available for the dose.
- Check that the dose selector is at "0," then dial the units of insulin for the dose.
- Put on gloves.
- Clean the injection site and administer the subcutaneous injection, holding the pen like a dart. Push the button on the pen all the way in.
- Keep the button depressed and count to 6 before removing from the skin.
- Remove the needle from the pen and dispose in a sharps container.
- Remove gloves and additional PPE, if used. Perform hand hygiene.
- Document administration on the CMAR/MAR, including the injection site.

Patient using an insulin pen. *(Photo by B. Proud.)*

Adapted from Moshang, J. (2005). Making a point about insulin pens. *Nursing, 35*(2), 46–47.

Insulin pens are also available for insulin administration. Insulin injection pens are prefilled devices that combine the insulin container and syringe. Patients attach a needle for each administration, dial a dose of insulin, and depress a plunger to administer the dose. See Guidelines for Nursing Care 28-1: Using an Insulin Injection Pen.

Heparin is also administered subcutaneously. The abdomen is the most commonly used site. Avoid the area 2″ around the umbilicus and the belt line. The manufacturer's directions for subcutaneous administration of low-molecular-weight heparin preparations, such as enoxaparin (Lovenox), include specific instructions regarding administration site and technique (Sanofi Aventis, 2012). Administer enoxaparin in an area on the abdomen between the left or right anterolateral and left or right posterolateral abdominal wall (Fig. 28-11). To administer the medication, pinch the tissue gently and insert the needle at a 90-degree angle. In addition, enoxa-

parin is packaged in a prefilled syringe with an air bubble. Do not expel the air bubble before administration.

Some medications, such as insulin and morphine, may be administered continuously via the subcutaneous route. Continuous subcutaneous insulin infusion (CSII or insulin pump) allows for multiple preset rates of insulin delivery. This system uses a small computerized reservoir that

Anterior view   Posterior view

FIGURE 28-11. Sites for administration of enoxaparin.

FIGURE 28-12. Patient wearing an insulin pump. *(Photo by B. Proud.)*

delivers insulin via tubing through a small plastic cannula or needle inserted into the subcutaneous tissue. The pump is programmed to deliver multiple preset rates of insulin delivery. The settings can be adjusted for exercise and illness, and bolus doses can be delivered related to meals. Sites are changed every 2 to 3 days. Figure 28-12 shows a patient wearing an insulin pump. Another example of a medication given via continuous subcutaneous infusion is morphine. Subcutaneous morphine infusion can be used for palliative dyspnea and pain management. Advantages of continuous subcutaneous medication infusion include the longer rate of absorption via the subcutaneous route and convenience for the patient.

ADMINISTERING MEDICATIONS INTRAMUSCULARLY

Intramuscular injections deliver medication through the skin and subcutaneous tissues into certain muscles. Muscles have larger and a greater number of blood vessels than does subcutaneous tissue, allowing faster onset of action than with subcutaneous injections. Some medications administered intramuscularly are formulated to have a longer duration of effect. The deposit of medication creates a depot at the site of injection, designed to deliver slow, sustained release over hours, days, or weeks. This route is used to administer drugs such as antibiotics, hormones, and vaccines, such as the pneumococcal and hepatitis vaccines. The accompanying box, Through the Eyes of a Student, relates one student's experience administering an intramuscular injection.

Intramuscular Injection Sites. Various sites may be used for intramuscular injections. To avoid complications, it is important to be able to identify anatomic landmarks and site boundaries and to use an accurate, careful technique when administering intramuscular injections. If care is not taken, possible complications include abscesses; cellulitis; injury to blood vessels, bones, and nerves; lingering pain; tissue necrosis; and periostitis (inflammation of the membrane covering a bone). Avoid any site that is bruised, tender, hard, swollen, inflamed, or scarred.

Consider the age of the patient, medication type, and medication volume when selecting a site for intramuscular

THROUGH THE EYES OF A STUDENT

I entered my patient's room, knowing that she had had surgery less than 12 hours before my arrival, and introduced myself. I asked how she was feeling, to which she immediately responded, "I feel really sick. I think I'm going to throw up. I need something—now!" I told her that I would check the medication orders and be back as soon as possible. I walked quickly to the medication administration record, and there it was glaring at me in black and white on the CMAR: "Prochlorperazine (Compazine), 10 mg IM q 6 hr PRN nausea or vomiting." My mind raced as I thought, "I have never given an IM injection. There has to be something else ordered." I knew there wasn't. I found my clinical instructor and announced, "My patient needs an IM injection." Given the anxiety I was feeling, everything went surprisingly well as we prepared the medication. I went over the procedure one last time before entering the patient's room.

We approached the patient just in time for her to look at us in sheer terror and cry, "I hope that shot isn't for me; I hate them," which did nothing for my already shaking hands. I explained that she couldn't take a pill because she could not have anything by mouth because of the nature of her surgery and that this would help. She was agreeable after hearing the rationale. My instructor and I positioned the patient on her side—a feat in itself—so that I could give her the shot in the ventrogluteal area. I marked the landmarks at least half

a dozen times, wiped the area with alcohol, and asked her if she was ready for the injection. *Big mistake!* She swiftly replied, "No, but get it over with." I took a minute to reassure her (and silently, me) again.

A little voice in my head repeated the words my *technologies* professor had said a million times, "Darting action is the key to a successful injection." So, I aimed at the bull's-eye that appeared in front of my eyes. My hand, which seemed to be moving in slow motion, propelled downward at a 90-degree angle. Secretly, I prayed that I would not hit my own hand. I looked down and it was a bull's-eye, thank goodness, but the needle had not penetrated the muscle! The patient successfully tensed her muscle tight enough to intercept the needle midflight. At that moment, she relaxed, probably because she thought the worst was over, and I pushed the needle into place. I slowly drew back the plunger to make sure no blood appeared in the syringe. I began injecting the prochlorperazine slowly, watching my hands shake. Then I withdrew the needle and gently applied pressure over the site. It was over and I wanted to scream, "I did it!" but I kept my composure to feign the experience I lacked. Giving my first IM injection was not as bad as I thought it would be!

Alison L. Moriarty
Georgetown University, Washington, DC

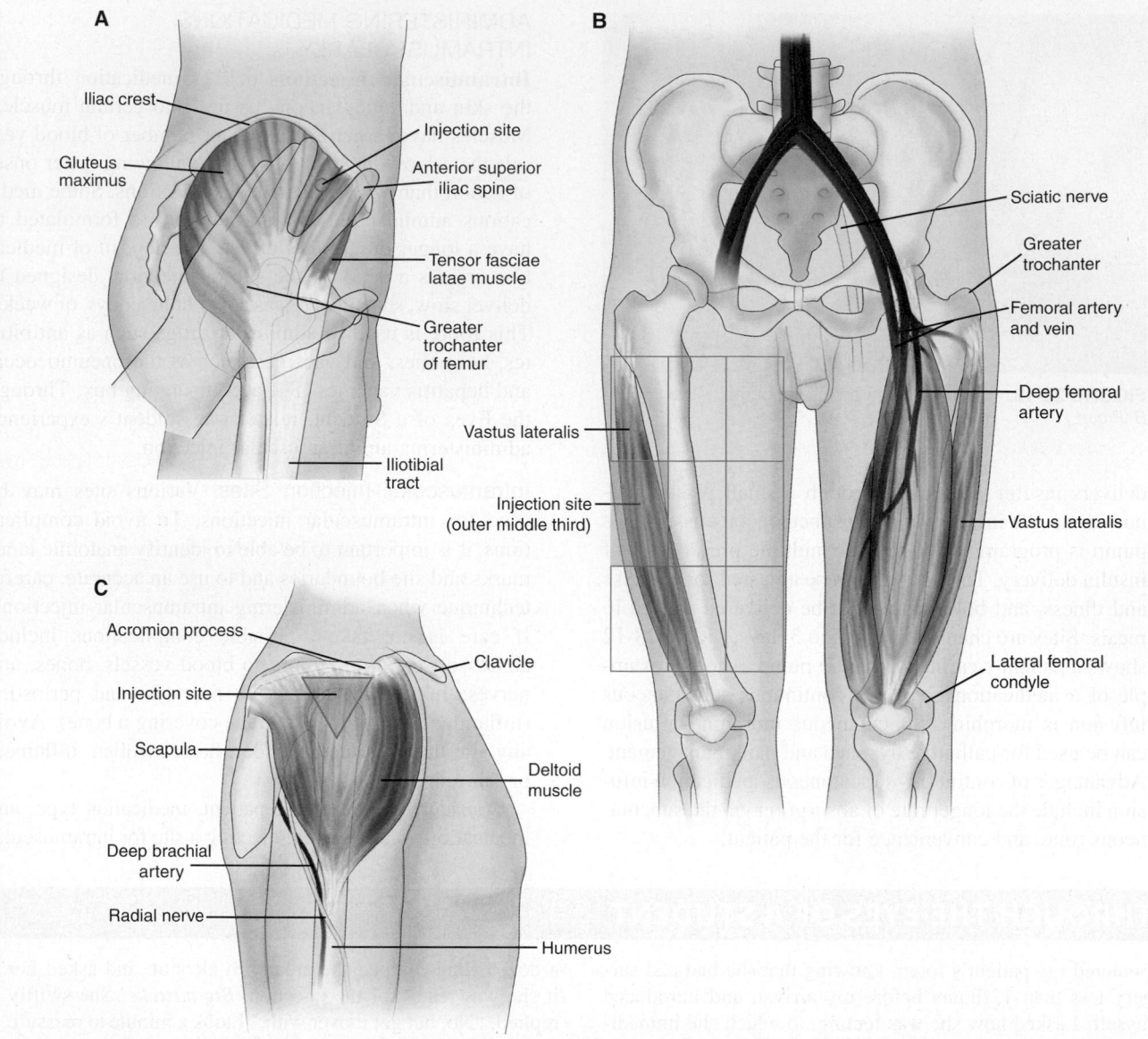

FIGURE 28-13. Sites for intramuscular injections. (**A**) The ventrogluteal site is located by placing the palm on the greater trochanter and the index finger toward the anterosuperior iliac spine. (**B**) The vastus lateralis site is identified by dividing the thigh into thirds, horizontally and vertically. (**C**) The deltoid muscle site is located by palpating the lower edge of the acromion process.

injection. See Table 28-4 for information related to intramuscular site selection. Rotate the sites used to administer intramuscular medications when therapy requires repeated injections. Whatever pattern of rotating sites is used, provide a description of it in the patient's plan of nursing care.

The *ventrogluteal site* (see Fig. 28-13A) involves the gluteus medius and gluteus minimus muscles in the hip area. This site offers a large muscle mass that is relatively free from major nerves and blood vessels, the area is clean (fecal contamination is rare at this site), and the patient can be on the back, abdomen, or side for the injection. To relax the gluteal muscle, the patient may flex the knees while lying on the back, point the toes inward while lying in the prone position, and flex the upper leg in front of the lower leg in the side-lying position. Although any of these three positions may be used when injecting

into the ventrogluteal site, nurses increasingly prefer the side-lying position.

To locate the ventrogluteal site, place the palm of your hand over the greater trochanter, with your fingers facing the patient's head. The right hand is used for the patient's left hip, or the left hand for the right hip, to identify landmarks. Place the index finger on the anterosuperior iliac spine and extend the middle finger dorsally, palpating the iliac crest. A triangle is formed, and the injection is given in the center of the triangle.

The *vastus lateralis* (see Fig. 28-13B) involves the quadriceps femoris muscle and is located along the anterolateral aspect of the thigh. There are no large nerves or vessels in its proximity, and it does not cover a joint. To locate the site, divide the thigh into thirds horizontally and vertically and administer the injection in the outer

Table 28-4 INTRAMUSCULAR SITE SELECTION

CRITERIA	RECOMMENDED SITE
Age of Patient	
Infants	Vastus lateralis
Toddlers and children	Vastus lateralis or deltoid
Adults	Ventrogluteal or deltoid
Medication Type	
Biologicals (infants and young children)	Vastus lateralis
Biologicals (older children and adults)	Deltoid
Hepatitis B/Rabies	Deltoid
Medications that are known to be irritating, Viscous, or oily solutions	Ventrogluteal

Adapted from Centers for Disease Control and Prevention (CDC). (2012). *The pink book: Appendices. Epidemiology and prevention of vaccine preventable diseases* (11th ed.). Appendix D. Vaccine administration. Vaccine administration guidelines. Available at http://www.cdc.gov/vaccines/pubs/pinkbook/index.html#appendices; and Nicoll, L., & Hesby, A. (2002). Intramuscular injection: An integrative research review and guideline for evidence-based practice. *Applied Nursing Research, 16*(2), 149–162.

middle third. This space provides a large number of injection sites. The vastus lateralis site is particularly desirable for infants and children, whose gluteal muscles are poorly developed. Restrain infants between the nurse's arm and body to safely administer an injection here.

The *deltoid muscle* is located in the lateral aspect of the upper arm (see Fig. 28-13C). It is the recommended site for vaccines for adults and may be used for children between 1 and 18 years of age for vaccine administration (CDC, 2012). The deltoid muscle is not developed enough in infants to absorb medication adequately.

Damage to the radial nerve and artery is a risk with use of the deltoid site. Intramuscular injections into the deltoid muscle should be limited to 1 mL of solution. Locate the deltoid muscle by palpating the lower edge of the acromion process. A triangle is formed at the midpoint in line with the axilla on the lateral aspect of the upper arm, with the base of the triangle at the acromion process. Hepatitis B virus vaccine is one medication that should be given in the deltoid muscle in adults to induce adequate levels of the antibody.

The dorsogluteal site has been previously identified as a possible site to be used for intramuscular medication administration. However, this site has been associated with inadvertent injection into subcutaneous tissue because the area is covered with subcutaneous tissue in many people; injection into subcutaneous tissue alters drug absorption and causes tissue irritation. More important, this site has been associated with significant injury, including pain and temporary or permanent paralysis, caused by damage to the sciatic nerve. Therefore, this site is no longer recommended for use for intramuscular

injections (Aschenbrener & Venable, 2012; Greenway, 2004; Nicoll & Hesby, 2002; Small, 2004; Zimmerman, 2010).

Equipment. It is important to choose the right equipment for a particular intramuscular injection. Needle length should be based on the site for injection and the patient's age (see Table 28-5 for intramuscular needle length recommendations). Patients who are obese may require a longer needle (Zaybak, Gunes, Tamsel, Khorshid, & Eser, 2007) and those who are emaciated may require a shorter needle. Appropriate gauge is determined by the medication being administered. Generally, biologic agents and medications in aqueous solutions should be administered with a 20- to 25-gauge needle. Medications in oil-based solutions should be administered with an 18- to 25-gauge needle. Many medications come in prefilled syringe units. If a needle is provided on the prefilled unit, ensure that the needle on the unit is the appropriate length for the patient and situation.

Procedure. The volume of medication that can be administered intramuscularly varies based on the intended site. Generally, 1 to 4 mL is the accepted volume range, with no more than 1 mL given at the deltoid site. The less-developed muscles of children and older adults limit the intramuscular injection to 1 to 2 mL.

Administer the intramuscular injection so that the needle is perpendicular to the patient's body. This should ensure that it is given using an angle of injection between 72 to 90 degrees (Katsma & Katsma, 2000). An outdated practice is the drawing up of an air bubble into the syringe after the medication has been prepared. This is not supported by research and should not be used (Nicoll & Hesby, 2002).

Many of the drugs given intramuscularly can cause irritation to subcutaneous tissues when backflow into

Table 28-5 INTRAMUSCULAR INJECTION NEEDLE LENGTH

SITE/AGE*	NEEDLE LENGTH
Vastus lateralis	5/8" to 1"
Deltoid (children)	5/8" to 1¼"
Deltoid (adults)	5/8" to 1½"
Ventrogluteal (adults)	1½"

*Patients who are obese may require a longer needle (Zaybak et al., 2007) and those who are emaciated may require a shorter needle.
Adapted from Centers for Disease Control and Prevention (CDC). (2012). *The pink book: Appendices. Epidemiology and prevention of vaccine preventable diseases* (11th ed.). Appendix D. Vaccine administration. Vaccine administration guidelines. Available http://www.cdc.gov/vaccines/pubs/pinkbook/index.html#appendices; and Nicoll, L., & Hesby, A. (2002). Intramuscular injection: An integrative research review and guideline for evidence-based practice. *Applied Nursing Research, 16*(2), 149–162.

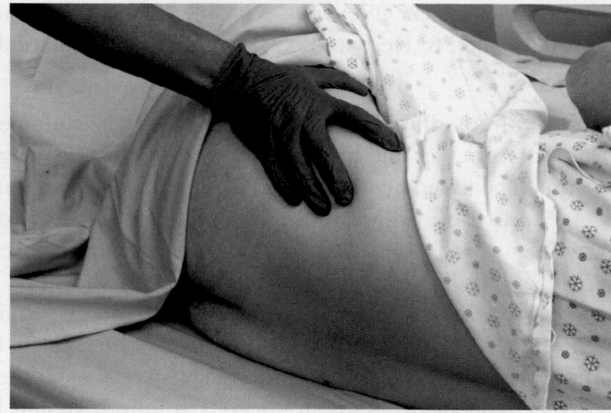

FIGURE 28-14. Spreading the skin taut at ventrogluteal site. *(Photo by Rick Brady.)*

the tissues occurs along the injection track. Therefore, the **Z-track technique** is recommended for all intramuscular injections to ensure that medication does not leak back along the needle track and into the subcutaneous tissue (Nicoll & Hesby, 2002; Zimmerman, 2010). This technique reduces pain and discomfort, particularly for patients receiving injections over an extended period. The Z-track method is also suggested for older patients who have decreased muscle mass. Some agents, such as iron, are best given via the Z-track method due to the irritation and discoloration associated with this agent.

In the Z-track technique, attach a clean needle to the syringe after the syringe is filled with the medication to prevent the injection of any residual medication on the needle into superficial tissues. Pull the skin down or to one side about 1″ (2.5 cm) and hold in this position with the nondominant hand. Insert the needle and inject the medication slowly. Withdraw the needle steadily and

release the displaced tissue to allow it to return to its normal position. Massage of the site is *not* recommended because it may cause irritation by forcing the medication to leak back into the needle track. However, gentle pressure may be applied with a dry sponge. The procedure for administering an intramuscular injection using the Z-track technique is outlined in Skill 28-7 on pages 827–831.

A previously included practice in intramuscular injection is aspiration (the process of pulling back on the plunger of the syringe before injection to ensure that the medication is not injected into a blood vessel). However, according to the CDC (2012) and current review of evidence (Crawford & Johnson, 2012), aspiration is not required. Some literature suggests that aspiration *may* be indicated when administering large-molecule medications such as penicillin (Crawford & Johnson). Consult facility policy and manufacturer recommendations to ensure safe administration.

An alternative method for intramuscular injection is to stretch the skin flat between two fingers and hold it taut for needle insertion. This technique for administering an intramuscular injection is illustrated in Figure 28-14. Figure 28-15 compares the angles for needle insertion for different forms of injections.

Several techniques have been suggested as interventions that can be used to reduce discomfort and pain associated with intramuscular injections. The application of manual pressure at the insertion site is one suggestion. Firmly press the insertion site for 10 seconds before needle insertion. This is thought to stimulate the surrounding nerve endings, leading to a reduction in the sensory input from the injection and decreased pain intensity (Chung, Ng, & Wong, 2002). Another suggested practice is to use separate needles to draw up and administer the medication. Changing the needle prior to administration of the

FIGURE 28-15. Comparison of the angles of insertion for intramuscular, subcutaneous, and intradermal injections.

medication ensures that the tip of the needle is sharp and free from medication residue, significantly reducing pain intensity associated with the injection (Ağaç & Güneş, 2010). Box 28-2 on page 779 provides additional techniques for reducing discomfort when injecting medications subcutaneously or intramuscularly.

ADMINISTERING MEDICATIONS INTRAVENOUSLY

Intravenous administration of medications delivers the drug directly into the bloodstream. Medications administered intravenously have an immediate effect. The **intravenous route** is the most dangerous route of administration because the drug is placed directly into the bloodstream, it cannot be recalled, and its actions cannot be slowed. Intravenous administration is the route used in most emergency situations when immediate onset of action is required. There also are many nonemergency clinical situations in which drugs are administered intravenously. Patient-controlled analgesia (PCA) allows the patient to control administration of an intravenous analgesic for pain management (refer to Chapter 34). Skill 39-1 on pages 1520–1527 describes the basic technique for administering an intravenous infusion. There are several ways to administer medications intravenously. Observe aseptic technique when administering medications intravenously to prevent introduction of microorganisms.

Medications via Intravenous Solution. Medications may be added to the patient's infusion solution. In most facilities, the pharmacist adds the prescribed drug to a large volume of intravenous solution.

When medication is administered by continuous infusion, the patient receives it slowly and over a long period. Although this can be an advantage when it is desirable to give the medication slowly, it is a disadvantage when the patient needs to receive the drug more quickly. Also, if for some reason not all of the solution can be infused, the patient will not receive the prescribed amount of the medication. Check the patient receiving medication by a continuous intravenous infusion for possible adverse effects at least every hour.

Medications via an Intravenous Bolus or Push. A medication can be administered as an intravenous bolus or push. This involves a single injection of a concentrated solution directly into an intravenous line (Skill 28-8, pp. 832–835). The drug is administered very slowly over at least 1 minute. Confirm exact administration times by consulting a pharmacist or drug reference.

Medications via Intermittent Intravenous Infusion. Medications can be administered by intermittent intravenous infusion. The drug is mixed with a small amount of the intravenous solution, such as 50 to 100 mL, and administered over a short period at the prescribed interval (e.g., every 4 hours). The administration is most often performed using an intravenous infusion pump, which requires the nurse to program the infusion rate into the pump. "Smart (computerized) pumps" are being used by many facilities for intravenous infusions, including intermittent infusions. Smart pumps also require programming of infusion rates by the nurse, but also are able to identify dosing limits and practice guidelines to aid in safe administration. More information about intravenous infusions and smart pumps is provided in Chapter 39. Administration may be achieved by gravity infusion, which requires the nurse to calculate the infusion rate in drops per minute. The best practice, however, is to use an intravenous infusion pump. The calculated flow rate of a medication administered via gravity can be altered when the patient bends the extremity proximal to the intravenous insertion site, lifts the extremity, or has an infiltration at the insertion site.

As mentioned, the CDC and the Occupational Safety and Health Administration (OSHA) recommend needleless devices. Needleless devices prevent needlesticks and provide access to the primary venous line. Access or connection ports are used to connect intermittent intravenous infusions. A patient with an intravenous line in place can receive the solution containing the medication by way of a piggyback setup, a volume-control administration set (e.g., Pediatrol or Volutrol), or a mini-infusion pump (syringe pump).

The intravenous **piggyback delivery system** requires the intermittent or additive solution to be placed higher than the primary solution container. An extension hook provided by the manufacturer provides for easy lowering of the main intravenous container. The port on the primary intravenous line has a back-check valve that automatically stops the flow of the primary solution, allowing the secondary or piggyback solution to flow when connected. A tandem delivery setup is similar, except that both solutions remain at the same height and there is no back-check valve at the secondary port on the primary line. This type of setup is used infrequently because the solution from the primary intravenous line will back up into the tandem line if this intermittent infusion is not clamped immediately after it is infused. Because manufacturers' designs vary, check the directions carefully for the systems used in the agency. Intravenous administration of medications using a piggyback setup is explained in Skill 28-9, pages 836–841.

Medications can also be placed in a **volume-control administration set** for intermittent intravenous infusion. The medication is diluted with a small amount of solution and administered through the patient's intravenous line (Fig. 28-16). This type of equipment may be used for infusing solutions into children, critically ill, and older patients when the volume of fluid infused is a concern.

The **mini-infusion pump** (syringe pump) for intermittent infusion is battery operated and allows medication mixed in a syringe to be connected to the primary

FIGURE 28-16. Volume-control administration set and IV solution for dilution of medication. *(Photo by B. Proud.)*

line (Fig. 28-17) and delivered by mechanical pressure applied to the syringe plunger.

A medication or drug infusion lock, also known as an intermittent peripheral venous access device, is used for patients who require intermittent intravenous medication, but not a continuous intravenous infusion. This device consists of a needle or catheter connected to a short length of tubing capped with a sealed injection port. A peripheral venous access device is shown in Skill 28-10 on pages 841–845. After the catheter is in place in the patient's vein, anchor the catheter and tubing to the patient's arm so that the catheter remains in place until the patient no longer requires the repeated medication intravenously.

An intermittent peripheral venous access device allows the patient more freedom than a continuous intravenous infusion. The patient is connected to the intravenous line when it is time to receive the medication and disconnected when the medication is completed. It is important to keep the device patent (working) by flushing with small amounts of saline pushed through the device on

a routine basis. Do not start intermittent infusion until intravenous placement is confirmed. Flush the peripheral venous access device before the infusion is begun and after the infusion is completed to clear the vein of any medication and to prevent clot formation in the needle. The procedure for flushing this device with saline is discussed in Skill 28-10. A medication prescribed as an intravenous bolus or push (discussed on page 785) may also be administered via a medication lock (refer to Skill 28-10). Assess the intravenous site for complications (see Chapter 39). If infiltration or phlebitis occurs, remove the device and replace in a new site.

In addition to a peripheral intravenous line, intermittent intravenous medication may be administered through a central venous access device (CVAD). Many of these devices have particular specifications to be followed when using for administration of fluids or medication. It is important to be aware of the specifics for the device being used. Facilities have specific policies in place for reference. CVADs are discussed in more detail in Chapter 39.

Administering Topical Medications

Medications delivered via the topical route are applied to the skin or mucous membranes, including the eyes, ears, nose, rectum, vagina, and lungs. **Topical applications** are usually intended for direct action at a particular site, although some can have systemic effects and are given for systemic effect. The action depends on the type of tissue and the nature of the agent.

If the site of application is readily accessible, such as the skin, an agent can easily be placed onto it. If it is a cavity, such as the nose, or is enclosed, such as the eye, a mechanical applicator may be needed to introduce the drug.

SKIN APPLICATIONS

The skin is a mechanical and chemical barrier that protects the underlying tissues. It is a sense organ, with receptors that respond to touch, pain, pressure, and temperature. The skin helps in excretion, in regulating body temperature, and in storing essentials to the body such as water, salts, and glucose.

When a drug is incorporated in an agent such as an ointment and rubbed into the skin for absorption, the procedure is referred to as an inunction. On normal skin, drugs are absorbed into the lining of the sebaceous glands. Absorption is hindered because of the protective outer layer of the skin, which makes penetration difficult and because of the fatty substances that protect the lining of the glands. Cleaning the skin thoroughly with soap or detergent and water before administration and then rubbing the medicated preparation into the skin can enhance absorption. Absorption can also be improved by using a drug mixed in an ointment or added to a liniment that will mix with the fat in the gland lining. When indicated, local heat applied to the application area can improve blood circulation and promote absorption. To prevent any absorption by the nurse's skin, wear gloves during the application of topical

FIGURE 28-17. Inserting syringe into mini-infusion pump.

BOX 28-3 TYPICAL PREPARATIONS APPLIED TO THE SKIN AREAS

Preparation	Use	Nursing Considerations
Powder	Promote drying of the skin Prevent friction on the skin	Use caution when applying to prevent inhalation of the powder. Apply powder to gauze square, then apply to the desired site to minimize inhalation of the airborne particles.
Ointment	Provide prolonged contact of a medication with the skin Soften the skin	Massage thoroughly into intact skin.
Creams and oils	Lubricate and soften skin Prevent drying of skin	When applying to large parts of the body, warm preparation in the hand or fingers to prevent the patient from experiencing chilling.
Lotions	Protect and soothe the skin	Shake thoroughly before using. Apply with cotton balls or gauze.
Transdermal: reservoirs, micro-reservoirs, adhesives, matrices	These systems are a "sandwich" of layers, each with a specific job. An impermeable backing prevents drug diffusion from the exposed portion. The drug layer of the system contains drug, with a rate-controlling layer to slow the release of the drug over time, ending with an adhesive layer to enhance the attachment of the system to the patient's skin (Ball & Smith, 2008).	Wear gloves. Handle by edges to avoid touching drug when handling system. Rotate application sites to avoid skin irritation.

medications. Refer to Box 28-3 for information related to typical preparations applied to the skin areas.

The transdermal route is being used more frequently to deliver medication. This involves applying to the skin a disk or patch that contains medication intended for daily use or for longer intervals. Transdermal patches are commonly used to deliver hormones, narcotic analgesics, cardiac medications, and nicotine. Transdermal patches that contain estrogen should not be applied to breast tissue due to the associated risks of breast cancer. Medication errors have occurred when patients applied multiple patches at once or failed to remove the overlay on the patch that exposes the skin to the medication. Opioid analgesic patches are associated with the most adverse drug effects. Clear patches have a cosmetic advantage but can be difficult to find on the patient's skin when they need to be removed or replaced. Despite a slow onset of action, transdermal drug patches maintain consistent serum drug levels. See Guidelines for Nursing Care 28-2: Applying Transdermal Patches (on page 788).

EYE INSTILLATIONS AND IRRIGATIONS
The receptors for the sense of sight are located in the eye. The outer layer of the eyeball is called the sclera. The cornea is the transparent part of the sclera in front of the eyeball. The sclera is fibrous and tough, but the cornea is injured easily by trauma. For this reason, applications to the eye seldom are placed directly onto the eyeball. Because direct application cannot be made onto the sensitive cornea, applications intended to act on the eye or the lids are placed onto, or instilled or irrigated into, the lower conjunctival sac.

The eye is a delicate organ, highly susceptible to infection and injury. Although the eye is never free of microorganisms, the secretions of the conjunctiva have a protective action against many pathogens. For maximum safety for the patient, the equipment, solutions, and ointments introduced into the conjunctival sac should be sterile. If this is not possible, follow the most careful guidelines for medical asepsis.

Eye Drops. Eye drops are instilled for their local effects, such as for pupil dilation or constriction when examining the eye, for treating an infection, or for controlling intraocular pressure in patients with glaucoma. The type and amount of solution depend on the purpose of the instillation. See Guidelines for Nursing Care 28-3: Instilling Eye drops (on page 789).

Ointments. Various types of medication in ointment form may be prescribed for the eye. These ointments are usually used for a local infection or irritation. Eye ointments are dispensed in a tube. A small amount of ointment is distributed along the exposed lower conjunctival sac after the eyelids and eyelashes have been cleansed. About 1/2″ of ointment is squeezed from the tube along the exposed sac moving from the inner canthus to the outer canthus of the eye. After the application, the eyes should be closed. The warmth helps to liquefy the ointment. Instruct the patient to move the eye because this helps to spread the ointment under the lids and over the surface of the eyeball. Explain that the ointment may temporarily blur vision; encourage the patient not to rub the eye.

GUIDELINES FOR NURSING CARE 28-2

APPLYING TRANSDERMAL PATCHES

- Perform hand hygiene and put on PPE, as indicated.
- **Identify the patient. Compare the information with the CMAR/MAR. The patient should be identified using at least two methods (TJC, 2013).**
- **Complete necessary assessments before administering medications. Check the patient's allergy bracelet or ask the patient about allergies. Explain the purpose and action of the medication to the patient.**
- Scan the patient's bar code on the identification band, if required.
- **Based on facility policy, the third check of the label may occur at this point. If so, recheck the labels with the CMAR/MAR before administering the medications to the patient.**
- Put on gloves.
- Assess patient's skin where patch is to be placed, looking for any signs of irritation or breakdown. Site should be clean, dry, and free of hair. Rotate application sites.
- **Remove any old transdermal patches from the patient's skin.** Fold patch in half with adhesive sides sticking together and discard according to facility policy.
- Gently wash the area where the old patch was with soap and water.
- Remove the patch from its protective covering.
- Remove the covering on the patch without touching the medication surface. Apply the patch to the patient's skin.

Use the palm of your hand to press firmly for about 10 seconds. Do not massage.
- Depending on facility policy, initial and write the date and time of administration on a piece of medical tape. Apply the tape to the patient's skin in close proximity to the patch. **Do not write directly on the medication patch.**
- Remove gloves and additional PPE, if used. Perform hand hygiene.
- Document the administration of medication immediately after administration including date, time, dose, route of administration, and site of administration on CMAR/MAR or record.
- Evaluate patient's response to medication within appropriate time frame for early detection of adverse effects.
- Check for dislodgement of the patch if the patient is active. Read information about the patch or consult with the prescriber or pharmacist to determine reapplication schedule and procedure.
- Assess for any skin irritation at application site. If necessary, remove the patch, wash the area carefully with soap and water, and allow skin to air dry. Apply a new patch at a different site. Assess the potential for adverse reaction.
- Aluminum backing on a patch necessitates precautions if defibrillation is required. Burns and smoke may result. These patches should be removed before an MRI is performed to avoid burning of the skin.

Eye Irrigation. Eye irrigation is performed to remove secretions or foreign bodies or to cleanse and soothe the eye. In an emergency, eye irrigation can be used to remove chemicals that may burn the eye. Copious amounts of tap water should be used to remove chemicals such as acid. The irrigation should continue for at least 15 minutes, and then professional help should be sought. Many emergency departments have eye flush stations to help with eye irrigations. Care should be taken so that the overflowing irrigation fluid does not contaminate the other eye.

Eye Medication Disks. An eye medication disk is flexible and resembles a contact lens. These disks contain medication that is released gradually into the conjunctival sac. Once applied, the disk remains in place for as long as a week before being removed and discarded. When properly placed, the disk is completely covered by the lower eyelid, allowing the patient to wear contact lenses, swim, and sleep with the disk in place. Eye medication disks are usually applied at bedtime because they initially cause blurring of vision.

EAR INSTILLATIONS AND IRRIGATIONS

The ear contains the receptors for hearing and equilibrium. It consists of the external ear, the middle ear, and the inner ear. The external ear consists of the auricle or pinna and the exterior auditory canal. The auditory canal serves as a passageway for sound waves. Drugs or irriga-

tions are instilled into the auditory canal for their local effect. They are used to soften wax, relieve pain, apply local anesthesia, destroy organisms, or destroy an insect lodged in the canal, which can cause almost intolerable discomfort. If the ear canal has swollen to the point that medication cannot pass, a long piece of cotton material called a wick is inserted so that one end is near the middle ear and the other end is external. This cotton then acts as a wick to help medication get into the canal.

The tympanic membrane separates the external ear from the middle ear. Normally, it is intact and closes the entrance to the middle ear completely. If it is ruptured or has been opened by surgical intervention, the middle ear and the inner ear have a direct passage to the external ear. When this occurs, instillations and irrigations should be performed with the greatest of care to prevent forcing materials from the outer ear into the middle ear and the inner ear. Sterile technique is used to prevent infection.

Ear Drops. Follow the techniques listed in Guidelines for Nursing Care 28-4: Instilling Ear Drops (on page 790) when placing drops in the external auditory canal.

Ear Irrigations. Irrigations of the external auditory canal are ordinarily done for cleaning purposes or for applying heat to the area. Typically, normal saline solution is used, although an antiseptic solution may be indicated for local action. To prevent pain, the irrigation solution should be

GUIDELINES FOR NURSING CARE 28-3

INSTILLING EYE DROPS

- Perform hand hygiene.
- **Identify the patient. Compare the information with the CMAR/MAR. The patient should be identified using at least two methods (TJC, 2013).**
- **Complete necessary assessments before administering medications. Check the patient's allergy bracelet or ask the patient about allergies. Explain the purpose and action of the medication to the patient.**
- Scan the patient's bar code on the identification band, if required.
- **Based on facility policy, the third check of the label may occur at this point. If so, recheck the labels with the CMAR/MAR before administering the medications to the patient.**
- Put on gloves.
- Offer the patient paper tissues to remove solution and tears that may spill from the eye during the procedure.
- Clean the eyelids and eyelashes of any drainage with cotton balls or gauze squares moistened with normal saline solution. Debris can be carried into the eye when the conjunctival sac is exposed. Use each area of the cleaning surface once, moving from the inner toward the outer canthus to prevent carrying debris to the lacrimal ducts.
- Tilt the patient's head back slightly if sitting, or place the patient's head over a pillow if lying down. **Tilting the patient's head should be avoided if the patient has a cervical spine injury.** The head may be turned slightly to the affected side to prevent solution or tears from flowing toward the opposite eye.
- Remove the cap from the medication bottle, being careful not to touch the inner side of the cap.
- Invert the monodrip plastic container that is commonly used to instill eye drops.
- Have the patient look up while focusing on something on the ceiling.
- Place the thumb or two fingers near the margin of the lower eyelid immediately below the eyelashes, and exert pressure downward over the bony prominence of the cheek. The lower conjunctival sac is exposed as the lower lid is pulled down.

- **Hold the dropper close to the eye but avoid touching the eyelids or lashes.** Touching the eye, eyelids, or lashes can contaminate the medication in the bottle; startle the patient, causing blinking; or injure the eye.
- Squeeze the container and allow the prescribed number of drops to fall in the lower conjunctival sac. Do not allow medication to fall onto the cornea. This may injure the cornea or cause the patient to have an unpleasant sensation.
- Release the lower lid after the eye drops are instilled. Ask the patient to close the eyes gently.
- Apply gentle pressure with your gloved finger over the inner canthus to prevent the eye drops from flowing into the tear duct. This minimizes the risk of systemic effects from the medication.
- Instruct the patient not to rub the affected eye.
- Remove gloves and additional PPE, if used. Perform hand hygiene.
- Document the administration of medication immediately after administration including date, time, dose, route of administration, and site of administration on CMAR/MAR or record.
- Evaluate the patient's response to the medication within the appropriate time frame.

With the lower lid pulled down, the nurse prepares to administer the eye drops on the lower conjunctival sac.

---

at least at room temperature. An irrigation syringe is used in most instances. An irrigating container with tubing and an ear tip may also be used, especially if the purpose of the irrigation is to apply heat to the area.

NASAL INSTILLATIONS

Besides serving as the olfactory organ, the nose functions as an airway to the lower respiratory tract and protects the tract by cleaning and warming the air taken in by inspiration. Cilia project on most of the surfaces of the nasal mucous membrane, which help remove particles of dirt and dust from the inspired air. The nose also serves as a resonator when speaking and singing.

Nasal instillations are used to treat allergies, sinus infections, and nasal congestion. Medications with a sys-

temic effect, such as vasopressin, may also be prepared as a nasal instillation. The nose is normally not a sterile cavity, but, because of its connection with the sinuses, it is important to observe medical asepsis carefully when using nasal instillations. See Guidelines for Nursing Care 28-5: Administering a Nasal Spray (on page 791).

Medications may also be applied to the nasal mucous membrane via nasal drops. The patient should blow the nose before instilling the drops. Have the patient sit up with head tilted well back and maintain this position for a few minutes after instillation. This position allows the solution to flow well back into the nares. Hold up the tip of the nose and place the dropper just inside the naris, about one third of an inch, without touching the nare. Instill the prescribed number of drops in one naris and

GUIDELINES FOR NURSING CARE 28-4

INSTILLING EAR DROPS

- Perform hand hygiene and put on PPE, as indicated.
- **Identify the patient. Compare the information with the CMAR/MAR. The patient should be identified using at least two methods (TJC, 2013).**
- **Complete necessary assessments before administering medications. Check the patient's allergy bracelet or ask the patient about allergies. Explain the purpose and action of the medication to the patient.**
- Scan the patient's bar code on the identification band, if required.
- **Based on facility policy, the third check of the label may occur at this point. If so, recheck the labels with the CMAR/MAR before administering the medications to the patient.**
- Put on gloves.
- Clean the external ear of drainage with cotton balls moistened with normal saline solution, as necessary.
- Place the patient on the unaffected side in bed, or if ambulatory, have the patient sit with the head well tilted to the side so that the affected ear is uppermost. This positioning prevents the drops from escaping from the ear.
- Draw up the amount of solution needed in the dropper. Excess medication should not be returned to a stock bottle. A monodrip plastic container may also be used.
- Straighten the auditory canal by pulling the cartilaginous portion of the pinna up and back in an adult (Fig. A),

straight back for a child older than 3 (Fig. B), and down and back in an infant or a child under age 3 years (Fig. C). Pulling on the pinna as described helps to straighten the canal properly for ear instillation.

- Hold the dropper in the ear with its tip above the auditory canal. For an infant or an irrational or confused patient, protect the dropper with a piece of soft tubing to help prevent injury to the ear.
- **Allow drops to fall on the side of the canal. Avoid instilling in the middle of the canal, to avoid instilling directly onto the tympanic membrane.**
- Release the pinna after instilling the drops, and have the patient maintain the position to prevent the medication from escaping.
- Gently press on the tragus a few times to help move the medication from the canal toward the tympanic membrane.
- If ordered, loosely insert a cotton ball to prevent medication from leaking out.
- Wait 5 minutes before instilling drops in the second ear, if ordered.
- Remove gloves and additional PPE, if used. Perform hand hygiene.
- Document the administration of medication immediately after administration including date, time, dose, route of administration, and site of administration on CMAR/MAR or record.

(**A**) Adult patient positioned for eardrop instillation; nurse straightens the auditory canal by pulling the cartilaginous portion of the pinna up and back. (**B**) School-aged child positioned for eardrop instillation; nurse straightens the auditory canal by pulling the cartilaginous portion of the pinna straight back. (**C**) Child under 3 years of age ready for eardrop instillation; nurse straightens the auditory canal by pulling the cartilaginous portion of the pinna down and back. Child can be held by parent.

GUIDELINES FOR NURSING CARE 28-5

INSTILLING NOSE SPRAY

- Perform hand hygiene and put on PPE, as indicated.
- **Identify the patient. Compare the information with the CMAR/MAR. The patient should be identified using at least two methods (TJC, 2013):**
- **Complete necessary assessments before administering medications. Check the patient's allergy bracelet or ask the patient about allergies. Explain the purpose and action of the medication to the patient.**
- Scan the patient's bar code on the identification band, if required.
- **Based on facility policy, the third check of the label may occur at this point. If so, recheck the labels with the CMAR/MAR before administering the medications to the patient.**
- Put on gloves.
- Provide the patient with paper tissues and ask that the patient blow the nose before instilling the nose drops.
- Have the patient sit up with head tilted back. **Tilting the patient's head should be avoided if the patient has a cervical spine injury.**
- Instruct the patient to inhale gently through the nose as the spray is being administered or not, depending on the medication being administered.
- Agitate the bottle gently, if required for specific medication. Insert the tip of the nose piece of the bottle into one nostril.
- Close the opposite nostril with a finger. Instruct the patient to breathe in gently through the nostril, if required. Compress or activate the bottle to release one spray at the same time the patient breathes in.
- Keep the medication container compressed and remove from the nostril. Release the container from the compressed

state. Do not allow the container to return to its original position until it is removed from the patient's nose.
- Have patient hold his or her breath for a few seconds, and then breathe out slowly through the mouth. Repeat in the other nostril, as prescribed or indicated.
- Wipe the outside of the bottle nose piece with a clean, dry tissue or cloth and replace the cap. Instruct the patient to avoid blowing the nose for 5 to 10 minutes, depending on the medication.
- Remove gloves and additional PPE, if used. Perform hand hygiene.
- Document the administration of medication immediately after administration including date, time, dose, route of administration, and site of administration on CMAR/MAR or record.

Inserting tip of bottle into nostril. (Craven, R.F. & Hirnle, C. J. (2009). *Fundamentals of Nursing* (6th ed). Lippincott Williams & Wilkins | Wolters Kluwer Health.)

---

then into the other. Avoid touching the nares with the dropper; inadvertent contact may cause the patient to sneeze and contaminate the dropper.

VAGINAL APPLICATIONS

A healthy vagina contains few pathogens, but many nonpathogenic organisms. The nonpathogens are important because they protect the vagina from the invasion of pathogens. The normal secretions in the vagina are acidic and further serve to protect the vagina from microbial invasion. Therefore, the normal mucous membrane is its own best protection.

Creams, foams, and tablets can be applied intravaginally using a narrow, tubular applicator with an attached plunger. Suppositories that melt when exposed to body heat are also administered by vaginal insertion. Refrigerate suppositories for storage.

Ask the patient to void before inserting the medication. Position the patient so that she is lying on her back with knees flexed. Maintain privacy with draping. Provide adequate light to visualize the vaginal opening. See Guidelines for Nursing Care 28-6: Inserting Vaginal Cream or Suppository (on page 792).

RECTAL INSTILLATIONS

Rectal suppositories are used primarily for their local action, such as laxatives and fecal softeners. Systemic effects are also achieved with rectal suppositories. Acetaminophen suppositories are used for an antipyretic effect, and many antiemetics are available in suppository form to relieve nausea and vomiting. Do not administer suppositories to patients who have had recent rectal or prostate surgery. Assess recent laboratory values, particularly the patient's white blood cell and platelet counts. Patients who are thrombocytopenic or neutropenic should not receive rectal suppositories. Do not administer rectal suppositories to patients at risk for cardiac arrhythmias.

Use clean disposable gloves to prevent contamination with feces and microorganisms. Refer to Guidelines for Nursing Care 28-7: Inserting a Rectal Suppository (on page 793). After the suppository is inserted, the patient should remain in that position for 5 minutes. If the suppository is for laxative purposes, it must remain in position for 35 to 45 minutes, or until the patient feels the urge to defecate.

GUIDELINES FOR NURSING CARE 28-6

INSERTING VAGINAL CREAM OR SUPPOSITORY

- Perform hand hygiene and put on PPE, if indicated.
- **Identify the patient. Compare the information with the CMAR/MAR. The patient should be identified using at least two methods (TJC, 2013).**
- **Complete necessary assessments before administering medications. Check the patient's allergy bracelet or ask the patient about allergies. Explain the purpose and action of the medication to the patient.**
- Scan the patient's bar code on the identification band, if required.
- **Based on facility policy, the third check of the label may occur at this point. If so, recheck the labels with the CMAR/MAR before administering the medications to the patient.**
- Ask the patient to void before inserting medication.
- Put on gloves.
- Position the patient so that she is lying on her back with knees flexed. Maintain privacy with draping. Provide adequate light to visualize vaginal opening.
- Spread labia with fingers and clean area at vaginal orifice with washcloth and warm water, using a different corner of the washcloth with each stroke. Wipe from front to back.
- Remove gloves and put on new gloves.

- Fill a vaginal applicator with the prescribed amount of cream, or have a suppository ready (Fig. A).
- Lubricate the applicator with lubricant, as necessary. The rounded end of a suppository may be lubricated with a water-soluble lubricant (Fig. B).
- For a vaginal cream, spread the labia and introduce the applicator gently in a rolling manner while directing it downward and backward to follow the normal contour of the vagina for its full length. Push the plunger to its full length, then gently remove the applicator with the plunger depressed. For a vaginal suppository, lubricate your gloved index finger on your dominant hand. Spread the labia and insert the rounded end of the suppository along the posterior wall of the canal to the length of your finger.
- **Ask the patient to remain in the supine position for 5 to 10 minutes after insertion.**
- Offer the patient a perineal pad to collect drainage.
- Remove gloves and additional PPE, if used. Perform hand hygiene.
- Document the administration of medication immediately after administration including date, time, dose, route of administration, and site of administration on CMAR/MAR or record.

(**A**) Filling vaginal applicator with cream. (**B**) Lubricating vaginal suppository.

Administering Medications by Inhalation

Drugs for **inhalation** are aerosolized, delivered in small particles, and breathed in by the patient. The lungs are supplied richly with blood and have a large surface area. These characteristics allow drugs to be absorbed easily from the lower respiratory tract. Inhalation may be used to administer several different classes of drugs with varying properties and indications. The smaller the particles of inhaled medication, the lower in the respiratory tract the medication tends to travel. A disadvantage of using this route is that the drug dosage is difficult to establish.

Drugs classified as bronchodilators are an example of a medication administered by inhalation. Bronchodilators act to decrease resistance to airflow by enlarging

air passageways. Bronchodilators promote relaxation of musculature in the tracheobronchial tree. The relaxed passages produce less resistance to airflow and provide an opened respiratory passageway. Bronchodilators are further discussed in Chapter 38.

Drugs for inhalation may be administered by a hand atomizer or a nebulizer. These devices break up the medication into a mist for more efficient inhalation. The hand-held, metered-dose inhaler (MDI) is often used incorrectly, and the correct dose of medication is not delivered. For better medication delivery, use a spacer whenever administering medication via an MDI, particularly with a child. Refer to Guidelines for Nursing Care 28-8: Using an Inhaled Medication Device.

GUIDELINES FOR NURSING CARE 28-7

INSERTING A RECTAL SUPPOSITORY

- Perform hand hygiene and put on PPE, if indicated.
- **Identify the patient. Compare the information with the CMAR/MAR. The patient should be identified using at least two methods (TJC, 2013).**
- **Complete necessary assessments before administering medications. Check the patient's allergy bracelet or ask the patient about allergies. Explain the purpose and action of the medication to the patient.**
- Scan the patient's bar code on the identification band, if required.
- **Based on facility policy, the third check of the label may occur at this point. If so, recheck the labels with the CMAR/MAR before administering the medications to the patient.**
- Put on gloves.
- Assist the patient to his left side in a Sims position. Drape accordingly to expose only the buttocks.
- Remove the suppository from its wrapper. Apply lubricant to the rounded end. Lubricate the index finger of your dominant hand.

- Separate the buttocks with your nondominant hand and instruct the patient to breathe slowly and deeply through the mouth while the suppository is being inserted.
- Using your index finger, insert the suppository, round end first, along the rectal wall. Insert about 3 to 4 inches.
- Use toilet tissue to clean any stool or lubricant from around the anus. Release the buttocks. Encourage the patient to remain on his side for at least 5 minutes and retain the suppository for the appropriate amount of time for the specific medication.
- Remove gloves and additional PPE, if used. Perform hand hygiene.
- Document the administration of medication immediately after administration including date, time, dose, route of administration, and site of administration on CMAR/MAR or record.

GUIDELINES FOR NURSING CARE 28-8

USING AN INHALED MEDICATION DEVICE

- Assess the patient's ability to manage a metered-dose inhaler, dry powder inhaler, or small-volume nebulizer.
- Explain, demonstrate, and encourage the patient to manipulate the inhaler or nebulizer apparatus.
- Encourage the patient to wash hands thoroughly before using device.
- Perform hand hygiene.
- **Identify the patient. Compare the information with the CMAR/MAR. The patient should be identified using at least two methods (TJC, 2013).**
- **Complete necessary assessments before administering medications. Check the patient's allergy bracelet or ask the patient about allergies. Explain the purpose and action of the medication to the patient.**
- Scan the patient's bar code on the identification band, if required.
- **Based on facility policy, the third check of the label may occur at this point. If so, recheck the labels with the CMAR/MAR before administering the medications to the patient.**

Metered-Dose Inhaler (MDI)

- Remove the mouthpiece cover and shake inhaler well.
- If a spacer is used, remove cover from the spacer. Attach the MDI to the spacer. Have the patient place the spacer's mouthpiece into mouth, grasping securely with teeth and lips.
- If no spacer is used, patient takes a deep breath, exhales, holds the inhaler 1 to 2 inches away from the mouth,

inhales slowly and deeply while depressing the medication canister and continues to inhale for a full breath.
- Have patient breathe normally through the spacer.
- Patient should depress the canister, releasing one puff into the spacer, then inhale slowly and deeply through the mouth.
- **Instruct patient to hold his or her breath for 5 to 10 seconds, or as long as possible, then to exhale slowly through pursed lips.**
- **Wait 1 to 5 minutes, as prescribed, before administering the next puff, as prescribed.**
- Have the patient gargle and rinse with tap water after using an MDI, as necessary. Clean the MDI according to the manufacturer's directions.

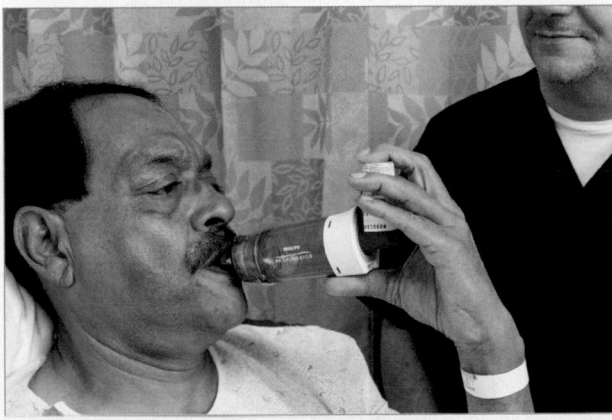

Patient using a metered-dose inhaler with a spacer.

(continued)

GUIDELINES FOR NURSING CARE 28-8 *continued*

Dry Powder Inhaler (DPI)

* Understand the specific instructions for individual DPI.
* Perform hand hygiene.
* **Identify the patient. Compare the information with the CMAR/MAR. The patient should be identified using at least two methods (TJC, 2013).**
* Explain the procedure to the patient.
* Remove the mouthpiece cover and load a dose if necessary. Alternately, activate the inhaler, if necessary, according to the manufacturer's directions.
* Have the patient breathe out slowly and completely, without breathing into the DPI. **The patient should place teeth over, and seal lips around, the mouthpiece. Do not block the opening with the tongue or teeth.**
* **Have the patient breathe in quickly and deeply through the mouth, for longer than 2 to 3 seconds.**
* Remove the inhaler from the mouth. Instruct the patient to hold his or her breath for 5 to 10 seconds, or as long as possible, and then to exhale slowly through pursed lips.
* Wait 1 to 5 minutes, as prescribed, before administering the next puff. After the prescribed amount of puffs has been administered, have the patient replace the cap or storage container.
* Have the patient gargle and rinse with tap water after using a DPI, as necessary. Clean the DPI according to the manufacturer's directions.

Small-Volume Nebulizer

* Perform all preparation steps for administering medications as described previously.
* Remove the nebulizer cup from the device and open it.
* Place premeasured unit dose medication in the bottom section of the cup or use a dropper to place concentrated dose of medication in the cup and add prescribed fluid to dilute it.
* Screw the top portion of the nebulizer cup back in place and attach the cup to the nebulizer.
* Attach one end of tubing to the stem on the bottom of the nebulizer cuff and the other end to the air compressor or oxygen source.
* Turn on the air compressor or oxygen.

Small-volume nebulizer.

* Check that a fine medication mist is produced by opening the valve.
* Have the patient place the mouthpiece into mouth and grasp securely with teeth and lips.
* **Have patient inhale slowly and deeply through the mouth and hold each breath for a slight pause before exhaling. (A nose clip may be necessary if the patient is also breathing through the nose.)**
* Have patient continue this inhalation technique until all medication in the nebulizer cup has been aerosolized (usually about 15 minutes).
* Have the patient gargle and rinse with tap water after using the nebulizer, as needed.
* Clean the nebulizer according to manufacturer's directions.

Special Considerations

* Patients should know how to tell when medication levels are getting low. The most reliable method is to look on the canister and see how many puffs the canister contains. Divide this number by the number of puffs used daily to ascertain how many days the MDI will last. For instance, if the MDI contains 200 puffs and the patient takes 6 puffs per day, the MDI should last for 33 days. Keep a diary or record of inhaler use and discard the inhaler on reaching the labeled number of doses. This method may be cumbersome and impractical for some patients, but it is a reliable way to determine how much medication remains in an MDI. Another accurate way to know when the canister is depleted is to use a dose counter, which counts down each time the canister is activated (Rubin, 2010). **Floating the canister in water is not reliable and is contraindicated. Immersion in water can cause valve obstruction and threatens product integrity (Rubin).**

Home Considerations

* Spacer and inhalers should be cleaned at least weekly with warm water or soaked in a vinegar solution (1 pint of water to 2 oz of vinegar) for 20 minutes. Rinse with clean water and allow to air dry.

Examples of metered-dose inhalers, spacer, and dry powder inhaler.

Dry powder inhalers (DPI) are another type of delivery method for inhaled medications. The medication is supplied in a powder form, either in a small capsule or disk inserted into the DPI, or in a compartment inside the DPI. DPIs are breath activated. A quick breath by the patient activates the flow of medication, eliminating the need to coordinate activating the inhaler (spraying the medicine) while inhaling the medicine at the same time. However, the drug output and size distribution of the aerosol from a DPI is more or less dependent on the flow rate through the device, thus the patient must be able to take a powerful, deep inspiration (Rubin, 2010). Many types of DPIs are available, with distinctive operating instructions. Some have to be loaded with a dose of medication each time they are used and some hold a preloaded number of doses. It is important to understand the particular instructions for the medication and particular delivery device being used. Refer to the Guidelines for Nursing Care 28-8.

Nebulization may also result from the force of an oxygen stream or compressed air passed through the fluid in a nebulizer or an atomizer. This method is valuable for patients who require inhalation of a drug several times a day when the hand atomizer is fatiguing. Infants and toddlers can also benefit from nebulized medications. With the use of an oxygen mask, children can receive medications with minimal interruption of their activities. Oxygen masks for the pediatric population come in a variety of sizes and also have dinosaurs or turtles to make the mask less intimidating for the child. The oxygen stream is also useful in the production of vapors when high humidity is needed continuously for long periods. Refer to the Guidelines for Nursing Care 28-8.

Documenting Medication Administration

The medication record is a legal document. Recording each dose of medication as soon as possible after it is given provides a documented record that can be consulted if there are any questions about whether the patient received the medication. Do not record medications before they are given. If the medication were then not given, the medication record would show falsely that the patient received the medication. Different forms are used for recording medications; an example of a computerized medication administration record (CMAR) is given in Figure 28-18.

The name of the medication, dosage, route of administration, time given, and name of the person administering the medication are noted in the record. Record the site used for an injection. The identity of the nurse completing the documentation is recorded based on the unique user ID and password assigned to each nurse when a CMAR is used. Other specific patient information may be required. For instance, record the pulse rate when administering some cardiac drugs or record a description of the effects on the patient's pain when administering analgesics.

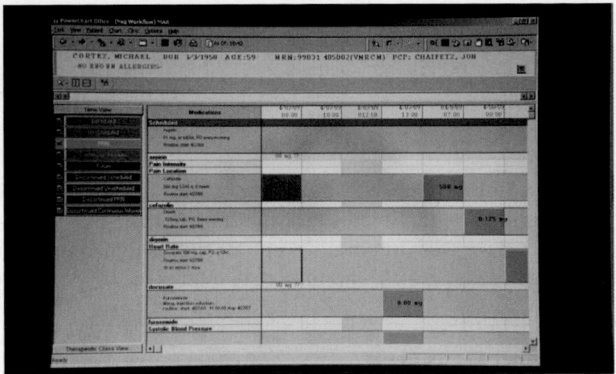

FIGURE 28-18. Example of a computerized medication administration record. *(Photo by B. Proud.)*

OMITTED DRUGS

Drugs may be omitted intentionally or inadvertently. The omission and the reason for it are documented on the patient's record. Drugs may be omitted intentionally for the following reasons:

- The patient is to have a diagnostic test and is required to fast before the test. Oral drugs may be omitted, or their administration may be delayed, depending on the primary care provider's orders.
- The problem for which the medication is intended no longer exists. For example, a laxative has been ordered for a patient. The patient has had a bowel movement and no longer needs the laxative. The laxative is then omitted.
- The patient is suspected of having an allergy to the medication. Any suspected allergy should be reported to the primary care provider.

REFUSED DRUGS

If the patient refuses to take a drug that is considered essential to the therapeutic regimen, report this promptly. It is important to determine the reason for the refusal and to help the patient accept needed drugs. If the patient is not persuaded by reasonable efforts and adamantly refuses to take a medication, it is unwise to continue urging the patient. Patients have the right to refuse therapy; recognize and respect that right. Describe the refusal to take prescribed drugs and the manner in which the situation was managed in the patient's record and report the refusal according to facility policy.

Preventing and Responding to Medication Errors

Nurses should take every precaution to avoid errors when administering therapeutic agents. The safe nurse does not allow automatic habits of preparing medications or technology to replace constant thinking, purposeful action, and repeated checking for accuracy. Nurses may lack knowledge about the medication, including the indication, usual dose, route, actions, adverse effects, contraindications, and drug–drug or food–drug interactions, which can lead to errors (Shane, 2009). It is important to make

RESEARCH IN NURSING

BRIDGING THE GAP TO EVIDENCE-BASED PRACTICE

Medication Errors

Medication administration is one of the highest risk areas in health care, and medication errors can have many causes. Nurses have very important responsibilities in the prevention of medication errors, and they play a key role in the medication process.

Related Research

Unver, V., Tastan, S., & Akbayrak, N. (2012). Medication errors: Perspectives of newly graduated and experienced nurses. *International Journal of Nursing Practice, 18*(4), 317–324.

This study investigated the perspectives of newly graduated (87) and experienced (82) nurses concerning medication errors. Data was collected on rates, causes, and reporting of medication errors. The two highest perceived causes of medication errors were nurse exhaustion and nurse distraction. A statistically significant difference was found between experienced nurses and newly graduated nurses in relation to

the identification of what constitutes a medication error. This indicated that increased professional experience might lead to an increased level of awareness concerning the occurrence of medication errors. It was shown that experienced nurses are better able to recognize the causes of drug errors compared with newly graduated nurses. Most medication errors were preventable.

Relevance to Nursing Practice

Nurses have a responsibility to maintain heightened awareness of the causes for medication errors in their practice. Training nurses to understand the causes of medication errors and related prevention should be provided to newly graduated nurses, and continuous training should continue for experienced nurses.

For additional research, visit thePoint.

use of appropriate references, including medication software, online medication databases, and consultation with a pharmacist (Dinescu et al., 2012).

Nurses need to understand the causes of medication errors and related prevention methods to reduce the incidence of error. Refer to the accompanying Research in Nursing display, "Medication Errors." Common types of medication errors include the following:

- Inappropriate prescribing of the drug (e.g., incorrect dose, quantity, or route; or inadequate instruction)
- Extra, omitted, or wrong doses
- Administration of a medication to a patient that was not ordered for that patient (see Focused Critical Thinking Guide 28-1)
- Administration of a drug by an incorrect route or at an incorrect rate
- Failure to give a medication within the prescribed time interval
- Incorrect preparation of a drug before administration
- Improper technique when administering a drug
- Giving a drug that has deteriorated

Medication errors often occur at points of transition in care: on admission to a hospital, at transfer from one department to another, and at discharge home or to another facility. The principal cause of medication error at these times is the incorrect or incomplete transfer of medication information (Barnsteiner, 2005). Nurses and other health care providers must be vigilant in order to minimize the high risk for harm from adverse drug events when communication about medications is not clear and in carefully checking that all medications that are appropriate are reordered. A medication reconciliation process that maintains a current, accurate list of medications

a patient has received has been shown to decrease the incidence of medication errors that occur at these points of transition in patient care (Aschenbrenner & Venable, 2012; Barnsteiner, 2005). Nurses are often responsible for management of these lists and need to be on heightened alert to watch for errors at these points of transition.

Prompt acknowledgment of errors may minimize their possible detrimental effect. The immediate priority is the safety of the patient. The following steps are recommended when a medication error occurs:

1. Check the patient's condition immediately when the error is noted. Observe for the development of adverse effects related to the error.
2. Notify the nurse manager and the primary care provider to discuss possible courses of action, depending on the patient's condition.
3. Write a description of the error on the patient's medical record, including remedial steps that are taken.
4. Complete the form used for reporting errors, as dictated by facility policy. These forms—called special event, event, or unusual occurrence reports—require an objective, complete account of the medication error. Include the steps taken after the error was recognized. For legal reasons, describe the error fully and accurately. Medication errors are a common allegation in nursing liability cases. Do not document in the patient's record the fact that an incident report was filed.

There are several voluntary external reporting programs that track medication errors. Nurses and other health care providers are encouraged to report medication errors to these organizations. Reporting errors to one of these programs assists in learning more about patient safety, enhancing patient safety standards, and implementing

FOCUSED CRITICAL THINKING GUIDE 28-1

MEDICATIONS

You are caring for two residents in a long-term care facility. One of your residents is scheduled to receive a B_{12} injection, and because it will be your first intramuscular injection, it has you more than a little apprehensive. You are eagerly waiting for the moment when your instructor will be free to supervise your injection. Meanwhile, she has cleared you to administer the 10 AM meds; you bring a multivitamin, a diuretic, and an anti-inflammatory agent to one of your assigned residents. When you go to record the medications you administered, you suddenly realize to your horror that you brought them to the wrong resident. When you grab your buddy and confide your error, she says, "Whatever you do, don't tell Miss McMullen [the clinical instructor]. She gets spastic about med errors and has a reputation for gleefully failing students!" You remember that the resident who received the wrong medications has no known drug allergies and you think that she probably wouldn't suffer any adverse effects from the meds she received. What should you do?

1. Identify goal of thinking

Determine how you ought to respond to the realization that you administered medications to the wrong resident.

2. Assess adequacy of knowledge

Pertinent circumstances: A resident has received three medications that were not ordered for her. *You are a nursing student in your first clinical rotation* and fear your clinical instructor's response should you inform her about your error. You are unsure of the harm that might result from the resident receiving the wrong medication.

Prerequisite knowledge: To decide how you should respond in this situation, you need to understand your professional obligations, which include your moral and legal accountability for having committed a medication error. You will need knowledge of the pharmacologic action of each of the medications you administered and their potential adverse effects on the resident who received them (possible interactions with other medications she is receiving, contraindications with related adverse effects, etc.). You recognize that there is no way for you to get the knowledge you need to make a morally and legally defensible response unless you admit your error to a responsible party.

Room for error/Time constraints: Because you do not know the effects of these medications, you are not in a position to judge how much room there is for error, nor are you able to make a prudent decision about how much time you have to act. The only defensible response is to seek help to clarify your position immediately because a resident's well-being is potentially at stake. No imagined personal costs would justify a delay in your admission of your error.

3. Address potential problems

The most serious obstacle to critical thinking in this situation would be an inability to think rationally about your obligation to report the error because of your fear of being censured by your clinical instructor. You will want to examine critically your friend's claim that your instructor will respond harshly because this may not, in fact, be the case. You will also want to test your friend's unstated assumption that your primary obligation in this sort of situation is to take care of yourself—even if this course of action results in harm to a patient. It would be helpful to think through the consequences of every health care professional behaving in this manner.

4. Consult helpful resources

Given that you are new to medication administration and are unable to assess the potential harm caused to the resident who received the wrong medications, you will find that your most helpful resource is your instructor, and you will need to enlist her assistance immediately. She will probably want to contact the resident's physician to determine whether there are any contraindications to this resident's receiving the medications you administered or possible interactions with other medications. A pharmacist may also need to be consulted. You will want to be familiar with the institution's policy on medication errors and will need to know how to complete an incident report. If the long-term care facility has a risk manager, you may want to consult that person.

5. Critique judgment/decision

You have two options here: Admit your error and initiate appropriate follow-up or attempt to cover up your error and "hope for the best." Your decision will basically be made on the strength of your moral conviction that your primary obligation is to safeguard patient well-being, even should this involve some self-sacrifice. Once you recognize the potentially disastrous consequences of patients not being able to trust health care professionals to act in their best interests, you decide that there really is only one professionally acceptable response in this situation, and you inform your instructor. It turns out that the resident who received the wrong medications suffered no adverse reactions. You, on the other hand, spend an awful morning following up on your error and even have to delegate your B_{12} injection to another student while you are admitting your error to the resident, her attending, and the charge nurse, as well as completing the special event report. At the end of the day, your instructor compliments you for your honesty and sense of responsibility and cautions you not to repeat the mistake. You are grateful that your worst fears (*failing*) weren't confirmed and leave the unit having learned a powerful lesson about the costs of being accountable.

practices to reduce errors. MEDWATCH (www.fda.gov/ Safety/MedWatch/default.htm) is administered by the FDA. The National Coordinating Council for Medication Error Reporting and Prevention (www.nccmerp.org) is a cooperative effort supported by organizations from a wide variety of backgrounds, including consumer, health system, trade and manufacturer, nursing, pharmacy, and medicine organizations, as well as government, licensing, and risk management agencies. MEDMARX (www.medmarx.com) is a subscription database operated by the U.S. Pharmacopeia (USP) used by hospitals and health care systems to track and trend adverse drug reactions and medication errors.

Although event reports often have a negative connotation for many nurses, event reports can provide vital information that can be used to prevent the error from being repeated. These tools can provide tracking of errors throughout the institution, providing information that may prevent future medication errors. The emphasis should be on the collaborative efforts necessary to provide safe patient care and decrease the incidence of errors. Peer review committees have proved effective in some health care settings.

Another effort to prevent medication errors involves the assignment of pharmacists to patient care areas in the hospital. The pharmacists spend time on the units and interact directly with the nurses, physicians, and other health care providers to ensure safe medication delivery. They review patient profiles, discuss adverse effects of drugs and potential drug interactions, and ensure that medications are administered at appropriate times across nursing shifts. This team approach has the potential to reduce medication errors significantly.

The health information technologies discussed previously—including computerized health records, computerized provider order entry, bar coding, automated drug-dispensing systems, and unit dosing—can potentially contribute to reducing medication errors. However, the person administering the medication, the nurse, needs to remain vigilant in preventing errors.

Teaching about Medications

Teaching about medications is an ongoing process and should begin as soon as the patient is admitted to the health care facility. Developing a plan of care related to medications is an important part of nursing care. See the

TEACHING TIPS 28-1

MEDICATIONS

Health Topic	Teaching Tip	Why Is This Important?
General information	• Medication name and dosage • Intended effects of medication • Expected adverse effects of medication	Patients should know the names and reasons for medications in case of medical emergencies. Patients should also know expected adverse effects of the medication so they do not stop taking the medication.
Taking the medication	• Medications should be taken at the same time every day. • Teach whether food, beverages, or other medications have any effect on the medication. • Teach what patient should do if a dose is missed. • Teach patient to take medications as prescribed for as long as prescribed. • Teach not to alter drug dosage without consulting health care provider.	If patients make taking medications a part of their daily routine, they are less likely to miss a dose. Some medications require food to prevent stomach irritation; absorption of other medications is impeded by food in the stomach. Patients are likely to miss a dose of medication and need to know what to do if this happens. Some medications have severe consequences if stopped abruptly; others need to be taken for a set period of time and at a recommended dosage to be effective.
Special instructions	• Teach what to do when adverse effects occur. • Keep medications with them when traveling. • Do not share medications with other people. • Proper storage • Keep a list of all medications, including OTC drugs, dietary supplements, herbs, and natural supplements.	Patients need to know whom to contact if any adverse effects occur. Luggage can be lost or misplaced. Teach patients that just because someone else has similar symptoms, it does not mean that the same medication should be taken. Medication should be kept out of the reach of children and pets. For labeling purposes, medications should be kept in the container in which they were dispensed. Some medications are sensitive to humidity and light; keep medications in a cool, dry place. Keep your health care providers up to date on your list of medications.

Nursing Plan of Care for Regina Sauder on pages 800–801. In many cases, patients continue a prescribed medication regimen at home after discharge from the hospital. A factor that affects the patient's compliance with the medication regimen at home is education about the prescribed medications. Teaching should be tailored to the patient's level of understanding and with an awareness of any cultural implications. Written instructions, based on an assessment of the patient's level of literacy, can be used as a reference for the patient. Well-educated patients can act as a final safety net in the medication process when nurses encourage patient participation in care (Popescu, 2011). Refer to Teaching Tips 28-1: Medications.

Explain the techniques of medication administration to the patient and family. Before being discharged from a health care facility, the patient should practice the necessary techniques under the supervision of a nurse to acquire sufficient skill for safe administration. Many patients have learned to give themselves injections, as well as many other medications, when the teaching was planned well and the patient was able and willing to learn.

Emphasize the importance of taking medications as prescribed and for as long as prescribed. A common error made by patients is simply omitting a drug, either through carelessness or because they believe that missing a dose is not important. Various aids are available to remind the patient to take medication on schedule. Medication containers that beep when a dose is due to be taken, scratch-off dots on a medication label, and an electronic cap that signals dosage time and records each time the cap is removed are available. Advise patients to keep their medications with them when they travel. If luggage is lost or misplaced, refilling the prescription may be difficult.

Instruct the patient not to alter the dosage without consulting the primary care provider. Also, teach the patient not to discontinue medications when symptoms disappear. Drugs used to maintain health, such as those used to control high blood pressure, need to be continued as ordered to avoid recurrence of symptoms.

Caution the patient not to share prescribed medications with other family members or with friends and neighbors. Inappropriate use of another person's drugs can have serious consequences.

The patient should be able to verbalize the following:

- How and when to administer the medication
- When to notify the health care provider
- Expected effects and adverse effects

Nurses have a responsibility to teach about drug abuse. Teaching may take place on an individual basis or on a family or community level. Drug abuse is a major public health concern worldwide, especially among teenagers and young adults. Refer to the Nursing Advocacy in Action box. Continued public and individual education is indicated, and nurses are also expected to set high standards for their own behavior and use of drugs. Because drug abuse is increasingly common in health care providers, nurses who suspect that a colleague is abusing drugs must observe, document, and intervene for the patients' safety.

Nurses working with patients to promote appropriate behaviors related to medication administration should examine their own behaviors as factors in the success of the plan. Nurses who role model good health behaviors are more effective teachers. Use the display, Promoting Health 28-1: Medications, (on page 800) for yourself before using it with others.

Evaluating

Assess the effectiveness of drugs in several ways. Clinical observation is the first method. Collect subjective data from the patient (e.g., "My pain has disappeared") and collect objective data (e.g., the patient's vital signs) to evaluate effectiveness of the medication. It is also important to assess the patient for adverse drug effects.

Measurement of drug levels in body fluids provides data about the patient's response to a particular medication. For many drugs—including digoxin, warfarin, anticonvulsants,

NURSING ADVOCACY IN ACTION

Substance abuse during pregnancy results in significant health problems for the mother, fetus, and newborn. Recently, OxyContin has become a popular alternative to other street drugs such as heroin. In utero exposure to opiates is associated with neonatal abstinence syndrome in as many as 55% to 94% of exposed infants. The onset and severity of the infant's withdrawal from the drug varies with the type and duration of the drug taken by the mother.

Patient Scenario

Jasmine is a 24-year-old single mother who is homeless. She has a history of injecting OxyContin (120–500 mg/day) intravenously for the past 2 years due to pain in her back. She has a history of barbiturate abuse during her last

pregnancy. She has delivered two other infants prematurely at 32 weeks and 36 weeks. Both of these children are in foster care.

Implications for Nursing Advocacy

How will you respond if you are Jasmine's clinic nurse? Talk with your classmates and experienced nurses about the questions that follow.

- If you elect to advocate for Jasmine and her baby, what practical steps can you take to ensure better health outcomes?
- What is reasonable to expect of a student nurse, a graduate nurse, and an experienced nurse in this situation?
- What advocacy skills are needed to effectively respond to this challenge?

PROMOTING HEALTH 28-1

MEDICATIONS

Use the assessment checklist to determine how well you are meeting your needs related to safe medication practices. Then develop a prescription for self-care by choosing appropriate behaviors from the list of suggestions.

Assessment Checklist

❏ almost always   ❏ sometimes   ❏ almost never

❏ ❏ ❏ 1. I store medications in a safe place (e.g., a cool, dry place, away from direct sunlight, out of the reach of children).

❏ ❏ ❏ 2. I discard medications that have passed their expiration date.

❏ ❏ ❏ 3. I wear a Medic-Alert tag or carry information that identifies a drug allergy or required medication.

❏ ❏ ❏ 4. I am cautious about combining prescribed medication with OTC drugs, herbal supplements, alcohol, or foods that can interact with the drug.

Self-Care Behaviors

1. Finish all prescriptions as ordered by physician or nurse practitioner.
2. Avoid foods, alcohol, or over-the-counter drugs and herbal supplements that may interact with a prescribed drug.
3. Use available resources (textbooks, pharmacist, physician) to verify the potential for drug interactions or possible adverse effects of a medication.
4. Use a reminder system to maintain medication schedule.
5. Avoid sharing medications or taking someone else's prescribed pills.
6. Complete any laboratory tests necessary for maintenance or adjustment of a medication regimen.
7. Practice safe behaviors when storing medications.
8. Purchase drugs from the same pharmacy as an additional safeguard with multiple medication regimens.

Information to promote safe medication practices, such as information about prescription and over-the-counter medications, medication safety, medication administration, and alternative medications, is available online. Visit thePoint for a list of Internet resources.

---

and aminoglycoside antibiotics—monitoring blood levels is an important component of therapy. Test the patient to determine whether the drug level in the blood is within the therapeutic range. Drug dosages may be adjusted based on the serum drug level. Monitoring systems can also assist the nurse in evaluating drug effectiveness. For the

patient with an arrhythmia, for example, a cardiac monitor can show a change in heart rhythm.

See the accompanying Nursing Plan of Care for Regina Sauder for an example of the nursing process for medication administration.

NURSING PLAN OF CARE 28-1

for Regina Sauder

Regina Sauder, 73 years old, presented to the emergency department with pain, swelling, and erythema of her left calf. She has a history of lymphoma. Vascular studies of the lower extremities show a left leg deep vein thrombosis. She was admitted to the hospital and started on intravenous heparin. After 3 days of heparin

therapy, she was started on warfarin, in addition to the heparin. Her warfarin dose is being adjusted based on her daily INR level. Daily assessment of her INR level will continue in the hospital until her level is therapeutic. Initially, weekly monitoring of the INR level will continue after discharge.

ASSESSMENT FINDINGS

- PTT is 60 seconds, within expected parameters for adequate hypercoagulation with heparin therapy.
- INR is 1.2, in the low end of expected parameter for adequate hypercoagulation with warfarin therapy.
- Patient's left lower leg is without swelling, tenderness, and erythema.
- Patient states, "It feels so much better. I had so much pain, but not now. But, why am I taking two different medications? Am I going to have to go home with this tube in my arm?" Mrs. Sauder appears anxious, is fidgeting, and becomes tearful during the conversation with the nurse. She states, "I think this new pill sounds scary." Her husband reports unease about his wife's ability "to keep track of everything."
- Patient and husband unable to verbalize knowledge regarding signs of bleeding, dosage, timing of administration, dietary guidelines, or need for scheduled follow-up blood work.
- Patient and her husband live in a two-story home, with the bathroom on the second floor.

NURSING PLAN OF CARE 28-1 *continued*

for Regina Sauder

NURSING DIAGNOSIS	Risk for Injury, bleeding, related to adverse effects of warfarin and falls
EXPECTED OUTCOME	By 3/20/15, the patient and her husband will:

- Be able to identify signs and symptoms of bleeding

NURSING INTERVENTIONS	RATIONALE	EVALUATIVE STATEMENT
Provide instruction identifying signs and symptoms of bleeding.	Focuses teaching session on a single idea, allowing the patient to concentrate more completely on the material. Older patients and highly anxious patients have reduced short-term memory and benefit from mastery of one concept at a time.	3/19/15 Outcome met. Mrs. Sauder and her husband are able to identify signs and symptoms of bleeding to report to their physician. *B. Huber, RN*
Give patient and husband written pamphlet from drug manufacturer.	Provide information using various media because different people take in information in different ways. Provides concrete reinforcement.	
Encourage questions.	Patients and family members often feel shy or embarrassed about asking questions. Gives permission to ask.	

EXPECTED OUTCOME	By 3/20/15, the patient's husband will:

- Remove from their home potential hazards that could lead to falls.

NURSING INTERVENTIONS	RATIONALE	EVALUATIVE STATEMENT
Review with patient and husband potential causes of falls at home.	Falls may cause internal bleeding.	3/18/15 Outcome met. Husband removed several loose rugs, repaired loose stairs, and improved the lighting at the stairs to the bathroom. *B. Clapp, RN*
Assist the patient and husband in evaluating their home environment to identify potential hazards.	Remove potential hazards to prevent falls and injury.	
Encourage the use of proper lighting, handrails on stairways, removal of scatter rugs, fastening loose carpet edges.	Remove potential hazards to prevent falls and injury.	

SAMPLE DOCUMENTATION	3/17/15 Nursing Patient, husband, and nurse met to discuss potential effects of warfarin therapy and risk for injury. Discussion centered on importance of preventing injury while on warfarin at home. See plan of care. Patient progress will be evaluated in 4 days, 3/21/15. *B. Clapp, RN*

SKILL 28-1 ADMINISTERING ORAL MEDICATIONS

DELEGATION CONSIDERATIONS

The administration of oral medications is not delegated to nursing assistive personnel (NAP) or unlicensed assistive personnel (UAP) in the acute care setting. The administration of specified oral medications to stable patients in some long-term care settings may be delegated to nursing assistive personnel (NAP) or unlicensed assistive personnel (UAP) who have received appropriate training. Depending on the state's nurse practice act and the organization's policies and procedures, the administration of oral medications may be delegated to licensed practical/vocational nurses (LPN/LVNs). The decision to delegate must be based on careful analysis of the patient's needs and circumstances, as well as the qualifications of the person to whom the task is being delegated. Refer to the Delegation Guidelines in Appendix A (found on thePoint).

EQUIPMENT

- Medication in disposable cup or oral syringe
- Liquid (e.g., water, juice) with straw, if not contraindicated
- Medication cart or tray
- Computer-generated medication administration record (CMAR) or medication administration record (MAR)
- PPE, as indicated

IMPLEMENTATION

ACTION	RATIONALE
1. Gather equipment. Check each medication order against the original in the medical record, according to facility policy. Clarify any inconsistencies. Check the patient's medical record for allergies.	This comparison helps to identify errors that may have occurred when orders were transcribed. The primary care provider's order is the legal record of medication orders for each facility.
2. Know the actions, special nursing considerations, safe dose ranges, purpose of administration, and adverse effects of the medications to be administered. Consider the appropriateness of the medication for this patient.	This knowledge aids the nurse in evaluating the therapeutic effect of the medication in relation to the patient's disorder and can also be used to educate the patient about the medication.
3. Perform hand hygiene.	Hand hygiene prevents the spread of microorganisms.
4. Move the medication cart to the outside of the patient's room or prepare for administration in the medication area.	Organization facilitates error-free administration and saves time.
5. Unlock the medication cart or drawer. Enter the pass code into the computer and scan employee identification, if required.	Locking the cart or drawer safeguards each patient's medication supply. Hospital accrediting organizations require medication carts to be locked when not in use. Entering the pass code and scanning ID allows only authorized users into the computer system and identifies the user for documentation by the computer.
6. **Prepare medications for one patient at a time.**	This prevents errors in medication administration.
7. Read the CMAR/MAR and select the proper medication from the unit stock or patient's medication drawer.	This is the *first* check of the medication label.
8. Compare the medication label with the CMAR/MAR (Figure 1). Check expiration dates and perform calculations, if necessary. Scan the bar code on the package, if required.	This is the *second* check of the label. Verify calculations with another nurse to ensure safety, if necessary.

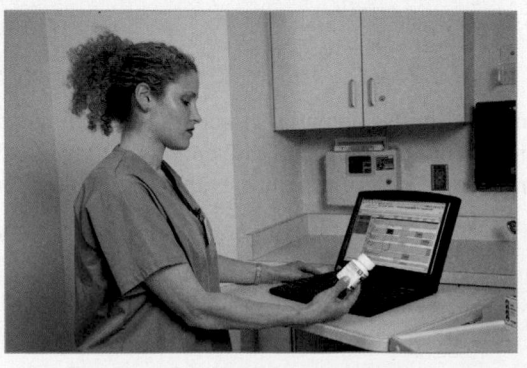

FIGURE 1. Comparing medication label with the CMAR.

ACTION

9. Prepare the required medications:

   a. *Unit dose packages:* Place unit dose-packaged medications in a disposable cup. **Do not open the wrapper until at the bedside.** Keep opioids and medications that require special nursing assessments in a separate container.

   b. *Multidose containers:* When removing tablets or capsules from a multidose bottle, pour the necessary number into the bottle cap and then place the tablets or capsules in a medication cup. Break only scored tablets, if necessary, to obtain the proper dosage. Do not touch tablets or capsules with hands.

   c. *Liquid medication in multidose bottle:* When pouring liquid medications out of a multidose bottle, hold the bottle so that the label is against the palm. Use the appropriate measuring device when pouring liquids, and read the amount of medication at the bottom of the meniscus at eye level (Figure 2). Wipe the lip of the bottle with a paper towel.

FIGURE 2. Measuring at eye level. *(Photo by B. Proud.)*

10. **Depending on facility policy, the third check of the label may occur at this point. If so, when all medications for one patient have been prepared, recheck the labels with the CMAR/MAR before taking the medications to the patient.**

11. Replace any multidose containers in the patient's drawer or unit stock. **Lock the medication cart before leaving it.**

12. Transport medications to the patient's bedside carefully, and keep the medications in sight at all times.

13. **Ensure that the patient receives the medications at the correct time.**

14. Perform hand hygiene and put on PPE, if indicated.

RATIONALE

Wrapper is kept intact because the label is needed for an additional safety check. Special assessments may be required before giving certain medications. These may include assessing vital signs and checking laboratory test results.

Pouring medication into the cap allows for easy return of excess medication to the bottle. Pouring tablets or capsules into your hand is unsanitary.

Liquid that may drip onto the label makes the label difficult to read. Accuracy is possible when the appropriate measuring device is used and then read accurately.

This *third* check ensures accuracy and helps to prevent errors. Note: Many facilities require the third check to occur at the bedside, after identifying the patient and before administration.

Locking the cart or drawer safeguards the patient's medication supply. Hospital accrediting organizations require medication carts to be locked when not in use.

Careful handling and close observation prevent accidental or deliberate disarrangement of medications.

Check agency policy, which may allow for administration within a period of 30 minutes before or 30 minutes after the designated time.

Hand hygiene and PPE prevent the spread of microorganisms. PPE is required based on transmission precautions.

(continued)

SKILL 28-1 ADMINISTERING ORAL MEDICATIONS *continued*

ACTION

15. **Identify the patient. Compare the information with the CMAR/MAR. The patient should be identified using at least two methods** (The Joint Commission [TJC], 2013):

    a. Check the name on the patient's identification band (Figure 3).

    b. Check the identification number on the patient's identification band.

    c. Check the birth date on the patient's identification band.

    d. Ask the patient to state name and birth date, based on facility policy.

16. **Complete necessary assessments before administering medications. Check the patient's allergy bracelet or ask the patient about allergies. Explain the purpose and action of each medication to the patient.**

17. Scan the patient's bar code on the identification band, if required (Figure 4).

RATIONALE

Identifying the patient ensures the right patient receives the medications and helps prevent errors. The patient's room number or physical location is not used as an identifier (TJC, 2013). Replace the identification band if it is missing or inaccurate in any way.

This requires a response from the patient, but illness and strange surroundings often cause patients to be confused.

Assessment is a prerequisite to administration of medications.

The bar code provides an additional check to ensure that the medication is given to the right patient.

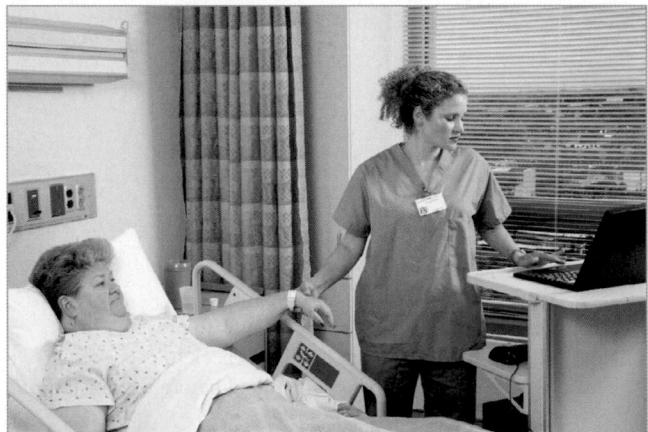

FIGURE 3. Checking patient's name and ID number with the CMAR.

FIGURE 4. Scanning the bar code on the patient's identification bracelet. *(Photo by B. Proud.)*

18. **Based on facility policy, the third check of the medication label may occur at this point. If so, recheck the labels with the CMAR/MAR before administering the medications to the patient.**

19. Assist the patient to an upright or lateral (side-lying) position.

20. Administer medications:

    a. Offer water or other permitted fluids with pills, capsules, tablets, and some liquid medications.

    b. Ask whether the patient prefers to take the medications by hand or in a cup.

Many facilities require the third check to occur at the bedside, after identifying the patient and before administration. If facility policy directs the third check at this time, this *third* check ensures accuracy and helps to prevent errors.

Swallowing is facilitated by proper positioning. An upright or side-lying position protects the patient from aspiration.

Liquids facilitate swallowing of solid drugs. Some liquid drugs are intended to adhere to the pharyngeal area, in which case liquid is not offered with the medication.

This encourages the patient's participation in taking the medications.

ACTION	RATIONALE
21. **Remain with the patient until each medication is swallowed. Never leave medication at the patient's bedside** (Figure 5).	Unless you have seen the patient swallow the drug, the drug cannot be recorded as administered. The patient's chart is a legal record. Medications can be left at the bedside only with a prescriber's order.

FIGURE 5. Remaining with the patient until each medication is swallowed.

ACTION	RATIONALE
22. Assist the patient to a comfortable position. Remove PPE, if used. Perform hand hygiene.	Promotes patient comfort. Proper removal of PPE prevents transmission of microorganisms. Hand hygiene deters the spread of microorganisms.
23. Document the administration of the medication immediately after administration. See Documentation section below.	Timely documentation helps to ensure patient safety.
24. Evaluate the patient's response to medication within the appropriate time frame.	The patient needs to be evaluated for therapeutic and adverse effects from the medication.

DOCUMENTATION

Guidelines

Record each medication immediately after it is administered on the CMAR/MAR or record using the required format. Include the date and time of administration (Figure 6). If using a bar-code system, medication administration is automatically recorded when the bar code is scanned. PRN medications require documentation of the reason for administration. Prompt recording avoids the possibility of accidentally repeating the administration of the drug. If the drug was refused or omitted, record this in the appropriate area on the medication record and notify the primary care provider. This verifies the reason that medication was omitted

FIGURE 6. Recording each medication administered on the CMAR.

(continued)

SKILL 28-1 | ADMINISTERING ORAL MEDICATIONS *continued*

and ensures that the primary care provider is aware of the patient's condition. Recording administration of an opioid may require additional documentation on a controlled-substance record, stating drug count and other specific information. A record of fluid intake and output measurement is required.

Sample Documentation

DocuCare Practice documenting medication administration in *Lippincott DocuCare*.

8/6/15 0835 Patient states he is having constant stabbing leg pains. Rates pain as an 8/10. Percocet 2 tabs administered.

—*K. Sanders, RN*

8/6/15 0905 Patient resting comfortably. Rates leg pain as a 1/10.

—*K. Sanders, RN*

8/6/15 1300 Patient states he does not want pain medication, despite return of leg pain. States, "It made me feel woozy last time." Feelings discussed with patient. Patient agrees to take Percocet 1 tab at this time.

—*K. Sanders, RN*

8/6/15 1320 Percocet 1 tab given PO.

—*K. Sanders, RN*

UNEXPECTED SITUATIONS AND ASSOCIATED INTERVENTIONS

- *Patient states that it feels like medication is lodged in throat:* Offer patient more fluids to drink. If allowed, offer the patient bread or crackers to help move the medication to the stomach.

- *It is unclear whether the patient swallowed the medication:* Check in the patient's mouth, under tongue, and between cheek and gum. Patients with altered mental status may not be aware that the medication was not swallowed. Also, patients may "cheek" medications to avoid taking the medication or to save it for later use. Watch patients requiring suicide precautions closely to ensure that they are not "cheeking" the medication or hiding it in the mouth. These patients may be trying to accumulate a large amount of medication to take all at once in a suicide attempt. Substance abusers may cheek medication to accumulate a large amount to take all at once so that they may feel a high from medication.

- *Patient vomits immediately or shortly after receiving oral medication:* Assess vomit, looking for pills or fragments. Do not re-administer medication without notifying primary care provider. If a whole pill is seen and can be identified, the primary care provider may ask that the medication be administered again. If a pill is not seen or medications cannot be identified, do not re-administer the medication in order to prevent the patient from receiving too large a dose.

- *Child refuses to take oral medications:* Some medications may be mixed in a small amount of food, such as pudding or ice cream. Do not add the medication to liquids because the medication may alter the taste of liquids; if child then refuses to drink the rest of the liquid, you will not know how much of the medication was ingested. Use creativity when devising ways to administer medications to a child. See the section Infant and Child Considerations for suggestions.

- *The capsule or tablet falls to the floor during administration.* Discard and obtain a new dose for administration. This prevents contamination and transmission of microorganisms.

- *Patient refuses medication.* Explore the reason for the patient's refusal. Review the rationale for using the drug and any other information that may be appropriate. If you are unable to administer the medication despite education and discussion, document the omission according to facility policy and notify the primary care provider.

SPECIAL CONSIDERATIONS

General Considerations

- Some liquid medication preparations, such as suspensions, require agitation to ensure even distribution of medication in the solution. Be familiar with the specific requirements for medications you are administering.

- Place medications intended for sublingual absorption under the patient's tongue. Instruct the patient to allow the medication to dissolve completely. Reinforce the importance of not swallowing the medication tablet.

- Some oral medications are provided in powdered forms. Verify the correct liquid in which to dissolve the medication for administration. This information is usually included on the package. Verify any unclear instructions with a pharmacist or medication reference. If there is more than one possible liquid in which to dissolve the medication, include the patient in the decision process; patients may find one choice more palatable than another.

- Ongoing assessment is an important part of nursing care for both evaluation of patient response to administered medications and early detection of adverse effects. If an adverse effect is suspected, withhold further medication doses and notify the patient's primary care provider. Additional intervention is based on type of reaction and patient assessment.

- If the patient questions a medication order or states that the medication is different from the usual dose, always recheck and clarify with the original order and/or primary care provider before giving the medication.

- If the patient's level of consciousness is altered or swallowing is impaired, check with the primary care provider to clarify the route of administration or alternative forms of medication. This may also be a solution for a pediatric or confused patient who is refusing to take a medication.

- Patients with poor vision can request large-type labels on medication containers. A magnifying lens also may be helpful.

- Provide written medication information to reinforce discussion and education in the appropriate language, if the patient is literate. If the patient is unable to read, provide written information to family or significant other, if appropriate. Written information should be at a 5th-grade level to ensure ease of understanding.

- If the patient has difficulty swallowing tablets, it may be appropriate to crush the medication to facilitate administration. However, not all medications can be crushed or altered; long-acting and slow-release drugs are examples of medications that cannot be crushed. Therefore, it is important to consult a medication reference and/or pharmacist. If the medication can be crushed, use a pill-crusher or mortar and pestle to grind the tablet into a powder. Crush each pill one at a time. Dissolve the powder with water or other recommended liquid in a liquid medication cup, keeping each medication separate from the others. Keep the package label with the medication cup for future comparison of information. Combine the crushed medication with a small amount of soft food, such as applesauce or pudding, to facilitate administration.

Infant and Child Considerations

- Special devices, such as oral syringes and calibrated nipples, are available in a pharmacy to ensure accurate dose calculations for young children and infants.

- Some creative ways to administer medications to children include the following: have a "tea party" with medicine cups; place oral syringe (without needle) or dropper in the space between the cheek and gum and slowly administer the medication; save a special treat for after the medication administration (e.g., movie, playroom time, or a special food, if allowed).

- The Institute for Safe Medication Practices (ISMP) and the U.S. Food and Drug Administration (FDA) have received reports of infants choking on the plastic caps that fit on the end of syringes when used to administer oral medications. They recommend the following: remove and dispose of caps before giving syringes to patients or families, caution family caregivers to dispose of caps on syringes they buy over the counter, and report any problems with syringe caps to the FDA. Companies manufacture syringes labeled "oral use" without the caps on them (ISMP, 2012; FDA, 2012c).

Older Adult Considerations

- Older patients with arthritis may have difficulty opening childproof caps. On request, the pharmacist can substitute a cap that is easier to open. A rubber band twisted around the cap may provide a more secure grip for older patients.

- Consider large-print written medication information, when appropriate.

(continued)

SKILL 28-1 ADMINISTERING ORAL MEDICATIONS *continued*

- Physiologic changes associated with the aging process—including decreased gastric motility, muscle mass, acid production, and blood flow—can affect the patient's response to medication, including drug absorption and increased risk of adverse effects. Older adults are more likely to take multiple drugs, thus drug interactions in the older adult are a very real and dangerous problem. Refer to Focus on the Older Adult: Nursing Strategies to Address Age-Related Changes in Drug Response, on page 758.

Home Care Considerations

- Encourage the patient to discard expired prescription medications based on label instructions or community guidelines.
- Discuss safe storage of medications when there are children and pets in the home environment.
- Discuss with parents the difference in over-the-counter medications made for infants and medications made for children. Many times parents do not realize that there are different strengths to the actual medications, leading to under- or overdosing.
- Encourage patients to carry a card listing all medications they take, including dosage and frequency, in case of an emergency.
- Discuss the importance of using an appropriate measuring device for liquid medications. Caution patients not to use eating utensils for measuring medications; use a liquid medication cup, oral syringe, or measuring spoon to provide accurate dosing.

SKILL 28-2 REMOVING MEDICATION FROM AN AMPULE

DELEGATION CONSIDERATIONS

The preparation of medication from an ampule is not delegated to nursing assistive personnel (NAP) or unlicensed assistive personnel (UAP). Depending on the state's nurse practice act and the organization's policies and procedures, the preparation of medication from an ampule may be delegated to a licensed practical/vocational nurse (LPN/LVN). The decision to delegate must be based on careful analysis of the patient's needs and circumstances, as well as the qualifications of the person to whom the task is being delegated. Refer to the Delegation Guidelines in Appendix A (found on thePoint).

EQUIPMENT

- Sterile syringe and filter needle
- Ampule of medication
- Small gauze pad

- Computer-generated medication administration record (CMAR) or medication administration record (MAR)

IMPLEMENTATION

ACTION	RATIONALE
1. Gather equipment. Check the medication order against the original order in the medical record, according to facility policy. Clarify any inconsistencies. Check the patient's chart for allergies.	This comparison helps to identify errors that may have occurred when orders were transcribed. The primary care provider's order is the legal record of medication orders for each facility.
2. Know the actions, special nursing considerations, safe dose ranges, purpose of administration, and adverse effects of the medications to be administered. Consider the appropriateness of the medication for this patient.	This knowledge aids the nurse in evaluating the therapeutic effect of the medication in relation to the patient's disorder and can also be used to educate the patient about the medication.
3. Perform hand hygiene.	Hand hygiene prevents the spread of microorganisms.

ACTION	RATIONALE
4. Move the medication cart to the outside of the patient's room or prepare for administration in the medication area.	Organization facilitates error-free administration and saves time.
5. Unlock the medication cart or drawer. Enter the pass code and scan employee identification, if required.	Locking the cart or drawer safeguards each patient's medication supply. Hospital accrediting organizations require medication carts to be locked when not in use. Entering the pass code and scanning ID allows only authorized users into the computer system and identifies the user for documentation by the computer.
6. **Prepare medications for one patient at a time.**	This prevents errors in medication administration.
7. Read the CMAR/MAR and select the proper medication from unit stock or the patient's medication drawer.	This is the *first* check of the label.
8. Compare the label with the CMAR/MAR. Check expiration dates and perform calculations, if necessary. Scan the bar code on the package, if required.	This is the *second* check of the label. Verify calculations with another nurse to ensure safety, if necessary.
9. Tap the stem of the ampule (Figure 1) or twist your wrist quickly (Figure 2) while holding the ampule vertically.	This facilitates movement of medication in the stem to the body of the ampule.
10. Wrap a small gauze pad around the neck of the ampule.	This will protect your fingers from the glass as the ampule is broken.
11. Use a snapping motion to break off the top of the ampule along the scored line at its neck (Figure 3). **Always break away from your body.**	This protects your face and fingers from any shattered glass fragments.
12. Attach the filter needle to the syringe. Remove the cap from the filter needle by pulling it straight off.	Use of a filter needle prevents the accidental withdrawing of small glass particles with the medication. Pulling the cap off in a straight manner prevents accidental needlestick.

FIGURE 1. Tapping stem of the ampule.

FIGURE 2. Twisting wrist quickly while holding the ampule vertically.

FIGURE 3. Using a snapping motion to break top of the ampule.

(continued)

SKILL 28-2 REMOVING MEDICATION FROM AN AMPULE *continued*

ACTION

13. Withdraw medication in the amount ordered plus a small amount more (approximately 30% more). **Do not inject air into the solution. While inserting the filter needle into the ampule, be careful not to touch the rim.** Use either of the following methods to withdraw the medication:

    a. Insert the tip of the needle into the ampule, which is upright on a flat surface, and withdraw fluid into the syringe (Figure 4). **Touch the plunger at the knob only.**

    b. Insert the tip of the needle into the ampule and invert the ampule. Keep the needle centered and not touching the sides of the ampule. Withdraw fluid into syringe (Figure 5). **Touch the plunger at the knob only.**

RATIONALE

By withdrawing an additional small amount of medication, any air bubbles in the syringe can be displaced once the syringe is removed while allowing ample medication to remain in the syringe. The contents of the ampule are not under pressure; therefore, air is unnecessary and will cause the contents to overflow. The rim of the ampule is considered contaminated.

Handling the plunger at the knob only will keep the shaft of the plunger sterile.

Surface tension holds the fluids in the ampule when inverted. If the needle touches the sides or is removed and then reinserted into the ampule, surface tension is broken, and fluid runs out. Handling the plunger at the knob only will keep the shaft of the plunger sterile.

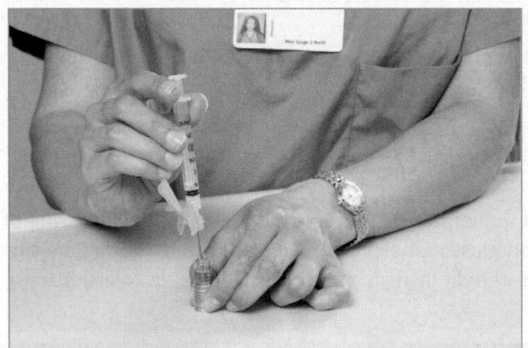

FIGURE 4. Withdrawing medication from upright ampule. *(Photo by B. Proud.)*

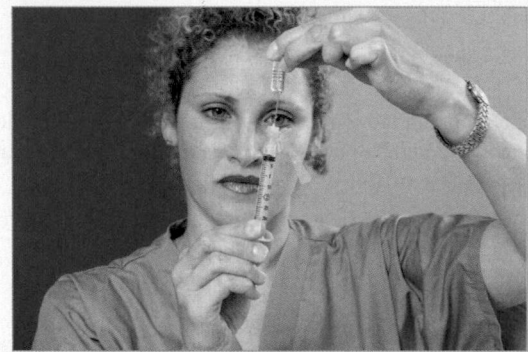

FIGURE 5. Withdrawing medication from inverted ampule. *(Photo by B. Proud.)*

14. Wait until the needle has been withdrawn to tap the syringe and expel the air carefully by pushing on the plunger. **Check the amount of medication in the syringe with the medication dose and discard any surplus according to facility policy.**

15. **Depending on facility policy, the third check of the label may occur at this point. If so, when all medications for one patient have been prepared, recheck the labels with the CMAR/MAR before taking the medications to the patient.**

16. **Engage the safety guard on the filter needle and remove the needle. Discard the filter needle in a suitable container. Attach the appropriate administration device to the syringe.**

17. Discard the ampule in a suitable container.

18. Lock the medication cart before leaving it.

19. Perform hand hygiene.

20. Proceed with administration, based on the prescribed route.

Ejecting air into the solution increases pressure in the ampule and can force the medication to spill out over the ampule. Ampules may have overfill. Careful measurement ensures that the correct dose is withdrawn.

This *third* check ensures accuracy and helps to prevent errors. *Note:* Many facilities require the *third* check to occur at the bedside, after identifying the patient and before administration.

The filter needle used to draw up medication should not be used to administer the medication. This will prevent any glass shards from entering the patient during administration.

Any medication that has not been removed from the ampule must be discarded because sterility of contents can not be maintained in an opened ampule.

Locking the cart or drawer safeguards the patient's medication supply. Hospital accrediting organizations require medication carts to be locked when not in use.

Hand hygiene deters the spread of microorganisms.

See appropriate skill for prescribed route.

DOCUMENTATION

Guidelines

It is not necessary to record the removal of the medication from the ampule. Prompt recording of administration of the medication is required immediately after it is administered.

UNEXPECTED SITUATIONS AND ASSOCIATED INTERVENTIONS

- *You cut yourself while trying to open the ampule:* Discard ampule in case contamination has occurred. Clean and bandage the wound and obtain a new ampule. Report according to facility policy.

- *All of the medication was not removed from the stem and insufficient medication remains in the body of the ampule for dose:* Discard the ampule and drawn medication. Obtain a new ampule and start over. Medication in the original ampule stem is considered contaminated once the neck of the ampule has been placed on a nonsterile surface.

- *You inject air into the inverted ampule, spraying medication:* Wash hands to remove any medication. If any medication has gotten into eyes, perform eye irrigation. Obtain a new ampule for medication dose. Report injury, if appropriate, according to facility policy.

- *Medication is drawn up without using a filter needle:* Replace the needle with a filter needle. Inject the medication through the filter needle into a new syringe, then administer to the patient.

- *Plunger becomes contaminated before inserted into the ampule:* Discard the needle and syringe and start over. If the plunger is contaminated after medication is drawn into the syringe, it is not necessary to discard and start over. The contaminated plunger will enter the barrel of the syringe when pushing the medication out and will not contaminate the medication.

SKILL 28-3 | REMOVING MEDICATION FROM A VIAL

DELEGATION CONSIDERATIONS

The preparation of medication from a vial is not delegated to nursing assistive personnel (NAP) or unlicensed assistive personnel (UAP). Depending on the state's nurse practice act and the organization's policies and procedures, the preparation of medication from a vial may be delegated to licensed practical/vocational nurses (LPN/LVN). The decision to delegate must be based on careful analysis of the patient's needs and circumstances, as well as the qualifications of the person to whom the task is being delegated. Refer to the Delegation Guidelines in Appendix A (found on thePoint).

EQUIPMENT

- Sterile syringe and needle or blunt cannula (size depends on medication being administered)
- Vial of medication
- Antimicrobial swab
- Second needle (optional)
- Filter needle (optional)
- Computer-generated medication administration record (CMAR) or medication administration record (MAR)

IMPLEMENTATION

ACTION	RATIONALE
1. Gather equipment. Check the medication order against the original order in the medical record, according to facility policy. Clarify any inconsistencies. Check the patient's chart for allergies.	This comparison helps to identify errors that may have occurred when orders were transcribed. The primary care provider's order is the legal record of medication orders for each facility.
2. Know the actions, special nursing considerations, safe dose ranges, purpose of administration, and adverse effects of the medications to be administered. Consider the appropriateness of the medication for this patient.	This knowledge aids the nurse in evaluating the therapeutic effect of the medication in relation to the patient's disorder and can also be used to educate the patient about the medication.
3. Perform hand hygiene.	Hand hygiene deters the spread of microorganisms.
4. Move the medication cart to the outside of the patient's room or prepare for administration in the medication area.	Organization facilitates error-free administration and saves time.

(continued)

SKILL 28-3 REMOVING MEDICATION FROM A VIAL *continued*

ACTION	**RATIONALE**
5. Unlock the medication cart or drawer. Enter pass code and scan employee identification, if required.	Locking the cart or drawer safeguards each patient's medication supply. Hospital accrediting organizations require medication carts to be locked when not in use. Entering the pass code and scanning ID allows only authorized users into the system and identifies the user for documentation by the computer.
6. **Prepare medications for one patient at a time.**	This prevents errors in medication administration.
7. Read the CMAR/MAR and select the proper medication from unit stock or the patient's medication drawer.	This is the *first* check of the label.
8. Compare the label with the CMAR/MAR. Check expiration dates and perform calculations, if necessary. Scan the bar code on the package, if required.	This is the *second* check of the label. Verify calculations with another nurse to ensure safety, if necessary.
9. Remove the metal or plastic cap on the vial that protects the rubber stopper.	Cap needs to be removed to access the medication in the vial.
10. **Swab the rubber top with the antimicrobial swab and allow to dry.**	Antimicrobial swab removes surface bacteria contamination. Allowing the alcohol to dry prevents it from entering the vial on the needle.
11. Remove the cap from the needle or blunt cannula by pulling it straight off. Touch the plunger at the knob only. Draw back an amount of air into the syringe that is equal to the specific dose of medication to be withdrawn. Some facilities require use of a filter needle when withdrawing premixed medication from multidose vials.	Pulling the cap off in a straight manner prevents accidental needle-stick injury. Handling the plunger at the knob only will keep the shaft of the plunger sterile. Because a vial is a sealed container, injection of an equal amount of air (before fluid is removed) is required to prevent the formation of a partial vacuum. If not enough air is injected, the negative pressure makes it difficult to withdraw the medication. Using a filter needle prevents any solid material from being withdrawn through the needle.
12. Hold the vial on a flat surface. Pierce the rubber stopper in the center with the needle tip and inject the measured air into the space above the solution (Figure 1). Do not inject air into the solution.	Air bubbled through the solution could result in withdrawal of an inaccurate amount of medication.
13. Invert the vial. **Keep the tip of the needle or blunt cannula below the fluid level (Figure 2).**	This prevents air from being aspirated into the syringe.
14. Hold the vial in one hand and use the other to withdraw the medication. **Touch the plunger at the knob only. Draw up the prescribed amount of medication while holding the syringe vertically and at eye level (Figure 3).**	Handling the plunger at the knob only will keep the shaft of the plunger sterile. Holding the syringe at eye level facilitates accurate reading, and the vertical position makes removal of air bubbles from the syringe easy.

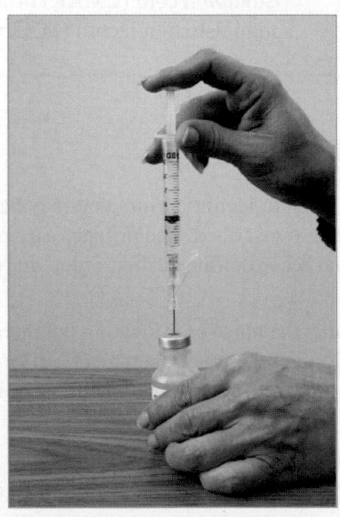

FIGURE 1. Injecting air with vial upright.

FIGURE 2. Positioning needle tip in solution.

FIGURE 3. Withdrawing medication at eye level.

ACTION	**RATIONALE**
15. If any air bubbles accumulate in the syringe, tap the barrel of the syringe sharply and move the needle past the fluid into the air space to reinject the air bubble into the vial. Return the needle tip to the solution and continue withdrawal of the medication.	Removal of air bubbles is necessary to ensure an accurate dose of medication.
16. After the correct dose is withdrawn, remove the needle from the vial and carefully replace the cap over the needle. **If a filter needle has been used to draw up the medication, remove it and attach the appropriate administration device.** Some facilities require changing the needle, if one was used to withdraw the medication, before administering the medication.	This prevents contamination of the needle and protects against accidental needlesticks. A one-handed recap method may be used as long as care is taken not to contaminate the needle during the process. A filter needle used to draw up medication should not be used to administer the medication to prevent any solid material from entering the patient. Changing the needle may be necessary because passing the needle through the stopper on the vial may dull the needle. In addition, it ensures that the tip of the needle is free from medication residue, significantly reducing pain intensity associated with the injection (Ağaç & Güneş, 2010).
17. **Check the amount of medication in the syringe with the medication dose and discard any surplus.**	Careful measurement ensures that the correct dose is withdrawn.
18. **Depending on facility policy, the third check of the label may occur at this point. If so, when all medications for one patient have been prepared, recheck the labels with the CMAR/MAR before taking the medications to the patient.**	This *third* check ensures accuracy and helps to prevent errors. *Note:* Many facilities require the *third* check to occur at the bedside, after identifying the patient and before administration.
19. **If a multidose vial is being used, label the vial with the date and time opened, and store the vial containing the remaining medication according to facility policy.**	Because the vial is sealed, the medication inside remains sterile and can be used for future injections. Labeling the opened vials with a date and time limits its use after a specific time period.
20. Lock the medication cart before leaving it.	Locking the cart or drawer safeguards the patient's medication supply. Hospital accrediting organizations require medication carts to be locked when not in use.
21. Perform hand hygiene.	Hand hygiene deters the spread of microorganisms.
22. Proceed with administration, based on the prescribed route.	See appropriate skill for prescribed route.

DOCUMENTATION

Guidelines

It is not necessary to record the removal of the medication from the ampule. Prompt recording of administration of the medication is required immediately after it is administered.

UNEXPECTED SITUATIONS AND ASSOCIATED INTERVENTIONS

- *A piece of rubber stopper is noticed floating in medication in syringe:* Discard the syringe, needle, and vial. Obtain a new vial, syringe, and needle, and prepare dose as ordered.
- *As needle attached to syringe filled with air is inserted into vial, the plunger is immediately pulled down:* If possible to withdraw medication, continue steps as explained previously. If such a vacuum has formed that this is impossible, remove syringe and inject more air into the vial. This is caused by previous withdrawal of medication without the addition of air into the vial.
- *Plunger is contaminated before injecting air into vial:* Discard needle and syringe and start over.
- *Plunger is contaminated after medication is drawn into syringe:* It is not necessary to discard needle and syringe and start over. The contaminated plunger will enter the barrel of the syringe when pushing the medication out and will not contaminate the medication.

SKILL 28-4 | MIXING MEDICATIONS FROM TWO VIALS IN ONE SYRINGE

DELEGATION CONSIDERATIONS

The preparation of medication from two vials is not delegated to nursing assistive personnel (NAP) or unlicensed assistive personnel (UAP). Depending on the state's nurse practice act and the organization's policies and procedures, the preparation of medication from two vials may be delegated to licensed practical/vocational nurses (LPN/LVN). The decision to delegate must be based on careful analysis of the patient's needs and circumstances, as well as the qualifications of the person to whom the task is being delegated. Refer to the Delegation Guidelines in Appendix A (found on the Point).

EQUIPMENT

The preparation of two types of insulin in one syringe is used as the example in the following procedure.

- Two vials of medication (insulin in this example)
- Sterile syringe (insulin syringe in this example)
- Antimicrobial swabs
- Computer-generated medication administration record (CMAR) or medication administration record (MAR)

IMPLEMENTATION

ACTION	RATIONALE
1. Gather equipment. Check the medication order against the original order in the medical record, according to facility policy.	This comparison helps to identify errors that may have occurred when orders were transcribed. The primary care provider's order is the legal record of medication orders for each facility.
2. Know the actions, special nursing considerations, safe dose ranges, purpose of administration, and adverse effects of the medications to be administered. Consider the appropriateness of the medication for this patient.	This knowledge aids the nurse in evaluating the therapeutic effect of the medication in relation to the patient's disorder and can also be used to educate the patient about the medication.
3. Perform hand hygiene.	Hand hygiene prevents the spread of microorganisms.
4. Move the medication cart to the outside of the patient's room or prepare for administration in the medication area.	Organization facilitates error-free administration and saves time.
5. Unlock the medication cart or drawer. Enter the pass code and scan employee identification, if required.	Locking the cart or drawer safeguards each patient's medication supply. Hospital accrediting organizations require medication carts to be locked when not in use. Entering the pass code and scanning ID allows only authorized users into the system and identifies the user for documentation by the computer.
6. **Prepare medications for one patient at a time.**	This prevents errors in medication administration.
7. Read the CMAR/MAR and select the proper medications from unit stock or the patient's medication drawer.	This is the *first* check of the label.
8. Compare the labels with the CMAR/MAR. Check expiration dates and perform dosage calculations, if necessary. Scan the bar code on the package, if required.	This is the *second* check of the labels. Verify calculations with another nurse to ensure safety, if necessary.
9. If necessary, remove the cap that protects the rubber stopper on each vial.	The cap protects the rubber top.
10. **If medication is a suspension (e.g., a modified insulin, such as NPH insulin), roll and agitate the vial to mix it well.**	There is controversy regarding how to mix insulin in suspension. Some sources advise rolling the vial; others advise shaking the vial. Consult facility policy. Regardless of the method used, it is essential that the suspension be mixed well to avoid administering an inconsistent dose.
11. **Cleanse the rubber tops with antimicrobial swabs.** Allow the top to dry.	Antimicrobial swab removes surface bacteria contamination. Allowing the alcohol to dry prevents it from entering the vial on the needle.

ACTION

12. Remove the cap from the needle by pulling it straight off. Touch the plunger at the knob only. Draw back an amount of air into the syringe that is equal to the dose of modified insulin to be withdrawn.

13. Hold the modified vial on a flat surface. Pierce the rubber stopper in the center with the needle tip and inject the measured air into the space above the solution (Figure 1). Do not inject air into the solution. Withdraw the needle.

14. Draw back an amount of air into the syringe that is equal to the dose of unmodified insulin to be withdrawn.

15. Hold the unmodified vial on a flat surface. Pierce the rubber stopper in the center with the needle tip and inject the measured air into the space above the solution (Figure 2). Do not inject air into the solution. Keep the needle in the vial.

16. Invert the vial of unmodified insulin. Hold the vial in one hand and use the other to withdraw the medication. **Touch the plunger at the knob only. Draw up the prescribed amount of medication while holding the syringe at eye level and vertically (Figure 3).** Turn the vial over, then remove the needle from the vial.

RATIONALE

Pulling the cap off in a straight manner prevents accidental needlestick. Handling the plunger by the knob only ensures sterility of the shaft of the plunger. Before fluid is removed, injection of an equal amount of air is required to prevent the formation of a partial vacuum, because a vial is a sealed container. If not enough air is injected, the negative pressure makes it difficult to withdraw the medication.

Unmodified insulin should never be contaminated with modified insulin. Placing air in the modified insulin first without allowing the needle to contact the insulin ensures that the second vial-entered (unmodified) insulin is not contaminated by the medication in the other vial. Air bubbled through the solution could result in withdrawal of an inaccurate amount of medication.

A vial is a sealed container. Therefore, injection of an equal amount of air (before fluid is removed) is required to prevent the formation of a partial vacuum. If not enough air is injected, the negative pressure makes it difficult to withdraw the medication.

Air bubbled through the solution could result in withdrawal of an inaccurate amount of medication.

Holding the syringe at eye level facilitates accurate reading, and the vertical position allows easy removal of air bubbles from the syringe. The first dose is prepared and is not contaminated by insulin that contains modifiers.

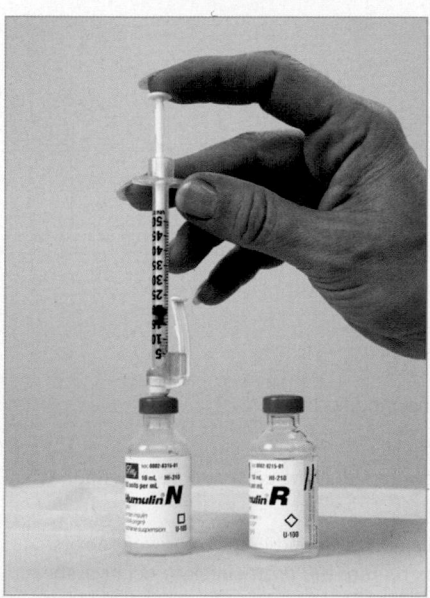

FIGURE 1. Injecting air into modified insulin preparation.

FIGURE 2. Injecting air into the unmodified insulin vial.

FIGURE 3. Withdrawing the prescribed amount of unmodified insulin.

(continued)

SKILL 28-4 · MIXING MEDICATIONS FROM TWO VIALS IN ONE SYRINGE *continued*

continued

ACTION	RATIONALE
17. Check that there are no air bubbles in the syringe.	The presence of air in the syringe would result in an inaccurate dose of medication.
18. **Check the amount of medication in the syringe with the medication dose and discard any surplus.**	Careful measurement ensures that the correct dose is withdrawn.
19. **Recheck the vial label with the CMAR/MAR.**	This is the *third* check to ensure accuracy and to prevent errors. It must be checked now for the first medication in the syringe, as it is not possible to ensure accuracy once the second drug is in the syringe.
20. Calculate the endpoint on the syringe for the combined insulin amount by adding the number of units for each dose together.	Allows for accurate withdrawal of the second dose.
21. Insert the needle into the modified vial and invert it, taking care not to push the plunger and inject medication from the syringe into the vial. Invert the vial of modified insulin. Hold the vial in one hand and use the other to withdraw the medication. **Touch the plunger at the knob only. Draw up the prescribed amount of medication while holding the syringe at eye level and vertically (Figure 4). Take care to withdraw only the prescribed amount.** Turn the vial over, then remove the needle from the vial. Carefully recap the needle. Carefully replace the cap over the needle.	Previous addition of air eliminates the need to create positive pressure. Holding the syringe at eye level facilitates accurate reading. Capping the needle prevents contamination and protects the nurse against accidental needlesticks. A one-handed recap method may be used as long as care is taken to ensure that the needle remains sterile.

FIGURE 4. Withdrawing modified insulin.

22. **Check the amount of medication in the syringe with the medication dose.**	Careful measurement ensures that the correct dose is withdrawn.
23. **Depending on facility policy, the third check of the label may occur at this point. If so, recheck the label with the CMAR/MAR before taking the medications to the patient.**	This *third* check ensures accuracy and helps to prevent errors. *Note:* Many facilities require the *third* check to occur at the bedside, after identifying the patient and before administration.

ACTION	RATIONALE
24. **Label the vials with the date and time opened, and store the vials containing the remaining medication according to facility policy.**	Because the vial is sealed, the medication inside remains sterile and can be used for future injections. Labeling the opened vials with a date and time limits its use after a specific time period. The CDC recommends that medications packaged as multiuse vials be assigned to a single patient whenever possible (CDC, 2011).
25. Lock the medication cart before leaving it.	Locking the cart or drawer safeguards the patient's medication supply. Hospital accrediting organizations require medication carts to be locked when not in use.
26. Perform hand hygiene.	Hand hygiene deters the spread of microorganisms.
27. Proceed with administration, based on the prescribed route.	See appropriate skill for prescribed route.

DOCUMENTATION

Guidelines

It is not necessary to record the removal of the medication from the ampule. Prompt recording of administration of the medication is required immediately after it is administered.

UNEXPECTED SITUATIONS AND ASSOCIATED INTERVENTIONS

- *You contaminate the plunger before injecting air into the insulin vial:* Discard the needle and syringe and start over. If plunger is contaminated after medication is drawn into the syringe, it is not necessary to discard and start over. The contaminated plunger will enter the barrel of the syringe when pushing the medication out and will not contaminate the medication.
- *You allow modified insulin to come in contact with the needle before entering the unmodified insulin vial:* Discard the needle and syringe and start over.
- *You notice that the combined amount is not the ordered amount (e.g., you have less or more units in the combined syringe than ordered):* Discard syringe and start over. There is no way to know for sure which dosage is wrong or which medication should be expelled.
- *You inject medication from the first vial (in the syringe) into the second vial:* Discard the vial and syringe and start over.

SPECIAL CONSIDERATIONS

General Considerations

- A patient with diabetes who is visually impaired may find it helpful to use a magnifying apparatus that fits around the syringe.
- Before attempting to explain or demonstrate devices that help low-vision diabetic patients to prepare their medication, attempt to use the device yourself under similar circumstances. To detect any difficulties the patient may experience, practice using the aid with your eyes closed or in a poorly lit room.

Infant and Child Considerations

School-aged children are generally able to prepare and administer their own injections, such as insulin, with supervision (Kyle & Carman, 2013). Parents/significant others and the child should be involved in the teaching.

SKILL 28-5 ADMINISTERING AN INTRADERMAL INJECTION

DELEGATION CONSIDERATIONS

The administration of an intradermal injection is not delegated to nursing assistive personnel (NAP) or unlicensed assistive personnel (UAP). Depending on the state's nurse practice act and the organization's policies and procedures, the administration of an intradermal injection may be delegated to licensed practical/vocational nurses (LPN/LVN). The decision to delegate must be based on careful analysis of the patient's needs and circumstances, as well as the qualifications of the person to whom the task is being delegated. Refer to the Delegation Guidelines in Appendix A (found on the Point).

EQUIPMENT

- Prescribed medication
- Sterile syringe, usually a tuberculin syringe calibrated in tenths and hundredths, and a needle, ¼- to ½-inch, 25- or 27-gauge
- Antimicrobial swab
- Disposable gloves
- Small gauze square
- Computer-generated medication administration record (CMAR) or medication administration record (MAR)
- PPE, as indicated

IMPLEMENTATION

ACTION	RATIONALE
1. Gather equipment. Check each medication order against the original order in the medical record according to facility policy. Clarify any inconsistencies. Check the patient's chart for allergies.	This comparison helps to identify errors that may have occurred when orders were transcribed. The primary care provider's order is the legal record of medication orders for each facility.
2. Know the actions, special nursing considerations, safe dose ranges, purpose of administration, and adverse effects of the medications to be administered. Consider the appropriateness of the medication for this patient.	This knowledge aids the nurse in evaluating the therapeutic effect of the medication in relation to the patient's disorder and can also be used to educate the patient about the medication.
3. Perform hand hygiene.	Hand hygiene deters the spread of microorganisms.
4. Move the medication cart to the outside of the patient's room or prepare for administration in the medication area.	Organization facilitates error-free administration and saves time.
5. Unlock the medication cart or drawer. Enter the pass code and scan employee identification, if required.	Locking the cart or drawer safeguards each patient's medication supply. Hospital accrediting organizations require medication carts to be locked when not in use. Entering the pass code and scanning ID allows only authorized users into the system and identifies the user for documentation by the computer.
6. **Prepare medications for one patient at a time.**	This prevents errors in medication administration.
7. Read the CMAR/MAR and select the proper medication from unit stock or the patient's medication drawer.	This is the *first* check of the label.
8. Compare the label with the CMAR/MAR. Check expiration dates and perform calculations, if necessary. Scan the bar code on the package, if required.	This is the *second* check of the label. Verify calculations with another nurse to ensure safety.
9. If necessary, withdraw medication from an ampule or vial as described in Skills 28-2 and 28-3 on pages 808–813.	
10. **Depending on facility policy, the third check of the label may occur at this point. If so, when all medications for one patient have been prepared, recheck the labels with the CMAR/MAR before taking the medications to the patient.**	This *third* check ensures accuracy and helps to prevent errors. *Note:* Many facilities require the *third* check to occur at the bedside, after identifying the patient and before administration.
11. Lock the medication cart before leaving it.	Locking the cart or drawer safeguards the patient's medication supply. Hospital accrediting organizations require medication carts to be locked when not in use.

ACTION

12. Transport medications to the patient's bedside carefully, and keep the medications in sight at all times.

13. **Ensure that the patient receives the medications at the correct time.**

14. Perform hand hygiene and put on PPE, if indicated.

15. **Identify the patient. Compare the information with the CMAR/MAR. The patient should be identified using at least two methods** (The Joint Commission [TJC], 2013):

    a. Check the name on the patient's identification band.

    b. Check the identification number on the patient's identification band.

    c. Check the birth date on the patient's identification band.

    d. Ask the patient to state his or her name and birth date, based on facility policy.

16. Close the door to the room or pull the bedside curtain.

17. **Complete necessary assessments before administering medications. Check the allergy bracelet or ask the patient about allergies. Explain the purpose and action of the medication to the patient.**

18. Scan the patient's bar code on the identification band, if required (Figure 1).

19. **Based on facility policy, the third check of the label may occur at this point. If so, recheck the labels with the CMAR/MAR before administering the medications to the patient.**

20. Put on clean gloves.

21. Select an appropriate administration site. Assist the patient to the appropriate position for the site chosen. Drape as needed to expose only the area of the site to be used.

RATIONALE

Careful handling and close observation prevent accidental or deliberate disarrangement of medications.

Check agency policy, which may allow for administration within a period of 30 minutes before or 30 minutes after the designated time.

Hand hygiene and PPE prevent the spread of microorganisms. PPE is required based on transmission precautions.

Identifying the patient ensures the right patient receives the medications and helps prevent errors. The patient's room number or physical location is not used as an identifier (TJC, 2013). Replace the identification band if it is missing or inaccurate in any way.

This requires a response from the patient, but illness and strange surroundings often cause patients to be confused.

This provides patient privacy.

Assessment is a prerequisite to administration of medications. Explanation provides rationale, increases knowledge, and reduces anxiety.

Provides an additional check to ensure that the medication is given to the right patient.

FIGURE 1. Scanning the bar code on the patient's identification bracelet.

Many facilities require the *third* check to occur at the bedside, after identifying the patient and before administration. If facility policy directs the *third* check at this time, this *third* check ensures accuracy and helps to prevent errors.

Gloves help prevent exposure to contaminants.

Appropriate site prevents injury and allows for accurate reading of the test site at the appropriate time. Draping provides privacy and warmth.

(continued)

SKILL 28-5 ADMINISTERING AN INTRADERMAL INJECTION *continued*

ACTION

22. Cleanse the site with an antimicrobial swab while wiping with a firm, circular motion and moving outward from the injection site. Allow the skin to dry.

23. Remove the needle cap with the nondominant hand by pulling it straight off.

24. Use the nondominant hand to spread the skin taut over the injection site (Figure 2).

25. Hold the syringe in the dominant hand, between the thumb and forefinger with the bevel of the needle up.

26. Hold the syringe at a 5- to 15-degree angle from the site. Place the needle almost flat against the patient's skin (Figure 3), bevel side up, and insert the needle into the skin. Insert the needle only about ⅛ inch with entire bevel under the skin.

27. Once the needle is in place, steady the lower end of the syringe. Slide your dominant hand to the end of the plunger.

28. Slowly inject the agent while watching for a small wheal or blister to appear (Figure 4).

RATIONALE

Pathogens on the skin can be forced into the tissues by the needle. Moving from the center outward prevents contamination of the site. Allowing skin to dry prevents introducing alcohol into the tissue, which can be irritating and uncomfortable.

This technique lessens the risk of an accidental needlestick.

Taut skin provides an easy entrance into intradermal tissue.

Using the dominant hand allows for easy, appropriate handling of the syringe. Having the bevel up allows for smooth piercing of the skin and introduction of the medication into the dermis.

The dermis is entered when the needle is held as nearly parallel to the skin as possible and is inserted about ⅛ inch.

Prevents injury and inadvertent advancement or withdrawal of the needle.

The appearance of a wheal indicates that the medication is in the dermis.

FIGURE 2. Spreading the skin taut over the injection site.

FIGURE 3. Inserting the needle almost level with the skin.

FIGURE 4. Observing for wheal while injecting medication.

ACTION	RATIONALE
29. Withdraw the needle quickly at the same angle that it was inserted. Do not recap the used needle. Engage the safety shield or needle guard.	Withdrawing the needle quickly and at the angle at which it entered the skin minimizes tissue damage and discomfort for the patient. Safety shields or needle guards prevent accidental needlestick injury.
30. **Do not massage the area after removing the needle. Tell the patient not to rub or scratch the site. If necessary, gently blot the site with a dry gauze square. Do not apply pressure or rub the site.**	Massaging the area where an intradermal injection is given may spread the medication to underlying subcutaneous tissue.
31. Assist the patient to a position of comfort.	This provides for the well-being of the patient.
32. Discard the needle and syringe in the appropriate receptacle.	Proper disposal of the needle prevents injury.
33. Remove gloves and additional PPE, if used. Perform hand hygiene.	Removing PPE properly reduces the risk for infection transmission and contamination of other items. Hand hygiene prevents the spread of microorganisms.
34. Document the administration of the medication immediately after administration. See Documentation section below.	Timely documentation helps to ensure patient safety.
35. Evaluate the patient's response to the medication within the appropriate time frame.	The patient needs to be evaluated for therapeutic and adverse effects from the medication.
36. Observe the area for signs of a reaction at determined intervals after administration. Inform the patient of the need for inspection.	With many intradermal injections, you need to look for a localized reaction in the area of the injection at the appropriate interval(s), determined by the type of medication and purpose. Explaining this to the patient increases compliance.

DOCUMENTATION

Guidelines

Record each medication administered on the CMAR/MAR or record using the required format—including date, time, and the site of administration—immediately after administration. Some facilities recommend circling the injection site with ink. Circling the injection site easily identifies the site of the intradermal injection and allows for future careful observation of the exact area. If using a bar-code system, medication administration is automatically recorded when the bar code is scanned. PRN medications require documentation of the reason for administration. Prompt recording avoids the possibility of accidentally repeating the administration of the drug. If the drug was refused or omitted, record this in the appropriate area on the medication record and notify the primary care provider. This verifies the reason that medication was omitted and ensures that the primary care provider is aware of the patient's condition.

UNEXPECTED SITUATIONS AND ASSOCIATED INTERVENTIONS

- *You do not note wheal or blister at site of injection:* Medication has been injected subcutaneously. Document according to facility policy and inform the primary care provider. You may need to obtain an order to repeat the procedure.

- *Medication leaks out of injection site before needle is withdrawn:* Needle was inserted less than ⅛ inch. Document according to facility policy and inform the primary care provider. You may need to obtain an order to repeat the procedure.

- *You stick yourself with the needle before injection:* Discard needle and syringe appropriately. Follow facility policy regarding needlestick injury. Prepare new syringe with medication and administer to the patient. Complete appropriate paperwork and follow facility policy regarding accidental needlestick injuries.

- *You stick yourself with the needle after injection:* Discard needle and syringe appropriately. Follow facility policy regarding needlestick injury. Complete appropriate paperwork and follow facility policy regarding accidental needlesticks.

(continued)

SKILL 28-5   ADMINISTERING AN INTRADERMAL INJECTION   *continued*

SPECIAL CONSIDERATIONS

- Ongoing assessment is an important part of nursing care for both evaluation of patient response to administered medications and early detection of adverse effects. If an adverse effect is suspected, withhold further medication doses and notify the patient's primary care provider. Additional intervention is based on type of reaction and patient assessment.
- Aspiration, pulling back on the plunger after insertion and before administration, is not recommended for an intradermal injection. The dermis does not contain large blood vessels.
- Some agencies recommend administering intradermal injections with the bevel down instead of the bevel up. Check facility policy.

SKILL 28-6   ADMINISTERING A SUBCUTANEOUS INJECTION

DELEGATION CONSIDERATIONS

The administration of a subcutaneous injection is not delegated to nursing assistive personnel (NAP) or unlicensed assistive personnel (UAP). Depending on the state's nurse practice act and the organization's policies and procedures, the administration of a subcutaneous injection may be delegated to licensed practical/vocational nurses (LPN/LVN). The decision to delegate must be based on careful analysis of the patient's needs and circumstances, as well as the qualifications of the person to whom the task is being delegated. Refer to the Delegation Guidelines in Appendix A (found on thePoint).

EQUIPMENT

- Prescribed medication
- Sterile syringe and needle. Needle size depends on the medication to be administered and patient body type (see previous discussion).
- Antimicrobial swab
- Non-latex, disposable gloves
- Small gauze square
- Computer-generated medication administration record (CMAR) or medication administration record (MAR)
- PPE, as indicated

IMPLEMENTATION

ACTION	RATIONALE
1. Gather equipment. Check each medication order against the original order in the medical record, according to facility policy. Clarify any inconsistencies. Check the patient's chart for allergies.	This comparison helps to identify errors that may have occurred when orders were transcribed. The primary care provider's order is the legal record of medication orders for each facility.
2. Know the actions, special nursing considerations, safe dose ranges, purpose of administration, and adverse effects of the medications to be administered. Consider the appropriateness of the medication for this patient.	This knowledge aids the nurse in evaluating the therapeutic effect of the medication in relation to the patient's disorder and can also be used to educate the patient about the medication.
3. Perform hand hygiene.	Hand hygiene prevents the spread of microorganisms.
4. Move the medication cart to the outside of the patient's room or prepare for administration in the medication area.	Organization facilitates error-free administration and saves time.
5. Unlock the medication cart or drawer. Enter the pass code and scan employee identification, if required.	Locking the cart or drawer safeguards each patient's medication supply. Hospital accrediting organizations require medication carts to be locked when not in use. Entering the pass code and scanning ID allows only authorized users into the computer system and identifies the user for documentation by the computer.
6. **Prepare medications for one patient at a time.**	This prevents errors in medication administration.

ACTION	RATIONALE
7. Read the CMAR/MAR and select the proper medication from unit stock or the patient's medication drawer.	This is the *first* check of the label.
8. Compare the label with the CMAR/MAR. Check expiration dates and perform calculations, if necessary. Scan the bar code on the package, if required.	This is the *second* check of the label. Verify calculations with another nurse to ensure safety, if necessary.
9. If necessary, withdraw medication from an ampule or vial as described in Skills 28-2 and 28-3 on pages 808–813.	
10. **Depending on facility policy, the third check of the label may occur at this point. If so, when all medications for one patient have been prepared, recheck the labels with the CMAR/MAR before taking the medications to the patient.**	This *third* check ensures accuracy and helps to prevent errors. *Note:* Many facilities require the *third* check to occur at the bedside, after identifying the patient and before administration.
11. Lock the medication cart before leaving it.	Locking the cart or drawer safeguards the patient's medication supply. Hospital accrediting organizations require medication carts to be locked when not in use.
12. Transport medications to the patient's bedside carefully, and keep the medications in sight at all times.	Careful handling and close observation prevent accidental or deliberate disarrangement of medications.
13. **Ensure that the patient receives the medications at the correct time.**	Check agency policy, which may allow for administration within a period of 30 minutes before or 30 minutes after the designated time.
14. Perform hand hygiene and put on PPE, if indicated.	Hand hygiene and PPE prevent the spread of microorganisms. PPE is required based on transmission precautions.
15. **Identify the patient. Compare the information with the CMAR/MAR. The patient should be identified using at least two methods** (The Joint Commission [TJC], 2013):	Identifying the patient ensures that the right patient receives the medications and helps prevent errors. The patient's room number or physical location is not used as an identifier (TJC, 2013). Replace the identification band if it is missing or inaccurate in any way.
a. Check the name on the patient's identification band.	
b. Check the identification number on the patient's identification band.	
c. Check the birth date on the patient's identification band.	
d. Ask the patient to state his or her name and birth date, based on facility policy.	This requires a response from the patient, but illness and strange surroundings often cause patients to be confused.
16. Close the door to the room or pull the bedside curtain.	This provides patient privacy.
17. **Complete necessary assessments before administering medications. Check the patient's allergy bracelet or ask the patient about allergies. Explain the purpose and action of the medication to the patient.**	Assessment is a prerequisite to administration of medications. Explanation provides rationale, increases knowledge, and reduces anxiety.
18. Scan the patient's bar code on the identification band, if required (Figure 1).	Scanning provides an additional check to ensure that the medication is given to the right patient.

FIGURE 1. Scanning the bar code on the patient's identification bracelet. *(Photo by B. Proud.)*

(continued)

SKILL 28-6 ADMINISTERING A SUBCUTANEOUS INJECTION *continued*

ACTION	RATIONALE
19. **Based on facility policy, the third check of the label may occur at this point. If so, recheck the labels with the CMAR/MAR before administering the medications to the patient.**	Many facilities require the *third* check to occur at the bedside, after identifying the patient and before administration. If facility policy directs the *third* check at this time, this *third* check ensures accuracy and helps to prevent errors.
20. Put on clean gloves.	Gloves help prevent exposure to contaminants.
21. Select an appropriate administration site.	Appropriate site prevents injury and allows for accurate reading of the test site at the appropriate time.
22. Assist the patient to the appropriate position for the site chosen. Drape, as needed, to expose only the area of the site to be used.	Appropriate site prevents injury. Draping helps maintain the patient's privacy.
23. Identify the appropriate landmarks for the site chosen.	Good visualization is necessary to establish the correct location of the site and to avoid tissue damage.
24. Cleanse the area around the injection site with an antimicrobial swab. Use a firm, circular motion while moving outward from the injection site (Figure 2). Allow the area to dry.	Pathogens on the skin can be forced into the tissues by the needle. Moving from the center outward prevents contamination of the site. Allowing the skin to dry prevents introducing alcohol into the tissue, which can be irritating and uncomfortable.
25. Remove the needle cap with the nondominant hand, pulling it straight off.	The cap protects the needle from contact with microorganisms. This technique lessens the risk of an accidental needlestick.
26. Grasp and bunch the area surrounding the injection site or spread the skin taut at the site (Figure 3).	Decision to create a skin fold is based on the nurse's assessment of the patient and needle length used. Pinching is advised for thinner patients and when a longer needle is used, to lift the adipose tissue away from underlying muscle and tissue. If pinching is used, once the needle is inserted, release the skin to avoid injecting into compressed tissue. If the skin is pulled taut, it provides easy, less painful entry into the subcutaneous tissue.

FIGURE 2. Cleaning injection site.

FIGURE 3. Bunching tissue at injection site.

27. Hold the syringe in the dominant hand between the thumb and forefinger. Inject the needle quickly at a 45- to 90-degree angle (Figure 4).	Inserting the needle quickly causes less pain to the patient. Subcutaneous tissue is abundant in well-nourished, well-hydrated people and spare in emaciated, dehydrated, or very thin persons. For a person with little subcutaneous tissue, it is best to insert the needle at a 45-degree angle.

ACTION

28. After the needle is in place, release the tissue. If you have a large skin fold pinched up, ensure that the needle stays in place as the skin is released. Immediately move your non-dominant hand to steady the lower end of the syringe. Slide your dominant hand to the end of the plunger. Avoid moving the syringe.

29. Inject the medication slowly (at a rate of 10 sec/mL).

30. Withdraw the needle quickly at the same angle at which it was inserted, while supporting the surrounding tissue with your nondominant hand.

31. Using a gauze square, apply gentle pressure to the site after the needle is withdrawn (Figure 5). **Do not massage the site.**

RATIONALE

Injecting the solution into compressed tissues results in pressure against nerve fibers and creates discomfort. If there is a large skin fold, the skin may retract away from the needle. The non-dominant hand secures the syringe. Moving the syringe could cause damage to the tissues and inadvertent administration into an incorrect area.

Rapid injection of the solution creates pressure in the tissues, resulting in discomfort.

Slow withdrawal of the needle pulls the tissues and causes discomfort. Applying counter traction around the injection site helps to prevent pulling on the tissue as the needle is withdrawn. Removing the needle at the same angle at which it was inserted minimizes tissue damage and discomfort for the patient.

Massaging the site can damage underlying tissue and increase the absorption of the medication. Massaging after heparin administration can contribute to hematoma formation. Massaging after an insulin injection may contribute to unpredictable absorption of the medication.

FIGURE 4. Inserting needle.

FIGURE 5. Applying pressure to the injection site.

32. Do not recap the used needle. Engage the safety shield or needle guard. Discard the needle and syringe in the appropriate receptacle.

33. Assist the patient to a position of comfort.

34. Remove gloves and additional PPE, if used. Perform hand hygiene.

35. Document the administration of the medication immediately after administration. See Documentation section on page 826.

36. Evaluate the patient's response to the medication within an appropriate time frame for the particular medication.

Safety shields or needle guards prevent accidental needlestick. Proper disposal of the needle prevents injury.

This provides for the well-being of the patient.

Removing PPE properly reduces the risk for infection transmission and contamination of other items. Hand hygiene prevents the spread of microorganisms.

Timely documentation helps to ensure patient safety.

The patient needs to be evaluated for therapeutic and adverse effects from the medication.

(continued)

SKILL 28-6 ADMINISTERING A SUBCUTANEOUS INJECTION *continued*

DOCUMENTATION
Guidelines

Record each medication given on the CMAR/MAR or record using the required format, including date, dose, time, and the site of administration, immediately after administration. If using a bar-code system, medication administration is automatically recorded when the bar code is scanned. PRN medications require documentation of the reason for administration. Prompt recording avoids the possibility of accidentally repeating the administration of the drug. If the drug was refused or omitted, record this in the appropriate area on the medication record and notify the primary care provider. This verifies the reason medication was omitted and ensures that the primary care provider is aware of the patient's condition.

UNEXPECTED SITUATIONS AND ASSOCIATED INTERVENTIONS

- *When skin fold is released, needle pulls out of skin:* Engage the safety shield or needle guard. Appropriately discard the needle. Attach a new needle to the syringe and administer injection.

- *Patient refuses to let you administer medication in a different location:* Explain the rationale behind rotating injection sites. Discuss other available injection sites with the patient. If the patient still will not allow injection in another area, administer medication to the patient, document patient's refusal of rotation of injection site and discussion, and notify primary care provider.

- *You stick yourself with needle before injection:* Discard the needle and syringe appropriately. Follow facility policy regarding needlestick injury. Prepare a new syringe with medication and administer to the patient. Complete appropriate paperwork and follow facility policy regarding accidental needlestick injuries.

- *You stick yourself with needle after injection:* Discard the needle and syringe appropriately. Complete appropriate paperwork and follow facility policy regarding accidental needlestick injuries.

- *During injection, patient pulls away from needle before medication is delivered fully:* Remove and appropriately discard the needle. Attach a new needle to the syringe and administer the remaining medication at a different site. Document events and interventions according to facility policy.

SPECIAL CONSIDERATIONS
General Considerations

- Ongoing assessment is an important part of nursing care for both evaluation of patient response to administered medications and early detection of adverse effects. If an adverse effect is suspected, withhold further medication doses and notify the patient's primary care provider. Additional intervention is based on type of reaction and patient assessment.

- Refer to the section on Drug-Specific Equipment and Techniques on pages 779–781 for important guidelines for administering heparin and low-molecular-weight heparin preparations such as enoxaparin (Lovenox) subcutaneously (see Fig. 28-11 on page 780).

Infant and Child Considerations

- Do not tell a child that an injection will not hurt. Describe the feel of the injection as a pinch or a sting. Children who believe that you have been dishonest with them are less likely to cooperate with future procedures.

Older Adult Considerations

- Many older patients have less adipose tissue. Adjust the length of the needle and angle of insertion accordingly. (Refer to discussion earlier in this Skill.) You do not want to inadvertently give a subcutaneous medication intramuscularly.

Home Care Considerations

- Reuse of syringes in the home setting is not recommended.

- Because absorption rates vary from site to site, it is recommended that patients administering their own insulin use the same area of the body at the same time every day to ensure more consistent absorption and prevent tissue changes from repeated use of the same site

(Aschenbrenner & Venable, 2012; ADA, 2004). Rotate injection sites within the area of the body being used.

- Changes and improvements to insulin syringes to make injections painless have resulted in thinner, shorter, sharper, and better lubricated needles. As a result, after one injection the tip of the fine needles can bend and form a hook that can tear tissue if reused. In addition, these fine needles can break and leave fragments in the skin and tissue if reused. Reuse results in more painful injections related to a reduction in needle lubricant and tip damage. Therefore, teach patients to use a new needle and syringe for each injection.

- Encourage patients to consult the policies of their local government regarding contaminated and sharps waste disposal. Teach patients to dispose of needles and syringes in a hard, plastic container. Liquid detergent or liquid fabric softener containers are good choices. Never use glass containers.

SKILL 28-7 ADMINISTERING AN INTRAMUSCULAR INJECTION

DELEGATION CONSIDERATIONS

The administration of an intramuscular injection is not delegated to nursing assistive personnel (NAP) or unlicensed assistive personnel (UAP). Depending on the state's nurse practice act and the organization's policies and procedures, the administration of an intramuscular injection may be delegated to licensed practical/vocational nurses (LPN/LVN). The decision to delegate must be based on careful analysis of the patient's needs and circumstances, as well as the qualifications of the person to whom the task is being delegated. Refer to the Delegation Guidelines in Appendix A (found on thePoint).

EQUIPMENT

- Gloves
- Additional PPE, as indicated
- Medication
- Sterile syringe and needle of appropriate size and gauge

- Antimicrobial swab
- Small gauze square
- Computer-generated medication administration record (CMAR) or medication administration record (MAR)

IMPLEMENTATION

ACTION	RATIONALE
1. Gather equipment. Check each medication order against the original order in the medical record according to facility policy. Clarify any inconsistencies. Check the patient's chart for allergies.	This comparison helps to identify errors that may have occurred when orders were transcribed. The primary care provider's order is the legal record of medication orders for each facility.
2. Know the actions, special nursing considerations, safe dose ranges, purpose of administration, and adverse effects of the medications to be administered. Consider the appropriateness of the medication for this patient.	This knowledge aids the nurse in evaluating the therapeutic effect of the medication in relation to the patient's disorder and can also be used to educate the patient about the medication.
3. Perform hand hygiene.	Hand hygiene prevents the spread of microorganisms.
4. Move the medication cart to the outside of the patient's room or prepare for administration in the medication area.	Organization facilitates error-free administration and saves time.

(continued)

SKILL 28-7 ADMINISTERING AN INTRAMUSCULAR INJECTION *continued*

ACTION	**RATIONALE**
5. Unlock the medication cart or drawer. Enter the pass code and scan employee identification, if required.	Locking the cart or drawer safeguards each patient's medication supply. Hospital accrediting organizations require medication carts to be locked when not in use. Entering the pass code and scanning ID allows only authorized users into the system and identifies the user for documentation by the computer.
6. **Prepare medications for one patient at a time.**	This prevents errors in medication administration.
7. Read the CMAR/MAR and select the proper medication from unit stock or the patient's medication drawer.	This is the *first* check of the label.
8. Compare the label with the CMAR/MAR. Check expiration dates and perform calculations, if necessary. Scan the bar code on the package, if required.	This is the *second* check of the label. Verify calculations with another nurse to ensure safety, if necessary.
9. If necessary, withdraw medication from an ampule or vial as described in Skills 28-2 and 28-3 on pages 808–813.	
10. **Depending on facility policy, the third check of the label may occur at this point. If so, when all medications for one patient have been prepared, recheck the labels with the CMAR/MAR before taking the medications to the patient.**	This *third* check ensures accuracy and helps to prevent errors. *Note:* Many facilities require the *third* check to occur at the bedside, after identifying the patient and before administration.
11. Lock the medication cart before leaving it.	Locking the cart or drawer safeguards the patient's medication supply. Hospital accrediting organizations require medication carts to be locked when not in use.
12. Transport medications to the patient's bedside carefully, and keep the medications in sight at all times.	Careful handling and close observation prevent accidental or deliberate disarrangement of medications.
13. **Ensure that the patient receives the medications at the correct time.**	Check agency policy, which may allow for administration within a period of 30 minutes before or 30 minutes after the designated time.
14. Perform hand hygiene and put on PPE, if indicated.	Hand hygiene and PPE prevent the spread of microorganisms. PPE is required based on transmission precautions.
15. **Identify the patient. Compare the information with the CMAR/MAR. The patient should be identified using at least two methods (The Joint Commission [TJC], 2013):**	Identifying the patient ensures that the right patient receives the medications and helps prevent errors. The patient's room number or physical location is not used as an identifier (TJC, 2013). Replace the identification band if it is missing or inaccurate in any way.
a. Check the name on the patient's identification band.	
b. Check the identification number on the patient's identification band.	
c. Check the birth date on the patient's identification band.	
d. Ask the patient to state name and birth date, based on facility policy.	This requires a response from the patient, but illness and strange surroundings often cause patients to be confused.
16. Close the door to the room or pull the bedside curtain.	This provides patient privacy.
17. **Complete necessary assessments before administering medications. Check the patient's allergy bracelet or ask the patient about allergies. Explain the purpose and action of the medication to the patient.**	Assessment is a prerequisite to administration of medications. Explanation provides rationale, increases knowledge, and reduces anxiety.
18. Scan the patient's bar code on the identification band, if required (Figure 1).	Provides an additional check to ensure that the medication is given to the right patient.
19. **Based on facility policy, the third check of the label may occur at this point. If so, recheck the labels with the CMAR/MAR before administering the medications to the patient.**	Many facilities require the *third* check to occur at the bedside, after identifying the patient and before administration. If facility policy directs the *third* check at this time, this *third* check ensures accuracy and helps to prevent errors.
20. Put on clean gloves.	Gloves help prevent exposure to contaminants.

ACTION

FIGURE 1. Scanning the bar code on the patient's identification bracelet. *(Photo by B. Proud.)*

21. Select an appropriate administration site.

22. Assist the patient to the appropriate position for the site chosen. Drape, as needed, to expose only the area of site being used.

23. Identify the appropriate landmarks for the site chosen.

24. Cleanse the area around the injection site with an antimicrobial swab. Use a firm, circular motion while moving outward from the injection site. Allow the area to dry.

25. Remove the needle cap by pulling it straight off. Hold the syringe in your dominant hand between the thumb and forefinger.

26. Displace the skin in a Z-track manner. Pull the skin down or to one side about 1 inch (2.5 cm) with your nondominant hand and hold the skin and tissue in this position (Figure 2).

RATIONALE

Selecting the appropriate site prevents injury.

Appropriate positioning for the site chosen prevents injury. Draping helps maintain the patient's privacy.

Good visualization is necessary to establish the correct site location and to avoid damage to tissues.

Pathogens on the skin can be forced into the tissues by the needle. Moving from the center outward prevents contamination of the site. Allowing the skin to dry prevents introducing alcohol into the tissue, which can be irritating and uncomfortable.

This technique lessens the risk of an accidental needlestick and also prevents inadvertently unscrewing the needle from the barrel of the syringe.

Z-track technique is recommended for all intramuscular injections to ensure that the medication does not leak back along the needle track and into the subcutaneous tissue (Nicoll & Hesby, 2002; Zimmerman, 2010). This technique reduces pain and discomfort, particularly for patients receiving injections over an extended period. The Z-track method is also suggested for older patients who have decreased muscle mass. Some agents, such as iron, are best given via the Z-track method due to the irritation and discoloration associated with this agent.

A   B   C   D

FIGURE 2. The Z-track, or zigzag, technique is recommended for intramuscular injections. (**A**) Normal skin and tissues. (**B**) Moving the skin to one side. (**C**) Needle is inserted at a 90-degree angle. (**D**) Once the needle is withdrawn, displaced tissue is allowed to return to its normal position, preventing the solution from escaping from the muscle tissue.

(continued)

SKILL 28-7 ADMINISTERING AN INTRAMUSCULAR INJECTION *continued*

ACTION	RATIONALE
27. Quickly dart the needle into the tissue so that the needle is perpendicular to the patient's body (Figure 3). This should ensure that the medication is administered using an injection angle between 72 and 90 degrees.	A quick injection is less painful. Inserting the needle at a 72- to 90-degree angle facilitates entry into muscle tissue.
28. As soon as the needle is in place, use the thumb and forefinger of your nondominant hand to hold the lower end of the syringe. Slide your dominant hand to the end of the plunger. Inject the solution slowly (10 sec/mL of medication).	Moving the syringe could cause damage to the tissues and inadvertent administration into an incorrect area. Rapid injection of the solution creates pressure in the tissues, resulting in discomfort. According to the CDC (2012) and current review of evidence (Crawford & Johnson, 2012), aspiration is not required for intramuscular injections. Some literature suggests that aspiration *may* be indicated when administering large-molecule medications such as penicillin (Crawford & Johnson). Consult facility policy and manufacturer recommendations to ensure safe administration.
29. Once the medication has been instilled, wait 10 seconds before withdrawing the needle.	Allows medication to begin to diffuse into the surrounding muscle tissue (Nicoll & Hesby, 2002).
30. Withdraw the needle smoothly and steadily at the same angle at which it was inserted, supporting tissue around the injection site with your nondominant hand.	Slow withdrawal of the needle pulls the tissues and causes discomfort. Applying counter traction around the injection site helps to prevent pulling on the tissue as the needle is withdrawn. Removing the needle at the same angle at which it was inserted minimizes tissue damage and discomfort for the patient.
31. Apply gentle pressure at the site with a dry gauze (Figure 4). **Do not massage the site.**	Light pressure causes less trauma and irritation to the tissues. Massaging can force medication into subcutaneous tissues.

FIGURE 3. Darting the needle into the tissue.

FIGURE 4. Applying pressure at the injection site.

ACTION	RATIONALE
32. Do not recap the used needle. Engage the safety shield or needle guard, if present. Discard the needle and syringe in the appropriate receptacle.	Proper disposal of the needle prevents injury.
33. Assist the patient to a position of comfort.	This provides for the well-being of the patient.
34. Remove gloves and additional PPE, if used. Perform hand hygiene.	Removing PPE properly reduces the risk for infection transmission and contamination of other items. Hand hygiene prevents the spread of microorganisms.
35. Document the administration of the medication immediately after administration. See Documentation section on page 831.	Timely documentation helps to ensure patient safety.
36. Evaluate the patient's response to medication within an appropriate time frame. Assess the site, if possible, within 2 to 4 hours after administration.	The patient needs to be evaluated for therapeutic and adverse effects from the medication. Visualization of the site allows for assessment of any untoward effects.

DOCUMENTATION

Guidelines

Record each medication given on the CMAR/MAR or record using the required format—including date, time, and the site of administration—immediately after administration. If using a bar-code system, medication administration is automatically recorded when the bar code is scanned. PRN medications require documentation of the reason for administration. Prompt recording avoids the possibility of accidentally repeating the administration of the drug. If the drug was refused or omitted, record this in the appropriate area on the medication record and notify the primary care provider. This verifies the reason medication was omitted and ensures that the primary care provider is aware of the patient's condition.

UNEXPECTED SITUATIONS AND ASSOCIATED INTERVENTIONS

- *You stick yourself with needle before injection:* Discard the needle and syringe appropriately. Follow agency policy regarding needlestick injury. Prepare a new syringe with medication and administer to the patient. Complete appropriate paperwork and follow facility policy regarding accidental needlesticks.

- *You stick yourself with needle after injection:* Discard the needle and syringe appropriately. Follow agency policy regarding needlestick injury. Complete appropriate paperwork and follow facility policy regarding accidental needlesticks.

- *During injection, patient pulls away from needle before medication is delivered fully:* Remove and appropriately discard the needle. Attach a new needle to the syringe and administer the remaining medication at a different site. Document events and interventions, according to facility policy.

- *While injecting needle into patient, you hit patient's bone:* Withdraw and discard the needle. Apply a new needle to the syringe and administer in an alternate site. Document incident in patient's medical record. Notify primary care provider. Complete appropriate paperwork related to special events according to facility policy.

SPECIAL CONSIDERATIONS

General Considerations

- Ongoing assessment is an important part of nursing care for both evaluation of patient response to administered medications and early detection of adverse effects. If an adverse effect is suspected, withhold further medication doses and notify the patient's primary care provider. Additional intervention is based on the type of reaction and patient assessment.

Infant and Child Considerations

- The vastus lateralis is the preferred site for intramuscular injections in infants.

Older Adult Considerations

- Muscle mass atrophies as a person ages. Take care to evaluate the patient's muscle mass and body composition. Use appropriate needle length and gauge for the patient's body composition. Choose the appropriate site based on the patient's body composition.

Home Care Considerations

- Encourage patients to consult the policies of their local government regarding contaminated and sharps waste disposal. Explain that needles and syringes should be disposed of in a hard plastic container. Liquid detergent or liquid fabric softener containers are good choices. Glass containers should not be used.

- Reuse of syringes in the home setting is not recommended.

SKILL 28-8 ADMINISTERING MEDICATIONS BY INTRAVENOUS BOLUS OR PUSH THROUGH AN INTRAVENOUS INFUSION

DELEGATION CONSIDERATIONS

The administration of medications by intravenous bolus is not delegated to nursing assistive personnel (NAP) or unlicensed assistive personnel (UAP). Depending on the state's nurse practice act and the organization's policies and procedures, the administration of specified intravenous medications in some settings may be delegated to licensed practical/vocational nurses (LPN/LVN) who have received appropriate training. The decision to delegate must be based on careful analysis of the patient's needs and circumstances, as well as the qualifications of the person to whom the task is being delegated. Refer to the Delegation Guidelines in Appendix A (found on thePoint).

EQUIPMENT

- Antimicrobial swab
- Watch with second hand, or stopwatch
- Disposable gloves
- Additional PPE, as indicated
- Prescribed medication

- Syringe with a needleless device or 23- to 25-gauge, 1-inch needle (follow facility policy)
- Syringe pump, if necessary
- Computer-generated medication administration record (CMAR) or medication administration record (MAR)

IMPLEMENTATION

ACTION	RATIONALE
1. Gather equipment. Check the medication order against the original order in the medical record, according to facility policy. Clarify any inconsistencies. Check the patient's chart for allergies. Verify the compatibility of the medication and IV fluid. Check a drug resource to clarify whether the medication needs to be diluted before administration. Check the administration rate.	This comparison helps to identify errors that may have occurred when orders were transcribed. The primary care provider's order is the legal record of medication orders for each facility. Compatibility of medication and solution prevents complications. Delivers the correct dose of medication as prescribed.
2. Know the actions, special nursing considerations, safe dose ranges, purpose of administration, and adverse effects of the medications to be administered. Consider the appropriateness of the medication for this patient.	This knowledge aids the nurse in evaluating the therapeutic effect of the medication in relation to the patient's disorder and can also be used to educate the patient about the medication.
3. Perform hand hygiene.	Hand hygiene prevents the spread of microorganisms.
4. Move the medication cart to the outside of the patient's room or prepare for administration in the medication area.	Organization facilitates error-free administration and saves time.
5. Unlock the medication cart or drawer. Enter the pass code and scan employee identification, if required.	Locking the cart or drawer safeguards each patient's medication supply. Hospital accrediting organizations require medication carts to be locked when not in use. Entering the pass code and scanning ID allows only authorized users into the system and identifies the user for documentation by the computer.
6. **Prepare medication for one patient at a time.**	This prevents errors in medication administration.
7. Read the CMAR/MAR and select the proper medication from unit stock or the patient's medication drawer.	This is the *first* check of the label.
8. Compare the label with the CMAR/MAR. Check expiration dates and perform calculations, if necessary. Scan the bar code on the package, if required.	This is the *second* check of the label. Verify calculations with another nurse to ensure safety, if necessary.
9. If necessary, withdraw medication from an ampule or vial as described in Skills 28-2 and 28-3 on pages 808–813.	
10. **Depending on facility policy, the third check of the label may occur at this point. If so, when all medications for one patient have been prepared, recheck the labels with the CMAR/MAR before taking the medications to the patient.**	This *third* check ensures accuracy and helps to prevent errors. *Note:* Many facilities require the *third* check to occur at the bedside, after identifying the patient and before administration.

ACTION	RATIONALE
11. Lock the medication cart before leaving it.	Locking the cart or drawer safeguards the patient's medication supply. Hospital accrediting organizations require medication carts to be locked when not in use.
12. Transport medications and equipment to the patient's bedside carefully, and keep the medications in sight at all times.	Careful handling and close observation prevent accidental or deliberate disarrangement of medications. Having equipment available saves time and facilitates performance of the task.
13. **Ensure that the patient receives the medications at the correct time.**	Check agency policy, which may allow for administration within a period of 30 minutes before or 30 minutes after designated time.
14. Perform hand hygiene and put on PPE, if indicated.	Hand hygiene and PPE prevent the spread of microorganisms. PPE is required based on transmission precautions.
15. **Identify the patient. Compare the information with the CMAR/MAR. The patient should be identified using at least two methods** (The Joint Commission [TJC], 2013):	Identifying the patient ensures that the right patient receives the medications and helps prevent errors. The patient's room number or physical location is not used as an identifier (TJC, 2013). Replace the identification band if it is missing or inaccurate in any way.
a. Check the name on the patient's identification band.	
b. Check the identification number on the patient's identification band.	
c. Check the birth date on the patient's identification band.	
d. Ask the patient to state name and birth date, based on facility policy.	This requires a response from the patient, but illness and strange surroundings often cause patients to be confused.
16. Close the door to the room or pull the bedside curtain.	This provides patient privacy.
17. Complete necessary assessments before administering medications. Check the patient's allergy bracelet or ask the patient about allergies. Explain the purpose and action of the medication to the patient.	Assessment is a prerequisite to administration of medications. Explanation provides rationale, increases knowledge, and reduces anxiety.
18. Scan the patient's bar code on the identification band, if required (Figure 1).	Provides an additional check to ensure that the medication is given to the right patient.

FIGURE 1. Scanning the bar code on the patient's identification bracelet.

(continued)

SKILL 28-8 ADMINISTERING MEDICATIONS BY INTRAVENOUS BOLUS OR PUSH THROUGH AN INTRAVENOUS INFUSION *continued*

ACTION	RATIONALE
19. **Based on facility policy, the third check of the label may occur at this point. If so, recheck the labels with the CMAR/MAR before administering the medications to the patient.**	Many facilities require the *third* check to occur at the bedside, after identifying the patient and before administration. If facility policy directs the *third* check at this time, this *third* check ensures accuracy and helps to prevent errors.
20. **Assess the IV site for presence of inflammation or infiltration.**	IV medication must be given directly into a vein for safe administration.
21. If IV infusion is being administered via an infusion pump, pause the pump.	Pausing prevents infusion of fluid during bolus administration and activation of pump occlusion alarms.
22. Put on clean gloves.	Gloves prevent contact with blood and body fluids.
23. Select an injection port on the tubing that is closest to the venipuncture site. Clean the port with an antimicrobial swab.	Using the port closest to the needle insertion site minimizes dilution of the medication. Cleaning deters entry of microorganisms when the port is punctured.
24. Uncap the syringe. Steady the port with your nondominant hand while inserting the syringe into the center of the port.	This supports the injection port and lessens the risk for accidentally dislodging the IV or entering the port incorrectly.
25. Move your nondominant hand to the section of IV tubing just above the injection port. Fold the tubing between your fingers.	This temporarily stops flow of gravity IV infusion and prevents medication from backing up the tubing.
26. Pull back slightly on the plunger just until blood appears in the tubing.	This ensures injection of medication into the bloodstream.
27. **Inject the medication at the recommended rate** (Figure 2). See Special Considerations on page 835.	This delivers correct amount of medication at proper interval according to manufacturer's directions.

FIGURE 2. Injecting medication while interrupting IV flow. *(Photo by B. Proud.)*

28. Release the tubing. Remove the syringe. Do not recap the used needle, if used. Engage the safety shield or needle guard, if present. Release the tubing and allow the IV fluid to flow. Discard the needle and syringe in the appropriate receptacle.	Proper disposal of the needle prevents injury.
29. Check IV fluid infusion rate. Restart the infusion pump, if appropriate.	Injection of bolus may alter the rate of fluid infusion, if infusing by gravity.
30. Remove gloves and additional PPE, if used. Perform hand hygiene.	Removing PPE properly reduces the risk for infection transmission and contamination of other items. Hand hygiene prevents the spread of microorganisms.
31. Document the administration of the medication immediately after administration. See Documentation section on page 835.	Timely documentation helps to ensure patient safety.
32. Evaluate the patient's response to the medication within the appropriate time frame.	The patient needs to be evaluated for therapeutic and adverse effects from the medication.

DOCUMENTATION
Guidelines

Document the administration of the medication immediately after administration—including date, time, dose, route of administration, site of administration, and rate of administration—on the CMAR/MAR or record using the required format. If using a bar-code system, medication administration is automatically recorded when the bar code is scanned. PRN medications require documentation of the reason for administration. Prompt recording avoids the possibility of accidentally repeating the administration of the drug. If the drug was refused or omitted, record this in the appropriate area on the medication record and notify the primary care provider. This verifies the reason medication was omitted and ensures that the primary care provider is aware of the patient's condition.

UNEXPECTED SITUATIONS AND ASSOCIATED INTERVENTIONS

- *Upon assessing IV site before administering medication, no blood return is aspirated:* If IV appears patent, without signs of infiltration, and IV fluid infuses without difficulty, proceed with administration. Observe closely for signs and symptoms of infiltration during and after administration.

- *Upon assessing patient's IV site before administering medication, you note that IV has infiltrated:* Stop IV fluid and remove the IV from the extremity. Restart the IV in a different location. Continue to monitor the new IV site as medication is administered.

- *While administering medication, you note a cloudy, white substance forming in IV tubing:* Stop the IV from flowing and stop administering the medication. Clamp the IV at site nearest to the patient. Change the administration tubing and restart the infusion. Check literature or consult the pharmacist regarding compatibility of the medication and IV fluid.

- *While you are administering medication, patient begins to complain of pain at IV site:* Stop the medication. Assess the IV site for any signs of infiltration or phlebitis. Flush the IV with normal saline to check for patency. If the IV site appears within normal limits, resume medication administration at a slower rate.

SPECIAL CONSIDERATIONS

- Facility policy may recommend the following variations when injecting a bolus IV medication:
  - Release the folded tubing after each increment of the drug has been administered at the prescribed rate to facilitate delivery of the medication.
  - Use a syringe with 1 mL normal saline to flush the tubing after an IV bolus is delivered to ensure that residual medication in the tubing is not delivered too rapidly.

- Consider how fast the IV fluid is flowing to determine whether a flush of normal saline is in order after administering the medication. If the IV fluid is flowing less than 50 mL per hour, it may take the medication up to 30 minutes to reach the patient. This depends on what type of tubing is being used in the agency.

- If the IV is a small gauge (22- to 24-gauge) placed in a small vein, a blood return may not occur even if IV is intact. Also, the patient may complain of stinging and pain at the site while the medication is being administered due to irritation of a vein. Placing a warm pack over the vein or slowing the rate may relieve discomfort.

- If the medication and IV solution are incompatible, a bolus may be given by flushing the tubing with normal saline before and after the medication bolus. Consult facility policy.

- Ongoing assessment is an important part of nursing care for both evaluation of patient response to administered medications and early detection of adverse effects. If an adverse effect is suspected, withhold further medication doses and notify the patient's primary care provider. Additional intervention is based on type of reaction and patient assessment.

SKILL 28-9 ADMINISTERING A PIGGYBACK INTERMITTENT INTRAVENOUS INFUSION OF MEDICATION

DELEGATION CONSIDERATIONS	The administration of medications by intermittent IV infusion is not delegated to nursing assistive personnel (NAP) or unlicensed assistive personnel (UAP). Depending on the state's nurse practice act and the organization's policies and procedures, the administration of specified IV medications in some settings may be delegated to licensed practical/vocational nurses (LPN/LVN) who have received appropriate training. The decision to delegate must be based on careful analysis of the patient's needs and circumstances, as well as the qualifications of the person to whom the task is being delegated. Refer to the Delegation Guidelines in Appendix A (found on thePoint).

EQUIPMENT

- Medication prepared in labeled small-volume bag
- Short secondary infusion tubing (microdrip or macrodrip)
- IV pump
- Needleless connector, if required, based on facility system
- Antimicrobial swab

- Metal or plastic hook
- IV pole
- Date label for tubing
- Computer-generated medication administration record (CMAR) or medication administration record (MAR)
- PPE, as indicated

IMPLEMENTATION

ACTION	RATIONALE
1. Gather equipment. Check each medication order against the original order in the medical record, according to facility policy. Clarify any inconsistencies. Check the patient's chart for allergies.	This comparison helps to identify errors that may have occurred when orders were transcribed. The primary care provider order is the legal record of medication orders for each facility.
2. Know the actions, special nursing considerations, safe dose ranges, purpose of administration, and adverse effects of the medications to be administered. Consider the appropriateness of the medication for this patient.	This knowledge aids the nurse in evaluating the therapeutic effect of the medication in relation to the patient's disorder and can also be used to educate the patient about the medication.
3. Perform hand hygiene.	Hand hygiene prevents the spread of microorganisms.
4. Move the medication cart to the outside of the patient's room or prepare for administration in the medication area.	Organization facilitates error-free administration and saves time.
5. Unlock the medication cart or drawer. Enter the pass code and scan employee identification, if required.	Locking the cart or drawer safeguards each patient's medication supply. Hospital accrediting organizations require medication carts to be locked when not in use. Entering the pass code and scanning ID allows only authorized users into the system and identifies the user for documentation by the computer.
6. **Prepare medications for one patient at a time.**	This prevents errors in medication administration.
7. Read the CMAR/MAR and select the proper medication from unit stock or the patient's medication drawer.	This is the *first* check of the label.
8. Compare the label with the CMAR/MAR. Check expiration dates. Confirm the prescribed or appropriate infusion rate. Calculate the drip rate if using the gravity system. Scan the bar code on the package, if required.	This is the *second* check of the label. Verify calculations with another nurse to ensure safety, if necessary. Infusing the medication at the appropriate rate prevents injury.
9. **Depending on facility policy, the third check of the label may occur at this point. If so, when all medications for one patient have been prepared, recheck the labels with the CMAR/MAR before taking the medications to the patient.**	This *third* check ensures accuracy and helps to prevent errors. *Note:* Many facilities require the *third* check to occur at the bedside, after identifying the patient and before administration.

ACTION	RATIONALE
10. Lock the medication cart before leaving it.	Locking the cart or drawer safeguards the patient's medication supply. Hospital accrediting organizations require medication carts to be locked when not in use.
11. Transport medications to the patient's bedside carefully, and keep the medications in sight at all times.	Careful handling and close observation prevent accidental or deliberate disarrangement of medications.
12. **Ensure that the patient receives the medications at the correct time.**	Check facility policy, which may allow for administration within a period of 30 minutes before or 30 minutes after designated time.
13. Perform hand hygiene and put on PPE, if indicated.	Hand hygiene and PPE prevent the spread of microorganisms. PPE is required based on transmission precautions.
14. **Identify the patient. Compare the information with the CMAR/MAR. The patient should be identified using at least two methods (The Joint Commission [TJC], 2013):**	Identifying the patient ensures that the right patient receives the medications and helps prevent errors. The patient's room number or physical location is not used as an identifier (TJC, 2013). Replace the identification band if it is missing or inaccurate in any way.
a. Check the name on the patient's identification band.	
b. Check the identification number on the patient's identification band.	
c. Check the birth date on the patient's identification band.	
d. Ask the patient to state name and birth date, based on facility policy.	This requires a response from the patient, but illness and strange surroundings often cause patients to be confused.
15. Close the door to the room or pull the bedside curtain.	This provides patient privacy.
16. **Complete necessary assessments before administering medications. Check the patient's allergy bracelet or ask the patient about allergies. Explain the purpose and action of the medication to the patient.**	Assessment is a prerequisite to administration of medications. Explanation provides rationale, increases knowledge, and reduces anxiety.
17. **Scan the patient's bar code on the identification band, if required (Figure 1).**	Scanning provides an additional check to ensure that the medication is given to the right patient.

FIGURE 1. Scanning the bar code on the patient's identification bracelet.

(continued)

SKILL 28-9 ADMINISTERING A PIGGYBACK INTERMITTENT INTRAVENOUS INFUSION OF MEDICATION *continued*

ACTION	**RATIONALE**
18. **Based on facility policy, the third check of the label may occur at this point. If so, recheck the labels with the CMAR/MAR before administering the medications to the patient.**	Many facilities require the third check to occur at the bedside, after identifying the patient and before administration. If facility policy directs the third check at this time, this *third* check ensures accuracy and helps to prevent errors.
19. Assess the IV site for the presence of inflammation or infiltration.	IV medication must be given directly into a vein for safe administration.
20. Close the clamp on the short secondary infusion tubing. Using aseptic technique, remove the cap on the tubing spike and the cap on the port of the medication container, taking care to avoid contaminating either end.	Closing the clamp prevents fluid from entering the system until the nurse is ready. Maintaining sterility of the tubing and the medication port prevents contamination.
21. Attach infusion tubing to the medication container by inserting the tubing spike into the port with a firm push and twisting motion, taking care to avoid contaminating either end.	Maintaining sterility of tubing and medication port prevents contamination.
22. Hang piggyback container on an IV pole, positioning it higher than the primary IV according to manufacturer's recommendations (Figure 2). Use metal or plastic hook to lower primary IV fluid container.	Position of the containers influences the flow of the IV fluid into the primary setup.
23. Place a label on the tubing with the appropriate date.	Tubing for the piggyback setup may be used for 48 to 96 hours, depending on agency policy. Label allows for tracking of the next date to change the medication.
24. Squeeze the drip chamber on the tubing and release. Fill to the line, or about half full. Open the clamp and prime the tubing. Close the clamp. Place the needleless connector on the end of the tubing, using sterile technique, if required.	This removes air from the tubing and preserves the sterility of the setup.
25. Use an antimicrobial swab to clean the access port or stopcock above the roller clamp on the primary IV infusion tubing (Figure 3).	This deters entry of microorganisms when the piggyback setup is connected to the port. The backflow valve in the primary line secondary port stops the flow of the primary infusion while the piggyback solution is infusing. Once completed, the backflow valves open and flow of the primary solution resumes.

FIGURE 2. Positioning piggyback container on IV pole. *(Photo by B. Proud.)*

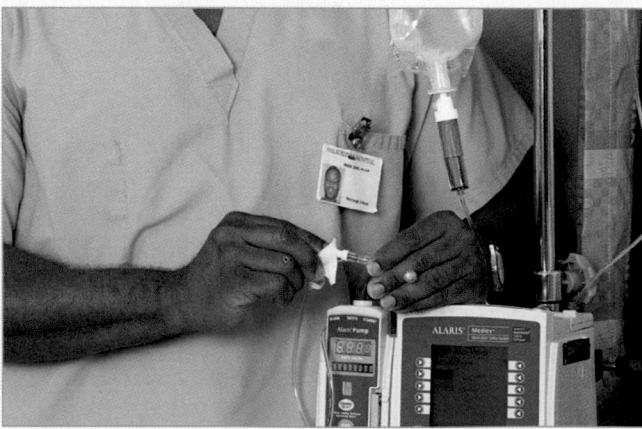

FIGURE 3. Cleaning access port. *(Photo by B. Proud.)*

ACTION	RATIONALE

ACTION

26. Connect the piggyback setup to the access port or stopcock (Figure 4). If using, turn the stopcock to the open position.

27. Open the clamp on the secondary tubing. Set the rate for the secondary infusion on the infusion pump and begin the infusion (Figure 5). If using gravity infusion, use the roller clamp on the primary infusion tubing to regulate flow at the prescribed delivery rate (Figure 6). Monitor medication infusion at periodic intervals.

RATIONALE

Needleless systems and the stopcock setup eliminate the need for a needle and are recommended by the CDC.

The backflow valve in the primary line secondary port stops the flow of the primary infusion while the piggyback solution is infusing. Once completed, the backflow valves open and flow of the primary solution resumes. It is important to verify the safe administration rate for each drug to prevent adverse effects.

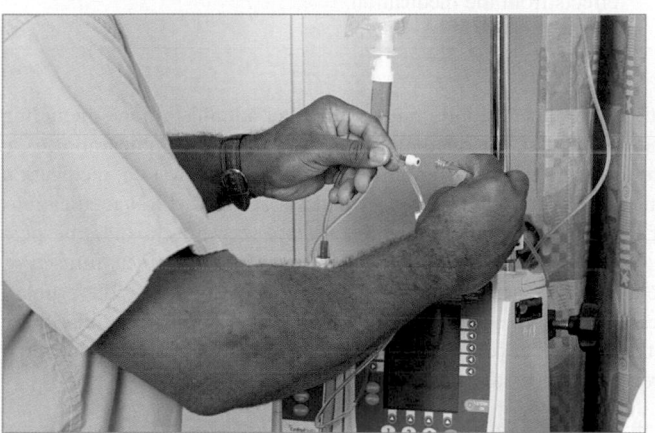

FIGURE 4. Connecting piggyback setup to access port. *(Photo by B. Proud.)*

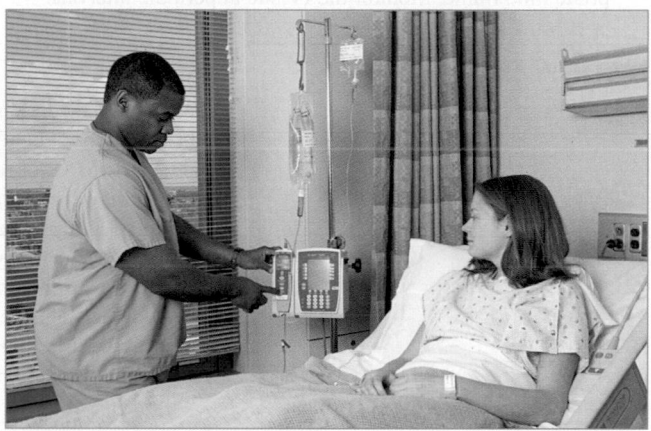

FIGURE 5. Setting rate on infusion pump. *(Photo by B. Proud.)*

FIGURE 6. Using roller clamp on primary infusion tubing to regulate gravity flow. *(Photo by B. Proud.)*

28. Clamp the tubing on the piggyback set when the solution is infused. Follow facility policy regarding disposal of equipment.

Most facilities allow the reuse of tubing for 48 to 96 hours. This reduces risk for contaminating the primary IV setup.

29. Raise primary IV fluid container to its original height. **Check the primary infusion rate on the infusion pump. If using gravity infusion, readjust the flow rate of the primary IV.**

Most infusion pumps automatically restart primary infusion at the previous rate after secondary infusion is completed. If using gravity infusion, piggyback medication administration may interrupt the normal flow rate of the primary IV. Rate readjustment may be necessary.

(continued)

SKILL 28-9 ADMINISTERING A PIGGYBACK INTERMITTENT INTRAVENOUS INFUSION OF MEDICATION *continued*

ACTION	**RATIONALE**
30. Remove PPE, if used. Perform hand hygiene.	Removing PPE properly reduces the risk for infection transmission and contamination of other items. Hand hygiene prevents the spread of microorganisms.
31. Document the administration of the medication immediately after administration. See Documentation section below. Document the volume of fluid administered on the intake and output record, if necessary.	Timely documentation helps to ensure patient safety.
32. Evaluate the patient's response to medication within the appropriate time frame. Monitor the IV site at periodic intervals.	The patient needs to be evaluated for therapeutic and adverse effects from the medication.

DOCUMENTATION

Guidelines

Document the administration of the medication immediately after administration—including date, time, dose, route of administration, site of administration, and rate of administration—on the CMAR/MAR or record using the required format. If using a bar-code system, medication administration is automatically recorded when the bar code is scanned. PRN medications require documentation of the reason for administration. Prompt recording avoids the possibility of accidentally repeating the administration of the drug. If the drug was refused or omitted, record this in the appropriate area on the medication record and notify the primary care provider. This verifies the reason medication was omitted and ensures that the primary care provider is aware of the patient's condition. Document the volume of fluid administered on the intake and output record, if necessary.

UNEXPECTED SITUATIONS AND ASSOCIATED INTERVENTIONS

- *Upon assessing the IV site before administering medication, you note that the IV has infiltrated:* Stop the IV fluid and remove the IV from the extremity. Restart the IV in a different location. Continue to monitor the new IV site as medication is administered.

- *While administering medication, you note a cloudy, white substance forming in the IV tubing:* Stop the IV from flowing and stop administering the medication to prevent precipitate from entering the patient's circulation. Clamp the IV at the site nearest to the patient. Replace the tubing on the primary and secondary infusions. Check the literature regarding incompatibilities of medications before administering. Medication infusion may require a second IV site or flushing of tubing before and after administration, using the tandem system.

- *While you are administering medication, the patient begins to complain of pain at the IV site:* Stop the medication. Assess the IV site for any signs of infiltration or phlebitis. Flush the IV with normal saline to check for patency. If the IV site appears within normal limits, resume medication administration at a slower rate.

SPECIAL CONSIDERATIONS

General Considerations

- An alternate way to prime the secondary tubing, particularly if an administration set is in place from a previous infusion, is to "backfill" the secondary tubing. Attach the medication bag to the secondary infusion tubing. Lower the medication bag below the main IV solution container and open the clamp on the secondary infusion tubing. This allows the primary IV solution to flow up the secondary tubing to the drip chamber, "backfilling" the tubing. Allow the solution to enter the drip chamber until the drip chamber is half full. Close the clamp on the secondary tubing and hang the medication container on the IV pole. Proceed with administration by lowering the primary IV container, as described previously. This "backfill" method keeps the infusion system intact, preventing both introduction of microorganisms and loss of medication when the tubing is primed. Check facility policy regarding the use of "backfilling."

- Ongoing assessment is an important part of nursing care for both evaluation of patient response to administered medications and early detection of adverse effects. If an adverse effect is suspected, withhold further medication doses and notify the patient's primary care provider. Additional intervention is based on type of reaction and patient assessment.

Infant and Child Considerations

- Infants and small children with fluid restrictions may not tolerate the added IV fluid needed for administration with piggyback or volume-control systems.

SKILL 28-10 INTRODUCING DRUGS THROUGH A MEDICATION OR DRUG-INFUSION LOCK (INTERMITTENT PERIPHERAL VENOUS ACCESS DEVICE) USING THE SALINE FLUSH

DELEGATION CONSIDERATIONS

The administration of medications through an intermittent peripheral venous access device is not delegated to nursing assistive personnel (NAP) or unlicensed assistive personnel (UAP). Depending on the state's nurse practice act and the organization's policies and procedures, the administration of specified IV medications in some settings may be delegated to licensed practical/vocational nurses (LPN/LVN) who have received appropriate training. The decision to delegate must be based on careful analysis of the patient's needs and circumstances, as well as the qualifications of the person to whom the task is being delegated. Refer to the Delegation Guidelines in Appendix A (found on thePoint).

EQUIPMENT

- Medication
- Saline flushes (2), volume according to facility policy usually 2 to 3 mL
- Antimicrobial swabs
- Watch with second hand or stopwatch feature
- Disposable gloves
- Computer-generated medication administration record (CMAR) or medication administration record (MAR)

IMPLEMENTATION

ACTION	RATIONALE
1. Gather equipment. Check the medication order against the original order in the medical record, according to agency policy. Clarify any inconsistencies. Check the patient's chart for allergies. Check a drug resource to clarify whether the medication needs to be diluted before administration. Verify the recommended administration rate.	This comparison helps to identify errors that may have occurred when orders were transcribed. The primary care provider's order is the legal record of medication orders for each facility. Compatibility of medication and solution prevents complications. Recommended infusion rate delivers the correct dose of medication as prescribed.
2. Know the actions, special nursing considerations, safe dose ranges, purpose of administration, and adverse effects of the medications to be administered. Consider the appropriateness of the medication for this patient.	This knowledge aids the nurse in evaluating the therapeutic effect of the medication in relation to the patient's disorder and can also be used to educate the patient about the medication.
3. Perform hand hygiene.	Hand hygiene prevents the spread of microorganisms.

(continued)

SKILL 28-10 INTRODUCING DRUGS THROUGH A MEDICATION OR DRUG-INFUSION LOCK (INTERMITTENT PERIPHERAL VENOUS ACCESS DEVICE) USING THE SALINE FLUSH *continued*

ACTION	**RATIONALE**
4. Move the medication cart to the outside of the patient's room or prepare for administration in the medication area.	Organization facilitates error-free administration and saves time.
5. Unlock the medication cart or drawer. Enter the pass code and scan employee identification, if required.	Locking the cart or drawer safeguards each patient's medication supply. Hospital accrediting organizations require medication carts to be locked when not in use. Entering the pass code and scanning ID allows only authorized users into the system and identifies the user for documentation by the computer.
6. **Prepare medication for one patient at a time.**	This prevents errors in medication administration.
7. Read the CMAR/MAR and select the proper medication from unit stock or the patient's medication drawer.	This is the *first* check of the label.
8. Compare the label with the CMAR/MAR. Check expiration dates and perform calculations, if necessary. Scan the bar code on the package, if required.	This is the *second* check of the label. Verify calculations with another nurse to ensure safety, if necessary.
9. If necessary, withdraw the medication from an ampule or vial as described in Skills 28-2 and 28-3 on pages 808–813.	Allows administration of the medication.
10. **Depending on facility policy, the third check of the label may occur at this point. If so, when all medications for one patient have been prepared, recheck the labels with the CMAR/MAR before taking the medications to the patient.**	This *third* check ensures accuracy and helps to prevent errors. *Note:* Many facilities require the *third* check to occur at the bedside, after identifying the patient and before administration.
11. Lock the medication cart before leaving it.	Locking the cart or drawer safeguards the patient's medication supply. Hospital accrediting organizations require medication carts to be locked when not in use.
12. Transport medications and equipment to the patient's bedside carefully, and keep the medications in sight at all times.	Careful handling and close observation prevent accidental or deliberate disarrangement of medications. Having equipment available saves time and facilitates performance of the task.
13. **Ensure that the patient receives the medications at the correct time.**	Check facility policy, which may allow for administration within a period of 30 minutes before or 30 minutes after designated time.
14. Perform hand hygiene and put on PPE, if indicated.	Hand hygiene and PPE prevent the spread of microorganisms. PPE is required based on transmission precautions.
15. **Identify the patient. Compare the information with the CMAR/MAR. The patient should be identified using at least two methods** (The Joint Commission [TJC], 2013):	Identifying the patient ensures that the right patient receives the medications and helps prevent errors. The patient's room number or physical location is not used as an identifier (TJC, 2013). Replace the identification band if it is missing or inaccurate in any way.
a. Check the name on the patient's identification band.	
b. Check the identification number on the patient's identification band.	
c. Check the birth date on the patient's identification band.	
d. Ask the patient to state name and birth date, based on facility policy.	This requires a response from the patient, but illness and strange surroundings often cause patients to be confused.
16. Close the door to the room or pull the bedside curtain.	This provides patient privacy.
17. **Complete necessary assessments before administering medications. Check the patient's allergy bracelet or ask the patient about allergies. Explain the purpose and action of the medication to the patient.**	Assessment is a prerequisite to administration of medications. Explanation provides rationale, increases knowledge, and reduces anxiety.

ACTION	**RATIONALE**

18 Scan the patient's bar code on the identification band, if required (Figure 1).

Scanning provides an additional check to ensure that the medication is given to the right patient.

19. **Based on facility policy, the third check of the label may occur at this point. If so, recheck the labels with the CMAR/MAR before administering the medications to the patient.**

Many facilities require the *third* check to occur at the bedside, after identifying the patient and before administration. If facility policy directs the *third* check at this time, this *third* check ensures accuracy and helps to prevent errors.

20. Assess the IV site for the presence of inflammation or infiltration.

IV medication must be given directly into a vein for safe administration.

21. Put on clean gloves.

Gloves protect the nurse's hands from contact with the patient's blood.

22. Clean the access port of the medication lock with an antimicrobial swab (Figure 2).

Cleaning removes surface contaminants at the lock entry site.

FIGURE 1. Scanning the bar code on the patient's identification bracelet.

FIGURE 2. Cleaning access port.

23. Stabilize the port with your nondominant hand and insert the syringe, or needleless access device, of normal saline into the access port (Figure 3).

This allows for careful insertion into the center circle of the lock.

24. Release the clamp on the extension tubing of the medication lock. Aspirate gently and check for blood return (Figure 4).

This ensures that the catheter of the medication lock is in a vein.

FIGURE 3. Inserting syringe into access port.

FIGURE 4. Aspirating for blood return.

(continued)

SKILL 28-10

INTRODUCING DRUGS THROUGH A MEDICATION OR DRUG-INFUSION LOCK (INTERMITTENT PERIPHERAL VENOUS ACCESS DEVICE) USING THE SALINE FLUSH *continued*

25. Gently flush with normal saline by pushing slowly on the syringe plunger. Observe the insertion site while inserting the saline. Remove the syringe.

Saline flush ensures that the IV line is patent. Puffiness or swelling as the site is flushed could indicate infiltration of the catheter.

26. Insert the syringe, or needleless access device, with the medication into the port and gently inject the medication, using a watch to verify correct administration rate. **Do not force the injection if resistance is felt.**

Easy installation of medication usually indicates that the lock is still patent and in the vein. If force is used against resistance, a clot may break away and cause a blockage elsewhere in the body.

27. Remove the medication syringe from the port. Stabilize the port with your nondominant hand and insert the syringe, or needleless access device, of normal saline into the port. Gently flush with normal saline by pushing slowly on the syringe plunger (Figure 5). If the medication lock is capped with a positive pressure valve/device, remove the syringe, then clamp the extension tubing (Figure 6). Alternately, to gain positive pressure if a positive pressure valve/device is not present, clamp the extension tubing as you are still flushing the last of the saline into the medication lock. Remove the syringe.

Positive pressure prevents blood from backing into the catheter and causing the medication lock to clot off.

FIGURE 5. Flushing port with normal saline.

FIGURE 6. Clamping the access port.

28. Discard the syringe in the appropriate receptacle.

Proper disposal prevents injury.

29. Remove PPE, if used. Perform hand hygiene.

Removing PPE properly reduces the risk for infection transmission and contamination of other items. Hand hygiene prevents the spread of microorganisms.

30. Document the administration of the medication immediately after administration. See Documentation section.

Timely documentation helps to ensure patient safety.

31. Evaluate the patient's response to the medication within the appropriate time frame.

The patient needs to be evaluated for therapeutic and adverse effects from the medication.

32. Check the medication lock site at least every 8 hours or according to facility policy.

This ensures patency of system.

DOCUMENTATION

Guidelines

Document the administration of the medication and saline flush—including date, time, dose, route of administration, site of administration, and rate of administration—on the CMAR/MAR or record using the required format, immediately after administration. If using a bar-code system, medication administration is automatically recorded when the bar code is scanned. PRN medications require documentation of the reason for administration. Prompt recording avoids the possibility of accidentally repeating the administration of the drug. If the drug was refused or omitted, record this in the appropriate area on the medication record and notify the primary care provider. This verifies the reason the medication was omitted and ensures that the primary care provider is aware of the patient's condition.

UNEXPECTED SITUATIONS AND ASSOCIATED INTERVENTIONS

- *Upon assessing the medication lock site before administering medication, you note that the medication lock has infiltrated:* Remove the medication lock from the extremity. Restart peripheral venous access in a different location. Continue to monitor the new site as the medication is administered.

- *While you are administering medication, patient begins to complain of pain at the site:* Stop the medication. Assess the medication lock site for signs of infiltration and phlebitis. Flush the medication lock with normal saline again to recheck patency. If the IV site appears within normal limits, resume medication administration at a slower rate. If pain persists, stop, remove the medication lock, and restart in a different location.

- *As you are attempting to access lock, tip of syringe touches patient's arm:* Discard the syringe. Prepare a new dose for administration.

- *No blood return is noted upon aspiration:* If medication lock appears patent, without signs of infiltration, and normal saline fluid infuses without difficulty, proceed with administration. Observe closely for signs and symptoms of infiltration during and after administration.

SPECIAL CONSIDERATIONS

General Considerations

- If a medication lock is not used, flush with saline every 8 to 12 hours to maintain patency, according to facility policy.

- Routinely change the medication lock site every 72 to 96 hours, according to facility policy. This reduces the risk of infection and emboli in the bloodstream.

- Intermittent infusions of small-volume IV medications can also be administered through the medication lock. Attach the IV medication container to infusion tubing and prime. After flushing the medication lock with saline as outlined previously, attach the infusion tubing to the medication lock. Set the infusion rate in the infusion pump. Alternately, adjust the infusion rate with a roller clamp on gravity infusion tubing. After infusion is completed, remove the tubing from the lock and flush with saline as outlined previously.

- Ongoing assessment is an important part of nursing care for evaluation of patient response to administered medications and early detection of adverse effects. If an adverse effect is suspected, withhold further medication doses and notify the patient's primary care provider. Additional intervention is based on type of reaction and patient assessment.

Infant and Child Considerations

- If the volume of medication being administered is small (less than 1.0 mL), always include the amount of flush solution as part of the total amount to be injected and take this into account when determining how fast to push a medication. For example, if the medication is to be injected at a rate of 1.0 mL per minute and the total amount of solution to be injected is 2.25 mL (0.25 mL medication volume plus 2.0 mL saline flush solution volume equals 2.25 mL), then the medication would be injected over a period of 2 minutes 15 seconds.

DEVELOPING CLINICAL REASONING

1. You are scheduled to give an intramuscular injection in the ventrogluteal site and remember learning that it should be administered using the Z-track technique. When you mention this to the nurse in the hospital who has been taking care of your patient, she tells you there is no reason to use the Z-track technique. You remember your instructor telling you to use the Z-track technique. What should you do?

2. You are caring for two patients and have just completed giving medications to the first when you realize that you gave her the medications ordered for your other patient. What should you do?

PRACTICING FOR NCLEX

1. A nurse administers a dose of an oral medication for hypertension to a patient who immediately vomits after swallowing the pill. What would be the appropriate initial action of the nurse in this situation?
   a. Readminister the medication and notify the primary care provider.
   b. Readminister the pill in a liquid form if possible.
   c. Assess the vomit, looking for the pill.
   d. Notify the primary care provider.

2. A nurse is administering an oral medication to a patient via a gastric tube. The nurse observes the medication enter the tube, and then the tube becomes clogged. What would be the appropriate initial action of the nurse in this situation?
   a. Attempt to dislodge the medication with a 10-mL syringe.
   b. Notify the primary care provider.
   c. Remove the tube and replace it with another tube.
   d. Flush the tube with 60 mL of water.

3. A nurse who is administering medications to patients in an acute care setting studies the pharmacokinetics of the drugs being administered. Which statements accurately describe these mechanisms of action? Select all that apply.
   a. Distribution occurs after a drug has been absorbed into the bloodstream and is made available to body fluids and tissues.
   b. Metabolism is the process by which a drug is transferred from its site of entry into the body to the bloodstream.
   c. Absorption is the change of a drug from its original form to a new form, usually occurring in the liver.
   d. During first-pass effect, drugs move from the intestinal lumen to the liver by way of the portal vein instead of going into the system's circulation.
   e. The gastrointestinal tract, as well as sweat, salivary, and mammary glands, are routes of drug absorption.
   f. Excretion is the process of removing a drug, or its metabolites (products of metabolism), from the body.

4. A nurse is reconstituting powdered medication in a vial. Which action is a recommended step in this process?
   a. The nurse draws up the proper amount of powered medication into the syringe.
   b. The nurse inserts the needle through the rubber stopper of the diluent vial.
   c. The nurse gently agitates the powdered medication vial to mix the powder and diluent completely.
   d. The nurse draws up the prescribed amount of medication while holding the syringe horizontally at eye level.

5. A medication order reads: "K-Dur, 20 mEq po b.i.d." When and how does the nurse correctly give this drug?
   a. Daily at bedtime by subcutaneous route
   b. Every other day by mouth
   c. Twice a day by the oral route
   d. Once a week by transdermal patch

6. A nurse is preparing medications for patients in the ICU. The nurse is aware that there are patient variables that may affect the absorption of these medications. Which statements accurately describe these variables? Select all that apply.
   a. Patients in certain ethnic groups obtain therapeutic responses at lower doses or higher doses than those usually prescribed.
   b. Some people experience the same response with a placebo as with the active drug used in studies.
   c. People with liver disease metabolize drugs more quickly than people with normal liver functioning.
   d. A patient who receives a pain medication in a noisy environment may not receive full benefit from the medication's effects.
   e. Oral medications should not be given with food as the food may delay the absorption of the medications.
   f. Circadian rhythms and cycles may influence drug action.

7. A physician orders a pain medication for a postoperative patient that is a PRN order. When would the nurse administer this medication?
   a. A single dose during the postoperative period
   b. Doses administered as needed for pain relief
   c. One dose administered immediately
   d. Doses routinely administered as a standing order

8. A nurse is administering a pain medication to a patient. In addition to checking his identification bracelet, the nurse correctly verifies his identity by:
   a. Asking the patient his name
   b. Reading the patient's name on the sign over the bed
   c. Asking the patient's roommate to verify his name
   d. Asking, "Are you Mr. Brown?"

9. The nurse is administering a medication to a patient via a nasogastric tube. Which are accurate guidelines related to this procedure? Select all that apply.
   a. Crush the enteric-coated pill for mixing in a liquid.
   b. Flush open the tube with 60 mL of very warm water.
   c. Check for proper placement of the nasogastric tube.
   d. Give each medication separately and flush with water between each drug.
   e. Lower the head of the bed to prevent reflux.
   f. Adjust the amount of water used if patient's fluid intake is restricted.

10. A medication order reads: "Hydromorphone, 2 mg IV every 3 to 4 hours PRN pain." The prefilled cartridge is available with a label reading "Hydromorphone 2 mg/1 mL." The cartridge contains 1.2 mL of hydromorphone. Which nursing action is correct?
    a. Give all the medication in the cartridge because it expanded when it was mixed.
    b. Call the pharmacy and request the proper dose.
    c. Refuse to give the medication.
    d. Dispose of 0.2 mL correctly before administering the drug.

11. A patient requires 40 units of NPH insulin and 10 units of regular insulin daily subcutaneously. What is the correct sequence when mixing insulins?
    a. Inject air into the regular insulin vial and withdraw 10 units; then, using the same syringe, inject air into the NPH vial and withdraw 40 units of NPH insulin.
    b. Inject air into the NPH insulin vial, being careful not to allow the solution to touch the needle; next, inject air into the regular insulin vial and withdraw 10 units; then, withdraw 40 units of NPH insulin.
    c. Inject air into the regular insulin vial, being careful not to allow the solution to touch the needle; next, inject air into the NPH insulin vial and withdraw 40 units; then, withdraw 10 units of regular insulin.
    d. Inject air into the NPH insulin vial and withdraw 40 units; then, using the same syringe, inject air into the regular insulin vial and withdraw 10 units of regular insulin.

12. Ms. Hall has an order for hydromorphone (Dilaudid), 2 mg, intravenously, q 4 hours PRN pain. The nurse notes that according to Ms. Hall's chart, she is allergic to Dilaudid. The order for medication was signed by Dr. Long. What would be the correct procedure for the nurse to follow in this situation?
    a. Administer the medication; the doctor is responsible for medication administration.
    b. Call Dr. Long and ask that she change the medication.
    c. Ask the supervisor to administer the medication.
    d. Ask the pharmacist to provide a medication to take the place of Dilaudid.

13. A nurse is administering heparin subcutaneously to a patient. What is the correct technique for this procedure?
    a. Aspirate before giving and gently massage after the injection.
    b. Do not aspirate; massage the site for 1 minute.
    c. Do not aspirate before or massage after the injection.
    d. Massage the site of the injection; aspiration is not necessary but will do no harm.

14. A nurse discovers that she made a medication error. What should be the nurse's first response?
    a. Record the error on the medication sheet.
    b. Notify the physician regarding course of action.
    c. Check the patient's condition to note any possible effect of the error.
    d. Complete an incident report, explaining how the mistake was made.

15. A nurse is teaching an adolescent patient how to use a meter-dosed inhaler to control his asthma. What are appropriate guidelines for this procedure? Select all that apply.
    a. Remove the mouthpiece cover and shake the inhaler well.
    b. Take shallow breaths when breathing through the spacer.
    c. Depress the canister releasing one puff into the spacer and inhale slowly and deeply.
    d. After inhaling, exhale quickly through pursed lips.
    e. Wait 1 to 5 minutes as prescribed before administering the next puff.
    f. Gargle and rinse with salt water after using the MDI.

ANSWERS WITH RATIONALES

1. *c.* If a patient vomits immediately after swallowing an oral pill, the nurse should assess the vomit for the pill or fragments of it. The nurse should then notify the primary care provider to see if another dosage should be administered.

2. *a.* If medication becomes clogged in a gastric tube, the nurse should attach a 10-mL syringe on the end of the tube and pull back and lightly apply pressure to the plunger in a repetitive motion to attempt to dislodge the medication. If the medication does not move through the tube, the nurse should notify the primary care provider, who may request the tube be replaced.

3. *a, d, f.* Distribution occurs after a drug has been absorbed into the bloodstream and the drug is distributed throughout the body, becoming available to body fluids and body tissues. Some drugs move from the intestinal lumen to the liver by way of the portal vein and do not go directly into the systemic circulation following oral absorption. This is called the first-pass effect, or hepatic first pass. Excretion is the process of removing a drug or its metabolites (products of metabolism) from the body. Absorption is the process by which a drug is transferred from its site of entry into the body to the bloodstream. Metabolism, or biotransformation, is the change of a drug from its original form to a new form. The liver is the primary site for drug metabolism. The gastrointestinal tract, as well as sweat, salivary, and mammary glands, are routes of drug excretion.

4. *c.* When reconstituting powdered medication in a vial, the nurse should draw up the appropriate amount of diluent into the syringe, insert the needle through the center of the self-sealing stopper on the powdered medication vial, inject the diluent into the powdered medication vial, remove the needle from the vial and replace the cap, and gently agitate the vial to mix the powdered medication and diluent completely. The nurse should then draw up the prescribed amount of medication while holding the syringe vertically and at eye level.

5. *c.* The abbreviation "b.i.d." refers to twice-a-day administration. po (by mouth) refers to administration by the oral route.

6. *a, b, d, f.* Nurses need to know about medications that may produce varied responses in patients from different ethnic groups. The patient's expectations of the medication may affect the response to the medication, for example, when a placebo is given and a patient has a therapeutic effect. The patient's environment may also influence the patient's response to medications, for example, sensory deprivation and overload may affect drug responses. Circadian rhythms and cycles may also influence drug action. The liver is the primary organ for drug breakdown, thus pathologic conditions that involve the liver may slow metabolism and alter the dosage of the drug needed to reach a therapeutic level. The presence of food in the stomach can delay the absorption of orally administered medications. Alternately, some medications should be given with food to prevent gastric irritation, and the nurse should consider this when establishing a patient's medication schedule. Other medications may have enhanced absorption if taken with certain foods.

7. *b.* When the prescriber writes a PRN order ("as needed") for medication, the patient receives medication when it is requested or required. With a single or one-time order, the directive is carried out only once, at a time specified by the prescriber. A stat order is a single order carried out immediately. A standing order (or routine order) is carried out as specified until it is canceled by another order.

8. *a.* The nurse should ask the patient to state his name. A sign over the patient's bed may not always be current. The roommate is an unsafe source of information. The patient may not hear his name but may reply in the affirmative anyway (e.g., a person with a hearing deficit).

9. *c, d, f.* The nurse should use the recommended procedure for checking tube placement prior to administering medications. The nurse should also give each medication separately and flush with water between each drug and adjust the amount of water used if fluids are restricted. Enteric-coated medications should not be crushed, the tube should be flushed with 15 to 30 mL of water, and the head of the bed should be elevated to prevent reflux.

10. *d.* Many cartridges are overfilled, and some of the medication needs to be discarded. Always check the volume needed to provide the correct dose with the volume in the syringe. Giving the excess medication in the cartridge may result in adverse effects for the patient. For this dose, it is not necessary to call the pharmacy or refuse to give the medication, provided the order is written correctly.

11. *b.* Regular or short-acting insulin should never be contaminated with NPH or any insulin modified with added protein. Placing air in the NPH vial first without allowing the needle to contact the solution ensures that the regular insulin will not be contaminated.

12. *b.* The nurse is responsible for any medications he or she gives and must contact the doctor to inform her of the patient's allergy to the drug. The nurse should not give the medication and might speak with the supervisor only if uncomfortable with the physician's answer once she is notified. The nurse is legally unable to order a replacement medication, as is the pharmacist.

13. *c.* When giving heparin subcutaneously, the nurse should not aspirate or massage, so as not to cause trauma or bleeding in the tissues.

14. *c.* The nurse's first responsibility is the patient—careful observation is necessary to assess for any effect of the medication error. The other nursing actions are pertinent, but only after checking the patient's welfare.

15. *a, c, e.* The correct procedure for using a meter-dosed inhaler is: remove the mouthpiece cover and shake the inhaler well; breathe normally through the spacer; depress the canister releasing one puff into the spacer and inhale slowly and deeply; after inhaling, hold breath for 5 to 10 seconds, or as long as possible, and then exhale slowly through pursed lips; wait 1 to 5 minutes as prescribed before administering the next puff; and gargle and rinse with tap water after using the MDI.

MEDICATION CALCULATION PROBLEMS

1. Metoprolol (Lopressor), 25 mg PO, is ordered. Metoprolol is available as 50-mg tablets. How many tablets would the nurse administer?

2. Phenytoin (Dilantin), 100 mg PO, is ordered to be given through a nasogastric tube. Phenytoin is available as 30 mg/5 mL. How much would the nurse administer?

3. Captopril (Capoten), 12.5 mg PO, is ordered. Captopril is available as 25-mg tablets. How many tablets would the nurse administer?

4. Potassium chloride (K-Dur), 20 mEq, is ordered. Potassium chloride is available as 10 mEq per tablet. How many tablets would the nurse administer?

5. Digoxin (Lanoxin), 0.0625 mg PO, is ordered. Digoxin is available as 0.125-mg tablets. How many tablets would the nurse administer?

6. Propantheline bromide (Pro-Banthine), 15 mg, is ordered. Propantheline bromide is available as 7.5-mg tablets. How many tablets would the nurse administer?

7. Ciprofloxacin (Cipro), 500 mg PO, is ordered. Ciprofloxacin is available as 250-mg tablets. How many tablets would the nurse administer?

8. Furosemide (Lasix), 20 mg PO, is ordered. Furosemide is available as 40-mg tablets. How many tablets would the nurse administer?

9. Theophylline elixir, 100 mg PO, is ordered by way of a percutaneous endoscopic gastrostomy tube. Theophylline elixir is available as 80 mg/15 mL. How much would the nurse administer?

10. Clonidine (Catapres), 0.1 mg PO, is ordered. Clonidine is available as 0.2-mg tablets. How many tablets would the nurse administer?

11. Vitamin K, 10 mg given IM, is ordered. Vitamin K is available as 5 mg/mL. How much would the nurse administer?

12. Morphine sulfate 10 mg IV is ordered. Morphine is available as 4 mg/mL. How much would the nurse administer?

13. Midazolam (Versed), 3 mg IM, is ordered. Midazolam is available as 5 mg/mL. How much would the nurse administer?

14. Ondansetron (Zofran) 0.15 mg/kg is ordered. Ondansetron is available as 2 mg/mL. The patient weighs 30 kg. How much would the nurse administer?

15. Epoetin alfa (Epogen), 2,000 units SC, is ordered. Epoetin alfa is available as 4,000 units/mL. How much would the nurse administer?

16. Nalbuphine (Nubain), 1.5 mg IM, is ordered. Nalbuphine is available as 1 mg/mL. How much would the nurse administer?

17. Octreotide acetate (Sandostatin), 50 mcg SC, is ordered. Octreotide is available as 100 mcg/mL. How much would the nurse administer?

18. Lisinopril (Zestril) 40 mg once a day is ordered. Zestril is available as an oral solution 8 mg/mL. How much should the nurse administer via the enteral feeding tube?

19. Prochlorperazine (Compazine), 7.5 mg IM, is ordered. Prochlorperazine is available as 5 mg/mL. How much would the nurse administer?

20. Glycopyrrolate (Robinul), 0.4 mg IM, is ordered. Glycopyrrolate is available as 0.2 mg/mL. How much would the nurse administer?

ANSWERS TO MEDICATION CALCULATION PROBLEMS

1. $$\frac{\text{dose on hand}}{\text{quantity on hand}} = \frac{\text{dose required}}{X \text{ (quantity desired)}}$$
$$\frac{50 \text{ mg}}{1 \text{ tablet}} = \frac{25 \text{ mg}}{X}$$
cross-multiply:
$$50X = 25$$
$$X = 0.5 \text{ or } \frac{1}{2} \text{ tablet}$$

2. $\dfrac{\text{dose on hand}}{\text{quantity on hand}} = \dfrac{\text{dose desired}}{X\,(\text{quantity desired})}$

$$\dfrac{30\ \text{mg}}{5\ \text{mL}} = \dfrac{100\ \text{mg}}{X}$$

cross-multiply:

$$30X = 500$$
$$X = 16.66\ \text{or}\ 17\ \text{mL}$$

3. $\dfrac{\text{dose on hand}}{\text{quantity on hand}} = \dfrac{\text{dose desired}}{X\,(\text{quantity desired})}$

$$\dfrac{20\ \text{mg}}{1\ \text{tablet}} = \dfrac{12.5\ \text{mg}}{X}$$

cross-multiply:

$$25X = 12.5$$
$$X = 0.5\ \text{or}\ \tfrac{1}{2}\ \text{tablet}$$

4. $\dfrac{\text{dose on hand}}{\text{quantity on hand}} = \dfrac{\text{dose desired}}{X\,(\text{quantity desired})}$

$$\dfrac{10\ \text{mEq}}{1\ \text{tablet}} = \dfrac{20\ \text{mEq}}{X}$$

cross-multiply:

$$10X = 20$$
$$X = 2\ \text{tablets}$$

5. $\dfrac{\text{dose on hand}}{\text{quantity on hand}} = \dfrac{\text{dose desired}}{X\,(\text{quantity desired})}$

$$\dfrac{0.125\ \text{mg}}{1\ \text{tablet}} = \dfrac{0.0625\ \text{mg}}{X}$$

cross-multiply:

$$0.125X = 0.0625$$
$$X = 0.5\ \text{or}\ \tfrac{1}{2}\ \text{tablet}$$

6. $\dfrac{\text{dose desired}}{\text{quantity on hand}} \times \dfrac{\text{quantity}}{\text{on hand}} = X\,(\text{desired quantity})$

$$\dfrac{15\ \text{mg}}{7.5\ \text{mg}} \times 1\ \text{tablet} = X$$

$$2 \times 1 = 2\ \text{tablets}$$

7. $\dfrac{\text{dose desired}}{\text{quantity on hand}} \times \dfrac{\text{quantity}}{\text{on hand}} = X\,(\text{desired quantity})$

$$\dfrac{500\ \text{mg}}{250\ \text{mg}} \times 1\ \text{tablet} = X$$

$$2 \times 1 = 2\ \text{tablets}$$

8. $\dfrac{\text{dose desired}}{\text{dose on hand}} \times \dfrac{\text{quantity}}{\text{on hand}} = X\,(\text{desired quantity})$

$$\dfrac{20\ \text{mg}}{250\ \text{mg}} \times 1\ \text{tablet} = X$$

$$2 \times 1 = 2\ \text{tablets}$$

9. $\dfrac{\text{dose desired}}{\text{dose on hand}} \times \dfrac{\text{quantity}}{\text{on hand}} = X\,(\text{desired quantity})$

$$\dfrac{100\ \text{mg}}{80\ \text{mg}} \times 15\ \text{mL} = X$$

$$\dfrac{1500}{80} = X$$

$$X = 18.75 = 19\ \text{mL}$$

10. $\dfrac{\text{dose desired}}{\text{dose on hand}} \times \dfrac{\text{quantity}}{\text{on hand}} = X\,(\text{desired quantity})$

$$\dfrac{0.1\ \text{mg}}{0.2\ \text{mg}} \times 1\ \text{tablet} = X$$

$$\tfrac{1}{2} \times 1 = X$$
$$X = \tfrac{1}{2}\ \text{tablet}$$

11. $\dfrac{\text{dose on hand}}{\text{quantity on hand}} = \dfrac{\text{dose desired}}{X\,(\text{quantity desired})}$

$$\dfrac{5\ \text{mg}}{1\ \text{mL}} = \dfrac{10\ \text{mg}}{X}$$

cross-multiply:

$$5X = 10$$
$$X = 2\ \text{mL}$$

12. $\dfrac{\text{dose on hand}}{\text{quantity on hand}} = \dfrac{\text{dose desired}}{(\text{quantity desired})}$

$$\dfrac{4\ \text{mg}}{1\ \text{mL}} = \dfrac{10\ \text{mg}}{X}$$

cross-multiply:

$$4X = 10$$
$$X = 2.5\ \text{mL}$$

13. $\dfrac{\text{dose on hand}}{\text{quantity on hand}} = \dfrac{\text{dose desired}}{X\,(\text{quantity desired})}$

$$\dfrac{5\ \text{mg}}{1\ \text{mL}} = \dfrac{3\ \text{mg}}{X}$$

cross-multiply:

$$5X = 3$$
$$X = 0.6\ \text{mL}$$

14.
$$\dfrac{0.15\ \text{mg}}{1\ \text{kg}} = \dfrac{x}{30\ \text{kg}}$$

$$1x = 4.5\ \text{mg dose}$$

$\dfrac{\text{dose on hand}}{\text{quantity on hand}} = \dfrac{\text{dose desired}}{(\text{quantity desired})}$

$$\dfrac{2\ \text{mg}}{1\ \text{mL}} = \dfrac{4.5\ \text{mg}}{X}$$

cross-multiply:

$$2X = 4.5$$
$$X = 2.25\ \text{mL}$$

15. $\dfrac{\text{dose on hand}}{\text{quantity on hand}} = \dfrac{\text{dose desired}}{X\,(\text{quantity desired})}$

$$\dfrac{4000\ \text{U}}{1\ \text{mL}} = \dfrac{2000\ \text{U}}{X}$$

cross-multiply:

$$4000X = 2000$$
$$X = \tfrac{1}{2}\ \text{mL}$$

16. $\dfrac{\text{dose desired}}{\text{dose on hand}} \times \dfrac{\text{quantity}}{\text{on hand}} = X\,(\text{desired quantity})$

$$\dfrac{1.5\ \text{mg}}{1\ \text{mg}} \times 1\ \text{mL} = X$$

$$1.5 \times 1 = X$$
$$X = 1.5\ \text{mL}$$

17. $\dfrac{\text{dose desired}}{\text{dose on hand}} \times \dfrac{\text{quantity}}{\text{on hand}} = X \text{ (desired quantity)}$

$$\dfrac{50 \text{ mg}}{100 \text{ mcg}} \times 1 \text{ mL} = X$$

$$\dfrac{1}{2} \times 1 = X$$

$$X = \frac{1}{2} \text{ mL}$$

18. $\dfrac{\text{dose on hand}}{\text{quantity on hand}} = \dfrac{\text{dose desired}}{\text{quantity desired}}$

$$\dfrac{8 \text{ mg}}{1 \text{ mL}} = \dfrac{40 \text{ mg}}{X}$$

cross-multiply:

$$8X = 40$$

$$X = 5 \text{ mL via enteral feeding tube}$$

19. $\dfrac{\text{dose desired}}{\text{dose on hand}} \times \dfrac{\text{quantity}}{\text{on hand}} = X \text{ (desired quantity)}$

$$\dfrac{7.5 \text{ mg}}{5 \text{ mg}} \times 1 \text{ mL} = X$$

$$1.5 \times 1 = X$$

$$X = 1.5 \text{ mL}$$

20. $\dfrac{\text{dose desired}}{\text{dose on hand}} \times \dfrac{\text{quantity}}{\text{on hand}} = X \text{ (desired quantity)}$

$$\dfrac{0.4 \text{ mg}}{0.2 \text{ mg}} \times 1 \text{ mL} = X$$

$$2 \times 1 = X$$

$$X = 2 \text{ mL}$$

TAYLOR SUITE RESOURCES

Explore these additional resources to enhance learning for this chapter:

- NCLEX-Style Questions and other resources on thePoint, http://thePoint.lww.com/Taylor8e
- *Study Guide for Fundamentals of Nursing, 8th edition*
- Adaptive Learning | Powered by prepU, http://thepoint.lww.com/prepu
- *Skill Checklists for Fundamentals of Nursing, 8th edition*
- *Taylor's Clinical Nursing Skills:* Chapter 5, Medication Administration
- *Taylor's Video Guide to Clinical Nursing Skills:* Oral and Topical Medications, Injectable Medications, and Intravenous Medications
- *Lippincott DocuCare* Fundamentals cases

Bibliography

Ackley, B. J., & Ladwig, G. B. (Eds.) (2011). *Nursing Diagnosis Handbook* (9th ed.). St. Louis: Elsevier/Mosby.

Ağaç, E., & Günes, Ü. Y. (2010). Effect on pain of changing the needle prior to administering medicine intramuscularly: a randomized controlled trial. *Journal of Advanced Nursing, 67*(3), 563–568.

Alsaleh, F. M., Smith, F. J., Keady, S., & Taylor, K. M. G. (2010). Insulin pumps: from inception to the present and toward the future. *Journal of Clinical Pharmacy and Therapeutics, 35*(2), 127–138.

American Diabetes Association (ADA). (2004). Insulin administration: Position statement. *Diabetes Care, 27*(Supplement 1), S106–S109.

American Society of Health-System Pharmacists (ASHP). (2009). ASHP statement on bar-code-enabled medication administration technology. *American Journal of Health-System Pharmacy, 66*(6), 588–590.

Annersten, M., & Willman, A. (2005). Performing subcutaneous injections: A literature review. *Worldviews on Evidence-Based Nursing, 2*(3), 122–130.

Arunthari, V., Bruinsma, R. S., Lee, A. S., & Johnson, M. M. (2012). A prospective, comparative trial of standard and breath-actuated nebulizer: Efficacy, safety, and satisfaction. *Respiratory Care, 57*(8), 1242–1247.

Aschenbrenner, D., & Venable, S. (2012). *Drug therapy in nursing* (4th ed.). Philadelphia: Wolters Kluwer Health/Lippincott Williams & Wilkins.

Aziz, A. M. (2012). Subcutaneous injections: preventing needlestick injuries in the community. *British Journal of Community Nursing, 17*(6), 258–264.

Bajaj, S., Whiteman, A., & Brandner, B. (2011). Transdermal drug delivery in pain management. *Continuing Education in Anaesthesia, Critical Care & Pain, 11*(2), 39–43.

Ball, A., & Smith, K. (2008). Optimizing transdermal drug therapy. *American Journal of Health-System Pharmacy, 65*(14), 1337–1346.

Balon, J., & Thomas, S. A. (2011). Comparison of hospital admission medication lists with primary care physician and outpatient pharmacy lists. *Journal of Nursing Scholarship, 43*(3), 292–300.

Barnsteiner, J. (2005). Medication reconciliation: Transfer of medication information across settings—keeping it free from error. *American Journal of Nursing, 105*(3 Suppl), 31–36.

Barrons, R., Pegram, A., & Borries, A. (2011). Inhaler device selection: Special considerations in elderly patients with chronic obstructive pulmonary disease. *American Journal of Health-System Pharmacy, 68*(13), 1221–1232.

Best, C., & Wilson, N. (2011). Advice on safe administration of medications via enteral feeding tubes. *Nutrition, Supplement,* S6–S8.

Boltz, M., Capezuti, E., Fulmer, T., & Zwicker, D. (Eds.) (2012). *Evidence-based geriatric nursing protocols for best practice* (4th ed.). New York: Springer Publishing Company.

Brown, S. (2012). Overcoming the pitfalls of medication reconciliation. *Nursing Management, 43*(1), 15–17.

Buchholz, S. (2012). *Henke's med-math. Dosage calculation, preparation & administration* (7th ed.). Philadelphia: Wolters Kluwer Health/Lippincott Williams & Wilkins.

Bulechek, G. M, Butcher, H. K., Dochterman, J. M., & Wagner, C. M. (Eds.). (2013). *Nursing interventions classification (NIC)* (6th ed.). St. Louis, MO: Elsevier/Mosby.

Burke, K. (2005). Executive summary: The state of the science on safe medication administration symposium. *American Journal of Nursing, 105*(3 Suppl), 4–9.

Carter-Templeton, H., & McCoy, T. (2008). Are we on the same page? A comparison of intramuscular injection explanations in nursing fundamental texts. *MEDSURG Nursing, 17*(4), 237–240.

Centers for Disease Control and Prevention (CDC). (2011). Injection safety. Safe injection practices to prevent transmission of infections to patients. Available at www.cdc.gov/injectionsafety/IP07_standardPrecaution.html

Centers for Disease Control and Prevention (CDC). (2012). *The pink book: Appendices. Epidemiology and prevention of vaccine preventable diseases* (11th ed.). Appendix D. Vaccine administration. Vaccine administration guidelines. Available at http://www.cdc.gov/vaccines/pubs/pinkbook/downloads/appendices/appdx-full-d.pdf

Choo, J., Hutchinson, A., & Bucknall, T. (2010). Nurses' role in medication safety. *Journal of Nursing Management, 18*(7), 853–861.

Chung, J. W., Ng, W. M., & Wong, T. K. (2002). An experimental study on the use of manual pressure to reduce pain in intramuscular injections. *Journal of Clinical Nursing, 11*(4), 457–461.

Cocoman, A., & Murray, J. (2010). Recognizing the evidence and changing practice on injection sites. *British Journal of Nursing, 19*(18), 1170–1174.

Cohen, M. R. (2012). Medication errors. *Nursing, 42*(9), 17.

Craig, G. (2009). *Clinical calculations made easy* (4th ed.). Philadelphia: Wolters Kluwer Health/Lippincott Williams & Wilkins.

Cranwell-Bruce, L. (2009). Update in diabetes management. *MEDSURG Nursing, 18*(1), 51–54.

Crawford, C. L., & Johnson, J. A. (2012). To aspirate or not: An integrative review of the evidence. *Nursing, 42*(3), 20–25.

Crawford, D. (2012). Maintaining good practice in the administration of medicines to children. *Nursing Children & Young People, 24*(4), 29–35.

Creadon Shanks, L. & Zelko Enlow, M. (2011). Medication calculation competency. *American Journal of Nursing, 111*(10), 67–69.

Dasqupta, A., Sansgiry, S. S., Jacob, S. M., Frost, C. P., Dwibedi, N., & Tipton, J. (2011). Descriptive analysis of workflow variables associated with barcode-based approach to medication administration. *Journal of Nursing Care Quality, 26*(4), 377–384.

Dinescu, L. I., Todorov, D., Biglow, M., Toderika, Y., Cohen, H., & Patel, K. (2012). Medication safety in rehabilitation medicine. *Physical Medicine & Rehabilitation Clinics of North America, 23*(2), 271–303.

Dougherty, L., Sque, M., & Crouch, R. (2012). Decision-making processes used by nurses during intravenous drug preparation and administration. *Journal of Advanced Nursing, 68*(6), 1302–1311.

Dudek, S. (2014). *Nutrition essentials for nursing practice* (7th ed.). Philadelphia: Wolters Kluwer Health/Lippincott Williams & Wilkins.

Durand, C., Alhammad, A., & Willett, K. C. (2012). Practical considerations for optimal transdermal drug delivery. *American Journal of Health-System Pharmacy, 69*(2), 116–124.

Dychter, S. S., Gold, D. A., & Haller, M. F. (2012). Subcutaneous drug delivery. A route to increased safety, patient satisfaction, and reduced costs. *Journal of Infusion Nursing, 35*(3), 154–160.

Elliott, M., & Liu, Y. (2010). The nine rights of medication administration: an overview. *British Journal of Nursing, 19*(5), 300–305.

Flynn, L., Liang, Y., Dickson, G. L., Xie, M., & Suh, D. C. (2012). Nurses' practice environments, error interception practices, and inpatient medication errors. *Journal of Nursing Scholarship, 44*(2), 180–186.

Gavriloff, C. (2012). A performance improvement plan to increase nurse adherence to use of medication safety software. *Journal of Pediatric Nursing, 27*(4), 375–382.

Gibney, M. A., Arce, C. H., Byron, K. J., & Hirsch, L. J. (2010). Skin and subcutaneous adipose layer thickness in adults with diabetes at sites used for insulin injections: implications for needle length recommendations. *Current Medical Research & Opinion, 26*(6), 1519–1530.

Greenway, K. (2004). Using the ventrogluteal site for intramuscular injection. *Nursing Standard, 18*(25), 39–42.

Grossman, S., & Porth, C.M. (2014). *Porth's pathophysiology: concepts of altered health states.* (9th ed.). Philadelphia: Wolters Kluwer Health/Lippincott Williams & Wilkins.

Hart Tipton, P., Aigner, M. J., Finto, D., Haislet, J. A., Pehl, L., Sanford, P., & Williams, M. (2012). Consider the accuracy of height and weight measurements. *Nursing, 42*(5), 50–52.

Hess, D. R., MacIntyre, N. R., Mishoe, S. C., Galvin, W. F., & Adams, A. B. (2012). *Respiratory Care. Principles and Practice* (2nd ed.). Sudbury, MA: Jones & Bartlett Learning.

Hinkle, J. L., & Cheever K. H. (2014). *Brunner & Suddarth's Textbook of Medical-Surgical Nursing* (13th ed.). Philadelphia: Wolters Kluwer Health/Lippincott Williams & Wilkins.

Hughes, L. (2012). Assessing a patient with an insulin pump. *Nursing, 42*(9), 62–64.

Hughes, R., & Ortiz, E. (2005). Medication errors. *American Journal of Nursing, 105*(3 Suppl), 14–24.

Hunter, J. (2008). Subcutaneous injection technique. *Nursing Standard, 22*(21), 41–44.

The Institute for Safe Medication Practices (ISMP). (2013). ISMP's list of error-prone abbreviations, symbols, and dose designations. Available at http://www.ismp.org/Tools/errorproneabbreviations.pdf

The Institute for Safe Medication Practices (ISMP). (2012). ISMP and FDA campaign to eliminate use of error-prone abbreviations. Available at www.ismp.org/tools/abbreviations

The Institute for Safe Medication Practices (ISMP). (2007). The five rights: A destination without a map. Available at http://www.ismp.org/newsletters/acutecare/articles/20070125.asp

Janda, S. M., & Fagan, N. L. (2010). Practical review of pharmacology concepts. *Urologic Nursing, 30*(1), 15–20.

The Joint Commission (TJC). (2014). 2014 National patient safety goals. Available at http://www.joint commission.org/standards_information/npsgs.aspx

Katsma, D. L., & Katsma, R. P. E. (2000). The myth of the 90°-angle intramuscular injection. *Nurse Educator, 25*(1), 34–37.

Kee, J. L., Hayes, E. R., & McCuistion, L. E. (2012). *Pharmacology: A Nursing Process Approach* (7th ed.). St. Louis: Elsevier/Saunders.

Kelly, J. & Wright, D. (2010). Administering medication to adult patients with dysphagia: part 2. *Nursing Standard, 24*(26), 61–68.

Klejka, D. E. (2012). Shhh! Conducting a Quiet Zone pilot study for medication safety. *Nursing, 42*(9), 18–21.

Kyle, T., & Carman, S. (2013). *Essentials of pediatric nursing* (2nd ed.). Philadelphia: Wolters Kluwer Health/Lippincott Williams & Wilkins.

Lareau, S. C., & Hodder, R. (2012). Teaching inhaler use in chronic obstructive pulmonary disease patients. *Journal of the American Academy of Nurse Practitioners, 24*(2), 113–120.

Lavery, I. (2011). Intravenous therapy: preparation and administration of IV medicines. *British Journal of Nursing, 20* (Intravenous Supplement), S28–34.

Lemoine, J. B., & Hurst, H. M. (2012). Using smart pumps to reduce medication errors in the NICU. *Nursing for Women's Health, 16*(2), 151–158.

Lenehan, G. (2012). The Emergency Nurses Association (ENA) "Weighs in" on pediatric medication safety: "Weigh children in kilograms only!" *Journal of Emergency Nursing, 38*(3), 205–206.

Leyshon, J. (2011). Improving inhaler technique in patients with asthma. *Nursing Standard, 26*(9), 49–56.

Love, G. (2006). Administering an intradermal injection. *Nursing, 36*(6), 20.

Lorenz, J. M. (2010). Polypharmacy in the elderly: increased use of medications raises risk of drug interactions, side effects and adverse reactions. *Advance for Nurses, 7*(12), 11–14, 17.

Macdonald, M. (2010). Patient safety. Examining the adequacy of the 5 rights of medication administration. *Clinical Nurse Specialist, 24*(4), 196–201.

Malarkey, L. M., & McMorrow, M. E. (2012). *Saunders nursing guide to laboratory and diagnostic tests* (2nd ed.). St. Louis: Elsevier/Saunders.

Mandrack, M., Cohen, M. R., Featherling, J., Gellner, L., Judd, K., Kienle, P. C., & Vanderveen, T. (2012). Nursing best practices using automated dispensing cabinets: Nurses' key role in improving medication safety. *MEDSURG Nursing, 21*(3), 134–144.

Marik, P. E. & Flemmer, M. (2012). Do dietary supplements have beneficial health effects in industrialized nations: what is the evidence? *Journal of Parenteral & Enteral Nutrition, 36*(2), 159–168.

Martin, D., Kripalani, S., & DuRapau, V. J. (2012). Improving medication management among at-risk older adults. *Journal of Gerontological Nursing, 38*(6), 24–34.

McRoberts, S. (2005). The use of bar code technology in medication administration. *Clinical Nurse Specialist, 19*(2), 55–56.

Meetoo, D., McAllister, G., West, A., & Turnbull, M. (2012). In pursuit of excellence in diabetes care: trends in insulin delivery. *British Journal of Nursing, 21*(10), 588–595.

Mishra, P., & Stringer, M. D. (2010). Sciatic nerve injury from intramuscular injection: a persistent and global problem. *International Journal of Clinical Practice, 64*(11), 1573–1579.

Moorhead, S., Johnson, M., Maas, M. L., & Swanson, E. (Eds). (2013). *Nursing Outcomes Classification (NOC).* (5th ed.). St. Louis: Elsevier/Mosby.

Moshang, J. (2005). Making a point about insulin pens. *Nursing, 35*(2), 46–47.

Muñoz, C., & Hilgenberg, C. (2005). Ethnopharmacology. *American Journal of Nursing, 105*(8), 40–47.

Murphy, M., & While, A. (2012). Medication administration practices among children's nurses: a survey. *British Journal of Nursing, 21*(15), 928–933.

NANDA International (NANDA-I). (2012). *Nursing diagnoses: Definitions & classification 2012–2014.* West Sussex, UK: Wiley-Blackwell.

Nicoll, L., & Hesby, A. (2002). Intramuscular injection: An integrative research review and guideline for evidence-based practice. *Applied Nursing Research, 16*(2), 149–162.

Perry, S. E., Hockenberry, M. J., Lowdermilk, D. L., & Wilson, D. (2010). *Maternal child nursing care* (4th ed.). Maryland Heights, MO: Elsevier/Mosby.

Pezzotti, W., & Freuler, M. (2012). Using anticoagulants to steer clear of clots. *Nursing, 42*(2), 26–35.

Popescu, A., Currey, J., & Botti, M. (2011). Multifactorial influences on and deviations from medication administration safety and quality in the acute medical/surgical context. *Worldviews on Evidence-based Nursing, 8*(1), 15–24.

Rack, L., Dudjak, L. A., & Wolf, G. A. (2012). Study of nurse workarounds in a hospital using bar code medication administration system. *Journal of Nursing Care Quality, 27*(3), 232–239.

Ritter, L. A., & Hoffman, N. A. (2010). *Multicultural health.* Boston: Jones and Bartlett.

Rubin, B. K. (2010). Air and soul: the science and application of aerosol therapy. *Respiratory Care, 55*(7), 911–921.

Rubin, B., & Durotoye, L. (2004). How do patients determine that their metered-dose inhaler is empty? *Chest, 126*(4), 1134–1137.

Sander, N., Fusco-Walker, S. Harder, J., & Chipps, B. E. (2006). Dose counting and the use of pressurized metered-dose inhalers: running on empty. *Annals of Allergy, Asthma & Immunology, 97*(1), 34–38.

Sanofi Aventis. (2012). How to Self-inject Lovenox®. Available at http://www.lovenox.com/consumer/prescribed-lovenox/self-inject/inject-lovenox.aspx

Scheiner, G., Sobel, R., Smith, D., Pick, A., Kruger, D., King, J., & Green, K. (2009). Insulin pump therapy: Guidelines for successful outcomes. *The Diabetes Educator, 35*(Suppl 2), 295–435.

Shane, R. (2009). Current status of administration of medications. *American Journal of Health-System Pharmacy, 66*(Suppl 3), S42–S47.

Shanks, L. C., & Enlow, M. Z. (2011). Medication calculation competency. *American Journal of Nursing, 111*(10), 67–69.

Sherriff, K., Wallis, M., & Burston, S. (2011). Medication calculation competencies for registered nurses: a literature review. *Australian Journal of Advanced Nursing, 28*(4), 75–83.

Simmons, D., Graves, K., & Flynn, E. (2009). Threading needles in the dark: The effect of the physical work environment on nursing practice. *Critical Care Nursing Quarterly, 32*(2), 70–74.

Small, S. (2004). Preventing sciatic nerve injury from intramuscular injections: Literature review. *Journal of Advanced Nursing, 47*(3), 287–296.

Spector, R. E. (2009). *Cultural diversity in health and illness* (7th ed.). Upper Saddle River, NJ: Pearson/Prentice Hall.

Spollett, G. R. (2012). Improved disposable insulin pen devices provide an alternative to vials and syringes for insulin administration. *Diabetes Spectrum, 25*(2), 117–122.

Sulosaari, V., Suhonen, R., & Leino-Kilpi, H. (2011). An integrative review of the literature on registered nurses' medication competence. *Journal of Clinical Nursing, 20*(3/4), 464–478.

Swanlund, S., Scherck, K., Metcalfe, S., & Jesek-Hale, S. (2008). Keys to successful self-management of medications. *Nursing Science Quarterly, 21*(3), 238–246.

Tabloski, P. (2010). *Gerontological nursing* (2nd ed.). Upper Saddle River, NJ: Pearson.

Tamura, B. K., Bell, C. L., Inaba, M., & Masaki, K. H. (2012). Outcomes of polypharmacy in nursing home residents. *Clinics in Geriatric Medicine, 28*(2), 217–236.

Toedter Williams, N. (2008). Medication administration through enteral feeding tubes. *American Journal of Health-System Pharmacy, 65*(24), 2347–2357.

Tran, M., Ciarkowski, S., Wagner, D., & Stevenson, J. G. A case study on the safety impact of implementing smart patient-controlled analgesic pumps at a tertiary care academic medical center. *Joint Commission Journal on Quality & Patient Safety, 38*(3), 112–119.

Unver, V., Tastan, S., & Akbayrak, N. (2012). Medication errors: Perspectives of newly graduated and experienced nurses. *International Journal of Nursing Practice, 18*(4), 317–324.

U.S. Food and Drug Administration (FDA). (2012a). Drugs—Information for Consumers. Available at http://www.fda.gov/Drugs/ResourcesForYou/Consumers/default.htm

U.S. Food and Drug Administration (FDA). (2012b). Drugs—Medication errors. Available at www.fda.gov/Drugs/DrugSafety/MedicationErrors/default.htm#abbreviations

U.S. Food and Drug Administration (FDA). (2012c). Safety—MedWatch: The FDA safety information and adverse event reporting program. Available at www.fda.gov/Safety/MedWatch/default.htm

U.S. Food and Drug Administration (FDA). (2010). Dietary Supplements. Available at www.fda.gov/AboutFDA/Transparency/Basics/ucm193949.htm

Van Leeuwen, A. M., Poelhuis-Leth, D., & Bladh, M. L. (2011). *Davis's Comprehensive Handbook of Laboratory & Diagnostic Tests with Nursing Implications* (4th ed.). Philadelphia: F. A. Davis.

Walsh, L., & Brophy, K. (2010). Staff nurses' sites of choice for administering intramuscular injections to adult patients in the acute care setting. *Journal of Advanced Nursing, 67*(5), 1034–1040.

Ward, H. (1988). *My friends' beliefs.* New York: Walker and Company.

Ward-Smith, P. (2010). Individual variations in drug responses. *Urologic Nursing, 30*(1), 22–27.

World Health Organization (WHO). (2014). *Medicines. Adverse drug reactions monitoring.* Available at http://www.who.int/medicines/areas/quality_safety/safety_efficacy/advdrugreactions/en/

Wright, D. & Kelly, J. (2012). Reducing drug administration errors in patients with dysphagia. *Nurse Prescribing, 10*(7), 357–360.

Zaybak, A., Gunes, U., Tamsel, S., Khorshid, L., & Eser, I. (2007). Does obesity prevent the needle from reaching muscle in intramuscular injections? *Journal of Advanced Nursing, 58*(6), 552–556.

Zimmerman, P. G. (2010). Revisiting IM injections. *American Journal of Nursing, 110*(2), 60–61.

29

Perioperative Nursing

MOLLY GREENBAUM

Molly, a 38-year-old woman who is scheduled for a vaginal hysterectomy later in the day, arrives at the hospital at 6:30 AM. With tears in her eyes and wringing her hands, she states, "I really didn't sleep very much last night. I kept thinking about the surgery."

MARCUS BENJAMIN

Marcus, a 73-year-old man, has just had a total hip replacement under general anesthesia and is transferred to the postanesthesia care unit (PACU). His vital signs are stable. He has an intravenous catheter in his right antecubital space, infusing at 125 mL/hr, and an indwelling urinary catheter in place, draining clear yellow urine. The dressing over the surgical site is clean and dry, without any drainage.

GABRIELLE MCALLISTER

Gabrielle McAllister is a 5-year-old girl scheduled for a tonsillectomy and adenoidectomy at a hospital-based same-day surgery unit. She was born with a congenital cardiac defect and has had 6 prior surgeries. She is small for her age and is allergic to latex, but is an otherwise healthy kindergarten student.

After completing the chapter, you will be able to accomplish the following:

1. Describe the surgical experience, including perioperative phases, classifications of surgery, types of anesthesia, informed consent and advance directives, and outpatient/same-day surgery.

2. Conduct a preoperative nursing history and physical assessment to identify patient strengths as well as factors that increase risks for surgical and postoperative complications.

3. Prepare a patient physically and psychologically for surgery.

4. Identify assessments and interventions specific to the prevention of complications in the immediate and early postoperative phases.

5. Use the nursing process to develop an individualized plan of care for the surgical patient during each phase of the perioperative period.

KEY TERMS

anesthesia	moderate sedation/ analgesia	phase
atelectasis		pneumonia
deep vein thrombosis (DVT)	never events	shock
	postanesthesia care unit (PACU)	thrombophlebitis
elective surgery		time-out
embolus	perioperative nursing	urgent surgery
emergency surgery	perioperative	
hemorrhage		

The treatment of many illnesses and injuries includes some type of surgical intervention. Surgery is an intervention in which the knowledge and skill of multiple care providers are combined to create the best possible care for the welfare of the patient. Surgery may be done for a variety of reasons: to cure or minimize disease; to diagnose the specific presence of a disease or condition; to reconstruct or eliminate a defect; to enhance form and function; to palliate, or offer comfort, when cure is not possible; to follow up or monitor an incurable disease process; and to offer a preventive option when disease is inevitable, such as an elective, prophylactic mastectomy for a woman at high risk for breast cancer. Surgery may be planned or unplanned, elective/optional or necessary, major or minor, and may involve any body part or system. Surgery is a stressor that requires physical and psy-chosocial adaptations for both the patient and the family. The patient's recovery from a surgical procedure requires skillful and knowledgeable nursing care, whether the surgery is done on an outpatient basis or in the hospital. (See the accompanying Reflective Practice box (on page 854) for an example of nursing care for a patient who has undergone surgery.)

Nursing care provided for the patient before, during, and after surgery is called **perioperative nursing**. All members of the interdisciplinary team use this term. The nursing process is used to make assessments and provide interventions to promote the recovery of health, prevent further injury or illness, and facilitate coping with alterations in physical structure and function.

A conceptual model for perioperative nursing care is shown in Figure 29-1 (on page 855). In this model, the patient is at the center of all care activities. Surrounding the patient are four domains. Three of these domains—safety, physiologic responses, and patient and family behavioral responses—are integral to patient care. The fourth domain, health system, represents the structure elements and other health system activities that must be present to support safe, effective, high-quality patient care.

With this model, each domain has desired outcomes. These outcomes are identified first in the model because perioperative nursing is preventive in nature. This is in contrast to the usual progression of the nursing process, which begins with assessment. Thus, perioperative nurses base their plans of care on recognized desired outcomes. Perioperative nurses assess the patient for the relevance of the outcome, then identify nursing diagnoses and plan interventions. One of the most significant roles of the perioperative nurse is that of advocate for patient safety; the nurse implements evidence-based strategies to protect vulnerable surgical patients (Lockhart, 2012).

The type of surgery scheduled influences the desired outcomes, nursing diagnoses, assessments, and interventions carried out by the nurse. The perioperative nurse's role in hospital-based surgery is usually specific to the intraoperative phase. The perioperative nurse's goal is to promote and assist the patient and family to achieve a level of wellness equal to or greater than what they had prior to the surgical procedure (Association of periOperative Registered Nurses [AORN], 2013a).

THE SURGICAL EXPERIENCE

Regardless of the surgical or interventional procedure required or the setting in which it is performed, all patients progress through specific phases, require some type of anesthesia and monitoring support, and must give an informed consent for surgery.

The Perioperative Phases

The patient who is having surgery progresses through several distinct periods, called the **perioperative phases**. The three phases of perioperative patient care are:

• The *preoperative phase*, beginning when the patient and surgeon mutually decide that surgery is necessary and will

REFLECTIVE PRACTICE: CULTIVATING QSEN COMPETENCIES

CHALLENGE TO ETHICAL AND LEGAL SKILLS

During a recent clinical experience on a level II ICU, I cared for Ron Johnson, a middle-aged male patient who had an extensive medical history that included gunshot wounds, bilateral leg amputations, paraplegia, and several surgeries. Because of this, he had lengthy hospital stays and was known by the staff as being a difficult and manipulative patient. During my encounter with him, he was first day postop from a surgical procedure for urinary diversion. He was ordered to be NPO for the first 2 to 3 days following the surgery. However, he claimed that his surgeon had told him that he would be able to eat the day after the surgery, and he was demanding that I give him food and fluids. "I want some food and I want it now!" I told the patient that I had to follow the orders in his chart and that it was unlikely that he would be able to have anything by mouth during my shift. He asked me to explain the reasons for being NPO after surgery, and I did my best under the time constraints by telling him that the bowel is affected by anesthesia and it is not ready to handle the intake of food and fluids. In all honesty, I didn't know the major consequences of eating or drinking after surgery; however, I didn't admit this to him. He was obviously not satisfied with my explanation because when I returned from my lunch break, he was sitting in front of a lunch tray. He had talked some of the nursing assistants into getting him the items. He made the decision to act against my instructions and the instructions of his surgeon, perhaps because I was not able to give him a clear, articulate explanation of his NPO status.

Thinking Outside the Box: Possible Courses of Action

- Tell the patient that I was unable to give him the best explanation of his NPO status, informing him that I would return in 5 to 10 minutes after consulting with a nurse, and deciding the best way to articulate to him the consequences of ignoring the order.
- Avoid giving him any explanation at all, assuming that because of his extensive surgical history he knew the reasons why he must not eat or drink.
- Ask another nurse or even the dietitian to explain the NPO order.
- Alert the surgeon that this patient was at risk for being noncompliant and ask him to come to see the patient as soon as possible.

Evaluating a Good Outcome: How Do I Define Success?

- The patient verbalizes an understanding of my explanation and the consequences of his actions.
- The patient complies with the physician's orders and with my instructions.
- The patient remains free of injuries/complications.
- I feel competent in my explanations and actions.
- I am able to take responsibility for the patient's actions.

Personal Learning: Here's to the Future!

This patient taught me a great deal. He taught me that sometimes, rather than giving an inadequate explanation, it would be better to admit that you do not know or that your knowledge is not up to par in a particular area. I should have been honest with Mr. Johnson, admitting that I was unsure about why he wasn't allowed to eat or drink. It would have been more advantageous to consult with someone else before giving him a more thorough explanation. I also should have recognized that Mr. Johnson was exhibiting extreme frustration and depression, placing him at high risk for noncompliance. All he needed was someone to take extra time with him, offering compassion and support. Unfortunately, the patient did not comply with the order and thus was at risk for developing serious complications, such as a bowel obstruction. I alerted the surgeon of the patient's actions and, luckily, the surgeon was understanding. In the future, I will make a major effort to gather the appropriate information to give patients a thorough, understandable explanation when they ask for specific information.

Colleen Kilcullen, Georgetown University

REFLECTION ON QUALITY AND SAFETY COMPETENCIES

How would you respond in a similar situation? Why? What does this tell you about yourself and about the adequacy of your skills for professional practice? Can you think of other ways to approach this situation? What *knowledge, skills,* and *attitudes* do you need to develop in order to continuously improve quality and safety when caring for patients like Mr. Johnson?

Patient-Centered Care: What information about his postoperative instructions needs to be clearly communicated to Mr. Johnson? How might his past history have influenced the nursing student's actions? Explain. If you were this nursing student, would Mr. Johnson's past history have influenced you? Why or why not? How could you involve Mr. Johnson as a partner in coordinating his care, thus minimizing his frustration? How could you provide emotional support?

Teamwork and Collaboration/Quality Improvement: What communication skills do you need to provide clear, comprehensive information to Mr. Johnson? Would collaboration with your instructor or Mr. Johnson's nurse have resulted in another approach to communicating and explaining the physician's orders in a timely manner?

Safety/Evidence-Based Practice: Can you obtain any resources/articles from the nursing literature that provide information and guidance regarding risks associated with intake of food and fluids in the immediate postoperative period? Do you think your response to Mr. Johnson provided a safe environment for him?

Informatics: What information should be electronically documented regarding your interaction with Mr. Johnson? Is there a better way to describe this patient or is "noncompliant" appropriate? Can you identify the essential information that must be noted in his electronic record to support safe patient care?

FIGURE 29-1. Perioperative Patient-Focused Model (Adapted from AORN Perioperative Patient-Focused Model. Copyright AORN, Inc., 2170 S. Parker Road, Suite 300, Denver, CO 80231.)

take place. It ends when the patient is transferred to the operating room (OR) or procedural bed.

- The *intraoperative phase,* beginning when the patient is transferred to the OR bed until transfer to the **postanesthesia care unit (PACU)**. The PACU is an area often adjacent to the surgical suite designed to provide care for patients recovering from anesthesia or moderate sedation/analgesia.
- The *postoperative phase,* beginning with admission to the PACU or other recovery area and ending with complete recovery from surgery and the last follow-up physician visit.

The postoperative phase can be further divided into phase I, providing patient care from a totally anesthetized state to one requiring less acute nursing interventions; phase II, preparing the patient for self-care or family care or for care in a phase III extended care environment; and phase III, providing ongoing care for patients requiring extended observation or intervention after transfer or discharge from phase I or II (American Society of PeriAnesthesia Nurses [ASPAN], 2010; Godden 2010).

With the increasing trend toward short-stay or same-day surgery, nursing interventions in each phase of perioperative nursing care may vary somewhat, but they remain basically the same. The nursing process is used during each phase to meet physical and psychosocial needs and to facilitate the patient's return to health. Each of these phases, with related patient needs and nursing activities, is described in detail in this chapter.

Surgical Procedure Classification

Surgical procedures usually are classified according to urgency, risk, and purpose. Table 29-1 (on page 856) lists each classification, with purposes and examples for each. No matter what the defined degree of risk, any surgical procedure imposes physical and psychological stress, and is seldom considered minor by the patient.

 RECALL Molly Greenbaum, the 38-year-old woman who is to undergo a vaginal hysterectomy. The nurse would incorporate knowledge about the various classifications of surgery to plan appropriate care before and after surgery. ●

Surgery Based on Urgency

Surgery based on urgency is further categorized into broad categories that cross specialty areas:

- *Elective surgery* is a procedure that is preplanned and based on the patient's choice and availability of scheduling

Table 29-1 CLASSIFICATION OF SURGICAL PROCEDURES

CLASSIFICATION	PURPOSE	EXAMPLES
Based on Urgency		
Elective: Delay of surgery has no ill effects; can be scheduled in advance based on patient's choice.	• To remove or repair a body part • To restore function • To improve health • To improve self-concept	Tonsillectomy, hernia repair, cataract extraction and lens implantation, hemorrhoidectomy, hip prosthesis, scar revision, facelift, mammoplasty
Urgent: Usually done within 24–48 hours.	• To remove or repair a body part • To preserve or restore health	Removal of gallbladder, coronary artery bypass, surgical removal of a malignant tumor, colon resection, amputation
Emergency: Done immediately.	• To prevent further tissue damage • To preserve life (plus purposes listed above)	Control of hemorrhage; repair of trauma, perforated ulcer, intestinal obstruction; tracheostomy
Based on Degree of Risk		
Major: May be elective, urgent, or emergency	• To preserve life • To remove or repair a body part • To restore function • To improve or maintain health	Carotid endarterectomy, cholecystectomy, nephrectomy, colostomy, hysterectomy, radical mastectomy, amputation, trauma repair
Minor: Primarily elective	• To remove skin lesions • To correct deformities	Teeth extraction, removal of warts, skin biopsy, dilation and curettage, laparoscopy, cataract extraction, arthroscopy
Based on Purpose		
Diagnostic	• To make or confirm a diagnosis	Breast biopsy, laparoscopy, bronchoscopy, exploratory laparotomy
Ablative	• To remove a diseased body part	Appendectomy, subtotal thyroidectomy, partial gastrectomy, colon resection, amputation
Palliative	• To relieve or reduce intensity of an illness; is not curative	Colostomy, nerve root resection, débridement of necrotic tissue, balloon angioplasties, arthroscopy
Reconstructive	• To restore function to traumatized or malfunctioning tissue • To improve self-concept	Scar revision, plastic surgery, skin graft, internal fixation of a fracture, breast reconstruction
Transplantation	• To replace organs or structures that are diseased or malfunctioning	Kidney, liver, cornea, heart, joints
Constructive	• To restore function in congenital anomalies	Cleft palate repair, closure of atrial–septal defect

for the patient, surgeon, and facility. This is a nonurgent procedure that does not have to be done immediately.

• *Urgent surgery* must be done within a reasonably short time frame to preserve health, but is not an emergency.

• *Emergency surgery* must be done immediately to preserve life, a body part, or function.

Surgery Based on Degree of Risk

Surgery is classified as minor or major based on the degree of risk for the patient. Minor surgery is almost always performed in settings such as a physician's office, an outpatient clinic, or a same-day, outpatient surgery setting (also referred to as ambulatory surgery). This classification means that the surgical procedure usually carries a low risk and results in few complications. In contrast, major surgery may require hospitalization and specialized care, has a higher degree of risk, involves major body organs or life-threatening situations, and has a greater risk for postoperative complications.

However, the major and minor nomenclature is not as descriptive of actual procedures today because of the remarkable evolution of surgical science and technology. Advances in the use of laser techniques and minimally inva-

sive approaches involving very small incisions make major surgery less traumatic, facilitating shortened hospital stays. New surgical approaches using minimally invasive techniques and robotic technology continue to evolve. Thus, many surgical procedures, even though they are classified as major, are now performed on an outpatient (same-day/ambulatory) basis or as a 23-hour hospital stay. Major procedures can be accomplished in short time frames with minimal anesthesia. The patient can return home on the same day with nominal pain, allowing a quick return to normal daily activities.

Surgery Based on Purpose

Surgery may also be classified according to its purpose. Some terms used to classify surgical procedures based on purpose include *diagnostic, curative, preventive, ablative, palliative, reconstructive, transplantation,* and *constructive* (see Table 29-1).

Anesthesia

Anesthesia is a method and technique of making potentially uncomfortable interventions tolerable and safe. Anesthetic agents can be administered systemically (to the whole body) or regionally (to a specific region of the body) to block nerve conduction. General, or systemic, anesthesia is a balance of loss of consciousness, analgesia (pain relief), relaxation, and loss of reflexes (temporary paralysis). In contrast, regional anesthesia does not cause narcosis (sleepiness), but results in analgesia and reflex loss. Moderate sedation involves intravenous administration of sedatives and analgesics to produce analgesia and a degree of amnesia that can be promptly reversed, whereas topical or local anesthesia targets a specific tissue of the body. Anesthesiologists (medical doctors) or certified registered nurse anesthetists (CRNAs) administer anesthetic agents while monitoring the patient's physiologic response and maintaining homeostasis throughout the procedure and recovery. Nurse anesthesia is an advanced nursing specialty. Both physicians and nurses who administer anesthesia perform preoperative physical assessments, conduct preoperative teaching, administer anesthesia during the surgical procedure, and oversee the patient's postoperative recovery from the anesthetic.

General (Systemic) Anesthesia

General anesthesia involves the administration of drugs by the inhalation or intravenous (IV) route to produce central nervous system depression. General anesthesia typically is a combination of both intravenous and inhalation anesthetics. The desired actions of general anesthesia are loss of consciousness, analgesia, relaxed skeletal muscles, and depressed reflexes. Choices of route and type of anesthesia are made primarily by the anesthesia provider after discussion with the patient. Many factors influence these choices, including the type and length of surgery and the physical and psychological status of the patient. Inhalation anesthesia is often used because it has the advantage of rapid induction, excretion, and reversal of effects.

The three phases of general anesthesia are induction, maintenance, and emergence. Induction begins with administration of the anesthetic agent and continues until the patient is ready for the incision. Maintenance continues from this point until near the completion of the procedure. Emergence starts as the patient begins to awaken from the altered state induced by the anesthesia and usually ends when the patient is ready to leave the operating room; the length of time depends on the depth and length of anesthesia. New anesthetic agents enable patients to emerge from anesthesia and "wake up" in a fraction of the time required in the past. When these agents are used, patients frequently bypass PACU stage 1 and move directly to PACU stage 2. This is referred to as "fast tracking." This enables more surgical procedures to be safely done in physicians' offices and in other ambulatory settings.

General anesthesia is advantageous because it can be used for patients of any age and for any surgical procedure, with the patient unaware of the physical trauma of the surgery. There are, however, major associated risks for circulatory and respiratory depression, postoperative nausea and vomiting (PONV), and alterations in thermoregulation. Postop-

erative bronchospasm is another risk, especially in patients with multiple comorbidities.

Children and young adults require greater attention as they emerge from general anesthesia because they may "wake up" disoriented and thrash about. The nurse may need to hold them securely to prevent injury to themselves and others.

 REMEMBER Marcus Benjamin, the 73-year-old man who had a total hip replacement. The nurse would need to incorporate knowledge about the risks associated with general anesthesia along with knowledge of the physiologic changes associated with aging when developing an appropriate plan of care for him. Key to this plan of care would be measures that prevent or minimize Mr. Benjamin's risk for complications. ●

Moderate Sedation/Analgesia

Moderate sedation/analgesia, also called *conscious* or *procedural sedation,* is used for short-term and minimally invasive procedures. The patient maintains cardiorespiratory function and can respond to verbal commands while the IV administration of sedatives and analgesics raises the pain threshold and produces an altered mood with some degree of amnesia (AORN, 2013b). The patient retains the ability to keep the airway open and can respond appropriately. In addition to anesthesiologists and CRNAs, perioperative, endoscopy, interventional radiology or interventional cardiology nurses with specialized training and competence in administering the medications and monitoring the patient's cardiac rate and rhythm, respiratory rate, oxygen saturation, level of consciousness, level of pain, blood pressure, and skin condition may administer this type of anesthesia.

Regional Anesthesia

Regional anesthesia occurs when an anesthetic agent is injected near a nerve or nerve pathway in or around the operative site, inhibiting the transmission of sensory stimuli to central nervous system receptors. The patient receiving regional anesthesia remains awake, but loses sensation in a specific area or region of the body. In some instances, reflexes may also be lost. Although regional anesthesia may be selected for numerous types of surgery and patients, it is especially useful in reducing postsurgical pain, bowel dysfunction, and length of hospital stay for older adult patients in addition to reducing risks associated with general anesthesia for this population.

Regional anesthesia may be accomplished through major nerve blocks or through spinal (subarachnoid block), caudal, or epidural blocks:

- *Nerve blocks* are accomplished by injecting a local anesthetic around a nerve trunk supplying the area of surgery such as the jaw, face, and extremities. Onset and duration of the block depend on the anesthetic drug, its concentration, the amount injected, and the addition of epinephrine, which prolongs the block.

- *Spinal anesthesia* is achieved by injecting a local anesthetic into the subarachnoid space through a lumbar puncture, causing sensory, motor, and autonomic blockage. This type of anesthesia is used for surgery of the lower abdomen, perineum, and legs. Adverse effects of spinal anesthesia may include hypotension, headache, and urine retention.
- *Caudal anesthesia* is the injection of the local anesthetic into the epidural space through the caudal canal in the sacrum; it may be used for procedures on the lower extremities or perineum.
- *Epidural anesthesia* involves the injection of the anesthetic through the intervertebral spaces, usually in the lumbar region (although it may also be used in the thoracic or cervical regions). It is used for surgeries of the chest, abdomen, pelvis, and legs.

Topical and Local Anesthesia

Local anesthesia is the injection of an anesthetic agent such as lidocaine, bupivacaine, or tetracaine to a specific area of the body. It bathes the tissue around a targeted nerve or infiltrates the underlying tissue in the operative area. The surgeon administers local anesthesia for minor, short-term surgical or diagnostic procedures such as tissue biopsy. Epinephrine may be mixed with the local anesthetic to minimize bleeding by causing local vasoconstriction. It also prolongs the length of analgesia by trapping the anesthetic in the tissue through slowed absorption that results from the vasoconstriction of the surrounding vessels. Local anesthesia may also be injected during general anesthetic procedures to prolong pain relief after the general anesthetic wears off.

Topical anesthesia is used on mucous membranes such as the moist linings of the nose and mouth, open skin surfaces, wounds, and burns. Cocaine in a 4% to 10% solution is the most commonly used agent; other common agents are lidocaine, tetracaine and bupivacaine. Some topical drugs can only be used on intact skin in order to avoid rapid absorption. Topical anesthetics may be sprayed, spread, or applied with a compress of drug-saturated gauze or cotton-tipped applicators. Loss of feeling and sensation occur in the specific area where the topical anesthesia is applied. This type of anesthesia can be used prior to repair of simple lacerations in children or to prevent pain from diagnostic procedures involving areas such as the nose and throat.

Informed Consent and Advance Directives

Informed consent is the patient's voluntary agreement to undergo a particular procedure or treatment (such as surgery). The procedural physician should provide the following information in understandable words (layman's terms):

- Description of the procedure or treatment (its name, site and side if applicable), along with potential alternative therapies
- The underlying disease process and its natural course
- Name and qualifications of the person performing the procedure or treatment

- Explanation of the common risks involved, including risk for damage, disfigurement, or death, and how often they occur
- Explanation that the patient has the right to refuse treatment and that consent can be withdrawn
- Explanation of expected outcome, recovery, and rehabilitation plan and course

Informed consent protects the patient, the physician, and the health care institution. The signed, dated, and timed form is a legal document as well as an ethical imperative (Mathias, 2012). The responsibility for securing informed consent from the patient lies with the person who will perform the procedure. This is usually the physician. The nurse may sign as a witness, signifying that the patient signed the consent form without coercion and was alert and aware of the act. The patient always has the right to refuse treatment.

Consent forms are not legal if the patient is confused, unconscious, sedated, mentally incompetent, or a minor (as determined by state laws). Consent may be given in those instances by a parent, spouse, next of kin, or legal guardian. Most states have a list prioritizing authorized next of kin for signing operative consents. It is important to know who is authorized so that the proper person can be contacted in case a question arises. In emergency situations, the physician may obtain consent over the telephone or by court order. More detailed information about informed consent is included in Chapter 7.

Advance directives, also legal documents, allow patients to specify instructions for health care treatment should they be unable to communicate these wishes postoperatively. This allows patients to discuss their wishes with family members in advance of the surgery. Two common forms of advance directive include living wills and durable power of attorney for health care. If the patient should experience a serious, life-threatening complication, such as intraoperative cardiac arrest, the family has previous knowledge of the patient's wishes regarding cessation of treatment, resuscitative efforts, or end-of-life decisions. It is important to discuss and document the exact wishes of the patient and family members before surgery, especially related to resuscitation (do-not-resuscitate [DNR]).

Outpatient/Same-Day Surgery

Surgical procedures performed in outpatient or same-day surgical settings are common. These include freestanding surgery centers, hospital-based surgery centers, interventional units, and physicians' offices. Some freestanding surgery centers specialize in selected types of surgery, such as orthopedics, repair of cataracts, or hernia repair. Others perform a wide variety of surgical interventions, including major surgical procedures that formerly required a stay in a hospital.

Typically, patients are admitted to the ambulatory surgery center the morning of surgery. Allowing the patient to spend the night before surgery at home and to return home to recover reduces much of the stress associated with surgery. Patients who are older, chronically ill or who do not have support systems or access to resources to provide the care needed after surgery may require additional teaching and referral for home care services. When possible, the nurse should arrange these types of referrals prior to the date of surgery.

THE NURSING PROCESS FOR PREOPERATIVE CARE

Patients who require surgical intervention and nursing care enter the health care setting due to a wide variety of situations, ranging from essentially healthy people who have planned elective procedures to emergency admissions for treatment of trauma or serious illness (such as a cardiac arrest or stroke). Surgical patients may be of any age and at any point on the health–illness continuum. It is the nurse's responsibility to identify factors that affect the risk of a surgical procedure. This includes assessing the physical and psychosocial needs of the patient and family and establishing a plan of care based on appropriate nursing diagnoses. Interventions are designed to meet the patient's physical and psychological needs and facilitate recovery as the patient progresses through the perioperative period.

CONSIDER Gabrielle McAllister, the 5-year-old girl scheduled for tonsillectomy and adenoidectomy (T & A). As a child with a history of cardiac defects, prior surgeries, and latex allergy, she is at risk for anesthesia complications related to her birth defects and allergic reaction if exposed to latex. The nurse would need to obtain a thorough history of her previous surgeries, what happens when she is exposed to latex, and how she responded after the surgeries to identify her risk for problems with the current surgical procedure and anesthesia. ●

Some outcomes that frame plans of care for surgical patients might include that patients:

- Receive respectful and culturally and age-appropriate care
- Be free from injury and adverse effects related to positioning, retained surgical items, or chemical, physical, or electrical hazards
- Be free from surgical site infection
- Maintain fluid and electrolyte balance and skin integrity
- Maintain normal body temperature
- Have their pain managed
- Demonstrate an understanding of the physiologic and psychological responses to their planned surgery
- Participate in their rehabilitation process following surgery

Assessing

The importance of preoperative assessment cannot be overemphasized. Surgery is a major trauma to the body, and preoperative assessments identify factors that may place the patient at greater risk for complications during and after surgery (see Examples of Nursing Interventions and Nursing Outcomes Classifications [NIC/NOC]: Risk Identification).

Assessment of the surgical patient includes:

- Obtaining a health history and performing a physical assessment to establish a baseline database
- Identifying risk factors and allergies that could cause surgical adverse events
- Identifying medications and treatments the patient is currently receiving
- Determining the teaching and psychosocial needs of the patient and family
- Determining postsurgical support and referral needs for recovery

EXAMPLES OF NURSING OUTCOMES AND NURSING INTERVENTIONS CLASSIFICATIONS (NIC/NOC)

RISK IDENTIFICATION

Nursing Interventions	Nursing Outcomes
• Review past health history and documents for evidence of existing or previous medical and nursing diagnoses and treatments. • Initiate referrals to health care personnel and/or agencies, as appropriate. • Determine availability and quality of resources (e.g., psychological, financial, education level, family and other social relationships, and community). • Determine status of basic living needs. • Use mutual goal setting as appropriate.	• Risk Detection • Risk Control

Data from Bulechek, G., Butcher, H., Dochterman, J. M., & Wagner, C. (Eds.). (2013). *Nursing interventions classification (NIC)* (6th ed.). St. Louis: Elsevier/Mosby; and Moorhead, S., Johnson, M., Maas, M., & Swanson, E. (Eds.). (2013). *Nursing outcomes classification (NOC)* (5th ed.). St. Louis: Elsevier/Mosby.

BOX 29-1 PREOPERATIVE INFORMATION FOR OUTPATIENT/SAME-DAY SURGERY

Using simple language the patient can understand, instruct the patient (verbally and in writing) as follows:

- List medications routinely taken, and ask the physician which should be taken or omitted the morning of surgery.
- Notify the surgeon's office if a cold or infection develops before surgery.
- List all allergies, and be sure the OR staff is aware of them.
- Follow all instructions from your surgeon regarding bathing or showering with a special soap solution.
- Remove nail polish and do not wear makeup on the day of the procedure.

- Leave all jewelry and valuables at home.
- Wear clothing that buttons in front; short-sleeved garments are better for surgery on the hands.
- Have someone available for transportation home after recovery from anesthesia.

Inform patient of:

- Limitations on eating or drinking before surgery, with a specific time to begin the limitations.
- When and where to arrive for the procedure, as well as the estimated time when the procedure will be performed.

The assessment is often conducted several days before surgery as part of preoperative laboratory screening and teaching; this is referred to as preadmission testing. It may be conducted in the hospital, a surgical clinic, an office, in the patient's home, or by phone.

Preoperative nursing assessments and teaching are key care activities for patients who will be having outpatient or same-day surgery. Preoperative teaching can often be combined with preoperative screening tests, which are usually done up to 30 days before the scheduled surgery. Preoperative assessment and teaching for outpatient/ same-day surgery includes providing important information and preoperative instructions to the patient and family (Box 29-1).

Health History

The health history identifies risk factors and strengths in the patient's physical and psychosocial status and helps the nurse to individualize the preoperative assessment. Health history information significant to the surgical experience includes the patient's developmental level; medical history, including allergies; medication history, including nonprescription drugs; previous surgeries; implants, extremity limitations, perceptions and knowledge of the surgery to be done; nutrition; use of alcohol, illicit drugs, or nicotine; activities of daily living and occupation; coping patterns and support systems; and sociocultural needs.

DEVELOPMENTAL CONSIDERATIONS

Infants and older adults are at a greater risk from surgery than are children and young or middle-aged adults. The infant has a lower total blood volume, making even a small loss of blood a serious concern because of the risk for dehydration and the inability to respond to the need for increased oxygen during surgery. In addition, an infant's airway is small, soft, and pliable; also, infants and small children frequently have upper respiratory infections, such as colds, that can cause airway obstruction and hypoxia. This patient population can quickly develop bronchospasm, stridor, and respiratory arrest. If a child exhibits signs of even mild respiratory infection

on the day of surgery, the child's procedure might be postponed until a later date.

Infants also have difficulty maintaining stable body temperature during surgery because the shivering reflex is not well developed, making hypothermia or hyperthermia more likely. Their lower glomerular filtration rate and creatinine clearance can lead to a slower metabolism of drugs that require renal biotransformation. Because the liver is immature until after the first year of life, the effects of muscle relaxants and narcotics may be prolonged.

Physiologic changes associated with aging (described in Chapter 19) increase the surgical risk for older patients. These changes, summarized in the Focus on the Older Adult display, decrease older adults' ability to respond to the stress of surgery, alter the effects of preoperative and postoperative medications and anesthesia, and prolong or alter wound healing processes. With an increasing older adult population, assessing physiologic changes is crucial to providing safe, quality nursing care to older surgical patients. Chronic illnesses, more common in the older population, also increase surgical risk and may require alterations in usual perioperative procedures. For example, a patient with congestive heart failure may be more easily fatigued and thus unable to be up and about as rapidly after surgery.

 CONSIDER Marcus Benjamin, the 73-year-old man who had a total hip replacement. Due to his age, the nurse would need to be alert to potential complications specifically associated with age-related changes, reduced mobility, and use of general anesthesia, IV therapy, and urinary catheterization. ●

MEDICAL HISTORY

The medical history provides information about past and current illnesses. Pathologic changes associated with past and current illnesses increase surgical risk as well as the risk for postoperative complications. Preoperative assessments and documentation are necessary to provide a database for individualized assessments and interventions

FOCUS ON THE OLDER ADULT

NURSING STRATEGIES TO ADDRESS AGE-RELATED CHANGES IN PERIOPERATIVE PATIENTS

Age-Related Changes	Nursing Strategies
Cardiovascular	
Decreased cardiac output, stroke volume, and cardiac reserve Decreased peripheral circulation Increased vascular rigidity	• Obtain and record baseline vital signs. • Assess peripheral pulses. • Teach leg exercises, turning, and explain the purpose of early ambulation after surgery. • Document normal activity levels and tolerance of fatigue. • Monitor fluid administration rate. • Allow sufficient time for effects of medications to occur.
Respiratory	
Reduced vital capacity Diminished cough reflex Decreased oxygenation of blood Decreased chest expansion and strength of intercostal muscles and diaphragm	• Obtain and record baseline respiratory depth and rate. • Teach coughing and deep-breathing exercises. • Teach use of incentive spirometer. • Assess color of skin. • Explain use of pulse oximeter for monitoring postoperative oxygenation.
Central Nervous System	
Decreased reaction time and coordination Reduced short-term memory Sensory deficits Decreased thermoregulation ability	• Orient to surroundings. • Institute safety measures, such as keeping environment clear of clutter and using a night-light. • Allow additional time for teaching, "teach-back" activities, and questions and answers. • Use appropriate measures to conserve body heat.
Renal	
Decreased renal blood flow Reduced bladder capacity	• Monitor amount and times of voiding. • Monitor fluid and electrolyte status. • Maintain and record intake and output.
Gastrointestinal	
Increased gastric pH Prolonged gastric-emptying time Decreased hepatic blood flow and enzyme function	• Obtain baseline weight. • Monitor nutritional status (weight, laboratory data). • Observe for prolonged effects of medications.
Integumentary	
Decreased vascularity Decreased skin moisture and elasticity Decreased subcutaneous fat	• Assess skin status. • Monitor fluid status. • Pad and protect bony prominences. • Monitor skin for pressure areas. • Use minimal amounts of tape on dressings and intravenous sites.

in the intraoperative and postoperative phases of care. Examples of diseases and associated risks may include:

- Cardiovascular diseases—such as thrombocytopenia, hemophilia, recent myocardial infarction or cardiac surgery, heart failure, and dysrhythmias—increase the risk for anesthesia complications, including hemorrhage and hypovolemic shock, hypotension, venous stasis, thrombophlebitis, and overhydration with IV fluids.
- Respiratory disorders—such as pneumonia, bronchitis, asthma, emphysema, and chronic obstructive pulmonary diseases—increase the risk for respiratory depression from anesthesia as well as postoperative

pneumonia, atelectasis, and alterations in acid–base balance.
- Kidney and liver diseases influence the patient's response to anesthesia, affect fluid and electrolyte as well as acid–base balance, alter the metabolism and excretion of drugs, and impair wound healing.
- Endocrine diseases, especially diabetes mellitus, increase the risk for hypoglycemia or acidosis, slow wound healing, and present an increased risk for postoperative cardiovascular complications.

SURGICAL HISTORY

Data about previous surgeries are important for meeting the patient's physical and psychological needs throughout the perioperative period. Physical implications of previous surgeries are important to the intraoperative and postoperative phases (e.g., previous heart or lung surgery may necessitate adaptations in anesthesia and in positioning during surgery). Previous surgical complications—such as malignant hyperthermia, latex sensitivity, pneumonia, thrombophlebitis, or **deep vein thrombosis (DVT)**, a formation of a blood clot ("thrombus") in a deep vein or surgical site infection—may put the patient at risk during this surgery, necessitating vigilant intraoperative and postoperative monitoring.

The patient's past experiences with surgery also affect the plan of care established in the preoperative phase, especially if a past experience was negative. When the interview elicits negative feelings about the surgical experience, pain management, or nursing interventions carried out to prevent complications during previous surgeries, teaching and mutual goal setting take on an even greater importance. For children, stressful events before surgery include the admission process, lab tests, injections, the timeframe before and during transport to the OR, and the recovery period in the PACU.

In addition to experiences with past surgery, the patient's perceptions and knowledge of the surgical procedure to be performed should be assessed. The patient's questions or statements about the surgery are important for meeting psychological and family needs when preparing the patient for surgery and planning for patient and family teaching and preparation for discharge.

MEDICATION HISTORY

The use of prescribed, over-the-counter, or herbal drugs can affect the patient's reaction to, and increase the risk from, the stress of surgery and the effects of the anesthetic agent. Some herbal products can increase bleeding while others may potentiate the actions of depressant anesthetic drugs. Drugs in the following categories increase surgical risk:

- Anticoagulants (may precipitate hemorrhage)
- Diuretics (may cause electrolyte imbalances, with resulting respiratory depression from anesthesia)
- Tranquilizers (may increase the hypotensive effect of anesthetic agents)
- Adrenal steroids (abrupt withdrawal may cause cardiovascular collapse in long-term users)
- Antibiotics in the mycin group (when combined with certain muscle relaxants used during surgery, may cause respiratory paralysis)

Although some medications are discontinued before surgery, the nurse should know the purposes and actions of the patient's drugs as well as the physician's orders. Specific medications may be given the morning of surgery with sips of water (e.g., patients with heart or cardiovascular problems or diabetes mellitus).

NUTRITIONAL STATUS

Both malnutrition and obesity increase surgical risk. Surgery increases the body's need for nutrients necessary for normal tissue healing and resistance to infection. A patient who is malnourished is at a higher risk for alterations in fluid and electrolyte balance, delay in wound healing, and wound infection. Obese patients are at increased risk for respiratory, cardiovascular, positional injury, DVT, and gastrointestinal problems. Overweight patients may have obstructive sleep apnea, putting them at risk for reduced respiratory function. They may also have gastroesophageal reflux disease (GERD), putting them at risk for aspiration of stomach contents. Fatty tissue has a poor blood supply and, therefore, has less resistance to infection. As a result, postoperative complications of delayed wound healing, wound infection, and disruption in the integrity of the wound are more common.

USE OF ALCOHOL, ILLICIT DRUGS, OR NICOTINE

Patients with a large habitual intake of alcohol require larger doses of anesthetic agents and postoperative analgesics, increasing the risk for drug-related complications. Patients who use illicit drugs are at risk for interactions with anesthetic agents. These are specific to the illicit drug used and should be noted on the medical record for safe anesthetic management. IV drug use may render veins hardened, inflamed, and unusable for anesthesia drug administration.

Patients who smoke are at higher risk for respiratory complications after surgery. All patients retain pulmonary secretions during anesthesia, but smokers, who already have increased mucous secretions and decreased ciliary action in the tracheobronchial tree, have more difficulty clearing the respiratory passages after surgery. In addition, the tracheobronchial mucosa is chronically irritated in people who smoke; anesthesia increases this irritation. Patients who smoke are at risk for hypoxia and postoperative pneumonia. Smoking compromises wound healing by constricting blood vessels, impairing blood flow to healing tissues.

ACTIVITIES OF DAILY LIVING AND OCCUPATION

Exercise, rest, and sleep habits are important for preventing postoperative complications and facilitating recovery. A patient with a well-established exercise program has improved cardiovascular, respiratory, metabolic, and musculoskeletal function, thereby lowering the risks of surgery. Rest and sleep are essential to physical and emotional adaptation and recovery from the stress of surgery. Information from the health history allows the nurse to individualize interventions to promote rest and sleep.

Many surgical procedures require a delay in returning to a career or occupation or may affect how the patient earns a living. Knowledge of a patient's usual work and concerns about returning to work helps the nurse plan necessary teaching and referrals.

COPING PATTERNS AND SUPPORT SYSTEMS

Assessing the patient's psychological, sociocultural, and spiritual dimensions is as important as the physical history and examination. Surgery is a major psychological stressor and affects coping patterns, support systems, and individual human needs. A surgical procedure, whether it is planned or unexpected, major or minor, causes anxiety and fear. While obtaining the health history, the nurse uses cues from the patient's and family's verbal and nonverbal communication to identify fears and concerns and to plan nursing interventions to provide the information and emotional support necessary to successful recovery from surgery.

Surgery is an unfamiliar experience over which a person has no control; the resulting anxiety and fear may be expressed in many ways such as anger, withdrawal, apathy, confrontation, or questioning. Patients often fear the unknown, pain or death, and changes in body image and self-concept. The patient typically has fears about the surgery itself—the anesthesia, the diagnosis, the future, financial and family responsibilities, response to pain, or possible disfigurement or disability. Common fears are that the anesthesia will not "put me to sleep," that death will occur during surgery, or that the patient will not be able to handle postoperative pain. Surgical procedures may leave the patient with permanent changes in body structure, function, or appearance. This may increase patients' fear of alterations in physical attractiveness, social relationships, lifestyle, and sexuality.

 REMEMBER Molly Greenbaum, the 38-year-old woman who is fearful of surgery? Her statements about the inability to sleep, in conjunction with the tears in her eyes and wringing of hands, would be cues that she is experiencing stress. Exploring Molly's fears, past coping mechanisms, and support systems would be valuable in developing the patient's plan of care, both before and after surgery. Doing so would help to promote a positive perioperative experience for her. In addition, the nurse would need to investigate what fears Molly may be experiencing related to a vaginal hysterectomy such as changes in physical attractiveness, marital relationship, sexuality, and end of reproductive capability. ●

Therapeutic communication skills are essential for establishing the trusting nurse–patient relationship that is necessary to identify and resolve fear. Encourage the patient to identify and verbalize fears; often simply talking about fears helps to diminish their magnitude. At the same time, incorrect knowledge can be identified and corrected, strengths can be noted, and teaching can be done. The reduction of anxiety is of major importance in preoperative preparation; emotional stress added to the physical stress of surgery increases the surgical risk. The nursing history should elicit the ways in which a patient provides self-support to reduce stress. These are discussed in Chapter 41 and range from listening to music to practicing active relaxation techniques. See the accompanying Research in Nursing box.

Coping with stress can be facilitated through the support systems identified in the assessment phase of preoperative

RESEARCH IN NURSING

BRIDGING THE GAP TO EVIDENCE-BASED PRACTICE

Effect of Music Intervention on Anxiety

Undergoing surgery is a stressful experience for most people. Patients have concerns about the procedure and its outcomes, possible pain, and other postoperative effects. A majority of patients admit to some degree of anxiety surrounding the surgery. The noise level in the operating room or PACU often contributes to or exacerbates the level of anxiety. Florence Nightingale, in her recordings, noted the negative effects of noise on patients. Music has been recognized since ancient times as having a positive effect on healing. The use of music in health care situations has been credited with reducing patient's anxiety and fear, promoting comfort, and providing distraction and pleasure.

Related Research

Johnson, B., Raymond, S., & Goss, J. (2012) Perioperative music or headsets to decrease anxiety. *Journal of PeriAnesthesia Nursing*, 27(3), 146–154.

This study explored the effects of music versus noise-blocking headphones on the level of anxiety in women undergoing same-day gynecologic surgery. The 119 women who participated in the study were randomly assigned to either a usual-care group, use of music with headphones, or headphones only. Preoperative and postoperative anxiety was rated using a Rapid Assessment Anxiety tool with a score ranging from 0 (no anxiety) to 10 (most anxiety possible). Music/headphones were continued throughout surgery and removed when the patients were alert and oriented. All three groups experienced a drop in anxiety from pre- to postoperative status, but the "usual-care" group had the least improvement. The music group experienced the lowest postoperative anxiety scores. However, the headphone group had a greater change overall possibly because they had a slightly higher preoperative anxiety score.

Relevance to Nursing Practice

Music has proved to be a noninvasive, inexpensive intervention that has a positive effect on anxiety levels for patients undergoing surgery. It distracts patients from surrounding noises from equipment and staff and provides some sense of control in an unfamiliar environment. Lowering anxiety levels via the use of music contributes to a restful, healing atmosphere for surgical patients.

FOCUSED ASSESSMENT GUIDE 29-1

PREOPERATIVE PHYSICAL ASSESSMENT

Factors to Assess	Questions and Approaches
General survey	• Note general state of health. • Note body posture and stature. • Take and record vital signs.
Skin	• Inspect skin for color, characteristics, and location and appearance of any lesions. • Assess skin over bony prominences. • Determine skin turgor.
Chest and lungs	• Observe chest excursion and diameter and shape of thorax. • Auscultate breath sounds. • Palpate for any pain or tenderness.
Cardiovascular system	• Inspect for jugular vein distention. • Auscultate apical rate, rhythm, and character. • Auscultate heart sounds. • Inspect for peripheral edema. • Palpate strength of peripheral pulses.
Abdomen	• Inquire about time of last bowel movement. • Inspect abdominal contour. • Auscultate bowel sounds.
Neurologic system	• Note orientation, level of consciousness, awareness, and speech. • Assess reflexes. • Assess motor and sensory ability. • Assess visual and hearing ability.
Musculoskeletal system	• Inspect and note joint range of motion. • Palpate muscle strength. • Assess ability to ambulate.

nursing care. As much as possible, family members or significant others should be part of the initial interview and should be included in discussions of fears and concerns. Encourage family members to provide support before and after surgery. When permitted, encourage parents to accompany their child to the preoperative waiting area and bring them to the recovery area when the patient is awake.

Identifying the patient's spiritual beliefs aids in meeting individual spiritual needs. These needs can be met through acceptance, participation in prayer or other rituals, and/or referral to a spiritual leader. Faith in a higher being or source of personal strength provides support and helps to reduce fears in many people.

The need for other support systems can also be identified in the initial interview. For example, a patient having a colostomy, heart transplant, or mastectomy may have many questions answered and anxieties reduced by a preoperative visit from a person who has had the same operation and adapted successfully.

SOCIOCULTURAL NEEDS

A person's perceptions of and reactions to the surgical experience are influenced by individual factors, including family health beliefs and practices, economic factors,

and cultural/ethnic background. A patient who requires surgery, but has grown up in a family that believes that surgical intervention is the last possible option for treating illness, may be hesitant about the surgery or may be convinced that death will result. The resulting anxiety may make this patient even more susceptible to surgical risk. Reactions to teaching, physical care, and pain are also influenced by family values and cultural/ethnic identity. For example, a male patient reared with the belief that it is unmanly to acknowledge pain may demonstrate a stoic acceptance of pain and refuse needed medications postoperatively.

Cultural and ethnic influences also affect the patient's responses to and perceptions of the surgical experience. The patient's cultural background may require that nursing interventions be individualized to meet needs in such areas as language, food preferences, family interactions and participation, personal space, and health beliefs and practices (see Chapter 5). For example, a patient from a culture that believes that bed rest is the most important treatment for illness or injury may have difficulty accepting the need for postoperative exercises and early ambulation. Language barriers require the use of interpreter services.

Physical Assessment

Assessing the patient's current physical status provides data for interventions to decrease surgical risk and potential postoperative complications. Depending on the situation, the physical assessment is conducted as described in Chapter 25. See also Focused Assessment Guide 29-1 for key areas to assess preoperatively.

Various presurgical screening tests provide objective data of normal body function. In cases of abnormalities, such tests provide data for medical interventions to improve the patient's physical status and thus decrease the risks for surgical complications. The nurse's role is to ensure that the tests are explained to the patient, appropriate specimens are collected, the results are documented in the patient's record before surgery, and abnormal findings are reported.

Usual presurgical screening tests include chest x-ray, electrocardiography, complete blood count, electrolyte levels, and urinalysis. Normal findings for laboratory tests are found in Appendix C on thePoint. Significant abnormal findings include an elevated white blood cell count (presence of infection), decreased hematocrit and hemoglobin level (presence of bleeding, anemia), hyperkalemia or hypokalemia (increased risk for cardiac problems, elevated blood urea nitrogen or urinalysis results. Additional cardiac clearance may be indicated for patients with a cardiac history or abnormal electrocardiographic (EKG) results. Glucose testing is done as part of presurgical screening and often repeated the morning of surgery.

Diagnosing

Nursing diagnoses for patients in the preoperative phase may be identified for various actual or potential problems for which a patient is at risk. These are derived from the analysis of subjective and objective data obtained from the health history and physical examination as well as information from other health team members and screening tests. Many diagnoses reflect assessment of risk and are made to guide interventions for patient needs in the intraoperative and postoperative phases. Nursing care throughout the perioperative period must be consistent and documented; the preoperative nursing diagnoses and desired outcomes provide the basis for consistent, coordinated care from admission through recovery. See Examples of NANDA-I Nursing Diagnoses appropriate to the preoperative period.

Outcome Identification and Planning

Preoperative nursing care is affected by the length of the preoperative phase. There may not be enough time for comprehensive assessments and teaching for patients who enter the hospital through the emergency department needing immediate surgery and those who have outpatient/same-day surgery. In such cases, the nurse uses standardized preoperative plans and individualizes the plan for the particular patient and family. Outcomes are standard for all patients having surgery, but nursing interventions are designed to meet the priority needs of individual patients and situations.

Planning for the entire perioperative period is done in the preoperative phase and includes expected outcomes that are discussed and mutually agreed on by the nurse, the patient, and the family. Specific appropriate outcomes include that the patient (Petersen, 2011):

- Is physically and emotionally prepared for surgery
- Demonstrates turning, coughing, and deep-breathing exercises
- Verbalizes expectations and understanding of postoperative pain management
- Maintains fluid intake and nutritional balance to meet needs

EXAMPLES OF NANDA-I NURSING DIAGNOSES

THE PREOPERATIVE PATIENT

Nursing Diagnoses	Related Factors	Sample Defining Characteristics
Anxiety	Any condition that is perceived as a threat or danger, such as effects of surgery on ability to carry out family roles and responsibilities. Any condition that is perceived as a danger, such as the possibility of dying while under anesthesia.	• Restlessness, poor eye contact, fidgeting, quivering voice, hand tremor • Increased pulse and respirations • Sweating, dry mouth, fatigue, nausea, urinary frequency • Preoccupation, forgetfulness, decreased attention span • Verbalizations of distress, worry, being afraid
Risk for Infection	Any condition that interferes with normal inflammatory healing process	*Risk Factors* • Obesity • Aging • Immunosuppression • Malnutrition

Implementing

Preoperative nursing interventions provide the patient with the necessary psychological and physical preparation for surgery and the postoperative phase. This section discusses implementing the plan of care to meet established patient goals. Skill 29-1 on pages 884–889 outlines the actions and rationale for preoperative patient care.

Preparing the Patient Psychologically Through Communicating

Surgery is almost always viewed as a life crisis and evokes anxiety and fear. Anxiety can be reduced and recovery facilitated by nursing actions that focus on therapeutic communication and patient and family teaching. Each patient is a unique individual who responds to the surgical experience in a unique way. One note of caution: Avoid false reassurance. In an attempt to allay anxiety and fear, the nurse may be tempted to reassure patients that they will be fine. Such a response denies patients' emotional needs, shuts off therapeutic communications and trust, and may not be true.

The nurse uses therapeutic communication skills and techniques, as described in Chapter 20, to establish a supportive and trusting nurse–patient relationship and to facilitate psychological safety and security. Nursing interventions to meet the psychological needs of the surgical patient through communication are outlined in Box 29-2.

Preparing the Patient Psychologically Through Teaching

Teaching about postoperative activities, a nursing responsibility, is implemented in the preoperative phase. Patients and families need to know about surgical events and sensations, how to manage pain, and how to perform the physical activities necessary to decrease the risk for postoperative complications and facilitate recovery. The teaching–learning process (see Chapter 21) is individualized to meet common and individual patient needs. The success of preoperative teaching varies with the timing of the teaching, the individual patient and that patient's support systems, the type of surgery, and group versus individual sessions. Preoperative teaching has proven beneficial in decreasing postoperative complications and length of stay as well as positively influencing recovery. Patients who are well prepared with detailed preoperative instruction deal more effectively with their surgery and are better prepared to manage their pain and engage in appropriate self-care activities.

The timing of teaching is a significant consideration: Teaching too far in advance of surgery or when the patient is anxious is less effective. In today's health care system, patients often enter the hospital the day of surgery and teaching must be adapted to this schedule. Many institutions provide teaching sessions before admission to prepare the patient for surgery. Whether done before or after admission, a preoperative teaching checklist gives nurses organized, comprehensive guidelines for instruction. Box 29-3 provides a sample of preoperative teaching with associated surgical events.

TEACHING ABOUT SURGICAL EVENTS AND SENSATIONS

When surgery is scheduled, explain to patients and their families how long the surgery and postanesthesia care will last, as well as what will be done before, during, and after surgery (e.g., procedures, medications, equipment). If the surgery is elective, an actual or computerized tour of the operating suite, or a video of the preoperative journey to the OR, may be helpful in reducing anxiety and fear of the unknown. This is especially helpful for children. Provide an explanation of surgical events, including a description of the various members of the health care team; where and when to report for admission; instructions for preoperative skin preparation, fasting, and bowel prep, if ordered; instructions for taking special medications; and the importance of bringing a responsible adult to drive the patient home. Explain to patients that they may not drive themselves home or take public transportation alone if they have had any anesthesia or sedation.

Patients also benefit from knowing what sensory alterations they may experience during the perioperative period. Although the sensations differ depending on the type of surgery, teaching should include information about dry mouth and drowsiness from preoperative medications, a sore throat from the insertion of an endotracheal tube, a gradual return of feeling and movement after spinal anesthesia, and pain from the surgical incision. It is also important to make sure that patients are aware of the coolness of the environment, firmness of the OR bed, the sounds and sights of multiple care providers

---

BOX 29-2 NURSING INTERVENTIONS TO MEET PSYCHOLOGICAL NEEDS OF PATIENTS HAVING SURGERY

- Establish and maintain a therapeutic relationship, allowing the patient to verbalize fears and concerns.
- Use active listening skills to identify and validate verbal and nonverbal messages revealing anxiety and fear.
- Use touch, as appropriate, to demonstrate genuine empathy and caring.
- Be prepared to respond to common patient questions about surgery, including:
  - Will I lose control of body functions while I'm having surgery?
  - How long will I be in the operating room and PACU?
  - Where will my family be?
  - Will I have pain when I wake up?
  - Will the anesthetic make me sick?
  - Will I need a blood transfusion?
  - How long will it be before I can eat?
  - What kind of scar will I have?
  - When will I be able to be sexually active?
  - When can I go back to work?

Box 29-3	**SAMPLE PREOPERATIVE TEACHING: ACTIVITIES AND EVENTS FOR IN-HOSPITAL SURGERY**

Preoperative Phase
- ❏ Exercises and physical activities
  - ❏ Deep-breathing exercises
  - ❏ Coughing
  - ❏ Incentive spirometry
  - ❏ Turning
  - ❏ Leg exercises
- ❏ Pain management
  - ❏ Meaning of PRN orders for medications
  - ❏ Timing for best effect of medications
  - ❏ Splinting incision
  - ❏ Nonpharmacologic pain management options
- ❏ Visit by anesthesiologist
- ❏ Physical preparation
  - ❏ NPO
  - ❏ Sleeping medication the night before
  - ❏ Preoperative checklist (review items)
- ❏ Visitors and waiting room
- ❏ Transported to operating room by stretcher

Intraoperative Phase
- ❏ Holding area
  - ❏ Skin preparation
  - ❏ Intravenous lines and fluids
- ❏ Medications
- ❏ Operating room
  - ❏ Operating room bed
  - ❏ Lights and common equipment (e.g., cardiac monitor, pulse oximeter, warming device)

- ❏ Safety belt
- ❏ Sensations
- ❏ Staff

Postoperative Phase
- ❏ Postanesthesia care unit
  - ❏ Frequent vital signs, assessments (e.g., orientation, movement of extremities, strength of grasp)
  - ❏ Dressings/drains/tubes/catheters
  - ❏ Intravenous lines
  - ❏ Pain medications/comfort measures
  - ❏ Family notification
  - ❏ Sensations
  - ❏ Airway/oxygen therapy/pulse oximetry
  - ❏ Staff
- ❏ Transfer to unit (on stretcher)
  - ❏ Frequent vital signs
  - ❏ Sensations
  - ❏ Pain medications/nonpharmacologic strategies
  - ❏ NPO, diet progression
  - ❏ Exercises
  - ❏ Early ambulation
- ❏ Family visits

wearing surgical masks, and the bright overhead lights. Assure patients that they are the most important person in the room and will be well cared for and comforted. It is likely that the patient will receive antianxiety medication, which is also an amnesic. However, this medication should not prevent the nurse from clarifying information with patients and answering their questions.

TEACHING ABOUT PAIN MANAGEMENT

Pain is a normal part of the surgical experience and a major concern for the patient and family. Evidence-based guidelines for the management of acute surgical pain have been established by several professional agencies. The guidelines are based on these principles: (1) the pain reported by the patient is the determining factor of pain control, (2) pain must be assessed as often as every 2 hours after major surgery, and (3) the older patient is at risk for both undertreatment and overtreatment of pain. Continuing or unresolved pain can increase the patient's length of recovery and delay discharge. Treat unrelieved postoperative pain as a serious complication of surgery, not as a normal expectation. The nurse is responsible for assessment, implementation, evaluation of a pain management plan, and for teaching the patient preoperatively how to communicate and report pain (see Chapter 34) so that it is manageable. Introduce children and their families to an age-specific pain scale preoperatively.

Teach the patient and family that medications to relieve pain will be ordered by the physician and administered by the nurse. The physician may order pain medications to be given on a regular basis or on an as-needed (PRN) basis. If medication is ordered PRN, there is a time restriction between doses (e.g., every 2 or 4 hours). Explain to patients that they need to ask for the medication before the pain becomes severe. If the medication does not control the pain or if the patient has unpleasant side effects (such as nausea and vomiting), a different medication can be ordered. There is little danger of addiction to pain medications used in the postoperative management of pain. The use of relaxation techniques (e.g., deep breathing, music, and guided imagery) enhances the effects of pain medications.

Alternative methods of pain control that may be used after surgery include transcutaneous electrical nerve stimulation (TENS), pressure-controlled pain pumps filled with local anesthetics with soaker drains placed inside the incision, patient-controlled analgesia (PCA), and patient-controlled epidural anesthesia (PCEA). PCA infusion pumps allow patients to self-administer doses of pain-relieving medication within physician-prescribed time and dose limits. Patients activate the delivery of the medication by pressing a button on a cord connected to the pump or a button directly on the pump. Teach the patient how to use these methods of pain control before surgery and monitor their effectiveness after surgery.

GUIDELINES FOR NURSING CARE 29-1

TEACHING DEEP BREATHING TECHNIQUES

- Place the patient in semi-Fowler's position, with the neck and shoulders supported.
- Ask the patient to place the hands over the rib cage, so that the patient can feel the chest rise as the lungs expand.
- Ask the patient to:
  - Exhale gently and completely.
  - Inhale through the nose gently and completely.
  - Hold the breath for 3 to 5 seconds and mentally count "one, one thousand, two, one thousand," and so forth.
- Exhale as completely as possible through the mouth with lips pursed (as if whistling).
- Repeat three times.
- This exercise should be done every 1 to 2 hours while the patient is awake for the first 24 hours after surgery and as necessary thereafter, depending on risk factors and pulmonary status.

A discussion of TENS and information about nursing interventions when using PCA are in Chapter 34.

TEACHING ABOUT PHYSICAL ACTIVITIES

The most common causes of postoperative complications are alterations in cardiovascular and respiratory function, including atelectasis, pneumonia, thrombophlebitis, and DVT. Physical activities to reduce the risk for these complications are deep breathing, coughing, incentive spirometry, leg exercises, and turning in bed. These, and other activities that will be required postoperatively, are taught in the preoperative period. The patient should be able to state the purpose and demonstrate the activities before going to surgery. This section gives the rationale for the activities; postoperative complications are discussed later in the chapter.

Deep Breathing. During surgery, the cough reflex is suppressed, mucus accumulates in the tracheobronchial passageways, and the lungs do not ventilate fully. After surgery, respirations often are less effective as a result of the anesthesia, pain medications, and pain from the incision. Patients who have thoracic or high abdominal incisions are especially prone to shallow breathing

because of incisional pain with deeper respirations. As a result, alveoli do not inflate and may collapse, and secretions are retained, increasing the risk for atelectasis and respiratory infection. Deep-breathing exercises hyperventilate the alveoli and prevent them from collapsing again, improve lung expansion and volume, help to expel anesthetic gases and mucus, and facilitate oxygenation of tissues. See Guidelines for Nursing Care 29-1 for how to teach the patient deep-breathing techniques.

Coughing. Coughing helps remove retained mucus from the respiratory tract and usually is taught in conjunction with deep breathing. Coughing is especially important in patients with an increased risk for respiratory complications. Because coughing is often painful, teach the patient how to splint the incision (i.e., support the incision with a pillow or folded bath blanket) and to use the period after pain medication has been administered to best advantage. See Guidelines for Nursing Care 29-2 on how to teach the patient how to cough effectively.

Incentive Spirometry. An incentive spirometer is often ordered for patients having surgery, and the proper technique for using it should be practiced preoperatively.

GUIDELINES FOR NURSING CARE 29-2

EFFECTIVE COUGHING

- Place the patient in a semi-Fowler's position, leaning forward.
- Provide a pillow or folded bath blanket to use in splinting the incision.
- Ask the patient to:
  - Inhale and exhale deeply and slowly through the nose three times.
  - Take a deep breath and hold it for 3 seconds.
  - "Hack" out for three short breaths.
  - With mouth open, take a quick breath.
  - Cough deeply once or twice.
  - Take another deep breath.
- Repeat the exercise every 2 hours while awake.

Encouraging patient to "hack" out three short coughs after holding breath.

This device helps to increase lung volume and inflation of alveoli and facilitates venous return. A gauge on the incentive spirometry device allows patients to measure their progress and provides immediate positive reinforcement for the breathing efforts. See Chapter 38 for more information.

Leg Exercises. During surgery, venous blood return from the legs slows. In addition, some surgical positions, such as having the legs elevated in the lithotomy position (see illustration in Box 25-2 on page 634) decrease venous return. With circulatory stasis in the legs, thrombophlebitis, DVT, and the risk for emboli are potential complications. Leg exercises increase venous return through flexion and contraction of the quadriceps and gastrocnemius muscles. Leg exercises must be individualized to patient needs, physical condition, physician preference, and agency protocol. Figure 29-2 highlights how to teach the patient to perform leg exercises.

Turning in Bed. Turning in bed improves venous return, respiratory function, and intestinal peristalsis and prevents the unrelieved skin pressure that would occur if the patient were to remain in only one position. Although turning in bed sounds like a simple procedure, incisional pain makes it difficult, underscoring the need for practicing it before surgery. To turn in bed, patients should raise one knee, reach across to grasp the side rail on the side toward which they are turning, and roll over while pushing with the bent leg and pulling on the side rail. A small pillow is useful for splinting the incision while turning. The patient should turn and change positions in bed every 2 hours when awake.

Preparing the Patient Physically

The physical preparation of the patient for surgery varies, depending on the patient's physical status and special needs, type of surgery, and physician's orders. Certain nursing interventions are appropriate for all surgical patients in the areas of hygiene and skin preparation, elimination, nutrition and fluids, and rest and sleep. The nurse is also responsible for the preparation and safety of the patient on the day of surgery.

HYGIENE AND SKIN PREPARATION

Intact skin is the body's first line of defense against microorganisms, and the surgical incision provides a potential entry for infection. Therefore, the skin is prepared to minimize skin contamination and decrease the risk for postoperative surgical site infection.

The skin is cleaned at the operative site with an antibacterial soap or solution to remove bacteria. The patient can do this while taking a bath or shower. Preoperative showers or baths are taken before the scheduled surgery using chlorhexidine gluconate (CHG) soap. Remind patients to use a three-step process when bathing or showering preoperatively: apply, lather, rinse (How-to-guide, 2012). The nurse may need to cleanse children and adult inpatients

Lie in a semi-Fowler's position. Bend the knee, raise the foot, and keep it elevated for a few seconds.

Extend the lower leg

Lower the leg to the bed. Do this 5 times with one leg, then repeat with the other leg.

A Point toes of both feet toward the foot of the bed. Relax both feet.

B Pull toes toward the chin. Relax both feet.

C Make circles with both ankles. First circle to the right, then to the left. Repeat 3 times. Relax both feet.

FIGURE 29-2. Leg exercises to increase venous return.

preoperatively with microfiber cloths impregnated with chlorhexidine gluconate antimicrobial skin antiseptic. This skin antiseptic eliminates skin microorganisms and leaves an antimicrobial film on their skin. Shampooing the hair and cleaning the fingernails also help to reduce the number of organisms present on the body.

Leave hair at the surgical site in place if possible. Removal of hair at the surgical site depends on the amount of hair, the location of the incision, and the type of surgical procedure being performed. If ordered, this

PICO IN PRACTICE

ASKING CLINICAL QUESTIONS

Scenario: You are a staff nurse who works in a same-day surgery center. You are asked to serve as a preceptor for a newly hired nurse, Terri, who has just finished a nurses' refresher course at the local community college. Terri worked as a perioperative nurse for over 12 years, but her practice was on hiatus while she stayed at home to raise two children for the past 15 years. One day, Terri asks you why it is no longer standard practice to shave patients' surgical sites to prepare them for surgery. She notes to you that this was standard protocol for patients 15 years ago, and was thought to diminish the incidence of surgical site infections.

• POPULATION: Perioperative patients
• INTERVENTION: Surgical site shaving of hair
• COMPARISON: No surgical site shaving of hair
• OUTCOME: Lower rates of surgical site infections

PICO Question: Does preoperative shaving of the surgical site result in lower rates of surgical site infections?

Finding: From the Cochrane Collaboration: Tanner, J., Norrie, P., & Melen, K. (2011). Preoperative hair removal to reduce surgical site infections. *Cochrane Database of Systematic Reviews, 11,* CD004122.

Findings from this systematic review indicate that routine shaving of surgical sites is not associated with lower rates of surgical site infections and may pose a surgical site infection risk. If hair must be removed preoperatively from a surgical site, clippers are associated with lower rates of surgical site infections than razors.

Level of Evidence: Level I

Recommendation: You note to Terri that though shaving surgical sites may have been standard practice 15 years ago, this practice actually may pose a surgical site infection risk and is no longer advocated. If hair must be removed from a surgical site preoperatively, then clippers should be used rather than razors.

may be done on the unit or in the surgical suite immediately before the operation, usually in the surgical holding area. If hair must be removed, AORN (AORN, 2013b) recommends removing only the hair that will interfere with the surgical procedure using hair clippers as close to the time of surgery as possible (see the accompanying box, PICO in Practice: Asking Clinical Questions). Document the condition of the skin, method of hair removal and skin preparation site and agent on the patient record. Instruct the patient not to shave the area of the surgical site prior to surgery unless so directed by the physician.

ELIMINATION

Emptying the bowel of feces is no longer a routine procedure before surgery. The nurse uses preoperative assessment to determine the need for an order to facilitate bowel elimination. If the patient has not had a bowel movement for several days or has had preoperative barium diagnostic tests, an enema helps prevent postoperative constipation.

If the patient is scheduled for surgery of the lower gastrointestinal tract, a prescribed bowel prep and cleansing enema may be ordered. Peristalsis does not return for 24 to 48 hours after the bowel is handled, so preoperative cleansing helps to decrease postoperative constipation. An empty bowel also prevents contamination of the surgical area during surgery.

Insertion of an indwelling urinary catheter may be ordered before surgery, especially in patients having pelvic surgery, to prevent bladder distention or accidental injury. If an indwelling catheter is not in place, instruct the patient to void immediately before receiving preoperative medications to ensure an empty bladder during surgery.

NUTRITION AND FLUIDS

Patients need to be well nourished and hydrated before surgery to counterbalance fluid, blood, and electrolyte loss during surgery; to facilitate anesthesia delivery; and to promote tissue healing after surgery. Preoperative assessments provide a baseline for physical preparation for surgery, including the need for supplemental nutrition, fluids, or electrolytes. A patient who is undernourished may require parenteral nutrition (see Chapter 35) and IV electrolyte replacements. If the patient's screening tests show a hemoglobin level of less than 10 g/dL and a hematocrit of less than 33%, blood or blood component therapy may be given preoperatively to maintain volume and increase the oxygenation of tissue during surgery.

Although maintaining a nothing by mouth (NPO) status for at least 8 hours prior to surgery was formerly the standard, the American Society of Anesthesiologists (2011) revised practice guidelines for preoperative fasting. The new practice guidelines allow patients to drink clear liquids up to 2 hours before surgery with the order of the physician. If clear liquids are allowed, they should be carefully defined for the patient, and include water, fruit juices without pulp, carbonated beverages, clear tea, and black coffee. These liquids do not include any alcohol. Patients, especially children, may be less anxious, better hydrated, and experience fewer headaches and nausea after surgery if permitted selected fluids (including breast milk for infants) up to within 2 to 4 hours before surgery. Light meals such as tea and toast may be consumed up to 6 hours before surgery; fatty meals should be consumed up to 8 hours before surgery. Instruct patients having a colonoscopy to refrain from eating prepared foods that contain Olestra, a synthetic-fat food additive used in fat-free snack foods like potato chips. This chemical is not always totally eliminated from the bowel and causes yellow adhesive plaques to form on colonoscopes and surgical instruments. It also may cover mucosal tissue lesions.

The nurse explains the reason for being NPO to the patient and, at the appropriate time, removes all food and fluids from the bedside and places a sign over the bed so that all health team members and visitors know about the restriction. If the patient eats or drinks, notify the physician at once; the procedure may have to be delayed or cancelled.

REST AND SLEEP

Rest and sleep are important in reducing the stress before surgery and for healing and recovery after surgery. The nurse can facilitate rest and sleep in the immediate preoperative period by meeting psychological needs, carrying out teaching, providing a quiet environment, encouraging relaxation or comfort measures that are personally effective for the individual patient, or administering the prescribed bedtime sedative medication for hospitalized surgical patients.

Preparing the Patient on the Day of Surgery

A preoperative checklist is often used to outline the nurse's responsibilities on the day of surgery; these activities must be completed and documented before the patient is transported to surgery. Some of these activities have already been described (e.g., NPO, preoperative teaching, informed consent, skin preparation, screening tests, bladder elimination).

Preoperative medications that might be prescribed are as follows:

- Sedatives, such as diazepam (Valium), midazolam (Versed), or lorazepam (Ativan) to alleviate anxiety and decrease recall of events related to surgery
- Anticholinergics, such as atropine and glycopyrrolate (Robinul), to decrease pulmonary and oral secretions and to prevent laryngospasm
- Narcotic analgesics, such as morphine, to facilitate patient sedation and relaxation and to decrease the amount of anesthetic agent needed
- Neuroleptanalgesic agents, such as fentanyl citrate–droperidol (Innovar), to cause a general state of calmness and sleepiness
- Histamine-2 receptor blockers, such as cimetidine (Tagamet) and ranitidine (Zantac), to decrease gastric acidity and volume

Guidelines for Nursing Care 29-3 provides further information about preoperative interventions the day of surgery for a hospitalized patient.

Evaluating

Evaluating the plan of care for the preoperative phase is based on the expected outcomes. The plan is effective if the patient is physically and emotionally prepared for surgery, verbalizes expected events and sensations of the perioperative period, and demonstrates postoperative exercises and activities.

GUIDELINES FOR NURSING CARE 29-3

PROVIDING PREOPERATIVE PATIENT CARE: HOSPITALIZED PATIENT (DAY OF SURGERY)

- Check that preoperative consent forms are signed and dated, witnessed, and correct; that advance directives are in the medical record (as applicable); and that the patient's chart is in order.
- Gather the needed equipment and supplies.
- Perform hand hygiene.
- **Check vital signs.** Notify physician of any pertinent changes (i.e., rise or drop in blood pressure, elevated temperature, cough, symptoms of infection).
- Provide hygiene and oral care. Assess for loose teeth. **Verify adherence to food and fluid restrictions before surgery.**
- Instruct the patient to remove all personal clothing, including underwear, and put on a hospital gown.
- Ask patient to remove cosmetics, jewelry including body piercing, nail polish, and prostheses (e.g., contact lenses, false eyelashes, dentures). Some facilities allow a wedding band to be left in place, depending on the type of surgery, provided it is secured to the finger with tape.
- If possible, give valuables to a family member or place valuables in an appropriate area, such as the hospital safe if this is not possible.

- **Have patient empty bladder before surgery.**
- Attend to any special preoperative orders, such as starting an IV line.
- Complete preoperative checklist and record of patient's preoperative preparation.
- **Administer preoperative medication as prescribed by physician/anesthesia provider.**
- Raise side rails of bed; place bed in lowest position. Instruct patient to remain in bed or on stretcher. If necessary, a safety belt may be used.
- Help move the patient from the bed to the transport stretcher if necessary. Reconfirm patient identification and ensure that all preoperative events and measures are documented.
- Tell the family of the patient where the patient will be taken after surgery and the location of the waiting area where the surgeon will come to explain the outcome of the surgery.
- After the patient leaves for the OR, prepare the room and make a postoperative bed for the patient. Anticipate any necessary equipment based on the type of surgery and the patient's history.

THE NURSING PROCESS FOR INTRAOPERATIVE CARE

The intraoperative phase of surgery begins with admission of the patient to the surgical area and lasts until the patient is transferred to the PACU or other recovery area. The perioperative nurse has critical responsibilities and roles in collaboratively meeting patient needs. The nursing process uses the preoperative data and plan as a basis for the intraoperative plan of care.

Assessing

The first room the patient enters when transferred to the surgical area is the preoperative holding area. Nurses in surgical scrub attire identify the surgical patient, assess the patient's emotional and physical status, and verify the information on the preoperative checklist including assessment data, lab reports, and consents for surgery and blood transfusion. They may also carry out required immediate preoperative care, including performing skin preparation, starting IV fluids, placing intermittent pneumatic compression devices (IPCDs) to prevent DVT, determining pain level, assuring patient and family, providing comfort, and giving preoperative medications. The nurse also assesses the patient's response to the procedures, and explains the events of surgery.

The Joint Commission (TJC), an independent accrediting agency for health care organizations and agencies, has established a standard universal protocol to prevent wrong-site, wrong-procedure, and wrong-person surgery. The universal protocol has three components (TJC, 2014):

1. Preoperative patient identification verification process
2. Marking the operative site
3. Final verification just prior to beginning the procedure, referred to as the **time-out**

The time-out occurs immediately before starting the surgical procedure and is initiated by a designated member of the team. The surgeon, the anesthesia provider, the circulating nurse, the operating room technician and any other active participants conduct the time-out assessment and ensure that there are no questions or concerns. During the time-out, all members of the surgical team must agree on the identity of the patient, the correct surgical site, and the procedure that will be performed. The completion of the time-out is documented appropriately.

When the operating room (OR) is ready, the patient is transported to the OR. Once the patient transfers from the stretcher to the OR bed, the patient is identified again with the operative team using at least two identifiers (such as name, birth date). The patient is then anesthetized, positioned, prepped, and draped. The perioperative nurse assesses the patient and reviews preoperative data, paying particular attention to factors that increase surgical risk. To maintain patient safety, the nurse also assesses the patient during positioning and monitors supplies used.

Diagnosing

Patient problems in the intraoperative period may occur as a result of the position of the patient, the effects of the anesthesia, equipment used, disruption of tissues during surgery, and the incision. See Examples of NANDA-I Nursing Diagnoses: The Intraoperative Patient.

Outcome Identification and Planning

The planning phase of the nursing process focuses on identifying interventions most effective for preventing complications, anticipating patient problems, and ensuring patient safety. Some expected outcomes are that the patient will:

- Remain free of neuromuscular injury
- Remain free from wrong-site, wrong-side, wrong-patient surgical procedure
- Maintain fluid and electrolyte balance
- Maintain skin integrity (other than for the incision)
- Have symmetric breathing patterns
- Be free of injury from burns, retained surgical items (inaccurate count of sharps, instruments, and soft goods such as surgical sponges used during the procedure), and medication errors
- Remain free from surgical-site infection
- Maintain normothermia

EXAMPLES OF NANDA-I NURSING DIAGNOSES

THE INTRAOPERATIVE PATIENT

Nursing Diagnoses	Related Factors	Sample Defining Characteristics
Risk for Imbalanced Fluid Volume	Hemorrhage Failure of regulatory mechanisms	• Increased pulse rate with decreased volume • Decreased blood pressure
Risk for Perioperative Positioning Injury	Any lengthy surgical procedure requiring special intraoperative positioning	*Risk Factors* • Aging • Obesity • Anesthesia, with resulting sensory/perceptual alterations • Emaciation

Implementing

During surgery, nurses function as scrub nurses and circulating nurses, in an expanded role as registered nurse first assistants (RNFAs), or as advanced practice registered nurses (APRNs).

The scrub nurse is a member of the sterile team who maintains sterile technique while draping and handling instruments and supplies. The circulating nurse identifies and assesses the patient on admission to the operating room, and collaborates with multiple surgical team members to provide safe patient care, including the following: carefully positioning the patient on the OR bed; using an approved antimicrobial agent to prepare the skin at the surgical site (prep); placing a Foley catheter (if indicated); assisting with monitoring the patient during surgery; providing additional supplies; anticipating needs of the surgical team to facilitate the procedure; maintaining environmental safety; and counting the number of instruments, sharp items such as needles, and soft goods such as sponges used during the surgery to prevent the accidental loss of an item in the surgical site. The RNFA actively assists the surgeon by providing exposure of the operative area, hemostasis (by using surgical clamps or other medical devices on bleeding tissue), and wound closure. The APRN coordinates care activities; collaborates with physicians and nurses in all phases of perioperative and postanesthesia care; and integrates case management, critical paths, and research into care of the surgical patient. Additional educational preparation is required for the roles of the RNFA and the APRN.

Recent information based on findings from the National Practitioner Data Bank that handles medical malpractice claims indicates the frequency that "never events" occur in the surgical setting. **Never events** are serious but preventable surgical errors that are reported about 4,000 times each year (Nordqvist, 2012). Examples of these errors include leaving a foreign object in the patient's body, performing the wrong surgery, or operating on the incorrect body site (Agency for Healthcare Research and Quality [AHRQ], 2012). Safety procedures implemented to prevent never events include the previously mentioned time-out checks, marking the surgical site, and using electronic bar codes to count sponges, towels, and surgical instruments before and after surgery (Nordqvist, 2012). These never events are considered sentinel events by the Joint Commission, and the Centers for Medicare and Medicaid Services (CMS) does not reimburse hospitals for any expenses incurred as a result of a preventable patient injury. Public reporting of these errors improves the quality of care and hospitals are under increased pressure to correct the problems that contribute to these events (AHRQ, 2012).

Positioning

The patient is placed in a specific operative position after anesthesia has produced loss of consciousness and reflexes. Ensure patient safety, comfort, good body alignment and padding of bony surfaces in positioning to prevent alterations in neuromuscular (Bouyer-Farullo, 2013), integumentary, respiratory, and vascular function. The risk for skin injury is avoided by lifting, rather than rolling or pulling, the patient into the surgical position. Rolling or pulling can cause a shearing force, in which two or more tissue layers slide on each other, stretching subcutaneous blood vessels, obstructing blood flow, and contributing to pressure ulcers. Preoperative assessment findings guide the nurse in knowing extremity limitations and other functional needs to individualize patient care.

Although all of the operative positions are not described here, perioperative nurses need to know the position to be used and significant nursing considerations for that position. Two examples are the Trendelenburg position and the lithotomy position. The Trendelenburg position requires lowering the upper torso and raising the feet. It is commonly used in minimally invasive surgery of the lower abdomen or pelvis. The displacement of the abdominal viscera toward the head decreases diaphragmatic movement and respiratory exchange; blood pools in the upper torso, and blood pressure increases; and hypotension can result with return to the supine position. Shearing with resultant tissue damage is also a significant risk in this position. The lithotomy position is used for gynecologic, rectal, and urologic procedures. The placement of legs in stirrups causes pooling of blood in the legs, increasing the risk of thrombophlebitis. Pressure can also damage the peroneal nerve, with resultant foot drop. Patients can experience lower back strain if they are not positioned slowly and carefully. Refer to Chapter 25 for additional information regarding body positions.

Draping

Drapes are used to create and maintain a sterile field around the operative site, preventing the passage of microorganisms, particulate matter, and fluids between sterile and nonsterile areas. The only area left exposed is the incision site. In some cases, plastic adhesive drapes may be used to form a complete seal over the skin. With these drapes, skin color is visible, and the incision is made through the impermeable adhesive drape.

Documenting

Throughout surgery, the perioperative nurse documents on the intraoperative record ongoing patient assessment, item counts (soft goods, sharps, instruments), monitoring data (e.g., vital signs, urine output, blood loss, pulse oximetry results, body temperature), positioning, medications, dressings and drains, specimens, equipment used (electrosurgery unit and settings, ultrasound, video, stirrups for positioning), and responses to care. This documentation includes planning and implementation of perioperative nursing activities and evaluation of the achievement of patient outcomes.

Transferring to the Postanesthesia Care Unit (PACU)

After completion of the surgical procedure and emergence from anesthesia, the patient is moved carefully from the operating bed to a stretcher or bed. This is a critical time: sudden or rough handling can cause severe hypotension or potentially lethal cardiac or respiratory arrest. The patient is then transported to the PACU, and the OR nurse provides a hand-off report to the PACU nurse containing relevant preoperative and intraoperative assessments and interventions. The primary objective of the hand-off report from OR nurse to PACU nurse is to provide accurate information about the patient's care, procedure, tourniquet time, drains, medications used, presenting condition, and any important events that occurred during the procedure. It allows for communication, clarification and questions, and continuity of care.

Evaluating

Evaluation of the effectiveness of the plan of care for the intraoperative phase is based on the expected outcomes. If met, the plan was effective.

POSTOPERATIVE NURSING CARE

The postoperative phase can be divided into two stages—immediate care (usually provided in the PACU in both in-hospital and outpatient/same-day surgery centers) and ongoing postoperative care (lasting from return to the unit through convalescence). Nursing assessments and interventions are consistent with those in the preoperative and intraoperative phases and are carried out to maintain function, promote recovery, and facilitate coping with alterations in structure or function. (See the accompanying Through the Eyes of a Student.) Assessments and nursing interventions are combined in discussing immediate postoperative care; the phases of the nursing process are used to describe ongoing postoperative care.

Immediate Postoperative Assessment and Care

Care in the PACU involves assessing the postoperative patient, with emphasis on preventing complications from anesthesia and/or the surgery. Assessments are continuous, using preoperative and intraoperative data as bases for comparison. The assessments made in the PACU include respiratory status (airway, pulse oximetry), cardiovascular status (blood pressure), temperature, central nervous system status (level of alertness, movement, shivering), fluid status, wound status, gastrointestinal status (nausea and vomiting), and general condition. These assessments initially are made every 10 to 15 minutes. Children can quickly lose their airway and go into a crisis. Therefore, they must be monitored at least every 5 minutes. Emergence delirium, waking up thrashing and disoriented, is common in children. Emergence delirium may start in the OR and may continue into PACU. It is important to safeguard patients from hurting themselves.

The average PACU stay is about 1 hour, but it will vary depending on the type of surgery, length of anesthesia, and patient response. Outpatient/same-day surgery patients return home after full recovery in the PACU or phase 2 recovery. The critical role functions of the PACU nurse include vigilant monitoring during emergence from anesthesia and the first hours after surgery, pain management, fluid and electrolyte balance, stabilization of physiologic parameters (such as heart and respiratory rate), and preparation for the next level of care.

 MR. Benjamin, the older adult who has had a total hip replacement, will require frequent assessments during his stay in the PACU, specifically vital signs, cardiovascular status, respiratory status, IV therapy, wound status, and urinary elimination. If he had spinal anesthesia, neurologic assessments would be done every 15 minutes. ●

Respiratory Status

The nurse assesses respiratory function by monitoring respiratory rate, rhythm, and depth; auscultating breath sounds;

THROUGH THE EYES OF A STUDENT

The first time I took care of a patient with "multiple tubes," I was horrified at the thought of actually touching the patient. I hadn't really been exposed to that many critically ill patients until my last semester as a student nurse. I remember being assigned a patient in the cardiothoracic intensive care unit. The patient was a "fresh heart"—a coronary artery bypass graft patient who had just been operated on that morning.

I remember walking into the room and thinking, "What do I do with all of these tubes?" and then with horror thinking, "What if one of them falls out?" Needless to say, I was overwhelmed and frightened but at the same time excited at the challenge that faced me. I asked my preceptor what

each tube was for and where it was hooked up and whether it would fall out if I touched it. She answered all my questions with patience and understanding and asked me if I wanted to handle the tubes. I looked at her as if she were insane, but went ahead and did it. Would you believe that nothing fell out! I must admit that the experience taught me a lot, but it also got me over the fear of tubes.

I now chuckle every time I see a nursing student's face with that same look of horror as I had, and I try to answer every question with the same degree of patience and understanding that my preceptor had for me.

—Lynda L. Ullmer, RN, Gaithersburg, MD

noting the oxygen saturation level and PCO_2 levels; assessing skin color; and observing cardiovascular and mental status. During a surgical procedure with general anesthesia, an endotracheal tube may be inserted to administer the anesthetic gases and maintain patent air passages. This artificial airway is not removed until the laryngeal and pharyngeal reflexes return, allowing the patient to control the tongue, cough, and swallow. If newer short-acting anesthetic agents are used, the endotracheal tube is usually removed in the OR. The nurse assesses the patient's airway for patency, administers oxygen, and initiates pulse oximetry. Ineffective respiratory function is indicated by restlessness and anxiety; unequal chest expansion with use of accessory muscles; shallow, noisy respirations; cyanosis; and tachycardia.

Respiratory obstruction is the most common PACU emergency. It may occur as a result of secretion accumulation, obstruction by the tongue, laryngospasm (a sudden, violent contraction of the vocal cords), or laryngeal edema. Respiratory obstruction is indicated by assessments of ineffective respiratory function plus observing for wheezing or crowing sounds with respiratory effort. Positioning, administering humidified oxygen, encouraging the patient to take deep breaths, and suctioning may be used to maintain a patent airway and tissue oxygenation. In case of laryngospasm, call for help. Jaw thrusts, positive pressure ventilation, emergency medications, and even reintubation may be necessary (Salem, Crystal, & Nimmagadda, 2012).

Cardiovascular Status

Assess cardiovascular function by taking vital signs, monitoring electrocardiogram rate and rhythm, and observing skin color and condition. Compare blood pressure findings with baseline data from the preoperative period. Transient hypertension can occur as a result of anesthetic effects, respiratory insufficiency, the surgical procedure, or the excitement phase of recovery from anesthesia.

Hypotension may be the result of varied factors, including anesthetic agents, preoperative medications, position changes, blood loss, respiratory alterations, and peripheral blood pooling. Oxygen administration, deep breathing, leg exercises, verbal stimulation (to help expel anesthetic gases and facilitate increasing level of consciousness), and maintaining accurate IV flow rates can raise low blood pressure.

Patients are at risk for altered body temperature related to the surgical procedure, its length, anesthetic agents, a cool surgical environment, age, and use of cool irrigating or infusion fluids. Inadvertent hypothermia (temperature below 36°C [96°F]) can lead to complications of poor wound healing, hemodynamic stress, cardiac disturbances, coagulopathy, delayed emergence from anesthesia, and shivering and its associated discomfort (AORN, 2013b). Measure the patient's body temperature, usually by the temporal or tympanic route, and initiate interventions if the patient complains of being cold or is hypothermic. Warmed blankets placed on the patient's body and forced warm-air devices are used for rewarming.

Assess all pulses for bilateral equality, rhythm, rate, and character. Of special significance are assessments of abnormal function—an irregular rhythm, absence of pulses, or tachycardia. Carefully evaluate for tachycardia, an early symptom of shock. Other related assessments for shock are a decreasing blood pressure, cyanosis, a cool skin temperature, and a decrease in urine output. After surgery on an extremity, closely monitor pulse checks, neurologic checks, color, temperature and sensation.

Central Nervous System Status

The return of central nervous system function is assessed through the patient's response to stimuli and orientation. Consciousness returns in reverse order, with the usual pattern being: (1) unconsciousness, (2) response to touch and sounds, (3) drowsiness, (4) awake but not oriented, and (5) awake and oriented. Nurses in the PACU verbally reorient the patient by gently touching and calling the patient by name. If the patient had spinal anesthesia, neurologic checks are done every 15 minutes for the first hour.

Fluid Status

Fluid imbalance may result from factors such as preoperative fluid restriction, fluid loss during surgery, wound drainage, or the surgical stress response (with retention of sodium and water). Imbalanced fluid volume (deficit or excess) is a risk for all surgical patients but is an especially important consideration in children and older adults. Assessing fluid status includes skin turgor, vital signs, urine output, wound drainage, and IV fluid intake and blood product administration. IV fluid administration assessments include the type of fluid infused, the rate, location of lines, condition of the IV insertion site, and the security and patency of the tubing.

Wound Status

The nurse in the PACU assesses the dressing over the incision for amount, consistency, and color of drainage as well as for any tubes or drains and the amount and type of drainage by that route. Large amounts of bright-red drainage, combined with other abnormal physical status assessments (restlessness, pallor, cool moist skin, decreasing blood pressure, increasing pulse and respiratory rates), may indicate hemorrhage and hypovolemic shock. Report these symptoms immediately.

 Concept Mastery Alert

If a large amount of fresh red drainage appears on a patient's dressing, the nurse should *not* remove the dressing and apply a new one. It is best to reinforce the dressing with additional bandages to reduce the possibility of hemorrhage resulting from dislodging clots that may be forming.

Pain Management

Pain is both a subjective and an objective experience. Pain management experts recommend the assessment of pain using a rating scale. The scale may be verbal (ranging from no pain to worst possible pain), numeric (with 10 on a scale of 0 to 10 being the worst possible pain), or a "faces" rating scale, ranging from a smiley face indicating no pain to a face that has frowns and tears for worst possible pain (see Chapter 34). Initial pain management, using nonsteroidal anti-inflammatory drugs (NSAIDs) and opiates, occurs in the PACU. Opiates may be delivered by PCA, allowing the patient to control the analgesic administration. Nonpharmacologic methods to decrease pain and improve comfort include positioning, verbal reassurance, and touch. Preoperative determination of methods that are personally effective for the patient assist in effective implementation in the PACU. These should supplement, not substitute for, pharmacologic pain relief.

General Condition

Other assessments and interventions are made to ensure physical and emotional comfort and safety. Constant reorientation and reassurance that the surgery is completed provide psychological comfort. Careful assessments, proper positioning, and use of side rails maintain physical safety. The patient is discharged from the PACU when physical status and level of consciousness are considered stable. The PACU nurse should notify the family that the patient is being transferred back to the patient's room, and give a

verbal and written hand-off report to the unit nurse about the assessments and interventions during the intraoperative and immediate postoperative phases.

Ongoing Postoperative Care

Ongoing postoperative care is planned to facilitate recovery from surgery and coping with alterations. The plan of care includes promoting physical and psychological health, preventing complications, and teaching self-care when the patient returns home. Skill 29-2 on pages 889–894 outlines initial and ongoing postoperative patient care.

THE NURSING PROCESS FOR ONGOING POSTOPERATIVE CARE

Assessing

The nurse on the unit assists PACU personnel in transferring the patient to the bed in the unit and makes an initial assessment using data from the preoperative and intraoperative phases. A postoperative checklist or flow sheet may be used. The initial assessment is often combined with the implementation of postoperative physician's orders. See Table 29-2 for focused assessments and interventions.

Table 29-2	POSTOPERATIVE ASSESSMENTS AND INTERVENTIONS ON RETURN TO THE UNIT
FACTORS TO ASSESS	**ASSESSMENTS AND INTERVENTIONS**
Vital signs and oxygen saturation	• Temperature, blood pressure, pulse and respiratory rates; oxygen saturation • Note, report, and document deviations from preoperative and PACU data as well as symptoms of complications.
Color and temperature of skin	• Skin color (pallor, cyanosis), skin temperature, and diaphoresis
Level of consciousness	• Orientation to time, place, and person • Reaction to stimuli and ability to move all four extremities
Intravenous fluids	• Type and amount of solution, flow rate, security and patency of tubing • Infusion site
Surgical site	• Dressing and dependent areas for drainage (color, amount, consistency) • Drains and tubes; be sure they are intact, patent, and properly connected to drainage systems.
Other tubes	• Assess indwelling urinary catheter, gastrointestinal suction, and others for drainage, patency, and amount of output. • Ensure that dependent drainage bags are hanging properly and suction drainage is attached and functioning. • If oxygen is ordered, ensure placement of ordered application and flow rate.
Comfort	• Assess pain (location, duration, intensity) and determine whether analgesics were given in the PACU. • Assess for nausea and vomiting. • Cover the patient with a blanket. • Reorient to the room as necessary. • Allow family members to remain with the patient after the initial assessment is completed.
Position and safety	• Place the patient in an ordered position, *or* • If the patient is not fully conscious, place in the side-lying position. • Elevate the side rails and place the bed in low position.

EXAMPLES OF NANDA-I NURSING DIAGNOSES

THE POSTOPERATIVE PATIENT

Nursing Diagnoses	Related Factors	Sample Defining Characteristics
Risk for Infection	Any condition that interferes with normal inflammatory healing process or provides an entry for infectious agents	*Risk Factors* • Obesity • Aging • Immunosuppression • Malnutrition • Presence of incision • Decreased ability to cough, deep breathe, use incentive spirometer • Presence of drains, tubes, and catheters • Insertion site for intravenous therapy
Acute Pain	Any condition that causes actual tissue damage, such as the surgical incision	• Rating pain as severe on a scale of 1 to 10 (i.e., as a 9) • Positioning or guarding self to avoid pain • Inability to sleep • Loss of appetite • Diaphoresis, changes in vital signs, dilated pupils • Moaning, crying, sighing

After conducting the assessment, document the time of arrival and all assessment data. Facility protocol is followed for assessment routines: Common time frames are every 15 minutes until stable, changing to every 1 to 2 hours for the first 24 hours, and every 4 hours thereafter. Although protocols are used as guidelines in the immediate postoperative period, the nurse is responsible for adjusting the frequency and priorities of assessment to the specific needs of each patient.

Diagnosing

Nursing diagnoses in the postoperative phase cover observed problems or those for which the patient is at risk. When making nursing diagnoses, the nurse uses assessment data and plans of care established before and during surgery, and may consult with the family for verification of nursing diagnosis. See Examples of NANDA-I Nursing Diagnoses appropriate to the postoperative period.

Outcome Identification and Planning

The plan of care in the postoperative phase begins in the preoperative phase, when nursing activities to reduce stress and teach postoperative activities are implemented. From admission, prepare the patient and family for uneventful recovery and self-care after discharge. Individualize specific expected outcomes based on risk factors, the surgical procedure, and the patient's unique needs. Examples of desired postoperative outcomes for a patient after major surgery are as follows:

The patient will:

• Carry out leg exercises every 2 to 4 hours.
• Deep breathe and cough effectively every 2 hours.
• Verbalize decreasing levels of pain.
• Have a balanced intake and output.
• Regain normal bowel and bladder elimination.

• Exhibit a healing surgical incision.
• Remain free of infection.
• Verbalize any concerns about appearance of wound.
• Verbalize and demonstrate wound self-care.

Implementing

Many nursing interventions in the postoperative phase have already been discussed in this chapter or are fully discussed in other chapters. Therefore, this section focuses on nursing interventions to meet the expected outcomes of the plan of care. Nursing care is discussed to prevent complications, promote a return to health, and facilitate coping with alterations in function and/or body image.

A wide variety of factors increase the risk of postoperative complications, including age, health habits, physical condition, medical history, psychological status, and surgical intervention (e.g., anesthesia, positioning, wound). Ongoing postoperative assessments and interventions are implemented to decrease the risk for postoperative complications. If they occur, provide physical assessments and care and emotional support to the patient and family, and carry out prescribed treatments. See Nursing Advocacy in Action (on page 878) for an example of a patient who may require an advocate.

Preventing Cardiovascular Complications

Nursing interventions to prevent or monitor for cardiovascular complications are listed in Box 29-4 (on page 878). Specific cardiovascular complications include hemorrhage, shock, thrombophlebitis, and pulmonary embolus.

HEMORRHAGE

Hemorrhage is an excessive internal or external blood loss, and may lead to hypovolemic shock. It may occur from any number of causes. Common manifestations

NURSING ADVOCACY IN ACTION

Patient Scenario

Alex is a 28-year-old man admitted to the surgical intensive care unit after undergoing a partial gastric bypass surgical procedure. He originally weighed 700 lbs but lost 100 lbs prior to being approved for the surgery. Patients like Alex are usually admitted to the intensive care unit for airway management and to ensure strict adherence to fluid intake restrictions needed to maintain the integrity of the suture line. You are assigned to care for Alex. The nurse giving the report says the following:

- "Alex is noncompliant with the fluid intake restrictions. He tries to sneak water. I don't know why we have to care for patients who are not willing to follow the medical treatment plan that they agreed to before surgery."
- "He should be repositioned hourly but since he's not motivated to participate with his ADLs, especially bathing and turning in bed, I wouldn't worry. Why should

we take a risk of hurting ourselves when he obviously doesn't care?"
- "His mother told the charge nurse yesterday that caregivers were making comments related to his size and were not providing the same quality of care as they gave to other patients."

Implications for Nursing Advocacy

How will you respond if you are Alex's nurse? Talk with your classmates and experienced nurses about the questions that follow.

- If you elect to advocate for Alex, what practical steps can you take to ensure better health outcomes?
- What is reasonable to expect of a student nurse, a graduate nurse, and an experienced nurse in this situation?
- What advocacy skills are needed to effectively respond to this challenge?

---

of hemorrhage include restlessness, anxiety, and frank bleeding as well as hypotension; cold, clammy skin; a weak, thready, and rapid pulse; cool, mottled extremities; deep, rapid respirations; decreased urine output; thirst; and apprehension. The primary priorities for the patient experiencing a hemorrhage is to stop the bleeding and replace blood volume. Nursing interventions include calling the medical intervention team, notifying the surgeon immediately, applying a pressure dressing to the bleeding site, and being prepared to have the patient return to the OR if bleeding cannot be stopped.

SHOCK

Shock is the body's reaction to acute circulatory failure as the result of an alteration in circulatory control or a loss of intravascular fluid. The type of shock most commonly seen in postoperative patients is hypovolemic shock, which occurs from a decrease in blood volume. Common manifestations of shock are the same as those for hemorrhage.

The primary priority for a patient in shock is to improve and maintain tissue perfusion by eliminating the cause

of the shock. Nursing interventions include calling for the medical intervention team and notifying the surgeon immediately; establishing and maintaining the airway; placing the patient in a flat position with the legs elevated 30 to 45 degrees; administering oxygen; monitoring vital signs, hematocrit, and blood gas results; maintaining body warmth with covers; and administering medications. The nurse must also be prepared to assist with the insertion of IV lines and to administer fluids as well as whole blood or its components.

 Concept Mastery Alert

Monitoring urine output is an important nursing intervention because adequate urine output indicates adequate tissue perfusion.

THROMBOPHLEBITIS

Thrombophlebitis is an inflammation of a vein associated with thrombus (blood clot) formation. Thrombophlebitis from venous stasis is most commonly seen

---

Box 29-4 NURSING INTERVENTIONS TO PREVENT OR MONITOR POSTOPERATIVE CARDIOVASCULAR COMPLICATIONS

- Assess and document vital signs as ordered and as the patient's status dictates, using preoperative assessments as a baseline.
- Provide covers, forced warm air, or other warming device or techniques as necessary to prevent shivering and hypothermia.
- Maintain fluid balance.
- Maintain accurate intake and output.
- Monitor rate, type, and access site of intravenous fluids.
- Assess skin turgor and hydration of mucous membranes.
- Monitor amount, color, and consistency of wound drainage (dressings and drains or tubes).
- Implement leg exercises and turning in bed every 2 hours.

- Assist with ambulation. Ambulation usually begins the evening of surgery and increases as tolerated; blood pressure and pulse and respiratory rates are used to monitor tolerance.
- Apply and follow protocols for graduated compression stockings or pneumatic compression devices, if ordered.
- Administer anticoagulant medications, if prescribed.
- Measure bilateral calf and thigh circumference daily.
- Assess for leg swelling, tenderness or palpable venous cord.
- Avoid positioning that impedes venous return (e.g., do not mechanically raise the knee portion of the bed or place pillows under the knees).

in the legs of postoperative patients. Manifestations of thrombophlebitis are pain and cramping in the calf or thigh of the involved extremity, redness and swelling in the affected area, elevated temperature, and an increase in the diameter of the involved extremity.

The primary priorities for the patient with thrombophlebitis are preventing a clot from breaking loose and becoming an embolus that travels to the lungs, heart, or brain, and preventing further clot formation. Nursing interventions include notifying the surgeon, administering medications (e.g., anti-inflammatory agents, anticoagulants, analgesics), maintaining the patient on bed rest, applying external heat, and applying graduated compression stockings or intermittent pneumatic compression (IPC) devices (Alexander-Magalee, 2013; Box 29-5). It is also important during every shift to assess the legs for swelling and tenderness; measure bilateral calf or thigh circumference; and determine if the patient experiences any chest pain or dyspnea (Zrelak, Utter, Cuny, & Romano, 2012). Instruct the patient not to massage the legs.

Preventing Respiratory Complications

Nursing interventions to prevent respiratory complications include monitoring vital signs; implementing deep breathing, coughing, and incentive spirometry; turning in bed every 2 hours; ambulating; maintaining hydration; avoiding positioning that decreases ventilation; and monitoring responses to narcotic analgesics. At the 2012 American College of Surgeons (ACS) Annual Clinical Congress, McAneny reported on a postoperative pulmonary care program known as I COUGH[SM], which reduced respiratory complications. I COUGH stands for (ACS, 2012):

- **I**ncentive spirometry
- **C**oughing/deep breathing
- **O**ral care
- **U**nderstanding (patient and staff education)
- **G**etting out of bed at least three times daily
- **H**ead of bed elevation

Specific respiratory complications include pulmonary embolus, pneumonia, and atelectasis.

PULMONARY EMBOLUS

An **embolus** is a blood clot or foreign substance that is dislodged and travels through the bloodstream until it lodges in a smaller vessel. In postoperative patients, the embolus is often part of a thrombus that breaks free from a vein wall. If the embolus lodges in the pulmonary vessels, it is called a pulmonary embolus. Manifestations of a pulmonary embolus include dyspnea, chest pain, cough, cyanosis, rapid respirations, tachycardia, and anxiety. This is a life-threatening condition and immediate treatment is necessary. The primary goals of care are to stabilize cardiovascular and respiratory function as well as prevent further emboli. Nursing interventions include notifying the physician immediately, calling the medical intervention team, maintaining the patient on bed rest in the semi-Fowler's position, assessing vital signs frequently, administering oxygen, administering medications (e.g., anticoagulants, analgesics), and instructing the patient to avoid Valsalva's maneuver (forced exhalation against a closed glottis, such as straining to have a bowel movement) to prevent

---

BOX 29-5 INTERMITTENT PNEUMATIC COMPRESSION (IPC) DEVICES

Pneumatic compression devices are composed of an air pump, connecting tubes, and an extremity sleeve. The sleeve may cover the entire leg or may extend from the foot to the knee. A variety of types are available; the accompanying figure provides one example. The devices apply brief pressure to the legs to enhance blood flow and venous return, thereby decreasing the risk for thrombophlebitis after surgery. The devices may apply either intermittent or sequential pressure. Intermittent pneumatic compression (IPC) devices fit over the entire leg, with inflation and deflation of the sleeve covering the leg alternating from one leg to the other by a preset timer. Sequential pneumatic compression devices are designed so that pressure moves up the leg in increments. They may inflate and deflate by alternating from one leg to the other, or they may do so for both legs at once.

Nursing Care

- Explain the purpose of the device to the patient.
- Apply the device according to the manufacturer's instructions, making sure that two fingers fit between the leg and the sleeve.
- Position the tubing so the patient can move about without interrupting the airflow.
- Remove the sleeves at least once a day for skin care and assessment.

- Assess the extremities for peripheral pulses, edema, changes in sensation, and movement on a regular schedule.
- Ensure that all chambers are inflating in proper sequence once per shift.

Intermittent or sequential pneumatic compression devices.

increased intrathoracic pressure and, possibly, increased emboli.

PNEUMONIA

Pneumonia is an inflammation of the alveoli as the result of an infectious process or the presence of foreign material. Pneumonia may occur postoperatively as a result of aspiration, infection, depressed cough reflex, increased secretions from anesthesia, dehydration, and immobilization. Manifestations of pneumonia include fever, chills, a cough that produces rusty or purulent sputum, crackles and wheezes, dyspnea, and chest pain. The primary goals of care are to treat the underlying infection, maintain respiratory function, and prevent the spread of microorganisms. Nursing interventions include those used to prevent or monitor for respiratory complications and promoting full aeration of the lungs by positioning the patient in semi-Fowler's or Fowler's position, administering oxygen, administering medications (e.g., antibiotics, expectorants, analgesics), providing frequent oral hygiene, and ensuring rest and comfort.

ATELECTASIS

Atelectasis is the incomplete expansion or collapse of alveoli with retained mucus, involving a portion of lung and resulting in poor gas exchange. Manifestations of atelectasis include decreased lung sounds over the affected area, dyspnea, cyanosis, crackles, restlessness, and apprehension. The primary goals of care are to ensure oxygenation of tissues, prevent further atelectasis, and expand involved lung tissues. Nursing interventions include those used to prevent or monitor for respiratory complications, and positioning the patient in semi-Fowler's position, administering oxygen, and administering analgesics for pain. For a sudden onset, notify the surgeon immediately and call the medical intervention team.

Preventing Surgical Site Complications

The nurse assesses and cares for the surgical site to promote healing and prevent complications such as infection, dehiscence (wound closure separation), and evisceration (protrusion of intra-abdominal organs). Wound care is discussed in Chapter 31. Nursing interventions to prevent surgical site complications are assessing vital signs (especially for fever); maintaining hydration; maintaining nutritional status; encouraging a diet high in proteins, carbohydrates, calories, and vitamins; using proper hand hygiene; and following aseptic technique when changing dressings at the surgical site and exit sites for tubes and drains. Dispose of soiled gloves and dressings following standard precautions. Surgical Care Improvement Project (SCIP) core measures recommend that antibiotics be discontinued within 24 hours after surgery end time to prevent proliferation of resistant bacteria. SCIP also states that blood glucose should be maintained at normal levels to promote wound healing and that Foley catheters should be discontinued on postoperative day 1 or 2 (TJC, 2012).

Promoting a Return to Health

Nurses provide interventions during postoperative recovery to promote physical and psychological functioning at as near a normal state as possible. The plan of care to achieve this objective includes activities to meet elimination, fluid and electrolyte balance, nutrition, rest and comfort, and pain management needs.

ELIMINATION NEEDS

Both urinary and bowel elimination are altered by anesthesia, manipulation of organs during surgery, inactivity, pain medication, and altered fluid and food intake during the perioperative period. Assessments and nursing interventions to promote the return of normal bowel and urinary elimination are outlined in Box 29-6.

BOX 29-6 NURSING ASSESSMENTS AND INTERVENTIONS TO MEET POSTOPERATIVE ELIMINATION NEEDS

Bowel Elimination

- Assess for the return of peristalsis by auscultating bowel sounds every 4 hours when the patient is awake.
- Assess abdominal distention, especially if bowel sounds are not audible or are high pitched (indicative of possible paralytic ileus, which is an absence of intestinal peristalsis).
- Assess ability to pass flatus and stool.
- Assist with movement in bed and ambulation to relieve gas pains, a common postoperative discomfort.
- Encourage food and fluid intake when ordered, especially fruit juices and high-fiber foods.
- Maintain privacy when patient is using the bedpan, urinal, commode, or bathroom.
- Administer suppositories, enemas, or medications, such as stool softeners, as prescribed.

Urinary Elimination

- Monitor patterns of intake and output.
- Assist in assuming normal position to void by using an upright position when on a bedpan and using a bedside commode or bathroom when able, or by assisting the male patient to stand upright to void with a urinal.
- Assess for bladder distention by palpating above the symphysis pubis if the patient has not voided within 8 hours after surgery or if the patient has been voiding frequently in amounts of less than 50 mL; notify the physician of abnormal assessment results.
- Maintain prescribed intravenous fluid infusion rates.
- Encourage oral fluid intake when prescribed.
- Provide privacy when the patient is using bedpan, bedside commode, urinal, or bathroom.
- Initiate urinary catheterization, if prescribed.

FLUID AND NUTRITION NEEDS

Nursing assessments and interventions to meet fluid needs include monitoring patterns of intake and output, maintaining prescribed IV fluid infusion rates, and assessing skin turgor and mucous membranes for dehydration. Nutrition needs are met by monitoring weight, providing oral hygiene before meals and as needed, monitoring postoperative dietary progression (often from clear to full liquids, then from soft to regular diet), maintaining an environment conducive to appetite (clean, neat, free of odors), encouraging the patient to sit up in bed or a chair for meals, and encouraging family presence during meals.

COMFORT AND REST NEEDS

Comfort is a priority after surgery. Factors that interfere with comfort include nausea, vomiting, thirst, hiccups, positioning in bed, room noise and temperature, and pain at the surgical site. Nursing interventions that promote rest and comfort by alleviating these problems are listed in Guidelines for Nursing Care 29-4. The nurse also promotes comfort by providing personal hygiene, keeping bed linens clean, maintaining a patient-preferred room temperature, providing quiet rest periods, and allowing family members to remain with the patient.

Helping the Patient Cope

Surgery may alter the patient's physical appearance as well as physiologic function, leading to the risk for or actual alterations in self-concept and body image. Changes in a person's self-perception can influence all of the human dimensions and areas of human functioning, including self-esteem, relationships with others, sexual identity, spiritual beliefs, sociocultural values, and independent and fulfilling engagement in activities of daily living.

Many surgical patients have the same reaction to loss of a body part as to a death (see Chapter 42). The response and adaptation to the loss are influenced by multiple factors, including age, cultural values and beliefs, sociocultural background, significance of the body part, visibility of the body part, time to prepare for the change, and support people available. A surgical patient's grief is a normal and appropriate response. It is unique to the person experiencing it, and although there are stages and phases of grief, there is no timetable for it. The nurse must be aware of the patient's needs and provide interventions to meet those needs in coping with change. Nursing interventions to facilitate coping and adaptation are outlined in Box 29-7.

BOX 29-7 NURSING INTERVENTIONS TO FACILITATE POSTOPERATIVE COPING AND ADAPTATION

- Accept each patient as a unique individual.
- Identify through verbal and nonverbal cues patients who are at risk for alteration in self-concept. The risk is increased if the patient has little support from others, a visible alteration, or an alteration that will seriously affect functional ability.
- Allow time for patients and families to verbalize their feelings about the alteration, and do not assume that all patients will have problems.
- Identify and support strengths and effective coping mechanisms.
- Encourage the patient and family to be part of goal setting and decision-making throughout the surgical experience.
- Provide teaching and honest information to the patient and family about all aspects of care.
- Work collaboratively with other members of the health care team to provide referrals and resources as necessary to meet physical, psychological, and spiritual needs.

GUIDELINES FOR NURSING CARE 29-4

PROMOTING POSTOPERATIVE REST AND COMFORT

Nausea and Vomiting
- Avoid giving large amounts of fluids or food at one time, especially after being NPO.
- Administer prescribed medications.
- Provide oral hygiene, as needed.
- Maintain clean environment.
- Avoid use of a straw.
- Avoid strong smelling food.
- Assess for possible allergy to medications, such as antibiotics or analgesics.
- Maintain bowel elimination.

Thirst
- Offer sips of water or ice chips when NPO (if permitted).
- Maintain oral hygiene.

Hiccups
- Have the patient do the following:
  - Take several swallows of water while holding the breath (if not NPO).
  - Rebreathe into a paper bag.
  - Eat a teaspoon of granulated sugar.

Surgical Pain
- Assess pain frequently; administer prescribed analgesics every 2 to 4 hours on a regular schedule during the first 24 to 36 hours after surgery.
- Reinforce preoperative teaching for pain management.
- Offer nonpharmacologic measures to supplement medications: massage, position changes, relaxation, guided imagery, meditation, music.

Providing Outpatient/Same-Day Surgery Postoperative Care

Evaluating the patient's postoperative status after outpatient/same-day surgery focuses on ensuring that the patient can be safely cared for at home. After surgery and recovery from the anesthetic, ask the patient to sit up and drink liquids. A patient who is no longer drowsy or dizzy, has stable vital signs, and has voided is allowed to go home accompanied by a responsible adult. The patient is not allowed to drive a car or go home alone on public transportation. The usual length of time from completion of surgery to discharge is 1 to 3 hours, provided that established criteria have been met. Give written and verbal instructions for home care to the patient and family. Ask the patient and family to "teach them back" to verify their understanding. The patient and nurse both sign and date that these instructions were received, reviewed, and understood.

Evaluating

The nurse may evaluate the achievement of desired outcomes for postoperative recovery and rehabilitation in a number of ways. Because the final resolution of some desired outcomes may not be apparent or measurable at the time of discharge, many institutions use follow-up telephone calls or mailed surveys to patients. It may also be possible to collaborate with the physician's office to have a patient complete a survey on the first postoperative visit. Whatever mechanism is selected, include the following important outcomes as part of evaluative criteria: absence of surgical site infection, patient satisfaction with pain management measures, return to former levels of mobility and activity, absence of postoperative discharge nausea and vomiting (PDNV), and absence of other complications for which the patient was at risk.

See Nursing Care Plan 29-1 for examples of the nursing process related to perioperative care.

NURSING PLAN OF CARE 29-1

for Gabrielle McAllister

Remember Gabrielle McAllister, the 5-year-old admitted for removal of her tonsils and adenoids in same-day surgery. When she arrived, she was clinging to her mother and crying. Her mother said, "I don't think I can stand this again, but I know it has to be done." The admitting nurse made the following assessments:

- Five-year-old female, small for age, with history of several previous surgeries for congenital cardiac defect.
- History of latex allergy.
- Crying, clinging to mother.
- Mother verbalizes fear of daughter having surgery again.

NURSING DIAGNOSIS Anxiety related to upcoming surgery manifested by child's crying and clinging to mother, mother's verbalization of fear

EXPECTED OUTCOME 1/29/15—Prior to surgery, child (and mother, as appropriate) will:

- Calmly sit on mother's lap
- Verbalize decreased anxiety (mother)
- Demonstrate knowledge of physiologic and psychological responses to surgery (mother)

NURSING INTERVENTIONS	RATIONALE	EVALUATIVE STATEMENT
Assess patient and family knowledge base.	Patient/family may be misinformed or unaware of patient's surgery or preop instructions. Prior surgery experience may have been different.	1/29/15 Outcome met: Patient/family understands expectations for surgery, is calm and cuddled on her mother's lap, clutching her toy bunny named "Bunny."
Review preop teaching.	Patient/family may need teaching or reinforcement.	*C. Smith, RN*
Clarify understanding of questions and preop instructions and teaching.	This ensures that the patient and family understand and conveys caring and compassion from the nurse.	

NURSING PLAN OF CARE 29-1 *continued*

for Gabrielle McAllister

NURSING INTERVENTIONS	RATIONALE	EVALUATIVE STATEMENT
Provide appropriate emotional support and calm environment.	Most patients respond positively to compassion and kindness.	1/29/15 Outcome met: Patient is calm and quiet. States that she is ready to have her tonsils taken out so that she will not have any more sore throats. She knows that her parents will be waiting "just next door" until she is done. States, "this is Bunny's 4th surgery."
Orient to OR environment with time and sensory information.	Information and positive interpersonal communication may decrease anxiety.	
Allow patient to take her stuffed toy bunny with her to the OR.	Favorite toys will bring comfort and sense of not being alone.	
Communicate unresolved issues to OR team.	OR team will be able to continue support measures.	*C. Smith, RN*

NURSING DIAGNOSIS Latex Allergy Response related to developed hypersensitivity to natural latex rubber from multiple exposures

EXPECTED OUTCOME 1/29/15—During the perioperative period, the child will:
- Remain free of signs and symptoms of latex allergy

NURSING INTERVENTIONS	RATIONALE	EVALUATIVE STATEMENT
Assess patient environment for latex-containing items.	Patients with a latex allergy may have allergic response to any object containing latex.	1/29/15 Outcome met. Latex allergy bracelet applied to left wrist. No signs or symptoms of latex reaction on transfer to OR.
Provide latex-free or latex-safe substitutes.	Safety for the patient with a latex allergy mandates the provision of latex-free objects and donning an allergy ID bracelet.	*C. Smith, RN*
Provide patient with allergy ID bracelet.		
Notify OR team of patient's latex allergy.	Anesthesia will have emergency drugs available if patient demonstrates intraoperative reaction. OR team will be able to continue to provide a latex-free intraoperative environment.	

NURSING DIAGNOSIS Acute pain (postoperative) related to effects of surgical removal of tonsils and adenoids

EXPECTED OUTCOME 1/29/15—Throughout the perioperative period, the child will:
- Verbalize decreased level of pain in her throat
- Demonstrate/report adequate pain control

(continued)

NURSING PLAN OF CARE 29-1   *continued*

for Gabrielle McAllister

NURSING INTERVENTIONS	RATIONALE	EVALUATIVE STATEMENT
Assess for pain using age-appropriate pain scale and report to physician or anesthesiologist.	Pain is subjective. Caregivers need to be aware of patient's perception. Preemptive (before the painful event) analgesia may protect the patient from awakening with severe postop pain, nausea, and vomiting.	1/29/15 Outcome met. CRNA gave 0.5 mg of midazolam IV before transfer to OR. Patient is sleeping quietly. *C. Smith, RN*
Implement pain control measures as needed.	Pain control measures may be necessary to ensure patient's comfort.	1/30/15 Outcome met. Pain medication administered as requested by child's mother; child reports decreasing pain in her throat. *C. Smith, RN*

SAMPLE DOCUMENTATION

1/29/15
Patient and parent identified on admission to preop holding area. Patient expressed mild fear of procedure and separation from parents. Patient made comfortable with warm blankets and sitting on mother's lap after donning OR pajamas. Assessed for knowledge of impending procedure. Preop teaching reinforced with mother. Assurance given about pain and latex allergy management protocol. Latex allergy armband applied and included in hand-off report to anesthesia provider and OR team. CRNA gave 0.2 mg midazolam IV before transfer to OR. Patient calm and sleeping quietly on transfer, accompanied by toy stuffed bunny named "Bunny." No signs or symptoms of latex reaction on transfer to OR.

C. Smith, RN

 # SKILL 29-1   PROVIDING PREOPERATIVE PATIENT CARE: HOSPITALIZED PATIENT

DELEGATION CONSIDERATIONS

Preoperative assessment and teaching is not delegated to nursing assistive personnel (NAP) or unlicensed assistive personnel (UAP). Depending on the state's nurse practice act and the organization's policies and procedures, preoperative teaching may be delegated to licensed practical/vocational nurses (LPN/LVN) after an assessment of education needs by the registered nurse. The decision to delegate must be based on careful analysis of the patient's needs and circumstances, as well as the qualifications of the person to whom the task is being delegated. Refer to the Delegation Guidelines in Appendix A (found on thePoint).

EQUIPMENT (varies, depending on the type of surgery)

- Blood pressure cuffs
- Electronic blood pressure monitor
- Pulse oximeter sensors
- IV pump
- Graduated compression stockings
- Pneumatic compression device
- Tubes, drains, vascular access tubing
- Incentive spirometer
- Small pillow
- Personal protective equipment (PPE), as indicated

IMPLEMENTATION

ACTION

RATIONALE

1. Check the patient's medical record for the type of surgery and review the medical orders. Review the nursing database, history, and physical examination. Check that the baseline data are recorded; report those that are abnormal.

These checks ensure that the care will be provided for the right patient and that any specific teaching based on the type of surgery will be addressed. Also, this review helps to identify patients who are at increased surgical risk.

2. **Check that all diagnostic testing has been completed and results are available; identify and report abnormal results.** Gather the necessary supplies.

This check may influence the type of surgery performed and anesthetic used, as well as the timing of surgery or the need for additional consultation. Preparation promotes efficient time management and an organized approach to the task.

3. Perform hand hygiene and put on PPE, if indicated.

Hand hygiene and PPE prevent the spread of microorganisms. PPE is required based on transmission precautions.

4. Identify the patient.

Identifying the patient ensures that the right patient receives the intervention and helps prevent errors.

5. Close the curtains around the bed and close the door to the room, if possible. Explain to the patient and significant other what you are going to do and why you are going to do it. Place necessary supplies on the bedside stand or overbed table, within easy reach.

This ensures the patient's privacy. Explanation relieves anxiety and facilitates cooperation. Bringing everything to the bedside conserves time and energy. Arranging items nearby is convenient, saves time, and avoids unnecessary stretching and twisting of muscles on the part of the nurse.

6. Explore the psychological needs of the patient and family related to the surgery.

Meeting the psychological needs of the patient and family before surgery can have a beneficial effect on the postoperative course.

   a. Establish a therapeutic relationship, encouraging the patient to verbalize concerns or fears.

   b. Use active listening skills, answering questions and clarifying any misinformation.

   c. Use touch, as appropriate, to convey genuine empathy.

   d. Offer to contact spiritual counselor (e.g., priest, minister, rabbi) to meet spiritual needs.

Spiritual beliefs for some patients and family can provide a source of support over the perioperative course.

7. **Identify learning needs of the patient and family.** Ensure that the informed consent of the patient for the surgery has been signed, timed, dated, and witnessed. Inquire if the patient has any questions regarding the surgical procedure (Figure 1). Check the patient's record to determine if an advance directive has been completed. If an advance directive has not been completed, discuss with the patient the possibility of completing it, as appropriate. If the patient has had surgery before, ask about this experience.

This enhances surgical recovery and allays anxiety by preparing the patient for postoperative convalescence, discharge plans, and self-care. The surgeon is responsible for explaining the details of the surgical procedure and potential risks and complications. The nurse is responsible for clarifying what the surgeon has explained to the patient and contacting the surgeon if the patient does not understand or has further questions. An advance directive provides written communication of the patient's wishes to the health care team related to the patient's desire for extraordinary life-sustaining treatments if the patient's condition is deemed unsalvageable. Previous surgical experience may impact preoperative care positively or negatively, depending on the patient's experience.

FIGURE 1. Identifying the needs of the patient and answering questions.

(continued)

SKILL 29-1   PROVIDING PREOPERATIVE PATIENT CARE: HOSPITALIZED PATIENT   *continued*

ACTION	RATIONALE
8. Teach deep breathing exercises (see Guidelines for Nursing Care 29-1, page 868 for specific technique).	Deep breathing exercises improve lung expansion and volume, help expel anesthetic gases and mucus from the airway, and facilitate the oxygenation of body tissues.
9. Teach coughing and splinting (see Guidelines for Nursing Care 29-2, p. 868 for specific technique).	Coughing helps remove retained mucus from the respiratory tract. Splinting minimizes pain while coughing or moving.
10. Teach use of incentive spirometer (Figure 2); also refer to Guidelines for Nursing 38-1 on page 1420 for specific information.	Incentive spirometry improves lung expansion, helps expel anesthetic gases and mucus from the airway, and facilitates oxygenation of body tissues.
11. Teach leg exercises, as appropriate.	Leg exercises assist in preventing muscle weakness, promote venous return, and decrease complications related to venous stasis. Leg exercises may be contraindicated for patients with certain conditions, such as lower extremity fractures.
12. Assist the patient in putting on graduated compression stockings and demonstrate how the pneumatic compression device operates (refer to Chapter 32 for specific information).	Graduated compression stockings and pneumatic compression devices are used postoperatively for patients who are at risk for a deep vein thrombosis (DVT) and pulmonary embolism.
13. Teach turning in the bed.	Turning and repositioning of the patient is important to prevent postoperative complications and to minimize pain.
a. Instruct the patient to use a pillow or bath blanket to splint where the incision will be. Ask the patient to raise the left knee and reach across to grasp the right side rail of the bed when turning toward the patient's right side (Figure 3). If turning to the left side, the patient will bend the right knee and grasp the left side rail.	
b. When turning the patient onto the right side, ask the patient to push with bent left leg and pull on the right side rail (Figure 4). Explain that you will place a pillow behind the patient's back to provide support, and that the call bell will be placed within easy reach (Figure 5).	
c. Explain to the patient that position change is recommended every 2 hours.	

FIGURE 2. An incentive spirometer helps increase lung volume and promotes inflation of the alveoli.

FIGURE 3. Instructing patient to raise the left knee and reach across to grasp the right side rail toward which she will be turning.

ACTION

FIGURE 4. Helping patient to roll over to her right side while she pushes with the left bent leg and pulls on the side rail.

14. Teach pain management.

   a. Discuss past experiences with pain and interventions that the patient has used to reduce pain.

   b. Discuss the availability of analgesic medication postoperatively.

   c. Discuss the use of patient-controlled analgesia (PCA), as appropriate (refer to Chapter 34).

   d. Explore the use of other alternative and nonpharmacologic methods to reduce pain, such as position change, massage, relaxation/diversion, guided imagery, and meditation.

15. Review equipment that may be used after surgery.

   a. Show the patient various types of equipment, such as IV pumps, electronic blood pressure cuff, tubes, and surgical drains.

16. Provide skin preparation.

   a. **Ask the patient to bathe or shower with the antiseptic solution. Remind the patient to clean the surgical site.**

RATIONALE

FIGURE 5. After patient is turned, provide support with pillows behind the patient's back.

Using prescribed analgesics to minimize pain helps prevent postoperative complications.

Past experiences with pain can impact the patient's ability to manage surgical pain. Pain is a subjective experience and the interventions effective in reducing pain vary from patient to patient.

Depending on the medical order, the patient may need to request analgesic medication as needed, or a patient-controlled analgesia (PCA) or epidural analgesia may be ordered, for which the patient will need specific instruction on how to use. (See Chapter 34 for more information.)

Patient understanding of the use of PCA is crucial for effective, safe administration.

These measures may reduce anxiety and may decrease the amount of pain medication that is needed. Analgesic therapy should involve a multimodal approach influenced by age, weight, and comorbidity.

Knowledge can reduce anxiety about equipment. The patient may need an indwelling urinary (Foley) catheter during and after surgery to keep the bladder empty and to monitor urinary output. Drains are frequently used to remove excess fluid around the surgical incision.

An antiseptic shower, bath, or cleansing with antimicrobial-impregnated wipes may be ordered the evening before surgery and repeated the morning of surgery to begin the process of preparing the skin before surgery and to prevent infection. Evidence-based practice advises against hair removal at the surgical site due to increased potential for infection. The Centers for Disease Control and Prevention (CDC) recommends that if shaving is necessary, it should be performed immediately before the surgery, using disposable supplies and aseptic technique. Follow facility policy regarding skin preparation of the surgical patient. In addition, immediately before the surgical procedure, the skin of the patient's operative site will be cleansed with a product that is compatible with the antiseptic used for showering.

(continued)

SKILL 29-1 PROVIDING PREOPERATIVE PATIENT CARE: HOSPITALIZED PATIENT *continued*

ACTION	RATIONALE
17. Provide teaching about and follow dietary/fluid restrictions. **Explain to the patient that both food and fluid will be restricted before surgery to ensure that the stomach contains a minimal amount of gastric secretions. This restriction is important to reduce the risk of aspiration. Emphasize to the patient the importance of avoiding food and fluids during the prescribed time period, because failure to adhere may necessitate cancellation of the surgery.**	Ensure that fluid and dietary restrictions (NPO), as ordered by the primary care provider or in facility protocol, have been followed. These restrictions assist in preventing regurgitation and aspiration.
18. Provide intestinal preparation, as appropriate. In certain situations, the bowel will need to be prepared by administering enemas or laxatives to evacuate the bowel and to reduce the intestinal bacteria.	This preparation will be needed when major abdominal, perineal, perianal, or pelvic surgery is planned.
a. As needed, provide explanation of the purpose of enemas or laxatives before surgery. If patient will be administering an enema, clarify the steps as needed.	Enemas can be stressful, especially when repeated enemas are required to obtain a clear fluid return. Repeated enemas may cause fluid and electrolyte imbalance, orthostatic hypotension, and weakness. Follow safety precautions to guard against patient falls. Anesthetic agents and abdominal surgery can interfere with normal elimination function during the initial postoperative period. (Refer to Chapter 37 to review skill for enema administration.)
19. **Check administration of regularly scheduled medications.** Review with the patient routine medications, over-the-counter medications, and herbal supplements that are taken regularly. Check the medical orders and review with the patient which medications will be permitted the day of surgery.	Many patients take medications for a variety of chronic medical conditions. Adjustments in taking these medications may be needed before surgery. Certain medications, such as aspirin, are stopped days before surgery due to their anticoagulant effect. Certain cardiac and respiratory drugs may be taken the day of surgery per medical order. If the patient is diabetic and takes insulin, the insulin dosage may be reduced.
20. Remove PPE, if used. Perform hand hygiene.	Removing PPE properly reduces the risk for infection transmission and contamination of other items. Hand hygiene prevents the spread of microorganisms.

DOCUMENTATION

Guidelines

Document that the patient's records were reviewed, including the history, physical assessment, and any laboratory values and diagnostic studies. Record that the surgeon was notified of any abnormal values. Document the components of perioperative teaching that were reviewed with the patient and family, if present, such as use of the incentive spirometer, deep breathing exercises, splinting, leg exercises, graduated compression stockings, and pneumatic compression devices. Record the patient's ability to demonstrate the skills and response to the teaching, and note if any follow-up instruction needs to be performed. Document other preoperative teaching, including pain management, intestinal preparation, medications, and preoperative skin preparation. Record any patient concerns about the surgery and whether the surgeon was contacted to provide any further explanations. Document the emotional support that was offered to the patient and if a spiritual counselor was notified per request of patient.

Sample Documentation

4/2/15 1030 Patient's records were reviewed and no abnormal results were identified. Perioperative teaching points reviewed with patient and his wife, including the rationale for each of these points. Patient demonstrated proper use of incentive spirometry, deep breathing, splinting while coughing, and leg exercises. Reviewed pain management, intestinal preparation, medications, and preoperative skin preparation. Patient stated that he was anxious about the surgery because this will be his first time to the operating room. Emotional support and reassurance were provided.

—J. Grabes, RN

UNEXPECTED SITUATIONS AND ASSOCIATED INTERVENTIONS

- *A patient's laboratory results are noted to be abnormal:"* Notify primary care provider. Some abnormalities, such as an elevated international normalized ratio (INR) or abnormalities in the complete blood count (CBC), may postpone the surgery.
- *A patient says to you, "I'm not sure I really want this surgery:"* Discuss with the patient why the patient feels this way. Notify primary care provider. Patients should not undergo surgery until they are sure that surgery is what they want.

SPECIAL CONSIDERATIONS

General Considerations

- Obese patients are at greater risk of surgical complications and death compared with optimal-weight patients. In taking an obese patient's history, be alert for other medical conditions, such as diabetes, hypertension, and sleep apnea that also increase risk.

Infant and Child Considerations

- Children have special needs related to their overall health, age, and size. Easing preoperative anxiety of the child is crucial, which includes using simple and concrete terms when providing information.
- The nurse needs to be sensitive to the anxiety level of the parent, providing support, explanations, and patient teaching, as needed.
- Accurate weights are essential for correct medication dosages.
- Developmentally appropriate pain assessment and therapy needs to be initiated to ensure adequate pain management.

Older Adult Considerations

- Age-related changes and pre-existing chronic conditions can affect the postoperative course of the older adult patient.
- It is important to present preoperative teaching information slowly with reinforcement, because processing of information can be slower.
- Pain assessment and therapy may be suboptimal due to communication barriers and any comorbidity present in many older adult patients. These patients may respond differently to pain medication; therefore, careful and individualized attention is required.

SKILL 29-2 | PROVIDING POSTOPERATIVE CARE WHEN PATIENT RETURNS TO ROOM

DELEGATION CONSIDERATIONS

Postoperative measurement of vital signs may be delegated to nursing assistive personnel (NAP) or unlicensed assistive personnel (UAP), as well as to licensed practical/vocational nurses (LPN/LVN). Postoperative assessment and teaching is not delegated to NAP or UAP. Depending on the state's nurse practice act and the organization's policies and procedures, postoperative teaching may be delegated to LPN/LVN after an assessment of education needs by the registered nurse. The decision to delegate must be based on careful analysis of the patient's needs and circumstances, as well as the qualifications of the person to whom the task is being delegated. Refer to the Delegation Guidelines in Appendix A (found on thePoint).

EQUIPMENT (varies, depending on the surgery)

- Electronic blood pressure monitor
- Blood pressure cuff
- Electronic thermometer
- Pulse oximeter
- Stethoscope
- IV pump, IV solutions
- Graduated compression stockings
- Pneumatic compression devices
- Tubes, drains, vascular access tubing
- Incentive spirometer
- PPE, as indicated
- Blankets, as needed

(continued)

SKILL 29-2 PROVIDING POSTOPERATIVE CARE WHEN PATIENT RETURNS TO ROOM *continued*

IMPLEMENTATION

ACTION	**RATIONALE**
Immediate Care	
1. When patient returns from the PACU, participate in hand-off report from the PACU nurse and review the operating room and PACU data. Gather the necessary supplies.	Obtaining a hand-off report ensures accurate communication and promotes continuity of care. Preparation promotes efficient time management and an organized approach to the task.
2. Perform hand hygiene and put on PPE, if indicated.	Hand hygiene and PPE prevent the spread of microorganisms. PPE is required based on transmission precautions.
3. Identify the patient.	Identifying the patient ensures that the right patient receives the intervention and helps prevent errors.
4. Close the curtains around the bed and close the door to the room, if possible. Explain to the patient or significant other what you are going to do and why you are going to do it. Place necessary supplies on the bedside stand or overbed table, within easy reach.	This ensures the patient's privacy. Explanation relieves anxiety and facilitates cooperation. Bringing everything to the bedside conserves time and energy. Arranging items nearby is convenient, saves time, and avoids unnecessary stretching and twisting of muscles on the part of the nurse.
5. **Place patient in safe position (semi- or high Fowler's or side-lying). Note level of consciousness.**	A sitting position (head of bed elevated) facilitates deep breathing; the side-lying position with neck slightly extended prevents aspiration and airway obstruction. Alternate positions may be appropriate based on the type of surgery.
6. **Obtain vital signs. Monitor and record vital signs frequently.** Assessment order may vary, but usual frequency includes taking vital signs every 15 minutes the first hour, every 30 minutes the next 2 hours, every hour for 4 hours, and finally every 4 hours.	Comparison with baseline preoperative vital signs may indicate impending shock or **hemorrhage.** Some institutions use a paper or computer flow sheet to record initial postoperative data.
7. Assess the patient's respiratory status. (refer to Chapter 25). Measure the patient's oxygen saturation level (Figure 1).	Comparison with baseline preoperative respiratory assessment may indicate impending respiratory complications.

FIGURE 1. Obtaining postoperative oxygen saturation level.

ACTION	**RATIONALE**
8. Assess the patient's cardiovascular status (refer to Chapter 25).	Comparison with baseline preoperative cardiovascular assessment may indicate impending cardiovascular complications.
9. Assess the patient's neurovascular status, based on the type of surgery performed (refer to Chapter 25).	Comparison with baseline preoperative neurovascular assessment may indicate impending neurovascular complications.

ACTION	RATIONALE
10. Provide for warmth, using heated or extra blankets, as necessary (Figure 2). Assess skin color and condition.	The operating room is a cold environment. Hypothermia is uncomfortable and may lead to cardiac arrhythmias and impaired wound healing.
11. Check dressings for color, odor, presence of drains, and amount of drainage (Figure 3). Mark the drainage on the dressing by circling the amount, and include the time. Turn the patient to assess visually under the patient for bleeding from the surgical site.	Hemorrhage and shock are life-threatening complications of surgery. Early recognition is essential.

FIGURE 2. Providing extra blankets for warmth.

FIGURE 3. Checking the dressings for color, odor, and amount of drainage.

12. Verify that all tubes and drains are patent and equipment is working; note amount of drainage in collection device. If an indwelling urinary (Foley) catheter is in place, note urinary output.	This ensures function of drainage devices.
13. Verify and maintain IV infusion at prescribed rate.	This replaces fluid loss and prevents dehydration and electrolyte imbalances.
14. Assess for pain and relieve it by administering medications ordered by the primary care provider. If the patient has been instructed in use of PCA for pain management, review its use. Check record to verify if analgesic medication was administered in the PACU.	Use a facility-approved pain scale. Observe for nonverbal behavior that may indicate pain, such as grimacing, crying, and restlessness. Analgesics and other nonpharmacologic pain strategies are used for relief of postoperative pain.
15. Provide for a safe environment. Keep bed in low position with side rails up, based on facility policy. Have call bell within patient's reach.	This prevents accidental injury. Easy access to call bell permits patient to call for nurse when necessary.
16. Remove PPE, if used. Perform hand hygiene.	Removing PPE properly reduces the risk for infection transmission and contamination of other items. Hand hygiene prevents transmission of microorganisms.

Ongoing Care

17. Promote optimal respiratory function.	Anesthetic agents may depress respiratory function. Patients who have existing respiratory or cardiovascular disease, have abdominal or chest incisions, who are obese, older (Shippee-Rice, Fetzer, & Long, 2012), or in a poor state of nutrition are at greater risk for respiratory complications.
a. Assess respiratory rate, depth, quality, color, and capillary refill. Ask if the patient is experiencing any difficulty breathing.	Postoperative analgesic medication can reduce the rate and quality of the respiratory effort.

(continued)

SKILL 29-2 | PROVIDING POSTOPERATIVE CARE WHEN PATIENT RETURNS TO ROOM *continued*

ACTION

    b. Assist with coughing and deep breathing exercises (refer to Guidelines for Nursing Care 29-1 and 29-2 on page 868).

    c. Assist with incentive spirometry.

    d. Assist with early ambulation.

    e. Provide frequent position changes.

    f. Administer oxygen as ordered.

    g. Monitor pulse oximetry.

18. Promote optimal cardiovascular function:

    a. Assess apical rate, rhythm, and quality, and compare with peripheral pulses, color, and blood pressure. Ask if the patient has any chest pains or shortness of breath.

    b. Provide frequent position changes.

    c. Assist with early ambulation.

    d. Apply graduated compression stockings or pneumatic compression devices, if ordered and not in place. If in place, assess for integrity.

    e. Provide leg and range-of-motion exercises if not contraindicated.

19. Promote optimal neurologic function:

    a. Assess level of consciousness, movement, and sensation.

    b. Determine the level of orientation to person, place, and time.

    c. Test motor ability by asking the patient to move each extremity.

    d. Evaluate sensation by asking the patient if your touch can be felt on the patient's extremity.

20. Promote optimal renal and urinary function as well as fluid and electrolyte status. Assess intake and output, evaluate for urinary retention, and monitor serum electrolyte levels.

    a. Promote voiding by offering bedpan at regular intervals, noting the frequency, amount, and if there are any burning or urgency symptoms.

    b. Monitor urinary catheter drainage if present.

    c. Measure intake and output.

21. Promote optimal gastrointestinal function and meet nutritional needs:

    a. Assess abdomen for distention and firmness. Ask if patient feels nauseated, had been vomiting, and if passing flatus.

    b. Auscultate for bowel sounds.

RATIONALE

Preventive measures can improve venous return and circulatory status.

Anesthetic and pain management agents can alter neurologic function.

Older patients may take longer to return to their level of orientation before surgery. Drugs and anesthetics will delay this return (Shippee-Rice et al., 2012).

Anesthesia alters motor and sensory function.

Anesthetic agents and surgical manipulation in the area may temporarily depress bladder tone and response, causing urinary retention.

Frequency, burning, or urgency may indicate possible urinary tract abnormality.

The primary care provider needs to be notified if the urinary output is < 30 mL/hr or 240 mL/8-hr period.

Intake and output are good indicators of fluid balance.

Anesthetic agents and narcotics depress peristalsis and normal functioning of gastrointestinal tract. Flatus indicates return of peristalsis.

Presence of bowel sounds indicates return of peristalsis.

ACTION	RATIONALE
c. Assist with diet progression; encourage fluid intake; monitor intake.	Patients may experience nausea after surgery, thus are encouraged to resume diet slowly, starting with clear liquids and advancing as tolerated.
d. Medicate for nausea and vomiting, as ordered.	Antiemetics are frequently ordered to alleviate postoperative nausea.
22. Promote optimal wound healing.	Alterations in nutritional, circulatory, and metabolic status may predispose patient to infection and delayed healing.
a. Assess condition of wound for presence of drains and any drainage.	
b. Use surgical asepsis for dressing changes and drain care.	Surgical asepsis reduces the risk of infection.
c. Inspect all skin surfaces for beginning signs of pressure ulcer development and use pressure-relieving supports to minimize potential skin breakdown.	Lying on the operating room table in the same position can predispose some patients to pressure ulcer formation, especially in patients who have undergone lengthy procedures.
23. Promote optimal comfort and relief from pain.	This shortens recovery period and facilitates return to normal function.
a. Assess for pain (location and intensity, using pain scale).	Control of postoperative pain promotes patient comfort and recovery.
b. Provide for rest and comfort; provide extra blankets, as needed, for warmth.	Patients may experience chills in the postoperative period.
c. Administer pain medications, as needed, and/or initiate nonpharmacologic methods, as appropriate.	
24. Promote optimal meeting of psychosocial needs:	This facilitates individualized care, anxiety reduction, and patient's return to normal health.
a. Provide emotional support to patient and family, as needed.	
b. Explain procedures and offer explanations regarding postoperative recovery, as needed, to both patient and family members.	

DOCUMENTATION

Guidelines

Document the time that the patient returns from PACU to the surgical unit. Record the patient's level of consciousness, vital signs, all assessments, and condition of dressing. If patient has oxygen running, an IV, or any other equipment, record this information. Document pain assessment, interventions that were instituted to alleviate pain, and the patient's response to the interventions. Document any patient teaching that is reviewed with the patient, such as use of incentive spirometer.

Sample Documentation

4/10/15 1330 Patient returned to room at 1315, drowsy but easily aroused; answers to name. Patient's temperature 98.8°F, pulse 78, BP 122/84, O$_2$ sat 96% on O$_2$ 2 L/min. Right lower abdominal dressing dry and intact. Rates pain at a "4" on scale of 1–10, was medicated in PACU with 10 mg morphine sulfate IV at 1030. Incentive spirometry completed × 10 cycles, 750 mL each. Patient deep breathing and coughing without production and turned to right side with HOB elevated. See flow sheet for additional system assessments.

—J. Grabbs, RN

(continued)

SKILL 29-2 PROVIDING POSTOPERATIVE CARE WHEN PATIENT RETURNS TO ROOM *continued*

UNEXPECTED SITUATIONS AND ASSOCIATED INTERVENTIONS

- *Vital signs are progressively increasing or decreasing from baseline:* Notify primary care provider. A continued decrease in blood pressure or an increase in heart rate could indicate internal bleeding.
- *Dressing was clean before but now has large amount of fresh blood:* Do not remove dressing. Reinforce dressing with more bandages. Removing the bandage could dislodge any clot that is forming and lead to further blood loss. Notify primary care provider.
- *Patient reports pain that is not relieved by ordered medication:* After fully assessing pain (location, description, alleviating factors, aggravating factors), notify primary care provider. Pain can be a clue to other problems, such as hemorrhage.
- *Patient is febrile within 12 hours of surgery:* Assist patient with coughing and deep breathing. If ordered, begin incentive spirometry. Continue to monitor vital signs and laboratory values such as complete blood count (CBC).
- *Adult patient has a urine output of less than 30 mL/hour:* Unless this is expected, notify primary care provider. Urine output is a good indicator of tissue perfusion. Patient may need more fluid or may need medication to increase blood pressure if it is low.

SPECIAL CONSIDERATIONS

General Considerations

- Be aware of baseline sensory deficits. Ensure that appropriate aids are in place, such as glasses or hearing aids. Lack of appropriate aids may impact postoperative assessments, such as level of consciousness.
- For patients undergoing throat surgery, such as a tonsillectomy, evaluate swallowing pattern. A patient who has had throat surgery and swallows frequently may be bleeding from the incision site.
- In the obese patient, medications may not perform as expected related to the lack of serum proteins that are needed to bind with drugs to support their effectiveness. Additionally, due to the larger kidney mass of the obese patient, renal elimination rates of certain drugs are increased, reducing the effectiveness of these drugs.
- Check to make sure that the mattress for the obese patient is of high quality, because this patient is at greater risk for skin breakdown due to the poor vascular supply of adipose tissue.
- Ensure that written postoperative instructions specific to the patient and follow-up appointments with the surgeon or other health care professionals are provided to each patient upon discharge from the hospital or outpatient center. Information, such as signs and symptoms to report to the primary care provider, as well as restrictions in activity and diet, are addressed. In addition, patients discharged the same day as their surgery are required to have a responsible individual accompany them home, and a contact telephone number is to be provided in case of emergency. The patient should be alert and oriented, or mental status should be at the patient's baseline. The vital signs of the patient should be stable. Have the patient "teach back" important information/instructions in the patient's own words.

Infant and Child Considerations

- Postoperative complications are often related to the respiratory system in this age group. After receiving general anesthesia, premature infants are at greater risk for apnea.
- Infants and children are at great risk for temperature-related complications because their body temperature can change rapidly. It is essential to have warmed blankets and other warming equipment available to avoid this complication.

Older Adult Considerations

- In the older adult patient, postoperative pneumonia can be a very serious complication, resulting in death. Therefore, it is especially important to encourage and assist the patient in using the incentive spirometer and with deep breathing exercises.
- Older patients may take longer to return to normothermia and their level of orientation before surgery. Drugs and anesthetics will delay this return.

DEVELOPING CLINICAL REASONING

1. You are providing the immediate preoperative care for a woman scheduled for surgery to remove a brain tumor. She tells you she does not want the surgery because she knows she is dying and just wants to go home to be with her husband and children. She also knows that her husband cannot accept the fact that she is dying and wants her to have the surgery. What do you do?

2. You are assigned to discharge a woman from your same-day surgery unit to her home. You strongly believe that she is not ready to go home, and there is no caregiver in her home. When you voice your concern to the surgeon, you are told that this is not your problem and that there is nothing anyone can do about the situation because her insurer will not approve hospitalization. How do you respond?

PRACTICING FOR NCLEX

1. A perioperative nurse is preparing a patient for surgery for treatment of a ruptured spleen as the result of an automobile crash. The nurse knows that this type of surgery belongs in what category?
   a. Minor, diagnostic
   b. Minor, elective
   c. Major, emergency
   d. Major, palliative

2. A nurse is preparing a patient for a cesarean section and teaches her the effects of the regional anesthesia she will be receiving. Which effects would the nurse expect? Select all that apply.
   a. Loss of consciousness
   b. Relaxation of skeletal muscles
   c. Reduction or loss of reflex action
   d. Localized loss of sensation
   e. Prolonged pain relief after other anesthesia wears off
   f. Infiltrates the underlying tissues in an operative area

3. A nurse has been asked to witness a patient signature on an informed consent form for surgery. For which of these patients would the document be valid? Select all that apply.
   a. A 92-year-old patient who is severely confused
   b. A 45-year-old patient who is oriented and alert
   c. A 10-year-old patient who is oriented and alert
   d. A 36-year-old patient who has had a narcotic premedication
   e. A 45-year-old mentally ill patient who has been ruled incompetent
   f. A 22-year old patient having an abortion against her partner's wishes

4. A 72-year-old woman who is scheduled for a hip replacement is taking several medications on a regular basis. Which drug category might create a surgical risk for this patient?
   a. Anticoagulants
   b. Antacids
   c. Laxatives
   d. Sedatives

5. A nurse is caring for an obese patient who has had surgery. The nurse monitors this patient for what postoperative complication?
   a. Hunger
   b. Impaired wound healing
   c. Hemorrhage
   d. Gas pains

6. A responsibility of the nurse is the administration of preoperative medications to patients. Which statements describe the action of these medications? Select all that apply.
   a. Diazepam is given to alleviate anxiety.
   b. Ranitidine is given to facilitate patient sedation.
   c. Atropine is given to decrease oral secretions.
   d. Morphine is given to depress respiratory function.
   e. Cimetidine is given to prevent laryngospasm.
   f. Fentanyl citrate–droperidol is given to facilitate a sense of calm.

7. A nurse is teaching a man scheduled to have same-day surgery. Which teaching method would be most effective in preoperative teaching for ambulatory surgery?
   a. Lecture
   b. Discussion
   c. Audiovisuals
   d. Written instructions

8. A 70-year-old male is scheduled for surgery. He says to the nurse, "I am so frightened—what if I don't wake up?" What would be the nurse's best response?
   a. "You have a wonderful doctor."
   b. "Let's talk about how you are feeling."
   c. "Everyone wakes up from surgery!"
   d. "Don't worry, you will be just fine."

9. A nurse is explaining pain control methods to a patient undergoing a bowel resection. The patient is interested in the PCA pump and asks the nurse to explain how it works. What would be the nurse's correct response?
   a. "The pump allows the patient to be completely free of pain during the postoperative period."
   b. "The pump allows the patient to take unlimited amounts of medication as needed."
   c. "The pump allows the patient to choose the type of medication given postoperatively."
   d. "The pump allows the patient to self-administer limited doses of pain medication."

10. A patient had a surgical procedure that necessitated a thoracic incision. The nurse anticipates that he will have a higher risk for postoperative complications involving which body system?
    a. Respiratory system
    b. Circulatory system
    c. Digestive system
    d. Nervous system

11. While assessing a patient in the PACU, a nurse notes increased wound drainage, restlessness, a decreasing blood pressure, and an increase in the pulse rate. The nurse interprets these findings as most likely indicating:
    a. Thrombophlebitis
    b. Atelectasis
    c. Infection
    d. Hemorrhage

12. A patient tells the nurse she is having pain in her right lower leg. How does the nurse assess for the presence of thrombophlebitis?
    a. By palpating the skin over the tibia and fibula
    b. By documenting daily calf circumference measurements
    c. By recording vital signs obtained four times a day
    d. By noting difficulty with ambulation

13. A scrub nurse is assisting a surgeon with a kidney transplant. What are the patient responsibilities of this surgical team member? Select all that apply.
   a. Maintaining sterile technique
   b. Draping and handling instruments and supplies
   c. Identifying and assessing the patient on admission
   d. Integrating case management
   e. Preparing the skin at the surgical site
   f. Providing exposure of the operative area

14. Older adults often have reduced vital capacity as a result of normal physiologic changes. Which nursing intervention would be most important for the postoperative care of an older surgical patient specific to this change?
   a. Take and record vital signs every shift.
   b. Turn, cough, and deep breathe every 4 hours.
   c. Encourage increased intake of oral fluids.
   d. Assess bowel sounds daily.

15. A nurse is explaining the rationale for performing leg exercises after surgery. Which reason would the nurse include in the explanation?
   a. Promote respiratory function
   b. Maintain functional abilities
   c. Provide diversional activities
   d. Increase venous return

ANSWERS WITH RATIONALES

1. *c.* This surgery would involve a major body organ, has the potential for postoperative complications, requires hospitalization, and must be done immediately to save the patient's life. Elective surgery is a procedure that is preplanned by essentially healthy people. Diagnostic surgery is performed to confirm a diagnosis. Palliative surgery is not curative, rather it is done to relieve or reduce the intensity of an illness.

2. *c, d.* A localized loss of sensation and possible loss of reflexes occurs with a regional anesthetic. Loss of consciousness and relaxation of skeletal muscles occurs with general anesthesia. Prolonged pain relief after other anesthesia wears off and infiltration of the underlying tissues in an operative area occur with topical anesthesia.

3. *b, f.* A consent form is not legal if the patient signing the form is confused, sedated, unconscious, or a minor.

4. *a.* Anticoagulant drug therapy would increase the risk for hemorrhage during surgery.

5. *b.* Fatty tissue is less vascular and, therefore, less resistant to infection and more prone to delayed wound healing.

6. *a, c, f.* Sedatives, such as diazepam (Valium), midazolam (Versed), or lorazepam (Ativan) are given to alleviate anxiety and decrease recall of events related to surgery. Anticholinergics, such as atropine and glycopyrrolate (Robinul) are given to decrease pulmonary and oral secretions and to prevent laryngospasm. Neuroleptanalgesic agents, such as fentanyl citrate–droperidol (Innovar) are given to cause a general state of calm and sleepiness. Histamine-2 receptor blockers, such as cimetidine (Tagamet) and ranitidine (Zantac) are given to decrease gastric acidity and volume. Narcotic analgesics, such as morphine, are given to facilitate patient sedation and relaxation and to decrease the amount of anesthetic agent needed.

7. *d.* Written instructions are most effective in providing information for same-day surgery.

8. *b.* This answer allows the patient to talk about his feelings and fears, and is therapeutic.

9. *d.* PCA infusion pumps allow patients to self-administer doses of pain-relieving medication within physician-prescribed time and dose limits. Patients activate the delivery of the medication by pressing a button on a cord connected to the pump or a button directly on the pump.

10. *a.* A thoracic incision makes it more painful for the patient to take deep breaths or cough. Shallow respirations and ineffective coughing increase the risk for respiratory complications.

11. *d.* Increased wound drainage, restlessness, decreasing blood pressure, and increasing pulse rate are assessment findings that indicate hemorrhage. Manifestations of thrombophlebitis are pain and cramping in the calf or thigh of the involved extremity, redness and swelling in the affected area, elevated temperature, and an increase in the diameter of the involved extremity. Manifestations of atelectasis include decreased lung sounds over the affected area, dyspnea, cyanosis, crackles, restlessness, and apprehension. Signs of infection include elevated white blood count and fever.

12. *b.* Inflammation from thrombophlebitis increases the size of the affected extremity and can be assessed by measuring circumference on a regular basis.

13. *a, b.* The scrub nurse is a member of the sterile team who maintains sterile technique while draping and handling instruments and supplies. Two duties of the circulating nurse are to identify and assess the patient on admission to the operating room and prepare the skin at the surgical site. The RNFA actively assists the surgeon by providing exposure of the operative area. The APRN coordinates care activities, collaborates with physicians and nurses in all phases of perioperative and postanesthesia care, and integrates case management, critical paths, and research into care of the surgical patient.

14. *b.* Reduced vital capacity in older adults increases the risk for respiratory complications, including pneumonia and atelectasis. Having the patient turn, cough, and deep breathe every 4 hours maintains respiratory function and helps to prevent complications.

15. *d.* Leg exercises in the postoperative period increase venous return. As a result, the patient has a decreased risk for thrombophlebitis and emboli.

TAYLOR SUITE RESOURCES

Explore these additional resources to enhance learning for this chapter:

- NCLEX-Style Questions and other resources on thePoint, http://thePoint.lww.com/Taylor8e
- *Study Guide for Fundamentals of Nursing, 8th edition*
- Adaptive Learning | Powered by prepU, http://thepoint.lww.com/prepu
- *Skill Checklists for Fundamentals of Nursing, 8th edition*
- *Taylor's Clinical Nursing Skills:* Chapter 6, Perioperative Nursing
- *Taylor's Video Guide to Clinical Nursing Skills:* Perioperative Nursing

Bibliography

Agency for Healthcare Research and Quality (AHRQ). (2012). Never Events. Available at http://www.psnet.ahrq.gov/primer.aspx?primerID=3

Alexander-Magalee, M. (2013). Mechanical and pharmacologic prophylaxis for DVT. *OR Nurse 7*(1), 45–47.

American College of Surgeons (ACS) Annual Clinical Congress (2012). New respiratory care program suggests promise in decreasing pulmonary complications in surgical patients. Available at http://www.facs.org/clincon2012/press/mcaneny.html

American Society of Anesthesiologists, Inc. (ASA) (2011). Practice guidelines for preoperative fasting and the use of pharmacologic agents to reduce the risk of pulmonary aspiration: Application to healthy patients undergoing elective procedures—An updated report by the American Society of Anesthesiologists Committee on Standards and Practice Parameters. *Anesthesiology, 114*(3), 495–511.

American Society of PeriAnesthesia Nurses (ASPAN). (2010). *Standards of perianesthesia nursing practice, 2010–2012.* Thorofare, NJ: American Society of PeriAnesthesia Nurses.

Association of periOperative Registered Nurses (AORN). (2013a). Standards of perioperative nursing. *Perioperative standards and recommended practices.* Denver: AORN, Inc.

Association of periOperative Registered Nurses (AORN). (2013b). Recommended Practices for Perioperative Nursing. In *AORN, Perioperative standards and recommended practices.* Denver: AORN, Inc.

Bouyer-Ferullo, S. (2013). Preventing perioperative peripheral nerve injuries. *AORN Journal 97*(1), 111–121.

Bulechek, G., Butcher, H., Dochterman, J., & Wagner, C. (Eds.). (2013). *Nursing interventions classification (NIC)* (6th ed.). St. Louis: Elsevier/Mosby.

Godden, B. (2010). Why should we care about the standards? *Journal of PeriAnesthesia Nursing, 25*(4), 255–257.

Institute for Healthcare Improvement (IHI). (2012). How-to Guide: Prevent Surgical Site Infection for Hip and Knee Arthroplasty. Available at http://www.ihi.org/resources/Pages/Tools/HowtoGuidePreventSSIforHip-KneeArthroplasty.aspx

The Joint Commission (TJC). (2014). 2014 National patient safety goals. Available at http://www.jointcommission.org/standards_information/npsgs.aspx

The Joint Commission (TJC). (2012). Surgical Care Improvement Project. Available at http://www.jointcommission.org/surgical_care_improvement_project/

Lockhart, L. (2012). Advocacy now: a perioperative imperative. *Perioperative Nursing Clinics 7*(4), 375–377.

Mathias, J. M. (2012). Tips, lessons from a recent Joint Commission survey. *OR Manager 28*(10), 18–22.

Moorhead, S., Johnson, M., Maas, M., & Swanson, E. (Eds.). (2013). *Nursing outcomes classification (NOC)* (5th ed.). St. Louis: Elsevier/Mosby.

NANDA International (NANDA-I). (2012). *NANDA Nursing Diagnoses: Definitions & Classification, 2012–2014.* West Sussex, UK: Wiley-Blackwell.

Nordqvist, J. (2012). Surgical errors occur more than 4,000 times a year in the U.S. *Medical News Today.* Available at http://www.medicalnewstoday.com/articles/254426.php

Petersen C. (2011) *Perioperative nursing data set* (3rd edition). Denver, CO: AORN.

Rothrock, J. (2011). *Alexander's care of the patient in surgery* (14th ed.). St. Louis: Elsevier/Mosby.

Salem, M. R., Crystal, G. J., & Nimmagadda, U. (2012). Understanding the mechanics of laryngospasm is crucial for proper treatment. *Anesthesiology, 117*(2), 441–442.

Sherwood, G., & Barnsteiner, J. (2012). *Quality and Safety in Nursing: A Competency Approach to Improving Outcomes.* West Sussex, UK: Wiley-Blackwell.

Shippee Rice, R. V., Fetzer, S. J., & Long, J. V. (2012). *Gerioperative nursing care.* New York: Springer.

Tanner, J., Norrie, P., & Melen, K. (2011). Preoperative hair removal to reduce surgical site infections. *Cochrane Database of Systematic Reviews, 11,* CD004122.

Zrelak, P. A., Utter, G. H., Cuny, J., Romano, P. S. (2012). Using the Agency for Healthcare Research and Quality Patient Safety Indicators for Targeting Nursing Quality Improvement, *Journal of Nursing Care Quality, 27*(2), 99–108.

UNIT
VII

Promoting Healthy Physiologic Responses

*T*he art and science of caring are blended when nurses implement actions to meet basic human needs and to promote healthy physiologic responses. The chapters in Unit VII focus on information and guidelines essential to nursing practice in a wide variety of clinical settings that involve both healthy and ill patients of all ages. Included are nursing interventions to promote comfort and pain management and to meet basic physiologic needs: hygiene, activity and rest, nutrition, elimination, oxygenation, and fluid–electrolyte balance.

Each basic physiologic need is discussed first with a review of concepts pertinent to the specific area of human function and response, then with an examination of factors that affect need satisfaction. The steps of the nursing process are used to provide guidelines and information necessary for making accurate assessments establishing outcomes; and planning, implementing, and evaluating specific nursing interventions to meet needs and promote wellness.

The chapters in Unit VII enable the beginning nurse to integrate the knowledge and skills necessary to promote healthy physiologic responses in patients in any practice setting. Nursing process skills are further refined to ensure that care is holistic, comprehensive, and individualized.

"

…what nursing has to do is to put the patient in the best condition for nature to act upon him."

Florence Nightingale (1820–1910) a philosopher, theorist, statistician, humanitarian, and inspirational leader who founded modern nursing through a systematic method of training well-qualified nurses; she also initiated important reforms in military sanitation and hospital construction that greatly improved patient survival

30

Hygiene

KYLIE SIMPSON

Kylie, age 20, is a student at a state university. After having vaginal itching and burning for 2 weeks, she visits the campus health clinic. She is diagnosed with a vaginal infection. She asks the nurse at the campus health clinic, "Is there something wrong with me? This is the second vaginal infection I have had in 7 months. Isn't there something I can do to keep this from happening again?"

SONYA DELAMORDO

Sonya is an older Hispanic woman who has had a stroke (brain attack) resulting in right-sided paralysis. She is being discharged from the hospital and will now live with her daughter, who will be her primary caregiver. Her daughter is eager to learn everything she can about caring for her mother and asks numerous questions, including the best way to keep her mother clean.

ANDREW CRAIG

Andrew, age 68, has multiple diagnoses and limited mobility. He lives in an extended-care facility. Andrew needs assistance with his daily morning care. This morning, however, he tells the nurse, "I've already had a complete bath."

LEARNING OBJECTIVES

After completing the chapter, you will be able to accomplish the following:

1. Identify factors affecting personal hygiene.
2. Assess the adequacy of hygiene practices and self-care behaviors using appropriate interview and physical assessment skills.
3. Assess the condition of the patient's skin, oral cavity, hair, and nails using appropriate interview and physical assessment skills.
4. Develop nursing diagnoses that identify hygiene problems amenable to nursing intervention.
5. Describe the priorities of scheduled hygiene care.
6. Demonstrate techniques for assisting patients with hygiene measures, including those used when administering various types of baths and those used in cleaning each part of the body.
7. Describe agents commonly used on the skin and scalp, including any precautions necessary for their use.
8. Plan, implement, and evaluate nursing care for common problems of the skin and mucous membranes.

KEY TERMS

alopecia	gingivitis	periodontitis
caries	glossitis	plaque
cerumen	halitosis	stomatitis
cheilosis	pediculosis	tartar

Measures for personal cleanliness and grooming, called *personal hygiene,* promote physical and psychological well-being. Personal hygiene practices vary widely among people. It is important that personal care be carried out conveniently and frequently enough to promote personal hygiene and wellness. Acute and chronic illness, hospitalization, and institutionalization may make it necessary to modify hygiene practices. In these situations, the nurse helps the patient to continue sound hygiene practices and can teach the patient and family members, when necessary, regarding hygiene. Nurses assisting patients with basic hygiene must respect individual patient preferences, providing only the care that patients cannot, or should not, provide for themselves. In addition, nurses should value each patient as an individual and take into consideration the patient's physical, mental, and emotional state of being while providing hygiene care (see the accompanying Reflective Practice box on page 902).

This chapter discusses multiple factors that affect personal hygiene and nursing measures that promote personal

hygiene. A practical guide for assessing the adequacy of personal hygiene is presented. The data collected when assisting with hygiene may lead to the identification of multiple nursing diagnoses and collaborative problems. Examples of such diagnoses and problems are provided in the chapter. In addition, patient outcomes are presented, as are specific nursing strategies used when performing care of the skin, mouth, eyes, ears, nose, feet, perineal areas, and vaginal areas. The concluding nursing plan of care related to feminine hygiene illustrates how the nurse uses knowledge of personal hygiene practices and the integumentary system, along with specific nursing interventions, to resolve nursing diagnoses and to promote the patient's general sense of well-being.

HYGIENE PRACTICES

Hygienic practices include caring for the skin, hair, nails, mouth, teeth, and perineal area. There are strong links between good hygiene practices and a person's health. Inadequate hygiene practices can contribute to alterations in a person's health.

The skin, or integument, is the largest organ of the body and has multiple functions. The integumentary system is made up of the skin, the subcutaneous layer directly under the skin, and the appendages of the skin, including the hair and nails. Chapter 31 provides a description of the anatomy and physiology of the integumentary system and factors that affect skin integrity.

Hair is an accessory structure of the skin. Good general health is essential for attractive hair and skin, and cleanliness is a positive influence. Illness affects the hair, especially when endocrine abnormalities, increased body temperature, poor nutrition, or anxiety and worry are present. Changes in the color or condition of the hair shaft are related to changes in hormonal activity or to changes in the blood supply to hair follicles.

The nails are an accessory structure of the skin composed of epithelial tissue. Healthy nailbeds are pink, convex, and evenly curved. With certain pathologic conditions, and to some extent with aging, the nails become ridged and areas become concave. Hygienic care includes keeping the nails trimmed and clean.

A person's general health influences the health of that person's mouth and teeth, and proper care of the mouth and teeth lends to overall health. There is an established relationship between healthy teeth and a diet sufficient in calcium and phosphorus, along with vitamin D, which is necessary for the body to make use of these minerals. Maintaining good oral hygiene and dental care has several benefits. There is esthetic value in having a clean and healthy mouth. Having one's own teeth in good condition contributes to an intact body image. In addition, the beginning of the digestive process and tasting pleasure are enhanced when the mouth and teeth are in good condition.

The perineal area is dark, warm, and often moist, providing conditions that favor bacterial growth. The patient who cannot clean the perineal area needs the nurse's assistance for this important part of personal hygiene. Neglecting

CHALLENGE TO INTERPERSONAL SKILLS

It was our first day of clinical, sophomore year, and we were instructed to do complete AM care with our patients. My patient, Andrew Craig, was a 68-year-old man with multiple diagnoses and limited mobility. As I entered the room, he told me he had just had a bed bath a few hours earlier. I wasn't sure what to do, so I asked the tech if my patient had already had a complete bed bath. The tech pulled me into the patient's room and proceeded to scream at the patient, telling him not to lie to me and threatening to make him sit in the chair all day. This patient did not have a hip and had antibi-otic beads in the area, so it was very painful for him to sit in a chair because the beads dug into his side. The tech then told me to do the bed bath and left the room. I was left in a very awkward position because the patient was mad at me and I was astounded by how the tech had treated this patient. I was extremely upset as a result of this confrontation.

The day was emotionally very difficult for me, and when I arrived home, I became even more upset. The manner in which the tech treated the patient, even though the patient had a tendency to be manipulative, was completely out of line.

Thinking Outside the Box: Possible Courses of Action

- Make the best of a bad situation, but do nothing to change the status quo: "Hey, I'm only a student, right?"
- Confront the tech and tell her about my outrage.
- Report the tech to her supervisor.
- Consult with my instructor about how a professional nurse should respond in a situation like this.
- Be prepared to "go to the top" if initial attempts to reform a bad system don't meet with success.

Evaluating a Good Outcome: How Do I Define Success?

- The patient's basic hygiene needs are met.
- The patient's humanity and integrity are respected.
- Health care professionals and technicians are held accountable for incompetent, unethical, and illegal behavior (the tech, nursing leadership, and administration in this long-term care facility).
- I learn how to be a successful patient advocate.

Personal Learning: Here's to the Future!

I proceeded to talk to my clinical instructor and the coordinator of the class about the incident. The coordinator contacted the long-term care facility and I had to give a formal statement about the incident. The nurse manager who took my statement was not very receptive and was actually very patronizing.

This entire experience helped me to recognize the type of nurse I want to be. First and foremost, I always want to ensure that I provide high-quality patient care. At the time of my unfortunate experience, I did not respond immediately to the tech's inappropriate comments. But now that I have gained more experience and become more confident, I would definitely respond immediately if a similar situation ever arose again. I realize that I can't let fear stand in my way when the quality of patient care is suffering. I would encourage any nurse who sees a colleague or anyone treating a patient without the utmost respect and care to speak up and contact appropriate personnel to discuss the situation.

In addition to this one tech's inappropriate behavior, the overall conditions of this long-term care facility were appall-ing. I learned a lot this semester about the shortage of nurses (1 RN for 40 patients) and, consequently, how patient care is being jeopardized. During the unfortunate episode to which I was exposed, I was astonished and outraged, but I didn't take any steps to change the conditions except reporting this one incident. At the end of the semester, we reported the conditions to the class coordinator. Now I realize that as an individual, I could have done more to change the conditions in the long-term care facility. In retrospect, I should have taken a leadership role and notified the outside licensing agency about these conditions (the long-term care facility ended up losing its accreditation that summer). All nurses are responsible for ensuring the quality of care given to patients, and we must contact whomever necessary to ensure changes are made.

This experience was very difficult for me, but in the end, I think it opened my eyes to the importance of nurses acting as advocates and leaders.

Catherine Barrell, Georgetown University

REFLECTION ON QUALITY AND SAFETY COMPETENCIES

How do you think you would respond in a similar situation? Why? What does this tell you about yourself and about the adequacy of your skills for professional practice? What *knowledge, skills,* and *attitudes* do you need to develop to continuously improve the quality and safety of care for patients like Mr. Craig?

Patient-Centered Care: What factors may have played a role in the tech's answer to the patient and nursing student? What interventions should the nursing student implement to provide care based on respect for the patient's preferences, values, and needs? How did the nursing student's actions adhere to ethical and legal principles? Did the nursing student act as an advocate for Mr. Craig?

Teamwork and Collaboration/Quality Improvement: How could the nursing staff and other care providers collabo-rate to provide respectful care for Mr. Craig? What communication skills do you need to improve to ensure you function as a member of the patient-care team and to obtain assistance when needed?

Safety/Evidence-Based Practice: Is it within the nursing student's scope of practice to individually contact a higher authority such as a licensing agency about the situation? What evidence in nursing literature provides guidance for decision making regarding providing culturally competent health care?

Informatics: Can you identify the essential information that should be documented in Mr. Craig's electronic record to support safe patient care and coordination of care? Is there other documentation that should be part of the student's response to this incident? Can you think of other ways to respond to or approach the situation?

perineal cleaning for the patient who cannot provide self-care often results in physical and psychological discomfort for the patient, skin breakdown, and offensive odors.

FACTORS AFFECTING PERSONAL HYGIENE

Hygiene activities and practices can protect health and prevent disease. However, hygiene practices vary widely among groups and people. It is important to respect differences in patient hygiene practices and provide care and information in a nonjudgmental manner. The following factors may influence personal hygiene behaviors.

Culture

It is important to identify cultural variations that could affect a patient's personal hygiene preferences, such as typical bathing habits, and behaviors, such as use of various hygiene-related products. For example, people from some cultures place a high value on personal cleanliness and feel unclean unless they shower or bathe at least once daily. Many consider bathing incomplete without the use of products to reduce or mask normal body odors. Other people often find a weekly bath sufficient and may feel no need to mask normal body odors. Culture may also influence whether bathing is a private or communal activity.

 CONSIDER Sonya Delamordo, the Hispanic woman being discharged to her daughter's home after experiencing a stroke. Although the daughter is very eager to take care of her mother, the nurse would need to investigate the patient's culture to determine how the patient might feel about being cared for by her daughter. Typically, hygiene is a personal matter. The nurse needs to discuss hygiene care with the patient and her daughter to ensure competent care. •

Socioeconomic Class

A person's socioeconomic class and financial resources often define the hygiene options available to that person. For example, someone renting a room in a boarding house may have limited or no access to a tub or shower and may have limited finances to buy soap, shampoo, shaving cream, and deodorant. Homeless people, who often carry all their belongings in a car or shopping cart, may welcome the warm running water and soap available in roadside or public restrooms.

Spiritual Practices

Spiritual practices, including religious beliefs, may dictate ceremonial washings and purifications, sometimes as a prelude to prayer or eating. For example, in the Orthodox Jewish tradition, ritual baths are required for women after childbirth and menstruation. In some religions, contact with a deceased person or a deceased animal may make a person "unclean." Other religions dictate that no modern facilities be installed in homes. This would prohibit some people from having running water and toilets in their homes. As a result, they may bathe infrequently.

Developmental Level

Children learn hygiene practices while growing up. Family practices often dictate hygiene habits, such as morning or evening baths; the frequency of shampooing, tooth brushing, and clothing changes; feelings about nudity; and so on. As adolescents become more concerned about their personal appearance, they may adopt new hygiene measures, such as taking showers more frequently and wearing deodorant. Bathing frequency commonly decreases as a person ages, possibly due to limitations in mobility and the natural tendency toward drier skin with age. Older adults may experience an increase in skin conditions or problems, increasing the need for education related to hygiene and skin care (Cowdell, 2011).

Health State

Disease, surgery, or injury may reduce a person's ability to perform hygiene measures or motivation to follow usual hygiene habits. Weakness, dizziness, and fear of falling may prevent a person from entering a tub or shower or from bending to wash the lower extremities. Illness may also create a demand for new or modified hygiene measures. For example, peripheral vascular complications that often accompany diabetes mellitus require meticulous foot care. The presence of pain with an acute condition or chronic pain can affect a person's ability to perform and/or tolerate personal hygiene measures.

 REMEMBER Sonya Delamordo, who has right-sided paralysis as a result of a stroke. She will have to adapt to caring for herself, dealing with the mobility limitations of her right side, especially if she is right handed. Both she and her daughter will have to learn how to adapt personal hygiene practices, based on Sonya's abilities. •

Personal Preferences

People have different preferences with regard to hygiene practices such as taking a shower versus a tub bath, using bar soap versus liquid soap, and washing to wake oneself or to relax before sleep. A person's self-concept and sexuality also influence personal hygiene practices. For example, in an effort to promote a positive self-image, older adults may use skin care products advertised to prevent wrinkles and diminish signs of aging. Women who are sexually active may use a variety of hygiene products following intercourse to promote cleanliness.

THE NURSING PROCESS FOR SKIN CARE AND PERSONAL HYGIENE
Assessing

The comprehensive nursing assessment uses interview and physical assessment skills to elicit data about the patient's hygiene status. When alterations in a patient's physical or mental health state result in impaired ability to maintain acceptable personal hygiene, additional specific assessment skills are needed to determine the patient's limitations.

Nursing History

Bathing practices and cleansing habits and rituals vary widely. A clear threat to health must exist before a nurse decides that a person's hygiene practices are inadequate. The nurse assessing the adequacy of a patient's hygiene practices determines whether the patient has the knowledge, attitude, skills, and resources to care for the skin and mucous membranes. Refer to Focused Assessment Guide 30-1.

FOCUSED ASSESSMENT GUIDE 30-1

HYGIENE PRACTICES

Factors to Assess	Questions and Approaches
Daily and weekly bathing habits	Tell me about your daily and weekly bathing habits. Are there special bathing or hygiene products you routinely use or can't use? How can the nurses best help you to meet your hygiene needs?
Factors interfering with hygiene practices (sensory, cognitive, endurance, mobility, or motivation)	What recently or in the past has interfered with your hygiene practices? Does anything interfere with your ability to be as clean as you would like?
Pain	Do you have pain? Describe characteristics, onset, location, duration, associated symptoms, and intensity. Does the pain interfere with your ability to perform personal hygiene tasks? Does caring for yourself cause pain or discomfort?
Exposure history	Do you sunbathe? How much sun or tanning-booth exposure do you get? Do you use sunscreen? Does your job or daily activities/hobbies expose you to chemicals, such as bleach, petroleum, paint, insecticides, or cleaning products?
History of skin or mucous membrane problems (nature, onset of problem and frequency, causes, severity, symptoms, interventions attempted, results)	Describe any skin problems with rashes, lumps, itching, dryness, lesions, ecchymosis, or masses. What have you used to relieve these symptoms?
Special hygiene practices • Mouth	How do you clean your teeth and gums? How often do you have a dental examination? Do you have any dental appliances? Are there any tender areas or lesions in your mouth?
• Eyes, ears, and nose	Do you wear glasses or contact lenses to improve your vision? Do you wear a hearing aid? Have you experienced any discharge or bleeding from or swelling of your eyes, ears, or nose?
• Hair	Have you noticed any unusual dryness of the scalp or changes in hair texture and amount?
• Feet and nails	Is the appearance of the nails normal? How do you normally care for and clean your nails? Is the skin intact on the feet? Have you noticed any swelling of one or both feet? Do you wear any special shoes?
• Perineum	Have you noticed any unusual discharge, swelling, itching, or inflammation? Are you able to complete your own perineal care? Do you follow any special hygiene practices during menstruation? What type of feminine hygiene products (e.g., pads, tampons, douches) do you use?
• Piercings/Tattoos	Do you have any body piercings on your face, neck, arms, legs, torso, navel, or genitals? Have you experienced any problems related to the procedure? Do you have any tattoos? Are the tattoos healed? How do you care for your piercing(s) and/or tattoo(s)?

Hygiene practices include bathing and care of the skin and specific body areas, including the oral cavity, eyes, ears, nose, hair, nails, feet, and perineal and vaginal areas. Ask if the patient has noticed changes in or problems with these areas. Ask the patient about personal hygiene routines and products used. Inquire about any problems the patient may be experiencing related to completion of personal hygiene.

SKIN

Question the patient about any past or current problems (e.g., rashes, lumps, itching, dryness, lesions). When skin problems are present, ask the patient the following:

- How long have you had this problem?
- Does it bother you?
- How does it bother you? Does it itch?
- Have you found anything that helps relieve these symptoms?

When documenting the nursing history, be specific, clearly describing the patient's typical hygiene practices and any complaints. The following are two examples of documentation of patients' personal practices related to hygiene and skin care:

> Hygiene: "Showers twice daily, once in the morning and after working out in the evening. Skin tends to be very dry, and moisturizing creams are used daily. Aveeno® Oilated baths as needed. Allergic to deodorant soaps."

> Integument: "History of athlete's foot since high school days with outbreaks every 2 to 3 months. Knowledgeable about appropriate foot care. Uses antifungal agent such as terbinafine hydrochloride (Lamisil DermaGel) or tolnaftate (Tinactin cream), a topical fungicidal agent."

ORAL CAVITY

Identify the patient's normal oral hygiene practices and the variables influencing these practices. Note the history of any oral problems and related treatments.

Identify any variables known to cause oral problems, such as deficient self-care abilities, poor nutrition or excessive intake of refined sugars, family history of periodontal disease, or ingestion of chemotherapeutic agents that produce oral lesions. Patients at increased risk for oral problems include those who are seriously ill, comatose, dehydrated, confused, depressed, or paralyzed. Patients with mental health problems are also at risk for alterations in oral health (Bloomfield & Pegram, 2012). Patients who are mouth breathers, those who can have no oral intake of nutrition or fluids, those with nasogastric tubes or oral airways in place, and those who have had oral surgery are also at increased risk.

EYES, EARS, AND NOSE

Ask the patient to identify any special eye, ear, or nose care that the patient performs. Also, address any specific care measures related to the use and care of visual aids or prosthetics (glasses, contact lenses, artificial eye) and hearing aids. Inquire about any history of eye, ear, and nose problems, and related treatments.

HAIR

Identify the patient's usual hair and scalp care practices, including styling preferences. Note any history of hair or scalp problems; possible causes of changes in the distribution, texture, or amount of hair; and related treatments. Be alert for any factors that are known to cause hair or scalp problems or that require special care such as deficient self-care abilities, immobility, malnutrition, and treatments known to result in hair loss (e.g., certain chemotherapeutic agents).

NAILS AND FEET

Gather information about the patient's normal nail and foot care practices. Include the type of footwear worn and any history of nail or foot problems and their treatments. Foot problems, particularly common in people with diabetes mellitus and peripheral vascular disease, often require hospitalization. A proactive educational approach can prevent many of the serious complications (e.g., ulcers, lower extremity amputations) associated with foot problems.

Identify any variables known to cause nail and foot problems, such as deficient self-care abilities, vascular disease, arthritis, diabetes mellitus, history of biting nails or trimming them improperly, frequent or prolonged exposure to chemicals or water, trauma, ill-fitting shoes, or obesity.

PERINEAL AND VAGINAL AREAS

Note any history of perineal or vaginal problems and related treatments. Identify any variables known to cause perineal or vaginal problems or to create a need for special care, such as urinary or fecal incontinence, an indwelling Foley catheter, childbirth, douching, rectal or genital surgery, and diseases such as urinary tract infection, diabetes mellitus, and certain sexually transmitted infections (STIs, e.g., herpes).

Physical Assessment

An assessment of pertinent body systems can provide data about the patient's hygiene status and the patient's ability to maintain acceptable personal hygiene.

MUSCULOSKELETAL SYSTEM

Impairment of the musculoskeletal system can interfere with a patient's ability to perform tasks related to personal hygiene. The skills used to assess the musculoskeletal system are described in detail in Chapters 25 and 32. Many conditions produce muscle weakness, decreased range of motion, impaired balance, fatigue, and/or lack of coordination.

SKIN

The inspection and palpation skills used to assess the integumentary system are described in detail in Chapters 25 and 31. Assisting patients with basic hygiene measures provides an excellent opportunity for examining a patient's skin. Many people are unaware that they have skin lesions, such as precancerous moles, that if untreated could prove fatal. Early detection and treatment of skin problems are important nursing functions.

When examining the skin, pay careful attention to cleanliness, color, texture, temperature, turgor, moisture, sensation, vascularity, and any lesions. Follow these general guidelines for assessing the skin:

- Proceed systematically in a head-to-toe fashion.
- Use a good source of light, preferably daylight.
- Compare bilateral parts for symmetry.
- Use standard terminology to report and record findings.
- Allow data obtained in the nursing history to direct the skin assessment.
- Identify any variables known to cause skin problems, such as deficient self-care abilities, immobility, malnutrition, decreased hydration, decreased sensation, sun exposure, vascular problems (altered tissue perfusion or venous return), or the presence of irritants (body

secretions or excretions on the skin, other chemicals, mechanical devices).

Because lifestyle factors, changes in health state, illness, and certain diagnostic and therapeutic measures may adversely affect the skin, be alert for patients who may be at high risk for skin problems, and perform the appropriate skin assessment. Assessment may reveal dry skin, acne, or skin rashes. Table 30-1 summarizes recommended treatments for these skin problems.

When documenting a physical assessment of the skin, describe exactly what is observed or palpated, including appearance, texture, size, location or distribution, and characteristics of any findings. The following are two examples of documentation of the physical assessment of the skin:

> *"Skin is light brown, even tone, warm, dry, and elastic; no petechiae, lesions, or excoriation; multiple moles of small size and regular border and surface."*
>
> *"Red, macular rash generalized over trunk and thighs; semi-confluent lesions measure 1 to 2 mm; abrupt onset."*

Table 30-1   SKIN CARE PROBLEMS

SKIN PROBLEM	DEFINITION	TREATMENT
Dry Skin	The skin loses moisture and may crack and peel, or become irritated and inflamed. Symptoms include scaling, flaking, itching, and cracks in the skin.	• Keep baths or showers short, and/or bathe less frequently. • Use warm, not hot water to bathe. • Use as little soap as possible. Try mild cleansers or soaps. • Dry skin thoroughly and gently. • Use moisturizers at least daily. • Drink plenty of water throughout the day. • Use a humidifier if the air is dry.
Acne	A skin condition that is characterized by clogged pores (blackheads, whiteheads, pimples), caused by dead skin cells and sebum (oil) sticking together in the pore. Sometimes bacteria that live on the skin also get inside the clogged pore. Inside the pore, the bacteria have a perfect environment for multiplying very quickly. With a large amount of bacteria inside, the pore becomes inflamed (red and swollen). If the inflammation goes deep into the skin, an acne cyst or nodule appears. Acne can appear on the face, back, chest, neck, shoulders, upper arms and buttocks.	• Avoid squeezing or picking infected areas because this can spread the infection and cause scarring. • Gently wash the face twice a day with a mild cleanser and warm (not hot) water. • Use oil-free, water-based moisturizers and make-up. Look for products that are "noncomedogenic" or "nonacnegenic." Use cosmetics sparingly to avoid further blockage of the sebaceous ducts. • Keep hair off the face and wash hair daily. • Some acne treatments (both over-the-counter and prescription) can increase the skin's sensitivity to sunlight and ultraviolet light. Avoid sun/tanning booth exposure; use sunscreen. • Patients with a lot of acne, cysts, or nodules should consider consulting a dermatologist.
Skin rashes	Eruptions or inflammations of the skin that may be found anywhere on the body. May be precipitated by skin contact with an allergen, overexposure to the sun, and/or systemic causes, like a reaction to a medication.	• Wash area thoroughly with a mild cleansing agent and rinse well. • Use a moisturizing lotion on a dry rash to prevent itching and promote healing. • Use a drying agent on a wet rash. • Try tepid baths to help relieve inflammation and itching. • Use antiseptic sprays or lotions to help lessen itching, promote healing, and prevent skin breakdown. • Avoid exposure to causative agent, if known. • See a health care provider if symptoms do not respond to treatment or become worse.

ORAL CAVITY

A physical assessment of the oral cavity involves inspection of the oral cavity and surrounding structures with attention to any unusual odors. When performing the physical assessment of the oral cavity, examine the following:

- *Lips:* color, moisture, lumps, ulcers, lesions, and edema
- *Buccal mucosa:* color, moisture, lesions, nodules, and bleeding
- *Color of the gums and surface of the gums:* lesions, bleeding, edema, and exudate
- *Teeth:* any loose, missing, or carious (decayed) teeth. Note the presence of dentures or other orthodontic devices.
- *Tongue:* color, symmetry, movement, texture, and lesions
- *Hard and soft palates:* intactness, color, patches, lesions, and petechiae
- *Oropharynx:* movement of the uvula and condition of tonsils, if present

Also, note unusual mouth odors and assess the adequacy of mastication and swallowing. Refer to Chapter 25 for further description of nursing assessment of the oral cavity.

When inspecting the oral cavity, observe for any oral problems. These problems may be benign or only mildly annoying to patients, but they may also be life threatening. Identifying the problem and its cause and initiating appropriate treatment are imperative. This may require consultation with a dentist or physician.

Dental Caries. The decay of teeth with the formation of cavities is called **caries.** Caries result from failure to remove **plaque,** an invisible, destructive, bacterial film that builds up on everyone's teeth and eventually leads to the destruction of tooth enamel. A successful plaque-fighting program includes limiting sweet snacks such as soft drinks, candy, gum, jams, and jellies between meals; thorough cleansing of the teeth; and regular dental check-ups. The use of antiplaque fluoride toothpastes, mouth rinses, and flossing also help prevent dental caries.

Periodontal Disease. The major cause of tooth loss in adults older than 35 years of age is gum disease. **Gingivitis** is an inflammation of the gingiva, the tissue that surrounds the teeth. **Periodontitis,** or periodontal disease, is a marked inflammation of the gums that also involves degeneration of the dental periosteum (tissues) and bone. Symptoms include bleeding gums; swollen, red, painful gum tissues; receding gum lines with the formation of pockets between the teeth and gums; pus that appears when gums are pressed; and loose teeth. If unchecked, plaque builds up and, along with dead bacteria, forms hard deposits called **tartar** at the gum lines. The tartar attacks the fibers that fasten teeth to the gums and eventually attacks bone tissue. The teeth then loosen and fall out. **Halitosis,** a strong mouth odor or a persistent bad taste in the mouth, may be the first indication of periodontal disease. Regular treatment by a dentist is imperative.

Other Oral Problems. Other oral problems that may be observed when inspecting the oral cavity include the following:

- **Stomatitis,** an inflammation of the oral mucosa, has numerous causes, such as bacteria, virus, mechanical trauma, irritants, nutritional deficiencies, and systemic infection. Symptoms may include heat, pain, increased flow of saliva, and halitosis.
- **Glossitis,** an inflammation of the tongue, can be caused by deficiencies of vitamin B_{12}, folic acid, and iron.
- **Cheilosis,** an ulceration and dry scaling of the lips with fissures at the angles of the mouth, is most often caused by vitamin B complex deficiencies (especially riboflavin).
- Dry oral mucosa may simply be related to dehydration or may be caused by mouth breathing, an alteration in salivary functioning, or certain medications (e.g., anticholinergic drugs).
- Oral malignancies, appearing as lumps or ulcers, must be distinguished from benign mouth problems because early detection may lead to cure; later detection can lead to radical surgery or death. Teach patients to see their dentist immediately if they notice white or red patches, persistent sores, swelling, bleeding, numbness, or pain in the mouth.

EYES, EARS, AND NOSE

During the eye examination, note the position, alignment, and general appearance of the eye. Check that eyelashes are distributed equally and curl outward. Note the presence of lesions, nodules, redness, swelling, crusting, flaking, excessive tearing, or discharge of eyelids. Check the color of the conjunctivae and test the patient's blink reflex.

When examining the ear, note its position, alignment, and general appearance. Pay particular attention to a build-up of **cerumen** (wax) in the canal, dryness, crusting, or the presence of any discharge or foreign body. Older adults can have a build-up of cerumen that can cause impaired hearing. This is a result of harder, drier cerumen and decreased motility of the cilia in the ear canal.

While examining the nose, note its position and general appearance, patency of the nostrils, and presence of tenderness, dryness, edema, bleeding, discharge, or secretions.

Refer to Chapter 25 for additional information related to nursing assessment of the eyes, ears, and nose.

HAIR

Assess the condition of the hair. Inspect it for texture, cleanliness, and oiliness. Inspect the scalp for any scaling, lesions, inflammation, or infection. Note any abnormalities such as dandruff, hair loss, or infestations. Patients of African American descent may have very dry scalps and dry, fragile hair. Patients of Asian descent tend to have straight hair that does not necessarily require special care. When in doubt, ask the patient, a family member, or significant other about the specific manner in which hair care is performed. Refer to Chapter 25 for additional information related to nursing assessment of hair.

Dandruff. Dandruff is a condition characterized by itching and flaking of the scalp and may be complicated by the embarrassment it causes. Persistent, severe cases usually require medical attention, but daily brushing and shampooing with a medicated shampoo may be all that is needed to keep the scalp free of dandruff.

Hair Loss. Hair growth and hair loss are ongoing, daily processes. Hair loss becomes a potential problem only when it exceeds hair growth. Absence or loss of hair is called **alopecia**. Alopecia on the head is also referred to as baldness. Alopecia can be a partial or complete, local or generalized, loss of hair. Patchy hair loss can result from infections of the scalp. Hair loss from plaiting, excessive backcombing and teasing, or the use of hair rollers is usually temporary; hair returns when the tension on the hair shaft is halted.

Excessive generalized hair loss may occur with infection, especially with high fever, nutritional deficiencies, hormonal disorders, childbirth, general anesthesia, drug toxicity, chemotherapy, thyroid disease, liver disease, hepatic and renal failure, and radiation. Alopecia can also occur as part of the aging process. Alopecia related to aging is more common in men than women. There is no known cure for baldness. Although some medications are currently in use and others are being developed, their long-term efficacy is unknown. For example, minoxidil (Rogaine), a cardiovascular and antihypertensive drug, has reversed balding to some degree when applied to the scalp. Hairpieces, frequently worn by people who are bald, require the same care as normal hair but less frequent washing.

Hair transplantation is a surgical procedure for baldness. Hair is taken from donor sites, usually from the back or sides of the scalp, and transplanted to areas with no hair. The procedure is long and expensive but reportedly has decided benefits for people who find baldness psychologically unpleasant. Complications include serious scalp infections.

Pediculosis. Infestation with lice is called **pediculosis**. There are three common types of lice: *Pediculus humanus capitis,* which infests the hair and scalp; *Pediculus humanus corporis,* which infests the body; and *Phthirus pubis,* which infests the shorter hairs on the body, usually the pubic and axillary hair. Lice lay eggs, called nits, on the hair shafts. Nits are white or light gray and look like dandruff but cannot be brushed or shaken off the hair. Frequent scratching and scratch marks on the body and the scalp suggest the presence of pediculosis.

Pediculosis can be spread directly by contact with the hair of infested persons. It is less common for transmission to occur indirectly through contact with clothing, bed linen, brushes, and combs of infested persons. Teaching patients, especially children, not to share personal items is a good way to prevent transmission. The importance of environmental measures is controversial. Clothing, headgear, pillowcases, and towels should be washed in hot water and dried on the hot cycle of the dryer.

Several commercial preparations, called pediculicides, are available for the treatment of pediculosis. These drugs destroy the lice and their eggs or nits. However, two treatments are usually necessary before all the nits are destroyed. The procedures and the medications used for the treatment of pediculosis vary among health agencies. The infested hair may be shaved, especially when pubic and axillary hair is infested. In addition, the partners of patients with pubic infestation must be notified.

When educating the patient, stress the importance of finishing the treatment. Many times the patient will shampoo the hair once and not follow through with a second washing. Failure to complete the treatment has produced lice that are now resistant to many of the pediculicides on the market. See Teaching Tips 30-1: Dealing With Head Lice.

Ticks. Ticks are an important problem because they can transmit serious diseases such as Lyme disease, Rocky Mountain spotted fever, and Colorado tick fever. Ticks attach themselves to a human host as the person brushes past leaves, brush, and tall grasses. Once on a person, ticks move to a warm and moist location, like the hairline, armpit, or groin, where they burrow into the host's skin and feed off the host's blood. Transmission of tick-borne diseases can be decreased if the tick is removed within 24 hours of becoming attached. To remove a tick, grasp it with clean tweezers close to the skin. Pull it straight out with a slow and steady motion (CDC, 2011b). Once the tick is removed, cleanse the area with soap and warm water. A person should seek medical attention if part of the tick remains after removal or if a rash or fever develops within several weeks of removing a tick.

The most important thing to consider regarding ticks is that prevention of tick bites is key. While in wooded areas, tall grass, or brush, consider wearing light-colored long pants and long sleeves. Spray clothing and exposed skin with insect repellant. Frequently check clothing and skin for ticks, which look like small black or brown spots (MedlinePlus, 2012a).

NAILS AND FEET

Examine nails for intactness and cleanliness. Assess capillary refill and the contour of the nail bed. Observe the nail base for redness, swelling, bleeding, discharge, and tenderness. Patients with dark skin tones may have freckles or pigmented streaks in their nails and nails may be thicker. Examine the feet for cleanliness and intactness of skin, and note any swelling, inflammation, lesions, tenderness, or orthopedic problems. Examine carefully the

TEACHING TIP 30-1

DEALING WITH HEAD LICE

Health Topic	Teaching Tip	Why Is This Important?
Who is at risk for getting head lice?	Preschool- and elementary-aged children (age 3–11 yr) and their families are most often infested; however, anyone coming in contact with someone who has lice can become infected.	Lice can infect any person, regardless of hygiene practices or social status.
How do you become infected with head lice?	Head lice move by crawling; they cannot hop or fly. Head lice are spread by direct contact with the hair of an infested person. Anyone who comes in head-to-head contact with someone who already has head lice is at greatest risk. Head-to-head contact is common during play at school, at home, and elsewhere (sports activities, playground, slumber parties, camp). Although uncommon, head lice can be spread by sharing clothing or belongings. This happens when lice crawl, or nits attached to shed hair hatch, and get on the shared clothing or belongings, such as sharing clothing (hats, scarves, coats, sports uniforms) or articles (hair ribbons, barrettes, combs, brushes, towels, stuffed animals) recently worn or used by an infested person. Head lice can also be spread by lying on a bed, couch, pillow, or carpet that has recently been in contact with an infested person.	Avoid head-to-head (hair-to-hair) contact during play and other activities at home, school, and elsewhere (sports activities, playground, slumber parties, camp). Do not share clothing such as hats, scarves, coats, sports uniforms, hair ribbons, or barrettes. Do not share combs, brushes, or towels.
What are the signs and symptoms of head lice infestation?	Tickling feeling on scalp; itching; sores on the head caused by scratching. Irritability and difficulty sleeping; head lice are most active in the dark. The lice may also be seen, especially behind the ears and near the neckline at the back of the neck.	The faster the lice are noticed, the easier they are to eradicate.
How is head lice infestation treated?	Apply a pediculicide* according to the manufacturer's directions. Hats, scarves, pillow cases, bedding, clothing, and towels worn or used by the infested person in the 2-day period just before treatment is started can be machine washed and dried using the hot water and hot air cycles because lice and eggs are killed by exposure for 5 minutes to temperatures greater than 128.3°F. Items that cannot be laundered may be dry-cleaned or sealed in a plastic bag for 2 weeks. Items such as hats, grooming aids, and towels that come in contact with the hair of an infested person should not be shared. Soak combs and brushes in hot water (at least 130°F) for 5–10 minutes. *Note: Women who are pregnant or breastfeeding should not use pediculicides. Consult a health care provider before using pediculicides on a person who has allergies, asthma, or other medical conditions.	All head lice must be killed or removed or a reinfestation may occur. Retreatment of head lice usually is recommended because no approved pediculicide completely kills all lice eggs.

Information obtained from Centers for Disease Control (CDC). (2010). Parasites—lice. Available at http://www.cdc.gov/parasites/lice/

skin between the toes. Refer to Chapter 25 for additional information on techniques for assessing the nails and feet.

PERINEAL AND VAGINAL AREAS

Examine the male genitalia for lesions, swelling, inflammation, excoriation, tenderness, and discharge (amount, color, odor, source). Examine the female genitalia for color, size, lesions, masses, swelling, inflammation, excoriation, tenderness, and discharge (amount, color, odor,

source). Inspect the anal area for cracks, nodules, distended veins, masses, or polyps. Note any perineal odors. Refer to Chapter 25 for additional information about perineal assessment.

Diagnosing

A careful assessment of the adequacy of a patient's hygiene practices and the assessment of the skin, mucous membranes, and other body areas may lead to the development of one or more nursing diagnoses related to alterations in hygiene. Each nursing diagnosis statement identifies a patient problem and suggests expected patient outcomes. The etiology of the problem directs nursing interventions. Problems concerning deficient hygiene are categorized as self-care deficits. Self-Care Deficit diagnoses address specific activities necessary to meet daily needs: feeding, bathing, dressing, and toileting. It is important to identify the cause of these problems correctly. If hygiene is deficient because of insufficient knowledge, health education may quickly remedy the problem. If, however, hygiene is viewed as a low priority by the individual or the person lacks the physical ability to perform hygiene measures, these problems must be addressed before health education can be effective. The following are examples of appropriate nursing diagnoses:

- Bathing Self-Care Deficit related to postoperative weakness
- Ineffective Health Maintenance: dental caries related to deficient oral hygiene practices
- Impaired Oral Mucous Membrane related to malnutrition and dehydration
- Impaired Social Interaction related to negative body image: acne

Examples of these diagnoses, etiologic factors, and defining characteristics appear in Examples of NANDA-I Nursing Diagnoses: Hygiene.

In certain situations, a wellness nursing diagnosis may be appropriate as the patient progresses toward an increased level of health awareness and wellness. An example of a wellness diagnosis may be Readiness for Enhanced Self-Care related to oral hygiene practices.

Data collected during the nursing assessment may also lead to the identification of a collaborative problem. For example, a patient receiving intravenous chemotherapy is at risk for developing phlebitis, a complication requiring a collaborative approach. Therefore, when caring for a patient receiving intravenous chemotherapy, checking the infusion site every shift is a priority based on the nurse's knowledge that this complication can occur. In addition, careful preparation and administration of the drug according to the manufacturer's instructions, adherence to nursing protocols for the maintenance of intravenous infusions, and ongoing nursing assessment are crucial to help reduce the risk for phlebitis. If redness, warmth, tenderness, or swelling is noted, immediate collaborative intervention is indicated.

Similarly, a nurse may notice a 1.5-cm mole with an irregular border on a patient's back during a bath. Prompt reporting of this finding to the physician may lead to the detection and early, successful treatment of the medical diagnosis of malignant melanoma.

Outcome Identification and Planning

The plan of nursing care identifies nursing measures to assist the patient to develop or maintain hygiene practices that contribute to a sense of well-being. Appropriate expected outcomes are listed here. The patient will:

- Verbalize feeling comfortable and clean
- Participate fully in necessary hygiene measures according to cognitive, sensory, mobility, and endurance abilities
- Maintain intact skin and mucous membranes

EXAMPLES OF NANDA-I NURSING DIAGNOSES

HYGIENE

Nursing Diagnoses	Related Factors	Sample Defining Characteristics
Bathing Self-Care Deficit	Sensory, cognitive, endurance, mobility, or motivation deficits; low value attached to regular bathing, brushing, flossing, and dental examinations; pain	"I don't need a bath. I'm not dirty." Seventy-year-old man 5 days after a left thoracotomy. Transient confusion, generalized postoperative weakness. Unable to ambulate more than a few steps with assistance of two caregivers.
Impaired Oral Mucous Membrane	Ineffective oral hygiene, immunosuppressed, malnutrition, NPO for more than 24 hours, dehydration	Fifty-year-old woman recently diagnosed with cancer, receiving chemotherapy. Resulting stomatitis. "My mouth is so painful! It's an 8 out of 10." Noted to have ulcers in mouth, inability to eat, oral liquid intake limited to tepid, nonacidic liquids. Leery of using soft Toothette for oral care. Unable to verbalize importance of and technique for oral saline rinses.
Impaired Social Interaction	Negative body image	"I hate the way I look. Everyone stares at me. I don't even feel like going to school." Sixteen-year-old boy has come to the pediatrician's office for a physical for his driver's license permit. He has severe acne, involving his face, neck, and back.

FOCUS ON THE OLDER ADULT

NURSING STRATEGIES TO ADDRESS AGE-RELATED CHANGES IN HYGIENE

Age-Related Changes	Nursing Strategies
Impaired Oral Mucous Membrane • Loss of elasticity, atrophy of epithelial cells, diminished blood supply to connective tissue • Decreased salivation • Use of medications for chronic conditions that may cause dry mouth	• Floss and brush teeth with fluoride toothpaste twice a day; rinse after meals. • Brush dentures twice a day and rinse with cool water; remove and rinse dentures and mouth after meals. • Avoid mouthwashes with alcohol content. • Inspect mouth daily for lesions and inflammation. • Use lubricant on lips. • Suck on sugar-free candies, chew sugarless gum, use salivary substitutes. • Continue with dental exams at the dentist every 6 months.
Impaired Physical Mobility • Decreased range of motion • Presence of chronic conditions that compromise functional ability • Decreased muscle strength and agility	• Use adaptive devices for hygiene such as toothbrush with a large handle or extended handle, long-handled body sponge, shower chair, and grab bars. • Provide for safety in the bathroom: use nonslip mats, grab bars.
Risk for Impaired Skin Integrity • Diminished secretion of natural oils and perspiration • Loss of elasticity • Thinning of epidermis, loss of elastin and subcutaneous fat	• Use safe water temperatures to bathe; warm water, not hot. • Avoid soap; use pH-balanced skin cleansers. • Shower instead of tub bath. • Use skin moisturizers and emollients at least daily. • Bath regularly, but less often (not every day).

Adapted from Boltz, M., Capezuti, E., Fulmer, T., & Zwicker, D. (Eds.) (2012). *Evidence-based geriatric nursing protocols for best practice* (4th ed.). New York: Springer Publishing Company; Tabloski, P. A. (2010). *Gerontological Nursing* (2nd ed.). Upper Saddle River, NJ: Pearson; and Cowdell, F. (2011). Older people, personal hygiene, and skin care. *MEDSURG Nursing, 20*(5), 235–240.

• Demonstrate correct skin care measures (when indicated) such as oral care; care of eyes, ears, and nose; nail and foot care; and perineal and vaginal care
• Demonstrate signs of healing in existing lesions (oral, scalp, or perineal)
• Exhibit lips, oral mucosa, gums, and tongue that are intact, moist, and free of inflammation and lesions
• Verbalize importance of good teeth-brushing habits, fluoride use, and regular dental examinations
• Demonstrate healthy functioning of eyes, ears, and nose
• Exhibit eyes, ears, and nose that appear clean
• Demonstrate proper use and care of visual or auditory aids
• Exhibit clean hair
• Verbalize satisfaction with appearance
• Participate in hair and scalp care as able
• Exhibit intact, clean, and manicured nails
• Demonstrate intact, clean, and lesion-free foot skin
• Report reduced or absent nail and foot problems (specify: calluses, corns, plantar warts, ingrown nails, athlete's foot)

Implementing

When performing general hygiene measures, respect the patient's personal preferences and encourage as much self-care as the patient can perform. Nurses should implement interventions to meet the patient's need for privacy, and promote physiologic and psychological wellness. The following sections discuss hygiene measures, including providing scheduled care; assisting with bathing and skin care; massaging; providing routine head-to-toe hygiene care; providing environmental care, including making the bed; and teaching patients about skin care. Refer to the accompanying Focus on the Older Adult display for interventions related to hygiene for this age group.

Nurses who role model good health behaviors are more effective teachers. Use the Promoting Health 30-1 display (on page 912) for yourself before using it with others.

Providing Scheduled Hygiene Care

When patients require nursing assistance with personal hygiene, provide this care at regular intervals. In most hospitals and long-term care settings, early morning care, morning care, afternoon care, hour of sleep care, and care as needed are provided. These are individualized according to the patient's personal and cultural preferences. Personal care assistance in the home and other community-based settings centers on patient preferences and routines.

PROMOTING HEALTH 30-1

HYGIENE

Use the assessment checklist to determine how well you are meeting your needs related to hygiene. Then develop a prescription for self-care by choosing appropriate behaviors from the list of suggestions.

Assessment Checklist

❏ almost always	❏ sometimes	❏ almost never

❏ ❏ ❏ 1. I keep my hair clean and neatly styled.

❏ ❏ ❏ 2. My skin is clean.

❏ ❏ ❏ 3. The condition of my mouth indicates satisfactory oral hygiene.

❏ ❏ ❏ 4. My nails are neatly manicured.

❏ ❏ ❏ 5. My body is free of unpleasant odors.

Self-Care Behaviors

1. Ensure that diet and exercise are appropriate, since this contributes to healthy skin.

2. Brush and floss teeth regularly and visit the dentist every 6 months.

3. Keep hair clean, combed, and brushed regularly.

4. Use certain hair care products (e.g., hair dyes) cautiously, since they may damage the hair.

5. Clean under nails and maintain nails at an appropriate length. Clip nails straight across and shape or smooth with an emery board or file, if necessary.

6. Bathe and cleanse skin regularly. Apply lotion or cream to dry skin, as necessary. Cleanse the axilla and perineal area thoroughly and apply deodorant or antiperspirant as needed.

7. Appreciate the relationship between hygiene and overall well-being.

Information to promote healthy hygiene practices is available online. Visit the Point for a list of Internet resources.

REMEMBER Andrew Craig, the older man in the extended-care facility who reported that he had already had a complete bath. The nurse would need to investigate this to determine if he had indeed received care. If he had not, then the nurse would need to seek additional information to explain his statement; perhaps the patient was too tired or did not like having to be helped with his care. This information is essential to plan the patient's care effectively. ●

EARLY MORNING CARE

Shortly after the patient awakens, assist with toileting if necessary and then provide comfort measures to refresh the patient and prepare him or her for breakfast (or diagnostic tests). Nursing measures include washing the face and hands and providing mouth care. If needed, supplies necessary for morning care can be ordered at this time.

MORNING CARE (AM CARE)

After breakfast, complete morning care. Depending on the patient's self-care abilities, offer assistance with toileting, oral care, bathing, back massage, special skin care measures (e.g., pressure ulcer), hair care (includes shaving if indicated), cosmetics, dressing, and positioning for comfort. Cosmetics, if desired, can enhance morale in an ill patient. Agency policies are followed for refreshing or changing bed linens, and the patient's bedside area is tidied. When morning care is completed, the patient should feel refreshed and should be in a comfortable and safe environment.

Morning care is often categorized as self-care, partial care, or complete care. Patients identified as self-care are capable of managing their personal hygiene independently once oriented to the bathroom. However, offer a back massage and spend time assessing the patient's day-to-day needs. Patients identified as partial care most often receive morning hygiene care at the bedside or seated near the sink in the bathroom. They usually require assistance with body areas that are difficult to reach. Patients identified as complete care require nursing assistance with all aspects of personal hygiene. A complete bed bath is done, or the patient is taken to the shower.

AFTERNOON CARE (PM CARE)

Hospitalized patients frequently receive visitors in the afternoon or evening or use this time to rest when not scheduled for tests or therapies. Ensure the patient's comfort after lunch and offer assistance to nonambulatory patients with toileting, hand washing, and oral care.

HOUR OF SLEEP CARE (HS CARE)

Shortly before the patient retires, again offer assistance with toileting, washing of the face and hands, and oral care. Because many patients find that a back massage helps them to relax and fall asleep, offer one routinely. Change any soiled bed linens or clothing, and position the patient comfortably. Ensure that the call light and any other objects the patient desires (e.g., urinal, radio, water glass) are within easy reach.

AS NEEDED CARE (PRN CARE)

In addition to scheduled care, offer individual hygiene measures as needed. Some patients require oral care every 2 hours. Patients who are diaphoretic (sweating profusely) may need their clothing and bed linens changed several times a shift. At other times, a nurse may decide to forego hygiene measures because the patient's need for undisturbed rest may be a higher priority.

Assisting with Bathing and Skin Care

Bathing serves a variety of purposes, including:

- Cleansing the skin
- Acting as a skin conditioner
- Helping to relax a restless person
- Promoting circulation by stimulating the skin's peripheral nerve endings and underlying tissues
- Serving as a musculoskeletal exercise through activity involved with bathing, thereby improving joint mobility and muscle tonus
- Stimulating the rate and depth of respirations
- Promoting comfort through muscle relaxation and skin stimulation
- Providing sensory input
- Helping to improve self-image
- Providing an excellent opportunity to strengthen the nurse–patient relationship, to thoroughly assess the patient's integumentary system, to observe the patient's physiologic and emotional status closely, to teach the patient as indicated, and to demonstrate care and interest in the patient's general welfare

The simple act of bathing a patient is a vital and caring intervention. The accompanying Examples of Nursing Interventions and Nursing Outcomes Classifications (NIC/NOC) box lists standardized nursing interventions and corresponding outcomes related to helping the patient promote cleaning of the body for relaxation, cleanliness, and healing. In recent years, this basic personal care measure has often been assigned to an unlicensed staff member rather than the professional nurse. It has become a task to be accomplished rather than an opportunity for therapeutic individualized intervention. Although unlicensed assistive personnel are increasingly performing hygiene measures, the nurse is responsible for ensuring that hygiene measures are performed sat-

isfactorily. Refer to Chapter 14 for a discussion of the nurse's accountability when care is delegated. Nurses whose primary focus is the patient, however, can use the time spent on assisting with bathing to establish a rapport with the patient and to further assess the patient's integumentary system. Refer to the accompanying Through the Eyes of a Student (on page 914). Bathing is performed in a matter-of-fact and dignified manner. If this approach is followed, patients generally do not find care by a person of the opposite gender to be offensive or embarrassing.

SHOWER AND TUB BATHS

A shower may be the preferred method of bathing for patients who are ambulatory and able to tolerate the activity. Tub baths may be an option, particularly in long-term care or other community-based settings, depending on facility policy. For the most part, even though many patients can bathe on their own, the following responsibilities apply:

- Check to see that the bathroom is available, clean, and safe. Showers should have mats or nonskid strips to prevent patients from slipping and falling.
- Ensure that necessary articles—such as skin cleanser, washcloth, towel, and gown—are available for the patient.
- Provide a place for a weak or physically disabled patient to sit in a shower. Most health agencies have a stool or chair that can be used in the shower, and handheld showerheads may facilitate the process. Some nurses have reported that a commode chair with the pan removed serves effectively as a shower chair and offers the patient more support than a stool or chair.
- Assist the patient to the shower or bathroom, as indicated. Patients who are beginning ambulation often need assistance to help prevent falling or fainting.
- Check to see that the water temperature is safe and comfortable—100°F to less than 120°F–125°F. The lower temperature is recommended for children and adults over 65 years of age (Burn Foundation, 2012).

EXAMPLES OF NURSING INTERVENTIONS AND NURSING OUTCOMES CLASSIFICATIONS (NIC/NOC)

BATHING

Nursing Interventions	Nursing Outcomes
• Monitor functional ability while bathing. • Offer hand washing after toileting and before meals. • Use fun bathing techniques with children, such as wash dolls or toys. • Bathe in water of a comfortable temperature. • Monitor skin condition while bathing. • Apply lubricating ointment and cream to dry skin areas.	• Self-care: Bathing • Patient Satisfaction: Functional assistance • Oral Hygiene • Motivation • Energy Conservation

From: Bulechek, G. M., Butcher, H. K., Dochterman, J. M., & Wagner, C. M. (Eds.). (2013). *Nursing interventions classification (NIC)*. (6th ed., p. 91). St. Louis: Elsevier/Mosby; and Moorhead, S., Johnson, M., Maas, M. L., & Swanson, E. (Eds.). (2013). *Nursing outcomes classification (NOC)*. (5th ed., pp. 146, 214, 387, 625). St. Louis: Elsevier/Mosby. A full listing of nursing activities for each nursing intervention and outcomes can be found in these books.

THROUGH THE EYES OF A STUDENT

I entered the room with a feeling of dread. How could I possibly bathe the sick, elderly, helpless woman lying in this hospital bed? I had never bathed anyone older than age 2 years, other than myself, of course. How would I be able to move her limp, seemingly lifeless old body? What would an 85-year-old body look like? I could not imagine. I've read all the manuals that describe this procedure, I know what to do; so why am I so nervous? I must be worried that I will hurt her in some way. Maybe she has not been cared for properly before and her hygiene is poor. Well, I might as well get this over with because I'll be doing it the rest of my life. I've got to learn sometime.

I've mustered up enough courage to enter my patient's room. Michelle, her primary nurse, offers to help me because the patient is so difficult to move. Boy, am I relieved! Right before Michelle and I are about to begin, my patient, Mrs. Ash, asks for her teeth. I assume this must mean her dentures and reassure her that I have not seen them but will be happy to look for them as soon as we have completed her bath. Michelle and I each take a side and begin to bathe her. It's truly amazing how those range-of-motion exercises come to mind so easily. I had thought they were long forgotten with the rest of the past semester. Wouldn't my instructors love to hear me now! Suddenly Mrs. Ash yells, "I need the bedpan!" "Oh no!" I thought, as I rushed to the bathroom with soapy gloved hands trying frantically to locate her bedpan before there could be an accident. Michelle, who remained calm

during my frenzy, simply stated, "Don't worry, she has an indwelling catheter. She says that every time I bathe her." I knew she had a catheter, how did I forget? Somewhat humbled, I returned to the procedure. I really wanted to put some lotion on her skin because it was so dry. When we were ready to do her back, we prepared to lift her. I pulled her toward me, and Michelle was to continue the bath. We were not prepared for what we saw underneath. Firmly cushioned in Mrs. Ash's lower left buttock were none other than her dentures! On removing them, Michelle and I had to smile at the periodontal grin implanted on Mrs. Ash's bottom. Michelle then asked her how her teeth had gotten to the location where we found them. All she seemed to know was that she needed those teeth back in her mouth NOW! She snatched the dentures from Michelle's hand and attempted to insert them. Michelle and I in unison blurted out, "No, Mrs. Ash, please wait until we clean your teeth before you put them back in your mouth!" Mrs. Ash, somewhat confused, begrudgingly handed over her teeth to be cleaned. Michelle had the honors while I finished the last touches of good hygiene for Mrs. Ash.

What a difference cleanliness can make, not only for the patient, but also for me, the student nurse. I felt better knowing that Mrs. Ash was clean and that this procedure was behind me. And to think that I was apprehensive! This was definitely an interesting learning experience.

—*Marilyn Johnson, Holy Family College, Philadelphia*

- Ensure privacy for patients who can safely shower or bathe independently. See that a call device is handy, and make sure the patient knows what the button is for, so that the patient can obtain help if necessary.
- Help the patient get in and out of the bathtub, as indicated. Have the patient grasp the handrails at the side of the tub, or place a chair at the side of the tub. The patient sits on the chair and eases to the edge of the tub. After putting both feet into the tub, it is then relatively easy for the patient to reach the opposite side and ease down into the tub. The patient may kneel first in the tub and then sit in it; this process can be reversed when leaving the tub. Use a hydraulic lift, when available, to lower and lift patients who are unable to maneuver safely or completely bear their weight. Some community-based settings have walk-in tubs available.
- Keep the bathroom door unlocked. Health personnel should be able to enter with ease if the patient needs help. A sign hung on the door ensures privacy. Never leave children or confused patients alone in the bathroom.
- Help to wash and dry areas of the body that the patient cannot reach, such as the back.
- Make any necessary adaptations. For example, if the patient is confused and becomes agitated as a result of overstimulation when bathing, reduce the stimuli. Turn down the lights and play soft music and/or warm the

room before taking the patient into it (Johnson, 2011). Box 30-1 outlines possible measures to implement to meet the bathing needs of patients with dementia.

Figure 30-1 illustrates several features that add to the safety of a patient taking a shower. Ensure proper cleaning of shower or tub between patient uses to comply with infection control measures, according to facility policy.

 RECALL Sonya Delamordo, the older Hispanic woman who is going to live at her daughter's home after a stroke. Although the responsibilities listed apply to a hospitalized patient, the nurse can incorporate these responsibilities into the teaching plan for Mrs. Delamordo's daughter to ensure the patient's safety with hygiene. ●

 BED BATHS

Some patients must remain in bed as a part of their therapeutic regimen but can still bathe themselves. Other patients are not on bed rest but require total or partial assistance with bathing in bed due to physical limitations, such as fatigue or limited range of motion. Implement the following nursing measures to help patients take a bath in bed:

- Provide the patient with articles for bathing and a basin of water that is a comfortable and safe temperature.

BOX 30-1 MEETING THE BATHING NEEDS OF PATIENTS WITH DEMENTIA

- Shift the focus of the interaction from the "task of bathing" to the needs and abilities of the patient. Focus on comfort, safety, autonomy, and self-esteem, in addition to cleanliness.
- Individualize patient care. Consult the patient, the patient's record, family members, and other caregivers to determine patient preferences.
- Consider what can be learned from the behaviors associated with dementia about the needs and preferences of the patient. A patient's behavior may be an expression of unmet needs; unwillingness to participate may be a response to uncomfortable water temperatures or levels of sound or light in the room.
- Ensure privacy and warmth.
- Consider other methods for bathing. Showers and tub baths are not the only options in bathing. Towel baths, washing under clothes, and bathing "body sections" one day at a time are other possible options.
- Maintain a relaxed demeanor. Use calming language. Use one-step commands. Try to determine phrases and terms the patient understands in relation to bathing and make use of them. Offer frequent reassurance.
- Encourage independence. Use hand-over-hand or a guided hand technique to cue the patient regarding the purpose of the interaction and allow the patient to perform some of the activities independently.
- Explore the need for routine analgesia before bathing. Move limbs carefully and be aware of signs of discomfort during bathing.
- Wash the face and hair at the end of the bath or at a separate time. Water dripping in the face and having a wet head are often the most upsetting parts of the bathing process for people with dementia.

Adapted from Jablonski, R. A., Therrien, B., & Kolanowski, A. (2011). No more fighting and biting during mouth care: Applying the theoretical constructs of threat perception to clinical practice. *Research and Theory for Nursing Practice: An International Journal, 25*(3), 163–175; Johnson, R. H. (2011). Practical care: creative strategies for bathing. *Nursing & Residential Care, 13*(8), 392–394; Keefe, S. (2010). Bath safety and dementia. Advance for Long-term Care Management. Available at https://nursing.advanceweb.com/Regional-Content/Articles/Bath-Safety-Dementia.aspx; and Papa, K. S. (2011). A dignified bathing experience. *Advance for Long-Term Care Management, 14*(6), 16.

Place these items conveniently for the patient on a bedside stand or overbed table.

- Provide privacy for the patient. Make sure the call device is within reach.
- Remove the top linens from the patient's bed and replace them with a bath blanket.
- Place cosmetics in a convenient place for the patient. Provide a mirror, a good light, and hot water for patients who wish to shave with a razor.
- Assist patients who cannot bathe themselves completely. For example, some patients can wash only the upper parts of the body. Nursing personnel then complete the remainder of the bath.

Bathing procedures for patients who require total nursing assistance vary among health agencies. Skill 30-1 on pages 932–937 offers one example as a guide. It assumes that the patient can be raised or lowered in bed and that, although the patient may have limited movement, the nurse can manage the patient alone.

THE BAG BATH OR DISPOSABLE BATH

Research has suggested, and some health care agencies recommend, use of the "bag bath" as an alternative to the traditional bed bath. There are several variations of this bath. In one system, 8 to 10 washcloths are contained in a plastic bag; cleanser and warm water are added to prepare the bath. Another self-contained bathing system consists of a package containing 8 to 10 premoistened, disposable washcloths (Fig. 30-2 on pagge 916). The unopened package is warmed in the microwave or stored in a warmer until use. Each part of the patient's body is cleansed with a fresh cloth. No rinsing is required. The skin is allowed to air dry (for about 30 seconds) so that the emollient ingredient of the cleaner remains on the skin.

Feedback about this procedure has been overwhelmingly positive. Nursing staff value the time savings when compared with a traditional bed bath and find it effective and easy to perform. These products also eliminate the cross-infection risk posed by soap, water, bath basins, and washcloths (Massa, 2012). Most patients have commented favorably on the disposable bath. Patients with mild to moderate skin impairments demonstrated an improved skin condition with consistent use of the disposable bath (Massa, 2010).

PROMOTING SKIN HEALTH

An easy and effective way to promote the barrier function of the skin and keep the skin healthy is the daily

FIGURE 30-1. Examples of features that add to the safety of a patient taking a shower or bath. (**A**) Call bell equipped with a pull cord. (**B**) Shower equipped with a safety seat and hand rail. *(Photo by B. Proud.)*

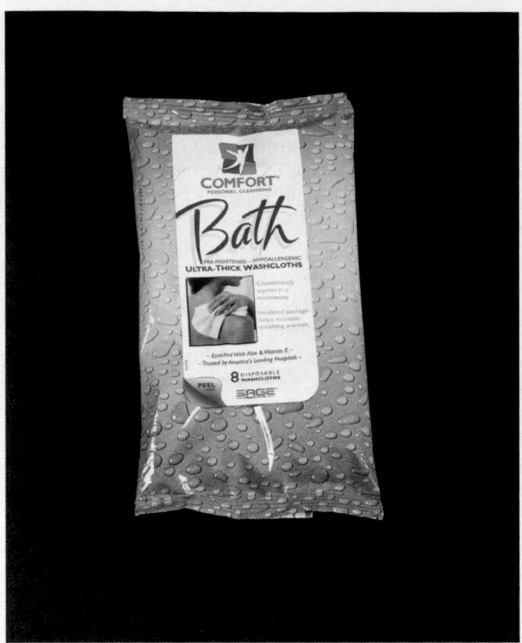

FIGURE 30-2. Commercial self-contained bathing system.

use of soap substitutes, topical emollients, and barrier products (Voegeli, 2010). Soap cleans the skin, but at the same time it removes dirt from the surface, it affects the lipids that are present on the skin and the skin pH. This contributes to drier skin, damaging the barrier function of the skin. The substitution of a nonsoap emollient cleaning agent is an easy way to prevent drying and damage to the skin. The rinseless products mentioned in the description of a bag bath are examples of nonsoap emollient cleaning agents.

The use of chlorhexidine gluconate for bathing has been shown to reduce colonization of skin with pathogens and is becoming part of personal hygiene policies in some facilities. Chlorhexidine can be added to bath water, but is also available, and easier to use, in prepackaged impregnated cloths. Bathing with chlorhexidine may be used to reduce the incidence of hospital-acquired infections, such as central line–associated bloodstream infections and surgical site infections, as well as to reduce the acquisition of or decolonization with multidrug-resistant organisms (Ritz, Pashnik, Padula, & Simmons, 2012; Sievert, Armola, & Halm, 2011). Refer to the accompanying Research in Nursing box below.

Topical emollient agents—also known as moisturizers—can be applied to the skin as a lotion, cream, gel, or ointment. They act to seal water into the skin and replace lipids in the skin, effectively hydrating the skin and recreating its waterproof barrier. Apply topical moisturizers after bathing. Ideally, they should be applied twice a day but may need more frequent application, depending on the skin condition and the product used.

Skin barrier products include creams, ointments, and films; they are used to protect vulnerable skin and to protect skin at risk for damage caused by excessive exposure to water and irritants, such as urine and feces. They are

RESEARCH IN NURSING

BRIDGING THE GAP TO EVIDENCE-BASED PRACTICE

Bathing and Health Care–Associated Infections

Prevention of health care–associated infections (HAIs) is a major challenge for health care providers. Health care agencies constantly strive to implement evidence-based practices to reduce the risk of HAIs for patients and promote patient health.

Related Research

Ritz, J., Pashnik, B., Padula, C., & Simmons, K. (2012). Effectiveness of 2 methods of chlorhexidine bathing. *Journal of Nursing Care Quality*, 27(2), 171–175.

This study examined the impact of chlorhexidine gluconate (CHG) bathing on the transmission of methicillin-resistant *Staphylococcus aureus* (MRSA) and vancomycin-resistant *Enterococcus* (VRE) on an inpatient oncology unit, using a convenience sample of 405 patients, over a 6-month period. The study also compared the cost of two chlorhexidine bath delivery methods, and evaluated nursing time and satisfaction related to bath administration. Specific protocols were developed for each type of bath, based on a review of the literature. Patients received a daily bath using two ounces of 4% CHG solution added to the bathing water or were bathed daily with prepackaged 2% CHG impregnated cloths. MRSA

and VRE transmission rates decreased from those during the pervious years. Costs associated with bathing increased, but the time to administer the bath decreased with the chlorhexidine cloths. The nursing staff reported satisfaction with the use of the chlorhexidine cloths; all of the 32 nursing staff reported that the product was easier to use, took less time, and required fewer supplies. The majority (94%) of the staff preferred the cloth bathing method.

Relevance to Nursing Practice

This study suggests that the implementation of a relatively simple procedure, daily bathing with a consistent dose of CHG, along with a continued emphasis on hand hygiene and transmission-based precautions, can reduce the risk of transmission of MRSA and VRE. These results can be useful to other facilities in decreasing HAIs. Nurses and nursing staff are the primary providers of bathing activities in many health care settings and should consider the implementation of interventions to break the chain of infection, improve patient health, and decrease health care costs.

For additional research, visit thePoint.

BOX 30-2 GENERAL SKIN CARE PRINCIPLES

- Assess the patient's skin daily.
- Cleanse the skin when indicated, such as when soiled, using a no-rinse, pH-balanced cleanser.
- Avoid using soap and hot water; avoid excessive friction and scrubbing.
- Minimize skin exposure to moisture (incontinence, wound leakage); use a skin barrier product as necessary.
- Use skin emollients after bathing and as needed.

Adapted from Voegeli, D. (2010). Care or harm: Exploring essential components in skin care regimens. *British Journal of Nursing, 19*(13), 812, 814, 816, 818–819; Wound Ostomy and Continence Nurses Society, 2003, as cited in Voegeli, 2010.

also used to prevent skin breakdown around stomas and wounds with excessive exudate. Application of one of these products forms a thin layer on the surface of the skin to repel potential irritants. Apply these products by following the manufacturer's recommendations and facility policy. Box 30-2 outlines general skin care principles.

MASSAGING THE BACK

A backrub generally follows the patient's bath. A backrub acts as a general body conditioner and can relieve muscle tension and promote relaxation. Some nurses forego giving backrubs to patients due to time constraints. However, giving a backrub allows the nurse to observe the skin for signs of breakdown. A backrub improves circulation; can decrease pain, distress, and anxiety; can improve sleep quality; and provides a means of communication with the patient through the use of touch.

Because some patients may consider the backrub a luxury and be reluctant to accept it, be sure to communicate its importance and value to the patient. An effective backrub should take 4 to 6 minutes to complete. If a lotion is used, warm it before use.

Be aware of the patient's medical diagnosis when considering giving a backrub. A backrub is contraindicated, for example, if the patient has had back surgery or has fractured ribs. Position the patient on the abdomen or, if this is contraindicated, on the side. Recommended techniques for administering a backrub are outlined in Skill 34-1 on pages 1188–1191.

Assisting with Oral Hygiene

The mouth requires care even during illness, but sometimes care must be modified to meet a patient's needs. Adequate oral hygiene care is imperative to promote the patient's sense of well-being and prevent deterioration of the oral cavity. Poor oral hygiene is reported to lead to the colonization of the oropharyngeal secretions by respiratory pathogens. Diligent oral hygiene care can improve oral health and limit the growth of pathogens in the oropharyngeal secretions, decreasing the incidence of

aspiration pneumonia, community-acquired pneumonia, ventilator-associated pneumonia, and other systemic diseases, such as diabetes, heart disease, and stroke (Tada & Miura, 2012; CDC, 2011a; Durgude & Cocks, 2011; AACN, 2010).

An oral assessment tool can assist with assessment of the status of the oral cavity, as well as help to determine the frequency and procedure for oral care. If the patient can assist with mouth care, provide the necessary materials (Skill 30-2, pp. 938–940). Physical limitations, such as those associated with aging, often lead to less than adequate oral hygiene. The dexterity required for adequate brushing and flossing may decrease with age or illness. Older patients may be dependent on caregivers for oral hygiene. Patients with cognitive impairment, such as dementia, are also at risk for inadequate oral hygiene (Jablonski, Therrien, & Kolanowski, 2011). If the patient is unable to perform oral hygiene, make certain that the mouth receives care as often as necessary to keep it clean and moist, as often as every 1 or 2 hours if necessary. This is especially important for patients who cannot drink or are not permitted fluids by mouth. Refer to Box 30-3 for suggestions to meet the oral hygiene needs for patients with cognitive impairments. Skill 30-3 on pages 941–943 gives techniques for administering oral hygiene to dependent patients. Moisten the mouth with water, if allowed, and lubricate the lips often enough to keep the membranes well moistened. Following the steps for cleaning the mouth thoroughly is more important than the agent used. This supports the personal experience of many people that no mouthwash, breath freshener, ointment, or paste replaces a thorough mechanical cleaning of the oral cavity.

The use of chlorhexidine gluconate as part of oral hygiene has been integrated into oral hygiene regiments and is available in an oral spray and dental gel (Ames et al., 2011; Kelly, Timmis, & Twelvetree, 2010). The

BOX 30-3 MEETING THE ORAL HYGIENE NEEDS OF PATIENTS WITH COGNITIVE IMPAIRMENTS

- Choose a time of day when the patient is most calm and accepting of care.
- Enlist the aid of a family member or significant other.
- Break the task into small steps.
- Provide distraction, such as playing favorite music, while providing care.
- Allow the patient to participate. The nurse can put a hand over the patient's to guide the activity.
- Start the activity, showing the patient what to do, then let the patient take over.
- Withdraw and try again later if the patient strongly refuses care.
- Document effective and ineffective interventions to provide appropriate information for staff to give consistent, effective care.

Adapted from Tabloski, P. A. [2010]. *Gerontological nursing* (2nd ed.). Upper Saddle River, NJ: Pearson.

use of chlorhexidine gluconate as part of protocols for systematic oral care for critically ill patients has been shown to reduce the incidence of health care–associated pneumonia (Ames et al., 2011).

TOOTH BRUSHING AND FLOSSING

Brush and floss teeth twice a day and rinse the mouth after meals. A soft-bristled toothbrush should be small enough to reach all teeth. Clean and dry all brushes between uses. Bacteria do most damage directly after eating, so make sure the patient brushes the teeth immediately after eating or drinking. In addition, clean the tongue with the toothbrush. Use a toothbrush even when the patient has no or few teeth. It is the only effective way to remove plaque and debris.

Automatic toothbrushes, electric or battery operated, are simple to use and are as good as manual brushes for removing debris and plaque. These devices are very useful for patients with arthritis or other conditions that make it difficult to brush effectively (Mayo Foundation for Medical Education and Research [MFMER], 2011d). Pressurized water spray units are available to assist with oral hygiene. However, if too much water pressure is used, particles of debris may be forced into tissue pockets, leading to gum damage. Therefore, discuss their use with a dentist.

The toothbrush cannot reach areas between the teeth where food lodges, so flossing twice a day is recommended. Flossing removes the debris that the toothbrush cannot and helps to break up colonies of bacteria.

Toothpastes and powders aid the brushing process and usually have a pleasant taste that encourages brushing, especially by children. Most dentifrices are safe to use, but those containing harsh abrasives may scratch the enamel of the teeth, thus are not recommended. Salt and sodium bicarbonate are far less expensive than proprietary products on the market and just as effective for short-term use. However, these products lack fluoride and should not be used exclusively. Dentifrices containing stannous fluoride and antitartar agents, as well as antiplaque rinses, decrease dental caries and thus are recommended by many dentists.

MOUTHWASHES

An offensive breath odor (halitosis) is often systemic in nature. For example, the odor of onions and garlic on the breath comes from the lungs, where the oils are being removed from the bloodstream and eliminated with respiration. A mouthwash cannot remove halitosis when odors are being eliminated by respiration.

If the cause of halitosis is poor oral hygiene, cleaning reduces the odor. Commercial mouthwashes may also be helpful. Therapeutic mouth rinses that reduce bacteria can help reduce plaque, gingivitis, and bad breath. Anticavity rinses with fluoride help protect tooth enamel and are often used with children (American Dental Association [ADA], 2012). If concentrated mouthwashes are used frequently in debilitated patients, however, they may injure oral tissue.

DENTURE CARE

Failing to wear dentures for a long period allows the gum line to change, thus affecting the fit of the dentures. If the patient has been instructed to remove dentures while sleeping, a disposable denture cup is convenient and easy to use. Advise the patient not to wrap dentures in toilet tissue or disposable wipes because these are likely to be thrown away.

Patients with dentures are more likely to keep them in the mouth if they are kept clean. If the patient cannot care for them, the nurse must ensure that the dentures are clean. Use care when handling a patient's dentures because they represent a considerable financial investment, and replacement for damage or loss is expensive. Brush dentures twice a day; remove and rinse dentures and mouth after meals.

When cleaning dentures, put on gloves and hold them over a basin of water or a sink lined with a washcloth or soft towel (Fig. 30-3) so that if they slip from your grasp, they will not fall onto a hard surface and break. If necessary, grasp the dentures with a 4" × 4" piece of gauze to help prevent them from slipping out of your gloved hands. Use cool or lukewarm water to cleanse them. Hot water may warp the plastic material of which most dentures are made. Use a soft toothbrush and toothpaste. Dentures may be soaked in commercial preparations to help remove stains and hardened particles and then rinsed well after cleaning. Give the patient the opportunity to brush the gums and tongue and rinse the mouth before the dentures are replaced. Assist the patient with care as necessary. Store dentures in cold water when not in the patient's mouth. Leaving dentures to dry can cause warping, leading to discomfort when worn.

Providing Eye Care

Normally, the eyes are kept clean with lacrimal secretions. During illness, the eyes may produce more secretions than normal and may appear glass-like. Use the following

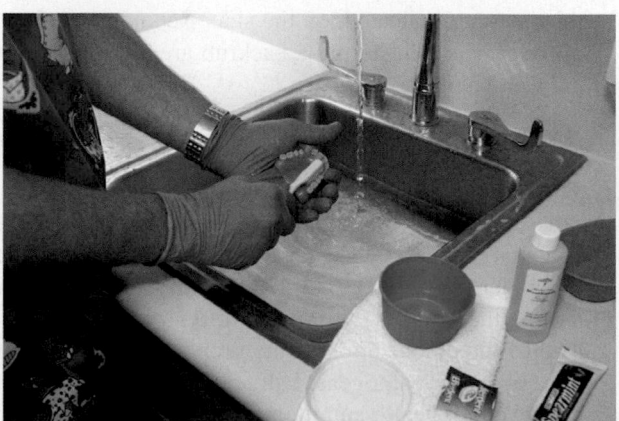

FIGURE 30-3. Proper method for cleaning dentures.

techniques when secretions adhere to the eyelashes and become dry and crusty or when discharge is present:

- Wear gloves during the cleaning procedure.
- Use water or normal saline and cotton balls or a clean washcloth or compress to clean the eyes. Never use soap to clean the eyes because soap is irritating to eye tissues.
- Position the patient on the same side as the eye to be cleaned so that solution and debris do not run across the bridge of the nose and contaminate the other eye.
- Dampen a washcloth or cotton ball with the solution of choice and wipe once while moving the cotton ball from the inner canthus to the outer canthus of the eye. This technique minimizes the risk for forcing debris into the area drained by the nasolacrimal duct. Turn the washcloth and use a different section for each stroke. Alternately, discard the used cotton ball.
- Continue this technique, using a different section of the washcloth or one cotton ball for each stroke, until the eye is clean.
- Turn the patient to the opposite side and clean the other eye in the same manner.
- Wipe the lashes dry with a paper tissue or a clean washcloth, exposing a clean area of the tissue or cloth with each stroke.
- If the eyelashes are matted with secretions or debris that cannot be removed by wiping, apply a warm, wet compress to the closed eye for 3 to 5 minutes to loosen the secretions so that they may be removed in a painless manner.

CARE OF THE UNCONSCIOUS PATIENT'S EYES

Patients with diminished or absent blink (corneal) reflexes and patients whose eyelids remain open require frequent eye care, at least every 4 hours. If the eye is not kept moist, corneal ulceration may result from excessive drying of the eye. Nursing measures include using saline or artificial tears, based on the medical orders, to lubricate the eye and a protective eye shield to keep the eye closed.

EYEGLASS CARE

Eyeglasses are essential for many people and represent a considerable financial investment. Take special precautions to prevent them from being broken or lost. Encourage patients who need glasses to wear them to avoid eyestrain.

Many eyeglasses have plastic lenses, which are considerably lighter in weight than glass lenses but correct vision just as well. Plastic lenses scratch easily. Whenever setting down glasses, make sure they are placed with the lenses up.

Clean eyeglasses over a terry towel, so that if they slip they will not become scratched or broken. Use warm water and soap or a special cleansing preparation. Hot water may warp plastic lenses and frames. Rinse the glasses well after cleaning them with soap and water; dry them with a clean, soft cotton cloth, such as a cotton handkerchief or a special eyeglass cleaning cloth. Paper products that are made of wood pulp increase the risk of scratching the lenses, so do not use a dry paper tissue to clean eyeglasses. Do not use silicone tissues to clean plastic lenses.

CONTACT LENS CARE

A contact lens is a small disc worn directly on the eyeball. It stays in place by surface tension of the eye's tears. Contact lenses are either rigid (hard) or soft. Rigid gas permeable (RGP) lenses are more rigid than soft lenses and therefore more durable for an active user (Cleveland Clinic, 2009a). Soft lenses are made of a plastic material that absorbs water to become soft and pliable. They are brittle when dehydrated and absorb water when placed in a solution, usually normal saline, or when in contact with tears. Soft lenses may be used for daily wear or extended wear. Disposable soft lenses are also available.

People who wear contact lenses, and the nurses caring for them, need to take special precautions to keep the lenses free of microorganisms that may lead to eye infections and to avoid injuring or scratching the surface of the eye. When providing contact lens care, always perform meticulous hand hygiene and put on gloves before touching eye surfaces and lenses. Caution lens wearers about eye irritation in the presence of noxious vapors or smoke. Also, remind lens wearers that lenses should not come into contact with cosmetics, soaps, or hair sprays because eye irritation may result. Urge the patient to report immediately to the prescribing physician any adverse reaction related to contact lens use.

The cornea, which consists of dense connective tissue, does not have its own blood supply. It is nourished primarily by oxygen from the atmosphere and from tears. In a patient who wears contact lenses, the cornea requires more than its normal supply of oxygen because its metabolic rate increases. To allow the cornea to receive a maximal supply of oxygen, hard lenses should not be worn for more than 12 to 16 hours and should be removed before sleeping. Extended-wear soft lenses can be left in place for 1 to 30 days, depending on the manufacturer. People wearing extended-wear lenses should clean them at least once a week. The time that disposable soft lenses should be worn also varies according to the type and manufacturer. A new type of disposable lens is replaced daily, whereas other options include lenses that can be worn day and night for 7 days or during waking hours only for 14 days. Excessive tearing, pain, and redness signal the need to remove lenses.

If a patient wears contact lenses but cannot remove them, the nurse is responsible for removing them. This may occur, for example, when the nurse is caring for an unconscious patient. Whenever an unconscious patient is admitted without any family present, always assess to determine whether the patient wears contact lenses. Leaving contact lenses in place for long periods could result in permanent eye damage.

Before removing rigid lenses, use gentle pressure to center the lens on the cornea. When removing soft lenses, use gentle pressure to move the lens down to the sclera and pinch to remove. A small suction device can also be used in an emergency situation to remove gas-permeable or hard lenses. Figure 30-4 demonstrates removal of RGP and soft lenses. Once the lens is removed, identify it as being for the right or left eye, because the two lenses are not necessarily identical. If an eye injury is present, do not try to remove lenses because of the danger of causing an additional injury.

ARTIFICIAL EYE CARE

Most patients who wear an artificial eye prefer to care for it themselves if they are able. Encourage them to do so when possible. The necessary equipment includes a

Removing Rigid Gas Permeable (RGP) Lenses

If the lens is not centered over the cornea, apply gentle pressure on the lower eyelid to center the lens.

Gently pull the outer corner of the eye toward the ear.

Position the other hand below the lens to receive it and ask the patient to blink.

Or

Gently spread the eyelids beyond the top and bottom edges of the lens.

Gently press lower eyelid up against the bottom of the lens.

After the lens is tipped slightly, move eyelids towards one another to cause the lens to slide out between the eyelids.

Removing Soft Contact Lenses

Storing Lenses

Have the patient look forward. Retract the lower lid with one hand. Using the pad of the index finger on the other hand, move the lens down the sclera.

Using the pads of the thumb and index finger, grasp the lens with a gentle pinching motion and remove.

Because lenses may be different for each eye, storage cases are marked L and R, designating left and right lenses. It is important to place the first lens in its designated cup in the storage case before removing the second lens to avoid mixing them up.

FIGURE 30-4. Removing contact lenses.

Behind the ear
(moderate to severe loss)

In the ear
(mild to severe loss)

In the canal
(mild to moderate loss)

FIGURE 30-5. Several types of hearing aids.

small basin, soap and water for washing, and solution for rinsing the prosthesis. Normal saline or tap water can be used for rinsing. Most people have their own method for cleaning the eye socket and the area around it. Ask how the patient does this, and enable the patient to continue with the usual practice. When the nurse is performing the care, the patient should be lying down so that the prosthesis does not accidentally fall to the floor. Flush the socket with normal saline before replacing the prosthesis.

Providing Ear Care

Other than cleaning the outer ears, little intervention is needed for routine hygiene of the ear. After the ears are washed, dry them carefully with a soft towel so that water and **cerumen** (wax) are removed by capillary action. Forcing the towel into the ear for drying or using a cotton-tipped applicator may aid in the formation of wax plugs. Using bobby pins, hairpins, paper clips, or fingernails to remove wax from the ear is extremely dangerous because these may injure or puncture the eardrum.

If the patient uses a hearing aid, check the batteries routinely and clean the earpieces or ear mold daily with mild soap and water. A whistling sound that is audible when the hearing aid is held in the hand with the power on and the volume high indicates that the battery is functioning properly. Refer to Chapter 20 for strategies nurses can use to promote communication with a hearing-impaired patient. If hearing loss is mild and the patient is not using a hearing aid, the following suggestions may help to improve hearing and should be included in any patient teaching:

- Avoid noisy places for conversation.
- Choose well-lit places where it is easier to look at the speaker's face, lips, and hands for cues to the conversation.
- Cup your hand behind your ear.
- Ask people to face you when they are speaking to you.

- Ask people to repeat what they said, if it was not clear to you, and to speak slowly.
- Consider buying amplitude devices so that you can hear your television and radio without turning up the sound.

Figure 30-5 illustrates three types of hearing aids.

Providing Nose Care

The best way to clean the nose is to blow it gently. Both nostrils should be open while doing this. Closing one nostril adds to the danger of forcing debris into the eustachian tubes. Irrigations are usually contraindicated because of the danger of forcing material into the sinuses.

If the external nares are crusted, applying a warm, moist compress helps to soften and remove the crusts. Disposable paper tissues are recommended for nasal secretions. A cotton-tipped applicator may be used to clean the nares, but with great care to avoid injury. Never introduce the applicator into the nares.

Providing Hair Care

Daily brushing of the hair helps keep it clean and distributes oil along the shaft of each hair. Brushing also stimulates blood circulation in the scalp. Hair that becomes entangled is difficult to comb. Combing tiny sections of hair at a time may be necessary if a patient's hair has not been combed for even 1 day. The best way to protect long hair from matting and tangling is to ask the patient for permission to braid it. Patients usually consent to the procedure if it increases their comfort. Parting the hair in the middle on the back of the head and making two braids, one on either side, prevents the discomfort of lying on one heavy braid on the back of the head. When braiding a patient's hair, ensure that the hair is not pulled too tightly.

Occasionally, a patient's hair is almost hopelessly matted, and cutting the hair may be necessary. Before a patient's hair is cut, usually the patient signs a written consent. Also, as appropriate, discuss with a member of the patient's immediate family the necessity of cutting the hair.

Tightly curled (kinky) hair usually requires special attention. It is normally dry and curly and becomes matted and tangled easily. Use a comb with wide-spaced teeth and work the hair through from the neckline upward toward the forehead.

Some people have their hair straightened, but even after this process, it may be difficult to untangle the hair when the person is confined to bed. Some African Americans style their hair in small braids. The braids are not undone for shampooing and may need to have a lubricant or oil applied daily to prevent hair strands from breaking. Demonstrate cultural consideration by grooming the patient's hair in the style preferred by the patient.

SHAMPOOING THE HAIR

The hair, which is exposed to the same dirt and oil as the skin, requires washing as often as necessary to keep it clean. Wash the comb and brush each time the hair is washed and as frequently as necessary between shampoos. Many health agencies have beauticians and barbers to assist with hair care, including shampooing, but this does not relieve the nurse of the responsibility.

Before shampooing the hair, brush or have the patient brush and comb the hair well to stimulate the scalp and undo tangled hair. The patient may then shampoo the hair while showering, if able. In some settings, a medical order is required for shampooing a patient's hair.

For patients on bed rest—whether at home or in the hospital—who are unable to shampoo their own hair, use the following as a guide:

- Prepare several pitchers of water of a suitably warm temperature for a thorough washing and rinsing, shampoo, one or two towels for drying, and a receptacle to receive wash and rinse water.
- Place a protective pad and a plastic hair-washing tray if one is available (Fig. 30-6) under the head.
- Place the patient in a position over the pad so that water drainage is directed into the receptacle.

FIGURE 30-6. The nurse uses a protective pad and plastic tray to prepare for shampooing a patient's hair.

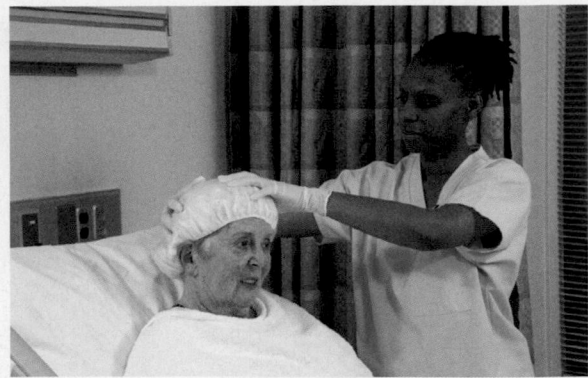

FIGURE 30-7. Using a shampoo cap to clean a patient's hair.

- Wet the hair, apply shampoo, and massage the scalp well while washing the hair.
- Rinse the hair and reapply shampoo for a second washing, if indicated.
- Rinse the hair thoroughly.
- Apply conditioner if requested or if the scalp appears dry.
- Dry the hair as quickly as possible to prevent the patient from becoming chilled, and arrange the hair according to the patient's preference.

If regular shampooing is inappropriate or is contraindicated by the patient's condition, other products for use at the bedside are available. Products for use at the bedside do not require rinsing and are available as foams, concentrates, and dry powders. After application of a foam or concentrate cleaner, lather the product and then towel-dry the hair. Comb and style the hair as per the patient's preference. Keep the head covered with a towel until the hair dries to help minimize chilling of the patient. Alternately, shampoo caps are available, and are being used with increasing frequency (Figure 30-7). These commercially prepared, disposable caps contain a rinseless shampoo product. Warm the cap in the microwave or store it in a warmer until use. Place the cap on the patient's head and massage the hair and scalp through the cap, to lather the shampoo. After shampooing for the manufacturer's suggested length of time, remove and discard the cap. Finally, towel dry the patient's hair and style it according to the patient's preference.

SHAVING

Grooming of body hair other than hair on the head can be an important part of a patient's self-esteem and well-being. Patients with beards or mustaches may require nursing assistance to keep the beard and mustache clean. Never trim or shave a patient's beard or mustache without the patient's consent. Female patients may require assistance with shaving underarm and leg hair, depending on the patient's personal preference and abilities. Blade razors tend to give a closer shave than do electric razors, but many patients find electric razors more convenient and practical. Electric shavers are usually recommended when the patient is receiving anticoagulant therapy or

GUIDELINES FOR NURSING CARE 30-1

SHAVING

- Perform hand hygiene.
- Identify patient. Explain procedure to the patient.
- Cover patient's chest with a towel or waterproof pad. Fill bath basin with comfortably warm (100°F to <120°F–125°F) water.
- Press a warm washcloth on the patient's skin to soften the hair.
- Dispense shaving cream into palm of hand. Rub hands together, then apply to area to be shaved in a layer approximately 0.5" thick.
- With one hand, pull the skin taut at the area to be shaved. Using a smooth stroke, begin shaving. *If shaving the face,* shave with the direction of hair growth in downward, short strokes. *If shaving a leg,* shave against the hair in upward, short strokes.
- Remove residual shaving cream with a wet washcloth.
- If patient requests, apply aftershave or lotion to area shaved.
- Remove and discard gloves and perform hand hygiene.

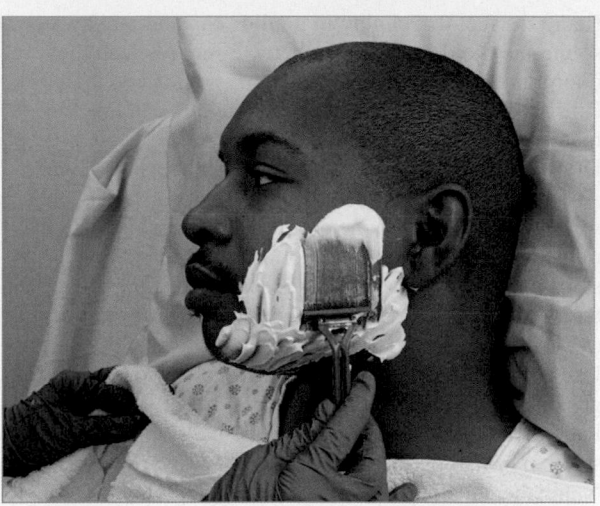

Shaving the face.

has a bleeding disorder and are especially convenient for ill and bedridden patients. Shaving after a warm bath or shower softens the hair, making the process easier. The technique for shaving patients who cannot shave themselves is described in Guidelines for Nursing Care 30-1.

Providing Fingernail Care

The following are recommended techniques for the care of fingernails:

- File the nails straight across, then round the tips in a gentle curve. Do not trim so far down on the sides that the skin and cuticle are injured.
- Remove hangnails, which are broken pieces of cuticle, by cutting them off. Avoid injury to tissue with the cuticle scissors.
- Gently push cuticles back off the nail when soft and pliable after washing in warm water.
- Push back cuticles with a blunt instrument or a terry cloth.
- Apply an emollient to the cuticle to help prevent hangnails.
- Clean under the nails with a blunt instrument, being careful not to injure the area where the nail is attached to the underlying tissue.

Splitting and peeling of the nails are usually caused by dryness. Teach the patient to avoid contact with soap and water as much as possible, use a good hand cream frequently, and avoid using polish remover with acetone, which tends to dry the nails (MFMER, 2011c).

Providing Foot Care

Proper foot care is important at any age. It becomes even more so with aging and when conditions such as circula-

tory disturbances or diabetes mellitus are present. Guidelines for Nursing Care 30-2 (on page 924) highlights the appropriate techniques related to foot care.

Cut toenails straight across the toes. Discourage patients with conditions such as diabetes and peripheral vascular diseases from doing nail care at home (Lyman & Vlahovic, 2010). Encourage patients with these diseases to see a podiatrist for treatment related to bunions, corns, or calluses (MFMER, 2012a).

Providing Perineal Care

Perineal cleaning is performed in a matter-of-fact and dignified manner. If this approach is followed, patients generally do not find care by a person of the opposite gender to be offensive or embarrassing.

 REMEMBER Sonya Delamordo, who is going home after a stroke to her daughter's home. The patient may be embarrassed to have her daughter help with perineal care. The nurse would encourage the patient to do as much as she is able, using her left side. By doing so, the patient maintains some control over the situation, thereby promoting her self-esteem and fostering personal hygiene and independence. ●

In some cases, a sitz bath may be used to clean and soothe the perineal and anal areas. The procedure associated with administering a sitz bath is discussed in Chapter 31.

Perineal care may be carried out while the patient remains in bed. When performing perineal care, follow these guidelines:

GUIDELINES FOR NURSING CARE 30-2

PROVIDING FOOT CARE

- Bathe the feet thoroughly in a mild soap and tepid water solution. Avoid soaking the feet. Be sure to clean the interdigital area.
- Rinse the feet to remove soap residue that can dry and irritate the skin.
- Dry feet thoroughly, including the area between the toes.
- Apply a moisturizer to feet if they are dry. Patients with diabetes and peripheral artery disease should apply moisturizer on the tops and bottoms of the feet to keep the skin soft. These patients should sprinkle talcum powder or cornstarch between the toes to keep the skin dry (MFMER, 2011a).
- Use an antifungal foot powder if necessary to prevent fungal infections, such as athlete's foot.
- Patients with diabetes should file the nails; avoid using scissors or nail clippers, which may slip and injure tissues. Nondiabetic patients should avoid digging into or cutting the toenails at the lateral corners when trimming the nails.
- Do not cut off corns or calluses. Avoid commercial removers because they may contain ingredients that can lead to development of infection and ulcers. Consult a *podiatrist,* a physician who treats foot disorders, when corns or calluses are present.

- Explain the dangers of going barefoot. Skin on the feet may be injured, or athlete's foot may be acquired in public showers.
- Advise patients to wear appropriate footwear. Break in new shoes gradually. Improperly fitting shoes can lead to corns, calluses, bunions, and blisters. The soles should be flexible and nonslippery and the heel heights should be safe and offer appropriate support. Shoes with rough ridges, wrinkles, or tears in the linings should be discarded or repaired.
- Advise patients to wear cotton socks, which provide warmth and absorb perspiration.
- Teach patients to avoid wearing knee-high stockings, and do not sit with the knees crossed because this can obstruct the circulation to the lower extremities and feet.
- Prop the feet up above the level of the hips a few minutes several times a day if the feet swell.
- Avoid using heating pads and hot-water bottles because of the danger of blistering and burning the feet.
- Report any signs of foot problems to your primary care provider. This is especially important for patients with diabetes.

- Assemble supplies, and provide for privacy.
- Explain the procedure to the patient, perform hand hygiene, and put on disposable gloves.
- Wash and rinse the groin area (both male and female patients). Use a small amount of mild, unscented soap and water.
- For a female patient, spread the labia and move the washcloth from the pubic area toward the anal area to prevent carrying organisms from the anal area back over the genital area (Fig. 30-8). Always proceed from the least contaminated area to the most contaminated area. Use a clean portion of the washcloth for each stroke. Rinse the washed areas well with plain water.

- For a male patient, clean the tip of the penis first, moving the washcloth in a circular motion from the meatus outward. Wash the shaft of the penis using downward strokes toward the pubic area (Fig. 30-8). Always proceed from the least contaminated area to the most contaminated area. Rinse the washed areas well with plain water. In an *uncircumcised male patient* (teenage or older), retract the foreskin (prepuce) while washing the penis. Pull the uncircumcised male patient's foreskin back into place over the glans penis to prevent constriction of the penis, which may result in edema and tissue injury. It is not recommended to retract the foreskin for cleaning during infancy and childhood, as

FIGURE 30-8 Performing normal perineal care.

injury and scarring could occur (MedlinePlus, 2012b). Wash and rinse the male patient's scrotum. Handle the scrotum, which houses the testicles, with care because the area is sensitive.

- Dry the cleaned areas and apply an emollient as indicated. Avoid the use of powder. Powder may become a medium for the growth of bacteria.
- Turn the patient on his or her side and continue with cleansing the anal area. Continue in the direction of least contaminated to most contaminated area. In the female, cleanse from the vagina toward the anus. In both female and male patients, change the washcloth with each stroke until the area is clean. Rinse and dry the area.
- Remove gloves and perform hand hygiene. Continue with additional care as necessary.

If the patient has an indwelling catheter and the agency recommends daily care for the catheter, this is usually done after perineal care. Care of an indwelling catheter is discussed in Chapter 36.

Incontinent patients require special attention to perineal care. Patients with urinary or fecal incontinence are at risk for perineal skin damage. This damage is related to moisture, changes in the pH of the skin, overgrowth of bacteria and infection of the skin, and erosion of perineal skin from friction on moist skin. Skin care for these patients should include measures to reduce overhydration (excess exposure to moisture), contact with ammonia and bacteria, and friction. Remove soil and irritants from the skin during routine hygiene, and clean the area when the skin becomes exposed to irritants. Avoid using soap and excessive force for cleaning. The use of perineal skin cleansers, moisturizers, and barriers is recommended for skin care for the incontinent patient. These products help promote healing and prevent further skin damage. Incontinence, and nursing care of the patient with incontinence, is discussed further in Chapters 31, 36, and 37.

 Concept Mastery Alert

For the patient who is incontinent, it is important to keep the area clean and dry. Do not use soap, and protect the area with moisture barriers.

Providing Vaginal Care

Vaginal mucous secretions are odor free until they combine with air and perspiration. Thus, for vaginal care, using plain soap and water is the most effective means to control odor. In normal, healthy women, daily douching is believed to be unnecessary and unwise because it tends to remove normal bacterial flora from the vagina, and an acidic solution may irritate or injure normal cells. Douching has also been linked to vaginal irritation, bacterial vaginosis, and pelvic inflammatory disease. Although douching is occasionally ordered to treat a vaginal infection, it is not recommended as a routine hygiene measure.

Deodorants to control odor around the vaginal orifice are unnecessary. No therapeutic benefit from their use has been proven to date. Use of these special deodorants is not a substitute for keeping the area clean; female patients often require teaching on this subject.

If patients insist on using them explain that, although these deodorants do not contain aluminum salts, which are irritating to the mucous membrane, they are intended for external use only. They should not be placed on sanitary napkins or tampons. Some sprays have been reported as possibly harmful when sprayed into the vagina. Repeated use is not generally recommended because of reported irritation and rashes. In addition, the sprays should not be used on broken skin areas.

Providing Care for Body Piercing

Body piercing has increased in popularity and acceptance over recent years, regardless of socioeconomic and cultural background. Piercings can be found on the face (tongue, lips, nose, eyebrows), ears, neck, arms, legs, torso, navel, and genitals of patients. Nurses and other health care providers need to provide safe and effective care for patients with body piercings, including accurate assessment and site care. Basic wound care used for body piercings is usually called "aftercare." Aftercare techniques are used for the new piercing and whenever the piercing fistula has become disrupted through injury or exhibits signs of infection or inflammation (MFMER, 2012b; Halliday, 2005). Guidelines for Nursing Care 30-3 provides appropriate techniques related to piercing site care.

GUIDELINES FOR NURSING CARE 30-3

PROVIDING BODY PIERCING CARE

- Perform hand hygiene before providing care. Explain what you are going to do. Put on gloves.
- Clean the jewelry and the piercing site of all crust and debris. Rinse the site with warm water and use a cotton swab to gently remove any crusting.
- Apply a dab of liquid medicated cleanser to the area. Turn the jewelry back and forth to work the cleanser around the opening. Rinse well. Remove gloves. Perform hand hygiene.

- Advise patients to avoid the use of alcohol, peroxide, and ointments at the site.
- Oral piercing aftercare includes rinsing with an antibacterial, alcohol-free mouthwash for 30 to 60 seconds after meals and at bedtime. The patient should brush the teeth with a new, soft-bristled toothbrush.
- Advise patients to avoid oral tobacco use.
- Most piercings take 6 to 8 weeks to heal, but some may take several months or a year to heal.

Piercing jewelry may cause difficulty with placement of treatment devices, and can interfere with diagnostic imaging, such as magnetic resonance imaging (MRI) or computerized axial tomography (CT scan), or contribute to patient injury during MRI or other procedures, such as surgery or Foley catheter placement (Durkin, 2012; DeBoer, et al., 2011). Some practitioners routinely recommend that all jewelry is removed, whereas others state that a selective approach to removal is appropriate (DeBoer, et al., 2011). Various devices are available to be used to keep the piercing tract open when removal is required. The use of intravenous catheter to maintain piercing patency has also been suggested (DeBoer, Seaver, Vidra, Robinson, & Klepacki, 2011). Nurses should consult facility policies related to removal of body piercing jewelry.

Providing Environmental Care

A person's environment can improve or detract from the patient's sense of well-being. The patient's environment can consist of a room in a facility, such as a hospital, one or more rooms in the patient's home or apartment, or something in-between. Regardless of the setting, ensure that this area is clean and clutter-free, safe, and pleasant.

The patient's environment in a hospital or other facility consists of the bedside unit and the furnishings and equipment in the space around the bed. Basic furniture includes the bed, overbed table, bedside stand, and chairs. Standard equipment in the health care environment includes the call light, oxygen, suction, and electrical outlets; light fixtures; bath basin; emesis basin; bedpan or urinal; water pitcher and glass; and bed linens. One nursing responsibility is ensuring that necessary equipment and items are in their proper place and functioning properly. Patients usually store personal items in the bedside stand. Always request permission from alert patients or family members before opening the stand to obtain the bath basin, lotion, or other items. When assisting with hygiene, respecting the patient's right to privacy and ownership of personal goods decreases the patient's sense of powerlessness.

Before leaving the bedside, get into the habit of saying to the patient, "Is there anything else I can do to make you more comfortable?" Checking with the patient communicates genuine caring and can correct for any oversights. In the case of manipulative patients, set limits regarding what comfort and hygiene measures can be performed.

Good ventilation in patient rooms is imperative to limit pathogens and unpleasant odors associated with body secretions and excretions, for example, urine, stool, vomitus, draining wounds, or body odors. Decrease odors by emptying bedpans, urinals, and emesis basins promptly. When the waste receptacle in the patient's room is used to dispose of soiled dressings or anything with a strong odor, be sure to remove the trash before leaving the room. Dispose of the trash according to facility policy. Room deodorizers may need to be used.

Patient preferences for room temperature often vary widely. Whenever possible, respect the patient's preference when determining the room temperature. In general, the room temperature should be between 68°F–74°F (20°C and 23°C).

Many patients find it difficult to sleep in a health care facility. Patients are often disturbed frequently for assessment or treatment purposes. Care should be taken to reduce harsh lighting and noises whenever possible, although adequate lighting is necessary for all nursing procedures. Whenever possible, avoid carrying on conversations immediately outside the patient's room. Many patients find this stressful because the noise disturbs them and because they believe whatever is being said involves them.

BED SAFETY AND COMFORT

Many people who are ill and hospitalized or are being cared for at home spend a large portion of the day—if not the entire day—in bed, so the bed is an important part of the patient's environment. Nursing responsibilities include ensuring a safe and comfortable bed.

The typical hospital bed has a motorized metal frame in three sections, which allows the height of the bed to be raised or lowered and the head and foot to be adjusted. Know how to operate the bed and be ready to explain it to the patient. Bed positions are described in Chapter 33.

Hospital beds can also be ordered for use in the home. Because certain positions may be harmful to some patients, instruct the patient and family about advisable bed positions and the use of the bed controls. Historically, hospital beds have been generally 26 inches (66 cm) from the floor. This is higher than most beds at home, enabling the nurse or caregiver to reach the patient without undue musculoskeletal strain. However, many manufacturers are making low-height beds available to health care facilities. These beds have a minimum height of 7 to 15 inches from the floor.

Side rails are used to provide assistance with moving in bed, and access to bed controls is often on the side rails. See Chapter 26 for additional discussion about the use of side rails. Use side rails when indicated and according to facility policy. Also, lock the wheels or casters on the hospital bed whenever the bed is stationary to prevent the bed from moving when the patient is moving from the bed to an upright position or being transferred. The headboard of most hospital beds is removable to allow close patient contact in an emergency situation.

Nurses are responsible for ensuring the safety and comfort of the patient at the bedside. To promote bed safety while maintaining patient comfort, ensure the following before leaving the patient's bedside:

- The bed is in its lowest position.
- The bed position is safe for the patient.
- The bed controls are functioning (bed is electrically safe).
- The call light is functioning and always within reach.

FIGURE 30-9. This special bed is an air-flotation, low-air-loss support surface that provides pressure relief. In this KinAir III, there is a microprocessor computer control panel that controls airflow and temperature precisely. A built-in digital scale and heater are included. The bed also has a quick-release level for CPR. *(Photo courtesy of KCI Therapeutic Services, San Antonio, TX.)*

- Side rails are raised if indicated.
- The wheels or casters are locked.

The hospital mattress is firm and generally covered with a water-repellent material that can be easily wiped with a bactericidal solution between patients. A variety of therapeutic beds and mattresses are available to reduce or relieve the effects of pressure on the skin (Fig. 30-9). These are discussed in more detail in Chapter 31.

Facility policies usually dictate the availability and use of bed linens. Bed linens include mattress covers, sheets, incontinence pads, pillowcases, blankets, bedspreads, and bath blankets. Changing the bed linen is often not the nurse's responsibility and is delegated. The nurse is responsible for coordinating with assistive personnel to ensure patient comfort. To promote bed comfort, ensure the following before leaving a patient:

- Linens are clean and free of crumbs and wrinkles.
- The patient feels comfortably warm.
- Pressure areas are protected from rough sheets, hem edges, and water-repellent material. This is especially important for patients with a nursing diagnosis of Risk for Impaired Skin Integrity.

 MAKING A BED

A comfortable bed and appropriate bedding contribute to a patient's sense of well-being. Usually bed linens are changed after the bath, but some agencies change linens only when soiled. The bed is made for the ambulatory patient, as described in Skill 30-4 on pages 943–946. If the patient is bedridden, the occupied bed is made, as described in Skill 30-5 on pages 946–950.

Although there are variations in the procedure for making an occupied bed, these minor differences have no real effect on the patient's comfort. In some instances, creativity and flexibility are necessary when changing linens because of the patient's condition, orthopedic appliances on the bed, or treatments that may be in progress. Refer to Through the Eyes of a Student.

Teaching Patients About Skin Care

Teaching about skin care can occur at different times. For example, teaching can be done informally during assessment and care procedures. Here, the nurse shares information about general skin care measures, including ways to prevent or reduce a patient's risk for skin problems. Teaching addressing a specific topic, such as dry skin, diabetic foot care, or acne, may be addressed as part of the nursing care plan. The following section describes common topics related to skin care and skin problems.

SOAPS AND DETERGENTS

A wide variety of soaps and detergents are available. Soaps are often made from vegetable and animal fats, whereas most detergents are made from petroleum derivatives. Studies have shown that expensive cleansing agents are no more effective than their less expensive counterparts. Patients who experience dry skin or other alterations in

THROUGH THE EYES OF A STUDENT

One of my first patients was a man in his late 60s who had suffered a stroke. I was assigned to care for him, and his care included a bed bath and complete linen change—with him in the bed. I was determined to complete this task totally on my own, without asking anyone for help. This was my first mistake.

The patient yelled out a lot and had very rough mannerisms. I kept thinking to myself, "I must treat him with gentle care and not show any fear." Inside I was shaking furiously.

I managed to complete his bath and then began to change the sheets. I helped the patient to turn to one side, tucking the dirty linens close to him. I applied the fitted sheets to the upper portion of the bed...so far, so good. Immediately

going to the foot of the bed, I applied the bottom portion. The top portion popped off—I ran to the top of the bed, reapplied the top portion—the bottom portion popped off—I reapplied it.... I must have spent 15 minutes running back and forth trying to get both ends to stay on. By this time, sweat was pouring off my face.

When I finally cried "Uncle," I discovered that certain fitted sheets just didn't fit all the mattresses. The usual routine in this case is to walk to the linen closet and get another fitted sheet. That probably takes about 15 seconds!

—*Linda A. Keough*
Delaware County Community College, Media, Pennsylvania

skin health may benefit from using nonsoap cleaning agents. Refer to the discussion of these agents earlier in this chapter in the Promoting Skin Health section on pages 915–917.

DEODORANTS AND ANTIPERSPIRANTS

Perspiration is essentially odorless, although it contains some waste products, such as uric acid and ammonia. The odor of perspiration results when bacteria, normally present on everyone's skin, act on the skin's normal secretions.

Inform patients that keeping the body and clothing clean is the best way to prevent body odors. Recommend the use of deodorants and antiperspirants after the skin is clean. Deodorants mask odor, and antiperspirants are intended to reduce the amount of perspiration. They act as astringents and tend to close the exits of the sweat glands. Advise patients to use antiperspirants and deodorants with care and according to directions to prevent skin irritation. Keep in mind that these products are contraindicated in some situations, such as before mammography and during the postoperative period for a patient who has had a mastectomy.

COSMETICS

Cosmetics frequently enhance the appearance of clean and healthy skin. Cosmetics can be used judiciously to help disguise blemishes, improve skin coloring, and make wrinkles appear less obvious. However, certain cultural and religious groups discourage their use.

Periodically, cosmetics containing harmful ingredients have appeared on the market. Be alert to such agents and help consumers avoid their use. The U.S. Department of Health and Human Services Food and Drug Administration (FDA) enforces federal laws on the purity of foods, drugs, and cosmetics and on the advertising claims of their manufacturers. The FDA is a good source of information regarding cosmetic safety.

Remind patients that cosmetics often become contaminated with bacteria and fungi. Teach patients not to share cosmetics and advise them to discard cosmetics after they are 2 to 4 months old, especially those applied near the eyes (U.S. Food and Drug Administration [FDA], 2012c). Encourage patients to keep makeup applicators and brushes immaculately clean.

SUNSCREEN

Spending time in the sun increases the risk of skin cancer and early skin aging (FDA, 2012b). Sun damage to the body is caused by invisible ultraviolet (UV) radiation. Patients of all skin tones are potentially susceptible to sunburn and other harmful effects of exposure to UV radiation. Everyone should take precautions to protect skin from sun damage. However, people who need to be especially careful in the sun are those who have pale skin; blond, red, or light brown hair; those who have been treated for skin cancer; or those who have a family member who's had skin cancer (FDA, 2010b). Others

BOX 30-4	SUN PROTECTION MEASURES

Patients of all skin tones are potentially susceptible to sunburn and other harmful effects of exposure to UV radiation from the sun. Everyone should take precautions to protect skin from sun damage. To reduce risk of sunburn and skin damage related to sun exposure, encourage patients to use the following sun protection measures:

- Use broad spectrum sunscreens with SPF (sun protection factor) values of 15 or higher regularly and as directed.
- Reapply sunscreen, even if labeled "water resistant," at least every 2 hours. Apply sunscreen more often if sweating or jumping in and out of the water. Refer to individual product directions.
- Limit time in the sun, especially between the hours of 10 AM and 2 PM, when the sun's rays are most intense.
- Wear clothing to cover skin exposed to the sun; for example, long-sleeved shirts, pants, sunglasses, and broad-brimmed hats.
- Avoid using sunscreen for infants less than 6 months old (FDA, 2012d).
- Keep infants under 6 months old out of the sun and in the shade (FDA, 2012d). Dress infants in clothing that covers their sensitive skin, as well as a wide brimmed hat.

Adapted from Printz, C. (2012). Dermatology community applauds new FDA sunscreen regulations: Labeling requirements aim to make it easier for consumers to select a sunscreen. *Cancer, 118*(1), 1–3; U.S. Food and Drug Administration (FDA). (2012a). Sun safety: Save your skin! Available at http://www.fda.gov/ForConsumers/ConsumerUpdates/ucm049090.htm; and U.S. Food and Drug Administration (FDA). (2012d). Should you put sunscreen on infants? Not usually. Available at http://www.fda.gov/ForConsumers/ConsumerUpdates/ucm309136.htm

who need to be especially aware of sun-care precautions are patients who are prescribed certain medications that increase sun sensitivity, such as furosemide (Lasix), glyburide (Micronase), and quinolone antibiotics (e.g., ciprofloxacin [Cipro]). To reduce risk of sunburn and skin damage related to sun exposure, encourage patients to use sun protection measures. Refer to Box 30-4 for a list of suggested sun protection measures.

Evaluating

Performing or assisting with the performance of hygiene measures provides a means of at least daily contact with the patient to determine whether the patient is achieving outcomes related to hygiene and skin care. Indicators that can be used to determine outcome achievement include the following:

- Level of patient's participation in hygiene program
- Elimination of, reduction in, or compensation for factors interfering with the patient's independent execution of hygiene measures, for example, weakness, decreased motivation, and lack of knowledge

- Changes related to specific skin problems, for example, healing of skin lesions, elimination or reduction in causative factors, and independent patient management of the prescribed treatment program

The following are examples of evaluation related to hygiene:

10/26/15—Outcome partially met. Patient's oral mucosa is intact, but thick, dry secretions continue to build up on oral mucosa and gums despite every-4-hour care.

   Revision: Increase frequency of oral hygiene to every 2 hours. Instruct family.

   —N. Glynn, RN

10/24/15—Outcome met. Patient demonstrated correct care (cleaning) of artificial eye for the past two mornings. States, "I guess I should be happy to be alive and still able to see."

   —N. Glynn, RN

10/27/15—Outcome partially met. Patient reports that she is uncomfortable wearing a wig but feels better since its purchase.

Revision: Patient still has many questions about effects of chemotherapy; continue teaching and use opportunities to build self-esteem.

   —A. Jones, RN

10/27/15—Expected outcome met. Patient correctly verbalized rationale for diabetic foot care program and expressed interest in attending the diabetic classes.

   —A. Diaz, RN

11/20/15—Outcome partially met. Child returned to clinic with clean perineal area and relief of painful urination. Mother reports child spends half the time with her and half with father (parents separated) and that father is not committed to hygiene practices.

   Revision: Continue to provide positive feedback for accomplishments and reinforce importance of perineal hygiene with child.

   —C. Moser, RN

Ongoing evaluation helps adjust the nursing plan of care. For examples of the nursing process for hygiene, see the accompanying Nursing Plan of Care 30-1 for Kylie Simpson and Female University Students.

NURSING PLAN OF CARE 30-1

for Kylie Simpson and Female University Students

Glenda Davis is a nurse practitioner who works in a campus health clinic at a state university. Kylie Simpson met with Glenda Davis at the clinic. Kylie had been having vaginal itching and burning for 2 weeks. She was diagnosed with a vaginal infection. She asks Glenda, "This is terrible. It's the second infection in 7 months. Is there something wrong with me? Isn't there something I can do to keep this from happening again?"

Frequently, women ask Glenda questions about feminine hygiene. Realizing that each woman who presents with a question probably represents many other women with similar unvoiced questions, Glenda talks with Kylie, including patient teaching regarding feminine hygiene in their discussion. Glenda decides to develop an insert entitled *Self-Care: Feminine Hygiene* for the campus newspaper. The information she plans to include and the population she will address in her checklist are based on the following assessment data:

- Diverse female population is of various ages, cultures, religions, sexual orientation, and family and lifestyle backgrounds.
- Knowledge about feminine hygiene varies widely from almost no knowledge to students who are well read or members of women's health professions.
- Students who present with questions are mostly concerned about the risk of acquiring a sexually transmitted infection (STI) or the dangers of certain products (e.g., tampons and toxic shock syndrome) or have questions related to intercourse and contraception.
- Numerous students report to the clinic with vaginal infections and urinary tract infections.
- Interest is high; ability to comprehend written materials is high.

NURSING DIAGNOSIS	Deficient Knowledge: Feminine Hygiene related to information misinterpretation, lack of exposure, and unfamiliarity with information resources as manifested by female students presenting to the campus clinic with questions about feminine hygiene; high incidence of vaginal and urinary tract infections; negative attitudes about feminine body frequently expressed
EXPECTED OUTCOME	Students will: • Express positive body image, valuing their uniqueness

(continued)

NURSING PLAN OF CARE 30-1 *continued*

for Kylie Simpson and Female University Students

NURSING INTERVENTIONS	RATIONALE	EVALUATIVE STATEMENT
With each student who presents at the clinic for help with a gynecologic concern or problem, take the time to assess her knowledge of the female body and her acceptance of her body and comfort with it.	The women's health movement has encouraged women to feel ownership of their bodies, to appreciate their uniqueness as women, and to increase their awareness of their physical bodies and the feelings associated with them. Many women still feel that the genital area and cyclic phenomena such as the menstrual cycle and the female sexual response cycle are "dirty"; and symptoms in this area may evoke fear, guilt, anxiety, and shame.	*Six-month evaluation:* 6/30/15 Outcome partially met: Students are beginning to discuss gynecologic concerns more freely, yet great hesitance persists. *Revision:* Continue to help women to know, understand, and accept their bodies and to talk about their bodies. Make this a priority of the nursing staff at the clinic. *G. Davis, RN*
Counsel appropriately.	It is important for nurses to provide women with information about their bodies.	

EXPECTED OUTCOME   Students will:

- Correctly describe feminine hygiene self-care behaviors they are willing to incorporate into their daily lifestyles.

NURSING INTERVENTIONS	RATIONALE	EVALUATIVE STATEMENT
Assess with each patient her knowledge of feminine hygiene practices (correct any misconceptions) and motivation to use them consistently.	Many women have never been instructed about feminine hygiene, and harmful practices may be "picked up" from the media and other sources (e.g., the use of frequent douching and deodorants to eliminate normal body odors).	6/30/15 Outcome met. Following publication of the *Self-Care: Feminine Hygiene* feature and one-on-one counseling using this printed handout, patients are knowledgeable about preventive hygiene measures. *G. Davis, RN*
Address specific concerns related to menstruation, intercourse, other maturational events.	Maturational events, such as menstruation, becoming sexually active, and pregnancy, may result in a need for new or modified hygiene practices.	
Teach the importance of using preventive hygiene measures to reduce the likelihood of acquiring a urinary tract or vaginal infection. Distribute the *Self-Care: Feminine Hygiene* handout and discuss this with the patient.	It is better to prevent a genitourinary infection than to treat it.	

NURSING PLAN OF CARE 30-1   *continued*

for Kylie Simpson and Female University Students

EXPECTED OUTCOME   Campus health clinic records will:

• Demonstrate a reduction in both new and recurrent genitourinary infections

NURSING INTERVENTIONS	RATIONALE	EVALUATIVE STATEMENT
Educate women regarding preventive hygiene measures (refer to the *Self-Care* handout).	It is better to prevent a genitourinary infection than to treat it.	6/30/15 Outcome met. Six months after publication and use of the *Self-Care: Feminine Hygiene* handout, the incidence of genitourinary infections is reduced 10%. Will continue to keep education in this regard a priority. *G. Davis, RN*
Educate women to distinguish normal from abnormal findings (vaginal discharge, pain, bleeding, problems with urination) and to seek help when appropriate. Nursing measures include teaching preventive measures, instructing in recognition of symptoms, and assisting with self-care activities to prevent and treat infections, including the securing of assistance when indicated.	Early treatment of genitourinary infections reduces the likelihood of residual problems.	
Document new and recurrent genitourinary infections; identify predisposing factors.	Documentation facilitates ongoing management of a recurring problem.	

SAMPLE DOCUMENTATION

6/15/15

Nursing student visited clinic and expressed need for information about feminine hygiene practices in general as well as those specific hygiene measures for use after intercourse. Also related concern about contracting an STI from partners. Reported that she became sexually active this year and has sexual intercourse once or twice weekly. Stated that "many of my friends use douches" and questioned whether any particular douche products are recommended. We discussed the *Self-Care: Feminine Hygiene* handout and reviewed various health care practices. Clarified for student her misconception regarding the advisability of douching. Also counseled her about her right to talk with a sexual partner about STIs and previous contacts with infected people. Advised that she refrain from contact or use a condom when she has intercourse. Student reported feeling more "in charge" of body and better able to care for it. Discussed all topics on plan of care and encouraged her to revisit clinic in 6 months for further clarification and evaluation.

G. Davis, RN

SKILL 30-1 | PROVIDING A BED BATH

DELEGATION CONSIDERATIONS

The implementation of a shower or tub bath may be delegated to nursing assistive personnel (NAP) or unlicensed assistive personnel (UAP), as well as to licensed practical/vocational nurses (LPN/LVN). The decision to delegate must be based on careful analysis of the patient's needs and circumstances, as well as the qualifications of the person to whom the task is being delegated. Refer to the Delegation Guidelines in Appendix A (found on thePoint).

EQUIPMENT

- Washbasin and warm water
- Personal hygiene supplies (deodorant, lotion, and others)
- Skin-cleaning agent
- Emollient and skin barrier, as indicated
- Towels (2)

- Washcloths (2)
- Bath blanket
- Gown or pajamas
- Bedpan or urinal
- Laundry bag
- Nonsterile gloves; other PPE as indicated

IMPLEMENTATION

ACTION	RATIONALE
1. Review the patient's health record for any limitations in physical activity.	Identifying limitations prevents patient discomfort and injury.
2. Perform hand hygiene and put on gloves and/or other PPE, if indicated.	Hand hygiene and PPE prevent the spread of microorganisms. PPE is required based on transmission precautions.
3. Identify the patient. Discuss the procedure with the patient and assess the patient's ability to assist in the bathing process, as well as personal hygiene preferences.	Identifying the patient ensures that the right patient receives the intervention and helps prevent errors. Discussion promotes reassurance and provides knowledge about the procedure. Dialogue encourages patient participation and allows for individualized nursing care.
4. Assemble equipment on overbed table within reach.	Organization facilitates performance of task.
5. Close the curtains around the bed and close the door to the room, if possible. Adjust the room temperature, if necessary.	This ensures the patient's privacy and lessens the risk for loss of body heat during the bath.
6. Adjust the bed to a comfortable working height; usually elbow height of the caregiver (VISN8 Patient Safety Center, 2009).	Having the bed at the proper height prevents back and muscle strain.
7. Remove sequential compression devices and antiembolism stockings from lower extremities according to agency protocol.	Most manufacturers and agencies recommend removal of these devices before the bath to allow for assessment.
8. Put on gloves. Offer the patient a bedpan or urinal.	Gloves are necessary for potential contact with blood or body fluids. Voiding or defecating before the bath lessens the likelihood that the bath will be interrupted, because warm bath water may stimulate the urge to void.
9. Remove gloves and perform hand hygiene.	Hand hygiene deters the spread of microorganisms.
10. Put on a clean pair of gloves. Lower the side rail nearer to you and assist the patient to the side of bed where you will work. Have the patient lie on his or her back.	Gloves prevent transmission of microorganisms. Having the patient positioned near the nurse and lowering the side rail prevent unnecessary stretching and twisting of muscles on the part of the nurse.
11. Loosen top covers and remove all except the top sheet. Place the bath blanket over the patient, then remove the top sheet while the patient holds the bath blanket in place. If the linen is to be reused, fold it over a chair. Place soiled linen in a laundry bag. Take care to prevent the linen from coming in contact with your clothing.	The patient is not exposed unnecessarily, and warmth is maintained. If a bath blanket is unavailable, the top sheet may be used in its place.

ACTION	RATIONALE
12. Remove the patient's gown and keep the bath blanket in place. If the patient has an IV line and is not wearing a gown with snap sleeves, remove the gown from the other arm first. Lower the IV container and pass the gown over the tubing and the container. **Rehang the container and check the drip rate.**	This provides uncluttered access during the bath and maintains warmth of the patient. IV fluids must be maintained at the prescribed rate.
13. **Raise side rails.** Fill the basin with a sufficient amount of comfortably warm water (100°F to 120°F to 125°F). Add skin cleanser, if appropriate, according to the manufacturer's directions. Change as necessary throughout the bath. Lower the side rail closer to you when you return to the bedside to begin the bath.	Side rails maintain patient safety. Adjusting the water temperature to 100°F to <120°F to 125°F decreases risk of burns and drying of the skin. The lower temperature is recommended for children and adults over 65 years of age (Burn Foundation, 2012). Warm water is comfortable and relaxing for the patient. It also stimulates circulation and provides for more effective cleansing.
14. Put on gloves, if necessary. If desired, fold the washcloth like a mitt on your hand so that there are no loose ends (Fig. 1 through Fig. 3).	Gloves are necessary if there is potential contact with blood or body fluids. Having loose ends of cloth drag across the patient's skin is uncomfortable. Loose ends cool quickly and feel cold to the patient.
15. Lay a towel across the patient's chest and on top of the bath blanket.	This prevents chilling and keeps the bath blanket dry.
16. **With no cleanser on the washcloth, wipe one eye from the inner part of the eye, near the nose, to the outer part (Fig. 4). Rinse or turn the cloth before washing the other eye.**	Soap is irritating to the eyes. Moving from the inner to the outer aspect of the eye prevents carrying debris toward the nasolacrimal duct. Rinsing or turning the washcloth prevents spreading organisms from one eye to the other.

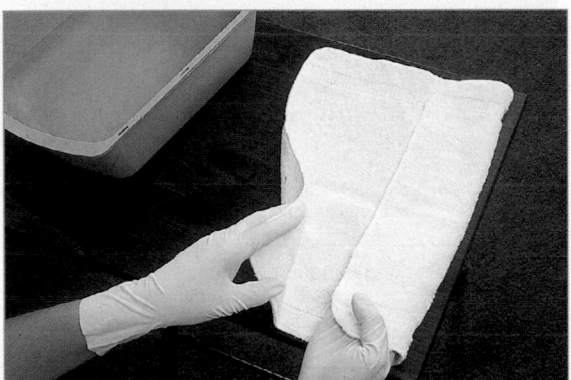

FIGURE 1. Folding washcloth in thirds around hand to make a bath mitt.

FIGURE 2. Straightening washcloth before folding into mitt.

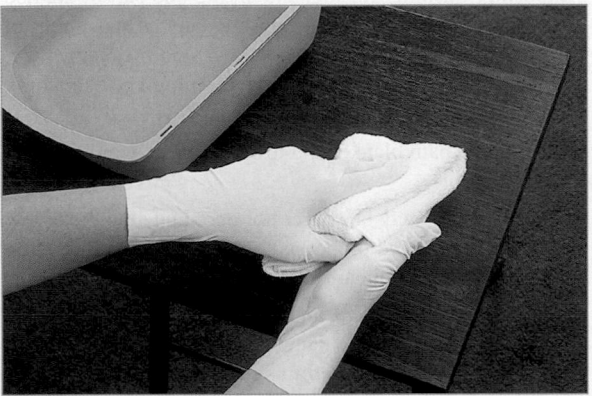

FIGURE 3. Folding ends over and tucking ends under folded washcloth over palm.

FIGURE 4. Washing from the inner corner of the eye outward.

(continued)

SKILL 30-1 PROVIDING A BED BATH *continued*

ACTION

17. Bathe the patient's face, neck, and ears. Apply appropriate emollient.

18. Expose the patient's far arm and place the towel lengthwise under it. Using firm strokes, wash the hand, arm, and axilla, lifting the arm as necessary to access axillary region (Fig. 5). Rinse, if necessary, and dry. Apply an appropriate emollient.

19. Place a folded towel on the bed next to the patient's hand and put the basin on it. Soak the patient's hand in the basin (Fig. 6). Wash, rinse if necessary, and dry the hand. Apply an appropriate emollient.

RATIONALE

Use of emollients is recommended to restore and maintain skin integrity (Voegeli, 2010).

The towel helps to keep the bed dry. Washing the far side first eliminates contaminating a clean area once it is washed. Gentle friction stimulates circulation and muscles and helps remove dirt, oil, and organisms. Long, firm strokes are relaxing and more comfortable than short, uneven strokes. Rinsing is necessary when using some cleansing products. Use of emollients is recommended to restore and maintain skin integrity (Voegeli, 2010).

Placing the hand in the basin of water is an additional comfort measure for the patient. It facilitates thorough washing of the hands and between the fingers, and aids in removing debris from under the nails. Use of emollients is recommended to restore and maintain skin integrity (Voegeli, 2010).

FIGURE 5. Exposing the far arm and washing it.

FIGURE 6. Soaking hand in basin.

20. Repeat Actions 18 and 19 for the arm nearer you. An option for the nurse who is shorter or susceptible to back strain might be to bathe one side of the patient first, then move to the other side of the bed to complete the bath.

21. Spread a towel across the patient's chest. Lower the bath blanket to the patient's umbilical area. Wash, rinse, if necessary, and dry the chest. Keep the chest covered with the towel between the wash and rinse. Pay special attention to the folds of skin under the breasts. Apply an appropriate emollient.

22. Lower the bath blanket to the perineal area. Place a towel over the patient's chest.

23. Wash, rinse, if necessary, and dry abdomen (Fig. 7). Carefully inspect and clean umbilical area and any abdominal folds or creases. Apply an appropriate emollient.

24. Return the bath blanket to its original position and expose the far leg. Place the towel under the far leg. Using firm strokes, wash, rinse if necessary, and dry the leg from the ankle to the knee and the knee to the groin (Fig. 8). Apply an appropriate emollient.

Exposing, washing, rinsing, and drying one part of the body at a time avoids unnecessary exposure and chilling. Areas of folds of skin may be sources of odor and skin breakdown if not cleaned and dried properly. Use of emollients is recommended to restore and maintain skin integrity (Voegeli, 2010).

Keeping the bath blanket and towel in place avoids exposure and chilling.

Skin-fold areas may be sources of odor and skin breakdown if not cleaned and dried properly. Use of emollients is recommended to restore and maintain skin integrity (Voegeli, 2010).

The towel protects linens and prevents the patient from feeling uncomfortable from a damp or wet bed. Washing from the ankle to the groin with firm strokes promotes venous return. Use of emollients is recommended to restore and maintain skin integrity (Voegeli, 2010).

ACTION	RATIONALE

FIGURE 7. Washing the abdomen, with perineal and chest areas covered.

FIGURE 8. Washing and drying far leg, keeping the other leg covered.

25. Wash, rinse if necessary, and dry the foot. Pay particular attention to the areas between the toes. Apply an appropriate emollient.

Drying the feet is important to prevent irritation, possible skin breakdown, and infections (National Institute on Aging, 2012). Use of emollients is recommended to restore and maintain skin integrity (Voegeli, 2010).

26. Repeat Actions 24 and 25 for the other leg and foot.

27. Make sure the patient is covered with the bath blanket. Change the water and washcloth at this point or earlier, if necessary.

The bath blanket maintains warmth and privacy. Clean, warm water prevents chilling and maintains patient comfort.

28. Assist the patient to a prone or side-lying position. Put on gloves, if not applied earlier. Position the bath blanket and towel to expose only the back and buttocks.

Positioning the towel and bath blanket protects the patient's privacy and provides warmth. Gloves prevent contact with body fluids.

29. Wash, rinse if necessary, and dry back and buttocks area (Fig. 9). **Pay particular attention to cleansing between the gluteal folds, and observe for any redness or skin breakdown in the sacral area.**

Fecal material near the anus may be a source of microorganisms. Prolonged pressure on the sacral area or other bony prominences may compromise circulation and lead to development of decubitus ulcer.

FIGURE 9. Washing the upper back.

(continued)

SKILL 30-1 PROVIDING A BED BATH *continued*

ACTION	RATIONALE
30. If not contraindicated, give patient a backrub. Alternatively, a back massage may be given after perineal care (see Skill 34-1 on pages 1188–1191). Apply an appropriate emollient and/or skin barrier product.	A backrub improves circulation to the tissues and is an aid to relaxation. A backrub may be contraindicated in patients with cardiovascular disease or musculoskeletal injuries. Use of emollients is recommended to restore and maintain skin integrity (Voegeli, 2010). Skin barriers protect the skin from damage caused by excessive exposure to water and irritants, such as urine and feces.
31. Raise the side rail. Refill the basin with clean water. Discard the washcloth and towel. Remove gloves and put on clean gloves.	The washcloth, towel, and water are contaminated after washing the patient's gluteal area. Changing to clean supplies decreases the spread of organisms from the anal area to the genitals.
32. Clean the perineal area or set the patient up to allow the patient to complete perineal self-care. If the patient is unable, lower the side rail and complete perineal care. Apply skin barrier, as indicated. Raise the side rail, remove gloves, and perform hand hygiene.	Providing for perineal self-care may decrease embarrassment for the patient. Effective perineal care reduces odor and decreases the risk for infection through contamination. Skin barriers protect the skin from damage caused by excessive exposure to water and irritants, such as urine and feces.
33. Help the patient put on a clean gown and assist with the use of other personal toiletries, such as deodorant or cosmetics.	This provides for the patient's warmth and comfort.
34. Protect the pillow with a towel and groom the patient's hair.	
35. **When finished, make sure that the patient is comfortable, with the side rails up and the bed in the lowest position.**	Proper positioning with raised side rails and proper bed height provides for patient comfort and safety.
36. Change the bed linens, as described in Skills 30-4 and 30-5 on pages 943–950. Dispose of soiled linens according to facility policy. Clean the bath basin according to facility policy before returning it to storage at the bedside. Remove gloves and any other PPE, if used. Perform hand hygiene.	Proper disposal of linens and cleaning of the bath basin reduces the risk for transmission of microorganisms. Removing PPE properly reduces the risk for infection transmission and contamination of other items. Hand hygiene prevents the spread of microorganisms.

DOCUMENTATION

Guidelines

Record any significant observations and communication. Document the condition of the patient's skin. Record the procedure, amount of assistance given, and patient participation. Document the application of skin care products, such as a skin barrier.

Sample Documentation

> 7/14/15 2130 Bath provided with complete assistance; reddened area (3 cm × 3 cm) noted on patient's sacral area; skin-care team consultation made.
> —C. Stone, RN

UNEXPECTED SITUATIONS AND ASSOCIATED INTERVENTIONS

• *Patient becomes chilled during bath:* If the room temperature is adjustable, increase it. Another bath blanket may be needed.

• *The patient becomes unstable during the bath:* Critically ill patients often need to be bathed in stages. For instance, the right arm is bathed, then the patient is allowed to rest for a short period before the left arm is bathed. The amount of rest time needed depends on how unstable the patient is and which parameter is being monitored. If the blood pressure drops when the patient is stimulated, the nurse may watch the blood pressure while bathing the patient and stop when it begins to decrease. Once the blood pressure returns to the previous level, the nurse can resume bathing the patient.

SPECIAL CONSIDERATIONS

General Considerations

• To remove the gown from a patient with an IV line, take the gown off the uninvolved arm first, then thread the IV tubing and bottle or bag through the arm of the gown. To replace the gown, place the clean gown on the unaffected arm first and thread the IV tubing and bottle or bag from inside the arm of the gown on the involved side. Never disconnect IV tubing to change a gown, because this causes a break in a sterile system and could introduce infection.

- Lying flat in bed during the bed bath may be contraindicated for certain patients. The position may have to be modified to accommodate their needs.

- Incontinent patients require special attention to perineal care. Patients with urinary or fecal incontinence are at risk for perineal skin damage. This damage is related to moisture, changes in the pH of the skin, overgrowth of bacteria and skin infection and erosion of perineal skin from friction on moist skin. Skin care for these patients should include measures to reduce overhydration (excess exposure to moisture), reduce contact with ammonia and bacteria, and reduce friction. Remove soil and irritants from the skin during routine hygiene, as well as cleansing when the skin becomes exposed to irritants. Avoid using soap and excessive force for cleaning. The use of perineal skin cleansers, moisturizers, and moisture barriers is recommended for skin care for the incontinent patient. These products help promote healing and prevent further skin damage.

- If the patient has an indwelling catheter, use mild soap and water or a perineal cleanser to clean the perineal area; rinse the area well. Do not use powders and lotions after cleaning. Do not use antibiotic or other antimicrobial cleaners or betadine at the urethral meatus (Herter & Wallace Kazer, 2010; Society of Urologic Nurses and Associates [SUNA], 2010). Facility policy may recommend use of an antiseptic cleaning agent or plain soap and water to clean the catheter. Put on clean gloves before cleaning the catheter. Clean 6 to 8 inches of the catheter, moving from the meatus downward. Be careful not to pull or tug on the catheter during the cleaning motion. Inspect the meatus for drainage and note the characteristics of the urine.

- The use of chlorhexidine gluconate for bathing has been shown to reduce colonization of the skin with pathogens and is becoming part of personal hygiene policies in some facilities. Chlorhexidine can be added to bath water, but is also available, and easier to use, in prepackaged impregnated cloths. Bathing with chlorhexidine may be used to reduce the incidence of hospital-acquired infections, such as central line–associated bloodstream infections and surgical site infections, as well as to reduce the acquisition of or decolonization with multidrug-resistant organisms (Ritz et al., 2012; Sievert et al., 2011).

- If applying lotion, warm the lotion in your hands before it is applied to the patient to prevent chilling.

Infant and Child Considerations

- When bathing an infant or young child, have supplies within easy reach, and support or hold the child securely at all times to ensure safety.
- Never leave the child alone.

Older Adult Considerations

- Check the temperature of the water carefully before bathing an older patient, because sensitivity to temperature may be impaired in older adults.
- An older, continent patient may not require a full bed bath with soap and water every day. If dry skin is a problem, water and skin lotion or bath oil may be used on alternate days.

Home Care Considerations

- Evaluate the safety of the bathing area in the home. Tub mats, adhesive strips, grab bars, and shower stools can help prevent falls.
- Use plastic trash bags or a plastic shower-curtain liner to protect the mattress when bathing or shampooing a patient in bed. Disposable washcloths may also be an option to consider. A large plastic container or baby bathtub can effectively serve as a shampoo basin.
- If linens are soiled with blood or body fluids, instruct family members to wear gloves when handling them. They should be rinsed first in cold water, then washed separately from other household wash, using hot water, laundry detergent, and bleach.
- Teach a family member or caregiver how to perform comfort measures, such as a backrub.
- For patients at home with an indwelling catheter, instruct them or their caregivers to wash the urinary meatus and perineal area twice daily with mild soap and water or a perineal cleanser.
- Teach patients to clean the anal area after each bowel movement. Careful hand washing is imperative.

SKILL 30-2 ASSISTING THE PATIENT WITH ORAL CARE

DELEGATION CONSIDERATIONS	The implementation of oral care may be delegated to nursing assistive personnel (NAP) or unlicensed assistive personnel (UAP), as well as to licensed practical/vocational nurses (LPN/ LVN). The decision to delegate must be based on careful analysis of the patient's needs and circumstances, as well as the qualifications of the person to whom the task is being delegated. Refer to the Delegation Guidelines in Appendix A (found on thePoint).

EQUIPMENT

- Toothbrush
- Toothpaste
- Emesis basin
- Glass with cool water
- Disposable gloves
- Additional PPE, as indicated
- Towel
- Mouthwash (optional)
- Washcloth or paper towel
- Lip lubricant (optional)
- Dental floss

IMPLEMENTATION

ACTION	RATIONALE
1. Perform hand hygiene and put on gloves if assisting with oral care, and/or other PPE, if indicated.	Hand hygiene and PPE prevent the spread of microorganisms. PPE is required based on transmission precautions.
2. Identify the patient. Explain the procedure to the patient.	Identifying the patient ensures that the right patient receives the intervention and helps prevent errors. Explanation facilitates cooperation.
3. Assemble equipment on the overbed table within the patient's reach.	Organization facilitates performance of task.
4. Close the room door or curtains. Place the bed at an appropriate and comfortable working height, usually elbow height of the caregiver (VISN8 Patient Safety Center, 2009).	Closing the door or curtains provides privacy. Proper bed height helps reduce back strain while performing the procedure.
5. Lower the side rail and assist the patient to a sitting position, if permitted, or turn the patient onto the side. Place the towel across the patient's chest.	The sitting or side-lying position prevents aspiration of fluids into the lungs. The towel protects the patient from dampness.
6. Encourage the patient to brush own teeth according to the following guidelines. Assist, if necessary.	
a. Moisten the toothbrush and apply toothpaste to the bristles.	Water softens the bristles.
b. Place the brush at a 45-degree angle to the gum line (Fig. 1) and brush from the gum line to the crown of each tooth (Fig. 2). Brush the outer and inner surfaces. Brush back and forth across the biting surface of each tooth.	Facilitates removal of plaque and tartar. The 45-degree angle of brushing permits cleansing of all surface areas of the tooth.

FIGURE 1. Placing brush at a 45-degree angle to the gum line.

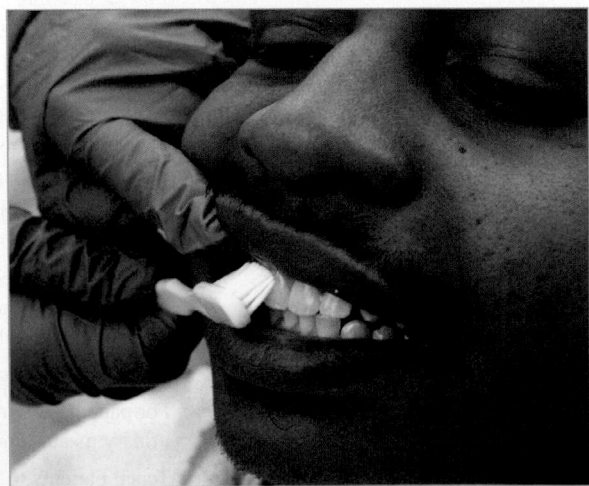

FIGURE 2. Brushing from the gum line to the crown of each tooth.

ACTION

RATIONALE

c. Brush the tongue gently with the toothbrush (Fig. 3).

Removes coating on the tongue. Gentle motion does not stimulate gag reflex.

d. Have the patient rinse vigorously with water and spit into the emesis basin (Fig. 4). Repeat until clear. Suction may be used as an alternative for removal of fluid and secretions from the mouth.

The vigorous swishing motion helps to remove debris. Suction is appropriate if the patient is unable to expectorate well.

FIGURE 3. Brushing the tongue.

FIGURE 4. Holding emesis basin for patient to rinse and spit.

7. Assist the patient to floss teeth, if appropriate:

Flossing aids in removal of plaque and promotes healthy gum tissue.

a. Remove approximately 6 inches of dental floss from the container or use a plastic floss holder. Wrap the floss around the index fingers, keeping about 1 to 1.5 inches of floss taut between the fingers.

The floss must be held taut to get between the teeth.

b. Insert the floss gently between the teeth, moving it back and forth downward to the gums.

Trauma to the gums can occur if floss is forced between teeth.

c. Move the floss up and down, first on one side of a tooth and then on the other side of the tooth, until the surfaces are clean (Fig. 5). Repeat in the spaces between all teeth.

This ensures that both sides of all teeth are cleaned.

d. Instruct the patient to rinse the mouth well with water after flossing.

Vigorous rinsing helps to remove food particles and plaque that have been loosened by flossing.

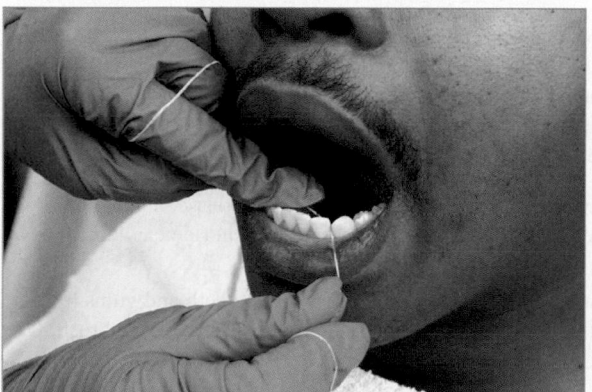

FIGURE 5. Flossing the teeth.

(continued)

SKILL 30-2 ASSISTING THE PATIENT WITH ORAL CARE *continued*

ACTION	RATIONALE
8. Offer mouthwash if the patient prefers.	Mouthwash leaves a pleasant taste in the mouth.
9. Offer lip balm or petroleum jelly.	Lip balm lubricates lips and prevents drying.
10. Remove equipment. Remove gloves and discard. Raise the side rail and lower the bed. Assist the patient to a position of comfort.	Removing gloves properly reduces the risk for infection transmission and contamination of other items. These actions promote patient comfort and safety.
11. Remove any other PPE, if used. Perform hand hygiene.	Removing PPE properly reduces the risk for infection transmission and contamination of other items. Hand hygiene prevents the spread of microorganisms.

DOCUMENTATION

Guidelines

Record oral assessment, significant observations, and unusual findings, such as bleeding or inflammation. Document any teaching done. Document procedure and patient response.

Sample Documentation

> 10/20/15 0930 Patient performed oral care with minimal assistance. Oral cavity mucosa pink and moist. No evidence of bleeding or ulceration. Lips slightly dry; lip moisturizer applied. Reinforcement provided related to importance of flossing teeth every day. Patient demonstrates appropriate flossing technique.
> —L. Schneider, RN

UNEXPECTED SITUATIONS AND ASSOCIATED INTERVENTIONS

- *While cleaning the teeth, you notice a large amount of bleeding from the gum line:* Stop brushing. Allow the patient to gently rinse the mouth with water and spit into the emesis basin. Before brushing again, check the patient's most recent platelet level. Consider the use of a softer toothbrush to provide oral hygiene.
- *Patient has braces on teeth:* Brush extra thoroughly. Braces collect food particles.

SPECIAL CONSIDERATIONS

General Considerations

- Use a soft-bristled toothbrush with a small head even when the patient has no or few teeth. It is the only effective way to remove plaque and debris from the teeth, gums, and tongue.
- A patient receiving chemotherapy medication may have bleeding gums and extremely sensitive mucous membranes. Use a soft sponge toothette for cleaning, and a saltwater rinse (half teaspoon salt in 1 cup of warm water; Polovich et al., 2009).
- Automatic toothbrushes, electric or battery operated, are simple to use and are as good as manual brushes for removing debris and plaque. These devices are very useful for patients with arthritis or other conditions that make it difficult to brush effectively (MFMER, 2011d).
- The use of chlorhexidine gluconate as part of oral hygiene has been integrated into oral hygiene regimens and is available in an oral spray and dental gel (Ames et al., 2011; Kelly et al., 2012). The use of chlorhexidine gluconate as part of protocols for systematic oral care for critically ill patients has been shown to reduce the incidence of health care–associated pneumonia (Ames et al., 2011).

Infant and Child Considerations

- When assisting small children with oral care, do not use toothpaste that contains fluoride if the child cannot spit out excess. Excessive amounts of ingested fluoride can lead to a discoloration of the teeth.
- Oral hygiene should begin as soon as an infant's teeth erupt. Clean teeth and gums by wiping with a damp cloth. As the infant gets more teeth, introduce a small toothbrush. Use water to clean an infant's teeth, not toothpaste.

SKILL 30-3   PROVIDING ORAL CARE FOR THE DEPENDENT PATIENT

DELEGATION CONSIDERATIONS	The implementation of oral care for a dependent patient may be delegated to nursing assistive personnel (NAP) or unlicensed assistive personnel (UAP) after assessment by the registered nurse, as well as to licensed practical/vocational nurses (LPN/LVN). The decision to delegate must be based on careful analysis of the patient's needs and circumstances, as well as the qualifications of the person to whom the task is being delegated. Refer to the Delegation Guidelines in Appendix A (found on the**Point**).

EQUIPMENT

- Toothbrush
- Toothpaste
- Emesis basin
- Glass with cool water
- Disposable gloves
- Additional PPE, as indicated
- Towel

- Mouthwash (optional)
- Dental floss (optional)
- Denture-cleaning equipment (if necessary)
- Denture cup
- Denture cleaner
- 4 × 4 gauze
- Washcloth or paper towel

- Lip lubricant (optional)
- Sponge Toothette
- Irrigating syringe with rubber tip (optional)
- Suction catheter with suction apparatus (optional)

IMPLEMENTATION

ACTION	**RATIONALE**
1. Perform hand hygiene and put on PPE, if indicated.	Hand hygiene and PPE prevent the spread of microorganisms. PPE is required based on transmission precautions.
2. Identify the patient. Explain the procedure to the patient.	Identifying the patient ensures that the right patient receives the intervention and helps prevent errors. Explanation facilitates cooperation.
3. Assemble equipment on the overbed table within reach.	Organization facilitates performance of task.
4. Close the room door or curtains. Place the bed at an appropriate and comfortable working height, usually elbow height of the caregiver (VISN8 Patient Safety Center, 2009). Lower one side rail and position the patient on the side, with the head tilted forward. Place the towel across the patient's chest and the emesis basin in position under the chin. Put on gloves.	Cleaning another person's mouth is invasive and may be embarrassing (Holman, et al., 2005). Closing the door or curtains provides privacy. Proper bed height helps reduce back strain while performing the procedure. The side-lying position with head forward prevents aspiration of fluid into the lungs. The towel and emesis basin protects the patient from dampness. Gloves prevent the spread of microorganisms.
5. Gently open the patient's mouth by applying pressure to the lower jaw at the front of the mouth. Remove dentures, if present. Brush the teeth and gums carefully with a toothbrush and paste (Fig. 1). Lightly brush the tongue.	Toothbrush provides friction necessary to clean areas where plaque and tartar accumulate.

FIGURE 1. Carefully brushing patient's teeth.

(continued)

SKILL 30-3   PROVIDING ORAL CARE FOR THE DEPENDENT PATIENT   *continued*

ACTION	RATIONALE
6. Use a Toothette dipped in water to rinse the oral cavity. If desired, insert the rubber tip of the irrigating syringe into the patient's mouth and rinse gently with a small amount of water (Fig. 2). **Position the patient's head to allow for return of water or use the suction apparatus to remove the water from the oral cavity (Fig. 3).**	Rinsing helps clean debris from the mouth. Forceful irrigation may cause aspiration.

FIGURE 2. Using irrigating syringe and a small amount of water to rinse mouth.

FIGURE 3. Using suction to remove excess fluid.

ACTION	RATIONALE
7. Clean the dentures before replacing.	Cleaning maintains dentures and oral hygiene. Plaque can accumulate on dentures and promote oropharyngeal colonization of pathogens.
8. Apply lubricant to the patient's lips.	This prevents drying and cracking of the lips.
9. Remove equipment and return the patient to a position of comfort. Remove your gloves. Raise the side rail and lower the bed.	Promotes patient comfort and safety. Removing gloves properly reduces the risk for infection transmission and contamination of other items.
10. Remove additional PPE, if used. Perform hand hygiene.	Removing PPE properly reduces the risk for infection transmission and contamination of other items. Hand hygiene prevents the spread of microorganisms.

DOCUMENTATION

Guidelines

Record oral assessment, significant observations, and unusual findings, such as bleeding or inflammation. Document any teaching done. Document the procedure and patient response.

Sample Documentation

7/10/15 0945 Oral care performed. Oral cavity mucosa pink and moist. Small amount of bleeding noted from gums after using soft-bristled toothbrush. Resolved spontaneously when brushing completed. No evidence of ulceration. Lips slightly dry; lip moisturizer applied.

—*C. Stone, RN*

UNEXPECTED SITUATIONS AND ASSOCIATED INTERVENTIONS	• *Patient begins to bite the toothbrush:* Do not jerk the toothbrush out. Wait for the patient to relax the mouth before removing the toothbrush and continuing with care. • *Mouth is extremely dry with crusts that remain after oral care provided:* Increase frequency of oral hygiene. Apply mouth moisturizer to oral mucosa.
SPECIAL CONSIDERATIONS	• Suction toothbrushes may be used with patients with dysphagia. • A patient receiving chemotherapy medication may have bleeding gums and extremely sensitive mucous membranes. Use a soft sponge Toothette for cleaning, and a saltwater rinse (half teaspoon salt in 1 cup of warm water) (Polovich et al., 2009). • Use a soft-bristled toothbrush with a small head even when the patient has no or few teeth. It is the only effective way to remove plaque and debris from the teeth, gums, and tongue.

SKILL 30-4 | MAKING AN UNOCCUPIED BED

DELEGATION CONSIDERATIONS	The making of an unoccupied bed may be delegated to nursing assistive personnel (NAP) or unlicensed assistive personnel (UAP), as well as to licensed practical/vocational nurses (LPN/LVN). The decision to delegate must be based on careful analysis of the patient's needs and circumstances, as well as the qualifications of the person to whom the task is being delegated. Refer to the Delegation Guidelines in Appendix A (found on thePoint).

EQUIPMENT	• One large flat sheet • One fitted sheet • Drawsheet (optional) • Blankets • Bedspread	• Pillowcases • Linen hamper or bag • Bedside chair • Waterproof protective pad (optional)	• Disposable gloves • Additional PPE, as indicated

IMPLEMENTATION

ACTION	RATIONALE
1. Perform hand hygiene. Put on PPE, as indicated.	Hand hygiene and PPE prevent the spread of microorganisms. PPE is required based on transmission precautions.
2. Explain to the patient what you are going to do and the reason for doing it, if the patient is present in the room.	Explanation facilitates cooperation.
3. Assemble necessary equipment on the bedside stand or overbed table.	Arranging items nearby is convenient, saves time, and avoids unnecessary stretching and twisting of muscles on the part of the nurse.
4. Adjust the bed to a comfortable working height, usually elbow height of the caregiver (VISN8 Patient Safety Center, 2009). Drop the side rails.	Having the bed at the proper height prevents back and muscle strain. Having the side rails down reduces strain on the nurse while working.
5. Disconnect call bell or any tubes from bed linens.	Disconnecting devices prevents damage to the devices.
6. Put on gloves. Loosen all linen as you move around the bed, from the head of the bed on the far side to the head of the bed on the near side.	Gloves prevent the spread of microorganisms. Loosening the linen helps prevent tugging and tearing on the linen. Loosening the linen and moving around the bed systematically reduce strain caused by reaching across the bed.

(continued)

SKILL 30-4   MAKING AN UNOCCUPIED BED   *continued*

ACTION	RATIONALE
7. Fold reusable linens, such as sheets, blankets, or spread, in place on the bed in fourths and hang them over a clean chair.	Folding saves time and energy when reusable linen is replaced on the bed. Folding linens while they are on the bed reduces strain on the nurse's arms. Some facilities change linens only when soiled.
8. Snugly roll all the soiled linen inside the bottom sheet and place directly into the laundry hamper (Fig. 1). **Do not place on the floor or furniture. Do not hold soiled linens against your uniform.**	Rolling soiled linens snugly and placing them directly into the hamper helps prevent the spread of microorganisms. The floor is heavily contaminated; soiled linen will further contaminate furniture. Soiled linen contaminates the nurse's uniform, which may spread organisms to another patient.
9. If possible, shift the mattress up to the head of bed. If the mattress is soiled, clean and dry according to facility policy before applying new sheets.	This allows more foot room for the patient.
10. Remove your gloves, unless indicated for transmission-based precautions. Place the bottom sheet with its center fold in the center of the bed. Open the sheet and fan-fold to the center (Fig. 2).	Gloves are not necessary to handle clean linen. Removing gloves properly reduces the risk for infection transmission and contamination of other items. Opening linens on the bed reduces strain on the nurse's arms and diminishes the spread of microorganisms. Centering the sheet ensures sufficient coverage for both sides of the mattress.

FIGURE 1. Bundling soiled linens in bottom sheet and holding them away from body.

FIGURE 2. Opening bottom sheet and fan-folding to center of bed.

ACTION	RATIONALE
11. Pull the bottom sheet over the corners at the head and foot of the mattress.	Making the bed on one side and then completing the bed on the other side saves time. Having bottom linens free of wrinkles reduces patient discomfort.
12. If using, place the drawsheet with its center fold in the center of the bed and positioned so it will be located under the patient's midsection. Open the drawsheet and fan-fold to the center of the mattress (Fig. 3). If a protective pad is used, place it over the drawsheet in the proper area and open to the center fold. Not all facilities use drawsheets routinely. The nurse may decide to use one. In some institutions, the protective pad doubles as a drawsheet. Tuck the drawsheet securely under the mattress.	If the patient soils the bed, the drawsheet and pad can be changed without the bottom and top linens on the bed. Having all bottom linens in place before tucking them under the mattress avoids unnecessary moving about the bed. A drawsheet can aid moving the patient in bed.
13. Move to the other side of the bed to secure the bottom linens. Pull the bottom sheet tightly and secure over the corners at the head and foot of the mattress. Pull the drawsheet tightly and tuck it securely under the mattress.	This removes wrinkles from the bottom linens, which can cause patient discomfort and promote skin breakdown.

ACTION	RATIONALE
14. Place the top sheet on the bed with its center fold in the center of the bed and with the hem even with the head of the mattress. Unfold the top sheet. Follow the same procedure with the top blanket or spread, placing the upper edge about 6 inches below the top of the sheet.	Opening linens by shaking them spreads organisms into the air. Holding linens overhead to open them causes strain on the nurse's arms.
15. Tuck the top sheet and blanket under the foot of the bed on the near side. Miter the corners (Fig. 4).	This saves time and energy and keeps the top linen in place.

FIGURE 3. Placing drawsheet on bed.

FIGURE 4. Mitering corner of top sheet and spread.

16. Fold the upper 6 inches of the top sheet down over the spread and make a cuff.	This makes it easier for the patient to get into bed and pull up the covers.
17. Move to the other side of the bed and follow the same procedure for securing top sheets under the foot of the bed and making a cuff (Fig. 5).	Working on one side of the bed at a time saves energy and is more efficient.
18. Place the pillows on the bed. Open each pillowcase in the same manner as you opened other linens. Gather the pillowcase over one hand toward the closed end. Grasp the pillow with the hand inside the pillowcase. Keep a firm hold on the top of the pillow and pull the cover onto the pillow. Place the pillow at the head of the bed (Fig. 6).	Opening linens by shaking them causes organisms to be carried on air currents. Covering the pillow while it rests on the bed reduces strain on the nurse's arms and back.

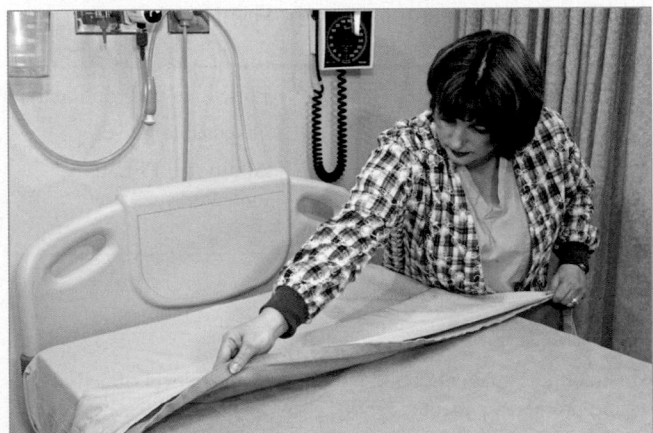

FIGURE 5. Cuffing top linens.

FIGURE 6. Placing pillow on bed.

(continued)

SKILL 30-4 MAKING AN UNOCCUPIED BED *continued*

ACTION	RATIONALE
19. Fan-fold or pie-fold the top linens.	Having linens opened makes it more convenient for the patient to get into bed.
20. Secure the signal device on the bed, according to facility policy	The patient will be able to call for assistance as necessary. Promotes patient comfort and safety.
21. Raise the side rail and lower the bed.	Promotes patient comfort and safety.
22. Dispose of soiled linen according to facility policy.	Deters the spread of microorganisms.
23. Remove any other PPE, if used. Perform hand hygiene.	Removing PPE properly reduces the risk for infection transmission and contamination of other items. Hand hygiene prevents the spread of microorganisms.

DOCUMENTATION	Changing of bed linens does not require documentation. The use of a specialty bed, or bed equipment, such as Balkan frame or foot cradle, should be documented.
UNEXPECTED SITUATIONS AND ASSOCIATED INTERVENTIONS	• *Drawsheet is not available:* A flat sheet can be folded in half to substitute for a drawsheet, but extra care must be taken to avoid wrinkles in the bed. • *Patient is frequently incontinent of stool or urine:* More than one protective pad can be placed under the patient to protect the bed, but take care to ensure that the patient is not lying on wrinkles from linens.
SPECIAL CONSIDERATIONS	• There are many different types of specialty beds available for use as part of treatment and prevention of many health issues, such as treatment of pressure ulcers. Refer to manufacturer's recommendations and instructions on use of specialty lines and products with this equipment.

SKILL 30-5 MAKING AN OCCUPIED BED

DELEGATION CONSIDERATIONS	The making of an occupied bed may be delegated to nursing assistive personnel (NAP) or unlicensed assistive personnel (UAP), as well as to licensed practical/vocational nurses (LPN/LVN). The decision to delegate must be based on careful analysis of the patient's needs and circumstances, as well as the qualifications of the person to whom the task is being delegated. Refer to the Delegation Guidelines in Appendix A (found on thePoint).

EQUIPMENT			
• One large flat sheet	• Bedspread	• Protective pad (optional)
• One fitted sheet	• Pillowcases	• Disposable gloves
• Drawsheet (optional)	• Linen hamper or bag	• Additional PPE, as indicated
• Blankets	• Bedside chair	

IMPLEMENTATION

ACTION	RATIONALE
1. Check health care record for limitations on patient's physical activity.	This facilitates patient cooperation, determines level of activity, and promotes patient safety.

ACTION	RATIONALE
2. Perform hand hygiene. Put on PPE, as indicated.	Hand hygiene and PPE prevent the spread of microorganisms. PPE is required based on transmission precautions.
3. Identify the patient. Explain what you are going to do.	Patient identification validates the correct patient and correct procedure. Discussion and explanation allay anxiety and prepare the patient for what to expect.
4. Assemble equipment on the overbed table within reach.	Organization facilitates performance of task.
5. Close the curtains around the bed and close the door to the room, if possible.	This ensures the patient's privacy.
6. Adjust the bed to a comfortable working height, usually elbow height of the caregiver (VISN8 Patient Safety Center, 2009).	Having the bed at the proper height prevents back and muscle strain.
7. Lower the side rail nearest you, leaving the opposite side rail up. Place the bed in the flat position unless contraindicated.	Having the mattress flat makes it easier to prepare a wrinkle-free bed.
8. Put on gloves. Check the bed linens for the patient's personal items. **Disconnect the call bell or any tubes/drains from the bed linens.**	Gloves prevent the spread of microorganisms. It is costly and inconvenient when personal items are lost. Disconnecting tubes from linens prevents discomfort and accidental dislodging of the tubes.
9. Place a bath blanket over the patient. Have the patient hold on to the bath blanket while you reach under it and remove the top linens (Fig. 1). Leave the top sheet in place if a bath blanket is not used. Fold the linen that is to be reused over the back of a chair. Discard soiled linen in the laundry bag or hamper. **Do not place on the floor or furniture. Do not hold soiled linens against your uniform.**	The blanket provides warmth and privacy. Placing linens directly into the hamper helps prevent the spread of microorganisms. The floor is heavily contaminated; soiled linen will further contaminate furniture. Soiled linen contaminates the nurse's uniform, which may spread organisms to another patient.
10. If possible, and another person is available to assist, grasp the mattress securely and shift it up to the head of the bed.	This allows more foot room for the patient.
11. Assist the patient to turn toward the opposite side of the bed, and reposition the pillow under the patient's head.	This allows the bed to be made on the vacant side.
12. Loosen all bottom linens from the head, foot, and side of the bed.	This facilitates removal of linens.
13. Fan-fold or roll soiled linens as close to the patient as possible (Fig. 2).	This makes it easier to remove linens when the patient turns to the other side.

FIGURE 1. Removing top linens from under bath blanket.

FIGURE 2. Moving soiled linen as close to patient as possible.

(continued)

SKILL 30-5 MAKING AN OCCUPIED BED *continued*

ACTION	RATIONALE

ACTION

14. Use clean linen and make the near side of the bed. Place the bottom sheet with its center fold in the center of the bed (Fig. 3). Open the sheet and fan-fold to the center, positioning it under the old linens (Fig. 4). Pull the bottom sheet over the corners at the head and foot of the mattress.

RATIONALE

Opening linens on the bed reduces strain on the nurse's arms and diminishes the spread of microorganisms. Centering the sheet ensures sufficient coverage for both sides of the mattress. Positioning under the old linens makes it easier to remove linens.

FIGURE 3. Placing bottom sheet with center fold in center of bed.

FIGURE 4. Fan-folding bottom sheet to the center, positioning it under the old linens.

15. If using, place the drawsheet with its center fold in the center of the bed and positioned so that it will be located under the patient's midsection. Open the drawsheet and fan-fold to the center of the mattress. Tuck the drawsheet securely under the mattress (Fig. 5). If a protective pad is used, place it over the drawsheet in the proper area and open to the center fold. Not all facilities use drawsheets routinely. The nurse may decide to use one.

If the patient soils the bed, drawsheet and pad can be changed without the bottom and top linens on the bed. A drawsheet can aid moving the patient in bed.

16. Raise the side rail. Assist the patient to roll over the folded linen in the middle of the bed toward you. Reposition the pillow and bath blanket or top sheet. Move to the other side of the bed and lower the side rail.

This ensures patient safety. The movement allows the bed to be made on the other side. The bath blanket provides warmth and privacy.

17. Loosen and remove all bottom linen (Fig. 6). Discard soiled linen in the laundry bag or hamper. **Do not place on the floor or furniture. Do not hold soiled linens against your uniform.**

Placing linens directly into the hamper helps prevent the spread of microorganisms. The floor is heavily contaminated; soiled linen will further contaminate furniture. Soiled linen contaminates the nurse's uniform, which may spread organisms to another patient.

FIGURE 5. Tucking drawsheet tightly.

FIGURE 6. Removing soiled bottom linens from other side of bed.

ACTION

18. Ease clean linen from under the patient. Pull the bottom sheet taut and secure at the corners at the head and foot of the mattress. Pull the drawsheet tight and smooth. Tuck the drawsheet securely under the mattress.

19. Assist the patient to turn back to the center of bed. Remove the pillow and change the pillowcase. Open each pillowcase in the same manner as you opened the other linens. Gather the pillowcase over one hand toward the closed end. Grasp the pillow with the hand inside the pillowcase. Keep a firm hold on the top of the pillow and pull the cover onto the pillow. Place the pillow under the patient's head.

20. Apply the top linens, sheet and blanket, if desired, so that it is centered. Fold the top linens over at the patient's shoulders to make a cuff. Have the patient hold on to the top linens and remove the bath blanket from underneath (Fig. 7).

RATIONALE

This removes wrinkles and creases in the linens, which are uncomfortable to lie on.

Opening linens by shaking them causes organisms to be carried on air currents.

This allows bottom hems to be tucked securely under the mattress and provides for privacy.

FIGURE 7. Removing bath blanket from under top linens.

21. Secure top linens under the foot of the mattress and miter corners. Loosen the top linens over the patient's feet by grasping them in the area of the feet and pulling gently toward the foot of the bed.

22. Return the patient to a position of comfort. Remove your gloves. Raise the side rail and lower the bed. Reattach the call bell.

23. Dispose of soiled linens according to agency policy.

24. Remove any other PPE, if used. Perform hand hygiene.

This provides for a neat appearance. Loosening linens over the patient's feet gives more room for movement.

Promotes patient comfort and safety. Removing gloves properly reduces the risk for infection transmission and contamination of other items.

Deters the spread of microorganisms.

Removing PPE properly reduces the risk for infection transmission and contamination of other items. Hand hygiene prevents the spread of microorganisms.

DOCUMENTATION

Changing of bed linens does not require documentation. The use of a specialty bed, or bed equipment, such as Balkan frame or foot cradle, should be documented. Document any significant observations and communication.

(continued)

SKILL 30-5 | MAKING AN OCCUPIED BED *continued*

UNEXPECTED SITUATIONS AND ASSOCIATED INTERVENTIONS

• *Dirty linens are grossly contaminated with urinary or fecal drainage:* Obtain an extra towel or protective pad. Place the pad under and over the soiled linens so that new linens will not be in contact with soiled linens. Clean and dry the mattress according to facility policy before applying new sheets.

SPECIAL CONSIDERATIONS

Older Adult Considerations

• Using a soft bath blanket or a flannelette blanket as a bottom sheet may solve the problem of "coldness" for older adult patients with vascular problems or arthritis.

DEVELOPING CLINICAL REASONING

1. Practice the art of back massage with a willing partner until you feel comfortable and confident including this nursing measure in your routine care. Discuss with other students the therapeutic benefits of massage, and identify nursing situations for which it may be the primary therapy.

2. Interview people of different ages and cultural backgrounds about their hygiene practices. Ask specific questions about the type of nursing assistance they would require if hospitalized and unable to meet their hygiene needs independently. Are there special products or equipment they would need? To what extent are nurses obliged to respect the hygiene preferences of patients?

PRACTICING FOR NCLEX

1. A nurse is scheduling hygiene for patients on her unit. What is the most important consideration when planning a patient's personal hygiene?
   a. When the patient had his or her most recent bath
   b. The patient's usual hygiene practices and preferences
   c. Where the bathing fits in the nurse's schedule
   d. The time that is convenient for the patient care assistant

2. A nurse caring for patients in a critical care unit knows that providing good oral hygiene is an essential part of nursing care. What are some of the benefits of providing this care? Select all that apply.
   a. It promotes the patient's sense of well-being.
   b. It prevents deterioration of the oral cavity.
   c. It contributes to decreased incidence of aspiration pneumonia.
   d. It eliminates the need for flossing.
   e. It decreases oropharyngeal secretions.
   f. It compensates for an inadequate diet.

3. A nurse assisting with a patient bed bath observes that an older female patient has dry skin. The patient states that her skin is always "itchy." Which nursing action would be the nurse's best response?
   a. Bathe the patient more frequently.
   b. Use an emollient on the dry skin.

   c. Massage the skin with alcohol.
   d. Discourage fluid intake.

4. A nurse caring for patients in a skilled nursing facility performs risk assessments on the patients for foot and nail problems. Which patients would be at a higher risk? Select all that apply.
   a. A patient who is taking antibiotics for chronic bronchitis
   b. A patient diagnosed with type II diabetes
   c. A patient who is obese
   d. A patient who has a nervous habit of biting his nails
   e. A patient diagnosed with prostate cancer
   f. A patient whose job involves frequent hand washing

5. Nurses performing skin assessments on patients must pay careful attention to cleanliness, color, texture, temperature, turgor, moisture, sensation, vascularity, and lesions. Which guidelines should nurses follow when performing these assessments? Select all that apply.
   a. Compare bilateral parts for symmetry.
   b. Proceed in a toe-to-head systematic manner.
   c. Use standard terminology to report and record findings.
   d. Do not allow data from the nursing history to direct the assessment.
   e. Document only skin abnormalities on the patient record.
   f. Perform the appropriate skin assessment when risk factors are identified.

6. A nurse is caring for an adolescent with severe acne. Which recommendations would be most appropriate to include in the teaching plan for this patient? Select all that apply.
   a. Wash the skin twice a day with a mild cleanser and warm water
   b. Use cosmetics liberally to cover blackheads.
   c. Use emollients on the area.
   d. Squeeze blackheads as they appear.
   e. Keep hair off the face and wash hair daily.
   f. Avoid sun-tanning booth exposure and use sunscreen.

7. A nurse observes a marked inflammation of the gums, along with recession and bleeding of the gums, and documents this observation using which term?
   a. Glossitis
   b. Caries
   c. Cheilosis
   d. Periodontitis

8. An unresponsive patient is wearing gas-permeable contact lenses. How would the nurse remove these lenses?
   a. Gently irrigate the eye with an irrigating solution from the inner canthus outward.
   b. Grasp the lens with a gentle pinching motion.
   c. Don sterile gloves before attempting the removal procedure.
   d. Ensure that the lens is centered on the cornea before gently manipulating the lids to release it.

9. Mr. James has an eye infection with a moderate amount of discharge. Which action would be most appropriate for the nurse to use when cleaning his eyes?
   a. Using hydrogen peroxide
   b. Wiping from the outer canthus to the inner canthus
   c. Positioning him on the same side as the eye to be cleansed
   d. Using only one cotton ball per eye

10. A nurse is providing foot care for patients in a long-term care facility. Which actions are recommended guidelines for this procedure? Select all that apply.
    a. Bathe the feet thoroughly in a mild soap and tepid water solution.
    b. Soak the feet in warm water and bath oil.
    c. Dry feet thoroughly, including the area between the toes.
    d. Use an alcohol rub if the feet are dry.
    e. Use an antifungal foot powder if necessary to prevent fungal infections.
    f. Cut the toenails at the lateral corners when trimming the nail.

11. A nurse is caring for an 80-year-old patient who has become weak and fatigues easily. He is unable to wash his body and always asks the nurse to brush his teeth. Based on this information, what is an appropriate nursing diagnosis for this patient?
    a. Risk for Impaired Skin Integrity related to immobility
    b. Bathing/Hygiene Self-Care Deficit related to decreased strength and endurance
    c. Social Isolation related to lack of visitors
    d. Impaired Oral Mucous Membrane related to inability to brush his teeth

12. A nurse is teaching a student nurse how to cleanse the perineal area of both male and female patients. What are accurate guidelines when performing this procedure? Select all that apply.
    a. For male and female patients, wash the groin area with a small amount of soap and water and rinse.
    b. For a female patient, spread the labia and move the washcloth from the anal area toward the pubic area.
    c. For male and female patients, always proceed from the most contaminated area to the least contaminated area.
    d. For male and female patients, use a clean portion of the washcloth for each stroke.
    e. For a male patient, clean the tip of the penis first, moving the washcloth in a circular motion from the meatus outward.
    f. In an uncircumcised male patient do not retract the foreskin (prepuce) while washing the penis.

13. An older patient with an unsteady gait requests a tub bath. Which action would be most appropriate?
    a. Add Alpha-Keri oil to the water to prevent dry skin.
    b. Allow the patient to lock the door to guarantee privacy.
    c. Assist the patient in and out of the tub to prevent falling.
    d. Keep the water temperature very warm because the patient chills easily.

14. A nurse is about to bathe a female patient who has an intravenous access in place in her forearm. The patient's gown, which does not have snaps on the sleeves, needs to be removed prior to bathing. What should the nurse do?
    a. Temporarily disconnect the IV tubing at a point close to the patient and thread it through the gown sleeve.
    b. Cut the gown with scissors to allow arm movement.
    c. Thread the bag and tubing through the gown sleeve, keeping the line intact.
    d. Temporarily disconnect the tubing from the IV container, threading it through the gown.

15. A nurse is caring for a 25-year-old male patient who is comatose following a head injury. The patient has several piercings in his ears and nose. The piercing in his nose appears to be new and is crusted and slightly inflamed. Which action would be appropriate when caring for this patient's piercings?
    a. Do not remove or wash the piercings without permission from the patient.
    b. Rinse the sites with warm water and remove crusts with a cotton swab.
    c. Wash the sites with alcohol and apply an antibiotic ointment.
    d. Remove the jewelry and allow the sites to heal over.

ANSWERS WITH RATIONALES

1. *b.* Bathing practices and cleansing habits and rituals vary widely. The patient's preferences should always be taken into consideration, unless there is a clear threat to health. The patient and nurse should work together to come to a mutually agreeable time and method to accomplish the patient's personal hygiene. The availability of staff to assist may be important, but the patient's preferences are a higher priority.

2. *a, b, c.* Adequate oral hygiene is essential for promoting the patient's sense of well-being and preventing deterioration of the oral cavity. Diligent oral hygiene care can also improve oral health and limit the growth of pathogens in oropharyngeal secretions, decreasing the incidence of aspiration pneumonia and other systemic diseases (AACN, 2006; AACN, 2010). Oral care does not eliminate the need for flossing, decrease oropharyngeal secretions, or compensate for poor nutrition.

3. *b.* An emollient soothes dry skin, whereas frequent bathing increases dryness, as does alcohol. Discouraging fluid intake leads to dehydration and, subsequently, dry skin.

4. *b, c, d, f.* Variables known to cause nail and foot problems include deficient self-care abilities, vascular disease, arthritis, diabetes mellitus, history of biting nails or trimming them improperly, frequent or prolonged exposure to chemicals or water, trauma, ill-fitting shoes, and obesity.

5. *a, c, f.* When performing a skin assessment, the nurse should compare bilateral parts for symmetry, use standard terminology to report and record findings, and perform the appropriate skin assessment when risk factors are identified. The nurse should proceed in a head-to-toe systematic manner, and allow data from the nursing history to direct the assessment. When

documenting a physical assessment of the skin, the nurse should describe exactly what is observed or palpated, including appearance, texture, size, location or distribution, and characteristics of any findings.

6. *a, e, f.* Washing the skin removes oil and debris, hair should be kept off the face and washed daily to keep oil from the hair off the face, and sunbathing should be avoided when using acne treatments. Liberal use of cosmetics and emollients can clog the pores. Squeezing blackheads is always discouraged because it may lead to infection.

7. *d.* Periodontitis is a marked inflammation of the gums, whereas caries refers to the presence of tooth decay. Cheilosis is ulceration of the lips, and glossitis is an inflammation of the tongue.

8. *d.* The lens must be situated on the cornea, not the sclera, before removal. To remove hard contact lenses, the upper and lower eyelids are gently maneuvered to help loosen the lens and slide it out of the eye. An attempt to grasp a hard lens might result in a scratch on the cornea. Clean, not sterile, gloves are used.

9. *c.* Positioning the patient on the same side as the involved eye discourages contamination of the other eye. Always cleanse from the inner canthus to the outer canthus to avoid forcing debris into the nasolacrimal duct. Water or normal saline should be used for cleansing the eye of any discharge, and one cotton ball should be used for each stroke.

10. *a, c, e.* The following are recommended guidelines for foot care: bathe the feet thoroughly in a mild soap and tepid water solution; dry feet thoroughly, including the area between the toes; and use an antifungal foot powder if necessary to prevent fungal infections. The nurse should avoid soaking the feet, use moisturizer if the feet are dry, and avoid digging into or cutting the toenails at the lateral corners when trimming the nails.

11. *b.* Risk for Impaired Skin Integrity, Social Isolation, and Impaired Oral Mucous Membrane may be appropriate nursing diagnoses for this patient. However, not enough is known, based on the information given, to formulate these diagnoses. The priority at this time, based on the given information, is Bathing/Hygiene Self-Care Deficit.

12. *a, d, e.* Wash and rinse the groin area (both male and female patients) with a small amount of soap and water, and rinse. For male and female patients, always proceed from the least con-

taminated area to the most contaminated area and use a clean portion of the washcloth for each stroke. For a male patient, clean the tip of the penis first, moving the washcloth in a circular motion from the meatus outward. For a female patient, spread the labia and move the washcloth from the pubic area toward the anal area. In an uncircumcised male patient (teenage or older), retract the foreskin (prepuce) while washing the penis.

13. *c.* Safe nursing practice requires that the nurse assist a patient with an unsteady gait in and out of the tub. Adding Alpha-Keri oil to the bath water is dangerous for this patient because it makes the tub slippery. Although privacy is important, if the patient locks the door, the nurse cannot help if there is an emergency. The water should be comfortably warm at 43°C to 46°C. Older patients have an increased susceptibility to burns due to diminished sensitivity.

14. *c.* Threading the bag and tubing through the gown sleeve keeps the system intact. Opening an IV line, even temporarily, causes a break in a sterile system and introduces the potential for infection. Cutting a gown is not an alternative except in an emergency.

15. *b.* When providing care for piercings, the nurse should perform hand hygiene and put on gloves, then cleanse the site of all crusts and debris by rinsing the site with warm water, removing the crusts with a cotton swab. The nurse should then apply a dab of liquid medicated cleanser to the area, turn the jewelry back and forth to work the cleanser around the opening, rinse well, remove gloves, and perform hand hygiene. The nurse should not use alcohol, peroxide, or ointments at the site or remove the piercings unless it is absolutely necessary (e.g., when an MRI is ordered.)

TAYLOR SUITE RESOURCES

Explore these additional resources to enhance learning for this chapter:

- NCLEX-Style Questions and other resources on thePoint, http://thePoint.lww.com/Taylor8e
- *Study Guide for Fundamentals of Nursing, 8th edition*
- Adaptive Learning | Powered by prepU, http://thepoint.lww.com/ prepu
- *Skill Checklists for Fundamentals of Nursing, 8th edition*
- *Taylor's Clinical Nursing Skills:* Chapter 7, Hygiene
- *Taylor's Video Guide to Clinical Nursing Skills:* Hygiene

Bibliography

Ackley, B. J., & Ladwig, G. B. (2011). *Nursing Diagnosis Handbook* (9th ed.). St. Louis: Elsevier/Mosby.

Agency for Healthcare Research and Quality (AHRQ). National Guideline Clearinghouse. (2011). Prevention of pressure ulcers. Available at http://guideline.gov/syntheses/synthesis.aspx?id=25078&search=prevent+pressure+ulcers

American Academy of Dermatology (AAD). (2012). Acne. Available at www.aad.org/skin-conditions/dermatology-a-to-z/acne

American Academy of Dermatology (AAD). (2012). 12 ways to get better results from acne treatment. Available at http://www.skincarephysicians.com/acnenet/twelve_results.html

American Association of Critical-Care Nurses (AACN). (2010). Practice Alert: Oral care in the critically ill. Available at http://aacn.org/WD/Practice/Content/practicealerts.content?menu=Practice

American Association of Critical-Care Nurses (AACN). (2010). Practice Alert. Venous thrombosis prevention. Available at http://aacn.org/WD/Practice/Docs/PracticeAlerts/VTE%20Prevention%2004–2010%20final.pdf

American Dental Association (ADA). (2012). Mouthrinses. Available at http://www.ada.org/1319.aspx

Ames, N. J., Sulima, P., Yates, J. M., McCullagh, L., Gollins, S. L., Soeken, K., & Wallen, G. R. (2011). Effects of systematic oral care in critically ill patients: A multicenter study. *American Journal of Critical Care, 20*(5), e103–e113. Available at http://ajcc.aacnjournals.org/content/20/5/e103.full.pdf+html

Bissett, S., & Preshaw, P. (2011). Guide to providing mouth care for older people. *Nursing Older People, 23*(10), 14–21.

Bloomfield, J., & Pegram, A. (2012). Physical healthcare needs: oral hygiene in the mental health setting. *Mental Health Practice, 15*(6), 32–38.

Bloomfield, J., Pegram, A., & Jones, A. (2008). Recommended procedure for bed making in hospital. *Nursing Standard, 22*(23), 41–44.

Boltz, M., Capezuti, E., Fulmer, T., & Zwicker, D. (eds.) (2012). *Evidence-based geriatric nursing protocols for best practice* (4th ed.). New York: Springer Publishing Company.

Brown, A., & Butcher, M. (2005). A guide to emollient therapy. *Nursing Standard, 19*(24), 68–75.

Bulechek, G. M., Butcher, H. K., Dochterman, J. M., & Wagner, C. M. (Eds.). (2013). *Nursing interventions classification (NIC)* (6th ed.). St. Louis: Elsevier/Mosby.

Burn Foundation. (2012). Burn prevention. Safety facts on scald burns. Available at http://www.burnfoundation.org/programs/resource.cfm?c=1&a=3

Centers for Disease Control and Prevention (CDC). (2011a). Oral health—Preventing cavities, gum disease, tooth loss, and oral cancers at a glance 2011. Available at http://www.cdc.gov/chronicdisease/resources/publications/AAG/doh.htm

Centers for Disease Control and Prevention (CDC). (2011b). Tick removal. Available at http://www.cdc.gov/ticks/removing_a_tick.html

Centers for Disease Control and Prevention (CDC). (2010). Parasites–Lice. Available at http://www.cdc.gov/parasites/lice/

Chan, E. Y., Lee, Y. K., Poh, T. H., Ng, I. H. L., & Prabhakaran, L. (2011). Translating evidence into nursing practice: oral hygiene for care dependent adults. *International Journal of Evidence-Based Healthcare, 9*(2), 172–183.

Ciancio, S. (2008). Mouth rinses and their impact on oral hygiene. *Access, 22*(5), 24–29.

Cleveland Clinic. (2009a). Soft contact lenses. Available at http://my.clevelandclinic.org/eye/patients/products/soft_contact_lenses.aspx

Cleveland Clinic. (2009b). Contact lens care. Available at http://my.clevelandclinic.org/devices/vision_correction/Contact_Lenses/hic_Contact_Lens_Care.aspx

Coate, D. (2010). The ABCs of bathing. *Advance for Long-Term Care Management, 13*(3), 21–22.

Cowdell, F. (2011). Older people, personal hygiene, and skin care. *MEDSURG Nursing, 20*(5), 235–240.

DeBoer, S., Seaver, M., Vidra, D., Robinson, B., & Klepacki, J. (2011). Breasts, bellies, below, and beyond: Body piercing jewelry and the transfer technique—when in doubt, don't necessarily take it out! *Journal of Emergency Nursing, 37*(6), 541–553.

Durgude, Y., & Cocks, N. (2011). Nurse's knowledge of the provision of oral care for patients with dysphagia. *British Journal of Community Nursing, 16*(12), 604–610.

Durkin, S. E. (2012). Tattoos, body piercing, and healthcare concerns. *Journal of Radiology Nursing, 31*(1), 20–25.

Dyble, T., & Ashton, J. (2011). Use of emollients in the treatment of dry skin conditions. *British Journal of Community Nursing, 16*(5), 214–220.

Halliday, K. (2005). Body piercing: Issues and challenges for nurses. *Journal of Forensic Nursing, 1*(2), 47–56.

Hennequin-Hoenderdos, N. L., Slot, D. E., & Van der Weijden, G. A. (2011). Complications of oral and peri-oral piercings: a summary of case reports. *International Journal of Dental Hygiene, 9*(2), 101–109.

Herter, R., & Wallace Kazer, M. (2010). Best practices in urinary catheter. *Home Healthcare Nurse, 28*(6), 342–349.

Hess, C. T. (2013). *Clinical guide to skin & wound care.* (7th ed.). Philadelphia: Wolters Kluwer Health/Lippincott Williams & Wilkins.

Hogan-Quigley, B., Palm, M. L., & Bickley, L. (2012). *Bates' Nursing Guide to Physical Examination and History Taking.* Philadelphia: Wolters Kluwer Health/Lippincott Williams & Wilkins.

Holman, C., Roberts, S., & Nicole, M. (2005). Practice update: Clinical skills with older people. Promoting oral hygiene. *Nursing Older People, 16*(10), 37–38.

Jablonski, R. A., Therrien, B., & Kolanowski, A. (2011). No more fighting and biting during mouth care: Applying the theoretical constructs of threat perception to clinical practice. *Research and Theory for Nursing Practice: An International Journal, 25*(3), 163–175.

Jarvis, C. (2012). *Physical Examination & Health Assessment.* (6th ed.). St. Louis: Elsevier/Saunders.

Jensen, S. (2011). *Nursing Health Assessment. A best practice approach.* Philadelphia: Wolters Kluwer Health/Lippincott Williams & Wilkins.

Johnson, R. H. (2011). Practical care: creative strategies for bathing. *Nursing & Residential Care, 13*(8), 392–394.

Johnstone, L., Spence, D., & Koziol-McClain, J. (2010). Oral hygiene care in the pediatric intensive care unit: Practice recommendations. *Pediatric Nursing, 36*(2), 85–97.

Kanjirath, P. P., Kim, S. E., & Inglehart, M. R. (2011). Diabetes and oral health: The importance of oral health-related behavior. *The Journal of Dental Hygiene, 85*(4), 264–272.

Keefe, S. (2010). Bath safety and dementia. *Advance for Long-term Care Management.* Available at https://nursing.advanceweb.com/Regional-Content/Articles/Bath-Safety-Dementia.aspx

Kelly, T., Timmis, S., & Twelvetree, T. (2010). Review of the evidence to support oral hygiene in stroke patients. *Nursing Standard, 24*(37), 35–38.

Kyle, T., & Carman, S. (2013). *Essentials of pediatric nursing* (2nd ed.). Philadelphia: Wolters Kluwer Health/Lippincott Williams & Wilkins.

Lyman, T. P., & Vlahovic, T. C. (2010). Foot care from A to Z. *Dermatology Nursing, 22*(5), 2–8.

Malkin, B., & Berridge, P. (2009). Guidance on maintaining personal hygiene in nail care. *Nursing Standard, 23*(41), 35–38.

Massa, J. (2010). Improving efficiency, reducing infection, and enhancing experience. *British Journal of Nursing, 19*(22), 1408–1414.

Mayo Foundation for Medical Education and Research (MFMER). (2012a). Peripheral artery disease (PAD). Lifestyle and home remedies. Available at http://www.mayoclinic.com/health/peripheral-arterial-disease/DS00537/DSECTION=lifestyle-and-home-remedies

Mayo Foundation for Medical Education and Research (MFMER). (2012b). Piercings: How to prevent complications. Available at http://www.mayoclinic.com/health/piercings/SN00049

Mayo Foundation for Medical Education and Research (MFMER). (2011a). Amputation and diabetes: How to protect your feet. Available at http://www.mayoclinic.com/health/amputation-and-diabetes/DA00140

Mayo Foundation for Medical Education and Research (MFMER). (2011b). Denture care: How do I clean dentures? Available at http://www.mayoclinic.com/health/denture-care/AN02028/

Mayo Foundation for Medical Education and Research (MFMER). (2011c). Fingernails: Do's and don'ts for healthy nails. Available at http://www.mayoclinic.com/health/nails/WO00020

Mayo Foundation for Medical Education and Research (MFMER). (2011d). Oral health: Brush up on dental care basics. Available at www.mayoclinic.com/health/dental/DE00003

MedlinePlus. (2012a). Tick bites. Available http://www.nlm.nih.gov/medlineplus/tickbites.html

MedlinePlus. (2012b). Penis care (uncircumcised). Available at http://www.nlm.nih.gov/medlineplus/ency/article/001917.htm

MedlinePlus. (2012c). Rashes. Available at http://www.nlm.nih.gov/medlineplus/rashes.html

Moorhead, S., Johnson, M., Maas, M. L., & Swanson, E. (Eds.). (2013). *Nursing Outcomes Classification (NOC).* (5th ed.). St. Louis: Elsevier/Mosby.

NANDA International (NANDA-I). (2012). *Nursing diagnoses: Definitions & classification 2012–2014.* West Sussex, UK: Wiley-Blackwell.

National Institute on Aging (NIA). (2012). Age page. Foot Care. Available at http://www.nia.nih.gov/health/publication/foot-care

Papa, K. S. (2011). A dignified bathing experience. *Advance for Long-Term Care Management, 14*(6), 16.

Pegram, A., Bloomfield, J., & Jones, A. (2007). Clinical skills: Bed bathing and personal hygiene needs of patients. *British Journal of Nursing, 16*(6), 356–358.

Pellatt, G. (2007). Clinical skills: Bed making and patient positioning. *British Journal of Nursing, 16*(5), 302–305.

Polovich, M., White, J., & Kelleher, L. (Eds). (2009). *Chemotherapy and biotherapy guidelines and recommendations for practice* (3rd ed.). Pittsburgh, PA: Oncology Nursing Society.

Printz, C. (2012). Dermatology community applauds new FDA sunscreen regulations: Labeling requirements aim to make it easier for consumers to select a sunscreen. *Cancer, 118*(1), 1–3.

Ritter, L. A., & Hoffman, N. A. (2010). *Multicultural health.* Boston: Jones and Bartlett.

Ritz, J., Pashnik, B., Padula, C., & Simmons, K. (2012). Effectiveness of 2 methods of chlorhexidine bathing. *Journal of Nursing Care Quality, 27*(2), 171–175.

Rönner, A. C., Berland, C. R., Runeman, B., & Kaijser, B. (2010). The hygienic effectiveness of 2 different skin cleansing procedures. *Journal of Wound, Ostomy, and Continence Nursing, 37*(3), 260–264.

Sievert, S. C., Armola, R., & Halm, M. A. (2011). Chlorhexidine gluconate bathing: Does it decrease hospital-acquired infections? *American Journal of Critical Care, 20*(2), 166–170.

Smeltzer, S. C., Bare, B. G., Hinkle, J. L., & Cheever, K. H. (2010). *Brunner & Suddarth's textbook of medical–surgical nursing.* (12th ed.). Philadelphia: Wolters Kluwer Health/Lippincott Williams & Wilkins.

Society of Urologic Nurses and Associates (SUNA). (2010). *Prevention & control of catheter-associated urinary tract infection (CAUTI). Clinical practice guideline.* Available at https://www.suna.org/sites/default/files/download/cautiGuideline.pdf.

Spector, R. E. (2009). *Cultural diversity in health and illness* (7th ed.). Upper Saddle River, NJ: Pearson/Prentice Hall.

Tabloski, P. A. (2010). *Gerontological nursing* (2nd ed.). Upper Saddle River, NJ: Pearson.

Tada, A., & Miura, H. (2012). Prevention of aspiration pneumonia with oral care. *Archives of Gerontology & Geriatrics, 55*(1), 16–21.

Taylor, J. J., & Cohen, B. J. (2013). *Memmler's structure and function of the human body* (10th ed.). Philadelphia: Wolters Kluwer Health/Lippincott Williams & Wilkins.

U.S. Department of Health and Human Services. (2004). *Cosmetics and your health fact sheet.* Available at http://womenshealth.gov/publications/our-publications/fact-sheet/cosmetics-your-health.cfm

U.S. Food and Drug Administration (FDA). (2010). A guide to bed safety. Bed rails in hospitals, nursing homes and home health care: The facts. Available at http://www.fda.gov/MedicalDevices/ProductsandMedicalProcedures/GeneralHospitalDevicesandSupplies/HospitalBeds/ucm123676.htm

U.S. Food and Drug Administration (FDA). (2012a). Sun safety: Save your skin! Available at http://www.fda.gov/ForConsumers/ConsumerUpdates/ucm049090.htm

U.S. Food and Drug Administration (FDA). (2012b). Sunscreen. Available at http://www.fda.gov/Drugs/ResourcesForYou/Consumers/BuyingUsingMedicineSafely/UnderstandingOver-the-CounterMedicines/ucm239463.htm

U.S. Food and Drug Administration (FDA). (2012c). Use eye cosmetics safely. Available at http://www.fda.gov/ForConsumers/ConsumerUpdates/ucm048943.htm

U.S. Food and Drug Administration (FDA). (2012d). *Should you put sunscreen on infants? Not usually.* Available at http://www.fda.gov/ForConsumers/ConsumerUpdates/ucm309136.htm

VISN8 Patient Safety Center. (2009). *Safe patient handling and movement algorithms.* Tampa, FL: Author. Available at www.visn8.va.gov/patientsafetycenter/safePthandling/default.asp

Voegeli, D. (2012). Moisture-associated skin damage: aetiology, prevention and treatment. *British Journal of Nursing, 21*(9), 517–521.

Voegeli, D. (2010). Care or harm: Exploring essential components in skin care regimens. *British Journal of Nursing, 19*(13), 812, 814, 816, 818–819.

31

Skin Integrity and Wound Care

MARY BIESICKER

Mary, who is 84 years of age, has been cared for at home by her daughter since being hospitalized last year for a cerebrovascular accident (stroke). She has been unable to take care of herself, finds it increasingly more difficult to get out of bed, and is having more frequent episodes of incontinence. According to her daughter, Mary has developed a "blister" on her back. She is being assessed by the home health care nurse at the request of her daughter, who is finding it increasingly difficult to care for her mother alone.

LUCIUS EVERLY

Lucius, a 52-year-old man who has a history of diabetes and circulatory problems, underwent abdominal surgery several days ago and is in the critical care unit. He is slouched down in bed; his abdominal dressing is moist and only part of the tape securing the dressing is adhering to the skin. His level of consciousness is decreased, and he responds only to moderate touch and pain. Further assessment reveals the beginning of a pressure ulcer on his heel.

SAM BENTZ

Sam, a 56-year-old man, has been admitted to the hospital for aggressive treatment of a bone infection that has not responded to usual treatment methods. Mr. Bentz is 5 feet 4 inches tall and weighs more than 300 pounds. He tells you, "Last time I was here, my skin got really irritated and I developed several skin wounds."

LEARNING OBJECTIVES

After completing the chapter, you will be able to accomplish the following:

1. Discuss the processes involved in wound healing.
2. Identify factors that affect wound healing.
3. Identify patients at risk for pressure ulcer development.
4. Describe the method of staging of pressure ulcers.
5. Accurately assess and document the condition of wounds.
6. Provide nursing interventions to prevent pressure ulcers.
7. Implement appropriate dressing changes for different kinds of wounds.
8. Provide information to patients and caregivers for self-care of wounds at home.
9. Apply hot and cold therapy effectively and safely.

KEY TERMS

bandage	fistula	sanguineous drainage
biofilm	friction	
débridement	granulation tissue	scar
dehiscence		serosanguine-ous drainage
dermis	ischemia	
desiccation	maceration	serous drainage
dressing	necrosis	
epidermis	negative-pressure wound therapy (NPWT)	shear
epitheliali-zation		sinus tract
		subcutaneous tissue
eschar	pressure ulcer	
evisceration	purulent drainage	wound
exudate		

The skin is the body's first line of defense, protecting the underlying structures from invasion by organisms. Maintaining an intact skin surface is important because a break or disruption in this integrity is potentially dangerous and possibly life threatening. The nurse plays a major role in maintaining the patient's skin integrity, in identifying risk factors that predispose a patient to a break in integrity, in intervening to prevent or reduce a patient's risk for impaired skin integrity, and in providing specific wound care when breaks in integrity arise. Additional information related to general skin care is discussed in Chapter 30.

Knowledgeable and skilled wound care is an essential component of nursing care. Using the nursing process, an individualized plan of care is developed to assess the patient and the wound, identify and prevent complications, implement and evaluate skills essential to wound care, and provide physical and emotional support to facilitate healing, adaptation, and self-care. Wound care may be required in any health care setting, and complex wound care at home is on the rise.

This chapter provides information about disruptions in skin and tissue integrity, including wounds and pressure ulcers. Because applications of heat and cold are used to treat altered skin integrity, a discussion of those treatment modalities is also included. Refer to the Reflective Practice display on pages 956–957 for an illustration of nursing care issues related to skin integrity.

ANATOMY AND PHYSIOLOGY OF THE INTEGUMENTARY SYSTEM

Knowledge of the basic anatomy and physiology of the integumentary system and an understanding of the role of this system in the body provides a foundation for assessment and for planning and implementing interventions to promote optimal skin integrity. This knowledge also helps nurses understand, interpret, and analyze assessment findings and provides the rationale for sound nursing interventions.

Structures of the Skin

The skin, or integument, is the largest organ of the body and has multiple functions. The skin covers the entire body and is continuous with mucous membranes at normal body orifices. It is essential for maintaining life.

The integumentary system is made up of the skin, the subcutaneous layer directly under the skin, and the appendages of the skin, including glands in the skin, hair, and nails. The integumentary system also includes the blood vessels, nerves, and sensory organs of the skin.

The skin has two layers, the epidermis and the dermis. An underlying layer, the subcutaneous layer (or hypodermis), is sometimes included in descriptions as the third layer of the skin (Jarvis, 2012; Stephen-Haynes, 2012; Grossman, 2014). A cross-section of normal skin is illustrated in Figure 31-1 (on page 957).

The top layer, or outermost portion, is the **epidermis**. The epidermis is composed of layers of stratified epithelial cells. These cells fuse to form a protective, waterproof layer of keratin material. Epithelial cells have no blood vessels of their own and depend on underlying tissues for nourishment and waste removal. When well nourished, epithelium regenerates relatively easily and quickly.

The second layer of skin, the **dermis**, consists of a framework of elastic connective tissue. Nerves, hair follicles, glands, and blood vessels are located in this layer. Each hair consists of the shaft, which projects through the dermis beyond the surface of the skin, and the hair follicle, which lies in the dermis.

The dermis rests on the **subcutaneous tissue**, the underlying layer that anchors the skin layers to the underlying tissues of the body. The subcutaneous tissue consists of adipose tissue, made up of lobules of fat cells, and connective tissue. This layer stores fat for energy, serves as a heat

CHALLENGE TO ETHICAL AND LEGAL SKILLS

I had a tough clinical 2 weeks ago while caring for Lucius Everly, a critical care postop patient with a history of diabetes and circulation problems. The nurse I was working with had floated to the unit on this day, but I didn't know that at the time. Mr. Everly appeared to be neglected by other caregivers, and because he was not communicating and had a decreased level of consciousness, he could not express his needs. I saw that he needed bathing, wound care, repositioning in bed, and some additional attention. While in the room, the nurse spoke about Mr. Everly as though he were deaf. In my opinion, the nurse did not respect his inability to communicate. I became frustrated because she did not share my sense of concern for him. I became irritated when I asked what we could do to care for the poor circulation to his feet. My irritation increased when I realized that he was developing a pressure sore on his heel.

Thinking Outside the Box: Possible Courses of Action

- Tell my clinical instructor of my frustrations earlier in the day so my patient's care could have been addressed earlier and my frustrations wouldn't have built up.
- Go to my nurse and tell her that I disagreed with the care she was providing, insisting that more needed to be done for this patient.
- Ask the charge nurse to assess the quality of care that my patient was getting compared to what he needed to be receiving.

Evaluating a Good Outcome: How Do I Define Success?

- Patient receives a higher quality of care.
- The nurse is not insulted by hearing feedback about the care she is providing.
- By addressing the problem earlier in the process, my frustrations do not interfere with the rest of my day.
- The patient is not discriminated against and neglected based on his inability to communicate and his decreased level of consciousness.

Personal Learning: Here's to the Future!

Happy and sad outcome. Although this patient was not verbally communicating, I held his hand, talked to him, and felt that he was able to recognize my caring presence. After our lunch break, I verbalized my frustration about the lack of care to my clinical instructor and I asked if she would come meet him and help me provide the care I saw was due. My clinical instructor agreed that this patient was in need of more care. She, unlike my nurse, did not speak about his condition in front of him as though he could not hear. My instructor also made sure we did everything possible so that this patient was as comfortable as possible. She talked to him as though he was able to hear. In addition, my instructor called in the charge nurse to point out the lack of care this patient had been receiving, wanting to ensure that his future level of care improved. My instructor and the charge nurse, in a professional, nondegrading way, expressed to the assigned nurse that this patient needed a higher quality of care due to his critical condition. Having my teacher agree with my concerns for this patient and address the nurse and charge nurse made me feel much better about the care my patient would then receive. I later told my teacher that I was frustrated because I felt all the nurse was concerned about was "giving all the medications, and signing off on the right pages," when in fact talk-ing to this patient, holding his hand, and making him more comfortable was definitely more important. Two days later the patient died. I was sad but so honored to have been able to care for him and hold his hand in his last days.

Although I think I should have gone to my clinical instructor earlier in the day to explain the problem I was having, telling her was the right decision. My instructor took my concerns seriously and first helped me care for the patient, then went straight to the charge nurse to ensure proper skin and wound care for the patient. Lastly, she was able to address the nurse without insulting her to make sure we were all on the same page about the care this patient needed but had not been getting. By speaking up, I was able to leave my clinical assignment feeling positive about my actions and advocating for this patient. I still felt frustrated with how he had been cared for and realized that all too often as care providers we get too involved in the routine of charting, distributing medications, and so on, and can forget how important some simple measures are such as offering a gentle touch, positioning, providing hygiene and wound care, and just spending time with the patient.

Carrie Staines, Georgetown University

REFLECTION ON QUALITY AND SAFETY COMPETENCIES

How do you think you would respond in a similar situation? Why? What does this tell you about yourself and about the adequacy of your skills for professional practice? What factors might have affected the assigned nurse's response to the patient? Would the student have been affected by any of these same factors? Do you agree with the criteria to evaluate a successful outcome? Did the nursing student validate the rationale for the outcome? What *knowledge, skills,* and *attitudes* do you need to develop to continuously improve the quality and safety of care for patients like Mr. Everly?

Patient-Centered Care: What evidence from the scenario would lead you to suspect that the patient is at risk for impaired skin integrity? What preventive measures might be appropriate? What measures might be appropriate to ensure therapeutic patient-centered care?

insulator for the body, and provides a cushioning effect for protection. This fatty tissue layer contains blood and lymph vessels, nerves, and fat cells.

Functions of the Skin and Mucous Membranes

The skin has multiple functions: protection, temperature regulation, psychosocial, sensation, vitamin D production, immunologic, absorption, and elimination. See Table 31-1 (on page 958) for details of each of these functions.

Mucous membranes line body cavities that open to the outside of the body, joining with the skin. They can also be found in the digestive tract, the respiratory passages, and the urinary and reproductive tracts. Epithelium covers the mucous membrane surfaces and contains cells that secrete mucus. Mucous membranes have receptors that offer

the body protection. For example, an irritating substance in the upper respiratory tract causes a person to sneeze, and food caught in the larynx or trachea causes a person to cough. Sneezing and coughing are protective mechanisms that help rid the body of foreign materials. Mucous membranes are insensitive to temperature, except in the mouth and rectum, but are sensitive to pressure. Mucous membranes also function to absorb substances from their surface. For example, digested food is absorbed through the mucous membrane in the small intestine.

Factors Affecting Skin Integrity

Basic principles related to integrity of the skin and mucous membranes include the following:

- Unbroken and healthy skin and mucous membranes serve as the first lines of defense against harmful agents.

FIGURE 31-1. A cross-section of normal skin.

Labels: Hair, Epidermis, Sebaceous gland, Dermis, Hair follicle, Papilla, Subcutaneous tissue, Sweat pore, Arrector pili muscle, Eccrine sweat gland, Nerve, Arteriole, Venule

Table 31-1 FUNCTIONS OF THE SKIN

FUNCTION	MECHANISMS
Protection	• Acts as a barrier to water, microorganisms, and damaging ultraviolet rays of the sun. • Protects against infection. • Injury to underlying tissues and organs is decreased by intact skin. • Prevents loss of moisture from the surface and underlying structures.
Temperature Regulation	• The evaporation of perspiration draws heat from the skin. • Blood vessels in the skin dilate to dissipate heat. • In cold conditions, blood vessels in the skin constrict to diminish heat loss. • In cold conditions, contraction of pilomotor muscles cause the hair to stand on end, forming a layer of air on the body for insulation (gooseflesh or goose bumps).
Psychosocial	• External appearance is a major contributor to self-esteem. • Skin plays an important role in identification and communication.
Sensation	• Millions of nerve endings in the skin provide the sense of touch, pain, pressure, and temperature. • Sensory impulses from the skin allow the body to adjust to the environment, in conjunction with the brain and spinal cord.
Vitamin D Production	• A precursor for vitamin D is present in the skin, which, in conjunction with ultraviolet rays from the sun, produces vitamin D.
Immunologic	• A breach in the surface of the skin triggers immunologic responses in the skin.
Absorption	• Substances, such as medications, can be absorbed through the skin for local and systemic effects.
Elimination	• Water, electrolytes, and nitrogenous wastes are excreted in small amounts in sweat.

• Resistance to injury of the skin and mucous membranes varies among people. Factors influencing resistance include the person's age, the amount of underlying tissues, and illness conditions.
• Adequately nourished and hydrated body cells are resistant to injury. The better nourished the cell is, the better able it is to resist injury and disease.
• Adequate circulation is necessary to maintain cell life. When circulation is impaired for any reason, cells receive inadequate nourishment and cannot remove wastes efficiently.

Table 31-2 identifies some factors that place a patient at risk for skin alterations.

Developmental Considerations

Specific characteristics of the skin are associated with different developmental stages. Hygiene practices at every age have a direct influence on the status and appearance of the skin.

• In children younger than 2 years, the skin is thinner and weaker than it is in adults.
• An infant's skin and mucous membranes are injured easily and are subject to infection. Careful handling of infants is required to prevent injury to and infection of the skin and mucous membranes.
• A child's skin becomes increasingly resistant to injury and infection.
• The structure of the skin changes as a person ages. In older adults, the maturation of epidermal cells is prolonged, leading to thin, easily damaged skin. Circulation and collagen formation are impaired, leading to decreased elasticity and increased risk for tissue damage from pressure.

Changes that occur in the skin with aging are discussed in Focus on the Older Adult (on page 960).

State of Health

The state of a person's health and therapeutic treatments have a direct effect on the condition of the skin. Proper nutrition, adequate circulation, and good overall health are important for healthy skin.

• Very thin and very obese people tend to be more susceptible to skin irritation and injury.
• Fluid loss through fever, vomiting, or diarrhea reduces the fluid volume of the body. This is termed *dehydration* and makes the skin appear loose and flabby.
• Excessive moisture such as perspiration, often associated with being ill, predisposes the skin to breakdown, especially in skin folds. Excessive moisture may also occur as a result of incontinence of urine and/or stool.
• Jaundice, a condition caused by excessive bile pigments in the skin, results in a yellowish skin color. The skin is often itchy and dry; patients with jaundice are more likely to scratch their skin and cause an open lesion, with the potential for infection.
• Diseases of the skin such as eczema and psoriasis may have a genetic predisposition and often cause lesions that require special care.

WOUNDS AND PRESSURE ULCERS

A **wound** is a break or disruption in the normal integrity of the skin and tissues. That disruption may range from a small cut on a finger to a third-degree burn covering almost all of the body. Wounds may result from mechanical forces

Table 31-2 FACTORS PLACING AN INDIVIDUAL AT RISK FOR SKIN ALTERATIONS

FACTOR	NURSING IMPLICATIONS
Lifestyle Variables	
Homosexuality, history of multiple sexual partners; intravenous drug users; hemophiliacs; bisexual male; partners of these demographics	• These patients are at high risk for infection with human immunodeficiency virus (HIV) and acquired immunodeficiency syndrome (AIDS). • Assessment needs to include careful examination of the skin for purple blotches that may be indicative of Kaposi's sarcoma.
Occupation or other activity that gives an individual prolonged exposure to the sun	• Places person at high risk for developing skin cancer, which has an excellent prognosis if detected and treated in its early stages but which may be fatal if treatment is delayed. • Assessment needs to include careful examination for a sore that does not heal or a change in size or color of a wart or mole.
Body piercing	• Potential interference with airway management. Potential risk for bacterial and viral infections, scarring, nerve damage, tissue trauma, and deformity. • Assess patient's knowledge of symptoms of infection at the site and when to seek medical care. • Assess piercing site(s) for redness, swelling, discharge, or excessive pain at the site.
Age	See text discussion regarding developmental issues related to skin and the Focus on the Older Adult feature on p. 960.
Changes in Health State	
Dehydration or malnutrition	• If fluid, protein, and vitamin C intake is deficient, skin loses elasticity and becomes prone to breakdown. • Nursing care is directed toward preventing skin breakdown: frequent changes of patient's position with skin assessment at each change, special mattresses and protection of bony prominences, use of lotions, and attention to fluid and nutritional status.
Reduced sensation (paralysis, local nerve damage, circulatory insufficiency)	• Patient's inability to sense temperature extremes, pressure, friction, and other such factors can easily result in injury. • Nursing care incorporates special attention to safety.
Illness	
Diabetes mellitus	• Numerous factors combine to cause skin problems in diabetic patients: cuts and sores that do not heal, lesions on the lower extremities that ulcerate and become necrotic, and recurrent bacterial and fungal infections. • The diabetic patient must be taught special hygiene measures to prevent trauma to the skin and learn to assess the skin carefully to detect any alteration.
Diagnostic Measures	
Gastrointestinal (GI) series	• The GI cleansing preparations administered to patients having GI studies done may result in diarrhea, which irritates the sensitive skin in the perianal area—especially if the patient had bouts of diarrhea before the studies; anticipating the problem, noting redness and inflammation, and beginning warm baths and ointments are welcome nursing measures that patients may be too embarrassed to seek.
Therapeutic Measures	
Bed rest	• Bed rest predisposes patients to skin breakdown; the harsh detergents used on hospital laundry compound this problem. • Pressure points need to be examined frequently and protected.
Casts	• Casts easily irritate the skin; careful assessment, covering the rough edges of the cast, and skin care are indicated.
Aquathermia unit	• Wet heat has therapeutic benefit but, if applied to the skin for too long, may macerate the skin; follow protocol in length of application, examine skin carefully between treatments, and allow to dry.
Medications	• Medications may cause allergic skin reactions, such as rashes. • When evaluating the patient's response to a new drug, examine the skin for redness and itching.
Radiation Therapy	• Radiation therapy exposes normal skin cells as well as cancer cells in treatment field to effects of radiation, with the potential for erythema and moist desquamation (loss of skin integrity).

FOCUS ON THE OLDER ADULT

NURSING STRATEGIES TO ADDRESS AGE-RELATED CHANGES IN SKIN

Age-Related Changes	Nursing Strategies
Subcutaneous and dermal tissue become thin: • Skin is more easily injured. • Skin has less capacity to insulate. • Skin wrinkles more easily. • Sensation of pressure and pain is reduced.	• Do not apply tape to skin unless necessary. • Check skin frequently to observe for any signs of a pressure ulcer. • Pad bony prominences if necessary. • Assess pressure tolerance by checking pressure points for redness after 30 minutes.
Activity of the sebaceous and sweat glands decreases: • Skin becomes dryer. • Pruritus (itching) may occur.	• Clean perineal area daily but do not bathe full body on a daily basis. • Apply lotions as needed. • Encourage adequate hydration.
Cell renewal is shorter: • Healing time is delayed.	• Perform careful skin assessments, looking for signs of skin breakdown.
Melanocytes (cells that make the pigment that colors hair and skin) decline in number: • Hair becomes gray-white. • Skin may be unevenly pigmented.	• Assist patient with skin checks, observing for any signs of melanoma or other skin abnormalities.
Collagen fiber is less organized: • Skin loses elasticity.	• Check skin frequently for tears, irritation, or breakdown.

(such as surgical incisions) or physical injury (such as a burn). Examples of types of wounds and their causes are highlighted in Table 31-3.

Wound Classification

Wounds are classified in many different ways, including intentional or unintentional (based on how they were acquired), open or closed, and acute or chronic (based on the length of time the patient has had the wound). Wounds may also be classified as partial-thickness (all or a portion of the dermis is intact), full-thickness (the entire dermis and sweat glands and hair follicles are severed), or complex (the dermis and underlying subcutaneous fat tissue are damaged or destroyed).

Intentional Wounds and Unintentional Wounds

An intentional wound is the result of planned invasive therapy or treatment. These wounds are purposefully created for therapeutic purposes. Examples of intentional wounds include those that result from surgery, intravenous therapy, and lumbar puncture. The wound edges are clean, and bleeding is usually controlled. Because the wound was made under sterile conditions with sterile supplies and skin preparation, the risk for infection is decreased, and healing is facilitated.

 THINK back to Lucius Everly, the patient who had abdominal surgery and is in the critical care unit. His postoperative treatments would

necessitate the placement of one or more intravenous accesses. His venous access and surgical wound would be considered intentional wounds. The nurse would incorporate an understanding of the principles of surgical asepsis when caring for these wound sites to prevent infection. ●

Unintentional wounds are accidental. These wounds occur from unexpected trauma, such as from accidents, forcible injury (such as a stabbing or a gunshot), and burns. Because the wounds occur in an unsterile environment, contamination is likely. Wound edges are usually jagged, multiple traumas are common, and bleeding is uncontrolled. These factors create a high risk for infection and a longer healing time.

Open and Closed Wounds

An open wound occurs from intentional or unintentional trauma. The skin surface is broken, providing a portal of entry for microorganisms. Bleeding, tissue damage, and increased risk for infection and delayed healing may accompany open wounds. Examples include incisions and abrasions.

A closed wound results from a blow, force, or strain caused by trauma such as a fall, an assault, or a motor vehicle crash. The skin surface is not broken, but soft tissue is damaged, and internal injury and hemorrhage may occur. Examples include ecchymosis and hematomas.

Table 31-3 TYPES OF WOUNDS

TYPE	CAUSE
Incision	Cutting or sharp instrument; wound edges in close approximation and aligned
Contusion	Blunt instrument, overlying skin remains intact, with injury to underlying soft tissue; possible resultant bruising and/or hematoma
Abrasion	Friction; rubbing or scraping epidermal layers of skin; top layer of skin abraded
Laceration	Tearing of skin and tissue with blunt or irregular instrument; tissue not aligned, often with loose flaps of skin and tissue
Puncture	Blunt or sharp instrument puncturing the skin; intentional (such as venipuncture) or accidental
Penetrating	Foreign object entering the skin or mucous membrane and lodging in underlying tissue; fragments possibly scattering throughout tissues
Avulsion	Tearing a structure from normal anatomic position; possible damage to blood vessels, nerves, and other structures
Chemical	Toxic agents such as drugs, acids, alcohols, metals, and substances released from cellular necrosis
Thermal	High or low temperatures; cellular necrosis as a possible result
Irradiation	Ultraviolet light or radiation exposure
Pressure ulcers	Compromised circulation secondary to pressure or pressure combined with friction
Venous ulcers	Injury and poor venous return, resulting from underlying conditions, such as incompetent valves or obstruction
Arterial ulcers	Injury and underlying ischemia, resulting from underlying conditions, such as atherosclerosis or thrombosis
Diabetic ulcers	Injury and underlying diabetic neuropathy, peripheral arterial disease, diabetic foot structure

Adapted from Hess, C. (2013). *Skin & wound care* (7th ed.). Philadelphia, Wolters Kluwer Health/Lippincott Williams & Wilkins; Baranoski, S., & Ayello, E. A. (2012). *Wound care essentials. Practice Principles.* (3rd ed.). Philadelphia: Wolters Kluwer Health/Lippincott Williams & Wilkins; Grossman, S. (2014). Porth's pathophysiology: Concepts of altered health states. (9th ed.). Philadelphia: Wolters Kluwer Health/Lippincott Williams & Wilkins and Hinkle J. L., & Cheever, K. H. (2014). *Brunner & Suddarth's Textbook of Medical-Surgical Nursing* (13th ed., p. 2528 [Chart 71-6]). Philadelphia: Wolters Kluwer Health/Lippincott Williams & Wilkins.

Acute and Chronic Wounds

Acute wounds, such as surgical incisions, usually heal within days to weeks. The wound edges are well approximated (edges meet to close skin surface) and the risk of infection is lessened. Acute wounds usually move through the healing process without difficulty. Chronic wounds, in contrast, do not progress through the normal sequence of repair. The healing process is impeded. The wound edges are often not approximated, the risk of infection is increased, and the normal healing time is delayed. Chronic wounds remain in the inflammatory phase of healing (discussed in the next section). Chronic wounds include any wound that does not heal along the expected continuum, such as wounds related to arterial or venous insufficiency, and pressure ulcers.

 Wound Healing

Wound healing is a process of tissue response to injury. Injured tissues are repaired by physiologic mechanisms that regenerate functioning cells and replace connective tissue cells with scar tissue. The healing process fills the gap caused by tissue destruction, restoring the structural integrity of the damaged tissue through the orderly release of growth factors and chemical mediators (Grossman, 2014). These substances help to increase the blood supply to the damaged area, wall off and remove cellular and foreign debris, and initiate cellular development.

Normally, the healing process occurs without assistance. However, interventions can help to support the process. For example, tissue healing is promoted by keeping the injured area free of debris through proper cleaning. Positioning the wounded area to promote circulation to that part helps to promote tissue healing. These interventions are based on the principles of wound healing outlined in Box 31-1 (on page 962).

Wound repair occurs by primary intention, secondary intention, or tertiary intention (Hess, 2013). Wounds healed by primary intention are well approximated (skin edges tightly together). Intentional wounds with minimal tissue loss, such as those made by a surgical incision with sutured approximated edges, usually heal by primary intention. Wounds healed by secondary intention have edges that are not well approximated. Large, open wounds, such as from burns or major trauma, which require more tissue replacement and are often contaminated, commonly heal by secondary intention. If a wound that is healing by primary intention becomes infected, it will heal by secondary intention. Wounds that heal by secondary intention take longer to heal and form more scar tissue (Grossman, 2014). Connective tissue healing and repair follow the same phases in healing. However, differences occur in the length of time required for each phase and in the extent of new tissue formed. Wounds healed by tertiary intention, or delayed primary closure, are those wounds left open for several days to allow edema or infection to resolve or fluid to drain, and then are closed (Hess, 2013).

BOX 31-1 PRINCIPLES OF WOUND HEALING

- Intact skin is the first line of defense against microorganisms. A break in the integrity of the skin increases the risk for infection. Careful hand hygiene before caring for a wound is probably the single most effective method for preventing wound infections.
- The body responds systemically to trauma in any of its parts. For example, a surgical incision can cause a variety of systemic reactions, including increased body temperature, increased heart and respiratory rates, anorexia or nausea and vomiting, musculoskeletal tension, and hormonal changes.
- An adequate blood supply is essential for the body's normal response to any injury. The blood transports increased numbers of leukocytes, erythrocytes, and platelets to the site of injury. Antibodies are carried by the plasma. Increased circulation to the injured part removes toxins and debris and provides nutrients and oxygen. Areas of the body with a good blood supply, such as the head and the neck, heal faster than areas in which the blood supply is not as great, such as the distal part of an extremity.
- Normal healing is promoted when the wound is free of foreign material, such as excessive exudate, dead or damaged tissue cells, pathogenic organisms, or embedded fragments of bone, metal, glass, or other substances. In some situations, a collection of pus or foreign body is walled off and healing occurs around it to form an abscess.
- The ability to handle altered skin integrity depends on the extent of the damage and the person's general state of health. The capacity to deal adequately with a wound is limited when a healthy person sustains a massive injury, when the patient has a chronic illness or a depressed immune system, or when the patient is very young or very old.
- The body's response to a wound is more effective if proper nutrition has been maintained.
  - Undernourished patients are at greater risk for developing a wound infection because they have difficulty mounting their cell-mediated defense system associated with T-lymphocyte activity, and some leukocytic functions are diminished in the presence of protein deficiency.
  - Although the role of fatty acids in wound healing is not well understood, certain quantities of glucose are necessary to meet the energy requirements for wound healing.
  - Various vitamins, minerals, and trace elements are also needed for efficient wound healing. Vitamin A is necessary for collagen synthesis and epithelialization. Vitamin B complex serves as a cofactor of enzyme reactions needed for wound healing. Vitamin C is needed for collagen synthesis, capillary formation, and resistance to infection. Vitamin K is needed for the synthesis of prothrombin. Zinc, copper, and iron assist in collagen synthesis. Manganese serves as an enzyme activator.

Phases of Wound Healing

The wound healing process can be divided into three or four phases, depending on the reference. In this chapter, four phases will be discussed: hemostasis, inflammation, proliferation, and maturation. These four phases systematically lead to repair of the injury (Baranoski & Ayello, 2013; Hess, 2013). If three stages are identified, hemostasis is included as part of the inflammatory stage.

HEMOSTASIS

Hemostasis occurs immediately after the initial injury. Involved blood vessels constrict and blood clotting begins through platelet activation and clustering. After only a brief period of constriction, these same blood vessels dilate and capillary permeability increases, allowing plasma and blood components to leak out into the area that is injured, forming a liquid called **exudate**. The accumulation of exudate causes swelling and pain. Increased perfusion results in heat and redness. If the wound is small, the clot loses fluid and a hard scab is formed to protect the injury. The platelets are also responsible for releasing substances that stimulate other cells to migrate to the injury to participate in the other phases of healing.

INFLAMMATORY PHASE

The inflammatory phase follows hemostasis and lasts about 4 to 6 days. White blood cells, predominantly leukocytes and macrophages, move to the wound. Leukocytes arrive first to ingest bacteria and cellular debris. About 24 hours after the injury, macrophages (a larger phagocytic cell) enter the wound area and remain for an extended period. Macrophages are essential to the healing process. They not only ingest debris, but also release growth factors that are necessary for the growth of epithelial cells and new blood vessels. These growth factors also attract fibroblasts that help to fill in the wound, which is necessary for the next stage of healing. Acute inflammation is characterized by pain, heat, redness, and swelling at the site of the injury. During the inflammatory phase, the patient has a generalized body response, including a mildly elevated temperature, leukocytosis (increased number of white blood cells in the blood), and generalized malaise.

PROLIFERATION PHASE

The proliferation phase is also known as the fibroblastic, regenerative, or connective tissue phase. The proliferation phase lasts for several weeks. New tissue is built to fill the wound space, primarily through the action of fibroblasts. Fibroblasts are connective tissue cells that synthesize and secrete collagen and produce specialized growth factors responsible for inducing blood vessel formation as well as increasing the number and movement of endothelial cells. Capillaries grow across the wound, bringing oxygen and nutrients required for continued healing. Fibroblasts form fibrin that stretches through the clot. A thin layer of epithelial cells forms across the wound, and blood flow across the wound is reinstituted. The new tissue, called **granulation tissue**, forms the foundation for scar tissue development.

It is highly vascular, red, and bleeds easily. In wounds that heal by first intention, epidermal cells seal the wound within 24 to 48 hours, thus the granulation tissue is not visible.

Collagen synthesis and accumulation continue, peaking in 5 to 7 days. Depending on the size of the wound, collagen deposit continues for several weeks or even years. By the end of the second week following the injury, the majority of white blood cells have left the wound area, and the wound is lighter in color. The systemic symptoms now typically disappear. During this phase, adequate nutrition and oxygenation, as well as prevention of strain on the suture line, are important patient care considerations.

Wounds that heal by secondary intention eventually follow the same process but take longer to heal and form more scar tissue (Grossman, 2014). Granulation tissue fills the wound and is then covered by skin cells that grow over the granulation tissue. Connective tissue healing and repair follow the same phases in healing. However, differences occur in the length of time required for each phase and in the extent of granulation tissue formed.

MATURATION PHASE

The final stage of healing, maturation (or remodeling) begins about 3 weeks after the injury, possibly continuing for months or years. Collagen that was haphazardly deposited in the wound is remodeled, making the healed wound stronger and more like adjacent tissue. New collagen continues to be deposited, which compresses the blood vessels in the healing wound, so that the **scar**, an avascular collagen tissue that does not sweat, grow hair, or tan in sunlight, eventually becomes a flat, thin line. Scar tissue is less elastic than uninjured tissue. The strength of the scar tissue remains less than that of normal tissue, even many years following injury and it is never fully restored (Baranoski & Ayello, 2012, p. 91). Wounds that heal by secondary intention take longer to remodel and form a scar smaller than the original wound. If the scar is over a joint or other body structure, it may limit movement and cause disability.

 RECALL Sam Bentz, the 56-year-old man admitted for treatment of a bone infection. The nurse would apply the knowledge about the phases of wound healing when reviewing this patient's past history (the wounds he developed during his last hospital admission). In addition, this knowledge would help form the basis for the patient's plan of care should another wound occur during this hospitalization. ●

Factors Affecting Wound Healing

A variety of factors affect wound healing. Local factors, those occurring directly in the wound, include pressure, **desiccation** (dehydration), **maceration** (overhydration), trauma, edema, infection, excessive bleeding, **necrosis** (death of tissue), and the presence of **biofilm** (a thick grouping of microorganisms). Systemic factors, those occurring throughout the body, include age, circulation to and oxygenation of tissues, nutritional status, wound condition, health status, immunosuppression, and medication use (Huether & McCance, 2012; Hess, 2013; Grossman, 2014).

LOCAL FACTORS

Factors occurring local to the wound itself can prolong wound healing. These factors are discussed in the following sections.

Pressure

Pressure disrupts the blood supply to the wound area. Persistent or excessive pressure interferes with blood flow to the tissue and delays healing.

Desiccation

Desiccation is the process of drying up. Cells dehydrate and die in a dry environment. This cell death causes a crust to form over the wound site and delays healing. Wounds that are kept moist (not wet) and hydrated experience enhanced epidermal cell migration, which supports **epithelialization** (epithelial cell migration to the wound bed; Hess, 2013).

Maceration

Maceration, softening and breakdown of skin, results from prolonged exposure to moisture. Overhydration of cells related to urinary and fecal incontinence can also lead to maceration and impaired skin integrity. This damage is related to moisture, changes in the pH of the skin, overgrowth of bacteria and infection of the skin, and erosion of skin from friction on moist skin.

Trauma

Repeated trauma to a wound area results in delayed healing or the inability to heal.

Edema

Edema at a wound site interferes with the blood supply to the area, resulting in an inadequate supply of oxygen and nutrients to the tissue.

Infection

Bacteria in a wound increase stress on the body, requiring increased energy to deal with the invaders. Infection requires large amounts of energy be spent by the immune system to fight the microorganisms, leaving little or no reserves to attend to the job of repair and healing. In addition, toxins produced by bacteria and released when bacteria die interfere with wound healing and cause cell death.

Excessive Bleeding

Excessive bleeding results in large clots. Large clots increase the amount of space that must be filled during healing and interferes with oxygen diffusion to the tissue. In addition, accumulated blood is an excellent place for growth of bacteria and promotes infection (Huether & McCance, 2012).

Necrosis

Dead tissue present in the wound delays healing. Dead tissue appears as slough—moist, yellow, stringy tissue—and eschar appears as dry, black, leathery tissue. Healing of the

FOCUS ON THE OLDER ADULT

NURSING STRATEGIES TO ADDRESS AGE-RELATED CHANGES IN WOUND HEALING

Age-Related Changes	Nursing Interventions
Skin loses turgor and is more fragile.	• Maintain hydration with intravenous fluids as prescribed. • Maintain record of intake and output. • Use caution when removing tape.
Decreased secretion of enzymes and absorption of nutrients and minerals may increase risk for delayed wound healing.	• Maintain intake of adequate kilocalories with oral, enteral, or parenteral feedings. • Ensure that diet is high in protein, vitamin A, vitamin C, and trace elements (zinc and copper). • Monitor lab results such as serum albumin, total protein.
Risk of infection increases from: • Slower inflammatory response • Reduced antibody production and endocrine system function • Increased incidence of chronic illnesses, such as diabetes mellitus and cardiovascular disease, that compromise circulation and tissue oxygenation	• Maintain careful hand hygiene and surgical asepsis with dressing changes and care of tubes or drains. • Take and record vital signs, noting and reporting increased temperature. • Monitor wound for manifestations of infection. • Administer medications as prescribed. • Administer supplemental oxygen as prescribed.

wound will not take place with necrotic tissue in the wound. Removal of the dead tissue must occur for healing to begin (Hess, 2013; Beitz, 2012).

Biofilm

Wound biofilms are the result of wound bacteria growing in clumps, imbedded in a thick, self-made, protective, slimy barrier of sugars and proteins. This barrier contributes to decreased effectiveness of antibiotics against the bacteria (antibiotic resistance) and decreases the effectiveness of the normal immune response by the patient (Beitz, 2012). The bacteria also produce a protective matrix that attaches the biofilm to the wound surface. Biofilms impair wound healing and contribute to chronic wound inflammation (Baranoski & Ayello, 2012).

SYSTEMIC FACTORS

Factors not related to the wound location itself also can prolong wound healing. These factors are discussed in the following sections.

Age

The major skin layers arise from different embryologic origins, resulting in poor adherence between the epidermis and the dermis. This loose binding between the layers causes the layers to separate easily during an inflammatory process, placing infants and small children at risk for impaired skin integrity. Epidermal stripping, the unintentional removal of the epidermis with tape removal, is one type of such injury. Care should be taken to minimize tension, traction, and wrinkles on the skin when using tape on these young patients.

Children and healthy adults, however, heal more rapidly than do older adults, in whom physiologic changes caused by aging result in diminished fibroblastic activity and circulation. Older adults are more likely to have one or more

chronic illnesses, with pathologic changes that impede the healing process. See the accompanying Focus on the Older Adult display for other age-related factors affecting wound healing.

Circulation and Oxygenation

Adequate blood flow to deliver nutrients and oxygen and to remove local toxins, bacteria, and other debris is essential for wound healing. Certain physical conditions, because of their effect on circulation and oxygenation, can affect wound healing. Circulation may be impaired in older adults and in people with peripheral vascular disorders, cardiovascular disorders, hypertension, or diabetes mellitus. Oxygenation of tissues is decreased in people with anemia or chronic respiratory disorders and in those who smoke.

 RECALL Lucius Everly, the patient described in the Reflective Practice display. The nurse's ability to integrate knowledge of the effects of diabetes on circulation would be important in planning measures to ensure adequate circulation to his extremities as a means to prevent skin breakdown. ●

In addition, large amounts of subcutaneous and tissue fat (which has fewer blood vessels) in people who are obese may slow wound healing because fatty tissue is more difficult to suture, is more prone to infection, and takes longer to heal.

 REMEMBER Sam Bentz, the middle-aged patient with a bone infection described at the beginning of the chapter. The nurse would incorporate an understanding of this patient's past history and large size to develop an appropriate plan of care to prevent future occurrences of skin breakdown. ●

Nutritional Status

Wound healing requires adequate proteins, carbohydrates, fats, vitamins, and minerals. Calories and protein are necessary to rebuild cells and tissues. Vitamins A and C are essential for epithelialization and collagen synthesis. Zinc plays a role in proliferation of cells. Fluids are necessary for optimal function of cells. All phases of the wound healing process are slowed or inadequate in the patient with poor nutritional status and fluid balance.

Some patients who are obese suffer from protein malnutrition, which interferes with healing. Patients who are undernourished may lack the nutritional stores to promote wound healing. Nutrition is further discussed in Chapter 35.

Medications and Health Status

Patients who are taking corticosteroid drugs or require postoperative radiation therapy are at high risk for delayed healing and wound complications. Corticosteroids decrease the inflammatory process, which may delay healing. Radiation depresses bone marrow function, resulting in decreased leukocytes and an increased risk of infection. The presence of a chronic illness (such as cardiovascular disease or diabetes mellitus) or impaired immune function can impair wound healing. Chemotherapeutic agents impair or stop proliferation of all rapidly growing cells, including cells involved in wound healing. Prolonged antibiotic therapy increases a patient's risk for secondary infection and superinfection.

Immunosuppression

Suppression of the immune system as a result of disease (e.g., AIDS, lupus), medication (e.g., chemotherapy), or age (e.g., changes associated with advancing age) can delay wound healing.

Wound Complications

Wound complications include infection, hemorrhage, dehiscence, evisceration, and fistula. These complications increase the risk for generalized illness and death, lengthen the patient's need for health care interventions, and add to health care costs.

INFECTION

Wound infection results when the patient's immune system fails to control the growth of microorganisms. Microorganisms can invade a wound at the time of trauma, during surgery, or at any time after the initial wound occurs. A contaminated wound is more likely to become infected than one that is not contaminated. Additionally, the risk of infection is increased in a surgical wound created during a procedure involving the intestines because the risk for contamination with fecal material is high. Wound infections also occur as a result of hospital-acquired infections (HAIs). Symptoms of wound infection usually become apparent within 2 to 7 days after the injury or surgery; often, the patient is at home. Symptoms of infection include purulent drainage; increased drainage, pain, redness, and swelling in and around the wound; increased body temperature; and increased white blood cell count. Additional signs and symptoms include

delayed healing and discoloration of granulation tissue in the wound (Baranoski & Ayello, 2012). In patients with infection in a chronic wound, pain and delayed healing may be the only symptoms (Baranoski & Ayello, 2012). Wound infections impair healing. Wound infections can lead to other complications, including development of chronic wounds, osteomyelitis (bone infection) and sepsis (presence of pathogenic organisms in the blood or tissues).

HEMORRHAGE

Hemorrhage may occur from a slipped suture, a dislodged clot at the wound site, infection, or the erosion of a blood vessel by a foreign body, such as a drain. Check the dressing and the wound under the dressing, if possible, frequently during the first 48 hours after the injury, and no less than every 8 hours thereafter. If excessive bleeding does occur, additional pressure dressings or packing may be necessary, fluid replacement is probably necessary, and surgical intervention may be required. Internal hemorrhage causes the formation of a hematoma. If the bleeding leads to a large accumulation of blood, it can put pressure on surrounding blood vessels and cause tissue ischemia (deficiency of blood to an area). See Chapter 29 for more information about hemorrhage.

DEHISCENCE AND EVISCERATION

Dehiscence and evisceration (Fig. 31-2) are the most serious postoperative wound complications. **Dehiscence** is the partial or total separation of wound layers as a result of excessive stress on wounds that are not healed. **Evisceration** is the most serious complication of dehiscence (Hinkle & Cheever, 2014; Harvey, 2005). The wound completely separates, with protrusion of viscera through the incisional area. Patients at

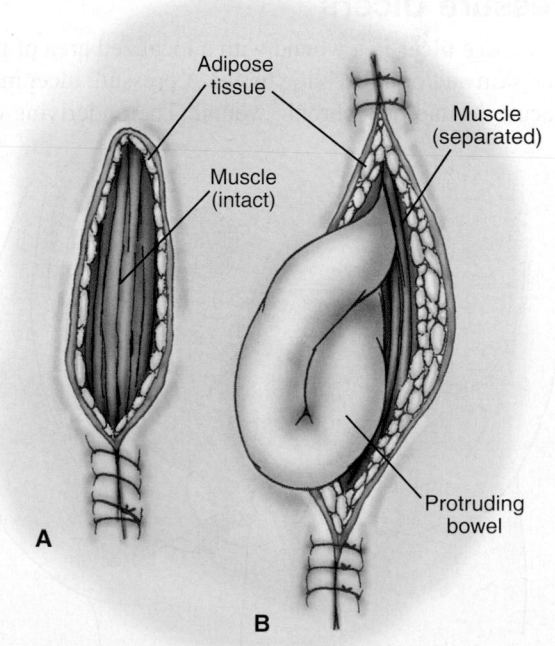

FIGURE 31-2. Wound complications. (**A**) Dehiscence. (**B**) Evisceration.

greater risk for these complications include those who are obese or malnourished, smoke tobacco, use anticoagulants, have infected wounds, or experience excessive coughing, vomiting, or straining (Hinkle & Cheever, 2014). An increase in the flow of fluid from the wound between postoperative days 4 and 5 may be a sign of an impending dehiscence. The patient may say that "something has suddenly given way." If dehiscence occurs, cover the wound area with sterile towels moistened with sterile 0.9% sodium chloride solution and notify the physician. Once dehiscence occurs, the wound is managed like any open wound. Dehiscence and evisceration of an abdominal incision is a medical emergency. Place the patient in the low Fowler's position and cover the exposed abdominal contents, as discussed previously. Do not leave the patient alone. Notify the primary care provider immediately. This situation is an emergency that requires prompt surgical repair (Harvey, 2005).

FISTULA FORMATION

A **fistula** is an abnormal passage from an internal organ or vessel to the outside of the body or from one internal organ or vessel to another. Fistulas may be created purposefully; for example, an arteriovenous fistula is created surgically to provide circulatory access for kidney dialysis. However, fistula formation is often the result of infection that has developed into an abscess, which is a collection of infected fluid that has not drained. Accumulated fluid applies pressure to surrounding tissues, leading to the formation of the unnatural passage. Figure 31-3 illustrates an enterovaginal fistula, which is an abnormal connection between the rectum and vagina. The presence of a fistula increases the risk for delayed healing, additional infection, fluid and electrolyte imbalances, and skin breakdown.

Pressure Ulcers

A **pressure ulcer** is a wound with a localized area of injury to the skin and/or underlying tissue. A pressure ulcer may be an acute wound or a chronic wound. The underlying cause is pressure. Most pressure ulcers develop when soft tissue is compressed between a bony prominence and an external surface for a prolonged period of time, or when soft tissue undergoes pressure in combination with shear and/or friction (Hess, 2013; National Pressure Ulcer Advisory Panel [NPUAP], 2012a). The terms *decubitus ulcer, pressure sore,* and *bedsore* are also used to refer to this type of wound. The term *pressure ulcer* is considered the most appropriate term because pressure is the most prominent underlying cause.

Pressure ulcers are costly in terms of patient discomfort, disfigurement, decreased quality of life, and health care expenditures (Hess, 2013; Baranoski & Ayello, 2012; O'Tuathall & Taqi, 2011). Most pressure ulcers occur in older adults as a result of a combination of factors, including aging skin, chronic illnesses, immobility, malnutrition, fecal and urinary incontinence, and altered level of consciousness. Other significant at-risk populations include people with spinal cord injuries, traumatic brain injuries, or neuromuscular disorders. When pressure ulcers occur, aggressive intervention and treatment can spare the patient unnecessary pain and discomfort, prevent further tissue deterioration, hasten wound healing, and save millions of health care dollars.

Factors in Pressure Ulcer Development

Pathologic changes at a pressure ulcer site result from blood vessel collapse caused by pressure, usually from body weight. Necrosis eventually occurs, leading to the characteristic ulcer. Two mechanisms contribute to pressure ulcer development: (1) external pressure that compresses blood vessels and (2) friction and shearing forces that tear and injure blood vessels and abrade the top layer of skin.

EXTERNAL PRESSURE

Pressure ulcers usually occur over bony prominences where body weight is distributed over a small area without much subcutaneous tissue to cushion damage to the skin. Common sites for pressure ulcers are illustrated in Figure 31-4. Of the susceptible areas, most pressure ulcers occur over the sacrum and coccyx, followed by the trochanter and the calcaneus (heel).

The major predisposing factor for a pressure ulcer is external pressure applied over an area, which results in occluded blood capillaries and poor circulation to tissues. Insufficient circulation deprives tissues of oxygen and nutrients, which leads to **ischemia** (deficiency of blood in a particular area), hypoxia (inadequate amount of oxygen available to cells), edema, inflammation, and, ultimately, necrosis and ulcer formation. A pressure ulcer may form in as little as 1 to 2 hours if the patient has not moved or been repositioned to allow circulation to flow to dependent areas. Patients with casts, orthopedic devices, or support stockings require routine assessment of areas where inadequate circulation may be a contributing factor to the development of a pressure ulcer.

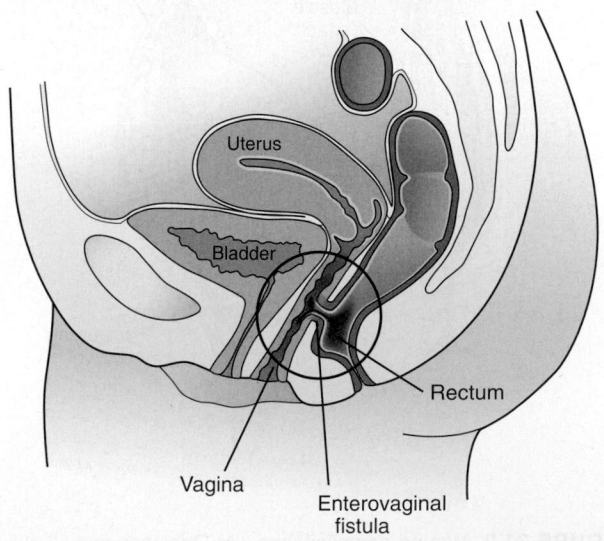

Uterus

Bladder

Rectum

Vagina

Enterovaginal fistula

FIGURE 31-3. Fistula.

CONSIDER Mr. Everly, the postoperative patient in the critical care unit described in the Reflective Practice display. The nurse would

FIGURE 31-4. Common sites for development of pressure ulcers.

integrate knowledge of the patient's condition, including his decreased level of consciousness and confinement in bed, to plan measures such as a turning schedule, proper positioning, and activities to promote movement in bed, thereby preventing body parts from exposure to prolonged pressure. ●

FRICTION AND SHEAR

Friction occurs when two surfaces rub against each other. The injury, which resembles an abrasion, also can damage superficial blood vessels directly under the skin. A patient who lies on wrinkled sheets is likely to sustain tissue damage as a result of friction. The skin over the elbows and heels often is injured due to friction when patients lift and help move themselves up in bed with the use of their arms and feet. Friction burns can also occur on the back when patients are pulled or slid over sheets while being moved up in bed or transferred onto a stretcher.

Shear results when one layer of tissue slides over another layer. Shear separates the skin from underlying tissues. The small blood vessels and capillaries in the area are stretched and possibly tear, resulting in decreased circulation to the tissue cells under the skin. Figure 31-5 illustrates how shearing forces occur. Patients who are pulled, rather than lifted, when being moved up in bed or from bed to chair or stretcher are at risk for injury from shearing forces. A patient who is partially sitting up in bed is susceptible to shearing force when the skin sticks to the sheet and underlying tissues move downward with the body toward the foot of the bed. This may also occur in a patient who sits in a chair but slides down.

Risks for Pressure Ulcer Development

In addition to pressure, friction, and shear, a combination of causes contributes to ulcer development. These include immobility, nutrition and hydration, skin moisture, mental

status, and age; these factors are addressed here. Additional risk factors are outlined in Box 31-2 (on page 968).

IMMOBILITY

Patients who spend long periods of time in bed or seated without shifting their body weight properly are at great risk for developing a pressure ulcer (Hess, 2013). People who are ambulatory usually do not develop this type of injury because no part of the body experiences prolonged pressure. In addition, when asleep, healthy people tend to move about in bed freely. Patients who are unconscious and paralyzed,

FIGURE 31-5. Shearing forces can occur when a patient is moved carelessly or slides down in bed.

BOX 31-2 **RISK FACTORS FOR PRESSURE ULCER DEVELOPMENT**

Immobility, nutrition and hydration, skin moisture, mental status, and age are factors in the development of pressure ulcers. In addition, patients compromised by the following conditions are at risk for pressure ulcer development:

- Dehydration
- Incontinence
- Skin hygiene
- Diabetes mellitus
- Diminished pain awareness
- Fractures
- History of corticosteroid therapy
- Immunosuppression
- Multisystem trauma
- Poor circulation
- Previous pressure ulcers
- Significant obesity or thinness

Adapted from Lloyd Jones, M. (2012b). Prevention and treatment of superficial pressure damage. *Nursing & Residential Care, 14*(1), 14, 16, 18, 20; Hess, C. (2013). *Wound care* (7th ed.). Philadelphia: Wolters Kluwer Health/Lippincott Williams & Wilkins; and National Pressure Ulcer Advisory Panel (NPUAP). (2012d). Pressure ulcer prevention points. Available at http://www.npuap.org/resources/educational-and-clinical-resources/pressure-ulcer-prevention-points/

those with cognitive impairments, or those with other physical limitations such as a fracture, are subject to pressure ulcers if they are allowed to remain in any one position for an extended period. People who are emotionally depressed ordinarily do not move around much, placing them at risk for pressure ulcer formation. Additional factors that cause immobility and may result in this serious problem include surgery and the use of tranquilizers or sedatives.

NUTRITION AND HYDRATION

Protein–calorie malnutrition predisposes a person to pressure ulcer formation because poorly nourished cells are damaged easily. Protein deficiency leading to a negative nitrogen balance, electrolyte imbalances, and insufficient caloric intake also predisposes the skin to injury. Other deficiencies can increase risk. For example, vitamin C deficiency causes capillaries to become fragile, with resultant poor circulation to the area. The condition of the teeth or fit of dentures may also exacerbate the problem of inadequate dietary intake. Dehydration as well as edema can interfere with circulation and subsequent cell nourishment.

MOISTURE

Primary sources of skin moisture include perspiration, urine, feces, and drainage from wounds (Voegeli, 2012). Prolonged moisture on the skin reduces the skin's resistance to trauma, particularly damage from friction and shear. When skin is damp, less friction is required to blister and abrade skin. Additionally, the moisture associated with urinary and fecal incontinence is believed to increase the risk for skin damage due to the chemical irritation from the ammonia in the urine. Ammonia also raises the alkalinity of the skin pH, altering

the function of the normally acidic skin. A more alkaline pH promotes premature shedding of skin cells and decreases the skin's defense against bacteria, which results in enhanced growth of pathogens, such as yeast and staphylococci.

MENTAL STATUS

The more alert a person is, the more likely the individual is to protect skin integrity by relieving pressure periodically and maintaining adequate skin hygiene. Apathy, confusion, or a comatose state can diminish these self-care abilities and increase the likelihood of skin breakdown.

AGE

Older adults are at a greater risk for pressure ulcer formation because the aging skin is more susceptible to injury. Chronic and debilitating diseases, more common in this age group, may adversely affect circulation and oxygenation of dermal structures. Other problems, such as malnutrition and immobility, compound the risk of pressure ulcer development in older adults.

Pressure Ulcer Staging

The first indication that a pressure ulcer may be developing is blanching (becoming pale and white) of the skin over the area under pressure. This ischemia makes the skin appear paler than in areas where circulation is adequate. When pressure is relieved, ischemia is rapidly followed by hyperemia. Reactive hyperemia is a blanchable reddening of the skin that occurs when pressure is removed. The body literally floods the area with blood to nourish and remove wastes from the cells. The area appears red and feels warm, but blanches when slight pressure is applied. Reactive hyperemia is not a pressure ulcer. After a patient who has been lying supine for 2 hours is repositioned onto the side, any reddened area due to reactive hyperemia should fade within 60 to 90 minutes. In patients with darkly pigmented skin, it may be best to assess for hyperemia by touch; the skin feels warm. Also, assess for some change in color relative to the surrounding skin.

If the pressure continues after ischemia occurs, circulation is further impaired and a pressure ulcer develops. Appropriate intervention depends on early recognition of the stage of development of the pressure ulcer. Pressure ulcers are commonly classified according to six stages (four numbered and two unnumbered)—suspected deep-tissue injury, stage I, stage II, stage III, stage IV, and unstageable (NPUAP, 2012a). See the accompanying Research in Nursing box, which highlights the importance of the nurse's role in accurate assessment of pressure ulcers, essential to providing appropriate and effective wound care.

Suspected deep-tissue injury presents as a purple or maroon, localized area of discolored intact skin or blood-filled blister due to damage of underlying soft tissue from pressure and/or shear. It may initially present as a painful, firm, mushy, boggy, warmer, or cooler area as compared to adjacent tissue (NPUAP, 2012a).

A stage I pressure ulcer is a defined area of intact skin with nonblanchable redness of a localized area usually over a bony prominence. Darkly pigmented skin may not have

RESEARCH IN NURSING

BRIDGING THE GAP TO EVIDENCE-BASED PRACTICE

Accurate Assessment of Pressure Ulcers

Pressure ulcers are costly in terms of patient discomfort, disfigurement, decreased quality of life, fatalities, and health care expenditures. Nurses play an important role in accurate assessment of pressure ulcers, which is essential to providing appropriate and effective wound care.

Related Research

Alvey, B., Heard, H., & Hennen, N. (2012). Improving accuracy of pressure ulcer staging and documentation using a computerized clinical decision support system. *Journal of Wound, Ostomy and Continence Nursing, 39*(6), 607–612.

The purpose of this study was to evaluate an algorithm designed to assess and document pressure ulcers (PUs), using a computerized clinical decision support (CCDS) system. Thirty-one RNs, LPNs, and student nurses volunteered to participate in this descriptive study. The CCDS program was built as an algorithm based on the National Pressure Ulcer Advisory Panel's definitions of PUs. Users of the CCDS document are required to provide descriptions of the wound using drop-down menus, defining the characteristics, depth, and color of the PU. The computer program then assigns a PU stage. Users can accept the CCDS-suggested stage or override the system to enter a stage. Participants used the CCDS to document the characteristics of 5 PUs presented in photographs and determine the stage of the PU. A total of 123 stagings were included in data analyses. Data were analyzed to determine the accuracy of the nurses' staging compared to that of the researcher. Data were also analyzed

to test for differences between PU groups, including overall accuracy, accuracy in accepting the CCDS suggested stage, and accuracy when the override function was used. Nurses accurately staged PU photographs 64% of the time (79 of 123) during the simulation exercise by either accepting the CCDS-suggested stage or overriding the suggestion. Within the accurately staged PUs, nurses agreed with the CCDS-suggested stage 55% of the time (68 of 123). In the other 9% of ratings (11 of 123), the nurses staged accurately by overriding the CCDS suggestion, which was based on incorrect descriptors selected. Nurses were significantly more accurate using CCDS-suggested stage as compared to PU staged by overriding the CDDS. The authors concluded these findings support a potential benefit in using the CCDS to improve nurses' accuracy in PU staging because the characteristics are already listed and once selected, the CCDS assigns the correct PU stage.

Relevance to Nursing Practice

In order to provide quality care for patients with pressure ulcers, nurses must be able to accurately identify and stage pressure ulcers. Use of technology, such as a computerized clinical decision support system, as well as knowledge and skills, can assist in providing accurate and effective wound care, which contributes to the patient's overall well-being and to prevention of complications related to pressure ulcers.

For additional research, visit thePoint.

---

visible blanching; its color may differ from the surrounding skin. The area may be painful, firm, soft, warmer, or cooler as compared to adjacent tissue (NPUAP, 2012a). A stage II pressure ulcer involves partial thickness loss of dermis and presents as a shallow, open ulcer (NPUAP). A stage III ulcer presents with full-thickness tissue loss. Subcutaneous fat may be visible, but bone, tendon, or muscle is not exposed. Slough that may be present does not obscure the depth of tissue loss. Ulcers at this stage may include undermining and tunneling (NPUAP). Stage IV ulcers involve full-thickness tissue loss with exposed bone, tendon, or muscle. Slough or eschar may be present on some part of the wound bed and often include undermining and tunneling.

Pressure ulcers are classified as unstageable when the base of the ulcer is covered by slough (yellow, tan, gray, green, or brown) and/or eschar (tan, brown, or black) in the wound bed. **Eschar** is a thick, leathery scab or dry crust that is necrotic (dead tissue) and must be removed before the stage can be determined accurately. However, stable (dry, adherent, intact, without erythema or fluctuance) eschar on the heels serves as "the body's natural (biological) cover" and should not be removed (NPUAP, 2012a).

Detailed descriptions of these stages and a visual representation are presented in Box 31-3 (on page 970).

Psychological Effects of Wounds and Pressure Ulcers

Because the skin is a sensory organ and plays a major role in communication with others and self-image, wounds and pressure ulcers require emotional as well as physical adaptation. Although stress and adaptation vary greatly among people, actual and potential emotional stressors are common in all patients with wounds. These stressors impact the quality of life of the patient and caregivers and include pain, anxiety, fear, activities of daily living, and changes in body image.

Pain

Pain is part of almost any trauma, from a small cut on the finger to a large incision made during abdominal surgery or a chronic arterial ulcer. Although pain can be considered a physical complication, it also has a large psychological component. Pain from wounds is often increased by activities such as ambulating, coughing, moving in bed, and dressing changes. The actual pain might be worsened by the patient's apprehension about such activities. Nursing interventions to reduce pain can greatly reduce emotional stress. See Chapter 34 for a more in-depth discussion of pain.

(text continues on page 972)

BOX 31-3 COMPARISON OF STAGES OF PRESSURE ULCERS

Suspected Deep Tissue Injury

Purple or maroon localized area of discolored intact skin or blood-filled blister due to damage of underlying soft tissue from pressure and/or shear. Deep tissue injury may be difficult to detect in individuals with dark skin tones. The area may be preceded by tissue that is painful, firm, boggy, warmer, or cooler as compared to adjacent tissue. Evolution may include a thin blister over a dark wound bed. The wound may further evolve and become covered by a thin eschar. Evolution may be rapid, exposing additional layers of tissue even with optimal treatment.

Stage I

Intact skin with nonblanchable redness of a localized area usually over a bony prominence. Darkly pigmented skin may not have visible blanching; its color may differ from the surrounding area. The area may be painful, firm, soft, warmer, or cooler as compared to adjacent tissue. Stage I may be difficult to detect in individuals with dark skin tones. Stage I may indicate "at risk" persons.

Stage II

Partial-thickness loss of dermis presenting as a shallow open ulcer with a red pink wound bed, without slough. Presents as a shiny or dry shallow ulcer without slough or bruising (which indicates suspected deep tissue injury). May also present as an intact or open/rupture serum-filled blister. This stage should not be used to describe skin tears, tape burns, perineal dermatitis, maceration, or excoriation.

BOX 31-3   COMPARISON OF STAGES OF PRESSURE ULCERS   *continued*

Stage III

Full-thickness tissue loss. Subcutaneous fat may be visible, but bone, tendon, or muscle are not exposed. Bone/tendon is not visible or directly palpable. Slough may be present but does not obscure the depth of tissue loss. May include undermining and tunneling. The depth of a stage III pressure ulcer varies by anatomic location. The bridge of the nose, ear, occiput, and malleolus do not have subcutaneous tissue, and stage III ulcers at these locations can be shallow. In contrast, areas with significant adipose tissue can develop extremely deep stage III pressure ulcers.

Stage IV

Full-thickness tissue loss with exposed bone, tendon, or muscle. Exposed bone/tendon is visible or directly palpable. Slough or eschar may be present on some parts of the wound bed. Often includes undermining and tunneling. The depth of a stage IV pressure ulcer varies by anatomic location. The bridge of the nose, ear, occiput, and malleolus do not have subcutaneous tissue and these ulcers can be shallow at these locations. Stage IV ulcers can extend into muscle and/or supporting structures (e.g., fascia, tendon, or joint capsule), making osteomyelitis possible.

Unstageable

Full-thickness tissue loss in which the base of the ulcer is covered by slough (yellow, tan, gray, green, or brown) and/or eschar (tan, brown, or black) in the wound bed. Until enough slough and/or eschar is removed to expose the base of the wound, the true depth, and therefore stage, cannot be determined. Stable (dry, adherent, intact, without erythema, or fluctuance) eschar on the heels serves as "the body's natural (biological) cover" and should not be removed.

Reprinted with permission from National Pressure Ulcer Advisory Panel (NPUAP) (2012a). Pressure ulcer stages/categories. Available at http://www.npuap.org/resources/educational-and-clinical-resources/npuap-pressure-ulcer-stagescategories/; and Grossman, S. (2014). Porth's pathophysiology: Concepts of altered health states. (9th ed.). Philadelphia: Wolters Kluwer Health/Lippincott Williams & Wilkins.

Illustrations reprinted with permission from National Pressure Ulcer Advisory Panel (NPUAP) (2012b). Pressure ulcer staging/illustrations. Available at http://www.npuap.org/resources/educational-and-clinical-resources/pressure-ulcer-categorystaging-illustrations/

FOCUSED CRITICAL THINKING GUIDE 31-1

WOUND CARE: PROMOTING ACCEPTANCE OF CHANGES IN BODY IMAGE

During both clinical days in 1 week, you (a female student) have been assigned to care for a middle-aged woman who has had a breast removed because of cancer. The patient, Mrs. Nola, is an attractive woman who is usually cheerful and eager to get better and return home. However, on both days, she turned her head away and would not look at the incision when her dressing was changed. She tells you that she "just can't stand to look at herself." Her husband has left the room during the dressing changes after telling you that "it makes me sick to see what happened to my wife." Mrs. Nola is to be discharged to her home the next day and needs to learn how to provide self-care for her wound. What do you do?

1. Identify goal of thinking

Determine the most effective way of ensuring wound care and at the same time assisting Mrs. Nola in accepting her altered self-image.

2. Assess adequacy of knowledge

Pertinent circumstances: The diagnosis of cancer was made only 1 day before the surgical removal of the breast. The patient is to be discharged to her home the next day. The wound from her mastectomy has not completely healed and will require dressing changes for another 3 or 4 days. Mrs. Nola has had a disfiguring surgery and is coping with not only a change in body image, but also the diagnosis of cancer. She has never been seriously ill or had surgery. She has a strong, loving relationship with her husband, but he is unable to deal with the physical disfigurement at this time.

Prerequisite knowledge: Before you decide what to do in this situation, you need to know at what level Mrs. Nola is in coping with the diagnosis of cancer. If she is still in denial about the disease, it is likely that she is also denying the surgical procedure and the changes in her body. You will need to review responses to the diagnosis of cancer as well as the stages of grief and loss. You will have to learn what her sources of support are and how she can best access and use them. You will need to assess how best to help her achieve wound care in the face of her continued refusal even to look at the wound.

Room for error: If she is forced to look at the wound or made to feel inadequate because of her inability to do so, she will feel threatened and most likely will become angry in response to the perceived threat.

Time constraints: Some decision about wound care must be made before her discharge the next day.

3. Address potential problems

There are several potential obstacles to critical thinking in this situation. As a student, you want to exhibit safe, knowledgeable care, and the importance of teaching for home care has been an emphasis in this course. As a woman, you have a sense of what the loss of a breast must mean. Having had a family member die of cancer, you find yourself wanting to do everything for Mrs. Nola. As a novice in nursing, you find it difficult to handle these emotional components of patient care and find yourself wanting to scold both the patient and her husband for being so silly about something as simple as a dressing.

4. Consult helpful resources

You must first understand the loss and grief Mrs. Nola is experiencing, and you must then relate that to her response to self-care of the wound. Your best source of information about her coping methods and sources of personal strength is Mrs. Nola herself. You also discuss the most effective way of providing wound care at home with your instructor and the case manager for Mrs. Nola.

5. Critique judgment/decision

After talking to Mrs. Nola, your instructor, and the case manager, you mutually agree that Mrs. Nola cannot be hurried into acceptance of her medical diagnosis or her body changes. The case manager consults with Mrs. Nola's physician, who writes an order for a home health care nurse to visit for the next 4 days and complete the dressing change. After talking with Mrs. Nola, you identify that she is still very much in denial. You discuss with her the possibility of having a visitor from "Reach to Recovery," a support group for women with breast cancer who have had a mastectomy. Mrs. Nola tells you that she thinks she would like to talk to someone with the same problem, and you call a referral for her. When you tell Mrs. Nola that a home health care nurse will be visiting her for the first few days at home to change her dressing, tears come into her eyes. She says "I am so scared, I just don't know what to do." You realize that insisting that Mrs. Nola do her own dressing would have been extremely stressful for her and that you would have considered the wound as more important than the patient. When you share the situation in post-conference, your clinical group supports your decision.

Anxiety and Fear

Anxiety and fear are common responses to a wound. Patients are apprehensive about the possibility of the wound opening, how much privacy will be lost as the wound is being cared for, and how they and others will react to the appearance and smell of the wound. When caring for patients with wounds, demonstrating acceptance and empathy, encouraging the expression of feelings, answering questions accurately and honestly, and avoiding excessive exposure of body parts when giving wound care are essential.

Activities of Daily Living

The presence of an acute or chronic wound or pressure ulcer can have an impact on the ability of the patient to perform activities of daily living. Physical, financial, and medical restrictions can result in limitations on a patient's ability to perform things normally done in daily living including any daily activity related to self-care (such as feeding oneself, bathing, dressing, grooming), work, homemaking, and leisure, restricting the patient's life.

Changes in Body Image

Body image reflects a person's view of oneself as a whole entity. When the skin and tissues are traumatized, that image is changed, requiring the person to adapt and reformulate the concept of self. Wounds and scars that are visible to others, especially on the face, can result in feelings of conspicuousness, ugliness, and diminished self-worth. Large scars, such as from removal of a breast or from creation of a colostomy opening, can seriously affect the person's sexuality, social relationships, and self-concept. Referral to support groups or counselors may be necessary to facilitate coping and acceptance of changes in body structure or function. See the Focused Critical Thinking Guide 31-1. In addition, Chapter 40 contains more information about self-concept.

THE NURSING PROCESS FOR WOUNDS AND PRESSURE ULCERS
Assessing

The patient's health history is an essential component for assessing the patient's integumentary status and identification of risk factors for problems with the skin. This information can be obtained from either the patient or a family member. The nursing examination combined with laboratory findings can provide information to identify a patient's strengths, the nature of any problems, their course, related signs and symptoms, and their onset, frequency, and effects on activities of daily living. The nurse decides, based on these findings, what problems can be treated independently by nursing. Other problems are referred to a physician and/or other collaborative professionals for decisions on treatment.

Nursing History

When obtaining the nursing history, include questions about the appearance of the skin and patient activities that may contribute to the development of a pressure ulcer. Often a combination of factors places the patient at greatest risk for a pressure ulcer.

Question the patient and family about recent changes in the appearance or condition of the skin and any skin care regimens. Also, assess activity status, nutritional state, elimination patterns, and cognitive state.

Evaluate the patient's general condition and laboratory test results. Be alert for signs and symptoms of infection, which may cause generalized malaise, increased pain, anorexia, and an elevated body temperature and pulse rate. Laboratory data indicating an infection include an elevated white blood cell count and, if a wound culture has been done, a causative organism.

The accompanying Focused Assessment Guide 31-1 (on page 974) provides additional suggestions for gathering a nursing history.

Skin Assessment

Skin assessment should be an integral part of every patient's care. Physical assessment of the skin is included as part of the initial database collection. Skin assessment provides needed information for developing an appropriate plan of care. The inspection and palpation skills used to assess the integumentary system are described in detail in Chapter 25. Be sure to inspect the skin systematically in a head-to-toe fashion, including bony prominences, on admission and then at regular intervals for all at-risk patients. Reassessment is recommended (NPUAP, 2012a), as follows:

- *Acute care setting:* On admission, then reassessed at least every 24 hours or if the patient's condition changes. Reassess stable patients in intensive care units daily; reassess unstable patients every shift.
- Long-term care setting: On admission, then reassess weekly for 4 weeks, then quarterly and whenever the resident's condition changes
- Home health care: On admission, then reassess at every visit

Early detection and treatment of skin problems are important nursing functions. It is important to provide patients with a proactive strategy for skin care. Many conditions and wounds, particularly pressure ulcers, can be prevented or minimized with early interventions. Interventions to promote skin health are discussed in Chapter 30.

Wound Assessment

Wound assessment involves inspection (sight and smell) and palpation for appearance, drainage, odor, and pain. Wound assessment determines the status of the wound, identifies barriers to the healing process, and identifies signs of complications. Accurate assessment provides essential baseline data and information to judge the effectiveness of treatment and wound healing progression. Skin integrity and wound assessment are performed at regular intervals, based on the nature of the wound and facility policy.

APPEARANCE OF THE WOUND

Note the location of the wound. Location is described in relation to the nearest anatomic landmark, such as bony prominences. Document the size of the wound. Measurements are taken in millimeters or centimeters, measuring length, width, and depth. Refer to Guidelines for Nursing Care 31-1 (on page 975) for details on measuring a wound.

FOCUSED ASSESSMENT GUIDE 31-1

SKIN INTEGRITY

Factors to Assess	Questions and Approaches
Appearance of skin	• Do you have any skin areas that are discolored? • Do some areas of skin on your body feel warmer or colder than others? • Describe the moisture in your skin: is it damp, dry, oily? • Have you noticed that your skin seems to be thinner? Where? • Have you noticed any swelling in your feet, ankles, or fingers? • Tell me about how you take care of your skin. For example, do you take a tub bath or shower? How often? Do you use oils or lotions?
Recent changes in skin	• Do you have any sores on your body? If so, how many, and where are they? Have they changed in size? Do you have any drainage from them? • Have you noticed that the skin over your hips or backbone gets red if you sit or lie in one position for a long time? Does this disappear in a short time when you are up? • Have you gotten a piercing or tattoo recently?
Activity/mobility	• Do you need assistance to walk or move? If so, how much? • Are you confined to your bed or a chair when up? • Can you change your position when you want to?
Nutrition	• Have you gained or lost weight recently? • Describe your usual meals each day. • How many glasses or cups of liquid do you drink each day? • Do you take any food supplements or vitamins? • Do you prepare your own meals? • Do you wear dentures? How do they fit? • Do you have any difficulty swallowing? • Has a doctor ever told you that you are anemic?
Pain	• If you have a sore, is it painful? • Do you take anything for pain? If so, what do you take, and how often? Does it help?
Elimination	• Have you noticed any problems with your bowels or urination? If so, describe. • Have you ever used pads or special pants because you can't control your urine or stools?

Assess wounds for the approximation of the wound edges (edges meet) and signs of dehiscence or evisceration. Assess the color of the wound and surrounding area. Note the presence of drains, tubes, staples, and sutures. The edges of a healthy healing surgical wound appear clean and well approximated, with a crust along the wound edges. Initially, the edges are reddened and slightly swollen. After approximately 1 week, the skin is closer to normal in appearance, with wound edges healing together. The skin surrounding the wound may at first be bruised, but this too returns to normal as blood is reabsorbed.

When infection is present, the wound is swollen and deep red. It feels hot on palpation, and drainage is increased and possibly purulent. If dehiscence is impending or present, the wound edges are separated. If the wound edges have separated and the wound is open, describe the type of tissue in the wound: granulation, slough, or eschar (see Box 31-4 on page 976).

Assess for the presence of odor, but only after the wound has been cleaned. The presence of odor can be indicative of certain types of bacteria.

DRAINAGE

The inflammatory response results in the formation of exudate, which then drains from the wound. The exudate is composed of fluid and cells that escape from blood vessels and are deposited in or on tissue surfaces. This exudate is called wound drainage and is described as serous, sanguineous, serosanguineous, or, if infected, purulent.

- **Serous drainage** is composed primarily of the clear, serous portion of the blood and from serous membranes. Serous drainage is clear and watery.
- **Sanguineous drainage** consists of large numbers of red blood cells and looks like blood. Bright-red sanguineous drainage is indicative of fresh bleeding, whereas darker drainage indicates older bleeding.
- **Serosanguineous drainage** is a mixture of serum and red blood cells. It is light pink to blood tinged.
- **Purulent drainage** is made up of white blood cells, liquefied dead tissue debris, and both dead and live bacteria. Purulent drainage is thick, often has a musty or foul odor, and varies in color (such as dark yellow or green), depending on the causative organism.

GUIDELINES FOR NURSING CARE 31-1

MEASURING WOUNDS AND PRESSURE ULCERS

Size of the Wound

- Draw the shape and describe it.
- Measure the length, width, and diameter (if circular).

Depth of the Wound

- Perform hand hygiene. Put on gloves.
- Moisten a sterile, flexible applicator with saline and insert it gently into the wound at a 90-degree angle with the tip down (Figure A).
- Mark the point on the swab that is even with the surrounding skin surface, or grasp the applicator with the thumb and forefinger at the point corresponding to the wound's margin (Figure B).
- Remove the swab and measure the depth with a ruler (Figure C).

Wound Tunneling

- Use standard precautions; use appropriate transmission-based precautions when indicated.
- Perform hand hygiene. Put on gloves.
- Determine direction: Moisten a sterile, flexible applicator with saline and gently insert a sterile applicator into the site where tunneling occurs. View the direction of the applicator as if it were the hand of a clock (Figure D). The direction of the patient's head represents 12 o'clock. Moving in a clockwise direction, document the deepest sites where the wound tunnels.
- Determine the depth: While the applicator is inserted into the tunneling, mark the point on the swab that is even with the wound's edge, or grasp the applicator with the thumb and forefinger at the point corresponding to the wound's margin. Remove the swab and measure the depth with a ruler (see Figure C).
- Document both the direction and depth of tunneling.

Adapted from Hess, C. (2013). *Clinical guide to skin & wound care* (7th ed., pp. 17–21). Philadelphia: Wolters Kluwer Health/Lippincott Williams & Wilkins.

FIGURE A

FIGURE B

FIGURE C

FIGURE D

Drains may be inserted in or near a wound to promote drainage, reducing the risk of abscess formation and promoting wound healing. Various types of drains are described in Table 31-4 and discussed later in this chapter.

Assess the amount, color, odor, and consistency of wound drainage. The amount and color depend on the wound location and size. Typically, larger wounds have more drainage than do smaller wounds. Assess wound drainage on the wound, on the dressings, in drainage

Table 31-4 COMMON TYPES OF DRAINS

TYPE	PURPOSE	EXAMPLE
Penrose	Provides sinus tract	After incision and drainage of abscess, in abdominal surgery
T-tube	For bile drainage	After gallbladder surgery
Jackson-Pratt	Decreases dead space by collecting drainage	After breast removal, abdominal surgery
Hemovac	Decreases dead space by collecting drainage	After abdominal, orthopedic surgery
Gauze, iodoform gauze, NuGauze	Allow healing from base of wound	Infected wounds, after removal of hemorrhoids

BOX 31-4 RYB WOUND CLASSIFICATION

A color classification system termed RYB (red yellow black) can be used for wound assessment and to help direct treatment for open wounds, or healing by secondary intention (Hess, 2013; Krasner, 1995; Stotts, 1990). This classification, with related interventions, is based on the assessment of wound color. However, many wounds have red, yellow, and black components and are categorized as mixed wounds (see Figure). When all colors are present, the wound is treated first for the most serious color: black, followed by yellow, and finally red.

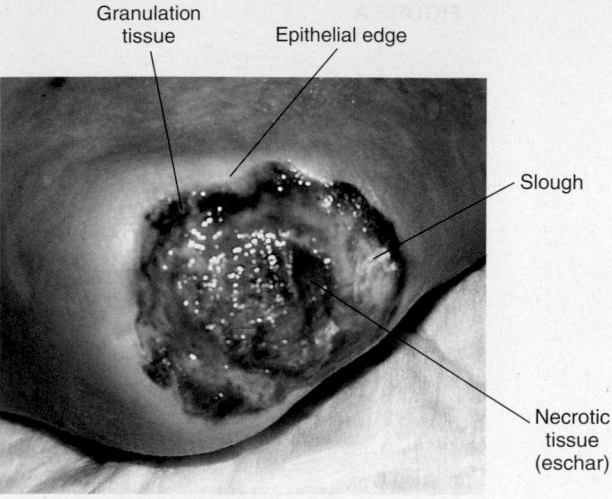

Granulation tissue
Epithelial edge
Slough
Necrotic tissue (eschar)

R = Red = Protect

Red wounds are in the proliferative stage of healing and reflect the color of normal granulation tissue. Wounds in this stage need protection with nursing interventions that include gentle cleansing, use of moist dressings, and changing of the dressing only when necessary, and/or based on product manufacturer's recommendations.

Y = Yellow = Cleanse

Yellow in the wound may indicate the presence of exudate (drainage) or slough, and requires wound cleaning. These wounds are characterized by oozing from the tissue covering the wound, often accompanied by purulent drainage. Drainage can be whitish yellow, creamy yellow, yellowish green, or beige. To cleanse these wounds, nursing interventions include the use of wound cleansers and irrigating the wound.

B = Black = Débride

Black in the wound may indicate the presence of an eschar (necrotic tissue), which is usually black but may also be brown, gray, or tan. The eschar requires débridement (removal) before the wound can heal. These wounds are often cared for by advanced practice nurses who are educated in the care of more complex wounds. After débridement, the wound is treated as a yellow wound and then, as healing progresses, a red wound.

---

bottles or reservoirs, or—depending on the location of the wound and the amount of drainage—under the patient.

SUTURES AND STAPLES

Skin sutures are used to hold tissue and skin together. Sutures may be black silk, synthetic material, or fine wire. Sutures are removed when enough tensile strength has developed to hold the wound edges together during healing. The time frame varies depending on the patient's age, nutritional status, and wound location. Frequently, after skin sutures are removed, small wound-closure strips of adhesive are applied across the wound to give additional support as it continues to heal. Figure 31-6 shows an example of an incision with sutures. Retention sutures are used to provide extra support for patients who are obese and for wounds with an increased risk for dehiscence.

Pressure Ulcer Assessment

Most pressure ulcers can be prevented (Black et al., 2011). It is a nursing priority to perform a comprehensive assessment in all settings and identify patients at risk for pressure ulcers, predisposing factors, or evidence of actual pressure ulcers.

RISK ASSESSMENT

An aggressive approach to prevent a pressure ulcer or manage the care of a patient who already has impaired skin integrity begins with a risk assessment form, which

should be simple to use, reliable, and cost effective. Use the assessment tool in conjunction with nursing judgment to ensure implementation of the most appropriate patient care (Braden, 2012). Several different scales are available to assess risk, such as the Norton scale (physical condition, mental condition, activity, mobility, incontinence) and the Braden scale (mental status, continence, mobility, activity, nutrition; Fig. 31-7). With these tools,

FIGURE 31-6. Incision with sutures.

Braden Scale for Predicting Pressure Sore Risk

Sensory Perception: Ability to respond meaningfully to pressure-related discomfort

SCORE

1. **Completely Limited:** Unresponsive (does not moan, flinch, or grasp) to painful stimuli, due to diminished level of consciousness or sedation, OR limited ability to feel pain over most of body surface.
2. **Very Limited:** Responds only to painful stimuli. Cannot communicate discomfort except by moaning or restlessness, OR has a sensory impairment which limits the ability to feel pain or discomfort over half of body.
3. **Slightly Limited:** Responds to verbal commands but cannot always communicate discomfort or need to be turned, OR has some sensory impairment which limits ability to feel pain or discomfort in 1 or 2 extremities.
4. **No Impairment:** Responds to verbal commands. Has no sensory deficit which would limit ability to feel or voice pain or discomfort.

Moisture: Degree to which skin is exposed to moisture

SCORE

1. **Constantly Moist:** Skin is kept moist almost constantly by perspiration, urine, etc. Dampness is detected every time patient is moved or turned.
2. **Very Moist:** Skin is often but not always moist. Linen must be changed at least once a shift.
3. **Occasionally Moist:** Skin is occasionally moist, requiring an extra linen change approximately once a day.
4. **Rarely Moist:** Skin is usually dry: linen requires changing only at routine intervals.

Activity: Degree of physical activity

SCORE

1. **Bedfast:** Confined to bed.
2. **Chairfast:** Ability to walk severely limited or non-existent. Cannot bear own weight and/or must be assisted into chair or wheelchair.
3. **Walks Occasionally:** Walks occasionally during the day, but for very short distances, with or without assistance. Spends majority of each shift in bed or chair.
4. **Walks Frequently:** Walks outside the room at least twice and inside room at least once every 2 hours during waking hours.

Mobility: Ability to change and control body position

SCORE

1. **Completely immobile:** Does not make even slight changes in body or extremity position without assistance.
2. **Very Limited:** Makes occasional slight changes in body or extremity position but unable to make frequent or significant changes independently.
3. **Slightly Limited:** Makes frequent though slight changes in body or extremity position independently.
4. **No Limitation:** Makes major and frequent changes in position without assistance.

Nutrition: Usual food intake pattern

SCORE

1. **Very Poor:** Never eats a complete meal. Rarely eats more than 1/3 of food offered. Eats 2 servings or less of protein (meat or dairy products) per day. Takes fluids poorly. Does not take a liquid dietary supplement, OR is NPO and/or maintained on clear liquids or IV for more than five days.
2. **Probably Inadequate:** Rarely eats a complete meal and generally eats only about half of any food offered. Protein intake includes only 3 servings of meat or dairy products per day. Occasionally will take a dietary supplement, OR receives less than optimum amount of liquid diet or tube feeding.
3. **Adequate:** Eats over half of most meals. Eats a total of 4 servings of protein (meat, dairy products) each day. Occasionally will refuse a meal, but will usually take a supplement if offered, OR is on a tube feeding or TPN regimen, which probably meets most of nutritional needs.
4. **Excellent:** Eats most of every meal. Never refuses a meal. Usually eats a total of 4 or more servings of meat and dairy products. Occasionally eats between meals. Does not require supplementation.

Friction and Shear

SCORE

1. **Problem:** Requires moderate to maximum assistance in moving. Complete lifting without sliding against sheets is impossible. Frequently slides down in bed or chair, requiring frequent repositioning with maximum assistance. Spasticity, contractures, or agitation leads to almost constant friction.
2. **Potential Problem:** Moves feebly or requires minimum assistance. During a move skin probably slides to some extent against sheets, chair, restraints, or other devices. Maintains relatively good position in chair or bed most of the time but occasionally slides down.
3. **No Apparent Problem:** Moves in bed and in chair independently and has sufficient muscle strength to lift up completely

3 or 4 = Moderate to Low Impairment	Risk Level	NPO: Nothing by Mouth	
Total Points Possible: 23	19-23 Not at risk	IV: Intravenously	**Total Score:**
Risk Predicting Score: 16 or Less	15-18 low risk	TPN: Total parenteral nutrition	
	13-14 moderate risk		
	10-12 high risk		
	≤ 9 very high risk		

FIGURE 31-7. Braden scale for predicting pressure ulcer risk. *(Copyright 1988 by Barbara Braden and Nancy Bergstrom. Reprinted with permission. All rights reserved.)*

a numeric score is assigned to each assessment area. The degree of risk is based on the patient's total score. Using the Braden scale, a score of 19 to 23 indicates no risk; 15 to 18, mild risk; 13 to 14, moderate risk; 10 to 12, high risk; and 9 or lower, very high risk (Braden & Maklebust, 2005). Patients may have additional risk factors and/or other health problems not measured by the chosen assessment scale. Therefore, good nursing judgment may reveal the need for a higher intensity of preventive intervention than what may be identified by the scale alone (Braden, 2012).

Once a patient's risk has been identified, agencies use different approaches. Appropriate interventions are initiated based on the patient's identified risk. Many health care facilities use a special pressure ulcer assessment form. Documenting assessments is essential to ensure continuity of care, providing the foundation on which to develop the skin plan of care. All caregivers in the home or health care agency need to be aware of specific assessments, including assessment of mobility, nutritional status, and moisture and incontinence.

MOBILITY

Assessing a patient's mobility status includes evaluating the patient's ability to move, turn, and reposition the body. A patient who is confined to bed or a chair or has limited range of motion is at increased risk for a pressure ulcer. This assessment of activity status is done upon admission to the health care facility or during the initial home care interview. The use of any assistive devices to maintain mobility and activity is noted. Additional suggestions for gathering information about mobility are described in Chapter 32.

NUTRITIONAL STATUS

The importance of sound nutrition in the prevention and treatment of a pressure ulcer is well established. Older adults, in particular, need adequate nutrition for optimal health and wound healing. Nutritional assessment is described in Chapter 35. The following laboratory criteria indicate that a patient is nutritionally at risk for development of a pressure ulcer:

- Albumin level <3.2 mg/dL (normal, 3.5–5 mg/dL).
- Prealbumin <19 mg/dL (normal 16–40 mg/dL)
- Body weight decrease of 5% to 10%

Additional laboratory tests to consider in patients at risk for or presenting with pressure ulcers include:

- Total lymphocyte count <1,800/mm^3 (normal, 1,000–4,000/mm^3)
- Hemoglobin A1C >8% (normal <6%)
- Glucose >120 mg/dL (normal 70–120 mg/dL)

MOISTURE AND INCONTINENCE

Many studies have documented that moisture makes the skin more susceptible to injury. Whether the moisture is from perspiration, wound drainage, urine, or stool, the skin is compromised. Moisture can create an environment in which microorganisms can multiply and the skin is more likely to blister, suffer abrasions, and become macerated (softening or disintegration of the skin in response to moisture). Chapters 36 and 37 have additional assessment information related to incontinence.

APPEARANCE OF EXISTING PRESSURE ULCER

Skin assessment for a pressure ulcer specifically includes inspection of the following (Baranoski & Ayello, 2012; NPUAP, 2012c; Hess, 2013):

- Location of any lesion or ulcer
- Identification of the stage (see Box 31-3, pp. 970–971)
- Size of the ulcer: length, width, depth (see Guidelines for Nursing Care 31-1, p. 975); presence of undermining, a hollow between the skin surface and the wound bed, resulting from death of the underlying tissue
- Color and type of wound tissue
- Presence of any abnormal pathways in the wound, such as a **sinus tract** (a cavity or channel underneath the wound that has the potential for infection) or tunneling (a passageway or opening that may be visible at skin level, but with most of the tunnel under the surface of the skin). See Guidelines for Nursing Care 31-1.
- Visible necrotic tissue; necrotic tissue that is in the process of separating from viable portions of the body is referred to as slough.
- Presence of an exudate or drainage (amount and type)
- Presence of odor
- Presence or absence of granulation tissue
- Visible evidence of epithelialization
- Periwound skin condition

The Pressure Ulcer Scale for Healing (PUSH Tool) was developed by the National Pressure Ulcer Advisory Panel (NPUAP, 2012c) as a quick, reliable tool to monitor the change in pressure ulcer status over time (Fig. 31-8). Graphing the PUSH Tool scores over time for each ulcer allows health care providers to "tell at a glance" whether the ulcer is healing, remains unchanged, or is deteriorating (NPUAP, 2012c).

The RYB Wound Classification (red yellow black; see Box 31-4, p. 976) can also be used to aid in assessment and description of the pressure ulcer appearance.

Pain Assessment

Nurses have long recognized that patients with alterations in skin integrity—including surgical wounds, traumatic wounds, and pressure ulcer wounds—experience pain. Focus assessment on whether dressing changes, positioning in bed or in a chair, or movement elicits any expressions of pain. Pain and associated stress may have a significant impact on wound healing, causing disruption of the healing process and prolonging healing (Woo, 2012). Perform a pain assessment at each dressing change; measure and document the level of pain before, during, and after a procedure (Woo, 2012; Benbow, 2011). Even if pain is never verbalized or expressed, always assume that pain is a definite possibility, and focus on comfort

Pressure Ulcer Scale for Healing (PUSH)
PUSH Tool 3.0

NATIONAL PRESSURE ULCER ADVISORY PANEL

Patient Name_____ Patient ID# _____

Ulcer Location _____ Date _____

Directions:

Observe and measure the pressure ulcer. Categorize the ulcer with respect to surface area, exudate, and type of wound tissue. Record a sub-score for each of these ulcer characteristics. Add the sub-scores to obtain the total score. A comparison of total scores measured over time provides an indication of the improvement or deterioration in pressure ulcer healing.

LENGTH X WIDTH (in cm²)	0	1	2	3	4	5	Sub-score
	0	< 0.3	0.3 – 0.6	0.7 – 1.0	1.1 – 2.0	2.1 – 3.0	
	6	7	8	9	10		
	3.1 – 4.0	4.1 – 8.0	8.1 – 12.0	12.1 – 24.0	> 24.0		
EXUDATE AMOUNT	0	1	2	3			Sub-score
	None	Light	Moderate	Heavy			
TISSUE TYPE	0	1	2	3	4		Sub-score
	Closed	Epithelial Tissue	Granulation Tissue	Slough	Necrotic Tissue		
							TOTAL SCORE

Length x Width: Measure the greatest length (head to toe) and the greatest width (side to side) using a centimeter ruler. Multiply these two measurements (length x width) to obtain an estimate of surface area in square centimeters (cm²). Caveat: Do not guess! Always use a centimeter ruler and always use the same method each time the ulcer is measured.

Exudate Amount: Estimate the amount of exudate (drainage) present after removal of the dressing and before applying any topical agent to the ulcer. Estimate the exudate (drainage) as none, light, moderate, or heavy.

Tissue Type: This refers to the types of tissue that are present in the wound (ulcer) bed. Score as a "4" if there is any necrotic tissue present. Score as a "3" if there is any amount of slough present and necrotic tissue is absent. Score as a "2" if the wound is clean and contains granulation tissue. A superficial wound that is reepithelializing is scored as a "1". When the wound is closed, score as a "0".

4 – **Necrotic Tissue (Eschar):** black, brown, or tan tissue that adheres firmly to the wound bed or ulcer edges and may be either firmer or softer than surrounding skin.

3 – **Slough:** yellow or white tissue that adheres to the ulcer bed in strings or thick clumps, or is mucinous.

2 – **Granulation Tissue:** pink or beefy red tissue with a shiny, moist, granular appearance.

1 – **Epithelial Tissue:** for superficial ulcers, new pink or shiny tissue (skin) that grows in from the edges or as islands on the ulcer surface.

0 – **Closed/Resurfaced:** the wound is completely covered with epithelium (new skin).

FIGURE 31-8. Pressure Ulcer Scale for Healing (PUSH) PUSH Tool 3.0 (©National Pressure Ulcer Advisory Panel) Available at http://www.npuap.org/wp-content/uploads/2012/03/push3.pdf

needs. Ask the patient about pain from the wound. If the patient experiences increased or constant pain from the wound, perform further assessments. Pain, especially when accompanied by an increased or purulent flow of drainage, may indicate delayed healing or an infection. Surgical incisional pain is usually most severe for the first 2 to 3 days and then progressively diminishes. Detailed assessment of pain is discussed in Chapter 34.

Diagnosing

Data that the nurse collects may lead to the development of several nursing diagnoses related to skin integrity and wound care. Each nursing diagnosis statement identifies a patient problem and suggests expected patient outcomes. The etiology of the problem directs nursing interventions. The following are examples of appropriate nursing diagnoses:

- Disturbed Body Image
- Deficient Knowledge related to wound care
- Impaired Tissue Integrity
- Impaired Skin Integrity
- Risk for Impaired Skin Integrity
- Risk for Infection

Examples of diagnoses, etiologic factors, and defining characteristics appear in Examples of NANDA-I Nursing Diagnoses: Patient With a Wound or Pressure Ulcer.

Outcome Identification and Planning

When nurses care for patients who have or are at risk for impaired skin and tissue integrity, nursing interventions are planned for returning the patient to health by facilitating wound healing, reducing the risk for complications, and promoting psychosocial adaptation. The following are examples of appropriate outcomes. The patient will:

- Maintain skin integrity
- Demonstrate self-care measures to prevent pressure ulcer development
- Demonstrate self-care measures to promote wound healing
- Demonstrate evidence of wound healing
- Demonstrate increase in body weight and muscle size, if appropriate
- Remain free of infection at the site of the wound or pressure ulcer
- Remain free of signs and symptoms of infection
- Experience no new areas of skin breakdown
- Verbalize that the pain management regimen relieves pain to an acceptable level
- Be discharged to home within established parameters
- Demonstrate appropriate wound care measures before discharge
- Verbalize understanding of signs and symptoms to report and necessary follow-up care

Implementing

Provide preventive measures for patients at risk. Teach patients about their health conditions and provide information and support to improve patients' health literacy. Refer to the accompanying Promoting Health Literacy display.

EXAMPLES OF NANDA-I NURSING DIAGNOSES

PATIENT WITH A WOUND OR PRESSURE ULCER

Nursing Diagnoses	Related Factors	Sample Defining Characteristics
Impaired Skin Integrity	Any condition that alters the dermis and/or epidermis, such as a surgical incision or traumatic wound; moisture, physical immobilization	• Presence of intentional or unintentional wound; disruption of skin surface • Presence of a pressure ulcer; destruction of skin layers
Risk for Infection	Any condition that interferes with the normal inflammatory healing process or provides an entry for infectious agents	Risk factors: • Disruption in skin integrity • Immunosuppression • Chronic disease (such as diabetes mellitus or obesity) • Extremes of age • Malnutrition • Presence of drains, tubes, or catheters
Disturbed Body Image	Any condition that causes confusion in the mental image of oneself, such as a surgical or traumatic wound	• "I just don't feel like I'm the same person I used to be." • "I'll never be able to do my job if this arm doesn't work." • Refusal to look at incision or area of surgical treatment • Actual change in one's body from surgery or trauma • Actual change in function of body part

PROMOTING HEALTH LITERACY

IN PATIENTS WITH BREAST CANCER

Patient Scenario

Tashana Douglas, 42, has been diagnosed with breast cancer. She had a modified mastectomy 3 weeks ago and has returned to the clinic to discuss the rest of her treatment. She is going to have several weeks of outpatient radiation therapy. She states, "I feel pretty good, and the surgeon said my cancer is gone. Why do I need more treatment? My neighbor told me her sister had radiation and had terrible side effects." Ms. Douglas appears anxious as she relates that the neighbor's sister was extremely tired and had a "terrible rash or burn with her treatment. It took a long time to get better and really hurt." She states, "I don't know if I want to risk having that happen to me!" Ms. Douglas verbalizes concern that she will "give the radiation to others in her home and make them sick." She asks, "Do you think I should have this radiation stuff?"

Nursing Considerations: *Tips for Improving Health Literacy*

Review with Ms. Douglas the appropriate interventions she should be using to ensure that her surgical site heals, including skin care. Provide Ms. Douglas with easy-to-read information about radiation therapy and potential side effects, as well as interventions she can implement to prevent and/or minimize the side effects of radiation therapy, particularly side effects related to skin integrity. Encourage her to ask her primary care provider, as well as the radiologist, as many questions as needed to understand her condition and the planned radiation treatment. Encourage Ms. Douglas to ask her primary care provider the following three questions:

- What is my main problem?
- What do I need to do?
- Why is it important for me to do this?

What additional measures can you take to help increase health literacy in this patient? What other measures would be helpful if Ms. Douglas does not speak English, cannot read, or has other learning deficits?

When caring for the patient with a wound or pressure ulcer, nursing interventions focus on preventing infection, promoting wound healing, preventing further injury or alteration in skin integrity, promoting physical and emotional comfort, and facilitating coping. The accompanying Nursing Interventions and Nursing Outcomes Classifications (NIC/NOC) box offers suggested nursing interventions and outcomes related to Risk for Impaired Skin Integrity. It is often appropriate and necessary to consult with the wound care specialist, often a wound certified nurse specialist, to plan and coordinate the most effective care for the patient.

Preventing Pressure Ulcers

Tissue load management refers to therapeutic means to manage pressure, friction, and shear on tissues (Baranoski & Ayello, 2012). Interventions to prevent injury to the skin and promote optimal health are outlined in Guidelines for Nursing Care 31-2 (on page 982). Additional interventions related to personal hygiene and maintaining skin health are discussed in Chapter 30. Implement interventions related to tissue load management as part of the nursing plan of care for patients at risk for developing pressure ulcers or who have a pressure ulcer. This includes interventions that can be implemented while the patient is in bed and sitting in chairs or wheelchairs.

To protect patients at risk from the adverse effects of pressure, implement turning and positioning schedules, as well as the use of appropriate support surfaces (tissue load management surfaces). Reposition bed-bound people at least every two hours and chair-bound people every hour (NPUAP, 2012d). Older adult patients tend to have less tissue tolerance, necessitating more frequent repositioning if redness on bony prominences is noted.

EXAMPLES OF NURSING INTERVENTIONS AND NURSING OUTCOMES CLASSIFICATIONS (NIC/NOC)

RISK FOR IMPAIRED SKIN INTEGRITY

Nursing Interventions	Nursing Outcomes
<ul><li>Bed Rest Care</li><li>Incision Site Care</li><li>Wound Care</li><li>Pressure Management</li><li>Pressure Ulcer Prevention</li><li>Skin Surveillance</li></ul>	<ul><li>Tissue Integrity: Skin and Mucous Membranes</li><li>Immobility Consequences: Physiological</li></ul>

Reprinted with permission from: Bulechek, G. M., Butcher, H. K., Dochterman, J. M., & Wagner, C. M. (Eds.). (2013). *Nursing interventions classification (NIC).* (6th ed., p. 546). St. Louis: Elsevier/Mosby; and Moorhead, S., Johnson, M., Maas, M. L., & Swanson, E. (Eds.). (2013). *Nursing outcomes classification (NOC)* (5th ed., pp. 269, 538). St. Louis: Elsevier/Mosby. A full listing of nursing activities for each nursing intervention and outcomes can be found in these books.

GUIDELINES FOR NURSING CARE 31-2

PREVENTING PRESSURE ULCERS

- Assess the skin of patients at risk on a daily basis. Pay particular attention to bony prominences.
- Cleanse the skin routinely and whenever any soiling occurs. Use a mild cleansing agent, minimal friction, and avoid hot water.
- Maintain higher humidity in the environment and use skin moisturizers for dry skin.
- Avoid massage over bony prominences.
- Protect the skin from moisture associated with episodes of incontinence or exposure to wound drainage.
- Minimize skin injury from friction and shearing forces by using proper positioning, turning, and transferring

techniques. Use lubricants, protective films, dressings, and padding to diminish the effects of friction on the skin.
- Use appropriate support surfaces (tissue load management surfaces).
- Investigate reasons for inadequate dietary intake of protein and calories. Administer nutritional supplements or more aggressive nutritional intervention as needed.
- Continue efforts to improve mobility and activity. If this is unrealistic, attempt to maintain current level of activity, mobility, and range of motion.
- Document measures used to prevent pressure ulcers and the results of these interventions.

The oblique position, an alternative to the side-lying position, results in significantly less pressure on the trochanter area. The best approach to turning and repositioning is to evaluate and reevaluate each patient to best determine an appropriate turning schedule (Baranoski & Ayello, 2012).

Positioning devices such as pillows, foam wedges, or pressure-reducing boots can prove helpful to keep body weight off bony prominences. For example, a standard pillow placed under the calves raises the heels off the bed and alleviates pressure. Never use ring cushions, or "donuts," because they increase venous pressure. Minimize the effects of shearing force by limiting the amount of time the head of the bed is elevated, when possible.

Support surfaces are an important part of managing pressure, friction, and shear on tissues (NPUAP, 2012d; Baranoski & Ayello, 2012; Hess, 2013). A support surface is a specialized device for pressure redistribution designed for management of tissue loads. Support surfaces are available in sizes and shapes to be used on beds, chairs, examination tables, and operating room tables. Support surfaces are pressure-reducing or pressure-relieving devices. The most common support surfaces are seating devices (air, fluid foam, or gel cushions), air-, gel-, or water-filled mattress overlays; static flotation mattresses; alternating air mattresses; low-air-loss beds; and air-fluidized beds. It is important to individualize the type of support surface based on the patient's needs. Some support surfaces allow for an extended length of time between position changes. Because none of these devices totally relieves pressure, continue to perform position changes at regular intervals.

The use of appropriate devices to ensure safe patient handling and movement is an important part of tissue load management. Use friction-reducing sheets and lifting devices with patients who cannot assist during transfers and position changes. These interventions and devices are discussed at length in Chapter 32.

Wound Care/Wound Management

The goal of wound care is to promote tissue repair and regeneration so that skin integrity is restored. Wounds can be treated by leaving them open to air; no **dressing** (protective covering placed over a wound) is applied. Wounds left open to the air heal more slowly because wound drying produces a dried eschar or scab. If the scab is removed accidentally before healing is complete, reinjury occurs, and the new delicate cells are exposed. Wounds left open are exposed to more environmental factors and potential injury.

Closed wound care uses dressings to keep the wound moist, promoting healing. A moist environment is best for wound healing. When a dressing is placed over a wound, the wound fluid keeps the surface of the wound moist. As a result, epidermal cells migrate more rapidly, maximizing healing. In addition, covered wounds can help patients cope with alterations in body image.

Generally, an ideal dressing should maintain a moist environment, be absorbent, provide thermal insulation, act as a bacterial barrier, reduce or eliminate pain at the wound site, and allow for pain-free removal (Baranoski & Ayello, 2012; Wound Healing and Management Node Group, 2011). Many different types of dressings are available, but all have essentially the same purposes:

- Provide physical, psychological, and aesthetic comfort
- Prevent, eliminate, or control infection
- Absorb drainage
- Maintain a moist wound environment
- Protect the wound from further injury
- Protect the skin surrounding the wound
- Remove necrotic tissue, if appropriate

There is no standard frequency for how often dressings should be changed. It depends on the amount of drainage, the primary practitioner's preference, the nature of the wound, and the particular wound care product being used. It is customary for the surgeon or other advanced practice professional to perform the first dressing change on a surgical wound, usually within 24 to 48 hours after surgery.

 CONSIDER the care needed by Lucius Everly, the patient in the critical care unit. Although he has multiple needs, performing incisional wound care cannot be overlooked; otherwise, his risk of infection may increase. ●

Wound contamination occurs through a moist medium. Microorganisms can move from the external surface through the dressing to the wound if a dressing remains in place until it is saturated. Microorganisms can also move from the wound to the outer surface of a saturated dressing. For these reasons, always replace dressings with fresh dressings or reinforce the dressing with additional dressings before drainage causes saturation.

Dressing changes provide an excellent opportunity for teaching, especially important when the patient will be changing dressings at home. Encourage the patient to help as much as possible, if appropriate.

The sight of the wound may disturb a patient. Listen carefully to what the patient is saying and observe nonverbal communication as well. In some instances, the patient may not want to look at the wound, particularly with a wound that involves a change in normal body functions or appearance, such as a wound resulting from the removal of a breast, the amputation of an extremity, or the placement of a tube in a draining wound. With patience and emotional support, patients can learn to cope with and adapt to their wound.

TYPES OF WOUND DRESSINGS

The items needed for a dressing change may be gathered individually or may be packaged in a sterile dressing tray, depending on the health care setting. Wound care in the home may depend on the supplies provided by the patient or family.

The number and type of dressings used depend on the location and size of the wound, type and depth of wound, the presence of infection, the need for **débridement** (removal of devitalized tissue and foreign material), and the amount and type of drainage. Dry gauze dressings can be used to cover wounds, commonly closed surgical wounds. These dressings come in various sizes (2 × 2 inches, 4 × 4 inches, 4 × 8 inches) and are commercially packaged as single units or in packs. Gauze dressings often consist of three layers. The first layer of dressing material applied directly to a draining wound is often nonabsorbent but hydrophilic (i.e., capable of carrying moisture). This type of material allows drainage from the wound to move into overlying absorbent layers of dressing, helping to prevent maceration and reinfection. Moreover, this type of dressing is less likely to stick to the wound, making dressing changes more comfortable for the patient.

Material to absorb and collect drainage is then placed over the first layer of nonabsorbent material. This mate-

FIGURE 31-9. Surgical pad applied as last layer of wound dressing.

rial acts as a wick, pulling drainage out by capillary action. Absorbent cotton has far greater capillarity than untreated cotton. Therefore, cotton-lined gauze sponges soak up more liquid than do unlined sponges. The number of gauze sponges used in the dressing depends on the amount of drainage. Loosely packed gauze, the threads of which act as numerous wicks, enhances capillarity and directs drainage upward and away from the wound. Fluffed and loosely packed dressings are more absorbent than tightly packed dressings. The top of the dressing may be further protected by surgical or abdominal pads, which are thick, absorbent pads that help to absorb profuse drainage (Fig. 31-9).

Nonadherent gauzes include sterile petrolatum gauze and Telfa gauze. Telfa's shiny outer surface is applied to the wound. These dressings allow drainage to pass through and be absorbed by the outer absorbent layer but prevent outer dressings from adhering to the wound and causing further injury when removed.

Special gauze dressings (e.g., Sof-Wick) are precut halfway to fit around drains or tubes (Fig. 31-10). Larger dressings (8 × 10 bandages, abdominal pads [ABDs], Surgi-Pads) are placed over the smaller gauze dressings and absorb drainage and protect the wound from contamination or injury.

FIGURE 31-10. Precut dressing placed around surgical drain.

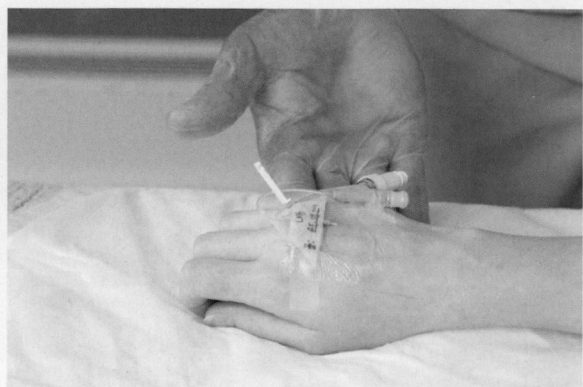

FIGURE 31-11. Transparent film dressing placed on intravenous access site.

FIGURE 31-12. Hydrocolloid dressing in place on wound.

Transparent films (e.g., OpSite) are semipermeable membrane dressings that are adhesive and waterproof. These dressings are occlusive, decreasing the possibility of contamination, while allowing visualization of the wound. This type of dressing is often used over peripheral intravenous sites, central venous access device insertion sites, and noninfected healing wounds (Fig. 31-11).

 THINK back to Lucius Everly, the patient in the critical care unit. The nurse most likely would use a transparent dressing on his venous access sites, thereby allowing frequent assessment of the sites. ●

When caring for open wounds and pressure ulcers, it is necessary to keep the wound tissue moist and the surrounding skin dry. Therefore, use dressings that continuously keep the wound moist, placing the moist dressing only on the wound surface and keeping the intact, healthy skin surrounding the ulcer dry because it is susceptible to damage. Select a dressing that absorbs exudate, if present, but still maintains a moist environment for healing. Use a skin sealant or moisture-barrier ointment on the surrounding skin and secure the dressing with the least amount of tape or other material to secure that is necessary.

The presence of foreign matter and/or devitalized, injured, infected tissue in a wound may indicate the need for débridement to promote wound healing (Hess, 2013; Baranoski & Ayello, 2012; Beitz, 2012). Débridement can be accomplished through several different methods. Autolytic débridement uses occlusive dressings, such as hydrocolloids (Fig. 31-12) or transparent films, and uses the body's own enzymes and defense mechanisms to loosen and liquefy necrotic tissue. Biosurgical débridement involves the use of sterile fly larvae. The larvae secrete an enzyme that liquefies dead tissue, which is ingested by the larvae, clearing the wound of bacteria and infection. Enzymatic débridement involves the application of commercially prepared enzymes to speed up the body's autolytic process. Mechanical débridement uses external physical force to dislodge and remove debris and necrotic tissue. This could be achieved by

wound irrigation with pulsed pressure lavage (washing), whirlpool therapy, ultrasound or laser treatment, or with surgical débridement. In the past, wet-to-dry gauze dressings have been used to débride wounds; this is no longer considered good practice. This type of dressing damages healthy wound bed tissue and can be painful (Baranoski & Ayello, 2012; Agency for Healthcare Research and Quality [AHRQ], 2011). Concern exists that complete drying of the gauze disrupts angiogenesis. However, despite concerns by wound care experts, these dressings are still prescribed by physicians for wound débridement.

There are many other wound care products/dressings available, each with distinctive actions, as well as indications, contraindications, advantages, and disadvantages. It is very important for the nurse to be aware of the products available in a particular facility and be familiar with the indications for, and correct use of, each type of dressing and wound care product. A wound with heavy exudate will need a more absorptive dressing and a dry wound will require rehydration with a dressing that keeps the wound moist. Table 31-5 outlines the purposes and uses for several wound dressing/product categories.

 CHANGING THE DRESSING

Prepare the patient for the dressing change before starting the procedure by explaining what will be done. If wound care is uncomfortable, administer a prescribed analgesic 30 to 45 minutes before changing the dressing. Also, plan to change the dressing midway between meals so that the patient's appetite and mealtimes are not disturbed.

Provide privacy by properly screening the patient; close the room door and curtain. Then help the patient into a position that is comfortable and also convenient for changing the dressing. Expose only the area necessary to perform the wound care while maintaining proper draping.

Using appropriate aseptic techniques when changing the dressing is crucial. Be especially vigilant in performing hand hygiene thoroughly before and after changing dressings and in adhering to standard precautions and transmission-based precautions, when necessary. Among the most common causes of hospital-acquired infections is

Table 31-5 EXAMPLES OF WOUND DRESSINGS/PRODUCTS

TYPE	PURPOSES	USE
Transparent films, such as: Bioclusive DermaView Mefilm Polyskin Uniflex OpSite Tegaderm	• Allow exchange of oxygen between wound and environment • Are self-adhesive • Protect against contamination; waterproof • Prevent loss of wound fluid • Maintain a moist wound environment • Facilitate autolytic débridement • No absorption of drainage • Allow visualization of wound • May remain in place for 24 to 72 hours, resulting in less interference with healing	• Wounds with minimal drainage • Wounds that are small; partial-thickness • Stage I pressure ulcers • Cover dressings for gels, foams, and gauze • Secure intravenous catheters, nasal cannulas, chest tube dressing, central venous access devices
Hydrocolloid dressings, such as: DuoDerm Comfeel PrimaCol Ultec Exuderm	• Are occlusive or semi-occlusive, limiting exchange of oxygen between wound and environment • Minimal to moderate absorption of drainage • Maintain a moist wound environment • Are self-adhesive • Provide cushioning • Facilitate autolytic débridement • Protect against contamination • May be left in place for 3 to 7 days, resulting in less interference with healing	• Partial- and full-thickness wounds • Wounds with light to moderate drainage • Wounds with necrosis or slough • Not for use with wounds that are infected
Hydrogels, such as: IntraSite Gel Aquasorb ClearSite Hypergel ActiFormCool	• Maintain a moist wound environment • Minimal absorption of drainage • Facilitate autolytic débridement • Do not adhere to wound • Reduce pain • Most require a secondary dressing to secure	• Partial- and full-thickness wounds • Necrotic wounds • Burns • Dry wounds • Wounds with minimal exudate • Infected wounds
Alginates, such as: Sorbsan Algicell Curasorb AQUACEL KALGINATE Melgisorb	• Absorb exudate • Maintain a moist wound environment • Facilitate autolytic débridement • Require secondary dressing • Can be left in place for 1 to 3 days	• Infected and noninfected wounds • Wounds with moderate to heavy exudate • Partial- and full-thickness wounds • Tunneling wounds • Moist red and yellow wounds • Not for use with wounds with minimal drainage or dry eschar
Foams, such as: Lyofoam Allevyn Biatain Mepilex Optifoam	• Maintain a moist wound environment • Do not adhere to wound • Insulate wound • Highly absorbent • Can be left in place up to 7 days • Some products need a secondary dressing to secure	• Absorb light to heavy amounts of drainage • Use around tubes and drains • Not for use with wounds with dry eschar
Antimicrobials, such as: SilvaSorb Acticoat Excilon Silverlon	• Antimicrobial or antibacterial action • Reduce infection • Prevent infection	• Draining, exuding, and nonhealing wounds to protect from bacterial contamination and reduce bacterial contamination • Acute and chronic wounds
Collagens, such as: BGC Matrix Stimulin PROMOGRAN Matrix	• Absorbent • Maintain a moist wound environment • Do not adhere to wound • Compatible with topical agents • Nonadherent • Conform well to the wound surface • Require secondary dressing to secure	• Partial- or full-thickness wounds • Infected and noninfected wounds • Skin grafts • Donor sites • Tunneling wounds • Moist red and yellow wounds • Wounds with minimal to heavy exudate

(continued)

Table 31-5   EXAMPLES OF WOUND DRESSINGS/PRODUCTS   *continued*

TYPE	PURPOSES	USE

Contact layers, such as:
   Adaptic Touch
   Profore WCL
   Telfa Clear
	• Placed in contact with base of wound, protecting base from trauma during dressing change
	• Allow exudate to pass to a secondary dressing
	• Not intended to be changed with every dressing change
	• May be used with topical medication, wound filler, or gauze dressings
	• Require secondary dressing
		• Partial- and full- thickness wounds
		• Shallow, dehydrated wounds
		• Wounds with eschar
		• Wounds with viscous exudate

Composites, such as:
   Alldress
   Covaderm
   StrataSorb
	• Combine two or more physically distinct products in a single dressing with several functions
	• Allow exchange of oxygen between wound and environment
	• May facilitate autolytic débridement
	• Provide physical bacterial barrier and absorptive layer
	• Semiadherent or nonadherent
	• Primary or secondary dressing
		• Partial- and full-thickness wounds
		• Wounds with minimal to heavy exudate
		• Necrotic tissue
		• Mixed (granulation and necrotic tissue) wounds
		• Infected wounds

Adapted from Anderson, I. (2010). Key principles involved in applying and removing wound dressings. *Nursing Standard, 25*(10), 51–57; White, R. (2010). Wound dressings and other topical treatment modalities in bioburden control. In K. F. Cutting & S. Percival (Eds.), *Microbiology of wounds*. Boca Raton, FL: CRC Press. In *Journal of Wound Care, 20*(9), 431–439; Baranoski, S., & Ayello, E. A. (2012). *Wound care essentials: Practice Principles* (3rd ed.). Wolters Kluwer Health/Lippincott Williams & Wilkins; and Hess, C. (2013). *Skin & wound care* (7th ed.). Philadelphia: Wolters Kluwer Health/Lippincott Williams & Wilkins.

carelessness in practicing asepsis during dressing changes. Surgical wounds that have dehisced require the use of sterile technique. Pressure ulcers are nonsterile wounds. There is no need to use sterile dressings on these wounds, and nonsterile gloves can be used for wound care (Pegram & Bloomfield, 2010).

 Concept Mastery Alert

A helpful way to remember which technique to use for wound care is this:
   Surgery occurs under sterile conditions, so surgical wounds = sterile technique; pressure ulcers = clean technique.

Removing a Dressing. Remove any dressing currently in place:

• Use standard precautions; use appropriate transmission-based precautions when indicated.
• Perform hand hygiene and put on clean (nonsterile) gloves.
• Remove tapes and dressings in the direction of hair growth to minimize trauma to the skin. Use a push–pull method; lift a corner of the dressing away from the skin, then gently push the skin away from the dressing.
• Carefully lift the adhesive barrier from the surrounding skin. If there is resistance, use a silicone-based adhesive remover, as this allows for the easy, rapid, and painless removal without the associated problems of skin stripping (Denyer, 2011; Benbow, 2011).

• Slowly remove the dressing, noting the amount, type, color, and odor of the drainage.
• Discard the dressing according to facility policy.
• Remove gloves and perform hand hygiene.

Cleaning the Wound. Perform wound cleaning to remove microorganisms and debris with as little chemical and mechanical force as possible and protect healthy granulation tissue. Normal saline solution (0.9% sodium chloride) is usually the agent of choice, particularly when cleaning pressure ulcer wounds. There are also commercially prepared cleansing sprays available for use.

Wounds are cleaned initially and before applying any new dressing. Guidelines for Nursing Care 32-3 outlines the techniques for cleaning a wound with approximated edges, such as a surgical incision, and for cleaning a wound with unapproximated edges, to remove cellular debris and drainage. It is also used to apply local heat or an antiseptic to an area. Wound irrigation is a directed flow of solution over tissues. Sterile equipment and solutions are required for irrigating an open wound, even in the presence of an existing infection. Sterile 0.9% sodium chloride or sterile water, a commercially prepared wound cleanser, an antiseptic, or an antibiotic solution may be used, depending on the condition of the wound and the primary practitioner's order. A sterile, large-volume syringe is used to direct the flow of the solution. After irrigation, open wounds may be packed with appropriate dressing materials to absorb additional drainage and allow

GUIDELINES FOR NURSING CARE 31-3

CLEANING WOUNDS

Cleaning Wounds with Approximated Edges

- Use standard precautions; use appropriate transmission-based precautions when indicated.
- Moisten a sterile gauze pad or swab with the prescribed cleansing agent.
- Use a new swab or gauze for each downward stroke.
- Clean from top to bottom.
- Work outward from the incision in lines parallel to it (Figure A).
- Wipe from the clean area toward the less clean area.

Cleaning Wounds with Unapproximated Edges

- Use standard precautions; use appropriate transmission-based precautions when indicated.
- Moisten a sterile gauze pad or swab with the prescribed cleansing agent and squeeze out excess solution.
- Use a new swab or gauze for each circle.
- Clean the wound in full or half circles, beginning in the center and working toward the outside (Figure B).
- Clean to at least 1 inch beyond the end of the new dressing.
- If a dressing is not being applied, clean to at least 2 inches beyond the wound margins.

FIGURE A

FIGURE B

Reprinted with permission from Hess, C. (2013). *Wound care* (7th ed.). Philadelphia: Wolters Kluwer Health/Lippincott Williams & Wilkins.

healing by secondary intention to take place. Nonsterile solutions are generally used to clean the skin surface if the wound edges are approximated.

Applying a New Dressing. Apply a skin protectant or barrier to the healthy skin around the wound. This is particularly important if there is drainage from the wound. The skin protectant prevents skin irritation and excoriation from tape, adhesives, and wound drainage.

The nurse should be familiar with and follow the manufacturer's guidelines for the specific dressing in use. General guidelines for applying a new dressing include (Hess, 2013):

- Check the wound care order or nursing care plan.
- Perform hand hygiene.
- Use standard precautions; use appropriate transmission-based precautions when indicated.
- Check the patient's identification.
- Explain what you are going to do to the patient.

- Provide privacy by closing the door to the room and pulling the bedside curtain.
- Put on gloves.
- Cleanse the wound, and periwound skin, as prescribed.
- Apply a skin barrier, such as Skin Prep, to the areas of skin where the dressing adhesive or tape will be placed and to areas around the wound where drainage may come in contact with skin.
- Gently place the dressing at the wound center and extend it at least 1 inch beyond the wound in each direction. Alternately, follow the manufacturer's directions for application.
- Remove gloves when the dressing is in place, before handling tape, if used.
- Do not apply tape under tension to prevent blisters and skin shearing.
- Perform hand hygiene.

Some wounds require packing with dressing material as part of treatment. It is important to be familiar with and follow the manufacturer's guidelines for the specific product in use. To pack a wound:

- Check the wound care order or nursing care plan.
- Perform hand hygiene.
- Use standard precautions; use appropriate transmission-based precautions when indicated.
- Check the patient's identification.
- Explain what you are going to do to the patient.
- Provide privacy by closing the door to the room and pulling the bedside curtain.
- Cleanse the wound and periwound skin, as prescribed.
- Apply a skin barrier, such as Skin Prep, to the areas of skin where the dressing adhesive or tape will be placed and to areas around the wound where drainage may come in contact with skin.
- Moisten packing material as necessary and as indicated by the manufacturer's directions or medical orders.
- Loosely pack the wound cavity just until the wound surfaces and edges are covered. If tunneling is present, pack the tunneling area first, then the base of the wound. Alternately, follow the manufacturer's directions for application.
- Ensure that all wound surfaces are covered and kept moist.
- Do not allow packing to overlap the wound edges; maceration of surrounding tissues could occur.
- Cover with appropriate top dressing.

Skill 31-1 on page 1004–1009 describes the process for cleaning a wound and applying a dry sterile dressing. Skill 31-2 on page 1009–1012 describes cleaning a wound and applying a saline-moistened dressing. Skill 31-3 on page 1013–1016 presents the technique for irrigating a wound.

Securing Wound Dressings. Many dressings are self-adhesive, thus no further material is needed to secure the dressing in place over the wound. However, other wound dressings require additional materials to hold the dressings in place, including tape, bandages and binders, and Montgomery straps.

Tape can be used to secure dressings in place. Tape comes in a wide variety of sizes and types, ranging in width from 1 to 4 inches (1-inch-wide tape is the most commonly used). Take care to protect the skin surrounding the wound from injury-related irritation or shearing,

Table 31-6 **TYPES OF TAPE**

TYPE	PURPOSE
Adhesive (can cause occlusion, allergy, skin maceration, shearing)	Used for strength, support, and economy • To secure dressings and splints • To strap joints to prevent athletic injuries • To immobilize or stabilize body parts • To provide pressure • To approximate wound edges
Paper, plastic, acetate	Increased comfort, decreased allergic and skin problems • To close small wounds • To secure dressings
Microfoam	Used for compression or pressure dressings

or tearing of the skin during tape removal. Table 31-6 summarizes the types and purposes of different tapes.

Bandages and binders are used to secure dressings, apply pressure, and support the wound. **Bandages** are strips of cloth, gauze (e.g., roller gauze, Kerlix, Kling), or elasticized material (e.g., ACE bandages) used to wrap a body part. They come packaged in rolls and vary in width from 1 to 6 inches. Binders are designed for a specific body part and include slings, abdominal binders, chest binders, and T-binders. They may be made of cloth (flannel, muslin) or of an elasticized material that fastens together with Velcro. The Guidelines for Nursing Care 31-4 highlights important principles for applying bandages and binders.

A *roller bandage* is a continuous strip of material wound on itself to form a cylinder or roll. Plain gauze, elastic webbing, and stretchable roller bandages are made in various widths and lengths. Begin applying the bandage to the distal part of the area. The free end is held in place with one hand while the other hand passes the roll around the body part. After the bandage is anchored, the roll is passed or rolled around the body part, taking care to exert equal tension in all turns and rolling toward the heart, to avoid causing venous stasis and resulting edema. Apply the bandage using a circular turn, spiral turn, or figure-of-eight turn (Fig. 31-13). For each technique, keep

GUIDELINES FOR NURSING CARE 31-4

APPLYING BANDAGES AND BINDERS

- Clean the area to be covered and dry it thoroughly before applying a bandage or binder, because prolonged heat and moisture on the skin may cause skin breakdown.
- Bandage the body part in the normal functioning position to prevent deformities and discomfort.
- Apply the bandage or binder with sufficient pressure to provide the amount of immobilization or support desired,

to remain in place, and to secure a dressing when present. Do not apply pressure to such a degree that circulation to the involved body part is impeded.
- Maintain equal tension with all bandage turns; avoid unnecessary and uneven overlapping of turns.
- After application, assess circulation and comfort at regular intervals.

FIGURE 31-13. Techniques for applying various bandages.

tension equal by unwinding the bandage gradually and only with as much length as is required. Evenly overlap one-half to two-thirds the width of the bandage with each turn, except for the circular turn. A circular turn is used primarily to anchor a bandage. In a circular turn, wrap the bandage around the body part, completely overlapping the previous bandage turn. Once the circular turn anchors the bandage, application continues, ascending in a spiral manner using a spiral turn. Each turn overlaps the preceding one by one-half or two-thirds the width of the bandage. The spiral turn is useful for the wrist, fingers, and trunk. The figure-of-eight turn consists of making oblique overlapping turns that ascend and descend alternately. It is effective for use around joints, such as the knee, elbow, ankle, and wrist. When removing a roller bandage, cut the bandage with bandage scissors to prevent excessive manipulation of the part. Cut on the side opposite the injury or the wound, from one end to the other, so that the bandage can be folded open for its entire length. If the bandage is to be reused, it may be unwound by keeping the loose ends together and passing it as a ball from one hand to the other while unwinding it.

When applying a *recurrent bandage,* make a few circular turns to anchor the bandage, and place the initial end of the bandage at the center of the body part being bandaged, well back from the tip to be covered. Pass the bandage back and forth over the tip, first on the one side and then on the other side of the centerpiece of the bandage. Figure 31-13 shows how to apply a recurrent bandage to a residual limb, using the figure-of-eight turn to finish the bandage. Recurrent bandages are used for fingers, for the head, and for a residual limb.

Of the many different kinds of *binders,* those used most commonly include straight binders, T-binders, and slings. A straight binder is a straight piece of material, usually about 15 to 20 cm (6 to 8 inches) wide and long enough to more than circle the torso. It is used for the chest and the abdomen. Straight binders may be pinned or, more commonly, fastened with Velcro.

A T-binder might be used to secure dressings on the rectum and perineum and in the groin. The single T-binder is used for female patients, the double T-binder for male patients. Pass the belt around the waist and secure it, then pass the tails between the legs and fasten them to the belt.

A sling is used to support an arm. Most health care agencies use commercial strap slings or sleeve slings. In the home, a large piece of cloth folded into a triangle can be used as a sling (see Fig. 31-13).

Montgomery straps use ties attached to an adhesive backing to hold dressings in place. Protect the patient's skin with a skin barrier, such as Skin Prep, or a hydrocolloid dressing, prior to applying the Montgomery straps. Apply the adhesive backing to the skin adjacent to the wound, with the ties extending over the wound area. When the dressing is changed, untie the strips and turn them back to allow for wound care. After applying the new dressing, tie the straps over the dressing to hold it

FIGURE 31-14. Montgomery straps make it possible to care for a wound without removing adhesive strips with each dressing change.

in place (Fig. 31-14). Montgomery straps can be useful in preventing skin irritation and damage due to constant retaping with dressing changes. Change Montgomery straps only when they become moist or soiled.

Caring for Patients with Wound Drains

A variety of drains, catheters, or tubes may be inserted into or near a wound when it is anticipated that a collection of fluid in a closed area would delay healing. After a surgical procedure, the surgeon places one end of the tube or drain in or near the area to be drained and passes the other end through the skin, either directly through the incision or through a separate opening called a stab wound. Wound drains are either open systems that drain into dressings or closed systems that drain into a suction device. Drains and tubes may or may not be sutured in place.

OPEN DRAINAGE SYSTEMS

A Penrose drain is soft and flexible. This drain does not have a collection device. It empties into absorptive dressing material. It promotes drainage passively, with the drainage moving from the area of greater pressure, in the wound or surgical site, to the area of less pressure,

FIGURE 31-15. Penrose drain.

FIGURE 31-16. Jackson-Pratt drain.

the dressing. It is not sutured in place. A sterile, large safety pin is often attached to the outer portion to prevent the drain from slipping back into the incised area (Fig. 31-15). Care is necessary to ensure that these drains are not dislodged during dressing changes. Sometimes the physician orders a Penrose drain that is to be shortened each day. To do so, grasp the end of the drain with sterile forceps, pull it out a short distance while using a twisting motion, and cut off the end of the drain with sterile scissors. Place a new sterile pin at the base of the drain, as close to the skin as possible.

CLOSED DRAINAGE SYSTEMS

Closed drainage systems consist of a drainage tube that may be connected to an electrical suction device or have a portable built-in reservoir to maintain constant low suction. Examples include Jackson-Pratt drainage tubes (Fig. 31-16) and Hemovacs (Fig. 31-17). These tubes are usually sutured to the skin. The closed drainage system prevents microorganisms from entering the wound from

saturated dressings. Closed drainage systems also allow accurate measurement of drainage. Be sure to know which type of drain or tube was inserted during surgery to ensure accurate assessments and interventions. These systems must be emptied and the suction reestablished according to the directions for each device. This usually involves compressing the container while the port is open, then closing the port after the device is compressed. Skills 31-4 on pages 1017–1019 and 31-5 on pages 1019–1022 outline the procedures for caring for Jackson-Pratt and Hemovac drains. Wear gloves when emptying the drainage and do not touch the open port to avoid contaminating the port.

Collecting a Wound Culture

If assessment of the wound indicates a possible infection, it is important to culture the wound. Culturing the wound allows identification of the infecting organism(s) and appropriate interventions. Skill 31-6 on pages 1022–1026 reviews the process for obtaining a wound culture.

FIGURE 31-17. Hemovac drain.

Using Additional Techniques to Promote Wound Healing

FIBRIN SEALANTS

Fibrin glues were initially mixtures of bovine or human fibrinogen, thrombin, and calcium. Newer fibrin sealants are concentrated human clottable proteins and human thrombin. The sealant is applied to tissues during an operative procedure to stop bleeding and glue together epidermal surfaces. This allows for wound closure with minimal drainage or scarring. The glue is eventually metabolized and absorbed by the body. Dressings are not needed over these wounds because the skin is closed completely (Harvey, 2005).

NEGATIVE-PRESSURE WOUND THERAPY (NPWT)

Negative-pressure wound therapy (NPWT, or topical negative pressure [TNP]) promotes wound healing and wound closure through the application of uniform negative pressure on the wound bed, reduction in bacteria in the wound, and the removal of excess wound fluid, while providing a moist wound healing environment. The negative pressure results in mechanical tension on the wound tissues, stimulating cell proliferation, blood flow to wounds, and the growth of new blood vessels. It is used to treat a variety of acute or chronic wounds, wounds with heavy drainage, wounds failing to heal, or wounds healing slowly. Examples of such wounds include pressure ulcers; arterial, venous, and diabetic ulcers; dehisced surgical wounds; infected wounds; skin graft sites; and burns. NPWT is not considered for use in the presence of active bleeding; wounds with exposed blood vessels, organs, or nerves; malignancy in wound tissue; presence of dry/necrotic tissue; wounds with exposed vessels, nerves, tendons and ligaments; or with fistulas of unknown origin (Hess, 2013; Martindell, 2012; Preston, 2008; Thompson, 2008). Cautious use is indicated in the presence of unrelieved pressure, anticoagulant therapy, poor nutritional status, and immunosuppressant therapy (Martindell; Preston). Assess candidates for pre-existing bleeding disorders or the use of anticoagulants and other medications or supplements that prolong bleeding times, such as aspirin or ginkgo biloba (Malli, 2005; Preston). Skill 31-7 on pages 1026–1029 outlines the procedure for applying NPWT.

GROWTH FACTORS

Growth factors are naturally occurring proteins. They are applied to the wound bed, where they bind to cells to promote granulation, cell proliferation, and cell migration. They are used during the proliferative phase of wound healing in patients with chronic nonhealing wounds.

OXYGEN THERAPY

Oxygen therapy is sometimes used to facilitate repair of slowly healing wounds. It involves placing patients in a hyperbaric, pressurized chamber, where they breathe 100% oxygen. The tissues are exposed to the high-concentration oxygen environment, which promotes cell proliferation, blood flow to wounds, and the growth of new blood vessels. The action of white blood cells is also enhanced.

HEAT AND COLD THERAPY

The application of heat or cold is sometimes used as part of the treatment of wounds. The application of heat accelerates the inflammatory response to promote healing. The local application of cold constricts peripheral blood vessels, reduces muscle spasms, and promotes comfort. The use of these therapies is discussed later in the chapter.

OTHER TREATMENT OPTIONS FOR PRESSURE ULCERS

When other treatment options have failed, surgery may be considered. Surgical procedures may include direct closure of the wound, skin grafting, or various skin flap procedures. The decision is based on the patient's condition and the severity of the ulcer. After surgery, vigilantly protect the surgical site from pressure and contamination.

Several other treatment modalities are being investigated. They include electrical stimulation, laser irradiation, ultrasound, and miscellaneous topical agents and systemic drugs.

Removing Sutures or Staples

Sutures are removed when the wound has developed enough tensile strength to hold the wound edges together during healing. This stage varies from patient to patient, depending on age, nutritional status, and wound location. Silk sutures typically are removed within 6 to 8 days to prevent suture marks, even though collagen formation and remodeling take a total of at least 21 days. This means the scar may still stretch and widen after the silk sutures have been removed. Special subcutaneous techniques have been developed to minimize this problem.

FIGURE 31-18. Applying Steri-Strips on an incision.

Sutures are removed with a suture removal set; staples are removed with a special staple remover. The steps in removing sutures and staples are summarized in the accompanying Guidelines for Nursing Care 31-5. After the removal of skin sutures, small adhesive wound-closure strips, that look something like tape, are sometimes applied across the healing wound to help hold it together and give additional support as it continues to heal (Fig. 31-18). Unless otherwise directed, these adhesive strips are not removed during wound care.

Teaching Wound Care at Home
GENERAL GUIDELINES

With the increase in ambulatory surgery and earlier discharge of patients from inpatient settings to home care, teaching patients and their families about wound care is important. Although a nurse may be needed to change dressings and provide wound care in complex situations, family members often are taught how to perform the procedure. To provide the continuity of care that is necessary to prevent infection and promote healing, be sure to

---

GUIDELINES FOR NURSING CARE 31-5

REMOVING STAPLES AND SUTURES

The removal of staples or sutures may be done by the physician, an advanced practice professional, or by the nurse with a medical order. Always follow agency protocol; keep in mind these general guidelines:

- Use sterile techniques, following recommended CDC guidelines for care of wounds.
- Perform hand hygiene before and after the procedure.
- Explain the procedure to the patient. Describe the sensation that will be experienced as a pulling or slightly uncomfortable experience.
- Use proper technique to remove and dispose of old dressings.
- Clean the incision from the center of the wound outward, according to agency policy and procedure for type of agent.
- Remove every other suture or staple to be sure wound edges are healed; if they are, remove remaining sutures or staples as ordered.
- Remove or reapply dressing, depending on physician preference and agency policy.
- Steri Strip application may be ordered for the healed wound after removal of staples or sutures to give additional support to the wound as it continues to heal. Follow agency protocol and primary care provider preference for placement of these tapes.

Specifics for Suture Removal

1. Use a sterile suture removal kit.
2. Using the sterile forceps, grasp the knot of the first suture and gently lift the knot.
3. Using the sterile scissors, cut one side of the suture below the knot close to the skin (Figure A).
4. Grasp the knot with the forceps and pull the cut suture through the skin (be sure to pull through the healed wound only the portion of the suture that has been inside the tissue).

Specifics for Staple Removal

1. As directed on the package, gently position the sterile staple remover under the staple to be removed.
2. Firmly close the staple remover to straighten the staple ends; do not lift upward while disengaging staple ends (Figure B).
3. Carefully lift upward with the closed staple remover to remove the staple from the incision line. It may be necessary to remove one end of the staple and then the other if it does not easily lift out.

FIGURE A. Removing sutures.

FIGURE B. Removing staples.

TEACHING TIPS 31-1

WOUND CARE AND HEALING

Health Topic	Teaching Tip	Why is This Important?
Supplies	• Methods for obtaining dressing supplies such as purchasing from pharmacies, drug stores, discount stores, and medical supply stores • Considerations for costs and ease of use • Investigation about reimbursement by insurance company or other source of health care financing for supplies	Patients need to be able to obtain appropriate supplies in order to perform prescribed care. Wound care will not be completed if patient cannot obtain supplies due to financial limitations, inability to obtain supplies, or if wound care plan is complex or not within patient's level of understanding.
Infection prevention	• Signs and symptoms of infection to be immediately reported to the health care provider • Need to watch for increased body temperature, flu-like symptoms, red or separated wound edges, increased pain in the wound, and increased drainage that is thick and has a foul odor • Wearing of disposable gloves when changing the dressing • Hand hygiene before putting on and after removing the gloves • Proper methods for disposal of old dressing, such as wrapping old dressing in several layers of newspaper or putting it in a plastic bag before disposal in a trash container	Early detection of possible complications promotes early intervention and prevention of further complications. Reduces transmission of microorganisms.
Wound healing	• Importance of eating well-balanced meals that are high in protein and vitamins • Need to drink 6 to 8 glasses of fluids each day • Rest periods during the day • Modifications in activities of daily living and exercise until healing is complete and approval is given by health care provider	Promotes optimal healing.

include teaching about wound care as part of discharge planning and in interactions with home care patients and families. A summary of teaching content is outlined in Teaching Tips 31-1: Wound Care and Healing.

PRESSURE ULCER PREVENTION AND CARE
Teaching patients and caregivers how to prevent pressure ulcers requires a comprehensive, organized educational effort. Initially, the health care provider presents basic information that explains the terminology, identifies risk factors, explains where and how pressure ulcers develop, and describes various prevention strategies and options. Illustrated instructions written at the level of the learner are a valuable resource. The protocols listed in the Guidelines for Nursing Care boxes serve as a model for development of a teaching plan that incorporates basic principles and targets individuals at risk. As new information becomes available, education for prevention of pressure ulcers requires updating.

Involve the patient and caregivers in the plan of care and provide them with a good understanding about causative factors for the pressure ulcer. Instruct them in proper

hand hygiene techniques and how to identify the signs and symptoms of infection. Provide the patient and caregivers with simple, easy-to-read instructions. Encourage frequent consultation with the primary health care provider about the progress of wound healing and products used. In addition, ensure that the patient, family, or caregivers understand the need for adequate nutrition to aid in wound healing. Assess the patient's nutritional status and suggest consultation with a dietitian for dietary deficiencies, if necessary.

If dressing changes or wound care is painful, teach the patient to use pain medication as prescribed 30 to 60 minutes before the procedure. Reinforce the importance of hand hygiene before and after the dressing change.

Documenting Wound Care
Documentation related to wound care is an important nursing responsibility. Clear and accurate documentation is essential for communication of wound status and tracking of the progression of healing. Precise documentation contributes to continuity of care, accurate evaluation of care, and appropriate changes in wound care, if necessary.

Left CVA Wound and skin assessment tool

Primary diagnosis ___Left CVA___

Secondary diagnosis ___Diabetes___

Pertinent medical history ___Right-side weakness, depression, IDDM___

WOUND ANATOMICAL LOCATION:

Site ___Right heel___   Date of outset ___10/18/11___

(circle affected area)

R L   L R   L   R

R   L   R

L   R   L   R

Classification	Terms	Type
Pressure ulcers	**ST1**—nonblanchable erythema of intact skin; heralding lesion of skin ulceration	**1.** Stage 1
	ST2—partial-thickness skin loss involving epidermis or dermis; ulcer is superficial; presents as an abrasion, blister, or shallow crater	**2.** Stage 2
	ST3—full-thickness skin loss involving damage or necrosis of subcutaneous tissue that may extend down to, but not through, underlying fascia; ulcer presents as a deep crater with or without tunneling of adjacent tissue	**3.** Stage 3
	ST4—full-thickness skin loss with extensive destruction, tissue necrosis, or damage to muscle, bone, or support structures	**4.** Stage 4
	U—wound completely covered with necrotic tissue; cannot be staged until wound base is visible	**5.** Unstageable
Wound	**PTW** (partial-thickness wound)—loss of epidermis and partial loss of dermis	**6.** Skin tear
	FTW (full-thickness wound)—tissue destruction extending through the dermis and involving the subcutaneous layer; may involve muscle or bone	**7.** Surgical
		8. Vascular ulcer
		9. Other
Color	**R**—clean, healthy, granulating tissue	**10.** Red
	Y—presence of slough or fibrinous tissue	**11.** Yellow
	B—presence of eschar	**12.** Black
	M—two or more colors present in wound (specify color by letters, such as R/Y)	**13.** Mixed
Skin condition	**SC** (skin condition)—an abnormal finding on the surface of the skin	**14.** Rash
		15. Incontinence-related
		16. Bruise
		17. Xerosis
		18. Other

DATE (M/D/Y)	TERM	TYPE #	LENGTH, WIDTH (cm)	DEPTH (cm)	TUNNELING (cm, o'clock)	COLOR (R/Y/B/M)	DRAINAGE (amount and type)	ODOR & TYPE (Y/N)		PAIN (Y*/N)	PHOTO (Y/N)	ADJUNCTIVE THERAPIES OR PRODUCTS AND ADDITIONAL COMMENTS	SIGNATURE, TITLE
10/1 8/04	ST 2	2	4 x 3	< 0. 1	Ø	10	Scant, serous	N		N	Y	☒ Support Surface ☒ Nutritional Intervention ☐ New Orders Obtained T & P 2 hours, heel protectors, heels elevated	B. Carey, RN
												☐ Support Surface ☐ Nutritional Intervention ☐ New Orders Obtained	

Patient's Name (Last, Middle, First)	Attending Physician	Room Number		ID Number
Brown, Ann	Dr. A. Dennis	123-2	0	1726

Hess, C.T. © Wound Care Strategies, Inc., 2004.

FIGURE 31-19. Wound and skin assessment/documentation tool. (Reprinted with permission from Hess, C. [2008]. *Wound care* [6th ed.; pp. 110–111]. Philadelphia: Wolters Kluwer Health/Lippincott Williams & Wilkins.)

Use a skin and wound assessment tool to accurately record assessment findings and treatment interventions. Photographs of a wound contribute to accurate assessment documentation and measurement of changes over time (Hess, 2013). Figure 31-19 shows an example of a paper skin and wound assessment/documentation tool. Figure 31-20 (on page 996) shows an example of an electronic documentation tool.

Evaluating

Evaluation of wound and pressure ulcer care involves reassessment at regular intervals to monitor response to the treatment, determine the effectiveness of the treatment, and allow for necessary changes in the plan of care. The plan of care for the patient with a wound is evaluated based on the expected outcomes. Evaluation is ongoing throughout the care of the patient, with the plan being effective if no complications have occurred during wound healing, wound is progressing through the healing stages, and the patient or family has the knowledge and skill necessary for wound care at home, if appropriate.

When evaluating the effectiveness of a plan of care designed to prevent the development of pressure ulcers or to treat pressure ulcers or other wounds already present, the nurse uses each nurse–patient interaction to determine if the patient has met the individualized expected outcomes in the plan of care. Nursing care is considered effective if the patient, family member, or caregiver expresses satisfaction with prevention and treatment measures and is able to accomplish the following:

• Participate effectively in preventive and treatment regimens
• Prevent development of any additional areas of skin breakdown
• Demonstrate progressive healing of pressure ulcer or other wound
• Improve overall physical condition (including nutritional state and mobility status)

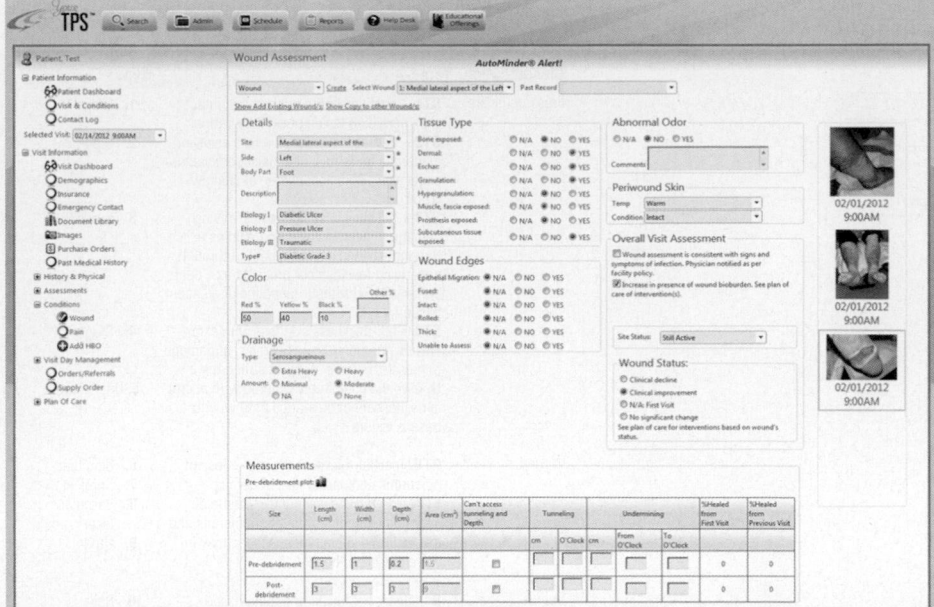

FIGURE 31-20. Electronic wound and skin assessment/documentation tool. (Reprinted with permission from Hess, C. [2013]. *Clinical Guide to Skin and Wound care* [7th ed.; p. 127]. Philadelphia: Wolters Kluwer Health/Lippincott Williams & Wilkins. Source: TPS EMR© Wound Care Strategies, Inc. 2012. www.wellcare strategies.com)

- Remain free of infection at any pressure ulcer or other wound site
- Communicate the need for additional support (environmental, physical, psychosocial)

Evaluation is a continuous process that involves ongoing assessment and revised plans and implementations. Color photographs are an excellent method of evaluating the progression of wound healing, allowing visual comparison of the wound at the initial assessment and throughout the plan of care through the recovery stages.

HEAT AND COLD THERAPY

Heat and cold are applied to a specific part or all of a patient's body to bring about a local or systemic change in body temperature for various therapeutic purposes. Physiologic responses to heat and cold are modified by the method and duration of application, the degree of heat and cold applied, the patient's age and physical condition, and the amount of body surface covered by the application. Nurses use heat and cold as nursing interventions in both hospital- and community-based settings.

Body temperature is regulated by cells in the hypothalamus in response to signals from thermal (heat and cold) receptors located close to the skin's surface. Stimulation of these receptors sends sensory messages to the anterior hypothalamus to initiate mechanisms to dissipate heat (through vasodilation and sweating) or to preserve warmth through vasoconstriction and piloerection ("goose bumps"). Pain receptors, also located near the skin's surface, are also affected by heat and cold as painful stimuli, with excessive heat perceived as burning and excessive cold experienced as numbness followed by pain.

Effects of Applying Heat

The application of local heat dilates peripheral blood vessels, increases tissue metabolism, reduces blood viscosity and increases capillary permeability, reduces muscle tension, and helps relieve pain. Vasodilation increases local blood flow. In turn, the supply of oxygen and nutrients to the area is increased, and venous congestion is decreased. As local blood flow increases, the viscosity of blood is reduced and increased capillary permeability improves the delivery of leukocytes and nutrients while also facilitating the removal of wastes and prolonging clotting time. These actions, combined with increased tissue metabolism, accelerate the inflammatory response to promote healing.

Heat reduces muscle tension to promote relaxation and helps to relieve muscle spasms and joint stiffness. Heat also helps relieve pain by stimulating specific nerve fibers, closing the gate that allows the transmission of pain stimuli to centers in the brain. Because of these local physiologic effects, heat in various forms is used to treat infections, surgical wounds, inflamed tissue, arthritis, joint and muscle pain, dysmenorrhea, and chronic pain.

The systemic effects of extensive, prolonged heat include increased cardiac output, sweating, increased pulse rate, and decreased blood pressure. This response occurs when heat is applied to a large body area, increasing the blood flow to that area while decreasing it to another part of the body, in effect, causing hypovolemic shock.

Effects of Applying Cold

The local application of cold constricts peripheral blood vessels, reduces muscle spasms, and promotes comfort. Cold reduces blood flow to tissues and decreases the local release of pain-producing substances such as histamine, serotonin, and bradykinin. This action in turn reduces the formation of edema and inflammation. Decreased metabolic needs and capillary permeability, combined with increased coagulation of blood at the wound site, facilitate the control of bleeding and reduce edema formation.

Cold also reduces muscle spasm, alters tissue sensitivity (producing numbness), and promotes comfort by slowing the transmission of pain stimuli. Cold, for these effects, is used after direct trauma, for dental pain, for muscle spasms, after sprains, and to treat some chronic pain syndromes.

Exposure to prolonged or extensive environmental cold produces systemic effects of increased blood pressure, shivering, and goose bumps. Although shivering is a normal body response to cold, prolonged cold may cause tissue injury.

Physiologic Considerations

The rebound phenomenon is important to the therapeutic value of heat and cold and to the safety of patients receiving such therapy. Heat produces maximum vasodilation in 20 to 30 minutes; if heat is continued beyond that time, tissue congestion and vasoconstriction occurs (for unknown reasons). With cold, maximum vasoconstriction occurs when the skin reaches 60°F (15°C); then vasodilation begins.

The ability of the body to adapt to heat and cold is an important consideration when applying heat or cold and when teaching patients and caregivers about heat and cold therapy. Initially, heat and cold skin receptors are stimulated strongly by sudden changes in temperature. For the first few seconds after being stimulated, the response decreases rapidly. It then decreases more slowly for the next 30 minutes, as the receptors adapt to the temperature. A hot application, even if the temperature remains constant, does not feel as warm after adaptation has taken place. Be sure to inform patients that increasing the temperature or lengthening the time of application can seriously damage tissues.

THE NURSING PROCESS FOR HEAT AND COLD THERAPY

Assessing

Before initiating heat or cold therapy, assess the patient's physical and mental status, the condition of the body area to be treated with heat or cold, and the condition of the equipment to be used. Carefully evaluate factors influencing the patient's ability to tolerate heat and cold applications. These factors are the basis for the following considerations:

- How long will the heat or cold be applied? Prolonged exposure increases tolerance, and rebound effects are undesirable.
- What body part is involved? Some body areas, such as the neck, perineum, and inner aspects of the wrist and forearm, are more sensitive to thermal changes.
- Is the skin intact? Open tissue or abraded skin is more sensitive to thermal changes.
- How large is the area? Applications of heat or cold to large areas of the body cause systemic responses and lower tolerance of temperature change.

- What is the patient's age? Infants, children, and older adults do not tolerate temperature changes as well as adults.
- What is the patient's physical condition? Patients with certain alterations in health, such as those with cardiovascular or peripheral vascular diseases, might have reduced response to or tolerance of thermal changes.

Assessing Overall Status

Assessing the patient's overall status includes obtaining a health history and completing a physical examination. A history of cardiovascular or peripheral vascular impairment, sensory impairment, and alterations in mental status, such as confusion or decreased level of consciousness, indicates the need for caution when using heat or cold because of the danger of tissue damage. Assessments include response to stimuli (sharp and dull), color and appearance of body tissues, circulation (pulses, blanching sign, temperature, color), level of consciousness, and orientation.

 CONSIDER Mr. Everly, the postoperative patient in the critical care unit. Imagine that the physician had ordered heat or cold applications for this patient. The nurse would need to obtain a thorough assessment of his physical status when planning this care because his history of diabetes and circulation problems, in conjunction with his decreased level of consciousness, would place him at high risk for injury and tissue damage. In addition, the nurse would need to assess him frequently during the application of heat or cold to ensure his safety. •

Do not apply heat to an open wound immediately after the trauma; during hemorrhage; over noninflammatory edema; to an acutely inflamed area, a localized malignant tumor, the testes, or the abdomen of a pregnant woman; or over metallic implants. Conversely, do not use cold for open wounds or for patients with impaired peripheral circulation or allergy to cold.

Assessing the Area of Application

Perform baseline assessments to ensure safety and to evaluate the outcomes of therapy. The risk for damage to tissues is increased if the area is traumatized or has altered integrity. Assess for open lesions, blisters, wounds, edema, bleeding, or drainage or evidence of altered circulation such as changes in color, temperature, pulses, and sensation. As with any assessment, compare body parts bilaterally for changes. Tissues with decreased or absent pulses, those that appear pale or cyanotic, and those that feel cold to the touch indicate a decrease in circulation. Subsequently, the risk for injury from heat and cold applications increases.

When the heat or cold is applied, make ongoing assessments to ensure patient safety and comfort. When heat is applied, assess the patient for undesired responses, including localized redness, blistering, and pain (symptoms of burning), along with possible systemic responses, such as hypotension and changes in consciousness. When cold is applied, assess for localized responses, including pallor, cyanosis, numbness, and pain.

Assessing the Condition of Equipment

The nurse is responsible for checking the equipment used and for maintaining patient safety. Included in this responsibility is checking the condition of cords, plugs, and heating or cooling elements. In addition, inspect the equipment for fluid leaks. Also, check to ensure that the equipment distributes and maintains the constant temperature. Do not use faulty equipment; if faulty equipment is found, it should be returned for repair.

Diagnosing

The patient's need for and response to the heat or cold suggest possible nursing diagnoses, including the following:

- Acute Pain
- Ineffective Tissue Perfusion
- Chronic Pain
- Risk for Injury

Outcome Identification and Planning

Heat and cold are used for a variety of therapeutic purposes that are an essential part of planning individualized care and forming the basis for patient outcomes. When applications of heat or cold are part of a plan of care, the following outcomes are appropriate; specific outcomes should be chosen based on the purpose of the application. The patient will:

- Verbalize increased comfort
- Demonstrate evidence of wound healing, decreased muscle spasms, decreased edema, and increased comfort
- Verbalize and demonstrate safe hot or cold application

Implementing

Heat and cold applications may be moist or dry, using many forms and methods. The prescription for the heat and cold application should include the type of application, the body area to be treated, and the frequency and length of time for the applications.

Explain to the patient the purpose and steps of the application and the sensations that will be experienced. In the hospital, provide a timer or clock and have the call bell within reach. In the home, teach the patient or family member to check the equipment each time to ensure that it is in good working order, avoid lying or leaning on the equipment, cover the heating device with a protective cloth, apply heat only for the prescribed time period, and report any changes in sensation or discomfort to the health care provider.

Applying Heat

Heat is applied by both dry and moist methods. Hot water bags, electric heating pads, aquathermia pads, or chemi-

cal heat packs provide local dry heat by conduction. Hot compresses or packs, sitz baths, or soaks provide moist heat by conduction.

DRY HEAT

Hot Water Bags. Hot water bags are a method of dry heat application. Although relatively easy and inexpensive to use, they have disadvantages. They may leak, and often the weight of the bag or bottle on the patient's body part can be uncomfortable. Moreover, there is a danger of burns from improper use.

Electric Heating Pads. An electric heating pad can be used to apply dry heat locally. It is easy to apply, is relatively safe to use, and provides constant and even heat. Improper use can, however, result in injury. When applying a heating pad, follow these recommendations:

- Avoid using pins to secure a heating pad. There is a danger of electric shock if a pin touches a wire.
- Place a covering over the pad, preferably one that is moisture proof. Also, prevent wet and moist conditions around the pad. Short-circuiting the heating element may cause an electric shock. Do not cover the heating pad with anything that might be heavy; heat may accumulate and burn the patient when it cannot dissipate normally from the pad.
- Place a heating pad anteriorly or laterally to, not under, the body part. If the heating pad is between the patient and the mattress, heat dissipation may be inadequate, leading to burning of the patient or the bed linens.
- Use a heating pad with a selector switch that cannot be turned up beyond a safe temperature. After heat has been applied and a certain amount of adaptation of heat receptors takes place, the patient often increases the heat when the switch is not permanently preset because the pad does not seem sufficiently warm. Many people have been burned by turning up the heat in an electric pad because they thought the pad was too cool.
- Assess the skin at regular intervals for the effects of excessive exposure to heat such as increased skin redness, changes in sensation, or discomfort.
- Check agency protocol for the use of heating pads; a release form may need to be signed.

Aquathermia Pads. Aquathermia (Aqua-K) pads are commonly used in health care agencies and homes for various health problems, including back pain, muscle spasms, thrombophlebitis, and mild inflammation. These devices are safer to use than a heating pad, but they too must be checked carefully. Guidelines for using an aquathermia pad are given in Skill 31-8 on pages 1030–1032.

Hot Packs. Commercial hot packs provide a specified amount of dry heat for a specific period. Instructions on the package describe how to activate the pack, either by striking it on a firm surface or by squeezing or kneading it. Follow the same precautions as for other types of dry heat applications.

MOIST HEAT

Warm Moist Compresses. Warm moist compresses are used to promote circulation and healing and to reduce edema. Because moist heat evaporates and cools rapidly, change these compresses frequently and cover them with a heating agent (hot water bottle, heating pad, Aqua-K pad).

Sitz Baths. Sitz baths are a method of applying tepid or warm water to the pelvic, perineal, or rectal areas by sitting in a tub, special chair, or basin filled with sufficient water to reach the umbilicus. Special basins that fit onto the toilet seat are available. They are designed so that the patient's buttocks fit into a rather deep seat that is filled with water of the desired temperature; the legs and feet remain out of the water. The basins are disposable and economical for home or health care agency use. A regular bathtub is not as satisfactory for a sitz bath because the heat causes generalized vasodilation, altering the effect desired. Techniques for administering a sitz bath are given in Guidelines for Nursing Care 31-6.

Warm Soaks. The immersion of a body area into warm water or a medicated solution is called a soak. The pur-

poses of soaks vary: to increase blood supply to a locally infected area; to aid in cleaning large, sloughing wounds, such as burns; to improve circulation; and to apply medication to a locally infected area. A soak has the added advantage of making manipulation of a painful area much easier because the body part is buoyed by the weight of water it displaces. If a warm soak is ordered, follow these general guidelines:

- If a soak is prescribed for a large wound (e.g., an entire arm or lower leg or even an area of the torso), expect to adapt sterile technique. For example, sterilize the container into which the body area is placed before use if possible; if not, clean the container scrupulously. Tap water may be used for soaks because it is accepted as being free from pathogens.
- Unless the temperature of the soak is prescribed otherwise, set the temperature of the water within a range of 105°F to 109°F (40.5°C to 43°C), which is considered to be physiologically effective and comfortable for the patient.
- Position the container holding the fluid so that the part to be immersed is comfortable and the patient is in good body alignment.
- During the treatment, which usually takes 15 to 20 minutes per soak, maintain the temperature of the soak

GUIDELINES FOR NURSING CARE 31-6

ASSISTING WITH A SITZ BATH

- Test the water in a sitz bath (Figure) with a thermometer before the patient enters the water.
- If the purpose of the sitz bath is to apply heat, use water at a temperature of 34°C to 37°C (93°F to 99°F) for

Sitz bath.

15 minutes to produce relaxation of the parts involved after a short initial period of contraction. Do not use warm water if considerable congestion is already present.
- If the purpose of the sitz bath is to produce relaxation or to promote healing in a wound by cleansing it of discharge and debris, use water at a temperature of 34°C to 37°C (93°F to 99°F). Check agency protocols for the correct temperature.
- Assist the patient into the tub or onto the sitz bath and position properly. The patient should be able to sit in the basin or tub with the feet flat on the floor without any pressure on the sacrum or thighs.
- Wrap a blanket around the shoulders to protect from chilling and exposure.
- Monitor the patient closely for signs of weakness and fatigue, and discontinue the bath if faintness, pallor, a rapid pulse rate, or nausea is noted.
- Test the water in the tub several times, and keep it at the desired temperature. Additional hot water may be added by pouring it slowly from a pitcher or by opening the hot water faucet slightly. Agitate the water by stirring it as the hot water is added to prevent burning the patient.
- Do not leave the patient alone if there are any questions about safety.
- Help the patient out of the tub when the bath is completed. A sitz bath should take 15 to 20 minutes. Help the patient dry, and cover him or her adequately.

as constant as possible. This may be done by discarding some of the fluid every 5 minutes and replacing it or by adding solutions at a higher temperature while agitating the water. When replacing or adding fluids, have the patient remove the extremity from the soak.

Applying Cold

Cold is applied by both dry and moist methods. Dry cold is provided with ice bags, cold packs, or a hypothermia blanket (or pad). Cold compresses are a method of applying moist cold.

DRY COLD

Ice Bags. An ice bag, like its counterpart hot water bottle or bag, is a relatively easy and inexpensive method for applying cold to an area. It has essentially the same disadvantages as the hot water bag. When using an ice bag, follow these recommendations:

- Fill the bag with small pieces of ice to about two-thirds full. This makes the bag lightweight. Using ice chips, rather than cubes, makes it easier to mold the bag to the body part.
- Remove air from the ice bag in the same manner as removing air from a hot water bag.
- After securing the cap, test the ice bag for leaks and wipe off excess moisture.
- Place a cover on the ice bag to provide comfort and to absorb moisture that may accumulate on the outside of the bag.
- Apply an ice bag for 30 minutes, then remove it for about an hour before reapplying it. This technique prevents the effects of prolonged exposure to cold (Fig. 31-21).

FIGURE 31-21. Cloth-wrapped ice bag. (Reprinted with permission from Craven & Hinkle. [2009]. *Fundamentals of Nursing* [6th ed.; pp. 1015]. Philadelphia: Wolters Kluwer Health/ Lippincott Williams & Wilkins.)

- In the home setting, a bag of frozen vegetables (such as peas) makes a good substitute for an ice bag.

Cold Packs. Commercially prepared ice packs are available in many health care agencies and may be purchased commercially. These bags are sealed containers filled with a chemical or a nontoxic substance. Depending on the type, the bags are frozen in the freezer or (if not frozen) are squeezed to activate the chemical that produces the cold. These packs are advantageous because the frozen solution remains pliable and can be easily molded to fit the body part. They are covered with a ribbed cotton sleeve so that the bag can be slipped onto an extremity, or the bag can simply be placed on a body part, such as the head. Assess the skin beneath the pack periodically for symptoms of numbness and pain.

MOIST COLD

Moist, cold local applications are called cold compresses. They might be used for an injured eye, a headache, a tooth extraction, and sometimes for hemorrhoids. The texture and thickness of the material used depend on the area to which it is applied. For example, eye compresses could be prepared from surgical gauze compresses, which have a small amount of cotton filling. A washcloth makes an excellent compress for the head or face.

Immerse the material used for the application in a clean basin that contains pieces of ice and a small amount of water. Wring the compress thoroughly before applying it to avoid dripping. Dripping is uncomfortable for the patient and may result in wetting the patient's clothing or bed linens. Change the compress frequently, continuing the application for 20 minutes. Repeat the application every 2 to 3 hours as ordered. Ice bags or commercial devices are available for keeping the compresses cold, helping to decrease the frequency with which they must be changed.

Evaluating

The expected outcomes for applying heat and cold when included as part of a plan of care are used to evaluate the effectiveness of the planned interventions. Although the specific outcomes depend on the purpose of the application, nursing care is considered effective if the patient is able to:

- Verbalize increased comfort
- Verbalize increased ability to rest and sleep
- Demonstrate evidence of wound healing
- Demonstrate a decrease in symptoms of muscle spasms, inflammation, and edema
- Verbalize and demonstrate safe hot and cold applications

Ongoing evaluation of skin integrity is needed to determine needs and the effectiveness of any interventions, including heat and cold therapy. (See the accompanying concept map for Lucius Everly and the Nursing Plan of Care 31-1 for Mary Biesicker, on pages 1002–1003.)

Lucius Everly, who has a history of diabetes and circulatory problems, underwent abdominal surgery several days ago and is now in the critical care unit. When you enter, he is slouched down in bed. Assessment reveals that his abdominal dressing is moist, and only part of the tape securing the dressing is adhering to the skin. His level of consciousness is decreased, and he responds only to moderate touch and pain. With repositioning, he moans. Further assessment reveals the beginning of a pressure ulcer on his heel. He is NPO and has a central intravenous catheter in place for administration of total parenteral nutrition (TPN). An indwelling catheter is in place to accurately measure intake and output. He is currently afebrile but has been prescribed antibiotics prophylactically.

Priority 1

Risk for Infection related to surgical incision and invasive therapy
Supporting Data:
- Abdominal surgical incision with moist dressing
- Pressure ulcer on heel
- Weakened defenses from chronic illness, such as diabetes and circulatory problems
- Central venous catheter
- Indwelling urinary catheter
- Afebrile
- IV antibiotics prescribed

Outcome:
Patient will remain afebrile with absence of redness or purulent drainage at surgical site. Urine will remain clear.

Nursing Interventions:
- Maintain aseptic technique with dressing change, parenteral therapy, and indwelling urinary catheter
- Use proper handwashing technique
- Dispose of soiled dressings appropriately
- Change dressing as needed
- Note appearance of pressure ulcer, incision, and IV insertion sites
- Monitor characteristics of urine
- Monitor temperature every 4 hours

Evaluation: Lucius is afebrile. His urine is clear. No drainage is noted from pressure ulcer. His surgical incision is draining serosanguineous material. Continue interventions.

Priority 2

Impaired Skin Integrity related to surgical incision and parenteral therapy
Supporting Data:
- Abdominal surgical incision
- Moist dressings, loosely secured
- History of factors impeding healing (diabetes and circulatory problems)
- Central venous catheter
- NPO receiving TPN

Outcome: Patient will demonstrate signs of a healing incision, absence of skin irritation, absence of IV infiltration, and will maintain optimal nutrition

Nursing Interventions:
- Change abdominal dressing daily and as needed to prevent saturated dressings
- Inspect surgical incision for signs of healing
- Cleanse surgical incision
- Use Montgomery straps to secure dressing and prevent skin irritation from tape
- Use transparent dressing to cover central venous catheter insertion site to allow inspection of insertion site
- Inspect insertion site frequently and administer TPN as prescribed to meet nutritional needs and promote healing

Evaluation: Surgical dressings have been changed as needed to minimize moisture against skin. Pink granulation tissue is noted at the surgical incision. Nutrition has been maintained as noted by stable weight and a prealbumen level within normal limits. Parenteral therapy maintained without signs of infiltration.

Priority 3

Impaired Tissue Integrity related to altered mobility and chronic illness
Supporting Data:
- Decreased level of consciousness
- Unable to turn independently
- Pressure ulcer on heel
- History of circulatory problems and diabetes

Outcome:
Patient will demonstrate signs of healing in pressure ulcer on heel; no further skin breakdown will occur.

Nursing Interventions:
- Inspect skin, noting areas that are reddened
- Use Braden scale to assess risk for pressure ulcer
- Turn and reposition patient at least every 2 hours, using padded devices
- Use linen to assist in position change to decrease shearing force
- Apply heel protectors
- Avoid pressure on heels by placing pillow under calves when patient in supine position
- Cover pressure ulcer on heel with appropriate protective dressing
- Consider consult with wound care specialist

Evaluation: Lucius has been consistently turned every 2 hours; healthy granulation tissue is noted in wound bed.

- - - - - Relationship   Assessment   Nursing Diagnosis   Outcome Identification   Interventions   Evaluation

Concept map displaying the nursing process for Lucius Everly.

NURSING PLAN OF CARE 31-1

for Mary Biesicker

Mary Biesicker, who is 84 years of age, has been cared for at home by her daughter since being hospitalized last year for a stroke. During the past several months, Mary has been confined to her bed, has had minimal appetite, and has occasionally been confused and disoriented. During the past week, she has had several episodes of bowel and bladder incontinence. Her daughter also reports that Mary has developed a "blister on her lower back at the end of her backbone." She is scheduled for an assessment visit by the nurse from a local home health care agency because her daughter is finding it increasingly difficult to care for her mother alone.

The nurse's initial assessment of Mary, relative to skin integrity, revealed the following:

Skin status: Presence of a nickel-sized open area on the sacrum (stage II pressure ulcer), 2 cm in diameter and 1 cm in depth. No abnormal pathways noted. Reddened area (0.5 cm) surrounding lesion. No drainage noted. Reddened area (2.5 cm) also noted on right elbow. Skin dry over all body surfaces.

Nutritional status: Daughter states, "usual weight is 115 to 120 lb, and she has definitely lost some weight." Poor skin turgor.

Elimination status: Wearing "adult diaper," diaper damp with urine and small amount of light brown liquid stool.

Activity status: Lying quietly in bed, moans when area around lesion is palpated.

NURSING DIAGNOSIS   Impaired Skin Integrity related to mechanical factors, inactivity, altered nutritional intake, and incontinence as manifested by stage II pressure ulcer on sacral area and reddened area on right elbow

EXPECTED OUTCOME   6/6/15—at weekly visit, the patient will:

- Experience reduction of pressure on bony prominences (absence of any additional reddened areas)

NURSING INTERVENTIONS	RATIONALE	EVALUATIVE STATEMENT
Assess skin for development of any pressure areas (use agency tool).	Pressure results in poor circulation that causes skin breakdown.	6/13/15 Outcome met. Patient has been turned from side to side every 2 hours. Reddened area on right elbow measures 1.25 cm in diameter. No new reddened areas observed.
Avoid sitting or lying on a pressure ulcer.	This facilitates pressure relief in the area and allows blood to reenter capillaries and provide oxygen to the area.	
Reposition from side to side at least every 2 hours.	The duration of pressure is more devastating to skin than the amount of pressure.	*Recommendation:* Arrange for delivery of hospital bed with over-bed trapeze setup. Secure a home health care aide for limited period of time to assist with repositioning during the night and allow daughter time to rest.
Use pillows to maintain side-lying or oblique position in bed and support right elbow off bed surface.	Pillows relieve pressure on lesion and areas at risk and promote improved circulation to those areas.	*M. Lieb, RN*
Place foam overlay mattress on bed.	Static device provides support and relieves pressure on skin surface.	

EXPECTED OUTCOME   6/6/15—at weekly visit, the patient will:

- Demonstrate a reduction in the size of the stage II pressure ulcer on sacrum

NURSING PLAN OF CARE 31-1 *continued*

for Mary Biesicker

NURSING INTERVENTIONS	RATIONALE	EVALUATIVE STATEMENT
Assess condition of pressure ulcer at time of dressing change (refer to previous assessments).	Signs of infection and deterioration can be recognized and treatment plan revised.	6/13/15 Outcome met. Pressure ulcer has decreased slightly in size—1.7 cm in diameter, depth remains the same. No apparent infection noted. Will continue with present treatment regimen.
Irrigate wound with normal saline using a 60-mL piston syringe with a catheter tip.	Normal saline cleanses the wound without harming tissues.	
Dry skin thoroughly surrounding the ulcer.	Moisture makes intact skin more susceptible to injury.	*M. Lieb, RN*
Apply moisture-retentive dressing (Tegasorb).	Moisture-retentive dressings create a healing environment by allowing epithelial cells to bridge the wound gap and close it.	
Use clean technique for the dressing change.	In the home, the risk is minimal for cross contamination of micro-organisms.	

EXPECTED OUTCOME 6/6/15—at weekly visit, the patient/caregiver will:

- Demonstrate skills required to promote skin integrity and care for a pressure ulcer

NURSING INTERVENTIONS	RATIONALE	EVALUATIVE STATEMENT
Assess caregiver's (daughter) motivation and ability to manage treatment regimen.	Motivation influences readiness to learn and contributes to positive learning outcomes.	6/13/15 Outcome partially met. Daughter able to recognize appearance of pressure areas on skin. Stated she would like to review treatment routine again. Daughter performed assessment and dressing change satisfactorily with nurse in attendance. Clarified and reviewed written instructions again. Daughter states, "I feel much more confident now."
Instruct daughter about causes, skin assessment techniques, and individualized treatment regimen. Provide written instructions and illustrations when possible.	A clear, concise teaching guide provides consistent education and is available for reinforcement.	
Provide information about community resources available for assistance with care of mother.	Resources provide opportunity for support and problem solving.	*M. Lieb, RN*

SAMPLE DOCUMENTATION

6/20/15

Home health care visit (nursing)

Mrs. Biesicker was revisited in her home for continued assessment and treatment of pressure ulcer. Nursing diagnosis: Impaired Skin Integrity related to pressure, inactivity, inadequate nutritional intake, and incontinence. According to daughter, patient was turned and repositioned every 2 hours. Foam mattress and pillow supports used for support and pressure reduction. Dressing on pressure ulcer changed. Wound cleansed with normal saline, intact skin surrounding wound, and Tegasorb dressing applied. Granulation tissue noted in wound bed, no evidence of drainage or reddened area around wound. Ulcer has decreased to 1½ cm in size. Reddened area not apparent on right elbow. Reviewed written instructions with daughter for 6/23/15 to discuss health care options. Will continue current plan of care and visits every other day.

M. Lieb, RN

SKILL 31-1 | CLEANING A WOUND AND APPLYING A DRY, STERILE DRESSING

DELEGATION CONSIDERATIONS

Wound care and procedures requiring the use of a sterile field and other sterile items are not delegated to nursing assistive personnel (NAP) or unlicensed assistive personnel (UAP). Depending on the state's nurse practice act and the organization's policies and procedures, these procedures may be delegated to licensed practical/vocational nurses (LPNs/LVNs). The decision to delegate must be based on careful analysis of the patient's needs and circumstances, as well as the qualifications of the person to whom the task is being delegated. Refer to the Delegation Guidelines in Appendix A (found on thePoint).

EQUIPMENT

- Sterile gloves
- Clean disposable gloves
- Additional PPE, as indicated
- Gauze dressings
- Surgical or abdominal pads
- Sterile dressing set or suture set (for the sterile scissors and forceps)
- Sterile cleaning solution as ordered (commonly 0.9% normal saline solution, or a commercially prepared wound cleanser)
- Sterile basin (may be optional)
- Sterile drape (may be optional)
- Plastic bag or other appropriate waste container for soiled dressings
- Waterproof pad and bath blanket
- Tape or ties
- Bath blanket or other linens for draping patient
- Additional dressings and supplies needed or required by the primary care provider's order

IMPLEMENTATION

ACTION	RATIONALE
1. Review the medical order for wound care or the nursing plan of care related to wound care. Gather necessary supplies.	Reviewing the order and plan of care validates the correct patient and correct procedure. Preparation promotes efficient time management and an organized approach to the task.
2. Perform hand hygiene and put on PPE, if indicated.	Hand hygiene and PPE prevent the spread of microorganisms. PPE is required based on transmission precautions.
3. Identify the patient.	Identifying the patient ensures that the right patient receives the intervention and helps prevent errors.
4. Assemble equipment on the overbed table within reach.	Organization facilitates performance of the task.
5. Close curtains around the bed and close the door to the room if possible. Explain to the patient what you are going to do and why you are going to do it.	This ensures the patient's privacy. Explanation relieves anxiety and facilitates cooperation.
6. Assess the patient for the possible need for nonpharmacologic pain-reducing interventions or analgesic medication before wound care dressing change. Administer appropriate prescribed analgesic. Allow enough time for the analgesic to achieve its effectiveness.	Pain is a subjective experience influenced by past experience. Wound care and dressing changes may cause pain for some patients.
7. Place a waste receptacle or bag at a convenient location for use during the procedure.	Having a waste container handy means the soiled dressing may be discarded easily, without the spread of microorganisms.
8. Adjust the bed to a comfortable working height, usually elbow height of the caregiver (VISN 8, 2009).	Having the bed at the proper height prevents back and muscle strain.
9. Assist the patient to a comfortable position that provides easy access to the wound area. Use the bath blanket to cover any exposed area other than the wound. Place a waterproof pad under the wound site.	Patient positioning and use of a bath blanket provide for comfort and warmth. Waterproof pad protects underlying surfaces.

ACTION

10. Check the position of drains, tubes, or other adjuncts before removing the dressing. Put on clean, disposable gloves and loosen tape on the old dressings (Fig. 1). If necessary, use an adhesive remover to help get the tape off.

11. Carefully remove the soiled dressings (Fig. 2). If there is resistance, use a silicone-based adhesive remover to help remove the tape. If any part of the dressing sticks to the underlying skin, use small amounts of sterile saline to help loosen and remove it (Fig. 3).

RATIONALE

Checking ensures that a drain is not removed accidentally if one is present. Gloves protect the nurse from contaminated dressings and prevent the spread of microorganisms. Adhesive-tape remover helps reduce patient discomfort during dressing removal.

Cautious removal of the dressing is more comfortable for the patient and ensures that any drain present is not removed. A silicone-based adhesive remover allows for the easy, rapid, and painless removal without the associated problems of skin stripping (Denyer, 2011; Benbow, 2011). Sterile saline moistens the dressing for easier removal and minimizes damage and pain.

FIGURE 1. Loosening dressing tape.

FIGURE 2. Removing soiled dressing.

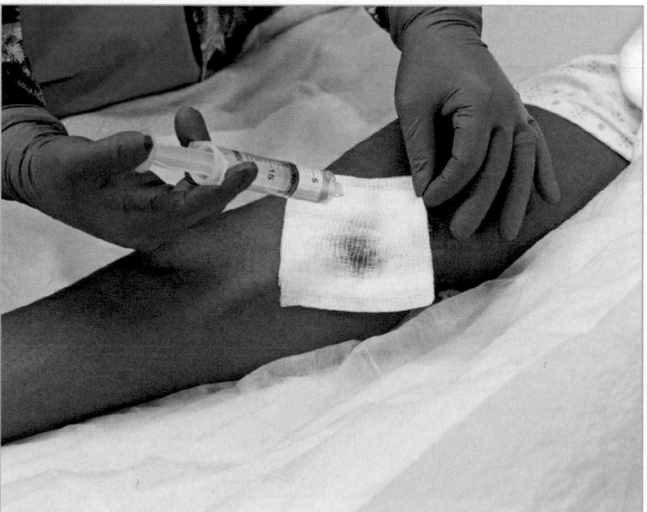

FIGURE 3. Using saline to aid in removing dressing.

(continued)

SKILL 31-1 CLEANING A WOUND AND APPLYING A DRY, STERILE DRESSING *continued*

ACTION	RATIONALE
12. After removing the dressing, note the presence, amount, type, color, and odor of any drainage on the dressings (Fig. 4). Place soiled dressings in the appropriate waste receptacle. Remove your gloves and dispose of them in an appropriate waste receptacle (Fig. 5).	The presence of drainage should be documented. Proper disposal of soiled dressings and used gloves prevents the spread of microorganisms.

FIGURE 4. Assessing dressing that has been removed.

FIGURE 5. Removing gloves.

ACTION	RATIONALE
13. Inspect the wound site for size, appearance, and drainage. Assess if any pain is present. Check the status of sutures, adhesive closure strips, staples, and drains or tubes, if present. Note any problems to include in your documentation.	Wound healing or the presence of irritation or infection should be documented.
14. **Using sterile technique, prepare a sterile work area and open the needed supplies (Fig. 6).**	Supplies are within easy reach and sterility is maintained.

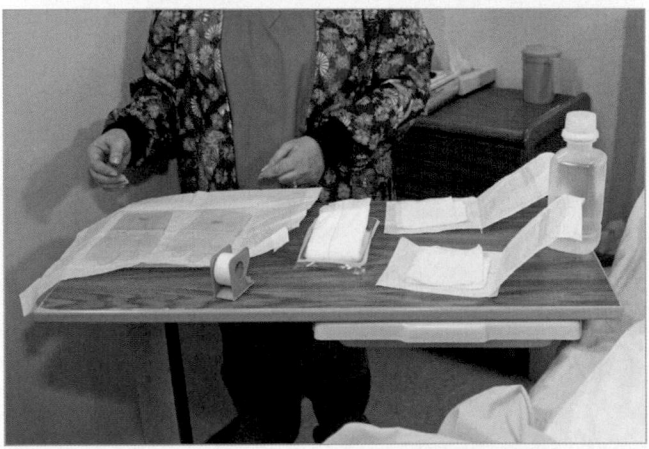

FIGURE 6. Setting up sterile field.

ACTION	RATIONALE
15. Open the sterile cleaning solution. Depending on the amount of cleaning needed, the solution might be poured directly over gauze sponges over a container for small cleaning jobs, or into a basin for more complex or larger cleaning.	Sterility of dressings and solution is maintained.

ACTION	RATIONALE
16. Put on sterile gloves (Fig. 7). Alternately, clean gloves (clean technique) may be used when cleaning a chronic wound or pressure ulcer.	Use of sterile gloves maintains surgical asepsis and sterile technique, and reduces the risk for spreading microorganisms. Clean technique is appropriate for cleaning chronic wounds or pressure ulcers.
17. Clean the wound. **Clean the wound from top to bottom and from the center to the outside (Fig. 8).** Following this pattern, use new gauze for each wipe, placing the used gauze in the waste receptacle. Alternately, spray the wound from top to bottom with a commercially prepared wound cleanser.	Cleaning from top to bottom and center to outside ensures that cleaning occurs from the least to most contaminated area and a previously cleaned area is not contaminated again. Using a single gauze for each wipe ensures that the previously cleaned area is not contaminated again.
18. Once the wound is cleaned, dry the area using a gauze sponge in the same manner. Apply ointment or perform other treatments, as ordered (Fig. 9).	Moisture provides a medium for growth of microorganisms. The growth of microorganisms may be inhibited and the healing process improved with the use of ordered ointments or other applications.
19. If a drain is in use at the wound location, clean around the drain.	Cleaning the insertion site helps prevent infection.
20. Apply a layer of dry, sterile dressing over the wound (Fig. 10). Forceps may be used to apply the dressing.	Primary dressing serves as a wick for drainage. Use of forceps helps ensure that sterile technique is maintained.

FIGURE 7. Putting on sterile gloves.

FIGURE 8. Cleaning wound with dampened gauze.

FIGURE 9. Applying antimicrobial ointment to wound with cotton applicator.

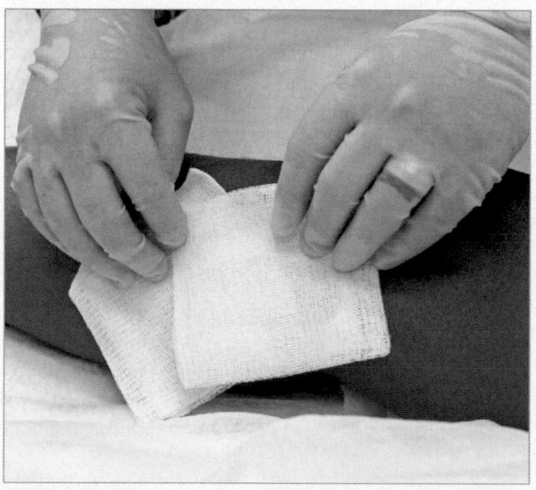

FIGURE 10. Applying dry dressing to site.

(continued)

SKILL 31-1   CLEANING A WOUND AND APPLYING A DRY, STERILE DRESSING   *continued*

ACTION	RATIONALE
21. Place a second layer of gauze over the wound site, as necessary.	A second layer provides for increased absorption of drainage.
22. Apply a surgical or abdominal pad (ABD) over the gauze at the site as the outermost layer of the dressing, as necessary (Fig. 11).	The dressing acts as additional protection for the wound against microorganisms in the environment and increased absorption of drainage.

FIGURE 11. Applying a surgical pad over dressing and securing with tape.

ACTION	RATIONALE
23. Remove and discard gloves. Apply tape, Montgomery straps or roller gauze to secure the dressings. Alternately, many commercial wound products are self-adhesive and do not require additional tape.	Proper disposal of gloves prevents the spread of microorganisms. Tape or other securing products are easier to apply after gloves have been removed.
24. After securing the dressing, label it with date and time. Remove all remaining equipment; place the patient in a comfortable position, with the side rails up and the bed in the lowest position.	Recording date and time provides communication and demonstrates adherence to the plan of care. Proper patient and bed positioning promotes safety and comfort.
25. Remove PPE, if used. Perform hand hygiene.	Removing PPE properly reduces the risk for infection transmission and contamination of other items. Hand hygiene prevents the spread of microorganisms.
26. Check all wound dressings every shift. More frequent checks may be needed if the wound is more complex or dressings become saturated quickly.	Checking dressings ensures the assessment of changes in patient condition and timely intervention to prevent complications.

DOCUMENTATION

Guidelines

Document the location of the wound and that the dressing was removed. Record your assessment of the wound, including approximation of wound edges; presence of sutures, staples, or adhesive closure strips; and the condition of the surrounding skin. Note if redness, edema, or drainage is observed. Document cleansing of the incision with normal saline and any application of antibiotic ointment as ordered. Record the type of dressing that was reapplied. Note pertinent patient and family education and any patient reaction to this procedure, including patient's pain level and effectiveness of nonpharmacologic interventions or analgesia if administered.

Sample Documentation

DocuCare Practice documenting wound care in *Lippincott DocuCare*.

> 9/8/15 0600 Dressing removed from left lateral calf incision. Scant purulent secretions noted on dressing. Incision edges approximately 1 mm apart, red, with ecchymosis and edema present. Small amount of purulent drainage from wound noted. Area cleansed with normal saline, dried, antibiotic ointment applied per order. Surrounding tissue red and ecchymotic. Redressed with nonadhering dressing, gauze, and wrapped with stretch gauze. Patient reports adequate pain control after preprocedure analgesic; states pain is dull ache, 1/10 on pain scale.
>
> —N. Joiner, RN

UNEXPECTED SITUATIONS AND ASSOCIATED INTERVENTIONS

- *The previous wound assessment states that the incision was clean and dry and the wound edges were approximated, with the staples and surgical drain intact. The surrounding tissue was without inflammation, edema, or erythema. After the dressing is removed, the nurse notes the incision edges are not approximated at the distal end, multiple staples are evident in the old dressing, the surrounding skin tissue is red and swollen, and purulent drainage is on the dressing and leaking from the wound:* Assess the patient for any other signs and symptoms, such as pain, malaise, fever, and paresthesias. Place a dry sterile dressing over the wound site. Report the findings to the primary care provider and document the event in the patient's record. Be prepared to obtain a wound culture and implement any changes in wound care as ordered.

- *After the nurse has put on sterile gloves, the patient moves too close to the edge of the bed and the nurse must support her with his hands to prevent the patient from falling:* If nothing else in the sterile field was touched, remove the contaminated gloves and put on new sterile gloves. If you did not bring a second pair, use the call bell to summon a coworker to provide a new pair of gloves.

- *The nurse has set up dressing supplies, removed the old dressing, and put on sterile gloves to clean the wound. The nurse then realizes that a necessary piece of dressing material has been forgotten:* Ask the patient to press the call bell to summon a coworker to provide the missing supplies.

SPECIAL CONSIDERATIONS

General Considerations

- Instruct the patient, if appropriate, and ancillary staff members to observe for excessive drainage that may overwhelm the dressing. They should also report when dressings become soiled or loosened from the skin.

Older Adult Considerations

- The skin of older adults is less elastic and more sensitive; use paper tape, Montgomery straps, or roller gauze (on extremities) to prevent tearing of the skin.

SKILL 31-2   APPLYING A SALINE-MOISTENED DRESSING

DELEGATION CONSIDERATIONS

Wound care and procedures requiring the use of a sterile field and other sterile items are not delegated to nursing assistive personnel (NAP) or to unlicensed assistive personnel (UAP). Depending on the state's nurse practice act and the organization's policies and procedures, these procedures may be delegated to licensed practical/vocational nurses (LPN/LVNs). The decision to delegate must be based on careful analysis of the patient's needs and circumstances, as well as the qualifications of the person to whom the task is being delegated. Refer to the Delegation Guidelines in Appendix A (found on thePoint).

(continued)

SKILL 31-2 APPLYING A SALINE-MOISTENED DRESSING *continued*

EQUIPMENT

- Clean, disposable gloves
- Sterile gloves, if indicated
- Additional PPE, as indicated
- Sterile dressing set or suture set (for the sterile scissors and forceps)
- Sterile thin-mesh gauze dressing for packing, if ordered
- Sterile gauze dressings
- Surgical or abdominal pads
- Skin-protectant wipes
- Sterile basin

- Sterile cleaning solution as ordered (commonly 0.9% normal saline solution)
- Sterile saline
- Tape or ties
- Plastic bag or other appropriate waste container for soiled dressings
- Sterile cotton-tipped applicators
- Supplies for wound cleansing or irrigation, as necessary
- Waterproof pad and bath blanket

IMPLEMENTATION

ACTION	RATIONALE
1. Review the medical orders for wound care or the nursing plan of care related to wound care. Gather necessary supplies.	Reviewing the order and plan of care validates the correct patient and correct procedure. Preparation promotes efficient time management and an organized approach to the task.
2. Perform hand hygiene and put on PPE, if indicated.	Hand hygiene and PPE prevent the spread of microorganisms. PPE is required based on transmission precautions.
3. Identify the patient.	Identifying the patient ensures that the right patient receives the intervention and helps prevent errors.
4. Assemble equipment on the overbed table within reach.	Organization facilitates performance of the task.
5. Close the curtains around the bed and close the door to the room if possible. Explain what you are going to do and why you are going to do it to the patient.	This ensures the patient's privacy. Explanation relieves anxiety and facilitates cooperation.
6. Assess the patient for possible need for nonpharmacologic pain-reducing interventions or analgesic medication before wound care dressing change. Administer the appropriate prescribed analgesic. Allow enough time for the analgesic to achieve its effectiveness.	Pain is a subjective experience influenced by past experience. Wound care and dressing changes may cause pain for some patients.
7. Place a waste receptacle or bag at a convenient location for use during the procedure.	Having a waste container handy means the soiled dressing may be discarded easily, without the spread of microorganisms.
8. Adjust the bed to a comfortable working height, usually elbow height of the caregiver (VISN 8, 2009).	Having the bed at the proper height prevents back and muscle strain.
9. Assist the patient to a comfortable position that provides easy access to the wound area. Position the patient so that the wound cleanser or irrigation solution will flow from the clean end of the wound toward the dirtier end, if being used (see Skill 31-1). Use the bath blanket to cover any exposed area other than the wound. Place a waterproof pad under the wound site.	Patient positioning and use of a bath blanket provide for comfort and warmth. Gravity directs the flow of liquid from the least contaminated to the most contaminated area. Waterproof pad protects underlying surfaces.
10. Put on clean gloves. Carefully and gently remove the soiled dressings. If there is resistance, use a silicone-based adhesive remover to help remove the tape. If any part of the dressing sticks to the underlying skin, use small amounts of sterile saline to help loosen and remove it.	Gloves protect the nurse from handling contaminated dressings. Cautious removal of the dressing is more comfortable for the patient and ensures that any drain present is not removed. A silicone-based adhesive remover allows for the easy, rapid, and painless removal without the associated problems of skin stripping (Denyer, 2011; Benbow, 2011). Sterile saline moistens the dressing for easier removal and minimizes damage and pain.
11. After removing the dressing, note the presence, amount, type, color, and odor of any drainage on the dressings. Place soiled dressings in the appropriate waste receptacle.	The presence of drainage should be documented. Discarding dressings appropriately prevents the spread of microorganisms.

ACTION

12. Assess the wound for appearance, stage, the presence of eschar, granulation tissue, epithelialization, undermining, tunneling, necrosis, sinus tract, and drainage. Assess the appearance of the surrounding tissue. Measure the wound.

13. Remove your gloves and put them in the receptacle.

14. Using sterile technique, open the supplies and dressings. Place the fine-mesh gauze into the basin and pour the ordered solution over the mesh to saturate it.

15. Put on sterile gloves. Alternately, clean gloves (clean technique) may be used to clean a chronic wound or pressure ulcer.

16. Clean the wound. Refer to Skill 31-1. Alternately, irrigate the wound, as ordered or required (see Skill 31-3, pp. 1013–1016).

17. Dry the surrounding skin with sterile gauze dressings.

18. Apply a skin protectant to the surrounding skin, if needed.

19. If not already on, put on sterile gloves. Squeeze excess fluid from the gauze dressing. Unfold and fluff the dressing.

20. Gently press to loosely pack the moistened gauze into the wound (Fig. 1). If necessary, use the forceps or cotton-tipped applicators to press the gauze into all wound surfaces (Fig. 2).

RATIONALE

This information provides evidence about the wound healing process and/or the presence of infection.

Discarding gloves prevents the spread of microorganisms.

Gauze touching the wound surface must be moistened to increase the absorptive ability and promote healing.

Sterile gloves maintain surgical asepsis. Clean technique is appropriate when cleaning chronic wounds and pressure ulcers.

Cleaning the wound removes previous drainage and wound debris.

Moisture provides a medium for growth of microorganisms.

A skin protectant prevents skin irritation and breakdown.

Sterile gloves prevent contamination of the dressing material. The gauze provides a thin, moist layer to contact all the wound surfaces.

The dressing provides a moist environment for all wound surfaces. Avoid overpacking the gauze; loosely pack to prevent too much pressure in the wound bed, which could impede wound healing.

FIGURE 1. Gently pressing gauze into wound.

FIGURE 2. Using a cotton-tipped applicator to press gauze into all wound surfaces.

21. Apply several dry, sterile gauze pads over the wet gauze.

22. Place the ABD pad over the gauze.

23. Remove and discard gloves. Apply tape, Montgomery straps or roller gauze to secure the dressings. Alternately, many commercial wound products are self-adhesive and do not require additional tape.

24. After securing the dressing, label the dressing with the date and time. Remove all remaining equipment; place the patient in a comfortable position, with the side rails up and the bed in the lowest position.

Dry gauze absorbs excess moisture and drainage.

The ABD pad prevents contamination.

Proper disposal of gloves prevents the spread of microorganisms. Tape or other securing products are easier to apply after gloves have been removed.

Recording the date and time provides communication and demonstrates adherence to the plan of care. Proper patient and bed positioning promotes safety and comfort.

(continued)

SKILL 31-2 APPLYING A SALINE-MOISTENED DRESSING *continued*

ACTION	**RATIONALE**
25. Remove PPE, if used. Perform hand hygiene.	Removing PPE properly reduces the risk for infection transmission and contamination of other items. Hand hygiene prevents the spread of microorganisms.
26. Check all wound dressings every shift. More frequent checks may be needed if the wound is more complex or dressings become saturated quickly.	Checking dressings ensures the assessment of changes in patient condition and timely intervention to prevent complications.

DOCUMENTATION

Guidelines

Document the location of the wound and that the dressing was removed. Record your assessment of the wound, including evidence of granulation tissue, presence of necrotic tissue, stage (if appropriate), and characteristics of drainage. Include the appearance of the surrounding skin. Document the cleansing or irrigation of the wound and solution used. Record the type of dressing that was reapplied. Note pertinent patient and family education and any patient reaction to this procedure, including patient's pain level and effectiveness of nonpharmacologic interventions or analgesia if administered.

Sample Documentation

11/20/15 1645 Healing abdominal incision with granulating tissue noted. Open area 2 cm × 4 cm × 0.5 cm depth in center of incision. No evidence of necrosis or tunneling. Scant amount of serous drainage. Saline-moistened dressing applied to open wound; covered loosely with ABD dressing. Patient denies pain from incision. Instructed patient that moist saline gauze will facilitate the healing process and to notify nurse for any discomfort related to incision.

—R. Dobbins, RN

UNEXPECTED SITUATIONS AND RELATED INTERVENTIONS

- *When removing a patient's dressing, the assessment reveals eschar in the wound:* Notify the primary care provider or wound care specialist; a different treatment modality and/or débridement may be necessary. The presence of eschar in a wound precludes the staging of the wound. The eschar must be removed for adequate pressure ulcer staging to be done. However, note that stable (dry, adherent, intact, without erythema or movement) eschar on the heels serves as "the body's natural (biological) cover" and should not be removed (NPUAP, 2012a).

- *The wound assessment reveals several depressions or crater-like areas on inspection of a wound:* Notify the primary care provider or wound care specialist, who may order the wound to be packed. Pack wound cavities loosely with dressing material. Overpacking may increase pressure and interfere with tissue healing.

- *The nurse notes that the wound dressing is dry upon removal:* Reduce the time interval between changes to prevent drying of the materials, which may disrupt healing tissue.

SPECIAL CONSIDERATIONS

- Make sure ancillary staff understand the importance of reporting excessive drainage from the dressing, and any soiled or loose dressings.

- Guidelines from the Wound, Ostomy and Continence Nurses Society (WOCN) recommend that clean gloves may be used to treat chronic wounds and pressure ulcers as long as infection-control procedures are followed. The *no-touch technique* may be used within these guidelines. Clean gloves are used to handle dressing material. Irrigants and dressings are sterile. The wound is redressed by picking up dressing materials by the corner and placing the untouched side over the wound (WOCN, 2012).

- Many products are available to treat chronic wounds and pressure ulcers. Treatment varies based on facility policy, nursing protocol, clinical specialist referrals, primary care provider orders, and product in use.

SKILL 31-3 PERFORMING IRRIGATION OF A WOUND

DELEGATION CONSIDERATIONS

Irrigation of a wound and procedures requiring the use of a sterile field and other sterile items are not delegated to nursing assistive personnel (NAP) or to unlicensed assistive personnel (UAP). Depending on the state's nurse practice act and the organization's policies and procedures, these procedures may be delegated to licensed practical/vocational nurses (LPN/LVNs). The decision to delegate must be based on careful analysis of the patient's needs and circumstances, as well as the qualifications of the person to whom the task is being delegated. Refer to the Delegation Guidelines in Appendix A (found on thePoint).

EQUIPMENT

- A sterile irrigation set, including a basin, irrigant container, and irrigation syringe
- Sterile irrigation solution as ordered, warmed to body temperature, commonly 0.9% normal saline solution
- Plastic bag or other waste container to dispose of soiled dressings
- Sterile gloves
- Sterile drape (may be optional)
- Clean, disposable gloves

- Moisture-proof gown, mask, and eye protection
- Additional PPE, as indicated
- Sterile dressing set or suture set (for the sterile scissors and forceps)
- Waterproof pad and bath blanket, as needed
- Sterile gauze dressings
- Sterile packing gauze, as needed
- Tape or ties
- Skin-protectant wipes

IMPLEMENTATION

ACTION	**RATIONALE**
1. Review the medical orders for wound care or the nursing plan of care related to wound care. Gather the necessary supplies.	Reviewing the order and plan of care validates the correct patient and correct procedure. Preparation promotes efficient time management and an organized approach to the task.
2. Perform hand hygiene and put on PPE, if indicated.	Hand hygiene and PPE prevent the spread of microorganisms. PPE is required based on transmission precautions.
3. Identify the patient.	Identifying the patient ensures that the right patient receives the intervention and helps prevent errors.
4. Assemble the equipment on the overbed table within reach.	Organization facilitates performance of the task.
5. Close the curtains around the bed and close the door to the room if possible. Explain what you are going to do and why you are going to do it to the patient.	This ensures the patient's privacy. Explanation relieves anxiety and facilitates cooperation.
6. Assess the patient for the possible need for nonpharmacologic pain-reducing interventions or analgesic medication before wound care and/or dressing change. Administer the appropriate prescribed analgesic. Allow enough time for the analgesic to achieve its effectiveness before beginning the procedure.	Pain is a subjective experience influenced by past experience. Wound care and dressing changes may cause pain for some patients.
7. Place a waste receptacle or bag at a convenient location for use during the procedure.	Having a waste container handy means the soiled dressing may be discarded easily, without the spread of microorganisms.
8. Adjust the bed to a comfortable working height, usually elbow height of the caregiver (VISN 8, 2009).	Having the bed at the proper height prevents back and muscle strain.
9. Assist the patient to a comfortable position that provides easy access to the wound area. Position the patient so that the irrigation solution will flow from the clean end of the wound toward the dirtier end. Use the bath blanket to cover any exposed area other than the wound. Place a waterproof pad under the wound site.	Patient positioning and the use of a bath blanket provide for comfort and warmth. Gravity directs the flow of liquid from the least contaminated to the most contaminated area. Waterproof pad protects underlying surfaces.

(continued)

SKILL 31-3 PERFORMING IRRIGATION OF A WOUND *continued*

ACTION	RATIONALE
10. Put on a gown, mask, and eye protection.	Using PPE such as gowns, masks, and eye protection is part of *Standard Precautions.* A gown protects clothes from contamination should splashing occur. Goggles protect mucous membranes of the eyes from contact with irrigant fluid or wound drainage.
11. Put on clean gloves. Carefully and gently remove the soiled dressings. If there is resistance, use a silicone-based adhesive remover to help remove the tape. If any part of the dressing sticks to the underlying skin, use small amounts of sterile saline to help loosen and remove it.	Gloves protect the nurse from handling contaminated dressings. Cautious removal of the dressing is more comfortable for the patient and ensures that any drain present is not removed. A silicone-based adhesive remover allows for the easy, rapid, and painless removal without the associated problems of skin stripping (Denyer, 2011; Benbow, 2011). Sterile saline moistens the dressing for easier removal and minimizes damage and pain.
12. After removing the dressing, note the presence, amount, type, color, and odor of any drainage on the dressings. Place soiled dressings in the appropriate waste receptacle.	The presence of drainage should be documented. Discarding dressings appropriately prevents the spread of microorganisms.
13. Assess the wound for appearance, stage, presence of eschar, granulation tissue, epithelialization, undermining, tunneling, necrosis, sinus tract, and drainage. Assess the appearance of the surrounding tissue. Measure the wound.	This information provides evidence about the wound healing process and/or the presence of infection.
14. Remove your gloves and put them in the receptacle.	Discarding gloves prevents the spread of microorganisms.
15. Set up a sterile field, if indicated, and wound cleaning supplies. Pour warmed sterile irrigating solution into the sterile container. Put on the sterile gloves. Alternately, clean gloves (clean technique) may be used when irrigating a chronic wound or pressure ulcer.	Using warmed solution prevents chilling the patient and may minimize patient discomfort. Sterile technique and gloves maintain surgical asepsis. Clean technique is appropriate for irrigating chronic wounds or pressure ulcers.
16. Position the sterile basin below the wound to collect the irrigation fluid.	Patient and bed linens are protected from contaminated fluid.
17. Fill the irrigation syringe with solution (Fig. 1). **Using your nondominant hand, gently apply pressure to the basin against the skin below the wound to form a seal with the skin (Fig. 2).**	The solution will collect in the basin and prevent the irrigant from running down the skin. Patient and bed linens are protected from contaminated fluid.

FIGURE 1. Drawing up sterile solution from sterile container into irrigation syringe.

FIGURE 2. Patient lying on side with wound exposed, sterile collection container placed against skin, bed protected with waterproof pad.

ACTION	RATIONALE
18. **Gently direct a stream of solution into the wound (Fig. 3). Keep the tip of the syringe at least 1 inch above the upper tip of the wound. When using a catheter tip, insert it gently into the wound until it meets resistance. Gently flush all wound areas.**	Debris and contaminated solution flow from the least contaminated to most contaminated area. High-pressure irrigation flow may cause patient discomfort as well as damage granulation tissue. A catheter tip allows the introduction of irrigant into a wound with a small opening or one that is deep.
19. Watch for the solution to flow smoothly and evenly. When the solution from the wound flows out clear, discontinue irrigation.	Irrigation removes exudate and debris.
20. Dry the surrounding skin with gauze dressings (Fig. 4).	Moisture provides a medium for growth of microorganisms. Excess moisture can contribute to skin irritation and breakdown.
21. Apply a skin protectant to the surrounding skin.	A skin protectant prevents skin irritation and breakdown.
22. Apply a new dressing to the wound (see Skills 31-1 and 31-2, Fig. 5).	Dressings absorb drainage, protect the wound, and promote healing.

FIGURE 3. Irrigating wound with a gentle stream of solution. Solution drains into collection container.

FIGURE 4. Drying around wound, not in wound, with sterile gauze pad.

FIGURE 5. Applying a new dressing.

(continued)

SKILL 31-3 PERFORMING IRRIGATION OF A WOUND *continued*

ACTION	**RATIONALE**
23. Remove and discard gloves. Apply tape, Montgomery straps, or roller gauze to secure the dressings. Alternately, many commercial wound products are self-adhesive and do not require additional tape.	Tape or other securing products are easier to apply after gloves have been removed. Proper disposal of gloves prevents the spread of microorganisms.
24. After securing the dressing, label it with date and time. Remove all remaining equipment; place the patient in a comfortable position, with side rails up and bed in the lowest position.	Recording the date and time provides communication and demonstrates adherence to the plan of care. Proper patient and bed positioning promotes safety and comfort.
25. Remove remaining PPE. Perform hand hygiene.	Removing PPE properly reduces the risk for infection transmission and contamination of other items. Hand hygiene prevents the spread of microorganisms.
26. Check all wound dressings every shift. More frequent checks may be needed if the wound is more complex or dressings become saturated quickly.	Checking dressings ensures the assessment of changes in patient condition and timely intervention to prevent complications.

DOCUMENTATION

Guidelines

Document the location of the wound and that the dressing was removed. Record your assessment of the wound, including evidence of granulation tissue, presence of necrotic tissue, stage (if appropriate), and characteristics of drainage. Include the appearance of the surrounding skin. Document the irrigation of the wound and solution used. Record the type of dressing that was applied. Note pertinent patient and family education and any patient reaction to this procedure, including patient's pain level and effectiveness of nonpharmacologic interventions or analgesia if administered.

Sample Documentation

> <u>3/5/15</u> 1700 Dressing removed from left outer heel area. Minimal serosanguineous drainage noted on dressings. Wound 4 × 5 × 2 cm, pink, with granulation tissue evident. Surrounding skin tone consistent with patient's skin, no edema or redness noted. Irrigated with normal saline, and hydrogel dressing applied.
>
> —J. Lark, RN

UNEXPECTED SITUATIONS AND ASSOCIATED INTERVENTIONS

- *The patient experiences pain when the wound irrigation is begun:* Stop the procedure and administer an analgesic as ordered. Obtain new sterile supplies and begin the procedure after an appropriate amount of time has elapsed to allow the analgesic to begin working. Note the patient's pain on the nursing plan of care so that pain medication can be given before future wound treatments.

- *During the wound irrigation, the nurse notes bleeding from the wound. This has not been documented as happening with previous irrigations:* Stop the procedure. Assess the patient for other symptoms. Obtain vital signs. Report the findings to the primary care provider and document the event in the patient's record.

SKILL 31-4 CARING FOR A JACKSON-PRATT DRAIN

DELEGATION GUIDELINES

Care for a Jackson-Pratt drain insertion site is not delegated to nursing assistive personnel (NAP) or to unlicensed assistive personnel (UAP). Depending on the organization's policies and procedures, the drain may be emptied and reconstituted by nursing assistive personnel (NAP) or unlicensed assistive personnel (UAP). Depending on the state's nurse practice act and the organization's policies and procedures, these procedures may be delegated to licensed practical/vocational nurses (LPN/LVNs). The decision to delegate must be based on careful analysis of the patient's needs and circumstances, as well as the qualifications of the person to whom the task is being delegated. Refer to the Delegation Guidelines in Appendix A (found on thePoint).

EQUIPMENT

- Graduated container for measuring drainage
- Clean, disposable gloves
- Additional PPE, as indicated
- Cleansing solution, usually sterile normal saline
- Sterile gauze pads
- Skin-protectant wipes
- Dressing materials for site dressing, if used

IMPLEMENTATION

ACTION	RATIONALE
1. Review the medical orders for wound care or the nursing plan of care related to wound/drain care. Gather necessary supplies.	Reviewing the order and plan of care validates the correct patient and correct procedure. Preparation promotes efficient time management and organized approach to the task.
2. Perform hand hygiene and put on PPE, if indicated.	Hand hygiene and PPE prevent the spread of microorganisms. PPE is required based on transmission precautions.
3. Identify the patient.	Identifying the patient ensures that the right patient receives the intervention and helps prevent errors.
4. Assemble equipment on the overbed table within reach.	Organization facilitates performance of the task.
5. Close the curtains around the bed and close the door to the room, if possible. Explain what you are going to do and why you are going to do it to the patient.	This ensures the patient's privacy. Explanation relieves anxiety and facilitates cooperation.
6. Assess the patient for possible need for nonpharmacologic pain-reducing interventions or analgesic medication before wound care dressing change. Administer the appropriate prescribed analgesic. Allow enough time for the analgesic to achieve its effectiveness before beginning the procedure.	Pain is a subjective experience influenced by past experience. Wound care and dressing changes may cause pain for some patients.
7. Place a waste receptacle at a convenient location for use during the procedure.	Having a waste container handy means that the soiled dressing may be discarded easily, without the spread of microorganisms.
8. Adjust the bed to a comfortable working height, usually elbow height of the caregiver (VISN 8, 2009).	Having the bed at the proper height prevents back and muscle strain.
9. Assist the patient to a comfortable position that provides easy access to the drain and/or wound area. Use a bath blanket to cover any exposed area other than the wound. Place a waterproof pad under the wound site.	Patient positioning and use of a bath blanket provide comfort and warmth. Waterproof pad protects underlying surfaces.
10. Put on clean gloves; put on a mask or face shield, as indicated.	Gloves prevent the spread of microorganisms; mask reduces the risk of transmission should splashing occur.

(continued)

SKILL 31-4 CARING FOR A JACKSON-PRATT DRAIN *continued*

ACTION	RATIONALE

11. Place the graduated collection container under the drain outlet. Without contaminating the outlet valve, pull off the cap. The chamber will expand completely as it draws in air. **Empty the chamber's contents completely into the container (Fig. 1). Use the gauze pad to clean the outlet. Fully compress the chamber with one hand and replace the cap with your other hand (Fig. 2).**

Emptying the drainage allows for accurate measurement. Cleaning the outlet reduces the risk of contamination and helps prevent the spread of microorganisms. Compressing the chamber reestablishes the suction.

FIGURE 1. Emptying contents of Jackson-Pratt drain into collection container.

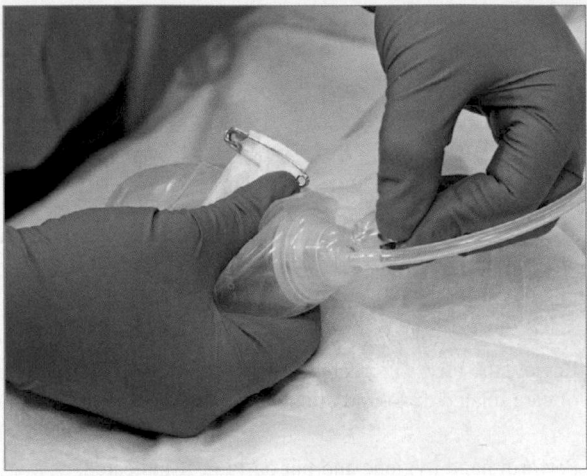

FIGURE 2. Compressing Jackson-Pratt drain and replacing cap.

12. Check the patency of the equipment. **Make sure the tubing is free from twists and kinks.**

Patent, untwisted, or unkinked tubing promotes appropriate wound drainage.

13. Secure the Jackson-Pratt drain to the patient's gown below the wound with a safety pin, **making sure that there is no tension on the tubing.**

Securing the drain prevents injury to the patient and accidental removal of the drain.

14. Carefully measure and record the character, color, and amount of the drainage. Discard the drainage according to facility policy. Remove gloves.

Documentation promotes continuity of care and communication. Appropriate disposal of biohazard material reduces the risk for microorganism transmission.

15. Put on clean gloves. If the drain site has a dressing, redress the site. Include cleaning of the sutures with the gauze pad moistened with normal saline. Dry sutures with gauze before applying the new dressing.

Dressing protects the site. Cleaning and drying sutures deters growth of microorganisms.

16. If the drain site is open to air, observe the sutures that secure the drain to the skin. Look for signs of pulling, tearing, swelling, or infection of the surrounding skin. Gently clean the sutures with the gauze pad moistened with normal saline. Dry with a new gauze pad. Apply skin protectant to the surrounding skin, if needed.

Early detection of problems leads to prompt intervention and prevents complications. Gentle cleaning and drying prevent the growth of microorganisms. Skin protectant prevents skin irritation and breakdown.

17. Remove and discard gloves. Remove all remaining equipment; place the patient in a comfortable position, with the side rails up and the bed in the lowest position.

Proper removal of gloves prevents spread of microorganisms. Proper patient and bed positioning promotes safety and comfort.

18. Remove additional PPE, if used. Perform hand hygiene.

Removing PPE properly reduces the risk for infection transmission and contamination of other items. Hand hygiene prevents the spread of microorganisms.

19. Check drain status at least every 4 hours. Check all wound dressings every shift. Perform more frequent checks if the wound is more complex or dressings become saturated quickly.

Checking the drain ensures proper functioning and early detection of problems. Checking dressings ensures the assessment of changes in patient condition and timely intervention to prevent complications.

DOCUMENTATION
Guidelines

Document the location of the wound and drain, the assessment of the wound and drain site, and patency of the drain. Note if sutures are intact. Document the presence and characteristics of drainage on the old dressing upon removal. Include the appearance of the surrounding skin. Document cleansing of the drain site. Record any skin care and the dressing applied. Note that the drain was emptied and recompressed. Note pertinent patient and family education and any patient reaction to the procedure, including patient's pain level and effectiveness of nonpharmacologic interventions or analgesia, if administered. Document the amount and characteristics of drainage obtained on the appropriate intake and output record.

Sample Documentation

2/7/15 2400 Right chest incision and drain open to air. Wound edges approximated, slight ecchymosis, no edema, redness, or drainage. Steri-Strips intact. J-P drain patent and secured with suture. Exit site without edema, drainage, or redness. Drain emptied and recompressed. 40 mL sanguineous drainage recorded.
—Carol White, RN

UNEXPECTED SITUATIONS AND ASSOCIATED INTERVENTIONS

- *A patient has a Jackson-Pratt drain in the right lower quadrant following abdominal surgery. The record indicates that it has been draining serosanguineous fluid, 40 to 50 mL every shift. While performing your initial assessment, you note that the dressing around the drain site is saturated with serosanguineous secretions and there is minimal drainage in the collection chamber:* Inspect the tubing for kinks or obstruction. Assess the patient for changes in condition. Remove the dressing and assess the site. Often, if the tubing becomes blocked with a blood clot or drainage particles, the wound drainage will leak around the exit site of the drain. Cleanse the area and redress the site. Notify the primary care provider of the findings and document the event in the patient's record.

- *Your patient calls you to the room and says, "I found this in the bed when I went to get up." He has his Jackson-Pratt drain in his hand. It is completely removed from the patient:* Assess the patient for any new and abnormal signs or symptoms, and assess the surgical site and drain site. Apply a sterile dressing with gauze and tape to the drain site. Notify the primary care provider of the findings and document the event in the patient's record.

SPECIAL CONSIDERATIONS

- Often patients have more than one Jackson-Pratt drain. Number or letter the drains for easy identification. Record the drainage from each drain separately, identified by the number or letter, on the intake and output record.

- When the patient with a drain is ready to ambulate, empty and compress the drain before activity. Secure the drain to the patient's gown below the wound, making sure there is no tension on the drainage tubing. This removes excess drainage, maintains maximum suction, and avoids strain on the drain's suture line.

SKILL 31-5 CARING FOR A HEMOVAC DRAIN

DELEGATION GUIDELINES

Care for a Hemovac drain insertion site is not delegated to nursing assistive personnel (NAP) or to unlicensed assistive personnel (UAP). Depending on the organization's policies and procedures, the drain may be emptied and reconstituted by nursing assistive personnel (NAP) or to unlicensed assistive personnel (UAP). Depending on the state's nurse practice act and the organization's policies and procedures, these procedures may be delegated to licensed practical/vocational nurses (LPN/LVNs). The decision to delegate must be based on careful analysis of the patient's needs and circumstances, as well as the qualifications of the person to whom the task is being delegated. Refer to the Delegation Guidelines in Appendix A (found on thePoint).

(continued)

SKILL 31-5 CARING FOR A HEMOVAC DRAIN *continued*

EQUIPMENT

- Graduated container for measuring drainage
- Clean, disposable gloves
- Additional PPE, as indicated
- Cleansing solution, usually sterile normal saline
- Sterile gauze pads
- Skin-protectant wipes
- Dressing materials for site dressing, if used

IMPLEMENTATION

ACTION	RATIONALE
1. Review the medical orders for wound care or the nursing plan of care related to wound/drain care. Gather necessary supplies.	Reviewing the order and plan of care validates the correct patient and correct procedure. Preparation promotes efficient time management and an organized approach to the task.
2. Perform hand hygiene and put on PPE, if indicated.	Hand hygiene and PPE prevent the spread of microorganisms. PPE is required based on transmission precautions.
3. Identify the patient.	Identifying the patient ensures that the right patient receives the intervention and helps prevent errors.
4. Assemble equipment on the overbed table within reach.	Organization facilitates performance of the task.
5. Close curtains around the bed and close the door to the room, if possible. Explain what you are going to do and why you are going to do it to the patient.	This ensures the patient's privacy. Explanation relieves anxiety and facilitates cooperation.
6. Assess the patient for the possible need for nonpharmacologic pain-reducing interventions or analgesic medication before wound care dressing change. Administer the appropriate prescribed analgesic. Allow enough time for the analgesic to achieve its effectiveness before beginning the procedure.	Pain is a subjective experience influenced by past experience. Wound care and dressing changes may cause pain for some patients.
7. Place a waste receptacle at a convenient location for use during the procedure.	Having a waste container handy means that the soiled dressing may be discarded easily, without the spread of microorganisms.
8. Adjust the bed to a comfortable working height, usually elbow height of the caregiver (VISN 8, 2009).	Having the bed at the proper height prevents back and muscle strain.
9. Assist the patient to a comfortable position that provides easy access to the drain and/or wound area. Use a bath blanket to cover any exposed area other than the wound. Place a waterproof pad under the wound site.	Patient positioning and use of a bath blanket provide comfort and warmth. Waterproof pad protects underlying surfaces.
10. Put on clean gloves; put on a mask or face shield, as indicated.	Gloves prevent the spread of microorganisms; mask reduces the risk of transmission should splashing occur.
11. Place the graduated collection container under the drain outlet. **Without contaminating the outlet, pull off the cap.** The chamber will expand completely as it draws in air. **Empty the chamber's contents completely into the container (Fig. 1). Use the gauze pad to clean the outlet. Fully compress the chamber by pushing the top and bottom together with your hands. Keep the device tightly compressed while you apply the cap (Fig. 2).**	Emptying the drainage allows for accurate measurement. Cleaning the outlet reduces the risk of contamination and helps prevent the spread of microorganisms. Compressing the chamber reestablishes the suction.
12. Check the patency of the equipment. **Make sure that the tubing is free from twists and kinks.**	Patent, untwisted, or unkinked tubing promotes appropriate drainage from the wound.
13. Secure the Hemovac drain to the patient's gown below the wound with a safety pin, **making sure that there is no tension on the tubing.**	Securing the drain prevents injury to the patient and accidental removal of the drain.
14. Carefully measure and record the character, color, and amount of the drainage. Discard the drainage according to facility policy.	Documentation promotes continuity of care and communication. Appropriate disposal of biohazard material reduces the risk for microorganism transmission. Proper disposal of gloves deters transmission of microorganisms.

ACTION

FIGURE 1. Emptying Hemovac drain into collection container.

RATIONALE

FIGURE 2. Compressing the Hemovac and securing the cap.

ACTION	RATIONALE
15. Put on clean gloves. If the drain site has a dressing, redress the site. Include cleaning of the sutures with the gauze pad moistened with normal saline. Dry sutures with gauze before applying new dressing.	Dressing protects the site. Cleaning and drying sutures deters growth of microorganisms.
16. If the drain site is open to air, observe the sutures that secure the drain to the skin. Look for signs of pulling, tearing, swelling, or infection of the surrounding skin. Gently clean the sutures with the gauze pad moistened with normal saline. Dry with a new gauze pad. Apply skin protectant to the surrounding skin, if needed.	Early detection of problems leads to prompt intervention and prevents complications. Gentle cleaning and drying prevent the growth of microorganisms. Skin protectant prevents skin irritation and breakdown.
17. Remove and discard gloves. Remove all remaining equipment; place the patient in a comfortable position, with the side rails up and the bed in the lowest position.	Proper removal and disposal of gloves prevents the spread of microorganisms. Proper patient and bed positioning promotes safety and comfort.
18. Remove additional PPE, if used. Perform hand hygiene.	Removing PPE properly reduces the risk for infection transmission and contamination of other items. Hand hygiene prevents the spread of microorganisms.
19. Check drain status at least every 4 hours. Check all wound dressings every shift. More frequent checks may be needed if the wound is more complex or dressings become saturated quickly.	Checking the drain ensures proper functioning and early detection of problems. Checking dressings ensures the assessment of changes in patient condition and timely intervention to prevent complications.

DOCUMENTATION

Guidelines

Document the location of the wound and drain, the assessment of the wound and drain site, and patency of the drain. Note whether sutures are intact. Document the presence and characteristics of drainage on the old dressing upon removal. Include the appearance of the surrounding skin. Document cleansing of the drain site. Record any skin care and any dressing applied. Note that the drain was emptied and recompressed. Note pertinent patient and family education and any patient reaction to this procedure, including patient's pain level and effectiveness of nonpharmacologic interventions or analgesia, if administered. Document the amount and characteristics of drainage obtained on the appropriate intake and output record.

(continued)

SKILL 31-5 | CARING FOR A HEMOVAC DRAIN *continued*

Sample Documentation

> 1/18/15 1000 Hemovac drain in place in left lower extremity, site open to air. Suture intact; exit site slightly pink, without redness, edema, or drainage. Surrounding skin without edema, ecchymosis, or redness. Exit site and suture cleansed with normal saline. Hemovac emptied of 90 mL sanguineous secretions and recompressed.
>
> —A. Smith, RN

UNEXPECTED SITUATIONS AND ASSOCIATED INTERVENTIONS

- *A patient has a Hemovac drain placed in the left knee following surgery. The record indicates it has been draining serosanguineous secretions, 40 to 50 mL every shift. While performing your initial assessment, you note that the collection chamber is completely expanded. The nurse empties the device and compresses to resume suction. A short time later, the nurse observes that the chamber is completely expanded again:* Inspect the tubing for kinks or obstruction. Inspect the device, looking for breaks in the integrity of the chamber. Make sure the cap is in place and closed. Assess the patient for changes in condition. Remove the dressing and assess the site. Make sure that the drainage tubing has not advanced out of the wound, exposing any of the perforations in the tubing. If you are not successful in maintaining the suction, notify the primary care provider of the findings and interventions and document the event in the patient's record.

SPECIAL CONSIDERATIONS

- When the patient with a drain is ready to ambulate, empty and compress the drain before activity. Secure the drain to the patient's gown below the wound, making sure there is no tension on the drainage tubing. This removes excess drainage, maintains maximum suction, and avoids strain on the drain's suture line.

SKILL 31-6 | COLLECTING A WOUND CULTURE

DELEGATION CONSIDERATIONS

Collection of a wound culture is not delegated to nursing assistive personnel (NAP) or to unlicensed assistive personnel (UAP). Depending on the state's nurse practice act and the organization's policies and procedures, collection of a wound culture may be delegated to licensed practical/vocational nurses (LPN/LVNs). The decision to delegate must be based on careful analysis of the patient's needs and circumstances, as well as the qualifications of the person to whom the task is being delegated. Refer to the Delegation Guidelines in Appendix A (found on thePoint).

EQUIPMENT

- A sterile Culturette kit (aerobic or anaerobic) with swab, or a culture tube with individual sterile swabs
- Sterile gloves
- Clean, disposable gloves
- Additional PPE, as indicated
- Plastic bag or appropriate waste receptacle
- Patient label for the sample tube
- Biohazard specimen bag
- Bath blanket (if necessary to drape the patient)
- Supplies to clean the wound and reapply a sterile dressing after obtaining the culture (Refer to Skills 31-1 and 31-2, pp. 1004–1012)

IMPLEMENTATION

ACTION	RATIONALE
1. Review the medical orders for obtaining a wound culture. Gather necessary supplies.	Reviewing the order and plan of care validates the correct patient and correct procedure. Preparation promotes efficient time management and an organized approach to the task.

ACTION	RATIONALE
2. Perform hand hygiene and put on PPE, if indicated.	Hand hygiene and PPE prevent the spread of microorganisms. PPE is required based on transmission precautions.
3. Identify the patient.	Identifying the patient ensures that the right patient receives the intervention and helps prevent errors.
4. Assemble equipment on the overbed table within reach.	Organization facilitates performance of the task.
5. Close curtains around the bed and close the door to the room if possible. Explain what you are going to do and why you are going to do it to the patient.	This ensures the patient's privacy. Explanation relieves anxiety and facilitates cooperation.
6. Assess the patient for the possible need for nonpharmacologic pain-reducing interventions or analgesic medication before obtaining the wound culture. Administer the appropriate prescribed analgesic. Allow enough time for the analgesic to achieve its effectiveness before beginning the procedure.	Pain is a subjective experience influenced by past experience. Wound care and dressing changes may cause pain for some patients.
7. Place an appropriate waste receptacle within easy reach for use during the procedure.	Having the waste container handy means that soiled materials may be discarded easily, without the spread of microorganisms.
8. Adjust the bed to a comfortable working height, usually elbow height of the caregiver (VISN 8, 2009).	Having the bed at the proper height prevents back and muscle strain.
9. Assist the patient to a comfortable position that provides easy access to the wound. If necessary, drape the patient with the bath blanket to expose only the wound area. Place a waterproof pad under the wound site. Check the culture label against the patient's identification bracelet (Fig. 1).	Patient positioning and use of a bath blanket provide for comfort and warmth. Checking the culture label with the patient's identification ensures that the correct patient undergoes the correct procedure.

FIGURE 1. Checking culture label with the patient's identification band.

10. If there is a dressing in place on the wound, put on clean gloves. Carefully and gently remove the soiled dressings. If there is resistance, use a silicone-based adhesive remover to help remove the tape. If any part of the dressing sticks to the underlying skin, use small amounts of sterile saline to help loosen and remove it.	Gloves protect the nurse from handling contaminated dressings. Cautious removal of the dressing is more comfortable for the patient and ensures that any drain present is not removed. A silicone-based adhesive remover allows for the easy, rapid, and painless removal without the associated problems of skin stripping (Denyer, 2011; Benbow, 2011). Sterile saline moistens the dressing for easier removal and minimizes damage and pain.
11. After removing the dressing, note the presence, amount, type, color, and odor of any drainage on the dressings. Place soiled dressings in the appropriate waste receptacle.	The presence of drainage should be documented. Discarding dressings appropriately prevents the spread of microorganisms.

(continued)

SKILL 31-6 | COLLECTING A WOUND CULTURE *continued*

ACTION	RATIONALE
12. Assess the wound for appearance, stage, presence of eschar, granulation tissue, epithelialization, undermining, tunneling, necrosis, sinus tract, and drainage. Assess the appearance of the surrounding tissue. Measure the wound.	This information provides evidence about the wound healing process and/or the presence of infection.
13. Remove your gloves and put them in the receptacle.	Discarding gloves prevents the spread of microorganisms.
14. Set up a sterile field, if indicated, and wound cleaning supplies. Put on the sterile gloves. Alternately, clean gloves (clean technique) may be used when cleaning a chronic wound.	Sterile gloves maintain surgical asepsis. Clean technique is appropriate when cleaning chronic wounds.
15. Clean the wound. Refer to Skill 31-1 on pp. 1004–1009. Alternately, irrigate the wound, as ordered or required (see Skill 31-3, pp. 1013–1016).	Cleaning the wound removes previous drainage and wound debris, which could introduce extraneous organisms into the collected specimen, resulting in inaccurate results.
16. Dry the surrounding skin with gauze dressings. Put on clean gloves.	Moisture provides a medium for growth of microorganisms. Excess moisture can contribute to skin irritation and breakdown. The use of a culture swab does not require immediate contact with the skin or wound, thus clean gloves are appropriate to protect the nurse from contact with blood and/or body fluids.
17. Twist the cap to loosen the swab on the Culturette tube, or open the separate swab and remove the cap from the culture tube. **Keep the swab and inside of the culture tube sterile (Fig. 2).**	Supplies are ready to use and within easy reach, and aseptic technique is maintained.
18. If contact with the wound is necessary to separate wound margins to permit insertion of the swab deep into the wound, put a sterile glove on one hand to manipulate the wound margins. Clean gloves may be appropriate for contact with pressure ulcers and chronic wounds.	If contact with the wound is necessary to collect the specimen, a sterile glove is necessary to prevent contamination of the wound.
19. **Carefully insert the swab into the wound. Press and rotate the swab several times over the wound surfaces. Avoid touching the swab to intact skin at the wound edges (Fig. 3). Use another swab if collecting a specimen from another site.**	Cotton tip absorbs wound drainage. Contact with skin could introduce extraneous organisms into the collected specimen, resulting in inaccurate results. Using another swab at a different site prevents cross-contamination of the wound.

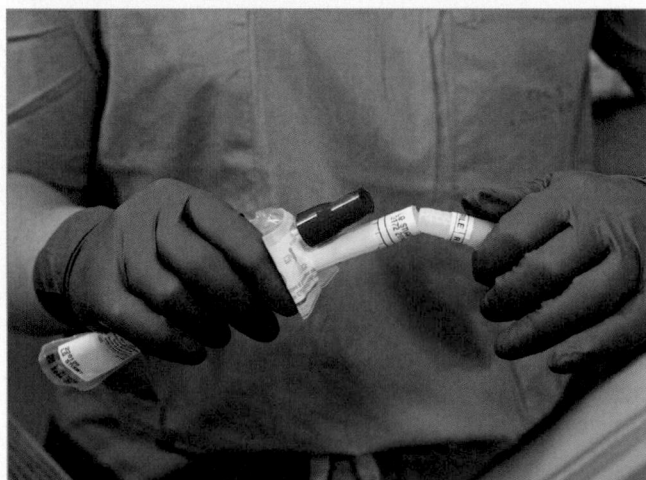

FIGURE 2. Removing cap from culture tube.

FIGURE 3. Rotating the swab several times over the wound surfaces.

ACTION	RATIONALE
20. Place the swab back in the culture tube (Fig. 4). **Do not touch the outside of the tube with the swab.** Secure the cap. Some swab containers have an ampule of medium at the bottom of the tube. It might be necessary to crush this ampule to activate. Follow the manufacturer's instructions for use.	The outside of the container is protected from contamination with microorganisms, and the sample is not contaminated with organisms not in the wound. Surrounding the swab with culture medium is necessary for accurate culture results.
21. Remove gloves and discard them accordingly.	Removing gloves properly reduces the risk for infection transmission and contamination of other items.
22. Put on gloves. Place a dressing on the wound, as appropriate, based on medical orders and/or the nursing plan of care. Refer to Skills 31-1 and 31-2, pp. 1004–1009. Remove gloves.	Wound dressings protect, absorb drainage, provide a moist environment, and promote wound healing. Removing gloves properly reduces the risk for infection transmission and contamination of other items.
23. After securing the dressing, label the dressing with the date and time. Remove all remaining equipment; place the patient in a comfortable position, with the side rails up and the bed in the lowest position.	Recording the date and time provides communication and demonstrates adherence to the plan of care. Proper patient and bed positioning promotes safety and comfort.
24. Label the specimen according to your institution's guidelines and send it to the laboratory in a biohazard bag (Fig. 5).	Proper labeling ensures proper identification of the specimen.
25. Remove PPE, if used. Perform hand hygiene.	Removing PPE properly reduces the risk for infection transmission and contamination of other items. Hand hygiene prevents the spread of microorganisms.

FIGURE 4. Placing swab in the culture tube.

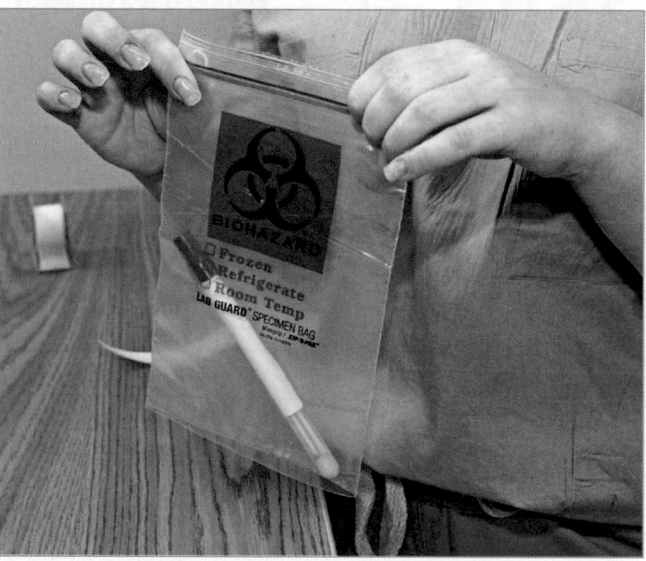

FIGURE 5. Labeled culture container in biohazard bag.

DOCUMENTATION

Guidelines

Document the location of the wound, the assessment of the wound, including type of tissue present, presence of necrotic tissue, stage (if appropriate), and characteristics of the drainage. Include the appearance of the surrounding skin. Document cleansing of the wound and the obtaining of the culture. Record any skin care and/or dressing applied. Note pertinent patient and family education and any patient reaction to this procedure, including patient's pain level and effectiveness of nonpharmacologic interventions or analgesia, if administered.

(continued)

SKILL 31-6 | COLLECTING A WOUND CULTURE *continued*

Sample Documentation

> <u>6/22/15</u> 2100 Wound noted on patient's hand; 2 cm × 3 cm × 1 cm, red, tender, with purulent drainage present. Edges macerated, without erythema and tenderness. Wound cleaned with normal saline, culture obtained. Skin barrier applied to surrounding area, wound packed with moist saline gauze, dressed with dry gauze and Kling. Hand elevated. Culture labeled and sent to lab.
> —J. Wentz, RN

UNEXPECTED SITUATIONS AND ASSOCIATED INTERVENTIONS

- *The nurse has inserted the culture swab into the patient's wound to obtain the specimen and realizes that the wound was not cleaned:* Discard this swab. Obtain the additional supplies needed to clean the wound according to facility policy and a new culture swab. Cleaning the wound prior to obtaining a specimen for culture removes previous drainage, wound debris, and skin flora, which could introduce extraneous organisms into the specimen, resulting in inaccurate results. Clean the wound and then proceed to obtain the culture specimen.

- *As the nurse prepares to insert the culture swab into the wound, the nurse inadvertently touches the swab to the patient's bedclothes:* Discard this swab, obtain a new culture swab, and collect the specimen.

SKILL 31-7 | APPLYING NEGATIVE-PRESSURE WOUND THERAPY

DELEGATION CONSIDERATIONS

The application of negative-pressure wound therapy is not delegated to nursing assistive personnel (NAP) or unlicensed assistive personnel (UAP). Depending on the state's nurse practice act and the organization's policies and procedures, the application of negative–pressure wound therapy may be delegated to licensed practical/vocational nurses (LPN/LVNs). The decision to delegate must be based on careful analysis of the patient's needs and circumstances, as well as the qualifications of the person to whom the task is being delegated. Refer to the Delegation Guidelines in Appendix A (found on thePoint).

EQUIPMENT

- Negative-pressure unit (V.A.C. ATS unit)
- Evacuation/collection canister
- V.A.C. Foam dressing
- V.A.C. Drape
- T.R.A.C. Pad
- Skin-protectant wipes
- Sterile gauze sponge
- A sterile irrigation set, including a basin, irrigant container, and irrigation syringe
- Sterile irrigation solution as ordered, warmed to body temperature

- Waste receptacle to dispose of contaminated materials
- Sterile gloves (2 pairs)
- Sterile scissors
- Clean, disposable gloves
- Gown, mask, eye protection
- Additional PPE, as indicated
- Sterile scissors
- Waterproof pad and bath blanket

IMPLEMENTATION

ACTION	RATIONALE
1. Review the medical order for the application of NPWT therapy, including the ordered pressure setting for the device. Gather necessary supplies.	Reviewing the order validates the correct patient and correct procedure. Preparation promotes efficient time management and an organized approach to the task.

ACTION	RATIONALE
2. Perform hand hygiene and put on PPE, if indicated.	Hand hygiene and PPE prevent the spread of microorganisms. PPE is required based on transmission precautions.
3. Identify the patient.	Identifying the patient ensures that the right patient receives the intervention and helps prevent errors.
4. Assemble equipment on the overbed table within reach.	Organization facilitates performance of the task.
5. Close curtains around the bed and close the door to the room, if possible. Explain what you are going to do and why you are going to do it to the patient.	This ensures the patient's privacy. Explanation relieves anxiety and facilitates cooperation.
6. Assess the patient for the possible need for nonpharmacologic pain-reducing interventions or analgesic medication before wound care dressing change. Administer the appropriate prescribed analgesic. Allow enough time for the analgesic to achieve its effectiveness before beginning the procedure.	Pain is a subjective experience influenced by past experience. Wound care and dressing changes may cause pain for some patients.
7. Adjust the bed to a comfortable working height, usually elbow height of the caregiver (VISN 8, 2009).	Having the bed at the proper height prevents back and muscle strain.
8. Assist the patient to a comfortable position that provides easy access to the wound area. Position the patient so that the irrigation solution will flow from the clean end of the wound toward the dirty end. Expose the area and drape the patient with a bath blanket if needed. Put a waterproof pad under the wound area.	Patient positioning and draping provide comfort and warmth. Gravity directs the flow of liquid from the least contaminated to the most contaminated area. Waterproof pad protects the patient and the bed linens.
9. Have the disposal bag or waste receptacle within easy reach for use during the procedure.	Having a waste container handy allows for easy disposal of the soiled dressings and supplies, without the spread of microorganisms.
10. Using sterile technique, prepare a sterile field and add all the sterile supplies needed for the procedure to the field. Pour warmed, sterile irrigating solution into the sterile container.	Proper preparation ensures that supplies are within easy reach and sterility is maintained. Warmed solution may result in less discomfort.
11. Put on a gown, mask, and eye protection.	Use of PPE is part of *Standard Precautions*. A gown protects your clothes from contamination if splashing should occur. Goggles protect mucous membranes of your eyes from contact with irrigant fluid.
12. Put on clean gloves. Carefully and gently remove the dressing. If there is resistance, use a silicone-based adhesive remover to help remove the dressing. **Note the number of pieces of foam removed from the wound. Compare with the documented number from the previous dressing change.**	Gloves protect the nurse from handling contaminated dressings. A silicone-based adhesive remover allows for the easy, rapid, and painless removal without the associated problems of skin stripping (Denyer, 2011; Benbow, 2011). Counting the number of pieces of foam assures the removal of all foam that was placed during the previous dressing change.
13. Discard the dressings in the receptacle. Remove your gloves and put them in the receptacle.	Proper disposal of dressings and used gloves prevents the spread of microorganisms.
14. Put on sterile gloves. Using sterile technique, irrigate the wound (see Skill 31-3, pp. 1013–1016).	Irrigation removes exudate and debris.
15. Clean the area around the wound with normal saline. Dry the surrounding skin with a sterile gauze sponge.	Moisture provides a medium for growth of microorganisms.
16. Assess the wound for appearance, stage, the presence of eschar, granulation tissue, epithelialization, undermining, tunneling, necrosis, sinus tract, and drainage. Assess the appearance of the surrounding tissue. Measure the wound.	This information provides evidence about the wound healing process and/or the presence of infection.
17. **Wipe intact skin around the wound with a skin-protectant wipe and allow it to dry well.**	Skin protectant provides a barrier against irritation and breakdown.

(continued)

SKILL 31-7 APPLYING NEGATIVE-PRESSURE WOUND THERAPY *continued*

ACTION	RATIONALE
18. **Using sterile scissors, cut the foam to the shape and measurement of the wound. Do not cut foam over the wound.** More than one piece of foam may be necessary if the first piece is cut too small. Carefully place the foam in the wound. **Ensure foam-to-foam contact if more than one piece is required. Note the number of pieces of foam placed in the wound.**	Aseptic technique maintains sterility of items to come in contact with the wound. Foam should fill the wound but not cover intact surrounding skin. Foam fragments may fall into the wound if cutting is performed over the wound. Foam-to-foam contact allows for even distribution of negative pressure. Recording the number of pieces of foam aides in assuring the removal of all foam with the next dressing change.
19. Trim and place the V.A.C. Drape to cover the foam dressing and an additional 3- to 5-cm border of intact periwound tissue. The V.A.C. Drape may be cut into multiple pieces for easier handling.	The occlusive air-permeable V.A.C. Drape provides a seal, allowing the application of the negative pressure.
20. Choose an appropriate site to apply the T.R.A.C. Pad.	T.R.A.C. Pad should be placed in the area where the greatest fluid flow and optimal drainage is anticipated. Avoid placing over bony prominences or within creases in the tissue.
21. Pinch the drape and cut a 2-cm hole through it. Apply the T.R.A.C. Pad (Fig. 1). Remove V.A.C. Canister from the package and insert into the V.A.C. Therapy Unit until it locks into place. Connect the T.R.A.C. Pad tubing to canister tubing (Fig. 2) and check that the clamps on each tube are open. Turn on the power to the V.A.C. Therapy Unit and select the prescribed therapy setting.	A hole in the drape allows for removal of fluid and/or exudate. The canister provides a collection chamber for the drainage.

FIGURE 1. Applying T.R.A.C. Pad.

FIGURE 2. Connecting T.R.A.C. tubing to collection canister tubing.

22. **Assess the dressing to ensure seal integrity. The dressing should be collapsed, shrinking to the foam and skin.**	Shrinkage confirms a good seal, allowing for accurate application of pressure and treatment.
23. Remove and discard gloves.	Proper disposal of gloves prevents the spread of microorganisms.
24. Label the dressing with the date and time. Remove all remaining equipment; place the patient in a comfortable position, with the side rails up and the bed in the lowest position.	Recording the date and time provides communication and demonstrates adherence to the plan of care. Proper patient and bed positioning promotes safety and comfort.
25. Remove PPE, if used. Perform hand hygiene.	Removing PPE properly reduces the risk for infection transmission and contamination of other items. Hand hygiene prevents the spread of microorganisms.
26. Check all wound dressings every shift. More frequent checks may be needed if the wound is more complex or dressings become saturated quickly.	Checking dressings ensures the assessment of changes in patient condition and timely intervention to prevent complications.

DOCUMENTATION

Guidelines

Record your assessment of the wound, including evidence of granulation tissue, presence of necrotic tissue, stage (if appropriate), and characteristics of drainage. Include the appearance of the surrounding skin. Document the cleansing or irrigation of the wound and solution used. Document the application of the NPWT, noting the pressure setting, patency, and seal of the dressing. Describe the color and characteristics of the drainage in the collection chamber. Record pertinent patient and family education and any patient reaction to this procedure, including the presence of pain and effectiveness or ineffectiveness of pain interventions.

Sample Documentation

<u>4/5/15</u> 0800 NPWT dressing intact with good seal maintained, V.A.C. system patent, pressure setting 50 mm Hg. Purulent, sanguineous drainage noted in collection chamber and tubing. Surrounding tissue without edema, redness, ecchymosis, or signs of irritation. Patient verbalizes an understanding of movement limitations related to the system.

—B. Clark, RN

UNEXPECTED SITUATIONS AND ASSOCIATED INTERVENTIONS

- *While assessing the patient, the nurse notes that the seal between the transparent dressing and the foam and skin is not tight:* Check the dressing seals, tubing connections, and canister insertion, and ensure that the clamps are open. If a leak in the transparent dressing is identified, the appropriate pressure is not being applied to the wound. Apply additional transparent dressing to reseal. If this application does not correct the break, change the dressing.

- *The patient complains of acute pain while NPWT is operating:* Assess the patient for other symptoms, obtain vital signs, assess the wound, and assess the vacuum device for proper functioning. Report your findings to the primary care provider and document the event in the patient's record. Administer analgesics as ordered. Continue or change the wound therapy as ordered.

SPECIAL CONSIDERATIONS

- Change the wound dressing initially 48 hours after beginning treatment, then two to three times per week for noninfected wounds, as indicated by the wound's response to the intervention (Baranoski & Ayello, 2012). Time dressing changes to allow for wound assessment by the other members of the health care team.

- Monitor infected wounds often; dressings may need to be changed more often than 48 to 72 hours (Hess, 2013).

- Measure and record the amount of drainage each shift as part of the intake and output record.

- Check the fluid level in the canister periodically. Depending on the particular device in use, replace the canister whenever full or nearly full.

- Be alert for audible and visual alarms on the vacuum device to alert you to problems, such as tipping of the device greater than 45 degrees, a full collection canister, an air leak in the dressing, or dislodgment of the canister.

- NPWT should operate for 24 hours a day. It should not be shut off for more than 2 hours in a 24-hour period. When NPWT is restarted, irrigate the wound per medical order or facility policy, and apply a new NPWT dressing.

- When maceration of the surrounding skin beneath the occlusive dressing occurs, this may be treated by placing a barrier/wafer dressing beneath the transparent dressing to protect the skin. Verify with facility policy as needed.

SKILL 31-8 | APPLYING AN EXTERNAL HEATING PAD

DELEGATION CONSIDERATIONS

The application of an external heating pad may be delegated to nursing assistive personnel (NAP) or to unlicensed assistive personnel (UAP), as well as to licensed practical/vocational nurses (LPN/LVNs). The decision to delegate must be based on careful analysis of the patient's needs and circumstances, as well as the qualifications of the person to whom the task is being delegated. Refer to the Delegation Guidelines in Appendix A (found on thePoint).

EQUIPMENT

- Aquathermia heating pad (or other brand) with electronic unit
- Distilled water
- Cover for the pad, if not part of pad
- Gauze bandage or tape to secure the pad
- Bath blanket
- PPE, as indicated

IMPLEMENTATION

ACTION	RATIONALE
1. Review the medical order for the application of heat therapy, including frequency, type of therapy, body area to be treated, and length of time for the application. Gather necessary supplies.	Reviewing the order and plan of care validates the correct patient and correct procedure. Preparation promotes efficient time management and an organized approach to the task.
2. Perform hand hygiene and put on PPE, if indicated.	Hand hygiene and PPE prevent the spread of microorganisms. PPE is required based on transmission precautions.
3. Identify the patient.	Identifying the patient ensures the right patient receives the intervention and helps prevent errors.
4. Assemble equipment on the overbed table within reach.	Organization facilitates performance of the task.
5. Close the curtains around the bed and the close door to the room, if possible. Explain what you are going to do and why you are going to do it to the patient.	This ensures the patient's privacy. Explanation relieves anxiety and facilitates cooperation.
6. Adjust the bed to a comfortable working height, usually elbow height of the caregiver (VISN 8, 2009).	Having the bed at the proper height prevents back and muscle strain.
7. Assist the patient to a comfortable position that provides easy access to the area where the heat will be applied; use a bath blanket to cover any other exposed area.	Patient positioning and use of a bath blanket provide comfort and warmth.
8. Assess the condition of the skin where the heat is to be applied.	Assessment supplies baseline data for post-treatment comparison and identifies conditions that may contraindicate the application.
9. Check that the water in the electronic unit (Fig. 1) is at the appropriate level. Fill the unit two-thirds full or to the fill mark, with distilled water, if necessary. Check the temperature setting on the unit to ensure that it is within the safe range.	Sufficient water in the unit is necessary to ensure proper function of the unit. Tap water leaves mineral deposits in the unit. Checking the temperature setting helps to prevent skin or tissue damage.

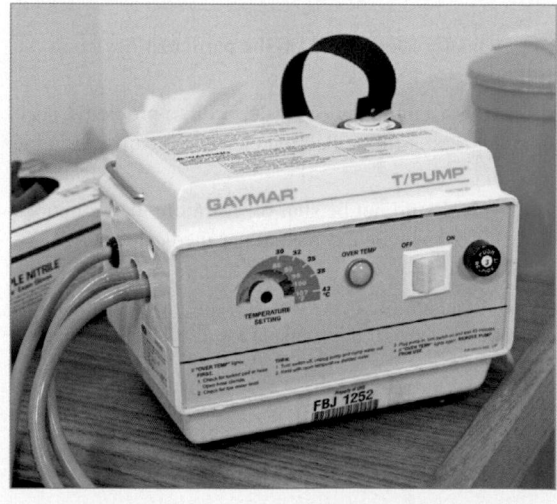

FIGURE 1. External heating pad electronic unit.

ACTION	RATIONALE
10. Attach the pad tubing to the electronic unit tubing (Fig. 2).	Allows flow of warmed water through the heating pad.
11. Plug in the unit and warm the pad before use. Apply the heating pad to the prescribed area (Fig. 3). Secure with gauze bandage or tape.	Plugging in the pad readies it for use. Heat travels by conduction from one object to another. Gauze bandage or tape holds the pad in position. **Do not use pins, as they may puncture and damage the pad.**

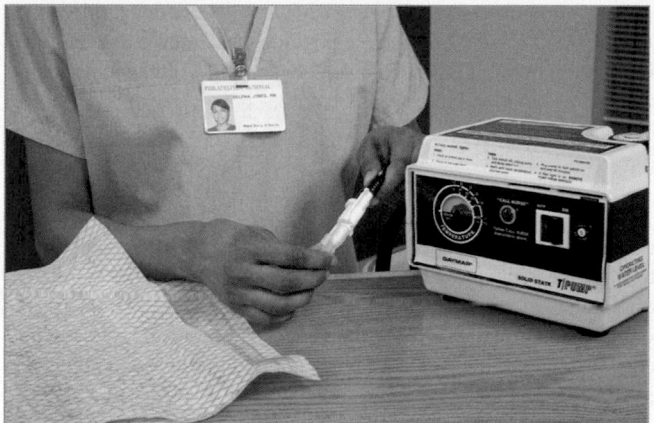

FIGURE 2. Attaching pad tubing to electronic unit tubing.

FIGURE 3. Applying the heating pad.

ACTION	RATIONALE
12. **Assess the condition of the skin and the patient's response to the heat at frequent intervals, according to facility policy. Do not exceed the prescribed length of time for the application of heat.**	Maximum vasodilation and therapeutic effects from the application of heat occur within 20 to 30 minutes. Using heat for more than 45 minutes results in tissue congestion and vasoconstriction, known as the rebound phenomenon. Also, prolonged heat application may result in an increased risk for burns.
13. Remove gloves and discard. Remove all remaining equipment; place the patient in a comfortable position, with the side rails up and the bed in the lowest position.	Proper removal of gloves prevents spread of microorganisms. Proper patient and bed positioning promotes safety and comfort.
14. Remove additional PPE, if used. Perform hand hygiene.	Removing PPE properly reduces the risk for infection transmission and contamination of other items. Hand hygiene prevents the spread of microorganisms.
15. **Monitor the time the heating pad is in place to prevent burns and skin/tissue damage. Monitor the condition of the patient's skin and the patient's response at frequent intervals.**	Extended use of heat results in an increased risk for burns from the heat. Impaired circulation may affect the patient's sensitivity to heat.
16. Remove the pad after the prescribed amount of time (up to 30 minutes). Reassess the patient and area of application, noting the effect and presence of adverse effects.	Removal reduces the risk of injury due to prolonged heat application. Heat applications are used to promote healing; reduce muscle tension; relieve muscle spasm, joint stiffness, and pain; and treat infections, surgical wounds, inflammation, arthritis, joint pain, muscle pain, and chronic pain. Assessment provides input as to the effectiveness of the treatment.

DOCUMENTATION

Guidelines

Document the rationale for application of heat therapy. If the patient is receiving heat therapy for pain, document the assessment of pain pre- and post-intervention. Specify the type of heat therapy and location where it is applied, as well as length of time. Record the condition of the skin, noting any redness or irritation before the heat application and after the application. Document the patient's reaction to the heat therapy. Record any appropriate patient or family education.

(continued)

SKILL 31-8 APPLYING AN EXTERNAL HEATING PAD *continued*

Sample Documentation

> 9/13/15 2300 Patient complaining of pain, rating it 5 out of 10. Aquathermia pad applied to patient's lower back for 30 minutes; now rating pain as 2 out of 10. Skin without signs of redness or irritation before and after application.
> —*M. Martinez, RN*

UNEXPECTED SITUATIONS AND ASSOCIATED INTERVENTIONS

- *When performing a periodic assessment of the site during the application of heat, the nurse notes excessive swelling and redness at the site and the patient complains of pain that was not present prior to the application of heat:* Remove the heat source. Assess the patient for other symptoms and obtain vital signs. Report your findings to the primary care provider and document the interventions in the patient's record.

SPECIAL CONSIDERATIONS

General Considerations

- Direct heat treatment is contraindicated for patients at risk for bleeding, patients with a sprained limb in the acute stage, or patients with a condition associated with acute inflammation. Use cautiously with children and older adults. Patients with diabetes, stroke, spinal cord injury, and peripheral neuropathy are at risk for thermal injury, as are patients with very thin or damaged skin. Be extremely careful when applying to heat-sensitive areas, such as scar tissue and stomas.
- Instruct the patient not to lean or lie directly on the heating device, as this reduces air space and increases the risk for burns.
- Check the water level in the Aquathermia unit periodically. Evaporation may occur. If the unit runs dry, it could become damaged. Refill with distilled water periodically.

Older Adult Considerations

- Older adults are more at risk for skin and tissue damage because of their thin skin, loss of heat sensation, decreased subcutaneous tissue, and changes in the body's ability to regulate temperature. Check these patients more frequently during therapy.

Home Care Considerations

- A hot water bag or commercially prepared hot pack may be used in the home to apply heat. If using a hot water bag, fill with hot tap water to warm the bag, then empty it to detect any leaks. Check the temperature of the water with a bath thermometer or test on your inner wrist, adjusting the temperature as ordered (usually 115°F to 125°F for adults). Checking the temperature ensures that the heat applied is within the acceptable range of temperatures. Fill the bag one-half to two-thirds full. Partial filling keeps the bag lightweight and flexible so that it can be molded to the treatment area. Squeeze the bag until the water reaches the neck; this expels air, which would make the bag inflexible and would reduce heat conduction. Fasten the top and cover the bag with an absorbent cloth. The covering protects the skin from direct contact with the bag. If using a commercially prepared hot pack, follow the manufacturer's directions and carefully assess the skin before and after heat application.

DEVELOPING CLINICAL REASONING

1. How would you individualize your teaching about needed supplies, wound care, and resources for the following patients?
   - A homeless man admitted to the hospital for gangrene of the big toe. The toe has been amputated.
   - A teenage gang member treated in the emergency department for a superficial (but long) knife wound
   - An infant who has had abdominal surgery and is now having diarrhea

- A frail, 80-year-old man who needs daily dressing changes on a draining wound and lives with his blind wife

2. Describe the nursing interventions you would include in a plan of care to prevent pressure ulcers in the following patients:
   - A middle-aged woman, 70 pounds over normal body weight, who has a fractured femur and is recovering at home (she lives alone)
   - A 90-year-old man with cognitive impairment who is confined to bed
   - A 17-year-old girl who is paralyzed from the waist down after a diving accident and is wheelchair dependent

PRACTICING FOR NCLEX

1. Thirty-six hours after having surgery, a patient has a slightly elevated body temperature and generalized malaise, as well as pain and redness at the surgical site. Which intervention is most important to include in this patient's nursing care plan?
   a. Document the findings and continue to monitor the patient.
   b. Administer antipyretics, as ordered.
   c. Increase the frequency of assessment to every hour and notify the patient's primary care provider.
   d. Increase the frequency of wound care and contact the primary care provider for an antibiotic order.

2. A nurse caring for patients in the PACU teaches a novice nurse how to assess and document wound drainage. Which statements accurately describe a characteristic of wound drainage? Select all that apply.
   a. Serous drainage is composed of the clear portion of the blood and serous membranes.
   b. Sanguineous drainage is composed of a large number of red blood cells and looks like blood.
   c. Bright red sanguineous drainage indicates fresh bleeding and darker drainage indicates older bleeding.
   d. Purulent drainage is composed of white blood cells, dead tissue, and bacteria.
   e. Purulent drainage is thin, cloudy, and watery and may have a musty or foul odor.
   f. Serosanguineous drainage can be dark yellow or green depending on the causative organism.

3. A patient who has a large abdominal wound suddenly calls out for help because she feels as though something is falling out of her incision. Inspection reveals a gaping open wound with tissue bulging outward. In which order should the nurse perform the following interventions? Arrange from first to last.
   a. Notify the physician immediately of the situation.
   b. Cover the exposed tissue with sterile towels moistened with sterile NSS.
   c. Place the patient in the low Fowler's position.

4. A patient, age 16, was in an automobile accident and received a wound across her nose and cheek. After surgery to repair the wound, the patient says, "I am so ugly now." Based on this statement, what nursing diagnosis would be most appropriate?
   a. Pain
   b. Impaired Skin Integrity
   c. Disturbed Body Image
   d. Disturbed Thought Processes

5. A patient is admitted with a nonhealing surgical wound. Which nursing action is most effective in preventing a wound infection?
   a. Using sterile dressing supplies
   b. Suggesting dietary supplements
   c. Applying antibiotic ointment
   d. Performing careful hand hygiene

6. A nurse who is changing dressings of postoperative patients in the hospital documents various phases of wound healing on the patient charts. Which statements accurately describe these stages? Select all that apply.
   a. Hemostasis occurs immediately after the initial injury.
   b. A liquid called exudate is formed during the proliferation phase.
   c. White blood cells move to the wound in the inflammatory phase.
   d. Granulation tissue forms in the inflammatory phase.
   e. During the inflammatory phase, the patient has generalized body response.
   f. A scar forms during the proliferation phase.

7. The nurse assesses the wound of a patient who cut himself on the upper thigh with a chain saw. The nurse then documents the presence of biofilms in the wound. What is the effect of this condition on the wound? Select all that apply.
   a. Enhanced healing due to the presence of sugars and proteins
   b. Delayed healing due to dead tissue present in the wound
   c. Decreased effectiveness of antibiotics against the bacteria
   d. Impaired skin integrity due to overhydration of the cells of the wound
   e. Delayed healing due to cells dehydrating and dying
   f. Decreased effectiveness of the patient's normal immune process

8. The nurse is cleaning an open abdominal wound that has unapproximated edges. What are accurate steps in this procedure? Select all that apply.
   a. Use standard precautions or transmission-based precautions when indicated.
   b. Moisten a sterile gauze pad or swab with the prescribed cleansing agent and squeeze out excess solution.
   c. Clean the wound in full or half circles beginning on the outside and working toward the center.
   d. Work outward from the incision in lines that are parallel to it from the dirty area to the clean area.
   e. Clean to at least one inch beyond the end of the new dressing if one is being applied.
   f. Clean to at least three inches beyond the wound if a new dressing is not being applied.

9. A nurse is developing a plan of care for an 86-year-old woman who has been admitted for right hip arthroplasty (hip replacement). Which assessment finding(s) indicate a high risk for pressure ulcer development for this patient? Select all that apply.
   a. The patient takes time to think about her responses to questions.
   b. The patient's age of 86 years.
   c. Patient reports inability to control urine.
   d. A scheduled hip arthroplasty
   e. Lab findings include BUN 12 (elderly normal 8–23 mg/dL) and creatinine 0.9 (adult female normal 0.61–1 mg/dL).
   f. Patient reports increased pain in right hip when repositioning in bed or chair.

10. A nurse is explaining to a patient the anticipated effect of the application of cold to an injured area. What response indicates that the patient understands the explanation?
    a. "I can expect to have more discomfort in the area where the cold is applied."
    b. "I should expect more drainage from the incision after the ice has been in place."
    c. "I should see less swelling and redness with the cold treatment."
    d. "My incision may bleed more when the ice is first applied."

11. A nurse is providing patient teaching regarding the use of negative-pressure wound therapy. Which explanation provides the most accurate information to the patient?
    a. The therapy is used to collect excess blood loss and prevent the formation of a scab.
    b. The therapy will prevent infection, ensuring that the wound heals with less scar tissue.
    c. The therapy provides a moist environment and stimulates blood flow to the wound.
    d. The therapy irrigates the wound to keep it free from debris and excess wound fluid.

12. After an initial skin assessment, the nurse documents the presence of a reddened area that has blistered. According to recognized staging systems, this ulcer would be classified as:
    a. Stage I
    b. Stage II
    c. Stage III
    d. Stage IV

13. The nurse uses the RYB wound classification system to assess the wound of a client who cut his arm on a factory machine. The nurse documents the wound as "red." What would be the priority nursing intervention for this type of wound?
    a. Irrigate the wound.
    b. Provide gentle cleansing of the wound.
    c. Débride the wound.
    d. Change the dressing frequently.

14. A nurse is developing a plan of care related to prevention of pressure ulcers for residents in a long-term care facility. Which action would be a priority in preventing a patient from developing a pressure ulcer?
    a. Keeping the head of the bed elevated as often as possible
    b. Massaging over bony prominences
    c. Repositioning bed-bound patients every 4 hours
    d. Using a mild cleansing agent when cleansing the skin

15. A nurse is measuring the depth of a patient's puncture wound. Which technique is recommended?
    a. Moisten a sterile, flexible applicator with saline and insert it gently into the wound at a 90-degree angle with the tip down.
    b. Draw the shape of the wound and describe how deep it appears in centimeters.
    c. Gently insert a sterile applicator into the wound and move it in a clockwise direction.
    d. Insert a calibrated probe gently into the wound and mark the point that is even with the surrounding skin surface with a marker.

ANSWERS WITH RATIONALES

1. *a.* The assessment findings are normal for this stage of healing following surgery. The patient is in the inflammatory phase of the healing process, which involves a response by the immune system. This acute inflammation is characterized by pain, heat, redness, and swelling at the site of the injury (surgery, in this case). The patient also has a generalized body response, including a mildly elevated temperature, leukocytosis, and generalized malaise.

2. *a, b, c, d.* Serous drainage is composed primarily of the clear, serous portion of the blood and serous membranes. Serous drainage is clear and watery. Sanguineous drainage

consists of large numbers of red blood cells and looks like blood. Bright-red sanguineous drainage is indicative of fresh bleeding, whereas darker drainage indicates older bleeding. Purulent drainage is made up of white blood cells, liquefied dead tissue debris, and both dead and live bacteria. Purulent drainage is thick, often has a musty or foul odor, and varies in color (such as dark yellow or green), depending on the causative organism. Serosanguineous drainage is a mixture of serum and red blood cells. It is light pink to blood tinged.

3. *c, b, a.* Dehiscence and evisceration is a postoperative emergency that requires prompt surgical repair. The correct order of implementation by the nurse is to place the patient in the low Fowler's position, cover the exposed tissue with sterile towels moistened with sterile NSS, and notify the physician immediately of the situation.

4. *c.* Wounds cause emotional as well as physical stress.

5. *d.* Although all of the answers may help in preventing wound infections, careful hand washing (medical asepsis) is the most important.

6. *a, c, e.* Hemostasis occurs immediately after the initial injury and exudate occurs in this phase due to the leaking out of plasma and blood components into the injured area. White blood cells, predominantly leukocytes and macrophages, move to the wound in the inflammatory phase to ingest bacteria and cellular debris. During the inflammatory phase, the patient has a generalized body response, including a mildly elevated temperature, leukocytosis (increased number of white blood cells in the blood), and generalized malaise. New tissue, called granulation tissue, forms the foundation for scar tissue development in the proliferation phase. New collagen continues to be deposited in the maturation phase, which forms a scar.

7. *c, f.* Wound biofilms are the result of wound bacteria growing in clumps, imbedded in a thick, self-made, protective, slimy barrier of sugars and proteins. This barrier contributes to decreased effectiveness of antibiotics against the bacteria (antibiotic resistance) and decreases the effectiveness of the normal immune response by the patient (Beitz, 2012). Necrosis (dead tissue) in the wound delays healing. Maceration or overhydration of cells related to urinary and fecal incontinence can lead to impaired skin integrity. Desiccation is the process of drying up, in which cells dehydrate and die in a dry environment.

8. *a, b, e.* The correct procedure for cleaning a wound with unapproximated edges is: (1) use standard precautions and appropriate transmission-based precautions when indicated, (2) moisten sterile gauze pad or swab with prescribed cleansing agent and squeeze out excess solution, (3) use a new swab or gauze for each circle, (4) clean the wound in full or half circles beginning in the center and working toward the outside, (5) clean to at least one inch beyond the end of the new dressing, and (6) clean to at least two inches beyond the wound margins if a dressing is not being applied.

9. *b, c, d, f.* Pressure, friction, and shear, as well as other factors, usually combine to contribute to pressure ulcer development. The skin of older adults is more susceptible to injury; incontinence contributes to prolonged moisture on the skin, as well as negative effects related to urine in contact with skin; hip surgery involves decreased mobility

during the postoperative period, as well as pain with movement, contributing to immobility; and increased pain in the hip may contribute to increased immobility. All these factors are related to an increased risk for pressure ulcer development. Apathy, confusion, and/or altered mental status are risk factors for pressure ulcer development. Dehydration (indicated by an elevated BUN and creatinine) is a risk for pressure ulcer development.

10. *c.* The local application of cold constricts peripheral blood vessels, reduces muscle spasms, and promotes comfort. Cold reduces blood flow to tissues, decreases the local release of pain-producing substances, decreases metabolic needs, and capillary permeability. The resulting effects include decreased edema, coagulation of blood at the wound site, promotion of comfort, decreased drainage from wound, and decreased bleeding.

11. *c.* Negative-pressure wound therapy (or topical negative pressure [TNP]) promotes wound healing and wound closure through the application of uniform negative pressure on the wound bed, reduction in bacteria in the wound, and the removal of excess wound fluid, while providing a moist wound healing environment. The negative pressure results in mechanical tension on the wound tissues, stimulating cell proliferation, blood flow to wounds, and the growth of new blood vessels. It is used to treat a variety of acute or chronic wounds, wounds with heavy drainage, wounds failing to heal, or healing slowly.

12. *b.* A stage II pressure ulcer involves partial thickness loss of dermis and presents as a shallow open ulcer with a red pink wound bed, without slough. It may also present as an intact or open/ruptured serum-filled blister.

13. *b.* Red wounds are in the proliferative stage of healing and reflect the color of normal granulation tissue. Wounds in this stage need protection with nursing interventions that include gentle cleansing, use of moist dressings, and changing of the dressing only when necessary, and/or based on product manufacturer's recommendations. To cleanse yellow wounds, nursing interventions include the use of wound cleansers and irrigating the wound. The eschar found in black wounds requires débridement (removal) before the wound can heal.

14. *d.* To prevent pressure ulcers, the nurse should cleanse the skin routinely and whenever any soiling occurs by using a mild cleansing agent with minimal friction, and avoiding hot water. The nurse should minimize the effects of shearing force by limiting the amount of time the head of the bed is elevated, when possible. Bony prominences should not be massaged, and bed-bound patients should be repositioned every 2 hours.

15. *a.* To measure the depth of a wound, the nurse should perform hand hygiene and put on gloves; moisten a sterile, flexible applicator with saline and insert it gently into the wound at a 90-degree angle with the tip down; mark the point on the swab that is even with the surrounding skin surface, or grasp the applicator with the thumb and forefinger at the point corresponding to the wound's margin; and remove the swab and measure the depth with a ruler.

TAYLOR SUITE RESOURCES

Explore these additional resources to enhance learning for this chapter:

- NCLEX-Style Questions and other resources on the**Point**, http://thePoint.lww.com/Taylor8e
- *Study Guide for Fundamentals of Nursing, 8th edition*
- Adaptive Learning | Powered by prepU, http://thepoint.lww.com/prepu
- *Skill Checklists for Fundamentals of Nursing, 8th edition*
- *Taylor's Clinical Nursing Skills:* Chapter 8, Skin Integrity and Wound Care
- *Taylor's Video Guide to Clinical Nursing Skills:* Skin Integrity and Wound Care
- *Lippincott DocuCare* Fundamentals cases

Bibliography

Ackley, B. J., & Ladwig, G. B. (2011). *Nursing Diagnosis Handbook* (9th ed.). St. Louis: Elsevier/Mosby.

Agency for Healthcare Research and Quality (AHRQ). National Guideline Clearinghouse. (2011). Pressure ulcer treatment recommendations. In: Prevention and treatment of pressure ulcers: clinical practice guideline. Available http://www.guideline.gov/content.aspx?id=25139&search=pressure+ulcer+treatment#Section420

Alvey, B., Heard, H., & Hennen, N. (2012). Improving accuracy of pressure ulcer staging and documentation using a computerized clinical decision support system. *Journal of Wound, Ostomy and Continence Nursing, 39*(6), 607–612.

Anderson, I. (2010). Key principles involved in applying and removing wound dressings. *Nursing Standard, 25*(10), 51–57.

Baranoski, S., & Ayello, E. A. (2012). *Wound care essentials: Practice Principles* (3rd ed.). Philadelphia: Wolters Kluwer Health/Lippincott Williams & Wilkins.

Beeson, T., Adams, G., Prickel, C., Treon, M. L., Mink, J., & Buelow, J. M. (2010). Thinking about the Braden Scale. *Clinical Nurse Specialist, 24*(2), 49–50.

Beitz, J. M. (2012). Wound debridement: Therapeutic options and care considerations. *Critical Care Nursing Clinics of North America, 24*(2), 239–253.

Benbow, M. (2011). Addressing pain in wound care and dressing removal. *Nursing & Residential Care, 13*(10), 474, 476, 478.

Benbow, M. (2008a). Exploring the concept of moist wound healing and its application in practice. *British Journal of Nursing, 17*(15) (Tissue viability supplement), S4–S16.

Benbow, M. (2008b). Pressure ulcer prevention and pressure-relieving surfaces. *British Journal of Nursing, 17*(13), 830–835.

Bergstrom, N., Braden, B., Laguzza, A., & Holman, V. (1987). The Braden scale for predicting pressure sore risk. *Nursing Research, 36*(4), 205–210.

Black, J., Berke, C., & Urzendowski, G. (2012). Pressure ulcer incidence and progression in critically ill subjects. *Journal of Wound, Ostomy and Continence Nursing, 39*(3), 267–273.

Black, J. M., Edsberg, L. E., Baharestani, M. M., Langemo, D., Goldberg, M., McNichol, L., Cuddigan, J., & the National Pressure Ulcer Advisory Panel. (2011). Pressure ulcers. Avoidable or unavoidable? Results of the National Pressure Ulcer Advisory Panel Consensus Conference. *Ostomy Wound Management, 57*(2), 24–37.

Black, J. M., Gray, M., Bliss, D. Z., Kennedy-Evans, K. L., Logan, S., Baharestani, M. M., Colwell, J. C., Goldberg, M., & Ratliff, C. R. (2011). MASD Part 2: Incontinence-associated dermatitis and intertriginous dermatitis. *Journal of Wound, Ostomy and Continence Nursing, 38*(4), 359–370.

Boltz, M., Capezuti, E., Fulmer, T., & Zwicker, D. (eds.) (2012). *Evidence-based geriatric nursing protocols for best practice* (4th ed.). New York: Springer Publishing Company.

Borgquist, O., Ingemansson, R., & Malmsjö, M. (2011). Individualizing the use of negative pressure wound therapy for optimal wound healing: A focused review of the literature. *Ostomy Wound Management, 57*(4), 44–54.

Braden, B. J. (2012). The Braden Scale for predicting pressure sore risk: Reflections after 25 years. *Advances in Skin & Wound Care, 25*(2), 61.

Braden, B., & Maklebust, J. (2005). Preventing pressure ulcers with the Braden scale. *American Journal of Nursing, 105*(6), 70–72.

Brunner, M., Droegemueller, C., Rivers, S., & Deuser, W. E. (2012). Prevention of incontinence-related skin breakdown for acute and critical care patients: Comparison of two products. *Urologic Nursing, 32*(4), 214–219.

Bulechek, G. M., Butcher, H. K., Dochterman, J. M., & Wagner, C. M. (Eds.). (2013). *Nursing interventions classification (NIC)* (6th ed.). St. Louis: Elsevier/Mosby.

Burr, S., & Penzer, R. (2005). Promoting skin health. *Nursing Standard, 19*(36), 57–65.

Centers for Disease Control and Prevention (CDC). (2010). Healthcare-associated infections (HAIs). Frequently asked questions about surgical site infections. Available at http://www.cdc.gov/HAI/ssi/faq_ssi.html

Cowdell, F. (2010). Promoting skin health in older people. *Nursing Older People, 22*(10), 21–26.

Demarré, L., Beeckman, D., Vanderwee, K., Defloor, T., Grypdonck, M., & Verhaeghe, S. (2012). Multi-stage versus single-stage inflation and deflation cycle for alternating low pressure air mattresses to prevent pressure ulcers in hospitalised patients: A randomised-controlled clinical trial. *International Journal of Nursing Studies, 49*(4), 416–426.

Denyer, J. (2011). Reducing pain during the removal of adhesive and adherent products. *British Journal of Nursing, 20*(15) (Tissue Viability Supplement), S28–35.

Downie, F., Egdell, S., Bielby, A., & Searle, R. (2010). Barrier dressings in surgical site infection prevention strategies. *British Journal of Nursing, 19*(20) (Tissue Viability Supplement), S42–S46.

Dudek, S. (2014). *Nutrition essentials for nursing practice* (7th ed.). Philadelphia: Wolters Kluwer Health/Lippincott Williams & Wilkins.

Durai, R., & Ng, P. C. H. (2010). Surgical vacuum drains: Types, uses and complications. *AORN Journal, 91*(2), 266–274.

Dyble, T., & Ashton, J. (2011). Use of emollients in the treatment of dry skin conditions. *British Journal of Community Nursing, 16*(5), 214–220.

Elliott, J. (2011). Applying pressure ulcer prevention theory to practice. *Nursing & Residential Care, 13*(6), 276–279.

Flores, A. (2008). Sterile versus non-sterile glove use and aseptic technique. *Nursing Standard, 23*(6), 35–39.

Geraghty, J. (2011). Introducing a new skin-care regimen for the incontinent patient. *British Journal of Nursing, 20*(7), 409–415.

Gould, D. (2012). Causes, prevention and management of surgical site infection. *Nursing Standard, 26*(47), 47–56.

Gross, S., Larsen, B. J., Mollo, J. A., Pilon, D., & Silfies, T. (2012). Back to basics: A medical–surgical orthopedic unit's quest to decrease pressure ulcers. *Med-Surg Matters, 21*(1), 16–19.

Grossman, S. (2014). *Porth's pathophysiology: concepts of altered health states*. (9th ed.). Philadelphia: Wolters Kluwer Health/Lippincott Williams & Wilkins.

Gupta, S., & Ichioka, S. (2010). Optimal use of negative pressure wound therapy in treating pressure ulcers. *International Wound Journal, 9*(Suppl. 1), 8–16.

Harvey, C. (2005). Wound healing. *Orthopaedic Nursing, 24*(2), 143–157.

He, W., Liu, P., & Chen, H.-L. (2012). The Braden Scale cannot be used alone for assessing pressure ulcer risk in surgical patients: A meta-analysis. *Ostomy Wound Management, 58*(2), 34–40.

Hess, C. (2013). *Clinical guide to skin & wound care* (7th ed.). Philadelphia: Wolters Kluwer Health/Lippincott Williams & Wilkins.

Hinkle, J. L., & Cheever, K. H. (2014). *Brunner & Suddarth's Textbook of Medical-Surgical Nursing* (13th ed.). Philadelphia: Wolters Kluwer Health/Lippincott Williams & Wilkins.

Hogan-Quigley, B., Palm, M. L., & Bickley, L. (2012). *Bates' nursing guide to physical examination and history taking*.Philadelphia: Wolters Kluwer Health/Lippincott Williams & Wilkins.

Huether, S. E., & McCance, K. L. (2012.) *Understanding pathophysiology* (5th ed.). St. Louis: Elsevier.

Jarvis, C. (2012). *Physical examination & health assessment* (6th ed.). St. Louis: Elsevier/Saunders.

Jensen, S. (2011). *Nursing health assessment. A best practice approach*.Philadelphia: Wolters Kluwer Health/Lippincott Williams & Wilkins.

Kee, J. L., Hayes, E. R., McCuistion, L. E. (2012). *Pharmacology: A nursing process approach* (7th ed.). St. Louis: Elsevier/Saunders.

Kelly, J. (2010). Methods of wound debridement: a case study. *Nursing Standard, 25*(25), 51–56, 58–59.

Korniewicz, D. M., Siegel, J., Fajardo, V., & El-Masri, M. (2011). Evaluation of the incidence of pressure ulcers using Hill-Rom VersaCare surfaces. *Advances in Skin & Wound Care, 24*(4), 160–166.

Krasner, D. (1995). Wound care: How to use the red-yellow-black system. *American Journal of Nursing, 5*(95), 44–47.

Kyle, T., & Carman, S. (2013). *Essentials of pediatric nursing* (2nd ed.). Philadelphia: Wolters Kluwer Health/Lippincott Williams & Wilkins.

Lloyd Jones, M. (2012a). Choosing the appropriate barrier product. *Nursing & Residential Care, 14*(4), 184–188.

Lloyd Jones, M. (2012b). Prevention and treatment of superficial pressure damage. *Nursing & Residential Care, 14*(1), 14, 16, 18, 20.

Lloyd Jones, M. (2008). Assessing and managing wound pain during dressing changes. *Nursing & Residential Care, 10*(7), 325–330.

Malarkey, L. M., & McMorrow, M. E. (2012). *Saunders nursing guide to laboratory and diagnostic tests* (2nd ed.). St. Louis: Elsevier/Saunders.

Malli, S. (2005). Device safety. Keep a close eye on vacuum-assisted wound closure. *Nursing, 35*(7), 25.

Martindell, D. (2012). Safety monitor. The safe use of negative-pressure wound therapy. *American Journal of Nursing, 112*(6), 59–63.

Medlin, S. (2012). Nutrition for wound healing. *British Journal of Nursing, 21*(12) (Tissue Viability Supplement), S511–S515.

Moorhead, S., Johnson, M., Maas, M. L., & Swanson, E. (Eds). (2013). *Nursing outcomes classification (NOC).* (5th ed.). St. Louis: Elsevier/Mosby.

NANDA International (NANDA-I). (2012). *Nursing diagnoses: Definitions & classification 2012–2014.* West Sussex, UK: Wiley-Blackwell.

National Pressure Ulcer Advisory Panel (NPUAP). (2012a). NPUAP Pressure ulcer stages/categories. Available at http://www.npuap.org/resources/educational-and-clinical-resources/npuap-pressure-ulcer-stagescategories/

National Pressure Ulcer Advisory Panel (NPUAP). (2012b). Pressure ulcer staging/illustrations. Available at http://www.npuap.org/resources/educational-and-clinical-resources/pressure-ulcer-categorystaging-illustrations/

National Pressure Ulcer Advisory Panel (NPUAP). (2012c). PUSH tool. Available at http://www.npuap.org/resources/educational-and-clinical-resources/push-tool/

National Pressure Ulcer Advisory Panel (NPUAP). (2012d). Pressure ulcer prevention points. Available at http://www.npuap.org/resources/educational-and-clinical-resources/pressure-ulcer-prevention-points/

Nilsson, S., & Renning, A.-C. (2012). Pain management during wound dressing in children. *Nursing Standard, 26*(32), 50–55.

O'Tuathall, C., & Taqi, R. (2011). Evaluation of three commonly used pressure ulcer risk assessment scales. *British Journal of Nursing, 20*(6) (Tissue Viability Supplement), S27–S34.

Parnham, A. (2012). Pressure ulcer risk assessment and prevention in children. *Nursing Children and Young People, 24*(2), 24–29.

Pegram, A., & Bloomfield, J. (2010). Wound care: Principles of aseptic technique. *Mental Health Practice, 14*(2), 14–18.

Perry, S. E., Hockenberry, M. J., Lowdermilk, D. L., & Wilson, D. (2010). *Maternal child nursing care* (4th ed.). Maryland Heights, MO: Elsevier/Mosby.

Peterson, M. J., Schwag, W., van Oostrom, J. H., Gravenstein, N., & Caruso, L. J. (2010). Effects of turning on skin-bed interface pressures in healthy adults. *Journal of Advanced Nursing, 66*(7), 1556–1564.

Posthauer, M. E. (2012). Nutrition strategies for wound healing. *Journal of Legal Nurse Consulting, 23*(1), 15–23.

Preston, G. (2008). An overview of topical negative pressure therapy in wound care. *Nursing Standard, 23*(7), 62–68.

Ritter, L. A., & Hoffman, N. A. (2010). *Multicultural health*.Boston: Jones and Bartlett.

Rush, A., & Muir, M. (2012). Maintaining skin integrity in bariatric patients. *British Journal of Community Nursing, 17*(4), 154–159.

Spear, M. (2012). Wound exudate—The good, the bad, and the ugly. *Plastic Surgical Nursing, 32*(2), 77–79.

Spector, R. E. (2009). *Cultural diversity in health and illness* (7th ed.). Upper Saddle River, NJ: Pearson/Prentice Hall.

Sprigle, S., & Sonenblum, S. (2011). Assessing the evidence supporting redistribution of pressure for pressure ulcer prevention: A review. *Journal of Rehabilitation Research & Development, 48*(3), 203–214.

Stephen-Hayes, J. (2012). Skin tears: achieving positive clinical and financial outcomes. *British Journal of Community Nursing,* (3 Suppl), S6-S16.

Stephen-Hayes, J. (2011). Managing exudate and the key requirements of absorbent dressings. *British Journal of Nursing, 16*(Supplement), S44–S49.

Stephen-Haynes, J. (2008). Skin integrity and silicone: APPEEL 'no-sting' medical adhesive remover. *British Journal of Nursing, 17*(12), 792–795.

Stotts, N. (1990). Seeing red, yellow and black: The three-color concept of wound care. *Nursing, 20*(2), 59–61.

Sullivan, J. M. (2011). Caring for older adults after surgery. *Nursing, 41*(4). 48–51.

Tabloski, P. (2010). *Gerontological nursing* (2nd ed.). Upper Saddle River, NJ: Pearson.

Taylor, J. J., & Cohen, B. J. (2013). *Memmler's structure and function of the human body* (10th ed.). Philadelphia: Wolters Kluwer Health/Lippincott Williams & Wilkins.

Thompson, G. (2008). An overview of negative pressure wound therapy (NPWT). *Wound Care, 13*(6), S23–4, S26, S28–30.

Timms, L. (2011). Effect of nutrition on wound healing in older people: a case study. *British Journal of Nursing, 20*(11) (Tissue Viability Supplement), S4–S10.

Tschannen, D., Bates, O., Talsma, A., & Guo, Y. (2012). Patient-specific and surgical characteristics in the development of pressure ulcers. *American Journal of Critical Care, 21*(2), 116–125.

Turns, M. (2011). The diabetic foot: an overview of assessment and complications. *British Journal of Nursing, 20*(15) (Tissue Viability Supplement), S19–S25.

Van Leeuwen, A. M., Poelhuis-Leth, D., & Bladh, M. L. (2011). *Davis's Comprehensive Handbook of Laboratory & Diagnostic Tests with Nursing Implications* (4th ed.). Philadelphia: F. A. Davis.

VISN 8 Patient Safety Center. (2009). Safe patient handling and movement algorithms. Tampa, FL: Author. Available at www.visn8.va.gov/patientsafety center/safePthandling/default.asp.

Voegeli, D. (2012). Moisture-associated skin damage: aetiology, prevention and treatment. *British Journal of Nursing, 21*(9), 517–518, 520–521.

Voegeli, D. (2010). Care or harm: Exploring essential components in skin care regimens. *British Journal of Nursing, 19*(13), 810, 812, 814, 816, 818–819.

Walker, J. (2007). Patient preparation for safe removal of surgical drains. *Nursing Standard, 21*(49), 39–41.

White, R. (2010). Wound dressings and other topical treatment modalities in bioburden control. In K. F. Cutting & S. Percival (Eds.), *Microbiology of wounds.* Boca Raton, FL: CRC Press. In *Journal of Wound Care, 20*(9), 431–439.

Woo, K. Y. (2012). Exploring the effects of pain and stress on wound healing. *Advances in Skin & Wound Care, 25*(1), 38–44.

The Wound Healing and Management Node Group. Joanna Briggs Institute. (2011). Wet-to-dry saline moistened gauze for wound dressing. *Wound Practice and Research, 19*(1), 48–49.

Wound, Ostomy and Continence Nurses Society (WOCN). (2012). Clean vs. sterile dressing techniques for management of chronic wounds. A fact sheet. *Journal of Wound, Ostomy and Continence Nursing, 39*(2S), S30–S34.

QUAN HONG NGUYEN

Mr. Nguyen is a 75-year-old man who had an ischemic stroke (cerebrovascular accident or brain attack) secondary to thrombosis (formation of a blood clot). His neurologic deficits have remained unchanged for the 2 days he has been in the hospital. He is alert, but has hemiplegia (weakness) on his left side. His wife states, "It will be quite a bit of work for me to care for Quan at home. My bones and joints hurt all the time. He needs a lot of help turning, moving, and getting out of bed. How will I manage?"

KELSI LESTER

Kelsi is a 10-year-old girl in the pediatric unit as a result of a skiing accident. Unconscious at present, she may or may not regain consciousness. Kelsi is on bedrest. She requires frequent positioning to maintain correct body alignment as well as passive range of motion exercises to maintain her range of motion.

MAGGIE WYATT

Maggie, a woman in her 30s, was hospitalized because the external fixation device used to treat her fractured right tibia caused an infection in her leg. Following therapy for the infection, the patient is being discharged and requires transfer from the wheelchair to her mother's car.

After completing the chapter, you will be able to accomplish the following:

1. Describe the role of the skeletal, muscular, and nervous systems in the physiology of movement.
2. Identify variables that influence body alignment and mobility.
3. Differentiate isotonic, isometric, and isokinetic exercise.
4. Describe the effects of exercise and immobility on major body systems.
5. Assess body alignment, mobility, and activity tolerance, using appropriate interview and assessment skills.
6. Develop nursing diagnoses that correctly identify mobility problems amenable to nursing interventions.
7. Utilize principles of body mechanics when appropriate.
8. Use safe patient handling and movement techniques and equipment when positioning, moving, lifting, and ambulating patients.
9. Design exercise programs.
10. Plan, implement, and evaluate nursing care related to select nursing diagnoses involving mobility problems.

KEY TERMS

active exercise
ankylosis
atrophy
body mechanics
cartilage
contractures
dangling
exercise
flaccidity
footdrop

isokinetic exercise
isometric exercise
isotonic exercise
ligaments
negative nitrogen balance
neurons
orthopedics

osteoporosis
paralysis
paresis
passive exercise
patient care ergonomics
range of motion
spasticity
tendons
tonus

This chapter describes the physiology of movement and factors affecting body alignment and mobility. A comprehensive section on exercise differentiates the types of exercise, explores the role of exercise in disease prevention and health promotion, notes risks related to exercise, and assists in the design of individualized exercise programs. The effects of immobility on body systems are discussed along with related nursing interventions. A practical guide for assessing body alignment and mobility states is included, with pertinent interview questions and physical assessment techniques. Analysis of patient mobility data may lead to the nursing diagnoses of Impaired Physical Mobility or Activity Intolerance or to diagnoses identifying effects of mobility problems on other areas of human functioning. Examples of nursing diagnoses are included, expected outcomes are identified, and specific nursing strategies are presented. The concluding Nursing Plan of Care illustrates how the nurse uses knowledge of mobility and of safe patient-handling techniques along with specific nursing interventions to promote fitness and to resolve mobility problems. The Reflective Practice box highlights important considerations to keep in mind when caring for patients with activity deficits.

PHYSIOLOGY OF MOVEMENT AND ALIGNMENT

Purposeful, coordinated movement of the body and maintenance of alignment require the integrated functioning of the musculoskeletal and nervous systems. The following sections review concepts related to movement and alignment.

Skeletal System

The framework of bones, the joints between them, and cartilage that protects our organs and allows us to move is called the skeletal system. Functions of this system include:

- Supporting the soft tissues of the body (maintains body form and posture)
- Protecting crucial components of the body (brain, lung, heart, spinal cord)
- Furnishing surfaces for the attachments of muscles, tendons, and ligaments, which, in turn, pull on the individual bones and produce movement
- Providing storage areas for minerals (such as calcium) and fat
- Producing blood cells (hematopoiesis)

The 206 bones in the human body are classified by their shape. Long bones, found in the upper and lower extremities (e.g., humerus and femur), contribute to height and length. Short bones, located in the wrist and ankle, contribute to movement. Flat bones are relatively thin (e.g., ribs and several of the skull bones) and contribute to shape (structural contour). Irregular bones are all those bones not included in the preceding classifications (e.g., bones of the spinal column and jaw).

Bones are too rigid to bend without damage. Therefore, all movements that change the positions of the bony parts of the body occur at joints. The terms *articulation* and *joint* refer to the area where a bone meets another bone. Joints are classified according to the amount of movement they permit and on the basis of the material between the adjoining bones. Types of joints are outlined in Table 32-1 (on page 1040). Diarthroses or synovial joints, joints in which there is a potential space containing lubricating synovial fluid between the articulating bones, are freely moving joints.

REFLECTIVE PRACTICE: CULTIVATING QSEN COMPETENCIES

CHALLENGE TO TECHNICAL SKILLS

Last year during my medical–surgical clinical experience, I was taking care of Maggie Wyatt, a female patient in her 30s, with an external fixation device on her right leg. The patient had broken her tibia, and had undergone three surgeries to try to correct the fracture. Maggie's current admission was for the treatment of an infection caused by the external device in place to treat the fracture. I was assigned to care for her on the day that she was being discharged. Throughout the day, I formed a close bond with her, and the nurse asked me to bring Maggie to her car when she was ready to leave. I was a little apprehensive about being able to help her into the car with the external fixator in place because she could not bend her leg at all. I had a couple of choices—I could take her down to the car myself and hope that there wouldn't be any problem helping her get into the car, or I could tell the nurse I didn't feel comfortable bringing the patient to the car because I didn't have any experience transferring patients with a device such as this one. However, I really wanted to bring this patient down and see her through the final stage of discharge.

Thinking Outside the Box: Possible Courses of Action

- Take the patient down to the car by myself and do the best I can to help transfer her to the car.
- Explain to the nurse that I don't feel that I have the skills to bring this patient down on my own and ask her to do it.
- Explain to the nurse that I would really like to bring the patient down to the car but that I do not feel that I have the experience to do it on my own; ask her to assist me.
- Ask the nurse about what the best way to transfer the patient to the car is, before taking the patient to the car.

Evaluating a Good Outcome: How Do I Define Success?

- Patient receives the highest quality of care and has the least amount of pain possible during the transfer.
- I learn from the experience and gain skills and knowledge for the future.
- Patient is at least not harmed and is possibly benefited by my action.

Personal Learning: Here's to the Future!

Unfortunately, in this case I did not make the right decision. I convinced myself that it could not be that difficult to transfer this very cooperative patient to her car with her mother's assistance. However, I was very wrong. I definitely should have asked for assistance. The car was extremely small, and it was hard to get her to sit across the back seat while keeping her leg completely straight. The patient was experiencing a fair amount of pain from the device. So, every time we tried to get her into the car, she experienced more pain. Fortunately, a physical therapist came outside to help another patient and then also helped us. I realized that not only did I not have the skills to transfer her myself, but also that this was really a two-person job. The physical therapist taught me the best way to transfer this patient, and I learned a great deal from the experience. I was lucky that my patient was very understanding and accommodating in this situation. I learned how to transfer a patient properly, but most importantly, I realized how important it is to trust your instincts and ask for help when you think you may need it—it's always better to be overprepared than underprepared.

Catherine Barrell, Georgetown University

REFLECTION ON QUALITY AND SAFETY COMPETENCIES

How do you think you would respond in a similar situation? Why? What does this tell you about yourself and about the adequacy of your skills for professional practice? Do you agree with the criteria that the nursing student used to evaluate a successful outcome? Are there any other criteria that would be appropriate to use? Did the nursing student meet the criteria? Why or why not? What *knowledge, skills,* and *attitudes* do you need to develop to continuously improve the quality and safety of care for patients like Ms. Wyatt?

Patient-Centered Care: What factors do you think might have influenced the nursing student's actions? Suppose that the patient was using crutches or a walker instead of having the fixation device in place. How might the nursing student's actions been different?

Teamwork and Collaboration/Quality Improvement: Imagine that the physical therapist did not arrive on the scene. What would have been the nursing student's next best action? What communication skills do you need to improve to ensure that you function as a member of the patient-care team?

Safety/Evidence-Based Practice: What resources could the student have accessed to ensure the safe transfer of the patient? What evidence in nursing literature provides guidance for decision making regarding care of this patient? Can you think of other ways to respond to or approach the situation?

Table 32-1   JOINTS

TYPE	MOVEMENT	MATERIAL BETWEEN THE BONES	EXAMPLES
Fibrous	Immovable (synarthrosis)	No joint cavity; fibrous connective tissue between bones	Sutures between bones of skull
Cartilaginous	Slightly movable (amphiarthrosis)	No joint cavity; cartilage between bones	Pubic symphysis; joints between bodies of vertebrae
Synovial	Freely movable (diarthrosis)	Joint cavity containing synovial fluid	Gliding, hinge, pivot, condyloid, saddle, ball-and-socket joints

Reprinted with permission from Taylor, J. J., & Cohen, B. J. (2013). *Memmler's structure and function of the human body* (10th ed.). Philadelphia: Wolters Kluwer Health/Lippincott Williams & Wilkins.

Freely movable joints are discussed here in relation to the topic of activity.

Several types of freely movable joints are found in the body. These include:

- *Ball-and-socket joint:* The rounded head of one bone fits into a cuplike cavity in the other; flexion–extension, abduction–adduction, and rotation can occur (e.g., shoulder and hip joints).
- *Condyloid joint:* The oval head of one bone fits into a shallow cavity of another bone; flexion–extension and abduction–adduction can occur (e.g., wrist joint and joints connecting fingers to palm).
- *Gliding joint:* Flat surfaces of the bone slide over one another; flexion–extension and abduction–adduction can occur (e.g., carpal bones of wrist and tarsal bones of feet).

- *Hinge joint:* A spool-like (rounded) surface of one bone fits into a concave surface of another bone; only flexion–extension can occur (e.g., elbow, knee, ankle joints).
- *Pivot joint:* A ring-like structure that turns on a pivot; movement is limited to rotation (e.g., joints between the atlas and axis of the neck and between the proximal ends of the radius and the ulna at the wrist).
- *Saddle joint:* Bone surfaces are convex on one side and concave on the other; movements include flexion–extension, adduction–abduction, circumduction, and opposition (e.g., joint between the trapezium and metacarpal of the thumb).

Movements possible at diarthrodial joints include abduction, adduction, flexion, extension, and rotation. Special movements of the forearm, ankle, and clavicle include supination, pronation, inversion, and eversion. The thumb is the only joint that can perform opposition. These movements

Table 32-2 TERMS COMMONLY USED TO DESCRIBE BODY POSITIONS AND MOVEMENTS

TERM	DEFINITION AND EXAMPLE
Abduction	Lateral movement of a body part away from the midline of the body. *Example:* A person's arm is abducted when it is moved away from the body.
Adduction	Lateral movement of a body part toward the midline of the body. *Example:* A person's arm is adducted when it is moved from an outstretched position to a position alongside the body.
Circumduction	Turning in a circular motion; combines abduction, adduction, extension, and flexion. *Example:* Circling the arm at the shoulder, as in bowling or a serve in tennis.
Flexion	The state of being bent. *Example:* A person's cervical spine is flexed when the head is bent forward, chin to chest.
Extension	The state of being in a straight line. *Example:* A person's cervical spine is extended when the head is held straight on the spinal column.
Hyperextension	The state of exaggerated extension. It often results in an angle greater than 180 degrees. *Example:* A person's cervical spine is hyperextended when looking overhead, toward the ceiling.
Dorsiflexion	Backward bending of the hand or foot. *Example:* A person's foot is in dorsiflexion when the toes are brought up as though to point them at the knee.
Plantar flexion	Flexion of the foot. *Example:* A person's foot is in plantar flexion in the footdrop position.
Rotation	Turning on an axis; the turning of a body part on the axis provided by its joint. *Example:* A thumb is rotated when it is moved to make a circle.
Internal rotation	A body part turning on its axis toward the midline of the body. *Example:* A leg is rotated internally when it turns inward at the hip and the toes point toward the midline of the body.
External rotation	A body part turning on its axis away from the midline of the body. *Example:* A leg is rotated externally when it turns outward at the hip and the toes point away from the midline of the body.
Special Movements	
Pronation	The assumption of the prone position. *Example:* A person is in the prone position when lying on the abdomen; a person's palm is prone when the forearm is turned so that the palm faces downward.
Supination	The assumption of the supine position. *Example:* A person is in the supine position when lying on the back; a person's palm is supine when the forearm is turned so that the palm faces upward.
Inversion	Movement of the sole of the foot inward (occurs at the ankle)
Eversion	Movement of the sole of the foot outward (occurs at the ankle)
Opposition	Rotation of the thumb around its long access (movement of the thumb across the palm to touch each fingertip of the same hand).

are defined in Table 32-2 and illustrated in Skill 32-6 on pages 1105–1113.

The strength and flexibility of the skeletal system also depend on ligaments, tendons, and cartilage. **Ligaments** are tough, fibrous bands of connective tissue that bind joints together and connect bones and cartilage. **Tendons** are strong, flexible, inelastic fibrous bands and flattened sheets of connective tissue that attach muscle to bone. **Cartilage** is hard, nonvascular connective tissue found in the joints as well as in the nose, ear, thorax, trachea, and larynx. Cartilage in joints functions as a shock absorber and provides a smooth surface that reduces friction between the moving parts of the joint. Fat may also provide padding at joints.

Muscular System

The muscular system is composed of three types of muscles: (1) skeletal, (2) cardiac, and (3) smooth or visceral muscles. Muscle tissue produces movement by contraction of its cells. Skeletal muscle works with tendons and bones to move the body. Cardiac muscle forms the bulk of the heart and produces the contractions that create the heartbeat. Smooth muscle forms the walls of the hollow organs (such as the stomach and intestines), and is in the walls of blood vessels and other hollow tubes (such as ureters) that connect

internal organs. Skeletal muscle is discussed here in relation to the topic of activity.

The skeletal muscle system includes the skeletal muscle tissue and connective tissue that comprise individual muscle organs, such as the biceps. Bones and joints provide form to the body and serve as the levers and fulcrums that make body movement possible. Movement results from a skeletal muscle contracting and exerting force on a tendon, which, in turn, pulls on a bone. Muscles have two differing points of attachment: (1) the attachment of a muscle to the more stationary bone is called the point of origin, and (2) the attachment to the more movable bone is the point of insertion. Between these two points is the fleshy "belly" of the muscle. The excitability, contractility, extensibility, and elasticity of muscles enable them to perform four important functions for the body through contraction:

* *Motion:* Skeletal muscle contractions pull on tendons and move the bones, creating movements as simple as extending the arm to as highly coordinated as swimming or skiing.
* *Maintenance of posture:* Skeletal muscle contractions hold the body in stationary positions.
* *Support:* Skeletal muscles support soft tissues in the abdominal wall and floor of the pelvic cavity.

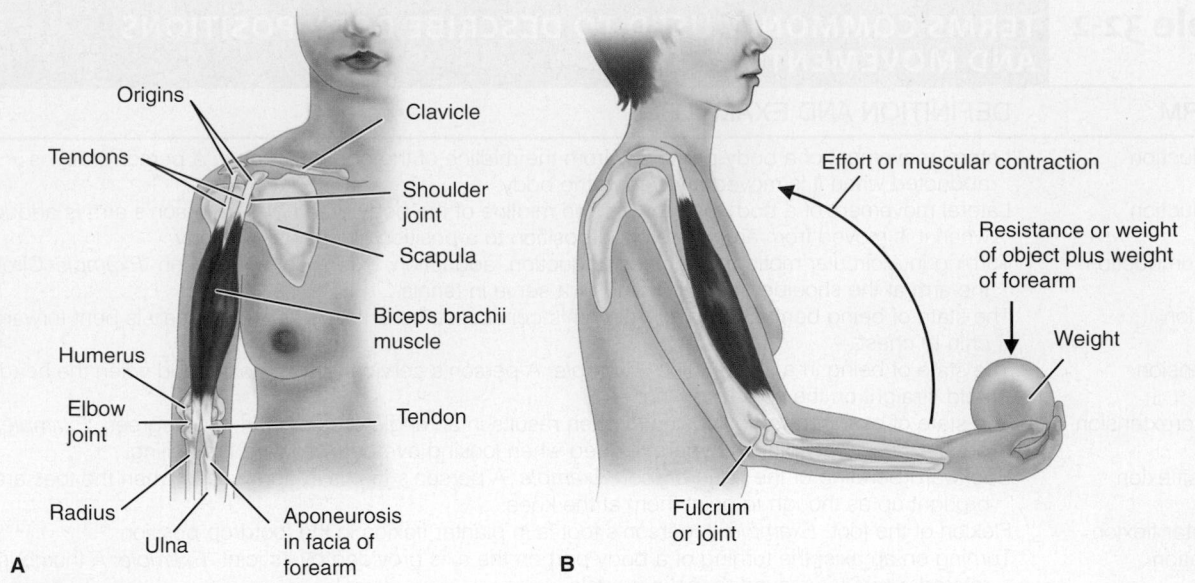

FIGURE 32-1. Relationship of skeletal muscles to bones. (**A**) Skeletal muscles produce movements by pulling on bones. (**B**) Bones serve as levers, and joints act as fulcrums for the levers. The lever and fulcrum principle is illustrated by the movement of the forearm lifting a weight.

• *Heat production:* Skeletal muscle contractions produce heat and help maintain body temperature.

Figure 32-1 illustrates the relationship of skeletal muscles to bones and the use of bones as levers and of joints as fulcrums to produce body movement.

Nervous System

The skeletal and muscular systems cannot produce purposeful movement without a functioning nervous system. Nerve impulses stimulate muscles to contract. More specifically:

• Nerve cells called **neurons** conduct impulses from one part of the body to another.
• The afferent neurons convey information from receptors in the periphery of the body to the central nervous system (CNS; e.g., light pressure on nose).
• This information is processed by the CNS, leading to a response (e.g., "There is a fly on my nose. I want to brush it off.").
• The efferent neurons convey the response from the CNS to skeletal muscles by way of the somatic nervous system (e.g., muscles in the arm, wrist, and hand contract, and the fingers brush the fly from the nose).

Normal Movement and Alignment

The following concepts are an important part of normal movement and musculoskeletal functioning, and contribute to a person's overall well-being.

Body Alignment or Posture

Good posture, or proper body alignment, is the alignment of body parts that permits optimal musculoskeletal balance and operation, and promotes healthy physiologic functioning. A person in correct alignment is experiencing no undue strain on the joints, muscles, tendons, or ligaments while balance is maintained.

 CONSIDER Maggie Wyatt, the woman being discharged with an external fixation device in place. Although the device is heavy and awkward and requires her to keep her right leg extended, body alignment is crucial for Maggie to prevent undue strain on other parts of her body. ●

The criteria for correct alignment in the standing, sitting, and reclining positions are described in the Assessing section later in this chapter.

Balance

A body in correct alignment is balanced. An object is balanced when its center of gravity is close to its base of support, the line of gravity goes through the base of support, and the object has a wide base of support. The center of gravity of an object is the point at which its mass is centered. When the human is standing, the center of gravity is located in the center of the pelvis about midway between the umbilicus and the symphysis pubis. The line of gravity is a vertical line that passes through the center of gravity. The base of support is the foundation that provides for an object's stability. The wider the base of support and the lower the center of gravity, the greater the stability of the object will be. Figure 32-2 illustrates the effect of the base of support and gravity on body balance.

Body balance increases when people spread the feet farther apart and flex the hips and knees. This broadens the base of support and lowers the center of gravity. These two simple maneuvers are important interventions that can decrease the musculoskeletal strain that occurs with excessive stretching

FIGURE 32-2. The effect of the base of support and gravity on balance is shown. (**A**) The line of gravity passes through the wide base of support. This person is the most stable of the three. **B**) The line of gravity also passes through the base of support, although the base is narrower. This person is less stable than the person in **A**. (**C**) The line of gravity does not pass through the base of support. This person is unstable.

or overexertion of a muscle or muscle–tendon unit. Musculoskeletal strain most commonly affects the lower back and cervical spine region. Trauma to the musculoskeletal system is discussed later in the chapter.

Coordinated Body Movement

Coordinated body movement is the ability of muscles to work together for purposeful movement. Using major and stronger muscle groups, rather than weaker ones, and taking advantage of the body's natural levers and fulcrums facilitates the actions of lifting, carrying, pushing, pulling, and moving objects. Major muscle groups include the flexors, extensors, and abductors of the thighs; flexors and extensors of the knees; and flexors and extensors of the upper and lower arms. For example, use of the arm bones as levers and the elbows as fulcrums facilitates lifting a weight against resistance, the force of gravity—the lever and fulcrum principle (see Fig. 32-1).

Postural Reflexes

Postural reflexes are the group of reflexes (automatic movements) that maintain body position and equilibrium, whether at rest or during movement. Integrated functioning of the musculoskeletal and nervous systems is essential for body alignment and balance. Postural tonus, the sustained

contraction of select skeletal muscles that keeps the human body in an upright position against the force of gravity, depends on the functioning of several postural reflexes:

- *Labyrinthine sense:* The sensory organs in the inner ear provide this sense of position, orientation, and movement. Body movement (e.g., changes in head position) stimulates the sensory organs, which then transmit these impulses to the cerebellum.
- *Proprioceptor or kinesthetic sense:* This informs the brain of the location of a limb or body part as a result of joint movements stimulating special nerve endings in muscles, tendons, and fascia.
- *Visual or optic reflexes:* Visual impressions contribute to posture by alerting the person to spatial relationships with the environment (nearness of ceilings, walls, furniture, condition of floor, etc.).
- *Extensor or stretch reflexes:* When extensor muscles are stretched beyond a certain point (e.g., when knees buckle under), their stimulation causes a reflex contraction that aids a person to reestablish erect posture (e.g., straighten the knee).

Body Mechanics

Body mechanics is the use of proper body positions to provide protection from the stress of movement and activity, specifically in regard to structure, function, and position of the body (Waters, Nelson, Hughes, & Menzel, 2009). It includes proper body movement in daily activities, the prevention and correction of problems associated with posture, and the enhancement of coordination and endurance. It is important to use the principles of body mechanics during activity and during rest periods, to prevent injury and to prevent sore muscles and joints. The principles of body mechanics are also used to assess and maintain the alignment of patients. The correct use of body mechanics is a part of illness prevention and health promotion. Many activities in which the nurse engages, from as simple an activity as moving a chair, repositioning the medication cart, or reaching to silence a monitor alarm, require understanding and using these principles. Nurses who consciously develop good habits can demonstrate to others proper ways of using the musculoskeletal system. The application of body mechanics is discussed in the Implementing section of the Nursing Process, later in the chapter.

Patient Care Ergonomics

Patient-handling tasks are the primary cause of musculoskeletal disorders among nurses (American Nurses Association [ANA], 2013). Nurses who retire from or leave nursing often cite back, shoulder, and neck injuries as an influencing factor. Of nurses in the United States, 52% have reported injuries to their back, and an estimated 12% leave the profession annually because of these injuries (Hunter, Branson, & Davenport, 2010; Waters et al., 2009). Many nurses say they have had episodes of occupation-related back problems and accept back pain as a routine consequence of the job—but this need not be. Variables that can lead to back injuries or back pain for health care workers include:

- Uncoordinated lifts
- Manual lifting and transferring of patients without assistive devices
- Lifting when fatigued
- Lifting after recent recovery from a back injury
- Repetitive movements such as lifting, transferring, and repositioning patients
- Standing for long periods of time
- Transferring patients from beds to stretchers and chairs, wheelchairs, or operating tables; repositioning patients in bed
- Repetitive tasks
- Transferring/repositioning uncooperative or confused patients (Nelson, Motacki, & Menzel, 2009; Waters et al., 2009)

Patient care ergonomics is the practice of designing equipment and work tasks to conform to the capability of the worker in relation to patient care. It is very important to incorporate patient care ergonomics into nursing practice and patient care. Frequently, it is necessary to move a patient who is weak or unable to move on one's own. However, as discussed, manual lifting, transferring, and repositioning of patients that involves lifting most or all of a patient's weight are high-risk activities for nurses and patients. Even routine repetitive care activities, such as changing bed linens and bathing patients, have the potential to cause back injury.

A more effective approach to safe patient transfers is thought to include patient assessment criteria; algorithms for patient handling and movement decisions; specialized patient handling equipment used properly and operated using good body mechanics; and the use of lift teams. The use of mechanical lifts and other patient handling devices reduces the effect of cumulative trauma and injuries in nursing that occur slowly over time because of repeated musculoskeletal stress and decreases health care worker fatigue (VISN 8 Patient Safety Center, 2009; Nelson et al., 2009). In addition, the use of assistive patient handling equipment contributes to patient comfort and protects patient dignity, while increasing safety. Patients are less subjected to awkward or forceful handling when nurses use assistive patient handling equipment compared to when lifting, transferring, or repositioning is done manually (VISN 8 Patient Safety Center; Nelson et al.).

Research conducted at the VISN 8 Patient Safety Center of Inquiry at the James A. Haley Veterans Hospital Veterans Administration Medical Center, and other institutions, supports the consistent use of standardized protocols and mechanical lifting devices as a more effective approach to decrease the risk of injury for health care workers, rather than just using proper body mechanics (Nelson et al., 2009). The Occupational Safety & Health Administration (OSHA, 2012) recommends a no-lift policy for all health care facilities.

Preventive measures should focus on careful assessment of the patient care environment so that patients can be moved safely and effectively. The use of a back belt does not prevent back injury. In some institutions, specially trained staff members who function as "back injury resource nurses" are responsible for assisting nurses to assess patients. Other institutions have created "lift teams" or "patient lift teams" as part of their institution's safe patient handling policy. Lift teams are groups of specially trained staff that provide safe patient transfers (VISN 8 Patient Safety Center, 2009; OSHA, 2012). The application of patient care ergonomics, specifically safe patient handling and movement, is discussed in detail later in this chapter, in the Implementation section of the Nursing Process.

Orthopedics

Orthopedics refers to the correction or prevention of disorders of body structures used in locomotion. Nurses have long recognized that basic orthopedic principles apply in all areas of nursing, not just to patients with bone fractures or other pathologic skeletal changes. For example, a person who has a sedentary occupation and engages in little physical activity may have poorly developed muscles. A patient who is on complete bed rest is in danger of losing muscle tonus. **Tonus** is the term used to describe the state of slight contraction—the usual state of skeletal muscles. If bed rest is prolonged, the patient is in danger of developing **contractures** (permanent contraction of a muscle) unless exercise, joint motion, and good posture is maintained. Position and movement, or lack thereof, also influence the functioning of various internal body processes.

FACTORS AFFECTING MOVEMENT AND ALIGNMENT

Numerous factors, including growth and development, physical health, mental health, lifestyle variables, attitude and values, fatigue and stress, and external factors such as weather, influence a person's posture, movement, and daily activity level.

Developmental Considerations

A person's age and degree of neuromuscular development markedly influence body proportions, posture, body mass, movements, and reflexes. To promote neuromuscular development in patients of all ages and to facilitate each patient's use of the body to perform self-care activities, nurses need to be familiar with developmental variations in body proportions and neuromuscular development. These variations are presented in Table 32-3 with related nursing assessment priorities and nursing interventions.

 RECALL Kelsi Lester, the 10-year-old girl in a coma. Typically, children of this age are highly active and mobile. However, Kelsi is confined to bed due to her accident. The nurse would obtain a history of Kelsi's activity level before the accident to determine her neuromuscular development. The nurse would then use this information to develop an age-appropriate plan of care to maximize Kelsi's level of function. ●

Table 32-3   ACTIVITY VARIATIONS BASED ON DEVELOPMENTAL LEVEL: ASSESSMENT PRIORITIES AND NURSING INTERVENTIONS

DEVELOPMENTAL LEVEL	ASSESSMENT PRIORITIES	NURSING INTERVENTIONS
Infant • Periods of activity and alertness alternate with quiet periods and sleep. • At 3 months: may raise chest and head when prone • By 5 months: head control usually achieved	Assess the following key developmental milestones at these ages: **3 to 6 mo** • Ability to sit • Head control **6 to 9 mo** • Sits steadily • Rolls over • Creeps on all fours • Pulls to a standing position • Has improved hand–eye coordination **9 to 12 mo** • Progresses toward unassisted walking • Is able to pick up small objects	• Encourage parents to examine their baby (e.g., count fingers and toes). • Respond to concerns that parents have about minor variations in newborn's appearance or behavior. • Emphasize that individual variation in activity patterns and neuromuscular development should be expected. • Account for any prematurity when discussing normal developmental progression of preterm infants.
Toddler • Gross and fine motor development continue rapidly. • By 15 months: most can walk unassisted. • At 18 months: most can run. • At 2 years: most can jump. • At 3 years: most can stack blocks, string large beads, work simple puzzles, and dress themselves.	• Assess progress in walking, running, and jumping. • Assess small-muscle coordination (e.g., ability to dress themselves, wash hands, brush teeth). • Distinguish slow developers who fall within normal range from those with developmental lags.	• Help parents to learn and accept their child's uniqueness. • Teach parents the importance of providing a safe environment. • Enthusiastically reinforce and praise toddler's mastery of new skills. • Set limits so that toddler does not overextend self in drive for mastery of skills.
Child • Muscles, bones, and nervous system develop, allowing greater gross and fine motor control. • By age 4: negotiate stairs, walk backward, and hop on one foot. • By age 5: skip, jump rope, and jump off heights of several steps. • Able to manipulate writing materials. • Has acquired all basic mechanisms for physical locomotion.	• Use developmental charts to assess gross and fine motor development. • Determine activity level and types of play that involve physical exertion.	• Teach parents that attitudes about the body and exercise are developed during this period. • Counsel as appropriate. • Assess safety issues and reinforce safety teaching at each stage.
Adolescent • Size increases: there is a growth spurt. • Secondary sex characteristics appear. • If physically fit: can be a time of boundless energy and great athletic performance. • If inactive: may begin a lifelong pattern of unhealthy behavior.	• Determine activity level and type of regular exercise. • Evaluate safety of recreational choices. • Screen for scoliosis (lateral curvature of the spine). • Examine muscle mass, tone, and strength and joint mobility.	• Encourage physical activity, regular exercise, and limitation of sedentary hobbies. • Lifestyle counseling regarding the importance of exercise and fitness is critical. • Encourage to exercise regularly if necessary. • Caution about gauging physical limits and not "pushing too hard."
Adult • Stands and sits erect and is capable of balanced and coordinated, purposeful movement. • During pregnancy: center of gravity shifts because of developing fetus. • Activity levels vary greatly.	• Assess balance between activity and rest in person's lifestyle. • Note any lifestyle factors or illnesses that interfere with mobility or ability to carry out activities of daily living.	• Fitness counseling is important. • Clarify misconceptions about exercise. • Design and monitor safe exercise programs. • Those with mobility alterations may require special care.
Older Adult • Increased convexity in the thoracic spine (kyphosis) from disk shrinkage and decreased height • Flexed posture • Loss of muscle tone • Subcutaneous fat loss • Arthritic joint changes may be present.	• Assess general ease of movement and gait. • Assess alignment. • Check joints and their function. • Assess muscle mass, tone, and strength.	Teach and counsel about: • Importance of regular exercise • Need to maintain proper weight • Need for high protein, calcium, and vitamin D–enriched diet • Pacing activities • Using assistive devices safely when needed • Safety-proof homes to reduce falls

Physical Health

Problems in the musculoskeletal or nervous systems can have a negative influence on body alignment and movement. Similarly, illness or trauma involving other body systems may interfere with movement because of either the underlying pathology or the treatment regimen. Nurses must be sensitive to how both acute and chronic health problems affect a patient's general appearance (posture, body proportions, and movements) and their ability to move purposefully to perform activities of daily living (ADLs). When assessing a patient's response to a mobility deficit, work to:

- Encourage attempts at behaviors that promote self-care activities despite limitations (e.g., offer supportive suggestions to patients who attempt to feed themselves despite having hemiparesis)
- Reinforce behaviors that promote healthy functioning (e.g., congratulate a patient who manages transfers well despite left-sided weakness or paralysis)
- Correct behaviors that compound the mobility deficit over time (e.g., teach successful adaptive strategies that can be shared with other patients and families to a patient with arthritis who severely restricts movement because of joint stiffness and tenderness; or teach energy-conservation measures to patients with emphysema who have greatly decreased activity tolerance)

Muscular, Skeletal, or Nervous System Problems

Problems with the musculoskeletal or nervous systems may involve one or more of the following health issues.

CONGENITAL OR ACQUIRED POSTURAL ABNORMALITIES

A newborn with developmental hip dysplasia, torticollis (inclining of head to affected side) or a clubfoot; a teenager with lordosis (exaggerated anterior convex curvature of the spine) or scoliosis (lateral curvature of the spine); and an older person with kyphosis (increased convexity in the curvature of the thoracic spine) are all experiencing postural abnormalities that affect their appearance and mobility. Nursing responsibilities may include the following:

- Early detection of and referral for these problems
- Exploration and selection of patient education, counseling, and support as treatment options
- Careful attention to positioning, transfers, and exercise
- Education of the patient and family regarding safe self-care activities

PROBLEMS WITH BONE FORMATION OR MUSCLE DEVELOPMENT

Problems with bone formation may include any of the following:

- Congenital problems, such as achondroplasia, in which premature bone ossification (bone tissue formation) leads to dwarfism, or osteogenesis imperfecta, which is characterized by excessively brittle bones and multiple fractures both at birth and later in life

- Nutrition-related problems, such as vitamin D deficiency, which results in deformities of the growing skeleton (rickets)
- Disease-related problems, such as Paget disease, in which excessive bone destruction and abnormal regeneration result in skeletal pain, deformities, and pathologic fractures
- Age-related problems, such as osteoporosis, in which bone destruction exceeds bone formation and in which the resultant thin, porous bones fracture easily

The muscular dystrophies are a group of genetically transmitted disorders that share a common progressive degeneration and weakness of skeletal muscles. They vary in terms of the muscle groups involved and their clinical course. Myasthenia gravis is a weakness of the skeletal muscles caused by an abnormality at the neuromuscular junction that prevents muscle fibers from contracting. Myotonic muscular dystrophy involves prolonged muscle spasms or stiffening after use. Duchenne muscular dystrophy involves a muscle decrease in size, as well as weakening of muscles over time.

Nursing responsibilities for patients with problems of bone formation and muscle development and functioning include the following:

- Careful collaboration with the physician and health care team to determine the motor capacities of the person
- Patient and family education aimed at developing optimal mobility
- Having a solid knowledge base about the underlying disease process
- The ability to position, transfer, and exercise the patient safely, with attention to patient comfort

PROBLEMS AFFECTING JOINT MOBILITY

Inflammation, degeneration, and trauma can all interfere with joint mobility. The term *arthritis* describes more than 100 different diseases that affect areas in or around joints. Arthritis is characterized by inflammation, pain, damage to joint cartilage, and/or stiffness (Arthritis Foundation, 2013b; Centers for Disease Control and Prevention [CDC], 2011). The most common type is osteoarthritis, also termed *degenerative joint disease*. Osteoarthritis is a noninflammatory, progressive disorder of movable joints, particularly weight-bearing joints, characterized by the deterioration of articular cartilage and pain with motion. Once the articular cartilage is damaged, bony deposits (bone spurs) may form in the joints, causing more pain with movement of the joint.

 REMEMBER Mrs. Nguyen, the older woman concerned about caring for her husband at home. The nurse would need to consider the impact of possible age-related problems as contributing to Mrs. Nguyen's current problems with bone and joint pain. Due to her older adult status, the likelihood of osteoporosis and degenerative joint disease is high. Therefore, teaching to minimize stress on the joints when assisting with her husband's care would be important in preventing possible bone and joint injuries and reducing pain. ●

Trauma to a joint may result in a sprain or a dislocation. A sprain occurs with the wrenching or twisting of a joint, resulting in a partial tear or rupture to its attachments. A dislocation is characterized by the displacement of a bone from a joint with tearing of ligaments, tendons, and capsules. Any condition restricting joint mobility has potentially crippling effects.

Nurses caring for patients with joint problems work collaboratively with physicians, physical therapists, and other health care professionals to maintain joint mobility. Patient education is directed to the patient's mastery of an exercise and care program, which fosters tissue repair and maximal independence in ADLs.

 THINK back to Maggie Wyatt, the woman being discharged after treatment for a fractured tibia. The nurse would need to work closely with other members of Maggie's health care team to ensure that joint mobility is maintained, even with the device in place. The discharge teaching plan would include measures to maintain function of the right leg while the external fixation device immobilizes the fractured area. ●

TRAUMA TO THE MUSCULOSKELETAL SYSTEM

Injury to the musculoskeletal system can result in fractures and soft-tissue injuries. A fracture, a break in the continuity of a bone or cartilage, may result from a traumatic injury or some underlying disease process. Healing requires realignment of the bone fragment, immobilization, and restoration of the bone's function. Soft-tissue injuries include sprains, strains, and dislocations (sprains and dislocations are discussed in the previous section, Problems Affecting Joint Mobility). A strain, the least serious of these injuries, is a stretching of a muscle. Nurses need to be knowledgeable in first-aid measures for musculoskeletal trauma as well as in acute and rehabilitative care.

PROBLEMS AFFECTING THE CENTRAL NERVOUS SYSTEM

A problem in any of the principal parts of the brain or spinal cord involved with skeletal muscle control can affect mobility. The cerebral motor cortex assumes the major role of controlling precise, discrete movements. A cerebrovascular accident (stroke) or head trauma may damage the motor cortex and produce temporary or permanent voluntary motor impairment. Basal ganglia integrate semivoluntary movements such as walking, swimming, and laughing. In Parkinson disease, there is progressive degeneration of the basal ganglia of the cerebrum, thus affecting walking and coordination. Unnecessary skeletal movements result in tremors and muscle rigidity, which interfere with voluntary movement. The cerebellum assists the motor cortex and basal ganglia by making body movements smooth and coordinated. In multiple sclerosis, the myelin sheaths of neurons in the CNS deteriorate to hardened scars or plaques. Plaque formation in the cerebellum may produce lack of coordination, tremors, and/or weakness.

The pyramidal pathways convey voluntary motor impulses from the brain through the spinal cord by way of two major pathways: (1) the pyramidal pathway and (2) the extrapyramidal pathway. With trauma to the spinal cord, transection (severing) of these motor pathways results in complete bilateral loss of voluntary movement below the level of the trauma.

Patients with injury to the CNS often verbalize that no one talks with them (or with their families) about how the disease may progress and affect their functioning. Nurses caring for these patients need to be knowledgeable about the pathology and clinical course of these diseases to provide appropriate patient education and counseling.

 RECALL Kelsi Lester, the 10-year-old in a coma after a skiing accident. Although Kelsi is unconscious, the nurse must communicate with her, making sure to explain all that is happening to her and all that is being done. In addition, the nurse would need to communicate with Kelsi's family to ensure that they understand what is happening. For example, the nurse needs to explain the reasons for frequent turning, position changes, and exercises while Kelsi is unconscious. ●

Problems Involving Other Body Systems

The pathology of numerous other acute and chronic illnesses may also affect mobility. Chronic obstructive pulmonary disease and conditions such as ascites may alter posture. Any illnesses that interfere with oxygenation at the cellular level decrease the amount of oxygen available to the muscles for work and thus decrease activity tolerance. These illnesses include anemia, angina, cardiac arrhythmias, heart failure, and chronic obstructive pulmonary disease. Diseases characterized by a larger breakdown of protein than that which is manufactured leads to a **negative nitrogen balance** (e.g., anorexia nervosa and certain cancers) that results in muscle wasting and decreased physical energy for movement and work. Symptoms accompanying many illnesses, such as fatigue, muscle aches, and pain, may also lead to immobility. Bed rest is an important component of treatment for many diseases or trauma states, such as myocardial infarction, surgery, and fractures. Although rest is essential for the healing process, immobility associated with bed rest may cause its own problems. Table 32-4 (on page 1048) outlines a comparison of the effects of immobility and exercise on body systems. Nurses need to be vigilant in determining the effects of any injury or illness on mobility and in providing care to facilitate optimal mobility as early as possible.

Mental Health

A person's mental health influences body appearance and movement as much as the person's physical health. Body processes tend to slow down in depression, and there is a lack of visible energy and enthusiasm. Body posture also may be affected. For example, the person with depression often sits with head bowed and shoulders slumped, and may lack the energy to eat or even to use the toilet. Even facial

Table 32-4 COMPARISON OF EFFECTS OF EXERCISE AND IMMOBILITY ON BODY SYSTEMS

BODY SYSTEM	EFFECTS OF EXERCISE	EFFECTS OF IMMOBILITY
Cardiovascular System	↑Efficiency of heart ↓Resting heart rate and blood pressure ↑Blood flow and oxygenation of all body parts	↑Cardiac workload ↑Risk for orthostatic hypotension ↑Risk for venous thrombosis
Respiratory System	↑Depth of respiration ↑Respiratory rate ↑Gas exchange at alveolar level ↑Rate of carbon dioxide excretion	↓Depth of respiration ↓Rate of respiration Pooling of secretions Impaired gas exchange
Gastrointestinal System	↑Appetite ↑Intestinal tone	Disturbance in appetite Altered protein metabolism Altered digestion and utilization of nutrients ↓Peristalsis
Urinary System	↑Blood flow to kidneys ↑Efficiency in maintaining fluid and acid–base balance ↑Efficiency in excreting body wastes	↑Urinary stasis ↑Risk for renal calculi ↓Bladder muscle tone
Musculoskeletal System	↑Muscle efficiency ↑Coordination ↑Efficiency of nerve impulse transmission	↓Muscle size, tone, and strength ↓Joint mobility, flexibility Bone demineralization ↓Endurance, stability ↑Risk for contracture formation
Metabolic System	↑Efficiency of metabolic system ↑Efficiency of body temperature regulation	↑Risk for electrolyte imbalance Altered exchange of nutrients and gases
Integument	Improved tone, color, and turgor, resulting from improved circulation	↑Risk for skin breakdown and formation of pressure ulcers
Psychological Well-Being	Energy, vitality, general well-being Improved sleep Improved appearance Improved self-concept Positive health behaviors	↑Sense of powerlessness ↓Self-concept ↓Social interaction ↓Sensory stimulation Altered sleep–wake pattern ↑Risk for depression Risk for learned helplessness

movement may be decreased to the point at which the person's face registers no emotion (termed a flat affect). Conversely, people who are not depressed are more likely to have erect posture, animated facial features, and energy for routine activities.

Lifestyle

Many variables—including occupation, leisure activity preferences, and cultural influences—influence a person's lifestyle, whether active or sedentary. Many occupations are sedentary (e.g., computer technician). Therefore, people in sedentary occupations wishing to exercise regularly need to plan ahead for these leisure activities by preparing to exercise before or after work hours or during a lunch break. People may also participate in leisure activities that are sedentary in nature such as reading, debating, crafts, and watching television. In addition, a person's diet and smoking history are other lifestyle variables that influence mobility. Culture and gender may also play a role, encouraging or discouraging exercise.

Nurses, particularly those involved in community health activities, need to consider appropriate forms of exercise

and geographic location before making recommendations to patients from diverse cultures. For example, walking is a commonly prescribed exercise. However, walking may pose a threat to the person who only has access to walk in unsafe environments, such as high-crime areas. Identifying culturally acceptable physical activities is an important step in planning a program of physical activity. Physical activities that are congruent with overall lifestyle and cultural context will be easier to incorporate into daily living (Lee & Im, 2010). The nurse must talk with the patient and family members to determine preferred activities. While the nurse must avoid stereotyping, an exercise prescription for a Native American might include suggestions for exploring nearby mountain areas, hunting, or even participating in Native American dances as more acceptable methods for increasing activity level.

Attitude and Values

In some families, such as those who hike, swim, or play ball together, children learn early to value regular exercise. As these children mature, they often continue to value exercise and find new ways to incorporate regular exercise into their daily routine. On the other hand, children may be raised in families who are sedentary and in which watching sports is the closest anyone comes to exercise. Attitudes and values learned early may be internalized for a lifetime. Individual values also influence the exercise options people make. People who place a high value on physical attractiveness may be highly committed to regular exercise because it helps produce the body they want. Another person may exercise because of the desire for physical strength, relating strength with power. However, someone more disposed to intellectual pursuits may perceive body development as simply wasting time that could be better used to develop the mind. Sometimes, people view exercise as too much of a chore, thus avoid it. It is important to offer suggestions for how to incorporate exercise into the person's daily routine, making exercise less of a chore.

Fatigue and Stress

Chronic stress may deplete body energy to the point that fatigue makes even the thought of exercise overwhelming. Ironically, regular exercise is energizing and can better equip a person to deal with daily stresses. Excessive exercise, however, may stress the body and lead to injury as well as to fatigue.

External Factors

Many external factors can influence activity and mobility. Among these, weather probably exerts the greatest influence over outside exercise. A brisk, clear day is invigorating and invites increased activity. However, high humidity, very hot and very cold temperatures, rain, and snow discourage outdoor exercise. Sufficient financial resources for gym memberships, access to exercise equipment, safe outdoor parks and sports areas, the availability of malls for early-morning walkers, support people, and occupational or insurance rewards for exercise can all encourage regular exercise. Discouraging factors include lack of free time, insufficient financial resources for equipment purchase or gym membership, air pollution, unsafe neighborhoods, and lack of support and reinforcement.

EXERCISE

Active exertion of muscles involving the contraction and relaxation of muscle groups is termed **exercise**. Each of the many different types of exercise can produce different physiologic and psychological benefits.

Types of Exercise

Exercise can be divided into two major types. One is based on the type of *muscle contraction* occurring during the exercise. The second is based on the type of *body movement* occurring and the health benefits achieved.

Muscle Contraction

Exercise may be categorized according to the type of muscle contraction involved as being isotonic, isometric, or isokinetic (Fig. 32-3).

Isotonic exercise

Isometric exercise

Isokinetic exercise

FIGURE 32-3. Three types of exercise. *Isotonic exercise* involves muscle shortening and active movement. *Isometric exercise* involves muscle contraction without shortening. *Isokinetic exercise* involves muscle contraction with resistance.

Isotonic exercise involves muscle shortening and active movement. Examples include carrying out ADLs, independently performing range-of-motion exercises, and swimming, walking, jogging, and bicycling. Potential benefits include increased muscle mass, tone, and strength; improved joint mobility; increased cardiac and respiratory function; increased circulation; and increased osteoblastic or bone-building activity. These benefits do not occur when the nurse or family member performs passive range-of-motion exercises for a patient because the patient's muscles do not exert effort. Therefore, although still beneficial, the overall potential benefits are reduced.

Isometric exercise involves muscle contraction without shortening (i.e., there is no movement or only a minimum shortening of muscle fibers). Examples include contractions of the quadriceps and gluteal muscles, such as what occurs when holding a Yoga pose. Potential benefits are increased muscle mass, tone, and strength; increased circulation to the exercised body part; and increased osteoblastic activity. Nurses should encourage both isotonic and isometric exercises for hospitalized patients with limited mobility.

Isokinetic exercise involves muscle contractions with resistance. The resistance is provided at a constant rate by an external device, which has a capacity for variable resistance. Examples include rehabilitative exercises for knee and elbow injuries and lifting weights. Using the device, the person takes the muscles and joint through a complete range of motion without stopping, meeting resistance at every point. A continuous passive motion (CPM) device used postoperatively after joint surgery (knee replacement, anterior cruciate ligament [ACL] repair) performs these same type exercises passively for the patient.

 CONSIDER Maggie Wyatt, the woman being discharged with an external fixation device in place. A specific exercise routine that includes isotonic and isometric exercises would most likely be prescribed for Maggie. Later in the course of Maggie's treatment, after her fracture has healed, isokinetic exercises may be included to strengthen her right leg. ●

Body Movement

Exercise activities may also be categorized according to the type of body movement involved and the health benefits they produce. Types of exercise involving body movement include aerobic exercises, stretching exercises, strength and endurance exercises, and movement and ADLs.

Aerobic exercise refers to sustained (often rhythmic) muscle movements that increase blood flow, heart rate, and metabolic demand for oxygen over time, promoting cardiovascular conditioning. Examples of aerobic activities include swimming, walking, jogging, cross-country skiing, aerobic dancing, bicycling, jumping rope, and racquetball. Aerobic exercise may be further distinguished as having high or low impact. The number of injuries, such as shin splints, related to high-impact aerobic workouts led to the development of low-impact workouts that place less stress on the musculoskeletal system. Low-impact aerobic exercises include those activities in which at least one foot is on the ground at all times, like walking, rowing, or riding a stationary bicycle. High-impact exercises include activities that are more apt to jar the spine, like running, jumping, or kick-boxing.

Stretching exercises involve movements that allow muscles and joints to be stretched gently through their full range of motion, increasing flexibility. Specific warm-up and cooldown exercises, Hatha yoga, and some forms of dance are examples. Benefits include increased range-of-joint movements, improved circulation and posture, and relaxation.

Strength and endurance exercises are components of a variety of muscle-building programs. Weight training, calisthenics, and specific isometric exercises can build both strength and endurance, increasing the power of the musculoskeletal system and generally improving the whole body. They may or may not have aerobic benefit.

Movement and ADLs include housecleaning, running after playful toddlers, climbing stairs instead of riding in elevators, and so on. Household activities can also contribute to an active lifestyle.

Effects of Exercise on Major Body Systems

The human body was designed for motion, and regular exercise is necessary for its healthy functioning. The effects of regular exercise on major body systems are explored in the following sections and outlined in Table 32-4 on page 1048. People differ in the benefits they receive from exercise based on the patient's age and overall health status. People who choose inactive lifestyles or who are forced into inactivity by illness or injury are at high risk for serious health problems (see Effects of Immobility on the Body section starting on page 1051).

Cardiovascular System

To meet the demand for oxygen created by the rhythmic contraction and relaxation of skeletal muscle groups, the supply of oxygenated blood to skeletal muscle needs to be increased. The cardiovascular system meets this challenge by increasing the heart rate, increasing the contractile strength of the myocardium, and increasing stroke volume (volume of blood ejected), thus increasing cardiac output. Arterial (systolic) blood pressure is increased, and blood is shunted from the nonexercising tissues to the heart and muscles. Exercise also improves venous return because the contracting muscles compress superficial veins and push blood back to the heart against gravity. Over time, regular exercise results in cardiovascular conditioning and produces the following benefits:

- Increased efficiency of the heart
- Decreased heart rate and blood pressure
- Increased blood flow to all body parts
- Improved venous return
- Increased circulating fibrinolysin (substance that breaks up small clots)

Respiratory System

The respiratory and cardiovascular systems work together to make increased oxygen available to the muscles. During exercise, the depth of respiration, respiratory rate, gas exchange at the alveolar level, and rate of carbon dioxide excretion are increased. Over time, regular exercise leads to improved pulmonary functioning. Improvements in pulmonary function include:

- Improved alveolar ventilation
- Decreased work of breathing
- Improved diaphragmatic excursion

Musculoskeletal System

The rhythmic contraction and relaxation of muscle groups during exercise result in increased muscle mass, tone, strength, and increased joint mobility. The more a person exercises, the more strength the individual has to exercise or work in the future. Regular exercise produces the following benefits:

- Increased muscle efficiency (strength) and flexibility
- Increased coordination
- Reduced bone loss
- Increased efficiency of nerve impulse transmission

Regular exercise is also believed to slow the effects of aging. For example, exercise has been shown to help prevent **osteoporosis** (the process of bone demineralization) associated with aging. Exercise has also been associated with minimizing bone loss during chemotherapy.

Metabolic Processes

The metabolic rate increases during exercise so that sufficient glucose and fatty acids can be converted to provide the energy needed for increased muscle function. During strenuous exercise, the metabolic rate can increase to up to 20 times the person's normal rate. Increased body heat and waste products are also produced. With regular exercise, the efficiency of metabolism and body temperature regulation is increased. Other benefits of exercise on the metabolic processes include:

- Increased triglyceride breakdown
- Increased gastric motility
- Increased production of body heat

Gastrointestinal System

During exercise, blood is shunted away from the stomach and intestines to the exercising muscles. With regular exercise:

- Appetite is increased.
- Intestinal tone is increased, which improves digestion and elimination.
- Weight may be controlled.

Urinary System

Regular exercise increases blood circulation, including improved blood flow to the kidneys. This allows the kidneys to maintain the body's fluid balance and acid–base balance more efficiently and to excrete body wastes.

Skin

Increased circulation resulting from regular exercise nourishes the skin. Thus, regular exercise aids in promoting the overall general health of the skin.

Psychosocial Outlook

Some of the most important benefits of regular exercise are psychological. These benefits include:

- Increased energy, vitality, and general well-being
- Improved sleep
- Improved appearance (body image)
- Improved self-concept
- Increased positive health behaviors

Risks Related to Exercise

A common reason many people give for not exercising is fear of experiencing personal harm. Personal harm can include cardiovascular events, muscle injuries, or falling. The nurse must be responsive to these fears with realistic knowledge of the risks associated with exercise and specific prevention strategies.

Precipitation of a Cardiac Event

Although the risk of exercise precipitating a major cardiac event in a healthy person is minimal, the risk is much higher for people with known or suspected cardiovascular disease. Thus, a pre-exercise medical examination, medical supervision during exercise, and an individually designed exercise plan are recommended for sedentary people older than 35 years of age and for any person with a past or current cardiovascular condition, diabetes, osteoporosis, asthma, or obesity (National Institutes of Health [NIH], 2005).

Orthopedic Discomfort and Disability

Orthopedic problems caused by irritation of bones, tendons, ligaments, and sometimes muscles are the most common injuries associated with exercise. This irritation may result from added weight-bearing stress or from collision with the ground, an object, or another person. Teach patients to follow the guideline of rest, ice, compression, and elevation (RICE) if injury occurs. While the injured area is resting, recommend the application of ice to minimize pain and edema, an elastic bandage for compression, and elevation of the injured area to help reduce edema. Advise the patient to contact a physician immediately to diagnose the extent of the injury and instruct the patient to discontinue exercise until the injury is healed.

Other Health Problems

Other types of health problems may be associated with different types of exercise, depending to a large extent on external factors (temperature on a given day, humidity, pollution index, safety of the neighborhood) as well as internal factors (age, history of previous injury, overuse, obesity, health history). Examples of other health problems related to exercise include heat exhaustion or heat stroke, exercise-induced asthma, and chest pain related to overexertion.

Effects of Immobility on the Body

Lack of exercise, inactivity, or immobility related to illness or injury place a person at high risk for serious health problems. Immobility can affect the major body systems and has been linked to a predisposition to many chronic health problems (Peterson, 2007). One in ten premature deaths worldwide are caused by inactivity, and physical inactivity has been found to be as equally damaging as smoking and obesity (Lee et al., 2012). Like the benefits a person receives from exercise, complications resulting from immobility differ in their occurrence and severity based on the patient's age and overall health status.

Cardiovascular System

The primary and serious effects of immobility on the cardiovascular system include increased cardiac workload, orthostatic hypotension, and venous stasis, with resulting venous thrombosis. Immobility results in an increased workload for the heart. With immobility, the skeletal muscles that normally compress valves in the leg veins and help to pump the blood back to the right side of the heart do not adequately contract. There is less resistance offered by the blood vessels and blood pools in the veins, thus increasing the venous blood pressure and changing the distribution of blood in the immobile person. As a result, the heart rate, cardiac output, and stroke volume increase.

Immobility predisposes the patient to thrombi formation because of venous stasis, especially in the legs, where normal muscular activity helps move blood toward the central circulatory system. During periods of immobility, calcium leaves the bones and enters the blood, where it influences blood coagulation, leading to an increased risk of thrombus formation.

A person who is immobile is more susceptible to developing orthostatic hypotension. The normal neurovascular adjustments that occur to maintain systemic blood pressure with position changes are not used during periods of inactivity and become inoperative. A drop in blood pressure may occur as a result of a lack of vasoconstriction when changing from a supine to an upright position. The person tends to feel weak and faint when this condition occurs. See Chapter 24 for additional discussion of orthostatic hypotension.

Respiratory System

The effects of immobility on the respiratory system are related to decreased ventilatory effort and increased respiratory secretions. Immobility causes a decrease in the depth and rate of respirations, in part because of a reduced need for oxygen by body cells. When areas of lung tissue are not used over time, atelectasis (incomplete expansion or collapse of lung tissue) may occur. Immobility results in a poor exchange of carbon dioxide and oxygen, upsets their balance in the body, and eventually causes an acid–base imbalance.

When a person is immobile, the movement of secretions in the respiratory tract is decreased, causing secretions to pool and leading to respiratory congestion. These conditions predispose the person to respiratory tract infections. Hypostatic pneumonia is a type of pneumonia that results from inactivity and immobility. The situation worsens when the person is dehydrated or using pharmacologic agents that increase the tenacity of secretions, depress the coughing mechanism, and/or depress respirations.

Decreased movement in the thoracic cage during respirations also occurs with immobility. This decrease may be due to loss of tonus in muscles involved with respirations, pressure on the chest wall because of the patient's position in bed, or depression of the respiratory system by various pharmaceutical agents.

Musculoskeletal System

Effects of immobility on the musculoskeletal system are rapidly seen in patients confined to bed. People attempting to walk after several days of bed rest are often surprised to find how weak their legs have become. Immobility (musculoskeletal disuse) leads to decreased muscle size (**atrophy**), tone, and strength; decreased joint mobility and flexibility; bone demineralization; and limited endurance, resulting in problems with ADLs.

Immobility is often the cause of contractures and **ankylosis**, a consolidation and immobilization of a joint. Contractures result from atrophy of muscles and from a decrease in the muscle's strength, coordination, and endurance, resulting in an inability to function. A joint can be permanently fixed when ankylosed.

The process of bone demineralization (osteoporosis) is also increased in immobile patients. Normally, the stress and strain of weight-bearing activity stimulate bone formation and balance it with the natural destruction of bone. With immobility, however, bone formation slows while breakdown increases, resulting in a net loss of bone calcium, phosphorus, and bone matrix. This condition, disuse osteoporosis, is characterized by bones that may be either spongy or brittle. Bone demineralization may result in pathologic fractures related to the bone's brittleness, bone deformities related to the bone's sponginess, arthropathy (joint disease) related to calcium depletion in the joints, or renal calculi (stones) related to the excessive excretion of calcium through the kidneys and urinary tract.

Metabolic Processes

Because the resting body requires less energy, the cellular demand for oxygen is decreased, leading to a decreased metabolic rate. In many immobilized patients, however, factors such as fever, trauma, chronic illness, or poor nutrition can actually increase the body's metabolic demands and increase catabolism (the breakdown of the body's protein stores to provide energy to meet the body's energy requirements). If unchecked, this process results in muscle wasting and a negative nitrogen balance. Anorexia, or decreased appetite, often accompanies and compounds this problem. Negative nitrogen balance and poor nutrition thus worsen the muscle atrophy and weakness already resulting from immobility. Numerous fluid and electrolyte imbalances, alterations in the exchange of nutrients and gases at the cellular level, and gastrointestinal (GI) problems can all result from metabolic disturbances.

Gastrointestinal System

Immobility leads to disturbances in appetite, decreased food intake, altered protein metabolism, and poor digestion and utilization of food. If people increase food intake while decreasing energy expenditure, weight gain will result. Normal muscular activity in the GI tract also slows down in an immobile person, which often results in constipation, poor defecation reflexes, and an inability to expel feces and gas adequately.

Urinary System

In a nonerect patient, the kidneys and ureters are level, and urine remains in the renal pelvis for a longer period of time before gravity causes it to move into the ureters and bladder. Urinary stasis favors the growth of bacteria that, when present in sufficient quantities, may cause urinary tract infections. Poor perineal hygiene, incontinence, decreased fluid intake, or an indwelling urinary catheter can increase the risk for urinary tract infection in an immobile patient.

Immobility also predisposes the patient to renal calculi, or kidney stones, which are a consequence of high levels of urinary calcium; urinary retention and incontinence resulting from decreased bladder muscle tone; the formation of alkaline urine, which facilitates growth of urinary bacteria; and decreased urine volume.

Skin

In patients who are immobile, especially those who are older or debilitated, the impaired circulation that accompanies immobility may result in serious skin breakdown. Prolonged pressure over bony prominences produces areas of breakdown, leading to pressure ulcers. Pressure ulcers are described in detail in Chapter 31.

Psychosocial Outlook

When a person can no longer move the body purposefully and needs to depend on someone else for assistance with simple self-care activities, the person's sense of self is often threatened. Skeletal deformities can influence body image, an inability to meet role expectations can decrease self-concept, and a prolonged period of lying dependent in bed can lead to feelings of worthlessness and diminished self-esteem.

Immobility can produce exaggerated emotional responses to the stresses of everyday living. Patients can become apathetic, possibly because of decreased sensory stimulation, and develop altered thought processes. Lack of mobility can also diminish a person's opportunities to interact socially and deprive that person of normal support systems. Coping difficulties are common for both immobilized patients and their families. Furthermore, the amount of time immobilized patients spend resting often disrupts their usual sleep–wake patterns and may interfere with both the quantity and quality of their sleep.

REMEMBER Kelsi Lester, the 10-year-old girl who is unconscious. Due to her current state, Kelsi is at high risk for developing any or all of the possible complications associated with immobility, including thrombi, pneumonia, constipation, urinary tract infection, and skin breakdown. Although she is unconscious, the effects of immobility ultimately can affect her psychosocial outlook. The nurse would integrate knowl-edge of the effects of immobility when developing Kelsi's plan of care that would include close frequent assessment, early detection, and prompt intervention to prevent any possible complications. Vigilant nursing care is essential. ●

THE NURSING PROCESS
Assessing

The comprehensive nursing assessment uses both interview and physical assessment skills to elicit data about the patient's mobility and activity status. When alterations in a patient's physical or mental health state result in impaired mobility, additional specific assessment skills are needed to determine the patient's physical limitations.

Nursing History

During the nursing history, interview patients regarding their daily activity level, endurance, exercise and fitness goals, mobility problems, physical or mental health alterations that affect mobility, and external factors affecting mobility. Questioning patients about their fitness goals is important to provide an indication of the patient's view of health. This interviewing strategy communicates to patients that you expect them to be exercising and is itself a powerful teaching tool.

The accompanying Focused Assessment Guide illustrates elements common to obtaining a mobility status history (on page 1054). When a problem exists, assess the nature of the problem, its onset and frequency, known causes, severity and symptoms, effects on everyday functioning, the interventions attempted by the patient, and the results.

Physical Assessment

Physical assessment of mobility status includes an assessment of general ease of movement and gait; alignment, joint structure, and function; muscle mass, tone, and strength; and endurance. Table 32-5 (on page 1055) provides normal findings and significant alterations. During this assessment, direct attention to both structure and function. The patient's ability to stand, walk, sit up, and grasp are important because these enable the patient to wash, dress, and feed oneself and perform other basic ADLs.

Older adults make up an increasingly larger part of the general population. Functional decline (inability to care for oneself by bathing, dressing, toileting, eating, transferring, and/or maintaining continence) in older adults can have severe consequences. Changes in mobility status contribute to this functional decline. Assessment of an older patient's ability to care for oneself is an important part of a mobility assessment. This assessment can provide clues to changes in health and prevent, or prevent further, functional decline. Refer to the accompanying Research

FOCUSED ASSESSMENT GUIDE 32-1

MOBILITY AND EXERCISE

Factors to Assess	Questions and Approaches
Daily activity level	Describe the activities you normally carry out during a routine day. What type of physical exercise is a part of your daily lifestyle? • Activities of daily living • Type, frequency, duration of physical exercise • Past history of activity and exercise; recent changes
Endurance	Describe how much and what type of activity makes you tired. • History of dizziness, dyspnea, frequent pauses in activity to rest, pounding heart, or marked increase in respiratory rate after moderate activity
Exercise/fitness goals	What exercise or fitness goals are you currently working on? • Attitudes about exercise and physical fitness • Knowledge of the benefits of exercise • Motivation to exercise • Current exercise and fitness goals
Mobility problems	Do you experience any problems with movement or with more vigorous activity or exercise? If yes, please describe these problems. • Nature of the problem (including symptoms) • Onset of disturbance and frequency • Known causes • Severity • Effect of problem on everyday functioning • Interventions attempted and results
Physical or mental health alterations	Are there any physical or mental health problems that may be affecting your mobility? Tell me about them. • Decrease of strength or endurance (e.g., myocardial infarction, congestive heart failure, cardiomyopathy, chronic obstructive pulmonary disease, cancer, gastrointestinal disorders) • Neuromuscular impairment (multiple sclerosis, Parkinson disease, spinal injuries) • Musculoskeletal impairment (arthritis, fractures, muscular dystrophy) • Perceptual or cognitive impairment (cerebrovascular accident, brain tumor or trauma, vision disorders, dementia) • Pain or discomfort (burns, rheumatoid arthritis, chronic pain syndrome, postoperative pain) • Depression or severe anxiety (neurosis, schizophrenia)
External factors affecting mobility	Is there anything else you can think of that limits your ability to get around? • Environmental factors (stairs, lack of railings or other assistive devices, poor lighting, unsafe neighborhood) • Financial resources

in Nursing display (on page 1056) regarding functional decline and nursing care. See the accompanying Focus on the Older Adult (on page 1057) for an example of a tool to use to measure the older adult's capacity to care for oneself and assist nurses to detect subtle changes in health and prevent functional decline.

GENERAL EASE OF MOVEMENT AND GAIT

Begin the physical assessment of an ambulatory patient the moment the patient walks into the room. Voluntarily controlled, fluid, and coordinated body movements are keys to the integrated functioning of the skeletal, muscular, and nervous systems. Note whether the patient's body movements are quick and sure or slow and deliberate. These observations communicate both a sense of the person's emotional status and self-care abilities.

Common involuntary movements that may be observed include tremors (continuous quivering of whole muscles or major portions of a muscle) and tics (irregularly occurring spasmodic movements such as winking, grimacing, or shoulder shrugging).

Note the gait of the patient who is ambulatory. The patient's movements while walking should be coordinated and the posture well balanced. The arms should swing freely in a rhythm alternating with the legs. Figure 32-4 (on page 1056) illustrates stance and swing, the two phases of the normal gait. The heel of the right foot strikes the ground (stance), while the toe of the left foot pushes off and leaves the ground, moving the leg from behind to in front of the body (swing). While one leg is in the stance phase, the other is in the swing phase. Detection of gait abnormalities is important because gait

Table 32-5 OVERVIEW OF THE PHYSICAL ASSESSMENT OF MOBILITY STATUS

COMPONENT	NORMAL FINDING	SIGNIFICANT ALTERATIONS
General ease of movement	Body movements are: • Voluntarily controlled (purposeful) • Fluid • Coordinated	Involuntary movements: • Tremors • Tics • Chorea • Athetosis • Dystonia • Fasciculations • Myoclonus • Oral–facial dyskinesias
Gait and posture	Head erect, vertebrae are straight. Knees and feet point forward. Arms at side with elbows flexed. Arms swing freely in alternation with leg swings. While one leg is in the stance phase, the other is in the swing phase.	Abnormalities of gait and posture: • Spastic hemiparesis • Scissors gait • Steppage gait • Sensory ataxia • Cerebellar ataxia • Parkinsonian gait • Gait of old age • Use of assistive devices for ambulation
Alignment	Independent maintenance of correct alignment: • In the standing and sitting position, a straight line can be drawn from the ear through the shoulder and hip. • In bed, the head, shoulders, and hips are aligned.	Abnormal spinal curvatures Inability to maintain correct alignment independently
Joint structure and function	Absence of joint deformities Full range of motion	Limitation in the normal range of motion Increased joint mobility Swelling or tenderness in or around the joint Heat or redness Crepitation Deformities Muscle atrophy, nodules, skin changes Asymmetry of involvement
Muscle mass, tone, and strength	Adequate muscle mass, tone, and strength to accomplish movement and work	Atrophy, hypertrophy Hypotonicity (flaccidity), spasticity Paresis or paralysis
Endurance	Ability to turn in bed, maintain correct alignment when sitting and standing, ambulate, and perform self-care activities	Physiologic or psychological inability to tolerate an increase in activity: • Significantly increased pulse, respiration, blood pressure after rest • Shortness of breath, dyspnea • Weakness • Pallor • Confusion • Vertigo • Pain

abnormalities may place the person at risk for injury and may indicate a neuromuscular disorder or intoxication.

Note whether the patient uses any assistive devices such as a wheelchair, brace, cane, walker, or crutches to aid in ambulation. Also, determine whether the assistive device is meeting the patient's needs, if it is required for mobility, and if it is being used safely.

ALIGNMENT

Correct body alignment permits optimal musculoskeletal balance and operation, and promotes optimal physiologic functioning. Deviations in body alignment may result from chronic poor posture, trauma, muscle damage, or nerve dysfunction. Pain, fatigue, and a person's mental and emotional status may also influence alignment.

Observe alignment when a patient is standing, sitting, or lying (Fig. 32-5 on page 1056). Note whether the patient is able to maintain correct alignment independently.

A patient's body is in correct body alignment in the standing position when:

• The head is held erect and in the midline
• The face is in the forward position, in the same direction as the feet

RESEARCH IN NURSING

BRIDGING THE GAP TO EVIDENCE-BASED PRACTICE

Functional Decline and Nursing Interventions

Functional decline (inability to care for oneself by bathing, dressing, toileting, eating, transferring, and/or maintaining continence) in hospitalized patients can have severe consequences. Changes in mobility status contribute to this functional decline. Nurses are in ideal positions to integrate a function-focused approach, including increased activity and exercise, into care interactions to support restoration of function and prevent complications of functional decline.

Related Research

Bolz, M., Resnick, B., Capezuti, E., Shuluk, J., & Secic, M. (2012). Functional decline in hospitalized older adults: Can nursing make a difference? *Geriatric Nursing, 33*(4), 272–279.

The demographic and clinical characteristics of patients who were provided function-focused care activities were examined in this prospective observational study of 93 older adults. The study also examined the relationship between change in physical activity and function-focused care activities. Function-focused care activities included interventions

by nurses to help patients engage in activities of daily living and physical activity: specifically, helping patients engage in eating, taking medication, bathing, dressing, turning in bed, and ambulating versus simply performing the tasks for the patient or limiting the amount of activity that patients perform. Patients who received function-focused care experienced less decrement in activities of daily living function during hospitalization. The authors concluded that hospitalized older adults can benefit from function-focused care.

Implications for Nurses

This study suggests that efforts by nurses to encourage older adults to participate as much as possible in the completion of activities of daily living and physical activity can prevent functional decline, allowing patients to maintain independence and prevent complications of immobility. Encouraging discussions about methods to assist older adults in maintaining or increasing physical activity during hospitalization should be a part of routine nursing care.

- The chest is held upward and forward
- The spinal column is upright, and the curves of the spine are within normal limits
- The abdominal muscles are held upward, with the abdomen comfortably tucked in and the buttocks downward

- The arms hang comfortably at the sides
- The knees are extended in a slightly flexed position—not bent or hyperextended in the knee-locked position
- The feet are at right angles to the lower legs
- The line of gravity goes through the midline, from the middle of the forehead to a midpoint between the feet;

Swing phase begins   Stance phase   Swing phase completed

Normal gait

FIGURE 32-4. The stance and swing phases of normal gait.

FIGURE 32-5. Adequate posture. In the sitting and standing positions, a straight line can be drawn from the ear through the shoulder and hip. In bed, the head, shoulders, and hips are aligned.

FOCUS ON THE OLDER ADULT

KATZ INDEX OF INDEPENDENCE IN ACTIVITIES OF DAILY LIVING

ACTIVITIES POINTS (1 OR 0)	INDEPENDENCE: (1 POINT)	DEPENDENCE: (0 POINTS)
	NO supervision, direction, or personal assistance	WITH supervision, direction, personal assistance, or total care
BATHING POINTS:____	(1 POINT) Bathes self completely or needs help in bathing only a single part of the body such as the back, genital area, or disabled extremity.	(0 POINTS) Needs help with bathing more than one part of the body, getting in or out of the tub or shower. Requires total bathing.
DRESSING POINTS:____	(1 POINT) Gets clothes from closets and drawers and puts on clothes and outer garments complete with fasteners. May have help tying shoes.	(0 POINTS) Needs help with dressing self or needs to be completely dressed.
TOILETING POINTS:____	(1 POINT) Goes to toilet, gets on and off, arranges clothes, cleans genital area without help.	(0 POINTS) Needs help transferring to the toilet, cleaning self, or uses bedpan or commode.
TRANSFERRING POINTS:____	(1 POINT) Moves in and out of bed or chair unassisted. Mechanical transferring aides are acceptable.	(0 POINTS) Needs help in moving from bed to chair or requires a complete transfer.
CONTINENCE POINTS:____	(1 POINT) Exercises complete self-control over urination and defecation.	(0 POINTS) Is partially or totally incontinent of bowel or bladder.
FEEDING POINTS:____	(1 POINT) Gets food from plate into mouth without help. Preparation of food may be done by another person.	(0 POINTS) Needs partial or total help with feeding or requires parenteral feeding.

TOTAL POINTS = _____ 6 = High (*patient independent*) 0 = Low (*patient very dependent*)

Adapted slightly from Katz, S., Down, T. D., Cash, H. R., & Grotz, R. C. (1970). Progress in the development of the index of ADL. *The Gerontologist*, 10(1), 20–30. Copyright © The Gerontological Society of America. Reproduced [adapted] by permission of the publisher.

laterally the line of gravity runs vertically from the middle of the skull to the posterior of the foot
- The base of support is on the soles of the feet, and weight is distributed through the soles and heels

Correct body alignment when sitting is similar to correct alignment when standing except that the hips are flexed, the knees are flexed and not crossed, and the base of support is on the buttocks and upper thighs. The weight is distributed evenly on the buttocks and thighs. The thighs are parallel and the popliteal area should be free of the edge of the chair to prevent circulatory stasis and possible nerve injury. The patient's forearms are supported either on the armrests, lap, or on a flat surface in front of the chair.

JOINT STRUCTURE AND FUNCTION
Use inspection and palpation to examine joints, their range of motion, and the surrounding tissue. **Range of motion** is the maximum degree of movement of which a joint is normally capable. (Skill 32-6 on pp. 1105–1113

illustrates the range of motion of selected joints.) When assessing joint mobility, note the following:
- Size, shape, color, and symmetry of joints: note any masses, deformities, or muscle atrophy
- Range of motion of each joint
- Any limitation in the normal range of motion or any unusual increase in the mobility of a joint (instability); range of motion varies among people and decreases with aging
- Muscle strength when performing range-of-motion exercises against resistance
- Any swelling, heat, tenderness, pain, nodules, or crepitation (palpable or audible crunching or grating sensation produced by motion of the joint)
- Comparison of findings in one joint with those of the opposite joint

MUSCLE MASS, TONE, AND STRENGTH
Adequate skeletal muscle mass, tone, and strength are prerequisites to appropriate body movement and work

performance. Mass refers to muscle size. Assess muscle mass throughout the body and compare one muscle group to another using tape measurements. Hypertrophy refers to increased muscle mass resulting from exercise or training. Atrophy describes muscle mass that is decreased through disuse or neurologic impairment. Patients experiencing muscle wasting as a result of a chronic disease process such as cancer may report visible changes in muscle mass.

The slight residual tension that remains in a resting normal muscle with an intact nerve supply is termed muscle tone. Assess muscle tone by flexing and extending the elbow or knee and noting the degree of resistance to these movements. Decreased tone, also known as hypotonicity or **flaccidity**, results from disuse or neurologic impairments, and is described as a weakness or paralysis of the involved area. **Spasticity**, or hypertonicity, increased tone that interferes with movement, is also caused by neurologic impairments, and is often described as a stiffness, tightness, or pulling of the muscle.

 THE nurse would need to assess closely the muscle tone of Kelsi Lester, the 10-year-old girl who is unconscious. Due to her current neurologic status of being unconscious, this assessment information would provide a means to evaluate her nervous system function. In addition, the nurse would be alert for evidence of flaccidity, which could result from lack of use or possibly impairment of her nervous system due to the accident. •

Muscle strength varies greatly from one person to another and even within the same person, and is affected by muscle use. Test muscle strength by asking the patient to move actively against resistance. For example, instruct the patient to push the examiner's palms apart or to push the foot against the examiner's palm. When comparing muscle groups, remember that a person's dominant side tends to be stronger.

Impaired muscle strength or weakness is termed **paresis**. The absence of strength secondary to nervous impairment is called **paralysis**. Hemiparesis refers to weakness of one half of the body, and hemiplegia is paralysis of one half of the body. Paraplegia is paralysis of the legs, and quadriplegia is paralysis of the arms and legs.

Assess whether the patient's muscle strength is adequate for the performance of tasks the patient deems necessary. For example, a patient whose primary means of ambulation is a wheelchair requires upper body strength.

ENDURANCE

When assessing endurance, evaluate the patient's ability to turn in bed, maintain correct alignment when sitting or standing, ambulate, and perform self-care activities. When a physical or psychological factor is believed to be affecting endurance, evaluate the following:

- Vital signs while the patient is at rest
- Ability to perform the activity (e.g., ambulation)

- Patient's response during and after the activity
- Vital signs immediately after the activity
- Vital signs after the patient has rested for 3 minutes

Significant findings indicating that a person's exercise tolerance has been reached include noticeably increased pulse, respirations, and blood pressure; shortness of breath; dyspnea; weakness; pallor; confusion; and vertigo.

Diagnosing

Recognizing cues that indicate both potential and actual problems is essential when analyzing data about a patient's mobility status. Because the problems associated with immobility can seriously undermine the patient's well-being and often require complex and costly treatment, prepare to direct interventions aimed at preventing these problems whenever possible. The plan of care for the patient with an alteration in mobility should include nursing diagnoses that identify the complications of immobility for which the patient is at greatest risk.

Nursing diagnoses specifically addressing problems of mobility include:

- Activity Intolerance
- Impaired Physical Mobility
- Risk for Injury

Examples of related factors and defining characteristics are listed in the accompanying Examples of NANDA-I Nursing Diagnoses box.

A patient's mobility status also may affect other areas of human functioning. Examples of nursing diagnoses related to problems of mobility may include:

- Impaired Transfer Ability related to generalized weakness
- Bathing, Feeding, Dressing, Toileting Self-Care Deficit related to physical weakness (decreased muscle mass and strength), altered mobility (upper or lower extremities)
- Sexual Dysfunction related to neuromuscular impairment
- Risk for Disuse Syndrome

Outcome Identification and Planning

If the patient is not experiencing any mobility problems, expected patient outcomes are directed toward the promotion of physical fitness. For example, the patient will:

- Follow a program of regular physical exercise that improves cardiovascular function, endurance, flexibility, and strength

To achieve this long-term expected outcome, numerous short-term expected outcomes may be needed. An example follows.

By the next visit, 8/20/15, the patient will:

- Identify four personal benefits of regular exercise
- Describe an exercise program (activities, frequency, duration) the patient is willing to follow
- Identify his/her target heart range

EXAMPLES OF NANDA-I NURSING DIAGNOSES

MOBILITY

Nursing Diagnoses	Related Factors	Sample Defining Characteristics
Activity Intolerance	• Any condition that interferes with the transport of oxygenated blood to tissue (e.g., cardiac problems such as congestive heart failure and arrhythmias; respiratory problems, especially chronic obstructive pulmonary disease; circulatory problems; diabetes mellitus) • Any condition that causes fatigue (depression, pain, sleep disturbances, prolonged bed rest, sedentary lifestyle) • Generalized weakness	• Decreased ability to perform basic self-care activities: turning in bed, changing position, ambulating, washing, dressing, eating, and so on • Altered response to activity: • Exertional dyspnea, shortness of breath, excessive increase in respiratory rate • Weak pulse, excessive increase in pulse rate, change in rhythm • Blood pressure that fails to increase with activity or that decreases • Weakness, pallor, confusion, vertigo • Reports of fatigue or pain with activity
Impaired Physical Mobility	• Musculoskeletal impairment (fracture, arthritis) • Neuromuscular impairment (muscular dystrophy, multiple sclerosis) • Decreased strength and endurance • Pain or discomfort • Depression or anxiety • Decreased muscle control, mass, or strength • Joint stiffness • Pharmaceutical agents (narcotics for pain, sedatives for rest) • Therapy-related restrictions on movement (e.g., an order for bed rest, traction, cast, or splints)	• Physical inability to move purposefully or a reluctance to move • Limited range of motion • Limited ability to perform fine or gross motor skills • Slowed, jerky, or uncoordinated movements • Postural instability

- Obtain medical clearance for the exercise program if at high risk for complications
- List support systems that will reinforce exercise efforts

Patients at high risk for specific mobility problems require different expected outcomes. For example, the patient will:

- Demonstrate correct body alignment whenever observed (alignment)
- Adhere to an every-2-hour positioning schedule (alignment)
- Demonstrate full range of joint motion (joint mobility)
- Demonstrate adequate muscle mass, tone, and strength to perform functional ADLs (muscle mass, tone, strength)

Patients who are immobile require outcomes directed toward preventing complications related to inactivity and its effects on the body systems. For example, the patient will:

- Be free from signs of skin breakdown
- Change from a lying to a standing position safely, without injury
- Show signs of adequate venous return
- Be free of contractures
- Maintain effective airway clearance

Individualize outcomes for more specific problems (e.g., for the patient learning to walk with crutches or needing to master transfer techniques with only upper body mobility).

 CONSIDER Maggie Wyatt, the woman being discharged after treatment for a fracture. An appropriate outcome for Ms. Wyatt would be that she demonstrates ability to transfer herself from the bed to the chair and then to the car, with the assistance of a support person. ●

Implementing

The use of body mechanics to reduce the risk of injury when providing patient care and safe patient handling and movement strategies are discussed in the following sections. Nursing strategies designed to promote correct body alignment, mobility, and fitness are described, as well as interventions to prevent complications from immobility. Techniques for the use of graduated compression stockings and pneumatic compression devices, as well as performing range-of-motion exercises, are discussed. It is important to remember that the Occupational Safety and Health Administration (OSHA, 2012) recommends a no-lift policy for all health care facilities. Instead, they advise using patient handling aids and mechanical lifting equipment for patients who are unable to assist in their transfer. Incorporating these safe patient handling and movement strategies, techniques for turning and moving a patient in bed, moving a patient from bed to stretcher and from bed to chair, and logrolling a patient are discussed later. Also included are sections on preparing and helping patients to ambulate after bed rest and nursing strategies to promote exercise.

Application of Body Mechanics to Prevent Injury

Providing patient care places demands on the nurse's musculoskeletal system. These demands are a result of the movements required and use of equipment necessary to provide patient care, as well as the handling of patients. Nurses lift, carry, push, pull, and move objects and people routinely in the course of their work. Performing these actions correctly is necessary to avoid musculoskeletal strain and injury. Body mechanics include proper body movement in daily activities, the prevention and correction of problems associated with posture, and the enhancement of coordination and endurance. The following guidelines for good body mechanics are important to anyone, including nurses, who are engaged in physical activity both at home and at work. Overexertion injuries to workers' necks, shoulders, and backs are the most costly work-related injury for health care facilities (June & Cho, 2011; OSHA, 2012).

Techniques to prevent back stress that should be included routinely in injury-prevention programs include the following:

- Develop a habit of erect posture (correct alignment). Slouching can strain neck and back muscles. When sitting, use the chair back to support the whole spine, keeping shoulders back but relaxed. Balance the head over the shoulders, avoid leaning forward, and hold in the stomach muscles.
- Use the longest and the strongest muscles of the arms and the legs to help provide the power needed in strenuous activities. The muscles of the back are less strong and more easily injured when used improperly.
- Use the internal girdle and a long midriff to stabilize the pelvis and to protect the abdominal viscera when stooping, reaching, lifting, or pulling. The internal girdle is made by contracting the gluteal muscles in the buttocks downward and the abdominal muscles upward. It is helped further by making a long midriff by stretching the muscles in the waist. Figure 32-6 illustrates the internal girdle.
- Work as closely as possible to an object that is to be lifted or moved. This brings the body's center of gravity close to that of the object being moved, permitting most of the burden to be borne by the leg and arm muscles, rather than the back. Figure 32-7 illustrates a proper and an improper way to pick up an object.

FIGURE 32-6. (*Left*) Internal girdle "on." Abdominal muscles contracted, giving a feeling of upward pull, and gluteal muscles contracted, giving a downward pull. (*Right*) Slouch position, showing abdominal muscles relaxed and body out of good alignment.

- Face the direction of your movement. Avoid twisting your body.
- Use the weight of the body as a force for pulling or pushing, by rocking on the feet or leaning forward or backward. This reduces the amount of strain placed on the arms and the back.
- Slide, roll, push, or pull an object, rather than lift it, to reduce the energy needed to lift the weight against the pull of gravity.

FIGURE 32-7. (*Left*) A good position for lifting is illustrated. This person is using the long and strong muscles of the arms and legs and holding the object so that the line of gravity falls within the base of support. (*Right*) This is an incorrect position for lifting because pull is exerted on the back muscles and leaning causes the line of gravity to fall outside the base.

- Use the weight of the body to push an object by falling or rocking forward and to pull an object by falling or rocking backward.
- Push rather than pull equipment when possible. Keep arms close to your body and push with your whole body, not just your arms.
- Begin activities by broadening your base of support. Spread the feet to shoulder width.
- Make sure that the surface is dry and smooth when moving an object to decrease the effects of friction. Rough, wet, or soiled surfaces can contribute to increased friction, increasing the amount of effort required to move an object.
- Flex the knees, put on the internal girdle, and come down close to an object that is to be lifted.
- Break up heavy loads into smaller loads. The National Institute for Occupational Safety and Health (NIOSH) recommends manual load lifting limits of 35 pounds (Waters, 2007). Take breaks from lifting or moving to relax and recover.

Ensuring Safe Patient Handling and Movement

Safe patient handling and transfers involve the use of patient assessment criteria, algorithms for patient handling decisions, and proper use of patient handling equipment. Keep the patient in good alignment and protect the patient from injury while being moved.

SAFE PATIENT TRANSFER

Follow these recommended guidelines when moving and lifting patients:

- Assess the patient. Know the patient's medical diagnosis, capabilities, and any movement not allowed. Apply braces or any device the patient wears before helping from bed.

- Assess the patient's ability to assist with the planned movement. Encourage patients to assist in their own transfers. Encouraging patients to perform tasks that are within their capabilities promotes independence. It is important to eliminate or reduce unnecessary tasks to reduce the risk of injury and increase the patient's self-esteem and mobility levels.
- Assess the patient's ability to understand instructions and cooperate with the staff to achieve the movement. Box 32-1 outlines general guidelines to consider related to mobility and safe handling of people with dementia.
- Use an assessment tool to aid in patient assessment and decision-making regarding safe patient handling and movement. An example of a tool can be found in Figure 32-8 (on page 1062).
- During any patient-transferring task, if any caregiver is required to lift more than 35 pounds of a patient's weight, consider the patient to be fully dependent and use assistive devices for the transfer.
- Ensure that enough staff is available and present to safely move the patient. See the Reflective Practice box at the beginning of the chapter.
- Assess the area for clutter, accessibility to the patient, and availability of devices. Remove any obstacles that may make moving and lifting inconvenient.
- Decide which equipment to use. Step-by-step protocols or algorithms are available to aid decision making to prevent injury to staff and patients (Fig. 32-9 on page 1063). Use handling aids, transfer equipment, and assistive devices (discussed later) whenever possible to help reduce risk of injury to yourself and the patient.
- Plan carefully what you will do before moving or lifting a patient. Assess the mobility of attached equipment. You may injure the patient or yourself if you

---

BOX 32-1 SAFE HANDLING OF PATIENTS WITH DEMENTIA

- Be aware that communication problems and weakness can make the handling of patients with dementia challenging.
- Face the patient when speaking.
- Use clear, short sentences.
- Call patient by name.
- Use calm, reassuring tone of voice.
- Offer simple, step-by-step instructions.
- Repeat verbal cues and prompts as necessary; this is helpful when thought processes are delayed.
- Determine if the patient experiencing dementia has receptive aphasia. This inability to understand what is being said results in noncompliance with verbal instructions.
- Phrase instructions positively. For example, remind the patient to "Stand up" until the chair is correctly positioned, instead of saying "Don't sit down." The patient may not register the "Don't" and will try to sit too early.

Positive instructions are more likely to result in successful maneuvers.
- Ask one question at a time, allow the patient to answer, and repeat the question if necessary.
- Allow the patient to focus on the task; avoid correcting the process of the action unless it would be dangerous to the patient not to do so.
- Identify the patient's established patterns of behavior, customs, traits, and everyday habits and try to incorporate these habits into desired activities. For instance, a patient with dementia may resist or become frightened when a morning shower is attempted if the patient was accustomed to evening baths. Another patient may have difficulty getting out of bed in the morning for the simple reason that he is being asked to get out on what he considers the wrong side of the bed.

(Adapted from Varnam, W. [2011] How to mobilize patients with dementia to a standing position. *Nursing Older People, 23*(8), 31–36; Miller, C. [2008]. Communication difficulties in hospitalized older adults with dementia: Try these techniques to make communicating with patients easier and more effective. *American Journal of Nursing, 108*[3], 58–66; and Wright, K. [2005]. Mobility and safe handling of people with dementia. *Nursing Times, 101*[17], 38–40.)

Assessment Criteria and Care Plan for Safe Patient Handling and Movement

I. Patient's Level of Assistance:

_____ Independent— Patient performs task safely, with or without staff assistance, with or without assistive devices.

_____ Partial Assist—Patient requires no more help than standby, cueing, or coaxing, or caregiver is required to lift no more than 35 lbs of a patient's weight.

_____ Dependent—Patient requires nurse to lift more than 35 lbs of the patient's weight, or patient is unpredictable in the amount of assistance offered. In this case assistive devices should be used.

An assessment should be made prior to each task if the patient has varying level of ability to assist due to medical reasons, fatigue, medications, etc. When in doubt, assume the patient cannot assist with the transfer/repositioning.

II. Weight-Bearing Capability
_____ Full
_____ Partial
_____ None

III. Bilateral Upper-Extremity Strength
_____ Yes
_____ No

IV. Patient's level of cooperation and comprehension:
_____ Cooperative—may need prompting; able to follow simple commands.
_____ Unpredictable or varies (patient whose behavior changes frequently should be considered as unpredictable), not cooperative, or unable to follow simple commands.

V. Weight: _____ Height: _____
Body Mass Index (BMI) [needed if patient's weight is over 300 lbs]¹:_____
If BMI exceeds 50, institute Bariatric Algorithms

The presence of the following conditions are likely to affect the transfer/repositioning process and should be considered when identifying equipment and technique needed to move the patient.

VI. Check applicable conditions likely to affect transfer/repositioning techniques.

_____ Hip/Knee/Shoulder Replacements	_____ Respiratory/Cardiac Compromise	_____ Fractures
_____ History of Falls	_____ Wounds Affecting Transfer/Positioning	_____ Splints/Traction
_____ Paralysis/Paresis	_____ Amputation	_____ Severe Osteoporosis
_____ Unstable Spine	_____ Urinary/Fecal Stoma	_____ Severe Pain/Discomfort
_____ Severe Edema	_____ Contractures/Spasms	_____ Postural Hypotension
_____ Very Fragile Skin	_____ Tubes (IV, Chest, etc.)	

Comments: _____

_____

_____

VII. Appropriate Lift/Transfer Devices Needed:

Vertical Lift: _____

Horizontal Lift: _____

_____

Other Patient Handling Devices Needed: _____

_____

Sling Type: Seated _____ Seated (Amputee) _____ Standing _____ Supine _____ Ambulation _____ Limb Support _____

Sling Size: _____

Signature: _____ **Date:** _____

¹If patient's weight is over 300 lbs, the BMI is needed. For Online BMI table and calculator see: http://www.nhlbi.nih.gov/guidelines/obesity/bmi_tbl.htm

FIGURE 32-8. Sample assessment tool for safe patient handling and movement. (VISN 8 Patient Safety Center. [2009]. Safe patient handling and movement algorithms. Available at http://www.visn8.va.gov/visn8/patientsafetycenter/safePtHandling/default.asp)

have not planned well. If necessary, enlist the support of another caregiver. This reduces the strain on everyone involved. Communicate the plan with staff and the patient to ensure coordinated movement.

• Explain to the patient what you plan to do. Then use what abilities the patient has to assist you. This tech-

nique often decreases the effort required and the possibility of injury to you.

• If the patient is in pain, administer the prescribed analgesic sufficiently in advance of the transfer to allow the patient to participate in the move more comfortably.

Algorithm 4: Reposition in Bed: From Side to Side or Up

Start here

↓

Can patient assist?

Fully able → Caregiver assistance not needed; may or may not use positioning aid.

Partially able → Encourage patient to assist using positioning aid or cues

No

↓

Use full-body sling lift and 2 or more caregivers.

< 200 pounds: Use a friction-reducing device and 2 to 3 caregivers.

> 200 pounds: Use a friction-reducing device and at least 3 caregivers.

General Notes:
- This is not a 1-person task; *do not pull from head of bed.*
- When pulling a patient up in bed, the bed should be flat or in a Trendelenburg position, with the side rail down.
- For patients with stage III or IV pressure ulcers, care must be taken to avoid shearing force.
- The height of the bed should be appropriate for staff safety (at the elbows).
- If the patient can assist when repositioning up in bed, ask him to flex the knees and push on the count of 3.
- During any patient-handling task, if the caregiver is required to lift more than 35 lbs. of a patient's weight, then the patient should be considered to be fully dependent and assistive devices should be used.

FIGURE 32-9. Step-by-step procedure or algorithm used to outline safe technique for repositioning a patient in bed. (VISN 8 Patient Safety Center. [2009]. Safe patient handling and movement algorithms. Available at http://www.visn8.va.gov/visn8/patientsafetycenter/safePtHandling/default.asp)

- Elevate the bed as necessary so that you are working at a height that is comfortable and safe for you.
- Lock the wheels of the bed, wheelchair, or stretcher so that they do not slide while you are moving the patient.
- Be sure the patient is in good body alignment while being moved and lifted to protect the patient from strain and muscle injury.
- Support the patient's body properly. Avoid grabbing and holding an extremity by its muscles.
- Avoid friction on the patient's skin during moving.
- Use friction-reducing devices whenever possible, especially during lateral transfers.
- Move your body and the patient in a smooth, rhythmic motion. Jerky movements tend to put extra strain on muscles and joints and are uncomfortable for the patient.
- Use mechanical devices such as lifts, slides, transfer chairs, or gait belts for moving patients. Be sure that you understand how the device operates and that the patient is properly secured and informed of what will

occur. If you are not comfortable with the operation of the equipment, obtain assistance from a caregiver who is. Patients who do not understand or are afraid may be unable to cooperate and may cause injury to the staff as well as suffer injury as a result.
- Ensure that the equipment used meets weight requirements. Bariatric patients (BMI >50) require bariatric transfer aids and equipment. Bariatric transfer aids and equipment are designed to be used with people who are obese.

 CONSIDER Mrs. Nguyen, the woman caring for her husband at home. The nurse would evaluate the need for assistive devices and secure the identified items for patient care. The nurse would incorporate safe patient handling and moving guidelines when role modeling the proper techniques for moving and lifting Mr. Nguyen. In addition, the nurse would use these guidelines to develop a teaching

FIGURE 32-10. Gait belts.

plan for Mrs. Nguyen to ensure safety for all involved when moving and lifting Mr. Nguyen. After teaching Mrs. Nguyen, the nurse would observe her performing the technique to ensure understanding. ●

EQUIPMENT AND ASSISTIVE DEVICES

Many devices and equipment are available to aid in transferring, repositioning, and lifting patients. It is important to use the right equipment and appropriate device based on patient assessment and desired movement.

Gait Belts. A gait belt is a device used for transferring patients and assisting with ambulation (Fig. 32-10). The belt, which often has handles, is placed around the patient's waist and secured by Velcro fasteners. The handles can be placed in a variety of configurations so that the caregiver can have better access to, improved grasp of, and control of the patient. Some belts are hand-held slings that go around the patient, providing a firm grasp for the caregiver and facilitating the transfer. The gait belt is used to help the patient stand and provides stabilization during pivoting. Gait belts also allow the nurse to assist in ambulating patients who have leg strength, can cooperate, and require minimal assistance. Do not use gait belts on patients with abdominal or thoracic incisions (OSHA, 2009).

Stand-Assist and Repositioning Aids. Some patients need minimal assistance to stand up. With an appropriate support to grasp, they can lift themselves. Many types of devices can help a patient to stand. These devices can be freestanding or attached to the bed or wheelchair. Other aids have a pull bar to assist the patient to stand, and then a seat unfolds under the patient. After the patient sits on the seat, the device can be wheeled to the toilet, chair, shower, or bed.

Lateral-Assist Devices. Lateral-assist devices reduce patient–surface friction during side-to-side transfers. Roller boards, slide boards, transfer boards, inflatable mattresses, and friction-reducing lateral-assist devices are examples of these devices, which make transfers safer and more comfortable for the patient. For example, an inflatable lateral-assist device is a flexible mattress that is placed under the patient. An attached, portable air supply then inflates the mattress, which provides a layer of air under the patient. This air cushion allows nursing staff to perform the move with much less effort (Baptiste, Boda, Nelson, Lloyd, & Lee, 2006), but has been found to place the care providers at an increased risk of injury because of the horizontal reach required, posture adopted during transfer, and lack of handles (Nelson & Baptiste, 2004). Another example is a transfer board, usually made of smooth, rigid, low-friction material (such as coated wood or plastic). The board, which is placed under the patient, provides a slick surface for the patient during transfers, reducing friction and the force required to move the patient. A third type of lateral sliding aid is made of a special fabric that reduces friction. Some devices have long handles that reduce reaching by staff to improve safety and make the transfer easier (Fig. 32-11).

Friction-Reducing Sheets. Friction-reducing sheets can be used under patients to prevent skin shearing when moving patients in bed and when assisting with lateral transfers. Their use reduces friction and the force required to move patients.

Mechanical Lateral-Assist Devices. Mechanical lateral-assist devices include specialized stretchers and eliminate the need to slide the patient manually. Some devices are motorized, whereas others use a hand crank. A portion of the device moves from the stretcher to the bed, sliding under

FIGURE 32-11. Lateral-assist device with long handles to reduce reaching by staff.

the patient, bridging the bed and stretcher (Fig. 32-12). The device is then returned to the stretcher, effectively moving the patient without any pulling by staff members.

Transfer Chairs. Chairs that can convert into stretchers are available. These are useful with patients who have no weight-bearing capacity, cannot follow directions, and/or cannot cooperate. The back of the chair bends back and the leg supports elevate to form a stretcher configuration, eliminating the need for lifting the patient. Some of these chairs have built-in mechanical aids to perform the patient transfer, as detailed previously.

Powered Stand-Assist and Repositioning Lifts. These devices can be used with patients who can bear weight on at least one leg, can follow directions, and are cooperative. A simple sling is placed around the patient's back and under the arms. Some devices come with breathable slings that can remain under the patient, reducing the risk for the nurse in turning the patient to position the sling. The patient rests the feet on the device's footrest and places the hands on the handle. The device mechanically assists the patient to stand, without any assistance from the nurse (Fig. 32-13). Once the patient is standing, the

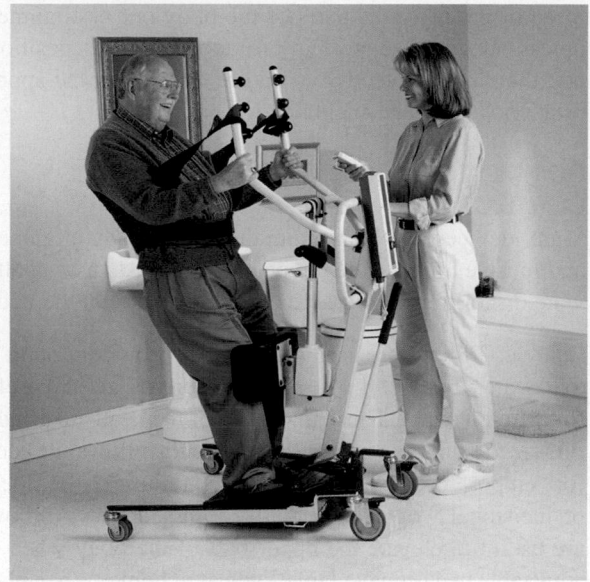

FIGURE 32-13. Stand-assist aid.

device can be wheeled to a chair, the toilet, or bed. Some devices have removable footrests and can be used as a walker. Some have scales incorporated into the device that can be used to weigh the patient.

Powered Full-Body Lifts. These devices are used with patients who cannot bear any weight to move them out of bed, into and out of a chair, and to a commode or stretcher. A full-body sling is placed under the patient's body, including head and torso, then the sling is attached to the lift (Fig. 32-14). As mentioned previously, some of these slings are made to stay under the patient to decrease strain on the staff during placement. The device slowly lifts the patient. Some devices can be lowered to the floor to pick up a patient who has fallen. These devices are available on portable bases and ceiling-mounted tracks.

Positioning Patients in Bed

Positioning that maintains correct body alignment and facilitates physiologic functioning contributes to the patient's psychological and physical well-being. The

FIGURE 32-12. Mechanical lateral-assist device.

FIGURE 32-14. Powered full-body lift.

force of gravity pulls parts of the body out of alignment unless adequate support is provided. Various positions are, therefore, protective in nature only when the appropriate positions are maintained.

COMMON DEVICES TO PROMOTE CORRECT ALIGNMENT

Many devices can help maintain proper body alignment and muscle tonus while the patient is in bed and can alleviate discomfort or pressure on various parts of the body.

Pillows. Pillows are used primarily to provide support or to elevate a body part. Pillows of different sizes are useful for different parts. Those intended for the head are usually full-sized or large-sized pillows. Small pillows are ideal for support or elevation of the extremities, shoulders, or incisional wounds. Specially designed heavy pillows are useful to elevate the upper part of the body when an adjustable bed is unavailable, such as at home. When placing the pillows, assess for proper alignment. For example, excess cervical flexion would not be comfortable or useful in maintaining adequate respiratory patterns.

Mattresses. For a mattress to be comfortable and supportive, it must be firm but have sufficient "give" to permit proper body alignment. A patient who must remain in a bed with a nonsupportive mattress may complain of backache and other discomforts.

Special mattresses, pads, and types of beds used to help prevent pressure ulcers are discussed in Chapter 31.

Adjustable Beds. The nurse can elevate the head and foot of an adjustable bed to the desired degree. This positioning is discussed later in the chapter. Some adjustable beds allow the bed to be "broken," or gatched, so that the mattress is flexed at the level of the knees. This position is rarely recommended because it can cause pressure on the popliteal space behind the knee, resulting in impaired circulation to the lower extremity and an increased risk for clot formation.

It is also possible to change the adjustable bed so that the distance from the bed to the floor can be altered. Position the bed at the height that will let the patient stand with the least amount of effort. Health care workers use the higher bed positions so that they do not strain their backs while providing bed care. However, a low bed position between treatments decreases the risk of injury if the patient were to fall out of bed. General guidelines for safe use of beds are discussed in Chapter 31.

Many beds used in patient care environments have improvements to support transfer and repositioning of the patient. Some beds easily convert to a chair, bypassing the need for bed-to-chair transfers. Other beds are designed to align the patient's hip with the pivot point in the bed, minimizing slippage toward the foot of the bed when the head of the bed is raised and reducing the need to reposition the patient. Many new mattress surfaces are designed to eliminate the need for frequent repositioning by the

FIGURE 32-15. A trapeze device makes it possible for the patient to lift part of the body from the bed, facilitating turning and moving up in bed.

nurse; some provide a cushion of air under the patient during movement, reducing friction; and others have surfaces that can rotate to move the patient as needed for care.

 CONSIDER Mrs. Nguyen, the older woman caring for her husband after his stroke. If necessary and not already in the home, an adjustable bed or pressure-relieving mattress pads or coverings could be recommended to help her provide care to her husband. This would be beneficial to both Mrs. Nguyen and her husband. ●

Trapeze Bar. A trapeze bar (Fig. 32-15) is a handgrip suspended from a frame near the head of the bed. A patient can grasp the bar with one or both hands and raise one's trunk from the bed. The trapeze makes moving and turning considerably easier for many patients and facilitates transfers into and out of bed. It can also be used when a patient needs to perform exercises that strengthen some muscles of the upper extremities (e.g., biceps).

Additional Equipment. The greatest danger to the feet occurs when they are unsupported in the dorsiflexion position. The toes drop downward, and the feet are in plantar flexion. Because of the pull of gravity, this position of the feet occurs naturally when the body is at rest. If maintained for extended periods, plantar flexion can cause an alteration in the length of muscles, and the patient may develop a complication called **footdrop**. In this position, the foot is unable to maintain itself in the perpendicular position, heel–toe gait is impossible, and the patient experiences extreme difficulty in walking. The use of a foot support, such as a foot board, foot boot, or high-top sneakers, helps avoid this complication. Figure 32-16 demonstrates a foot in plantar flexion versus the dorsiflexion position maintained by wearing a high-top canvas sneaker.

If top bedding must be kept off the patient's lower extremities, a device called a cradle is used. A cradle is usually a metal frame that supports the bed linens away

FIGURE 32-16. (**A**) Plantar flexion occurs when the foot is not supported. (**B**) When high-top sneakers support the feet, the dorsiflexion position is maintained.

A   B

from the patient while providing privacy and warmth. There are a number of sizes and shapes of cradles. If used, securely fasten the cradle to the bed so that it does not slide or fall on the patient.

Sandbags, available in various sizes, can be used to immobilize an extremity and support body alignment. When properly filled, they should be pliable enough to be shaped to body contours to provide support. Avoid hard or firmly packed sandbags. Position a sandbag to avoid creating pressure on a bony prominence.

Trochanter rolls are used to support the hips and legs so that the femurs do not rotate outward. Figure 32-17 illustrates and describes how to use trochanter rolls. Properly placed pillows can also be used to help prevent the thighs from turning outward, but they tend to slip out of place and require frequent adjustment to be effective.

If a patient is paralyzed or unconscious, hand–wrist splints or hand rolls may be necessary to provide a means for keeping the thumb in the correct position, that is, slightly adducted and in apposition to the fingers. A hand roll can be created by folding a washcloth, rolling it, and securing it in place with tape. Once placed against the palm of the hand, it can effectively keep the hand in a functional position (Fig. 32-18). A commercial plastic or aluminum splint also may be used to hold the thumb in place regardless of the hand position. Encourage patients who are not moving their fingers to do finger exercises, with special attention to having the thumb touch the tip of each finger.

Side rails can assist the patient in rolling from one side to the other or to sitting up without calling for assistance. Using the side rails can help the patient retain or regain muscle efficiency. When using side rails, be sure to explain their use to patients and their families and follow the protocol of the health care agency. If a patient requests that side rails be raised for additional security, the patient must have the ability to raise and lower the side rails independently. Safe use of side rails is discussed in Chapter 26.

PROTECTIVE POSITIONING

Patients accustomed to an active lifestyle who generally use a bed only for sleep are often unaware of the importance of correct body alignment and regular position changes when on prescribed bed rest. Whenever possible, teach both the patient and family the following:

- Correct positioning techniques
- The need to change positions frequently, at least every 2 hours

FIGURE 32-17. Trochanter rolls prevent external rotation of the hips of a bedridden patient. The patient is placed on a folded sheet so that the top edge is at the hips and the lower edge is about one-third of the way down the thighs. Towels or bath blankets are rolled under each side until the roll is snugly against the patient's hips and thighs. The support cannot unroll, and the weight of the patient keeps it secure.

FIGURE 32-18. A hand roll holds the hand in functional position.

Table 32-6 COMMON BED POSITIONS AND PROTECTIVE NURSING ACTIONS

POSITION	COMPLICATION TO BE PREVENTED	SUGGESTED PREVENTIVE ACTIONS
Fowler's Position	Flexion contracture of the neck	Allow the head to rest against the mattress or be supported by a small pillow only.
	Exaggerated curvature of the spine	Use a firm support for the back; position the patient so that the angle of elevation starts at the hips.
	Dislocation of the shoulder	Support the forearms on pillows to elevate them sufficiently so that no pull is exerted on the shoulders.
	Flexion contracture of the wrist	Support the hand on pillows so that it is in natural alignment with the forearm.
	Edema of the hand	Support the hand so that it is slightly elevated in relation to the elbow.
	Flexion contractures of the fingers and abduction of the thumbs	Provide hand–wrist splints if necessary.
	Impaired lower extremity circulation and knee contracture, pressure on heels	Elevate the knees for only brief periods; place one or two pillows under the lower legs from below the knees to the ankles; avoid pressure on the popliteal vessels; avoid using the knee gatch.
	External rotation of the hips	Use trochanter roll.
	Footdrop	Support the feet in dorsal flexion. Use footboard; high-top sneakers can also be used.
Protective Supine Position	Exaggerated curvature of the spine and flexion of the hips	Provide a firm, supportive mattress; use a bed board if necessary.
	Flexion contracture of the neck	Place pillows under the upper shoulders, neck, and head so that the head and neck are held in the correct position.
	Internal rotation of the shoulders and extension of the elbows (hunch shoulders)	Place pillows or arm supports under the forearms so that the upper arms are alongside the body and the forearms are pronated slightly.
	Flexion of the lumbar curvature	Place rolled towel or small pillow under lumbar curvature if needed.
	Extension of the fingers and abduction of the thumbs (clawhand deformities)	Use hand–wrist splints if appropriate.
	External rotation of the femurs	Place sandbags or a trochanter roll alongside the hips and the upper half of the thighs.
	Hyperextension of the knees	Place a pillow under the lower legs from below the knees to the ankles.
	Footdrop	Use a footboard or make an improvised firm foot support to hold the feet in dorsal flexion; high-top sneakers may also be recommended.
Protective Side-Lying or Lateral Position	Lateral flexion of the neck	Place a pillow under the head and the neck.
	Inward rotation of the arm and interference with respiration	Place a pillow under the upper arm; lower arm should be flexed and positioned comfortably.
	Extension of the finger and abduction of the thumbs	Provide hand–wrist splint if necessary.
	Internal rotation and adduction of the femur	Use one or two pillows as needed to support the leg from the groin to the foot.
	Twisting of the spine	Ensure that both shoulders are aligned with both hips.

Table 32-6 COMMON BED POSITIONS AND PROTECTIVE NURSING ACTIONS *continued*

POSITION	COMPLICATION TO BE PREVENTED	SUGGESTED PREVENTIVE ACTIONS
Protective Sims' Position	Lateral flexion of the neck	Place a small pillow under the head unless the drainage of oral secretions is desired.
	Damage to nerves and blood vessels in the axillae of the lower arm	Carefully position lower arm behind and away from the patient's back.
	Internal shoulder rotation and adduction	Abduct the upper shoulder slightly so that the shoulder and elbow are flexed; place a pillow between the chest and upper arm.
	Internal rotation and adduction of the hip; lumbar lordosis	Place a pillow under the upper flexed leg from the groin to the foot.
	Twisting of the spine	Ensure that both shoulders are aligned with both hips.
	Footdrop	Support the lower foot in dorsiflexion with a sandbag.
Protective Prone Position	Flexion on the cervical spine	Place a small pillow under the head.
	Hyperextension of the spine; impaired respirations	Place some suitable support under the patient between the end of the rib cage and the upper abdomen if this facilitates breathing and space is available.
	Footdrop	Move the patient down in bed so that the feet are over the mattress, or support the lower legs on a pillow just high enough to keep the toes from touching the bed.

- The importance of using the time allotted to position changes to exercise the extremities and to assess and massage pressure areas (reddened areas should not be massaged)

When the patient is unable to change position independently, use a turn schedule, posted at the bedside to assist with and document the rotation of positions. Table 32-6 describes common bed positions and nursing measures to prevent complications associated with these positions.

Fowler's Position. The semi-sitting position, or Fowler's position, calls for the head of the bed to be elevated 45 to 60 degrees. This position is often used to promote cardiac and respiratory functioning because abdominal organs drop in this position, providing maximal space in the thoracic cavity. This is also the position of choice for eating, conversation, and urinary and intestinal elimination.

Variations of Fowler's position include high Fowler's and low Fowler's or semi-Fowler's position. In the high Fowler's position, the head of the bed is elevated 90 degrees. When a bedside table with a pillow on top of it is placed in front of the patient in high Fowler's position, the patient can lean forward and rest the arms on the pillow, assuming a posture that allows for maximal lung expansion. In low Fowler's or semi-Fowler's position, the head of the bed is elevated only 30 degrees.

In Fowler's position, the buttocks bear the main weight of the body. In this position, the heels, sacrum, and scapulae are at risk for skin breakdown and require frequent assessment. See Table 32-6 for information about correct positioning and nursing actions to prevent complications associated with this position.

Supine or Dorsal Recumbent Position. In the supine position, the patient lies flat on the back with the head and shoulders slightly elevated with a pillow unless contraindicated, such as spinal anesthesia or surgery on the spinal vertebrae. Correct alignment in the supine position is illustrated in Table 32-6.

Side-Lying or Lateral Position. In the side-lying position, the patient lies on the side and the main weight of the body is borne by the lateral aspect of the lower scapula and the lateral aspect of the lower ilium. Because many people routinely fall asleep in the side-lying position, this is a comfortable alternative to the supine position for the patient on bed rest. Although it relieves pressure on the scapulae, sacrum, and heels and allows the legs and feet to be comfortably flexed, support pillows are needed for correct positioning (see Table 32-6).

The oblique position, a variation of the side-lying position, is recommended as an alternative to the side-lying position because it places significantly less pressure on the trochanter region. The patient turns toward the side with the hip of the top leg flexed at a 30-degree angle and the knee flexed at 35 degrees. The calf of the upper leg is positioned slightly behind the body's midline. Pillows support the patient's back and calf of the top leg (Fig. 32-19 on page 1070).

FIGURE 32-19. Modified lateral position (oblique position) is an alternative to the side-lying position and results in significantly less pressure on the trochanter area.

Another variation of the lateral position is Sims' position. In this position, the patient again lies on the side, but the lower arm is behind the patient and the upper arm is flexed at both the shoulder and the elbow. In this position, the main body weight is borne by the anterior aspects of the humerus, clavicle, and ilium. Thus, the major pressure points differ from those in the lateral and other bed-lying positions (see Table 32-6).

Prone Position. In the prone position, the person lies on the abdomen with the head turned to the side. The body is straight in the prone position because the shoulders, head, and neck are in an erect position, the arms are easily placed in correct alignment with the shoulder girdle, the hips are extended, and the knees can be prevented from flexing or hyperextending. When patients on bed rest use this position periodically, it helps to prevent flexion contractures of the hips and knees. However, the pull of gravity on the trunk when the patient lies prone produces a marked lordosis or forward curvature of the lumbar spine. The position is thus contraindicated for people with spinal problems. The pull of gravity on the feet may result in plantar flexion unless the legs and feet are positioned carefully (see Table 32-6).

Using Graduated Compression Stockings and Pneumatic Compression Devices

Venous stasis and the development of venous thrombosis are potential complications of immobility. Graduated compression stockings and pneumatic compression devices are passive interventions prescribed to aid in the prevention of these common complications of inactivity.

GRADUATED COMPRESSION STOCKINGS

Graduated compression stockings are often used for patients at risk for deep vein thrombosis, pulmonary embolism, and to help prevent phlebitis (described in Chapter 29). Manufactured by several companies, they are made of elastic material and are available in either knee-high or thigh-high length. By applying pressure, graduated compression stockings increase the velocity of blood flow in the superficial and deep veins and improve venous valve function in the legs, promoting venous return to the heart. By preventing pooling of the blood, clot formation is less likely. An order is required from the patient's primary care provider for their use. When assisting with graduated compression stockings, follow these general nursing guidelines:

- Measure the patient's legs to determine the proper size of stocking. Each leg should have a correct fitting stocking; if measurements are different, then two different sizes of stocking need to be ordered to ensure correct fitting on each leg (Walker & Lamont, 2008). The manufacturer whose stockings are being used gives directions for measuring. Some stockings fit either leg; others are designated right or left. An improperly fitting stocking is uncomfortable and ineffective and possibly even harmful (Miller, 2011).
- Assess the skin condition and neurovascular status of the legs. Report abnormalities before continuing with the application of the stockings.
- Be prepared to apply the stockings in the morning before the patient is out of bed and while the patient is supine. If the patient is sitting or has been up and about, have the patient lie down with legs and feet elevated for at least 15 minutes before applying the stockings. Otherwise, the leg vessels are congested with blood, reducing the effectiveness of the stockings.
- Do not massage the legs. If a clot is present, it may break away from the vessel wall and circulate in the bloodstream.
- Check the legs regularly for redness, blistering, swelling, and pain. Some recommend checking the legs at least once every 8 hours; others recommend twice a day. Remove the stockings completely once a day to bathe the legs and feet.
- Launder the stockings as necessary, but at least every 3 days. Soiled stockings irritate the skin. Dry the stockings on a flat surface to prevent them from stretching. If using a clothes dryer, set on low heat and remove as soon as the cycle is complete. The patient may need two pairs of stockings to wear one pair while the second pair is being cleaned.

Always remove graduated compression stockings during morning care and inspect the legs. Then reapply the stockings before the patient is out of bed, as shown in Skill 32-1 on pages 1090–1093.

PNEUMATIC COMPRESSION DEVICES

Intermittent pneumatic compression devices may be used in conjunction with graduated compression stockings or alone. They are composed of an air pump, connecting tubes, and extremity sleeves that apply intermittent or sequential pressure to the legs to enhance blood flow and venous return, stimulating the normal muscle-pumping action in the legs. They require a prescriber's order and are often prescribed for high-risk surgical patients, those with decreased mobility or chronic venous disease, and patients at risk for deep-vein disorders.

Turning the Patient in Bed

Frequently, a patient cannot turn in bed without assistance. Nurses need to use their knowledge of correct alignment to turn the patient from the back onto the side, from the back onto the abdomen, and from the abdomen onto the back. A suggested decision-making strategy is outlined in Figure 32-9 on page 1063 (VISN 8, 2009). If the patient is unable to assist with movement, a full-body sling and two or more caregivers are required. When turning the patient, the bed should be at the height of the caregivers' elbows to ensure a comfortable working height. The technique for turning a patient in bed is described and illustrated in Skill 32-2 on pages 1093–1095. Mastering this turning technique helps nurses adhere to an every-2-hour turn schedule for an immobile patient.

CONSIDER Mrs. Nguyen, the older woman who will be caring for her husband at home, and Kelsi Lester, the 10-year-old girl who is unconscious. Teaching Mrs. Nguyen how to properly turn her husband in bed and assist him to get out of bed will be crucial to minimize stress and strain on her back and legs. Turning Kelsi every 2 hours would be essential to prevent alterations in her skin integrity. ●

Moving a Patient Up in Bed

A suggested decision-making strategy is outlined in Figure 32-9 on page 1063 (VISN 8, 2009). The first decision point is whether the patient can assist. If the patient is fully able, caregiver assistance is not needed and the patient may or may not use a positioning aid. If the patient is fully able to assist in moving up in the bed, allow the patient to complete the movement independently, with safe supervision. The patient assists movement either by pushing with the feet flat against the bed or by using an overbed trapeze. If only partially able, encourage the patient to assist using a positioning aid or cues. If the patient is less than 200 pounds, use a friction-reducing device and two to three caregivers. If the patient is over 200 pounds, use a friction-reducing device and at least three caregivers. If the patient is not able to assist, use a full-body sling lift and two or more caregivers. Friction-reducing sheets or other devices should be used to minimize shearing forces and work effort. A technique used to move a patient up in bed when the patient is partially able to assist and two caregivers are available is described and illustrated in Skill 32-3 on pages 1095–1098.

Moving a Patient From Bed to Stretcher

Considerable care must be taken when moving a patient from a bed to a stretcher, or vice versa, to prevent injury to the patient and caregivers. A suggested decision-making strategy is outlined in Figure 32-20 (VISN 8, 2009).

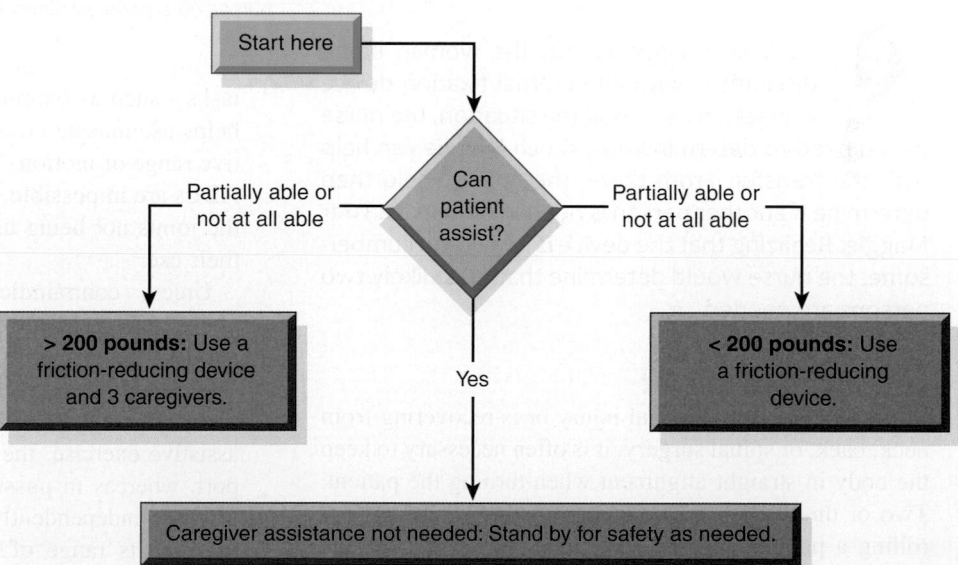

FIGURE 32-20. Step-by-step procedure used to make decisions for safely transferring a patient from bed to stretcher. (VISN 8 Patient Safety Center. [2009]. Safe patient handling and movement algorithms. Available at http://www.visn8.va.gov/visn8/patientsafetycenter/safePtHandling/default.asp)

If the patient is fully able to assist in the transfer, allow the patient to complete the movement independently, with supervision for safety. If the patient is partially able or not able to assist at all and weighs less than 200 pounds, use a friction-reducing device. If the patient weighs more than 200 pounds, a friction-reducing device and three caregivers are required. If the patient is unconscious or weakened, additional nurses are needed to support the extremities and the head. These actions are described in Skill 32-4 on pages 1098–1101. When returning the patient to the bed from the stretcher, the same techniques are used.

Moving a Patient From Bed to Chair

Safety and comfort are key concerns when assisting the patient out of bed. Preliminary assessment of vital signs provides baseline data; subsequent recordings determine the effect of this activity on the patient. The position of the nurse when preparing to move the patient and during placement of the chair are critical elements in the transfer. The patient's apparel should be sufficient to prevent embarrassment and provide warmth yet not impede movement.

Assess the patient's ability to bear weight when determining the appropriate method for transfer and the appropriate transfer aid. Patients who are unable to bear partial weight or full weight or who are uncooperative should be transferred using a full-body sling lift with two caregivers. The technique for assisting a patient to transfer from bed to chair is described in Skill 32-5 on pages 1101–1105.

 RECALL Maggie Wyatt, the woman being discharged with an external fixation device in place. In assessing the situation, the nurse would need to determine how much Maggie can help with the transfer. From there, the nurse would then determine if another person is needed to help transfer Maggie. Realizing that the device is heavy and cumbersome, the nurse would determine that most likely two persons are needed. ●

Logrolling a Patient

When a patient has a spinal injury or is recovering from neck, back, or spinal surgery, it is often necessary to keep the body in straight alignment when turning the patient. Two or three nurses can accomplish this safely by logrolling a patient (Fig. 32-21). Do not try to logroll the patient without enough help. Do not twist the patient's head, spine, shoulders, knees, or hips while logrolling. Refer to the accompanying Guidelines for Nursing Care 32-1: Logrolling a Patient.

Assisting with Range-of-Motion Exercises

Range of motion is the complete extent of movement of which a joint is normally capable. Engaging in routine

FIGURE 32-21. Logrolling by two or three nurses aids in turning a patient with a spinal injury. One nurse stands on the side, holding the drawsheet taut. The patient is moved toward the other two nurses on a predetermined signal.

tasks—such as bathing, eating, dressing, and writing—helps use muscle groups that keep many joints in effective range of motion. When all or some of one's normal ADLs are impossible, it is important to give attention to the joints not being used or to those that are limited in their use.

Unless contraindicated, encourage active, active-assistive, or passive range-of-motion exercises regularly and include them in the patient's plan of care. In **active exercise**, the patient independently moves joints through their full range of motion (isotonic exercise). In active-assistive exercise, the nurse may provide minimal support, whereas in **passive exercise**, the patient is unable to move independently, and the nurse moves each joint through its range of motion. Both active and passive exercises improve joint mobility and increase circulation to the affected part, but only active exercise increases muscle mass, tone, and strength and improves cardiac and respiratory functioning. Thus, exercises should be as active as the patient's physical condition permits. It is also helpful to teach isometric exercises to patients to increase muscle mass, tone, and strength.

Include directives in the nursing plan of care for range-of-motion exercises, specifying what, how, and when, so

GUIDELINES FOR NURSING CARE 32-1

LOGROLLING A PATIENT

- Ensure that adequate personnel are available—three to four, depending on the stability of the patient's neck.
- Use a friction-reducing sheet, or if not available, a drawsheet, to facilitate smooth movement. Ensure that the sheet extends from above the patient's shoulders to below the hips.
- Perform hand hygiene.
- Provide privacy by closing the door and/or pulling the bedside curtain.
- Explain what you are going to do to the patient.
- Perform a baseline assessment of the patient's neurologic status.
- Raise the bed to a comfortable working height and lower the side rails, if in raised position.
- Have the patient cross the arms on the chest.
- Place a pillow between the knees.
- Have two nurses stand on one side of the bed opposite the direction the patient will be turned. The third helper

stands on the other side, and if necessary, the fourth at the head of the bed/stretcher to stabilize the neck.
- Fanfold or roll the drawsheet tightly against the patient and carefully slide the patient to the side of the bed toward the two nurses.
- Have one helper then move to the other side of the bed, so that two nurses are on the side to which the patient is turning.
- Face the patient. Everyone moves on a predetermined signal. Holding the rolled drawsheet taut to support the body, turn the patient as a unit toward the two nurses. The patient's head, shoulders, spine, hips, and knees should turn simultaneously.
- Use pillows to support the patient's back, buttocks, and legs in straight alignment in a side-lying position.
- Raise the side rails, lower the bed, and place the call bell within the patient's reach.
- Reassess the patient's neurologic status and comfort level.
- Document the procedure and the patient's response.

that all who care for the patient observe the same routine. In some institutions, nurses work closely with physiotherapists in designing and implementing exercise programs. Refer to Table 32-2 on page 1041 for an explanation of terms related to movement. The following are basic guidelines to follow when helping to put the patient's joints through range of motion:

- Teach the patient what exercise is being undertaken, why, and how it will be done. A show-and-tell technique is often helpful.
- Avoid overexertion and continuing exercises to the point that the patient develops fatigue. The exercises are not meant to exhaust or tax the patient. It may be necessary to delay certain exercises until the patient's condition allows.
- Avoid neck hyperextension and attempts to achieve full range of motion in all joints with older patients. These movements may prove painful. Encourage adequate range of motion in those joints necessary to perform ADLs.
- Start gradually and work slowly. All movements should be smooth and rhythmic. Irregular and jerky movements are uncomfortable for patients.
- Move each joint until there is resistance but not pain. Report uncomfortable reactions and stop exercises until further instructions are obtained.

Concept Mastery Alert

Caution is necessary when performing range of motion exercises with patients who are unresponsive because these patients are unable to report complaints of pain.

- While exercising joints, use a variety of support measures to prevent muscle strain or injury to the patient, as demonstrated in Figure 32-22:
  - *Cupping:* placing a cupped hand under the joint to support it (e.g., under the elbow)
  - *Cradling:* supporting the joint with one hand while cradling the distal portion of the extremity with the remaining arm (e.g., the calf or forearm might be cradled while the knee or elbow is supported)
  - *Supporting* the joint by holding the adjacent distal and proximal muscular areas (indicated when a joint is painful); grasping muscle groups or major tendons is likely to cause injury to the tissues
- Return the joint to a neutral position, that is, its normal position of alignment, when finishing each exercise.
- Keep friction at a minimum when moving extremities to avoid injuring the skin.
- Use range-of-motion exercises twice a day, and do the exercises regularly to build up muscle and joint capabilities. Perform each exercise two to five times. It is possible to perform many of the exercises when the patient is being bathed as part of that procedure. Encourage routine tasks such as eating, dressing, self-bathing, and writing to help to put certain joints through range of motion.
- Expect the patient's respiratory and heart rate to increase during exercising, which is good. These rates should return to usual resting levels within 3 minutes. If they do not, the exercises are probably too strenuous for the patient.
- Use passive exercises as necessary, but encourage active exercises of the same kind when the patient is able to do so independently. Exercises should continue at home after a period of hospitalization, as necessary.

FIGURE 32-22. Support measures used to prevent muscle strain or injury to the patient during range-of-motion exercises. (**A**) Using a cupped hand to support a joint. (**B**) Supporting the joint by holding the distal and proximal areas adjacent to the joint. (**C**) Cradling the distal portion of a lower extremity.

 THINK back to Maggie Wyatt, the woman being discharged after treatment for a fracture. Range-of-motion exercises are essential for Maggie to maintain function. Although physical therapy would probably develop the exercise regimen, the nurse would need to reinforce these instructions with Maggie before discharge. In addition, the nurse would observe Maggie performing the active range-of-motion exercises, giving encouragement and correcting any misunderstandings, and would assist with the passive exercises until she goes home. ●

The goal of range-of-motion exercises is to keep the patient in the best possible physical state when bed rest is necessary or movement is restricted. When range-of-motion exercises are not considered as routine measures, consult the primary care provider physician. Skill 32-6 on pages 1105–1113 illustrates the normal movements incorporated in passive range-of-motion exercises.

Helping Patients Ambulate

Fortunately, for most patients, prolonged periods of bed rest are no longer considered necessary during most illnesses. Activity, even as mild as a short walk around the room, down the hall, from the bedroom to the living room, or out into the yard, is a protective measure for the body.

PHYSICAL CONDITIONING TO PREPARE FOR AMBULATION

Patients who are not confined to bed for long periods, who sleep well, and who experience possibly short periods of rest during the day may not require special considerations for increased physical activity in preparation for ambulation. However, others have to be prepared for the day when ambulation is resumed. Certain exercises that strengthen the overall efficiency of the musculoskeletal system can be done in bed. Check for physical activity restrictions or other contraindications before beginning any exercises.

Quadriceps and Gluteal Setting Drills (Sets). Quadriceps drills are an isometric exercise—an exercise in which muscle tension occurs without a significant change in the length of the muscle. One of the most important muscle groups used in walking is the quadriceps femoris. This muscle group helps extend the leg and flex the thigh. To help reduce weakness and make first attempts at walking easier, encourage bedridden patients to contract this muscle group frequently. Following are techniques for quadriceps drills:

- Have the patient contract or tighten the muscles on the front of the thighs. The patient has the feeling of pushing the knees downward into the mattress and pulling the feet upward.
- Have the patient hold the position just described while counting slowly to four, and then relax the muscles for an equal count. Emphasize that relaxation is important to prevent muscle fatigue.
- Caution the patient not to hold the breath during these exercises to avoid straining the heart.
- Teach the patient to do quadriceps drills two or three times each hour, four to six times a day, or as ordered by the health care provider.
- Instruct the patient to stop the exercise short of muscle fatigue.

The muscles in the buttocks can be exercised in the same way by pinching the buttocks together and then relaxing them. This is called gluteal setting. Tightening and holding the abdominal muscles for six seconds and then relaxing them also strengthens this muscle group to facilitate walking.

Pushups. The muscles of the arms and shoulders may also need strengthening before the patient is ready to be out of bed. Exercises should improve the strength needed to hold onto or get into a chair and to move about with greater ease. They are part of the preparation for patients who must learn to walk on crutches.

A trapeze attached to the bed of a patient who has limited use of the lower part of the body helps the patient to move about in bed and strengthens muscles in the upper part of the body. However, this does not strengthen the triceps, which is the muscle group necessary for crutch walking or for moving from a bed to a chair. More suitable exercises are pushups, which are done as follows:

- While sitting up in bed without support, the patient can do pushup exercises to strengthen the triceps. Instruct the patient to lift the hips off the bed by pushing down with the hands on the mattress. If the mattress is too soft, a block of books can be placed on the bed under the patient's hands.
- Pushups may also be done with the patient lying in bed on the abdomen. Instruct the patient to place the hands near the outstretched body at about shoulder level, with palms down on the mattress and elbows bent sharply. Then have the patient straighten the elbows to lift the head and shoulders off the bed.
- Pushups may also be done when the patient sits in an armchair or wheelchair. The patient places the hands on the arms of the chair and then raises the body out of the seat.
- Pushups should be done three or four times a day at first, with the number increased as upper body strength is increased.

 REMEMBER Maggie Wyatt, the woman with a fracture being discharged? Due to bed rest, her physical conditioning may be less than what it was before the fracture. Therefore, exercises—such as quadriceps and gluteal setting exercises and pushups in bed—could help to improve Maggie's conditioning, allowing her to participate more fully in her care. These exercises will prepare Maggie for transferring from the bed to the chair or from the chair to the car. ●

Dangling. **Dangling** refers to the position in which the person sits on the edge of the bed with legs and feet over the side of the bed. This exercise helps prepare patients for being out of bed. It is carried out as follows:

- Place the patient in the sitting position in bed for a few minutes. This will accustom the patient to this position and help prevent feelings of faintness.
- Place the bed in the low position or have a footstool handy on which the patient can rest the feet while dangling.
- Move the patient toward the side of the bed near you so that you do not stretch and strain while turning the patient.
- Pivot the patient a quarter of a turn by supporting the shoulders and legs. Swing the patient's legs over the side of the bed. The patient may place hands on your shoulders.
- Rest the patient's feet on the floor or on a footstool. This gives a sense of security, and lessens the likelihood that the patient will slide off the bed.
- Have the patient move the feet using an up-and-down, marching motion. This promotes circulation in the legs.
- Assess for lightheadedness or other signs of orthostatic hypotension (dizziness, nausea, tachycardia, or pallor).
- Remain with the patient and be ready to place the patient back to a lying position if feeling faint, to prevent falling out of bed.

Daily Activities for Purposeful Exercise. Many activities can be carried out in ways that encourage patients to move and gain the benefit of exercise, improving physical conditioning. When patients understand the purpose, they often adopt other exercises for themselves. For example, position the bedside stand so that the patient must use shoulder and arm muscles to reach it, instead of placing it so that little effort is required to take things from it. Place the signal cord (call light) so that the patient must move either the arm or shoulder to reach it, as long as it is definitely within reach. Encourage patients to sit up and reach for the overbed table, to pull it close, and then to push it back in place. In addition, encourage patients to try to carry out self-care activities, including washing their back independently or putting on socks while still in bed.

In a hospital setting, ADLs may be one of the few independent activities that a patient can perform. Allowing patients to do as much as they can independently is vital. Be sure to offer encouragement and praise. "Learned dependency," which often occurs with the older adult population, can lead to a decrease in self-esteem and depression. Collaborate with the occupational therapist when necessary to determine types of adaptive equipment that would help the patient achieve maximal functional independence. Box 32-2 (on page 1076) provides examples of available adaptive equipment. Providing the necessary adaptive tools, coupled with encouraging independence, will create the optimal outcome.

PROVIDING ASSISTANCE WITH WALKING

Many patients who have been confined to bed for an extended period find that they must almost learn to walk

BOX 32-2 — ADAPTIVE EQUIPMENT TO ASSIST WITH ACTIVITIES OF DAILY LIVING

- Long-handled bath sponges
- Reachers
- Long-handled shoehorns and sock aids
- Elastic shoelaces
- Utensils that are enlarged, specially angulated, or have special grips
- Velcro devices
- Universal cuffs (to hold silverware, comb, toothbrush, and the like, in palm)
- Feeding devices such as plates or bowls with suction-cup bottoms and/or lips to help with scooping food
- Splints and positioning equipment
- Shower chairs
- Transfer benches
- Environmental adaptations (grab bars, ramps)

all over again. Often, nurses play a major role in the patient's recovery, mental outlook, hope, and faith, especially when the patient must adhere to a rigid and often difficult schedule of re-educating muscle groups.

Because muscle re-education is a major task, the patient needs the assistance of experts in physical medicine. However, nurses can assist patients out of bed and help them walk when a physical therapist is not present. Plan to walk with a patient who is walking for the first few times after a period of bed rest.

Before getting the patient out of bed, do the following:

- Assess the patient's ability to walk and the need for assistance (one nurse, two nurses, walker, cane, walking belt, or crutches).
- Explain to the patient exactly what is to be done: transfer technique from bed to erect position, projected distance to be ambulated, assistance available, and the correct manner of using it. Instruct the patient to alert the nurse immediately if feeling dizzy or weak.
- Ensure that the patient has a clear path for ambulation.
- Provide skid-proof footwear.

Assist the patient to an erect position for ambulation, pausing after the patient is seated at the edge of the bed and again after the patient first stands to ensure that the patient feels steady. Use a gait belt, if necessary, to prevent injury to the nurse and patient. Reinforce the need to stand erect and to hold the head high to achieve the full benefits of walking. Patients who are fearful of walking often tend to look at their feet. Remind the patient to take deep breaths to aerate the lungs while walking. Because patients who are walking for the first time after prolonged bed rest often feel faint or weak, plan ambulation for a short distance, gradually increasing the distance as tolerated. As this distance is increased, have chairs readily available should the patient need to rest. Should a patient faint or begin to fall while walking, stand with feet apart to create a wide base of support and rock the pelvis out on the side facing the patient. With arms under the patient's axillae and encircling the patient, slide the patient down one's body to the floor, carefully protecting the patient's head (Fig. 32-23A). If the patient is wearing a gait belt, use the belt to ease the patient backward against one's own body and gently ease the patient to the floor while protecting the patient's head. When two nurses are assisting a patient who starts to fall or faint, they both should use one hand to grasp the gait belt to support the patient and grasp the patient's hand or wrist with their other hand. After they have steadied the patient, they can slowly lower the patient to a chair or the floor (Fig. 32-23B). Practice these maneuvers before they are needed in an emergency situation.

One-Nurse Assist. Patients who require minimal nursing assistance may walk well with the nurse walking

FIGURE 32-23. (**A**) One nurse guiding a patient to the floor. (**B**) Two nurses lowering a patient to the floor.

A   B

FIGURE 32-24. Assistance with ambulation. The nurse stands on the patient's weaker side and grasps the gait belt.

alongside. Provide support by standing at the patient's side and placing both hands at the patient's waist. Supporting the patient at the waist helps the patient to maintain an erect posture and prevents unintentionally pulling the patient to one side. Use of a gait belt snugly secured around the patient's waist also provides this type of support. Grasp the belt securely in the back, and walk behind and slightly to the side of the patient (Fig. 32-24).

Frequently, it is necessary to assist the patient with intravenous (IV) therapy equipment to walk. Secure a portable IV pole that moves easily. The patient walks with the assistance of the nurse and the portable IV pole. Ensure that all the equipment is secure before walking and be alert for any tension or sudden action that might dislodge or interfere with the infusion. Also, consider reviewing this technique with family members who are assisting with ambulation and are unfamiliar with how to steady the patient, maneuver equipment, and navigate through crowded or narrow areas.

When a patient has weakness or paralysis on one side, stand on the weaker or affected side and stabilize the patient by grasping the gait belt. Support the patient's weak arm by using one hand to support the patient's forearm and hand.

Two-Nurse Assist. A two-nurse assist is the safer method to use when there is uncertainty about the patient's ability to walk. Use of a gait belt snugly secured around the patient's waist provides a safe method for the nurses to support the patient. Each nurse should grasp the belt securely with the hand nearest the patient at the handle on each side of the patient. Support the patient's near arm by holding the patient's lower arm or hand. Walk slightly behind and to the side of the patient.

MECHANICAL AIDS FOR WALKING

Various devices can assist a patient with walking. These devices enhance the patient's balance and ability to bear weight. The most common are walkers, canes, braces, and crutches. Typically, a patient is fitted for a device and instructed in its use in the department of physical medicine or physical therapy. In this instance, the nurse's concern is chiefly to reinforce the teaching the patient has received and to ensure that the patient continues to use the device properly to assist in safe ambulation. In some health care settings, however, nurses may be responsible for fitting patients with the device and teaching them the appropriate way to use the device. Whenever you assess a patient who has been using a walker, cane, brace, or crutches for a period of time, determine whether the device is still needed, whether it continues to meet the patient's needs, and whether the patient continues to use it properly.

Some older patients consider the use of a mobility aid a visible symbol of weakness or an indication of decline in capabilities and loss of independence. Many patients refuse to use them and keep them out of sight. If the mobility aid is intended for short-term use (e.g., after hip replacement surgery), the response is usually more positive. Be sensitive to a patient's perspective regarding these devices and focus on the meaning the aid has for the patient, rather than simply emphasizing how to use it. Allow patients some control over their mobility decisions while still ensuring a safe environment. General guidelines for helping patients who need the assistance of a walker, cane, brace, or crutches include the following:

- Whenever possible, instruct the patient and family members in the correct use of the device before it is needed (e.g., before surgery). If family members are knowledgeable, they can reinforce the teaching as needed.
- When ready to begin walking with the new device, make sure the patient is wearing rubber-soled, well-fitting shoes and that there is a clear path for ambulation (clean, flat, dry, well lit). Use a gait belt, especially if the patient is at high risk for falls.
- Before moving, make sure the patient is steady on the feet when standing; instruct the patient to stand erect, looking straight ahead. The nurse should walk behind and slightly to one side of the patient (in cases of hemiparesis or hemiparalysis, walk on the patient's affected side). Should the patient lose balance, be prepared to grasp the patient's shoulder and the gait belt to steady the patient.

Walker. A walker is a lightweight metal frame (usually aluminum) with four legs (see Fig. 32-25A on page 1078). Walkers improve balance by increasing the patient's base of support, enhancing lateral stability, and supporting the patient's weight. The walker provides a sense of security and support. There are several types of walkers, specified according to the arm strength and balance of the patient. Most walkers have four legs with rubber tips. Some walkers have wheels on the front legs. These

FIGURE 32-25. Mechanical aids to walking. (**A**) A walker is a lightweight metal frame with a broad, four-point base of support. The walker should be adjusted to the height of the patient's hip joint so that the patient's elbows are flexed about 30 degrees. (**B**) Three types of canes. Single-ended canes with half-circle handles are recommended for patients requiring minimal support. Single-ended canes with straight handles are recommended for patients with hand weakness. Three- or four-prong canes are recommended for patients with poor balance.

walkers are best for patients with a gait that is too fast for a walker without wheels and for patients who have difficulty lifting a walker. Because lifting repeatedly is not required, energy expenditure and stress to the back and upper extremities is lower than with a standard walker (Mayo, 2011c). Walkers also are available with wheels on all four legs. Patients who require a larger base of support and do not rely on the walker to bear weight can use these. If full body weight is applied to this type of walker, it could roll away, resulting in a fall. Wheeled walkers are best for patients who need minimal weight bearing from the walker. Walkers often prove to be difficult to maneuver through doorways and congested areas. They should not be used on stairs (Mayo).

When the patient stands between the back legs of the walker with arms relaxed at the side, the top of the walker should line up with the crease on the inside of the patient's wrist. When the patient's hands are placed on the grips, elbows should be flexed about 30 degrees (Mayo, 2011c). The walker's rubber tips should be intact to prevent slipping. Generally, patients lift the walker without wheels ahead of themselves and step into it. Instruct a patient using a walker to do the following:

- Wear nonskid shoes or slippers.
- When rising from a seated position, use the chair arms for support. Once standing, place one hand at a time on the walker and move forward into it.
- Begin by pushing the walker forward, keeping the back upright. Place one leg inside the walker, keeping the

walker in place. Then, step forward with the remaining leg into the walker, keeping the walker still. Repeat the process by moving the walker forward again.
- Caution the patient to avoid pushing the walker out too far in front and leaning over it. Patients should always step into the walker, rather than walking behind it, staying upright as they move (Mayo, 2011c).
- Never attempt to use a walker on stairs.

Canes. Canes widen a person's base of support, providing increased balance (Nolen, Liu, Liu, McGee, & Grando, 2010). Canes come in three variations (see Fig. 32-25B): single-ended canes with half-circle handles (recommended for patients requiring minimal support and those who will be using stairs frequently), single-ended canes with straight handles (recommended for patients with hand weakness because the handgrip is easier to hold, but not recommended for patients with poor balance), canes with three (tripod) or four prongs (quad cane) or legs to provide a wide base of support (recommended for patients with poor balance).

Many canes are adjustable; fit them so that when the patient stands with the cane's tip 4 inches (10 cm) to the side of the foot, the cane extends from the floor to the patient's hip joint. The elbow should be flexed 30 degrees when holding the cane. Rubber tips on the cane prevent slipping and accidents. Inspect these regularly to ensure that they are intact. Teach patients to stand erect when walking with a cane and not to lean out over the cane.

When walking with a cane, instruct patients to hold the cane in the opposite hand from the leg with the most severe deficit (Mayo, 2011c). Ambulation proceeds in the following fashion:

1. The patient stands with weight evenly distributed between the feet and the cane.
2. The cane is held on the patient's stronger side and is advanced 4 to 12 inches (10–30 cm).
3. Supporting weight on the stronger leg and the cane, the patient advances the weaker foot forward, parallel with the cane.
4. Supporting weight on the weaker leg and the cane, the patient next advances the stronger leg forward ahead of the cane (heel slightly beyond the tip of the cane).
5. The weaker leg is moved forward until even with the stronger leg, and the cane is once again advanced as in step 2.

When less support is required from the cane, the patient can advance the cane and weaker leg forward while the stronger leg supports the patient's weight. Teach patients to position their canes within easy reach when they sit down so that they can rise easily.

Braces. Braces that support weakened leg muscles are available in many variations. Nursing responsibilities include knowing when the brace is to be worn and the correct technique for applying the brace, monitoring

FIGURE 32-26. Axillary (*left*) and forearm (*right*) support crutches.

to ensure correct use of the brace by the patient, and observing for any untoward problems the brace might cause (e.g., skin irritation). Muscle changes such as those occurring with growth and development or brought about by illness (atrophy) may require the brace to be refitted to maintain its effectiveness.

Crutches. Sometimes it is necessary for patients to use crutches for a time to avoid using one leg or to help strengthen one or both legs. The two types of crutches most commonly used are axillary crutches and forearm crutches (Fig. 32-26).

Forearm crutches are used for patients requiring long-term support for ambulation (Mincer, 2007). A supportive frame extends beyond the handgrip for the lower arm to help guide the crutch. These crutches are more likely to be used by patients who have permanent limitations and will always need crutch assistance for ambulation.

Axillary crutches are used to provide support for patients who have temporary restrictions on ambulation. These crutches require significant upper body and arm strength to use. The procedure for crutch walking is usu-

ally taught by a physical therapist, but it is important for the nurse to be knowledgeable about the patient's progress and the gait being taught. Be prepared to guide the patient at home or in the hospital after the initial teaching is completed. Remind the patient that the support of body weight should come primarily on the hands and arms while using the crutches, not in the axillary areas, where pressure may damage nerves and cut off circulation. Also, the crutches should not be forced into the axillae each time the body moves forward. Teaching Tips 32-1 (on page 1080) summarizes the important content to reinforce regarding crutch walking.

Promoting Exercise
PREVENTING ILLNESS AND PROMOTING WELLNESS THROUGH EXERCISE

According to *Healthy People 2020,* regular physical activity helps prevent certain chronic diseases such as hypertension, type 2 diabetes, and cardiovascular disease (U.S. Department of Health and Human Services [USDHHS], 2012). Vigorous physical activity is not always needed to achieve positive results. Studies have shown that moderate physical activity can be beneficial when incorporated into daily routines (Mayo, 2011b). Current recommendations encourage children and adolescents to be physically active for 60 minutes or more a day and adults to engage in activity that requires moderate effort, such as brisk walking for two and a half hours or more a week (USDHHS, 2008).

Nurses who role model healthy behaviors are more effective teachers. Use Promoting Health 32-1 (on page 1080) to assess yourself before using it with others. This display reflects on self-care behaviors vital for maintaining a healthy level of activity. Promoting exercise and emphasizing wellness behaviors are challenging opportunities for nurses. It is important to be committed to assisting and supporting patients to make lifestyle changes that improve the patients' health and well-being.

Advanced age has traditionally been associated with a decline in muscle strength and reluctance to exercise. Maintaining balance during exercise is frequently a concern of patients and caregivers. The accompanying Examples of Nursing Interventions and Nursing Outcomes Classifications (NIC/NOC) box (on page 1081) lists standardized nursing interventions and corresponding outcomes related to helping the patient with impaired physical mobility. As researchers focus on the potential of regular exercise activities to slow the aging process, nurses intervene to prevent the deleterious effects associated with decreased physical activity. See the accompanying Focus on the Older Adult display (on page 1081) for a summary of the benefits of exercise and specific precautions related to exercise for this age group.

An ongoing program of exercise for older patients also promotes confidence, improves outlook, offers opportunities for socialization, and fosters continued independence,

CRUTCH WALKING

Health Topic	Teaching Tip	Why Is This Important?
Safety measures	Routinely inspect crutch tips. Replace worn crutch tips. Crutch tips need to remain dry. Inspect the structure of your crutches routinely for cracks in a wooden crutch or bends in an aluminum crutch.	Rubber crutch tips increase surface tension and help prevent slipping. Water decreases surface friction and increases the risk of slipping. Cracks in a wooden crutch decrease its ability to support weight. Bends in aluminum crutches alter body alignment.
Correct positioning for use of crutches	Prevent pressure on the axillae. Keep elbows close to sides. Prevent crutches from getting closer than 12 inches to feet.	Pressure placed on the axillae can cause damage to nerves and circulation. This helps stabilize the crutches to prevent the patient from falling. This prevents the patient from tripping over the crutches.
Functioning at home	*To rise from a chair:* Slide forward to the edge of the chair. Extend the injured leg to prevent any weight bearing. Place crutches on unaffected side, lean forward, and push off using the crutches. *To climb stairs:* Advance unaffected leg past crutches, then place weight on unaffected leg. Advance affected leg and then crutches to the step. Continue with this order until top of stairs is reached. *To descend stairs:* Move crutches and affected leg first, followed by the unaffected leg.	Patient needs to learn that everyday occurrences may be challenging and, if not done correctly, may end up with injury to affected leg.

ACTIVITY

Use the assessment checklist to determine how well you are meeting your needs related to oxygenation. Then develop a prescription for self-care by choosing appropriate behaviors from the list of suggestions.

Assessment Checklist

❑ almost always   ❑ sometimes   ❑ almost never

❑ ❑ ❑   1. My lifestyle demonstrates that I place a high value on exercise as a component of wellness (e.g., I use stairs instead of elevators).

❑ ❑ ❑   2. I exercise for 30 to 45 minutes three or four times per week.

❑ ❑ ❑   3. I have sufficient energy for each day's tasks.

❑ ❑ ❑   4. I maintain my target weight/BMI.

Self-Care Behaviors

1. Decide to make the most of everyday opportunities for exercise: use stairs instead of elevators, walk instead of ride, park the car farther from your destination than usual and walk the distance briskly, and so forth.

2. Choose exercise activities you enjoy and plan three or four 30- to 45-minute exercise sessions weekly.

3. Obtain medical clearance for exercise if you fall in a high-risk group. Learn and observe the appropriate exercise safeguards (e.g., wear running shoes with the proper support).

4. Alternate types of exercise to avoid boredom.

5. Use part of your lunchtime for brisk walking or other exercise.

6. Invite a friend to exercise with you so you have the added support of a buddy or join a spa, health club, or exercise group.

7. Consistently use principles of body mechanics in both leisure and work activities.

8. Build up exercise sessions gradually to avoid overexertion and injury to muscles.

9. Evaluate your lifestyle to see what prevents you from exercising regularly and address these factors (low value attached to health or exercise, low motivation, lack of time, lack of rest, or faulty nutrition).

Information to promote cardiovascular health and oxygenation is available online. Visit thePoint for a list of Internet resources.

FOCUS ON THE OLDER ADULT

NURSING STRATEGIES TO PROMOTE EXERCISE AND ACTIVITY FOR AGE-RELATED CHANGES

Age-Related Changes	Nursing Strategies
Activity Intolerance • Decreased respiratory vital capacity • Decreased transport of oxygenated blood to tissue (as in chronic obstructive pulmonary disease or decreased cardiac output)	• Encourage patient to gradually increase physical activity and to listen to cues from one's own body. • Teach effective breathing techniques. • Instruct patient to avoid sudden position changes that may cause dizziness. • Instruct patient to avoid extreme temperatures if exercising. • Provide for sufficient hydration. • Encourage patient to avoid exercise if weak or ill. • Instruct patient to stop exercising if chest pain occurs, and consult with physician before resuming activity. • Instruct patient to respect fatigue. Do not push to the point of exhaustion.
Impaired Physical Mobility • Decreased range of motion • Decreased stability of gait	• Encourage patient to warm up before beginning exercises and to cool down after exercising. • Encourage patient to modify exercises versus forcing joints beyond the natural range of motion. • Discuss safety precautions that patient may take when exercising, such as walking in a gym or mall versus on an uneven sidewalk, and walking with a partner. • Recommend that patient wear proper footwear when exercising.

while lessening the potential for falls and other injuries. Older people who integrate a planned exercise regimen into their daily routine benefit physiologically and report improved self-esteem.

DESIGNING EXERCISE PROGRAMS

The benefits of exercise for each of the major body systems are so significant that designing individualized exercise programs for patients is an important nursing responsibility, often in conjunction with the physical therapist. Such a program should incorporate ADLs and planned exercise sessions. Depending on the patient's physical condition, exercise is designed to promote optimal fitness.

The individual's commitment to a program of regular exercise depends on the following:

• Knowledge of the benefits of exercise and the problems related to immobility

EXAMPLES OF NURSING INTERVENTIONS AND NURSING OUTCOMES CLASSIFICATIONS (NIC/NOC)

EXERCISE THERAPY: BALANCE

Nursing Interventions	Nursing Outcomes
• Determine the patient's ability to participate in activities requiring balance. • Evaluate sensory functions (e.g., vision, hearing, proprioception). Provide assistive devices. • Provide a safe environment for practice of exercises. • Encourage the patient to maintain a wide base of support, if needed. • Assist to stand (or sit) and rock the body from side to side to stimulate balance mechanisms. • Assist the patient to practice standing with eyes closed for short periods at regular intervals to stimulate proprioception. • Monitor the patient's response to balance exercises.	• Activity tolerance • Coordinated movement • Patient satisfaction: Functional assistance

Reprinted with permission from Bulechek, G. M., Butcher, H. K., Dochterman, J. M., & Wagner, C. M. (Eds.). (2013). *Nursing interventions classification (NIC)* (6th ed., p. 184–185). St. Louis: Elsevier/Mosby; and Moorhead, S., Johnson, M., Maas, M. L., & Swanson, E. (Eds). (2013). *Nursing Outcomes Classification (NOC)*. (5th ed., p. 79, 146, 187). St. Louis: Elsevier/Mosby. A full listing of nursing activities for each nursing intervention and outcomes can be found in these books.

- Appreciation of the fact that in society, sedentary lifestyles are common and most people must consciously choose to exercise
- Belief that each person is responsible for one's own health and that exercise is essential to one's well-being

Foster a commitment to regular exercise by teaching and counseling patients about exercise. To do this, be knowledgeable about the types and benefits of exercise as well as the risks associated with exercise.

When working with a patient to develop an individualized exercise prescription, use the following guidelines:

- Explore the patient's fitness goals, interests, skills, exercise opportunities, and exercise capacity.
- Assist the patient in obtaining medical clearance for exercise.
- Explore feasible exercise activities with the patient, considering the health benefits sought, the time involved, cost, any need for special equipment, precautions, and risks.
- Develop an exercise program that specifies warm-up and cool-down activities (walking, stretching) and three or four major exercise activities from which the patient can choose.
- Specify the frequency, duration, and intensity of the exercise activity. The recommended frequency for activity that requires moderate effort, such as brisk walking, is two and a half hours or more a week (USDHHS, 2008).
- Encourage the patient to complement the exercise program with everyday activities that require exercise.

- Try to identify with the patient any potential threats to the exercise program's successful implementation. Plan support strategies.
- Use ongoing evaluation to determine whether the exercise prescription is meeting the patient's needs and whether the patient is adhering to the prescription.
- Encourage the patient to have an exercise partner; they will encourage each other as well as keep each other company during the exercise.

Box 32-3 identifies characteristics of a successful exercise program and prevention strategies to avoid the risks associated with exercise.

Evaluating

When evaluating the effectiveness of a plan of care designed to help patients enhance, maintain, or regain mobility and fitness goals, use each nurse–patient interaction to evaluate the patient in the following respects:

- General ease of movement and gait
- Body alignment
- Joint structure and function
- Muscle mass, tone, and strength
- Endurance

An excellent time to assess these essential ingredients of well-being is when the patient is performing simple everyday tasks such as walking, undertaking hygiene measures, dressing, and eating. Because illness and enforced inactivity can affect these tasks negatively, ongoing evaluation is necessary if serious problems are to be avoided. For examples of the nursing process for activity, see the accompanying concept map for Kelsi Lester and Nursing Plan of Care 32-1 for Quan Hong Nguyen on pages 1084–1089.

BOX 32-3   CHARACTERISTICS OF A SUCCESSFUL EXERCISE PROGRAM

- The program is individually designed (considers the person's fitness goals, interests, skills, exercise opportunities, and exercise capacity).
- The program specifies warm-up and cool-down activities and a variety of major exercise activities—variety is preferable to a single-exercise activity.
- The program specifies frequency, intensity, and duration of exercise.
- The program is convenient to perform, compatible with the person's lifestyle, and fun!
- The person in such a program should understand the program and feel confident that exercise will result in definite health benefits.

Prevention Strategies to Avoid Risks Associated with Exercise

People beginning exercise programs should be familiar with the following guidelines:

- Obtain a pre-exercise medical examination and medical supervision during exercise if older than age 35 years and sedentary or if there is any past or current cardiovascular condition.
- Begin a new exercise program slowly and allow your body's support structure time to accommodate to the new stress.
- Know your body and respect its limitations. Never force a joint beyond its natural range of motion.
- Respect fatigue. Whenever you feel tingling, pain, or burning in a muscle, stop and rest the muscle for 15 minutes before continuing to exercise.
- Follow the safety guidelines for specific exercises; for example, joggers are advised to run on soft surfaces as opposed to cement or asphalt, to wear well-constructed shoes with thick soles and arch supports, and to run in a safe environment with a low pollution index.

Kelsi Lester is a 10-year-old girl in the pediatric unit as a result of a skiing accident. She is unconscious and may or may not regain consciousness. She is on complete bed rest. She requires frequent positioning to maintain correct body alignment and attention to her ROM. She responds to painful stimuli with slight nonpurposeful withdrawal. No spontaneous movements are noted. Ultrasound of lower extremities was negative for deep vein thrombosis (DVT). Subcutaneous heparin administration has been prescribed to prevent thrombus formation. Continuous tube feedings and intravenous therapy are prescribed to meet Kelsi's fluid and nutritional needs. Kelsi has been incontinent of stool and has an indwelling urinary catheter. Her heels are reddened, but otherwise her skin is intact. Kelsi's mother is at the bedside; she states, "I feel so helpless."

Priority 1	Priority 2	Priority 3
Nursing Diagnosis: Ineffective Tissue Perfusion: Potential for Thrombus Formation related to altered mobility.	**Nursing Diagnosis: Impaired Physical Mobility related to altered neurological functioning.**	**Nursing Diagnosis: Impaired Skin Integrity related to altered mobility from skiing accident.**
Supporting Data:	**Supporting Data:**	**Supporting Data:**
• Unconscious	• Unconscious	• No spontaneous movements
• No spontaneous movements	• No spontaneous movements noted	• Heels reddened
• No swelling or redness areas noted in calf	• Responds to painful stimuli with nonpurposeful withdrawal	• Incontinent of stool
• Ultrasound of lower extremities was negative for DVT	• Complete bed rest	• Continuous tube feedings
		• Foley catheter and IV in place
		• Complete bed rest
Outcome: Patient will remain free of DVT.	**Outcome:** Patient will maintain neurological function and be free from muscular contractures.	**Outcome:** Patient will maintain intact skin integrity.
Nursing Interventions:	**Nursing Interventions:**	**Nursing Interventions:**
• Maintain anti-embolism stockings and sequential pneumatic compression devices	• Assess motor function	• Assess skin every 8 hours
• Turn and reposition at least every 2 hours	• Turn and reposition at least every 2 hours	• Use Braden scale to assess risk for pressure ulcer
• Perform passive ROM exercises 3 times a day	• Support proper body alignment using positioning devices	• Maintain nutrition by monitoring tube feedings as prescribed
• Maintain adequate hydration with parenteral therapy and tube feedings as prescribed	• Use foot boot to prevent foot drop	• Use alternating pressure mattress
• Monitor for side effects of anticoagulant therapy	• Use wrist splints and hand rolls to maintain functional position	• Turn and reposition every 2 hours
	• Perform passive ROM 3 times a day; teach parents to assist with exercises	• Remove protective devices and splints periodically to assess for skin irritation
	• Consult physical therapy and occupational therapy	• Assess IV insertion site for any redness or swelling
	• Explain procedures to Kelsi prior to performing activity	• Document any areas of skin breakdown
		• Check for incontinence frequently and cleanse perirectal area; apply barrier cream
		• Use bed linens to reposition to avoid shearing pressure force
Evaluation: Kelsi has no occurrences of DVT. Anti-embolism stockings, sequential pneumatic compression devices, and activity have been maintained.	**Evaluation:** Kelsi is being turned every 2 hours. Positioning devices are being used. No contractures or foot drop is noted. Parents are assisting in turning and ROM exercises.	**Evaluation:** Kelsi's heels are no longer reddened. She shows no signs of skin breakdown.

- - - - - **Relationship**   ■ **Assessment**   ■ **Nursing Diagnosis**   ■ **Outcome Identification**   ■ **Interventions**   ■ **Evaluation**

Concept map displaying the nursing process for Kelsi Lester.

NURSING PLAN OF CARE 32-1

for Quan Hong Nguyen

Quan Hong Nguyen is an alert, 75-year-old married man who was admitted to the hospital with a diagnosis of an ischemic stroke (cerebrovascular accident or brain attack [Hinkle & Cheever, 2014]) secondary to thrombosis (formation of a blood clot). He has a history of hypertension. This is his second hospital day, and the attending physicians have termed the stroke a *completed stroke;* that is, Mr. Nguyen's neurologic deficits have been unchanged for 2 days, and he is believed to be ready for more aggressive rehabilitative treatment. On hospital day 2, an assessment of Mr. Nguyen's mobility status and ability to participate in activities of daily living revealed the following data:

- *Mental status*—basically alert and able to follow simple commands; expresses his needs verbally when encouraged, but speech is slow; seems forgetful of usual routine for basic self-care activities
- *Neuromuscular status*—hemiplegia; severe motor and sensory deficits of the left side of the face and the left arm and leg

- *Muscle mass, tone, and strength*—well-developed muscles in all extremities; history of a lifetime of sports, most recently played tennis two to four times weekly; decreased muscle tone (hypotonicity, flaccidity) in left arm and leg motor function is absent in left arm and very weak in left leg; strong motor function on right extremities; incapable of weight-bearing on left side; incapable of independent turning, sitting, standing, transferring, or ambulation
- *Joint mobility*—decreased on left side; otherwise full range of motion; no contractures
- *Endurance*—fatigues quickly (e.g., during complete bath)
- Some deficit in spatial–perceptual orientation (e.g., ignores objects on his left side), but it is difficult to assess this completely yet

NURSING DIAGNOSIS Impaired Physical Mobility (turning in bed, sitting, standing, transferring, ambulating) related to left hemiplegia and weakness as manifested by: motor function absent in left arm and weak in left leg, decreased joint mobility in left extremities, fatigue

EXPECTED OUTCOME 1/25/15 Whenever observed, the patient will:

- Be in correct body alignment with (1) each joint on the left side higher than the joint proximal to it and (2) supportive devices in place (bed board, footboard, trochanter roll, hand–wrist splint, shoulder sling, pillows)

NURSING INTERVENTIONS	**RATIONALE**	**EVALUATIVE STATEMENT**
At each position change (as dictated by every-2-hour turn schedule posted at the bedside), make sure that the patient is in correct alignment. Follow agency positioning guidelines for the supine, side-lying (lies on unaffected side), and prone positions.	Correct positioning prevents contractures, relieves pressures, and maintains alignment. • Positioning each joint higher than the preceding one prevents edema and its resulting fibrosis. • Placing the patient in the prone position for 30 minutes two or three times daily helps prevent knee and hip flexion contractures.	1/27/15 Outcome being met. Every-2-hour positioning schedule being followed with patient in correct body alignment to prevent contractures. *S. Beecher, RN*
Use the following supportive devices: firm mattress, footboard, trochanter roll, shoulder sling when the patient is in the upright position, volar resting splint, and pillows.	Support devices aid in maintaining the patient in correct positioning. • Firm mattress provides skeletal support. • Footboard during flaccid period prevents footdrop, heel cord shortening, and plantar flexion.	

NURSING PLAN OF CARE 32-1 *continued*

for Quan Hong Nguyen

NURSING INTERVENTIONS	RATIONALE	EVALUATIVE STATEMENT
	• Trochanter roll prevents external rotation of the hip when the patient is in the dorsal position. • Shoulder sling during the flaccid period prevents shoulder subluxation and shoulder–hand syndrome. • Volar resting splint supports the wrist and hand in a functional position. • A pillow in the axilla of the left side prevents adduction of the affected side.	
Teach both the patient and family the importance of correct positioning.	Teaching promotes self-care and lays the foundation for successful rehabilitation.	
Allow the family to participate in helping the patient to get comfortable in the different positions.	Involving the family in the patient's care facilitates the coping process.	

EXPECTED OUTCOME   By hospital day 7, 1/30/15, the patient will:

- Replace the passive range-of-motion exercises the nurse is now performing four times daily to all joints with (1) the patient's active exercise of the left arm and left leg and (2) the patient's active range-of-motion exercises for all other joints.

NURSING INTERVENTIONS	RATIONALE	EVALUATIVE STATEMENT
Assess the patient's knowledge of the importance of exercise and ability and motivation to exercise.	Unless the patient understands the reason for exercise and is physically, mentally, and attitudinally capable of exercise, he will not follow through.	1/30/15 Outcome partially met. Patient has successfully demonstrated complete set of range-of-motion exercises (to both left and right sides); however, he tires during the exercises and stops unless verbally encouraged.
Teach the patient how to exercise his left arm and leg by using his unaffected (right) extremities.	Active exercise maintains joint mobility, prevents contracture development in the paralyzed extremity, prevents further deterioration of the neuromuscular system, helps to regain motor control, and increases circulation. Involving the patient in self-care improves self-esteem and aids in regaining independence.	*Revision:* Monitor patient's exercise four times daily; continue to enlist family's support. *S. Beecher, RN*
Demonstrate a complete set of range-of-motion exercises to the patient and family and have the patient return the demonstrations.	Involving the family helps ensure the success of the exercise program because it requires a big time and effort commitment.	

(continued)

NURSING PLAN OF CARE 32-1 *continued*

for Quan Hong Nguyen

EXPECTED OUTCOME By hospital day 7, 1/30/15, the patient will:

- Perform quadriceps, gluteal, and abdominal settings five times daily

NURSING INTERVENTIONS	RATIONALE	EVALUATIVE STATEMENT
Teach the patient and family how to tighten the quadriceps, gluteal, and abdominal muscles and hold them for 6 seconds (slow count to 4) before relaxing. A 2-minute rest should be allowed between contractions and the patient should be cautioned not to hold his breath during these exercises. The exercises should be stopped short of muscle fatigue.	These exercises will maintain muscle mass, tone, and strength (while the patient is on bed rest); and prevent atrophy. They also increase circulation to the exercised body parts. Holding the breath places a strain on the heart.	1/30/15 Outcome partially met. Patient has demonstrated exercises correctly; however, he needs to be reminded to perform them. Family is effective in this regard. *Revision:* Compliment family on excellent job they are doing and reinforce importance of exercise to maximize rehabilitative potential. *S. Beecher, RN*

EXPECTED OUTCOME By hospital day 7, 1/30/15, the patient will:

- Participate in the every-2-hour positioning schedule by assisting with turning to the degree he is able

NURSING INTERVENTIONS	RATIONALE	EVALUATIVE STATEMENT
Teach the patient how he can help to reposition himself by grabbing onto the side rail with his right hand and also by placing his unaffected leg under the left one to move himself.	The more the patient can do independently, the more in control he will feel. These activities will pave the way to increasing independence in self-care activities.	1/27/15 Outcome met. Patient consistently assists in repositioning. Seems pleased to be able to help the nurses in this way. *S. Beecher, RN*

EXPECTED OUTCOME By hospital day 7, 1/30/15, the patient will:

- Demonstrate a safe pivot transfer from bed to chair and chair to bed

NURSING INTERVENTIONS	RATIONALE	EVALUATIVE STATEMENT
Demonstrate the pivot transfer technique. Assess the stage of recovery of muscle function.	Most patients will begin to show signs of spasticity with exaggerated reflexes within 48 hours—this denotes progress. If muscles are still flaccid after several weeks, prognosis for regaining function is poor.	1/30/15 Outcome met. Patient can safely transfer from bed to chair and chair to bed using pivot technique but requires nursing assistance. *S. Beecher, RN*

EXPECTED OUTCOME By hospital day 7, 1/30/15, the patient will:

- Demonstrate standing balance

NURSING PLAN OF CARE 32-1 *continued*

for Quan Hong Nguyen

NURSING INTERVENTIONS	RATIONALE	EVALUATIVE STATEMENT
Assess activity tolerance by taking vital signs before attempting balance training and transfers.	Vital signs and the patient's physical condition should be assessed before a new activity, during the activity, and shortly afterward to assess activity tolerance.	1/30/15 Outcome not met. Patient has not demonstrated standing balance; falls to left side without nursing support.
Precede transfers with balance training. Assist the patient to a sitting position at the edge of the bed and observe for steadiness and the ability to maintain an erect posture.	The patient needs sitting and standing balance before progressing to harder tasks. Dizziness or syncope may signal vasomotor instability.	*Revision:* Allow more time for goal achievement. *S. Beecher, RN*
Place the chair by the bed on the patient's unaffected side and assist the patient to dress. Initially, the nurse helps the patient to stand by placing the right knee against the patient's strong knee, grasping the patient around the waist with both arms, and pulling the patient forward while rocking back on the left leg (nurse's knees are slightly flexed).	This prevents the patient's knees from buckling and the pressure of the nurse's knee forces the patient to straighten the strong knee and bear weight on it. In this position, the patient's feet cannot slip forward. In this position, the nurse is using good principles of body mechanics.	
Once the patient is standing, assess standing balance and observe for signs of activity intolerance (pallor, shortness of breath, excessive increase in pulse rate, perspiration). Direct the patient to (1) grab the far arm of the chair with his strong arm, (2) turn on his strong foot, and (3) sit down. The nurse's right leg and the patient's strong leg are used as a pivot.	Using the unaffected extremity facilitates movement and provides stability.	
Pivot the patient out of bed to chair three times a day (may pivot out of bed to bedside commode). Gradually increase time in the chair based on the patient's tolerance. Correctly align the patient in the chair using supportive devices as necessary.	Increasing exercise to the patient's tolerance level promotes improved muscle strength and maintenance of range of motion.	

EXPECTED OUTCOME On discharge to rehabilitation center, the patient will:
- Be free of contractures

(continued)

NURSING PLAN OF CARE 32-1 *continued*

for Quan Hong Nguyen

NURSING INTERVENTIONS	RATIONALE	EVALUATIVE STATEMENT
Implement previously stated nursing actions.	These actions maintain joint mobility and decrease likelihood of contractures. These actions promote independence and return to activities of daily living.	1/30/15 Outcome met. Patient has no contractures. *S. Beecher, RN*

NURSING DIAGNOSIS Self-Care Deficit (all basic self-care activities) related to decreased alertness and left-sided motor and sensory deficits as manifested by: inability to use left arm (is right-handed), inability to ambulate, forgetfulness, fatigue.

EXPECTED OUTCOME By hospital day 7, 1/30/15, the patient will:

- Demonstrate beginning ability to resume self-care activities despite motor and sensory deficits of left side; use right arm to (1) assist in morning hygiene; (2) feed himself (finger foods, beverages); and (3) exercise.

NURSING INTERVENTIONS	RATIONALE	EVALUATIVE STATEMENT
Continue to assess extent of the patient's motor and sensory deficits and ability to perform self-care activities.	This facilitates recognition of any recovery of function and allows setting of appropriate goals.	1/29/15 Outcome met. For the past 2 days, patient has washed his left arm, abdomen, and legs; combed his hair; fed himself; and performed range-of-motion exercises. *S. Beecher, RN*
Set realistic short-term goals for each session with patient and reward progress: "This morning we'll see how much of your bath you are able to manage yourself!" "It must feel good to be able to do this for yourself again."	Adding *realistic* new tasks for each day gives the patient a goal to work toward; a pattern of *noticed* success encourages continued efforts.	
Approach the patient from his unaffected side, and place call bell, bedside table, phone, and so on, on this side.	This helps the patient to compensate for alterations in sensory perception.	
Teach patient how to transfer all self-care activities to the unaffected side and how to use one-handed techniques and adaptive equipment.	There is never only one way to do anything.	
Encourage the patient to brush his teeth, comb his hair, bathe and feed himself, and to assist in toileting. Explain to the family why it is critical to allow him to do these things himself, even if movements are tiring, clumsy, and initially frustrating.	This improves the patient's sense of control of his own activities of daily living and improves morale.	

NURSING PLAN OF CARE 32-1 *continued*

for Quan Hong Nguyen

NURSING INTERVENTIONS	RATIONALE	EVALUATIVE STATEMENT
Continually re-evaluate the patient's need for gentle care versus firm, directive encouragement. Involve the family in this process.	Emotional lability is common after stroke. Patients fluctuate between heroic efforts toward independent self-care and whining demands to be totally cared for. The appropriate nursing response varies from moment to moment and runs the range of tender care to unrelenting firm direction. All nursing responses need to communicate the nurse's sincere care for the patient and commitment to developing his best potential.	

EXPECTED OUTCOME   On discharge to rehabilitation center, the patient will:

- Show signs of physical and mental readiness to acquire increasing independence in self-care

NURSING INTERVENTIONS	RATIONALE	EVALUATIVE STATEMENT
Implement previously stated nursing actions.	These actions help the patient toward regaining control of his daily living and improve morale.	1/31/15 Outcome met. Patient's muscle strength and joint mobility maintained during hospitalization. Patient is now participating in self-care activities and is eager to learn skills to become more independent. *S. Beecher, RN*

SAMPLE DOCUMENTATION

1/25/15 1500, Nursing

Dr. Steel examined the patient at 1300 and noted he is now in "completed stroke stage and ready for more aggressive rehabilitative treatment." This was explained to patient, his wife, and son. The patient smiled and seemed to understand that he is out of immediate danger. Initial instructions given to the patient on how he can assist with position changes and actively exercise his left arm and leg. Correctly demonstrated these maneuvers with verbal cueing. Motor function still absent in left arm and weak in left leg. Plan of care revised to incorporate new exercise goals.

S. Beecher, RN

SKILL 32-1 APPLYING AND REMOVING GRADUATED COMPRESSION STOCKINGS

DELEGATION CONSIDERATIONS

The application and removal of graduated compression stockings may be delegated to nursing assistive personnel (NAP) or unlicensed assistive personnel (UAP), as well as to licensed practical/vocational nurses (LPN/LVNs). The decision to delegate must be based on careful analysis of the patient's needs and circumstances, as well as the qualifications of the person to whom the task is being delegated. Refer to the Delegation Guidelines in Appendix A (found on thePoint).

EQUIPMENT

- Elastic graduated compression stockings in ordered length in correct size.
- Measuring tape
- Talcum powder (optional)
- Skin cleanser, basin, towel
- PPE, as indicated

IMPLEMENTATION

ACTION	RATIONALE
1. Review the medical record and medical orders to determine the need for graduated compression stockings.	Reviewing the medical record and order validates the correct patient and correct procedure.
2. Perform hand hygiene. Put on PPE, as indicated.	Hand hygiene and PPE prevent the spread of microorganisms. PPE is required based on transmission precautions.
3. Identify the patient. Explain what you are going to do and the rationale for use of elastic stockings.	Patient identification validates the correct patient and correct procedure. Discussion and explanation allay anxiety and prepare the patient for what to expect.
4. Close the curtains around the bed and close the door to the room, if possible.	This ensures the patient's privacy.
5. Adjust the bed to a comfortable working height, usually elbow height of the caregiver (VISN 8 Patient Safety Center, 2009).	Having the bed at the proper height prevents back and muscle strain.
6. Assist the patient to the supine position. If the patient has been sitting or walking, have the patient lie down with legs and feet well elevated for at least 15 minutes before applying stockings.	Dependent position of legs encourages blood to pool in the veins, reducing the effectiveness of the stockings if they are applied to congested blood vessels.
7. Expose legs one at a time. Wash and dry legs, if necessary. Powder the leg lightly unless the patient has a respiratory problem, dry skin, or sensitivity to the powder. If the skin is dry, a lotion may be used. Powders and lotions are not recommended by some manufacturers; check the package material for manufacturer specifications.	Helps maintain patient's privacy. Powder and lotion reduce friction and make application of stockings easier.
8. Stand at the foot of the bed. Place a hand inside the stocking and grasp the heel area securely. Turn the stocking inside-out to the heel area, leaving the foot inside the stocking leg (Fig. 1).	Inside-out technique provides for easier application; bunched elastic material can compromise extremity circulation.

FIGURE 1. Pulling graduated compression stocking inside-out.

ACTION

9. With the heel pocket down, ease the stocking foot over the foot and heel (Fig. 2). Check that the patient's heel is centered in the heel pocket of the stocking (Fig. 3).

FIGURE 2. Putting foot of stocking onto patient.

10. Using your fingers and thumbs, carefully grasp the edge of the stocking and pull it up smoothly over the ankle and calf, toward the knee (Fig. 4). Make sure it is distributed evenly.

11. Pull forward slightly on the toe section. If the stocking has a toe window, make sure it is properly positioned. Adjust if necessary to ensure that the material is smooth.

12. If the stockings are knee-length, make sure each stocking top is 1 to 2 inches below the patella. Make sure the stocking does not roll down.

13. If applying thigh-length stocking, continue the application. Flex the patient's leg. Stretch the stocking over the knee.

14. Pull the stocking over the thigh until the top is 1 to 3 inches below the gluteal fold (Fig. 5). Adjust the stocking, as necessary, to distribute the fabric evenly. Make sure the stocking does not roll down.

FIGURE 4. Pulling the stocking up the leg.

RATIONALE

Wrinkles and improper fit interfere with circulation.

FIGURE 3. Ensuring that heel is centered after stocking is on foot.

Easing the stocking carefully into position ensures proper fit of the stocking to the contour of the leg. Even distribution prevents interference with circulation.

Ensures toe comfort and prevents interference with circulation.

Prevents pressure and interference with circulation. Rolling stockings may have a constricting effect on the veins.

This ensures even distribution.

Prevents excessive pressure and interference with circulation. Rolling stockings may have a constricting effect on the veins.

FIGURE 5. Pulling the stocking up over the thigh.

(continued)

SKILL 32-1 APPLYING AND REMOVING GRADUATED COMPRESSION STOCKINGS *continued*

ACTION	RATIONALE
15. Remove equipment and return the patient to a position of comfort. Remove gloves. Raise the side rail and lower the bed. Place the call bell and other essential items within reach.	Promotes patient comfort and safety. Removing gloves properly reduces the risk for infection transmission and contamination of other items. Having the call bell and other essential items within reach promotes safety.
16. Remove any other PPE, if used. Perform hand hygiene.	Removing PPE properly reduces the risk for infection transmission and contamination of other items. Hand hygiene prevents the spread of microorganisms.

Removing Stockings

17. To remove a stocking, grasp the top of the stocking with your thumb and fingers and smoothly pull the stocking off inside out to heel. Support the foot and ease the stocking over it.	This preserves the elasticity and contour of the stocking. It allows assessment of circulatory status and condition of the skin on the lower extremity and allows for skin care.

DOCUMENTATION

Guidelines

Document the patient's leg measurements as a baseline. Document the application of the stockings, size of stocking applied, skin and leg assessment, and neurovascular assessment.

Sample Documentation

> 7/22/15 0945 Leg measurements: calf 14½ inches, length heel to knee 16 inches. Measurements equal bilaterally. Knee-high graduated compression stockings (medium/regular) applied bilaterally. Posterior tibial and dorsalis pedal pulses +2 bilaterally; capillary refill less than 2 seconds and skin on toes consistent with rest of skin and warm. Skin on lower extremities is intact bilaterally.
> —C. Stone, RN

UNEXPECTED SITUATIONS AND ASSOCIATED INTERVENTIONS

- *Patient's leg measurements are outside the guidelines for the available sizes:* Notify the prescriber. The patient may require custom-fitted stockings.
- *Patient has a lot of pain with application of stockings:* If pain is expected (e.g., if the patient has a leg incision), it may be necessary to premedicate the patient and apply the stockings once the medication has had time to take effect. If the pain is unexpected, notify the primary care provider because the patient may be developing a deep vein thrombosis.
- *Patient has an incision on the leg:* When applying and removing stockings, be careful not to hit the incision. If the incision is draining, apply a small bandage to the incision so that it does not drain onto the stockings. If the stockings become soiled by drainage, wash and dry according to instructions.
- *Patient is to ambulate with stockings:* Place skid-resistant socks or slippers on before the patient attempts to ambulate.

SPECIAL CONSIDERATIONS

General Considerations

- Remove stockings once every shift for 20 to 30 minutes. Wash and air dry, as necessary, according to manufacturer's directions.
- Assess the patient at least every shift for skin color, temperature, sensation, swelling, and the ability to move. If complications are evident, remove the stockings and notify the primary care provider.
- Evaluate stockings to ensure that the top or toe opening does not roll with movement. Rolled stocking edges can cause excessive pressure and interfere with circulation.
- Despite the use of elastic stockings, a patient may develop deep vein thrombosis or phlebitis. Unilateral swelling, redness, tenderness, pain, and warmth are possible indicators of these complications. Notify the primary care provider of the presence of any symptoms.

Home Care Considerations

- Make sure that the patient has an extra pair of stockings ordered during hospitalization before discharge (for payment and convenience purposes).
- Stockings may be laundered with other "white" clothing. Avoid excessive bleach. Remove from dryer as soon as "low heat" cycle is complete to avoid shrinkage. Stockings may also be air dried. Check manufacturer's directions.

SKILL 32-2   ASSISTING A PATIENT WITH TURNING IN BED

DELEGATION CONSIDERATIONS

Assisting a patient to turn in bed may be delegated to nursing assistive personnel (NAP) or unlicensed assistive personnel (UAP), as well as to licensed practical/vocational nurses (LPN/LVNs). The decision to delegate must be based on careful analysis of the patient's needs and circumstances, as well as the qualifications of the person to whom the task is being delegated. Refer to the Delegation Guidelines in Appendix A (found on thePoint).

EQUIPMENT

- Friction-reducing sheet or draw sheet
- Bed surface that inflates to aid in turning
- Pillows or other supports to help the patient maintain the desired position after turning and to maintain correct body alignment for the patient
- Additional caregivers and/or safe handling equipment to assist, based on assessment
- Nonsterile gloves, if indicated; other PPE as indicated

IMPLEMENTATION

ACTION	RATIONALE
1. Review the medical orders and nursing plan of care for patient activity. Identify any movement limitations and the ability of the patient to assist with turning. **Consult patient handling algorithm, if available, to plan appropriate approach to moving the patient.**	Checking the medical orders and plan of care validates the correct patient and correct procedure. Identification of limitations and ability along with use of an algorithm helps to prevent injury and aids in determining the best plan for patient movement.
2. Gather any positioning aids or supports, if necessary.	Having aids readily available promotes efficient time management.
3. Perform hand hygiene. Put on PPE, as indicated.	Hand hygiene and PPE prevent the spread of microorganisms. PPE is required based on transmission precautions.
4. Identify the patient. Explain the procedure to the patient.	Patient identification validates the correct patient and correct procedure. Discussion and explanation help allay anxiety and prepare the patient for what to expect.
5. Close the curtains around the bed and close the door to the room, if possible. Position at least one nurse on either side of the bed. Place pillows, wedges, or any other support to be used for positioning within easy reach. Place the bed at an appropriate and comfortable working height, usually elbow height of the caregiver (VISN 8 Patient Safety Center, 2009). Lower both side rails.	Closing the door or curtain provides privacy. Proper bed height helps reduce back strain while performing the procedure. Proper positioning and lowering of the side rails facilitates moving the patient and minimizes strain on the nurses.
6. If not already in place, position a friction-reducing sheet under the patient.	Friction-reducing sheets aid in preventing shearing and in reducing friction and the force required to move the patient.
7. Using the friction-reducing sheet, move the patient to the edge of the bed, opposite the side to which the patient will be turned. Raise the side rails.	With this placement, the patient will be on the center of the bed after turning is accomplished. Raising side rails ensures patient safety.

(continued)

SKILL 32-2 ASSISTING A PATIENT WITH TURNING IN BED *continued*

<table>
<tr><td>

ACTION

</td><td>

RATIONALE

</td></tr>
<tr><td>

8. If the patient is able, have the patient grasp the side rail on the side of the bed toward which the patient is turning (Fig. 1). Alternately, place the patient's arms across his or her chest and cross his or her far leg over the leg toward which they are turning.

</td><td>

This encourages the patient to assist as much as possible with the movement. This facilitates the turning motion and protects the patient's arms during the turn.

</td></tr>
</table>

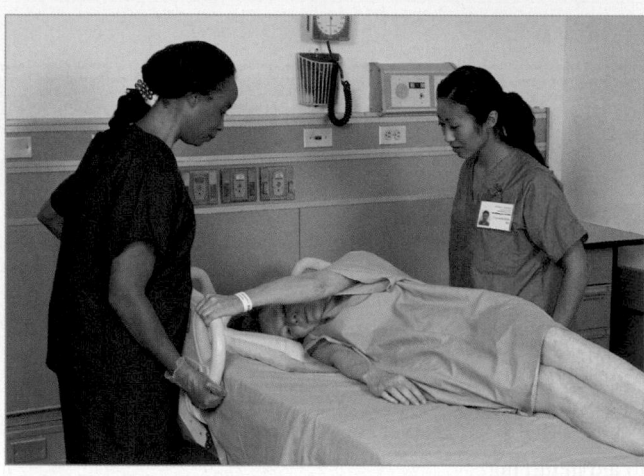

FIGURE 1. Having the patient grasp the side rail on the side of the bed toward which he or she is turning. *(Note: Patient's covers have been pulled back in this series of photos to show skill action. Covers should be folded back just enough to work, not expose patients unnecessarily.) (Photo by B. Proud.)*

9. If available, activate the bed turn mechanism to inflate the side of the bed behind the patient's back.

Activating the turn mechanism inflates the side of the bed for approximately 10 seconds, aiding in propelling the patient to turn, and reducing the work required by the nurse. This helps avoid straining the nurse's lower back.

10. The nurse on the side of the bed toward which the patient is turning should stand opposite the patient's center with feet spread about shoulder width and with one foot ahead of the other (Fig. 2). Tighten your gluteal and abdominal muscles and flex your knees. Use your leg muscles to do the pulling. The other nurse should position hands on the patient's shoulder and hip, assisting to roll the patient to the side. Instruct the patient to pull on the bed rail at the same time. Use the friction-reducing sheet to gently pull the patient over on his or her side (Fig. 3).

Each nurse is in a stable position with good body alignment and prepared to use large muscle masses to turn the patient. These maneuvers support the patient's body and use the nurses' weight to assist with turning.

FIGURE 2. Standing opposite the patient's center with feet spread about shoulder width and with one foot ahead of the other. *(Photo by B. Proud.)*

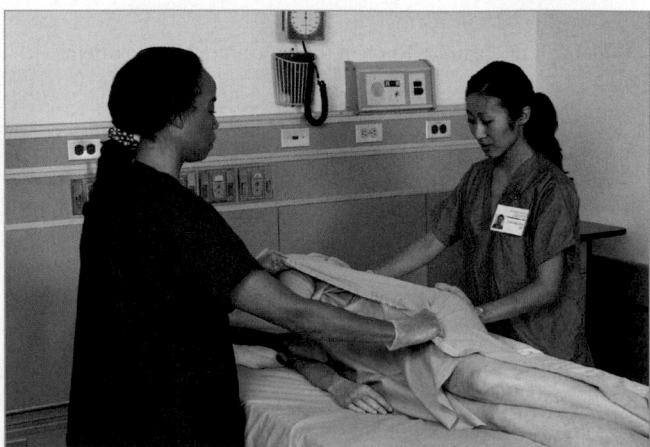

FIGURE 3. Using friction reducing sheet to pull the patient over on her side. *(Photo by B. Proud.)*

ACTION	RATIONALE

11. Use a pillow or other support behind the patient's back. Pull the shoulder blade forward and out from under the patient.

Pillow will provide support and help the patient maintain the desired position. Positioning the shoulder blade removes pressure from the bony prominence.

12. Make the patient comfortable and position in proper alignment, using pillows or other supports under the leg and arm, as needed. Readjust the pillow under the patient's head. Elevate the head of the bed as needed for comfort.

Positioning in proper alignment with supports ensures that the patient will be able to maintain the desired position and will be comfortable.

13. Place the bed in the lowest position, with the side rails up, as indicated. Make sure the call bell and other necessary items are within easy reach.

Adjusting the bed height ensures patient safety. Having the call bell and essential items readily available helps promote safety.

14. Clean transfer aids, per facility policy, if not indicated for single patient use. Remove gloves and other PPE, if used. Perform hand hygiene.

Proper cleaning of equipment between patient use prevents the spread of microorganisms. Removing PPE properly reduces the risk for infection transmission and contamination of other items. Hand hygiene prevents the spread of microorganisms.

DOCUMENTATION

Guidelines

Many facilities provide areas on the bedside flow sheet to document repositioning. Be sure to document the time the patient's position was changed, use of supports, and any pertinent observations, including skin assessment. Document the patient's tolerance of the position change. Document aids used to facilitate movement.

Sample Documentation

11/10/15 1130 Patient repositioned from right side to left side; alignment maintained with wedge support behind back and pillow between legs. Skin on pressure points on right side without signs of irritation, edema, or redness. Patient reports no pain with movement. Friction-reducing sheet used to facilitate transfer and left in place under patient. Three caregivers required for repositioning.
—B. Clapp, RN

UNEXPECTED SITUATIONS AND ASSOCIATED INTERVENTIONS

• *You are turning a patient by yourself, but you realize that the patient cannot help as much as you thought and is heavier than you anticipated:* Use the call bell to summon assistance from a coworker. Alternatively, cover the patient, make sure all rails are up, lower the bed to the lowest position, and get someone to assist you. Consider using a friction-reducing sheet and two to three additional caregivers.

SPECIAL CONSIDERATIONS

• Calculate the body mass index (BMI) for patients weighing over 300 pounds. If BMI exceeds 50, institute Bariatric Algorithms.

SKILL 32-3 MOVING A PATIENT UP IN BED WITH THE ASSISTANCE OF ANOTHER CAREGIVER

DELEGATION CONSIDERATIONS

Moving a patient up in bed may be delegated to nursing assistive personnel (NAP) or unlicensed assistive personnel (UAP), as well as to licensed practical/vocational nurses (LPN/LVNs). The decision to delegate must be based on careful analysis of the patient's needs and circumstances, as well as the qualifications of the person to whom the task is being delegated. Refer to the Delegation Guidelines in Appendix A (found on thePoint).

(continued)

SKILL 32-3 MOVING A PATIENT UP IN BED WITH THE ASSISTANCE OF ANOTHER CAREGIVER *continued*

EQUIPMENT

- Friction-reducing sheet or other friction-reducing device
- Nonsterile gloves, if indicated; other PPE as indicated
- Additional caregivers to assist, based on assessment
- Full-body sling lift and cover sheet, if necessary, based on assessment

IMPLEMENTATION

ACTION	RATIONALE
1. Review the medical record and nursing plan of care for conditions that may influence the patient's ability to move or to be positioned. Assess for tubes, IV lines, incisions, or equipment that may alter the positioning procedure. Identify any movement limitations. **Consult patient handling algorithm, if available, to plan appropriate approach to moving the patient.**	Reviewing the order and plan of care validates the correct patient and correct procedure. Identification of limitations and ability and use of an algorithm helps to prevent injury and aids in determining the best plan for patient movement.
2. Perform hand hygiene and put on PPE, if indicated.	Hand hygiene and PPE prevent the spread of microorganisms. PPE is required based on transmission precautions.
3. Identify the patient. Explain the procedure to the patient.	Patient identification validates the correct patient and correct procedure. Discussion and explanation help allay anxiety and prepare the patient for what to expect.
4. Close the curtains around the bed and close the door to the room, if possible. Place the bed at an appropriate and comfortable working height, usually elbow height of the caregiver (VISN 8 Patient Safety Center, 2009). Adjust the head of the bed to a flat position or as low as the patient can tolerate. Place the bed in slight Trendelenburg position, if the patient is able to tolerate it.	Closing the door or curtain provides for privacy. Proper bed height helps reduce back strain while you are performing the procedure. Flat positioning helps to decrease the gravitational pull of the upper body. Placing the bed in slight Trendelenburg position aids movement.
5. Remove all pillows from under the patient. Leave one at the head of the bed, leaning upright against the headboard.	Removing pillows from under the patient facilitates movement; placing a pillow at the head of the bed prevents accidental head injury against the top of the bed.
6. Position at least one nurse on either side of the bed, and lower both side rails.	Proper positioning and lowering the side rails facilitate moving the patient and minimize strain on the nurses.
7. If a friction-reducing sheet (or device) is not in place under the patient, place one under the patient's midsection.	A friction-reducing device supports the patient's weight and reduces friction during the repositioning.
8. Ask the patient (if able) to bend the legs and put feet flat on the bed to assist with the movement.	Patient can use major muscle groups to push. Even if the patient is too weak to push on the bed, placing the legs in this position will assist with movement and prevent skin shearing on the heels.
9. Have the patient fold the arms across the chest. Have the patient (if able) lift the head, with the chin on the chest.	Positioning in this manner provides assistance, reduces friction, and prevents hyperextension of the neck.
10. One nurse should be positioned on each side of the bed, at the patient's midsection, with feet spread shoulder width apart and one foot slightly in front of the other.	Doing so positions each nurse opposite the center of the body mass, lowers the center of gravity, and reduces the risk for injury.
11. If available on the bed, engage the mechanism to make the bed surface firmer for repositioning.	Decreases friction and effort needed to move the patient.
12. Grasp the friction-reducing sheet securely, close to the patient's body.	Having the sheet close to the body brings the patient's center of gravity closer to each nurse and provides a secure hold.
13. Flex your knees and hips. Tighten your abdominal and gluteal muscles, and keep your back straight.	Using the legs' large muscle groups and tightening muscles during transfer prevent back injury.

ACTION

14. If possible, the patient can assist with the move by pushing with the legs. Shift your weight back and forth from your back leg to your front leg and count to three (Fig. 1). On the count of three, move the patient up in bed (Fig. 2). Repeat the process, if necessary, to get the patient to the right position.

15. Assist the patient to a comfortable position and readjust the pillows and supports, as needed. Take the bed out of Trendelenburg position and return the bed surface to the normal setting, if necessary. Raise the side rails. Place the bed in the lowest position (Fig. 3). Make sure the call bell and other necessary items are within easy reach.

16. Clean transfer aids per facility policy, if not indicated for single-patient use. Remove gloves or other PPE, if used. Perform hand hygiene.

RATIONALE

If the patient assists, the nurses exert less effort.

The rocking motion uses the nurses' weight to counteract the patient's weight. Rocking develops momentum, which provides a smooth lift with minimal exertion by the nurses.

Readjusting the bed and adjusting the bed height ensures patient safety and comfort. Having the call bell and essential items readily available helps promote safety.

Proper cleaning of equipment between patient use prevents the spread of microorganisms. Removing PPE properly reduces the risk for infection transmission and contamination of other items. Hand hygiene prevents the spread of microorganisms.

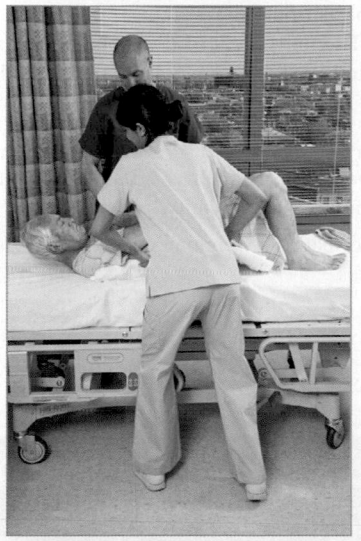

FIGURE 1. Nurses positioned at the patient's midsection, shifting weight from back leg to front leg in preparation for move. *(Note: Patient's covers have been pulled back in this series of photos to show skill action. Covers should be folded back just enough to work, not expose patients unnecessarily.)*

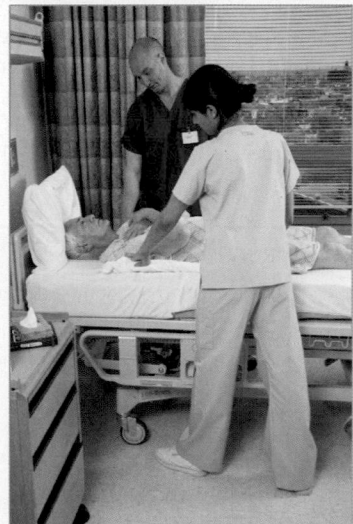

FIGURE 2. Patient moved up in bed.

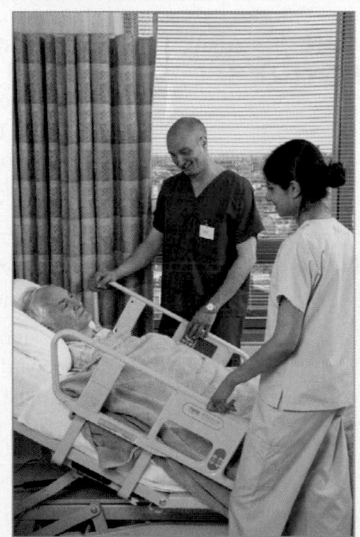

FIGURE 3. Adjusting bed to a safe and comfortable position.

(continued)

SKILL 32-3

MOVING A PATIENT UP IN BED WITH THE ASSISTANCE OF ANOTHER CAREGIVER *continued*

DOCUMENTATION

Guidelines

Many facilities provide areas on the bedside flow sheet to document repositioning. Document the time the patient's position was changed, use of supports, and any pertinent observations, including skin assessment. Document the patient's tolerance of the position change. Document aids used to facilitate movement.

Sample Documentation

> 11/10/15 1130 Patient repositioned from right side to left side; alignment maintained with wedge support behind back and pillow between legs. Skin on pressure points on right side without signs of irritation, edema, or redness. Patient reports no pain with movement.
>
> —B. Clapp, RN

UNEXPECTED SITUATIONS AND ASSOCIATED INTERVENTIONS

- *You are attempting to move a patient up in the bed with another nurse. Your first attempt is unsuccessful, and you realize the patient is too heavy for only two people to move:* Obtain the assistance of at least two other coworkers. Make use of available friction-reducing devices. Use full-body lift, if available. Position opposing pairs at the patient's shoulders and buttocks to distribute the weight. If necessary, have a fifth person lift the patient's legs or heels. The movement of a very large patient is aided by putting the bed in a slight Trendelenburg position temporarily, provided the patient can tolerate it.

SPECIAL CONSIDERATIONS

- When moving a patient with a leg or foot problem, such as a cast, wound, or fracture, one assistant should be assigned to lift and move that extremity.
- Calculate the body mass index (BMI) for patients weighing over 300 pounds. If BMI exceeds 50, institute Bariatric Algorithms.

SKILL 32-4

TRANSFERRING A PATIENT FROM THE BED TO A STRETCHER

DELEGATION CONSIDERATIONS

The transfer of a patient from bed to stretcher may be delegated to nursing assistive personnel (NAP) or unlicensed assistive personnel (UAP), as well as to licensed practical/vocational nurses (LPN/LVNs). The decision to delegate must be based on careful analysis of the patient's needs and circumstances, as well as the qualifications of the person to whom the task is being delegated. Refer to the Delegation Guidelines in Appendix A (found on thePoint).

EQUIPMENT

- Transport stretcher
- Friction-reducing sheet
- Lateral-assist device, such as a transfer board, roller board, or mechanical lateral-assist device, if available
- Bath blanket
- Regular blanket
- At least two assistants, depending on the patient's condition
- Nonsterile gloves and/or other PPE, as indicated

IMPLEMENTATION

ACTION	RATIONALE
1. Review the medical record and nursing plan of care for conditions that may influence the patient's ability to move or to be positioned. Assess for tubes, IV lines, incisions, or equipment that may alter the positioning procedure. Identify any movement limitations. **Consult patient handling algorithm, if available, to plan appropriate approach to moving the patient.**	Reviewing the medical record and plan of care validates the correct patient and correct procedure. Checking for interfering equipment helps reduce the risk for injury. Identification of limitations and ability along with use of an algorithm helps to prevent injury and aids in determining best plan for patient movement.
2. Perform hand hygiene and put on PPE, if indicated.	Hand hygiene and PPE prevent the spread of microorganisms. PPE is required based on transmission precautions.
3. Identify the patient. Explain the procedure to the patient.	Patient identification validates the correct patient and correct procedure. Discussion and explanation help allay anxiety and prepare the patient for what to expect.
4. Close curtains around the bed and close the door to the room, if possible. Adjust the head of the bed to a flat position or as low as the patient can tolerate. Raise the bed to a height that is even with the transport stretcher (VISN 8 Patient Safety Center, 2009). Lower the side rails, if in place.	Closing the door or curtain provides privacy. Proper bed height and lowering side rails make transfer easier and decrease the risk for injury.
5. Place the bath blanket over the patient and remove the top covers from underneath.	Bath blanket provides privacy and warmth.
6. If a friction-reducing transfer sheet is not in place under the patient, place one under the patient's midsection. Have the patient fold the arms against the chest and move the chin to the chest. Use the friction-reducing sheet to move the patient to the side of the bed where the stretcher will be placed. Alternately, place a lateral-assist device under the patient. Follow the manufacturer's directions for use.	A friction-reducing sheet supports the patient's weight, reduces friction during the lift, and provides a secure hold. Positioning with chin to chest and arms folded provides assistance, reduces friction, and prevents hyperextension of the neck. A transfer board or other lateral-assist device makes it easier to move the patient and minimizes the risk for injury to the patient and nurses.
7. Position the stretcher next to (and parallel) to the bed. **Lock the wheels on the stretcher and the bed.**	Positioning equipment makes the transfer easier and decreases the risk for injury. Locking the wheels keeps the bed and stretcher from moving.
8. Two nurses should stand on the stretcher side of the bed. A third nurse should stand on the side of the bed without the stretcher.	Team coordination facilitates patient safety during transfer.
9. Use the friction-reducing sheet to roll the patient away from the stretcher (Fig. 1). Place the transfer board across the space between the stretcher and the bed, partially under the patient (Fig. 2). Roll the patient onto his or her back, so that the patient is partially on the transfer board.	The transfer board or other lateral-assist device reduces friction, easing the workload to move the patient.

FIGURE 1. Using sheet to roll patient away from stretcher.

FIGURE 2. Positioning transfer board under patient.

(continued)

SKILL 32-4   TRANSFERRING A PATIENT FROM THE BED TO A STRETCHER *continued*

ACTION	RATIONALE
10. The nurse on the side of the bed without the stretcher should grasp the friction-reducing sheet at the head and chest areas of the patient. The nurse on the stretcher side of the bed should grasp the friction-reducing sheet at the head and chest, and the other nurse on that side should grasp the friction-reducing sheet at the chest and leg areas of the patient.	Grasping the friction-reducing sheet at these locations evenly supports the patient.
11. **At a signal given by one of the nurses, have the nurses standing on the stretcher side of the bed pull the friction-reducing sheet. At the same time, the nurse (or nurses) on the other side push, transferring the patient's weight toward the transfer board, and pushing the patient from the bed to the stretcher (Fig. 3).**	Working in unison distributes the work of moving the patient and facilitates the transfer.
12. Once the patient is transferred to the stretcher, remove the transfer board, and secure the patient until the side rails are raised (Fig. 4). Raise the side rails. To ensure the patient's comfort, cover the patient with a blanket and remove the bath blanket from underneath. Leave the friction-reducing sheet in place for the return transfer. Make sure the call bell and other necessary items are within easy reach.	Side rails promote safety. Blanket promotes comfort and warmth. Having the call bell and essential items readily available helps promote safety.
13. Clean the transfer aids per facility policy, if not indicated for single-patient use. Remove gloves and any other PPE, if used. Perform hand hygiene.	Proper cleaning of equipment between patient use prevents the spread of microorganisms. Removing PPE properly reduces the risk for infection transmission and contamination of other items. Hand hygiene prevents the spread of microorganisms.

FIGURE 3. Transferring patient onto stretcher.

FIGURE 4. Securing the patient on the stretcher.

DOCUMENTATION

Guidelines

Document the time and method of transport, and patient's destination, according to facility policy. Document the use of transfer aids and number of staff required for the transfer.

Sample Documentation

> 5/12/15 1005 Patient transferred to stretcher via three-person assistance and lateral-assist transfer sheet. Transported to radiology for chest x-ray.
>
> —M. Joliet, RN

UNEXPECTED SITUATIONS AND ASSOCIATED INTERVENTIONS	• *Your patient needs to be transported to another department by stretcher. The patient is very heavy and somewhat confused, so you are concerned about his ability to cooperate with the transfer:* Consult a Bariatric Algorithm. Obtain the assistance of three or more additional coworkers. Use a mechanical lateral-transfer device or air-assisted transfer device to move the patient.
SPECIAL CONSIDERATIONS	• Some mechanical lateral-transfer aids are motorized and others use a hand crank. If a mechanical lateral-assist device is used, follow the manufacturer's directions for safe movement of the patient. Be familiar with weight restrictions for individual pieces of equipment.
	• Keep in mind that the transfer of patients is often delegated to unlicensed personnel. Before moving patients, all personnel need to complete instructions about this skill and must be able to provide return demonstrations of transfer skills. When a patient is being transferred, communicate clearly any mobility restrictions or special care needs.
	• Calculate the body mass index (BMI) for patients weighing over 300 pounds. If BMI exceeds 50, institute Bariatric Algorithms.

SKILL 32-5   TRANSFERRING A PATIENT FROM THE BED TO A CHAIR

DELEGATION CONSIDERATIONS	The transfer of a patient from the bed to a chair may be delegated to nursing assistive personnel (NAP) or unlicensed assistive personnel (UAP), as well as to licensed practical/vocational nurses (LPN/LVNs). The decision to delegate must be based on careful analysis of the patient's needs and circumstances, as well as the qualifications of the person to whom the task is being delegated. Refer to the Delegation Guidelines in Appendix A (found on thePoint).

EQUIPMENT	
• Chair or wheelchair	• Additional staff person to assist
• Gait belt	• Blanket to cover the patient in the chair
• Stand-assist aid, if available	• Nonsterile gloves and/or other PPE, as indicated

IMPLEMENTATION

ACTION	RATIONALE
1. Review the medical record and nursing plan of care for conditions that may influence the patient's ability to move or to be positioned. Assess for tubes, IV lines, incisions, or equipment that may alter the positioning procedure. Identify any movement limitations. **Consult patient-handling algorithm, if available, to plan appropriate approach to moving the patient.**	Reviewing the medical record and plan of care validates the correct patient and correct procedure. Identification of limitations and ability and use of an algorithm help to prevent injury and aid in determining the best plan for patient movement.
2. Perform hand hygiene and put on PPE, as indicated.	Hand hygiene and PPE prevent spread of microorganisms. PPE is required based on transmission precautions.

(continued)

SKILL 32-5 TRANSFERRING A PATIENT FROM THE BED TO A CHAIR *continued*

ACTION	RATIONALE
3. Identify the patient. Explain the procedure to the patient.	Patient identification validates the correct patient and correct procedure. Discussion and explanation help allay anxiety and prepare the patient for what to expect.
4. If needed, move equipment to make room for the chair. Close the curtains around the bed and close the door to the room, if possible.	A clear pathway from the bed to the chair facilitates the transfer. Closing the door or curtain provides for privacy.
5. Place the bed in the lowest position. Raise the head of the bed to a sitting position, or as high as the patient can tolerate.	Proper bed height and positioning facilitate the transfer. The amount of energy needed to move from a sitting position or elevated position to a sitting position is decreased.
6. **Make sure the bed brakes are locked. Put the chair next to the bed. If available, lock the brakes of the chair. If the chair does not have brakes, brace the chair against a secure object.**	Locking brakes or bracing the chair prevents movement during transfer and increases stability and patient safety.
7. Encourage the patient to make use of a stand-assist aid, either freestanding or attached to the side of the bed, if available, to move to the side of the bed and to a side-lying position, facing the side of the bed on which the patient will sit.	Encourages independence, reduces strain for staff, and decreases risk for patient injury.
8. Lower the side rail, if necessary, and stand near the patient's hips. Stand with your legs shoulder width apart with one foot near the head of the bed, slightly in front of the other foot.	The nurse's center of gravity is placed near the patient's greatest weight to assist the patient to a sitting position safely.
9. Encourage the patient to make use of the stand-assist device. Assist the patient to sit up on the side of the bed; ask the patient to swing the legs over the side of the bed. At the same time, pivot on your back leg to lift the patient's trunk and shoulders. Keep your back straight; avoid twisting.	Gravity lowers the patient's legs over the bed. The nurse transfers weight in the direction of motion and protects his or her back from injury.
10. **Stand in front of the patient, and assess for any balance problems or complaints of dizziness (Fig. 1). Allow the patient's legs to dangle a few minutes before continuing.**	Standing in front of the patient prevents falls or injuries from orthostatic hypotension. The sitting position facilitates transfer to the chair and allows the circulatory system to adjust to a change in position.
11. Assist the patient to put on a robe, as necessary, and nonskid footwear.	Robe provides warmth and privacy. Nonskid soles reduce the risk for falling.
12. Wrap the gait belt around the patient's waist, based on assessed need and facility policy (Fig. 2).	Gait belts improve the caregiver's grasp, reducing the risk of musculoskeletal injuries to staff and the patient. Provides firmer grasp for the caregiver if patient should lose his or her balance.
13. Stand facing the patient. Spread your feet about shoulder width apart and flex your hips and knees.	This position provides stability and allows for smooth movement using the legs' large muscle groups.

FIGURE 1. Standing in front of the patient, and assessing for any balance problems or complaints of dizziness.

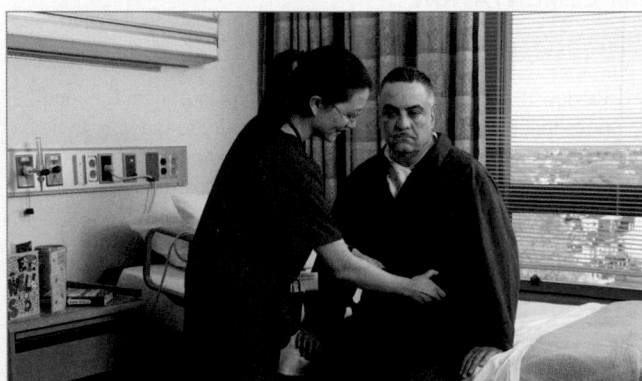

FIGURE 2. Wrapping the gait belt around the patient's waist.

ACTION	RATIONALE
14. Ask the patient to slide the buttocks to the edge of the bed until the feet touch the floor. Position yourself as close as possible to the patient, with your foot positioned on the outside of the patient's foot. If a second staff person is assisting, have that staff person assume a similar position. Grasp the gait belt (Fig. 3).	Doing so provides balance and support.
15. Encourage the patient to make use of the stand-assist device. If necessary, have the second staff person grasp the gait belt on the opposite side. Rock back and forth while counting to three. **On the count of three, using the gait belt and your legs (not your back), assist the patient to a standing position (Fig. 4).** If indicated, brace your front knee against the patient's weak extremity as the patient stands. Assess the patient's balance and leg strength. If the patient is weak or unsteady, return the patient to bed.	Holding at the gait belt prevents injury to the patient. Bracing your knee against a weak extremity prevents a weak knee from buckling and the patient from falling. Assessing balance and strength helps to identify the need for additional assistance to prevent falling.

FIGURE 3. Standing close to patient and grasping gait belt.

FIGURE 4. Nurse using the gait belt and her legs to help raise the patient to a standing position.

16. Pivot on your back foot and assist the patient to turn until the patient feels the chair against his or her legs.	This action ensures proper positioning before sitting.
17. Ask the patient to use his arm to steady himself on the arm of the chair while slowly lowering to a sitting position. Continue to brace the patient's knees with your knees and hold the gait belt. Flex your hips and knees when helping the patient sit in the chair (Fig 5).	The patient uses his or her own arm for support and stability. Flexing hips and knees uses major muscle groups to aid in movement and reduce strain on the nurse's back.

FIGURE 5. Assisting the patient to sit.

(continued)

SKILL 32-5

TRANSFERRING A PATIENT FROM THE BED TO A CHAIR *continued*

ACTION	RATIONALE
18. Assess the patient's alignment in the chair. Remove the gait belt, if desired. Depending on patient comfort, it could be left in place to use when returning to bed. Cover with a blanket, if needed. Make sure the call bell and other essential items are within easy reach.	Assessment promotes comfort; blanket provides warmth and privacy; having the call bell and other essential items readily available helps promote safety.
19. Clean transfer aids per facility policy, if not indicated for single-patient use. Remove gloves and any other PPE, if used. Perform hand hygiene.	Proper cleaning of equipment between patient use prevents the spread of microorganisms. Removing PPE properly reduces the risk for infection transmission and contamination of other items. Hand hygiene prevents the spread of microorganisms.

DOCUMENTATION

Guidelines

Document the activity, including the length of time the patient sat in the chair, any other pertinent observations, and the patient's tolerance of and reaction to the activity. Document the use of transfer aids and number of staff required for transfer.

Sample Documentation

5/13/15 1135 Patient dangled at side of bed for 5 minutes without complaints of dizziness or lightheadedness. Patient assisted out of bed to chair with minimal difficulty; gait belt in place. Tolerated sitting in chair for 30 minutes. Assisted back to bed, in semi-Fowler's position. Both upper side rails up.
—J. Minkins, RN

UNEXPECTED SITUATIONS AND ASSOCIATED INTERVENTIONS

• *You are assisting a patient out of bed. The previous times the patient has gotten up, you have not had any difficulty helping him by yourself, so you are working alone this time. The patient is positioned on the side of the bed. You flex your hips and knees to help him stand. As you move to pivot to the chair, the patient becomes very lightheaded and weak and his knees buckle. The patient is too heavy for you to lift to the chair:* Do not continue the move to the chair. Lower the patient back to the side of the bed. Pivot him back into bed, cover him, and raise the side rails. Check vital signs and assess for any other symptoms. After his symptoms have subsided and you are ready to get him up again, arrange for the assistance of another staff member. Have the patient dangle his legs for a longer period of time before standing. Assess for lightheadedness or dizziness before helping him stand up. Notify the primary care provider if there are any significant findings or if his symptoms persist.

SPECIAL CONSIDERATIONS

• Transfer of a patient to a chair or toilet can be accomplished using a powered stand-assist and repositioning lift, if available. These devices can be used with patients who have weight-bearing ability on at least one leg and who can follow directions and are cooperative. A simple sling is placed around the patient's back and under the arms. The patient rests feet on the device's footrest and places the hands on the handle. The device mechanically assists the patient to stand, without any lifting by the nurse (see page 1065). Once the patient is standing, the device can be wheeled to a chair, the toilet, or bed. Some devices have removable footrests and can be used as a walker. Some have scales incorporated into the device that can be used to weigh the patient.

• Patients who are unable to bear partial weight or full weight or who are uncooperative, as well as bariatric patients, should be transferred using a full-body sling lift.

- Calculate the body mass index (BMI) for patients weighing over 300 pounds. If BMI exceeds 50, institute Bariatric Algorithms.
- The transfer of patients is often delegated to unlicensed personnel. Before moving patients, all personnel need to complete instructions about this skill and must be able to provide return demonstrations of transfer skills. Before the transfer, communicate clearly any mobility restrictions or special care needs.

SKILL 32-6 PROVIDING RANGE-OF-MOTION EXERCISES

DELEGATION CONSIDERATIONS

Patient teaching regarding range-of-motion exercises cannot be delegated to nursing assistive personnel (NAP) or unlicensed assistive personnel (UAP). Reinforcement or implementation of range-of-motion (ROM) exercises may be delegated to NAP or UAP, as well as to licensed practical/vocational nurses (LPN/LVNs). The decision to delegate must be based on careful analysis of the patient's needs and circumstances, as well as the qualifications of the person to whom the task is being delegated. Refer to the Delegation Guidelines in Appendix A (found on thePoint).

EQUIPMENT

No special equipment or supplies are necessary to perform ROM exercises. Wear nonsterile gloves and/or other PPE, as appropriate.

IMPLEMENTATION

ACTION	RATIONALE
1. Review the medical orders and nursing plan of care for patient activity. Identify any movement limitations.	Reviewing the order and plan of care validates the correct patient and correct procedure. Identification of limitations prevents injury.
2. Perform hand hygiene and put on PPE, if indicated.	Hand hygiene and PPE prevent the spread of microorganisms. PPE is required based on transmission precautions.
3. Identify the patient. Explain the procedure to the patient.	Patient identification validates the correct patient and correct procedure. Discussion and explanation help allay anxiety and prepare the patient for what to expect.
4. Close the curtains around the bed and close the door to the room, if possible. Place the bed at an appropriate and comfortable working height, usually elbow height of the caregiver (VISN 8 Patient Safety Center, 2009). Adjust the head of the bed to a flat position or as low as the patient can tolerate.	Closing the door or curtains provides privacy. Proper bed height helps reduce back strain while performing the procedure.
5. Stand on the side of the bed where the joints are to be exercised. Lower the side rail on that side, if in place. Uncover only the limb to be used during the exercise.	Standing on the side to be exercised and lowering the side rail prevent strain on the nurse's back. Proper draping provides for privacy and warmth.
6. Perform the exercises slowly and gently, providing support by holding the areas proximal and distal to the joint. Repeat each exercise two to five times, moving each joint in a smooth and rhythmic manner. **Stop movement if the patient complains of pain or if you meet resistance.**	Slow, gentle movements with support prevent discomfort and muscle spasms resulting from jerky movements. Repeated movement of muscles and joints improves flexibility and increases circulation to the body part. Pain may indicate that the exercises are causing damage.
7. While performing the exercises, begin at the head and move down one side of the body at a time. **Encourage the patient to do as many of these exercises independently as possible.**	Proceeding from head to toe, one side at a time, promotes efficient time management and an organized approach to the task. Both active and passive exercises improve joint mobility and increase circulation to the affected part, but only active exercise increases muscle mass, tone, and strength and improves cardiac and respiratory functioning.

(continued)

SKILL 32-6 PROVIDING RANGE-OF-MOTION EXERCISES *continued*

ACTION	RATIONALE
8. Move the chin down to rest on the chest (Fig. 1). Return the head to a normal upright position (Fig. 2). Tilt the head as far as possible toward each shoulder (Fig. 3).	These movements provide for flexion, extension, and lateral flexion of the head and neck.
9. Move the head from side to side, bringing the chin toward each shoulder (Fig. 4).	These movements provide for rotation of neck.
10. Start with the arm at the patient's side (Fig. 5) and lift the arm forward to above the head (Fig. 6). Return the arm to the starting position at the side of the body.	These movements provide for flexion and extension of the shoulder.

FIGURE 1. Moving patient's chin down to rest on chest.

FIGURE 2. Holding patient's head upright and centered.

FIGURE 3. Moving patient's head to one shoulder.

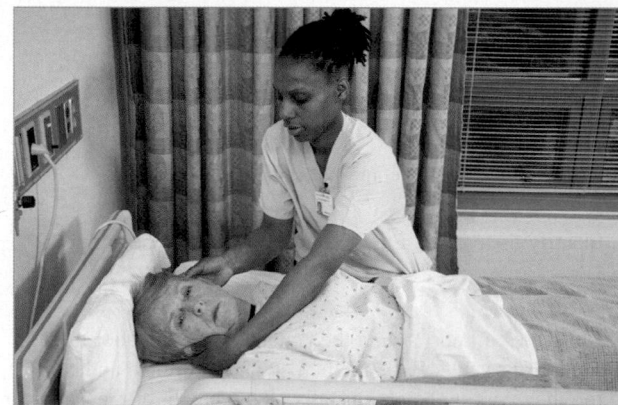

FIGURE 4. Moving patient's chin toward one shoulder.

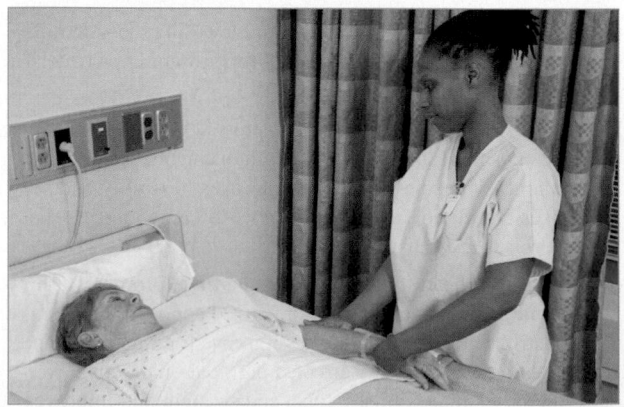

FIGURE 5. Holding patient's arm at side.

FIGURE 6. Lifting patient's arm above patient's head.

ACTION

11. With the arm back at the patient's side, move the arm laterally to an upright position above the head (Fig. 7), and then return it to the original position. Move the arm across the body as far as possible (Fig. 8).

12. Raise the arm at the side until the upper arm is in line with the shoulder. Bend the elbow at a 90-degree angle (Fig. 9) and move the forearm upward and downward, then return the arm to the side.

13. Bend the elbow and move the lower arm and hand upward toward the shoulder (Fig. 10). Return the lower arm and hand to the original position while straightening the elbow.

RATIONALE

These movements provide for abduction and adduction of the shoulder.

These movements provide for internal and external rotation of the shoulder.

These movements provide for flexion and extension of the elbow.

FIGURE 7. Moving patient's arm laterally to an upright position above patient's head.

FIGURE 8. Moving arm across patient's body as far as possible.

FIGURE 9. Raising patient's arm until upper arm is in line with patient's shoulder, with elbow bent.

FIGURE 10. Bending patient's elbow, lower arm, and hand upward toward shoulder.

(continued)

SKILL 32-6 PROVIDING RANGE-OF-MOTION EXERCISES *continued*

ACTION	RATIONALE
14. Rotate the lower arm and hand so that the palm is up (Fig. 11). Rotate the lower arm and hand so that the palm of the hand is down.	These movements provide for supination and pronation of the forearm.
15. Move the hand downward toward the inner aspect of the forearm (Fig. 12). Return the hand to a neutral position even with the forearm (Fig. 13). Then move the dorsal portion of the hand backward as far as possible.	These movements provide for flexion, extension, and hyperextension of the wrist.

FIGURE 11. Rotating patient's lower arm and hand so that palm is up.

FIGURE 12. Moving patient's hand downward toward inner aspect of forearm.

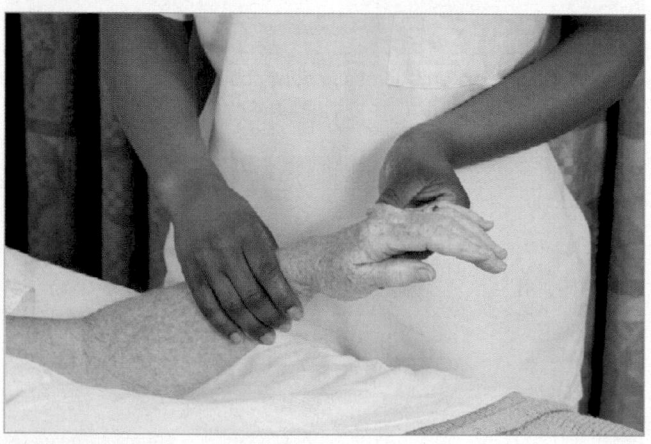

FIGURE 13. Returning hand to the neutral position.

ACTION	RATIONALE
16. Bend the fingers to make a fist (Fig. 14), then straighten them out (Fig. 15). Spread the fingers apart (Fig. 16) and return them back together. Touch the thumb to each finger on the hand (Fig. 17).	These movements provide for flexion, extension, abduction, and adduction of the fingers.
17. Extend the leg and lift it upward (Fig. 18). Return the leg to the original position beside the other leg.	These movements provide for flexion and extension of the hip.

ACTION

RATIONALE

FIGURE 14. Bending patient's fingers to make a fist.

FIGURE 15. Straightening out patient's fingers.

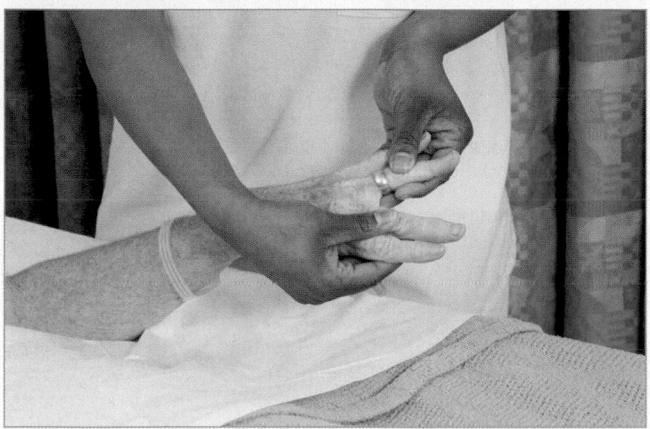

FIGURE 16. Spreading patient's fingers apart.

FIGURE 17. Assisting patient to touch thumb to each finger.

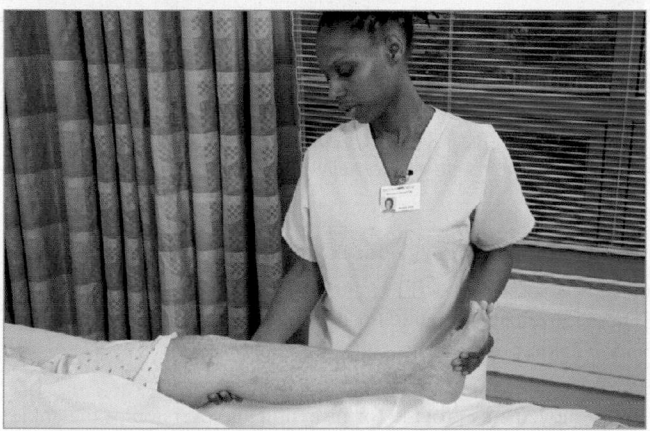

FIGURE 18. Extending and lifting patient's leg.

(continued)

SKILL 32-6   PROVIDING RANGE-OF-MOTION EXERCISES   *continued*

ACTION	RATIONALE
18. Lift the leg laterally away from the patient's body (Fig. 19). Return the leg back toward the other leg and try to extend it beyond the midline (Fig. 20).	These movements provide for abduction and adduction of the hip.
19. Turn the foot and leg toward the opposite leg to rotate it internally (Fig. 21). Turn the foot and leg outward, away from the opposite leg, to rotate it externally (Fig. 22).	These movements provide for internal and external rotation of the hip.

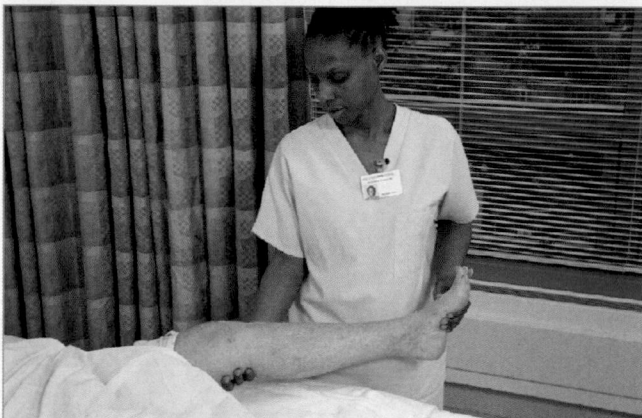

FIGURE 19. Lifting the patient's leg laterally away from body (abduction).

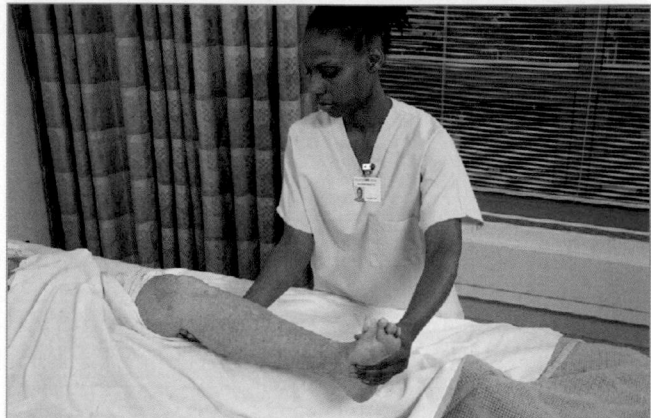

FIGURE 20. Returning leg back toward the other leg and trying to extend it beyond the midline, if possible.

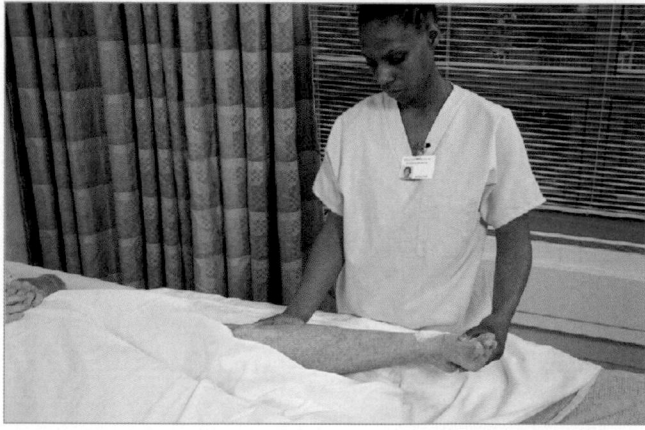

FIGURE 21. Turning patient's foot and leg toward the opposite leg to rotate it internally.

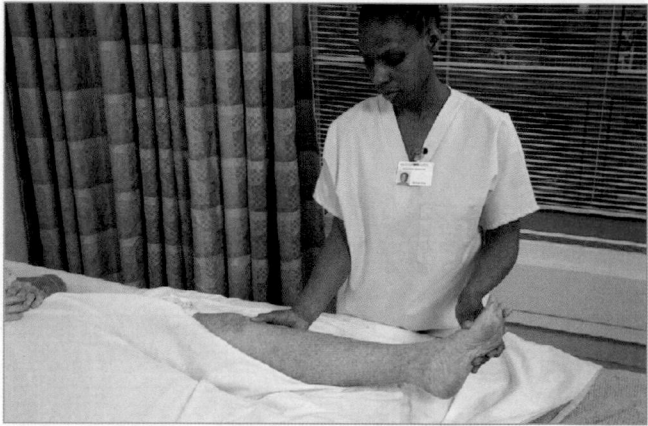

FIGURE 22. Turning patient's foot and leg outward, away from the opposite leg, to rotate it externally.

ACTION	RATIONALE
20. Bend the leg and bring the heel toward the back of the leg (Fig. 23). Return the leg to a straight position (Fig. 24).	These movements provide for flexion and extension of the knee.
21. At the ankle, move the foot up and back until the toes are upright (Fig. 25). Move the foot, with the toes pointing downward (Fig. 26).	These movements provide for dorsiflexion and plantar flexion of the ankle.
22. Turn the sole of the foot toward the midline (Fig. 27). Turn the sole of the foot outward (Fig. 28).	These movements provide for inversion and eversion of the ankle.

ACTION

RATIONALE

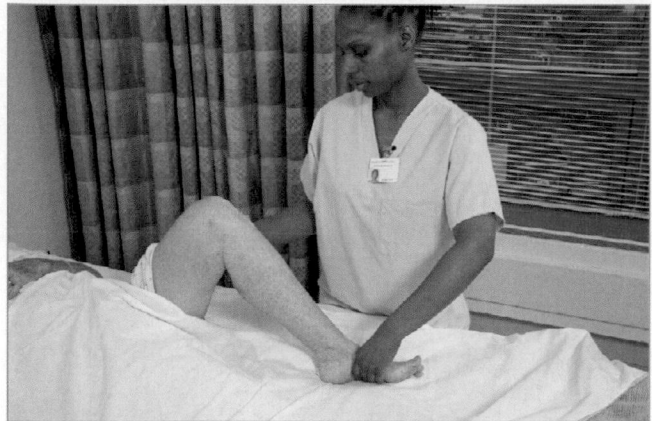

FIGURE 23. Bending patient's leg and bringing the heel toward the back of the leg.

FIGURE 24. Returning leg to a straight position.

FIGURE 25. At the ankle, moving patient's foot up and back until toes are upright.

FIGURE 26. Moving patient's foot with toes pointing down.

FIGURE 27. Turning sole toward the midline.

FIGURE 28. Turning sole outward.

(continued)

SKILL 32-6 PROVIDING RANGE-OF-MOTION EXERCISES *continued*

ACTION

23. Curl the toes downward (Fig. 29), then straighten them out (Fig. 30). Spread the toes apart (Fig. 31) and bring them together (Fig. 32).

RATIONALE

These movements provide for flexion, extension, abduction, and adduction of the toes.

FIGURE 29. Curling patient's toes downward.

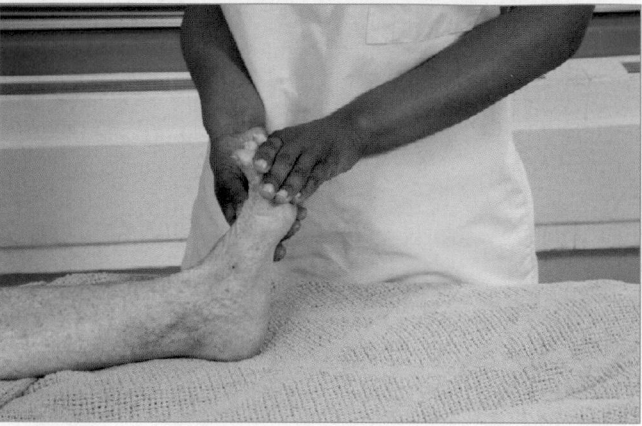

FIGURE 30. Straightening patient's toes.

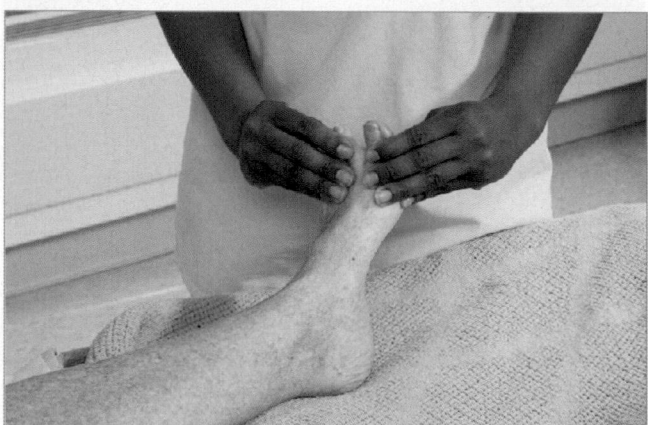

FIGURE 31. Spreading patient's toes apart.

FIGURE 32. Bringing patient's toes together.

24. Repeat these exercises on the other side of the body. Encourage the patient to do as many of these exercises independently as possible.

25. When finished, make sure that the patient is comfortable, with the side rails up and the bed in the lowest position. Place the call bell and other essential items within reach.

26. Remove gloves and any other PPE, if used. Perform hand hygiene.

Repeating motions on the other side provides exercise for the entire body. Self-esteem, self-care, and independence are encouraged through the patient performing the exercises on his or her own.

Proper positioning with raised side rails and proper bed height provides patient comfort and safety. Having the call bell and other essential items within reach promotes safety.

Removing PPE properly reduces the risk for infection transmission and contamination of other items. Hand hygiene prevents the spread of microorganisms.

DOCUMENTATION

Guidelines

Document the exercises performed, any significant observations, and the patient's reaction to the activities.

Sample Documentation

<u>5/1/15</u> 0945 Range-of-motion exercises performed to all joints. Patient able to perform active ROM of head, neck, shoulders, and arms. Required moderate assistance with ROM to lower extremities. Denied any complaints of pain during exercises. Patient tolerated exercise session well. Sitting in semi-Fowler's position with side rails up, watching television.

—*J. Chrisp, RN*

UNEXPECTED SITUATIONS AND ASSOCIATED INTERVENTIONS

- *While you are performing range-of-motion exercises, the patient complains of feeling tired:* Stop the activity for that time. Re-evaluate the nursing plan of care. Space the exercises out at different times of the day. Schedule exercise times for the parts of the day the patient is typically feeling more rested.
- *While exercising your patient's leg, he complains of sudden, sharp pain:* Stop the exercises. Assess the patient for other symptoms. Notify the primary care provider of the event, the patient's uncomfortable reactions, and your assessment findings. Joints should be moved until there is resistance, but not pain. Report uncomfortable reactions and halt exercises. Revise activity plan if necessary.

SPECIAL CONSIDERATIONS

General Considerations

- Incorporate the exercises when possible into daily activities, such as during bathing.
- Obtain a medical order and specific instructions to perform ROM exercises for patients with acute arthritis, fractures, torn ligaments, joint dislocation, acute myocardial infarction, and bone tumors or metastases.

Older Adult Considerations

- Avoid neck hyperextension and attempts to achieve full range of motion in all joints with older patients.

DEVELOPING CLINICAL REASONING

1. Pretend that you have a mobility impairment (i.e., you have to use crutches or a walker, cane, or wheelchair), and attempt to perform your usual daily activities, ideally including visiting a public place, such as a school or mall. How did you feel about the restriction of your movement? How can nurses best assist patients who are coping with these restrictions? How did the public respond to your impairment, and what effects might such responses have on individuals with mobility impairments? Are public spaces adequately adapted to meet the needs of those with mobility impairments? What measures are needed to address any deficiencies? Did you identify any safety needs?

2. Suppose a friend is confined to bed for several months after a motorcycle accident that resulted in severe orthopedic and internal injuries. What nursing measures would you recommend to avoid the hazards of immobility?

PRACTICING FOR NCLEX

1. A nurse is preparing an exercise program for a 65-year-old male patient who has COPD. Which instructions would the nurse include in a teaching plan for this patient? Select all that apply.
   a. Instruct the patient to avoid sudden position changes that may cause dizziness.
   b. Recommend that the patient restrict fluid until after exercising is finished.
   c. Instruct the patient to push a little further beyond fatigue each session.
   d. Instruct the patient to avoid exercising in very cold or very hot temperatures.
   e. Encourage the patient to modify exercise if weak or ill.
   f. Recommend that the patient consume a high-carb, low protein diet.

2. A nurse is providing range-of-motion exercises for a 53-year-old female patient who is recovering from a stroke. During the session, the patient complains that she is "too tired to go on." What would be priority nursing actions for this patient? Select all that apply.
   a. Stop performing the exercises.
   b. Decrease the number of repetitions performed.
   c. Re-evaluate the nursing plan of care.
   d. Move to the patient's other side to perform exercises.
   e. Encourage the patient to finish the exercises and then rest.
   f. Assess the patient for other symptoms.

3. A nurse is ambulating a 48-year-old female patient for the first time following surgery for a knee replacement. Shortly after beginning to walk, the patient tells the nurse that she is dizzy and feels like she might fall. Place these nursing actions in the order in which the nurse should perform them to protect the patient:
   a. Grasp the gait belt.
   b. Stay with the patient and call for help.
   c. Place feet wide apart with one foot in front.
   d. Gently slide patient down to the floor, protecting her head.
   e. Pull the weight of the patient backward against your body.
   f. Rock your pelvis out on the side of the patient.

4. A nurse caring for patients in a pediatrician's office assesses infants and toddlers for physical developmental milestones. Which patient would the nurse refer to a specialist based on failure to achieve these milestones?
   a. A 4-month-old infant who is unable to roll over
   b. A 6-month-old infant who is unable to hold his head up himself
   c. An 11-month-old infant who cannot walk unassisted
   d. An 18-month-old toddler who cannot jump

5. A nurse is caring for a 26-year-old male patient who has been hospitalized for a spinal cord injury following a motor vehicle accident. Which action would the nurse perform when logrolling the patient to reposition him on his side?
   a. Have the patient extend his arms outward and cross his legs on top of a pillow.
   b. Stand at the side of the bed in which the patient will be turned while another nurse gently pushes the patient from the other side.
   c. Have the patient cross his arms on his chest and place a pillow between his knees.
   d. Place a cervical collar on the patient's neck and gently roll him to the other side of the bed.

6. A nurse is caring for an 82-year-old woman in a long-term care facility who has had two urinary tract infections in the past year related to immobility. Which finding would the nurse expect in this patient?
   a. Improved renal blood supply to the kidneys
   b. Urinary stasis
   c. Decreased urinary calcium
   d. Acidic urine formation

7. A nurse is caring for a 73-year-old male patient who is hospitalized with pneumonia and is experiencing some difficulty breathing. The nurse most appropriately assists him into which position to promote maximal breathing in the thoracic cavity?
   a. Dorsal recumbent position
   b. Lateral position
   c. Fowler's position
   d. Sims' position

8. A nurse is assisting a postoperative patient with conditioning exercises to prepare for ambulation. The nurse correctly instructs the patient to do which actions? Select all that apply.
   a. Do full-body pushups in bed six to eight times daily.
   b. Breathe in and out smoothly during quadriceps drills.
   c. Place the bed in the lowest position or use a footstool for dangling.
   d. Dangle on the side of the bed for 30 to 60 minutes.

e. Allow the nurse to bathe the patient completely to prevent fatigue.
f. Perform quadriceps 2 to 3 times per hour, 4 to 6 times a day.

9. A nurse is caring for a patient who is on bed rest following a spinal injury. In which position would the nurse place the patient's feet to prevent footdrop?
   a. Supination
   b. Dorsiflexion
   c. Hyperextension
   d. Abduction

10. A nurse is instructing a patient who is recovering from a stroke how to use a cane. Which step would the nurse include in the teaching plan for this patient?
    a. Support weight on stronger leg and cane and advance weaker foot forward.
    b. Hold the cane in the same hand of the leg with the most severe deficit.
    c. Stand with as much weight distributed on the cane as possible.
    d. Do not use the cane to rise from a sitting position, as this is unsafe.

11. A 17-year-old has a fractured left leg, which has been casted. Following teaching from the physical therapist for using crutches, the nurse reinforces which teaching point with the patient?
    a. Use the axillae to bear body weight.
    b. Keep elbows close to the sides of the body.
    c. When rising, extend the uninjured leg to prevent weight bearing.
    d. To climb stairs, place weight on affected leg first.

12. A nurse working in a long-term care facility uses proper patient-care ergonomics when handling and transferring patients to avoid back injury. Which action should be the focus of these preventive measures?
    a. Carefully assessing the patient care environment
    b. Using two nurses to lift a patient who cannot assist
    c. Wearing a back belt to perform routine duties
    d. Properly documenting the patient lift

13. A nurse is assisting a patient who is 2 days postoperative from a cesarean section to sit in a chair. After assisting the patient to the side of the bed and to stand up, the patient's knees buckle and she tells the nurse she feels faint. What should the nurse do in this situation?
    a. Wait a few minutes and then continue the move to the chair.
    b. Call for assistance and continue the move with the help of another nurse.
    c. Lower the patient back to the side of the bed and pivot her back into bed.
    d. Have the patient sit down on the bed and dangle her feet before moving.

14. A 49-year-old who injured his spine in a motorcycle accident is receiving rehabilitation services in a short-term rehabilitation center. The nurse caring for him correctly tells the aide not to place him in which position?
    a. Side-lying
    b. Fowler's
    c. Sims'
    d. Prone

15. A nurse is using the Katz Index of Independence in Activities of Daily Living to assess the mobility of an 80-year-old hospitalized female patient. During the patient interview the nurse documents the following patient data: "Patient bathes self completely but needs help with dressing. Patient toilets independently and is continent. Patient needs help moving from bed to chair. Patient follows directions and can feed self." Based on this data, which score would the patient receive on the Katz index?
    a. 2
    b. 4
    c. 5
    d. 6

ANSWERS WITH RATIONALES

1. *a, d.* Teaching points for exercising for a patient with COPD include avoiding sudden position changes that may cause dizziness and avoiding extreme temperatures. The nurse should also instruct the patient to provide for adequate hydration, respect fatigue by not pushing to the point of exhaustion, and avoid exercise if weak or ill. Older adults should consume a high-protein, high-calcium, and vitamin D–enriched diet.

2. *a, c, f.* When a patient complains of fatigue during range-of-motion exercises, the nurse should stop the activity, re-evaluate the nursing plan of care, and assess the patient for further symptoms. The exercises could then be scheduled for times of the day when the patient is feeling more rested, or spaced out at different times of the day.

3. *c, f, a, e, d, b.* If a patient being ambulated starts to fall, you should place your feet wide apart with one foot in front, rock your pelvis out on the side nearest the patient, grasp the gait belt, support the patient by pulling her weight backward against your body, gently slide her down your body toward the floor, protecting her head, and stay with the patient and call for help.

4. *b.* By 5 months, head control is usually achieved. An infant usually rolls over by 6 to 9 months. By 15 months, most toddlers can walk unassisted. By 2 years, most toddlers can jump.

5. *c.* The procedure for logrolling a patient is: (1) Have the patient cross the arms on the chest and place a pillow between the knees; (2) have two nurses stand on one side of the bed opposite the direction the patient will be turned with the third helper standing on the other side and if necessary, a fourth helper at the head of the bed to stabilize the neck; (3) fanfold or roll the drawsheet tightly against the patient and carefully slide the patient to the side of the bed toward the nurses; (4) have one helper move to the other side of the bed so that two nurses are on the side to which the patient is turning; (5) face the patient and have everyone move on a predetermined time, holding the drawsheet taut to support the body, and turn the patient as a unit toward the two nurses.

6. *b.* In a nonerect patient, the kidneys and ureters are level. In this position, urine remains in the renal pelvis for a longer period of time before gravity causes it to move into the ureters and bladder, resulting in urinary stasis. Urinary stasis favors the growth of bacteria that may cause urinary tract infections.

Regular exercise, not immobility, improves blood flow to the kidneys. Immobility predisposes the patient to *increased* levels of urinary calcium and alkaline urine, contributing to renal calculi and urinary tract infection, respectively.

7. *c.* Fowler's position promotes maximal breathing space in the thoracic cavity and is the position of choice when someone is having difficulty breathing. Lying flat on the back or side or Sims' position would not facilitate respiration and would be difficult for the patient to maintain.

8. *b, c, f.* Breathing in and out smoothly during quadriceps drills maximizes lung inflation. The patient should perform quadriceps 2 to 3 times per hour, 4 to 6 times a day, or as ordered. The patient should never hold their breath during exercise drills because this places a strain on the heart. Pushups are usually done three or four times a day and involve only the upper body. Dangling for 30 to 60 minutes is unsafe. The nurse should place the bed in the lowest position or use a footstool for dangling. The nurse should also encourage the patient to be as independent as possible to prepare for return to normal ambulation and ADLs.

9. *b.* For a patient who has footdrop, the nurse should support the feet in dorsiflexion, and use a footboard or high-top sneakers to further support the foot. Supination involves lying patients on their back or facing a body part upward, and hyperextension is a state of exaggerated extension. Abduction involves lateral movement of a body part away from the midline of the body. These positions would not be used to prevent footdrop.

10. *a.* The proper procedure for using a cane is to (1) stand with weight distributed evenly between the feet and cane; (2) support weight on the stronger leg and the cane and advance the weaker foot forward, parallel with the cane; (3) support weight on the weaker leg and cane and advance the stronger leg forward ahead of the cane; (4) move the weaker leg forward until even with the stronger leg and advance the cane again as in step 2. The patient should keep the cane within easy reach and use it for support to rise safely from a sitting position.

11. *b.* The patient should keep the elbows at the sides, prevent pressure on the axillae to avoid damage to nerves and circulation, extend the injured leg to prevent weight bearing when rising from a chair, and advance the unaffected leg first when climbing stairs.

12. *a.* Preventive measures should focus on careful assessment of the patient care environment so that patients can be moved safely and effectively. Using lifting teams and assistive patient handling equipment rather than two nurses to lift increases safety. The use of a back belt does not prevent back injury. The methods used for safe patient handling and movement should be documented but are not the primary focus of interventions related to injury prevention.

13. *c.* If a patient becomes faint and knees buckle when moving from bed to a chair, the nurse should not continue the move to the chair. The nurse should lower the patient back to the side of the bed, pivot her back into bed, cover her, and raise the side rails. Assess the patient's vital signs and for the presence of other symptoms. Another attempt should be made with the assistance of another staff member if vital signs are stable. Instruct the patient to remain in the sitting position on the

side of the bed for several minutes to allow the circulatory system to adjust to a change in position, and avoid hypotension related to a sudden change in position.

14. *d.* The prone position is contraindicated in patients who have spinal problems because the pull of gravity on the trunk when the patient lies prone produces a marked lordosis, or forward curvature of the lumbar spine.

15. *b.* The total score for this patient is 4. On the Katz Index of Independence in ADLs, one point is awarded for independence in each of the following activities: bathing, dressing, toileting, transferring, continence, and feeding.

TAYLOR SUITE RESOURCES

Explore these additional resources to enhance learning for this chapter:

- NCLEX-Style Questions and other resources on thePoint, http://thePoint.lww.com/Taylor8e
- *Study Guide for Fundamentals of Nursing, 8th edition*
- Adaptive Learning | Powered by prepU, http://thepoint.lww.com/prepu
- *Skill Checklists for Fundamentals of Nursing, 8th edition*
- *Taylor's Clinical Nursing Skills:* Chapter 9, Activity
- *Taylor's Video Guide to Clinical Nursing Skills:* Activity

Bibliography

Ackley, B. J., & Ladwig, G. B. (2011). *Nursing diagnosis handbook* (9th ed.). St. Louis: Elsevier/Mosby.

American Association of Critical-Care Nurses (AACN). (2010). Practice alert. Venous thromboembolism prevention. Available at http://www.aacn.org/WD/Practice/Docs/PracticeAlerts/VTE%20Prevention%2004-2010%20final.pdf

American Geriatric Society. (2012). Choosing the right cane or walker. Available at http://www.healthinaging.org/files/documents/tipsheets/canes_walkers.pdf

American Nurses Association (ANA). (2013). Safe patient handling and mobility. Available at http://www.nursingworld.org/MainMenuCategories/Occupationaland Environmental/occupationalhealth/handlewithcare.aspx

Arthritis Foundation. (2013a). What is osteoarthritis? Available at http://www.arthritis.org/what-is-osteoarthritis.php

Arthritis Foundation. (2013b). Understanding arthritis. Available at http://www.arthritis.org/conditions-treatments/understanding-arthritis/

Baptiste, A. (2011). An evaluation of nursing tasks. *Work, 40*(2), 115–124.

Baptiste, A., Boda, S., Nelson, A., Lloyd, J., & Lee, W. (2006). Friction-reducing devices for lateral patient transfers: A clinical evaluation. *AAOHN Journal, 54*(4), 173–180.

Black, T. R., Shah, S. M., Busch, A. J., Metcalfe, J., & Lim, H. J. (2011). Effect of transfer, lifting, and repositioning (TLR) injury prevention program on musculoskeletal injury among direct care workers. (2011). *Journal of Occupational and Environmental Hygiene, 8*(4), 226–235.

Boltz, M., Capezuti, E., Fulmer, T., & Zwicker, D. (Eds.) (2012). *Evidence-based geriatric nursing protocols for best practice* (4th ed.). New York: Springer Publishing Company.

Bolz, M., Resnick, B., Capezuti, E., Shuluk, J., & Secic, M. (2012). Functional decline in hospitalized older adults: Can nursing make a difference? *Geriatric Nursing, 33*(4), 272– 279.

Bulechek, G. M., Butcher, H. K., Dochterman, J. M., & Wagner, C. M. (Eds.). (2013). *Nursing interventions classification (NIC)* (6th ed.). St. Louis, MO: Elsevier/Mosby.

Centers for Disease Control and Prevention (CDC). (2011a). Healthy weight—it's not a diet, it's a lifestyle! Physical activity for a healthy weight. Available at http://www.cdc.gov/healthyweight/physical_activity/

Centers for Disease Control and Prevention (CDC). (2011b). Arthritis basics. Available at http://www.cdc.gov/arthritis/basics.htm

de Castro, A. B. (2004). "Handle With Care®: The American Nurses Association's Campaign to Address Work-Related Musculoskeletal Disorders" *Online Journal of Issues in Nursing, 9*(3), Manuscript 2. Available at www.nursingworld.org/MainMenuCategories/ANAMarketplace/ANAPeriodicals/OJIN/TableofContents/Volume92004/No3Sept04/HandleWithCare.aspx

Esposito, E. M., & Fitzpatrick, J. J. (2011). Registered nurses' beliefs of the benefits of exercise, their exercise behavior and their patient teaching regarding exercise. *International Journal of Nursing Practice, 17*(4), 351–356.

Fernandes, T. (2006a). Moving and handling: Hoists and slings. *Nursing and Residential Care, 8*(12), 548–551.

Fernandes, T. (2006b). Suitable moving and handling equipment: A guide. *International Journal of Therapy and Rehabilitation, 13*(10), 477–481.

Gait belt handle helps during transfers. (2010). *Journal of Gerontological Nursing, 36*(12), 8.

Geerts, W. H., Bergqvist, D., Pineo, G. F., Heit, J. A., Samama, C. M., Lassen, M. R., & Colwell, C. W. (2008). Prevention of venous embolism: American College of Chest Physicians Evidence-based clinical practice guidelines (8th ed.). *CHEST, 133*(6 Suppl), S381–S453.

Green, D. (2012). Moving and positioning individuals. *Nursing & Residential Care, 14*(10), 506–509.

Grossman, S. (2014). Porth's pathophysiology: concepts of altered health states. (9th ed.). Philadelphia: Wolters Kluwer Health/Lippincott Williams & Wilkins.

Haglund, K., Kyle, J., & Finkelstein, M. (2010). Pediatric safe patient handling. *Journal of Pediatric Nursing, 25*(2), 98–107.

Hinkle, J. L., & Cheever, K. H. (2014). *Brunner & Suddarth's textbook of medical–surgical nursing* (13th ed.). Philadelphia: Wolters Kluwer Health/Lippincott Williams & Wilkins.

Hinton, M. V. (2010). Establishing a safe patient handling/minimal lift program. *Orthopaedic Nursing, 29*(5), 325–330.

Hobbs, T., Wolverton, C., & Clevenger, K. (2007). Lift team technologies elevate positive outcomes. *Nursing Management, 38*(7), 50–52.

Hogan-Quigley, B., Palm, M. L., & Bickley, L. (2012). *Bates' nursing guide to physical examination and history taking.* Philadelphia: Wolters Kluwer Health/Lippincott Williams & Wilkins.

Howard, N. L. (2010). Patient handling: Fact vs. fiction. *American Nurse Today, 5*(7), 32–34.

Huether, S. E., & McCance, K. L. (2012.) *Understanding pathophysiology* (5th ed.). St. Louis: Elsevier.

Hunter, B., Branson, M., & Davenport, D. (2010). Saving costs, saving health care providers' backs, and creating a safe patient environment. *Nursing Economics, 28*(2), 130–134.

Jarvis, C. (2012). *Physical examination & health assessment* (6th ed.). St. Louis: Elsevier/Saunders.

Jensen, S. (2011). *Nursing Health Assessment. A best practice approach.* Philadelphia: Wolters Kluwer Health/Lippincott Williams & Wilkins.

Jitramontree, N. (2010). Exercise promotion: walking in elders. *Journal of Gerontological Nursing, 36*(11), 10–18.

June, K., & Cho, S. (2011). Low back pain and work-related factors among nurses in intensive care units. *Journal of Clinical Nursing, 20*(3/4), 479–487.

Krill, C., Baven, C., & Staffileno, B. A. (2012). Moving from a clinical question to research: The implementation of a safe patient handling program. *MEDSURGNursing, 21*(2), 104–106, 116.

Kyle, T., & Carman, S. (2013). *Essentials of pediatric nursing* (2nd ed.). Philadelphia: Wolters Kluwer Health/Lippincott Williams & Wilkins.

Lee, I. M., Shiroma, E. J., Lobelo, F., Puska, P., Blair, S. N., & Katzmarzyk, P. T. (2012). Effect of physical inactivity on major non-communicable diseases worldwide: an analysis of burden of disease and life expectancy. *Lancet, 380*(9838), 219–229.

Lee, S., & Im, E. (2010). Ethnic differences in exercise and leisure time physical activity among midlife women. *Journal of Advanced Nursing, 66*(4), 814–827.

Marcus, B., Williams, D., Dubbert, P., Sallis, J., King, A., Yancey, A., et al. (2006). Physical activity intervention studies: What we know and what we need to know: A scientific statement from the American Heart Association Council on nutrition, physical activity, and metabolism. *Circulation, 114*(24), 2739–2752.

Mayo Clinic. (2011a). Back pain at work: Preventing pain and injury. Available at www.mayoclinic.com/health/back-pain/HQ00955

Mayo Clinic. (2011b). Exercise: 7 benefits of regular physical activity. Available at www.mayoclinic.com/health/exercise/HQ01676

Mayo Clinic. (2011c). Slide show: Tips for choosing and using walkers. Available at www.mayoclinic.com/health/walker/HA00060

Menzel, N. N., & Nelson, A. L. (2010). Strengthening your evidence base: Focus on safe patient handling. *American Nurse Today, 5*(7), 38–40.

Miller, C. (2008). Communication difficulties in hospitalized older adults with dementia: Try these techniques to make communicating with patients easier and more effective. *American Journal of Nursing, 108*(3), 58–66.

Miller, J. A. (2011). Use and wear of anti-embolism stockings: A clinical audit of surgical patients. *International Wound Journal, 8*(1), 74–83.

Mincer, A. (2007). Assistive devices for the adult patient with orthopaedic dysfunction: Why physical therapists choose what they do. *Orthopaedic Nursing, 26*(4), 226–233.

Moorhead, S., Johnson, M., Maas, M. L., & Swanson, E. (Eds). (2013). *Nursing outcomes classification (NOC).* (5th ed.). St. Louis: Elsevier/Mosby.

Murphy Dawson, J., & Harrington, S. (2012). Regulatory readiness: Embracing safe patient handling. *Nursing Management, 43*(10), 15–17.

NANDA International (NANDA-I). (2012). *Nursing diagnoses: Definitions & classification 2012–2014.* West Sussex, UK: Wiley-Blackwell.

National Institutes of Health (NIH), & National Heart, Lung and Blood Institute (NHLBI). (2005). *Aim for a healthy weight.* NIH Publication No. 05-5213. Bethesda, MD: Author.

National Osteoporosis Foundation. (2013). Learn about osteoporosis. Available at http://nof.org/learn/basics

Nelson, A., & Baptiste, A. (2004). Evidence-based practices for safe patient handling and movement. *Online Journal of Issues in Nursing, 9*(3), Manuscript 3.

Nelson, A., Motacki, K., & Menzel, N. (2009). *The illustrated guide to safe patient handling and movement.* New York: Springer Publishing Company.

NIOSH sets 35-lb limit as the max for safe lifts. (2007). *Hospital employee health, 26*(12), 136–137.

Nolen, J., Liu, H., Liu, H., McGee, M., & Grando, V. (2010). Comparison of gait characteristics with a single-tip cane, tripod cane, and quad cane. *Physical & Occupational Therapy in Geriatrics, 28*(4), 387–395.

Occupational Safety & Health Administration (OSHA), U.S. Department of Labor. (2009). Guidelines for Nursing Homes. Ergonomics for the Prevention of Musculoskeletal Disorders. Available at www.osha.gov/ergonomics/guidelines/nursinghome/final_nh_guidelines.pdf

Occupational Safety & Health Administration (OSHA), U.S. Department of Labor. (2012). Safe patient handling. Available at www.osha.gov/SLTC/healthcarefacilities/safepatienthandling.html

Pellatt, G. (2005). Safe handling. The safety and dignity of patients and nurses during patient handling. *British Journal of Nursing, 14*(21), 1150–1156.

Peterson, J. (2007). Get moving! Physical activity counseling in primary care. *Journal of the American Academy of Nurse Practitioners, 19*(7), 349–357.

Perry, S. E., Hockenberry, M. J., Lowdermilk, D. L., & Wilson, D. (2010). *Maternal child nursing care* (4th ed.). Maryland Heights, MO: Elsevier/Mosby.

Ritter, L. A., & Hoffman, N. A. (2010). *Multicultural health.* Boston: Jones and Bartlett.

Spector, R. E. (2009). *Cultural diversity in health and illness* (7th ed.). Upper Saddle River, NJ: Pearson/Prentice Hall.

Tabloski, P. (2010). *Gerontological nursing* (2nd ed.). Upper Saddle River, NJ: Pearson.

Taylor, J. J., & Cohen, B. J. (2013). *Memmler's structure and function of the human body* (10th ed.). Philadelphia: Wolters Kluwer Health/Lippincott Williams & Wilkins.

U.S. Department of Agriculture (USDA). (2012). ChooseMyPlate.gov. Available at http://www.choosemyplate.gov/index.html

U.S. Department of Health and Human Services (DHHS). (2012). *Healthy People 2020.* Physical Activity. Available at http://www.healthypeople.gov/2020/topicsobjectives2020/overview.aspx?topicid=33

U.S. Department of Health and Human Services (DHHS). (2008). Physical activity guidelines for Americans. Available at http://www.health.gov/paguidelines/default.aspx

Varnam, W. (2011). How to mobilize patients with dementia to a standing position. *Nursing Older People, 23*(8), 31–36.

VISN 8 Patient Safety Center. (2009). Safe patient handling and movement. Available at http://www.visn8.va.gov/visn8/patientsafetycenter/safePtHandling/default.asp

Wallace, M., & Shelkey, M. (2008). Monitoring functional status in hospitalized older adults. *American Journal of Nursing, 108*(4), 64–71.

Walker, L., & Lamont, S. (2008). Graduated compression stockings to prevent deep vein thrombosis. *Nursing Standard, 22*(40), 35–38.

Wanless, S., & Wanless, S. (2012). Hoisting a patient: principles and advice for safer practice. *Nursing & Residential Care, 14*(6), 306–310.

Waters, T. R. (2007). When is it safe to manually lift a patient? *American Journal of Nursing, 107*(8), 53–58.

Waters, T. R., Nelson, A., Hughes, N., & Menzel, N. (2009). *Safe patient handling training for schools of nursing. Curricular materials.* Available at http://www.cdc.gov/niosh/docs/2009–127/pdfs/2009–127.pdf

Winslow, E. H., & Brosz, D. L. (2010). Unraveling the mystery of graduated compression stockings. *OR Nurse, 4*(3), 56.

Wright, K. (2005). Mobility and safe handling of people with dementia. *Nursing Times, 101*(17), 38–40.

Zisberg, A., Shadmi, E., Sinoff, G., Gur-Yaish, N., Srulovici, E., & Admi, H. (2011). Low mobility during hospitalization and functional decline in older adults. *Journal of the American Geriatrics Society, 59*(2), 266–273.

33 Rest and Sleep

JEANETTE AND ABBY CLARK

Jeanette accompanies her 15-year-old daughter, Abby, to the clinic. While the daughter is having some routine laboratory testing done in another department, Mrs. Clark says, "She always seems to be tired. When she was small, I could never get her to sleep. Now all she wants to do is sleep. It's all I can do to get her up for school each morning."

CHARLIE BITNER

Charlie is an 86-year-old man who has recently been admitted to a long-term care facility. He tells his daughter that "even though I go to bed around 9 pm, I don't fall asleep until after midnight and then I'm up twice to go to the bathroom and have a lot of trouble falling back to sleep." His daughter has mentioned to the nurse that her father spends a lot of time napping during the day.

THE OMEARA FAMILY

Lydia Omeara asks whether she should let her infant twins sleep in bed with her and her husband. "They have their own beds, of course, but at night, when they get up, they like to be in bed with us. Plus, I still breastfeed my babies, so having them nearby would really make it easier for me."

After completing the chapter, you will be able to accomplish the following:

1. Describe the functions and physiology of sleep.
2. Identify variables that influence rest and sleep.
3. Describe nursing implications that address age-related differences in the sleep cycle.
4. Perform a comprehensive sleep assessment using appropriate interview questions, a sleep diary when indicated, and physical assessment skills.
5. Describe common sleep disorders, noting key assessment criteria.
6. Develop nursing diagnoses that correctly identify sleep problems that may be treated through independent nursing interventions.
7. Describe nursing strategies to promote rest and sleep based on scientific rationale.
8. Plan, implement, and evaluate nursing care related to selected nursing diagnoses involving sleep problems.

KEY TERMS

circadian rhythm	non–rapid eye movement (NREM) sleep	restless leg syndrome (RLS)
delta sleep	parasomnias	sleep
dyssomnias	rapid eye movement (REM) sleep	sleep apnea
enuresis		sleep cycle
hypersomnia		sleep deprivation
insomnia	rest	sleep hygiene
melatonin		somnambulism
narcolepsy		

In this chapter, **rest** connotes a condition in which the body is in a decreased state of activity, with the consequent feeling of being refreshed. Many factors affect a person's ability to rest. Adults juggling the demands of their job and family responsibilities often find little opportunity for rest and relaxation during the course of a day. Children involved in numerous extracurricular activities, as well as trying to excel academically, also do not have the opportunity to rest and relax during the day. Even when rest is possible, one's environment is not always conducive to physical and mental relaxation. Suggestions for preparing a restful environment and promoting relaxation are discussed later in the chapter.

Sleep is a state of rest accompanied by altered consciousness and relative inactivity. It is a complex rhythmic state involving a progression of repeated cycles, each representing different phases of body and brain activity. Although sensitivity to external stimuli is diminished during sleep, this sensitivity can be reversed readily.

Most people can fall asleep easily and remain asleep until the desired waking time. Conversely, others rarely fall asleep without a struggle; then when they do, sleep is fragmented. Insufficient sleep can seriously affect a person's physical and psychological health (see Physical and Psychological Effects of Insufficient Sleep on pages 1124–1125). Consequently, nurses need to be vigilant in detecting and treating sleep disturbances. See the accompanying Reflective Practice display on page 1120.

This chapter provides the nurse with knowledge of the functions and physiology of sleep and factors affecting sleep. Practical suggestions for performing a comprehensive sleep assessment are included. Sample interview questions for a general sleep history are presented, along with information on sleep diaries and pertinent physical assessment data. The importance of analyzing these data is explained, and numerous examples of nursing diagnoses are given. Expected patient outcomes and specific nursing strategies for promoting rest and sleep are described. The concluding nursing plan of care illustrates how the nurse's knowledge of rest and sleep, combined with skilled nursing interventions and caring, can resolve sleep problems.

PHYSIOLOGY OF SLEEP

Two systems in the brainstem, the reticular activating system (RAS) and the bulbar synchronizing region, are believed to work together to control the cyclic nature of sleep. The RAS extends upward through the medulla, the pons, the midbrain, and into the hypothalamus. It facilitates reflex and voluntary movements as well as cortical activities related to a state of alertness. The RAS comprises many nerve cells and fibers. The fibers have connections that relay impulses into the cerebral cortex and spinal cord.

During sleep, the RAS experiences few stimuli from the cerebral cortex and the periphery of the body. Wakefulness occurs when this system is activated with stimuli from the cerebral cortex and from periphery sensory organs and cells (see Fig. 33-1 on page 1122). For example, an alarm clock awakens us from sleep to a state of consciousness, in which we realize that we must prepare for the day. Sensations such as pain, pressure, and noise produce wakefulness by means of peripheral organs and cells.

The hypothalamus has control centers for several involuntary activities of the body, one of which concerns sleeping and waking. Injury to the hypothalamus may cause a person to sleep for abnormally long periods.

Various neurotransmitters are involved with the sleeping process. Norepinephrine and acetylcholine—in addition to dopamine, serotonin, and histamine—are involved with excitation. Gamma-aminobutyric acid (GABA) appears to be necessary for inhibition. However, research has yet to prove exactly how biochemical changes and hormones function in sleep.

REFLECTIVE PRACTICE: CULTIVATING QSEN COMPETENCIES

CHALLENGE TO ETHICAL AND LEGAL SKILLS

I was working in our well-baby clinic today when a mother, Lydia Omeara, asked my advice about letting her infant twins sleep in bed with her and her husband: "They have their own beds, of course, but at night, when they get up, they seem to like to be in bed with us. Plus, I still breastfeed my babies, so having them nearby would really make it easier for me." She mentioned reading an article recently about this, noting that while this custom is usual in other countries, it had been discouraged until recently in the United States.

According to the article, she said that it seems that more and more U.S. parents are doing this now. She asked for my advice, and I had no idea how to respond. Clearly, anything that resulted in better rest for the parents—who are up many times each night if the babies aren't sleeping well—would seem to be a good idea. However, I vaguely remembered learning that small children are at increased risk for sudden infant death syndrome in an adult bed. I needed to find the best way to respond to Mrs. Omeara.

Thinking Outside the Box: Possible Courses of Action

- Make up an answer: "Yes, it's OK" or "No way! What are you, crazy?"
- Refer her to a nurse with more experience.

- Tell her that I honestly don't know the answer but I will find out more about this and then get back to her.

Evaluating a Good Outcome: How Do I Define Success?

- A decision is made about where the children sleep that protects them and promotes rest, health, and well-being for each member of the family.
- I learn more about what science dictates is the best recommendation.

- I am faithful to my professional obligations to be knowledgeable about matters like this.

Personal Learning: Here's to the Future!

Since I don't have children myself and couldn't ever remember spending the night in my parents' bed or having a conversation with them about this, I certainly couldn't draw on personal experience in responding to this mother. In addition, we had never studied anything about this topic. I did remember a recent article in *Newsweek* magazine raising the issue, but I didn't remember this article proposing a scientifically grounded recommendation. As a result, I did some research on this issue and learned that there is a wide range of opinion on this matter. I did my best to

summarize the arguments, pro and con, and then I shared these with Mrs. Omeara so that she and her husband could make an informed decision.

This little experience has taught me a lot about the power of my profession to influence—literally—how people are born, live, and die. I want to have enough knowledge to help people make the best possible life choices, never leading them astray by virtue of my ignorance!

Amy Norris, Georgetown University

REFLECTION ON QUALITY AND SAFETY COMPETENCIES

How do you think you would respond in a similar situation? Why? What does this tell you about yourself and about the adequacy of your skills for professional practice? Do you agree with the criteria that the nursing student used to evaluate a successful outcome? Why or why not? What *knowledge, skills,* and *attitudes* do you need to develop to continuously improve quality and safety when caring for patients like Lydia Omeara?

Patient-Centered Care: What information would be necessary for the nursing student to obtain from the patient to provide an overall picture of the family situation? How can you provide clear, reliable, and unbiased information to Ms. Omeara in a timely manner? What is the best way to communicate emotional support to Ms. Omeara as she struggles with making the right decision for her and her family?

Teamwork and Collaboration/Quality Improvement: What communication skills do you need to continue to

function as a resource and advocate for your patient? Could collaboration with other nurses in the well-baby clinic result in a sleep history tool that you could use to assess Ms. Omeara's sleep needs and pattern?

Safety/Evidence-Based Practice: Can you secure any evidence in nursing literature that provides information related to the risk of sudden infant death syndrome when infants share a bed with their parents? How do you think your response contributed to a safe environment for Ms. Omeara and her twins?

Informatics: What information should be electronically documented regarding your assessment of Ms. Omeara's sleep needs? Can you identify essential information that was provided in order for Ms. Omeara and her husband to make an informed decision?

Circadian Rhythms

Rhythmic biologic clocks are known to exist in plants, animals, and humans. Influenced by both internal and external factors, they regulate certain biologic and behavioral functions in humans. Some cycles are monthly, such as a woman's menstrual cycle. **Circadian rhythms** complete a full cycle every 24 hours. "Circa" in Latin means "approximately" and "diem" is the Latin word for "day"; circadian represents approximately 1 day (Porth, 2011). Fluctuations in a person's heart rate, blood pressure, body temperature, hormone secretions, metabolism, and performance and mood depend in part on circadian rhythms.

Sleep is one of the body's most complex biologic rhythms. Circadian synchronization exists when a person's sleep–wake patterns follow the inner biologic clock located in the hypothalamus. When physiologic and psychological rhythms are high or most active, the person is awake; when these rhythms are low, the person is asleep. Light and dark are powerful regulators of the sleep–wake circadian rhythm; when there is interference with the normal cycle, circadian disruption, or chronodisruption, occurs. For example, nurses who work the night shift may routinely sleep from 2 PM to 8 PM, and peak physiologic activity may occur between 10 PM and 6 AM during work. The exposure to light at night during normal sleeping hours is termed *night shift chronodisruption* (Stokowski, 2012). Problems of desynchronization occur when sleep–wake patterns are frequently altered and the person attempts to sleep during high-activity rhythms or to work when the body is physiologically prepared to rest. A person's individual biologic clock also responds to numerous influences such as occupational demands and social pressures.

THINK back to Charlie Bitner, the older man living in a long-term care facility. The nurse would need to assess Mr. Bitner, gathering data about his circadian rhythm. This knowledge would be important in developing an individualized plan of care for the patient to promote adequate sleep. ●

Stages of Sleep

Research reveals that there are two major stages of sleep: **non–rapid eye movement (NREM) sleep** and **rapid eye movement (REM) sleep**. These stages have been studied and analyzed with the help of the electroencephalograph (EEG), which receives and records electrical currents from the brain; the electrooculogram (EOG), which records eye movements; and the electromyograph (EMG), which records muscle tone. This combination of diagnostic recordings is referred to as a sleep study or polysomnogram. It is a noninvasive, pain-free study usually conducted over one or two nights in a sleep study facility. Once a physician interprets the results, any sleep disorder detected can be treated (National Sleep Foundation [NSF], 2011h).

NREM Sleep

NREM sleep (comprising about 75% of total sleep) consists of four stages. Stages I and II, consuming about 5% and 50% of a person's sleep time, respectively, are light-sleep states. During these stages, the person can be aroused with relative ease. Stages III and IV, each representing about 10% of total sleep time, are deep-sleep states, termed **delta sleep** or slow-wave sleep. The arousal threshold (intensity of stimulus required to awaken) is usually greatest in stage IV NREM. Throughout the stages of NREM sleep, the parasympathetic nervous system dominates, and decreases in pulse, respiratory rate, blood pressure, metabolic rate, and body temperature are observed. Characteristics of the four stages of NREM sleep are summarized in Box 33-1.

REM Sleep

It is more difficult to arouse a person during REM sleep than during NREM sleep. In normal adults, the REM state consumes 20% to 25% of a person's nightly sleep time. People who are awakened during the REM state almost always report that they have been dreaming. They can usually vividly recall their dreams even if they were absurd or have no sensible meaning for them. Everyone dreams.

During REM sleep, the pulse, respiratory rate, blood pressure, metabolic rate, and body temperature increase, whereas general skeletal muscle tone and deep tendon reflexes are depressed. REM sleep is believed to be essential to mental and emotional equilibrium and to play a role in learning, memory, and adaptation.

A person who is deprived of REM sleep for several nights generally will spend more time in REM sleep on successive nights. This phenomenon, termed REM rebound, allows the total amount of REM sleep to remain fairly constant over time. See Box 33-1 for characteristics of REM sleep.

Sleep Cycle

Normally during a **sleep cycle**, a person passes consecutively through the four stages of NREM sleep. This pattern is then reversed, and the person returns from stage IV to stage III to stage II. Instead of reentering stage I and awakening, the person enters into the REM stage of sleep, after which the person reenters NREM sleep at stage II and returns to stages III and IV. A person awakened from sleep at any time will return to sleep by starting at stage I of NREM sleep.

CONSIDER Charlie Bitner, the long-term care resident described at the beginning of the chapter. When evaluating Mr. Bitner's sleep cycle, the nurse would need to keep in mind that each time Mr. Bitner awakes, his sleep cycle is starting all over again. Subsequently, he is experiencing light sleep, characteristic of sleep stages I and II. ●

Most people go through four or five cycles of sleep each night. On average, each cycle lasts about 90 to 100 minutes. The term *sleep architecture* is used to describe this alternating

Box 33-1 CHARACTERISTICS OF NREM AND REM SLEEP

NREM Sleep

Stage I
- The person is in a transitional stage between wakefulness and sleep.
- The person is in a relaxed state but still somewhat aware of the surroundings.
- Involuntary muscle jerking may occur and waken the person.
- The stage normally lasts only minutes.
- The person can be aroused easily.
- This stage constitutes only about 5% of total sleep.

Stage II
- The person falls into a stage of sleep.
- The person can be aroused with relative ease.
- This stage constitutes 50% to 55% of sleep.

Stage III
- The depth of sleep increases, and arousal becomes increasingly difficult.
- This stage composes about 10% of sleep.

Stage IV
- The person reaches the greatest depth of sleep, which is called *delta sleep*.

- Arousal from sleep is difficult.
- Physiologic changes in the body include the following:
  - Slow brain waves are recorded on an EEG.
  - Pulse and respiratory rates decrease.
  - Blood pressure decreases.
  - Muscles are relaxed.
  - Metabolism slows and the body temperature is low.
  - This constitutes about 10% of sleep.

REM Sleep
- Eyes dart back and forth quickly.
- Small muscle twitching, such as on the face
- Large muscle immobility, resembling paralysis
- Respirations irregular; sometimes interspersed with apnea
- Rapid or irregular pulse
- Blood pressure increases or fluctuates
- Increase in gastric secretions
- Metabolism increases; body temperature increases
- Encephalogram tracings active
- REM sleep enters from stage II of NREM sleep and reenters NREM sleep at stage II: arousal from sleep difficult
- Constitutes about 20% to 25% of sleep

between REM and NREM sleep during these cycles (Yoder, Staisiunas, Meltzer, Knutson, & Arora, 2012). The cycles tend to become longer as morning approaches. Ordinarily, more deep sleep occurs in the delta stage (NREM stages III and IV) in the first half of the night, especially if one is tired or has lost sleep.

Figure 33-1 illustrates the normal sleep pattern of young adults. Variations in the sleep cycle occur according to age, as Figure 33-2 illustrates.

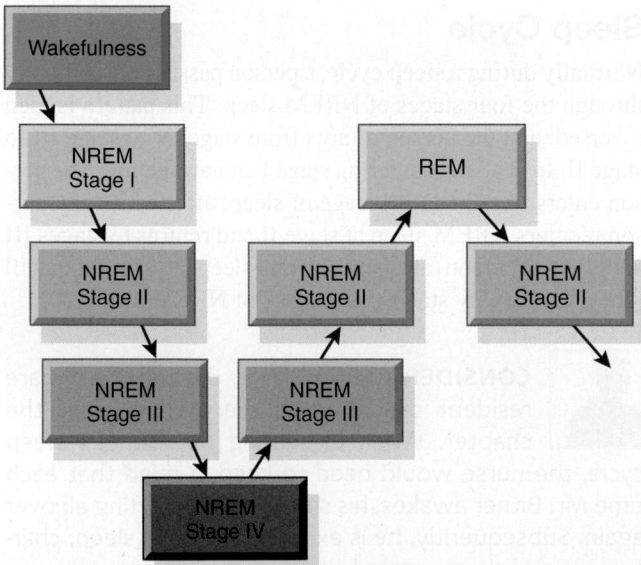

FIGURE 33-1. A single normal sleep cycle. In the normal nocturnal pattern, the shaded cycle is repeated four or five times. Periods of REM sleep generally increase in duration; periods of deep sleep (stage IV) progressively decrease as morning approaches.

Sleep Requirements and Patterns

For no known reason, an average of 8 hours of sleep per night has been the accepted standard for adults, despite

FIGURE 33-2. A comparison of developmental differences in NREM and REM cycles during nocturnal sleep for children, young adults, and older people.

BOX 33-2 DEVELOPMENTAL PATTERNS OF SLEEP

Newborns and Infants

Sleep Pattern

- *Newborn:* Sleeps an average of 16 hours/24 hours; averages about 4 hours at a time.
- Each infant's sleep pattern is unique. On average, infants sleep 10 to 12 hours at night, with several naps during the day.
- Usually by 8 to 16 weeks of age, an infant sleeps through the night.
- REM sleep constitutes much of the sleep cycle of a young infant.

Nursing Implications

- Teach parents to position infant on the back. This is the only safe sleeping position for infants less than 1 year old. Sleeping in the prone position increases the risk for sudden infant death syndrome (SIDS).
- Advise parents that eye movements, groaning, grimacing, and moving are normal activities at this age.
- Encourage parents to have infant sleep in a separate area rather than their bed.
- Caution parents about placing pillows, crib bumpers, quilts, stuffed animals, and so on in the crib because this may pose a suffocation risk.

Toddlers

Sleep Pattern

- Need for sleep declines as this stage progresses. May initially sleep 12 hours at night with two naps during the day and end this stage sleeping 8 to 10 hours a night and napping once during the day.
- Toddlers may begin to resist naps and going to bed at night.
- They may move from crib to youth bed or regular bed at around 2 years.

Nursing Implications

- Establish a regular bedtime routine (e.g., reading a story, singing a lullaby, saying prayers).
- Advise parents of the value of a routine sleeping pattern with minimal variation.
- Encourage attention to safety once child moves from crib to bed. If child attempts to wander out of room, a folding gate may be necessary across the door of the room.

Preschoolers

Sleep Pattern

- Children in this stage generally sleep 9 to 16 hours at night, with 12 hours being the average.
- The REM sleep pattern is similar to that of an adult.
- Daytime napping decreases during this period, and by the age of 5 years, most children no longer nap.
- This age group may continue to resist going to bed at night.

Nursing Implications

- Encourage parents to continue bedtime routines.
- Advise parents that waking from nightmares or night terrors (awakening screaming about 20 minutes after falling asleep) are common during this stage. Waking the child and comforting the child generally helps. Sometimes use of a night light is soothing.

School-Aged Children

Sleep Pattern

- Younger school-aged children may require 10 to 12 hours nightly, whereas older children in this stage may average 8 to 10 hours.
- Sleep needs usually increase when physical growth peaks.

Nursing Implications

- Discuss the fact that the stress of beginning school may interrupt normal sleep patterns.
- Advise that a relaxed bedtime routine is most helpful at this stage.
- Inform parents about child's awareness of the concept of death possibly occurring at this stage. Encourage parental presence and support to help alleviate some of the child's concerns.

Adolescents

Sleep Pattern

- Sleep needs of teenagers vary widely, but the average requirement is 9 to 10 hours. The growth spurt that normally occurs at this stage may necessitate the need for more sleep; however, the stresses of school, activities, and part-time employment may cause adolescents to have a restless sleep. Adolescents tend to go to bed later than younger children and adults, but early morning start times for high school frequently require an early awakening time. This can result in an average of only 7 to 7.5 hours of sleep a night.
- Many adolescents do not get enough sleep.

Nursing Implications

- Advise parents that their adolescents' complaints of fatigue or inability to do well in school may be related to not enough sleep. *Excessive daytime sleepiness (EDS)* may also make the teenager more vulnerable to accidents and behavioral problems.

Young Adults

Sleep Pattern

- The average amount of sleep required is 8 hours, but in fact, many young adults require less sleep.
- Sleep is affected by many factors: physical health, type of occupation, exercise. Lifestyle demands may interfere with sleep patterns.
- REM sleep averages about 20% of sleep.

Nursing Implications

- Reinforce that developing good sleep habits has a positive effect on health, particularly as a person ages.
- If loss of sleep is a problem, explore lifestyle demands and stress as possible causes.
- Suggest use of relaxation techniques and stress-reduction exercises rather than resorting to medication to induce sleep. Sleep medications decrease REM sleep, may be habit forming, and frequently lose their effectiveness over time.

Middle-Aged Adults

Sleep Pattern

- Total sleep time decreases during these years, with a decrease in stage IV sleep.

(continued)

BOX 33-2 DEVELOPMENTAL PATTERNS OF SLEEP *continued*

- The percentage of time spent awake in bed begins to increase.
- People become more aware of sleep disturbances during this period.

Nursing Implications

- Encourage adults to investigate consistent sleep difficulties to exclude pathology or anxiety and depression as causes.
- Encourage adults to avoid use of sleep-inducing medication on a regular basis.

Older Adults

Sleep Pattern

- An average of 7 to 9 hours of sleep is usually adequate for this age group.
- Sleep is less sound, and stage IV sleep is absent or considerably decreased. Periods of REM sleep shorten.

- Elderly people frequently have great difficulty falling asleep and have more complaints of problems sleeping.
- Decline in physical health, psychological factors, effects of drug therapy (e.g., nocturia), or environmental factors may be implicated as causes of inability to sleep.

Nursing Implications

- A comprehensive nursing assessment and individualized interventions may be effective in the long-term care of this age group.
- Emphasize concern for a safe environment because it is not uncommon for older people to be temporarily confused and disoriented when they first awake.
- Use sedatives with extreme caution because of declining physiologic function and concerns about polypharmacy.
- Encourage people to discuss sleep concerns with their physicians.

obvious variations seen in the general population (see Box 33-2). No rigid formula exists for the regular intervals and duration of sleep. It is important, however, that each person follow a pattern of rest that maintains one's own well-being.

Despite individual variations, some generalities can be stated. On average, infants require 14 to 20 hours each day. Growing children, including adolescents, require from 10 to 14 hours of sleep.

 RECALL Jeanette Clark, the mother of an adolescent girl who seems to want to sleep all the time. When discussing this issue with Mrs. Clark, the nurse would need to integrate information about the adolescent's developmental stage—that is, that adolescence is a period of tremendous growth, which requires an increased amount of sleep. •

The recommended amount of sleep for adults is 7 to 9 hours. Those who are able to relax and rest easily, even while awake, often find that less sleep is needed, whereas others may find that more sleep is required to overcome fatigue. Fatigue can be considered a normal, protective body mechanism and nature's warning that sleep is necessary. Chronic fatigue, however, is abnormal and is often a symptom of illness.

Sleep patterns of older adults vary, but the optimal recommendation for this age group is also 7 to 9 hours. They may sleep less, however, because of insomnia and medical conditions that interrupt their sleep. In addition, the quality of their sleep changes.

Patterns of sleep periodicity appear to be learned. For example, most people learn to sleep at night and to be awake and work during the day. However, many night workers learn to sleep equally well during the day.

Physical and Psychological Effects of Insufficient Sleep

Many people have sleep disturbances that go undetected for years, progressively undermining their energy and destroy-

ing their sense of self. Hedges and Ruggiero (2012) summarized the physical, emotional, and cognitive consequences of insomnia and predict that by the middle of the 21st century approximately 100 million Americans will suffer from this disorder.

The term *short sleeper* refers to someone who sleeps less than 6 hours a night. Over the past 30 years, there has been a significant increase in short sleepers in the United States. Some 25% of adults in the United States report that they get insufficient sleep approximately 15 days of each month (*Healthy People 2020,* 2012). Insufficient sleep in children may affect normal growth and development and could be a contributing factor in performance deficits and behavioral problems. Furthermore, short sleep duration in childhood is associated with an increased risk of obesity during childhood or later in life (Hart, 2012). The NSF (2011b) has also identified a possible link between insufficient sleep and obesity in adults and children. Various studies confirm that adults and children who slept less than the recommended hours per night were more likely to be overweight. This sleep–weight link is possibly related to two hormones: leptin and ghrelin. Leptin signals the brain to stop eating, whereas ghrelin promotes continued eating. Research suggests that sleep deprivation lowers leptin levels and elevates ghrelin levels, thus increasing one's appetite. To compound the problem, the brain may interpret a drop in leptin as a sign of starvation. Unfortunately, the brain then signals the body to eat more while it simultaneously lowers the body's metabolic rate. When this happens, people are more likely to gain weight, even if food intake is decreased (Schardt, 2012).

People who suffer sleep difficulties caused by working night shifts or constantly changing work shifts may experience adverse effects, including anxiety, personal conflicts, loneliness, depression, gastrointestinal symptoms, an increased risk for breast and colorectal cancer, increase in type 2 diabetes, hypertension, higher rates of cardiovascular disease including strokes, and substance abuse (Stokowski,

2012; Fuller & Bain, 2010). Data indicate that breast cancer occurs 30% more frequently in women who work nights compared to those who have never worked the night shift (NSF, 2012). According to multiple studies, the performance of a person awake for 17 hours or more resembles that of someone intoxicated with alcohol (Caruso, 2012a).

Sleep loss that results in fatigue and decreased competence increases the risk of a sleep-related motor vehicle accident. The National Sleep Foundation (2011c) reports that 60% of Americans admitted driving while feeling drowsy during the past year and 37% state that they actually fell asleep while driving. A large study of critical care nurses reported that 43% of the nurses stated that they fell asleep while stopped at a traffic light and 20% had a traffic accident or a near miss directly associated with their fatigue (Johnson, 2011).

In addition, studies of physicians' and nurses' work habits have concluded that shiftwork sleep disorders (SWSD) from extended work schedules are a causative factor in a substantial number of adverse medical events and errors. Fatigue and sleepiness can compromise patient safety and increase the risk for adverse events such as medication errors. Sleep deprivation and the resulting consequences of decreased alertness and ability to perform tasks competently are well documented. *Healthy People 2020* recognizes that improved attention to sleep health promotes a safer environment for health care workers and their patients. In their 2010 report, they include a focus on increasing the number of people who get 7 or more hours of sleep daily, expanding the number of people with sleep apnea who get treatment, and decreasing the rate of motor vehicle accidents related to drowsy driving (Caruso, 2012b). The Joint Commission (TJC) issued a Sentinel Alert in 2011 acknowledging the impact of fatigue on health care workers and listed suggestions for health care agencies to reduce fatigue-related risks. These include (TJC, 2011):

- Assess work schedules and staffing to address extended work shifts and hours.
- Review hand-off processes and procedures to ensure safe transfer of information.
- Request staff input in designing work schedules to minimize staff fatigue.
- Develop and implement a fatigue management plan.
- Educate staff about sleep hygiene and the effects of fatigue on patient safety.
- Address staff concerns about fatigue.
- Encourage teamwork to support staff who work extended shifts.
- Keep the effects of fatigue in mind when reviewing adverse events.

FACTORS AFFECTING SLEEP

A variety of factors influence both the quality and quantity of sleep.

Developmental Considerations

Variations in sleep patterns are related to age. Box 33-2 on pages 1123–1124 highlights these variations and associated nursing implications. Routine assessment of sleepiness or short sleep patterns in children is a first step in identifying the existence of a sleep problem and factors interfering with a child's sleep. Parents report that physicians do not routinely query them during childhood health examinations about their child's sleep patterns and habits. However, with a growing body of evidence linking inadequate sleep with obesity in children, more health care practitioners are concerned about patterns of sleep in children and are reviewing them with parents.

A majority of people ages 65 and older report difficulty falling asleep, early awakening or waking frequently during the night, napping, or not feeling rested after a night's sleep (Hedges & Ruggiero, 2012). Older people often need more time to fall asleep and are less able to cope with changes in their usual sleep patterns compared to younger people. Many older people nap during the day, which often results in sleeping fewer hours at night. Chronic illnesses in older adults may also affect their sleep patterns. For instance, many older men have enlargement of the prostate gland, which may cause them to awaken throughout the night to use the bathroom.

Motivation

A desire to be wakeful and alert helps overcome sleepiness and sleep. For example, a tired person may be wakeful and alert when at a party or when attending an interesting play or concert. The opposite is also true: When there is minimal motivation to be awake, sleep generally follows. For example, a student who is bored and disinterested in a lecture or class may doze during the lecture.

Culture

A person's cultural beliefs and practices can influence rest and sleep. Although developmental stages are similar, children's bedtime rituals, sleeping position and place, and pattern of sleep may vary based on culture. Methods to enhance or foster sleep may also be culturally influenced. For example, an older Asian patient may choose herbal tea rather than a sleeping medication to promote relaxation and sleep. A cultural orientation toward privacy and quiet makes sleep difficult in a busy special care unit where male and female patients sleep in close proximity. Sensitivity to a patient's culture must be included in the plan of care for preparing the patient for an evening's sleep.

 THINK back to Mrs. Omeara, the mother of infant twins. She is wondering whether she should let her twins sleep in her and her husband's bed. The nurse would need to investigate the family's cultural background to determine any influences it may have on the patient's question. The nurse would then use this information to develop an individualized, culturally appropriate plan of care for dealing with this question. ●

Lifestyle and Habits

Various lifestyle factors can affect a person's ability to sleep well. People working a shift other than the day shift must reorganize their priorities, or sleep difficulties may occur. Based on the circadian cycle, the body prepares for sleep at night by decreasing the body temperature and releasing **melatonin** (a natural chemical produced at night that decreases wakefulness and promotes sleep). Working the night shift disrupts this natural process and can result in loss of sleep and other adverse effects (see Physical and Psychological Effects of Insufficient Sleep on pages 1124–1125), The following website offers tips to help a person on night shift adjust to a reversal of circadian rhythms: www.cdc.gov/niosh/topics/workschedules.

Developing a sleep pattern is especially difficult if the shift changes periodically. Nurses who work long hours and varying shifts have difficulty finding time to exercise, which can promote weight gain. Longer work hours have also been identified as a factor in an increase in the number of errors while at work (Fuller & Bain, 2010).

The duration and quality of sleep can be affected by watching some types of television shows, participating in stimulating outside activities, and taking part in activity or exercise within 3 hours of the person's normal bedtime. One's abilities to relax from work-related pressures and to put aside home stresses are also important factors in the ability to fall asleep. Nurses who role model good health behaviors are more effective teachers. Use the Promoting Health 33-1: Rest and Sleep display for yourself before using it with others.

Physical Activity and Exercise

Activity and exercise increase fatigue and, in many instances, promote relaxation that is followed by sleep. It appears that physical activity increases both REM and NREM sleep.

Moderate exercise is a healthy way to promote sleep, but exercise that occurs within a 3-hour interval before normal bedtime can hinder sleep. The fatigue that results from nor-mal work activities or exercise is believed to contribute to a restful sleep, whereas excessive exercise or exhaustion can decrease the quality of sleep.

 REMEMBER Jeanette Clark, the mother of the adolescent girl who seems to be sleeping all the time. As part of the health promotion teaching plan, the nurse would need to explain to Mrs. Clark about the significant changes occurring during adolescence. In addition to this stage being a period of rapid growth, it is also a time of increased activity—physically, emotionally, and socially. All of these may be affecting her daughter's sleep patterns. ●

Dietary Habits

It has long been believed that the dietary amino acid L-tryptophan acts to promote sleep. A small protein-containing snack before bedtime used to be recommended for patients with insomnia. However, as nutritionists have studied the effects of various foods on mood, new information has emerged. Carbohydrates make tryptophan more available to the brain. This explains why meals heavy in carbohydrate content tend to cause drowsiness. Therefore, a small protein- and carbohydrate-containing snack such as peanut butter on toast or cheese and crackers may be more effective (NSF, 2011e).

ALCOHOL INTAKE

Alcoholic beverages, when used in moderation, appear to induce sleep in some people. However, large quantities have been found to limit REM and delta sleep. Initially, alcohol consumption may help to induce sleep but once the alcohol is cleared from the body, sleep is fragmented and disrupted often. Women and older adults are more vulnerable to the effects of alcohol. Most recommendations to promote effective sleep recommend that alcohol and products containing

---

PROMOTING HEALTH 33-1

REST AND SLEEP

Use the assessment checklist to determine how well you are meeting needs for rest and sleep. Then develop a prescription for self-care by choosing appropriate behaviors from the list of suggestions.

Assessment Checklist

❑ almost always	❑ sometimes	❑ almost never

❑ ❑ ❑ 1. I feel rested and refreshed when I get up in the morning.

❑ ❑ ❑ 2. I have energy to carry out normal activities of daily living.

❑ ❑ ❑ 3. I understand the normal changes in sleep and rest requirements and patterns that occur with aging.

❑ ❑ ❑ 4. I set aside time for quiet recreation and restful activities each day.

Self-Care Behaviors

1. Follow a regular routine for bedtime and morning awakening.
2. Accept individual differences in need for sleep.
3. Use relaxation exercises to relax before bedtime, especially if feeling stressed.
4. Avoid caffeine, smoking, and alcohol before bedtime.
5. Adjust bedcoverings, room temperature, and lighting to your preferences.
6. Eat a small carbohydrate snack before going to bed.
7. Be aware of the potential dangers of sleeping pills.
8. Use some part of each day for quiet, enjoyable activities such as crafts, hobbies, reading, watching television, listening to music, and visiting with friends.
9. Incorporate three or four periods of regular exercise into each week.

alcohol should not be used within 6 hours of sleep (Schardt, 2012).

CAFFEINE-CONTAINING BEVERAGES

Caffeine is a central nervous system stimulant. For many people, beverages containing caffeine interfere with the ability to fall asleep. Caffeine is thought to interfere with the action of adenosine, which is a compound found in every cell in the body. It binds to adenosine receptors in the brain, thus preventing the adenosine from entering nerve cells and causing drowsiness. Many people avoid caffeine in the evening so as not to disrupt sleep but caffeine consumed earlier in the day can also lengthen the time needed to fall asleep (Schardt, 2012). Examples of beverages containing caffeine include coffee, tea, and most cola drinks. Chocolate also contains caffeine.

SMOKING

Nicotine has a stimulating effect; smokers usually have a more difficult time falling asleep. They are more easily aroused once asleep and may describe themselves as light sleepers. Eliminating cigarette smoking after the evening meal appears to improve the smoker's ability to fall asleep. People usually report improved sleep patterns after discontinuing nicotine use.

Total withdrawal from smoking may be associated with temporary sleep disturbances. Patients who stop smoking often have more daytime sleepiness and report significantly more restlessness at night. Whether this is a short-term effect or is related to nicotine's effect on the central nervous system is uncertain.

Environmental Factors

Most people sleep best in their usual home environments. Sleeping in a strange or new environment tends to influence both REM and NREM sleep. People accustomed to sleeping in a noisy environment, such as a busy large city, actually have a hard time falling asleep in an area that is extremely quiet. By turning on a radio or other noise, the person may actually be able to rest in the new environment. Likewise, if a patient is accustomed to sleeping in a quiet environment, a room next to a high-traffic area, such as the nurse's desk, may not be the best place for this patient to rest.

Psychological Stress

Psychological stress, such as from illness and various life situations, tends to disturb sleep. Generally, psychological stress affects sleep in two ways: (1) the person experiencing stress may find it difficult to obtain the amount of sleep needed; and (2) REM sleep decreases in amount, which tends to add to anxiety and stress.

 CONSIDER Mrs. Omeara, the mother described in the beginning of the chapter and in the Reflective Practice display. The nurse would need to gather additional information about Mrs. Omeara's current situation to determine if any stressors might be affecting her ability to obtain adequate rest and sleep. Areas to address may include her typical daily activities, amount of time spent caring for each child, employment, and amount of assistance and support from others. In addition, the nurse would need to investigate the reasons underlying Mrs. Omeara's question about the babies sleeping in the parents' bed. ●

Illness

Illness, a physiologic as well as a psychological stressor, influences sleep. Certain illnesses are more closely related to sleep disturbances than others. For example:

- Gastric secretions increase during REM sleep. Many people with gastroesophageal reflux (GERD) awaken at night with heartburn or pain. They find that using antacids to neutralize stomach acidity often relieves discomfort and promotes sleep.
- The pain associated with coronary artery disease and myocardial infarction is more likely with REM sleep.
- Epilepsy seizures are most likely to occur during NREM sleep and appear to be depressed by REM sleep.
- Liver failure and encephalitis tend to cause a reversal in day–night sleeping habits.
- Hypothyroidism tends to decrease the amount of NREM sleep, especially stages II and IV, while hyperthyroidism may result in difficulty falling asleep.
- End-stage renal disease (ESRD) disrupts nocturnal sleep and leads to excessive daytime sleepiness. Patients with ESRD who receive dialysis also have a higher incidence of restless leg syndrome (discussed later in the chapter), which possibly is related to the iron deficiency common in ESRD.

Medications

Health care practitioners must also take into account the effect that drugs used to treat medical or psychological disorders have on sleep. Drugs that decrease REM sleep include barbiturates, amphetamines, and antidepressants. Diuretics, antiparkinsonian drugs, some antidepressants and antihypertensives, steroids, decongestants, caffeine, and asthma medications are seen as additional common causes of sleep problems.

Chronotherapeutics is a growing field of study that involves the strategic use of time in the administration of medicine. Researchers have determined that certain treatments for disease are more effective when circadian rhythms are taken into account. For example, a larger midafternoon dose of asthma medication may be more effective in preventing attacks that commonly occur at night during sleep. The timing of antihypertensive medication administration may need to be adjusted to provide peak protection during early-morning hours, when heart attacks are more common. Cancer chemotherapy appears to be less toxic when administered at certain times of the day. Paying attention to biologic rhythms may influence drug tolerance and medication effectiveness.

COMMON SLEEP DISORDERS

A nurse who interviews a patient to obtain a sleep history needs to understand common sleep disturbances to recognize significant data. The most recent classification of sleep disorders categorized by the International Classification of Sleep Disorders includes four major categories of disturbances:

- Dyssomnias
- Parasomnias
- Sleep disorders associated with medical or psychiatric disorders
- Other proposed disorders

The more common sleep disorders are the dyssomnias and parasomnias. **Dyssomnias** are sleep disorders characterized by insomnia or excessive sleepiness. **Parasomnias** are patterns of waking behavior that appear during sleep. A brief description of these disturbances follows, with the major focus on specific symptoms associated with the sleep disorder.

Dyssomnias

Insomnia

Insomnia is characterized by difficulty falling asleep, intermittent sleep, or early awakening from sleep. It is the most common of all sleep disorders. People older than 60 years of age, women (especially after menopause), and people with a history of depression are more likely to experience insomnia. Many cases of insomnia are related to disruptions in circadian rhythms. This sleep disorder can also occur during periods of stress, in situations involving some change in the normal environment such as shift work, after traveling across time zones (jet lag), and as a result of the side effects of medications. Common medications that may result in insomnia include those taken for hypertension and cardiovascular disease, cold and allergies, thyroid disease, asthma, and depression (NSF, 2011a).

Usually, people reporting insomnia have been observed to fall asleep more quickly and sleep more than they report they do. However, the condition can lead to such distress that further wakefulness results. A person with insomnia often reports feeling tired, lethargic, and irritable during the day. Difficulty concentrating is also a common manifestation. Older adults who experience insomnia while in an acute care setting may manifest delirium as a symptom of sleep deprivation. It is a challenge for health care providers to understand the effects of age-related changes on sleep and be alert for the potential complications associated with insomnia in this growing population.

Treatment of transient insomnia is usually unnecessary because most episodes last for only a short period. Insomnia that lasts less than 4 weeks is termed short-term while chronic insomnia persists for more than 1 month and even years. Chronic insomnia is frequently listed as the motivating factor for a visit to a sleep disorder clinic.

According to the NSF (2011a), 10% to 15% of the U.S. population suffer from chronic insomnia and up to 40% of adults admit they have experienced some symptoms of insomnia during the past year. A growing number of health conditions have been associated with chronic insomnia. They include obesity; type 2 diabetes; psychiatric disorders,

such as depression; and cardiovascular disorders such as heart failure, stroke, hypertension, and myocardial infarction (heart attack). The misuse of alcohol or caffeine can have an adverse effect on sleep; stopping these behaviors may reduce or eliminate the insomnia.

Nonpharmacologic approaches should be attempted initially to resolve the insomnia. Cognitive behavioral therapy (CBT) is a safe, effective means of managing chronic insomnia and may include progressive muscle relaxation measures, stimulus control, and sleep restriction therapy (Hedges & Ruggiero, 2012). CBT involves meeting with a therapist and working through maladaptive sleep beliefs. It may also include biofeedback, additional relaxation techniques, and sleep hygiene measures (see Teaching About Rest and Sleep). When used in conjunction with these other complementary therapies, CBT is very successful. Research involving behavioral therapy for older adults with insomnia has provided positive results for a larger percentage of the participants in the study. Interventions included education about the mechanism of sleep as well as instructions to get up at the same time every day, retire at night only when sleepy, eliminate any napping during the day, and remain in bed only when sleeping. Two meetings with each participant accompanied by two phone calls appeared to provide improved sleep and meaningful improvement in insomnia for this population (Buysse et al., 2011).

If, however, these measures prove ineffective, pharmacologic treatment may be necessary. Pharmacologic options include the use of sedatives and hypnotics. However, only short-term use, at the lowest dose, is recommended (see Using Medications to Produce Sleep). Over-the-counter preparations such as melatonin and valerian have not proved to be particularly effective remedies for insomnia. Melatonin is a hormone that is produced in the brain and released prior to the onset of sleep. Researchers have concluded that it is not effective in treating most sleep disorders. The results have been similar for research involving the effects of valerian on sleep (Schardt, 2012; Hedges & Ruggiero, 2012).

Hypersomnia

Hypersomnia is a condition characterized by excessive sleep, particularly during the day. This disorder is also referred to as idiopathic hypersomnia and is a debilitating condition. A person may fall asleep for intervals during work, while eating, or even during conversations. These naps do not usually relieve their symptoms. When they awake, they are often disoriented, irritated, restless, and have slower speech and thinking processes.

Causes of hypersomnia are unknown but may include:

- Another sleep disorder, such as sleep apnea
- Drug or alcohol abuse
- Head trauma or other injury to the central nervous system
- Effect of certain medications
- Depression
- Obesity
- Other medical conditions (multiple sclerosis, epilepsy)

Some people may have a genetic predisposition to hypersomnia. It appears most often in adolescents and young adults. Although not usually life threatening, hypersomnia can have some serious consequences, such as motor vehicle accidents that occur because of drowsiness or falling asleep while driving. These attacks may occur indefinitely (NSF, 2011d).

Treatment of hypersomnia is symptomatic in nature. Stimulant drugs may prove effective, or in some cases, antidepressants may be prescribed. Attention to diet (avoidance of alcohol and caffeine) and behavioral changes (avoidance of night work and social activities later in the evening) may offer some relief from such episodes.

Narcolepsy

Narcolepsy is a condition characterized by an uncontrollable desire to sleep. A person with narcolepsy can literally fall asleep standing up, while driving a car, in the middle of a conversation, or while swimming. People with narcolepsy tend to fall asleep quickly, find it difficult to wake up, sleep fewer hours than others, and sleep restlessly. Narcolepsy is considered a neurologic disorder. The condition usually begins in susceptible people during adolescence or early adulthood and continues through life. Epidemiologic data indicate that approximately 550 per 1,000,000 people are narcoleptics (NSF, 2011f).

Sleepiness during the day is often the first symptom of narcolepsy, which usually occurs several years before experiencing any difficulty with nighttime sleep. Common features of narcolepsy include the following:

- Sleep attacks: irresistible urge to sleep, regardless of the type of activity in which the patient is engaged
- Cataplexy: sudden loss of motor tone that may cause the person to fall asleep; usually experienced during a period of strong emotion
- Hypnagogic hallucinations: nightmares or vivid hallucinations
- Sleep-onset REM periods: during a sleep attack, the person moves directly into REM sleep
- Sleep paralysis: skeletal paralysis that occurs during the transition from wakefulness to sleep

Because narcolepsy is a rare disorder, diagnosis is lengthy and difficult. Most people with narcolepsy have low hypocretin levels. This is a chemical in the brain that causes alertness and wakefulness. It is unknown at this time what causes this low hypocretin level (National Heart Lung & Blood Institute [NHLBI], 2010). Undiagnosed, a person with narcolepsy is potentially dangerous to self and others. In some countries, a person with a diagnosis of narcolepsy is not permitted to drive a motor vehicle. A sleep study is important to confirm the diagnosis of narcolepsy. At present, there is no cure. However, medications that restore alertness allow near-normal functioning for most patients.

A central nervous system stimulant (e.g., methylphenidate [Ritalin]) that causes wakefulness may be used to control narcolepsy. Additional medications such as modafinil (Provigil), a wakefulness-promoting compound, and sodium oxybate (Xyrem), a sedative used for treating disturbed nocturnal sleep, have proved effective in treating narcoleptic symptoms (Lehne, 2013). People using such drugs should take them faithfully because with discontinuation of use, the uncontrollable desire to sleep returns. In addition to medications, behavioral therapies may help to control the symptoms of narcolepsy. Avoidance of heavy meals and alcohol may also prove helpful (NSF, 2011f).

Sleep Apnea

Sleep apnea, generally referred to as sleep-disordered breathing (SDB), is a condition in which a person experiences the absence of breathing (apnea) or diminished breathing efforts (hypopnea) during sleep between snoring intervals. Breathing may cease for 10 to 20 seconds, possibly as long as 2 minutes. During long periods of apnea, the oxygen level in the blood drops, the pulse usually becomes irregular, and the blood pressure often increases. This decrease in ventilation and associated physiologic response activates the fight or flight response of the sympathetic nervous system and the sleeper startles and awakens (Simmons & Pruitt, 2012). Many people experience sleep apnea without symptoms, but excessive daytime sleepiness is commonly reported. Although it occurs most commonly in middle-aged men who are obese and have short, thick necks, women and people of other ages may also experience it.

Obstructive sleep apnea (OSA) can result when the airway is occluded because of the collapse of the hypopharynx (Fig. 33-3) or from other structural abnormalities such as enlarged tonsils and adenoids, a deviated nasal septum,

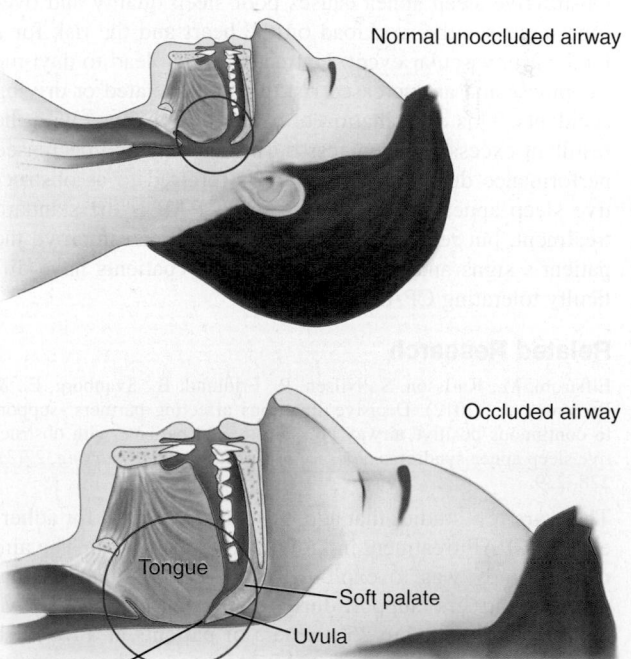

FIGURE 33-3. Obstructive sleep apnea occurs when the airway is occluded due to collapse of the hypopharynx. Normally, the airway remains open during sleep (see inset).

and thyroid enlargement. Narrowing of nasal passageways caused by allergic rhinitis or nasal polyps is another factor contributing to OSA. Sleep apnea affects more than 18 million American adults, but most are never diagnosed and treated. Approximately 3% of children may also have OSA (Simmons & Pruitt, 2012).

Some investigators have theorized that sleep apnea may explain certain cases of death that occur during sleep. People with severe, untreated OSA are 2.5% more likely to suffer a fatal cardiovascular event (Simmons & Pruitt, 2012). In healthy people, OSA may impair cardiac function over time and lead to the development of heart failure. If heart failure has already been diagnosed, OSA may result in progression of this condition. Sleep apnea and heart failure are a dangerous combination, making it even more important to recognize and treat OSA.

Clinical information and polysomnography can confirm the diagnosis of sleep apnea. This overnight sleep study also includes a video recording of sleep awakenings and movements. Cardiopulmonary monitoring of the arterial oxygen saturation and an electrocardiogram (ECG) to detect any cardiac arrhythmias can also assist in the diagnosis of obstructive sleep apnea. Based on the sleep study findings, including the number of apneic episodes per hour, OSA is classified as mild, moderate, or severe.

People with obstructive sleep apnea may become irritable during the day, fall asleep during monotonous activities, have difficulty concentrating, and exhibit slower reaction times. They are also more likely to be involved in motor vehicle accidents. Alcohol, tobacco, and sleeping pills increase the breathing disruption that occurs in sleep apnea, thus should be avoided.

The definitive treatment of moderate or severe obstructive sleep apnea involves use of a continuous positive airway pressure machine (CPAP). CPAP is noninvasive and consists of a mask connected to an air pump that is worn during sleep. This device delivers positive air pressure that holds the airway open. It can significantly improve the manifestations of OSA but adherence and continued use of the CPAP device is inconsistent. Many patients discontinue use of CPAP because of a sensation of claustrophobia, discomfort exhaling against air inflow, or dryness and skin irritation (see the accompanying Research in Nursing display). Mild OSA can be managed with a custom-made oral appliance (OA), also known as a mandibular advancement device (MAD). These hard, plastic devices are fitted by a dentist or orthodontist based on a mold of the patient's mouth. If a person is unable to tolerate CPAP, an oral appliance is an alternative treatment. Both CPAP and MAD must be used every sleep event to be effective (Agency for Healthcare Research

RESEARCH IN NURSING

BRIDGING THE GAP TO EVIDENCE-BASED PRACTICE

Influence of Partners' Support on Patient Adherence to CPAP Treatment

Obstructive sleep apnea causes poor sleep quality and over time increases the workload on the heart and the risk for a fatal cardiovascular event. Untreated, it can lead to daytime sleepiness and an increased risk for work-related or driving accidents. This combination of apnea or hypopnea with the resultant excessive sleepiness during the day and decreased performance during awake hours is referred to as obstructive sleep apnea syndrome (OSAS). CPAP is the standard treatment, but requires some adaptation. It can improve the patient's signs and symptoms, but many patients have difficulty tolerating CPAP.

Related Research

Elfstrom, M., Karlsson, S., Nilsen, P., Fridlund, B., Svanborg, E., & Brostrom, A. (2012). Decisive situations affecting partners' support to continuous positive airway pressure-treated patients with obstructive sleep apnea syndrome. *Journal of Cardiovascular Nursing, 27*(3), 228–239.

There are few studies that address partner support for adherence to CPAP treatment in individuals with OSAS. The aim of this study was to explore and describe situations that affected partners' support during the initial phase of CPAP treatment. There were 25 partners of patients at a Swedish hospital clinic who participated in this study. These patients were diagnosed with OSAS and using CPAP for treatment. Two researchers conducted two interviews with the partners that lasted from 12 to 60 minutes each. These interviews

focused on positive and negative factors or decisive situations that influenced the patient's adherence to CPAP and partner support. Findings of this study indicated that adverse effects (both physical and psychological), a negative initial response to the CPAP treatment, practical problems (humidifier issues, traveling with the device), and limited partner involvement were negative influencers of partner support. Positive partner support resulted when the CPAP treatment functioned appropriately, improvements in the patient's condition were noted, motivation was high, and support from others was present. In addition, these findings should positively impact and guide the development of education programs for new CPAP users and the involvement and participation of their partners.

Relevance to Nursing Practice

As patient teachers and educators, nurses need an awareness of factors that positively influence adherence to CPAP treatment. Despite the significant improvement that patients experience when CPAP is used as prescribed, the treatment requires some adaptation and commitment as well as intensive support from health care providers. Nurses also initially can identify patients at risk, assess rest and sleep issues, discuss lifestyle changes that might prove helpful, and address patient and partner concerns about CPAP treatment.

For additional research, visit thePoint.

and Quality, 2011). If conservative treatment methods fail, surgery to remove soft tissue at the back of the mouth may be an option. This surgery is not without risks and poses significant postoperative issues for the patient. People who opt for the procedure need continued support and comprehensive teaching, including coping strategies, for the immediate postoperative period.

The American Academy of Pediatrics has revised recommendations for diagnosis and treatment of obstructive sleep apnea syndrome in children. According to their guidelines, children and adolescents with symptoms of OSA, including snoring, should have polysomnography to confirm the diagnosis. Severe complications can occur if this disorder is untreated or ignored. Options for treatment in children include weight loss if obesity is present, adenotonsillectomy (removal of tonsils and adenoids), CPAP, or intranasal corticosteroids (Marcus et al., 2012).

Restless Leg Syndrome

Restless leg syndrome (RLS) is a common sleep disorder that affects up to 15% of the population, most often middle-aged and older adults. Approximately 2% of children also suffer from RLS, and there appears to be a strong genetic component. Almost 75% of these children have a parent with RLS (NSF, 2011g). People with **restless leg syndrome (RLS)**

cannot lie still and report unpleasant creeping, crawling, or tingling sensations in the legs. Usually, these sensations are in the calf, but they may occur anywhere from the ankle to the thigh. Occasionally, RLS can occur in the arms, face, or torso. Patients describe an irresistible urge to move the legs when these sensations occur, usually during the evening and night. In some cases, symptoms may affect both sides of the body. RLS is seen in patients with end-stage renal disease (ESRD), diabetes, iron deficiency, peripheral neuropathy, and pregnancy. Over-the-counter medications such as antihistamines can exacerbate the symptoms of RLS. This disorder has no specific diagnostic test and no known cure.

Nonpharmacologic measures to prevent or alleviate this discomfort include massaging the legs, walking, doing knee bends, and moving or gently stretching the legs. Research continues into additional treatment options, but the following may prove effective:

- Eliminating use of caffeine, tobacco, and alcohol
- Taking a mild analgesic at bedtime (provided it is compatible with the current medical regimen)
- Applying heat or cold to the extremity
- Using relaxation techniques. Biofeedback and transcutaneous electrical nerve stimulation (TENS) may also relieve symptoms (see the accompanying Promoting Health Literacy display).

PROMOTING HEALTH LITERACY

IN PATIENTS WITH RESTLESS LEG SYNDROME

Patient Scenario

Mary Weymouth is a 40-year-old woman who has an appointment to see her primary physician because of a "strange sensation in her legs that is keeping her awake at night." When asked by the nurse to further describe her symptoms, Mary explains that she has this feeling that "something is crawling up her lower leg." She keeps moving her leg from side to side until she finally just gets out of bed and walks around for a while. She states that movement seems to "make it better" but this does not work all the time. Sometimes, she also gets "pretty severe cramping pain" that can last several hours. Mary relates that this has been happening 2 or 3 nights a week for at least 1 month and she finds that she is "very sleepy" the following day. At times when she is at work, she said that she finds herself starting to "nod off" and is afraid that someone might notice and she could lose her job. She's tried drinking a few glasses of wine at night to relax her and has also occasionally taken some Tylenol PM to see if that will help her sleep through the night. Nothing seems to help. After the physician examined her, he asked if anyone in her family had similar symptoms. Mary remembered that her mother used to tell her that she sometimes had "nervous legs" at night. The physician reviews her history and tells Mary that her symptoms indicate that she has Restless Leg Syndrome. At this time, he prefers not to prescribe medication for her but wants her to try some nonpharmacologic measures to see if they ease her symptoms. As Mary is making another appointment, she tells the nurse that "she doesn't know how much longer she can manage without a good night's sleep most nights. I may just have to give Tylenol PM another try."

Nursing Considerations: *Tips for Improving Health Literacy*

Provide Mary with some specific information about measures that may ease her symptoms of RLS and allow her to get a restful sleep. Recommend that she avoid alcohol, caffeine, and any over-the-counter sleeping medications because they contain antihistamines that may aggravate the symptoms of RLS. Encourage her to participate in and incorporate into her daily life any regular, moderate physical activity to promote better sleep at night. Suggest using a heating pad or warm bath or an ice pack to possibly help with these sensations. Explain to Mary that there is no specific diagnostic test for RLS, but if her symptoms are not relieved by these other measures, there is a medication that the physician might prescribe. Also, give her information about the website that is specifically for patients with RLS. When Mary returns for her follow-up appointment, she needs to be prepared to ask her physician the following questions:

- What is my main problem? Can anything else be associated with this Restless Leg Syndrome?
- What else do I need to do?
- Why is it important for me to do this?
- What can you do if you prescribe a medication and it does not help with my symptoms?

What additional measures can you take to help increase health literacy in this patient? What other measures would be helpful if Mary did not speak English, could not read, or had other learning deficits?

Ropinirole (Requip) and pramipexole dihydrochloride (Mirapex) are drugs that have been approved by the U.S. Food and Drug Administration (FDA) to treat restless leg syndrome. Two additional medications have been approved for treatment of moderate to severe RLS: gabapentin enacarbil (Horizant extended-release tablets) and rotigotine transdermal system (Neupro). Both are sustained-release medications that have proved effective for relief of the symptoms of RLS (FDA, 2011; Restless Legs Syndrome Foundation, 2012).

A process has been started to change the name of restless leg syndrome to Willis-Ekbom disease (RLS Foundation, 2011). A task force considered the original designation confusing since other body parts, including the legs, can be involved. The Restless Legs Syndrome Foundation (http://www.rls.org) is a support group available for the millions of people with this disorder who experience chronic sleep loss.

Sleep Deprivation

Sleep deprivation refers to a decrease in the amount, consistency, or quality of sleep. It may result from decreased REM sleep or NREM sleep. Total sleep deprivation is rarely seen, other than in experimental settings. There are many causes, and the manifestations progress from irritability and impaired mental abilities to a total disintegration of personality. In general, the effects of sleep deprivation become increasingly apparent after 30 hours of continual wakefulness.

Partial sleep deprivation may result in loss of concentration, inattention, and impaired information processing, and poses serious safety risks. Excessive daytime sleepiness, a form of partial sleep deprivation, impairs performance at times when people need to be alert. The strange environment of the hospital, physical discomfort and pain, the effects of medications, and the need for 24-hour nursing care may also contribute to sleep deprivation in hospitalized patients.

It is unclear whether irreversible damage to body tissue results from prolonged or chronic sleep deprivation. As mentioned earlier in this chapter, recent research has indicated the possibility of a causal relationship between sleep deprivation and obesity, cancer, diabetes, and cardiovascular conditions. However, sleep deprivation clearly produces changes in physical and mental functioning, supporting the belief that sleep is essential for well-being. Sleep deprivation may be caused by shorter periods of sleep, which over time can cause impairment. Whether it occurs as a result of a disorder or is due to voluntary sleep curtailment, sleep deprivation has wide-ranging negative consequences for human health and well being (see the earlier section, Physical and Psychological Effects of Insufficient Sleep, p. 1123).

RECALL Charlie Bitner, the long-term care facility resident complaining of sleep problems. From the patient's statements, the nurse would identify that Mr. Bitner is at risk for developing sleep deprivation. Therefore, the nurse would work with Mr. Bitner to establish measures that would promote effective sleep patterns. ●

Parasomnias

Parasomnias are patterns of waking behavior that appear during REM or NREM stages of sleep. They are more commonly seen in children. Although parasomnias are commonly outgrown before adulthood, safety and prevention of injury are paramount concerns. These sleep disorders can occur rarely or on a regular basis. Examples of parasomnias include:

- **Somnambulism** or sleepwalking may range from sitting up in bed to walking around the room or the house to walking outside the house. The sleepwalker is unaware of his environment.
- *REM Behavior Disorder (RBD)* is characterized by "acting out" dreams while asleep. While experiencing the dream episode, the sleeper can moan and thrash around in the bed, possibly causing harm to a bed partner or oneself (American Sleep Association, 2010).
- *Sleep terrors* are more common in children and occur during the deepest stages of sleep. Typical behavior involves waking up screaming and sitting up in bed. They may appear to be awake and reasonable but are unable to communicate when they awaken from a sleep terror.
- *Nightmares* are frightening dreams that are vivid and disturbing. They occur more frequently in children and represent a normal developmental process.
- *Bruxism* is grinding of one's teeth and frequently is an indicator of stress.
- **Enuresis** is urinating during sleep or bedwetting. It occurs most commonly in males who are over three years of age.
- *Sleep-related eating disorder* occurs when a person eats while sleeping but has no recollection of eating in the morning. It can occur during sleepwalking and those affected can gain weight and experience injury either from cooking in their sleep or eating potentially dangerous raw food. They may also exhibit signs of sleep disruption during waking hours.

THE NURSING PROCESS FOR REST AND SLEEP

Assessing

Sleep History

Interview questions help identify the patient's sleep–wakefulness patterns, the effect of these patterns on everyday functioning, the patient's use of sleep aids, and the presence of sleep disturbances and contributing factors. If the patient's sleep is adequate and poses no problems, the sleep history may be brief (four questions), or it may be more detailed. When the patient's response to any of the interview questions indicates a potential problem, open-ended questions may be used to gather more data (Focused Assessment Guide 33-1).

If the patient is being admitted to a care facility, assess the patient's usual times for retiring and waking, bedtime rituals, and preferences regarding sleep environment so that

FOCUSED ASSESSMENT GUIDE 33-1

REST AND SLEEP

Factors to Assess	Questions and Approaches
Usual sleep–wakefulness pattern: Recent changes Usual sleeping and waking times	Do you set an alarm and hit "snooze" before getting up? How many hours of sleep do you usually get in a day? Do you wake up earlier in the morning than you would like and find it difficult to fall back asleep? Have there been any recent changes in your usual sleep–wake patterns? If yes, describe them and tell me if they are causing any problems for you. Do you usually go to bed and wake up about the same time each day?
Number of hours of undisturbed sleep	How have you been sleeping? Do you have any difficulty falling asleep? Do you wake up frequently during the night? Do you dream at night? Are your dreams frightening?
Quality of sleep Number and duration of naps	How much sleep do you think you need to feel rested? Do you take naps throughout the day?
Effect of sleep pattern on everyday functioning Energy level (ability to perform activities of daily living)	In what way does the sleep you get each day affect your everyday living? Has this sleep disturbance caused any change in your sex life? Do you feel rested and ready to start the day when you wake up? Are there times during the day or certain activities when you feel especially tired? What happens when you don't get enough sleep? Are you having difficulty concentrating?
Sleep aids Means of relaxing before bedtime Bedtime rituals Sleep environment Pharmacologic aids	What do you do to relax before you get ready for bed? Describe what you usually do to help yourself fall asleep. Tell me how you like your room (lights, noises, ventilation, position of door, temperature) and bed (mattress, pillows, blankets) when you are sleeping. Do you take any medications to help you sleep? Are you taking any medicine at all?
Sleep disturbances and contributing factors Nature of the sleep disturbance Onset of disturbance Causes (physical, psychosocial, medicine related) Severity Symptoms Interventions attempted and results	Tell me about your sleep problem. How often does it occur? Are you doing anything differently now that might be causing the problem? Do you wake up gasping for air? Do you snore? Do you recall changing your position frequently during the night? What have you been doing to deal with the problem? How effective were these measures?

these can be incorporated into the plan of care, if possible. Patients in hospitals often receive fragmented sleep. Their sleep may be disrupted by routine care measures, noise in the environment, and lighting (see the accompanying Nursing Advocacy in Action display on page 1134). Paying attention to small matters can make the difference between a patient's having a good night of sleep or no sleep.

When a sleep disturbance is noted, ask about the following when obtaining the history:

• The nature of the problem
• The cause of the problem
• The related signs and symptoms
• When the problem began and how often it occurs
• How the problem affects everyday living
• The severity of the problem and whether it can be treated independently by nurses or needs to be referred to another health care professional

• How the patient is coping with the problem and the success of any treatments attempted

 THINK back to Lydia Omeara, the mother of twin infants who was asking about allowing the infants to sleep in their parents' bed. The nurse would need to obtain a sleep history from Mrs. Omeara to ascertain her sleep pattern. This information would be helpful in determining the reasons for allowing the children to sleep in their parents' bed. ●

Assistance from the patient's bed partner may be needed to aid in data collection and provide more accurate information regarding the patient's sleep patterns. The patient's record may also contain pertinent information (e.g., a history of illnesses that influence sleep).

NURSING ADVOCACY IN ACTION

Patient Scenario

Maria was born premature. After surgery on her bowel, she was placed on the transplantation list for a new liver and small bowel and started on total parenteral nutrition. She is now 9 months old but has spent the last 4 weeks in the hospital with fungemia, a fungus infection spread throughout the bloodstream. Her single mother, Ms. Gomez, practically lives at the hospital and in recent days has annoyed the nurses with her complaints about the nursing care. Her English is limited, but she is able to express her annoyance at the many times Maria is awakened during the night for treatment and care. "Why can't the nurses do several things at once so Maria can at least get a few hours of uninterrupted sleep?!" Recently the nurses complained to the medical director and he informed Ms. Gomez that if she doesn't stop interfering with Maria's care, the doctors will take Maria off the transplantation list. The nurse giving you the report repeats this story and tells you "not to take any complaints or grief from the mom." When you meet Ms.

Gomez and listen to her story, you admire her love for Maria and willingness to advocate for her. You also sense the mother's frustration with the system. She asks you tearfully, "They can't take Maria off the list, can they? I am only trying to be a good mother." Ms. Gomez appears to have no family or other support network.

Implications for Nursing Advocacy

How would you respond if you were the nurse assigned Maria as a patient? Talk with your classmates and experienced nurses about the questions that follow.

- Is it fair to say that Ms. Gomez is being threatened for trying to advocate for her baby? If you elect to advocate for Maria and her mother, what practical steps can you take to remedy this situation?
- What is it reasonable to expect of a student nurse, graduate nurse, and an experienced nurse in this situation?
- What advocacy skills are needed to effectively respond to this challenge?

Sample records of a sleep history in a comprehensive nursing assessment are as follows:

- *"Reports needs 8 to 9 hours of sleep to feel his best and usually gets this without problem. Generally retires at 11:30 PM and rises at 7:30 AM. No special sleep rituals."*
- *"Mother reports toddler has erratic sleep patterns. May nap at any time in the afternoon or evening and sleep from 1 to 3 hours. Depending on nap, goes to bed anywhere from 7 to 11 PM and sleeps about 11 to 13 hours. Resists falling asleep and wants "water, story, snack, kisses, etc." Parents' lifestyle is constantly changing—little consistency for the child regarding sleep expectations."*

In outpatient settings and physicians' offices, the issue of healthy sleep practices and the presence of sleep disorders are not routinely assessed. Given that the need for adequate sleep has become a national health problem, it can be expected that this will become a focus in future patient interactions.

Sleep Diary

A sleep diary or log provides more specific data on the patient's sleep–wakefulness patterns over a period of time. It summarizes information about these patterns, possibly indicating activities and behaviors that affect the quality and quantity of sleep. Generally, the diary is kept for 14 days and typically includes a graph of the total number of hours of sleep per day. Depending on the nature of the problem, graphs may be made of the number of undisturbed hours of sleep, number of awakenings, and so forth. In addition, a daily record is completed addressing the following:

- Time patient retires
- Time patient tries to fall asleep
- Approximate time patient falls asleep
- Time of any awakenings during the night and when sleep was resumed

- Time of awakening in the morning
- Presence of any stressors patient believes are affecting his or her sleep
- A record of any food, drink, or medication patient believes has positively or negatively influenced his or her sleep (include time of ingestion)
- Record of physical activities—type, duration, and time
- Record of mental activities—type, duration, and time
- Record of activities performed 2 to 3 hours before bedtime, bedtime rituals, changes in sleep environment
- Presence of any worries or anxieties patient believes are affecting his or her sleep

 REMEMBER Jeanette Clark, the mother of the adolescent girl who seems to be sleeping all the time. Having Mrs. Clark's daughter complete a sleep diary might be helpful in obtaining a better picture of what is happening and helping rule out other causes for the daughter's increased fatigue and sleeping. These underlying causes could be wide ranging, including such conditions as depression, physical illness, or increased activity or schoolwork. ●

It is helpful if the patient has a bed partner who can assist with the diary. The patient needs to understand that the diary is simply a diagnostic tool. If keeping the diary causes too much stress for the patient and further interferes with the ability to sleep restfully, it should be discontinued.

There are additional screening tools that can be used to assess sleep disturbances and the quality of sleep. Some examples include:

- The Epworth Sleepiness Scale
- The Pittsburgh Sleep Quality Index (PSQI)
- Sleep Disturbance Questionnaire

See the Internet Resources available on thePoint to access these sites.

Physical Assessment

The findings in the physical assessment may either confirm that the patient is getting sufficient rest to provide energy for the day's activities or validate the existence of a sleep disturbance that is decreasing the quantity or quality of sleep. Key findings include energy level (presence of physical weakness, fatigue, lethargy, or decreased energy), facial characteristics (narrowing or glazing of eyes, swelling of eyelids, decreased animation), or behavioral characteristics (yawning, rubbing eyes, slow speech, slumped posture). Physical data suggestive of potential sleep problems (e.g., obesity, enlarged neck, deviated nasal septum) may also be noted.

If the nurse or a bed partner can observe the patient sleeping, other sleep characteristics to assess include restlessness, sleep postures, and sleep activities such as snoring or leg jerking (restless leg syndrome). Snoring is caused by an obstruction to airflow through the nose and mouth. Other than disturbing others in the same bedroom, snoring is not ordinarily a sleeping disorder. However, snoring accompanied by apnea can present a problem. When snoring changes from the characteristic sawing-wood sound to a more irregular silence followed by a snort, this indicates obstructive apnea. As mentioned earlier, the recently revised clinical practice guideline from The American Academy of Pediatrics states that snoring in children needs to be evaluated as a possible indication of OSA.

Diagnosing
Disturbed Sleep Pattern as the Problem

When assessment data point to a sleep problem that is amenable to nursing therapy, it receives the label Disturbed Sleep Pattern if the problem is time limited or Sleep Deprivation if the problem is prolonged. Common etiologies for these nursing diagnoses may include the following:

- Impaired comfort or pain
- Changes in bedtime rituals or sleep environment
- Disruption of circadian rhythm
- Exercise just before sleep
- Caffeine, nicotine, or alcohol intake after dinner
- Drug dependency and withdrawal
- Symptoms of physical illness

Examples of nursing diagnoses in which the disturbed sleep pattern is the primary problem are presented in the accompanying Examples of NANDA-I Nursing Diagnoses box.

EXAMPLES OF NANDA-I NURSING DIAGNOSES

SLEEP

Nursing Diagnoses	Related Factors	Sample Defining Characteristics
Disturbed Sleep Pattern: Difficulty Falling Asleep	Worries about family and lack of destressing rituals	• "At least 4 or 5 nights a week, I lay in bed awake for 3 or 4 hours before I finally fall asleep. Sometimes it is 2 or 3 in the morning and I'm still awake worrying about the kids. I've tried getting up and reading or paying my bills, but even that doesn't make me sleepy." • Reports problem falling asleep for past 6 months; is widowed and very concerned about two teenage sons. Never sleeps until both sons are home. States she does nothing special to relax. Feels her worries are "her business"—no support person with whom she shares these.
Disturbed Sleep Pattern: Difficulty Remaining Asleep	Noise of hospital environment and need for periodic treatments	• Admitted to hospital 3/6/14; cholecystectomy 3/7/14 • "I don't think I've had one decent night's sleep since my surgery. I've been falling asleep about 9 PM and then someone wakes me up for my medicine. I just about get back to sleep and someone's putting the light on to poke at my dressing or to check this tube. I know I'm getting grouchy." • Orders include every-4-hour vital signs; nursing assessment of the incision, nasogastric tube, intravenous therapy; and medication for pain and for sleep.
Disturbed Sleep Pattern: Altered Sleep–Wake Patterns	Frequent rotations of shift and overtime	• Graduate nurse, 24 years old, who has been working on a busy medical floor for 6 months; rotates 11–7 and 7–3 shifts; recently a problem with staffing has necessitated frequent rotations. Patient often volunteers (two or three times a week) for overtime. • "I don't know what is wrong with me. I'm so tired anymore and don't feel at all like myself. All I want to do when I'm off is to sleep—but often I can't fall asleep when I lay down. Please help!"

Disturbed Sleep Pattern as the Etiology

The disturbed sleep pattern may affect many other areas of human functioning. In the nursing diagnoses that follow, the disturbed sleep pattern is the cause of another problem:

- Anxiety related to inability to fall asleep, inability to control behavior while asleep, and sleep apnea (threat of death)
- Activity Intolerance related to sleep deprivation
- Fatigue related to prolonged excessive role demands
- Ineffective Coping related to insomnia: insufficient quantity and quality of sleep
- Impaired Gas Exchange related to sleep apnea (oxygen saturation of the blood)
- Risk for Injury related to somnambulism, narcolepsy, sleep apnea
- Deficient Knowledge (e.g., nonpharmacologic remedies for insomnia) related to misinformation, lack of interest in learning, cognitive limitation
- Impaired Social Interaction related to excessive daytime sleeping, sleep deprivation

Important Distinctions

Because the problem statement of the nursing diagnosis identifies what is wrong with the patient and suggests the expected outcomes and the etiology of the problem directs nursing interventions, analysis of the assessment data is essential when deciding whether the sleep data indicate the problem, contribute to a different problem, or are signs or symptoms of the problem. Sleep data potentially fit in all three categories. For example, when a disturbed sleep pattern involving altered sleep–wake patterns is assessed in a graduate nurse who is getting adjusted to a new full-time job, shift work, and increased independence, three different diagnoses might be written:

- *Disturbed Sleep Pattern associated with altered sleep–wake patterns related to shift work and stress of new job as manifested by complaints of always feeling tired and not getting enough sleep:* The disturbed sleep pattern involving the altered sleep–wake pattern is the problem statement; priority nursing energies are directed toward changing this pattern and helping the patient achieve both the necessary quantity and quality of sleep.
- *Ineffective Coping related to multiple stresses of new job and altered sleep–wake pattern (sleep deprivation) as manifested by statements such as, "I don't know how much longer I can do this," "I'm always tired, and all I want to do is sleep," "I'm so grouchy—people must hate me!"* Here, the altered sleep–wake pattern is just one of the factors contributing to the patient's problem of ineffective coping; priority nursing energies are directed toward improving the patient's coping skills by teaching the patient how to increase the quantity and quality of sleep.
- *Ineffective Coping related to multiple stressors and lack of stress-relieving rituals as manifested by inability to fall asleep, excessive fatigue, and feelings*

that personality is changing: In this instance, the altered sleep–wake pattern is merely a symptom of the patient's actual problem—ineffective coping. The expectation is that when the coping problem is resolved, the symptom will disappear.

None of the preceding diagnoses is more correct than the others. With each patient, the nurse must review each cluster of significant data and identify the key problem, contributing factors, and related signs and symptoms. The exact nature of the nursing diagnosis directs the nursing interventions.

Outcome Identification and Planning

Rest and sleep are essential components of well-being. Planning for patient care, especially in a health care facility, involves planning with the patient suitable measures to promote rest and sleep. Whenever nurses care for a patient, nursing measures support the following expected patient outcomes: The patient will:

- Maintain a sleep–wake pattern that provides sufficient energy for the day's tasks
- Demonstrate self-care behaviors that provide a healthy balance between rest and activity
- Identify stress-relieving rituals that enable the patient to fall asleep more easily
- Demonstrate decreased signs of sleep deprivation
- Verbalize feeling less fatigued and more in control of life activities

Implementing

In most cases, sleep problems are not the primary reason for a patient's interaction with the health care system. Communicating with the patient while displaying a non-judgmental, caring attitude often is the key to detecting a patient's sleep problem. Patients who believe the nurse is generally concerned about their well-being are not reluctant to discuss their insomnia. In order to correct a sleep problem, the patient needs to believe that the nurse cares and will provide extra help to promote rest and sleep. The accompanying box, Examples of Nursing Interventions and Nursing Outcomes Classifications (NIC/NOC), lists interventions that aid in sleep promotion.

Preparing a Restful Environment

A comfortable bed helps promote rest and sleep. The bottom linen should be tight and clean. The upper linen, while secure, should allow freedom of movement and should not exert pressure, especially over the legs and feet. Good body alignment is conducive to relaxation. For patients who must assume unusual positions because of their illness, ingenuity and skill are necessary to minimize muscle strain and discomfort. For example, patients who must remain in the orthopneic position to aid breathing should be well supported in a manner that relieves muscle strain.

A quiet and darkened room with privacy is relaxing for nearly everyone. In a strange environment, unfamiliar noises, such as people walking by or entering and leaving

EXAMPLES OF NURSING INTERVENTIONS AND NURSING OUTCOMES CLASSIFICATIONS (NIC/NOC)

SLEEP ENHANCEMENT

Nursing Interventions	Nursing Outcomes
Approximate patient's regular sleep–wake cycle in planning care. • Determine the effects of the patient's medications on sleep pattern. • Adjust environment (e.g., light, noise, temperature, mattress, bed) to promote sleep. • Encourage patient to establish a bedtime routine to facilitate transition from wakefulness to sleep. • Facilitate maintenance of patient's usual bedtime routines, presleep cues/props, and familiar objects (e.g., for children, a favorite blanket/toy, rocking, pacifier, or story; for adults, a book to read, etc.) as appropriate. • Instruct patient to avoid bedtime foods and beverages that interfere with sleep. • Instruct patient how to perform autogenic muscle relaxation or other nonpharmacologic forms of sleep inducement. • Initiate/implement comfort measures of massage, positioning, and affective touch. • Discuss with patient and family sleep-enhancing techniques	• Motivation • Rest • Sleep • Health Promoting Behavior • Medication Response

Bulechek, G., Butcher, H., Dochterman, J., & Wagner, C. (2013). *Nursing interventions classification (NIC)* (6th ed., p. 349). St. Louis: Elsevier/Mosby. A full listing of nursing activities for each nursing intervention can be found in this book.

Moorhead, S., Johnson, M., Maas, M., & Swanson, E. (2013). *Nursing outcomes classification (NOC)* (5th ed., p. 697). St. Louis: Elsevier/Mosby. A full listing of nursing outcomes for each nursing diagnosis can be found in this book.

the room and the sounds of elevator doors, bring complaints from most hospitalized patients. Although some of these sounds are difficult to control, make every effort to reduce disturbances and to promote relaxation and sleep. Many health care facilities have made attempts to transform their patient care areas into quieter settings that facilitate rest and sleep. Attention to design features with a focus on eliminating environmental noise, providing patients with private rooms, and formal quiet times on units all are aimed at creating a more supportive environment that is conducive to good sleep.

The temperature of the room, the amount of ventilation, and the amount of bed covering are matters of individual choice. Meet the patient's wishes when at all possible.

Many older patients cannot sleep if they feel cold. Thermal blankets or comforters, insulated bed socks, cotton flannel sheets, leg warmers, long underwear, and a stockinette cap help patients stay warm and promote comfort and sleep. See Focus on the Older Adult for additional suggestions.

 RECALL Charlie Bitner, the older man living in a long-term care facility. The nurse would work with Mr. Bitner to ensure that his sleeping area is as comfortable and restful as possible. Making sure that he is warm enough, dimming the lights, closing the door (as much as allowed), and minimizing disturbances outside his room would be key. •

FOCUS ON THE OLDER ADULT

AGE-RELATED CHANGES AND NURSING STRATEGIES FOR REST AND SLEEP

Age-Related Changes	Nursing Strategies
Disturbed Sleep Pattern: Initiation of Sleep • Decreased physical activities	• Encourage patient to engage in some type of physical activity, such as walking or water aerobics.
• Tired and fatigued throughout day • Depression • Polypharmacy	• Discourage napping throughout day. • Arrange for assessment for depression and treatment. • Review medications that patient is taking and assess for any side effects of sleep pattern disturbances.
Disturbed Sleep Pattern: Maintaining Sleep • Nocturia	• Decrease fluids during the evening. • Take diuretics in the morning or early evening.
• Sleep-related movement disturbances (e.g., restless leg syndrome)	• Discuss problems with health care provider.

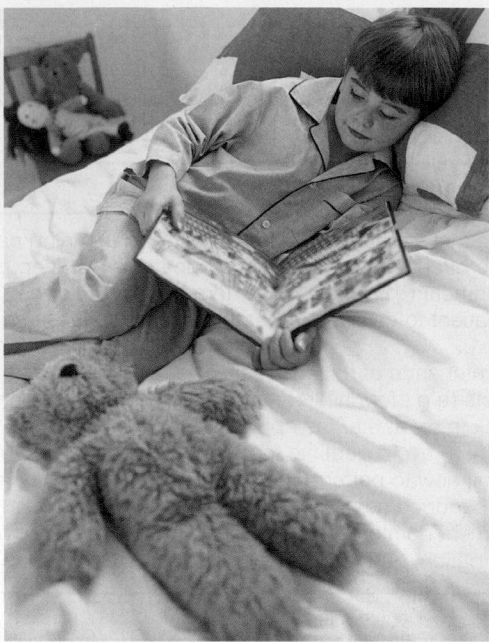

FIGURE 33-4. A bedtime routine helps promote sleep in children.

Promoting Bedtime Rituals

Most people have bedtime rituals to help them relax and promote sleep. Reading, listening to the radio, watching television, talking to a family member, and praying are common before-sleep activities. Children may take a favorite doll, stuffed toy, or blanket to bed; listen to a bedtime story; kiss everyone good night; and say prayers before bed (Fig. 33-4). Readiness for sleep follows a personal hygiene routine for many people, such as brushing teeth, washing hands and face, voiding, or taking a bath or shower. Snacks are important elements in the bedtime rituals of many children and adults. Although eating the wrong foods may produce a bad night's sleep, going to bed hungry may also interfere with sleep.

 TEACHING Mrs. Omeara about the importance of bedtime rituals for her twin infants may promote the children's sleep. In addition, the nurse would need to reinforce the need for Mrs. Omeara's bedtime rituals to ensure that the sleep she obtains is restful. •

To promote relaxation and sleep, be alert to the patient's bedtime rituals and observe them as much as possible. Include these rituals in the patient's plan of care so that all health personnel can observe them.

Offering Appropriate Bedtime Snacks and Beverages

Because carbohydrates seem to promote sleep, there appears to be justification for offering a snack or beverage high in carbohydrates before bedtime, such as toast, a small bagel, crackers, or a glass of fruit juice, if this is allowed in the patient's regimen. An alcoholic beverage helps to promote sleep for some people. However, alcohol after dinner generally should be avoided because it may interrupt the normal sleep cycle and interfere with deep sleep. For most patients, beverages containing caffeine should be avoided for at least 4 to 5 hours before bedtime. Recommend that the patient take fluids during the day but avoid excessive fluid intake before bedtime to prevent the need to use the bathroom during the night.

Promoting Relaxation

One can relax without sleeping, but sleep rarely occurs until one is relaxed. Stress and anxiety interfere with a person's ability to relax, rest, and sleep. Means for dealing with worries include dealing with problems as they arise, conditioning yourself to consider stressful issues only at certain times, teaching yourself that worrying never solves problems and is counterproductive, and giving the worries over to another (e.g., a trusted family member, friend, caregiver, or God). The distraction and relaxation techniques described in Chapters 34 and 41 may be beneficial for a patient whose worries are contributing to a sleep disturbance. A backrub, a warm bath, and washing the face if the patient is bedridden are typical nursing measures to help patients relax. The technique for back massage is described in Skill 34-1 on pages 1188–1191.

Promoting Comfort

One of the greatest deterrents to rest and sleep is pain, which commonly occurs in illness. Depending on the cause and severity of the discomfort or pain, appropriate nursing measures include remaining with a lonely and frightened child or adult, using the simple strategy of caring presence and touch, offering a back massage, obtaining an extra blanket, or administering an analgesic. These and other nursing techniques to promote comfort are described in Chapter 34. Be sensitive to the patient's discomfort to recognize and relieve it.

Respecting Normal Sleep–Wake Patterns

Make every effort to allow patients to experience their normal period of sleep. In many instances, insisting that all patients retire and awaken at specific times is not necessary. For example, is there a good reason to wake a patient at 7 AM if the patient ordinarily sleeps until 9 AM? The patient's normal napping habits should also be followed when possible. REM sleep is more common during morning naps, whereas NREM sleep is more common during naps later in the day. With this knowledge, help patients plan napping periods that best fit their needs and interfere the least amount with nighttime sleeping.

Scheduling Nursing Care to Avoid Unnecessary Disturbances

Many patients complain that they are awakened to take sleeping pills and are aroused in the early morning to prepare for breakfast long before it is served. Consider these common complaints when developing the patient's plan of care to promote rest and sleep.

Whenever possible, provide care during periods when the patient is normally awake. When this is not feasible, avoid awakening the patient during REM sleep, when the rapid eye movements can be observed. Because a patient's need for sleep is important, examine priorities for nursing care. For example, consider whether checking a vital sign or carrying out a particular nursing measure is more important than the patient's sleep (see Focused Critical Thinking Guide 33-1 on page 1140).

Minimizing Sleep Disturbances in a Hospital Setting

Studies have demonstrated that excessive noise on patient care units interferes with sleep and that these noise-related disruptions can increase blood pressure, decrease oxygen saturation, and delay wound healing (Haupt, 2012). Behavioral manifestations such as disorientation, restlessness and irritability are also possible consequences, particularly in older patients. Patient surveys consistently report that noise and sleep deprivation are among the top concerns during a hospitalization. The most commonly implicated sources of noise include staff conversations, roommates, and electronic sounds such as IV alarms and phones (Anderson, 2012). Researchers have reported that the patient's stage of sleep can affect the patient's response to hospital noises. Sleep disruption is more common during non-REM stage II sleep. One group of researchers reported that hospital noise levels during the day were above World Health Organization recommendations and at times even approached the sound level produced by a chain saw (Wallis, 2012). In an ICU setting, sleep is even further challenged by the level of light in the unit. Nighttime light can range

from a level similar to that at twilight and peak at a level brighter than lighting in some television studios (Moye, 2010). Nursing interventions to manage the level of light and sound, thus facilitating a more restful environment, include:

- Maintaining a brighter room environment during daylight hours and dim lights in the evening
- Decreasing the volume on alarms, telephones, overhead paging, and staff conversations
- Closing doors to patient rooms
- Scheduling procedures together so as not to awaken patients multiple times for vital signs, blood draws, bathing, or medication administration that can safely be postponed for a short time
- Medicating for pain if needed
- Keeping the room cool and providing earplugs and eye masks if requested (Moye, 2010).

Some health care facilities have implemented specific efforts to minimize noise levels. These initiatives include campaigns titled "Shhh" (Silent Hospitals Help Healing) and "Hush" (Help Us Support Healing) and institution of a Quiet Hour (Chen, 2012; Haupt, 2012). It is difficult to guarantee a good night's sleep during a hospitalization but recognizing and listening to patients' concerns are critical to delivery of individualized, quality nursing care.

Using Medications to Promote Sleep

Medications for sleep are often ordered for patients. A thorough sleep history and assessment is required prior to the use of medications to induce sleep. The underlying cause for the sleep deprivation must be determined; nondrug interventions are usually the first treatment choice. When insomnia cannot be managed by these other means, hypnotic drugs are often prescribed. Hypnotics induce sleep; antianxiety drugs reduce anxiety and tension. However, the sleep produced by hypnotics is an unnatural sleep. All these drugs disturb either REM or NREM sleep to some degree. Although most hypnotics provide several nights of excellent sleep, the medication often loses its effect after 1 or 2 weeks. Hypnotics should only be used when the cause of the insomnia is unknown or has not been managed by other means. At this point, many people increase the dosage of the medication or complement the drug with alcohol. Vigorous nursing intervention is needed to prevent a patient from developing a pattern of drug dependency and alcohol abuse.

The most commonly prescribed sleep aids are discussed here. For short-term use, the benzodiazephine-like drugs, zaleplon (Sonata) and zolpidem tartrate (Ambien), are often prescribed to promote sleep in older adults because there is less residual sleepiness. Zolpidem tartrate sublingual tablets (Intermezzo) have recently been approved by the FDA for insomnia associated with middle-of-the-night awakening. It is intended for use when at least 4 hours of sleep time remain and is a lower dose formation of Ambien (Jeffrey, 2011). Eszopiclone (Lunesta) is

FOCUSED CRITICAL THINKING GUIDE 33-1

SLEEP

You have just arrived on the unit and checked your clinical assignment. You have two patients today and about 30 minutes before preconference. Your routine is to review their charts for pertinent information, go and introduce yourself to them, and take their morning vital signs before preconference. With 10 minutes to spare, you visit your second patient and find that he is sound asleep. Remembering that he had a fractured hip repaired 2 days ago and that the night nurse had stated in his note that the patient was restless and awake until 4:00 AM, you are reluctant to awaken him. On the other hand, at your midterm conference your instructor commented that you need to improve your organizational skills. If you don't have your vital signs recorded until after preconference, then breakfast arrives, doctors make rounds, and you're that much further behind in your morning care and documentation. When you look at the flow sheet at the foot of the bed, you note that the last set of vitals were taken at midnight and were within normal limits. You're attempting to reconcile several things—the importance of these morning vital signs, the patient's need for sleep, and your need to accomplish your tasks on time and receive a good evaluation. What should you do?

1. Identify goal of thinking

Determine whether it is more important to awaken your patient for morning vital signs or let him sleep at least until after your preconference.

2. Assess adequacy of knowledge

Pertinent circumstances: Your patient had major surgery 2 days ago, did not have a restful night, but is sleeping peacefully now. You realize that his vital signs can be an important indicator of a complication. You also need to accomplish your tasks in a timely and organized manner.

Prerequisite knowledge: To make your decision, you need knowledge about his postoperative condition and assessment data that indicate he is recovering or developing a complication. You are aware that sleep is vital to promote tissue repair, physical recovery, and mental well-being. You also need to review the tasks that you need to accomplish this morning and decide how and if priorities could be shifted.

Room for error/time constraints: Will a delay in taking vital signs cause injury to this patient? You are not planning to omit this task but just questioning whether to postpone it and allow the patient to have some additional sleep.

3. Address potential problems

Waking your patient for vital signs may be disturbing for him and interfere with his need for rest. A decision to postpone morning vital signs might also cause several problems. If the patient has developed a complication, such as an infection, his elevated temperature may go undetected for at least another hour. By the time you come out of preconference, the patient may be eating his breakfast, which further delays recording of vital signs. You perceive that you are already falling behind on your schedule and are really intent on completing your responsibilities on time today.

4. Consult helpful resources

Before you make your decision, you should check the patient's flow sheet and note whether the previous set of vital signs were within normal limits. The primary nurse and your instructor may also help you sort through your priorities in this situation.

5. Critique judgment/decision

You have two choices here. If you wake your patient and take his vital signs, you are disturbing him when he is sleeping soundly, risking the fact that he may be angry with you, but you are on schedule for the day's activities. By postponing his vital signs at least until after postconference, you provide additional rest for the patient but know that you are already behind schedule and worry that your instructor will view you as disorganized. After reviewing your options and checking his chart again, you decide to allow him to sleep and plan to take them as soon as possible after your preconference. During preconference, when your instructor reviews your priorities for the day, she comments positively that you have individualized care based on your particular patient's needs at the moment. In your mind, you determine that the vital signs are your next priority and will take minimal time, and you should still be able to complete care and documentation in a competent manner and on time.

---

prescribed for longer-term treatment of chronic insomnia. Ramelteon (Rozerem) is prescribed to facilitate the onset of sleep but is not intended for sleep maintenance. It may be used long-term and activates receptors for melatonin (Lehne, 2013).

Sleep medications are often ordered on a PRN (as needed) basis. Administer these medications only when indicated and always with the full knowledge of their limitations. Provide thorough patient education about these medications. In addition, help patients develop other self-care strategies, including developing healthy sleep and lifestyle behaviors. Use alternative nonpharmacologic measures to promote sleep when appropriate. Over-the-counter (OTC) sleep medications most often contain antihistamines and should only be used on a short-term basis because of the potential for adverse effects and their lack of effectiveness over a lengthy time period.

 REMEMBER Charlie Bitner, the older man living in the long-term care facility. Nonpharmacologic measures would be helpful to promote sleep. Having Mr. Bitner consume a warm beverage before bedtime, listen to soft music, or receive a backrub may promote relaxation, thereby enhancing the effectiveness of the prescribed sleep medication. •

Teaching About Rest and Sleep

A well-informed person is better able to cope with distressing situations. Teach patients and their families about the nature of rest and sleep and their importance to well-being. For example, the fact that children and adults are getting less sleep has been implicated as a contributing factor to the obesity epidemic in the United States. This information appears to verify that lack of sleep affects not just the brain, but also the entire body (see Physical and Psychological Effects of Insufficient Sleep).

Also teach patients about normal variations in sleep patterns and common measures to promote relaxation and sleep (Teaching Tips 33-1). Discuss sleep hygiene recommendations with the patient. **Sleep hygiene** refers to nonpharmacologic recommendations that help a person get a better night's sleep. These entail reviewing and changing lifestyles and environment. Sleep hygiene suggestions include the following:

• Restricting the intake of caffeine, nicotine, and alcohol, especially later in the day

• Avoiding mental and physical activities after 5 PM that are stimulating
• Avoiding daytime naps
• Eating a light carbohydrate/protein snack before bedtime
• Avoiding high fluid intake in the evening so as to minimize trips to the bathroom during the night
• Sleeping in a cool, dark room
• Eliminating use of a bedroom clock
• Taking a warm bath before bedtime
• Trying to keep the sleep environment as quiet and stress-free as possible (Hedges & Ruggiero, 2012)

Stimulus control involves using the bedroom for sex and sleep only. People with insomnia who have problems initiating sleep should stay in the bedroom for only 15 to 20 minutes. If after this time they cannot fall asleep, they should leave the room and return only when they feel sleepy. Getting up at the same time every day, no matter what time the person fell asleep, and refraining from napping during the day are recommended.

Sleep restriction is based on the theory of limiting the time in bed to actual sleep time. It is thought that excessive time in bed may result in fragmented sleep, which may exacerbate the insomnia. A sleep diary helps to determine sleep patterns. The focus of sleep restriction is to avoid naps and early bedtimes and actually change the way a person sleeps.

Relaxation therapy involves any type of relaxation, such as progressive muscle relaxation, imagery training, or meditation. Not all relaxation methods are beneficial for all patients. Relaxation therapy and biofeedback are discussed in detail in Chapter 41.

TEACHING TIPS 33-1

REST AND SLEEP

Health Topic	Teaching Tip	Why Is This Important?
Activity	• Find an activity that can be done daily and involves physical exertion, such as walking. • Do not participate in any physical activities right before bedtime.	• Sleep is easier to obtain if some physical activity has been completed. • Many people find it hard to rest and sleep right after a physical activity.
Diet	• Avoid food, beverages, or OTC medications that contain caffeine in the evening. • Eat a light dinner. • Eat a light carbohydrate-containing snack at bedtime if hungry.	• Caffeine is a stimulant and may prolong the time it takes to fall asleep. • Eating a large meal before bedtime may produce heartburn, delaying sleep. • Carbohydrates may affect the serotonin levels in the brain and thus promote sleep.
Sleep Patterns	• Keep to usual waking time every day, even if previous night's bedtime was later than usual or sleep was restless. • Get out of bed if unable to fall asleep within 30 minutes, and go into another room.	• Keeping the same pattern helps the body's circadian rhythms. • By using the bedroom for only sleep and sexual activity, the mind begins to associate this room with sleep.

Discuss the plan of care with the patient to make sure that the patient deems it acceptable. If a sleep disorder becomes a problem and common nursing measures are inadequate, the nurse may need to refer the patient to a health practitioner with the expertise to deal with it.

Evaluating

Evaluate the effectiveness of the plan of care to promote rest and sleep by checking whether the patient has met the individualized expected outcomes specified in the plan. See Nursing Plan of Care 33-1 for Mr. Bitner.

Nursing care is considered effective if the patient is able to:

- Verbalize feeling rested or having had a restful night's sleep
- Identify factors that interfere with or disrupt the normal sleep pattern
- Use techniques that promote sleep and provide a restful environment
- Concentrate and function effectively during waking hours
- Eliminate behaviors related to sleep deprivation

NURSING PLAN OF CARE 33-1

for Mr. Bitner

Mr. Bitner is an alert, widowed, 86-year-old man who was admitted to a long-term care facility 2 months ago. He is ambulatory and performs most of his self-care. His admitting medical diagnoses include diabetes mellitus and hypertension. He adds to this list "a touch of arthritis." His daughter complains to the charge nurse that her father seems to be spending more and more time during the day napping and that he says he does not sleep well at night. A comprehensive sleep assessment of Mr. Bitner after his daughter's expression of concern reveals the following data.

SLEEP–WAKEFULNESS PATTERN

- Patient goes to bed between 8 and 9 PM and gets out of bed between 7 and 8 AM because the staff are getting his roommate out of bed at this time. He states he never falls asleep before midnight because he always watched the late news at home. He usually wakes twice during the night to void and often cannot go back to sleep.
- During the day, patient is frequently observed dozing in his chair. If not discouraged, he returns to his room midmorning and afternoon for a 1-hour nap.

EFFECT OF SLEEP PATTERN ON EVERYDAY LIVING

- Patient states: "I'm always tired. I don't seem to have much energy anymore."

- Patient has not socialized yet with other residents and, without strong encouragement, does not participate in group activities.
- From his point of view, life holds little reason for him to be awake. "I worked for the railroad for almost 50 years and I never overslept once."

SLEEP AIDS

- Patient denies ever using medication to fall asleep. States he often relaxed at home in the evening with a couple of beers.
- Patient likes a dim light on during the night so that he can find the bathroom easily and likes his bedroom door ajar.
- Patient sleeps with two blankets and is often still cold.

SLEEP DISTURBANCES AND CONTRIBUTING FACTORS

- Patient states: "Ever since my wife died, I'm just not getting enough sleep, and since I came here it's worse. I don't know why I don't fall asleep when I go to bed or why I wake up so much. It sure makes the nights long."
- Patient has no regular periods of exercise and drinks black coffee with every meal as well as one or two diet colas in the evening.

NURSING DIAGNOSIS	Disturbed Sleep Pattern: involving difficulty falling asleep and remaining asleep related to new sleep environment and schedule, evening caffeine intake, and insufficient meaningful daytime activity
EXPECTED OUTCOME	By the next monthly assessment, 1/20/14, the patient will: • Retire after viewing the 11 PM news in the TV room with Mr. Sparter

NURSING PLAN OF CARE 33-1 *continued*

for Mr. Bitner

NURSING INTERVENTIONS	RATIONALE	EVALUATIVE STATEMENT
Assess advisability of reestablishing Mr. Bitner's usual retiring pattern of going to bed after the 11 PM news. Assess how patient spends the time from the evening meal to 11 PM— explore relaxing alternatives with him. Investigate possibility that he and Mr. Sparter might become social partners.	Strengthens the natural rhythm of his sleep–wake cycle. Elimination of evening naps will facilitate his falling asleep more easily.	1/18/14 Outcome met. Patient does not go to bed until after the news and has been observed talking with Mr. Sparter. *Recommendation:* Continue to develop evening activities with him—he finds that the time after supper "drags." *M. LeBon, RN*

EXPECTED OUTCOME By the next monthly assessment, 1/20/14, the patient will:

- Report that he falls asleep within 1 hour of getting into bed

NURSING INTERVENTIONS	RATIONALE	EVALUATIVE STATEMENT
Continue to assess how long it takes patient to fall asleep after getting into bed. Explore with patient means to relax before falling asleep—deep breathing, imagery, prayer. Teach the importance of using the bed only as a place to sleep. Advise patient when he cannot sleep to get out of bed and to go to another room where he can perform some monotonous activity (watching television, listening to radio).	In elderly patients, stage I time is increased. Activities that calm and relax the person prepare the body for sleep. This maintains the bed as a powerful stimulus for sleep and helps to prevent "conditioned" insomnia ("Well, here I am in bed now and I know sleep won't come").	1/18/14 Outcome partially met. Three or four nights a week, he falls asleep within 30 minutes of going to bed. States he really misses comfort of his wife. *Revision:* Investigate patient's sense of loss and need for touch. May be a good candidate for pet therapy program. *M. LeBon, RN*

EXPECTED OUTCOME By the next monthly assessment, 1/20/14, the patient will:

- Decrease nighttime awakenings to one, after which he returns to a sound sleep

NURSING INTERVENTIONS	RATIONALE	EVALUATIVE STATEMENT
Assess and manipulate factors that contribute to nighttime awakenings: • Need to void (time of day diuretic is taken, amounts of fluid intake in the evening) • Roommate's wakefulness, snoring, or need for care • Uncomfortableness in strange environment • Comfort (e.g., temperature) Teach patient how, on awakening, to concentrate on breathing until he falls back to sleep.	Individualizing the patient's bedtime environment and meeting comfort needs (warmth, soft light, and so forth) promote sleep onset and maintenance. This uses the power of positive thinking to facilitate return to sleep.	1/18/14 Outcome partially met. Nighttime awakenings vary from none to three nightly. See previous revision. *M. LeBon, RN*

(continued)

NURSING PLAN OF CARE 33-1 *continued*

for Mr. Bitner

EXPECTED OUTCOME By the next monthly assessment, 1/20/14, the patient will:

- Attend the center's exercise sessions Monday through Friday at 10 AM.

NURSING INTERVENTIONS	RATIONALE	EVALUATIVE STATEMENT
Assess whether patient understands the relation between daily exercise and his ability to sleep.	Regular exercise throughout the day is known to increase physical fatigue and to promote sleep. Exercise or stimulating activities immediately before retiring interfere with sleep's onset.	1/20/14 Outcome met. Patient has become an enthusiastic participant in exercise sessions—attends daily. *M. LeBon, RN*
Determine how his exercise needs can best be met (i.e., through a group program or an individualized program of walking, or other program).	Exercise program must be individualized based on physical state and interests of patient.	
Use positive verbal reinforcement to communicate to patient that someone cares that he is using positive means to remedy his sleep disturbance and increase his well-being.	Activity provides the opportunity for socialization and improvement of a self-image. Positive reinforcement promotes continued participation.	
Encourage patient's daughter to go for walks with him when she visits and to question him about his exercise program.	Communications and interaction with family members helps the elderly patient to maintain self-esteem and to feel valuable and loved.	

EXPECTED OUTCOME By the next monthly assessment, 1/20/14, the patient will:

- Substitute caffeine-free beverages for coffee and cola at supper and evening snack

NURSING INTERVENTIONS	RATIONALE	EVALUATIVE STATEMENT
Assess patient's willingness to substitute caffeine-free beverages for coffee and cola.	Caffeine is a stimulant that can cause difficulty sleeping.	1/20/14 Outcome met. Patient now drinks decaffeinated coffee with meals and milk in the evening. Dislikes caffeine-free sodas. *M. LeBon, RN*
Consult with dietary department and his daughter about options. Experiment with options until his preferences are determined.	Caffeine-free versions of beverages are often available and can be used based on patient acceptance.	
Gradually reduce his caffeine intake, especially from evening meal onward. Offer a carbohydrate evening snack.	Carbohydrate snack appears to promote sleep.	

NURSING PLAN OF CARE 33-1 *continued*

for Mr. Bitner

SAMPLE DOCUMENTATION	12/20/13 Nursing Family conference to discuss Mr. Bitner's sleep disturbance—initiated by daughter's concern. Present were Mr. Bitner and his daughter (A. Jelner), K. Behner (social worker), W. Quing (activity director), and M. LeBon (primary nurse). Primary nurse presented findings from comprehensive sleep assessment: Nursing diagnosis: Disturbed Sleep Pattern: difficulty falling asleep and remaining asleep related to new sleep environment and schedule, evening caffeine intake, and insufficient meaningful daytime activity. Discussion centered on strategies to help Mr. Bitner develop interests in the center, including possibilities for increased physical exercise, decrease his evening caffeine intake (daughter to bring noncaffeinated colas), and reestablish usual retiring and waking times. See plan of care. Patient's progress will be evaluated at next monthly assessment, 1/20/14. *M. LeBon, RN*

DEVELOPING CLINICAL REASONING

1. Interview three adults of varying ages (young, middle, elderly) about their sleep and rest patterns, using the Focused Assessment Guide in this chapter. Explore the special problems experienced by each of the adults, the efficacy of the self-help measures they use to cope, and helpful nursing interventions.

2. Interview three practicing nurses who are recent graduates. Using the Focused Assessment Guide in the text, ask them: if they are getting adequate rest, what factors are compromising their rest (e.g., working double or rotating shifts), how any lack of rest is affecting their practice, and what self-help measures have they used or would be appropriate. Discuss with your classmates the situation of practicing nurses with sleep alterations, the factors that place nurses at risk for sleep alterations, and what students can learn to lower their risk.

PRACTICING FOR NCLEX

1. A nurse assesses a patient's body temperature in the late afternoon as 37.2°C (99°F). What would be the nurse's best action related to this slight elevation in temperature?
   a. Assess the patient for infection.
   b. Record the temperature as a normal finding.
   c. Call the physician for an order for antipyretics.
   d. Decrease the room temperature.

2. A nurse observes some involuntary muscle jerking in a sleeping patient. The nurse determines that the patient is most likely in which stage of sleep?
   a. Stage I NREM sleep
   b. Stage II NREM sleep
   c. Stage IV NREM sleep
   d. REM sleep

3. A nurse observes a slight increase in a patient's vital signs while he is sleeping during the night. According to the patient's stage of sleep, the nurse expects what conditions to be true? Select all that apply.
   a. He is aware of his surroundings at this point.
   b. He is in delta sleep at this time.
   c. It would be most difficult to awaken him at this time.
   d. This is most likely an NREM stage.
   e. This stage constitutes around 20% to 25% of total sleep.
   f. The muscles are relaxed in this stage.

4. A nurse working the night shift at a hospital observes the developmental factors that may affect sleep. Which statements accurately describe these variations? Select all that apply.
   a. REM sleep constitutes much of the sleep cycle of a preschool child.
   b. By the age of 8 years, most children no longer take naps.
   c. Sleep needs usually decrease when physical growth peaks.
   d. Many adolescents do not get enough sleep.
   e. Total sleep decreases in adults with a decrease in stage IV sleep.
   f. Sleep is less sound in older adults and stage IV sleep may be absent.

5. A nurse is discussing with an older female patient the factors that affect sleep. What fact does the nurse teach her?
   a. Drinking a cup of regular tea at night induces sleep.
   b. Using alcohol moderately promotes a deep sleep.
   c. Aging decreases the amount of REM sleep a person experiences.
   d. Exercising decreases REM and NREM sleep.

6. A nurse is assessing patients in a skilled nursing facility for sleep deficits. Which patients would be considered at a higher risk for having sleep disturbances? Select all that apply.
   a. A patient who has uncontrolled hypothyroidism
   b. A patient with coronary artery disease
   c. A patient who has gastroesophageal reflux (GERD)
   d. A patient who is HIV positive
   e. A patient who is taking corticosteroids for arthritis
   f. A patient with a urinary tract infection

7. A nurse is providing discharge teaching for patients regarding their medications. For which patients would the nurse recommend actions to promote sleep? Select all that apply.
   a. A patient who is taking iron supplements for anemia
   b. A patient with Parkinson disease who is taking dopamine
   c. An elderly patient taking diuretics for congestive heart failure
   d. A patient who is taking antibiotics for an ear infection
   e. A patient who is prescribed antidepressants
   f. A patient who is taking low-dose aspirin prophylactically

8. A nurse working the night shift in a pediatric unit observes a 10-year-old male patient walking the hallway in a sleep state. The child is unaware of his environment and doesn't recall the incident in the morning. Which sleep disorder would the nurse expect?
   a. Bruxism
   b. Cataplexy
   c. Restless leg syndrome
   d. Somnambulism

9. A nurse is performing a sleep assessment on a patient being treated for a sleep disorder. During the assessment, the patient falls asleep in the middle of a conversation. The nurse would suspect which disorder?
   a. REM behavior disorder
   b. Narcolepsy
   c. Enuresis
   d. Sleep apnea

10. A nurse is teaching a patient with a sleep disorder how to keep a sleep diary. Which data would the nurse have the patient document? Select all that apply.
    a. Daily mental activities
    b. Daily physical activities
    c. Morning and evening body temperature
    d. Daily measurement of fluid intake and output
    e. Presence of anxiety or worries affecting sleep
    f. Morning and evening blood pressure readings

11. To promote sleep in a patient, a nurse suggests what intervention?
    a. Follow the usual bedtime routine if possible.
    b. Drink two or three glasses of water at bedtime.
    c. Have a large snack at bedtime.
    d. Take a sedative-hypnotic every night at bedtime.

12. A nurse formulates the following diagnosis for an elderly patient who is having trouble getting to sleep at night: Disturbed Sleep Pattern: Initiation of Sleep. Which of the following nursing interventions would the nurse perform related to this diagnosis? Select all that apply.
    a. Arrange for assessment for depression and treatment.
    b. Discourage napping during the day.
    c. Decrease fluids during the evening.
    d. Administer diuretics in the morning.
    e. Encourage patient to engage in some type of physical activity.
    f. Assess medication for side effects of sleep pattern disturbances.

13. A nurse is caring for a patient who states he has had trouble sleeping ever since his job at a factory changed from the day shift to the night shift. Which diagnosis would be most appropriate for this patient?

   a. Ineffective Coping: Multiple Stressors of New Job
   b. Sleep Deprivation: Difficulty Falling Asleep
   c. Disturbed Sleep Pattern: Altered Sleep–Wake Pattern
   d. Risk for Injury: Activity Intolerance/Sleep Deprivation

14. A nurse caring for patients in a busy hospital environment should implement which recommendation to promote sleep?
    a. Keep the room light dimmed during the day.
    b. Keep the room cool.
    c. Keep the door of the room open.
    d. Offer a sleep aid medication to patients on a regular basis.

15. A nurse caring for patients in a long-term care facility is implementing interventions to help promote sleep in elderly patients. Which action is recommended for these patients?
    a. Increase physical activities during the day.
    b. Encourage short periods of napping during the day.
    c. Increase fluids during the evening.
    d. Dispense diuretics during the afternoon hours.

ANSWERS WITH RATIONALES

1. **b.** A slight increase in body temperature in the late afternoon is the result of a normal circadian rhythm and does not need to be reported unless it becomes higher. This slight variation from normal does not necessarily mean an infection is present. A warm environment might cause an elevation in body temperature, but the most likely cause is normal circadian rhythm.

2. **a.** Involuntary muscle jerking occurs in stage I NREM sleep. In the other stages, the muscles proceed from a relaxed state to large muscle immobility.

3. **c, e.** This scenario describes REM sleep. During REM sleep, it is difficult to arouse a person, and the vital signs increase. REM sleep constitutes about 20% to 25% of sleep. In stage I NREM sleep, the person is somewhat aware of surroundings. Delta sleep is NREM stages III and IV sleep. In stage IV NREM sleep, the muscles are relaxed, whereas small muscle twitching may occur in REM sleep.

4. **d, e, f.** Many adolescents do not get enough sleep due to the stresses of school, activities, and part-time employment causing restless sleep. Total sleep time decreases during adult years, with a decrease in stage IV sleep. Sleep is less sound in older adults, and stage IV sleep is absent or considerably decreased. REM sleep constitutes much of the sleep cycle of a young infant, and by the age of 5 years, most children no longer nap. Sleep needs usually increase when physical growth peaks.

5. **c.** The nurse would teach the patient that the amount of REM sleep decreases with age. Regular tea contains caffeine and increases alertness. Large quantities of alcohol limit REM and delta sleep. Physical activity increases both REM and NREM sleep.

6. **a, b, c.** A patient who has uncontrolled hypothyroidism tends to have a decreased amount of NREM sleep, especially stages II and IV. The pain associated with coronary artery disease and myocardial infarction is more likely with REM sleep, and a patient who has gastroesophageal reflux (GERD) may awaken at night with heartburn pain. Being HIV positive, taking corticosteroids, and having a urinary tract infection does not usually change sleep patterns.

7. **b, c, e.** Drugs that decrease REM sleep include barbiturates, amphetamines, and antidepressants. Diuretics, antiparkinsonian drugs, some antidepressants and antihypertensives, steroids, decongestants, caffeine, and asthma medications are seen as additional common causes of sleep problems.

8. **d.** Somnambulism (sleepwalking) may range from sitting up in bed to walking around the room or the house to walking outside the house. The sleepwalker is unaware of the environment. Bruxism is grinding of one's teeth and frequently is an indicator of stress. Cataplexy is a sudden loss of motor tone that may cause the person to fall asleep; it is usually experienced during a period of strong emotion. People with restless leg syndrome (RLS) cannot lie still and report unpleasant creeping, crawling, or tingling sensations in the legs.

9. **b.** Narcolepsy is an uncontrollable desire to sleep; the person may fall asleep in the middle of a conversation. REM Behavior Disorder (RBD) is characterized by "acting out" dreams while asleep. Enuresis is urinating during sleep or bedwetting. Sleep apnea is a condition in which breathing ceases for a period of time between snoring.

10. **a, b, e.** A sleep diary includes mental and physical activities performed during the day and the presence of any anxiety or worries the patient may be experiencing that affect sleep. A record of fluid intake and output, body temperature, and blood pressure is not usually kept in a sleep diary.

11. **a.** Keeping the same bedtime schedule helps promote sleep. Drinking two or three glasses of water at bedtime will probably cause the patient to awaken during the night to void. A large snack may be uncomfortable right before bedtime; instead, a small protein and carbohydrate snack is recommended. Taking a sedative-hypnotic every night disturbs REM and NREM sleep, and sedatives also lose their effectiveness quickly.

12. **a, b, e, f.** For patients who are having trouble initiating sleep, the nurse should arrange for assessment for depression and treatment, discourage napping, promote activity, and assess medications for sleep disturbance side effects. Limiting fluids and administering diuretics in the morning are appropriate interventions for Disturbed Sleep Pattern: Maintaining Sleep.

13. **c.** When assessment data point to a sleep problem that is amenable to nursing therapy, it receives the label Disturbed Sleep Pattern if the problem is time limited (such as changing shifts) or Sleep Deprivation if the problem is prolonged. The labels Ineffective Coping and Risk for Injury have not yet been determined.

14. **b.** The nurse should keep the room cool and provide earplugs and eye masks. The nurse should also maintain a brighter room environment during daylight hours and dim lights in the evening, and keep the door of the room closed. Sleep aid medications should only be offered as prescribed.

15. **a.** In order to promote sleep in the elderly patient, the nurse should encourage daily physical activity such as walking or water aerobics, discourage napping during the day, decrease fluids at night, and dispense diuretics in the morning or early evening.

TAYLOR SUITE RESOURCES

Explore these additional resources to enhance learning for this chapter:

- NCLEX-Style Questions and other resources on **thePoint**, http://thePoint.lww.com/Taylor8e
- *Study Guide for Fundamentals of Nursing, 8th edition*
- Adaptive Learning | Powered by prepU, http://thepoint.lww.com/prepu

Bibliography

Agency for Healthcare Research and Quality (AHRQ). (2011). Treating sleep apnea. Available at http://effectivehealthcare.ahrq.gov/ehc/products/117/684/sleep_ap_consumer.pdf

American Sleep Association (ASA). (2010). Parasomnias. Available at http://www.sleepassociation.org/index.php?p=aboutparasomnias

Anderson, P. (2012). Hospital noise, especially alarms, most disruptive to sleep. Available at http://www.medscape.com/viewarticle/767459

Bulechek, G., Butcher, H., Dochterman, J., & Wagner, C. (2013). *Nursing interventions classification (NIC)* (6th ed., p. 349). St. Louis: Elsevier/Mosby.

Buysse, D., Germain, A., Moul, D., Franzen, P., Brar, L., Fletcher, M., ... Monk, T. (2011). Efficacy of brief behavioral treatment for chronic insomnia in older adults. *Archives of Internal Medicine, 171*(10), 887–895.

Caruso, C. (2012a). Better sleep: Antidote to on-the-job fatigue. *American Nurse, 7*(5), 45–46.

Caruso, C. (2012b). Running on empty: Fatigue and healthcare professionals. Available at http://www.medscape.com/viewarticle/768414

Chen, P. (2012). The clatter of the hospital room. Available at http://well.blogs.nytimes.com/2012/08/02/the-clatter-of-the-hospital-room/?ref=health&pagewanted=print

Elfstrom, M., Karlsson, S., Nilsen, P., Fridlund, B., Svanborg, E. & Brostrom, A. (2012). Decisive situations affecting partners' support to continuous positive airway pressure-treated patients with obstructive sleep apnea syndrome. *Journal of Cardiovascular Nursing, 27*(3), 228–239.

Fuller, T., & Bain, E. (2010). Shift workers give sleep short shrift. *American Journal of Nursing, 110*(2), 28–30.

Hart, C. (2012). Sleep and obesity in children: A review. Available at http://www.medscape.org/viewarticle/766237

Haupt, B. (2012). Instituting Quiet Hour improves patient satisfaction. *Nursing, 42*(4), 14–15.

Healthy People 2020. (2012). Sleep health. Available at http://www.healthypeople.gov/2020/topicsobjectives2020/overview.aspx?topicid=38

Hedges, C., & Ruggiero, J. (2012). Treatment options for insomnia. *The Nurse Practitioner: The American Journal of Primary Health Care, 37*(1), 14–19.

Jeffrey, S. (2011). FDA approves Intermezzo, first drug for early awakening. Available at http://www.medscape.com/viewarticle/754201

Johnson, K. (2011). Sleep deprivation in medical caregivers has deadly results. Available at http://www.medscape.com/viewarticle/745022?src=mp&spon=24

The Joint Commission (TJC). (2011). Sentinel Event Alert, 48. Available at www. http://jointcommission.org/assets/1/18/sea_48.pdf

Lehne, R. (2013). *Pharmacology for Nursing Care* (8th ed.). St. Louis: Elsevier/Saunders.

Marcus, C., Brooks, L., Draper, K., Gozal, D., Halbower, A., Jones, J., ... Shiffman, R. (2012). Diagnosis and management of childhood obstructive sleep apnea syndrome. Available at http://pediatrics.aappublications.org/content/early/2012/08/22/peds.2012-1671

Moorhead, S., Johnson, M., Maas, M., & Swanson, E. (2013). *Nursing outcomes classification (NOC)* (5th ed., p. 697). St. Louis: Elsevier/Mosby.

Moye, M. (2010). Sleep deprivation in the ICU. *Advance for Nurses, 12*(20), 12(20), 7–13.

NANDA International (NANDA-I). (2012). *NANDA nursing diagnoses: Definitions & classification: 2012–2014.* West Sussex, UK: Wiley-Blackwell.

National Heart Lung and Blood Institute (NHLBI). (2010). What is narcolepsy? Available at http://www.nhlbi.nih.gov/health/health-topics/topics/nar/

National Sleep Foundation (NSF). (2012). Does night work put women's health at risk? Available at http://sleepfoundation.org/alert/does-night-work-put-womens-health-risk

National Sleep Foundation (NSF). (2011a). Insomnia and sleep. Available at http://sleepfoundation.org/sleep-disorders-problems

National Sleep Foundation (NSF). (2011b). Diet, exercise and sleep. Available at http://www.sleepfoundation.org/article/sleep-topics/diet-exercise-and-sleep

National Sleep Foundation (NSF). (2011c). Drowsy driving. Available at http://www.sleepfoundation.org/article/sleep-topics/drowsy-driving

National Sleep Foundation (NSF). (2011d). Extreme sleepiness. Available at http://www.sleepfoundation.org/article/sleep-related-problems/idiopathic-hypersomnia-and-sleep

National Sleep Foundation (NSF). (2011e). Food and sleep. Available at http://www.sleepfoundation.org/article/sleep-topics/food-and-sleep

National Sleep Foundation (NSF). (2011f). Narcolepsy and cataplexy. Available at http://sleep-foundation.org/sleep-disorders-problems/excessive-daytime-sleepiness-disorders/narcolepsy-and-cataplexy

National Sleep Foundation (NSF). (2011g). Restless legs syndrome (RLS) and sleep. Available at http://www.sleepfoundation.org/article/sleep-related-problems/restless-legs-syndrome-rls-and-sleep

National Sleep Foundation (NSF). (2011h). Sleep studies. Available at http://www.sleepfoundation.org/article/sleep-topics/sleep-studies

Porth, C. (2011). *Essentials of pathophysiology: Concepts of altered health states* (3rd ed.). Philadelphia: Wolters Kluwer Health/Lippincott Williams & Wilkins.

Restless Legs Syndrome Foundation (RLS). (2012). FDA approves new medication for restless legs syndrome. Available at https://www.rls.org/document.doc?id=2201

Restless Legs Syndrome Foundation (RLS). (2011). Changing the name of RLS. Available at http://www.rls.org/namechange

Schardt, D. (2012). (2012). Sleep on it. *Nutrition Action Newsletter, 39*(3), 9–11.

Sherwood G., & Barnsteiner, J. (2012). *Quality and Safety in Nursing*. West Sussex, UK: Wiley-Blackwell.

Simmons, S., & Pruitt, B. (2012). Sounding the alarm for patients with obstructive sleep apnea. *Nursing, 42*(4), 34–41.

Stokowski, L. (2012). Help me make it through the night (shift). Available at http://www.medscape.com/viewarticle/757050

U.S. Food and Drug Administration (FDA). (2011). FDA approves Horizant to treat restless legs syndrome. Available at http://www.fda.gov/NewsEvents/Newsroom/PressAnnouncements/ucm250188.htm

Wallis, I. (2012). Hospital noise puts patients at risk. *American Journal of Nursing, 112*(4), 17.

Yoder, J., Staisiunas, P., Meltzer, D., Knutson, K., & Arora, V. (2012). Noise and sleep among adult medical inpatients: far from a quiet night. *Archives of Internal Medicine, 172*(1), 68–70.

34

Comfort and Pain Management

CARLA POTTER

Carla is a 26-year-old woman. She reports "bad cramps" and periodic fatigue, anxiety, irritability, and mood swings approximately 1 week before the start of her menses. She told the nurse practitioner that her job as a computer programmer is stressful and these monthly symptoms are affecting her job performance and relationships.

SHEREE LINCOLN

Sheree, a 42-year-old woman who has just undergone abdominal surgery, returns to the medical–surgical unit. Patient-controlled analgesia (PCA) is prescribed. Approximately 2 hours after returning from surgery, the patient is complaining of pain. Assessment reveals that she has not been using the PCA device.

XAVIER MALTON

Xavier, a 5-year-old boy diagnosed with ulcerative colitis, is in the bathroom with his mother. He suddenly grabs his belly while on the toilet and starts to scream, "Something hurts really bad!" His mother pulls the emergency call bell. He is doubled over in pain and can't get off the toilet. After being assisted back to his bed and receiving the smallest dose of pain medication possible as per the physician's order, Xavier continues to scream for half an hour more as he curls up in a fetal position on his bed. "The pain is so bad, it will never go away!"

LEARNING OBJECTIVES

After completing the chapter, you will be able to accomplish the following:

1. Describe specific elements in the pain experience.

2. Compare and contrast acute and chronic pain.

3. Identify factors that may affect a person's pain experience.

4. Obtain a complete pain assessment using appropriate interviewing and physical assessment skills.

5. Develop nursing diagnoses that correctly identify pain problems and demonstrate the relationship between pain and other areas of human functioning.

6. Demonstrate the correct use of nonpharmacologic pain relief measures.

7. Administer analgesic agents safely to produce the desired level of analgesia without causing undesirable side effects.

8. Collaborate with the members of other health disciplines, using different treatment modalities to promote pain relief.

9. Use teaching and counseling skills to empower patients to direct their own pain management programs.

KEY TERMS

acute pain	intractable	phantom pain
addiction	modulation	
adjuvant	neuromodula-tors	physical dependence
analgesic		placebo
breakthrough pain	neuropathic pain	psychogenic pain
chronic pain	neurotransmit-ters	referred pain
cutaneous pain	nociceptors	
dynorphin	nociceptive pain	remission
endorphins		somatic pain
enkephalins	opioid	tolerance
ethnocentrism	pain threshold	transduction
exacerbation	pain tolerance	transmission
gate control theory	perception	visceral pain

Pain is a common reason for seeing a physician and for taking medication. It is estimated that approximately 116 million Americans suffer from chronic pain and as much as $635 million is spent annually to treat it (Pfeifer, 2011).

Additional costs of inadequately treated pain include physiologic and psychological effects, caregiver burden, social isolation, disability and lost work productivity, and spiritual implications (Westbrook & D'Arcy, 2012; Galloway, Buckenmaier, & Polomano, 2011). Physiologic and psychological effects of pain include hyperglycemia, immune system dysfunction, altered coagulation, gastrointestinal (GI) ileus, urinary retention, decreased lung volume, sympathetic nervous system stimulation, and psychological distress (Smeltzer, Bare, Hinkle, & Cheever, 2010).

Scientists and clinicians have united in their efforts to ensure that pain management is a high priority in our health care system. New advances in understanding and treating pain have focused on the real possibility of controlling most human pain. The Joint Commission (TJC) supports the patient's right to pain management and has published standards for assessment and management of pain in hospitals, ambulatory care settings, long-term care, and home care settings (TJC, 2012b). The Joint Commission recommendations for health care organizations include teaching all patients to rate their pain using a pain rating scale, determining a pain rating goal with each patient, and providing appropriate care to treat the pain (TJC, 2012a).

A person in pain often experiences the pain as an all-consuming reality and wants only one intervention—pain relief. If pain relief were as simple as rubbing a back or administering a prescribed analgesic, the nurse's task would be easy. However, no two people experience pain exactly the same way. Differences in individual pain perception and response to pain, as well as the multiple and diverse causes of pain, require the nurse to have and use highly specialized knowledge and abilities to promote comfort and to relieve pain. The most essential of these are the nurse's knowledge and understanding that the patient's pain is real, the willingness to become involved in the patient's pain experience, and a competence in developing effective pain management regimens. (See the accompanying Reflective Practice box for an example.)

Although pain is often all consuming for patients, it can be missed or misjudged easily because it is intangible. As a result, it is often easier to overlook or minimize a patient's poorly communicated pain than it is to ignore a dressing that needs to be changed, the need for assistance with walking, or the administration of a prescribed medication. Nurses who somehow manage to practice nursing while remaining insensitive to the comfort needs of their patients do a grave disservice to these patients and to the nursing profession itself.

This chapter discusses the pain experience and factors that influence it. A detailed guide to assessing pain is presented, along with numerous examples of nursing diagnoses and specific nursing strategies for promoting comfort and assisting patients to achieve pain management goals. The concluding nursing plan of care illustrates how to use specific nursing interventions based on knowledge of and sensitivity to the patient's pain experience to resolve pain problems successfully.

REFLECTIVE PRACTICE: CULTIVATING QSEN COMPETENCIES

CHALLENGE TO ETHICAL AND LEGAL SKILLS

While working as a childcare technician one summer, I took my job quite seriously. As a nurse-in-training, I saw this job as an extension of my nursing education. I believed that the standards of care to which I held myself in my clinical rotations, and to which my professors held me, applied just as diligently in this job. I quickly found that I was the only childcare technician on the floor who held myself, let alone everyone else, to such high standards. In addition, I was quite dismayed to find that my standards for quality were actually higher than those of most of the registered nurses (RNs) employed on that unit. Nonetheless, I did not let that dissuade me. I sought out the few RNs whose standards were on par with mine, and I tried to work with them as often as possible.

One particular evening, about 15 minutes before our 12 1/2-hour shift was finally over, I was very grateful to be working with one such nurse. The quality of care that one of my patients was receiving from the physicians during an episode of acute pain was what I could only kindly call substandard.

I was caring for Xavier Malton, a 5-year-old boy diagnosed with ulcerative colitis, a form of inflammatory bowel disease (IBD). Suddenly, at the end of this relatively quiet shift, the emergency call bell alarm sounded. Frantically searching the switchboard for the source of the alarm, I realized that it was coming from Xavier's bathroom. As I ran the 10 feet to his room, thoughts of him bleeding internally or perforating his bowel ran through my head. I got there at the same time his nurse did, only to discover that his mother had pulled the alarm because her son had suddenly grabbed his belly while on the toilet and had started screaming that something was hurting very much. He was so doubled over in pain that he could not even get off the toilet. Having Crohn's disease myself, another form of IBD, I knew that the pain this boy was experiencing was excruciating and not imagined.

Over the course of the next half hour, his physicians reluctantly allowed us to drag them into his room, but they would only examine him after we insisted it was necessary because they could be dealing with an obstruction or a perforated bowel that might need surgery. Their attitude was that since he had IBD, abdominal pain was part of that, and that we should just "Let it pass" uneventfully, giving him the smallest dose of pain medication possible—which we did.

However, Xavier continued to scream, literally, for half an hour more, as he lay curled up in a fetal position on his bed. From across the hallway, I could hear him screaming that the pain was "so bad" and that it would never go away.

Thinking Outside the Box: Possible Courses of Action

- I can "give up" and try not to care since this system clearly is not committed to meeting comfort needs. But this means abandoning my patients.
- I could be persistent about advocating for this patient until his pain is relieved—trying to get as many health care professionals on my side as possible.
- I can consult with a colleague whom I respect about the best way to accomplish the above, since I don't want to alienate caregivers with whom I will need to continue to work.

Evaluating a Good Outcome: How Do I Define Success?

- Patient's pain is relieved and patient reports feeling comfortable.
- Colleagues are newly committed to the responsibility of *everyone* to adequately manage pain.
- My working relationships with other professional caregivers are not compromised by my fierce advocacy for this patient.
- My personal and professional integrity remains intact.

Personal Learning: Here's to the Future!

Forty-five minutes after our shift had ended, Xavier's nurse and I were still following the physicians around, demanding that they reassess the patient and prescribe additional pain medication for him. Finally, we simply refused to leave the hospital until Xavier's pain was properly treated. We threatened to report them to The Joint Commission for substandard care, for allowing a 5-year-old child to scream and writhe in pain when all they needed to do was write a PRN order for additional pain medication.

Finally, they wrote the order. Unfortunately, the narcotic they ordered was in short supply in the hospital, and we had none on the floor. The pharmacy had none to give. We spent the next 15 minutes tracking some down. Finally, we did give Xavier additional pain medication—and ultimately, it did relieve his pain and he was able to fall asleep. However, we left the hospital almost an hour and a half after our shift had ended, time that was lost to Xavier and time for which we would not receive compensation.

Transforming the culture of health care is a daunting task. Challenging the traditionally all-powerful physician takes courage and commitment. Demanding an unacceptable situation be remedied requires an absolute belief in the rights of the patient. The situation was indeed unacceptable—even when everyone else thinks it is acceptable. Any RN facing a situation that has the potential to transform the culture of health care for the better has the responsibility to take advantage of that situation, no matter what the professional risk. I would recommend that any RN in a similar situation take the same steps that Xavier's nurse and I did. Fight for what you believe is right. Do not be afraid to challenge others who you think are wrong, even physicians. Be confident in your opinions. Refuse to back down. Remember that if you do not ensure that your patient's needs are met, maybe no one else will either. Advocate at all times for high-quality care, never settling for less.

Tracey Sara Miller, Georgetown University

(continued)

THE PAIN EXPERIENCE

Pain is an elusive and complex phenomenon, and despite its universality, its exact nature remains a mystery. It is one of the human body's defense mechanisms that indicates the person is experiencing a problem. Margo McCaffery (1979, p. 11) offers the classic definition of pain that is probably of greatest benefit to nurses and their patients: "Pain is whatever the experiencing person says it is, existing whenever he (or she) says it does." This definition rests on the belief that the only one who can be a real authority on whether, and how, a person is experiencing pain is that person. The International Association for the Study of Pain (IASP) further defines pain as an unpleasant sensory and emotional experience associated with actual or potential tissue damage (IASP, 1994).

Pain is present whenever a person says it is, even when no specific cause of the pain can be found. Health practitioners must rely on the patient's description of the pain because it is a subjective symptom that only the patient can identify and describe.

 CONSIDER Xavier Malton, the 5-year-old boy with ulcerative colitis who suddenly develops acute pain. The nurse demonstrates understanding that Xavier is indeed experiencing pain because of his screaming that something hurts. Furthermore, his screaming is validated by his body posture and inability to get off the toilet. ●

The Pain Process

The four specific physiologic processes involved in nociception (the ability to feel painful stimuli) include transduction, transmission, perception, and modulation of pain (Pasero & McCaffery, 2011).

Transduction

The activation of pain receptors is referred to as **transduction**. It involves conversion of painful stimuli into electrical impulses that travel from the periphery to the spinal cord at the dorsal horn. The **nociceptors**, or peripheral receptors, respond selectively to specific noxious stimuli. Additionally, when the threshold of perception for pain has been reached and when there is injured tissue, it is believed that the injured tissue releases chemicals that excite or activate nerve endings. For example, a damaged cell releases histamine, which excites nerve endings. Lactic acid accumulates in tissues injured by lack of blood supply and is believed to excite nerve endings, causing pain, or to lower the threshold of nerve endings to other stimuli (e.g., heat or pressure). The prolonged effect of pain stimuli acting on the central nervous system (CNS) can lead to sensitization, meaning that the threshold for activation of pain is lowered. At that point, even harmless stimuli can trigger pain; pain signals are faster and feel more intense.

Other substances are also released that stimulate nociceptors or pain receptors. These include bradykinin, prostaglandins, and substance P:

- Bradykinin, a powerful vasodilator that increases capillary permeability and constricts smooth muscle, plays an important role in the chemistry of pain at the site of an injury even before the pain message gets to the brain. It also triggers the release of histamine and, in combination with it, produces the redness, swelling, and pain typically observed when an inflammation is present.
- Prostaglandins are important hormone-like substances that send additional pain stimuli to the CNS.
- Substance P sensitizes receptors on nerves to feel pain and also increases the rate of firing of nerves.

Prostaglandins, substance P, and serotonin (a hormone that can act to stimulate smooth muscles, inhibit gastric secretion, and produce vasoconstriction) are **neurotransmitters**, substances that either excite or inhibit target nerve cells.

Receptors in the skin and superficial organs are incapable of responding selectively. However, mechanical, thermal, chemical, and electrical agents may stimulate them. Friction from bed linens and pressure from a cast are mechanical stimulants. Sunburn and cold water on a tooth with caries are thermal stimulants. An acid burn is the result of a chemical stimulant. The jolt of a static charge is an electrical stimulant.

Transmission of Pain Stimuli

Pain sensations from the site of an injury or inflammation are conducted along pathways to the spinal cord and then on to higher centers. These pathways are clearly defined in certain areas, but are still somewhat unclear in other areas. The overall process is known as **transmission**. No specific pain organs or cells exist in the body. Rather, an interlacing network of undifferentiated free nerve endings receives painful stimuli. Free nerve ending pain receptors include the afferent (those fibers carrying impulses from the pain receptors toward the brain) fast-conducting A-delta-fibers and the slow-conducting C-fibers. The larger A-delta-fibers transmit acute, well-localized pain; the smaller C-fibers convey diffuse, visceral pain that is often described as burning and aching. It is estimated that there are several million of these nerve endings in the body, numerous in the layers of the skin and in some internal tissues, such as the joint surfaces. In the deeper tissues of the body, the pain receptors are diffusely but unevenly spread.

A protective pain reflex is responsible for withdrawal of an endangered tissue from a damaging stimulus. Sensory impulses travel over A-fibers through the dorsal root ganglion to the dorsal horn of the spinal cord. At this point, the sensory nerve impulse synapses with a motor neuron, and the impulse is carried along efferent nerve pathways back to the site of the painful stimulus in a reflex arc. This results in an immediate muscle contraction that removes the injured part from the source of the pain. Figure 34-1 illustrates the transmission of the pain sensation, the initiation of the protective reflex response, and conscious awareness of the location, intensity, and quality of the pain after the impulse reaches the cortex.

Perception of Pain

The **perception** of pain involves the sensory process that occurs when a stimulus for pain is present. It includes the person's interpretation of the pain. The threshold of perception, the **pain threshold**, is the lowest intensity of a stimulus that causes the subject to recognize pain. This threshold is remarkably similar for everyone, but some studies have reached the conclusion that women have lower thresholds than men (Smeltzer et al., 2010). The possibility that men and women have different expectations relative to pain perception may be a contributing factor to pain threshold. Still, it is theorized by at least some authorities that the

FIGURE 34-1. Pain sensation and relief. (1) Pain's path begins as a message and is received by nerve endings in a burned finger. (2) The pain signal from the burned finger travels as an electrochemical impulse along the length of the nerve to the dorsal horn on the spinal cord, a region that runs the length of the spine and receives signals from all over the body. (3) The message is relayed to the thalamus, a sensory center in the brain where sensations such as heat, cold, pain, and touch first become conscious. (4) It then travels on to the cortex, where the intensity and location of pain are perceived. (5) Pain relief begins as a signal from the brain and descends by way of the spinal cord. (6) In the dorsal horn, chemicals such as endorphins are released to diminish the pain message from the injured finger.

phenomenon of adaptation does occur, that is, the pain threshold can be changed within a certain range. This phenomenon has been studied, for example, when prisoners of war reported that the pain of repeated torture was not as acute as it would have been under different circumstances. Many factors might well have played a role, but at least some adaptation appears likely.

Adaptation may also be demonstrated when a person's hand is immersed in warm water. A sensation of pain eventually occurs as the water is heated. However, the person can tolerate a higher temperature as water is gradually heated to the pain level than if the hand had been plunged into hot water without any preparation.

Modulation of Pain

The process by which the sensation of pain is inhibited or modified is referred to as **modulation**. The sensation of pain appears to be regulated or modified by substances called neuromodulators. These **neuromodulators** are endogenous opioid compounds, meaning they are naturally present, morphine-like chemical regulators in the spinal cord and brain. They appear to have analgesic activity and alter the perception of pain. These endogenous opioid compounds are believed to produce their analgesic effects by binding to specific opioid receptor sites throughout the CNS, blocking the release or production of pain-transmitting substances. Both pain and stress appear capable of activating the endogenous opiate system.

Endorphins and enkephalins are opioid neuromodulators. **Endorphins** are produced at neural synapses at various points along the CNS pathway. They are powerful pain-blocking chemicals that have prolonged analgesic effects and produce euphoria. It is suggested that endorphins may be released when certain measures are used to relieve pain, such as skin stimulation and relaxation techniques, and when certain pain-relieving drugs are used. The endorphin, **dynorphin**, has the most potent analgesic effect. However, many questions remain about endorphins.

Enkephalins, which are widespread throughout the brain and dorsal horn of the spinal cord, are considered less potent than endorphins. **Enkephalins** are thought to reduce pain sensation by inhibiting the release of substance P from the terminals of afferent neurons.

The Gate Control Theory of Pain

Many theories have attempted to explain the mechanism of pain. However, the **gate control theory** provides the most practical model regarding the concept of pain. It describes the transmission of painful stimuli and recognizes a relation between pain and emotions. The theory states that certain nerve fibers, those of small diameter, conduct excitatory pain stimuli toward the brain, but nerve fibers of a large diameter appear to inhibit the transmission of pain impulses from the spinal cord to the brain. There is a gating mechanism that is believed by some to be located in substantia gelatinosa cells in the dorsal horn of the spinal cord. The exciting and inhibiting signals at the gate in the spinal cord determine the impulses that eventually reach the brain. Thus, only a limited amount of sensory information can be processed by the nervous system at any given moment. When too much information is sent through, certain cells in the spinal column interrupt the signal as if closing a gate.

The brain can also influence the gating mechanism. Past experiences and learned behaviors, which are interpreted by the brain, regulate or adjust the eventual behavioral responses to pain. Thus, the gating mechanism appears to be influenced by the amount of activity in large and small afferent fibers in addition to nerve impulses that descend from the brain.

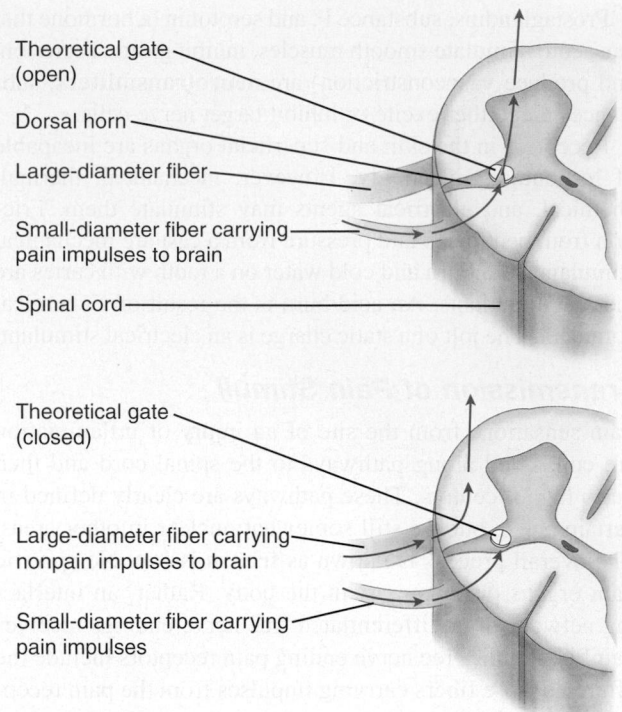

FIGURE 34-2. An illustration of the gate control theory of pain.

This helps explain why different people interpret similar painful stimuli differently. Although not everyone accepts the gate control theory, it appears to explain why mechanical and electrical interventions or heat and pressure may provide effective pain relief. Nursing measures, such as massage or a warm compress to a painful lower back area, stimulate large nerve fibers to close the gate, thus blocking pain impulses from that area. Figure 34-2 illustrates the gate control theory of pain.

Types of Pain

Pain may be classified according to its duration, its location or source, its mode of transmission, or its etiology.

Duration of Pain

Perhaps the most common distinction involves the duration of pain. **Acute pain** is generally rapid in onset and varies in intensity from mild to severe. It is protective in nature; that is, it warns the person of tissue damage or organic disease. After its underlying cause is resolved, acute pain disappears. It should end once healing occurs. Causes of acute pain include a pricked finger, sore throat, or surgery.

Chronic pain is pain that may be limited, intermittent, or persistent but that lasts beyond the normal healing period. The most recent definition of chronic pain no longer mentions the previous guideline of 3 to 6 months duration for pain to be considered chronic. Commonly, people with chronic pain experience periods of **remission** (when the disease is present but the person does not experience symptoms) or **exacerbation** (the symptoms reappear). Pain associated with cancer, or other progressive disorders, is termed chronic malignant pain. Pain in people whose tissue injury is non-progressive or healed is termed chronic nonmalignant pain. Recently, both cancer pain and chronic nonmalignant pain have been grouped together and referred to as prolonged or persistent pain.

Patients have difficulty describing chronic pain because it may be poorly localized. Moreover, health care personnel have difficulty assessing it accurately because of the unique responses of individual patients to persistent pain. Unlike acute pain, chronic pain is often perceived as meaningless and may lead to withdrawal, depression, anger, frustration, and dependency. In addition, the misconceptions and personal biases of caregivers can adversely affect the management of patients with chronic pain. Health care personnel may view people with chronic pain, in general, as hysterical personalities, malingerers, or hypochondriacs. Pain that is associated with a disease process, such as cancer, is more likely to be viewed as valid while pain that is not well defined may be misinterpreted or dismissed by health care providers. On the other hand, nurses who have experienced chronic pain or struggled through the experience with a loved one have a special awareness of its debilitating, destructive nature.

Nurses need an awareness of their own personal feelings toward pain (especially chronic pain) and the factors that affect pain if they are to assess and manage their patient's pain creatively and effectively. See Promoting Health 34-1 for a checklist of behaviors to foster one's self-awareness of comfort needs and pain.

Source of Pain

Pain can also be categorized according to its location. **Cutaneous pain** (superficial pain) usually involves the skin or subcutaneous tissue. A paper cut that produces sharp pain with a burning sensation is an example of cutaneous pain. Deep **somatic pain** is diffuse or scattered and originates in tendons, ligaments, bones, blood vessels, and nerves. Strong pressure on a bone or damage to tissue that occurs with a sprain causes deep somatic pain. **Visceral pain** is poorly localized and originates in body organs in the thorax, cranium, and abdomen. This pain occurs as organs stretch abnormally and become distended, ischemic, or inflamed. A reflex contraction or spasm of the abdominal wall, called guarding, may occur as a protective mechanism to prevent additional trauma to underlying structures. A person automatically tenses the abdomen when an acute abdominal pain condition is present. This prevents underlying tissues and organs from being palpated or touched.

 THINK back to Sheree Lincoln, the woman who has had abdominal surgery. Based on the nurse's understanding of the sources of pain, the nurse would identify that Sheree is most likely experiencing visceral pain, secondary to the effects of surgery on the abdominal organs. ●

Mode of Transmission

Pain also can be classified based on its mode of transmission. Pain can originate in one part of the body but be perceived in an area distant from its point of origin. This is known as **referred pain**. Pain associated with a myocardial infarction (heart attack) is frequently referred to the neck, shoulder, or arms (often the left arm). Referred pain is transmitted to a cutaneous (skin) site different from where it originated. This is possible because the pain can travel to other areas of the body innervated by the affected nerve root.

PROMOTING HEALTH 34-1

COMFORT

Use the assessment checklist to determine how well you are meeting comfort needs. Then, develop a prescription for self-care by choosing appropriate behaviors from the list of suggestions.

Assessment Checklist

❑ almost always	❑ sometimes	❑ almost never

❑ ❑ ❑ 1. Obtain a medical evaluation when acute or chronic pain is present.

❑ ❑ ❑ 2. Respect pain as the body's means of signaling that all is not well.

❑ ❑ ❑ 3. Control stress in the environment.

❑ ❑ ❑ 4. Avoid excessive fatigue.

❑ ❑ ❑ 5. Practice stress reduction or diversionary behaviors when pain is present.

❑ ❑ ❑ 6. Become aware of personal preconceived notions that affect your perception of pain in others.

Self-Care Behaviors

1. I seek medical attention when pain persists.
2. I am aware of my usual behavioral responses to pain.
3. I use stress reduction techniques regularly.
4. I am able to have a restful sleep at night.
5. I have a positive outlook about my present situation.
6. I am aware of how to use distraction strategies to deal with pain.

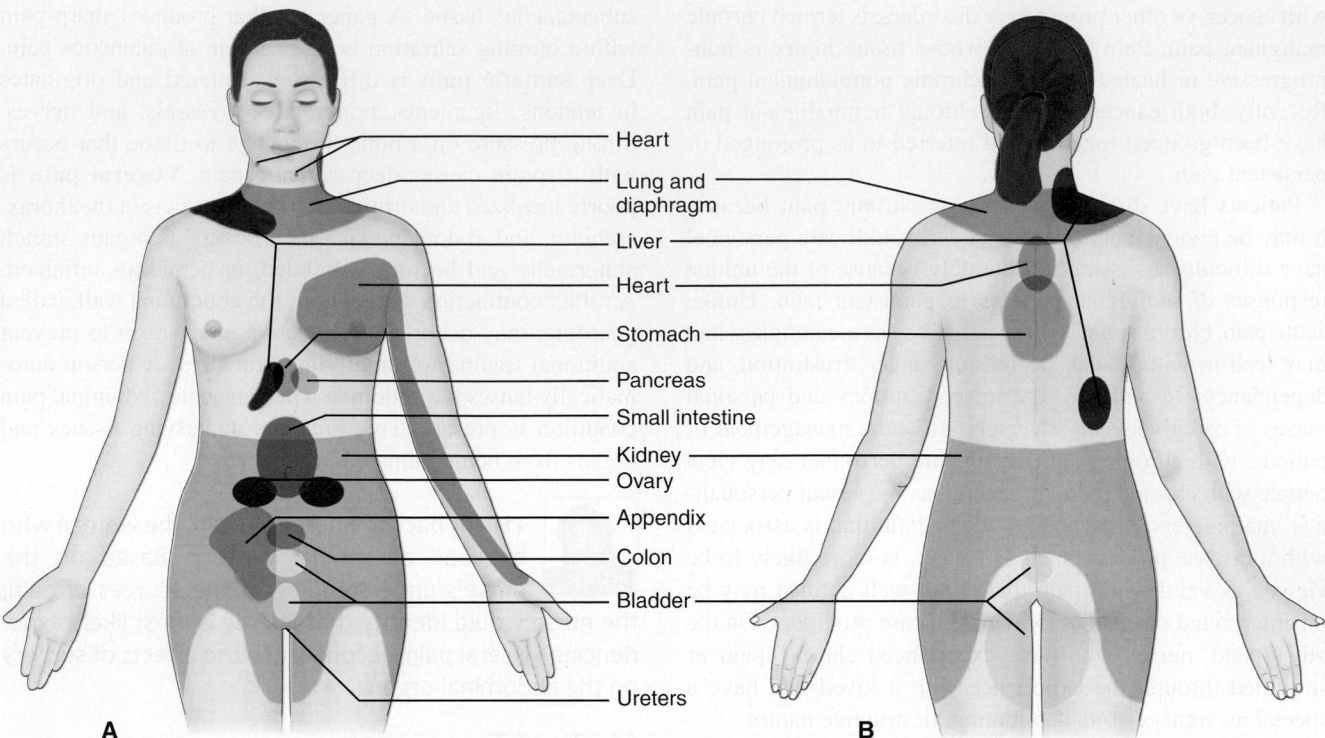

FIGURE 34-3. These drawings representing the anterior (**A**) and posterior (**B**) views of the body illustrate areas to which various organs refer pain.

Figure 34-3 illustrates cutaneous areas to which pain from various organs is usually referred.

Etiology

Pain also is classified by its cause, which can be highly varied. **Nociceptive pain** refers to the normal process that results in noxious stimuli being perceived as painful. **Nociceptors** are the peripheral nerve fibers that transmit pain from somatic and visceral sites. **Neuropathic pain** results as a direct consequence of a lesion or disease affecting abnormal functioning of the peripheral nervous system (PNS) or the CNS (D'Arcy, 2011a). The exact cause of neuropathic pain is unknown but it can originate either peripherally (e.g., phantom leg pain) or centrally (e.g., pain from spinal cord injury). Neuropathic pain can be of short duration but frequently is chronic. It is often described as burning, electric, tingling, or stabbing. Allodynia, a characteristic feature of neuropathic pain, is pain that occurs after a weak or nonpainful stimuli, such as a light touch or a cold drink, which normally should not cause pain. Numerous pain syndromes have been identified that produce neuropathic pain. Several common examples are included in Table 34-1. All of these pain syndromes are capable of causing severe pain. Appropriate treatment of these syndromes is often delayed as a result of misdiagnosis and can prove difficult to treat. Nursing can play an important role in their early detection.

When pain is resistant to therapy and persists despite a variety of interventions, it is referred to as **intractable**. Nurses and physicians together need to determine the appropriate pain treatment for each case of intractable pain so that a person can regain a healthy quality of life.

The pain that is often referred to an amputated leg where receptors and nerves are clearly absent is a real experience for the patient. This type of pain is called **phantom pain** or phantom limb pain and is without demonstrated physiologic or pathologic substance. One theory suggests that sensory misrepresentations from the missing limb may still remain in the brain, thereby causing phantom pain.

Pain may originate from physical causes, that is, a physical cause for the pain can be identified. Pain may also have a psychogenic origin (**psychogenic pain**), meaning that a physical cause for the pain cannot be identified. However, it has been observed that a pure origin is probably rare, and pain usually has both physical and psychogenic components. Furthermore, pain that results from a mental event can be just as intense as pain that results from a physical event.

Responses to Pain

The three types of responses to pain are physiologic, behavioral, and affective. Examples of these responses are listed in Box 34-1. The severity of pain and its duration affect responses to pain. Increases in vital signs may occur briefly in acute pain and may be absent in chronic pain states (Pasero & McCaffery, 2011).

 Concept Mastery Alert

Physiologic responses are involuntary body responses; behavioral responses reflect body movements; affective responses reflect mood and emotions.

Table 34-1   COMMON PAIN SYNDROMES PRODUCING NEUROPATHIC PAIN

PAIN SYNDROME	DESCRIPTION
Complex regional pain syndrome (causalgia)	Pain occurs in the area of a partially injured peripheral nerve (the most common lesions are of the brachial plexus or median or sciatic nerve). The pain is described as burning, severe, diffuse, and persistent and is elicited by minimal movement or touch of the affected area. It increases with repeated stimulation and continues even after stimulation ceases.
Postherpetic neuralgia	Pain syndrome follows an acute central nervous system infection, such as herpes zoster (shingles). The herpes syndrome is characterized by a vesicular eruption and neuralgic pain, which is usually unilateral and encircles the body in band-like clusters. The severity of the pain may be mild to severe. Intractable pain may persist for months to years.
Phantom limb pain	Pain that may occur in any person who has had a body part amputated either surgically or traumatically. Pain varies and may be a severe, burning, fiery sensation; crushing; cramping; a sense that the limb is edematous; or a sensation that the limb is being twisted and distorted. It may be triggered by the sensation of touching the stump, the occurrence of another illness, fatigue, atmospheric changes, and emotional stress.
Trigeminal neuralgia	Paroxysms of lightning-like stabs of intense pain in the distribution of one or more divisions of the trigeminal nerve, the fifth cranial nerve. Pain is usually experienced in the mouth, gums, lips, nose, cheek, chin, and surface of the head and may be triggered by everyday activities like talking, eating, shaving, or brushing one's teeth.
Diabetic neuropathy	A common complication of long-term diabetes mellitus. Metabolic and vascular changes result in damage to peripheral and autonomic nerves. Sensory loss can result when peripheral nerves are involved and eventually lead to injury progressing to infection and gangrene. Symptoms include sensations of numbness, prickling, or tingling (paresthesias).

 RECALL Xavier Malton, the child with ulcerative colitis experiencing an acute episode of pain. The nurse is initially able to assess that Xavier is in pain by his screams. Additionally, the nurse interprets his behavioral and affective responses, such as his body posture, inability to get off of the toilet, and later his fetal position in bed. Moreover, the nurse would validate these findings with physiologic responses such as skin color, muscle tension, and possibly vital signs. •

Mild pain experienced briefly may produce little or no behavioral response; intense pain experienced briefly usually results in reflex action to escape the cause. The patient often is able to accept pain that continues for a relatively

BOX 34-1   COMMON RESPONSES TO PAIN

Behavioral (Voluntary) Responses

Moving away from painful stimuli

Grimacing, moaning, and crying

Restlessness

Protecting the painful area and refusing to move

Physiologic (Involuntary) Responses

Typical Sympathetic Responses When Pain Is Moderate and Superficial

Increased blood pressure*

Increased pulse and respiratory rates*

Pupil dilation

Muscle tension and rigidity

Pallor (peripheral vasoconstriction)

Increased adrenalin output

Increased blood glucose

Typical Parasympathetic Responses When Pain Is Severe and Deep

Nausea and vomiting

Fainting or unconsciousness

Decreased blood pressure

Decreased pulse rate

Prostration

Rapid and irregular breathing

Affective (Psychological) Responses

Exaggerated weeping and restlessness

Withdrawal

Stoicism

Anxiety

Depression

Fear

Anger

Anorexia

Fatigue

Hopelessness

Powerlessness

*An increase in vital signs may occur briefly in acute pain but may not occur when chronic pain is present.

short time, such as for a few days or a week, without it being all-consuming. The patient expects relief and believes the cause is self-limiting. However, anxiety is ordinarily present. On the other hand, chronic pain tends to consume the entire person. It demands total attention so that the patient has limited resources to take care of other matters of daily living. It is physically and emotionally exhausting and tends to result in depression and irritability. Chronic fatigue usually accompanies chronic pain.

Lack of an obvious response to pain does not mean the patient is without pain. Careful assessment is especially important to understand what the patient is experiencing.

FACTORS AFFECTING THE PAIN EXPERIENCE

Pain is a highly personal experience. Many factors influence the comfort status of a person at any given moment. When a person experiences pain, almost anything can influence how the painful stimulus is transmitted to the brain, how it is perceived, and the response that is made to it.

A person learns to know what causes unpleasantness and what to interpret as pain. Each person's interpretation is influenced by background, such as how he or she has experienced and dealt with pain in the past, and what culture has taught the person about pain. Through past experiences, each person also learns to differentiate among the various types of pain and to associate pain with certain descriptive words. Table 34-2 lists common definitions for additional terms used by patients to describe pain.

Cultural and Ethnic Variables

Cultural norms dictate much of our daily behavior, attitudes, and values. Therefore, it is natural that culture influences the person's response to pain. **Ethnocentrism** refers to the tendency to believe that one's cultural norms are correct and are the standard used to evaluate other's beliefs (Narayan, 2010). Nurses, as a subculture, value self-control and the ability to function under stress. As a result, nurses may expect patients in pain to display a similarly calm, objective, uncomplaining approach to pain. Nurses need to understand that there are ways other than their own of responding to pain. It is particularly important to avoid stereotyping responses to pain because the nurse frequently encounters patients who are in pain or anticipating that it will develop. A form of pain expression that is frowned on in one culture may be desirable in another cultural group. Be knowledgeable about cultural variations and develop an understanding of cultural influences on pain tolerance, expressions of pain, and alternative practices used to manage pain.

By 2050, it is predicted that the minority population in the United States will increase from the current 30% to 54% (Narayan, 2010). This increase in cultural diversity and the accompanying different languages poses many challenges for pain assessment and management. When the patient's language differs from that of the nurse, assessment becomes even more difficult given the potential for misunderstanding

Table 34-2 | **ADDITIONAL TERMS USED TO DESCRIBE PAIN**

TERM	DESCRIPTION
Quality	
Sharp	Pain that is sticking in nature and that is intense.
Dull	Pain that is not as intense or acute as sharp pain, possibly more annoying than painful. It is usually more diffuse than sharp pain.
Diffuse	Pain that covers a large area. Usually, the patient is unable to point to a specific area without moving the hand over a large surface, such as the entire abdomen.
Shifting	Pain that moves from one area to another, such as from the lower abdomen to the area over the stomach.
Other terms used to describe the quality of pain include sore, stinging, pinching, cramping, gnawing, cutting, throbbing, shooting, and vise-like pressure.	
Severity	
Severe or excruciating Moderate Slight or mild	These terms depend on the patient's interpretation of pain. Behavioral and physiologic signs help assess the severity of pain. On a scale of 1 to 10, slight pain could be described as being between about 1 and 3; moderate pain, between about 4 and 7; and severe pain, between about 8 and 10.
Periodicity	
Continuous	Pain that does not stop.
Intermittent	Pain that stops and starts again.
Brief or transient	Pain that passes quickly.

the level of pain. People from different cultures may describe pain as an ache or a hurt. Each of these terms can reflect varying levels of intensity, with the term *pain* usually describing the most severe discomfort and *ache* the least pain.

Western cultures prefer medicinal approaches to control pain, whereas Eastern cultures gravitate toward medicinal herbs or energy therapies such as acupuncture as an attempt to balance yin and yang (Narayan, 2010). Health care providers increase their respect and sensitivity for diversity if they understand the effects of culture and ethnicity on the pain experience. Table 34-3 describes typical pain responses in selected ethnocultural groups. The nurse working with other ethnic groups can find pertinent studies in the literature and on various websites. However, it is important to note that the mixed ethnic heritage that is common today makes it more difficult to anticipate individual responses to pain.

Even though culture and ethnicity affect a patient's behavioral response to pain, consistent pain assessment is possible. Pain assessment tools have been translated into multiple languages and the assessment results can be similar across various cultures. A cultural accommodation such as

Table 34-3 PAIN EXPRESSION IN SELECTED ETHNOCULTURAL GROUPS

ETHNIC GROUP	RESPONSE TO PAIN
African Americans	Often viewed as a sign of illness or disease. Some believe that suffering and pain are inevitable. Spiritual and religious beliefs may contribute to high tolerance for pain. Some believe that praying and laying on of hands may aid in deliverance from pain and suffering.
Arab Americans	Often view pain as unpleasant and something that should be controlled. Tend to express pain openly with family members but may act in a more restrained manner in the presence of health professionals. Usually expect positive response from Western medical interventions to control pain.
Chinese Americans	Expressions of pain are usually similar to those of Americans. Often believe pain is related to the influence of imbalances in the yin and yang. The whole body's balance of yin and yang rather than just the area where pain is present is vital to one's wellness. The whole body must be treated and not just the symptoms. Usually cope with pain by using externally applied oils and massage as well as warmth, sleeping on the area of pain, relaxation, and aspirin.
Greek Americans	Ponos (pain) is viewed by most as an evil that needs to be eradicated. Physical and emotional pain are usually shared with the family. Family is considered a resource for pain relief because they act as advocates and provide emotional support.
Mexican Americans	Most delay seeking medical help for pain and hope, instead, that it will go away; consider it a necessary part of life. Seem to experience more pain than other ethnic groups but report it less frequently. Often see a direct relationship between pain and suffering and immoral behavior.
Navajo Indians	Do not usually openly express their pain or request pain medication. Adequate pain control is often difficult because they may mask the actual intensity of their pain. May prefer herbal medicines and use them without the knowledge of the health care provider.

Adapted from Purnell, L., & Paulanka, B. (2008). *Transcultural health care: A culturally competent approach* (3rd ed.). Philadelphia: F. A. Davis.

transposing a horizontal numeric pain rating scale to a vertical presentation may simplify pain assessment for a Chinese patient since this is the format in which the Chinese language is read (Pasero & McCaffery, 2011). Pain rating scales are discussed later in this chapter.

Recent research has confirmed that low-income and minority populations are less likely to receive the recommended treatments for pain in all health care settings. Although pain is undertreated in the general population, minority patients often experience pain for a lengthy period of time before seeking treatment for it. Their location in geographic areas that may not be easily accessible to health care facilities or pharmacies with insufficient supplies of pain medications may also be implicated as reasons for inadequate assessment and treatment. Language problems, culturally inappropriate pain assessment tools, and prejudice and misconceptions may contribute to unsatisfactory pain outcomes. There is agreement that health care providers need a focused awareness of these inequities and a concerted effort to confront these disparities (Meghani & Gallagher, 2012). Additional information on cultural influences on pain is presented in Chapter 5.

Family, Gender, and Age Variables

Other culturally related variables are family, gender, and age. A person's response to pain or symptoms may be affected or influenced by the response of family members. Spouses also may reinforce pain behavior in their partners.

Children growing up in different families may learn to "be brave" and ignore pain or to use the pain experience to secure attention and service from family members. Family size and birth order do not appear to be significant in distinguishing chronic pain sufferers.

Similarly, children may learn that there are gender differences in pain expression. It may be acceptable for a little girl to run home crying with a scraped knee, but a little boy may be told that he should be brave and not cry. Adult men and women may hold on to gender expectations regarding pain communication and incorrectly interpret the presence or absence of pain expressions in others. Women are more comfortable communicating the discomfort associated with pain, but this ability to verbalize may cause some to view the pain as emotionally or psychologically based. Several studies report that pain in women needs to be addressed more aggressively because their pain management is consistently reported as inadequate.

In addition, different age groups have different beliefs and norms regarding pain sensation and response. At one time, the infant's inability to communicate pain led health care practitioners to the erroneous assumption that pain sensation was diminished or absent. More recently, it has been demonstrated that infants and small children are sensitive to and experience pain. Among older people, pain has often been viewed as a natural component of the aging process, being ignored or undertreated by health care providers.

On the other hand, conditions normally painful in young adults (e.g., myocardial infarction) may result in minimal pain complaints in older people. That an older person does not complain of pain may indicate that the person fears the treatment for the pain or just refuses to give in to the pain. For many older adults, pain has become accepted as a daily occurrence and is regarded as part of the normal aging process. These variables, which influence pain sensation, perception, and response, make pain assessment a complex task for the nurse.

Religious Beliefs

Religious beliefs can be a powerful influence on the person's experience of pain. In some religions, people view pain and suffering as a "lack of goodness" in themselves. Thus, pain and suffering are viewed as a means of purification or of making up for individual and community sin. This meaning helps the person to cope with pain, thus becoming a source of strength. Patients with this belief may refuse analgesics and other pain relief measures, feeling that this lessens their suffering. On the other hand, illness and pain may also be viewed as punishment from a vengeful God. People may find their faith shaken and question the existence of a loving God. How can belief in a loving God be compatible with their present experience of pain? Anger, resentment, and depression may compound the pain experience. Patients may find it helpful to confer with a spiritual adviser about their pain experience.

Environment and Support People

A person's environment and the presence or absence of caring support people may also influence the experience of pain. Many people find that the strangeness of the health care environment, especially the lights, noise, lack of sleep, and constant activity of a critical care unit, compounds the experience of pain. The sense of powerlessness that accompanies admission to a health care facility may decrease the person's ability to cope with pain.

RECALL Sheree Lincoln, the postoperative patient in pain described at the beginning of the chapter. In addition to the pain related to surgery, the nurse would need to assess the effect of the environment on Sheree's pain. For example, she may be frightened by equipment being used postoperatively. Additionally, she may feel alone and powerless due to her current condition. Assessment also would need to include information about past experiences with pain, support persons available, and teaching she received preoperatively. ●

Depersonalization or separation from a favorite pillow, pet, or source of music may further decrease the person's sense of comfort. For some, the presence of a loved family member or friend is essential to their sense of well-being. Others prefer to be alone when in pain and may become agitated in the presence of a family member.

Some patients may use their pain to acquire secondary gains, such as special attention and services from their families. If unchecked, this tendency usually leads to resentment and anger in family members and their eventual avoidance of the patient. Intervening and attempting an honest discussion of this problem is important.

Anxiety and Other Stressors

Anxiety, which is almost always present when pain is anticipated or being experienced, tends to increase the perceived intensity of pain. The threat of the unknown is ordinarily more devastating and anxiety producing than a threat for which one has been prepared. Many studies have focused on the relationship between anxiety and pain or depression and pain, but the results are conflicting and unclear regarding these relationships. Until this has been confirmed, it is best to assume that pain is the responsible cause when anxiety or depression is also present (Pasero & McCaffery, 2011).

Although a cause-and-effect relationship has not clearly been verified, pain may be aggravated with anxiety, muscular tension, and fatigue. The rested and relaxed person can often cope with more discomfort than someone who is suffering from a lack of sleep.

THINK back to Carla Potter, the young woman experiencing "bad cramps" prior to her menses. She also reports anxiety, fatigue, and mood swings in addition to other symptoms. In order to individualize her plan of care, the nurse needs to gather additional data and investigate the possibility of specific relaxation measures that may effectively help Carla Potter to reduce some of the anxiety that she reports. ●

A person who is greatly fatigued and who has no competing demands requiring attention may experience pain more acutely. For example, many people have discovered that the pain of a foot ache or an ingrown toenail that was only mildly annoying during the day's work becomes unbearable at night when there is nothing else to distract the mind from the pain.

Past Pain Experience

A person's experience of pain in the past and the qualities of that experience profoundly affect new pain experiences:

- Some patients have never known severe pain and have no fear of pain, not realizing how intense the sensation can be.
- Some patients have experienced severe acute or chronic pain in the past but received immediate and adequate pain relief. These patients are generally unafraid of pain and initiate appropriate requests for assistance.
- Some patients have known severe pain in the past and were unable to secure relief. Even the suggestion of new pain can lead to acute feelings of fear, despair, and hopelessness.
- A person whose past pain experience led to correction of unhealthy behavior and produced a greater sense of health and well-being may respect and value pain and consider the meaning and significance of a new pain carefully.

- In general, people who have experienced more pain than usual in their lifetimes tend to anticipate more pain and to exhibit increased sensitivity to pain.
- Some pain memories are virtually unerasable; new contact with conditions similar to those that caused the earlier pain can provoke a violent response.

THE NURSING PROCESS FOR COMFORT AND PAIN MANAGEMENT

Assessing

Because the pain experience is unique to each person, the nurse who wants to help the patient achieve comfort and pain control needs sophisticated pain assessment skills. Assessing all factors that affect the pain experience—psychological, emotional, and sociocultural, as well as physiologic—is essential. Pain is complex and difficult to interpret and requires a reliable assessment tool.

Pain as the Fifth Vital Sign

In an effort to improve patients' quality of life and make pain management a priority, the American Pain Society, in 1995, encouraged caregivers to include assessment for pain as the fifth vital sign. Routine measurement of vital signs accompanied by a pain assessment raises awareness of the existence of pain, places additional emphasis on optimizing pain relief, and moves patients more quickly toward comfort and recovery.

The Joint Commission (TJC), in an effort to improve pain management, also developed accreditation standards that included emphasis on the patient's right to effective assessment and treatment of pain. These standards include the following:

- Patients have the right to appropriate assessment and management of their pain.
- Initial assessment and ongoing assessment of the existence of pain should also include the nature and intensity of the pain in all patients.
- Assessment results should be recorded in a manner that promotes regular reassessment and follow-up.
- Staff, including new clinical staff, must be oriented and competent in assessment and management of pain.
- The effect of oral analgesics must be evaluated 45 to 60 minutes after they are administered.
- IV analgesics should be reevaluated 15 to 30 minutes after administration.
- Policies and procedures that support prescription or ordering of pain medications must be in place.
- Pain must be managed so that it does not interfere with a patient's participation in rehabilitation.
- Patients and families require education about effective pain management.
- Discharge planning should address the patient's needs for management of pain symptoms.

- Data must be collected to monitor the appropriateness and effectiveness of the facility's pain management plan.

Common Misconceptions

Many patient misconceptions interfere with the patient's ability to communicate pain. It is important to assess for the following common patient beliefs related to pain and communicating it:

- The doctor has ordered pain-relieving medication for me, which I will be given routinely.
- If I ask for something for my pain, I may become addicted to the medication.
- Sometimes it is better to put up with the pain than to deal with the side effects of the pain medication.
- I should somehow be able to control my pain. It is immature to talk about pain.
- It is better to wait until the pain gets really bad before asking for help. If I take the medication now for moderate pain, it won't relieve severe pain later on.
- I don't want to bother anyone—I know how busy everyone is.
- It's natural for me to have pain after surgery. After a few days, I should notice it lessening.

 RECALL Sheree Lincoln, the woman who has undergone abdominal surgery. It would be important for the nurse to investigate Sheree's understanding of her postoperative pain and what her expectations are. Doing so would provide clues for the nurse indicating possible patient misconceptions about pain and pain relief, thereby providing a basis for teaching and correcting these misconceptions. ●

Pasero and McCaffery (2011) summarize additional misconceptions and prejudices about pain and pain relief that hamper the nurse's assessment and treatment of the patient with pain (available on thePoint).

Components of a Pain Assessment

The nurse will generally assess the following characteristics of pain:

- Patient's verbalization and description of the pain
- Duration of the pain
- Location of the pain
- Quantity and intensity of the pain
- Quality of the pain
- Chronology of the pain
- Aggravating factors
- Alleviating factors
- Physiologic indicators of the pain
- Behavioral responses
- Effect of the pain experience on activities and lifestyle

When assessing a person's pain, Pasero and McCaffery (2011) discuss these basic methods:

- Patient's self-report
- Report of family member, other person close to the patient, or caregiver who is familiar with the patient

FOCUSED ASSESSMENT GUIDE 34-1

THE PAIN EXPERIENCE

Factors to Assess	Questions and Approaches
Characteristics of the pain Location	*"Where is your pain? Is it external or internal?"* (Asking the patient with acute pain to point to the painful area with one finger may help to localize the pain. Patients with chronic pain may have difficulty trying to localize their pain, however.)
Duration	*"How long have you been experiencing pain? How long does a pain episode last? How often does a pain episode occur?"*
Quantity	Ask the patient to indicate the degree (amount) of pain currently experienced on the following scale:

0	1	2	3	4	5	6	7	8	9	10
No pain		Mild pain		Moderate pain			Severe pain			Pain as bad as it can be

It is also helpful to ask how much pain the patient has (on the same scale) when the pain is at its least and at its worst:

Least _____ Worst _____

Quality	*"What words would you use to describe your pain?"*
Chronology	*"How does the pain develop and progress?"* (If pattern can be identified, interventions early in a pain sequence will often be far more effective than those used after the pain is well established.) *"Has the pain changed since it first began? If so, how?"*
Aggravating factors	*"What makes the pain occur or increase in intensity?"*
Alleviating factors	*"What makes the pain go away or lessen? What methods of relief have you tried in the past? How long were they used? How effective were they?"* (Methods of relief currently in effect for hospitalized patients should be apparent from the chart. It is important to verify the use of current orders and their effectiveness with the patient. Outpatients may need to be asked to record a medication profile, a thorough and accurate account of all medications they are taking.)
Associated phenomena	*"Are there any other factors that seem to relate consistently to your pain? Any other symptoms that occur just before, during, or after your pain?"*
Physiologic responses Vital signs (blood pressure, pulse, respirations) Skin color Perspiration Pupil size Nausea	Signs of sympathetic stimulation may occur with acute pain but need not be present to verify the presence of pain. Signs of parasympathetic stimulation (decreased blood pressure and pulse, rapid and irregular respirations, pupil constriction, nausea and vomiting, and warm, dry skin) may occur, especially in prolonged, severe, visceral, or deep pain.
Muscle tension	Observe. Ask the patient whether he or she is aware of any tight, tense muscles.
Anxiety	Are signs of anxiety evident? (May include decreased attention span or ability to follow directions, frequent asking of questions, shifting of topics of conversation, avoidance of discussion of feelings, acting out, somatizing.)
Behavioral responses Posture, gross motor activities	Does patient rub or support a particular area? Make frequent position changes? Walk, pace, kneel, or assume a rolled-up position? Does patient rest a particular body part? Protect an area from stimulation? Lie quietly? (In acute pain, postural and gross motor activities are often altered; in chronic pain, the only signs of change may be postures characteristic of withdrawal.)
Facial features	Does the patient have a pinched look? Are there facial grimaces? Knotted brow? Overall taut, anxious appearance? (A look of fatigue is more characteristic of chronic pain.)
Verbal expressions	Does the patient sigh, moan, scream, cry, repetitively use the same words?

FOCUSED ASSESSMENT GUIDE 34-1 *continued*

THE PAIN EXPERIENCE

Factors to Assess	Questions and Approaches
Affective responses	
Anxiety	*"Do you feel anxious? Are you afraid? If so, how bad are these feelings?"*
Depression	*"Do you feel depressed, down, or low? If so, how bad are these feelings? Are your feelings about yourself mostly good or bad? Do you have feelings of failure? Do you see yourself or your illness as a burden to those you care about?"*
Interactions with others	How does the patient act when in pain in the presence of others? How does the patient respond to others when not in pain? How do significant others and caregivers respond to the patient when the patient is in pain? When the patient is not in pain?
Degree to which pain interferes with patient's life (use past performance as baseline)	*"Does the pain interfere with sleep? If so, to what extent? Is fatigue a major factor in the pain experience? Is the conduct of intimate or peer relationships affected by the pain? Is work function affected? Participation in recreational–diversional activities?"* (An activity diary is often helpful—sometimes crucial. One to several weeks of hourly activity recorded by the patient may be necessary. Levels of pain, intake of food, and sleep–rest periods are noted along with activities performed. Separate diaries for inpatient and outpatient episodes may be necessary because hospitalization markedly affects the nature and type of activities performed.)
Perception of pain and meaning to patient	*"Are you worried about your illness? Do you see any connection between your pain and the nature or course of illness? If so, how do you see them as related? Do you find any meaning in your pain? If so, is this beneficial or detrimental to you? Are you struggling to find some meaning for your pain?"*
Adaptive mechanisms used to cope with pain	*"What do you usually do to relieve stress? How well do these things work? What techniques do you use at home to help cope with the pain? How well have they worked? Do you use these in the hospital? If not, why not?"*
Outcomes	*"What would you like to be doing right now, this week, this month, if the pain were better controlled? How much would the pain have to decrease (on the 0–10 scale) for you to begin to accomplish these goals?"*

- Nonverbal behaviors (restlessness, grimacing, crying, clenching fists, protecting the painful area)
- Physiologic measures (increased blood pressure and pulse). However, most research verifies that reliance on vital signs to indicate the presence of pain should be minimized. The absence of an increase in vital signs does not mean that pain is not present.

Focused Assessment Guide 34-1 suggests questions and approaches helpful in assessing pain factors.

 Concept Mastery Alert

Assessment of pain requires information from a variety of sources. However, patients are the expert on their pain and their rating of the pain is most important.

Various forms used to help guide the assessment of pain have been described in the nursing literature. The primary purposes of using a guide to assess pain are to eliminate guesswork and biases when dealing with the patient's pain, to understand what the person is experiencing, to analyze findings that will help prepare an appropriate nursing response to the patient's pain, and to facilitate improved outcomes, such as fewer complications, shorter hospital stays, and improved quality of life.

For continued assessment of pain and evaluation of pain control measures, a pain scale allows the patient to rate effectively pain experienced on a continual basis. A numerical pain scale that is currently the national standard is displayed in the Focused Assessment Guide 34-1. This scale is best for use with verbally communicative patients.

Do not overlook pain in patients who have difficulty with communication. Their pain requires adequate treatment. Examples of pain rating scales that can be used with patients who are nonverbal or have difficulty communicating verbally include the Payen behavioral pain scale for use with critically ill patients who are intubated and the Face Legs Activity Cry and Consolability (FLACC) pain scale for use with infants and young children (from ages 2 months to 7 years) and with older adults who can't speak. Information about these pain-rating scales is included in Table 34-4. Whichever scale is used, it is best to use the same scale to rate a patient's pain throughout a hospital stay.

A comprehensive pain assessment must also include discussion of the patient's expectations for pain relief. The patient and health care team need to select a realistic goal or a number on the pain scale that is acceptable and satisfactory and that facilitates recovery. This helps the patient recognize and report pain that is unacceptable and

Table 34-4 PAIN ASSESSMENT SCALES

RESOURCE	WEBSITE	INDICATIONS
COMFORT Scale	http://pain.about.com/od/testingdiagnosis/ig/pain-scales/Comfort-Scale.htm	Infants, children, adults who are unable to use NRS or Wong–Baker FACES Pain Rating Scale
CRIES Pain Scale	http://pain.about.com/od/testingdiagnosis/ig/pain-scales/Cries-Scale.htm	Neonates (ages 0–6 months)
FLACC Scale	http://pain.about.com/od/testingdiagnosis/ig/pain-scales/Flacc-Scale.ht	Infants and children (2 months–7 years) who are unable to validate the presence of or quantify the severity of pain
Wong–Baker FACES Pain Rating Scale	http://www.wongbakerfamces.org/	Adults and children (>3 years old) in all patient care settings
0–10 Numeric Rating Scale	www.rehabmeasures.org/PDF%20Library/Numeric%20Pain%20Rating%20Scale%20Instructions.pdf	Adults and children (>9 years old) in all patient care settings who are able to use numbers to rate the intensity of their pain
Checklist of Nonverbal Indicators	http://prc.coh.org/PainNOA/CNPI_Tool.pdf	Adults who are unable to validate the presence of or quantify the severity of pain using either the Numeric Rating Scale or Wong–Baker FACES Pain Rating Scale
Oucher Pain Scale	http://www.oucher.org/history.html	Young children who can point to a face to indicate their level of pain
PAINAD Scale	http://web.missouri.edu/~proste/tool/cog/painad.pdf	Patients whose dementia is so advanced that they cannot verbally communicate
FPS-R (Faces Pain Scale – Revised)	www.iasp-pain.org/Content/NavigationMenu/GeneralResourceLinks/FacesPainScaleRevised/default.htm	Young children in parallel with numerical self-rating scales (0–10). Patients choose the depiction of a facial expression that best corresponds with their pain.
Payen Behavioral Pain Scale	http://www.consensus-conference.org/data/Upload/Consensus/1/pdf/1670.pdf	Useful with intubated, critically ill patients; measurement of bodily indicators of pain; and tolerance of intubation.

also allows caregivers to evaluate more readily the effectiveness of their pain management techniques.

Assessment of Special Populations

Pain rating scales attempt to confirm and, if possible, quantify the presence of pain in a variety of populations and situations. Alternative approaches to pain assessment for special populations ensure that unacceptable levels of pain are addressed and treated.

CHILDREN

In recent years, health care personnel have become much more concerned about addressing pain and pain relief in infants and children. Previously, it was believed that young children lacked the neurologic development to sense pain the way adults do. Thus, pain relief was not a priority when children were hospitalized. Young children frequently received no treatment for pain for medical or surgical procedures during their entire hospital stay. Yet, infants, particularly premature infants, are as sensitive to painful stimuli as older children and adults.

Despite advances in knowledge about pain in children, a recent study documented that pain was undertreated in children recovering at home following tonsillectomy or adenoidectomy. Parents used various pain rating scales to indicate when their children were experiencing pain, but only 24% of the 86% who were experiencing significant pain were medicated or received even one dose of the prescribed analgesic. This may have been due to the fact that parents did not recognize that their children were in pain or were reluctant to administer pain medication to young children for fear they may become dependent on it (Potera, 2010).

Current thinking is that inadequately controlled pain during infancy and childhood may alter a person's response to pain in adulthood. Children who learn unhealthy responses to chronic pain are more likely to become adults with chronic pain (Institute of Medicine [IOM], 2011). Pain is frustrating for children because they are unable to understand the concept and cause of pain and may have difficulty describing it. Depending on age, children may see the pain as a form of punishment for something that they have done. Therefore, assessment and management of pain in children is critical.

Current methods of assessing and measuring children's pain frequently involve use of more than one technique for assessment. A pain history provides information about the language the child uses to indicate pain, how and to whom this pain is usually reported, and indications of previous pain experiences and coping strategies. Self-report by the child is usually the most reliable account of pain. Communication with parents, guardians, or other important family members is also vital for accurate pediatric pain assessment and management. In addition, the following observations may provide an indication of the presence and severity of pain in a child:

- Irritability and restlessness
- Crying, screaming, or other verbal expression of pain
- Grimacing, grinding of teeth, or clenching fists
- Touching or grabbing of painful body part
- Kicking, thrashing, or attempting to move away from a painful stimulus

Numerous scales and tools can be used to assess a child's pain. One commonly used pain assessment scale, the Wong-Baker FACES pain rating scale (Fig. 34-4), asks children to compare their pain to a series of faces ranging from a broad smile to a tearful grimace. The Oucher pain scale, developed by Beyer and colleagues (1992) for use in young patients, combines a 0-to-100 scale with six photographic images of children in pain. This scale is helpful for use with older children. Adaptations of the Oucher pain scale are also available for various ethnic groups.

The CRIES Pain Scale is a tool intended for use with neonates and infants from 0 to 6 months. The COMFORT Scale, used to assess pain and distress in critically ill pediatric patients, relies on six behavioral and two physiologic factors that determine the level of analgesia needed to adequately relieve pain in these children. The FLACC scale (F—Faces, L—Legs, A—Activity, C—Cry, C—Consolability), designed for infants and children from age 2 months to 7 years who are unable to validate the presence or severity of pain, rates each of the five categories on a 0-to-2 scale. Additionally, children may be asked to record their pain experiences in a daily diary. Detecting

and accurately assessing pediatric pain have resulted in new and innovative approaches toward pain control in children.

 THINK back to Xavier Malton, the 5-year-old with acute pain. Incorporating the use of an age-appropriate pain assessment tool would be crucial in assessing Xavier's pain. Because Xavier is 5 years old, he may have difficulty describing his pain and its severity. For example, according to Xavier, "Something was hurting very much." Using the FACES scale or the Oucher scale would help the nurse to quantify the severity of Xavier's pain, providing objective evidence from which to intervene appropriately. The tool also would be extremely useful in determining the effectiveness of pain relief interventions, providing objective evidence denoting any changes in the pain's severity. This evaluation would serve as a basis for continuing pain management. ●

COGNITIVELY IMPAIRED PATIENTS

Assessment of pain in people who are cognitively impaired presents special challenges to nurses. It is generally recognized that people who are cognitively impaired are frequently undertreated because they may be unable to report pain verbally or describe the dimensions of their pain. Pain has been demonstrated as a possible cause of aggressive behavior in cognitively impaired older adults. Currently, some of these patients may be located in community-based settings rather than long-term care facilities and a variety of health care professionals may interact with these people. In order to manage their pain effectively, knowledge about accurate assessment of their pain is imperative (Baldridge & Andrasik, 2010).

To manage pain effectively, nurses must rely on their own careful assessments, their empathic qualities, and the expectation that a cognitively impaired patient will experience pain if a verbal patient usually reports this event as painful. Some common behaviors that can be

FIGURE 34-4. Wong-Baker FACES Pain Rating Scale. Instructions: Explain to the person that each face is for a person who feels happy because he has no pain (hurt) or sad because he has some or a lot of pain. *Face 0* doesn't hurt at all. *Face 2* hurts just a little bit. *Face 4* hurts a little more. *Face 6* hurts even more. *Face 8* hurts a whole lot. *Face 10* hurts as much as you can imagine, although you don't have to be crying to have this worst pain. Ask the person to choose the face that best describes how much pain he or she has. Rating scale is recommended for persons aged 3 years and older. (Reprinted with permission from Hockenberry, M. J., Wilson, D. [2013]. *Wong's essentials of pediatric nursing* (9th ed.]. St. Louis: Elsevier/Mosby.)

assessed for indicators of pain in this population include (Pasero & McCaffery, 2011):

- Facial expressions
- Verbalizations and vocalizations
- Body movements
- Changes in interpersonal interactions
- Changes in activity patterns or routines
- Changes in mental status

The combination of a history of pain, observations of a patient's pain by families and caregivers, and the presence of medical diagnoses associated with pain also facilitates pain assessment in this population. Moreover, special efforts are needed to identify accurate methods for assessing pain in this population. The Pain Assessment in Advanced Dementia (PAINAD) scale has been developed to assess pain in this population. It relies on observation of five specific items: breathing, vocalization, facial expression, body language, and consolability (Pasero & McCaffery, 2011). Refer to Table 34-4 on page 1164 for additional information regarding the PAINAD scale.

OLDER ADULTS

Assessing pain in the older adult population can be challenging. Adults over the age of 65 years experience pain more frequently than do younger adults and endure moderate to severe pain for twice as long as younger adults (Eliopoulos, 2010). Approximately 80% of older adults suffer with at least one chronic illness and experience varying degrees of discomfort (Jablonski, DuPen, & Ersek, 2011). Untreated chronic pain in older adults can result in disrupted sleep patterns, altered social activities, and a decline in their ability to complete the routine activities of daily living (Brown, Kirkpatrick, Swanson, & McKenzie, 2011). However, many see pain in the elderly as part of the normal aging process. Another myth held by many is that older patients have a decreased sensitivity to pain and, therefore, a heightened pain tolerance. Because many older people have chronic disease, pain is a common occurrence.

Assessment of pain in the older adult can be problematic. Vision or hearing impairments may influence the assessment format. Multiple-drug regimens that are common in older people can also affect reliable reporting of pain. Many older adults view pain as a forecast of serious illness or death, thus are reluctant to admit its occurrence or report it. Boredom, loneliness, and depression may affect an older adult's perception and report of pain.

Experts agree that pain can be adequately assessed in older adults using common rating scales. The Wong-Baker FACES Pain Rating Scale (see Fig. 34-4), recommended for pain assessment in children, may also be effective for this age group because a 0-to-5 scale is easier to use. The Numeric Rating Scale, the verbal descriptor scale, and the Faces Pain Scale–Revised (FPS-R; see Table 34-4 on page 1164) are additional pain rating scales that are also widely used for assessing pain in older adults. Some research has indicated that older adults prefer a vertical

Iowa Pain Thermometer (IPT)

FIGURE 34-5. Iowa Pain Thermometer (IPT).

pain scale such as the Iowa Pain Thermometer shown in Figure 34-5, rather than the horizontal numeric pain scales (McGuire, 2011). Special attention and consideration of an older patient's pain can positively affect the nurse's ability to assess pain accurately.

Diagnosing

Pain is such a complex phenomenon that its analysis often requires multidisciplinary collaboration. Although nursing has much to offer people experiencing both acute and chronic pain, the data collected by the nurse during the comprehensive pain assessment benefit the patient most when shared with physicians and other members of the health care team.

Attempting to intervene before an accurate assessment has been completed may mask the real cause of the patient's pain and lead to false assumptions and even further progression of symptoms and the disease process. The nurse who notes a pattern of headaches in a patient and relates this to the patient's description of recent stress (divorce, relocation, new job) may erroneously assume that the headaches are merely stress related and devise and implement a plan of relaxation exercises. A more careful analysis of patient data, however, may reveal that the headaches are of vascular origin, are migraine in nature, and that medical intervention is indicated. The headaches may also be symptomatic of intracranial disease such as a brain tumor, in which case delay in diagnosis could decrease the possibility of treatment and cure.

When a nursing diagnosis of acute or chronic pain is developed, the diagnostic statement and plan of care should identify the following:

- Type of pain
- Etiologic factors, to the extent that they are known and understood
- Patient's behavioral, physiologic, and affective responses
- Other factors affecting pain stimulus, transmission, perception, and response

Pain or Chronic Pain as the Problem

Many diagnoses can be developed for pain problems. The importance of identifying these problems and including them as priorities in the plan of care cannot be overstated. See the accompanying box, Examples of NANDA-I Nursing Diagnoses.

Pain or Chronic Pain as the Etiology

Because the experience of pain affects so many other aspects of human functioning, pain may be the etiology of numerous other nursing diagnosis statements, including but not limited to:

- Ineffective Airway Clearance related to postoperative incisional pain
- Anxiety related to pain anticipation and inadequate pain management in the past
- Constipation related to chronic use of narcotic analgesics
- Ineffective Health Maintenance related to loss of will to live secondary to prolonged chronic pain
- Hopelessness related to belief that present pain means imminent death
- Risk for Injury related to decreased pain sensation
- Fatigue related to lack of relief from chronic pain
- Fear related to possible significance of pain
- Disturbed Sleep Pattern from inability to fall asleep related to pain's worsening at night
- Risk for Spiritual Distress related to belief that God is unfairly causing this pain as some sort of undeserved punishment
- Risk for Self-Directed Violence related to loss of will to live with unrelieved chronic pain

Outcome Identification and Planning

After the diagnosis of a pain problem is made, developing and implementing a plan of care that demonstrates

EXAMPLES OF NANDA-I NURSING DIAGNOSES

PAIN

Nursing Diagnoses	Related Factors	Sample Defining Characteristics
Pain: Acute Postoperative	Fear of taking prescribed analgesics	• Recent cholecystectomy • Face is pale and drawn; vital signs elevated from baseline • States, "I don't like to ask for anything for pain because I know people often get addicted."
Pain	Prolonged labor (dystocia) and commitment to natural childbirth	• Admitted to labor unit 18 hours ago with moderate contractions 2 minutes apart • Strength of contractions weakening; progress of dilation and effacement slow; failure to progress • "I'll feel like a failure if I take anything for pain. I want to 'go natural.' I know I can do it. Besides, the drugs would only hurt my baby."
Chronic Pain: Headaches	Inadequate pain management secondary to belief that somehow patient "deserves this pain"	• Reports history of migraine headaches for past 5 years • Never sought treatment • "My mother told me that we all get the pain in life that we deserve—goodness, I've been no saint."
Chronic Pain	Inadequate pain management of metastatic cancer involving bone	• "I can't help feeling, though, that no one is meant to live like this." • Diagnosed with cancer of bladder 2 years ago; presently metastatic spread to spine • Rates pain 10 on a scale of 1 (minimal) to 10 (greatest) • "I haven't been taking as much of this pain medicine as the doctor said I could because if I get used to it now nothing will work when the pain gets even worse later." • "When I told the nurse in the hospital about my pain she said I'd have to get used to it." • "I don't want to burden my wife and kids with my pain."

nursing's commitment to assist the patient in developing effective pain management strategies is crucial.

Nursing measures are directed toward the achievement of the following patient outcomes for people whose pain is acute in nature (i.e., it is expected that with healing the pain will subside and eventually disappear). The patient will:

- Describe a gradual reduction of pain, using a scale ranging from 0 (no pain) to 10 (pain as bad as it can be)
- Demonstrate competent execution of successful pain management program (specify)

When pain or chronic pain is the etiology in nursing diagnosis statements, outcomes will be specific to the underlying interference with health that is associated with the pain.

For patients whose pain is chronic in nature, an expected outcome may be contacting a hospice or a pain clinic. Hospice care (also mentioned in Chapters 8 and 9) addresses the physical, spiritual, social, and economic needs of terminally ill patients and their families in either the home or a hospice center. Pain relief is a priority in this setting. Numerous outpatient centers are also available to support patients with chronic pain and to improve their pain management through a variety of approaches. The physician, nurse, and other members of the health care team collaborate to develop the optimal pain-treatment plan for each patient with chronic pain.

Implementing

After the plan of care is developed, the nurse implements the nursing strategies that are most likely to assist the patient to achieve pain relief outcomes, whether at home or in a health care facility. Nursing interventions described in this chapter include establishing a trusting nurse–patient relationship, manipulating factors that affect the pain experience, initiating nonpharmacologic pain relief measures, managing pharmacologic interventions, review-

ing additional pain control measures, ensuring ethical and legal responsibility to relieve pain, and teaching the patient about pain. See the accompanying box, Examples of Nursing Intervention and Nursing Outcome Classifications (NIC/NOC), for management of pain.

Establishing a Trusting Nurse–Patient Relationship

Most patients with pain feel better, suffer less, and experience less anxiety when they believe that a competent nurse cares about their experience of pain and is available for help and support. Without the confidence developed in a good nurse–patient relationship, nothing seems to work. With it, amazing results have been obtained by using measures that ordinarily are only modestly effective. Measures that help strengthen the nurse–patient relationship and promote pain relief include discussing pain with the patient, allowing the patient to help choose a method of pain relief, and visiting and remaining with the patient in pain. These measures promote a collaborative relationship in which the patient's pain is treated with respect (see the accompanying box, Through the Eyes of a Patient).

Manipulating Factors Affecting the Pain Experience

There are many ways to manage pain. In addition to pharmacologic and nonpharmacologic measures, simple nursing interventions can positively alter patients' pain experience and speed their recovery.

REMOVING OR ALTERING THE CAUSE OF PAIN

Removing or altering the cause of the pain is ideal and sometimes possible. Possible measures that promote comfort and help in pain relief include removing or loosening a tight binder, if permissible; seeing to it that a distended bladder is emptied; taking steps to relieve constipation and flatus; changing body positions and ensuring correct body alignment; and changing soiled linens and dressings

EXAMPLES OF NURSING INTERVENTION AND NURSING OUTCOME CLASSIFICATIONS (NIC/NOC)

PAIN MANAGEMENT

Nursing Interventions	Nursing Outcomes
• Perform a comprehensive assessment of pain to include location, characteristics, onset/duration, frequency, quality, intensity, and precipitating factors. • Consider cultural influences on pain response. • Explore with patient factors to relieve/worsen pain. • Assure patient attentive analgesic care.	• Pain: disruptive effects • Anxiety level • Pain level • Pain control • Self management: Acute illness • Self-management: Chronic disease

Bulechek, G., Butcher, H., Dochterman, J., & Wagner, C. (2013). *Nursing Interventions Classification (NIC)* (6th ed., pp. 285–286). St. Louis: Elsevier/Mosby. A full listing of nursing activities for each nursing intervention can be found in this book.

Moorhead, S., Johnson, M., Maas, M., & Swanson, E. (2013). *Nursing Outcomes Classification (NOC)* (5th ed., p. 719). St. Louis: Elsevier/Mosby. A full listing of nursing outcomes for each nursing diagnosis can be found in this book.

THROUGH THE EYES OF A PATIENT

I've always thought of myself as a "take charge" kind of person. It's important for me in my business to be calm and always in control of my emotions. The "big C" changed everything for me. A recent hospitalization made me take time to think about what's happening to me.

Even in the hospital, I had a steady stream of visitors—some friends and some business associates. Even the mayor stopped by to see me! For all of them, I was my usual self—smiling, joking, and acting as if everything was normal. I made sure I took my pain medicine before they came. I kept all my fears about cancer and dying hidden behind my smiling face. I never broke down—not even in front of my wife! Men aren't supposed to cry, you know!

One nurse's simple gesture changed all that. One evening after all my visitors, my wife, and my son had left, she must have sensed something. She came over, stood next to me, put her arm around my shoulders and quietly said, "You know, Bob, it's alright to cry." It was like the dam opened up. I looked at her, my face cracked, and all of a sudden I couldn't stop sobbing. She must have known that I needed to talk about what was happening to me. I needed to say those words out loud to someone—"I'm afraid the pain will get too bad! I'm afraid of dying. I can't let my family see me this way!" She just let me cry, kept holding my hands, and just by being there and listening, helped me at that particular moment in ways that you will never know.

that may be irritating the skin. A hungry or thirsty patient may need a snack or a drink to feel more comfortable.

Certain drugs are useful for removing or altering the intensity of painful stimuli. For example, drugs that decrease smooth-muscle spasms in the GI tract and those that decrease contractions of skeletal muscles reduce discomfort.

ALTERING FACTORS AFFECTING PAIN TOLERANCE

As a result of the pain assessment and the trusting relationship the nurse has established, the nurse is better able to identify those factors that are increasing the patient's pain experience and decreasing the patient's pain tolerance. **Pain tolerance** is the point beyond which a person is no longer willing to endure pain. Alleviate these factors whenever possible. For example, patients whose families have never acknowledged their pain and who have repeatedly been told that their pain is all in their head may experience a greater ability to deal with their pain when someone finally takes the pain seriously. Nursing measures include communication to the patient that responses to pain are acceptable and providing education to the patient's family.

Fatigue tends to increase pain, thus promoting rest is helpful. The patient in pain usually feels more comfortable when the environment is quiet and restful. Although sensory restrictions—such as eliminating unnecessary noise and bright lights—are usually indicated, it is rarely helpful to leave the patient alone in an environment with little sensory input. The patient is then more likely to focus on self and the discomfort.

Lack of knowledge, finding no meaning in the pain, being pessimistic about its relief, and fear may also interfere with the patient's ability to deal with pain. Common fears include a loss of control and embarrassment by being unable to deal with the pain maturely. Another fear may be a fear of taking pain relief medication. The patient may view the need for medication as a sign of weakness or may fear addiction or loss of the effectiveness at a later date. Older patients, in particu-

lar, are frequently frustrated by similar concerns about pain management.

Initiating Complementary and Alternative Relief Measures

Although analgesics are usually the primary treatment measure for pain, a growing trend is seen involving integration of complementary alternative medicine (CAM) therapies. These nonpharmacologic interventions are varied—they can be practiced in all health care settings and combined with conventional medical treatment. Refer to Chapter 27 for additional discussion of complementary and alternative relief measures.

USING DISTRACTION

Conscious attention often appears to be necessary to experience pain, whereas preoccupation with other things has been observed to distract the patient from pain. Distraction requires the patient to focus attention on something other than the pain. It is not entirely clear whether distraction raises the threshold of pain or increases pain tolerance. Many patients whose pain is relieved by distraction report being able to place pain in the periphery of awareness. This is compatible with the theory that if the reticular formation in the brainstem receives sufficient sensory input, it can ignore or block out select sensations such as pain. The Lamaze method of childbirth is one common example involving the use of distraction.

Distraction alone may relieve mild pain. However, it is most effective when used before pain begins or soon thereafter. It has also been proven effective when used with analgesics for treatment of a brief episode of severe pain (e.g., pain that accompanies a diagnostic procedure). Distraction may also be used successfully with children.

 RECALL Xavier Malton, the child with ulcerative colitis in severe pain. The nurse could incorporate the use of nonpharmacologic measures for pain relief, such as distraction, to enhance the effectiveness of analgesics. ●

Techniques that distract attention include the following:

- Visual distractions: counting objects, reading, or watching TV
- Auditory distractions: listening to music
- Tactile kinesthetic distractions: holding or stroking a loved person, pet, or toy; rocking; slow rhythmic breathing
- Interactive video games
- Project distractions: playing a challenging game, performing meaningful play or work

EMPLOYING HUMOR

Humor can be an effective distraction, can help a person cope with pain, and may even have a positive effect on the immune system. It has been proven beneficial in relieving acute painful procedural pain in children. Many pain, cancer, and ambulatory care centers encourage patients to view humorous videos before a painful, tedious procedure (IOM, 2011). Facente (2006) discussed the potential effects of laughter on a patient's ability to cope with pain and discomfort. These are highlighted in Box 34-2.

Remember to use humor only with patients who are responsive to its use and wish to use it. Humor should not be used in patients with moderate to severe pain, nor should it be a replacement for pharmacologic analgesia. In addition, humor must be patient specific. Thus, the nurse will need to determine what makes a patient laugh, how the patient has used humor or play in the past, and how it helped. Let the patient select the humorous materials, and when possible, incorporate strategies that include the patient's family and friends.

LISTENING TO MUSIC

Listening to music can relax, soothe, decrease pain, and provide distraction. By stimulating the release of endorphins, music enhances one's sense of well-being and decreases the need for pain medication. Recent studies have confirmed that postoperative music therapy resulted in a 50% reduction in pain intensity and patients needed less analgesia following surgery. Most of the music sessions were 30 minutes in duration. Patients can select the music they prefer for relaxation before, during, and after surgical experiences, or to help focus on breathing techniques during labor. Acute pain guidelines recommend music and relaxation as interventions that, in combination with opioids, help to relieve moderate postoperative pain. Music therapy has the potential to be an integral component of pain management therapies (Whitaker, 2010).

USING IMAGERY

Patients who use imagery (an example of mind–body interaction) to decrease pain sensation imagine something that involves one or all of the senses, concentrate on that image, and gradually become less aware of the pain. Imagery may be as simple as a child thinking of "happy things" (a beloved pet, lollipops, Christmas morning, Grandmom's lap) or as involved as an adult recreating a favorite place and then experiencing the healing presence or touch of a loved person or the healing energies of nature in that setting. The imagery technique has also been used to create an image in which the cause of the pain is visualized and then overcome or counteracted by some more powerful image.

Imagery has been found to be more effective for patients with chronic pain than for patients with acute, severe pain. General techniques for successfully guiding a patient to use imagery include the following:

- Help the patient to identify the problem or goal.
- Suggest that the patient begin the imagery with several minutes of focused breathing, relaxation, or meditation.
- Help the patient to develop images of the problem, as well as personal internal resources (e.g., coping strategies) and external healing therapies (e.g., medications, treatments).
- Encourage images of the desired state of well-being at the end of the session.

If the patient becomes restless or upset, the imagery experience is terminated and attempted later when the patient seems better disposed. See PICO in Practice 34-1. Guided imagery is also discussed in Chapter 41.

EMPLOYING RELAXATION

Relaxation techniques reduce skeletal muscle tension and lessen anxiety. By assisting the patient with relaxation techniques, the nurse acknowledges the patient's pain and expresses a willingness to help the patient relieve the distress caused by that pain. The positive effects of relaxation for the person with pain include the following (LeMone, Burke, & Bauldoff, 2011):

- Improved quality of sleep
- Distraction from the pain
- Decreased fatigue
- Increased confidence and sense of self-control in coping with pain
- Lessening of the detrimental physiologic effects of continued or repeated stress from pain

---

BOX 34-2 THERAPEUTIC EFFECTS OF LAUGHTER

Laughter causes the following physiologic and psychological effects:

- Decreases levels of epinephrine (the stress hormone)
- Activates the immune system
- Elevates the threshold for pain and can minimize the pain sensation
- Promotes spiritual and psychological coping
- Helps one to face difficult or unpleasant procedures
- Creates a more positive atmosphere
- Increases heart rate and stimulates circulation
- Deepens respirations
- Causes muscles to contract

Adapted from Facente, A. (2006). Humor in health care: Irreverent or invaluable? *Nursing, 36*(4), 64hn6–64hn7.

PICO IN PRACTICE

ASKING CLINICAL QUESTIONS

Scenario: You and your next-door neighbor Sarah walk your dogs together every day after work. Several times over the past few months, Sarah has sent you text messages during the work day, telling you that she cannot go walking with you because she is going home sick from work with migraine headaches. One evening during a walk, Sarah expresses her frustration to you. She tells you she has been diagnosed by her primary provider with chronic migraine headaches that are precipitated by work-related stress. She has been prescribed sumitriptan (Imitrex) for her migraines and it does provide relief. However, she wonders if there may be another nonpharmacologic therapy she may try instead that could help relieve her pain.

- POPULATION: Adult woman with chronic migraine headaches
- INTERVENTION: Nonpharmacologic intervention
- COMPARISON: Sumitriptan
- OUTCOME: Relief of migraine headache–associated pain

PICO Question: Among adult women with chronic migraine headaches, is there a nonpharmacologic intervention that may be as effective as sumitriptan in relieving the pain associated with migraine headaches?

Finding: From the Joanna Briggs Institute: Joanna Briggs Institute (2011). Nursing intervention for adult patients experiencing chronic pain. *Best practice: Evidence-based information sheets for health professionals, 15*(10), 1–4.

Within this best-practice information sheet, it is noted that guided imagery may be effective in managing chronic tension headaches with or without migraines. However, this therapy is noted to be effective only when used in tandem with conventional pharmacologic management. This recommendation was based on findings from one randomized controlled trial.

Level of Evidence: Level II

Recommendation: You tell Sarah that best practices at this time indicate that guided imagery may be effective at providing her with relief, but only if it is done while she continues to take her sumitriptan. She is unfamiliar with guided imagery, so you describe this complementary therapy to her and direct her to the National Center for Complementary and Alternative Medicine (NCCAM) of the National Institutes of Health (NIH) for further information, at http://nccam.nih.gov.

- Increased effectiveness of other pain relief measures
- Improved ability to tolerate pain
- Decreased distress or fear during anticipation of pain
- Reassurance that the nurse is aware of the person's problem and wants to help

Relaxation is most effective as a pain relief measure when combined with slow, deep, easy breathing from the abdomen or diaphragm, with the patient's eyelids closed or with the person focusing on a real or imagined fixed spot. Progressive muscle relaxation seems to have a positive effect on arthritis pain. Relaxation techniques are also discussed in Chapters 27 and 41.

 CONSIDER Carla Potter, the young woman with reported symptoms of premenstrual syndrome (PMS). Relaxation techniques may help her to better manage her periods of anxiety. The first step is to assess her familiarity with relaxation techniques and discuss which of these measures are adaptable to her work environment and are acceptable to her. ●

USING CUTANEOUS STIMULATION

The success of cutaneous stimulation (techniques that stimulate the skin's surface) in relieving pain is often explained using the gate control theory. The gate control theory of pain involves cutaneous nerve fibers, which are large-diameter fibers carrying impulses to the CNS. When the skin is stimulated, pain is believed to be controlled by closing the gating mechanism in the spinal cord. This decreases the number of pain impulses that reach the brain for perception. These techniques can be used in all health care settings to supplement a pain-control regimen. Some forms of cutaneous stimulation include the following:

- Massage (with or without analgesic ointments or liniments containing menthol); see Skill 34-1 on pages 1188–1191
- Application of heat or cold, or both intermittently (see detailed discussion in Chapter 31)
- Acupressure
- Transcutaneous electrical nerve stimulation (TENS)

Acupressure, a modern-day Western descendant of acupuncture, involves the use of the fingertips to create gentle but firm pressure to usual acupuncture sites. This technique of holding and releasing various pressure points has a calming effect, most likely related to the body's release of endorphins and enkephalins. Acupressure is easily taught to patients and families. Because patients can perform acupressure on themselves, it gives them a feeling of control in their care.

TENS is a noninvasive alternative technique that involves electrical stimulation of large-diameter fibers to inhibit transmission of painful impulses carried over small-diameter fibers. The TENS unit consists of a battery-powered portable unit, lead wires, and cutaneous electrode pads that are applied to the painful area (Fig. 34-6 on page 1172). The use of TENS requires a physician's order.

FIGURE 34-6. (A) TENS unit. **(B)** Applying TENS electrodes.

TENS therapy has reportedly been effective in reducing postoperative pain and improving mobility after surgery. Positive results have also been noted when it is used as an adjunct to physical therapy and for patients with low back pain. The TENS unit may be applied intermittently throughout the day or worn for extended periods of time, depending on the physician's order.

Use of cutaneous stimulation is limited because the pain must be localized. Otherwise, it is most likely too diffuse to be effective. In addition, most people cannot tolerate stimulation of the painful area; however, they may be helped by stimulation of the surrounding or contralateral area.

USING ACUPUNCTURE

Acupuncture is a technique that uses needles of various lengths inserted into specific parts of the body to produce insensitivity to pain. The technique was developed in China and has been used for centuries in many Asian countries. It has gained acceptance in the Western world as an alternative intervention to help control discomfort from disorders such as headaches, menstrual cramps, postoperative dental pain, fibromyalgia, osteoarthritis, low back pain, and carpal tunnel syndrome. The relief of pain by acupuncture is generally explained on the basis of the gate control theory. Chiropractors or doctors of oriental medicine (DOMs) administer acupuncture most often. This therapy is considered safe when an experienced practitioner who uses sterile acupuncture needles performs it. Self-hypnosis may also account for some of acupuncture's success. Repeated treatments are often needed (Simmons, 2011; NCCAM, 2010).

USING HYPNOSIS

Hypnosis, a technique that produces a subconscious state accomplished by suggestions made by a hypnotist, has been used successfully in many instances to control pain. The person's state of consciousness is altered by suggestions so that pain is not perceived as it normally would be. According to many hypnotists, it also alters the physical signs of pain. Many people can be taught autohypnosis, that is, self-induced hypnosis, for the control of pain. It is generally believed that a successful response to hyp-

nosis is related to the person's openness to suggestion, belief that hypnosis will work, and emotional readiness.

EMPLOYING BIOFEEDBACK

Biofeedback is a technique that uses a machine to monitor physiologic responses through electrode sensors on the patient's skin. The feedback signal or unit transforms the physiologic data into a visual display. Upon seeing pain-related responses, such as increased muscle tension or elevated blood pressure, the patient is taught to regulate this physiologic response and control pain by practicing techniques such as deep-breathing exercises, progressive relaxation exercises, or visual imagery. Biofeedback decreases the person's pain by reducing the anxiety associated with lack of control over bodily functions, distracts the person's attention from the pain to concentration on the person's inner state and the feedback signal, and reduces the cause of the pain. Eventually, the desired effect is for a person to produce the expected effect without the use of the biofeedback machinery. Limitations of this method include the high degree of motivation needed and difficulty of maintaining control after the training program.

PROVIDING HEALING/THERAPEUTIC TOUCH

Healing Touch is an energy therapy that has proved valuable as an adjunct to traditional medicine. Studies have indicated that it has been effective in reducing pain and anxiety in hospitalized patients and is recognized as an alternative therapy in end-of-life care (Sammons, 2011). It requires no equipment, uses light touch, and is appropriate for every level of care. Acceptance has been an obstacle for Healing Touch therapy but practitioners feel certain that the movement toward evidence-based practice will help Healing Touch gain credibility. See Research in Nursing box.

Therapeutic Touch is an alternative therapy that involves using one's hands to direct an energy exchange consciously from the practitioner to the patient to facilitate healing or pain relief. It is viewed by many as a powerful adjunct to pain relief therapy. Patients who have received therapeutic touch state that it helps with feelings of

RESEARCH IN NURSING

BRIDGING THE GAP TO EVIDENCE-BASED PRACTICE

The Effect of Healing Touch on Persistent Pain In Older Adults

It is common knowledge that pain is underassessed and undertreated, particularly in older adults residing in long-term care facilities. A majority of this population suffers from chronic pain, with estimates varying from 20% to 80%. Analgesics used to treat chronic pain can have adverse effects on older adults and their medication regimens are more complicated, leading to the potential for drug interactions. Many factors affect a person's reaction to pain including previous pain experiences and their effect on quality of life. The addition of a complementary nonpharmacologic approach to pain management, such as Healing Touch, addresses the subjective component of pain and provides an additional method to use to ease pain for people in this setting.

Related Research

Wardell, D., Decker, S., & Engebretson, J. (2012). Healing touch for older adults with persistent pain. *Holistic Nursing Practice*, 26(4), 194–202.

The goal of this research was to explore the effect that Healing Touch had on older adults with chronic pain living in a long-term care facility. Healing Touch is an alternative energy therapy that is thought to rebalance the system and promote healing. This was a secondary study meant as a follow-up to previous research. Twelve residents of five long-term care facilities participated in this study and had a Healing Touch intervention 3 times per week for 30 minutes over 2 weeks followed by a closing session with one of the three certified Healing Touch practitioners (CHTPs) who each had at least 5 years of experience and conducted the research sessions. The residents were at least 60 years old, were able to complete self-report data instruments, and had multiple painful chronic conditions and multiple medication regimens. Pain assessments including quality of life were completed pre- and postintervention. A participant's level of pain was measured using the Verbal Descriptor Scale. A tool for observational behavioral assessment of pain was also utilized. Only one of the participants did not have a positive response to the HT and none of the older adults had an adverse or negative response. There were varying degrees of response to Healing Touch in regard to pain relief. Initially, all the participants believed that HT would not help their "long-standing problems" but usually by the third session, they verified that it did provide some level of a positive effect on their pain. The researchers concluded that since pain has a subjective component and is an individualized experience, it is difficult to measure objectively the effects of Healing Touch on pain. They concur, however, that HT may offer a benefit to this population and provide positive outcomes.

Relevance to Nursing Practice

Healing Touch is just one of the nonpharmacologic, non-traditional nursing measures that might individualize care and take into account the varying complexities of aging and pain. Many patients as well as health care practitioners are unaware of the potential benefits of alternative approaches to pain management. Although it is difficult to measure and quantify, Healing Touch may offer a benefit to older adults with chronic pain issues. Coupled with nursing assessments, observations, and traditional treatments for pain, this complementary therapy provides an additional treatment modality as nurses strive to provide holistic care to their patients.

For additional research, visit thePoint.

---

comfort, calmness, and well-being. It is derived from the ancient practice of laying on of hands, but nurses skilled in Therapeutic Touch never actually touch their patients when using this technique. Therapeutic Touch was developed by nurses, does not require a physician's order, and can be used in any setting. Nurses caring for patients with terminal diseases relate that therapeutic touch complements their efforts to alleviate suffering and can be used to promote comfort during the final stages of life.

PROVIDING ANIMAL-FACILITATED THERAPY

Either a patient's own pet or an animal with an experienced handler can be used as complementary therapy to help relieve pain and provide a degree of comfort to people in various health care settings. The Delta Society is a relatively new organization that is responsible for providing the animal visits. These visits are either casual (*animal-assisted activities*—AAA) or more focused with a stated goal and documented results (*animal-assisted therapy*—AAT). Animals that visit patients include dogs, rabbits, guinea pigs, birds, and cats. AAT has been used to relieve pain in children in acute care settings and also has been effective in reducing pain and fatigue in adults with dementia. Specific Centers for Disease Control and Prevention (CDC) guidelines must be followed when animals are brought into a health care facility (D'Arcy, 2011b).

Managing Pharmacologic Relief Measures

Whether pain is acute or chronic, measures exist to control most pain experiences. However, many misconceptions still exist about pain relief, and because of this, many people still receive inadequate pain treatment and suffer needlessly. To make informed decisions and individualize care, nurses need updated information and ongoing education about drug therapy, the cornerstone of many pain-treatment regimens.

ADMINISTERING ANALGESICS

An **analgesic** is a pharmaceutical agent that relieves pain. Analgesics function to reduce the person's perception of pain and to alter the person's responses to discomfort.

There are three general classes of drugs used for pain relief:

- **Opioid** analgesics (all controlled substances; e.g., morphine, codeine, oxycodone, meperidine, hydromorphone, methadone)
- Nonopioid analgesics (acetaminophen and nonsteroidal anti-inflammatory drugs [NSAIDs])
- Adjuvant analgesics (anticonvulsants, antidepressants, multipurpose drugs)

The nurse administering analgesics needs to combine a healthy respect for the drug being administered with a thorough knowledge of its mechanism of action, side effects, and administration guidelines. This combination of knowledge of and respect for the drug should result in analgesics being used wisely to produce their desired effect.

Knowledge of common analgesics enables the nurse to tailor the patient's regimen and communicate professionally with physicians about a patient who is being undermedicated or who needs a different drug or a different route of administration. Nurses should not refrain from using analgesics or reduce their doses because of an unrealistic fear of their potency and side effects.

Repeated studies have confirmed improvement in pain assessment and documentation but not in pain relief. Pain is still undertreated and frequently unrelieved. Physician, nurse, and patient variables all contribute to this situation. Physicians often prescribe insufficient analgesic doses because of a tendency to overestimate the efficacy and duration of analgesics, underestimate the pain experience, and worry excessively about the possibility of respiratory problems and addiction. Nurses, who ideally spend the most time with the patient and who are supposed experts in human responses (e.g., the response to pain), often compound this problem by further reducing the insufficient analgesic dose or by not administering the medication at all. Nurse variables include the low priority given to pain management, arbitrary pain assessments and erroneous judgments about a patient's pain and need for analgesia, and fear of being the person who administers the drug that causes respiratory depression or another serious side effect. According to Pasero and McCaffery (2011), health care providers need to be held accountable for their failure to provide optimum pain relief for all people. The inability of many patients to discuss their pain and to request pain assistance perpetuates this problem.

Opioid Analgesics. Opioids, formerly called narcotic analgesics, are generally considered the major class of analgesics used in the management of moderate to severe pain because of their effectiveness. In sufficient dosage, they are considered capable of relieving pain of virtually every nature. Opioids produce analgesia by attaching to opioid receptors in the brain. Pasero and McCaffery (2011) compare this attachment as similar to a key fitting in a lock. New research on opioid analgesics also indicates that opioid receptors are present on peripheral terminals of sensory nerves and cells of the immune system (Pasero & McCaffery, 2011). Opioid receptor sites are further classified as mu, delta, and kappa types. The difference in opioid effects is related to their interaction with these three opioid types of receptors. Opioids that produce analgesia (agonists) can compete for binding sites on the receptors with opioids that do not produce analgesia (antagonists). An opioid agonist such as morphine binds to the mu site and produces analgesia that is also associated with unwanted side effects. An opioid antagonist such as naloxone (Narcan) also competes for binding on the mu site but it blocks the analgesic effect of morphine as well as its side effects. Most of the opioid analgesics commonly used in a clinical setting bind primarily to mu receptor sites. Patients also differ in their sensitivity to morphine because of genetic variability of the mu receptor site (Overdyk & Guerra, 2011). This is referred to as opioid polymorphism.

Morphine, the prototype opioid, is available in multiple dosage forms, has a fairly predictable action, and is relatively inexpensive. The most common side effects associated with opioid use are sedation, nausea, and constipation. Most side effects disappear with prolonged use, but if constipation persists, it usually responds to treatment with increased fluids and fiber and use of a mild laxative or stool softener. An opioid-naïve person can experience the side effects but has not taken opioids with enough frequency to become tolerant. This contrasts with an opioid-tolerant person who has taken opioids long enough and at sufficient levels to develop tolerance to the analgesic effect of the opioid and most of the side effects except constipation.

Respiratory depression is a commonly feared side effect of opioid use. In reality, it is an uncommon occurrence in long-term therapy because patients have usually developed a tolerance to the drug and its respiratory-depressant effects. However, studies have indicated that approximately half of the patients in an acute care medical–surgical setting who had a cardiopulmonary arrest had been receiving opioids. The most common events preceding these arrests are usually respiratory in nature. Opioid-induced respiratory depression is difficult to treat and is usually preceded by sedation. Nursing assessment using the numeric sedation scale can determine those patients at risk for respiratory depression more so than assessing the respiratory rate (Overdyk & Guerra, 2011). The Pasero Opioid-Induced Sedation Scale that can be used to assess respiratory depression is as follows (Pasero & McCaffery, 2011):

- S = sleep, easy to arouse: no action necessary
- 1 = awake and alert; no action necessary
- 2 = occasionally drowsy but easy to arouse; requires no action
- 3 = frequently drowsy and drifts off to sleep during conversation; decrease the opioid dose
- 4 = somnolent with minimal or no response to stimuli; discontinue the opioid and consider use of naloxone

If respiratory depression is suspected and the opioid dose is withheld, the patient may be physically stimulated by shaking or using a loud sound, along with reminders every few minutes to breathe deeply. If this is ineffective, naloxone (Narcan), an opioid antagonist that reverses the respiratory-depressant effect of an opioid, can be used. Naloxone is administered intravenously at a very slow rate. Within 1 to 2 minutes, the patient usually opens the eyes and is able to respond to the nurse. When the patient is alert again and the respiratory rate is greater than 9 breaths/min, the opioid may be resumed.

Many myths and irrational fears persist concerning the use of opioid analgesics. Patients and caregivers cite fear of addiction as a reason for ineffective treatment of pain. Because of this, nurses are concerned about administering prescribed doses of opioids, physicians underprescribe pain medication, and patients refuse or take less than prescribed doses of the drugs. Addiction in primary care practices is thought to number approximately 5% even though many of the remaining patients may be taking opioids on a regular basis (Westbrook & D'Arcy, 2012). Physical dependence and tolerance are frequently confused with addiction. **Physical dependence** is a phenomenon in which the body physiologically becomes accustomed to long-term opioid therapy and suffers withdrawal symptoms if the opioid is suddenly removed or the dose is rapidly decreased. **Tolerance** occurs when the body becomes accustomed to the opioid and needs a larger dose each time for pain relief. The side effects diminish along with the pain relief. Tolerance does not indicate addiction. **Addiction** is a pattern of compulsive opioid use for means other than pain control. According to D'Arcy (2010a), the four characteristics that define addiction are a craving for the substance, compulsive use, lack of control over the drug, and continued use despite harm. Less than 1% of patients with pain become addicted to opioids, yet many nurses surveyed seriously overestimated the likelihood of addiction when opioids are used for pain relief. In reality, physical dependence and tolerance are expected responses; patients treated with opioids for pain rarely develop addiction (D'Arcy, 2010a). *Pseudoaddiction* occurs when pain is undertreated and behaviors associated with addiction are observed. This response is due to a lack of sufficient pain control (Dunn & Neuman, 2012). This tolerance and physical dependence (resulting in a decrease in analgesic effect) that can occur after 4 weeks of regular opioid use can be treated by increasing the opioid dose until pain control is again apparent.

When people report that pain is present, research confirms that each patient's expression and self-report of pain are unique even if they have the same degree of pain. Important factors to consider when administering an opioid analgesic include:

- The patient's pain rating
- The sedation level
- The patient's comfort-function goal (the pain rating that allows a patient to perform necessary or desired activities)

Continuous intravenous infusion of opioids has proved effective for the relief of acute postoperative pain. In 2004, the American Society for Pain Management recommended the development of guidelines for the practice of using range orders to administer IV opioids to patients in acute pain. Pasero and McCaffery (2011) define a range order as "a medication order in which the selected dose varies over a prescribed range according to the patient's situation and status." The only variable in a range order is the dosage; the dosage interval should not be stated as a range (Rosier, 2012). An example of a range order is: morphine 2 to 8 mg IV every 2 hours as needed for pain.

A wide variety of nurses' interpretations of these range orders still persists for the delivery of IV opioids. The Joint Commission includes an accreditation criterion stating that hospitals must have a clear policy regarding range orders and there must be input from nursing, medicine, and pharmacy to ensure that interpretation of range orders is consistent and in agreement with TJC requirements. However, if hospitals have a clear protocol regarding range orders, nurses have the opportunity to address each patient's individual pain experience while protecting against adverse effects. Although there are many parameters to consider, ultimately, a nurse requires excellent assessment skills and good clinical judgment to use range orders safely and effectively.

Morphine is considered the gold standard of opioids. It is effective, inexpensive, available in multiple dosage forms, and prescribed more often than any other opioid. Opioid rotation is a common practice—physicians switch to other opioids to minimize side effects and continue to provide effective pain management. In opioid rotation, the current opioid is discontinued and immediately replaced with an equianalgesic dose of an alternative drug. An *equianalgesic* dose is one equivalent to the same degree of analgesia as that produced by 10 mg of parenteral morphine. Equianalgesic charts list other analgesic doses and routes that are interchangeable (Lehne, 2013). Methadone must be used cautiously because it has a long duration of action, allowing it to accumulate to dangerous levels that result in respiratory depression and sedation. It is difficult to calculate the most effective dose of methadone in an acute pain situation. However, a recent study found methadone effective in reducing postoperative pain when administered prior to complex spinal surgery (Power, 2011). Meperidine (Demerol) was used extensively in the past, but its use is now discouraged because significant accumulation of a toxic metabolite from the breakdown of meperidine can lead to altered mental status, delirium, seizures, and psychosis. When used, it is primarily for prevention and treatment of postoperative shivering and in short-term pain management in patients who cannot tolerate other opioids (Dobbins, 2010).

Nonopioid Analgesics. Nonopioid analgesics, such as acetaminophen and nonsteroidal anti-inflammatory drugs (NSAIDs), are usually the drugs of choice for both acute and persistent moderate chronic pain. The simplest dosage schedules and least invasive pain management modalities should be used first. Many times, these drugs alone can provide adequate pain relief. Many of these medications are over-the-counter (OTC) products, whereas some are available by prescription only. Some can cause gastric side effects, but these symptoms may be preventable if the drug is taken with food or antacids.

Acetaminophen has long been viewed as one of the safest and best-tolerated analgesics. It has proved to be an effective drug for acute pain treatment and is the most commonly used analgesic in the United States (Lehne, 2013). It has a low incidence of adverse effects, but the risk of hepatotoxicity must be considered when acetaminophen is used for a lengthy period or at larger than the recommended dose. If pain is not controlled using the recommended dose of acetaminophen, NSAIDs or an opioid analgesic may be required to achieve pain relief.

NSAIDs also have an anti-inflammatory effect. Individual responses to NSAIDs vary, but these agents are contraindicated in patients with bleeding disorders (their action may interfere with platelet function) or probable infections (NSAIDs can mask the signs of an infection). An FDA advisory committee has recommended that the labels on all NSAIDs warn the consumer about the potential for gastric bleeding if certain risk factors are present and the caution that NSAIDs should be taken for the shortest times needed. The combination of nonopioid analgesics and opioids provides more analgesia than either drug taken alone. Multimodal analgesic therapy is a relatively recent approach to pain management. It combines two or more classes of analgesics that target different sites in the peripheral and central nervous systems to maximize pain relief with fewer adverse effects. The most common multimodal approach is a combination of nonopioid, opioid, and adjuvant analgesics. The patient and family will require an explanation regarding why multiple medications have been prescribed and how they work to relieve pain (Arnstein, 2011; McGuire, 2011; Pasero & McCaffery, 2011).

The COX-2 inhibitors, a class of NSAIDs, have a lower risk of gastrointestinal bleeding but are thought to significantly increase cardiovascular risks. Two of the COX-2 inhibitors, rofecoxib (Vioxx) and valdecoxib (Bextra), have been withdrawn from the market because of increased evidence of adverse cardiac events. Celecoxib (Celebrex), another COX-2 inhibitor, is available in the United States and used for treatment of osteoarthritis and rheumatoid arthritis (Lehne, 2013). The recommendation is that NSAIDs appear to be safe in low doses for short periods of time.

Adjuvant Analgesics. Adjuvant drugs are typically used for other purposes but are also used to enhance the effect of opioids by providing additional pain relief. They may also reduce side effects from prescribed opioids or lessen anxiety about the pain experience. Adjuvant analgesics include antidepressants, anticonvulsants, corticosteroids, and biophosphonates. They may be used to treat acute pain resulting from surgery, burns, or trauma but are also effective for persistent neuropathic pain syndromes such as fibromyalgia, diabetic neuropathy, and postherpetic neuralgia (Pasero & McCaffery, 2011).

APPLYING GENERAL PRINCIPLES FOR ANALGESIC ADMINISTRATION

When using medications for pain relief, the nurse must first assess the patient's pain and understand the patient's goals for pain relief. In the home as well as in acute care settings, nurses provide quality nursing care when they empower patients to take charge of their own pain relief measures. The following guidelines are recommended for effective, individualized pain management in any setting:

- Review the pain scale of choice thoroughly.
- Discuss the benefits of using a pain scale.
- Try various pain control measures.
- Use pain control measures before pain increases in severity.
- Ask the patient what has proved effective for pain relief in the past.
- Select and modify pain control measures based on the patient's response.
- Encourage the patient to try the pain treatment several times before labeling it ineffective.
- Be open-minded about alternative pain relief strategies.
- Be persistent.
- Be a safe practitioner.

In the home, oral morphine is still the drug of choice to control chronic pain and to control moderate to severe acute pain. This method is less expensive and easy to administer, but requires that the patient is able to swallow and retain food and fluids.

Accurate documentation is imperative to determine effectiveness of the current regimen or the need to change pain control measures if relief is not obtained. Pain diaries or flow sheets provide a method for people to document their particular pain experience, list medication or alternative therapies that were used to treat the pain, and record their effectiveness. Attempts to recall particular aspects of a painful experience are not always accurate. Pain diaries can be used in a variety of settings and help improve the overall management of pain. Since more patients with acute and chronic pain are cared for in their home environment, effective patient and family teaching is the cornerstone of pain relief therapy.

Ongoing Assessment. Just as the pain experience of each patient is unique, so too is the response of each patient to a prescribed analgesic. The nurse continually needs to evaluate whether the medication is producing the desired analgesic effect; identify changes in the patient's condition (correction or worsening of pathology, increased drug tolerance) that necessitate changes in the analgesic agent, dose, or route of administration; and identify the development of side effects of the analgesic that may warrant its discontinuance. As long as the patient's pain exists, ongoing assessment and documentation of pain control is imperative. Fundamental to this assessment is the knowledge of the basic action, doses, and routes of administration; side effects; and administration guidelines of the analgesic being administered.

Timing is an important consideration when administering analgesics. To time analgesics appropriately, know the average duration of action for the drug and time administration so that the peak analgesic effect occurs when the pain is expected to be most intense. For example, an analgesic would be offered before ambulating a patient postoperatively.

A PRN (as needed) drug regimen has not been proven effective for people experiencing acute pain. In the early postoperative period, when pain is expected, this protocol may result in an intense pain experience for the patient. Later, however, in the postoperative course, a PRN schedule may be acceptable to relieve occasional pain episodes. Continuous intravenous infusion has proved effective for the relief of acute postoperative pain. Patient-controlled analgesia (PCA) and epidural analgesia are discussed later in the chapter.

The PRN protocol is totally inadequate for patients experiencing chronic pain. Regular administration of analgesics, or around-the-clock (ATC) administration (at regularly scheduled intervals), has been shown to offer superior pain management for chronic cancer pain. Long-acting, controlled-release oral morphine or oxycodone or use of a fentanyl patch have been proven effective for this type of pain. The U.S. Food and Drug Administration (FDA) issued its second warning regarding safe use of the fentanyl patch. It is intended for use in patients who are opioid-tolerant and have chronic pain; it should not be used to treat acute pain. Patients need instruction to apply the patch according to the time interval prescribed, avoid the application of heat in areas where the patch is in place, and dispose of used patches appropriately (FDA, 2010). After a series of pediatric accidental exposures to fentanyl patches, the FDA again alerted the public regarding proper disposal. They recommend folding together the adhesive side of the patch and flushing the patch down the toilet (Jeffrey, 2012).

Management of Breakthrough Pain.
Breakthrough pain (BTP) is a temporary flare-up of moderate to severe pain that occurs even when the patient is taking ATC medication for persistent pain. As many as 50% to 90% of cancer patients experience breakthrough pain. This pain is often not diagnosed correctly and is frequently undertreated. Breakthrough pain can be classified as incident pain (e.g., pain caused by movement), idiopathic (spontaneous pain due to an unknown cause), or end-of-dose pain, when the pain occurs before the next dose of

analgesic is due. Although it usually occurs in patients with chronic pain, it can occur in acute situations, such as in a patient with postoperative pain. Incident BTP is treated more effectively with supplemental doses of a short-acting opioid taken on a PRN basis, rather than with an increase in the dose of the ATC medication or shortening of the interval between doses, which typically is more effective with end-of-dose pain. However, the treatment for idiopathic BTP is more difficult and usually requires adjustment of the dose and dosing interval to relieve this pain. Effective management of BTP requires a medication with a mu opioid analgesic that has a rapid onset and short duration of effect such as morphine, hydromorphone, or fentanyl. The oral, buccal, and sublingual routes of administration are frequently used for treatment of breakthrough pain (Pasero, 2012).

Concern About Prescription Analgesic Abuse.
In the past decade, nearly 15,000 people in the United States have died every year from an overdose of prescription pain medications. Unintended drug overdose is now the second leading cause of accidental death. This number exceeds the total number of overdose deaths from heroin and cocaine combined. The FDA reported that opioids, including oxycodone, fentanyl, morphine, methadone, and acetaminophen-hydrocodone were among the drugs most frequently involved in fatal outcomes (Anderson, 2012). Many Americans 12 years and older have reported that they use prescription analgesics for nonmedical purposes. Practitioners have responded to the need for improved pain relief by prescribing more opioids for patients; in some cases, the substance abuse that subsequently occurs is an unintended consequence. The segment of the population who abuse opioids are sensitive to this concern on the part of physicians to address pain more vigorously. They visit multiple doctors and request opioid prescriptions for high daily doses. This group is at high risk for a drug overdose, but they also distribute drugs to others who are using them without a prescription. A significant number of people who died of opioid overdose did not have a prescription in their medical record for the drug that killed them (CDC, 2012).

The CDC has referred to this abuse as a public health epidemic. Efforts are underway to combat prescription drug abuse. States are encouraged to develop electronic drug monitoring programs to track all prescriptions and patients using opioid analgesics as well as those patients who shop various doctors or order medication fraudulently from various "pill mills." The overriding goal is to have uniform pain management guidelines that are safe and effective. An additional strategy involves pain management education for physicians regarding the risks of high-dose opioid therapy. In an effort to address national prescription drug abuse, the FDA announced a risk evaluation and mitigation strategy (REMS) that is required for prescribers of extended-release and long-acting opioid medications. The emphasis of this ground-breaking program is the education of health care professionals in the safe use of these drugs. Drug manufacturers also must develop educational information that prescribers can use to educate their patients about the risks and benefits of opioid use. The FDA requires that pharmaceutical firms provide and fund the plan, but the training is not yet mandatory for physicians (Gandey, 2011).

USING ACUTE PAIN MANAGEMENT TREATMENT REGIMENS

As a patient's advocate, ensure that a strong emphasis is placed on the need for aggressive, individualized strategies that can minimize or eliminate acute pain and promote positive patient outcomes. Preventing pain is easier than treating it once it has occurred. Discuss pain control options with patients before surgery, and address the patient's responsibility regarding reporting pain. Additional nursing interventions that can eliminate acute postoperative pain include maintaining a steady serum level of the analgesic (PCA or epidural analgesia can help here), treating side effects quickly and aggressively, encouraging use of nonpharmacologic complementary therapies as adjuncts to the medical regimen, and expecting incident pain and dealing with it.

Undertreatment of pain that accompanies procedures, whether performed in a hospital, home, or outpatient clinic, is a common occurrence. If there is any doubt about the likelihood of pain resulting from a procedure, provide analgesia. In situations in which the patient is unable to report the presence of pain (e.g., an unconscious patient), it is important to consider pain relief if a procedure is planned that normally elicits a complaint of pain. This could include turning a patient or a dressing change. In this case, the acronym APP (assume pain present) should be documented (McGuire, 2011). In some instances, for example, if the patient is unable to communicate verbally but capable of some response, it may be necessary to provide a method for the patient to indicate that pain is occurring during a procedure. The simple raising of a finger or hand or squeeze of a squeak toy can alert the caregiver that analgesia is needed.

EMPLOYING CANCER OR CHRONIC PAIN MANAGEMENT TREATMENT REGIMENS

People with cancer sometimes suffer needlessly from pain. This pain, surprisingly, remains undertreated in both children and adults; nurses need to act as advocates for pain relief for these patients. The major principles that guide treatment for cancer or chronic pain include:

• Giving medications orally, if possible, for ease and convenience of administration
• Administering medication ATC rather than on a PRN basis
• Adjusting the dose to achieve maximum benefits with minimal side effects
• Allowing patients as much control as possible over their medication regimen

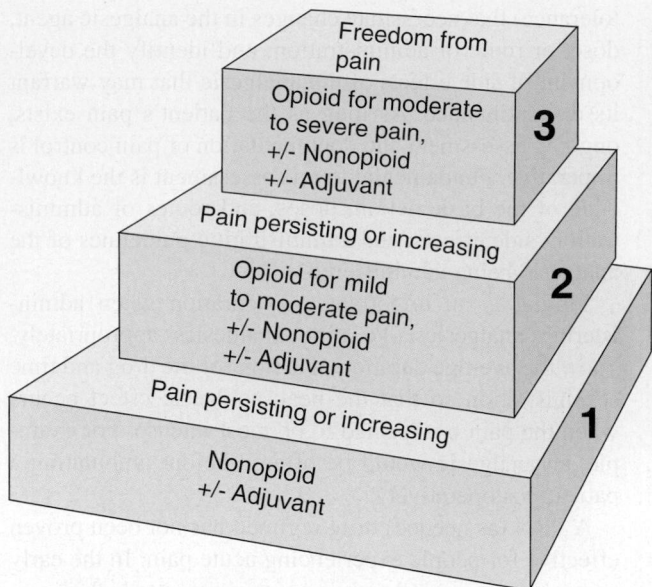

FIGURE 34-7. The WHO three-step pain relief ladder. (© World Health Organization. Redrawn with permission.)

In an effort to alleviate unnecessary pain and suffering, the World Health Organization (WHO) devised a three-step analgesic ladder (Fig. 34-7) that recommends the appropriate progression of drugs and dosages that should be used to manage chronic pain effectively. Emphasis is on individualizing treatment and using the analgesic ladder to provide attentive, aggressive pain relief. The effectiveness of the WHO analgesic ladder is widely acknowledged; this regimen provides relief to 70% to 90% of patients with cancer pain. Movement through the analgesic ladder may not always progress through all steps in an orderly manner depending on the intensity of the cancer patient's pain (Vargas-Schaffer, 2010). Some clinicians have suggested that the WHO three-step analgesic ladder may require some adjustment based on the clinical experience that has occurred in the 20 years since the ladder was proposed. The 10% to 30% of patients with severe pain who do not obtain satisfactory pain relief using this guideline may require alternative routes of drug administration, nerve blocks, or other invasive procedures to relieve their pain. The WHO ladder approach to pain management has also proved effective in treatment of patients with phantom limb pain and end-stage renal disease (Pasero & McCaffery, 2011).

PROVIDING PAIN TREATMENT IN SPECIAL POPULATIONS

Children and older adults need accurate assessment and treatment of pain. Their behavioral indicators of pain are unique, which necessitates special approaches to determine the presence and level of pain as well as individualized techniques to relieve the pain.

Children. Effective pain management in children requires careful assessment; good communication among patient, family, and caregivers; and a thorough understanding of the actions and side effects of drugs used to relieve pain. The child is still the best source of information about the pain; various assessment tools mentioned previously help to measure the intensity of the pain.

 THINK back to Xavier Malton, the child with ulcerative colitis in acute pain. The nurse needs to assess Xavier continually for effectiveness of the prescribed analgesic and request changes in any orders if the analgesic is not effective. Considering Xavier's current state, suggesting that the physician change the analgesic administration from PRN dosing to around-the-clock dosing may be appropriate for a short period of time. ●

In postoperative situations, children need analgesics ATC or by continuous infusion. Opioids are the drug of choice for moderate to severe pain. Pain management for cancer pain or chronic pain in children follows the prescription outlined in the WHO analgesic ladder. Withholding opioid drugs from children with cancer because of fear of addiction is unjustified because current knowledge does not indicate that they are vulnerable to this problem.

Children also require pain management to minimize or alleviate the pain and distress associated with some procedures. The misconception persists that children experience pain differently. It is important to understand that if a procedure is painful for an adult, then it is also painful for a child. Adequate education before the procedure and using drug and nondrug therapies to complement each other can take the pain and fear out of the experience. This is especially important for children with a chronic disease who must undergo multiple procedures as part of the treatment regimen.

Older Adults. Research on pain management in older adults has focused on pain associated with chronic illness and acute postoperative pain. Little is known about pain in well older adults living in the community. However, residents of long-term care facilities are a vulnerable population who experience a high prevalence of pain. Many health care providers, and older people as well, expect that pain is a natural outcome of the aging process. As stated previously, pain is routinely undertreated in this population. Recommendations for analgesic administration for older adults include the following (Westbrook & D'Arcy, 2012):

- Use acetaminophen cautiously for mild to moderate pain. NSAIDs also have the potential for renal and gastric complications; a proton pump inhibitor may be prescribed to decrease gastric side effects.
- Administer medications, if possible, via the oral route.
- Use IV analgesics cautiously because decreased circulation poses a risk for reduced absorption of opioids. The recommendation is to "start low and go slow."

Opioid drugs can be used safely for older adult patients as long as appropriate precautions are taken, pain is conscientiously assessed, and potential side effects are monitored. Adjust dosage and dosing intervals for the older adult based on therapeutic response to the drug and the presence of adverse effects. The accompanying Focus on the Older Adult box describes additional strategies pertinent to this age group.

ADMINISTERING ANALGESICS BY OTHER METHODS

In addition to the variety of drugs used to treat pain, multiple options exist for drug delivery systems. Patient-controlled analgesia, epidural analgesia, and other advanced

---

FOCUS ON THE OLDER ADULT

NURSING STRATEGIES TO ADDRESS AGE-RELATED CHANGES AFFECTING COMFORT

Age-Related Changes	Nursing Strategies
Communication Difficulties	• Observe carefully for any behavioral manifestations or indications of pain (e.g., change in activity level or grimacing with movement). • Use open-ended questions to solicit information about pain. • Rely on family or caregiver to assist with information-gathering process. • Monitor for any behavior changes or confusion after medication has been taken.
Denial of Pain	• Clarify terms used to describe pain or discomfort. • Emphasize importance of reporting pain to caregivers. • Express concern about pain and a willingness to help. Explain that pain is not a normal consequence of aging.
Altered Physiologic Response to Analgesics	• Be aware of dosage and frequency to avoid oversedation and toxicity. • Monitor carefully for oversedation and respiratory depression. • Explain side effects of analgesics to patient. • Use memory aid if necessary to avoid overdosing. • Discourage self-medication. • Caution about use of alcohol with analgesics. • Caution about driving or operating machinery when taking analgesics.

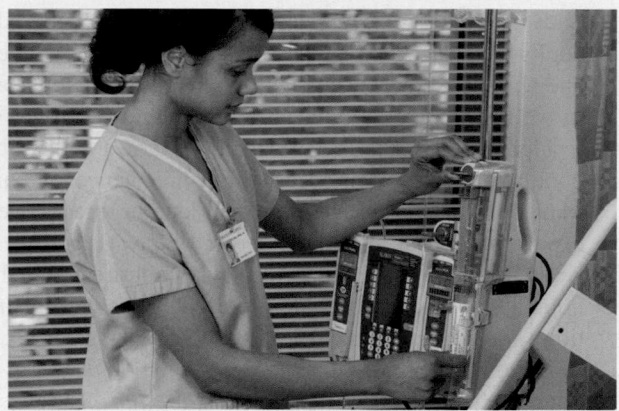

FIGURE 34-8. A patient-controlled analgesia unit allows the patient to regulate the intravenous infusion of small amounts of analgesic as needed.

interventions have improved pain management and the quality of life for many people.

Patient-Controlled Analgesia. Patient-controlled analgesia (PCA) provides effective individualized analgesia and comfort (Figure 34-8). This method of analgesia therapy may be used to manage acute and chronic pain in a health care facility or the home. It is used less frequently with cancer pain, for which oral medication is the preferred route. This device is most commonly used to deliver analgesics intravenously, subcutaneously, or via the epidural route. The most frequently prescribed drugs for PCA administration are morphine, fentanyl, and hydromorphone.

The PCA system consists of a computerized, portable infusion pump containing a chamber for a syringe that is prefilled with the prescribed opioid analgesic. Both The Joint Commission (TJC) and the Institute for Safe Medication Practices (ISMP) recommend standard doses and concentrations prepared in prefilled syringes. Initially, a loading dose is administered to raise blood levels to a therapeutic level and control the pain. When the sensation of pain reoccurs, the patient pushes a button that activates the PCA device to deliver a small preset bolus dose of the analgesic. A dose interval that is programmed into the PCA unit (usually, 6–8 minutes) prevents reactivation of the pump and administration of another dose during that period of time. The pump mechanism can also be programmed to deliver only a specified amount of analgesic within a given time interval (the lock-out interval). This is most commonly every hour or, occasionally, every 4 hours. The 1-hour lock-out is viewed more favorably in opioid-naïve patients. These safeguards limit the possibility of possible overmedication. In addition, time is provided for the patient to evaluate the effect of the previous dose. PCA pumps also have a locked safety system that prohibits any tampering with the device (Pasero & McCaffery, 2011).

The proper selection of patients for PCA is vital for a positive experience. Suitable candidates for this type of delivery system include people who are alert and capable of controlling the unit. The Joint Commission and ISMP both identify people who are not recommended for this type of pain relief. These include confused older patients, infants and very young children, cognitively impaired patients, patients with conditions for which oversedation poses a significant health risk (e.g., asthma and sleep apnea), and patients who are taking other medications that potentiate opioids. PCA has proven safe for use in developmentally normal children as young as 4 years of age (Pasero & McCaffery, 2011).

PCA has many advantages:

- Consistent analgesic blood level is maintained rather than the inconsistent analgesia obtained with periodic injections, which results in sharp rises and falls of serum opioid levels.
- The analgesic is delivered intravenously or epidurally so that absorption is faster and more predictable than with the intramuscular route.
- The patient is in charge of the pain management program.
- The patient tends to use less medication because it is self-administered before the pain becomes too severe.
- The patient is able to ambulate earlier, which promotes less pulmonary complications.
- The patient is more satisfied and has improved pain relief.

PCA by proxy, which means that someone other than the patient activates the pump, continues to be a controversial issue. Unauthorized family members or caregivers (instead of the patient) who administer PCA by pushing the dosage button can cause serious analgesic overdoses resulting in oversedation, respiratory depression, and death. Some clinicians argue that in a pediatric setting, nurse-controlled analgesia or caregiver-controlled analgesia is appropriate. For this to be safe, rigid agency protocols need to be in place. The Joint Commission issued a sentinel event alert on PCA and does not recommend PCA by proxy. Institutions must verify that they have protocols in place to protect against unauthorized PCA delivery. It also recommends that warning labels stating, "Only the patient should press this button" be attached to PCA pumps (Pasero & McCaffery, 2011). Refer to Chapter 26 for a discussion of sentinel event alerts. The Joint Commission also advises that caregivers need to carefully monitor patients for respiratory depression using pulse oximetry and capnography (measurement of carbon dioxide concentrations) as appropriate. The carbon dioxide level in a patient's expirations can be measured by a sensor contained in a mask or nasal cannula that the patient is wearing. This provides a more reliable measure of impending respiratory depression.

Setting up the PCA system and ensuring that it is functioning properly are nursing responsibilities. Improper programming of the pump is the most common human error associated with this therapy. Both The Joint

Commission and the ISMP recommend that another nurse checks the patient ID, drug dose and concentrations, PCA pump settings, and the infusion tubing and site prior to the initiation of PCA.

 RECALL Sheree Lincoln, the postoperative woman who is to use the PCA system for pain control. Two hours after surgery, the patient is complaining of pain but has not used the PCA system. The nurse would need to determine the underlying reasons for not using the device. This assessment would include investigation of Sheree's knowledge base and what, if any, teaching she received preoperatively. For example, Sheree may have received teaching on how to use PCA but may not have understood when or why to use it. Possibly she may want to avoid use of any medication. The nurse would use this opportunity to reinforce instructions for using PCA and also for other nonpharmacologic measures for pain relief such as distraction, relaxation, massage, or imagery ●

An oral patient-controlled analgesia device is available that allows patients to self-administer doses of opioid analgesics. The Medication on Demand (MOD) device is an oral PCA device attached to an IV pole and requires that the patient wear a "radio frequency identification" wristband that allows access to the MOD. In order to receive a dose of medication, patients record their level of pain, swipe their wristband over the device, and remove a single dose once the drawer is opened. The interval between medication doses is programmed into the MOD as per the physician's order. When this lock-out interval has passed, a green "ready light" appears on the device. The MOD device is loaded with a cartridge containing 8 doses of the prescribed opioid. Increased patient satisfaction is an expected outcome with MOD (Stett, 2010).

Opioid analgesia via a continuous subcutaneous infusion (CSI) is a safe, effective alternative when IV access is not available and oral analgesia is no longer possible. Candidates for CSI are often patients requiring hospice and palliative care. Equipment consists of a small butterfly needle inserted subcutaneously and an infusion pump and administration set that is clearly labeled "subcutaneous infusion." This set-up delivers the opioid in a small amount of fluid (typically 2–3 mL/hr) and can be programmed with a lock-out feature and options for bolus dosing. Morphine is usually the opioid of choice. Nurses can initiate CSI therapy once the Infusion Nursing Society has validated their competence. Assessment of CSI includes monitoring of vital signs, pain level, and the insertion site for leakage or bleeding. It is a valid pain management option that delivers individualized care (D'Arcy, 2010b).

Epidural Analgesia. Epidural analgesia can be used to provide pain relief during the immediate postoperative phase (particularly after thoracic, abdominal, orthopedic, and vascular surgery) and for chronic pain situations. Epidural pain management is also being used for children with terminal cancer and for children undergoing hip, spinal, or lower extremity surgery. It is contraindicated if the patient is unable to give an informed consent, takes systemic anticoagulants, has a systemic or local infection, has increased intracranial pressure, is allergic to opioids or local anesthetics, or has a history of long-term use of aspirin products or NSAIDs (Sawhney, 2012). The anesthesiologist usually inserts the catheter in the mid-lumbar region into the epidural space between the walls of the vertebral canal and the dura mater or outermost connective tissue membrane surrounding the spinal cord. For temporary therapy, the catheter exits directly over the spine, and the tubing is positioned over the patient's shoulder, with the end of the catheter taped to the person's chest. For long-term therapy, the catheter is usually tunneled subcutaneously and exits on the side of the body or on the abdomen (Fig. 34-9).

The opioid and/or local anesthetic acts directly on the opiate receptors in the spinal cord; pain relief is achieved with smaller doses and less severe side effects. The epidural analgesia can be administered as a bolus dose (either one time or intermittent) via a continuous infusion pump or by means of a patient-controlled epidural analgesia (PCEA) pump. The drug of choice is usually preservative-free morphine or fentanyl. Because the epidural space contains blood vessels, nerves, and fat,

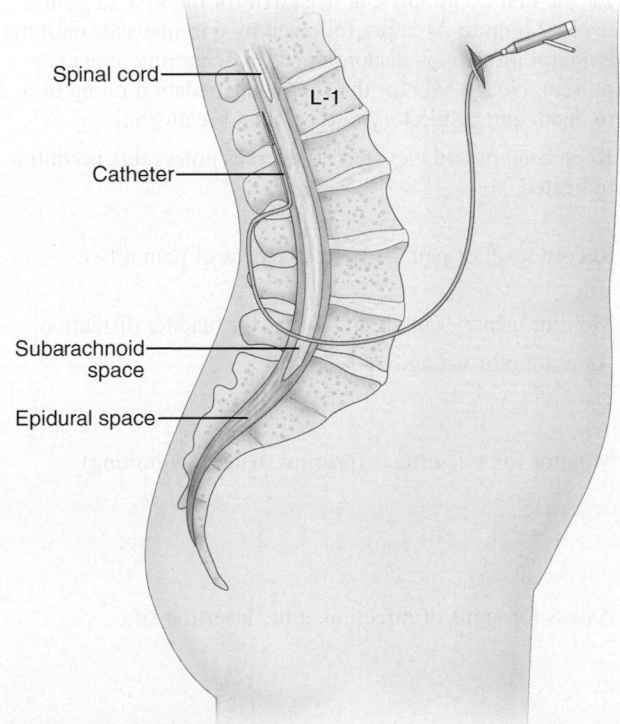

FIGURE 34-9. Placement of an epidural catheter for long-term use.

lipid-soluble fentanyl is readily dissolved and has a rapid onset of action (5 minutes) but a short duration of action (approximately 2 hours). Hydromorphone has a 15- to 30-minute onset and a duration of action up to 18 hours. Morphine is a hydrophilic opioid, meaning that this drug has a high affinity for water. It has a slower onset of action but may exert its analgesic effect for as long as 24 hours because it remains longer in the cerebrospinal fluid (CSF) and spinal tissue (Sawhney, 2012). Epidural catheters used for the management of acute pain are typically removed between 36 and 72 hours after surgery, when oral medication can be substituted for relief of pain.

Nursing responsibilities vary among institutions but must include careful monitoring of the patient's response to therapy, with particular attention to the respiratory rate and pattern (Guidelines for Nursing Care 34-1). Too much narcotic or a displaced catheter may allow the medication to have a depressant effect on the brainstem center, causing life-threatening respiratory depression. Other potential side effects include hypotension, pruritus, urinary retention, nausea and vomiting, and infection or contamination.

Local Anesthesia. Anesthetic agents may be applied topically to the skin or mucous membranes or injected into the body to produce a temporary loss of sensation and motor and autonomic function in a localized area. The agents work by chemically blocking the nerve pathways involved in pain sensation and response, and are sometimes called nerve blocks. Many people have experienced nerve blocks during dental work, when having a wound sutured, during delivery of a newborn, or for some minor surgical procedures. Nursing measures include noting any

GUIDELINES FOR NURSING CARE 34-1

CARING FOR PATIENTS RECEIVING EPIDURAL OPIOIDS

Nursing Action	*Rationale*
Verify the physician's order for analgesia, drug preparation, and rate of infusion with another RN.	Verification provides for safe administration of the correct dose at the correct rate.
Keep an ampule of 0.4 mg of naloxone (Narcan) available on the unit.	Naloxone reverses the respiratory depressant effect of opioids.
Label solution, tubing, and pump apparatus "For Epidural Infusion Only."	Labeling prevents inadvertent administration of other intravenous medications through this setup.
Assess and record sedation level (using a sedation scale) and respiratory status, including pulse oximetry continually for the first 20 minutes, at least q1h for the first 12 hours, every 2 h up to 24 hours followed by q4h intervals until the epidural infusion is discontinued (or according to agency policy). Notify MD for the following: sedation rating of 3, ↓ in depth and respiratory rate below 8 breaths/min.	Opioids can depress respiratory center in the medulla. Change in level of consciousness is usually the first sign of altered respiratory function.
Keep head of bed elevated 30 degrees unless this is contraindicated.	Elevation of the patient's head minimizes upward migration of opioid in the spinal cord, thus decreasing risk for respiratory depression.
Record level of pain and effectiveness of pain relief.	Referencing helps in determining need for subsequent "breakthrough" pain medication.
Monitor urinary output and assess for bladder distention.	Opioids can cause urinary retention.
Assess motor strength q4h.	Catheter may migrate into the intrathecal space and allow opioids to block transmission of nerve impulses completely through the spinal cord to the brain.
Monitor for side effects (pruritus, nausea, vomiting).	Opioids may spread into the trigeminal nerve, causing itching or resulting in nausea and vomiting due to slowed gastrointestinal function or stimulation of a chemoreceptor trigger zone in the brain. Medications are available to treat these side effects.
Assess for signs of infection at the insertion site.	Inflammation or local infection may develop at the catheter insertion site. Strict aseptic technique and sterile dressing and tubing changes according to agency policy can prevent this complication.
Do not administer any other narcotics or adjuvant drugs without approval of clinician responsible for epidural injection.	Additional medication may potentiate the action of the opioid, increasing the risk for respiratory depression.

allergic responses the patient has had in the past to anesthetic agents, alerting the patient to the pain associated with the initial injection of the anesthetic if the physician does not numb the area first, offering emotional support to the patient during the procedure, observing for any untoward effects, and protecting the patient from injury until sensory and motor functions return. Two topical anesthetic creams (EMLA, which contains 2.5% lidocaine and 2.5% prilocaine, and L.M.X.4, formerly ELA-Max, a 4%-lidocaine cream) provide safe, effective analgesia for children before painful procedures such as phlebotomy, lumbar puncture, or bone marrow aspiration. EMLA cream is prescribed by the physician and must be covered by an occlusive dressing for at least 1 hour before the procedure to provide local pain relief. After the time period, the cream is removed. ELA-MAX is an OTC preparation that takes effect in 30 minutes or less (Pasero & McCaffery, 2011).

Teaching the Patient and Family About Pain

Often, a well-informed person can cope better with the distress of pain and tends to experience less anxiety about pain. See the Promoting Health Literacy box for suggestions regarding communicating with your health care practitioner to ensure improved outcomes related to pain management.

Teaching about pain should include family members so that they understand the concept of pain and are able to help the person in pain. The patient and family need information about the nature and causes of pain, explanation about a pain scale that can be used easily, practice with this assessment tool, and assistance to set goals for comfort and either optimal function or recovery. Teaching Tips 34-1 (on page 1184) includes specific suggestions related to safety concerns about pain control in the home setting. In addition, provide the patient and family with information about available resources, including reputable online sources for pain control and treatment, and encourage them to use them.

Play may be used effectively to discover a child's experience of pain and to teach the child how to cope with pain. Children are usually receptive to using dolls to act out pain experiences.

Ensuring the Ethical and Legal Responsibility to Relieve Pain

Quality pain management results when patients have access to safe, effective pain relief measures. Health care providers, in addition to monitoring, delivering, and documenting administration of analgesics, also have responsibility to inform patients that effective pain relief is vital to their treatment. Patients also have the right to expect that

PROMOTING HEALTH LITERACY

IN PATIENTS WITH PAIN

Patient Scenario

Jennifer Tyler, 44, has had several visits to her primary physician about her pain. She told the office nurse that she "doesn't know how much more of this I can take." Her history reveals that she has had an "aching pain, literally all over my body" for the last 3 months. Jennifer states that "It's taking over my life now. Everything I do hurts, and to make it worse, I don't sleep well at night and I can't even think straight." Additional symptoms she reported include fatigue, occasional muscle spasms in her legs, headaches that are occurring on a more frequent basis, and general anxiety about her health. Jennifer reports that initially she tried Advil off and on with some mild relief and even admits taking some "old muscle relaxants" that her husband had from a back injury. Despite the antidepressants and sleeping pills that were prescribed for her, she has not been able to get much in the way of pain relief. After his initial examination, her physician has ordered a variety of laboratory studies to try and determine exactly what is causing Ms. Tyler's pain. At this visit, he told Ms. Tyler that he suspects fibromyalgia may be the cause of her pain and other symptoms. He prescribes pregabalin (Lyrica) and wants to see her again in 3 weeks to see how this medication is working for her. As she is making the next appointment, Jennifer tells the nurse, "I sure hope this new medicine works. I'm running out of hope here. What kind of a life is this?"

Nursing Considerations: *Tips for Improving Health Literacy*

Provide Ms. Tyler with printed literature about fibromyalgia. Explain that this disease is difficult to diagnose and that this medication has recently been approved by the Food and Drug Administration (FDA) to treat fibromyalgia. Tell Ms. Tyler that the doctor may adjust her dose depending on how she tolerates the medicine and what kind of results she is getting from the drug. Caution her that dizziness and blurred vision may occur as side effects. Tell her if she has any signs of an allergic reaction, she should immediately stop taking the medication and report this to the physician. Inform her that she should avoid alcohol consumption while taking Lyrica and not to drive if she experiences any dizziness and blurred vision. Explain to her that the doctor may prescribe additional therapies to help her deal with rehabilitation as she recovers from this disease. Encourage Ms. Tyler when she returns for her next visit to be prepared to ask her physician the following questions:

- What is my main problem?
- What do I need to do?
- Why is it important for me to do this?
- What can you do if this new medication is not working?
- What else can you or I do to treat my pain?

What additional measures can you take to help maintain health literacy in this patient? What other measures would be helpful if Ms. Tyler did not speak English, could not read, or had other learning deficits?

TEACHING TIPS 34-1

COMFORT

Health Topic	Teaching Tip	Why Is This Important?
Safety	Do not drive vehicle or operate heavy machinery after taking pain medication.	Reflexes may be slowed and cognitive thinking decreased due to pain medications.
	Avoid alcohol and other CNS depressants while taking pain medication.	Alcohol may interact with the pain medication and further depress the CNS, leading to respiratory failure.
	Do not smoke without someone else present while taking pain medication.	The patient may become tired due to the medication, fall asleep while smoking, and start a house fire.
	Do not walk without assistance while taking pain medication.	Some pain medications can cause drowsiness, dizziness, and blurred vision.
	Keep record or pain diary of level of pain, medication taken, and effect of medication.	Provides more accurate documentation of pain experience and prevents overdoses.
Diet	Do not take pain medication on an empty stomach.	Many patients become nauseated if pain medication is taken on an empty stomach.
Miscellaneous	Do not breastfeed without checking with your physician while taking pain medication.	Many pain medications can be found in breast milk and may harm the baby.

their statements of pain will be heeded quickly. Institutions must assign and educate clinicians to address these issues in a timely, knowledgeable manner. The rights of patients with pain highlighted in Box 34-3 recognize the multidimensional aspects of the pain experience and a person's right to have pain controlled as soon as possible. Also, as mentioned previously in this chapter, a patient's right to effective pain control is a focus of The Joint Commission.

 CONSIDER Xavier Malton, the child with acute pain. The nurses in the scenario advocated for Xavier, reinforcing his rights to have pain controlled as soon as possible. ●

Many health care institutions recognizing the need to individualize and prioritize interventions for specific populations have developed clinical experts. Since pain assessment and management can pose a challenge to many nurses, health care institutions have committed to a focus on best practices and improved patient outcomes

Box 34-3 A BILL OF RIGHTS FOR PEOPLE WITH PAIN

1. I have the right to have my reports of pain accepted and acted on by health care professionals.
2. I have the right to have my pain controlled, no matter what its cause or how severe it may be.
3. I have the right to be treated with respect at all times. When I need medication for pain, I should not be treated like a drug abuser.

May be duplicated for use in clinical practice. Reprinted with permission from McCaffery, M., & Pasero, C. (1999). *Pain: Clinical manual* (p. 13). Copyright © 1999, Mosby, Inc. St. Louis.

on their individual units. The Pain Resource Nurse (PRN) has an expressed interest in pain management, is an effective communicator, and acts as a coach or mentor for colleagues. The PRN is usually a staff nurse involved with direct patient care. The role is multifaceted and PRNs foster implementation of evidenced-based practice. They may also be involved in developing or refining patient education materials, reviewing and updating documentation requirements, and selecting the appropriate pain assessment tools (Quinn-O'Neil, Kilgallen, & Terlizzi, 2011).

Understanding the Placebo Controversy

The term **placebo** comes from the Latin word meaning "I shall please." According to Pasero and McCaffery (2011), a placebo is defined as "any medication or procedure, including surgery, that may produce an effect in a patient because of its implicit or explicit intent and not because of its specific physical or chemical properties." The person, unaware of the placebo's properties, may find it to be effective for the relief of pain because of the perception that it will provide comfort and because of belief in the person administering it. It is an injustice to judge a person experiencing relief from pain after the use of a placebo as a malingerer or as mentally ill. Various researchers have reported that a positive placebo effect may be related to a physiologic response (release of endorphins) or the patient's cultural expectations, attitudes, health beliefs, or anticipation of a positive response. Use of a placebo also has the potential to cause a harmful or undesirable response referred to as a nocebo. This negative outcome may involve mild discomforts such as nausea and pruritis or life-threatening complications.

The use of placebos, however, raises serious ethical questions. Is lying to a patient justifiable? A nurse who administers a placebo must be willing to risk the possible consequence of the patient becoming aware of the duplicity and then refusing to trust the nurse or any other health care professional again. Patients who feel themselves to be in pain are vulnerable. If such patients discover a seeming plot to trick them into feeling better, it is unlikely that those patients will respect or appreciate the intentions of the physicians and nurses involved. The long-term negative effects of this practice far outweigh any of its benefits. The Oncology Nursing Society and the American Nurses Association, in addition to other professional organizations, oppose placebo use. The American Society for Pain Management Nursing (ASPMN) agrees that placebo use is fraudulent and deceptive when used to assess and treat pain but supports placebo use in clinical trials in which the patient has signed an informed consent and the institutional review board has approved the research (Arnstein, Broglio, & Wuhrman, 2011). The nurse has firm legal and ethical grounds for refusing to administer a placebo.

Evaluating

As soon as a pain problem is identified and a treatment plan developed and implemented, evaluation becomes ongoing. Evaluation is directed toward the changing nature of the pain experience, the treatment modalities (pain management program), and the patient's and family's response to the plan of care, all of which overlap.

The Pain Experience

The pain the patient is experiencing may change in many ways, thus the nurse must be careful not to make a judgment about this too quickly. For example, if the pain lessens in intensity or disappears, it may mean that the underlying cause of the pain is diminished or absent and that treatment should be stopped, or it may mean that the pain management program is effective and should be continued. When pain intensity increases, it may simply indicate the need for more aggressive therapy, or it may be a warning that the underlying pathology has changed or worsened and that new medical intervention is required. Often, a new problem amenable to treatment is masked by "old pain," and its detection may be delayed to the point that treatment is useless.

Management Regimens

The use of both noninvasive and invasive therapies must be continually evaluated to determine whether they are the best possible means the patient could use to obtain pain relief and whether they are effective with only minimal risk to the patient. Too often, a patient stays with the first analgesic prescribed without questioning whether it is the most effective drug for the particular pain, whether the dosage and timing guidelines are correct for the patient, and whether the analgesic is perhaps producing annoying or even harmful side effects that another drug would not produce.

Similarly, one patient may take to progressive relaxation exercises and find them helpful, whereas another patient may obtain similar benefits from a daily walking program. Nursing time spent evaluating the effectiveness of each pain relief therapy is well spent and results in a pain management program that is truly individualized to the patient.

Patient and Family Response

Ultimately, the plan of care is unsuccessful unless the patient and family are satisfied with the results. A successful plan of care results in the achievement of specified patient outcomes valued by the patient. Whenever possible, nursing care should terminate when the patient and family can independently direct the pain management program with the assistance of appropriate resources.

Nursing Plan of Care 34-1 highlights the nursing process related to pain for Carla Potter.

NURSING PLAN OF CARE 34-1

for Carla Potter

Carla Potter is a 26-year-old white woman. She is unmarried and has no children. She is employed at a large company as a computer programmer. During the past 7 months, she has been experiencing periodic fatigue, anxiety, irritability, depression, and mood swings. Her general health is excellent. The nurse practitioner at the gynecologist's office believes Ms. Potter may be suffering from premenstrual syndrome. The nurse practitioner who interviewed Ms. Potter noted the following data:

• Patient has generalized discomfort—fatigue, anxiety, irritability, depression, and mood swings—about

1 week before her menses; discomfort subsides after onset of menses.
• Discomforts are believed to be heightened by stress at work but do not depend on this. Patient denies any new or unusual stress in life but believes symptoms are affecting her job performance and relationships.
• Patient relates history of "bad cramps" ever since periods started. Patient lacks knowledge of appropriate dietary and stress management techniques.
• Patient relates she has occasionally taken some of her friend's "tranquilizers" to ease her through a bad day—but she prefers not to take medication.

(continued)

NURSING PLAN OF CARE 34-1 *continued*

for Carla Potter

NURSING DIAGNOSIS	Ineffective Coping related to discomforts of premenstrual symptoms as manifested by reports of fatigue, anxiety, irritability, depression, and mood swings	
EXPECTED OUTCOME	By the next monthly assessment, 10/30/14, patient will:	
	• Use relaxation techniques during periods of anxiety	

NURSING INTERVENTIONS	**RATIONALE**	**EVALUATIVE STATEMENT**
Assess patient's knowledge of relaxation techniques and motivation to use them.	Effective use of relaxation techniques requires a motivated patient.	10/30/14 Outcome partially met, patient used relaxation techniques during two periods of anxiety. Was driving on expressway during another period of anxiety, which made relaxation difficult.
Instruct patient regarding the use of progressive relaxation exercises and controlled breathing during periods of anxiety. For example, "Find a quiet, comfortable place and sit down. Consciously contract and relax the muscles of the whole body starting at the head and neck and working down to the feet until completely relaxed. At the same time, take slow, rhythmic breaths. Continue until anxiety passes."	Relaxation and controlled breathing are used to decrease anxiety and increase coping mechanisms.	*R. Gordon, RNC*

EXPECTED OUTCOME	By the next monthly assessment, 10/30/14, the patient will:	
	• Use a meal plan that includes three balanced meals per day and excludes caffeine, sugar, and sodium	

NURSING INTERVENTIONS	**RATIONALE**	**EVALUATIVE STATEMENT**
Assess patient's nutritional intake. Have patient identify current food preferences high in caffeine, sugar, and sodium and discuss substitutes. Teach patient rationale for decreasing intake of caffeine, sugar, and sodium.	Refined sugar and caffeine contribute to feelings of tension and irritability. Sodium contributes to water retention in the body.	10/30/14 Outcome met. Patient used meal plan for three balanced meals per day and eliminated all sugar, caffeine, and sodium from diet.
Instruct patient in developing a meal plan that includes three balanced meals per day.	Balanced meals provide optimal nutrition.	*R. Gordon, RNC*

EXPECTED OUTCOME	By the next monthly assessment, 10/30/14, the patient will:	
	• Incorporate exercise into routine	

NURSING PLAN OF CARE 34-1 *continued*

for Carla Potter

NURSING INTERVENTIONS	RATIONALE	EVALUATIVE STATEMENT
Assess value patient attaches to physical fitness and regular periods of aerobic exercise; explore preferences.	Exercise can alleviate symptoms of depression, tension, anxiety, fatigue, and irritability. Exercise also serves as a distraction from discomforts.	10/30/14 Outcome met. Patient includes daily brisk walk around her neighborhood in her routine. *R. Gordon, RNC*
Instruct patient in use of regular daily exercise; design exercise prescription.	The fitness produced by regular exercise contributes to self-esteem.	

EXPECTED OUTCOME   By the next monthly assessment, 10/30/14, the patient will:

- Supplement her diet with 50 mg of vitamin B_6 daily

NURSING INTERVENTIONS	RATIONALE	EVALUATIVE STATEMENT
Instruct patient on daily use of vitamin B_6.	Vitamin B_6 may be effective in relieving symptoms of irritability, fatigue, and depression.	10/30/14 Outcome met. Patient supplements her diet daily with 50 mg of vitamin B_6. *R. Gordon, RNC*

EXPECTED OUTCOME   By the next monthly assessment, 10/30/14, the patient will:

- Continue use of daily record of premenstrual syndrome (PMS) symptoms

NURSING INTERVENTIONS	RATIONALE	EVALUATIVE STATEMENT
Instruct patient to continue use of daily record of PMS symptoms throughout the menstrual cycle.	Record keeping allows evaluation of the effectiveness of care plan.	10/30/14 Outcome met. Patient continued daily record, which illustrated drastic reduction in occurrence of PMS symptoms. Patient expressed delight in greater feeling of control she now has over how she feels. "I never realized that so many things affect my comfort level and health." *R. Gordon, RNC*

SAMPLE DOCUMENTATION	8/13/14 Nursing
	Consultation with patient regarding apparent symptoms of PMS. She stated she experiences fatigue, anxiety, irritability, depression, and mood swings about 1 week before her menses. She states these symptoms interfere with her job performance and relationships. She also states that these symptoms seem to subside after onset of her menses. Patient admits to use of tranquilizers but prefers not to use medication. Advised patient to keep daily record of symptoms for one complete menstrual cycle. Patient indicated understanding of all instructions. She will return to office after completion of daily record for its analysis and to begin treatment, if indicated. *R. Gordon, RNC*

Courtesy of Ruth E. Gordon, RNC, CRNP, DEd, Assistant Professor, Department of Nursing, Millersville University, Millersville, PA.

SKILL 34-1 GIVING A BACK MASSAGE

DELEGATION CONSIDERATIONS	Providing a back massage may be delegated to nursing assistive personnel (NAP) or unlicensed assistive personnel (UAP), as well as to licensed practical/vocational nurses (LPN/LVNs). The decision to delegate must be based on careful analysis of the patient's needs and circumstances, as well as the qualifications of the person to whom the task is being delegated. Refer to the Delegation Guidelines in Appendix A (found on thePoint).

EQUIPMENT	• Pain assessment tool and pain scale	• Towel
	• Powder, if not contraindicated	• Nonsterile gloves, if indicated
	• Bath blanket	• Additional PPE, as indicated

IMPLEMENTATION

ACTION	RATIONALE
1. Perform hand hygiene and put on PPE, if indicated.	Hand hygiene and PPE prevent the spread of microorganisms. PPE is required based on transmission precautions.
2. Identify the patient.	Identifying the patient ensures that the right patient receives the intervention and helps prevent errors.
3. Offer a back massage to the patient and explain the procedure.	Explanation encourages patient understanding and cooperation and reduces apprehension.
4. Put on gloves, if indicated.	Gloves are not usually necessary. Gloves prevent contact with blood and body fluid.
5. Close the room door and/or the curtain around the bed.	Closing the door or curtain provides privacy, promotes relaxation, and reduces noise and stimuli that may aggravate pain and reduce comfort.
6. Assess the patient's pain, using an appropriate assessment tool and measurement scale (see Table 34-4, p. 1164).	Accurate assessment is necessary to guide treatment and pain relief interventions and to evaluate the effectiveness of pain control measures.
7. Raise the bed to a comfortable working position, usually elbow height of the caregiver (VISN 8 Patient Safety Center, 2009), and lower the side rail.	Having the bed at the proper height prevents back and muscle strain.
8. Assist the patient to a comfortable position, preferably the prone or side-lying position. Remove the covers and move the patient's gown just enough to expose the patient's back from the shoulders to sacral area. Drape the patient, as needed, with the bath blanket.	This position exposes an adequate area for massage. Draping the patient provides privacy and warmth.
9. Warm the lubricant or lotion in the palm of your hand, or place the container in a small basin of warm water. **During massage, observe the patient's skin for reddened or open areas. Pay particular attention to the skin over bony prominences.** (See Chapter 31 for detailed information regarding skin assessment.)	Cold lotion causes chilling and discomfort. Pressure may interfere with circulation and lead to pressure ulcers.
10. Using light, gliding strokes (*effleurage*), apply lotion to patient's shoulders, back, and sacral area (Figure 1).	Effleurage relaxes the patient and lessens tension.

ACTION

RATIONALE

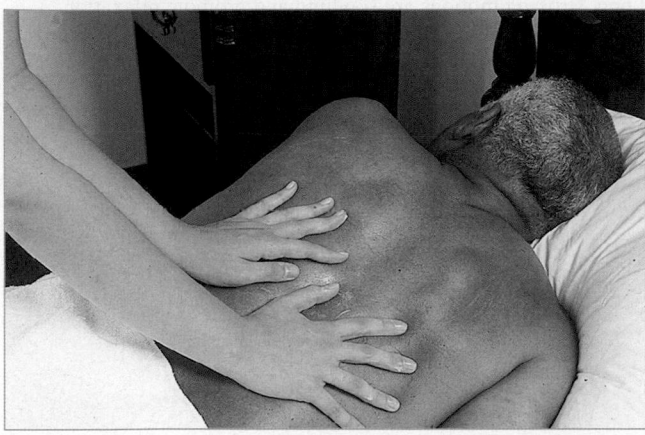

FIGURE 1. Using effleurage on a patient's back.

11. Place your hands beside each other at the base of the patient's spine and stroke upward to the shoulders and back downward to the buttocks in slow, continuous strokes (Figure 2). Continue for several minutes.

Continuous contact is soothing and stimulates circulation and muscle relaxation.

12. Massage the patient's shoulder, entire back, areas over the iliac crests, and sacrum with circular stroking motions. **Keep your hands in contact with the patient's skin.** Continue for several minutes, applying additional lotion, as necessary.

A firm stroke with continuous contact promotes relaxation

13. Knead the patient's skin by gently alternating grasping and compression motions (*pétrissage*) (Figure 3).

Kneading increases blood circulation.

FIGURE 2. Stroking upward to the shoulders.

FIGURE 3. Using pétrissage.

(continued)

SKILL 34-1 GIVING A BACK MASSAGE *continued*

ACTION	RATIONALE
14. Complete the massage with additional long, stroking movements that eventually become lighter in pressure (Figure 4).	Long, stroking motions are soothing and promote relaxation; continued stroking with gradual lightening of pressure helps extend the feeling of relaxation.

FIGURE 4. Using light strokes with lessening pressure.

ACTION	RATIONALE
15. Use the towel to pat the patient dry and to remove excess lotion.	Drying provides comfort and reduces the feeling of moisture on the back.
16. Remove gloves, if worn. Reposition the patient's gown and covers. Raise the side rail and lower the bed. Assist the patient to a position of comfort.	Repositioning bedclothes, linens, and the patient helps to promote patient comfort and safety.
17. Remove additional PPE, if used. Perform hand hygiene.	Removing PPE properly reduces the risk for infection transmission and contamination of other items. Hand hygiene prevents transmission of microorganisms.
18. Evaluate the patient's response to interventions. Reassess the level of discomfort or pain using original assessment tools. Reassess and alter plan of care, as appropriate.	Reassessment allows for individualization of the patient's plan of care and promotes optimal patient comfort.

DOCUMENTATION

Guidelines

Document pain assessment and other significant assessments. Document massage use, length of time of massage, and patient response. Record alternative treatments to consider, if appropriate.

Sample Documentation

> 12/6/15 2330 Patient reports inability to sleep and increased pain at surgical site, rated 3/10. Medicated with propoxyphene 100 mg and acetaminophen 650 mg, as ordered. Back massage administered ×10 minutes. Skin intact without redness. Patient reports increased comfort and relaxation; "I feel like I could sleep now."
>
> —B. Black, RN
>
> 12/6/15 2400 Patient reports pain level 0/10.
>
> —B. Black, RN

UNEXPECTED SITUATIONS AND ASSOCIATED INTERVENTIONS

• *The patient cannot lie prone, so you are giving him a back massage while he is lying on his side. However, as you begin to massage the back, the patient cannot maintain the side-lying position:* If possible, have the patient hold on to the side rail on the side to which he is facing. If this is not possible or the patient cannot assist, use pillows and bath blankets to prevent the patient from rolling. If necessary, enlist the help of another person to maintain the patient's position. If possible, experiment with other positions based on the patient's condition and comfort, such as leaning forward against a pillow on the bedside table while sitting in a chair.

• *While massaging the patient's back, you notice a 2 inch reddened area on the patient's sacrum:* Note this observation in the patient's medical record and report it to the physician. Do not massage the area. When the back massage is completed, position the patient off the sacral area, using pillows to maintain the patient's position, and institute a turning schedule.

SPECIAL CONSIDERATIONS

General Considerations

• Before giving a back massage, assess the patient's body structure and skin condition, tailoring the duration and intensity of the massage accordingly. If you are giving a back massage at bedtime, have the patient ready for bed beforehand so the massage can help the patient fall asleep.

• If the patient has oily skin, substitute a talcum powder or lotion of the patient's choice. However, to avoid aspiration, do not use powder if the patient has an endotracheal or tracheal tube in place. Avoid using powder and lotion together because this can lead to skin maceration.

• When massaging the patient's back, stand with one foot slightly forward and your knees slightly bent to allow effective use of your arm and shoulder muscles.

Infant and Child Considerations

• Hold infants and small children in a comfortable, well-supported position, such as against the chest or across the lap.

Older Adult Considerations

• Be gentle with massage. The skin on older adults is often fragile and dry.

DEVELOPING CLINICAL REASONING

1. Interview a nurse who specializes in pain management. Ask the nurse to describe the various physiologic and emotional responses to pain that the nurse has observed in patients with acute and chronic pain. Question the nurse about the different nursing interventions most likely to be effective for patients, in general, experiencing either acute or chronic pain. Inquire about specific pain management information and guidelines that the nurse usually includes in discharge planning and teaching.

2. Consider what you personally believe about pain: what it is, what causes it, what is most likely to relieve it. Determine how pain is currently being managed within the tradition of Western medicine and what role nursing plays in keeping patients pain free. Visit nontraditional health centers where practitioners use a variety of noninvasive pain relief modalities, such as acupressure, relaxation techniques, imagery, and massage. In what ways, if any, has this new learning experience modified your beliefs about pain? Will it change your ability to design effective pain management regimens for your patients?

PREPARING FOR NCLEX

1. A nurse instructor is teaching a class of student nurses about the nature of pain. Which statements accurately describe this phenomenon? Select all that apply.
   a. Pain is whatever the physician treating the pain says it is.
   b. Pain exists whenever the person experiencing it says it exists.
   c. Pain is an emotional and sensory reaction to tissue damage.
   d. Pain is a simple, universal, and easy-to-describe phenomenon.
   e. Pain that occurs without a known cause is psychological in nature.
   f. Pain is classified by duration, location, source, transmission, and etiology.

2. One of the most common distinctions of pain is whether it is acute or chronic. Which examples describe chronic pain? Select all that apply.
   a. A patient is receiving chemotherapy for bladder cancer.
   b. An adolescent is admitted to the hospital for an appendectomy.
   c. A patient is experiencing a ruptured aneurysm.
   d. A patient who has fibromyalgia requests pain medication.
   e. A patient has back pain related to an accident that occurred last year.
   f. A patient is experiencing pain from second-degree burns.

3. A patient complains of abdominal pain that is difficult to localize. The nurse documents this as which type of pain?
   a. Cutaneous
   b. Visceral
   c. Superficial
   d. Somatic

4. A female patient who is having a myocardial infarction complains of pain that is situated in her jaw. The nurse documents this as what type of pain?
   a. Transient pain
   b. Superficial pain
   c. Phantom pain
   d. Referred pain

5. The three types of responses to pain are physiologic, behavioral, and affective. Which are examples of behavioral responses to pain? Select all that apply.
   a. A patient cradles a wrist that was injured in a car accident.
   b. A child is moaning and crying due to a stomachache.
   c. A patient's pulse is increased following a myocardial infarction.
   d. A patient in pain strikes out at a nurse who attempts to bathe him.
   e. A patient who has chronic cancer pain is depressed and withdrawn.
   f. A child pulls away from a nurse trying to give him an injection.

6. An elderly patient is confined to bedrest following cervical spine surgery to treat nerve pinching. The nurse is vigilant about turning the patient and assessing the patient regularly to prevent the formation of pressure ulcers. What type of agent is the stimulus for pressure ulcers?
   a. Mechanical
   b. Thermal
   c. Chemical
   d. Electrical

7. A nurse uses a whirlpool to relax a patient following intense physical therapy to restore movement in her legs. What is a potent pain-blocking neuromodulator, released through relaxation techniques?
   a. Prostaglandins
   b. Substance P
   c. Endorphins
   d. Serotonin

8. A patient is postoperative following an emergency cesarean section birth. The patient asks the nurse about the use of pain medications following surgery. What would be a correct response by the nurse?
   a. "It's not a good idea to ask for pain medication regularly as it can be addictive."
   b. "It is better to wait until the pain gets unbearable before asking for pain medication."
   c. "It's natural to have to put up with pain after surgery and it will lessen in intensity in a few days."
   d. "Your doctor has ordered pain medications for you, which you should not be afraid to request any time you have pain."

9. Applying the gate control theory of pain, what would be an effective nursing intervention for a patient with lower back pain?
   a. Encouraging regular use of analgesics
   b. Applying a moist heating pad to the area at prescribed intervals
   c. Reviewing the pain experience with the patient
   d. Ambulating the patient after administering medication

10. The nurse is assessing the pain of a neonate who is admitted to the NICU with a heart defect. Which pain assessment scale would be the best tool to use with this patient?
   a. CRIES scale
   b. COMFORT scale
   c. FLACC scale
   d. FACES scale

11. Mr. Wright is recovering from abdominal surgery. When the nurse assists him to walk, she observes that he grimaces, moves stiffly, and becomes pale. She is aware that he has consistently refused his pain medication. What would be a priority nursing diagnosis for this patient?
   a. Acute Pain related to fear of taking prescribed postoperative medications
   b. Impaired Physical Mobility related to surgical procedure
   c. Anxiety related to outcome of surgery
   d. Risk for Infection related to surgical incision

12. When developing the plan of care for a patient with chronic pain, the nurse plans interventions based on the knowledge that chronic pain is most effectively relieved when analgesics are administered in what matter?
   a. On a PRN (as needed) basis
   b. Conservatively
   c. Around the clock (ATC)
   d. Intramuscularly

13. When assessing pain in a child, the nurse needs to be aware of what considerations?
   a. Immature neurologic development results in reduced sensation of pain.
   b. Inadequate or inconsistent relief of pain is widespread.
   c. Reliable assessment tools are currently unavailable.
   d. Narcotic analgesic use should be avoided.

14. A pregnant woman is receiving an epidural analgesic prior to delivery. The nurse provides vigilant monitoring of this patient to prevent the occurrence of:
   a. Pruritus
   b. Urinary retention
   c. Vomiting
   d. Respiratory depression

15. When assessing a patient receiving a continuous opioid infusion, the nurse immediately notifies the physician when the patient has:
   a. A respiratory rate of 10/min with normal depth
   b. A sedation level of 4
   c. Mild confusion
   d. Reported constipation

ANSWERS WITH RATIONALES

1. **b, c, f.** Margo McCaffery (1979, p. 11) offers the classic definition of pain that is probably of greatest benefit to nurses and their patients: "Pain is whatever the experiencing person says it is, existing whenever he (or she) says it does." The International Association for the Study of Pain (IASP) further defines pain as an unpleasant sensory and emotional experience associated with actual or potential tissue damage (IASP, 1994). Pain is an elusive and complex phenomenon, and despite its universality, its exact nature remains a mystery. Pain is present whenever a person says it is, even when no specific cause of the pain can be found. Pain may be classified according to its duration, its location or source, its mode of transmission, or its etiology.

2. **a, d, e.** Chronic pain is pain that may be limited, intermittent, or persistent but that lasts beyond the normal healing period. Examples are cancer pain, fibromyalgia pain, and back pain. Acute pain is generally rapid in onset and varies in intensity from mild to severe, as occurs with an emergency appendectomy, a ruptured aneurysm, and pain from burns.

3. *b.* The patient's pain would be categorized as visceral pain, which is poorly localized and can originate in body organs in the abdomen. Cutaneous pain (superficial pain) usually involves the skin or subcutaneous tissue. A paper cut that produces sharp pain with a burning sensation is an example of cutaneous pain. Deep somatic pain is diffuse or scattered and originates in tendons, ligaments, bones, blood vessels, and nerves. Strong pressure on a bone or damage to tissue that occurs with a sprain causes deep somatic pain.

4. *d.* Referred pain is perceived in an area distant from its point of origin, whereas transient pain is brief and passes quickly. Superficial pain originates in the skin or subcutaneous tissue. Phantom pain may occur in a person who has had a body part amputated, either surgically or traumatically.

5. *a, b, f.* Protecting or guarding a painful area, moaning and crying, and moving away from painful stimuli are behavioral responses. Examples of a physiologic or involuntary response would be increased blood pressure or dilation of the pupils. Affective responses, such as anger, withdrawal, and depression, are psychological in nature.

6. *a.* Receptors in the skin and superficial organs may be stimulated by mechanical, thermal, chemical, and electrical agents. Friction from bed linens causing pressure sores and pressure from a cast are mechanical stimulants. Sunburn is a thermal stimulant. An acid burn is the result of a chemical stimulant. The jolt from a lightening bolt is an electrical stimulant.

7. *c.* Endorphins are produced at neural synapses at various points along the CNS pathway. They are powerful pain-blocking chemicals that have prolonged analgesic effects and produce euphoria. It is thought that endorphins are released through pain relief measures, such as relaxation techniques. Prostaglandins, substance P, and serotonin (a hormone that can act to stimulate smooth muscles, inhibit gastric secretion, and produce vasoconstriction) are neurotransmitters or substances that either excite or inhibit target nerve cells.

8. *d.* Many pain medications are ordered on a PRN (as needed) basis. Therefore, nurses must be diligent to assess patients for pain and administer medications as needed. A patient should not be afraid to request these medications and should not wait until the pain is unbearable. Few people become addicted to the medications if used for a short period of time. Pain following surgery can be controlled and should not be considered a natural part of the experience that will lessen in time.

9. *b.* Nursing measures such as applying warmth to the lower back stimulate the large nerve fibers to close the gate and block the pain. The other choices do not involve attempts to stimulate large nerve fibers that interfere with pain transmission as explained by the gate control theory.

10. *a.* The CRIES Pain Scale is a tool intended for use with neonates and infants from 0 to 6 months. The COMFORT Scale, used to assess pain and distress in critically ill pediatric patients, relies on six behavioral and two physiologic factors that determine the level of analgesia needed to adequately relieve pain in these children. The FLACC scale (F—Faces, L—Legs, A—Activity, C—Cry, C—Consolability) was designed for infants and children from age 2 months to 7 years who are unable to validate the presence or severity of pain. The FACES scale is used for children who can compare their pain to the faces depicted on the scale.

11. *a.* Mr. Wright's immediate problem is his pain that is unrelieved because he refuses to take his pain medication for an unknown reason. The other nursing diagnoses are plausible, but not a priority in this situation.

12. *c.* The PRN protocol is totally inadequate for patients experiencing chronic pain. ATC doses of analgesics are more effective, whereas conservative pain management for whatever reason may also prove ineffective. Intramuscular administration is not practical on a long-range basis for a patient with chronic pain.

13. *b.* Health care personnel are only now becoming aware of pain relief as a priority for children in pain. The evidence supports the fact that children do indeed feel pain and reliable assessment tools are available specifically for use with children. Opioid analgesics may be safely used with children as long as they are carefully monitored.

14. *d.* Too much of an opioid drug given by way of an epidural catheter or a displaced catheter may result in the occurrence of respiratory depression. Pruritus, urinary retention, and vomiting may occur but are not life threatening.

15. *b.* Sedation level is more indicative of respiratory depression because a drop in level usually precedes it. A sedation level of 4 calls for immediate action because the patient has minimal or no response to stimuli. A respiratory level of 10 with normal depth of breathing is usually not a cause for alarm. Mild confusion may be evident with the initial dose and then disappear; additional observation is necessary. Constipation should be reported to the physician, but is not the priority in this situation.

TAYLOR SUITE RESOURCES

Explore these additional resources to enhance learning for this chapter:

- NCLEX-Style Questions and other resources on thePoint, http://thePoint.lww.com/Taylor8e
- *Study Guide for Fundamentals of Nursing, 8th edition*
- Adaptive Learning | Powered by prepU, http://thepoint.lww.com/prepu
- *Skill Checklists for Fundamentals of Nursing, 8th edition*
- *Taylor's Clinical Nursing Skills:* Chapter 10, Comfort and Pain Management
- *Taylor's Video Guide to Clinical Nursing Skills:* Comfort
- *Lippincott DocuCare* Fundamentals cases

Bibliography

Anderson, P. (2012). Opioid rotation practices linked to fatalities. Available at http://www.medscape.com/viewarticle/761577

Arnstein, P. (2010). Is my patient drug-seeking or in need of pain relief? *Nursing, 40*(5), 60–61.

Arnstein, P. (2011). Multimodal approaches to pain management. *Nursing, 41*(3), 60–61.

Arnstein, P., Broglio, K., & Wuhrman, E. (2011). Placebos: No place in pain management. *Nursing, 41*(1), 66–67.

Baldridge, K., & Andrasik, F. (2010). Pain assessment in people with intellectual or developmental disabilities. *American Journal of Nursing, 110*(12), 29–37.

Beyer, J., Denyes, M. J., & Villarruel, A. M. (1992). The creation, validation, and continuing development of the Oucher: A measure of pain intensity in children. *Journal of Pediatric Nursing, 7*(5), 335–346.

Brown, S., Kirkpatrick, M., Swanson, M., & McKenzie, I. (2011). Pain experience of the elderly. Available at http://www.medscape.com/viewarticle/754762

Bulechek, G., Butcher, H., Dochterman, J., & Wagner, C. (2013). *Nursing Interventions Classification (NIC)* (6th ed., pp. 285–286). St. Louis: Elsevier/Mosby.

Centers for Disease Control and Prevention (CDC). (2012). Prescription painkiller overdoses in the U.S. Available at http://www.cdc.gov/Features/VitalSigns/PainkillerOverdoses/

D'Arcy, Y. (2010a). How to manage pain in addicted patients. *Nursing, 40*(8), 60–64.

D'Arcy, Y. (2010b). Is continuous subcutaneous infusion a good route for pain medication? *Nursing, 40*(10), 59–60.

D'Arcy, Y. (2010c). Managing chronic pain in acute care: Getting it right. *Nursing, 40*(4), 49–51.

D'Arcy, Y. (2011a). New criteria for assessing and treating neuropathic pain. *Nursing, 41*(12), 61–62.

D'Arcy, Y. (2011b). "Paws" to provide comfort, relieve pain. *Nursing, 41*(4), 67–68.

Dobbins, E. (2010). Where has all the meperidine gone? *Nursing, 40*(1), 65–66.

Dunn, D., & Neuman, J. (2012). How substance abuse impacts pain management in acute care. *Nursing, 42*(8), 66–68.

Eliopoulos, C. (2010). *Gerontological nursing.* Philadelphia: Wolters Kluwer Health/Lippincott Williams & Wilkins.

Facente, A. (2006). Humor in health care: Irreverent or invaluable? *Nursing, 36*(4), 64hn6–64hn7.

Galloway, K, Buckenmaier, C., & Polomano, R. (2011). Understanding pain and pain responses. *American Pain Today,* Sept (Suppl), 3–7.

Gandey, A. (2011). Pain specialists back plan for opioid education. Available at http:// www.medscape.com/viewarticle/743476

Hockenberry, M., & Wilson, D. (2013). *Wong's Essentials of Pediatric Nursing* (9th ed.). St. Louis: Elsevier/Mosby.

Institute of Medicine (IOM). 2011. *Relieving pain in America.* Washington, DC: The National Academies Press.

International Association for the Study of Pain (IASP). (1994). Part III: Pain terms, a current list with definitions and notes on usage. In H. Merskey & N. Bogduk (Eds). *Classification of chronic pain,* 2nd ed., pp. 209–214). Seattle: IASP Press.

International Association for the Study of Pain. (2012). *IASP taxonomy.* Available at http://www.iasp-pain.org/Education/Content.aspx?ItemNumber=1698.

Jablonski, A., DuPen, A., & Ersek, M. (2011). The use of algorithms in assessing and managing persistent pain in older adults. *American Journal of Nursing, 111*(3), 34–45.

Jeffrey, S. (2012). FDA issues warning on fentanyl patches. Available at http://www.medscape.com/viewarticle/762326

Joanna Briggs Institute (2011). Nursing intervention for adult patients experiencing chronic pain. *Best practice: Evidence-based information sheets for health professionals, 15*(10), 1–4.

The Joint Commission (TJC). (2012a). Facts about pain management. Available at http://www.jointcommission.org/pain_management/

The Joint Commission (TJC). (2012b). Nutritional, functional, and pain assessments and screens. Available at http://www.jointcommission.org/standards_information/jcfaqdetails.aspx?StandardsFaqid=208&Programid=1

Lehne, R. (2013). *Pharmacology of nursing care* (8th ed.). St. Louis: Elsevier/Saunders.

LeMone, P., Burke, K., & Bauldoff, G. (2011). *Medical–surgical nursing: Critical thinking in patient care* (5th ed.). Upper Saddle River, NJ: Pearson/Prentice Hall.

McCaffery, M. (1979). *Nursing management of the patient in pain* (2nd ed.). Philadelphia: J. B. Lippincott.

McGuire, L. (2011). Evidenced-based pain management. *Nurse.com NurseWeek,* 42–47.

Meghanis, S., & Gallagher, R. (2012). Time to take stock: A meta-analysis and systemic review of pain treatment disparities in the United States. *Pain Medicine, 13,* 150–174.

Moorhead, S., Johnson, M., Maas, M., & Swanson, E. (2013). *Nursing Outcomes Classification (NOC)* (5th ed., p. 719). St. Louis: Elsevier/Mosby.

NANDA International. (2012). *NANDA nursing diagnosis: Definitions & classification: 2012–2014.* West Sussex, UK: Wiley-Blackwell.

Narayan, M. C. (2010). Culture's effects on pain assessment and management. *American Journal of Nursing, 110*(4), 38–49.

National Center for Complementary and Alternative Medicine (NCCAM). (2010). Acupuncture for pain. Available at http://nccam.nih.gov/health/acupuncture/acupuncture-for-pain.htm

Overdyk, F. J., & Guerra, J. J. (2011). Improving outcomes in med–surg patients with opioid-induced respiratory depression. *American Nurse Today, 6*(11), 26–31.

Pasero, C., & McCaffery, M. (2011). *Pain assessment and pharmacological management.* St. Louis: Elsevier/Mosby.

Pasero, C. (2012). Breaking the cycle of breakthrough pain. Available at http://www.medscape.com/viewarticle/767957

Pfeifer, G. (2011). Transforming pain care: An IOM report. *American Journal of Nursing, 111*(9), 18.

Potera, C. (2010). Postoperative childhood pain undertreated at home. *American Journal of Nursing, 110*(1), 18.

Power, I. (2011). An update on analgesics. Available at http://www.medscape.com/viewarticle/745129

Purnell, L., & Paulanka, B. (2008). *Transcultural health care: A culturally competent approach* (3rd ed.). Philadelphia: F. A. Davis.

Quinn-O'Neil, B., Kilgallen, M., & Terlizzi, J. (2011). Creating a unit-based resource nurse program. *American Journal of Nursing, 111*(9), 46–51.

Rosier, P. (2012). Facing up to the challenge of range orders. *Nursing, 42*(12), 64–65.

Sammons, M. (2011). The healing power of touch. Available at http://news.nurse.com/article/20110818/ED02/110818002#.U2fDoyjA5UQ.

Sawhney, M. (2012). Epidural analgesia: What nurses need to know. *Nursing, 42*(8), 36–42.

Sherwood, G., & Barnsteiner, J. (2012). *Quality and safety in nursing.* West Sussex, UK: Wiley-Blackwell.

Simmons, S. (2011). Complementary and alternative therapies for low-back pain. *Nursing, 41*(5), 54–55.

Smeltzer, S., Bare, B., Hinkle, J., & Cheever, K. (2010). *Textbook of medical–surgical nursing* (12th ed.). Philadelphia: Wolters Kluwer Health/Lippincott Williams & Wilkins.

Stett, G. (2010). About the MOD. Available at http://www.avancen.com/about_the_mod.php

U.S. Food and Drug Administration (FDA). (2010). Second safety warning on fentanyl skin patch. Available at http://www.fda.gov/ForConsumers/ConsumerUpdates/ucm100223.htm

Vargas-Schaffer, G. (2010). Is the WHO analgesic ladder still valid? *Canadian Family Practice, 56*(6), 514–517.

VISN 8 Patient Safety Center. (2009). Safe patient handling and movement. Available at http://www.visn8.va.gov/visn8/patientsafetycenter/safePtHandling/default.asp

Wardell, D., Decker, S., & Engebretson, J. (2012). Healing touch for older adults with persistent pain. *Holistic Nursing Practice, 26*(4), 194–202.

Westbrook, G., & D'Arcy, Y. (2012). Pain management basics. *Nurse.com, 21*(3), 28–33.

Whitaker, M. (2010). Sounds soothing: Music therapy for postoperative pain. *Nursing, 40*(12), 53–54.

35

Nutrition

SUSAN OAKLAND

Susan Oakland, a 21-year-old student, is pregnant with her first child. Susan is in the ninth week of her pregnancy. She is experiencing persistent nausea, vomiting, and fatigue. She has had difficulty eating, with a resulting weight loss of 3 pounds since her first prenatal visit at 5 weeks gestation.

WILLIAM JOHNSTON

William Johnston, a 42-year-old executive, is newly diagnosed with high blood pressure and high cholesterol. He confides that his health has been the last thing on his mind and that his health habits are less than admirable. "I usually eat on the run, often fast food, or big dinners with lots of alcohol. I can't remember the last time I worked out or did any exercise, unless running from my car to the train counts! I guess it's no wonder I've gained a few pounds over the years!"

CHARLES GALLAGHER

Charles Gallagher is the husband of a 67-year-old woman who is in the end stages of advanced dementia. She had a percutaneous endoscopic gastrostomy (PEG) inserted during her last hospitalization 6 weeks ago due to recurrent episodes of aspiration pneumonia from an inability to swallow. He states, "I was talking to the chaplain at the long-term care facility, and he questioned the wisdom of this tube. I respect him but we really don't have an option here, do we? I mean, if they take the tube out she'll starve to death—right?"

DocuCare | Additional patient scenarios available in *Lippincott DocuCare*.

KEY TERMS

absorption	gastrostomy	peripheral parenteral nutrition (PPN)
anorexia	ketosis	
anthropometric	lipid	
aspiration	minerals	protein
basal metabolism	nasogastric (NG) tube	recommended dietary allowance (RDA)
body mass index (BMI)	nasointestinal (NI) tube	
calorie	NPO	total parenteral nutrition (TPN)
carbohydrate	nutrient	
cholesterol	nutrition	trans fat
digestion	obesity	triglycerides
dysphagia	parenteral nutrition	vitamins
enteral nutrition	percutaneous endoscopic gastrostomy tube (PEG)	waist circumference
gastric residual		

Nutrition is vital for life and health. Poor nutrition can seriously decrease one's level of wellness, which makes it a vital component of nursing. This chapter provides information about the basic principles of nutrition, focusing on the six classes of nutrients, energy balance, choices for an adequate diet, food patterns and habits, and factors affecting nutrition. In addition, components of simple screening and in-depth nutritional assessments are outlined. Two sets of nursing diagnoses are provided, and patient outcomes for healthy nutrition are discussed. The accompanying plan of care illustrates the significance of nutrition in nursing care. Nurses incorporate nutrition into all aspects of patient-centered nursing care and are involved in all aspects of nutritional care. Refer to the accompanying Reflective Practice box.

PRINCIPLES OF NUTRITION

The science of **nutrition** is the study of how food nourishes the body. It encompasses the study of nutrients and how they are handled by the body as well as the impact of human behavior and environment on the process of nourishment. As such, this discipline involves physiology, psychology, and socioeconomics.

Nutrients are specific biochemical substances used by the body for growth, development, activity, reproduction, lactation, health maintenance, and recovery from illness or injury. The metabolic processes involved in these functions are complex. Subsequently, most nutrients work better together than they do alone. Also, nutrient needs change throughout the life cycle in response to changes in body size, activity, growth, development, and state of health.

Some nutrients are considered *essential* because either they are not synthesized in the body or are made in insufficient amounts. Essential nutrients must be provided in the diet or through supplements. Essential nutrients that supply energy and build tissue (such as carbohydrates, fats, protein) are referred to as *macronutrients. Micronutrients*, such as vitamins and minerals, are required in much smaller amounts to regulate and control body processes.

Nonessential nutrients do not have to be supplied through dietary sources because they either are not required for body functioning or are synthesized in the body in adequate amounts. Some nutrients can be converted to others in the body. For instance, the body converts excess carbohydrates and protein into fat and stores them as triglycerides.

Of the six classes of nutrients, three supply energy (carbohydrates, protein, lipids [fats]) and three are needed to regulate body processes (vitamins, minerals, water).

Energy Balance

The body needs energy to function. Energy is derived or obtained from foods consumed. Energy in the diet is measured in the form of kilocalories, commonly abbreviated as **calories**, or cal. Only carbohydrates, protein, and fat provide energy. Vitamins and minerals, needed for the metabolism of energy, do not provide calories.

Total energy intake for a meal, a day, or longer, can be calculated by using food composition tables: The values given for total calories for each food item eaten can simply be added, or the grams of carbohydrate, protein, and fat for

REFLECTIVE PRACTICE: CULTIVATING QSEN COMPETENCIES

CHALLENGE TO LEGAL AND ETHICAL SKILLS

Mrs. Constance Gallagher is only 67 years old, but she is in the end stages of advanced dementia. She can no longer swallow and has had several hospitalizations in the past year for aspiration pneumonia. She lives in a long-term care facility (where I am doing a clinical rotation for my gerontologic nursing experience) and has a devoted family—husband, son, and daughter—who all visit regularly. For the last 6 weeks, she has received enteral feedings from a percutaneous

endoscopic gastrostomy (PEG) tube that was placed during her last hospitalization. Mrs. Gallagher's husband confided to me that the chaplain at the long-term care facility, whom he respects and likes, questioned the wisdom of the feeding tube. He then asked me, "But we really don't have an option here, do we? I mean, if they take the tube out, she'll starve to death, no?" I had no idea how to respond.

Thinking Outside the Box: Possible Courses of Action

- Simply refer Mr. Gallagher to someone more experienced about these things (since I am clearly over my head).
- Find out more about this myself and then get back to him.

- Request an ethics consult to explore how we can best respond to the husband's questions about what is in his wife's best interests, taking into consideration the role the long-term care facility's chaplain is playing.

Evaluating a Good Outcome: How Do I Define Success?

- The patient's medical goals are met, including, if the family wishes, a dignified death.
- The Gallagher family feels at peace with their decisions and the results of these decisions.
- An ethically justified decision is made about continuing or withdrawing artificial nutrition and hydration that is

respectful of Mrs. Gallagher's wishes (to the extent that these are known) and compatible with her beliefs and interests.
- I develop skill in assisting with tough end-of-life decisions and learn more about how an ethics consult functions.

Personal Learning: Here's to the Future!

When I reported my exchange with Mr. Gallagher to the charge nurse, she said we might want to call an ethics consult because there were actually a few similar situations pending and not everyone on the unit seemed comfortable with the lead role the chaplain was taking in recommending the withdrawal of nutritional support. The consult was a great experience. All of the patient's family members attended, plus the medical director of the home, the nurses on the patient's unit, the chaplain, the social worker, the long-term care facility's ethicist, and myself. After the medical director described the natural progression of advanced dementia, the ethicist noted that there is a difference between dying of starvation (which only happens if food is withdrawn but fluids continue to hydrate) and dying of dehydration (which will happen if we pull the PEG tube and discontinue all enteral

feedings, and which is not believed to be painful). The ethicist then asked the family if they knew what the patient would want done if she could be asked if the benefits of continuing nutritional support outweighed the accompanying burdens of having her wrists restrained so she wouldn't pull out the tube, skin problems, and the like. After some discussion, they were in agreement that she would not want to live this way. Since the Gallaghers were Catholic, the Catholic chaplain was invited to describe what the Roman Catholic Church teaches about this. After a rather lengthy discussion, a decision was made to withdraw enteral feedings. The family seemed at peace with their decision.

Through this experience, I learned how an ethics consult works and can see the advantages of utilizing this resource in the future.

REFLECTION ON QUALITY AND SAFETY COMPETENCIES

How do you think you would respond in a similar situation? Why? What does this tell you about yourself and about the adequacy of your skills for professional practice? Do you agree with the criteria that the nursing student used to evaluate a successful outcome? Are there any other criteria that would be appropriate to use? Did the nursing student meet the criteria? Why or why not? What *knowledge, skills,* and *attitudes* do you need to develop to continuously improve the quality and safety of care for patients like Mrs. Gallagher?

Patient-Centered Care: What resources could you or the nurses offer to provide compassionate and coordinated care based on respect for the patient's preferences, values, and needs? How did the ethics consult facilitate decision making? What ethical and legal principles were maintained? How did the nursing student act as a patient advocate? Was the human dignity of the patient and the patient's family maintained?

Teamwork and Collaboration/Quality Improvement: What communication skills do you need to improve to ensure

that you function as a member of the patient-care team? What skills do you need to implement effective strategies for communicating and resolving conflict? What skills do you need to assert your own position/perspective in discussions about patient care? What other services or resources might be available to aid in this type of decision-making process?

Safety/Evidence-Based Practice: What skills do you need to improve to ensure that patients in your care receive the best nursing care possible? What evidence in nursing literature provides guidance for decision making regarding care of this patient?

Informatics: Can you identify the essential information that must be available in Mrs. Gallagher's electronic health record to support safe patient care and coordination of care? Can you identify the appropriate process to protect confidentiality of protected health information in the patient's health records? Can you think of other ways to respond to or approach the situation?

each food item eaten can be added and multiplied by the appropriate calorie level (4, 4, and 9 calories, respectively).

Energy in the body is used to carry on any kind of activity, whether voluntary or involuntary. A person's total daily energy expenditure is the sum of all the calories used to perform physical activity, maintain basal metabolism, and digest, absorb, and metabolize food.

If a person's daily energy intake is equal to total daily energy expenditure, the person's weight will remain stable. However, if the energy intake is less than the energy expended, the person's weight will decrease. If the energy intake exceeds energy expenditure, weight will increase.

Metabolic Requirements

Basal metabolism is the energy required to carry on the involuntary activities of the body at rest—the energy needed to sustain the metabolic activities of cells and tissues (Grossman & Porth, 2014). These activities include actions such as maintaining body temperature and muscle tone, producing and releasing secretions, propelling food through the gastrointestinal (GI) tract, inflating the lungs, and contracting the heart muscle. As the amount of energy used on physical activity declines, the proportion of calories used for basal metabolism increases; it accounts for more than half of most people's total energy requirements. Because of their larger muscle mass, men have a higher basal metabolic rate (BMR) than women. BMR is about 1 cal/kg of body weight per hour for men and 0.9 cal/kg per hour for women.

 THINK back to William Johnston, the middle-aged man with hypertension and high cholesterol. Based on the patient's gender, the nurse would expect his BMR to be greater than that for a woman. The nurse would need to consider this fact when planning the patient's care. ●

Other factors that increase BMR include growth, infections, fever, emotional tension, extreme environmental temperatures, and elevated levels of certain hormones, especially epinephrine and thyroid hormones. Aging, prolonged fasting, and sleep all decrease BMR. Most nutritionists agree that fasting or following a very–low-calorie diet defeats a weight-loss plan because the body interprets this eating pattern as starvation and compensates by slowing down the resting metabolic rate, making it even more difficult to lose weight.

Body Weight Standards

As previously discussed, if a person's energy intake does not equal energy expenditure, weight will fluctuate. Ideal body weight (IBW) or healthy body weight is an estimate of optimal weight for optimal health. A general guideline, often called the rule-of-thumb method, determines ideal weight based on height. This formula is as follows:

For adult females:

> 100 lb. (for height of 5 ft.) ± 5 lb. for each additional inch over 5 ft.

For adult males:

> 106 lb. (for height of 5 ft.) ± 6 lb. for each additional inch over 5 ft.

Add or deduct 10% from this figure based on body frame size. However, note that using this method can result in unrealistically low figures for adults who are very short or very tall, which must be taken into consideration. Height and weight tables are commonly used for infants and children.

The more preferred methods to establish ideal body weight include **body mass index (BMI)** for adults and children and measurement of **waist circumference** for adults only (National Institutes of Health [NIH], 2012a).

The BMI, or Quetelet Index (W/H^2), is a ratio of weight (in kilograms) to height (in meters). The BMI is a reliable indicator of total body fat stores in the general population. Health practitioners use this more accurate weight calculation as an initial assessment of nutritional status. The BMI does not differentiate according to gender and is calculated for adults in the following manner:

Using kilograms and meters:

$$BMI = \frac{\text{weight in kilograms}}{(\text{height in meters}) \times (\text{height in meters})}$$

Using pounds and inches:

$$BMI = \frac{\text{weight in pounds}}{(\text{height in inches}) \times (\text{height in inches})} \times 703$$

According to the most recent BMI guidelines published by the National Heart, Lung, and Blood Institute (NHLBI), a person with a BMI below 18.5 is underweight, a BMI of 18.5 to 24.9 is a healthy weight, a BMI of 25 to 29.9 indicates an overweight person, a BMI of 30 or greater indicates obesity, and a BMI of 40 or greater indicates extreme obesity (NIH, 2012a).

BMI also provides an estimation of relative risk for diseases such as heart disease, diabetes, and hypertension. However, it is important to note that BMI may not be accurate for certain groups of people, such as athletes, with a large muscle mass, people with edema or dehydration, and older people and others who have lost muscle mass (NIH, 2012a; Dudek, 2014). In addition, ethnic differences exist in the relationship between BMI and health risks (Dudek).

Overweight and obesity are defined differently for children and teens than for adults. Children are still growing, and boys and girls mature at different rates. BMIs for children and teens compare their heights and weights against growth charts that take age and gender into account. This is called BMI-for-age percentile. A child or teen's BMI-for-age percentile shows how the individual's BMI compares with other boys and girls of the same age (NIH, 2012a). Additional information about BMI-for-age and growth charts for children can be found at the BMI-for-age calculator from the Centers for Disease Control and Prevention (CDC, 2011). Refer to Box 35-1 for information to interpret the results of a BMI-for-age calculation.

Box 35-1 | BMI-FOR-AGE PERCENTILE (CHILDREN AND TEENS)

Less than 5th percentile	Underweight
5th percentile to less than the 85th percentile	Healthy weight
85th percentile to less than the 95th percentile	Overweight
95th percentile or greater	Obese

(Reprinted from National Institutes of Health [NIH]. National Heart, Lung and Blood Institute. [2012a]. How are overweight and obesity diagnosed? Available at http://www.nhlbi.nih.gov/health/health-topics/topics/obe/diagnosis.html; and Centers for Disease Control and Prevention [CDC]. [2011]. Healthy weight. Assessing your weight. BMI percentile calculator for child and teen. Available at http://apps.nccd.cdc.gov/dnpabmi/.)

A significant intentional or unintentional change in the patient's weight can also indicate poor nutritional status and/or health problems. Significant weight change is determined by how much weight is lost per unit of time. To calculate the percent of weight change, use the following formula.

$$\text{usual body weight} - \text{current body weight} \div \text{usual body weight} \times 100$$

Unintentional weight loss is considered significant if it falls into the following guidelines (Dudek, 2014):

- Greater than 2% in 1 week
- Greater than 5% in 1 month
- Greater than 7.5% in 3 months
- Greater than 10% in 6 months

Waist circumference is measured by placing a measuring tape snugly around the patient's waist at the level of the umbilicus (Fig. 35-1). This measurement is a good indicator of abdominal fat. Where excess body fat is deposited is thought to be an important and reliable indicator of risk for disease, such as type 2 diabetes, dyslipidemia, hypertension,

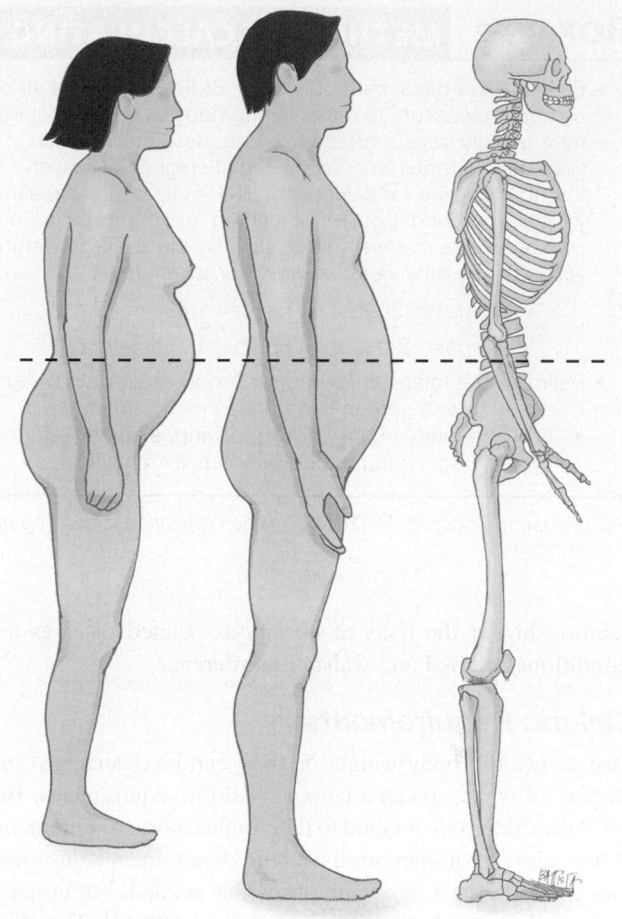

FIGURE 35-1. Positioning of measuring tape at the level of the umbilicus for waist circumference.

and cardiovascular disease (Dudek, 2014). This risk increases with a waist measurement of 40 inches or more for men and 35 inches or more for women (NIH, 2012a). As with BMI, ethnic groups differ in regard to where risk begins in relation to waist circumference (Dudek). Table 35-1 displays the

Table 35-1 | RISK OF OBESITY-ASSOCIATED DISEASES AND CONDITIONS BY BMI AND WAIST CIRCUMFERENCE RELATIVE TO NORMAL WEIGHT AND WAIST CIRCUMFERENCE

		WAIST CIRCUMFERENCE	
	BMI (kg/m²)	Men ≤40 Inches (102 cm) Women ≤35 Inches (88 cm)	Men >40 Inches (102 cm) Women >35 Inches (88 cm)
Underweight	<18.5	NA	NA
Normal	18.5–24.9	NA	NA
Overweight	25.0–29.9	Increased	High
Obesity, Class I	30.0–34.9	High	Very high
Obesity, Class II	35.0–39.9	Very high	Very high
Extreme Obesity	40.0+	Extremely high	Extremely high

*Increased waist circumference can also be a marker for increased risk even in persons of normal weight.

(Reprinted from National Institutes of Health [NIH], National Heart, Lung and Blood Institute [NHLBI]. [2000]. *The practical guide: Identification, evaluation, and treatment of overweight and obesity in adults.* Available at www.nhlbi.nih.gov/guidelines/obesity/prctgd_c.pdf)

BOX 35-2 METHOD OF CALCULATING CALORIC REQUIREMENTS

- Estimate the basal metabolic rate (BMR) or the amount of calories necessary to maintain the body at rest. Because men usually have a greater muscle mass than women, their caloric requirements are slightly higher. A rule-of-thumb guideline for calculating BMR is to multiply healthy weight (in pounds) by 10 for women and 11 for men. For a person who is overweight, multiply by the average weight within the healthy weight range. For example:

    Male: 130 lb × 11 cal/lb = 1,430 cal/day

    Female: 130 lb × 10 cal/lb = 1,300 cal/day

- Estimate the total calories according to usual activity level. Choose the category that describes usual activities.
    - 20% Sedentary: mostly sitting, driving, sleeping, standing, reading, typing, other low-intensity activities
- 30% Light activity: light exercise, such as walking not more than 2 hours per day
- 40% Moderate activity: moderate exercise such as heavy housework, gardening, and very little sitting
- 50% High activity: active in physical sports or a labor-intensive occupation, such as construction work
- Multiply the BMR by the percentage associated with the activity level. For example, the above female's BMR = 1,300 calories per day. She engages in light activity.

    1,300 × 30% = 390

    1,300 + 390 = 1,690 total daily calories

(Adapted from Dudek, S. G. [2014]. *Nutrition essentials for nursing practice* [7th ed.]. Philadelphia: Lippincott Williams & Wilkins/Wolters Kluwer Health.)

relationship of the risks of obesity-associated diseases and conditions by BMI and waist circumference.

Caloric Requirements

Just as healthy body weight or IBW can be determined in a variety of ways, so can a person's calorie requirements. Box 35-2 illustrates one method to determine calorie requirements. After calorie requirements have been determined, adjustments can be made for weight gain or loss, as needed. For instance, 1 lb (0.45 kg) of body fat equals about 3,500 cal. Therefore, to gain or lose 1 lb (0.45 kg) in a week, it is necessary to increase or decrease, respectively, daily calorie intake by 500 cal (3,500 cal divided by 7 days = 500 cal/day). Similarly, a weight gain or loss of 2 lb (0.9 kg) per week would require an adjustment of 1,000 cal/day. Because it becomes increasingly difficult to plan an adequate diet as the calorie level drops, diets that result in more than a 2-lb (0.9-kg) weight loss per week are not recommended.

 CONSIDER William Johnston, the man with poor health habits. The nurse would work with Mr. Johnston to develop an appropriate weight-loss plan that would contain adequate calories yet still foster a weight loss of 1 to 2 lb/week. Doing so would promote weight loss while still allowing for adequate nutritional intake. ●

Energy Nutrients

Carbohydrates, protein, and fats are potential sources of energy for the body.

Carbohydrates

Carbohydrates, commonly known as sugars and starches, are organic compounds composed of carbon, hydrogen, and oxygen. They serve as the structural framework of plants. The only animal source of carbohydrate in the diet is lactose, or "milk sugar."

The significance of carbohydrates cannot be overstated. They are relatively easy to produce and store, making them the most abundant and least expensive source of calories in the diet worldwide. In countries where grains are the dietary staple, carbohydrates may contribute as much as 90% of total calories. Table 35-2 summarizes the sources, functions, and significance of dietary carbohydrates. Carbohydrate intake is often correlated to income. As income increases, carbohydrate intake decreases and protein intake, a more expensive form of energy, increases.

CLASSIFICATION AND METABOLISM

The number of molecules within the structure determines the classification of carbohydrates. They are classified as simple (monosaccharide and disaccharide) or complex (polysaccharide) sugars.

Carbohydrates are more easily and quickly digested than protein and fat. Ninety percent of carbohydrate intake is digested. This percentage decreases as fiber intake increases. All carbohydrates are converted to glucose for transport through the blood or for use as energy. Glucose is an efficient fuel that certain tissues, particularly the central nervous system, rely on almost exclusively for energy. Glucose is transported from the GI tract, through the portal vein, to the liver. The liver stores glucose and regulates its entry into the blood. Hormones, especially insulin and glucagon, are responsible for keeping serum glucose levels fairly constant during both feasting and fasting.

Through a series of steps, cells oxidize (burn) glucose to provide energy, carbon dioxide, and water. Depending on a person's state of energy balance, the period between when carbohydrate is consumed and when it is used for energy may vary from minutes to months or longer. Unlike protein and fat, glucose is burned efficiently and completely and does not leave a toxic product for the kidneys to excrete.

When the supply of glucose exceeds what is needed for energy and for maintaining serum levels, it is stored. If muscle or liver glycogen stores are deficient, glucose

Table 35-2 SOURCES, FUNCTIONS, AND SIGNIFICANCE OF CARBOHYDRATES, PROTEIN, AND FAT

NUTRIENT	SOURCES	FUNCTIONS	SIGNIFICANCE
Carbohydrates			
Simple sugars and starch	Fruits Vegetables Grains: rice, pasta, breads, cereals Dried peas and beans Milk (lactose) Sugars: white and brown sugar, honey, molasses, syrup	Provide energy Spare protein so it can be used for other functions Prevent ketosis from inefficient fat metabolism	An adequate intake for total fiber is 25 g/day (women) and 38 g/day (men); maximum level of 25% of total calories or less from added sugars. Low carbohydrate intake can cause ketosis; high simple sugar intake increases the risk for dental caries.
Cellulose and other water-insoluble fibers	Whole wheat flour and wheat bran Vegetables: cabbage, peas, green beans, wax beans, broccoli, brussel sprouts, cucumber skins, peppers, carrots Apples	Absorb water to increase fecal bulk Decrease intestinal transit time	Are nondigestible; therefore, are excreted Help relieve constipation North Americans are urged to eat more of all types of fiber. Excess intake can cause gas, distention, and diarrhea.
Water-soluble fibers	Oat bran and oatmeal Dried peas and beans Vegetables Prunes, pears, apples, bananas, oranges	Slow gastric emptying Lower serum cholesterol level Delay glucose absorption	Help improve glucose tolerance in diabetics
Protein	Milk and milk products Meat, poultry, fish Eggs Dried peas and beans Nuts	Tissue growth and repair Component of body framework: bones, muscles, tendons, blood vessels, skin, hair, nails Component of body fluids: hormones, enzymes, plasma proteins, neurotransmitters, mucus Helps regulate fluid balance through oncotic pressure Helps regulate acid–base balance Detoxifies harmful substances Forms antibodies Transports fat and other substances through the blood Provides energy when carbohydrate intake is inadequate	Experts recommend that we eat less animal protein and more vegetable protein. Protein deficiency is characterized by edema, retarded growth and maturation, muscle wasting, changes in the hair and skin, permanent damage to physical and mental development (in children), diarrhea, malabsorption, numerous secondary nutrient deficiencies, fatty infiltration of the liver, increased risk for infections, and high mortality. Protein malnutrition occurs secondary to chronic diseases, such as cancer, AIDS, and COPD; it may also result from acute critical illnesses such as trauma and sepsis. It may also be seen in the homeless, the elderly, fad dieters, adults addicted to drugs or alcohol, and people with eating disorders.
Fat	Butter, oils, margarine, lard, salt pork, salad dressings, mayonnaise, bacon Whole milk and whole milk products High-fat meats Nuts	Provides energy Provides structure Insulates the body Cushions internal organs Necessary for the absorption of fat-soluble vitamins	High-fat diets increase the risk for heart disease and obesity and are correlated with an increased risk for colon and breast cancers.

(Adapted from Dudek, S. G. [2014]. *Nutrition essentials for nursing practice* [7th ed.]. Philadelphia: Wolters Kluwer Health/ Lippincott Williams & Wilkins.)

is converted to glycogen and stored (glycogenesis). Conversely, glycogen is broken down in time of need to supply a ready source of glucose (glycogenolysis). When glycogen stores are adequate, the body converts excess glucose to fat and stores it as triglycerides in adipose tissue.

FUNCTIONS AND RECOMMENDED DIETARY ALLOWANCE

The primary function of carbohydrates is to supply energy. Except for indigestible fiber, all carbohydrates provide 4 calories per gram, regardless of the source.

The **recommended dietary allowance (RDA)** of essential nutrients refers to recommendations for average daily amounts that healthy population groups should consume over time. Although an exact requirement for carbohydrates has not been established, at least 50 to 100 g are needed daily to prevent **ketosis** (an abnormal accumulation of ketone bodies that is frequently associated with acidosis). The *Dietary Guidelines for Americans 2010* (U.S. Department of Agriculture [USDA] & Department of Health and Human Services [DHHS], 2010) recommends that carbohydrates provide 45% to 65% of total calories for adults, mostly in the form of complex carbohydrates. Sugars added to foods supply calories but few or no nutrients. Refer to Table 35-2 for more information regarding the sources, functions, and significance of carbohydrates.

Protein

Protein is a vital component of every living cell. Within the human body, more than 1,000 different proteins are made by combining various amounts and proportions of the 22 basic building blocks known as amino acids. Although amino acids, like carbohydrates, contain carbon, hydrogen, and oxygen, they differ in that amino acids also contain nitrogen. Nine amino acids are classified as essential because they cannot be synthesized in the body; they must be obtained from the diet. The remaining 13 amino acids are no less important, but because the body can make them as long as a supply of nitrogen is available, they are termed nonessential. Proteins are required for the formation of all body structures, including genes, enzymes, muscle, bone matrix, skin, and blood.

CLASSIFICATION AND METABOLISM

Dietary proteins may be labeled complete (high quality) or incomplete (low quality), based on their amino acid composition. Complete proteins contain sufficient amounts and proportions of all the essential amino acids to support growth, whereas incomplete proteins are deficient in one or more essential amino acids. Generally, animal proteins (eggs, dairy products, meats) are complete, and plant proteins (grains, legumes, vegetables) are incomplete. The only exception is soy, a plant protein that is considered a complete protein. Because different sources of plant proteins lack different amino acids, a plant protein can be complemented by combining it with a different plant protein or by adding a small amount of an animal protein to supply a complete protein. Examples of complementary vegetable

proteins include corn tortilla with refried beans and lentil rice soup. Complementary proteins that use a small amount of animal protein include cereal with milk, rice pudding, and a cheese sandwich.

 Concept Mastery Alert

Complete protein = animal protein *or* plant protein + small amount of animal protein.

Dietary protein is broken down into amino acid particles by pancreatic enzymes in the small intestine. These are absorbed through the intestinal mucosa to be transported to the liver. In the liver, amino acids are recombined into new proteins or are released into the bloodstream for use in protein synthesis by tissues and cells. Excess amino acids are converted to fatty acids, ketone bodies, or glucose and are stored or used as metabolic fuel.

The body's protein tissues are in a constant state of flux. Tissues are continuously being broken down (catabolism) and replaced (anabolism). Nitrogen balance, a comparison between catabolism and anabolism, can be measured by comparing nitrogen intake (protein intake) and nitrogen excretion (nitrogen lost in urine, urea, feces, hair, nails, skin). When catabolism and anabolism are occurring at the same rate, as in healthy adults, the body is in a state of neutral nitrogen balance (i.e., nitrogen intake equals nitrogen excretion). A positive nitrogen balance occurs when nitrogen intake is greater than excretion, and indicates tissue growth—for example, during childhood, pregnancy, lactation, and recovery from illness. A negative nitrogen balance occurs when more nitrogen is excreted than is ingested, and indicates tissue is breaking down faster than it is being replaced. This undesirable state occurs in situations such as starvation and the catabolism that immediately follows surgery, illness, trauma, and stress. This can result in the wasting of muscle tissue as it is converted to glucose for energy.

FUNCTIONS AND RECOMMENDED DIETARY ALLOWANCE

The major function of protein is to maintain body tissues that break down from normal wear and tear and to support the growth of new tissue. Protein can be oxidized to provide 4 calories per gram. Using protein for energy is more expensive both financially and physiologically than using carbohydrates. The nitrogen remaining after protein is metabolized burdens the kidneys. In addition, energy must be used to excrete the nitrogen. Like carbohydrates, protein consumed in excess of need can be converted to and stored as fat.

The recommended daily intake for protein for adults is 0.8 g/kg of desirable body weight, or about 46 g for a woman weighing 127 pounds and 56 g for a man weighing 154 pounds. Protein intake should contribute 10% to 35% of total caloric intake for adults (Dudek, 2014). Refer to Table 35-2 for more information about the sources, functions, and significance of protein.

Fats

Fats in the diet, or **lipids**, are insoluble in water and, therefore, insoluble in blood. Like carbohydrates, they are composed of carbon, hydrogen, and oxygen. Ninety-five percent of the lipids in the diet are in the form of **triglycerides**, the predominant form of fat in food and the major storage form of fat in the body. Compound lipids (such as phospholipids, in which a lipid is combined with another substance) and derived lipids (such as cholesterol) constitute the remainder of the lipids ingested.

CLASSIFICATION AND METABOLISM

Food fats contain mixtures of saturated and unsaturated fatty acids. The difference in degree of saturation depends on the amount of hydrogen in fat molecules. Saturated fats contain more hydrogen than unsaturated fats. Most animal fats are considered saturated and have a solid consistency at room temperature. Conversely, most vegetable fats are considered unsaturated, remain liquid at room temperature, and are referred to as oils. Saturated fats tend to raise serum cholesterol levels, whereas unsaturated fats lower serum cholesterol levels. When manufacturers partially hydrogenate liquid oils, they become more solid and more stable. This substance is referred to as **trans fat**. Trans fat raises serum cholesterol. Therefore, it is to be counted in with the total number of saturated fats in a day. The U.S. Food and Drug Administration (FDA) requires that food nutrition labels list trans fat so that consumers may make healthy choices in their diet (FDA, 2012a).

Cholesterol is a fatlike substance found only in animal products. It is not an essential nutrient; the body makes sufficient amounts (Dudek, 2014). Cholesterol is an important component of cell membranes and is especially abundant in brain and nerve cells. It also is used to synthesize bile acids and is a precursor of the steroid hormones and vitamin D. Although cholesterol serves many important functions in the body, high serum levels are clearly associated with an increased risk for atherosclerosis. To help lower serum cholesterol levels, researchers recommend limiting cholesterol intake, eating less total fat—especially saturated and trans fat—eating more unsaturated fat, and increasing fiber intake, which increases fecal excretion of cholesterol.

 REMEMBER William Johnston, the middle-aged executive with hypertension and high cholesterol? Due to Mr. Johnston's "on-the-run" lifestyle, developing an individualized nutritional plan might be somewhat challenging. Based on an assessment of Mr. Johnston's eating habits, likes, and dislikes, the nurse would work with him to develop a plan that promotes weight loss and includes limiting cholesterol and total fat intake and consuming more foods containing unsaturated fats and fiber. Adapting the plan will help to promote adherence to it, thereby increasing the chances for success. ●

Fat digestion occurs largely in the small intestine. Bile, secreted by the gallbladder, emulsifies fat to increase the surface area so that pancreatic lipase can break down fat more effectively. Through a complex series of events, most fats are absorbed into the lymphatic circulation with the help of a protein carrier and are transported to the liver. Of 100 grams eaten, only about 3 grams are excreted in the feces.

FUNCTIONS AND RECOMMENDED DIETARY ALLOWANCE

Fats are the most concentrated source of energy in the diet, providing 9 calories for every gram. Fat increases the palatability of the diet (e.g., to most people, filet mignon tastes better than flank steak) and has a high satiety value because it delays gastric emptying time. In the body, fat aids in the absorption of the fat-soluble vitamins and provides insulation, structure, and temperature control. Refer to Table 35-2 on page 1201 for more information about the sources, functions, and significance of fat.

The *Dietary Guidelines for Americans 2010* recommends that fat intake be no more than between 20% and 35% of total caloric intake, with less than 10% of fat calories from saturated fats and less than 300 mg/day of cholesterol (USDA & DHHS, 2010).

Regulatory Nutrients

Vitamins, minerals, and water are regulatory nutrients because the body needs them for the metabolism of energy nutrients.

Vitamins

Vitamins are organic compounds needed by the body in small amounts. Most vitamins are active in the form of coenzymes, which, together with enzymes, facilitate thousands of chemical reactions in the body. Although vitamins do not provide energy (calories), they are needed for the metabolism of carbohydrates, protein, and fat. Vitamins are essential in the diet because most are not synthesized in the body or are made in insufficient quantities. The absence or insufficient use of vitamins in the body causes specific deficiency syndromes.

Vitamins are present in foods in only small amounts. Fresh foods are higher in vitamins than processed foods because vitamins may be destroyed by light, heat, air, and during preparation. The exception is when vitamins not naturally occurring in a food are added, such as vitamin D–fortified milk. This process is called fortification.

In the United States, severe vitamin deficiencies are uncommon. Mild or subclinical deficiencies of vitamin A, vitamin C, folate, and vitamin B_6, however, may affect a significant proportion of the population, especially those who (1) are members of certain age groups or patient groups (infants, adolescents, pregnant and lactating women, older people); (2) smoke, abuse alcohol, or use medications on a long-term basis; (3) are chronically ill, either physically or psychologically; or (4) are poor or finicky eaters, such as chronic dieters and food faddists.

Vitamins are classified as either water soluble or fat soluble. Water-soluble vitamins include vitamin C and the B-complex vitamins (ascorbic acid, thiamin, riboflavin,

Table 35-3 SUMMARY OF VITAMINS*

NUTRIENT	SOURCES	FUNCTIONS	SIGNS AND SYMPTOMS OF DEFICIENCY	SIGNS AND SYMPTOMS OF EXCESS
Water-Soluble Vitamins				
Vitamin C (ascorbic acid)	Citrus fruits, broccoli, green pepper, strawberries, greens	Collagen formation, antioxidant, enhances iron absorption	Scurvy, hemorrhaging, delayed wound healing	Hot flashes, headache, nausea, diarrhea
Vitamin B complex				
Thiamin	Pork, liver, whole and enriched grains, legumes	Coenzyme in key reactions that produce energy from glucose	Beriberi, mental confusion, fatigue	None known
Riboflavin	Milk, organ meats, enriched grains, greens	Carbohydrate, protein, and fat metabolism	Dermatitis, glossitis, photophobia	None known
Niacin	Kidney, grains, lean meat, nuts	Carbohydrate, protein, and fat metabolism	Pellagra, dermatitis	Flushing and itching, nausea, vomiting, liver damage
B_6 (pyridoxine)	Yeast, banana, cantaloupe, broccoli, spinach	Coenzyme in protein, fat, carbohydrate metabolism	Microcytic anemia, CNS problems	Difficulty walking, numbness of feet and hands
Folate	Green leafy vegetables, liver	RNA and DNA synthesis, formation and maturation of RBC	Macrocytic anemia: fatigue, weakness, pallor	None known
B_{12} (cyanocobalamin)	Animal products: organ meats, seafood	Coenzyme in protein metabolism and formation of heme portion of hemoglobin	Pernicious anemia (B_{12} deficiency related to impaired absorption due to lack of intrinsic factor)	None known
Pantothenic acid	Widespread in foods; meat, poultry, fish, whole grain cereals	Carbohydrate, protein, and fat metabolism	None known	None known
Biotin	Liver, egg yolk	Carbohydrate, protein, and fat metabolism	Rare; dry skin, anorexia, fatigue	None known
Fat-Soluble Vitamins				
Vitamin A (retinol, retinal, retinoic acid)	Liver, carrots, egg yolk, fortified milk	Visual acuity in dim light, formation and maintenance of skin and mucous membranes; immune function	Night blindness, rough skin, bone growth ceases	Anorexia, loss of hair, dry skin, bone pain, vomiting, birth defects during pregnancy
Vitamin D (cholecalciferol, ergosterol)	Sunlight, fortified milk, fish liver oils	Calcium and phosphorus metabolism, stimulates calcium absorption	Retarded bone growth, bone malformation	Excessive calcification of bones, renal calculi, nausea, headache
Vitamin E (tocopherol)	Vegetable oils, wheat germ, whole grain products	Antioxidant, protects vitamin A, heme synthesis	Increased RBC hemolysis and macrocytic anemia in premature infants	Relatively nontoxic, although large doses can cause fatigue, diarrhea, and enhance action of anticoagulant medications
Vitamin K	Dark, green leafy vegetables; synthesized in intestines from gut bacteria	Synthesis of certain proteins necessary for blood clotting	Hemorrhagic disease of newborn, delayed blood clotting	Hemolytic anemia and liver damage with synthetic vitamin K

*The Dietary Reference Intakes (DRI) and other information regarding these vitamins can be found at http://www.nutrition.gov/smart-nutrition-101/dietary-reference-intakes-rdas

(Adapted from Dudek, S. G. [2014]. *Nutrition essentials for nursing practice* [7th ed.]. Philadelphia: Wolters Kluwer Health/ Lippincott Williams & Wilkins; and U.S. Food and Drug Administration (US FDA). (2012c). *Smart nutrition 101. Dietary reference intakes*. Available at http://www.nutrition.gov/smart-nutrition-101/dietary-reference-intakes-rdas)

niacin, pyridoxine, biotin pantothenic acid, folate, cobalamin). They are absorbed through the intestinal wall directly into the bloodstream. Although some tissues are able to hold limited amounts of water-soluble vitamins, they usually are not stored in the body. Deficiency symptoms are apt to develop quickly when intake is inadequate; therefore, a daily intake is recommended. However, because water-soluble vitamins are not stored, amounts consumed in excess of need are excreted in the urine. Toxicities are not likely, although megadoses of certain water-soluble vitamins can be harmful.

Vitamins A, D, E, and K, the fat-soluble vitamins, are absorbed with fat into the lymphatic circulation. Like fat, they must be attached to a protein to be transported through the blood. Secondary deficiencies of the fat-soluble vitamins can occur anytime fat digestion or absorption is altered, such as during malabsorption syndromes and pancreatic and biliary diseases. The body stores excesses of the fat-soluble vitamins mostly in the liver and adipose tissue. Because they are stored, a daily intake is not imperative and deficiency symptoms may take weeks, months, or years to develop. Excessive intake, particularly of vitamins A and D, is toxic.

Many studies have attempted to evaluate the relationship of vitamin intake to diseases ranging from cardiovascular disease, osteoporosis, and neural tube defects to some types of cancers (NIH, 2007). Although scrutiny and research continue about vitamin supplements and their long-term effects, most nutritionists agree that vitamins will never be a substitute for good nutrition and healthy lifestyle practices (Dudek, 2014; Lichtenstein & Russell, 2005; USDA & DHHS, 2010). The *Dietary Guidelines for Americans 2010* (USDA & DHHS, 2010) recommends that nutrient needs be met primarily through consuming foods. Supplements may be useful when they fill a specific identified nutrient gap that cannot or is not otherwise being met by the person's intake of food (NIH, 2007; USDA & DHHS, 2010). Supplementation can ensure adequate intakes of specific nutrients because of physiologic limitations or changes (Lichtenstein & Russell, 2005). For example, folate (folic acid) supplementation during pregnancy has significantly decreased the risk of children born with neural tube defects (USDA & DHHS, 2010). Table 35-3 summarizes water- and fat-soluble vitamins.

 THINK back to Susan Oakland, the young woman who is pregnant. She will be advised to take a daily multivitamin supplement as part of her prenatal care. Supplements are used in conjunction with an optimal diet, to meet the increased nutrient requirements of pregnancy. ●

Minerals

Minerals are inorganic elements found in all body fluids and tissues in the form of salts (e.g., sodium chloride) or combined with organic compounds (e.g., iron in hemoglobin). Some minerals function to provide structure within the body, whereas others help to regulate body processes. Minerals, which are elements, are not broken down or rearranged in the body but, rather, are contained in the ash that remains after digestion. Excessive soaking and cooking in water can cause loss of minerals from food. However, minerals are commonly not destroyed by food processing.

Macrominerals (bulk minerals), minerals needed by the body in amounts greater than 100 mg/day, include calcium, phosphorus (phosphates), sulfur (sulfate), sodium, chloride, potassium, and magnesium. Microminerals, or trace elements, are minerals needed by the body in amounts less than 100 mg/day. Microminerals that have recommended dietary intake established include iron, zinc, manganese, chromium, copper, molybdenum, selenium, fluoride, and iodine. Additional trace elements included arsenic, boron, nickel, silicon, cobalt, and vanadium. Dietary guidelines for these elements have not been established. Ultratrace elements are elements that are consumed in microgram quantities each day. They occur in very low quantities in human tissues and their essentiality is uncertain. These elements include aluminum, lithium, nickel, silicon, tin, and vanadium. Macrominerals and microminerals that have recommended intake guidelines are summarized in Table 35-4 (on page 1206).

Water

As the major body constituent present in every body cell, water accounts for between 50% and 60% of the adult's total weight. Infants have proportionately more water accounting for body weight. About two thirds of the body's water is contained within the cells (intracellular fluid [ICF]); the remainder is called extracellular fluid (ECF), which includes all other body fluids, such as plasma and interstitial fluid. Total body water and ECF decrease with age; ICF increases with an increase in body mass. Refer to Chapter 39 for more information on water in the body.

Water is more vital to life than food because it provides the fluid medium necessary for all chemical reactions, it participates in many reactions, and it is not stored in the body. Water acts as a solvent that dissolves many solutes, thereby aiding digestion, absorption, circulation, and excretion. Through evaporation from the skin, water helps to regulate body temperature. As a lubricant, water is needed both for mucous secretions and for movement between joints.

 THINK back to Charles Gallagher, husband of the woman with advanced dementia receiving enteral nutrition. During the group meeting about continuing or withdrawing the enteral nutrition, Mr. Gallagher learns that withdrawal of the feedings would also involve limited water intake. This information is important in helping Mr. Gallagher and his family arrive at an informed decision about whether or not to continue the enteral feedings. ●

Sources of water in the diet include not only beverages but also solid foods, which contain between 10% and 98% water. Water is also produced through the metabolism of

Table 35-4 SUMMARY OF MACROMINERALS AND MICROMINERALS*

NUTRIENT	SOURCES	FUNCTIONS	SIGNS AND SYMPTOMS OF DEFICIENCY	SIGNS AND SYMPTOMS OF EXCESS
Macrominerals				
Calcium	Milk and dairy products, canned fish with bones, greens	Bone and tooth formation, blood clotting, nerve transmission, muscle contraction	Tetany, osteoporosis	Renal calculi in susceptible people
Phosphorus	Milk and milk products, soft drinks, processed foods	Bone and tooth formation, acid–base balance, energy metabolism	Hypophosphatemia: anorexia, muscle weakness	Hyperphosphatemia: symptoms of hypocalcemic tetany
Magnesium	Green leafy vegetables, nuts, beans, grains	Bone and tooth formation, protein synthesis, carbohydrate metabolism	Hypomagnesemia: weakness, muscle pain, poor heart function	Hypermagnesemia: CNS depression, coma, hypotension
Sulfur (provided by adequate amounts of protein)	Meat, eggs, milk, dried peas and beans, nuts	Promotes certain enzyme reactions and detoxification reactions	None known	None known
Sodium	Salt, processed foods	Major ion of extracellular fluid, fluid balance, acid–base balance	Hyponatremia: muscle cramps, cold and clammy skin	Edema, weight gain, high blood pressure if susceptible
Potassium	Whole grains, fruits, leafy vegetables	Major ion of intracellular fluid, fluid balance, acid–base balance	Hypokalemia: muscle cramps and weakness, irregular heartbeat	Hyperkalemia: irritability, anxiety, cardiac arrhythmia, heart block
Chloride	Salt	Component of HCl in stomach, fluid balance, acid–base balance	Hypochloremia: muscle spasms, alkalosis, depressed respirations	Hyperchloremia: acidosis
Microminerals				
Iron	Liver, lean meats, enriched and whole grain breads and cereals	Oxygen transport by way of hemoglobin, constituent of enzyme systems	Microcytic anemia, pallor, decreased work capacity, fatigue, weakness	Hemosiderosis; acute iron poisoning from accidental overdose leads to GI symptoms and possible shock
Iodine	Iodized salt, seafood, food additives	Component of thyroid hormones	Goiter	Acne-like lesions
Zinc	Oysters, liver, meats, dried peas and beans, nuts	Tissue growth, sexual maturation, immune response	Impaired growth, sexual maturation, immune system functioning	Anorexia, nausea, vomiting, diarrhea, muscle pain, lethargy
Copper	Liver, shellfish, grains, dried peas and beans	Aids in iron metabolism and activity of some enzymes	Anemia, altered bone formation, hypercholesterolemia	Nervous system disturbances, vomiting
Manganese	Whole grains, nuts, dried peas and beans, fruit	Part of enzymes needed for protein and energy metabolism	Poor reproductive performance, growth retardation	None known
Fluoride	Fluoridated water, fish, tea	Tooth formation and integrity, bone formation and integrity	Tooth decay; may increase risk for osteoporosis	Mottling and discoloration of tooth enamel
Chromium	Whole grains, meats	Cofactor for insulin, proper glucose metabolism	Impaired glucose tolerance, insulin resistance	None known
Selenium	Wheat (if grown in high-selenium soil), organ meats	Antioxidant	None known	Loss of hair, brittle fingernails, fatigue
Molybdenum	Liver, whole grains, dried peas and beans, organ meats	Oxidizes sulfur and products of sulfur metabolism	None known	Interferes with copper metabolism
Cobalt	Organ meats	Essential component of vitamin B_{12}	None known	None known

*The Dietary Reference Intakes (DRI) and other information regarding these minerals can be found at http://www.nutrition.gov/smart-nutrition-101/dietary-reference-intakes-rdas

(Adapted from Dudek, S. G. [2014]. *Nutrition essentials for nursing practice* [7th ed.]. Philadelphia: Wolters Kluwer Health/Lippincott Williams & Wilkins; and U.S. Food and Drug Administration (US FDA). (2012c). *Smart nutrition 101. Dietary reference intakes.* Available http://www.nutrition.gov/smart-nutrition-101/dietary-reference-intakes-rdas.)

carbohydrates, protein, and fat. It leaves the body through urine, feces, expired air, and perspiration. Water intake (an average of 2,200 to 3,000 mL/day for adults [Dudek, 2014]) usually equals water output. Water balance may be seriously affected when intake (such as in older adults or people in comatose states) or output (such as in patients with altered renal function, profuse perspiration, diarrhea, vomiting, fistulas, drainage tubes, hemorrhage, severe burns) is altered.

 ## Digestion

The food consumed by a person supplies the essential nutrients needed for cells to perform their necessary functions, but the cells cannot use food in its consumed form. The gastrointestinal system breaks down the food into particles small enough to pass into the cells and be used by the cells. This breakdown process is called **digestion**. Digestion begins in the mouth where food is taken in, mixes with saliva, is pushed into the pharynx by the tongue, and then continues into the esophagus. Peristalsis moves the food through the esophagus and into the stomach. The stomach churns the ingested food, mixing it with substances to break down the food and convert it to a semiliquid mixture. The food leaves the stomach and enters the small intestine. The small intestine secrets enzymes, which, along with secretions from the liver and pancreas, digest the food. The digested nutrients are then transferred into the person's circulation (**absorption**), to be transported throughout the body. Most absorption of digested food and minerals, and some absorption of water, occurs through the walls of the small intestine. Undigested waste materials continue through the gastrointestinal tract and are eliminated. Elimination of these waste products is discussed in Chapter 37. Figure 37-1 on page 1346 illustrates the organs of the gastrointestinal tract.

Adequate Diet Selection

An adequate diet provides a balanced intake of all essential nutrients in appropriate amounts. However, what constitutes an adequate diet is less obvious. Tools for planning or evaluating a diet for adequacy include dietary recommendations and guidelines issued from health and U.S. governmental agencies, the Dietary Reference Intakes (DRIs), and the "MyPlate" food guidance system. These tools are discussed later in this chapter in detail. The task of promoting health through proper nutrition has been made easier by labeling regulations that mandate specific information about food contents and their comparison to recommended daily intakes.

Dietary Recommendations

The *Dietary Guidelines for Americans* are science-based strategies compiled by the Public Health Service of the Department of Health and Human Services and the U.S. Department of Agriculture. These guidelines provide advice to promote health and to reduce risk for major chronic diseases through diet and physical activity. Although these diet recommendations are not guaranteed to prevent diseases, many experts believe that most Americans can reduce their risk for chronic diet-related diseases, such as diabetes, certain types of cancer, and heart disease, by modifying the typical American or Western diet. The Public Health Service of the Department of Health and Human Services and the U.S. Department of Agriculture together update the *Dietary Guidelines for Americans* every 5 years. A summary of the Dietary Guidelines 2010 appears in Box 35-3 (on page 1208). The complete guidelines are available at http://www.health.gov/dietaryguidelines/2010.asp (USDA & DHHS, 2010).

Dietary Reference Intakes

The Dietary Reference Intakes (DRIs) provide recommended nutrient intakes for use in a variety of settings. The DRIs are actually a set of four reference values. The DRIs include:

- Recommended Dietary Allowance (RDA) is the average daily dietary intake of a nutrient that is sufficient to meet the requirement of nearly all (97%–98%) healthy people.
- Adequate Intake (AI) for a nutrient is established when an RDA cannot be determined. Therefore a nutrient either has an RDA or an AI. The AI is based on observed intakes of the nutrient by a group of healthy people.
- Tolerable Upper Intake Level (UL) is the highest daily intake of a nutrient that is likely to pose no risks of toxicity for almost all individuals. As intake above the UL increases, risk increases.
- Estimated Average Requirement (EAR) is the amount of a nutrient that is estimated to meet the requirement of half of all healthy people in the population.

Each of these reference values distinguishes between gender and different life stages. RDAs, AIs and ULs are dietary guidelines for individuals, whereas EARs provide guidelines for groups and populations (FDA, 2012c). Links to the DRIs, including RDAs and the ULs, as well as vitamin and mineral fact sheets, can be found at http://www.nutrition.gov/smart-nutrition-101.

MyPlate Food Guide

In June 2011, the U.S. Department of Agriculture (USDA) replaced the MyPyramid with the MyPlate food guidance graphic. MyPlate is part of a communication initiative based on *2012 Dietary Guidelines for Americans* to help consumers make better food choices. MyPlate is designed to remind Americans to eat healthfully. MyPlate illustrates the five food groups using a familiar mealtime visual, a place setting (Fig. 35-2 on page 1208). The goals of the recommendations are to balance calories by encouraging consumers to enjoy food, but eat less, and avoid oversized portions. Consumers are also advised to increase the intake of vitamins, minerals, and dietary fiber by making half the plate fruits and vegetables, at least half of grains consumed whole grains, and switching to fat-free or low-fat (1%) milk. Consumers are encouraged to reduce sodium consumption by comparing sodium in foods like soup, bread, and frozen meals and choose foods with lower numbers. MyPlate also encourages the consumption of water instead of sugary drinks. The importance of activity and exercise

BOX 35-3 SUMMARY OF DIETARY GUIDELINES FOR AMERICANS 2010

To achieve adequate nutrients within energy needs:

- Maintain calorie balance over time to achieve and sustain a healthy weight.
- Focus on consuming nutrient-dense foods and beverages.

To balance calories to manage weight:

- Prevent and/or reduce overweight and obesity through improved eating and physical activity behaviors.
- Control total calorie intake to manage body weight. For people who are overweight or obese, this will mean consuming fewer calories from foods and beverages.
- Increase physical activity and reduce time spent in sedentary behaviors.
- Maintain appropriate calorie balance during each stage of life—childhood, adolescence, adulthood, pregnancy and breastfeeding, and older age.

Guidelines for physical activity include:

- Engage in regular physical activity and reduce sedentary activities to promote health, psychological well-being, and a healthy body weight.
- To achieve and maintain a healthy body weight, adults should do the equivalent of 150 minutes of moderate-intensity aerobic activity each week. If necessary, adults should increase their weekly minutes of aerobic physical activity gradually over time and decrease calorie intake to a point at which they can achieve calorie balance and a healthy weight. Some adults will need a higher level of physical activity than others to achieve and maintain a healthy body weight. Some may need more than the equivalent of 300 minutes per week of moderate-intensity activity.

Foods and nutrients to increase:

- Increase vegetable and fruit intake.
- Eat a variety of vegetables, especially dark-green and red and orange vegetables and beans and peas.
- Consume at least half of all grains as whole grains. Increase whole-grain intake by replacing refined grains with whole grains.
- Increase intake of fat-free or low-fat milk and milk products, such as milk, yogurt, cheese, or fortified soy beverages.
- Choose a variety of protein foods, which include seafood, lean meat and poultry, eggs, beans and peas, soy products, and unsalted nuts and seeds.

- Increase the amount and variety of seafood consumed by choosing seafood in place of some meat and poultry.
- Replace protein foods that are higher in solid fats with choices that are lower in solid fats and calories and/or are sources of oils.
- Use oils to replace solid fats where possible.
- Choose foods that provide more potassium, dietary fiber, calcium, and vitamin D, which are nutrients of concern in American diets. These foods include vegetables, fruits, whole grains, and milk and milk products.

Foods and food components to reduce:

- Reduce daily sodium intake to less than 2,300 milligrams (mg) and further reduce intake to 1,500 mg among persons who are 51 and older and those of any age who are African American or have hypertension, diabetes, or chronic kidney disease. The 1,500-mg recommendation applies to about half of the U.S. population, including children, and the majority of adults.
- Consume less than 10 percent of calories from saturated fatty acids by replacing them with monounsaturated and polyunsaturated fatty acids.
- Consume less than 300 mg per day of dietary cholesterol.
- Keep trans fatty acid consumption as low as possible by limiting foods that contain synthetic sources of trans fats, such as partially hydrogenated oils, and by limiting other solid fats.
- Reduce the intake of calories from solid fats and added sugars.
- Limit the consumption of foods that contain refined grains, especially refined grain foods that contain solid fats, added sugars, and sodium.

If alcohol is consumed, it should be consumed in moderation—up to one drink per day for women and two drinks per day for men—and only by adults of legal drinking age.
  To build healthy eating patterns:

- Select an eating pattern that meets nutrient needs over time at an appropriate calorie level.
- Account for all foods and beverages consumed and assess how they fit within a total healthy eating pattern.
- Follow food safety recommendations when preparing and eating foods to reduce the risk of foodborne illnesses.

(Adapted from United States Department of Agriculture [USDA] & Department of Health and Human Services [DHHS]. [2010]. Dietary guidelines for Americans 2010. Available at http://www.health.gov/dietaryguidelines/2010.asp)

are emphasized, including the recommendations for children and adolescents to be physically active for 60 minutes or more a day and adults to engage in activity that requires moderate effort, such as brisk walking for two and a half hours or more a week (USDA, 2012). Visitors to the website can personalize nutritional and physical activity plans, track foods consumed and physical activities, and get support to help make healthier choices. Additional information regarding the MyPlate guidelines is available at http://www.choosemyplate.gov/ (USDA, 2012).

Food Labeling

Food labels provide a significant amount of nutritional information for the consumer. Regulations that control

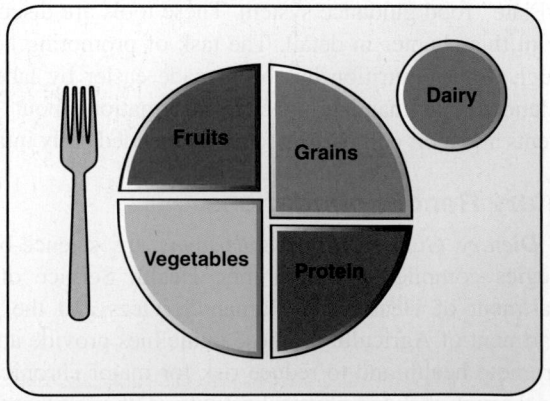

FIGURE 35-2. The MyPlate food guidance graphic. (Source: U.S. Department of Agriculture [USDA]. [2008]. Available at http://www.choosemyplate.gov/index.html)

food labels have always been controversial. In 1975, the FDA, a federal agency charged with protecting the U.S. food and drug supply, enacted legislation for a standardized label format that was considered a positive step toward educating the consumer about nutrition. Confusion and misinformation resulted as food manufacturers oversimplified or exaggerated health claims for their products. In 1990, Congress passed the Nutritional Labeling and Education Act, which required all foods, including fruits and vegetables, to be clearly labeled. Four broad categories are addressed in this legislation. They include nutrition labeling, serving sizes, descriptors, and health claims. Starting January 1, 2006, labels were required to include information related to the amount of trans fat (trans fatty acids) on nutrition fact labels. Consumers should be easily able to identify the amount of saturated fat, trans fat, cholesterol, and dietary fiber included in a product, and the number of calories from fat, in addition to viewing a listing of other nutritional information. Figure 35-3 illustrates a sample label with explanation of terms. The food label is a tool to educate the public about nutrition and aid in choosing foods wisely.

FACTORS AFFECTING NUTRITION

A person's food patterns and habits have a great impact on overall food intake. Food habits are a product of many evolving variables, such as physiologic and physical factors that influence nutrient requirements (e.g., stage of development, state of health, medications) and physical, sociocultural, and psychosocial factors that influence food choices (e.g., economics, culture, religion, tradition, education, politics, social status, food ideology [the meaning of food for an individual], learned aversions). These variables alone or in combination also can affect food intake and overall nutrition.

Physiologic and Physical Factors That Influence Nutrient Requirements

There are various reasons a person's nutrient requirements may differ. Some are permanent, such as gender, whereas others are temporary, such as pregnancy.

Developmental Considerations

Throughout the life cycle, nutrient needs change in relation to growth, development, activity, and age-related changes in

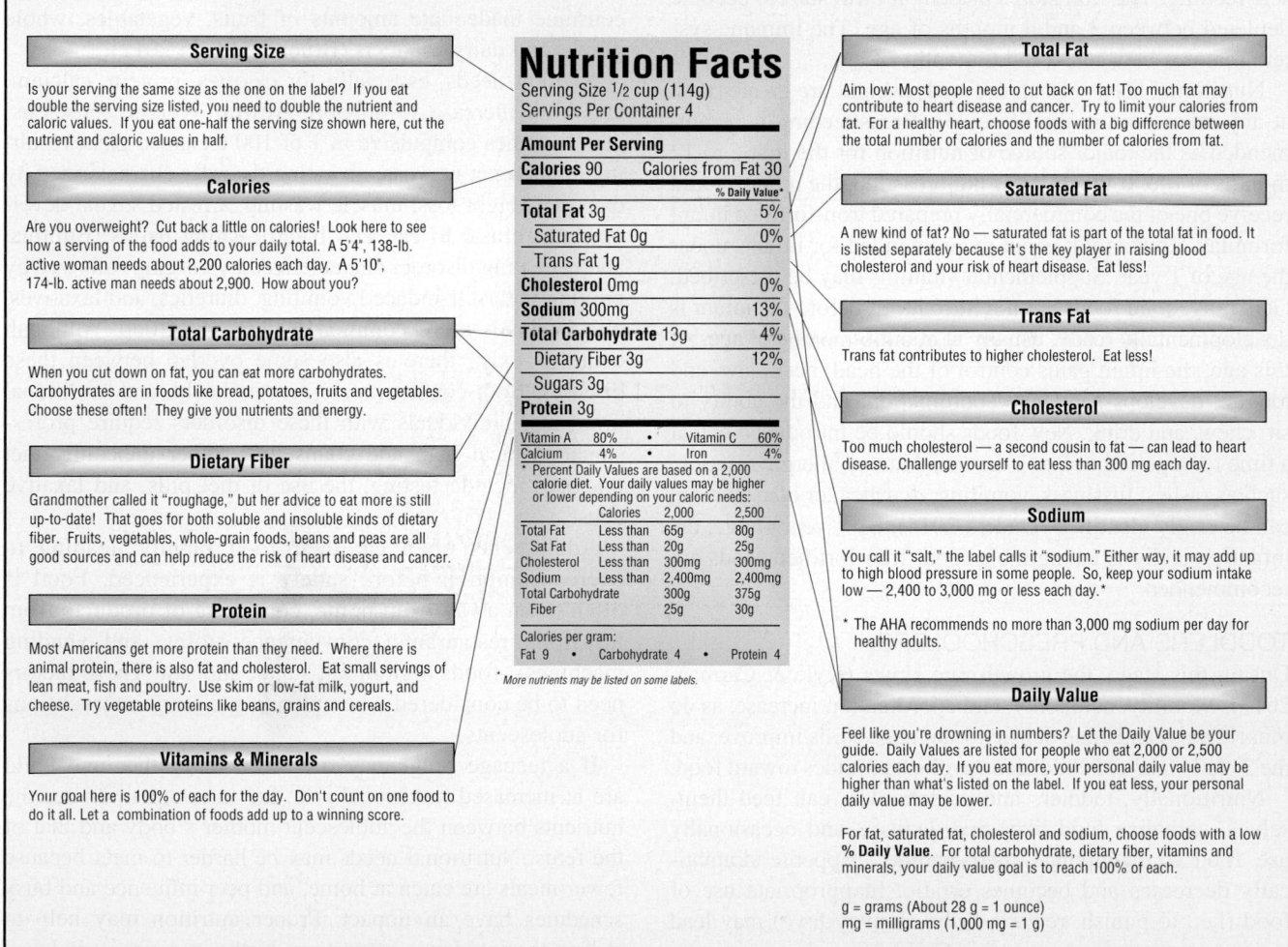

FIGURE 35-3. Sample nutritional label with explanation of terms. (Source: U.S. Food and Drug Administration [FDA]. [2012]. How to understand and use the nutrition facts label. Available at http://www.fda.gov/Food/ResourcesForYou/Consumers/NFLPM/ucm274593.htm)

metabolism and body composition. Periods of intense growth and development, such as during infancy, adolescence, pregnancy, and lactation, cause an increase in nutrient needs. Nutrient needs stabilize during adulthood, although older people may need more or less of some nutrients. Age influences not only nutrient requirements, but also food intake. The consistency of food consumed, eating patterns, and the significance of food change with physical and psychosocial development.

 REMEMBER Susan Oakland, the student who is pregnant, and William Johnston, the executive with hypertension and high cholesterol, described at the beginning of the chapter. The nurse would need to incorporate knowledge of each patient's developmental level when planning care. •

INFANTS

The period from birth to 1 year of age is the most rapid period of growth. Birth weight doubles in 4 to 6 months and triples by 1 year of age. Length increases 50% in the first year. Muscle control and the development of hand–eye coordination allow the infant to progress to sitting upright and self-feeding. The iron stores present at birth start to become depleted between 3 and 4 months of age. The immune system matures between 4 and 6 months of age.

Nutritional needs per unit of body weight are greater than at any other time in the life cycle. Breastfeeding is recommended as the major source of nutrition for the first 6 to 12 months of life. If the infant is not breastfed, the infant should receive one of the commercially prepared iron-fortified infant formulas. Cow's milk is not recommended for infants under the age of 1 year. Supplemental vitamins may be prescribed. Generally, solid foods are not introduced before the infant is developmentally ready, usually at about 6 months of age. At this age, the infant gains control of the head, neck, jaw, and tongue; develops hand–eye coordination; and the ability to sit, chew, and drink. New foods should be introduced one at a time for a period of 5 to 7 days so that any allergic reaction, such as rashes, fussiness, vomiting, diarrhea, or constipation, can be easily identified (Dudek, 2014). By 1 year of age, the infant typically is eating table food. Iron-fortified foods are recommended.

TODDLERS AND PRESCHOOLERS

During this stage, the growth rate slows (Kyle & Carman, 2013). Mobility, autonomy, and coordination increase, as do muscle mass and bone density. Language skills improve, and the 3- to 5-year-old child also develops attitudes toward food.

Nutritionally, toddlers and preschoolers can feed themselves, verbalize food likes and dislikes, and occasionally use food to manipulate their parents. Appetite dramatically decreases and becomes erratic. Inappropriate use of food (i.e., to punish, reward, bribe, convey love) may lead to inappropriate food attitudes. Children in this age group often experience an inadequate intake of fruits and vegetables and/or excessive intake of sweetened fruit drinks.

SCHOOL-AGED CHILDREN

The 6- to 12-year-old child has an uneven, individualized, sometimes erratic growth pattern. Permanent teeth erupt as the digestive system matures. Socialization and independence increase. At this stage, the body accumulates reserves in preparation for the upcoming adolescent growth spurt.

Nutritional implications for the school-aged child focus on health promotion. Increasing energy requirements need to be balanced with foods of high nutritional value. The appetite improves but still may be irregular. The parents' role as the primary regulator of food intake diminishes, and advertising has more of an impact on the child's food choices.

ADOLESCENTS

Adolescence is a period of rapid physical, emotional, social, and sexual maturation. The growth spurt begins at different ages among individuals. Girls begin menstruation and experience fat deposition, whereas males experience an increase in muscle mass, lean body tissue, and bones. Adolescence is also marked by intense psychosocial growth, family conflict, and social and peer pressure. Childhood nutrition problems often worsen during adolescence. Adolescents tend to skip breakfast, contributing to a lower-quality diet and decreased performance in school. Children in this age group tend to consume inadequate amounts of fruits, vegetables, whole grains, and dairy products (Bruening et al., 2012).

Nutrient needs, especially for calories, protein, calcium, and iron, increase to support growth. Weight consciousness becomes compulsive in 1 of 100 teenaged girls, resulting in anorexia nervosa, an eating disorder characterized by extreme weight loss, muscle wasting, arrested sexual development, refusal to eat, and bizarre eating habits. Bulimia, another eating disorder characterized by gorging followed by purging with self-induced vomiting, diuretics, and laxatives, also becomes more common in this age group. Although contrasts exist, there is also some overlap between these diseases. Both conditions are serious health and nutritional problems; individuals with these disorders require professional medical help and counseling. Other unhealthy diet practices include fasting, the use of diet pills, and laxative abuse.

Adolescents often eat their food rapidly, leading to overconsumption before satiety is experienced. Food is often eaten away from home, consisting of products from fast food restaurants, convenience stores, and vending machines—foods high in fat, sugar, and salt. These factors need to be considered when planning dietary interventions for adolescents.

If a teenage pregnancy occurs, both mother and child are at increased nutritional risk due to competition for the nutrients between the adolescent mother's body and that of the fetus. Nutritional needs may be harder to meet because fewer meals are eaten at home, and peer influence and busy schedules have an impact. Proper nutrition may help to reduce the incidence of preterm births, pregnancy-induced hypertension, and anemia, which are common in adolescent pregnancies (Dudek, 2014).

ADULTS

With adulthood, growth ceases. This age is also marked by a decline in the BMR with each decade. Adults may become more aware of the preventive role of exercise, or pressures of work and family may lead to a decline in physical activity and exercise.

Nutritional needs level off in adulthood, and fewer calories are required because of the decrease in BMR. Weight gain results if adjustments in caloric intake are not made.

PREGNANT AND LACTATING WOMEN

During pregnancy, the fetus, maternal tissues, and placenta grow dramatically. Weight gain occurs, and GI changes as a result of the pregnancy may result in nausea, vomiting, heartburn, or constipation. The quantity of breast milk produced depends on an adequate supply of nutrients.

Nutrient needs during pregnancy increase to support growth and maintain maternal homeostasis, particularly during the second and third trimesters. During the second trimester, normal-weight women need approximately 340 extra calories per day and 450 extra calories per day in the third trimester (Academy of Nutrition and Dietetics, 2012). Key nutrient needs include protein, calories, iron, folic acid, calcium, and iodine. Caloric needs are higher for lactation than pregnancy, and the nutritional quality of breast milk is maintained at the expense of maternal nutrition if dietary intake is inadequate.

OLDER ADULTS

Because of the decreases in BMR and physical activity and loss of lean body mass, energy expenditure decreases. Loss of teeth and periodontal disease may make chewing more difficult. A decrease in peristalsis can result in constipation. Loss of taste between sweet and salty begins between 55 and 59 years of age, but discrimination between bitter and sour remains intact. The sensation of thirst also decreases. Degenerative diseases and the use of medications are more common with aging. It is not uncommon for social isolation, poor self-esteem, or loss of independence to affect nutritional intake negatively.

Because of the changes related to aging, the caloric needs of the body decrease. The need for nutrients, however, stays the same or increases (Dudek, 2014). Foods that are difficult to chew may need to be eliminated, whereas an increase in fiber and fluid intake can relieve constipation. Older adults are also prone to dehydration, and lack of interest in eating is common. Nutrient intake, digestion, absorption, metabolism, or excretion may be altered because of the physiologic changes common to this age. Dietary restrictions related to chronic illness, limited income, isolation, and age-related physiologic changes place persons in this age group at risk for malnutrition (Tabloski, 2010).

Gender

Men differ from women in their nutrient requirements due to differences in body composition and reproductive function. Their larger muscle mass translates into higher caloric and protein requirements (therefore, slightly higher needs for B vitamins that metabolize calories and protein) because muscle is more metabolically active than adipose tissue (women have proportionately more adipose tissue). Women of childbearing age have higher iron requirements related to menstruation.

State of Health

The alteration in nutrient requirements that results from illness and trauma varies with the intensity and duration of the stress. For instance, fevers increase the need for calories and water. Unlike fevers related to septicemia, however, fevers caused by a mild case of the flu require few dietary adjustments.

Trauma, like major surgery, burns, and crush injuries, is followed by hormonal changes that profoundly affect the body's use of nutrients. To preserve or replenish body nutrient stores and to promote healing and recovery, nutrient requirements increase dramatically in the adaptive phase after stress. In some cases of severe trauma, such as major burns, the rehabilitative phase of recovery, characterized by the gradual normalization of nutrient needs, may last for years.

Chronic disorders—for example, diabetes mellitus, renal disease, hypertension, heart disease, GI disorders, and cancer—can alter nutrient requirements by influencing nutrient intake, digestion, absorption, metabolism, utilization, or excretion.

Mental health problems, such as depression and confusion, can cause a patient to forget to eat or lack the motivation to eat, leading to malnutrition.

Alcohol Abuse

Alcohol can alter the body's use of nutrients, and thereby its nutrient requirements, by numerous mechanisms. The toxic effect of alcohol on the intestinal mucosa interferes with normal nutrient absorption; thus, requirements increase as the efficiency of absorption decreases. Need for B vitamins increases because they are used to metabolize alcohol. Alcohol can also influence nutrient metabolism by impairing nutrient storage, increasing nutrient catabolism, and increasing nutrient excretion. Alcohol abuse that results in liver damage has profound effects on the body's nutrient metabolism and requirements.

Medication

Many drugs have the potential to influence nutrient requirements. Nutrient absorption may be altered by drugs that (1) change the pH of the GI tract, (2) increase GI motility, (3) damage the intestinal mucosa, or (4) bind with nutrients, rendering them unavailable to the body. Nutrient metabolism can be altered by drugs that (1) act as nutrient antagonists, (2) alter the enzyme systems that metabolize nutrients, or (3) alter nutrient degradation. Some drugs alter the renal reabsorption of nutrients and, therefore, may increase or decrease nutrient excretion.

Megadoses of Nutrient Supplements

Because some nutrients compete against each other for absorption, an excess of one nutrient can lead to a deficiency (or increase the requirement) of another, especially if one is absorbed preferentially. For instance, a delicate balance exists between zinc and copper. People who take therapeutic levels of zinc run the risk of developing a copper deficiency—which is otherwise rare—unless they also increase their intake of copper.

Dietary supplements can have drug-like effects and may interact with food and medication (Zelig & Rigassio Radler, 2012). Accurate information regarding the patient's use of dietary supplements is imperative to provide safe and appropriate care. The use of herbs, vitamins, minerals, and other supplements can impact a patient's plan of care and must be considered by all members of the health care team. For example, a patient taking gingko biloba (an herbal), aspirin, and vitamin E (dietary supplement) may have to have surgery postponed due to an increased risk for excessive bleeding, because each of these substances have anticoagulant properties (Marik & Flemmer, 2012). A list of accurate, reliable sources for the latest information about specific herbs and supplements based on scientific evidence is included in the Internet Resources found on thePoint website.

Physical, Sociocultural, and Psychosocial Factors That Influence Food Choices

Dietary choices or restrictions also are influenced by economics, culture, religion, and personal feelings and meanings associated with food. The financial income of the patient or the patient's household can directly impact the ability to purchase sufficient food and/or food of high nutritional value. Diverse lifestyles and eating habits directly impact a person's nutritional health and well-being. Religious restrictions and beliefs or cultural practices may affect the patient's acceptance of, response to, and compliance with dietary therapies. Health care providers need an understanding of a patient's cultural values, beliefs, and practices to provide culturally acceptable care.

Economic Factors

The adequacy of a person's food budget affects dietary choices and patterns. The increasing cost of food, coupled with limited purchasing power, may result in a decrease in the nutritional quality of the diet. Many variables influence the types of foods purchased. Creative use of the food dollar means using unit pricing to determine cost per serving (e.g., comparing the unit price of 39¢ per serving with a similar product's 45¢ per serving), selecting foods that contain adequate nutrients, and buying seasonal foods that are more economical and can be prepared easily at home. Avoiding convenience foods and meals purchased away from home can save food dollars.

Religion

Dietary restrictions associated with religions might affect a patient's nutritional requirements. Many religions eschew certain types of food products. For example, Mormons do

not use coffee, tea, or alcohol, and are encouraged to limit meat consumption. Hindus do not eat beef because cows are considered sacred. Many Hindus are vegetarian, adhering to the concept of nonviolence as applied to animal sources of food (Ritter & Hoffman, 2010; Dudek, 2014). Therefore, alternative food choices or meal patterns may be necessary. Kosher dietary laws require special food preparation techniques and prohibit intake of pork and shellfish. Thus, a patient's religious affiliation may affect that individual's nutritional regimen. Question patients regarding any preferences or restrictions. Vegetarian, kosher, and other special diets are available in hospitals, long-term care facilities, retirement homes, and programs, such as Meals on Wheels.

Meaning of Food

Food means different things to different people, with food playing multiple roles in the lives of most people. In addition to satisfying hunger and providing nutrition, food may signify a celebration, a social gathering, or a reward. Some people use various foods to indicate caring or to give comfort and reassurance during times of stress or unhappiness. Mealtime may evoke memories of family discussions, laughter, and enjoyable times. Some may remember conflicts associated with eating or avoid eating because it reminds them of their loneliness and isolation. Others, because of society's emphasis on being thin, may resort to fad or crash weight-reduction diets to resolve eating conflicts and lose weight rapidly. This initial weight reduction seldom is sustained for an extended period, and a cycle of yo-yo dieting frequently results. Drastic weight loss is followed by an eating binge that causes the dieter to regain all the lost weight and, possibly, some additional weight each time the sequence occurs. Nutritional deficiencies may occur and place the person at risk for other diseases. Losing weight and keeping it off require a change in eating habits as part of the overall commitment to health.

Culture

Nutritional diversity is common among cultural or ethnic groups. The variety and selections are unique to each group and represent their personal beliefs and customs. Culture influences what is eaten or considered edible, how it is prepared, and what combinations of food are permitted. Herbal treatments that are popular in some cultures may interfere with or counteract the action of prescribed medication. The variations in food choices within a culture also depend on income levels and availability of foods. General and specific cultural knowledge allows the health care provider to ask the right questions when interacting with patients of varying backgrounds. Nurses who are aware of the specific needs and beliefs of culturally diverse patient populations are better able to communicate effectively and provide optimal care. Box 35-4 suggests guidelines for effective communication about nutrition with culturally diverse patients.

If a patient of a different culture is to be placed on a specific diet, discussing food choice options is necessary to customize the diet to meet the person's cultural demands.

| BOX 35-4 | COMMUNICATING EFFECTIVELY ABOUT NUTRITION WITH CULTURALLY DIVERSE PATIENTS |

- Acquire basic information about health beliefs and practices of various cultural groups in your health care setting. This provides a basis for assessing patients' beliefs and practices. Recognize, however, that within all cultures and ethnic groups, there are members who do not hold all the values of the group.
- Ask specifically about the use of folk or home remedies prescribed by a nontraditional healer.
- Determine the patient's language preferences for spoken and written communication.
- Utilize printed or audiovisual information that is in the language spoken by your patients.
- Promote healthy food choices by identifying healthy traditional food practices and encourage their use.

- Support healthy new food practices.
- Discourage the adoption of less healthy American dietary practices.
- Encourage cultural sensitivity in health care workers in your particular setting.
- Recognize that diversity exists within cultural groups. For example, the Hispanic population includes Mexicans, Cubans, Puerto Ricans, and other Latino groups.
- Emphasize threads or messages in health teaching that are common to all cultures (e.g., concern about family, faith, home).
- Help culturally diverse patients to value and understand the importance of communicating concerns and asking questions about prescribed dietary practices.

(Adapted from Ritter, L. A., & Hoffman, N. A. [2010]. *Multicultural health.* Boston: Jones and Bartlett; and Dudek, S. [2014]. *Nutrition essentials for nursing practice* [7th ed.]. Philadelphia: Wolters Kluwer Health/Lippincott Williams & Wilkins.)

Discussing ways to integrate cultural food preferences into current nutrition guidelines is an important part of nursing care.

Additional Sociocultural Factors Affecting Nutritional Intake

In addition to the previously mentioned factors, consider the following issues to determine their impact on a patient's nutritional status (Dudek, 2014):

- Illiteracy
- Language barriers
- Knowledge of nutrition
- Lack of caregiver or social support
- Social isolation
- Limited ability to obtain or purchase food
- Lack of or inadequate cooking and/or food preparation arrangements

Food Intake

At times, a combination of physiologic and physical factors that influence nutrient requirements and, or in combination with, sociocultural and psychosocial factors can affect a person's nutritional intake. Subsequently, these factors can result in a decrease or increase in food intake.

Decreased Food Intake

Food intake may decrease for various reasons. Patients with a BMI of less than 18.5 are considered underweight. **Anorexia**, or the lack of appetite, may be related to systemic and local diseases; numerous psychosocial causes, such as fear, anxiety, depression, or pain; and impaired ability to smell and taste—or it may occur secondary to drug therapy or medical treatments. Others who may have limited food intake include those who have difficulty chewing and swallowing, those who experience chronic GI problems or undergo certain surgical procedures, those with certain chronic illnesses (such as cancer), and those with inadequate food budgets.

 Concept Mastery Alert

Anorexia is different from anorexia nervosa. Anorexia is a general term that involves a lack of appetite that results from numerous causes. Anorexia nervosa is an eating disorder that involves varied issues including extreme weight loss, muscle wasting, arrested sexual development, refusal to eat, and bizarre eating habits.

 CONSIDER Charles Gallagher, whose wife is receiving enteral feedings. The underlying reason for insertion of the PEG tube was her inability to swallow and subsequent development of aspiration pneumonia that required numerous hospitalizations. The nurse would need to communicate this information to Mr. Gallagher to ensure that he understands the rationale for the feeding. This understanding is important for decision making. •

Increased Food Intake

Increased food intake may lead to obesity. Obesity presents a serious health problem physically, socially, and emotionally. **Obesity** is defined as body weight 20% or more above ideal weight or having a BMI of 30 or more. A positive caloric balance, resulting from an excess caloric intake or a decrease in energy expenditure, leads to the gradual accumulation of weight. This excess weight increases the risk for numerous medical problems; increases the risks associated with surgery; increases the risk for complications during pregnancy, labor, and delivery; and increases morbidity and mortality. People who are obese are often discriminated against in social, educational, and employment settings. In a society that values thinness, obesity can cause one to feel desperate, frustrated, depressed, and rejected, and to perceive oneself as a failure. About two thirds of adults in the United States are overweight and nearly one-third are considered obese (have a BMI ≥30; Weight-control Information

Network [WIN], 2012b). In addition, approximately 31.8% of young people between the ages of 2 and 19 are considered to be either overweight or obese, and 16.9% are considered to be obese (WIN).

Numerous theories about the cause of obesity have been proposed. According to genetic theories, a low resting metabolic rate or an inherited family tendency contribute to obesity. Physiologic factors that have been implicated include an increased number of fat cells, a lowered basal metabolic rate set point, a decreased amount of brown fat that burns kilocalories, insulin resistance, and hormone imbalance. A food and family environment that encourages overeating, a lifestyle in which exercise is minimal, and the availability of foods in a multitude of settings at all times are environmental factors that contribute to obesity (WIN, 2012a). Additionally, many identify psychological reasons for obesity, including compulsiveness, using food to satisfy emotional needs, relying on food for compensation for lack of affection and companionship, and overeating as a release mechanism for boredom, anxiety, and feelings of inadequacy. Obesity is resistant to treatment, and weight loss is temporary at best unless behavior modification and exercise are incorporated into the dietary plan.

BOX 35-5 NUTRITIONAL ASSESSMENT CONSIDERATIONS FOR OLDER ADULTS*

Biochemical Data
- Low serum albumin level (<3.5 mg/dL) may be a reflection of the aging process rather than a nutritional risk factor. Albumin synthesis declines with age.
- Hemoglobin levels that are lower than normal may only reflect anemia observed in older people as part of the aging process.

Anthropometric Data
- Because of age-related changes in body composition, skin-fold measurements, if used, should be taken from several body sites.

Dietary Data
- Dietary recall may be inaccurate because of vision and memory problems.
- Question use of vitamin and mineral supplements.
- Gather information concerning medication regimen (prescribed and over-the-counter) to assess for food–drug interactions and adverse effects of medications.

*Specific clinical data for older adults may be found in the Focus on the Older Adult display.

THE NURSING PROCESS
Assessing

Nutritional status has a significant impact on both health and disease. For well patients, good nutritional status can help to maintain health, promote normal growth and development, and protect against disease. During illness, good nutritional status can reduce the risk for complications and speed recovery time. Conversely, poor nutritional status can increase the risk for illness or death.

Like other aspects of nursing care, nutritional assessment is a systematic approach used to identify the patient's actual or potential needs, formulate a plan to meet those needs, initiate the plan or assign others to implement it, and evaluate the effectiveness of the plan. The level of assessment may range from simple screening to a comprehensive, in-depth assessment, depending on individual circumstances. Regardless of the level of assessment, nutritional assessment is appropriate for all patients. Nurses can collect assessment data through history taking (dietary, medical, socioeconomic data), physical assessments (anthropometric and clinical data), and laboratory data. When performing a nutritional assessment, nurses need to be aware of the specific changes in older people that may reflect on the accuracy of the assessment process (Box 35-5).

Nurses working with patients to promote appropriate behaviors related to nutrition should examine their own behaviors as factors in the success of the plan. Nurses who role model good health behaviors are more effective

teachers. Use the display, Promoting Health 35-1: Nutrition, for yourself before using it with others.

Dietary Data

Collect dietary data from the patient or family or caregivers and evaluate it according to the *Dietary Guidelines,* DRI, or the MyPlate food guide, depending on the purpose of the assessment.

NUTRITIONAL SCREENING

Nutritional screening is an important part of the nursing assessment. Screening looks for cues associated with nutrition problems to determine if a person is malnourished or at risk for malnutrition. The Mini Nutritional Assessment tool (MNA) is an example of a screening tool used to detect older adults at risk for malnutrition before changes in albumin level and the BMI. The MNA is a combination of screening questions followed by anthropometric measurements, including BMI, midarm and calf circumference, and weight loss. The MNA is fast and easy, and recommended for use with all older adult patients, whether they are community dwelling, hospitalized, or in long-term care settings (DiMaria-Ghalili & Guenter, 2008).

After a screening tool identifies a patient at risk, such as in a group of older adults, it is imperative to complete a nutritional assessment as a follow-up. These patients are usually referred to a dietitian for a comprehensive nutritional assessment (Dudek, 2014). When this is combined with other methods of assessing nutritional status, the nurse is better prepared to coordinate a focused strategy to combat malnutrition.

PROMOTING HEALTH 35-1

NUTRITION

Use the assessment checklist to determine how well you are meeting your needs related to nutrition practices. Then develop a prescription for self-care by choosing appropriate behaviors from the list of suggestions.

Assessment Checklist

☐ almost always   ☐ sometimes   ☐ almost never

☐ ☐ ☐   1. I know and use the recommended dietary guidelines and servings.

☐ ☐ ☐   2. My weight is within 10% of the ideal for my height and body frame.

☐ ☐ ☐   3. I maintain an appropriate balance between exercise and food intake.

☐ ☐ ☐   4. I limit my fat, sugar, salt, and red meat intake.

☐ ☐ ☐   5. I limit my caffeine intake.

☐ ☐ ☐   6. I use alcoholic beverages in moderation.

☐ ☐ ☐   7. I make an effort to eat high-fiber foods.

Self-Care Behaviors

1. Maintain desirable weight, eating a variety of foods in adequate amounts from each of the food groups.

2. Eat slowly, take smaller portions, and avoid second helpings if trying to control overeating.

3. Eat a variety of foods low in calories and high in nutrients to lose weight.

4. Obtain medical clearance before starting a weight-loss program.

5. Avoid too many foods high in cholesterol (milk, egg yolk, organ meats, fats, oils); instead choose lean meat, fish, poultry, and beans.

6. Eat foods high in fiber: whole-grain breads and cereals, fruits, vegetables, dry beans.

7. Avoid excess use of salt and sugar.

8. Begin an exercise program and maintain it.

9. Learn healthy eating habits; read labels, become familiar with healthy fast-food and restaurant menus; and drink alcohol moderately (if at all).

10. Substitute healthy rewards for yourself that do not include high-caloric, low nutrition snacks and beverages

Information to promote effective nutrition, dietary supplement use and safety; nutrient recommendations; and database resources are available online. Visit thePoint for a list of Internet resources.

ASSESSING DIETARY INTAKE

Many different methods can be used to assess actual dietary intake.

24-Hour Recall Method. The easiest way to collect dietary data is to obtain a 24-hour recall of all food and beverages the patient normally consumes during an average day. Ask the patient to recall details related to nutritional intake from the prior 24 hours. This method includes the patient's portion sizes, meal and snack patterns, meal timing, and location where food is eaten. Because this method relies on memory and accurate interpretation of portion sizes, the information may not be reliable.

Food Diaries/Calorie Counts. Food diaries and calorie counts require documentation of actual intake for a specified period of time. In an outpatient setting, ask the patient to record everything the patient has had to eat or drink, including portion size, over a set period of time. In the hospital setting, documentation is usually completed by the nursing staff. These tools may provide a better overall picture of nutrient intake because all food and beverages consumed in a specified period, usually 3 to 7 days, are recorded.

Food Frequency Record. Food frequency records give a general picture of nutritional consumption. Ask patients questions to elicit an average number of times certain foods or food groups are consumed in a given period of time: per day, per week, or per month. For example, ask, "How many times in the last week have you eaten fresh fruit or fish?" or "How many times in the last week have you had a glass of milk?"

Diet History. A more comprehensive approach to diet assessment is a full diet history. In addition to a 24-hour food recall, calorie counts/food diaries, and food-frequency record, interview questions are geared to provide information on past and present food intake and habits. Sample questions are included in the accompanying Focused Assessment Guide 35-1 (on page 1216).

 CONSIDER William Johnston, the man who has less-than-healthful dietary and health habits. The nurse could use a diet history to obtain specific information about Mr. Johnston's actual intake. Analysis of this information would reveal his actual dietary intake and identify potential and actual nutritional problems. ●

MEDICAL AND SOCIOECONOMIC DATA

Medical, social, and economic factors, as well as cultural and psychological influences, require evaluation for their impact on nutritional requirements and food choices. A nutritional assessment should include the following medical, social, and economic information (DiMaria-Ghalili & Amella, 2005; Dudek, 2014). Medical data include:

• Current illness as well as medical and surgical history
• Past and current drug history
• History of drug dependence or abuse

FOCUSED ASSESSMENT GUIDE 35-1

NUTRITION

Factors to Assess	Questions and Approaches
Usual dietary intake	Does your current intake differ from your usual intake? If so, is the reason a loss of appetite, changes in smell or taste, difficulty chewing and swallowing, hospitalization, a modified diet? With whom do you usually eat meals?
Food allergies or intolerances	Do you have any food allergies or intolerances?
Food preparation and storage	Who does the food shopping? Who prepares the meals? How is the food normally prepared? For instance, is food usually fried, baked, or broiled? Do you have adequate food storage space and preparation equipment?
Type of dietary practices	Do you now or have you in the past followed a modified diet prescribed by a physician? Do you now or have you in the past used a fad diet, health foods, or self-prescribed supplements?
Eating disorder patterns	Do you view yourself as overweight? Do you weigh yourself frequently during one day? How is your appetite? Do you binge on large amounts of food in a short period? Have you ever caused yourself to vomit after eating a meal? Have you used laxatives, diuretics, herbal supplements, or over-the-counter weight-loss pills to lose weight?

- Ability to chew and swallow, including condition of mouth, missing teeth, or dentures
- Appetite, food intolerance and allergies, and bowel habits

Social data include:

- Age, gender, family history, lifestyle (e.g., those at extremes in age are most at risk)
- Educational background
- Information about occupation, exercise, and sleep patterns
- Religious affiliation, cultural and ethnic background
- Use of alcohol and tobacco

Economic Data include:

- Source of income
- Food budget

ANTHROPOMETRIC DATA

Anthropometric measurements are used to determine body dimensions. In children, anthropometric measurements are used to assess growth rate; in adults, they can give indirect measurements of body protein and fat stores. For the data to be accurate and reliable, use standardized equipment and procedures, and compare the data with the appropriate reference standards for the patient's age and gender.

Obtain height and weight, the most common anthropometric measurements, when the patient is admitted to the health care facility and periodically thereafter or assess height and weight in a home care environment. Weigh a

patient on the same scale each time and at the same time of day, preferably before breakfast. Height and weight are used to calculate the patient's BMI. Because actual weight may be increased if the patient has edema, consider hydration status. Although self-reported weight may be recorded when actual weight is unobtainable, it is highly inaccurate and must be noted. Record an actual weight as soon as feasibly possible. Self-reported height in the older adult can be inaccurate related to shortening of the spine (DiMaria-Ghalili & Amella, 2005). Record an actual height as soon as possible.

Additional anthropometric measurements include triceps skin-fold measurements, a measure of subcutaneous fat stores; midarm circumference, a measure of skeletal muscle mass; and midarm muscle circumference, a measure of both skeletal muscle mass and fat stores.

BODY MASS INDEX AND WAIST CIRCUMFERENCE

Calculate the patient's body mass index (BMI) and measure waist circumference, as discussed earlier in the chapter. Compare results with the established guidelines to determine the patient's ideal body weight and identify potential health risks. Refer to Table 35-1 on page 1199.

CLINICAL DATA

Although signs and symptoms of altered nutrition may be observed during a physical assessment (Table 35-5), they usually do not appear until the condition is advanced. In addition, further investigation is necessary to determine

Table 35-5 CLINICAL OBSERVATIONS FOR NUTRITIONAL ASSESSMENT

BODY AREA	SIGNS OF GOOD NUTRITIONAL STATUS	SIGNS OF POOR NUTRITIONAL STATUS
General appearance	Alert, responsive	Listless, apathetic, and cachetic
General vitality	Endurance, energetic, sleeps well, vigorous	Easily fatigued, no energy, falls asleep easily, looks tired, apathetic, depressed mood
Weight	Normal for height, age, body build	Overweight or underweight
Hair	Shiny, lustrous, firm, not easily plucked, healthy scalp	Dull and dry, brittle, loss of color, easily plucked, thin and sparse
Face	Uniform skin color; healthy appearance, not swollen	Dark skin over cheeks and under eyes, flaky skin, facial edema (moon face), pale skin color
Eyes	Bright, clear, moist, no sores at corners of eyelids, membranes moist and healthy pink color, no prominent blood vessels	Pale eye membranes, dry eyes (xerophthalmia); Bitot's spots, increased vascularity, cornea soft (keratomalacia), small yellowish lumps around eyes (xanthelasma), dull or scarred cornea
Lips	Good pink color, smooth, moist, not chapped or swollen	Swollen and puffy (cheilosis), angular lesion at corners of mouth or fissures or scars (stomatitis)
Tongue	Deep red, surface papillae present	Smooth appearance, beefy red or magenta colored, swollen, hypertrophy or atrophy
Teeth	Straight, no crowding, no cavities, no pain, bright, no discoloration, well-shaped jaw	Cavities, mottled appearance (fluorosis), malpositioned, missing teeth
Gums	Firm, good pink color, no swelling or bleeding	Spongy, bleed easily, marginal redness, recessed, swollen and inflamed
Glands	No enlargement of the thyroid, face not swollen	Enlargement of the thyroid (goiter), enlargement of the parotid (swollen cheeks)
Skin	Smooth, good color, slightly moist, no signs of rashes, swelling, or color irregularities	Rough, dry, flaky, swollen, pale, pigmented, lack of fat under the skin, fat deposits around the joints (xanthomas), bruises, petechiae
Nails	Firm, pink	Spoon shaped (koilonychia), brittle, pale, ridged
Skeleton	Good posture, no malformations	Poor posture, beading of the ribs, bowed legs or knock-knees, prominent scapulas, chest deformity at diaphragm
Muscles	Well developed, firm, good tone, some fat under the skin	Flaccid, poor tone, wasted, underdeveloped, difficulty walking
Extremities	No tenderness	Weak and tender, edema of lower extremities
Abdomen	Flat	Swollen
Nervous system	Normal reflexes, psychological stability	Decrease in or loss of ankle and knee reflexes, psychomotor changes, mental confusion, depression, sensory loss, motor weakness, loss of sense of position, loss of vibration, burning and tingling of the hands and feet (paresthesia)
Cardiovascular system	Normal heart rate and rhythm, no murmurs, normal blood pressure for age	Cardiac enlargement, tachycardia, abnormal blood pressure
GI system	No palpable organs or masses (liver edge may be palpable in children)	Enlarged liver or spleen

(Adapted from Dudek, S. G. [2014]. *Nutrition essentials for nursing practice* [7th ed.]. Philadelphia: Wolters Kluwer Health/Lippincott Williams & Wilkins; and Mahan, L., & Jarvis, C. [2012]. *Physical examination & health assessment* [6th ed.]. St. Louis: Elsevier/Saunders.)

whether abnormal findings are actually caused by a nutritional deficiency, are possibly related to a nutritional deficiency, or are unrelated to nutritional status.

Assess for barriers to eating. **Dysphagia** (difficulty swallowing or the inability to swallow) can be the result of poor dental health, cancer, or a neurologic disease, such as stroke, Parkinson's disease, or dementia, and may reduce the patient's nutritional intake. Dysphagia also is associated with an increased risk for **aspiration**, the misdirection of oropharyngeal secretions or gastric contents into the larynx and lower respiratory tract (Eisenstadt, 2010). Dental problems are associated with impaired chewing and avoidance of foods that may be difficult to chew, such as meat, fruit, and vegetables. Patients who experience weakness and fatigue may find eating to be a chore to avoid. Diminished sensor abilities, such as sight, taste, smell, and hearing, may also impact a patient's nutritional intake.

BIOCHEMICAL DATA

Laboratory tests, which measure blood and urine levels of nutrients or biochemical functions that depend on an adequate supply of nutrients, can objectively detect nutritional problems in their early stages. Most routine biochemical tests measure protein status; measures of body vitamin, mineral, and trace element status are also available.

Hemoglobin, the oxygen-carrying protein of the red blood cells, and hematocrit, the volume of red blood cells packed by centrifugation in a given volume of blood, are measures of plasma protein that also reflect a person's iron status. Protein status can also be determined by measuring serum albumin and transferrin levels and by a total lymphocyte count. Serum albumin levels are a good indicator of a patient's nutritional status a few weeks prior to when the blood is drawn and can help identify chronic nutrition problems (Van Leeuwen, Poelhuis-Leth, & Bladh, 2011). The albumin level does not change with increasing age, but malnutrition and various disease states cause its level to decrease. Serum albumin levels can also be affected by the patient's hydration status; overhydration can cause a low albumin level and dehydration may cause a very high level. Prealbumin levels indicate short-term nutritional status, can be used to detect daily changes in a patient's protein status, and are an excellent marker for malnutrition (Van Leeuwen et al.). Transferrin acts as an iron-transporting protein, but because it is related to iron levels may not always be an accurate indicator of nutritional status. The total lymphocyte count reflects immune status and is directly affected by impaired nutritional states.

Blood glucose, blood cholesterol, and blood triglycerides are additional laboratory tests relative to nutritional status. Twenty-four-hour urine tests used to measure protein metabolism include urine creatinine excretion and urine urea nitrogen. Urea, a breakdown product of amino acids, can be measured in the urine and blood. It reflects protein intake and the body's ability to detoxify and excrete this metabolic byproduct. Creatinine levels are directly proportional to the body's muscle mass; a reduction in this value reflects severe malnutrition. These biochemical indicators with nutritional implications are summarized in Box 35-6.

Diagnosing

Assessment data may reveal actual or potential nutritional problems. As soon as problems are identified, refer the patient to appropriate services, including a dietitian.

Imbalanced Nutrition as the Problem

Data that the nurse collects may lead to the development of several nursing diagnoses related to nutrition. The following nursing diagnoses may be made when imbalanced nutrition is the cause of the patient's disorder:

BOX 35-6 | **BIOCHEMICAL DATA WITH NUTRITIONAL IMPLICATIONS**

- Hemoglobin (normal = 12–18 g/dL)
  decreased → anemia
- Hematocrit (normal = 40%–50%)
  decreased → anemia
  increased → dehydration
- Serum albumin (normal = 3.5–5.5 g/dL)
  decreased → malnutrition (prolonged protein depletion), malabsorption
- Prealbumin (normal = 23–43 mg/dL)
  decreased → protein depletion, malnutrition
- Transferrin (normal = 240–480 mg/dL)
  decreased → anemia, protein deficiency
- Blood urea nitrogen (normal = 17–18 mg/dL)
  increased → starvation, high protein intake, severe dehydration
  decreased → malnutrition, overhydration
- Creatinine (normal = 0.4–1.5 mg/dL)
  increased → dehydration
  decreased → reduction in total muscle mass, severe malnutrition

(Adapted from Dudek, S. [2014]. *Nutrition essentials for nursing practice* [7th ed.]. Philadelphia: Wolters Kluwer Health/Lippincott Williams & Wilkins; and Van Leeuwen, A. M., Poelhuis-Leth, D., & Bladh, M. L. [2011]. *Davis's Comprehensive Handbook of Laboratory & Diagnostic Tests with Nursing Implications* [4th ed.]. Philadelphia: F. A. Davis.)

- Imbalanced Nutrition: Less Than Body Requirements related to nothing by mouth (NPO), inadequate tube feeding, prolonged use of a clear liquid diet, numerous food intolerance or allergies, excessive dieting, anorexia, chewing or swallowing difficulties, nausea, vomiting, chronic diarrhea, malabsorption, psychological eating disorders (anorexia nervosa, bulimia), alcoholism, metabolic and endocrine disorders, inappropriate use of supplements
- Imbalanced Nutrition: More Than Body Requirements related to overeating, inactivity, metabolic and endocrine disorders, inappropriate use of supplements
- Risk for Imbalanced Nutrition: More Than Body Requirements related to inappropriate eating, closely spaced pregnancies, metabolic and endocrine disorders, inappropriate use of supplements

See specific examples in the accompanying Examples of NANDA-I Nursing Diagnoses box.

Imbalanced Nutrition as the Etiology

Data that the nurse collects may lead to the development of several nursing diagnoses related to nutrition. Nutritional problems may affect other areas of human functioning. In the following nursing diagnoses, the nutritional problem is the cause of another problem.

- Ineffective Health Maintenance related to lack of knowledge about adequate nutrition

EXAMPLES OF NANDA-I NURSING DIAGNOSES

NUTRITION

Nursing Diagnoses	Related Factors	Sample Defining Characteristics
Imbalanced Nutrition: Less Than Body Requirements	Malabsorption	• "I seem to eat all day long and yet I keep losing weight." • Reports losing 15 lb within the past 3 weeks. Has 8 to 10 bowel movements daily of frothy, odorous stools that float. Fecal fat excretion test indicates steatorrhea. Patient appears fatigued and undernourished; muscle wasting is evident. Laboratory data reveal low serum albumin level (protein deficiency) and iron-deficiency anemia.
Imbalanced Nutrition: More Than Body Requirements	Excessive intake in relation to physical activity	• "I don't have time to eat at work." "I don't eat that much, but it is at night when I get home from work, usually around 7 PM, sometimes later." • Patient reports a 10-lb weight gain within the past month and 50-lb weight gain in last year. Patient reports large food portion size in relation to suggested food guidelines. • BMI 45; waist circumference 54 inches • Patient reports job involves sitting at desk for most of day. Limited physical exercise. States: "Walking makes my back hurt, so I cannot walk for long periods of time."
Impaired Swallowing	Neuromuscular impairment	• "Food seems to get stuck." "Sometimes I can't finish eating because I cough too much." • Swallowing evaluation study reports abnormality in oral and pharyngeal phases. Patient observed to have difficulty chewing; delayed swallow; gags and coughs during meal; gurgly voice quality noted after meal.

• Constipation related to inadequate fluid or fiber intake
• Deficient Fluid Volume related to inadequate fluid intake
• Risk for Infection related to inadequate calorie intake, inadequate protein intake
• Impaired Home Maintenance Management related to inability to purchase, store, or prepare food for family

Wellness Diagnosis

Data that the nurse collects may lead to the development of several nursing diagnoses related to nutrition. For patients who are incorporating sound nutritional practices in their daily routine, the following wellness diagnosis may be appropriate: Readiness for Enhanced Nutrition associated with food safety.

Outcome Identification and Planning

Expected outcomes are derived from the actual or potential nutritional problems diagnosed. The goal is to maintain or restore optimal nutritional status using foods the patients like and tolerate as appropriate for their situation. Goals should also include those to alleviate symptoms or side effects of disease or treatment and to prevent complications or diet-related chronic diseases. General patient outcomes are listed here. Actual patient outcomes should list specific behaviors and criteria individualized for the patient situation. The patient will:

• Attain and maintain ideal body weight, as indicated by BMI and waist circumference
• Eat a diet adequate but not excessive, in all nutrients, based on the MyPlate food guideline system, the DRIs, and dietary recommendations and guidelines issued from health and U.S. governmental agencies
• Eat a variety of food in each of three or more meals
• Follow the appropriate modified diet, when necessary, to restore health, avoid disease recurrences, and prevent or delay potential complications.

 REMEMBER Charles Gallagher, the husband of the woman receiving enteral nutrition. Initially, outcomes would focus on maintaining his wife's nutritional status. However, the informed decision made to withdraw the nutritional support would lead the nurse to revise the outcomes. Therefore, the outcomes then would focus on emotional comfort for the Gallagher family and a peaceful, dignified death for Mrs. Gallagher. ●

Implementing

Providing proper and adequate nourishment to the patient is a team effort implemented in a variety of settings. Diet orders may be written by the primary care provider in the inpatient setting, confirmed by the dietitian, and frequently explained to the patient by the nurse. The

EXAMPLES OF NURSING INTERVENTION AND NURSING OUTCOME CLASSIFICATIONS (NIC/NOC)

NUTRITION

Nursing Interventions	Nursing Outcomes
• Nutrition Management • Weight Management • Nutritional Counseling • Nutritional Monitoring	• Nutritional Status • Appetite • Weight: Body Mass • Self Care: Eating

Reprinted from Bulechek, G. M., Butcher, H. K., Dochterman, J. M., & Wagner, C. M. (Eds.). (2013). *Nursing interventions classification (NIC)* (6th ed., pp. 274–277, 415). St. Louis: Elsevier/Mosby; and Moorhead, S., Johnson, M., Maas, M. L., & Swanson, E. (Eds.). (2013). *Nursing Outcomes Classification (NOC)* (5th ed., pp. 95, 384, 467, 551). A full listing of nursing activities for each nursing intervention and outcome can be found in these books.

nurse may also be responsible for screening patients at home who are at nutritional risk, observing intake and appetite, evaluating the patient's tolerance, assisting the patient with eating, administering enteral and parenteral feedings, consulting with the dietitian and primary care provider when dietary problems arise, addressing the potential for drug–nutrient reactions, obtaining more food or snacks for the patient when appropriate, monitoring food brought by visitors, and participating in nutrition education efforts. The accompanying Examples of Nursing Intervention and Nursing Outcome Classifications (NIC/NOC) box lists standardized nursing interventions and corresponding outcomes related to nutrition.

Teaching Nutritional Information

For the greatest chance of success, tailor diet instructions individually to the patient's lifestyle, culture, intellectual ability, and level of motivation. Although strict guidelines and printed handouts may seem ideal, in practice, simplicity and compromise are often the keys to patient compliance.

 RECALL William Johnston, the patient with hypertension and high cholesterol. The nurse would need to consider Mr. Johnston's lifestyle when developing a teaching plan for him. As a result of his "on-the-run" lifestyle, the nurse would need to adapt the teaching plan, making sure that it is realistic for his needs. For example, the nurse might teach Mr. Johnston about reading food labels to ensure that his selections, when he is "on the run" are low in fat and cholesterol. In addition, the nurse would also provide Mr. Johnston with appropriate suggestions for choices when dining out. Doing so will help communicate to him that the plan is workable, enhancing the chances of Mr. Johnston complying with the plan, thereby achieving success. •

Include information about food safety issues in patient teaching. This includes safe handling of foods, food storage, and preventing food-borne illness. Encourage patients to wash hands and clean food contact surfaces frequently when handling and preparing foods. Wash fruits and vegetables before eating or preparation. This helps prevent contamination of food with bacteria and viruses. Teach patients to cook foods to a safe temperature to kill microorganisms. Also, explain that raw, cooked, and ready-to-eat foods should be separated during shopping and preparation and should be stored separately. This prevents cross-contamination with microorganisms. Chill (refrigerate) perishable food promptly and keep cold foods at 41°F or lower to prevent the growth of pathogens. Advise patients to avoid raw (unpasteurized) milk and products made from unpasteurized milk and raw eggs. Teach patients to avoid undercooked meat and poultry, unpasteurized juices, and raw sprouts (USDA & DHHS, 2010).

Monitoring Nutritional Status

Malnourished patients are more likely to have slower wound healing and to develop complications. Prevention of malnutrition can have a positive effect on patient outcomes. In the hospital, shortened stays limit the time available for nutritional screening and intervention. Patients are often acutely ill and uninterested or unable to absorb and retain any nutritional instruction. It may also be difficult to include a family member or caregiver responsible for food preparation in scheduled teaching sessions. In many situations, the home health care nurse has the opportunity to have a significant impact on nutritional health. Provide instruction in a relaxed setting that allows insight into a patient's cultural orientation and family patterns and traditions. This type of environment also encourages modification and adjustments in the nurse's approach to nutritional instruction. Investigate the variety of community services and programs that are available to provide nutritional support to patients at home. The accompanying box, Focus on the Older Adult, includes teaching content and strategies for the specific nutritional challenges facing the older adult.

Nurses are often involved in the process of diet progression. The decision to advance a patient's diet

FOCUS ON THE OLDER ADULT

NURSING STRATEGIES TO ADDRESS AGE-RELATED CHANGES AFFECTING NUTRITION

Age-Related Changes	Nursing Strategies
Altered ability to chew related to loss of teeth, ill-fitting dentures, and gingivitis	• Encourage and instruct patient to care for and retain own teeth and dentures. • Encourage proper tooth brushing and use of special toothpaste if gums and teeth are sensitive. • Chop, shred, or puree foods that are difficult to chew. • Select ground meat, fish, or poultry as protein sources more easily chewed.
Loss of senses of smell and taste	• Serve food that is attractive and at proper temperature. • Serve one food at a time rather than mixing foods. • Serve foods with different textures and aromas.
Decreased peristalsis in the esophagus	• Avoid cold liquids. • Avoid emotional upsets and stress-producing situations. • Take anticholinergic drugs as ordered by physician.
Gastroesophageal reflux	• Avoid overeating. • Avoid juices, chocolate, and fat. • Avoid alcohol and smoking. • Elevate the head of the bed 30 to 40 degrees when sleeping. • Lose weight if necessary. • Avoid bending over. • Take antacids or other medications as ordered by physician. • Avoid eating right before bedtime.
Decreased gastric secretions	• Chew food thoroughly. • Eat meals on a regular schedule. • Use antacids or other medications as prescribed by physician. • Be alert for symptoms of deficiency of nutrients, particularly iron, calcium, fat, protein, and vitamin B_{12}.
Slowed intestinal peristalsis	• Eat a high-fiber diet. • Remain as active as possible. • Increase fluid intake. • Avoid laxative use. • Eat meals at a regular time. • Drink prune juice or eat prunes every morning.
Lowered glucose tolerance	• Eat more complex carbohydrates. • Avoid sugar-rich foods.
Reduction in appetite and thirst sensation	• Offer fluids at regular intervals and at preferred temperature. • Be alert for symptoms of dehydration and electrolyte imbalance. • Offer small meals at frequent intervals.
Nutritional deficiencies related to alcohol intake	• Encourage diet high in protein and carbohydrates. • Offer small, frequent meals to maintain caloric intake. • Restrict sodium and fluids if edema is present. • Take multivitamin supplements, as ordered by physician.
Loss of appetite associated with depression and loneliness	• Promote mealtime as a social event. • Set an attractive table in a pleasant setting. • Eat outdoors whenever possible. • Invite guests as often as possible. • Participate in special programs for senior citizens.
Physical handicaps	• Open cartons and assist with setup of meal. • Arrange for home-delivered meals. • Conserve energy when preparing meals (sit on a stool, etc.). • Provide transportation and assistance to obtain food.

(continued)

FOCUS ON THE OLDER ADULT *continued*

NURSING STRATEGIES TO ADDRESS AGE-RELATED CHANGES AFFECTING NUTRITION

Age-Related Changes	Nursing Strategies
Low income	• Buy specials when available at food store. • Use generic brands. • Use coupons. • Cook larger quantities than necessary and freeze the leftovers for future use. • Substitute eggs, skim milk powder, and beans for meat. • Check for any community resources available to elderly.
Malnutrition	• Eat essential foods first. • Select nutrient-dense foods. • Monitor for signs of nutritional deficiencies. • Encourage eating by planning special events.
Increased risk for drug–nutrient interactions	• Avoid unnecessary drugs; monitor for polypharmacy. • Be aware of drug actions and interactions. • Check with pharmacist to determine if medication may or may not be taken with food. • Assess for confusion and inability to manage medication regimen.

is based on the return of gastrointestinal function, the absence of symptoms related to a particular disease process, or the resolution of whatever prompted the dietary restriction. Often, medical orders are written to begin the patient on one diet and advance to another diet as tolerated. This allows the nurse to assess the patient's tolerance of the beginning diet and change, or advance, the diet based on the assessments. Tolerance of diet can be assessed by the following: absence of nausea, vomiting, and diarrhea; absence of feelings of fullness; absence of abdominal pain and distention; feelings of hunger; and the ability to consume at least 50% to 75% of the food on the meal tray. For example, a postoperative patient may have an order to begin a clear liquid at breakfast and advance to a house diet as tolerated. The patient would receive a clear liquid diet for breakfast. The nurse would assess the patient's ability to ingest the clear liquids and then make a decision regarding progression of the diet.

Stimulating Appetite

Pain, illness, anxiety, and medications can contribute to anorexia and poor intake when in a health care facility or in the home. To the hospitalized patient, food and eating may take on much greater meaning. Loss of control over food choices, the way food is prepared, when and how food is served, and eating alone may do little to encourage normal eating. Make every effort to ensure that the proper food is not only served, but also eaten. The additional time and attention spent when encouraging a person to eat may have a positive effect on dietary intake. The following measures may help to stimulate appetite in any setting:

• Serve small, frequent meals to avoid overwhelming the person with large amounts of food.
• Solicit food preferences and encourage favorite foods from home or prepared when at home, if possible.

• Provide encouragement and a pleasant eating environment.
• Be sure that any prepared food looks attractive.
• Schedule procedures and medications at times when they are least likely to interfere with appetite.
• Control pain, nausea, or depression with medications.
• Offer alternatives for items that a person cannot or will not eat.
• Encourage or provide good oral hygiene. Ensure that the patient's dentures are well-fitting and in place, if applicable.
• Remove clutter from the eating area.
• Keep eating area free from irritating odors.
• Arrange food tray so that a person can easily reach food.
• Provide a comfortable position.
• Ask about any rituals during mealtimes at home and include them if possible.
• If patients are absent from their rooms during mealtime, order a late food tray or keep food warm until they return.
• Do not disturb mealtime; don't interrupt patients for non-urgent procedures during mealtime.

Assisting With Eating

The loss of independence that comes with the inability to self-feed can be a severe blow to a person's self-esteem. The following measures may help a person maintain dignity while being fed:

• Involve the person as much as possible. Solicit the patient's preferences regarding the order of items eaten and the eating pace.
• Provide appropriate drinks.
• Sit at the patient's eye level and make eye contact to create a more relaxed atmosphere.
• Engage the person in pleasant conversation to ease tension.

BOX 35-7 SPECIAL CONSIDERATIONS AND INTERVENTIONS FOR FEEDING PATIENTS WITH DEMENTIA OR OTHER ALTERATIONS IN COGNITION

- Change the environment in which meals occur.
- Assess the area where meals are served. Create a home-like environment by preparing food close to the place where it will be served to stimulate senses.
- Observe as many former rituals as possible, such as handwashing and saying a blessing.
- Avoid clutter and distractions.
- Maintain a pleasant, well-lighted room. Play calming music.
- Keep food as close to its original form as possible.
- Serve meals in the same place at the same time.
- Closely supervise mealtime.
- Check food temperatures to prevent accidental mouth burns.
- Assist as needed. Be alert for cues from the patient. Turning away may signal that the patient has had enough to eat or that the patient needs to slow down. Leaning

- forward with an open mouth usually means the patient is ready for more food.
- Stroking the underside of the chin may help promote swallowing.
- Provide one food item at a time. Offer small, frequent eating opportunities. A whole tray of food may be overwhelming.
- Ensure that the patient's glasses and hearing aid are working properly.
- Demonstrate what you want the patient to do. State the goal clearly, and then mimic the action with exaggerated motions.
- Provide between-meal snacks that are easy to consume using the hands.
- Use adaptive feeding equipment as needed such as weighted utensils, large-handled cups, and larger or smaller silverware than standard.
- Promote family involvement to encourage eating.

(Adapted from Cole, D. [2012]. Optimising nutrition for older people with dementia. *Nursing Standard, 26*[20], 41–48; Dudek, S. [2014]. *Nutrition essentials for nursing practice* [7th ed.]. Philadelphia: Wolters Kluwer Health/Lippincott Williams & Wilkins; Lin, L., Watson, R., & Wu, S. [2010]. What is associated with low food intake in older people with dementia? *Journal of Clinical Nursing, 19*[1–2], 53–59; Tabloski, P. [2010]. *Gerontological nursing* [2nd ed.]. Upper Saddle River, NJ: Pearson; and Dunne, A. [2010]. Nutrition and dementia. *Nursing & Residential Care, 12*[3], 112, 114, 116.)

- Place a napkin, not a bib, over the person's clothes for protection.
- Use straws or special eating utensils whenever possible.
- Ensure that if a person wears dentures, hearing aids, or glasses, they are in place before mealtime.
- Open containers, cut meat, or apply condiments to the prepared food only if the person wishes.

When assisting visually impaired patients:

- Explain placement of foods on plates and food tray. Relating items on plate to the location on a clock face may be helpful.
- Provide special plate guards, utensils, double handles, and compartmentalized plates.

- Place foods and dishes in similar locations at each meal.
- Use straws for beverages, if not contraindicated by the presence of dysphagia.
- Provide supervision as needed.

Box 35-7 outlines special considerations and interventions for feeding patients with dementia or other alterations in cognition. Box 35-8 highlights nursing considerations for feeding patients with dysphagia.

Providing Oral Nutrition

A variety of oral diets are available in health care settings and may be prescribed for use at home. Oral diets

BOX 35-8 SPECIAL CONSIDERATIONS AND INTERVENTIONS FOR FEEDING PATIENTS WITH DYSPHAGIA

- Provide at least a 30-minute rest period prior to mealtime. A rested person will likely have less difficulty swallowing.
- Sit the patient upright, preferably in a chair. If bedrest is mandatory, elevate the head of the bed to a 90-degree angle.
- Provide mouth care immediately before meals to enhance the sense of taste.
- Avoid rushed or forced feeding. Adjust the rate of feeding and size of bites to the patient's tolerance.
- Collaborate to obtain a speech therapy consult for swallowing evaluation.
- Initiate a nutrition consult for appropriate diet modification such as chopping, mincing, or pureeing of foods and liquid consistency (thin, nectar-thick, honey-like, spoon-thick).

- Keep in mind that some patients may find thickened liquids unpalatable and thus drink insufficient fluids.
- Reduce or eliminate distractions at mealtime so that the patient can focus attention on swallowing.
- Alternate solids and liquids.
- Assess for signs of aspiration during eating: sudden appearance of severe coughing; choking; cyanosis; voice change, hoarseness, and/or gurgling after swallowing; frequent throat clearing after meals; or regurgitation through the nose or mouth.
- Inspect oral cavity for retained food.
- Avoid or minimize the use of sedatives and hypnotics since these agents may impair the cough reflex and swallowing.

(Adapted from Metheny, N. [2012]. Preventing aspiration in older adults with dysphagia. Available at http://consultgerirn.org/uploads/File/trythis/try_this_20.pdf; Eisenstadt, E. S. [2010]. Dysphagia and aspiration pneumonia in older adults. *Journal of the American Academy of Nurse Practitioners, 22*[1], 17–22; and Dudek, S. [2014]. *Nutrition essentials for nursing practice* [7th ed.]. Philadelphia: Wolters Kluwer Health/Lippincott Williams & Wilkins.)

Table 35-6 SELECTED THERAPEUTIC DIETS

DIET AND DESCRIPTION	INDICATIONS
Consistent-Carbohydrate Diet: Total daily carbohydrate content is consistent; emphasizes general nutritional balance. Calories based on attaining and maintaining healthy weight. High-fiber and heart-healthy fats encouraged; sodium and saturated fats are limited.	Type I and type 2 diabetes, gestational diabetes, impaired glucose tolerance
Fat-Restricted Diet: Low-fat diets are intended to lower the patient's total intake of fat.	Chronic cholecystitis (inflammation of the gallbladder) to decrease gallbladder stimulation; cardiovascular disease, to help prevent atherosclerosis.
High-fiber: Emphasis on increased intake of foods high in fiber.	Prevent or treat constipation; irritable bowel syndrome; diverticulosis
Low-fiber: Fiber limited to <10 g/day.	Before surgery; ulcerative colitis; diverticulitis; Crohn's disease
Sodium-restricted: Sodium limit may be set at 500–3000 mg/day	Hypertension; heart failure; acute and chronic renal disease, liver disease
Renal diet: Reduce workload on kidneys to delay or prevent further damage; control accumulation of uremic toxins. Protein restriction 0.6–1 g/kg/day; sodium restriction 1,000–3,000 mg/day; Potassium and fluid restrictions dependent on patient situation	Nephrotic syndrome; chronic kidney disease; diabetic kidney disease

may be categorized as regular, modified consistency, or therapeutic (Dudek, 2014). Regular, regular vegetarian, and modified consistency diets are outlined here. Information regarding common therapeutic diets is outlined in Table 35-6.

NORMAL OR HOUSE DIETS
Normal, regular, or house diets are designed to achieve or maintain optimal nutritional status by providing adequate amounts of all nutrients. The diet's actual composition and nutritional value varies with the quantity and types of food selected by the patient. No foods are excluded. Portion sizes are not limited. Regular diets are adjusted to meet age-specific needs throughout the life cycle and may also be altered to meet vegetarian or kosher eating (Dudek, 2014).

VEGETARIAN DIETS
Some patients may prefer a vegetarian diet for a variety of reasons, such as religious preference, ethical belief that killing animals for food is unjust, fear of contamination with pesticides, or health concerns about the cholesterol and saturated fats found in meats. There are many different forms of vegetarianism, ranging from avoidance of red meat to complete elimination of all animal products. Meats are usually replaced with legumes, grains, and vegetables, and, if well planned, this type of diet can satisfy all nutritional requirements. Because fewer or no animal products are consumed, vegetarians consume less saturated fat, cholesterol, and animal protein and greater amounts of carbohydrates, fiber, and other important nutrients. Vitamin B_{12}, vitamin A, and iron are nutrients that may require supplementation in some vegetarian diets, but most vegetarian diets are not deficient in

any nutrients. Support patients who follow a vegetarian diet by assisting them or their caregiver to select nutritious food items from the large variety of foods available within their dietary framework.

MODIFIED CONSISTENCY DIETS
Liquid diets are used most often as transitional diets when eating resumes after acute illness, surgery, or parenteral nutrition. Because clear liquid diets are inadequate in calories, protein, and most nutrients, progression to more nutritious alternatives is recommended as soon as possible.

Full liquid diets contain all the items on a clear liquid diet. Additional items allowed include milk and milk drinks, puddings, custards, plain frozen desserts, pasteurized eggs, cereal gruels, vegetable juices, and milk and egg substitutes in addition to clear liquids. A full liquid diet contains liquids that can be poured at room temperature. High-calorie, high-protein supplements are recommended if a full liquid diet is used for more than 3 days.

Mechanically altered diets are adequate in calories and nutrients, and may be used on a long-term basis. Additional information regarding modified consistency diets and dysphagia diets (a variation of the modified consistency diet) can be found in Table 35-7.

NOTHING BY MOUTH
In some cases, such as before surgery to prevent aspiration related to anesthesia and after surgery until bowel sounds return, patients may be given nothing by mouth (**NPO**). NPO may also be necessary for patients undergoing certain medical tests; for patients experiencing severe nausea and vomiting, an inability to chew or swallow, or various acute or chronic GI abnormalities; for those who are comatose; and for women during labor and delivery.

Table 35-7 | MODIFIED CONSISTENCY DIETS

DIET AND DESCRIPTION	INDICATIONS
Clear Liquid Diet: Composed only of clear fluids or foods that become fluid at body temperature. Requires minimal digestion and leaves minimal residue. Includes clear broth, coffee, tea, clear fruit juices (apple, cranberry, grape), gelatin, popsicles, commercially prepared clear liquid supplements.	Preparation for bowel surgery and lower endoscopy; acute gastrointestinal disorders; initial postoperative diet
Pureed Diet: Also known as a blenderized liquid diet because the diet is made up of liquids and foods blenderized to liquid form. All foods are allowed.	After oral or facial surgery; chewing and swallowing difficulties
Mechanically Altered Diet: Regular diet with modifications for texture. Excludes most raw fruits and vegetables and foods with seeds, nuts, and dried fruits. Foods are chopped, ground, mashed or soft.	Chewing and swallowing difficulties; after surgery to the head, neck, or mouth.

The following measures may provide comfort to patients who are ordered NPO:

- Encourage or provide good oral hygiene.
- Provide the patient with ice chips or sips of water as allowed.
- Urge the patient to avoid watching others eat. Suggest alternate activities at mealtimes.

Well-nourished patients can easily withstand the stress of NPO for a short period, but being NPO for an extended period of time poses a nutritional challenge for many people. Patients with increased nutritional requirements and those who will be NPO for more than 2 days may require nutritional support from **enteral nutrition**, administering nutrients directly into the stomach, or **parenteral nutrition**, providing nutrition via IV therapy. These therapies are discussed in the following sections.

Providing Enteral Nutrition

Oral feeding is the preferred and most effective method of feeding patients. However, at times, a patient will be unable to meet nutritional needs through oral intake of an adequate diet. In this circumstance, an alternate feeding method may be necessary. Selection of a feeding tube may be appropriate, because the next best method of feeding is via the enteral route. Enteral nutrition involves passing a tube into the GI tract to administer a formula containing adequate nutrients. Gastric feedings have the advantage of allowing the stomach to be used as a natural reservoir, regulating the amount of foods and liquids released into the small intestine. This alternate feeding method may deliver total or supplemental nutrition over a short-term period or for longer intervals. Consider factors related to selection of a feeding tube, including aspiration risk, the anticipated duration of the feeding tube, the function of the gastrointestinal (GI) tract, and the patient's overall condition and prognosis. Also, it is important to consider the ethical implications surrounding initiation of tube feedings, which entail knowledge of the patient's wishes concerning this intervention.

The decision to place, maintain, and/or discontinue feeding tubes can be a source of much turmoil in the lives of patients and their families. There are many emotional, physical, psychological, and cultural aspects to the institution, maintenance, and withdrawal of nutrition. Nurses can be a source of great support and information to aid patients and their families in making nutrition-related health care decisions.

SHORT-TERM NUTRITIONAL SUPPORT

For short-term use (less than 4 weeks), a nasogastric or nasointestinal route is usually selected. A **nasogastric (NG) tube** is inserted through the nose and into the stomach. However, the patient is at risk for aspirating the tube feeding solution into the lungs, a disadvantage for using this route. Patients with a dysfunctional gag reflex, high risk of aspiration, gastric stasis, gastroesophageal reflux, nasal injuries, and those who are unable to have the head of the bed elevated during feedings are not candidates for nasogastric feeding (American Society for Parenteral and Enteral Nutrition (A.S.P.E.N.), 2011; Best, 2005).

Traditional nasogastric tubes are firm and large in diameter. One example is a Levin tube. A Levin tube is a flexible rubber or plastic single-lumen tube with holes at the stomach end and a connector at the opposing end (Fig. 35-4). The connector allows for attachment to a

FIGURE 35-4. Levin tube.

FIGURE 35-5. Dobbhoff tube.

feeding apparatus and medication administration. Occasionally, a smaller, softer, more pliable polyurethane tube may be inserted via the nose into the stomach or small intestine. This type of tube is advantageous, providing greater patient comfort and less trauma to the nares. A Dobbhoff tube is an example of this type of tube (Fig. 35-5). However, the smaller tube diameter makes checking tube placement and medication administration more difficult than with the larger-diameter tubes. The method of inserting a nasogastric tube is described in Skill 35-1 on pages 1240–1246. Insertion of this tube requires skill and accuracy and is frequently done by the nurse.

A **nasointestinal (NI) tube** is passed through the nose and into the upper portion of the small intestine. It may be indicated for a patient with increased risk for aspiration due to a diminished gag reflex or slow gastric motility. Administration of the feeding solution into the small intestine also avoids the potential for gastric reflex. Some medical conditions (delayed gastric emptying, gastric tumor) also necessitate the use of a nasointestinal tube. However, when formula is delivered directly into the intestine, a type of dumping syndrome may develop because the pyloric valve in the stomach, which normally slows transit of food into the intestine, is bypassed. Rapid administration of hypertonic feeding solution into the proximal small intestine causes the movement of extracellular fluid from the vascular system into the small intestine. Distention of the small intestine occurs, with accompanying gas, bloating, nausea, diarrhea, cramping, and lightheadedness.

CONFIRMATION OF NG FEEDING TUBE PLACEMENT

Verify correct placement of the nasogastric tube after the initial insertion, before beginning a feeding or instilling liquids, and at regular intervals during continuous feedings. This ensures that the tip of the tube is situated in the stomach or intestine, preventing inadvertent administration of substances into the wrong place. A misplaced feeding tube in the lungs or pulmonary tissue places the patient at risk for aspiration. Radiographic examination, measurement of aspirate pH, visual assessment of aspi-

rate, measurement of tube length and measurement of tube marking, and monitoring of carbon dioxide are used to confirm feeding tube placement. With the exception of radiographic examination, the use of several of these techniques in conjunction with each other increases the likelihood of correct tube placement. An old technique of auscultation of air injected into a feeding tube has proved unreliable and may result in tragic consequences if used as an indicator of tube placement (Stepter, 2012; AACN, 2010; Best, 2005; Khair, 2005). Therefore, do not use it to confirm feeding tube placement.

Radiographic Examination. This is the standard procedure to verify initial placement of a feeding tube (A.S.P.E.N., 2011; AACN, 2010; Best, 2005; Ellet, 2004; Khair, 2005; Metheny & Meert, 2004). However, radiographs expose the patient to radiation, must be interpreted by a physician, are costly if done on a routine basis, and may be inaccessible. A radiograph only confirms the position of the tube at the time it was taken. The tube may have moved at any point thereafter. Also, as previously stated, placement must be checked frequently while the tube is in place.

Measurement of Aspirate pH and Visual Assessment of Aspirate. The recommended method for checking placement, other than radiograph, is measuring the pH of the aspirate (AACN, 2010; Best, 2005; Hinkle & Cheever, 2014; Khair, 2005; May, 2007). However, when continuous feedings are in use, pH becomes less helpful, because the nutritional formula buffers the pH of gastrointestinal secretions (Metheny et al., 2005). Visual assessment of aspirated gastric contents is also suggested as a tool to check placement (Hinkle & Cheever, 2014; A.S.P.E.N., 2009a; Stepter, 2012). Refer to Guidelines for Nursing Care 35-1.

Aspiration of fluid through the feeding tubes is sometimes difficult, especially if a smaller diameter tube is used. Because they are less rigid, they may be more likely to collapse when negative pressure is applied during aspiration. More than likely, the difficulty is a result of a blocked tube. Additionally, the ports on the tip of the tube may not be positioned in fluid. Research by clinicians has demonstrated that aspiration is easier in small-bore tubes if there are multiple ports rather than a single port. Several attempts may be necessary to aspirate gastric contents. If repeated instillations of 30 mL of air and repositioning prove ineffective, tube placement should be checked by radiograph after obtaining an order from the primary care provider.

Measurement of Tube Length and Measurement of Tube Marking. Another way to verify tube placement is to measure the length of the exposed tube after insertion and document this measurement. Then, before each feeding, check tube length and compare findings with the initial measurement in conjunction with pH measurement and visual assessment of aspirate. Any increase in the length of the exposed tube may indicate dislodgement

GUIDELINES FOR NURSING CARE 35-1

VISUAL ASSESSMENT AND pH MEASUREMENT OF GASTRIC CONTENTS

Allow 1-hour interval after patient has received medication or completed an intermittent feeding before testing pH of gastric fluid. If feeding is continuous, plan pH testing at a time when feeding can be withheld.

- Insert 30 mL of air into tube before aspirating GI contents to flush out contents of tube.
- Withdraw small amount (5–10 mL) of gastric secretions.
- If unable to obtain specimen, reposition the patient and flush tube again with 30 mL of air. It may be necessary to retry several times.
- Place drop of gastric secretions onto pH paper or place small amount in plastic cup and dip pH paper into it. Within 30 seconds, compare color on paper with chart supplied by manufacturer. (A pH meter and color chart is also an option.)
- Document results on patient's flow sheet. The following are indications of placement:

pH

- Stomach: pH less than 5.5 (If patient is taking an acid-inhibiting agent, range may be 4.0–6.0)
- Intestines: pH 7.0 or higher
- Respiratory tract: pH 6.0 or higher

Color of Aspirate

- Stomach: grassy green, tan, off-white, bloody, or brown
- Intestines: medium to deep golden-yellow (may be greenish-brown if stained with bile)
- Respiratory tract: off-white and tinged with mucus

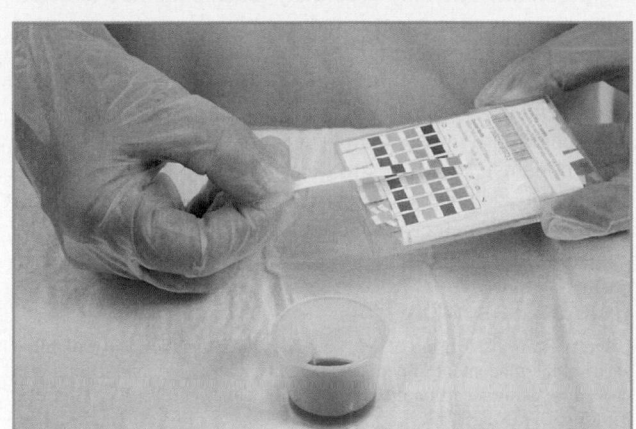

(Adapted from American Association of Critical-Care Nurses [AACN]. [2010]. *Practice alert: Verification of feeding tube placement*. Available at http://aacn.org/WD/Practice/Docs/PracticeAlerts/Verification_of_Feeding_Tube_Placement_05–2005.pdf; Best, C. [2005]. Caring for the patient with a nasogastric tube. *Nursing Standard, 20*[3], 59–65; Khair, J. [2005]. Guidelines for testing the placing of nasogastric tubes. *Nursing Times, 101*[20], 26–27; Stepter, C. R. [2012]. Maintaining placement of temporary enteral feeding tubes in adults: A critical appraisal of the evidence. *MedSurgNursing, 21*[2], 61–69; and Turgay, A. S., & Khorshid, L. [2010]. Effectiveness of the auscultatory and pH methods in predicting feeding tube placement. *Journal of Clinical Nursing, 19*[11–12], 1553–1559.

(AACN, 2010; Bourgault, Ipe, Weaver, Swartz, & O'Dea, 2007; Hinkle & Cheever, 2014). Marking the tube with an indelible marker at the nostril and then assessing this marking each time the tube is used ensures that the tube has not become displaced.

Carbon Dioxide Monitoring. Monitoring for carbon dioxide to determine nasogastric tube position and/or dislodgement has been evaluated (Gilbert & Burns, 2012; Chau, Lo, Thompson, Fernandez, & Griffiths, 2011; Munera-Seeley et al., 2008). This involves the use of a capnograph or a colorimetric end-tidal CO_2 detector to detect the presence of carbon dioxide, which would indicate tube positioning in the patient's airway. However, a carbon dioxide sensor cannot determine where a feeding tube's tip ends in the gastrointestinal tract (esophagus, stomach, or small bowel; AACN, 2010). See the accompanying Research in Nursing display (on page 1228) regarding the use of one of these devices.

Confirming Nasointestinal Tube Placement. After an initial x-ray for placement, the nurse can validate that the tube is still in the small intestine by checking the pH of the aspirate (pH ≥6 and bile-stained, ranging in color from light to golden yellow or brownish-green; AACN, 2010).

LONG-TERM NUTRITIONAL SUPPORT

When enteral feeding is required for a long-term period, an enterostomal tube may be placed through an opening created into the stomach (gastrostomy) or into the jejunum (jejunostomy). A gastrostomy is also the preferred route to deliver enteral nutrition in the patient who is comatose because the gastroesophageal sphincter remains intact, making regurgitation and aspiration less likely than with NG tube feedings (Hinkle & Cheever, 2014). Placement of a tube into the stomach can be accomplished by a surgeon or gastroenterologist via a **percutaneous endoscopic gastrostomy (PEG)** or a surgically (open or laparoscopically) placed **gastrostomy** tube. PEG tube insertion is often used because, unlike a traditional, surgically placed gastrostomy tube, it usually does not require general anesthesia. Use of a PEG tube or other type of gastrostomy tube requires an intact, functional GI tract. Insertion of a PEG tube involves local anesthesia, passage of an endoscope into the stomach, a small incision or stab wound through the skin of the abdomen, pushing a cannula through the small incision, insertion of a guide wire or suture material through the cannula, and introduction and placement of the PEG tube through one of several methods. Figure 35-6 (on page 1229) illustrates a PEG tube in place in the stomach.

RESEARCH IN NURSING

BRIDGING THE GAP TO EVIDENCE-BASED PRACTICE

Confirmation of Nasogastric Tube Placement

Inadvertent placement of nasogastric feeding tubes into the tracheopulmonary system during insertion and displacement at a time following initial insertion are potential life-threatening problems. The only absolutely reliable method to determine accurate placement is radiography. However, repeated radiographic testing is not practical or safe. Several methods of bedside testing, including evaluation of tube aspirate, measurement of aspirate pH, and measurement of exposed tube length, are in use; there is a continued need to strive for more conclusive methods to determine tube placement. Can the use of a device to detect the presence of carbon dioxide be used to detect inadvertent placement into the airway instead of the stomach?

Related Research

Gilbert, R. T., & Burns, S. M. (2012). Increasing the safety of blind gastric tube placement in pediatric patients: The design and testing of a procedure using a carbon dioxide detection device. *Journal of Pediatric Nursing, 27*(5), 528–532.

This study evaluated the use of a new commercial CO_2 sensor that was developed to assist in evaluating the placement of nasogastric feeding tubes. Prior to each feeding tube placement, the nurse took two measurements of tube length. One was from the point of entry (nose or mouth) to the ear to the level of the carina. The other was from the point of entry to the ear to the xiphoid process. The data collector then placed a CO2nfirm Now device on the distal end of the feeding tube prior to placement. As the tube was placed, both the bedside nurse and the study investigator monitored for signs of respiratory distress; if any signs of distress were observed, then the tube was immediately removed. If there were no signs of distress, then the tube was placed to the premeasured depth of the carina. The CO2nfirm Now was assessed for color change from purple to yellow, which indicated the presence of carbon dioxide. If there was color change from purple to yellow but the patient was clinically stable, the investigator disconnected the CO2nfirm Now from the feeding tube and flushed the device with room air using a 5-ml syringe until the purple color returned. This step was necessary due to the potential for carbon dioxide being in the mouth or back of

the throat during feeding tube placement. CO2nfirm Now was then reattached to the gastric tube. The data collector flushed the feeding tube through the CO2nfirm Now with 3 ml room air, and a small volume of air was aspirated from the gastric tube through the CO2nfirm Now device. This process was necessary because the pediatric gastric tubes used in this population have smaller internal diameters than those used in the adult population. Total reliance on the passive flow of gases entering or exiting the tubes was not possible. Thus, our procedure required both the active flushing and then aspiration of gases past the CO2nfirm Now device as described. If having done this flushing step, there continued to be a yellow color change on the device, it was determined that the gastric tube had been inadvertently placed into the airway and the tube was withdrawn. If there was no color change, the bedside nurse continued to advance the tube to the premeasured gastric level. The tube was secured, and an abdominal x-ray was obtained to determine if tube placement was in the esophagus, stomach, or postpyloric. This step was done to verify tube placement per a standing PICU guideline. Sixty devices were tested on 42 patients over a period of 15 months. Three of the feeding tubes were removed as a result of a color change, indicating the detection of carbon dioxide during tube placement, and three were removed for other reasons. The ability of the colorimetric device to detect the presence of carbon dioxide was 100% accurate in all cases in which the tube was in contact with carbon dioxide. The authors concluded the use of a carbon dioxide sensing device during the blind placement of gastric tubes in pediatric patients may be a beneficial innovation to pediatric practices. The procedure presents little to no additional risk and increased the safety of the procedure.

Relevance to Nursing Practice

The CO_2 sensor is a helpful bedside tool to use in conjunction with clinical methods during nasogastric feeding tube insertions. Nurses should consider investigating the use of these devices for use in their individual clinical facilities.

For additional research, visit the**Point**.

In long-term feeding situations in which gastric problems exist, the jejunostomy is an alternate method through which nutrition can be delivered. These tubes may be inserted surgically or with endoscopic or laparoscopic guidance. Figure 35-7 illustrates a PEG/J tube in the jejunum. Gastrostomy or jejunostomy tubes are not easily dislodged.

For patients who are active yet require long-term continuous or intermittent feedings, a low-profile gastrostomy device (LPGD) may be an option (Fig. 35-8). Children are also excellent candidates for LPGDs. The external apparatus is minimal and consists of a button or skin disk that is

stable, less irritating to the skin, and has no external tubing, making it easier to conceal with clothing. Additional advantages include the fact that it can be immersed in water, is less noticeable, and is less likely to migrate or become dislodged. The device has a cap, which is opened to access the feeding tube and connect with the administration set.

Checking placement of a gastrostomy or jejunostomy tube requires regular comparisons (according to facility policy) of the tube length to the measurement (inches or centimeters) that was documented after insertion. An indelible marker can be used to identify the exit point of the tube from the abdominal wall.

FIGURE 35-6. Percutaneous endoscopic gastrostomy tube in place in the stomach. (Reprinted with permission from Hinkle, J. L., & Cheever, K. H. [2014]. *Brunner & Suddarth's textbook of medical-surgical nursing* [13th ed., p. 1032]. Philadelphia: Wolters Kluwer Health/Lippincott Williams & Wilkins.)

ADMINISTRATION OF ENTERAL FEEDING

Feeding Schedule. Based on the patient's physical, medical, and nutritional condition, the nutritionist usually makes recommendations concerning the feeding pattern or schedule. Continuous feedings allow gradual introduction of the formula into the GI tract, promoting maximal absorption. They require use of an enteral feeding pump, which limits the patient's mobility and increases cost. Continuous feeding into the stomach, however, is controversial because of the risk for reflux and aspiration.

Feedings into the intestine are always continuous to avoid triggering dumping syndrome, as the natural res-

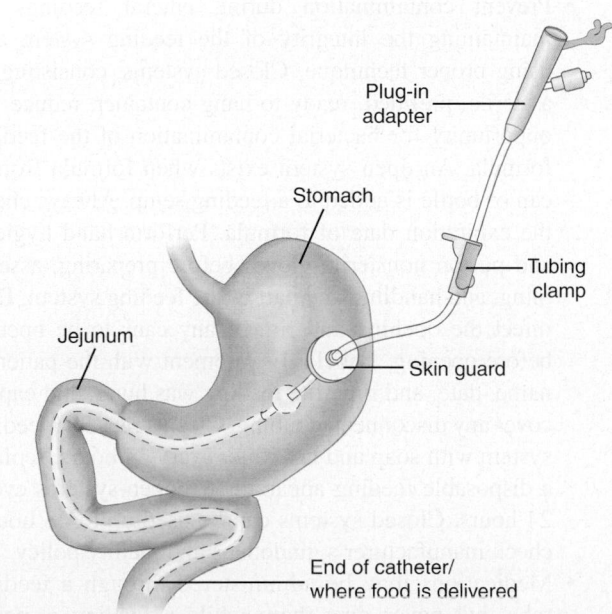

FIGURE 35-7. PEG/J tube inserted in the jejunum.

FIGURE 35-8. Low-profile gastrostomy device (LPGD).

ervoir of the stomach is bypassed. Dumping syndrome is caused by overdistention of the small intestine. The use of intermittent or bolus feedings would provide larger-than-normal amounts of food and liquid in the proximal small intestine, causing overdistention, leading to nausea, diarrhea, cramping, and lightheadedness (Dudek, 2014).

Intermittent feedings are the preferred method for gastric feeding. Intermittent feedings are delivered at regular intervals in equal portions, introducing the formula gradually over a set period of time via gravity or a feeding pump. Alternately, bolus intermittent feedings, for which a syringe is used to deliver the formula quickly into the stomach, may place the patient at risk for aspiration or cause distention. They are usually not recommended but may be used in long-term situations if tolerated by the patient. Intermittent feedings resemble a more normal pattern of intake and allow the patient freedom of movement between feedings (Dudek, 2014).

Another option is cyclic feeding. This involves administering continuous feeding for a portion of the 24-hour period. The usual routine is to feed the patient for 12 to 16 hours, most often overnight. Cyclic feeding allows the patient to attempt eating regular meals during the day, if this is possible, making ambulation and activity easier. Skill 35-2 on pages 1247–1253 describes administration of a tube feeding.

Enteral Feeding Formulas. Many enteral feeding formulas are available. The nutritional composition of tube feedings depends on the feeding route, the patient's ability to digest and absorb nutrients, and the patient's nutrient and fluid requirements. Other considerations include the availability and cost of the formula, medical conditions that require diet modifications, food intolerance, and allergies. Standard formulas contain intact molecules of protein, carbohydrates, and fats, requiring the patient to have normal digestion and absorption. Hydrolyzed formulas contain proteins and other nutrients in simple forms that require little or no digestion. These formulas are used with patients with impaired digestion or absorption. In addition to being nutritionally balanced, formulas may be high in calories; contain fiber; contain additional protein; or be especially formulated for patients with respiratory, renal, or other health problems. Detailed information about their composition and caloric value (most routine formulas contain 1 to 1.2 cal/mL, although 2 cal/mL concentrations are available) can be obtained from the product label.

Feedings are initiated at full strength. The rate of infusion begins at 25 to 50 mL per hour, depending on facility policy. The rate is then advanced by 10 to 25 mL per hour every 8 to 12 hours until the desired rate is achieved. Rate advancement is based on patient tolerance. Starting the feeding at a slower rate and progressing slowly improves tolerance. The previous practice of diluting feedings has not been shown to improve feeding tolerance and prolongs the period of inadequate nutrition support (Dudek, 2014). Criteria to consider when evaluating patient feeding tolerance includes:

- Absence of nausea, vomiting
- Minimal or no gastric residual
- Absence of diarrhea and constipation
- Absence of abdominal pain and distention
- Presence of bowel sounds within normal limits

Enteral Feeding Pumps. An enteral feeding pump regulates the amount of feeding solution that is delivered to the patient. A pump should be used when slow rates of enteral formula are required (A.S.P.E.N., 2009b). The newer pumps are user friendly, have built-in safeguards that protect the patient from complications, and can be used in both institutions and the home. Safety features include automatic tube flush, cassettes that prevent free flow of formula, safety tips that prevent accidental attachment to an IV setup, and various audible and visible alarms. Most pumps can operate for up to 8 hours on battery. However, manufacturers recommend using the pump plugged into an electrical outlet for recharging whenever the patient is seated or resting for a period of time.

NURSING CONSIDERATIONS FOR ENTERAL FEEDING

Facility and agency protocols may differ and should be followed, but nursing actions that contribute to successful tube feedings focus on patient safety, monitoring for complications, comfort, and education.

Promoting Patient Safety. To promote patient safety when administering a tube feeding, be sure to include the following interventions as part of patient care:

- Check tube placement before administering any fluids, medications, or feeding, using multiple techniques: x-ray, pH testing, aspirate characteristics, external length marking, and carbon dioxide monitoring (refer to Guidelines for Nursing Care 35-1, p. 1227).
- Check **gastric residual** (feeding remaining in the stomach) before each feeding or every 4 to 6 hours during a continuous feeding (according to institution policy). High

gastric residual volumes (200 to 250 mL or greater) can be associated with high risk for aspiration and aspiration-related pneumonia (Bourgault et al., 2007; Metheny, 2008). Record residuals on flow sheet or in progress notes. Follow the clinician's order or facility policy for withholding feedings based on the residual. Some experts now recommend that the patient's pattern of residual is more important than the amount (A.S.P.E.N., 2011; Bourgault et al.; Metheny). Hold feedings if residual volumes exceed 200 mL on two successive assessments (A.S.P.E.N.). It is important to note that it is important to flush the feeding tube with water after checking gastric residual, to help prevent tube occlusions (A.S.P.E.N.; Bourgault et al.; Metheny). Refer to the accompanying Through the Eyes of a Student display for a student nurse's experience with residual and a tube feeding.

- Assess the abdomen for abnormalities. Assess for bowel sounds at least once per shift to check for the presence of peristalsis and a functional intestinal tract. Experts, however, have recently concluded that it is common for acutely ill patients to have delayed gastric emptying; therefore, delaying enteral feedings based on hypoactive bowel sounds may place a patient at risk for malnutrition. Gastric distention, abdominal girth, nausea, vomiting, bloating, or pain are better indicators of how well a patient is tolerating a tube feeding (Metheny, Mills, & Stewart, 2012; AACN, 2012; Palmer & Metheny, 2008).
- Make sure the patient is as upright as possible during feeding. If the patient is in bed during feedings, elevate the head of the bed at least 30 degrees during feeding and for 1 hour afterward to prevent reflux and aspiration. Pause the feeding if the patient has to be repositioned or temporarily laid flat. Resume the feeding only after the patient's head is returned to at least a 30-degree elevation.
- Prevent contamination during enteral feedings by maintaining the integrity of the feeding system and using proper technique. Closed systems, consisting of a sterile, prefilled, ready-to-hang container, reduce the opportunity for bacterial contamination of the feeding formula. An open system exists when formula from a can or bottle is added to a feeding setup. Always check the expiration date of formula. Perform hand hygiene and put on nonsterile gloves before preparing, assembling, and handling any part of the feeding system. Disinfect the opening and rim of any cans to be opened before opening. Label all equipment with the patient's name, date, and time the feeding was hung, and cap or cover any disconnected tubing. Clean a reusable feeding system with soap and hot water every 24 hours; replace a disposable feeding apparatus for open systems every 24 hours. Closed systems can be used up to 48 hours; check manufacturer's guidelines and facility policy.
- Medications may be administered through a feeding tube, but never give them while a feeding is being infused. Administer liquid forms of medications

THROUGH THE EYES OF A STUDENT

She looked lost in that big hospital bed, so thin and frail. Her hair was as white as her pillowcase and blankets, and her skin looked almost transparent. And then, I saw it. Snaking under her blankets into her belly was the feeding tube surrounded by thick, green, smelly discharge.

During preconference, my instructor had told me that I needed to check residual every 2 hours to monitor her absorption rate. The first time, with my instructor standing beside me like my guardian angel (or my patient's guardian angel, I'm not sure which), the procedure naturally went off without a hitch. I could do this, I thought, feeling more confident.

Because my patient had chronic diarrhea as well as skin breakdown at her sacrum, the next 2 hours flew by in a whirlwind of bathing. But now, the time had come. This is it, I thought. I'm on my own for the second residual check. And, again, I breathed a sigh of relief when the procedure was completed with no problems.

As the day progressed, I got myself a little behind schedule because I was determined to remove the hardened crusts from underneath her nails. Before I knew it, I got the message from another student that it was post-conference time. Oh no! I didn't do my last residual check yet. Quickly, I emptied the basin I was using on her fingernails and grabbed the plunger. I reached into my pocket for my hemostat to clamp off the line and the next thing I saw was feeding formula squirting all over the bed, my patient, the clean Chux, and me! I had cut the line instead of clamping it!

I quickly pinched both ends to stop the formula from squirting and frantically called for help. While waiting for rescue, I checked on my patient's response, not knowing how she was going to react. Thankfully, she was sound asleep, soothed by her recent nail massage. It seemed like forever before my instructor rushed in. With my eyes filling up, I attempted to explain that I had grabbed the scissors from my pocket instead of the hemostat. Guardian angel that she was (I think she was both of ours), my instructor calmly and efficiently proceeded to attach both ends of the tube together with the use of an adapter. Then we let the patient's physician know what happened.

Many lessons were learned that day, such as don't attempt a procedure in haste, and have all your supplies readily at hand. But the one thing I'll never, ever forget is that the scissors are the crooked ones!

—Eileen Cooper
Delaware County Community College, Media, PA

---

whenever possible. Never add medications directly to the formula; some drugs become ineffective when mixed with feeding formulas; medications mixed in feeding formulas may cause clogging of the feeding tube. It is very important to flush the tube with water before, between, and after the administration of medications. Administering medications through an enteral feeding tube is discussed in depth in Chapter 28.

Monitoring for Complications. Patients receiving tube feedings are at risk for several complications. Table 35-8 (on page 1232) summarizes nursing measures to prevent selected complications. In addition, prevent the tube from becoming clogged or obstructed. Common causes of clogged enteral tubes include aspirated stomach contents, residue from medications, slow feeding flow rate, infrequent or inadequate addition of water to the system, and using a tube with a small lumen (A.S.P.E.N., 2009b; Dudek, 2014). After checking placement, flush tube with 30 to 50 mL of water before and after each feeding or introduction of medications, at least every 4 hours during a continuous feeding, and after aspirating a tube for gastric contents (A.S.P.E.N.; Dudek, 2014). After flushing the tube, be sure to document the amount on the intake and output record. Use of a feeding pump helps to prevent clogging. If an occlusion occurs, use a 60-mL syringe containing 30 to 60 mL of warm water to attempt to unclog the tube.

Providing Comfort Measures. Patients with nasogastric tubes often experience discomfort related to irritation to nasal and throat mucosa and drying of the oral mucous membranes. Implement several nursing interventions to ensure the patient's comfort and prevent alterations in the integrity of these tissues.

- Administer oral hygiene frequently (every 2 to 4 hours) to prevent drying of tissues and to relieve thirst. Offer the patient the opportunity to rinse the mouth with warm water and mouthwash solution frequently. Lubricate the lips generously.
- Keep the nares clean, especially around the tube, where secretions tend to accumulate. Using a lubricant after cleaning the nares is recommended.
- Help control local irritation from the tube in the throat. Analgesic throat lozenges or anesthetic sprays may be effective.
- Encourage the patient, if able, to verbalize concerns about tube feeding and presence of the tube. A visit from another person who has learned to cope with this alternate feeding method may prove helpful.
- Ensure that the tube is secured to the patient's nose and gown to prevent tension and tugging on the tube, causing trauma to the nares, and potential displacement.

 RECALL Charles Gallagher, the husband of the woman with advanced dementia receiving enteral nutrition. The nurse could teach Mr. Gallagher how to provide oral hygiene for his wife, including lubricating her lips. Doing so would allow Mr. Gallagher to feel some control over the situation. In addition, he would be helping to meet his wife's comfort needs and his own needs. ●

Table 35-8 PREVENTING COMPLICATIONS OF ENTERAL FEEDING

POTENTIAL COMPLICATION	PREVENTIVE INTERVENTIONS
Aspiration	• Use appropriate measures to check tube placement. • Elevate head of bed at least 30–45 degrees during feeding and for 1 hour afterward. • Give small, frequent feedings. • Avoid oversedation of patient. • Check residual volume per policy.
Clogged tube	• Flush tube before and after feeding, every 4 hours during continuous feeding, and after withdrawing aspirate. • Instill 30 mL of warm water with 50-mL or 60-mL syringe to attempt to unclog tube.
Nasal erosion with nasogastric or nasointestinal tubes	• Check nostrils every shift for signs of pressure. • Clean and moisten nares every 4 to 8 hours. • Start feeding at slow rate.
Diarrhea	• Prevent contamination in both open and closed systems. • Change delivery set every 12 to 24 hours according to agency policy. • Refrigerate opened cans of formula and discard after 24 hours. • Limit hang time to 8 hours when using open system. • Use aseptic technique for patients who are immunosuppressed or acutely ill. • Assess for fecal impaction.
Other GI symptoms (nausea, vomiting, distention)	• Check residual prior to intermittent feedings and every 4 hours during continuous feedings. • Avoid oversedating client (delays gastric emptying). • Administer GI motility medications (metoclopramide), as ordered.
Unplanned extubation	• Anchor tube adequately with commercial device, elastic net, or tape. • Check on patient frequently. • Measure external length of tubing at regular intervals.
Stoma infection	• Clean skin every shift with soap and warm water. Dry thoroughly. • Use topical antibiotics and/or antifungals, as ordered. • Assess for signs of infection. • Request consult with wound care specialist, as needed.

Providing Instruction. Often, patients will continue to receive enteral feedings at home. Teaching Tips 35-1 outlines important points to review with patients and families in the home setting. Provide the patient and family with individualized instructions in written form as a reference for the patient and caregivers. Be sure to include the following in the teaching plan:

• Information about the administration of feedings, operation of the pump, formula, instructions regarding rate and how to check for tube placement, as well as what to do if the tube becomes dislodged
• Care of the tube insertion site and possible complications that need to be reported
• Proper preparation, cleaning, and disposal of equipment
• Emergency telephone numbers, including the number for the home health care agency and the physician
• Arrangements for follow-up from the home health care nurse as soon as possible after discharge

REMOVAL OF NASOGASTRIC TUBE
Removing the nasogastric tube as carefully as it is inserted is important to avoid causing the patient undue discomfort. After the tube is removed, provide for oral hygiene to remove disagreeable tastes and odors. Thorough oral hygiene is crucial when the tube has been in

the intestinal tract and in contact with intestinal contents. Directions for removing the nasogastric tube are given in Skill 35-3 on pages 1253–1255.

NASOENTERIC TUBES FOR DECOMPRESSION
In addition to providing enteral feedings, nasogastric tubes can be used for other purposes. They may be inserted to decompress or drain the stomach of fluid, unwanted stomach contents, such as poison or medication and air, allowing it to rest, or before or after surgery, to promote healing. Nasogastric tubes may also be used to monitor GI bleeding and prevent intestinal obstruction. Tubes used for these purposes and associated nursing care are discussed in detail in Chapter 38.

Providing Parenteral Nutrition
Parenteral nutrition is the administration of nutritional support via the intravenous route. Patients who can't meet their nutritional needs by the oral or enteral routes may require intravenous nutritional supplementation. Intravenous supplementation may be prescribed for patients who have nonfunctional gastrointestinal (GI) tracts, who are comatose, or those who have high caloric and nutritional needs due to illness or injury—patients undergoing aggressive cancer therapy and

TEACHING TIPS 35-1

HOME ENTERAL FEEDINGS

Health Topic	Teaching Tip	Why Is This Important?
Cleaning around a gastric tube insertion site	Use of soap and water, making sure that area is adequately rinsed	If soap is left under the gastric tube guard, it can lead to skin irritation.
	Rotation of the guard after cleaning around it	The guard can put pressure on the skin, leading to skin breakdown.
Checking residuals	Method and reason for checking residual contents, as well as what to do with residual contents	Residual contents should not be routinely discarded to prevent an acid–base imbalance; however, the patient or caregiver should know when discarding is appropriate to prevent aspiration of stomach contents.
Delivering tube feedings	Head elevation while delivering a gastric feeding and for approximately an hour after the feeding	Keeping the head elevated helps to prevent aspiration of gastric tube feedings.
	Method of administration such as delivering the feedings via continuous or bolus method, and steps for carrying out the feeding	Some patients do not tolerate the bolus method without vomiting. The patient or caregiver should know how to operate the machinery if it is to be delivered via continuous method or how to set up for a bolus feeding.
Leaking of gastric contents	Method of checking for problems (is guard too loose or balloon not filled adequately) if gastric tube is leaking stomach contents around insertion site	If gastric tube is leaking acidic stomach contents, the area around the insertion site can quickly break down.
Placement check	Methods to check placement to ensure that tube has not migrated inward or outward	Gastrostomy tubes can be marked with an indelible marker. The mark should be checked to make sure it is at the level of the abdominal wall. If the mark is not visible, the tube may have migrated inward. If the mark is away from the abdominal wall, the tube may no longer be in the stomach.
		Patients may also measure the length of the tube from the skin and record the measurement. This measurement should be confirmed to ensure that the tube has not migrated (Tracey & Patterson, 2006).

those recovering from extensive burns, surgery, sepsis, or multiple fractures, for instance. Parenteral nutrition can be administered centrally, through a central venous access device (TPN), or peripherally (PPN), through a short-term intravenous access in a peripheral vein. The basic difference between the two types is the concentration of the solutions infused.

Total parenteral nutrition (TPN) is a highly concentrated, hypertonic nutrient solution. TPN provides calories; restores nitrogen balance; and replaces essential fluids, vitamins, electrolytes, minerals, and trace elements. TPN can also promote tissue and wound healing and normal metabolic function. It provides the bowel a chance to heal and reduces activity in the gallbladder, pancreas, and small intestine. TPN may be used to improve a patient's response to surgery (Worthington & Gilbert, 2012). TPN meets the patient's nutritional needs by way of nutrient-filled solutions administered intravenously through a central venous access device,

such as a multilumen, nontunneled catheter into the subclavian vein, or a peripherally inserted central catheter (PICC).

Assessment criteria used to determine the need for TPN include an inability to achieve or maintain enteral access; motility disorders; intractable diarrhea; impaired absorption of nutrients from the GI tract and when oral intake has been or is expected to be inadequate over a 7- to 14-day period (Worthington & Gilbert; A.S.P.E.N. & SCCM, 2009).

Peripheral parenteral nutrition (PPN) is a less concentrated nutrient solution sometimes prescribed for patients who have a malfunctioning gastrointestinal tract and need short-term nutrition lasting less than 2 weeks (Worthington & Gilbert, 2012). PPN is administered through a peripheral vein. Peripheral veins cannot tolerate highly concentrated solutions, thus the solution is not as nutrient dense as TPN and is not widely used (Dudek, 2014).

Table 35-9 COMMON COMPONENTS OF TPN

ADDITIVE	PURPOSE
Dextrose (carbohydrate)	Calories for metabolism
Amino acids	Protein for tissue repair
Lipids	Essential fatty acids and calories for metabolism, wound healing, red blood cell production
Acetate	Prevents metabolic acidosis
Calcium	Development of bones and teeth; aids in blood clotting
Chloride	Regulates acid–base balance; maintains osmotic pressure
Folic acid	DNA formation; promotes growth and development
Magnesium	Carbohydrate and protein absorption
Phosphorus	Cell energy and calcium balance
Potassium	Cellular activity and cardiac function
Sodium	Controls water distribution; maintains normal fluid balance
Vitamin B complex	Carbohydrate absorption
Vitamin C	Wound healing
Vitamin D	Bone metabolism; maintains serum calcium levels
Vitamin K	Prevents bleeding disorders
Micronutrients, such as zinc, cobalt, and manganese	Wound healing; red blood cell synthesis

(Adapted from Metheny, N. M. [2012]. *Fluid and electrolyte balance. Nursing Considerations* (5th ed.). Sudbury, MA: Jones & Bartlett Learning; *Fluids & electrolytes made incredibly easy*. [2011]. [5th ed.]. Philadelphia: Wolters Kluwer Health/Lippincott Williams & Wilkins; and Dudek, S. [2014]. *Nutrition essentials for nursing practice* (7th ed.). Philadelphia: Wolters Kluwer Health/Lippincott Williams & Wilkins.)

PARENTERAL NUTRITION SOLUTIONS AND ADMINISTRATION

TPN solutions are hypertonic. TPN contains the three primary components necessary to maintain nutrition: proteins, carbohydrates, and fats. Additional components of parenteral nutrition include electrolytes, vitamins, and trace elements. The TPN formula is tailored to the individual patient's specific needs. Common components of TPN are listed in Table 35-9. Fat or lipid emulsions and dextrose add caloric value that the body needs to meet energy requirements. Because of the high glucose concentration, usually about 25% (thus, a hypertonic solution), it is important to monitor blood glucose levels (Skill 35-4, pp. 1256–1259).

PPN solutions are isotonic. PPN solutions contain components similar to those of TPN but in lesser concentrations and amounts. They contain low concentrations of dextrose and amino acids. PPN solutions provide fewer calories and supplement a patient's inadequate oral intake. This solution usually contains 10% glucose or lower, which is suitable for administration into a peripheral vessel (Infusion Nurses Society [INS], 2011).

Physical incompatibility between the intravenous nutrition formula and other intravenous solutions, especially medications, is a potential problem that must be addressed. If the patient has a multilumen catheter in place, dedicate one lumen for the administration of the parenteral nutrition. Do not use that lumen or administration set for any other purpose, to prevent incompatibility problems. If the patient's intravenous catheter has only one lumen, attempt to obtain a peripheral intravenous access for the administration of additional solutions. Consider discussing the potential for a midline or peripherally inserted central catheter with the patient's health care team. If an additional access is not available, research the compatibility of the solutions to be administered. Little research exists on the stability and compatibility of parenteral nutrition solutions and most medications. If compatible medications or other solutions must be given through the same lumen as parenteral nutrition, attach the administration set as close to the catheter hub as possible to limit the amount of contact between the drug (or solution) and the parenteral nutrition solution.

Avoid adding medications to the parenteral nutrition solution because of the potential incompatibilities of medication and nutrients in the solution (Dudek, 2014). A pharmacist can add insulin if the patient's glucose level is above 150 to 200 mg/dL. Heparin may be added to reduce fibrin buildup on the tip of the intravenous catheter (Dudek). Never add medication to parenteral nutrition solutions after they are dispensed from the pharmacy (INS, 2011).

PREVENTING COMPLICATIONS

TPN therapy is costly, requires constant monitoring, and has the potential for causing infections as well as

GUIDELINES FOR NURSING CARE 35-2

MONITORING ADMINISTRATION OF PARENTERAL NUTRITION

- Use the same catheter lumen for administration of parenteral nutrition each time the tubing is changed.
- Use a pump to administer infusion of parenteral nutrition.
- Infusion rate changes are made incrementally to avoid severe hyperglycemia or hypoglycemia. Wean patients gradually from parenteral nutrition to prevent rebound hypoglycemia, based on facility policy.
- Discard unused parenteral nutrition solution within 24 hours of starting its administration.
- Check vital signs every 4 hours to monitor for development of infection or sepsis.
- Monitor blood glucose levels every 6 hours.
- Use aseptic technique when changing solution, tubing, filter, or dressings according to agency policy.
- Infusion administration sets should include an in-line filter. Change infusion administration sets every 24 hours.

- Change site dressings according to agency protocol. Transparent semipermeable dressings are changed once per week. Gauze dressings do not allow for inspection of exit site without dressing removal and are changed every 48 hours. In addition, change dressings immediately if they become wet, soiled, or nonocclusive.
- Check that all connections are securely taped, catheter is clamped before opening the system, and insertion site is covered with sterile dressing.
- Compare the patient's daily weight to fluid intake and output. Total weight gain should not be greater than 3 lb per week. Weight gain greater than 1 lb per day indicates fluid retention.
- Assess serum protein and electrolyte levels for signs of imbalance.

---

metabolic and mechanical complications. It should be used only when enteral intake is inadequate or contraindicated, and should be gradually discontinued as soon as possible. Prevention of potential complications associated with TPN requires vigilance and careful monitoring by the nurse. Potential complications include the following (Hinkle & Cheever, 2014; Worthington & Gilbert, 2012):

- Complications related to the use of central venous access devices, such as pneumothorax and thromboembolism (inflammation of a blood vessel and formation of a thrombus [blood clot])
- Infection and sepsis
- Metabolic alterations, such as hyperglycemia or hypoglycemia
- Fluid, electrolyte, and acid–base imbalances
- Phlebitis
- Hyperlipidemia
- Liver and gallbladder disease

Guidelines for Nursing Care 35-2 lists nursing guidelines for monitoring administration of parenteral nutrition.

PARENTERAL NUTRITION IN THE HOME SETTING

Many patients require long-term parenteral nutrition and continue such therapy in the home. Individuals with acquired immunodeficiency syndrome (AIDS), advanced cancer, difficulty swallowing, or chronic bowel problems are candidates for this type of nutritional support. Nurses are involved in educating the patient and caregiver about the techniques and responsibilities associated with parenteral nutrition, providing technical and psychological support, and documenting the assessments that allow

parenteral nutrition to be continued in the home. Patient education should specifically include:

- Basic information about what TPN is and what it is used for
- Adverse reactions or catheter complications
- Circumstances that require contacting the primary care provider
- Basic care of the venous access device used to administer
- Maintenance of equipment
- Frequency for measuring the patient's weight, intake and output, and monitoring glucose levels

Evaluating

The effectiveness of the plan of care is evaluated as the last step in the nursing process. On an ongoing basis, the nurse accomplishes the following:

- Evaluates the patient's progress toward meeting nutritional outcomes
- Evaluates the patient's tolerance and adherence to the diet, when appropriate
- Assesses the patient's level of understanding of the diet and/or dietary-related interventions and the need for further instruction or reinforcement
- Communicates findings to other members of the health care team
- Revises the plan of care, as needed, or terminates nursing care

For samples of the nursing process for nutrition, see the accompanying concept map for William Johnston and the Nursing Plan of Care 35-1 for Susan Oakland on pages 1237–1240.

William Johnston, a 42-year-old executive, is newly diagnosed with high blood pressure and high cholesterol. He confides that his health habits are less than admirable. "I usually eat on the run, often fast food, or big dinners with lots of alcohol. I can't remember the last time I worked out or did any exercise, unless running from my car to the train counts! I guess it's no wonder I've gained a few pounds over the years." He reports that he is 6 feet tall and currently weighs 213 lbs. His body mass index (BMI) is 29. During this office visit, the physician prescribes an antihypertensive medication and an antihyperlipidemic medication for his hypertension (HTN) and high cholesterol.

Priority 1

Nursing Diagnosis: Imbalanced Nutrition: More Than Body Requirements related to overeating and lack of exercise.
Supporting Data:
• Weight, 213 lbs; Height, 6 feet
• BMI is 29
• Diet consists of fast foods & big dinners
• Does not exercise
• Heavy alcohol use

Outcome:
Patient will identify ideal body weight and safely reduce weight towards this goal.

Nursing Interventions:
• Identify desired caloric intake
• Teach patient to weigh self weekly
• Assess typical dietary choices by having patient keep a food diary for 3 days
• Review dietary intake with the patient and compare to ideal meal plan using food pyramid guidelines
• Encourage gradual weight loss of 1–2 lbs/week
• Encourage/assist in plan of exercise (30–45 minutes, 5 days per week)
• Discuss ways of reducing stress

Evaluation: William stated he is committed to losing weight. He is walking briskly for 30 minutes at lunch time, 5 days a week. He has lost 2 lbs the first week.

Priority 2

Nursing Diagnosis: Ineffective Health Maintenance related to lack of knowledge about dietary restrictions to modify heart risk.
Supporting Data:
• Newly diagnosed HTN and high cholesterol
• Eating fast foods
• Heavy alcohol use
• Eats out frequently

Outcome:
Patient will demonstrate appropriate food choices within dietary restrictions.

Nursing Interventions:
• Assess willingness and motivation to learn
• Note patient's support systems
• Provide information regarding a diet low in sodium, cholesterol, and saturated fat
• Discuss strategies to maintain dietary restrictions when eating out
• Limit alcohol intake to decrease triglycerides
• Identify high nutritional value snacks that are portable when on the run
• Consult dietitian
• Provide printed instructions for ongoing reference

Evaluation: William developed a sample meal plan for a busy day, picking appropriate food choices, but states he might be too busy to think about this every day. Encourage consultation with dietitian.

Priority 3

Nursing Diagnosis: Deficient Knowledge related to newly diagnosed hypertension and hypercholesterolemia.
Supporting Data:
• Hypertension
• Hypercholesterolemia
• Poor health habits
• Hectic lifestyle
• Antihypertensive and antihyperlipidemic medications

Outcome:
Patient will verbalize understanding of management of HTN and hypercholesterolemia and will demonstrate behaviors to maintain health.

Nursing Interventions:
• Assess level of current knowledge
• Assess preferences for method of learning
• Provide printed material for future reference
• Teach the names, dose, times, actions, and side effects of medications he is taking
• Teach patient to take pulse and blood pressure every day and report significant changes to healthcare provider
• Teach patient the impact of hypertension and high cholesterol on the development of heart disease

Evaluation: William states his father died from heart disease; he doesn't want of follow in his footsteps. During a 2-week follow-up visit, you note he recorded his daily BP and pulse. His BP today is 123/82 mm Hg.

- - - - - **Relationship**   **Assessment**   **Nursing Diagnosis**   **Outcome Identification**   **Interventions**   **Evaluation**

Concept map displaying the nursing process for William Johnston.

NURSING PLAN OF CARE 35-1

for Susan Oakland

Susan Oakland, a 21-year-old student, was seen at the prenatal clinic for her first pregnancy at 5 weeks' gestation. On her next visit, 4 weeks later, she complained of nausea and vomiting and had lost 3 lb (1.4 kg).

ASSESSMENT FINDINGS

A comprehensive nutritional assessment revealed the following data:

ANTHROPOMETRIC DATA

Usual body weight: 112 lb (50.8 kg)
Weight at 9 weeks' gestation: 109 lb (49.4 kg)
Height: 5 feet 5 inches (165.1 cm)
BMI: 18.6
Ideal body weight: 125 lb. (56.7 kg; range is 113–137 lb. [51.3–62.1 kg])
Expected weight gain for 9 weeks' gestation: 1 to 2 lb (0.45–0.9 kg)

BIOCHEMICAL DATA

Laboratory data revealed low hemoglobin level and hematocrit.

MEDICAL AND SOCIOECONOMIC DATA

- Patient complains of nausea and vomiting, which begin in the morning and continue until midafternoon. Her appetite is poor. She also states, "I'm always tired."
- Patient and her husband are first-semester graduate students; their source of income is graduate assistantships, and their food budget is limited.
- Patient states that she did not intend to become pregnant, but both she and her husband are excited about becoming parents. She plans to take a leave of absence from school for one semester when the baby is born; she wants to breastfeed.

CLINICAL DATA

Patient appears pale. No other abnormal physical findings were noted.

DIETARY DATA

- Patient's 24-hour recall revealed an inadequate intake from the milk group and a marginal intake from the grain and meat groups. She skips breakfast because of a hurried schedule, which is now complicated by nausea. Lunch comprises soup, salad, and fruit. Dinner usually comprises chicken; cooked vegetables; pasta, rice, or potatoes; and fruit. Patient dislikes red meat and eats it only once or twice a month. She also dislikes milk and substitutes sugar-free soft drinks and water. Before becoming pregnant, she drank five or six cups of black coffee a day, but now she avoids it. Her snacks usually consist of fresh fruit and vegetables.
- Patient is very weight conscious; she periodically crash diets to maintain her weight at 112 lb (50.8 kg).
- Patient does not take vitamins, medications, or drugs; she drinks socially, one or two times per month.
- Nutritional problems and contributing factors include the following:
  - Inadequate intake of milk and calories contributed to by nausea and vomiting, dislike for milk, limited food budget, weight consciousness
  - Poor iron intake contributed to by lack of good sources of iron in her diet, no supplemental iron intake
  - Meal-skipping contributed to by nausea and vomiting, hurried schedule
  - Underweight or weight loss contributed to by weight consciousness, nausea, and vomiting

NURSING DIAGNOSIS *Imbalanced Nutrition:* Less Than Body Requirements related to increased requirements imposed by pregnancy, nausea and vomiting, weight consciousness, hurried schedule, food dislikes as manifested by: reports of anorexia, fatigue, 3-lb weight loss in 4 weeks' time, pale color, and low hemoglobin and hematocrit values.

EXPECTED OUTCOME By the next monthly assessment, 6/26/15, the patient will:
- Eat 6 small meals per day

(continued)

NURSING PLAN OF CARE 35-1 *continued*

for Susan Oakland

NURSING INTERVENTIONS	RATIONALE	EVALUATIVE STATEMENT
Determine how the patient's schedule may be altered to allow time for meals. Encourage the patient to have easy-to-eat foods available for quick snacks, like cartons of yogurt, cheese and crackers, muffins, and fresh fruit. Advise the patient that nausea may be lessened by avoiding periods of hunger, and that later in the pregnancy, avoiding hunger will help ensure a steady supply of nutrients to the fetus.	Patient complained that her current schedule prevents regular meals. Easy-to-eat foods may be more acceptable and can be nutritionally comparable to traditional meals. Low blood glucose may contribute to nausea early in pregnancy; later in pregnancy, low blood glucose and resultant ketosis may be harmful to the fetus.	6/26/15 Outcome met. Patient eats three meals daily. Tries snacking on easy-to-eat foods when possible. *Recommendation:* Encourage more snacking to increase overall food intake. *L. Swift, RN*

EXPECTED OUTCOME By the next monthly assessment, 6/26/15, the patient will:

- Eat dry crackers, bread sticks, or dry cereal 30 minutes before rising

NURSING INTERVENTIONS	RATIONALE	EVALUATIVE STATEMENT
Advise the patient to eat a source of dry carbohydrates before getting up in the morning.	Eating dry carbohydrates 30 minutes before rising helps avoid nausea.	6/26/15 Outcome met. Patient eats dry crackers every morning 30 minutes before getting out of bed. Reports that it prevents morning nausea. *L. Swift, RN*

EXPECTED OUTCOME By the next monthly assessment, 6/26/15, the patient will:

- Avoid diet soft drinks

NURSING INTERVENTIONS	RATIONALE	EVALUATIVE STATEMENT
Advise the patient to avoid diet soft drinks. Recommend acceptable nutritional alternatives to the patient.	Saccharin and aspartame have not been proved safe for the fetus. Diet sodas are filling but offer no calories for the fetus.	6/26/15 Outcome partially met. Patient reports that she drinks two or three cans of diet soft drinks a week at school to relieve thirst because nothing else is available. *Recommendation:* Encourage the patient to bring something to drink during the day from home, such as frozen drink boxes of 100% fruit juice, which will thaw at room temperature, or an insulated container of ice water or milk flavored with vanilla (dislikes plain milk). *L. Swift, RN*

NURSING PLAN OF CARE 35-1 *continued*

for Susan Oakland

EXPECTED OUTCOME By the next monthly assessment, 6/26/15, the patient will:
- Eat the recommended number of servings from each food group as suggested by the daily food guide for pregnancy

NURSING INTERVENTIONS	RATIONALE	EVALUATIVE STATEMENT
Provide the patient with a daily food guide for pregnancy, and explain the rationale for the increased recommendations. Investigate acceptable alternatives for red meat and milk, which the patient normally does not consume.	Because this is the patient's first pregnancy, she is not aware of the recommendations for eating during pregnancy. Although no single particular food is essential during pregnancy, red meat is essential during pregnancy and an excellent source of iron, and milk is an excellent source of calcium, two minerals important for the developing fetus. If the patient is not provided with nutritionally equivalent alternatives, her diet may not be optimal, even if she consumes the recommended number of servings from the meat and milk groups (i.e., patient may not be getting as much iron as she can from her diet if she relies on fish, cheese, and white-meat poultry to satisfy the meat group recommendations).	6/26/15 Outcome partially met. Patient's intake is improved: Intake from the grain and meat groups is adequate instead of marginal. However, the patient still has difficulty consuming enough items from the milk group. *Recommendation:* Continue encouraging the patient to consume more items from the milk group such as cheese, yogurt, and pudding. Will advise the patient to add skim milk powder whenever possible to fortify home-cooked and home-baked products. Will recommend that the patient increase her intake of nondairy sources of calcium, such as broccoli, spinach, and greens or breakfast cereal, fruit juice, and soy beverages with added calcium. Iron may also be consumed through turkey dark meat, shellfish, or spinach. *L. Swift, RN*

EXPECTED OUTCOME By the next monthly assessment, 6/26/15, the patient will:
- Gain 1 to 2 lb

NURSING INTERVENTIONS	RATIONALE	EVALUATIVE STATEMENT
Advise the patient on the recommended rate and amount of weight gain. Stress the importance of quality weight gain.	Patient needs to understand that a 28- to 40-lb gradual weight gain (based on her BMI using the patient's usual weight) is considered optimal for fetal development, and results in little gain in maternal fat tissue. However, because the fetus and maternal tissues require nutrients along with calories, it is essential that the weight gain comes from eating nutrient-dense calories instead of empty calories.	6/26/15 Outcome met. Noting a relief from nausea and an increase in the number of daily meals, the patient gained 2 lb. *L. Swift, RN*

(continued)

NURSING PLAN OF CARE 35-1 *continued*

for Susan Oakland

EXPECTED OUTCOME By the next monthly assessment, 6/26/15, the patient will:
- Take prenatal vitamins as prescribed by the physician

NURSING INTERVENTIONS	RATIONALE	EVALUATIVE STATEMENT
Advise the patient to take the supplement as prescribed and that the supplements are not a substitute for an adequate diet.	Supplements are intended to be used in conjunction with an optimal diet, not in place of one, because they do not provide optimal amounts of all required nutrients. Because the requirements for folic acid and iron during pregnancy are usually not met through diet alone, supplements of these two nutrients in particular are necessary.	6/26/15 Outcome met. Patient reports taking supplement as prescribed. No adverse effects noted. *Recommendation:* Will continue to monitor patient's tolerance of supplement. Will continue to implement plan and reassess at next monthly appointment, 7/28/15. *L. Swift, RN*
Advise the patient that the iron content in the supplements may cause constipation and the stools to become black.	Common adverse effects of large iron doses are constipation and black stools.	

SAMPLE DOCUMENTATION

5/22/15 Nursing

Mrs. Oakland was seen for routine prenatal checkup at 9 weeks' gestation. Assessment findings reveal that the patient is underweight, has lost 3 lb (1.4 kg) in the past 4 weeks, is experiencing nausea and vomiting, has a deficient hemoglobin and hematocrit, and is fatigued. Other contributing factors include weight consciousness, hurried schedule, and food dislikes. Discussion centered on maintaining good dietary habits, improving overall intake and meal patterns to meet the demands of pregnancy and subsequent lactation, initiating dietary changes aimed at avoiding nausea and vomiting, and increasing iron intake. See plan of care. Patient's progress will be evaluated at the next monthly visit, 6/26/15.

L. Swift, RN

SKILL 35-1 INSERTING A NASOGASTRIC (NG) TUBE

DELEGATION CONSIDERATIONS

The insertion of a nasogastric (NG) tube is not delegated to nursing assistive personnel (NAP) or unlicensed assistive personnel (UAP). Depending on the state's nurse practice act and the organization's policies and procedures, insertion of an NG tube may be delegated to licensed practical/vocational nurses (LPN/LVNs). The decision to delegate must be based on careful analysis of the patient's needs and circumstances, as well as the qualifications of the person to whom the task is being delegated. Refer to the Delegation Guidelines in Appendix A (found on thePoint).

EQUIPMENT

- Nasogastric tube of appropriate size (8–18 French)
- Stethoscope
- Water-soluble lubricant
- Normal saline solution or sterile water, for irrigation, depending on facility policy

- Tongue blade
- Irrigations set, including a Toomey (20–50 mL)
- Flashlight
- Nonallergenic tape (1 inch wide)
- Tissues
- Glass of water with straw
- Topical anesthetic—lidocaine spray or gel (optional)
- Clamp

- Suction apparatus (if ordered)
- Bath towel or disposable pad
- Emesis basin
- Safety pin and rubber band
- Nonsterile disposable gloves
- Additional PPE, as indicated
- Tape measure or other measuring device
- Skin barrier
- pH paper

IMPLEMENTATION

ACTION	RATIONALE
1. Verify the medical order for insertion of an NG tube. Gather equipment, including selection of the appropriate NG tube.	Ensures that the patient receives the correct treatment. Assembling equipment provides for an organized approach to task. NG tubes should be radiopaque, contain clearly visible markings for measurement, and may have multiple ports for aspiration.
2. Perform hand hygiene and put on PPE, if indicated.	Hand hygiene and PPE prevent the spread of microorganisms. PPE is required based on transmission precautions.
3. Identify the patient.	Identifying the patient ensures that the right patient receives the intervention and helps prevent errors.
4. Explain the procedure to the patient and provide the rationale as to why the tube is needed. Discuss the associated discomforts that may be experienced and possible interventions that may allay this discomfort. Answer any questions as needed.	Explanation facilitates patient cooperation. Some patient surveys report that of all routine procedures, the insertion of an NG tube is considered the most painful. Lidocaine gel or sprays are possible options to decrease discomfort during NG tube insertion.
5. Assemble equipment on the overbed table within reach.	5. Arranging items nearby is convenient, saves time, and avoids unnecessary stretching and twisting of muscles on the part of the nurse.
6. Close the patient's bedside curtain or door. Raise the bed to a comfortable working position, usually elbow height of the caregiver (VISN 8, 2009). Assist the patient to high Fowler's position or elevate the head of the bed 45 degrees if the patient is unable to maintain an upright position (Fig. 1). Drape the chest with a bath towel or disposable pad. Have an emesis basin and tissues handy.	Closing the curtains or door provides for patient privacy. Having the bed at the proper height prevents back and muscle strain. The upright position is more natural for swallowing and protects against bronchial intubation aspiration if the patient should vomit. Passage of tube may stimulate gagging and tearing of eyes.

FIGURE 1. Placing patient in semi- to high Fowler's position in preparation for tube insertion.

(continued)

SKILL 35-1 INSERTING A NASOGASTRIC (NG) TUBE *continued*

ACTION	RATIONALE
7. **Measure the distance to insert the tube by placing the tip of the tube at the patient's nostril and extending the tube to the tip of the earlobe (Fig. 2) and then to the tip of the xiphoid process (Fig. 3).** Mark the tube with an indelible marker.	Measurement ensures that the tube will be long enough to enter patient's stomach.

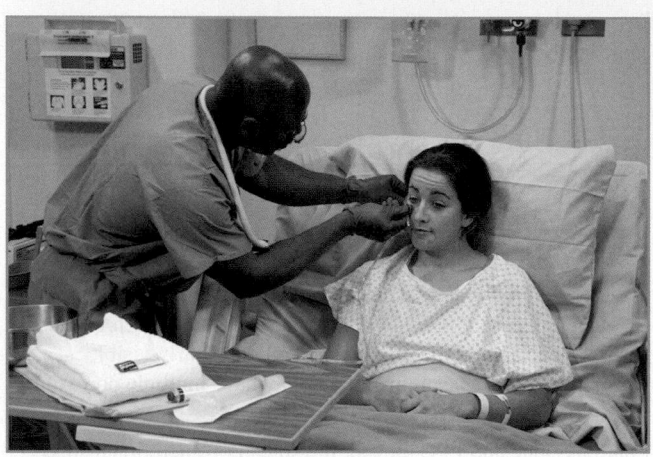

FIGURE 2. Measuring NG tube from nostril to tip of earlobe.

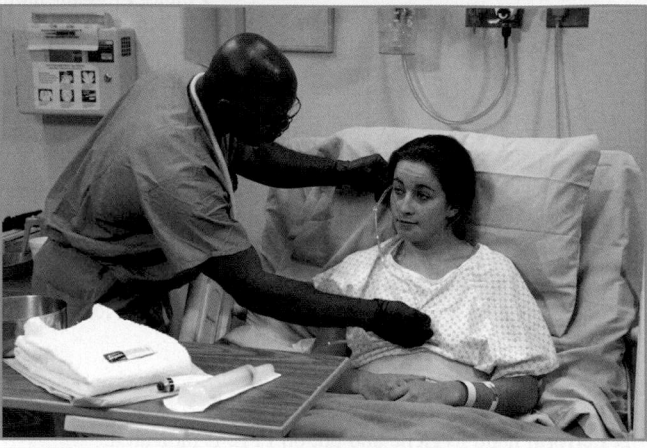

FIGURE 3. Measuring NG tube from tip of earlobe to xiphoid process.

8. Put on gloves. Lubricate the tip of the tube (at least 2 to 4 inches) with water-soluble lubricant. Apply a topical anesthetic to the nostril and oropharynx, as appropriate.	Lubrication reduces friction and facilitates passage of the tube into the stomach. Water-soluble lubricant will not cause pneumonia if the tube accidentally enters the lungs. Topical anesthetics act as local anesthetics, reducing discomfort. Consult the physician for an order for a topical anesthetic such as lidocaine gel or spray if needed.
9. After selecting the appropriate nostril, ask the patient to slightly flex the head back against the pillow. Gently insert the tube into the nostril while directing the tube upward and backward along the floor of the nose (Fig. 4). The patient may gag when the tube reaches the pharynx. Provide tissues for tearing or watering of eyes. Offer comfort and reassurance to the patient.	Following the normal contour of the nasal passage while inserting the tube reduces irritation and the likelihood of mucosal injury. The tube stimulates the gag reflex readily. Tears are a natural response as the tube passes into the nasopharynx. Many patients report that gagging and throat discomfort can be more painful than the tube passing through the nostrils.

FIGURE 4. Beginning insertion with patient positioned with head slightly flexed back.

ACTION	RATIONALE

10. When the pharynx is reached, instruct the patient to touch the chin to the chest. Encourage the patient to sip water through a straw or swallow even if no fluids are permitted. Advance the tube in a downward and backward direction when the patient swallows (Fig. 5). Stop when the patient breathes. **If gagging and coughing persist, stop advancing the tube and check placement of the tube with tongue blade and flashlight.** If the tube is curled, straighten the tube and attempt to advance again. Keep advancing the tube until pen marking is reached. **Do not use force.** Rotate tube if it meets resistance.

Bringing the head forward helps close the trachea and open the esophagus. Swallowing helps advance the tube, causes the epiglottis to cover the opening of the trachea, and helps to eliminate gagging and coughing. Excessive coughing and gagging may occur if the tube has curled in the back of throat. Forcing the tube may injure mucous membranes.

FIGURE 5. Advancing tube after patient drops chin to chest and while swallowing.

11. **Discontinue the procedure and remove the tube if there are signs of distress, such as gasping, coughing, cyanosis, and inability to speak or hum.**

The tube is in the airway if the patient shows signs of distress and cannot speak or hum. If after three attempts, nasogastric insertion is unsuccessful, another nurse may try or the patient should be referred to another health care professional.

12. Secure the tube loosely to the nose or cheek until it is determined that the tube is in the patient's stomach:

Securing with tape stabilizes the tube while position is being determined.

   a. Attach a syringe to the end of the tube and aspirate a small amount of stomach contents.

The tube is in the stomach if its contents can be aspirated: pH of aspirate can then be tested to determine gastric placement. If unable to obtain a specimen, reposition the patient and flush the tube with 30 mL of air. This action may be necessary several times. Current literature recommends that the nurse ensure proper placement of the NG tube by relying on multiple methods and not one method alone.

   b. Measure the pH of the aspirated fluid using pH paper or a meter. Place a drop of gastric secretions onto pH paper or place a small amount in a plastic cup and dip the pH paper into it. Within 30 seconds, compare the color on the paper with the chart supplied by the manufacturer (Fig. 6).

Current research demonstrates that the use of pH is predictive of correct placement. The pH of gastric contents is acidic (less than 5.5). If the patient is taking an acid-inhibiting agent, the range may be 4.0 to 6.0. The pH of intestinal fluid is 7.0 or higher. The pH of respiratory fluid is 6.0 or higher. This method will not effectively differentiate between intestinal fluid and pleural fluid.

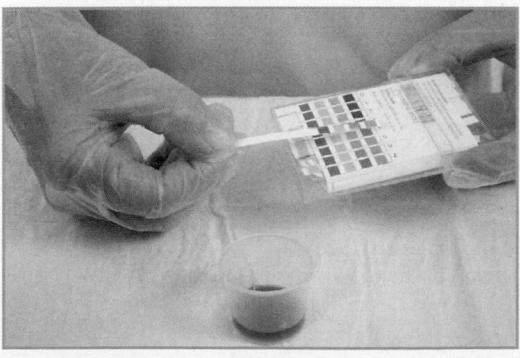

FIGURE 6. Checking pH of gastric fluid.

(continued)

SKILL 35-1 INSERTING A NASOGASTRIC (NG) TUBE *continued*

ACTION	RATIONALE
c. Visualize aspirated contents, checking for color and consistency.	Gastric fluid can be green with particles, off-white, or brown if old blood is present. Intestinal aspirate tends to look clear or straw-colored to a deep golden-yellow color. Also, intestinal aspirate may be greenish-brown if stained with bile. Respiratory or tracheobronchial fluid is usually off-white to tan and may be tinged with mucus. A small amount of blood-tinged fluid may be seen immediately after NG insertion.
d. Obtain a radiograph (x-ray) of placement of the tube, based on facility policy (and ordered by physician).	The x-ray is considered the most reliable method for identifying the position of the NG tube.
13. Apply skin barrier to the tip and end of the nose and allow to dry. Remove gloves and secure the tube with a commercially prepared device (follow manufacturer's directions) or tape to the patient's nose. To secure with tape:	Skin barrier improves adhesion and protects skin. Constant pressure of the tube against the skin and mucous membranes may cause tissue injury. Securing tube prevents migration of the tube inward and outward.

a. Cut a 4-inch piece of tape and split the bottom 2 inches (Fig. 7) or use packaged nose tape for NG tubes.

b. Place the unsplit end over the bridge of the patient's nose (Fig. 8).

c. Wrap split ends under and around the NG tube (Fig. 9). **Be careful not to pull the tube too tightly against the nose.**

FIGURE 7. Making a 2″ cut into a 4″ strip of tape.

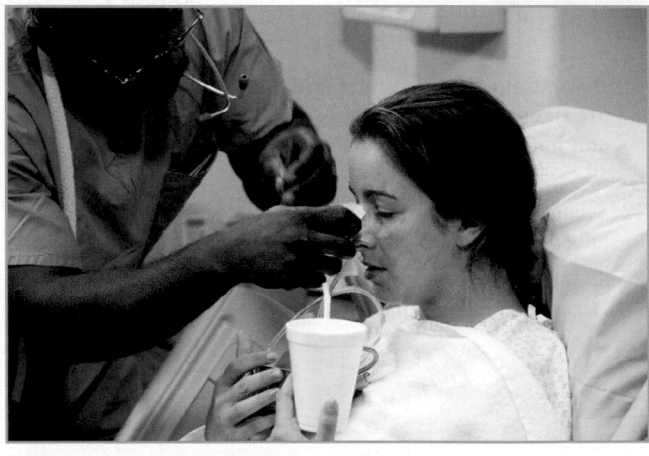

FIGURE 8. Applying tape to patient's nose.

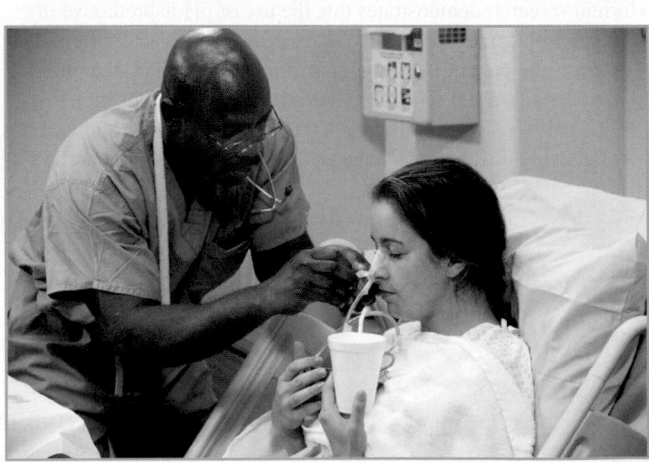

FIGURE 9. Wrapping split ends around NG tube.

ACTION

14. Put on gloves. Clamp the tube and remove the syringe. Cap the tube or attach it to suction (Fig. 10) according to the medical orders.

15. Measure length of the exposed tube. Reinforce the marking on the tube at the nostril with indelible ink. Ask the patient to turn the head to the side opposite the nostril in which the tube is inserted. Secure the tube to the patient's gown by using a rubber band or tape and safety pin. For additional support, tape the tube onto the patient's cheek using a piece of tape. **If a double-lumen tube (e.g., Salem sump) is used, secure the vent above the stomach level.** Attach the vent at shoulder level (Fig. 11).

RATIONALE

Suction provides for decompression of stomach and drainage of gastric contents.

Tube length should be checked and compared with this initial measurement, in conjunction with pH measurement and visual assessment of aspirate. An increase in the length of the exposed tube may indicate dislodgement (AACN, 2010; Bourgault et al., 2007; Hinkle & Cheever, 2014). The tube should be marked with an indelible marker at the nostril. This marking should be assessed each time the tube is used to ensure that the tube has not become displaced. Securing prevents tension and tugging on the tube. Turning the head ensures adequate slack in the tubing to prevent tension when the patient turns the head. Securing the double-lumen tube above stomach level prevents seepage of gastric contents and keeps the lumen clear for venting air.

FIGURE 10. NG tube attached to wall suction.

FIGURE 11. Patient with Salem sump tube (NG) secured. Note blue vent at patient's shoulder.

16. Assist with or provide oral hygiene at 2- to 4-hour intervals. Lubricate the lips generously and clean nares and lubricate as needed. Offer analgesic throat lozenges or anesthetic spray for throat irritation if needed.

17. Remove equipment and return the patient to a position of comfort. Remove gloves. Raise the side rail and lower the bed.

18. Remove additional PPE, if used. Perform hand hygiene.

Oral hygiene keeps mouth clean and moist, promotes comfort, and reduces thirst.

Promotes patient comfort and safety. Removing gloves properly reduces the risk for infection transmission and contamination of other items.

Removing PPE properly reduces the risk for infection transmission and contamination of other items. Hand hygiene prevents transmission of microorganisms.

DOCUMENTATION

Guidelines

Document the size and type of NG tube that was inserted and the measurement from the tip of the nose to the end of the exposed tube. Also, document the results of the x-ray that was taken to confirm the position of the tube, if applicable. Record a description of the gastric contents, including the pH of the contents. Document the naris where the tube is placed and the patient's response to the procedure. Include assessment data, both subjective and objective, related to the abdomen. Record the patient teaching that was discussed.

(continued)

SKILL 35-1 INSERTING A NASOGASTRIC (NG) TUBE *continued*

Sample Documentation

DocuCare Practice documenting NG tube insertion in *Lippincott DocuCare*.

> 10/4/15 0945 Abdomen slightly distended and taut; hypoactive bowel sounds. Patient reports transient nausea. 14-Fr Levin tube inserted via R naris, 20 cm of tube from naris to end of tube; gastric contents aspirated, pH 4, contents light green; patient tolerated without incident.
>
> —S. Essner, RN

UNEXPECTED SITUATIONS AND ASSOCIATED INTERVENTIONS

- *As a tube is passing through the pharynx, patient begins to retch and gag:* This is common during placement of an NG tube. Ask the patient if he or she wants the nurse to stop the procedure, which will allow the patient to gain composure from the gagging episode. Continue to advance the tube when the patient relates that he or she is ready. Have the emesis basin nearby in case the patient begins to vomit.

- *The nurse is unable to pass the tube after trying a second time down the one nostril:* If the patient's condition permits, inspect the other nostril and attempt to pass the nasogastric tube down this nostril. If unable to pass down this nostril, consult another health professional.

- *As tube is passing through pharynx, patient begins to cough and shows signs of respiratory distress:* **Stop advancing the tube.** The tube is most likely entering the trachea. Pull tube back into nasal area. Support the patient as the patient regains normal breathing ability and composure. If patient feels able to tolerate another attempt, ask the patient to keep the chin on the chest and swallow as the tube is advanced to help prevent the tube from entering the trachea. Begin to advance the tube, watching for any signs of respiratory distress.

- *No gastric contents can be aspirated:* If the patient is comatose, check the oral cavity. If the tube is in the gastric area, small air boluses may need to be given until gastric contents can be aspirated.

SPECIAL CONSIDERATIONS

General Considerations

To promote patient safety when administering a tube feeding, be sure to do the following:

- Check tube placement before administering any fluids, medications, or feedings. Use multiple techniques: x-ray, external length marking/measurement, pH testing, and aspirate characteristics.

- Some patients require a **nasointestinal tube**. To insert a nasointestinal tube:
  - Measure the tube from the tip of the nose to the ear lobe and from the ear lobe to the xiphoid process. Add 8 to 10 inches for intestinal placement. Mark tubing at the desired point.
  - Place patient on the right side. The nasointestinal tube is usually placed in the stomach and allowed to advance through peristalsis through the pyloric sphincter (may take up to 24 hours).
  - Administer medications to enhance GI motility, such as metoclopramide (Reglan), if ordered.
  - Test pH of the aspirate when the tube has advanced to the marked point to confirm placement in the intestine. Confirm the position by radiograph. Secure with tape once placement is confirmed.

- Monitoring for carbon dioxide to determine nasogastric tube position and/or dislodgement has been investigated (Gilbert & Burns, 2012; Munera-Seeley et al., 2008). This involves the use of a capnograph or a colorimetric end-tidal CO_2 detector to detect the presence of carbon dioxide, which would indicate tube positioning in the patient's airway instead of the stomach.

Infant and Child Considerations

- Infants are obligate nose breathers; insertion of the tube via the mouth may be appropriate (orogastric tube; Perry, Hockenberry, Lowdermilk, & Wilson, 2010).

- Age-specific equations are available to predict insertion distance and are the best method to determine insertion distance based on age and height for infants and children 2 weeks to 19 years of age. Other methods to determine insertion distance include the nose or mouth to ear-mid-xiphoid-umbilicus span. The accuracy of these methods has been challenged, however (Freeman et al., 2012).

SKILL 35-2   **ADMINISTERING A TUBE FEEDING**

DELEGATION CONSIDERATIONS

The administration of a tube feeding is not usually delegated to nursing assistive personnel (NAP) or unlicensed assistive personnel (UAP) in the acute care setting. The administration of a tube feeding in some settings may be delegated to NAP or UAP who have received appropriate training, after assessment of tube placement and patency by the registered nurse. Depending on the state's nurse practice act and the organization's policies and procedures, the administration of a tube feeding may be delegated to licensed practical/vocational nurses (LPN/LVNs). The decision to delegate must be based on careful analysis of the patient's needs and circumstances, as well as the qualifications of the person to whom the task is being delegated. Refer to the Delegation Guidelines in Appendix A (found on thePoint).

EQUIPMENT

- Prescribed tube feeding formula at room temperature
- Feeding bag or prefilled tube feeding set
- Stethoscope
- Nonsterile gloves
- Additional PPE, as indicated
- Alcohol preps
- Disposable pad or towel
- Asepto or Toomey syringe

- Enteral feeding pump (if ordered)
- Rubber band
- Clamp (Hoffman or butterfly)
- IV pole
- Water for irrigation and hydration as needed
- pH paper
- Tape measure, or other measuring device

IMPLEMENTATION

ACTION	RATIONALE
1. Gather equipment. Check amount, concentration, type, and frequency of tube feeding in the patient's medical record. Check expiration date of formula.	This provides for organized approach to task. Checking ensures that correct feeding will be administered. Outdated formula may be contaminated.
2. Perform hand hygiene and put on PPE, if indicated.	Hand hygiene and PPE prevent the spread of microorganisms. PPE is required based on transmission precautions.
3. Identify the patient.	Identifying the patient ensures that the right patient receives the intervention and helps prevent errors.
4. Explain the procedure to the patient and why this intervention is needed. Answer any questions as needed.	Explanation facilitates patient cooperation.
5. Assemble equipment on the overbed table within reach.	Organization facilitates performance of task.
6. Close the patient's bedside curtain or door. Raise the bed to a comfortable working position, usually elbow height of the caregiver (VISN 8, 2009). Perform key abdominal assessments.	Closing curtains or door provides for patient privacy. Having the bed at the proper height prevents back and muscle strain. Due to changes in the patient's condition, assessment is vital before initiating the intervention.
7. **Position the patient with the head of the bed elevated at least 30 to 45 degrees or as near normal position for eating as possible.**	This position minimizes the possibility of aspiration into the trachea. Patients who are considered at high risk for aspiration should be assisted to at least a 45-degree position.
8. Put on gloves. Unpin the tube from the patient's gown. Verify the position of the marking on the tube at the nostril. Measure the length of the exposed tube and compare with the documented length.	Gloves prevent contact with blood and body fluids. The tube should be marked with an indelible marker at the nostril. This marking should be assessed each time the tube is used to ensure that the tube has not become displaced. Tube length should be checked and compared with this initial measurement, in conjunction with pH measurement and visual assessment of the aspirate. An increase in the length of the exposed tube may indicate dislodgement (AACN, 2010; Bourgault et al., 2007; Hinkle & Cheever, 2014).

(continued)

SKILL 35-2 ADMINISTERING A TUBE FEEDING *continued*

ACTION

9. Attach a syringe to the end of the tube and aspirate a small amount of stomach contents, as described in Skill 35-1 (Fig. 1).

10. Check the pH as described in Skill 35-1 (Fig. 2).

RATIONALE

The tube is in the stomach if its contents can be aspirated: pH of the aspirate can then be tested to determine gastric placement. If unable to obtain a specimen, reposition the patient and flush the tube with 30 mL of air. This action may be necessary several times. Current literature recommends that the nurse ensure proper placement of the NG tube by relying on multiple methods and not one method alone.

Current research demonstrates that the use of pH is predictive of correct placement. The pH of gastric contents is acidic (less than 5.5). If the patient is taking an acid-inhibiting agent, the range may be 4.0 to 6.0. The pH of intestinal fluid is 7.0 or higher. The pH of respiratory fluid is 6.0 or higher. This method will not effectively differentiate between intestinal fluid and pleural fluid.

Testing for pH before the next feeding in intermittent feedings is conducted since the stomach has been emptied of the feeding formula. However, if the patient is receiving continuous feedings, the pH measurement is not as useful, since the formula raises the pH.

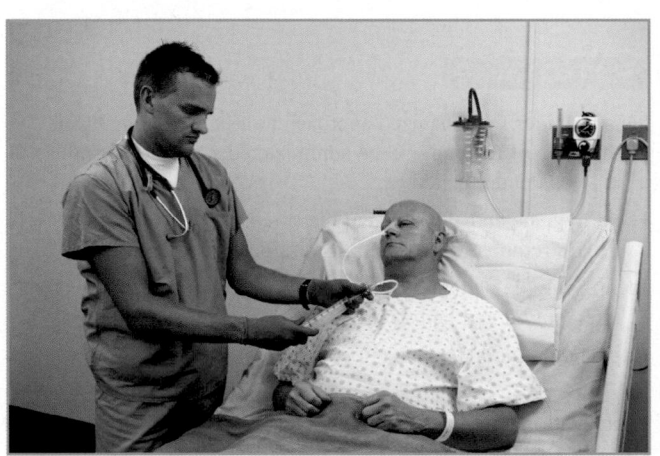

FIGURE 1. Aspirating gastric contents.

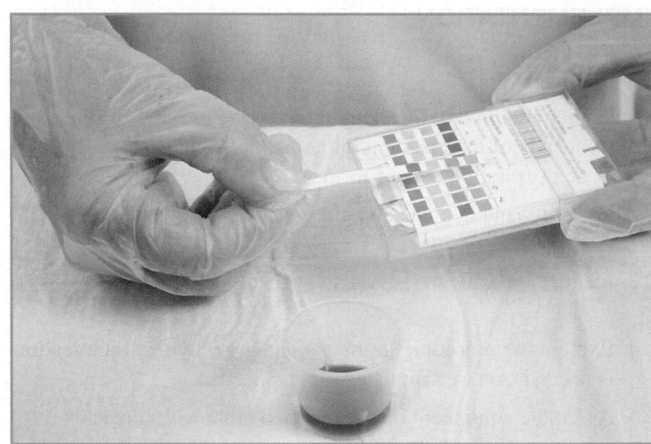

FIGURE 2. Checking pH of gastric fluid.

11. Visualize aspirated contents, checking for color and consistency.

12. If it is not possible to aspirate contents, assessments to check placement are inconclusive, the exposed tube length has changed, or there are any other indications that the tube is not in place, check placement by x-ray.

Gastric fluid can be green with particles, off-white, or brown if old blood is present. Intestinal aspirate tends to look clear or straw-colored to a deep golden-yellow color. Also, intestinal aspirate may be greenish-brown if stained with bile. Respiratory or tracheobronchial fluid is usually off-white to tan and may be tinged with mucus. A small amount of blood-tinged fluid may be seen immediately after NG insertion.

The x-ray is considered the most reliable method for identifying the position of the NG tube.

ACTION	RATIONALE

13. After multiple steps have been taken to ensure that the feeding tube is located in the stomach or small intestine, **aspirate all gastric contents with the syringe and measure to check for gastric residual—the amount of feeding remaining in the stomach.** Return the residual based on facility policy. Proceed with feeding if amount of residual does not exceed agency policy or the limit indicated in the medical record.

Checking for residual before each feeding or every 4 to 6 hours during a continuous feeding according to institutional policy is implemented to identify delayed gastric emptying. High gastric residual volumes (200 to 250 mL or greater) can be associated with high risk for aspiration and aspiration-related pneumonia (Bourgault et al., 2007; Metheny, 2008). Some experts now recommend that the patient's pattern of residual is more important than the amount (A.S.P.E.N., 2011; Bourgault et al.; Metheny). Feedings should be held if residual volumes exceed 200 mL on two successive assessments (A.S.P.E.N.). Research findings are inconclusive on the benefit of returning gastric volumes to the stomach or intestine to avoid fluid or electrolyte imbalance, which has been accepted practice. Consult facility policy concerning this practice.

14. Flush tube with 30 mL of water for irrigation. Disconnect syringe from tubing and cap end of tubing while preparing the formula feeding equipment. Remove gloves.

Flushing tube prevents occlusion (A.S.P.E.N., 2011; Bourgault et al., 2007; Metheny, 2008). Capping the tube deters the entry of microorganisms and prevents leakage onto the bed linens.

15. Put on gloves before preparing, assembling, and handling any part of the feeding system.

Gloves prevent contact with blood and body fluids and deter transmission of contaminants to feeding equipment and/or formula.

16. Administer feeding.

When Using a Feeding Bag (Open System)

a. Label the bag and/or tubing with date and time. Hang the bag on an IV pole and adjust to about 12 inches above the stomach. Clamp the tubing.

Labeling date and time of first use allows for disposal within 24 hours, to deter growth of microorganisms. Proper feeding bag height reduces risk of the formula being introduced too quickly.

b. Check the expiration date of the formula. Cleanse the top of the feeding container with a disinfectant before opening it (Fig. 3). Pour the formula into the feeding bag and allow the solution to run through the tubing. Close the clamp.

Cleansing the container top with the alcohol minimizes risk for contaminants entering the feeding bag. The formula displaces air in the tubing.

c. Attach the feeding setup to the feeding tube (Fig. 4), open the clamp, and regulate the drip according to the medical order, or allow the feeding to run in over 30 minutes.

Introducing the formula at a slow, regular rate allows the stomach to accommodate the feeding and decreases GI distress.

FIGURE 3. Cleaning top of feeding container with alcohol before opening it.

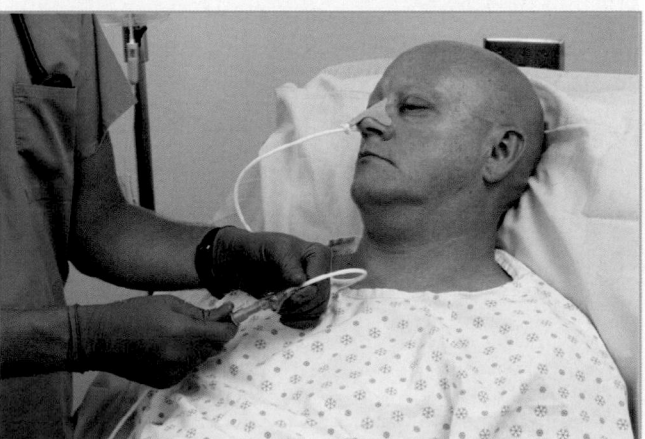

FIGURE 4. Attaching feeding bag tubing to NG tube.

(continued)

SKILL 35-2 ADMINISTERING A TUBE FEEDING *continued*

ACTION	RATIONALE

ACTION

d. **Add 30 to 60 mL (1 to 2 oz) of water for irrigation to the feeding bag when the feeding is almost completed (Fig. 5) and allow it to run through the tube.**

e. Clamp the tubing immediately after water has been instilled. Disconnect the feeding setup from the feeding tube. Clamp the tube and cover the end with the cap (Fig. 6).

RATIONALE

Water rinses the feeding from the tube and helps to keep it patent.

Clamping the tube prevents air from entering the stomach. Capping the tube deters entry of microorganisms and covering the end of the tube protects the patient and linens from fluid leakage from the tube.

FIGURE 5. Pouring water into feeding bag.

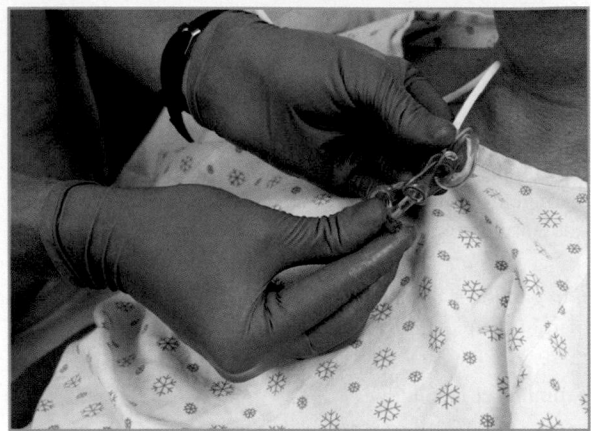

FIGURE 6 Capping NG tube after it is clamped.

When Using a Large Syringe (Open System)

a. Remove the plunger from a 30- or 60-mL syringe (Fig. 7).

b. Attach a syringe to the feeding tube, pour a premeasured amount of tube feeding formula into the syringe (Fig. 8), open the clamp, and allow the food to enter the tube. Regulate the rate, fast or slow, by height of the syringe. **Do not push formula with syringe plunger.**

Introducing the formula at a slow, regular rate allows the stomach to accommodate the feeding and decreases GI distress. The higher the syringe is held, the faster the formula flows.

FIGURE 7. Removing plunger from a 60-mL syringe.

FIGURE 8. Pouring formula into syringe.

ACTION	RATIONALE

c. **Add 30 to 60 mL (1 to 2 oz) of water for irrigation to the syringe (Fig. 9) when feeding is almost completed, and allow it to run through the tube.**

Water rinses the feeding from the tube and helps to keep it patent.

d. When the syringe has emptied, hold the syringe high and disconnect it from tube. Clamp the tube and cover the end with the cap.

By holding the syringe high, the formula will not backflow out of tube and onto the patient. Clamping the tube prevents air from entering the stomach. Capping the end of tube deters entry of microorganisms. Covering the end protects the patient and linens from fluid leakage from the tube.

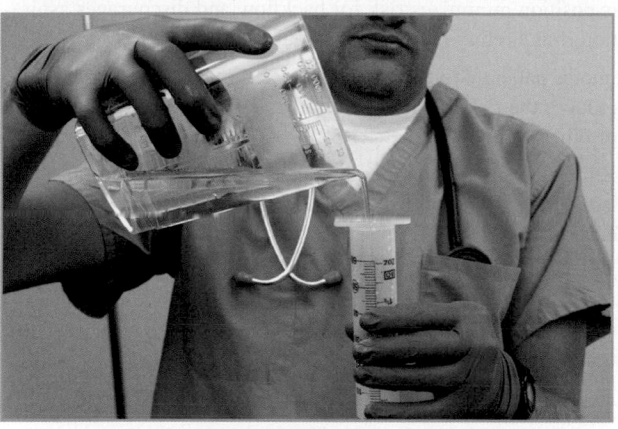

FIGURE 9. Pouring water into almost-empty syringe.

When Using an Enteral Feeding Pump

a. Close the flow-regulator clamp on the tubing and fill the feeding bag with prescribed formula. Amount used depends on agency policy. Place a label on the container with the patient's name, date, and time the feeding was hung.

Closing the clamp prevents formula from moving through the tubing until the nurse is ready. Labeling date and time of first use allows for disposal within 24 hours, to deter growth of microorganisms.

b. Hang the feeding container on an IV pole. Allow the solution to flow through the tubing.

This prevents air from being forced into the stomach or intestines.

c. Connect to the feeding pump following the manufacturer's directions. Set the rate (Fig. 10). Maintain the patient in the upright position throughout the feeding. If the patient needs to temporarily lie flat, pause the feeding. Resume the feeding after the patient's position has been changed back to at least 30 to 45 degrees.

Feeding pumps vary. Some of the newer pumps have built-in safeguards that protect the patient from complications. Safety features include cassettes that prevent free-flow of formula, automatic tube flush, safety tips that prevent accidental attachment to an IV setup, and various audible and visible alarms. Feedings are started at full strength rather than diluted which was recommended previously. A smaller volume, 10 to 40 mL, of feeding infused per hour and gradually increased has been shown to be more easily tolerated by patients.

FIGURE 10. Setting up feeding pump with feeding bag and primed tubing.

SKILL 35-2 ADMINISTERING A TUBE FEEDING *continued*

ACTION	RATIONALE
d. **Check placement of the tube and gastric residual every 4 to 6 hours.**	Checking placement (Steps 9–12) verifies that the tube has not moved out of the stomach. Checking gastric residual (Step 13) monitors absorption of the feeding and prevents distention, which could lead to aspiration.
17. Observe the patient's response during and after tube feeding and assess the abdomen at least once per shift.	Pain or nausea may indicate stomach distention, which may lead to vomiting. Physical signs such as abdominal distention and firmness or regurgitation of tube feeding may indicate intolerance.
18. **Have the patient remain in the upright position for at least 1 hour after feeding.**	This position minimizes risk for backflow and discourages aspiration if any reflux or vomiting should occur.
19. Remove equipment and return the patient to a position of comfort. Remove gloves. Raise the side rail and lower the bed.	Promotes patient comfort and safety. Removing gloves properly reduces the risk for infection transmission and contamination of other items.
20. Put on gloves. Wash and clean equipment or replace according to agency policy. Remove gloves.	This prevents contamination and deters spread of microorganisms. Reusable systems are cleansed with soap and water with each use and replaced every 24 hours. Refer to agency policy and manufacturer guidelines for specifics on equipment care.
21. Remove additional PPE, if used. Perform hand hygiene.	Removing PPE properly reduces the risk for infection transmission and contamination of other items. Hand hygiene prevents transmission of microorganisms.

DOCUMENTATION

Guidelines

Document the type of nasogastric tube or gastrostomy/jejunostomy tube that is present. Record the criteria that were used to confirm proper placement before feeding was initiated, such as the tube length in inches or centimeters compared to the length on initial insertion. Document the aspiration of gastric contents and pH of the gastric contents when intermittent feeding is used. Note the components of the abdominal assessment, such as observation of the abdomen, presence of distention or firmness, and presence of bowel sounds. Include subjective data, including any reports from the patient such as abdominal pain or nausea or any other patient response. Record the amount of gastric residual volume that was obtained. Document the position of the patient, the type of feeding, and the method and amount of feeding. Include any relevant patient teaching.

Sample Documentation

10/29/15 1015 Position of NG tube was compared with initial measurement on insertion. Abdomen nondistended and soft; patient denies pain or nausea. HOB raised to 45 degrees. Thirty (30) mL residual aspirated prior to feeding; pH 3.9. Aspirate returned to stomach; aspirate yellow with dark flecks. 150 mL of Jevity 1.2 Cal. administered via bolus feeding. Tube flushed with 60 mL water with ease. Patient instructed to call for nurse for pain or nausea or other concerns related to feeding.

—S. Essner, RN

UNEXPECTED SITUATIONS AND ASSOCIATED INTERVENTIONS

• *Tube is found not to be in stomach or intestine:* Tube must be in stomach before feeding. If tube is in esophagus, patient is at increased risk for aspiration. See Skill 35-1 for steps to replace tube.

• *When checking for residual, the nurse aspirates a large amount:* Before discarding or replacing residual, check with the primary care provider and facility policy. Replacing a large amount may increase patient's risk for vomiting and aspiration, while discarding a large amount may increase patient's risk for metabolic alkalosis. At times, the primary care provider may instruct the nurse to replace half of the residual and recheck in a set amount of time.

• *Patient complains of nausea after tube feeding:* Ensure that the head of the bed remains elevated and that suction equipment is at bedside. Check the medication record to see if any antiemetics have been ordered for the patient. Consider notifying the primary care provider for an order for an antiemetic.

• *When attempting to aspirate contents, the nurse notes that tube is clogged:* Most obstructions are caused by coagulation of formula. Try using warm water and gentle pressure to remove the clog. Carbonated sodas, such as colas, and meat tenderizers have not been shown effective in removing clogs in feeding tubes. Never use a stylet to unclog tubes. The tube may have to be replaced. To prevent clogs, ensure that adequate flushing is completed after feedings.

SPECIAL CONSIDERATIONS	• Checking for the residual amount of feeding in the stomach is explained in Step 13. High gastric residual volumes (200 to 250 mL or greater) can be associated with high risk for aspiration and aspiration-related pneumonia (Bourgault et al., 2007; Metheny, 2008). For patients who are experiencing gastric dysfunction or decreased level of consciousness, feedings may be held for smaller residual amounts (less than 400 mL) (Bourgault et al.; Metheny). Also, research findings are inconclusive on the benefit of returning gastric volumes to the stomach or intestine to avoid fluid or electrolyte imbalance, which has been accepted practice. Consult agency policy concerning this practice. Some researchers point out that high residual volumes are not indicative of intolerance to the tube feeding. In contrast, low residual volumes do not guarantee that patients are tolerating enteral tube feedings and are not at risk for aspiration (McClave et al., 2005). Monitoring for trends in gradually increasing amounts of residual volumes and assessing for other signs of intolerance such as gastric pain or distention should be implemented (A.S.P.E.N., 2011; Bourgault et al.; Metheny). Feedings should be held if residual volumes exceed 200 mL on two successive assessments (A.S.P.E.N.).

• When the patient with dementia and/or family is deciding on whether to agree to tube-feeding nutrition, inform them that research is recommending that tube feedings not be used for this population of patients since they do not increase survival or prevent malnutrition or aspiration. It is suggested to use such methods as increasing feeding assistance and changing food consistency, as well as respecting patient preferences, as needed (American Dietetic Association [ADA], 2008).

• Some feeding equipment allows for the addition of water for flushes to a second feeding container, which enters the system through a second set of tubing. The feeding pump will automatically administer the preset volume of flush at the preset frequency.

SKILL 35-3   REMOVING A NASOGASTRIC TUBE

DELEGATION CONSIDERATIONS	The removal of a nasogastric (NG) tube is not delegated to nursing assistive personnel (NAP) or unlicensed assistive personnel (UAP). Depending on the state's nurse practice act and the organization's policies and procedures, removal of an NG tube may be delegated to licensed practical/vocational nurses (LPN/LVNs). The decision to delegate must be based on careful analysis of the patient's needs and circumstances, as well as the qualifications of the person to whom the task is being delegated. Refer to the Delegation Guidelines in Appendix A (found on thePoint).

EQUIPMENT	• Tissues	• Stethoscope	• Normal saline solution for irrigation (optional)
	• 50-mL syringe	• Disposable plastic bag	
	• Nonsterile gloves	• Bath towel or disposable pad	• Emesis basin
	• Additional PPE, as indicated		

(continued)

SKILL 35-3 REMOVING A NASOGASTRIC TUBE *continued*

IMPLEMENTATION

ACTION	RATIONALE
1. Check the medical record for the order for removal of the NG tube.	This ensures correct implementation of the primary care provider's order.
2. Perform hand hygiene and put on PPE, if indicated.	Hand hygiene and PPE prevent the spread of microorganisms. PPE is required based on transmission precautions.
3. Identify the patient.	Identifying the patient ensures that the right patient receives the intervention and helps prevent errors.
4. Explain the procedure to the patient and why this intervention is warranted. Describe that it will entail a quick few moments of discomfort. Perform key abdominal assessments.	Patient cooperation is facilitated when explanations are provided. Due to changes in the patient's condition, assessment is vital before initiating the intervention.
5. Pull the patient's bedside curtain. Raise the bed to a comfortable working position, usually elbow height of the caregiver (VISN 8, 2009). Assist the patient into a 30- to 45-degree position. Place a towel or disposable pad across the patient's chest (Fig. 1). Give tissues and the emesis basin to the patient.	Provides for privacy. Appropriate working height facilitates comfort and proper body mechanics for the nurse. Towel or pad protects the patient from contact with gastric secretions. Emesis basin is helpful if the patient vomits or gags. Tissues are necessary if the patient wants to blow the nose when the tube is removed.
6. Put on gloves. Discontinue suction and separate the tube from the suction. Unpin the tube from the patient's gown and carefully remove the adhesive tape from the patient's nose.	Gloves prevent contact with blood and body fluids. Disconnecting the tube from the suction and the patient allows for its unrestricted removal.
7. Check placement (as outlined in Skill 35-1) and attach syringe and **flush with 10 mL of water or normal saline solution (optional) or clear with 30 to 50 mL of air (Fig. 2).**	Air or saline solution clears the tube of secretions, feeding, or debris.

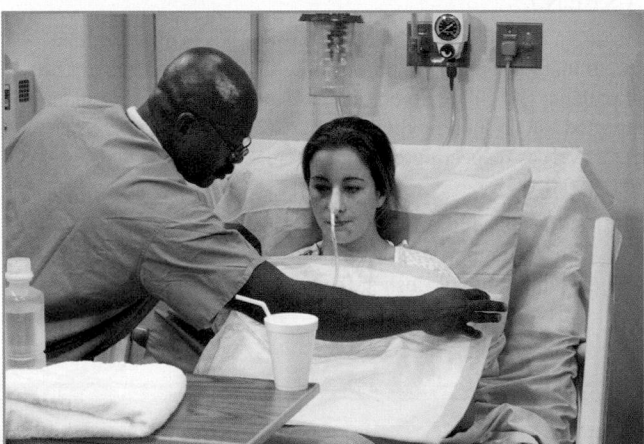

FIGURE 1. Placing towel or disposable pad across patient's chest.

FIGURE 2. Flushing NG tube with 10 mL saline.

8. Clamp tube with fingers by doubling tube on itself (Fig. 3). **Instruct the patient to take a deep breath and hold it. Quickly and carefully remove the tube while the patient holds breath.** Coil the tube in the disposable pad as you remove it from the patient.	Clamping prevents drainage of the gastric contents into the pharynx and esophagus. The patient holds the breath to prevent accidental aspiration of gastric secretions in the tube. Careful removal minimizes trauma and discomfort for patient. Containing the tube in a pad while removing prevents leakage onto the patient.
9. Dispose of the tube per facility policy. Remove gloves. Perform hand hygiene.	This prevents contamination with microorganisms.
10. Offer mouth care to the patient and facial tissue to blow the nose. Lower the bed and assist the patient to a position of comfort as needed.	These interventions promote patient comfort.

ACTION	RATIONALE
11. Remove equipment, and raise the side rail and the lower bed.	Promotes patient comfort and safety.
12. Put on gloves and measure the amount of nasogastric drainage in the collection device. Record the measurement on the output flow record, subtracting irrigant fluids if necessary (Fig. 4). Add a solidifying agent to the nasogastric drainage and dispose of the drainage according to facility policy.	Irrigation fluids are considered intake. To obtain the true nasogastric drainage, irrigant fluid amounts are subtracted from the total nasogastric drainage. Nasogastric drainage is recorded as part of the output of fluids from the patient. Solidifying agents added to liquid nasogastric drainage facilitate safe biohazard disposal.

FIGURE 3. Doubling tube on itself.

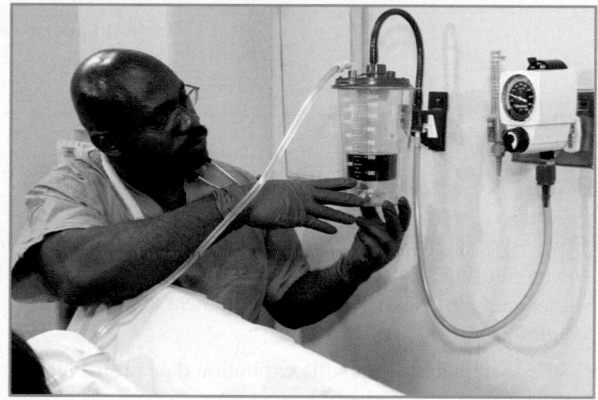

FIGURE 4. Measuring the amount of nasogastric drainage in the collection device.

13. Remove additional PPE, if used. Perform hand hygiene.	Removing PPE properly reduces the risk for infection transmission and contamination of other items. Hand hygiene prevents transmission of microorganisms.

DOCUMENTATION

Guidelines

Document assessment of the abdomen. If an abdominal girth reading was obtained, record this measurement. Document the removal of the nasogastric tube from the naris where it had been placed. Note if there is any irritation to the skin of the naris. Record the amount of NG drainage in the suction container on the patient's intake-and-output record as well as the color of the drainage. Record any pertinent teaching, such as instruction to the patient to notify the nurse if experiencing any nausea, abdominal pain, or bloating.

Sample Documentation

10/29/15 1320 NG tube removed from L naris without incident. 600 mL of dark brown liquid emptied from NG tube. Patient's abdomen is 66 cm; abdomen is soft, nontender with hypoactive bowel sounds in all 4 quadrants.

—S. Essner, RN

UNEXPECTED SITUATIONS AND ASSOCIATED INTERVENTIONS

- *Within 2 hours after NG tube removal, patient's abdomen is showing signs of distention:* Notify the primary care provider. Anticipate an order to reinsert the NG tube.
- *Epistaxis occurs with removal of NG tube:* Occlude both nares until bleeding has subsided. Ensure that the patient is in the upright position. Document epistaxis in the patient's medical record.

SKILL 35-4 OBTAINING A CAPILLARY BLOOD SAMPLE FOR GLUCOSE TESTING

DELEGATION CONSIDERATIONS

Obtaining a capillary blood sample for glucose testing may be delegated to nursing assistive personnel (NAP) or unlicensed assistive personnel (UAP), as well as licensed practical/vocational nurses (LPN/LVNs). The decision to delegate must be based on careful analysis of the patient's needs and circumstances, as well as the qualifications of the person to whom the task is being delegated. Refer to the Delegation Guidelines in Appendix A (found on thePoint).

EQUIPMENT

- Blood glucose meter
- Sterile lancet
- Cotton balls or gauze squares
- Testing strips for meter

- Nonsterile gloves
- Additional PPE, as indicated
- Skin cleanser and water or alcohol swab

IMPLEMENTATION

ACTION	RATIONALE
1. Check the patient's medical record or nursing plan of care for the monitoring schedule. You may decide that additional testing is indicated based on nursing judgment and the patient's condition.	This confirms scheduled times for checking blood glucose. Independent nursing judgment may lead to the decision to test more frequently, based on the patient's condition.
2. Gather equipment. Check the expiration date on the blood test strips.	This provides an organized approach to the task. Blood test strips that are past the expiration date could cause inaccurate results and should not be used.
3. Perform hand hygiene and put on PPE, if indicated.	Hand hygiene and PPE prevent the transmission of microorganisms. PPE is required based on transmission precautions.
4. Identify the patient. Explain the procedure to the patient and instruct the patient about the need for monitoring blood glucose.	Identifying the patient ensures that the right patient receives the intervention and helps prevent errors. Explanation helps to alleviate anxiety and facilitate cooperation.
5. Close the curtains around the bed and close the door to the room, if possible.	Closing the curtain or door provides patient privacy.
6. Turn on the monitor.	The monitor must be on for use.
7. Enter the patient's identification number or scan the patient's identification bracelet, if required, according to facility policy.	Use of identification number allows for electronic storage and accurate identification of patient data.
8. Put on nonsterile gloves.	Gloves protect the nurse from exposure to blood or body fluids.
9. Prepare the lancet using aseptic technique.	Aseptic technique maintains sterility.
10. Remove the test strip from the vial. **Recap the container immediately.** Test strips also come individually wrapped. **Check that the code number for the strip matches the code number on the monitor screen.**	Immediate recapping protects strips from exposure to humidity, light, and discoloration. Matching code numbers on the strip and glucose monitor ensures that the machine is calibrated correctly.
11. Insert the strip into the meter according to directions for that specific device. Alternately, the strip may be placed in the meter after collection of a sample on the test strip, depending on meter in use.	Correctly inserted strip allows the meter to read the blood glucose level accurately.
12. **Have the patient wash hands with skin cleanser and warm water and dry thoroughly. Alternately, cleanse the skin with an alcohol swab. Allow skin to dry completely.**	Washing with skin cleanser and water or alcohol cleanses the puncture site. Warm water also helps to cause vasodilation. Alcohol can interfere with accuracy of results if not completely dried.
13. Choose a skin site free of lesions and calluses. Make sure there is no edema, and that the site is warm (Van Leeuwen et al., 2011).	Areas with lesions are not suitable for capillary sampling. Calluses, edema, and vasoconstriction (cool to palpation) interfere with the ability to obtain a blood sample.

ACTION	**RATIONALE**
14. Hold the lancet perpendicular to the skin and pierce the site with the lancet (Fig. 1).	Holding the lancet in the proper position facilitates proper skin penetration.
15. Wipe away the first drop of blood with a gauze square or cotton ball if recommended by the manufacturer of the monitor.	Manufacturers recommend discarding the first drop of blood, which may be contaminated by serum or cleansing product, producing an inaccurate reading.
16. Encourage bleeding by lowering the hand, making use of gravity. Lightly stroke the finger, if necessary, until a sufficient amount of blood has formed to cover the sample area on the strip, based on monitor requirements (check instructions for the monitor). Take care not to squeeze the finger, not to squeeze at the puncture site, or not to touch the puncture site or blood.	An appropriate-sized droplet facilitates accurate test results. Squeezing can cause injury to the patient and alter the test result (Ferguson, 2005).
17. Gently touch a drop of blood to the pad to the test strip without smearing it (Fig. 2). Depending on the meter in use, insert the strip in the meter after collection of the sample on the test strip.	Smearing blood on the strip may result in inaccurate test results.

FIGURE 1. Piercing patient's finger with lancet.

FIGURE 2. Applying blood to test strip.

18. Press the time button if directed by the manufacturer.	Correct timing produces accurate results.
19. Apply pressure to the puncture site with a cotton ball or dry gauze. **Do not use an alcohol wipe.**	Pressure causes hemostasis. Alcohol stings and may prolong bleeding.
20. Read the blood glucose results and document appropriately at bedside. Inform the patient of the test result.	Timing depends on type of meter.
21. Turn off the meter, remove the test strip, and dispose of supplies appropriately. Place the lancet in a sharps container.	Proper disposal prevents exposure to blood and accidental needlestick.
22. Remove gloves and any other PPE, if used. Perform hand hygiene.	Removing PPE properly reduces the risk for infection transmission and contamination of other items. Hand hygiene reduces the transmission of microorganisms.

DOCUMENTATION

Guidelines

Document blood glucose level on a flow sheet in the medical record, according to facility policy. Document pertinent patient assessments, any intervention related to glucose level, and any patient teaching. Report abnormal results and/or significant assessments to primary health care provider.

(continued)

SKILL 35-4 OBTAINING A CAPILLARY BLOOD SAMPLE FOR GLUCOSE TESTING *continued*

Sample Documentation

DocuCare **Practice documenting blood glucose testing in *Lippincott DocuCare*.**

11/1/15 0800 Patient performed own fingerstick blood glucose test with minimal guidance. Verbalized rationale for fasting measurement and able to state symptoms of hypoglycemia. Patient's fingerstick blood glucose level 168. Four units regular Humulin insulin given per sliding scale, in addition to 10 units NPH Humulin insulin scheduled for 0800. Patient encouraged to review written guidelines for subcutaneous insulin administration; will review procedure and plan to have patient administer insulin at dinnertime. Patient verbalized an understanding.

—B. Clapp, RN

UNEXPECTED SITUATIONS AND ASSOCIATED INTERVENTIONS

- *Extremity is pale and cool to the touch:* Begin by warming the extremity. Have adult patients warm their hands by rubbing them together. Warm, moist compresses also may be used.

- *Blood glucose level results are above or below normal parameters:* Assess the patient for signs of hyperglycemia or hypoglycemia, respectively. Check the medical record for ordered interventions, such as insulin dosage or carbohydrate administration. Notify the health care provider of results and assessment.

SPECIAL CONSIDERATIONS

General Considerations

- In adults, the middle or ring finger is the preferred site for a capillary blood sample (Malarkey & McMorrow, 2012; Van Leeuwen et al., 2011).

- If the selected site feels cool or appears pale, warm compresses can be applied for 3 to 5 minutes to dilate the capillaries.

- Sampling of blood from an alternative site other than fingertips may have limitations. Blood in the fingertips shows changes in glucose levels more quickly than blood in other parts of the body. This means that alternative site test results may differ from fingertip test results when glucose levels are changing rapidly (e.g., after a meal, taking insulin, or during or after exercise) because the results may be inaccurate. Caution patients to use a fingertip sample if it is less than 2 hours after eating, less than 2 hours after injecting rapid-acting insulin, during exercise or within 2 hours of exercise, when sick or under stress, when having symptoms of hypoglycemia, if unable to recognize symptoms of hypoglycemia, or if site results do not agree with the way the patient feels (FDA, 2013).

- Meters require calibration at least monthly or according to the manufacturer's recommendation, and when a new bottle of test strips is opened. Manufacturer's directions for calibration should be followed. After calibration, the meter is checked for accuracy by testing a control solution containing a known amount of glucose.

- Inadequate sampling can cause errors in the results. It is very important to be aware of requirements for the specific monitor used.

- Continuous glucose monitoring systems have become available. These devices use sensors placed just below the skin in the subcutaneous tissue and electrical stimulation to draw interstitial fluid through intact skin into the sensor. A transmitter sends information about glucose levels from the sensor to a pager-like wireless monitor. These devices provide real-time measurements of glucose levels at 1-minute or 5-minute intervals (NDIC, 2012). These systems supplement standard fingerstick meters and provide a way to see glucose trends and track patterns.

Infant and Child Considerations

- Heel sticks, using the outer aspect of the heel, may be used for infants. Warming the heel before the sample is taken dilates the blood vessels in the area and aids in sampling (Perry et al., 2010). This technique is not without controversy, as it is painful and can lead to fibrosis, scarring, and necrotizing osteochondritis (from puncture of the heel bone; Shah & Ohlsson, 2012; Perry et al.).

Older Adult Considerations

- Meters are available with large digital readouts or audio components for patients with visual impairments.

Home Care Considerations

- Patients monitor blood glucose levels routinely at home. Provide education focusing on important elements of diabetes education to assist patients in managing their diabetes, including the signs, symptoms, and management of hypoglycemia and hyperglycemia; correct administration of oral hypoglycemic agents and/or insulin; fingerstick blood glucose monitoring; and the accurate use of fingerstick blood glucose monitoring equipment (Hughes, 2012).
- Many different types of monitors are available. Assist patients to identify desirable features for individual use.

DEVELOPING CLINICAL REASONING

1. Prepare a diet for an economically disadvantaged family consisting of a single working mother and her three children, ages 3 to 14 years, taking into consideration the family's culture (specify a minority culture in your locale) and yearly income (below poverty level).

2. Prepare a 1-day menu that meets the recommended daily allowance of essential nutrients for the following patients:
   - An obese teenager
   - A child vegetarian
   - An executive with high blood pressure who dines out frequently with clients
   - A woman running a minimum of 12 miles daily as she trains for a marathon

PRACTICING FOR NCLEX

1. A nurse is calculating the body mass index (BMI) of a 35-year-old male patient who is extremely obese. The patient's height is 5′6″ and his current weight is 325 pounds. What would the nurse document as his BMI?
   a. 50.5
   b. 52.4
   c. 54.5
   d. 55.2

2. A nurse is helping an overweight female patient to devise a meal plan to lose 2 pounds per week. How many calories would the patient need to delete per day in order to accomplish this goal?
   a. 250 calories
   b. 500 calories
   c. 750 calories
   d. 1000 calories

3. A nurse is feeding an elderly patient who has dementia. Which intervention should the nurse perform to facilitate this process?
   a. Stroke the underside of the patient's chin to promote swallowing.
   b. Serve meals in different places and at different times.
   c. Offer a whole tray of various foods to choose from.
   d. Avoid between-meal snacks to ensure hunger at mealtime.

4. A 56-year-old male patient who has COPD is refusing to eat. Which intervention would be most helpful in stimulating his appetite?
   a. Administering pain medication after meals.
   b. Encouraging food from home when possible.
   c. Scheduling his respiratory therapy before each meal.
   d. Reinforcing the importance of his eating exactly what is delivered to him.

5. A nurse is feeding a patient who is experiencing dysphagia. Which nursing intervention would the nurse initiate for this patient?
   a. Feed the patient solids first and then liquids last.
   b. Place the head of the bed at a 30-degree angle during feeding.
   c. Puree all foods to a liquid consistency.
   d. Provide a thirty-minute rest period prior to mealtime.

6. A nurse is evaluating patients to determine their need for total parenteral nutrition (TPN). Which patients would be the best candidates for this type of nutritional support? Select all that apply.
   a. A patient with irritable bowel syndrome who has intractable diarrhea
   b. A patient with celiac disease not absorbing nutrients from the GI tract
   c. A patient who is underweight and needs short-term nutritional support
   d. A patient who is comatose and needs long-term nutritional support
   e. A patient who has anorexia and refuses to take foods via the oral route
   f. A patient with burns who has not been able to eat adequately for 5 days

7. A nurse is feeding a patient who states that she is feeling nauseated and can't eat what is being offered. What would be the most appropriate initial action of the nurse in this situation?
   a. Remove the tray from the room.
   b. Administer an antiemetic and encourage the patient to take small amounts.
   c. Explore with the patient why she does not want to eat her food.
   d. Offer high-calorie snacks such as pudding and ice cream.

8. A 62-year-old male patient has been admitted to the alcoholic referral unit in the local hospital. Based on an understanding of the effects of alcohol on the GI tract, which is a priority concern related to nutrition?
   a. Vitamin B malnutrition
   b. Obesity
   c. Dehydration
   d. Vitamin C deficiency

9. A nurse is caring for a newly placed gastrostomy tube of a postoperative patient. Which nursing action is performed correctly?
   a. The nurse dips a cotton-tipped applicator into sterile saline solution and gently cleans around the insertion site.
   b. The nurse wets a washcloth and washes the area around the tube with soap and water.
   c. The nurse adjusts the external disk every 3 hours to avoid crusting around the tube.
   d. The nurse tapes a gauze dressing over the site after cleansing it.

10. A nurse is assessing a patient who has been NPO (nothing by mouth) prior to abdominal surgery. The patient is ordered a clear liquid diet for breakfast, to advance to a house diet as tolerated. Which assessments would indicate to the nurse that the patient's diet should not be advanced?
    a. The patient consumed 75% of the liquids on her breakfast tray.
    b. The patient tells you she is hungry.
    c. The patient's abdomen is soft, nondistended, with bowel sounds.
    d. The patient reports fullness and diarrhea after breakfast.

11. A patient who is moved to a hospital bed following throat surgery is ordered to receive continuous tube feedings through a small-bore nasogastric tube. Following placement of the tube, which nursing action would the nurse initiate to ensure correct placement of the tube?
    a. Auscultate the bowel sounds.
    b. Measure the gastric aspirate pH.
    c. Measure the amount of residual in the tube.
    d. Order radiographic examination of the tube.

12. Which of the following nursing diagnoses would be most appropriate for a patient with a body mass index (BMI) of 18?
    a. Risk for Imbalanced Nutrition: More Than Body Requirements
    b. Imbalanced Nutrition: More Than Body Requirements
    c. Readiness for Enhanced Nutrition
    d. Imbalanced Nutrition: Less Than Body Requirements

13. A nurse is inserting a nasogastric tube ordered for a patient to monitor bleeding in his GI tract. When the tube is being passed through the pharynx, the patient begins to cough and show signs of respiratory distress. What would be the priority action of the nurse upon this assessment?
    a. Keep the tube in place and notify the primary care provider immediately.
    b. Stop advancing the tube and pull it back into the nasal area.
    c. Ask the patient if he wants the nurse to stop the procedure.
    d. Call for help to perform CPR.

14. A nurse is administering a tube feeding for a patient who is post bowel surgery. When attempting to aspirate the contents, the nurse notes that the tube is clogged. What would be the nurse's next action following this assessment?
    a. Use warm water and gentle pressure to remove the clog.
    b. Use a stylet to unclog the tubes.
    c. Administer cola to remove the clog.
    d. Replace the tube with a new one.

15. A nurse performs presurgical assessments of patients in an ambulatory care center. Which patient would the nurse report to the surgeon as possibly needing surgery to be postponed?
    a. A 19-year-old patient who is a vegan
    b. An elderly patient who takes daily nutritional drinks
    c. A 43-year-old patient who takes ginko bilboa and an aspirin daily
    d. An infant who is breast-feeding

ANSWERS WITH RATIONALES

1. **b.** $$BMI = \frac{weight\ in\ pounds\ (325)}{(height\ in\ inches)(66) \times (height\ in\ inches)(66)} \times 703$$
   $$BMI = 52.4$$

2. **d.** 1 lb (0.45 kg) of body fat equals about 3,500 cal. Therefore, to gain or lose 1 lb (0.45 kg) in a week, daily calorie intake should be increased or decreased, respectively, by 500 cal (3,500 cal divided by 7 days = 500 cal/day). Similarly, a weight gain or loss of 2 lb (0.9 kg) per week would require an adjustment of 1,000 cal/day.

3. **a.** To feed a patient with dementia, the nurse should stroke the underside of the patient's chin to promote swallowing, serve meals in the same place and at the same time, provide one food item at a time since a whole tray may be overwhelming, and provide between-meal snacks that are easy to consume using the hands.

4. **b.** Food from home that the patient enjoys may stimulate him to eat. Pain medication should be given before meals, respiratory therapy should be scheduled after meals, and telling the patient what he must eat is no guarantee that he will comply.

5. **d.** When feeding a patient who has dysphagia, the nurse should provide a 30-minute rest period prior to mealtime to promote swallowing; alternate solids and liquids when feeding the patient; sit the patient upright or, if on bedrest, elevate the head of the bed at a 90-degree angle; and initiate a nutrition consult for diet modification and food size and/or consistency.

6. **a, b, f.** Assessment criteria used to determine the need for TPN include an inability to achieve or maintain enteral access; motility disorders; intractable diarrhea; impaired absorption of nutrients from the GI tract (patient with celiac disease) and when oral intake has been or is expected to be inadequate over a 7- to 14-day period (Worthington & Gilbert, 2012; A.S.P.E.N., 2002). TPN promotes tissue healing and is a good choice for a patient with burns who has an inadequate diet. Oral intake is the best method of feeding; the second best method is via the enteral route. For short-term use (less than 4 weeks), a nasogastric or nasointestinal route is usually selected. A gastrostomy (enteral feeding) is the preferred route to deliver enteral nutrition in the patient who

is comatose because the gastroesophageal sphincter remains intact, making regurgitation and aspiration less likely than with NG tube feedings. Patients who refuse to take food should not be force fed nutrients against their will.

7. *a.* The first action of the nurse when a patient has nausea is to remove the tray from the room. The nurse may then offer small amounts of foods and liquids such as crackers or ginger ale. The nurse may also administer a prescribed antiemetic and try small amounts of food when it takes effect.

8. *a.* The need for B vitamins is increased in alcoholics because these nutrients are used to metabolize alcohol, thus depleting their supply. Alcohol abuse specifically affects the B vitamins. Obesity, dehydration, and vitamin C deficiency may be present, but these are not directly related to the effect of alcohol on the GI tract.

9. *a.* When caring for a new gastrostomy tube, the nurse would use a cotton-tipped applicator dipped in sterile saline to gently cleanse the area, removing any crust or drainage. The nurse would not use a washcloth with soap and water on a new gastrostomy tube, but may use this method if the site is healed. Also, once the sutures are removed, the nurse should rotate the external bumper 90 degrees once a day. The nurse should leave the site open to air unless there is drainage. If there is drainage, one thickness of precut gauze should be placed under the external bumper and changed as needed to keep the area dry.

10. *d.* Tolerance of diet can be assessed by the following: absence of nausea, vomiting, and diarrhea; absence of feelings of fullness; absence of abdominal pain and distention; feelings of hunger; and the ability to consume at least 50% to 75% of the food on the meal tray.

11. *d.* Although a radiographic examination exposes the patient to radiation and is costly, it is still the most accurate method to check correct tube placement. Other methods that can be used are aspiration of gastric contents and measurement of the pH of the aspirate. The recommended method for checking placement, other than a radiograph, is measuring the pH of the aspirate. Visual assessment of aspirated gastric contents is also suggested as a tool to check placement. In addition, the length of the exposed tube is measured after insertion and documented. Tube length should be checked and compared with this initial measurement, in conjunction with the previous two methods for checking tube placement. The auscultatory method is considered inaccurate and unre-

liable. Measurement of residual amount does not confirm placement.

12. *d.* A patient with a body mass index (BMI) of 18 is considered underweight, therefore a diagnosis of Imbalanced Nutrition: Less than Body Requirements is appropriate. The patient is not at risk for imbalanced nutrition because it is already a problem and certainly is not experiencing nutrition that is more than body requirements. Readiness for Enhanced Nutrition is appropriate when there is a healthy pattern of nutrient intake that is sufficient for meeting metabolic needs and can be strengthened and enhanced.

13. *b.* As the tube is passing through the pharynx and the patient begins to cough and show respiratory distress, the nurse should stop advancing the tube and pull it back into the nasal area. The nurse should also support the patient as he regains normal breathing ability and composure and have him try again if he feels able to.

14. *a.* In order to remove a clog in a feeding tube, the nurse should try using warm water and gentle pressure to unclog it. A stylet should never be used to unclog a tube, and cola and meat tenderizers have not been shown effective in removing clogs. The nurse should first attempt to remove the clog, and if unsuccessful, the tube should be replaced.

15. *c.* A patient taking gingko biloba (an herbal), aspirin, and vitamin E (dietary supplement) may have to have surgery postponed due to an increased risk for excessive bleeding, because each of these substances have anticoagulant properties. Being a vegan should not affect surgery unless the patient has serious nutritional deficiencies. Drinking nutritional drinks and breastfeeding do not adversely affect the outcomes of surgery.

TAYLOR SUITE RESOURCES

Explore these additional resources to enhance learning for this chapter:

- NCLEX-Style Questions and other resources on the**Point**, http://thePoint.lww.com/Taylor8e
- *Study Guide for Fundamentals of Nursing, 8th edition*
- Adaptive Learning | Powered by prepU, http://thepoint.lww.com/prepu
- *Skill Checklists for Fundamentals of Nursing, 8th edition*
- *Taylor's Clinical Nursing Skills:* Chapter 11, Nutrition; Chapter 18, Skill 18-8
- *Taylor's Video Guide to Clinical Nursing Skills:* Nutrition
- *Lippincott DocuCare* Fundamentals cases

Bibliography

Academy of Nutrition and Dietetics. (2012). Healthy weight during pregnancy. Available at http://www.eatright.org/Public/content.aspx?id=10933

Ackley, B. J., & Ladwig, G. B. (2011). *Nursing Diagnosis Handbook* (9th ed.). St. Louis: Elsevier/Mosby.

Amella, E. J., & Lawrence, J. F. (2007). Eating and feeding issues in older adults with dementia. *Part II: Interventions.* Available at http://consultgerirn.org/uploads/File/trythis/try_this_d11_2.pdf

American Association of Critical-Care Nurses (AACN). (2010). Practice alert: Verification of feeding tube placement. Available at http://aacn.org/WD/Practice/Docs/PracticeAlerts/Verification_of_Feeding_Tube_Placement_05-2005.pdf.

American Association of Critical-Care Nurses (AACN). (2012). Practice alert. Prevention of aspiration. *CriticalCareNurse, 32*(3), 71–73.

American Dietetic Association (ADA). (2008). Position of the American Dietetic Association: Ethical and legal issues in nutrition, hydration, and feeding. *Journal of the American Dietetic Association, 108*(5), 873–82.

American Society for Parenteral and Enteral Nutrition (A.S.P.E.N.) (2011). Guidelines: Access for administration of nutrition support. Available at http://www.nutritioncare.org/Professional_Resources/Guidelines_and_Standards/Guidelines/Access_for_Administration_of_Nutrition_Support/

American Society for Parenteral and Enteral Nutrition (A.S.P.E.N.) (2009a). Enteral nutrition practice recommendations. Enteral Access Devices: Selection, Insertion, and Maintenance Considerations. Available at http://www.nutritioncare.org/Professional_Resources/Guidelines_and_Standards/Guidelines/2009_ENPR_-_Section_V_Enteral_Access_Devices/#Section_C

American Society for Parenteral and Enteral Nutrition (A.S.P.E.N.) (2009b). Enteral nutrition practice recommendations. Enteral nutrition administration.

Available at http://www.nutritioncare.org/Professional_Resources/Guidelines_and_Standards/Guidelines/2009_ENPR_-_Section_VI_Enteral_Nutrition_Administration/

American Society for Parenteral and Enteral Nutrition (A.S.P.E.N.) (2009c). Enteral nutrition practice recommendations. Medication administration. Available at http://www.nutritioncare.org/Professional_Resources/Guidelines_and_Standards/Guidelines/2009_ENPR_-_Section_VII_Medication_Administration/

American Society for Parenteral and Enteral Nutrition (A.S.P.E.N.) and Society of Critical Care Medicine (SCCM). (2009). Guidelines for the provision and assessment of nutrition support therapy in the adult critically ill patient. *Journal of Parenteral and Enteral Nutrition, 33*(3), 277–316.

Aselage, M. B. (2012). Measuring mealtime difficulties: eating, feeding and meal behaviours in older adults with dementia. *Journal of Clinical Nursing, 19*(5–6), 621–631.

Beckstrand, J., Cirgin Ellet, M., & McDaniel, A. (2007). Predicting internal distance to the stomach for positioning nasogastric and orogastric feeding tubes in children. *Journal of Advanced Nursing, 59*(3), 274–289.

Best, C., & Summers, J. (2010). Strategies for nutritional care in acute settings. *Nursing Older People, 22*(6), 27–31.

Best, C., & Wilson, N. (2011). Advice on safe administration of medications via enteral feeding tubes. *British Journal of Community Nursing, Nutrition Supplement* (Nov), S6–S10.

Best, C. (2005). Caring for the patient with a nasogastric tube. *Nursing Standard, 20*(3), 59–65.

Bloomfield, J., & Pegram, A. (2012). Improving nutrition and hydration in the hospital: the nurse's responsibility. *Nursing Standard, 26*(34), 52–56.

Boltz, M., Capezuti, E., Fulmer, T., & Zwicker, D. (eds.) (2012). *Evidence-based geriatric nursing protocols for best practice* (4th ed.). New York: Springer Publishing Company.

Bourgault, A., Ipe, L., Weaver, J., Swartz, S., & O'Dea, P. J. (2007). Development of evidence-based guidelines and critical care nurses' knowledge of enteral feeding. *Critical Care Nurse, 27*(4), 17–29.

Brown, A. W. (2008). Clinician's guide to diabetes gadgets and gizmos. *Clinical Diabetes, 26*(2), 66–71.

Bruening, M., Eisenberg, M., MacLehose, R., Nanney, M. S., Story, M., & Neumark-Sztainer, D., (2012). relationship between adolescents' and their friends' eating behaviors: Breakfast, fruit, vegetables, whole-grain, and dairy intake. *Journal of the Academy of Nutrition and Dietetics, 112*(10), 1608–1613.

Bulechek, G. M, Butcher, H. K., Dochterman, J. M., & Wagner, C. M. (Eds.). (2013). *Nursing interventions classification (NIC)* (6th ed.). St. Louis: Elsevier/ Mosby.

Centers for Disease Control and Prevention (CDC). (2011). Healthy weight. Assessing your weight. BMI percentile calculator for child and teen. Available at http://apps.nccd.cdc.gov/dnpabmi/

Chau, J. P. C., Lo, S. H. S., Thompson, D. R., Fernandez, R., & Griffiths (2011). Use of end-tidal carbon dioxide detection to determine correct placement of nasogastric tube: A meta-analysis. *International Journal of Nursing Studies, 48*(4), 513–521.

Cole, D. (2012). Optimising nutrition for older people with dementia. *Nursing Standard, 26*(20), 41–48.

Dale, L. (2006). Make a point about alternate site blood glucose sampling. *Nursing, 36*(2), 52–53.

DiMaria-Ghalili, R., & Amella, E. (2005). Nutrition in older adults. *American Journal of Nursing, 105*(3), 40–51.

DiMaria-Ghalili, R., & Guenter, P. (2008). The mini nutritional assessment. *American Journal of Nursing, 108*(2), 50–59.

Dudek, S. (2014). *Nutrition essentials for nursing practice* (7th ed.). Philadelphia: Wolters Kluwer Health/Lippincott Williams & Wilkins.

Dunne, A. (2010). Nutrition and dementia. *Nursing & Residential Care, 12*(3). 112, 114, 116.

Eisenstadt, E.S. (2010). Dysphagia and aspiration pneumonia in older adults. *Journal of the American Academy of Nurse Practitioners, 22*(1), 17–22.

Ellet, M. (2004). What is known about methods of correctly placing gastric tubes in adults and children. *Gastroenterology Nursing, 27*(6), 253–261.

Ferguson, A. (2005). Blood glucose monitoring. *Nursing Times, 101*(38), 28–29.

Freeman, D., Saxton, V., & Holberton, J. (2012). Estimation of gastric tube insertion length in newborns. *Advances in Neonatal Care, 12*(3), 179–182.

Forest-Lalande, L. (2012). The management of feeding gastrostomies. *Gastrointestinal Nursing, 10*(3), 28–35.

Gilbert, R. T., & Burns, S. M. (2012). Increasing the safety of blind gastric tube placement in pediatric patients: The design and testing of a procedure using a carbon dioxide detection device. *Journal of Pediatric Nursing, 27*(5), 528–532.

Grossman, S., & Porth, C.M. (2014). Porth's pathophysiology: concepts of altered health states. (9th ed.). Philadelphia: Wolters Kluwer Health/Lippincott Williams & Wilkins.

Hadaway, L. (2005). Administering parenteral nutrition with other I.V. drugs. *Nursing, 35*(2), 26.

Hinkle, J. L., & Cheever, K. H. (2014). *Brunner & Suddarth's textbook of medical-surgical nursing* (13th ed.). Philadelphia: Wolters Kluwer Health/Lippincott Williams & Wilkins.

Hogan-Quigley, B., Palm, M. L., & Bickley, L. (2012). *Bates' nursing guide to physical examination and history taking.* Philadelphia: Wolters Kluwer Health/Lippincott Williams & Wilkins.

Huether, S. E., & McCance, K. L. (2012.) *Understanding pathophysiology* (5th ed.). St. Louis: Elsevier.

Hughes, L. (2012). Think "SAFE." Four crucial elements for diabetes education. *Nursing, 42*(1), 58–61.

Hughes, S. M. (2011). Management of dysphagia in stroke patients. *Nursing Older People, 23*(3), 21–24.

Infusion Nurses Society (INS). (2011). Infusion nursing standards of practice. *Journal of Infusion Nursing, 34*(Suppl: 1S).

Jarvis, C. (2012). *Physical examination & health assessment* (6th ed.). St. Louis: Elsevier/Saunders.

Jeejeebhoy, K. N. (2012). Parenteral nutrition in the intensive care unit. *Nutrition Reviews, 70*(11), 623–630.

Kaiser, M. J., Bauer, J. M., Uter, W., Donini, L. M., Stange, I., Volkert, D., Diekmann, R., ... Sieber, C. C. (2011). Prospective validation of the modified Mini Nutritional Assessment Short-Forms in the community, nursing home, and rehabilitation setting. *Journal of the American Geriatrics Society, 59*(11), 2124–2128.

Kee, J. L., Hayes, E. R., & McCuistion, L. E. (2012). *Pharmacology: A Nursing Process Approach* (7th ed.). St. Louis: Elsevier/Saunders.

Kenny, D. J., & Goodman, P. (2010). Care of the patient with enteral tube feeding. An evidence-based practice protocol. *Nursing Research, 59*(1S), S22–S31.

Khair, J. (2005). Guidelines for testing the placing of nasogastric tubes. *Nursing Times, 101*(20), 26–27.

Kyle G. (2011). Managing dysphagia in older people with dementia. *British Journal of Community Nursing, 16*(1), 6–10.

Kyle, T., & Carman, S. (2013). *Essentials of pediatric nursing* (2nd ed.). Philadelphia: Wolters Kluwer Health/Lippincott Williams & Wilkins.

Lichtenstein, A., & Russell, R. (2005). Essential nutrients: Food or supplements? Where should the emphasis be? *JAMA: Journal of the American Medical Association, 294*(3), 351–358.

Lin, L., Watson, R., & Wu, S. (2010). What is associated with low food intake in older people with dementia? *Journal of Clinical Nursing, 19*(1–2), 53–59.

Malarkey, L. M., & McMorrow, M. E. (2012). *Saunders nursing guide to laboratory and diagnostic tests* (2nd ed.). St. Louis: Elsevier/Saunders.

Marik, P. E., & Flemmer, M. (2012). Do dietary supplements have beneficial health effects in industrialized nations: What is the evidence? *Journal of Parenteral and Enteral Nutrition, 36*(2), 159–168.

McClave, S., Lukan, J., Stefater, J., Lowen, C., Looney, S., Matheson, P., Gleeson, K., & Spain, D. (2005). Poor validity of residual volumes as a marker for risk of aspiration in critically ill patients. *Critical Care Medicine, 33*(2), 324–330.

McGinnis, C. M., Worthington, P., & Lord, L. M (2010). Nasogastric versus feeding tubes in critically ill patients. *CriticalCareNurse, 30*(6), 80–82.

Medlin, S. (2012). Recent developments in enteral feeding for adults: an update. *British Journal of Nursing, 21*(18), 1061–1067.

Meetoo, D. D., McAllister, G., & West, A. (2011). Assessing glycaemic control: self-monitoring of blood glucose. *British Journal of Nursing, 20*(15), 919–925.

Metheny, N. (2012). Preventing aspiration in older adults with dysphagia. Available at http://consultgerirn.org/uploads/File/trythis/try_this_20.pdf

Metheny, N. (2008). Residual volume measurement should be retained in enteral feeding protocols. *American Journal of Critical Care, 17*(1), 62–64.

Metheny, N. A., Mills, A. C., & Stewart, B. J. (2012). Monitoring for intolerance to gastric tube feedings: a national survey. *American Journal of Critical Care, 21*(2), e33–e40.

Metheny, N., & Meert, K. (2004). Monitoring feeding tube placement. *Nutrition in Clinical Practice, 19*(5), 487–542.

Metheny, N., Schnelker, R., McGinnis, J., Zimmerman, G., Duke, C., Merritt, B., ... Oliver, D. A. (2005). Indicators of tube site during feedings. *Journal of Neuroscience Nursing, 37*(6), 320–325.

Metheny, N., & Stewart, B. (2002). Testing feeding tube placement during continuous tube feedings. *Applied Nursing Research, 15*(4), 254–258.

Metheny, N. M. (2012). *Fluid and electrolyte balance: Nursing considerations* (5th ed.). Sudbury, MA: Jones & Bartlett Learning.

Miller, C. (2008). Communication difficulties in hospitalized older adults with dementia: Try these techniques to make communicating with patients easier and more effective. *American Journal of Nursing, 108*(3), 58–66.

Miller, S. (2011). Capnometry vs pH testing in nasogastric tube placement. *Gastrointestinal Nursing, 9*(2), 30–33.

Moorhead, S., Johnson, M., Maas, M. L., & Swanson, E. (Eds.). (2013). *Nursing Outcomes Classification (NOC)* (5th ed.). St. Louis: Elsevier/Mosby.

Munera-Seeley, V., Ochoa, J., Brown, N., Bayless, A., Correia, M., Bryk, J., et al. (2008). Use of a colorimetric carbon dioxide sensor for nasoenteric feeding tube placement in critical care patients compared with clinical methods and radiography. *Nutrition in Clinical Practice, 23*(3), 318–321.

NANDA International (NANDA-I). (2012). *Nursing diagnoses: Definitions & classification 2012–2014.* West Sussex, UK: Wiley-Blackwell.

National Diabetes Information Clearinghouse (NDIC). (2012). *Continuous glucose monitoring.* Available http://diabetes.niddk.nih.gov/dm/pubs/glucose-monitor/index.aspx#continue.

National Institutes of Health (NIH), National Heart, Lung and Blood Institute (NHLBI). (2012a). How are overweight and obesity diagnosed? Available at http://www.nhlbi.nih.gov/health/health-topics/topics/obe/diagnosis.html

National Institutes of Health (NIH), National Heart, Lung and Blood Institute (NHBLI). (2012b). What are overweight and obesity? Available at http://www.nhlbi.nih.gov/health/health-topics/topics/obe/.

National Institutes of Health (NIH), National Heart, Lung and Blood Institute (NHLBI). (2005). Aim for a healthy weight. NIH publication no. 05-5213. Bethesda, MD: Author. Available at www.nhlbi.nih.gov/health/public/heart/obesity/aim_hwt.htm

National Institutes of Health (NIH), NIH State-of-the-Science Panel. (2007). NIH State-of-the-Science Conference Statement: Multivitamin/mineral supplements and chronic disease prevention. *Journal of Clinical Nutrition, 85*(1), Supplement: 257S–264S.

National Institutes of Health (NIH), National Heart, Lung and Blood Institute (NHLBI). (2000). NHLBI Obesity Education Initiative. The practical guide: Identification, evaluation, and treatment of overweight and obesity in adults. NIH publication no. 00-4084. Available at www.nhlbi.nih.gov/guidelines/obesity/prctgd_c.pdf

Ojo, O., & Bowden, J. (2012). Infection control in enteral feed and feeding systems in the community. *British Journal of Nursing, 21*(18), 1070–1075.

Palmer, J., & Metheny, N. (2008). Preventing aspiration during nasogastric, nasointestinal, or gastrostomy tube feedings. *American Journal of Nursing, 108*(2), 40–44, 47–49.

Perry, S. E., Hockenberry, M. J., Lowdermilk, D. L., & Wilson, D. (2010). *Maternal child nursing care* (4th ed.). Maryland Heights, MO: Elsevier/Mosby.

Ritter, L. A., & Hoffman, N. A. (2010). *Multicultural health.* Boston: Jones and Bartlett.

Schiavone, P. A., Stoner, N. E., Compher, C. W., Kinosian, B. P., & Boullata, J. I. (2010). Management of catheter-related infection in patients receiving home parenteral nutrition. Available at http://www.medicine.virginia.edu/clinical/departments/medicine/divisions/digestive-health/nutrition-support-team/nutrition-articles/SchiavoneArticle.pdf

Shah, V., & Ohlsson, A. (2012). *Venepuncture versus heel lance for blood sampling in term neonates. Cochrane Database of Systematic Reviews.* Available http://summaries.cochrane.org/CD001452/venepuncture-versus-heel-lance-for-blood-sampling-interm-neonates.

Skates, J. J., & Anthony, P. (2012). Identifying geriatric malnutrition in nursing practice: The Mini Nutritional Assessment (MNA)—An evidence-based screening tool. *Journal of Gerontological Nursing, 38*(3), 18–27.

Söderhamn, U., Flateland, S., Jessen, L., & Söderhamn, O. (2011). Perceived health and risk of undernutrition: a comparison of different nutritional screening results in older patients. *Journal of Clinical Nursing, 20*(15/16), 2162–2171.

Spector, R. E. (2009). *Cultural diversity in health and illness* (7th ed.). Upper Saddle River, NJ: Pearson/Prentice Hall.

Stayner, J. L., Bhatnagar, A., McGinn A. N., & Fang, J. C. (2012). Feeding tube placement: Errors and complications. *Nutrition in Clinical Practice, 27*(6), 738–748.

Stepter, C. R. (2012). Maintaining placement of temporary enteral feeding tubes in adults: A critical appraisal of the evidence. *MedSurgNursing, 21*(2), 61–69.

Tabloski, P. (2010). *Gerontological nursing* (2nd ed.). Upper Saddle River, NJ: Pearson.

Taylor, J. J., & Cohen, B. J. (2013). *Memmler's structure and function of the human body* (10th ed.). Philadelphia: Wolters Kluwer Health/Lippincott Williams & Wilkins.

Tracey, D., & Patterson, G. (2006). Care of the gastrostomy tube in the home. *Home Healthcare Nurse, 24*(6), 381–386.

Turgay, A. S., & Khorshid, L. (2010). Effectiveness of the auscultatory and pH methods in predicting feeding tube placement. *Journal of Clinical Nursing, 19*(11–12), 1553–1559.

U.S. Department of Agriculture (USDA). (2012). ChooseMyPlate.gov. Available at http://www.choosemyplate.gov/index.html

U.S. Department of Agriculture (USDA) and Department of Health and Human Services (DHHS). (2010). Dietary guidelines for Americans 2010. Available at http://www.health.gov/dietaryguidelines/2010.asp

U.S. Food and Drug Administration (FDA). (2013). *Medical devices. Blood glucose monitoring devices.* Available http://www.fda.gov/%20medicaldevices/productsandmedicalprocedures/invitrodiagnostics/glucosetestingdevices/default.htm.

U.S. Food and Drug Administration (FDA). (2012a). Food. Trans fat now listed with saturated fat and cholesterol. Available at http://www.fda.gov/food/ingredientspackaginglabeling/labelingnutrition/ucm274590.htm

U.S. Food and Drug Administration (FDA). (2012b). How to understand and use the nutrition facts label. Available at http://www.fda.gov/food/ingredients packaginglabeling/labelingnutrition/ucm274593.htm

U.S. Food and Drug Administration (FDA). (2012c). Smart nutrition 101. Dietary reference intakes. Available at http://www.nutrition.gov/smart-nutrition-101/dietary-reference-intakes-rdas

Van Leeuwen, A. M., Poelhuis-Leth, D., & Bladh, M. L. (2011). *Davis's Comprehensive Handbook of Laboratory & Diagnostic Tests with Nursing Implications* (4th ed.). Philadelphia: F. A. Davis.

VISN 8 Patient Safety Center. (2009). Safe patient handling and movement algorithms. Available at http://www.visn8.va.gov/patientsafetycenter/safepthandling/

Weight-control Information Network (WIN): National Institute of Diabetes and Digestive and Kidney Diseases (NDDK). (2012a). Eating healthy & physical activity across your lifespan. Better health and you: Tips for adults. Available at http://win.niddk.nih.gov/publications/PDFs/tipsforadults804bw.pdf

Weight-control Information Network (WIN): National Institute of Diabetes and Digestive and Kidney Diseases (NDDK). (2012b). Overweight and obesity statistics. Prevalence of overweight and obesity. Available at http://win.niddk.nih.gov/statistics/index.htm#b

Whitmore, C. (2012). Blood glucose monitoring: an overview. *British Journal of Nursing, 21*(10), 583–587.

Wilson, N., & Blackett, B. (2012). Parenteral nutrition: considerations for practice. *British Journal of Community Nursing, Nutrition Supplement* (May), S16–S19.

Worthington, P. H., & Gilbert, K. A. (2012). Parenteral nutrition. Risks, complications, and management. *Journal of Infusion Nursing, 35*(1), 52–64.

Zelig, R., & Rigassio Radler, D. (2012). Understanding the properties of common dietary supplements: Clinical implications for healthcare practitioners. *Nutrition in Clinical Practice, 27*(6), 767–776.

36

Urinary Elimination

ELANA JASPERS

Elana Jaspers, age 83, is experiencing a decreased ability to perform activities of daily living (ADLs) related to arthritis. After being hospitalized for pneumonia, she moved into an extended-care facility. A short time after her arrival in her new home, Mrs. Jaspers began having difficulty with urinary incontinence.

ANNA GALINSKI

Anna Galinski, age 85, is frail and has numerous medical problems. She lives in a long-term care facility and, like many of the residents, was on a toileting regimen. Not long after a new charge nurse arrived, Anna, and the other residents who used to be on toileting regimens, had indwelling catheters inserted.

MIDORI MORITA

Midori Morita, age 69, is taking care of her 70-year-old husband at home. She asks, "Should I talk with my husband's doctor about getting him a urinary catheter? Ever since he came home from the hospital this last time, he seems unable to use the urinal. He dribbles urine constantly and I can't keep up with the laundry. He had a catheter in the hospital."

KEY TERMS

autonomic bladder	intermittent urethral catheter	stress incontinence
bacteriuria	Kegel exercises	suprapubic catheter
continent urinary reservoir	micturition	total incontinence
cutaneous ureterostomy	mixed incontinence	transient incontinence
enuresis	nephrotoxic	urge incontinence
external condom catheter	nocturia	urinary diversion
functional incontinence	overflow incontinence	urinary incontinence
hematuria	postvoid residual (PVR)	urinary retention
ileal conduit	reflex incontinence	urination
indwelling urethral catheter	specific gravity	voiding

Elimination from the urinary tract helps to rid the body of waste products and materials that exceed bodily needs. This chapter describes the anatomy and physiology of the urinary system and factors that affect **urination**, the process of emptying the bladder. In addition, a practical guide for assessing urinary elimination is included, along with detailed information on specific assessment measures, such as monitoring fluid intake, collecting urine specimens, testing urine, and assisting with other diagnostic procedures. Analysis of urinary assessment data may lead the nurse to identify one or more nursing diagnoses or to detect a medical problem early. When planning care, the nurse establishes expected patient outcomes. This chapter presents specific nursing strategies to address these patient outcomes. The chapter concludes with a patient care study that illustrates how the nurse's knowledge of the urinary system and urinary pathology forms the foundation for specific nursing interventions to resolve urinary problems.

Problems involving urinary elimination can be so embarrassing to patients that they may no longer participate in activities outside the home. Nurses assisting patients with urinary elimination problems or intervening to resolve health problems related to urination utilize many specialized skills. Refer to the Reflective Practice box (on page 1266).

ANATOMY AND PHYSIOLOGY
Kidneys and Ureters

The kidneys are located on either side of the vertebral column behind the peritoneum, in the upper abdominal cavity. One of the more significant functions of the kidneys is to help maintain the composition and volume of body fluids. About once every 30 minutes, the body's total blood volume passes through the kidneys for waste removal. The kidneys filter and excrete blood constituents that are not needed and retain those that are. Despite varying kinds and amounts of food and fluids ingested, body fluids remain relatively stable if the kidneys are functioning properly. Urine, the waste product excreted by the kidneys, contains organic, inorganic, and liquid wastes.

The nephron is the basic structural and functional unit of the kidneys. There are about 1 million nephrons in each kidney. Each nephron consists of a complicated system of arterioles, capillaries, and tubules. Nephrons remove the end products of metabolism, such as urea, creatinine, and uric acid from the blood plasma and form urine. The nephrons maintain and regulate fluid balance through the mechanisms of selective reabsorption and secretion of water, electrolytes, and other substances.

Once formed, urine from the nephrons empties into the pelvis of each kidney. From each kidney, urine is transported by rhythmic peristalsis through the ureters to the urinary bladder. The ureters enter the bladder obliquely. A fold of membrane in the bladder closes the entrance to the ureters so that urine is not forced up the ureters to the kidneys when pressure exists in the bladder. Figure 36-1 (on page 1267) shows the male and female urinary systems and the position of the kidneys and ureters in the abdomen.

REFLECTIVE PRACTICE: CULTIVATING QSEN COMPETENCIES

CHALLENGE TO ETHICAL SKILLS

We had a strange experience during our rotation in a community long-term care facility. I was assigned to care for Anna Galinski, an 85-year-old frail woman with numerous medical problems. She, like many of the residents, was on a toileting regimen. In the middle of our 7-week experience, a new charge nurse started working on our unit. All of a sudden, Anna and the other residents who

used to be on toileting regimens were given indwelling catheters. Knowing the greatly increased risk of infections with indwelling catheters, we suspected that the decision to rely on indwelling catheters was more a matter of convenience for the staff than what was in the best interests of the residents. The problem, how do you challenge a charge nurse?

Thinking Outside the Box: Possible Courses of Action

- Don't rock the boat! In 3 weeks, we'd be out of there. Keep our mouths shut and don't challenge authority.
- Ask for a meeting with the new charge nurse to explain our concerns, bringing our instructor for support. Be

willing to go higher if the charge nurse cannot justify her decision and refuses to respond to our concerns.
- Work around the problem and try to get the residents' families to raise the issue.

Evaluating a Good Outcome: How Do I Define Success?

- Decisions are made about indwelling catheters that benefit and do not harm residents.
- I am faithful to my advocacy responsibilities within the current scope of my practice as a third-year student.

- I learn how to make the health care system work for patients/residents.
- I learn how to constructively challenge a physician or colleague.

Personal Learning: Here's to the Future!

This turned into a painful experience that made me realize just how difficult it can be to be an effective advocate for patients and residents. I am also newly aware of just how vulnerable long-term care facility residents are. A group of four students and myself asked to meet with the charge nurse. When we told her our concerns, she tried to justify her decision, but we still couldn't see any proof that the decision was made to benefit residents. Regrettably, she didn't respond to our concerns about infections at all. Because she was adamant about keeping the catheters,

we told her that we would take the matter higher. Ultimately, we had to go all the way to the medical director, after thoroughly researching our concerns and getting lots of support for the argument we were making. In the process, the charge nurse made horrible accusations about us, threatening to ensure that students from our school would never work in this facility again. Eventually, all was well that ended well. The charge nurse was "relieved of her administrative responsibilities" and our good names were restored. However, the process that we went through was difficult.

REFLECTION ON QUALITY AND SAFETY COMPETENCIES

How do you think you would respond in a similar situation? Why? What does this tell you about yourself and about the adequacy of your skills for professional practice? Do you agree with the criteria that the nursing student used to evaluate a successful outcome? Are there any other criteria that would be appropriate to use? Did the nursing student meet the criteria? Why or why not? What knowledge, skills, and attitudes do you need to develop to continuously improve the quality and safety of care for patients like Anna Galinski?

Patient-Centered Care: What resources could you or the nurses use as a basis to provide compassionate and appropriate care based on respect for the patient's needs? How did the nursing student act as a patient advocate? Was the human dignity of the patient maintained?

Did the nursing students act appropriately? Legally? Ethically? Why or why not?

Teamwork and Collaboration/Quality Improvement: What communication skills do you need to improve to ensure that you function as a member of the patient-care

team? What skills do you need to implement effective strategies for communicating and resolving conflict? What skills do you need to assert your own position/perspective in discussions about patient care? What other services or resources might be available to aid in this type of decision-making process?

Safety/Evidence-Based Practice: What skills do you need to improve to ensure that patients in your care receive the best nursing care possible? What evidence in nursing literature provides guidance for decision making regarding care of this patient? What issues or factors might have played a role in the charge nurse's response? The students' responses? Do you think that the charge nurse would have responded differently if the students had included their instructor in the meeting?

Informatics: Can you identify the essential information that must be available in Mrs. Galinski's electronic health record to support safe patient care and coordination of care? Can you think of other ways to respond to or approach the situation?

FIGURE 36-1. Frontal view of the female urinary tract (*left*) and lateral view of the male urinary tract (*right*).

Bladder

The urinary bladder is a smooth muscle sac that serves as a temporary reservoir for urine. It is composed of three layers of muscle tissue: the inner longitudinal layer, the middle circular layer, and the outer longitudinal layer. These three layers are called the detrusor muscle. At the base of the bladder, the middle circular layer of muscle tissue forms the internal, or involuntary, sphincter, which guards the opening between the urinary bladder and the urethra. The urethra conveys urine from the bladder to the exterior of the body.

The urinary bladder muscle is innervated by the autonomic nervous system. The sympathetic system carries inhibitory impulses to the bladder and motor impulses to the internal sphincter. These impulses cause the detrusor muscle to relax and the internal sphincter to constrict, retaining urine in the bladder. The parasympathetic system carries motor impulses to the bladder and inhibitory impulses to the internal sphincter. These impulses cause the detrusor muscle to contract and the sphincter to relax. The urinary bladder is shown in Figure 36-2.

The bladder normally contains urine under very little pressure. As the volume of urine increases, the pressure increases only slightly. The bladder wall is able to adapt to this pressure because of the muscle tissue in the bladder. This makes it possible for urine to continue to enter the bladder from the ureters against low pressure. When the pressure becomes sufficient to stimulate nerves in the bladder wall (stretch receptors), the person feels a desire to empty the bladder.

Urethra

The urethra's function is to transport urine from the bladder to the exterior of the body. The anatomy of the urethra differs in males and females. The male urethra functions in the excretory system and the reproductive system. It is about 5 1/2″ to 6 1/4″ (13.7 to 16.2 cm) long and consists of three parts: the prostatic, the membranous, and the cavernous portions (Fig. 36-3 on page 1268). The external urethral sphincter consists of striated muscle and is located just beyond the prostatic portion of the urethra. The external sphincter is under voluntary control.

In contrast, the female urethra is about 1 1/2″ to 2 1/2″ (3.7 to 6.2 cm) long. The external, or voluntary, sphincter is located in the middle of the urethra. No portion of the female urethra is external to the body, as in the male, although the muscle at the meatus is usually called the external sphincter.

Act of Urination

The process of emptying the bladder is known as urination, **micturition**, or **voiding**. The nerve centers for urination are situated in the brain and the spinal cord. Urinating, or voiding, is largely an involuntary reflex act, but its control can be learned. The voluntary control of urination develops as the higher nerve centers develop after infancy. Until that time, voiding is purely a reflex action. People whose bladders are no longer controlled by the brain because of injury or disease also void by reflex only. This is called **autonomic bladder**.

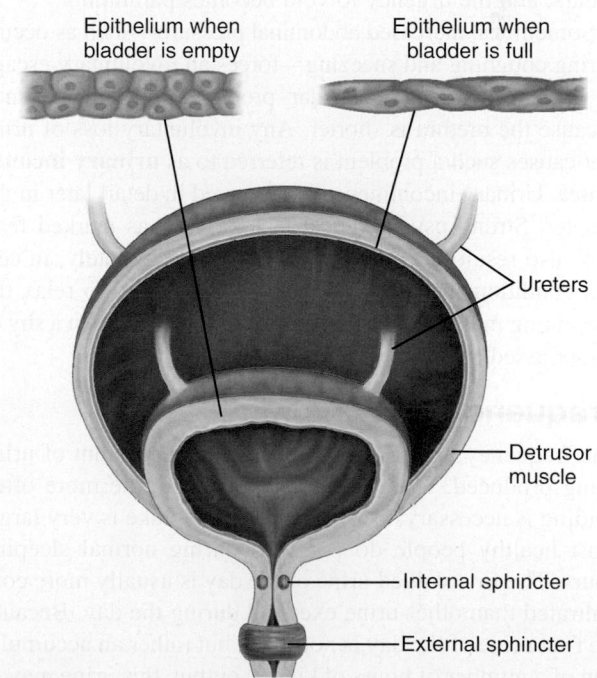

FIGURE 36-2. The urinary bladder.

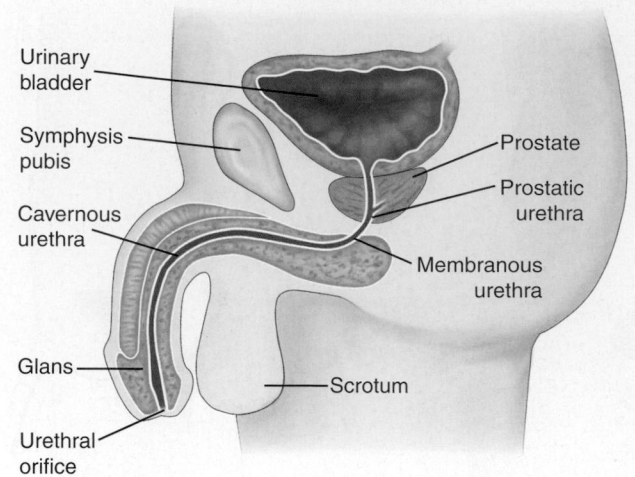

FIGURE 36-3. Parts of the male urethra.

Stretch receptors in the bladder are stimulated as the urine collects. The person feels a desire to void, usually when the bladder fills to about 150 to 250 mL in an adult. The pressure within the bladder is many times greater during urination than it is during the time the bladder is filling. When urination is initiated, the detrusor muscle contracts, the internal sphincter relaxes, and urine enters the posterior urethra. The muscles of the perineum and the external sphincter relax, the muscle of the abdominal wall contracts slightly, the diaphragm lowers, and urination occurs.

The act of urination is normally painless. The voluntary control of voiding is limited to initiating, restraining, and interrupting the act. Restraint of voiding is thought to occur subconsciously when the volume of urine in the bladder is small. If voiding is delayed, however, the bladder continues to fill. Discomfort may then be felt when undue distention occurs, and the urgency to void becomes paramount.

Sometimes, increased abdominal pressure—such as occurs during coughing and sneezing—forces an involuntary escape of urine. This is a particular problem for some women because the urethra is shorter. Any involuntary loss of urine that causes such a problem is referred to as **urinary incontinence**. Urinary incontinence is discussed in detail later in the chapter. Strong psychological factors, such as marked fear, may also result in involuntary urination. Alternately, in certain conditions, it may be difficult for a person to relax the restraining muscles sufficiently to void, such as when a shy or embarrassed person needs to give a urine specimen.

Frequency of Urination

The frequency of urination depends on the amount of urine being produced. The more urine produced, the more often voiding is necessary. Except when fluid intake is very large, most healthy people do not void during normal sleeping hours. The first voided urine of the day is usually more concentrated than other urine excreted during the day. Because the first urine of the day is not fresh, but rather an accumulation of a number of hours of kidney output, this urine may or may not be used as a specimen for certain tests.

Some people normally void small amounts at frequent intervals because they habitually respond to the first early urge to void. This habit usually is meaningless and is not necessarily an indication of disease. On the other hand, if this pattern occurs as a change in urination routine, it may indicate illness. Other people have habits of infrequent voiding. For example, some people go 8 to 12 waking hours or longer without urinating. A habitual low fluid intake or a decrease in the sensation of thirst associated with aging may be one reason. The inaccessibility of toilet facilities owing to travel, work circumstances, or illness, as well as limitations in mobility, can also lead to infrequent urination. People who habitually urinate infrequently develop more urinary tract infections and kidney disorders than those who urinate at least every 3 to 4 hours. The reason for this is believed to be stagnation of urine in the bladder, which serves as a good medium for bacterial growth. Newly occurring infrequent voiding can also indicate a decreased production of urine caused by a kidney or circulatory disorder. **Urinary retention** occurs when urine is produced normally but is not excreted completely from the bladder. Factors associated with urinary retention include medications, an enlarged prostate, or vaginal prolapse.

FACTORS AFFECTING URINATION

Numerous factors affect the amount and quality of urine produced by the body and the manner in which it is excreted.

Developmental Considerations

Infants are born without voluntary control of urination and with little ability to concentrate urine. An infant's urine is usually very light in color and without odor. At about 6 weeks of age, the infant's nephrons are able to control reabsorption of fluids in the tubules and effectively concentrate urine. As a child grows, the bladder gradually enlarges, with an increase in capacity. Most children develop urinary control between the ages of 2 and 5 years. Daytime control precedes nighttime control, and girls generally develop control earlier than boys. Older children and adults control urination voluntarily. They seldom wake to void at night because their kidneys are able to concentrate urine and produce less urine at night as a result of decreased renal blood flow.

Toilet Training

Voluntary control of the urethral sphincters occurs between 18 and 24 months of age. However, many other factors are required to achieve conscious control of bladder function. Toilet training usually begins at about 2 to 3 years of age.

Toilet training should not begin until the child is able to:

- Hold urine for 2 hours
- Recognize the feeling of bladder fullness
- Communicate the need to void and control urination until seated on the toilet

The child's desire to gain control is also important. Wanting to be like a parent or older sibling often provides adequate motivation. Lifelong attitudes toward urination, the body, and cleanliness may develop during the time of toilet training.

Cultures approach toilet training differently. In some cultures, toilet training begins before the child is 1 year old; in other cultures, it may not be considered until the child is near 5 years of age. It is important to recognize cultural influences on this parenting responsibility while promoting flexibility. Reassure parents that any regression of toileting skills that occurs during a child's hospitalization is to be expected and is usually short-lived.

Occasional daytime incontinence of urine in a child is usually not a cause for concern. Continued incontinence of urine past the age of toilet training is termed **enuresis**. Nocturnal enuresis (nighttime bedwetting) usually subsides by 6 years of age (Kyle & Carman, 2013).

Effects of Aging

Physiologic changes that accompany normal aging may affect urination in older adults. These changes include the following:

- The diminished ability of the kidneys to concentrate urine may result in **nocturia** (urination during the night).
- Decreased bladder muscle tone may reduce the capacity of the bladder to hold urine, resulting in increased frequency of urination.
- Decreased bladder contractility may lead to urine retention and stasis, which increases the likelihood of urinary tract infection.
- Neuromuscular problems, degenerative joint problems, alterations in thought processes, and weakness may interfere with voluntary control and the ability to reach a toilet in time.

Medications prescribed for other health problems in the older adult may interfere with bladder function. For example, diuretics cause increased urine production, resulting in the need for increased urination and possibly **urge incontinence** (the involuntary loss of urine that occurs soon after feeling an urgent need to void). Sedatives and tranquilizers may diminish awareness of the need to void.

People who view themselves as old, powerless, and neglected may cease to value voluntary control over urination and simply find toileting too much bother no matter what the setting. Incontinence may be the result.

 CONSIDER Midori Morita's 70-year-old husband who has been experiencing urinary problems since his last hospitalization. The nurse would need to keep in mind age-related changes during assessment of Mr. Morita in order to determine if he is experiencing urinary problems related to these changes or if they are due to another cause. •

Food and Fluid Intake

When the body is functioning well, the kidneys help the body maintain a careful balance of fluid intake and output, which should be about equal. When the body is dehydrated, the kidneys reabsorb fluid. The urine produced is more concentrated and is decreased in amount. Conversely, with fluid overload, the kidneys excrete a large quantity of dilute urine.

Alcohol produces a diuretic effect by inhibiting the release of antidiuretic hormone, increasing urine production. Foods high in water may increase urine production. Foods and beverages with high sodium content cause sodium and water reabsorption and retention, thereby decreasing urine formation. Certain foods may affect the odor of the urine (asparagus, onions) or its color (beets).

Psychological Variables

Many individual, family, and sociocultural variables influence a person's normal voiding habits. For some people, voiding is a personal and private act—something one does not talk about. Needing assistance with a bedpan or urinal provokes great embarrassment and anxiety, especially when the bedpan is offered by a nurse of the opposite gender. For others, voiding is a natural act that does not cause embarrassment; these people readily excuse themselves to void whenever the urge presents.

Some people who experience stress void smaller amounts of urine at more frequent intervals. Stress can also interfere with the ability to relax the perineal muscles and the external urethral sphincter. When this happens, the person may feel an urge to void, but emptying the bladder completely becomes difficult or impossible.

Activity and Muscle Tone

Among the many benefits of regular exercise are increased metabolism and optimal urine production and elimination. During prolonged periods of immobility, decreased bladder and sphincter tone can result in poor urinary control and urinary stasis. People with indwelling urinary catheters lose bladder tone because the bladder muscle is not being stretched by the bladder filling with urine. Other causes of decreased muscle tone include childbearing, muscle atrophy due to decreased estrogen levels as seen with menopause, and damage to muscles from trauma.

Pathologic Conditions

Certain renal or urologic problems can affect both the quantity and the quality of urine produced. Diseases associated with renal problems include congenital urinary tract abnormalities, polycystic kidney disease, urinary tract infection, urinary calculi (kidney stones), hypertension, diabetes mellitus, gout, and certain connective tissue disorders. Renal failure is a condition in which the kidneys fail to remove metabolic end products from the blood and are unable to regulate fluid, electrolyte, and pH balance. Acute renal failure is a sudden decline in kidney function, and may be caused by conditions such as severe dehydration, anaphylactic shock, pyelonephritis, and ureteral obstruction. Chronic kidney disease is the end result of irreparable damage to the kidneys, developing slowly over many years. Chronic renal failure is caused by conditions such as diabetes, hypertension, and glomerulonephritis.

Diseases that reduce physical activity or lead to generalized weakness, such as arthritis, Parkinson's disease, and degenerative joint disease, may interfere with toileting. Cognitive deficits and certain psychiatric problems can interfere with a person's ability or desire to control urination voluntarily. Fever and diaphoresis (profuse perspiration) result in body fluid conservation by the kidneys. Urine production is decreased, and the urine is highly concentrated. Other pathologic conditions, such as congestive heart failure, may lead to fluid retention and decreased urine output. High blood glucose levels, such as with diabetes mellitus, may lead to an increase in urine output secondary to an osmotic diuretic effect.

Medications

Medications have numerous effects on urine production and elimination. Of gravest concern are the many prescription and nonprescription drugs known to be **nephrotoxic** (capable of causing kidney damage). Abuse of analgesics, such as aspirin or ibuprofen (Advil), can cause nephrotoxicity; some antibiotics, such as gentamicin, can be nephrotoxic.

Diuretics, which commonly are used in the treatment of hypertension and other disorders, prevent the reabsorption of water and certain electrolytes in the tubules. Depending on their strength, they cause moderate to severe increases in production and excretion of dilute urine. Cholinergic medications stimulate contraction of the detrusor muscle and produce urination. Some analgesics and tranquilizers suppress the central nervous system, interfering with urination by diminishing the effectiveness of the neural reflex.

Certain drugs cause urine to change color, including the following:

- Anticoagulants may cause **hematuria** (blood in the urine), leading to a pink or red color.
- Diuretics can lighten the color of urine to pale yellow.
- Phenazopyridine (Pyridium), a urinary tract analgesic, can cause orange or orange-red urine.
- The antidepressant amitriptyline (Elavil) or B-complex vitamins can turn urine green or blue-green.
- Levodopa (L-dopa), an antiparkinson drug, and injectable iron compounds can lead to brown or black urine.

THE NURSING PROCESS FOR URINARY ELIMINATION

Assessing

A comprehensive nursing assessment of the functioning of a patient's urinary system includes the following:

- Collection of data about the patient's voiding patterns, habits, and difficulties and a history of current or past urinary problems
- Physical examination of the bladder, if indicated, and urethral meatus; assessment of skin integrity and hydration; and examination of the urine
- Correlation of these findings with the results of diagnostic tests and procedures for examining the urine and the urinary tract

 RECALL Anna Galinski, the 85-year-old frail woman living in a long-term care facility. Initially, she was placed on a toileting regimen, but now she and other patients on the unit have indwelling catheters. In determining how to respond to the situation, it would be helpful for the nurse to perform a comprehensive assessment of the patient. Doing so would provide information to substantiate whether or not catheter insertion was indicated. ●

Nursing History

In the nursing history, question the patient (or caregiver) about usual voiding habits and any current or past voiding difficulties. Box 36-1 lists some additional terms that can be used to describe several urinary problems. When interacting with patients, use terminology that the patient and/or the caregiver understands. The accompanying Focused Assessment Guide 36-1 lists elements of a urinary elimination history that should be incorporated into the initial nursing assessment.

With infants, assess the number of wet diapers per day that the infant produces. Newborns should have six to eight wet diapers per day (Kyle & Carman, 2013). With young children, assess whether the child has achieved bladder control during both day and nighttime. Be sure to indicate on the nursing history and care plan the words that the child uses to indicate the need to void.

With older adults, decreased bladder tone may be a problem. Note on the nursing history any problems, how the person normally handles these problems, and your judgment of the adequacy of the solution.

BOX 36-1 ADDITIONAL TERMS USED TO DESCRIBE URINARY PROBLEMS

Anuria: 24-hour urine output is less than 50 mL; synonyms are complete *kidney shutdown* or *renal failure*

Dysuria: Painful or difficult urination

Frequency: Increased incidence of voiding

Glycosuria: Presence of sugar in the urine

Nocturia: Awakening at night to urinate

Oliguria: Scanty or greatly diminished amount of urine voided in a given time; 24-hour urine output is less than 400 mL

Polyuria: Excessive output of urine (diuresis)

Proteinuria: Protein in the urine; indication of kidney disease

Pyuria: Pus in the urine; urine appears cloudy

Suppression: Stoppage of urine production; normally, the adult kidneys produce urine continuously at the rate of 60 to 120 mL/h

Urgency: Strong desire to void

Urinary incontinence: Involuntary loss of urine

URINARY ELIMINATION

Factors to Assess	Questions and Approaches
Usual patterns of urinary elimination	How often do you urinate (pass your water) during the day? Do you awaken at night to empty your bladder? How would you describe your urine?
Recent changes in urinary elimination	Have you noticed any changes in your usual voiding patterns (frequency, amount, force of stream, difficulty, comfort)? Do you ever leak urine (e.g., on your way to the bathroom or when you sneeze or cough)? Do you ever notice that your undergarments are wet or damp?
Aids to elimination	Is there anything you do that helps you to urinate?
Present or past occurrence of voiding difficulties (nature of problem, onset, frequency, causes, severity, symptoms, intervention attempted, results)	Tell me about any problems you are having now when you urinate (urgency, pain or burning, difficulty starting or stopping stream, dribbling, incontinence). If there is a problem, describe what you feel like before you urinate and while you are urinating. Have you had any urinary problems in the past (any history of urinary tract infections, kidney or bladder disease or problems)? Do you use any type of absorbent pad or product to protect your clothes?
Presence of artificial orifices (normal routine, history of problems)	Tell me about your usual routine with your ileal conduit.

Patients with urinary diversions may have established individualized personal care routines. A **urinary diversion** involves the surgical creation of an alternate route for excretion of urine and is discussed later in the chapter. Assess the procedures and equipment used by patients to make sure they follow accepted guidelines and do not predispose themselves to infection or other risk. Record in both the history and the nursing plan of care any special routine, equipment, or supplies the patient uses for urinary elimination.

When a patient (or caregiver) reports a problem with voiding, explore its duration, severity, and precipitating factors. Also, note the patient's perception of the problem and the adequacy of the patient's self-care behaviors.

 REMEMBER Midori Morita, the wife of the 70-year-old man experiencing problems with "dribbling." The nurse would need to question Mrs. Morita about the problem, obtaining specific information such as when it started, how often it occurs, how much the patient is voiding, events of the previous hospitalization, and any factors associated with it such as use of medications, increased fluid intake, or changes in mobility. ●

Physical Assessment

The physical assessment of urinary functioning includes an examination of the urinary bladder, if indicated, urethral meatus, skin, and urine. The kidneys are normally well protected by considerable fat and connective tissue,

making palpation difficult. Palpation of the kidneys is usually performed as part of a more detailed assessment. This technique requires deep palpation and is generally assessed by advanced health care professionals, such as an advanced practice nurse or physician.

BLADDER

Assessment of the bladder may be indicated when patients experience difficulty voiding or other alterations in elimination. The bladder is normally positioned below the symphysis pubis and cannot be palpated or percussed when empty. When the bladder is distended, it rises above the symphysis pubis and may reach to just below the umbilicus (Fig. 36-4 on page 1272). Before palpating the bladder, always ask when the patient voided last. Observe the lower abdominal wall, noting any swelling, and palpate this area for tenderness. Note the smoothness and roundness of the bladder. Measure the height of the edge of the bladder above the symphysis pubis.

A bedside scanner is another way to assess the bladder. These portable bladder ultrasound devices create an image of the patient's bladder and calculate urine volume present in the bladder. This method is noninvasive and painless. A bladder scan can be performed at the bedside, poses no risk for infection, and is a safer alternative to catheterization to determine bladder urine volume. Results are most accurate when the patient is in the supine position during the scanning. Skill 36-1 on pages 1302–1305 outlines the procedure for assessing bladder volume using an ultrasound bladder scanner.

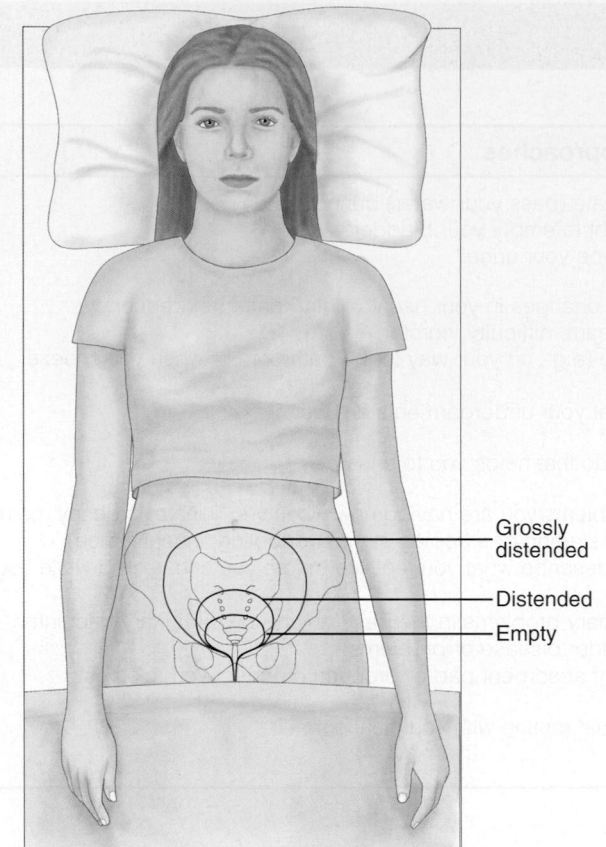

FIGURE 36-4. Position of bladder when empty and distended.

URETHRAL ORIFICE

Inspect the urethral orifice for any signs of inflammation, discharge, or foul odor. In females, the urethral meatus is a slit-like opening below the clitoris and above the vaginal orifice. Place female patients in the dorsal recumbent position with the inner labia retracted for good visualization of the meatus. In males, the meatus is at the tip of the penis. If the male patient is uncircumcised, retract the foreskin to visualize the meatus.

SKIN INTEGRITY AND HYDRATION

Because problems with urinary functioning may result in disturbances in hydration and excretion of body wastes, assess the skin carefully for color, texture, and turgor. Assess the integrity of the skin in the perineal area. Problems with incontinence may result in severe excoriation (abrasion of the epidermis).

 INSPECTING the perineal area would be extremely important when assessing Mrs. Jaspars. Her problems with urinary incontinence places the patient at risk for changes in skin integrity. ●

Urine Characteristics

Assess the patient's urine for color, odor, clarity, and the presence of any sediment. Note any abnormalities.

In select patients, monitor the pH and **specific gravity** of the urine (which is a measure of the density of urine compared with the density of water) and check the urine for abnormal constituents such as protein, blood, glucose, ketone bodies, and bacteria (see the section entitled Point of Care Urine Testing on p. 1277). The normal characteristics of urine are detailed in Table 36-1.

Special Assessment Techniques

In addition to the nursing history and physical examination, the nurse gathers data about urinary elimination through the following assessment measures: measuring urine output, collecting urine specimens, performing point of care urine testing, and assisting with diagnostic procedures. These are discussed in the following sections.

MEASURING URINE OUTPUT

Measuring the patient's fluid intake and output is an important nursing responsibility. Accuracy of the total fluid intake and output from all sources aids in identifying potential alterations in fluid balance and is essential for planning the patient's nursing and medical care. The measurement of fluid intake and output is described further in Chapter 39. Gloves are required when handling urine to prevent exposure to pathogenic microorganisms or blood that may be present in the urine. Goggles also are worn whenever there is a concern of urine splashing. The measurement of fluid intake and output may be delegated to unlicensed personnel. However, the nurse is responsible for ensuring that staff members understand the required procedures, and the nurse must validate the accuracy of the measurements.

Measuring Urine Output in Patients Who Are Continent. Patients who have self-control over urination are continent. The procedure for measuring the urine output of a patient who is continent and voiding is as follows:

1. Ask the patient to void into a bedpan, urinal, or specimen hat, either in bed or in the bathroom. Urinary devices used to collect or measure urine are shown in Figure 36-5 (on page 1274).
2. Pour the urine from the collection device into the appropriate measuring device provided by the agency. The devices are calibrated in milliliters. Collection devices may be calibrated for measurement, eliminating the need for an additional measuring device.
3. Place the calibrated container on a flat surface, such as a shelf, for an accurate reading. Reading at eye level, note the amount of urine voided and record it in the patient's electronic record. Record the total amount voided during each shift. The total for the 24-hour period is usually calculated by the electronic record computer software. Alternately, the information may be recorded in a paper form at the bedside. Figure 36-6 (on page 1275) shows a paper form used for recording urine output.

Table 36-1 CHARACTERISTICS OF URINE

CHARACTERISTIC	NORMAL FINDINGS	SPECIAL CONSIDERATIONS
Color	A freshly voided specimen is pale yellow, straw-colored, or amber, depending on its concentration.	Urine is darker than normal when it is scanty and concentrated. Urine is lighter than normal when it is excessive and diluted. Certain drugs, such as cascara, L-dopa, and sulfonamides, alter the color of urine. Some foods can alter the color; for example, beets can cause urine to appear red.
Odor	Normal urine smell is aromatic. As urine stands, it often develops an ammonia odor because of bacterial action.	Some foods cause urine to have a characteristic odor; for example, asparagus causes urine to have a strong, musty odor. Urine high in glucose content has a sweet odor. Urine that is heavily infected has a fetid odor.
Turbidity	Fresh urine should be clear or translucent; as urine stands and cools, it becomes cloudy.	Cloudiness observed in freshly voided urine is abnormal and may be due to the presence of red blood cells, white blood cells, bacteria, vaginal discharge, sperm, or prostatic fluid.
pH	The normal pH is about 6.0, with a range of 4.6 to 8. (Urine alkalinity or acidity may be promoted through diet to inhibit bacterial growth or urinary stone development or to facilitate the therapeutic activity of certain medications.) Urine becomes alkaline on standing when carbon dioxide diffuses into the air.	A high-protein diet causes urine to become excessively acidic. Certain foods tend to produce alkaline urine, such as citrus fruits, dairy products, and vegetables, especially legumes. Certain foods such as meats tend to produce acidic urine. Certain drugs influence the acidity or alkalinity of urine; for example, ammonium chloride produces acidic urine, and potassium citrate and sodium bicarbonate produce alkaline urine.
Specific gravity	This is a measure of the concentration of dissolved solids in the urine. The normal range is 1.015 to 1.025.	Concentrated urine will have a higher than normal specific gravity; diluted urine will have a lower than normal specific gravity. In the absence of kidney disease, a high specific gravity usually indicates dehydration and a low specific gravity indicates overhydration.
Constituents	*Organic* constituents of urine include urea, uric acid, creatinine, hippuric acid, indican, urine pigments, and undetermined nitrogen. *Inorganic* constituents are ammonia, sodium, chloride, traces of iron, phosphorus, sulfur, potassium, and calcium.	*Abnormal constituents* of urine include blood, pus, albumin, glucose, ketone bodies, casts, gross bacteria, and bile.

4. Discard the urine in the toilet unless a specimen is required. If a specimen is required, pour the urine into an appropriate specimen container.

To ensure that all voided urine is measured, be sure to tell ambulatory patients when their urine output is to be measured and recorded. A specimen hat is a valuable device that can be placed under the toilet seat to collect and measure voided urine for ambulatory patients (see Fig. 36-5). Patients who are willing and able can be taught to measure and record their own output.

Measuring Urine Output in Patients Who Are Incontinent.
Urinary incontinence is the involuntary or uncontrolled loss of urine from the bladder. It is difficult to accurately measure urinary output for incontinent patients. Note the number of times the patient is incontinent and any notable urine characteristics, such as color and odor. Additional nursing interventions are required to collect urine for measurement. Use of scheduled toileting (assisting the patient to the toilet to attempt to void on a regular basis, such as every 2 hours) can assist in obtaining urine for measurement, for required laboratory specimens, and prevent incontinence. Urinary incontinence is discussed in more detail later in the chapter.

Measuring Urine Output in Patients With an Indwelling Catheter.
For patients with an indwelling catheter, the procedure for measuring urine output is as follows:

1. Put on clean gloves.
2. Place a calibrated measuring device beneath the urine collection bag at the bedside. To prevent the spread of infection, patients should have their own calibrated measuring device.

Bedpan and fracture pan: containers used to collect urine from nonambulatory patients.
Urinal container used to collect urine from nonambulatory male patients.

Specimen hat: container that is placed anteriorly on the toilet, underneath the seat. Used to collect urine.
Specimen cup: container that holds urine.
Calibrated measuring device: makes possible the recording of an accurate urine output.

FIGURE 36-5. Devices for collecting and measuring urine.

Large urine collection bag with urimeter for use with patients who have indwelling urinary catheters and require frequent urine output measurements, such as hourly.
Small urine collection bag, commonly called a leg bag, for use by ambulatory patients who have an indwelling urinary catheter.
Large urine collection bag.

3. Place the drainage spout from the collection bag above, but not touching, the calibrated measuring device, and open the clamp.
4. Allow the urine to flow from the collection bag into the measuring device.
5. Reclamp the drainage tube, wipe the spout of the tube with an alcohol pad, and replace the tube into the slot on the drainage bag. Proceed with measurement of urine as described earlier.

Catheterized patients who are acutely ill may require hourly measurements of urine. This is facilitated by using a special collection bag that has a built-in calibrated measuring chamber called a urimeter (see Fig. 36-5). After assessing and recording the amount of urine produced hourly, tilt the measuring chamber so that this urine flows into the general collection bag. This empties the measuring chamber, making it ready to collect the next hour's urine.

COLLECTING URINE SPECIMENS

Different techniques are used for collecting urine specimens. The nurse needs to understand the rationale for the specific test ordered, as well as the correct collection procedure associated with the required test in order to ensure obtaining the appropriate urine sample.

Routine Urinalysis. A sterile urine specimen is not required for a routine urinalysis. Collect urine by having the patient void into a clean bedpan, urinal, or receptacle (e.g., a specimen hat in the toilet bowl). Take care to avoid contamination with feces. If a woman is menstruating when a urine sample is obtained, note this on the laboratory slip because red blood cells may appear in the urine. When patients are voiding into a bedpan or collection device on the toilet, instruct them not to place toilet tissue into the urine because this makes analysis more difficult. Using aseptic technique, pour the urine into an appropriate container; label it with the patient's name, date, and time of collection; package it appropriately; and send it to the laboratory for examination. Do not leave urine standing at room temperature for a long period before sending it to the laboratory because this may alter both the appearance and chemistry of the urine.

Clean-Catch or Midstream Specimen. A clean-catch specimen of urine is required in some situations. Most health care agencies specify that a clean-catch specimen be collected during midstream. This means that the patient voids and discards a small amount of urine; continues voiding in a sterile specimen container to collect the urine; stops voiding into container; removes container

Intake and Output Chart

7:00 AM _11-18-12_ to 7:00 AM _11-19-12_

	Intake					Output						
	Oral	I.V.	Blood	Other	Comments	Urine	Stool	Gastric tube	Drainage tubes	Vomitus	Other	Comments
7-8	250				Force fluids to 1100cc/shift	300						
8-9												
9-10	120											
10-11	60											
11-12	100					250						
12-1	300											
1-2	240											
2-3	100					200						
8 hr Tot	1170					750						voiding 5 discomfort
3-4												
4-5												
5-6												
6-7												
7-8												
8-9												
9-10												
10-11												
8 hr Tot												
11-12												
12-1												
1-2												
2-3												
3-4												
4-5												
5-6												
6-7												
8 hr Tot												
24 hr Tot												

Total intake	Total output

FIGURE 36-6. An example of a paper form used for recording intake and output.

and continues voiding; then discards the last amount of urine in the bladder. The first small amount of urine voided helps to flush away any organisms near the meatus because the findings may be inaccurate if these organisms enter the specimen. Additionally, it is generally thought that urine voided at midstream is most characteristic of the urine the body is producing.

 Concept Mastery Alert

A clean-catch midstream urine specimen is considered a sterile specimen.

A patient who can carry out the technique properly may collect one's own clean-catch midstream urine specimen and often prefers to do so. The nurse provides the appropriate equipment and instructions for the procedure. Refer to Guidelines for Nursing Care 36-1: Obtaining a Clean-Catch or Midstream Urine Specimen (on page 1276).

Sterile Specimen. Sterile urine specimens may be obtained by catheterizing the patient's bladder or by taking the specimen from an indwelling catheter already in place. (Refer to the Catheterizing the Patient's Bladder

discussion on pages 1287–1295 and Guideline 36-2 on pages 1289–1290.)

When it is necessary to collect a urine specimen from a patient with an indwelling catheter, always obtain it from the catheter itself using the special port for specimens. A specimen from the collecting receptacle (drainage bag) may not be fresh urine and could result in an inaccurate analysis. Always observe sterile technique while collecting a urine specimen from an indwelling catheter. Gather equipment, including a syringe, an antiseptic swab, a sterile specimen container, nonsterile gloves, and possibly a clamp. The size of the syringe for the specimen depends on the specific laboratory test. A urine culture requires about 3 mL, whereas routine urinalysis requires at least 10 mL of urine. Also, check the catheter to determine if an access port for specimen removal is present. Wearing gloves protects the nurse from any contact with the specimen.

If urine is not present in the tube, clamp the tube below the access port briefly (not to exceed 30 minutes) to allow urine to accumulate. Clean the access port with an antiseptic swab, and carefully attach the syringe to the port (Fig. 36-7 on page 1276). Aspirate urine into the syringe, remove the syringe, release the clamp if one was used,

GUIDELINES FOR NURSING CARE 36-1

OBTAINING A CLEAN-CATCH OR MIDSTREAM URINE SPECIMEN

Female

- Perform hand hygiene.
- Wear clean gloves.
- Separate the labia. Clean the area at the meatus with soap and water, or according to policy.
- Have the patient void about 30 mL into the toilet or bedpan and discard this urine.
- Position the sterile specimen container near, but not touching, the meatus, and collect at least 10 mL of urine in the container. If the specimen is being collected while the patient is lying down, ask her to void forcibly to prevent urine from dribbling across the perineum.
- Stop collecting urine before the patient empties the bladder. Allow patient to continue voiding into a bedpan or the commode and discard this urine.
- Remove gloves and perform hand hygiene.
- Label the specimen container, package it appropriately, and send the specimen to the laboratory.

Male

- Perform hand hygiene.
- Wear clean gloves.
- Retract the foreskin to expose the glans penis in the uncircumcised male patient.
- Clean the area of the external meatus with soap and water.
- Have the patient void about 30 mL into the toilet or urinal and discard this urine.
- Have the patient void directly into the sterile container and collect at least 10 mL of urine in the container.
- Stop collecting urine before the patient empties his bladder. Allow the patient to void the remaining urine into the toilet or urinal and discard it.
- Return the foreskin to its normal position in an uncircumcised patient to prevent swelling and irritation of the glans penis.
- Remove gloves and perform hand hygiene.
- Label the specimen container appropriately and send the specimen to the laboratory.

and transfer the specimen to the appropriate container. Label the specimen with the patient's name, date, and time of collection; then package and transport the specimen according to facility policy.

Urine Specimens from a Urinary Diversion. Urine specimens can be obtained from urinary diversions. Clean urine specimens can be obtained from a urinary diversion appliance into a clean container for a routine urinalysis (Williams, 2012). If a urine sample is needed for culture and sensitivity, it can be obtained by two methods. The preferred method is to catheterize the stoma. Remove the stoma appliance and clean the stoma site with warm water. Using sterile technique, insert the urinary catheter into the stoma site and advanced 2 to 2.25 inches. If there is resistance, rotate the catheter gently until it slides forward. If there is continued resistance, do not force the catheter any further (Williams). After collection of a

sufficient amount of urine, remove the catheter and reapply the stoma appliance.

24-Hour Urine Specimens. For some laboratory studies, 24-hour specimen collection is required. The patient and the entire nursing team must understand the importance of collecting all the urine voided in a 24-hour period. Post a sign on the patient's bathroom door as a helpful reminder not to discard urine. Initiate a collection at a specific time (which is recorded) by asking the patient to empty the bladder. Discard this urine and then collect all urine voided for the next 24 hours. At the end of the 24 hours, ask the patient to void. Add this urine to the previously collected urine, and then send the entire specimen to the laboratory.

Depending on the type of examination, the urine from each voiding may be kept in a separately marked container and the time of each voiding recorded, or all urine

FIGURE 36-7. Obtaining a urine specimen from an indwelling urinary catheter. (**A**) Use an antiseptic swab to clean the access port. (**B**) Attach syringe and aspirate urine into the syringe. *(Photos by B. Proud.)*

FIGURE 36-8. Disposable urine collection device for infants and young children.

voided may be collected in a common receptacle. The laboratory usually specifies whether a preservative is used to retard decomposition and whether the specimen is to be refrigerated or kept on ice. In some situations, the patient may be required to collect the specimen at home. Many laboratories have a transport service that picks up specimens from a patient's home and returns them to the laboratory within the appropriate time frame.

Specimens From Infants and Children. Plastic disposable collection bags are available for collecting urine specimens from infants and young children who have not achieved voluntary bladder control (Fig. 36-8). Follow the manufacturer's instructions and take care when applying and removing the bag to avoid irritating the sensitive perineal skin.

POINT-OF-CARE URINE TESTING

In some situations, the nurse may perform tests to detect abnormal constituents in urine specimens at the bedside or in the office setting. This is especially true when urine specimens are being tested repeatedly for known abnormalities, when screening tests are being used, or when laboratory facilities are not readily available. For example, a nurse may test urine for the presence of glucose, protein, bilirubin, bacteria, and blood. The results of the test are recorded on the patient's record. Many commercially prepared diagnostic kits are available for such tests and can be used in the home or the health care facility. Although these tests are economical and fast, laboratory analysis is recommended when precise results are needed.

Most commercially prepared diagnostic kits contain all needed equipment and the appropriate reagent (a substance used in a chemical reaction to detect another substance). Reagents are available as tablets, fluids, impregnated paper, and plastic strips with a special coating. When the urine comes in contact with the reagent, a chemical reaction occurs, causing a color change. This color is then compared with an accompanying chart that describes the significance of the color.

The precise directions for the amount of the specimen, the time allowed for the chemical reaction, and the interpretation of the color vary with the manufacturer. Therefore, always follow the directions accompanying the diagnostic kit exactly.

The nurse may also determine the specific gravity of urine, which is a measure of the density of urine compared with the density of water (see Table 36-1, p. 1273). The higher the number, the more concentrated the urine is, unless there are abnormal components, such as glucose or protein, in the urine. Specific gravity can be determined with manufactured plastic reagent strips, as described previously.

ASSISTING WITH DIAGNOSTIC PROCEDURES

Nurses also assist with diagnostic procedures. Various diagnostic procedures, which can be performed in a hospital or outpatient facility, are used to study the urinary system. Common diagnostic procedures related to the urinary system include urodynamic studies, cystoscopy, intravenous pyelogram, retrograde pyelogram, computed tomography (CT) scans, renal biopsy, and ultrasound examination. Nurses are responsible for preparing the patient for the procedure and giving appropriate aftercare. Explaining the procedure helps reduce the patient's anxieties. The preparation and aftercare of the patient for each of these procedures are described in Box 36-2 (on page 1278).

Diagnosing

The data collected about the patient's urinary functioning may lead to one or more nursing diagnoses. Some data are appropriately reported to the primary care provider and may contribute to the identification of a medical diagnosis.

Urinary Functioning as the Problem

Nursing diagnoses that specifically address problems in urinary functioning include problems of incontinence, pattern alteration, and urinary retention. Sample defining characteristics for these diagnoses appear in the accompanying Examples of NANDA-I Nursing Diagnoses box (on page 1279).

Urinary Functioning as the Etiology

Difficulty with urination or changes in normal voiding patterns may affect other areas of human functioning. Examples of nursing diagnoses related to urinary problems include the following:

- Caregiver Role Strain related to incontinence of family member
- Impaired Skin Integrity (Actual, Risk for) related to incontinence
- Acute Pain related to bladder spasms, dysuria, urinary retention, cancer of the bladder, diagnostic procedures
- Disturbed Body Image related to urinary diversion
- Disturbed Sleep Pattern related to nocturia
- Toileting Self-Care Deficit related to parent's lack of knowledge or motivation to toilet train child, neuromuscular impairment or musculoskeletal disorders, immobility, trauma or surgical procedures, confusion, disorientation

(text continues on page 1280)

BOX 36-2 COMMON DIAGNOSTIC PROCEDURES USED TO STUDY THE URINARY TRACT

Urodynamic Studies

Urodynamic studies are a group of tests that measure how urine flows, is stored, and is eliminated in the lower urinary tract. They are used to identify abnormal voiding patterns in persons with incontinence or the inability to void normally.

Preparation
- Usually, no fluid or food restrictions are necessary before the test.
- Bladder should be full before the test.
- Inform the patient that a catheter will be inserted during the test.

Aftercare
- Teach the patient to drink eight to ten 8-oz glasses of water in the 24 hours after the test.
- Teach the patient the signs and symptoms of a urinary tract infection and to report any symptoms immediately.

Cystoscopy

Cystoscopy is the direct visual examination of the bladder, ureteral orifices, and urethra with a cystoscope. It is used to view, diagnose, and treat disorders of the lower urinary tract, interior bladder, urethra, male prostatic urethra, and ureteral orifices.

Preparation
- The patient is allowed liquids on the morning of the examination.
- Sedation and analgesics are usually prescribed before the procedure.
- Obtain a signed consent form (required for the procedure).
- Tell the patient that the procedure is ordinarily painless.

Aftercare
- Know that tissue swelling, dysuria, and hematuria may occur because of trauma from the procedure.
- Encourage a generous fluid intake, and observe and measure urine output for at least 24 hours.
- Observe the patient for urinary retention and for signs of infection; nosocomial infection after a cystoscopy is common.

Intravenous Pyelogram (Excretory Urography)

Intravenous pyelogram is the radiographic examination of the kidney and ureter after a contrast material is injected intravenously. It is used to diagnose kidney and ureter disease and impaired renal function.

Preparation
- Withhold or limit fluids or foods before testing. Obtain patient's allergy history, focusing on sensitivity to iodine, shellfish, or seafood (contrast may contain iodine).
- This test is contraindicated for patients with elevated BUN and creatinine levels and pregnant patients.
- Older, debilitated, or young patients may not tolerate this dehydration; compromises may need to be made for those patients.
- Give a laxative the evening before the examination and an enema the morning of the examination so that stool and gas do not interfere with visualization.

- Obtain a signed consent form (required for the procedure).
- Tell the patient to void before the examination.

Aftercare
- Offer fluids and food immediately after the examination.
- Provide sufficient fluids to replace those lost during the pretest period.
- Observe the patient for signs of a reaction to the contrast material, such as a rash, nausea, and hives. Contrast may initiate acute renal failure. Monitor intake and output.

Retrograde Pyelogram

Retrograde pyelogram is the radiographic and endoscopic examination of the kidneys and ureters after a contrast material is injected into the renal pelvis through the ureter.

Preparation
- Do not give fluids or food after midnight before the examination.
- This test is contraindicated for pregnant patients and those with an iodine allergy.
- Give a laxative the evening before the examination and an enema the morning of the examination so that stool and gas do not interfere with visualization.
- Tell the patient to void before the examination.
- Obtain a signed consent form (required for the procedure).

Aftercare
- Offer foods and fluids immediately if no anesthesia has been used. If anesthesia has been used, delay offering foods and fluids for several hours.
- Check the vital signs regularly if anesthesia has been used.
- Observe the patient for signs of a reaction to the contrast material, such as a rash, nausea, and hives.
- Monitor urine output and appearance for at least 24 hours. Hematuria and dysuria can occur.
- Be aware that ureteral catheters may be in place and should be connected to drainage receptacles so that the amount and character of drainage from each catheter can be noted.

Renal Ultrasound

A renal ultrasound is a noninvasive procedure that involves the use of ultrasound to visualize the renal parenchyma and renal blood vessels. It is used to characterize renal masses and infections, visualize large calculi; detect malformed kidneys; provide guidance during other procedures, such as biopsy; and monitor the status of renal transplants and kidney development in children with congenital processes.

Preparation
- Obtain a signed consent form (required).
- Restrict food and fluids for 8 to 12 hours before renal ultrasound.
- Tell the patient not to smoke or chew gum before the procedure to prevent swallowing air.
- Inform the patient that the procedure is painless.

Aftercare
- Know that no special care is required after the test.
- Inform the patient that results are usually available 1 to 2 days after the study.

BOX 36-2   COMMON DIAGNOSTIC PROCEDURES USED TO STUDY THE URINARY TRACT   *continued*

Computed Tomography (CT Scanning)

CT scanning is a noninvasive radiographic procedure whereby a body part can be scanned from different angles with an x-ray beam and a computer that calculates varying tissue densities and records a cross-sectional image.

Preparation

- Obtain a signed consent form (required).
- The patient is usually NPO for 8 hours before the test if a contrast dye is used.
- Obtain patient's history of any allergic reaction or hypersensitivity to shellfish, iodine, or any contrast dyes (contrast may contain iodine).
- Remove all metal objects from the patient before the test.
- Medications may usually be taken until 2 hours before the test.

Aftercare

- Observe for a delayed reaction to the contrast dye (skin rash, urticaria, headache, vomiting). An oral antihistamine may be given for mild reactions.
- Be supportive to patient and family. The test can be frightening.
- Instruct the patient to resume usual diet and activity unless otherwise indicated.

Renal Biopsy

It is an invasive procedure that involves obtaining a small piece of renal tissue for microscopic examination. Tissue sample may be obtained by needle and syringe through a skin puncture or small incision, during an open surgical procedure during which a wedge of tissue is removed, or through a cystoscope during which a brush is used to obtain a tissue fragment.

Preparation

- Obtain coagulation studies and hematocrit.
- Obtain baseline vital signs.
- Withhold food and fluid before the procedure.
- Obtain a signed consent form (required).
- Sedation may be necessary, depending on the type of procedure.

Aftercare

- Instruct the patient to lie quietly for 4 hours.
- Monitor urine for hematuria during the first 24 hours. Collect each voided specimen in a separate cup labeled with the time.
- Monitor vital signs and dressing for any indication of shock or bleeding.
- Instruct the patient to avoid strenuous activities or heavy lifting for several days and to report any flank pain, hematuria, or dizziness.

EXAMPLES OF NANDA-I NURSING DIAGNOSES

URINARY ELIMINATION

Nursing Diagnoses	Related Factors	Sample Defining Characteristics
Impaired Urinary Elimination	Sensory motor impairment Urinary tract infection Anatomic obstruction	Postvoid residual of 450 mL via bladder scanner "It hurts when I pass my water and I have to go every hour!" "I have to get up frequently at night to urinate."
Functional Urinary Incontinence	Altered environmental factors Sensory, cognitive, or mobility deficits	"I don't know why Johnny started wetting since he's been hospitalized. He has been toilet trained for 6 months now." "When I remember to take Mother to the toilet she urinates fine. But if I don't remember, I find her wet." "After my hip surgery, I walk so slow, I just can't get to the bathroom in time!"
Stress Urinary Incontinence	Overdistention between voiding Weak pelvic muscles and structural supports	Obese mother of four reports involuntary dribbling of urine with coughs, sneezes, hearty laughter. Patient "too busy to void" during day reports involuntary leakage of urine with sudden movement, coughing, sneezing, and laughing.
Urinary Retention	High urethral pressure caused by weak detrusor Inhibition of reflex arc Strong sphincter Blockage	Elderly man diagnosed with benign prostatic hypertrophy complains of inability to urinate despite feeling bladder is full. Woman 6 hours after delivery has had no urine output since labor; 800 mL IV fluids infused; fundus of uterus is displaced to the right by a full bladder.

EXAMPLES OF NURSING INTERVENTIONS AND NURSING OUTCOMES CLASSIFICATIONS (NIC/NOC)

FUNCTIONAL URINARY INCONTINENCE

Nursing Interventions	Nursing Outcomes
• Prompted Voiding • Self-Care Assistance: Toileting • Urinary Elimination Management • Urinary Habit Training	• Self-Care: Toileting • Urinary Continence • Urinary Elimination

Adapted from Moorhead, S., Johnson, M., Maas, M. L., & Swanson, E. (Eds). (2013). *Nursing Outcomes Classi-fication (NOC)* (5th ed., pp. 314, 377–378, 407). St. Louis: Mosby Elsevier/Mosby; and Bulechek, G. M, Butcher, H. K., Dochterman, J. M., & Wagner, C. M. (Eds.). (2013). *Nursing interventions classification (NIC)* (6th ed.). St. Louis: Mosby Elsevier/Mosby. A full listing of nursing activities for each nursing outcome and intervention can be found in these books.

The nurse's challenge is to identify human responses to alterations in urinary elimination that pose specific health problems for the patient and family.

Outcome Identification and Planning

When the patient is ambulatory and not experiencing difficulties with the urinary system, normal voiding is usually not a problem. Trauma or illness, however, may result in the patient's need for nursing assistance with voiding. Nursing interventions should support planned patient outcomes. The patient will:

- Produce urine output about equal to fluid intake
- Maintain fluid and electrolyte balance
- Empty the bladder completely at regular intervals
- Report ease of voiding
- Maintain skin integrity

Implementing

Nursing interventions focus on maintaining and promoting normal urinary patterns, improving or controlling urinary incontinence, preventing potential problems associated with bladder catheterization, and assisting with care of urinary diversions. Nurses can assist the patient and family to achieve desirable outcomes for their urination needs.

 THINK back to Anna Galinski, the frail woman in a long-term care facility. The toileting program focused on maintaining and promoting the patient's normal urinary patterns. However, now that the patient has an indwelling catheter, the nurse needs to focus on preventing problems associated with catheterization. Weighing the risks and benefits of catheterization for this patient would be crucial. •

The accompanying Examples of Nursing Intervention and Nursing Outcome Classifications (NIC/NOC) box offers suggested nursing outcomes and interventions related to functional urinary incontinence.

Promoting Normal Urination

Nursing care to promote normal urination includes interventions to support normal voiding habits, fluid intake, strengthening of muscle tone, stimulating urination and resolving urinary retention, and assisting with toileting. Nurses working with patients to promote appropriate behaviors related to urine elimination should examine their own behaviors as factors in the success of the plan. Nurses who role model good health behaviors are more effective teachers. Use the display, Promoting Health 36-1, for yourself before using it with others.

MAINTAINING NORMAL VOIDING HABITS

If the patient's voiding habits are adequate, provide care or teach the patient to maintain these habits to ensure comfort and satisfactory urine output. Attention to the following variables is helpful:

- *Schedule:* Some patients report urinating on demand in no apparent pattern. Others have inflexible patterns that have developed over the years and become anxious if these are interrupted. Some patients need assistance to urinate and may experience urgency. Nursing actions should support the patient's usual urinating pattern as much as possible.

- *Urge to void:* Assist the patient to void when the patient first feels the urge to void. Routinely delaying urination may result in difficulty initiating a stream and/or urinary stasis. Urinary stasis can contribute to the development of urinary tract infections.

- *Privacy:* Many adults and children cannot urinate in the presence of another person. Unless the patient is extremely weak and requires assistance, provide privacy in the health care facility and in the home.

- *Position:* Helping patients assume their usual voiding position may be all that is necessary to resolve an inability to urinate. Some male patients cannot use a urinal while lying down or sitting; encourage them to void while standing at the bedside unless this is contraindicated. Similarly, some female patients cannot void easily on a bedpan but respond favorably with a bedside commode.

PROMOTING HEALTH 36-1

URINE ELIMINATION

Use the assessment checklist to determine how well you are meeting your needs related to urinary elimination. Then develop a prescription for self-care by choosing appropriate behaviors from the list of suggestions.

Assessment Checklist

☐ almost always	☐ sometimes	☐ almost never

☐ ☐ ☐ 1. I urinate at regular intervals throughout the day.

☐ ☐ ☐ 2. I have an adequate fluid intake.

☐ ☐ ☐ 3. I limit my sodium intake.

☐ ☐ ☐ 4. My urine volume remains relatively constant.

Self-Care Behaviors

1. Maintain a normal voiding pattern and volume.
2. Respond as soon as possible to the urge to void.
3. Drink eight to ten 8-oz glasses of water daily.
4. Avoid foods that contain excess sodium.
5. Monitor use of caffeine, alcohol, or medication schedules that promote voiding and may interfere with sleep.
6. Seek medical assistance for any change in the characteristics of urine or presence of pain on urination.

Information to promote effective urinary elimination—such as information about elimination problems, urinary incontinence, and renal and bladder diseases—is available online. Visit thePoint for a list of Internet resources.

• *Hygiene:* Patients who are confined to bed find it difficult to perform their usual genital hygiene. Careful cleansing of the perineal and genital areas is needed for patient comfort and to prevent infection. This is easily accomplished for patients on bedrest by using warmed, moistened disposable washcloths and skin cleanser or by pouring warm, soapy water over the perineal area while the patient is still on the bedpan, followed by clear water. Families providing care for ill members at home may be taught this technique.

Because people customarily wash their hands after toileting, offer patients confined to bed a moistened towelette or soap and water to wipe their hands after removing the bedpan or urinal. Specific recommendations for urinary elimination problems that affect older adults are listed in the accompanying Focus on the Older Adult box (on page 1282).

 RECALL Anna Galinski, the frail older woman in the long-term care facility. Ideally, before the charge nurse had inserted the catheter into Mrs. Galinski, strategies to promote normal urinary elimination should have been attempted to determine their effectiveness in promoting urinary elimination. In addition, when advocating for the patient, the nurse would strongly urge incorporating strategies to promote normal urinary elimination into the patient's plan of care to determine their effectiveness, ultimately substantiating that catheterization was not necessary. ●

PROMOTING FLUID INTAKE

Many people routinely drink less fluid than is optimal to promote healthy urinary functioning. Adults with no disease-related fluid restrictions should drink 2,000 to 2,400 mL (eight to ten 8-oz glasses) of fluid daily. A common misperception is that drinking this much fluid causes water retention and contributes to weight gain. If a good proportion of the daily fluid intake is water,

the kidneys and urinary structures are well flushed, and waste products, including potentially harmful bacteria, are removed. Monitor fluid intake for excessive amounts of caffeine-containing beverages, high-sodium beverages, and high-sugar beverages.

Provide fresh water, juices, and fluids of preference to patients confined to bed. Remind children and patients who are confused to drink. Fluid restrictions may be ordered for patients with certain diseases. For others, forced fluids (above-average intake of fluids) are prescribed. Incorporate this information in the plan of care and explain it to the patient.

STRENGTHENING MUSCLE TONE

Weakening of the pelvic floor muscles is a common cause of urinary continence problems in women and men (Perry, 2011). Pelvic floor muscle training (PFMT) can improve voluntary control of urination and significantly reduce or eliminate problems with **stress incontinence** (involuntary loss of urine related to an increase in intra-abdominal pressure) by strengthening perineal and abdominal muscle tone (Huebner et al., 2011). PFMT, more commonly called **Kegel exercises**, targets the inner muscles that lie under and support the bladder. These muscles can be toned, strengthened, and actually made larger by a regular routine of tightening and relaxing. Often patients have difficulty determining which muscles to exercise. These are the same muscles that the patient contracts to stop urinating in midstream or to control defecation. Instruct patients to contract the pelvic floor muscles for 10 seconds and to relax them for 10 seconds. Encourage the patient to perform Kegel exercises without involving the muscles in the abdomen, inner thigh, and buttocks. When the patient is familiar with these sensations, these exercises should be performed multiple times a day for at least 3 months, and possibly longer, depending on the response (Perry; Huebner et al.). The exercises can be done anywhere. Assist patients to incorporate them into their daily activities.

FOCUS ON THE OLDER ADULT

NURSING STRATEGIES TO ADDRESS AGE-RELATED CHANGES AFFECTING URINARY ELIMINATION

Age-Related Changes	Nursing Strategies
Nocturia, Frequency, and Urgency	• Ensure easy access to the bathroom or commode. • Discourage fluid intake at bedtime. • Discourage alcohol use before bedtime. • Evaluate medication regimen and schedule, particularly diuretics and drugs that produce sedation or confusion. • Use a night light. • Use clothing that is easily removed for voiding. • Keep assistive ambulatory devices (walkers, canes, and the like) readily available. • Evaluate gait and ability to ambulate safely. • Assess for urinary tract infection.
Incontinence	• Maintain a fluid intake of 1,500 to 2,000 mL/day. • Discourage use of alcohol, artificial sweeteners, and caffeine. • Provide easy access to the bathroom. • Assess factors that influence voiding. • Use assistive devices when necessary (raised toilet seat, grab bars, walker). • Use collection devices when necessary (urinal or bedpan). • Ensure safety when ambulating (e.g., skid-proof slippers). • Encourage use of whole, unprocessed, coarse wheat bran to prevent constipation and fecal impaction. • Perform Kegel exercises several times daily. • Encourage participation in a bladder retraining program.
Urinary Tract Infections	• Consider insertion of an indwelling catheter as the last resort. • Maintain a liberal fluid intake. • Encourage shower instead of tub bath to decrease opportunity for bacteria in bath water to enter urethra. • Void at frequent intervals; every 2 hours if possible. • Void immediately after sexual intercourse. • Assess for signs of urinary tract infection (may be nonspecific in an older adult patient). • Continue antimicrobial therapy as ordered.

PFMT can also be accomplished by using vaginal weights. The patient inserts a small weighted cone into her vagina. She then contracts her pelvic floor musculature to prevent the cone from falling out. The cones can be gradually increased in weight as the muscles are strengthened.

ASSISTING WITH TOILETING

The amount of assistance provided to a patient in relation to toileting varies, depending on the patient's abilities and health status.

Toilet. Even when the patient can use the bathroom toilet, the nurse may be responsible for noting any abnormalities of urinary elimination. In some instances, patients may be taught to report abnormalities to the nurse and instructed not to flush the toilet until the nurse checks the urine. In other instances, when the urine volume is to be calculated, the patient may need to urinate in a bedpan or a specimen hat placed in the toilet so that the urine can be measured before it is discarded. Although many patients can easily be taught to measure their urine output, the nurse is responsible for observing urine at least once during a shift and more frequently if warranted.

Assist weakened patients to the bathroom. If there is any danger of the patient falling, remain in attendance. Never lock the bathroom door. Also, ensure that a signal bell is within easy reach so that the patient can summon help easily if feeling weak and needing assistance. A handrail near the toilet also is helpful.

Commode. Commodes are chairs—straight-back chairs or wheelchairs with open seats and a shelf or a holder underneath that holds a bedpan or bucket (Fig. 36-9). They can be used for patients who can get out of bed but cannot use the bathroom toilet. The commode can be placed adjacent to the bed, and the patient can be assisted to it with minimal exertion. If the patient has a roommate, any visitors may be asked to exit the room while the patient uses the commode. Remember to pull the curtain in the room and close the door to provide for patient privacy.

Bedpan and Urinal. Male patients confined to bed usually use the urinal for voiding and the bedpan for defecation; female patients use the bedpan for both (see Fig. 36-5, p. 1274). Many patients find it embarrassing and difficult to use the bedpan and/or the urinal. When

FIGURE 36-9. Bedside commode.

a patient uses a bedpan or urinal, maintain the patient's privacy.

A special bedpan called a fracture bedpan is frequently used by people with fractures of the femur or lower spine. Smaller and flatter than the ordinary bedpan, it is helpful for patients who cannot easily raise themselves onto the regular bedpan. Very thin or elderly patients often find it easier and more comfortable to use the fracture bedpan. Skills 36-2 and 36-3 on pages 1306–1310 show how to assist a patient with using a bedpan and urinal.

Caring for Patients with Urinary Tract Infections

Urinary tract infections (UTIs) are a leading cause of morbidity and health care expenditures in persons of all ages, accounting for up to 40% of infections reported by acute care hospitals (Edward et al., 2007; Klevans et al., 2007 in AACN, 2011). UTIs are the leading cause of systemic infections in older adults. Women are especially vulnerable to UTIs because the female urethra is shorter and in closer proximity to the vagina and rectum. UTIs can affect both the upper urinary tract, involving the kidneys and ureters (pyelonephritis) and lower urinary tract, involving the bladder and urethra (cystitis). *Escherichia coli,* bacteria commonly found in the gastrointestinal tract, are the most common causal organism (National Kidney Foundation [NKF], 2010).

RISK FACTORS

Those at greatest risk for a UTI include the following:

- *Sexually active women:* During intercourse, perineal bacteria can migrate into the urethra and bladder.
- *Women who use diaphragms for contraception:* The spermicide used with a diaphragm decreases the amount of normally protective vaginal flora.
- *Postmenopausal women:* Urinary stasis, which is common at this age, provides an optimal environment for bacteria to multiply; in addition, decreased estrogen contributes to loss of protective vaginal flora.
- *People with an indwelling urinary catheter in place:* Up to 80% of UTIs are associated with the presence of an indwelling urinary catheter (Apisarnthanark et al., 2007 in AACN, 2011). A catheter-associated urinary

tract infection (CAUTI) increases hospital cost and is associated with increased morbidity and mortality. CAUTIs are considered by the Centers for Medicare and Medicaid Services to represent a reasonably preventable complication of hospitalization. As such, no additional payment is provided to hospitals for CAUTI treatment-related costs (Klevans et al., 2007 in AACN, 2011; Wald & Kramer, 2007, in AACN, 2011; CMS, 2012). Although a break in sterile technique during placement can lead to an infection, most pathogens are introduced via handling of the catheter and drainage device after placement.

- *People with diabetes mellitus:* Glucose in the urine acts as an excellent medium for bacteria to proliferate.
- *Older adults:* The physiologic changes associated with aging (listed earlier in the chapter) predispose older people to the development of UTIs. In addition, enlargement of the prostate as men age can contribute to the development of UTIs in older men (NKF, 2013).

 CONSIDER Anna Galinski, the frail older adult woman in the long-term care facility. Her risk for developing a UTI is increased due to her age. This risk now is further increased because of the catheter insertion. ●

DIAGNOSTIC EVALUATION

In addition to the nursing history and physical examination, laboratory findings can identify the presence of a UTI. A urine sample from a clean-catch or sterile specimen should be sent to the laboratory for a culture and sensitivity (C&S) test. A C&S is positive if it shows at least 100,000 organisms per milliliter of urine. Lower counts may be considered clinically significant if the patient has signs and symptoms of a UTI (Van Leeuwen, Poelhuis-Leth, & Bladh, 2011). The presence of bacteria in a clean-catch midstream or sterile urine specimen, accompanied by symptoms (e.g., dysuria, urinary frequency or urgency, or cloudy urine with a foul odor), indicates a UTI. Red blood cells and nitrates also may be present in the urine.

TREATMENT

Various protocols are used to treat UTIs. A short-course antibiotic regimen (1 large dose vs. 3 or 7 days of smaller doses) usually eradicates infections of the lower urinary tract; longer antimicrobial therapy is required for upper UTIs. Patient education can help prevent UTI recurrence. Teaching the patient about measures that promote health and decrease the severity and incidence of UTIs is a major nursing responsibility. Instruct the patient to:

- Drink eight to ten 8-oz glasses of water daily.
- Observe the urine for color, amount, odor, and frequency. Report any sign of infection to your health care provider.
- Dry the perineal area after urination or defecation from the front to the back, or from the urethra toward the rectum.

- Drink two glasses of water before and after sexual intercourse and void immediately after intercourse.
- Take showers rather than baths.
- Wear underwear with a cotton crotch, and avoid clothing that is tight and restrictive on the lower half of the body.
- Drink 10 oz of cranberry or blueberry juice daily. These juices contain chemicals that may help prevent **bacteriuria** (bacteria in the urine) by inhibiting bacteria from adhering to the bladder wall and urinary catheters (NKF, 2010). Daily cranberry juice should not be recommended for patients with a personal or family history of kidney stones (MedlinePlus, 2013).

Nursing interventions to prevent UTIs for a patient with an indwelling catheter are discussed later in the chapter.

Caring for an Incontinent Patient

Urinary incontinence, any involuntary leakage of urine, is widely underreported and underdiagnosed. It is one of the most common chronic health problems. However, it is not an inevitable result of growing old or bearing children. Many people self-manage this life-altering condition for many years before seeking assistance from a health care provider.

Urinary incontinence is more prevalent in women and increases with age. It is a special problem for older adults who may experience decreasing control over urination and who may find it more difficult to reach a toilet in time to void because of mobility problems or dexterity problems in undressing. The discomfort, odor, and embarrassment of urine-soaked clothing can greatly diminish a person's self-concept, causing the individual to feel like a social outcast.

Age-related changes do affect urinary function, but urinary incontinence can be treated and individualized interventions can help the patient lead a normal life. Of those who seek treatment, 80% are cured or have their symptoms improved notably.

Patients frequently turn to absorbent products for protection when they are incontinent of urine if they have not had this condition properly diagnosed and treated. These products absorb or contain urine leakage. Many types of disposable and reusable products are available, including perineal pads or liners, protective underwear, guards and drip collection pouches, and adult briefs. When used improperly, such products may cause skin breakdown and place the patient at risk for a UTI. Long-term use of these products is not recommended until the following factors have been considered and discussed with a health care provider:

- Functional disability of the patient
- Type and severity of incontinence
- Gender
- Availability of caregivers
- Failure of previous treatment programs
- Patient preference

Advertisements for adult disposable undergarments have increased public awareness about urinary incontinence, but they fail to mention possible treatment strategies (see Focused Critical Thinking Guide 36-1).

 REVIEW the scenario at the beginning of the chapter describing Midori Morita and her husband. The nurse should assess the feelings of Midori and her husband related to the problems associated with his urinary dribbling and incontinence. Midori may be feeling overwhelmed and possibly upset or angry. Her husband most likely would be feeling embarrassed and possibly disgusted. Helping them resolve these feelings is essential for effective care. •

TYPES OF URINARY INCONTINENCE

The National Association for Continence (NAFC, 2013a) and the U.S. Department of Health and Human Services (USDHHS, 2010) identify numerous types of urinary incontinence. **Transient incontinence** appears suddenly and lasts for 6 months or less. It is usually caused by treatable factors, such as confusion secondary to acute illness, infection, and as a result of medical treatment, such as the use of diuretics or intravenous fluid administration. Stress incontinence (discussed earlier in the chapter) occurs when there is an involuntary loss of urine related to an increase in intra-abdominal pressure. This commonly occurs during coughing, sneezing, laughing, or other physical activities. Childbirth, menopause, obesity, or straining from chronic constipation can also result in urine loss. The leakage usually does not occur when the person is supine. Urge incontinence is the involuntary loss of urine that occurs soon after feeling an urgent need to void (urgency). These patients experience a loss of urine before getting to the toilet and an inability to suppress the need to urinate. A diagnosis of **mixed incontinence** indicates that there is urine loss with features of two or more types of incontinence. **Overflow incontinence**, or chronic retention of urine, is the involuntary loss of urine associated with overdistention and overflow of the bladder. The signal to empty the bladder may be underactive or absent, the bladder fills, and dribbling occurs. It may be due to a secondary effect of some drugs, fecal impaction, or neurologic conditions. **Functional incontinence** is urine loss caused by the inability to reach the toilet because of environmental barriers, physical limitations, loss of memory, or disorientation.

Patients with **reflex incontinence** experience emptying of the bladder without the sensation of the need to void. Spinal cord injuries may lead to this type of incontinence. **Total incontinence** is a continuous and unpredictable loss of urine, resulting from surgery, trauma, or physical malformation. Urination cannot be controlled due to an anatomic abnormality.

Urinary incontinence is treatable. Appropriate interventions can significantly reduce the symptoms of urinary incontinence and even prevent its occurrence.

FOCUSED CRITICAL THINKING GUIDE 36-1

URINARY INCONTINENCE

You have been assigned to care for an 80-year-old patient, Mrs. Bartowski, who was admitted with a recurrent leg ulcer and is due to be discharged the following day. Her nursing notes indicate that she has had two or three episodes of urinary incontinence every day while in the hospital and her plan of care states "use adult diapers." You go into the room to answer Mrs. Bartowski's call bell and help her into the bathroom. She is wearing an adult disposable undergarment, and a half-used package is on the chair. After voiding 150 mL of urine, she tearfully begs, "Please don't put that diaper back on me; I'm not a child." According to her chart, Mrs. Bartowski is mentally alert, lives at home with her daughter who has visited her in the hospital frequently, and appears able to identify her need to urinate. You're aware that there are effective alternative therapies to resolve or minimize urinary incontinence rather than relying on absorbent products. However, the nurses have obviously made a decision to use disposable undergarments in this situation. You prefer to leave the diaper off, try some other measures, and possibly discuss this with the patient's daughter, but as a student nurse, you are here for only 2 days. You want to be a patient advocate and do the right thing. What should you do?

1. Identify goal of thinking

Determine whether it is more important to replace the diaper against the patient's wishes or leave it off and discuss the possibility of using behavioral strategies with the staff.

2. Assess adequacy of knowledge

Pertinent circumstances: Mrs. Bartowski is alert and oriented and obviously upset that diapers are being used. She has used her call bell when she feels the urge to urinate, but incontinent episodes have also been documented. The nursing staff has decided that diapers are appropriate for this patient. Her daughter, with whom she lives, appears supportive and attentive. Discharge is scheduled for tomorrow.

Prerequisite knowledge: Before you decide what to do in this situation, you need to discuss your options with your instructor. Of primary importance is whether the patient and her daughter are interested in pursuing alternatives. They can also provide invaluable information about her elimination pattern at home. The primary care provider must be consulted to determine the etiology of the incontinence and validate that her urinary tract is intact and functioning adequately. You will also need to review the various treatment options for incontinence because these will have to be communicated to the patient and her daughter before discharge.

Room for error/time constraints: Absorbent products can provide a sense of security and are widely used for incontinence. There is, however, the possibility that continence can be restored once incontinence is assessed, recognized, and addressed. Early dependence on absorbent products can remove the motivation to seek treatment and promote acceptance of the condition. The treatment options should be discussed with Mrs. Bartowski and her daughter before discharge tomorrow.

3. Address potential problems

Continuing to use absorbent products offers a temporary solution to the problem. They may protect the patient from embarrassment and provide a sense of security, although they do nothing to prevent incontinent episodes. Explore the patient's feelings regarding the use of these products. The use of these products can communicate expectations of an acceptance of incontinence as an inevitable part of aging, which is not true. Absorbent products can also interfere with the patient's ability to use the toilet independently. Using behavioral techniques to control incontinence will require health teaching before discharge and a long-term commitment to follow-up in the home.

4. Consult helpful resources

The patient's motivation to restore continence is your most valuable resource. The primary nurse or case manager, the primary care provider, and your instructor can also help you sort through your priorities in this situation. The latest research recommends use of behavioral techniques first to treat incontinence.

5. Critique judgment/decision

If you decide to reapply a diaper against the patient's wishes, you may, in fact, be supporting the myth that incontinence is inevitable and untreatable. Long-term use of absorbent products can place the patient at risk for skin breakdown and a urinary tract infection if used improperly. You decide to leave the diaper off and establish regular intervals for voiding for the 2 days you will be caring for Mrs. Bartowski. In this short time, you hope to demonstrate to the patient, her daughter, and the staff that it is possible for Mrs. Bartowski to maintain a pattern of continence. Because she will most likely be discharged tomorrow, you also discuss the possibility of referral to home care or a continence expert who will instruct, support, and follow through with the necessary components of care. When you discuss your situation at postconference, your clinical group supports your decision.

ASSESSMENT

Through careful assessment and planned interventions (see upcoming discussion), continence may be restored. Carefully assess environmental factors for their potential impact on urinary incontinence. Equipment that gives the person better access to toileting facilities, such as a walker, cane, wheelchair, and Velcro closings on clothing, may be necessary. Dietary habits, such as excess caffeine intake or insufficient fluid intake, both of which can irritate the bladder and contribute to incontinence, indicate the need for teaching about nutrition (NAFC, 2013b).

A voiding record or diary provides information about the frequency, timing, and amount of voiding. By noting any patterns to voiding, either continent or incontinent, the nurse may find correlations with medications, fluid intake, or other causes of incontinence and may be able to prevent any further incontinent episodes. Voiding diaries can also be used to evaluate the effectiveness of interventions.

Physical examination and specific diagnostic tests also aid in identifying urinary incontinence. Palpate the patient's abdomen for a distended bladder, any masses, or tenderness. The **postvoid residual (PVR)** urine (the amount of urine remaining in the bladder immediately after voiding) can be measured by the use of a portable ultrasound device that scans the bladder. Bladder ultrasound poses no risk for infection and is considered a safer alternative to catheterization. This measurement can also be obtained by catheterizing the patient. Catheterization, however, involves the increased risk for introduction of microorganisms into the bladder and resulting UTI. A PVR of less than 50 mL indicates adequate bladder emptying. A PVR of greater than 150 mL is often recommended as the guideline for catheterization because residual urine volumes of greater than 100 mL have been associated with the development of UTIs (National Kidney and Urologic Diseases Information Clearinghouse [NKUDIC], 2012). Refer to Skill 36-1 on pages 1302–1305 for the procedure for assessing bladder volume using an ultrasound bladder scanner.

 THINK back to Midori Morita, the woman caring for her husband, who is experiencing urinary problems at home. The nurse would need to carefully assess all aspects of Mr. Morita's current status, including the environment, and develop a patient-specific teaching plan for Mrs. Morita and her husband. ●

TREATMENT

Noninvasive, low-risk behavioral interventions are the first line of therapy for urinary incontinence. Community settings are ideally suited for using many of these interventions. Nurses can identify patients who are incontinent and use these techniques or refer them to nurse or advanced practice continence experts in the community. All nurses caring for older adults need to be familiar with education about urinary incontinence. Many possible treatment interventions for urinary incontinence fall within the nurse's scope of practice. (See Box 36-3 for a summary of behavioral and treatment interventions.)

Many patients incorrectly believe that surgery is the only treatment option for urinary incontinence. Surgical intervention is considered only if behavioral and pharmacologic measures prove ineffective. Nursing skills and creativity can help patients become continent again before surgery is used.

Applying an External (Condom) Catheter

When voluntary control of urination is not possible for male patients, an alternative to an indwelling catheter is the **external condom catheter**. This soft, pliable sheath made of silicone material is applied externally to the

---

BOX 36-3 TREATMENT OPTIONS FOR URINARY INCONTINENCE

Behavioral Techniques

- *Pelvic floor exercises:* Kegel exercises to strengthen pelvic floor muscles and sphincter muscles. Kegel exercises can be done alone, with weighted cones, or with biofeedback.
- *Biofeedback:* Measuring devices are used to help patient become aware of when pelvic floor muscles are contracting.
- *Electrical stimulation:* Electrodes are placed in the vagina or rectum that then stimulate nearby muscles to contract.
- *Timed voiding or bladder training:* May be used with biofeedback. Patient keeps track of when voiding and leaking occur to enable oneself to plan when to void, with increasing length of voiding intervals. Bladder training involves biofeedback and muscle training. Urgency control is addressed using distraction and relaxation techniques.

Pharmacologic Treatment

- Treatment is dependent on type of incontinence. Some medications inhibit contractions of the bladder, others

may relax muscles, and some tighten muscles at the bladder neck and urethra.
- Topical estrogen may be used in postmenopausal women to relieve atrophy of involved muscles.
- Collagen may be injected into the tissue around the urethra to add bulk and help close the urethral opening.

Mechanical Treatment

- Pessaries: A stiff ring that is inserted into the vagina, where it helps to reposition the urethra. The pessary may be placed by the patient or by a nurse.
- External barriers: Adhere to the urethral opening to stop urine leakage. The barrier is a small foam pad placed over the urethral opening. It seals against the body to keep urine from leaking. It is removed and discarded before the patient voids.
- Urethral insert: Small device, like a plug, that fits into the urethra. Removed to void, the insert is replaced until the patient needs to void again.
- Surgical intervention: Used as a last resort. Type of surgery depends on cause of incontinence.

penis. Most devices are self-adhesive. The catheter is connected to drainage tubing and a collection bag, and can be used with a leg bag.

 THINK back to Midori Morita, the woman described at the beginning of the chapter who is caring for her husband at home. The nurse might suggest using a condom catheter for Mrs. Morita's husband as a possible alternative, rather than an indwelling catheter, which would increase his risk for infection. ●

Nursing care of a patient with a condom catheter includes vigilant skin care to prevent excoriation. Remove the condom daily and wash the penis with soap and water, dry it carefully, and inspect the skin for irritation. In hot and humid weather, more frequent changing may be required. Always follow the manufacturer's instructions for applying the condom because there are several variations. In all cases, care must be taken to fasten the condom securely enough to prevent leakage, yet not so tightly as to constrict the blood vessels in the area. The tip of the tubing should be kept 1″ to 2″ (2.5–5 cm) beyond the tip of the penis to prevent irritation to the sensitive glans area. Maintaining free urinary drainage is another nursing priority. Institute measures to prevent the tubing from becoming kinked and urine from backing up in the tubing. Urine can lead to excoriation of the glans; position the tubing that collects the urine from the condom to draw urine away from the penis. Steps for applying a condom catheter are described in Skill 36-4 on pages 1311–1313.

For some men, the condom catheter may not be an option because of penis retraction. For these patients, the retracted penis pouch may be appropriate. This is a bag-like appliance in which the penis is placed. The pouch can then be connected to a leg bag.

Catheterizing the Patient's Bladder

Urinary catheterization is the introduction of a catheter (tube) through the urethra into the bladder for the purpose of withdrawing urine. Catheter-associated UTIs are the most common hospital-acquired infection in the United States and is one reason catheterization should be avoided whenever possible. When it is deemed necessary, it should be performed using strict aseptic technique and left in place for the shortest length of time possible (Hooton et al., 2010). The duration of catheterization is the most important risk factor for the development of a UTI (Bernard, Hunter, & Moore, 2012). See the accompanying PICO in Practice box.

PICO IN PRACTICE

ASKING CLINICAL QUESTIONS

Scenario: You are a staff nurse who works on a medical–surgical unit that specializes in orthopedics. One day, you attend an in-service training session on how to use a portable bladder scanner. The hospital has just purchased six, one for use on each of the six medical–surgical units. The nurse educator who conducts the in-service tells your class that the bladder scanner is useful in detecting when patients have significant urinary retention that may require intermittent catheterization, typically when there is at least 400 milliliters (mL) of urine present in the bladder. She asserts that routine use of indwelling urinary catheters (i.e., Foley catheters) can lead to more catheter-associated urinary tract infections (CAUTIs) than intermittent catheterization. You note that most of your patients who have total knee or hip replacements keep their indwelling urethral catheters until their second postoperative day. Now that a portable bladder scanner is available for use on your orthopedics unit, you wonder whether patients who have had either total knee or hip replacements would have reduced rates of CAUTIs if their indwelling urinary catheters are discontinued before they are admitted to the unit.

- POPULATION: Postoperative patients with total knee and hip replacements
- INTERVENTION: Intermittent urethral catheterization as needed
- COMPARISON: Routine use of indwelling urethral catheters
- OUTCOME: CAUTIs

PICO Question: Among patients who have had total knee and hip replacement surgery, is intermittent urethral catheterization on an as-needed basis associated with reduced rates of CAUTIs as compared with use of indwelling urethral catheters?

Finding: From the Cochrane Collaboration: Niel-Weise, B. S., & van den Broek, P. J. (2009). Urinary catheter policies for short-term bladder drainage in adults. *Cochrane Database of Systematic Reviews, 1*, CD004203.

This systematic review found that using urethral catheters intermittently as needed rather than leaving indwelling urethral catheters in place reduced the chances of having CAUTIs in patients who had either knee or hip surgery.

Level of Evidence: Level I

Recommendation: You propose implementation of a new postoperative protocol to your interdisciplinary unit-based quality improvement committee, which includes members that represent nursing, infection control, and orthopedic surgery. Specifically, you propose that indwelling urethral catheters be removed within the first few hours postoperatively in patients who have total knee or hip replacement surgery. You propose a protocol for use of intermittent catheters when these patients note an urge to void but an inability to do so, and there is at least 400 mL of urine present that is confirmed by the portable bladder scanner. You propose that the effectiveness of this new protocol be verified through monitoring the rates of CAUTIs in these patients to determine if they are less after the new policy is implemented.

REASONS FOR URINARY CATHETERIZATION
Common reasons for urinary catheterization include:

- Relieving urinary retention. Retention is often temporary and is common after surgery involving the lower abdomen, pelvis, bladder, or urethra, especially if ambulation is delayed, fluid intake is minimal, or epidural analgesia is used for pain control. Any mechanical obstruction, such as swelling at the meatus, which can occur after childbirth, or an enlarged prostate in men, may cause retention. Some patients who are unable to use any other bladder management method, such as those with neurogenic bladder dysfunction related to a disability (e.g., spinal cord injury), require long-term use of an indwelling catheter.
- Obtaining a sterile urine specimen
- Obtaining a urine specimen when a specimen cannot be secured satisfactorily by other means. Examples include collecting an uncontaminated specimen from a woman who is menstruating or from an incontinent patient.
- Emptying the bladder before, during, or after surgery and before certain diagnostic examinations.
- Monitoring renal function of critically ill patients
- Increasing comfort for terminally ill patients

IMPORTANT CONSIDERATIONS ABOUT THE LOWER URINARY TRACT
When catheterization is planned, consider the following about the lower urinary tract:

- The bladder is normally a sterile cavity.
- The external opening to the urethra can never be sterilized.
- The bladder has defense mechanisms. It empties itself of urine regularly and maintains an acidic environment, which has antibacterial advantages. These help to maintain a sterile bladder under normal circumstances and also help in clearing an infection if it occurs.

- Pathogens introduced into the bladder can ascend the ureters and cause bladder and kidney infections.
- A healthy bladder is not as susceptible to infection as an injured one. A state of lowered resistance, present in many diseases and stressful situations, predisposes the patient to urinary infection.

TYPES OF CATHETERS
Intermittent urethral catheters, or straight catheters, are used to drain the bladder for shorter periods. Intermittent catheterization should be considered as an alternative to short-term or long-term indwelling urethral catheterization to reduce catheter-associated UTIs (Hooton et al., 2012). Intermittent catheterization is becoming the gold standard for the management of bladder-emptying dysfunctions and following surgical interventions. Certain advantages to intermittent catheterization, including the lower risks of catheter-associated UTI and complications, may make it a more desirable and safer option than indwelling catheterization (Herter & Wallace Kazer, 2010, pp. 343–344). Intermittent catheterization, performed by the patient or a caregiver in the home, may be necessary for patients with spinal cord injuries or other neurologic conditions. Although the risk for UTI is always present, most research supports the use of clean, rather than sterile, technique in this environment. Patients can be taught to insert and remove intermittent catheters themselves. The procedure for self-catheterization is essentially the same as that used by the nurse to catheterize a patient. Initially, a female patient may use a mirror to locate the meatus, but eventually she can learn to insert the catheter using just touch. Self-catheterization is recommended at regular intervals to prevent overdistention of the bladder and decreased blood flow through the wall of the bladder (Hinkle & Cheever, 2014). Intermittent catheters and catheterization are discussed in Guidelines for Nursing Care 36-2. Box 36-4 outlines important information related to patient self-catheterization.

Box 36-4   PATIENT INTERMITTENT SELF-CATHETERIZATION

- Explain the reason for self-catheterization and corresponding health issues related to the need for catheterization.
- Explain the consequences of not doing intermittent self-catheterization, such as upper urinary tract problems, urinary tract infections and incontinence.
- Explain potential complications, such as bleeding and the risk of urinary tract infections and what to do if they occur.
- Ensure privacy and dignity.
- Include discussion regarding the frequency of intermittent catheterization and how to incorporate into usual daily routine.
- Explain the anatomy of the urinary tract, hygiene, and preparation of the catheter.
- Demonstrate how to open, hold, and use the catheter.

- Explain catheterization process, demonstrate process, and observe return demonstration by patient.
- Explore process to obtain supplies, cleaning of reusable catheters, and storage.
- Provide information in an appropriate format (such as written materials or video, in appropriate language) to reinforce instruction.
- Allow the patient adequate time to ask questions.
- Provide information about how to recognize a urinary tract infection and other signs/symptoms to report to primary health care provider.
- Aids are available to help meet the challenges of intermittent self-catheterization for patients with poor eyesight, reduced mobility, and/or reduced manual dexterity.

(Adapted from Logan, K. [2012]. An overview of male intermittent self-catheterisation. *British Journal of Nursing, 21*[18], S18–S22; Mangnall, J. [2012]. Key considerations of intermittent catheterisation. *British Journal of Nursing, 21*[7], 392, 394, 396–398; Newman, D. K., & Willson, M. M. [2011]. Review of intermittent catheterization and current best practices. *Urologic Nursing, 31*[1], 12–28; Rantell, A. [2012]. Intermittent self-catheterisation in women. *Nursing Standard, 26*[42], 61–68; and Stewart, E. [2011]. Intermittent self-catheterization and infection reduction. *British Journal of Neuroscience Nursing, 7*[5], S4–S7.)

GUIDELINES FOR NURSING CARE 36-2

INTERMITTENT URETHRAL CATHETERIZATION

Female

- Identify the patient. Discuss the procedure with the patient and assess the patient's ability to assist with the procedure. Discuss any allergies with the patient, especially to iodine and latex. Review the chart for any limitations in physical activity.
- Bring the catheter kit and other necessary equipment to the bedside. Obtain assistance from another staff member, if necessary. Perform hand hygiene. Put on disposable gloves.
- Close curtains around the bed and close the door to the room if possible.
- Provide for good light. Artificial light is recommended (use of a flashlight requires an assistant to hold and position it). Place a trash receptacle within easy reach.
- Raise the bed to a comfortable working height. Stand on the patient's right side if you are right handed, the patient's left side if you are left handed.
- Assist the patient to the dorsal recumbent position with knees flexed, feet about 2 feet apart, with her legs abducted. Drape the patient. Alternately, use the Sims, or lateral, position. Place the patient's buttocks near the edge of the bed with her shoulders at the opposite edge and her knees drawn toward her chest. Slide waterproof drape under the patient.
- Put on clean gloves. Clean the perineal area with washcloth, skin cleanser, and warm water, using a different corner of the washcloth with each stroke. Wipe from above orifice downward toward sacrum (front to back). Rinse and dry. Remove gloves. Perform hand hygiene again.
- Open sterile catheterization tray on a clean overbed table using sterile technique.
- Put on sterile gloves. Grasp upper corners of the drape and unfold the drape without touching unsterile areas. Fold back a corner on each side to make a cuff over gloved hands. Ask the patient to lift her buttocks and slide the sterile drape under her with gloves protected by cuff.
- Place a fenestrated sterile drape over the perineal area, exposing the labia, if appropriate.
- Place sterile tray on drape between the patient's thighs.
- Open all the supplies. Fluff cotton balls in tray before pouring antiseptic solution over them. Alternately, open package of antiseptic swabs. Open specimen container if specimen is to be obtained.
- Lubricate 1 to 2 inches of catheter tip.
- With thumb and one finger of nondominant hand, spread labia and identify meatus. If the patient is in the side-lying position, lift the upper buttock and labia to expose the urinary meatus. Be prepared to maintain separation of labia with one hand until the catheter is inserted and urine is flowing well and continuously.
- Use your dominant hand to pick up a cotton ball. Clean one labial fold, top to bottom (from above the meatus down toward the rectum), then discard the cotton ball. Using a new cotton ball for each stroke, continue to clean the other labial fold, then directly over the meatus.
- With your uncontaminated, dominant hand, place drainage end of catheter in receptacle. If a specimen is

required, place the end into the specimen container in the receptacle.
- Using your dominant hand, hold the catheter 2 to 3 inches from the tip and insert it slowly into the urethra. Advance the catheter until there is a return of urine—approximately 2 to 3 inches (4.8–7.2 cm). Do not force the catheter through the urethra into the bladder. Ask the patient to breathe deeply, and rotate the catheter gently if slight resistance is met as the catheter reaches the external sphincter.
- Hold the catheter securely at the meatus with your nondominant hand while the bladder empties. If a specimen is being collected, remove the drainage end of the tubing from the specimen container after the required amount is obtained and allow urine to flow into receptacle. Set specimen container aside and place lid on container.
- Allow the bladder to empty. Withdraw the catheter slowly and smoothly after urine has stopped flowing. Remove equipment and dispose of according to facility policy. Wash and dry the perineal area as needed.
- Remove your gloves. Assist the patient to a comfortable position. Cover the patient with bed linens. Place the bed in the lowest position.
- Put on clean gloves. Secure the container lid and label specimen. Send urine specimen to the laboratory promptly or refrigerate it.
- Remove gloves. Perform hand hygiene.

Male

- Identify the patient. Discuss the procedure with the patient and assess the patient's ability to assist with the procedure. Discuss any allergies with the patient, especially to iodine and latex. Review the chart for any limitations in physical activity.
- Bring the catheter kit and other necessary equipment to the bedside. Obtain assistance from another staff member, if necessary. Perform hand hygiene. Put on disposable gloves.
- Close curtains around the bed and close the door to the room if possible.
- Provide for good light. Artificial light is recommended. Place a trash receptacle within easy reach.
- Raise the bed to a comfortable working height. Stand on the patient's right side if you are right handed, the patient's left side if you are left handed.
- Position the patient on his back with thighs slightly apart. Drape the patient so that only the area around the penis is exposed. Slide waterproof pad under the patient.
- Put on clean gloves. Clean the genital area with washcloth, skin cleanser, and warm water. Clean the tip of the penis first, moving the washcloth in a circular motion from the meatus outward. Wash the shaft of the penis using downward strokes toward the pubic area. Rinse and dry. Remove gloves. Perform hand hygiene again.
- Open sterile catheterization tray on a clean overbed table using sterile technique.
- Put on sterile gloves. Open sterile drape and place on the patient's thighs. Place fenestrated drape with opening over penis.

(continued)

GUIDELINES FOR NURSING CARE 36-2 *continued*

INTERMITTENT URETHRAL CATHETERIZATION

- Place catheter set on or next to the patient's legs on sterile drape.
- Open all the supplies. Fluff cotton balls in tray before pouring antiseptic solution over them. Alternately, open package of antiseptic swabs. Open specimen container if specimen is to be obtained.
- Remove cap from syringe prefilled with lubricant.
- Lift penis with nondominant hand. Retract foreskin in uncircumcised patient. Be prepared to keep this hand in this position until the catheter is inserted and urine is flowing well and continuously.
- Using your dominant hand and the forceps, pick up a cotton ball. Using a circular motion, clean the penis, moving from the meatus down the glans of the penis. Repeat this cleansing motion two more times, using a new cotton ball each time. Discard each cotton ball after one use.
- Hold penis with slight upward tension and perpendicular to the patient's body. Use your dominant hand to pick up the lubricant syringe. Gently insert tip of syringe with lubricant into urethra and instill the 10 mL of lubricant.
- With your uncontaminated, dominant hand, place drainage end of catheter in receptacle. If a specimen is required, place the end into the specimen container in the receptacle.

- Use your dominant hand to pick up the catheter and hold it an inch or two from the tip. Ask patient to bear down as if voiding. Insert catheter tip into meatus. Ask the patient to take deep breaths as you advance the catheter 6 to 8 inches (14.4–19.2 cm) or until urine flows.
- Hold the catheter securely at the meatus with your nondominant hand while the bladder empties. If a specimen is being collected, remove the drainage end of the tubing from the specimen container after the required amount is obtained and allow urine to flow into receptacle. Set specimen container aside.
- Allow the bladder to empty. Withdraw the catheter slowly and smoothly after urine has stopped flowing. Remove equipment and dispose of according to facility policy. Wash and dry the genital area as needed. Replace foreskin in forward position if necessary.
- Remove your gloves. Assist the patient to a comfortable position. Cover the patient with bed linens. Place the bed in the lowest position.
- Put on clean gloves. Cover and label specimen. Send urine specimen to the laboratory promptly or refrigerate it.
- Remove gloves. Perform hand hygiene.

If a catheter is to remain in place for continuous drainage, an **indwelling urethral catheter** is used. Indwelling catheters are also called retention or Foley catheters. The indwelling urethral catheter is designed so that it does not slip out of the bladder. A balloon is inflated to ensure that the catheter remains in the bladder once it is inserted. Indwelling catheters are used for the gradual decompression of an overdistended bladder, for intermittent bladder drainage and irrigation, and for continuous bladder drainage. Several types of indwelling catheters are available, but the principles on which they operate are similar.

The indwelling catheter has more than one lumen (open tube) within the catheter. In a double-lumen catheter, one lumen is connected directly to the balloon, which is inflated with sterile water; the other is the lumen through which the urine drains. The triple-lumen catheter provides an additional lumen for the instillation of irrigating solution. Figure 36-10 illustrates a triple-lumen, double-lumen, and straight catheter.

A **suprapubic catheter** is used for long-term continuous drainage. This type of catheter is inserted surgically through a small incision above the pubic area (Fig. 36-11). Suprapubic bladder drainage diverts urine from the urethra when injury, stricture, prostatic obstruction, or gynecologic or abdominal surgery has compromised the flow of urine through the urethra. A suprapubic catheter is often preferred over indwelling urethral catheters for long-term urinary drainage. Suprapubic catheters are associated with decreased risk of contamination with

organisms from fecal material, elimination of damage to the urethra, a higher rate of patient satisfaction, and lower risk of catheter-associated UTIs (Rew & Smith, 2011; Hooton et al., 2010). The drainage tube is secured with sutures or tape. Care of the patient with a suprapubic catheter includes skin care around the insertion site; care of the drainage tubing and drainage bag is the same as for an indwelling catheter (see Caring for Patients With an Indwelling Catheter on pages 1293–1294).

Concept Mastery Alert

Continuous drainage can be achieved with either an indwelling urinary catheter or a suprapubic catheter. However, if the continuous drainage is long term, a suprapubic catheter would be best.

Urinary catheters are available in several different types of materials, with varying benefits and problems. The newest technology involves the use of antimicrobial coatings—such as silver alloy—on the catheter to reduce bacterial attachment, colonization, and migration, which result in catheter-associated UTIs (Hooton et al., 2010).

HAZARDS OF URETHRAL CATHETERIZATION
Sepsis and trauma are the two major hazards of introducing an instrument such as a catheter into the bladder. The male urethra is especially vulnerable to injury because of its longer length. An object forced through a stricture

FIGURE 36-10. (**A**) Triple-lumen indwelling catheter. (**B**) Double-lumen indwelling catheter. (**C**) Straight catheter.

or an irregular opening from the wrong angle can seriously damage the urethra. Although the female urethra is shorter than the male urethra, it is also susceptible to damage if a catheter is forced through it. The mucous membrane lining the urethra is delicate and damaged easily by the friction resulting from the insertion of a catheter. Bacteria can enter the bladder when the catheter is inserted. When the catheter is left in place, the organisms may move up the catheter lumen or the space between the catheter and the urethral wall. This asymptomatic condition in which bacteria are present in the urine is known as bacteriuria.

EQUIPMENT

The equipment used for catheterization is usually prepackaged in a sterile, disposable tray and is the same for both male and female patients. Most kits already contain a standard-sized catheter. Catheters are graded on the French (F) scale according to lumen size. For long-term use in an adult, a 14F to 16F catheter with a 5- to 10-mL balloon is commonly used (Newman, 2008). Smaller catheters usually are not necessary. A smaller lumen would be so small that it would increase the time necessary for emptying the bladder. Larger catheters distend the urethra and increase the discomfort of the procedure. Large-size catheters (18F or larger) can increase erosion of the bladder neck and urethral mucosa and cause the formation of strictures (Herter & Wallace Kazer, 2010). Sizes 5F to 8F are used for infants and young children. Sizes 8F to 12F catheters are commonly used for older children (Perry, Hockenberry, Lowdermilk, & Wilson, 2010).

PATIENT PREPARATION

Before the catheterization, explain to the patient the procedure and the reason for it. Tell the patient that catheter

FIGURE 36-11. A suprapubic catheter positioned in the bladder.

insertion produces a sensation of pressure and some discomfort. Explain that measures will be taken to avoid exposure and embarrassment. The more relaxed the patient is, the easier it will be to insert the catheter.

The most common patient position for catheter insertion is the dorsal recumbent position, with the patient preferably on a solid surface, such as a firm mattress or a treatment table. Catheterizing a patient in a bed with a soft mattress, especially a female patient, is not as satisfactory because the patient's pelvic surfaces are not firmly supported and visualization of the meatus is difficult. Also, the patient may sink into the bed, causing the bladder to be lower than the outlet of the catheter. If the patient is in bed, supporting the buttocks on a firm cushion is helpful.

The Sims, or lateral, position is an alternate position for catheter insertion in female patients. This position may allow better visualization and be more comfortable for the patient, especially if hip and knee movements are difficult. The smaller area of exposure is also less stressful for the patient. Allow the patient to lie on either side, depending on which position is easiest for the nurse and best for the patient's comfort. Place the patient's buttocks near the edge of the bed with her shoulders at the opposite edge and her knees drawn toward her chest. Lift the upper buttock and labia to expose the urinary meatus (Fig. 36-12).

URETHRAL CATHETER INSERTION

Nurses are responsible for inserting indwelling catheters and caring for the patient. Skill 36-5 on pages 1313–1319 describes catheterization of the female urinary bladder, and Skill 36-6 on pages 1319–1324 describes catheter-

ization of the male urinary bladder. Adhering to surgical asepsis is of utmost importance to help prevent UTIs. An inflated balloon holds the indwelling catheter in position in the bladder. The prefilled syringe included in the catheter kit contains the amount of sterile water needed to inflate the balloon to the desired spherical shape. It is important to use the entire amount provided by the manufacturer to avoid underinflation of the catheter balloon. A balloon that is only partially inflated could cause irritation and erosion to the mucosa in the bladder.

Insert indwelling catheters for male patients to the catheter bifurcation to avoid inadvertent inflation of the balloon in the urethra. The technique of applying lubricant to the catheter before inserting it in a male patient is not recommended. Lubricant applied externally to the catheter remains at the meatus, essentially allowing an unlubricated catheter to cause trauma to the lining of the urethra. The recommendation is to gently insert the tip of a syringe prefilled with lubricant into the male urethra before inserting the catheter (see Skill 36-6, pp. 1319–1324). If the prepackaged kit does not contain a syringe with lubricant, the nurse may need assistance in filling a syringe while keeping the lubricant sterile. Some institutions use lidocaine jelly for lubrication before insertion of the catheter. The jelly comes prepackaged in a sterile syringe and serves a dual purpose of lubricating and numbing the urethra. A medical order is necessary for the use of lidocaine jelly.

Properly secure an indwelling catheter to the thigh or abdomen to prevent movement and excessive force on the bladder neck or urethra, which leads to injury (Gray, 2008). The indwelling catheter is connected to a drainage and collection system that must be properly positioned and secured to minimize the risk for infection. The following

FIGURE 36-12. Demonstration of the side-lying position (*left*) and of how to expose the urinary meatus when catheterizing a female patient in the side-lying position (*right*).

technique is used to complete the closed urinary drainage system:

- Check to see that the patient is not lying on the drainage tubing and compressing it.
- Keep the catheter drainage bag below the level of the bladder at all times.
- Keep the drainage bag off the floor at all times to reduce the risk of infection. The floor is grossly contaminated.
- Check that all connections are secure and that no leakage is occurring.

See the accompanying Through the Eyes of a Student for a student's account of her experience with urinary catheterization.

CARING FOR PATIENTS WITH AN INDWELLING CATHETER

The following are nursing measures used to care for patients with an indwelling catheter:

- Wash hands before and after caring for a patient with an indwelling catheter.
- Clean the perineal area thoroughly, especially around the meatus, daily and after each bowel movement.
- Cleanse the catheter by cleaning gently from the meatus outward.
- Use mild soap and water or a perineal cleanser to clean the perineal area; rinse the area well. Do not use powders and lotions after cleaning. Do not use antibiotic or other antimicrobial cleaners or betadine at the urethral meatus (Herter & Wallace Kazer, 2010; Society of Urologic Nurses and Associates [SUNA], 2010).
- Make sure that the patient maintains a generous fluid intake, unless contraindicated by other health concerns. This helps prevent infection and irrigates the catheter naturally by increasing urine output.

- Encourage the patient to be up and about, as ordered.
- Note the volume and character of urine, and record observations carefully. Observe the urine through the drainage tubing and in the collecting container. Note and record the amount of urine on the patient's intake-and-output record every 8 hours. The collecting container is calibrated, but the volume markings are only approximations. Empty the urine into a graduated container that is calibrated accurately for correct determination of output.
- Do not open the drainage system to obtain urine specimens or to measure urine. If the tubing becomes disconnected and the sterile closed drainage system has been compromised, replace the catheter and collecting system (SUNA, 2010). When emptying the drainage bag, make sure the drainage spout does not touch a contaminated surface.
- Teach the patient the importance of personal hygiene—especially the importance of careful cleaning after having a bowel movement—and thorough, frequent hand hygiene.
- Promptly report any signs or symptoms of infection. These include a burning sensation and irritation at the meatus, cloudy urine, a strong odor to the urine, an elevated temperature, and chills.
- Help the patient take a shower bath if possible. Remember to keep the collecting bag lower than the bladder to promote drainage.
- Consider evidence-based practice guidelines and facility policy to ensure that the catheter is removed at the earliest time possible, to limit use to the shortest duration possible (Adams, Bucior, Day, & Rimmer, 2013; Bernard et al., 2012; Gokula et al., 2012; Hooton et al., 2010).

THROUGH THE EYES OF A STUDENT

Remembering my first hospital experiences, I would have to say that doing my first catheterization was the scariest. I was working with a nurse on the maternity floor. Our patient had not voided in more than 8 hours and seemed to be in great discomfort. We palpated her abdomen to see if her bladder was distended, and it was. Because she didn't have an urge to void, we decided to straight cath her to lessen her discomfort. The nurse I was working with turned and handed me the kit. She said, "You know what to do, right?" Automatically I replied, "Sure."

My heart began to race. Of course, I knew the procedure, but I never actually did it on a real person. Not only was I nervous about doing the procedure, but I also didn't want to make her labor more painful. The nurse, out of courtesy, asked the patient if she minded if I did the procedure. Thank God, the patient had a soft side for a beginner. Smiling, she looked at me and said, "You know what you're doing, right?" Again, I said, "Sure." I began setting up to begin my mission. To my amazement, I really

did remember how to prepare for a catheterization. I even was amazed that my sterile procedure wasn't bad for the first time. When it was time to insert the catheter, I took a deep breath. Thankfully, it went in nice and smooth, and I reached the bladder in seconds. The urine began flowing through rapidly. It seemed like it would never stop. Amazingly, it filled the container. I removed the catheter, cleaned up, and let out my breath.

In summary, I was glad that I had the experience to do a catheterization. The nurse told me that I did a good job, which made me feel good. Also, my patient thanked me for relieving some of her discomfort and gave me a reassuring smile. As I look back now, it wasn't as bad as I had myself believed it would be. Even though it's invasive to the patient, sometimes it's necessary. I want to do everything I can to help my patients. Now, I look at all my new adventures as helping my patients feel better.

—*Alysia Paxson, Holy Family College, Philadelphia*

RESEARCH IN NURSING

BRIDGING THE GAP TO EVIDENCE-BASED PRACTICE

Postoperative Urinary Catheters

Preventing catheter-associated urinary tract infection (CAUTI) is a health care priority. Routine placement of a urinary catheter for longer than 2 days postoperative had been found to increase the risk of infection. What factors may be contributing to increased duration of use?

Related Research

Bhardwaj, R., Pickard, R., Carrick-Sen, D., & Britain, K. (2012). Patients' perspectives on timing of urinary catheter removal after surgery. *British Journal of Nursing, 21*(18), S4, S6–S9.

The aims of this study were to explore patients' perceptions of the care process relating to perioperative catheterization to identify patient factors that encourage early removal, reducing the number of postoperative catheter-associated urinary tract infections. In this qualitative study, patients were asked about attitudes towards, and beliefs surrounding, perioperative catheterization and timing of catheter removal in terms of their past and current experience and future perception. Interviews were audio recorded and transcribed for analysis. Catheter duration ranged from 1 to 10 days. Major themes elicited included: lack of understanding of the purpose and catheterization process, loss of patient autonomy and dignity,

and impact of environmental factors. The authors concluded that a lack of knowledge of the catheterization process among participants led to fears and concerns that may have contributed to delayed catheter removal. The authors suggest changes to patient care to reduce catheter duration, including ensuring the provision of preoperative information, greater patient involvement in catheter removal decisions, and provision of easily accessible toilet facilities.

Relevance to Nursing Practice

Lack of awareness among patients concerning the association between catheter duration and CAUTI risk may contribute to increased duration of postoperative catheter use. Once armed with relevant knowledge, patients could be more involved in decisions related to catheter use and could be motivated to contribute to planning the removal of their catheter. Nurses have a responsibility to provide accurate and appropriate patient education, and should consider this an important part of the plan of care whenever possible, resulting in improved patient care and decreased CAUTIs.

For additional research, visit thePoint.

- Refer to the accompanying Research in Nursing: Postoperative Urinary Catheters display.
- Change indwelling catheters only as necessary. The interval between catheter changes varies and should be individualized for the patient, based on clinical symptoms: catheter encrustations, obstruction, leakage, bleeding, and catheter-associated UTIs (Herter & Wallace Kazer, 2010; SUNA, 2010).

  Patients who required long-term use of an indwelling catheter for persistent urinary retention may experience self-care practice and catheter challenges. See the accompanying display, Research in Nursing: Long-Term Urinary Catheters, for a discussion of catheter practices and problems.

PATIENT EDUCATION

Teach patients who have an indwelling catheter how the system functions and how they can assist with their care. Teaching points include keeping the tubing free of kinks, maintaining a constant downward flow of urine, maintaining an adequate fluid intake, and promptly reporting any unusual symptoms.

If the patient is ambulatory, connect the indwelling catheter to a smaller drainage bag that can be secured to the leg. Instruct the patient to do the following:

- Empty the leg bag at regular intervals. A full drainage bag may cause reflux of urine into the bladder or may pull away from its attachment on the leg.

- Wash hands before and after emptying the leg bag. Use an antiseptic solution to cleanse the connections.
- Care for the drainage bag daily, using a vinegar solution (1 part vinegar to 3 parts water). Clean the tubing and bag and allow to air dry before using again (SUNA, 2005a).

IRRIGATING THE INDWELLING CATHETER OR BLADDER

The flushing of a tube, canal, or area with solution is called irrigation. Natural irrigation of the catheter through increased fluid intake by the patient is preferred. The purpose of an external catheter irrigation is to restore or maintain its patency. A bladder irrigation rinses out the bladder and can also instill medication that acts directly on the bladder wall. Routine intermittent irrigation of long-term catheters is not recommended (SUNA, 2010). Avoid catheter irrigation unless necessary to relieve or prevent obstruction (Herter & Wallace Kazer, 2010). Skill 36-7 on pages 1325–1327 describes the procedure to perform an intermittent irrigation for an indwelling catheter using a closed system.

Continuous or frequent irrigations may be ordered when a blood clot or other debris threatens to block the catheter. Closed-system irrigation is recommended to prevent the introduction of pathogens into the bladder. Preferably, the patient who needs frequent irrigation so that the catheter and tubing remain patent will have a triple-lumen catheter using continuous irrigation (Fig. 36-13 on page 1296). Skill 36-8 on pages 1328–1330 describes continuous bladder irrigation.

RESEARCH IN NURSING

BRIDGING THE GAP TO EVIDENCE-BASED PRACTICE

Long-Term Urinary Catheters

Long-term urinary catheters may be appropriate for patients unable to use other bladder management methods, patients with a disability that makes it difficult to use the bathroom, and for patients with neurogenic bladder dysfunction. Living with an indwelling urinary catheter presents challenges that must be addressed on a daily basis. What issues do patients using a long-term indwelling catheter encounter?

Related Research

Catheter problems may include blockage, urinary tract infection, accidental dislodgement, and leakage of urine. Catheter management challenges may include drainage bag replacement and/or cleaning and caregiver assistance.

Wilde, M. H., McDonald, M. V., Brasch, J., McMahon, J. M., Fairbanks, E., Shah, S.,…Scheid, E. (2013). Long-term urinary catheter users self-care practices and problems. *Journal of Clinical Nursing*, 22(3/4), 356–367.

The aims of this study were to describe self-care practices and catheter problems in adult community-living long-term indwelling urinary catheter users and to explore relationships among catheter practices and problems. This descriptive and exploratory analysis utilized home interviews conducted with catheter users who provided information by self-reported recall over the previous 2 months. Data was analyzed by descriptive statistics and tests of association between demographics, catheter practices, and catheter problems. The sample was widely diverse in age, race, and medical diagnosis. Urethral catheters were used slightly more often than suprapubic catheters. Many participants were highly disabled, having difficulty in bathing,

dressing, toileting, and getting out of bed. Participants also required assistance with eating. A high percentage of catheter problems were reported, including bypass leakage of urine, urinary tract infections, blockage of the catheter, catheter-associated pain, and accidental dislodgement of the catheter. Treatment of catheter-related problems contributed to additional health care utilization, including extra nurse or clinic visits, visits to the emergency department or hospitalization. Symptoms of catheter-associated urinary tract infection most often included changes in the color or character of urine or generalized symptoms. The authors concluded that catheter-related problems contribute to excess health problems and health care utilization and costs.

Relevance to Nursing Practice

Many of the catheter-related problems reported in this study could be prevented or minimized with more attention to catheter management, early identification of problems and more evidence-based catheter practices. Nurses are often in the position of being the primary care provider and advocate for patients with long-term indwelling catheters. Nurses are in strategic positions to plan interventions to address the persistent catheter-related problems that affect large proportions of long-term indwelling urinary catheter users. Nurses have a responsibility to provide accurate and appropriate patient education, and should consider this an important part of the plan of care whenever possible, which will result in improved patient care.

For additional research, visit thePoint.

REMOVING THE INDWELLING CATHETER

The removal of an indwelling catheter and the after-care of the patient should include the following nursing measures:

- Wash hands before and after the procedure, and wear gloves.
- Deflate the balloon before attempting to remove the catheter by inserting a syringe into the balloon valve and aspirating all of the sterile water used to inflate it. Do not cut the tubing with scissors.
- Ask the patient to take several deep breaths to relax while you gently remove the catheter. Wrap the catheter in a towel or disposable waterproof drape.
- Clean the perineal area after the catheter is removed.
- Ensure that the patient's fluid intake is generous, and record the patient's fluid intake as well as time and amount of fluid output for at least 24 hours (or according to facility policy) following catheter removal. Instruct the patient to void into a bedpan, urinal, or specimen hat, either in bed or in the bathroom. If patient does not void within 8 to 10 hours of removal of the indwelling catheter, notify the primary care provider.

- Inform the patient that it may take a little while for the bladder to reestablish voluntary control and that an accident at this time is not unusual.
- Tell the patient that there may be a slight burning sensation when voiding the first one or two times after catheter removal.
- Observe the urine carefully for any abnormalities. Document the volume of the first void to validate adequate emptying of the bladder post removal.
- Record and report any unusual signs or symptoms, such as discomfort, a burning sensation when voiding, bleeding, or changes in vital signs, especially the patient's temperature. Be alert to any signs or symptoms of infection, and report them promptly.

Caring for a Patient With a Urologic Stent

When a patient has a urinary tract obstruction, a urologic stent may be inserted. The stent may be temporary (when placed in the ureters) or permanent (when positioned in the urethra). Temporary stents are usually made of a pliable material such as radiopaque silicone. Permanent

- Irrigation bag
- Drip chamber
- Clamp
- Bladder
- Tubing to irrigation port
- Port for inflation of catheter balloon
- Tubing from bladder
- Drainage bag

FIGURE 36-13. A continuous bladder irrigation (CBI) setup.

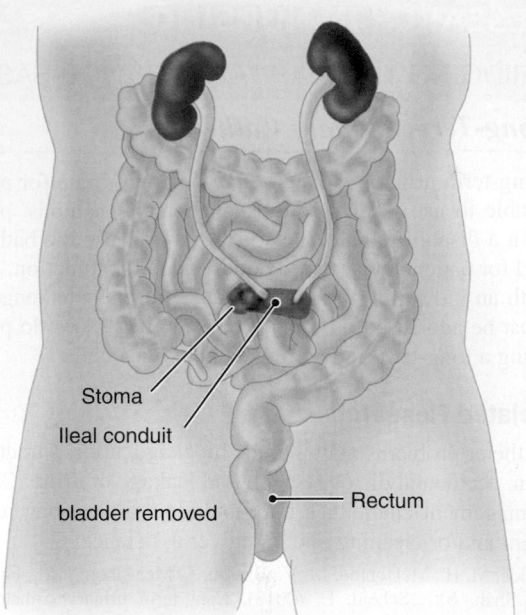

- Stoma
- Ileal conduit
- bladder removed
- Rectum

FIGURE 36-14. An ileal conduit. The ureters are brought to the separated segment of the ileum of the small intestine and a stoma is made where the urine is excreted.

stents are stronger and typically are made of a flexible metal mesh. They are commonly inserted during a cystoscopic procedure; in most cases, the patient receives only a local anesthetic and sedation. Urologic stents relieve urinary obstructions and provide a path for the flow of urine. Major nursing responsibilities include assessment, measurement, and documentation of urinary output. Never irrigate a blocked stent. Instruct the patient with a urologic stent to notify the primary care provider immediately if the urine becomes bright red, severe pain occurs, the drainage pattern changes, or any sign of infection is present. Also, encourage the patient to wear a medical alert bracelet at all times.

Caring for a Patient With a Urinary Diversion

Obstructions or tumors in the urinary tract may require some patients to have urinary flow diverted surgically.

Urinary diversions may also be used as part of the treatment for patients with a neurogenic bladder, radiation cystitis, or congenital anomalies of the lower urinary tract. An **ileal conduit** is a type of incontinent cutaneous urinary diversion. An ileal conduit involves a surgical resection of the small intestine, with transplantation of the ureters to the isolated segment of small bowel. This separated section of the small intestine is then brought to the abdominal wall, where urine is excreted through a stoma, a surgically created opening on the body surface. Figure 36-14 shows how the ureters are diverted in an ileal conduit. A **cutaneous ureterostomy** is another type of incontinent cutaneous urinary diversion in which the ureters are directed through the abdominal wall and attached to an opening in the skin. These cutaneous diversions are usually permanent, and the patient wears an external appliance to collect the urine because elimination of the urine from the stoma cannot be controlled voluntarily.

Another option for diversion of urine is a **continent urinary reservoir** (e.g., the Indiana pouch and the Kock pouch). Figure 36-15 shows how the ureters are diverted into a segment of ileum and cecum in an Indiana pouch. This is a surgical alternative that uses a section of the intestine to create an internal reservoir that holds urine, with the creation of a catheterizable stoma. The external stoma or outlet must be catheterized at regular intervals to drain the urine that has collected in this reservoir.

GENERAL CARE GUIDELINES

Creation of a urinary diversion is a surgical procedure. Therefore, the patient needs physical and psychological support before and after surgery. This support can come

FIGURE 36-15. An Indiana pouch. The ureters are diverted into a segment of ileum and cecum to create an internal reservoir that holds urine and a catheterizable stoma. (Reprinted with permission from Hinkle, J. L., & Cheever, K. H. [2014]. *Brunner & Suddarth's textbook of medical–surgical nursing* [13th ed.]. Philadelphia: Wolters Kluwer Health/Lippincott Williams & Wilkins.)

from the patient's significant others as well as from members of the health care team and people who have had similar experiences. The ostomy created for the diversion requires specific physical care for which the nurse is initially responsible. The following guidelines help to promote the patient's physical and psychological comfort related to stoma care:

- Inspect the patient's stoma regularly. It should be dark pink to red and moist (Fig. 36-16). A pale stoma may indicate anemia, and a dark or purple-blue stoma may reflect compromised circulation or ischemia. Bleeding around the stoma and its stem should be minimal. Notify the primary care provider promptly if bleeding persists or is excessive, or if color changes occur in the stoma.

FIGURE 36-16. The appearance of a normal stoma is red and smooth, with a mucous membrane surface.

- Note the size of the stoma, which usually stabilizes within 6 to 8 weeks. Most stomas protrude 1/2″ to 1″ from the abdominal surface and may initially appear swollen and edematous. The edema usually subsides after 6 weeks. If an abdominal dressing is in place over the surgical incision, check it frequently for drainage and bleeding. The dressing is usually removed after 24 hours.
- Keep the skin around the stoma site (peristomal area) clean and dry. If care is not taken to protect the skin around the stoma, irritation or infection may occur. A leaking appliance frequently causes skin erosion. Candida or yeast infections can also occur around the stoma if the area is not kept dry.
- Measure the patient's fluid intake and output. Careful monitoring of the patient's urinary output is necessary to detect fluid imbalances and adequate functioning of the diversion.
- Keep the patient as free of odors as possible. If the patient has an external appliance, empty the appliance frequently.
- Monitor the return of intestinal function and peristalsis. Initially after surgery, peristalsis is inhibited. Remember, the patient had a bowel resection as part of the urinary diversion procedure.
- If the patient has an ileal conduit, mucus may appear in the urine as a normal finding because the isolated segment of small intestine continues to produce mucous, as part of its normal functioning.
- Explain each aspect of care to the patient and explain what the patient's role will be when beginning self-care. Patient teaching is one of the most important aspects of care and should include family members when appropriate. Teaching can begin before surgery so that the patient has adequate time to absorb information.
- Encourage the patient to participate in care and to look at the stoma. Patients normally experience emotional depression during the early postoperative period. Help the patient to cope by listening, explaining, and being available and supportive. A visit from a representative of the local ostomy support group may be helpful. Patients usually begin to accept their altered body image when they are willing to look at the stoma, make neutral or positive statements concerning the ostomy, and express interest in learning self-care.

EXTERNAL APPLIANCES

The external appliance to collect the urine for patients with incontinent urinary diversions is typically a soft pouch that is either reusable or disposable. The upper part of the pouch has a firm faceplate several inches in diameter, with an opening the size of the stoma. Some faceplates are detachable from the pouch, while other appliances are one piece (Fig. 36-17 on page 1298). The plate surface is secured firmly around the stoma opening with a moisture-proof adherent so that no urine leakage occurs. Many patients also wear an elasticized belt that

Two-piece pouches

FIGURE 36-17. Two-piece appliances.

FIGURE 36-18. During hemodialysis, a machine does the work of the kidneys to filter wastes, electrolytes, and fluid from the body. (Reprinted with permission from Craven, R., & Hirnle, C. (2009). *Fundamentals of nursing: Human health and function* [6th ed.]. Philadelphia: Wolters Kluwer Health/Lippincott Williams & Wilkins.)

goes around the waist and connects to each side of the faceplate for added support. The lower end of the appliance has a drainage valve, which is used for emptying.

The patient needs to empty the appliance frequently. This is to prevent the pouch from becoming heavy with the weight of urine, causing tension on the faceplate, and possibly loosening the seal. For most people, this means emptying the appliance several times a day. The pouch can also be attached to drainage tubing and a large collection bag to avoid having to frequently empty the appliance, such as during the night or when confined to bed. In home situations, urine collection tubing and receptacles designed to be placed under the bed can be used at night.

URINARY APPLIANCE APPLICATION AND REMOVAL

The frequency of changing the appliance depends on the type being used. The appliance usually is changed after a time of low fluid intake, such as in the early morning. Urine production is less at this time, making changing the appliance easier. Skill 36-9 on pages 1330–1334 describes how to change an appliance worn over an ileal conduit.

PATIENT EDUCATION

Patient education is essential for independence in self-care. As the patient assumes responsibility for self-care, teach the patient how to make the necessary observations, to be aware of indications of problems, and to recognize when to seek assistance. For these goals to be met, the patient and/or family member needs to be able to do the following:

- Explain the reason for the urinary diversion and the rationale for treatment.
- Demonstrate self-care behaviors that effectively manage the diversion.
- Describe follow-up care and existing support resources.
- Report where supplies may be obtained in the community.
- Verbalize related fears and concerns.
- Demonstrate a positive body image.

The assistance of a wound, ostomy, and continence nurse (WOCN) can help the patient achieve these outcomes. Also, refer the patient to the United Ostomy Association for further information and helpful periodicals.

Caring for a Patient Receiving Dialysis

Dialysis is used to treat patients who experience severely decreased or total loss of kidney function. Dialysis is a mechanical way of filtering waste from the blood. There are two categories of dialysis: hemodialysis and peritoneal dialysis.

Hemodialysis involves a machine that does the work healthy kidneys normally perform by filtering harmful wastes, electrolytes, and fluid from the blood that would normally be eliminated in the patient's urine (Fig. 36-18). Patients receive a vascular access in order to receive hemodialysis. This vascular access, an arteriovenous (AV) fistula (a surgically created connection between an artery and a vein; Fig. 36-19A) or AV graft (a surgically created path between an artery and a vein using a flexible, synthetic tube; Fig. 36-19B) allows for easy access to the bloodstream. A temporary or permanent double-lumen central venous catheter can also be used to provide vascular access for hemodialysis (Richard, 2011). These vascular accesses are the point at which blood is removed from the patient's body for dialysis and then returned (Mayo, 2011a).

Peritoneal dialysis involves using blood vessels in the abdominal lining (peritoneum) to fill in for the kidneys, with the help of a fluid (dialysate) washed in and out of the peritoneal space. Diffusion and osmosis occur as waste products move from an area of higher concentration (the blood stream) to an area of lesser concentration (the dialysate fluid) through the peritoneum (Hinkle & Cheever, 2014). Patients receive a catheter (a thin, soft plastic tube) surgically placed through the abdomen into the peritoneal cavity (Fig. 36-20). It is used to carry the dialysis solution in and out of the patient's abdomen (Mayo, 2011b).

Care of either catheter site is a nursing responsibility. Care involves assessment of the catheter sites. Skill 36-10 on pages 1335–1336 outlines nursing care related to caring for a hemodialysis access. Refer to Skill 36-11

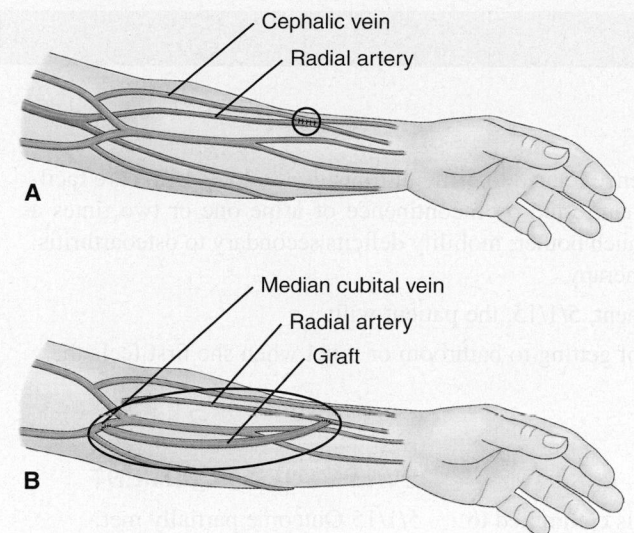

FIGURE 36-19. (**A**) Arteriovenous fistula, created by connecting an artery and vein. (**B**) Arteriovenous graft, created by using a synthetic tube to form a path between an artery and vein. (Reprinted with permission from Hinkle, J. L., & Cheever, K. H. [2014]. *Brunner & Suddarth's textbook of medical surgical nursing* [13th ed.]. Philadelphia: Wolters Kluwer Health/ Lippincott Williams & Wilkins.)

FIGURE 36-20. Peritoneal dialysis. (Reprinted with permission from Hinkle, J. L., & Cheever, K. H. [2014]. *Brunner & Suddarth's textbook of medical surgical nursing* [13th ed.]. Philadelphia: Wolters Kluwer Health/Lippincott Williams & Wilkins.)

on pages 1336–1338 for nursing care related to caring for a patient with a peritoneal dialysis catheter.

Evaluating

The nurse evaluates the effectiveness of a plan of care to promote healthy urinary functioning by checking whether the patient has met the individualized patient goals specified in the plan. See the Nursing Plan of Care 36-1 for Mrs. Jaspers. Nursing care is considered effective if the patient expresses satisfaction with the regular voiding pattern and is able to:

- Produce a sufficient quantity of urine to maintain fluid, electrolyte, and acid–base balance

- Empty the bladder completely at regular intervals without discomfort
- Provide care for urinary diversion and know when to notify the primary care provider
- Develop a plan to modify any factors that contribute to current urinary problems or that might impair urinary functioning in the future
- Correct unhealthy urinary habits, such as delaying voiding, drinking insufficient fluids, or abusing diuretics

NURSING PLAN OF CARE 36-1

for Elana Jaspers

Mrs. Elana Jaspers is an alert, 83-year-old woman whose husband of 59 years died 6 months ago. Although Mrs. Jaspers was adamant about wanting to live independently in her own home, arthritis severely restricted her movement and ability to manage. After a hospitalization for pneumonia, she was transferred to a long-term care facility 1 month ago. The admitting medical diagnoses included hypertension, osteoarthritis, and depression. A comprehensive nursing assessment of Mrs. Jaspers performed 1 month after her admission to a long-term care facility included the following notations:

- Continent of urine on admission
- At present, incontinent of urine one or two times a day; often found wet in the morning; states it is "too much bother to get into the bathroom"
- Sits in chair in room unless encouraged and assisted to walk, although capable of independent ambulation with care; progressive muscle atrophy and joint stiffness
- No identifiable pathology underlying incontinence
- Medications include a diuretic for hypertension and a tricyclic antidepressant
- Reddened skin in the perineal area

(continued)

NURSING PLAN OF CARE 36-1 *continued*

for Elana Jaspers

NURSING DIAGNOSIS	Functional Urinary Incontinence related to difficult transition to long-term care facility and mobility deficit as manifested by incontinence of urine one or two times a day; feeling toileting is too much bother; mobility deficits secondary to osteoarthritis; diuretic and antidepressant therapy
EXPECTED OUTCOME	By the next monthly assessment, 5/1/15, the patient will:

- Verbalize the importance of getting to bathroom or toilet when she first feels the need to void

NURSING INTERVENTIONS	**RATIONALE**	**EVALUATIVE STATEMENT**
Assess the value the patient attaches to voluntary control of urination and urinary continence; counsel appropriately.	Unless the patient is committed to the plan of care, goal achievement is impossible.	5/1/15 Outcome partially met. Patient has commented on the importance of regular toileting but still finds this "too much trouble" some days.
Teach the importance of complete bladder emptying at regular intervals and the harmful effects of ignoring the urge to void.	Patient understanding of the causes and harmful effects of urinary incontinence may motivate desire for reestablishment of voluntary control.	*Revision:* Reinforce value.
		D. Mora, RN
Assess patient's normal voiding habits at home and assist her to reestablish these. Initial reminders to toilet herself may be necessary.	Respect for the patient's normal voiding schedule and patterns communicates nursing's sincere concern for the individual and encourages patient achievement of goals.	

EXPECTED OUTCOME	By the next monthly assessment, 5/1/15, the patient will:

- Demonstrate the ability to walk to the bathroom using cane to toilet herself

NURSING INTERVENTIONS	**RATIONALE**	**EVALUATIVE STATEMENT**
Assess the patient's ability to toilet herself independently. Work consistently with her to increase activity tolerance: encourage short walks throughout the day to increase mobility.	One response to experiencing the multiple losses associated with aging is to surrender all control and become increasingly dependent. Nonpathology-based incontinence is less likely to occur if the daily living of the person keeps her more mobile, flexible, oriented, and motivated. An older person who seeks to take control and has a positive self-image is more continent.	5/1/15 Outcome met. Patient can safely walk to bathroom using cane and toilet herself when she wants to.
		D. Mora, RN

NURSING PLAN OF CARE 36-1 *continued*

for Elana Jaspers

NURSING INTERVENTIONS	RATIONALE	EVALUATIVE STATEMENT
Refer patient to occupational therapy for assistance with diagnosis and treatment if necessary.	The specialized skills of the occupational therapist may facilitate relearning toileting skills.	5/1/15 Outcome not met. Patient repeatedly neglects AM perineal care.
Communicate clearly that the patient is expected to use the toilet to urinate. Refrain from using incontinent briefs or pads. Talk with family about patient's having sufficient undergarments to allow changes as needed until control is reestablished.	Understanding that the staff expects continence and is committed to working with the patient to achieve it is a powerful patient motivator.	*Revision:* Reteach both the importance and procedure of perineal care. Assess each AM. *D. Mora, RN*
Assess patient's motivation and ability to be clean, dry, and comfortable.	Patient may not understand how easily skin irritation can occur and danger of pressure ulcers.	
Teach perineal hygiene.	Keeping the perineal area clean and dry promotes intact skin around the urinary meatus and the perineal area. Proper hygiene measures also decrease the possibility of bacteria or organisms migrating into the bladder.	

EXPECTED OUTCOME By the next monthly assessment, 5/1/15, the patient will:

- Decrease urinary incontinent episodes to less than three or four per week

NURSING INTERVENTIONS	RATIONALE	EVALUATIVE STATEMENT
Communicate to patient that the nurses *care* about her reestablishing urinary continence and believe she can do this. Use verbal reinforcement to reward "dry" days.	A common feeling of recently institutionalized older adults is *abandonment* and the sense that no one cares; response: "Why should I?" Communicating that the patient's progress toward goal achievement is valued by the nurses is an excellent encouragement to continue progress.	5/1/15 Outcome met. Patient in last week was completely dry for 4 of 7 days. Recorded four incontinent episodes. *D. Mora, RN*
Chart incontinent episodes and monitor progress; discuss this with patient.	This records progress with incontinent episodes and provides positive reinforcement.	

NURSING DIAGNOSIS Impaired Skin Integrity related to functional urinary incontinence as manifested by reddened perineal area (skin still intact)

EXPECTED OUTCOME By the next monthly assessment, 5/1/15, the patient will:

- Demonstrate healing of reddened perineal area

(continued)

NURSING PLAN OF CARE 36-1 *continued*

for Elana Jaspers

NURSING INTERVENTIONS	RATIONALE	EVALUATIVE STATEMENT
Assess skin for breakdown each AM and PM and after each incontinent episode.	Perineal care is often neglected or assigned to the least trained personnel in care settings. Skin irritation not detected and treated early may progress to serious pressure ulcers.	5/1/15 Outcome partially met. Perineal area is less inflamed. *Revision:* Continue to monitor perineal hygiene. No need for protective ointment. D. Mora, RN
Teach the patient the importance of washing this area carefully with soap and water each AM and after incontinent episodes. Teach the importance of always cleaning and wiping the perineum from front to back to prevent autoinfection. Until incontinent episodes are eliminated, a protective waterproof ointment may be indicated.	The woman who is doing self-care may neglect it entirely or use incorrect technique.	
Encourage use of cotton underwear and avoidance of nylon pantyhose, girdles, tight-fitting pants.	Nylon products tend to hold moisture and may minimize airflow to the perineal area.	

SAMPLE DOCUMENTATION

4/3/15 Nursing

This AM, after an incontinent episode, Mrs. Jaspers began to talk about how hard it is to get adjusted to living here, and commented, "I feel like just giving up." We talked about the importance of being as independent as possible and the dangers of becoming passively dependent. Nursing teaching and counseling included values of independently adhering to usual toileting schedule and importance of perineal hygiene. Two hours later, after lunch, Mrs. Jaspers walked to bathroom and toileted herself. Progress with urinary incontinence will continue to be monitored. Ability definitely present but encouragement needed.

D. Mora, RN

SKILL 36-1 ASSESSING BLADDER VOLUME USING AN ULTRASOUND BLADDER SCANNER

DELEGATION CONSIDERATIONS

The assessment of bladder volume using an ultrasound bladder scanner is not delegated to nursing assistive personnel (NAP) or unlicensed assistive personnel (UAP). Depending on the state's nurse practice act and the organization's policies and procedures, this procedure may be delegated to licensed practical/vocational nurses (LPN/LVNs). The decision to delegate must be based on careful analysis of the patient's needs and circumstances, as well as the qualifications of the person to whom the task is being delegated. Refer to the Delegation Guidelines in Appendix A (found on thePoint).

EQUIPMENT

- Bladder scanner
- Ultrasound gel or bladder scan gel pad
- Alcohol wipe or other sanitizer recommended by the scanner manufacturer and/or facility policy
- Clean gloves
- Additional PPE, as indicated
- Paper towel or washcloth

IMPLEMENTATION

ACTION	RATIONALE
1. Review the patient's medical record for any limitations in physical activity. Gather equipment.	Physical limitations may require adaptations in performing the skill. Assembling equipment provides an organized approach to task.
2. Perform hand hygiene and put on PPE, if indicated.	Hand hygiene and PPE prevent the spread of microorganisms. PPE is required based on transmission precautions.
3. Identify the patient.	Identifying the patient ensures that the right patient receives the intervention and helps prevent errors.
4. Close the curtains around the bed and close the door to the room, if possible. Discuss the procedure with the patient and assess the patient's ability to assist with the procedure, as well as personal hygiene preferences.	This ensures the patient's privacy. This discussion promotes reassurance and provides knowledge about the procedure. Dialogue encourages patient participation and allows for individualized nursing care.
5. Adjust the bed to a comfortable working height; usually elbow height of the caregiver (VISN 8 Patient Safety Center, 2009). Place the patient in a supine position. Drape patient. Stand on the patient's right side if you are right-handed, patient's left side if you are left-handed.	Having the bed at the proper height prevents back and muscle strain. Proper positioning allows accurate assessment of bladder volume. Keeping the patient covered as much as possible promotes patient comfort and privacy. Positioning allows for ease of use of dominant hand for the procedure.
6. Put on clean gloves.	Gloves prevent contact with blood and body fluids.
7. Press the ON button. Wait until the device warms up. Press the SCAN button to turn on the scanning screen.	Many devices require a few minutes to prepare the internal programs.
8. Press the appropriate gender button. The appropriate icon for male or female will appear on the screen (Fig. 1).	The device must be programmed for the gender of the patient by pushing the correct button on the device. If a female patient has had a hysterectomy, the male button is pushed (Altschuler & Diaz, 2006).
9. Clean the scanner head with the appropriate cleaner (Fig. 2).	Cleaning the scanner head deters transmission of microorganisms.

FIGURE 1. Identifying the icon for the patient's gender. (*Photo by B. Proud.*)

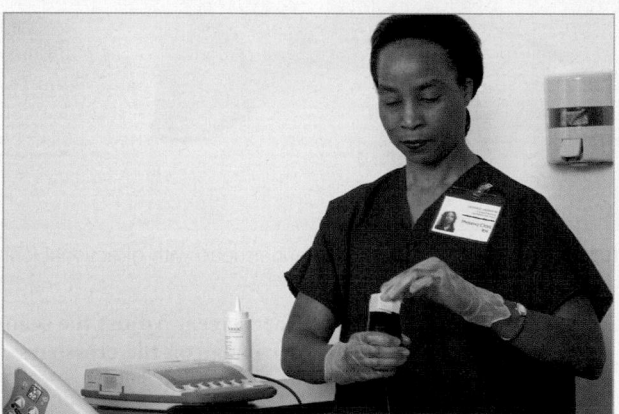

FIGURE 2. Cleaning scanner head. (*Photo by B. Proud.*)

(continued)

SKILL 36-1 ASSESSING BLADDER VOLUME USING AN ULTRASOUND BLADDER SCANNER *continued*

ACTION	RATIONALE
10. Gently palpate the patient's symphysis pubis (anterior midline junction of pubic bones). Place a generous amount of ultrasound gel or gel pad midline on the patient's abdomen, about 1 to 1.5 inches above the symphysis pubis (Fig. 3).	Palpation identifies the proper location and allows for correct placement of scanner head over the patient's bladder.

FIGURE 3. (**A**) Placing ultrasound gel about 1 to 1½ inches above symphysis pubis. (*Photo by B. Proud.*) (**B**) Gel pad.

ACTION	RATIONALE
11. Place the scanner head on the gel or gel pad, **with the directional icon on the scanner head toward the patient's head. Aim the scanner head toward the bladder (point the scanner head slightly downward toward the coccyx; Patraca, 2005).** Press and release the scan button (Fig. 4).	Proper placement allows for accurate reading of urine in bladder.

FIGURE 4. (**A**) Positioning the scanner head with directional icon toward the patient's bladder. (**B**) Scan button. (*Photos by B. Proud.*)

ACTION	RATIONALE
12. Observe the image on the scanner screen. **Adjust the scanner head to center the bladder image on the crossbars (Fig. 5).**	This action allows for accurate reading of urine in bladder.
13. Press and hold the DONE button until it beeps. Read the volume measurement on the screen. Print the results, if required, by pressing PRINT.	This action provides accurate documentation of reading.

ACTION	RATIONALE

Aiming icon

BladderScan™

150ml

READY TO SCAN
CURRENT = 143ml
[DONE] [RE] [F] [SCAN]

FIGURE 5. Centering the image on the crossbars. (Reprinted with permission from Patraca, K. [2005]. Measure bladder volume without catheterization. *Nursing, 35*[4], 4.)

14. Use a washcloth or paper towel to remove remaining gel from the patient's skin. Alternately, gently remove gel pad from patient's skin. Return the patient to a comfortable position. Remove your gloves and ensure that the patient is covered.

Removal of the gel promotes patient comfort. Removing contaminated gloves prevents spread of microorganisms.

15. Lower bed height and adjust head of bed to a comfortable position. Reattach call bell, if necessary.

These actions promote patient safety.

16. Remove additional PPE, if used. Perform hand hygiene.

Removing PPE properly reduces the risk for infection transmission and contamination of other items. Hand hygiene prevents the spread of microorganisms.

DOCUMENTATION

Guidelines

Document the assessment data that led to the use of the bladder scanner, relevant symptoms, the urine volume measured, and the patient's response.

Sample Documentation

7/06/15 1130 Patient has not voided 8 hours after catheter removal. Patient denies feelings of discomfort, pressure, and pain. Bladder not palpable. Bladder scanned for 120 mL of urine. Patient encouraged to increase oral fluid intake to eight 6-oz glasses today. Dr. Liu notified of assessment. Orders received to rescan in 4 hours if patient does not void.

—B. Clapp, RN

UNEXPECTED SITUATIONS AND ASSOCIATED INTERVENTIONS

• *You press wrong icon for patient's gender when initiating scanner:* Turn scanner off and back on. Re-enter information using correct gender button.

• *You have reason to believe bladder is full, based on assessment data, but scanner reveals little to no urine in bladder:* Ensure proper positioning of scanner head. Place a generous amount of ultrasound gel or gel pad midline on the patient's abdomen, about 1 to 1.5 inches above the symphysis pubis. Place the scanner head on the gel or gel pad, with the directional icon on the scanner head toward the patient's head. Aim the scanner head toward the bladder (point the scanner head slightly downward toward the coccyx). Ensure that the bladder image is centered on the crossbars.

SKILL 36-2 | ASSISTING WITH THE USE OF A BEDPAN

DELEGATION CONSIDERATIONS	Assisting a patient with the use of a bedpan may be delegated to nursing assistive personnel (NAP) or unlicensed assistive personnel (UAP), as well as to licensed practical/vocational nurses (LPN/LVNs). The decision to delegate must be based on careful analysis of the patient's needs and circumstances, as well as the qualifications of the person to whom the task is being delegated. Refer to the Delegation Guidelines in Appendix A (found on thePoint).

EQUIPMENT	• Bedpan (regular or fracture) • Toilet tissue • Disposable clean gloves • Additional PPE, as indicated	• Cover for bedpan or urinal (disposable waterproof pad or cover) • Disposable washcloths and skin cleanser • Moist towelettes, skin cleanser and water, or hand sanitizer

IMPLEMENTATION

ACTION	RATIONALE
1. Review the patient's medical record for any limitations in physical activity. Gather equipment.	Activity limitations may contraindicate certain actions by the patient. Assembling equipment provides an organized approach to task.
2. Perform hand hygiene and put on PPE, if indicated.	Hand hygiene and PPE prevent the spread of microorganisms. PPE is required based on transmission precautions.
3. Identify the patient.	Identifying the patient ensures that the right patient receives the intervention and helps prevent errors.
4. Assemble equipment on the chair next to the bed within reach.	Arranging items nearby is convenient, saves time, and avoids unnecessary stretching and twisting of muscles on the part of the nurse.
5. Close curtains around the bed and close the door to the room, if possible. Discuss the procedure with the patient and assess the patient's ability to assist with the procedure, as well as personal hygiene preferences.	This ensures the patient's privacy. This discussion promotes reassurance and provides knowledge about the procedure. Dialogue encourages patient participation and allows for individualized nursing care.
6. Unless contraindicated, apply powder to the rim of the bedpan. Place bedpan and cover on the chair next to the bed. Put on gloves.	Powder helps keep the bedpan from sticking to the patient's skin and makes it easier to remove. Powder is not applied if the patient has respiratory problems, is allergic to powder, or if a urine specimen is needed (could contaminate the specimen). The bedpan on the chair allows for easy access. Gloves prevent contact with blood and body fluids.
7. Adjust bed to comfortable working height, usually elbow height of the caregiver (VISN 8 Patient Safety Center, 2009). Place the patient in a supine position, with the head of the bed elevated about 30 degrees, unless contraindicated.	Having the bed at the proper height prevents back and muscle strain. Supine position is necessary for correct placement of the patient on the bedpan.
8. Fold the top linen back just enough to allow placement of the bedpan. If there is no waterproof pad on the bed and time allows, consider placing a waterproof pad under the patient's buttocks before placing the bedpan.	Folding back the linen in this manner minimizes unnecessary exposure while still allowing the nurse to place the bedpan. The waterproof pad will protect the bed should there be a spill.
9. Ask the patient to bend the knees. Have the patient lift the hips upward. Assist the patient, if necessary, by placing your hand that is closest to the patient palm up, under the lower back, and assist with lifting. Slip the bedpan into place with the other hand (Fig. 1).	The nurse uses less energy when the patient can assist by placing some of his or her weight on the heels.
10. **Ensure that the bedpan is in proper position and the patient's buttocks are resting on the rounded shelf of the regular bedpan or the shallow rim of the fracture bedpan.**	Having the bedpan in the proper position prevents spills onto the bed, ensures patient comfort, and prevents injury to the skin from a misplaced bedpan.

ACTION

FIGURE 1. Assisting patient to raise self in bed to position the bedpan. *(Note: Covers should only be folded back just enough to work, not expose patient unnecessarily. Covers in this series of photos have been pulled back to show action.)*

11. Raise the head of the bed as near to sitting position as tolerated, unless contraindicated. Cover the patient with bed linens.

12. **Place the call bell and toilet tissue within easy reach. Place the bed in the lowest position.** Leave the patient if it is safe to do so. Use side rails appropriately (Fig. 2).

FIGURE 2. Placing call bell within patient's reach and handing patient toilet tissue.

13. Remove gloves and additional PPE, if used. Perform hand hygiene.

Removing the Bedpan

14. Perform hand hygiene and put on gloves and additional PPE, as indicated. Adjust the bed to a comfortable working height, usually elbow height of the caregiver (VISN 8 Patient Safety Center, 2009). Have a receptacle, such as a plastic trash bag, handy for discarding tissue.

15. Lower the head of the bed, if necessary, to about 30 degrees. Remove the bedpan in the same manner in which it was offered, being careful to hold it steady. Ask the patient to bend the knees and lift the buttocks up from the bedpan. Assist the patient, if necessary, by placing your hand that is closest to the patient palm up, under the lower back, and assist with lifting. Place the bedpan on the bedside chair and cover it.

RATIONALE

This position makes it easier for the patient to void or defecate, avoids strain on the patient's back, and allows gravity to aid in elimination. Covering promotes warmth and privacy.

Falls can be prevented if the patient does not have to reach for needed items. Placing the bed in the lowest position promotes patient safety. Leaving the patient alone, if possible, promotes self-esteem and shows respect for privacy. Side rails assist the patient in repositioning.

Proper removal of PPE prevents transmission of microorganisms. Hand hygiene deters the spread of microorganisms.

Hand hygiene deters the spread of microorganisms. Gloves prevent exposure to blood and body fluids. Having the bed at the proper height prevents back and muscle strain. Proper disposal of soiled tissue prevents transmission of microorganisms.

Holding the bedpan steady prevents spills. The nurse uses less energy when the patient can assist by placing some of his or her weight on the heels. Covering the bedpan helps to prevent the spread of microorganisms.

(continued)

SKILL 36-2 ASSISTING WITH THE USE OF A BEDPAN *continued*

ACTION	**RATIONALE**
16. If the patient needs assistance with hygiene, wrap tissue around the hand several times, and wipe the patient clean, using one stroke from the pubic area toward the anal area. Discard tissue. Use warm, moist, disposable washcloth and skin cleanser to clean perineal area. Place the patient on his or her side and spread buttocks to clean the anal area.	Cleaning area from front to back minimizes fecal contamination of the vagina and urinary meatus. Cleaning the patient after the patient has used the bedpan prevents offensive odors and irritation to the skin.
17. Do not place toilet tissue in the bedpan if a specimen is required or if output is being recorded. Place toilet tissue in the appropriate receptacle.	Mixing toilet tissue with a specimen makes laboratory examination more difficult and interferes with accurate output measurement.
18. Return the patient to a comfortable position. Make sure the linens under the patient are dry. Replace or remove pad under the patient, as necessary. Remove your gloves and ensure that the patient is covered.	Positioning helps to promote patient comfort. Removing contaminated gloves prevents spread of microorganisms.
19. Raise the side rail. Lower the bed height and adjust the head of the bed to a comfortable position. Reattach the call bell.	These actions promote patient safety.
20. Offer patient supplies to wash and dry the hands, assisting as necessary.	Washing hands after using the urinal helps prevent the spread of microorganisms.
21. Put on clean gloves. Empty and clean the bedpan, measuring the urine in a graduated container, as necessary. Discard trash receptacle with used toilet paper per facility policy.	Gloves prevent exposure to blood and body fluids. Cleaning reusable equipment helps prevent the spread of microorganisms.
22. Remove additional PPE, if used. Perform hand hygiene.	Removing PPE properly reduces the risk for infection transmission and contamination of other items. Hand hygiene prevents the spread of microorganisms.

DOCUMENTATION

Guidelines

Document the patient's tolerance of the activity. Record the amount of urine voided on the intake and output record, if appropriate. Document any other assessments, such as unusual urine characteristics or alterations in the patient's skin.

Sample Documentation

> <u>12/06/15</u> 0730 Patient placed on fracture bedpan with a two-person assist. Voided 400 mL dark yellow urine; strong odor noted. Perineal skin intact, without redness or irritation. Specimen sent for urinalysis as ordered.
> —S. Barnes, RN

SPECIAL CONSIDERATIONS

- A fracture bedpan is usually more comfortable for the patient, but it does not hold as large a volume as the regular bedpan.
- Very thin or elderly patients often find it easier and more comfortable to use the fracture bedpan.
- Bedpan should not be left in place for extended periods because this can result in excessive pressure and irritation to the patient's skin.

SKILL 36-3   ASSISTING WITH THE USE OF A URINAL

DELEGATION CONSIDERATIONS

Assisting a patient with the use of a urinal may be delegated to nursing assistive personnel (NAP) or unlicensed assistive personnel (UAP), as well as to licensed practical/vocational nurses (LPN/LVNs). The decision to delegate must be based on careful analysis of the patient's needs and circumstances, as well as the qualifications of the person to whom the task is being delegated. Refer to the Delegation Guidelines in Appendix A (found on thePoint).

EQUIPMENT

- Urinal with end cover (usually attached)
- Toilet tissue
- Clean gloves
- Additional PPE, as indicated
- Disposable washcloths and skin cleanser
- Moist towelettes, skin cleanser and water, or hand sanitizer

IMPLEMENTATION

ACTION	RATIONALE
1. Review the patient's medical record for any limitations in physical activity. Gather equipment.	Activity limitations may contraindicate certain actions by the patient. Assembling equipment provides an organized approach to the task.
2. Perform hand hygiene and put on PPE, if indicated.	Hand hygiene and PPE prevent the spread of microorganisms. PPE is required based on transmission precautions.
3. Identify the patient.	Identifying the patient ensures that the right patient receives the intervention and helps prevent errors.
4. Assemble equipment on the chair next to the bed within reach.	Arranging items nearby is convenient, saves time, and avoids unnecessary stretching and twisting of muscles on the part of the nurse.
5. Close the curtains around the bed and close the door to the room, if possible. Discuss the procedure with the patient and assess the patient's ability to assist with the procedure, as well as personal hygiene preferences.	This ensures the patient's privacy. This discussion promotes reassurance and provides knowledge about the procedure. Dialogue encourages patient participation and allows for individualized nursing care.
6. Put on gloves.	Gloves prevent exposure to blood and body fluids.
7. Assist the patient to an appropriate position, as necessary: standing at the bedside, lying on one side or back, sitting in bed with the head elevated, or sitting on the side of the bed.	These positions facilitate voiding and emptying of the bladder.
8. If the patient remains in the bed, fold the linens just enough to allow for proper placement of the urinal.	Folding back the linen in this manner minimizes unnecessary exposure while still allowing the nurse to place the urinal.
9. If the patient is not standing, have him spread his legs slightly. **Hold the urinal close to the penis and position the penis completely within the urinal (Fig. 1). Keep the bottom of the urinal lower than the penis. If necessary, assist the patient to hold the urinal in place.**	Slight spreading of the legs allows for proper positioning of the urinal. Placing penis completely within the urinal and keeping the bottom lower than the penis avoids urine spills.
10. Cover the patient with the bed linens.	Covering promotes warmth and privacy.

FIGURE 1. Positioning urinal in place for a male patient. (*Note: Covers should only be folded back just enough to work, not expose patient unnecessarily. Covers have been pulled back to show action.*)

(continued)

SKILL 36-3 ASSISTING WITH THE USE OF A URINAL *continued*

ACTION	RATIONALE
11. Place the call bell and toilet tissue within easy reach. Have a receptacle, such as a plastic trash bag, handy for discarding tissue. Ensure that the bed is in the lowest position. Leave the patient if it is safe to do so. Use the side rails appropriately.	Falls can be prevented if the patient does not have to reach for needed items. Placing the bed in the lowest position promotes patient safety. Leaving the patient alone, if possible, promotes self-esteem and shows respect for privacy. Side rails assist the patient in repositioning.
12. Remove gloves and additional PPE, if used. Perform hand hygiene.	Proper removal of PPE reduces transmission of microorganisms. Hand hygiene deters the spread of microorganisms.

Removing the Urinal

ACTION	RATIONALE
13. Perform hand hygiene. Put on gloves and additional PPE, as indicated.	Hand hygiene and PPE prevent the spread of microorganisms. Gloves prevent exposure to blood and body fluids. PPE is required based on transmission precautions.
14. Pull back the patient's bed linens just enough to remove the urinal. Remove the urinal. Cover the open end of the urinal. Place on the bedside chair. If patient needs assistance with hygiene, wrap tissue around the hand several times, and wipe patient dry. Place tissue in receptacle. Use warm, moist, disposable washcloth and skin cleanser to clean perineal area as necessary, and as per patient request.	Covering the end of the urinal helps to prevent the spread of microorganisms. Cleaning the patient after he has used the bedpan prevents offensive odors and skin irritation.
15. Return the patient to a comfortable position. Make sure the linens under the patient are dry. Remove your gloves and ensure that the patient is covered.	Proper positioning promotes patient comfort. Removing contaminated gloves prevents the spread of microorganisms.
16. Ensure that the patient call bell is in reach.	Promotes patient safety.
17. Offer the patient supplies to wash and dry his hands, assisting as necessary.	Washing hands after using the urinal helps prevent the spread of microorganisms.
18. Put on clean gloves. Empty and clean the urinal, measuring the urine in a graduated container, as necessary. Discard the trash receptacle with used toilet paper per facility policy.	Measurement of urine volume is required for accurate intake and output records.
19. Remove gloves and additional PPE, if used, and perform hand hygiene.	Gloves prevent exposure to blood and body fluids. Removing PPE properly reduces the risk for infection transmission and contamination of other items. Hand hygiene prevents the spread of microorganisms.

DOCUMENTATION

Guidelines

Document the patient's tolerance of the activity. Record the amount of urine voided on the intake and output record, if appropriate. Document any other assessments, such as unusual urine characteristics or alterations in the patient's skin.

Sample Documentation

12/06/15 0730 Patient using urinal at bedside to void. Voided 600 mL yellow urine. Perineal skin intact, without redness or irritation. Reinforced need for continued use of urinal for recording accurate output. Patient verbalized an understanding of instructions.

—S. Barnes, RN

Special Considerations

- Urinal should not be left in place for extended periods because pressure and irritation to the patient's skin can result. If patient is unable to use alone or with assistance, consider other interventions, such as assisting the patient to use a bedside commode or applying an external condom catheter.
- It may be necessary to assist patients who have difficulty holding the urinal in place, such as those with limited upper extremity movement or alteration in mentation, to prevent spillage of urine.
- The urinal may also be used standing or sitting at the bedside or in the patient's bathroom, if the patient is able to do so.

SKILL 36-4   APPLYING AN EXTERNAL CONDOM CATHETER

DELEGATION CONSIDERATIONS	The application of an external condom catheter may be delegated to nursing assistive personnel (NAP) or unlicensed assistive personnel (UAP), as well as to licensed practical/vocational nurses (LPN/LVNs). The decision to delegate must be based on careful analysis of the patient's needs and circumstances, as well as the qualifications of the person to whom the task is being delegated. Refer to the Delegation Guidelines in Appendix A (found on the Point).

EQUIPMENT

- Condom sheath in appropriate size
- Skin protectant, such as Cavilon™ or Skin Prep™
- Velcro leg strap, catheter securing device, or tape
- Bath blanket
- Reusable leg bag with tubing or urinary drainage setup

- Basin of warm water and skin cleanser
- Disposable gloves
- Additional PPE, as indicated
- Washcloth and towel
- Scissors

IMPLEMENTATION

ACTION	RATIONALE
1. Gather equipment.	Assembling equipment provides an organized approach to task.
2. Perform hand hygiene and put on PPE, if indicated.	Hand hygiene and PPE prevent the spread of microorganisms. PPE is required based on transmission precautions.
3. Identify the patient.	Identifying the patient ensures that the right patient receives the intervention and helps prevent errors.
4. Close curtains around the bed and close the door to the room, if possible. Discuss the procedure with the patient. Ask the patient if he has any allergies, especially to latex.	This ensures the patient's privacy. This discussion promotes reassurance and provides knowledge about the procedure. Dialogue encourages patient participation and allows for individualized nursing care. Some condom catheters are made of latex.
5. Assemble equipment on the overbed table within reach.	Arranging items nearby is convenient, saves time, and avoids unnecessary stretching and twisting of muscles on the part of the nurse.
6. Adjust the bed to a comfortable working height, usually elbow height of the caregiver (VISN 8 Patient Safety Center, 2009). Stand on the patient's right side if you are right-handed, or on patient's left side if you are left-handed.	Having the bed at the proper height prevents back and muscle strain. Positioning on one side allows for ease of use of dominant hand for catheter application.
7. Prepare the urinary drainage setup or reusable leg bag for attachment to the condom sheath.	Provides an organized approach to the task.
8. Position the patient on his back with thighs slightly apart. Drape the patient so that only the area around the penis is exposed. Slide a waterproof pad under the patient.	Positioning allows access to the site. Draping prevents unnecessary exposure and promotes warmth. The waterproof pad will protect bed linens from moisture.
9. Put on disposable gloves. Trim any long pubic hair that is in contact with the penis.	Gloves prevent contact with blood and body fluids. Trimming pubic hair prevents pulling of hair by adhesive without the risk of infection associated with shaving.
10. Clean the genital area with a washcloth, skin cleanser, and warm water. If the patient is uncircumcised, retract the foreskin and clean the glans of the penis. Replace the foreskin. Clean the tip of the penis first, moving the washcloth in a circular motion from the meatus outward. Wash the shaft of the penis using downward strokes toward the pubic area. Rinse and dry. Remove gloves. Perform hand hygiene again.	Washing removes urine, secretions, and microorganisms. The penis must be clean and dry to minimize skin irritation. If the foreskin is left retracted, it may cause venous congestion in the glans of the penis, leading to edema.
11. Apply skin protectant to the penis and allow to dry.	Skin protectant minimizes the risk of skin irritation from adhesive and moisture and increases the adhesive's ability to adhere to the skin.

(continued)

SKILL 36-4 | APPLYING AN EXTERNAL CONDOM CATHETER *continued*

ACTION	RATIONALE
12. Roll the condom sheath outward onto itself. Grasp the penis firmly with your nondominant hand. **Apply the condom sheath by rolling it onto the penis with your dominant hand (Fig. 1). Leave 1 to 2 inches (2.5 to 5 cm) of space between the tip of the penis and the end of the condom sheath.**	Rolling the condom sheath outward allows for easier application. The space prevents irritation to the tip of the penis and allows free drainage of urine.
13. **Apply pressure to the sheath at the base of the penis for 10 to 15 seconds.**	Application of pressure ensures good adherence of the adhesive with the skin.
14. Connect the condom sheath to the drainage setup (Fig. 2). Avoid kinking or twisting the drainage tubing.	The collection device keeps the patient dry. Kinked tubing encourages backflow of urine.

FIGURE 1. Unrolling sheath onto penis.

FIGURE 2. Connecting condom sheath to drainage setup.

15. Remove gloves. Secure drainage tubing to the patient's inner thigh with a Velcro leg strap or tape. Leave some slack in the tubing for leg movement.	Proper attachment prevents tension on the sheath and potential inadvertent removal.
16. Assist the patient to a comfortable position. Cover the patient with bed linens. Place the bed in the lowest position.	Positioning and covering provide warmth and promote comfort. Bed in the lowest position promotes patient safety.
17. Secure the drainage bag below the level of the bladder. Check that drainage tubing is not kinked and that movement of the side rails does not interfere with the drainage bag.	This facilitates drainage of urine and prevents the backflow of urine.
18. Remove equipment. Remove gloves and additional PPE, if used. Perform hand hygiene.	Proper disposal of equipment prevents transmission of microorganisms. Removing PPE properly reduces the risk for infection transmission and contamination of other items. Hand hygiene prevents the spread of microorganisms.

DOCUMENTATION

Guidelines

Document the assessment data supporting the decision to use a condom catheter, the application of the condom catheter, and the condition of the patient's skin. Record urine output on the intake and output record.

Sample Documentation

7/12/15 1910 Patient incontinent of urine; states: "It just comes too fast. I can't get to the bathroom in time." Perineal skin slightly reddened. Discussed rationale for use of condom catheter. Patient and wife agreeable to trying condom catheter. Medium-sized condom catheter applied; 200 mL of clear urine returned. Leg bag in place for daytime use. Patient verbalized understanding of need to call for assistance to empty drainage bag.

—B. Clapp, RN

UNEXPECTED SITUATIONS AND ASSOCIATED INTERVENTIONS

- *Condom catheter leaks with every voiding:* Check size of condom catheter. If it is too big or too small, it may leak. Check space between tip of penis and end of condom sheath. If this space is too small, the urine has no place to go and will leak out.

- *Condom catheter will not stay on patient:* Ensure that condom catheter is correct size and that penis is thoroughly dried before applying condom catheter. Remind patient that condom catheter is in place, so that patient does not tug at tubing. If the patient has a retracted penis, a condom catheter may not be the best choice; there are pouches made for patients with a retracted penis.

- *When assessing patient's penis, you find a break in skin integrity:* Do not reapply condom catheter. Allow skin to be open to air as much as possible. If institution has a wound, ostomy, and continence nurse, arrange for a consult.

SKILL 36-5   CATHETERIZING THE FEMALE URINARY BLADDER

DELEGATION CONSIDERATIONS

The catheterization of the female urinary bladder is not delegated to nursing assistive personnel (NAP) or unlicensed assistive personnel (UAP). Depending on the state's nurse practice act and the organization's policies and procedures, catheterization of the female urinary bladder may be delegated to licensed practical/vocational nurses (LPN/LVNs). The decision to delegate must be based on careful analysis of the patient's needs and circumstances, as well as the qualifications of the person to whom the task is being delegated. Refer to the Delegation Guidelines in Appendix A (found on thePoint).

EQUIPMENT

- Sterile catheter kit that contains:
  - Sterile gloves
  - Sterile drapes (one of which is fenestrated)
  - Sterile catheter (use the smallest appropriate-size catheter, usually a 14F to 16F catheter with a 5- to 10-mL balloon [Newman, 2008]).
  - Antiseptic cleansing solution and cotton balls or gauze squares; antiseptic swabs
  - Lubricant
  - Forceps
  - Prefilled syringe with sterile water (sufficient to inflate indwelling catheter balloon)

- Sterile specimen container (if specimen is required)
- Flashlight or lamp
- Waterproof, disposable pad
- Sterile, disposable urine collection bag and drainage tubing (may be connected to catheter in catheter kit)
- Velcro® leg strap, catheter securing device, or tape
- Disposable gloves
- Additional PPE, as indicated
- Washcloth, skin cleanser, and warm water to perform perineal hygiene before and after catheterization

IMPLEMENTATION

ACTION	RATIONALE
1. Review the patient's chart for any limitations in physical activity. Confirm the medical order for indwelling catheter insertion.	Physical limitations may require adaptations in performing the skill. Verifying the medical order ensures that the correct intervention is administered to the right patient.
2. Gather equipment. Obtain assistance from another staff member, if necessary.	Assembling equipment provides an organized approach to task. Assistance from another person may be required to perform the intervention safely.

(continued)

SKILL 36-5 CATHETERIZING THE FEMALE URINARY BLADDER *continued*

ACTION	**RATIONALE**
3. Perform hand hygiene and put on PPE, if indicated.	Hand hygiene and PPE prevent the spread of microorganisms. PPE is required based on transmission precautions.
4. Identify the patient.	Identifying the patient ensures that the right patient receives the intervention and helps prevent errors.
5. Close curtains around the bed and close the door to the room, if possible. Discuss the procedure with the patient and assess the patient's ability to assist with the procedure. Ask the patient if she has any allergies, especially to latex or iodine.	This ensures the patient's privacy. This discussion promotes reassurance and provides knowledge about the procedure. Dialogue encourages patient participation and allows for individualized nursing care. Some catheters and gloves in kits are made of latex. Some antiseptic solutions contain iodine.
6. Provide good lighting. Artificial light is recommended (use of a flashlight requires an assistant to hold and position it). Place a trash receptacle within easy reach.	Good lighting is necessary to see the meatus clearly. A readily available trash receptacle allows for prompt disposal of used supplies and reduces the risk of contaminating the sterile field.
7. Assemble equipment on the overbed table within reach.	Arranging items nearby is convenient, saves time, and avoids unnecessary stretching and twisting of muscles on the part of the nurse.
8. Adjust the bed to a comfortable working height, usually elbow height of the caregiver (VISN 8 Patient Safety Center, 2009). Stand on the patient's right side if you are right-handed, on the patient's left side if you are left-handed.	Having the bed at the proper height prevents back and muscle strain. Positioning allows for ease of use of dominant hand for catheter insertion.
9. Assist the patient to a dorsal recumbent position with knees flexed, feet about 2 feet apart, with her legs abducted. Drape the patient (Fig. 1). Alternately, the Sims', or lateral, position can be used. Place the patient's buttocks near the edge of the bed with her shoulders at the opposite edge and her knees drawn toward her chest (Fig. 2). Allow the patient to lie on either side, depending on which position is easiest for the nurse and best for the patient's comfort. Slide a waterproof pad under the patient.	Proper positioning allows for adequate visualization of the urinary meatus. Embarrassment, chilliness, and tension can interfere with catheter insertion; draping the patient will promote comfort and relaxation. The Sims' position may allow better visualization and be more comfortable for the patient, especially if hip and knee movements are difficult. The smaller area of exposure is also less stressful for the patient. The waterproof pad will protect bed linens from moisture.

FIGURE 1. Patient in dorsal recumbent position and draped properly.

FIGURE 2. Demonstration of side-lying position.

10. Put on clean gloves. Clean the perineal area with a washcloth, skin cleanser, and warm water, using a different corner of the washcloth with each stroke. Wipe from above the orifice downward toward sacrum (front to back). Rinse and dry. Remove gloves. Perform hand hygiene again.	Gloves reduce the risk of exposure to blood and body fluids. Cleaning reduces microorganisms near the urethral meatus and provides an opportunity to visualize the perineum and landmarks before the procedure. Hand hygiene reduces the spread of microorganisms.

ACTION

11. Prepare a urine drainage setup if a separate urine collection system is to be used. Secure to the bed frame according to the manufacturer's directions.

12. Open sterile catheterization tray on a clean overbed table using sterile technique.

13. Put on sterile gloves. Grasp the upper corners of the drape and unfold the drape without touching nonsterile areas. Fold back a corner on each side to make a cuff over gloved hands. Ask the patient to lift her buttocks and slide a sterile drape under her with gloves protected by the cuff.

14. Based on facility policy, position the fenestrated sterile drape. Place a fenestrated sterile drape over the perineal area, exposing the labia (Fig. 3). (**Note:** the fenestrated drape is not shown in the remaining illustrations in order to provide a clear view of the procedure.)

15. Place a sterile tray on the drape between the patient's thighs.

16. Open all the supplies. Open a package of antiseptic swabs. Alternately, fluff cotton balls in the tray before pouring antiseptic solution over them. Open a specimen container if a specimen is to be obtained.

17. Lubricate 1 to 2 inches of catheter tip.

18. With thumb and one finger of your nondominant hand, spread the labia and identify the meatus. **Be prepared to maintain separation of the labia with one hand until the catheter is inserted and urine is flowing well and continuously (Fig. 4).** If the patient is in the side-lying position, lift the upper buttock and labia to expose the urinary meatus.

RATIONALE

This facilitates connection of the catheter to the drainage system and provides easy access.

Placement of equipment near the worksite increases efficiency. Sterile technique protects the patient and prevents transmission of microorganisms.

The drape provides a sterile field close to the meatus. Covering the gloved hands will help keep the gloves sterile while placing the drape.

The drape expands the sterile field and protects against contamination. Use of a fenestrated drape may limit visualization and is considered optional by some practitioners and/or facility policies.

This provides easy access to supplies.

It is necessary to open all supplies and prepare for the procedure while both hands are sterile.

Lubrication facilitates catheter insertion and reduces tissue trauma.

Smoothing the area immediately surrounding the meatus helps to make it visible. Allowing the labia to drop back into position may contaminate the area around the meatus, as well as the catheter. The nondominant hand is now contaminated.

FIGURE 3. Patient with fenestrated drape in place over perineum.

FIGURE 4. Using dominant hand to separate and hold labia open.

(continued)

SKILL 36-5 · CATHETERIZING THE FEMALE URINARY BLADDER *continued*

ACTION	RATIONALE
19. Use your dominant hand to pick up an antiseptic swab or use forceps to pick up a cotton ball. **Clean one labial fold, top to bottom (from above the meatus down toward the rectum), then discard the cotton ball. Using a new cotton ball/swab for each stroke, continue to clean the other labial fold, then directly over the meatus (Fig. 5).**	Moving from an area where there is likely to be less contamination to an area where there is more contamination helps prevent the spread of microorganisms. Cleaning the meatus last helps reduce the possibility of introducing microorganisms into the bladder.
20. With your noncontaminated, dominant hand, place the drainage end of the catheter in receptacle. If the catheter is pre-attached to sterile tubing and a drainage container (closed drainage system), position the catheter and setup within easy reach on the sterile field. Ensure that the clamp on the drainage bag is closed.	This facilitates drainage of urine and minimizes risk of contaminating sterile equipment.
21. **Using your dominant hand, hold the catheter 2 to 3 inches from the tip and insert slowly into the urethra (Fig. 6). Advance the catheter until there is a return of urine— approximately 2 to 3 inches (4.8 to 7.2 cm). Once urine drains, advance the catheter another 2 to 3 inches (4.8 to 7.2 cm). Do not force the catheter through the urethra into the bladder.** Ask the patient to breathe deeply, and rotate the catheter gently if slight resistance is met as the catheter reaches the external sphincter.	The female urethra is about 1.5 to 2.5 inches (3.6 to 6.0 cm) long. Applying force on the catheter is likely to injure mucous membranes. The sphincter relaxes and the catheter can enter the bladder easily when the patient relaxes. Advancing an indwelling catheter an additional 2 to 3 inches (4.8 to 7.2 cm) ensures placement in the bladder and facilitates inflation of the balloon without damaging the urethra.

FIGURE 5. Wiping perineum with cotton ball held by forceps. Wipe in one direction—from top to bottom.

FIGURE 6. Inserting catheter with dominant hand while nondominant hand holds labia apart.

ACTION	RATIONALE
22. Hold the catheter securely at the meatus with your nondominant hand. Use your dominant hand to inflate the catheter balloon (Fig. 7). Inject the entire volume of sterile water supplied in the prefilled syringe.	Bladder or sphincter contraction could push the catheter out. The balloon anchors the catheter in place in the bladder. Manufacturer provides appropriate amount of sterile water for the size of catheter in the kit; thus, use entire syringe provided in the kit.
23. Pull gently on the catheter after the balloon is inflated to feel resistance.	Improper inflation can cause patient discomfort and malpositioning of the catheter.
24. Attach the catheter to the drainage system if not already pre-attached (Fig. 8).	Closed drainage system minimizes the risk for microorganisms being introduced into the bladder.

ACTION

FIGURE 7. Inflating balloon of indwelling catheter.

25. Remove equipment and dispose of it according to facility policy. Discard the syringe in a sharps container. Wash and dry the perineal area, as needed.

26. Remove gloves. **Secure the catheter tubing to the patient's inner thigh with a Velcro® leg strap, catheter securing device, or tape (Fig. 9).** Leave some slack in catheter for leg movement.

FIGURE 9. Catheter secured to leg.

27. Assist the patient to a comfortable position. Cover the patient with bed linens. Place the bed in the lowest position.

28. Secure the drainage bag below the level of the bladder. Check that the drainage tubing is not kinked and that movement of the side rails does not interfere with the catheter or drainage bag.

29. Put on clean gloves. Obtain urine specimen immediately, if needed, from the drainage bag. Label the specimen. Send the urine specimen to the laboratory promptly or refrigerate it.

30. Remove gloves and additional PPE, if used. Perform hand hygiene.

RATIONALE

FIGURE 8. Attaching catheter to drainage bag.

Proper disposal prevents the spread of microorganisms. Placing the syringe in a sharps container prevents reuse. Cleaning promotes comfort and appropriate personal hygiene.

Proper attachment prevents trauma to the urethra and meatus from tension on the tubing. Whether to tape the drainage tubing over or under the leg depends on gravity flow, patient's mobility, and patient's comfort.

Positioning and covering provides warmth and promotes comfort.

This facilitates drainage of urine and prevents the backflow of urine.

Catheter system is sterile. Obtaining a specimen immediately allows access to a sterile system. Keeping urine at room temperature may cause microorganisms, if present, to grow and distort laboratory findings.

Removing PPE properly reduces the risk for infection transmission and contamination of other items. Hand hygiene prevents the spread of microorganisms.

(continued)

SKILL 36-5 | CATHETERIZING THE FEMALE URINARY BLADDER *continued*

DOCUMENTATION

Guidelines

Document the type and size of catheter and balloon inserted, as well as the amount of fluid used to inflate the balloon. Document the patient's tolerance of the activity. Record the amount of urine obtained through the catheter and any specimen obtained. Document any other assessments, such as unusual urine characteristics or alterations in the patient's skin. Record urine amount on intake and output record, if appropriate.

Sample Documentation

DocuCare Practice documenting catheterization of the female urinary bladder in *Lippincott DocuCare.*

7/14/15 0915 Primary care provider notified of palpable bladder (3 cm below umbilicus) and patient's inability to void; 750 mL of urine noted with bladder scan. A 16F Foley catheter inserted without difficulty; 10 mL of sterile water injected into balloon port; 700 mL clear yellow urine returned. Patient states, "Oh, I feel much better now." Bladder is no longer palpable. Patient tolerated procedure without adverse event.

—B. Clapp, RN

UNEXPECTED SITUATIONS AND ASSOCIATED INTERVENTIONS

- *No urine flow is obtained, and you note that catheter is in vaginal orifice:* Leave catheter in place as a marker. Obtain new sterile gloves and catheter kit. Start the procedure over and attempt to place a new catheter directly above the misplaced catheter. Once the new catheter is correctly in place, remove the catheter in the vaginal orifice. Because of the risk of cross-infection, never remove a catheter from the vagina and insert it into the urethra.

- *Patient moves legs during procedure:* If no supplies have been contaminated, ask the patient to hold still and continue with the procedure. If supplies have been contaminated, stop the procedure and start over. If necessary, get an assistant to remind the patient to hold still.

- *Urine flow is initially well established and urine is clear, but after several hours flow dwindles:* Check tubing for kinking. If the patient has changed position, the tubing and drainage bag may need to be moved to facilitate drainage of urine.

- *Patient complains of extreme pain when you are inflating balloon:* Stop inflation of balloon. Balloon is most likely still in urethra. Withdraw the solution from the balloon. Insert the catheter an additional 0.5 to 1 inch (1.2 to 2.4 cm) and slowly attempt to inflate the balloon again.

- *Urine leaks out of meatus around the catheter:* Do not increase the size of the indwelling catheter. Make sure the smallest sized catheter with a 10-mL balloon is used. Large catheters cause bladder and urethral irritation and trauma. Large balloon-fill volumes occupy more space inside the bladder and put added weight on the base of the bladder. Irritation of the bladder wall and detrusor muscle can cause leakage. If leakage persists, consider an evaluation for urinary tract infection. Ensure that the correct amount of solution was used to inflate the balloon. Underfilling the balloon can cause the catheter to dislodge into the urethra, causing urethral spasm, pain, and discomfort. If you suspect underfill, do not attempt to push the catheter further into the bladder. Remove the catheter and replace. Assess the patient for constipation. Bowel full of stool can cause pressure on the catheter lumen and prevent the drainage of urine. Implement interventions to prevent/treat constipation.

SPECIAL CONSIDERATIONS

General Considerations

- Be familiar with facility policy and/or primary practitioner guidelines for the maximum amount of urine to remove from bladder at the time of insertion.

- If the patient is unable to lift the buttocks or maintain the required position for the procedure, the assistance of another staff member may be necessary to place the drape under the patient and to help the patient maintain the required position.

- Supplies can be opened and prepared on the overbed table, moving the tray onto the bed just before cleansing the patient.

- If there is not an immediate flow of urine after the catheter has been inserted, several measures may prove helpful:

  - Have the patient take a deep breath, which helps to relax the perineal and abdominal muscles.

  - Rotate the catheter slightly, because a drainage hole may be resting against the bladder wall.

  - Raise the head of the patient's bed to increase pressure in the bladder area.

  - Assess the patient's intake to ensure adequate fluid intake for urine production.

  - Assess the catheter and drainage tubing for kinks and occlusion.

- If the catheter cannot be advanced, have the patient take several deep breaths. Rotate the catheter half a turn and try to advance. If you are still unable to advance, remove the catheter. Notify the primary care provider.

- Some catheter kits do not contain the catheter. This allows you to select a catheter and balloon size separately.

Infant and Child Considerations

- Sizes 5F to 8F are used for infants and young children. Sizes 8F to 12F catheters are commonly used for older children (Perry et al., 2010).

- Distraction, such as blowing bubbles, deep breathing, or singing a song, can help the child relax.

- Lidocaine jelly is often used to anesthetize and lubricate the area before insertion of the catheter, decreasing the child's discomfort and anxiety.

Home Care Considerations

- Intermittent catheterization, performed by the patient or a caregiver in the home, may be necessary for patients with spinal cord injuries or other neurologic conditions. Although the risk for UTI is always present, most research supports the use of clean, rather than sterile, technique in this environment. The procedure for self-catheterization is essentially the same as that used by the nurse to catheterize a patient. Self-catheterization is recommended at regular intervals to prevent overdistention of the bladder and decreased blood flow through the wall of the bladder (Hinkle & Cheever, 2014; SUNA, 2010; see Box 36-4, p. 1288).

SKILL 36-6 | CATHETERIZING THE MALE URINARY BLADDER

DELEGATION CONSIDERATIONS

The catheterization of the male urinary bladder is not delegated to nursing assistive personnel (NAP) or unlicensed assistive personnel (UAP). Depending on the state's nurse practice act and the organization's policies and procedures, catheterization of the male urinary bladder may be delegated to licensed practical/vocational nurses (LPN/LVNs). The decision to delegate must be based on careful analysis of the patient's needs and circumstances, as well as the qualifications of the person to whom the task is being delegated. Refer to the Delegation Guidelines in Appendix A (found on thePoint).

EQUIPMENT

- Sterile catheter kit that contains:
  - Sterile gloves
  - Sterile drapes (one of which is fenestrated)
  - Sterile catheter (use the smallest appropriate-size catheter, usually a 14F to 16F catheter with a 5- to 10-mL balloon [Newman, 2008]).

- Antiseptic cleansing solution and cotton balls or gauze squares; antiseptic swabs
- Lubricant
- Forceps
- Prefilled syringe with sterile water (sufficient to inflate indwelling catheter balloon)

(continued)

SKILL 36-6 CATHETERIZING THE MALE URINARY BLADDER *continued*

- Sterile basin (usually base of kit serves as this)
- Sterile specimen container (if specimen is required)
- Flashlight or lamp
- Waterproof, disposable pad
- Sterile, disposable urine collection bag and drainage tubing (may be connected to catheter in catheter kit)

- Velcro® leg strap, catheter securing device, or tape
- Disposable gloves
- Additional PPE, as indicated
- Washcloth, skin cleanser, and warm water to perform perineal hygiene before and after catheterization

IMPLEMENTATION

ACTION	RATIONALE
1. Review chart for any limitations in physical activity. Confirm the medical order for indwelling catheter insertion.	Physical limitations may require adaptations in performing the skill. Verifying the medical order ensures that the correct intervention is administered to the right patient.
2. Gather equipment. Obtain assistance from another staff member, if necessary.	Assembling equipment provides an organized approach to the task. Assistance from another person may be required to perform the intervention safely.
3. Perform hand hygiene and put on PPE, if indicated.	Hand hygiene and PPE prevent the spread of microorganisms. PPE is required based on transmission precautions.
4. Identify the patient.	Identifying the patient ensures that the right patient receives the intervention and helps prevent errors.
5. Close curtains around the bed and close the door to the room, if possible. Discuss the procedure with the patient and assess the patient's ability to assist with the procedure. Ask the patient if he has any allergies, especially to latex or iodine.	This ensures the patient's privacy. This discussion promotes reassurance and provides knowledge about the procedure. Dialogue encourages patient participation and allows for individualized nursing care. Some catheters and gloves in kits are made of latex. Some antiseptic solutions contain iodine.
6. Provide good lighting. Artificial light is recommended (use of a flashlight requires an assistant to hold and position it). Place a trash receptacle within easy reach.	Good lighting is necessary to see the meatus clearly. A readily available trash receptacle allows for prompt disposal of used supplies and reduces the risk of contaminating the sterile field.
7. Assemble equipment on the overbed table within reach.	Arranging items nearby is convenient, saves time, and avoids unnecessary stretching and twisting of muscles on the part of the nurse.
8. Adjust the bed to a comfortable working height, usually elbow height of the caregiver (VISN 8 Patient Safety Center, 2009). Stand on the patient's right side if you are right-handed, on the patient's left side if you are left-handed.	Having the bed at the proper height prevents back and muscle strain. Positioning allows for ease of use of the dominant hand for catheter insertion.
9. Position the patient on his back with thighs slightly apart. Drape the patient so that only the area around the penis is exposed. Slide a waterproof pad under the patient.	This prevents unnecessary exposure and promotes warmth. The waterproof pad will protect bed linens from moisture.
10. Put on clean gloves. Clean the genital area with a washcloth, skin cleanser, and warm water. Clean the tip of the penis first, moving the washcloth in a circular motion from the meatus outward. Wash the shaft of the penis using downward strokes toward the pubic area. Rinse and dry. Remove gloves. Perform hand hygiene again.	Gloves reduce the risk of exposure to blood and body fluids. Cleaning the penis reduces microorganisms near the urethral meatus. Hand hygiene reduces the spread of microorganisms.
11. Prepare a urine drainage setup if a separate urine collection system is to be used. Secure to the bed frame according to the manufacturer's directions.	This facilitates connection of the catheter to the drainage system and provides easy access.
12. Open the sterile catheterization tray on a clean overbed table, using sterile technique.	Placement of equipment near the worksite increases efficiency. Sterile technique protects the patient and prevents the spread of microorganisms.

ACTION	RATIONALE

ACTION

13. Put on sterile gloves. Open a sterile drape and place on the patient's thighs. Place the fenestrated drape with the opening over the penis (Fig. 1).

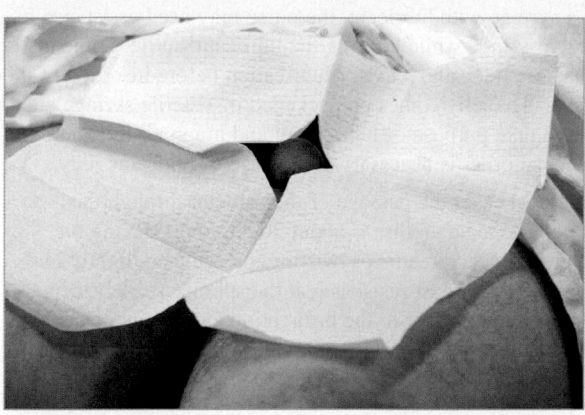

RATIONALE

This maintains a sterile working area.

FIGURE 1. Patient lying supine with fenestrated drape over penis.

14. Place the catheter set on or next to the patient's legs on a sterile drape.

15. Open all the supplies. Open a package of antiseptic swabs. Alternately, fluff cotton balls in the tray before pouring antiseptic solution over them. Open a specimen container if a specimen is to be obtained. Remove the cap from a syringe prefilled with lubricant.

16. Place the drainage end of the catheter in the receptacle. If the catheter is pre-attached to the sterile tubing and drainage container (closed drainage system), position the catheter and setup within easy reach on a sterile field. Ensure that the clamp on the drainage bag is closed.

17. Lift the penis with your nondominant hand. Retract the foreskin in the uncircumcised patient. **Be prepared to keep this hand in this position until the catheter is inserted and urine is flowing well and continuously. Use your dominant hand to pick up an antiseptic swab or use forceps to pick up a cotton ball. Using a circular motion, clean the penis, moving from the meatus down the glans of the penis (Fig. 2). Repeat this cleansing motion two more times, using a new cotton ball/ swab each time. Discard each cotton ball/swab after one use.**

Sterile setup should be arranged so that the nurse's back is not turned to it, nor should it be out of the nurse's range of vision.

It is necessary to open all supplies and prepare for the procedure while both hands are sterile.

This facilitates drainage of urine and minimizes the risk of contaminating sterile equipment.

The hand touching the penis becomes contaminated. Cleansing the area around the meatus and under the foreskin in the uncircumcised patient helps prevent infection. Moving from the meatus toward the base of the penis prevents bringing microorganisms to the meatus.

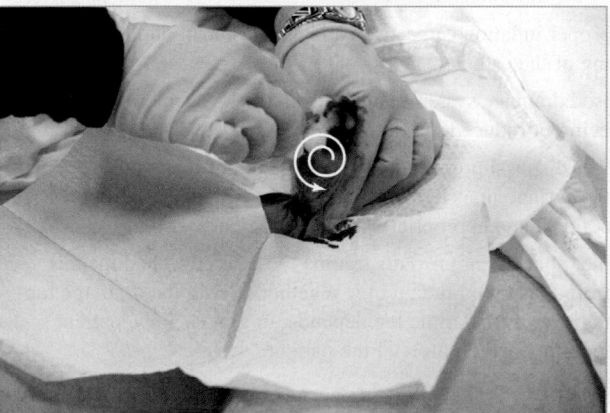

FIGURE 2. Lifting penis with gloved nondominant hand and cleaning meatus with cotton ball held with forceps in gloved dominant hand.

(continued)

SKILL 36-6 | CATHETERIZING THE MALE URINARY BLADDER *continued*

ACTION	RATIONALE
18. Hold the penis with a slight upward tension and perpendicular to the patient's body. Use the dominant hand to pick up the lubricant syringe. **Gently insert the tip of the syringe with lubricant into the urethra and instill the 10 mL of lubricant** (Fig. 3).	The lubricant causes the urethra to distend slightly and facilitates passage of the catheter without traumatizing the lining of the urethra (SUNA, 2005c). If the prepackaged kit does not contain a syringe with lubricant, the nurse may need assistance in filling a syringe while keeping the lubricant sterile. Some institutions use lidocaine jelly for lubrication before insertion of the catheter. The jelly comes prepackaged in a sterile syringe and serves a dual purpose of lubricating and numbing the urethra. A medical order is necessary for the use of lidocaine jelly.
19. Use your dominant hand to pick up the catheter and hold it an inch or two from the tip. Ask the patient to bear down as if voiding. **Insert catheter tip into meatus (Fig. 4). Ask the patient to take deep breaths. Advance the catheter to the bifurcation or "Y" level of the ports. Do not use force to introduce the catheter.** If the catheter resists entry, ask the patient to breathe deeply and rotate the catheter slightly.	Bearing down eases the passage of the catheter through the urethra. The male urethra is about 20 cm long. Having the patient take deep breaths or twisting the catheter slightly may ease the catheter past resistance at the sphincters. Advancing an indwelling catheter to the bifurcation ensures its placement in the bladder and facilitates inflation of the balloon without damaging the urethra.

FIGURE 3. Inserting syringe into urethra and instilling lubricant.

FIGURE 4. Inserting catheter using dominant hand.

ACTION	RATIONALE
20. Hold the catheter securely at the meatus with your nondominant hand. Use your dominant hand to inflate the catheter balloon. **Inject the entire volume of sterile water supplied in the prefilled syringe. Once the balloon is inflated, the catheter may be gently pulled back into place. Replace the foreskin over the catheter.** Lower the penis.	Bladder or sphincter contraction could push the catheter out. The balloon anchors the catheter in place in the bladder. Manufacturer provides the appropriate amount of solution for the size of catheter in the kit; thus, use the entire syringe provided in the kit.
21. Pull gently on the catheter after the balloon is inflated to feel resistance.	Improper inflation can cause patient discomfort and malpositioning of the catheter.
22. Attach the catheter to the drainage system, if necessary.	Closed drainage system minimizes the risk for microorganisms being introduced into the bladder.
23. Remove equipment and dispose of it according to facility policy. Discard the syringe in a sharps container. Wash and dry the perineal area as needed.	Proper disposal prevents the spread of microorganisms. Placing the syringe in a sharps container prevents reuse. Promotes comfort and appropriate personal hygiene.
24. Remove gloves. Secure the catheter tubing to the patient's inner thigh or lower abdomen (with the penis directed toward the patient's chest) with a Velcro® leg strap, catheter securing device, or tape. Leave some slack in the catheter for leg movement.	Proper attachment prevents trauma to the urethra and meatus from tension on the tubing. Whether to take the drainage tubing over or under the leg depends on gravity flow, patient's mobility, and comfort of the patient.

ACTION	RATIONALE
25. Assist the patient to a comfortable position. Cover the patient with bed linens. Place the bed in the lowest position.	Positioning and covering provides warmth and promotes comfort.
26. Secure the drainage bag below the level of the bladder. Check that the drainage tubing is not kinked and that movement of the side rails does not interfere with the catheter or drainage bag.	This facilitates drainage of urine and prevents the backflow of urine.
27. Put on clean gloves. Obtain a urine specimen immediately, if needed, from the drainage bag. Label the specimen. Send the urine specimen to the laboratory promptly or refrigerate it.	Catheter system is sterile. Obtaining a specimen immediately allows access to a sterile system. Keeping urine at room temperature may cause microorganisms, if present, to grow and distort laboratory findings.
28. Remove gloves and additional PPE, if used. Perform hand hygiene.	Removing PPE properly reduces the risk for infection transmission and contamination of other items. Hand hygiene prevents the spread of microorganisms.

DOCUMENTATION

Guidelines

Document the type and size of catheter and balloon inserted, as well as the amount of fluid used to inflate the balloon. Document the patient's tolerance of the activity. Record the amount of urine obtained through the catheter and any specimen obtained. Document any other assessments, such as unusual urine characteristics or alterations in the patient's skin. Record urine amount on intake and output record, if appropriate.

Sample Documentation

DocuCare Practice documenting catheterization of the male urinary bladder in *Lippincott DocuCare*.

7/14/15 1830 Patient unable to void for 8 hours and reports, "I feel like I have to go to the bathroom." Bladder scanned for 540 mL urine. Primary care provider notified; 10 mL 2% lidocaine jelly instilled before catheterization per order; 14F Foley catheter inserted without difficulty; 10 mL of sterile water injected into 5-mL balloon port; 525 mL clear yellow urine returned. Patient reports decreased bladder pressure. Patient tolerated procedure without adverse event.

—B. Clapp, RN

UNEXPECTED SITUATIONS AND ASSOCIATED INTERVENTIONS

- *Patient complains of intense pain when you begin to inflate balloon:* Stop inflation. Be sure to insert the catheter all the way into the bifurcation. The balloon is probably still in the urethra. Damage to the urethra can result if the balloon is inflated in urethra.

- *You cannot insert catheter past 3 to 4 inches; rotating the catheter and having patient breathe deeply are of no help:* If still unable to place catheter, notify primary care provider. Repeated catheter placement attempts can traumatize the urethra. Primary care provider may order and insert a Coude catheter.

- *Patient is obese or has retracted penis:* Have an assistant available to place fingers on either side of the pubic area and press backward to bring the penis out of the pubic cavity. Hold the patient's penis up and forward. The catheter still needs to be inserted to the bifurcation; the length of the urethra has not changed.

- *Urine flow initially contains a large amount of sediment and then suddenly stops; bladder remains palpable:* Catheter may be plugged with sediment. After obtaining an order from the primary care provider, gently irrigate the catheter to restore flow.

- *Urine leaks out of the meatus around the catheter:* Do not increase the size of the indwelling catheter. Make sure the smallest sized catheter with a 10-mL balloon is used. Large catheters cause bladder and urethral irritation and trauma. Large, balloon-fill volumes occupy more space inside the bladder and put added weight on the base of the bladder. Irritation of the bladder wall and detrusor muscle can cause leakage. If leakage persists, consider an evaluation for urinary tract infection. Ensure that the correct amount of solution was used to inflate the balloon. Underfilling the balloon can cause the catheter to dislodge into the urethra,

(continued)

SKILL 36-6 CATHETERIZING THE MALE URINARY BLADDER *continued*

causing urethral spasm, pain, and discomfort. If underfill is suspected, do not attempt to push the catheter further into the bladder. Remove the catheter and replace. Assess the patient for constipation. Bowel full of stool can cause pressure on the catheter lumen and prevent the drainage of urine. Implement interventions to prevent/treat constipation.

- *Urine flow is initially well established and urine is clear, but after several hours urine flow dwindles:* Check tubing for kinking. If the patient has changed position, the tubing and drainage bag may need to be moved to facilitate drainage of urine.

SPECIAL CONSIDERATIONS

General Considerations

- Be familiar with facility policy and/or primary practitioner guidelines for the maximum amount of urine to remove from the bladder at the time of insertion.
- Supplies can be opened and prepared on the overbed table, moving the tray onto the bed just before cleansing the patient.
- If there is not an immediate flow of urine after the catheter has been inserted, several measures may prove helpful:
  - Have the patient take a deep breath, which helps to relax the perineal and abdominal muscles.
  - Rotate the catheter slightly, because a drainage hole may be resting against the bladder wall.
  - Raise the head of the patient's bed to increase pressure in the bladder area.
  - Assess the patient's intake to ensure adequate fluid intake for urine production.
  - Assess the catheter and drainage tubing for kinks and occlusion.
  - Urethral strictures, false passages, prostatic enlargement, and postsurgical bladder-neck contractures can make urethral catheterization difficult and may require the services of a urologist. With any question regarding the location of the catheter, such as no return of urine, do not inflate the balloon. Remove the catheter and notify the physician (SUNA, 2005c).
- If the catheter cannot be advanced, having the patient take several deep breaths may be helpful. Rotate the catheter half a turn, and try to advance. If you are still unable to advance, remove the catheter. Notify the primary care provider.
- Some catheter kits do not contain the catheter. This allows you to select a catheter and balloon size separately.

Infant and Child Considerations

- Sizes 5F to 8F are used for infants and young children. Sizes 8F to 12F catheters are commonly used for older children (Perry et al., 2010).
- Distraction, such as blowing bubbles, deep breathing, or singing a song, can help the child relax.
- Lidocaine jelly is often used to anesthetize and lubricate the area before insertion of the catheter, decreasing the child's discomfort and anxiety.

Older Adult Considerations

- If resistance is met while inserting a catheter and rotating does not help, it is important to never force the catheter. The resistance may be caused by enlargement of the prostate gland, which is commonly seen in men over age 50 years. A special crook-tipped catheter called a Coude catheter, inserted by the physician or advanced practice nurse, may be required to maneuver past the prostate gland.

Home Care Considerations

- Intermittent catheterization, performed by the patient or a caregiver in the home, may be necessary for patients with spinal cord injuries or other neurologic conditions. Although the risk for UTI is always present, most research supports the use of clean, rather than sterile, technique in this environment. The procedure for self-catheterization is essentially the same as that used by the nurse to catheterize a patient. Self-catheterization is recommended at regular intervals to prevent overdistention of the bladder and decreased blood flow through the wall of the bladder (Hinkle & Cheever, 2014; SUNA, 2010; see Box 36-4, p. 1288).

SKILL 36-7 PERFORMING INTERMITTENT CLOSED CATHETER IRRIGATION

DELEGATION CONSIDERATIONS	Intermittent closed catheter irrigation is not delegated to nursing assistive personnel (NAP) or unlicensed assistive personnel (UAP). Depending on the state's nurse practice act and the organization's policies and procedures, intermittent closed catheter irrigation may be delegated to licensed practical/vocational nurses (LPN/LVNs). The decision to delegate must be based on careful analysis of the patient's needs and circumstances, as well as the qualifications of the person to whom the task is being delegated. Refer to the Delegation Guidelines in Appendix A (found on the Point).

EQUIPMENT

- Sterile basin or container
- Sterile irrigating solution (at room temperature or warmed to body temperature)
- 30- to 60-mL syringe (with 18- or 19-gauge blunt-end needle, if catheter access port is not a needleless system)
- Clamp for drainage tubing
- Bath blanket
- Disposable gloves
- Additional PPE, as indicated
- Waterproof pad
- Alcohol or other disinfectant swab

IMPLEMENTATION

ACTION	RATIONALE
1. Confirm the order for catheter irrigation in the medical record.	Verifying the medical order ensures that the correct intervention is administered to the right patient.
2. Gather equipment.	Assembling equipment provides an organized approach to the task.
3. Perform hand hygiene and put on PPE, if indicated.	Hand hygiene and PPE prevent the spread of microorganisms. PPE is required based on transmission precautions.
4. Identify the patient.	Identifying the patient ensures that the right patient receives the intervention and helps prevent errors.
5. Close curtains around the bed and close the door to the room, if possible. Discuss the procedure with the patient.	This ensures the patient's privacy. This discussion promotes reassurance and provides knowledge about the procedure. Dialogue encourages patient participation and allows for individualized nursing care.
6. Assemble equipment on the overbed table within reach.	Arranging items nearby is convenient, saves time, and avoids unnecessary stretching and twisting of muscles on the part of the nurse.
7. Adjust the bed to a comfortable working height, usually elbow height of the caregiver (VISN 8 Patient Safety Center, 2009).	Having the bed at the proper height prevents back and muscle strain.
8. Put on gloves. Empty the catheter drainage bag and measure the amount of urine, noting the amount and characteristics of the urine. Remove gloves.	Gloves prevent contact with blood and body fluids. Emptying the drainage bag allows for accurate assessment of drainage after the irrigation solution is instilled. Assessment of urine provides a baseline for future comparison. Proper removal of PPE prevents transmission of microorganisms.
9. Assist patient to a comfortable position and expose the access port on the catheter setup. Place a waterproof pad under the catheter and aspiration port. Remove the catheter from the device or tape the anchoring catheter to the patient.	This provides adequate visualization. Waterproof pad protects the patient and bed from leakage. Removing the catheter from the anchoring device or tape allows for manipulation of the catheter.
10. Open supplies, using aseptic technique. Pour the sterile solution into a sterile basin. Aspirate the prescribed amount of irrigant (usually 30 to 60 mL) into sterile syringe. Put on gloves.	Use of aseptic technique ensures sterility of irrigating fluid and prevents spread of microorganisms. Gloves prevent contact with blood and body fluids.

(continued)

SKILL 36-7 PERFORMING INTERMITTENT CLOSED CATHETER IRRIGATION *continued*

ACTION	**RATIONALE**
11. **Cleanse the access port on the catheter with antimicrobial swab (Fig. 1).**	Cleaning the port reduces the risk of introducing organisms into the closed urinary system.
12. Clamp or fold the catheter tubing below the access port (Fig. 2).	This directs the irrigating solution into the bladder, preventing flow into the drainage bag.

FIGURE 1. Cleansing access port on catheter.

FIGURE 2. Clamping catheter below access port.

13. Attach the syringe to the access port on the catheter using a twisting motion (Fig. 3). **Gently instill solution into the catheter (Fig. 4).**	Gentle irrigation prevents damage to the bladder lining. Instillation of fluid dislodges material blocking the catheter.

FIGURE 3. Attaching syringe to access port with twisting motion.

FIGURE 4. Gently instilling irrigation solution.

14. Remove the syringe from the access port (Fig. 5). **Unclamp or unfold tubing and allow irrigant and urine to flow into the drainage bag.** Repeat procedure, as necessary.	Gravity aids drainage of urine and irrigant from the bladder.
15. Remove gloves. Secure catheter tubing to the patient's inner thigh or lower abdomen (if a male patient) with anchoring device or tape. Leave some slack in the catheter for leg movement.	Proper attachment prevents trauma to the urethra and meatus from tension on the tubing. Whether to take the drainage tubing over or under the leg depends on gravity flow and patient's mobility and comfort.
16. Assist the patient to a comfortable position. Cover the patient with bed linens. Place the bed in the lowest position.	Positioning and covering provide warmth and promote comfort. Lowering the bed contributes to patient safety.

ACTION

RATIONALE

FIGURE 5. Removing syringe from access port.

17. Secure drainage bag below the level of the bladder. Check that drainage tubing is not kinked and that movement of the side rails does not interfere with the catheter or drainage bag.

This facilitates drainage of urine and prevents the backflow of urine.

18. Remove equipment and discard syringe in appropriate receptacle. Remove gloves and additional PPE, if used. Perform hand hygiene.

Proper disposal of equipment prevents transmission of microorganisms. Removing PPE properly reduces the risk for infection transmission and contamination of other items. Hand hygiene prevents the spread of microorganisms.

19. Assess the patient's response to the procedure and the quality and amount of drainage after the irrigation.

This provides accurate assessment of the patient's response to the procedure.

DOCUMENTATION

Guidelines

Document baseline assessment of the patient. Document the amount and type of irrigation solution used and the amount and characteristics of drainage returned after the procedure. Document the ease of irrigation and the patient's tolerance of the procedure. Record urine amount emptied from the drainage bag before the procedure and the amount of irrigant used on the intake and output record. Subtract the irrigant amount from the urine output when totaling output to provide accurate recording of urine output.

Sample Documentation

> 7/22/15 1630 Urinary catheter irrigated with 60 mL of normal saline without difficulty. All of irrigation returned plus 200 mL of cloudy yellow urine. Patient tolerated procedure without adverse effect. Order received to notify physician if urine output is less than 30 mL/hour.
>
> —B. Clapp, RN

UNEXPECTED SITUATIONS AND ASSOCIATED INTERVENTIONS

- *Irrigation solution will not enter the catheter:* Do not force the solution into the catheter. Notify the primary care provider. Prepare to change the catheter.
- *Tubing was not clamped before introducing irrigation solution:* Repeat irrigation, making sure to clamp the tube before introducing irrigation solution. If the tubing is not clamped, the irrigation solution will drain into the urinary drainage bag and not enter the catheter.

SPECIAL CONSIDERATIONS

- If irrigant is a medication intended for action in the bladder, be aware of specific dwell time included in the order or determined by the action of the medication. Allow the appropriate amount of time to lapse before unclamping the drainage tubing after instillation of the irrigant.

SKILL 36-8 ADMINISTERING A CONTINUOUS CLOSED BLADDER OR CATHETER IRRIGATION

DELEGATION CONSIDERATIONS

The administration of continuous closed bladder irrigation is not delegated to nursing assistive personnel (NAP) or unlicensed assistive personnel (UAP). Depending on the state's nurse practice act and the organization's policies and procedures, administration of continuous closed bladder irrigation may be delegated to licensed practical/vocational nurses (LPN/LVNs). The decision to delegate must be based on careful analysis of the patient's needs and circumstances, as well as the qualifications of the person to whom the task is being delegated. Refer to the Delegation Guidelines in Appendix A (found on thePoint).

EQUIPMENT

- Sterile irrigating solution (at room temperature or warmed to body temperature)
- Sterile tubing with drip chamber and clamp for connection to irrigating solution
- IV pole
- IV pump (if bladder is being irrigated with a solution containing medication)
- Three-way indwelling catheter in place in patient's bladder
- Indwelling catheter drainage setup (tubing and collection bag)
- Alcohol or other disinfectant swab
- Bath blanket
- Disposable gloves
- Additional PPE, as indicated

IMPLEMENTATION

ACTION	RATIONALE
1. Confirm the order for catheter irrigation in the medical record, including infusion parameters. If irrigation is to be implemented via gravity infusion, calculate the drip rate. Often, orders are to infuse to keep the urine clear of blood.	Verifying the medical order ensures that the correct intervention is administered to the right patient. Solution must be administered via gravity at the appropriate rate as prescribed.
2. Gather equipment.	Assembling equipment provides an organized approach to task.
3. Perform hand hygiene and put on PPE, if indicated.	Hand hygiene and PPE prevent the spread of microorganisms. PPE is required based on transmission precautions.
4. Identify the patient.	Identifying the patient ensures that the right patient receives the intervention and helps prevent errors.
5. Close the curtains around the bed and close the door to the room, if possible. Discuss the procedure with the patient.	This ensures the patient's privacy. This discussion promotes reassurance and provides knowledge about the procedure. Dialogue encourages patient participation and allows for individualized nursing care.
6. Assemble equipment on the overbed table within reach.	Arranging items nearby is convenient, saves time, and avoids unnecessary stretching and twisting of muscles on the part of the nurse.
7. Adjust the bed to a comfortable working height, usually elbow height of the caregiver (VISN 8 Patient Safety Center, 2009).	Having the bed at the proper height prevents back and muscle strain.
8. Empty the catheter drainage bag and measure the amount of urine, noting the amount and characteristics of the urine.	Emptying the drainage bag allows for accurate assessment of drainage after the irrigation solution is instilled. Assessment of urine provides a baseline for future comparison.
9. Assist the patient to a comfortable position and expose the irrigation port on the catheter setup. Place a waterproof pad under the catheter and aspiration port.	This provides adequate visualization. Waterproof pad protects the patient and bed from leakage.

ACTION

10. Prepare a sterile irrigation bag for use as directed by the manufacturer. Clearly label the solution as "Bladder Irrigation." Include the date and time on the label. Hang bag on an IV pole 2.5 to 3 feet above the level of the patient's bladder. Secure the tubing clamp and insert the sterile tubing with drip chamber to the container using aseptic technique (Fig. 1). Release the clamp and remove the protective cover on the end of the tubing without contaminating it. Allow the solution to flush the tubing and remove air (Fig. 2). Clamp the tubing and replace the end cover.

RATIONALE

Proper labeling provides accurate information for caregivers. Sterile solution not used within 24 hours of opening should be discarded. Aseptic technique prevents contamination of solution irrigation system. Priming the tubing before attaching irrigation clears air from the tubing that might cause bladder distention.

FIGURE 1. Inserting tubing into solution bag.

FIGURE 2. Removing air from irrigation tubing.

11. Put on gloves. **Cleanse the irrigation port on the catheter with an alcohol swab. Using aseptic technique, attach irrigation tubing to the irrigation port of the three-way indwelling catheter (Fig. 3).**

Aseptic technique prevents the spread of microorganisms into the bladder.

12. Check the drainage tubing to make sure clamp, if present, is open.

An open clamp prevents accumulation of solution in the bladder.

13. **Release the clamp on the irrigation tubing and regulate the flow at the determined drip rate, according to the ordered rate (Fig. 4).** If the bladder irrigation is to be done with a medicated solution, use an electronic infusion device to regulate the flow.

This allows for continual gentle irrigation without causing discomfort to the patient. An electronic infusion device regulates the flow of the medication.

FIGURE 3. Attaching irrigation tubing to irrigation port on catheter.

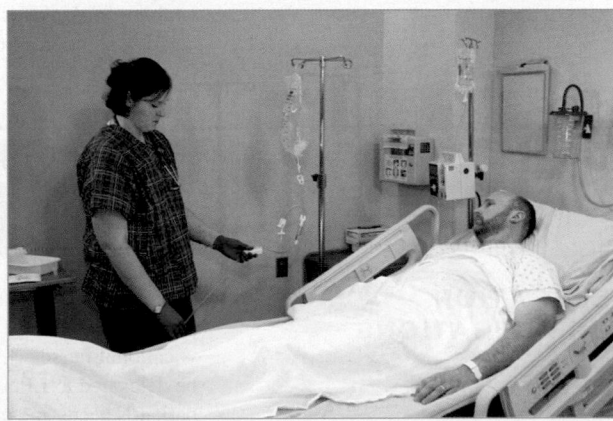

FIGURE 4. Regulating irrigation flow rate using flow clamp.

(continued)

SKILL 36-8 ADMINISTERING A CONTINUOUS CLOSED BLADDER OR CATHETER IRRIGATION *continued*

ACTION	RATIONALE
14. Remove gloves. Assist the patient to a comfortable position. Cover the patient with bed linens. Place the bed in the lowest position.	Positioning and covering provide warmth and promote comfort and safety.
15. Assess the patient's response to the procedure, and quality and amount of drainage.	Assessment is necessary to determine effectiveness of the intervention and to detect adverse effects.
16. Remove equipment. Remove gloves and additional PPE, if used. Perform hand hygiene.	Proper disposal of equipment prevents transmission of microorganisms. Removing PPE properly reduces the risk for infection transmission and contamination of other items. Hand hygiene prevents the spread of microorganisms.
17. As irrigation fluid container nears empty, clamp the administration tubing. Do not allow the drip chamber to empty. Disconnect the empty bag and attach a new full irrigation solution bag.	This eliminates the need to separate tubing from the catheter and clear air from the tubing. Opening the drainage system provides access for microorganisms.
18. Put on gloves and empty drainage collection bag as each new container is hung and recorded.	Gloves protect against exposure to blood, body fluids, and microorganisms.

DOCUMENTATION

Guidelines

Document baseline assessment of the patient. Document the amount and type of irrigation solution used and the patient's tolerance of the procedure. Record urine amount emptied from the drainage bag before the procedure and the amount of irrigant used on the intake and output record. Record the amount of urine and irrigant emptied from the drainage bag. **Subtract the amount of irrigant instilled from the total volume of drainage to obtain the volume of urine output.**

Sample Documentation

12/14/15 1330 Foley catheter replaced with 3-way Foley catheter. Bladder nonpalpable. Continuous bladder irrigation with normal saline initiated at 100 mL/hour. Patient tolerated procedure without adverse effect. Drainage from bladder slightly cloudy, light cherry colored. No evidence of clots.
—B. Clapp, RN

UNEXPECTED SITUATIONS AND ASSOCIATED INTERVENTIONS

• *Continuous bladder irrigation begins and hourly drainage is less than amount of irrigation being given:* Palpate for bladder distention. If patient is lying supine, rolling the patient onto his or her side may help increase the amount of drainage. Check to make sure that the tubing is not kinked. If return flow remains decreased, notify the primary care provider.

• *Bladder irrigation is not flowing at ordered rate, even with clamp wide open:* Check the tubing for kinks or pressure points. Raise the bag 3 to 6 inches and then check flow of irrigation solution. Frequently check flow rate of irrigation solution.

SKILL 36-9 EMPTYING AND CHANGING A STOMA APPLIANCE ON AN ILEAL CONDUIT

DELEGATION CONSIDERATIONS

The emptying of a stoma appliance on an ileal conduit may be delegated to nursing assistive personnel (NAP) or unlicensed assistive personnel (UAP), as well as to licensed practical/vocational nurses (LPN/LVNs). The changing of a stoma appliance on an ileal conduit may be delegated to LPN/LVNs. The decision to delegate must be based on careful analysis of the patient's needs and circumstances, as well as the qualifications of the person to whom the task is being delegated. Refer to the Delegation Guidelines in Appendix A (found on thePoint).

EQUIPMENT

- Basin with warm water
- Skin cleanser, towel, washcloth
- Silicone-based adhesive remover
- Gauze squares
- Skin protectant, such as SkinPrep
- Ostomy appliance
- Stoma measuring guide

- Graduated container
- Ostomy belt (optional)
- Disposable gloves
- Additional PPE, as indicated
- Waterproof, disposable pad
- Small plastic trash bag

IMPLEMENTATION

ACTION	RATIONALE
1. Gather equipment.	Assembling equipment provides an organized approach to task.
2. Perform hand hygiene and put on PPE, if indicated.	Hand hygiene and PPE prevent the spread of microorganisms. PPE is required based on transmission precautions.
3. Identify the patient.	Identifying the patient ensures that the right patient receives the intervention and helps prevent errors.
4. Close the curtains around the bed and close the door to the room, if possible. Explain what you are going to do and why you are going to do it to the patient. Encourage the patient to observe or participate, if possible.	This ensures the patient's privacy. Explanation relieves anxiety and facilitates cooperation. Discussion promotes cooperation and helps to minimize anxiety. Having the patient observe or assist encourages self-acceptance.
5. Assemble equipment on the overbed table within reach.	Arranging items nearby is convenient, saves time, and avoids unnecessary stretching and twisting of muscles on the part of the nurse.
6. Assist the patient to a comfortable sitting or lying position in bed or a standing or sitting position in the bathroom. If the patient is in bed, adjust the bed to a comfortable working height, usually elbow height of the caregiver (VISN 8 Patient Safety Center, 2009). Place a waterproof pad under the patient at the stoma site.	Either position should allow the patient to view the procedure in preparation for learning to perform it independently. Lying flat or sitting upright facilitates smooth application of the appliance. Having the bed at the proper height prevents back and muscle strain. A waterproof pad protects linens and the patient from moisture.

Emptying the Appliance

7. Put on gloves. Hold the end of the appliance over a bedpan, toilet, or measuring device. Remove the end cap from the spout. Open the spout and empty the contents into the bedpan, toilet, or measuring device (Fig. 1).	Gloves protect the nurse from exposure to blood and body fluids. Emptying the pouch before handling it reduces the likelihood of spilling the excretions.

FIGURE 1. Emptying urine into graduated container.

(continued)

SKILL 36-9 EMPTYING AND CHANGING A STOMA APPLIANCE ON AN ILEAL CONDUIT *continued*

ACTION	**RATIONALE**
8. Close the spout. Wipe the spout with toilet tissue. Replace the cap.	Drying the spout removes any urine.
9. Remove equipment. Remove gloves. Assist the patient to a comfortable position.	Proper removal of PPE prevents the transmission of microorganisms. Ensures patient comfort.
10. If appliance is not to be changed, place the bed in the lowest position. Remove additional PPE, if used. Perform hand hygiene.	Lowering the bed promotes patient safety. Removing PPE properly reduces the risk for infection transmission and contamination of other items. Hand hygiene prevents the spread of microorganisms.

Changing the Appliance

ACTION	**RATIONALE**
11. Place a disposable waterproof pad on the overbed table or other work area. Set up the washbasin with warm water and the rest of the supplies. Place a trash bag within reach.	The pad protects the surface. Organization facilitates performance of procedure.
12. Put on clean gloves. Place waterproof pad under the patient at the stoma site. Empty the appliance if necessary as described in steps 6–8.	Waterproof pad protects linens and the patient from moisture. Emptying the contents before removal prevents accidental spillage of fecal material.
13. Gently remove the appliance, starting at the top and keeping the abdominal skin taut (Fig. 2). Remove the appliance faceplate from the skin by pushing the skin from the appliance rather than pulling the appliance from the skin (Fig. 3). Apply a silicone-based adhesive remover by spraying or wiping with the remover wipe as needed.	The seal between the surface of the faceplate and the skin must be broken before the faceplate can be removed. Harsh handling of the appliance can damage the skin and impair the development of a secure seal in the future. Silicone-based adhesive remover allows for the rapid and painless removal of adhesives and prevents skin stripping (Rudoni, 2008; Stephen-Haynes, 2008).

FIGURE 2. Gently removing appliance faceplate from skin.

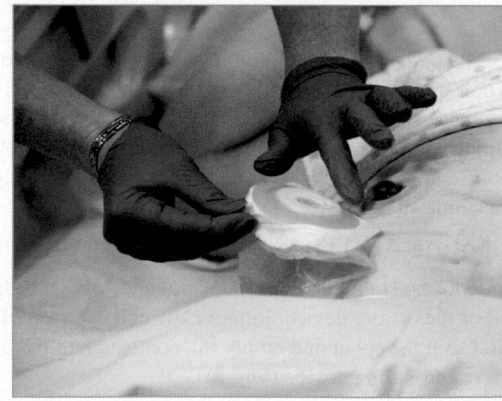

FIGURE 3. Pushing skin from appliance rather than pulling appliance from skin.

ACTION	**RATIONALE**
14. Place the appliance in the trash bag, if disposable. If reusable, set aside to wash in lukewarm soap and water and allow to air dry after the new appliance is in place.	Thorough cleaning and airing of the appliance reduce odor and deterioration of appliance. For aesthetic and infection-control purposes, used appliances should be discarded appropriately.
15. Clean the skin around the stoma with mild skin cleanser and water or a cleansing agent and a washcloth (Fig. 4). Remove all old adhesive from the skin; additional adhesive remover may be used. Do not apply lotion to the peristomal area.	Cleaning the skin removes excretions and old adhesive and skin protectant. Excretions or a buildup of other substances can irritate and damage the skin. Lotion will prevent a tight adhesive seal.
16. Gently pat the area dry. **Make sure the skin around the stoma is thoroughly dry.** Assess the stoma and condition of the surrounding skin.	Careful drying prevents trauma to the skin and stoma. An intact, properly applied urinary collection device protects skin integrity. Any change in color and size of the stoma may indicate circulatory problems.

ACTION

RATIONALE

FIGURE 4. Cleaning stoma with cleansing agent and washcloth.

FIGURE 5. Placing one or two gauze squares over stoma opening.

17. Place one or two gauze squares over the stoma opening (Fig. 5).

18. Apply skin protectant to a 2-inch (5-cm) radius around the stoma, and allow it to dry completely, which takes about 30 seconds.

19. Lift the gauze squares for a moment and measure the stoma opening, using the measurement guide. Replace the gauze. Trace the same size opening on the back center of the appliance. Cut the opening 1/8-inch larger than the stoma size (Fig. 6). Use a finger to gently smooth the wafer edges after cutting. Check that the spout is closed and the end cap is in place.

20. Remove the paper backing from the appliance faceplate. Quickly remove the gauze squares and discard appropriately; ease the appliance over the stoma. Gently press onto the skin while smoothing over the surface (Fig. 7). Apply gentle, even pressure to the appliance for approximately 30 seconds.

Continuous drainage must be absorbed to keep the skin dry during appliance change.

The skin needs protection from the potentially excoriating effect of the appliance adhesive. The skin must be perfectly dry before the appliance is placed to get good adherence and to prevent leaks.

The appliance should fit snugly around the stoma, with only 1/8 inch of skin visible around the opening. A faceplate opening that is too small can cause trauma to the stoma. If the opening is too large, exposed skin will be irritated by urine. Wafer edges may be uneven after cutting and could cause irritation to and/or pressure on the stoma. A closed spout and secured end cap prevent urine from leaking from the appliance.

The appliance is effective only if it is properly positioned and adhered securely. Pressure on the faceplate allows the faceplate to mold to the patient's skin and improve the seal.

FIGURE 6. Cutting the faceplate opening 1/8 inch larger than stoma size.

FIGURE 7. Applying faceplate over stoma.

(continued)

SKILL 36-9 EMPTYING AND CHANGING A STOMA APPLIANCE ON AN ILEAL CONDUIT *continued*

ACTION	RATIONALE
21. Secure the optional belt to the appliance and around the patient.	An elasticized belt helps support the appliance for some people.
22. Remove gloves. Assist the patient to a comfortable position. Cover the patient with bed linens. Place the bed in the lowest position.	Removing gloves reduces the risk of transmission of microorganisms. Positioning and covering provide warmth and promote comfort. Bed in the lowest position promotes patient safety.
23. Put on clean gloves. Remove or discard any remaining equipment and assess the patient's response to the procedure.	The patient's response may indicate acceptance of the ostomy as well as the need for health teaching.
24. Remove gloves and additional PPE, if used. Perform hand hygiene.	Removing PPE properly reduces the risk for infection transmission and contamination of other items. Hand hygiene prevents the spread of microorganisms.

DOCUMENTATION

Guidelines

Document the procedure, including the appearance of the stoma, condition of the peristomal skin, characteristics of the urine, the patient's response to the procedure, and pertinent patient teaching.

Sample Documentation

7/23/15 1245 Ileal conduit appliance changed. Mr. Jones present. Mrs. Jones asking questions about care for ileal conduit, states, "I don't know if I'll ever be able to care for this thing at home." Tearful at times. Patient encouraged to express feelings. Patient agreed to talk with wound, ostomy, and continence nurse about concerns. Mr. Jones very supportive, also asking appropriate questions. Patient states would like to watch change one more time before she attempts to do it. Stoma is moist and red, peristomal skin intact, draining yellow urine with small amount of mucus.

—B. Clapp, RN

UNEXPECTED SITUATIONS AND ASSOCIATED INTERVENTIONS

- *You remove appliance and find area of skin excoriated:* Make sure that the appliance is not cut too large. Skin that is exposed inside of the ostomy appliance will become excoriated. Assess for the presence of a fungal skin infection. If present, consult with the primary care provider to obtain appropriate treatment. Cleanse the skin thoroughly and pat dry. Apply products made for excoriated skin before placing the appliance over the stoma. Frequently check the faceplate to ensure that a seal has formed and that there is no leakage. Confer with the primary care provider for a wound, ostomy, and continence nurse (WOCN) consult to manage these issues. Document the excoriation in the patient's chart.

- *Faceplate is leaking after applying new appliance:* Remove the appliance, clean the skin, and start over.

- *You are ready to place faceplate and notice that opening is cut too large:* Discard the appliance and begin over. A faceplate that is cut too big may lead to excoriation of the skin.

- *Stoma is dark brown or black:* Stoma should appear pink to red, shiny and moist. Alterations indicate compromised circulation. If the stoma is dark brown or black, suspect ischemia and necrosis. Notify the primary care provider immediately.

SKILL 36-10 CARING FOR A HEMODIALYSIS ACCESS (ARTERIOVENOUS FISTULA OR GRAFT)

DELEGATION CONSIDERATIONS

The assessment of and care for a hemodialysis access is not delegated to nursing assistive personnel (NAP) or unlicensed assistive personnel (UAP). Depending on the state's nurse practice act and the organization's policies and procedures, these procedures may be delegated to licensed practical/vocational nurses (LPN/LVNs). The decision to delegate must be based on careful analysis of the patient's needs and circumstances, as well as the qualifications of the person to whom the task is being delegated. Refer to the Delegation Guidelines in Appendix A (found on the Point).

EQUIPMENT

- Stethoscope
- PPE, as indicated

IMPLEMENTATION

ACTION	RATIONALE
1. Perform hand hygiene and put on PPE, if indicated.	Hand hygiene and PPE prevent the spread of microorganisms. PPE is required based on transmission precautions.
2. Identify the patient.	Identifying the patient ensures that the right patient receives the intervention and helps prevent errors.
3. Close the curtains around the bed and close the door to the room, if possible. Explain what you are going to do, and why you are going to do it, to the patient.	This ensures the patient's privacy. Explanation relieves anxiety and facilitates cooperation. Discussion promotes cooperation and helps to minimize anxiety.
4. Question the patient about the presence of muscle weakness and cramping; changes in temperature; sensations, such as numbness, tingling, burning, itchiness; and pain.	Aids in determining the patency of the hemodialysis access, as well as the presence of complications.
5. Inspect the area over the access site for continuity of skin color. Inspect for any redness, warmth, tenderness, edema, rash, blemishes, bleeding, tremors, and twitches. Inspect the muscle strength and the patient's ability to perform range of motion in the extremity/body part with the hemodialysis access.	Inspection aids in determining the patency of the hemodialysis access; the status of the patient's circulatory, neurologic, and muscular function; and presence of infection. Compare with the opposite body area/part.
6. Palpate over the access site, feeling for a thrill or vibration (Fig. 1). Palpate pulses above and below the site. Palpate the continuity of the skin temperature along and around the extremity. Check capillary refill in the fingers or toes of the extremity with the fistula or graft.	Palpation aids in determining the patency of the hemodialysis access; the status of the patient's circulatory, neurologic, and muscular function; and presence of infection. Compare with the opposite body area/part.

FIGURE 1. Palpating access site for thrill.

ACTION	RATIONALE
7. Auscultate over the access site with the bell of the stethoscope, listening for a bruit or vibration.	Palpation aids in determining the patency of the hemodialysis access.
8. Ensure that a sign is placed over the head of the bed informing the health care team which arm is affected. **Do not measure blood pressure, perform a venipuncture, or start an IV on the access arm.**	The affected arm should not be used for any other procedures, such as obtaining blood pressure, which could lead to clotting of the graft or fistula. Venipuncture or IV access could lead to an infection of the affected arm and could cause the loss of the graft or fistula.

(continued)

SKILL 36-10 CARING FOR A HEMODIALYSIS ACCESS (ARTERIOVENOUS FISTULA OR GRAFT) *continued*

ACTION	RATIONALE
9. Instruct the patient not to sleep with the arm with the access site under the head or body.	This could lead to clotting of the fistula or graft.
10. Instruct the patient not to lift heavy objects with, or put pressure on, the arm with the access site. Advise the patient not to carry heavy bags (including purses) on the shoulder of that arm.	This could lead to clotting of the fistula or graft.
11. Remove PPE, if used. Perform hand hygiene.	Removing PPE properly reduces the risk for infection transmission and contamination of other items. Hand hygiene prevents the spread of microorganisms.

DOCUMENTATION

Guidelines

Document assessment findings, including the presence or absence of a bruit and thrill. Document any patient education and patient response.

Sample Documentation

> 5/10/15 0830 Arteriovenous fistula patent in left upper arm. Area without redness, pain, and edema; skin at site similar to surrounding skin tone. Patient denies pain and tenderness. Positive bruit and thrill noted. Patient verbalized understanding of importance of avoiding venipuncture in left arm.
>
> —B. Clapp, RN

UNEXPECTED SITUATIONS AND ASSOCIATED INTERVENTIONS

- *Thrill is diminished or not palpable and/or bruit is diminished or not audible:* Notify the primary care provider immediately. The thrill and bruit are caused by arterial blood flowing into the vein. If these signs are not present, the access may be clotting off.
- *Site is warm to touch, erythematous, or painful, or has a skin blemish:* Notify the primary care provider. These signs can indicate a site infection.

SKILL 36-11 CARING FOR A PERITONEAL DIALYSIS CATHETER

DELEGATION CONSIDERATIONS

The care of a peritoneal dialysis catheter is not delegated to nursing assistive personnel (NAP) or unlicensed assistive personnel (UAP). Depending on the state's nurse practice act and the organization's policies and procedures, care of a peritoneal dialysis catheter may be delegated to licensed practical/vocational nurses (LPN/LVNs). The decision to delegate must be based on careful analysis of the patient's needs and circumstances, as well as the qualifications of the person to whom the task is being delegated. Refer to the Delegation Guidelines in Appendix A (found on thePoint).

EQUIPMENT

- Face masks (2)
- Sterile gloves
- Nonsterile gloves
- Additional PPE, as indicated
- Antimicrobial cleansing agent, per facility policy
- Sterile gauze squares (4)
- Sterile basin
- Sterile drain sponge
- Transparent, occlusive site dressing
- Topical antibiotic, such as mupirocin or gentamicin,
- depending on order and policy
- Sterile applicator
- Plastic trash bag
- Bath blanket

IMPLEMENTATION

ACTION	RATIONALE
1. Review the patient's medical record for orders related to catheter site care. Gather equipment.	Ensures appropriate interventions for the patient. Assembling equipment provides an organized approach to the task.
2. Perform hand hygiene and put on PPE, if indicated.	Hand hygiene and PPE prevent the spread of microorganisms. PPE is required based on transmission precautions.
3. Identify the patient.	Identifying the patient ensures that the right patient receives the intervention and helps prevent errors.
4. Close the curtains around the bed and close the door to the room, if possible. Explain what you are going to do and why you are going to do it to the patient. Encourage the patient to observe or participate if possible.	This ensures the patient's privacy. Explanation relieves anxiety and facilitates cooperation. Discussion promotes cooperation and helps to minimize anxiety. Having the patient observe or assist encourages self-acceptance.
5. Assemble equipment on the overbed table within reach.	Arranging items nearby is convenient, saves time, and avoids unnecessary stretching and twisting of muscles on the part of the nurse.
6. Adjust bed to comfortable working height, usually elbow height of the caregiver (VISN 8 Patient Safety Center, 2009). Assist the patient to a supine position. Expose the abdomen, draping the patient's chest with the bath blanket, exposing only the catheter site.	Having the bed at the proper height prevents back and muscle strain. The supine position is usually the best way to gain access to the peritoneal dialysis catheter. Use of a bath blanket provides patient warmth and avoids unnecessary exposure.
7. Put on unsterile gloves. Put on one of the facemasks; have the patient put on the other mask.	Gloves protect the nurse from contact with blood and bodily fluids. Use of facemasks deters the spread of microorganisms.
8. Gently remove old dressing, noting odor, amount, and color of drainage, leakage, and condition of the skin around the catheter. Discard the dressing in an appropriate container.	Drainage, leakage, and skin condition can indicate problems with the catheter, such as infection.
9. Remove gloves and discard. Set up a sterile field. Open packages. Using aseptic technique, place two sterile gauze squares in a basin with an antimicrobial agent. Leave two sterile gauze squares opened on the sterile field. Alternately (based on facility's policy), place sterile antimicrobial swabs on the sterile field. Place a sterile applicator on the field. Squeeze a small amount of the topical antibiotic on one of the gauze squares on the sterile field.	Until the catheter site has healed, aseptic technique is necessary for site care to prevent infection.
10. Put on sterile gloves. Pick up the dialysis catheter with your nondominant hand. **With the antimicrobial-soaked gauze/ swab, cleanse the skin around the exit site using a circular motion, starting at the exit site and then slowly going outward 3 to 4 inches. Gently remove crusted scabs, if necessary.**	Aseptic technique is necessary to prevent infection. The antimicrobial agent cleanses the skin and removes any drainage or crust from the wound, reducing the risk for infection.
11. **Continue to hold the catheter with your nondominant hand. After the skin has dried, clean the catheter with an antimicrobial-soaked gauze, beginning at the exit site, going around the catheter, and then moving up to the end of the catheter. Gently remove crusted secretions on the tube, if necessary.**	Antimicrobial agents cleanse the catheter and remove any drainage or crust from the tube, reducing the risk for infection.
12. Using the sterile applicator, apply the topical antibiotic to the catheter exit site, if prescribed.	Application of mupirocin and gentamicin at the catheter exit site prevents exit site infection and peritonitis (Bernardini et al., 2005).
13. Place a sterile drain sponge around the exit site. Then place a 4 × 4 gauze over the exit site. Cover with transparent, occlusive dressing. Remove masks.	The drain sponge and 4 × 4 gauze are used to absorb any drainage from the exit site. Occlusion of the site with a dressing deters contamination of the site. Once the site is covered, masks are no longer necessary.

(continued)

SKILL 36-11 CARING FOR A PERITONEAL DIALYSIS CATHETER *continued*

ACTION	RATIONALE
14. Label the dressing with date, time of change, and your initials.	Other personnel working with the catheter will know information related to site care.
15. Coil the exposed length of tubing and secure to the dressing or the patient's abdomen with tape.	Anchoring the catheter absorbs any tugging, preventing tension on and irritation to the skin or abdomen.
16. Assist the patient to a comfortable position. Cover the patient with bed linens. Place the bed in the lowest position.	Positioning and covering provide warmth and promote comfort. A bed in the lowest position promotes patient safety.
17. Put on clean gloves. Remove or discard equipment and assess the patient's response to the procedure.	These actions deter the spread of microorganisms. The patient's response may indicate acceptance of the catheter or the need for health teaching.
18. Remove gloves and additional PPE, if used. Perform hand hygiene.	Removing PPE properly reduces the risk for infection transmission and contamination of other items. Hand hygiene prevents the spread of microorganisms.

DOCUMENTATION

Guidelines

Document the dressing change, including condition of the skin surrounding the exit site, drainage, or odor, as well as the patient's reaction to procedure, and any patient teaching provided.

Sample Documentation

> 8/22/15 1530 Peritoneal dialysis catheter dressing changed; skin surrounding catheter slightly erythematous, but remains intact. Small amount of clear drainage approximately the size of a dime without odor noted on drain sponge. Patient asking appropriate questions regarding dressing change. Verbalized an understanding of explanations.
>
> —B. Clapp, RN

UNEXPECTED SITUATIONS AND ASSOCIATED INTERVENTIONS

• *Patient complains of pain when you palpate the abdomen; purulent or cloudy drainage is present, or foul odor is noted when old dressing is removed:* Notify the primary care provider immediately. Any of these signs could indicate a site infection or peritonitis.

• *You note that the old dressing is saturated with clear fluid:* Replace the dressing to prevent skin breakdown. Notify the primary care provider. A frequent complication is leakage from the exit site. Frequently check the dressing, especially after the patient has had solution placed in the abdominal cavity.

SPECIAL CONSIDERATIONS

General Considerations

• Instruct patients to avoid showering for 2 to 3 weeks, until the site has healed (Lee & Park, 2012).

• Instruct patients with a peritoneal dialysis catheter to avoid tub baths and public pools.

• Remind patients performing own site care of the importance of good handwashing before self-care. The use of alcohol-based hand gels or washing with antimicrobial soap is recommended (Hain & Chan, 2013).

• Discourage patients from wearing tight clothes and belts around the exit site.

Home Care Considerations

• Often, clean technique, instead of sterile technique, is used by the patient and caregivers in the home.

• Teach patients the signs of exit site infection and encourage them to contact their primary care provider for prompt intervention.

DEVELOPING CLINICAL REASONING

1. The daughter of an older patient who is about to be discharged to the daughter's home requests that a catheter be inserted in her mother to make home care easier. The mother knows when she needs to void but needs assistance to get to the bathroom. How do you respond to the daughter's request?

2. If you noted the following when assessing a patient, what would you do?
   - A 6-year-old refuses to give a urine sample.
   - Frank blood appears in urine of a patient who has no history of urinary problems.
   - When you ask for a urine sample, a teenager asks, "This won't reveal drugs, will it?"
   - A young woman complains of painful urination with burning.
   - An older man reports frequency and pain when voiding.

PRACTICING FOR NCLEX

1. A nurse caring for patients in a long-term care facility is often required to collect urine specimens from patients for laboratory testing. Which techniques for urine collection are performed correctly? Select all that apply.
   a. The nurse catheterizes a patient to collect a sterile urine sample for routine urinalysis.
   b. The nurse collects a clean-catch urine specimen in the morning from a patient and stores it at room temperature until an afternoon pick-up.
   c. The nurse collects a sterile urine specimen from the collection receptacle of a patient's indwelling catheter.
   d. The nurse collects about 3 mL of urine from a patient's indwelling catheter to send for a urine culture.
   e. The nurse collects a urine specimen from a patient with a urinary diversion by catheterizing the stoma.
   f. The nurse discards the first urine of the day when performing a 24-hour urine specimen collection on a patient.

2. A nurse caring for patients in an extended-care facility performs regular assessments of the patients' urinary functioning. Which patients would the nurse screen for urinary retention? Select all that apply.
   a. A 78-year-old male patient diagnosed with an enlarged prostate
   b. An 83-year-old female patient who is on bedrest
   c. A 75-year-old female patient who is diagnosed with vaginal prolapse
   d. An 89-year-old male patient who has dementia
   e. A 73-year-old female patient who is taking antihistamines to treat allergies
   f. A 90-year-old male patient who has difficulty walking to the bathroom

3. A nurse is preparing a brochure to teach patients how to prevent urinary tract infections. Which teaching points would the nurse include? Select all that apply.
   a. Wear underwear with a synthetic crotch.
   b. Take baths rather than showers.
   c. Drink eight to ten 8-oz glasses of water per day.
   d. Drink a glass of water before and after intercourse and void afterwards.
   e. Limit caffeine-containing beverages.
   f. Drink 10 oz of cranberry or blueberry juice daily.

4. A patient who has pneumonia has had a fever for 3 days. What characteristics would the nurse anticipate related to the patient's urine output?
   a. Decreased and highly concentrated
   b. Decreased and highly dilute
   c. Increased and concentrated
   d. Increased and dilute

5. The physician has ordered an indwelling catheter inserted in a hospitalized male patient. What consideration would the nurse keep in mind when performing this procedure?
   a. The male urethra is more vulnerable to injury during insertion.
   b. In the hospital, a clean technique is used for catheter insertion.
   c. The catheter is inserted 2″ to 3″ into the meatus.
   d. Since it uses a closed system, the risk for urinary tract infection is absent.

6. A nurse is performing intermittent closed-catheter irrigation for a patient with an indwelling catheter. After attaching the syringe to the access port on the catheter, the nurse finds that the irrigant will not enter the catheter. What intervention would the nurse appropriately perform next?
   a. Apply pressure to the catheter to force the solution into the catheter.
   b. Disconnect and reconnect the drainage system quickly.
   c. Notify the primary care provider.
   d. Change the catheter.

7. A nurse is caring for a 56-year-old male patient diagnosed with bladder cancer who has a urinary diversion. Which actions would the nurse take when caring for this patient? Select all that apply
   a. Measure the patient's fluid intake and output.
   b. Keep the skin around the stoma moist.
   c. Empty the appliance frequently.
   d. Report any mucous in the urine to the primary care provider.
   e. Encourage the patient to look away when changing the appliance.
   f. Monitor the return of intestinal function and peristalsis.

8. A nurse is changing the stoma appliance on a patient's ileal conduit. Which characteristic of the stoma would alert the nurse that the patient is experiencing ischemia?
   a. The stoma is hard and dry.
   b. The stoma is a pale pink color.
   c. The stoma is swollen.
   d. The stoma is a purple-blue color.

9. After surgery, a patient is having difficulty voiding. Which nursing action would most likely lead to an increased difficulty with voiding?
   a. Pouring warm water over the patient's fingers.
   b. Having the patient ignore the urge to void until her bladder is full.
   c. Using a warm bedpan when the patient feels the urge to void.
   d. Stroking the patient's leg or thigh.

10. A nurse caring for a patient's hemodialysis access documents the following: "5/10/15 0930 Arteriovenous fistula patent in right upper arm. Area is warm to touch and edematous. Patient denies pain and tenderness. Positive bruit and thrill

noted." Which documented finding would the nurse report to the primary care provider?
a. Positive bruit noted.
b. Area is warm to touch and edematous.
c. Patient denies pain and tenderness.
d. Positive thrill noted.

11. A nurse is caring for an alert, ambulatory, older resident in a long-term care facility who voids frequently and has difficulty making it to the bathroom in time. Which nursing intervention would be most helpful for this patient?
a. Teach the patient that incontinence is a normal occurrence with aging.
b. Ask the patient's family to purchase incontinence pads for the patient.
c. Teach the patient to perform Kegel exercises at regular intervals daily.
d. Insert an indwelling catheter to prevent skin breakdown.

12. A nurse is caring for a patient who is taking phenazopyridine (Pyridium, a urinary tract analgesic). The patient questions the nurse: "My urine was bright orangish-red today; is there something wrong with me?" What would be the nurse's best response?
a. "This is a normal finding when taking phenazopyridine."
b. "This may be a sign of blood in the urine."
c. "This may be the result of an injury to your bladder."
d. "This is a sign that you are allergic to the medication and must stop it."

13. A nurse is caring for a male patient who had a condom catheter applied following hip surgery. What action would be a priority when caring for this patient?
a. Preventing the tubing from kinking to maintain free urinary drainage
b. Not removing the catheter for any reason
c. Fastening the condom tightly to prevent the possibility of leakage
d. Maintaining bedrest at all times to prevent the catheter from slipping off

14. A nurse forms the following nursing diagnosis for a patient: Impaired Urinary Elimination related to maturational enuresis. Based on this diagnosis, for which patient is the nurse caring?
a. An adult older than 65 years of age who is incontinent
b. A child older than 4 years of age who has involuntary urination
c. A 12-month-old child who has involuntary urination
d. A patient with neurologic damage resulting in bladder dysfunction

15. Data must be collected to evaluate the effectiveness of a plan to reduce urinary incontinence in an older adult patient. Which information is least important for the evaluation process?
a. The incontinence pattern
b. State of physical mobility
c. Medications being taken
d. Age of the patient

ANSWERS WITH RATIONALES

1. *d, e, f.* A urine culture requires about 3 mL of urine, whereas routine urinalysis requires at least 10 mL of urine. The

preferred method of collecting a urine specimen from a urinary diversion is to catheterize the stoma. For a 24-hour urine specimen, the nurse should discard the first voiding, then collect all urine voided for the next 24 hours. A sterile urine specimen is not required for a routine urinalysis. Urine chemistry is altered after urine stands at room temperature for a long period of time. A specimen from the collecting receptacle (drainage bag) may not be fresh urine and could result in an inaccurate analysis.

2. *a, c, e.* Urinary retention occurs when urine is produced normally but is not excreted completely from the bladder. Factors associated with urinary retention include medications such as antihistamines, an enlarged prostate, or vaginal prolapse. Being on bedrest, having dementia, and having difficulty walking to the bathroom may place patients at risk for urinary incontinence.

3. *c, e, f.* It is recommended that a healthy adult drink eight to ten 8-oz glasses of fluid daily, limit caffeine because it is irritating to the bladder mucosa, and drink 10 oz of cranberry or blueberry juice daily to help prevent bacteriuria. It is also recommended to wear underwear with a cotton crotch, take showers rather than baths, and drink two glasses of water before and after sexual intercourse and void immediately after intercourse.

4. *a.* Fever and diaphoresis cause the kidneys to conserve body fluids. Thus, the urine is concentrated and decreased in amount.

5. *a.* Because of its length, the male urethra is more prone to injury and requires that the catheter be inserted 6″ to 8″. This procedure requires surgical asepsis to prevent introducing bacteria into the urinary tract. The presence of an indwelling catheter places the patient at risk for a UTI.

6. *c.* If the irrigation solution will not enter the catheter, the nurse should not force the solution into the catheter; instead, the nurse should notify the primary care provider and prepare to change the catheter.

7. *a, c, f.* When caring for a patient with a urinary diversion, the nurse should measure the patient's fluid intake and output to monitor fluid balance, change the appliance frequently, monitor the return of intestinal function and peristalsis, keep the skin around the stoma dry, watch for mucous in the urine as a normal finding, and encourage the patient to participate in care and look at the stoma.

8. *d.* A purple-blue stoma may reflect compromised circulation or ischemia. A pale stoma may indicate anemia. The stoma may be swollen at first, but that condition should subside with time. A normal stoma should be moist and dark pink to red in color.

9. *b.* Ignoring the urge to void makes urination even more difficult and should be avoided. The other activities are all recommended nursing activities to promote voiding.

10. *b.* The nurse would report a site that is warm and edematous as this could be a sign of a site infection. The thrill and bruit are normal findings caused by arterial blood flowing into the vein. If these are not present, the access may be cutting off. No report of pain is a normal finding.

11. *c.* Kegel exercises may help a patient regain control of the micturition process. Incontinence is not a normal consequence

of aging. Using absorbent products may remove motivation from the patient and caregiver to seek evaluation and treatment of the incontinence; they should be used only after careful evaluation by a health care provider. An indwelling catheter is the last choice of treatment.

12. *a.* Pyridium is noted for turning the urine orange-red; the patient needs to be aware of this.

13. *a.* The catheter should be allowed to drain freely through tubing that is not kinked. It also should be removed daily to prevent skin excoriation and should not be fastened too tightly or restriction of blood vessels in the area is likely. Confining a patient to bedrest increases the risk for other hazards related to immobility.

14. *b.* Maturational enuresis is involuntary urination after an age when continence should be present. A 12-month-old child is not expected to be continent, and incontinence and neurologic damage are not maturational problems.

15. *d.* Incontinence is not a natural consequence of the aging process. All the other factors are necessary information for the plan of care.

TAYLOR SUITE RESOURCES

Explore these additional resources to enhance learning for this chapter:

* NCLEX-Style Questions and other resources on thePoint, http://thePoint.lww.com/Taylor8e
* *Study Guide for Fundamentals of Nursing,* 8th edition
* Adaptive Learning | Powered by prepU, http://thepoint.lww.com/prepu
* *Skill Checklists for Fundamentals of Nursing,* 8th edition
* *Taylor's Clinical Nursing Skills:* Chapter 12, Urinary Elimination
* *Taylor's Video Guide to Clinical Nursing Skills:* Urinary Elimination and Urinary Catheters
* *Lippincott DocuCare* Fundamentals cases

Bibliography

Ackley, B. J., & Ladwig, G. B. (2011). *Nursing Diagnosis Handbook* (9th ed.). St. Louis: Elsevier/Mosby.

Adams, D., Bucior, H., Day, G., & Rimmer, J. A. (2012). HOUDINI: make that urinary catheter disappear—nurse-led protocol. *Journal of Infection Prevention, 13*(2), 44–46.

Altschuler, V., & Diaz, L. (2006). Bladder ultrasound. *MEDSURG Nursing, 15*(5), 317–318.

American Association of Critical-Care Nurses (AACN). (2011). *AACN practice alert. Catheter-associated urinary tract infections.* Available at http://www.aacn.org/WD/practice/docs/practicealerts/catheter-associated-uti-practice-alert.pdf

Avent, Y. (2012). Wound wise: Understanding urinary diversions. *Nursing Made Incredibly Easy!, 10*(4), 47–52.

Bentley, A. (2012). Recommended practice. Stoma care: Older adults. *PACEsetterS, 9*(1), 23–25.

Bernard, M. S., Hunter, K. F., & Moore, K. N. (2012). Decrease the duration of indwelling urethral catheters and potentially reduce the incidence of catheter-associated urinary tract infections. *Urologic Nursing, 32*(1), 29–37.

Bhardwaj, R., Pickard, R., Carrick-Sen, D., & Britain, K. (2012). Patients' perspectives on timing of urinary catheter removal after surgery. *British Journal of Nursing, 21*(18), S4, S6–S9.

Boltz, M., Capezuti, E., Fulmer, T., & Zwicker, D. (Eds.) (2012). *Evidence-based geriatric nursing protocols for best practice* (4th ed.). New York: Springer Publishing Company.

Bradway, C., & Cacchione, P. (2010). Teaching strategies for assessing and managing urinary incontinence in older adults. *Journal of Gerontological Nursing, 36*(7), 18–26.

Bulechek, G. M, Butcher, H. K., Dochterman, J. M., & Wagner, C. M. (Eds.). (2013). *Nursing interventions classification (NIC)* (6th ed.). St. Louis: Elsevier/Mosby.

Bullman, S. (2011). Ins and outs of suprapubic catheters—a clinician's experience. *Urologic Nursing, 31*(5), 259–264.

Burch, J. (2011). Peristomal skin care and the use of accessories to promote skin health. *British Journal of Nursing, 20*(7), S4–S10.

Burch, J. (2010). Caring for peristomal skin: what every nurse should know. *British Journal of Nursing, 19*(3), 166–172.

Carrion, J. (2012). Vascular access devices for hemodialysis. *OR Nurse, 6*(1), 28–33.

Centers for Medicare & Medicaid Services (CMS). (2012). Hospital-acquired conditions. Available at http://www.cms.gov/Medicare/Medicare-Fee-for-Service-Payment/HospitalAcqCond/Hospital-Acquired_Conditions.html

Cipa-Tatum, J., Kelly-Signs, M., & Afsart, K. (2011). Urethral erosion: a case for prevention. *Journal of Wound Ostomy & Continence Nursing, 38*(5), 581–558.

Collia Pellatt, G. (2012). Promoting male urinary continence. *British Journal of Nursing, Supplement* (May), S5–S11.

Cutright, J. (2011). The effect of the bladder scanner policy on the number of urinary catheters inserted. *Journal of Wound Ostomy Continence Nursing, 38*(1), 71–76.

Dailly, S. (2012). Auditing urinary catheter care. *Nursing Standard, 26*(20), 35–40.

De Jaeger, M. (2011). Exploring urinary catheters: the perspectives of patients and nurses. *British Journal of Nursing, 20*(7), 400, 402, 404, 406, 408.

Denyer, J. (2011). Reducing pain during the removal of adhesive and adherent products. *British Journal of Nursing, 20*(15) (Tissue Viability Supplement), S28–S35.

Edward, J. R., Peterson, K. D., Andrus, M. L., Tolson, T. S., Goulding, J. S., Dudeck, M. A., ... Horan T. C. (2007). National Healthcare Safety Network (NHSN) report, data summary for 2006, issued June 2007. *American Journal of Infection Control 35*:290–301.

Ehlman, K., Wilson, A., Dugger, R., Eggleston, B., Coudret, N., & Mathis, S. (2012). Nursing home staff members' attitudes and knowledge about urinary incontinence: The impact of technology and training. *Urologic Nursing, 32*(4), 205–213.

Flynn Makic, M. B., VonRueden, K. T., Rauen, C. A., & Chadwick, J. (2011). Evidence-based practice habits: Putting more sacred cows out to pasture. *CriticalCareNurse, 31*(2), 38–61.

Foxley, S. (2011). Indwelling urinary catheters: accurate monitoring of urine output. *British Journal of Nursing, 20*(9), 564, 566–569.

Gokula, M., Smolen, D., Gaspar, P. M., Hensley, S. J., Benninghoff, M. C., & Smith, M. (2012). Designing a protocol to reduce catheter-associated urinary tract infections. *American Journal of Infection Control, 40*(10), 1002–1004.

Gray, M. L. (2008). Securing the indwelling catheter. *American Journal of Nursing, 108*(12), 44–50.

Grossman, S., & Porth, C. M. (2014). *Porth's pathophysiology: concepts of altered health states.* (9th ed.). Philadelphia: Wolters Kluwer Health/Lippincott Williams & Wilkins.

Hägglund, D. (2010). A systematic literature review of incontinence care for persons with dementia: the research evidence. *Journal of Clinical Nursing, 19*(3–4), 303–312.

Hain, D., & Chan, J. (2013). Best available evidence for peritoneal dialysis catheter exit-site care. *Nephrology Nursing Journal, 40*(1), 63–69.

Herter, R., & Wallace Kazer, M. (2010). Best practices in urinary catheter. *Home Healthcare Nurse, 28*(6), 342–349.

Hinkle, J. L., & Cheever, K. H. (2014). *Brunner & Suddarth's Textbook of Medical–Surgical Nursing* (13th ed.). Philadelphia: Wolters Kluwer Health/Lippincott Williams & Wilkins.

Hogan-Quigley, B., Palm, M. L., & Bickley, L. (2012). *Bates' nursing guide to physical examination and history taking.* Philadelphia: Wolters Kluwer Health/Lippincott Williams & Wilkins.

Hooton, T. M., Bradley, S. F., Cardenas, D. D., Colgan, R., Geerlings, S. E., Rice, J. C., ... Nicolle, L. E. (2010). Diagnosis, prevention, and treatment of catheter-associated urinary tract infection in adults: 2009 international clinical practice guidelines from the Infectious Diseases Society of America. *Clinical Infectious Diseases, 50*(5), 625–663. Available at http://www.idsociety.org/uploadedFiles/IDSA/Guidelines-Patient_Care/PDF_Library/Comp%20UTI.pdf

Huebner, M., Riegel, K., Hinninghofen, H., Wallwiener, D., Tunn, R., & Reisenauer, C. (2011). Pelvic floor muscle training for stress urinary incontinence: A randomized, controlled trial comparing different conservative therapies. *Physiotherapy Research International, 16*(3), 133–40.

Huether, S. E., & McCance, K. L. (2012.) *Understanding pathophysiology* (5th ed.). St. Louis: Elsevier.

Jarvis, C. (2012). *Physical examination & health assessment* (6th ed.). St. Louis: Elsevier/Saunders.

Kannankeril, A. J., Lam, H. T., Reyes, E. B., & McCartney, J. (2011). Urinary tract infection rates associated with re-use of catheters in clean intermittent catheterization of male veterans. *Urologic Nursing, 31*(1), 41–48.

Kee, J. L., Hayes, E. R., & McCuistion, L. E. (2012). *Pharmacology: A nursing process approach* (7th ed.). St. Louis: Elsevier/Saunders.

Keyock, K. L., & Newman, D. K. (2011). Understanding stress incontinence. *The Nurse Practitioner, 36*(10), 24–36.

Klevans, R. M., Edwards, J. R, Richards, C. L., Horan, T. C. (2007). Estimating health care-associated infections and deaths in US hospitals, 2002. *Public Health Reports 122*:160–166.

Kyle, G. (2011). Reducing urethral catheterization trauma with urethral gels. *British Journal of Neuroscience Nursing, 7*(5), S8–S12.

Kyle, T., & Carman, S. (2013). *Essentials of pediatric nursing* (2nd ed.). Philadelphia: Wolters Kluwer Health/Lippincott Williams & Wilkins.

Lee, A., & Park, Y. (2012). Reducing peritoneal dialysis catheter exit site infections by implementing a standardized postoperative dressing protocol. *Renal Society of Australasia Journal, 8*(1), 18–22.

Lever, R. B. (2011). Essential guide to urinary incontinence. *Practice Nurse, 41*(8), 33–36.

Logan, K. (2012). An overview of male intermittent self-catheterisation. *British Journal of Nursing, 21*(18), S18–S22.

Malarkey, L. M., & McMorrow, M. E. (2012). *Saunders nursing guide to laboratory and diagnostic tests* (2nd ed.). St. Louis: Elsevier/Saunders.

Mangnall, J. (2012). Key considerations of intermittent catheterisation. *British Journal of Nursing, 21*(7), 392, 394, 396–398.

Mangnall, J. (2012). Promoting patient safety in continence care. *Nursing Standard, 26*(23), 49–56.

Mangnall, J. (2011). Selecting the right urinary leg bag drainage system for patient needs. *British Journal of Nursing, 20*(13), 797–798, 800–802.

Matteucci, R., & Walsh, K. (2013). Evidence-based care sheet. Urinary catheter use and prevention of infection. *CINAHL Information Systems.* Glendale, CA: EBSCO Publishing.

Mayo Clinic. (2011a). Hemodialysis. Available at http://www.mayoclinic.com/health/hemodialysis/MY00281.

Mayo Clinic. (2011b). Peritoneal dialysis. Available at http://www.mayoclinic.com/health/peritoneal-dialysis/MY00282

MedlinePlus. (2013). Urinary tract infection—adults. Available at http://www.nlm.nih.gov/medlineplus/ency/article/000521.htm

Moorhead, S., Johnson, M., Maas, M. L., & Swanson, E. (Eds.). (2013). *Nursing Outcomes Classification (NOC)* (5th ed.). St. Louis: Elsevier/Mosby.

NANDA International (NANDA-I). (2012). *Nursing diagnoses: Definitions & classification 2012–2014.* West Sussex, UK: Wiley-Blackwell.

National Association For Continence (NAFC). (2013a). The basic types of urinary incontinence. Available at http://www.nafc.org/index.php?page=types-of-incontinence

National Association For Continence (NAFC). (2013b). Diet and daily habits: Can this affect your bladder or bowel control? Available at http://www.nafc.org/bladder-bowel-health/frequently-asked-questions/diet-and-daily-habits/

National Kidney Foundation (NKF). (2013). Urinary tract infections. Available at http://www.kidney.org/atoz/content/uti.cfm

National Kidney Foundation (NKF). (2010). Urinary tract infections. Available at http://www.kidney.org/atoz/pdf/uti.pdf

National Kidney Foundation (NKF). (2006). Peritoneal dialysis. Available at http://www.kidney.org/atoz/pdf/peritonealdialysis.pdf

National Kidney and Urologic Diseases Information Clearinghouse (NKUDIC). (2012). Urodynamic testing. Available at http://kidney.niddk.nih.gov/KUDiseases/pubs/urodynamic/index.aspx

National Kidney and Urologic Diseases Information Clearinghouse (NKUDIC). (2011; updated 2012). Urinary tract infections in adults. Available at http://kidney.niddk.nih.gov/KUDiseases/pubs/utiadult/index.aspx

National Kidney and Urologic Diseases Information Clearinghouse (NKUDIC). (2010). Bladder control for women. Available at http://kidney.niddk.nih.gov/kudiseases/pubs/bladdercontrol/.

National Kidney and Urologic Diseases Information Clearinghouse (NKUDIC). (2007a). Urinary retention. Available at http://kidney.niddk.nih.gov/Kudiseases/pubs/UrinaryRetention/UrinaryRetention_508.pdf

National Kidney and Urologic Diseases Information Clearinghouse (NKUDIC). (2007b; updated 2012). Urinary incontinence in men. Available at http://kidney.niddk.nih.gov/KUDiseases/pubs/uimen/index.aspx

National Kidney and Urologic Diseases Information Clearinghouse (NKUDIC). (2007c; updated 2010). Urinary incontinence in women. Available at http://kidney.niddk.nih.gov/kudiseases/pubs/uiwomen/index.aspx

Nazarko, L. (2012). Evaluating clinical indications for continued catheterisation. *Nursing & Residential Care, 14*(9), 450, 452, 454–455.

Newman, D. K., & Willson, M.M. (2011). Review of intermittent catheterization and current best practices. *Urologic Nursing, 31*(1), 12–28.

Newman, D. (2008). Internal and external urinary catheters: A primer for clinical practice. *Ostomy Wound Management, 54*(12), 18–20, 22–26, 28–38.

Palese, A., Buchini, S., Deroma, L., & Barbone, F. (2010). The effectiveness of the ultrasound bladder scanner in reducing urinary tract infections: a meta-analysis. *Journal of Clinical Nursing, 19*(21/22), 2970–2979.

Patraca, K. (2005). Measure bladder volume without catheterization. *Nursing, 35*(4), 4.

Perry, M. (2011). Assessing and treating stress incontinence. *Practice Nursing, 22*(8), 434–437.

Perry, S. E., Hockenberry, M. J., Lowdermilk, D. L., & Wilson, D. (2010). *Maternal child nursing care* (4th ed.). Maryland Heights, MO: Elsevier/Mosby.

Rantell, A. (2012). Intermittent self-catheterisation in women. *Nursing Standard, 26*(42), 61–68.

Rew, M., & Smith, R. (2011). Reducing infection through the use of suprapubic catheters. *British Journal of Neuroscience Nursing, 7*(5), S13–S16.

Richard, C. J. (2011). Preservation of vascular access for hemodialysis in acute care settings. *Critical Care Nursing Quarterly, 34*(1), 76–83.

Ritter, L. A., & Hoffman, N. A. (2010). *Multicultural health.* Boston: Jones and Bartlett.

Rudoni, C. (2008). A service evaluation of the use of silicone-based adhesive remover. *British Journal of Nursing, Stoma Care Supplement, 17*(2), 54, 56, 58–59.

Schneider, M. A. (2012). Prevention of catheter-associated urinary tract infections in patients with hip fractures through education of nurses to specific catheter protocols. *Orthopaedic Nursing, 31*(1), 12–18.

Society of Urologic Nurses and Associates (SUNA). (2010). Prevention & control of catheter-associated urinary tract infection (CAUTI). Clinical practice guideline. Available at https://www.suna.org/sites/default/files/download/cautiGuideline.pdf

Society of Urologic Nurses and Associates (SUNA). (2005a). Care of the patient with an indwelling catheter: Clinical practice guideline. Available at http://www.suna.org/resources/indwellingCatheter.pdf

Society of Urologic Nurses and Associates (SUNA). (2005b). Female urethral catheterization: Clinical practice guideline. Available at http://www.suna.org/resources/femaleCatheterization.pdf

Society of Urologic Nurses and Associates (SUNA). (2005c). Male urethral catheterization: Clinical practice guideline. Available at http://www.suna.org/resources/maleCatheterization.pdf

Spector, R. E. (2009). *Cultural diversity in health and illness* (7th ed.). Upper Saddle River, NJ: Pearson/Prentice Hall.

Stephen-Hayes, J. (2008). Skin integrity and silicone: APPEEL 'nosting' medical adhesive remover. *British Journal of Nursing, 17*(2), 792–795.

Stewart, E. (2011). Intermittent self-catheterization and infection reduction. *British Journal of Neuroscience Nursing, 7*(5), S4–S7.

Stewart, E. (2010). Treating urinary incontinence in older women. *British Journal of Community Nursing, 15*(11), 526–532.

Tabloski, P. (2010). *Gerontological nursing* (2nd ed.). Upper Saddle River, NJ: Pearson.

Taylor, J. J., & Cohen, B. J. (2013). *Memmler's structure and function of the human body* (10th ed.). Philadelphia: Wolters Kluwer Health/Lippincott Williams & Wilkins.

The Joanna Briggs Institute (JBI). (2011). The Joanna Briggs Institute best practice information sheet: The effectiveness of pelvic floor muscle exercises on urinary incontinence in women following childbirth. *Nursing and Health Sciences, 13*(3), 378–381.

The Joanna Briggs Institute (JBI). (2004). Clinical effectiveness of different approaches to peritoneal dialysis catheter exit-site care. *BestPractice, 8*(1), 1–7.

Turner, B., & Dickens, N. (2010). Long-term urethral catheterisation. *Primary Health Care, 21*(4), 32–38.

Uberoi, V., Calixte, N., Coronel, V. R., Furlong, D. J., Orlando, R. P., & Lerner, L.B. (2013). Reducing urinary catheter days. *Nursing, 43*(1), 16–20.

U.S. Department of Health and Human Services (USDHHS), Office on Women's Health. (2010). *Urinary incontinence fact sheet.* Available at http://www.womenshealth.gov/publications/our-publications/fact-sheet/urinary-incontinence.html

Van Leeuwen, A. M., Poelhuis-Leth, D., & Bladh, M. L. (2011). *Davis's comprehensive handbook of laboratory & diagnostic tests with nursing implications* (4th ed.). Philadelphia: F. A. Davis.

VISN 8 Patient Safety Center. (2009). *Safe patient handling and measurement algorithms.* Available at www.visn8.va.gov/patientsafetycenter/safePtHandling

Wilde, M. H., McDonald, M. V., Brasch, J., McMahon, J. M., Fairbanks, E., Shah, S., … Scheid, E. (2013). Long-term urinary catheter users self-care practices and problems. *Journal of Clinical Nursing, 22*(3/4), 356–367.

Williams, J. (2012). Stoma care: obtaining a urine specimen from a urostomy. *Gastrointestinal Nursing, 10*(5), 11–12.

Wilson, M. (2011). Addressing the problems of long-term urethral catheterization: part 2. *British Journal of Nursing, 21*(1), 16, 18–20, 22, 24–25.

Wilson, M. (2011). Addressing the problems of long-term urethral catheterization: part 1. *British Journal of Nursing, 20*(22), 1418, 1420–1424.

Winder, A. (2012). Good practice in catheter care. *Journal of Community Nursing, 26*(6), 15–16, 19–20.

Yates, A. (2012). Management of long-term urinary catheters. *Nursing & Residential Care, 14*(4), 172, 174, 176–178.

37

Bowel Elimination

JEREMY GREEN

Jeremy, age 4, has been attending daycare since his mother returned to work 6 months ago. He presents at the hospital with a history of liquid stools, six to seven times a day, for the last 3 days.

ALBERTA FRANKLIN

Alberta, age 55, has recently undergone abdominal surgery that resulted in the creation of a sigmoid colostomy. Her stoma is bright red and moist and draining semisoft brown stool. Her ostomy appliance needs to be changed.

LEROY COBBS

Leroy, newly diagnosed with cancer, is taking acetaminophen (Tylenol) with codeine for pain. He is hospitalized for fecal impaction. "Nobody told me I would get so constipated," he says. "It's been almost a week and I'm still not moving my bowels normally. I didn't know anything could hurt so bad. I'll take my chances with the cancer pain in the future rather than take more pain meds and have this happen again."

KEY TERMS

anus	enema	laxative
bowel incontinence	fecal impaction	occult blood
bowel-training program	fecal incontinence	ostomy
cathartic	feces	paralytic ileus
colostomy	fissure	peristalsis
constipation	flatulence	stoma
defecation	flatus	stool
diarrhea	hemorrhoids	suppository
endoscopy	ileostomy	Valsalva maneuver

Expectations about bowel elimination, usual patterns of defecation, and the ease with which a person speaks about bowel problems differ widely among people. Although most people have experienced minor acute bouts of diarrhea or constipation, some people experience severe or chronic alterations in bowel elimination that affect their fluid and electrolyte balance, hydration, nutritional status, skin integrity, comfort, and self-concept. Moreover, many illnesses, diagnostic tests, medications, and surgical treatments can affect bowel elimination.

This chapter discusses the physiology of bowel elimination and the multiple factors that influence this process. A guide for assessing bowel elimination, including diagnostic studies of the gastrointestinal tract and their associated nursing responsibilities, is presented. Numerous examples of nursing diagnoses are included. In addition, included in this chapter are goals for both the nurse and the patient and nursing strategies to meet those goals. The accompanying Reflective Practice display illustrates nursing strategies addressing bowel diversions. The concluding nursing plan of care illustrates the use of specific nursing interventions to resolve bowel elimination problems.

ANATOMY AND PHYSIOLOGY

The gastrointestinal tract, also known as the alimentary tract or canal, extends from the mouth to the **anus**, the outlet of the gastrointestinal tract. The anatomy of the gastrointestinal tract is shown in Figure 37-1 (on page 1346). The stomach and small intestine are discussed briefly. The major organ involved with bowel elimination is the large intestine, which will be discussed in greater detail.

Stomach

The stomach is a hollow, J-shaped, muscular organ located in the left upper portion of the abdomen. The stomach stores food during eating, secretes digestive fluids, churns food to aid in digestion, and pushes the partially digested food, called chyme, into the small intestine. The pyloric sphincter, a muscular ring that regulates the size of the opening at the end of the stomach, controls the movement of chyme from the stomach into the small intestine.

Small Intestine

The small intestine is about 20 feet (6 m) long and about 1 inch (2.2 cm) wide. The small intestine is made up of three parts: the first is the duodenum, the middle section is the jejunum, and the distal section that connects with the large intestine is the ileum (Fig. 37-2 on page 1346). The small intestine secretes enzymes that digest proteins and carbohydrates. Digestive juices from the liver and pancreas enter the small intestine through a small opening in the duodenum. The small intestine is responsible for digestion of food and absorption of nutrients into the bloodstream.

Large Intestine

The connection between the ileum of the small intestine and the large intestine is the ileocecal, or ileocolic, valve. This valve normally prevents contents from entering the large intestine prematurely and prevents waste products from returning to the small intestine.

REFLECTIVE PRACTICE: CULTIVATING QSEN COMPETENCIES

CHALLENGE TO TECHNICAL SKILLS

Although nursing students learn the technologies in the simulation practice laboratory, it is often quite a different situation when they are asked to perform the technology for the first time independently. I found this to be true the first time that I had to perform colostomy care independently.

I met Alberta Franklin while working as a nursing extern this summer. She was a 55-year-old woman who had recently undergone abdominal surgery and creation of a sigmoid colostomy. She required a new colostomy bag, and I was asked to change the bag. Although colostomies do not require the computerized technology found in an ICU, they do require technical skills. I had practiced changing colostomy bags in the nursing skills lab and had observed nurses changing the colostomy bag in the hospital. I had even previously changed a colostomy bag while being supervised by a nurse. Although I was not completely comfortable with the situation, I agreed to change the bag. I quickly reviewed the steps in the protocol book and went into the patient's room. I measured the colostomy and then cut the bag to the appropriate size. Unfortunately, I had measured the colostomy incorrectly, and the bag was too large, so I had to leave the room and get more supplies. After a few more obstacles, I was able to adhere a properly fitting bag to the patient—but not before the patient correctly guessed that this was the first time I had performed this skill! Her ability to guess that I had never performed this skill before illustrates my technical incompetence.

Thinking Outside the Box: Possible Courses of Action

- Refuse to provide the care and ask another nurse to change the colostomy bag.
- Observe a nurse performing the care one more time.
- Check protocol and perform the care, knowing that I could call a nurse if needed.
- "Wing it" and hope that I remember what I had learned in lab.

Evaluating a Good Outcome: How Do I Define Success?

- Patient receives safe care.
- Patient's needs are met.
- Nurse demonstrates technical competency with the skill.

Personal Learning: Here's to the Future!

I think that my actions were appropriate. Although I was unsure about my technical skills regarding colostomy care, I performed the skill adequately. In addition, I reviewed the appropriate steps and I knew that I could summon the assistance of a nurse in case I needed to do so. I also made sure that I knew where the nurse was so that if I did need help, I wouldn't waste any time looking for help. Therefore, I ensured that the patient's safety would not be compromised. Although at that time I would have preferred to have another nurse perform the colostomy change, I am glad that I completed this technical skill independently. Observing another person performing a skill can be beneficial, but there comes a point when you must "spread your wings" and complete the skill on your own. Of course, this philosophy regarding spreading your wings applies only to certain technologies: It would be inappropriate to use this philosophy if it compromised patient safety. However, in instances like this one, where patient safety is not compromised and the appropriate teaching and training have been completed, I think it is appropriate to take action. If you don't, the various technologies in the hospital can become extremely intimidating and overwhelming. As a result, fear increases, which can possibly threaten a patient's safety and lead to injury.

Elizabeth Nalli, Georgetown University

REFLECTION ON QUALITY AND SAFETY COMPETENCIES

How do you think you would respond in a similar situation? Why? What does this tell you about yourself and about the adequacy of your skills for professional practice? Do you agree with the criteria that the nursing student used to evaluate a successful outcome? Are there any other criteria that would be appropriate to use? Did the nursing student meet the criteria? Why or why not? What *knowledge, skills,* and *attitudes* do you need to develop to continuously improve the quality and safety of care for patients like Ms. Franklin?

Patient-Centered Care: How could you involve the patient as a partner in coordinating her care to minimize frustration on the part of the patient and student? What interventions should the nursing student implement to provide care based on respect for the patient's preferences, values, and needs? What might you have done to prevent the numerous trips in and out of the patient's room? Did the nursing student's actions adhere to ethical and legal principles? If not, describe what principles were violated.

Teamwork and Collaboration/Quality Improvement: What communication skills do you need to improve to ensure that you function as a member of the patient-care team? What skills do you need to initiate requests for help and to obtain assistance when needed?

Safety/Evidence-Based Practice: What actions or behaviors by the nursing student might have provided clues to the patient that this was the nursing student's first independent attempt at the skill? What skills do you need to improve to ensure that patients in your care receive the best nursing care possible?

Informatics: Can you identify the essential information that must be available in Ms. Franklin's electronic health record to support safe patient care and coordination of care? What information should be documented in the electronic health record regarding the student's assessment and interventions? Can you think of other ways to respond to or approach the situation?

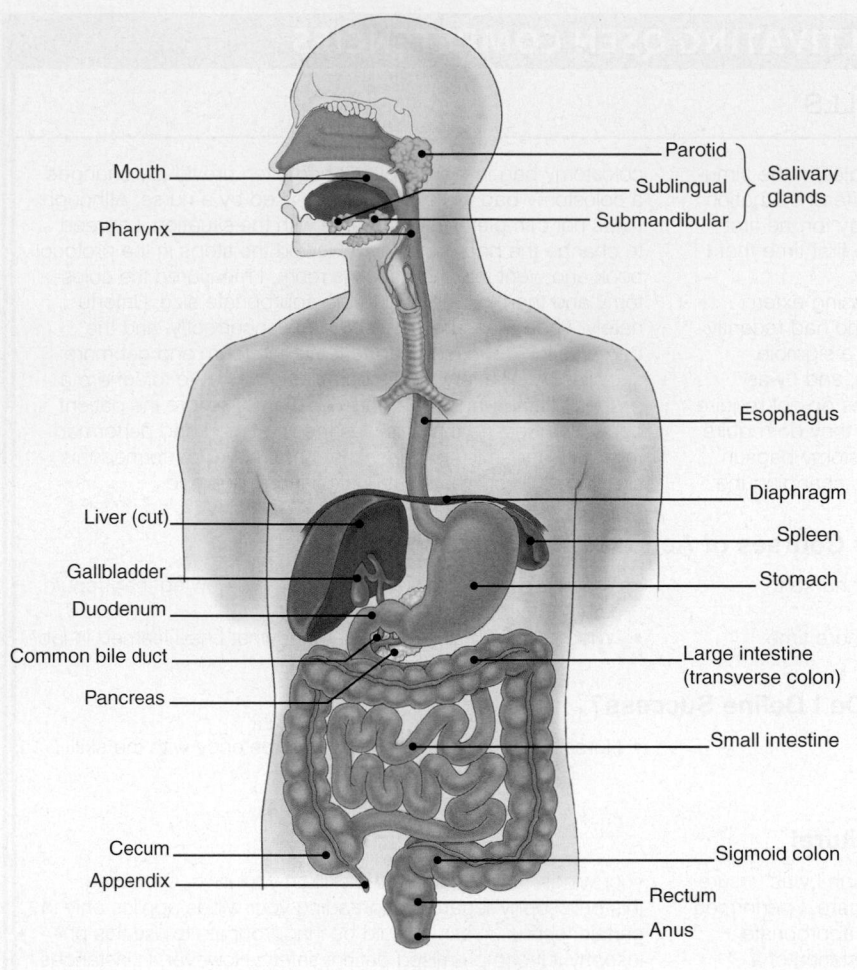

Mouth

Pharynx

Parotid

Sublingual — Salivary glands

Submandibular

Esophagus

Diaphragm

Liver (cut)

Spleen

Gallbladder

Stomach

Duodenum

Common bile duct

Pancreas

Large intestine (transverse colon)

Small intestine

Cecum

Appendix

Sigmoid colon

Rectum

Anus

FIGURE 37-1. Organs of the gastrointestinal tract.

Duodenum

Right colic (hepatic) flexure

Ascending colon

Jejunum

Ilium

Ileocecal valve

Appendix

Left colic (splenic) flexure

Transverse colon

Descending colon

Tenia coli

Sigmoid colon

Rectum

Anal canal

Anal Sphincter

Anus

FIGURE 37-2. The small and large intestines.

The large intestine, the primary organ of bowel elimination, is the lower, or distal, part of the gastrointestinal tract. The large intestine, also known as the colon, extends from the ileocecal valve to the anus. The colon in adults is about 5 feet (1.5 m) long, but variations in length are normal. Width also varies; at its narrowest point, the colon is about 1 inch (2.5 cm) wide; at its widest point, it is about 3 inches (7.5 cm). The diameter of the colon decreases from the cecum to the anus (see Fig. 37-2).

From the cecum, the first part of the large intestine, the digestive contents enter the colon, which consists of several segments. The ascending colon extends from the cecum upward toward the liver, where it turns to cross the abdomen. This turn is called the hepatic flexure. Upon turning, this portion of the colon becomes the transverse colon, crossing the abdomen from right to left. The colon then turns at the splenic flexure to become the descending colon. The descending colon passes down the left side of the body to the sigmoid, or pelvic, colon.

The sigmoid colon contains **feces**, solid waste products that have reached the distal end of the colon and are ready for excretion. Once excreted, feces are called **stool**. The sigmoid colon empties into the rectum, the last part of the large intestine. The rectum is about 12 cm (5 inches) long, 2.5 cm (1 inch) of which is the anal canal. In the rectum, three transverse folds of tissue are present that may help to hold the fecal material in the rectum temporarily. Vertical folds also are present, each of which contains an artery and a vein. If the veins become abnormally distended, **hemorrhoids** occur.

The rectum is empty except immediately before and during **defecation** (the process of bowel elimination; a bowel movement). Feces are excreted from the rectum through the anal canal, which is approximately 2.5 to 3.8 cm (1–1.5 inches) long, and out an opening called the anus.

Functions of the large intestine include the absorption of water, the formation of feces, and the expulsion of feces from the body. Bacteria that reside in the large intestine act on food residue while it makes its way through the large intestine. Bacterial action produces vitamin K and some of the B-complex vitamins. The products of digestion, chyme, move from the small intestine, passing through the ileocecal valve, and enter the cecum. Approximately 1,500 mL of chyme enters the large intestine daily. Its contents are liquid or watery. While passing through the large intestine, most water is absorbed. About 800 to 1,000 mL of liquid is absorbed daily by the intestinal tract, allowing for the formed, semisolid consistency of the normal stool. When absorption does not occur properly, such as when the waste products pass through the large intestine rapidly, the stool is soft and watery. Conversely, if the stool remains in the large intestine too long, or if too much water is absorbed, the stool becomes dry and hard.

 RECALL Alberta Franklin, the woman who had surgery that resulted in the creation of a sigmoid colostomy. Knowledge of normal gastrointestinal function would help the nurse in developing a

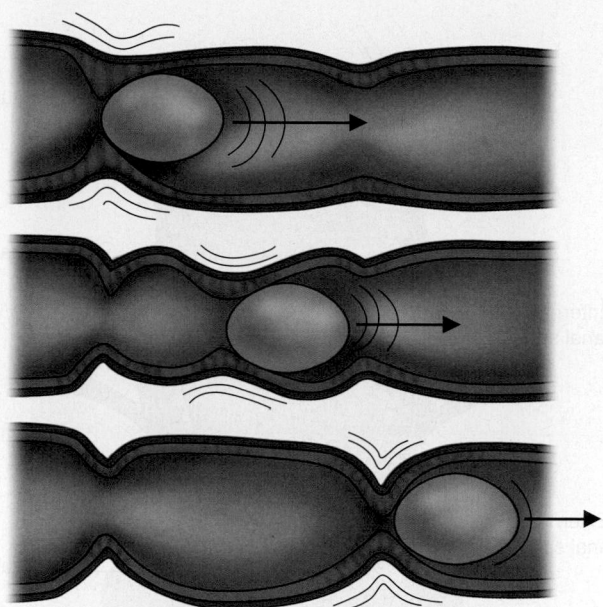

FIGURE 37-3. Peristaltic movements in the intestine.

teaching plan for this patient about her ostomy and what to expect in relation to bowel function. ●

Nervous System Control

The autonomic nervous system innervates the muscles of the colon. The parasympathetic nervous system stimulates movement, while the sympathetic system inhibits movement. Contractions of the circular and longitudinal muscles of the intestine, **peristalsis**, occur every 3 to 12 minutes, moving waste products along the length of the intestine continuously (Fig. 37-3). Mass peristaltic sweeps occur one to four times each 24-hour period in most people, propelling the fecal mass forward. This movement is different from the frequent peristaltic rushes that occur in the small intestine. Mass peristalsis often occurs after food has been ingested, accounting for the urge to defecate that often occurs after meals. Timing nursing interventions to evacuate bowel contents with this natural urge to defecate is helpful. One-third to one-half of ingested food waste is normally excreted in the stool within 24 hours, and the remainder within the next 24 to 48 hours.

After passing through the sigmoid colon, the waste products enter the rectum, where they are stopped from exiting by the anal sphincters (Fig. 37-4 on page 1348). The internal sphincter in the anal canal and the external sphincter at the anus control the discharge of feces and **flatus** (intestinal gas). The internal sphincter consists of involuntary smooth muscle tissue that is innervated by the autonomic nervous system. Motor impulses are carried by the sympathetic system (thoracolumbar) and inhibitory impulses by the parasympathetic system (craniosacral). These two divisions of the autonomic nervous system function antagonistically in a dynamic equilibrium. The external sphincter at the anus has striated muscle tissue and is under voluntary control. The levator ani muscle reinforces the action of the external sphincter and is controlled voluntarily.

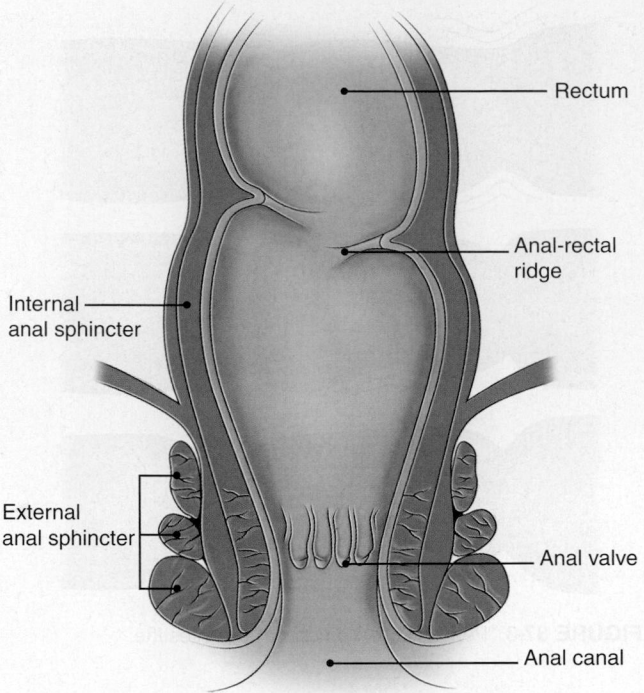

FIGURE 37-4. Interior view of the rectum and anal canal.

Labels (clockwise): Rectum · Anal-rectal ridge · Anal valve · Anal canal · External anal sphincter · Internal anal sphincter

Defecation

Defecation refers to the emptying of the large intestine. Two centers govern the reflex to defecate, one in the medulla and a subsidiary one in the spinal cord. When parasympathetic stimulation occurs, the internal anal sphincter relaxes and the colon contracts, allowing the fecal mass to enter the rectum.

The rectum becomes distended by the fecal mass, the primary stimulus for the defecation reflex. Rectal distention leads to an increase in intrarectal pressure, causing the muscles to stretch and thereby stimulating the defecation reflex and subsequently the urge to eliminate.

The external anal sphincter, which is under voluntary control, is constricted or relaxed at will. If the urge to defecate is ignored, defecation often can be delayed voluntarily. During the act of defecation, several additional muscles aid in the process. Voluntary contraction of the muscles of the abdominal wall by holding one's breath, contracting the diaphragm, and closing the glottis increases intra-abdominal pressure up to four or five times the normal pressure, which helps expel feces. Simultaneously, the muscles on the pelvic floor contract and aid in expulsion of the fecal mass. Defecation is eased by flexing the thigh muscles, which increases abdominal pressure, and by the sitting position, which increases downward pressure on the rectum.

When a person bears down to defecate, the increased pressures in the abdominal and thoracic cavities result in a decreased blood flow to the atria and ventricles, thus temporarily lowering cardiac output. Once bearing down ceases, the pressure is lessened, and a larger than normal amount of blood returns to the heart. This act may dangerously elevate the blood pressure in a person with hypertension (Hinkle & Cheever, 2014). Therefore, this technique of bearing down,

termed the **Valsalva maneuver**, may be contraindicated in people with cardiovascular problems and other illnesses.

The act of defecation is usually painless. If the bowels move at regular intervals and the stools are formed and soft, functional problems involving frequency of elimination seldom occur. Many people become concerned if they do not have a daily bowel movement. However, normal elimination patterns can vary widely among people. Although many adults pass one stool each day, other healthy people have more frequent or less frequent bowel movements. Some people have a bowel movement two or three times a week; others, two or three times a day.

FACTORS AFFECTING BOWEL ELIMINATION

Various factors can affect bowel elimination. Interference with the normal functioning of elimination from the intestines can occur in health as well as during illness. Elimination can be affected by a person's developmental stage, daily patterns, the amount and quality of fluid or food intake, the level of activity, lifestyle, emotional states, pathologic processes, medications, and procedures, such as diagnostic tests and surgery.

Developmental Considerations

Age affects what a person eats and the body's ability to digest nutrients and eliminate wastes. The stools of an infant are markedly different from those of an older person. Because patients are often reluctant to discuss their bowel habits and stool characteristics, nurses need to be familiar with bowel concerns pertinent to each developmental group.

Infant

The stool characteristics depend on whether the infant is being fed breast milk or formula. Breast milk is easier for the infant's intestines to break down and absorb. Breastfed babies have more frequent stools; the stools are yellow to golden and loose, and usually have little odor. The stools of formula-fed infants vary from yellow to brown, are paste-like in consistency, and have a stronger odor because of the decomposition of protein. The stools of both breastfed and formula-fed infants may have curds and mucus. Infants have no voluntary control over bowel elimination.

The number of stools infants pass varies greatly. For example, breastfed infants can pass from 2 to 10 stools daily, whereas bottle-fed infants typically pass 1 or 2 stools daily. At the age of 1 year, all infants commonly pass one or two stools a day. Parents may mistakenly interpret the infant's liquid stool as **diarrhea** (passage of more than three loose stools a day). Loose stools may be related to overfeeding. Diarrhea is an increase in frequency, and a change in consistency, of stools. True diarrhea requires evaluation. Some children have bowel movements only once every 2 to 3 days. Teach parents that as long as the stools are soft, the child is not constipated. If **constipation** (dry, hard stool; persistently difficult passage of stool; and/or the incomplete

FOCUS ON THE OLDER ADULT

NURSING STRATEGIES TO ADDRESS AGE-RELATED CHANGES AFFECTING BOWEL ELIMINATION

Age-related Changes	Nursing Strategies
Slowing of gastrointestinal motility with increased stomach-emptying time	• Encourage small, frequent meals. • Discourage heavy activity after eating. • Encourage a high-fiber, low-fat diet. • Encourage adequate fluid intake. • Discourage regular use of laxatives. • Evaluate medication regimen for possible adverse effects.
Decreased muscle tone/incontinence	• Provide easy access to the bathroom. • Use assistive devices when necessary (raised toilet seat, grab bars, walker). • Ensure safety when ambulating (e.g., skid-proof slippers). • Encourage participation in a bowel-retraining program.
Weakening of intestinal walls with greater incidence of diverticulitis	• Encourage a high-fiber diet and adequate fluid intake. • Teach patients not to ignore the urge to have a bowel movement. • Encourage regular exercise.

passage of stool) occurs, dietary manipulation is the initial treatment. The consistent use of suppositories and laxatives is discouraged. Infants with persistent constipation require evaluation for structural defects.

Toddler

Between the ages of 18 and 24 months, the nerve fibers innervating the internal and external anal sphincters become fully developed, at which point voluntary control of defecation becomes possible. Voluntary defecation requires intact muscular, sensory, and nervous structures. Successful bowel training also includes awareness by the toddler of the need to defecate, the ability to communicate this need, the wish to please the significant person involved in bowel training, and praise and reinforcement for the toddler's successful behavior. Daytime bowel control is normally attained by 30 months of age, but the age varies with each child.

Help parents to understand that physiologic maturity is the first priority for successful bowel training. Discourage the use of punishment or shame for a lack of readiness to become toilet-trained or for elimination accidents. Toddlers who are toilet-trained often regress and experience soiling when hospitalized; scolding or acting disgusted only reinforces this behavior. Use a constructive approach by seeking the underlying cause.

School-Aged Child, Adolescent, and Adult

From childhood into adulthood, defecation patterns vary in quantity, frequency, and rhythmicity. Many people worry needlessly about normal stool characteristics or bowel habits; others may not understand the significance of changes in bowel habits. Emphasize that the use of over-the-counter laxatives and enemas can have serious consequences and that any problems prompting such use need to be evaluated.

Older Adult

Constipation is often a chronic problem for older adults. Diarrhea, **fecal impaction** (prolonged retention or an accumulation of fecal material that forms a hardened mass in the rectum), or **fecal incontinence** (involuntary or inappropriate passing of stool or flatus) can also result from physiologic or lifestyle changes. See the accompanying Focus on the Older Adult box above and PICO in Practice box on page 1350.

Daily Patterns

Most people have individual patterns of bowel elimination involving frequency, timing considerations, position, and place. Changes in any of these patterns may upset a person's routine and lead to constipation. For example, many people defecate after breakfast, when the gastrocolic and duodenocolic reflexes cause mass propulsive movements in the large intestine. If this urge to defecate is ignored because the person finds the time or place inconvenient, the feces remain in the rectum until the defecation reflex is initiated again. Meanwhile, water continues to be absorbed from the unexpelled feces, which makes the stool dry, hard, and painful to pass.

Most people assume the squatting or slightly forward-sitting position with the thighs flexed. In either position, increased pressure is placed on the abdomen, as well as downward pressure on the rectum; both facilitate defecation. Obtaining the same results when seated on a bedpan is difficult. Embarrassment may further inhibit defecation. In addition, for most people, defecation is a private affair experienced easily only in the comfort of one's own bathroom. Defecation may be difficult in a shared hospital room with only a curtain for privacy.

Food and Fluid

Both the type and the amount of foods eaten and the amount of fluids ingested affect elimination. A high-fiber diet and a daily fluid intake of 2,000 to 3,000 mL facilitate bowel

PICO IN PRACTICE

ASKING CLINICAL QUESTIONS

Scenario: You are the nurse manager of an assisted-living facility. You know all of the 50 older adult residents of this facility quite well. Knowing that you are a nurse, they are comfortable asking your advice when they experience various physical ailments. Several of them have recently voiced complaints of constipation and ask you to recommend an over-the-counter laxative. You wonder what type of laxative might be best for this population of patients.

- POPULATION: Older adult residents of an assisted-living facility
- INTERVENTION: Over-the-counter laxative
- COMPARISON: None
- OUTCOME: Relief of constipation

PICO Question: What type of over-the-counter laxative is best at providing relief of constipation among older adult residents of an assisted-living facility?

Finding: From the Joanna Briggs Institute: Chen, Z. (2013). Constipation management. *Evidence Summary.*

This evidence-based summary recommends that the first choice of laxative for ambulatory older adults with constipation should be a bulking agent, such as psyllium (Metamucil); an osmotic agent such as magnesium hydroxide (Milk of Magnesia) or stimulant agent such as docusate (Correctol) should be recommended as first choice for older adults on bedrest.

Level of Evidence: Level I

Recommendation: You recommend that the older adult residents who complain of constipation and wish to use a laxative should preferentially try a bulking agent first, such as psyllium (Metamucil).

elimination. High-fiber foods, such as whole grains and bran, dried peas and beans, and fresh fruits and vegetables, increase the bulk in fecal material. Bulkier feces increase pressure on the intestinal wall, which serves as a stimulus for peristalsis. As a result, feces move more quickly through the colon, allowing less time for water to be reabsorbed. Subsequently, the stool is soft and easy to pass. When the stool moves quickly through the colon there is also less time for toxins to be absorbed from feces by the colon. Many believe that these toxins play an important role in promoting the development of colon cancer. Therefore, preventing their absorption by the colon is a key part of colon cancer prevention.

People digest and tolerate foods differently. This variation is determined in part by one's culture. For example, travelers to a foreign country who eat native foods or drink the water may suffer severe indigestion and elimination problems, such as diarrhea.

Food intolerance may alter bowel elimination, possibly resulting in diarrhea, gaseous distention, and cramping. For example, people who lack the enzyme lactase, which helps to break down the simple sugar lactose found in milk and milk products, cannot digest milk; this is called lactose intolerance. These people often experience excessive intestinal gas and diarrhea when they ingest milk.

Certain foods have been associated with specific effects on bowel elimination. These include:

- Constipating foods: processed cheese, lean meat, eggs, pasta
- Foods with laxative effect: certain fruits and vegetables (e.g., prunes), bran, chocolate, spicy foods, alcohol, coffee
- Gas-producing foods: onions, cabbage, beans, cauliflower

Activity and Muscle Tone

Regular exercise improves gastrointestinal motility and muscle tone, whereas inactivity decreases both. Adequate tone in the abdominal muscles, the diaphragm, and the perineal muscles is essential for ease of defecation. Patients on prolonged bedrest or those with decreased mobility are prime candidates for constipation.

Lifestyle

Many individual, family, and sociocultural variables influence a person's usual elimination habits. The long-term effects of bowel training may result in a person's (1) acceptance of bowel elimination as a normal life process, (2) preoccupation with bowel elimination, or (3) feeling that bowel elimination is a "dirty" process. Rituals associated with bowel elimination, cleanliness considerations, the language used to talk about bowel elimination or reluctance to discuss it, individual responses to involuntary passage of flatus (gas), and so on, vary widely among people. A person's daily schedule, occupation, and leisure activities may contribute to a habit of defecating at regular times or to an irregular pattern. Nurses who role model good health behaviors are more effective teachers. Use the Promoting Health 37-1 display for yourself before using it with others.

Psychological Variables

Psychological stress affects the body in many ways. In some people, anxiety seems to have a direct effect on gastrointestinal motility, and diarrhea accompanies periods of high anxiety. In the fight-or-flight response, when the body mobilizes itself for intense action, blood is shunted away from the stomach and intestines, resulting in a slowing of gastrointestinal motility. People who chronically worry and those with certain personality types who tend to hold onto problems and negative feelings may experience frequent constipation.

Pathologic Conditions

Numerous pathologic processes may change a person's usual bowel elimination habits. Changes in stool characteristics or frequency may be one of the first clinical manifestations of a disease; their evaluation may lead to the diagnosis of the disease. For example, when a patient reports stool has become narrower or ribbon-like, a tumor may be obstructing normal stool passage through the colon. The nurse should report this finding to the physician. Similarly, a parent's report that a child's stools are frequent, bulky, greasy, and foul smelling suggests cystic fibrosis. This requires further evaluation, especially if other clinical manifestations are present.

Diarrhea may result from pathologic conditions such as diverticulitis (inflammation of a diverticulum from obstruction [by fecal matter], resulting in abscess formation), infection, malabsorption syndromes (the inability of the digestive system to absorb one or more of the major vitamins, minerals, or nutrients), neoplastic diseases (tumors), diabetic neuropathy (damage to nerve cells), hyperthyroidism, and uremia (retention of urea in the blood).

Constipation may be the result of conditions such as diseases within the colon or rectum and injury to, or degeneration of, the spinal cord and megacolon (extremely dilated colon). Changes in color, contents, odor, and appearance of stool may be related to conditions that traumatize the stomach or intestines, or that interfere with normal digestion. Thus, stool assessment is an important diagnostic task for the nurse.

Outbreaks of food poisoning can result in severe gastrointestinal symptoms, including diarrhea. For example, infections caused by certain types of *Escherichia coli*, particularly dangerous for young children (under 10 years of age) and older adults, can progress quickly to life-threatening hematologic and renal complications (Grossman & Porth, 2014).

Severe abdominal cramping followed by watery or bloody diarrhea may signal a microbial infection, which can be confirmed by a stool sample. Supportive treatment, careful monitoring, and attentive nursing care are essential.

Intestinal obstruction occurs when blockage prevents the normal flow of intestinal contents through the intestinal tract (Hinkle & Cheever, 2014). Mechanical obstructions result from pressure on the intestinal walls. Examples of causes of mechanical obstruction include tumors, stenosis, adhesions, hernias, and strictures. Functional obstructions result from an inability of the intestinal musculature to move the contents through the bowel. Examples of causes of functional obstruction include muscular dystrophy, diabetes mellitus, Parkinson disease, and manipulation of the bowel during surgery. The effects of surgery are further detailed later in the chapter.

Medications

Medications are available that can promote peristalsis (**cathartics** and **laxatives**) or inhibit peristalsis (antidiarrheal medications). These are discussed later in the chapter.

Other types of medications may affect bowel elimination and stool characteristics. Opioids, antacids containing aluminum, iron sulfate, and anticholinergic medications decrease gastrointestinal motility, with the potential to cause constipation.

 REMEMBER Leroy Cobbs, the patient described at the beginning of the chapter who developed fecal impaction resulting from the narcotic analgesics he was using to control his cancer pain. Had the possible adverse effects of narcotics for pain control been addressed in the patient's medication teaching plan when the drug was first prescribed, the risk for fecal impaction could have been reduced. Additionally, the teaching plan could have addressed measures to counteract the effects of the medication. ●

Many medications can cause diarrhea as a side effect. For example, diarrhea is a potential adverse effect of treatment with amoxicillin clavulanate (Augmentin), an antibiotic. In this situation, using antidiarrheal drugs is not recommended because its use would prolong the exposure of the intestinal mucosa to the irritating effect of the antibiotic. Medications with magnesium, such as over-the-counter antacids, can cause diarrhea. If diarrhea is severe enough, the drug may need to be discontinued.

Medications may also influence the appearance of the stool, for a variety of reasons. Any drug with the potential to cause gastrointestinal bleeding (e.g., anticoagulants, aspirin products) may cause the stool to appear pink to red to black. Iron salts result in a black stool from the oxidation of iron. Antacids may cause a white discoloration or speckling in the stool. Antibiotics may cause a green-gray color related to impaired digestion.

Because antibiotics are used so extensively in the health care setting, many patients are at risk for infection with *Clostridium difficile* (Hinkle & Cheever, 2014), a hospital-acquired infection. When a patient is receiving treatment with broad-spectrum antibiotics, there is a disruption in the normal intestinal flora, allowing microorganism to flourish within the intestine. *C. difficile* causes intestinal mucosal damage and inflammation, resulting in diarrhea and abdominal cramping. *C. difficile* spores are shed in feces and are relatively resistant to disinfectants. These microorganisms can be spread on the hands of health care providers after contact with equipment or surfaces contaminated with the microorganism. Institute contact precautions for infected patients. Consider environmental surfaces and items close to the patient, such as the side rails and overbed table, to be contaminated. Intensified environmental cleaning is required (Hinkle & Cheever, 2014; Centers for Disease Control and Prevention [CDC], 2010).

Diagnostic Studies

Diagnostic studies may affect a patient's usual bowel elimination pattern. For example, patients may need to fast for diagnostic studies. The ingestion of barium during diagnostic procedures, such as a barium enema, may result in constipation or impaction if it is not completely eliminated after the procedure. Additionally, the stress of hospitalization and waiting for the results of studies, combined with changes in food intake, can severely alter a patient's usual elimination patterns. The cathartics or enemas used for bowel cleansing before certain diagnostic studies of the gastrointestinal tract can interfere with the normal timing of a patient's bowel movements. Refer to Table 37-2 on page 1362 for additional information related to laxatives.

Surgery and Anesthesia

Abdominal incisions and direct manipulation of the bowel during abdominal surgery inhibit peristalsis, causing a con-

dition termed **paralytic ileus** (postoperative ileus). This temporary stoppage of peristalsis normally lasts 3 to 5 days. During this time, food and oral fluids are usually withheld. Many times, the patient is receiving narcotics for pain relief, which can exacerbate the situation. If this condition persists, distention and symptoms of acute obstruction may occur, possibly resulting in the need for surgical intervention. Inhaled general anesthetic agents also inhibit peristalsis by blocking the parasympathetic impulses to the intestinal musculature. However, local and regional anesthetics have little effect on peristalsis.

THE NURSING PROCESS FOR BOWEL ELIMINATION

Assessing

Assessment of the gastrointestinal tract and bowel elimination includes pertinent patient history, physical assessment, and diagnostic studies.

Nursing History

Because many patients are reluctant to initiate a conversation about their bowel status, include pertinent bowel elimination questions in each comprehensive nursing history. The accompanying Focused Assessment Guide 37-1 provides some appropriate questions for health history assessment related to bowel elimination.

If the patient is experiencing any disturbance in bowel elimination, conduct a more detailed assessment, directing attention to the factors described earlier that may influence bowel elimination.

Patients who are critically ill or who have impaired cognition may be incapable of reporting their bowel status accurately. Record the patient's daily bowel status to look for clues to impending problems. While making daily rounds, ask patients who can give reliable answers when they moved their bowels last and chart the response. If the patient cannot provide this information, the nurse or ancillary staff who assists the patient with bowel elimination records any bowel movement.

Physical Assessment

Examination of the abdomen is discussed in Chapter 25. Refer to this chapter for details and additional information related to the assessment of the gastrointestinal system. An overview of examination techniques that may be helpful when assessing the functioning of the gastrointestinal tract is described here.

ABDOMEN

The sequence for abdominal assessment proceeds from inspection, auscultation, and percussion to palpation. Inspection and auscultation are performed before palpation because palpation may disturb normal peristalsis and bowel motility. Advanced practice professionals perform percussion and deep palpation of the abdomen. Refer

FOCUSED ASSESSMENT GUIDE 37-1

BOWEL ELIMINATION

Factors to Assess	Questions and Approaches
Usual patterns of bowel elimination	How often do you move your bowels? Any special time of the day? What does your stool look like: • Frequency • Time of day • Description of usual stool characteristics (amount, consistency, shape, color, odor)
Aids to elimination	Do you use anything to help move your bowels? • Natural aids (liquids, food) • Pharmacologic aids (laxatives) • Enemas
Recent changes in bowel elimination	Have you noticed any changes in your stool recently? Have you noticed any blood in your stool? (May need to ask patient about color blindness.) Have you noted a difference in the appearance of your stool (narrowing, presence of mucus)?
Problems with bowel elimination	Are your bowels causing you any problem now? • Nature of disturbance • Onset and frequency • Causes (*physical:* food and fluid intake, exercise status, history of surgery or illnesses influencing gastrointestinal tract; psychosocial; medicine related) • Severity • Symptoms • Interventions attempted and results
Presence of artificial orifices (normal routine, history of problems)	What is your usual routine with your colostomy or ileostomy? Do you have any problems with it?

to a health assessment text for details. Place the patient comfortably in the supine position with the abdomen exposed, the chest and pubic area draped, and the knees slightly flexed. Encourage the patient to urinate prior to the examination so that the bladder is empty.

Inspection. First, observe the contour of the abdomen, noting any masses, scars, or areas of distention. Peristalsis is usually not visible except in very thin patients. When an intestinal obstruction is present, the visible waves of peristalsis to the point of the obstruction may be observed on the abdomen. Observe the contour of the abdomen. Significant findings may include the presence of distention (inflation) or protrusion (projection).

Auscultation. Using the diaphragm of a warmed stethoscope, listen for bowel sounds in all abdominal quadrants, using a systematic, clockwise approach. If the patient has a nasogastric tube in place, disconnect it from suction during this assessment to allow for accurate interpretation of sounds. Keep in mind that the timing of the patient's most recent meal or a full bladder may also affect the examination.

Note the frequency and character of bowel sounds, intermittent audible clicks and gurgles produced by the movement of air and flatus in the gastrointestinal tract.

They are usually high-pitched, gurgling, and soft, indicating bowel motility and peristalsis. Their frequency may range from 5 to 30 bowel sounds per minute, depending on the rate of peristalsis (Jensen, 2011). Significant findings include hypoactive bowel sounds, a diminished rate of sounds; hyperactive bowel sounds, intense with increased frequency; and absent or infrequent bowel sounds. Hypoactive bowel sounds indicate diminished bowel motility, commonly caused by abdominal surgery or late bowel obstruction. Hyperactive bowel sounds indicate increased bowel motility, commonly caused by diarrhea, gastroenteritis, or early bowel obstruction. Decreased or absent bowel sounds, evidenced only after listening for 5 minutes (Jensen), signify the absence of bowel motility, commonly associated with peritonitis, paralytic ileus, and/or prolonged immobility. Describe bowel sounds as audible, hyperactive, hypoactive, or inaudible.

Palpation. Next, perform light palpation in each quadrant. Watch the patient's face for nonverbal signs of pain during palpation. Palpate each quadrant in a systematic manner, noting muscular resistance, tenderness, enlargement of the organs, or masses. If the patient complains of abdominal pain, palpate the area of pain last. If the patient's abdomen is distended, note the presence of firmness or tautness.

ANUS AND RECTUM

Perform a superficial examination each time you wash a patient's anal area or assist with bowel evacuation. The nurse's skill level determines the extent of further rectal examination. Physicians or advanced practiced nurses primarily conduct physical assessments of the rectum and anus. Refer to a health assessment text for details.

Inspection is used to assess the anal area, which normally has increased pigmentation and some hair growth.

Assess for lesions, ulcers, **fissures** (linear break on the margin of the anus), inflammation, and external hemorrhoids (dilated veins appearing as reddened protrusions). Ask the patient to bear down as though having a bowel movement. Assess for the appearance of internal hemorrhoids or fissures. Normally, there is no protrusion of tissue. Observe for a fecal mass, which may distend the anus. Inspect the perineal area for areas of skin irritation or breakdown secondary to diarrhea or fecal incontinence.

Table 37-1 THE STOOL: NORMAL CHARACTERISTICS AND SPECIAL CONSIDERATIONS FOR OBSERVATION

CHARACTERISTIC	NORMAL FINDING	SPECIAL CONSIDERATIONS FOR OBSERVATION
Volume	Variable	The volume of the stool depends on the amount the person eats and the nature of the diet. For example, a diet high in roughage produces more feces than a soft, bland diet. Consistently large diarrheal stools suggest a disorder in the small bowel or proximal colon; small, frequent stools with urgency to pass them suggest a disorder of the left colon or rectum.
Color	Infant: Yellow to brown Adult: Brown	The brown color of the stool is due to stercobilin, a bile pigment derivative. The rapid rate of peristalsis in the breast-fed infant causes the stool to be yellow. The color of the stool is influenced by diet. For example, the stool will be almost black if the person eats red meat and dark green vegetables, such as spinach. The stool will be light brown if the diet is high in milk and milk products and low in meat. The absence of bile may cause the stool to appear white or clay-colored. Certain drugs influence the color of the stool. For example, iron salts cause the stool to be black. Antacids cause it to be whitish. Bleeding high in the intestinal tract causes a stool to be black owing to the digestion of the blood. Bleeding low in the intestinal tract results in fresh blood in the stool. The stool darkens with standing.
Odor	Pungent; may be affected by foods ingested	The characteristic odor of the stool is due to indole and skatole, caused by putrefaction and fermentation in the lower intestinal tract. The odor of the stool is influenced by its pH value, which normally is neutral or slightly alkaline. Excessive putrefaction causes a strong odor. The presence of blood in the stool causes a unique odor.
Consistency	Soft, semisolid, and formed	The consistency of the stool is influenced by fluid and food intake and gastric motility. The less time stool spends in the intestine (or the shorter the intestine), the more liquid the stool. Many pathologic conditions influence consistency.
Shape	Formed stool is usually about 1 inch (2.5 cm) in diameter and has the tubular shape of the colon, but may be larger or smaller, depending on the condition of the colon.	A gastrointestinal obstruction may result in a narrow, pencil-shaped stool. Rapid peristalsis thins the stool. Increased time spent in the large intestine may result in a hard, marble-like fecal mass.
Constituents	Waste residues of digestion: bile, intestinal secretions, shed epithelial cells, bacteria, and inorganic material (chiefly calcium and phosphates); seeds, meat fibers, and fat may be present in small amounts	Internal bleeding, infection, inflammation, and other pathologic conditions may result in abnormal constituents. These include blood, pus, excessive fat, parasites, ova, and mucus. Foreign bodies also may be found in the stool.

Stool Characteristics

Nurses are responsible for observing and recording information about the patient's stool. Table 37-1 describes the characteristics of a normal stool, along with special considerations used when observing a stool. Report and record anything unusual, including the passage of little or no gas or unusual amounts of gas.

Note and record, usually on the patient's bedside flow sheet, the frequency, amount, and characteristics of the patient's bowel movements. Describe any additional unusual observations, such as lightheadedness or straining, on the patient's medical record. When assistive personnel or the patient assumes this responsibility, check with the patient at regular intervals to see that the recording is accurate.

Ideally, populations at high risk for bowel elimination problems are identified before problems occur, and such problems are prevented or minimized through vigilant nursing care. Be aware of the clinical manifestations of colon cancer because early detection significantly improves survival. Refer to Box 37-1, Warning Signs of Colon Cancer.

Diagnostic Studies

The nurse is often responsible for caring for patients with elimination problems who are undergoing diagnostic testing. Specific guidelines for the nurse's role in stool collection and direct and indirect visualization studies follow.

STOOL COLLECTION

The nurse is responsible for obtaining the specimen according to facility procedure, labeling the specimen, and ensuring that the specimen is transported to the laboratory in a timely manner. The institution's policy and procedure manual or laboratory manual identifies specific information about the amount of stool needed, the time frame during which stool is to be collected, and the type of specimen container to use.

Use of medical aseptic techniques is imperative. Always wear disposable gloves when any contact or handling of a stool specimen is likely. Hand hygiene before and after glove use is essential. Also, take care not to contaminate the outside of the specimen container with stool. Package, label, and transport specimens according to facility policy to ensure that no leakage of the specimen occurs. Patients may need specific instructions about

collecting a stool specimen. These instructions may include the following:

- Void first, because the laboratory study may be inaccurate if the stool contains urine.
- Defecate into the required container, such as clean or sterile bedpan or the bedside commode (depending on the specimen required), rather than the toilet, because the water in the toilet bowl may affect the analysis results.
- Do not place toilet tissue in the bedpan or specimen container because contents in the paper may influence laboratory results.
- Notify the nurse when the specimen is available, so that it may be collected and transported to the laboratory as required.

When placing a specimen in a laboratory container, put on gloves and use two clean tongue blades. Usually, 1 inch (2.5 cm) of formed stool or 15 to 30 mL of liquid stool is sufficient. If portions of the stool include visible blood, mucus, or pus, include these with the specimen. Also, be sure that the specimen is free of any barium or enema solution. Because a fresh specimen produces the most accurate results, send the specimen to the laboratory immediately. If this is not possible, refrigerate it unless contraindicated.

Stool Culture. Culture of stool is indicated when there is suspected infection from bacteria, virus, fungi, or parasites. Obtain stool cultures before initiation of anti-infective therapy. If antibiotic or antifungal therapy has already begun, identify the specific medication in the laboratory request (Jessee, 2010).

Occult Blood. **Occult blood** in the stool (blood that is hidden in the specimen or cannot be seen on gross examination) can be detected with screening tests. Certain conditions, such as ulcer disease, inflammatory bowel disorders, and colon cancer, place the patient at high risk for intestinal bleeding. The color of the stool may reflect the source of the bleeding. Generally, black stools indicate upper gastrointestinal bleeding, such as from a peptic ulcer, due to a reaction between hemoglobin and gastric acid. Lower gastrointestinal bleeding, such as from hemorrhoids or a polyp, may produce bright-red blood in the stool. Certain foods and medications can also cause a black or reddish stool.

To test the stool for blood, use a commercial product according to the manufacturer's directions. The Hematest and guaiac test are chemical tests commonly used to determine occult blood in the stool. These simple tests use reagent substances to detect the enzyme peroxidase in the hemoglobin molecule. Nurses may perform tests for occult blood in the stool at the bedside within an institution or outpatient setting, or by patients at home, allowing for low-cost inpatient and outpatient screening (Jesse, 2010). More commonly, the sample is sent to a medical laboratory for processing.

BOX 37-1   WARNING SIGNS OF COLON CANCER

- Change in the bowel elimination pattern
- Blood in the stools
- Rectal or abdominal pain
- Change in the character of the stool
- Sensation of incomplete emptying after bowel movement

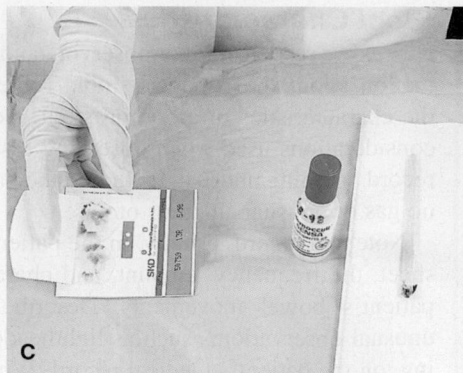

A   B   C

FIGURE 37-5. Testing a stool specimen for occult blood. (**A**) Applying a stool specimen to the test paper. (**B**) Adding developing solution to the back side of the paper according to directions. (**C**) Blue coloration indicating positive results. *(Photos by B. Proud.)*

Ingestion of certain foods and medications before the specimen collection can result in *false-positive* results. Foods that may cause a false-positive result include red meat, animal liver and kidneys, salmon, tuna, mackerel and sardines, tomatoes, cauliflower, horseradish, turnips, melon, bananas, and soybeans. Certain medications, such as a salicylate intake of more than 325 mg daily, steroids, and iron preparations, also may lead to false-positive readings (Leeuwen, Poelhuis-Leth, & Bladh, 2011). The ingestion of vitamin C can produce *false-negative* results even if bleeding is present. The following are recommendations for the patient preparing for a fecal occult blood test:

- Before stool testing, avoid the foods (for 4 days) and drugs (for 7 days) that may alter test results. Do not use laxatives, enemas, or suppositories for 3 days before testing.
- Postpone the test until 3 days after her period has ended if a woman is menstruating.
- Postpone the test if hematuria or bleeding hemorrhoids are present.
- Postpone the test if the patient has had a recent nose or throat bleed.
- Caution a person who is color-blind to the color blue not to attempt to interpret the test results.

In clinical settings, these restrictions are usually not practical. It is important to note the presence of any of the aforementioned conditions in the clinical setting. Guidelines for Nursing Care 37-1 gives additional nursing considerations for fecal occult blood testing. Figure 37-5 demonstrates the procedure for a Hemoccult test.

Timed Specimens. Consider the first stool passed by the patient as the start of the collection period. Depending on the test, it may require saving the entire stool passed or only a sample. Collect the required volume of every stool passed within the designated period. Follow laboratory instructions for sending stools to the laboratory.

Specimens for Pinworms. Adult pinworms, parasitic intestinal worms, live in the cecum. Pinworms migrate to the anal area during the night to deposit eggs and retreat into the anal canal during the day. The most common symptom of a pinworm infection is perianal itching. Collect this specimen in the morning, immediately after the patient awakens and before the patient urinates, has a bowel movement, or a bath. Use clear cellophane tape to collect a specimen for pinworms; frosted tape makes examination difficult. Apply gloves and press the tape against the anal opening, remove it immediately, and then place it on a slide. Pinworm eggs can usually be

GUIDELINES FOR NURSING CARE 37-1

TESTING FOR FECAL OCCULT BLOOD

- Instruct the patient about food and drug restrictions for at least 4 days before the test, if applicable.
- Review manufacturer's directions for collecting the specimen. Equipment may include a specimen card, collection tissues, or test paper.
- Avoid mixing the specimen with urine or water.
- Inform the patient that multiple or serial specimens are usually collected from different bowel movements to verify results.
- Collect the amount recommended for the particular test (usually only a small amount is required).

- Wear gloves and perform hand hygiene if collecting a specimen from a bedpan, commode, or plastic receptacle.
- Use tongue blades to transfer the stool to the test tape or folder.
- Follow instructions based on type of test. Hemoccult slide test requires placing 2 drops of developer solution on the back side of the specimen paper.
- Document the test results according to facility policy. *A blue color is a positive result and needs to be reported.*
- Inform the patient of the test results.

detected on the tape under a microscope. For accurate results, this test may need to be repeated on consecutive days.

DIRECT VISUALIZATION STUDIES

Endoscopy is the direct visual examination of body organs or cavities. Most commonly, this is done using a fiberoptic endoscope, a long, flexible tube containing glass fibers that transmit light into the organ and return an image that can be viewed. Pincers may be inserted through the tube to obtain a tissue sample for biopsy. An endoscope enables the practitioner to view the integrity of the mucosa, blood vessels, and specific organ parts and is helpful for diagnosing inflammatory, ulcerative, and infectious diseases; benign and malignant neoplasms; and other lesions of the esophageal, gastric, and intestinal mucosa. Endoscopic studies include the following:

- *Esophagogastroduodenoscopy (EGD):* visual examination of the esophagus, the stomach, and the duodenum
- *Colonoscopy:* visual examination of the large intestine from the anus to the ileocecal valve
- *Sigmoidoscopy:* visual examination of the sigmoid colon, the rectum, and the anal canal

Nursing responsibilities before and after these studies are described in Box 37-2 (on page 1358).

A newer procedure is wireless capsule endoscopy. In this procedure, the patient swallows a capsule, about the size of a vitamin, which contains a small camera that emits a radio signal. The capsule is propelled through the small intestine via peristalsis, taking two pictures per second. Several wires on the patient's abdomen pick up the radio signal from the capsule, and the data are recorded on a data recorder, which the patient wears on a belt. The system captures about 55,000 images in an 8-hour exam. The patient returns to the facility after 8 hours, and the external sensors and data recorder are removed. The information is downloaded from the recorder to a computer and can be transferred to a videotape for easy viewing by the physician. The capsule is excreted during the process of normal defecation in 24 to 48 hours and is intended for one-time use only (Van Leeuwen et al., 2011).

The patient is normally NPO (fasting) for 10 to 12 hours the evening before capsule ingestion. During the first 2 hours of the study, the patient is not allowed to eat or drink anything. After the first 2 hours, the patient may consume small amounts of liquids. After 4 hours, the patient may have a small meal. The patient may resume normal activities while the camera is passing through the small intestine. Because there is no sedation or discomfort and a normal day can be planned, many patients prefer this method of endoscopy. Additionally, no air is needed to expand the small intestine, as it is in traditional endoscopy; therefore, the patient does not feel uncomfortable and bloated. This method, however, does not allow for obtaining biopsies of any suspicious area, so additional endoscopic studies may be required, based on the results.

INDIRECT VISUALIZATION STUDIES

Indirect visualization of the gastrointestinal tract is commonly performed through radiography. The passage of x-rays through the patient creates a radiograph or film depicting body structures. This technique is useful for detecting obstructions, strictures, inflammatory disease, tumors, ulcers, and other lesions, and for diagnosing a hiatal hernia and other structural changes in the gastrointestinal tract. Use of a radiopaque contrast medium, such as barium sulfate, accentuates the body structures being visualized. In the upper gastrointestinal examination and small-bowel series, the patient drinks the barium sulfate like a milkshake. The barium coats the esophagus, stomach, and small intestine to enhance visualization. In the barium enema or lower gastrointestinal examination, barium sulfate is instilled into the large intestine through a rectal tube inserted through the anus. Fluoroscopy projects consecutive x-ray images onto a screen for continuous observation of the flow of the barium. During a computerized tomography (CT) scan, thin beams of x-rays are directed at and move around the abdomen, resulting in computer-manipulated pictures that are not obscured by overlying anatomy. Contrast may be given orally or intravenously to enhance the images. Magnetic resonance imaging (MRI) provides physiologic information and detailed anatomic views of tissues using a superconducting magnet and radiofrequency signals. Computers use the signals to construct detailed sectional images of the abdomen. Intravenous contrast can be given to enhance the images. Abdominal ultrasound visualizes all solid upper abdominal organs, including the liver, bile ducts, gallbladder, appendix, pancreas, kidneys, adrenals, spleen, and the abdominal aorta and vena cava. The specific nursing responsibilities related to these studies are included in Box 37-2.

SCHEDULING FOR DIAGNOSTIC STUDIES

Nurses are commonly involved in scheduling diagnostic studies when a patient is to undergo multiple studies. Use the following guidelines for scheduling studies of the gastrointestinal tract:

1. Follow a logical sequence when more than one test is required for accurate diagnosis:
   - Fecal occult blood tests: to detect gastrointestinal bleeding
   - Barium studies: to visualize gastrointestinal structures and reveal any inflammation, ulcers, tumors, strictures, or other lesions
   - Endoscopic examinations: to visualize an abnormality, locate a source of bleeding, and if necessary provide biopsy tissue samples
2. A barium enema and routine radiography should precede an upper gastrointestinal series because retained barium from an upper gastrointestinal series could take several days to pass through the gastrointestinal tract and cloud anatomic detail on the barium enema studies.
3. Noninvasive procedures usually take precedence over invasive procedures, such as endoscopic studies, when

BOX 37-2 | COMMON DIAGNOSTIC STUDIES FOR THE GASTROINTESTINAL TRACT

Esophagogastroduodenoscopy (EGD)

It allows visual examination of the esophagus, stomach, and upper duodenum by means of a long, flexible, fiber-optic–lighted scope.

Preparation

- A signed consent form is required for this procedure.
- Fasting is required 6 to 12 hours before the test (check agency policy).
- Dentures need to be removed before the test.
- Remind patients that they will be awake but sedated and that a local anesthetic will be sprayed into the mouth and throat to depress the gag reflex.

Aftercare

- Withhold food and fluids until the gag reflex returns.
- Check vital signs according to the protocol.
- Observe for signs of perforation: pain, persistent difficulty swallowing, vomiting blood, or black, tarry stools.
- Explain to the patient that it is normal to sense throat soreness and hoarseness for several days; saline gargles and lozenges may be helpful.

Colonoscopy

It allows visual examination of the rectum, colon, and distal small bowel using a long, flexible, fiber-optic–lighted scope.

Preparation

- Ensure that an informed consent is signed.
- Preparation prior to test may involve:
  - Clear liquid diet (24–48 h before test)
  - 2-day bowel preparation—strong cathartic and Dulcolax on day 1 and enema the day of the test, or
  - 1-day bowel preparation—ingestion of a gallon of bowel cleanser, such as GoLytely, in a short period of time
  - Sedation will be given before the test.

Aftercare

- Patient may experience flatulence or gas pains because air was used to distend the intestines for better visibility.
- Usual diet may be resumed once patient recovers from the sedation.
- Check vital signs according to agency protocol.
- Observe for signs of bowel perforation: rectal bleeding, abdominal pain and distention, fever, malaise.

Sigmoidoscopy

It allows visual examination of the distal sigmoid colon, the rectum, and the anal canal through a flexible or rigid sigmoidoscope.

Preparation

- Ensure that an informed consent is signed.
- Preparation usually consists of a light meal before the test and two Fleet enemas.
- Sedation is not usually required.

Aftercare

- Patient may experience flatulence or gas pains because air was used to distend the intestines for better visibility.
- Observe for signs of bowel perforation.
- If biopsy was performed, patient should be informed that slight rectal bleeding may occur.

Upper Gastrointestinal (UGI) and Small-Bowel Series

This involves fluoroscopic examination of the esophagus, stomach, and small intestine after ingestion of barium sulfate.

Preparation

- Ensure that an informed consent is signed.
- Keep patient NPO after midnight the day of the test.
- Inform patient that a chalky-tasting barium contrast mixture will be given to drink before the test.

Aftercare

- A post-test cathartic (e.g., Milk of Magnesia) is usually prescribed to prevent fecal impaction from barium sulfate that has hardened. Notify the physician or primary care provider if barium is not passed, usually within 2 days.
- Explain that the barium may lighten the color of stools for the next several days. After the barium is expelled, the stool color will return to normal.

Barium Enema

This involves a series of radiographs that examine the large intestine after rectal instillation of barium sulfate.

Preparation

- An informed consent must be signed.
- Preparation may consist of dietary modifications, increased fluid intake, a cathartic, NPO after midnight, and enemas until clear before the test.
- Review the patient's history for any history of ulcerative colitis or active GI bleeding that would prohibit the use of the standard bowel preparation.

Aftercare

- Encourage fluids to prevent dehydration.
- Inform the patient that the barium may lighten the color of the stools. A cathartic may be prescribed. Notify the physician or primary care provider if barium is not passed, usually within 2 days.
- Encourage rest because the bowel preparation and the test exhaust many patients.

Abdominal Ultrasound

Uses ultrasound waves to visualize organs via a small transducer placed against the skin.

Preparation

- Assure the patient that no radiation is employed and that the test is painless.
- Patient must be NPO for a minimum of 8 hours before the examination.
- Explain that gel will be applied to the skin and that a sensation of warmth or wetness may be felt. The gel does not stain, but avoid wearing nonwashable clothing.
- Abdominal ultrasound must be performed before studies involving barium, as retained barium may compromise the study.

Aftercare

- Ensure that any residual gel is removed from the skin.
- Normal diet and fluids may be resumed, unless contraindicated by the test results.

Magnetic Resonance Imaging (MRI)

This test provides physiologic information and detailed anatomic views of tissues using a superconducting magnet and radiofrequency signals.

Preparation

- Evaluate the patient for need for sedation. Patients who are claustrophobic or unable to lie still during study may benefit from sedation.

BOX 37-2 COMMON DIAGNOSTIC STUDIES FOR THE GASTROINTESTINAL TRACT *continued*

- Patient may need to fast or consume only clear liquids prior to study. Patient should avoid alcohol, nicotine, caffeine, and iron supplements prior to the study.
- Patients with implanted surgical clips or other metallic structures and those with implanted electromechanical devices, such as cardiac pacemakers, drug infusion pumps, and cochlear implants, should not be exposed to MRI procedures.
- An informed consent is required.
- Pregnant patients are not routinely scanned because an increase in amniotic fluid/fetal temperature may be harmful.

Aftercare
- If intravenous contrast is used during study, monitor for sensitivity and adverse reactions.
- Monitor contrast injection site for signs of irritation, infection, and bruising.
- If prestudy sedation was given, monitor patient closely until sedation wears off to prevent injury.

Abdominal CT Scan
Thin beams of x-rays are directed at and move around the abdomen, resulting in computer-manipulated pictures that are not obscured by overlying anatomy.

Preparation
- An oral contrast is consumed before the study if the upper gastrointestinal tract is to be examined.
- Intravenous iodine contrast is usually administered.
- Assess for patient allergies to iodine, IV contrast, and/or shellfish. Prestudy preparation may be required if allergies are present.
- Assess for renal impairment; check laboratory values for elevated BUN and creatinine levels.
- Patient should be NPO for at least 4 hours before study.
- CT scan is contraindicated for pregnant patients.
- An informed consent is required.
- Metformin (Glucophage) must be discontinued prior to study and held after study to prevent renal failure. Consult with physician for patient medication modifications.

Aftercare
- If intravenous contrast is used during study, monitor for sensitivity and adverse reactions.
- Monitor contrast injection site for signs of irritation, infection, and bruising.
- If prestudy sedation was given, monitor patient closely until sedation wears off to prevent injury.

Adapted from Hinkle, J.L., & Cheever, K.H. (2014). *Brunner & Suddarth's textbook of medical–surgical nursing* (13th ed.). Philadelphia: Wolters Kluwer Health/Lippincott Williams & Wilkins; Malarkey, L.M., & McMorrow, M. E. (2012). *Saunders nursing guide to laboratory and diagnostic tests* (2nd ed.). St. Louis: Elsevier/Saunders.; and Van Leeuwen, A. M., Poelhuis-Leth, D., & Bladh, M. L. (2011). *Davis's comprehensive handbook of laboratory & diagnostic tests with nursing implications* (4th ed.). Philadelphia: F. A. Davis.

sufficient diagnostic data can be obtained from them. In some instances, endoscopic studies may be done before barium studies to ensure visualization.

Diagnosing
Nursing Diagnoses for bowel elimination can be divided into two categories: Bowel elimination as the problem and bowel elimination as the etiology.

Bowel Elimination as the Problem
When the analysis of assessment data points to a bowel elimination problem that can be prevented or resolved by independent nursing intervention, a nursing diagnosis is developed. If alterations in bowel elimination require new self-care behaviors—for example, colostomy management—Deficient Knowledge may be an appropriate nursing diagnosis. See the accompanying box, Examples of NANDA-I Nursing Diagnoses: Bowel Elimination (on page 1360).

Bowel Elimination as the Etiology
Problems of bowel elimination may also affect other areas of human functioning. In the nursing diagnoses that follow, problems of bowel elimination are the etiology for other problems:

- Delayed Growth and Development related to child's inability to attain bowel control secondary to inconsistency and lack of adequate parental knowledge

- Deficient Fluid Volume related to prolonged diarrhea
- Impaired Skin Integrity related to prolonged diarrhea, fecal incontinence
- Ineffective Coping related to inability to accept permanent ostomy

Outcome Identification and Planning
Interventions for patients without specific bowel elimination problems are directed toward the patient's achievement of the following outcomes. The patient will:

- Have a soft, formed bowel movement every 1 to 3 days without discomfort
- Explain the relationship between bowel elimination and dietary fiber, fluid intake, and exercise
- Relate the importance of seeking medical evaluation if changes in stool color or consistency persist

Interventions for patients with specific bowel elimination problems are directed to appropriate outcomes based on the specific problem. Examples of problem-based outcomes include the following: The patient will:

- Describe the functioning and purpose of the ostomy
- Ingest an adequate amount of fiber
- Monitor the amount and consistency of stools
- Express acceptance of the ostomy
- Demonstrate skin care for the ostomy
- Respond to the urge to defecate in a timely manner
- Maintain the integrity of perineal skin

EXAMPLES OF NANDA-I NURSING DIAGNOSES

BOWEL ELIMINATION

Nursing Diagnoses	Related Factors	Sample Defining Characteristics
Constipation	Decreased fiber in diet Decreased fluid intake Inactivity Delaying defecation when urge is present Abuse of laxatives Use of constipating medications (antacids, opioid analgesics, anticholinergics) Change in routine Pain associated with defecation	*"I feel bloated and know I have to move my bowels but I can't."* *"Whenever I'm constipated I feel lethargic and lose my appetite."* • Reports straining during defecation with little result • Passes small "marbles" of dry, hard stool • Decreased frequency • Decreased frequency of bowel sounds or changes in abdominal growling • Straining often results in small amount of bleeding from swollen external hemorrhoids • Reports feeling rectal fullness or pressure in rectum • Headache
Diarrhea	Adverse effects of pharmaceutical agents Abuse of laxatives Emotional stress Intestinal infection Colon disease and other diseases Radiation	• At least three loose liquid stools per day, increased frequency • Urgency • Reports of abdominal pain and/or cramping • Hyperactive bowel sounds
Bowel Incontinence	Dietary habits General decline in muscle tone Laxative abuse Rectal sphincter abnormality Cognitive impairment	• Involuntary passage of stool (stool characteristics vary) • *"I'm sorry, I couldn't get into the bathroom (or onto the bedpan) quickly enough."* • *"It came so fast I couldn't hold it back."* • Constant dribbling of soft stool

Implementing

Nursing care related to bowel elimination includes interventions to promote regular bowel habits, prevent and treat constipation, prevent and treat diarrhea, decrease flatulence, promote elimination of feces, manage bowel incontinence, and implement **bowel-training programs**. Nursing care related to caring for a patient with a nasogastric tube for gastric decompression is also discussed in the following sections.

Promoting Regular Bowel Habits

Promote regular bowel habits in well and ill patients by attention to timing, positioning, privacy, nutrition, and exercise.

TIMING

Encourage toileting at the patient's usual time during the day. Offer whatever assistance is needed to help the patient to the bathroom, commode, or bedpan at the time that a patient usually experiences the urge to defecate. This is often about an hour after meals, when mass colonic peristalsis occurs. Because many patients feel uncomfortable about requesting time for elimination, inform all patients about the importance of heeding this natural urge, explaining that postponing it could result in constipation and other problems.

POSITIONING

Sitting upright on a toilet or commode promotes defecation. Most patients who are able to use the bedside commode or bathroom toilet have little difficulty assuming this position, although they may need support. An elevated toilet seat may be ordered for patients with orthopedic problems who cannot lower themselves to a toilet seat. Sitting upright promotes a sense of normalcy and the effects of gravity help to promote regular bowel movements.

Patients who need to use a bedpan in bed often benefit from having the head of the bed elevated to as close to a sitting position as possible, at least 30 degrees, unless this is contraindicated. An overhead trapeze may be helpful for patients with weak lower extremities. Refer to Skill 37-2 on pp. 1382–1385 for more information about positioning a patient on a bedpan. Offer the patient moistened hand wipes at the bedside to substitute for hand-washing after toileting. Always empty, clean, and return bedpans to the patient's bedside stand or store according to facility policy.

PRIVACY

Because most people consider elimination a private act, always respect the patient's need to be alone while defecating, unless the patient's condition makes this impossible. Pull the bedside drapes around a patient who is using a bedside commode or bedpan. If any visitors are present, ask them to step outside for a few minutes. For well patients who cannot defecate in a public restroom (with multiple toilets) or strange environment, suggest that they use a private restroom with only one toilet.

NUTRITION

Patients with bowel elimination problems may need a dietary analysis to determine which foods and fluids are contributing to their problem and which may help in its treatment. General dietary recommendations to promote regular defecation include a fluid intake of 2,000 to 3,000 mL and high fiber intake. Water is recommended as the fluid of choice because fluids containing large amounts of caffeine and sugar may have a diuretic effect. Increasing fiber intake without sufficient fluid intake can result in severe gastrointestinal problems, including fecal impaction. Specific recommendations for treating constipation, diarrhea, and excessive flatulence follow.

EXERCISE

Regular exercise improves gastrointestinal motility and aids in defecation. Encourage well patients to exercise regularly for two and a half hours or more a week (U.S. Department of Health and Human Services, 2008). Ambulate patients who are ill as soon as possible, instructing them about how inactivity can lead to constipation, distention, and impaction. Bedside exercises may be helpful for patients who are immobile.

Teach the following exercises to help patients with weak abdominal and perineal muscles who are using a bedpan:

- Abdominal setting: The patient, lying in a supine position, tightens and holds the abdominal muscles for 6 seconds and then relaxes them. Repeat several times each waking hour.
- Thigh strengthening: The thigh muscles are flexed and contracted by slowly bringing the knees up to the chest one at a time and then lowering them to the bed. Perform this exercise several times for each knee each waking hour.

Providing Comfort Measures

Comfort measures related to defecation include working with the patient to develop a bowel elimination routine that results in the easy passage of a soft, formed stool; being attentive to perineal hygiene and the maintenance of skin integrity; and using warm, moist heat (sitz bath or tub bath) to soothe the perineal area. Additional non-surgical treatment options include the following (Hinkle & Cheever, 2014):

- Encouraging recommended diet (if pertinent) and exercise
- Using medications, such as laxatives and antidiarrheals, only as needed
- Applying ointments or astringents (witch hazel)
- Using suppositories that contain anesthetics

Preventing and Treating Constipation

Constipation is dry, hard stool; persistently difficult passage of stool; and/or the incomplete passage of stool. Decreased gastric motility slows the passage of feces through the large intestine, resulting in increased fluid absorption from the fecal mass and causing dry, hard stool. Straining often accompanies defecation. Some people may be constipated and yet have a daily bowel movement, whereas others who regularly defecate no more than three times a week are not constipated. People at high risk for constipation include patients on bedrest or with decreased mobility who take medications that cause constipation (e.g., opioids, anticholinergics), patients with reduced fluids, bulk, or fiber in their diet, people who are depressed, and patients with central nervous system disease or local lesions that cause pain while defecating.

TEACHING ABOUT NUTRITION

Promoting healthy behaviors can assist the patient and family to achieve mutually desirable outcomes for preventing constipation. A combination of high-fiber foods (20–35 g of fiber), 60 to 80 oz (1.8–2.4 L) of fluid daily, and exercise has been shown to be effective in controlling constipation in patients with deficiencies in dietary intake of fiber and/or fluid and reduced amounts of exercise (Toner & Claros, 2012). Caution the patient to avoid increasing fiber intake without drinking enough fluids; this can lead to a bowel obstruction. Foods that contain high amounts of fiber include bran, fruits, vegetables, and whole grains.

 THINK back to Leroy Cobbs, the patient who developed fecal impaction while using narcotic analgesics. The nurse should list in the teaching plan foods that stimulate peristalsis to prevent future episodes of constipation. If the patient knows to include these foods in his diet, he will be less worried about future problems and may be more amenable to using the medication to control his pain. ●

TEACHING ABOUT LAXATIVES

Cathartics and **laxatives** are drugs that induce emptying of the intestinal tract. Although these terms are sometimes used interchangeably, cathartics exert a stronger effect on the intestines than do laxatives. Some of these drugs, such as castor oil, cascara, senna, and phenolphthalein, and bisacodyl (Dulcolax), act chemically by stimulating peristalsis. Others, such as psyllium hydrophilic mucilloid (Metamucil), act by increasing the intestinal bulk, which promotes additional mechanical stimulation on the intestine. Still others, such as mineral oil and docusate sodium (Colace), soften the fecal material. Other frequently used laxatives are the saline-osmotics, such as magnesium hydroxide (Milk of Magnesia [MOM]) and sodium phosphate (Phospho-Soda). These act by drawing water into the intestines, stimulating peristalsis.

Table 37-2 CLASSIFICATION OF LAXATIVES

TYPE	ACTION	ADVANTAGES	CAUTION
Bulk-forming (e.g., Metamucil)	Psyllium, grain, or synthetic product that causes stool to absorb water and swell, thus stimulating peristalsis	Usually acts within 24 hours	May interfere with absorption of calcium and iron and certain drugs Should not be given to bedridden patients or those with intestinal strictures May be expensive
Stool softener (e.g., Colace)	Agents with detergent activity that allow water and fat to penetrate and lubricate the stool	Recommended for those who must avoid straining	Has lubricant component of drug that may interfere with absorption of fat-soluble vitamins
Emollient (lubricant, e.g., mineral oil)	Lubricates the intestinal tract and retards colonic absorption of water, softening the stool, making it easier to pass	Usually effective within 8 hours	May interfere with absorption of fat-soluble vitamins Can be aspirated, possibly resulting in a lipid pneumonia
Stimulant (e.g., Dulcolax)	Drug promotes peristalsis by irritating the intestinal mucosa or stimulating nerve endings in intestinal wall	Works more quickly than bulking agents	Are the most abused laxatives on the market Causes lazy bowel syndrome May affect absorption of vitamin D and calcium Not recommended for elderly patients because of prolonged action Alters electrolyte transport
Osmotic (e.g., Miralax)	Drug draws water into intestine, resulting in a softer stool and inducing more frequent bowel movements	Is used when rapid cleansing desired	May cause bloating and/or diarrhea Can produce dehydration Not recommended in patients with kidney disease or heart failure

Magnesium hydroxide has antacid properties in small dosages and laxative properties in larger doses. Table 37-2 summarizes the types of laxatives.

Laxatives are sometimes necessary for people with limited activity or poor food intake. They are also used to empty the intestinal tract in preparation for surgery or diagnostic tests. Laxatives such as docusate sodium (Colace) may be used in conjunction with some prescribed medications to counteract the medications' constipating properties. Occasional use of laxatives is not harmful for most people, but people should not become dependent on them. Because many laxatives are available as nonprescription drugs, and advertising promotes their use, many people take them frequently on their own initiative, whether they need them or not.

Because of their chemical action, laxatives should not be taken when there is abdominal pain because an intestinal pathologic condition could be harmed by the increased peristalsis. Although many people take laxatives because they believe they are constipated, most are unaware that habitual use of laxatives may be the cause of chronic constipation.

Nurses play a key role in helping patients who abuse laxatives. Breaking the physical and psychological habit of using laxatives is not easy for a person who has come to depend on them; it often requires much patience, support, and teaching. The person also frequently needs assistance with diet, fluid intake, activity, and regularity of habits.

Preventing and Treating Diarrhea

Diarrhea, in adults, is the passage of more than three loose stools a day. Frequent bowel movements are not always indicative of diarrhea, but patients with diarrhea usually pass stools more frequently. Diarrhea is often associated with intestinal cramps. Nausea and vomiting may occur; blood also may be noted. Diarrhea is a protective response when the cause is irritants in the intestinal tract. Regardless of the cause, however, large amounts of fluids and electrolytes may be lost relatively quickly through diarrhea, especially in infants, young children, and older adults. If diarrhea is untreated, this loss of fluids and electrolytes places the person at high risk for life-threatening complications. If oral intake is possible, teach patients to avoid cold fluids and rich foods, especially sweets.

Additional nursing measures for the patient with diarrhea include the following:

- Answer the patient's call bell immediately or ensure that a bedpan or commode is within easy reach. Diarrhea can be embarrassing, and the patient needs to know that the nurse is there to help.
- Whenever possible, remove the cause of the diarrhea. Discontinuing medications that cause diarrhea usually results in a return to normal defecation within 1 to 3 days.
- If there is any indication of a fecal impaction, further evaluation is necessary before using antidiarrheal medications.

- Give special care to the region around the anus, where skin irritation is common. Keep the area clean and dry. Use skin creams, moisture barriers, ointments, or powders as necessary.

 SKIN care measures would be important to include in the plan of care for Jeremy Green, the young boy experiencing episodes of diarrhea. Doing so reduces his risk for perianal excoriation and breakdown, which could further impair his body image and cause additional discomfort and pain. ●

TEACHING ABOUT FOOD SAFETY

The first precaution is to ensure that food is safe for consumption and prepared and stored properly. Food poisoning, and the diarrhea that frequently accompanies it, can be prevented. The U.S. Department of Health and Human Services (2013) and the Centers for Disease Control (2011) recommend these measures:

- Never purchase food with damaged packaging.
- Take items that require refrigeration home immediately. Refrigerate perishable foods and leftovers within 2 hours (1 hour in summer). Refrigerator temperatures should be between 40°F and 32°F. Freezer temperatures should be 0°F or below.
- Wash hands and surfaces often. Wash surfaces and utensils after each use to prevent the spread of microorganisms.
- Use separate cutting boards and plates for produce and for meat, poultry, seafood, and eggs. Never cut meat on a wooden surface.
- Thoroughly wash all vegetables and fruit before preparing or eating.
- Do not wash meat, poultry, or eggs to prevent spreading microorganisms to the sink, countertops, and other kitchen surfaces.
- Never use raw eggs in any form because of the danger of infection with *Salmonella bacillus*. When cooking eggs, use only fresh ones that have been purchased within 3 to 5 weeks and kept in the refrigerator.
- Do not eat seafood raw. Do not eat seafood if it has a strong, unpleasant odor.
- Use a food thermometer to ensure cooking food to the safe internal temperature. Cook whole meats to 145°F, ground meats to 160°F, and poultry to 165°F. Microwave food thoroughly; cook to the safe temperature of 165°F or above.
- Keep food hot after cooking; maintain the safe temperature of 140°F or above.
- Give only pasteurized fruit juices to small children.

PREVENTING AND MANAGING TRAVELER'S DIARRHEA

There has been a significant increase in the numbers of people traveling outside their native countries, including overseas travel. Traveler's diarrhea, caused by bacterial enteropathogens, viruses, or parasites, is the most predict-

able travel-related illness. The most important determinant of risk is travel to high-risk destinations, including the countries of Mexico, Central and South America, Africa, the Middle East, and Asia (Connor, 2012). Symptoms include more than three loose stools in a 24-hour period, fever, nausea, vomiting, and abdominal cramps and/or pain.

Management includes education about prevention and self-treatment strategies. Advise patients to peel fruits and vegetables, and consume dry foods and foods that are piping hot and cooked thoroughly. Tell travelers to avoid tap water, ice cubes, fruit juice, unpeeled raw fruits and vegetables, unpasteurized dairy products, open buffets, and undercooked or reheated foods. Safe beverages include those that are bottled and sealed or carbonated. Boiled beverages and those appropriately treated with iodine or chorine are also safe to drink (Connor, 2012).

Treatment strategies include maintaining hydration with bottled water and/or fluids, use of antimotility agents, such as loperamide (Imodium), and antibiotics. For more severe fluid loss, replacement is best accomplished with oral rehydration salts (ORS; Connnor, 2012). Encourage patients considering travel to underdeveloped countries to discuss their personal risks and the provision of prescription medication with their physician or health care provider before beginning their travels.

TEACHING ABOUT TREATMENT FOR DIARRHEA

Treatment for diarrhea typically depends on whether the problem is acute or chronic. Acute diarrhea may result from a viral or bacterial infection, a reaction to medication, or alterations in diet. It is characterized by its sudden onset and lasts several hours to several days. Rehydration is key with acute diarrhea. Oral liquids may be used if the patient can tolerate them; otherwise, intravenous fluid replacement may be necessary. Stress the importance of hand hygiene with the patient and family. Avoid antidiarrheal agents in acute diarrhea until a bacterial causative agent has been ruled out.

Chronic diarrhea typically lasts for more than 3 to 4 weeks. Investigate chronic diarrhea to determine the underlying cause. Chronic diarrhea has many possible causes, such as irritable bowel syndrome (e.g., Crohn disease, ulcerative colitis), malabsorption syndromes, bowel tumor, metabolic disease (diabetes, hyperthyroidism), parasitic infection, side effects of drugs, laxative abuse, surgery, alcohol abuse, and radiation and chemotherapeutic agents. Chronic diarrhea usually necessitates pharmacologic intervention along with fluid and electrolyte replacement. Antidiarrheal medications are usually reserved for treatment of chronic diarrhea. Whatever the type of diarrhea, make every effort to identify and eliminate the underlying cause.

Several types of antidiarrheal medications are available. Medications such as camphorated opium tincture (Paregoric), loperamide (Imodium), and diphenoxylate hydrochloride (Lomotil) act directly on the smooth muscle of the gastrointestinal tract. Kaolin and pectin (Kaopectate)

Table 37-3	CLASSIFICATION OF ANTIDIARRHEAL MEDICATIONS			
CATEGORY	NAME	ACTION	ADVANTAGES	CAUTIONS
Action on gastro-intestinal smooth muscle	Opium (Paregoric)	Increases smooth muscle tone Decreases GI motility Diminishes GI secretions	Effective	May be addictive due to morphine content May cause drowsiness and lightheadedness Should be discontinued as soon as diarrhea has diminished
	Diphenoxylate and atropine (Lomotil)	Slows gastric motility through local effect on gastrointestinal wall	Effective	Is chemically related to morphine; atropine added to prevent addiction but in high doses can become addictive May cause drowsiness
	Loperamide (Imodium)	Inhibits peristalsis via direct effect on gastrointestinal wall muscles	Not addictive Longer duration than Lomotil	May cause drowsiness Must be discontinued if no improvement in 48 hours with acute cases
Absorbent	Kaolin-pectin (Kaopectate)	Absorbs and soothes	No drowsiness	May interfere with absorption of other oral medications May interfere with absorption of nutrients with prolonged use
Antisecretory/antimicrobial	Bismuth sub-salicylate (Pepto-Bismol)	Decreases gastrointestinal tract secretion Has antimicrobial action against bacterial and viral pathogens	No drowsiness	Contains salicylates; check with physician before giving to children or administering with aspirin May decrease absorption of some medications

is thought to act as an absorbent and demulcent. Bismuth subsalicylate (Pepto-Bismol) has an antimicrobial action and an antisecretory effect. Table 37-3 highlights the major antidiarrheal agents.

The focus of nursing care is on eliminating the cause of the diarrhea and replacing lost fluids as well as treating the symptoms. Some commercial fluid and electrolyte replacement products, such as Gatorade, may be helpful. Oral rehydration therapy using fluid and electrolyte replacement and water for adults is cost-effective and replaces fluid loss without the challenges associated with intravenous fluid therapy. Replace lost fluids and electrolytes with weak tea, water, bouillon, clear soup, and gelatin. It is particularly important to maintain fluid balance in older patients because of their increased risk for dehydration, fluid overload, and electrolyte imbalances.

Additional measures for preventing or treating diarrhea include avoiding highly spiced foods and foods with laxative effects, such as raw fruits and vegetables. Encourage the patient to eat foods with low fiber content. Foods low in fiber include eggs; well-cooked meat, fish, and poultry; juices without pulp; refined bread and cereal products; and well-cooked fruits and vegetables. The use of probiotics (live microorganisms that are similar to beneficial microorganisms found in the human gastrointestinal tract) to prevent, limit, and control diarrhea has been suggested as an effective dietary intervention for diarrhea, particularly antibiotic-associated diarrhea and *C. difficile*–associated disease. Examples of foods containing probiotics include cheese, yogurt, tempeh, miso, soymilk, and some commer-

cial dairy drinks (Salfi & Holt, 2012; Avadhani & Miley, 2011). Probiotics can also be ingested through the use of commercially prepared supplements.

Alterations in fluid and electrolyte balance occur faster and more often in infants and children compared to adults. Therefore, infants and children experiencing diarrhea require more fluid and electrolyte replacement compared to adults. Encourage fluids, especially oral rehydration solutions containing sodium chloride, potassium, and glucose (Pedialyte®, Infalyte®, and Ricelyte®), and make them accessible for the child. Special diets for dehydration such as the BRAT diet (bananas, rice cereal, applesauce, and toast) are no longer recommended because they lack sufficient calories.

Decreasing Flatulence

Excessive formation of gases in the stomach or intestines is known as **flatulence**. When the gas is not expelled but accumulates in the intestinal tract, the condition is referred to as intestinal distention or tympanites. Gas-producing foods, such as beans, cabbage, onions, cauliflower, and beer, often predispose a person to flatulence and distention.

 RECALL Alberta Franklin, the patient described in the Reflective Practice display. The nurse should include information about eliminating gas-producing foods in this patient's teaching plan to avoid excess gas formation and accumulation, which could cause her colostomy bag to overfill and possibly lead to detachment and leakage. ●

In addition to teaching about the avoidance of irritating foods, explain to the patient that reclining should be avoided after meals and one should move around in bed and ambulate in order to promote peristalsis and the escape of flatus.

Emptying the Colon of Feces

Several methods are used to help promote elimination of feces: enemas, suppositories, oral intestinal lavage, and digital removal of stool. Discussion of each of these methods follows.

ENEMAS

An **enema** is the introduction of a solution into the large intestine, usually to remove feces. The instilled solution distends the intestine and irritates the intestinal mucosa, thus increasing peristalsis. Enemas are classified as cleansing or retention enemas. Rectal agents and manipulation, including enemas, are discouraged for use with myelosuppressed patients and/or patients at risk for myelosuppression and mucositis, because they can lead to development of bleeding, anal fissures, or abscesses, which are portals for infection (National Cancer Institute [NCI], 2012).

Cleansing Enemas. Cleansing enemas are given to remove feces from the colon, commonly to:

- Relieve constipation or fecal impaction
- Prevent involuntary escape of fecal material during surgical procedures
- Promote visualization of the intestinal tract by radiographic or instrument examination
- Help establish regular bowel function during a bowel-training program

The most common types of solutions used for cleansing enemas are tap water, normal saline solution, soap solution, and hypertonic solution. Commonly used enema solutions are described in Table 37-4.

Hypotonic (tap water) and isotonic (normal saline solution) enemas are large-volume enemas that result in rapid colonic emptying. However, using such large volumes of solution (adults, 500–1,000 mL; infants, 150–250 mL) may be dangerous for patients with weakened intestinal walls, such as those with bowel inflammation or bowel infection. These solutions often require special preparation and equipment.

Hypertonic solution preparations are available commercially and are administered in smaller volumes (adult, 70–130 mL). These solutions draw water into the colon, which stimulates the defecation reflex. They may be contraindicated in patients for whom sodium retention is a problem. They are also contraindicated for patients with renal impairment or reduced renal clearance because such patients have compromised ability to excrete phosphate adequately, with resulting hyperphosphatemia (Jacobson, Peery, Thompson, Kanapka, & Caswell, 2010; Bowers, 2006).

Retention Enemas. Retention enemas are retained in the bowel for a prolonged period for different reasons:

- Oil-retention enemas: lubricate the stool and intestinal mucosa, making defecation easier. About 150 to 200 mL of solution is administered to adults.
- Carminative enemas: help to expel flatus from the rectum and provide relief from gaseous distention. Common solutions include the milk and molasses enema (equal parts) and the magnesium sulfate–glycerin–water (MGW) enema (30 mL of magnesium sulfate, 60 mL of glycerin, and 90 mL of warm water).
- Medicated enemas: provide medications that are absorbed through the rectal mucosa.
- Anthelmintic enemas: destroy intestinal parasites.

Equipment. Commercially prepared enema kits include a flexible bottle containing hypertonic solution with an attached prelubricated firm tip about 5 to 7.5 cm (2–3 inches) long. Its ease of use makes it particularly convenient in the home. Patients can readily administer their own enema in many instances.

For tap water, saline solution, or soap solution enema, a container, rubber or plastic tubing with side openings

Table 37-4 COMMONLY USED ENEMA SOLUTIONS

SOLUTION	AMOUNT	ACTION	TIME TO TAKE EFFECT	ADVERSE EFFECTS
Tap water (hypotonic)	500–1,000 mL	Distends intestine, increases peristalsis, softens stool	15 min	Fluid and electrolyte imbalance, water intoxication
Normal saline (isotonic)	500–1,000 mL	Distends intestine, increases peristalsis, softens stool	15 min	Fluid and electrolyte imbalance, sodium retention
Soap	500–1,000 mL (concentrate at 3–5 mL/1,000 mL)	Distends intestine, irritates intestinal mucosa, softens stool	10–15 min	Rectal mucosa irritation or damage
Hypertonic	70–130 mL	Distends intestine, irritates intestinal mucosa	5–10 min	Sodium retention
Oil (mineral, olive, or cottonseed oil)	150–200 mL	Lubricates stool and intestinal mucosa	30 min	

near its distal end, a tubing clamp, lubricant, and the solution are necessary. Regardless of the type of enema to be given, clean or medically aseptic technique is used. Always wear or have the caregiver wear disposable gloves to protect from exposure to blood, body fluids, and microorganisms.

Patient Preparation. Because enemas are a common procedure, some patients already know why they are used and how they are administered. Reinforce this information and correct any misconceptions that they may have. For patients who have not previously had an enema, explain the purpose, what they can expect, and how they can participate. In all cases, provide for patient privacy. The procedure offers an excellent opportunity for health teaching because many people are unfamiliar with or uncomfortable talking about the functioning of the intestinal tract. Failure to provide explanations and protect privacy may result in an uncomfortable and disagreeable situation for the patient.

A reclining position for enema administration—specifically left side-lying or the knee–chest position—is recommended, but if the patient has a respiratory disorder or is having difficulty breathing, elevate the head of the bed slightly. Avoid the Fowler's position because the solution will remain in the rectum and expulsion will occur rapidly, resulting in minimal cleansing. Some patients think the solution should be expelled as soon as possible. Reinforce the need to retain the solution to achieve the desired results.

Administration Using a Hypotonic or Isotonic (Large-Volume) Solution. The procedure for administering a cleansing enema using a large volume of solution is described in Skill 37-1 on pages 1377–1381.

Administration Using a Hypertonic (Small-Volume) Solution. Administering a cleansing enema using a hypertonic solution differs from the procedure described in Skill 37-1 in the following ways:

- The equipment is included in the commercially prepared set. The only additional equipment needed is a bedpan for a bedridden patient and a disposable waterproof pad to protect bed linens.
- Do not warm the hypertonic solution. Administer it at room temperature, and warm it only if it is very cold.
- Place the patient in the left side-lying position or the knee-chest position, which helps to distribute the solution throughout the lower intestinal tract and is recommended if the patient can assume it. Additional lubrication of the rectal tip is recommended, even though it is prelubricated.
- Instill the solution into the rectum by applying gentle pressure on the collapsible solution container (Fig. 37-6). It should take 1 to 2 minutes to administer the enema.
- Administer the hypertonic enema solution cautiously to a patient with hemorrhoids. The rigid tip may tear frag-

FIGURE 37-6 Technique for compressing a small-volume enema container.

ile rectal mucosa that is enlarged and inflamed, causing pain, torn rectal tissue, and necrosis. Generous lubrication is recommended before inserting the enema tip.

Administration of an Oil-Retention Enema. The procedure for giving an oil-retention enema differs from that for giving a cleansing enema in the following respects:

- A small rectal tube is used. The small size helps to reduce intestinal contractions so that the patient can retain the oil more easily. Oil enemas are available in commercial kits similar to those for hypertonic-solution enemas. The kits contain a small rectal tube.
- Administer the oil-retention enema at body temperature to minimize muscle contractions caused by a warmer or cooler solution.
- Instruct the patient to retain the oil for at least 30 minutes for best cleansing results.
- A cleansing enema is often ordered after an oil-retention enema to facilitate emptying of the bowel.

RECTAL SUPPOSITORIES

A **suppository** is a conical or oval solid substance shaped for easy insertion into a body cavity and designed to melt at body temperature. Various rectal suppositories are available. Some are fecal softeners, others have a direct action on the nerve endings in the rectal mucosa, and some liberate carbon dioxide when moistened. Fecal softeners are useful when the stool is very hard. Substances that stimulate the rectal nerves are helpful for people with weak muscle tone or poor innervation. The carbon dioxide suppositories liberate about 200 mL of gas, which causes distention, causing stimulation and elimination impulses. Refer to Chapter 28 for Guidelines for Nursing Care 28-7: Inserting a Rectal Suppository on page 793.

ORAL INTESTINAL LAVAGE

An oral solution, such as GoLYTELY® or Colyte®, can be used to cleanse the intestine of feces. This solution is prescribed by the physician and can be administered before diagnostic tests that require a clear bowel for visualization purposes or as a "bowel prep" before intestinal surgery. Evacuation of feces usually begins within 1 hour after the first glass and is completed within 4 to 6 hours. As with an enema, a clear return indicates that the bowel preparation is complete. A clear diet for 24 hours before taking this solution lessens the time needed for completion of the bowel prep, but potassium replacement may be required before surgery because of the limited potassium in a clear diet. The solution has a slightly salty taste and is easier to tolerate if it is cold and consumed quickly. Carefully assess older patients using oral intestinal lavage because older adults are more prone to electrolyte imbalances.

DIGITAL REMOVAL OF STOOL

Fecal impaction often prevents the passage of normal stools. Small amounts of fluid may pass around the impacted mass; liquid fecal seepage with no passage of normal feces is a sign of an impaction.

Include dietary interventions, adequate fluids, and adjustment of medication in the patient's plan of care before considering digital removal of feces (Kyle, Prynn, & Oliver, 2004). Increasing dietary fiber content to 30 g/day, increased water intake, and discontinuation of medications that can contribute to colonic hypomotility can help manage and prevent fecal impaction (Obokhare, 2012). If a patient with a fecal impaction cannot expel the fecal mass voluntarily and oil and cleansing enemas fail to break up the mass, the impaction must be broken up manually. An order from the primary health care provider is required. This procedure is very uncomfortable and may cause great discomfort to the patient as well as irritation of the rectal mucosa and bleeding. Digital removal of a fecal mass can stimulate the vagus nerve, resulting in a slowed heart rate. If this occurs, stop the procedure immediately, monitor the patient's heart rate and blood pressure, and notify the physician. Many patients find that a sitz bath or tub bath after this procedure soothes the irritated perineal area. The primary health care provider may order an oil-retention enema to be given before the procedure to soften stool. The procedure for digital (manual) removal of a fecal impaction is outlined in the Guidelines for Nursing Care 37-2; Digital Removal of Fecal Impaction (on page 1368).

 IT is important for the nurse caring for Leroy Cobbs, the patient with fecal impaction described at the beginning of the chapter, to demonstrate competency and care when performing manual disimpaction to decrease the patient's discomfort and embarrassment. Additionally, the nurse may need to adapt the procedure to ensure that the patient experiences relief as quickly as possible without any undue harm or injury. ●

Managing Bowel Incontinence

Bowel incontinence is the inability of the anal sphincter to control the discharge of fecal and gaseous material. The cause of incontinence is usually an organic disease, resulting either in a mechanical condition that hinders the proper functioning of the anal sphincter or an impairment in the nerve supply to the anal sphincter. Mental illness may also cause a patient to be indifferent to the passage of stool. Although bowel incontinence is seldom life-threatening, patients with bowel incontinence suffer embarrassment, may become depressed, and pose a challenge for nurses because of the risk for skin breakdown.

The following nursing interventions are helpful for a patient who suffers from bowel incontinence:

- Note when incontinence is most likely to occur, and place the patient on a bedpan at those times. If there is no pattern, offer a bedpan at regular intervals, such as every few hours.
- Keep the skin clean and dry by using proper hygienic measures. Apply a protective skin barrier after cleaning the skin, according to manufacturer's directions. Impaired skin integrity may develop when such measures are overlooked.
- Change bed linens and clothing as necessary to avoid odor, skin irritation, and embarrassment. Disposable bed pads and moisture-proof undergarments can be considered but should not be used until other measures have been tried. These materials often worsen any skin irritation or breakdown present as a result of skin contact with stool by retaining moisture against the skin, raising the pH of the skin, and prolonging contact of the stool against the skin, increasing damage from digestive enzymes present in the stool (Voegeli, 2012).
- Confer with the physician about using a suppository or a daily cleansing enema. These measures empty the lower colon regularly and often help to decrease incontinence. Bowel-training programs may also be helpful. (Bowel-training programs are discussed later in the chapter.)

INDWELLING RECTAL TUBE

In some health care agencies, a rectal indwelling catheter is used for patients with uncontrollable diarrhea. However, relatively little research supports the safety of this procedure and use should be avoided (Flynn Makic, VonRueden, Rauen, & Chadwick, 2011). Disadvantages of indwelling rectal tubes include leakage and perirectal skin damage, injury to the rectal mucosa, and injury of the anal sphincter. The fecal incontinence device, discussed in the next section, is a safer alternative.

FECAL INCONTINENCE DEVICE

An alternative measure to protect perianal skin from repeated episodes of fecal incontinence is the fecal incontinence device. This device can be secured via adhesive around the anal opening and attached to gravity drainage, allowing liquid stool to accumulate in a collection bag (Fig. 37-7 on page 1369). It is best applied before the perianal area becomes excoriated. If excoriation is already present, application of a skin barrier prior to applying the pouch can be effective.

Nursing responsibilities include careful regular assessment and documentation of the perianal skin condition and

GUIDELINES FOR NURSING CARE 37-2

DIGITAL REMOVAL OF FECAL IMPACTION

To manually remove a fecal impaction, the following technique is recommended:

- Explain the procedure to the patient.
- Have a second person assist with the procedure. The second person can reassure and comfort the patient while the first person works to break up the mass.
- Place the patient in a side-lying position. Drape the patient to preserve privacy yet provide easy access. Place a protective pad under the patient.
- Place a bedpan on the bed for depositing removed feces. Have toilet paper and personal cleaning supplies on hand for use after the procedure is completed.
- Use nonsterile gloves for the procedure because the intestinal tract is not sterile.
- Lubricate the index finger generously to reduce irritating the rectum, and insert the finger gently into the anal canal (Figure A). The presence of the finger added to the mass

tends to cause discomfort for the patient if the work is not done slowly and gently.

- Slowly and gently, work the finger around and into the hardened mass to break it up (Figures B and C), then remove pieces of it (Figure D). Instruct the patient to bear down, if possible, while extracting feces to ease in removal.
- Remove the impaction at intervals if it is severe. This helps to avoid discomfort as well as irritation, which can injure intestinal mucosa.
- Use an oil-retention enema if necessary. The enema may be given before attempts are made to break up and remove the impaction digitally, or it may be ordered after digital attempts fail. A cleansing enema is often ordered after an oil-retention enema.
- Wash and dry the patient's buttocks and anal area. Assist the patient to a comfortable position.

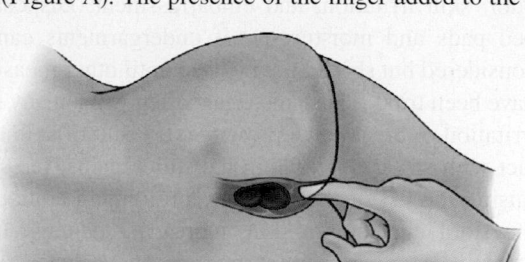

A
Inserting gloved, lubricated finger into fecal mass.

B
Slowly and gently, using finger to break up some of the hardened mass.

C
Breaking off a section of the impaction.

D
Removing a section of the impaction.

attentive management of the drainage system. Change the pouch at least every 72 hours, or sooner if it is not intact or leakage has occurred. Provide explanations and support to the patient and family members so that they understand the benefits of this system.

Designing and Implementing Bowel-Training Programs

Patients with a history of chronic constipation and impaction and those who are incontinent of stool may benefit

from a bowel-training program. The purpose of this program is to manipulate factors within the person's control (food and fluid intake, exercise, time for defecation) to produce the elimination of a soft, formed stool at regular intervals without a laxative. This effort to regain bowel control may be initiated in the health care setting or the patient's home. The accompanying Nursing Intervention and Nursing Outcome Classifications (NIC/NOC) box lists standardized nursing interventions and corresponding outcomes related to bowel management and training.

Removing paper backing from adhesive of rectal pouch.

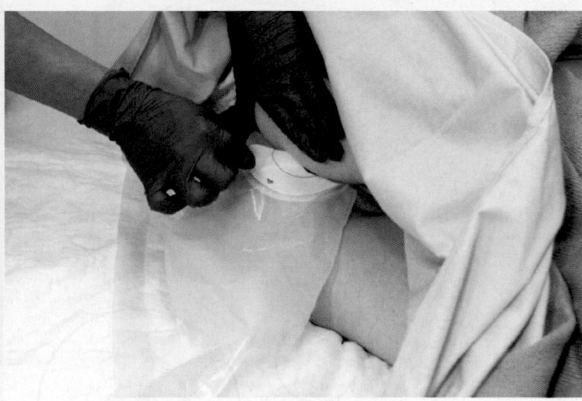

Applying pouch over anal opening.

Attaching connector of fecal pouch to tubing of drainage bag.

FIGURE 37-7. Applying a fecal incontinence device.

When the patient has established a regular pattern of defecation, continue to offer assistance with toileting at the successful time.

Maintaining a Nasogastric Tube

Nasogastric tubes may be inserted to decompress or drain the stomach of fluid or unwanted stomach contents such as poison or medication and air, and when conditions are present in which peristalsis is absent. Several of these conditions have been detailed previously in the chapter. Examples include paralytic ileus and intestinal obstruction by tumor or hernia. Nasogastric tubes (NGTs) are also used to allow the gastrointestinal tract to rest before or after abdominal surgery to promote healing and are

EXAMPLES OF NURSING INTERVENTIONS AND NURSING OUTCOMES CLASSIFICATIONS (NIC/NOC)

BOWEL MANAGEMENT

Nursing Interventions	Nursing Outcomes
• Plan bowel program with patient and appropriate others. • Monitor bowel movements including frequency, consistency, shape, volume, and color, as appropriate. • Monitor bowel sounds. • Teach patient about specific foods that are assistive in promoting bowel regularity. • Teach about foods that are assistive in promoting bowel regularity. • Ensure privacy. • Encourage adequate fluid intake.	• Bowel Elimination • Hydration • Gastrointestinal Function

Adapted from Bulechek, G. M, Butcher, H. K., Dochterman, J. M., & Wagner, C. M. (Eds.). (2013). *Nursing interventions classification (NIC)* (6th ed., p. 107). St. Louis: Elsevier/Mosby; and Moorhead, S., Johnson, M., Maas, M. L., & Swanson, E. (Eds.). (2013). *Nursing Outcomes Classification (NOC).* (5th ed., pp. 108–109, 239, 253). St. Louis: Elsevier/Mosby. A full listing of nursing activities for each nursing intervention and outcomes can be found in these books.

FIGURE 37-8. Levine tube and Salem sump nasogastric tubes. Insert on right shows close up of a one-way antireflux valve for Salem sump tube.

inserted to monitor gastrointestinal bleeding. Historically, a nasogastric tube has often been used postoperatively as a routine part of care after major abdominal surgery, to rest the intestinal tract and promote healing. Some research has suggested that the routine use of NGTs after abdominal surgery may serve no beneficial purpose and may actually delay the patient's progress, increasing the time required for flatus to occur and increasing pulmonary complications (Lafon & Lawson, 2012). It is suggested that selective decompression should be reserved for patients with nausea, vomiting, and abdominal distention after surgery (Brennan, 2008; Gannon, 2007; Nelson, Edwards, & Tse, 2007).

A nasogastric tube is a pliable single- or double-lumen (inner open space) tube that is hollow, allowing for the removal of gastric secretions and instillation of solutions into the stomach. The tube is passed through the nasopharynx into the stomach (Fig. 37-8). Refer to Chapter 35, Skill 35-1 on pages 1240–1246, for the procedure for nasogastric tube insertion and Skill 35-3 on pages 1253–1255 for the procedure for removal of a nasogastric tube. Tubes for decompression typically are attached to suction. Suction can be applied intermittently or continuously.

The Levine tube is a common single-lumen tube. It lacks a venting system, and mucosal damage can occur when suction is applied continuously. Therefore, suction usually is applied intermittently. Salem sump nasogastric tubes are double-lumen tubes. One lumen empties the stomach, and the other provides for a continuous flow of air. The airflow lumen controls suction by preventing the drainage lumen from pulling stomach mucosa into the tube's openings and irritating the stomach lining. A one-way antireflux valve may be used in the airflow lumen to prevent reflux of gastric contents through the airflow lumen (see Fig. 37-8). When pressure from gastric con-

tents enters the airflow tubing, the valve closes to prevent secretions from exiting the tube.

Nasogastric tubes used for decompression require irrigation with 30 to 60 mL of normal saline solution to maintain patency. Skill 37-2 on pages 1382–1385 describes the procedure for irrigating a nasogastric tube connected to suction.

To promote patient safety when instilling solutions into a nasogastric tube, tube placement must be verified before administration of any fluids or medications. Radiographic examination, measurement of aspirate pH, visual assessment of aspirate, measurement of tube length and measurement of tube marking, and monitoring of carbon dioxide are used to confirm nasogastric tube placement. With the exception of radiographic examination, the use of several of these techniques in conjunction with each other increases the likelihood of correct tube placement. An old technique of auscultation of air injected into a nasogastric tube has proved unreliable and may result in tragic consequences if used as an indicator of tube placement (American Association of Critical-Care Nurses [AACN], 2010; Best, 2005; Khair, 2005). Therefore, do not use it to confirm nasogastric tube placement.

Radiographic examination to confirm placement is the most accurate method for checking if the NG tube is in the stomach, but is often only ordered on initial placement, and many times is not prescribed for nasogastric tubes inserted for decompression. Two methods recommended for checking placement, other than radiograph, are visual assessment of aspirated gastric contents and measuring the pH of the aspirate (AACN, 2010; Best, 2005; Hinkle & Cheever, 2014). Refer to Chapter 35, Guidelines for Nursing Care 35-1; Visual Assessment and pH Measurement of Gastric Contents on page 1227. In addition, the length of the exposed tube is measured and marked after insertion and documented. Check and compare tube length with this initial measurement, in conjunction with the previous two methods for checking tube placement. An increase in the length of the exposed tube may indicate dislodgement (AACN, 2010; Hinkle & Cheever, 2014). Marking the tube with an indelible marker at the nostril and then assessing this marking each time the tube is used ensures that the tube has not become displaced.

Monitoring for carbon dioxide to determine nasogastric tube position and/or dislodgement has been evaluated (Gilbert & Burns, 2012; Chau, Lo, Thompson, Fernandez, & Griffiths, 2011; Munera-Seeley et al., 2008). This involves the use of a capnograph or a colorimetric end-tidal CO_2 detector to detect the presence of carbon dioxide, which would indicate tube positioning in the patient's airway. However, a carbon dioxide sensor cannot determine where a nasogastric tube's tip ends in the gastrointestinal tract (esophagus, stomach, or small bowel; AACN, 2010).

Patients with nasogastric tubes often experience discomfort related to irritation to nasal and throat mucosa, and drying of the oral mucous membranes. Administer oral hygiene frequently, as often as every 2 to 4 hours, to prevent drying of tissues and to relieve thirst. Frequently offer the patient the opportunity to rinse the mouth with warm water and mouthwash solution. Lubricate the lips generously. Keep the nares clean, especially around the tube, where secretions tend to accumulate. Use a lubricant after cleaning the nares. Help control local irritation from the tube in the throat by offering analgesic throat lozenges or anesthetic sprays, as prescribed. Ensure that the tube is secured to the patient's nose and gown to prevent tension and tugging on the tube, causing trauma to the nares and potential displacement.

Meeting the Needs of Patients With Bowel Diversions

Sometimes patients undergo surgical procedures to create an opening into the abdominal wall for fecal elimination. The word **ostomy** is a term for a surgically formed opening from the inside of an organ to the outside. The intestinal mucosa is brought out to the abdominal wall, and a **stoma**, the part of the ostomy that is attached to the skin, is formed by suturing the mucosa to the skin. An **ileostomy** allows liquid fecal content from the ileum of the small intestine to be eliminated through the stoma. A **colostomy** permits formed feces in the colon to exit through the stoma. Colostomies are further classified by the part of the colon from which they originate. Figure 37-9 shows the location of an ileostomy and various colostomies. In many institutions, if the ostomy surgery is not emergent, patients meet with a specially trained registered nurse called a wound, ostomy, and continence nurse (WOCN). Together, they determine the ideal location for the stoma.

An ileostomy or colostomy may be either temporary or permanent. Temporary ostomies are performed to allow the intestine to repair itself after inflammatory disease, some types of intestinal surgery, or injury. The patient

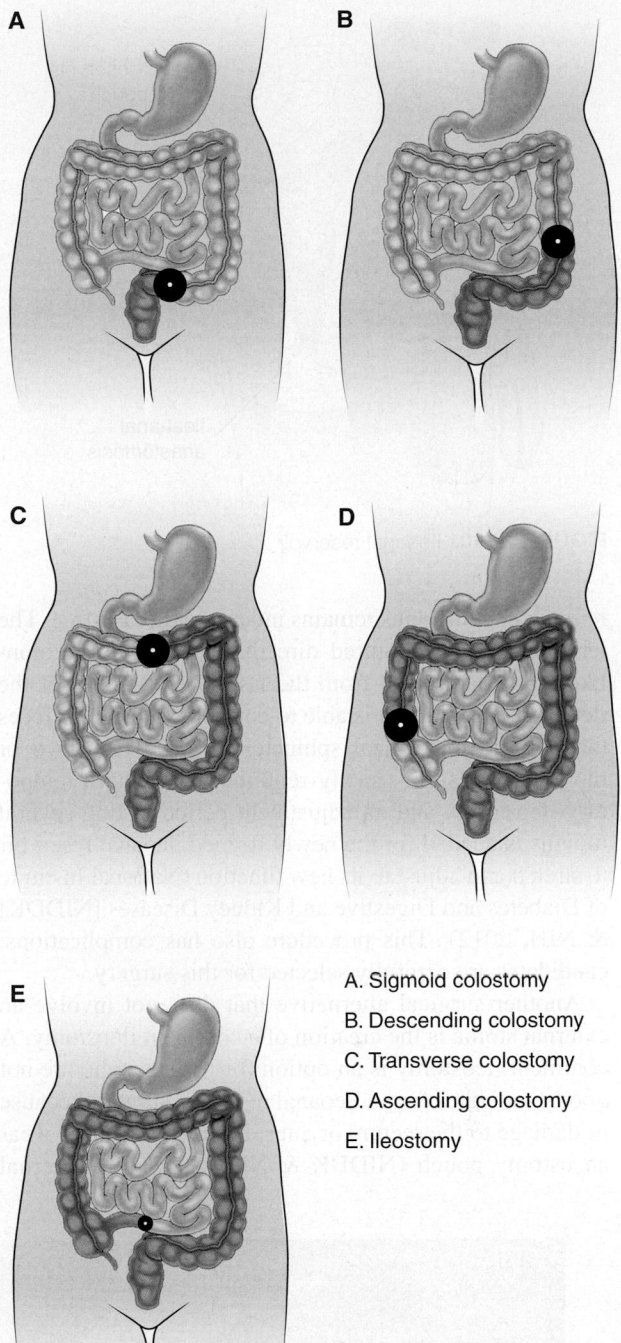

A. Sigmoid colostomy

B. Descending colostomy

C. Transverse colostomy

D. Ascending colostomy

E. Ileostomy

FIGURE 37-9. (**A–D**) Location of various colostomies, and (**E**) location of an ileostomy. The shaded portions represent the sections of the bowel that have been removed or are currently inactive.

returns for a second surgery in several weeks, and the intestine is reconnected. Permanent ostomies are performed for debilitating intestinal diseases or cancer of the colon or rectum. Patients will have these ostomies for the rest of their lives.

A surgical intervention that does not involve an external stoma is the creation of an ileoanal reservoir. Ileoanal reservoir surgery is an option when the large intestine is

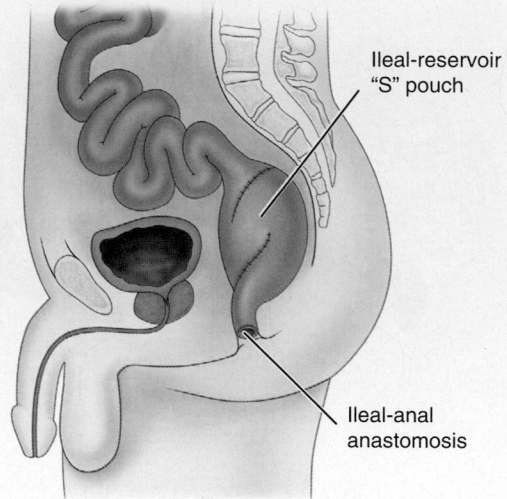

FIGURE 37-10. Ileoanal reservoir.

removed but the anus remains intact and disease-free. The terminal ileum is sutured directly to the anus, a colon-like pouch is created from the last several inches of the ileum, and the patient is able to control expulsion of feces through the intact anal sphincter (Fig. 37-10). Two or more surgeries are usually required, including a temporary ileostomy, and an adjustment period lasting several months is needed for the newly formed ileoanal reservoir to stretch and adjust to its new function (National Institute of Diabetes and Digestive and Kidney Diseases [NIDDK] & NIH, 2012). This procedure also has complications; candidates are carefully selected for this surgery.

Another surgical alternative that does not involve an external stoma is the creation of a continent ileostomy. A continent ileostomy is an option for patients who are not good candidates for an ileoanal reservoir surgery because of damage to the rectum or anus, but do not want to wear an ostomy pouch (NIDDK & NIH, 2012). An internal pouch is created that the patient can access through a nipple-like valve constructed from the ileum on the abdominal wall. The patient does not need to wear an external collection device, but because the valve malfunctions frequently, this procedure has limited use at this time.

COLOSTOMY AND ILEOSTOMY CARE

The patient with an ostomy needs physical and psychological support both preoperatively and postoperatively. This support can come from the patient's significant others, members of the health care team, and from people who have had similar experiences. The ostomy requires specific physical care for which the nurse is responsible initially. The following guidelines help to promote the ostomy patient's physical and psychological comfort:

• Keep the patient as free of odors as possible. Empty the ostomy appliance frequently.

• Inspect the patient's stoma regularly. It should be dark pink to red and moist. A pale stoma may indicate anemia, and a dark or purple-blue stoma may reflect compromised circulation or ischemia (Fig. 37-11). Bleeding around the stoma and its stem should be minimal. Notify the primary care provider promptly if bleeding persists or is excessive or if color changes occur in the stoma.

• Note the size of the stoma, which usually stabilizes within 6 to 8 weeks. Most stomas protrude ½ to 1 inch from the abdominal surface and may initially appear swollen and edematous. After 6 weeks, the edema has usually subsided. Depending on the surgical technique, the final stoma may be flush with the skin. Erosion of skin around the stoma area can also lead to a flush stoma (see Fig. 37-11). If an abdominal dressing is in place at the surgical incision, check it frequently for drainage and bleeding. The dressing is usually removed after 24 hours.

• Keep the skin around the stoma site (peristomal area) clean and dry. If care is not taken to protect the skin

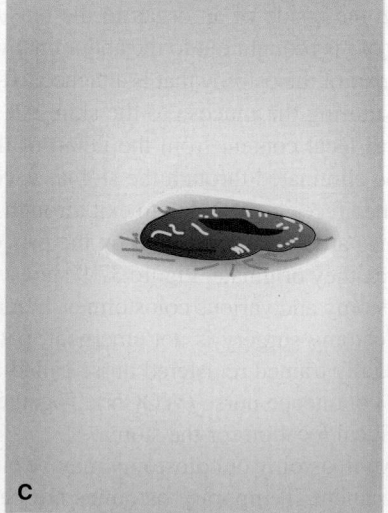

FIGURE 37-11. Comparison of stomal appearance. (**A**) Normal-appearing stoma is bright red, moist, and rounded. (**B**) A pale stoma indicates severe anemia. (**C**) Eroded skin around the area may lead to a flush stoma.

One-piece pouch   Two-piece pouch   Cut-to-fit pouch

FIGURE 37-12. Examples of ostomy pouches and closures. This equipment comes in various models and sizes. Convex pouches, belts, and other devices to prevent leaks and irritation are also available. (Courtesy of Hollister, Incorporated, Libertyville, Illinois.)

around the stoma, irritation or infection may occur. A leaking appliance frequently causes skin erosion. Candida or yeast infections can also occur around the stoma if the area is not kept dry.

- Measure the patient's fluid intake and output. Check the ostomy appliance for the quality and quantity of discharge. Initially after surgery, peristalsis may be inhibited. As peristalsis returns, stool will be eliminated from the stoma.
- Record intake and output every 4 hours for the first 3 days after surgery. If the patient's output decreases while intake remains stable, report the condition promptly.
- Explain each aspect of care to the patient and explain what the patient's role will be when beginning self-care. Patient teaching is one of the most important aspects of colostomy care and should include family members and/or people identified by the patient to include in care, when appropriate. Teaching can begin before surgery so that the patient has adequate time to absorb information.
- Encourage the patient to participate in care and to look at the ostomy. Patients normally experience emotional depression during the early postoperative period. Help the patient cope by listening, explaining, and being available and supportive. A visit from a representative of the local ostomy support group may be helpful. Patients usually begin to accept their altered body image when they are willing to look at the stoma, make neutral or positive statements concerning the ostomy, and express interest in learning self-care.

Changing the Ostomy Appliance. The ostomy appliance should protect the skin, collect the fecal discharge, and control odor. Typically, a colostomy does not produce drainage until normal peristalsis returns, usually within 2 to 5 days. An ileostomy drains within 24 to 48 hours because of the liquid contents in the small intestine.

For the first few days after surgery, most patients wear an open-ended appliance that allows for drainage of fecal material without removing the appliance. The skin barrier has an adhesive barrier that protects the surrounding skin from the stoma output. Appliances are either one-piece (barrier backing already attached to the pouch) or two-piece (separate pouch that fastens to the barrier backing). A transparent one-piece appliance is used in the initial postoperative period to allow for visualization of the stoma.

Appliances can be either drainable or closed. Empty a pouch that can be drained when it is one-third full and replace it every 3 to 7 days, or whenever the seal comes away from the skin. Remove and change nondrainable pouches when they are half full. Types of ostomy equipment are illustrated in Figure 37-12 and include various types of one-piece and two-piece pouches.

 RECALL Alberta Franklin, the patient with the new colostomy requiring a change of her appliance. The nurse needs to demonstrate competence and dexterity when changing this patient's bag by being adequately prepared and organized. Additionally, the nurse can use the time during bag changes to teach the patient about self-care measures and to assess the patient's acceptance of the colostomy. ●

If an appliance is leaking from underneath the skin barrier, ring, or wafer, remove the bag, cleanse the skin, and apply a new bag. Changing or emptying an ostomy appliance is shown in Skill 37-3 on pages 1385–1390. The act of removing an appliance from the skin can result in skin stripping, removal of the outer, loosely bound, epidermal cell layers. This can be uncomfortable or even very painful for the patient. The cumulative effects of skin stripping over time can result in peristomal skin breakdown. The use of a silicone-based adhesive remover allows for the easy, rapid, and painless removal of a stoma pouch without the associated problems of skin stripping (Rudoni, 2008; Stephen-Haynes, 2008). A skin sealant may be used to protect the skin under the skin wafer or barrier (Jones, Springfield, Brudwich, & Ladd, 2011).

Irrigating a Colostomy. Colostomy irrigation is a way of achieving fecal continence and control (Perston, 2010). Irrigations are used to promote regular evacuation of some colostomies. Colostomy irrigation may be indicated in patients who have a left-sided end colostomy in the descending or sigmoid colon, are mentally alert, have adequate vision, and have adequate manual dexterity needed to perform the procedure. Contraindications include irritable bowel syndrome, peristomal hernia, post-radiation damage to the bowel, diverticulitis, and Crohn disease (Carlsson et al., 2010). Various factors, such as the site of the colostomy in the colon (descending or sigmoid colostomy) and the patient's and physician's preferences, determine whether a colostomy is irrigated. Ileostomies are not irrigated because the fecal content of the ileum is liquid and cannot be controlled.

Water is inserted into the colostomy, and the water and feces are expelled from the colostomy into the irrigation sleeve and then the toilet. Once the patient has established a routine and has established bowel continence, a small appliance can be worn over the stoma. These "stoma caps" are small-capacity appliances with a pad to soak up discharge and a flatus filter (Perston, 2010). If a colostomy irrigation is to be implemented, consult facility policy regarding the accepted procedure and, ideally, consult the WOCN for patient education and support.

Long-Term Ostomy Care. The patient can return to an active and full life with an ostomy. Make the patient aware of community resources available for assistance, such as home health care nurses, special clinics, and ostomy support groups. Encourage the patient to seek medical follow-up care on a regular basis.

Patient education is essential for independence in self-care. As the patient assumes responsibility for self-care, teach the patient how to make the necessary observations, to be aware of indications of problems, and to recognize when to seek assistance. For these goals to be met, the patient and/or family member needs to be able to do the following:

- Explain the reason for bowel diversion and the rationale for treatment.
- Demonstrate self-care behaviors that effectively manage the ostomy.
- Describe follow-up care and existing support resources.
- Report where supplies may be obtained in the community.
- Verbalize related fears and concerns.
- Demonstrate a positive body image.

The assistance of a wound, ostomy, and continence nurse (WOCN) can help the patient achieve these outcomes. Also, refer the patient to the United Ostomy Association for further information and helpful periodicals.

During the first 6 to 8 weeks after surgery, encourage the patient with an ostomy to avoid foods high in fiber (e.g., foods with skins, seeds, shells) as well as any other foods that cause diarrhea or excessive flatus. By gradually adding new foods, the ostomy patient can progress to a normal diet. Urge patients to drink at least 2 quarts of fluids, preferably water, daily. Additional dietary considerations for patients with an ileostomy or colostomy are outlined in Box 37-3.

Patients with ileostomies need to be aware they may experience a tendency to develop food blockages, especially when high-fiber foods are consumed. This is because scar tissue from the place where the intestine passes through the abdominal muscle tightens the inside

---

BOX 37-3 **DIETARY CONSIDERATIONS FOR PATIENTS WITH AN ILEOSTOMY OR COLOSTOMY**

Foods That May Cause Gas

Alcohol and beer	Fried food (some)
Carbonated beverages	Melon
Chewing gum	Onions
Chives	Peppers
Cucumbers	Pickles
Dried peas, beans, and lentils	Sauerkraut
Eggs	

Vegetables from the cabbage family such as broccoli, Brussels sprouts, cabbage, cauliflower, and turnip

Foods That May Cause Stomal Blockage

Bean sprouts	Nuts
Cabbage	Olives
Carrots (raw)	Peas
Celery	Pickles
Coconut	Pineapple
Corn	Popcorn
Cucumbers	Seeds
Dried fruit	Skins and seeds from
Green pepper skin	fruits and vegetables
Lettuce	Spinach
Mushrooms	

Foods That May Help To Control Diarrhea

Applesauce	Soda crackers
Bananas	Starchy foods (rice, pasta,
Cheese	barley)
Creamy peanut butter	Tapioca
Oatmeal or oat bran	Yogurt
Potatoes	

Foods That Produce Odor

Asparagus	Garlic
Dried peas, beans, and lentils	Onions
Eggs	Some spicy foods
Fish	Turnip

Foods That Are Natural Intestinal Deodorizers

Buttermilk
Parsley
Yogurt

diameter of the ileum and can narrow it to much less than its normal 1-inch diameter. Fiber blockages can cause foul-smelling watery output, abdominal cramping, and distention, along with nausea and vomiting.

Health teaching about medication use is frequently overlooked for patients with ostomies. Some medications may discolor the stool and cause unusual odors, some may cause constipation, and some may not dissolve or be absorbed completely because the small bowel is where most absorption occurs. The use of liquid, chewable, or injectable forms rather than long-acting, enteric-coated, or sustained-release medications is recommended. Laxatives and enemas are dangerous because they may cause severe fluid and electrolyte imbalance.

Many times, patients are embarrassed when they have to use public restrooms to empty their bag. Teach patients with ostomies about the various methods of odor control. Remind them that if the bag is clean and sealed well, odor usually is not a problem during normal activity. Encourage the intake of dark green vegetables. These vegetables contain chlorophyll, which helps to deodorize the feces. Buttermilk, cranberry juice, parsley, and yogurt can also prevent odor. Crackers, toast, and yogurt can help to reduce gas, which in turn aids in odor control. Commercial odor-control products also are available for purchase. The WOCN can help with the selection of odor-control strategies.

The patient with an ostomy can resume normal activity, including work and sexual relations. However, the patient should avoid direct physical contact sports and heavy lifting. The patient can go swimming. When traveling, the patient should carry a 1- to 2-day supply of equipment in a carry-on bag in case checked luggage is lost. Nurses play a significant role in helping patients, their families, and significant others adjust to this major life change. These surgeries result in physical discomfort, changes in body image, loss of body function, and changes in personal hygiene. Patients need significant physical and psychological support to adjust to these changes. See the accompanying display, Research in Nursing: Living With a Colostomy.

Evaluating

The nurse evaluates the effectiveness of the plan of care to promote regular bowel elimination by checking to see if the patient has met the individualized patient outcomes specified in the plan. Nursing care is considered effective if the patient expresses satisfaction with regular pattern of defecation and the ability to pass a soft, formed stool comfortably without the use of medications or laxatives. The plan of care is most successful when the patient is able to accomplish the following:

- Verbalize the relationships among bowel elimination and nutrition, fluid intake, exercise, and stress management.
- Develop a plan to modify any factors that contribute to current bowel problems or that might adversely affect bowel functioning in the future.

See the accompanying Nursing Plan of Care 37-1.

RESEARCH IN NURSING

BRIDGING THE GAP TO EVIDENCE-BASED PRACTICE

Living With a Colostomy

A stoma operation causes major changes in a patient's life because of the resulting physical damage, disfigurement, loss of bodily function, and change in personal hygiene. Such changes are a cause of major concern for patients and raise important issues for the provision of quality care.

Related Research

Notter, J., & Chalmers, F. (2012). Living with a colostomy: a pilot study. *Gastrointestinal Nursing, 10*(6), 16, 18, 20, 22–24.

This survey explored issues impacting on coping and quality of life for those living with a colostomy. Questionnaires were sent to 1,000 patients with ostomies who volunteered to participate in research studies. The response rate was 47%; of the 469 questionnaires returned, 369 were used for descriptive data analysis. The remaining 100 responses could not be analyzed, as they were incomplete. Over 97% of the respondents were over 50 years of age; almost 30% reported complications necessitating further admissions and/or more surgery. Restrictions on activities of daily living, including social activities with family and friends, were present for 40% of respondents. Problems with leakage were reported by 50% of the participants and 33% found emptying and/or dis-

posal of used appliances to be a problem. Thirty-five percent of men and 37% of women reported experienced emotional problems, such as body image and self-confidence, adjustment to the impact of major surgery, and depression. In addition, participants (30% of men and 27% of women) reported that intimacy with their partner had been adversely affected.

Relevance to Nursing Practice

Patients experiencing life-altering surgeries, such as colostomies and ileostomies, require much information and support to adapt and achieve an adequate standard of living. Nurses are the members of the health care team who typically spend the most time in direct contact with these patients. Nurses have a unique opportunity to provide the education and support these patients need, and improve the care provided to these patients. In addition to assisting patients to learn the physical care needs related to a stoma, nurses must address the psychosocial concerns of patients with ostomies as part of their nursing interventions. Assisting patients to adjust and encouraging social interactions should be part of the care routinely given to stoma patients.

For additional research, visit thePoint.

NURSING PLAN OF CARE 37-1

for Jeremy Green

Jeremy Green, 4 years of age, was placed in daycare when his mother returned to work 6 months ago. He presents at the hospital with a diagnosis of viral gastro-enteritis. A comprehensive nursing assessment included the following notations:

- Admitted with complaints of diarrhea beginning 3 days ago.
- Seen today by pediatrician who recommended admission and work-up to exclude causes other than viral.
- Mother reports liquid stools (no observable blood, pus, or mucus) six to seven times daily beginning 3 days ago with amounts of "one to two cups."
- Urgency results in soiling of pants.

- Child has sipped boiled skim milk and cola and eaten a small amount of broth and a few pretzels, but has no appetite.
- Complained of nausea and vomited twice 3 days ago.
- Child is pale and eyes are sunken.
- Skin is warm and dry, with decreased turgor and dry mucous membranes.
- Hyperactive bowel sounds (52/minute)
- Height, 45 inches; weight, 36 lb; temperature, 99.8°F (rectally); pulse, 88 beats/min; respiratory rate, 18 breaths/min
- Mother reported several other children in same day-care center are out sick with diarrhea.

NURSING DIAGNOSIS Diarrhea related to unknown cause (possibly viral, rule out malabsorption of lactose and other causes) as manifested by passage of liquid stools (1–2 cups) for 3 days; urgency with fecal soiling.

EXPECTED OUTCOME At the time of discharge, the patient will:

- Voluntarily pass a formed stool of usual consistency (experience less or no diarrhea)

NURSING INTERVENTIONS	RATIONALE	EVALUATIVE STATEMENT
Assess and chart frequency and amount of diarrhea, stool characteristics, precipitating factors, and accompanying manifestations (gastrointestinal symptoms, hyperactive bowel sounds).	This assists in identifying the cause of the diarrhea.	5/8/15 Outcome partially met. No recurrence of liquid stools for 24 hours. Revision: Continue to monitor. *D. Lentsky, RN*

EXPECTED OUTCOME At the time of discharge, the patient will:

- Exhibit decreased bowel sounds (5–34/min)

NURSING INTERVENTIONS	RATIONALE	EVALUATIVE STATEMENT
Work collaboratively with the physician to identify the cause of the diarrhea. Obtain stool specimens and send to laboratory.	Correct treatment depends on identification of the cause of the diarrhea. Viral diarrhea is usually self-limiting and lasts 24 to 72 hours. Prolonged diarrhea after acute viral illness may be from temporary malabsorption of lactose or other simple sugars.	5/8/15 Outcome met. Bowel sounds are normal. *D. Lentsky, RN*
Instruct Jeremy and his parents (if they want to participate in care) on correct infection control precautions for handling stool.	Proper precautions prevent transmissions of infectious diarrhea to others.	

NURSING PLAN OF CARE 37-1   *continued*

for Jeremy Green

NURSING INTERVENTIONS	RATIONALE	EVALUATIVE STATEMENT
Increase frequency and length of rest periods and discourage strenuous activity.	Exercise and activity stimulate peristalsis.	
Administer prescribed antidiarrheal medication and observe for adverse effects.	Antidiarrheal medications may cause drowsiness and dizziness. These agents may be used in diarrhea due to viruses to slow peristalsis and passage of stool.	

SAMPLE DOCUMENTATION	
	5/7/15 Nursing Liquid stools have decreased to two in the past 24 hours. Negative report on stool culture; Dr. Simpson notified of results. Normal bowel sounds auscultated in all four quadrants. Patient denies pain, nausea, and cramping. *D. Lentsky, RN*

SKILL 37-1   ADMINISTERING A LARGE-VOLUME CLEANSING ENEMA

DELEGATION CONSIDERATIONS

The administration of some types of enemas may be delegated to nursing assistive personnel (NAP) or unlicensed assistive personnel (UAP) who have received appropriate training. The administration of a large-volume cleansing enema may be delegated to licensed practical/vocational nurses (LPN/LVNs). The decision to delegate must be based on careful analysis of the patient's needs and circumstances, as well as the qualifications of the person to whom the task is being delegated. Refer to the Delegation Guidelines in Appendix A (found on the Point).

EQUIPMENT

- Enema solution as ordered at a temperature of 105°F to 110°F (40°C to 43°C) for adults in the prescribed amount. (Amount will vary depending on type of solution, patient's age, and patient's ability to retain the solution. Average cleansing enema for an adult may range from 750 to 1,000 mL.)
- Disposable enema set, which includes a solution container and tubing
- Water-soluble lubricant
- IV pole
- Necessary additives, as ordered
- Waterproof pad
- Bath thermometer (if available)
- Bath blanket
- Bedpan and toilet tissue
- Disposable gloves
- Additional PPE, as indicated
- Paper towel
- Washcloth, skin cleanser, and towel

IMPLEMENTATION

ACTION	RATIONALE
1. Verify the order for the enema. Gather equipment.	Verifying the medical order is crucial to ensuring that the proper enema is administered to the right patient. Assembling equipment provides for an organized approach to the task.
2. Perform hand hygiene and put on PPE, if indicated.	Hand hygiene and PPE prevent the spread of microorganisms. PPE is required based on transmission precautions.

(continued)

SKILL 37-1 ADMINISTERING A LARGE-VOLUME CLEANSING ENEMA *continued*

ACTION	RATIONALE
3. Identify the patient.	Identifying the patient ensures that the right patient receives the intervention and helps prevent errors.
4. Explain the procedure to the patient and provide the rationale as to why the tube is needed. Discuss the associated discomforts that may be experienced and possible interventions that may allay this discomfort. Answer any questions as needed.	Explanation facilitates patient cooperation and reduces anxiety.
5. Assemble equipment on the overbed table within reach.	Arranging items nearby is convenient, saves time, and avoids unnecessary stretching and twisting of muscles on the part of the nurse.
6. Close the curtains around the bed and close the door to the room, if possible. Discuss where the patient will defecate. Have a bedpan, commode, or nearby bathroom ready for use.	This ensures the patient's privacy. Explanation relieves anxiety and facilitates cooperation. The patient is better able to relax and cooperate if familiar with the procedure and knowing everything is in readiness when the urge to defecate is felt. Defecation usually occurs within 5 to 15 minutes.
7. Warm the enema solution in the amount ordered, and check the temperature with a bath thermometer, if available. If a bath thermometer is not available, warm to room temperature or slightly higher, and test on the inner wrist. If tap water is used, adjust temperature as it flows from the faucet (Fig. 1).	Warming the solution prevents chilling the patient, adding to the discomfort of the procedure. Cold solution could cause cramping; a too-warm solution could cause trauma to the intestinal mucosa.
8. Add the enema solution to the container. Release the clamp and allow the fluid to progress through the tube before reclamping.	This causes any air to be expelled from the tubing. Although allowing air to enter the intestine is not harmful, it may further distend the intestine.
9. Adjust the bed to a comfortable working height, usually elbow height of the caregiver (VISN 8 Patient Safety Center, 2009). Position the patient on the left side (Sims position), as dictated by patient comfort and condition. Fold top linen back just enough to allow access to the patient's rectal area. Drape the patient with the bath blanket as necessary to maintain privacy and warmth. Place a waterproof pad under the patient's hip.	Having the bed at the proper height prevents back and muscle strain. Sims' position facilitates flow of solution via gravity into the rectum and colon, optimizing solution retention. Folding back the linen in this manner minimizes unnecessary exposure and promotes the patient's comfort and warmth. The waterproof pad will protect the bed.
10. Put on gloves.	Gloves prevent contact with contaminants and body fluids.
11. Elevate solution so that it is no higher than 18 inches (45 cm) above level of anus (Fig. 2). Plan to give the solution slowly over a period of 5 to 10 minutes. Hang the container on an IV pole or hold it at the proper height.	Gravity forces the solution to enter the intestine. The amount of pressure determines the rate of flow and pressure exerted on the intestinal wall. Giving the solution too quickly causes rapid distention and pressure, poor defecation, or damage to the mucous membrane.

FIGURE 1. Preparing enema bag.

FIGURE 2. Adjusting the height of the solution container until it is no more than 18 inches above the patient.

ACTION

12. Generously lubricate the end of the rectal tube 2 to 3 inches (5–7 cm). A disposable enema set may have a prelubricated rectal tube.

13. Lift the buttock to expose the anus. Ask the patient to take several deep breaths. Slowly and gently insert the enema tube 3 to 4 inches (7–10 cm) for an adult. Direct it at an angle pointing toward the umbilicus, not the bladder (Fig. 3).

14. If resistance is met while inserting the tube, permit a small amount of solution to enter, withdraw tube slightly, and then continue to insert it. **Do not force entry of the tube.** Ask the patient to take several deep breaths.

15. Introduce solution slowly over a period of 5 to 10 minutes. Hold the tubing all the time that the solution is being instilled. Assess for dizziness, lightheadedness, nausea, diaphoresis, and clammy skin during administration. **If the patient experiences any of these symptoms, stop the procedure immediately, monitor the patient's heart rate and blood pressure, and notify the primary care provider.**

16. Clamp the tubing or lower container if the patient has the urge to defecate or cramping occurs (Fig. 4). Instruct the patient to take small, fast breaths or to pant.

RATIONALE

Lubrication facilitates passage of the rectal tube through the anal sphincter and prevents injury to the mucosa.

Good visualization of the anus helps prevent injury to tissues. Deep breathing helps relax the anal sphincters. The anal canal is about 1 to 2 inches (2.5–5 cm) long. Insertion 3 to 4 inches ensures that the tube is inserted past the external and internal anal sphincters; further insertion may damage the intestinal mucous membrane. The suggested angle follows the normal intestinal contour and thus will help to prevent perforation of the bowel. Slow insertion of the tube minimizes spasms of the intestinal wall and sphincters.

Resistance may be due to spasms of the intestine or failure of the internal sphincter to open. The solution may help to reduce spasms and relax the sphincter, thus making continued insertion of the tube safe. Forcing a tube may injure the intestinal mucosa wall. Taking deep breaths helps relax the anal sphincter.

Introducing the solution slowly helps prevent rapid distention of the intestine and a desire to defecate. Assessment allows for detection of a vagal response. The enema may stimulate a vagal response, which increases parasympathetic stimulation, causing a decrease in heart rate.

These techniques help relax muscles and prevent premature expulsion of the solution.

FIGURE 3. Inserting enema tip into anus, directing tip toward umbilicus.

FIGURE 4. Holding bag lower to slow flow of enema solution.

(continued)

SKILL 37-1 ADMINISTERING A LARGE-VOLUME CLEANSING ENEMA *continued*

ACTION	RATIONALE
17. After solution has been given, clamp the tubing (Fig. 5) and remove the tube. Have a paper towel ready to receive the tube as it is withdrawn.	Wrapping tube in a paper towel prevents dripping of solution.
18. Return the patient to a comfortable position. Encourage the patient to hold the solution until the urge to defecate is strong, usually in about 5 to 15 minutes. Make sure the linens under the patient are dry. Remove your gloves and ensure that the patient is covered.	This amount of time usually allows muscle contractions to become sufficient to produce good results. Promotes patient comfort. Removing contaminated gloves prevents spread of microorganisms.
19. Raise the side rail. Lower the bed height and adjust the head of the bed to a comfortable position.	Promotes patient safety.
20. Remove additional PPE, if used. Perform hand hygiene.	Removing PPE properly reduces the risk for infection transmission and contamination of other items. Hand hygiene prevents the spread of microorganisms.
21. When the patient has a strong urge to defecate, place the patient in a sitting position on a bedpan or assist to the commode or bathroom. Offer toilet tissues, if not in the patient's reach (Fig. 6). Stay with the patient or have the call bell readily accessible.	The sitting position is most natural and facilitates defecation. Fall prevention is a high priority due to the urgency of reaching the commode.

FIGURE 5. Clamping tubing before removing.

FIGURE 6. Offering toilet tissue to patient on bedside commode.

ACTION	RATIONALE
22. Remind the patient not to flush the commode before you inspect the results of the enema.	The results need to be observed and recorded. Additional enemas may be necessary if the physician has ordered enemas "until clear." Refer to "Special Considerations," on p. 1381.
23. Put on gloves and assist the patient, if necessary, with cleaning of the anal area. Offer washcloths, skin cleanser, and water for handwashing. Remove gloves.	Cleaning the anal area and proper hygiene deter the spread of microorganisms. Gloves prevent contact with contaminants and body fluids.
24. Leave the patient clean and comfortable. Care for equipment properly.	Bacteria that grow in the intestine can be spread to others if equipment is not properly cleaned.
25. Perform hand hygiene.	Hand hygiene deters the spread of microorganisms.

DOCUMENTATION

Guidelines

Document the amount and type of enema solution used; amount, consistency, and color of stool; pain assessment rating; assessment of perineal area for any irritation, tears, or bleeding; and the patient's reaction to the procedure.

Sample Documentation

> 7/22/15 1310 800 mL warm tap water enema given via rectum. Large amount of soft, brown stool returned. No irritation, tears, or bleeding noted in perineal area. Patient complained of "stomach cramping," relieved when enema was released. Rates pain as 0 after evacuation of enema.
>
> —*K. Sanders, RN*

UNEXPECTED SITUATIONS AND ASSOCIATED INTERVENTIONS

- *Solution does not flow into rectum:* Reposition rectal tube. If solution will still not flow, remove tube and check for any fecal contents.
- *Patient cannot retain enema solution for adequate amount of time:* Patient may need to be placed on a bedpan in the supine position while receiving the enema. The head of the bed may be elevated 30 degrees for the patient's comfort.
- *Patient cannot tolerate large amount of enema solution:* Amount and length of administration may have to be modified if the patient begins to complain of pain.
- *Patient complains of severe cramping with introduction of enema solution:* Lower solution container and check temperature and flow rate. If the solution is too cold or flow rate too fast, severe cramping may occur.

SPECIAL CONSIDERATIONS

General Considerations

- Do not use rectal agents and rectal manipulation, including enemas, with patients who are myelosuppressed and/or patients at risk for myelosuppression and mucositis. These interventions can lead to development of bleeding, anal fissures, or abscesses, which are portals for infection (NCI, 2012).
- If the patient experiences fullness or pain or if fluid escapes around the tube, stop administration. Wait 30 seconds to a minute and then restart the flow at a slower rate. If symptoms persist, stop administration and contact the patient's physician.
- If the order states that the enema is to be given "until clear," check with the primary care provider before administering more than three enemas. Severe fluid and electrolyte imbalances may occur if the patient receives more than three cleansing enemas. Results are considered clear whenever there are no more pieces of stool in enema return. The solution may be colored but still considered a clear return.

Infant and Child Considerations

- When administering an enema to a child, use isotonic solutions. Plain water is not used because it is hypotonic and can cause rapid fluid shift and fluid overload (Perry, Hockenberry, Lowdermilk, & Wilson, 2010).
- Appropriate fluid volume for an enema (Perry et al., 2010):

  Infant: 120 to 240 mL

  2 to 4 yr: 240 to 360 mL

  4 to 10 yr: 360 to 480 mL

  11 yr: 480 to 720 mL
- Insert tubing into the rectum 2 to 3 inches for children, 1 inch for infants.

Older Adult Considerations

- If the older adult patient cannot retain the enema solution, administer the enema with the patient on the bedpan in the supine position. For comfort, elevate the head of the bed 30 degrees, if necessary, and use pillows appropriately.

SKILL 37-2 IRRIGATING A NASOGASTRIC TUBE CONNECTED TO SUCTION

DELEGATION CONSIDERATIONS

The irrigation of a nasogastric (NG) tube is not delegated to nursing assistive personnel (NAP) or unlicensed assistive personnel (UAP). Depending on the state's nurse practice act and the organization's policies and procedures, irrigation of an NG tube may be delegated to licensed practical/vocational nurses (LPN/LVNs). The decision to delegate must be based on careful analysis of the patient's needs and circumstances, as well as the qualifications of the person to whom the task is being delegated. Refer to the Delegation Guidelines in Appendix A (found on thePoint).

EQUIPMENT

- NG tube connected to continuous or intermittent suction
- Water or normal saline solution for irrigation (based on facility policy)
- Nonsterile gloves
- Additional PPE, as indicated
- Irrigation set (or a 60-mL catheter-tip syringe and cup for irrigating solution)
- Clamp

- Disposable waterproof pad or bath towel
- Emesis basin
- Tape measure or other measuring device
- pH paper and measurement scale

IMPLEMENTATION

ACTION	RATIONALE
1. Gather equipment. Verify the medical order or facility policy and procedure regarding frequency of irrigation, solution type, and amount of irrigant. Check expiration dates on irrigating solution and irrigation set.	Assembling equipment provides an organized approach to the task. Verification ensures that the patient receives the correct intervention. Facility policy dictates a safe interval for reuse of equipment.
2. Perform hand hygiene and put on PPE, if indicated.	Hand hygiene and PPE prevent the spread of microorganisms. PPE is required based on transmission precautions.
3. Identify the patient.	Identifying the patient ensures that the right patient receives the intervention and helps prevent errors.
4. Explain the procedure to the patient and why this intervention is needed. Answer any questions as needed. Perform key abdominal assessments.	Explanation facilitates patient cooperation. Due to potential changes in the patient's condition, assessment is vital before initiating the intervention.
5. Assemble equipment on the overbed table within reach.	Organization facilitates performance of the task.
6. Pull the patient's bedside curtain. Raise the bed to a comfortable working position, usually elbow height of the caregiver (VISN 8 Patient Safety Center, 2009). Assist the patient to a 30- to 45-degree position, unless this is contraindicated. Pour the irrigating solution into a container.	Provide for privacy. Appropriate working height facilitates comfort and proper body mechanics for the nurse. This position minimizes risk for aspiration. Preparing the irrigation provides an organized approach to the task.
7. Put on gloves. Place a waterproof pad on the patient's chest, under the connection of the nasogastric tube and suction tubing. **Check placement of the NG tube.**	Gloves prevent contact with body fluids. Waterproof pad protects the patient's clothing and bed linens from accidental leakage of gastric fluid. Checking placement before the instillation of the fluid is necessary to prevent accidental instillation into the respiratory tract if the tube has become dislodged.

ACTION

8. Draw up 30 mL of irrigation solution (or the amount indicated in the order or policy) into a syringe (Fig. 1).

9. Clamp the nasogastric tube near the connection site. Disconnect the tube from the suction apparatus (Fig. 2) and lay on disposable pad or towel, or hold both tubes upright in your nondominant hand (Fig. 3).

10. Place the tip of the syringe in the tube. **If a Salem sump or double-lumen tube is used, make sure that the syringe tip is placed in the drainage port and not in the blue air vent.** Hold the syringe upright and gently insert the irrigant (Fig. 4), or allow the solution to flow in by gravity if facility policy or medical order indicates. **Do not force the solution into the tube.**

RATIONALE

This delivers a measured amount of irrigant through the tube. Saline solution (isotonic) may be used to compensate for electrolytes lost through nasogastric drainage.

Clamping prevents leakage of gastric fluid.

Gentle insertion of saline solution (or gravity insertion) is less traumatic to the gastric mucosa.

The blue air vent acts to decrease pressure built up in the stomach when the Salem sump is attached to suction. It is not to be used for irrigation.

FIGURE 1. Preparing syringe with 30 mL of irrigation solution.

FIGURE 2. Clamping nasogastric tube while disconnecting.

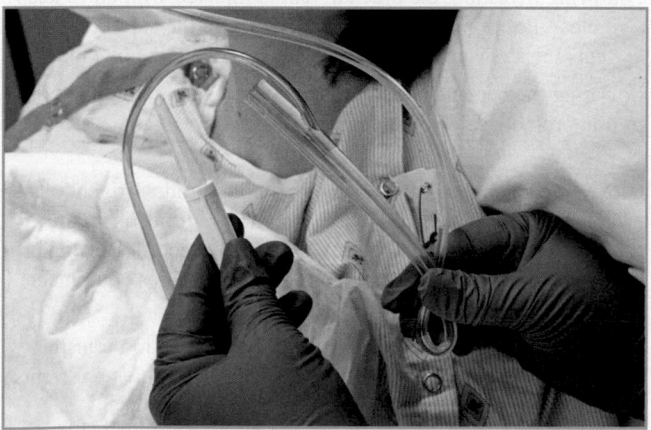

FIGURE 3. Holding both tubes upright to prevent leakage of gastric fluid.

FIGURE 4. Gently instilling irrigation.

(continued)

SKILL 37-2   IRRIGATING A NASOGASTRIC TUBE CONNECTED TO SUCTION *continued*

ACTION

11. **If unable to irrigate the tube, reposition the patient and attempt irrigation again. Inject 10 to 20 mL of air and aspirate again (Fig. 5). If repeated attempts to irrigate the tube fail, consult with the primary care provider or follow facility policy.**

12. After irrigant has been instilled, hold the end of the NG tube over an irrigation tray or emesis basin. Observe for return flow of NG drainage into an available container. Alternately, you may reconnect the NG tube to suction and observe the return drainage as it drains into the suction container.

13. If not already done, reconnect the drainage port to the suction, if ordered.

14. Inject air into the blue air vent after irrigation is complete. Position the blue air vent above the patient's stomach.

15. Remove gloves. Lower the bed and raise the side rails, as necessary. Assist the patient to a position of comfort. Perform hand hygiene.

16. Put on gloves. Measure the returned solution, if collected outside of the suction apparatus. Rinse equipment if it will be reused. Label with the date, patient's name, room number, and purpose (for NG tube/irrigation).

17. Remove gloves and additional PPE, if used. Perform hand hygiene.

RATIONALE

Tube may be positioned against the gastric mucosa, making it difficult to irrigate. Injection of air may reposition the end of the tube.

FIGURE 5. Injecting 10 to 20 mL of air into tube.

Return flow may be collected in an irrigating tray or other available container and measured. This amount will need to be subtracted from the irrigant to record the true NG drainage. A second method involves subtracting the total irrigant from the shift from the total NG drainage emptied over the entire shift, to find the true NG drainage. Check agency policy for guidelines.

Observation determines patency of the tube and the correct operation of the suction apparatus.

Allows for continued removal of gastric contents as ordered.

Following irrigation, the blue air vent is injected with air to keep it clear. Positioning the blue air vent above the stomach prevents the stomach contents from leaking from the NG tube.

Lowering the bed and assisting the patient to a comfortable position promote safety and comfort.

Gloves prevent contact with blood and body fluids. Irrigant placed in the tube is considered intake; solution returned is recorded as output. Record on the intake and output record. Rinsing promotes cleanliness, infection control, and prepares equipment for the next irrigation.

Removing PPE properly reduces the risk for infection transmission and contamination of other items. Hand hygiene prevents transmission of microorganisms.

DOCUMENTATION
Guidelines

Document assessment of the patient's abdomen. Record if the patient's NG tube is clamped or connected to suction, including the type of suction. Document the color and consistency of the NG drainage. Record the solution type and amount used to irrigate the NG tube, as well as ease of irrigation or any difficulty related to the procedure. Record the amount of returned irrigant, if collected outside of the suction apparatus. Alternately, record the irrigant amount so it can be subtracted from the total NG drainage amount at the end of the shift. Record the patient's response to the procedure and any pertinent teaching points that were reviewed, such as instructions for the patient to contact the nurse for any feelings of nausea, bloating, or abdominal pain.

Sample Documentation

> 10/15/15 1100 Abdomen slightly distended but soft; absent bowel sounds, denies nausea. NG tube placement confirmed; gastric contents clear with brown flecks, pH 4; exposed NG tube 20 cm, consistent with documented length. NG tube irrigated with 30 mL of normal saline. NG tube reconnected to low intermittent suction. Clear drainage with brown flecks noted from tube. Patient tolerated irrigation without incident.
>
> —S. Essner, RN

UNEXPECTED SITUATIONS AND ASSOCIATED INTERVENTIONS

- *Flush solution is meeting a lot of force when plunger is pushed:* Inject 20 to 30 mL of free air into the abdomen in an attempt to reposition the tube and enable flushing of the tube.

- *Tube is connected to suction as ordered, but nothing is draining from tube:* First check the suction canister to ensure that the suction is working appropriately. Disconnect the NG tube from suction and place your gloved thumb over the end of the suction tubing. If there is suction present, the problem lies in the NG tube itself. Next, attempt to flush the tube to ensure its patency.

- *After flushing the tube, the tube is not reconnected to suction as ordered:* Reconnect the tube to suction as soon as the error is noticed. Assess the abdomen for distention and ask the patient if he or she is experiencing any nausea or any abdominal discomfort. Complete any paperwork per institutional policy, such as an incident report.

SPECIAL CONSIDERATIONS

- A one-way, anti-reflux valve may be used in the airflow lumen to prevent reflux of gastric contents through the airflow lumen (see Fig. 5). When pressure from gastric contents enters the airflow tubing, the valve closes to prevent secretions from exiting the tube. This valve is removed before flushing the lumen with air, and then replaced.

- Monitoring for carbon dioxide to determine NG tube position and/or dislodgement has been investigated (Gilbert & Burns, 2012; Munera-Seeley et al., 2008). This involves the use of a capnograph or a colorimetric end-tidal CO_2 detector to detect the presence of carbon dioxide, which would indicate tube positioning in the patient's airway instead of the stomach.

SKILL 37-3 CHANGING AND EMPTYING AN OSTOMY APPLIANCE

DELEGATION CONSIDERATIONS

The empting of a stoma appliance on an ostomy may be delegated to nursing assistive personnel (NAP) or unlicensed assistive personnel (UAP), as well as to licensed practical/vocational nurses (LPN/LVNs). The changing of a stoma appliance on an ostomy may be delegated to an LPN/LVN. The decision to delegate must be based on careful analysis of the patient's needs and circumstances, as well as the qualifications of the person to whom the task is being delegated. Refer to the Delegation Guidelines in Appendix A (found on thePoint).

(continued)

SKILL 37-3 CHANGING AND EMPTYING AN OSTOMY APPLIANCE *continued*

EQUIPMENT

- Basin with warm water
- Skin cleanser, towel, washcloth
- Toilet tissue or paper towel
- Silicone-based adhesive remover
- Gauze squares
- Washcloth
- Skin protectant, such as SkinPrep
- One-piece ostomy appliance

- Closure clamp, if required, for appliance
- Stoma measuring guide
- Graduated container, toilet or bedpan
- Ostomy belt (optional)
- Disposable gloves
- Additional PPE, as indicated
- Small plastic trash bag
- Waterproof disposable pad

IMPLEMENTATION

ACTION	RATIONALE
1. Gather equipment.	Assembling equipment provides an organized approach to the task.
2. Perform hand hygiene and put on PPE, if indicated.	Hand hygiene and PPE prevent the spread of microorganisms. PPE is required based on transmission precautions.
3. Identify the patient.	Identifying the patient ensures that the right patient receives the intervention and helps prevent errors.
4. Close curtains around the bed and close the door to the room, if possible. Explain what you are going to do and why you are going to do it to the patient. Encourage the patient to observe or participate, if possible.	This ensures the patient's privacy. Explanation relieves anxiety and facilitates cooperation. Discussion promotes cooperation and helps to minimize anxiety. Having the patient observe or assist encourages self-acceptance.
5. Assemble equipment on the overbed table within reach.	Arranging items nearby is convenient, saves time, and avoids unnecessary stretching and twisting of muscles on the part of the nurse.
6. Assist the patient to a comfortable sitting or lying position in bed or a standing or sitting position in the bathroom. If the patient is in bed, adjust the bed to a comfortable working height, usually elbow height of the caregiver (VISN 8 Patient Safety Center, 2009). Place a waterproof pad under the patient at the stoma site.	Either position should allow the patient to view the procedure in preparation to learn to perform it independently. Lying flat or sitting upright facilitates smooth application of the appliance. Having the bed at the proper height prevents back and muscle strain. A waterproof pad protects linens and the patient from moisture.

Emptying an Appliance

ACTION	RATIONALE
7. Put on disposable gloves. Remove the clamp and fold the end of the appliance or pouch upward like a cuff (Fig. 1).	Gloves prevent contact with blood, body fluids, and microorganisms. Creating a cuff before emptying prevents additional soiling and odor.
8. Empty contents into a bedpan, toilet, or measuring device (Fig. 2).	Appliances do not need rinsing because rinsing may reduce appliance's odor barrier.

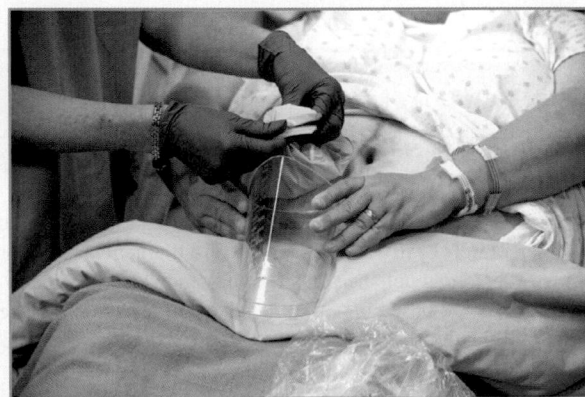

FIGURE 1. Removing clamp, getting ready to empty pouch.

FIGURE 2. Emptying contents of appliance into a measuring device.

ACTION

9. Wipe the lower 2 inches of the appliance or pouch with toilet tissue or paper towel (Fig. 3).

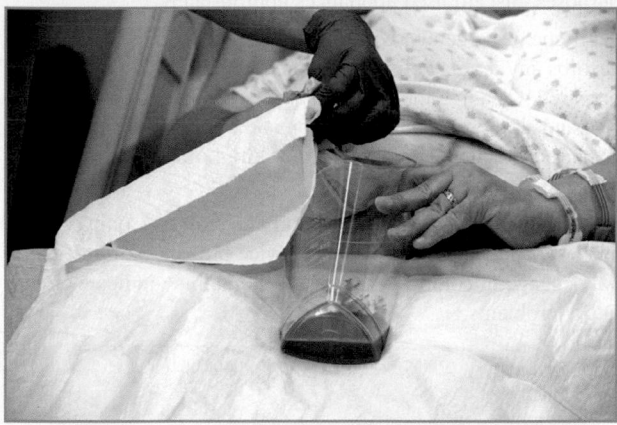

10. Uncuff the edge of the appliance or pouch and apply the clip or clamp, or secure the Velcro closure. Ensure that the curve of the clamp follows the curve of the patient's body. Remove gloves. Assist the patient to a comfortable position.

11. If the appliance is not to be changed, remove additional PPE, if used. Perform hand hygiene.

Changing an Appliance

12. Place a disposable pad on the work surface. Set up the washbasin with warm water and the rest of the supplies. Place a trash bag within reach.

13. Put on clean gloves. Place a waterproof pad under the patient at the stoma site. Empty the appliance as described previously.

14. Start at the top of the appliance and keep the abdominal skin taut. Gently remove the pouch faceplate from the skin by pushing the skin from the appliance rather than pulling the appliance from the skin (Fig. 4). Apply a silicone-based adhesive remover by spraying or wiping with the remover wipe.

RATIONALE

Drying the lower section removes any additional fecal material, thus decreasing odor problems.

FIGURE 3. Wiping lower 2 inches of pouch with paper towel.

The edge of the appliance or pouch should remain clean. The clamp secures closure. Hand hygiene deters spread of microorganisms. Ensures patient comfort.

Removing PPE properly reduces the risk for infection transmission and contamination of other items. Hand hygiene prevents the spread of microorganisms.

Protects surface. Organization facilitates performance of procedure.

Protects linens and the patient from moisture. Emptying the contents before removal prevents accidental spillage of fecal material.

The seal between the surface of the faceplate and the skin must be broken before the faceplate can be removed. Harsh handling of the appliance can damage the skin and impair the development of a secure seal in the future. Silicone-based adhesive remover allows for the rapid and painless removal of adhesives and prevents skin stripping (Rudoni, 2008; Stephen-Haynes, 2008).

FIGURE 4. Removing appliance.

(continued)

SKILL 37-3 CHANGING AND EMPTYING AN OSTOMY APPLIANCE *continued*

ACTION	RATIONALE
15. Place the appliance in the trash bag, if disposable. If reusable, set aside to wash in lukewarm soap and water, and allow to air dry after the new appliance is in place.	Thorough cleaning and airing of the appliance reduce odor and deterioration of appliance. For esthetic and infection-control purposes, discard used appliances appropriately.
16. Use toilet tissue to remove any excess stool from the stoma (Fig. 5). Cover the stoma with a gauze pad. Clean the skin around the stoma with skin cleanser and water or a cleansing agent and a washcloth. Remove all old adhesive from the skin; use an adhesive remover, as necessary. Do not apply lotion to the peristomal area.	Toilet tissue, used gently, will not damage the stoma. The gauze absorbs any drainage from the stoma while the skin is being prepared. Cleaning the skin removes excretions and old adhesive and skin protectant. Excretions or a buildup of other substances can irritate and damage the skin. Lotion will prevent a tight adhesive seal.
17. Gently pat area dry. **Make sure that the skin around the stoma is thoroughly dry.** Assess the stoma and the condition of the surrounding skin (Fig. 6).	Careful drying prevents trauma to skin and stoma. An intact, properly applied fecal collection device protects skin integrity. Any change in color and size of the stoma may indicate circulatory problems.

FIGURE 5. Using toilet tissue to wipe around stoma.

FIGURE 6. Assessing stoma and peristomal skin.

18. Apply skin protectant to a 2-inch (5-cm) radius around the stoma, and allow it to dry completely, which takes about 30 seconds.	The skin needs protection from the excoriating effect of the excretion and appliance adhesive. The skin must be perfectly dry before the appliance is placed to get good adherence and to prevent leaks.
19. Lift the gauze squares for a moment and measure the stoma opening, using the measurement guide (Fig. 7). Replace the gauze. Trace the same-size opening on the back center of the appliance (Fig. 8). Cut the opening 1/8 inch larger than the stoma size (Fig. 9). Use a finger to gently smooth the wafer edges after cutting.	The appliance should fit snugly around the stoma, with only 1/8 inch of skin visible around the opening. A faceplate opening that is too small can cause trauma to the stoma. If the opening is too large, exposed skin will be irritated by stool. Wafer edges may be uneven after cutting and could cause irritation to and/or pressure on the stoma.

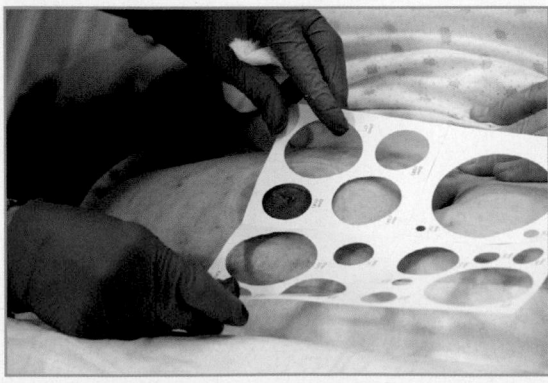

FIGURE 7. Using measurement guide to measure size of stoma.

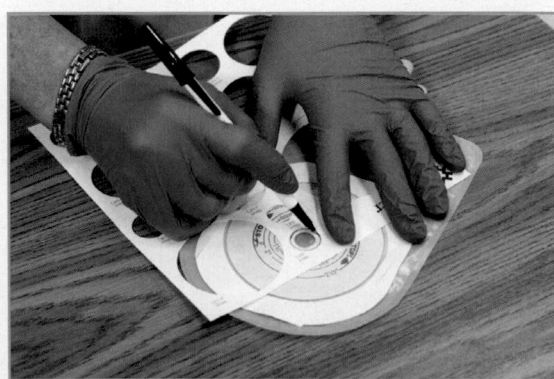

FIGURE 8. Tracing same-sized circle on the back and center of skin barrier.

ACTION	RATIONALE

FIGURE 9. Cutting the opening 1/8 inch larger than the stoma size.

20. Remove the paper backing from the appliance faceplate (Fig. 10). Quickly remove the gauze squares and ease the appliance over the stoma (Fig. 11). Gently press onto the skin while smoothing over the surface. Apply gentle, even pressure to the appliance for approximately 30 seconds.

The appliance is effective only if it is properly positioned and adhered securely. Pressure on the wafer allows the wafer to mold to the patient's skin and improve the seal (Jones et al., 2011).

FIGURE 10. Removing paper backing on faceplate.

FIGURE 11. Easing appliance over the stoma.

21. Close the bottom of the appliance or pouch by folding the end upward and using the clamp or clip that comes with the product (Fig. 12), or secure the Velcro closure. Ensure that the curve of the clamp follows the curve of the patient's body.

A tightly sealed appliance will not leak and cause embarrassment and discomfort for the patient.

FIGURE 12. Using clip to close bottom of appliance.

(continued)

SKILL 37-3 CHANGING AND EMPTYING AN OSTOMY APPLIANCE *continued*

ACTION	RATIONALE
22. Remove gloves. Assist the patient to a comfortable position. Cover the patient with bed linens. Place the bed in the lowest position.	Provides warmth and promotes comfort and safety.
23. Put on clean gloves. Remove or discard equipment and assess the patient's response to the procedure.	Gloves prevent contact with blood, body fluids, and microorganisms that contaminate the used equipment. The patient's response may indicate acceptance of the ostomy as well as the need for health teaching.
24. Remove gloves and additional PPE, if used. Perform hand hygiene.	Removing PPE properly reduces the risk for infection transmission and contamination of other items. Hand hygiene prevents the spread of microorganisms.

DOCUMENTATION

Guidelines

Document the appearance of the stoma, condition of peristomal skin, characteristics of drainage (amount, color, consistency, unusual odor), patient's reaction to procedure, and pertinent patient teaching.

Sample Documentation

DocuCare Practice documenting changing and emptying an ostomy appliance in *Lippincott DocuCare.*

> 7/22/15 1630 Colostomy appliance changed due to leakage. Stoma is pink, moist, and flat against abdomen. No erythema or excoriation of surrounding skin. Moderate amount of pasty, brown stool noted in bag. Patient asking appropriate questions during appliance application. States, "I'm ready to try changing the next one."
>
> —B. Clapp, RN

UNEXPECTED SITUATIONS AND ASSOCIATED INTERVENTIONS

- *Peristomal skin is excoriated or irritated:* Make sure that the appliance is not cut too large. Skin that is exposed inside of the ostomy appliance will become excoriated. Assess for the presence of a fungal skin infection. If present, consult with primary care provider to obtain appropriate treatment. Thoroughly cleanse the skin and apply skin barrier. Allow to dry completely. Reapply the pouch. Monitor pouch adhesion and change the pouch as soon as there is a break in adhesion. Confer with the primary care provider for a wound, ostomy, and continence nurse (WOCN) consult to manage these issues.

- *Patient continues to notice odor:* Check the system for any leaks or poor adhesion. Clean the outside of the bag thoroughly when emptying.

- *Bag continues to come loose or fall off:* Thoroughly cleanse the skin and apply skin barrier. Allow to dry completely. Reapply the pouch. Monitor pouch adhesion and change the pouch as soon as there is a break in adhesion.

- *Stoma is protruding into bag:* This is called a prolapse. Have the patient rest for 30 minutes. If the stoma is not back to normal size within that time, notify the primary care provider. If the stoma stays prolapsed, it may twist, resulting in impaired circulation to the stoma.

- *Stoma is dark brown or black:* Stoma should appear pink to red, shiny, and moist. Alterations indicate compromised circulation. If the stoma is dark brown or black, suspect ischemia and necrosis. Notify the primary care provider immediately (Avent, 2012).

DEVELOPING CLINICAL REASONING

1. Discuss the appropriate nursing intervention if an assessment revealed the following:
   - Patient has frank blood in stool.
   - Parent reports that child's stool is unusually foul smelling and greasy.
   - Patient's stool is ribbon-like.
   - Patient receiving cancer pain medication reports chronic constipation.
   - Teenager reports frequent episodes of diarrhea that leave her weak and dehydrated.

2. A 52-year-old man presents with acute stomach pain and altered bowel elimination: diarrhea. Role play with another student the interview you would use to assess his bowel elimination status. Identify variables that make you, as either the nurse or patient, uncomfortable talking about elimination. Discuss how you can best address your discomfort.

PRACTICING FOR NCLEX

1. A nurse is assessing the abdomen of a patient who is experiencing frequent bouts of diarrhea. The nurse first observes the contour of the abdomen, noting any masses, scars, or areas of distention. What action would the nurse perform next?
   a. Auscultate the abdomen using an orderly clockwise approach in all abdominal quadrants.
   b. Percuss all quadrants of the abdomen in a systematic clockwise manner to identify masses, fluid, or air in the abdomen.
   c. Lightly palpate over the abdominal quadrants; first checking for any areas of pain or discomfort.
   d. Deeply palpate over the abdominal quadrants, noting muscular resistance, tenderness, organ enlargement, or masses.

2. A nurse is administering a large-volume cleansing enema to a patient prior to surgery. Once the enema solution is introduced, the patient complains of severe cramping. What would be the appropriate nursing intervention in this situation?
   a. Elevate the head of the bed 30 degrees and reposition the rectal tube.
   b. Place the patient in a supine position and modify the amount of solution.
   c. Lower the solution container and check the temperature and flow rate.
   d. Remove the rectal tube and notify the primary care provider.

3. A nurse working in a hospital includes abdominal assessment as part of patient assessment. In which patients would a nurse expect to find decreased or absent bowel sounds after listening for 5 minutes? Select all that apply.
   a. A patient diagnosed with peritonitis
   b. A patient who is on prolonged bedrest
   c. A patient who has diarrhea
   d. A patient who has gastroenteritis
   e. A patient who has an early bowel obstruction
   f. A patient who has paralytic ileus caused by surgery

4. A nurse assesses the stool of patients who are experiencing gastrointestinal problems. In which patients would diarrhea be a possible finding? Select all that apply.
   a. A patient who is taking narcotics for pain
   b. A patient who is taking laxatives
   c. A patient who is taking diuretics
   d. A patient who is dehydrated
   e. A patient who is taking amoxicillin for an infection
   f. A patient taking over-the-counter antacids

5. A patient has a fecal impaction. The nurse correctly administers an oil-retention enema by:
   a. Administering a large volume of solution (500–1,000 mL)
   b. Mixing milk and molasses in equal parts for an enema
   c. Instructing the patient to retain the enema for at least 30 minutes
   d. Administering the enema while the patient is sitting on the toilet

6. A nurse prepares to assist a patient with her newly created ileostomy. Which recommended patient teaching points would the nurse stress? Select all that apply.
   a. "When you inspect the stoma, it should be dark purple-blue."
   b. "The size of the stoma will stabilize within 2 weeks."
   c. "Keep the skin around the stoma site clean and moist."
   d. "The stool from an ileostomy is normally liquid."
   e. "You should eat dark green vegetables to control the odor of the stool."
   f. "You may have a tendency to develop food blockages."

7. A nurse is preparing a hospitalized patient for a colonoscopy. Which nursing action is the recommended preparation for this test?
   a. Have the patient follow a clear liquid diet 24 to 48 hours before the test.
   b. Have the patient take Dulcolax and ingest a gallon of bowel cleaner on day 1.
   c. Prepare the patient for the use of general anesthesia during the test.
   d. Explain that barium contrast mixture will be given to drink before the test.

8. A nurse is performing digital removal of stool on a 74-year old female patient with a fecal impaction. During the procedure the patient tells the nurse she is feeling dizzy and nauseated, and then she vomits. What should be the nurse's next action?
   a. Reassure the patient that this is a normal reaction to the procedure.
   b. Stop the procedure, prepare to administer CPR, and notify the physician.
   c. Stop the procedure, assess vital signs, and notify the physician.
   d. Stop the procedure, wait five minutes, and then resume the procedure.

9. A nurse is scheduling tests for a patient who has been experiencing epigastric pain. The physician ordered the following tests: (a) barium enema, (b) fecal occult blood test, (c) endoscopic studies, and (d) upper gastrointestinal series. Which is the correct order in which the tests would normally be performed?
   a. c, b, d, a
   b. d, c, a, b
   c. a, b, d, c
   d. b, a, d, c

10. A nurse is caring for a patient who has a nasogastric tube in place for gastric decompression. Which nursing actions are appropriate when irrigating a nasogastric tube connected to suction? Select all that apply.
    a. Draw up 30 mL of saline solution into the syringe.
    b. Unclamp the suction tubing near the connection site to instill solution.

c. Place the tip of the syringe in the tube to gently insert saline solution.

d. Place syringe in the blue air vent of a Salem sump or double-lumen tube.

e. After instilling irrigant, hold the end of the NG tube over an irrigation tray.

f. Observe for return flow of NG drainage into an available container.

11. A nurse is teaching a patient with frequent constipation how to implement a bowel-training program. What is a recommended teaching point?
   a. Using a diet that is low in bulk
   b. Decreasing fluid intake to 1,000 mL
   c. Administering an enema once a day to stimulate peristalsis
   d. Allowing ample time for evacuation

12. A nurse caring for patients with bowel alterations formulates a nursing diagnosis for a patient with a new ileostomy. Which diagnosis is most appropriate?
   a. Disturbed Body Image
   b. Constipation
   c. Delayed Growth and Development
   d. Excess Fluid Volume

13. A nurse is irrigating the colostomy of a patient and is unable to get the irrigation solution to flow. What would be the nurse's next action in this situation?
   a. Assist the patient to a prone position on a waterproof pad and try again.
   b. Check the clamp on the tubing to make sure that the tubing is open.
   c. Quickly pull the cone from the stoma and check for bleeding.
   d. Remove the equipment and call the primary care provider.

14. A nurse is assisting a patient to empty and change an ostomy appliance. When the procedure is finished, the nurse notes that the stoma is protruding into the bag. What would be the nurse's first action in this situation?
   a. Reassure the patient that this is a normal finding with a new ostomy.
   b. Notify the primary care provider that the stoma is prolapsed.
   c. Have the patient rest for 30 minutes to see if the prolapse resolves.
   d. Remove the appliance and redo the procedure using a larger appliance.

15. A nurse is caring for a postpartum patient who has stitches in the perineum from an episiotomy (surgically planned incision to prevent vaginal tears). Which medication would the nurse most likely administer to this patient?
   a. A stool softener (Colace)
   b. An osmotic laxative (Miralax)
   c. A bulk-forming laxative (Metamucil)
   d. An emollient laxative (mineral oil)

ANSWERS WITH RATIONALES

1. *a.* The sequence for abdominal assessment proceeds from inspection, auscultation, percussion, and then palpation. Inspection and auscultation are performed before palpation because palpation may disturb normal peristalsis and bowel motility. Percussion and deep palpation are usually performed by advanced practice professionals.

2. *c.* If the patient complains of severe cramping with introduction of an enema solution, the nurse should lower the solution container and check the temperature and flow rate. If the solution is too cold or the flow rate too fast, severe cramping may occur.

3. *a, b, f.* Decreased or absent bowel sounds—evidenced only after listening for 5 minutes (Jensen, 2011)—signify the absence of bowel motility, commonly associated with peritonitis, paralytic ileus, and/or prolonged immobility. Hyperactive bowel sounds indicate increased bowel motility, commonly caused by diarrhea, gastroenteritis, or early bowel obstruction.

4. *b, e, f.* Diarrhea is a potential adverse effect of treatment with amoxicillin clavulanate (Augmentin), laxatives, or over-the-counter antacids. Narcotics, diuretics, and dehydration may lead to constipation.

5. *c.* The patient should be instructed to retain the enema solution for at least 30 minutes or as indicated in the manufacturer's instructions. The usual amount of solution administered with a retention enema is 150 to 200 mL for an adult. The milk and molasses mixture is a carminative enema that helps to expel flatus. The patient should be instructed to lie on the left side of the bed as dictated by patient condition and comfort.

6. *d, e, f.* Ileostomies normally have liquid, foul-smelling stool. The nurse should encourage the intake of dark green vegetables because they contain chlorophyll, which helps to deodorize the feces. Patients with ileostomies need to be aware they may experience a tendency to develop food blockages, especially when high-fiber foods are consumed. The stoma should be dark pink to red and moist. Stoma size usually stabilizes within 4 to 6 weeks, and the skin around the stoma site (peristomal area) should be kept clean and dry.

7. *a.* Preparation for a colonoscopy includes a clear liquid diet 24 to 48 hours before the test along with a 2-day bowel prep of a strong cathartic and Dulcolax on day 1 and enema on day 2 of the test, or a 1-day bowel prep that consists of ingestion of a gallon of bowel cleanser in a short period of time. Conscious sedation, not general anesthesia, will be given for the colonoscopy. A chalky-tasting barium contrast mixture is given to drink before an upper gastrointestinal and small-bowel series of tests.

8. *c.* When a patient complains of dizziness or lightheadedness and has nausea and vomiting during digital stool removal, the nurse should stop the procedure, assess heart rate and blood pressure, and notify the physician. The vagal nerve may have been stimulated.

9. *d.* A fecal occult blood test should be done first to detect gastrointestinal bleeding. Barium studies should be performed next to visualize gastrointestinal structures and reveal any inflammation, ulcers, tumors, strictures, or other lesions. A barium enema and routine radiography should precede an upper gastrointestinal series because retained barium from an upper gastrointestinal series could take several days to pass through the gastrointestinal tract and cloud anatomic detail on the barium enema studies. Noninvasive procedures usually take precedence over invasive procedures, such as endoscopic studies, when sufficient diagnostic data can be obtained from them.

10. *a, c, e, f.* The nurse irrigating a nasogastric tube connected to suction should draw up 30 mL of saline solution (or amount indicated in the order or policy) into the syringe, clamp the suction tubing near the connection site to protect the patient from leakage of NG drainage, place the tip of the syringe in the tube to gently insert the saline solution, then place the syringe in the drainage port, not in the blue air vent of a Salem sump or double-lumen tube (the blue air vent acts to decrease pressure built up in the stomach when the Salem sump is attached to suction). After instilling irrigant, hold the end of the NG tube over an irrigation tray or emesis basin, and observe for return flow of NG drainage into an available container.

11. *d.* For a bowel-training program to be effective, the patient must have ample time for evacuation (usually 20–30 minutes). Fluid intake is increased to 2,500 to 3,000 mL, food high in bulk is recommended as part of the program, and a daily enema is not administered in a bowel-training program. A cathartic suppository may be used 30 minutes before the patient's usual defecation time to stimulate peristalsis.

12. *a.* An ileostomy may cause disturbed body image due to the invasive nature of the procedure and the presence of the stoma. Constipation does not normally occur with an ileostomy because the drainage is liquid. Growth and development are not generally affected by the formation of an ileostomy. Excess fluid volume is unlikely to occur because the drainage is liquid and probably continual.

13. *b.* If irrigation solution is not flowing, the nurse should first check the clamp on the tubing to make sure the tubing is open. Next, the nurse should gently manipulate the cone in the stoma and check for a blockage of stool. If there is a blockage, the nurse should remove the cone from the stoma, clean the area, and gently reinsert. Alternately, the nurse could assist the patient to a side-lying or sitting position in bed, place a waterproof pad under the irrigation sleeve, and place the drainage end of the sleeve in a bedpan.

14. *c.* If the stoma is protruding into the bag after changing the appliance on an ostomy, the nurse should have the patient rest for 30 minutes. If the stoma is not back to normal size within that time, notify the physician. If the stoma stays prolapsed, it may twist, resulting in impaired circulation to the stoma.

15. *a.* Although all the choices are laxatives that would soften the stool and make it easier to expel, a stool softener, such as Colace, is the one recommended for a patient who must avoid straining. In this case, it would help to prevent disturbing the stitches in the perineum.

TAYLOR SUITE RESOURCES

Explore these additional resources to enhance learning for this chapter:

- NCLEX-Style Questions and other resources on the Point, http://thePoint.lww.com/Taylor8e
- *Study Guide for Fundamentals of Nursing, 8th edition*
- Adaptive Learning | Powered by prepU, http://thepoint.lww.com/prepu
- *Skill Checklists for Fundamentals of Nursing, 8th edition*
- *Taylor's Clinical Nursing Skills:* Chapter 13, Bowel Elimination
- *Taylor's Video Guide to Clinical Nursing Skills:* Bowel Elimination
- *Lippincott DocuCare* Fundamentals cases

Bibliography

Ackley, B. J., & Ladwig, G. B. (2011). *Nursing Diagnosis Handbook* (9th ed.). St. Louis: Elsevier/Mosby.

American Association of Critical-Care Nurses (AACN). (2010). Practice alert: Verification of feeding tube placement. Available at http://aacn.org/WD/Practice/Docs/PracticeAlerts/Verification_of_Feeding_Tube_Placement_05-2005.pdf

Avadhani, A., & Miley, H. (2011). Probiotics for prevention of antibiotic-associated diarrhea and *Clostridium difficile*–associated disease in hospitalized adults—a meta-analysis. *Journal of the American Academy of Nurse Practitioners, 23*(6), 269–274.

Avent, Y. (2012). Understanding fecal diversions. *Nursing made incredibly easy! 10*(5), 11–16.

Best, C. (2005). Caring for the patient with a nasogastric tube. *Nursing Standard, 20*(3), 59–65.

Bisanz, A., Tucker, A. M., Amin, D. M., Patel, D., Calderon, B. B., Joseph, M. M., & Curry, E. A. (2010). Summary of the causative and treatment factors of diarrhea and the use of a diarrhea assessment and treatment tool to improve patient outcomes. *Gastroenterology Nursing, 33*(4), 269–281.

Boltz, M., Capezuti, E., Fulmer, T., & Zwicker, D. (Eds.) (2012). *Evidence-based geriatric nursing protocols for best practice* (4th ed.). New York: Springer Publishing Company.

Bowers, B. (2006). Evaluating the evidence for administering phosphate enemas. *British Journal of Nursing, 15*(7), 378–381.

Brennan, M. (2008). Review: Routine NG decompression after abdominal surgery delays return of bowel function and increases pulmonary complications. *Evidence-Based Nursing, 11*(2), 55.

Bulechek, G. M, Butcher, H. K., Dochterman, J. M., & Wagner, C. M. (Eds.). (2013). *Nursing interventions classification (NIC)* (6th ed.). St. Louis: Elsevier/Mosby.

Burch, J. (2011). Stoma management: enhancing patient knowledge. *British Journal of Community Nursing, 16*(4), 162, 164, 166.

Burton, J., Allison, J., Smart, N., & Francis, N. (2011). Impact of stoma care on enhanced recovery after colorectal surgery. *Gastrointestinal Nursing, 9*(8), 15–16, 18–19.

Carlsson, E., Gylin, M., Nilsson, L., Svensson, K., Alverslid, I., & Persson, E. (2010). Positive and negative aspects of colostomy irrigation. *Journal of Wound, Ostomy, and Continence Nursing, 37*(5), 511–518.

Centers for Disease Control and Prevention (CDC). (2011). Making food safer to eat. Reducing contamination from the farm to the table. Available at http://www.cdc.gov/vitalsigns/FoodSafety/

Centers for Disease Control and Prevention (CDC). (2010). Frequently asked questions about *Clostridium difficile* for healthcare providers. Available at http://www.cdc.gov/HAI/organisms/cdiff/Cdiff_faqs_HCP.html

Chau, J. P. C., Lo, S. H. S., Thompson, D. R., Fernandez, R., & Griffiths, R. (2011). Use of end-tidal carbon dioxide detection to determine correct placement of nasogastric tube: A meta-analysis. *International Journal of Nursing Studies, 48*(4), 513–521.

Connor, B. A. (2012). *Travelers' Health. Chapter 2. The pre-travel consultation. Self-treatable conditions. Travelers' diarrhea.* Available at http://wwwnc.cdc.gov/travel/yellowbook/2012/chapter-2-the-pre-travel-consultation/travelers-diarrhea.htm

Denyer, J. (2011). Reducing pain during the removal of adhesive and adherent products. *British Journal of Nursing, 20*(15) (Tissue Viability Supplement), S28–35.

Dudek, S. (2014). *Nutrition essentials for nursing practice* (7th ed.). Philadelphia: Wolters Kluwer Health/Lippincott Williams & Wilkins.

Ellett, M. (2004). What is known about methods of correctly placing gastric tubes in adults and children. *Gastroenterology Nursing, 27*(6), 253–261.

Flynn Makic, M. B., VonRueden, K. T., Rauen, C. A., & Chadwick, J. (2011). Evidence-based practice habits: Putting more sacred cows out to pasture. *Critical Care Nurse, 31*(2), 38–44, 47–61.

Gannon, R. (2007). Current strategies for preventing or ameliorating postoperative ileus: A multimodal approach. *American Journal of Health-System Pharmacy, 64*(20), S8–12.

Geraghty, J. (2011). Introducing a new skin-care regimen for the incontinent patient. *British Journal of Nursing, 20*(7), 409–415.

Gilbert, R. T., & Burns, S. M. (2012). Increasing the safety of blind gastric tube placement in pediatric patients: The design and testing of a procedure using a carbon dioxide detection device. *Journal of Pediatric Nursing, 27*(5), 528–532.

Goldberg, M., Aukett, L. K., Carmel, J., Fellows, J., Folkedahl, B., & Pittman, J. (2010). Management of the patient with a fecal ostomy. Best practice guideline for clinicians. *Journal of Wound, Ostomy, and Continence Nursing, 37*(6), 596–598.

Grossman, S., & Porth, C. M. (2014). Porth's pathophysiology: concepts of altered health states. (9th ed.). Philadelphia: Wolters Kluwer Health/Lippincott Williams & Wilkins.

Hägglund, D. (2010). A systematic literature review of incontinence care for persons with dementia: the research evidence. *Journal of Clinical Nursing, 19*(3–4), 303–312.

Hinkle, J. L., & Cheever, K. H. (2014). *Brunner & Suddarth's textbook of medical–surgical nursing* (13th ed.). Philadelphia: Wolters Kluwer Health/Lippincott Williams & Wilkins.

Huether, S. E., & McCance, K. L. (2012.) *Understanding Pathophysiology* (5th ed.). St. Louis: Elsevier.

Higgins, D. (2008a). Patient assessment Part 3—Measurement of gastric fluid pH. *Nursing Times, 104*(9), 26–27.

Higgins, D. (2008d). Specimen collection Part 3—Collecting a stool specimen. *Nursing Times, 104*(19), 22–23.

Hogan-Quigley, B., Palm, M. L., & Bickley, L. (2012). *Bates' nursing guide to physical examination and history taking.* Philadelphia: Wolters Kluwer Health/Lippincott Williams & Wilkins.

Jacobson, R. M., Peery, J., Thompson, W. O., Kanapka, J. A., & Caswell, M. (2010). Serum electrolyte shifts following administration of sodium phosphates enema. *Gastroenterology Nursing, 33*(3), 191–201.

Jarvis, C. (2012). *Physical examination & health assessment* (6th ed.). St. Louis: Elsevier/Saunders.

Jensen, S. (2011). *Nursing health assessment. A best practice approach.* Philadelphia: Wolters Kluwer Health/Lippincott Williams & Wilkins.

Jessee, M. A. (2010). Stool studies: Tried, true, and new. *Critical Care Nursing Clinics of North America, 22*(1), 129–145.

Jones, K. (2010). Probiotics: preventing antibiotic-associated diarrhea. *Journal for Specialists in Pediatric Nursing, 15*(2), 160–162.

Jones, T., Springfield, T., Brudwich, M., & Ladd, A. (2011). Fecal ostomies: Practical management for the home health clinician. *Home Healthcare Nurse, 29*(5), 306–317.

Kee, J. L., Hayes, E. R., & McCuistion, L. E. (2012). *Pharmacology: A nursing process approach* (7th ed.). St. Louis: Elsevier/Saunders.

Khair, J. (2005). Guidelines for testing the placing of nasogastric tubes. *Nursing Times, 101*(20), 26–27.

Kyle, G., Prynn, P., & Oliver, H. (2004). An evidence-based procedure for the digital removal of feces. *Nursing Times, 100*(48), 71.

Kyle, T., & Carman, S. (2013). *Essentials of pediatric nursing* (2nd ed.). Philadelphia: Wolters Kluwer Health/Lippincott Williams & Wilkins.

Lafon, C., & Lawson, L. (2010). Postoperative ileus in GI surgical patients; pathogenesis and interventions. *Gastrointestinal Nursing, 10*(2), 45–49.

Leung, L., Riutta, T., Kotecha, J., & Rosser, W. (2011). Chronic constipation: An evidence-based review. *Journal of the American Board of Family Medicine, 24*(4), 436–451.

Levin, B., Lieberman, D. A., McFarland, B., Smith, R. A., Brooks, D., Andrews, K. S., … Winawer, S. J. (2008). Screening and surveillance for the early detection of colorectal cancer and adenomatous polyps, 2008: A joint guideline from the American Cancer Society, the US Multi-Society Task Force on Colorectal Cancer, and the American College of Radiology. *CA—A Cancer Journal for Clinicians, 58*(3), 130–160.

Malarkey, L. M., & McMorrow, M. E. (2012). *Saunders nursing guide to laboratory and diagnostic tests* (2nd ed.). St. Louis: Elsevier/Saunders.

Massey, R. L. (2012). Return of bowel sounds indicating an end of postoperative ileus: Is it time to cease this long-standing nursing tradition? *MEDSURG Nursing, 21*(3), 146–150.

Mayo Foundation for Medical Education and Research (MFMER). (2011). Constipation: Symptoms. Available at http://www.mayoclinic.com/health/constipation/DS00063/DSECTION=symptoms

Miller, S. (2011). Capnometry vs pH testing in nasogastric tube placement. *Gastrointestinal Nursing, 9*(2), 30–33.

Moorhead, S., Johnson, M., Maas, M. L., & Swanson, E. (Eds). (2013). *Nursing Outcomes Classification (NOC)* (5th ed.). St. Louis: Elsevier/Mosby.

Munera-Seeley, V., Ochoa, J., Brown, N., Bayless, A., Correia, M., Bryk, J., Zenati, M. (2008). Use of a colorimetric carbon dioxide sensor for nasoenteric feeding tube placement in critical care patients compared

with clinical methods and radiography. *Nutrition in Clinical Practice, 23*(3), 318–321.

NANDA International (NANDA-I). (2012). *Nursing diagnoses: Definitions & classification 2012–2014.* West Sussex, UK: Wiley-Blackwell.

National Association for Continence (NAFC). (2013). *Diet and daily habits: Can this affect your bladder or bowel control?* Available at http://www.nafc.org/bladder-bowel-health/frequently-asked-questions/diet-and-daily-habits/

National Cancer Institute (NCI). (2012). Gastrointestinal complications (PDQ®). Constipation. Available at http://www.cancer.gov/cancertopics/pdq/supportivecare/gastrointestinalcomplications/HealthProfessional/page2#top

National Institute of Diabetes and Digestive and Kidney Diseases (NIDDK), (2012). Bowel diversion surgeries: Ileostomy, colostomy, ileoanal reservoir, and continent ileostomy. Available at http://digestive.niddk.nih.gov/ddiseases/pubs/ileostomy/

National Institutes of Health. Clinical Center. (2007). Patient education. Managing bowel dysfunction. Available http://www.cc.nih.gov/ccc/patient_education/pepubs/bowel.pdf.

Nelson, R., Edwards, S., & Tse, B. (2007). Prophylactic nasogastric decompression after abdominal surgery. *Cochrane Database Systematic Review,* Issue 3. DOI: 10.1002/14651858.CD004929.pub3.

Ness, W., Hibberts, F., & Miles, S. (2012). Management of lower bowel dysfunction, including DRE and DRF. RCN guidance for nurses. Available at https://www.rcn.org.uk/__data/assets/pdf_file/0007/157363/003226.pdf

Notter, J., & Chalmers, F. (2012). Living with a colostomy: a pilot study. *Gastrointestinal Nursing, 10*(6), 16, 18, 20, 22–24.

Nutter, M., Dunston, D., Ieyoub, J., Hart, A., Harper, J., & Burke, M. S. (2010). A retrospective analysis comparing small bowel follow-through with wireless capsule endoscopy in the evaluation of obscure gastrointestinal bleeding. *Gastroenterology Nursing 33*(4), 298–302.

Obokhare, I. (2012). Fecal impaction: A cause for concern? *Clinics in Colon and Rectal Surgery, 25*(1), 53–57.

Perry, S. E., Hockenberry, M. J., Lowdermilk, D. L., & Wilson, D. (2010). *Maternal child nursing care* (4th ed.). Maryland Heights, MO: Elsevier/Mosby.

Person, B., Ifargan, R., Lachter, J., Duek, S., Kluger, Y., & Assalia, A. (2012). The impact of preoperative stoma site marking on the incidence of complications, quality of life, and patient's independence. *Diseases of the Colon & Rectum, 55*(7), 783–787.

Perston, Y. (2010). Ensuring effective technique in colostomy irrigation to improve quality of life. *Gastrointestinal Nursing, 8*(4), 18–22.

Qaseem, A., Denberg, T. D., Hopkins, R., Humphrey, L. L., Levine, J., Sweet, D. E., & Shekelle, P. (2012). Screening for colorectal cancer: A guidance statement from the American College of Physicians. *Annals of Internal Medicine, 156*(5), 378–386.

Ritter, L. A., & Hoffman, N. A. (2010). *Multicultural health.* Boston: Jones and Bartlett.

Rogers, J. (2012). Assessment, prevention and treatment of constipation in children. *Nursing Standard, 26*(29), 46–52.

Rudoni, C. (2008). A service evaluation of the use of silicone-based adhesive remover. *British Journal of Nursing, Stoma Care Supplement, 17*(2), S4, S6, S8–S9.

Rust, J. (2011). Complications arising from poor stoma siting. *Gastrointestinal Nursing, 9*(5), 17–18, 20, 22.

Salfi, S. F., & Holt, K. (2012). The role of probiotics in diarrheal management. *Holistic Nursing Practice, 26*(3), 142–149.

Simons, S. R., & Abdallah, L. M. (2012). Bedside assessment of enteral tube placement: Aligning practice with evidence. *American Journal of Nursing, 112*(2), 40–46.

Stephen-Haynes, J. (2008). Skin integrity and silicone: APPEEL 'no-sting' medical adhesive remover. *British Journal of Nursing, 17*(12), 792–795.

Stewart, M. L., & Schroeder, N. M. (2013). Dietary treatments for childhood constipation: efficacy of dietary fiber and whole grains. *Nutrition Reviews, 71*(2), 98–109.

Tabloski, P. (2010). *Gerontological nursing* (2nd ed.). Upper Saddle River, NJ: Pearson.

Taylor, J. J., & Cohen, B. J. (2013). *Memmler's structure and function of the human body* (10th ed.). Philadelphia: Wolters Kluwer Health/Lippincott Williams & Wilkins.

Toner, F., & Claros, E. (2012). Preventing, assessing, and managing constipation in older adults. *Nursing, 42*(12), 32–40.

U.S. Department of Health and Human Services (DHHS). (2013). Keep food safe: Check your steps. Available at http://www.foodsafety.gov/keep/basics/index.html

U.S. Department of Health and Human Services (DHHS). (2008). Physical activity guidelines for Americans. Available at http://www.health.gov/paguidelines/default.aspx

U.S. National Library of Medicine (NLM), Medline Plus. (2013). *Bowel retraining.* Available at http://www.nlm.nih.gov/medlineplus/ency/article/003971.htm

Van Leeuwen, A. M., Poelhuis-Leth, D., & Bladh, M. L. (2011). *Davis's comprehensive handbook of laboratory & diagnostic tests with nursing implications* (4th ed.). Philadelphia: F. A. Davis.

Voegeli, D. (2012). Moisture-associated skin damage: aetiology, prevention and treatment. *British Journal of Nursing, 21*(9), 517–518, 520–521.

Visich, K. L., & Pluth Yeo, T. (2010). The prophylactic use of probiotics in the prevention of radiation therapy-induced diarrhea. *Clinical Journal of Oncology Nursing, 14*(4), 467–473.

VISN 8 Patient Safety Center. (2009). *Safe patient handling and movement algorithms.* Tampa, FL: Author. Available http://www.visn8.va.gov/visn8/patientsafetycenter/safePtHandling/default.asp

Walker, C. A., & Lachman, V. D. (2013). Gaps in the discharge process for patients with an ostomy: An ethical perspective. *MEDSURG Nursing, 22*(1), 61–64.

Ward, C. W. (2012). Fast track program to prevent postoperative ileus. *MEDSURG Nursing, 21*(4), 214–220, 232.

Williams, J. (2012). Considerations for managing stoma complications in the community. *British Journal of Community Nursing, 17*(6), 266, 268–269.

Williams, J. (2011). Choosing devices for stoma patients. *Practice Nursing, 22*(12), 646, 648–649.

Williams, J., Gwillam, B., Sutherland, N., Matten, J., Hemmingway, J., Ilsey, H., Somerville, M., … Parker, T. (2010). Evaluating skin care problems in people with stomas. *British Journal of Nursing, 19*(17), S6, S8, S10, S12–S15.

Woodward, S. (2012). Assessment and management of constipation in older people. *Nursing Older People, 24*(5), 21–26.

Zimmaro Bliss, D., & Norton, C. (2010). Conservative management of fecal incontinence. An evidence-based approach to controlling this life-altering condition. *American Journal of Nursing, 110*(9), 30–38.

38

Oxygenation and Perfusion

TYRONE JACOBS

Tyrone, age 12, is brought to the emergency department gasping for breath. His parents are frantic. "It just seemed like he had a really bad cold," his mother says. An acute asthma attack is suspected, and measures are instituted immediately to protect the child's airway.

YAN KIM

Yan, age 57, developed respiratory failure from complications associated with pulmonary surgery. He is receiving oxygen therapy and mechanical ventilation via an endotracheal tube (airway into the trachea) and undergoing continuous cardiac monitoring.

JOAN McINTYRE

Joan, age 72, has been admitted to your medical unit with an acute exacerbation of chronic obstructive pulmonary disease (COPD). This is the fifth time she has been in the hospital this year. She is receiving supplemental oxygen and multiple medications to support her breathing. She is very weak, unable to perform activities of daily living (ADLs) for herself, and becomes extremely short of breath with minimal exertion. She has verbalized feelings of despair and has asked the staff, "to let me go if I should stop breathing."

DocuCare Additional patient scenarios available in *Lippincott DocuCare.*

After completing the chapter, you will be able to accomplish the following:

1. Describe the principles of respiratory and cardiovascular anatomy and physiology.

2. Describe the function and role of the respiratory and cardiovascular systems in oxygenation.

3. Describe age-related differences that influence the care of patients with oxygenation problems.

4. Identify factors that affect respiratory and cardiovascular function.

5. Perform a cardiopulmonary assessment using appropriate interview questions and physical assessment skills.

6. Develop nursing diagnoses that correctly identify problems that may be treated by independent nursing interventions.

7. Describe nursing strategies to promote adequate oxygenation and identify their rationale.

8. Plan, implement, and evaluate nursing care related to select nursing diagnoses involving oxygenation problems.

KEY TERMS

adventitious	dry powder inhaler (DPI)	nebulizer
alveoli		oxygenation
angina	dyspnea	pacemaker
arterial blood gas	dysrhythmia	perfusion
atelectasis	electrocardiogram (ECG)	pleural effusion
atria	endotracheal tube	pleural friction rub
atrioventricular bundle	expiration	pneumothorax
atrioventricular (AV) node	heart failure	pulmonary ventilation
bradypnea	hemothorax	pulse oximetry
bronchial	hyperventilation	respiration
bronchodilator	hypoventilation	sinoatrial (SA) node
bronchovesicular	hypoxemia	spirometer
capnography	hypoxia	sputum
cardiopulmonary	inspiration internal respiration	surfactant
cardiovascular	ischemia	tachypnea
cilia	metered-dose inhaler (MDI)	thoracentesis
circulation	myocardial infarction	tracheostomy
crackles	nasal cannula	ventricles
diffusion		vesicular
		wheezes

Life depends on a constant supply of oxygen. This demand for oxygen is met by the function of the respiratory and cardiovascular systems, also known as the **cardiopulmonary** system. This chapter describes the anatomy and physiology of the respiratory system. Also included is a discussion of the anatomy and physiology of the **cardiovascular** (heart and blood vessels) system as it pertains to its role in **oxygenation**, the process of providing life-sustaining oxygen to the body's cells. Additional information related to the cardiovascular system—including pulse, pulse physiology, blood pressure, and the physiology of blood pressure—is discussed in Chapter 24. In addition, this chapter explores general factors affecting cardiopulmonary functioning and oxygenation. Suggestions for performing a comprehensive assessment related to oxygenation are presented, including sample interview questions for both a general and focused history, a description of the nursing examination, and laboratory and radiologic studies related to oxygenation. After analyzing the data collected, nurses decide whether the data lead to a problem statement, indicate another problem, or are the possible cause of a problem. The chapter provides numerous examples of nursing diagnoses. Expected patient outcomes and specific nursing strategies for implementation are described. The concluding patient care study illustrates how, with knowledge of cardiopulmonary functioning and skilled nursing interventions, the nurse cares for a patient with oxygenation problems. Refer also to the accompanying Reflective Practice box.

ANATOMY AND PHYSIOLOGY OF OXYGENATION

Oxygenation of body tissues depends on several factors. One is the integrity of the airway system to transport air to and from the lungs. A properly functioning alveolar system in the lungs to oxygenate venous blood and to remove carbon dioxide from the blood is also important. A properly functioning cardiovascular system and blood supply to carry nutrients and wastes to and from body cells is a necessary component of oxygenation.

Knowledge of the basic anatomy and physiology of the respiratory and cardiovascular systems and an understanding of the role of these systems in oxygenation of body tissues provides a foundation for assessing oxygenation in patients and for planning and implementing interventions to promote optimal oxygenation. This knowledge also helps nurses understand, interpret, and analyze assessment findings and provides the rationale for sound nursing interventions.

Respiratory System

Oxygen and carbon dioxide must move through the alveoli as part of the oxygenation process. Thus, an adequately functioning respiratory system is vital for the exchange of gases.

Anatomy of the Respiratory System

The airway, which begins at the nose and ends at the terminal bronchioles, is a pathway for the transport and exchange

REFLECTIVE PRACTICE: CULTIVATING QSEN COMPETENCIES

CHALLENGE TO TECHNICAL SKILLS

Ventilators and telemetry have always intimidated me, so having a patient like Yan Kim was overwhelming. Mr. Kim was a 57-year-old man who had developed respiratory failure from complications secondary to pulmonary surgery. He was receiving oxygen therapy and mechanical ventilation via an endotracheal tube (airway into the trachea) and was also undergoing continuous cardiac monitoring. Providing care for him with all his equipment and so many alarms that could sound seemed insurmountable. The monitor had several different values on it and the continuous electrocardiogram (ECG) monitor always made me feel like the patient was on the verge of dying. We had not covered these skills yet in class, and I felt incompetent for the first 2 weeks of my critical care clinical experience. I could have voiced my concerns with these two machines, and I should have asked the first day what I should and shouldn't be worried about with critical care patients. But I didn't.

Thinking Outside the Box: Possible Course of Action

- Ask my instructor if there was any danger in having a patient who was receiving mechanical ventilation and being monitored by telemetry.
- Ask for someone to explain the ECG waveforms on the monitor and what to be concerned with when looking at them.
- Avoid caring for patients on ventilators and telemetry as part of their care.

Evaluating a Good Outcome: How Do I Define Success?

- Patient is safe and receives care by a competent care provider promoting his health.
- I am confident in my technical skills and able to use technology to deliver the most helpful care.
- I continue to ask questions, challenge my practice, and learn to contribute to improved care, which will lead to enhanced nursing.

Personal Learning: Here's To the Future!

Fortunately, our clinical rotations are planned so that we do not actually assume responsibility for taking care of critical care patients until we learn the necessary skills (telemetry and ventilation). This semester in my critical care clinical experiences, my fears have dissipated. I have learned that having patients that are being monitored continuously via telemetry is quite reassuring: tt serves as a constant monitor for me. Although I still assess the patient on my own, having continuous values to check is reassuring. As for the ventilator, I realized I knew a lot more than I thought. My instructor gave me a lesson on the ventilator during my clinical experience and connected the class lectures and book work with what I was seeing with my patient. I asked many questions and checked to see if I knew which settings would change with different scenarios. There are several settings and several values constantly being measured with the machine. Once I was able to see what all of these numbers meant and realized that I understood what each was for, I felt much more comfortable with patients on a ventilator. I realized my concerns and made sure that I provided unbiased care so that my concerns did not force me to neglect a patient.

Before, I would have been scared to get too close to the machine for fear of hitting the wrong button, fearing I would harm the patient. Now I am learning how the settings are specific to each patient. I feel comfortable reading the values and setting the controls. Still, I ask questions about the ventilator and telemetry readings because I want to know that I am interpreting them correctly. I feel it is my responsibility to obtain as much understanding and knowledge as I can so that I can provide the best care to these patients. This is very relieving and rewarding: now critical care patients don't seem so critical! My care for these patients is enhanced since I am more confident in my skills, and this enhances the care I deliver. Next time there is something new to me, I will voice my concern early on even if I am not "supposed to know" it yet.

Overall, although I still do not have much experience, I feel technically competent as a senior nursing student. I am confident because I challenge myself and I am self-motivated when it comes to searching for more information when needed.

Carrie Staines, Georgetown University

REFLECTION ON QUALITY AND SAFETY COMPETENCIES

How do you think you would respond in a similar situation? Why? Do you agree with the criteria that the nursing student used to evaluate a successful outcome? Are there any other criteria that would be appropriate to use? Did the nursing student meet the criteria? Why or why not? What *knowledge, skills,* and *attitudes* do you need to develop to continuously improve the quality and safety of care for patients like Mr. Kim?

Patient-Centered Care: What information should be communicated to the patient about the care provided? What interventions should the nursing student implement to provide care based on respect for the patient's preferences, values, and needs?

Teamwork and Collaboration/Quality Improvement: What communication skills do you need to improve to ensure that you function as a member of the patient-care team?

What skills do you need to initiate requests for help and to obtain assistance when needed?

Safety/Evidence-Based Practice: What information did the nursing student receive from the monitors? How did the nursing student use this information? How did the nursing student apply the knowledge obtained through the lessons given by the instructor? What evidence in nursing literature provides guidance for decision making regarding care of this patient? What does this tell you about yourself and about the adequacy of your skills for professional practice? How do you think the nursing student would have responded if the clinical experience were strictly observational?

Informatics: Can you identify the essential information that must be available in Mr. Kim's electronic health record to support safe patient care and coordination of care? Can you think of other ways to respond to or approach the situation?

FIGURE 38-1. The organs of the respiratory tract. (**A**) Overview. (**B**) Alveoli (air sacs) of the lungs and the blood capillaries. (**C**) Transverse section through the lungs.

of oxygen and carbon dioxide. The airway is divided into the upper and the lower airways.

The upper airway is composed of the nose, pharynx, larynx, and epiglottis. Its main function is to warm, filter, and humidify inspired air. The lower airway, known as the tracheobronchial tree, includes the trachea, right and left main stem bronchi, segmental bronchi, and terminal bronchioles (Fig. 38-1). Its major functions are conduction of air, mucociliary clearance, and production of pulmonary surfactant.

The airways are lined with mucus, which traps cells, particles, and infectious debris. This mucus covering also helps to protect the underlying tissues from irritation and infection. **Cilia**, which are microscopic hair-like projections, propel trapped material and accompanying mucus toward the upper airway so they can be removed by coughing. Removal is facilitated when mucus is watery in consistency. An adequate fluid intake is necessary for ciliary action and for the production of watery mucus normally present in the respiratory tract.

The lungs, the main organs of respiration, are located within the thoracic cavity on the right and left sides (see Fig. 38-1). The lungs extend from the base at the level of the diaphragm to the apex (top), which is above the first rib. The heart lies between the right and left lung.

Each lung is divided into lobes. The right lung has three lobes; the left has two. Each lobe is subdivided into segments or lobules. The main bronchus branches to each lung from the trachea. It immediately subdivides into secondary

bronchi, one to each lobe. The bronchi subdivide again and again, becoming smaller and smaller as they branch through the lung. The smallest of these branches are the bronchioles, ending at the terminal bronchioles. The lungs are composed of elastic tissue that can stretch or recoil.

At the end of the terminal bronchioles there are clusters of **alveoli** (singular, alveolus), small air sacs. The alveoli are the site of gas exchange. The wall of each alveolus is made of a single-cell layer of squamous epithelium (see Fig. 38-1). This thin wall allows for exchange of gases with the capillaries covering the alveoli. The average adult has more than 300 million alveoli. **Surfactant**, a detergent-like phospholipid, reduces the surface tension between the moist membranes of the alveoli, preventing their collapse. When surfactant production is reduced, the lung becomes stiff and the alveoli collapse.

The lungs and thoracic cavity are lined with a serous membrane called the pleura. The visceral pleura covers the lungs, and the parietal pleura lines the thoracic cavity. These two membranes are continuous with each other and form a closed sac. The pleural space lies between the two layers. Pleural fluid between the membranes acts as a lubricant and as an adhesive agent to hold the lungs in an expanded position. A few milliliters of fluid between the pleural surfaces allows the lungs to move easily along the chest wall as they expand and contract. Without this fluid, filling and emptying of the lungs are difficult.

Pressure within the pleural space (intrapleural pressure) is always subatmospheric (a negative pressure). This constant negative intrapleural pressure, along with the pleural fluid, holds the lungs in an expanded position.

Physiology of the Respiratory System

Living cells require oxygen and the removal of carbon dioxide, a byproduct of oxidation. Gas exchange, the intake of oxygen and the release of carbon dioxide, is made possible by pulmonary ventilation, respiration, and perfusion. **Pulmonary ventilation** refers to the movement of air into and out of the lungs. **Respiration** involves gas exchange between the atmospheric air in the alveoli and blood in the capillaries. **Perfusion** is the process by which oxygenated capillary blood passes through body tissues.

PULMONARY VENTILATION

Pulmonary ventilation (breathing) is the movement of air into and out of the lungs. The process of ventilation has two phases: inspiration (inhalation) and expiration (exhalation). **Inspiration**, the active phase, involves movement of muscles and the thorax to bring air into the lungs. **Expiration**, the passive phase, is the movement of air out of the lungs.

During inspiration, the following events occur: the diaphragm contracts and descends, lengthening the thoracic cavity; the external intercostal muscles contract, lifting the ribs upward and outward; and the sternum is pushed forward, enlarging the chest from front to back. This combination of an increased lung volume and decreased intrapulmonic pressure allows atmospheric air to move from an area of greater pressure (outside air) into an area of lesser pressure (within the lungs). The relaxation, or recoil, of these structures then results in expiration. The diaphragm relaxes and moves up, the ribs move down, and the sternum drops back into position. This causes a decreased volume in the lungs and an increase in intrapulmonic pressure. As a result, air in the lungs moves from an area of greater pressure to one of lesser pressure and is expired (Fig. 38-2).

Other physical factors contribute to airflow in and out of the lungs. These factors include the condition of the musculature, compliance of lung tissue, and airway resistance. The condition of the body's musculature can affect the process of respiration. Weakening of the muscles involved in respiration can contribute to less effective inhalation and exhalation. The accessory muscles of the abdomen, neck, and back are used to maintain respiratory movements at times when

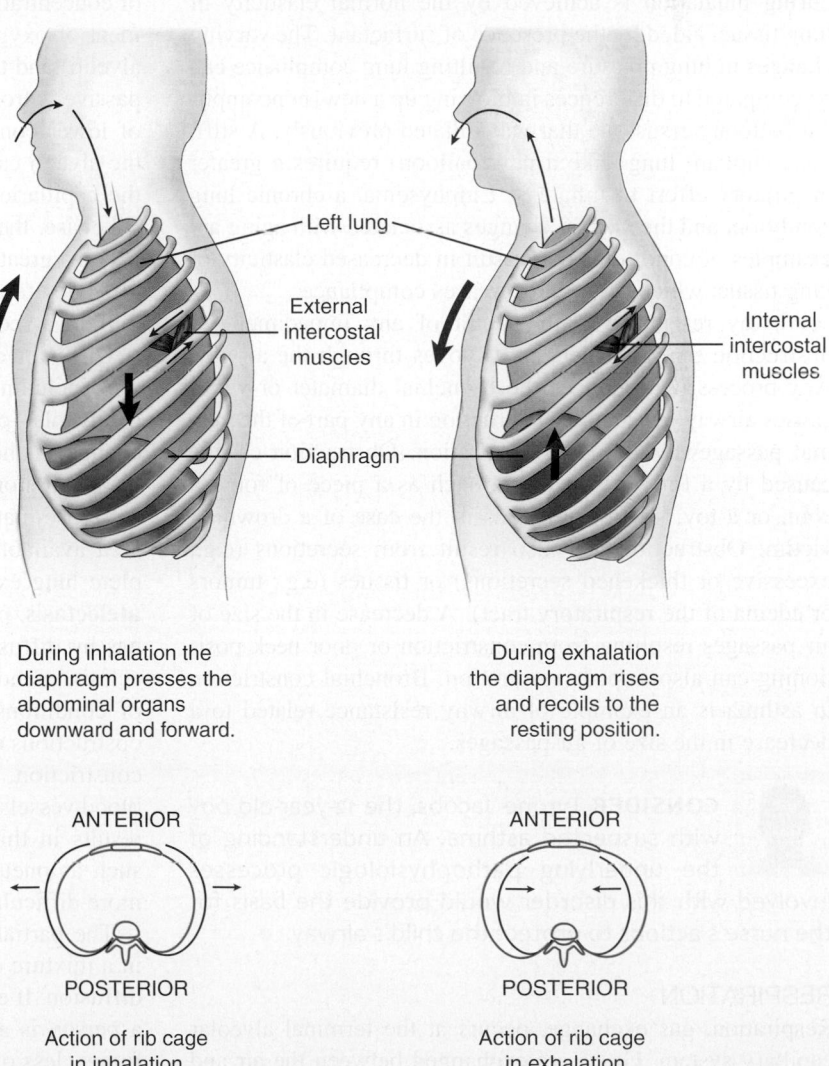

During inhalation the diaphragm presses the abdominal organs downward and forward.

During exhalation the diaphragm rises and recoils to the resting position.

Action of rib cage in inhalation

Action of rib cage in exhalation

FIGURE 38-2. Pulmonary ventilation.

FIGURE 38-3. Gas exchange in the alveolus. The greater pressure of the oxygen in the air inhaled into the alveoli causes the oxygen to move into the capillaries, which contain unoxygenated blood. The carbon dioxide in the returning venous blood moves from the capillaries (area of greater concentration) into the alveoli (area of lesser concentration).

breathing is difficult. These muscles are used to facilitate breathing; the movement is called retraction.

Lung compliance refers to the ease with which the lungs can be inflated. The compliance of lung tissue affects lung volume. The ability of the lungs to adequately fill with air during inhalation is achieved by the normal elasticity of lung tissue, aided by the presence of surfactant. The varying changes in lung pressure and resulting lung compliance can be compared to differences in blowing up a new, noncompliant balloon versus one that was inflated previously. A stiff, noncompliant lung (like a new balloon) requires a greater inspiratory effort to inflate it. Emphysema, a chronic lung condition, and the normal changes associated with aging are examples of conditions that result in decreased elasticity of lung tissue, which, in turn, decreases compliance.

Airway resistance is the result of any impediment or obstruction that air meets as it moves through the airway. Any process that changes the bronchial diameter or width causes airway resistance. Obstruction in any part of the normal passageways impedes respiration. Obstruction can be caused by a foreign substance, such as a piece of food, a coin, or a toy, or by liquids, as in the case of a drowning victim. Obstruction can also result from secretions (e.g., excessive or thickened secretions) or tissues (e.g., tumors or edema of the respiratory tract). A decrease in the size of air passages resulting from constriction or poor neck positioning can also impede respiration. Bronchial constriction in asthma is an example of airway resistance related to a decrease in the size of air passages.

 CONSIDER Tyrone Jacobs, the 12-year-old boy with suspected asthma. An understanding of the underlying pathophysiologic processes involved with this disorder would provide the basis for the nurse's actions to protect the child's airway. ●

RESPIRATION
Respiration, gas exchange, occurs at the terminal alveolar capillary system. Gases are exchanged between the air and

blood via the dense network of capillaries in the respiratory portion of the lungs and the thin alveolar walls (see Fig. 38-1, p. 1398 and Fig. 38-3). Gas exchange occurs via **diffusion**. Diffusion is the movement of gas or particles from areas of higher pressure or concentration to areas of lower pressure or concentration. In respiration, diffusion refers to the movement of oxygen and carbon dioxide between the air (in the alveoli) and the blood (in the capillaries). These gases move passively from an area of higher concentration to an area of lower concentration. The greater pressure of oxygen in the alveoli causes the oxygen to move from the alveoli into the capillaries containing the unoxygenated venous blood. Likewise, the carbon dioxide in the returning venous blood exerts a greater pressure than the carbon dioxide in the alveoli. Therefore, carbon dioxide diffuses across the capillary into the alveoli and ultimately is exhaled.

Diffusion of gases in the lung is influenced by several factors, including changes in surface area available, thickening of alveolar–capillary membrane, and partial pressure. Any change in the surface area available for diffusion hinders diffusion. For example, removal of a lung or the presence of a disease that destroys lung tissue can decrease the surface area available, ultimately affecting gas exchange. Incomplete lung expansion or the collapse of alveoli, known as **atelectasis**, prevents pressure changes and the exchange of gas by diffusion in the lungs. Areas of the lung with atelectasis cannot fulfill the function of respiration. Examples of conditions that predispose a patient to atelectasis are obstructions of the airway by foreign bodies, mucus, airway constriction, external compression by tumors or enlarged blood vessels, and immobility. Any disease or condition that results in thickening of the alveolar–capillary membrane, such as pneumonia or pulmonary edema, makes diffusion more difficult.

The partial pressure, or pressure resulting from any gas in a mixture depending on its concentration, can also affect diffusion. If environmental oxygen is reduced, such as when a person is at higher altitudes or in the presence of toxic fumes, less oxygen is available for diffusion. When oxygen is administered, an increased amount of oxygen is available, resulting in greater diffusion across capillary membranes.

PERFUSION

Oxygenated capillary blood passes through the tissues of the body in the process called perfusion. The amount of blood flowing through the lungs is a factor in the amount of oxygen and other gases that are exchanged. The amount of blood present in any given area of lung tissue depends partially on whether the person is sitting, standing, or lying down. Perfusion is greater in dependent areas. The perfusion of lung tissue also depends on the person's activity level. Greater activity results in an increased need for cellular oxygen by the body's tissues and a subsequent increase in cardiac output and consequently in increased blood return to the lungs. In addition, perfusion to the body's tissues depends on an adequate blood supply and proper cardiovascular functioning to carry oxygen and carbon dioxide to and from the lungs (discussed later).

Regulation of the Respiratory System

The respiratory center is located in the medulla in the brainstem, immediately above the spinal cord. It is stimulated by an increased concentration of carbon dioxide and hydrogen ions and, to a lesser degree, by the decreased amount of oxygen in the arterial blood. In addition, chemoreceptors in the aortic arch and carotid bodies are sensitive to the same **arterial blood gas** (measurement of blood pH, and arterial oxygen and carbon dioxide) levels and blood pressure, and can activate the medulla. Proprioceptors in the muscles and joints respond to body movements, such as exercise, and cause an increase in ventilation.

Stimulation of the medulla increases the rate and depth of ventilation (both inspiration and expiration) to blow off carbon dioxide and hydrogen and increase oxygen levels (the patient is breathing faster and more deeply). The medulla sends an impulse down the spinal cord to the respiratory muscles to stimulate a contraction leading to inhalation. If a

condition causes a chronic change in the oxygen and carbon dioxide levels, these chemoreceptors may become desensitized and not regulate ventilation adequately.

Alterations in Respiratory Function

If a problem exists in ventilation, respiration, or perfusion, **hypoxia** may occur. Hypoxia is a condition in which an inadequate amount of oxygen is available to cells. The most common symptoms of hypoxia are **dyspnea** (difficulty breathing), an elevated blood pressure with a small pulse pressure, increased respiratory and pulse rates, pallor, and cyanosis. Anxiety, restlessness, confusion, and drowsiness also are common signs of hypoxia. Hypoxia is often caused by **hypoventilation** (decreased rate or depth of air movement into the lungs). Hypoxia can also be a chronic condition. The effects of chronic hypoxia can be detected in all body systems and are manifested as altered thought processes, headaches, chest pain, enlarged heart, clubbing of the fingers and toes, anorexia, constipation, decreased urinary output, decreased libido, weakness of extremity muscles, and muscle pain. Additional information related to alterations in respiratory function is discussed in Chapter 24.

Cardiovascular System

Oxygen and carbon dioxide must move through the alveoli and be carried to and from body cells by the blood. Thus, an adequately functioning cardiovascular system is vital for exchange of gases.

Anatomy of the Cardiovascular System

The cardiovascular system is composed of the heart and the blood vessels. The heart is the main organ of **circulation**, the continuous one-way circuit of blood through the blood vessels, with the heart as the pump (Taylor & Cohen, 2013). The heart lies in the thoracic cavity between the lungs, in the center and somewhat to the left of the body's midline (Fig. 38-4).

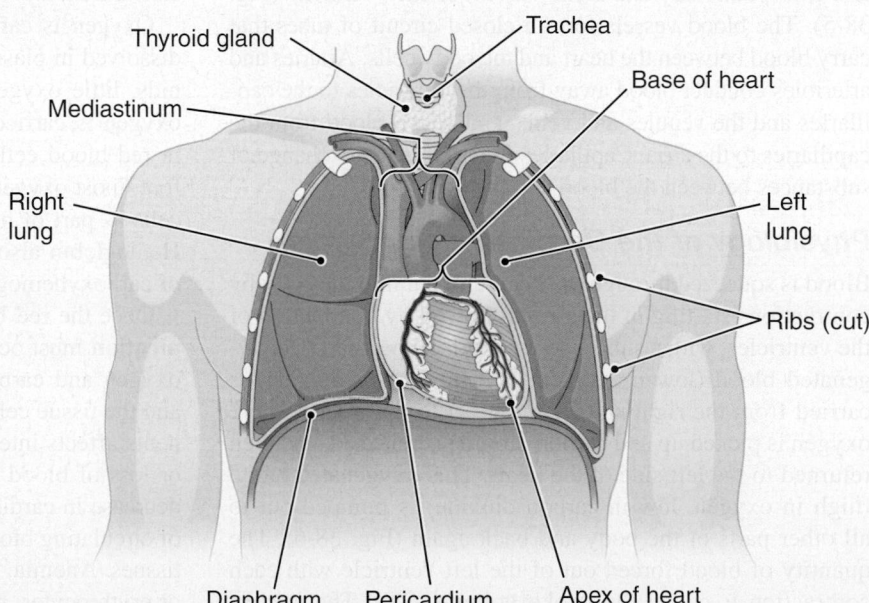

FIGURE 38-4. The heart in position in the thoracic cavity. (Reprinted with permission from Taylor, J. J., & Cohen, B. J. [2013]. *Memmler's structure and function of the human body* [10th ed.]. Wolters Kluwer Health/Lippincott Williams & Wilkins.)

Pulmonary valve

Superior vena cava

Aortic arch

Right pulmonary artery (branches)

Left pulmonary artery (branches)

Ascending aorta

Left pulmonary veins

Right pulmonary veins

Left atrium

Aortic valve

Left AV (mitral) valve

Right atrium

Right AV (tricuspid) valve

Left ventricle

Right ventricle

Inferior vena cava

Apex

Interventricular septum

■ Blood high in oxygen

■ Blood low in oxygen

FIGURE 38-5. The heart, valves, and vessels. (Adapted from Taylor, J. J., & Cohen, B. J. [2013]. *Memmler's structure and function of the human body* [10th ed.]. Wolters Kluwer Health/Lippincott Williams & Wilkins.)

The heart is a cone-shaped, muscular pump, divided into four hollow chambers. The upper chambers, the **atria** (singular, atrium), receive blood from the veins (the superior and inferior vena cava and the left and right pulmonary veins). The lower chambers, the **ventricles**, force blood out of the heart through the arteries (the left and right pulmonary arteries and the aorta). One-way valves that direct blood flow through the heart are located at the entrance (tricuspid and mitral valves) and exit (pulmonary and aortic valves) of each ventricle (Fig. 38-5). The blood vessels form a closed circuit of tubes that carry blood between the heart and the body cells. Arteries and arterioles conduct blood away from the ventricles to the capillaries and the venules and veins, and return blood from the capillaries to the atria. Capillaries function in the exchange of substances between the blood and the body cells.

Physiology of the Cardiovascular System

Blood is squeezed through the heart and out into the body by contractions starting in the atria, followed by contraction of the ventricles, with a subsequent resting of the heart. Deoxygenated blood (low in oxygen, high in carbon dioxide) is carried from the right side of the heart to the lungs, where oxygen is picked up and carbon dioxide is released, and then returned to the left side of the heart. This oxygenated blood (high in oxygen, low in carbon dioxide) is pumped out to all other parts of the body and back again (Fig. 38-6). The quantity of blood forced out of the left ventricle with each contraction is called the stroke volume (SV). The cardiac

output (CO) is the amount of blood pumped per minute, which averages from 3.5 L/min to 8.0 L/min in a healthy adult (Grossman & Porth, 2014). This volume is determined by using the following formula: cardiac output = stroke volume × heart rate. Thus, the cardiac output of an adult with a stroke volume of 70 mL and a heart rate of 70 beats/min is 4.9 L/min. Cardiac output increases during physical activity and decreases during sleep; it also varies depending on body size and metabolic needs.

Oxygen is carried via plasma and red blood cells. It is dissolved in plasma, but because oxygen is insoluble in liquids, little oxygen is carried in this way. The majority of oxygen is carried by the red blood cells. The hemoglobin in red blood cells has a strong affinity for oxygen. Therefore, most oxygen (97%) is carried in the body by red blood cells as part of hemoglobin in the form of oxyhemoglobin. Hemoglobin also carries carbon dioxide easily in the form of carboxyhemoglobin.

Once the red blood cells reach the tissues, **internal respiration** must occur. Internal respiration is the exchange of oxygen and carbon dioxide between the circulating blood and the tissue cells. Any abnormality in the blood's components affects internal respiration. For example, hemorrhage or loss of blood can cause a decrease in cardiac output. A decrease in cardiac output causes a reduction in the amount of circulating blood that is available to deliver oxygen to the tissues. Anemia, a decrease in the amount of red blood cells or erythrocytes, results in insufficient hemoglobin available

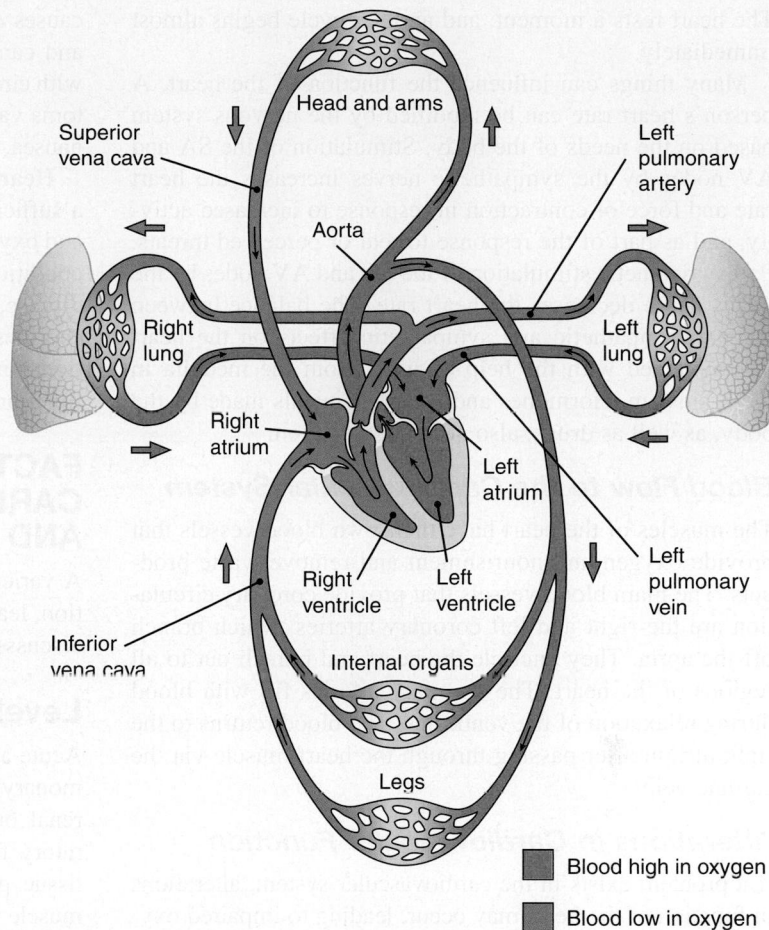

FIGURE 38-6. The right side of the heart pumps deoxygenated blood to the lungs, where oxygen is picked up and carbon dioxide released. The left side of the heart pumps oxygenated blood out to all other parts of the body. (Reprinted with permission from Taylor, J. J., & Cohen, B. J. [2013]. *Memmler's structure and function of the human body* [10th ed.]. Wolters Kluwer Health/Lippincott Williams & Wilkins.)

to transport oxygen. This may lead to an inadequate supply of oxygen to the tissues of the body. Alternately, exercise can improve the transport of oxygen. Regular exercise contributes to more effective pumping of the heart muscle, and improved oxygen transport to cells.

Regulation of the Cardiovascular System

Electrical impulses produced in and carried over specialized tissue within the heart control contraction of the muscles of the heart. These tissues make up the heart's conduction system (Fig. 38-7). The **sinoatrial (SA) node** is a mass of tissue in the upper right atrium, just below the opening of the superior vena cava. This node initiates the transmission of electrical impulses, causing contraction of the heart at regular intervals. It is also referred to as the **pacemaker**. After initiation, the electrical impulse travels throughout the muscle of each atrium, causing contraction of the atrium. The impulse also travels at the same time to the **atrioventricular (AV) node**, located at the bottom of the right atrium. When the impulse reaches the AV node, it enters a group of fibers called the **atrioventricular bundle**, or bundle of His. This bundle divides into right and left branches. Smaller conduction myofibers (Purkinje fibers) branch off, traveling throughout the ventricles. The right branch extends to the walls of the right ventricle and the left branch travels through the left ventricle. The electrical impulse continues

through the atrioventricular bundle and the Purkinje fibers, causing contraction of the ventricles. The contraction of the ventricles, which occurs just a moment after the atrial contractions, completes a cardiac cycle, or singe heartbeat.

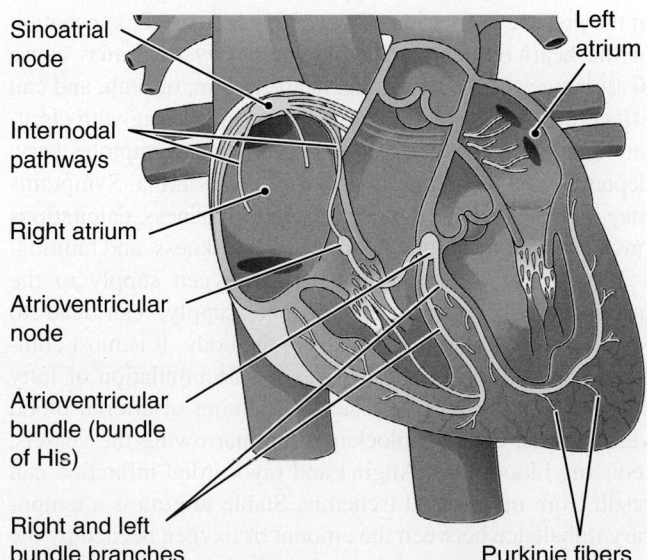

FIGURE 38-7. The conduction system of the heart. (Reprinted with permission from Taylor, J. J., & Cohen, B. J. [2013]. *Memmler's structure and function of the human body* [10th ed.]. Wolters Kluwer Health/Lippincott Williams & Wilkins.)

The heart rests a moment, and another cycle begins almost immediately.

Many things can influence the function of the heart. A person's heart rate can be modified by the nervous system based on the needs of the body. Stimulation of the SA and AV nodes by the sympathetic nerves increases the heart rate and force of contraction in response to increased activity, and as part of the response to real or perceived threats. Parasympathetic stimulation of the SA and AV nodes by the vagus nerve decreases the heart rate. The balance between the parasympathetic and sympathetic effects on the heart is maintained with the help of input from the medulla in the brainstem. Hormones and other chemicals made by the body, as well as drugs, also affect heart action.

Blood Flow to the Cardiovascular System

The muscles of the heart have their own blood vessels that provide oxygen and nourishment and remove waste products. The main blood vessels that provide coronary circulation are the right and left coronary arteries, which branch off the aorta. They encircle the heart and branch out to all regions of the heart. The coronary arteries fill with blood during relaxation of the ventricles. The blood returns to the right atrium after passing through the heart muscle via the cardiac veins.

Alterations in Cardiovascular Function

If a problem exists in the cardiovascular system, alterations in function of the heart may occur, leading to impaired oxygenation. A **dysrhythmia** or arrhythmia is a disturbance of the rhythm of the heart. Dysrhythmias are caused by an abnormal rate of electrical impulse generation from the SA node, or from impulses originating from a site or sites other than the SA node. They can also be caused by the abnormal conduction of electrical impulses through the heart. They can occur with heart disease, hypertension, damage to the heart, in the presence of various drugs, with decreased oxygenation of the heart tissues, and with trauma. Dysrhythmias cause disturbances of the heart rate, heart rhythm, or both, and can affect the pumping action of the heart, interfering with circulation, leading to alterations in oxygenation. Symptoms vary, depending on the cause and type of dysrhythmia. Symptoms may include decreased blood pressure, dizziness, palpitations (awareness of throbbing heart beats), weakness, and fainting.

Myocardial **ischemia**, decreased oxygen supply to the heart caused by insufficient blood supply, can lead to impaired oxygenation of tissues in the body. It is most commonly caused by atherosclerosis, the accumulation of fatty substances and fibrous tissue in the lining of arterial blood vessel walls, creating blockages and narrowing the vessels, reducing blood flow. Angina and myocardial infarction can result from myocardial ischemia. Stable **angina** is a temporary imbalance between the amount of oxygen needed by the heart and the amount delivered to the heart muscles. **Myocardial infarction**, one type of acute coronary syndrome characterized by the death of heart tissue due to lack of oxygen, is also known as a heart attack. Myocardial ischemia

causes disturbances of the heart rate, heart rhythm, or both, and can affect the pumping action of the heart, interfering with circulation, leading to alterations in oxygenation. Symptoms vary, based on the problem, but include pain, anxiety, nausea, vomiting, indigestion, and shortness of breath.

Heart failure occurs when the heart is unable to pump a sufficient blood supply, resulting in inadequate perfusion and oxygenation of tissues. It can be the result of many heart conditions, including chronic hypertension, coronary artery disease, and disease of the heart valves. Symptoms include shortness of breath, edema (swelling), and fatigue. Additional information related to alterations in cardiovascular function is discussed in Chapter 24.

FACTORS AFFECTING CARDIOPULMONARY FUNCTIONING AND OXYGENATION

A variety of factors affect adequate cardiopulmonary function, leading to impaired oxygenation. Important factors are discussed in the following sections.

Level of Health

Acute and chronic illnesses can affect a person's cardiopulmonary function dramatically. For example, people with renal or cardiac disorders often have compromised respiratory functioning because of fluid overload and impaired tissue perfusion. People with chronic illnesses often have muscle wasting and poor muscle tone. These problems affect all the muscles, including those of the respiratory system. Alterations in muscle function contribute to inadequate pulmonary ventilation and respiration, as well as inadequate functioning of the heart. Anemia can result in impaired respiratory function. As discussed previously, anemia may lead to an inadequate supply of oxygen to the tissues of the body. Because hemoglobin also carries carbon dioxide to the lungs, anemia results in diminished carbon dioxide exchange. Myocardial infarction causes a lack of blood supply to the heart muscle. Damage to the heart muscle interferes with effective contractions of the heart muscle, leading to decreased perfusion of tissues and decreased gas exchange. Physical changes such as scoliosis (curvature of the spine) influence breathing patterns and may cause air trapping. Research reveals a statistically significant correlation between obesity and chronic bronchitis. Moreover, people who are obese are often short of breath during activity, ultimately leading to less participation in exercise. As a result, the alveoli at the base of the lungs are rarely stimulated to expand fully.

 RECALL Yan Kim, the 57-year-old patient who developed respiratory failure from complications associated with pulmonary surgery. The acuity of the situation played a major role in the patient's current condition. The pulmonary surgery most likely reduced his respiratory function. The effects of anesthesia on his lungs and subsequently the development of complications compounded his situation. ●

Table 38-1 RESPIRATORY VARIATIONS IN THE LIFE CYCLE

	INFANT (BIRTH–1 YEAR)	EARLY CHILDHOOD (1–5 YEARS)	LATE CHILDHOOD (6–12 YEARS)	AGED ADULT (65+ YEARS)
Respiratory rate	30–55 breaths/min	20–40 breaths/min	18–26 breaths/min	16–24 breaths/min
Respiratory pattern	Abdominal breathing, irregular in rate and depth	Abdominal breathing, irregular	Thoracic breathing, regular	Thoracic, regular
Chest wall	Thin, little muscle, ribs and sternum easily seen	Same as infant's but with more subcutaneous fat	Further subcutaneous fat deposited, structures less prominent	Thin, structures prominent
Breath sounds	Loud, harsh crackles at end of deep inspiration	Loud, harsh expiration longer than inspiration	Clear inspiration is longer than expiration	Clear
Shape of thorax	Round	Elliptical	Elliptical	Barrel shaped or elliptical

Developmental Considerations

There are many age-related developmental considerations affecting respiratory function. Table 38-1 summarizes respiratory variations in the life cycle. Age-related variations in pulse rate and blood pressure can be found in Chapter 24, Table 24-1 on page 581.

Infants

The normal infant's chest is small, the airways are short, and aspiration is a potential problem. The respiratory rate is more rapid in infants than at any other age (see Table 38-1). As the alveoli increase in number and size, adequate oxygenation is accomplished at lower respiratory rates. Surfactant is formed in utero between 34 and 36 weeks. An infant born before 34 weeks may not have produced sufficient surfactant, leading to collapse of the alveoli and poor alveolar exchange. Synthetic surfactant can be given to the infant to help reopen the alveoli. Infants are at risk for upper respiratory tract infections and asthma as a result of exposure to secondhand smoke. Respiratory activity is primarily abdominal in infants. The pulse rate is more rapid in infancy than in adulthood, limiting the infant's ability to increase cardiac output by increasing the heart rate (Kyle & Carman, 2013).

Toddlers, Preschoolers, School-Aged Children, and Adolescents

The preschool child's eustachian tubes, bronchi, and bronchioles are elongated and less angular. Thus, the average number of routine colds and infections decreases until the child enters daycare or school and is exposed more frequently to pathogens. Young children who are not placed in daycare usually have not had the opportunity to develop antibodies for the variety of viruses and bacteria they may encounter in a school setting. Encourage good hand hygiene and tissue etiquette. Most children at this age have colds or upper respiratory infections, but some have more serious problems of otitis media, bronchitis, and pneumonia. Children in this age group are also at risk for asthma as a result of exposure to secondhand smoke. By the end of late childhood and during adulthood, the immune system is prepared to protect the person from most infections. A child's blood vessels widen and increase in length over time. The blood pressure increases over time, reaching the adult level in adolescence.

Older Adults

Specific physical changes occur in older adults that are unrelated to any pathology. Refer to the Focus on the Older Adult Box (on page 1406). The tissues and airways of the respiratory tract (including the alveoli) become less elastic. The power of the respiratory and abdominal muscles is reduced, therefore the diaphragm moves less efficiently. The chest is unable to stretch as much, resulting in a decline in maximum inspiration and expiration. Airways collapse more easily. These alterations increase the risk for disease, especially pneumonia and other chest infections.

THINK back to Joan McIntyre, the 72-year-old woman who is having an exacerbation of her chronic COPD. The nurse needs to incorporate information about age-related changes when planning the patient's care. The nurse also needs to consider that some of these age-related changes may be intensifying some of her symptoms and contributing to her decreased ability to care for herself. ●

The normal aging heart can maintain adequate cardiac output under ordinary circumstances, but may have a limited ability to respond to situations that cause physical or emotional stress (Hinkle & Cheever, 2014). Decreased physical activity, physical deconditioning, decreased elasticity of the blood vessels, and stiffening of the heart valves can lead to a decrease in the overall function of the heart.

Medication Considerations

Many medications affect the function of the cardiopulmonary system. Patients receiving drugs that affect the central nervous system need to be monitored carefully for respiratory complications. For example, opioids are chemical agents that depress the medullary respiratory center. As a result, the rate and depth of respirations decrease. Be alert

FOCUS ON THE OLDER ADULT

NURSING STRATEGIES TO ADDRESS AGE-RELATED CHANGES IN OXYGENATION

Age-Related Changes	Nursing Strategies
Decreased Gas Exchange and Increased Work of Breathing • Decreased elastic recoil of the lungs • Expiration requiring use of accessory muscles • Fewer functional capillaries and more fibrous tissue in alveoli • Decreased skeletal muscle strength in thorax • Reduction in vital capacity and increase in residual volume	• Encourage rest periods, as necessary. • Encourage cessation or moderation of smoking and second-hand smoke exposure. • Teach breathing exercises. • Remind about avoiding air pollutants. • Caution about effect of extreme weather conditions. • Instruct to avoid narcotics and sleeping pills. • Discuss home management with patient and family. • Teach avoidance of infection and preventive measures (i.e., pneumococcal and flu vaccination). • Use pillows as necessary to sleep.
Decreased Ventilation and Ineffective Cough • Less air exchange; more secretions remain in lungs • Drier mucous membranes • Altered pain sensation • Different norms for body temperature; fever may be atypical • Greater risk for aspiration due to slower gastric motility • Impaired mobility and inactivity, effects of medication	• Encourage increased fluid intake, especially water, as allowed. • Use cool-mist humidifier (teach proper cleaning technique). • Encourage attendance at pulmonary exercise rehabilitation program. • Discourage use of over-the-counter medications. • Teach how to splint thorax and cough effectively. • Instruct in use of supplemental oxygen. • Teach avoidance of milk products if they are troublesome.
Decreased Cardiac Output and Ability to Respond to Stress • Reduction in the elasticity of the heart's tissues • Heart muscle becomes less efficient—working harder to pump the same amount of blood through the body. • Progressive atherosclerosis (fatty buildup or plaques, thickening) in arterial walls and loss of elasticity • Capillary walls thicken slightly, leading to a slower rate of exchange of gases, nutrients, and waste.	• Encourage the inclusion of physical activity in the daily routine; pace activities. • Encourage a healthy low-fat, low-salt diet, including plenty of fruits, vegetables and whole grains. • Assist with smoking cessation and/or avoid the use of tobacco. • Teach the importance of regular check-ups • Assist with weight control. • Teach the importance of medication compliance. • Teach stress-reduction activities.

for the possibility of respiratory depression or arrest when administering any narcotic or sedative. Other medications decrease heart rate, with the potential to alter the flow of blood to body tissues.

Lifestyle Considerations

Activity levels and habits can dramatically affect a person's cardiopulmonary status. For example, sedentary activity patterns do not encourage the expansion of alveoli and the development of pulmonary exercise patterns (deep breathing). People who exercise (e.g., aerobics, walking, swimming) three to six times per week can better respond to stressors to respiratory health. Regular physical activity provides many health benefits, including increased heart and lung fitness, improved muscle fitness, and reducing the risk of heart disease.

Cultural influences can also play a role in a person's lifestyle, encouraging or discouraging healthy choices. Culture is a strong force in the determinants of health and behavior

change. An understanding of a patient's cultural background is necessary to promote health and disease prevention in any population (Ritter & Hoffman, 2010). For example, consider the implications of the use of traditional methods for health restoration, such as cupping by patients of Chinese descent to treat lung congestion (Spector, 2009). An important part of care would be to assess the impact of this practice and belief on a patient's readiness to participate in the proposed plan of care related to the treatment of pneumonia.

Cigarette smoking (active or passive) is a major contributor to lung disease and respiratory distress, heart disease, and lung cancer. Cigarette smoking is the most important risk factor for chronic COPD (Macnee, 2007). Smoking causes coronary heart disease, the leading cause of death in the United States (Centers for Disease Control and Prevention [CDC], 2010).

Nurses working with patients to initiate changes in health habits that affect oxygenation must also examine themselves as a factor in the success of the plan. Nurses who role model

PROMOTING HEALTH 38-1

OXYGENATION

Use the assessment checklist to determine how well you are meeting your needs related to oxygenation. Then develop a prescription for self-care by choosing appropriate behaviors from the list of suggestions.

Assessment Checklist

❑ almost always   ❑ sometimes   ❑ almost never

❑ ❑ ❑   1. I breathe easily, without discomfort and without feeling short of breath.

❑ ❑ ❑   2. I exercise regularly.

❑ ❑ ❑   3. I maintain normal weight for my height and body frame.

❑ ❑ ❑   4. I live in an environment free of pollution.

❑ ❑ ❑   5. I avoid substances (tobacco, chemicals) that cause respiratory problems.

❑ ❑ ❑   6. I arrange to receive recommended immunizations.

Self-Care Behaviors

1. Follow a regular exercise program with at least 150 minutes of moderate-intensity aerobic activity, 75 minutes of

vigorous-intensity aerobic activity, or an equivalent mix of the two each week (CDC, 2011).

2. Maintain normal body weight.

3. Obtain medical evaluation for chest pain, problems with breathing, and/or chronic cough with sputum or blood.

4. Evaluate personal use of tobacco.

5. Incorporate a plan to reduce smoking, then stop smoking on a specific target date.

6. Avoid exposure to secondhand smoke when possible.

7. Arrange to have a tuberculin test (PPD) done annually.

8. Receive a yearly influenza vaccine and a pneumococcal vaccine.

9. Avoid chemical substances that cause respiratory depression.

10. Maintain a pollution-free environment (as much as possible).

11. Support federal and community efforts to keep the air free of pollution.

Information to promote cardiovascular health and oxygenation is available online. Visit thePoint for a list of Internet resources.

---

good health behaviors are more effective teachers. Use the display, Promoting Health 38-1: Oxygenation, for yourself before using it with others.

Environmental Considerations

Although it is impossible to pinpoint all the effects of air pollution, researchers have demonstrated a high correlation between air pollution and cancer and lung diseases. For example, a person with adequate respiratory functioning who is exposed to air pollution may experience stinging of eyes and nasal passages, coughing, choking, headache, and dizziness. Occupational exposure to asbestos, silica, or coal dust, as well as environmental pollution, can lead to chronic pulmonary disease. Chronic exposure to radon, radiation, asbestos, and arsenic can lead to lung cancer. Additionally, people who have experienced an alteration in respiratory functioning in the past often have difficulty continuing to perform self-care activities in a polluted environment.

Psychological Health Considerations

Many psychological factors and conditions can affect the respiratory system. People responding to stress may sigh excessively or exhibit **hyperventilation** (increased rate and depth of ventilation, above the body's normal metabolic requirements). Hyperventilation can lead to a lowered level of arterial carbon dioxide. Generalized anxiety has been shown to cause enough bronchospasm to produce an episode of bronchial asthma. In addition, patients with respiratory problems often develop some anxiety as a result of the hypoxia caused by the respiratory problem.

 THINK back to Tyrone Jacobs, the young boy described at the beginning of the chapter. The patient is gasping for breath, which is extremely frightening and anxiety producing. In addition, his parents are frantic; this would increase Tyrone's anxiety level, further limiting his ability to breathe. The nurse needs to incorporate an understanding of this situation and plan interventions that promote oxygenation while reducing anxiety in both Tyrone and his parents. ●

THE NURSING PROCESS FOR OXYGENATION

Assessing

The patient's health history is an essential component for assessing the patient's cardiopulmonary function and ability to maintain adequate oxygenation. This information can be obtained from either the patient or a family member. The nursing examination combined with laboratory findings can provide information to identify a patient's strengths; the nature of any problems; their course; related signs and symptoms; and onset, frequency, and effects on activities of daily living. The nurse decides, based on these findings, what problems can be treated independently by nursing. Other problems are referred to a physician and/or other collaborative professionals for decisions on treatment.

FOCUSED ASSESSMENT GUIDE 38-1

OXYGENATION

Factors to Assess	Questions and Approaches
Usual patterns of respiration	How would you describe your breathing? Do you have allergies? What type(s) of allergies do you have? What relief measures do you use?
Medications	Are you taking any medications for your breathing, your heart, or for your blood pressure? What other medications are you taking?
Health history	Do you have any heart, lung, or breathing conditions? Does anyone in your family/home have any breathing conditions or respiratory infections?
Recent changes	Have you noticed any changes in your breathing (out of breath, cough, wheezing)? Have you noticed any changes in your ability to perform activities of daily living? Do you have any swelling or redness in your arms or legs? Do you have a respiratory infection? If so, what type? What relief measures are you using?
Lifestyle and environment	Do you smoke? If so, how many years have you smoked? How much do you smoke (i.e., how many packs per day or year)? Do you live with a smoker or are there smokers in your workplace? Are you exposed to respiratory irritants in your workplace? Are there other pollutants in your workplace?
Cough	How much and how often do you cough? What is it like (dry, bubbly, hoarse)? Do you cough up mucus? If so, how much and what does it look like? Do you have a history of allergies? Do you ever wheeze? Are you exposed to dust? Fumes?
Sputum	Do you ever cough up and spit out mucus? How much do you spit out and do you associate it with anything (time of day, environment)? What color is it? Is it ever blood tinged? What is its odor?
Pain	Do you have any chest pain? Do you have pain with breathing? Do you have pain in the arms or legs? When did it start? On a scale of 0 to 10 (10 being very painful), how severe is the pain? Where is the pain? Is the pain worse with inspiration? Expiration? Cough? Activity? Does the pain radiate? What measures are you using to relieve the pain?
Dyspnea	Is it constant or remittent or related to any activity? How do different positions affect it? How does it affect your daily activities? Can you sleep lying flat? How many pillows do you use?
Fever	Have you had pneumonia recently? Do you have any contact with people who have tuberculosis? Do you have night sweats? Are others in your household well or ill? Have you traveled anywhere recently?
Fatigue	Have you noticed you feel more tired lately? Are you getting your normal amount of sleep at night? Has your sleep at night been affected by any difficulty breathing? Do you become easily fatigued when you climb stairs?

Nursing History

The nursing history, an important clinical tool in the early steps of the nursing process, always includes a cardiopulmonary component. The information gained provides data about why the patient needs nursing care and what kind of care is required to maintain sufficient oxygenation of tissues. Interview questions help identify current or potential health deviations, actions performed by the patient for meeting cardiopulmonary needs, and the effects of such actions. They also help identify any contributing factors, the use of any aids to improve oxygenation, and effects of health problems on the patient's lifestyle and relationships with others.

Before starting the interview, make certain that the patient is not in acute distress. If the patient is experiencing any respiratory distress, initiate appropriate actions immediately to help relieve symptoms. Enlist the aid of family members or others to help answer questions. Interview the patient at a later point, when the patient is able, to expand the initial database. If no emergency interventions are necessary for the patient's clinical condition, obtain a comprehensive history at this time.

When a health deviation is noted during the data collection, collect as much descriptive information as possible, including whether the problem evolved suddenly or slowly. The accompanying Focused Assessment Guide 38-1 provides some appropriate questions for health history assessment related to oxygenation.

Physical Assessment

Examinations of the cardiopulmonary systems are discussed in Chapter 25. Refer to this chapter for details and additional information related to the assessment of these systems. Always proceed in a well-organized manner through a sequence of inspection, palpation, percussion, and auscultation. Note the patient's vital sign measurements, particularly the pulse and respiratory rate, as well as the blood pressure.

 RECALL Mr. Kim, the 57-year-old man who is receiving oxygen therapy and mechanical ventilation via an endotracheal tube (airway into the trachea). A complete assessment is necessary to identify specific problems related to oxygenation as well as to determine the effectiveness of current treatments. •

INSPECTION

Observe the patient's general appearance. Does the patient appear to be in any distress? Is the patient restless or anxious? Note the patient's level of consciousness and orientation to person, place, and time. Alterations in oxygenation to body tissues can be a result of respiratory or cardiac distress and lead to altered mental status. Inspect the patient's skin, mucous membranes, and general circulation, which can be a general indicator of the patient's health status, as well as indicating problems with oxy-genation. Pallor (lack of color) of skin and mucous membranes can indicate less than optimal oxygenation. Cyanosis (bluish discoloration) of these areas indicates decreased blood flow or poor blood oxygenation.

Note any abnormalities in the structures of the chest. The adult chest contour is slightly convex, with no sternal depression. The anteroposterior diameter should be less than the transverse diameter. Kyphosis (curvature of the spine) contributes to the older person's appearance of leaning forward and can limit respiratory ventilation. Barrel chest deformity may be a result of aging or COPD (chronic obstructive pulmonary disease). Note the contour of the intercostal spaces, which should be flat or depressed, and the movement of the chest, which should be symmetrical. Observe the respiratory rate, rhythm, and depth. Normally, respirations are quiet and nonlabored, and occur at a rate of 12 to 20 times each minute in healthy adults. Note any flaring of the nostrils, muscular retractions, **tachypnea** (rapid breathing), or **bradypnea** (slow breathing), which are suggestive of a health deviation requiring further evaluation.

Refer to Chapter 25 for a detailed discussion of inspection as part of the assessment of the respiratory and cardiovascular systems.

PALPATION

Palpate the chest. Note skin temperature and color. Skin temperature in this area is typically the same as the rest of the body. Assess chest expansion (thoracic excursion), which should be symmetrical. Note the presence or absence of masses, edema, or tenderness on palpation. Palpate the point of maximal impulse (PMI). Note pulsations in any other area of the chest. Abnormal size or location of the PMI or the presence of vibrations can indicate heart failure, myocardial infarction, disease of the heart valves, or other cardiac diseases. Palpate the patient's extremities. Assess skin temperature and color, pulses, and capillary refill. Note the presence or absence of edema, or tenderness on palpation. The presence of decreased skin temperature, pallor, cyanosis, decreased pulses, and prolonged capillary refill can indicate less than optimal cardiac function and oxygenation. The presence of edema an also indicate alterations in cardiovascular function.

Refer to Chapter 25 for a detailed discussion of palpation as part of the assessment of the respiratory and cardiovascular systems.

PERCUSSION

Percussion is used to assess the position of the lungs, density of lung tissue, and identify changes in the tissue. This assessment skill is not used frequently. When used, it is usually included in examinations performed by advanced practice nurses and other advanced practice professionals. Refer to Chapter 25 for a detailed discussion of percussion as part of the assessment of the respiratory and cardiovascular systems.

Table 38-2 COMMON LABORATORY STUDIES USED TO ASSESS CARDIOPULMONARY FUNCTION

STUDY	PREPARATION	AFTERCARE
Arterial Blood Gas and pH Analysis These examine arterial blood to determine the pressure exerted by oxygen and carbon dioxide in the blood and blood pH. This test measures the adequacy of oxygenation, ventilation, and perfusion. Normal results are: pH, 7.35 to 7.45; PCO_2, 35 to 45 mm Hg; PO_2, 80 to100 mm Hg; HCO_3, 22 to 26 mEq/L; and base excess or deficit, −2 to +2 mmol/L.	• Explain to the patient that this test requires an arterial puncture and collection of a blood specimen. • The radial, brachial, or femoral arteries are usually the sites of choice. • Perform Allen's test to ensure adequate ulnar blood flow when using the radial artery.	• Record supplemental oxygen or respirator settings on specimen information. • The arterial specimen is immediately placed on ice and taken to the laboratory. • Apply pressure for 5 to 10 minutes and watch for evidence of bleeding. If the patient is taking anticoagulants, pressure must be applied for a longer interval.
Cardiac Biomarkers CK and isoenzymes are enzymes that are released as a result of injury to tissues, including the heart muscle. Troponin is a protein found in skeletal and cardiac muscle fibers and is also released after injury to the heart. These biomarkers are used to monitor cardiac injury and myocardial infarction. Measuring the levels of these enzymes can help determine the extent and timing of the damage.	• Review the procedure with the patient. Inform the patient that this test can assist in assessing for heart damage. • Inform the patient that a series of samples will be required; based on facility protocol, samples could be taken three to four times, in 3- to 4-hour intervals. • Inform the patient that specimen collection takes approximately 5 to 10 minutes. • Address concerns about pain and explain that there may be some discomfort during the venipuncture (puncture of the vein). • There are no food, fluid, or medication restrictions unless ordered by the primary health care provider.	• Recognize anxiety related to test results. Provide teaching and information regarding the implications of the test results. • Reinforce information given by the patient's primary health care provider regarding further testing, treatment, or referral to another health care provider. • Depending on the results of this procedure, additional testing may be performed to evaluate or monitor progression of illness. • Evaluate test results in relation to the patient's symptoms, health care problems, and other tests performed.
Complete Blood Count (CBC)	• Review the procedure with the patient. Inform the patient that this test can assist in evaluating the body's response to illness. • Inform the patient that specimen collection takes approximately 5 to 10 minutes. • Address concerns about pain and explain that there may be some discomfort during the venipuncture (puncture of the vein). • There are no food, fluid, or medication restrictions unless ordered by the primary health care provider.	• Reinforce information given by the patient's primary health care provider regarding further testing, treatment, or referral to another health care provider. • Depending on the results of this procedure, additional testing may be performed to evaluate or monitor progression of illness. • Evaluate test results in relation to the patient's symptoms, health care problems, and other tests performed.
Cytologic Study This involves a microscopic examination of sputum and the cells it contains. It is done primarily to detect cells that may be malignant, determine organisms causing infection, and identify blood or pus in the sputum.	• Collect the specimen, if possible, in the morning before breakfast. The test usually involves 3 successive days of sputum collection. About 1 teaspoon of sputum is needed for a specimen. • The patient should take a deep breath, then expel the air with a deep cough. • Expectorate the specimen into a sterile specimen container with the appropriate preservative, if indicated. • Close the container with a tight-fitting lid.	• Advise the patient to inform the nurse when the specimen has been obtained. • Label and package the specimen and send it to the laboratory as soon as possible.

Adapted from Malarkey, L. M., & McMorrow, M. E. (2012). *Saunders nursing guide to laboratory and diagnostic tests* (2nd ed.). St. Louis: Elsevier/Saunders; VanLeeuwen, A. M., Poelhuis-Leth, D., & Bladh, M. L. (2011). *Davis's comprehensive handbook of laboratory & diagnostic tests with nursing implications* (4th ed.). Philadelphia: F. A. Davis.; and Hinkle, J. L., & Cheever, K. H. (2014). *Brunner & Suddarth's textbook of medical–surgical nursing* (13th ed.). Philadelphia: Wolters Kluwer Health/Lippincott Williams & Wilkins.

AUSCULTATION

Auscultation of the lungs assesses air flow through the respiratory passages and lungs. Listen for normal and abnormal lung sounds. Normal breath sounds include **vesicular** (low-pitched, soft sounds heard over peripheral lung fields), **bronchial** (loud, high-pitched sounds heard primarily over the trachea and larynx), and **bronchovesicular** (medium-pitched blowing sounds heard over the major bronchi) sounds. Auscultate as the patient breathes slowly through an open mouth. Breathing through the nose can produce falsely abnormal breath sounds.

In addition to air flow, listen for **adventitious** sounds (extra, abnormal sounds of breathing), such as wheezing or crackles. Abnormal lung sounds can occur as a result of alterations in the respiratory and cardiovascular systems and lead to impaired oxygenation. **Crackles**, frequently heard on inspiration, are soft, high-pitched discontinuous (intermittent) popping sounds. They are produced by fluid in the airways or alveoli and delayed reopening of collapsed alveoli. They occur due to inflammation or congestion and are associated with pneumonia, heart failure, bronchitis, and COPD. **Wheezes** are continuous musical sounds, produced as air passes through airways constricted by swelling, narrowing, secretions, or tumors. They are often heard in patients with asthma, tumors, or a buildup of secretions.

Auscultation of the heart assesses function of the heart, heart valves, and blood flow. Listen for normal and abnormal heart sounds. Listen to the rhythm of the beat and the characteristic "lub-dub." The first sound, the lub, is followed by the second sound, the dub, with a pause before the next lub-dub. These sounds are made by the closure of valves in the heart during the cardiac cycle. The lub correlates with the beginning of systole, the contraction of the ventricles, and is called S_1. The dub correlates with the end of systole and the beginning of diastole, the relaxation of the ventricles, and is called S_2.

In addition to S_1 and S_2, listen for extra and abnormal heart sounds. Abnormal heart sounds occur as a result of alterations in the cardiovascular system that may lead to impaired oxygenation. Refer to Chapter 25 for a detailed discussion of auscultation as part of the assessment of the respiratory and cardiovascular systems.

Common Diagnostic Tests

In addition to the nursing history and physical examination, the laboratory and diagnostic studies described in Table 38-2 and Table 38-3 (on pages 1412–1413) provide further assessment data that can aid in the formation of nursing diagnoses.

 THE nurse might anticipate diagnostic procedures such as arterial blood gas and pH analysis (ABG) for Joan McIntyre, the older woman with the acute exacerbation of COPD. This diagnostic test would provide information regarding the adequacy of her oxygenation and ventilation and help titrate (adjust) the administration of supplemental oxygen. It would also be used to evaluate her response to treatment and therapies. ●

The tests described in the next sections are not distinctive for a particular disease but reflect how well the cardiopulmonary systems are functioning.

ELECTROCARDIOGRAPHY

One of the most valuable and frequently used diagnostic tools, electrocardiography, measures the heart's electrical activity. Impulses moving through the heart's conduction system create electric currents that can be monitored on the body's surface. Electrodes attached to the skin can detect these electric currents and transmit them to an instrument that produces a record—the **electrocardiogram (ECG)**—of cardiac activity. The data are graphed as waveforms. ECG can be used to identify myocardial ischemia and infarction, heart damage, rhythm and conduction disturbances, chamber enlargement, electrolyte imbalances, and drug toxicity.

The standard 12-lead ECG uses a series of electrodes placed on the extremities and the chest wall to assess the heart from 12 different viewpoints (leads) by attaching ten cables with electrodes to the patient's limbs and chest; four limb electrodes and six chest electrodes. Each lead provides an electrographic snapshot of electrochemical activity of the myocardial cell membrane. The ECG device measures and averages the differences between the electrical potential of the electrode sites for each lead and graphs them over time, creating the standard ECG complex, called PQRST. These electrodes provide views of the heart from the frontal plane as well as the horizontal plane. It is essential that connection or placement of the ECG electrodes/leads is accurate to prevent misdiagnosis. The ECG tracing needs to be clear to enable accurate and reliable interpretation (Jevon, 2010).

An ECG is typically accomplished using a multichannel method. All electrodes are attached to the patient at once and the machine prints a simultaneous view of all leads. It is important to reassure the patient that the leads just sense and record and do not transmit any electricity. The patient must be able to lie still and refrain from speaking to prevent body movement from creating artifacts in the ECG. Variations of standard ECG include exercise ECG (stress ECG) and ambulatory ECG (Holter monitoring). Refer to Table 38-3 for information regarding these tests.

PULMONARY FUNCTION STUDIES

Pulmonary function studies encompass a group of tests used to assess respiratory function to assist in evaluating respiratory disorders. They provide an evaluation of lung dysfunction, diagnose disease, assess disease severity, assist in management of disease, and evaluate respiratory interventions. Most tests are administered by a respiratory therapist, technician, nurses with specialized training, or physicians. Several tests commonly encountered

(text continues on page 1414)

Table 38-3 COMMON DIAGNOSTIC STUDIES USED TO ASSESS CARDIOPULMONARY FUNCTION

STUDY	PREPARATION	AFTERCARE
Cardiac Coronary Catheterization (Angiography)		
A cardiac catheterization is an invasive study performed to evaluate coronary artery disease, visualize the coronary blood vessels, assess cardiac output, diagnose chest pain and complications of myocardial infarction, evaluate the need for coronary artery surgery, and assess the function of heart valves. Catheters are introduced into blood vessels of the right and left sides of the heart. Contrast dye is injected through the catheters and allows for x-ray visualization of the heart.	• Verify that an informed consent was obtained. Check for allergies and elevated blood urea nitrogen (BUN) or creatinine levels. • The patient is NPO after midnight before the procedure; if the study is late in the afternoon, the patient may have a clear liquid breakfast. • Inform the patient that when dye is given, a feeling of warmth or flushing, or a metallic taste, may occur.	• Assess the catheter insertion site for bleeding. Apply pressure to the site as needed, based on facility policy. Assess pulses distal to the insertion site. Monitor vital signs and electrocardiogram according to facility policy. • Bedrest should be maintained according to facility policy, usually for 4 to 6 hours after the study. • Instruct the patient not to drive or climb stairs for 24 hours; avoid heavy lifting, sports, and strenuous housework for 3 days; and to take no baths until the wound is healed. Patients may shower and change the site dressing after 24 hours.
Cardiac Exercise Stress Testing		
This procedure is a noninvasive way to evaluate the response of the cardiovascular system to physical stress, helping to identify the presence of coronary artery disease, the cause of chest pain, the functional capacity of the heart, the effectiveness of some cardiac medications, and evaluate dysrhythmias that occur during exercise. The patient exercises on a treadmill or pedals a stationary bicycle while the patient's electrocardiogram and blood pressure are monitored. The study is performed in a series of stages, gradually increasing the speed or resistance, until the patient reaches 85% of the maximum heart rate, becomes symptomatic, or displays changes on the electrocardiogram consistent with ischemia.	• The patient should be NPO for 4 hours before the test and should avoid stimulants such as tobacco and caffeine. Medications may be taken with a sip of water; however, patients should follow the directions given by their health care provider regarding taking certain cardiac medications before the test. Instruct the patient to wear comfortable clothing and shoes. • Inform the patient that this study can assist in assessing the heart's ability to respond to an increasing workload. • Question the patient about chest pain within the past 48 hours or a history of angina. • Inform the patient that the study takes approximately 30 to 60 minutes, and to report any symptoms, such as dizziness, breathlessness, or pain, that occur during the test.	• Recognize anxiety related to test results. Provide teaching and information regarding the implications of the test results. • Instruct the patient to report any angina or other discomfort experienced after the test. • Reinforce information given by the patient's primary health care provider regarding further testing, treatment, or referral to another health care provider.
Echocardiogram		
Echocardiography is a noninvasive ultrasound test used to evaluate abnormal heart sounds; size of the heart; size and function of the heart's structures; direction and speed of blood flow through the heart; and presence of abnormalities, such as tumors.	• Inform the patient that the test is painless. • The patient should be told to remove jewelry from the chest area.	• Reinforce information given by the patient's primary health care provider regarding further testing, treatment, or referral to another health care provider. • No special care is required after the echocardiogram.
Endoscopic Studies		
These involve direct visualization of a body cavity. A bronchoscope is used to examine the larynx, bronchi, and trachea. Bronchoscopy is used to view lesions, obtain a biopsy, improve drainage, remove foreign substances, evaluate trauma, and drain abscesses.	• Verify that an informed consent was obtained. • The patient should be NPO for 6 to 8 hours before the test. • An analgesic, sedative, and/or anticholinergic may be administered before the test. • Local anesthetic is sprayed into the throat.	• Withhold food and fluids until the gag reflex returns. • Check vital signs according to facility protocol. • Observe carefully for signs of respiratory impairment. Emergency resuscitation equipment should be available. • Warm saline gargles may relieve throat irritation once the gag reflex has returned.

Table 38-3 COMMON DIAGNOSTIC STUDIES USED TO ASSESS CARDIOPULMONARY FUNCTION *continued*

STUDY	PREPARATION	AFTERCARE
Holter Monitor This noninvasive study records the electric activity of the heart over a period of time, usually 24 to 48 hours, with an electronic recording device. It allows the patient to perform normal daily activities so that the response of the heart to these activities can be evaluated. It is also used to detect and evaluate dysrhythmias, evaluate chest pain and other symptoms, effectiveness of heart medications, and pacemaker function.	• Inform the patient of the purpose of the study and the importance of the patient's role in obtaining the needed information. • Instruct the patient to keep a diary of activities. Instruct the patient to trigger the event marker on the device whenever pain or other symptoms occur. Demonstrate and have the patient give a return demonstration regarding how to trigger the event marker. • Inform the patient that the recorder should remain dry; avoid bathing and showering. Contact with electrical devices—such as shavers, toothbrushes, and electric blankets—should be avoided.	• Instruct the patient to immediately report symptoms such as fast heart rate or difficulty breathing. • Reinforce information given by the patient's primary health care provider regarding further testing, treatment, or referral to another health care provider.
Lung Scan A lung scan is the recording on a photographic plate of the emissions of radioactive waves from a substance injected into a vein as it circulates through the lung. A *perfusion scan* (Q scan) is done to measure integrity of pulmonary blood vessels and evaluate blood flow abnormalities (e.g., pulmonary emboli). A *ventilation scan* (V scan) is done to detect ventilation abnormalities (especially in patients with emphysema). Both scans used together provide greater and more accurate diagnostic information than either test used alone.	• Verify that an informed consent was obtained, if required by facility. • Explain that no fasting is required. • The patient should be told to remove jewelry from the chest area.	• No special care is required after the lung scan. • Reassure the patient that no radiation precautions are necessary.
Skin Tests These determine antigen–antibody reactions and are used to identify exposure to diseases such as tuberculosis. In intradermal tests, antigens (to which the patient may have previously been exposed) are injected into the superficial layer of the skin with a needle and syringe to evaluate immune response.	• Check the patient's history for hypersensitivity to any of the test antigens. If positive, notify the physician before performing the test. • Cleanse the test area with alcohol and allow it to dry.	• Instruct the patient to have the test results read at the appropriate time. • After reading the results, document the reaction, noting the amount of erythema and induration. Note the presence of a positive result (elevated, red area), recording the diameter and elevation in millimeters. Record the test, time, date, method, and site of administration on the patient record.
Radiography Radiography is an x-ray examination of the lungs and the thoracic cavity. Radiographic examinations of the lungs are done to help diagnose pulmonary diseases and to determine the progress or development of disease.	• Instruct the patient to remove clothing to the waist and put on a gown. All metal jewelry should be removed. • The patient will be required to take a deep breath and hold it during the radiograph.	• No special care is required after a chest radiograph.

Adapted from Malarkey, L. M., & McMorrow, M. E. (2012). *Saunders nursing guide to laboratory and diagnostic tests* (2nd ed.). St. Louis: Elsevier/ Saunders; Van Leeuwen, A. M., Poelhuis-Leth, D., & Bladh, M. L. (2011). *Davis's comprehensive handbook of laboratory & diagnostic tests with nursing implications* (4th ed.). Philadelphia: F. A. Davis; and Hinkle, J. L., & Cheever, K. H. (2014). *Brunner & Suddarth's textbook of medical–surgical nursing* (13th ed.). Philadelphia: Wolters Kluwer Health/Lippincott Williams & Wilkins.

Box 38-1 COMMONLY MEASURED VALUES FROM PULMONARY FUNCTION TESTS

- Tidal volume (TV): Total amount of air inhaled and exhaled with one breath
- Vital capacity (VC): Maximum amount of air exhaled after maximum inspiration
- Forced vital capacity (FVC): Maximum amount of air that can be forcefully exhaled after a full inspiration
- Forced expiratory volume (FEV): The amount of air exhaled in the first second after a full inspiration; can also be measured at 2 or 3 seconds
- Total lung capacity (TLC): The amount of air contained within the lungs at maximum inspiration
- Residual volume (RV): The amount of air left in the lungs at maximal expiration
- Peak expiratory flow rate (PEFR): The maximum flow attained during the FVC

Adapted from Malarkey, L. M., & McMorrow, M. E. (2012. *Saunders nursing guide to laboratory and diagnostic tests* (2nd ed.). St. Louis: Elsevier/Saunders; and VanLeeuwen, A. M., Poelhuis-Leth, D., & Bladh, M. L. (2011). *Davis's comprehensive handbook of laboratory & diagnostic tests with nursing implications* (4th ed.). Philadelphia: F. A. Davis.

are described in the next section. More specialized tests and their purposes include:

- Diffusion capacity estimates the patient's ability to absorb alveolar gases and determine if a gas exchange problem exists.
- Maximal respiratory pressures help evaluate neuromuscular causes of respiratory dysfunction.
- Exercise testing helps evaluate dyspnea during exertion.

Refer to Box 38-1: Commonly Measured Values From Pulmonary Function Tests.

Spirometry. Spirometry measures the volume of air in liters exhaled or inhaled by a patient over time. It evaluates lung function and airway obstruction through respiratory mechanics. Spirometry can be used to measure the degree of airway obstruction and evaluates response to inhaled medications. The patient inhales deeply and exhales forcefully into a **spirometer**, an instrument that measures lung volumes and airflow. Patients also use spirometers to promote deep breathing while recovering from surgery, and to monitor health status in management of chronic asthma. A discussion regarding the use of incentive spirometers can be found later in this chapter.

Peak Expiratory Flow Rate. Peak expiratory flow rate (PEFR) refers to the point of highest flow during forced expiration. PEFR reflects changes in the size of pulmonary airways and is measured using a peak flow meter. It is routinely used for patients with moderate or severe asthma to measure the severity of the disease and degree of disease control. With the patient standing or sitting with the back positioned as straight as possible, the patient takes a deep breath and places the peak flow meter in the mouth, closing the lips tightly around the mouthpiece.

The patient forcibly exhales into the peak flow meter, and an indicator on the meter rises to a number. The patient is asked to repeat this three times, and the highest number is recorded. This produces a measurement in liters indicating the maximum flow rate during a forced expiration. Normal values are established in regard to height, age, and gender, as well as individual baseline values for patients with disease. Patients with asthma commonly measure PEFR at home to monitor airflow. The results are used to track disease progression and regulate treatment by the patient and clinician.

PULSE OXIMETRY

Pulse oximetry is a noninvasive technique that measures the arterial oxyhemoglobin saturation (SaO_2 or SpO_2) of arterial blood. The reported result is a ratio, expressed as a percentage, between the actual oxygen content of the hemoglobin and the potential maximum oxygen-carrying capacity of the hemoglobin (Van Leeuwen, Poelhuis-Leth, & Bladh, 2011). Pulse oximetry is useful for monitoring patients receiving oxygen therapy, titrating oxygen therapy, monitoring those at risk for hypoxia, and monitoring postoperative patients. Pulse oximetry does not replace arterial blood gas analysis. Desaturation (decreased level of SpO_2) indicates gas exchange abnormalities. Oxygen desaturation is considered a late sign of respiratory compromise in patients with reduced rate and depth of breathing (Johnson, Schweitzer, & Ahrens, 2011).

Be aware of the patient's hemoglobin level before evaluating oxygen saturation because the test measures only the percentage of oxygen carried by the available hemoglobin. Thus, even a patient with a low hemoglobin level could appear to have a normal SpO_2 because most of that hemoglobin is saturated. However, the patient may not have enough oxygen to meet body needs. A range of 95% to 100% is considered normal SpO_2; values ≤90% are abnormal, indicate that oxygenation to the tissues is inadequate, and should be investigated for potential hypoxia or technical error.

 CONSIDER Tyrone Jacobs, the young boy with asthma described at the beginning of the chapter. The nurse would use pulse oximetry initially to obtain baseline information about the patient's oxygen saturation level and then as a means to evaluate the effectiveness of therapy. ●

Figure 38-8 shows a nurse using a pulse oximetry unit, and Skill 38-1 on pages 1440–1444 outlines nursing responsibilities when using a pulse oximetry unit.

CAPNOGRAPHY

Capnography is a method to monitor ventilation and, indirectly, blood flow through the lungs. Exhaled air passes through a sensor that measures the amount of carbon dioxide (CO_2) exhaled with each breath. The reported results also provide information about the respiratory rate and depth, the presence of apnea, and efficiency of gas

FIGURE 38-8. Portable pulse oximetry unit, used to measure oxygen saturation (SpO$_2$) of arterial blood.

FIGURE 38-9. Position of the patient for thoracentesis.

exchange. When carbon dioxide levels are abnormal, either high or low, adverse effects, including death, can occur. It is useful for confirming placement of advanced airways and nasogastric tubes, as well as identifying patients with low cardiac output and hypoventilation. Capnography can detect signs of hypoventilation earlier than pulse oximetry (Johnson, Schweitzer, & Ahrens, 2011). The use of capnography to verify nasogastric tube placement is discussed in Chapter 37.

THORACENTESIS

Thoracentesis is the procedure of puncturing the chest wall and aspirating pleural fluid. The pleural cavity is a potential cavity because it is normally not distended with fluid or air. The physician or other advanced practice professional can perform a thoracentesis at the bedside with the nurse assisting, or it can be performed in the radiology department. The patient is required to sign a permit for this procedure. A thoracentesis may be performed to obtain a specimen for diagnostic purposes or to remove fluid that has accumulated in the pleural cavity and is causing respiratory difficulty and discomfort. Because the cavity being entered is sterile, surgical asepsis is required. Standard precautions also are used.

Procedure. A thoracentesis is usually carried out with the patient sitting on a chair or the edge of the bed with the legs supported and the arms folded and resting on a pillow on the bedside table (Fig. 38-9). If unable to sit up, the patient may lie on the unaffected side with the hand of the affected side raised above the shoulder.

The location where the needle is inserted depends on where the fluid is present and where the practitioner can best aspirate it. Once this spot is identified, the skin is cleansed with an antimicrobial agent. A local anesthetic is administered and then the needle is inserted between the ribs through the intercostal muscles and fascia and into the pleura. After the procedure, the needle or plastic catheter is removed and a small sterile dressing is placed over the entry site.

During thoracentesis, fluid or air can be removed from the pleural cavity with a syringe. Another method for removing fluid is to drain the fluid into a bottle in which a partial vacuum has been created. With this technique, a small plastic catheter may be threaded through the needle, allowing the needle to be withdrawn. This catheter reduces the possibility of puncturing the lung. When this method is used, the tubing connecting the needle and the bottle must be sterile. Commonly, a calibrated bottle is used to collect the drainage, allowing the amount of fluid removed to be determined. The maximum amount of fluid removed is generally 1,000 mL.

Nursing Responsibilities. The nurse is responsible for collecting baseline data before the procedure and for preparing the patient physically and emotionally for the procedure. Instruct the patient not to cough or breathe deeply during the procedure. Urge the patient to remain as still as possible to diminish the risk for accidental injury to the lung. Administer analgesics before the procedure as ordered.

During the procedure, observe the patient's reactions. Monitor the patient's color, pulse, and respiratory rates, reporting immediately to the primary care provider any deviation from the patient's baseline. Fainting, nausea, and vomiting may occur. Ensure that specimens, if obtained, are taken to the laboratory immediately.

After the procedure, assess the patient for changes in vital signs, particularly respirations. If a large amount of fluid was removed, respirations usually become easier. If the lung was punctured, respiratory distress becomes acute. If blood appears in the sputum or the patient has severe coughing, notify the primary care provider promptly. A chest radiograph is usually done after the procedure to verify the absence of complications.

Diagnosing

The data collected about the patient's cardiopulmonary status may lead to the development of one or more nursing diagnoses related to alterations in oxygenation. The etiology of the problem directs nursing interventions. Data collected during the nursing assessment may also lead to the identification of a collaborative problem.

Alterations in Oxygenation as the Problem

After the assessment is completed and the data are examined, the nurse concludes either that there is no problem at this time or that there is an actual or potential oxygenation problem that is amenable to independent or interdependent nursing actions. Examples of nursing diagnoses indicating alterations in oxygenation include:

- Ineffective Airway Clearance
- Decreased Cardiac Output
- Impaired Gas Exchange

Examples of these diagnoses, etiologic factors, and defining characteristics appear in Examples of NANDA-I Nursing Diagnoses: Oxygenation.

Alterations in Oxygenation as the Etiology

An alteration in oxygenation may affect other areas of human functioning. Examples of nursing diagnoses for which problems with oxygenation are the etiology for other problems include:

- Activity Intolerance related to imbalance between oxygen supply and demand
- Anxiety related to feeling of suffocation
- Fatigue related to impaired oxygen transport system
- Imbalanced Nutrition: Less Than Body Requirements, related to difficulty breathing
- Disturbed Sleep Pattern related to orthopnea and bronchodilators

Outcome Identification and Planning

When caring for patients with an alteration in oxygenation, nursing measures support the following general expected outcomes. The patient will:

- Demonstrate improved gas exchange in the lungs by an absence of cyanosis or chest pain and a pulse oximetry reading more than 95%
- Relate the causative factors, if known, and demonstrate a method of coping with these factors
- Preserve cardiopulmonary function by maintaining an optimal level of activity
- Demonstrate self-care behaviors that provide relief from symptoms and prevent further cardiopulmonary problems

When the patient's physical, psychosocial, and spiritual dimensions contribute to alterations in oxygenation, individualized expected outcomes are developed with the patient's input (e.g., "By March 15, the patient will be able to walk up one flight of steps at home without dyspnea.").

Implementing

Oxygen deficits, particularly in older people, impair all aspects of daily living. Going to get the mail or cleaning the house may become a monumental task for people with oxygen deficits. Nursing interventions related to oxygenation aim to promote optimal functioning of the cardiopulmonary systems, to promote comfort, and to promote and control coughing. Nurses may also need to intervene by performing chest physiotherapy, suctioning the airway, meeting respiratory needs with medications, providing supplemental oxygen, managing chest tubes, using artificial airways, clearing an obstructed airway, and administering CPR.

EXAMPLES OF NANDA-I NURSING DIAGNOSES

OXYGENATION

Nursing Diagnoses	Related Factors	Sample Defining Characteristics
Ineffective Airway Clearance	Fatigue; decreased intake of fluids; poor nutrition, a 20-year history of COPD, with recent development of pneumonia	• "I never feel as though I am getting enough air." • Thick, yellow secretions • Pale skin with circumoral cyanosis; respiratory rate is 40 breaths/min and shallow. Coarse crackles are auscultated bilaterally. • Cannot sit quietly in chair or on bed. • Ineffective cough
Impaired Gas Exchange	Smokes one pack of cigarettes per day; works with asbestos in auto factory; has had a cold for 7 days	• Cyanosis; using pursed-lip breathing • Sitting hunched forward with overbed table supporting arms. • Altered blood gases show respiratory acidosis. • Reports shortness of breath, nausea, and ankle edema for 1 week.
Ineffective Breathing Pattern	Anxious about results of cardiac catheterization and possible cardiac surgery	• Hyperventilating, tachypneic (40 breaths/minute) • "I have a tingling feeling in my fingers." • "I can't catch my breath and I can't lie down in bed."

Promoting Optimal Function

Healthy lifestyle choices and behaviors are an important part of preventing and managing cardiopulmonary diseases, which can have an impact on level of health and oxygenation. Vaccination is an important part of preventing respiratory infections. Teaching patients with problems of oxygenation about pollution-free environments is an important part of respiratory management. Many people with altered oxygenation experience anxiety as a result of their symptoms and the actual or potential loss of independence. It is important to minimize anxiety in patients with alterations in oxygenation in order to promote optimal functioning. Promoting good nutrition is another vital part of promoting optimal cardiopulmonary functioning.

Teach patients about their health conditions and provide information and support to improve patient health literacy. Refer to the accompanying Promoting Health Literacy box.

HEALTHY LIFESTYLE

Patients who practice good health-related behaviors can reduce their risk for many cardiopulmonary diseases. Explain that beneficial behaviors should be incorporated into their daily and weekly activities. Encourage patients to eat a healthy diet (see discussion later in the chapter). Encourage patients to maintain a healthy weight. Regular exercise should also be part of a patient's daily activities. Current recommendations suggest 150 minutes of moderate-intensity aerobic activity, 75 minutes of vigorous-intensity aerobic activity, or an equivalent mix of the two each week (CDC, 2011a). Teach patients to monitor their cholesterol, triglyceride, lipoprotein (HDL) and low-density lipoprotein levels, (LDL), as well as their blood pressure. Encourage patients to limit alcohol intake and stop smoking (see discussion later in the chapter).

VACCINATION

Influenza. Influenza (the flu) is a contagious respiratory illness that causes mild to severe illness, and even death. People at high risk for serious flu complications include young children; pregnant women; people with chronic health conditions like asthma, diabetes, or heart and lung disease; and people 65 years and older. The best way to prevent the flu is by getting vaccinated. All people 6 months of age and older should be vaccinated each year (CDC, 2012).

Pneumococcal Disease. Pneumococcal disease is an infection caused by a type of bacteria called pneumococcus. There are different types of pneumococcal disease, such as pneumococcal pneumonia, meningitis, and otitis media. Pneumococcal disease can be fatal. In some cases, it can result in long-term problems, like brain damage, hearing loss, and limb loss. Pneumococcal vaccine is very good at preventing severe disease, hospitalization, and death. Pneumococcal vaccine is recommended for all children less than 59 months of age. Children aged more than 24 months who are at high risk for pneumococcal disease and adults with risk factors should receive this vaccine. Risk factors for children and adults include those with long-term health problems, with a disease or condition that lowers the body's resistance to infection, or who are taking a drug or undergoing a treatment that lowers the body's resistance to infection. All adults 65 years of age and older, any adult 19 through 64 years of age who is a smoker or has asthma, and residents of long-term care facilities should also receive this vaccine (CDC, 2011b).

PROMOTING HEALTH LITERACY

IN PATIENTS WITH COPD

Patient Scenario

Nickoli Romanov, age 69, has been experiencing a morning cough for "several years," but states, "It wasn't too bad, so I lived with it." He reports increasing shortness of breath and fatigue over the last few months, with mucous production. He states that he has noticed increased amounts of mucous during the last few weeks, and significantly increased difficulty breathing with activity. Mr. Romanov reports smoking cigarettes for 40 years, but has recently been thinking about quitting. After having a medical workup, including pulmonary function studies, Mr. Romanov was diagnosed with chronic obstructive pulmonary disease (COPD). He tells the nurse that he doesn't really think that he can use "all these medications, especially that breathing thing," and doesn't really understand what COPD is. He asks, "Do you think my smoking is making me worse?"

Nursing Considerations: *Tips for Improving Health Literacy*

Provide Mr. Romanov with easy-to-read information about COPD. Encourage him to ask his primary care provider as many questions as needed to understand his condition. Explain that it is a breathing problem that comes on over a long time, but there are things he can do to feel better and help keep from getting worse. Reinforce that it is important to take the medications every day and learn the right way to use inhaled medications. Provide information and resources to help him quit smoking. Encourage Mr. Romanov to ask his primary care provider the following three questions:

• What is my main problem?
• What do I need to do?
• Why is it important for me to do this?

What additional measures can you take to help increase health literacy in this patient? What other measures would be helpful for Mr. Romanov if he did not speak English, could not read, or had other learning deficits?

TEACHING ABOUT POLLUTION-FREE ENVIRONMENTS

A pollution-free environment is particularly important for people with cardiopulmonary problems. Teach the patient to assess the environment and make adjustments, whenever possible, to factors that impair respiratory functioning ("triggers"). The patient must actively plan to prevent exposure to pollutants and triggers. This might involve a job change, use of protective equipment, requesting enforcement of laws by government agencies, or subcontracting jobs. In order to minimize triggers in the home, dusting and vacuuming the office and home must be done at least twice per week. In some situations, the patient may be asked to wear a mask to prevent some symptoms of respiratory distress. Explain to the patient that exposure to industrial or occupational hazards (e.g., paint, varnish, gaseous fumes, asbestos) must also be restricted.

In the United States, fine pollutants—including carbon monoxide, sulfur dioxide, total suspended particulates, ozone, and nitrogen dioxide—that pose a hazard to health are monitored closely. On days when pollutant levels are elevated significantly, morbidity and mortality rates among people with pre-existing pulmonary disease are increased greatly. Thus, on days when pollution alerts are announced, people with altered respiratory function should reduce their activities, stay indoors, and use an air conditioner, electronic air cleaner, or air filter. If pollen alters the patient's respiratory function, the same principles apply.

Cigarette smoking is a major risk factor in cardiopulmonary diseases. The inhalation of cigarette smoke increases airway resistance, reduces ciliary action, increases mucus production, causes thickening of the alveolar–capillary membrane, and causes bronchial walls to thicken and lose their elasticity. Smoking is the most common cause of chronic obstructive pulmonary disease (COPD), and increases the risk for many types of cancer, including cancers of the oral cavity, esophagus, lung, urinary bladder, and kidneys. In addition, cigarette smoking causes reduced circulation by narrowing the blood vessels (arteries). Smoking causes coronary heart disease, the leading cause of death in the United States, and causes a much greater risk for stroke, peripheral vascular disease, and abdominal aortic aneurysm (abnormal dilation of blood vessels). These effects occur in both smokers and nonsmokers (children and adults) who live with smokers (CDC, 2010). Habitual smokers usually have great difficulty quitting or reducing their smoking and need much encouragement. The American Lung Association and the American Heart Association (AHA) offer many free educational materials to aid and support patients who are trying to stop smoking. Their addresses and phone numbers are listed in local telephone directories; both agencies offer extensive information online. As a nurse, it is important to play a key role in presenting accurate information about the effects of smoking. Encourage the decision to never start smoking or to stop smoking. Provide appropriate information, counseling, support, and resources to assist patients to be successful with smoking cessation.

REDUCING ANXIETY

It is important to create an environment that is likely to reduce anxiety. Help institute measures to alleviate discomfort immediately. Use effective listening skills and accurate observation to display a caring attitude. Attempt to understand the patient's life experiences and habits without judging them. Patients with harmful health habits often fear they will be judged, which impedes the use of nursing interventions. Patients who believe nurses are genuinely concerned about them and their families are more willing to work toward achieving mutually desirable outcomes.

 THINK back to Joan McIntyre, the woman requesting to be "let go" if she should stop breathing. The nurse needs to provide support to the patient, showing genuine concern for her welfare. In addition, the nurse needs to act ethically and legally to ensure the patient's rights. ●

MAINTAINING GOOD NUTRITION

Beneficial behaviors, such as a healthy diet, should be incorporated into a patient's daily activities. Encourage patients to eat a diet that includes foods low in saturated fat and cholesterol, low in sodium (salt), and high in fiber. This diet can help patients reduce their risk for chronic disease such as cardiopulmonary diseases, improve health, and reduce the prevalence of overweight and obesity (U.S. Department of Agriculture [USDA], 2012).

Patients with cardiovascular diseases, such as hypertension, benefit from eating a diet rich in fruit, vegetables, low-fat dairy products, and nuts and legumes, with reduced amounts of fat, red meat, sweets, and beverages with sugar. This diet provides a high intake of potassium, magnesium, calcium, protein, and fiber, along with a low intake of saturated fat, sodium, cholesterol, total fat, and extra sugars.

People who work hard at breathing often do not have much energy for eating. Many of the medications used for treatment can cause anorexia and nausea. However, maintaining an adequate nutritional intake is crucial. Interventions should focus on ensuring an adequate intake of proteins, vitamins, and minerals. Consider the use of six small meals distributed over the course of the day instead of the usual three larger meals. Provide frequent oral hygiene and rest periods before eating to help improve the patient's intake. Encourage patients to eat their meals 1 to 2 hours after breathing treatments and exercises.

Patients who have COPD require a high-protein/high-calorie diet to counter malnutrition. Encourage obese patients to lose weight using a calorie-controlled diet. Diets should be 40% to 55% carbohydrates, 30% to 40% fat, and 12% to 20% protein. A diet rich in antioxidants, vitamins A and C, and the B vitamins is important. If supplemental oxygen is used, reinforce the importance of wearing the cannula during and after meals. Eating and digestion require energy, which causes the body to use more oxygen.

Promoting Comfort

Interventions to promote patient comfort are an important part of nursing care for patients with alterations in cardiopulmonary function. Promoting proper positioning, adequate fluid intake, humidification of inspired air, and appropriate breathing techniques are used to maximize the patient's sense of well-being. In addition, encourage the patient to pace physical activities and schedule frequent rest periods to conserve energy.

POSITIONING

Proper positioning is important to ease respirations. A proper position for breathing is a position that allows free movement of the diaphragm and expansion of the chest wall. Alternately, sitting in a slumped position permits the abdominal contents to push upward on the diaphragm, decreasing lung expansion during inspiration. People with dyspnea and orthopnea are most comfortable in a high Fowler's position because accessory muscles can easily be used to promote respiration. Research has demonstrated that, in patients with pulmonary disease who are acutely ill, turning to the prone position on a regular basis promotes oxygenation (Dirkes et al., 2012; Rickelmann, 2012). In this position, the posterior dependent sections of the lungs are better ventilated and perfused.

MAINTAINING ADEQUATE FLUID INTAKE

Patients can help keep their secretions thin by drinking 2 to 3 quarts (1.9–2.9 L) of clear fluids daily. Fluid intake should be increased to the maximum that the patient's health state can tolerate. Increased fluids are needed by patients who have an elevated temperature, who are breathing through the mouth, who are coughing, or who are losing excessive body fluids in other ways. However, encourage patients with heart failure and low sodium levels to limit their fluid intake to 1.5 L/day (Dudek, 2014).

PROVIDING HUMIDIFIED AIR

Inspiring dry air removes the normal moisture in the respiratory passages that protect against irritation and infection. This is especially troublesome for patients who cannot breathe through their nose. When air humidity is low, it may be necessary to humidify the air with room humidifiers or vaporizers. Electric vaporizers that produce steam or cool mist are also useful, but neither device has been demonstrated to have greater therapeutic value than the other. Although a cool-mist vaporizer reduces the danger of burns because it does not generate heat or hot water, it can be a medium for pathogen growth if it is not cleaned adequately. A steam vaporizer does not present this risk for infection because the heat kills most pathogens.

Promoting Proper Breathing

Many people, both well and ill, have breathing habits that are not conducive to maximal respiratory functioning. Some people develop a pattern of shallow breathing or walk with a posture that makes the chest wall appear caved in, affecting chest expansion. Ill people may limit their respiratory efforts to compensate for disease symptoms or an illness. Breathing exercises are designed to help patients achieve more efficient and controlled ventilations, to decrease the work of breathing, and to correct respiratory deficits. The accompanying box, Examples of Nursing Intervention and Nursing Outcome Classifications (NIC/NOC), lists standardized nursing interventions

EXAMPLES OF NURSING INTERVENTIONS AND NURSING OUTCOMES CLASSIFICATIONS (NIC/NOC)

VENTILATION ASSISTANCE

Nursing Interventions	Nursing Outcomes
• Maintain a patent airway. • Auscultate breath sounds, noting areas of decreased or absent ventilation and presence of adventitious sounds. • Initiate and maintain supplemental oxygen, as prescribed. • Administer appropriate pain medication to prevent hypoventilation. • Ambulate three to four times per day, as appropriate. • Monitor respiratory and oxygenation status. • Administer medications (e.g., bronchodilators and inhalers) that promote airway patency and gas exchange. • Teach pursed-lip breathing techniques, as appropriate. • Initiate a program of respiratory muscle strength and/or endurance training, as appropriate.	• Respiratory Status: Gas Exchange • Tissue Perfusion: Pulmonary • Respiratory Status: Ventilation • Vital Signs • Cardiopulmonary Status • Tissue Perfusion: Cellular

Reprinted from Bulechek, G. M., Butcher, H. K., Dochterman, J. M., & Wagner, C. M. (Eds.). (2013). *Nursing interventions classification (NIC)* (6th ed., pp. 411–412). St. Louis: Elsevier/Mosby; and Moorhead, S., Johnson, M., Maas, M. L., & Swanson, E. (Eds.). (2013). *Nursing outcomes classification (NOC)* (5th ed., pp. 431, 545, 550). St. Louis: Elsevier/Mosby. A full listing of nursing activities for each nursing intervention and outcomes can be found in these books.

and corresponding outcomes related to maximizing oxygen and carbon dioxide exchange in the lungs. Descriptions of specific techniques follow.

DEEP BREATHING

When hypoventilation occurs, a decreased amount of air enters and leaves the lungs. However, deep-breathing exercises can be used to overcome hypoventilation.

Instruct the patient to make each breath deep enough to move the bottom ribs. Unless the patient has a nasal condition that prohibits or prevents normal breathing, have the patient start slowly taking deep ventilations nasally and then expiring slowly through the mouth. Breathing through the nose warms, filters, and humidifies the air. The patient's respiratory status, motivation, and general clinical condition dictate the timing of this exercise, which should be done hourly while awake or four times daily.

USING INCENTIVE SPIROMETRY

Incentive spirometry provides visual reinforcement for deep breathing by the patient. An incentive spirometer assists the patient to breathe slowly and deeply and to sustain maximal inspiration. The gauge on the spirometer allows the patient to measure one's own progress, providing immediate positive reinforcement. It encourages the patient to maximize lung inflation and prevent or reduce atelectasis. Optimal gas exchange is supported and secretions can be cleared and expectorated. Before using incentive spirometry equipment, the patient needs instructions on using the equipment properly. Validate the patient's correct use of this equipment in both health care and home environments. See Guidelines for Nursing Care 38-1 for information regarding teaching patients to use this device.

PURSED-LIP BREATHING

Patients who experience dyspnea and feelings of panic can often reduce these symptoms by using pursed-lip breathing. Exhaling through pursed lips creates a smaller opening for air movement, effectively slowing and prolonging expiration. Prolonged expiration is thought to result in decreased airway narrowing during expiration and prevent the collapse of small airways. This results in improved air exchange and decreased dyspnea. Pursed-lip breathing also helps the patient to control the rate and depth of respiration, helping to reduce feelings of dyspnea. It also encourages relaxation, which aids the patient to gain control of dyspnea and reduce feelings of panic. Encourage patients with COPD to try this breathing technique to help manage their daily activities (Corbridge, Wilken, Kapella, & Gronkiewicz, 2012; Hinkle & Cheever, 2014).

While sitting upright, the patient inhales through the nose while counting to three, then exhales slowly and evenly against pursed lips while tightening the abdominal muscles. During exhalation, the patient counts to seven. To purse the lips, the patient should position the lips as though sucking through a straw or whistling. When walking and using pursed-lip breathing, the patient should inhale while taking two steps and then exhale through pursed lips while taking the next four steps, then repeat the cycle.

DIAPHRAGMATIC BREATHING

Many people with COPD breathe in a shallow, rapid, and exhausting pattern. Teach the patient with COPD to change this type of upper chest breathing to another form, diaphragmatic breathing. Diaphragmatic breathing reduces the respiratory rate, increases alveolar ventilation, and sometimes helps expel as much air as possible during expiration (Hinkle & Cheever, 2014).

GUIDELINES FOR NURSING CARE 38-1

TEACHING PATIENTS TO USE AN INCENTIVE SPIROMETER

- Assist the patient to an upright or semi-Fowler's position if possible.
- Remove dentures if they fit poorly.
- Assess for pain. Administer pain medication, as prescribed, if needed. **If the patient has recently undergone abdominal or chest surgery, place a pillow or folded blanket over a chest or abdominal incision for splinting.**
- Demonstrate how to steady the device with one hand and hold the mouthpiece with the other hand.
- Instruct the patient to exhale normally and then place lips securely around the mouthpiece.
- Instruct the patient not to breathe through the nose. Use a nose clip if necessary. **Instruct the patient to inhale slowly and as deeply as possible through the mouthpiece without using the nose (a nose clip may be used).**
- Instruct the patient to remove the lips from the mouthpiece and exhale normally. **If patient becomes light-headed during the process, tell him or her to stop and take a few normal breaths before resuming incentive spirometry.**

- Encourage the patient to complete breathing exercises about 5 to 10 times every 1 to 2 hours, if possible. Rest in between breaths as necessary.

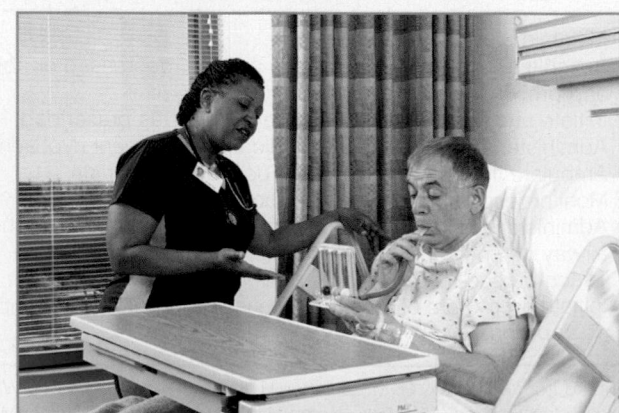

To do this, the patient places one hand on the stomach and the other on the middle of the chest. The patient breathes in slowly through the nose, letting the abdomen protrude as far as it will go, then breathes out through pursed lips while contracting the abdominal muscles, with one hand pressing inward and upward on the abdomen. The patient repeats these steps for 1 minute, followed by a rest for 2 minutes. Encourage the patient to practice this breathing pattern several times during the day, so that eventually it becomes automatic.

Promoting and Controlling Coughing

A cough is a cleansing mechanism of the body. It is a means of helping to keep the airway clear of secretions and other debris. A cough that is dry is termed a nonproductive cough. A cough that produces respiratory secretions is termed a productive cough. The respiratory secretion expelled by coughing or clearing the throat is called **sputum**.

When there are excessive fluids or secretions in an organ or body tissue, the patient is said to be congested. Thus, a person with secretions or fluid in the lungs is said to have congested lungs. If the cough is dry, the patient is said to be congested with a nonproductive cough. If the cough produces sputum, the patient is said to be congested with a productive cough. Thick respiratory secretions are sometimes called phlegm. A patient who is coughing and does not have any congestion or secretions produced is said to be noncongested with a nonproductive cough.

A series of events produce a cough. The cough mechanism (Fig. 38-10) consists of an initial irritation; a deep inspiration; a quick, tight closure of the glottis together with a forceful contraction of the expiratory intercostal muscles; and an upward push of the diaphragm. This causes an explosive movement of air from the lower to the upper respiratory tract. To be effective, a cough should have enough muscle contraction to force air to be expelled and to propel a liquid or a solid on its way out of the respiratory tract. Coughing is most effective when the patient is sitting upright with feet flat on the floor. Coughing can be voluntary or involuntary.

VOLUNTARY COUGHING

When a cough does not occur as a result of reflex stimulation of the cough-sensitive areas, it can be induced voluntarily. Teaching the patient to cough voluntarily is an important aspect of preoperative and postoperative care. Coughing is more effective when combined with deep breathing. Although teaching a patient to cough and deep breathe is relatively easy, experience has shown that it is difficult to motivate patients to follow through and perform coughing on their own. Refer to Guidelines for Nursing Care 29-2: Effective Coughing, on page 868, for detailed instructions for teaching this intervention. Frequently remind patients to perform effective coughing throughout the day. Develop a specific schedule for coughing on the patient's plan of care. Coughing early in the morning after rising removes secretions that have accumulated during the night. Coughing before meals improves the taste of food and oxygenation. At bedtime, coughing removes any buildup of secretions and improves sleep patterns. For a patient who is unable to cough voluntarily, manual stimulation over the trachea and prolonged exhalation can be helpful. If neither of these methods is successful, mechanical endotracheal suctioning with a catheter may be necessary.

If the patient has a neuromuscular disorder and is unable to cough physically, an assisted cough may be used. For an assisted cough, firm pressure is placed on the abdomen below the diaphragm in rhythm with exhalation. This pressure is similar to the Heimlich maneuver, but with less force. This pressure is used to substitute for the weakened or paralyzed abdominal muscles.

INVOLUNTARY COUGHING

Involuntary coughing often accompanies respiratory tract infections and irritations. Many times respiratory infections lead to the production of respiratory secretions. These secretions can trigger the cough mechanism. When the cough is productive, it helps clear the airway. However, when the cough is nonproductive, it can be fatiguing and irritating. Medications may control involuntary coughing. Refer to the next section, Cough Suppressants. Observation of the patient's breathing and coughing characteristics is necessary to determine the appropriate type of medication.

USING COUGH MEDICATIONS

Various medications can be used to promote coughing, aiding in the movement of mucus through the respiratory tract, and in controlling coughing to allow the patient to rest.

Expectorants. Expectorants are drugs that facilitate the removal of respiratory tract secretions by reducing the viscosity of the secretions. Patients with extremely tenacious (thick) secretions may need the secretions liquefied for their cough to be effective. In that way, the nonproductive

FIGURE 38-10. (**A**) A cough begins with a deep inspiration, distending the trachea and hyperinflating the lungs. (**B**) After inspiration, the glottis closes while intercostal and abdominal muscles contract forcibly. (**C**) When intrathoracic pressure reaches a high level, the glottis opens slightly, and the diaphragm is pushed up, producing an explosive movement of air.

cough of a person with lung congestion can become productive. Use of an expectorant by a person without congestion is inappropriate. Guaifenesin is widely used as an expectorant in cold and cough medications (e.g., Robitussin). Some health care providers consider adequate fluid intake and air humidification as effective expectorants.

Cough Suppressants. Suppressants are drugs that depress a body function—in this case, the cough reflex. Codeine, which is present in many cough preparations, is generally considered the preferred cough suppressant ingredient. However, codeine can be addictive, and because of possible abuse, most states require a prescription for its use. Drowsiness is a side effect, thus it may not be safe to use codeine when the person must remain alert, such as when driving a car. A suppressant that is not addictive is dextromethorphan, which can be found in many over-the-counter cold and cough remedies.

An irritating, nonproductive cough in people without congestion may be treated appropriately with suppressants. Suppression of the productive cough is usually not recommended unless the patient is trying to sleep. If a productive cough is suppressed, secretions can be retained, leading to a pulmonary infection.

Lozenges. Cough lozenges can often relieve mild, nonproductive coughs in people without congestion. A lozenge is a small, solid medication intended to be held in the mouth until it dissolves. Lozenges generally control coughs by the local anesthetic effect of benzocaine. The local anesthetic acts on sensory and motor nerves, controlling the primary irritation and inhibiting afferent and efferent impulses.

Teaching about Cough Medications. Cough medications are readily available, and people who purchase them are usually eager for relief. Often, consumers take excessive amounts of more than one type. Teach about the appropriate choice of expectorants and suppressants and about misuse of cough mixtures. For example, cough syrups with a high sugar or alcohol content can disturb the metabolic balance of patients with diabetes mellitus or can trigger a relapse for recovering alcoholics. Preparations containing antihistamines have an anticholinergic action, which can cause serious problems for people with

glaucoma or cause urinary retention in men with prostate enlargement. Other cough preparations can be detrimental to people with hypertension or thyroid or cardiac diseases. In addition, prolonged use of self-prescribed cough preparations can conceal more serious health problems. If a cough lasts more than 7 days, urge the person to contact the primary care provider. In addition, encourage the person to increase fluid intake if the secretions become too thick to expectorate.

Performing Chest Physiotherapy

Chest physiotherapy helps loosen and mobilize secretions, increasing mucous clearance. This is especially helpful for patients with large amounts of secretions or an ineffective cough. Chest physiotherapy includes percussion, vibration, and postural drainage.

PERCUSSION

Percussion of lung areas involves the use of a cupped palm to loosen pulmonary secretions so that they can be expectorated with greater ease. With the hand held in a rigid, dome-shaped position (Fig. 38-11), strike the area over the lung lobes to be drained in a rhythmic pattern. Position the patient in a lateral, supine, or prone position, based on the lobes to be treated. Proper hand and patient positioning will ensure that the patient does not experience any pain with this procedure. Percussion is never done on bare skin or performed over surgical incisions, below the ribs, or over the spine or breasts because of the danger of tissue damage. Typically, each area is percussed for 30 to 60 seconds several times a day. If the patient has tenacious secretions, the area may be percussed for up to 3 to 5 minutes several times per day. Patients may learn how to percuss the anterior surfaces of their own chest wall. In addition, it is a good idea to teach family members how to percuss posterior surfaces. Mechanical devices as well as manual handheld cupping devices also are available for percussion on the chest wall.

VIBRATING

Vibration uses manual compression and tremor on the patient's chest wall to help loosen respiratory secretions. Loosened secretions can be expectorated more easily. The practitioner uses rhythmic contraction and relaxation of

FIGURE 38-11. **(A)** The cupping position and action of the hand on manual percussion of the lung area. **(B)** The position and action of the hands necessary to use vibration to loosen respiratory secretions in the lungs. *(Photos by B. Proud.)*

arm and shoulder muscles while holding the hands flat on the patient's chest wall as the patient exhales. Vibration can be done for several minutes, several times a day. To avoid causing patient discomfort, vibration is never done over the patient's breasts, spine, sternum, and lower rib cage. Vibration (see Fig. 38-11) can also be taught to family members or accomplished using a mechanical device.

PROVIDING POSTURAL DRAINAGE

Postural drainage makes use of gravity to drain secretions from the lungs. Position the patient in a way that promotes the drainage of secretions from smaller pulmonary branches into larger ones, where they can be removed by coughing (Fig. 38-12). Vibration, percussion, or both often precede postural drainage.

When implementing postural drainage, have tissues and an emesis basin close at hand for the patient to use when coughing and expectorating secretions. Place the patient in an appropriate position to promote drainage from the lobes of the lungs. Postural drainage should be done two to four times a day for 20 to 30 minutes. Discontinue the drainage if the patient begins to feel weak or faint. Delay postural drainage for 1 to 2 hours after meals to avoid provoking vomiting. Appropriate positioning to achieve postural drainage is as follows:

- Use high Fowler's position to drain the apical sections of the upper lobes of the lungs.
- Place the patient in a lying position, half on the abdomen and half on the side, right and left, to drain the posterior sections of the upper lobes of the lungs.

- Place the patient lying on the left side with a pillow under the chest wall to drain the right lobe of the lung.
- Place the patient in the Trendelenburg position to drain the lower lobes of the lungs.

 ### Suctioning the Airway

Suctioning of the pharynx is indicated to maintain a patent airway and to remove saliva, pulmonary secretions, blood, vomitus, or foreign material from the pharynx. Suctioning of the oropharynx or nasopharynx may be indicated if the patient is able to raise secretions from the airways but unable to clear from the mouth. Refer to Skill 38-2 on pages 1444-1449. The frequency of suctioning varies with the amount of secretions present but should be done often enough to keep ventilation effective and as effortless as possible. If the patient is unable to raise secretions from the airways, tracheal suctioning may be indicated. Tracheal suctioning is discussed later in the chapter.

Suctioning irritates the mucosa and removes oxygen from the respiratory tract, possibly causing **hypoxemia** (insufficient oxygen in the blood). Thus, it is important to preoxygenate the patient before suctioning. This is accomplished by applying or increasing supplemental oxygen and having the patient take several deep breaths before inserting the catheter.

When performed correctly, suctioning provides comfort by relieving respiratory distress. When performed incorrectly, it can increase anxiety and pain and cause respiratory arrest. At minimum, it is an uncomfortable procedure and it can be a very painful and/or distressing

The lungs

Anterior view

Posterior view

Posterior lower lobes

Anterior lower lobes

Right lower lobe

Left lower lobe

FIGURE 38-12. Postural drainage. Shown are four positions that use the force of gravity to assist the drainage of secretions from the smaller bronchial airways into the main bronchi and trachea to enable the patient to cough them up.

experience. Individualized pain management must be performed in response to the patient's needs (Arroyo-Novoa et al., 2008). Anticipate the administration of analgesic medication to a patient who has had surgery or other trauma before suctioning, because the cough reflex will be stimulated. Possible complications of suctioning include infection, cardiac arrhythmias, hypoxia, mucosal trauma, and death.

Wear gloves on both hands, goggles, and a mask—and a gown, if necessary—for protection from microorganisms. Continuously monitor the patient's color and heart rate and the color, amount, and consistency of secretions. If cyanosis, an excessively slow or rapid heart rate, or suddenly bloody secretions are noted, stop suctioning immediately, administer oxygen, and notify the physician. Cyanosis and a change in heart rate can indicate hypoxemia. Blood can indicate damage to the mucosa.

Meeting Oxygenation Needs With Medications

Although treating patients with medications is a dependent nursing intervention, monitoring the patient's response and development of side effects to medications is an independent nursing action. Table 38-4 lists some common medications for improving respiratory functioning, their side effects, and nursing implications. Many of the drugs used to dilate bronchial airways interact with caffeine. Encourage patients to avoid caffeine, which may potentiate the side effects of bronchodilators.

ADMINISTERING INHALED MEDICATIONS

Inhaled medications may be administered to open narrowed airways (**bronchodilators**), to liquefy or loosen thick secretions (mucolytic agents), or to reduce inflammation in airways (corticosteroids). These medications typically are administered via nebulizer, metered-dose inhaler, or dry powder inhaler. Refer to Guidelines for Nursing Care 28-8 on pages 793–794 for pictures of these devices.

Nebulizers disperse fine particles of liquid medication into the deeper passages of the respiratory tract, where absorption occurs. The treatment continues until all the medication in the nebulizer cup has been inhaled.

A **metered-dose inhaler (MDI)** delivers a controlled dose of medication with each compression of the canister. Common mistakes that patients make when using MDIs include the following:

• Failing to shake the canister
• Holding the inhaler upside down
• Inhaling through the nose rather than the mouth
• Inhaling too rapidly
• Stopping the inhalation when the cold propellant is felt in the throat
• Failing to hold their breath after inhalation
• Inhaling two sprays with one breath

To use an MDI, the patient must activate the device while continuing to inhale. For some patients, especially young children and older adults, a spacer or extender device may be necessary to aid delivery of medication by the inhalation route. The spacer acts as a reservoir. When the MDI is compressed, the medication is deposited in the reservoir, and the patient then inhales the medication from the spacer device. This makes administration less complicated, the dose more predictable, and enhances the delivery of medication to the lungs.

Dry powder inhalers (DPI) are another type of delivery method for inhaled medications. DPIs are breath activated. A quick deep breath by the patient activates the flow of medication, eliminating the need to coordinate activating the inhaler (spraying the medicine) while inhaling the medicine at the same time. DPIs require less manual dexterity than do MDIs. DPIs are actuated by the patient's inspiration, so there is no need to coordinate the delivery of puffs with inhalation. Many types of DPIs are available with distinctive operating instructions. Some have to be loaded with a dose of medication each time they are used. Some hold a preloaded number of doses. It is important to understand the particular instructions for the medication being used. One disadvantage of DPIs is that the medication in DPIs will clump if exposed to humidity.

 REMEMBER Tyrone, the 12-year-old boy with suspected asthma. During this acute attack, the nurse would anticipate administering bronchodilators via a nebulizer. The physician may order bronchodilators to be administered at home using a nebulizer or possibly an MDI with a spacer, or dry powder inhaler. ●

TEACHING PATIENTS ABOUT INHALED MEDICATIONS

Patients need repeated instruction on how to use inhalers and nebulizers effectively and safely. Overuse may result in serious side effects and eventual ineffectiveness of the medication. Nebulizers require cleaning after use, thus patients must understand how to do this correctly. Patients must understand that it is important to keep track of dosing with MDIs. A few MDIs have integrated dose counters, but most do not, and it can be difficult to know when the canister is empty. Patients must understand the importance of keeping track of dosing to ensure that they are not using an empty canister. Most DPIs have a dose counter, so patients have accurate information about when to refill the medication. Patients should not exhale into the DPI, as they risk blowing out the medication. Information about how to use MDIs, DPIs, and small-volume nebulizers properly, including patient teaching information, is provided in Chapter 28, Guidelines for Nursing Care 28-8 on page 793. Package inserts with the medication also reinforce correct technique for using inhalers.

To ensure correct administration when a spacer is used, slow, deep inspirations are necessary. To prevent inhaling too quickly, some spacers are equipped with a whistle device that sounds if inhalation is too rapid. A spacer is also recommended for patients using corticosteroid

Table 38-4   SELECTED MEDICATIONS USED TO IMPROVE RESPIRATORY FUNCTION

MEDICATIONS	ACTIVITY	ROUTE	SIDE EFFECTS	NURSING IMPLICATIONS
Zafirlukast (Accolate)	Bronchodilator	PO	Headache, dizziness, nausea, vomiting	Not used to treat acute attacks. Do not give Accolate with meals.
Montelukast (Singulair)	Also inhibits leuko-triene release as well as inflamma-tory reaction			Singulair should be given before bedtime.
Albuterol	Bronchodilator	PO, inhalation	Tremors, anxiety, insomnia, headache, palpitations, hyper-tension, vomiting	Caution the patient not to increase dosage without con-sulting the primary care pro-vider. Be aware that children 2–6 years of age more fre-quently exhibit CNS stimulation.
Theophylline (aminophylline)	Bronchodilator	PO, IV, rectally	Nausea, vomiting, tachycardia, diure-sis, irritability, ver-tigo, convulsions, nervousness	Monitor vital signs closely. Force fluids as clinical status allows. Monitor serum theophylline levels, especially if the patient does not respond to the drug or if severe side effects develop.
Corticosteroids (prednisone, dexamethasone, budesonide, triamcinolone acetonide)	Reduces inflam-mation	PO, IV, inhalation, intranasal	Fluid retention, hyper-tension, mood swings, weight gain, gastritis, hyperglyce-mia, insomnia	Reduce sodium intake. Make the patient and family aware of potential for labile emotions. Weigh daily in the morning. Monitor blood pressure and blood sugar.
Diphenhydramine (Benadryl)	Antihistamine H1-receptor antagonist	PO	Drowsiness, anorexia, dry mouth, constipa-tion, blurred vision, urinary retention	Warn the patient to use only with the primary health care pro-vider's advice in the presence of bronchial asthma.
Cetrizine (Zyrtec)	Antihistamine H1-receptor antagonist	PO	Headache with limited sedative effect, not associated with anti-cholinergic effects	Monitor effectiveness of the drug. Contraindicated while breast-feeding.
Fexofenadine (Allegra)	Antihistamine H1-receptor antagonist	PO	Headache, not associ-ated with anticholiner-gic or sedative effects	
Cromolyn sodium (Intal)	Mast cell stabilizer Asthma prophy-lactic agent—no bronchodilator, antihistamine, or vasoconstrictor properties	Inhalation—MDI or nasal solution	Cough, nausea, nasal stinging and burn-ing, throat irritation	Remind the patient that this medication is used to prevent asthma attacks, not to treat acute episodes. Inform the patient that the drug is effective only if taken routinely (2–4 times per week). Safety is not established during pregnancy and breastfeeding.

CNS, central nervous system; PO, orally; IV, intravenously.

inhaled agents because it reduces the risk of acquiring an oral fungal infection.

Providing Supplemental Oxygen

Oxygen therapy, which provides supplemental oxygen, can increase the amount of oxygen transported in the blood. Oxygen is considered a medication and must be ordered by a health care provider. However, in an emer-gency situation the absence of a prescription should not delay the administration of oxygen to the patient (Hig-

ginson, Jones, & Davies, 2010). Oxygen therapy can be intimidating or frightening for patients. Therefore, pro-vide clear explanations about the procedures and purpose to help reduce anxiety. Encourage patients to discuss concerns. If oxygen is given in an emergency, explana-tions concurrent with administration are appropriate.

SOURCES OF OXYGEN

Therapeutic oxygen is supplied from a wall outlet or a por-table cylinder or tank. A specially designed flow meter is attached to the wall outlet (see Skill 38-3, pp. 1449–1452, for an illustration of a flow meter). A valve regulates the oxygen flow in liters per minute. To release oxygen safely and at the desired rate from a cylinder or tank, a regulator is used. The regulator has two gauges. The one nearest the tank shows the pressure or amount of oxygen in the tank. The other gauge indicates the number of liters per minute of oxygen being released. In patients with chronic respiratory insufficiency who use oxygen on a daily basis at home, having to transport an oxygen canister can impede their functional exercise capacity. The portable canister's weight and increased respiratory and skeletal muscle load contributes an additional burden for these patients. A small walking aid may be suggested to reduce the patient's burden. Oxygen concentrators are another way to provide oxygen. This oxygen delivery system concentrates room air to provide the appropriate concentration of oxygen to the patient. They are used frequently in home situations.

OXYGEN FLOW RATE

The flow rate of oxygen, measured in liters per minute, determines the amount of oxygen delivered to the patient. The rate varies depending on the condition of the patient and the route of administration of the oxygen. The flow rate does not necessarily reflect the oxygen concentration actually inspired by the patient because there is leaking and mixing with atmospheric air. If more precise doses are necessary, they are usually prescribed in terms of percentage of inspired oxygen. To regulate the oxygen percentage concentration accurately, samples of the air mixture the patient is actually inhaling may be analyzed every 4 hours. Several types of commercial oxygen analyzers are available.

The medical order prescribes the rate of oxygen administration. Closely monitor the flow rate to verify that the patient is receiving the prescribed concentration. Normally, excessive levels of carbon dioxide in the blood stimulate the patient to breathe. However, the chemoreceptors of some, but not all, patients with chronic lung disease, such as emphysema, become insensitive to carbon dioxide and respond to hypoxia to stimulate breathing (Hinkle & Cheever, 2014; McGlolin, 2008). If excessive oxygen is given, the stimulus to breathe is removed; as a result, the patient may stop breathing completely. Monitor respiratory rate and arterial blood gas results closely for changes. Many times, continuous pulse oximetry also is used to monitor the patient receiving oxygen.

HUMIDIFICATION

Most institutions do not require humidification with very-low-flow oxygen (2 L/min or less) delivered by nasal cannula (see oxygen delivery systems to follow) when administered to adults. However, because oxygen dries and dehydrates the respiratory mucous membranes, humidifying devices (supplying 20%–40% humidity) are commonly used when oxygen is delivered at higher flow rates. Distilled or sterile water is commonly used to humidify oxygen. When moving patients receiving humidified oxygen, make sure that water from the humidifier does not enter the tubing through which the oxygen is flowing. Additional suggestions for transporting a patient with a portable oxygen tank are given in Guidelines for Nursing Care 38-2.

PRECAUTIONS FOR OXYGEN ADMINISTRATION

Oxygen, which constitutes 21% of normal air, is a tasteless, odorless, and colorless gas. It supports combustion. To prevent fires and injuries, take the following precautions:

- Avoid open flames in the patient's room.
- Place "no smoking" signs in conspicuous places in the patient's home. Instruct the patient and visitors about the hazard of smoking when oxygen is in use.
- Check to see that electrical equipment used in the room, such as electric bell cords, razors, radios, and suctioning equipment, is in good working order and emits no sparks.
- Avoid wearing and using synthetic fabrics that build up static electricity.
- Avoid using oils in the area. Oil can ignite spontaneously in the presence of oxygen.

OXYGEN DELIVERY SYSTEMS

Oxygen can be administered by many different delivery systems: nasal cannula, nasopharyngeal catheter, transtracheal catheter, simple mask, partial rebreather mask, non-rebreather mask, Venturi mask, and tent. Table 38-5 (on page 1428) compares several oxygen delivery systems.

Nasal Cannula. A **nasal cannula**, also called nasal prongs, is the most commonly used oxygen delivery device. The cannula is a disposable plastic device with two protruding prongs that are inserted into the nostrils. The cannula is connected to an oxygen source with a flow meter and, many times, a humidifier. The cannula does not impede eating or speaking and is used easily in the home. Disadvantages of this system are that it can be dislodged easily and can cause dryness of the nasal mucosa. In addition, if a patient breathes through the mouth, it is difficult to determine the amount of oxygen the patient is actually receiving. Skill 38-3 describes oxygen administration by nasal cannula.

Nasopharyngeal Catheter. A nasopharyngeal catheter is another efficient means for administering oxygen, but it is infrequently used because it is uncomfortable for the patient and may cause trauma to respiratory mucous membranes. It is inserted into the nose through one nostril, with the end of the catheter resting in the oropharynx. It is important to remove the catheter for cleaning and change it to the other nostril every 12 to 24 hours (Eastwood, Gardner, & O'Connell, 2007). Gastric distention often occurs because the gas flow can be misdirected into the stomach.

Face masks. Disposable and reusable face masks are available. Fit the mask carefully to the patient's face to

GUIDELINES FOR NURSING CARE 38-2

TRANSPORTING A PATIENT WITH A PORTABLE OXYGEN CYLINDER

Before the Transfer

- Check that an additional oxygen source is available where the patient is being transferred.
- Check the amount of oxygen in the cylinder (place the cylinder key or wrench on the valve stem and turn fully counterclockwise until the needle on the gauge indicates the amount of available oxygen; turn the key back a half turn; use the cylinder only if the gauge indicates more than 500 psi).
- If available, use a table that gives the estimated minutes of available oxygen according to the amount of oxygen in the cylinder and the rate of flow ordered for the patient. This can help to determine whether the supply of oxygen is adequate for the transfer (Davis & Johnston, 2008).
- Connect the oxygen tubing to the flow meter adapter and adjust the flow-control dial to the prescribed setting.
- Attach the patient's oxygen cannula to transport oxygen.
- Ensure that the cylinder is secured in a holder before transporting the patient (it is a dangerous practice to place the cylinder between the patient's legs or next to the patient during transfer because injury to the patient may result).
- Place the coiled tubing under a pillow or attach it to linen or a patient's gown.

After the Transfer

- Attach the patient's oxygen cannula to wall oxygen.
- Turn off the oxygen flow from the cylinder by turning the cylinder key clockwise until it is tight.
- Remove any excess oxygen in the pressure gauge by "bleeding" it. Turn the flow-control dial back on until the hissing sound stops and the needle on the gauge has fallen to zero. Turn the flow-control dial off.

Cylinder pressure gauge

Flow-control gauge

Valve stem

Flow meter adapter

Flow-control dial

Humidifier bottle

Transport cart

---

avoid leakage of oxygen. It should be comfortably snug but not tight against the face. The most commonly used types of masks are the simple face mask, the partial rebreather mask, the nonrebreather mask, and the Venturi mask. Skill 38-4 on pages 1452–1455 describes the actions and rationales involved in using face masks.

The simple face mask is connected to oxygen tubing, a humidifier, and a flow meter, just like the nasal cannula. This mask has vents on its sides that allow room air to leak in at many places, thereby diluting the source oxygen. The vents also allow exhaled carbon dioxide to escape. Often a simple mask is used when an increased delivery of oxygen is needed for short periods (e.g., less than 12 hours). The mask should fit closely to the face to deliver this higher concentration of oxygen effectively. Patients may have difficulty keeping the mask in position over the nose and mouth, and because of this pressure and the presence of moisture, skin breakdown is a possibility. Eating or talking with the mask in place can be difficult. Because of the risk of retaining carbon dioxide, never apply the simple face mask with a delivery flow rate of less than 5 liters per minute.

The partial rebreather mask is similar to a simple face mask, but is equipped with a reservoir bag for the collection of the first part of the patient's exhaled air. The remaining exhaled air exits through vents. The air in the reservoir is mixed with 100% oxygen for the next inhalation. Thus, the patient rebreathes about one-third of the expired air from the reservoir bag. This type of mask permits the conservation of oxygen. An additional advantage is that the patient can inhale room air through openings in the mask if the oxygen supply is briefly interrupted. The disadvantages are those of any mask: eating and talking are difficult, a tight seal is required, and there is the potential for skin breakdown. Monitor the reservoir bag carefully. It should deflate slightly with inspiration; if it deflates completely, the flow rate should be increased until only a slight deflation is noted.

The nonrebreather mask delivers the highest concentration of oxygen via a mask to a spontaneously breathing patient. It is similar to the partial rebreather mask except that two one-way valves prevent the patient from rebreathing exhaled air. The reservoir bag is filled with oxygen that enters the mask on inspiration. Exhaled air escapes through

Table 38-5 OXYGEN DELIVERY SYSTEMS

METHOD	AMOUNT DELIVERED FiO$_2$ (FRACTION INSPIRED OXYGEN)	PRIORITY NURSING INTERVENTIONS
Nasal cannula	*Low Flow* 1–2 L/min = 23%–30% 3–5 L/min = 30%–40% 6 L/min = 42%	Check frequently that both prongs are in the patient's nares. For patients with chronic lung disease, limit rate to the minimum needed to raise arterial oxygen saturation to a level that provides adequate oxygen delivery to tissues (88%–92%), and no higher; usually 2–3 L/min. via nasal cannula (Austin et al., 2010).
Simple mask	*Low Flow* 6–8 L/min = 40%–60% (5 L/min is minimum setting)	Monitor the patient frequently to check placement of the mask. Support the patient if claustrophobia is a concern. Secure a medical order to replace the mask with a nasal cannula during mealtime.
Partial rebreather mask	*Low Flow* 8–11 L/min = 50%–75%	Set flow rate so that the mask remains two-thirds full during inspiration. Keep the reservoir bag free of twists or kinks.
Nonrebreather mask	*Low Flow* 12 L/min = 80%–100%	Maintain flow rate so that the reservoir bag collapses only slightly during inspiration. Check that the valves and rubber flaps are functioning properly (open during expiration and closed during inhalation). Monitor SaO$_2$ with pulse oximeter.
Venturi mask	*High Flow* 4–10 L/min = 24%–40%	Requires careful monitoring to verify FiO$_2$ at flow rate ordered. Check that air intake valves are not blocked.

Reprinted with permission from Hinkle, J. L., & Cheever, K. H. (2014). *Brunner & Suddarth's textbook of medical–surgical nursing* (13th ed.). Philadelphia: Wolters Kluwer Health/Lippincott Williams & Wilkins.

side vents. A malfunction of the bag could cause carbon dioxide buildup and suffocation. This mask can also be used to administer other gases, such as heliox. Heliox is a mixture of helium and oxygen, used to reduce the work of breathing, deliver aerosols, and reduce fear and anxiety for patients in respiratory distress. Helium has a very low density that allows it to flow easily into narrow or twisty air passages, delivering nebulized medications into the lower airways. In addition, carbon dioxide diffuses through helium at four to five times the rate it diffuses through room air, thus it can exit the body faster and easier (Hess, MacIntyre, Mishoe, Galvin, & Adams, 2012; Pruitt, 2007a).

The Venturi mask gets its name from the Venturi effect, which allows the mask to deliver the most precise concentrations of oxygen. This mask has a large tube with an oxygen inlet. As the tube narrows, the pressure drops, causing air to be pulled in through side ports. These ports are adjusted according to the prescription for oxygen concentration. Be sure that the ports are always open. If these are occluded by linens, clothing, or a patient rolling on the mask, the oxygen delivered might be at an unsafe (too high or too low) concentration.

Oxygen Tent. Oxygen also can be administered by way of an oxygen tent. An oxygen tent is a light, portable structure made of clear plastic and attached to a motor-driven unit. The motor helps to circulate and cool the air in the tent. The cooling device functions like an electric refrigeration unit. A thermostat in the unit keeps the tent at the temperature considered most comfortable for the patient. The tent fits either over the top part of the bed so that the patient's head and thorax are inside, or over the entire bed.

It has side openings through which nursing care can be administered. An oxygen tent is commonly used with children who need a cool and highly humidified airflow (e.g., children with pneumonia). Since the tent does not allow the maintenance of a satisfactory or precise oxygen concentration, it is rarely used with other patients. In addition, it is difficult to maintain a consistent level of oxygen and to deliver oxygen at a rate higher than 30% to 50% (Kyle & Carman, 2013). The humidified airflow quickly creates moisture, leading to damp clothing and linens, and, possibly, hypothermia. Therefore, frequent assessment of the child's temperature, pajamas, and bedding is necessary.

OXYGEN THERAPY IN THE HOME
Liquid oxygen and oxygen concentrators, rather than cylinders, are used more commonly in the home setting. Liquid oxygen is kept inside a small thermal container that can be refilled from a larger storage tank kept in the home. An oxygen concentrator removes nitrogen from the room air and concentrates the oxygen left in the air. The oxygen concentrator needs a power source such as an electrical outlet or battery pack. Oxygen concentrators are portable, cost-effective, and easy to use but cannot deliver oxygen flow at greater than 5 L/min (fraction of inspired oxygen [FiO$_2$] of about 40%; Stoller, 2011).

Patients using continuous supplemental oxygen therapy in the home have another alternative: transtracheal oxygen delivery (Fig. 38-13). With this type of delivery system, a small catheter is inserted into the trachea under local anesthesia, then the catheter is attached to the oxygen source. A transtracheal catheter does not interfere with talking, eating, or drinking and delivers oxygen

FIGURE 38-13. A transtracheal oxygen setup.

throughout the respiratory cycle rather than just at inspiration. The patient or family must assume responsibility for daily catheter care. Patients usually report improved mobility, comfort, and appearance, and lower cost with this delivery system.

Oxygen-conserving devices are also available for use outside the hospital setting. Reservoir cannulas have a reservoir space that stores oxygen during exhalation. On subsequent inhalation, the patient receives that stored oxygen, essentially adding a bolus volume to the continuous-flow oxygen delivery. The patient receives the same oxygen therapy at a lower continuous-oxygen flow rate, conserving oxygen use. Intermittent-flow devices operate by turning oxygen delivery on during some portion of inhalation and off for the balance of the breathing cycle. Patient-exhaled oxygen is conserved, allowing a supply of oxygen to last two to four times as long as if it was delivered continuously (Hess et al., 2012).

Patients using oxygen at home need instruction regarding safety precautions. See Teaching Tips 38-1 for information regarding the use of oxygen in the home setting.

Positive Airway Pressure (PAP)

Positive airway pressure (PAP) therapy uses mild air pressure to keep airways open. This treatment can help the body better maintain carbon dioxide and oxygen levels in the blood. PAP therapy may be used to treat many adult disorders, such as sleep apnea, obstructive sleep apnea, obesity hypoventilation syndrome, and heart failure. It also may be used to treat preterm infants whose lungs have not fully developed.

Continuous positive airway pressure (CPAP) provides continuous mild air pressure to keep airways open. Bilevel positive airway pressure (BiPAP) changes the air pressure while the patient breathes in and out. Both therapies use a mask or other device that fits over the nose or nose and mouth. Straps keep the mask in place. A tube connects the mask to the machine's motor, which blows air into the tube (National Heart Blood and Lung Institute [NHLBI], 2011).

Adjusting to the therapy and machine can take time. Patients report feeling strange wearing a mask on the

TEACHING TIPS 38-1

USING OXYGEN AT HOME

Health Topic	Teaching Tip	Why Is This Important?
Safety	• Do not smoke or use open flames within 10 feet of the oxygen source. • Do not use electrical equipment near oxygen administration set (e.g., space heaters, blow dryers). • Use caution with gas or electric appliances. • Ground oxygen concentrators. • Secure the oxygen tank in a holder and away from direct sunlight or heat. • Allow adequate airflow around the oxygen concentrator (avoid placing flush against the wall). • Notify local fire department of the oxygen in the home.	Oxygen is a combustible gas; a spark may ignite the oxygen.
Administration	• Follow the prescription for the oxygen flow rate. • Have the health care provider's and nurse's phone number readily available. • Ensure enough available oxygen prior to leaving the house for errands or trips. • Know how to reach the oxygen equipment vendor and the reasons for contacting the vendor. • Know signs and symptoms that indicate the need to call for emergency assistance.	Too much or too little oxygen may be detrimental to the patient.

face at night or feeling the flow of air. Some people feel confined by the mask. Nurses can assist patients by reinforcing accurate information about treatment; encourage patients to ease into use of the device. It may help for patients to start by practicing wearing just the mask for short periods of time while awake, for example, while watching TV. Then patients should try wearing the mask and hose with the air pressure on, still during the daytime, while awake. Once patients become accustomed to how the equipment feels, they should shift to using the device every time they sleep—at night and during naps. Inconsistently wearing the device may delay getting used to it.

Provide support and encouragement so that the patient persists with the therapy; it may take several weeks or more to see if the mask and pressure settings will work for the patient. In addition, relaxation exercises help some people adjust to using these therapies (NHLBI, 2012a). If the device is used in the hospital or other facility, nursing responsibilities also may include monitoring the settings, ensuring correct use by the patient, and assessment of respiratory status. Careful assessment of the patient's skin on the face, in the areas the mask sits, is an important part of care. Pressure from the mask can cause alterations in skin integrity.

Managing Chest Tubes

Patients with fluid (**pleural effusion**), blood (**hemothorax**), or air (**pneumothorax**) in the pleural space require a chest tube to drain these substances and allow the compressed lung to re-expand. A chest tube is a firm plastic tube with drainage holes in the proximal end that is inserted in the pleural space. Once inserted, the tube is secured with a suture and tape, covered with an airtight dressing, and attached to a drainage system that may or may not be attached to suction. Other components of the system may include a closed water-seal drainage system that prevents air from re-entering the chest once it has escaped and a suction control chamber that prevents excess suction pressure from being applied to the pleural cavity. The suction chamber may be a water-filled or a dry chamber. A water-filled suction chamber is regulated by the amount of water in the chamber, whereas dry suction has a one-way mechanical valve system that allows air to leave the chest and prevents air from moving back into the chest and is automatically regulated to changes in the patient's pleural pressure. Most health care agencies use a molded plastic, three-compartment disposable chest drainage unit for management of chest tubes (Fig. 38-14). There are also portable drainage systems that utilize gravity for drainage. Table 38-6 compares different types of chest drainage systems.

The type of drainage determines the placement of the chest tube. When air is to be drained, the tube is placed higher in the chest. If fluid needs to be drained, the tube is inserted lower in the lung because fluids settle at the base of the lung.

Nursing responsibilities include assisting with insertion and removal of a chest tube. Once the tube is in

FIGURE 38-14. A chest drainage system attached to a patient. *(Photo by Rick Brady.)*

place, monitor the patient's respiratory status and vital signs, check the dressing, and maintain the patency and integrity of the drainage system. Guidelines for monitoring a patient with a chest tube are shown in Guidelines for Nursing Care 38-3.

Removal of chest tubes can be a painful and stressful process for patients. Whenever possible, administer analgesics prior to the tube removal, at a sufficient interval to allow for the medication to take effect, based on the medication prescribed. The application of cold to the chest prior to removal has also been shown to decrease patient discomfort during chest tube removal. Refer to the accompanying Research in Nursing box on page 1432. Nursing responsibilities related to chest tube removal also include providing emotional support for the patient, as well as monitoring the patient's status after removal. Monitor the patient's respiratory status, vital signs, pain, and site dressing.

Using Artificial Airways

Artificial airways are used to preserve a functioning airway in patients who are unable to maintain a patent airway without assistance. Communicating effectively with patients with artificial airways, such as endotracheal tubes or tracheostomies, is essential. Patients with endotracheal tubes, and most tracheostomies, are unable to speak. The communication needs of these patients must be part of the nursing assessment. Identify appropriate alternate communication strategies to ensure that the patient's needs are conveyed. Consider the patient's impaired ability to communicate and keep communication tools (e.g., writing board, letters, vocabulary cards) close at hand, along with the call light or bell. To prevent anxiety, offer frequent reassurance and explanations and anticipate the patient's needs.

Table 38-6	COMPARISON OF CHEST DRAINAGE SYSTEMS	
TYPE	**DESCRIPTION**	**COMMENTS**
Traditional water-seal (also referred to as wet-suction) chamber	Has three chambers: a collection chamber, water-seal chamber (middle chamber), and wet-suction control chamber.	• Requires that sterile fluid be instilled into the water-seal and suction chambers. • Has positive and negative pressure–release valves. • Intermittent bubbling indicates that the system is functioning properly. • Additional suction can be added by connecting the system to a suction source.
Dry-suction water seal (also referred to as dry suction)	Has three chambers: a collection chamber, water-seal chamber (middle chamber), and wet-suction control chamber.	• Requires that sterile fluid be instilled in the water-seal chamber at the 2-cm level. • No need to fill the suction chamber with fluid. • Suction pressure is set with a regulator. • Has positive and negative pressure–release valves. • Has an indicator to signify that the suction pressure is adequate. • Quieter than traditional water-seal systems.
Dry-suction (also referred to as one-way valve system)	Has a one-way mechanical valve that allows air to leave the chest and prevents air from moving back into the chest.	• No need to fill suction chamber with fluid; can be set up quickly in an emergency. • Works even if knocked over, making it ideal for patients who are ambulatory.

Adapted from Hinkle, J. L., & Cheever, K. H. (2014). *Brunner & Suddarth's textbook of medical–surgical nursing* (13th ed.). Philadelphia: Wolters Kluwer Health/Lippincott Williams & Wilkins.

GUIDELINES FOR NURSING CARE 38-3

MONITORING A PATIENT WITH A CHEST TUBE

• Assess the patient's vital signs, respiratory status, oxygen saturation, and breath sounds. Assess for pain. Monitor for any indication of change in respiratory status.

• Observe the dressing around the chest tube insertion site and ensure that it is occlusive. Gently palpate around the insertion site, feeling for crepitus, a result of air or gas collecting under the skin (subcutaneous emphysema). Tape all connections securely.

• Check that the drainage tube has no dependent loops or kinks. Make sure the drainage collection device is positioned below the tube insertion site to facilitate drainage.

• Observe the water-seal chamber for fluctuations of the water level with the patient's inspiration and expiration (tidaling). If suction is used, temporarily disconnect the suction to observe for fluctuation. Assess for the presence of bubbling in the water-seal chamber. Add water, if necessary, to maintain the level at the 2-cm mark, or the mark recommended by the manufacturer.

• Assess the suction control chamber if suction is in use. If water suction is used, ensure that water is at the appropriate level; add water to ensure that suction is adequate. Gentle bubbling in the suction chamber indicates that suction is being applied to assist drainage.

• Keep the drainage collection device secure so that it does not tip over.

• Check that two padded Kelly clamps are available and secured at the bedside. If the drainage unit requires changing, position one clamp 1½ to 2½ inches from the insertion site; position the second clamp 1 inch down from the first one until the unit has been switched. Alternately, many systems have integrated clamps on the tubing. The chest tube may be clamped before its removal to observe the patient's tolerance when it is discontinued or the chest tube may be clamped to assess for an air leak.

• Keep a bottle of sterile saline or water at the bedside. If the chest tube disconnects from drainage unit, submerge the end in water. This is done instead of clamping to prevent another pneumothorax. Air is still allowed to escape.

• Never clamp the tube if the patient leaves the unit for a test or moves away from the bed. Disconnect the suction tubing from the drainage system, allowing the unit to continue to collect drainage by gravity.

• Avoid milking or stripping the tube to promote drainage. This creates excessive negative pressure that can damage delicate lung tissue.

• Measure drainage output at the end of each shift by marking the level on the container or placing a small piece of tape at the drainage level to indicate date and time. Drainage is never emptied from the collection chamber. Document the color and consistency of the drainage. Drainage that dramatically increases or becomes bright red indicates fresh bleeding. Notify the primary care provider immediately.

RESEARCH IN NURSING

BRIDGING THE GAP TO EVIDENCE-BASED PRACTICE

Chest Tube Removal and Pain

Removal of chest tubes can be a painful and stressful process for patients. Whenever possible, an analgesic should be provided prior to tube removal and sufficient time should be provided for it to take effect. The application of cold to the chest prior to removal has also been suggested to decrease patient discomfort during chest tube removal.

Related Research

Ertuğ, N., & Ülker, S. (2011). The effect of cold application on pain due to chest tube removal. *Journal of Clinical Nursing, 21*(5/6), 784–790.

The objective of this study was to determine the effect of application of cold to the chest wall on the pain related to chest tube removal. The study was conducted with 140 patients, divided evenly between an experimental group and a control group. Data was collected regarding the patient's demographic and health history. Skin temperature and pain intensity, using a visual analog scale, was measured at various points before and after the tube removal process. There were significant differences related to pain between the two groups. Age, gender, and the number of days the chest tube was inserted had no effect on the pain related to chest tube removal. This study concluded that the application of cold is effective in reducing the pain related to removal of a chest tube.

Relevance to Nursing Practice

Nursing interventions related to decreasing pain and increasing patient comfort are an important nursing responsibility. Interventions should include the use of nonpharmacologic interventions in addition to the administration of analgesics. The application of cold to the chest wall could significantly decrease the pain and discomfort experienced by a patient during removal of a chest tube. Nurses could easily incorporate this simple intervention as part of nursing care for these patients.

For additional research, visit thePoint.

OROPHARYNGEAL AND NASOPHARYNGEAL AIRWAYS

An oropharyngeal or nasopharyngeal airway is a semi-circular tube of plastic or rubber inserted into the back of the pharynx through the mouth (oro) or nose (naso) in a patient who is breathing spontaneously. The oropharyngeal airway is used to keep the tongue clear of the airway. It is often used for postoperative patients until they regain consciousness. Once the patient regains consciousness, remove the oropharyngeal airway. Do not use tape to hold the airway in place because the patient should be able to expel the airway once he or she becomes alert.

A nasopharyngeal airway is inserted through the nare and protrudes into the back of the pharynx. The nasal trumpet allows for frequent nasotracheal suctioning without trauma to the nasal passageway. This airway may be left in place, without much discomfort, in the patient who is alert and conscious. Techniques to use when inserting an artificial airway are outlined in Guidelines for Nursing Care 38-4.

ENDOTRACHEAL TUBE

An **endotracheal tube** is a polyvinylchloride airway that is inserted through the nose or mouth into the trachea, using a laryngoscope as a guide. It is used to administer oxygen by mechanical ventilator, to suction secretions easily, or to bypass upper airway obstructions (e.g., tongue or tracheal edema). Although uncomfortable and easy to manipulate with the tongue, orotracheal insertion is often the method of choice, especially in an emergency, because insertion is easier and a larger tube can be used, making ventilation easier. Placement of the tube through the nasotracheal route, although tolerated better by patients, is more difficult and requires the use of a narrower tube. Most commonly, a cuffed endotracheal tube is used (Fig. 38-15). This type of tube prevents air leakage and bronchial aspiration of foreign material while allowing more precise control of oxygen and mechanical ventilation. However, careful monitoring of cuff pressure is necessary to decrease the risk for tracheal necrosis. The smallest amount of air that results in an airtight seal between the trachea and the tube is desirable and less likely to result in complications.

Patients with endotracheal tubes often require suctioning via the endotracheal tube to remove secretions from the airway. Refer to the discussion related to tracheal suctioning later in the chapter. Routine oral suctioning to aspirate secretions that accumulate above the cuff of the tube is also necessary to reduce the risk of pneumonia (Sole, Penoyer, Bennett, Bertrand, & Talbert, 2011).

 CONSIDER Mr. Kim, the 57-year-old man receiving oxygen therapy and mechanical ventilation via an endotracheal tube. When developing the patient's plan of care, the nurse needs to assess him closely and frequently for signs and symptoms indicating an increase in secretions. If secretions increase, the nurse needs to suction the patient to maintain a patent airway and minimize his risk for hypoxemia and infection. ●

TRACHEOSTOMY

A tracheostomy tube is inserted for a variety of reasons. It may be used to replace an endotracheal tube, to provide a method for mechanical ventilation of the patient, to bypass an upper airway obstruction, or to remove tracheobronchial secretions.

GUIDELINES FOR NURSING CARE 38-4

INSERTING AN ARTIFICIAL AIRWAY

Inserting an Oropharyngeal Airway

- Use an airway that is the correct size. Airway should reach from the opening of the mouth to the back angle of the jaw.
- Wash your hands and put on PPE, as indicated.
- Identify the patient.
- Explain what you are going to do and the reason for doing it, even though the patient does not appear to be alert.
- Put on gloves; put on mask and goggles or face shield as indicated. Check for loose teeth, dentures or other foreign material. Use caution to prevent aspiration of loose teeth or pushing of object to the throat during insertion. Remove dentures if present.
- Position the patient in the semi-Fowler's position.
- Open the patient's mouth by using your thumb and index finger to gently pry teeth apart.
- **Insert the airway with the curved tip pointing up toward the roof of the mouth.**
- Slide the airway across the tongue to the back of the mouth.
- Rotate the airway 180 degrees as it passes the uvula (a flashlight can confirm the position of the airway with the curve fitting over the tongue).
- Ensure adequate ventilation by auscultating breath sounds.
- Position the patient on his or her side when the airway is in place.
- Remove the airway for a brief period every 4 hours, or according to facility policy. Provide mouth care and a clean airway before reinserting it.

Inserting a Nasopharyngeal Airway (Nasal Trumpet)

- Use an airway that is the correct size. Airway should reach from the tragus of the ear to the nostril plus 1 inch. The diameter should be slightly smaller than the diameter of the nostril.
- Wash your hands and put on PPE, as indicated.
- Identify the patient.
- Explain what you are going to do and the reason for doing it, even though the patient does not appear to be alert.

- Put on gloves; put on mask and goggles or face shield as indicated.
- **If the patient is awake and alert, position in the semi-Fowler's position. If the patient is not conscious or alert, position in a side-lying position.**
- Lubricate the airway with the water-soluble lubricant.
- **Gently insert the airway into the naris, narrow end first, until the rim is touching the naris. If resistance is met, stop and try inserting in the other naris.**
- Check placement by closing the patient's mouth and placing your fingers in front of the tube opening to check for air movement. Assess the pharynx to visualize the tip of the airway behind the uvula. Assess the nose for blanching or stretching of the skin.
- Remove the airway, clean it, and place it in the other naris at least every 8 hours, or according to facility policy. Assess for any evidence of skin breakdown.
- The airway may be used for suctioning to prevent trauma to the mucosa.

Airway
Tongue
Epiglottis
Trachea
Esophagus

Tracheostomy Procedure and Tubes. A **tracheostomy** is an artificial opening made into the trachea, usually at the level of the second or third cartilaginous ring. A curved tube, called a tracheostomy tube, is inserted through the opening. It is inserted in the operating room or intensive care unit under sterile conditions using local anesthesia, and can be temporary or permanent.

Adapter for connection to oxygen source

Valve connection to add air via syringe to inflate cuff

Cuff

Tube
Trachea
Inflated cuff
Deflated cuff

1   2   3

A   B

FIGURE 38-15. Endotracheal tube. (**A**) (1) Parts of a cuffed endotracheal tube; (2) tube in place with the cuff inflated; (3) tube in place with the cuff deflated. (**B**) Endotracheal tube in place.

FIGURE 38-16. Two types of tracheostomy sets: cuffless and cuffed.

The tube is made of semi-flexible plastic (polyurethane or silicone), rigid plastic, or metal and is available in different sizes with varied angles. The condition and needs of the patient determine the selection of either a metal or plastic tracheostomy tube. Although metal tubes are more cost-effective for long-term use, most do not have an adapter at the neck plate that permits connection to respiratory therapy equipment (e.g., an oxygen delivery system, Ambu bag, or mechanical ventilator).

A tracheostomy tube consists of an outer cannula or main shaft, an inner cannula, and an obturator. An obturator, which guides the direction of the outer cannula, is inserted into the tube during placement and removed once the outer cannula of the tube is in place (Fig. 38-16). Many tubes also have inner cannulas that may or may not be disposable. The outer cannula remains in place in the trachea, and the inner cannula is removed for cleaning or replaced with a new one. Periodic cleaning or replacement of the inner cannula prevents airway obstruction from secretions that have accumulated on the tube's inner surface. A tube with an inner cannula is necessary when patients have excessive secretions or have difficulty clearing their secretions. It also may be recommended for a patient who will be discharged with a tracheostomy tube in place.

Tracheostomy tubes may be either cuffed or cuffless (see Fig. 38-16). The inflated cuff seals the opening around the tube to create a tight fit in the trachea. This prevents air leakage and aspiration, and permits mechanical ventilation. Newer tracheal cuffs are low pressure, do not require deflating for short intervals every few hours, and can be maintained at lower than tracheal capillary pressure. If a cuffed tube is used, always deflate it before oral feeding unless the patient is at high risk for aspiration. If left cuffed, the balloon can cause pressure that extends through the trachea and onto the esophagus, possibly impeding swallowing or causing erosion of the tissue.

A fenestrated tracheostomy tube has one large or several small openings or windows on its outer curve, has an inner cannula, and can be cuffed or cuffless. When the patient is being mechanically ventilated, the inner cannula is in place, blocking the small openings. After

the patient is no longer connected to the ventilator, the inner cannula can be removed, the cuff deflated, and the tube plugged, allowing the patient to speak. Because the tube has these openings, it is not recommended for use in patients with a history of aspiration.

The tracheostomy tube is held in place by twill tapes or a Velcro strip fastened around the patient's neck. When the tracheostomy is new, a sterile, square gauze pad that has been precut by the manufacturer may be placed between the skin and outer wings of the tube. This tracheostomy dressing must be kept dry to prevent infection and skin irritation.

Regularly check cuff pressure, although some tubes have a pressure-release valve that prevents pressure from increasing to damaging levels. Also, because the tracheostomy tube bypasses the natural humidifying and heating mechanisms in the nose and mouth, administer heated, humidified oxygen to prevent secretions from becoming dry. Keep the tracheostomy tube free from foreign objects and nonsterile materials, such as cotton balls, loose threads from dressings, needles, and other small objects, to reduce the risk of obstruction and infection. Artificial noses, small pieces that attach over the end of the tracheostomy tube, are available to filter and warm the air before it enters the trachea.

Preparation for emergency situations is an important part of nursing care for these patients. The tracheostomy is the patient's only airway, and measures to maintain its patency need to be readily available. Standard bedside equipment for emergency use should include the obturator from the current tube, suction equipment, oxygen, a spare tracheostomy tube of the same size, and one a size smaller (Freeman, 2011; Roman, 2005).

Patients with tracheostomies frequently have an ineffective cough mechanism and copious secretions, which necessitate tracheal suctioning to remove secretions. Refer to the discussion related to tracheal suctioning later in the chapter.

Providing Tracheostomy Care. The nurse is responsible for replacing a disposable inner cannula or cleaning a nondisposable one. The inner cannula requires cleaning or replacement to prevent accumulation of secretions that can interfere with respiration and occlude the airway. Because soiled tracheostomy dressings place the patient at risk for the development of skin breakdown and infection, regularly change dressings and ties. Use gauze dressings that are not filled with cotton to prevent aspiration of foreign bodies (e.g., lint or cotton fibers) into the trachea. Clean the skin around a tracheostomy to prevent buildup of dried secretions and skin breakdown. Exercise care when changing the tracheostomy ties to prevent accidental decannulation or expulsion of the tube. Have an assistant hold the tube in place during the change or keep the soiled tie in place until a clean one is securely attached. Agency policy and patient condition determine specific procedures and schedules, but a newly inserted tracheostomy may require attention every 1 to 2 hours. Skill 38-5 on pages 1455–1459 outlines tracheostomy care.

TRACHEAL SUCTIONING

When performed correctly, suctioning provides comfort by relieving respiratory distress. When performed incorrectly, it can increase anxiety and pain and cause respiratory arrest. Tracheal suctioning may be performed by passing a sterile catheter through a tracheostomy or endotracheal tube. Suctioning to remove secretions is performed using the sterile technique as described in Chapter 23. The frequency of suctioning varies with the amount of secretions present but should be done often enough to keep ventilation effective and as effortless as possible. The suction catheter should be small enough not to occlude the airway being suctioned but large enough to remove secretions. Several sizes of catheters are available. Wear gloves on both hands, goggles, and a mask—and a gown, if necessary—for protection from microorganisms.

Tracheal suctioning is an uncomfortable procedure at minimum, and it can be a very painful and/or distressing experience. Therefore, anticipate assessing for the need for the administration of analgesic medication to a patient before suctioning (Arroyo-Novoa et al., 2008). However, only perform suctioning when clinically necessary because there are many potential risks. Risks include hypoxia, infection, tracheal tissue damage, dysrhythmias, and atelectasis. Sterile technique is used for tracheal suctioning, to reduce the risk of introduction of disease-causing organisms. In the home setting, clean technique is used, as the patient is not exposed to disease-causing organisms that may be found in health care settings, such as hospitals (American Association for Respiratory Care [AARC], 1999). Closely assess the patient before, during, and after the procedure to limit negative effects. In order to prevent hypoxia, hyperoxygenate the patient before and after suctioning and limit the application of suction to 10 to 20 seconds. Monitor the patient's pulse frequently to detect potential effects of hypoxia and stimulation of the vagus nerve. Using an appropriate suction pressure (80–150 mm Hg) will help prevent atelectasis related to the use of high negative pressure (Hess, et al., 2012). Research suggests that insertion of the suction catheter should be limited to a predetermined length (no further than 1 cm past the length of the tracheal or endotracheal tube) to avoid tracheal mucosal damage, including epithelial denudement, loss of cilia, edema, and fibrosis (Hess et al., 2012; Pate, 2004). Skill 38-6 on pages 1460–1465 describes suctioning a tracheostomy with an open system. The procedure is similar for an endotracheal tube.

A closed airway suction system can be used to keep the airway patent for a patient with an endotracheal or tracheostomy tube who is receiving continuous mechanical ventilation, and reduce the risk of hypoxemia or, possibly, infection (Fig. 38-17). The catheter, encased in a plastic sleeve, remains connected to the patient's airway or ventilator tubing for up to 24 hours. This closed system is cost-effective because only one catheter is used daily, and the caregiver has additional protection from exposure to the patient's secretions. Some systems have an access valve, a safety feature that completely closes off access between the suction catheter and the endotracheal tube.

T-piece

Suction catheter

Catheter sleeve

A   B

FIGURE 38-17. Closed airway suction system. (**A**) Closed tracheal suction system. (**B**) Closed system connected by a T-piece to the endotracheal tube and ventilator.

ASSISTING VENTILATION

Mechanical ventilators are used to assist or completely control ventilation. These machines are used with patients who have endotracheal or tracheostomy tubes in place. Mechanical ventilation can be performed in acute care facilities, in extended care settings, and in the home. Mechanical ventilation improves oxygenation and ventilation and supports the patient's breathing function during emergency or acute care episodes as well as long-term situations.

Many types of ventilators are available. The nurse is responsible for addressing the physical and psychological concerns of the patient and family. In addition, key interventions include evaluating the patient's response to ventilation therapy, using safe practices and techniques, and monitoring the patient carefully for complications. (See clinical texts and literature that discuss the use of mechanical ventilators in greater detail.)

Another mechanical device used to assist ventilation is intermittent positive-pressure breathing (IPPB). This is a method of providing a specific amount of air, oxygen, and aerosolized medication under increased pressure to the respiratory tract. The patient receiving IPPB inhales the aerosol therapy through a mouthpiece or face mask. IPPB forces deeper inspiration by positive-pressure inhalation and then permits passive exhalation. The amount of pressure varies with each patient. It is now recognized as an alternative therapy when the patient is unable or unwilling to make the effort to ventilate one's lungs. However, conservative methods must be attempted first, such as deep-breathing and coughing exercises, percussion, vibration, and postural drainage.

In emergency situations, the manual resuscitation bag (or Ambu bag) can be used to assist ventilation in patients whose respirations have ceased (Fig. 38-18). With the patient's head tilted back, jaw pulled forward, and airway cleared, the mask is held tightly over the patient's nose and mouth. The bag also fits easily over tracheostomy and endotracheal tubes. The operator's other hand compresses the bag at a rate that approximates normal respiratory rate (16–20 breaths/minute in adults). The one-way valve in the mask allows exhaled air to escape. Artificial ventilation can be sustained until spontaneous breathing starts, until other mechanical assistance is available, or until death is confirmed. The bag is self-inflating and may be attached to supplemental oxygen if needed.

Clearing an Obstructed Airway

Foreign-body obstruction of the airway often occurs during eating. In adults, meat is the most common food-related cause. In children, any variety of foods or objects can obstruct the upper airway. A patient who is semiconscious or unconscious develops airway obstruction as the tongue falls back, covering the pharynx. In fact, the tongue is the most common cause of airway obstruction.

Foreign bodies can cause a partial or complete airway obstruction. In partial airway obstruction with good air exchange, the patient can cough forcefully. Allow the person to cough, and encourage spontaneous breathing. Do not interfere with the patient's efforts to expel the object. With a partial airway obstruction, good air exchange can progress to poor air exchange. Poor air exchange may be indicated by a weak, ineffective cough, high-pitched noises while inhaling, increased breathing difficulties, and cyanosis. When this occurs, it is managed in the same way as complete airway obstruction.

With a complete airway obstruction, the victim is unable to speak or cough and may demonstrate the universal distress signal (clutching the throat with both hands; Fig. 38-19). Immediate action is necessary, or the patient will become unconscious as the brain becomes hypoxic. After complete airway obstruction has been determined, perform the Heimlich maneuver (abdominal thrusts). Follow the American Heart Association (AHA) protocols for obstructed airways and cardiopulmonary resuscitation (see next section). These protocols are continually being developed and updated.

FIGURE 38-18. Manual resuscitation bag (Smeltzer, S.C, et al. [2010]. Brunner & Suddarth's textbook of medical-surgical nursing (12th ed.). Wolters Kluwer Health/Lippincott Williams & Wilkins.)

FIGURE 38-19. Universal choking sign.

FIGURE 38-20. Placement of the automated external defibrillator (AED). (**A**) AED device. (**B**) Place the AED pad attached to the red cable connector to the left of the heart apex. To help remember where to place the pads, think "white right, red ribs." Placement of both electrode pads is the same as it is for manual defibrillation or cardioversion. *(Photo by B. Proud.)*

Administering Cardiopulmonary Resuscitation

Cardiopulmonary resuscitation (CPR) is the combination of chest compressions, which circulate blood, and mouth-to-mouth breathing, which supplies oxygen to the lungs. After checking the victim for a response, activate the emergency response system, get an automated external defibrillator (AED) or defibrillator, and begin CPR with the CAB sequence:

- **Chest Compressions:** Check the pulse. If the victim has no pulse, initiate chest compressions to provide artificial circulation.
- **Airway:** Tilt the head and lift the chin; check for breathing. The respiratory tract must be opened so that air can enter.
- **Breathing:** If the victim does not start to breathe spontaneously after the airway is opened, give two breaths lasting 1 second each.
- **Defibrillation:** Apply the AED as soon as it is available.

Start CPR in any situation in which either breathing alone or breathing and a heartbeat are absent. The brain is sensitive to hypoxia and will sustain irreversible damage after 4 to 6 minutes of no oxygen. The faster CPR is initiated, the greater the chance of survival.

During CPR, standard precautions are followed even though contact with a patient's blood or body fluids does not always occur. Occupational Safety and Health Administration (OSHA) standards require health care facilities to provide an ample supply of ventilation masks along with other protective barriers for staff to use during resuscitation efforts.

The automated external defibrillator (AED) has also proved effective in reducing deaths attributed to cardiac arrest. This easy-to-use, computer-based device is designed to deliver a shock to the heart muscle quickly to interrupt ventricular fibrillation, the most common initial rhythm occurring in cardiac arrest. The AED has the ability to analyze the heart's rhythm, direct the operator to deliver a shock when appropriate or deliver one automatically, and then reanalyze the rhythm to determine

whether it has returned to normal (Fig. 38-20). Using the AED is an integral part of resuscitation.

Most professional organizations recommend and support widespread efforts to teach CPR to laypeople and all health professionals. Mannequins for practice can be obtained from the AHA, the American Red Cross, and health agencies. The nurse is professionally responsible for maintaining proficiency in CPR skills. This necessitates periodic practice with mannequins (adult and infant). CPR must be administered quickly and accurately, without hesitation, when cardiac or pulmonary arrest occurs. In 2008, the AHA instituted changes in their suggestions regarding emergency interventions outside of health care facilities. Learning conventional CPR is still recommended. However, the AHA alternately recommends that when a teen or adult suddenly collapses, people near the victim should call 911 (activate the emergency response system) and push hard and fast in the center of the victim's chest. Studies of real emergencies that have occurred in homes, at work, or in public locations show that these two steps, called Hands-Only CPR, can be as effective as conventional CPR. Providing Hands-Only CPR to an adult who has collapsed from a sudden cardiac arrest can more than double or triple that person's chance of survival (AHA, 2012).

Evaluating

Evaluation is the final step of the nursing process; the accompanying concept map on page 1438 illustrates the nursing process for the care of Tyrone Jacobs. Evaluation is an ongoing and deliberate part of the nursing process that involves the nurse, patient, family, and other health care team members. It compares the patient's health status with previously defined expected outcomes and examines the patient's projected progress in meeting those outcomes. Everyone involved in the evaluation process needs to identify effective interventions and reasons for any failures in achieving the expected outcomes. Adjustments in the nursing plan of care are made accordingly. See Nursing Plan of Care 38-1 for Joan McEntyre on page 1439.

Tyrone Jacobs, age 12, is admitted to the pediatric unit after having a cold for 4 days. He is diagnosed with acute asthma and upper respiratory infection. His vital signs are as follows: BP 100/60 mm Hg, pulse 140 beats per minute, respiratory rate 40 breaths/minute, temperature of 101° F, and oxygen saturation of 90%. While listening to his lungs, you hear diffuse inspiratory and expiratory wheezes and scattered coarse crackles. You note an occasional cough, productive for thick yellow mucus. He is sitting upright in bed in a tripod position. He states, "Help me I can't breathe." Tyrone is placed on O₂ 2 liters/minute via nasal cannula and is receiving albuterol nebulizer treatments and IV antibiotics. His sputum culture reveals Gram-positive cocci. His mother appears very anxious and is pacing in the room. Tyrone is not making eye contact with mother or caregivers.

Priority 1

Nursing Diagnosis: Impaired Gas Exchange related to bronchoconstriction and inflammation of airways.
Supporting Data:
• Oxygen saturation is 90%
• O₂ @ 2 L/min via nasal cannula
• Respiratory rate is 40 breaths/min
• Sitting in tripod position
• Had cold for 4 days prior to admission
• Wheezes and coarse crackles auscultated
• Receiving albuterol nebulizer treatments

Outcome:
Patient will maintain oxygen saturation within normal limits on supplemental oxygen.

Nursing Interventions:
• Monitor pulse oximetry every 4 hrs
• Monitor and evaluate vital signs every 4hrs
• Maintain patient in position of comfort (tripod position)
• Evaluate effectiveness of albuterol nebulizer treatments
• Auscultate lungs every 4 hrs

Evaluation: Tyrone continues to have oxygen saturation below normal limits, tachypnea, and wheezing. Continue to monitor response to collaborative interventions. Notify physician for an increase in respiratory distress and a decrease in pulse oximetry.

Priority 2

Nursing Diagnosis: Ineffective Airway Clearance related to increased mucous production due to upper respiratory infection and asthma.
Supporting Data:
• Expectorating yellow mucus
• Temperature is 101° F
• Receiving IV antibiotics
• Sputum culture reveals Gram-positive cocci
• Receiving albuterol nebulizer treatments
• Has frequent bouts of coughing
• Wheezing and coarse crackles auscultated

Outcome:
Patient will readily expectorate secretions; lung sounds will clear.

Nursing Interventions:
• Encourage and instruct in coughing and pursed-lip breathing techniques
• Monitor effectiveness of bronchodilators in increasing expectoration of secretions
• Note characteristics of sputum
• Evaluate respiratory rate and effort
• Encourage increased fluid intake
• Auscultate breath sounds every 4 hrs

Evaluation: Tyrone continues to have audible adventitious sounds. He is readily expectorating secretions. Continue to monitor.

Priority 3

Nursing Diagnosis: Anxiety related to difficulty breathing and parental reaction to acute illness of child.
Supporting Data:
• Tyrone states, "Help me. I can't breathe."
• Mother pacing back and forth in room
• Heart rate is 140 beats/min
• Respiratory rate is 40 breaths/min
• Tyrone is not making eye contact with mother or caregivers

Outcome:
Patient will appear relaxed with reduced heart rate and respiratory rate; will interact with family and caregivers.

Nursing Interventions:
• Assess level of anxiety
• Provide calm, reassuring presence
• Utilize Therapeutic Touch
• Keep patient and family informed of actions taken to improve breathing
• Use brief, simple explanations
• Maintain quiet, calm environment
• Encourage pursed-lip breathing to manage dyspnea

Evaluation: Tyrone made eye contact with nurse as she explained the actions of his bronchodilators. Mother stopped pacing and sat beside son to provide comfort and reassurance. Continue interventions.

- - - - - **Relationship**   ■ **Assesment**   ■ **Nursing Diagnosis**   ■ **Outcome Identification**   ■ **Interventions**   ■ **Evaluation**

Concept map displaying nursing process for Tyrone Jacobs.

NURSING PLAN OF CARE 38-1

for Joan McIntyre

Mrs. McIntyre, age 72, has been admitted to your medical unit with an acute exacerbation of chronic obstructive pulmonary disease (COPD). This is the fifth time she has been in the hospital this year. She is receiving supplemental oxygen and multiple medications to support her breathing. She is very weak, unable to perform ADLs for herself, and becomes extremely short of breath with minimal exertion. Mrs. McIntyre has been eating only small amounts and states, "It is just too much!" She has verbalized feelings of despair and has asked the staff "to let me go if I should stop breathing." A comprehensive assessment revealed the following findings:

Respiratory rate, 32 breaths/min

Frequent weak cough, difficulty raising secretions, occasionally productive for yellow sputum; patient states, "I just can't get it out."

Dyspnea with minimal exertion; patient states, "I can't even eat or brush my teeth without feeling like I can't catch my breath!"

Lungs with decreased breath sounds, scattered sonorous wheezing

Oxygen saturation on oxygen at 3 L/min = 90%–92%

Picks at breakfast; consumes less than ¼ of breakfast tray

NURSING DIAGNOSIS Ineffective Airway Clearance related to bronchoconstriction, increased mucous production, and ineffective cough as manifested by frequent weak cough, inability to consistently expectorate sputum, presence of sonorous wheezes (rhonchi)

EXPECTED OUTCOME By 3/20/15, the patient will:

• Cough effectively and expectorate sputum

NURSING INTERVENTIONS	RATIONALE	EVALUATIVE STATEMENT
Assess respiratory status at least every 4 hours.	Establishes standards to detect early signs of compromise.	3/19/15 Outcome met. Mrs. McIntyre is able to consistently cough up and expectorate sputum. Patient states feelings of improved ability to clear sputum.
Teach importance of adequate hydration.	Patient understanding increases compliance and involves the patient in care.	
Offer patient a choice of preferred liquids every 2 hours	Liquids help to liquefy secretions and prevent dehydration.	*M. Jones, RN*
Teach and encourage the use of diaphragmatic breathing and coughing techniques.	Helps to improve ventilation and mobilize secretions without causing breathlessness and fatigue.	

NURSING DIAGNOSIS Self-Care Deficit: Hygiene, related to fatigue secondary to increased work of breathing as manifested by an inability to bathe and dress

EXPECTED OUTCOME By 3/20/15, the patient will:

• Meet self-care needs and demonstrate improved ability to participate in bathing and personal hygiene measures

(continued)

NURSING PLAN OF CARE 38-1 *continued*

for Joan McIntyre

NURSING INTERVENTIONS	RATIONALE	EVALUATIVE STATEMENT
Observe patient's functional level every shift.	Careful assessment guides adjustment of actions to meet patient's needs.	3/19/15 Continue interventions. Patient able to perform ¾ of bath before becoming too fatigued and weak. Patient requires continued reinforcement regarding diaphragmatic breathing during activity. Continue guidance to break activity into smaller tasks and utilize rest between activities. Patient states frustration with inability to accomplish entire personal care tasks in short period of time.
Encourage patient to voice feelings and concerns about self-care deficits.	Assists patient to achieve highest functional level possible.	
Teach patient to coordinate diaphragmatic breathing with activity.	Helps avoid excessive fatigue and dyspnea during activity.	
Group personal care activities into smaller steps; allow rest periods between activities.	Promotes energy conservation and helps avoid excessive fatigue and dyspnea.	
Assist with bathing and hygiene tasks as needed and only when patient has difficulty	Promotes feeling of independence	*M. Jones, RN*

SAMPLE DOCUMENTATION	3/17/15 1500 Nursing Patient verbalizes frustration with length of time required to complete personal care activities. Patient states, "I just want to be able to take care of myself without having to take an entire day to do it." Possible consult with occupational therapy/physical therapy discussed with patient, husband, and Dr. Miller. Patient expresses an interest in working with the occupational/physical therapist. *M. Jones, RN*

SKILL 38-1 USING A PULSE OXIMETER

DELEGATION CONSIDERATIONS	The measurement of oxygen saturation using a pulse oximeter may be delegated to nursing assistive personnel (NAP) or unlicensed assistive personnel (UAP), as well as to licensed practical/vocational nurses (LPN/LVNs). The decision to delegate must be based on careful analysis of the patient's needs and circumstances, as well as the qualifications of the person to whom the task is being delegated. Refer to the Delegation Guidelines in Appendix A (found on thePoint).

EQUIPMENT	• Pulse oximeter with an appropriate sensor or probe • Alcohol wipe(s) or disposable cleansing cloth	• Nail polish remover (if necessary) • PPE, as indicated

IMPLEMENTATION

ACTION	RATIONALE
1. Review the health record for any health problems that would affect the patient's oxygenation status.	Identifying influencing factors aids in interpretation of results.
2. Bring necessary equipment to the bedside stand or overbed table.	Bringing everything to the bedside conserves time and energy. Arranging items nearby is convenient, saves time, and avoids unnecessary stretching and twisting of muscles on the part of the nurse.

ACTION	RATIONALE

3. Perform hand hygiene and put on PPE, if indicated.

Hand hygiene and PPE prevent the spread of microorganisms. PPE is required based on transmission precautions.

4. Identify the patient.

Identifying the patient ensures that the right patient receives the intervention and helps prevent errors.

5. Close the curtains around the bed and close the door to the room, if possible. Explain what you are going to do and why you are going to do it to the patient.

This ensures the patient's privacy. Explanation relieves anxiety and facilitates cooperation.

6. Select an adequate site for application of the sensor.

Inadequate circulation can interfere with the oxygen saturation (SpO$_2$) reading.

   a. Use the patient's index, middle, or ring finger (Fig. 1).

Fingers are easily accessible.

   b. Check the proximal pulse (Fig. 2) and capillary refill (Fig. 3) at the pulse closest to the site.

Brisk capillary refill and a strong pulse indicate that circulation to the site is adequate.

   c. If circulation at the site is inadequate, consider using the earlobe, forehead, or bridge of the nose. Use the appropriate oximetry sensor for the chosen site.

These alternate sites are highly vascular alternatives. Correct use of appropriate equipment is vital for accurate results. The appropriate ear oximetry sensor should be used to obtain measurements from a patient's ear. The use of a finger sensor should be limited to use on the finger (Johnson, Anderson, & Hill, 2012).

   d. Use a toe only if lower extremity circulation is not compromised.

Peripheral vascular disease is common in lower extremities.

FIGURE 1. Selecting an appropriate finger.

FIGURE 2. Assessing pulse.

FIGURE 3. Assessing capillary refill.

(continued)

SKILL 38-1 | USING A PULSE OXIMETER *continued*

ACTION	RATIONALE
7. Select proper equipment:	
a. If one finger is too large for the probe, use a smaller finger.	Inaccurate readings can result if the probe or sensor is not attached correctly.
b. Use probes appropriate for the patient's age and size. Use a pediatric probe for a small adult, if necessary.	Probes come in adult, pediatric, and infant sizes.
c. Check if the patient is allergic to adhesive. A nonadhesive finger clip or reflectance sensor is available.	A reaction may occur if the patient is allergic to an adhesive substance.
8. Prepare the monitoring site. Cleanse the selected area with an alcohol wipe or disposable cleansing cloth (Fig. 4). Allow the area to dry. If necessary, remove nail polish and artificial nails after checking the pulse oximeter's manufacturer instructions.	Skin oils, dirt, or grime on the site can interfere with the passage of light waves. Research is conflicting regarding the effect of dark-color nail polish and artificial nails. It is prudent to remove nail polish (Hess et al., 2012). Refer to facility policy and pulse oximeter's manufacturer instructions regarding nail polish and artificial nails for additional information (Collins & Andersen, 2007; DeMeulenaere, 2007).
9. **Apply probe securely to skin (Fig. 5). Make sure that the light-emitting sensor and the light-receiving sensor are aligned opposite each other (not necessary to check if placed on the forehead or bridge of the nose).**	Secure attachment and proper alignment promote satisfactory operation of the equipment and accurate recording of the SpO_2.

FIGURE 4. Cleaning area.

FIGURE 5. Attaching probe to patient's finger.

10. Connect the sensor probe to the pulse oximeter (Fig. 6), turn the oximeter on, and check operation of the equipment (audible beep, fluctuation of bar of light or waveform on face of oximeter).	Audible beep represents the arterial pulse, and fluctuating waveform or light bar indicates the strength of the pulse. A weak signal will produce an inaccurate recording of the SpO_2. The tone of the beep reflects the SpO_2 reading. If the SpO_2 drops, the tone becomes lower in pitch.

FIGURE 6. Connecting sensor probe to unit.

ACTION	RATIONALE
11. Set the alarms on the pulse oximeter. Check the manufacturer's alarm limits for high and low pulse rate settings (Fig. 7).	Alarm provides additional safeguard and signals when high or low limits have been surpassed.

FIGURE 7. Checking alarms.

ACTION	RATIONALE
12. Check oxygen saturation at regular intervals, as ordered by the primary care provider, nursing assessment, and signaled by alarms. Monitor hemoglobin level.	Monitoring SpO_2 provides ongoing assessment of the patient's condition. A low hemoglobin level may be satisfactorily saturated yet inadequate to meet a patient's oxygen needs.
13. Remove the sensor on a regular basis and check for skin irritation or signs of pressure (every 2 hours for a spring-tension sensor or every 4 hours for an adhesive finger or toe sensor).	Prolonged pressure may lead to tissue necrosis. An adhesive sensor may cause skin irritation.
14. Clean nondisposable sensors according to the manufacturer's directions. Remove PPE, if used. Perform hand hygiene.	Cleaning equipment between patient use reduces the spread of microorganisms. Removing PPE properly reduces the risk for infection transmission and contamination of other items. Hand hygiene prevents the spread of microorganisms.

DOCUMENTATION

Guidelines

Documentation should include the type of sensor and location used; assessment of the proximal pulse and capillary refill; pulse oximeter reading; the amount of oxygen and delivery method if the patient is receiving supplemental oxygen; lung assessment, if relevant; and any other relevant interventions required as a result of the reading.

Sample Documentation

9/03/15 Pulse oximeter placed on patient's index finger on right hand. Radial pulse present with brisk capillary refill. Pulse oximeter reading 98% on oxygen at 2 L via nasal cannula. Heart rate measured by oximeter correlates with the radial pulse measurement.

—C. Bausler, RN

UNEXPECTED SITUATIONS AND ASSOCIATED INTERVENTIONS

- *Absent or weak signal:* Check vital signs and patient condition. If satisfactory, check connections and circulation to site. Hypotension makes an accurate recording difficult. Equipment (restraint, blood pressure cuff) may compromise circulation to site and cause venous blood to pulsate, giving an inaccurate reading. If the extremity is cold, cover with a warm blanket.
- *Inaccurate reading:* Check prescribed medications and history of circulatory disorders. Try the device on a healthy person to see if the problem is equipment-related or patient-related. Drugs that cause vasoconstriction interfere with accurate recording of oxygen saturation.
- *A bright light (sunlight or fluorescent light) is suspected of causing equipment malfunction:* Turn off the light or cover the probe with a dry washcloth. Bright light can interfere with operation of light sensors and cause unreliable report.

(continued)

SKILL 38-1 USING A PULSE OXIMETER *continued*

SPECIAL CONSIDERATIONS

General Considerations

- Accuracy of readings can be influenced by conditions that decrease arterial blood flow, such as peripheral edema, hypotension, and peripheral vascular disease.
- Correlate the pulse reading on the pulse oximeter with the patient's heart rate. Variation between pulse and heart rate may indicate that not all pulsations are being detected and another sensor site may be required (Pullen, 2010).
- Excessive motion of sensor probe site, such as with extremity tremors or shivering, can also interfere with obtaining an accurate reading.
- Bradycardia and irregular cardiac rhythms may also cause inaccurate readings.
- In patients with low cardiac index (cardiac output in liters per minute divided by body surface area in square meters), the forehead sensor may be better than the digit sensor for pulse oximetry (Fernandez et al., 2007).

Infant and Child Considerations

- For infants, the oximeter probe may be placed on the toe or foot.

Older Adult Considerations

- Careful attention to the patient's skin integrity and condition is necessary to prevent injury. Pressure or tension from the probe, as well as any adhesive used, can damage older, dry, thin skin.

Home Care Considerations

- Portable units are available for use in the home or in an outpatient setting.

SKILL 38-2 SUCTIONING THE OROPHARYNGEAL AND NASOPHARYNGEAL AIRWAYS

DELEGATION CONSIDERATIONS

The suctioning of the oropharyngeal airway may be delegated to nursing assistive personnel (NAP) or unlicensed assistive personnel (UAP) who have received appropriate training. Depending on the state's nurse practice act and the organization's policies and procedures, the suctioning of the oropharyngeal and nasopharyngeal airways may be delegated to licensed practical/vocational nurses (LPN/LVNs). The decision to delegate must be based on careful analysis of the patient's needs and circumstances, as well as the qualifications of the person to whom the task is being delegated. Refer to the Delegation Guidelines in Appendix A (found on thePoint).

EQUIPMENT

- Portable or wall suction unit with tubing
- A commercially prepared suction kit with an appropriate size catheter or
- Sterile suction catheter with Y-port in the appropriate size (Adult: 10F to 16F)
- Sterile disposable container
- Sterile gloves
- Sterile water or saline
- Towel or waterproof pad
- Goggles and mask or face shield
- Disposable, clean gloves
- Water-soluble lubricant
- Additional PPE, as indicated

IMPLEMENTATION

ACTION	RATIONALE
1. Bring necessary equipment to the bedside stand or overbed table.	Bringing everything to the bedside conserves time and energy. Arranging items nearby is convenient, saves time, and avoids unnecessary stretching and twisting of muscles on the part of the nurse.

ACTION	RATIONALE
2. Perform hand hygiene and put on PPE, if indicated.	Hand hygiene and PPE prevent the spread of microorganisms. PPE is required based on transmission precautions.
3. Identify the patient.	Identifying the patient ensures that the right patient receives the intervention and helps prevent errors.
4. Close the curtains around the bed and close the door to the room, if possible.	This ensures the patient's privacy.
5. Determine the need for suctioning. Verify the suction order in the patient's medical record, if necessary. **Assess for pain or the potential to cause pain. Administer pain medication, as prescribed, before suctioning.**	To minimize trauma to the airway mucosa, suctioning should be done only when secretions have accumulated or adventitious breath sounds are audible. Some facilities require an order for naso- and oropharyngeal suctioning. Suctioning stimulates coughing, which is painful for patients with surgical incisions and other conditions.
6. Explain what you are going to do and the reason for suctioning to the patient, even if the patient does not appear to be alert. Reassure the patient that you will interrupt procedure if the patient indicates respiratory difficulty.	Explanation alleviates fears. Even if the patient appears unconscious, explain what is happening. Any procedure that compromises respiration is frightening for the patient.
7. Adjust the bed to a comfortable working height, usually elbow height of the caregiver (VISN 8 Patient Safety Center, 2009). Lower the side rail closest to you. **If the patient is conscious, place him or her in a semi-Fowler's position. If patient is unconscious, place him or her in the lateral position, facing you.** Move the bedside table close to your work area and raise it to waist height.	Having the bed at the proper height prevents back and muscle strain. A sitting position helps the patient to cough and makes breathing easier. Gravity also facilitates catheter insertion. The lateral position prevents the airway from becoming obstructed and promotes drainage of secretions. The bedside table provides a work surface and helps maintain sterility of objects on the work surface.
8. Place a towel or waterproof pad across the patient's chest.	This protects the bed linens.
9. **Adjust suction to the appropriate pressure (Fig. 1).** For a wall unit for an adult: 100–150 mm Hg; neonates: 60–80 mm Hg; infants: 80–125 mm Hg; children: 80–125 mm Hg; adolescents: 80–150 mm Hg (Hess, 2012). For a portable unit for an adult: 10–15 cm Hg; neonates: 6–8 cm Hg; infants: 8–10 cm Hg; children: 8–10 cm Hg; adolescents: 8–15 cm Hg. **Put on a disposable, clean glove and occlude the end of the connecting tubing to check suction pressure.** Place the connecting tubing in a convenient location.	Higher pressures can cause excessive trauma, hypoxemia, and atelectasis.

FIGURE 1. Adjusting wall suction.

(continued)

SKILL 38-2 SUCTIONING THE OROPHARYNGEAL AND NASOPHARYNGEAL AIRWAYS *continued*

ACTION	RATIONALE
10. Open a sterile suction package using aseptic technique. The open wrapper or container becomes a sterile field to hold other supplies. Carefully remove the sterile container, touching only the outside surface. Set it up on the work surface and pour sterile saline into it.	Sterile normal saline or water is used to lubricate the outside of the catheter, minimizing irritation of mucosa during introduction. It is also used to clear the catheter between suction attempts.
11. Place a small amount of water-soluble lubricant on the sterile field, taking care to avoid touching the sterile field with the lubricant package.	Lubricant facilitates passage of the catheter and reduces trauma to the mucous membranes.
12. Increase the patient's supplemental oxygen level or apply supplemental oxygen per facility policy or primary care provider order.	Suctioning removes air from the patient's airway and can cause hypoxemia. Hyperoxygenation can help prevent suction-induced hypoxemia.
13. Put on a face shield or goggles and mask. Put on sterile gloves. **The dominant hand will manipulate the catheter and must remain sterile. The nondominant hand is considered clean rather than sterile and will control the suction valve (Y-port) on the catheter.** In the home setting and other community-based settings, maintenance of sterility is not necessary.	Gloves and other PPE protect the nurse from microorganisms. Handling the sterile catheter using a sterile glove helps prevent introducing organisms into the respiratory tract. In the home setting and other community-based settings, clean (instead of sterile) technique is used because the patient is not exposed to disease-causing organisms that may be found in health care settings, such as hospitals.
14. With your dominant gloved hand, pick up the sterile catheter. Pick up the connecting tubing with your nondominant hand and connect the tubing and suction catheter (Fig 2).	Sterility of the suction catheter is maintained.
15. Moisten the catheter by dipping it into the container of sterile saline (Fig. 3). Occlude the Y-tube to check suction.	Lubricating the inside of the catheter with saline helps move secretions in the catheter. Checking the suction ensures that the equipment is working properly.

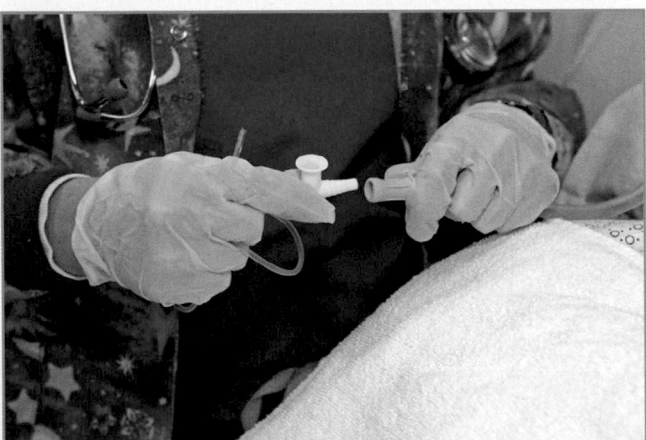

FIGURE 2. Connecting catheter to tubing.

FIGURE 3. Dipping catheter into sterile saline.

16. Encourage the patient to take several deep breaths.	Hyperventilation can help prevent suction-induced hypoxemia.
17. Apply lubricant to the first 2 to 3 inches of the catheter, using the lubricant that was placed on the sterile field.	Lubricant facilitates passage of the catheter and reduces trauma to the mucous membranes.
18. Remove the oxygen delivery device, if appropriate. Do not apply suction as the catheter is inserted. Hold the catheter between your thumb and forefinger.	Suctioning removes air from the patient's airway and can cause hypoxemia. Using suction while inserting the catheter can cause trauma to the mucosa and remove excessive oxygen from the respiratory tract.

ACTION

19. Insert the catheter:

   a. **For nasopharyngeal suctioning,** gently insert the catheter through the naris and along the floor of the nostril toward the trachea (Fig. 4). Roll the catheter between your fingers to help advance it. Advance the catheter approximately 5 to 6 inches to reach the pharynx.

   b. **For oropharyngeal suctioning,** insert the catheter through the mouth, along the side of the mouth toward the trachea. Advance the catheter 3″ to 4″ to reach the pharynx. (For nasotracheal suctioning, see the accompanying Skill Variation display.)

20. **Apply suction by intermittently occluding the Y-port on the catheter with the thumb of your nondominant hand and gently rotating the catheter as it is being withdrawn (Fig. 5). Do not suction for more than 10 to 15 seconds at a time.**

FIGURE 4. Inserting catheter into naris.

21. Replace the oxygen delivery device using your nondominant hand, if appropriate, and have the patient take several deep breaths.

22. Flush the catheter with saline (Fig. 6). Assess effectiveness of suctioning and repeat, as needed, according to the patient's tolerance. Wrap the suction catheter around your dominant hand between attempts.

RATIONALE

Correct distance for insertion ensures proper placement of the catheter. The general guideline for determining insertion distance for nasopharyngeal suctioning for an individual patient is to estimate the distance from the patient's earlobe to the nose.

Turning the catheter as it is withdrawn minimizes trauma to the mucosa. Suctioning for longer than 10 to 15 seconds robs the respiratory tract of oxygen, which may result in hypoxemia. Suctioning too quickly may be ineffective at clearing all secretions.

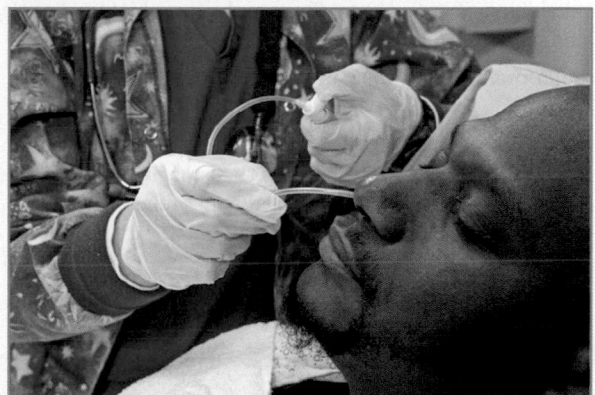

FIGURE 5. Suctioning nasopharynx.

Suctioning removes air from the patient's airway and can cause hypoxemia. Hyperventilation can help prevent suction-induced hypoxemia.

Flushing clears the catheter and lubricates it for next the insertion. Reassessment determines the need for additional suctioning. Wrapping prevents inadvertent contamination of the catheter.

FIGURE 6. Rinsing catheter.

(continued)

SKILL 38-2 SUCTIONING THE OROPHARYNGEAL AND NASOPHARYNGEAL AIRWAYS *continued*

ACTION	RATIONALE
23. **Allow at least a 30-second to 1-minute interval if additional suctioning is needed. No more than three suction passes should be made per suctioning episode. Alternate the nares, unless contraindicated, if repeated suctioning is required.** Do not force the catheter through the nares. Encourage the patient to cough and deep breathe between suctioning. **Suction the oropharynx after suctioning the nasopharynx.**	The interval allows for reventilation and reoxygenation of airways. Excessive suction passes contribute to complications. Alternating nares reduces trauma. Suctioning the oropharynx after the nasopharynx clears the mouth of secretions. More microorganisms are usually present in the mouth, so it is suctioned last to prevent transmission of contaminants.
24. When suctioning is completed, remove gloves from your dominant hand over the coiled catheter, pulling them off inside out. Remove the glove from your nondominant hand and dispose of gloves, catheter, and container with solution in the appropriate receptacle. Assist the patient to a comfortable position. Raise the bed rail and place the bed in the lowest position.	This technique reduces transmission of microorganisms. Proper positioning with raised side rails and proper bed height provide for patient comfort and safety.
25. Turn off suction. Remove the supplemental oxygen placed for suctioning, if appropriate. Remove the face shield or goggles and mask. Perform hand hygiene.	Proper removal of PPE and hand hygiene reduces risk of transmission of microorganisms.
26. Offer oral hygiene after suctioning.	Respiratory secretions that are allowed to accumulate in the mouth are irritating to mucous membranes and unpleasant for the patient.
27. Reassess the patient's respiratory status, including respiratory rate, effort, oxygen saturation, and lung sounds.	This assesses effectiveness of suctioning and the presence of complications.
28. Remove additional PPE, if used. Perform hand hygiene.	Removing PPE properly reduces the risk for infection transmission and contamination of other items. Hand hygiene prevents the spread of microorganisms.

DOCUMENTATION

Guidelines

Document the time of suctioning, your assessments before and after intervention, reason for suctioning, route used, and the characteristics and amount of secretions.

Sample Documentation

9/17/15 1440 Patient with gurgling on inspiration and weak cough; unable to clear secretions. Lungs with rhonchi (sonorous wheezes) in upper airways. Nasopharyngeal suction completed with 12F catheter. Large amount of thick, yellow secretions obtained. After suctioning, lung sounds clear in all lobes, respirations 18 breaths per min, no gurgling noted.

—C. Bausler, RN

UNEXPECTED SITUATIONS AND ASSOCIATED INTERVENTIONS

• *The catheter or sterile glove touches an unsterile surface:* Stop the procedure. If the gloved hand is still sterile, call for assistance and have someone open another catheter or remove the gloves and start the procedure over.

• *Patient vomits during suctioning:* If the patient gags or becomes nauseated, remove the catheter; it has probably entered the esophagus inadvertently. If the patient needs to be suctioned again, change catheters, because it is probably contaminated. Turn the patient to the side and elevate the head of the bed to prevent aspiration.

• *Secretions appear to be stomach contents:* Ask the patient to extend the neck slightly. This helps to prevent the tube from passing into the esophagus.

• *Epistaxis is noted with continued suctioning:* Notify the primary care provider and anticipate the need for a nasal trumpet (see Guidelines for Nursing Care 38-4, p. 1433). The nasal trumpet will protect the nasal mucosa from further trauma related to suctioning.

SPECIAL CONSIDERATIONS

Infant and Child Considerations

• For infants, use a 5F to 6F catheter.

• For children, use a 6F to 10F catheter.

SKILL 38-3 ADMINISTERING OXYGEN BY NASAL CANNULA

DELEGATION CONSIDERATIONS

The administration of oxygen by nasal cannula is not delegated to nursing assistive personnel (NAP) or unlicensed assistive personnel (UAP). Reapplication of the nasal cannula during nursing care activities, such as during bathing, may be performed by NAP or UAP. Depending on the state's nurse practice act and the organization's policies and procedures, administration of oxygen by nasal cannula may be delegated to licensed practical/vocational nurses (LPN/LVNs). The decision to delegate must be based on careful analysis of the patient's needs and circumstances, as well as the qualifications of the person to whom the task is being delegated. Refer to the Delegation Guidelines in Appendix A (found on thePoint).

EQUIPMENT

• Flow meter connected to oxygen supply
• Humidifier with sterile, distilled water (optional for low-flow system)
• Nasal cannula and tubing
• Gauze to pad tubing over ears (optional)
• PPE, as indicated

IMPLEMENTATION

ACTION	RATIONALE
1. Bring necessary equipment to the bedside stand or overbed table.	Bringing everything to the bedside conserves time and energy. Arranging items nearby is convenient, saves time, and avoids unnecessary stretching and twisting of muscles on the part of the nurse.
2. Perform hand hygiene and put on PPE, if indicated.	Hand hygiene and PPE prevent the spread of microorganisms. PPE is required based on transmission precautions.
3. Identify the patient.	Identifying the patient ensures that the right patient receives the intervention and helps prevent errors.
4. Close the curtains around the bed and close the door to the room, if possible.	This ensures the patient's privacy.
5. Explain what you are going to do and the reason for doing it to the patient. Review safety precautions necessary when oxygen is in use.	Explanation relieves anxiety and facilitates cooperation. Oxygen supports combustion; a small spark could cause a fire.

(continued)

SKILL 38-3 ADMINISTERING OXYGEN BY NASAL CANNULA *continued*

ACTION	RATIONALE

6. Connect nasal cannula to oxygen setup with humidification, if humidification is in use (Fig. 1). Adjust flow rate as ordered (Fig. 2). Check that oxygen is flowing out of the prongs.

Oxygen forced through a water reservoir is humidified before it is delivered to the patient, preventing dehydration of the mucous membranes. Low-flow oxygen does not require humidification.

FIGURE 1. Connecting cannula to oxygen source.

FIGURE 2. Adjusting flow rate.

7. Place the prongs in the patient's nostrils (Fig. 3). Place the tubing over and behind each ear with the adjuster comfortably under the chin. Alternately, the tubing may be placed around the patient's head, with the adjuster at the back or base of the head. Place gauze pads at the ear beneath the tubing, as necessary (Fig. 4).

Correct placement of the prongs and fastener facilitates oxygen administration and patient comfort. Pads reduce irritation and pressure and protect the skin.

FIGURE 3. Applying cannula to nares.

FIGURE 4. Placing gauze pad at ears.

8. Adjust the fit of the cannula, as necessary (Fig. 5). Tubing should be snug but not tight against the skin.

Proper adjustment maintains the prongs in the patient's nose. Excessive pressure from the tubing could cause irritation and pressure to the skin.

9. **Encourage patients to breathe through the nose, with the mouth closed.**

Nose breathing provides for optimal delivery of oxygen to the patient. The percentage of oxygen delivered can be reduced in patients who breathe through the mouth.

10. Reassess the patient's respiratory status, including respiratory rate, effort, and lung sounds. Note any signs of respiratory distress, such as tachypnea, nasal flaring, use of accessory muscles, or dyspnea.

Assesses the effectiveness of oxygen therapy.

ACTION	RATIONALE

FIGURE 5. Adjusting cannula, if needed.

11. Remove PPE, if used. Perform hand hygiene.

Removing PPE properly reduces the risk for infection transmission and contamination of other items. Hand hygiene prevents the spread of microorganisms.

12. Put on clean gloves. Remove and clean the cannula and assess nares at least every 8 hours, or according to agency recommendations (Fig. 6). Check nares for evidence of irritation or bleeding.

The continued presence of the cannula causes irritation and dryness of the mucous membranes.

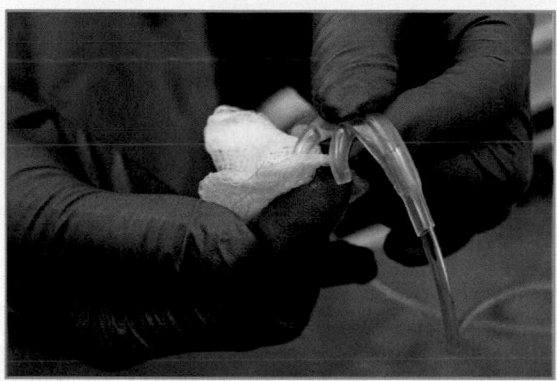

FIGURE 6. Cleaning cannula, when indicated.

DOCUMENTATION

Guidelines

Document your assessment before and after intervention. Document the amount of oxygen applied, the patient's respiratory rate, oxygen saturation, and lung sounds.

Sample Documentation

DocuCare Practice documenting the administration of oxygen by nasal cannula in *Lippincott DocuCare*.

9/17/15 1300 Oxygen via nasal cannula applied at 2 L/min. Humidification in place. Pulse oximeter before placing oxygen 92%; after oxygen at 2 L/min 98%. Respirations even and unlabored. Chest rises symmetrically. No nasal flaring or retractions noted. Lung sounds clear and equal all lobes.

—*C. Bausler, RN*

UNEXPECTED SITUATIONS AND ASSOCIATED INTERVENTIONS

• *Patient was fine on oxygen delivered by nasal cannula but now is cyanotic, and the pulse oximeter reading is less than 93%:* Check to see that the oxygen tubing is still connected to the flow meter and the flow meter is still on the previous setting. Someone may have stepped on the tubing, pulling it from the flow meter, or the oxygen may have accidentally been turned off. Assess lung sounds to note any changes. Report changes and assessment findings to the primary care provider.

(continued)

SKILL 38-3 ADMINISTERING OXYGEN BY NASAL CANNULA *continued*

- *Areas over ear or back of head are reddened:* Ensure that the areas are adequately padded and that the tubing is not pulled too tight. If available, a skin-care team may be able to offer some suggestions.
- *When dozing, patient begins to breathe through the mouth:* Temporarily place the nasal cannula near the mouth. If this does not raise the pulse oximeter reading, you may need to obtain an order to switch the patient to a mask while sleeping.

SPECIAL CONSIDERATIONS
Home Care Considerations

- Oxygen administration may need to be continued in the home setting. Portable oxygen concentrators are used most frequently. Instruct caregivers about safety precautions with oxygen use and make sure they understand the rationale for the specific liter flow of oxygen.
- To prevent fires and injuries, take the following precautions:
  - Avoid open flames.
  - **Place "No Smoking" signs in conspicuous places in the patient's home.** Instruct the patient and visitors about the hazard of smoking when oxygen is in use.
  - Check to see that electrical equipment used in the room is in good working order and emits no sparks.
  - Avoid using oils in the area. Oil can ignite spontaneously in the presence of oxygen.

SKILL 38-4 ADMINISTERING OXYGEN BY MASK

DELEGATION CONSIDERATIONS

The administration of oxygen by a mask is not delegated to nursing assistive personnel (NAP) or unlicensed assistive personnel (UAP). Reapplication of the mask during nursing care activities, such as during bathing, may be performed by NAP or UAP. Depending on the state's nurse practice act and the organization's policies and procedures, administration of oxygen by a mask may be delegated to licensed practical/vocational nurses (LPN/LVNs). The decision to delegate must be based on careful analysis of the patient's needs and circumstances, as well as the qualifications of the person to whom the task is being delegated. Refer to the Delegation Guidelines in Appendix A (found on thePoint).

EQUIPMENT

- Flow meter connected to oxygen supply
- Humidifier with sterile distilled water, if necessary, for the type of mask prescribed
- Face mask, specified by medical order
- Gauze to pad elastic band (optional)
- PPE, as indicated

IMPLEMENTATION

ACTION	RATIONALE
1. Bring necessary equipment to the bedside stand or overbed table.	Bringing everything to the bedside conserves time and energy. Arranging items nearby is convenient, saves time, and avoids unnecessary stretching and twisting of muscles on the part of the nurse.
2. Perform hand hygiene and put on PPE, if indicated.	Hand hygiene and PPE prevent the spread of microorganisms. PPE is required based on transmission precautions.
3. Identify the patient.	Identifying the patient ensures that the right patient receives the intervention and helps prevent errors.

ACTION

4. Close the curtains around the bed and close the door to the room, if possible.

5. Explain what you are going to do and the reason for doing it to the patient. Review safety precautions necessary when oxygen is in use.

6. Attach the face mask to the oxygen source (with humidification, if appropriate, for the specific mask; Fig. 1). Start the flow of oxygen at the specified rate. For a mask with a reservoir, be sure to allow oxygen to fill the bag (Fig. 2) before proceeding to the next step.

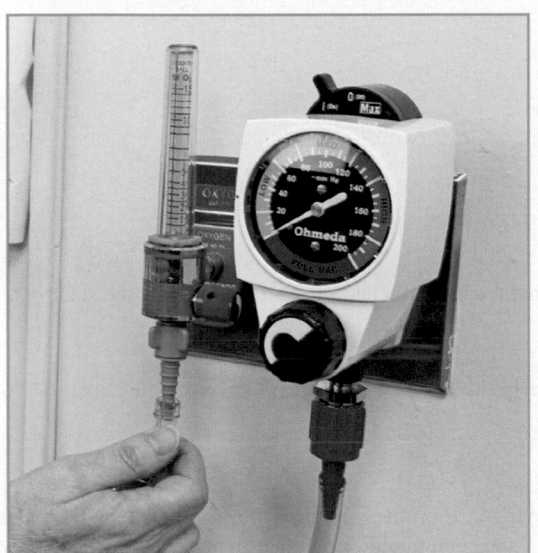

FIGURE 1. Connecting face mask to oxygen source.

7. Position the face mask over the patient's nose and mouth (Fig. 3). Adjust the elastic strap so that the mask fits snugly but comfortably on the face (Fig. 4). Adjust the flow rate to the prescribed rate (Fig. 5, p. 1454).

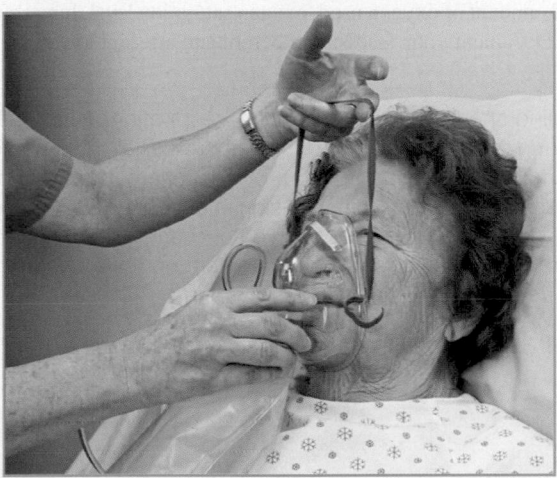

FIGURE 3. Applying face mask over nose and mouth.

RATIONALE

This ensures the patient's privacy.

Explanation relieves anxiety and facilitates cooperation. Oxygen supports combustion; a small spark could cause a fire.

Oxygen forced through a water reservoir is humidified before it is delivered to the patient, thus preventing dehydration of the mucous membranes. A reservoir bag must be inflated with oxygen because the bag is the oxygen supply source for the patient.

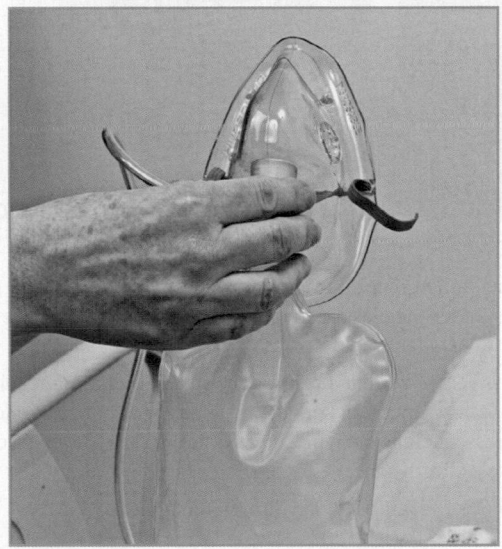

FIGURE 2. Allowing oxygen to fill bag.

A loose or poorly fitting mask will result in oxygen loss and decreased therapeutic value. Masks may cause a feeling of suffocation, and the patient needs frequent attention and reassurance.

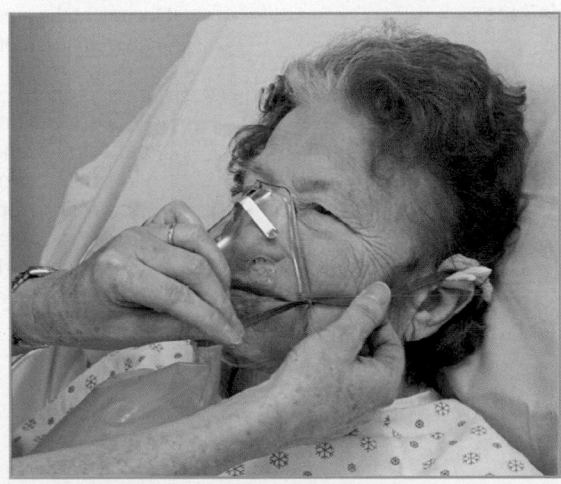

FIGURE 4. Adjusting elastic straps.

(continued)

SKILL 38-4   ADMINISTERING OXYGEN BY MASK   *continued*

ACTION	RATIONALE

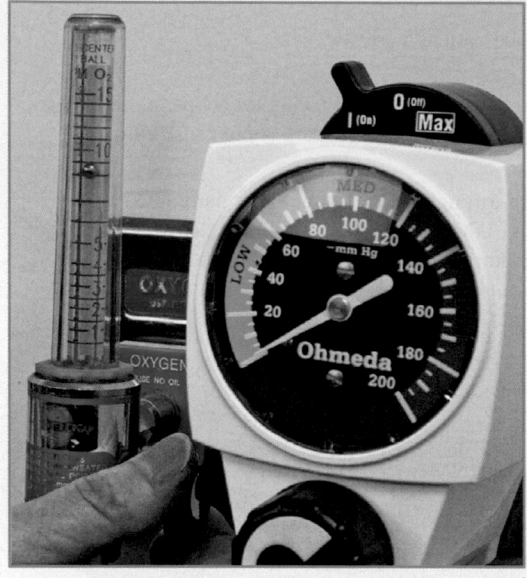

FIGURE 5. Adjusting flow rate.

ACTION	RATIONALE
8. If the patient reports irritation or you note redness, use gauze pads under the elastic strap at pressure points to reduce irritation to ears and scalp.	Pads reduce irritation and pressure and protect the skin.
9. Reassess the patient's respiratory status, including respiratory rate, effort, and lung sounds. Note any signs of respiratory distress, such as tachypnea, nasal flaring, use of accessory muscles, or dyspnea.	This helps assess the effectiveness of oxygen therapy.
10. Remove PPE, if used. Perform hand hygiene.	Removing PPE properly reduces the risk for infection transmission and contamination of other items. Hand hygiene prevents the spread of microorganisms.
11. **Remove the mask and dry the skin every 2 to 3 hours if the oxygen is running continuously. Do not use powder around the mask.**	The tight-fitting mask and moisture from condensation can irritate the skin on the face. There is a danger of inhaling powder if it is placed on the mask.

DOCUMENTATION

Guidelines

Document the type of mask used, amount of oxygen used, oxygen saturation level, lung sounds, and rate/pattern of respirations. Document your assessment before and after intervention.

Sample Documentation

9/22/15 Patient reports feeling short of breath. Skin pale, respirations 30 breaths per minute and labored. Lung sounds decreased throughout. Oxygen saturation via pulse oximeter 88%. Findings reported to Dr. Lu. Oxygen via nonrebreather face mask applied at 12 L/min as ordered. Patient's skin is pink after O_2 applied. Oxygen saturation increased to 98%. Respirations even and unlabored. Chest rises symmetrically. Respiratory rate 18 breaths per minute. Lungs remain with decreased breath sounds throughout. Patient denies dyspnea.

—C. Bausler, RN

UNEXPECTED SITUATIONS AND ASSOCIATED INTERVENTIONS

- *Patient was previously fine but now is cyanotic, and the pulse oximeter reading is less than 93%:* Check to see that the oxygen tubing is still connected to the flow meter and the flow meter is still on the previous setting. Someone may have stepped on the tubing, pulling it from the flow meter, or the oxygen may have accidentally been turned off. Assess lung sounds for any changes. Report changes and assessment findings to the primary care provider.
- *Areas over ear or back of head are reddened:* Ensure that the areas are adequately padded and that the tubing is not pulled too tight. If available, a skin-care team may be able to offer some suggestions.

SPECIAL CONSIDERATIONS

General Considerations

- Different types of face masks are available for use (see Table 38-5, p. 1428).
- It's important to ensure that the mask fits snugly around the patient's face. If it is loose, it will not effectively deliver the right amount of oxygen.
- The mask must be removed for the patient to eat, drink, and take medications. Obtain an order for oxygen via nasal cannula for use during meal times and limit the amount of times the mask is removed to maintain adequate oxygenation.

SKILL 38-5 PROVIDING CARE OF A TRACHEOSTOMY TUBE

DELEGATION CONSIDERATIONS

Care of a tracheostomy tube is not delegated to nursing assistive personnel (NAP) or unlicensed assistive personnel (UAP). Depending on the state's nurse practice act and the organization's policies and procedures, care of a tracheostomy tube in a stable situation, such as long-term care and other community-based care settings, may be delegated to licensed practical/vocational nurses (LPN/LVNs). The decision to delegate must be based on careful analysis of the patient's needs and circumstances, as well as the qualifications of the person to whom the task is being delegated. Refer to the Delegation Guidelines in Appendix A (found on thePoint).

EQUIPMENT

- Disposable gloves
- Sterile gloves
- Goggles and mask or face shield
- Additional PPE, as indicated
- Sterile normal saline
- Sterile cup or basin
- Sterile cotton-tipped applicators
- Sterile gauze sponges

- Disposable inner tracheostomy cannula, appropriate size for patient
- Sterile suction catheter and glove set
- Commercially prepared tracheostomy or drain dressing
- Commercially prepared tracheostomy holder
- Plastic disposal bag
- Additional nurse

IMPLEMENTATION

ACTION	RATIONALE
1. Bring necessary equipment to the bedside stand or overbed table.	Bringing everything to the bedside conserves time and energy. Arranging items nearby is convenient, saves time, and avoids unnecessary stretching and twisting of muscles on the part of the nurse.

(continued)

SKILL 38·5 PROVIDING CARE OF A TRACHEOSTOMY TUBE *continued*

ACTION	**RATIONALE**
2. Perform hand hygiene and put on PPE, if indicated.	Hand hygiene and PPE prevent the spread of microorganisms. PPE is required based on transmission precautions.
3. Identify the patient.	Identifying the patient ensures that the right patient receives the intervention and helps prevent errors.
4. Close the curtains around the bed and close the door to the room, if possible.	This ensures the patient's privacy.
5. Determine the need for tracheostomy care. **Assess the patient's pain and administer pain medication, if indicated.**	If the tracheostomy is new, pain medication may be needed before performing tracheostomy care.
6. Explain what you are going to do and the reason for doing it to the patient, even if the patient does not appear to be alert. Reassure the patient that you will interrupt procedure if he or she indicates respiratory difficulty.	Explanation alleviates fears. Even if the patient appears unconscious, the nurse should explain what is happening. Any procedure that compromises respiration is frightening for the patient.
7. Adjust the bed to a comfortable working position, usually elbow height of the caregiver (VISN 8 Patient Safety Center, 2009). Lower the side rail closest to you. **If the patient is conscious, place him or her in a semi-Fowler's position. If patient is unconscious, place him or her in the lateral position, facing you.** Move the overbed table close to your work area and raise it to waist height. Place a trash receptacle within easy reach of the work area.	Having the bed at the proper height prevents back and muscle strain. A sitting position helps the patient to cough and makes breathing easier. Gravity also facilitates catheter insertion. The lateral position prevents the airway from becoming obstructed and promotes drainage of secretions. The overbed table provides work surface and maintains sterility of objects on the work surface. A trash receptacle within reach prevents reaching over the sterile field or turning back to the field to dispose of trash.
8. Put on a face shield or goggles and mask. Suction the tracheostomy, if necessary. If the tracheostomy has just been suctioned, remove the soiled site dressing and discard before removal of gloves used to perform suctioning.	PPE prevents contact with contaminants. Suctioning removes secretions to prevent occluding the outer cannula while the inner cannula is removed.

Cleaning the Tracheostomy: Disposable Inner Cannula

9. Carefully open the package with the new disposable inner cannula, taking care not to contaminate the cannula or the inside of the package (Fig. 1). Carefully open the package with the sterile cotton-tipped applicators, taking care not to contaminate them. Open a sterile cup or basin and fill 0.5 inch deep with saline. Open the plastic disposable bag and place within reach on the work surface.	Inner cannula must remain sterile. Saline and applicators will be used to clean the tracheostomy site. A plastic disposable bag will be used to discard the removed inner cannula.
10. Put on disposable gloves.	Gloves protect against exposure to blood and body fluids.

FIGURE 1. Carefully opening package with new disposable inner cannula. *(Photo by B. Proud.)*

ACTION

11. Remove the oxygen source if one is present. Stabilize the outer cannula and faceplate of the tracheostomy with your nondominant hand. Grasp the locking mechanism of the inner cannula with your dominant hand. Press the tabs and release the lock (Fig. 2). Gently remove the inner cannula and place in a disposal bag. If not already removed, remove the site dressing and dispose of it in the trash.

12. Discard gloves and put on sterile gloves. Pick up the new inner cannula with your dominant hand, stabilize the faceplate with your nondominant hand, and gently insert the new inner cannula into the outer cannula. Press the tabs to allow the lock to grab the outer cannula (Fig. 3). Reapply the oxygen source, if needed.

RATIONALE

Stabilizing the faceplate prevents trauma to, and pain from, the stoma. Releasing the lock permits removal of the inner cannula.

Sterile gloves are necessary to prevent contamination of the new inner cannula. Locking to the outer cannula secures the inner cannula in place. Maintains oxygen supply to the patient.

FIGURE 2. Releasing lock on inner cannula.

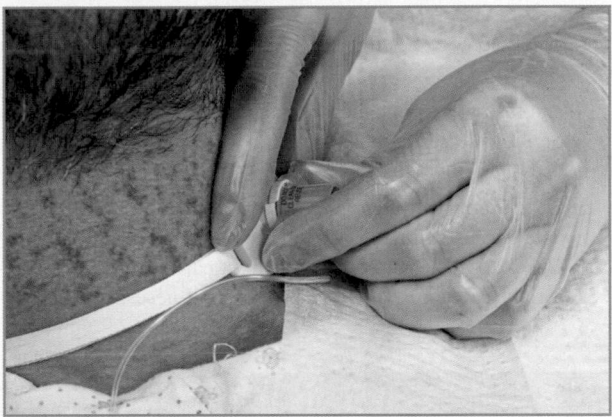

FIGURE 3. Locking new inner cannula in place.

Applying Clean Dressing and Holder

13. Remove the oxygen source, if necessary. Dip a cotton-tipped applicator or gauze sponge in a cup or basin with sterile saline and clean the stoma under the faceplate. Use each applicator or sponge only once, moving from the stoma site outward (Fig. 4).

Saline is nonirritating to tissue. Cleansing from the stoma outward and using each applicator only once promotes aseptic technique.

FIGURE 4. Cleaning from stoma site, outward.

(continued)

SKILL 38-5 PROVIDING CARE OF A TRACHEOSTOMY TUBE *continued*

ACTION	RATIONALE
14. Pat skin gently with a dry 4 × 4 gauze sponge.	Gauze removes excess moisture.
15. Slide a commercially prepared tracheostomy dressing or prefolded non–cotton-filled 4 × 4-inch dressing under the faceplate.	Lint or fiber from a cut cotton-filled gauze pad can be aspirated into the trachea, causing respiratory distress, or can embed in the stoma and cause irritation or infection.
16. Change the tracheostomy holder:	
a. **Obtain the assistance of a second person to hold the tracheostomy tube in place while the old collar is removed and the new collar is placed.**	Holding the tracheostomy tube in place ensures that the tracheostomy will not inadvertently be expelled if the patient coughs or moves.
b. Open the package for the new tracheostomy collar.	Doing so provides attachment for one side of the faceplate.
c. Both nurses should put on clean gloves.	Allows access to the new collar.
	Gloves prevent contact with blood, body fluids, and contaminants.
d. One nurse holds the faceplate while the other pulls up the Velcro tabs. Gently remove the collar.	Holding the tracheostomy tube in place ensures that the tracheostomy will not inadvertently be expelled if the patient coughs or moves. Pulling up the Velcro tabs loosens the collar.
e. The first nurse continues to hold the tracheostomy faceplate.	Prevents accidental extubation.
f. The other nurse places the collar around the patient's neck and inserts first one tab, then the other, into the openings on the faceplate and secures the Velcro tabs on the tracheostomy holder (Fig. 5).	Securing the Velcro tabs holds the tracheostomy in place and prevents accidental expulsion of the tracheostomy tube.
g. Check the fit of the tracheostomy collar. You should be able to fit one finger between the neck and the collar. Check to make sure that the patient can flex the neck comfortably. Reapply the oxygen source, if necessary (Fig. 6).	Allowing one fingerbreadth under the collar permits neck flexion that is comfortable and ensures that the collar will not compromise circulation to the area. Maintains oxygen supply to the patient.

FIGURE 5. Securing tabs on tracheostomy holder.

FIGURE 6. Reapplying oxygen source.

ACTION	RATIONALE
17. Remove gloves. Remove the face shield or goggles and mask. Assist the patient to a comfortable position. Raise the bed rail and place the bed in the lowest position.	Removing PPE properly reduces the risk for infection transmission and contamination of other items. Ensures patient comfort. Proper positioning with raised side rails and proper bed height provide for patient comfort and safety.
18. Reassess patient's respiratory status, including respiratory rate, effort, oxygen saturation, and lung sounds.	Assessments determine the effectiveness of interventions and for the presence of complications.
19. Remove additional PPE, if used. Perform hand hygiene.	Removing PPE properly reduces the risk for infection transmission and contamination of other items. Hand hygiene prevents the spread of microorganisms.

DOCUMENTATION

Guidelines

Document your assessments before and after interventions, including site assessment, presence of pain, lung sounds, and oxygen saturation levels. Document the presence of skin breakdown that may result from irritation or pressure from the tracheostomy collar. Document care given.

Sample Documentation

> 9/26/15 1300 Tracheostomy care completed; lung sounds clear in all lobes; respirations even/unlabored; site without erythema or edema; small amount of thick, yellow secretions noted at site.
>
> —C. Bausler, RN

UNEXPECTED SITUATIONS AND ASSOCIATED INTERVENTIONS

- *Patient coughs hard enough to dislodge tracheostomy:* Keep a spare tracheostomy and obturator at the bedside. Insert the obturator into the new tracheostomy and insert the tracheostomy into the stoma. Remove the obturator. Secure the ties and auscultate lung sounds. Palpate for any subcutaneous emphysema.

- *Tracheostomy becomes dislodged and is not easily replaced:* Notify the primary care provider immediately. This is an emergency situation. Cover the tracheostomy stoma. Assess the patient's respiratory status. Anticipate the possible need for maintaining ventilation using a manual resuscitation device.

- *On palpating around insertion site, you note a moderate amount of subcutaneous emphysema in tissue:* Assess for dislodgement of the tracheostomy tube. If the tube has become displaced, a buildup of air in the subcutaneous portion of the skin is likely. Notify the primary care provider if the subcutaneous emphysema is a change in the status of the tracheostomy.

SPECIAL CONSIDERATIONS

General Considerations

- One nurse working alone should always place new tracheostomy ties in place before removing old ties to prevent accidental extubation of the tracheostomy. If it is necessary to remove old ties first, obtain the assistance of a second person to hold the tracheostomy tube in place while the old tie is removed and the new tie is replaced.

- Make sure emergency equipment is easily accessible at the bedside. Keep a bag-valve mask, oxygen, the obturator from the current tracheostomy, spare tracheostomy of the same size, spare tracheostomy one size smaller, and suction equipment at the bedside of a patient with a tracheostomy tube at all times.

- If the patient is currently using a tracheostomy without a cuff, keep a spare tracheostomy of the same size with a cuff at the bedside for emergency use.

Home Care Considerations

- Instruct the patient and home caregiver on how to perform tracheostomy care. Observe a return demonstration and provide feedback.

- Clean, rather than sterile, technique can be used in the home setting.

- Sterile saline can be made by mixing 1 teaspoon of table salt in 1 quart of water and boiling for 15 minutes. The solution is cooled and stored in a clean, dry container. Discard saline at the end of each day to prevent growth of bacteria.

- Instruct the patient who is performing self-care to use a mirror to view the steps in the procedure.

SKILL 38-6 SUCTIONING A TRACHEOSTOMY: OPEN SYSTEM

DELEGATION CONSIDERATIONS

Suctioning a tracheostomy is not delegated to nursing assistive personnel (NAP) or unlicensed assistive personnel (UAP). Depending on the state's nurse practice act and the organization's policies and procedures, suctioning of a tracheostomy in a stable situation, such as long-term care and other community-based care settings, may be delegated to licensed practical/vocational nurses (LPN/LVNs). The decision to delegate must be based on careful analysis of the patient's needs and circumstances, as well as the qualifications of the person to whom the task is being delegated. Refer to the Delegation Guidelines in Appendix A (found on thePoint).

EQUIPMENT

- Portable or wall suction unit with tubing
- A commercially prepared suction kit with an appropriate-size catheter (See General Considerations, p. 1465) or
- Sterile suction catheter with Y-port in the appropriate size
- Sterile, disposable container
- Sterile gloves
- Towel or waterproof pad
- Goggles and mask or face shield
- Additional PPE, as indicated
- Disposable, clean gloves
- Resuscitation bag connected to 100% oxygen

IMPLEMENTATION

ACTION	RATIONALE
1. Bring necessary equipment to the bedside stand or overbed table.	Bringing everything to the bedside conserves time and energy. Arranging items nearby is convenient, saves time, and avoids unnecessary stretching and twisting of muscles on the part of the nurse.
2. Perform hand hygiene and put on PPE, if indicated.	Hand hygiene and PPE prevent the spread of microorganisms. PPE is required based on transmission precautions.
3. Identify the patient.	Identifying the patient ensures that the right patient receives the intervention and helps prevent errors.
4. Close curtains around the bed and close the door to the room, if possible.	This ensures the patient's privacy.
5. Determine the need for suctioning. Verify the suction order in the patient's medical record. **Assess for pain or the potential to cause pain. Administer pain medication, as prescribed, before suctioning.**	To minimize trauma to airway mucosa, suctioning should be done only when secretions have accumulated or adventitious breath sounds are audible. Suctioning can cause moderate to severe pain for patients. Individualized pain management is imperative (Arroyo-Novoa, et al., 2008). Suctioning stimulates coughing, which is painful for patients with surgical incisions.
6. Explain to the patient what you are going to do and the reason for doing it, even if the patient does not appear to be alert. Reassure the patient that you will interrupt the procedure if the patient indicates respiratory difficulty.	Explanation alleviates fears. Even if the patient appears unconscious, the nurse should explain what is happening. Any procedure that compromises respiration is frightening for the patient.
7. Adjust the bed to a comfortable working position, usually elbow height of the caregiver (VISN 8 Patient Safety Center, 2009). Lower the side rail closest to you. **If the patient is conscious, place the patient in a semi-Fowler's position (Fig. 1). If unconscious, place him or her in the lateral position, facing you.** Move the overbed table close to your work area and raise it to waist height.	Having the bed at the proper height prevents back and muscle strain. A sitting position helps the patient to cough and makes breathing easier. Gravity also facilitates catheter insertion. The lateral position prevents the airway from becoming obstructed and promotes drainage of secretions. The overbed table provides a work surface and maintains sterility of objects on the work surface.
8. Place a towel or waterproof pad across the patient's chest.	This protects the bed linens and the patient.

ACTION

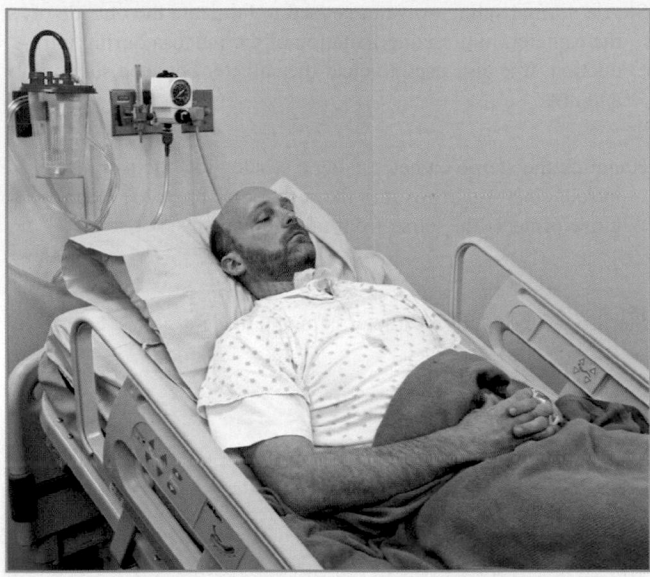

FIGURE 1. Patient in semi-Fowler's position.

9. Turn the suction to the appropriate pressure (Fig. 2).

For a wall unit for an adult: 100–150 mm Hg; neonates: 60–80 mm Hg; infants: 80–125 mm Hg; children: 80–125 mm Hg; adolescents: 80–150 mm Hg (Hess, 2012).

For a portable unit for an adult: 10–15 cm Hg; neonates: 6–8 cm Hg; infants: 8–10 cm Hg; children: 8–10 cm Hg; adolescents: 8–15 cm Hg.

Put on a disposable, clean glove and occlude the end of the connecting tubing to check suction pressure. Place the connecting tubing in a convenient location. If using, place the resuscitation bag connected to the oxygen within convenient reach.

RATIONALE

Higher pressures can cause excessive trauma, hypoxemia, and atelectasis. Glove prevents contact with blood and body fluids. Checking pressure ensures that equipment is working properly. Allows for an organized approach to procedure.

FIGURE 2. Turning suction device to appropriate pressure.

(continued)

SKILL 38-6 SUCTIONING A TRACHEOSTOMY: OPEN SYSTEM *continued*

ACTION	RATIONALE

10. Open a sterile suction package using aseptic technique. The open wrapper or container becomes a sterile field to hold other supplies. Carefully remove the sterile container, touching only the outside surface. Set it up on the work surface and pour sterile saline into it.

Sterile normal saline or water is used to lubricate the outside of the catheter, minimizing irritation of the mucosa during introduction. It is also used to clear the catheter between suction attempts.

11. Put on a face shield or goggles and mask (Fig. 3). Put on sterile gloves. **The dominant hand will manipulate the catheter and must remain sterile. The nondominant hand is considered clean rather than sterile and will control the suction valve (Y-port) on the catheter.**

Handling the sterile catheter using a sterile glove helps prevent introducing organisms into the respiratory tract; the clean glove protects the nurse from microorganisms.

12. With your dominant gloved hand, pick up the sterile catheter. Pick up the connecting tubing with your nondominant hand and connect the tubing and suction catheter (Fig. 4).

Sterility of the suction catheter is maintained.

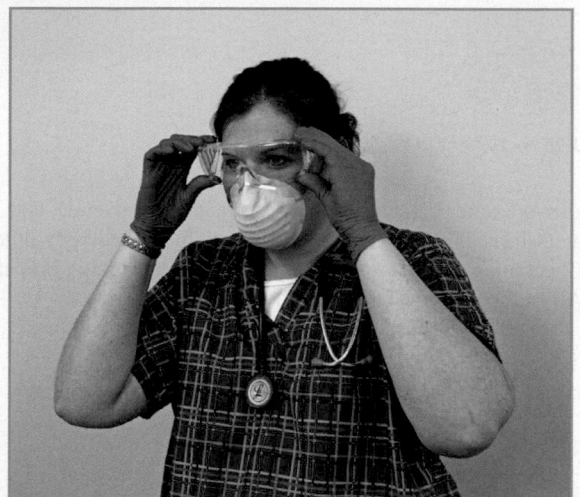

FIGURE 3. Putting on goggles and mask.

FIGURE 4. Connecting suction catheter to suction tubing.

13. Moisten the catheter by dipping it into the container of sterile saline, unless it is a silicone catheter (Fig. 5). Occlude the Y-tube to check the suction (Fig. 6).

Lubricating the inside of the catheter with saline helps move secretions in the catheter. Silicone catheters do not require lubrication. Checking ensures that equipment is working properly.

FIGURE 5. Moistening catheter in saline solution.

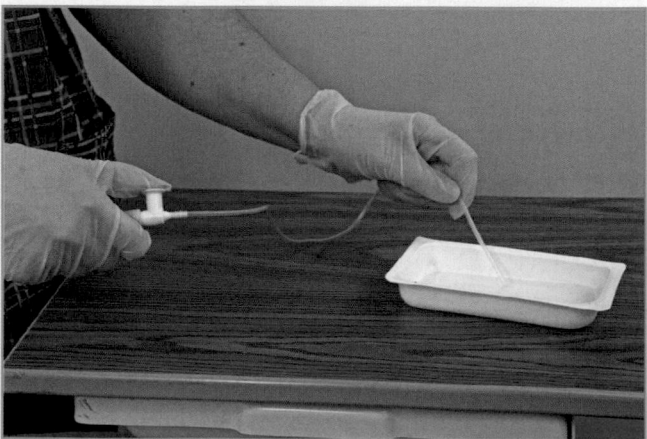

FIGURE 6. Occluding Y-port to check for proper suction.

ACTION

14. Using your nondominant hand and a manual resuscitation bag, hyperventilate the patient, delivering three to six breaths or use the sigh mechanism on a mechanical ventilator.

15. Open the adapter on the mechanical ventilator tubing or remove the oxygen delivery setup with your nondominant hand.

16. Using your dominant hand, gently and quickly insert the catheter into the trachea. **Advance the catheter to the predetermined length. Do not occlude the Y-port when inserting the catheter.**

17. Apply suction by intermittently occluding the Y-port on the catheter with the thumb of your nondominant hand, and gently rotate the catheter as it is being withdrawn (Fig. 7). **Do not suction for more than 10 to 15 seconds at a time.**

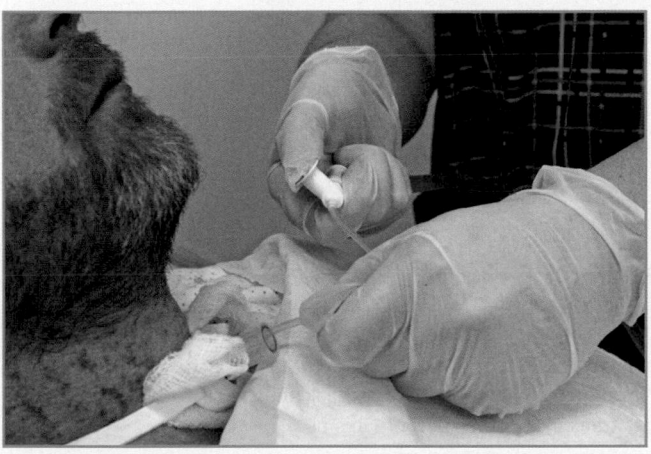

18. Hyperventilate the patient using your nondominant hand and a manual resuscitation bag, delivering three to six breaths. Replace the oxygen delivery device, if applicable, using your nondominant hand and have the patient take several deep breaths. If the patient is mechanically ventilated, close the adapter on the mechanical ventilator tubing and use the sigh mechanism on a mechanical ventilator.

19. Flush the catheter with saline. Assess the effectiveness of suctioning and repeat, as needed, according to the patient's tolerance. Wrap the suction catheter around your dominant hand between attempts.

RATIONALE

Hyperoxygenation and hyperventilation aid in preventing hypoxemia during suctioning.

This exposes the tracheostomy tube without contaminating your sterile gloved hand.

Catheter contact and suction cause tracheal mucosal damage, loss of cilia, edema, and fibrosis, and increase the risk of infection and bleeding for the patient. Insertion of the suction catheter to a predetermined distance, no more than 1 cm past the length of the endotracheal tube, avoids contact with the trachea and carina, reducing the effects of tracheal mucosal damage (Hahn, 2010; Ireton, 2007; Pate, 2004; Pate & Zapata, 2002). If resistance is met, the carina or tracheal mucosa has been hit. Withdraw the catheter at least ½ inch before applying suction. Suctioning when inserting the catheter increases the risk for trauma to the airway mucosa and increases the risk of hypoxemia.

Turning the catheter as it is withdrawn minimizes trauma to the mucosa. Suctioning for longer than 10 to 15 seconds robs the respiratory tract of oxygen, which may result in hypoxemia. Suctioning too quickly may be ineffective at clearing all secretions.

FIGURE 7. Applying intermittent suction while withdrawing catheter.

Suctioning removes air from the patient's airway and can cause hypoxemia. Hyperventilation can help prevent suction-induced hypoxemia.

Flushing clears the catheter and lubricates it for the next insertion. Reassessment determines the need for additional suctioning. Prevents inadvertent contamination of the catheter.

(continued)

SKILL 38-6 SUCTIONING A TRACHEOSTOMY: OPEN SYSTEM *continued*

ACTION	RATIONALE
20. Allow at least a 30-second to 1-minute interval if additional suctioning is needed. Do not make more than three suction passes per suctioning episode. Encourage the patient to cough and deep breathe between suctioning attempts. Suction the oropharynx after suctioning the trachea. Do not reinsert in the tracheostomy after suctioning the mouth.	The interval allows for reventilation and reoxygenation of airways. Excessive suction passes contribute to complications. Clears the mouth of secretions. More microorganisms are usually present in the mouth, so it is suctioned last to prevent transmission of contaminants.
21. When suctioning is completed, remove the glove from your dominant hand over the coiled catheter, pulling it off inside out (Fig. 8). Remove the glove from your nondominant hand and dispose of gloves, catheter, and container with solution in the appropriate receptacle. Assist the patient to a comfortable position. Raise the bed rail and place the bed in the lowest position.	This technique reduces transmission of microorganisms. Ensures patient comfort. Proper positioning with raised side rails and proper bed height provide for patient comfort and safety.

FIGURE 8. Removing gloves while keeping catheter inside.

ACTION	RATIONALE
22. Turn off the suction. Remove the supplemental oxygen placed for suctioning, if appropriate. Remove the face shield or goggles and mask. Perform hand hygiene.	Removing PPE properly reduces the risk for infection transmission and contamination of other items. Hand hygiene prevents transmission of microorganisms.
23. Offer oral hygiene after suctioning.	Respiratory secretions that are allowed to accumulate in the mouth are irritating to mucous membranes and unpleasant for the patient.
24. Reassess the patient's respiratory status, including respiratory rate, effort, oxygen saturation, and lung sounds.	These assess effectiveness of suctioning and the presence of complications.
25. Remove additional PPE, if used. Perform hand hygiene.	Removing PPE properly reduces the risk for infection transmission and contamination of other items. Hand hygiene prevents the spread of microorganisms.

DOCUMENTATION
Guidelines

Document the time of suctioning, your assessments before and after intervention, reason for suctioning, and the characteristics and amount of secretions.

Sample Documentation

> 9/1/15 1515 Lungs auscultated for wheezes in upper and lower lobes bilaterally. Respirations at 24 breaths per minute. Weak, ineffective cough noted. Tracheal suction completed with 12F catheter. Large amount of thick, yellow secretions obtained. Specimen for culture collected and sent, as ordered. After suctioning, lung sounds clear in all lobes, oxygen saturation at 97%, respirations 18 breaths per minute.
>
> —C. Bausler, RN

UNEXPECTED SITUATIONS AND ASSOCIATED INTERVENTIONS

- *Patient coughs hard enough to dislodge tracheostomy:* Keep a spare tracheostomy and obturator at the bedside. Insert the obturator into the tracheostomy tube and reinsert the tracheostomy into the stoma. Remove the obturator. Secure the ties and auscultate lung sounds. Palpate for any subcutaneous emphysema.

- *Tracheostomy becomes dislodged and is not easily replaced:* Notify the primary care provider immediately. This is an emergency situation. Cover the tracheostomy stoma. Assess the patient's respiratory status. Anticipate the possible need for maintaining ventilation using a manual resuscitation device.

- *Lung sounds do not improve greatly and oxygen saturation remains low after three suctioning attempts:* Allow the patient time to recover from the previous suctioning. If needed, hyperoxygenate again. Suction the patient again and assess whether the oxygen saturation increases, lung sounds improve, and secretion amount decreases.

SPECIAL CONSIDERATIONS

General Considerations

- Determine the size catheter to use by the size of the tracheostomy. The external diameter of the suction catheter should not exceed half of the internal diameter of the tracheostomy. Larger catheters can contribute to trauma and hypoxemia.

- Make sure emergency equipment is easily accessible at the bedside. Keep bag-valve mask, oxygen, and suction equipment at the bedside of a patient with a tracheostomy tube at all times.

DEVELOPING CLINICAL REASONING

1. Using the Focused Assessment Guide in this chapter, work with a partner to assess the respiratory functioning of the following patients. Discuss ways in which you would modify your assessment to meet the specific needs of individual patients:
   - A 6-year-old who presents in the pediatrician's office with asthma and is experiencing difficulty breathing
   - A 12-year-old who is brought to the emergency department after illicit use of inhalants ("huffing")
   - An adult dying of cancer receiving hospice care at home who is receiving increasing doses of narcotics, which depress respiratory functioning
   - A hospitalized young adult with a 24-pack/year history of smoking who is noted to have a persistent, hacking cough

2. A postoperative patient who is at high risk for pulmonary complications because of a long history of smoking refuses to use the incentive spirometer or to cooperate with instructions to breathe deeply. How would you respond to this patient? Discuss with other students what nursing response is most likely to secure his cooperation in necessary self-care measures.

PRACTICING FOR NCLEX

1. A nurse caring for a patient with chronic obstructive pulmonary disease (COPD) knows that hypoxia may occur in patients with respiratory problems. What are signs of this serious condition? Select all answers that apply.
   a. Dyspnea
   b. Hypotension
   c. Small pulse pressure
   d. Decreased respiratory rate
   e. Pallor
   f. Increased pulse rate

2. A nurse is suctioning the nasopharyngeal airway of a patient to maintain a patent airway. For which condition would the nurse anticipate the need for a nasal trumpet?
   a. The patient vomits during suctioning.
   b. The secretions appear to be stomach contents.
   c. The catheter touches an unsterile surface.
   d. Epistaxis is noted with continued suctioning.

3. A nurse is inserting an oropharyngeal airway for a patient who vomits when it is inserted. Which action would be the first that should be taken by the nurse related to this occurrence?
   a. Quickly position the patient on his or her side.
   b. Put on disposable gloves and remove the oral airway.
   c. Check that the airway is the appropriate size for the patient.
   d. Put on sterile gloves and suction the airway.

4. A nurse is choosing a catheter to use to suction a patient's endotracheal tube via an open system. On which variable would the nurse base the size of the catheter to use?
   a. The age of the patient
   b. The size of the endotracheal tube
   c. The type of secretions to be suctioned
   d. The height and weight of the patient

5. A nurse is caring for a 16-year-old male patient who has been hospitalized for an acute asthma exacerbation. Which testing methods might the nurse use to measure the patient's oxygen saturation? Select all that apply.
   a. Thoracentesis
   b. Spirometry
   c. Pulse oximetry
   d. Peak expiratory flow rate
   e. Diffusion capacity
   f. Maximal respiratory pressure

6. A patient with COPD is unable to perform activities of daily living (ADLs) without becoming exhausted. Which nursing diagnosis best describes this alteration in oxygenation as the etiology?
   a. Decreased Cardiac Output related to difficulty breathing
   b. Impaired Gas Exchange related to use of bronchodilators
   c. Fatigue related to impaired oxygen transport system
   d. Ineffective Airway Clearance related to fatigue

7. A nurse working in a long-term care facility is providing teaching to patients with altered oxygenation due to conditions such as asthma and COPD. Which measures would the nurse recommend? Select all that apply.
   a. Refrain from exercise.
   b. Reduce anxiety.
   c. Eat meals 1 to 2 hours prior to breathing treatments.
   d. Eat a high-protein/high-calorie diet.
   e. Maintain a high-Fowler's position when possible.
   f. Drink 2 to 3 pints of clear fluids daily.

8. A nurse is providing postural drainage for a patient with cystic fibrosis. In which position should the nurse place the patient to drain the right lobe of the lung?
   a. High Fowler's position
   b. Left side with pillow under chest wall
   c. Lying position/half on abdomen and half on side
   d. Trendelenberg position

9. A nurse is teaching a patient how to use a meter-dosed inhaler for her asthma. Which comments from the patient assure the nurse that the teaching has been effective? Select all that apply.
   a. "I will be careful not to shake up the canister before using it."
   b. "I will hold the canister upside-down when using it."

c. "I will inhale the medication through my nose."
   d. "I will continue to inhale when the cold propellant is in my throat."
   e. "I will only inhale one spray with one breath."
   f. "I will activate the device while continuing to inhale."

10. When planning care for a patient with chronic lung disease who is receiving oxygen through a nasal cannula, what does the nurse expect?
    a. The oxygen must be humidified.
    b. The rate will be no more than 2 to 3 L/min or less.
    c. Arterial blood gases will be drawn every 4 hours to assess flow rate.
    d. The rate will be 6 L/min or more.

11. A nurse is securing a patient's endotracheal tube with tape and observes that the tube depth changed during the retaping. Which action would be appropriate related to this incident?
    a. Instruct assistant to notify the primary care provider.
    b. Assess the patient's vital signs.
    c. Remove the tape, adjust the depth to ordered depth and reapply the tape.
    d. No action is required as depth will adjust automatically.

12. What action does the nurse perform to follow safe technique when using a portable oxygen cylinder?
    a. Checking the amount of oxygen in the cylinder before using it
    b. Using a cylinder for a patient transfer that indicates available oxygen is 500 psi
    c. Placing the oxygen cylinder on the stretcher next to the patient
    d. Discontinuing oxygen flow by turning cylinder key counterclockwise until tight

13. A nurse providing care of a patient's chest drainage system observes that the chest tube has become separated from the drainage device. What would be the first action that should be taken by the nurse in this situation?
    a. Notify the physician.
    b. Apply an occlusive dressing on the site.
    c. Assess the patient for signs of respiratory distress.
    d. Put on gloves and insert the chest tube in a bottle of sterile saline.

14. An emergency department nurse is using a manual resuscitation bag (Ambu bag) to assist ventilation in a patient with lung cancer who has stopped breathing on his own. What is an appropriate step in this procedure?
    a. Tilt the patient's head forward.
    b. Hold the mask tightly over the patient's nose and mouth.
    c. Pull the patient's jaw backward.
    d. Compress the bag twice the normal respiratory rate for the patient.

15. Which assessments and interventions should the nurse consider when performing tracheal suctioning? Select all that apply.
    a. Closely assess the patient before, during, and after the procedure.
    b. Hyperoxygenate the patient before and after suctioning.
    c. Limit the application of suction to 20 to 30 seconds.

d. Monitor the patient's pulse frequently to detect potential effects of hypoxia and stimulation of the vagus nerve.

e. Use an appropriate suction pressure (80–150 mm Hg).

f. Insert the suction catheter no further than 1 cm past the length of the tracheal or endotracheal tube.

ANSWERS WITH RATIONALES

1. *a, c, e, f.* If a problem exists in ventilation, respiration, or perfusion, hypoxia may occur. Hypoxia is a condition in which an inadequate amount of oxygen is available to cells. The most common symptoms of hypoxia are dyspnea (difficulty breathing), an elevated blood pressure with a small pulse pressure, increased respiratory and pulse rates, pallor, and cyanosis.

2. *d.* When epistaxis is noted with continued suctioning, the nurse should notify the physician and anticipate the need for a nasal trumpet. The nasal trumpet will protect the nasal mucosa from further trauma related to suctioning.

3. *a.* When a patient vomits upon insertion of an oropharyngeal airway, the nurse should immediately position the patient on his or her side to prevent aspiration, remove the oral airway, and suction the mouth if needed.

4. *b.* The nurse would base the size of the suctioning catheter on the size of the endotracheal tube. The external diameter of the suction catheter should not exceed half of the internal diameter of the endotracheal tube. Larger catheters can contribute to trauma and hypoxemia.

5. *b, c, d.* Spirometers are used to monitor the health status of patients with respiratory disorders, such as asthma. Pulse oximetry is used to obtain baseline information about the patient's oxygen saturation level and is also performed for patients with asthma, along with PEFR to monitor airflow. These three tests may be administered by the nurse. Diffusion capacity estimates the patient's ability to absorb alveolar gases and determines if a gas exchange problem exists. Maximal respiratory pressures help evaluate neuromuscular causes of respiratory dysfunction. Both tests are usually performed by a respiratory therapist. The physician or other advanced practice professional can perform a thoracentesis at the bedside with the nurse assisting, or in the radiology department.

6. *c.* Fatigue related to an impaired oxygen transport system is an example of a nursing diagnosis with alteration in oxygenation as the etiology or cause of other problems. Ineffective Airway Clearance, Decreased Cardiac Output and Impaired Gas Exchange are examples of nursing diagnoses indicating alterations in oxygenation as the problem.

7. *b, d, e.* When caring for patients with COPD, it is important to create an environment that is likely to reduce anxiety and ensure that they eat a high-protein/high-calorie diet. People with dyspnea and orthopnea are most comfortable in a high Fowler's position because accessory muscles can easily be used to promote respiration. Patients with COPD should pace physical activities and schedule frequent rest periods to conserve energy. Meals should be eaten 1 to 2 hours after breathing treatments and exercises, and drinking 2 to 3 quarts (1.9–2.9 L) of clear fluids daily is recommended.

8. *b.* For postural drainage, the nurse should place the patient lying on the left side with a pillow under the chest wall to drain the right lobe of the lung, use high Fowler's position to drain the apical sections of the upper lobes of the lungs, place the patient in a lying position, half on the abdomen and half on the side, right and left, to drain the posterior sections of the upper lobes of the lungs, and place the patient in the Trendelenburg position to drain the lower lobes of the lungs.

9. *d, e, f.* Common mistakes that patients make when using MDIs include failing to shake the canister, holding the inhaler upside down, inhaling through the nose rather than the mouth, inhaling too rapidly, stopping the inhalation when the cold propellant is felt in the throat, failing to hold their breath after inhalation, and inhaling two sprays with one breath.

10. *b.* A rate higher than 3 L/min may destroy the hypoxic drive that stimulates respirations in the medulla in a patient with chronic lung disease. Oxygen delivered at low rates does not necessarily have to be humidified, and arterial blood gases are not required at regular intervals to determine the flow rate.

11. *c.* The tube depth should be maintained at the same level unless otherwise ordered by the physician. If the depth changes, the nurse should remove the tape, adjust the tube to ordered depth, and reapply the tape.

12. *a.* The cylinder must always be checked before use to ensure that enough oxygen is available for the patient. It is unsafe to use a cylinder that reads 500 psi or less because not enough oxygen remains for a patient transfer. A cylinder that is not secured properly may result in injury to the patient. Oxygen flow is discontinued by turning the valve clockwise until it is tight.

13. *d.* When a chest tube becomes separated from the drainage device, the nurse should first put on gloves, open a sterile bottle of normal saline or water, and insert the chest tube into the bottle without contaminating the chest tube. This creates a water seal until a new drainage unit can be attached. Then the nurse should assess vital signs and notify the physician.

14. *b.* With the patient's head tilted back, jaw pulled forward, and airway cleared, the mask is held tightly over the patient's nose and mouth. The bag also fits easily over tracheostomy and endotracheal tubes. The operator's other hand compresses the bag at a rate that approximates normal respiratory rate (e.g., 16–20 breaths/min in adults).

15. *a, b, d, e.* Close assessment of the patient before, during, and after the procedure is necessary to limit negative effects. Risks include hypoxia, infection, tracheal tissue damage, dysrhythmias, and atelectasis. The nurse should hyperoxygenate the patient before and after suctioning and limit the application of suction to 10 to 20 seconds. The nurse should also take the patient's pulse frequently to detect potential effects of hypoxia and stimulation of the vagus nerve. Using an appropriate suction pressure (80–150 mm Hg) will help prevent atelectasis related to the use of high negative pressure. Research suggests that insertion of the suction catheter should be limited to a predetermined length (no further than 1 cm past the length of the tracheal or endotracheal tube) to avoid tracheal mucosal damage, including epithelial denudement, loss of cilia, edema, and fibrosis (Roman, 2005).

TAYLOR SUITE RESOURCES

Explore these additional resources to enhance learning for this chapter:

• NCLEX-Style Questions and other resources on thePoint, http://thePoint.lww.com/Taylor8e

• *Study Guide for Fundamentals of Nursing, 8th edition*
• Adaptive Learning | Powered by prepU, http://thepoint.lww.com/prepu
• *Skill Checklists for Fundamentals of Nursing, 8th edition*
• *Taylor's Clinical Nursing Skills:* Chapter 14, Oxygenation
• *Taylor's Video Guide to Clinical Nursing Skills:* Oxygenation
• *Lippincott DocuCare* Fundamentals cases

Bibliography

Ackley, B. J., & Ladwig, G. B. (2011). *Nursing Diagnosis Handbook* (9th ed.). St. Louis: Elsevier/Mosby.

ACLS review made incredibly easy (2nd ed.). (2012). Philadelphia: Wolters Kluwer Health/Lippincott Williams & Wilkins.

American Association for Respiratory Care (AARC) Clinical Practice Guideline. (2004). Nasotracheal suctioning—2004 revision & update. *Respiratory Care, 49*(9), 1080–1084.

American Association for Respiratory Care (AARC) Clinical Practice Guideline. (1999). Suctioning of the patient in the home. *Respiratory Care, 44*(1), 99–104.

American Heart Association (AHA). (2011). *BLS for healthcare providers. Student manual. Professional.* Dallas: Author.

American Heart Association (AHA). (2012). *CPR & ECC. Two steps to staying alive with Hands-only CPR.* Available at http://www.heart.org/HEARTORG/CPRAndECC/HandsOnlyCPR/Hands-Only-CPR_UCM_440559_SubHomePage.jsp

Arroyo-Novoa, C., Figueroa-Ramos, M., Puntillo, K., Stanik-Hutt, J., Thompson, C. L., White, C., & Rietman Wild, L. (2008). Pain related to tracheal suctioning in awake acutely and critically ill adults: A descriptive study. *Intensive & Critical Care Nursing, 24*(1), 20–27.

Austin, M.A., Blizzard, L., Walters, E.H., Wood-Baker, R. (2010). Effect of high flow oxygen on mortality in chronic obstructive pulmonary disease patients in prehospital setting: Randomised controlled trial. *British Medical Journal,* (Overseas & Retired Doctors Edition), 341c5462. doi:10.1136/bmj.c5462.

Barrons, R., Pegram, A., & Borries, A. (2011). Inhaler device selection: Special considerations in elderly patients with chronic obstructive pulmonary disease. *American Journal of Health-System Pharmacy, 68*(13), 1221–1232.

Boltz, M., Capezuti, E., Fulmer, T., & Zwicker, D. (Eds.) (2012). *Evidence-based geriatric nursing protocols for best practice* (4th ed.). New York: Springer Publishing Company.

Bulechek, G. M., Butcher, H. K., Dochterman, J. M., & Wagner, C. M. (Eds.). (2013). *Nursing interventions classification (NIC)* (6th ed.). St. Louis: Elsevier/Mosby.

Cardiovascular care made incredibly visual (2nd ed.). (2010). Philadelphia: Wolters Kluwer Health/Lippincott Williams & Wilkins.

Centers for Disease Control and Prevention (CDC). (2012). Seasonal influenza (flu). Available at http://www.cdc.gov/flu/index.htm

Centers for Disease Control and Prevention (CDC). (2011a). Healthy weight- it's not a diet, it's a lifestyle! Physical activity for a healthy weight. Available at http://www.cdc.gov/healthyweight/physical_activity/

Centers for Disease Control and Prevention (CDC). (2011b). Vaccines and preventable diseases: Pneumococcal vaccination. Available at http://www.cdc.gov/vaccines/vpd-vac/pneumo/default.htm#disease

Centers for Disease Control and Prevention (CDC). (2010). Smoking and tobacco use. Health effects: Heart disease and stroke. Available at http://www.cdc.gov/tobacco/basic_information/health_effects/heart_disease/index.htm

Centers for Disease Control and Prevention (CDC). (2009). Heart disease. Prevention: What you can do. Available at http://www.cdc.gov/heartdisease/what_you_can_do.htm

Chaney, S. E., & Sheriff, S. (2012). Evidence-based treatments for smoking cessation. *The Nurse Practitioner, 37*(4), 24–31.

Christopher, K. L., & Schwartz, M. D. (2011). Transtracheal oxygen therapy. *Chest, 139*(2), 435–440.

Collins, C., & Anderson, C. (2007). Deceptive simplicity: systemic oxygen delivery and pulse oximetry. *Journal of Paediatrics & Child Health, 43,* 510–512.

Corbridge, S., Wilken, L., Kapella, M. C., & Gronkiewicz, C. (2012). An evidence-based approach to COPD: Part 1. *American Journal of Nursing, 112*(3), 46–59.

Crawford, J., & Doherty, L. (2010). Ten steps to recording a standard 12-lead ECG. *Practice Nurse, 21*(12), 622–630.

Crisafulli, E., Costi, S., DeBlasio, F., Biscione, G., Americi, F., Penza, S., et al. (2007). Effects of a walking aid in COPD patients receiving oxygen therapy. *CHEST, 131*(4), 1068–1074.

Day, M. W. (2011). On alert for iatrogenic pneumothorax. *Nursing, 41*(6), 66–67.

Davis, M., & Johnston, J. (2008). Maintaining supplemental oxygen during transport. *American Journal of Nursing, 108*(1), 35–36.

DeMeulenaere, S. (2007). Pulse oximetry: uses and limitations. *The Journal of Nurse Practitioners, 3*(5), 312–317.

Dirkes, S., Dickinson, S., Havey, R., & O'Brien, D. (2012). Prone Positioning. Is it safe and effective? *Critical Care Nursing Quarterly, 35*(1), 64–75.

Dudek, S. (2014). *Nutrition essentials for nursing practice* (7th ed.). Philadelphia: Wolters Kluwer Health/Lippincott Williams & Wilkins.

Eastwood, G., Gardner, A., & O'Connell, B. (2007). Low-flow oxygen therapy: Selecting the right device. *Australian Nursing Journal, 15*(4), 27–30.

Ertuğ, N., & Ülker, S. (2011). The effect of cold application on pain due to chest tube removal. *Journal of Clinical Nursing, 21*(5/6), 784–790.

Fernandez, M., Burns, K., Calhoun, B., George, S., Martin, B., & Weaver, C. (2007). Evaluation of a new pulse oximeter sensor. *American Journal of Critical Care, 16*(2), 146–152.

Field, J. M., Hazinski, M. F., Sayre, M. R., Chameides, L., Schexnayder, S. M., Hemphill, R., Samson, R. A., et al. (2010). 2010 American Heart Association Guidelines for cardiopulmonary resuscitation and emergency cardiovascular care. Part 1: Executive summary. *Circulation, 122*(supp 3), S640–S656.

Freeman, S. (2011). Care of adult patients with a temporary tracheostomy. *Nursing Standard, 26*(2), 49–56.

Grossbach, I., Stranberg, S., & Chlan, L. (2011). Promoting effective communication for patients receiving mechanical ventilation. *CriticalCareNurse, 31*(3), 46–61.

Grossman, S., & Porth, C.M. (2014). Porth's pathophysiology: concepts of altered health states. (9th ed.). Philadelphia: Wolters Kluwer Health/Lippincott Williams & Wilkins.

Hahn, M. (2010). 10 considerations for endotracheal suctioning. *The Journal for Respiratory Care Practitioners, 23*(7), 32–33.

Hess, D. R., MacIntyre, N. R., Mishoe, S. C., Galvin, W. F., & Adams, A. B. (2012). *Respiratory care: Principles and practice* (2nd ed.). Sudbury, MA: Jones & Bartlett Learning.

Higginson, R., Jones, B, & Davies, K. (2010). Airway management for nurses: Emergency assessment and care. *British Journal of Nursing, 19*(16), 1006–1014.

Hinkle, J. L., & Cheever, K. H. (2014). *Brunner & Suddarth's textbook of medical–surgical nursing* (13th ed.). Philadelphia: Wolters Kluwer Health/Lippincott Williams & Wilkins.

Hogan-Quigley, B., Palm, M. L., & Bickley, L. (2012). *Bates' nursing guide to physical examina-*

tion and history taking. Philadelphia: Wolters Kluwer Health/Lippincott Williams & Wilkins.

Huether, S. E., & McCance, K. L. (2012.) *Understanding pathophysiology* (5th ed.). St. Louis: Elsevier.

Ireton, J. (2007). Tracheostomy suction: a protocol for practice. *Paediatric Nursing, 19*(10), 14–18.

Jarvis, C. (2012). *Physical examination & health assessment* (6th ed.). St. Louis: Elsevier/Saunders.

Jensen, S. (2011). *Nursing health assessment: A best practice approach.* Philadelphia: Wolters Kluwer Health/Lippincott Williams & Wilkins.

Jevon, P. (2010). Procedure for recording a standard 12-lead electrocardiogram. *British Journal of Nursing, 19*(10), 649–651.

Johnson, A., Schweitzer, D., & Ahrens, T. (2011). Time to throw away your stethoscope? Capnography: Evidence-based patient monitoring technology. *Journal of Radiological Nursing, 30*(1), 25–34.

Johnson, C. L., Anderson, M. A., & Hill, P. D. (2012). Comparison of pulse oximetry measures in a healthy population. *MEDSURGNursing, 21*(2), 70–76.

Jongerden, I., Rovers, M., Grypdonck, M., & Bonten, M. J. (2007). Open and closed endotracheal suction systems in mechanically ventilated intensive care patients: A meta-analysis. *Critical Care Medicine, 35*(1), 260–270.

Kee, J. L., Hayes, E. R., McCuistion, L. E. (2012). *Pharmacology: A nursing process approach* (7th ed.). St. Louis: Elsevier/Saunders.

Kyle, T., & Carman, S. (2013). *Essentials of pediatric nursing* (2nd ed.). Philadelphia: Wolters Kluwer Health/Lippincott Williams & Wilkins.

Lamar, J. (2012). Relationship of respiratory care bundle with incentive spirometry to reduced pulmonary complications in a medical general practice unit. *MEDSURGNursing, 21*(1), 33–36.

Lynes, D. (2010). Diagnosis and management of patients with COPD in primary care. *Nursing Standard, 25*(8), 49–57.

Macnee, W. (2007). Pathogenesis of chronic obstructive pulmonary disease. *Clinics in Chest Medicine, 28*(3), 479–513.

Malarkey, L. M., & McMorrow, M. E. (2012). *Saunders nursing guide to laboratory and diagnostic tests* (2nd ed.). St. Louis: Elsevier/Saunders.

Maliakal, M. (2011). Chest tubes. *Nursing, 41*(7), 33.

Massey, D. (2010). Respiratory assessment 1: Why do it and how to do it? *British Journal of Cardiac Nursing, 6*(11), 537–541.

Mayo Foundation for Medical Education and Research (MFMER). (2011). CPAP machines: Tips for avoiding 10 common problems. Available at http://www.mayoclinic.com/health/cpap/SL00017

McCool, F., & Rosen, M. (2006). Nonpharmacologic airway clearance therapies: ACCP evidence-based clinical practice guidelines. *Chest, 129*(1): Supplement, 250S–259S.

McGloin, S. (2008). Administration of oxygen therapy. *Nursing Standard, 22*(21), 46–48.

Meredith, T., & Massey, D. (2011). Respiratory assessment 2: More key skills to improve care. *British Journal of Cardiac Nursing, 6*(2), 63–68.

Moorhead, S., Johnson, M., Maas, M. L., & Swanson, E. (Eds.). (2013). *Nursing Outcomes Classification (NOC)* (5th ed.). St. Louis: Elsevier/Mosby.

Morton, P. G., & Fontaine, D. K. (2013). *Essentials of critical care nursing: A holistic approach.* Philadelphia: Wolters Kluwer Health/Lippincott Williams & Wilkins.

NANDA International (NANDA-I). (2012). *Nursing diagnoses: Definitions & classification 2012–2014.* West Sussex, UK: Wiley-Blackwell.

National Heart Lung and Blood Institute (NHLBI). (2012a). How is obesity hypoventilation syndrome treated? Available at http://www.nhlbi.nih.gov/health/health-topics/topics/ohs/treatment.html

National Heart Lung and Blood Institute (NHLBI). (2012b). Who is at risk for COPD? Available at http://www.nhlbi.nih.gov/health/health-topics/topics/copd/atrisk.html

National Heart Lung and Blood Institute (NHLBI). (2011). What is CPAP? Available at http://www.nhlbi.nih.gov/health/health-topics/topics/cpap/

Osadnik, C. R., McDonald, C. F., Jones, A. P., & Holland, A. E. (2012). Airway clearance techniques for chronic obstructive pulmonary disease. *Cochrane Database of Systematic Reviews,* Issue 3. Art. No.: CD008328. DOI: 10.1002/14651858.CD008328.pub2.

Parkes, R. (2011). Rate of respiration: The forgotten vital sign. *Emergency Nurse, 19*(2), 12–17.

Pate, M. (2004). Placement of endotracheal and tracheostomy tubes. *Critical Care Nurse, 24*(3), 13–14.

Pate, M., & Zapata, T. (2002). Ask the experts: How deeply should I go when I suction an endotracheal or tracheostomy tube? *Critical Care Nurse, 22*(2), 130–131.

Perry, S. E., Hockenberry, M. J., Lowdermilk, D. L., & Wilson, D. (2010). *Maternal child nursing care* (4th ed.). Maryland Heights, MO: Elsevier/Mosby.

Pruitt, B. (2007a). Latest advances in respiratory care. *Nursing, 37*(7), 56cc1, 56cc3.

Pruitt, B. (2007b). Take an evidence-based approach to treating acute lung injury. *Nursing, 37*(Supplement), 14–18.

Pullen, R. L. (2010). Using pulse oximetry accurately. *Nursing: Journal of Clinical Excellence, 40*(4), 63.

Rickelmann, C. (2012). EB 109 Standardized approach to safe, effective prone positioning in the surgical intensive care unit. *Critical Care Nurse, 32*(2), e62–e63.

Ritter, L. A., & Hoffman, N. A. (2010). *Multicultural health.* Boston: Jones and Bartlett.

Roman, M. (2005). Tracheostomy tubes. *MEDSURGNursing, 14*(2), 143–144.

Rubin, B. K. (2010). Air and soul: The science and application of aerosol therapy. *Respiratory Care, 55*(7), 911–921.

Rushing, J. (2007). Clinical do's and don'ts: Managing a water-seal chest drainage unit. *Nursing, 37*(12), 12.

The Society for Cardiological Science & Technology (SCST). (2010). Clinical guidelines by consensus: Recording a standard 12-lead electrocardiogram. Available at http://www.scst.org.uk/resources/consensus_guideline_for_recording_a_12_lead_ecg_Rev_072010b.pdf

Sole, M. L., Penoyer, D. A., Bennett, M., Bertrand, J., & Talbert, S. (2011). Oropharyngeal secretion volume in intubated patients: The importance of oral suctioning. *American Journal of Critical Care, 20*(6), e141–e145.

Spector, R. E. (2009). *Cultural diversity in health and illness* (7th ed.). Upper Saddle River, NJ: Pearson/Prentice Hall.

Stoller, J. K. (2011). An overview of home oxygen delivery devices and prescribing practices. *Canadian Journal of Respiratory Therapy, 47*(4), 22–27.

Subirana, M., Solà, I., & Benito, S. (2007). Closed tracheal suction systems versus open tracheal suction systems for mechanically ventilated adult patients. *Cochrane Database of Systematic Reviews, Issue 4.* Art. No.: CD004581.DOI: 10.1002/14651858.CD004581.pub2.

Sultan, P., Carvalho, B., Rose, B. O., & Cregg, R. (2011). Endotracheal tube cuff pressure monitoring: A review of the evidence. *Journal of Perioperative Practice, 21*(11), 379–386.

Tabloski, P. (2010). *Gerontological nursing* (2nd ed.). Upper Saddle River, NJ: Pearson.

Taylor, J. J., & Cohen, B. J. (2013). *Memmler's structure and function of the human body* (10th ed.). Philadelphia: Wolters Kluwer Health/Lippincott Williams & Wilkins.

U.S. Department of Agriculture. Center for Nutrition Policy and Promotion. (2012). *Dietary Guidelines for Americans.* Available at http://www.cnpp.usda.gov/DietaryGuidelines.htm

Van Leeuwen, A. M., Poelhuis-Leth, D., & Bladh, M. L. (2011). *Davis's Comprehensive Handbook of Laboratory & Diagnostic Tests with Nursing Implications* (4th ed.). Philadelphia: F. A. Davis.

Vates, S. (2011). Delivering oxygen therapy in acute care: Part 2. *Nursing Times, 107*(22), 21–23.

VISN 8 Patient Safety Center. (2009). *Safe patient handling and movement algorithms.* Tampa, FL: Author. Available http://www.visn8.va.gov/visn8/patientsafetycenter/safePtHandling/default.asp.

39

Fluid, Electrolyte, and Acid-Base Balance

GRACE GILLIGAN

Grace, a 28-year-old woman, arrives at the emergency department with complaints of severe episodes of nausea and vomiting over the last 48 hours. She has a past medical history of Crohn's disease, a gastrointestinal (GI) problem for which she underwent bowel resection surgery 1 month ago. "I thought the surgery would help my problems," she says. IV therapy was ordered to restore her fluid balance.

JEREMIAH STEIN

Jeremiah, a 22-year-old student, comes to the campus health center because he has been having two or three loose, watery bowel movements a day for the past week. "I kept thinking I would get better. I didn't have time to come to the clinic because of exams and I have been so busy, but now I don't feel good and I'm weak." Fluid volume deficit and electrolyte imbalances are a concern.

JACK SOO PARK

Jack, a 78-year-old man receiving intravenous (IV) therapy with antibiotics, states, "I'm having trouble breathing. It just started a little while ago." Physical examination reveals a bounding pulse, distended neck veins, and crackles and wheezes in the lungs. Excess fluid volume is suspected. Further checking reveals an IV fluid-administration error that has resulted in overhydration.

LEARNING OBJECTIVES

After completing the chapter, you will be able to accomplish the following:

1. Describe the location and functions of body fluids, including the factors that affect variations in fluid compartments.

2. Describe the functions, regulation, sources, and losses of the main electrolytes of the body.

3. Explain the principles of osmosis, diffusion, active transport, and filtration.

4. Describe how thirst and the organs of homeostasis (kidneys, heart and blood vessels, lungs, adrenal glands, pituitary gland, parathyroid glands) function to maintain fluid homeostasis.

5. Describe the role of buffer systems and respiratory and renal mechanisms in achieving and maintaining acid–base balance.

6. Identify the etiologies and defining characteristics for common fluid, electrolyte, and acid–base imbalances.

7. Perform a fluid, electrolyte, and acid–base balance assessment.

8. Describe the role of dietary modification, modification of fluid intake, medication administration, IV therapy, blood replacement, and parenteral nutrition (TPN) in resolving fluid, electrolyte, and acid–base imbalances.

9. Assess, plan, implement, and evaluate nursing care related to select nursing diagnoses involving fluid, electrolyte, and acid–base imbalances.

KEY TERMS

acid	cation	hypermagne-semia
acidosis	colloid osmotic pressure	
active transport		hypernatremia
	cross-matching	hyperphospha-temia
agglutinin	dehydration	hypertonic
alkalosis	diffusion	hypervolemia
anions	edema	hypocalcemia
antibody	electrolytes	hypochloremia
antigen	Extracellular fluid (ECF)	hypokalemia
autologous transfusion		hypomagnese-mia
base	hydrostatic pressure	
blood typing	hypercalcemia	hyponatremia
buffer	hyperchloremia	hypophospha-temia
capillary filtration	hyperkalemia	hypotonic

hypovolemia	isotonic	pH
intracellular fluid (ICF)	osmolarity	solutes
	osmosis	solvents
ion		

This chapter discusses the principles of fluid, electrolyte, and acid–base balance and common disturbances. Sample interview questions for performing a fluid-balance assessment are included, with information on specific physical assessment techniques and laboratory studies. Numerous examples of nursing diagnoses are provided and expected outcomes and specific nursing interventions to promote fluid and electrolyte balance are described. Appropriate nursing interventions include ongoing assessments, modifying dietary and fluid intake, administering medications, assisting with IV therapy, and blood replacement. The concluding plan of care illustrates how nurses combine their knowledge of fluid, electrolyte, and acid–base balance with skilled nursing assessments and interventions to resolve alterations in health status and to improve patient outcomes (Refer to the accompanying Reflective Practice box on page 1472).

PRINCIPLES OF FLUID, ELECTROLYTES, AND ACID–BASE BALANCE

Fluids and electrolytes are vital to life; adequate balance is imperative to maintain healthy functioning of the body. Fluids and electrolytes are involved in almost every cellular reaction and function. Chemical reactions that occur in the body depend on a careful acid and base balance.

Body Fluids

The primary body fluid is water, making it the most important nutrient of life. Although life can be sustained for many days without food, humans can survive for only a few days without water. Water in the body functions primarily to:

- Transport nutrients to cells and wastes from cells
- Transport hormones, enzymes, blood platelets, and red and white blood cells
- Facilitate cellular metabolism and proper cellular chemical functioning
- Act as a solvent for electrolytes and nonelectrolytes
- Help maintain normal body temperature
- Facilitate digestion and promote elimination
- Act as a tissue lubricant

The term *total body water* or *fluid* refers to the total amount of water, which is approximately 50% to 60% of body weight in a healthy person.

Body Fluid Compartments

Body fluid is located in two fluid compartments—the intracellular fluid or extracellular fluid, based on its location in the body. **Intracellular fluid (ICF)** is the fluid within cells,

REFLECTIVE PRACTICE

CHALLENGE TO INTERPERSONAL SKILLS

During my clinical rotation in the emergency department, I met Grace Gilligan. She was a 28-year-old woman who came to the emergency department with complaints of severe episodes of nausea and vomiting over the last 48 hours. She has a past medical history of Crohn's disease, a gastrointestinal (GI) problem for which she underwent bowel resection surgery 1 month ago. "I thought the surgery would help my problems." The patient was dehydrated and needed IV fluid therapy.

My co-assigned nurse attempted to start a peripheral venous access not once, but six times. The patient was already upset by her recurrent abdominal symptoms, but now had to deal with the continuous painful stick of a needle. During the course of attempts to start the IV, the patient stated that a nurse on the IV team always had to be called to insert her IVs. Although my nurse acknowledged the information, she continued trying to start the IV. Finally, on the sixth try, as the patient was in tears, the nurse was successful. It seemed as if the nurse was out to prove her abilities without caring for the patient. By the end, I had difficulty even watching.

Thinking Outside the Box: Possible Courses of Action

- While assisting the nurse to obtain more supplies (outside the patient's room), mention to the nurse that maybe the IV team should be called, since "enough is enough!"
- Tell my clinical instructor that the patient is being abused.
- Ask the doctor if he or she could address the situation.
- Tell the patient when the nurse was out of the room to refuse any more sticks until the IV team was called.

Evaluating a Good Outcome: How Do I Define Success?

- Patient is benefited by my actions....or at least not harmed.
- All actions are supported by rationale.
- The patient's wishes are respected.
- Personal integrity is not compromised.

Personal Learning: Here's to the Future!

Unfortunately, I did not take any actions to protect this patient. This was my first time in the emergency department as well as my first introduction to the nurse. I was intimidated by her. Furthermore, I was scared when she continued to attempt the catheter insertion with the patient in tears. I know that it is my responsibility to advocate for the needs of my patients. In the future, I hope that I will never compromise my integrity, beliefs, and values to prove something to a student. If I fail or am not confident in my skills, I will admit this and stop before my patient is put at risk.

Amy Persinger, Georgetown University

REFLECTION ON QUALITY AND SAFETY COMPETENCIES

How do you think you would respond in a similar situation? What does this tell you about yourself and about the adequacy of your skills for professional practice? Why? Do you agree with the criteria that the nursing student used to evaluate a successful outcome? Are there any other criteria that would be appropriate to use? Did the nursing student meet the criteria? Why or why not? What *knowledge, skills,* and *attitudes* do you need to develop to continuously improve the quality and safety of care for patients like Ms. Gillian?

Patient-Centered Care: How could you involve Ms. Gillian as a partner in coordinating her care to minimize frustration on the part of the patient, student, and nurse? What might have prompted the emergency department nurse to act as she did? The nursing student? How could the nursing student have advocated for the patient? What other barriers (other than those listed) might have interfered with the nursing student acting as an advocate?

Teamwork and Collaboration/Quality Improvement: What communication skills do you need to improve to ensure that you function as a member of the patient-care team? What skills do you need to implement effective strategies for communicating and resolving conflict? What skills do you need to assert your own position/perspective in discussions about patient care?

Safety/Evidence-based Practice: What evidence in nursing literature provides guidance for decision making regarding professional practice and venipuncture?

Informatics: Can you identify the essential information that must be available in Ms. Gillian's electronic record to support safe patient care and coordination of care? Can you think of other ways to respond to or approach the situation?

---

constituting about 70% of the total body water or 40% of the adult's body weight. **Extracellular fluid (ECF)** is all the fluid outside the cells, accounting for about 30% of the total body water or 20% of the adult's body weight. ECF includes two major areas, the intravascular and interstitial compartments. A third, usually minor, compartment is the transcellular fluid.

Intravascular fluid, or plasma, is the liquid component of the blood (i.e., fluid found within the vascular system). Interstitial fluid is the fluid that surrounds tissue cells and includes lymph (Hinkle & Cheever, 2014). Transcellular fluids include cerebrospinal, pericardial, synovial, intraocular, and pleural fluids, as well as sweat and digestive secretions. The capillary

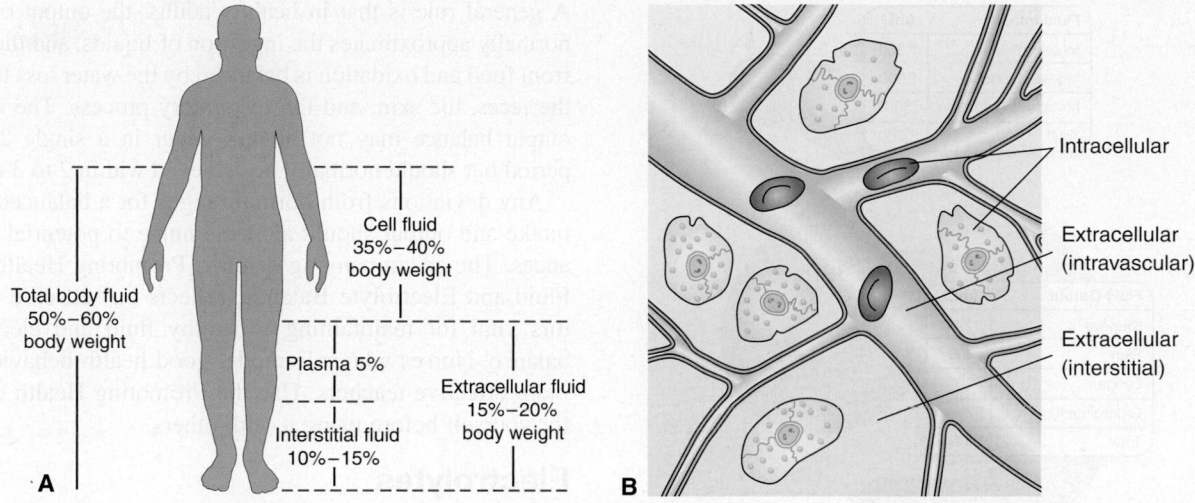

FIGURE 39-1. (**A**) Total body fluid represents 50% to 60% of body weight of a normal adult. (**B**) Primary fluid compartments.

walls and cell membranes separate the intracellular and extracellular compartments. Figure 39-1 illustrates the components of total body fluid and the primary fluid compartments.

Variations in Fluid Content

Variations in the fluid content from the normal 50% to 60% of the body's weight can occur, depending on such factors as the person's age, body fat, and gender. Table 39-1 illustrates age-related differences in total body water and in the various water compartments of the body. Infants have considerably more total body fluid and ECF than adults. Because ECF is more easily lost from the body than ICF, infants are more prone to fluid volume deficits.

Total body water also differs by gender and the amount of fat cells in the body. Fat cells contain little water, whereas lean tissue is rich in water. Thus, the more obese a person is, the smaller the person's percentage of total body water is when compared with body weight. Because women tend to have proportionally more body fat than men do, they also have less body fluid than men. Similarly, the decreasing percentage of body fluid in older people is related to an increase in fat cells. In addition, older adults lose muscle mass as a part of aging. The combined increase of fat and loss of muscle results in reduced total body water; after the age of 60, total body water is about 45% of a person's body weight. This decrease in water increases the risk for fluid imbalance in older adults.

Fluid Balance

The human body obtains water from several sources, including ingested liquids, food, and as a byproduct of metabolism. The ingestion of liquids provides the largest amount of water normally taken into the body. Fluid intake is regulated primarily by the thirst mechanism. Located within the hypothalamus, the thirst control center is stimulated by intracellular **dehydration** (the loss of or deprivation of water from the body or tissues) and decreased blood volume. The water contained in food is the second largest source of water for the body. The amount of water ingested depends on the diet. For example, melons and citrus fruit are high in water content, whereas cereal and dried fruits have relatively low water content. Water is an end product of the oxidation that occurs during the metabolism of food substances, specifically carbohydrates, fats, and protein. This amount of water obtained varies among the different types of nutrients. Generally, fluid intake averages 2,600 mL per day, with approximately 1,300 mL coming from ingested water, 1,000 mL coming from ingested food, and 300 mL from metabolic oxidation. Figure 39-2 illustrates daily fluid balance in a healthy person.

Fluid is lost from the body through *sensible* and *insensible* losses. Sensible losses can be measured and include fluid lost during urination, defecation, and wounds. Insensible losses cannot be measured or seen and include fluid lost from evaporation through the skin and as water vapor from the lungs during respiration. Water losses vary according to the person and

Table 39-1   WATER AS A PERCENTAGE OF BODY WEIGHT

WATER COMPARTMENT	INFANT	ADULT		ELDERLY PERSON
		Man	*Woman*	
Extracellular				
Intravascular	4	4	5	5
Interstitial	25	11	10	15
Intracellular	48	45	35	25
Total body water	77	60	50	45

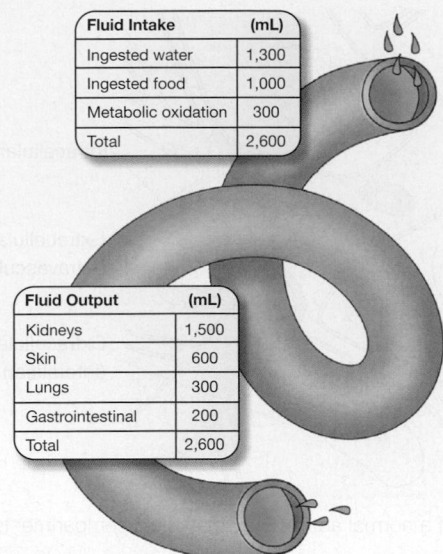

Fluid Intake	(mL)
Ingested water	1,300
Ingested food	1,000
Metabolic oxidation	300
Total	2,600

Fluid Output	(mL)
Kidneys	1,500
Skin	600
Lungs	300
Gastrointestinal	200
Total	2,600

FIGURE 39-2. In health, fluid intake and fluid losses are about equal. The amounts indicated are average adult daily fluid sources and losses.

the circumstances. Fluid output averages 2,500 to 2,900 mL per day (average 2,600 mL), with approximately 1,500 mL as urine from the kidneys, 600 mL fluid loss from the skin, 300 mL from the lungs, and 200 mL in feces via the gastrointestinal tract (see Fig. 39-2).

The desirable amount of fluid intake and loss in adults ranges from 1,500 to 3,500 mL each 24 hours, with most people averaging 2,500 to 2,600 mL per day. Although these figures are helpful guidelines, the person's health state as well as balance between actual intake and loss must be considered when assessing nursing needs. A person's intake should normally be approximately balanced by output or fluid loss.

A general rule is that in healthy adults, the output of urine normally approximates the ingestion of liquids, and the water from food and oxidation is balanced by the water loss through the feces, the skin, and the respiratory process. The intake–output balance may not always occur in a single 24-hour period but should normally be achieved within 2 to 3 days.

Any deviations from normal ranges for a balanced water intake and output should alert the nurse to potential imbalances. The accompanying display, Promoting Health 39-1: Fluid and Electrolyte Balance, reflects on self-care behaviors vital for maintaining a healthy fluid and electrolyte balance. Nurses who role model good health behaviors are more effective teachers. Use the Promoting Health display for yourself before using it with others.

Electrolytes

Electrolytes are substances that are capable of breaking into particles called ions. An **ion** is an atom or molecule carrying an electrical charge. Some ions develop a positive charge and are called **cations**. The major cations in body fluid are sodium, potassium, calcium, hydrogen, and magnesium ions. Other ions develop a negative charge and are called **anions**. The major anions in body fluid are chloride, bicarbonate, and phosphate. These charged particles are the basis of chemical interactions in the body necessary for metabolism and other functions. Molecules in the body that remain intact, without a charge, are called nonelectrolytes. In the human body, urea and glucose are examples of nonelectrolytes.

The electrolyte content of the fluids in various compartments of the body differ significantly. Major electrolytes in the ECF include sodium, chloride, calcium, and bicarbonate. Major electrolytes in the ICF include potassium, phosphorus, and magnesium. The functions, sources, means of loss, and regulation of these electrolytes are highlighted in Table 39-2

PROMOTING HEALTH 39-1

FLUID AND ELECTROLYTE BALANCE

Use the assessment checklist to determine how well you are meeting your fluid and electrolyte needs. Then develop a prescription for self-care by choosing appropriate behaviors from the list of suggestions.

Assessment Checklist

❏ almost always	❏ sometimes	❏ almost never

❏ ❏ ❏ 1. I drink six to eight glasses of water every day.

❏ ❏ ❏ 2. I am aware of early signs of dehydration or fluid retention.

❏ ❏ ❏ 3. I limit sugar, alcohol, and caffeine in my diet.

❏ ❏ ❏ 4. I am alert for any sudden variations in my weight.

❏ ❏ ❏ 5. I am aware of fluid and electrolyte imbalances that may be associated with intake of certain medications.

❏ ❏ ❏ 6. I diet sensibly when I need to lose weight.

Self-Care Behaviors

1. Consume about 1½ quarts of water daily.

2. Maintain normal body weight.

3. Avoid consuming excess amounts of products high in salt, sugar, and caffeine.

4. Limit alcohol intake because of its diuretic effect.

5. Obtain medical evaluation for any ongoing indications of fluid imbalance.

6. Monitor side effects of medications, especially diuresis and diarrhea.

7. Identify situations of high risk for fluid and electrolyte imbalance and intervene appropriately.

Information to promote fluid and electrolyte balance is available online. Visit thePoint for a list of Internet resources.

Table 39-2 MAJOR ELECTROLYTES

ELECTROLYTE	FUNCTIONS	SOURCES AND LOSSES	REGULATION
Sodium (Na^+): chief electrolyte of ECF; the normal serum concentration of sodium: 135–145 mEq/L	Regulates extracellular fluid volume; Na+ loss or gain accompanied by a loss or gain of water Affects serum osmolality Role in muscle contraction and transmission of nerve impulses Regulation of acid–base balance as sodium bicarbonate	Normally enters the body through the gastrointestinal tract from dietary sources, such as salt added to processed foods, sodium preservatives added to processed foods Lost from gastrointestinal tract, kidneys, and skin	Transported out of the cell by the sodium-potassium pump Regulated by renin-angiotensin-aldosterone system Elimination and reabsorption regulated by the kidneys Sodium concentrations affected by salt and water intake
Potassium (K^+): major cation of ICF; the normal serum concentration of potassium: 3.5–5.0 mEq/L	Controls intracellular osmolality Regulator of cellular enzyme activity Role in the transmission of electrical impulses in nerve, heart, skeletal, intestinal, and lung tissue; protein and carbohydrate metabolism; and cellular building Regulation of acid–base balance by cellular exchange with H^+	Adequate quantities via a well-balanced diet Leading food sources: fruits and vegetables, dried peas and beans, whole grains, milk, meats Lost via kidneys, stool, sweat, emesis Gastrointestinal (GI) secretions contain potassium in large quantities, so can be lost through vomitus	Regulated by aldosterone Eliminated by the kidneys (no effective method of conserving potassium) Additional regulation via transcellular shift between the ICF and ECF compartments
Calcium (Ca^{2+}): most abundant electrolyte in the body; 99% of body calcium is stored in bone; 1% inside cells; 0.1% in ECF; normal total serum calcium level: 8.6–10.2 mg/dL; normal ionized serum calcium level: 4.5–5.1 mg/dL	Role in blood coagulation and in transmission of nerve impulses Helps regulate muscle contraction and relaxation Activates enzymes that stimulate essential chemical reactions in the body Major component of bones and teeth	Absorbed from foods in the presence of normal gastric acidity and vitamin D Lost via feces and urine Sources include milk, milk products, and cheese; dried beans; fortified orange juice; green, leafy vegetables; small fish with bones; and dried peas and beans	Primarily excreted by gastrointestinal tract; lesser extent by kidneys Regulated by parathyroid hormone and calcitonin High serum phosphate results in decreased serum calcium level; low serum phosphate leads to increased serum calcium
Magnesium (Mg^{2+}): second most abundant ICF cation after potassium; normal serum concentration of magnesium: 1.3–2.3 mEq/L	Metabolism of carbohydrates and proteins Activator for many intracellular enzyme systems Role in neuromuscular function Acts on cardiovascular system, producing vasodilation	Enters the body via gastrointestinal tract Magnesium found in green, leafy vegetables; nuts; seafood; whole grains; dried peas and beans; cocoa Lost via urine with use of loop diuretics	Eliminated by kidneys Regulated by parathyroid hormone
Chloride (Cl^-): major ECF anion; normal serum level of chloride: 97–107 mEq/L	Major component of interstitial and lymph fluid; gastric and pancreatic juices, sweat, bile, and saliva Acts with sodium to maintain the osmotic pressure Role in the body's acid–base balance; combines with hydrogen ions to produce hydrochloric acid	Enters body via gastrointestinal tract Almost all chloride in diet comes from salt Found in foods high in sodium, processed foods	Normally paired with sodium; excreted and conserved with sodium by the kidneys Regulated by aldosterone alongside sodium Low potassium level leads to low chloride level
Bicarbonate (HCO_3^-): an anion that is the major chemical base buffer within the body; found in both ECF and ICF; normal serum bicarbonate level: 25–29 mEq/L	Regulates acid–base balance	Losses possible via diarrhea, diuretics, and early renal insufficiency Excess possible via overingestion of acid neutralizers, such as sodium bicarbonate	Bicarbonate levels regulated primarily by the kidneys Bicarbonate readily available as a result of carbon dioxide formation during metabolism
Phosphate (PO_4^-): major ICF anion; a buffer anion in both ICF and ECF; normal serum phosphate level: 2.5–4.5 mg/dL	Role in acid–base balance as a hydrogen buffer Promotes energy storage; carbohydrate, protein, and fat metabolism Bone and teeth formation Regulation of hormone and coenzyme activity Role in muscle and red blood cell function	Enters body via gastrointestinal tract Sources include all animal products (meat, poultry, eggs, milk, bread, ready-to-eat cereal) Absorption is diminished by concurrent ingestion of calcium, magnesium, and aluminum	Eliminated by kidneys Regulation by parathyroid hormone and by activated vitamin D Phosphate and calcium are inversely proportional; an increase in one results in a decrease in the other

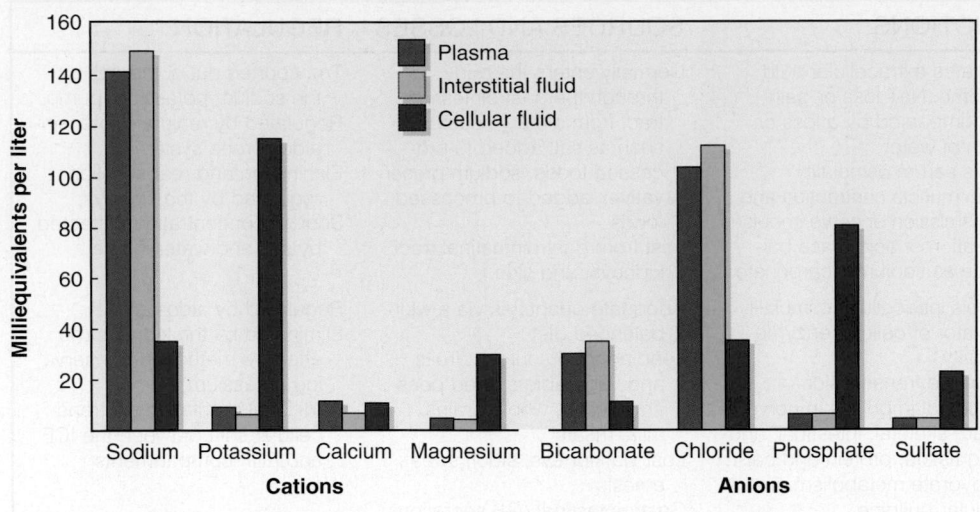

FIGURE 39-3. Electrolyte composition of body fluids according to compartment.

(hydrogen is discussed as part of acid–base balance). Figure 39-3 illustrates differences in the electrolyte composition of body fluids according to the compartments in which the fluids are found.

Electrolytes are measured in terms of their chemical combining power, or chemical activity. The milliequivalent (mEq) is the unit of measure that describes the chemical activity of electrolytes. One milliequivalent of either a cation or an anion is chemically equivalent to the activity of 1 mg of hydrogen. Therefore, 1 mEq of any cation is equivalent to 1 mEq of any anion. The total cations in the body are normally equal to the total anions, maintaining homeostasis (balanced state). In healthy people, the milliequivalents per liter for electrolytes in the body vary within a relatively narrow range. When electrolytes are not in balance, the person is at risk for alterations in health.

 CONSIDER Grace Gilligan, the young woman described in one of the beginning chapter scenarios. The nurse would need to be alert for electrolyte imbalances and possible acid–base imbalance due to the loss of gastric secretions from vomiting. ●

Regulation and Homeostatic Mechanisms of Fluid and Electrolyte Balance

Maintaining homeostasis of fluid volume and electrolytes is essential to healthy body functioning. Fluid and electrolyte homeostasis normally functions automatically and effectively.

Fluid and electrolyte balance is maintained by a number of mechanisms to facilitate fluid and electrolyte movement within the body. **Solvents** are liquids that hold a substance in solution; **solutes** are substances that are dissolved in a solution. Water is the primary solvent in the body. The solutes are electrolytes and nonelectrolytes. The body produces balance by shifting fluids and solutes between the ECF and the ICF. The mechanisms responsible for regulating this shift of fluids and transporting materials to and from intracellular compartments include organs and body systems, osmosis,

diffusion, active transport, and capillary filtration, and are described in the following sections.

Organs and Body Systems

Almost every organ and system in the body helps in some way to maintain fluid homeostasis. The specific functions of these organs and body systems related to the regulation of fluid and electrolyte balance are highlighted in Table 39-3.

Osmosis

Cell membranes are semipermeable, allowing some, but not all, solutes to pass through the cell membranes. The cell membrane is permeable to water or fluids. **Osmosis** is the major method of transporting body fluids. Water shifts and balance depend heavily on this route of transport (Fig. 39-4).

Through the process of osmosis, water (the solvent) passes from an area of lesser solute concentration and more water to an area of greater solute concentration and less water until

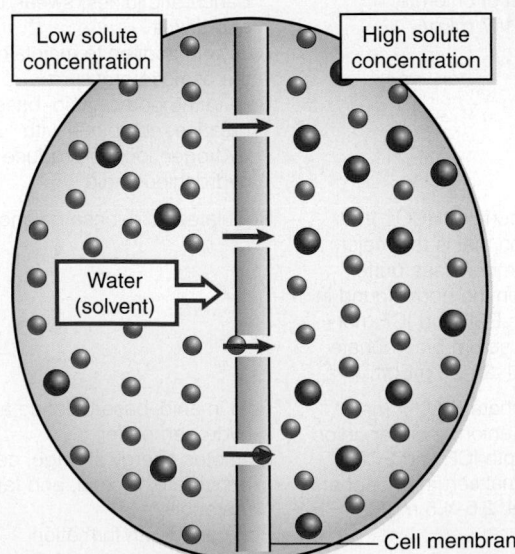

FIGURE 39-4. Osmosis. Body fluids are transported through cell membranes through the process of osmosis. Water, a solvent, moves from an area of lesser solute concentration to one of greater solute concentration, until equilibrium is established.

Table 39-3 ORGANS AND BODY SYSTEMS RELATED TO THE REGULATION OF FLUID AND ELECTROLYTE BALANCE

ORGAN/BODY SYSTEM	FUNCTIONS
Kidneys	• Regulate extracellular fluid (ECF) volume and osmolality by selective retention and excretion of body fluids • Regulate electrolyte levels in the ECF by selective retention of needed substances and excretion of unneeded substances • Regulate pH of ECF by excretion or retention of hydrogen ions • Excrete metabolic wastes (primarily acids) and toxic substances • Normally filter 180 L of plasma daily in the adult, while excreting only 1.5 L of urine
Heart and blood vessels	• Circulate nutrients and water throughout the body • Circulate blood through the kidneys under sufficient pressure for urine to form (pumping action of the heart) • React to hypovolemia by stimulating fluid retention (stretch receptors in the atria and blood vessels)

Lungs	• Remove approximately 300 mL of water daily through exhalation (insensible water loss) in the normal adult
	• Eliminate about 13,000 mEq of hydrogen ions (H^+) daily, as opposed to only 40 to 80 mEq excreted daily by the kidneys
	• Act promptly to correct metabolic acid–base disturbances; regulate H^+ concentration (pH) by controlling the level of carbon dioxide (CO_2) in the extracellular fluid as follows:
	  1. Metabolic alkalosis causes compensatory hypoventilation, resulting in CO_2 retention (increases acidity of the extracellular fluid).
	  2. Metabolic acidosis causes compensatory hyperventilation, resulting in CO_2 excretion (decreases acidity of the extracellular fluid).

Adrenal glands	• Regulate blood volume and sodium and potassium balance by secreting aldosterone, a mineral corticoid secreted by the adrenal cortex
	  1. The primary regulator of aldosterone appears to be angiotensin II, which is produced by the renin–angiotensin system. A decrease in blood volume triggers this system and increases aldosterone secretion, which causes sodium retention (and thus water retention) and potassium loss.
	  2. Decreased secretion of aldosterone causes sodium and water loss and potassium retention.
	• Cortisol, another adrenocortical hormone, has only a fraction of the potency of aldosterone.
	• However, secretion of cortisol in large quantities can produce sodium and water retention and potassium deficit.

Pituitary gland	• Stores and releases the antidiuretic hormone (ADH) (manufactured in the hypothalamus), which acts to allow the body to retain water. It acts chiefly to regulate sodium and water intake and excretion. Functions of ADH include:
	  1. Maintains osmotic pressure of the cells by controlling renal water retention or excretion
	    a. When osmotic pressure of the ECF is greater than that of the cells (as in hypernatremia—excess sodium—or hyperglycemia), ADH secretion is increased, causing renal retention of water.
	    b. When osmotic pressure of the ECF is less than that of the cells (as in hyponatremia), ADH secretion is decreased, causing renal excretion of water.
	  2. Controls blood volume (less influential than aldosterone)
	    a. When blood volume is decreased, an increased secretion of ADH results in water conservation.
	    b. When blood volume is increased, a decreased secretion of ADH results in water loss.

Thyroid gland	• Increases blood flow in the body by releasing thyroxine, leading to increased renal circulation and resulting in increased glomerular filtration and urinary output.
Nervous system	• Inhibits and stimulates mechanisms influencing fluid balance; acts chiefly to regulate sodium and water intake and excretion • Regulates oral intake by sensing intracellular dehydration, which triggers thirst (thirst center located in the hypothalamus) • Neurons, called osmoreceptors, are sensitive to changes in the concentration of ECF, sending appropriate impulses to the pituitary gland to release ADH or inhibit its release to maintain ECF volume concentration.
Gastrointestinal tract	Absorbs water and nutrients that enter the body through this route.

Parathyroid glands	• Regulate calcium (Ca^{2+}) and phosphate (HPO_4^{2-}) balance by means of parathyroid hormone (PTH); PTH influences bone reabsorption, calcium absorption from the intestines, and calcium reabsorption from the renal tubules.
	  1. Increased secretion of PTH causes:
	    a. Elevated serum calcium concentration
	    b. Lowered serum phosphate concentration
	  2. Conversely, decreased secretion of PTH causes:
	    a. Lowered serum calcium concentration
	    b. Elevated serum phosphate concentration

Data from Metheny, N. M. (2012). *Fluid and electrolyte balance. Nursing Considerations* (5th ed.). Sudbury, MA: Jones & Bartlett Learning; Grossman, S., & Porth, C.M. (2014). Porth's pathophysiology: concepts of altered health states. (9th ed.). Philadelphia: Wolters Kluwer Health/Lippincott Williams & Wilkins.

equilibrium is established. As a result, the volume of the more concentrated solution increases, and the volume of the weaker solution decreases. The process of osmosis stops when the concentration of solutes has been equalized on both sides of the cell membrane. The greater the difference in the concentration of the two solutions on each side of a semipermeable membrane, the greater the osmotic pressure or drawing power of water.

The concentration of particles in a solution, or its pulling power, is referred to as the **osmolarity** of a solution. A solution that has about the same concentration of particles, or osmolarity, as plasma (between 275 and 295 mOsm/L) is considered an **isotonic** solution.

An isotonic fluid remains in the intravascular compartment without any net flow across the semipermeable membrane. In contrast, a **hypertonic** solution has a greater osmolarity than plasma (>295 mOsm/L). Because a hypertonic solution has a greater osmolarity, water moves out of the cells and is drawn into the intravascular compartment, causing the cells to shrink. A **hypotonic** solution has less osmolarity than plasma (<275 mOsm/L). Because of a lower osmolarity, a hypotonic solution in the intravascular space moves out of the intravascular space and into intracellular fluid, causing cells to swell and possibly burst. In addition, electrolytes have "osmotic potential," which refers to the electrolytes' affinity for water (i.e., the capacity to pull water into a fluid compartment). Sodium, for example, has a high osmotic potential.

Diffusion

Diffusion is the tendency of solutes to move freely throughout a solvent. The solute moves from an area of higher concentration to an area of lower concentration (i.e., "downhill") until equilibrium is established (Fig. 39-5). Gases also move by diffusion. Oxygen and carbon dioxide exchange in the lung's alveoli and capillaries occurs by diffusion.

FIGURE 39-5. Diffusion. Solutes move from an area of higher concentration to an area of lower concentration until the concentration is equal in both areas.

FIGURE 39-6. Active transport. Solutes are moved ("pumped") from an area of lower concentration to an area of higher concentration.

Active Transport

Active transport is a process that requires energy for the movement of substances through a cell membrane, against the concentration gradient, from an area of lesser solute concentration to an area of higher solute concentration. Adenosine triphosphate (ATP), which is stored in all cells, supplies energy for solute movement in and out of the cell. Although this process is not entirely understood, the energy requirements for active transport are affected by characteristics of the cell membrane, specific enzymes, and concentrations of ions. This process explains the so-called pump mechanism (Fig. 39-6). If diffusion can be called "coasting downhill," active transport can be called "pumping uphill." Substances believed to use active transport include amino acids, glucose (in certain places only, such as in the kidneys and intestines), and ions of sodium, potassium, hydrogen, and calcium (*Fluids & electrolytes made incredibly easy*, 2011).

Capillary Filtration

Filtration is the passage of fluid through a permeable membrane. Fluids move from an area of high pressure to one of lower pressure. **Capillary filtration** results from the force of blood "pushing" against the walls of the capillaries. At the arterial end of the capillaries, filtration is dependent primarily on arterial blood pressure; at the venular side of the capillaries, filtration is dependent on venous blood pressure. The "pushing" force is referred to as **hydrostatic pressure**. When the hydrostatic pressure inside the capillary exceeds the surrounding interstitial space, fluids and solutes are forced out of the capillary wall into the interstitial space. In contrast, when the pressure inside the capillary is less than the pressure in the interstitial space, the fluids and solutes will move back into the capillary. Reabsorption is the process that acts to prevent too much fluid from leaving the capillaries no matter how high the hydrostatic pressure. Plasma proteins, particularly albumin, concentrated in the intravascular space or plasma facilitate this reabsorption

FIGURE 39-7. Capillary filtration.

process by "pulling" the fluid back into the capillaries. This "pulling" force is known as **colloid osmotic pressure**, or oncotic pressure. Under normal conditions, hydrostatic pressure in the arteriole end of a capillary exceeds plasma colloid pressure. Hydrostatic pressure at the venule end of the capillary is less than plasma colloid pressure. As a result, capillary filtration occurs along the first half of the vessel, and reabsorption occurs along the second half (Metheny, 2012). Filtration pressure is the difference between colloid osmotic pressure and blood hydrostatic pressure.

These pressures are important in understanding how fluid leaves arterioles, enters the interstitial compartment, and eventually returns to the venules. The filtration pressure is positive in the arterioles, helping to force or filter fluids into interstitial spaces; it is negative in the venules and thus helps fluid enter the venules. This is illustrated in Figure 39-7. Filtration is also involved in the proper functioning of the glomeruli of the kidneys.

Acid–Base Balance

Body fluids must maintain an acid–base balance to sustain health, homeostasis, and life. Specific chemical reactions are constantly occurring within the body that influence metabolism and the functions of various bodily systems. These chemical reactions are dependent on a balance of acids and bases. Conditions such as infection or trauma may alter this delicate acid–base balance. Acidity or alkalinity of a solution is determined by its concentration of hydrogen ions (H^+). An **acid** is a substance containing H^+ that can be liberated or released, such as carbonic acid. An alkali, or **base**, is a substance that can accept or trap H^+ ions, such as the bicarbonate ion.

An acid releases H^+, as follows:

$$\underset{\substack{\text{Carbonic}\\\text{acid}}}{H_2CO_3} \xrightarrow{\text{releases}} \underset{\substack{\text{hydrogen}\\\text{ion}}}{H^+} + \underset{\substack{\text{to form}\\\text{bicarbonate}\\\text{base}}}{HCO_3^-}$$

A base traps H^+, as follows:

$$\underset{\substack{\text{bicarbonate}\\\text{base}}}{HCO_3^-} + \underset{\substack{\text{traps hydrogen}\\\text{ion}}}{H^+} \xrightarrow{\text{to form}} \underset{\substack{\text{Carbonic}\\\text{acid}}}{H_2CO_3}$$

A strong acid dissociates (separates) completely in solution and releases all of its H^+ ions, whereas a weak acid releases only a small number. A base that binds or accepts H^+ ions easily is considered a strong base, whereas one that accepts H^+ ions less readily is considered weak.

The unit of measure used to describe acid–base balance is **pH**, which is an expression of H^+ ion concentration and the resulting acidity or alkalinity of a substance. The pH scale ranges from 1 to 14. A neutral solution measures 7; an example is pure water. Because pH is based on a negative logarithm, as the H^+ ions increase and a solution becomes more acid, the pH becomes less than 7. When the concentration of H^+ ions in a solution is reduced or accepted by another substance and the solution contains more base than acid, it is alkaline, and the pH is greater than 7. Gastric secretions that are strongly acidic have an approximate pH of 1 to 1.3, whereas strongly alkaline pancreatic secretions have an approximate pH of 10.

Normal blood plasma is slightly alkaline and has a normal pH range of 7.35 to 7.45. When the blood plasma pH exceeds the normal pH range in either direction, signs and symptoms of illness develop, and if the condition goes on unabated, death results. **Acidosis** is the condition characterized by an excess of H ions or loss of base ions (bicarbonate) in ECF in which the pH falls below 7.35. **Alkalosis** occurs when there is a lack of H ions or a gain of base (bicarbonate) and the pH exceeds 7.45 (see the section, Acid–Base Imbalances). Figure 39-8 illustrates normal pH, acidosis,

FIGURE 39-8. Acid–base balance. Note that acidosis is used to describe the condition of the pH falling below 7.35, and alkalosis describes a pH above 7.45. When the normal pH is exceeded in either direction, death can occur.

and alkalosis and shows the points at which death typically occurs. The narrow range of normal pH is achieved through three major homeostatic regulators of hydrogen ions: (1) chemical buffer systems, (2) respiratory mechanisms, and (3) renal mechanisms. There are alterations in these systems related to the developmental stage of an individual. Newborns are not able to acidify urine as well as older people. As people age, the effectiveness of both the lungs and kidneys can vary. In an older adult, if there is underlying lung disease, the regulation of acid–base balance may be less efficient. In addition, the kidneys of the older adult can have difficulty handling excess amounts of acid (*Fluids & electrolytes made incredibly easy*, 2011).

Chemical Buffer Systems

A **buffer** is a substance that prevents body fluids from becoming overly acidic or alkaline. Buffers combine with excess acids or bases to prevent major changes in pH, keeping the pH of body fluids as close as possible to normal (7.35–7.45). Buffers work in one of two ways. A buffer can function like a base and bind or soak up free hydrogen ions. Alternately, it may function like an acid and release hydrogen ions when too few are present in a solution. The body has three buffer systems: (1) the carbonic acid–sodium bicarbonate buffer system, (2) the phosphate buffer system, and (3) the protein buffer system.

CARBONIC ACID–SODIUM BICARBONATE BUFFER SYSTEM

The ratio of carbonic acid (H_2CO_3), the most common acid in human body fluid, to the body's most common base, bicarbonate (HCO_3^-), is important for acid–base balance and is the most important buffer system of the body. Normal ECF has a ratio of 20 parts bicarbonate to 1 part carbonic acid. The exact quantities are unimportant for acid–base balance as long as they remain in a 20:1 ratio. Carbonic acid and bicarbonate must be carefully controlled to maintain this ratio; if either is increased or decreased, the 20:1 ratio is no longer in effect and pH will change. This system buffers as much as 90% of the H^+ of ECF. The lungs help by regulating the production of carbonic acid resulting from the combination of carbon dioxide and water. The kidneys assist the bicarbonate system by regulating the production of bicarbonate.

PHOSPHATE BUFFER SYSTEM

The phosphate buffer system is active in intracellular fluids, especially in the renal tubules. It converts alkaline sodium phosphate (Na_2HPO_4), a weak base, to acid–sodium phosphate (NaH_2PO_4) in the kidneys.

PROTEIN BUFFER SYSTEM

The third buffer system is a mixture of plasma proteins and the globin portion of hemoglobin in red blood cells. Because plasma proteins and hemoglobin possess chemical groups that can combine with or liberate hydrogen ions, they tend to minimize changes in pH and serve as excellent buffering agents over a wide range of pH values working both inside and outside the cells. For example, excess hydrogen ions in

the blood cross over the plasma membrane of red blood cells and bind to the hemoglobin molecules that are plentiful in each red blood cell.

Respiratory Regulation of Hydrogen Ions

Due to the huge surface area from which CO_2 can readily diffuse, the lungs can bring about rapid changes in H^+ when needed. Carbon dioxide, constantly produced by cellular metabolism (carbonic acid [H_2CO_3] yields CO_2 and H_2O), is excreted by exhalation. When the amount of CO_2 in the blood increases, the sensitive chemoreceptors in the respiratory center in the medulla are stimulated to increase the rate and depth of respirations to eliminate more CO_2. As more CO_2 is exhaled, the H_2CO_3 level in the blood decreases, and the pH of the blood becomes more alkaline. When the blood level of CO_2 decreases, the respiratory center decreases the rate and depth of respirations to retain the CO_2 so that carbonic acid can be formed, thereby maintaining the delicate balance. As a result, the lungs are the primary controller of the body's carbonic acid supply. This total respiratory process occurs almost as rapidly as the buffering action in the carbonic acid–sodium bicarbonate system. The respiratory system is able to respond quickly in a healthy individual to restore the normal pH. However, this response is short term, and the response of the kidneys is needed for long-term adjustment (*Fluids & electrolytes made incredibly easy*, 2011).

Renal Regulation of Hydrogen Ions

Essentially, the kidneys excrete or retain hydrogen ions and form or excrete bicarbonate ions in response to the pH of the blood. In the presence of acidosis, the kidneys excrete hydrogen ions and form and conserve bicarbonate ions, thus raising the pH to the normal range. If alkalosis is present, the kidneys retain hydrogen ions and excrete bicarbonate ions in an effort to return to a balanced state. As a result, the concentration of bicarbonate in the plasma is regulated by the kidneys.

Acid–base regulation by the kidneys occurs more slowly than that which occurs by the carbonic acid–sodium bicarbonate system or by respiratory regulation. It may take as long as 3 days for a normal fluid pH to be restored by the kidneys. The pH of urine varies, depending on the ions that are being excreted, but it is generally between 4.5 and 8.2.

DISTURBANCES IN FLUID, ELECTROLYTE, AND ACID–BASE BALANCE

Nurses commonly encounter disturbances in fluid, electrolyte, and acid–base balance while caring for acutely or chronically ill patients. Although many of these disturbances are interrelated and may occur together, they are described here separately for learning purposes.

Fluid Imbalances

Fluid imbalances occur when the body's compensatory mechanisms are unable to maintain a homeostatic state. Fluid imbalances involve either the volume or distribution of water or electrolytes. Nursing implications related to fluid volume disturbances—including risk factors, nursing assessments, and interventions—are discussed later in the chapter.

Fluid Volume Deficit

Fluid volume deficit (FVD) is caused by a loss of both water and solutes in the same proportion from the ECF space. This state is commonly known as **hypovolemia** or isotonic fluid loss. Both osmotic and hydrostatic pressure changes force the interstitial fluid into the intravascular space in an effort to compensate for the loss of volume in the blood vessels. As the interstitial space is depleted, its fluid becomes hypertonic, and cellular fluid is then drawn into the interstitial space, leaving cells without adequate fluid to function properly. Fluid volume deficits result from the loss of body fluids, especially if fluid intake is decreased simultaneously.

Young children, older adults, and people who are ill are especially at risk for hypovolemia. Fluid volume deficit can rapidly result in a weight loss of 5% in adults and 10% in infants. A 5% weight loss is considered a pronounced fluid deficit; an 8% loss or more is considered severe. A 15% weight loss caused by fluid deficiency usually is life threatening.

 RECALL Jeremiah Stein, the college student with an increased number of loose, watery stools for a week. His assessment reveals that he has been limiting his oral intake, further compounding his risk for deficient fluid volume. Weighing Jeremiah would be an important intervention to include as part of the nursing assessment to help determine the extent of fluid loss. •

Third-space fluid shift refers to a distributional shift of body fluids into the transcellular compartment, such as the pleural, peritoneal (ascites), or pericardial areas; joint cavities; the bowel; or an excess accumulation of fluid in the interstitial space. The fluid moves out of the intravascular spaces (plasma) to any of these spaces. Once trapped in these spaces, the fluid is not easily exchanged with ECF. With third-space fluid shift, a deficit in ECF volume occurs. The fluid has not been lost but is trapped in another body space for a period of time and is essentially unavailable for use. These fluid shifts may be related to a disruption in the colloid osmotic pressure (decreased albumin), increased fluid volume (excess IV fluid replacement, renal dysfunction), increased capillary hydrostatic pressure (heart failure), hyponatremia, or an increase in the permeability of the capillary membrane (gross tissue trauma). A third-space shift may occur as a result of a severe burn, a bowel obstruction, surgical procedures, pancreatitis, ascites, or sepsis (Metheny, 2012). Decreased body weight does not occur as it does with an ECF volume deficit (vomiting or diarrhea), and the fluid loss cannot be measured.

 ### Fluid Volume Excess

Excessive retention of water and sodium in ECF in near-equal proportions results in a condition termed *fluid volume*

excess (FVE). It is also called **hypervolemia** or excess of isotonic fluid (Metheny, 2012; *Fluids & electrolytes made incredibly easy,* 2011). Common causes include malfunction of the kidneys, causing an inability to excrete the excesses, and failure of the heart to function as a pump, resulting in accumulation of fluid in the lungs and dependent parts of the body.

Due to the increased extracellular osmotic pressure from the retained sodium and water, fluid is pulled from the cells to equalize the tonicity. By the time the intracellular and extracellular spaces are isotonic to each other, an excess of both water and sodium is in the ECF, whereas the cells are nearly depleted. The excessive ECF may accumulate in either the intravascular compartments or interstitial spaces. Accumulation of fluid in the interstitial space is known as **edema**. Edema can be observed around the eyes, fingers, ankles, and sacral space, and can also accumulate in or around body organs. Accumulation of fluid may result in a weight gain in excess of 5%. The amount or severity of edema is typically graded (Fig. 39-9 on page 1482). Interstitial-to-plasma shift is the movement of fluid from the space surrounding the cells to the blood. Although the body attempts to maintain normal balance in all fluid spaces, the intravascular fluid is usually protected at the expense of interstitial fluid and ICF.

 REMEMBER Jack Soo Park, the patient who inadvertently received too much IV fluid? In Mr. Park's case, fluid accumulation involved his lungs and heart, exhibited by his bounding pulse, distended neck veins, and abnormal lung sounds. •

Electrolyte Imbalances

Electrolyte imbalances commonly involve a deficit or excess of the electrolyte. Abnormalities in electrolyte levels can indicate fluid or acid–base imbalance, or neuromuscular, cardiac, renal endocrine, or skeletal dysfunction. Results from venous blood will provide essential information related to possible electrolyte imbalances. When patients present with deficits or excesses of sodium, potassium, calcium, magnesium, phosphate, or chloride, careful nursing assessment depends on an understanding of the effects of these imbalances.

Hyponatremia and Hypernatremia

Sodium is the most abundant electrolyte in the ECF. Refer to Table 39-2 on page 1475. **Hyponatremia** refers to a sodium deficit in ECF (serum sodium <135 mEq/L) caused by a loss of sodium or a gain of water. Sodium may be lost through vomiting, diarrhea, fistulas, sweating, or as the result of the use of diuretics. The decrease in sodium causes fluid to move by osmosis from the less concentrated ECF compartment to the ICF space. This shift of fluid leads to swelling of the cells, with resulting confusion, hypotension, edema, muscle cramps and weakness, and dry skin. Cerebral edema can lead to seizures. Permanent neurologic damage and death can result from severe hyponatremia (Hinkle & Cheever, 2014).

1+ Pitting Edema

- Slight indentation (2 mm)
- Normal contours
- Associated with interstitial fluid volume 30% above normal

2 mm

2+ Pitting Edema

- Deeper pit after pressing (4 mm)
- Lasts longer than 1+
- Fairly normal contour

4 mm

3+ Pitting Edema

- Deep pit (6 mm)
- Remains several seconds after pressing
- Skin swelling obvious by general inspection

6 mm

4+ Pitting Edema

- Deep pit (8 mm)
- Remains for a prolonged time after pressing, possibly minutes
- Frank swelling

8 mm

Brawny Edema

- Fluid can no longer be displaced secondary to excessive interstitial fluid accumulation
- No pitting
- Tissue palpates as firm or hard
- Skin surface shiny, warm, moist

FIGURE 39-9. System for grading edema.

Hypernatremia refers to a surplus of sodium in ECF (serum sodium >145 mEq/L) caused by excess water loss or an overall excess of sodium. Fluid deprivation, lack of fluid consumption (such as in patients who cannot perceive, respond to, or communicate thirst [Grossman & Porth, 2014]), diarrhea, and excess insensible water loss (hyperventilation, burns) lead to excess sodium. Fluids move from the cells because of the increased extracellular osmotic pressure, causing them to shrink and leaving them without sufficient fluid. The cells of the central nervous system are especially affected, resulting in signs of neurologic impairment, including restlessness, weakness, disorientation, delusion, and hallucinations. Permanent brain damage, especially in children, can occur (Grossman & Porth, 2014).

Hypokalemia and Hyperkalemia

Potassium is the major intracellular electrolyte. Refer to Table 39-2 on page 1475. **Hypokalemia** refers to a potassium deficit in ECF (serum potassium <3.5 mEq/L) and is a common electrolyte abnormality. Potassium may be lost through vomiting, gastric suction, alkalosis, diarrhea, or as the result of

the use of diuretics. When the extracellular potassium level falls, potassium moves from the cell, creating an intracellular potassium deficiency. Sodium and hydrogen ions are then retained by the cells to maintain isotonic fluids. These electrolyte shifts influence normal cellular functioning, the pH of ECF, and the functions of most body systems, including the cardiovascular system. Skeletal muscles are generally the first to demonstrate a potassium deficiency. Typical signs of hypokalemia include muscle weakness and leg cramps, fatigue, paresthesias, and dysrhythmias.

Hyperkalemia refers to an excess of potassium in ECF (serum potassium >5 mEq/L). Excess potassium may result from renal failure, hypoaldosteronism, or the use of certain medications such as potassium chloride, heparin, angiotensin-converting enzyme (ACE) inhibitors, nonsteroidal anti-inflammatory drugs (NSAIDs), and potassium-sparing diuretics. Although this condition occurs less frequently than hypokalemia, it can be much more dangerous. Nerve conduction as well as muscle contractility can be affected. Skeletal muscle weakness and paralysis may occur. A variety of cardiac irregularities may result, including cardiac arrest if hyperkalemia is not corrected.

Hypocalcemia and Hypercalcemia

Calcium is a major component of bones and teeth. Refer to Table 39-2 on page 1475. **Hypocalcemia** refers to a calcium deficit in ECF (serum calcium <8.9 mg/dL, ionized calcium <4.5 mg/dL). Common causes related to a calcium deficit involve inadequate calcium intake, impaired calcium absorption, and excessive calcium loss. Manifestations of hypocalcemia include numbness and tingling of fingers, mouth, or feet; tetany; muscle cramps; and seizures.

Hypercalcemia refers to an excess of calcium in ECF (serum calcium >10.1 mg/dL, ionized calcium >5.1 mg/dL). Two major causes of hypercalcemia are cancer and hyperparathyroidism. Manifestations of hypercalcemia include nausea, vomiting, constipation, bone pain, excessive urination, thirst, confusion, lethargy, and slurred speech. Severe hypercalcemia (serum calcium ≥17 mg/dL) is an emergency situation because cardiac arrest may result.

Hypomagnesemia and Hypermagnesemia

Magnesium is the most abundant intracellular cation after potassium. Refer to Table 39-2 on page 1475. **Hypomagnesemia** refers to a magnesium deficit in the ECF (serum magnesium <1.5 mEq/L). Magnesium loss may occur with nasogastric suction, diarrhea, withdrawal from alcohol, administration of tube feedings or parenteral nutrition, sepsis, or burns. This abnormality may lead to muscle weakness, tremors, tetany, seizures, heart block, change in mental status, hyperactive deep tendon reflexes (DTRs), and respiratory paralysis.

Hypermagnesemia refers to a magnesium excess in the ECF (serum magnesium >2.5 mEq/L). It usually occurs with renal failure when the kidneys fail to excrete magnesium or from excessive magnesium intake (use of magnesium-containing antacids or laxatives). Clinical manifestations include nausea, vomiting, weakness, flushing, lethargy, loss of DTRs, respiratory depression, coma, and cardiac arrest.

Hypophosphatemia and Hyperphosphatemia

Phosphorus is a critical element of all the body's tissues. Refer to Table 39-2 on page 1475. **Hypophosphatemia** refers to a below-normal concentration of phosphorus in the ECF (serum phosphate <2.5 mg/dL or 1.8 mEq/L). Although this may indicate phosphorus deficiency, multiple factors may lower serum phosphate levels while total body phosphorus stores are normal. Hypophosphatemia can result from administration of calories to malnourished patients, alcohol withdrawal, diabetic ketoacidosis, hyperventilation, insulin release, absorption problems, and diuretic use. Manifestations include irritability, fatigue, weakness, paresthesias, confusion, seizures, and coma.

Hyperphosphatemia refers to above-normal concentrations of phosphorus in the ECF (serum phosphate >4.5 mg/dL or 2.6 mEq/L). Common causes are impaired kidney excretion and hypoparathyroidism. Hyperphosphatemia can result in tetany, anorexia, nausea, muscle weakness, and tachycardia.

Hypochloremia and Hyperchloremia

Chloride is the major anion of the ECF. Refer to Table 39-2 on page 1475. **Hypochloremia** refers to below-normal level of chloride in the ECF (serum chloride <96 mEq/L). A low level of chloride can result from severe vomiting and diarrhea, drainage of gastric fluid (GI tube), metabolic alkalosis, diuretic therapy, and burns. Manifestations include hyperexcitability of muscles, tetany, hyperactive DTRs, weakness, and muscle cramps.

Hyperchloremia refers to an above-normal level of chloride in the ECF (serum chloride >106 mEq/L). Hyperchloremia can result from metabolic acidosis, head trauma, increased perspiration, excess adrenocortical hormone production, and decreased glomerular filtration. Signs and symptoms include tachypnea, weakness, lethargy, diminished cognitive ability, hypertension, decreased cardiac output, dysrhythmias, and coma.

Acid–Base Imbalances

Acid–base imbalances occur when the carbonic acid or bicarbonate levels become disproportionate. When there is a single primary cause, these disturbances are known as respiratory acidosis or alkalosis and metabolic acidosis or alkalosis, which are described in the sections that follow. Some references use the term *nonrespiratory* to refer to metabolic disturbances. Although these disturbances are discussed separately, combined disturbances frequently occur. Complicated clinical situations may occur when respiratory and metabolic imbalances coexist.

Metabolic Acidosis and Alkalosis

Metabolic acidosis and alkalosis occur as the result of metabolic processes. A metabolic or nonrespiratory disturbance alters the bicarbonate level in the ECF. It is reflected in the HCO_3^- level of an arterial blood gas (ABG). Both the lungs and the kidneys attempt to compensate for this disorder by either excreting or retaining $PaCO_2$ (the lungs) and/or HCO_3^- and H^+ ions (the kidneys).

Metabolic acidosis or nonrespiratory acidosis is a proportionate deficit of bicarbonate in ECF. The deficit can occur as the result of an increase in acid components or an excessive loss of bicarbonate. It can be produced by a gain of hydrogen ion or loss of bicarbonate. The lungs attempt to increase carbon dioxide excretion by increasing the rate and depth of respirations, which occurs within a short time. However, respiratory compensation is generally not adequate, and the kidneys attempt to compensate by retaining bicarbonate and by excreting more hydrogen. In summary: Metabolic acidosis = low pH (increased hydrogen ion concentration) and a low plasma bicarbonate concentration due to a gain of hydrogen or loss of bicarbonate.

Metabolic alkalosis or nonrespiratory alkalosis is associated with an excess of HCO_3, a decrease in H^+ ions, or both, in the ECF. This may be the result of excessive acid losses or increased base ingestion or retention. The body attempts to compensate by retaining carbon dioxide. The respirations become slow and shallow, and periods of no breathing may occur. The kidneys attempt to excrete excess H_2O and Na ions with the excessive bicarbonate and retain H^+ ions. In summary: Metabolic alkalosis = high pH and a high plasma bicarbonate concentration due to a gain of bicarbonate or a loss of hydrogen.

Respiratory Acidosis and Alkalosis

Respiratory acidosis and alkalosis occur as a result of respiratory disturbances. A respiratory disturbance alters the carbonic acid level in the ECF. It is reflected in the $PaCO_2$ level of an ABG. Compensation for a respiratory disturbance occurs when the lungs attempt to either retain or eliminate $PaCO_2$ from the body or when the kidneys attempt to restore balance through the conservation, formation, or excretion of bicarbonate (HCO_3).

Respiratory acidosis is a primary excess of carbonic acid in the ECF. It is produced by inadequate excretion of CO_2 with inadequate ventilation, resulting in elevated plasma CO_2 and increased levels of carbonic acid. Any decrease in alveolar ventilation that results in retention of carbon dioxide can cause respiratory acidosis. Initially, the increased amounts of CO_2 stimulate the medulla in the respiratory center to increase the respiratory rate. Due to the increase in respiratory rate, CO_2 is expelled and the CO_2 level of the blood is reduced. If the respiratory response is not effective, the increasing CO_2 levels will stimulate the kidneys to eliminate H^+ ions (acids) and conserve bicarbonate and sodium ions. The $NaHCO_3$ acts to buffer the free acids and ultimately reduce the CO_2 levels and restore acid–base balance. In summary: Respiratory acidosis = high $PaCO_2$ due to alveolar hypoventilation.

Respiratory alkalosis is a primary deficit of carbonic acid in the ECF. It is the result of alveolar hyperventilation, breathing that is faster and deeper, and the consequent increase in the elimination of CO_2. This loss of CO_2 leads to a decrease in the carbonic acid level in the plasma and an increase in the pH. The chemoreceptors in the medulla sense the increase in pH and the presence of less carbonic acid and stimulate the body to breathe either more slowly or less deeply. If this condition lasts for about 6 hours or longer, the kidneys attempt to alleviate the imbalance by increasing the bicarbonate excretion and by retaining more hydrogen to correct the imbalance. In summary: Respiratory alkalosis = low $PaCO_2$ due to alveolar hyperventilation.

THE NURSING PROCESS FOR FLUID, ELECTROLYTE, AND ACID–BASE BALANCE
Assessing

Acute and chronic illness, trauma, and certain therapeutic interventions may place a patient at high risk for fluid, electrolyte, and acid–base imbalances. Such imbalances can seriously compromise the patient's health status and

may prove life threatening. The nursing assessment is directed toward the following:

- Identifying patients at high risk for fluid, electrolyte, and acid–base imbalances
- Determining specific imbalances by identifying the nature of the imbalances to include their severity, etiology, and defining characteristics or assessment findings
- Determining the plan of care, including the appropriate nursing diagnoses or collaborative problems, followed by the identification of specific outcomes and associated interventions
- Evaluating the effectiveness of the plan of care

Nursing assessment related to fluid, electrolyte, and acid–base balance should include a nursing history, physical assessment, fluid intake and output, daily weights, and laboratory studies. When an imbalance in fluid, specific electrolytes, or acid–base balance is suspected, the nurse needs to incorporate the associated assessments into the patient's care. Physical assessment and clinical assessment parameters, nursing considerations, normal findings in a healthy adult, and possible abnormal or significant findings are outlined in Tables 39-4 and 39-5 (on page 1487).

Nursing History

A comprehensive nursing history includes questions related to the patient's fluid and electrolyte status and acid–base balance. The accompanying Focused Assessment Guide 39-1 (on page 1488) includes interview questions to help identify the patient's usual pattern of fluid intake and elimination and the patient's self-evaluation of hydration status and awareness of particular problems.

Interview questions are also directed toward identifying patients with health conditions that increase the risk for imbalances. Risk factors include the following:

- Acute and chronic illnesses (e.g., diabetes mellitus, congestive heart failure, renal failure)
- Abnormal losses of body fluids (e.g., prolonged or severe vomiting or diarrhea, draining wounds, fistulas). Table 39-6 (on page 1488) lists imbalances that result from loss of specific body fluids.
- Burns
- Trauma
- Surgery
- Therapies that may disrupt fluid and electrolyte balance, e.g., medications such as diuretics and steroids, treatments such as IV therapy and total parenteral nutrition (TPN)

Physical Assessment

Physical assessment related to fluid, electrolyte, and acid–base balance includes the assessment of multiple body systems. Include assessment of the skin and mucous membranes, vital signs, and a neurologic assessment, as well as identification of relative symptoms or conditions such as excessive thirst, nausea, vomiting, diarrhea, draining wounds, or other fluid losses. Refer

Table 39-4 | PARAMETERS TO BE CONSIDERED IN PHYSICAL ASSESSMENT FOR FLUID, ELECTROLYTE, AND ACID–BASE BALANCE

ASSESSMENT PARAMETERS	NURSING CONSIDERATIONS	FINDINGS IN HEALTHY ADULT	SIGNIFICANT FINDINGS
Skin turgor (elasticity)	• The patient's skin over the sternum, inner aspect of the thighs, or forehead is pinched. • Some prefer to test skin turgor in children over the abdominal area and on the medial aspect of the thighs. • Skin turgor can vary with age, nutritional state, ethnicity, and complexion.	• Pinched skin immediately falls back to its normal position when released. • Reduced skin turgor is common in older patients (those more than 55–60 years of age) because of a primary decrease in skin elasticity.	• In a person with a fluid volume deficit, the skin flattens more slowly after the pinch is released; the skin may remain elevated for many seconds. • Severe malnutrition, particularly in infants, can cause depressed skin turgor even in the absence of fluid depletion.
Tongue turgor	• Unlike skin turgor, tongue turgor is not affected appreciably by age and thus is a useful assessment for all age groups. (In an arid climate, this may not be a reliable parameter.)	• Tongue has one longitudinal furrow.	• In the person with fluid volume deficit, there are additional longitudinal furrows and the tongue is smaller. • Sodium excess causes the tongue to look red and swollen.
Moisture and oral cavity	• A dry mouth may be the result of fluid volume deficit or of mouth breathing. (Exposure to an arid climate may result in a dry mouth.)	• Mucous membranes in oral cavity are moist.	• Dryness of the membrane where the cheek and gum meet indicates fluid volume deficit. • Dry sticky mucous membranes are noted in sodium excess. (The oral cavity feels like flypaper.)
Tearing and salivation		• Tearing and salivation decrease normally with age.	• The absence of tearing and salivation in a child is a sign of fluid volume deficit; it becomes obvious with a fluid loss of 5% of TBW.
Appearance of skin and skin temperature			• Metabolic acidosis can cause warm, flushed skin (due to peripheral vasodilation).
Facial appearance			• A person with a severe fluid volume deficit may have a pinched and drawn facial expression. • A fluid volume deficit of 10% of body weight causes decreased intraocular pressure, causing the eyes to appear sunken and to feel soft to the touch.
Edema (excessive accumulation of interstitial fluid)	• Pitting edema (see Fig. 39-9) • Measurement of an extremity or body part with a millimeter tape, in the same area each day, is a more exact method of measurement. • An excess of interstitial fluid may accumulate predominantly in the lower extremities of ambulatory patients and in the presacral region of bedridden patients. • The presence of periorbital (around the eyes) edema or pedal edema should prompt one to look for edema in other parts of the body.	• No edema	• Clinically, edema is not usually apparent in the adult until the retention of 5–10 lb of excess fluid occurs. • Pitting edema is not evident until at least a 10% increase in weight has occurred. • Formation of edema may be localized (as in thrombophlebitis) or generalized (as in heart failure, cirrhosis of the liver, or nephrotic syndrome). Edema of congestive heart failure, liver cirrhosis, or nephrotic syndrome is the result of sodium retention.

Table 39-4 **PARAMETERS TO BE CONSIDERED IN PHYSICAL ASSESSMENT FOR FLUID, ELECTROLYTE, AND ACID–BASE BALANCE** *continued*

ASSESSMENT PARAMETERS	NURSING CONSIDERATIONS	FINDINGS IN HEALTHY ADULT	SIGNIFICANT FINDINGS
Body temperature	• Because fever increases the loss of body fluids, it is important that temperature elevations be detected early and appropriate interventions be taken. • Body temperature and other vital signs should be assessed as ordered and at the nurse's discretion.	• Baseline temperature: diurnal variations	• There is an elevation of body temperature in hypernatremia (dehydration) probably related to lack of available fluid for sweating. • There is a decrease in body temperature in fluid volume deficit, when uncomplicated by infection. • Fever increases the loss of body fluids. • A temperature elevation between 101°F (38.3°C) and 103°F (39.4°C) increases the 24-hour fluid requirement by at least 500 mL, and a temperature above 103°F increases it by at least 1,000 mL.
Pulse		• Baseline pulse rate, rhythm, and volume	• Tachycardia is usually the earliest sign of the decreased vascular volume associated with fluid volume deficit. • Irregular pulse rates also occur with potassium imbalances and magnesium deficit. • Pulse quality/amplitude is decreased in fluid volume deficit and increased in fluid volume excess.
Respirations		• Baseline respiratory rate, rhythm, and qualities	• Deep, rapid respirations may be a compensatory mechanism for metabolic acidosis or a primary disorder causing respiratory alkalosis. • Slow, shallow respirations may be a compensatory mechanism for metabolic alkalosis or a primary disorder causing respiratory acidosis. • Moist crackles, in the absence of cardiopulmonary disease, indicate fluid volume excess.
Blood pressure	• Whenever a fluid imbalance is suspected, the patient's blood pressure is measured in the supine, sitting, and standing position to determine the presence of orthostatic changes	• Baseline blood pressure	• A fall in systolic pressure greater than 15 mm Hg from the lying to the sitting or standing position (postural hypotension) usually indicates fluid volume deficit.

Adapted from Hinkle, J.L., & Cheever K.H. (2014). *Brunner & Suddarth's textbook of medical–surgical nursing* (13th ed.). Philadelphia: Wolters Kluwer Health/Lippincott Williams & Wilkins; Metheny, N. M. (2012). *Fluid and electrolyte balance: Nursing Considerations* (5th ed.). Sudbury, MA: Jones & Bartlett Learning; and Grossman, S., & Porth, C.M. (2014). *Porth's pathophysiology: concepts of altered health states.* (9th ed.). Philadelphia: Wolters Kluwer Health/Lippincott Williams & Wilkins.

to Tables 39-4 and 39-5. Assessment of other body systems is included based on the patient's underlying health conditions.

Fluid Intake and Output

If monitoring of a patient's intake and output is required, alert the patient, family, and all caregivers to the need to measure all fluids entering and leaving the body. Refer

to Guidelines for Nursing Care 39-1: Measuring Fluid Intake and Output (on page 1489) for an explanation of correct measurement of a patient's intake and output.

Daily Weights

The record of a patient's daily weight may more accurately depict fluid balance status, due to possible numerous sources of inaccuracies in fluid intake and output

Table 39-5	**PARAMETERS TO BE CONSIDERED IN CLINICAL ASSESSMENT FOR FLUID, ELECTROLYTE, AND ACID–BASE BALANCE**			
ASSESSMENT PARAMETERS	**NURSING CONSIDERATIONS**	**FINDINGS IN HEALTHY ADULT**	**SIGNIFICANT FINDINGS**
Comparison of total intake and output of fluids	• Records may be initiated by the nurse for any patient with a real or potential water or electrolyte problem. • Intake should include all fluids taken into the body. • Output should include urine, vomitus, diarrhea, drainage from fistulas, and drainage from suction apparatus. Perspiration and drainage from lesions should be noted and estimated. Prolonged hyperventilation should also be noted because it is an important route of water vapor loss.	• Fluid intake approximately equals fluid output—when averaged over 2 or 3 days. • Range of 1,500–3,500 mL fluid intake and loss; 2,000 mL is average adult intake and loss per day. • Output of urine normally approximates the ingestion of liquids; water from food and oxidation is balanced by the water loss through feces, the skin, and the respiratory process.	• When the total intake is substantially less than the total output, the patient is in danger of fluid volume deficit. • When the total intake is substantially more than the total output, the patient is in danger of fluid volume excess.

Urine volume and concentration	• All fluid losses are measured according to routes.
	• A device calibrated for small volumes of urine is used when hourly urine volumes need to be measured.
	• Factors that can alter urinary output must be accounted for:
	  1. Amount of fluid intake
	  2. Losses from skin, lungs, and GI tract
	  3. Amount of waste products for excretions
	  4. Renal concentrating ability
	  5. Blood volume
	  6. Hormonal influences (primarily aldosterone and ADH)
		• Normal urinary output is about 1 mL/kg of body weight per hour (for the average adult: 1,500 mL/24 hr, which is equivalent to about 40–80 mL/hr).
		• Stress may diminish the 24-hour urine volume in the adult to 750–1,000 mL (or 30–50 mL/hr) because of increased aldosterone and ADH secretion.
		• The range of specific gravity is from 1.003 to 1.035. Urine osmolality ranges between 500 and 800 mOsm/kg (mmol/kg).
			• A low urine volume with a high specific gravity indicates fluid volume deficit.
			• A low urine volume with a low specific gravity indicates renal disease.
			• A high urine volume suggests fluid volume excess.
			• Urine volume is increased in conditions with high solute loads, such as diabetes mellitus.
			• Hypovolemia causes decreased renal perfusion, thus oliguria; hypervolemia causes increased urinary volume if the kidneys are functioning normally.

Body weight	• Because of the common inaccuracies in recording intake and output, body weight is believed to be a more accurate indicator of fluid gained and lost.
	• Guidelines for weighing a patient:
	  1. Use the same scale each time.
	  2. Measure weight at the same time each day: in the morning before breakfast and after voiding.
	  3. Ensure that the patient is wearing the same or similar clothing (clothing should be dry).
	  4. Use a bed scale if the patient is unable to stand on a small, portable scale.
	• A patient may have a severe fluid volume deficit even though body weight is essentially unchanged when there is a third-space loss of body fluid.
		• A patient's dry weight should remain relatively stable.	• Rapid variations in weight closely reflect changes in body fluid volume.
			• A rapid loss of body weight occurs when the total fluid intake is less than the total fluid output.
			  1. Rapid loss of 2% total body weight (TBW) indicates mild fluid volume deficit.
			  2. Rapid loss of 5% TBW indicates moderate fluid volume deficit.
			  3. Rapid loss of 8% or more of TBW indicates severe fluid volume deficit.
			• A rapid gain of body weight occurs when the total fluid intake is greater than the total fluid output.
			  1. Rapid gain of 2% TBW indicates mild fluid volume excess.
			  2. Rapid gain of 5% TBW indicates moderate fluid volume excess.
			  3. Rapid gain of 8% or more of TBW indicates severe fluid volume excess.
			• A rapid gain or loss of 1 kg (2.2 lb) of body weight is about equal to the gain or loss of 1 L of fluid.

Adapted from Hinkle, J.L., & Cheever, K.H. (2014). *Brunner & Suddarth's textbook of medical–surgical nursing* (13th ed.). Philadelphia: Wolters Kluwer Health/Lippincott Williams & Wilkins; Metheny, N. M. (2012). *Fluid and electrolyte balance: Nursing Considerations* (5th ed.). Sudbury, MA: Jones & Bartlett Learning; and Grossman, S., & Porth, C.M. (2014). Porth's pathophysiology: concepts of altered health states. (9th ed.). Philadelphia: Wolters Kluwer Health/Lippincott Williams & Wilkins.

FOCUSED ASSESSMENT GUIDE 39-1

FLUID, ELECTROLYTE, AND ACID–BASE BALANCE

Factors to Assess	Questions and Approaches
Usual patterns of fluid intake	Describe the amount and types of fluids you usually drink in a 24-hour period. Have there been any recent changes?
Usual pattern of fluid elimination	Describe your usual voiding/urination habits. Any recent changes in frequency or amount? Is your body losing fluids in any other major way? • Vomiting • Diarrhea • Excessive perspiration • Fistula
Patient's evaluation of hydration status	Do you think there is an approximate balance between your fluid intake and output? Have you noticed any signs that your body is experiencing too much or too little hydration (difficulty breathing, edema, dry skin and mucous membranes, thirst)?
History of disease process	Is there any history of disease process or injury that might disrupt fluid and electrolyte balance (e.g., diabetes mellitus, cancer, burns)?
Medication/nutrition history	Do you take any medications or treatments that might disrupt fluid and electrolyte balance (e.g., steroids, diuretics, parenteral nutrition, dialysis)? Have you been trying to lose weight by dieting, using diuretics, laxatives, or diet aids? Have you been following a high-protein, low-carbohydrate diet?
Fluid, electrolyte, and acid–base imbalances and contributing factors	Are you aware of any other fluid balance problems you may be experiencing? • Nature • Onset of problem and frequency • Causes • Severity • Symptoms • Intervention attempted and results

measurement. Weigh the patient at the same time every day. Be alert for other factors that may affect a patient's weight, such as using a different scale and weighing with the patient wearing different clothing. Refer to the accompanying Research in Nursing box.

Laboratory Studies

Laboratory tests are helpful in determining whether fluid, electrolyte, and acid–base balance exist. Descriptions of standard tests follow; tables of normal values are given in Appendix C available on thePoint.

Table 39-6 IMBALANCES RESULTING FROM LOSS OF SPECIFIC BODY FLUID

FLUID LOST	IMBALANCES LIKELY TO OCCUR	FLUID LOST	IMBALANCES LIKELY TO OCCUR
Gastric secretions	Extracellular fluid volume deficit Metabolic alkalosis Sodium deficit Potassium deficit Tetany (if metabolic alkalosis is present) Ketosis of starvation Magnesium deficit	Pancreatic juice	Metabolic acidosis Sodium deficit Calcium deficit Extracellular fluid volume deficit
		Sensible perspiration	Extracellular fluid volume deficit Sodium deficit
Intestinal secretions	Extracellular fluid volume deficit Metabolic acidosis Sodium deficit Potassium deficit	Insensible water loss	Water deficit (dehydration) Sodium excess
		Wound exudate	Protein deficit Sodium deficit Extracellular fluid volume deficit
Bile	Sodium deficit Metabolic acidosis	Ascites	Protein deficit Sodium deficit Plasma-to-interstitial fluid shift Extracellular fluid volume deficit

GUIDELINES FOR NURSING CARE 39-1

MEASURING FLUID INTAKE AND OUTPUT

- Instruct the patient and family regarding the need for a record of all fluids entering the body and all fluid output. Provide an explanation of the rationale along with instructions for how the patient can help keep measurements accurate. Some patients may need to be reminded each morning that this measurement will continue.
- Use the patient's plan of care to communicate to other nursing personnel the need to measure fluid intake and output.

A sign posted in the patient's room and a bedside form for recording intake and output are helpful reminders for both the patient and nurses.

- Measure both intake and output whenever possible, rather than estimate.
- Record intake and output totals for each 8-hour shift and total each 24 hours. If the nurse suspects a large difference between intake and output, total the columns earlier so that the primary care provider can be notified.

The Patient's Fluid Intake Includes the Following

- All fluids and foods that are liquid at room temperature (ice cream, gelatin dessert [Jell-O], and the like)
- Use the agency's designation of specific volumes for common food containers (e.g., juice glass = 90 mL;

milk carton = 240 mL). Remind the patient that sips of water or other fluids in between meals need to be recorded; small, disposable calibrated cups at the bedside facilitate accurate measurement. Remember that liquid medications or water taken with pills may significantly increase the fluid intake of some patients.
- All parenteral fluids
- Other fluids taken into the body: subcutaneous fluids, gastrointestinal tube feedings and flushes; IV flushes

The Patient's Fluid Output Includes the Following

- Urine; vomitus; diarrhea; drainage from fistulas, wounds, and ulcers; and drainage from suctioning devices or other tubes. Calibrated measuring devices should be readily available for accurate measurement. Disposable, calibrated urine collection containers that fit under the toilet seat are available for ambulatory patients. Urine or liquid feces in diapers or bed clothes, vomitus on clothing or bed linens, wound drainage saturating dressings, and so forth, need to be estimated.
- Heavy perspiration, noted on the output record, especially when the patient's clothing or bed linens are soaked
- Hyperventilation (water vapor loss) also noted on the output record. Record the rate and depth of respirations.

RESEARCH IN NURSING

BRIDGING THE GAP TO EVIDENCE-BASED PRACTICE

Monitoring Intravenous Infusions and Fluid Balance

Complications of intravenous fluid administration include electrolyte abnormalities and fluid overload, which can be detected by appropriate monitoring practices. Do nurses adequately assess and monitor patients receiving administration of intravenous fluids?

Related Research

Eastwood, G. M., Peck, L., Young, H., Prowle, J., Vasudevan, V., Jones, D., & Bellomo, R. (2012). Intravenous fluid administration and monitoring for adult ward patients in a teaching hospital. *Nursing and Health Sciences, 14*(2), 265–271.

This prospective clinical audit describes the administration and monitoring of maintenance intravenous (IV) fluid in patients in a tertiary teaching hospital. The authors examined the use of serum electrolyte and renal function measurements, the use of fluid balance charts, and the use of regular body weight measurements to detect and avoid complications related to IV fluid infusions. Serum electrolyte and renal function measurement were obtained in 85% versus 65% of patients receiving IV fluids versus no IV fluids. Fluid balance charts were maintained for 94% versus 44% of patients receiving IV fluids versus no IV fluids. Body weight mea-

surements were documented for 15% versus 14% for patients receiving IV fluids versus no IV fluids. Approximately 25% (85/332) of adult patients received IV fluids. Monitoring of these patients with regular blood tests and fluid balance charts was high (84%), but patient weight measurements were low (not documented in 85% of patients). The authors concluded that additional research was needed to identify the reasons for the lack of the use of this important assessment in this patient population.

Relevance to Nursing Practice

The use of appropriate assessments—including monitoring of electrolyte and renal function, fluid balance charts, and regular weight measurement—is an important part of nursing care to monitor patients receiving intravenous fluid infusions. Early identification of complications of IV fluid infusions leads to prompt interventions to prevent and/or correct complications/imbalances. Increased awareness of the need for appropriate assessments may contribute to prompt and effective intervention.

For additional research, visit thePoint.

COMPLETE BLOOD COUNT

The complete blood count determines the total number of red blood cells and values for hemoglobin and hematocrit. Significant values include the following:

- Increased hematocrit values: found in severe fluid volume deficit and shock (when hemoconcentration rises considerably)
- Decreased hematocrit values: found with acute, massive blood loss, and with hemolytic reaction after transfusion of incompatible blood or with fluid overload
- Increased levels of hemoglobin: found in hemoconcentration of the blood
- Decreased levels of hemoglobin: found with anemia states, severe hemorrhage, and after a hemolytic reaction

SERUM ELECTROLYTES, BLOOD UREA NITROGEN, AND CREATININE LEVELS

This screening test determines plasma levels of certain electrolytes such as sodium, potassium, chloride, and bicarbonate ions. In addition, the blood urea nitrogen (BUN) and creatinine levels can provide information related to the fluid status and the renal function of the patient. Significant values include the following:

- Below normal or above normal levels of sodium, potassium, calcium, magnesium, phosphate, and chloride. Refer to the electrolyte imbalance discussion earlier in the chapter.
- Below normal or above normal levels of bicarbonate ions. Refer to the acid–base discussion earlier in the chapter.
- Increased BUN: found with impaired renal function (such as associated with shock, heart failure, salt and water depletion), diabetic ketoacidosis, burns
- Increased creatinine: found with impaired renal function, heart failure, shock, dehydration

 RECALL Grace Gilligan, the woman described in one of the beginning scenarios. Although she needs IV therapy, it would be important for the nurse to determine the patient's electrolyte levels to establish a baseline to aid in determining the best IV solution for the patient and to determine the need for electrolyte replacement. •

URINE pH AND SPECIFIC GRAVITY

Both the urine pH and specific gravity may be obtained by dipstick measurement, using a fresh voided specimen or through laboratory analysis. The pH of urine usually ranges between 4.6 and 8.2. Lower than normal urinary pH can occur with metabolic acidosis, diabetic ketosis, and diarrhea. Higher than normal urinary pH can occur with respiratory alkalosis, potassium depletion, and chronic renal failure. Specific gravity is a measure of the urine's concentration. The range depends on the patient's state of hydration and varies with urine volume and the load of solutes to be excreted. Normal values range from 1.005 to 1.030

(concentrated urine: ≥1.025; dilute urine: ≤1.001–1.010). Increased urine specific gravity can occur with dehydration, vomiting, diarrhea, and heart failure. Decreased urine specific gravity can occur with renal damage.

ARTERIAL BLOOD GASES

Arterial blood gases (ABGs) are laboratory tests commonly used to determine the adequacy of oxygenation and ventilation, as well as in the assessment and treatment of acid–base imbalance. The ABG findings are obtained through analysis of an arterial blood sample. The pH of the plasma or blood indicates balance or impending acidosis or alkalosis. The blood's oxygen and carbon dioxide gas values are also reported, providing information regarding the effectiveness of the respiratory system. The partial pressures (indicated by "P") of these gases, or their tensions, are determined by the use of a nomogram, which reflects the chemical and physical activities of the two gases. The partial pressure of carbon dioxide is abbreviated $PaCO_2$; for oxygen, it is PaO_2. The "a" indicates an arterial specimen. When the PaO_2 is low, hemoglobin carries less than normal amounts of oxygen; when the PaO_2 is high, the hemoglobin carries more oxygen. The $PaCO_2$ is influenced almost entirely by respiratory activity. When the $PaCO_2$ is low, carbonic acid leaves the body in excessive amounts; when the $PaCO_2$ is high, there are excessive amounts of carbonic acid in the body. Oxygen saturation readings (SaO_2) reveal the percentage of oxygen in the blood that combines with hemoglobin.

The bicarbonate level (HCO_3^-) of the ABG report reflects the bicarbonate level of the body. The kidneys are involved in either reabsorbing bicarbonate or excreting bicarbonate, depending on what is needed to maintain the delicate acid–base balance.

Although compensation is the body's natural attempt to restore balance, correction may also be required. Correction involves using medical and nursing interventions to promote a return to homeostasis (e.g., pharmacologic agents, mechanical ventilation, monitor intake/output, dietary teaching). Table 39-7 outlines acid–base parameters for arterial blood gas studies.

Additional ABG values exist but are not included in this simple interpretation of acid–base imbalances. Partial pressure of oxygen (PaO_2) and oxygen saturation (SaO_2) results also directly reflect the adequacy of oxygenation

Table 39-7	ACID–BASE PARAMETERS FOR ARTERIAL BLOOD GAS STUDIES		
	NORMAL	**ACID**	**BASE**
pH	7.35–7.45	<7.35	>7.45
$PaCO_2$	35–45 mm Hg	>45 mm Hg	<35 mm Hg
HCO_3^-	22–26 mEq/L	<22 mEq/L	>26 mEq/L

and ventilation. When interpreting ABGs, follow these necessary steps:

1. Determine whether the pH is alkalotic or acidotic.
2. Check for the cause of the change in pH. Is it respiratory ($PaCO_2$) or metabolic (HCO_3^-)? In respiratory acid–base imbalances, the pH and $PaCO_2$ values are inversely abnormal (move in opposite directions):

   Respiratory acidosis:
   $\downarrow$ pH <7.35 $\uparrow$ $PaCO_2$ Normal HCO_3^-

   Respiratory alkalosis:
   $\uparrow$ pH >7.45 $\downarrow$ $PaCO_2$ Normal HCO_3^-

   In metabolic acid–base imbalances, the pH and HCO_3^- values are both high or both low:

   Metabolic acidosis:
   $\downarrow$ pH <7.35 $\downarrow$ HCO_3^- Normal $PaCO_2$

   Metabolic alkalosis:
   $\uparrow$ pH >7.45 $\uparrow$ HCO_3^- Normal $PaCO_2$

3. Determine whether the body is compensating for the pH change. When the problem is respiratory, the renal system assists in compensation either by increasing or by decreasing HCO_3^-. In contrast, the respiratory system assists in compensating for a metabolic acid–base imbalance by regulating CO_2 levels. When compensation occurs, the $PaCO_2$ and the HCO_3^- will always point in the same direction. The focus of compensation efforts is to return the pH to the normal range:

   Respiratory acidosis:
   $\downarrow$ pH <7.35 $\uparrow$ $PaCO_2$ $\uparrow$ HCO_3^-
   (compensation attempt)

   Respiratory alkalosis:
   $\uparrow$ pH >7.45 $\downarrow$ $PaCO_2$ $\downarrow$ HCO_3^-
   (compensation attempt)

   Metabolic acidosis:
   $\downarrow$pH <7.35 $\downarrow$ $HCO_3^-$$\downarrow$ $PaCO_2$
   (compensation attempt)

   Metabolic alkalosis:
   $\uparrow$ pH >7.45 $\uparrow$ $HCO_3^-$$\uparrow$ $PaCO_2$
   (compensation attempt)

4. Look at the total picture and determine whether compensation has occurred. Compensation is classified as follows:

   Absent if:
   pH abnormal
   One component abnormal
   Second component within normal range
   Partial if:
   pH abnormal
   One component abnormal
   Second component beginning to change
   Complete if:
   pH within normal range
   One component abnormal
   Second changed to move pH within normal range

Table 39-8 (on page 1492) lists assessments and nursing interventions related to these acid–base disturbances.

Diagnosing

Nursing diagnoses related to fluid, electrolyte, and acid–base balance can reflect a disturbance as the problem and result in nursing diagnoses that identify a fluid volume problem. Nursing diagnoses may also reflect the impact the imbalance has on other areas of functioning for the patient.

Fluid, Electrolyte, and Acid–Base Disturbances as the Problem

When assessment data point to fluid and electrolyte problems amenable to nursing therapy, appropriate nursing diagnoses include:

- Excess Fluid Volume
- Deficient Fluid Volume
- Risk for Deficient Fluid Volume
- Risk for Imbalanced Fluid Volume

Excess fluid volume may result from increased fluid intake or from decreased excretion, such as occurs with progressive renal disease, dysfunctions of the heart, and certain cancers. Fluid volume deficits may result from decreased intake or increased excretion of fluids as well as fluid shifts. In addition, fluid and electrolyte deficiencies may be related to situations involving strenuous exercise, extreme heat or dryness, and conditions that increase the metabolic rate, such as fever. The accompanying Examples of NANDA-I Nursing Diagnoses: Fluid and Electrolyte Balance (on page 1493) presents contributing factors and defining characteristics for these diagnoses.

Fluid and Electrolyte Disturbances as the Etiology

Disturbances in fluid, electrolyte, and acid–base balance may affect many other areas of human functioning. Examples of nursing diagnoses that may be appropriate include the following:

- Ineffective Breathing Pattern related to compensatory mechanism by lungs (hypoventilation or hyperventilation)
- Anxiety related to hyperventilation
- Risk for Injury related to neuromuscular irritability, cardiac arrhythmia
- Impaired Oral Mucous Membrane related to fluid volume deficit
- Risk for Impaired Skin Integrity related to fluid volume deficit or fluid volume overload
- Disturbed Thought Processes related to cerebral edema, mental confusion or disorientation, or convulsions

Outcome Identification and Planning

Nursing care supports the following expected outcomes. The healthy adult patient will:

- Maintain an approximate balance between fluid intake and fluid output (average about 2,500 mL fluid intake and output over 3 days)

Table 39-8 ACID–BASE DISTURBANCES

RISK FACTORS	ASSESSMENTS	NURSING INTERVENTIONS
Respiratory Acidosis		

Acute respiratory disease
    Pulmonary edema
    Aspiration of a foreign body
    Atelectasis
    Overdose of sedative or anesthetic
    Cardiac arrest
Chronic respiratory disease
    Emphysema
    Bronchial asthma
    Cystic fibrosis
Inadequate mechanical ventilation
CNS depression
Neuromuscular disease
	Acute respiratory acidosis
	    Mental cloudiness
	    Dizziness
	    Muscular twitching
	    Unconsciousness
	    ABGs
	        pH <7.35
	        $PaCO_2$ >45 mm Hg (primary)
	        HCO_3^- normal or only slightly elevated
	Chronic respiratory acidosis
	    Weakness
	    Dull headache
	    ABGs
	        pH <7.35 or low N
	        $PaCO_2$ >45 mm Hg (primary)
	        HCO_3^- >26 mEq/L (compensatory)
		Treatment is directed at improving
		    ventilation
		    Pharmacologic measures
		    Pulmonary hygiene measures
		    Adequate hydration
		    Supplemental oxygen
		Mechanical ventilation may be nec-
		    essary to correct disorder but must
		    be used cautiously to decrease
		    $PaCO_2$ slowly.

Respiratory Alkalosis		

Hyperventilation
Extreme anxiety (most common cause)
Hypoxemia
High fever
Early sepsis
Excessive ventilation by mechanical
    ventilator
CNS lesion involving the respiratory
    center
Thyrotoxicosis
	Lightheadedness
	Inability to concentrate
	Hyperventilation syndrome
	Tinnitus
	Palpitations
	Sweating
	Dry mouth
	Tremulousness
	Convulsions and loss of consciousness
	ABGs
	    pH >7.45
	    $PaCO_2$ <35 mm Hg (primary)
	    HCO_3^- <22 mEq/L (compensatory)
		If anxiety is the cause, encourage
		    the patient to breathe more slowly
		    (causes accumulation of CO_2)
		    or breathe into a closed system
		    (paper bag). Sedative may also be
		    necessary in extreme anxiety.
		Treatment of other causes is
		    directed at correcting the
		    underlying problem.

Metabolic Acidosis		

Diarrhea
Intestinal fistulas
Ureterosigmoidostomy
Parenteral nutrition
Excessive intake of acids, such as
    salicylates
Diabetic ketoacidosis
Renal failure
Starvational ketoacidosis
	Headache
	Confusion
	Drowsiness
	Increased respiratory rate and depth
	Nausea and vomiting
	Peripheral vasodilation
	ABGs
	    pH <7.35
	    HCO_3^- <22 mEq/L (primary)
	    $PaCO_2$ <35 mm Hg
	    Hyperkalemia frequently present
		Treatment is directed toward cor-
		    recting the metabolic deficit. If the
		    cause of the problem is excessive
		    intake of chloride, treatment obvi-
		    ously focuses on eliminating the
		    source. When necessary, bicar-
		    bonate is administered.

Metabolic Alkalosis		

Vomiting or gastric suction
Hypokalemia
Potassium-wasting diuretics
Alkali ingestion (bicarbonate-containing
    antacids)
Renal loss of H^+ (e.g., from steroid or
    diuretic use)
	Dizziness
	Tingling of fingers and toes
	Hypertonic muscles
	Depressed respirations (compensatory)
	ABGs
	    pH >7.45
	    HCO_3^- >26 mEq/L (primary)
	    $PaCO_2$ >45 mm Hg (compensatory)
	    Hypokalemia may be present
		Treatment is aimed at reversal of
		    the underlying disorder. Sufficient
		    chloride must be supplied for the
		    kidney to absorb sodium with
		    chloride (allowing the excretion of
		    excess bicarbonate). Treatment
		    also includes administration of
		    NaCl fluids to restore normal fluid
		    volume.

Adapted from *Fluids & electrolytes made incredibly easy!* (5th ed.). (2011). Philadelphia: Wolters Kluwer Health/Lippincott Williams & Wilkins; and Metheny, N. M. (2012). *Fluid and electrolyte balance: Nursing Considerations* (5th ed.). Sudbury, MA: Jones & Bartlett Learning.

EXAMPLES OF NANDA-I NURSING DIAGNOSES

FLUID AND ELECTROLYTE BALANCE

Nursing Diagnoses	Related Factors	Sample Defining Characteristics
Excess Fluid Volume	Renal failure, decreased cardiac output, liver disease, hormonal problems, excessive IV infusion/fluid intake, excessive sodium intake	• "I've noticed that my wedding ring is tight…also my clothes don't fit as well as they used to. I guess I've gained some weight." • Reports dyspnea with exertion, feeling weak and fatigued • Pitting edema in feet, ankles, lower legs • Taut, shiny skin • Jugular venous distention • Adventitious breath sounds • Increased blood pressure • 10-lb (4.5-kg) weight gain over past month • Fluid intake greater than output
Deficient Fluid Volume; Risk for Deficient Fluid Volume	Imposed fluid restrictions, inability to obtain or swallow fluids (debilitation, oral pain), extremes of age, vomiting, diarrhea, burns, excessive use of laxative, excessive diaphoresis, fever	• "I'm thirsty all the time." • "I've been vomiting and I have diarrhea— several times a day." • Change in mental status • Increased body temperature and pulse rate • Dry oral mucosa, cracked lips, furrowed tongue • Scanty, dark urine output • Sudden weight loss: 5 lb (2–3 kg) • Fluid output greater than fluid intake • Decreased skin turgor • Dry skin • Decreased blood pressure

• Maintain a urine specific gravity within normal range (1.005 to 1.030)

• Practice self-care behaviors to promote fluid, electrolyte, and acid–base balance; maintain adequate intake of fluid and electrolytes; respond appropriately to the body's signals of impending fluid, electrolyte, or acid–base imbalance

When an imbalance exists, the patient will:

• Relate relief of symptoms (specify) after implementation of treatment regimen (e.g., 1 month after decreasing sodium intake patient reports weight loss of 4 lb [1.8 kg])

• Exhibit signs and symptoms of restored balance or homeostasis after initiation of treatment

• Identify signs and symptoms of recurrence of imbalance with need to notify the primary health care provider

Implementing

Nursing interventions to prevent or correct fluid, electrolyte, and acid–base imbalances include dietary modification, modification of fluid intake, medication administration, IV therapy, blood and blood products replacement, administration of parenteral nutrition (TPN), allaying of anxiety as needed, and appropriate patient and family teaching. The accompanying box, Examples of Nursing Interventions and Nursing Outcomes Classifications (NIC/NOC) on page 1494, offers suggested nursing interventions and outcomes related to Deficient Fluid Volume.

Preventing Fluid and Electrolyte Imbalances

An adequate fluid intake and a well-balanced, nutritious diet with appropriate adjustments throughout the life cycle are essential to promoting fluid balance. The following are general measures to consider that will help prevent fluid imbalances:

• Be familiar with common life events that can lead to fluid imbalances, and observe the patient carefully. Infants are particularly vulnerable to fluid imbalances because body water accounts for a greater percentage of their weight, and fluid fluctuations are more common. Loss of fluid because of an illness can cause serious and life-threatening problems in infants.

• Note the patient's present fluid and food intake, and obtain a history of the patient's previous eating and drinking patterns. Learn whether the patient has been using a fad diet, which may lead to imbalances.

• Note whether the patient experiences excessive thirst or little or no thirst. Thirst, a subjective sensation, is an important factor determining water intake and, eventually, output through the kidneys. Although the thirst mechanism is poorly understood, both psychological and physiologic factors appear to be involved. An older patient is more susceptible to fluid-deficient conditions related to a less effective thirst mechanism (Tabloski, 2010). Be aware of excessive losses of fluids from the body, and attempt to prevent losses when

EXAMPLES OF NURSING INTERVENTIONS AND NURSING OUTCOMES CLASSIFICATIONS (NIC/NOC)

DEFICIENT FLUID VOLUME

Nursing Interventions	Nursing Outcomes
• Electrolyte management • Electrolyte monitoring • Fluid management • Fluid monitoring • Hypovolemia management • Intravenous therapy • Nutrition management	• Fluid balance • Hydration • Nutritional status: Food and fluid intake • Electrolyte and acid–base balance

Adapted from Moorhead, S., Johnson, M., Maas, M. L., & Swanson, E. (Eds). (2013). *Nursing Outcomes Classification (NOC)* (5th ed., pp. 495–496). St. Louis: Elsevier/Mosby; and Bulechek, G. M., Butcher, H. K., Dochterman, J. M., & Wagner, C. M. (Eds.). (2013). *Nursing interventions classification (NIC)* (6th ed., pp. 209–210, 236, 253, 386). St. Louis: Elsevier/Mosby. A full listing of nursing activities for each nursing outcome and intervention can be found in these books.

possible. Vomiting, pronounced perspiration, diarrhea, draining wounds, and excessive urinary output, for example, may cause excessive losses.

• Consider ways in which the patient's medical regimen may lead to fluid and electrolyte imbalances. For example, diuretics that stimulate urine formation may increase the elimination of both fluid and potassium. If food supplements high in potassium are not included in the diet or if potassium supplement drug therapy is not started, hypokalemia often follows.

• Learn whether the patient has been self-administering a treatment that may threaten fluid balance. Common practices that threaten fluid balance include the indiscriminate use of enemas, laxatives, antacids, and over-the-counter drugs or herbal medications to promote urination.

• Consider conditions with destructive effects on the body as threats to fluid balance. Examples include immobilization, trauma, burns, surgical procedures, and exposure to toxic agents.

• Teach patients to observe for signs and symptoms of fluid imbalances and to report them promptly. Examples include rapid weight gains and losses; swollen fingers, feet, and ankles; puffy eyelids; muscle weakness; change in skin sensations; and scanty or profuse urine production.

• Help patients and their families understand the significance of maintaining fluid balance and preventing imbalances.

• Be aware that normal physiologic changes associated with aging affect older patients' ability to maintain fluid balance. Fluid volume deficit is a common fluid

FOCUS ON THE OLDER ADULT

NURSING STRATEGIES TO ADDRESS AGE-RELATED CHANGES AFFECTING FLUID BALANCE

Age-Related Changes	Nursing Strategies
• Decreased sense of thirst • Medical conditions, e.g., heart failure or hypertension, requiring medications such as diuretics	• Ensure that oral intake is at least 1,500 mL for 24 hours. • Be aware of schedule for diagnostic tests (and associated dietary and fluid restrictions). • Offer fluids at regular intervals. • Replace fluids as necessary, either orally or intravenously. • Investigate individual fluid preferences. • Provide assistance or assistive devices for encouraging fluid intake.
Alterations in Renal Functioning • Loss of nephrons • Decreased renal blood flow	• Record accurate intake and output. • Note appearance and specific gravity of urine. • Check laboratory values for abnormal levels.
Alterations in Cardiac Functioning • Decreased efficiency as a pump • Volume intolerance	• Monitor breath sounds. • Assess for shortness of breath, wet productive cough, increased respiratory rate and work of breathing. • Monitor chest radiograph.

Table 39-9 | FLUID VOLUME DISTURBANCES

RISK FACTORS	ASSESSMENTS	NURSING INTERVENTIONS
Fluid Volume Deficit (Hypovolemia)		
GI: Vomiting, diarrhea, suction, fistulas	Thirst	Assess for presence or worsening of FVD.
Hemorrhage	Weight loss over short period	Administer oral fluids if indicated.
Excessive sweating	Weakness, fatigue, anorexia	If patient unable to eat and drink,
Skin trauma, burns, draining wounds	Dry mucous membranes	anticipate TPN or tube feedings to be
Third-space fluid shifts	Poor skin and tongue turgor	ordered.
Excessive laxative or diuretic use	Sunken eyes	Monitor patient's response to fluid intake,
Polyuria from renal disease or diuretics	Flat neck veins	either oral or parenteral.
Hyperglycemia	Urine output <30 mL/hr	Be alert for signs of fluid overload.
Change in mental status (unable to	Postural hypotension	Provide appropriate skin care.
gain access to fluids, depression,	Weak, rapid pulse	
confusion)	↑Urine specific gravity	
	↑Hematocrit	
	↑BUN	
	↑Serum sodium	
	Altered sensorium	
Fluid Volume Excess (Hypervolemia)		
Compromised regulatory mechanisms:	Weight gain over short period	Assess for presence or worsening of FVE.
renal failure, CHF, cirrhosis of liver,	Peripheral edema (may be pitting)	Encourage adherence to sodium-restricted
Cushing syndrome	Increased BP	and fluid-restricted diet, if ordered.
GI irrigation with hypotonic fluid	Shortness of breath	Avoid OTC drugs or check with primary
Excess IV fluids with sodium	Crackles and wheezes in lungs	care provider or pharmacist about
Corticosteroid therapy	Full, bounding pulse	sodium content.
Excessive ingestion of sodium-containing	Neck vein distention	Encourage rest periods.
substances in diet or sodium-containing	Polyuria if renal function is normal	Monitor patient's response to diuretics.
medications	Ascites, pleural effusion	Teach self-monitoring of weight and intake
	Pulmonary edema	and output.
	↓BUN (due to plasma dilution)	Attentive skin care.
	↓Hematocrit	Monitor respiratory status.
	↓Serum sodium	
	↓Urine specific gravity	

GI, gastrointestinal; BUN, blood urea nitrogen; FVD, fluid volume deficit; TPN, total parenteral nutrition; CHF, congestive heart failure; IV, intravenous; BP, blood pressure; FVE, fluid volume excess; OTC, over-the-counter.

and electrolyte disorder in this population. The accompanying Focus on the Older Adult box suggests specific nursing strategies to prevent and correct fluid and electrolyte imbalances.

Table 39-9 lists the risk factors, related assessments, and specific nursing interventions for fluid volume disturbances. Table 39-10 (on page 1496–1497) lists the risk factors, related assessments, and specific nursing interventions for electrolyte disturbances.

Developing a Dietary Plan

Teach patients about their health conditions and provide information and support to improve health literacy in patients. Refer to the accompanying Promoting Health Literacy box (on page 1498). Simple dietary changes may help to resolve fluid and electrolyte disturbances. After obtaining a nutritional assessment to identify actual or potential imbalances and food preferences (refer to Chapter 35), initiate teaching based on a nutritional plan that involves both the patient and the person who prepares the patient's meals. Include foods that help to resolve the fluid or electrolyte imbalance and that are acceptable to the patient. For example, for fluid volume deficit, increase foods with high water content (e.g., citrus fruit, melons, celery); for hypokalemia, increase foods with high potassium content (e.g., bananas, citrus fruits, apricots, melons, broccoli, potatoes, raisins, lima beans); and for hypernatremia, avoid foods high in sodium (e.g., processed cheese, lunch meats, canned soups and vegetables, salted snack foods) and eliminate the use of table salt.

When teaching the patient about foods to include or avoid, provide the patient with a written list for reference. Evaluate the patient's understanding of the teaching by having the patient identify foods that can be eaten freely or moderately as well as those to be avoided. Both the patient and person responsible for the patient's food preparation should be able to describe a 24-hour diet plan compatible with the recommended modifications.

Modifying Fluid Intake

Depending on the nature of the fluid or electrolyte imbalance, a patient's fluid intake may need to be increased,

(text continues on page 1498)

Table 39-10 ELECTROLYTE DISTURBANCES

RISK FACTORS	ASSESSMENTS	NURSING INTERVENTIONS
Hyponatremia		
Loss of sodium, as in:	Anorexia	Monitor fluid losses and gains.
Loss of GI fluids	Nausea and vomiting	Monitor for presence of GI and CNS symptoms.
Use of diuretics	Lethargy	Monitor serum Na levels.
Adrenal insufficiency	Confusion	Check urine specific gravity.
Gains of water, as in:	Muscle cramps	If able to eat, encourage foods and fluids with
Excessive administration of D_5W	Muscular twitching	high sodium content.
Water intoxication	Seizures	Be aware of sodium content of common IV fluids.
Disease states associated with	Coma	Avoid giving large water supplements to patients
SIADH (a form of hyponatremia)	Serum Na below 135 mEq/L	receiving isotonic tube feedings.
Pharmacologic agents that may	Urine specific gravity <1.010	Take seizure precautions when hyponatremia is
impair water excretion		severe.
Hypernatremia		
Water deprivation	Thirst	Monitor fluid losses and gains.
Increased sensible and insensible	Elevated body temperature	Observe for excessive intake of high sodium
water loss	Tongue dry and swollen, sticky	foods.
Ingestion of large amount of salt	mucous membranes	Monitor sodium content of prescriptions and OTC
Excessive parenteral administration	Severe hypernatremia	drugs.
of sodium-containing solutions	Disorientation	Monitor for changes in behavior such as restless-
Profuse sweating	Hallucinations	ness, lethargy, and disorientation.
Diabetes insipidus	Lethargy when undisturbed	Look for excessive thirst and elevated body
	Irritable and hyperactive	temperature.
	Focal or grand mal seizures	Monitor serum Na levels.
	Coma	Check urine specific gravity.
	Serum Na above 145 mEq/L	Give sufficient water with tube feedings to keep
	Urine specific gravity >1.015	serum Na and BUN at normal limits.
Hypokalemia		
Diarrhea	Fatigue	Monitor for occurrence of hypokalemia.
Vomiting or gastric suction	Anorexia, nausea, and vomiting	Assess digitalized patients at risk for hypokalemia,
Potassium-wasting diuretics	Muscle weakness	which potentiates the action of digitalis
Steroid administration and certain	Decreased bowel motility	Prevent hypokalemia by:
antibiotics	Cardiac arrhythmias	Encouraging extra K intake if possible
Poor intake as in anorexia nervosa,	Increased sensitivity to digitalis	Educating about abuse of laxatives and diuretics
alcoholism, potassium-free paren-	Polyuria, nocturia, dilute urine	Administer oral K supplements if ordered.
teral fluids	Postural hypotension	Be knowledgeable about danger of IV potassium
Polyuria	Serum K below 3.5 mEq/L	administration.
	ECG changes	
	Paresthesias or tender muscles	
Hyperkalemia		
Decreased potassium excretion	Vague muscle weakness	Monitor for hyperkalemia, which is life threatening.
Oliguric renal failure	Cardiac arrhythmias	Prevent hyperkalemia by:
Potassium-sparing diuretics	Paresthesias of face, tongue,	Following rules for safe administration of K
Hypoaldosteronism	feet, and hands	Avoiding giving patients with renal insufficiency
High potassium intake, especially in	Flaccid muscle paralysis	K-saving diuretics, K supplements, or salt
presence of renal insufficiency	GI symptoms such as nausea,	substitutes
Shift of potassium out of cells (aci-	intermittent intestinal colic, or	Cautioning about foods high in potassium content
dosis, tissue trauma, malignant	diarrhea may occur	
cell lysis)	Serum K >5.0 mEq/L	
Hypocalcemia		
Surgical hypoparathyroidism	Trousseau and Chvostek signs	Take seizure precautions when hypocalcemia is
Malabsorption	Numbness and tingling of fingers	severe.
Vitamin D deficiency	and toes	Monitor condition of airway.
Acute pancreatitis	Mental changes	Take safety precautions if confusion is present.
Excessive administration of citrated	Seizures	Educate people at risk for osteoporosis about the
blood	Spasm of laryngeal muscles	need for dietary calcium intake.
Alkalotic states	ECG changes	Discuss calcium-losing aspects of nicotine and
	Cramps in muscles of extremities	alcohol use.
	Total serum calcium <8.5 mg/dL	

Table 39-10   ELECTROLYTE DISTURBANCES *continued*

RISK FACTORS	ASSESSMENTS	NURSING INTERVENTIONS
Hypercalcemia		
Hyperparathyroidism	Muscular weakness	Increase mobilization when feasible.
Malignant neoplastic disease	Tiredness, lethargy	Encourage sufficient oral intake.
Prolonged immobilization	Constipation	Discourage excessive consumption of milk
Large doses of vitamin D	Anorexia, nausea, and vomiting	products.
Overuse of calcium supplements	Decreased memory and attention	Encourage bulk in the diet.
Thiazide diuretics	span	Take safety precautions if confusion is present.
	Polyuria and polydipsia	Be alert for signs of digitalis toxicity in hypercalce-
	Renal stones	mic patients.
	Neurotic behavior	Force fluids to prevent formation of renal stones.
	Cardiac arrest	
	Serum calcium >10.5 mg/dL	
Hypomagnesemia		
Chronic alcoholism	Neuromuscular irritability	Assess for magnesium deficit because it predis-
Intestinal malabsorption	Increased reflexes	poses patient to digitalis toxicity.
Diarrhea	Coarse tremors	Take seizure precautions if necessary.
Nasogastric suction	Seizures	Monitor condition of airway because laryngeal
Drugs	Cardiac manifestations	stridor can occur.
Thiazide diuretics	Tachyarrhythmias	Educate the patient if abuse of diuretics or laxa-
Aminoglycoside antibiotics	Increased susceptibility to digi-	tives is a problem.
Excessive doses of vitamin D	talis toxicity	Educate about intake of foods rich in magnesium.
Citrate preservative in blood	Mental changes	
	Disorientation	
	Mood changes	
	Serum magnesium <1.3 mEq/L	
Hypermagnesemia		
Renal failure	Early sign is serum magnesium	If hypermagnesemia is present, be alert for low BP
Adrenal insufficiency	level of 3–5 mEq/L	and shallow respirations, lethargy, drowsiness,
Excessive magnesium administra-	Flushing and sense of skin warmth	and coma.
tion during treatment of eclampsia	Hypotension	Do not give magnesium-containing medications to
Hemodialysis with hard water or	Depressed respirations	patient with renal failure or compromised renal
dialysate high in magnesium	Drowsiness, hypoactive reflexes,	function.
content	and muscular weakness	Be cautious of OTC drugs.
	Cardiac abnormalities	Check deep tendon reflexes frequently.
Hypophosphatemia		
Glucose administration	Cardiomyopathy	Be aware that severely hypophosphatemic
Refeeding after starvation	Acute respiratory failure	patients are at greater risk for infection.
Parenteral nutrition	Seizures	Administer IV phosphate products cautiously.
Alcohol withdrawal	Decreased tissue oxygenation	Introduce parenteral nutrition cautiously in patients
Diabetic ketoacidosis	Joint stiffness	who are malnourished.
Respiratory alkalosis	Serum phosphate <2.5 mg/dL	Monitor for diarrhea when taking oral supplements.
		Sudden increase in serum phosphate level can
		cause hypocalcemia.
Hyperphosphatemia		
Renal failure	Short-term consequences:	Monitor for signs of tetany.
Chemotherapy	Symptoms of tetany, such as	Be aware that soft tissue calcification can be a
Large intake of milk	tingling of the fingertips and	long-term complication of chronically elevated
Excessive intake of phosphate-	around the mouth, numbness,	serum phosphate levels.
containing laxatives (Fleet	and muscle spasms	Instruct patients that use of phosphate-containing
phosphosoda)	Long-term consequences:	laxatives can result in hyperphosphatemia.
Large vitamin D intake	Precipitation of calcium phos-	Avoid foods high in phosphorus content.
Hyperthyroidism	phate in nonosseous sites such	
	as the kidneys, joints, arteries,	
	skin, or cornea.	
	Serum phosphate >4.5 mg/dL	

CNS, central nervous system; ECG, electrocardiographic; OTC, over-the-counter; SIADH, syndrome of inappropriate antidiuretic hormone.
Adapted from Hinkle, J.L., & Cheever, K.H. (2014). *Brunner & Suddarth's textbook of medical–surgical nursing* (13th ed.). Philadelphia: Wolters Kluwer Health/Lippincott Williams & Wilkins; Metheny, N. M. (2012). *Fluid and electrolyte balance: Nursing Considerations* (5th ed.). Sudbury, MA: Jones & Bartlett Learning; and Grossman, S., & Porth, C.M. (2014). Porth's pathophysiology: concepts of altered health states. (9th ed.). Philadelphia: Wolters Kluwer Health/Lippincott Williams & Wilkins.

PROMOTING HEALTH LITERACY

IN PATIENTS WITH FLUID OR ELECTROLYTE IMBALANCES

Patient Scenario

Shamala Johnson, 58, had been experiencing complications from diabetes for the previous 10 years. She tells the nurse, "I really thought that I had things under control until lately. I can't believe one more thing has happened." Ms. Johnson was admitted to the hospital with end-stage renal failure. "I guess I knew this was coming eventually, but did not expect it so soon!" She initially received dialysis via a temporary dialysis catheter, but had surgery yesterday for an A-V shunt. Her current plan of care includes dietary modifications, including potassium, sodium, protein, and fluid restrictions. The nurse has assisted her with making dietary choices based on the hospital menus, and has arranged a consult with the dietitian. The patient asks, "Do you think I will have to keep this up at home? How will I manage to get the right food? And liquids, can I drink anything? I don't understand this at all!"

Nursing Considerations: *Tips for Improving Health Literacy*

Confirm her dietary modifications for after discharge. Provide Ms. Johnson with easy-to-read information about living with renal disease, and managing fluid and electrolytes, as well as protein restrictions. Encourage her to ask her primary care provider as many questions as needed to understand her condition. Explain that there are things she can do to feel in control and follow the suggested regimen. Provide information and resources for support at home. Encourage Ms. Johnson to ask her primary care provider the following three questions:

- What is my main problem?
- What do I need to do?
- Why is it important for me to do this?

What additional measures can you take to help increase health literacy in this patient? What other measures would be helpful for this patient if she did not speak English, could not read, or had other learning deficits?

---

decreased, or modified in terms of types of fluids ingested. Nursing responsibilities include:

- Identifying the appropriate fluid modification (e.g., with certain illnesses, the primary care provider may order fluid directives, such as "Restrict fluids to 1,000 mL daily")
- Determining whether the patient understands the rationale for the fluid modification, is motivated to follow the modification, and is capable of adhering to the plan (e.g., a bedridden patient who needs to increase fluid intake cannot do this independently)
- Developing and implementing a plan of care based on the preceding information

The accompanying PICO in Practice box highlights an example of evidence-based decision-making regarding nursing intervention for a patient with a fluid imbalance.

INCREASING FLUIDS

Increasing fluids involves an above-average intake of fluids. The usual order reads, "Encourage fluids" and indicates the amount of fluid the patient is to have in each 24-hour period. Typically, the plan of care specifies the amount of fluid to be ingested in 24 hours (for hospitalized patients, shift totals are helpful [e.g., 7–3, 1,200 mL, 3–11, 900 mL; 11–7, 300 mL]) and the patient's food preferences. Choose or assist with choosing fluids that best provide the calories and electrolytes needed by the patient.

Several techniques are recommended to help the patient take more than average amounts of fluids. Begin by explaining to the patient in understandable terms the rationale for the increased fluids and the specific goal of taking the daily amount of fluid prescribed. This explanation provides the patient with a greater understanding of

the reason for the increase in fluid intake. In addition, this information helps motivate the patient to comply with the treatment. Together with the patient, develop short-term goals for accomplishing the increased fluid intake. For example, the patient will drink a glass of water every hour, a particular beverage by the time a television program is finished, or a pitcher of water by lunch. In general, patients are more likely to reach set goals when they have been involved in setting these goals.

Ensure that a proportionately larger amount of fluid is offered during the early hours of the patient's waking day, rather than large amounts before bedtime. The patient can usually take fluids relatively easily after having few or no fluids during sleeping hours. However, large amounts of fluid at night interferes with the patient's ability to rest and sleep by being awakened during the night with the need to urinate.

Offering a variety of fluids served at the appropriate temperature is helpful, as is allowing the patient to indicate a preference; these measures help the patient comply with the treatment regimen. The likelihood for success also is increased because the patient is more likely to drink more when some liquids are iced and cold and when coffee or tea is hot. Variety also adds interest and makes increasing fluids more palatable. If patients dislike taking fluids (a common problem with children) or have swallowing difficulties, offering a gelatin dessert, flavored frozen water (Popsicles), water ice, or the like may meet with more success.

Always have fluids readily available for the patient. Take care to avoid a situation in which patients are unable to secure their own fluids (left with an unfilled water pitcher, an empty glass, a full pitcher out of reach, or a pitcher too heavy to lift). In addition, use attractive, clean,

PICO IN PRACTICE

ASKING CLINICAL QUESTIONS

Scenario: You are a staff nurse who works in an emergency department (ED) on the evening shift. One evening, a 3-year-old child is brought to the ED by her mother with complaints of 3 days of diarrhea and vomiting. The child's mother states that several children at her child's daycare center have been sick with a similar "stomach bug" over the course of the past week. The child's mother reports that the child last vomited 8 hours ago when she tried giving her some milk to drink and the child has not had anything to eat or drink since that time. The last episode of diarrhea was this past hour, and the child's mother reports that there may have been some urine mixed with the stool. The child's mucous membranes appear dry and she is lethargic but responds appropriately and lucidly to a variety of stimuli. The mother tells you: "When my oldest child was sick like this a few years ago, I took him here and the doctor gave him an IV (*sic*—peripheral intravenous line) and that seemed to perk him right up. I want you to ask the doctor if you can do that for my daughter." You believe the child is only mildly dehydrated based on your assessment findings and wonder whether oral rehydration should be tried as first-line therapy in treating this child.

- POPULATION: 3-year-old mildly dehydrated children
- INTERVENTION: Oral rehydration
- COMPARISON: IV rehydration
- OUTCOME: Effective rehydration

PICO Question: Is oral rehydration as effective as IV rehydration as a first-line intervention in treating mildly dehydrated 3-year-old children?

Finding: From the National Guidelines Clearinghouse: Cincinnati Children's Hospital Medical Center. (2011). Evidence-based clinical care guideline for prevention and management of acute gastroenteritis (AGE) in children aged 2 months through 18 years. Cincinnati, OH: Cincinnati Children's Hospital Medical Center.

This guideline specifies that children aged 2 months through 18 years of age with mild dehydration be treated with commercial oral rehydration solutions if tolerated and if losses of bodily fluids are greater than oral intake until rehydration is achieved. Milk should not be used as a rehydration fluid. Intravenous hydration is only indicated in severely dehydrated children or if the child's estimated fluid output continues to exceed oral intake after oral rehydration is tried. A clinical algorithm for assessing and treating children with acute gastroenteritis is included in this guideline.

Level of Evidence: Level I

Recommendation: You recommend to the ED physician that this child be treated first with commercial oral rehydration solutions as specified in this guideline. You also recommend that the ED Policy and Procedure Committee adopt the tenets of the clinical algorithm for management of children with acute gastroenteritis that are found within this guideline.

---

and easy-to-handle cups, glasses, and straws and practices that help to encourage the patient's desire to take fluids.

Patient participation in care promotes autonomy and self-esteem. Therefore, have the patient help keep a record of intake when possible. This often serves as a motivating factor to increase fluid intake. Offer support, understanding, and encouragement in providing nursing care because forcing fluid intake for the person experiencing no thirst can be uncomfortable.

Increasing the fluid intake of patients is among the most common nursing interventions. Use creativity to assist the patient and family to reach desired goals. Having a tea party may be a helpful strategy to use when encouraging a child to increase fluids. When determining the patient's increased fluid intake, be sure to include fluids replaced through nasogastric, gastrostomy, or jejunostomy tubes in the fluid balance summary.

RESTRICTING FLUIDS

Restricting the patient's fluid intake is sometimes necessary. The usual order reads, "Restrict fluids" and indicates the amount of fluid the patient is to have in each 24-hour period.

Several techniques are recommended to help patients restrict their intake of fluids. As with the method for increasing fluids, begin by explaining to the patient in understandable terms the rationale for the fluid restriction and the specified daily amount of fluid prescribed. Then work with the patient to develop short-term outcomes for accomplishing the overall task. Discuss with the patient the time intervals at which fluids will be served. Usually, offering fluids at 1- or 2-hour intervals and between meals is best because food often helps to relieve some feelings of thirst. Provide the fluid in small glasses or cups so that the container appears to contain more fluid than it actually does. Using ice chips also is helpful. Ice chips are about twice the volume of water in its liquid state and help to quench thirst. Remember to include the ice chips as part of the patient's fluid intake. If appropriate, encourage the patient to participate in one's own care by helping to keep a record of intake.

 CONSIDER Mr. Park, the patient who received too much IV fluid. As a result of this excess fluid intake and his subsequent development of problems, the nurse would be alert to the possibility that fluid restriction may be ordered. If this occurs, the nurse needs to ensure that Mr. Park understands the reason for the restriction. ●

Patients who need to restrict fluid intake often report thirst or dry mouth. Avoid offering patients dry, salty, or sweet foods and fluids because such items tend to increase thirst. Also, attempt to divert the patient's attention from thirst by involving the patient in activities, and keep fluids not intended for the patient out of sight. Provide understanding, support, and encouragement because limiting fluid intake is uncomfortable for a thirsty person.

Provide oral hygiene at regular intervals so that the patient's mouth remains clean and moist. Lubricate the lips and mucous membranes as indicated. If the patient is capable and cooperative, allow the patient to rinse the mouth with water without swallowing the fluid, to avoid exceeding the intake limit. Avoid hard candy and gum, as these actually contribute to drying of the mouth membranes.

Just as with fluid increases, fluid limits should also have shift totals set. This prevents one shift from taking all of the patient's allotted fluid and prepares the patient ahead of time for the fluid limits.

Administering Medications

Patients with fluid, electrolyte, and acid–base imbalances are often prescribed medications as part of the therapeutic regimen. Be knowledgeable about and understand the therapeutic effects of mineral–electrolyte preparations and diuretics, and appreciate the risk for life-threatening adverse effects. It is also important to consider the impact of other medications, such as steroids and hormone replacements, on fluid and electrolyte balance.

MINERAL–ELECTROLYTE PREPARATIONS

Mineral–electrolyte preparations are frequently prescribed to correct electrolyte imbalances. Nursing responsibilities include:

- Accurate administration of the medications, following manufacturer's guidelines: for example, dilute potassium supplements to disguise the unpleasant taste and decrease gastric irritation, monitor ABGs for increased pH after each 50–100 mEq of sodium bicarbonate to avoid overtreatment and metabolic alkalosis.
- Understand the intended therapeutic effect and evaluate the effectiveness of the therapy through patient assessment: for example, with magnesium sulfate, assess for decreased restlessness and irritability, decreased muscle tremors, control of convulsions.
- Assess for adverse effects: for example, with sodium chloride injection, observe for hypernatremia).
- Understand and appreciate the risks associated with administration and the appropriate precautions to avoid adverse outcomes: for example, intravenous potassium is never administered via intravenous bolus and the infusion rate for intravenous potassium chloride solutions requires careful monitoring. The maximum rate should be 10 mEq/hr for patients without cardiac monitoring. An administration error can result

in sudden hyperkalemia, leading to a fatal cardiac arrhythmia (Vallerand, Sanoski, & Deglin, 2013).
- Assess for drug interactions: for example, drugs that increase the effects of minerals and electrolytes include acidifying agents, alkalinizing agents, cation exchange resin, iron salts, and potassium salts Also, some minerals and electrolytes will enhance the effects of other medications, such as muscle relaxants.
- Teach patients about their prescribed mineral and electrolyte preparations and associated self-care behaviors.

DIURETICS

Diuretics are drugs that increase renal excretion of water, sodium, and other electrolytes. Although helpful in treating patients with fluid volume excess, they increase the risk for fluid volume deficit and serious electrolyte deficiencies. Careful monitoring of fluid intake, urine output, and serum electrolytes is essential for patient safety. Direct particular attention toward the patient's serum potassium level. It is important to provide patient education to any patient receiving diuretic therapy, including the rationale for the therapy, precautions, and side effects.

Administering Intravenous (IV) Therapy

A relatively common form of therapy for handling fluid disturbances is the use of infused intravenous solutions. The physician or other licensed health care professional with prescriptive privileges is responsible for prescribing the type and volume of solution to be administered. The nurse is responsible for initiating, monitoring, and discontinuing the therapy. The nurse is also responsible for critically evaluating all patient orders prior to administration. Any concerns regarding the type or amount of therapy prescribed should be immediately and clearly communicated to the prescribing practitioner. For example, if a patient's potassium level is noted to be elevated and the patient is prescribed a potassium-containing intravenous solution such as lactated Ringer's, the nurse should notify the prescribing practitioner of the laboratory result and request a revision of the patient order. Refer to the Reflective Practice box on page 1472.

As with other therapeutic agents, the nurse must understand the patient's need for intravenous therapy, the type of solution being used, its desired effect, and potential adverse reactions. The contents of selected IV solutions are listed, along with comments about their use, in Table 39-11.

 THINK back to Grace Gilligan, the woman with nausea and vomiting. The nurse could expect that this patient is high risk for fluid and electrolyte imbalances. What would be benefits and risks of administering the various IV solutions in Table 39-11 to this patient? How would you assess if the IV therapy were having its desired effect (improving the patient's condition)? ●

Table 39-11 SELECTED IV SOLUTIONS

SOLUTION	COMMENTS
Isotonic Solutions	
Total osmolality close to that of the ECF; replace the ECF	
5% dextrose in water (D_5W)	Supplies about 170 cal/L and free water (contains 50 g of glucose)
	Used in fluid loss, dehydration, hypernatremia
	Should not be used in excessive volumes because it does not contain any sodium; thus the fluid dilutes the amount of sodium in the serum. Brain swelling, or *hyponatremic encephalopathy*, can develop rapidly and cause death unless it is promptly recognized and treated.
0.9% NaCl (normal saline)	Not desirable as routine maintenance solution because it provides only Na^+ and Cl^-, which are provided in excessive amounts.
	May be used to expand temporarily the extracellular compartment if circulatory insufficiency is a problem; also used to treat hypovolemia, metabolic alkalosis, hyponatremia, hypochloremia.
	Used with administration of blood transfusions
Lactated Ringer's solution	Contains multiple electrolytes in about the same concentrations as found in plasma (note that this solution is lacking in Mg^{2+} and PO_4^{3-})
	Used in the treatment of hypovolemia, burns, and fluid lost from gastrointestinal sources
	Useful in treating metabolic acidosis
Hypotonic Solutions	
Hypotonic to plasma; replace ICF	
0.33% NaCl (⅓-strength normal saline)	Provides Na^+, Cl^-, and free water
	Na^+ and Cl^- allows kidneys to select and retain needed amounts
	Free water desirable as aid to kidneys in elimination of solutes
	Used in treating hypernatremia
0.45% NaCl (½-strength normal saline)	A hypotonic solution that provides Na^+, Cl^-, and free water
	Used as a basic fluid for maintenance needs
	Often used to treat hypernatremia (because this solution contains a small amount of Na^+, it dilutes the plasma sodium while not allowing it to drop too rapidly)
Hypertonic Solutions	
Hypertonic to plasma	
5% dextrose in 0.45% NaCl	Used to maintain fluid intake
10% dextrose in water ($D_{10}W$)	Supplies 340 cal/L
	Used in peripheral parenteral nutrition (PPN)
5% dextrose in 0.9% NaCl	Used to treat SIADH
	Can temporarily be used to treat hypovolemia if plasma expander is not available

Adapted from Hinkle, J.L., & Cheever, K.H. (2014). *Brunner & Suddarth's textbook of medical–surgical nursing* (13th ed.). Philadelphia: Wolters Kluwer Health/Lippincott Williams & Wilkins; Metheny, N. M. (2012). *Fluid and electrolyte balance: Nursing Considerations* (5th ed.). Sudbury, MA: Jones & Bartlett Learning; and *Fluids & electrolytes made incredibly easy!* (5th ed.). (2011). Philadelphia: Wolters Kluwer Health/Lippincott Williams & Wilkins.

EQUIPMENT

Sterile technique must be observed when accessing a vein to avoid possible catheter-related infection. Disposable infusion tubing and needles are used to help eliminate many possible sources of contamination and to reduce the cost of equipment aftercare.

Equipment varies according to the manufacturer. Be familiar with the equipment used in the facility or home setting. Typically, most solutions for infusions are dispensed in 1-L or 500-mL flexible or rigid plastic containers. Because plastic bags collapse under atmospheric pressure as the solution enters the patient's vein, they do not require a vent for air to enter to replace fluid flowing from the container. Small 50-, 100-, and 250-mL solution bags are available to administer intermittent IV medications (such as antibiotics given by IV piggyback).

Some medications bond with the plastic in IV bags. Therefore, glass bottles are required for these medications. Glass bottles do not collapse under atmospheric pressure and thus require a vent to allow air to enter the bottle as the fluid leaves the bottle.

IV administration tubing is used to attach the IV container to the patient's venous access. A basic administration set is illustrated in Figure 39-10. Infusion pumps usually require tubing specific for the device. Pump tubing shares many of the same features as tubing used for gravity infusion. Normally, an IV administration set includes a spike or piercing pin to access the IV container, a drip chamber for observing fluid drops, a slide clamp to stop fluid flow, a roller clamp to manually regulate the rate of flow, a filter, several injection ports for administration of medications or additional IV fluids, and a connector at the end of the tubing to connect with the venous access (preferably Luer lock design, with threads that securely screw on). Pump tubing also includes a mechanism that fits into the electronic device to control the infusion rate.

FIGURE 39-10. Basic administration tubing for intravenous therapy. *(Photo by B. Proud.)*

A variety of needles and catheters are commonly used for peripheral IV infusions. IV catheters are plastic tubes that have been mounted on a needle or are threaded through a needle for insertion. Once inserted, the needle is withdrawn, and the flexible catheter remains in the vein. The over-the-needle catheter is easy to insert and stable. Single- or double-winged infusion needles (butterflies) are short-beveled, thin-walled needles with plastic flaps. They may be used with short-term therapy or single-dose administration (Infusion Nurses Society [INS], 2011). Butterfly or scalp vein needles are not flexible, thus are more likely to infiltrate. Other equipment necessary to start an IV infusion is listed in Skill 39-1 on pages 1520–1527.

Many devices are available that minimize the potential for injury and promote safety when connecting, accessing, or disposing of IV equipment, including needleless systems and needle-housing systems in which the needle is recessed and protected. Refer to Chapters 26 and 28 for additional information about protective measures and use of IV equipment related to medication administration.

VASCULAR ACCESS DEVICES

Many different options for vascular access devices (IV catheters) are available for delivery of solutions and medications into a vein. The length of time the infusion therapy is needed, the type of medication or product that will be delivered intravenously, and the patient's health status as well as individualized needs determine which option is used. In addition, decisions on insertion site and catheter type should be guided by what will pose the least risk for IV complications (Dychter, Gold, Carson & Haller, 2012; INS, 2011; Koshy, 2011). The nursing care that is required will depend on the type of device or IV catheter that is utilized. Vascular access devices fall into three main categories: peripheral venous catheters, midline catheters, and central venous access devices (CVADs).

Peripheral Venous Catheters. Over-the-needle catheters, previously discussed, are the most common type of peripheral vascular catheter used. When infusion therapy will be brief, a short (<3 inches) peripheral catheter is placed in a peripheral vein. The tip of a short peripheral catheter terminates in the peripheral vein. This device is not appropriate for certain therapies—vesicant chemotherapy, drugs that are classified as irritants, or TPN, for example. Rotate the insertion site every 72 to 96 hours for an adult (O'Grady et al., 2011). For a child, the site can remain in place until the IV intervention is completed unless a complication develops (Centers for Disease Control and Prevention [CDC], 2011). The smallest-gauge device is usually selected to minimize trauma to the vein (see Chapter 28 for more discussion on gauges).

Midline Peripheral Catheters. Midline catheters are inserted peripherally, normally just above or below the antecubital fossa into the proximal basilica or cephalic veins. These catheters are longer (>3 inches) than peripheral venous catheters, and the distal tip terminates in the basilic, cephalic, or brachial vein, at or below the axillary level and distal to the shoulder (INS, 2011). These are not considered to be central lines and should not be used to infuse vesicants, hyperosmolar, or irritating solutions. Recommendations for dwell time at a particular insertion site vary from 1 to 4 weeks (Alexandrou et al., 2011; INS; 2011). Replace midline catheters only when there is a specific indication, such as phlebitis or system compromise (O'Grady et al., 2011). Follow facility policy for rotation of midline catheter insertion site.

Central Venous Access Devices. Central venous (vascular) access devices (CVADs) are an integral component of patient care in acute, ambulatory, and subacute care settings, as well as in the home and long-term care facilities. They provide access for a variety of IV fluids, medications, blood products, and TPN solutions and allow a means for hemodynamic monitoring and blood sampling. CVADs are devices where the tip of the catheter terminates in the central venous circulation, usually in the superior vena cava near its junction with the right atrium (INS, 2011). The use of ultrasound technology during insertion can increase success rates and decrease insertion-related complications, and is being used more frequently in practice (INS). The CDC (2011) recommends the use of ultrasound guidance, by those fully trained in its technique, to place central venous catheters (if this technology is available) to reduce the number of cannulation attempts and mechanical complications. All CVADs require radiographic confirmation of position after insertion and before use. The patient's diagnosis, the type of care that is required, and other factors (e.g., limited venous access, irritating drugs, patient request, or the need for long-term intermittent infusions) determine the type of CVAD used. Midline catheters, peripherally inserted central catheter (PICC) lines, and other central venous devices are not routinely changed in order to reduce the risk of infection (O'Grady et al., 2011). Changing these catheters may pose a greater risk than leaving the catheter in place. However, any central venous catheter may

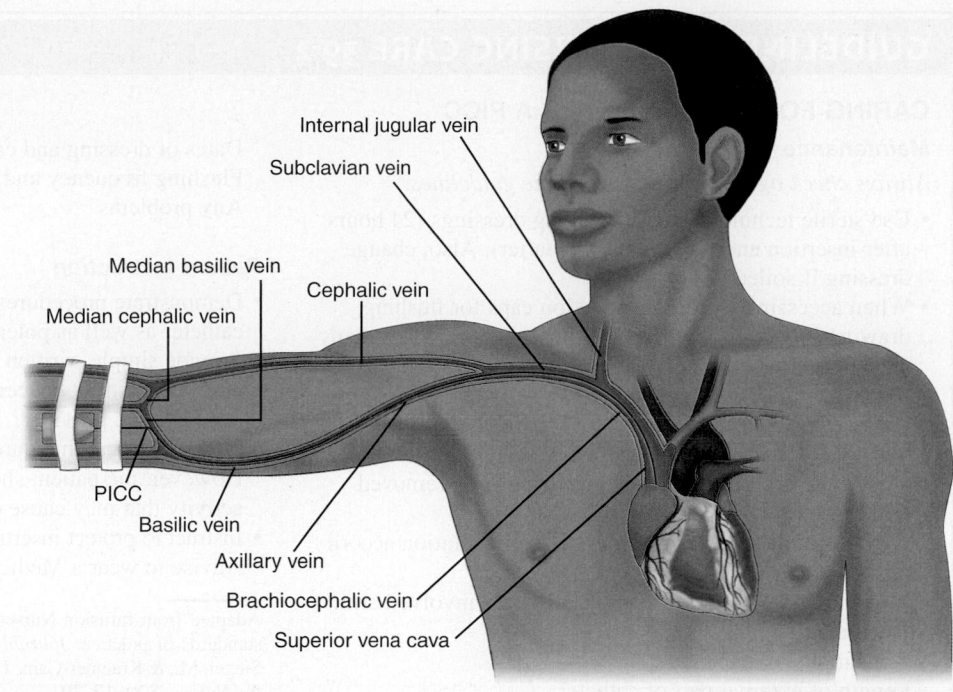

FIGURE 39-11. Placement of a peripherally inserted central catheter (PICC).

be replaced if suspicion of a catheter-related bloodstream infection exists. Types of CVADs include the following:

- PICCs
- Nontunneled percutaneous central venous catheters
- Tunneled central venous catheters
- Implanted ports

PICCs are a type of CVAD, >20 cm depending on patient size, that can be introduced into a peripheral vein (usually the basilic, median cubital, brachial, or cephalic veins (Fig. 39-11). A specially trained registered nurse or physician can insert this type of catheter. A PICC may be inserted in interventional radiology units or, in some institutions, at the bedside. Radiographic verification is always required before use. PICCs may have single or multiple lumens. They are used extensively in the home for IV therapy and have become an increasingly popular venous access device in acute-care settings, especially for patients requiring long-term IV therapy (6 weeks to 6 months). PICCs are replaced only as needed, that is, when the catheter is no longer patent or the site looks infected.

Indications for use of PICCs include administration of IV antibiotics for an extended period (2–6 weeks), infusion of parenteral nutrition, chemotherapy, continuous narcotic infusions, vesicants, hyperosmolar solutions, blood components, other specific medications (e.g., vasopressors, anticoagulants), and long-term rehydration. Advantages of using a PICC include less risk of complications, such as infection and pneumothorax, because the catheter is inserted peripherally (Hammond, 2004). PICCs are also cost effective and provide adequate hemodilution for medications. Guidelines for Nursing Care 39-2 (on page 1504) provides information related to nursing care for a patient with a PICC.

Nontunneled percutaneous central venous catheters (Fig. 39-12) have a shorter dwell time (3–10 days). These catheters can have double, triple, or quadruple lumens and are >8 cm, depending on patient size. They are introduced through the skin into the internal jugular, subclavian, or femoral veins. Catheters inserted via the femoral vein should have the distal tip dwell in the thoracic inferior vena cava above the level of the diaphragm (INS, 2011). They are mainly used in emergency settings (Gabriel, 2008a); the CDC (2011) recommends avoiding the femoral vein for central venous access in adult patients. This type of central venous catheter is associated with a high

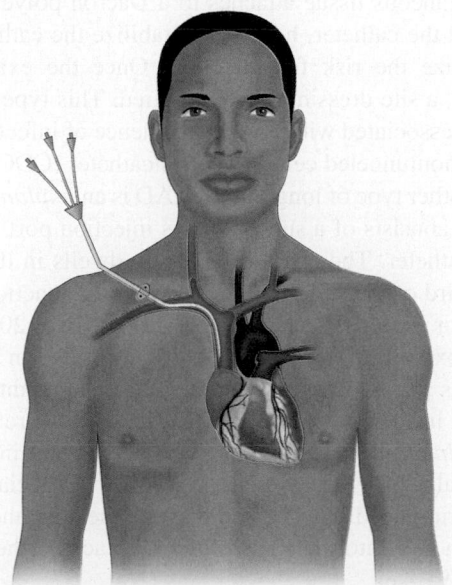

FIGURE 39-12. Placement of a triple-lumen nontunneled percutaneous central venous catheter.

GUIDELINES FOR NURSING CARE 39-2

CARING FOR A PATIENT WITH A PICC

Maintenance

Always check agency policy for specific guidelines.

- Use sterile technique when changing dressings (24 hours after insertion and 3 to 7 days thereafter). Also, change dressing if soiled or loose.
- When accessing lumens or injection caps for flushing, drawing blood, or changing the dressing, know that many agencies require the nurse and patient to wear a mask.
- Keep external portion of catheter coiled under dressing.
- Change catheter caps every 3 to 7 days based on frequency of access and facility policy. Many agencies have a policy to replace caps once they have been removed (e.g., when blood is drawn).
- Flush using normal saline and/or heparin solution according to facility policy.
- Avoid blood pressure measurement in the involved arm.
- Document:
  Appearance of site
  Length of external part of catheter

Dates of dressing and cap change
Flushing frequency and routine
Any problems

Patient Instruction

- Demonstrate procedures, care, and maintenance of PICC catheter as well as potential complications.
- Provide simple, written instructions for patient/caregiver at home. Instruct concerning reasons to notify nurse or primary care provider.
- Emphasize that there are minimal activity restrictions. However, the patient should avoid strenuous physical activity that may cause displacement of the catheter.
- Instruct to protect insertion site when showering or bathing.
- Advise to wear a Medic-Alert tag if use is long term.

Adapted from Infusion Nurses Society (INS). (2011). Infusion nursing standards of practice. *Journal of Infusion Nursing, 34*(Suppl: 1S); and Siegel, M., & Kraemer-Cain, J. (2011). PICC line care at home. *Advance for Nurses, 8*(8), 17–20.

---

risk for complications, particularly infection, accounting for most catheter-related bloodstream infections (CDC, 2011). Pneumothorax is another potential complication when the catheter is placed in the subclavian vein.

A *tunneled central venous catheter,* intended for long-term use, is implanted into the internal or external jugular or subclavian vein. The length of this catheter is >8 cm (approximately 90 cm, on average), depending on patient size, and is tunneled in subcutaneous tissue under the skin (usually the mid-chest area) for 3 to 6 inches to its exit site (Fig. 39-13). This device is initially sutured into place, but after 7 to 14 days, the sutures are removed. Subcutaneous tissue attaches to a Dacron polyester cuff around the catheter, helping to stabilize the catheter and minimize the risk for infection. Once the exit site is healed, a site dressing is not required. This type of catheter is associated with a lower incidence of infection than is the nontunneled central venous catheter (CDC, 2011).

Another type of long-term CVAD is an *implanted port,* which consists of a subcutaneous injection port attached to a catheter. The distal catheter tip dwells in the lower one-third of the superior vena cava to the junction of the superior vena cava and the right atrium (INS, 2011), and the proximal end or port is usually implanted in a subcutaneous pocket of the upper chest wall. Implanted ports placed in the antecubital area of the arm are referred to as *peripheral access system ports.* When not in use, no external parts of the system are visible. A special angled noncoring needle is inserted through the skin and rubber septum and into the port reservoir to access the system (Fig. 39-14).

Implanted ports require minimal care, but the discomfort related to accessing the port may be a disadvan-

tage for some patients. According to the CDC (2011), implanted ports are associated with the lowest risk for catheter-related bloodstream infections, and patients report improved self-image. Surgery is required for catheter removal.

PERIPHERAL VENOUS CATHETER SITE SELECTION

The nurse initiating a peripheral venous access needs to assess for the safest, most appropriate location for each particular patient. The suitability of particular

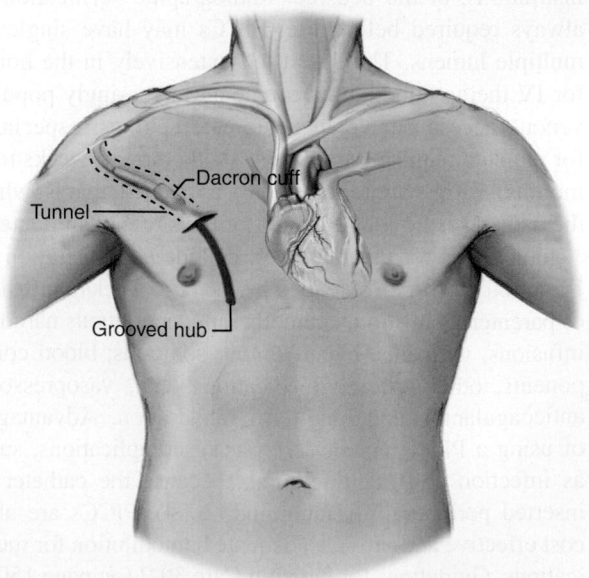

FIGURE 39-13. Placement of a tunneled central venous catheter.

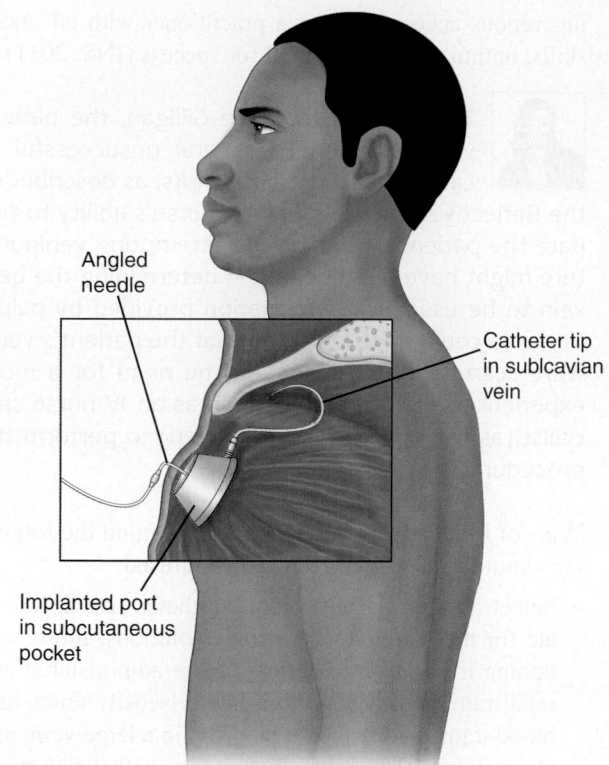

FIGURE 39-14. Placement of an implanted port with the tip in the subclavian vein. An angled needle is inserted through the skin and septum into the port.

veins for peripheral IV infusions varies with individual circumstances. Determine selection after considering the following factors.

Accessibility of a Vein.

Keep in mind the following guidelines related to peripheral venous catheters and access sites:

- Determine the most desirable accessible vein. The dorsal and ventral surfaces of the upper extremities are appropriate sites for infusion (INS, 2011). The superficial veins on the dorsal aspect of the hand can also be used successfully for some people, but can be more painful (I.V. Rounds, 2008). Avoid the ventral surface of the wrist and the lateral surface of the wrist for approximately 4 to 5 inches because of the potential risk for nerve damage. Initiate venous access in the distal areas of the upper extremities, as this allows for future sites proximal to the previous insertion site (INS, 2011). Figure 39-15A illustrates common infusion sites on the arm and hand.
- Generally, either arm may be used for IV therapy. Usually the nondominant arm is selected for patient comfort and to limit movement in the impacted extremity. For example, if the patient is right handed, the IV is preferably placed on the left extremity to improve the patient's ability to complete activities of daily living. This is particularly important if the duration of infusion is expected to be prolonged.

- The use of an extremity for intravenous therapy may be contraindicated in some circumstances. For example, patients with a history of breast cancer with same-side surgical axillary lymph node removal; patients with burns, infections, or traumatic injury to the extremity; and patients with upper extremity arteriovenous fistulas or catheters for dialysis treatment will not be able to have an intravenous catheter placed on the impacted extremity.
- Do not use the antecubital veins if another vein is available. They are not a good choice for infusion because flexion of the patient's arm can displace the IV catheter

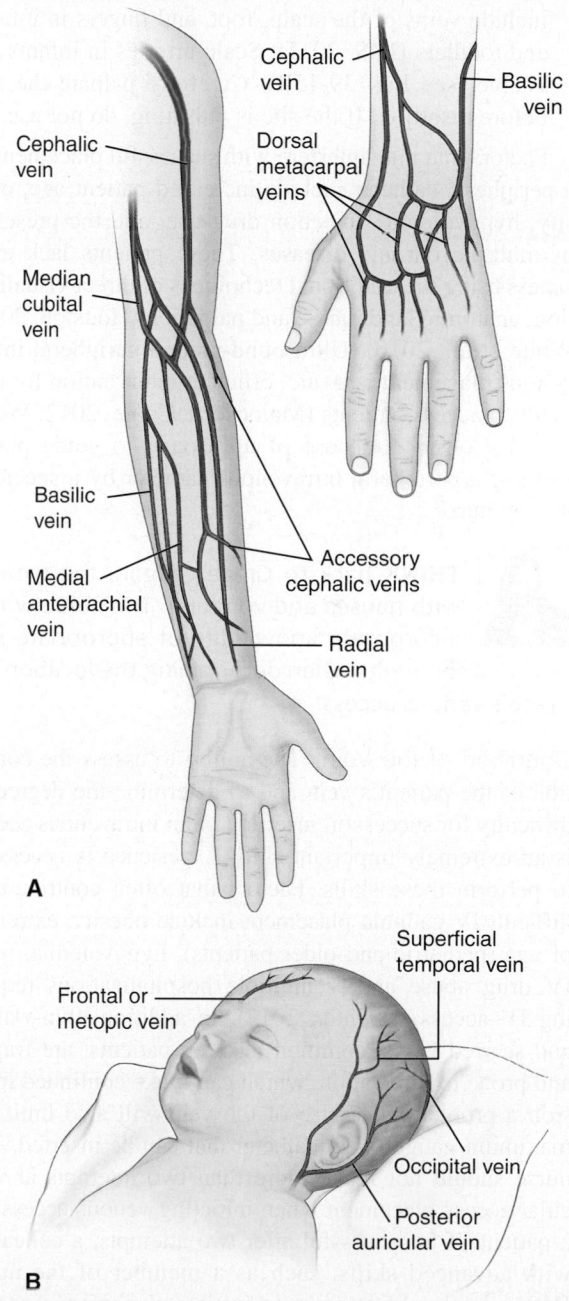

A

B

FIGURE 39-15. Peripheral venous access sites. (**A**) Infusion sites on the ventral and dorsal aspects of the lower arm and hand. (**B**) Infusion sites on the scalp of an infant.

over time. In addition, by avoiding the antecubital veins for peripheral venous catheters, a PICC line may be inserted at a later time, if needed.

- Do not use veins in the leg of an adult, unless other sites are inaccessible, because of the danger of stagnation of peripheral circulation and possible serious complications. The cannulation of the lower extremities is associated with risk of tissue damage, thrombophlebitis, and ulceration (INS, 2011). Some institutions require a medical order to insert an IV catheter in an adult patient's lower extremity.
- If the potential site is pulsating, it is likely to be an arterial vessel and you should not use it.
- Additional potential sites for neonates and children include veins of the scalp, foot, and fingers in infants and toddlers (INS, 2011). Scalp arteries in infants are visible (see Fig. 39-15B). Carefully palpate the site before insertion. If the site is pulsating, do not use.

Factors that may interfere with successful placement of a peripheral catheter include increased patient age, obesity, hypovolemia, injection drug use, and the presence of multiple chronic diseases. These patients lack easy access using the traditional techniques of direct visualization, anatomic landmarks, and palpation (Houston, 2013; White et al., 2010). Ultrasound-guided peripheral intravenous placement is a safe, efficient intervention for difficult-to-access patients (Maiocco & Coole, 2012; White et al.). Consider the use of ultrasound to guide placement of a peripheral intravenous catheter by a specially trained nurse.

 THINK back to Grace Gilligan, the woman with nausea and vomiting. The nurse would incorporate knowledge of appropriate site selection for adults when determining the location for Grace's venous access. ●

Condition of the Vein. The ability to assess the condition of the patient's vein and to determine the degree of difficulty for successful insertion of an intravenous access is an extremely important skill. Experience is necessary to perform these skills. Factors that often contribute to difficult IV cannula placement include obesity, extremes of age (pediatric and older patients), hypovolemia, prior IV drug abuse and/or multiple hospitalizations requiring IV access (Dychter, 2012). In addition, thin-walled and scarred veins, common in older patients, are fragile and prone to infiltration, which can make continued infusion a problem. The size of the vein will also limit the maximum gauge (size) catheter that can be inserted. The nurse should not make more than two attempts at vascular access placement when initiating venous access for a patient. If unsuccessful after two attempts, a colleague with advanced skills, such as a member of the nurse IV team, should attempt to initiate the venous access (Arbique & Arbique, 2007). In addition to promoting patient comfort, this practice preserves the limited remain-

ing venous access sites for a practitioner with advanced skills, optimizing the potential for success (INS, 2011).

 THINK back to Grace Gilligan, the patient who experienced several unsuccessful IV catheter insertion attempts, as described in the Reflective Practice box. The nurse's ability to palpate the patient's veins before attempting venipuncture might have been helpful in determining the best vein to be used. The information provided by palpation also could have indicated that the patient's veins were scarred, thus suggesting the need for a more experienced team member, such as an IV nurse specialist (as the patient had requested) to perform the procedure. ●

Type of Fluid to Be Infused. Keep in mind the following about the type of IV fluid to be infused:

- Select a vein and intravenous catheter size appropriate for the solution. Hypertonic solutions, those containing irritating medications, those administered at a rapid rate, and those with a high viscosity (such as a blood transfusion) should be given in a large vein, ideally using a large-gauge intravenous catheter to minimize vessel trauma and to facilitate the rate of flow.
- Advise the patient that some medications administered intravenously in a peripheral vein (e.g., potassium chloride and certain antibiotics) may cause irritation and pain; urge the patient to report any discomfort.

INITIATION OF AN IV INFUSION

Treat the administration of intravenous solutions in the same manner as medications, utilizing the same system of checks and rights of administration (refer to Chapter 28). Before the infusion is started, perform a final check of the solution to ensure that it is clear and contains no particles or precipitates. This check is especially important when substances have been added to the solution because some additives create precipitates. Commercially available in-line filters help reduce the risk for contamination by filtering the solution immediately before it enters the patient's vein. Skill 39-1 on pages 1520–1527 outlines the procedure for initiating an IV infusion.

Some adults and young children have a fear of needles. Provide information about the venipuncture process in an age-appropriate manner to decrease distress and anxiety (Hughes, 2012). Also, it may be advisable to use a product that eases the physical discomfort of venipuncture. Local anesthetic agents include intradermal agents, iontophoresis, low-frequency ultrasonification, pressure-accelerated lidocaine, and topical transdermal agents. The nurse needs to have knowledge of the anesthetic agent used and correct method of administration, based on manufacturer's recommendations and facility policy. The use of a local anesthetic requires monitoring for potential allergic reactions, tissue damage, or inadvertent injection of the drug into the vascular system (INS, 2011). Oral sucrose has been shown to be effective as a procedural analgesia for newborns and infants (Stevens et al., 2013); Kassab, Roydhouse, Fowler, & Foureur, 2012; Pasek & Huber, 2012) and should be used prior to initiation of venipuncture for these patients.

INFUSION REGULATION AND MONITORING
The nurse is responsible for maintaining the proper flow rate while ensuring the comfort and safety of the patient. The primary health care provider prescribes the amount of solution to be infused within a specified period. The nurse determines the rate based on the amount of solution to be infused over 1 hour. If the order is unclear or does not seem appropriate based on the patient's condition, it is the nurse's responsibility to ask the prescribing practitioner for clarification prior to beginning administration. Maintenance of the flow rate is important because it can directly affect the patient's fluid balance. Too slow a flow may result in a fluid volume deficit because fluid intake is not balancing fluid lost or it may delay the restoration of the balance. Infusing IV fluid too rapidly can overtax the body's capacities to adjust to the increase in the water volume or the electrolytes it contains and may lead to fluid volume excess. Allowing an infusion to get behind schedule and then increasing the rate to catch up might seriously jeopardize the patient's compensatory mechanisms and lead to serious complications, such as in a patient with heart failure. Skill 39-2 on pages 1528–1530 discusses the monitoring of an IV infusion.

The use of electronic infusion-control devices (e.g., IV pumps) has become a common, if not required, practice in acute care settings. These devices can be programmed to infuse a certain amount of fluid over a given time, usually milliliters per hour. When using an electronic device, it is not necessary to calculate the drops per minute, as is necessary with a gravity or free-flowing IV. The pump automatically regulates the flow rate at preset limits. An alarm sounds when air is in the tubing, the flow is obstructed, the solution level of the bottle or bag is getting low, or there is increased pressure in the system, such as occurs when an IV infiltrates and fluid flows into the tissues. "Smart pumps," computerized pumps, are beginning to be used in many facilities for IV infusions. Smart pumps also require programming of infusion rates by the nurse, but, in addition, are able to identify dosing limits and practice guidelines to aid in safe administration. The Institute for Safe Medication Practices (ISMP, 2013) states, "Smart pumps can provide a great deal of data that is useful in driving safe practices." Although the design of these pumps may enhance patient safety, it is important that nurses always remember that they are ultimately responsible for proper programming of the pump and fluid administration. Check the infusion every hour or more frequently, if indicated, to determine if the solution is being infused at the proper hourly rate.

Administration may be achieved by gravity infusion, which requires the nurse to calculate the infusion rate in drops per minute. If using a gravity or free-flowing IV, calculate the drip rate required to achieve the desired infusion rate. A method for determining flow rate is described in the accompanying Guidelines for Nursing Care 39-3. This method requires the nurse to know the amount of solution to be delivered, the total infusion time (in minutes), and the drop factor for the infusion tubing

GUIDELINES FOR NURSING CARE 39-3

REGULATING IV FLOW RATE
Follow facility guidelines to determine if infusion should be administered by electronic infusion device or by gravity.

- Check medical order for IV solution.
- Check patency of IV access.

If the infusion is to be administered by gravity infusion:

- Verify drop factor (number of drops in 1 mL) of the equipment in use.
- Calculate the flow rate:

EXAMPLE—Administer 1,000 mL D$_5$W over 10 hours (set delivers 60 gtt (drops)/ 1 mL).

a. **Standard formula**

$$\text{gtt (drops)/min} = \frac{\text{volume (mL)} \times \text{drop factor (gtt (drops)/mL)}}{\text{time (in minutes)}}$$

$$\text{gtt (drops)/min} = \frac{1,000 \text{ mL} \times 60}{600 \text{ (60 min} \times 10 \text{ h)}}$$

$$= \frac{60,000}{600}$$

$$= 100 \text{ gtt (drops)/min}$$

b. **Short formula using milliliters per hour**

$$\text{gtt (drops)/min} = \frac{\text{milliliters per hour} \times \text{drop factor (gtt (drops)/mL)}}{\text{time (60 min)}}$$

Find milliliters per hour by dividing 1,000 mL by 10 hours:

$$\frac{1000}{10} = 100 \text{ mL} \times 60$$

$$\text{gtt (drops)/min} = \frac{100 \text{ mL/60}}{60 \text{ min}}$$

$$= \frac{6,000}{60}$$

$$= 100 \text{ gtt (drops)/min}$$

FIGURE 39-16. Volume-control set.

in use. The drop factor, or drops per milliliter of solution, is determined by the size of the opening in the infusion apparatus. It varies among different products from different companies. Most health agencies use the products of a single company. The most common drop factors are macrodrop systems (10, 15, 20 drops/mL), a microdrip (60 drops/mL), and a blood administration set (10 drops/mL). Microdrip is used most often when small fluid volumes are administered, such as a rate less than 75 mL per hour. Macrodrop tubing is commonly used for rates greater than 75 mL per hour.

A less commonly used device, a volume-control device, or a buretrol (Fig. 39-16), may be used to reduce the risk for fluid overload or medication overdose. These devices are particularly important in pediatric settings in which catastrophic fluid overload is possible if adult fluid doses are inadvertently administered. Buretrols may also be used to deliver intermittent medications that need to be further diluted and given over a specific time.

Place a time tape (Fig. 39-17) on the container of solution to provide a quick reference for the nurse to monitor the rate at which the solution is entering the patient. The tape gives an hourly indication of where the fluid level should be at a given time.

 CONSIDER Jack Soo Park, the patient who received too much IV fluid. When planning Mr. Park's care, the nurse would need to include frequent assessments of the IV infusion to ensure that it is infusing at the proper flow rate. Placing the infusion on an infusion pump would have significantly reduced the potential for an infusion error. •

 SOLUTION AND TUBING CHANGES

If more than one container of solution is ordered for the patient, attach additional containers using the method

determined by the facility. One method for changing the solution and tubing is presented in Skill 39-3 on pages 1530–1534.

The frequency of administration set tubing changes varies. The Infusion Nurses Society provides guidelines related to administration set change. These Standards of Practice recommend the changing of administration set tubing based on the type of solution administered via the tubing and the type of infusion (continuous or intermittent). In addition, change administration set tubing immediately upon suspected contamination or when the integrity of the administration product or system has been compromised. Also, change tubing whenever the peripheral catheter site is rotated or when a new central vascular access device is placed (INS, 2011, p. S55). Box 39-1 outlines additional recommended administration set changes based on the type of infusion and device, according to INS Standards. See also the accompanying

FIGURE 39-17. Sample time tape for an IV solution container.

BOX 39-1 RECOMMENDED ADMINISTRATION SET CHANGE SCHEDULE

Type of Infusion/Type of Device	Recommended Frequency
• Primary and secondary continuous administration sets used to administer fluids other than lipid, blood, or blood products	• Change no more frequently than every 96 hours.
• Anti-infective CVAD	• Change every 7 days.
• Primary intermittent administration sets	• Change every 24 hours.
• Secondary intermittent administration sets detached from the primary administration set	• Change every 24 hours.
• Administration sets used to administer nonlipid-containing parenteral nutrition	• Change no more frequently than every 96 hours.
• Administration sets used to administer parenteral nutrition containing fat emulsions	• Change every 24 hours.
• Administration sets used to administer blood and blood components	• Change after the completion of each unit or every 4 hours.

Adapted from Infusion Nurses Society (INS). (2011). Infusion nursing standards of practice. *Journal of Infusion Nursing, 34* (Suppl: 1S); and O'Grady, N. P., Alexander, M., Burns, L. A., Dellinger, E. P., Garland, J., Heard, S. O., Lipsett, P.A., ... & the Healthcare Infection Control Practices Advisory Committee (HICPAC). Guidelines for the prevention of intravascular catheter-related infections. *American Journal of Infection Control, 39*(4 Supplement), S1–S34.

PICO in Practice box. It is important to be familiar with the particular policies and procedures of a given facility.

COMPLICATIONS OF IV THERAPY

Regularly assess venous access sites to detect common complications of intravenous therapy including infiltration (inadvertent leakage of intravenous solution into surrounding tissue), extravasation (inadvertent leakage of vesicant intravenous solution into surrounding tissue), phlebitis (inflammation of the wall of a vein), thrombophlebitis (blood clot in a vein, causing inflammation), and infection. Venous access device-related infections are a potentially serious complication related to intravenous therapy. The development of venous access device–related infection can range from the minor irritation of a localized site infection to a potentially life-threatening bloodstream infection or septicemia (Dychter et al., 2012).

PICO IN PRACTICE

ASKING CLINICAL QUESTIONS

Scenario: You are a staff nurse who works on a surgical step-down unit. Patients who are transferred to your unit from the surgical intensive care unit have IV lines in place. It has long been policy on this unit to routinely change IV tubing every 48 hours. Your hospital has instituted a program that encourages staff to make suggestions that could reduce unnecessary costs. You know that costs would be reduced if IV tubing were changed less frequently. However, you wonder if by doing so, your patients could experience more IV catheter–related infections.

- POPULATION: Hospital patients who have recently had surgery
- INTERVENTION: IV tubing changes every 48 hours
- COMPARISON: IV tubing changes longer than every 48 hours
- OUTCOME: IV catheter–related infections

PICO Question: Among patients who have recently had surgery, are IV tubing changes every 48 hours associated with less IV catheter–related infections than less frequent IV tubing changes?

Finding: From the National Guidelines Clearinghouse: O'Grady, N. P., Alexander, M., Burns, L. A., Dellinger, E. P.,

Garland, J., Heard, S. O., Lipsett, P. A., ... Healthcare Infection Control Practices Advisory Committee (HICPAC). (2011). *Guidelines for the prevention of intravascular catheter-related infections, 2011. American Journal of Infection Control, 39* (4 Supplement), S1–S34.

IV administration sets, including IV tubing, should be changed no more frequently than every 96 hours and at least every 7 days.

Strength of Evidence: Level I

Recommendation: You write a proposal that you send to your Nurse Manager and the Nursing Department Policy and Procedure Committee to change the interval for changing IV tubing from 48 hours to between 96 hours and 7 days. You cite the strength of the evidence in the guideline you found, and note that this guideline does not specify that there is an optimal time period for changing IV administration sets, including IV tubing, between 96 hours and 7 days. You suggest in your proposal that the Policy and Procedure Committee develop a clinical decision-making algorithm that may be used by staff nurses to assess IV setups daily between days 4 and 7 to determine whether or not they should be changed.

Local complications, such as infiltration, phlebitis, and thrombophlebitis, occur more frequently than do systemic complications. However, systemic complications (e.g., fluid overload, embolus, sepsis) are more serious and may be life threatening. Catheters are now available that are impregnated with antiseptics and coated with antibiotics; their use is recommended for patients at high risk for acquiring a catheter-related infection. Consult facility policy for guidance concerning catheter site care as well as the manufacturer's recommendations and precautions. An additional recommendation to prevent intravascular catheter-related infections is the use of a 2% chlorhexidine wash for daily skin cleansing (Lopez, 2011; O'Grady et al., 2011). Table 39-12 defines complications of IV

Table 39-12 COMPLICATIONS ASSOCIATED WITH INTRAVENOUS INFUSIONS

COMPLICATION/CAUSE	SIGNS AND SYMPTOMS	NURSING CONSIDERATIONS
Infiltration: the escape of fluid into the subcutaneous tissue Dislodged needle Penetrated vessel wall	Swelling, pallor, coldness, or pain around the infusion site; significant decrease in the flow rate	Check the infusion site every hour for signs/symptoms. Discontinue the infusion if symptoms occur. Restart the infusion at a different site. Use site-stabilization device.
Venous access device–related infection: Improper hand decontamination/hand hygiene Frequent disconnection of tubing, access ports, and/or access caps Poor insertion technique, multiple insertion attempts Multilumen catheters Long-term catheter insertion Frequent dressing changes Inadequate/improper decontamination of hub prior to use An IV solution that becomes contaminated when solutions are changed, a medication is added, or the solution is allowed to infuse for too long a period Inappropriate administration set changes	Erythema, edema, induration, drainage at the insertion site Fever, malaise, chills, other vital sign changes	Perform hand hygiene before and after palpating catheter insertion sites; before and after inserting, replacing, accessing, and dressing a venous access device. Assess catheter site at least daily. Notify primary care provider immediately if any signs of infection. Use scrupulous aseptic technique when starting an infusion. Follow best-practice guidelines for site care, changing of administration tubing sets, connectors, caps and other administration equipment. Follow facility protocol for culture of drainage. Consider use of 2% chlorhexidine wash for daily skin cleansing.
Phlebitis: an inflammation of a vein Mechanical trauma from needle or catheter Chemical trauma from solution	Local, acute tenderness; redness, warmth, and slight edema of the vein above the insertion site	Discontinue the infusion immediately. Apply warm, moist compresses to the affected site. Avoid further use of the vein. Restart the infusion in another vein.
Thrombus: a blood clot Tissue trauma from needle or catheter	Symptoms similar to phlebitis IV fluid flow may cease if clot obstructs needle.	Stop the infusion immediately. Apply warm compresses as ordered by the primary care provider. Restart the IV at another site. *Do not rub or massage the affected area.*
Speed shock: the body's reaction to a substance that is injected into the circulatory system too rapidly Too rapid a rate of fluid infusion into circulation	Pounding headache, fainting, rapid pulse rate, apprehension, chills, back pains, and dyspnea	Use the proper IV tubing. Carefully monitor the rate of fluid flow. Check the rate frequently for accuracy. A time tape is useful for this purpose.
Fluid overload: the condition caused when too large a volume of fluid infuses into the circulatory system Too large a volume of fluid infused into circulation	Engorged neck veins, increased blood pressure, and difficulty in breathing (dyspnea)	If symptoms develop, slow the rate of infusion. Notify the primary care provider immediately. Monitor vital signs. Carefully monitor the rate of fluid flow. Check the rate frequently for accuracy.
Air embolus: air in the circulatory system Break in the IV system above the heart level, allowing air in the circulatory system as a bolus	Respiratory distress Increased heart rate Cyanosis Decreased blood pressure Change in level of consciousness	Pinch off catheter or secure system to prevent entry of air. Place patient on left side in Trendelenburg position. Call for immediate assistance. Monitor vital signs and pulse oximetry.

infusions, noting common causes, signs and symptoms, and pertinent nursing considerations.

The patient can be an important source of information regarding the possibility of complications associated with IV therapy. If the patient is uncomfortable, check that the infusion is entering the vein as intended, the flow rate is not too rapid, the patient's position is satisfactory, and the circulatory status of the patient is intact. Anxiety about receiving an infusion can also cause discomfort for the patient. Provide appropriate and accurate information to the patient regarding the infusion to help decrease anxiety.

Assess for any deviation from the normal skin temperature of the site. For example, cool skin can indicate infiltration while warm skin can indicate phlebitis or infection. Also note the color of the skin at the venous access site. Pale or blanched skin can be a sign of infiltration, whereas red skin can indicate inflammation related to phlebitis or infection. Pus at the intravenous site indicates infection while leaking fluid at the site indicates infiltration. A palpable venous cord often is indicative of phlebitis (Dychter, 2012). Finally, fully investigate discomfort, pain, swelling or edema at the site as these symptoms

are associated with all of the five major complications listed earlier. Encourage patients to report any changes in the catheter site or any new discomfort (O'Grady et al., 2011). Use a standardized scale for assessing and documenting infiltration/extravasation from all types of vascular access devices (INS, 2011). Box 39-2 and Box 39-3 identify scales that can be used to grade and document infiltration and phlebitis if they occur.

VENOUS ACCESS SITE CARE

Scrupulous care of the infusion site is necessary to help control contamination and to help prevent the introduction of microorganisms into the bloodstream. Appropriate skin antisepsis, maintenance of an intact and patent dressing at the insertion site, use of appropriate dressing change regimens, and appropriate administration tubing replacements (previously discussed) are important means of preventing infection. Use of chlorhexidine, 70% alcohol, iodine, or povidone-iodine is recommended for skin antisepsis for peripheral venous catheters (INS, 2011; O'Grady et al., 2011). Chlorhexidine is not recommended for infants under 2 months of age (INS, 2011). Use of a >0.5% chlorhexidine preparation with alcohol is recommended for skin antisepsis for central venous catheter site care (CDC, 2011; O'Grady et al., 2011). The use of topical antibiotic ointments or creams on insertion sites is not recommended because of their potential to promote fungal infections and antimicrobial resistance (O'Grady et al., 2011). Transparent semipermeable membrane (TSM) dressings are used most commonly to protect the insertion site. TSM dressings (e.g., Tegaderm or OpSite IV) allow easy inspection of the IV site and permit evaporation of moisture that accumulates under the dressing. Sterile gauze may also be used to cover the catheter site. A gauze dressing is recommended if the patient is diaphoretic or if the site is bleeding or oozing;

BOX 39-2 INFILTRATION SCALE

Grade and document infiltration according to the most severe presenting indicator.

Grade	Clinical Criteria
0	No symptoms
1	Skin blanched Edema <1 inch in any direction Cool to touch With or without pain
2	Skin blanched Edema 1–6 inches in any direction Cool to touch With or without pain
3	Skin blanched, translucent Gross edema >6 inches in any direction Cool to touch Mild–moderate pain Possible numbness
4	Skin blanched, translucent Skin tight, leaking Skin discolored, bruised, swollen Gross edema >6 inches in any direction Deep pitting tissue edema Circulatory impairment Moderate–severe pain (Infiltration of any amount of blood product, irritant or vesicant)

Infusion Nurses Society (INS). (2006). *Infusion nursing standards of practice. Journal of Infusion Nursing, 29*(1S), S60, with permission.

BOX 39-3 PHLEBITIS SCALE

Grade and document phlebitis according to the most severe presenting indicator.

Grade	Clinical Criteria
0	No symptoms
1	Erythema at access site with or without pain
2	Pain at access site with erythema and/or edema
3	Pain at access site with erythema and/or edema Streak formation Palpable venous cord
4	Pain at access site with erythema and/or edema Streak formation Palpable venous cord >1 inch in length Purulent drainage

Infusion Nurses Society (INS). (2011). *Infusion nursing standards of practice. Journal of Infusion Nursing, 34*(1S), p. S65, with permission.

replace it with a TSM once this is resolved (O'Grady et al., 2011). Facility policy generally determines the type of dressing and the intervals for dressing change. Routine site care and dressing changes are not performed on peripheral catheters unless the dressing is soiled or no longer intact (INS, 2011). Perform site care and replace TSM dressings on CVADs every 5 to 7 days and every 2 days for CVAD sites with gauze dressings (INS, 2011; O'Grady et al., 2011). Change any dressing that is damp, loosened, or soiled immediately. In the event of drainage, site tenderness, or other signs of infection, change the dressing. This allows for the opportunity to assess, cleanse, and disinfect the site (INS, 2011, p. S63). Do not submerge venous catheters and catheter sites in water; showering is permitted with use of impermeable coverings to protect the catheter and connecting device (O'Grady et al., 2011).

Additional manufactured venous catheter securement/stabilization systems are commercially available. These systems are recommended for use on all venous access sites, particularly central venous access sites, to preserve the integrity of the access device, minimize catheter movement at the hub, and to prevent catheter migration and loss of access (INS, 2011, p. S46; O'Grady et al., 2011). The use of a stabilization device can also decrease the risk of infiltration, phlebitis, skin damage, occlusion, leaking, and unscheduled restart rates (Smith & Hannum, 2008). These devices include plastic shields and adhesive anchors. Hard plastic shields (Fig. 39-18) that are ventilated and secured with tape are often used in pediatric settings. In addition, they are helpful in minimizing venous access complications with geriatric patients (Smith & Hannum, 2008). Adhesive anchors eliminate the need for tape but are more costly and involve the use of strong adhesives that might make it difficult to change the dressing without dislodging the catheter. Skill 39-2 on pages 1528–1530 reviews how to monitor an IV site. Skill 39-4 on pages 1535–1538 explains how to change a dressing for a peripheral venous access device.

FIGURE 39-18. IV shield in place on the hand.

CAPPING A PRIMARY LINE FOR INTERMITTENT USE

When a continuous IV is no longer necessary, the primary IV line (short peripheral venous catheter or CVAD) can be capped and converted to an intermittent infusion device. A capped line consists of the IV catheter connected to a short length of extension tubing sealed with a cap. Capping of a short peripheral venous catheter is commonly referred to as a medication or saline lock. Capping of a vascular access device provides venous access for intermittent infusions or emergency medications. Vascular access devices used for intermittent infusions should be flushed with normal saline solution prior to each infusion as part of the assessment of catheter function. Flushing of the device is also required after each infusion to clear the infused medication or other solution from the catheter lumen. Vascular access devices should also be "locked" after completion of the flush solution at each use to decrease the risk of occlusion. According to the guidelines from the INS (2011), short peripheral catheters are locked with normal saline solution; CVADs should be locked with a heparin solution (10 units/mL) after each intermittent use. If the device is not in use, periodic flushing according to facility policy is required to keep the catheter patent. Skill 39-5 on pages 1538–1539 describes capping and flushing a peripheral venous access device.

DISCONTINUATION OF THE INFUSION

When the peripheral venous access is no longer required, or when the insertion site shows signs of local complications, the nurse assumes responsibility for discontinuing the access device. After performing hand hygiene, put on gloves, clamp the IV tubing, and remove the tape and sterile dressing. Avoid bending the catheter while it is withdrawn to prevent breakage. Apply pressure immediately to the area just above the insertion site until hemostasis is achieved. Apply pressure using a dry, sterile gauze pad rather than using an alcohol preparation; alcohol tends to burn and does not stop blood flow from the puncture wound. Apply an occlusive dressing to the site. Document the date and time of removal, the name of the person removing the device, and the assessment of the site.

Nurses or specialized IV team nurses may be responsible for removing a mid-line or PICC line. Other CVADs are usually removed by advanced practice professionals. Specific protocols must be followed to prevent breakage or fracture of the catheter. Guidelines for removal of a PICC are as follows:

- Wear clean gloves.
- Place the patient in the supine position, with the arm straight and the catheter insertion site at or below heart level (to prevent the risk for an air embolus).
- Remove the dressing carefully while stabilizing the hub of the catheter with one hand.
- Instruct the patient to hold the breath, and perform a Valsalva maneuver as the last portion of the catheter is removed; if unable to do so, time the removal

during patient expiration. Use of the Valsalva maneuver or removal during expiration reduces the risk for air embolism (Feil, 2012).

- Remove the catheter slowly. Grasp the catheter close to the insertion site and slowly ease the catheter out, keeping it parallel to the skin. Continue removing in small increments, using a smooth and gentle motion.
- Apply pressure to the site with a sterile dressing until hemostasis is achieved, then apply a petroleum-based ointment and a sterile dressing to the access site to seal the skin-to-vein tract and decrease the risk of air embolus (INS, 2011).
- Measure the catheter and compare it with the length listed in the chart when it was inserted. This ensures that the entire catheter was removed.
- Document the procedure, catheter length, site assessment, and how the patient tolerated the procedure.
- If resistance is felt when removing a catheter, stop removal. Resistance typically is caused by smooth muscle spasm inside the vein wall. Encourage the patient to relax and take deep breaths. Wait a few minutes and try again (Hadaway, 2009). Do not forcibly remove the catheter (INS, 2011). Replace the sterile dressing and notify the patient's primary care provider.

HOME INFUSION

Many patients return to their home from a health care facility with IV infusions. Portable infusion pumps and the availability of home care nurses have made this an acceptable alternative. After a patient has been identified as a candidate for home infusion therapy, begin assessment

and education to ensure a successful outcome. Candidates for infusion pump IV therapy in the home should meet certain criteria. They should be medically stable, have a full- or part-time caregiver, have access to a telephone, and have a refrigerator available for storage of prefilled medication cartridges. Patients can receive insulin infusions, pain medication, antibiotic therapy, chemotherapy, or TPN through portable infusion pumps at home.

PICCs and other CVADs are the most common type of catheter used for home health care patients. Home health care nurses play a crucial role in educating patients concerning successful management of IV catheters and observing for potential complications. The patient and any caregivers must be able to perform necessary skills independently before discharge from the health care facility. See Teaching Tips 39-1.

Administering Blood and Blood Products

A blood transfusion is the infusion of whole blood or a blood component such as plasma, red blood cells, cryoprecipitate, or platelets into the patient's venous circulation. Red blood cells have the important role of carrying oxygen from the lungs to all body tissues. Oxygen is essential to maintain normal cellular metabolism and cellular integrity. Platelets and the coagulation factors found in cryoprecipitate and plasma are essential for establishing homeostasis following an injury or invasive procedure. These blood components promote normal blood clotting, thus are important in the prevention of excessive blood loss. A blood product transfusion is given when a patient's red blood cells, platelets, or coagulation

TEACHING TIPS 39-1

IV THERAPY

Health Topic	Teaching Tip	Why Is This Important?
Sterile technique	• Proper handwashing technique • Dressing changes and care of site/device • Proper technique for infusing medications	Prevent local and systemic infection
Equipment use	• Proper technique for using all equipment and flushing of CVAD • Safe storage, maintenance, and disposal of solutions, supplies, and equipment • Protection of device/insertion site when showering or bathing	Prevent medication/infusion therapy error and complications such as bleeding, embolus, and/or infection related to improper use of equipment and flushing of CVAD.
Assessment Skills	Assessing for any indications of an infection or other complications and how to report such problems	Understanding of signs of infection and other complications promotes early detection and intervention.
Supplies	Obtaining supplies to continue home infusions	Continued supplies are needed to maintain prescribed home therapy.
Resources	How and why to contact the primary care provider, nurse, or home health care agency if questions or problems arise	Understanding of available resources and when it is appropriate to use these resources promotes compliance and maintenance of prescribed therapy.

factors decrease to levels that compromise a patient's health. Blood transfusions are not without risk, however. Life-threatening complications include a severe allergic reaction (anaphylaxis), hemolytic reaction, transfusion-related acute lung injury, and circulatory overload, and transmission of infectious diseases are a risk associated with blood product transfusion (Ead, 2011). It is always important that the potential benefits of the transfusion be considered against the potential risks. The person receiving the blood is the recipient. The person giving the blood is the donor. Steps in administering blood transfusions are described in Skill 39-6 on pages 1540–1544.

BLOOD TYPING AND CROSS-MATCHING

Before a blood product can be given to a patient, it must be determined that the blood of the donor is compatible with that of the patient. If incompatible, clumping and hemolysis of the recipient's blood cells result and death can occur. The laboratory examination to determine a person's blood type is called **blood typing**. The process of determining compatibility between blood specimens is **cross-matching**.

Blood Types. The four main blood types or groups in the ABO system of blood typing are A, B, AB, and O. Some groups are further broken down into subgroups.

Blood type, an inherited trait, is determined by the type of antigens and antibodies present in the blood. An **antigen** is a substance that causes the formation of antibodies. An **antibody** is a protein substance developed in the body in response to the presence of an antigen that has entered the body. An **agglutinin** is an antibody that causes a clumping of specific antigens. People who have type A blood have an A antigen on their red blood cells, those with type B blood have B antigens on their cells, those in the AB group have both A and B antigens, and people with type O blood have neither A nor B antigens on their red blood cells. People in each blood group have the agglutinins to the red blood cell antigens that they lack. Group A people have the agglutinin for B; group AB people have no agglutinins for A and B, whereas group O people have both A and B agglutinins in their blood serum. If a person with type O blood is transfused with blood from a person with either group A or group B blood, there would be destruction of the recipient's red blood cells because the recipient's anti-A or anti-B agglutinins would react with the A or B antigens in the donor's red blood cells. This explains why people with type AB blood are often called universal recipients (because people in this blood group have no agglutinins for either A or B antigens), and group O people are often called universal donors (because they have neither A nor B antigens).

Rh Factor. The Rh factor is an inherited antigen in human blood. There are five antigens in the Rh system, but the one designated D is of first concern. A person whose blood contains a D antigen is called Rh positive; an Rh-negative person lacks this D antigen. An Rh-negative person must receive blood from another Rh-negative person. If Rh-positive blood is administered to an Rh-negative person, the recipient develops anti-Rh agglutinins. Subsequent transfusion with Rh-positive blood may cause serious reactions with clumping and hemolysis of red blood cells.

BLOOD DONORS

Blood donors must be selected with care. Not only must the donor's blood be typed accurately, but it is also important to determine that the donor is free of infectious disease. The blood will be tested for human immunodeficiency virus (HIV), hepatitis B and C virus (HBV and HBC), syphilis, West Nile virus, and other viruses that can be transmitted to the recipient. The screening process is not perfect, however. After the proper testing process has been followed, the risk of HIV with blood transfusion is 1 in 1.4 million; the risk of West Nile Virus is 1 in 1 million, the risk of hepatitis C is 1 in 3.1 million; and the risk of hepatitis B is 1 in 82,000 (Ead, 2011).

The donor is examined carefully at the time of donation and receives specific information about eligibility and a confidential method to allow or disallow the distribution of the donated blood. Prospective donors must meet minimum requirements for age, height, and weight (American Red Cross, 2013). Prospective donors are questioned about their lifestyle and health history, including questions about diseases, medical conditions, past surgeries, tattoos, body piercing, travel, sexual habits, and medication/drug use. People may give blood only if their blood count (hemoglobin or hematocrit), temperature, pulse, and blood pressure are within normal ranges.

Some patients who know in advance that they will need blood can donate their own blood for transfusion (**autologous transfusion**), also called autotransfusion. Autotransfusion eliminates the danger of transmitting cross-infection from donor to recipient and decreases the risk for complications from mismatched blood. However, this technique requires advance planning (the blood must be donated 5 weeks before the surgery) and is not complication free. For example, catastrophic administration errors and infection are still possible even with autologous transfusion.

An additional transfusion technique related to autologous transfusion is utilized frequently in surgical settings. It is called intraoperative blood salvage. With this technique, a patient's own blood can be collected from specialized suction canisters, tubes and drains to allow for autologous transfusions.

BLOOD COMPONENTS

Whole blood is rarely used unless blood loss has been massive. This is because whole blood can be easily separated into its components. This allows patients to receive only the blood product they need, decreasing the risk for fluid overload and promoting blood product availability to more patients. For example, a patient may need red blood cells but not the blood plasma and its constituents.

Red blood cells can therefore be administered in concentrated form, called packed red blood cells (PRBCs). Examples of indications for PRBCs include:

- Patients demonstrating symptomatic anemia, which is a reduction in red blood cells or hemoglobin, resulting in symptoms of tachycardia and excessive fatigue (reflecting reduced oxygen delivery to tissues). This anemia may be related to disease conditions (e.g., end-stage renal disease, cancer, GI bleeding, and the like), surgical bleeding, or trauma.
- Patients with cardiovascular failure, with a need to increase blood volume and red blood cells while avoiding fluid overload

In situations in which there is a deficit in plasma proteins and/or components of the blood important for normal functioning of coagulation and fibrinolysis (including complement), administration of plasma may be a more appropriate option. Fresh-frozen plasma (FFP) is particularly useful in emergencies that involve massive blood loss because it will restore both coagulation factors and blood volume. It is also an excellent protein containing blood-volume expander when a patient develops a sudden critical fluid deficit: for example, in a patient who is severely burned and losing plasma rapidly from burn areas. Separate components of plasma that are also used therapeutically include human albumin (used for hypovolemic shock, albuminemia, liver failure), cryoprecipitate (used to treat bleeding due to hemophilia, disseminated intravascular coagulation, or depletion of coagulation factors such as fibrinogen following massive blood loss), and gammaglobulins, the antibody-containing part of plasma (used for gammaglobulin deficiencies).

Platelet infusion is indicated for the treatment or prevention of bleeding associated with deficiencies in the number or quality of a patient's platelets. The demand for platelets has risen noticeably during the past several decades; specialized products and preparation methods have been developed to reduce the risk for complications and improve the patient's response to platelet therapy.

INITIATION OF TRANSFUSION
Researchers have determined that the majority of fatal acute hemolytic transfusion reactions are a result of preventable human errors (Ead 2011). Thus, the importance of consistently following routine safety checks cannot be overemphasized. The nurse should always follow facility blood product transfusion policies and protocols. Two licensed practitioners (e.g., registered nurses and/or physicians) should perform pretransfusion safety checks together prior to blood product administration. The nurse should always confirm the patient's identity with at least two patient identifiers (e.g., full name, birthdate) and confirm that this information matches the information on the patient's identification band. The patient's blood type and Rh factor should also be checked against the blood type and Rh factor of the transfusion product. In

addition, the nurse should always confirm the expiration date of the blood product. Bar codes on blood products are currently being implemented to identify, track, and assign data to transfusions as an additional safety measure. In addition, the facility that prepared the blood and a code to track the blood back to its donor must be identified. While such systems offer the potential for improved safety, the nurse must always recognize that there is no replacement for vigilant and consistent safety checks. Clinicians (including nurses) are more likely to commit an error when they are fatigued, stressed, or in a rush (Ead, 2011). It is important for the nurse to recognize this and avoid the temptation to cut corners when performing pretransfusion safety checks.

The procedure for administering a blood transfusion (see Skill 39-6, pp. 1540–1544) is similar to the procedure for starting an intravenous infusion of fluids, with a few differences. Blood or blood components may be transfused via a 14- to 24-gauge peripheral venous access device. Transfusion for neonate or pediatric patients is usually given using a 22-top, 24-gauge peripheral venous access device (INS, 2011). Administer blood components using an in-line filter or an add-on filter that is appropriate for the prescribed component, following the manufacturer's directions for use (INS). It is generally recommended to start the infusion slowly and carefully monitor for complications after getting baseline vital signs. Facility policies vary on the frequency of vital signs during the infusion, but in general the most intense monitoring is required in the first 15 minutes of the infusion. Institution policies vary on the frequency of vital signs. If the patient's temperature is 100°F (37.8°C) or higher, notify the primary care provider. Return blood that has not been used within 30 minutes after its arrival from the blood bank. In addition, to prevent the risk for bacterial contamination, discontinue blood that has been infusing for more than 4 hours. Nurses are responsible for monitoring the patient for adverse reactions to the blood transfusion. Transfusion reactions can occur during or within 24 hours after administration of a blood product (acute reactions) or 1 day to several days after transfusion (delayed reactions). Table 39-13 (on page 1516) describes potential transfusion reactions that can be serious and/or life threatening.

Administering Parenteral Nutrition
Parenteral nutrition is the administration of nutritional support via the intravenous route. Patients who cannot meet their nutritional needs by the oral or enteral routes may require intravenous nutritional supplementation. Intravenous supplementation may be prescribed for a variety of patients, including those who have nonfunctional gastrointestinal (GI) tracts, who are comatose, or those who have high caloric and nutritional needs due to illness or injury; patients undergoing aggressive cancer therapy; and those recovering from extensive burns, surgery, sepsis, or multiple fractures. Parenteral nutrition can be administered centrally, through a central

Table 39-13 TRANSFUSION REACTIONS

REACTION	SIGNS AND SYMPTOMS	NURSING ACTIVITY
Allergic reaction: allergy to transfused blood	Hives, itching Anaphylaxis	• Stop transfusion immediately and keep vein open with normal saline. • Notify primary care provider immediately. • Administer antihistamine parenterally as necessary.
Febrile reaction: fever develops during infusion	Fever and chills Headache Malaise	• Stop transfusion immediately and keep vein open with normal saline. • Notify primary care provider. • Treat symptoms.
Hemolytic transfusion reaction: incompatibility of blood product	Immediate onset Facial flushing Fever, chills Headache Low back pain Shock	• Stop infusion immediately and keep vein open with normal saline. • Notify primary care provider immediately. • Obtain blood samples from site. • Obtain first voided urine. • Treat shock if present. • Send unit, tubing, and filter to lab. • Draw blood sample for serologic testing and send urine specimen to lab.
Circulatory overload: too much blood administered	Dyspnea Dry cough Pulmonary edema	• Slow or stop infusion. • Monitor vital signs. • Notify primary care provider. • Place in upright position with feet dependent.
Bacterial reaction: bacteria present in blood	Fever Hypertension Dry, flushed skin Abdominal pain	• Stop infusion immediately. • Obtain culture of patient's blood and return blood bag to lab. • Monitor vital signs. • Notify primary care provider. • Administer antibiotics stat.

venous access device (total parenteral nutrition [TPN]), or peripherally (peripheral parenteral nutrition [PPN]), through a short-term intravenous access in a peripheral vein. The basic difference between the two types is the concentration of the solutions infused. Assess for potential complications of TPN such as catheter-related infection and electrolyte imbalances. The procedure for TPN administration and related nursing responsibilities are described in Chapter 35.

Evaluating

Ongoing evaluation is integral. Throughout nursing care, evaluate and readjust your plans and interventions. Refer to the accompanying concept map for an illustration of the Nursing Process for Grace Gilligan. Evaluate the effectiveness of the plan of care to promote healthy fluid, electrolyte, and acid–base balance based on the following parameters:

• Are the patient's drinking and eating patterns supplying the needed fluid and electrolytes? Are food and fluid likes and dislikes interfering with the implementation of the care plan? Is the patient having any difficulties with oral fluids, tube feedings, IV therapy, or TPN?
• Is the patient's urine output about equal to the fluid intake? Does the patient void at least once each shift (except when sleeping)? Do urine characteristics

(color, odor, specific gravity) indicate healthy functioning of the kidneys and excretion of fluids?
• Are abnormal sources of fluid loss (e.g., vomiting, diarrhea, draining wounds, fistula) responding to treatment? Are these fluid losses effectively being replaced by the designated therapy? Are the signs of fluid volume deficit improving?
• Do the patient's weight and record of fluid intake and output indicate fluid balance?
• Are the signs and symptoms that initially manifested the fluid, electrolyte, or acid–base imbalances absent or improved? Has therapy led to any troublesome new signs or symptoms?
• Is the patient now able to practice self-care behaviors to maintain fluid, electrolyte, and acid–base balance? Can the patient describe appropriate responses to potential future problems?

This evaluation should be ongoing as the plan of care is implemented. As the patient achieves the expected outcomes, these should be noted and reinforced. Before nursing care is terminated, the patient and family should be able to independently promote fluid, electrolyte, and acid–base balance. Refer to the Nursing Plan of Care 39-1 for Jeremiah Stein on pages 1518–1519.

Grace Gilligan, 28-years-old, is admitted to the ER with complaints of severe episodes of nausea and vomiting over the last 48 hours. She has a past medical history of Crohn's disease, a gastrointestinal (GI) problem for which she underwent bowel resection surgery one month ago. Her admission assessment reveals that she is awake, alert, and oriented to person, place and time. Grace complains of dizziness when she sits up suddenly. Assessment reveals poor skin turgor and dry oral mucous membranes. Respirations are even, unlabored at 22 breaths/minute. Lungs are clear. Pulse is 132 beats/minute and weak. BP is 106/52 and temperature is 98.9°F. Abdomen is firm, distended, slightly tender with absent bowel sounds. A nasogastric tube was inserted. She reports a six pound weight loss over the past two days. She has not voided in the past 8 hours. Intravenous therapy is prescribed to restore fluid balance. An abdominal X-ray study reveals an intestinal obstruction. She tearfully relates, "I thought the surgery would help my problems."

Priority 1

Deficient Fluid Volume related to nausea and vomiting
Supporting Data:
• Recent abdominal surgery
• Severe episodes of nausea and vomiting
• NPO
• Nasogastric tube in place
• Abdomen firm, distended without bowel sounds
• X-ray confirmation of bowel obstruction
• Intravenous therapy
• Recent 6 pound weight loss
• Has not voided in past 8 hours
• Dry oral mucous membranes
• C/o orthostatic dizziness
• BP 106/52, pulse 132 beats/minute, respiratory rate 22 breaths/minute

Priority 2

Risk for Imbalanced Nutrition: Less Than Body Requirements related to nausea and vomiting, inability to tolerate, oral foods and fluids
Supporting Data:
• Six pound weight loss in 2 days
• NPO with nasogastric tube
• Abdomen distended and firm with absent bowel sounds
• Recent abdominal surgery

Priority 3

Anxiety related to change in health status
Supporting Data:
• Severe episodes of nausea and vomiting after recent abdominal surgery
• Uncertainty about health status
• Tearfully states, "I thought the surgery would help my problems."

Outcome:
Patient will achieve normal fluid volume, adequate urine output, stable vital signs, good skin turgor, moist mucous membranes, and normal electrolytes.

Outcome:
Patient will have nutritional needs addressed. Weight will stabilize.

Outcome:
Patient will report a reduction in anxiety to a manageable level and verbalize feelings surrounding anxiety.

Nursing Interventions:
• Monitor prescribed intravenous therapy
• Monitor intake and output balance
• Weigh daily
• Vital signs every 4 hours
• Irrigate nasogastric tube every 4 hours with normal saline as prescribed
• Note characteristics and amount of nasogastric drainage
• Perform abdominal assessment
• Provide mouth care every 2 hours
• Assess skin turgor, mucous membranes
• Monitor results of labwork

Nursing Interventions:
• Consult dietitian
• Weigh daily
• Perform an abdominal assessment to assist in determining return of bowel function
• Evaluate current weight and compare to ideal body weight
• Prepare to initiate and monitor total parenteral nutrition (TPN)
• Provide frequent mouth care

Nursing Interventions:
• Assist patient in identifying support systemS and previous coping techniques
• Encourage verbalization of feelings
• Active listening
• Relay accurate information regarding health status, correcting any misperceptionS
• Utilize comfort measures such as Therapeutic Touch
• Maintain calm, quiet environment

Evaluation: Intravenous therapy is maintained. Grace voided 250 mL of urine after 4 hours of IV therapy. Vital signs stabilized. Her abdomen remains distended without bowel sounds. A surgical consult was prescribed to evaluate the need for abdominal surgery.

Evaluation: Grace's abdomen remains distended with absent bowel sounds. She remains NPO and is being evaluated for surgery. Collaborate with dietitian and physician to determine need for TPN.

Evaluation: Grace verbalizes an understanding of rationales for interventions. She is participating in the plan of care and asking questions regarding plan of care.

- - - - - Relationship ☐ Assessment ☐ Nursing Diagnosis ☐ Outcome Identification ☐ Interventions ☐ Evaluation

Concept map illustrating the nursing process for Grace Gilligan.

NURSING PLAN OF CARE 39-1

for Jeremiah Stein

Jeremiah Stein is a 22-year-old man who is a senior in the premed program at a large state university. He is currently an honors student and plans to take the MCAT examination in 2 weeks. His overwhelming ambition is to be accepted into a prestigious medical school and to become a psychiatrist. He presents at the campus health clinic with the following assessment findings:

- History of occasional problems with diarrhea since his junior year in high school; self-treatment with kaolin and pectin (Kaopectate) and limiting his food and fluid intake; believes diarrhea is stress related; no medical evaluation to date.

- Has had two or three loose, watery bowel movements per day for the past week, with urgency and occasional fecal incontinence; believes this is related to anxiety about performance on MCAT and his need for good grades; always thirsty but afraid to drink much; urine output is decreased, and he noted that urine is darker in color and has a stronger odor.

  Nursing examination: temperature, 99.8°F (37.6°C); pulse, 92 beats/min; respirations, 18 breaths/min; blood pressure, 100/60 mm Hg; skin and mucous membranes are pale and dry; weight is 4 lb. less than usual (current weight, 170 lb.)

NURSING DIAGNOSIS Deficient Fluid Volume related to prolonged diarrhea and decreased fluid intake secondary to poor stress management as evidenced by 4-lb weight loss, dry skin and mucous membranes, and report of decreased urine output and concentrated urine

EXPECTED OUTCOME By next week's visit, 3/24/15, the patient will:
- Describe two effective means he has used to cope with stress

NURSING INTERVENTIONS	RATIONALE	EVALUATIVE STATEMENT
Explore with the patient (1) what he finds most stressing at present, (2) the control he believes he has over these stressors, and (3) the adequacy of his past and present stress management strategies.	Assisting the patient to eliminate and reduce stress where possible and learn to cope better with unavoidable stress (identify and eliminate causative factors) is critical in controlling stress-related diarrhea.	3/24/12 Outcome not met. Patient reports little progress in coping with stress. With MCATs 1 week away, he feels more tense than ever before. Reports no time to explore stress management techniques.
Assess for other factors contributing to diarrhea and fluid volume deficit.	Diarrhea may have a functional basis.	*Revision:* Goal is appropriate. Encourage visit to counseling center, if not before MCATs then as soon as possible afterward.
Teach relation between stress and bouts of diarrhea.	Stress may result in increased intestinal mobility.	*C. Ryan, RN*
Refer to counseling center on campus for assistance with stress management.	Professional assistance may facilitate identification and management of stressful situation.	

EXPECTED OUTCOME By the next week's visit, 3/31/15, the patient will:
- Report that his diarrhea is eliminated or decreased to one or two episodes per day

NURSING INTERVENTIONS	RATIONALE	EVALUATIVE STATEMENT
Teach the patient to link causative factors with diarrhea and to note anything that brings relief or assists in establishment of usual pattern of defecation.	Being able to make these connections helps the patient to assume charge of his own condition and to reinforce preventive strategies and successful relief measures.	3/31/15 Outcome met. Patient reports diarrhea decreased to one or two episodes per day.

NURSING PLAN OF CARE 39-1   *continued*

for Jeremiah Stein

NURSING INTERVENTIONS	RATIONALE	EVALUATIVE STATEMENT
Make sure the patient understands diet: chemically and mechanically nonirritating diet high in calories, protein, and minerals; exclude foods such as cocoa, chocolate, alcohol, cold or carbonated beverages, citrus juices; try frequent, small meals.	Some patients fear eating because it stimulates the gastrocolic reflex and may result in a stool. Eating the proper diet actually reduces bowel irritation and decreases peristalsis.	*Recommendation:* Advise patient that it is important to keep the appointment with his gastroenterologist because relief may only be temporary. *C. Ryan, RN*
Teach the patient proper use of prescribed medications	Loperamide hydrochloride controls diarrhea, and methylcellulose increases consistency of stool.	

EXPECTED OUTCOME   By next week's visit, 3/31/15, the patient will:

- Demonstrate improved fluid and electrolyte balance as evidenced by (1) maintenance of present weight (170 lb), (2) moist mucous membranes, and (3) report of increased urinary output

NURSING INTERVENTIONS	RATIONALE	EVALUATIVE STATEMENT
Explore with the patient a workable plan for oral replacement of fluids.	Collaboration with the patient to determine acceptable sources of fluid intake may allay his fear that fluid intake causes diarrheal episodes.	3/31/15 Outcome partially met. Patient reports diarrhea decreased to once or twice a day. Two days there was no diarrhea. Weight, 169 lb.
Have the patient note which calorie- and electrolyte (sodium and potassium)–rich fluids he can tolerate. Increase fluid intake to maintain a normal urine specific gravity.	Increased fluid intake is necessary to compensate for excessive loss in diarrhea and to reestablish fluid balance.	Mucous membranes are moist. Urine output is increased. *C. Ryan, RN*
Instruct the patient to weigh himself every other day and to note changes in the volume or appearance of his urine.	All other things being equal, weight loss is a good indicator of continued fluid volume deficit. Other signs include decreased urinary output and high specific gravity.	
Teach the patient the defining characteristics of electrolyte imbalances associated with prolonged diarrhea—hyponatremia and hypokalemia.	Excreted stool pulls electrolytes with it, especially sodium and potassium.	

SAMPLE DOCUMENTATION   3/31/15, Nursing

Mr. Stein returned to the clinic reporting that his diarrhea is decreased to one to two episodes per day and that he has an appointment with a gastroenterologist. He believes that modifying his diet, increasing rest periods, and medications (loperamide hydrochloride to control diarrhea and methylcellulose to increase the consistency of stool) were of great help. He still does not know how he can reduce his stress level. Nursing examination revealed temperature, 98.9°F (37.1°C); pulse, 88 beats/min; respirations, 18 breaths/min; blood pressure, 110/60 mm Hg; weight, 169 lb.; skin and mucous membranes less dry than on previous visit. States he has not noted much change in urine output but possibly less concentrated.

C. Ryan, RN

SKILL 39-1 INITIATING A PERIPHERAL VENOUS ACCESS IV INFUSION

DELEGATION GUIDELINES

The initiation of a peripheral venous access IV infusion is not delegated to nursing assistive personnel (NAP) or unlicensed assistive personnel (UAP). Depending on the state's nurse practice act and the organization's policies and procedures, initiation of a peripheral venous access IV infusion may be delegated to licensed practical/vocational nurses (LPN/LVNs). The decision to delegate must be based on careful analysis of the patient's needs and circumstances, as well as the qualifications of the person to whom the task is being delegated. Refer to the Delegation Guidelines in Appendix A (found on the Point).

EQUIPMENT

- IV solution, as prescribed
- Medication administration record (MAR) or computer-generated MAR (CMAR)
- Towel or disposable pad
- Nonallergenic tape
- IV administration set
- Label for infusion set (for next change date)
- Transparent site dressing
- Electronic infusion device (if appropriate)
- Tourniquet
- Time tape and/or label (for IV container)
- Cleansing swabs (chlorhexidine preferred; 70% alcohol, iodine, or povidone-iodine are also acceptable)

- IV securement/stabilization device, as appropriate
- Clean gloves
- Additional PPE, as indicated
- IV pole
- Local anesthetic (if ordered)
- IV catheter
- Short extension tubing
- End cap for extension tubing
- Alcohol or other disinfectant wipes
- Skin protectant wipe (e.g., SkinPrep)
- Prefilled 2-mL syringe with sterile normal saline for injection

IMPLEMENTATION

ACTION	RATIONALE
1. Verify the IV solution order on the MAR/CMAR with the medical order. Consider the appropriateness of the prescribed therapy in relation to the patient. Clarify any inconsistencies. Check the patient's chart for allergies. Check for color, leaking, and expiration date. Know techniques for IV insertion, precautions, purpose of the IV administration, and medications if ordered. Gather necessary supplies.	This ensures that the correct IV solution and rate of infusion and/or medication will be administered. The nurse is responsible for critically evaluating all patient orders prior to administration. Any concerns regarding the type or amount of therapy prescribed should be immediately and clearly communicated to the prescribing practitioner. This knowledge and skill is essential for safe and accurate IV and medication administration. Preparation promotes efficient time management and an organized approach to the task.
2. Perform hand hygiene and put on PPE, if indicated.	Hand hygiene and PPE prevent the spread of microorganisms. PPE is required based on transmission precautions.
3. Identify the patient.	Identifying the patient ensures that the right patient receives the intervention and helps prevent errors.
4. Close the curtains around the bed and close the door to the room, if possible. Explain what you are going to do and why you are going to do it to the patient. Ask the patient about allergies to medications, tape, or skin antiseptics, as appropriate. If considering using a local anesthetic, inquire about allergies for these substances as well.	This ensures the patient's privacy. Explanation relieves anxiety and facilitates cooperation. Possible allergies may exist related to medications, tape, or local anesthetic. Injectable anesthetic can result in allergic reactions and tissue damage.
5. If using a local anesthetic, explain the rationale and procedure to the patient. Apply the anesthetic to a few potential insertion sites. Allow sufficient time for the anesthetic to take effect.	Explanations provide reassurance and facilitate the patient's cooperation. Local anesthetic decreases the degree of pain felt at the insertion site. Some of the anesthetics take up to an hour to become effective.

ACTION

Prepare the IV Solution and Administration Set

6. Compare the IV container label with the MAR/CMAR. Remove the IV bag from the outer wrapper, if indicated. Check expiration dates. Scan the bar code on the container, if necessary. Compare the patient identification band with the MAR/CMAR. Alternately, label the solution container with the patient's name, solution type, additives, date, and time. Complete a time strip for the infusion and apply to the IV container.

7. Maintain aseptic technique when opening sterile packages and the IV solution. Remove the administration set from the package (see Fig. 39-10, p. 1502). Apply the label to the tubing, reflecting the day/date for next set change, per facility guidelines.

8. Close the roller clamp or slide clamp on the IV administration set (Fig. 1). Invert the IV solution container and remove the cap on the entry site, taking care not to touch the exposed entry site. Remove the cap from the spike on the administration set. Using a twisting and pushing motion, insert the administration set spike into the entry site of the IV container (Fig. 2). Alternately, follow the manufacturer's directions for insertion.

9. Hang the IV container on the IV pole. Squeeze the drip chamber and fill at least halfway (Fig 3).

RATIONALE

Checking the label with MAR/CMAR ensures that the correct IV solution will be administered. Identifying the patient ensures that the right patient receives the medications and helps prevent errors. Time strip allows for a quick visual reference by the nurse to monitor infusion accuracy.

Asepsis is essential for preventing the spread of microorganisms. Labeling tubing ensures adherence to facility policy regarding administration set changes and reduces the risk of the spread of microorganisms (see Box 39-1, p. 1509).

Clamping the IV tubing prevents air and fluid from entering the IV tubing at this time.

Inverting the container allows easy access to the entry site. Touching the opened entry site on the IV container and/or the spike on the administration set results in contamination and the container/administration set would have to be discarded. Inserting the spike punctures the seal in the IV container and allows access to the contents.

Suction causes fluid to move into drip chamber. Fluid prevents air from moving down the tubing.

FIGURE 1. Closing clamp on administration set.

FIGURE 2. Inserting administration set spike into entry site of IV fluid container.

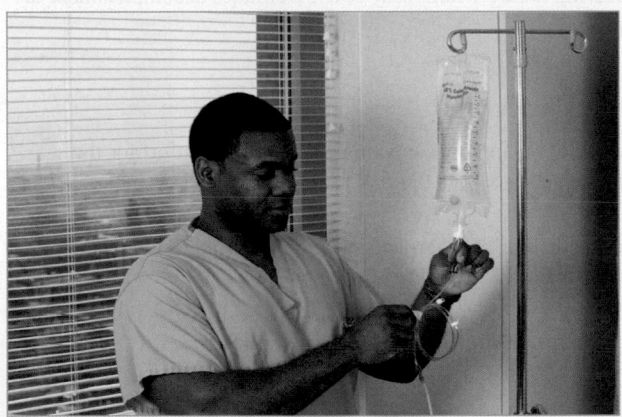

FIGURE 3. Squeezing drip chamber to fill at least halfway.

(continued)

SKILL 39-1 INITIATING A PERIPHERAL VENOUS ACCESS IV INFUSION *continued*

ACTION	RATIONALE
10. Open the IV tubing clamp, and allow fluid to move through tubing. Follow additional manufacturer's instructions for specific electronic infusion pump, as indicated. **Allow fluid to flow until all air bubbles have disappeared and the entire length of the tubing is primed (filled) with IV solution** (Fig. 4). Close the clamp. Alternately, some brands of tubing may require removal of the cap at the end of the IV tubing to allow fluid to flow. Maintain its sterility. After fluid has filled the tubing, recap the end of the tubing.	This technique prepares for IV fluid administration and removes air from the tubing. If not removed from the tubing, large amounts of air can act as an embolus. Touching the open end of the tubing results in contamination and the administration set would have to be discarded.
11. If an electronic device is to be used, follow the manufacturer's instructions for inserting tubing into the device (Fig. 5).	This ensures proper use of equipment.

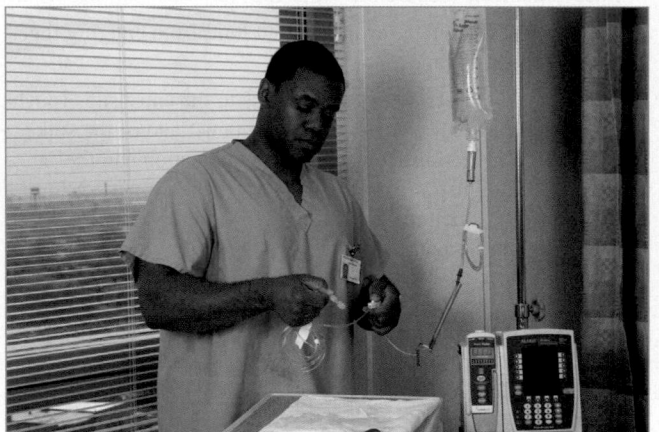

FIGURE 4. Priming administration set.

FIGURE 5. Inserting administration set into electronic infusion device.

Initiate Peripheral Venous Access

12. Place the patient in low-Fowler's position in bed. Place protective towel or pad under patient's arm.	The supine position permits either arm to be used and allows for good body alignment. Towel protects the underlying surface from blood contamination.
13. Provide emotional support, as needed.	Patient may experience anxiety due to fear of needlestick or IV infusion.
14. Open the short extension tubing package. Attach the end cap, if not in place. Clean the end cap with an alcohol wipe. Insert the syringe with normal saline into the extension tubing. Fill the extension tubing with normal saline and apply the slide clamp. Remove the syringe and place the extension tubing and syringe back on the package, within easy reach.	Priming the extension tubing removes air from the tubing and prevents administration of air when connected to venous access. Having tubing within easy reach facilitates accomplishment of procedure.
15. Select and palpate for an appropriate vein. Refer to the guidelines on page 1505. If the intended insertion site is visibly soiled, clean the area with soap and water.	The use of an appropriate vein decreases discomfort for the patient and reduces the risk for damage to body tissues.
16. If the site is hairy and agency policy permits, clip a 2-inch area around the intended entry site.	Hair can harbor microorganisms and inhibit adhesion of the site dressing. Shaving causes microabrasions and increases risk for infection (INS, 2011, p. S44).
17. Put on gloves.	Gloves prevent contact with blood and body fluids.

ACTION

18. Apply a tourniquet 3 to 4 inches above the venipuncture site to obstruct venous blood flow and distend the vein (Fig. 6). Direct the ends of the tourniquet away from the entry site. Make sure the radial pulse is still present.

FIGURE 6. Applying tourniquet.

19. Instruct the patient to hold the arm lower than the heart.

20. Ask the patient to open and close the fist. Observe and palpate for a suitable vein. Try the following techniques if a vein cannot be felt:

    a. Lightly stroke the vein downward.

    b. Remove the tourniquet and place warm, dry compresses over the intended vein for 10 to 15 minutes.

21. **Cleanse site with an antiseptic solution such as chlorhexidine or according to facility policy. Press the applicator against the skin and apply chlorhexidine, using a gentle back-and-forth motion. Do not wipe or blot. Allow to dry completely.**

22. Alternately, for patients who bruise easily, are at risk for bleeding, or have fragile skin, **apply the chlorhexidine without scrubbing for at least 30 seconds. Allow to dry completely. Do not wipe or blot.**

23. Using your nondominant hand placed about 1 or 2 inches below the entry site, hold the skin taut against the vein. **Avoid touching the prepared site.** Ask the patient to remain still while performing the venipuncture.

RATIONALE

Interrupting the blood flow to the heart causes the vein to distend. Distended veins are easy to see, palpate, and enter. The end of the tourniquet could contaminate the area of injection if directed toward the entry site. Tourniquet may be applied too tightly, thus assessment for radial pulse is important. Checking radial pulse ensures that the arterial supply is not compromised.

Lowering the arm below the heart level helps distend the veins by filling them.

Contracting the muscles of the forearm forces blood into the veins, thereby distending them further.

Massaging and tapping the vein help distend veins by filling them with blood.

Warm compresses help dilate veins. The use of dry heat increases the likelihood of successful peripheral catheter insertion (INS, 2011).

Cleansing is necessary because organisms on the skin can be introduced into the tissues or the bloodstream with the needle. Chlorhexidine is the preferred antiseptic solution, but iodine, povidone-iodine, and 70% alcohol are considered acceptable alternatives (INS, 2011). Scrubbing motion creates friction and lets the solution more effectively penetrate the epidermal layers (Hadaway, 2006).

Cleansing is necessary because organisms on the skin can be introduced into the tissues or the bloodstream with the needle. Avoiding use of scrubbing decreases risk of injury. A minimum of 30 seconds is the length of time that is necessary for chlorhexidine to be effective (Hadaway, 2006).

Pressure on the vein and surrounding tissues helps prevent movement of the vein as the needle or catheter is being inserted. The planned IV insertion site is not palpated after skin cleansing unless sterile gloves are worn to prevent contamination (INS, 2011). Patient movement may prevent proper technique for IV insertion.

(continued)

SKILL 39-1 INITIATING A PERIPHERAL VENOUS ACCESS IV INFUSION *continued*

ACTION	**RATIONALE**
24. Enter the skin gently, holding the catheter by the hub in your dominant hand, bevel side up, at a 10- to 15-degree angle (Fig. 7). Insert the catheter from directly over the vein or from the side of the vein. While following the course of the vein, advance the needle or catheter into the vein. A sensation of "give" can be felt when the needle enters the vein.	This allows the needle or catheter to enter the vein with minimal trauma and deters passage of the needle through the vein.
25. When blood returns through the lumen of the needle or the flashback chamber of the catheter, advance either device into the vein until the hub is at the venipuncture site. The exact technique depends on the type of device used.	The tourniquet causes increased venous pressure, resulting in automatic backflow. Placing the access device well into the vein helps to prevent dislodgement.
26. Release the tourniquet. Quickly remove the protective cap from the extension tubing and attach it to the catheter or needle. Stabilize the catheter or needle with your nondominant hand.	Bleeding is minimized and the patency of the vein is maintained if the connection is made smoothly between the catheter and tubing.
27. Continue to stabilize the catheter or needle and flush gently with the saline, observing the site for infiltration and leaking.	Infiltration and/or leaking and patient reports of pain and/or discomfort indicate that the insertion into the vein is not successful and should be discontinued.
28. Open the skin protectant wipe. Apply the skin protectant to the site, making sure to apply—at minimum—the area to be covered with the dressing. Place a sterile transparent dressing or catheter securing/stabilization device over the venipuncture site. Loop the tubing near the site of entry, and anchor with tape (nonallergenic) close to the site.	Skin protectant aids in adhesion of the dressing and decreases the risk for skin trauma when the dressing is removed. Transparent dressing allows easy visualization and protects the site. Stabilization/securing devices preserve the integrity of the access device, minimize catheter movement at the hub, and prevent catheter dislodgement and loss of access (INS, 2011, p. S46). Some stabilization devices also act as a site dressing. The weight of the tubing is sufficient to pull it out of the vein if it is not well anchored. Nonallergenic tape is less likely to tear fragile skin.
29. Label the IV dressing with the date, time, site, and type and size of catheter or needle used for the infusion (Fig. 8).	Other personnel working with the infusion will know the site, type of device being used, and when it was inserted. Peripheral venous catheter IV insertion sites are changed every 72 to 96 hours for an adult (O'Grady et al., 2011).

FIGURE 7. Stretching skin taut and inserting needle.

FIGURE 8. Venous access site with labeled dressing.

ACTION

30. Using an antimicrobial swab, cleanse the access cap on the extension tubing. Remove the end cap from the administration set. Insert the end of the administration set into the end cap (Fig. 9). Loop the administration set tubing near the site of entry, and anchor with tape (nonallergenic) close to the site. Remove gloves.

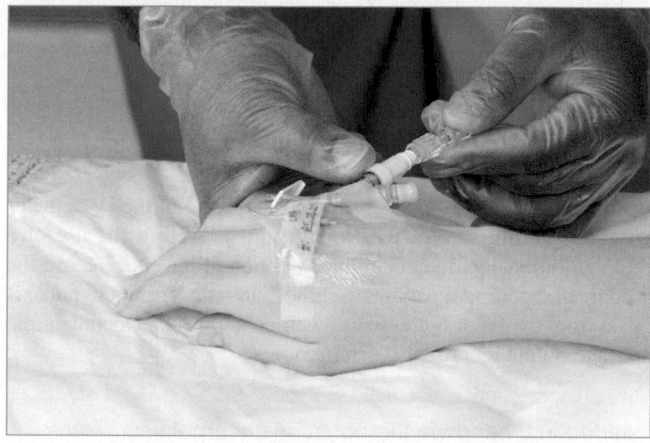

RATIONALE

Inserting the administration set allows initiation of the fluid infusion. The weight of the tubing is sufficient to pull it out of the vein if it is not well anchored. Nonallergenic tape is less likely to tear fragile skin. Removing gloves properly reduces the risk for infection transmission and contamination of other items.

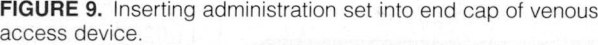

FIGURE 9. Inserting administration set into end cap of venous access device.

31. Open the clamp on the administration set. Set the flow rate and begin the fluid infusion (Fig. 10). Alternately, start the flow of solution by releasing the clamp on the tubing and counting the drops. Adjust until the correct drop rate is achieved. Assess the flow of the solution and function of the infusion device. Inspect the insertion site for signs of infiltration (Figure 11).

Verifying the rate and device settings ensures that the patient receives the correct volume of solution. If the catheter slips out of the vein, the solution will accumulate (infiltrate) into the surrounding tissue.

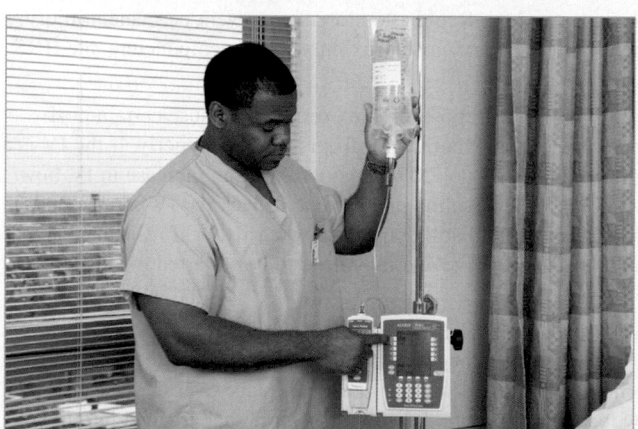

FIGURE 10. Initiating IV fluid infusion.

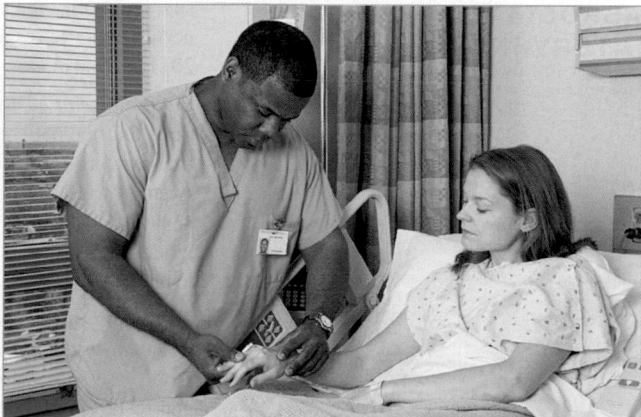

FIGURE 11. Inspecting insertion site.

32. Apply an IV securement/stabilization device if not already in place as part of the dressing, as indicated, based on facility policy. Explain to the patient the purpose of the device and the importance of safeguarding the site when using the extremity.

These systems are recommended for use on all venous access sites, and particularly central venous access sites, to preserve the integrity of the access device, minimize catheter movement at the hub, and prevent catheter dislodgement and loss of access (INS, 2011, p. S46). Some devices also act as a site dressing and may already have been applied.

(continued)

SKILL 39-1 INITIATING A PERIPHERAL VENOUS ACCESS IV INFUSION *continued*

ACTION	**RATIONALE**
33. Remove equipment and return the patient to a position of comfort. Lower the bed, if not in the lowest position.	Promotes patient comfort and safety.
34. Remove additional PPE, if used. Perform hand hygiene.	Removing PPE properly reduces the risk for infection transmission and contamination of other items. Hand hygiene prevents transmission of microorganisms.
35. Return to check flow rate and observe IV site for infiltration and/or other complications 30 minutes after starting infusion, and at least hourly thereafter. Ask the patient if he or she is experiencing any pain or discomfort related to the IV infusion.	Continued monitoring is important to maintain correct flow rate. Early detection of problems ensures prompt intervention.

DOCUMENTATION

Guidelines

Document the location where the IV access was placed, as well as the size of the IV catheter or needle, the type of IV solution, and the rate of the IV infusion, as well as the use of a securing or stabilization device. Additionally, document the condition of the site. Record the patient's reaction to the procedure and pertinent patient teaching, such as alerting the nurse if the patient experiences any pain from the IV or notices any swelling at the site. Document the IV fluid solution on the intake and output record.

Sample Documentation

DocuCare Practice documenting peripheral venous access infusion in *Lippincott DocuCare*.

> 11/02/15 0830 20G IV started in L hand via the dorsal metacarpal vein. Transparent dressing and peripheral stabilization device applied. Site without redness, drainage, or edema. D$_5$1/2 NS with 20 mEq KCl begun at 110 mL/hour. Patient instructed to call with any pain, discomfort, or swelling.
> —S. Barnes, RN

UNEXPECTED SITUATIONS AND ASSOCIATED INTERVENTIONS

- *An artery is inadvertently accessed or the patient complains of paresthesias, numbness, or tingling upon insertion:* Immediately remove the catheter, apply pressure to the insertion site, and notify the primary care provider. Rapid attention may prevent permanent injury; nerves and arteries are often located in very close proximity to the venipuncture site (INS, 2011, p. S44).

- *Fluid does not easily flow into the vein:* Reposition the extremity because certain positions that the patient may assume may prevent the IV from infusing properly. If the IV is a free-flowing IV, raise the height of the IV pole. This may promote an increase in IV flow. Attempt to flush the IV with 2 to 3 mL of saline in a syringe. Check the IV connector to ensure that the clamp is fully open. If fluid still does not flow easily, or if resistance is met while flushing, the IV may be against a valve and may need to be restarted in a different location.

- *Fluid does not flow easily into the vein and the skin around the insertion site is edematous and cool to the touch:* IV has infiltrated. Put gauze on gloves and remove the catheter. Apply pressure with a sterile gauze pad. Secure the gauze with tape over the insertion site and restart the IV in a new location. Estimate the volume of fluid that escaped into the tissue based on the rate of infusion and length of time since last assessment. Large volumes (greater than 25 to 50 mL) increase the risk of tissue damage (INS, 2011).

- *A small hematoma is forming at the site while you are inserting the catheter:* The vein is "blowing," which means a small hole has been made in the vein and blood is leaking out into the tissues. Remove and discard the catheter and choose an alternate insertion site.

- *Fluids are leaking around the insertion site:* Change the dressing on the IV. If the site continues to leak, remove the IV and restart it in a new location.

- *IV infusion set becomes disconnected from IV:* Discard the IV tubing to prevent infection. Attempt to flush the IV with 3 mL of normal saline. If the IV is still patent, the site may still be used, as long as the catheter hub has not been contaminated.

- *IV catheter is partially pulled out of insertion site (migrates externally):* Do not reinsert the catheter. Whether the IV is salvageable depends on how much of the catheter remains in the vein. Assess for proper placement in the vein before further use (INS, 2011). If this catheter is not removed, monitor it closely for signs of infiltration.

SPECIAL CONSIDERATIONS

General Considerations

- No more than two attempts at vascular access placement should be made by any one nurse when initiating venous access for a patient. If unsuccessful after two attempts, a colleague with advanced skills, such as a member of the nurse IV team, should attempt to initiate the venous access (Arbique & Arbique, 2007).

- Factors that may interfere with successful placement of a peripheral catheter include increased patient age, obesity, hypovolemia, injection drug use, and the presence of multiple chronic diseases. These patients lack easy access using the traditional techniques of direct visualization, anatomic landmarks, and palpation (Houston, 2013; White et al., 2010). Ultrasound guided peripheral intravenous placement is a safe, efficient intervention for patients who are difficult to assess (Maiocco & Coole, 2012; White et al.). Consider the use of ultrasound to guide placement of a peripheral intravenous catheter by a specially trained nurse.

- Closed IV catheter systems are available. These systems have the short extension tubing integrated into the catheter, eliminating the need to attach extension tubing to the IV catheter before insertion, which reduces potential contamination.

Infant and Child Considerations

- Do not choose hand insertion sites as the first choice for children because nerve endings are very close to the surface of the skin, and such an insertion is more painful. Once the child can walk, do not use the feet as insertion sites.

- Additional potential sites for neonates and children include veins of the scalp, foot, and fingers in infants and toddlers (INS, 2011). Scalp arteries in infants are visible (see Fig. 39-15B, p. 1505). Carefully palpate the site before insertion. If the site is pulsating, do not use.

- Do not replace peripheral catheters in children unless a complication develops (CDC, 2011).

- Chlorhexidine is not recommended for infants under 2 months of age (INS, 2011). Use of chlorhexidine (in infants and children older than 2 months), 70% alcohol, iodine, or povidone-iodine is recommended for skin antisepsis for peripheral venous catheters (INS, 2011; O'Grady et al., 2011).

- For infants under 2 months of age or pediatric patients with compromised skin integrity, remove dried povidone-iodine with normal saline wipes or sterile water (INS, 2011).

Older Adult Considerations

- Avoid using vigorous friction at the insertion site, which can traumatize fragile skin and veins in older adults.

- To decrease the risk for trauma to the vessel, experienced nurses may omit use of a tourniquet if the patient has prominent but especially fragile veins.

SKILL 39-2 MONITORING AN IV SITE AND INFUSION

DELEGATION CONSIDERATIONS	The monitoring of an IV site and infusion is not delegated to nursing assistive personnel (NAP) or unlicensed assistive personnel (UAP). Depending on the state's nurse practice act and the organization's policies and procedures, these procedures may be delegated to licensed practical/vocational nurses (LPN/LVNs). The decision to delegate must be based on careful analysis of the patient's needs and circumstances, as well as the qualifications of the person to whom the task is being delegated. Refer to the Delegation Guidelines in Appendix A (found on the Point).

EQUIPMENT	• PPE, as indicated

IMPLEMENTATION

ACTION

1. Verify the IV solution order on the MAR/CMAR with the medical order. Consider the appropriateness of the prescribed therapy in relation to the patient. Clarify any inconsistencies. Check the patient's chart for allergies. Check for color, leaking, and expiration date. Know the purpose of the IV administration and medications, if ordered.

2. **Monitor IV infusion every hour or per facility policy. More frequent checks may be necessary if medication is being infused.**

3. Perform hand hygiene and put on PPE, if indicated.

4. Identify the patient.

5. Close the curtains around the bed and close the door to the room, if possible. Explain what you are going to do and why you are going to do it to the patient.

6. If an electronic infusion device is being used, check settings, alarm, and indicator lights. Check set infusion rate (Fig. 1). Note the position of the fluid in the IV container in relation to the time tape. Teach the patient about the alarm features on the electronic infusion device.

7. If the IV is infusing via gravity, check the drip chamber and time the drops (Fig. 2). See Guidelines for Nursing Care 39-3, p. 1507 to review calculations.

RATIONALE

This ensures that the correct IV solution and rate of infusion, and/or medication, will be administered. The nurse is responsible for critically evaluating all patient orders. Any concerns regarding the type or amount of therapy prescribed should be immediately and clearly communicated to the prescribing practitioner. This knowledge and skill is essential for safe and accurate IV and medication administration.

Promotes safe administration of IV fluids and medication.

Hand hygiene and PPE prevent the spread of microorganisms. PPE is required based on transmission precautions.

Identifying the patient ensures that the right patient receives the intervention and helps prevent errors.

This ensures the patient's privacy. Explanation relieves anxiety and facilitates cooperation.

Observation ensures that the infusion control device and the alarm are functioning. Lack of knowledge about alarms may create anxiety for patient.

This ensures that the flow rate is correct. Use a watch with a second hand for counting the drops in regulating a gravity drip IV infusion.

FIGURE 1. Checking settings of infusion device.

FIGURE 2. Checking drip chamber and timing drops.

ACTION

8. Check the tubing for anything that might interfere with the flow (Fig. 3). Be sure clamps are in the open position.

9. Observe the dressing for leakage of IV solution.

10. Inspect the site for swelling, leakage at the site, coolness, or pallor, which may indicate infiltration (Fig. 4). Ask if the patient is experiencing any pain or discomfort. If any of these symptoms are present, the IV will need to be removed and restarted at another site. Check facility policy for treating infiltration. (Refer to Table 39-12, p. 1510 and Box 39-2, p. 1511.)

FIGURE 3. Checking tubing for anything that might interfere with flow rate.

11. Inspect the site for redness, swelling, and heat. Palpate for induration. Ask if the patient is experiencing pain. These findings may indicate phlebitis. Notify the primary care provider if phlebitis is suspected. The IV will need to be discontinued and restarted at another site. Check facility policy for treatment of phlebitis. (Refer to Table 39-12, p. 1510 and Box 39-3, p. 1511.)

12. Check for local manifestations (redness, pus, warmth, induration, and pain) that may indicate an infection is present at the site. Also check for systemic manifestations (chills, fever, tachycardia, hypotension) that may accompany local infection at the site. If signs of infection are present, discontinue the IV and notify the primary care provider. Be careful not to disconnect the IV tubing when putting on the patient's hospital gown or assisting the patient with movement.

13. Be alert for additional complications of IV therapy, such as fluid overload bleeding.

   a. Fluid overload can result in signs of cardiac and/or respiratory failure. Monitor intake and output and vital signs. Assess for edema and auscultate lung sounds. Ask if the patient is experiencing any shortness of breath.

   b. Check for bleeding at the site.

RATIONALE

Any kink or pressure on the tubing may interfere with the flow.

Leakage may occur at the connection of the tubing with the hub of the needle or the catheter and allow for loss of IV solution.

Catheter may become dislodged from the vein, and IV solution may flow into subcutaneous tissue.

FIGURE 4. Inspecting IV site.

Chemical irritation or mechanical trauma causes injury to the vein and can lead to phlebitis. Phlebitis is the most common complication related to IV therapy (Lavery, 2005).

Poor aseptic technique may allow bacteria to enter the needle, catheter insertion site, or tubing connection and may occur with manipulation of equipment.

Infusing too much IV solution results in an increased volume of circulating fluid volume.

Older patients are most at risk for this complication due to possible decrease in cardiac and/or renal functions.

Bleeding may be caused by anticoagulant medication. Bleeding at the site is most likely to occur when the IV is discontinued.

(continued)

SKILL 39-2 MONITORING AN IV SITE AND INFUSION *continued*

ACTION	RATIONALE
14. If appropriate, instruct the patient to call for assistance if any discomfort is noted at the site, the solution container is nearly empty, the flow has changed in any way, or if the electronic pump alarm sounds.	This facilitates patient cooperation and safe administration of the IV solution.
15. Remove PPE, if used. Perform hand hygiene.	Removing PPE properly reduces the risk for infection transmission and contamination of other items. Hand hygiene prevents transmission of microorganisms.

DOCUMENTATION

Guidelines

Document the type of IV solution as well as the infusion rate. Note the insertion site location and site assessment. Document the patient's reaction to the IV therapy as well as the absence of subjective reports that the patient is not experiencing any pain or other discomfort, such as coolness or heat associated with the infusion. Additionally, record that the patient is not demonstrating any other IV complications, such as signs or symptoms of fluid overload. Document the IV fluid solution on the intake and output record.

Sample Documentation

> <u>11/6/15</u> 1020 IV site right forearm/cephalic vein intact without swelling, redness, or drainage. D$_5$ 0.9% NS with 20 mEq KCl continues to infuse at 110 mL/hour. Patient instructed to call nurse with any swelling or pain.
> —S. Barnes, RN

UNEXPECTED SITUATIONS AND ASSOCIATED INTERVENTIONS

• *Patient's lung sounds were previously clear, but now some crackles in the bases are auscultated:* Notify the primary care provider immediately. The patient may be exhibiting signs of fluid overload. Be prepared to tell the health care provider what the past intake and output totals were, as well as the vital signs and pulse oximetry findings of the patient.

• *IV is not flowing as easily as it previously had been:* Check all clamps on the tubing and check tubing for any kinking. Check that the patient is not lying on the tubing. If the IV is over a joint, reposition the extremity and see if this helps the flow. You may need to apply an arm board. Attempt to flush the IV with 2 to 3 mL of normal saline. If the IV is painful or you meet resistance when attempting to flush, discontinue the IV and restart in another place.

SKILL 39-3 CHANGING AN IV SOLUTION CONTAINER AND ADMINISTRATION SET

DELEGATION CONSIDERATIONS

The changing of an IV solution container and administration set is not delegated to nursing assistive personnel (NAP) or unlicensed assistive personnel (UAP). Depending on the state's nurse practice act and the organization's policies and procedures, these procedures may be delegated to licensed practical/vocational nurses (LPN/LVNs). The decision to delegate must be based on careful analysis of the patient's needs and circumstances, as well as the qualifications of the person to whom the task is being delegated. Refer to the Delegation Guidelines in Appendix A (found on thePoint).

EQUIPMENT

For solution container change:
- IV solution, as prescribed
- MAR/CMAR
- Time tape and/or label (for IV container)
- PPE, as indicated

For tubing change:
- Administration set
- Label for administration set (for next change date)

- Sterile gauze
- Nonallergenic tape
- IV securement/stabilization device, as appropriate
- Clean gloves
- Additional PPE, as indicated
- Alcohol or other disinfectant wipes

IMPLEMENTATION

ACTION	RATIONALE
1. Verify the IV solution order on the MAR/CMAR with the medical order. Consider the appropriateness of the prescribed therapy in relation to the patient. Clarify any inconsistencies. Check the patient's chart for allergies. Check for color, leaking, and expiration date. Know the purpose of the IV administration, and medications if ordered. Gather necessary supplies.	This ensures that the correct IV solution and rate of infusion, and/or medication, will be administered. The nurse is responsible for critically evaluating all patient orders prior to administration. Any concerns regarding the type or amount of therapy prescribed should be immediately and clearly communicated to the prescribing practitioner. This knowledge and skill is essential for safe and accurate IV and medication administration. Preparation promotes efficient time management and organized approach to the task.
2. Perform hand hygiene and put on PPE, if indicated.	Hand hygiene and PPE prevent the spread of microorganisms. PPE is required based on transmission precautions.
3. Identify the patient.	Identifying the patient ensures that the right patient receives the intervention and helps prevent errors.
4. Close the curtains around the bed and close the door to the room, if possible. Explain what you are going to do and why you are going to do it to the patient. Ask the patient about allergies to medications or tape, as appropriate.	This ensures the patient's privacy. Explanation relieves anxiety and facilitates cooperation. Possible allergies may exist related to IV solution additive or tape.
5. Compare the IV container label with the MAR/CMAR (Fig. 1). Remove the IV bag from the outer wrapper, if indicated. Check expiration dates. Scan the bar code on the container, if necessary. Compare the patient identification band with the MAR/CMAR. Alternately, label the solution container with the patient's name, solution type, additives, date, and time. Complete a time strip for the infusion and apply to the IV container.	Checking the label with the MAR/CMAR ensures that the correct IV solution will be administered. Identifying the patient ensures that the right patient receives the medications and helps prevent errors. Time strip allows for a quick visual reference by the nurse to monitor infusion accuracy.

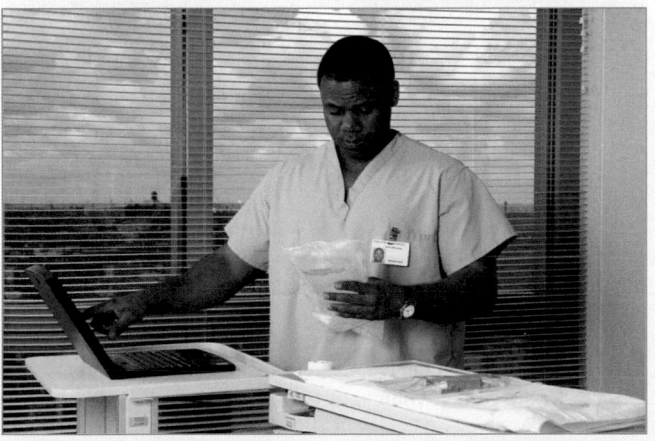

FIGURE 1. Comparing IV fluid container label with MAR/CMAR.

(continued)

SKILL 39-3 CHANGING AN IV SOLUTION CONTAINER AND ADMINISTRATION SET *continued*

ACTION	RATIONALE
6. Maintain aseptic technique when opening sterile packages and the IV solution. Remove the administration set from the package. Apply the label to the tubing, reflecting the day/date for next set change, per facility guidelines.	Asepsis is essential for preventing the spread of microorganisms. Labeling the tubing ensures adherence to facility policy regarding administration set changes and reduces the risk of spread of microorganisms. Refer to Box 39-1, p. 1509 for recommended administration set change guidelines.

To Change IV Solution Container

ACTION	RATIONALE
7. If using an electronic infusion device, pause the device or put on "hold." Close the slide clamp on the administration set closest to the drip chamber. If using gravity infusion, close the roller clamp on the administration set.	The action of the infusion device needs to be paused while the solution container is changed. Closing the clamps prevents the fluid in the drip chamber from emptying and air from entering the tubing during the procedure.
8. Carefully remove the cap on the entry site of the new IV solution container and expose the entry site, **taking care not to touch the exposed entry site.**	Touching the opened entry site on the IV container results in contamination and the container would have to be discarded.
9. Lift the empty container off the IV pole and invert it. Quickly remove the spike from the old IV container, **being careful not to contaminate it.** Discard the old IV container.	Touching the spike on the administration set results in contamination and the tubing would have to be discarded.
10. Using a twisting and pushing motion, insert the administration set spike into the entry site of the IV container. Alternately, follow the manufacturer's directions for insertion. Hang the container on the IV pole.	Inserting the spike punctures the seal in the IV container and allows access to contents.
11. Alternately, hang the new IV fluid container on an open hook on the IV pole. Carefully remove the cap on the entry site of the new IV solution container and expose the entry site, **taking care not to touch the exposed entry site.** Lift the empty container off the IV pole and invert it. Quickly remove the spike from the old IV container, **being careful not to contaminate it (Fig. 2).** Discard the old IV container. Using a twisting and pushing motion, insert the administration set spike into the entry port of the new IV container as it hangs on the IV pole (Fig. 3).	Touching the opened entry site on the IV container or the administration set spike results in contamination and both would have to be discarded. Inserting the spike punctures the seal in the IV container and allows access to contents.

FIGURE 2. Removing administration spike from old IV fluid container.

FIGURE 3. Inserting administration set spike into entry port of new IV fluid container.

ACTION	RATIONALE
12. If using an electronic infusion device, open the slide clamp, check the drip chamber of the administration set, verify the flow rate programmed in the infusion device, and turn the device to "run" or "infuse."	Verifying the rate and device settings ensures that the patient receives the correct volume of the solution.

ACTION

13. If using gravity infusion, slowly open the roller clamp on the administration set and count the drops. Adjust until the correct drop rate is achieved (Fig. 4).

FIGURE 4. Reopening clamp and adjusting flow rate.

To Change the IV Solution Container and Administration Set

14. Prepare the IV solution and administration set. Refer to Skill 39-1, Steps 6–10 on pages 1521–1522.

15. Hang the IV container on an open hook on the IV pole. Close the clamp on the existing IV administration set. Also, close the clamp on the short extension tubing connected to the IV catheter in the patient's arm.

16. If using an electronic infusion device, remove the current administration set from the device. Following the manufacturer's directions, insert a new administration set into the infusion device.

17. Put on gloves. Remove the current infusion tubing from the access cap on the short extension IV tubing. Using an antimicrobial swab, cleanse the access cap on the extension tubing. Remove the end cap from the new administration set. Insert the end of the administration set into the access cap. Loop the administration set tubing near the entry site, and anchor with tape (nonallergenic) close to the site (Fig. 5).

RATIONALE

Opening the clamp regulates the flow rate into the drip chamber. Verifying the rate ensures that the patient receives the correct volume of solution.

Clamping the existing IV tubing prevents leakage of fluid from the administration set after it is disconnected. Clamping the tubing on the extension set prevents introduction of air into the extension tubing.

Administration set has to be removed in order to insert new tubing into the device.

Cleansing the cap or port reduces the risk of contamination. Inserting the administration set allows initiation of the fluid infusion. The weight of the tubing is sufficient to pull it out of the vein if it is not well anchored. Nonallergenic tape is less likely to tear fragile skin.

FIGURE 5. Making sure clamp is open on new tubing, with short extension tubing taped in place.

(continued)

SKILL 39-3 CHANGING AN IV SOLUTION CONTAINER AND ADMINISTRATION SET *continued*

ACTION	**RATIONALE**
18. Open the clamp on the extension tubing. Open the clamp on the administration set.	Opening clamps allows the solution to flow to the patient.
19. If using an electronic infusion device, open the slide clamp, check the drip chamber of the administration set, verify the flow rate programmed in the infusion device, and turn the device to "run" or "infuse."	Verifying the rate and device settings ensures that the patient receives the correct volume of solution.
20. If using gravity infusion, slowly open the roller clamp on the administration set and count the drops. Adjust until the correct drop rate is achieved.	Opening the clamp regulates the flow rate into the drip chamber. Verifying the rate ensures that the patient receives the correct volume of solution.
21. Remove equipment. Ensure patient's comfort. Remove gloves. Lower the bed if not in the lowest position.	Promotes patient comfort and safety. Removing gloves properly reduces the risk for infection transmission and contamination of other items.
22. Remove additional PPE, if used. Perform hand hygiene.	Removing PPE properly reduces the risk for infection transmission and contamination of other items. Hand hygiene prevents transmission of microorganisms.
23. Return to check the flow rate and observe the IV site for infiltration and/or other complications 30 minutes after starting infusion, and at least hourly thereafter. Ask if the patient is experiencing any pain or discomfort related to the IV infusion.	Continued monitoring is important to maintain the correct flow rate. Early detection of problems ensures prompt intervention.

DOCUMENTATION

Guidelines

Document the type of IV solution and the rate of infusion (this is often done in the CMAR/MAR) as well as the assessment of the access site. Record the patient's reaction to the procedure and pertinent patient teaching, such as alerting the nurse if the patient experiences any pain from the IV or notices any swelling at the site. Document the IV fluid solution on the intake and output record.

Sample Documentation

> <u>11/3/15</u> 1015 IV fluid changed from $D_5$1/2 NS with 20 mEq KCl/L at 125 mL/hour to D_5 0.9% NS with 20 mEq KCl/L at 80 mL/hour. IV site intact; no swelling, redness, or drainage noted.
>
> —S. Barnes, RN

UNEXPECTED SITUATIONS AND ASSOCIATED INTERVENTIONS

- *Infusion does not flow or flow rate changes after bag and tubing are changed:* Make sure that the flow clamp is open and the drip chamber is approximately half full. Check the electronic device for proper functioning. Check the IV site for possible problems with the catheter, such as bending of the catheter or position of the patient's extremity, and inspect the IV site for signs and symptoms of complications. Readjust the flow rate.
- *After attaching new IV tubing, you note air bubbles in the tubing:* If the bubbles are above the roller clamp, you can easily remove them by closing the roller clamp, stretching the tubing downward, and tapping the tubing with your finger so that the bubbles rise to the drip chamber. If there is a larger amount of air in the tubing, swab the medication port on the tubing below the air with an antimicrobial solution and attach a syringe to the port below the air. Clamp the tubing below the access port. Aspirate the air from the tubing via the syringe. Remember that air bubbles in the tubing can be reduced if the tubing is primed slowly with fluid instead of allowing a wide-open flow of the solution.

SKILL 39-4 CHANGING A PERIPHERAL VENOUS ACCESS DRESSING

DELEGATION CONSIDERATIONS

The changing of a peripheral venous access dressing is not delegated to nursing assistive personnel (NAP) or unlicensed assistive personnel (UAP). Depending on the state's nurse practice act and the organization's policies and procedures, the changing of a peripheral venous access dressing may be delegated to licensed practical/vocational nurses (LPN/LVNs). The decision to delegate must be based on careful analysis of the patient's needs and circumstances, as well as the qualifications of the person to whom the task is being delegated. Refer to the Delegation Guidelines in Appendix A (found on thePoint).

EQUIPMENT

- Transparent occlusive dressing
- Cleansing swabs (chlorhexidine preferred; 70% alcohol, iodine, or povidone-iodine are also acceptable)
- Adhesive remover (optional)
- Alcohol or other disinfectant wipes
- Skin protectant wipe (e.g., SkinPrep)
- IV securement/stabilization device, as appropriate
- Tape
- Clean gloves
- Towel or disposable pad
- Additional PPE, as indicated

IMPLEMENTATION

ACTION	RATIONALE
1. Determine the need for a dressing change. Check facility policy. Gather equipment.	The particular facility's policies determine the type of dressing used and when these dressings are changed. Dressing changes might be required more often, based on nursing assessment and judgment. Immediately change any access site dressing that is damp, loosened, or soiled. Preparation promotes efficient time management and an organized approach to the task.
2. Perform hand hygiene and put on PPE, if indicated.	Hand hygiene and PPE prevent the spread of microorganisms. PPE is required based on transmission precautions.
3. Identify the patient.	Identifying the patient ensures that the right patient receives the intervention and helps prevent errors.
4. Close the curtains around the bed and close the door to the room, if possible. Explain what you are going to do and why you are going to do it to the patient. Ask the patient about allergies to tape and skin antiseptics.	This ensures the patient's privacy. Explanation relieves anxiety and facilitates cooperation. Possible allergies may exist related to tape or antiseptics.
5. Put on gloves. Place a towel or disposable pad under the arm with the venous access. If solution is currently infusing, temporarily stop the infusion. Hold the catheter in place with your nondominant hand and **carefully remove old dressing and/or stabilization/securing device** (Fig. 1). Use adhesive remover as necessary. Discard the dressing.	Gloves prevent contact with blood and body fluids. Pad protects the underlying surface. Proper disposal of dressing prevents transmission of microorganisms.

FIGURE 1. Carefully removing old dressing.

(continued)

SKILL 39-4 | CHANGING A PERIPHERAL VENOUS ACCESS DRESSING *continued*

ACTION

6. **Inspect the IV site for presence of phlebitis (inflammation), infection, or infiltration. Discontinue and relocate the IV, if noted. (Refer to Table 39-12, p. 1510; Boxes 39-2 and 39-3 on p. 1511.)**

7. **Cleanse the site with an antiseptic solution such as chlorhexidine or according to facility policy. Press an applicator against the skin and apply chlorhexidine using a gentle back-and-forth motion. Do not wipe or blot. Allow to dry completely.**

8. Open the skin protectant wipe. Apply the skin protectant to the site, making sure to cover at minimum the area to be covered with the dressing (Fig. 2). Allow to dry. Place a sterile transparent dressing or catheter securing/stabilization device over the venipuncture site (Fig. 3).

RATIONALE

Inflammation (phlebitis), infection, or infiltration causes trauma to tissues and necessitates removal of the venous access device.

Cleansing the skin is necessary because organisms on the skin can be introduced into the tissues or the bloodstream with the venous access. Chlorhexidine is the preferred antiseptic solution, but iodine, povidone-iodine, and 70% alcohol are considered acceptable alternatives (INS, 2011). A scrubbing motion creates friction and lets the solution more effectively penetrate the epidermal layers (Hadaway, 2006).

Skin protectant aids in adhesion of the dressing and decreases the risk for skin trauma when the dressing is removed. Transparent dressing allows easy visualization and protects the site. Stabilization/securing devices preserve the integrity of the access device, minimize catheter movement at the hub, and prevent catheter dislodgement and loss of access (INS, 2011, p. S46). Some stabilization devices also act as a site dressing.

FIGURE 2. Applying skin protectant to site.

FIGURE 3. Applying transparent dressing to site.

9. Label the dressing with the date, time of change, and initials. Loop the tubing near the entry site and anchor with tape (non-allergenic) close to the site (Fig. 4). Resume fluid infusion, if indicated. Check that IV flow is accurate and system is patent. Refer to Skill 39-2 on pages 1528–1530.

Other personnel working with the infusion will know what type of device is being used, the site, and when it was inserted. Peripheral venous catheter IV insertion sites are changed every 72 to 96 hours for an adult (O'Grady et al., 2011).

FIGURE 4. Site dressing with label and anchored tubing.

ACTION	RATIONALE
10. Apply an IV securement/stabilization device if not already in place as part of the dressing, as indicated, based on facility policy. Explain to the patient the purpose of the device and the importance of safeguarding the site when using the extremity.	These systems are recommended for use on all venous access sites, particularly central venous access sites, to preserve the integrity of the access device, minimize catheter movement at the hub, and prevent catheter dislodgement and loss of access (INS, 2011, p. S46). Some devices also act as a site dressing and may already have been applied.
11. Remove equipment. Ensure patient's comfort. Remove gloves. Lower the bed if not in the lowest position.	Promotes patient comfort and safety. Removing gloves properly reduces the risk for infection transmission and contamination of other items.
12. Remove additional PPE, if used. Perform hand hygiene.	Removing PPE properly reduces the risk for infection transmission and contamination of other items. Hand hygiene prevents transmission of microorganisms.

DOCUMENTATION

Guidelines

Document the location of the venous access as well as the condition of the site. Include the presence or absence of signs of erythema, redness, swelling, or drainage. Document the clinical criteria for site complications. (Refer to Table 39-12, p. 1510 and Boxes 39-2 and 39-3 on p. 1511.) Record the subjective comments of the patient regarding the absence or presence of pain at the site. Record the patient's reaction to the procedure and pertinent patient teaching, such as alerting the nurse if the patient experiences any pain from the IV or notices any swelling at the site.

Sample Documentation

11/15/15 1120 Dressing change to IV site in L hand (dorsal metacarpal) complete. Transparent dressing and peripheral stabilization device applied. Site without erythema, redness, edema, or drainage. D$_5$ NS infusing at 75 mL/hour. Patient instructed to call nurse with any pain, discomfort, swelling, or questions.

—S. Barnes, RN

UNEXPECTED SITUATIONS AND ASSOCIATED INTERVENTIONS

- *Patient complains that IV site feels "funny" and hurts:* Observe venous access site for redness, edema, and warmth. If present, clamp the tubing to stop the IV solution flow, remove the catheter, and apply a gauze dressing. Initiate a new venous access in a different site. Record site assessment and interventions, as well as the site for new venous access.

- *IV catheter is partially pulled out of insertion site (migrates externally):* Do not reinsert the catheter. Whether the IV is salvageable depends on how much of the catheter remains in the vein. Assess for proper placement in the vein before further use (INS, 2011). If this catheter is not removed, monitor it closely for signs of infiltration.

SPECIAL CONSIDERATIONS

General Considerations

- Use of chlorhexidine, 70% alcohol, iodine, or povidone-iodine is recommended for skin antisepsis for peripheral venous catheters (INS, 2011; O'Grady et al., 2011).

- The use of topical antibiotic ointments or creams on insertion sites is not recommended because of their potential to promote fungal infections and antimicrobial resistance (O'Grady et al., 2011).

- Do not submerge venous catheters and catheter sites in water; showering is permitted with use of impermeable coverings to protect the catheter and connecting device (O'Grady et al., 2011).

(continued)

SKILL 39-4 CHANGING A PERIPHERAL VENOUS ACCESS DRESSING *continued*

Infant and Child Considerations	• Chlorhexidine is not recommended for infants under 2 months of age (INS, 2011).
	• For infants under 2 months of age or pediatric patients with compromised skin integrity, remove dried povidone-iodine with normal saline wipes or sterile water (INS, 2011).
Older Adult Considerations	• Avoid using vigorous friction at the insertion site, which can traumatize fragile skin and veins in older adults.

SKILL 39-5 CAPPING FOR INTERMITTENT USE AND FLUSHING A PERIPHERAL VENOUS ACCESS DEVICE

DELEGATION CONSIDERATIONS

The capping and flushing of a peripheral venous access device is not delegated to nursing assistive personnel (NAP) or unlicensed assistive personnel (UAP). Depending on the state's nurse practice act and the organization's policies and procedures, these procedures may be delegated to licensed practical/vocational nurses (LPN/LVNs). The decision to delegate must be based on careful analysis of the patient's needs and circumstances, as well as the qualifications of the person to whom the task is being delegated. Refer to the Delegation Guidelines in Appendix A (found on the**Point**).

EQUIPMENT

- End cap device
- Clean gloves
- Additional PPE, as indicated
- 4 × 4 gauze pad

- Normal saline flush prepared in a syringe (1 to 3 mL) according to facility policy
- Alcohol or other disinfectant wipes
- Tape

IMPLEMENTATION

ACTION	**RATIONALE**
1. Determine the need for conversion to an intermittent access. Verify the medical order. Check facility policy. Gather equipment.	Ensures the correct intervention for the correct patient. Preparation promotes efficient time management and an organized approach to the task.
2. Perform hand hygiene and put on PPE, if indicated.	Hand hygiene and PPE prevent the spread of microorganisms. PPE is required based on transmission precautions.
3. Identify the patient.	Identifying the patient ensures that the right patient receives the intervention and helps prevent errors.
4. Close the curtains around the bed and close the door to the room, if possible. Explain what you are going to do and why you are going to do it to the patient. Ask the patient about allergies to tape and skin antiseptics.	This ensures the patient's privacy. Explanation relieves anxiety and facilitates cooperation. Possible allergies may exist related to tape or antiseptics.
5. Assess the IV site. Refer to Skill 39-2 on pages 1528–1530.	Complications, such as infiltration, phlebitis, or infection, necessitate discontinuation of the IV infusion at that site.
6. If using an electronic infusion device, stop the device (Fig. 1). Close the roller clamp on the administration set. If using gravity infusion, close the roller clamp on the administration set.	The action of the infusion device needs to be stopped and clamp closed to prevent leaking of fluid when tubing is disconnected.
7. Put on gloves. Close the clamp on the short extension tubing connected to the IV catheter in the patient's arm.	Clamping the tubing on the extension set prevents introduction of air into the extension tubing.
8. Remove the administration set tubing from the extension set. Cleanse the end cap with an antimicrobial swab.	Removing the infusion tubing discontinues the infusion. Cleaning the cap reduces the risk for contamination.

ACTION

9. Insert the saline flush syringe into the cap on the extension tubing. Pull back on the syringe to aspirate the catheter for positive blood return. If positive, instill the solution over 1 minute or flush the line according to facility policy (Fig. 2). Remove the syringe and reclamp the extension tubing.

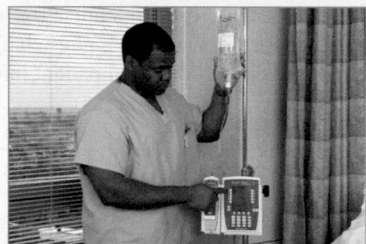

FIGURE 1. Stopping IV fluid infusion.

10. If necessary, loop the extension tubing near the entry site and anchor it with tape (nonallergenic) close to the site.

11. Remove equipment. Ensure patient's comfort. Remove gloves. Lower the bed if not in the lowest position.

12. Remove additional PPE, if used. Perform hand hygiene.

RATIONALE

Positive blood return confirms patency before administration of medications and solutions (INS, 2011, p. S60). Flushing maintains patency of the IV line. Action of the positive-pressure end cap is maintained with removal of the syringe before the clamp is engaged. Clamping prevents air from entering the extension set.

FIGURE 2. Flushing venous access device.

The weight of the tubing is sufficient to pull it out of the vein if it is not well anchored. Nonallergenic tape is less likely to tear fragile skin.

Promotes patient comfort and safety. Removing gloves properly reduces the risk for infection transmission and contamination of other items.

Removing PPE properly reduces the risk for infection transmission and contamination of other items. Hand hygiene prevents transmission of microorganisms.

DOCUMENTATION

Guidelines

Document discontinuation of IV fluid infusion. Record the condition of the venous access site. Document the flushing of the venous access device. This is often done in the CMAR/MAR. Record the patient's reaction to the procedure and any patient teaching that has occurred.

Sample Documentation

> 12/13/15 1720 IV infusion capped per order. Peripheral site right forearm (cephalic) flushed without resistance using 3 mL of saline. Dressing remains intact. Site without redness, swelling, drainage, or heat. Patient denies discomfort. Patient verbalized an understanding of the need to maintain IV access.
> —A. Lynn, RN

UNEXPECTED SITUATIONS AND ASSOCIATED INTERVENTIONS

- *Peripheral venous access site leaks fluid when flushed:* To prevent infection and other complications, remove from the site and restart in another location.

- *IV does not flush easily:* Assess insertion site. Infiltration and/or phlebitis may be present. If present, remove and restart in another location. In addition, the catheter may be blocked or clotted due to a kinked catheter at the insertion site. Aspirate and attempt to flush again. If resistance remains, do not force. Forceful flushing can dislodge a clot at the end of the catheter. Remove and restart in another location.

- *IV catheter is partially pulled out of insertion site (migrates externally):* Do not reinsert the catheter. Whether the IV is salvageable depends on how much of the catheter remains in the vein. Assess for proper placement in the vein before further use (INS, 2011). If this catheter is not removed, monitor it closely for signs of infiltration.

SPECIAL CONSIDERATIONS

- Some facilities may use end caps for venous access devices that are not positive-pressure devices. In this case, flush with the recommended volume of saline, ending with 0.5 mL of solution remaining in the syringe. While maintaining pressure on the syringe, clamp the extension tubing. This provides positive pressure, preventing backflow of blood into the catheter, decreasing the risk for occlusion.

SKILL 39-6 ADMINISTERING A BLOOD TRANSFUSION

DELEGATION CONSIDERATIONS

The administration of a blood transfusion is not delegated to nursing assistive personnel (NAP), unlicensed assistive personnel (UAP), or licensed practical/vocational nurses (LPN/LVNs).

EQUIPMENT

- Blood product
- Blood administration set (tubing with in-line filter, or add-on filter, and Y for saline administration)
- 0.9% normal saline for IV infusion
- IV pole
- Venous access; if peripheral site, preferably initiated with a 20-gauge catheter or larger

- Alcohol or other disinfectant wipes
- Clean gloves
- Additional PPE, as indicated
- Tape (hypoallergenic)
- Second registered nurse (or other licensed practitioner; e.g., a physician) to verify blood product and patient information

IMPLEMENTATION

ACTION	RATIONALE
1. Verify the medical order for transfusion of a blood product. Verify the completion of informed consent documentation in the medical record. Verify any medical order for pretransfusion medication. If ordered, administer medication at least 30 minutes before initiating transfusion.	Verification of order ensures that the patient receives the correct intervention. Premedication is sometimes administered to decrease the risk for allergic and febrile reactions for patients who have received multiple previous transfusions.
2. Gather all equipment.	Preparation promotes efficient time management and organized approach to the task.
3. Perform hand hygiene and put on PPE, if indicated.	Hand hygiene and PPE prevent the spread of microorganisms. PPE is required based on transmission precautions.
4. Identify the patient.	Identifying the patient ensures that the right patient receives the intervention and helps prevent errors.
5. Close the curtains around the bed and close the door to the room, if possible. Explain what you are going to do and why you are going to do it to the patient. Ask the patient about previous experience with transfusion and any reactions. Advise the patient to report any chills, itching, rash, or unusual symptoms.	This ensures the patient's privacy. Explanation relieves anxiety and facilitates cooperation. Previous reactions may increase the risk for reaction to this transfusion. Any reaction to the transfusion necessitates stopping the transfusion immediately and evaluating the situation.
6. Prime the blood administration set with the normal saline IV fluid. Refer to Skill 39-3 on pages 1530–1534.	Normal saline is the solution of choice for blood product administration. Solutions with dextrose may lead to clumping of red blood cells and hemolysis.
7. Put on gloves. If patient does not have a venous access in place, initiate peripheral venous access. (Refer to Skill 39-1, pp. 1520–1527.) Connect the administration set to the venous access device via the extension tubing. (Refer to Skill 39-1.) Infuse the normal saline per facility policy.	Gloves prevent contact with blood and body fluids. Infusion of fluid via venous access maintains patency until the blood product is administered. Start an IV before obtaining the blood product in case the initiation takes longer than 30 minutes. Blood must be stored at a carefully controlled temperature (4°C) and transfusion must begin within 30 minutes of release from the blood bank.
8. Obtain the blood product from the blood bank according to agency policy. Scan for bar codes on blood products if required.	Bar codes on blood products are currently being implemented in some agencies to identify, track, and assign data to transfusions as an additional safety measure.
9. Two nurses compare and validate the following information with the medical record, patient identification band, and the label of the blood product: • Medical order for transfusion of the blood product • Informed consent • Patient identification number • Patient name • Blood group and type • Expiration date • Inspection of blood product for clots, clumping, gas bubbles	Most states/agencies require two registered nurses to verify the following information: unit numbers match; ABO group and Rh type are the same; expiration date (after 35 days, red blood cells begin to deteriorate). Blood is never administered to a patient without an identification band. If clots or signs of contamination (clumping, gas bubbles) are present, return the blood to the blood bank.

ACTION	RATIONALE
10. **Obtain a baseline set of vital signs before beginning transfusion.**	Any change in vital signs during the transfusion may indicate a reaction.
11. Put on gloves. If using an electronic infusion device, put the device on "hold." Close the roller clamp closest to the drip chamber on the saline side of the administration set. Close the roller clamp on the administration set below the infusion device. Alternately, if using infusion via gravity, close the roller clamp on the administration set.	Gloves prevent contact with blood and body fluids. Stopping the infusion prevents blood from infusing to the patient before completion of preparations. Closing the clamp to saline allows the blood product to be infused via the electronic infusion device.
12. Close the roller clamp closest to the drip chamber on the blood product side of the administration set. Remove the protective cap from the access port on the blood container. Remove the cap from the access spike on the administration set. Using a pushing and twisting motion, insert the spike into the access port on the blood container, taking care not to contaminate the spike. Hang the blood container on the IV pole. Open the roller clamp on the blood side of the administration set. Squeeze the drip chamber until the in-line filter is saturated (Fig. 1). Remove gloves.	Filling the drip chamber prevents air from entering the administration set. The filter in the blood administration set removes particulate material formed during storage of blood. If the administration set becomes contaminated, the entire set would have to be discarded and replaced.

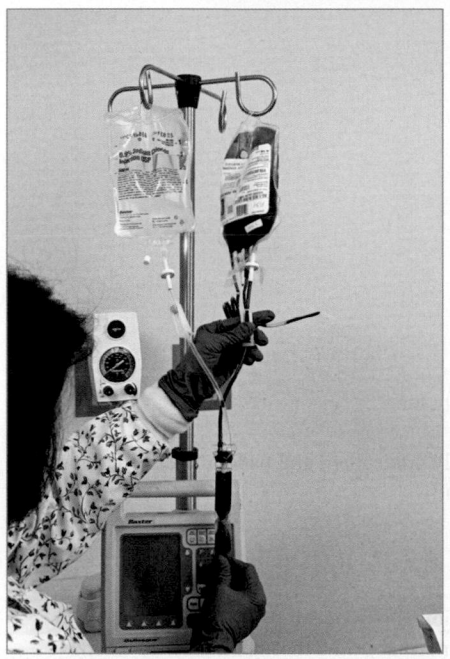

FIGURE 1. Squeezing the drip chamber to saturate the filter.

ACTION	RATIONALE
13. **Start administration slowly (no more than 25 to 50 mL for the first 15 minutes). Stay with the patient for the first 5 to 15 minutes of transfusion.** Open the roller clamp on the administration set below the infusion device. Set the flow rate and begin the transfusion. Alternately, start the flow of solution by releasing the clamp on the tubing and counting the drops. Adjust until the correct drop rate is achieved. Assess the flow of the blood and function of the infusion device. Inspect the insertion site for signs of infiltration.	Transfusion reactions typically occur during this period, and a slow rate will minimize the volume of red blood cells infused. Verifying the rate and device settings ensures that the patient receives the correct volume of solution. If the catheter or needle slips out of the vein, the blood will accumulate (infiltrate) into the surrounding tissue.
14. Observe the patient for flushing, dyspnea, itching, hives or rash, or any unusual comments.	These signs and symptoms may be an early indication of a transfusion reaction.

(continued)

SKILL 39-6 | ADMINISTERING A BLOOD TRANSFUSION *continued*

15. After the observation period (5 to 15 minutes), increase the infusion rate to the calculated rate to complete the infusion within the prescribed time frame, no more than 4 hours.

16. Reassess vital signs after 15 minutes (Fig. 2). Obtain vital signs thereafter according to facility policy and nursing assessment.

FIGURE 2. Assessing vital signs after 15 minutes.

17. Maintain the prescribed flow rate as ordered or as deemed appropriate based on the patient's overall condition, keeping in mind the outer limits for safe administration. Ongoing monitoring is crucial throughout the duration of the blood transfusion for early identification of any adverse reactions.

18. **During transfusion, assess frequently for transfusion reaction. Stop blood transfusion if you suspect a reaction. Quickly replace the blood tubing with a new administration set primed with normal saline for IV infusion. Initiate an infusion of normal saline for IV at an open rate, usually 40 mL/hour. Obtain vital signs. Notify the primary care provider and blood bank.**

19. When transfusion is complete, close the roller clamp on the blood side of the administration set and open the roller clamp on the normal saline side of the administration set. Initiate infusion of normal saline. When all of the blood has infused into the patient, clamp the administration set. Obtain vital signs. Put on gloves. Cap the access site or resume the previous IV infusion. (Refer to Skill 39-1, pp. 1520–1527 and Skill 39-5, pp. 1538–1539.) Dispose of blood-transfusion equipment or return it to the blood bank, according to facility policy.

If no adverse effects occurred during this time, the infusion rate is increased. If complications occur, they can be observed and the transfusion can be stopped immediately. Verifying the rate and device settings ensures that the patient receives the correct volume of solution. Transfusion must be completed within 4 hours due to the potential for bacterial growth in blood product at room temperature.

Vital signs must be assessed as part of monitoring for a possible adverse reaction. Facility policy and nursing judgment will dictate frequency.

Rate must be carefully controlled, and patient's reaction must be monitored frequently.

If a transfusion reaction is suspected, the blood must be stopped. Do not infuse the normal saline through the blood tubing because you would be allowing more of the blood into the patient's body, which could complicate a reaction. Besides a serious life-threatening blood transfusion reaction, the potential for fluid–volume overload exists in older patients and patients with decreased cardiac function.

Saline prevents hemolysis of red blood cells and clears the remainder of the blood in the IV line. Proper disposal of equipment reduces transmission of microorganisms and potential contact with blood and body fluids.

ACTION	RATIONALE
20. Remove equipment. Ensure the patient's comfort. Remove gloves. Lower the bed if not in the lowest position.	Promotes patient comfort and safety. Removing gloves properly reduces the risk for infection transmission and contamination of other items.
21. Remove additional PPE, if used. Perform hand hygiene.	Removing PPE properly reduces the risk for infection transmission and contamination of other items. Hand hygiene prevents transmission of microorganisms.
22. Monitor and assess the patient for one hour after the transfusion for signs and symptoms of delayed transfusion reaction. Provide patient education about signs and symptoms of delayed transfusion reactions.	Ensures early detection and prompt intervention. Delayed transfusion reactions can occur one day to several days after transfusion.

DOCUMENTATION

Guidelines

Document that the patient received the blood transfusion; include the type of blood product. Record the patient's condition throughout the transfusion, including pertinent data, such as vital signs, lung sounds, and the subjective response of the patient to transfusion. Document any complications or reactions and whether the patient had received the transfusion without any complications or reactions. Document the assessment of the IV site, and any other fluids infused during the procedure. Document transfusion volume and other IV fluid intake on the patient's intake and output record.

Sample Documentation

> 11/2/15 1100 T 97.6°F P 82 R 14 B/P 116/74. 1 unit of packed blood red cells initiated via left forearm (basilic) 18-gauge venous access without difficulty. Patient states "no discomfort." IV site intact, no swelling, redness, or pain.
> —S. Barnes, RN
>
> 11/2/15 1115 T 97.6°F P 78 R 16 B/P 118/68. 1 unit of packed blood red cells infusing via left forearm (basilic) 18-gauge venous access without difficulty. Patient states "no discomfort." IV site intact, no swelling, redness, or pain.
> —S. Barnes, RN
>
> 11/2/15 1445 T 97.6°F P 82 R 14 B/P 120/74. 1 unit of packed blood red cells completed via left forearm (basilic) 18-gauge venous access without difficulty. Patient denies symptoms of complications. IV site intact, no swelling, redness, or pain.
> —S. Barnes, RN

UNEXPECTED SITUATIONS AND ASSOCIATED INTERVENTIONS

- *Patient is becoming febrile but is exhibiting no other signs of a transfusion reaction:* Notify the primary care provider. The primary care provider may order acetaminophen and an antihistamine for the patient.

- *Patient reports shortness of breath; on auscultation you note crackles bilaterally in the bases:* Compare vital signs with normal vital sounds for this patient. Obtain a pulse oximetry reading. Notify the primary care provider. The primary care provider may order a dose of a diuretic or may decrease the rate of the transfusion. Continue to assess the patient for signs and symptoms of fluid overload.

- *Patient is febrile, tachycardic, and complaining of back pain:* The patient is having a transfusion reaction. Stop the transfusion immediately. Obtain new IV tubing with 0.9% sodium chloride. Notify the primary care provider and blood bank. Send the blood unit, tubing, and filter to the laboratory. Obtain additional diagnostic tests, such as blood and urine tests, based on facility policy.

(continued)

SKILL 39-6 ADMINISTERING A BLOOD TRANSFUSION *continued*

SPECIAL CONSIDERATIONS

General Considerations

- If an electronic infusion device is used to maintain the prescribed rate, ensure that it is designed for use with blood transfusions before initiating transfusion.
- Never warm blood in a microwave. Use a blood-warming device, if indicated or ordered, especially with rapid transfusions through a CVAD. Blood warmers should also be used for large-volume transfusions, exchange transfusions, patients with clinically significant conditions, and the neonate/pediatric population (INS, 2011, p. S93). Rapid administration of cold blood can result in cardiac arrhythmias.
- External compression devices, if used for rapid transfusions, should be equipped with a pressure gauge, should totally encase the blood bag, and should apply uniform pressure against all parts of the blood container. Do not use blood pressure cuffs (INS, 2011, p. S93).

Home Health Care Considerations

- Home health care agencies evaluate patients who are candidates for a blood transfusion at home.
- Home transfusion is not appropriate for patients who are actively bleeding or who recently had a reaction to a blood transfusion.
- The nurse transports the blood product to the patient's home in a special cooler. The nurse and competent adult check the serial number and other identification information together (INS, 2011).

DEVELOPING CRITICAL THINKING

1. Assess a healthy person and a patient whose fluid and electrolyte or acid–base balance is altered using Tables 39-4 and 39-5, which describe parameters to be considered in physical and clinical assessments for fluid, electrolyte, and acid–base balance. Compare and contrast your findings.

2. Review the record of a patient who has been receiving IV fluids over a period of 3 or more days. Note the daily intake and output records, pertinent laboratory values, and clinical behaviors, and make a judgment about the patient's fluid, electrolyte, and acid–base balance. What factors complicate a hospitalized patient's usual ability to remain in balance?

PRACTICING FOR NCLEX

1. A nurse is caring for an older patient with type II diabetes who is living in a long-term care facility. The nurse determines that the patient's fluid intake and output is approximately 1200 mL daily. What patient teaching would the nurse provide for this patient? Select all that apply.
   a. "Try to drink at least six to eight glasses of water each day."
   b. "Try to limit your fluid intake to one quart of water daily."
   c. "Limit sugar, salt, and alcohol in your diet."
   d. "Report side effects of medications you are taking, especially diarrhea."
   e. "Temporarily increase foods containing caffeine for their diuretic effect."
   f. "Weigh yourself daily and report any changes in your weight."

2. A nurse is performing a physical assessment of a patient who is experiencing fluid volume excess. Upon examination of the patient's legs, the nurse documents: "Pitting edema; 6 mm pit; pit remains several seconds after pressing with obvious skin swelling." What grade of edema has this nurse documented?
   a. 1+ pitting edema
   b. 2+ pitting edema
   c. 3+ pitting edema
   d. 4+ pitting edema

3. A nurse is preparing an IV solution for a patient who has hypernatremia. Which solutions are the best choices for this condition? Select all that apply.
   a. 5% dextrose in water (D_5W)
   b. 0.9% NaCl (normal saline)
   c. Lactated Ringer's solution
   d. 0.33% NaCl (⅓-strength normal saline)
   e. 0.45% NaCl (½-strength normal saline)
   f. 10% dextrose in water ($D_{10}W$)

4. A nurse is assessing infants in the NICU for fluid balance status. Which nursing action would the nurse depend on as the most reliable indicator of a patient's fluid balance status?
   a. Recording intake and output
   b. Testing skin turgor
   c. Reviewing the complete blood count
   d. Measuring weight daily

5. Which acid–base imbalance would the nurse suspect after assessing the following arterial blood gas values: pH, 7.30; $PaCO_2$, 36 mm Hg; HCO_3^-, 14 mEq/L?
   a. Respiratory acidosis
   b. Respiratory alkalosis
   c. Metabolic acidosis
   d. Metabolic alkalosis

6. A patient has been encouraged to increase fluid intake. Which measure would be most effective for the nurse to implement?
   a. Explaining the mechanisms involved in transporting fluids to and from intracellular compartments
   b. Keeping fluids readily available for the patient
   c. Emphasizing the long-term outcome of increasing fluids when the patient returns home
   d. Planning to offer most daily fluids in the evening

7. A nurse is caring for a patient who has fluid imbalance related to the development of ascites. Which imbalances would the nurse monitor for in this patient? Select all that apply.
   a. Extracellular fluid volume deficit
   b. Protein deficit
   c. Metabolic alkalosis
   d. Sodium deficit
   e. Plasma-to-interstitial fluid shift
   f. Metabolic acidosis

8. A nurse is monitoring a patient who is receiving an IV infusion of normal saline. The patient is apprehensive and presents with a pounding headache, rapid pulse rate, chills, and dyspnea. What would be the nurse's priority intervention related to these symptoms?
   a. Discontinue the infusion immediately, monitor vital signs, and report findings to primary care provider immediately.
   b. Slow the rate of infusion, notify the primary care provider immediately and monitor vital signs.
   c. Pinch off the catheter or secure the system to prevent entry of air, place the patient in the Trendelenburg position, and call for assistance.
   d. Discontinue the infusion immediately, apply warm, moist compresses to the site, and restart the IV at another site.

9. A nurse carefully assesses the acid–base balance of a patient who is unable to effectively control his carbonic acid supply. This is most likely a patient with damage to which of the following?
   a. Kidneys
   b. Lungs
   c. Adrenal glands
   d. Blood vessels

10. A nurse is monitoring a patient who is diagnosed with hypokalemia. Which nursing intervention would be appropriate for this patient?
    a. Encourage foods and fluids with high sodium content.
    b. Administer oral K supplements as ordered.
    c. Caution the patient about eating foods high in potassium content.
    d. Discuss calcium-losing aspects of nicotine and alcohol use.

11. A nurse is administering 500 mL of saline solution to a patient over 10 hours. The administration set delivers 60 gtts/min. Determine the infusion rate to administer via gravity infusion.
    Place your answer on the line provided below.

    _____

12. A nurse is initiating a peripheral venous access IV infusion for a patient. Following the procedure, the nurse observes that the fluid does not flow easily into the vein and the skin around the insertion site is edematous and cool to the touch. What would be the nurse's next action related to these findings?
    a. Reposition the extremity and raise the height of the IV pole.
    b. Apply pressure to the dressing on the IV.
    c. Pull the catheter out slightly and reinsert it.
    d. Put on gloves; remove the catheter; apply pressure with a sterile pad.

13. When monitoring an IV site and infusion, a nurse notes pain at the access site with erythema and edema. What grade of phlebitis would the nurse document?
    a. 1
    b. 2
    c. 3
    d. 4

14. A nurse is administering a blood transfusion for a patient following surgery. During the transfusion, the patient displays signs of dyspnea, dry cough, and pulmonary edema. What would be the nurse's priority actions related to these symptoms?
    a. Slow or stop the infusion; monitor vital signs, notify the physician, place the patient in upright position with feet dependent.
    b. Stop the transfusion immediately and keep the vein open with normal saline, notify the physician stat, administer antihistamine parenterally as needed.
    c. Stop the transfusion immediately and keep the vein open with normal saline, notify the physician, and treat symptoms.
    d. Stop the infusion immediately, obtain a culture of the patient's blood, monitor vital signs, notify the physician, administer antibiotics stat.

15. A nurse is flushing a patient's implanted port after administering medications. The nurse observes that the port flushes, but does not have a blood return. What would be the nurse's next action based on these findings?
    a. Gently push down on the needle and flush it a second time.
    b. Stop flushing and remove the needle; notify the primary care provider.
    c. Ask the patient to perform a Valsalva maneuver; change the patient position.
    d. Close the clamp; wait 3 minutes, try flushing the port again.

ANSWERS WITH RATIONALES

1. *a, c, d, f.* Generally, fluid intake and output averages 2,600 mL per day. This patient is experiencing dehydration and should be encouraged to drink more water, maintain normal body weight, avoid consuming excess amounts of products high in salt, sugar, and caffeine, limit alcohol intake, and monitor side effects of medications, especially diarrhea and water loss from diuretics.

2. *c.* 3+ pitting edema is represented by a deep pit (6 mm) that remains seconds after pressing with skin swelling obvious by general inspection. 1+ is a slight indentation (2 mm) with normal contours associated with interstitial fluid volume 30% above normal. 2+ is a 4-mm pit that lasts longer than 1+ with fairly normal contour. +4 is a deep pit (8 mm) that remains for a prolonged time after pressing with frank swelling.

3. *a, d, e.* 5% dextrose in water (D$_5$W), 0.33% NaCl (⅓-strength normal saline), and 0.45% NaCl (½-strength normal saline) are used to treat hypernatremia. 0.9% NaCl (normal saline) is used to treat hypovolemia, metabolic alkalosis, hyponatremia, and hypochloremia. Lactated Ringer's solution is used in the treatment of hypovolemia, burns, and fluid lost from gastrointestinal sources. 10% dextrose in water (D$_{10}$W) is used in peripheral parenteral nutrition (PPN).

4. *d.* Daily weight is the most reliable indicator of a person's fluid balance status. Intake and output are not always as accurate and may involve a subjective component. Measurement of skin turgor is subjective, and the complete blood count does not necessarily reflect fluid balance.

5. *c.* A low pH indicates acidosis. This, coupled with a low bicarbonate, indicates metabolic acidosis. The pH and bicarbonate would be elevated with metabolic alkalosis. Decreased PaCO$_2$ in conjunction with a low pH indicates respiratory acidosis; increased PaCO$_2$ in conjunction with an elevated pH indicates respiratory alkalosis.

6. *b.* Having fluids readily available helps promote intake. Explanation of the fluid transportation mechanisms (*a*) is inappropriate and does not focus on the immediate problem of increasing fluid intake. Meeting short-term outcomes rather than long-term ones (*c*) provides further reinforcement, and additional fluids should be taken earlier in the day.

7. *a, b, d, e.* Patients with fluid loss due to ascites are at risk for extracellular fluid volume deficit, protein deficit, sodium deficit, and plasma–interstitial fluid shift.

8. *a.* The nurse is observing the signs and symptoms of speed shock: the body's reaction to a substance that is injected into the circulatory system too rapidly. The nursing interventions for this condition are: discontinue the infusion immediately, report symptoms of speed shock to primary care provider immediately, and monitor vital signs once signs develop. Answer (b) is interventions for fluid overload, answer (c) is interventions for air embolus, and answer (d) is interventions for phlebitis.

9. *b.* The lungs are the primary controller of the body's carbonic acid supply and thus, if damaged, can affect acid–base balance. The kidneys are the primary controller of the body's bicarbonate supply. The adrenal glands secrete catecholamines and steroid hormones. The blood vessels act only as a transport system.

10. *b.* Nursing interventions for a patient with hypokalemia include encouraging foods high in potassium and administering oral K as ordered. Encouraging foods with high sodium content is appropriate for a patient with hyponatremia. Cautioning the patient about foods high in potassium is appropriate for a patient with hyperkalemia, and discussing the

calcium-losing aspects of nicotine and alcohol use is appropriate for a patient with hypocalcemia.

11. Ans: 50 gtts/min. When administering 500 mL of solution over 10 hours, and the set delivers 60 gtts/mL, the nurse would use the following formula:

$$\text{gtt/min} = \frac{500 \times 60}{600}$$

$$500 \times 60 = 30,000/600 = 50 \text{ gtts/min}$$

12. *d.* This IV has been infiltrated. The nurse should put on gloves and remove the catheter. The nurse should also apply pressure with a sterile gauze pad, secure the gauze with tape over the insertion site, and restart the IV in a new location.

13. *b.* Grade 2 phlebitis presents with pain at access site with erythema and/or edema. Grade 1 presents as erythema at access site with or without pain. Grade 3 presents as grade 2 with a streak formation and palpable venous cord. Grade 4 presents as grade 3 with a palpable venous cord >1 inch and with purulent drainage.

14. *a.* The patient is displaying signs and symptoms of circulatory overload: too much blood administered. In answer (b) the nurse is providing interventions for an allergic reaction. In answer (c) the nurse is responding to a febrile reaction, and in answer (d) the nurse is providing interventions for a bacterial reaction.

15. *c.* If a port flushes but does not have a blood return, the nurse should ask the patient to perform a Valsalva maneuver, have the patient change position or place the affected arm over the head, or raise or lower the head of the bed. If these measures do not work, the nurse should remove the needle and reaccess the device with a new needle.

TAYLOR SUITE RESOURCES

Explore these additional resources to enhance learning for this chapter:

- NCLEX-Style Questions and other resources on thePoint, http://thePoint.lww.com/Taylor8e
- *Study Guide for Fundamentals of Nursing, 8th edition*
- Adaptive Learning | Powered by prepU, http://thepoint.lww.com/prepu
- *Skill Checklists for Fundamentals of Nursing, 8th edition*
- *Taylor's Clinical Nursing Skills:* Chapter 15, Fluid, Electrolyte, and Acid–Base Balance
- *Taylor's Video Guide to Clinical Nursing Skills:* Intravenous Therapy and Central Venous Access Devices
- *Lippincott DocuCare* Fundamentals cases

Bibliography

Ackley, B. J., & Ladwig, G. B. (2011). *Nursing Diagnosis Handbook* (9th ed.). St. Louis: Elsevier/Mosby.

Adams, D. (2012). Needlestick and sharps injuries: practice update. *Nursing Standard, 26*(37), 49–57.

Alexandrou, E., Ramjan, L. M., Spencer, T., Frost, S. A., Salamonson, Y., Davidson, P. M., & Hillman, K. M. (2011). The use of midline catheters in the adult acute care setting: Clinical implications and recommendations for practice. *Journal of the Association for Vascular Access, 16*(1), 35–41.

American Red Cross. (2013). Donating blood. Eligibility requirements. Available at http://www.redcross blood.org/donating-blood/eligibility-requirements

Anderson, S., Cockrell, J., Beller, P., Murphy, E., Nelson, P., & Cederna-Moss, J. (2010). Administration of local anesthetic agents to decrease pain associated with peripheral vascular access. *Journal of Infusion Nursing, 33*(6), 353–361.

Arbique, J., & Arbique, D. (2007). IV rounds. Reducing the risk of nerve injuries. *Nursing, 37*(11), 20–21.

Ayers, P., & Dixon, C. (2012). Simple acid-base tutorial. *Journal of Parenteral and Enteral Nutrition, 36*(1), 18–23.

Barnette, L., & Kautz, D. D. (2013). Creative ways to teach arterial blood gas interpretation. *Dimensions of Critical Care Nursing, 32*(2), 84–87.

Baxter, A. L., Ewing, P. H., Young, G. B., Ware, A., Evans, N., & Manworren, R. C. B. (2013). EMLA application exceeding two hours improves pediatric

emergency department venipuncture success. *Advanced Emergency Nursing Journal, 35*(1), 67–75.

Bulechek, G. M., Butcher, H. K., Dochterman, J. M., & Wagner, C. M. (Eds.). (2013). *Nursing interventions classification (NIC)* (6th ed.). St. Louis, MO: Elsevier/Mosby.

Casey, A. L., Elliott, T. S. J. (2010). Prevention of central venous catheter-related infection: update. *British Journal of Nursing, 19*(2), 78, 80, 82, 84, 86–87.

Centers for Disease Control and Prevention (CDC). (2011). Guidelines for the prevention of intravascular catheter-related infections. Available at www.cdc.gov/hicpac/pdf/guidelines/bsi-guidelines-2011.pdf

Charron, K. (2012). Decreasing central line infections and needlestick injury rates. *Journal of Infusion Nursing, 35*(6), 370–375.

Collins, M., & Claros, E. (2011). Recognizing the face of dehydration. *Nursing, 41*(8), 26–32.

Cook, L. S. (2013). Infusion-related air embolism. *Journal of Infusion Nursing, 36*(1), 26–36.

Cook, L., Bellini, S., & Cusson, R. (2011). Heparinized saline vs normal saline for maintenance of intravenous access in neonates: An evidence-based practice change. *Advances in Neonatal Care, 11*(3), 208–215.

Crawford, A., & Harris, H. (2012a). Balancing act: Calcium & phosphorus. *Nursing, 42*(1), 36–42.

Crawford, A., & Harris, H. (2012b). SIADH: Fluid out of balance. *Nursing, 42*(9), 50–58.

Crawford, A., & Harris, H. (2011a). Balancing act: Hypomagnesemia & hypermagnesemia. *Nursing, 41*(10), 52–55.

Crawford, A., & Harris, H. (2011b). Balancing act: Sodium & potassium. *Nursing, 41*(7), 44–50.

Culleiton, A. L., & Simko, L. C. (2011). Keeping electrolytes & fluids in balance: Part 1. *Nursing 2011CriticalCare, 6*(2), 30–31, 33–35.

da Silva, G. A., Priebe, S., & Dias, F. N. (2010). Benefits of establishing an intravenous team and the standardization of peripheral intravenous catheters. *Journal of Infusion Nursing, 33*(3), 156–160.

Dudek, S. (2014). *Nutrition essentials for nursing practice* (7th ed.). Philadelphia: Wolters Kluwer Health/Lippincott Williams & Wilkins.

Dychter, S., Gold, D., Carson, D., & Haller, M. (2012). Intravenous therapy: A review of complications and economic considerations of peripheral access. *Journal of Infusion Nursing, 35*(2), 84–91.

Ead, H. (2011). Blood products and the phases of perianesthesia care: Reviewing the implications. *Journal of PeriAnesthesia Nursing, 26*(4), 262–276.

Eastwood, G. M., Peck, L., Young, H., Prowle, J., Vasudevan, V., Jones, D., & Bellomo, R. (2012). Intravenous fluid administration and monitoring for adult ward patients in a teaching hospital. *Nursing and Health Sciences, 14*(2), 265–271.

Feil, M. (2012). Pennsylvania patient safety advisory. Reducing risk of air embolism associated with central venous access devices. Available at http://patientsafetyauthority.org/ADVISORIES/Advisory Library/2012/Jun;9(2)/Pages/58.aspx

Fluids & electrolytes made incredibly easy! (5th ed.). (2011). Philadelphia: Wolters Kluwer Health/Lippincott Williams & Wilkins.

Gabriel, J. (2008a). Infusion therapy part one: Minimising the risks. *Nursing Standard, 22*(31), 51–56.

Gabriel, J. (2008b). Infusion therapy part two: Prevention and management of complications. *Nursing Standard, 22*(32), 41–48.

Gabriel, J. (2012). Venepuncture and cannulation: Considering the ageing vein. *British Journal of Nursing (Intravenous Supplement), 21*(2), S22–S28.

Ganter-Ritz, V., Speroni, K. G., & Atherton, M. (2012). A randomized double-blind study comparing intradermal anesthetic tolerability, efficacy, and cost-effectiveness of lidocaine, buffered lidocaine, and bacteriostatic normal saline for peripheral intravenous insertion. *Journal of Infusion Nursing, 35*(2), 93–99.

Grossman, S., & Porth, C.M. (2014). Porth's pathophysiology: concepts of altered health states. (9th ed.). Philadelphia: Wolters Kluwer Health/Lippincott Williams & Wilkins.

Hadaway, L. (2006). 5 steps to preventing catheter-related bloodstream infections. *LPN2009, 2*(5), 50–55.

Hadaway, L. C. (2010). Extra! Extra! Preventing extravasation. *Nursing made incredibly easy, 8*(2), 13–14.

Hadaway, L. C. (2009). Central venous access devices. *Nursing2009 Critical Care, 3*(5), 26–33.

Hammond, T. (2004). Choice and use of peripherally inserted central catheters by nurses. *Professional Nurse, 19*(9), 493–497.

Hess, C. T. (2009). Practice points. Monitoring laboratory values: Protein and albumin. *Advances in Skin & Wound Care, 22*(1), 48.

Higginson, R. (2011). IV therapy and infection control in patients in the community. *British Journal of Nursing, 20*(3), 152–155.

Hinkle, J.L., & Cheever, K.H. (2014). *Brunner & Suddarth's textbook of medical–surgical nursing* (13th ed.). Philadelphia: Wolters Kluwer Health/Lippincott Williams & Wilkins.

Hogan-Quigley, B., Palm, M. L., & Bickley, L. (2012). *Bates' nursing guide to physical examination and history taking.* Philadelphia: Wolters Kluwer Health/Lippincott Williams & Wilkins.

Holcomb, S. (2008). Third-spacing: When body fluid shifts. *Nursing, 38*(7), 50–53.

Houston, P. A. (2013). Obtaining vascular access in the obese patient population. *Journal of Infusion Nursing, 36*(1), 52–56.

Huether, S. E., & McCance, K. L. (2012.) *Understanding Pathophysiology* (5th ed.). St. Louis: Elsevier.

Hughes, T. (2012). Providing information to children before and during venepuncture. *Nursing Children and Young People, 24*(5), 23–28.

Infusion Nurses Society (INS). (2011). Infusion nursing standards of practice. *Journal of Infusion Nursing, 34*(Suppl: 1S).

Infusion Nurses Society (INS). (2006). Infusion nursing standards of practice. *Journal of Infusion Nursing, 29*(1S), S60.

Institute for Safe Medication Practices (ISMP). (2013). ISMP summit on the use of smart infusion pumps: Guidelines for safe implementation and use. Available at http://www.ismp.org/tools/guidelines/smartpumps/default.asp#benefits

I.V. Rounds. Comparing short peripheral cannula insertion sites. (2008). *Nursing, 38*(5), 60.

Jarvis, C. (2012). *Physical examination & health assessment* (6th ed.). St. Louis: Elsevier/Saunders.

The Joint Commission (TJC). (2014). *National patient safety goals.* Available at http://www.jointcommission.org/standards_information/npsgs.aspx

Julian, M. K. (2013). Caring for your patient receiving TPN. *Nursing made Incredibly Easy!, 11*(1), 8–11.

Kassab, M. I., Roydhouse, J. K., Fowler, C., & Foureur, M. (2012). The effectiveness of glucose in reducing needle-related procedural pain in infants. *Journal of Pediatric Nursing, 27*(1), 3–17.

Kee, J. L., Hayes, E. R., & McCuistion, L. E. (2012). *Pharmacology: A nursing process approach* (7th ed.). St. Louis: Elsevier/Saunders.

Koshy, R. (2011). Vascular access device selection for intravenous therapy. *Journal of Illinois Nursing, 109*(3), 24–28.

Kyle, T., & Carman, S. (2013). *Essentials of pediatric nursing* (2nd ed.). Philadelphia: Wolters Kluwer Health/Lippincott Williams & Wilkins.

Lavery, I. (2005). Peripheral intravenous therapy: key risks and implications for practice. *Nursing Standard, 19*(46), 55–64.

Liu, M. F., Lin, K. C., Chou, Y. H., & Lee, T. Y. (2010). Using non-nutritive sucking and oral glucose solution with neonates to relieve pain: a randomized controlled trial. *Journal of Clinical Nursing, 19*(11–12), 1604–1611.

Lopez, A. C. (2011). A quality improvement program combining maximal barrier precaution compliance monitoring and daily chlorhexidine gluconate baths resulting in decreased central line bloodstream infections. *Dimensions of Critical Care Nursing, 30*(5), 293–298.

Maiocco, G., & Coole, C. (2012). Use of ultrasound guidance for peripheral intravenous placement in difficult-to-access patients: Advancing practice with evidence. *Journal of Nursing Care Quality, 27*(1), 51–55.

Malarkey, L. M., & McMorrow, M. E. (2012). *Saunders nursing guide to laboratory and diagnostic tests* (2nd ed.). St. Louis: Elsevier/Saunders.

Mathers, D. (2011). Evidence-based practice: Improving outcomes for patients with a central venous access device. *Journal of the Association for Vascular Access, 16*(2), 64–72.

Metheny, N. M. (2012). *Fluid and electrolyte balance: Nursing Considerations* (5th ed.). Sudbury, MA: Jones & Bartlett Learning.

Micheletti, L. (2010). Arterial blood gas. *Advance for Nurses, 12*(1), 18.

Moorhead, S., Johnson, M., Maas, M. L., & Swanson, E. (Eds). (2013). *Nursing Outcomes Classification (NOC)* (5th ed.). St. Louis: Elsevier/Mosby.

Moureau, N. (2013). Safe patient care when using vascular access devices. *British Journal of Nursing, 22*(2), S14–S21.

Moureau, N.L. (2008). Tips for inserting an I.V. device in an older adult. *Nursing, 38*(12), 12.

NANDA International (NANDA-I). (2012). *Nursing diagnoses: Definitions & classification 2012–2014.* West Sussex, UK: Wiley-Blackwell.

O'Grady, N. P., Alexander, M., Burns, L. A., Dellinger, E. P., Garland, J., Heard, S. O., Lipsett, P. A., … the Healthcare Infection Control Practices Advisory Committee (HICPAC). (2011). Guidelines for the prevention of intravascular catheter-related infections. *American Journal of Infection Control, 39*(4 Supplement), S1–S34.

Ogston-Tuck, S. (2012). Intravenous therapy: guidance on devices, management and care. *British Journal of Community Nursing, 17*(10), 474–484.

Park, T. A., & Huber, J. M. (2012). Hospitalized infants who hurt: A sweet solution with oral sucrose. *Critical Care Nurse, 32*(1), 61–69.

Pasek, T.A., & Huber, J.M. (2012). Hospitalized infants who hurt: a sweet solution with oral sucrose. *Critical Care Nurse, 32*(1), 61–69.

Perry, S. E., Hockenberry, M. J., Lowdermilk, D. L., & Wilson, D. (2010). *Maternal child nursing care* (4th ed.). Maryland Heights, MO: Elsevier/Mosby.

Peterson, K. (2013). The development of central venous access device flushing guidelines utilizing an evidence-based practice process. *Journal of Pediatric Nursing, 28*(1), 85–88.

Richardson, D., & Kaufman, L. (2011). Reducing blood exposure risks and costs associated with SPIVC insertion. *Nursing Management, 42*(12), 31–34.

Scales, K. (2008). Intravenous therapy: A guide to good practice. *British Journal of Nursing, 17*(19) Supplement, S4–S12.

Schiavone, P. A., Stoner, N. E., Compher, C. W., Kinosian, B. P., & Boullata, J. I. (2010). Management of catheter-related infection in patients receiving home parenteral nutrition. *Practical Gastroenterology,* Nutrition Issues in Gastroenterology, Series #88. Available at http://www.mcdicine.virginia.edu/clinical/departments/medicine/divisions/digestive-health/nutrition-support-team/nutrition-articles/SchiavoneArticle.pdf

Schrieber, M. (2013). Understanding hyponatremia. *Nursing2013Critical Care, 8*(2), 8–10.

Siegel, M., & Kraemer-Cain, J. (2011). *PICC line care at home. Advance for Nurses, 8*(8), 17–20.

Stevens, B., Yamada, J., Lee, G.Y., & Ohlsson, A. (2013). Sucrose for analgesia in newborn infants undergoing painful procedures. *Cochrane Database of Systematic Reviews,* 2013, Issue 1. Art. No.: CD001069. DOI: 10.1002/14651858.CD001069.pub4.

Smith, J., & Hannum, F. (2008). Optimizing IV therapy in the elderly. *Advance for Nurses, 10*(18), 27–28.

Tabloski, P. (2010). *Gerontological nursing* (2nd ed.). Upper Saddle River, NJ: Pearson.

Taylor, J. J., & Cohen, B. J. (2013). *Memmler's structure and function of the human body* (10th ed.). Philadelphia: Wolters Kluwer Health/Lippincott Williams & Wilkins.

Thayer, D. (2012). Skin damage associated with intravenous therapy. *Journal of Infusion Nursing, 35*(6), 390–401.

Vallerand, A. H., Sanoski, C. A., & Deglin, J. H. (2013). *Davis's drug guide for nurses* (13th ed.). Philadelphia: F. A. Davis Company.

Van Leeuwen, A. M., Poelhuis-Leth, D., & Bladh, M. L. (2011). *Davis's comprehensive handbook of laboratory & diagnostic tests with nursing implications* (4th ed.). Philadelphia: F. A. Davis.

VISN 8 Patient Safety Center. (2009). *Safe patient handling and movement algorithms.* Tampa, FL: Author. Available at http://www.visn8.va.gov/visn8/patientsafetycenter/safePtHandling/default.asp

White, A., Lopez, F., & Stone, P. (2010). Developing and sustaining an ultrasound-guided peripheral intravenous access program for emergency nurses. *Advanced Emergency Nursing Journal, 32*(2), 173–188.

White, M. L., Crawley, J., Rennie, W. A., & Lewandowski, L. A. (2011). Examining the effectiveness of 2 solutions used to flush capped pediatric peripheral intravenous catheters. *Journal of Infusion Nursing, 34*(4), 260–270.

Wilkins, R. G., & Unverdorben, M. (2012). Accidental intravenous infusion of air. A concise review. *Journal of Infusion Nursing, 35*(6), 404–408.

Wilson, N., & Blackett, B. (2012). Parenteral nutrition: considerations for practice. *British Journal of Community Nursing, Nutrition Supplement* (May), S16–S19.

Worthington, P. H., & Gilbert, K. A. (2012). Parenteral nutrition. Risks, complications, and management. *Journal of Infusion Nursing, 35*(1), 52–64.

Wunderlich, R. (2013). Principles in the selection of intravenous solutions replacement: Sodium and water balance. *Journal of Infusion Nursing, 36*(2), 126–130.

Promoting Healthy Psychosocial Responses

*E*very person is a composite of interrelated physiologic, psychosocial, and spiritual *dimensions; alterations in one dimension affect the others.* Unit VIII discusses psychosocial considerations in holistic, person-centered care, focusing on sense of self; stress and adaptation; loss, grief, and dying; sensory stimulation; sexuality; and spirituality.

Each individual's sense of self is critical to that person's attitudes toward health and may affect self-care abilities positively or negatively. Additionally, developmental or experiential stressors can motivate or thwart psychosocial growth and self-actualization. Nursing interventions to promote healthy psychosocial responses—including maintaining, strengthening, or changing self-concept—are basic to all aspects of patient care. Because a person's sense of self shapes one's ability to respond to health care interventions, nurses include assessment and intervention to promote a positive sense of self.

Loss, grief, and dying are universal human experiences that most nurses encounter in some form on a daily basis. Effective nurses are competent and willing to assist people struggling with loss, grief, and dying.

Intact, functioning senses are necessary for life, normal growth and development, communication, and pleasurable experiences. Alterations in any of the senses require caring, knowledgeable, and individualized nursing interventions to meet needs, enhance individual independence, and prevent further overload or deprivation.

Sexuality and spirituality are also important components of human functioning. These dimensions are an integral part of each person's identity and are critical elements in holistic patient care. Nurses recognize the importance of these areas for optimal health and use their knowledge and skills to assist patients to enhanced wellness in these areas.

To facilitate wellness in each of these psychosocial spheres, nurses must develop self-awareness, including knowledge of their own personal attitudes, values, perceptions, and practices, as well as understand how others differ in these characteristics. Nurses' own personal biases, including the ability to accept others who have cultural, spiritual, racial, ethnic, or sexual identity characteristics that differ from their own, affect their ability to plan and provide optimal care. Nursing interventions and therapeutic interpersonal skills are used to elicit concerns, identify needs, implement teaching, make referrals, and demonstrate empathic caring and acceptance.

"The unique function of the nurse is to assist the individual ... in the performance of those activities contributing to health or its recovery (or to peaceful death) that he would perform unaided if he had the necessary strength, will or knowledge ... in such a way as to help him gain independence as rapidly as possible."

Virginia Henderson (1897–1996) the "first lady of nursing," whose career spanned almost 70 years as both author and researcher; her works on nursing principles are research based and have been translated into 25 languages

40

Self-Concept

ANTHONY SANTORINI

Anthony is a middle-aged man with a history of diabetes. He recently underwent a below-the-knee amputation due to complications resulting from poor glucose control. One morning, he states, "I feel like damaged goods. I'm not a whole man anymore."

MELISSA MOTSKY

Melissa is a 31-year-old married mother of three children ages 12, 10, and 8 who is a third-year nursing student in academic jeopardy. Melissa cries and calls herself a failure when she speaks to her academic advisor. She sees no way to work herself out of her current predicament.

DELORES SPARKS

Delores is a 72-year-old African American widow, diagnosed with advanced lung cancer 14 months ago. She was living alone in a small apartment until 9 months ago, when she had to move in with her daughter after a lengthy hospital stay because she was no longer capable of living alone, and had a probable prognosis of 3 months to live at most. A recent home visit revealed that the patient was increasingly depressed and feeling like a burden to her daughter. She stated, "I'm just an old dish rag, not good for anything anymore."

LEARNING OBJECTIVES

After completing the chapter, you will be able to accomplish the following:

1. Identify three dimensions of self-concept: self-knowledge, self-expectations, and self-evaluation (self-esteem).

2. Describe major steps in the development of self-concept.

3. Differentiate positive and negative self-concept and high and low self-esteem.

4. Identify six variables that influence self-concept.

5. Use appropriate interview questions and observations to assess a patient's self-concept.

6. Develop nursing diagnoses to identify disturbances in self-concept (body image, self-esteem, role performance, personal identity).

7. Describe nursing strategies that are effective in resolving self-concept problems.

8. Plan, implement, and evaluate nursing care related to select nursing diagnoses for disturbances in self-concept.

KEY TERMS

body image	identity diffusion	self-actualization
depersonalization	personal identity	self-concept
false self	role performance	self-esteem
global self		
ideal self		

Self-concept, or self-image, is crucial to a person's health and well-being throughout life. One's **self-concept**, which is the mental image or picture of self, has the power to either encourage or thwart personal growth. People with deficient self-concept might lack the motivation to learn self-care behaviors in response to illness, injury, or trauma. Nursing efforts aimed at teaching new health behaviors might fail until the patient values him/herself enough to want to invest energy in self-care. Some patients observing aspects of their negative self-concept that affect their health behaviors might desperately want to make modifications but have no idea how to do so. The experience of illness, diagnostic testing, and treatment can severely threaten a patient's self-concept. Nurses sensitive to patients' expressions of self-concept can use each nurse–patient interaction to enhance a patient's sense of self and to assist the patient in resolving self-concept disturbances. (See the accompanying Reflective Practice box for an example on page 1552.)

Several variables contribute to self-concept. For example, as discussed in Chapter 4, as people move through the hierarchy of human needs to higher levels, needs for self-esteem and self-actualization arise. The need for **self-esteem** is the need to feel good about oneself and to believe that others hold one in high regard. The need for **self-actualization** is the need to reach one's potential through full development of one's unique capability. At the other end of the spectrum are identity diffusion, dissociation, and depersonalization. **Identity diffusion** is the failure to integrate various childhood identifications into a harmonious adult psychosocial identity, which can lead to disruptions in relationships and problems of intimacy. **Depersonalization** is the subjective experience of the partial or total disruption of one's ego and the disintegration and disorganization of one's self-concept (Stuart, 2013). Figure 40-1 illustrates the continuum of self-concept responses.

OVERVIEW OF SELF-CONCEPT
Dimensions of Self-Concept

All of the feelings, beliefs, and values associated with "I" or "me" compose self-concept. Specific components of self-concept include personal identity, body image, self-esteem, and role performance. Crucial to each component are the dimensions of self-concept, which include self-knowledge, self-expectations, and self-evaluation.

People with a positive self-concept usually have greater and more diversified self-knowledge, more realistic perceptions and expectations, and a higher evaluation of themselves or higher self-esteem, whereas those with negative self-concept tend to exhibit poorer self-knowledge, less realistic perceptions and expectations, and lower self-esteem.

FIGURE 40-1. Continuum of self-concept responses. (Reprinted with permission from Stuart, G. W. [2013]. *Principles and practice of psychiatric nursing* [10th ed., p. 264]. St. Louis: Elsevier/Mosby.)

REFLECTIVE PRACTICE: CULTIVATING QSEN COMPETENCIES

CHALLENGE TO INTERPERSONAL SKILLS

Mrs. Delores Sparks is a 72-year-old, widowed, African American woman. Before her diagnosis of advanced lung cancer 14 months ago, she lived alone in a small apartment. Nine months ago, following a lengthy hospital stay, she moved in with her daughter when it was determined that she was no longer capable of living alone and probably had, at most, 3 months to live. I was visiting her during my home health care nursing experience and growing more and more concerned with her depression. Mrs. Sparks verbalized that she felt like a burden to her daughter, who has three children herself and was currently taking care of a granddaughter born to her eldest, unmarried daughter. Mrs. Sparks was being treated for her depression, but I was concerned about the effects all this was having on her self-concept. She told me she was like "an old dish rag" that wasn't good for anything anymore.

Thinking Outside the Box: Possible Courses of Action

- Try to cheer her up at each visit.
- Ignore her deteriorating self-concept, since focusing on it may only make her feel worse; it is certainly true that she has enough bad stuff going on in her life to make her feel bad.
- Explore sources of positive affirmations of her worth; try to use my professional relationship with her to communicate "You are a person of worth and I care about you!"

Evaluating a Good Outcome: How Do I Define Success?

- Mrs. Sparks' self-concept improves.
- I learn how to communicate a sense of worth to vulnerable patients.
- I learn how to address problems with self-concept.

Personal Learning: Here's to the Future!

Unfortunately, this situation got worse before it got better. Mrs. Sparks did not always take her meds for depression, and her daughter voiced increasing frustration with her mother's mood. "Mom talks all the time now about how even God doesn't want her. She says that she may have to take her own life since God doesn't seem to be doing it!" The daughter also said that Mrs. Sparks apologized to her constantly for being such a bother. Things didn't start to change until I learned that Mrs. Sparks used to be a very important member of her Baptist church community. She stopped attending services when she got too weak to go out. This was clearly a major loss for her. When I successfully got her minister to visit, he literally turned her life around, providing her with lots of positive reinforcement for how she could use her illness to do God's work. She seems much more peaceful now. I've also encouraged her to tell me stories about the church work she did in the past and these reminiscences seem to be helpful.

REFLECTION ON QUALITY AND SAFETY COMPETENCIES

Do you agree with the criteria that the nursing student used to evaluate a successful outcome? Why or why not? What *knowledge, skills,* and *attitudes* do you need to develop to continuously improve the quality and safety of care for patients like Mrs. Sparks?

Patient-Centered Care: How would you develop a respectful and successful partnership with Mrs. Sparks and her daughter? How might your interpersonal skills influence her self-concept?

Teamwork and Collaboration/Quality Improvement: What special competence did the minister bring to Mrs. Sparks? What other members of your caregiving team can you consult with? What does quality care for this family "look like"?

Safety/Evidence-Based Practice: Describe the patient's self-concept in the dimensions of self-knowledge, self-expectations, and self-evaluation. What does the evidence point to as "best practice" for Mrs. Sparks? What safety needs does she have, and how can you meet them?

Informatics: Can you identify the essential information that must be available in Mrs. Spark's electronic record to support safe patient care and coordination of care? Can you think of other ways to respond to or approach the situation? What else might the nursing student have done to ensure a successful outcome?

CONSIDER Anthony Santorini, the patient with a below-the-knee amputation. Analysis of this patient's comments would indicate that he is experiencing a negative self-concept. The nurse would need to assess Mr. Santorini more closely to determine his self-knowledge, self-expectations, and self-evaluation for each component of self-concept. This would help the nurse identify possible factors contributing to his status and gain a fuller picture of his current condition. ●

Self-Knowledge: "Who Am I?"

Global self is the term used to describe the composite of all the basic facts, qualities, traits, images, and feelings one holds about oneself. These strongly influence a person's ability to manage life events and ensure emotional stability. A person's self-knowledge includes:

- Basic facts (sex, age, race, occupation, cultural background, sexual orientation)
- Person's position within social groups
- Qualities or traits that describe typical behaviors, feelings, moods, and other characteristics (e.g., generous, hot-headed, ambitious, intelligent, sexy)

Although some labels cannot be changed (e.g., age and race), most are subjective and sensitive to change. Some conditions associated with alterations in self-concept or global self-worth include developmental changes, life crisis, illness, and loss.

 THINK back to Delores Sparks, the older woman with advanced lung cancer who feels like a burden. When assessing her global self-worth, the nurse would need to identify any developmental changes that Mrs. Sparks is experiencing that may be contributing to her current status, such as changes related to her increasing age. In addition, information about role changes, including the inability to care for herself and the need to be dependent due to her illness, in conjunction with the knowledge of her terminal condition and anticipatory grieving related to her death, would be essential for determining her feelings of global self-worth. ●

Self-Expectations: "Who or What Do I Want to Be?"

Expectations for the self flow from various sources. The **ideal self** constitutes the self one wants to be. These self-expectations develop unconsciously early in childhood and are based on images of role models such as parents, other caregiving figures, and public figures. These personal expectations might be healthy or unhealthy. Contrast the significance of a child's identifying a television "bad boy" or drug dealer as his hero rather than parents, government leaders, or other professional people. A **false self** might develop in people who have an emotional need to respond to the needs and ambitions significant people, such as parents, have for them.

Self-Evaluation: "How Well Do I Like Myself?"

Self-esteem is the evaluative and affective component of the self-concept, sometimes termed *self-respect, self-approval,* or *self-worth*. According to Maslow (1954, p. 90), all people "have a need or desire for a stable, firmly based, usually high evaluation of themselves, for self-respect or self-esteem, and for the esteem of others." Accordingly, he identified two subsets of esteem needs: (1) self-esteem needs (strength, achievement, mastery and competence, confidence in the face of the world, independence, freedom) and (2) respect needs or the need for esteem from others (status, dominance, recognition, attention, importance, appreciation). For Maslow, self-esteem comes from two major sources: how competent children think they are in various

aspects of life and how much social support they receive from other people. One's self-esteem, like the various self-images that make up one's self-concept, varies considerably depending on a specific relationship or situation.

Coopersmith (1967) identified the four bases of self-esteem as (1) significance—the way people feel they are loved and approved of by the people important to them, (2) competence—the way tasks that are considered important are performed, (3) virtue—the attainment of moral–ethical standards, and (4) power—the extent to which people influence their own and others' lives. According to Coopersmith, people with high, medium, and low self-esteem differ in their expectations of the future, in their affective reactions, and in their basic styles of adapting to environmental demands. People with high self-esteem, for example, are accustomed to being well received and successful. They are able to approach people, tasks, and new situations freely, with confidence in their ability to interact and to get along with people and to respond successfully to life's challenges.

Three major self-evaluation feelings or affects found in people are (1) pride, based on a positive self-evaluation, (2) guilt, based on behaviors incongruent with ideal self, and (3) shame, associated with low global self-worth. These affects are learned in early childhood within relationships with significant others and maintained through practice.

Sullivan (1953) proposed the self-representations of "good-me" and "bad-me" based on reflected appraisals of the self, learned in the context of a child's early relationship with significant others, especially parents. The child's feelings of self-esteem and self-worth develop out of that child's perceptions of the parenting figure's feelings, or affects, expressed in caring for the child. Sullivan posited that children perceived their parents' relative anxiety through a process he termed "empathy." Children exposed to higher levels of parental anxiety are at risk for developing lower self-esteem and a greater self-representation of "bad-me." As the child developed further, that child would begin to behave in ways that confirmed the earlier self-appraisals.

Sullivan and his most important interpreter within nursing, Hildegarde Peplau (1952; 1997), emphasized the fluidity of self-appraisals throughout the lifespan. They taught that positive interaction at any point in a person's life with new significant others (such as nurses) who are less anxious and more accepting and nurturing than prior figures can have a positive, growth-promoting effect on that person's self-esteem and self-concept.

Bowlby (1969) developed attachment theory, which describes modes by which a young child develops and maintains feelings about the self as well as values and beliefs about the world. Attachment is a process by which the child maintains felt security via an interpersonal bond with close caregivers, most notably parents. Through a learning process based on children's perception of their caregivers' thoughts and reactions toward them, children forms a sense of self as secure or insecure, calm or anxious, likable or not. Through this process, a child also develops beliefs and feelings about others as well as individual perceptions of situations and

FIGURE 40-2. Interaction between caregivers and the infant are important to the child's development. Feeding, holding, cuddling, and cooing are forms of interaction.

events. Depending on how healthy the child's attachment experience is with the early caregiver, the growing child's self-esteem might vary greatly. The child's thoughts and feelings about events might closely match reality or might be distorted and out of touch with reality. Such patterns tend to remain relatively fixed into adulthood.

Formation of Self-Concept

Although self-concept is largely considered to be a social creation that develops as a result of interactions with others (Fig. 40-2), contemporary nursing researchers and others recognize that certain inborn tendencies, such as temperament, when interacting with social and interpersonal experiences, are crucial in the formation of self-concept (McClowry, 2003). Psychoanalysts have also emphasized the importance of inborn traits, such as innate aggression, because they affect a child's interpersonal experiences and shape self-concept (Freud, 1961). According to the theoretical formulations previously stated, the formation of self-concept includes the following:

1. An infant learns that the physical self is different from the environment. If basic needs are met, warmth and affection are experienced, and the caregivers' anxiety is minimized, then the child begins life with positive feelings about self.
2. The child next internalizes (incorporates into self) other people's attitudes toward self, including attitudes directed toward the child's innate tendencies, such as temperament and aggression. This internalization forms the foundation of self-concept. Parents or other direct caregivers play the most influential role; peers play the second most influential role. Later, the child continues to behave in ways that confirm this early self-concept.
3. The child or adult internalizes the standards of society.

Stages in the development of the self include self-awareness (infancy), self-recognition (18 months), self-definition (3 years), and self-concept (6–7 years). Psychological conditions that foster healthy development of the self in children include:

- Emotional warmth and acceptance
- Effective structure and discipline
- Clearly defined standards and limits, so that children understand what goals, procedures, and conduct are approved
- Adequately defined roles for both older and younger members of the family
- Established methods of handling children that produce the desired behavior, discourage misbehavior, and deal with infractions when they occur
- Encouragement of competence and self-confidence (Fig. 40-3)
- Helping children meet challenges
- Appropriate role models
- A stimulating and responsive environment

Formation of self-concept is further described in developmental theories, especially in Erikson's stages of development, Piaget's cognitive developmental stages, and Havighurst's developmental tasks (see Chapters 17 and 18).

Factors Affecting Self-Concept

Almost any life experience can influence a person's self-concept. Key factors include developmental considerations, culture, internal and external resources, history of success and failure, stressors, and illness or trauma.

Developmental Considerations

As a person matures, the criteria that mark the experiences necessary for a positive self-concept change. Although the infant needs a supportive environment in which all human needs are met, the growing child needs the freedom to

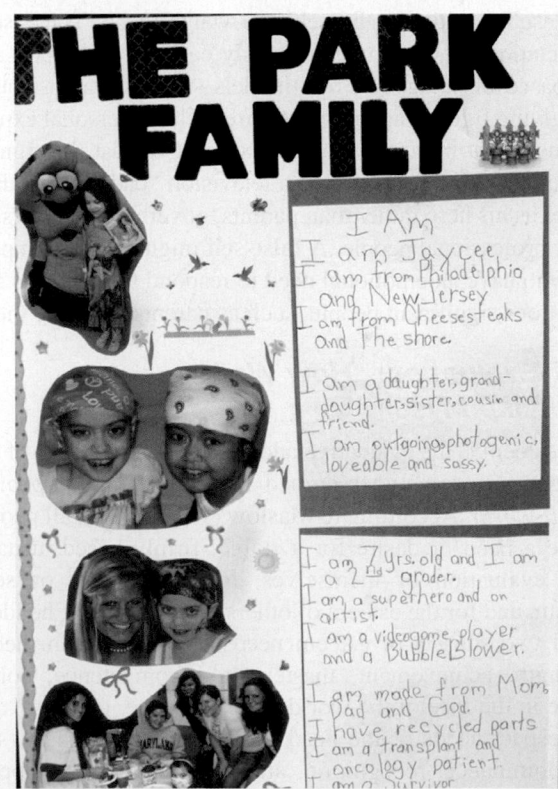

FIGURE 40-3. Jaycee's artwork illustrates her healthy self-concept. (Used with permission.)

explore and develop the ability to meet increasing personal needs. Table 40-1 highlights developmental changes affecting self-concept, related implications for nursing, and potential causes of self-concept disturbances.

Culture

As a child internalizes the values of parents and peers, culture begins to influence a sense of self. If the culture is relatively stable, little tension might be experienced between

Table 40-1 DEVELOPMENTAL CHANGES AFFECTING SELF-CONCEPT

DEVELOPMENTAL PERIOD	CHANGES AFFECTING SELF-CONCEPT	IMPLICATIONS FOR NURSING	POTENTIAL CAUSES OF DISTURBANCES IN SELF-CONCEPT
Infancy	• No self-concept at birth • Beginning differentiation of self and nonself	• Teach parents the critical importance of providing consistent and affectionate parenting. • Assess whether the parents have reasonable expectations of the infant: sleeping, eating, other awake behaviors.	• Unmet basic human needs • Lack of adequate body and sensory stimulation • Parents' lack of acceptance of the infant's appearance or behavior • Poor match between parent's and child's temperament or needs
Childhood	• An intact body is important to the young child who fears bodily mutilation. • During middle childhood, a sense of being trusted and loved, of being competent and trustworthy develops. • Differences between self and others are strong.	• If invasive procedures are indicated, explain simply to the child what is being done and offer the child support. • Assess the parents' ability to provide the type of developmental environment in which the child's self-concepts can evolve positively.	• Dysfunctional family • Too much or too little structure • Sensory perceptual impairments
Adolescence	• Development of secondary sex characteristics; rapid body changes • Sense of self is consolidated. • Emphasis on sexual identity • Parental influences on self-concept are often rejected; peers become more important; movement is toward development of own identity.	• Assess adolescent's self-knowledge and understanding of body changes. • Counsel adolescent regarding mature and healthy use of independence he or she craves. • Provide anticipatory guidelines regarding hazards to life, health, human functioning.	• Inability to accept body • Inability to resolve competing pulls to be both a child and an adult • Unhealthy peer pressure • Identity confusion
Adulthood	• Society places emphasis on intactness of body, fitness, energy, sexuality, style, productivity, sophistication, beauty. • Important to meet role expectations well	• Assess how realistic the adult's expectations are and the incentive they provide for growth and development. • Assist patient to deal constructively with negative influences in self-image. • Preretirement counseling	• Inability to fulfill conflicting role expectations • Failure to accept role responsibility (e.g., parenting responsibilities) • Unreasonable expectations • Irreversible body change related to trauma, illness • Unsatisfying job • Failure to develop new goals to give meaning and purpose to life • Multiple stressors
Later years	• Declining physical and possibly mental abilities • Multiple losses • Increasing dependency • Impending death • Diminished choices/options	• Assess how the older person is adjusting to effects of aging. • Counsel regarding meaningful use of time. • Explore resources. • Assess depression, substance abuse. • Recognize and value older adults' life experience.	• Loss of significant work (retirement); feelings of uselessness • Death of spouse, significant others • Diminished physical attractiveness, strength, overall health • Multiple stressors • Fear of dependency • Change may be more difficult.

what culture expects of the child and what the child expects of self. When parents, peers, and the adult world confront the child with different cultural expectations, however, the sense of self might be confused. For example, an adolescent might realize his or her parents live by the work ethic and believe it is necessary to rise early every day and put in a full day's work. That adolescent's peer group, however, has few demands placed on it and encourages the adolescent to hang out with the group. The adolescent's vocational aptitudes, meanwhile, are leading him or her to consider a music career in a rock group, which will keep the adolescent out late many nights doing something the parents do not classify as work.

Children of immigrants whose values and practices of their culture of origin vary from the culture of adoption face cultural dissonance. Parents might expect children to behave according to their own cultural norms; peers and society, as well as the adolescent's desire to "belong," may create the desire to abandon old cultural beliefs, attitudes, and practices among many of these children. Conflict between parents and children, as well as cultural confusion, might occur.

Internal and External Resources

The personal strengths a person recognizes, develops, and uses are powerful but subjective determinants of self-concept. For example, one person might use humor as both an effective coping mechanism and a successful interpersonal tool. Another person might use humor to avoid facing conflict but might feel badly about being known as a joker or clown. The degree to which a person integrates healthy, useful internal resources or personal strengths is associated with how well a person has been able to establish a positive self-concept in the context of nurturing experiences. Self-concept is also associated with the ability to identify and use external resources such as a network of support people, adequate finances, and organizational supports. People who feel more positively about themselves tend to feel connected to others and to society; they can identify and use more external resources. On the other hand, people who feel disconnected and alone tend to perceive and use fewer environmental resources.

History of Success and Failure

People with a history of repeated failure (in school, friendships, work, or marriage) might perceive themselves as failures and actually perpetuate this image by unconsciously encouraging others to treat them this way. They might come to fear success and actually find it easier to fail even though they do not like themselves that way. Thus, failure influences a person's self-concept negatively (e.g., Sullivan's "bad-me" self-representation), and one's self-concept causes a person to continue to fail. On the other hand, a series of successful experiences—especially when occurring in the context of an accepting, nurturing, caring relationship—might condition a person to strive for the next success, and a positive self-concept might be forged that expects success and makes it happen.

 THINK back to Melissa Motsky, the struggling nursing student. Consider how multiple less-than-satisfactory life experiences may culminate in Ms. Motsky's sense of personal failure in areas such as academics, relationships, role performance in her family and work experience. ●

Crises or Life Stressors

Life stressors or crises (e.g., marriage, divorce, acute or chronic illness, an exam, a new job or job loss, a gray hair, a fire) might call forth a personal response and mobilize a person's talents, resulting in good feelings about oneself, or it might result in emotional paralysis with diminished self-concept. People vary greatly in their perception of what constitutes a crisis or stressor, as well as the degree to which such experiences might disrupt or diminish self-concept. However, major stressors place anyone at relative risk for maladaptive responses such as withdrawal, isolation, depression, extreme anxiety, substance abuse, or exacerbation of physical illness. How the person perceives the stressor (threat, challenge, defeat) and the individual's ability to mobilize personal strengths and other resources are determined largely by that person's self-concept, which, in turn, is influenced by the response the person chooses.

Aguilera (1998) described three factors that determine a person's response to crisis: (1) the person's perception of the event or situation, (2) the person's situational supports (external resources), and (3) the coping mechanisms the person possesses (internal resources). All of these factors are related to self-concept. The degree of strength a person has in each area is related to one's precrisis self-concept. Similarly, each of these conditions can alter self-concept either positively or negatively during or after the crisis. Intervention to strengthen any of these three areas can help people better cope with crisis and emerge with enhanced self-concept.

 RECALL Anthony Santorini, the patient who had an amputation. To promote an enhanced self-concept, the nurse would need to assess his perception of the situation and his coping mechanisms to gain further insight into Mr. Santorini's self-concept. In addition, the nurse would need to investigate the support systems available to Mr. Santorini such as family, friends, and community resources that might be helpful in fostering a more positive self-concept. ●

Aging, Illness, or Trauma

Many people take a healthy body for granted. Society encourages a kind of denial of the eventuality of aging, chronic illness, and the necessity to integrate crisis and change throughout each person's lifetime. Society emphasizes and rewards youth, health, and narrow norms for physical attractiveness while devaluing seniors, those with chronic illness, and those whose appearance does not correspond to movie-star standards. Thus, even the suggestion of disease; the sudden impact of illness, trauma, or bodily disfigurement;

FIGURE 40-4. An illness or alteration in function may present a crisis situation, which affects the patient's self-concept. Changes may be positive or negative.

or signs of the aging process might pose serious threats to the self (Fig. 40-4). People vary greatly in their response to aging, illness, and trauma. This is due to the threats to self-concept and internal beliefs about the self that these conditions may pose. Refer to the Research in Nursing box.

 CONSIDER Delores Sparks, the woman described in the Reflective Practice display. Aging, by itself, can influence one's self-concept. However, the patient also is faced with the loss of independence and personal space, reliance on others for daily care, knowledge that she has a terminal illness, and the prospect of death in the near future. All of these factors are contributing to Mrs. Sparks' current status. •

THE NURSING PROCESS

Nurses who role model good health behaviors are more effective teachers. Use the display, Promoting Health 40-1, (on page 1558) for yourself before using it with others. Before nurses can successfully identify and resolve self-concept disturbances in patients, they must be comfortable with themselves and possess an adequate self-concept.

RESEARCH IN NURSING

BRIDGING THE GAP TO EVIDENCE-BASED PRACTICE

Promoting Positive Self-Concept

The experience of illness, diagnostic testing, and treatment can severely threaten self-concept. Social support, positive role function, and satisfaction with health care have been demonstrated to have a positive influence on the experience of dealing with illness. As an external resource for patients, nurses can help promote a positive self-concept.

Related Research

Lee, M-Y, Mu, P.-F., Tsay, S.-F., Chou, S.-S., Chen, Y.-C. & Wong, T.-W. 2012. Body image of children and adolescents with cancer: A metasynthesis on qualitative research findings. *Nursing & Health Sciences*, *14*(3), 381–390. DOI: 10.1111/j.1442–2018.2012.00695.x

Children and adolescents with cancer are confronted with many challenges. Repeated courses of treatment lead to loss of a normal, orderly life, and might even result in changes in interpersonal interactions. The derived four metasyntheses included being distanced from the body, loss of self-identity, self-protective strategies and support, and getting rid of the shackles of the body. In response to body image change, people with cancer develop self-protective, coping strategies. Children and adolescents who experience life-threatening cancer come to face body image change positively and might hold a confident attitude toward their future.

Relevance to Nursing Practice

Nurses should incorporate body image work into the daily care of children and adolescents with cancer patients. Not only is it an essential part of their recuperation process, but it will also aid them in returning to their lives, potentially negating or lessening the negative impact.

Related Research

Buxton, B., & Snethen, J. (July/August 2013). Obese women's perceptions and experiences of health care and primary care providers: A phenomenological study. *Nursing Research*, *62*(4), 252–259. doi: 10.1097/NNR.0b013e318299a6ba

The aim of this study was to describe the experiences and perceptions of obese women with regard to stigma in health care and from their health care provider. Four themes emerged from the analysis of the data: (a) perceptions of health and health care, (b) respect me as a person, (c) establishing a health care connection, and (d) assertiveness is necessary. Although stigma was not named by women in this study, all acknowledged some negative treatment by health care providers.

Relevance to Nursing Practice

Nearly two thirds of the adult population in the United States is overweight or obese. Adults who are overweight or obese require the same high-quality health care from their providers as any other adult. Unfortunately, stigma is a reality experienced by people who are overweight or obese, and health care professionals' views have sometimes been reported to be biased against people who are overweight or obese.

For additional research, visit thePoint.

PROMOTING HEALTH 40-1

SELF-CONCEPT

Use the assessment checklist to determine how well you are meeting your need for positive self-concept. Then develop a prescription for self-care by choosing appropriate behaviors from the list of suggestions.

Assessment Checklist

❏ almost always	❏ sometimes	❏ almost never

❏ ❏ ❏ 1. I have established appropriate expectations and goals for myself.

❏ ❏ ❏ 2. I have effective and satisfying relationships with others.

❏ ❏ ❏ 3. I cope effectively with change and loss.

❏ ❏ ❏ 4. I accept and feel good about myself.

Self-Care Behaviors

1. Accept normal variations in physical appearance and capabilities.
2. Use problem-solving and decision-making strategies to define expectations and set goals.
3. Set priorities and accept that no one person can be all things to all people.
4. Learn from past mistakes and then forget them; carrying around "excess baggage" is unhealthy.
5. Emphasize strengths and abilities in self.
6. Take an active part in group activities in school, work, church, or the community.
7. Volunteer time, talents, or services.
8. Avoid excessive alcohol and drugs.
9. Live life one day at a time.
10. Get help for self-concept disturbances that interfere with healthy social and professional activities.

Assessing

The nurse assessing a patient's self-concept focuses on personal identity, body image, self-esteem, and role performance. A general assessment of self-concept should be included in every comprehensive nursing assessment. It is as important to identify and label a patient's positive self-concept as it is to note problems.

Patients experiencing illness or trauma resulting in body disfigurement, altered functioning, or life crises that arrest development and thwart the achievement of life goals are at high risk for problems related to self-concept and should be assessed more carefully. If potential problems surface during the interview, a more thorough assessment should be carried out.

The accompanying Focused Assessment Guide highlights elements common to any self-concept assessment and high-risk factors.

When conducting this assessment, be aware of the limitations of self-reporting. Patients might give what they believe are the desired or socially acceptable responses to interview questions. "Why, of course I like myself. I'm a pretty good person. Yes, I have friends." For this reason, evaluate the patient's responses in relation to your observations about the patient and what you know about the patient from other sources. When the nursing assessment reveals a clustering of these behaviors, discuss this finding with the patient. This is especially true when there is a discrepancy between the patient's words and behavior. "You've told me that you feel in control of your situation right now and are committed to the treatment plan, but I notice you're not taking your medications regularly and you did mention that you are drinking more heavily...."

Personal Identity

When assessing self-concept, the information needed first is the patient's description of self. **Personal identity** describes a person's conscious sense of who he or she is. "How would you describe yourself to others?" Pay special attention to the labels used by the patient and the order in which they appear. A simple exercise consists of asking patients to "Make a list of 10 labels that you believe identify yourself (e.g., gay man, student, Italian American, opera fan, premed major). Put the most important label first, and then list the others in order of decreasing importance. (What if the order were reversed?) To what extent do you think your way of organizing information about yourself affects your behavior?"

It is important to discover whether individuals are comfortable with their perceived identity. Developmental changes, trauma, and cultural and gender dissonance might all place a patient at risk for personal identity disturbances.

Personal Strengths

Many patients focus naturally on their deficiencies; asking pointed questions about personal strengths can help a patient identify positive factors:

"What are some of your personal strengths...qualities you are proud of...things you do well?"

"What has helped you cope in the past when things were tough?"

Body Image

Body image is the person's subjective view of one's physical appearance. Body image disturbances can be expected with any alteration in bodily appearance, structure, or function.

FOCUSED ASSESSMENT GUIDE 40-1

SELF-CONCEPT

Factors to Assess	High-Risk Factors	Questions and Approaches
Personal identity	• Developmental changes • Trauma • Gender dissonance • Cultural dissonance	How would you describe yourself to others? • Personal characteristics and traits • Strengths • Fears
Body image	• Loss of body part or function • Disfigurement • Developmental changes	Describe your body to me. What do you like most/least about your body? Is there anything about your body that you would like to change?
Self-esteem	• Unhealthy interpersonal relationships • Failure to achieve developmental milestones • Failure to achieve life goals • Failure to live up to personal moral code • Sense of powerlessness	Tell me something about your sense of satisfaction with yourself. Tell me about your relationship with others. Who would you like to be? Who or what has influenced your self-expectations? Are these expectations realistic? • *Significance:* What is your response when you feel unloved or unappreciated by those who are important to you? • *Competence:* How do you feel about your ability to do the things in life that are important to you? • *Virtue:* To what degree are you satisfied with the way you are able to live up to your moral standards? • *Power:* To what extent do you feel able to control what happens to you in life? How does this make you feel?
Role performance	• Loss of valued role • Ambiguous role expectations • Conflicting role expectations • Inability to meet role expectations	Many of us "wear many hats." What roles (spouse, parent, student, athlete, nursing aide, dancer) are most important to you? How do you feel about your ability to do all the things your roles demand of you? Are these roles satisfying for you?

When a disturbed body image is suspected, carefully interview and observe the patient to identify the nature of the threat to the person's body image (functional significance of the part involved, importance of physical appearance, visibility of the part involved), the meaning the patient attaches to the threat, the adequacy of the patient's coping abilities, response of family members and significant others, and help available to the patient and patient's family.

Assess the patient's response to the deformity or limitation, including changes in independence–dependence patterns and in socialization and communication.

 RECALL Anthony Santorini, the middle-aged man who had an amputation. The patient voiced concerns that he was not "whole" anymore. The nurse would need to assess the underlying factors associated with this feeling. Is the feeling related to the actual loss of a body part, fear of further disfiguration due to continued complications, inability to function independently, or fear of how others will react to the loss? Additional inquiry is needed to deter-

mine the value Mr. Santorini places on physical appearance and the meaning he attaches to his extremities, such as ability to walk, work, or just get around the house or his environment. The nurse could then work with the patient and assist with adapting to the loss of his leg. Incorporating information about the use of a prosthesis may be helpful as he begins to adapt to his body change. •

RESPONSE TO DEFORMITY OR LIMITATION

Adaptive and maladaptive responses to deformity or limitation follow:

• *Adaptive responses:* Patient exhibits signs of grief and mourning (shock, disbelief, denial, anger, guilt, acceptance).

• *Maladaptive responses:* Patient continues to deny and to avoid dealing with the deformity or limitation, engages in self-destructive behavior, talks about feelings of worthlessness or insecurity, equates deformity or limitation with whole person, shows a change in ability to estimate relationship of body to environment.

INDEPENDENCE–DEPENDENCE PATTERNS

Adaptive and maladaptive responses to changes in independence–dependence patterns follow:

- *Adaptive responses:* Patient assumes responsibility for care (makes decisions), develops new self-care behaviors, uses available resources, interacts in a mutually supportive way with family.
- *Maladaptive responses:* Patient assigns responsibility for his or her care to others, becomes increasingly dependent, or stubbornly refuses necessary help.

Self-Esteem

When patients share their self-perceptions, use the opportunity to ask questions about whether patients like themselves, whether they are pleased with their expectations, and the progress they are making to realize these expectations. For example, you might state:

> *"Tell me what you like about yourself."*
> *"What would you change about yourself if you could?"*

You can obtain a quick indication of a patient's self-esteem by using a graphic description of self-esteem as the discrepancy between the "real self" (what we think we really are) and the "ideal self" (what we think we would like to be). Have the patient plot two points on a line—real self and ideal self (Fig. 40-5). The greater the discrepancy, the lower the self-esteem; the smaller the discrepancy, the higher the self-esteem.

A person's ideal self may differ dramatically from the current sense of self and positively or negatively influence behavior and personal development. If indicated, question the patient about self-expectations:

> *"You've told me something about who you are and how you view yourself now. Tell me who you would like to be in the future."*
> *"What life goals are important to you?"*
> *"Where do you see yourself 5 years from now? In 10 years?"*
> *"Are these expectations realistic?"*

FIGURE 40-5 Patients who perceive their real self as relatively close to the ideal self have high self-esteem. Patients who perceive their real self as far from the ideal self have low self-esteem.

> *"Are your expectations stemming from who you would like to be or from who you think you should be?"*
> *"Who or what has influenced your self-expectations?"*

Such questions help assess whether the patient possesses life goals that are positively motivating personal development. Identify any unrealistic expectations and explore their source with the patient. For example:

> *"You seem to feel that it is necessary to be all things to all people—no matter what this costs you. How might this belief have developed? Is it helpful to you?"*
> *"What I'm hearing is that your performance must always be perfect, that although you allow others to make mistakes, you cannot allow yourself this luxury. Tell me more about this."*
> *"You state you have no goals for the future. When you wake up each morning, what gets you out of bed? What keeps you moving?"*

If a more detailed assessment is needed, the concepts of socialization and communication, significance, competence, virtue, and power should be explored next.

SOCIALIZATION AND COMMUNICATION

Adaptive and maladaptive responses to socialization and communication follow:

- *Adaptive responses:* Maintains usual social patterns, communicates needs and accepts offers of help, serves as support for others
- *Maladaptive responses:* Isolates oneself, exhibits superficial self-confidence, is unable to express needs (becomes hostile, ashamed, frustrated, depressed)

To assess the quantity and quality of the patient's interpersonal relationships, which helps identify the person's level of social support and relatedness, you might ask:

> *"Who do you feel is important to you?"*
> *"Is there anyone you feel you can depend on for help if you need it?"*
> *"How do you feel about your relationships?"*
> *"Tell me about changes you've noticed in your ways of meeting and interacting with others."*
> *"Many people have 'people' problems. Are your relationships causing you any problems right now?"*

SIGNIFICANCE

To assess the patient's feelings of significance, you might ask:

> *"Are there people in your life with whom you share a close relationship?"*
> *"To what extent do you feel loved and approved of by the key people in your life?"*
> *"Does it bother you when you feel unloved or when others fail to appreciate you?"*
> *"In what ways do you let family members and friends know that you like them or are proud of their accomplishments?"*

COMPETENCE

To assess the patient's feelings of competence, you might ask:

"What are the things you need to do to feel important?"

"Is anything interfering with your ability to execute these tasks?" ("How does this make you feel?")

"How important to you is it to feel that others value your work?"

VIRTUE

To assess the patient's sense of virtue, you might ask:

"Tell me something about the moral–ethical principles that govern your life."

"How must you live to describe yourself as a 'good' person?"

"Describe any difficulties you experience in living up to your moral principles that you would like to discuss."

"In what ways can the nurses help you to live better according to your moral standards?"

POWER

To assess the patient's sense of power, you might ask:

"How important is it to you to 'be in control' of your life (health)?"

"To what extent did you feel 'in control' of your life (health) before this illness (trauma, crisis, and so forth)?"

"To what extent do you feel 'in control' of your life (health) currently?"

"What is it that makes you feel not in control?"

"How might you change this? How can nurses help you to develop and gain more control?"

Role Performance

We all play many roles. Life roles such as our occupation or profession can constitute a major portion of our identity. Our ability to successfully live up to societal as well as our own expectations regarding role-specific behaviors, or our **role performance** is easily compromised by illness and injury. Often, illness or developmental processes such as aging make it necessary to alter or relinquish previous roles. Generally, people experience such alterations as major losses. Thus, all people whose roles are altered or compromised are at risk for disturbances in self-concept. Role performance may also be affected by role ambiguity (failure to completely and accurately understand what a role demands), role stress (disparity between what one believes the role demands and what one is able to offer), and role overload (limited time because of other commitments makes it impossible to meet realistic role expectations). With any patient who has experienced compromised role performance, use the following questions:

"What major roles describe you—son, daughter, spouse, parent, employer or employee, student, club member, and so on?"

"How important is it to you to be good in each of these roles?"

"Tell me how successful you think you are in each of these roles."

"What roles or expectations would you change if you could?"

"What new skills or behaviors might be necessary to help you resume or modify current roles?"

"What is it like for you to lose a role that's been important to you?"

"How can I help you identify other role options or direction?"

 THINK back to Delores Sparks, the woman with advanced lung cancer now living with her daughter. The change in living situation and dependence on her daughter for everyday activities has definitely affected the patient's role performance. Once living alone and fairly self-sufficient, Mrs. Sparks now relies on her daughter. The role-performance questions would be extremely important to ask Mrs. Sparks to determine the actual impact her illness and change in living situation has had on her self-concept. ●

Diagnosing

Specific disturbances in self-concept that can be treated by independent nursing interventions receive one of four nursing diagnostic labels:

- *Disturbed Body Image:* The state in which one experiences confusion in the mental picture of one's physical self
- *Chronic (or Risk for Chronic) Low Self-Esteem* or *Situational (or Risk for Situational) Low Self-Esteem:* The state in which an individual experiences or is at risk for experiencing negative self-evaluation about self or capabilities
- *Ineffective Role Performance:* The state in which an individual experiences or is at risk for experiencing a disruption in the way that individual perceives one's role performance
- *Disturbed (or Risk for Disturbed) Personal Identity:* The state in which an individual experiences or is at risk for experiencing an inability to distinguish between self and nonself (NANDA International, 2012)

Common etiologies and defining characteristics for these diagnoses are found in the accompanying box, Examples of NANDA-I Nursing Diagnoses: Disturbances in Self-Concept (on pages 1562–1563).

In addition, *Readiness for Enhanced Self-Concept* is a pattern of perceptions and ideas about the self that is sufficient for well-being and can be strengthened (NANDA International, 2012). This is a wellness diagnosis.

Important Distinctions

When assessment data point to an alteration in self-concept, the first task is to determine whether the altered

EXAMPLES OF NANDA-I NURSING DIAGNOSES

DISTURBANCES IN SELF-CONCEPT

Nursing Diagnoses	Related Factors	Sample Defining Characteristics
Disturbed Body Image	Irreversible changes in body image such as amputation, mastectomy, hysterectomy, colostomy, scars, burns, disfiguring skin disorder	"Look at me. Nothing can ever be the same again. I feel less whole. When I look in the mirror, all I see is my (stump, missing breast, scar). I know when others look at me they feel repulsed or, at the very least, pity me."
	Effects of treatment (e.g., braces, casts)	Thirteen-year-old adolescent girl with scoliosis wearing a Milwaukee brace (covers pelvic area and has rods in the front and back that extend up to the chin): "I feel dumb in this thing... it's bad enough that my back is crooked but this makes me look like a freak. Besides, it's hot. Must I wear it to school?"
	Difficulty accepting development of secondary sex characteristics or delayed development of same	Fifteen-year-old adolescent boy, sophomore in high school, height 5'1", weight 88 lb: "When am I going to grow up and start looking like the other guys in my class?" No pubic hair; penis, testes, and scrotum are the same size and proportion as in childhood.
	Extreme thinness or obesity	Twenty-year-old woman, height 5'7", weight 200 lb: "I hate my body... I've been fat all my life and I'm always on a diet. Why can't I be like everyone else?"
Low Self-Esteem	Feeling unloved or unapproved of by significant others	Twelve-year-old son of parents in the process of getting a divorce: "No matter what I do to make my dad like me, he acts like I don't exist. When he's home, he fights with mom, but mostly he's away. I wouldn't even care if he yelled at me so long as he noticed me. I wonder why he doesn't like me?"
	Feelings of incompetence	Forty-two-year-old car salesperson, with company for 18 years: "What's wrong with me? I do my job, I'm never absent, I have a good sales record, but I keep getting passed over for promotions. I think I'm too old to move to a different company, but I don't want to just sell cars for someone else for the rest of my life!"
	Failure to live according to personal moral ethical code	Thirty-three-year-old single computer programmer: "I should have known I'd get pregnant—I deserve it. I knew I was wrong to go to bed with this guy. Basically, I've tried to live the way I think I should all my life up until now. What if something's wrong with the baby because of my sin?"
	Powerlessness	Sixty-seven-year-old alert widow with degenerative joint disease: "It may be hard for me to move around now, but darn it—there's nothing wrong with my mind. The kids think they are helping me by making all my decisions, but they aren't. I'm not a doddering old lady in a nursing home."
Ineffective Role Performance	Rejection of role	Twenty-two-year-old mother 2 days after birth of her second son (first son is 15 months old): "I don't know who my husband got to watch our son. I never wanted to be a mother anyway. My husband and I have never had any time for ourselves—and things aren't going to get any better."
	Role conflict Role fatigue Multiple life stressors	Twenty-one-year-old, full-time junior nursing student who failed a major exam; is married and the mother of an 18-month-old daughter; works every other weekend in a hospital as an ECG technician: "I'm trying so hard to get my grades up, but I don't know what else I can do. My husband seems to be losing patience with me more and more, and I sometimes feel awful about neglecting my daughter. I'd stop working but we need the money. I want nursing so bad but I'm getting awfully tired."

EXAMPLES OF NANDA-I NURSING DIAGNOSES *continued*

DISTURBANCES IN SELF-CONCEPT

Nursing Diagnoses	Related Factors	Sample Defining Characteristics
	Changing personal resources (physical health, mental abilities, motivation)	Fifty-year-old college chemistry teacher begins exhibiting signs of early Alzheimer disease; forgets where she is and what she is doing; began rambling in class and saying things that made no sense—much to the class's amusement. Later cried and called herself "stupid."
Disturbed Personal Identity	Unresolved crisis	Eighty-eight-year-old man who lost his wife 6 months ago; wife took care of all his needs; sits alone in the house all day: "We always did everything together. I wish I had died first. What shall I do?"
	Declining physical, mental, or sensory abilities	Same 88-year-old man 3 months after admission to long-term care institution, medical diagnosis "rule out depression/dementia"; has become increasingly withdrawn, never initiates conversation; responses to questions are sometimes inappropriate: "What do you mean, what's my name? Who cares? I want to go home to my wife."
	Rejection of membership in minority group	Fifteen-year-old Cambodian girl recently emigrated to the United States with family; in constant conflict with parents as she rejects her family's culture in hopes of fitting in with a peer group: "Sometimes I feel like I no longer know who I am or how I should act. I feel lonely inside and afraid."

self-concept is the problem, the cause of the problem (etiology), or merely a sign that a problem exists (defining characteristics). Self-concept data seem to fit well in all three categories. It is important to make an accurate determination because this directs the outcomes developed for the patient and related nursing interventions.

 CONSIDER Delores Sparks and the following nursing diagnoses:

SITUATIONAL LOW SELF-ESTEEM related to perceived failure in role of mother and grandmother manifested by feelings of being a bother and not good for anything anymore. Assessment data point to a disturbance in self-esteem as the priority problem. Nursing energies will be directed to helping the patient evaluate herself positively despite the stress of the illness and loss of independence.

INEFFECTIVE HEALTH MAINTENANCE related to decreased self-esteem as manifested by feelings of depression. Here, low self-esteem is contributing to the patient's problem of failing to maintain her health as much as possible by following through with actions, and by voicing thoughts of ending her own life. Nursing energies will be best directed to improving the patient's use of health resources, including helping her to value herself enough to choose healthy behaviors.

INEFFECTIVE COPING related to difficulty accepting changes in health status and role resulting from

terminal illness as manifested by low self-esteem statements ("I feel like an old dish rag, not good for anything anymore") and thoughts about ending her life ("since God isn't doing it"). Here, low self-esteem statements are the cues that led to the identification of the problem statement. One of the criteria used to evaluate nursing intervention to increase the patient's coping skills will be a reduction in or elimination of low self-esteem statements. ●

Outcome Identification and Planning

With all patients, nursing interventions need to be supportive of the following patient outcomes. The patient will achieve the following:

- Describe self realistically, identifying both strengths and deficiencies.
- Verbalize realistic expectations for self based on who the patient would like to be.
- Verbalize that self is liked, or at least "OK."
- Communicate feelings and needs in a way that is comfortable and effective in meeting needs.
- Nurture relationships in which needs for love and worth are mutually met (significance).
- Assume role-related responsibilities with confidence (competence).
- Express satisfaction with ability to live according to one's moral–ethical standards (virtue).
- Demonstrate confidence in ability to accomplish what is desired (power).

Sample outcomes for patients with specific disturbances in self-concept follow:

- Describe the relation between self-concept and behavior.
- Identify faulty thinking that reinforces a negative self-concept (distortions and denials, faulty categorizing, inappropriate standards).
- Integrate positive self-knowledge into self-concept.
- Report feeling better about oneself.

Implementing

Nursing interventions to assist patients to develop and maintain a positive self-concept can vary tremendously from one patient to another. You must be comfortable with your own self-concept before you can address problems in patients. Specific nursing strategies addressed in this section include helping patients identify and use personal strengths, helping at-risk patients maintain a sense of self, enhancing or modifying the self-concept, developing a positive body image, and working with parents and educators to develop self-esteem in children, adolescents, and older adults. These and other nursing interventions are summarized in the accompanying Examples of Nursing Interventions and Nursing Outcome Classifications (NIC/NOC) box.

Helping Patients Identify and Use Personal Strengths

When confronted with a major stressor, many people forget that they have histories of successful coping and numerous personal strengths. Patients at high risk for giving up are those with low self-esteem or multiple stressors they perceive as overwhelming.

Although attributing strength to a patient sounds like something nurses would do naturally, nurses frequently fall into the trap of "doing" for patients (i.e., solving their problems rather than helping them to identify and tap their personal power and strengths). Moreover, patients

FIGURE 40-6. The nurse helps the patient recognize his self-worth and strengths.

continually instruct nurses about how they should be perceived, and some patients successfully communicate a manipulative helplessness that encourages the nurse to take charge. An appropriate nursing response in this case is, "I wonder why you want me to speak with your physician about treatment alternatives. I'm sure you would feel much better hearing this information firsthand. If you'd like, I will stay here while you talk with the physician."

Patients experiencing powerlessness might need help to recognize their strengths (Fig. 40-6). Examples of personal strengths that might better equip a person to respond to life's challenges include:

- Healthy, functioning body
- Ability to adjust to/function with chronic bodily malfunction
- Cognitive abilities
- Positive self-concept
- Interpersonal skills
- Sense of meaning and purpose in life
- Belief system

EXAMPLES OF NURSING INTERVENTIONS AND NURSING OUTCOME CLASSIFICATIONS (NIC/NOC)

SELECTED SELF-AWARENESS ENHANCEMENT ACTIVITIES

Nursing Interventions	Nursing Outcomes
• Encourage patient to recognize and discuss thoughts and feelings. • Assist patient to realize that everyone is unique. • Assist patient to realize the impact of illness on self-concept. • Assist patient to change view of self as victim by defining own rights, as appropriate. • Assist patient to be aware of negative self-statements. • Assist patient to identify guilty feelings. • Explore with patient the need to control. • Assist patient to identify positive attributes of self.	• Differentiates self from environment. • Differentiates self from others. • Maintains awareness of internal signals to situations. • Maintains awareness of thoughts. • Maintains awareness of feelings. • Expresses feelings to others. • Reflects on interactions with others. • Remembers oneself in the past. • Imagines oneself in the future.

Adapted from Bulechek, G. M., Butcher, H. K., Dochterman, J., & Wagner, C. M. (Eds.). (2013). *Nursing interventions classification (NIC)*, (6th ed., pp. 334–335). St. Louis: Elsevier/Mosby; and Moorhead, S., Johnson, M., Maas, M. L., & Swanson, E. (2013). *Nursing outcomes classification (NOC)*, (5th ed., p. 463). St. Louis: Elsevier/Mosby. A full listing of nursing activities for each nursing outcome and intervention can be found in these books.

- Social support network
- Meaningful work
- Hobbies and other interests
- Education
- Life experience and a past history of effective coping
- Good sense of humor
- Spirituality
- Healthy nutritional state
- Ability to make decisions

Specific strategies that can be used to help patients identify and use personal strengths include the following:

- Encourage patients to identify their strengths.
- Replace self-negation with positive thinking.
- Notice and reinforce patient strengths.
- Encourage patients to will for themselves the strengths they desire and to try them on.
- Help patients cope with necessary dependency resulting from aging or illness.

Helping At-Risk Patients Maintain a Sense of Self

People who are acutely ill are often separated not only from their strengths, but also from any real sense of self. This occurs largely because, as patients in health care facilities, they are removed from their personal roles, environments, and belongings, and stripped of their individuality by staff caring for them. One patient, a college president who was recovering from serious complications after surgery for ovarian cancer, shared the following:

> When I first got sick, it didn't matter how people treated me because I knew who I was. As I've grown sicker and weaker, I become whomever people make me. If a nurse walks in here and moves me like meat, I become a slab of meat. My sense of self seems more and more dependent on how people respond to me.

Help patients maintain a sense of self and worth by doing the following:

- Use looks, speech, and judicious touch to communicate worth.
- Acknowledge the patient's status, roles, individuality.
- Speak to the patient respectfully and in a nonpatronizing manner.
- Converse with the patient about the patient's life experience.
- Address the patient by preferred name whenever entering the patient's room.
- Offer the patient a simple explanation before initiating any procedure.
- Move the patient's body respectfully if the patient is unable to do this.
- Respect the patient's privacy and sensibilities.
- Acknowledge and allow expression of negative feelings.
- Help the patient to recognize strengths and explore alternatives.

Always keep in mind that patients are people first and foremost. A person's illness does not define who that person is. Too often, health care professionals tend to focus primarily on a patient's illness, and the whole person is forgotten or ignored, with potential negative consequences for that patient's sense of self, such as lack of motivation to learn or execute important health care behaviors. The way nurses care for patients can directly impact self-concept; self-concept, in turn, directly impacts health. This type of caring does not require additional nursing time or energy. It does require from the nurse continual reaffirmation that nursing is a thoughtful, person-centered profession and that nothing is more important at any moment of a nurse's workday than the person being served.

Modifying a Negative Self-Concept

The time is ripe for change when a patient realizes that a negative self-concept is hindering personal development related to health care. One option is using a cognitive–behavioral approach to assist the patient in modifying self-concept. The general principle is to help the patient alter one's perspective of a situation from a more negative view to a more positive view, a process known as "reframing." Once a person can view one's situation more positively, a wider variety of behavioral options, coping mechanisms, or internal or external supports can be identified and activated. While any person's self-concept is usually firmly entrenched and naturally resists change, you should remain optimistic that change is possible, if even in small increments. Helpful nursing interventions include the following:

- Help the patient identify and describe in detail how the patient thinks and feels about situations related to self-concept (identify the patient's faulty thinking patterns).
- Explore with the patient alternative ways of viewing the same situation (reframe the patient's thinking about the situation).
- Teach the patient to "red flag" faulty thinking behavior as soon as the patient is aware of it. The goal is to replace the negative thinking and self-talk with thinking and self-talk that will develop a more positive self-image.
- Help the patient explore the positive dimensions of oneself that the patient wishes to develop, and incorporate this new knowledge into the self-concept.

Developing a Positive Body Image

Interventions for body image disturbances vary according to the nature of the disturbance. Interventions may include any combination of the following:

- Express interest in and acceptance of the patient through verbal and nonverbal expression. Allow the patient to share one's feelings openly. Sitting quietly by the patient for a few minutes, with a few words such as "How are things?" or "Tell me what's going on with you" communicates to the patient your willingness and readiness to share the patient's experience.
- Explore with the patient his or her feelings about altered body image and the patient's perceptions about the meaning and consequences of such alteration.

- Support the patient through the various stages of loss, grief, and mourning (shock, disbelief, denial, anger, guilt, acceptance), remembering that there is no one right way to proceed through these stages. Rather, patients may move fluidly in and out of various stages, sometimes returning to earlier stages. Some patients may need to learn that it is okay to cry, to be angry, or to feel depressed.
- Use play therapy with children so that they can describe their feelings and work through their grief using the nonthreatening medium of dolls or animals.
- Use self-reflection to gain awareness of your attitudes and feelings toward the patient. Be careful not to let facial expressions, words, or body positioning communicate to the patient disgust, fear, or rejection.
- While communicating support to the patient who is slow to develop and use appropriate self-care behaviors, firmly insist that the patient participate in his or her care to the extent that the patient is able. Whenever possible, provide the patient with honest answers to questions or put the patient in touch with the appropriate person to give the answers.
- Strengthen the decision-making ability of the patient by honestly exploring alternatives; help the patient to imagine living with the consequences of different courses of action.
- Reinforce the patient's personal strengths and help the patient and family to identify all possible resources.
- Assess the response of the patient's significant others and intervene if they negatively influence the patient.

Developing Self-Esteem in Children and Adolescents

Nurses who work in practice settings where they have access to groups of parents, adult caregivers, or teachers

---

BOX 40-1 BUILDING SELF-ESTEEM IN CHILDREN

Strategy One: Looking at the Positive and the Negative

Instruct parents to write an honest description of their child for a stranger. Next, have the parents underline the child's positive and negative qualities.

To reinforce the positive qualities, (1) notice examples of ability in many different circumstances and point this out to the child, (2) find occasion to frequently and honestly praise the child, and (3) give the child an opportunity to show ability frequently.

To address the negative qualities constructively, ask: (1) What need is being expressed by this behavior? (2) Can I see a positive quality being expressed by this behavior? (3) How can I help my child express this quality and meet her needs in a more positive way?

Reexamine the list of negative qualities and ignore those that are merely a matter of taste, preference, or personal style—and not really negative in a harmful manner.

Strategy Two: Listening

The following guidelines can help parents to use listening to communicate to a child, "You are important. What you say matters to me. You matter to me."

1. Make sure that you are ready to listen.
2. Give your child your full attention.
3. Minimize distractions.
4. Be an active listener.
5. Invite your child to talk.

Listen for the point of a child's story ("What is she trying to tell me? Why is this important to him?"). Don't feel that you have to fix things. Listen for and respond to the feelings.

Strategy Three: Using the Language of Self-Esteem

Feedback that enhances self-esteem has three components: (1) a description of the behavior (describe the behavior without judging it), (2) your reaction to the behavior (language that shares something about yourself), and (3) acknowledgment of the child's feelings. For example, "Thanks for playing with your brother tonight [description].

I was wondering how I was going to pay attention to our guests if he got fussy and was really grateful when I noticed that you kept him occupied and happy [reaction]. I know that there were other things you might have enjoyed doing more [acknowledgment]."

To give correction using the language of self-esteem, (1) describe the problematic behavior, (2) state a reason for the behavior change, (3) acknowledge the child's feelings, and (4) offer a clear statement of what is expected.

Attacking communications: "Don't let me ever hear you talk that way to your mother again."

Language of self-esteem: "I overheard you telling your mom that she should 'Get a life and get off your case.' [description]. When you talk like that it just makes people angry or sad, which isn't very helpful [reason for behavior change]. You probably feel like you are being picked on, and we may have some expectations that are different from those of your friends' parents. I hope you know that this is because we love you and want the best for you [acknowledgment]. In the future, try to talk to others with the same respect you'd like others to show you [statement of expectation]."

Avoid using the following destructive language styles, which tear down self-esteem: overgeneralizations ("You *never* come home on time!"), the silent treatment, and vague or violent threats.

Strategy Four: Helping Children Meet Expectations

To help children meet expectations, (1) be sure that your expectations are reasonable and appropriate for your child's age, (2) plan ahead, (3) be clear about your expectations, (4) focus on the positive, (5) provide choices when possible, and (6) provide rewards.

Strategy Five: Promoting a Feeling of Success

To help children have the courage to try new types of experiences, which results from successfully meeting challenges: (1) let a child know what to expect, (2) let your child practice the necessary skills, (3) be patient, and (4) make it safe to fail.

Adapted from McKay, M., & Fanning, P. (2000). *Self-esteem* (3rd ed.). Oakland, CA: New Harbinger Publications.

can offer specific guidelines for creating developmental environments that build high self-esteem. Box 40-1 offers five strategies for building self-esteem in children. Because some parents and educators may not have experienced these aids to personal growth themselves, it is beneficial to role model these behaviors when interacting with children.

Important learning tasks for children include understanding and accepting oneself, feelings, and others; independence; goals and purposeful behavior; mastery, competence, and resourcefulness; emotional maturity; and choices and consequences.

Enhancing Self-Esteem in Older Adults

The many losses associated with aging (e.g., diminished strength and physical health, interpersonal losses, retirement, shrinking income) make older adults especially vulnerable to disturbances in self-concept, particularly chronic low self-esteem. Society's generally negative view of aging compounds the problem. When interacting with older adults, employ the following interventions to enhance and maintain self-esteem in this population:

- Identify one's own attitudes and feelings about aging and older adults.
- Address seniors respectfully, communicating that you take their concerns seriously.
- Respect and affirm seniors' intellect, individuality, personal strengths, culture, and spirituality.
- Adjust communication style to accommodate any sensory or cognitive deficits.
- Encourage sharing of life experiences.
- Assist the person to identify strengths and coping mechanisms to deal with problems.
- Provide a safe environment for older adults to communicate such concerns as interpersonal or physical loss, feelings about illness and death, sexuality, or financial issues.
- Advocate for seniors needing help in attaining services necessary to meet their health care needs.
- Explore the personal meaning of dependency for the person, and help seniors adapt both physically and emotionally to any necessary dependency.

The Focus on the Older Adult box describes nursing interventions to promote self-esteem in older adults.

FOCUS ON THE OLDER ADULT

PROMOTING SELF-ESTEEM IN OLDER ADULTS

Area of Concern	Nursing Strategies
Personal identity	• When an older person's sense of self is threatened, assist the individual to find meaning in the experience, to regain mastery to the extent that this is possible, and to evaluate realistically the adequacy of the person's coping strategy. • Teach older people to identify and develop a game plan for confronting anxiety-producing situations. • Help to identify and secure intervention for treatable depressions. • Treat causes of self-identity disturbances such as pain, abusive living arrangements, and substance abuse.
Body image	• Notice and affirm positive physiologic characteristics of older adults. • Teach preventive self-care measures that reduce discomforting signs of aging (e.g., exercise, which maintains muscle mass and joint flexibility; proper nutrition; basic hygiene and skin care measures). • Explore new activities (including hobbies) that are within the changing physical capabilities of the older person.
Self-Esteem	• Assist older adults to identify and use personal strengths. • Communicate that you value older people simply for who they are (unconditional affirmation); know and use the name they prefer; ask them questions about their life, interests, or values. • When appropriate, use the expertise of older adults and ask their advice; let them know you value their life experiences. • Engage older people in activities in which they can be successful. • Allow older people to make tough decisions and confront challenging situations when appropriate; teach protective family members the value of older adults confronting situations that invite continued growth. • Empower older people to meet their own needs; provide necessary knowledge, teach new behaviors, instill the belief that they "can manage."
Role performance	• Explore with older people the many roles they have fulfilled throughout their lifetime; invite reminiscences. • Facilitate grieving over valued roles that can no longer be performed. • Remedy, whenever possible, factors that prevent older patients from engaging in valued roles. • Explore new roles.

Evaluating

Nurses who are sensitive to the relationship between self-concept and general well-being consistently evaluate the effect the nursing plan of care has on the patient's self-concept. When the plan of care includes specific interventions to assist patients with disturbances in body image, self-esteem, role performance, and personal identity, listen carefully to the patient's self-report and observe patient behaviors to see if the disturbances are being resolved. Basically, the patient should be able to meet the following outcomes:

- Is comfortable with body image and able to use it effectively to meet human needs
- Is able to describe self positively
- Is able to meet realistic role expectations without undue anxiety and fatigue
- Is capable of interacting appropriately with environment while recognizing self to be a separate and distinct entity

See the accompanying Nursing Plan of Care 40-1 for Ms. Motsky.

NURSING PLAN OF CARE 40-1

for Melissa Motsky

PATIENT CARE STUDY

Melissa Motsky is a 31-year-old married woman, mother of three children (aged 12, 10, and 8 years), and junior-level nursing student. She works every other weekend as a nurse's aide. She has just received a letter from the nursing division head informing her that she is in academic jeopardy and will fail out of the program unless her grades improve. She presents this to her adviser.

After talking with Ms. Motsky, who calls herself a failure and who cries as she describes her situation at home, her faculty adviser suspects a serious self-esteem problem and helps her to list factors contributing to her current sense of failure and low self-esteem. The following list is generated:

SIGNIFICANCE

- Receives little understanding, affection, approval from husband. "I stay with him because of the kids. I started back to school because I had to get out of the house and want to make something of myself. He doesn't understand this."
+ "The children are very supportive but get impatient when I have to study and can't spend time with them."
- Feels a failure in all the roles that are important to her—wife, mother, and, now, student. "I jeopardized everything to go back to school—if I fail, it's all

over for me. There just isn't enough time or energy to do anything well."
+ "They do love me at work, though, which makes me feel like nursing is what I should be doing."

VIRTUE

- "I've always believed that hard work pays off and that if you were faithful to your duty you'd be rewarded by the good life—I'm beginning to doubt that. Maybe I'm a fool for trying so hard."
+ "I do still try to live according to my beliefs and feel okay about this. I treat others as I'd like to be treated."

POWER

- "I always believed I could do anything I put my heart and soul into. But I can't seem to change my marriage, and if I fail out of school, that will be the end of all my dreams."

Key indicators of low self-esteem that also surfaced in the interview include overeating (10-lb weight gain during the past year), difficulty sleeping, fatigue, new sensitivity to criticism, and expressions of feeling unloved, alone, and no longer able to manage. Personal strengths include history of "can do" mentality, high motivation to succeed, and past history of success as mother and nurse's aide.

NURSING DIAGNOSIS	Situational Low Self-Esteem related to decreased sense of significance, competence, virtue, and power as manifested by expressions of being a failure, powerlessness, fatigue, tears, weight gain, low academic performance (test grades 68, 74)
EXPECTED OUTCOME	By this time next month, 11/2/15, the client will demonstrate increased self-esteem by: • Expressing positive statements about herself

NURSING PLAN OF CARE 40-1 *continued*

for Melissa Motsky

NURSING INTERVENTIONS	RATIONALE	EVALUATIVE STATEMENT
Assist the patient to rediscover her "own" personal strengths: identify personal qualities and strengths that have pleased her in the past and explore why this has changed; recommend that she make at least one positive statement about herself each morning and evening.	Patients can lose touch with their strengths, especially when multiple stressors seem to create impossible demands.	11/3/15 Outcome partially met. Patient's statements are of the "This is good, *but…*" variety. "I think I'm doing better in school but I don't know if it will continue." *Recommendation:* Continue to identify and reinforce personal strengths.
Consistently interact with the patient as if she had the power to weather the crisis successfully (i.e., "will" strength to her). Role model positive self-concept behaviors.	Once the patient senses that an authority believes in her power and expects her to use it, she may internalize this knowledge and act on it.	*C. Taylor, RN*

EXPECTED OUTCOME By this time next month, 11/2/15, the patient will demonstrate increased self-esteem by:

• Reporting ability to receive negative feedback without falling apart

NURSING INTERVENTIONS	RATIONALE	EVALUATIVE STATEMENT
Explore with the patient to what degree she allows the opinions of others to influence her self-concept.	Significance—sense of being loved and approved of by significant others—is a critical component of self-esteem.	11/3/15 Outcome partially met. Patient reports being able to handle everything except putdowns from her husband.
Teach how self-concept filters life experiences; thus, if I feel that I am a failure, I may interpret the words and behaviors of others as confirming this, even though that was not their intention.	Principle of self-consistency: once I am down, I may reinforce this by distorting what I feel, hear, and experience.	*Recommendation:* Explore origin of power she has given to her husband to influence her sense of self and what she wants to do about this. *C. Taylor, RN*
Explore with the patient ways she can enhance her self-concept independently of others (e.g., take time each day for herself). Encourage the patient to draw on personal strengths.	This facilitates internal locus of control versus external. Spending time on self communicates that self is valuable.	
Teach the patient how to analyze feedback constructively and respond appropriately; *cancel negative thinking.* For example, the patient receives care plan back with many corrections and the notation, "sloppy work." *Maladaptive response:* "She hates me. See, this proves I'll never be a good nurse. I wasted my time even doing this."	It is important to break the cycle of negative thinking, which reinforces negative self-concept.	

(continued)

NURSING PLAN OF CARE 40-1 *continued*

for Melissa Motsky

NURSING INTERVENTIONS	RATIONALE	EVALUATIVE STATEMENT
Adaptive response: "I spent as much time as I had on this…now let me see what I did wrong. Maybe I should make an appointment with my instructor so she can show me how to improve."		

EXPECTED OUTCOME By this time next month, 11/2/15, the patient will demonstrate increased self-esteem by:
- Getting a passing grade on her next quarterly examination

NURSING INTERVENTIONS	RATIONALE	EVALUATIVE STATEMENT
Explore study skills with the patient; recommend a study group.	Poor study skills may also be contributing to her low academic performance. A study group will meet both her social and academic needs.	11/3/15 Outcome met. Grade: 82 *C. Taylor, RN*
Discuss the importance of how she *perceives* present situation. If present failures are equated with *defeat,* she may be unable to mobilize her resources to succeed; if present failures represent *challenge,* it may call forth her best efforts and result in success.	The meaning given to present stressor can dramatically affect the patient's response to it and condition her for success or failure.	
Discuss the importance of breaking the cycle of failure leading to another failure.	If this short-term goal is met, it will set the stage for future successes and contribute to the patient's positive self-concept.	

EXPECTED OUTCOME By this time next month, 11/2/15, the patient will demonstrate increased self-esteem by:
- Verbalizing that the way she is living her life is okay

NURSING INTERVENTIONS	RATIONALE	EVALUATIVE STATEMENT
Assist the patient to examine her moral–ethical standards; explore sources of these standards and whether the patient feels comfortable with them.	Moral–ethical standards may be uncritically internalized and place the patient in conflict.	11/3/15 Outcome met. Patient stated: "I guess I'm living the best way I know how right now. If things are meant to be different, someone is going to have to show me how." *Recommendations:* Reinforce self-acceptance. *C. Taylor, RN*
Identify unrealistic standards; the patient may need "permission" to be human.	Unrealistic standards (perfectionism, conventionality) may constantly undermine the patient's self-esteem.	

NURSING PLAN OF CARE 40-1 *continued*

for Melissa Motsky

NURSING INTERVENTIONS	RATIONALE	EVALUATIVE STATEMENT
Refer for counseling, if appropriate.	Support groups on campus (counseling centers, ministries) may be able to meet the patient's needs.	

EXPECTED OUTCOME By this time next month, 11/2/15, the patient will demonstrate increased self-esteem by

- Reporting two recent instances when personal power was effective in accomplishing desired goals

NURSING INTERVENTIONS	RATIONALE	EVALUATIVE STATEMENT
Identify and affirm the patient's use of personal power to accomplish goals.	A negative self-concept may deny or distort personal successes; outside intervention may be necessary to bring these to consciousness.	11/3/15 Outcome met…with difficulty. Needed considerable prompting to identify successful use of her personal power. Was ready to attribute passing grade to luck rather than her own efforts. *Recommendations:* Have patient make daily record of her use of personal power and results. *C. Taylor, RN*

SAMPLE DOCUMENTATION

10/2/15 Nursing

Melissa Motsky presented today after receiving academic jeopardy letter. She is strongly motivated to complete nursing program successfully and seems to have the ability to do this. Current multiple life stressors—lack of support from husband, need to mother three children (12, 10, 8), part-time nurse's aide job (necessary for financial reasons), and current academic jeopardy (test grades 68, 74) are all contributing to her low self-esteem and overwhelming sense of being a failure. We together developed a care plan that it is hoped will help her to do better academically, as well as begin to feel better about herself. See attached. She will return 11/2/15 at 10 AM for follow-up.

C. Taylor, RN

SOAP Format

10/2/15, 12:30 PM, nursing

Academic jeopardy—Melissa Motsky

S: "I jeopardized everything to go back to school—if I fail, it's all over for me." Reports lack of support from husband, grief that she does not have enough time for children, failure of personal work ethic ("hard work pays off"), and sense of powerlessness.

O: Nursing II quarterly exam grades: 68, 74; weight gain of 10 lb during past year; facial and body expressions of fatigue, profuse tears

A: Low Self-Esteem related to decreased sense of significance, competence, virtue, and power

P: See attached plan of care.

C. Taylor, RN

DEVELOPING CLINICAL REASONING

1. The personal strengths a person recognizes, develops, and uses are powerful but subjective determinants of self-concept. Identify the strengths that have been major determinants of your self-concept (e.g., power, intelligence, physical attractiveness, goodness, humor, "can-do" attitude), and explore how these help you to succeed in nursing. Discuss with another student ways that nurses can assist patients to recognize, develop, and use personal strengths to cope better with the stress of injury and illness.

2. Role play with another student your responses to the following patients, then reverse roles. Reflect on the effects different types of nursing presence and response have on a patient's self-concept. Discuss the nursing responses that would be most helpful to patients at risk for self-concept disturbances.
   - A male patient who was recently passed over for a promotion states, "I can't believe I've got to deal with this ulcer. It's just one more thing holding me back from succeeding in this business."
   - An anorexic teenager tells you that she can't possibly eat the dinner you brought her and states, "I can't do my usual workout in here, and look how fat I'm getting."
   - A middle-aged male patient confides, "I need to talk with someone about how it feels to be a woman trapped in a man's body."
   - A woman, after mastectomy, refuses to look at the incision site and notes, "If I can't bring myself to look at this, how can I ever expect my husband to want me again?"
   - A resident in a long-term care facility says, "Don't trouble yourself about me. I'm sure you have lots of people to take care of who are more deserving of your time and attention."

PRACTICING FOR NCLEX

1. A nurse is performing a psychological assessment of a 19-year-old male patient who has Down syndrome. The patient is mildly developmentally disabled with an intelligence quotient of 82. He told his nurse, "I'm a good helper. You see I can carry these trays because I'm so strong. But I'm not very smart, so I have just learned to help with the things I know how to do." The patient most likely has which of the following?
   a. Negative self-concept and low self-esteem
   b. Negative self-concept and high self-esteem
   c. Positive self-concept and fairly high self-esteem
   d. Positive self-concept and low self-esteem

2. A nurse asks a 25-year-old patient to make a list of 20 words that describe him. After 15 minutes, the patient listed the following: 25 years old, male, named Joe; then declared he couldn't think of anything else. The nurse documents that the patient has demonstrated:
   a. Lack of self-esteem
   b. Deficient self-knowledge
   c. Unrealistic self-expectation
   d. Inability to evaluate himself

3. A nurse asks the same patient in question 2 to list facts, traits, or qualities that he would like to be descriptive of himself. The patient quickly lists 25 traits, all of which are characteristic of a successful man. When asked if he knows anyone like

this, he replies, "My father." This discrepancy between the patient's description of himself as he is and as he would like to be indicates:
   a. Negative self-concept
   b. Joe's modesty (lack of conceit)
   c. Body image disturbance
   d. Low self-esteem

4. A nurse is counseling a husband and wife who have decided that the wife will get a job so that the husband can go to pharmacy school, as he has wanted to do for some time. Their three teenagers, who were involved in the decision, are also getting jobs to buy their own clothes. The husband plans to work 12 to 16 hours weekly and states, "I was always an A student, but I may have to settle for Bs now because I don't want to neglect my family, and I need to work a few hours so that my wife won't have to work overtime." How would the nurse document the husband's self-expectations?
   a. Realistic and positively motivating his development
   b. Unrealistic and negatively motivating his development
   c. Unrealistic but positively motivating his development
   d. Realistic but negatively motivating his development

5. A school nurse is teaching parents how to foster a healthy development of self in their children. Which statement made by one of the parents needs to be followed up with further teaching?
   a. "I love my child so much I 'hug him to death' every day."
   b. "I think children need challenges, don't you?"
   c. "My husband and I both grew up in very restrictive families. We want our children to be free to do whatever they want."
   d. "My husband and I have different ideas about discipline, but we're talking this out because we know it's important for Johnny that we be consistent."

6. A mother of a 10-year-old daughter tells the nurse: "I feel incompetent as a parent and don't know how to discipline my daughter." What should be the nurse's first intervention when counseling this patient?
   a. Recommend that she discipline her daughter more strictly and consistently.
   b. Make a list of things her husband can do to give her more time and help her improve her parenting skills.
   c. Assist the mother to identify both what she believes is preventing her success and what she can do to improve.
   d. Explore with the mother what the daughter can do to improve her behavior and make the mother's role as a parent easier.

7. A nurse is counseling parents attending a parent workshop on how to build self-esteem in their children. Which teaching points would the nurse include to help parents achieve this goal? Select all that apply.
   a. Teach the parents to reinforce their child's positive qualities.
   b. Teach the parents to overlook occasional negative behavior.
   c. Teach parents to ignore neutral behavior that is a matter of personal preference.
   d. Teach parents to listen and "fix things" for their children.
   e. Teach parents to describe the child's behavior and judge it.
   f. Teach parents to let their children practice skills and make it safe to fail.

8. A nurse practicing in a physician's office assesses self-concept in patients during the patient interview. Which patient is least likely to develop problems related to self-concept?
   a. A 55-year-old woman television news reporter undergoing a hysterectomy (removal of uterus)
   b. A young clergyperson whose vocal cords are paralyzed after a motorbike accident
   c. A 32-year-old accountant who survives a massive heart attack
   d. A 23-year-old model who just learned that she has breast cancer

For questions 9 to 12, read the patient data and use the following letters to indicate the nursing diagnosis that the data suggest (each response may be used only once):
a. Personal Identity Disturbance
b. Body Image Disturbance
c. Self-Esteem Disturbance
d. Altered Role Performance

9. A patient has been in the United States only 3 months and has recently suffered the loss of her husband and job. She states that nothing feels familiar... "I don't know who I am supposed to be here" and she misses home (Nicaragua) terribly.
   Answer: _____

10. A sophomore in high school has missed a lot of school this year because of leukemia. He said he feels like he is falling behind in everything and misses "hanging out at the mall" with his friends most of all.
    Answer: _____

11. A college freshman away from home for the first time says, "Why did I have to be born into a family of big bottoms and short fat legs! No one will ever ask me out for a date. Oh, why can't I have long thin legs like everyone else in my class? What a frump I am."
    Answer: _____

12. A 33-year-old businessperson is now in counseling attempting to deal with a long-repressed history of sexual abuse by her father. "I guess I should feel satisfied with what I've achieved in life, but I'm never content, and nothing I achieve makes me feel good about myself... I hate my father for making me feel like I'm no good. This is an awful way to live."
    Answer: _____

13. A 36-year-old female who was divorced 5 years earlier enters the emergency department with severe burns and cuts on her face after an auto accident in a car driven by her fiancé of 3 months. Three weeks later, her fiancé has not yet contacted her. The patient states that he is very busy and she is too tired to have visitors anyway. The patient frequently lies with her eyes closed and head turned away. These data suggest that:
    a. There is no disturbance in self-concept.
    b. This patient has ego strength and high self-esteem but may have a disturbance of body image.
    c. The area of self-esteem has very low priority at this time and should be ignored until much later.
    d. It is probable that there are disturbances in self-esteem and body image.

14. A nurse is performing patient care for a severely ill patient who has cancer. Which nursing interventions are likely to assist a severely ill patient with cancer to maintain a positive sense of self? Select all that apply.
    a. The nurse makes a point to address the patient by name upon entering the room.
    b. The nurse avoids fatiguing the patient by performing all procedures in silence.
    c. The nurse performs care in a manner that respects the patient's privacy and sensibilities.
    d. The nurse offers the patient a simple explanation before moving her in any way.
    e. The nurse ignores negative feelings from the patient since they are part of the grieving process.
    f. The nurse avoids conversing with the patient about her life, family, and occupation.

15. A 16-year-old patient has a nursing diagnosis of Body Image Disturbance related to severe acne. In planning nursing care, what is an appropriate goal for this nursing diagnosis?
    a. The patient will make above-B grades in all tests at school."
    b. The patient will demonstrate by diet control and skin care increased interest in control of acne.
    c. The patient reports that she feels more self-confidence in her music and art, which she enjoys.
    d. The patient expresses that she is very smart in school.

ANSWERS WITH RATIONALES

1. *c.* The data point to the patient having a positive self-concept ("I'm a good helper") and fairly high self-esteem (realizes his strengths and limitations). The statement "But I'm not very smart" is accurate and is not an indication of a negative self-concept.

2. *b.* The patient's inability to list more than three items about himself indicates deficient self-knowledge. There are not enough data provided to determine whether he lacks self-esteem, has unrealistic self-expectations, or is unable to evaluate himself.

3. *d.* Low self-esteem is characterized by great discrepancy between the ideal and real selves. There are no data given here that suggest that Joe has either a negative self-concept or a body image disturbance. The data do indicate something more serious than modesty.

4. *a.* The patient's self-expectations are realistic, given his multiple commitments, and seem to be positively motivating his development.

5. *c.* Each option with the exception of *c* correctly addresses some aspect of fostering healthy development in children. Because children need effective structure and development, giving them total freedom to do as they please may actually hinder their development.

6. *c.* The first intervention priority with a mother who feels incompetent to parent a daughter is to assist the mother to identify what is preventing her from being an effective parent and then to explore solutions aimed at improving her parenting skills. The other interventions may prove helpful, but they do not directly address the mother's problem with her feelings of incompetence.

7. **a, c, f.** The nurse should include the following teaching points for parents: (1) reinforce their child's positive qualities; (2) address negative qualities constructively; (3) ignore neutral behavior that is a matter of taste, preference, or personal style; (4) don't feel they have to "fix things" for their children; (5) describe the child's behavior in a nonjudgmental manner; and (6) let their child know what to expect, practice the necessary skills, be patient, and make it safe to fail.

8. **a.** Based simply on the facts given, the 55-year-old news reporter would be least likely to experience body image or role performance disturbance because she is beyond her childbearing years, and the hysterectomy should not impair her ability to report the news. The young clergyperson's inability to preach (*b*), the 32-year-old's massive myocardial infarction (*c*), and the model's breast resection (*d*) have much greater potential to result in self-concept problems.

9. **a.** An unfamiliar culture, coupled with traumatic life events and loss of husband and job, result in this patient's total loss of her sense of self: "I don't know who I am supposed to be here." Her very sense of identity is at stake, not merely her body image, self-esteem, or role performance.

10. **d.** Important roles for this patient are being a student and a friend. His illness is preventing him from doing either of these well. This self-concept disturbance is basically one that concerns role performance.

11. **b.** Clearly, this patient's concern is with body image.

12. **c.** This patient's self-concept disturbance is mainly one of devaluing herself and thinking that she is no good. This is a self-esteem disturbance.

13. **d.** The traumatic nature of this patient's injuries, her fiancé's failure to contact her, and her withdrawal response all point to potential problems with both body image and self-esteem. It is not true that self-esteem needs are of low priority.

14. **a, c, d.** When assisting the patient to maintain a positive sense of self, the nurse should address the patient by name when entering the room; perform care in a manner that respects the patient's privacy; offer a simple explanation before moving the patient's body in any way; acknowledge the patient's status, role, and individuality; and converse with the patient about the patient's life experiences.

15. **b.** All of these patient goals may be appropriate for the patient but the only goal that directly addresses her body image disturbance is *b*.

TAYLOR SUITE RESOURCES

Explore these additional resources to enhance learning for this chapter:

- NCLEX-Style Questions and other resources on thePoint, http://thePoint.lww.com/Taylor8e
- *Study Guide for Fundamentals of Nursing, 8th edition*
- Adaptive Learning | Powered by prepU, http://thepoint.lww.com/prepu

Bibliography

Aguilera, D. C. (1998). *Crisis intervention: Theory and methodology* (7th ed.). St. Louis: Elsevier/Mosby.

Bowlby, J. (1969). *Attachment and loss: Vol I: Attachment.* New York: Basic Books.

Bulechek, G. M., Butcher, H. K., Dochterman, J., & Wagner, C. M. (Eds.) (2013). *Nursing interventions classification (NIC)* (6th ed.). St. Louis: Elsevier/Mosby.

Coopersmith, S. (1967). *The antecedents of self-esteem.* San Francisco: Freeman.

Freud, S. (1961). The ego and the id. In J. Strachey (Ed.), *The standard edition of the complete psychological works of Sigmund Freud* (Vol. XIX, pp. 3–63). London: The Hogarth Press.

Harter, S. (1999). *The construction of the self.* New York: Guilford.

LeMone, P. (1991). Analysis of a human phenomenon: Self concept. *Nursing Diagnosis, 2*(3), 126–130.

Maslow, A. (1954.) *Motivation and personality.* New York: Harper and Row.

McClowry, S. G. (2003). *Your child's unique temperament: Insights and strategies for responsive parenting.* Champaign, IL: Research Press.

McKay, M., & Fanning, P. (2000). *Self-esteem* (3rd ed.). Oakland, CA: New Harbinger Publications.

Moorhead, S., Johnson, M., Maas, M. L., & Swanson, E. (2013). *Nursing outcomes classification (NOC)* (5th ed.). St. Louis: Elsevier/Mosby.

NANDA International (NANDA-I). (2012). *Nursing diagnoses: Definitions & classification, 2012–2014.* West Sussex, UK: Wiley-Blackwell.

Peplau, H. E. (1952). *Interpersonal relations in nursing.* New York: G. P. Putnam & Sons.

Peplau, H. E. (1997). Peplau's theory of interpersonal relations. *Nursing Science Quarterly, 10*(4), 162–167.

Stuart, G. W. (2013). *Principles and practice of psychiatric nursing,* (10th ed.). St. Louis: Elsevier/Mosby.

Sullivan, H. S. (1953). *The interpersonal theory of psychiatry.* New York: W. W. Norton & Co.

41

Stress and Adaptation

Stress (a word taken from the term "distress") is a part of life: Everyone feels stress at one time or another. Books and magazines are full of articles about stress, discussing everything from the stressful effects of performing one's job to the positive (or negative) stress of holidays. Television and online advertisements for over-the-counter remedies promise fast relief from stress headaches and upset stomachs. Stress is blamed for obesity, drug and alcohol use, divorce, and child abuse. Feeling "stressed out" is common, and taking "stress breaks" to do physical exercise is recommended in many work settings. With stress such a part of everyday life, it is easy to see that an additional health problem, such as an illness or injury, can increase the physical and psychological effects of stress.

The experience of stress and the responses to it are unique to each person. The process of responding to stress is constant and dynamic and is essential to a person's physical, emotional, and social well-being. Stress is a major component in health and illness. Nurses need to understand the concepts and levels of stress when providing nursing care to patients in all settings. Nurses themselves are subject to stress from the demands of their career, and need to know healthy ways of responding (see the accompanying Reflective Practice display for an example).

BASIC CONCEPTS OF STRESS AND ADAPTATION

The basic concepts of stress and adaptation include stress, stressors, adaptation, and homeostasis.

Stress

Stress is a condition in which the human system responds to changes in its normal balanced state. Stress results from a change in one's internal or external environment that is perceived as a challenge, a threat, or a danger. The major sources of stress in our society arise from interpersonal relationships and performance demands rather than from actual physical threats (Pender, Murdaugh, & Parsons, 2011). Not only is stress a part of everyday experience, but a person's responses to stress are also necessary to life. Stress affects the whole person in all the human dimensions (physical, emotional, intellectual, social, spiritual), positively or negatively.

 THINK back to Sarah Keller, the nursing student complaining of feeling ill. By her own reports, she was feeling overwhelmed and extremely anxious about her upcoming critical care clinical rotation. The stresses included lack of confidence in manipulating the equipment and machines of the unit and the demands that might be placed on her by the instructor. As a result, she exhibited physiologic responses to these stresses. These stresses could also affect her ability to function intellectually and socially. ●

The perception of stress and the responses to it are highly individualized, not only from person to person, but also from one time to another in the same person. In addition, each person's perception of and responses to stress are structured by that person's culture, family, genetic inheritance, and life experiences.

Stressors

A stressor is anything that is perceived as challenging, threatening, or demanding. Stressors may be internal (e.g., an illness, a hormonal change, or fear) or external (e.g., loud noise or cold temperature). As with stress, the perception and effects of the stressor are highly individualized. Stressors themselves

REFLECTIVE PRACTICE: CULTIVATING QSEN COMPETENCIES

CHALLENGE TO ETHICAL AND LEGAL SKILLS

I went to the student health center this afternoon because I was feeling sick. Tomorrow I am supposed to begin my critical care rotation. My instructor is the same one that I had for health assessment, and that rotation was really a disaster. She has the reputation for being the hardest instructor in the school. She terrifies me. But I'm just as terrified of the tubes and machines that I'm going to be faced with in the critical care unit. Skilled with my hands I am definitely not! I'm not even in the unit and already I am quaking. I tried to switch rotations but no luck. Now, I have to decide what to do tomorrow. I already feel a migraine coming on!

Thinking Outside the Box: Possible Courses of Action

- Call in sick! Obviously, this can't be a long-term strategy.
- Grin and bear it! Just try to do my job and for the most part fade into the woodwork.
- Try to find a preceptor in critical care to whom I can explain my fears and have her or him help me develop the skills (and comfort!) I definitely need.
- Be honest with my instructor about my fears and the stress I am experiencing and ask for *help*!

Evaluating a Good Outcome: How Do I Define Success?

- I develop the skills (and comfort) I need to effectively provide care in a high-tech environment.
- No patient is harmed because of my lack of skill.
- I learn to manage my stress and use it to my advantage.
- I pass this rotation with flying colors!

Personal Learning: Here's to the Future!

After some hard reflection (and the wise counsel of my mother), I decided I was giving my fear of this rotation (and instructor!) way too much power over me! I realized that nursing would continue to put me in new and frightening situations. But escape just couldn't be my "modus operandi." So urging myself to "bite the bullet," I got to the clinical area. Immediately after preconference, I literally grabbed my instructor and told her I had to talk to her before I began giving care. While she'll never be called "warm and fuzzy," she surprised me by being understanding. Then she spent some extra time orienting me to the unit and helping me develop comfort with a lot of equipment I'd be using that day. I learned an important lesson in confronting fear and not letting it get the best of me. Hopefully, I can remember this the next time "flight" seems more attractive than "fight"!

Sarah Keller, Georgetown University

REFLECTION ON QUALITY AND SAFETY COMPETENCIES

How do you think you would respond in a similar situation? Why? What does this tell you about yourself and about the adequacy of your skills for professional practice? Can you think of other ways to respond? What *knowledge, skills,* and *attitudes* do you need to develop to continuously improve quality and safety in situations like the one experienced by this student nurse?

Patient-Centered Care: Can you identify a beneficial aspect of the stress experienced by this student nurse? Did her handling of this stressful situation facilitate her ability to deliver effective care and treatment to her patients in a new environment? Did this student nurse's interaction with her instructor reinforce her commitment to treating patients with dignity and respect?

Teamwork and Collaboration/Quality Improvement: How important are effective communication skills when collaborating with team members? Did the acknowledgment of the student's personal stress and her decision to share these concerns with her instructor facilitate her understanding of the value of working in a nonpunitive environment?

Explain the autonomic nervous system responses the nursing student was experiencing. How did the nursing student use task-oriented reactions and attack behavior? Propose some strategies that would be appropriate for her to use in the future to cope with stress and facilitate her role as an effective team member.

Safety/Evidence-Based Practice: Is there anything more the nursing student could have done to confront her fears, contribute to a safe patient care environment, and promote a positive outcome? Do you agree with her criteria to evaluate a successful outcome? Did the nursing student meet the criteria? What evidence in nursing literature provides guidance for managing stress in the work environment and finding effective methods to deal with it and care for yourself?

Informatics: Can you think of other ways to respond or to approach this situation? Do you think self-confidence gained from dealing effectively with stressful situations improves your ability to care for patients effectively and accurately document this care?

are neither positive nor negative, but they can have positive or negative effects as the person responds to change.

 CONSIDER Joan Rogerrio, the middle-aged woman who is returning to the workforce and experiencing a recurrence of her inflammatory bowel disease. The decision to return to work was fostered by the family's financial need, which could also be a stressor for her. The stress of returning to work after a 15-year absence exerted a negative effect, resulting in frequent episodes of diarrhea. ●

Types of Stressors

Stressors are both physiologic and psychosocial. A physiologic stressor may in turn cause psychosocial stress, and vice versa.

PHYSIOLOGIC STRESSORS

Physiologic stressors have both a specific effect and a general effect. The specific effect is an alteration of normal body structure and function. The general effect is the stress response. Primary physiologic stressors include chemical agents (drugs, poisons), physical agents (heat, cold, trauma), infectious agents (viruses, bacteria), nutritional imbalances, hypoxia, and genetic or immune disorders.

PSYCHOSOCIAL STRESSORS

There are an almost infinite variety of psychosocial stressors, which become so much a part of our daily lives that we often overlook them. To illustrate the many types of psychosocial stressors, consider those listed in Box 41-1. Psychosocial stressors include both real and perceived threats. The person's responses are continuous and include individualized coping mechanisms for responding to anxiety, guilt, fear, frustration, and loss. The mechanisms serve to maintain psychological homeostasis.

Adaptation

When a person is in a threatening or otherwise stressful situation, immediate responses occur. Those responses, which are

---

BOX 41-1 EXAMPLES OF PSYCHOSOCIAL STRESSORS

- Accidents, causing stress for the victim, the person who caused the accident, and the families of both
- Stressful or traumatic experiences of family members and friends
- Horrors of history, such as Nazi concentration camps, the dropping of the atomic bomb on Hiroshima, and the September 11, 2001 terrorist attacks
- Fear of aggression or mutilation, such as muggings, rape, murder, and terrorism
- Events of history that are brought into our homes through television such as wars, earthquakes, and violence in schools
- Rapid changes in our world and the way we live, including changes in economic and political structures and rapid advances in technology

---

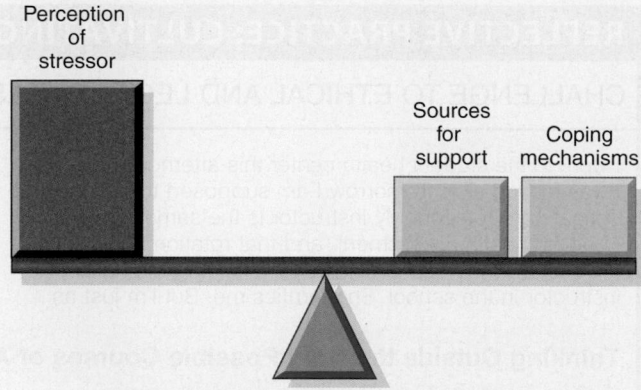

A balance is achieved when the perception of the stressful event is realistic and support and coping mechanisms are adequate

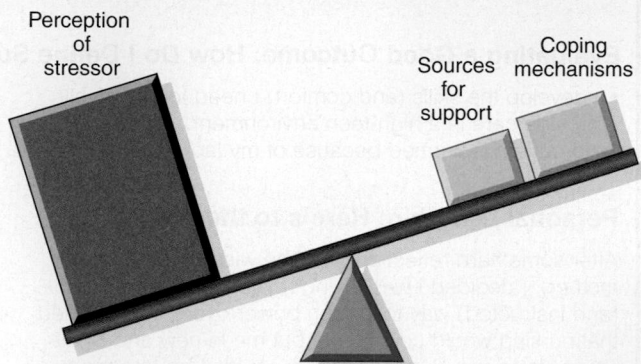

An imbalance can occur if the perception of the event is exaggerated or if sources for support or coping mechanisms are inadequate

FIGURE 41-1. A realistic perception of a stressful event, sources for emotional support, and appropriate coping mechanisms are components of a system of balances during stress.

often involuntary, are called coping responses. The change that takes place as a result of the response to a stressor is **adaptation**. Adaptation is, to some degree, an ongoing process as a person strives to maintain balance in his or her internal and external environments (Fig. 41-1). Adaptation also occurs in families and groups. Adaptation is necessary for normal growth and development, the ability to tolerate changing situations, and the ability to respond to physical and emotional stressors.

Homeostasis

Our bodies are always interacting with a constantly changing environment, including the external environment that surrounds our bodies and the internal environment that includes the mechanisms that regulate body functions and the fluids that surround body cells. To maintain health, the body's internal environment must remain in a balanced state. Various physiologic mechanisms within the body respond to internal changes to maintain relative constancy in the internal environment, a process called **homeostasis**.

Throughout history, people have believed that health is the result of a balanced state. Some of the most important people in medical history, including Hippocrates (the father of medicine) and Claude Bernard (the father of physiology), believed in and wrote about this balanced state. Originally, the focus was on life processes that occur within the body such as heart rate, blood pressure, and water balance. The concept of homeostasis has been expanded to include both physiologic and psychological balance.

MAINTENANCE OF PHYSIOLOGIC AND PSYCHOLOGICAL HOMEOSTASIS

The effects of physiologic and psychological stress are interrelated, as are the mechanisms that are consciously or unconsciously used to maintain homeostasis in response to stress. For example, the mechanisms described later, including the general adaptation syndrome (GAS) and mind–body interaction, are physiologic responses to either physical or emotional stressors.

Physiologic Homeostasis

The autonomic nervous system and the endocrine system primarily control homeostatic mechanisms. Involved to a lesser degree are the respiratory, cardiovascular, gastrointestinal, and renal systems. These mechanisms are self-regulating, occur without conscious thought, and usually function to correct abnormal conditions. On a simple level, these self-regulating mechanisms are like a thermostat regulating a furnace. When the temperature in a house falls below the preset temperature on the thermostat, the thermostat turns on the furnace, which heats the house to the desired temperature and then shuts off.

The regulatory mechanisms of the body are reacting constantly to internal changes to maintain homeostasis and health. The homeostatic mechanisms of the body systems are summarized in Table 41-1 (on page 1580). They are important in understanding the consequences of both short-term and long-term stress, which can threaten physiologic homeostasis and result in illness. In the 1980s, some investigators began using the term **allostasis** to describe this process of achieving stability or homeostasis through physiologic or behavioral change. The cumulative negative effects of these body responses to prolonged environmental and psychosocial stressors are referred to as an *allostatic load*. This represents the consequences of ongoing stress on the body with its resultant risks for a variety of diseases (Pender, Murdaugh & Parsons, 2011; Porth, 2011). Box 41-2 provides examples of illnesses known to be associated with stress.

Local Adaptation Syndrome (LAS)

The **local adaptation syndrome (LAS)** is a localized response of the body to stress. It involves only a specific body part (such as a tissue or organ) instead of the whole body. The stress precipitating the LAS may be traumatic or pathologic. LAS is a primarily homeostatic, short-term adaptive response. Although the body has many localized stress

---

BOX 41-2 EXAMPLES OF PHYSICAL ILLNESSES ASSOCIATED WITH STRESS

Autoimmune disorders
Graves disease (hyperthyroidism)
Rheumatoid arthritis
Ulcerative colitis
Psoriasis
Myasthenia gravis
Systemic lupus erythematosus (SLE)

Cardiovascular disorders
Hypertension
Coronary artery disease

Respiratory disorders
Asthma

Gastrointestinal disorders
Esophageal reflux
Constipation
Diarrhea
Ulcerative colitis

---

responses, the two most common responses that influence nursing care are the reflex pain response and the inflammatory response.

REFLEX PAIN RESPONSE

The **reflex pain response** is a response of the central nervous system to pain. It is rapid and automatic, serving as a protective mechanism to prevent injury. The reflex depends on an intact, functioning neurologic reflex arc and involves both sensory and motor neurons. For example, if you step into a bathtub of dangerously hot water, sensors in your skin detect the heat and immediately send a message to the spinal cord. A message is then sent to a motor nerve, which activates the muscles in your leg to pull back your foot. All of this happens before you consciously realize that the water is too hot to be safe.

INFLAMMATORY RESPONSE

The **inflammatory response** is a local response to injury or infection. It serves to localize and prevent the spread of infection and promote wound healing. When you cut your finger, for example, you often develop the symptoms of the inflammatory response—pain, swelling, heat, redness, and changes in function. The inflammatory response is discussed in Chapter 31.

General Adaptation Syndrome (GAS)

The **general adaptation syndrome (GAS)** is a biochemical model of stress developed by Hans Selye (1976). The GAS describes the body's general response to stress, a concept essential in all areas of nursing care. The three stages in the GAS are alarm reaction, stage of resistance, and stage

Table 41-1 HOMEOSTATIC REGULATORS OF THE BODY

SYSTEM	ACTION	EFFECT
Autonomic Nervous		
Parasympathetic—Functions under normal conditions and at rest (cranial and sacral nerves)		
	• Regulates heart rate	• Slows rate
	• Stimulates secretion of digestive juices and digestive tract smooth muscle	• Improves digestion, increases peristalsis
	• Stimulates insulin secretion	• Increases uptake of glucose by cells
Sympathetic—Functions under stress conditions to bring about the fight-or-flight response		
	• Stimulates heart rate and force	• Increases rate, strengthens contractions, increases cardiac output
	• Dilates skeletal muscle blood vessels	• Increases muscle strength
	• Dilates blood vessels to the brain	• Increases mental alertness
	• Stimulates release of glycogen stores	• Increases blood glucose levels
Endocrine		
Pituitary	• Secretes hormones: Adrenocorticotropic hormone (ACTH) Thyroid-stimulating hormone (TSH)	• Stimulates the adrenal cortex • Stimulates the thyroid
Adrenals	• Medulla produces epinephrine and norepinephrine	• Prepares the person for emergencies; supports the sympathetic system
	• Cortex secretes mineralocorticoids, glucocorticoids, and androgens	• Mineralocorticoid aldosterone regulates fluid and electrolytes • Glucocorticoids raise glucose levels (for energy) and increase resistance to physical stress • Androgens control the development and maintenance of male characteristics and are the primary precursor of natural estrogens
Thyroid	• Secretes thyroid hormone and calcitonin	• Regulates metabolic rate and growth
Other		
Cardiovascular	• Serves as transport system and pump	• Provides oxygen and nutrients and removes carbon dioxide and wastes from cells
Renal	• Filters, excretes, and reabsorbs metabolic products and water	• Maintains fluid, electrolyte, and acid–base balance
Respiratory	• Intake and output of oxygen and carbon dioxide	• Necessary for metabolism; helps maintain acid–base balance
Gastrointestinal	• Takes in food and fluids • Eliminates waste products	• Energy sources; maintains fluids and electrolytes

of exhaustion (Fig. 41-2). Although the alarm stage is short term (minutes to hours), the length of the resistance and exhaustion stages varies greatly, depending on such variables as the severity and duration of the stressor, the person's previous health and coping mechanisms, and the immediacy and effectiveness of health care interventions.

The GAS is a physiologic response to stress, but it is important to remember that the response results from either physical or emotional stressors. The stages occur with either physical or psychological damage to the person. Obvious examples are seen in patients with severe injury or an illness, but GAS is also a factor in mental illness, social isolation, and loss (or lack) of human relationships.

ALARM REACTION

Alarm is initiated when a person perceives a specific stressor and various defense mechanisms are activated. The perception of threat may be conscious or unconscious. The autonomic nervous system initiates the **fight-or-flight response**,

preparing the body to either fight off the stressor or to run away from it (usually not literally in the modern world). Hormone levels rise to prepare the body to react. This phase of the alarm reaction, called the shock phase, is characterized by an increase in energy levels, oxygen intake, cardiac output, blood pressure, and mental alertness. (If you recall the last time you almost had a car crash, you can easily identify these body reactions!) During the second phase of the alarm reaction, countershock, there is a reversal of body changes.

STAGE OF RESISTANCE

Having perceived the threat and mobilized its resources, the body now attempts to adapt to the stressor. Vital signs, hormone levels, and energy production return to normal. If the stress can be managed or confined to a small area (LAS), the body regains homeostasis. If the damage to the body is too great (e.g., with severe injury and bleeding or a major illness such as cancer or a heart attack), the adaptive mechanisms become exhausted.

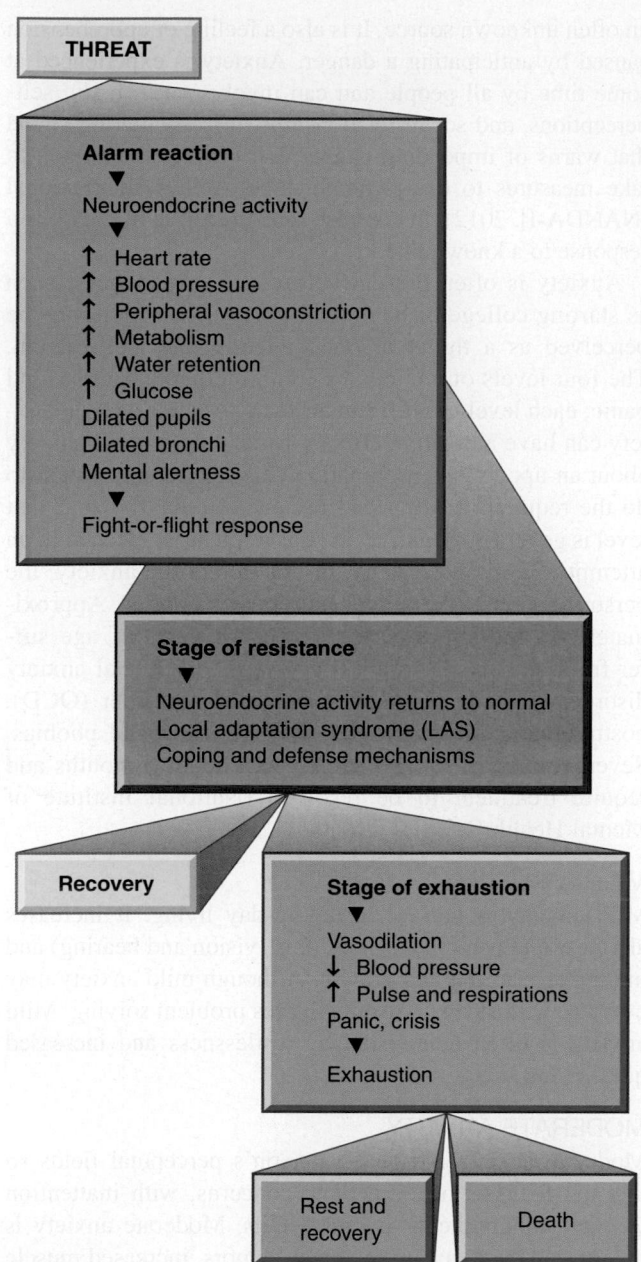

FIGURE 41-2. The general adaptation syndrome (general response to stress).

STAGE OF EXHAUSTION

Exhaustion results when the adaptive mechanisms can no longer provide defense. Without defense against the stressor, the body may either rest and mobilize its defenses to return to normal or reach total exhaustion and die.

Psychological Homeostasis

To maintain mental well-being, humans also must maintain psychological homeostasis. As discussed in Chapter 4, each person needs to feel loved and a sense of belonging, to feel safe and secure, and to have self-esteem. When these needs are not met or a threat to need fulfillment occurs, homeostatic measures in the form of coping or defense mechanisms help return the person to emotional balance.

Everyone frequently encounters physical, psychological, and social changes in their internal and external environments. A person's perception of these changes may be conscious or unconscious. If the person has the necessary resources, adaptation takes place and balance is maintained. If the resources cannot reestablish balance, a state of stress results. The person's responses and the degree of stress depend in part on the nature, intensity, timing, number, and duration of stressors. Adaptation to stress also depends on a person's age, developmental level, past experiences, support systems, and coping mechanisms (see Box 41-3 for age-related effects). Adaptive responses include the mind–body interaction, anxiety, and coping/defense mechanisms.

Mind–Body Interaction

Consider the following examples of mind–body interaction:

• Tomorrow, you are scheduled to take a final examination, and you must make a passing score to pass the course and remain in the nursing program. After being awake most of the night, you cannot swallow any food at breakfast, you have a rapid heartbeat, you are filled with feelings of apprehension, and you have diarrhea.
• Since his wife was killed in a car crash, Tom Green has been the sole support of his 4-year-old son, who is developmentally disabled and hyperactive. Tom has been coming to the neighborhood health clinic with increasing frequency over the past 5 months, complaining of weight loss, headaches, and stomach pain.

These examples illustrate the relationship between psychological stressors and the physiologic stress response (the general adaptation syndrome). In the first example, as you begin the test and discover that you know most of the answers, your stress decreases and your symptoms disappear rapidly. Tom's stress, however, is always present and is long term, increasing his risk for developing an illness.

BOX 41-3 SOURCES OF STRESS WITH AGING

Stress, with resultant anxiety, is a risk in the older population. As the number of older adults increases in the population, anxiety is now, and increasingly will be, a significant problem. Not all older patients will experience stress to the point of anxiety, but the following possible causes should always be considered when providing nursing care:

• Invasive or health-related tests or examinations
• Surgical procedures
• Diagnosis of chronic illnesses, including diabetes, cancer, and cardiovascular diseases
• Declining physical and/or mental capabilities
• Retirement
• Loss of spouse and/or significant others
• Increased social isolation
• Chronic pain
• Alcohol abuse
• Loss of independence in living arrangements, driving, and activities of daily living

BOX 41-4 PHYSIOLOGIC INDICATORS OF STRESS

Backache
Constipation or diarrhea
Dilated pupils
Dry mouth
Headache
Increased urination
Increased pulse, blood pressure, and respirations
Nausea
Sleep disturbances
Stiff neck
Increased perspiration
Chest pain
Weight gain or loss
Decreased sex drive

 REMEMBER Sarah Keller, the nursing student who said she felt she was getting sick from fears about her upcoming clinical rotation in the critical care unit and anticipation of having a strict instructor. As a result of her anticipated fears and lack of confidence, she physiologically responded to the stressors by feeling sick. ●

What causes this link between psychological stressors and the physiologic stress response? Although the exact cause is not well understood, it is thought that humans react to threats of danger as if they were physiologic threats. A person perceives the threat on an emotional level, and the body prepares itself either to resist the danger or to run away from it (the fight-or-flight response). Box 41-4 lists the physiologic indicators of stress.

Each person reacts in her or his own way. With prolonged stress, some may develop chronic diarrhea while others may develop nausea or heart palpitations. Such illnesses are real and are called **psychosomatic disorders** because the physiologic alterations are thought to be at least partially caused by psychological influences.

Another component of mind–body interaction is the effect of life changes on a person. Researchers have found that the number of changes a person has in one's life (both positive and negative) can be correlated with illness. A life change is defined as an event in a person's life that requires energy for adaptation. When energy is expended to adapt to the event, the person's resistance to illness is lowered. For example, although a holiday celebration with family and friends is considered a positive event in one's life, factors including the time necessary to prepare for the party, worrying about how everyone will get along, and trying to decide how much money to spend can generate stress.

Anxiety

The most common human response to stress is **anxiety**. Anxiety is a vague, uneasy feeling of discomfort or dread from an often unknown source. It is also a feeling of apprehension caused by anticipating a danger. Anxiety is experienced at some time by all people and can involve one's body, self-perceptions, and social relationships. It is an altering signal that warns of impending danger and enables the person to take measures to deal with threat (NANDA International [NANDA-I], 2012). In contrast, **fear** (a feeling of dread) is a response to a known threat.

Anxiety is often present before new experiences, such as starting college or beginning a new job, which may be perceived as a threat to one's identity and self-esteem. The four levels of anxiety are mild, moderate, severe, and panic; each level has different effects. At a mild level, anxiety can have a positive effect—for example, mild anxiety about an upcoming examination can motivate a student to do the required reading and review. Anxiety beyond that level is generally negative and has unpleasant effects. In an attempt to neutralize, deny, or counteract the anxiety, the person develops individual patterns of coping. Approximately 40 million Americans over 18 years of age suffer from anxiety disorders every year. Additional anxiety disorders include obsessive-compulsive disorder (OCD), posttraumatic stress disorder (PTSD) and social phobias. Severe anxiety disorders usually last about 6 months and require treatment to be resolved (National Institute of Mental Health [NIMH], 2013).

MILD ANXIETY

Mild anxiety is present in day-to-day living. It increases alertness and perceptual fields (e.g., vision and hearing) and motivates learning and growth. Although mild anxiety may interfere with sleep, it also facilitates problem solving. Mild anxiety is often manifested by restlessness and increased questioning.

MODERATE ANXIETY

Moderate anxiety narrows a person's perceptual fields so that the focus is on immediate concerns, with inattention to other communications and details. Moderate anxiety is manifested by a quavering voice, tremors, increased muscle tension, a complaint of "butterflies in the stomach," and slight increases in respirations and pulse.

SEVERE ANXIETY

Severe anxiety creates a very narrow focus on specific details, causing all behavior to be geared toward getting relief. The person has impaired learning ability and is easily distracted. Severe anxiety is characterized by extreme fear of a danger that is not real, by emotional distress that interferes with everyday life, and by avoiding situations that cause anxiety. It is manifested by difficulty communicating verbally, increased motor activity, a fearful facial expression, headache, nausea, dizziness, tachycardia, and hyperventilation. At this point, anxiety is no longer functioning as a signal for danger or motivation for a needed change, but results in maladaptive behaviors and emotional disability that signal the presence of an anxiety disorder (Videbeck, 2011).

PANIC

Panic causes the person to lose control and experience dread and terror. The resulting disorganized state is characterized by increased physical activity, distorted perception of events, and loss of rational thought. Panic is manifested by difficulty communicating verbally, agitation, trembling, poor motor control, sensory changes, sweating, tachycardia, hyperventilation, dyspnea, palpitations, a choking sensation, and sensations of chest pain or pressure. The person is unable to learn, concentrates only on the present situation, and often experiences feelings of impending doom. This level of anxiety can lead to exhaustion and death.

Coping Mechanisms

Anxiety often is managed without conscious thought by **coping mechanisms**, which are behaviors used to decrease stress and anxiety. Many coping behaviors are learned, based on one's family, past experiences, and sociocultural influences and expectations. As illustrated in the list that follows, coping behaviors may be positive or negative in terms of how they affect health. Typical coping behaviors include the following:

- Crying, laughing, sleeping, cursing
- Physical activity, exercise
- Smoking, drinking
- Lack of eye contact, withdrawal
- Limiting relationships to those with similar values and interests

Moderate, severe, and panic levels of anxiety are greater threats and involve more complex coping mechanisms as the person strives to reduce the stress and anxiety. Coping mechanisms often used at higher levels of anxiety are categorized as task-oriented reactions. Task-oriented reactions involve consciously thinking about the stress situation and then acting to solve problems, resolve conflicts, or satisfy needs. These reactions include attack behavior, withdrawal behavior, and compromise behavior.

Attack behavior occurs when a person attempts to overcome obstacles to satisfy a need; it may be constructive, with assertive problem solving, or destructive, with feelings and actions of aggression and hostility. Withdrawal behavior involves physical withdrawal from the threat, or emotional reactions such as admitting defeat, becoming apathetic, or feeling guilty and isolated. Compromise behavior is usually constructive, often involving the substitution of goals or negotiation to partially fulfill one's needs.

Defense Mechanisms

Other unconscious reactions to stressors, called **defense mechanisms**, often occur. These mechanisms protect one's self-esteem and are useful in mild to moderate anxiety. When extreme, however, they distort reality and create problems with relationships. At that point, the mechanisms become maladaptive instead of adaptive. Common defense mechanisms are summarized in Table 41-2 (on page 1584).

EFFECTS OF STRESS

Physiologic and psychological stress affects all of the human dimensions. It strongly influences how one attains basic human needs, it is a factor in health and illness, and it is a component in family reactions to illness. Both long-term stress and crisis situations may seriously affect a person's physical and emotional health.

Stress and Basic Human Needs

Basic human needs, described in Chapter 4, are common to all people. Stress, too, is common to all people. Both the attainment of these needs and the adaptation to stress require energy and motivate behaviors. As a person strives to meet basic human needs at each level, stress can be either a stimulus or a barrier.

How basic human needs are met and responses to stress are unique to the person, depending on the individual's sociocultural background, priorities, and past experiences (Box 41-5). In all people, the failure to meet needs results in an imbalance in homeostatic mechanisms and, eventually, illness.

Stress in Health and Illness

The health–illness continuum (described in Chapter 3) is affected by stress. Health and homeostatic balance are at one extreme of the continuum; exhaustion and death are at the other extreme.

Stress in a healthy person may promote health and prevent illness. For example, the fear of developing lung cancer

---

BOX 41-5 EFFECTS OF STRESS ON BASIC HUMAN NEEDS

Physiologic
Change in appetite, activity, or sleep
Change in elimination patterns
Increased pulse, respirations, blood pressure

Safety/Security
Feels threatened or nervous
Uses ineffective coping mechanisms
Is inattentive

Love/Belonging
Is withdrawn and isolated
Blames others for own faults
Demonstrates aggressive behaviors
Becomes overly dependent on others

Self-Esteem
Becomes a workaholic
Exhibits attention-seeking behaviors

Self-Actualization
Refuses to accept reality
Centers on own problems
Demonstrates lack of control

Table 41-2 COMMONLY OCCURRING DEFENSE MECHANISMS

DEFENSE MECHANISM	CAUSES	EXAMPLE
Compensation	A person attempts to overcome a perceived weakness by emphasizing a more desirable trait or overachieving in a more comfortable area.	A student who has difficulty with academics may excel in sports.
Denial	A person refuses to acknowledge the presence of a condition that is disturbing.	Despite finding a lump in her breast, a woman does not seek medical treatment.
Displacement	A person transfers (displaces) an emotional reaction from one object or person to another object or person.	An employee who is angry with a coworker kicks a chair.
Introjection	A person incorporates qualities or values of another person into one's own ego structure. This mechanism is important in the formation of conscience during childhood.	An older sibling tells his preschool sister not to talk to strangers, expressing his parents' values to his younger sister.
Projection	A person attributes thoughts or impulses to someone else.	A person who denies any sexual feelings for a coworker accuses him of sexual harassment.
Rationalization	A person tries to give a logical or socially acceptable explanation for questionable behavior ("behavior justification").	A patient who forgot to keep a health care appointment says, "If patients didn't have to wait 3 months to get an appointment, they wouldn't forget them."
Reaction formation	A person develops conscious attitudes and behavior patterns that are opposite to what he or she would really like to do.	A married woman is attracted to her husband's best friend but is constantly rude to him.
Regression	A person returns to an earlier method of behaving.	Children often regress to soiling diapers or demanding a bottle when they are ill.
Repression	A person voluntarily excludes an anxiety-producing event from conscious awareness.	A father may not remember shaking his crying baby.
Sublimation	A person substitutes a socially acceptable goal for one whose normal channel of expression is blocked.	A person who is aggressive toward others may become a star football player.
Undoing	A person uses an act or communication to negate a previous act or communication.	A husband who was physically abusive to his wife may bring her an expensive present the next day.

may motivate a person to stop smoking, or anxiety about baby care may prompt prospective parents to attend prenatal classes and read childcare books. Stressors in health also facilitate normal growth and development, provide the stimulus for learning constructive adaptive behaviors, stimulate problem-solving abilities, encourage social relationships, and help develop spiritual strength.

The effects of stress on a sick or injured person are, in contrast, usually negative. Stress can cause illness, and illness causes stress. The presence of an illness or a disability demands new coping skills at a time when homeostasis is challenged.

 REMEMBER Joan Rogerrio, the woman experiencing an exacerbation of her bowel disease. The negative effects of stress exacerbated her illness. As a result, Joan needs to develop new coping skills to deal with the demands of working to minimize the effects of this stressor on her illness. ●

People who enter health care settings as patients are also subjected to situational stressors.

Adaptation to acute and chronic illness or to traumatic injury involves two sets of adaptive tasks:

1. General tasks (as in the case of any situational stress) involve maintaining self-esteem and personal relationships and preparing for an uncertain future.
2. Illness-related tasks include such stressors as losing independence and control, handling pain and disability, and carrying out the prescribed medical regimen.

Every situation is different, and each person perceives and reacts to stressors in an individual manner. There is no one "best" way to cope with a given situation. Nursing considerations include the person's major concern, specific illness, sociocultural background, and available resources. For example, an older woman may be anxious about the cost of treatment for her hip fracture, whereas another woman, with the same injury, is seriously worried about the care of her cats while she is in the hospital. As another example,

Mary and Jane have both entered the hospital for treatment of breast cancer. Mary is worried about possible disfigurement and death, but she believes that with the help of surgery and chemotherapy, she can overcome the cancer. Jane, on the other hand, comes from a community that has strong fundamental religious beliefs. She believes that the cancer is a punishment from God and refuses treatment, even though she fears death.

Long-Term Stress

Long-term stress is a serious threat to physical and emotional health. As the duration, intensity, or number of stressors increases, a person's ability to adapt is lessened. The failure of adaptive mechanisms is also influenced by a person's state of health and past experiences with stress.

Long-term stress affects physical status, increasing the risk for disease or injury. Recovery and return to normal function are also compromised. High levels of ongoing stress are associated with multiple health disorders (see Box 41-2, p. 1579). Alcoholism and drug abuse, depression, suicide, accidents, and eating disorders have also been associated with chronic stress (Porth, 2011). It is believed that these diseases are the result of various factors, including the effects of the fight-or-flight response, eating patterns, lifestyle, and coping mechanisms. Stress alone does not cause autoimmune diseases such as rheumatoid arthritis but is believed to contribute to the progression of these diseases. Researchers have confirmed that chronic stress affects the ability of immune cells to respond to the hormones that normally regulate inflammation, thus allowing the development and progression of some diseases (Carnegie Mellon University, 2012). Under normal circumstances, cortisol, an anti-inflammatory hormone released by the adrenal glands, regulates the inflammatory response, but prolonged stress may decrease the effectiveness of the cortisol or the immune cells may be resistant to its effects (Sternberg, 2013). A person who reacts to stress by overeating, smoking, using alcohol or illegal drugs, or becoming hyperactive puts additional strain on the body. See the Promoting Health Literacy box for tips useful for patients experiencing long-term stress.

Family Stress

The stress that affects an ill person also affects the person's family members or significant others. When the family is viewed as a system, the behavior of the individual is influenced by his or her family, and any alterations in the individual's behavior in turn affect the family. Stressors for the family include changes in family structure and roles, anger and feelings of helplessness and guilt, loss of control over normal routines, and concern for financial stability. People who were neglected or abused as children are more vulnerable to stress as adults. They are 1.5 times more likely to experience serious health problems, including the development of autoimmune disease (Wilson & Severson, 2012). When the abuse occurs early in a child's life and is ongoing, changes in the brain's structure and function can occur, resulting in an altered immune response to inflammation and wound healing. The family thus is an integral part in the assessment, planning, nursing interventions, and evaluation of actions to promote adaptation to stress.

PROMOTING HEALTH LITERACY

IN PATIENTS EXPERIENCING LONG-TERM STRESS

Patient Scenario

Eva Weber is a 34-year-old single mother of twin boys. Both boys, now age 6, have had problems with developmental delays and have been diagnosed with attention-deficit disorder. Eva has a job at a dry cleaners but worries constantly that she won't be able to keep it since she has been late frequently because her car is old and breaks down often. Her former husband only pays child support about half the time, often because he has lost his construction job due to chronic alcoholism. When he drinks, he calls her constantly and sometimes comes to her house, beating on the door until she calls the police. She has problems sleeping and has lost 25 pounds, down from 145 to 120 on her 5 foot 9 inch frame. She admits she drinks and smokes too much, but says, "It's the only thing that makes me feel better for a while." Although the nurse practitioner at the local clinic has talked to her about stopping smoking and gaining weight, Eva has not been able to do so.

Nursing Considerations: *Tips for Improving Health Literacy*

Ask Eva to keep a "stress diary," noting when and how often something triggers her stress, how it makes her feel, and listing the things in her life that make her happy. Teach her how to take one day at a time, encouraging her to believe that she has control over some aspects of her life, but acknowledging that other aspects are uncontrollable. Suggest that she ask her primary health care provider for some help in stopping smoking in the form of medications and a definite plan for a time to stop. Explain and provide written guidelines for relaxation exercises. Discuss methods of reducing stress other than through alcohol and nicotine, including taking time to relax, talking with a friend, and learning to keep a positive outlook on life. Suggest other activities that are known to reduce stress, such as regular exercise, eating a nutritious diet, learning to say "no," avoiding people who are stressful, being more assertive, and doing something enjoyable each day. Encourage Eva to make an appointment at the clinic and to be prepared to ask her provider the following three questions:

- What is my main problem?
- What do I need to do?
- Why is it important for me to do this?

What additional measures can you take to help maintain health literacy in this patient? What other measures would be helpful for Eva if she did not speak English, could not read, or had other learning deficits?

CONSIDER Joan Rogerrio, the woman with an exacerbation of her bowel disease. Her family is already experiencing changes related to her return to work. These changes could be possible stressors for the family. These family stressors are increased by Joan's illness, which may ultimately affect her role performance. Thus, the nurse would need to assess the family situation for the effect of these stressors on the family. •

The family, both as individuals and as a unit, uses many of the same coping and defense mechanisms described previously. Family members may be overly protective, deny the seriousness of the illness, or blame health care providers for the patient's condition or behaviors. On the other hand, the family can provide the social support necessary to help the patient manage and adapt to stress. Emotional support from family members allows open expression of feelings and helps meet love and belonging needs. The inclusion of family members in problem solving, teaching and learning activities, and physical care helps both the patient and the family to maintain their self-esteem and feeling of worth.

Caring for a family member at home for long periods can also cause prolonged stress. Called **caregiver burden**, this stress response includes chronic fatigue, sleep problems, and an increased incidence of stress-related illnesses, such as high blood pressure and heart disease.

Prolonged stress can seriously threaten mental health. As coping or defense mechanisms become ineffective, a person may try less effective coping patterns or maladaptive defense mechanisms. As anxiety increases despite these measures, the person may experience difficulties on the job, with personal relationships, and with self-esteem.

Crisis

A **crisis** is a disturbance caused by a precipitating event, such as a perceived loss, a threat of loss, or a challenge, that is perceived as a threat to self. Crises may be maturational, situational, or adventitious. Maturational crises occur during developmental events that require role change, such as when a teenager transitions into adulthood. Situational crises occur when a life event disrupts a person's psychological equilibrium, such as loss of a job or death of a loved family member. Adventitious crises are accidental and unexpected events, resulting in multiple losses and major environmental changes—such as fires, earthquakes, and floods—that involve not only individuals but also entire communities.

In a crisis, the person's usual methods of coping are ineffective, resulting in increasingly greater levels of anxiety. This failure produces high levels of anxiety, disorganized behavior, and an inability to function adequately. After the precipitating event, the person's anxiety increases, and phases of the crisis emerge. The anxiety initially activates the person's usual methods of coping. If these are not effective, the person experiences more anxiety because the coping mechanisms are not working. As the crisis continues, the person tries new methods of coping or redefines the threat. This may lead to resolution of the crisis or, if not effective,

may result in severe or panic levels of anxiety. The crisis is more likely to be successfully resolved if the person views the event realistically, if effective coping mechanisms are present, and if situational support systems are available.

FACTORS AFFECTING STRESS AND ADAPTATION

Stress and adaptation are affected by the sources of stress, the types of stressors experienced, and personal factors.

Sources of Stress

Although there are an almost infinite number of sources of stress, they can be categorized into two broad areas: developmental stress and situational stress. Both require adaptive responses.

Developmental Stress

Developmental stress occurs as a person progresses through the normal stages of growth and development from birth to old age (described in Chapters 18 and 19). Within each stage, certain tasks must be resolved to reduce the stress. Examples associated with developmental stress include the following:

• The infant learning to trust others
• The toddler learning to control elimination
• The school-aged child socializing with peers
• The adolescent striving for independence
• The middle-aged adult accepting physical signs of aging
• The older adult reflecting on past life experiences with satisfaction

Situational Stress

Situational stress is different from developmental stress. It does not occur in predictable patterns as one progresses through life. Rather, situational stress can occur at any time, although the person's ability to adapt may be strongly influenced by his or her developmental level. Examples of situational stress, which may be either positive or negative, include the following:

• Illness or traumatic injury
• Marriage or divorce
• Loss (belongings, relationships, family member)
• New job
• Role change

RECALL the three individuals described at the beginning of the chapter. All three are experiencing situational stress, but each is responding differently; Mei is having headaches and diarrhea, Joan is experiencing an exacerbation of her bowel disease, and Sarah is feeling sick and shaky. •

Consider pregnancy as an example. A young married couple may be overjoyed at the prospect of becoming parents, whereas an unmarried adolescent may be panic-stricken when she discovers she is pregnant. The situations and the developmental levels of the young couple and the adolescent will have a major effect on the adaptations they will make. A person's physical and psychosocial capacities to cope with the situation depend not only on stage of maturation, but also on the support systems available.

Personal Factors

A person's adaptation to stress, whether positive or negative, is influenced by a number of personal factors. One's physiologic reserve and genetic inheritance are important in maintaining homeostasis and adapting to stressors. The ability to adapt is lower in the very young, the very old, and those with altered physical or mental health, who do not have the necessary physiologic reserve to cope with physical changes such as dehydration or fluid excess. Adequate nutrition and sleep are necessary for enzyme function, immune responses, wound healing, and energy production and restoration. Malnutrition, dietary deficits or excess, and sleep deprivation all impair one's ability to adapt to stress. Social factors and life events also affect one's adaptation to stress, with people who have strong support systems and relationships better able to adapt to stress and remain healthy.

STRESS AND ADAPTATION IN NURSING

Nursing involves activities and interpersonal relationships that are often stressful (Fig. 41-3). Activities identified as highly stressful include the following:

- Assuming responsibilities for which one is not prepared
- Working with unqualified personnel
- Working in an environment in which supervisors and administrators are not supportive
- Caring for a patient during a cardiac arrest or for a patient who is dying
- Experiencing conflict with a peer

This kind of stress is even greater for two groups of nurses: new graduates, who must adjust to an environment different from that experienced as students, and nurses who work in settings such as intensive care and emergency care. Patients

FIGURE 41-3. Some nursing specialties can be more stressful than others. To prevent burnout and alleviate personal stress, a nurse may need to work in another area of nursing temporarily or permanently.

in hospitals are more acutely ill. This, combined with a shortage of nurses, the increasing number of people over the age of 65, and the health care reforms that will allow greater access to health care, has resulted in more stressful conditions in the workplaces for nurses. They often need to work longer hours or more overtime and may have concerns about workplace violence or incidents of **lateral violence** (ANA, 2013). Lateral violence includes verbal, emotional, or physically abusive behavior of an RN toward another staff member; it may also include aggressive behavior or incivility and can involve overt responses such as shouting at another health care worker or more subtle responses such as failing to help another coworker (Major, 2013). Violent acts against health care workers and other episodes of workplace violence have increased, profoundly influencing nurses' feeling of safety and control over their environment (Strickler, 2013). Nurses may worry not only about the future of their positions but also about the safety of their patients, as well as harbor concerns about their own personal safety. The anxiety is complicated by the expectations of nurses. Even though they may have strong negative feelings and reactions, their role does not allow behaviors and verbal expressions that are less than positive and supportive.

Student nurses also experience stress and may have difficulty adapting to the requirements and responsibilities of caring for others. Factors causing stress in student nurses include the following:

- Fear of failing the classroom or clinical laboratory components of each course
- Fear of failing the licensure examination after graduation
- The demands of the nursing program
- Fear of injuring patients
- The need to balance work and study
- The need to meet financial and family responsibilities

 RECALL Sarah Keller, the nursing student described in the Reflective Practice display. She was feeling overwhelmed with the responsibilities of caring for patients in a high-tech environment. This feeling was compounded by her concerns about the assigned instructor. Subsequently, Sarah began to feel ill. ●

Most nurses and student nurses enjoy their education and work, coping with physical and emotional demands effectively. Some, however, become overwhelmed and develop symptoms of stress. The complex of behaviors is called **burnout**. Burnout can be compared with the exhaustion stage of anxiety and is characterized by a wide range of behaviors. Some nurses try to become "supernurses," expecting perfection in themselves and others. Some withdraw and do only minimal work, while still others resort to drugs or alcohol. Many nurses who cannot handle the stress leave the profession. Refer to the Research in Nursing box (on page 1588) for a study of proactive nursing strategies to cope with the trauma experienced by nurses in an emergency department setting.

RESEARCH IN NURSING

BRIDGING THE GAP TO EVIDENCE-BASED PRACTICE

Helping Nurses Develop Coping Strategies in Stressful Situations

Nurses who work in an emergency care setting respond to trauma cases on a regular basis. They may be prone to developing traumatic stress after their involvement in caring for traumatically injured patients. One recent national survey noted that over 50% of emergency nurses admitted symptoms of traumatic stress after caring for traumatically injured patients, and over 25% reported a decrease in their work productivity following this type of care. The purpose of this study was to determine the effect of proactive coping strategies that decrease traumatic stress for nurses involved in the emergency nursing care of trauma patients.

Related Research

Gates, D., & Gillespie, G. (2013). Using proactive coping to manage the stress of trauma patient care. *Journal of Trauma Nursing*, *20*(1), 44–50.

Nurses have identified threat-provoking situations that occur in the workplace. They include providing disaster management care, experiencing workplace violence, dealing with the death of a patient, and providing care to trauma patients. Nurses' personal experience with trauma, such as being the victim of a robbery or a sexual assault, can also negatively impact their stress response to trauma. Participants in this study were 137 practicing emergency nurses who completed five survey instruments. They included a Trauma Patient Event Questionnaire, an event survey that measured trau-

matic stress; a Proactive Coping Inventory, a survey that measured the participant's personal experience with trauma; and a demographic questionnaire. The most common proactive coping strategies that participants identified were getting feedback from friends, planning strategies, and being a "take charge" person. Results of this study indicated that emergency nurse participants did consistently use proactive coping strategies while experiencing personal traumatic stress. The correlation of proactive coping measures to the diminishment of traumatic stress was significant. Researchers theorized that the coping techniques proved effective in lowering the traumatic stress scores and without their use, the scores might have been significantly higher. It may be impossible in this setting to completely prevent these traumatic stress symptoms.

Relevance to Nursing Practice

The failure of emergency nurses to use proactive coping strategies can negatively affect both their personal life and professional performance. Since the environment can be stressful when dealing with trauma events, future interventions might prove most effective if they involve the entire health care team rather than an individual nurse. Nurses also need to be involved in any determination as to what strategies can be most effective.

What can graduate and student nurses do to help reduce stress and prevent burnout? The first step in preventing a stress level high enough to cause burnout is to identify and accept the stress. The same stress reduction techniques that are used for patients have positive benefits for nurses as well (see Encouraging Use of Stress Management Techniques in the Nursing Process section). Nurses must accept that they have the same needs and are as individual as their patients. Dickerson (2013) has developed a tool, the Stress Management Algorithm, to help nurses assess and cope with various stressors in their daily practice. By recognizing the early signs of stress and taking steps to reduce it, nurses can continue to be effective and productive as well as satisfied in the profession. (See Focused Critical Thinking Guide 41-1).

THE NURSING PROCESS FOR THE PATIENT WITH STRESS AND ANXIETY

Self-awareness of stress and anxiety is essential when caring for patients. Nurses who role model good health behaviors are more effective teachers. Use the tool found in Promoting Health 41-1 (on page 1590) for yourself before using it with others.

 REMEMBER Joan Rogerrio, the woman returning to work after an absence of 15 years. The nurse could use the tool in Promoting Health 41-1 (on page 1590) as part of the patient's assessment. Then the nurse could use those items identified as "sometimes" and "almost never" as a basis for teaching Joan measures to adapt and cope with her stressors. ●

Assessing

Stress and anxiety are problems that nurses encounter in patients of all ages and in all settings. Stress is assessed through a health assessment, including a nursing history and physical assessment. Risk factors for, or indicators of, stress may be identified through standardized tests or open-ended questions to elicit information. The patient's willingness to share information is affected by the level of stress experienced as well as the coping or defense mechanisms in use.

Nursing History

The nursing history assists the nurse in identifying stressors and how the person perceives and copes with stress. Manifestations of anxiety, as well as questions and leading statements to identify stress and anxiety, are listed in Focused Assessment Guide 41-1 (on page 1590).

FOCUSED CRITICAL THINKING GUIDE 41-1

STRESS AND ANXIETY

You are a senior nursing student in your community health course. You have been assigned to visit and provide ongoing assessments for Charles Obedide, a 28-year-old man who was involved in a serious motorcycle crash a year ago and is paralyzed from the waist down. Charles initially participated fully in his rehabilitation and has been living independently in an apartment that is wheelchair accessible. However, a month ago, Charles was ill for 2 weeks, lost his job, and broke up with his girlfriend. When you made your last home visit, Charles was restless, had an increased pulse, and did little talking. At this visit, Charles is wearing dirty clothes and has a strong body odor, and there are several empty beer cans on the table in the kitchen. Charles begins to cry, saying, "I am so upset—I can't sleep or eat—I need help." What would you do?

1. Identify goal of thinking

Identify the level of anxiety experienced by Charles and begin interventions to help Charles decrease his level of anxiety.

2. Assess adequacy of knowledge

Pertinent circumstances: Charles has had numerous losses in the past year, including loss of body function and changes in body image. He has recently lost his job, a major source of economic support and self-concept. He lost his girlfriend, a major source of support. Previously, Charles was clean and well groomed. There was no previous evidence of drinking. His parents live nearby and are supporting and loving.

Prerequisite knowledge: Before you decide what to do in this situation, you need to assess the level of anxiety experienced by Charles. You need to know the typical behaviors of each level and be able to recognize that Charles has severe anxiety. You must recognize that Charles needs interventions to regain equilibrium.

Room for error: Charles requires and has asked for help. You are unsure of your abilities to help him to deal effectively with his anxiety. You realize that his frustration with the situation could make him angry. You also know that depression and the potential for self-violence are risks unless something is done to reduce his anxiety.

Time constraints: Although you are not certain about how serious his problem is, you understand that Charles needs help in reducing his anxiety soon. There is time for you to ask for guidance from your instructor.

3. Address potential problems

There are several potential barriers to critical thinking in this situation. You realize Charles needs help in reducing his level of stress, which in turn causes you anxiety. You are also somewhat frightened about his appearance and behavior. You do not believe your own abilities are developed well enough to help Charles adequately, but at the same time, you do know he needs help.

4. Consult helpful resources

Your best source of information is Charles himself. You ask him what you can do to help him. He replies, "Just get someone here to help me." You ask his permission to call his mother and he agrees. His mother says she will be there in 5 minutes. You call your instructor, and she tells you to call the home health care agency for further instructions.

5. Critique judgment/decision

When his mother arrives, she says she had no idea he was so distressed. She talks to the home health care agency staff, who report that they have called Charles's physician and will continue to follow up on needed care and referrals for professional counseling. You believe you made the right decisions: you identified that Charles needed help, you contacted his mother to provide support, you contacted your instructor, and you contacted the home health care agency. You also remained calm during the situation, despite your own anxiety.

Physical Assessment

There are no specific guidelines for the physical assessment of stress. Physical indicators of stress, in addition to those listed in the Focused Assessment Guide, may include cardiac dysrhythmias, chest pain, headache, hyperventilation, diarrhea, tense muscles, and skin lesions, such as eczema. These manifestations are the result of the mind–body interaction described earlier.

Diagnosing

Assessment data may reveal stress to be the problem or the etiology of a problem.

Stress as the Problem

The following nursing diagnoses may be made when stress is the cause of the problem:

- Anxiety related to conflicts about values and goals in life, threat to self-concept, threat of death, threat of or change in health status, threat to or change in environment or role, situational/maturational crisis, or unmet needs
- Stress Overload related to single parenthood, inadequate economic resources, and chronic illness
- Moral Distress related to cultural conflicts, end-of-life decisions, conflicting information about ethical decision making, or treatment decisions

PROMOTING HEALTH 41-1

STRESS AND ADAPTATION

Nurses who design care plans for patients to reduce stress must also examine themselves as a factor in the success of that plan of care. The nurse who wishes to encourage healthy adaptation to stress must demonstrate behaviors that support a healthy lifestyle. Use the assessment checklist to determine how well you are adapting to stress. Then develop a prescription for self-care by choosing the appropriate behaviors from the list of suggestions.

Assessment Checklist

☐ almost always	☐ sometimes	☐ almost never

☐ ☐ ☐ 1. I have realistic perceptions of new situations, self, and others.

☐ ☐ ☐ 2. I understand my own personal physical and emotional responses to stress.

☐ ☐ ☐ 3. I anticipate and prepare for change.

☐ ☐ ☐ 4. I have the ability to satisfactorily solve problems and make decisions.

Self-Care Behaviors

1. Accept as positive indicators of growth the changes that come with different parts and stages of life.
2. Maintain an open mind about change—change what you can, and accept what you cannot change.
3. Avoid self-defeating behaviors to cope with stress such as smoking, alcohol, and drugs.
4. Avoid confrontational and unprofessional interactions with other staff members.
5. Develop a greater awareness of potential risks in the workplace that can result in violence.
6. Practice methods of stress management that work best for you: relaxation techniques, exercise, hobbies.
7. Set realistic goals.
8. Develop problem-solving strategies for use in stressful situations.
9. Accept help from others.
10. Take life one day at a time.

FOCUSED ASSESSMENT GUIDE 41-1

ANXIETY

Factors to Assess	Questions and Approaches
Subjective data: Heart palpitations Difficulty breathing Problems with appetite or sleep Feelings of sadness, apprehension, anger, mistrust, helplessness, hopelessness Changes in sexual desire	• "Have you noticed that you sometimes feel your heart beating or have difficulty breathing?" • "Tell me about your appetite and sleep." • "Of the following, which best describes how you are feeling: sad, apprehensive, angry, mistrustful, helpless, hopeless?" • "Tell me about any changes you have noticed in your sexual desire." • "How does your body feel when you are upset?"
Objective data: Dry mouth Increased perspiration Tremors Tachycardia Increased blood pressure Dilated pupils Crying Restlessness Rapid speech Pacing around the room Lack of facial expression	• Note body posture and movements. • Inspect skin and mucous membranes. • Take and record vital signs. • Note general affect.
Ability to verbalize anxiety	• "You have been very quiet today. Has something happened since our last visit?" • "It must be very frightening to be told that you have cancer." • "I notice you seem upset. Would you like to talk about it?" • "What has caused you to feel stressed in the past?" • "What do you do to feel better when you feel anxious?"

EXAMPLES OF NANDA-I NURSING DIAGNOSES

STRESS AND ADAPTATION

Nursing Diagnoses	Related Factors	Sample Defining Characteristics
Anxiety	Unmet needs, situational/maturational crises, threat to self-concept, stress, threat to or change in role status, health status, interaction patterns, role function, environment, economic status	**Behavioral:** • Restlessness, fidgeting, insomnia • "I am so worried about my son getting married." **Affective:** • Irritable, jittery, focused on self, worried, apprehensive • "I just know I won't be able to do what I have to in this new job." **Physiologic:** • Tremors, increased pulse and respirations, urinary urgency, perspiration, diarrhea, dry mouth, nausea, respiratory difficulties • "I can't eat or sleep, and my heart feels like it's going to jump out of my chest." **Cognitive:** • Preoccupation, confusion, decreased attention and concentration, tendency to blame others • "What did you just tell me? I can't seem to remember, and it's all my husband's fault for leaving me."
Ineffective Denial	A conscious or unconscious attempt to disavow the knowledge or meaning of an event to reduce anxiety, but leading to detriment of health	• "I do have a lot of heartburn, but I take something I bought at the store and it feels better." • "I have noticed some bright red blood when I have a bowel movement, but I figure it's just my hemorrhoids."

• Ineffective Denial related to continued smoking behavior
• Decisional Conflict related to placement of parent in long-term care facility

Examples of two of these diagnoses are highlighted in the accompanying box, Examples of NANDA-I Nursing Diagnoses.

Stress as the Etiology

Stress and anxiety may affect many other areas of human functioning. In the following nursing diagnoses, stress and anxiety are involved in the etiologies of other problems:

• Imbalanced Nutrition: Less Than Body Requirements related to inadequate caloric intake while striving to excel in gymnastics
• Caregiver Role Strain related to long-term stress of care for parent with Alzheimer disease
• Social Isolation related to feelings of worthlessness and apprehension following failure in school
• Spiritual Distress related to inability to accept diagnosis of terminal illness
• Hopelessness related to presence of disabling physical injuries

Outcome Identification and Planning

The nurse plans and implements care to decrease anxiety and facilitate adaptation in the patient with stress. The expected outcomes of the plan must be mutually determined with the patient or family members. Examples of the expected outcomes of the plan of care may include that the patient will achieve the following:

• Decrease the level of anxiety by verbalizing feelings and using support systems.
• Develop effective coping skills through problem-solving skills and anxiety-reducing techniques.
• Describe a reduction in anxiety and an increase in comfort.

Implementing

Nurses may use a variety of interventions to help patients decrease stress and to facilitate coping. If the patient's anxiety seems too great or the nurse is uncomfortable with the interventions, a referral should be made. Referrals may be made, for example, to a professional counselor; to people who have experienced the same type of surgery or health problem; or to the patient's rabbi, minister, or priest.

The nursing interventions discussed in this section include teaching healthy activities of daily living, encouraging use of support systems, and practicing stress management techniques. See the accompanying box, Examples of Nursing Interventions and Nursing Outcomes Classifications (NIC/NOC) (on page 1592), for activities and related outcomes for anxiety reduction.

EXAMPLES OF NURSING INTERVENTIONS AND NURSING OUTCOMES CLASSIFICATIONS (NIC/NOC)

ANXIETY REDUCTION

Nursing Interventions	Nursing Outcomes
• Use a calm, reassuring approach. • Explain all procedures, including sensations likely to be experienced during the procedure. • Stay with the patient to promote safety and reduce fear. • Listen attentively. • Encourage verbalizations of feelings, perceptions, and fears. • Instruct the patient on the use of relaxation techniques. • Assess for verbal and nonverbal signs of anxiety.	• Anxiety Level • Anxiety Self-Control • Coping • Information Processing • Stress Level

Adapted from Bulechek, G., Butcher, H., Dochterman, J. M., & Wagner, C. (Eds). (2013). *Nursing interventions classification (NIC)* (6th ed., p. 83). St. Louis: Elsevier/Mosby; and Moorhead, S., Johnson, M., Maas, M., & Swanson, E. (Eds). (2013). *Nursing outcomes classification (NOC)* (5th ed., p. 573). St. Louis: Elsevier/Mosby. A full listing of nursing activities for each nursing intervention and outcomes can be found in these books.

Methods should be selected carefully, based on the person's physical and emotional characteristics, family and social structure, and previously used successful coping mechanisms. Guidelines for Nursing Care 41-1 lists nursing interventions to reduce stress and anxiety for patients as they enter a health care setting.

Teaching Healthy Activities of Daily Living

A person's usual lifestyle greatly influences that individual's perceptions of and reactions to stressors. For example, a person who is overweight, sedentary, and chronically tired is at increased risk for developing an illness as a result of stress. These factors are also stressors and further increase the risk. Exercise, rest, and good nutrition are important components of stress reduction.

THINK about Sarah Keller's lifestyle as a nursing student. The workload involved with school and the factors associated with stress in nursing students described previously place Sarah at risk for stress. In addition, other factors, such as demands from family members or a need to work part-time, decrease her ability to maintain a healthy lifestyle with exercise, rest, and good nutrition. •

EXERCISE

Regular exercise helps maintain physical and emotional health. The benefits of exercise include an improved musculoskeletal system, more effective cardiovascular function, weight control, and relaxation. Exercise improves one's general sense of well-being, relieves tension, and enables coping with day-to-day stressors. General health guidelines recommend that an exercise program consist of 30 to 45 minutes of moderate activity above usual activity on most days of the week. People who are overweight, chronically ill, or older than 35 years of age should have a physical examination before beginning such a program. The type of exercise depends on what the person enjoys—for example, walking, jogging, bicycling, swimming, or sports such as golf or tennis.

GUIDELINES FOR NURSING CARE 41-1

REDUCING ANXIETY ON ADMISSION TO A HEALTH CARE FACILITY

1. Assess physical status, sensory status, and cognitive status.
2. Assess cultural/ethnic background, including beliefs about health care, dietary restrictions, and language spoken.
3. Assess past experiences with the health care system, including medical–surgical treatment for illness or injury.
4. Assess concerns and stressors.
5. Assess amount and type of support systems available.
6. Provide information about the environment:
   a. Ensure that all health care providers introduce themselves by name and title.
   b. Explain policies and routines.
   c. If the hospital is the setting, provide verbal and written guidelines for use of equipment, telephone, television, meals, and visiting hours.
7. Provide and discuss the patient's rights specific to care in the agency or institution.
8. Mutually determine expected outcomes of the plan of care.
9. Provide information about all diagnostic procedures, surgical procedures, activity, and diet.

REST AND SLEEP

Rest and sleep help the body maintain homeostasis and restore energy levels. Adequate rest can provide "insulation" against stress, but stress may interfere with one's ability to sleep. Although each person has individual needs, 7 to 9 hours of sleep a day is recommended. Relaxation techniques can be used during both health and illness to facilitate rest and sleep. Hospitalized patients may require additional nursing interventions to relieve pain and promote comfort to get needed rest.

NUTRITION

Nutrition plays an active role in maintaining the body's homeostatic mechanisms and in increasing resistance to stress. (Nutrition is discussed in detail in Chapter 35.) Obesity and malnutrition are major stressors and greatly increase the risk for illness. People of all ages should maintain a normal body weight and should follow these guidelines established by Dietary Guidelines for Americans (2010).

- Reduce intake of salt, refined sugar, animal fat, and cholesterol.
- Eat more fruit, vegetables, and whole grains.
- Eat less red meat and more fish and poultry.

Encouraging Use of Support Systems

Support systems provide emotional support that helps a person identify and verbalize feelings associated with stress. Other valuable contributions include providing information and services, maintaining a positive self-concept, and establishing an avenue for new relationships and social roles. In addition, families and support groups provide an accepting environment, allowing the person to explore problem-solving methods and try out new coping skills. There are support groups for almost every situation; examples are listed in Box 41-6.

Encouraging Use of Stress Management Techniques

Stress creates emotional distress that often produces physical signs and symptoms. One person may have tension headaches, another becomes irritable, another clenches the fists. Many people take legal or illegal drugs, smoke,

---

BOX 41-6 EXAMPLES OF SUPPORT GROUPS

Alcoholics Anonymous
Overeaters Anonymous
Weight Watchers
Parents Without Partners
Reach to Recovery (cancer)
Ostomy clubs
Child abuse support groups
Sudden infant death support groups
Stroke clubs
Assertiveness training groups

---

drink to excess, or eat compulsively. These behaviors can be modified and adaptive mechanisms strengthened through specific techniques aimed at managing stress. Only a few techniques are included here, but the literature describes many stress reduction methods, including exercise, prayer, art therapy, music therapy, massage, and therapeutic touch. Chapter 27 provides more information. Students should learn different methods they can use for themselves and in varied clinical situations.

RELAXATION

Relaxation techniques are useful in many situations, such as childbirth, pain, anxiety, sleeplessness, illness, and anger, and other uses are being discovered. Relaxation promotes a body reaction opposite to that of the fight-or-flight response: respiratory, pulse, and metabolic rates; blood pressure; and energy use are all decreased.

Relaxation can be taught to individuals or groups. It is especially helpful because it allows people to control their feelings and behaviors. Various techniques can be used, but most involve rhythmic breathing, reduced muscle tension, and an altered state of consciousness (National Center for Complementary and Alternative Medicine [NCCAM], 2013). Relaxation is discussed as a comfort measure in Chapter 34. Two helpful relaxation activities, to be practiced three or four times at each session, are deep breathing and progressive muscle relaxation (Guidelines for Nursing Care 41-2).

GUIDELINES FOR NURSING CARE 41-2

RELAXATION ACTIVITIES

Deep Breathing

1. Sit comfortably and place your hands on your stomach. Inhale slowly and deeply, letting your abdomen expand as much as possible. Hold your breath for a few seconds.

2. Exhale slowly through your mouth, blowing through puckered lips. When your abdomen feels empty, begin again with a deep inhalation.

Progressive Muscle Relaxation

1. Tighten your hand into a fist and notice how it feels. Hold the tension for a few seconds.

2. Loosen your grip, relax the muscles in your hand, and let the tension slip away.

3. Continue to tighten–hold–relax each muscle group: hands, arms, shoulders, face, chest, back, abdomen, legs, feet.

MEDITATION

Meditation has four components: quiet surroundings, a passive attitude, a comfortable position, and a word or mental image on which to focus. A person practicing meditation sits comfortably with closed eyes, relaxes the major muscle groups, and repeats the selected word silently with each exhalation. Alternatively, a person may focus on a pleasant scene and mentally place oneself in it while breathing slowly in and out. This exercise should be performed for 20 to 30 minutes twice a day.

 SARAH Keller, the nursing student, could learn to perform relaxation exercises or practice meditation. Both techniques would be helpful in reducing her stress. •

ANTICIPATORY GUIDANCE

Anticipatory guidance focuses on psychologically preparing a person for an unfamiliar or painful event. Nurses use this technique to teach patients about procedures and the surgical experience. When patients know what to expect, their anxiety is reduced and their coping mechanisms are more effective. For example, before performing a painful procedure (such as ambulating for the first time after surgery), teaching would include information about the pain involved—onset, severity, cause, and methods of relief. With this knowledge, the patient feels less threatened and tolerates the procedure more easily.

A related process is anticipatory socialization, in which people prepare themselves for roles to which they aspire but do not yet occupy. This process may be used, for example, to prepare expectant parents for the role of parenting, thereby enhancing the potential for the child to experience normal growth and development.

GUIDED IMAGERY

In guided imagery, a person creates a mental image, concentrates on the image, and becomes less responsive to other stimuli (including pain). The nurse sits by the patient and reads a description of a scene or an experience that the patient has described as happy, pleasant, or peaceful. The patient is then "guided" through the image. For example, using a soothing, soft voice, the nurse might start as follows: "You are floating in your swimming pool. The water is cool and comfortable. Birds are singing in the trees. The roses are perfuming the air." As the patient becomes more and more focused on the scene, the nurse needs only to verbally "paint the picture" at intervals.

BIOFEEDBACK

Biofeedback is a method of gaining mental control of the autonomic nervous system and thus regulating body responses, such as blood pressure, heart rate, and headaches. A measurement device (e.g., skin temperature sensors) is used, and the patient tries to control the readings through relaxation and conscious thought. Over a period of time, the feedback of the change in readings teaches the person to control physiologic functions that normally are considered involuntary responses.

Providing Crisis Intervention

A crisis is a situation that cannot be resolved by usual coping mechanisms. As a result, the person cannot function normally and requires interventions to regain equilibrium. **Crisis intervention** is a five-step problem-solving technique designed to promote a more adaptive outcome, including improved abilities to cope with future crises. The steps are as follows:

1. *Identify the problem.* This may be more difficult than it appears, as the cause of the crisis is often difficult for the person to identify accurately. Until it is clear, a solution is impossible.
2. *List alternatives.* All possible solutions to the problem need to be listed. An appropriate solution to a problem is much more likely if many options are considered.
3. *Choose from among alternatives.* Each option needs to be carefully considered, using a "what would happen if" approach. The alternative chosen will be highly individualized, based on the person's priorities and values.
4. *Implement the plan.* The alternative chosen is put into action. The nurse may need to provide support and encouragement so that action is taken.
5. *Evaluate the outcome.* In this final step, the effectiveness of the plan needs to be carefully considered. If it did not work as well as expected, another alternative should be tried. If it did work, it has the positive benefit of improving self-confidence and future problem-solving efforts.

The major factor in helping patients adapt to high levels of stress is to identify and plan individually for situations causing the stress. Facilitate the patient's recognition of his or her own stress level and specific responses to stress. Encourage adoption of a philosophy of accepting what cannot be changed and changing what cannot be accepted. Emphasize the importance of accepting help from others and giving support to others when needed, as well as being actively involved in problem solving and decision making. Nurses must use therapeutic communication skills in all interactions.

Evaluating

The evaluation of the plan of care is based on the mutually established expected outcomes. Be sure to observe both verbal and nonverbal cues when evaluating the usefulness of the plan. In general, the plan is considered successful if the patient and family achieve the following:

- Verbalize causes and effects of stress and anxiety
- Identify and use sources of support
- Use problem solving to find solutions to stressors
- Practice healthy lifestyle habits and anxiety-reducing techniques
- Verbalize a decrease in anxiety and an increase in comfort

See the accompanying Nursing Plan of Care 41-1 for Mei Fu.

NURSING PLAN OF CARE 41-1

for Mei Fu

Remember Mei Fu, the 24-year-old graduate student with a husband and two small children. At her clinic appointment, the nurse conducted a health history and physical assessment of Mrs. Fu and noted the following data:

- Patient is a thin woman who appears her stated age. She is currently in school and expects herself to make the highest grades. She also cares for her two children and her husband. Although her husband encourages her to go to school, he believes it is the wife's responsibility to provide all child and house care. She has had no previous serious illnesses or surgery.
- Patient reports having frequent headaches, rating the pain as a 3 on a scale of 0 (no pain) to 10 (worst

possible pain). She also reports having 4 to 6 bowel movements each day, sometimes with abdominal cramping. The diarrhea does not seem to be related to any type of foods eaten. Both the headaches and the diarrhea have been present for the past 2 months. During the interview, the patient appeared restless and talked rapidly. Questions often had to be repeated.
- Physical assessment reveals slight tachycardia, a fine hand tremor, and visible perspiration. Large muscle groups are tense and fists clenched. No tenderness is noted on abdominal palpation. Pupils are equal in size and react to light and accommodation. Nasal mucosa is normal.

NURSING DIAGNOSIS	Anxiety related to stress of achievement in school and care of family as manifested by rapid speech, tachycardia, tremor, tense muscles, headache, and diarrhea
EXPECTED OUTCOME	By her return appointment in 2 weeks, 10/20/15, Mrs. Fu will: • Identify sources of and responses to stress

NURSING INTERVENTIONS	**RATIONALE**	**EVALUATIVE STATEMENT**
Ask Mrs. Fu to keep a diary of hours spent in school-related activities and family care, number and times of headaches, and circumstances that occurred before diarrhea.	Identifying sources of stress and the physical responses to stress is the first step in planning coping strategies to reduce stress.	10/20/15 Outcome met. Mrs. Fu kept a diary as requested. She identified that she does not have any time for herself. Her headaches are worse during the week. She often has diarrhea when papers are due or when her husband and children are demanding of her time. *S. Aird, RN, FNP*

EXPECTED OUTCOME	By her return appointment, 10/20/15, Mrs. Fu will: • Identify sources of personal strength and support

NURSING INTERVENTIONS	**RATIONALE**	**EVALUATIVE STATEMENT**
Ask Mrs. Fu to make a list of the people who are important to her and provide her comfort. Ask her to discuss how these people can help her cope with her situation. Ask Mrs. Fu to describe her strengths as a woman, a mother, a wife, and a student.	Identifying support people and areas of personal strength provides the patient with the means to manage stress and enhances self-concept.	10/20/15 Outcome met. Mrs. Fu stated that her family is her greatest source of support, but they are in China and she misses them very much. She does have a very good friend who is also a good listener. She identified her strengths as being a person who cares for others and a good student. She said she is also a good artist, but has not had time for art for months. *S. Aird, RN, FNP*

(continued)

NURSING PLAN OF CARE 41-1 *continued*

for Mei Fu

EXPECTED OUTCOME By her return appointment, 10/20/15, Mrs. Fu will:

- Describe lifestyle changes that include eating a well-balanced diet with three meals a day, walking for 20 to 30 minutes four times a week, and sleeping restfully 7 hours a night

NURSING INTERVENTIONS	RATIONALE	EVALUATIVE STATEMENT
Discuss with Mrs. Fu the MyPlate guidelines and the importance of eating foods from each group. Also, discuss why she should eat three meals a day.	Adequate nutrition helps maintain the homeostatic mechanisms of the body and increases resistance to stress.	10/20/15 Outcome met. Mrs. Fu was given a copy of the MyPlate guidelines, and food preparations were discussed. Although the Fus have a healthy diet, Mrs. Fu often was too busy to eat more than a few bites. She said that she is making a big effort to eat three times a day.
Discuss with Mrs. Fu the benefits of regular exercise in reducing stress.	Exercise improves well-being, relieves tension, and facilitates coping with daily stressors.	She is walking to school and enjoys the time by herself. She arranged this time by asking her husband to take the children to school.
Discuss with Mrs. Fu the importance of sleep in reducing stress.	Adequate rest and sleep restore energy and facilitate coping with stressors.	She is sleeping better, and averages 7 hours most nights.

S. Aird, RN, FNP |

EXPECTED OUTCOME By her return appointment, 10/20/15, Mrs. Fu will:

- Practice relaxation for 20 minutes each day

NURSING INTERVENTIONS	RATIONALE	EVALUATIVE STATEMENT
Teach and have Mrs. Fu practice progressive muscle relaxation. Suggest that she buy a video to facilitate the technique (videos for relaxation are widely available). Recommend that she plan a time when she can be alone and use 20 minutes to complete the technique.	Relaxation promotes a response opposite to the stress response; it decreases heart rate, respiratory rate, blood pressure, and metabolic processes.	10/20/15 Outcome met. Mrs. Fu said that at first she had difficulty in finding time to be alone, but she feels so much better after she relaxes that she insists on the time. She did buy a video and says it helps her very much.

S. Aird, RN, FNP |

EXPECTED OUTCOME By her return appointment, 10/20/15, Mrs. Fu will:

- Report a decrease in headaches and diarrhea and an increase in her ability to provide self-care to manage stress

NURSING PLAN OF CARE 41-1 *continued*

for Mei Fu

NURSING INTERVENTIONS	RATIONALE	EVALUATIVE STATEMENT
Assess frequency and severity of headaches and bowel movements. Assess the patient's self-report of coping with stressors.	Decreasing stress in daily life often is effective in decreasing physical responses. Self-care of stress is critical in effective management.	10/20/15 Outcome met. Mrs. Fu reports she has noticed fewer headaches in the past week, and the diarrhea is almost gone. Mrs. Fu verbalized the importance of continuing to practice a healthy lifestyle and relaxation. She said she has spent time with her friend and has gotten out her sketchpad. She stated that she believes she can manage her life much better now. *S. Aird, RN, FNP*

SAMPLE DOCUMENTATION

10/06/15, 10 AM, nursing

Initial visit to student health center by Mrs. Fu to discuss physical problems of headache and diarrhea. History and physical assessment findings indicated large number of personal stressors, manifested by physical signs and symptoms. Assessment data supported nursing diagnosis: Anxiety related to stress of achievement in school and care of family. Discussion centered on identifying sources of stress, physical responses to stress, sources of support, and personal strength. Teaching strategies included diet, exercise, sleep, and progressive muscle relaxation. Patient's progress will be monitored at next visit on 10/20/15.

S. Aird, RN, FNP

DEVELOPING CLINICAL REASONING

1. Identify the nursing activities and relationships that cause you the most stress. What are your personal warning signs that a situation is becoming stressful? What do you do to decrease your level of stress? Who is most important in helping you do this?

2. List nursing interventions you would use to reduce stress in the following situations:
   - A newly married young woman who found a lump in her breast and is undergoing a breast biopsy
   - The parents of a 2-year-old who are sitting in the surgical waiting room as their child undergoes brain surgery
   - The daughter (and caregiver) of a woman with severe Alzheimer disease

PRACTICING FOR NCLEX

1. A nurse is assessing a 49-year-old male patient who complains of migraines that have become "unbearable." The patient tells the nurse, "I just got laid off from my job last week and I have two kids in college. I don't know how I'm going to pay for it all." Which physiologic effects of stress would be expected findings in this patient? Select all that apply.
   a. Changes in appetite
   b. Changes in elimination patterns
   c. Decreased pulse and respirations
   d. Use of ineffective coping mechanisms

   e. Withdrawal
   f. Attention-seeking behaviors

2. A nurse caring for patients in a hospital setting uses anticipatory guidance to prepare them for painful procedures. Which instruction would the nurse provide in this type of stress management?
   a. The nurse teaches patients rhythmic breathing to perform prior to the procedure.
   b. The nurse tells patients to focus on a pleasant place, mentally place themselves in it, and breathe slowly in and out.
   c. The nurse teaches patients about the pain involved in the procedure and methods to cope with it.
   d. The nurse teaches patients to create and focus on a mental image during the procedure to become less responsive to the pain.

3. A nurse witnesses a street robbery and is assessing a 26-year-old female patient who is the victim. The patient has minor scrapes and bruises and tells the nurse, "I've never been so scared in my life." What other symptoms would the nurse expect to find related to the fight-or-flight response to stress? Select all that apply.
   a. Increased heart rate
   b. Decreased muscle strength
   c. Increased mental alertness
   d. Increased blood glucose levels
   e. Decreased cardiac output
   f. Decreased peristalsis

4. A nurse is assessing the developmental levels of patients in a pediatric office. Which individual would a nurse document as experiencing developmental stress?
   a. An infant who learns to turn over
   b. A school-aged child who learns how to add and subtract
   c. An adolescent who is a "loner"
   d. A young adult who has a variety of friends

5. A nurse is caring for an older male patient in a long-term care facility who has a spinal cord injury affecting his neurologic reflex arc. Based on this patient data, what would be a priority intervention for this patient?
   a. Monitoring food and drink temperatures to prevent burns
   b. Providing adequate pain relief measures to reduce stress
   c. Monitoring for depression related to social isolation
   d. Providing meals high in carbohydrates to promote healing

6. A nurse is caring for a patient in the shock or alarm reaction phase of the GAS. Which response by the patient would be expected?
   a. Decreasing pulse
   b. Increasing sleepiness
   c. Increasing energy levels
   d. Decreasing respirations

7. A nurse interviews a woman who was abused by her partner and is staying at a women's shelter with her three children. She tells the nurse, "I'm so worried that my husband will find me and try to make me go back home." Which data would the nurse most appropriately document?
   a. "Patient displays moderate anxiety related to her situation."
   b. "Patient manifests panic related to feelings of impending doom."
   c. "Patient describes severe anxiety related to her situation."
   d. "Patient expresses fear of her husband."

8. A college student visits the school's health center with vague complaints of anxiety and fatigue. The student tells the nurse, "Exams are right around the corner and all I feel like doing is sleeping." The student's vital signs are within normal parameters. What would be an appropriate question to ask in response to these complaints?
   a. "Are you worried about failing your exams?"
   b. "Have you been staying up late studying?"
   c. "Are you using any recreational drugs?"
   d. "Do you have trouble managing your time?"

9. A nurse is interviewing a patient who just received news that he has pancreatic cancer. The patient tells the nurse that getting cancer could never happen to him. Which defense mechanism is this patient demonstrating?
   a. Projection
   b. Denial
   c. Displacement
   d. Repression

10. A visiting nurse is performing a family assessment of a young couple caring for their newborn who was diagnosed with cerebral palsy. The nurse notes that the mother's hair and clothing are unkempt, the house is untidy, and the mother states that she is "so busy with the baby that I don't have time to do anything else." What would be the priority intervention for this family?
    a. Arrange to have the infant removed from the home.
    b. Inform other members of the family of the situation.

c. Increase the number of visits by the visiting nurse.
d. Notify the care provider and recommend respite care for the mother.

11. A nurse is teaching a patient a relaxation technique. Which statement demonstrates the need for more teaching?
    a. "I must breathe in and out in rhythm."
    b. "I should take my pulse and expect it to be faster."
    c. "I can expect my muscles to feel less tense."
    d. "I will be more relaxed and less aware."

12. A certified nurse midwife is teaching a pregnant woman techniques to reduce the pain of childbirth. Which stress reduction activities would be most effective? Select all that apply.
    a. Progressive muscle relaxation
    b. Meditation
    c. Anticipatory socialization
    d. Biofeedback
    e. Rhythmic breathing
    f. Guided imagery

13. A nurse teaches problem solving to a college student who is in a crisis situation. What statement best illustrates the student's understanding of the process?
    a. "I need to identify the problem first."
    b. "Listing alternatives is the initial step."
    c. "I will list alternatives after I develop the plan."
    d. "I do not need to evaluate the outcome of my plan."

14. A nurse is performing an assessment of a female patient who is 8 months pregnant. The woman states, "I worry all the time about being able to handle becoming a mother." Which nursing diagnosis would be most appropriate for this patient?
    a. Ineffective Coping related to the new parenting role
    b. Ineffective Denial related to ability to care for a newborn
    c. Anxiety related to change in role status
    d. Situational Low Self-Esteem related to fear of parenting

15. A nurse is responsible for preparing patients for surgery in an ambulatory care center. Which technique for reducing anxiety would be appropriate for these patients?
    a. Discouraging over-verbalization of fears and anxieties
    b. Focusing on the outcome as opposed to the details of the surgery
    c. Providing time alone for reflection on personal strengths and weaknesses
    d. Mutually determining expected outcomes of the plan of care

ANSWERS WITH RATIONALES

1. **a, b.** Physiologic effects of stress include changes in appetite and elimination patterns as well as increased pulse and respirations. Using ineffective coping mechanisms, becoming withdrawn and isolated, and exhibiting attention-seeking behaviors are psychological effects of stress.

2. **c.** Anticipatory guidance focuses on psychologically preparing a person for an unfamiliar or painful event. When patients know what to expect, their anxiety is reduced, which occurs when teaching about the pain involved and related pain relief measures. Rhythmic breathing is a relaxation technique, focusing on a pleasant place and breathing slowly in and out is a meditation technique, and focusing on a mental image to reduce responses to stimuli is a guided imagery technique.

3. *a, c, d.* The sympathetic nervous system functions under stress to bring about the fight-or-flight response by increasing the heart rate, increasing muscle strength, increasing cardiac output, increasing blood glucose levels, and increasing mental alertness. Increased peristalsis is brought on by the parasympathetic nervous system under normal conditions and at rest.

4. *c.* The adolescent who is a loner is not meeting a major task (being a part of a peer group) for that level of growth and development.

5. *a.* A patient with a damaged neurologic reflex arc would have a diminished pain reflex response, which would put the patient at risk for burns as the sensors in the skin would not detect the heat of the food or liquids. All patients should be provided adequate pain relief, but this is not the priority intervention in this patient. Monitoring for depression would be an intervention for this patient but is not related to the damaged neurologic reflex arc. A patient who is immobile should eat a balanced diet based on the ChooseMyPlate dietary guidelines.

6. *c.* The body perceives a threat and prepares to respond by increasing the activity of the autonomic nervous and endocrine systems. The initial or shock phase is characterized by increased energy levels, oxygen intake, cardiac output, blood pressure, and mental alertness.

7. *d.* Fear is a response (feeling of dread) to a known threat. Anxiety, on the other hand, is a vague, uneasy feeling of discomfort or dread from an often unknown source. Panic causes a person to lose control and experience dread and terror, which can lead to exhaustion and death; that is not the case in this situation.

8. *a.* Mild anxiety is often handled without conscious thought through the use of coping mechanisms, such as sleeping, which are behaviors used to decrease stress and anxiety. Based on the complaints and normal vital signs, it would be best to explore the patient's level of stress and physiologic response to this stress.

9. *b.* Denial occurs when a person refuses to acknowledge the presence of a condition that is disturbing.

10. *d.* Reactions of family members to home health care for long periods of time, called caregiver burden, include chronic fatigue, sleep disorders, and an increased incidence of stress-related illnesses, such as hypertension and heart disease. The nurse should address the issue with the primary care provider and recommend a visit from a social worker and/or arrange for respite care for the family.

11. *b.* No matter what the technique, relaxation involves rhythmic breathing, a slower pulse, reduced muscle tension, and an altered state of consciousness.

12. *a, b, e, f.* Relaxation techniques are useful in many situations, including childbirth, and consist of rhythmic breathing and progressive muscle relaxation. Meditation and guided imagery could also be used to distract a patient from the pain of childbirth. Anticipatory socialization helps to prepare people for roles they don't have yet but aspire to, such as parenthood. Biofeedback is a method of gaining mental control of the autonomic nervous system and thus regulating body responses, such as blood pressure, heart rate, and headaches.

13. *a.* Although identifying the problem may be difficult, a solution to a crisis situation is impossible until the problem is identified.

14. *c.* The nursing diagnosis of Anxiety indicates situational/maturational crises or changes in role status. Ineffective coping refers to the inability to appraise stressors or use available resources. Ineffective denial is a conscious or unconscious attempt to disavow the knowledge or meaning of an event to reduce anxiety, and leads to detriment of health. Situational Low Self-Esteem diagnoses feelings of worthlessness related to the current situation the person is experiencing, not related to the fear of role changes.

15. *d.* Nurses preparing patients for surgery should mutually determine expected outcomes of the care, as well as encourage verbalizations of feelings, perceptions, and fears. Explain all procedures including sensations likely to be experienced during the procedure, and stay with the patient to promote safety and reduce fear.

TAYLOR SUITE RESOURCES

Explore these additional resources to enhance learning for this chapter:

- NCLEX-Style Questions and other resources on thePoint, http://thePoint.lww.com/Taylor8e
- *Study Guide for Fundamentals of Nursing, 8th edition*
- Adaptive Learning | Powered by prepU, http://thepoint.lww.com/prepu

Bibliography

American Nurses Association (ANA). (2013). *Nursing shortage.* Available at http://www.nursingworld.org/MainMenuCategories/ThePracticeofProfessionalNursing/workforce/NursingShortage

Bulechek, G., Butcher, H., Dochterman, J. M., & Wagner, C. (Eds.). (2013). *Nursing interventions classification (NIC)* (6th ed.). St. Louis: Elsevier/Mosby.

Carnegie Mellon University (2012). How stress influences disease: Study reveals inflammation as the culprit. *Science Daily.* Available at http://www.sciencedaily.com/releases/2012/04/120402162546.htm

Centers for Disease Control and Prevention (CDC). (2012a). Coping with stress. Available at http://www.cdc.gov/violenceprevention/pub/coping_with_stress_tips.html

Centers for Disease Control and Prevention (CDC). (2012b). Managing stress. Available at http://www.cdc.gov/Features/HandlingStress/

Dickerson, P. (2013). An algorithm to help you manage your stress. *American Nurse Today, 8*(3), 28–31.

Gates, D., & Gillespie, G. (2013). Using proactive coping to manage the stress of trauma patient care. *Journal of Trauma Nursing, 20*(1), 44–50.

Major, K. (2013). Crucial conversations in the workplace. *American Journal of Nursing, 113*(4), 66–70.

Moorhead, S., Johnson, M., & Maas, M., & Swanson E. (Eds.). (2013). *Nursing outcomes classification (NOC)* (5th ed.). St. Louis: Elsevier/Mosby.

NANDA International (NANDA-I). (2012). *Nursing diagnoses: Definitions & classification 2012–2014.* Oxford, UK: Wiley-Blackwell.

National Center for Complementary and Alternative Medicine (NCCAM). (2013). Relaxation techniques for health: An introduction. Available at http://nccam.nih.gov/health/stress/relaxation.htm

National Institute of Mental Health (NIMH). (2013). Anxiety disorders. Available at http://www.nimh.nih.gov/health/publications/anxiety-disorders/complete-index.shtml

Pender, N., Murdaugh, C., & Parsons, M. (2011). *Health promotion in nursing practice* (6th ed.). Upper Saddle River, NJ: Pearson Education, Inc.

Porth, C. (2011). *Essentials of Pathophysiology: Concepts of altered health states* (3rd ed.). Philadelphia: Wolters Kluwer Health/Lippincott Williams & Wilkins.

Seyle, H. (1976). *The stress of life.* New York: McGraw-Hill.

Sherwood, G., & Barnsteiner, J. (2012). *Quality and safety in nursing.* West Sussex, UK: Wiley-Blackwell.

Smith, Y. (2013). How to love and care for yourself unconditionally. *American Nurse Today, 8*(1), 30–33.

Sternberg, E. (2013). The stress response and autoimmune disease—what have we learned? *American Autoimmune Related Diseases Association, Inc.* Available at https://www.aarda.org/infocus_article.php?ID=31

Strickler, J. (2013). When it hurts to care: Workplace violence. *Nursing 43*(4), 58–62.

U.S. Department of Agriculture. (2010). Dietary Guidelines for Americans 2010. Available at http://www.cnpp.usda.gov/publications/dietaryguidelines/2010/policydoc/policydoc.pdf

Videbeck, S. (2011). *Psychiatric-mental health nursing* (5th ed.). Philadelphia: Wolters Kluwer Health/Lippincott Williams & Wilkins.

Wilson, D., & Severson, M. (2012). Long-term health outcomes of childhood sexual abuse. *American Nurse Today, 7*(10). Available at http://www.americannursetoday.com/Popups/ArticlePrint.aspx?id=11782

42

Loss, Grief, and Dying

YVONNE MALIC

Yvonne, a 20-year-old single woman, has just given birth to a baby, 11 weeks premature. The newborn weighs 2 lb 2 oz (1,021 g) and is immediately admitted to the neonatal intensive care unit because of severe respiratory distress. Up until this point, Yvonne had a normal pregnancy and was expecting a healthy baby girl. "I was so happy to be pregnant and I wanted to be a mother so much. But my baby is so tiny! And now the doctors are telling me that she has less than a 50% chance of surviving the next 24 hours."

ANNA MARIA ESPOSITA

The Espositas have been married for 19 years and have two children, Jorge, who is 16, and Marita, who is 13. It has been 2 years since Mrs. Esposita was diagnosed with ovarian cancer, and this period has been difficult for the entire family. At present, she is extremely cachexic (thin) and in the end stage of her illness. She initially tried aggressive treatment, and several chemotherapy regimens failed. During her last hospitalization 2 months ago, a decision was made not to continue treatment, and Mrs. Esposita told her family she wanted to die at home.

MANUEL PEREZ

Manuel is a 68-year-old man who moved to a retirement community with his 69-year-old wife 2 months ago. "We were looking forward to traveling and playing lots of golf. But she had this stroke, and now she has massive irreversible brain damage." Mr. Perez is sitting at his wife's bedside, holding her hand, and crying. "The doctors are asking me if I want to continue treatments that are keeping her alive. They mentioned donating her organs. I don't know what to do. We never talked about what we would want."

LEARNING OBJECTIVES

After completing the chapter, you will be able to accomplish the following:

1. Explain the concepts of loss and grieving, including types of loss and grief reactions.

2. Describe the signs of impending death.

3. Compare and contrast the five emotional stages of dying defined by Kübler-Ross.

4. Identify ethical and legal issues in end-of-life care, including advance directives, physician orders, and euthanasia.

5. Articulate and defend a personal response to a patient's plea, "Please help me die."

6. Explain six factors that affect loss, grief, and dying.

7. Describe physiologic, psychological, and spiritual care of a dying patient and family.

8. Use the nursing process to plan and implement care for dying patients and their families.

9. Outline nursing interventions when providing postmortem care.

10. Discuss the role of the nurse in caring for the family of a dying patient.

KEY TERMS

active euthanasia	do-not-resuscitate (DNR) order	mourning
actual loss		palliative care
advance directive	dysfunctional grief	palliative sedation
allow natural death (AND) order	euthanasia	perceived loss
	grief	physician order for life-sustaining treatment (POLST) form
anticipatory loss	hospice	
	loss	
bereaved	medical order for life-sustaining treatment (MOLST) form	terminal illness
comfort-measures-only order		terminal weaning
death		

There is the potential for loss, grief, and death at any stage of one's life. This is especially true for people experiencing altered health and for members of their family. A wide variety of losses may occur, including loss of a body part or function, loss of one's ability to care for oneself or to perform valued family or work roles, and death, which may

be the most difficult loss of all. Death may be as difficult for health care professionals as it is for surviving family members. The goals of nursing include promoting a peaceful death through compassionate palliative care and facilitating the patient's and family's coping with disability and death. The nurse is often the person providing support and care when loss or death occurs. To provide effective care, the nurse must have accepted his or her own feelings about death and understand the stages of grieving and dying. (For an example, see the Reflective Practice box on page 1602.)

CONCEPTS OF LOSS AND GRIEF

The types of loss as well as the varied responses to a loss are important concepts when planning and implementing nursing interventions to facilitate effective coping and adaptation.

Loss

Loss occurs when a valued person, object, or situation is changed or becomes inaccessible such that its value is diminished or removed. There are several types of loss, all of which everyone may experience at some time. **Actual loss** can be recognized by others as well as by the person sustaining the loss, for example, loss of a limb, a child, a valued object such as money, and a job. **Perceived loss**, such as loss of youth, financial independence, and a valued environment, is experienced by the person but is intangible to others. Directly related to actual and perceived loss are physical and psychological loss. A person who loses an arm in an automobile crash suffers from both the physical loss of the arm and the psychological loss that may be caused by an altered self-image and the inability to return to one's occupation or other activities. These losses are simultaneously physical, psychological, and actual. A person who is scarred but does not lose a limb may suffer a perceived and psychological loss of self-image.

 REMEMBER Mr. Perez, whose wife has brain damage from a recent stroke. The nurse could use knowledge of the types of losses to help Mr. Perez deal with all the recent changes in his life, including the loss of his wife as a partner. ●

Other types of loss are maturational loss, situational loss, and anticipatory loss. Maturational loss is experienced as a result of natural developmental processes. As examples, a first child may experience a loss of status when a sibling is born, and the parent of a single child may experience a sense of loss when the child begins school. Situational loss is experienced as a result of an unpredictable event, including traumatic injury, disease, death, or national disaster. **Anticipatory loss** occurs when a person displays loss and grief behaviors for a loss that has yet to take place (Fig. 42-1 on page 1603). Anticipatory loss is often seen in the families of patients with serious and life-threatening illnesses and may lessen the effect of the actual loss of a family member.

REFLECTIVE PRACTICE: CULTIVATING QSEN COMPETENCIES

CHALLENGE TO ETHICAL AND LEGAL SKILLS

Anna Maria Giordano was a 49-year-old female attorney who had recently suffered a major cerebral hemorrhage. I came in contact with Ms. Giordano on one of my off-site clinical rotations when I accompanied a social worker for a day at a large medical center. According to most of the nurses and physicians, and the documentation in her chart, her prognosis looked very poor. Due to the fact that she was a lawyer, her advance directives were very clear, appearing to say exactly what she wanted. In essence, her advance directives stated that if she was in a comatose condition and that it appeared as if there was no hope for recovery, she did not want life-sustaining treatment. Although testing did not reveal brain death, almost all the physicians agreed that her condition had little to no hope for improvement. However, one neurosurgeon felt that her condition was improving, with hopes for her recovery; therefore, he had no intention of stopping the life-sustaining treatment. Her family members from Boston had come earlier in the week to discuss treatment options and were given two points of view by two different physicians. Upon hearing the determination of a poor prognosis, seeing no improvement in the patient's condition over the past few weeks, and being familiar with her expressed preferences in the advance directive, I felt certain that she would not want life-sustaining treatment continued.

Thinking Outside the Box: Possible Courses of Action

- Ignore the entire situation: It didn't entirely concern me, since I was only observing as a nursing student for 1 day.
- Talk to the social worker about what I thought was stated in the advance directives, and ask why it wasn't being followed.
- Challenge the doctor as to why he was telling the family that the patient was improving when her assessments for the past 3 weeks had shown no improvement.

Evaluating a Good Outcome: How Do I Define Success?

- The patient is properly diagnosed and her wishes from her advance directives are followed as clearly as they are stated.
- Since the patient is unable to speak, her power of attorney is able to convey what the patient would want.
- The family and the patient's power of attorney are fully informed about the patient's condition so that they can make an educated decision based on what the patient would want.
- My personal and professional integrity are affirmed.

Personal Learning: Here's to the Future!

I chose to talk to the social worker about the patient's advance directives. The social worker was very aware of the situation, explaining that in the past, this neurosurgeon had given other patients' families more optimistic views of the situation, refusing to stop life-sustaining treatment. The social worker explained that she was in the process of bringing this issue to an ethics committee to discuss the situation and hoped that something would be resolved. She also explained that advance directives are often difficult to follow precisely. If the patient is unable to communicate, then the power of attorney takes over, trying his or her best to do what the patient would want. At these times, it can become very subjective. Therefore, following the advance directives is not as simple as one would think it would be.

Although my actions were not extraordinary in this situation, I felt that I learned quite a bit about advance directives, especially trying to honor the patient's and family's wishes. I had learned about advance directives in the past in my previous classes. However, this was the first time I had ever had to deal with them in actual practice. I was able to see how difficult it can be when making such an important decision. I was impressed by the way that the social worker was handling the case; I only hope that I would act in a similar fashion if I were ever faced with a situation like this in the future.

Kathryn Southerton, Georgetown University

REFLECTION ON QUALITY AND SAFETY COMPETENCIES

How do you think you would respond in a similar situation? Why? Are there any factors that might affect your response? If so, explain what these factors are and their possible effect. Do you agree with the criteria that the nursing student used to evaluate a successful outcome? Why or why not? What *knowledge, skills,* and *attitudes* do you need to develop to continuously improve the quality and safety of care for patients like Ms. Giordano? Was professional integrity affirmed? Explain.

Patient-Centered Care: How can you deliver thoughtful, patient-centered care for patients with whom you cannot communicate? How can you best communicate empathy and respect for this patient and her family?

Teamwork and Collaboration/Quality Improvement: What do you think might be influencing the neurosurgeon's refusal to end the life-sustaining treatment? How would you respond to this neurosurgeon? What does this tell you about yourself and about the adequacy of your skills for professional practice? The neurosurgeon is in what stage of grief, in your opinion? The nursing student? The social worker? What communication and interpersonal skills do you need to improve to ensure that you function as a member of the patient-care team and to obtain assistance when needed? What does quality care for Ms. Giordano "look like"?

Safety/Evidence-Based Practice: What does the evidence point to as "best practice" for Ms. Giordano? What safety needs does Ms. Giordano have and how can you meet them? Have you ever been involved in a situation involving an advance directive? If so, were the patient's wishes followed? If not, why not?

Informatics: Can you identify the essential information that must be available in Ms. Giordano's electronic record to support safe patient care and coordination of care? Can you think of other ways to respond to or approach the situation? What else might the nursing student have done to ensure a successful outcome?

FIGURE 42-1. A terminally ill patient's husband begins the grieving process.

 THINK back to Yvonne Malic, the 20-year-old single mother of the premature neonate described at the beginning of the chapter. The nurse could use knowledge of anticipatory loss to assist Yvonne in coping with the seriousness of her neonate's condition. •

Grief

Grief is an internal emotional reaction to loss. It occurs with loss caused by separation or by death. For example, many people who divorce experience grief. Loss of a body part, job, house, or pet may also cause grief. Normal expressions of grief may be physical (crying, headaches, difficulty sleeping, fatigue), emotional (feelings of sadness and yearning), social (feeling detached from others and isolating oneself from social contact), and spiritual (questioning the reason for your loss, the purpose of pain and suffering, the purpose of life and the meaning of death). **Mourning** is the actions and expressions of that grief, including the symbols and ceremonies (e.g., a funeral or final celebration of life) that make up the outward expressions of grief. People who are **bereaved** are in a state of grieving from loss of a loved one.

Grief Reactions

Reactions to grief and dying are similar. The stages of these reactions overlap and vary among people (see Factors That Affect Grief and Dying, later in this chapter). One person may skip a reaction stage, whereas another may repeat an earlier stage. Each person is different, and patients and family members may be at different reaction stages. Several theories explain the stages of reactions to grief and death. Two discussed here are by Engel and Kübler-Ross. More important than the actual stages of any given grief reaction is the idea that grief is a process that varies from person to person.

Engel (1964) was among the first to define stages of grief. Engel's six stages are 1) shock and disbelief, 2) developing awareness, 3) restitution, 4) resolving the loss, 5) idealization, and 6) outcome. Shock and disbelief are usually defined as refusal to accept the fact of loss, followed by a stunned or numb response: "No, not me." Developing awareness is characterized by physical and emotional responses such as anger, feeling empty, and crying: "Why me?" Restitution involves the rituals surrounding loss—with death, it includes religious, cultural, or social expressions of mourning, such as funeral services. Resolving the loss involves dealing with the void left by the loss. Idealization is the exaggeration of the good qualities that the person or object had, followed by acceptance of the loss and a lessened need to focus on it. Outcome, the final resolution of the grief process, includes dealing with loss as a common life occurrence.

Kübler-Ross (1969), a pioneer in the study of grief and death reactions, defined five stages of reaction similar to Engel's. These stages—(1) denial and isolation, (2) anger, (3) bargaining, (4) depression, and (5) acceptance—are discussed later in the chapter.

Dysfunctional Grief

Dysfunctional grief is abnormal or distorted; it may be either unresolved or inhibited. In unresolved grief, a person may have trouble expressing feelings of loss or may deny them; unresolved grief also describes a state of bereavement that extends over a lengthy period. With inhibited grief, a person suppresses feelings of grief and may instead manifest somatic (body) symptoms, such as abdominal pain or heart palpitations.

DYING AND DEATH

Dying may occur suddenly as a result of an accident, injury, or illness or it may occur after a prolonged experience of debilitating disease such as cancer, acquired immunodeficiency syndrome (AIDS), or Alzheimer disease.

Definitions of Death

The accurate definition of death has proven difficult over time, as technological advances, such as cardiopulmonary resuscitation, have been able to restore lost functions and "bring a person back to life." The Uniform Definition of Death Act (1981) provides a legal definition of **death** as follows: A person who has sustained either (1) irreversible cessation of all functions of circulatory and respiratory functions, or (2) irreversible cessation of all functions of the entire brain, including the brainstem, is dead. A determination of death must be made in accordance with accepted medical standards.

A Harvard University Medical School committee later added that the irreversible loss of brain function, accompanied by the more traditional signs, should be the definitive definition of death. These "Harvard criteria" are generally accepted with the understanding that errors in certification of death could occur in conditions that might not permanently suspend life processes, such as from hypothermia (extreme cold), drug or metabolic intoxication, or circulatory shock. In addition, special attention must be paid when a child under the age of 5 is involved. Most protocols require two separate clinical examinations. The medical criteria used to certify a death are:

- cessation of breathing
- no response to deep painful stimuli
- lack of reflexes (such as the gag or corneal reflex) and spontaneous movement

These clinical signs may be further confirmed by an electroencephalogram and/or cerebral blood flow study.

Signs of Impending Death

The clinical signs of impending or approaching death include:

- Difficulty talking or swallowing
- Nausea, flatus, abdominal distention
- Urinary and/or bowel incontinence or constipation
- Loss of movement, sensation, and reflexes
- Decreasing body temperature with cold or clammy skin
- Weak, slow, or irregular pulse
- Decreasing blood pressure
- Noisy, irregular, or Cheyne-Stokes respirations
- Restlessness and/or agitation
- Cooling, mottling, and cyanosis of the extremities and dependent areas

As death nears, the patient may have a decreased level of consciousness or agitated delirium. Although decreased consciousness and agitation are both normal at the end of life, they are very distressing to the patient's family.

Good Death

A good death is one that allows a person to die on one's own terms, relatively free of pain, and with dignity. It is free from avoidable distress and suffering for patients, families, and caregivers; in general accord with patients' families wishes; and reasonably consistent with clinical, cultural, and ethical standards (Institute of Medicine [IOM], 1997). The characteristics of a good death vary for each patient, but several factors are important for a good death. These factors include control of symptoms, preparation for death, opportunity to have a sense of completion of one's life, and a good relationship with health care professionals. Although the indicators for care that promote a good death listed in Box 42-1 were developed by the American Geriatrics Society (2007), they apply to people of all ages. Nurses play a critical role in focusing the health care team's attention on meeting the needs of dying people and their families.

Responses to Dying and Death

People have varying attitudes about death. Increasing numbers are choosing to die at home surrounded by loved ones. Others die alone or in intensive care units surrounded by health care professionals and technological equipment. Although each person reacts to the knowledge of impending death or to loss in his or her own way, there are similarities in the psychosocial responses to the situation. Kübler-Ross (1969) studied the emotional responses to death and dying in depth, and nursing and other helping professions have used her findings extensively.

BOX 42-1 | PROVIDING CARE TO FACILITATE A GOOD DEATH

Although death occurs at any age, the probability of death increases as one grows older. These selected position statements by The American Geriatrics Society Ethics Committee (2007) provide guidance for all health care providers in providing excellent care for dying patients of any age.

- The care of the dying patient should be guided by the values and preferences of the individual patient. Independence and dignity are central issues for many dying patients, particularly in older adults. Maintaining control and not being a burden can also be relevant concerns.
- Palliative care of dying patients is an interdisciplinary undertaking that attends to the needs of both patient and family.
- Care for dying patients should focus on the relief of symptoms, not limited to pain, and should use both pharmacologic and nonpharmacologic means.
- Physicians and other health care professionals, at all levels of training, should receive in-depth, insightful, and culturally sensitive instruction in the optimal care of dying patients.
- Adequate funding for research on the optimal care of dying patients is essential to improving end-of-life care.

The stages of dying, much like the stages of grief, may overlap, and the duration of any stage may range from as little as a few hours to as long as months. The process varies from person to person. Some people may be in one stage for such a short time that it seems as if they skipped that stage. Sometimes a person returns to a previous stage. According to Kübler-Ross, the five stages of dying, with common reactions, are:

1. *Denial:* The patient denies the reality of death and may repress what is discussed. The patient may think, "They made a mistake in the diagnosis. Maybe they mixed up my records with someone else's."
2. *Anger:* The patient expresses rage and hostility and adopts a "why me?" attitude: "Why me? I quit smoking and I watched what I ate. Why did this happen to me?"
3. *Bargaining:* The patient tries to barter for more time: "If I can just make it to my son's graduation I'll be satisfied. Just let me live until then." Many patients put their personal affairs in order, make wills, and fulfill last wishes, such as trips, visiting relatives, and so forth. It is important to meet these wishes, if possible, because bargaining helps patients move into later stages of dying.
4. *Depression:* The patient goes through a period of grief before death. The grief is often characterized by crying and not speaking much: "I waited all these years to see my daughter get married. And now I may not be here to see her walk down the aisle. I can't bear the thought of not being there for the wedding—and of not seeing my grandchildren."
5. *Acceptance:* When the stage of acceptance is reached, the patient feels tranquil. The patient has accepted the reality of death and is prepared to die. The patient may think, "I've

tied up all the loose ends: made the will, made arrangements for my daughter to live with her grandparents. Now I can go in peace knowing everyone will be fine."

Terminal Illness

In the case of a **terminal illness**, an illness in which death is expected within a limited period of time, the physician is usually responsible for deciding what, when, and how the patient should be told. The nurse, along with members of the clergy and other health care professionals, may be involved with these decisions and in discussing the condition with the patient. Most patients want to know their diagnosis and prognosis as soon as possible so that they can begin appropriate planning and take care of business and personal affairs. It is critical for terminally ill patients and their families to have some sense of how the disease is most likely to progress and what this will mean for the patient. All who are involved with the patient's care should know exactly what the patient and the family have been told; members of the patient's health care team need to communicate among themselves. *Cultural influences may dictate how much information is desired and which family members are to be informed.* For example, in many traditional Asian families, the patient's family is told the diagnosis and prognosis, not the patient. Since this is now changing, nurses must check local practice standards and policies as well as the preferences of individual patients and families.

Effect on the Patient

Many patients realize without being told that they have a terminal illness, picking up this knowledge from nonverbal communication by their families and by health care professionals. Patients must be allowed to go through the stages of the grieving process and supported in their decision making. Competent patients have the right to consent to and/or refuse any and all indicated medical treatment—even life-sustaining treatment—and should be made aware of this right. In the

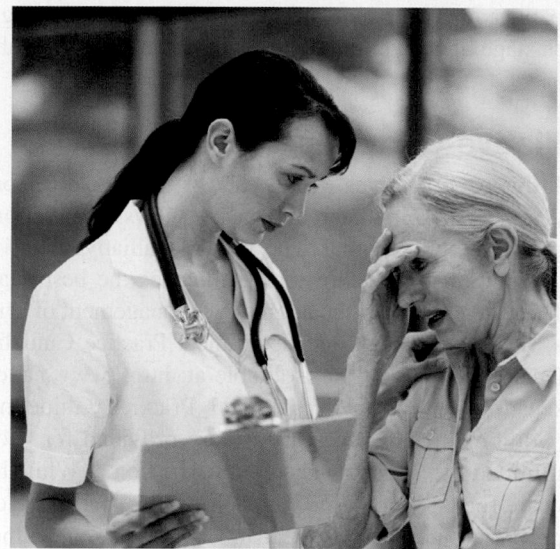

FIGURE 42-2. A nurse offers support to a patient's grieving spouse.

past, patients and family members complained about receiving care they did not want and of not being allowed to die. In today's climate of cost-conscious decision making, some patients and family members are complaining that they are being denied costly life-sustaining treatment because of inadequate personal funds or insurance or because they are deemed a poor "investment" of scarce resources. Remember that a patient's wishes should, if possible, be followed. Box 42-2 lists the rights of people who are dying.

Effect on the Family

The family and significant others of terminally ill patients should be encouraged to participate in planning the patient's care. Health care personnel should be available to discuss the patient's condition with family members and should offer support and care as the family begins the grieving process (Fig. 42-2). The family may want to make arrangements with

BOX 42-2 THE DYING PERSON'S BILL OF RIGHTS

I have the right to be treated as a living human being until I die.

I have the right to maintain a sense of hopefulness, however changing its focus may be.

I have the right to be cared for by those who can maintain a sense of hopefulness, however changing this might be.

I have the right to express my feelings and emotions about my approaching death in my own way.

I have the right to participate in decisions concerning my care.

I have the right to expect continuing medical and nursing attention even though "cure" goals must be changed to "comfort" goals.

I have the right not to die alone.

I have the right to be free from pain.

I have the right to have my questions answered honestly.

I have the right not to be deceived.

I have the right to have help from and for my family in accepting my death.

I have the right to die in peace and dignity.

I have a right to retain my individuality and not be judged for my decisions, which may be contrary to beliefs of others.

I have the right to discuss and enlarge my religious and/or spiritual experiences, whatever these may mean to others.

I have the right to expect that the sanctity of the human body will be respected after death.

I have the right to be cared for by caring, sensitive, knowledgeable people who will attempt to understand my needs and will be able to gain some satisfaction in helping me face my death.

Reprinted with permission from *American Journal of Nursing*, 75(1), 99.

the patient for funeral or memorial services, depending on which stage of grief both the patient and the family members are in.

Palliative Care and Hospice

Palliative care involves taking care of the whole person—body, mind, and spirit, heart and soul. It views dying as something natural and personal. The goal of palliative care is to give patients with life-threatening illnesses the best quality of life they can have by the aggressive management of symptoms. Be sure to check out the Clinical Practice Guidelines for Quality Palliative Care available at: http://www.national consensusproject.org/NCP_Clinical_Practice_Guidelines_ 3rd_Edition.pdf. **Hospice** care is care provided for people with limited life expectancy, often in the home. While hospice care focuses on the needs of the dying, palliative care is appropriate across the spectrum of disease and illness. Both palliative care and hospice are discussed in Chapter 8. Established in 1986, the Hospice and Palliative Care Nurses Association is the nation's largest and oldest professional organization dedicated to promoting excellence in palliative nursing care. Among its aims are assisting members of the nursing team with ensuring quality nursing care delivery, managing complex symptoms along with grief and bereavement, and having difficult conversations (www.hpna.org).

Ethical and Legal Dimensions

Multiple treatment options and sophisticated life-support technologies may make it difficult to draw the line between promoting life and needlessly prolonging the dying process. In these cases, health care decision making is complicated for patients and health care professionals alike. Patients have a legally and morally protected right to consent to or refuse medical therapies. Legal foundations for the patient's freedom to choose include the common law right of self-determination and the constitutionally supported right of privacy (discussed in Chapters 6 and 7). Discussions about legalizing physician-assisted suicide and physician-administered lethal injections ("aid in dying") pose new ethical challenges. As patients and families struggle with end-of-life treatment decisions, they are increasingly looking to nurses for information, advice, and support.

Advance Care Planning

Decisions about health care are becoming increasingly complex. Patients, family members, and health care professionals are voicing frustration as they grapple with complex decisions about prolonging life. Some of the most difficult cases involve patients who are no longer able (competent) to indicate their treatment preferences. Two kinds of written **advance directives** can minimize difficulties by allowing people to state in advance what their choices would be for health care should certain circumstances develop. Living wills provide specific instructions about the kinds of health care that should be provided or foregone in particular situations. A durable power of attorney for health care appoints an agent the person trusts to make decisions in the event of subsequent incapacity. A combination directive is illustrated in Figure 42-3. One popular directive in the United States titled *Five Wishes* (*Aging with Dignity,* 2013) allows people to specify:

1. The person I want to make care decisions for me when I can't
2. The kind of medical treatment I want or don't want
3. How comfortable I want to be
4. How I want people to treat me
5. What I want my loved ones to know

Many means have been suggested to ensure that adult patients have an opportunity to learn about and use advance directives to indicate their wishes about life-prolonging treatment and to appoint surrogate decision makers should they lose decision-making capacity. Nurses play an important role in facilitating this dialogue. In the United States, the Patient Self-Determination Act of 1990 requires all hospitals to inform patients about advance directives. **Because the status of advance directives varies from state to state, nurses must be familiar with federal and state laws concerning these directives.** Nurses can also be instrumental in developing institutional policies that ensure that patients on admission are encouraged to talk with family, significant others, and health care professionals about their treatment preferences (see the Research in Nursing box on page 1609). Important resources for advance care planning include Caring Connections (www.caringinfo.org) and the Consumer's Tool Kit for Health Care Advance Planning (http://apps. americanbar.org/aging/publications/docs/consumer_tool_ kit_bk.pdf).

A **physician order for life-sustaining treatment (POLST) form** is a medical order indicating a patient's wishes regarding treatments commonly used in a medical crisis. Because it is a medical order, a POLST form must be completed and signed by a health care professional and cannot be filled out by a patient. These forms are always completed in close consultation with the patient to ensure that the patient's values and goals of care are accurately represented. These brightly colored forms always remain with the patient, regardless of whether the patient is in the hospital, at home, or in a long-term care facility (www.polst.org). See Box 42-3 (on page 1609) for a description of the differences between an advance directive and POLST form. POLST forms are not available in every state. In some states, such as Maryland, these are called **medical orders for life-sustaining treatment (MOLST) forms.**

Allow Natural Death, Do-Not-Resuscitate, or No-Code Orders

To prevent the improper use of cardiopulmonary resuscitation, which is designed to prevent unexpected death, some physicians write do not resuscitate (DNR), or no code, on the chart of a patient if the patient or surrogate has expressed a wish that there be no attempts to resuscitate the patient. A **do-not-resuscitate order** means that no attempts are to be

D.C., Maryland and Virginia

ADVANCE DIRECTIVE

My Durable Power of Attorney for Health Care, Living Will and Other Wishes

I, _____ , write this document as a directive regarding my medical care.

Put the initials of your name by the choices you want.

PART 1. MY DURABLE POWER OF ATTORNEY FOR HEALTH CARE.

_____ I appoint this person to make decisions about my medical care if there ever comes a time when I cannot make those decisions myself:

NAME _____ PHONE HOME _____ WORK _____

ADDRESS _____

_____

If the person above cannot or will not make decisions for me, I appoint this person:

NAME _____ PHONE HOME _____ WORK _____

ADDRESS _____

_____

_____ I have not appointed anyone to make health care decisions for me in this or any other document.

I want the person I have appointed, my doctors, my family, and others to be guided by the decisions I have made below:

PART 2. MY LIVING WILL.

These are my wishes for my future medical care if there ever comes a time when I can't make these decisions for myself.

A. **These are my wishes if I have a *terminal condition*:**
   Life-Sustaining Treatments

   _____ I do not want life-sustaining treatments (including CPR) started. If life-sustaining treatments are started, I want them stopped.
   _____ I want life-sustaining treatments that my doctors think are best for me.

   _____ Other wishes: _____

   Artificial Nutrition and Hydration

   _____ I do not want artificial nutrition and hydration started if it would be the main treatment keeping me alive. If artificial nutrition and hydration is started, I want it stopped.
   _____ I want artificial nutrition and hydration even if it is the main treatment keeping me alive.

   _____ Other wishes: _____

   Comfort Care

   _____ I want to be kept as comfortable and free of pain as possible, even if such care prolongs my dying or shortens my life.

   _____ Other wishes: _____

B. **These are my wishes if I am ever in a *persistent vegetative state*:**

   Life-Sustaining Treatments

   _____ I do not want life-sustaining treatments (including CPR) started. If life-sustaining treatments are started, I want them stopped.
   _____ I want life-sustaining treatments that my doctors think are best for me.

   _____ Other wishes: _____

FIGURE 42-3. Example of an advance directive (Used with permission of District of Columbia Hospital Association, Washington, DC.) *(continued)*

Artificial Nutrition and Hydration

_____ I do not want artificial nutrition and hydration started if it would be the main treatment keeping me alive.
If artificial nutrition and hydration is started, I want it stopped.
_____ I want artificial nutrition and hydration even if it is the main treatment keeping me alive.
_____ Other wishes: _____

Comfort Care

_____ I want to be kept as comfortable as possible, even if such care prolongs my dying or shortens my life
_____ Other wishes: _____

C. **Other Direction**

You have the right to be involved in all decisions about your medical care, even those parts not dealing with terminal conditions or persistent vegetative states. If you have wishes not covered in other parts of this document, please indicate them here.

_____

_____

PART 3. OTHER WISHES.

A. **Organ Donation**

_____ I do not wish to donate any of my organs or tissues.
_____ I want to donate all of my organs and tissues.
_____ I only want to donate these organs and tissues: _____
_____ Other wishes: _____

Autopsy

_____ I do not want an autopsy.
_____ I agree to an autopsy if my doctors wish it.
_____ Other wishes: _____

If you wish to say more about any of the above choices, or if you have any other statements to make about your medical care, you may do so on a separate sheet of paper. If you do so, put here the number of pages you are adding: _____

PART 4. SIGNATURES.

You and two witnesses must sign this document for it to be legal.

A. **Your Signature**

By my signature below I show that I understand the purpose and the effect of this document.

SIGNATURE _____ DATE _____

ADDRESS _____

B. **Your Witnesses' Signatures**

I believe the person who has signed this advance directive to be of sound mind, that he/she signed or acknowledged this advance directive in my presence, and that he/she appears not to be acting under pressure, duress, fraud or undue influence. I am not related to the person making this advance directive by blood, marriage or adoption, nor, to the best of my knowledge, am I named in his/her will. I am not the person appointed in this advance directive. I am not a health care provider or an employee of health care provider who is now, or has been in the past, responsible for the care of the person making this advance directive.

Witness #1

SIGNATURE _____ DATE _____

ADDRESS _____

Witness #2

SIGNATURE _____ DATE _____

ADDRESS _____

FIGURE 42-3. _(continued)_

RESEARCH IN NURSING

BRIDGING THE GAP TO EVIDENCE-BASED PRACTICE

Quality End-of-Life Care for Patients Receiving Dialysis

Many studies have been done about what constitutes a "good death" and quality end-of-life care in the United States and Canada. Advance care planning has been shown to improve end-of-life care as it allows patients to receive information on their prognosis, treatment options, and burdens, then decide and communicate what care they wish to receive as their health deteriorates. A group of Irish nurses realized that advance directives have no legal standing in Ireland and very few people are aware of their existence. They decided to interview patients receiving hemodialysis to elicit their views about death, dying, and advance care planning.

Related Research

Collins, M., & Lehane, E. (2013). Perspectives on death, dying and advance care planning from patients receiving haemodialysis. *Journal of Renal Care, 39*(1), 5–11. DOI: 10.1111/j.1755–6686.2013.00340.x

A cross-sectional, quantitative, descriptive design was used with a convenience sample of 50 patients receiving hemodialysis. Data were collected by means of a researcher-administered questionnaire and analyzed using descriptive statistics. The majority of participants interviewed were comfortable talking about death, but not necessarily among family, with most desiring medical interventions to prolong life. The control of pain and other symptoms, being physically comfortable, and being at peace spiritually were the most important issues at end of life. This study provided insight into what is important to patients in relation to death, dying, and advance care planning.

Relevance to Nursing Practice

A group of nurses caring for a particular understudied population, patients receiving dialysis, used data from U.S. and Canadian sources to test its applicability in Ireland. What they discovered from their interviews will guide nursing's efforts to plan and deliver quality end-of-life care for patients receiving dialysis in Ireland. Since advance care planning is important for this population, nurses will need to support efforts to achieve legal standing for advance care planning in Ireland.

For additional research, visit thePoint.

---

made to resuscitate a patient whose breathing or heart stops. Some facilities use the term **allow natural death (AND) order** for do not resuscitate order since it is easier for families to authorize doing something positive rather than preventing something (resuscitative efforts) that is usually perceived to be helpful. You may also see a do not intubate or (DNI) order. Many physicians are reluctant to write these orders, however, especially when this issue is a source of conflict between the patient and family or between individual family members.

In some cases, a physician who believes the patient will not benefit from resuscitative measures may indicate verbally to the nurse that only a slow-code (or "show-code") should be called; that is, in the case of cardiopulmonary or respiratory arrest, calling a code and resuscitating the patient are to be delayed until these measures will be ineffectual. Many health care institutions have policies forbidding this, and a nurse could be charged with negligence in the event of a slow-code and resulting patient death. Be sure to check your agency's policies.

The standard of care still obligates health care professionals to attempt resuscitation if a patient's breathing or heart stops (cardiopulmonary arrest) and there is no AND or DNR order to the contrary. For this reason, nurses must clarify a patient's code status if the probable benefits of resuscitation are negligible or if the nurse has reason to believe a patient would not want to be resuscitated. Many states now allow patients living at home to craft POLST/MOLST orders that allow emergency medical technicians called to the home in the event of cardiopulmonary arrest to respect the patient's wishes not to be resuscitated.

Comfort Measures Only and Other Special Orders

When a discussion is taking place about resuscitation, it is appropriate to question also the use of other life-sustaining

---

BOX 42-3 PRIMARY DIFFERENCES BETWEEN AN ADVANCE DIRECTIVE AND A POLST FORM

Advance Directive

- For anyone 18 and older
- Provides instructions for **future** treatment
- Appoints a Health Care Representative
- Does not guide Emergency Medical Personnel
- Guides inpatient treatment decisions when made available

POLST

For persons with serious illness — at any age

- Provides medical orders for **current** treatment
- Guides actions by Emergency Medical Personnel when made available
- Guides inpatient treatment decisions when made available

Used with permission. POLST and Advance Directives. Available at http://www.polst.org/advance-care-planning/polst-and-advance-directives/

interventions, such as dialysis, ventilatory support, artificial nutrition and hydration, blood transfusions, antibiotics and other medications, and surgery. Whereas some patients may want aggressive life-sustaining treatment and such treatment may be medically beneficial, other patients may be at a point in their illness at which they choose to terminate all life-sustaining measures and allow the disease to progress naturally to death. There is no moral obligation to initiate or continue the use of life-sustaining treatment that is minimally effective or is a burden. However, laws may place constraints on those who decide to withhold or withdraw life-sustaining treatment for incompetent patients. Nurses should know pertinent federal and state laws and the policies in their institution or agency concerning the withholding or withdrawing of life-sustaining treatment. Nurses should also be familiar with the forms used to indicate patient preferences about end-of-life care.

Patients or their surrogates may request a **comfort-measures-only order**, which indicates that the goal of treatment is a comfortable, dignified death and that further life-sustaining measures are no longer indicated. A do-not-hospitalize order is often used for patients in long-term care and other residential settings who have elected not to be hospitalized for further aggressive treatment.

Terminal Weaning

Terminal weaning is the gradual withdrawal of mechanical ventilation from a patient with a terminal illness or an irreversible condition with a poor prognosis. In some cases, competent patients wish their ventilatory support to be ended; more often, the surrogate decision makers for an incompetent patient determine that continued ventilatory support is futile. Although it may be expected that a patient will not survive the weaning, death is never a certain outcome, and it is not unusual for a patient to begin spontaneous respirations once ventilatory support is withdrawn and live for several hours to several days. Competent patients and family members should be prepared for all possibilities. A nurse's role in terminal weaning is to participate in the decision-making process by offering helpful information about the benefits and burdens of continued ventilation and a description of what to expect if terminal weaning is initiated. Supporting the patient's family and managing sedation and analgesia are critical nursing responsibilities. Unfortunately, many agencies and institutions do not have policies covering this issue. Nurses involved in terminal weaning should consult the literature and be familiar with the latest research.

Voluntary Cessation of Eating and Drinking

As seriously ill, competent patients make end-of-life treatment decisions, they may also choose to refuse food and fluid with the intention of hastening death. It is important to distinguish the voluntary act of a patient who is still capable of eating and drinking making the decision to refuse food and fluids from the natural anorexia and loss of thirst that frequently accompany the end stages of dying. While some consider this to be a form of suicide, others view this as a decision to forego life-sustaining treatment. When nurses care for patients who want to refuse food and fluids, they must ensure that this is an informed and voluntary choice and remember that honoring this preference requires the support of the family, physician, and health care team who focus on palliative measures as the dying process unfolds (Quill & Byrock, 2000, p. 410).

Active and Passive Euthanasia

Euthanasia literally means "good dying." **Active euthanasia** is taking specific steps to cause a patient's death, while *passive euthanasia* is defined as withdrawing medical treatment with the intention of causing the patient's death. In other words, active euthanasia is *doing something* to end a patient's life, whereas passive euthanasia is *not doing something* to preserve a patient's life. In assisted suicide (which could be considered a form of active euthanasia), the clinician provides the patient with the means to cause one's own death (e.g., provides a prescription for a lethal dose of barbiturates). In active euthanasia, the clinician acts directly to cause the death of the patient (e.g., administers a lethal dose of medication).

Until recently, most societies maintained that the distinction between "killing" and "allowing to die" was morally relevant. This meant that passive euthanasia, the withholding or withdrawing of medically ineffective or disproportionately burdensome therapies, was morally and legally justified even when this hastened or directly caused a patient's death. On the other hand, making a lethal combination of drugs available to a patient wishing to die (assisted suicide) or administering a lethal injection or carbon monoxide, even when performed with compassionate intent at the request of a patient (active euthanasia), was deemed both immoral and illegal. Some are questioning this distinction today, and efforts are underway to legalize assisted suicide and active euthanasia in numerous countries. In the United States, at the time this text went to press, physician-assisted suicide was legal in Oregon, Washington, Montana, and Vermont. Nurses should understand the arguments for and against assisted suicide and active euthanasia and clarify what they believe (Box 42-4).

The American Nurses Association (ANA, 1994, 2013) issued position statements stating that assisting in suicide and participating in active euthanasia are in violation of the Code for Nurses, the ethical traditions and goals of the profession, and its covenant with society. Yet nurses may be confronted by patients who seek assistance in ending their lives. Unless you think through this issue carefully, you will be unprepared to respond to the request, "Nurse, please help me die." The American Nurses Association's Position Statement on Euthanasia, Assisted Suicide, and Aid in Dying can be reviewed at http://www.nursingworld.org/MainMenu Categories/EthicsStandards/Ethics-Position-Statements/ Euthanasia-Assisted-Suicide-and-Aid-in-Dying.pdf.

BOX 42-4 ETHICAL CHALLENGES: THINKING CRITICALLY ABOUT ASSISTED SUICIDE AND ACTIVE EUTHANASIA

Nurses are often the first to hear a patient's plea, "Please help me die." It is critical for nurses to reflect carefully on what they believe about assisted suicide and active euthanasia and how this influences the responses they make to patients. In 2013, assisted suicide is illegal in all states in the United States except Oregon, Washington, Montana, and Vermont.

- Should the principle of respect for autonomy be expansive enough to embrace respect for, and acquiescence to, a competent patient's request for assistance in dying?
- Does the right to privacy entail a right, in effect, to decide the time and manner of one's death and to gain assistance in implementing that decision?
- Is there such a thing as *rational* suicide?
- If assisted suicide and active euthanasia were to become accepted practices, would this simply represent a logical, defensible extension of the well-established moral basis for refusal of treatment and withholding/withdrawing treatment?

- Are assisted suicide and active euthanasia acts of mercy, morally grounded in the principles of benefiting and not harming patients and expressive of the virtues of compassion and beneficence?
- Is it possible to conceive of situations in which a nurse or a physician has a duty to help a patient die (specifically via active euthanasia or assisted suicide)?
- Is refusal to accede to a patient's request for assisted suicide or active euthanasia a form of abandonment, or are there limits to the duty to respect autonomy, right to privacy, and self-determination?
- Are calls for assisted suicide and active euthanasia emblematic of failure to provide adequate palliative care and to address the suffering of the dying?
- If medicine and nursing possess an "internal" morality, are assisted suicide and active euthanasia consistent with that morality?

Palliative Sedation

Palliative sedation is the lowering of patient consciousness using medication for the express purpose of limiting patient awareness of suffering that is intractable and intolerable (Kirk & Mahon, 2010). When patients who are imminently dying have pain and suffering that is unresponsive to other palliative interventions, palliative sedation to unconsciousness may be considered. Some are concerned that palliative sedation to unconsciousness offers a "back door" to euthanasia, since death is hastened for an unconscious patient who is not being artificially fed. Be sure to check your agency policies. Most restrict palliative sedation to unconsciousness to the imminently dying and exclude patients asking for such sedation for existential suffering or angst.

Death Certificate

U.S. law requires that a death certificate be prepared for each person who dies and specifies what information must be included. Death certificates are sent to local health departments, which compile many statistics from the information. The mortician assumes responsibility for handling and filing the death certificate with proper authorities. A clinician's signature is required on the certificate (check your state law to see if nurses can sign death certificates), as well as that of the pathologist, the coroner, and others in special cases. The nurse is responsible to ensure that the death certificate is signed.

Organ Donation

Patients who express a wish to donate functional organs, such as heart, corneas, liver, lungs, and kidneys, can fill out an organ donor consent card. In addition, depending on state law, signing the back of one's driver's license indicates approval of organ donation. The family of a deceased patient also may decide to donate the patient's functional organs. The nurse should be able to review options and provide consent forms to interested patients and their families. Until recently, most organs were retrieved from totally brain-dead patients. New protocols for retrieving organs from non–heart-beating cadavers are raising multiple practice concerns. Comprehensive attention to optimal patient and family care at the time of withdrawal of life-sustaining therapy needs to remain the nurse's priority. The scarcity of organs has resulted in legislation mandating hospitals and other health care agencies to notify transplantation programs of potential donors. Consult the United Network for Organ Sharing (UNOS), the private, nonprofit organization that manages the nation's organ transplant system under contract with the federal government, to learn more about donation and transplantation (www.unos.org).

 THINK back to Mr. Perez, who was asking about advance directives and organ donation after his wife was found to have massive, irreversible brain damage. The nurse could incorporate knowledge of organ donation to provide appropriate information for Mr. Perez so that he can make the most informed decision possible. ●

Autopsy

An autopsy is an examination of the organs and tissues of a human body after death. Consent for autopsy is legally required. The closest surviving family member or members usually have the authority to give or refuse consent. Some religious groups prohibit autopsies except for legal purposes.

It is usually the physician's responsibility to obtain permission for an autopsy. Sometimes the patient may grant this permission before death. The nurse can assist by explaining the reasons for an autopsy. Many relatives find comfort when they are told that the knowledge gained from an autopsy may contribute to advances in medical science as well as establish the exact cause of death.

If death is caused by accident, suicide, homicide, or illegal therapeutic practice, the coroner must be notified, according to law. The coroner may decide that an autopsy is advisable and can order that one be performed, even if the patient's family has refused consent. In some cases, a death that occurs within 24 hours of admission to the hospital must be reported to the coroner.

FACTORS THAT AFFECT GRIEF AND DYING

Many factors, including age, family relationships, socioeconomic position, and cultural and religious influences, affect a person's reaction to and expression of grief. Like the stages of grief reaction, these factors vary from person to person.

Developmental Considerations

Children do not understand death on the same level as adults do, but their sense of loss is just as great. Both terminally ill children and their siblings are likely to talk about and ask questions about death in an attempt to understand it. Terminally ill children require parental love and support as well as social interaction with other children. Death of a parent or another significant person can retard a child's development or may cause the child to regress developmentally. Children need to go through the same grief reactions as adults to accept such a loss and maintain emotional well-being.

The loss of a parent by a middle-aged adult helps to prepare the adult for the loss of a spouse or significant other and to accept one's own eventual death. Older people may lose a spouse or friends and relatives their own age. As this happens, they reminisce about life, put their lives and the purpose of living in perspective, and prepare themselves for their own inevitable death.

Family

Family roles have an important effect on a person's reactions to and expressions of grief. For example, the eldest sibling may feel a need to "be strong" and, therefore, may not grieve openly; a person who loses a spouse may display the same type of behavior to "protect the children."

The death of a child is a devastating experience for the family. The family needs time to accept the reality of the situation, opportunities to talk and to be listened to, and the experience of being able to express themselves behaviorally in a nonjudgmental environment. For example, the family of a terminally ill child may express feelings of guilt by wondering if they were responsible for the impending death. A sibling may suppress a guilt feeling for having wished the ill child (or a parent) dead.

Socioeconomic Factors

A bereaved family may suffer more acutely if there is no health or life insurance or pension after the death of the family provider. Such families face not only the loss of a loved one, but also an economic loss that may further disrupt family life. Older people especially may be placed in a difficult position because the death of a spouse may result in the decrease or even elimination of a source of retirement income for the surviving spouse. This reduction in income may lead to loss of home, community, and support systems.

Cultural, Gender, and Religious Influences

Culture influences a person's expression of grief. In many families in the Western culture, grief is a private matter shared only with the family. As such, many people internalize their feelings of grief and may not express their feelings of loss to others. On the other hand, cultural background may necessitate that the patient's and family's public display be emotional and distressed, with loud weeping and moaning.

Although gender roles have become less differentiated in the past few decades, male and female reactions to death may differ. Whereas men are often expected to be stoic and not cry in public, women may be judged as "cold" if they do not grieve publicly. A widow who has a job may not be as emotionally distraught as a woman who needed her husband for financial and other support. Likewise, a widower who has not taken care of the children or the house may view the future more bleakly than a man who has cooked meals and changed diapers. Some ethnic traditions may be ingrained in certain people. For example, the woman may be expected to be weak and need support, whereas the man may be expected to be emotionally supportive. This varies from culture to culture and from person to person.

Faith and religious practices play an important role in the expression of grief and provide comfort and solace to the person experiencing loss. At the same time, others may blame God for their suffering and the death of their loved one and turn away from God. Many people who have put spiritual matters in the background of their lives have found death to be an impetus for a return to earlier practices of religion. The thought of death also invites many to contemplate life's big questions: Is there life after death? Is there a supreme being? And if there is a supreme being, where do I stand in relationship to that being? What is the ultimate source of meaning in my life? See Chapter 45 for a discussion of spiritual care.

Cause of Death

The grief response often depends on the cause of death. Many deaths are sudden and involve shock as well as normal grieving in the survivors. Death from disease may generate several types of responses, including the belief that the death is a punishment (e.g., when AIDS was first diagnosed in homosexuals and drug users), terror and panic (e.g., when people are reminded of the devastation caused by plagues of earlier centuries), and guilt (e.g., when family and friends believe that they could have prevented the death).

Accidental death is often associated with feelings of bad luck. The guilt response can be enormous, especially when children die as the result of an accident. Death while

PROMOTING HEALTH 42-1

GRIEVING

If a past or current loss is influencing your everyday functioning, use the assessment checklist to see how well you are responding to the losses in your life. Then develop a prescription for self-care by choosing appropriate behaviors from the list of suggestions.

Assessment Checklist

❑ almost always	❑ sometimes	❑ almost never

❑ ❑ ❑ 1. I can name the personal losses that are currently influencing my state of well-being.

❑ ❑ ❑ 2. I have a plan for coping with these losses that is in place and helping me to cope.

❑ ❑ ❑ 3. I understand the importance of grieving, and I actually set time aside for this self-care measure.

❑ ❑ ❑ 4. I am comfortable with my feelings and am able to give them expression.

❑ ❑ ❑ 5. There is someone who knows and accepts me well enough to allow me to share openly and honestly.

❑ ❑ ❑ 6. I value being a supportive presence for people with life-threatening illnesses.

❑ ❑ ❑ 7. I respond genuinely to the concerns and feelings of dying patients and their families; I am not afraid to cry with patients and to allow my feelings to show.

Self-Care Behaviors

1. Make a list of the losses that are interfering with your present state of well-being. These may include the loss of health, valued role, image/reputation, relationship, material object, job, or person.

2. Determine whether or not you are addressing these losses in a conscious fashion, and identify coping strategies that may be of help.

3. Try implementing a "tried and true" or new coping strategy.

4. Talk about one of these losses with a friend, religious leader, or counselor/therapist. Assess your comfort level in sharing your feelings openly. Ask the person you are sharing with how that person thinks you are responding.

5. Be honest about any maladaptive coping strategies you may be using to cope such as addictions, apathy ("Who cares?"), withdrawal and passivity, depression, and acting out. Got any help you need to replace these maladaptive coping measures.

6. Reflect on what your level of comfort in being with people who are dying reveals about your own acceptance of the fact that we will all die.

---

defending a country usually is viewed by most of society as honorable and necessary. Violent deaths occur daily, especially in larger cities. Suicide accounts for a great number of violent deaths; in fact, among teenagers, it has become a major concern. It is also believed that many accidental deaths are actually suicides.

THE NURSE AS ROLE MODEL

Holistic care of the terminally ill patient and family almost always involves some personal emotional investment. It is unrealistic and unfair to expect nurses to handle circumstances surrounding death without feelings. The best policy seems to be taking the time to explore one's own feelings and express them (see Promoting Health 42-1).

A nurse who neglects to deal with personal feelings about life, dying, and death is in a questionable position for analyzing and considering the needs of patients facing death. A nurse's own feelings play a major role in determining the care given to a patient with a terminal illness. Some questions nurses should use to help clarify their thinking and feelings about dying and death follow:

- If I could control the events that result in my own death, where would I want to be? What cause of death would I choose? Whom would I want to have present during my terminal illness?
- What fears do I have about death?

- How would I answer these same questions for a patient for whom I have been caring?
- How could I improve the quality of care for a terminally ill patient for whom I am caring?
- If I were a member of the patient's family, what things would I want a nurse to do for me?

Nurses who care for a patient for an extended period may undergo a grief reaction when the patient dies (Fig. 42-4).

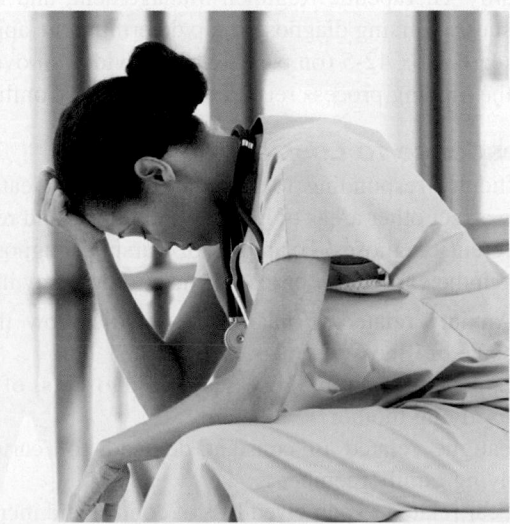

FIGURE 42-4. A nurse grieves the loss of a patient.

Grief after the death of a patient is natural; nurses should allow themselves to go through the grieving process rather than shut off the grief. Nurses should also address their personal health needs.

THE NURSING PROCESS FOR GRIEVING OR DYING PATIENTS AND FAMILIES

The nursing process is a helpful tool when caring for patients who are grieving or dying as well as caring for their families and significant others.

Assessing

Focused assessment for those experiencing loss, grief, and dying is directed toward determining the adequacy of the patient's and family's knowledge, perceptions, coping strategies (see Chapter 41), and resources. Pertinent interview questions are highlighted in Focused Assessment Guide 42-1. Physical assessment of both the dying patient and of concerned family, friends, and family caregivers is essential to diagnosing problems.

Diagnosing

The data the nurse collects about how a patient or the patient's caregivers are responding to an actual or impending loss or to impending death may support several different nursing diagnoses. Samples of these diagnoses and their defining characteristics are provided in the Examples of NANDA-I Nursing Diagnoses box (on page 1616).

Response to Loss as the Problem

Nursing diagnoses that specifically address human responses to loss and impending death in the problem statement include Caregiver Role Endurance, Decisional Conflict, Ineffective Denial, Ineffective Coping, Grieving or Complicated Grieving, Hopelessness, Ineffective Family Therapeutic Regimen Management, and Powerlessness. Nursing diagnoses help determine the appropriate care. Box 42-5 (on page 1617) provides an overview of the nursing process related to Decisional Conflict.

Response to Loss as the Etiology

Difficulty responding to loss or impending death may also affect other areas of human functioning and result in different diagnoses. Examples of nursing diagnoses for which the experience of loss as the etiology may include:

- Anxiety related to inability to predict how the last stage of illness will play itself out
- Interrupted Family Processes related to stress of caring for dying mother
- Fatigue related to constant demands of caring for dying family member
- Fear related to perceived loss of control and increasing need to be dependent in final stages of illness

- Deficient Knowledge related to lack of experience in caring for dying family member at home
- Situational Low Self-Esteem related to inability to accept need for assistance as disease progresses
- Spiritual Distress related to inability to reconcile diagnosis and pain with belief in a loving God
- Bathing, dressing, or feeding Self-Care Deficits related to decreasing strength as terminal illness progresses

Outcome Identification and Planning

Nursing care should be directed toward the achievement of the following goals or outcomes for grieving and dying patients and their families. The patient or family will:

- Demonstrate freedom to express feelings, needs, fears, and concerns
- Identify and use effective coping strategies
- Accept need for help as appropriate and use available resources
- Make health care decisions reflecting personal values and goals; ultimately feel peaceful about role in decision making
- Declare preferences regarding treatment options
- Report sufficient relief of pain to interact meaningfully with family and to attend to everyday concerns
- Experience a dignified and comfortable death
- Resolve grief after a suitable period of mourning and resume meaningful roles and daily activities (family or significant others)

The patient and the family should take an active role in planning for care. Such planning takes the patient's preferences into consideration, facilitates the acceptance of death by the patient and the family, and provides interventions to meet holistic needs.

Implementing

In addition to promoting a comfortable, dignified death, the nurse's aims in caring for dying patients and their families include facilitating coping of the dying person and family and promoting health and preventing illness of the family. The accompanying display, Focus on the Older Adult, (on page 1618) provides indicators for a comfortable, dignified, and peaceful death.

Developing a Trusting Nurse–Patient/Family Relationship

Communication is a lifelong need up to the moment of death and should be maintained at all times with the patient and family. To develop meaningful communication, the nurse must develop a trusting relationship with the patient. The nurse needs listening skills and the ability to recognize both verbal and nonverbal cues given by the patient and family. These skills are discussed in Chapter 20.

Be willing to discuss the patient's fears and doubts openly and to serve as a nonjudgmental listener. However, talking with dying patients is often difficult. The

(text continues on page 1618)

FOCUSED ASSESSMENT GUIDE 42-1

THE EXPERIENCE OF LOSS, GRIEF, DYING, AND DEATH

Assessment Priorities

- Patient and family's understanding of medical condition, prognosis, and dying process
- Patient and family's attitude toward death and dying and knowledge of the dying process
- Patient's preferences for end-of-life treatment and care: desire to be at home or in a hospital; decisions concerning treatment, resuscitation, advanced life support, organ donation, and the like
- Documented evidence of advance care planning
- Existence of advance directive **(It is critical that the authorized decision maker be known to all members of the health care team.)**
- Religious beliefs
- Cultural influences
- Stage of grief and death reaction
- Adequacy of coping behaviors
- Adequacy of resources
- Physiologic needs of the patient, for example, personal hygiene, pain control, nutritional and fluid needs
- Psychological needs of the patient and family, for example, fear of the unknown, pain, separation
- Spiritual needs of the patient and family: need for meaning and purpose, for love and relatedness, for forgiveness, for hope

Factors to Assess	Questions and Approaches
Adequacy of knowledge base	What have you been told about your condition? What do you know about this condition? Please describe what you have been told about your treatment options. Is there anything you don't understand about what your doctor is recommending? What else would you like to know about your present condition and treatment options? Do you know how to contact your doctor and to get the information you need/desire? *Objective is to identify whether or not the patient's and family's knowledge will allow them to make informed decisions that will serve their best interests.*
Realism of expectations/ perceptions	Have you had any previous experiences with this condition or with the death of someone you love? What are your expectations in this case? How do you see the next few weeks (days) playing out? What are your fears, hopes, concerns, worries? What good do you think might be happening in the midst of all this? *Objective is to discover whether the patient and family have unrealistic expectations or misperceptions about the diagnosis, prognosis, and care options that will interfere with their decision making and coping.*
Adequacy of coping strategies	Dealing with our own dying is a once-in-a-lifetime experience, and sometimes we begin the process feeling totally unprepared. Tell me something about how you think you are coping with all this. How well do you think those around you are coping? How can I help you develop or tap the resources that will help you to cope better? *Objective is to identify whether the patient and family are using effective coping strategies. If you detect problems, try to identify coping strategies they have used effectively in the past. Also, identify and address destructive habits that have not served them well in the past such as addictions, destructive relationships, passivity, and acting out. Creatively problem solve about new strategies they might try.*
Adequacy of resources	What is helping you to get through this? Do you think the resources available to you are adequate? If the sky was the limit, what help would you wish for? What is interfering with your getting the help you need? What community resources might be of help to you? Are you using these? *Objective is to assess the adequacy of the human, financial, spiritual, and psychological resources available to the patient. Questions should be directed to determining what, if anything, is interfering with the patient using whatever resources are available to facilitate coping.*
Physical response	A physical assessment of the patient and the patient's family and caregivers should be performed. *Objective is to detect problems with coping that result in fatigue, decreased energy, decreased self-care (deficient grooming, unplanned weight loss), and other maladaptive responses.*

EXAMPLES OF NANDA-I NURSING DIAGNOSES

LOSS AND IMPENDING DEATH

Nursing Diagnoses	Related Factors	Sample Defining Characteristics
Death Anxiety	Newly diagnosed terminal illness	"This can't be happening to me.... I know I'm going to die.... Why should I try and fight this? Mother fought this same diagnosis and died, why should I hope to be any different?"
Caregiver Role Endurance	Hospital discharged dying patient because of inadequate insurance	Spouse has dark circles under eyes, reports inability to sleep through the night, decreased appetite, and general lack of energy. "I want to do everything I can for Tony, but I feel so overwhelmed.... I don't think anyone prepared me for everything I now find myself needing to do for him.... I'm always afraid that I'll hurt him or do something wrong." "I don't want to complain, but I miss being able to go out with my friends. Last week, I didn't even get to church because Tony wasn't feeling well Sunday morning and asked me not to leave.... Sometimes I think I'll just go crazy."
Decisional Conflict	Repeat hospitalizations for aspiration pneumonia and new inability to swallow	Family members have requested ethics consult because they are split about pending decisions for initiation of artificial nutrition and hydration as well as advisability of future hospitalizations and continued aggressive treatment; the patient has Alzheimer disease and has been in a long-term care facility for the last 5 years.
Ineffective Coping	Inability to accept death of 42-year-old son who died of a heart attack 2 years ago; failure of coping mechanisms that worked in the past	70-year-old widow who lived alone with son until his death 2 years ago has become a recluse and eats just enough to keep herself alive; seems to exist on gin, cigarettes, and chocolate. "Mothers aren't supposed to outlive their children... why didn't God take me first? I just want to die and be with Bernie...."
Ineffective Denial	Inability to believe that she has AIDS and that husband was bisexual	Patient who is just "getting her life back in order" (left abusive husband 1 year ago and is newly happily remarried) learns that she has AIDS. "This can't be happening to me... after all I've been through... I hear what you are saying but I don't believe you... there must be some mistake...." Breaks next appointment and refuses to respond to repeated urgings to seek treatment.
Grieving	Knowledge that fetus is anencephalic	"I don't know how this can be happening to us.... We've tried to do everything right.... We've waited for this baby for so long.... It's hard to believe that our baby won't be normal and that if what the doctors say is true she will only live for a few hours or days at most...."
Complicated Grieving	Inability to accept death of anencephalic infant; no grief resolution	Two years after birth of anencephalic infant who died 3 days after delivery, couple has failed to come to peace with the child's death; divorce pending; the wife has lost 15 pounds, and her husband complains that she "really let herself go, she quit her job, mopes around the house all day, and isn't interested in anything anymore."
Hopelessness	Inability to accept son's diagnosis of leukemia and favorable prognosis linked to knowledge of death of neighbor's son who had similar diagnosis	"Don't be leading us on.... We know what leukemia means, we have neighbors who lost a son to leukemia.... It's not true that you can treat this...." Parents refuse to believe favorable prognosis; after hearing diagnosis, they become apathetic and withdrawn. "Marge and Joe tried to do everything to save their son and failed, why should we even try? Nothing else in our lives has worked out."

BOX 42-5 NURSING PROCESS RELATED TO DECISIONAL CONFLICT

Patients and the surrogate decision makers for incompetent patients frequently feel overwhelmed when they need to make life-and-death decisions about end-of-life care. The NANDA-I diagnosis for this response follows:

> Decisional Conflict: The state of uncertainty about course of action to be taken when choice among competing actions involves risk, loss, or challenge to values and beliefs (NANDA-I, 2009, p. 293)

Assessment Priorities

The objective of assessment is to identify patients and families who are at high risk for decisional conflict and to provide the support they need to make appropriate end-of-life care decisions that advance the patient's interests before problems develop. Potential problems when this need is overlooked include postponement of decision making, which interferes with the patient receiving optimal care; vacillation in decision making, which disturbs continuity of care for the patient; and escalation of conflict concerning decision making, which may result in a standoff between participating parties—the patient, individual family members, and health care professionals.

- Detect difficulties with making decisions: fear; insufficient or erroneous information; inadequate support; conflict between religious convictions, personal moral beliefs, and choice one wants to make; and reluctance to assume responsibility for making life-and-death decision.
- Identify what is causing the decision making to be hard for the patient or family and what type of information or support could reverse this.
- Identify potential conflicts between what the patient wants and what the patient's family or caregivers believe should be done.
- Observe the patient or the patient's surrogate decision makers for physical signs of distress that reflect feeling overwhelmed by the decision that needs to be made: signs of fatigue and general exhaustion, signs of agitation and distress, and signs of growing anger and alienation.
- Read the chart carefully to identify decisions that are pending and note the lack of movement toward a decision or toward resolution of existing conflict.

Expected Outcomes

The morally and legally valid decision maker will achieve the following:

- Describe care options (including the option of nontreatment), listing the advantages and disadvantages of each
- Seek clarification of options, if necessary, and whatever support is needed
- Express fears, concerns, and hopes
- Make an informed and voluntary choice
- Make end-of-life decisions that reflect the patient's values and goals, advancing the patient's interests
- Make end-of-life decisions that are consistent with the aims of medicine and nursing

Interventions

Nursing measures revolve around identifying and supporting the morally and legally valid decision maker. The following should be considered:

- Competent patients—those who can (1) understand the information needed to make the decision, (2) reason in accord with a relatively consistent set of values, and (3) communicate a preference—have the right to consent to and to refuse any and all indicated medical treatment.
- Surrogates of previously competent patients are to be guided by what is known about the patient's values and preferences. These surrogates may be designated in an advance directive, or there may be state or province law designating a hierarchy of surrogates, such as spouse, parent, adult child, sibling; the morally valid surrogate is the one who best knows the patient and the patient's preferences.
- Surrogates deciding for a never-competent patient (child or profoundly retarded adult) must be guided by a determination of what is in the patient's best interests by referring to more objective and socially shared values.

The nurse clarifies the goal of treatment (cure, stabilization of functioning, preparation for a comfortable and dignified death) and makes sure that treatment decisions are consistent with this goal. Nursing intervention may be helpful in making sure that everyone is clear about the goal of care and changes in the goal of care as the patient's condition changes. Because some physicians are reluctant to accept preparation for a comfortable, dignified death as an appropriate goal of medicine, some patients have received unwanted care that needlessly prolonged their dying. Conversely, decisions are being made today for financial and other reasons that deprive patients of wanted end-of-life care.

The nurse serves as an advocate for the patient and the family unless what the patient or family wants violates the profession of nursing and nursing's code of ethics or one's own conscience. If your beliefs and convictions do not allow you to advocate for a patient or family when what the patient wants is legal and clinically appropriate, you should immediately seek the advice of your supervisor. Interventions include the following:

- Providing whatever information and support the patient or family needs to make an informed and voluntary decision
- Referring the patient or family to sources that can clarify problematic aspects of the decision, such as religious authority, ethicist, legal counsel
- Identifying and addressing coercive influences on decision making, being sensitive to cultural norms; for example, whereas a controlling husband may be violating his wife's freedom to make autonomous choices in one culture, in another, it is customary for the husband (or male elder in the family) to make choices for a woman.

Documentation of end-of-life care preferences of competent, or previously competent, patients is important. This includes a written record of communication, a living will, durable power of attorney for health care, and a medical advance directive. These preferences must be communicated to those who are ordering care.

- Mediating sources of conflict
- Referring patient or family to an ethics consult team or ethics committee if conflict cannot be resolved

FOCUS ON THE OLDER ADULT

MEASURING QUALITY OF CARE AT THE END OF LIFE

The American Geriatrics Society developed the following statement of principles about quality care at the end of life, but these indicators work well for persons of all ages:

1. *Physical and emotional symptoms.* Pain, shortness of breath, fatigue, depression, fear, anxiety, nausea, skin breakdown, and other physical and emotional problems often destroy the quality of life at its end. Symptom management is regularly deficient. Care systems should focus on these needs and ensure that people can count on a comfortable and meaningful end of their lives.

2. *Support of function and autonomy.* Even with an inevitable and progressive decline with fatal illness, much can be done to maintain personal dignity and self-respect. Achieving better functional outcomes and greater autonomy should be valued.

3. *Advance care planning.* Often, the experience of patient and family can be improved just by planning ahead for likely problems, so that decisions can reflect the patient's preferences and circumstances rather than responding to crises.

4. *Aggressive care near death—site of death, CPR, and hospitalization.* Although aggressive care is often justified, most patients would prefer to have avoided it when short-term outcome is death. High rates of medical interventions near death should prompt further examination of provider judgment and care system design.

5. *Patient and family satisfaction.* The dying patient's peace of mind and the family's perception of the patient's care and comfort are extremely important. In the long run, we can hope that the time at the end of life will be especially precious, not merely tolerable. We must measure both patient and family satisfaction with these elements: the decision-making process, the care given, the out-

comes achieved, and the extent to which opportunities were provided to complete life in a meaningful way.

6. *Global quality of life.* Often a patient's assessment of overall well-being illuminates successes and shortcomings in care, which are not apparent in more specific measures. Quality of life can be good despite declining physical health, and care systems that achieve this should be valued.

7. *Family burden.* How health care is provided affects whether families have serious financial and emotional effects from the costs of care and the challenges of direct caregiving. Current and future pressures on funding health care are likely to displace more responsibility for services and payment onto families.

8. *Survival time.* With pressures upon health care resources likely to increase, there is new reason to worry that death will be accepted too readily. Purchasers and patients need to know survival times vary across plans and provider systems. In conjunction with information about symptoms, satisfaction, and the other domains listed here, such measures will allow insights into the priorities and trade-offs within each care system.

9. *Provider continuity and skill.* Only with enduring relationships with professional caregivers can patient and family develop trust, communicate effectively, and develop reliable plans. The providers also must have the relevant skills, including rehabilitation, symptom control, and psychological support. Care systems must demonstrate competent performance on continuity and provider skill.

10. *Bereavement.* Often health care stops with the patient's death, but the suffering of the family goes on. Survivors may benefit with relatively modest interventions.

Used with permission, *The American Geriatrics Society.*

following suggestions by Rancour (personal communication) are helpful:

- Often, when patients initiate conversations about dying, you may feel unprepared for their questions. They can take you by surprise, and can often lead you to believe that the patient expects a crystal ball response. Remember that the purpose of all such discussions is to keep the lines of communication open with the patient. The idea is to keep the subject of dying open to discussion and to communicate to the patient that it does not make you afraid to talk about it. An open-ended statement, such as "Tell me what concerns you the most" provide a means of encouraging communication.

- Some patients may be too fearful to ask physicians such questions. They often approach staff whom they perceive as less intimidating or more approachable. The question often comes in the middle of the night, when there are no distractions, when anxiety or pain may keep the patient awake, when the patient may feel most alone with psycho-spiritual distress. In any case, it is often on the nurse's watch when questions about dying may arise.

- Because of the surprising nature of such questions, you may feel tempted to escape ("I've got to go take that patient's vital signs right now."), or pass the buck ("That sounds like a question for your doctor.") Be vigilant to prevent such behavior and realize that it would only help reduce your own anxiety but would do nothing to assist with the patient's anxiety. It is well within the scope of your professional practice as a competent nurse to provide counseling and death education, especially when the patient asks you for it or indicates an unmet need for such information and support. *When in doubt, ask a question in response, such as* "What do you feel about that?" *or* "What have you been told already?" This will accomplish several things. It will help you regain your composure and will give you more information about what is on the patient's mind so that your intervention can be as specific and responsive to that patient as possible.

- Do not provide false reassurance. Remember that avoiding discussions about death robs the patient of precious time to accomplish goals that produce hope (Box 42-6). People who are dying hope for many

BOX 42-6   ENABLING HOPE IN THE TERMINALLY ILL

These guidelines are the product of an interdisciplinary team of those providing care for the terminally ill. They are presented to encourage anyone providing care for the terminally ill to consider the crucial place of hope in their caring and also their own potential to enable such hope.

Hope

Hope is the ingredient in life that enables an individual both to consider a future and to actively bring that future into being. Hope originates in imagination but must become a valued and realistic possibility for that individual in order to energize action. Hope has the capacity to embrace the reality of an individual's suffering without escaping from it (false hope) or being suffocated by it (despair, helplessness, hopelessness).

Hope is unique to each person. During terminal illness, the future being considered will become more focused, yet hope is essential for an individual to transcend despair and complete crucial life tasks.

Enabling Hope

Acknowledging Individual Uniqueness

To enable such hope, the care provider must acknowledge *the uniqueness of the individual* and take seriously the dreams of the terminally ill person within the changing nature of the illness. Steps that can be taken to translate hope into accomplishment must be considered. For this to happen, care providers need to do the following:

- Consider all language used, and appreciate how easily hopes can be disabled by such terms as "hopeless situation" or "nothing more can be done."
- Encounter the individual's feelings at his or her own level; be willing to stay at that individual's level and allow him or her to lead.
- Be willing to take the necessary time to establish rapport with the individual in order that his or her hopes can be shared in a supportive atmosphere. Where appropriate, use physical contact to build trust.
- Realize the changing nature both of the disease and the accompanying hopes. At one point, a hope for a cure may be the necessary activating force for an individual to undergo treatment; at another, a hope to consider one's dying may give the energy to complete crucial life tasks or endure the many losses of terminal illness.

Granting Control

A factor crucial to the nourishing of hope within an individual is that of *control*. An individual must be willing to take the necessary action to achieve what is hoped for. Terminal illness places many restrictions upon an individual and often robs that person of a feeling of being able to control the situation, thus leading to increasing helplessness and hopelessness. To counter this, efforts must be made not only to support an individual in hoping, but also to grant the person control in bringing realistic hopes into being.

To help support an individual's sense of control in order to enable active hoping, care providers need to do the following:

- Provide honest and accessible information regarding the progress of the illness.

- Allow an individual to express and work through many hopes in order to develop those hopes appropriate to him or her in the present context.
- Allow for freedom of choice regarding treatment options to the degree possible within the setting.
- Maximize the present possibilities for achieving hopes while allowing for the changing realities of terminal illness.

Being Aware of One's Own Feelings

Hope is strengthened by those who care for and support a terminally ill individual. Within the context of illness and suffering, hope may be fragile and must be nurtured in relationships with professional caregivers, family, and friends. To enable hope, care providers must be aware of their own hope for that individual.

Care providers need to do the following:

- Recognize their own assumptions regarding that particular individual and how those assumptions may inhibit the enabling of hope for that person.
- Be aware of how their own hope for that individual may differ from the hope being expressed by that person.
- Resist judging expressed hope and be willing to explore such hope further.
- Accept the individual's present suffering. Avoid giving "false hope" that minimizes the reality of the situation ("It can't be that bad," or "Don't worry, everything will be fine") or encouraging despair by focusing only upon the illness ("God can't possibly heal you now. That cancer's all through you!").

Supporting Spirituality

A component of hope is *spirituality*. Supported by faith in God, hope is the capacity to transcend present suffering, to lift one's perspective to future possibilities, and so to enable that individual to accomplish important life tasks. This capacity to transcend is facilitated by one's belief in the presence of God within the changing context of terminal illness.

To enable this spiritual aspect of hope, care providers need to do the following:

- Accept the individual's own spiritual journey and present level of faith (or lack of).
- Be open to expressed hopes that link with religious belief (e.g., "God will cure me" or "I pray that God will take me home soon").
- Allow for spiritual struggle and its resultant emotions (e.g., anger when "the cancer is back and God has failed to cure me!"). Recognize that the level of spiritual struggle during terminal illness may increase to enable the accomplishment of crucial hope for life tasks such as reconciliation and forgiveness.
- Be prepared to accept the reality of death as an aspect of hope. Accept an individual who has shifted hope to how he or she wishes to die, to life after death, to a meeting with deceased loved ones, and so on.
- Enable an individual to have access to whatever means and rites of religion that will encourage his or her hope.

Courtesy of Ted Creen, D.Min., Palliative Care Pastoral Consultant, 865 2nd Ave. West, Owen Sound, Ontario, Canada; 519-376-7886.

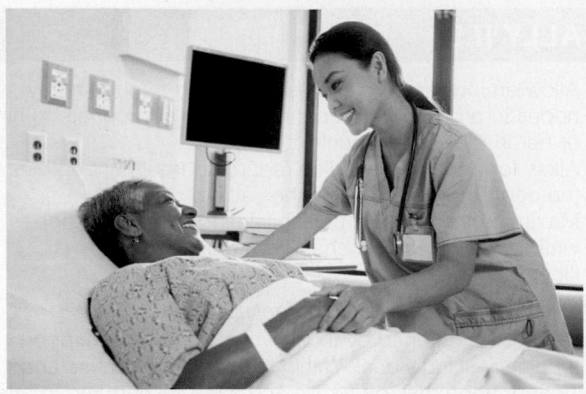

FIGURE 42-5. A nurse displays empathy and compassion.

things even when they cannot hope for a cure, such as hope for freedom from pain, to be surrounded by loved ones, and for the rest of their allotted time to be spent in meaningful pursuits.

A caring nurse feels at ease in crying with the grieving person and sharing experiences with fears, loneliness, and death. This allows the griever the freedom to express one's deepest concerns. Nonverbal communication is equally important. A smile, holding a hand, and eye-to-eye contact are all meaningful (Fig. 42-5). The warmth behind the gesture and the honest concern of the nurse are what count.

Hearing is believed to be the last sense to leave the body; many patients retain their hearing almost to the moment of death. Demonstrate kindness and thoughtfulness by speaking to a comatose patient and encouraging family members to do likewise. Explain to the patient the nursing care being given and the noises in the unit.

Explaining the Patient's Condition and Treatment

All involved health care personnel should know exactly what the patient and family have been told. Telling them different things puts the nurse and other team members at cross-purposes and sets up distrust in the family. Because patients and families often direct questions about the patient's prognosis to the nurse, the nurse should take the initiative in ensuring that terminology, prognosis, and the description of the progress are consistently presented and explained.

Explain the patient's condition and treatment to both the patient and the family. Patience is required during explanations. The patient and family members may be so overwhelmed by the diagnosis that they do not hear all the information that is shared with them. Question them to learn how much they have retained, then repeat the information they missed. Explain care options, as well as the expected outcomes of each option, fully.

Sadly, many health care professionals do not embrace "good dying" as a legitimate aim of medical and nursing care. As a result, the dying of many patients is painfully prolonged because no one initiates a patient/family conference to clarify the treatment goals when cure is no longer an option (see Promoting Health Literacy in Caregivers of Terminally Ill Patients). The nurse plays a key

PROMOTING HEALTH LITERACY

IN CAREGIVERS OF TERMINALLY ILL PATIENTS

Patient Scenario

Marlene Bough is a 47-year-old wife of a 49-year-old man who is nearing the end of his life as a result of widely metastasized thyroid cancer. Mr. Bough was initially diagnosed almost 5 years ago, but treatment is no longer able to control the growth of malignant tumors throughout his body. He has almost constant pain, is unable to walk, and has severe pulmonary and cardiovascular impairments. The doctors have told the couple that no more can be done to prolong Mr. Bough's life and that he has, at the most, less than 6 months to live. Mrs. Bough has taken a family leave from her job as a third-grade teacher so she can care for Mr. Bough at home, even though she is very concerned about being able to care for him and afraid she will cause him further pain.

Nursing Considerations: *Tips for Improving Health Literacy*

Schedule a home care planning meeting for Marlene and others who have indicated a desire to be helpful (daughter, sister-in-law, brother, colleagues at her school) and discuss how each person can help. Include times for family and friends to stay with Mr. Bough so that Marlene can have some time away from the care responsibilities. Demonstrate and have Marlene practice moving Mr. Bough in bed, providing hygiene, and administering pain medications. Discuss the responsibilities of the hospice provider and the goals of palliative care. Provide a written list of phone numbers for health care providers, including those that would be available at any time. Encourage Marlene to ask her husband, "What concerns you most?" and then to talk openly about what kind of treatment he wants for his final days. Include the following questions: "Where do you want to die?", "What kind of medical treatment do you want and do not want?", "What do you consider a good death?", "What kind of funeral service do you want?", and "Where do you want to be buried?" Ensure that advanced planning documents are completed. Encourage Marlene to take some time for herself, to recognize the stress of her husband's care, to welcome the help of others, and to use support people and groups after her husband's death. At that time, ask her to be prepared to ask the following three questions of herself and her health care provider:

• What is my main problem?
• What do I need to do?
• Why is it important for me to do this?

What additional measures can you take to help maintain health literacy in this woman? What other measures would be helpful for Marlene if she did not speak English, could not read, or had other learning disabilities?

role in helping the patient and family prepare for a comfortable and dignified death. Here, the primary focus is palliative, such that the patient and/or family accepts that death is inevitable and now focuses on how to spend the remaining days. For some, this means a referral to hospice or a palliative care program. Nurses play an important role in ensuring that timely prognostic information is given to patients and families so that they can decide how to spend their last days together. Some patients want to "die fighting" and will insist on intensive, life-sustaining treatment until every system fails. Others will choose not to have further treatment and want to spend their last days in a comfortable setting.

Teaching Self-Care and Promoting Self-Esteem

Encourage the patient to retain independence and make decisions as long as possible. Allow the patient to manage personal hygiene practices and self-feeding for as long as possible. After the patient is confined to bed, the creative nurse and family caregivers should attempt to find self-care activities the patient can perform. When physical abilities fail, determining when to take medication, for example, may be all the control the patient can retain.

Having familiar objects in view can help make the patient feel more comfortable and secure. Whether the patient is at home or in a health care agency, it is desirable to have the environment reflect personal preferences. This gives the patient some degree of control when health and other activities of daily living have slipped out of the patient's reach. It also supports self-esteem.

In the transition from independence to interdependence and ultimately to dependence, the patient may experience depression and express frustration and grief about "being a burden." It is crucial for professional

and nonprofessional caregivers to respond to the dying patient as a person of worth whose life has meaning and value. Chapter 20 discusses practical ways in which nurses can use looks, touch, words, and actions to communicate respect and caring.

Teaching Family Members to Assist in Care

Preparing family members to help provide care yields benefits to both the patient and family members. Having loved ones near comforts the patient. Family members, too, are comforted by knowing that they helped comfort the patient. Teach family members how to provide care to the patient. Family members may not want to provide physical care themselves but may want to know what to expect and how they can psychologically aid the patient. Provide assistance in this area by explaining the patient's condition, what treatment the patient is undergoing, and what result the family can expect from the treatment. Knowing the facts may help family members to cope better with impending loss.

Meeting the Needs of Dying Patients

Nursing interventions to meet the needs of dying patients are discussed in this section; examples of dying care activities are provided in the accompanying Examples of Nursing Interventions and Nursing Outcomes Classifications (NIC/NOC) box.

ADDRESSING PHYSIOLOGIC NEEDS

Physiologic care of the patient involves meeting physical needs such as personal hygiene, pain control, nutritional and fluid needs, movement, elimination, and respiratory care. Personal hygiene includes cleanliness of the skin, hair, mouth, nose, and eyes. Frequent baths and linen changes

EXAMPLES OF NURSING INTERVENTIONS AND NURSING OUTCOMES CLASSIFICATIONS (NIC/NOC)

GRIEF RESOLUTION

Nursing Interventions	Nursing Outcomes
• Assist the patient to identify the initial reaction to the loss. • Encourage expression of feelings about the loss. • Listen to expressions of grief. • Make empathetic statements about grief. • Encourage identification of greatest fears concerning loss. • Support progression through personal grieving stages. • Include significant others in discussions and decisions as appropriate. • Communicate acceptance of discussing loss. • Encourage the patient to implement cultural, religious, and social customs associated with the loss. • Assist in identifying modifications needed in lifestyle.	• Resolves feelings about loss • Verbalizes acceptance of loss • Maintains personal grooming and hygiene • Reports adequate sleep • Seeks social support

Bulechek, G., Butcher, H., Dochterman, J., & Wagner, C. M. (Eds.). (2013). *Nursing interventions classification (NIC)* (6th ed., p. 205). St. Louis. Elsevier/Mosby. Moorhead, S., Johnson, M., Maas, M., & Swanson, E. (Eds.) (2013). *Nursing outcomes classification (NOC)* (5th ed., p. 240). St. Louis: Elsevier/Mosby. A full listing of nursing activities for each nursing intervention and outcomes can be found in these books.

may be necessary. The mouth and nose should be kept free of mucus, and secretions should be wiped from the eyes.

The physician determines the medication and dosage needed for pain control, but the patient's wishes should be considered. (See Chapter 34 for a further discussion of pain control.) Some patients prefer and are able to control their own medication. A patient requiring nutritional support should be encouraged to take sips of water or ice chips if still able to swallow. The dying patient may elect to forego artificial nutrition and hydration because the burdens of feeding and hydrating artificially may outweigh the benefits. Problems with elimination include the development of incontinence, constipation, and/or urinary retention. Absorbent pads or a nearby bedpan may be used for patients experiencing incontinence, laxatives or enemas may be used for relieving constipation, and catheterization may be required for urinary retention. Bed linens should be changed often. Periodic movement should also be assisted; regular changes of position help prevent pressure ulcers. Repositioning the conscious patient in semi-Fowler's position can facilitate respirations; positioning the unconscious patient in a semiprone position allows drainage of saliva and mucus. Oxygen therapy may be necessary for some patients.

ADDRESSING PSYCHOLOGICAL NEEDS

When people speak of their fears of death, responses typically include fear of the unknown, pain, separation, leaving loved ones, loss of dignity, loss of control, and unfinished business. Kübler-Ross believes that there is still another, more overwhelming and more significant fear that often is repressed and unconscious: that of the catastrophic, destructive force that has befallen a person and that the person cannot change. Kübler-Ross points out that terminally ill people communicate this fear of a destructive force but do so largely through symbolic language. A person may use nonverbal language, such as a facial expression, a particular kind of handclasp, or, in the case of children, drawings and manner of play with toys. Verbal communication may also be used symbolically.

A fear of isolation, of having to face death alone, is a primary concern of the dying patient. Support the patient by indicating your presence, giving full attention, and showing that you care. Encourage the presence of family members in the room and sharing of reminiscences.

ADDRESSING NEEDS FOR INTIMACY

Terminally ill patients and their sexual partners may feel uncomfortable discussing their needs for intimacy. Partners may wish to be physically intimate with the dying person but are afraid of "hurting" him or her and may also be afraid that an open expression of sexuality is somehow "inappropriate" when someone is dying. Encourage discussion and suggest ways to be physically intimate that will meet the needs of both partners. A loving foot massage or a tender, cradling body embrace may be exactly what a dying person needs in one's last moments.

ADDRESSING SPIRITUAL NEEDS

Although not all patients follow specific spiritual or religious beliefs, most require some form of spiritual care. Many terminally ill patients find great comfort in the support they receive from their religious faith. Help obtain the services of clergy or pastoral care workers as the situation indicates. Most patients need to feel that their lives have meaning; many feel a need for hope in the face of death. Spiritual needs are discussed more fully in Chapter 45.

Meeting the Needs of the Family

The nurse can provide care for the family facing loss by listening to their concerns. Family members need to verbalize their worries and fears; nurses and other health care personnel can provide support by being nonjudgmental listeners. Likewise, nursing care of the grieving family involves communication and listening. Use the communication skills discussed in Chapter 20 and earlier in this section to be a nonjudgmental listener. Feedback to the family can be provided by summarizing or paraphrasing, without questioning the validity of the family's emotions. Be sure that all family members, including children, are able to participate in the grieving process. Family members may need to be reminded to get rest and to eat. Too many visitors may tire the patient; when explanations are offered, most relatives readily understand this.

The reality of death can be made less painful by preparing the family ahead of time. When the process has been explained to the family, they are better prepared to understand the needs of the dying person and how to support the individual.

Explain the steps of the grieving process to all family members ahead of time so that they will recognize the specific stages as they experience them and understand that the process is normal. They can then recognize that other members of the family are going through the same stages, perhaps at different times. This preparation promotes better understanding and communication within the family.

Death creates a change in family roles. As one person (the dying person) leaves a role, adjustments must be made within the family to compensate. Each member plays a part in that compensation, and the nurse can help with these adjustments.

Providing Postmortem Care

When a patient dies, the nurse's responsibilities include caring for the patient's body, caring for the family, and discharging specific legal responsibilities. The last involves ensuring that a death certificate is issued and signed, labeling the body, and reviewing organ donation arrangements, if any.

CARING FOR THE BODY

After the patient has been pronounced dead, the nurse is responsible for preparing the body. The body is placed in normal anatomic position to avoid pooling of blood, soiled dressings are replaced, and tubes are removed. In most cases, it is unnecessary to wash the body; the mortician normally attends to this. Some religions strictly forbid washing of the body, whereas in others a special person must perform it. In cultures in which the family's washing of the deceased's body is considered the last service a family can give a loved one, the family should be given the necessary supplies and left alone in the room with the body. If an autopsy is to be performed, any tubes that were in place should not be removed. In such cases, the nurse should follow the agency's policy.

The nurse is legally responsible for placing identification tags on either the shroud or garment the body is clothed in and the ankle to ensure that the body can be identified even if it is separated from its shroud. The nurse also places an identification tag on the patient's dentures or other prostheses to ensure that the mortician receives these. The importance of proper and complete identification cannot be overemphasized. The patient's body may be placed in the hospital's morgue refrigerator if mortuary arrangements were not made before the patient's death. If the patient died of a communicable disease, the body may require special handling to prevent the spread of disease. Requirements for such handling are usually specified by local laws and depend on the disease-causing organism, mode of transmission, and other characteristics.

CARING FOR THE FAMILY

After a patient has died, the nurse provides support and care to the patient's family (see Through the Eyes of a Student). In most cases, this involves listening to the family's expressions of grief, loss, and helplessness. Because comforting words are often difficult to find, offer solace and support by being an attentive listener. Family members may need to see the patient's body to accept the death fully; in such cases, arrange for family members to view the body before it is discharged to the mortician.

Sudden death creates unique problems for the family. In the case of sudden injury or illness, the physical needs of the patient are paramount to the health care team. This means that family members are not provided as much emotional support or information as they would be if the patient's illness were prolonged, nor are they permitted to exercise as many options regarding the patient's care. The family that loses a member unexpectedly has not had an opportunity to begin the grieving process or to share in grieving with the deceased person. Allow family members to express grief and provide emotional support. Often the family is in the emergency department waiting room when death is confirmed. They are stunned, bewildered, and numb. Do not rush them from the waiting room, but rather provide them with a private place to begin their grieving. Acknowledge their shock and listen to their grief. The family needs guidance in making plans and help in making decisions.

It is appropriate for the nurse who was caregiver or who took care of the patient for a prolonged period to attend the funeral. It also is appropriate for the nurse to make a follow-up call to the patient's family after the funeral or memorial service to offer both concern and care for the family's well-being. Follow-up visits are important to give support to the family. If the nurse assesses that the family is not coping well, appropriate referrals should be made. If the patient was cared for by

THROUGH THE EYES OF A STUDENT

We had had several day-shift clinical rotations, but this was our first evening clinical experience. We were unsure as to what the evening would be like. We knew the evening would provide us with a new outlook on nursing, but we were not prepared for what unfolded.

I had been taking care of a patient when another nursing student asked if I would check in on her patient while she had her dinner break. Each of the students knew this patient because we all had the pleasure of caring for him. I was told he was lying in bed watching television and that he had changed his code status to "DNR" (do not resuscitate) just that day. When I went to check on him, I found him lying in bed but not watching television. His eyes were closed as if he were sleeping peacefully. His mouth was open and his respirations were slow. I spoke his name several times without a response. At the same time, I was also checking for a radial pulse. When I couldn't find his pulse, I swiftly walked to find the instructor. Together we went back to him and assessed his condition. There were no radial or carotid pulses. His chest was now not rising and the instructor listened to his heart with a stethoscope. There wasn't a heartbeat. I stood there feeling helpless and low spirited. This was a man to whom we had all grown close. His family came to see him and to say a few final words. Tears were shed not only by his family but also by those of us who had cared for him.

Our first evening clinical was an extremely emotional night. We were all quiet as we walked down the hallway to go home. The student who was caring for him that night was stopped by his daughter and two young granddaughters. One granddaughter was wearing his hat and the other was carrying his belt. This man's daughter was broken-hearted by his death, yet needed to know that he wasn't alone when he died. The student told her that I had been the one with him. The daughter seemed relieved to know that he was not by himself when he died.

As I look back on that evening, I'm sad that this man is no longer with us. I did not know him for very long, but he touched me in a way that helped me understand the true meaning of nursing: not only to care for the sick, disabled, or enfeebled, but also to be human and offer support for grieving families.

—*Joyce A. Shearman, Delaware County
Community College, Media, Pennsylvania*

a hospice, the family is offered grief support for up to a year following the death.

CARING FOR OTHER PATIENTS

Because nurses in institutional settings often provide care to more than one patient at a time, after the death of one patient, the nurse must continue to provide care to the other patients. Other patients are often aware of a death and may need to be consoled; this is particularly true of a patient who has shared a room with the deceased patient. Other patients may have grief reactions and should be supported through the grief process. Death of a patient may cause depression in other patients and may make them more aware of their own future deaths.

Evaluating

The plan of nursing care for dying patients is effective if patients meet the outcome of a comfortable, dignified death and family members resolve their grief after a suitable time of mourning and resume meaningful life roles and activities. See Nursing Plan of Care 42-1 for Mrs. Esposita and her family.

NURSING PLAN OF CARE 42-1

for Mrs. Esposita and Her Family

Remember Mrs. Esposita, the woman with terminal cancer who is dying at home. The nurse who has been visiting Mrs. Esposita at home asked for assistance from her colleagues in devising a plan of care for Mr. Esposita. Until now, Mrs. Esposita wanted nothing to do with the local hospice because of a reported "bad experience" a neighbor had. Her insurance will not provide for all the home nursing care she needs, and her husband and children have been trying to meet her needs for nursing as well as run the house and meet their own needs. A demanding woman, Mrs. Esposita never seems satisfied with anything anyone does, and the family is looking utterly frustrated, angry, and fatigued. Jorge is coping by "opting out"; he frequently spends the night with friends and doesn't even call home to report on his whereabouts. Marita's grades have fallen, and she has dropped out of cheerleading and other school activities so that she can take care of her mother. Mr. Esposita, who has been silent until now, recently confided that he doesn't know how much longer he can go on this way, and seemed horrified to hear himself say, "I just wish she would die already and get this all over with!" He is very concerned about the changes in his children and feels powerless to change what is happening. For her part, Mrs. Esposita seems oblivious to her family's needs and, even in her weakened state, multiplies pleas for assistance. She seems to be afraid of dying and never wants to be left alone.

NURSING DIAGNOSIS	Caregiver Role Endurance related to multiple losses and burdens associated with caregiving responsibilities as manifested by self-report, breakdown in family relationships, fatigue, and anger
EXPECTED OUTCOME	By the next home visit on 10/17/2015, Mr. Esposita will: • Talk openly about his feelings and share his frustrations about his present situation

NURSING INTERVENTIONS	**RATIONALE**	**EVALUATIVE STATEMENT**
Plan visits for when there is time for private conversation with Mr. Esposita; initiate conversations by telling him that it is not unusual for family caregivers to feel fatigued, powerless, frustrated, angry, and emotionally distant. Encourage him to talk about what he is feeling: "You seemed surprised at yourself when you said that you wished your wife would 'just die.' This isn't an unusual wish for someone in your situation….Tell me more about what you are feeling now…."	This will normalize what Mr. Esposita is experiencing and communicate that someone cares about him and about what he is experiencing. Simply giving voice to what he is feeling and sharing this with a health care professional may help him to accept and address what he takes to be negative and possibly shameful feelings.	10/17/15 Outcome partially met. Mr. Esposita states that he feels better now that he is sharing some of what he's been holding in for such a long time, but he still believes that if he was really a good husband he wouldn't feel this way. Also, states that it is hard for him to find words to express everything that he is feeling. *Revision:* Continue to encourage Mr. Esposita to talk about what he is experiencing and provide a private opportunity for this to happen. *E. McLoughlin, RN*

NURSING PLAN OF CARE 42-1 *continued*

for Mrs. Esposita and Her Family

EXPECTED OUTCOME By 10/17/15, the patient will

- Develop a realistic caregiving plan that matches his ability to care with his wife's need for care and that identifies other resources for his wife's unmet needs

NURSING INTERVENTIONS	RATIONALE	EVALUATIVE STATEMENT
Assist Mr. Esposita to identify what his wife's actual needs for care are, how much of this care it is reasonable to expect the family to provide, and other potential caregiving sources.	Mr. Esposita may need "permission" to not meet his wife's unrealistic expectations. The nurse's authority may be useful in helping him to believe that he can be a good and faithful husband and still fail to meet her expectations. Identifying other caregiving resources will ensure that Mrs. Esposita's needs will be met.	10/17/15 Outcome not met. To date, Mr. Esposita has been unable to identify any additional caregivers for Mrs. Esposita and continues to feel the need to assume all responsibility for her care when he is home.

Revision: Bring list of community resources to Mr. Esposita, including church group, and plan with him to contact these sources. Reinforce that it is OK to ask for help.

E. McLoughlin, RN |
| Explain to Mrs. Esposita that her family may not be able to meet all her needs for care but that every effort will be made to ensure that these needs are met by other caregivers. | Even if the nurse's sympathies are with the family, it is critical to communicate to the patient that you are committed to her and intent on doing all in your power to ensure that her needs are met. If the patient's needs are met, it will improve her relationships with her family. | |
| Assist Mr. Esposita to identify and use new resources: identify at least one new support person who can sit with Mrs. Esposita and relieve the family of some of this burden; explore the family's reluctance to use hospice and evaluate other community resources. Use appropriate referrals. | The family members may be feeling unnecessarily overwhelmed because they have failed to explore the availability of other resources. A gentle push may be needed to make this happen. If a "sitter" can be obtained for several hours in the evening, this would give Mr. Esposita time after work to do something with his children or for himself. | |

EXPECTED OUTCOME By 10/24/15 Mr. Esposita will

- Report feeling more in control and less depressed and angry

(continued)

NURSING PLAN OF CARE 42-1   *continued*

for Mrs. Esposita and Her Family

NURSING INTERVENTIONS	RATIONALE	EVALUATIVE STATEMENT
Lead Mr. Esposita in a discussion that aims to identify everything that is making him feel powerless; then list those factors over which he has no control and those he can influence or change.	This will break the cycle of his thinking that there is nothing at present over which he can exert control. Simply making the list is a first step toward taking action.	10/24/15 Outcome met. Mr. Esposita reports that even though most of his situation remains unchanged, he no longer feels powerless and is less depressed and angry. He expressed gratitude for this intervention and says it has given him new energy.
Provide opportunities for Mr. Esposita to control decision making over those aspects of his life and his wife's care for which he can exert control. Affirm constructive decision making and ask him how it feels to be "back in control" of at least some aspects of his life. Discuss with Mr. Esposita those factors he can change, and assist him in making decisions.	This is an example of "guided discovery"; you are allowing Mr. Esposita to experience himself as once again in charge and to allow this experience to define his self-image. Reinforcement of his success affirms his self-image of one who is in charge. Types of support that can be given to caregivers include emotional (concern, trust), appraisal (affirms self-worth), informational (useful advice), and instrumental assistance or tangible goods.	*E. McLoughlin, RN*

SAMPLE DOCUMENTATION	
	10/24/15, 12 PM, Nursing

Met with Mr. Esposita this morning and talked about the plan to identify other caregivers who might be able to "sit" with his wife on some evenings in order to give him time to do things for his children and himself. He reported no progress in identifying anyone but also stated that he hadn't really made any efforts to locate someone: "Who would want to help us? Besides, I wouldn't want to inflict my wife and her moods on anyone right now." Explained that there are many individuals and groups who provide exactly this type of assistance and that his wife's moods were not uncommon for someone in her situation. Jointly, made a list of possible caregiver resources, including some family members who had earlier expressed an interest in helping out, the parish nurse service from his church, and finally the local hospice. If the first two sources do not work out, will explore family reluctance to use hospice resources more carefully because this may be their best hope. Will evaluate progress made on 10/24/15.

E. McLoughlin, RN

DEVELOPING CLINICAL REASONING

1. Recall personal losses (death of a family member or friend; loss of a significant relationship, job, or opportunity) and recollect what you were experiencing at the time. Try to remember what your expectations were for those to whom you looked for support and how your ability to cope was influenced by whether those expectations were met. Remembering that no two people respond to loss in exactly the same way, develop a list of nursing measures to help patients dealing with loss. Compare your list with those of other students and incorporate their ideas.

2. Compare and contrast the care a patient dying of cancer would receive in a critical care unit and at home with hospice care. Identify the advantages and disadvantages of each. Talk with family members and friends about their preferences. Use your analysis to help describe these options to prospective patients.

3. Role play a situation with a peer in which you counsel a woman with cancer who is told that cure is no longer an option and that she has less than 6 months to live. Reflect on how your experiences, beliefs, and values might affect what you say to patients and how you say it.

PRACTICING FOR NCLEX

1. A nurse midwife is assisting a patient to deliver a full-term baby. The patient is firmly committed to natural childbirth and has attended each natural childbirth class in preparation for labor and delivery. A cesarean delivery becomes necessary when her fetus displays signs of distress. Inconsolable, the patient cries and calls herself a failure as a mother. The nurse notes that the patient is experiencing what type of loss? Select all that apply.
   a. Actual
   b. Perceived
   c. Psychological
   d. Anticipatory
   e. Physical
   f. Maturational

2. A nurse who cared for a dying patient and his family documents that the family is experiencing a period of mourning. Which behaviors would the nurse expect to see at this stage? Select all that apply.
   a. The family arranges for a funeral for their loved one.
   b. The family arranges for a memorial scholarship for their loved one.
   c. The coroner pronounces the patient's death.
   d. The family arranges for hospice for their loved one.
   e. The patient is diagnosed with terminal cancer.
   f. The patient's daughter writes a poem expressing her sorrow.

3. A nurse interviews an 82-year-old resident of a long-term care facility who says that she has never gotten over the death of her son 20 years ago. She reports that her life fell apart after that and she never again felt like herself or was able to enjoy life. What type of grief is this woman experiencing?
   a. Abbreviated
   b. Anticipatory
   c. Dysfunctional
   d. Inhibited

4. A home health care nurse has been visiting a patient with AIDS who says, "I'm no longer afraid of dying. I think I've made my peace with everyone, and I'm actually ready to move on." This reflects the patient's progress to which stage of death and dying?
   a. Acceptance
   b. Anger
   c. Bargaining
   d. Denial

5. A nurse is visiting a male patient with pancreatic cancer who is dying at home. During the visit, he breaks down and cries and tells the nurse that it is unfair that he should have to die now when he's finally made peace with his family and wants to live. Which response by the nurse would be most appropriate?
   a. "You can't be feeling this way. You know you are going to die."
   b. "It does seem unfair. Tell me more about how you are feeling."
   c. "You'll be all right; who knows how much time any of us has"
   d. "Tell me about your pain. Did it keep you awake last night?"

6. A nurse is caring for a terminally ill patient during the 11 PM to 7 AM shift. The patient says, "I just can't sleep. I keep thinking about what my family will do when I am gone." What response by the nurse would be most appropriate?
   a. "Oh, don't worry about that now. You need to sleep."
   b. "What seems to be concerning you the most?"
   c. "I have talked to your wife and she told me she will be fine."
   d. "I have to go and give medicines, you should discuss this with your wife."

7. A patient tells a nurse that he has no one he trusts to make health care decisions for him should he become incapacitated. What should the nurse suggest he prepare?
   a. Combination advance medical directive
   b. Durable power of attorney for health care
   c. Living will
   d. Proxy for health care

8. A hospice nurse is caring for a patient who is terminally ill and who is on a ventilator. After a restless night, the patient hands the nurse a note with the request: "Please help me end my suffering." Which response by a nurse would best reflect adherence to the position of the American Nurses Association regarding assisted suicide?
   a. The nurse promises the patient that he or she will do everything possible to keep the patient comfortable but cannot administer an injection or overdose to cause the patient's death.
   b. The nurse tells the patient that under no condition can he be removed from the ventilator because this is active euthanasia and is expressly forbidden by the Code for Nurses.
   c. After exhausting every intervention to keep a dying patient comfortable, the nurse says, "I think you are now at a point where I'm prepared to do what you've been asking me. Let's talk about when and how you want to die."
   d. The nurse responds: "I'm personally opposed to assisted suicide, but I'll find you a colleague who can help you."

9. A patient diagnosed with breast cancer who is in the end stages of her illness has been in the medical intensive care unit for 3 weeks. Her husband tells the nurse caring for the patient that he and his wife often talked about the end of her life and that she was very clear about not wanting aggressive treatment that would merely prolong her dying. The nurse and husband both agree that this seems to be all that therapy is now doing for her. The nurse would suggest that the husband speak to his wife's physician about which type of order?
   a. Comfort-measures-only
   b. Do-not-hospitalize
   c. Do-not-resuscitate
   d. Slow-code-only

10. A nurse is preparing a family for a terminal weaning of a loved one. Which nursing actions would facilitate this process? Select all that apply.
   a. Participate in the decision-making process by offering the family information about the advantages and disadvantages of continued ventilatory support.
   b. Explain to the family what will happen at each phase of the weaning and offer support.
   c. Check the orders for sedation and analgesia, making sure that the anticipated death is comfortable and dignified.

d. Tell the family that death will occur almost immediately after the patient is removed from the ventilator.

e. Tell the family that the decision for terminal weaning of a patient must be made by the primary care provider.

f. Set up mandatory counseling sessions for the patient and family to assist them in making this end-of-life decision.

11. All of the following diagnoses may apply to a young couple who gave birth to a premature infant with serious respiratory problems who has been in the neonatal intensive care unit for the last 3 months. The couple has a 22-month-old son at home. Which diagnosis would be most appropriate based on the following assessment data: report of chronic fatigue and decreased energy, guilt about neglecting son at home, shortness of temper with one another, and apprehension about continued ability to go on this way?
    a. Grieving
    b. Ineffective Coping
    c. Caregiver Role Strain
    d. Powerlessness

12. A nurse is caring for terminally ill patients in a hospital setting. Which example describes appropriate end-of-life care?
    a. To eliminate confusion, taking care not to speak too much when caring for a comatose patient
    b. Sitting on the side of the bed of a dying patient, holding the patient's hand, and crying with the patient
    c. Referring to a counselor the daughter of a dying patient who is complaining about the care associated with artificially feeding her father
    d. Telling a dying patient to sit back and relax and performing patient hygiene for the patient because it is easier than having the patient help

13. A nurse is providing postmortem care. Which nursing action violates the standards of caring for the body after a patient has been pronounced dead and is not scheduled for an autopsy?
    a. The nurse places the patient in a sitting position while the family visits.
    b. The nurse places identification tags on both the shroud and the ankle.
    c. The nurse removes soiled dressings and tubes.
    d. The nurse makes sure a death certificate is issued and signed.

14. The family of a patient who has just died asks to be alone with the body and asks for supplies to wash the body. The nurse providing care knows that the mortician usually washes the body. Which response would be most appropriate?
    a. Inform the family that there is no need for them to wash the body since the mortician typically does this.
    b. Explain that hospital policy forbids their being alone with the deceased patient and that hospital supplies are to be used only by hospital personnel.
    c. Give the supplies to the family but maintain a watchful eye to make sure that nothing unusual happens.
    d. Provide the requested supplies, checking if this request is linked to their religious or cultural customs and asking if there is anything else you can do to help.

15. A 70-year-old female patient who has had a number of strokes refuses further life-sustaining interventions, including artificial nutrition and hydration. She is competent, understands the consequences of her actions, is not depressed, and

persists in refusing treatment. Her doctor is adamant that she cannot be allowed to die this way, and her daughter agrees. An ethics consult has been initiated. Who would be the appropriate decision maker?
    a. Patient
    b. Daughter
    c. Doctor
    d. Ethics consult team

ANSWERS WITH RATIONALES

1. **a, b, c.** The loss experienced by the woman is actual, perceived, and psychological. Actual loss can be recognized by others as well as by the person sustaining the loss, perceived loss is experienced by the person but is intangible to others, and psychological loss is a loss that is felt mentally as opposed to physically. Anticipatory loss occurs when one grieves prior to the actual loss, physical loss is loss that is tangible and perceived by others, and maturational loss is experienced as a result of natural developmental processes.

2. **a, b, f.** Mourning is defined as the period of acceptance of loss and grief, during which the person learns to deal with loss. It is the actions and expressions of that grief, including the symbols and ceremonies (e.g., a funeral or final celebration of life), that make up the outward expressions of grief. People who are bereaved are in a state of grieving from loss of a loved one.

3. **c.** Dysfunctional grief extends the mourning period for an abnormally long time, characterized by abnormal or distorted expressions of grief.

4. **a.** The patient's statement reflects the acceptance stage of death and dying defined by Kübler-Ross.

5. **b.** The nurse would want to validate that what the patient is saying has been heard and invite him to share more of his feelings, concerns, and fears.

6. **b.** Using an open-ended question allows the patient to continue talking. False reassurances are not helpful. Also, the patient's feelings and restlessness should be addressed as soon as possible.

7. **c.** The living will is a document whose precise purpose is to allow individuals to record specific instructions about the type of health care they would like to receive in particular end-of-life situations. A durable power of attorney for health care appoints an agent (proxy) the person trusts to make decisions in the event of subsequent incapacity. The combination advance medical directive also appoints a proxy for the patient.

8. **a.** The American Nurses Association (ANA, 1994, 2013) issued position statements stating that assisting in suicide and participating in active euthanasia are in violation of the Code for Nurses, the ethical traditions and goals of the profession, and its covenant with society.

9. **a.** Comfort-measures-only order. The wife would want all aggressive treatment to be stopped at this point and all care to be directed to a comfortable, dignified death.

10. **a, b, c.** A nurse's role in terminal weaning is to participate in the decision-making process by offering helpful information about the benefits and burdens of continued ventilation and a

description of what to expect if terminal weaning is initiated. Supporting the patient's family and managing sedation and analgesia are critical nursing responsibilities. In some cases, competent patients decide that they wish their ventilatory support ended; more often, the surrogate decision makers for an incompetent patient determine that continued ventilatory support is futile. Because there are no guarantees how any patient will respond once removed from a ventilator, and because it is possible for the patient to breathe on one's own and live for hours, days, and, rarely, even weeks, the family should not be told that death will occur immediately. Counseling sessions may be arranged if requested but are not mandatory to make this decision.

11. **c.** The defining characteristics for the NANDA diagnosis Caregiver Role Strain fit the set of assessment data provided.

12. **b.** The nurse should not be afraid to show compassion and empathy for the dying person, including crying with the patient if it occurs. The sense of hearing is believed to be the last sense to leave the body; many patients retain a sense of hearing almost to the moment of death; therefore nurses should explain to the comatose patient the nursing care being given. The nurse should address caregiver role endurance by actively listening to family members who are experiencing it. Because it is good to encourage dying patients to be as active as possible for as long as possible, it is generally not good

practice to perform basic self-care measures the patient can perform simply because it is "easier" to do it this way.

13. **a.** Because the body should be placed in normal anatomic position to avoid pooling of blood, leaving the body in a sitting position is contraindicated. The other actions are appropriate nursing responsibilities related to postmortem care.

14. **d.** The family may want to wash the body for personal, religious, or cultural reasons and should be allowed to do so.

15. **a.** Because this patient is competent, she has the right to refuse therapy that she finds to be disproportionately burdensome, even if this hastens her death. Neither her daughter nor her doctor has the authority to assume her decision-making responsibilities unless she asks them to do this. The ethics consult team is not a decision-making body; it can make recommendations but has no authority to order anything.

TAYLOR SUITE RESOURCES

Explore these additional resources to enhance learning for this chapter:

- NCLEX-Style Questions and other resources on thePoint, http://thePoint.lww.com/Taylor8e
- *Study Guide for Fundamentals of Nursing, 8th edition*
- Adaptive Learning | Powered by prepU, http://thepoint.lww.com/prepu

Bibliography

Aging with Dignity. (2013). *Five wishes.* Available at www.agingwithdignity.org/five-wishes.php

American Geriatrics Society (AGS) Ethics Committee. (2007). *Position Statement: The care of dying patients.* New York: Author.

American Nurses Association (ANA). (1991). *Position statement on promotion of comfort and relief of pain in dying patients.* Washington, DC: Author.

American Nurses Association (ANA). (1994). *Position statement on assisted suicide.* Washington, DC: Author.

American Nurses Association (ANA). (2013). Position Statement on Euthanasia, Assisted Suicide, and Aid in Dying. Available at http://www.nursingworld.org/MainMenuCategories/EthicsStandards/Ethics-Position-Statements/Euthanasia-Assisted-Suicide-and-Aid-in-Dying.pdf

Barclay, L., & Lie, D. (2008). End-of-life discussions may reduce aggressive care in terminally ill patients. Available at http://cme.medscape.com/viewarticle/581679

Beckstand, R. L., Callister, L. C., & Kirchoff, K. T. (2006). Providing a "good death": Critical care nurses' suggestions for improving end-of-life care. *American Journal of Critical Care, 15*(1), 38–46.

Bulechek, G., Butcher, H., Dochterman, J., & Wagner, C. M. (Eds.). (2013). *Nursing interventions classification (NIC)* (6th ed.). St. Louis: Elsevier.

Collins, M., & Lehane, E. (2013). Perspectives on death, dying and advance care planning from patients receiving haemodialysis. *Journal of Renal Care, 39*(1), 5–11. DOI: 10.1111/j.1755–6686.2013.00340.x

Emanuel, L., Ferris, F., von Gunten, C., & Von Roenn, J. (2008). The last hours of living: Practical advice for clinicians. Available at http://cme.medscape.com/viewprogram/5808?src=top10

Engel, G. L. (1964). Grief and grieving. *American Journal of Nursing, 64*(9), 93–98.

Ferrell, B., & Coyle, N. (2008). *The nature of suffering and the goals of nursing.* Cary, NC: Oxford University Press.

Holtslander, L. (2008). Ways of knowing hope: Carper's fundamental patterns as a guide for hope research with bereaved palliative caregivers. *Nursing Outlook, 56*(1), 25–30.

Institute of Medicine (IOM). (1997). *Approaching death: Improving care at the end of life.* Washington, DC: National Academy Press.

Johnson, J., & Johnson, M. (2003). *Grief: What it is and what you can do.* Omaha: Centering Corporation

Kirk, T. W. & Mahon, M. M. (2010). National Hospice and Palliative Care Organization (NHPCO) Position Statement and Commentary on the Use of Palliative Sedation in Imminently Dying Terminally Ill Patients. *Journal of Pain and Symptom Management, 39*(5), 914–923.

Kübler-Ross, E. (1969). *On death and dying.* New York: Macmillan.

Kübler-Ross, E. (1978). *To live until we say goodbye.* Englewood Cliffs, NJ: Prentice Hall.

Kübler-Ross, E. (1997). *On death and dying: What the dying have to teach doctors, nurses, clergy, and their own families.* New York: Simon & Schuster.

Love, A. W. (2007). Progress in understanding grief, complicated grief, and caring for the bereaved. *Contemporary Nurse, 27*(1), 73–83.

Lowery, S. (2008). Communication between the nurse and family caregiver in end-of-life care: A review of the literature. *Journal of Hospice and Palliative Nursing, 10*(1), 35–45.

Moorhead, S., Johnson, M., Maas, M., & Swanson, E. (Eds.) (2013). *Nursing outcomes classification (NOC)* (5th ed.). St. Louis: Elsevier/Mosby.

NANDA International (NANDA-I). (2012). *Nursing diagnoses: Definitions & classification 2012–2014.* West Sussex: Wiley-Blackwell.

National Consensus Project for Quality Palliative Care. (2013). Clinical practice guidelines for quality palliative care, 3rd ed. Available at http://www.nationalconsensusproject.org/NCP_Clinical_Practice_Guidelines_3rd_Edition.pdf

President's Commission for the Study of Ethical Problems in Medicine and Biomedical and Behavioral Research. (1981). *Defining death.* [Publication No. 81–600150]. Washington, DC: U.S. Government Printing Office.

Quill, T. E., & Byrock, I. R. (2000). Responding to intractable terminal suffering: The role of terminal sedation and voluntary refusal of food and fluids. *Annals of Internal Medicine, 132*(5): 408–414.

Rancour, P. (2008). Personal communication.

Rancour, P. (2008). *Tales from the pager chronicles.* Indianapolis: Sigma Theta Tau International.

Stajduhar, K. (2008). Factors influencing family caregivers' ability to cope with providing end-of-life cancer care at home. *Cancer Nursing, 31*(1), 77–85.

Thomas, R., Wilson, D., Justice, C., Birch, S., & Sheps, S. (2008). A literature review of preferences for end-of-life care in developed countries by individuals with different cultural affiliations and ethnicity. *Journal of Hospice and Palliative Nursing, 10*(3). Available at http://www.medscape.com/viewarticle/575049

Ufema, J. (2007). *Insights on death & dying.* Philadelphia: Wolters Kluwer Health/Lippincott Williams & Wilkins.

Williams, B. R., Lewis, D. R., Burgio, K. L. & Goode, P. S. (2012). Next-of-kin's perceptions of how hospital nursing staff support family presence before, during, and after the death of a loved one. *Journal of Hospice and Palliative Nursing, 14*(8), 541–550.

Watson, L. A. (2008). Informing critical care patients of a loved one's death. *Critical Care Nurse, 28*(3), 52–64.

43 | Sensory Functioning

ORI SOLTES

Ori, a 28-year-old man, is in the intensive care unit after a motor vehicle crash that resulted in multiple internal injuries as well as fractures. He is being monitored continuously and receiving mechanical ventilation. On the 5th day after the crash, he begins to exhibit transient episodes of acute confusion.

MURIEL HAO

Muriel is a 56-year-old woman who had surgery 2 days ago. She denies any complaints of pain or discomfort. She is receiving intravenous therapy via an infusion pump. She states, "Please stop that beeping. It's driving me nuts and I can't rest."

DOLORES PIROLLA

Dolores, a 74-year-old woman, comes to the older adult clinic with her 77-year-old husband who was diagnosed with macular degeneration and progressive vision loss. She states, "Now I've noticed he's also having difficulty hearing me. I'm worried because he doesn't want to leave the house and we hardly see any of our friends anymore. We used to go out to the movies or dinner at least once a week. Lately, if we get out once a month, that's a lot!"

LEARNING OBJECTIVES

After completing the chapter, you will be able to accomplish the following:

1. Describe the four conditions that must be met in each sensory experience.
2. Explain the role of the reticular activating system in sensory experience.
3. Identify etiologies and perceptual, cognitive, and emotional responses to sensory deprivation and sensory overload.
4. Perform a comprehensive assessment of sensory functioning using appropriate interview questions and physical assessment skills.
5. Develop nursing diagnoses that correctly identify sensory/perceptual alterations that may be treated by independent nursing interventions.
6. Describe specific nursing interventions to prevent sensory alterations, stimulate the senses, promote health literacy, and assist patients with sensory difficulties.
7. Develop, implement, and evaluate a plan of nursing care to help patients safely meet individualized sensory/perceptual outcomes.

KEY TERMS

adaptation	proprioception	sensory perception
arousal	reticular activating system (RAS)	sensory poverty
auditory		sensory reception
disturbed sensory perception	sensoristasis	
	sensory deficit	stereognosis
gustatory	sensory deprivation	stimulus
kinesthesia		tactile
olfactory	sensory overload	visceral

A person's senses are vital to survival, growth and development, and the experience of bodily pleasure. Nurses encounter many patients who have impaired sensory functioning that places them at risk for injury, disturbed growth and development, and decreased well-being. Moreover, the stress of illness or trauma and the need for diagnosis and treatment may quickly result in sensory deprivation or overload, with serious disturbances in visual, perceptual, cognitive, or emotional functioning (see the accompanying Reflective Practice box for an example on page 1632). Nurses are in the position to use knowledge of sensory functioning to support positive outcomes for patients (see Box 43-1 on page 1633). For

example, awareness of the intensities and sources of sound, ways to control noise, and the assessment of patients' perceptions of and responses to sound can provide nurses with a basis for therapeutic manipulation of the environment.

THE SENSORY EXPERIENCE
Components and Conditions

The sensory experience consists of two components: reception and perception. **Sensory reception** is the process of receiving data about the external or internal environment through the senses. The senses by which people maintain contact with the external environment are vision (visual), hearing (**auditory**), smell (**olfactory**), taste (**gustatory**), and touch (**tactile**). In addition, **stereognosis** is the sense that perceives the solidity of objects and their size, shape, and texture.

People orient themselves internally by the kinesthetic and visceral senses. (**Kinesthesia** refers to awareness of positioning of body parts and body movement; **visceral** pertains to inner organs.) The kinesthetic and visceral senses arise internally from muscles and hollow organs, respectively, and are the body's basic orienting systems. **Proprioception** is the term used to describe the sense, usually at a subconscious level, of the movements and position of the body and especially its limbs, independent of vision. This sense is gained primarily from input from sensory nerve terminals in muscles and tendons and the fibrous capsules of joints combined with input from the vestibular apparatus.

Sensory perception is the conscious process of selecting, organizing, and interpreting data from the senses into meaningful information. Perception is influenced by the intensity, size, change, or representation of stimuli, as well as by past experiences, knowledge, and attitudes.

For a person to receive the necessary data to experience the world, four conditions must be met:

- A **stimulus**—an agent, act, or other influence capable of initiating a response by the nervous system—must be present.
- A receptor or sense organ must receive the stimulus and convert it to a nerve impulse.
- The nerve impulse must be conducted along a nervous pathway from the receptor or sense organ to the brain.
- A particular area in the brain must receive and translate the impulse into a sensation.

 THINK back to Muriel Hao, the 56-year-old woman unable to rest because of the machine's beeping. The nurse would incorporate knowledge of sensory reception and perception to determine that the patient is experiencing a continuous and large amount of auditory stimuli from the beeping of the machine. In addition, the nurse would need to keep in mind other sources of stimuli, such as possible visual stimuli from the lighted numbers on the machine, tactile stimuli from being touched to determine the possible problem associated with the machine, and internal stimuli associated with pain and discomfort from surgery. ●

REFLECTIVE PRACTICE: CULTIVATING QSEN COMPETENCIES

CHALLENGE TO TECHNICAL SKILLS

All throughout nursing school, we are taught theory, and from that theory we are to use clinical reasoning to determine how to care for a particular patient, focusing on the patient, not the machines surrounding them. "You'll learn that later," they say.

I was assigned to care for Muriel Hao, a 56-year-old woman who had surgery 2 days ago. As I walk into her room, I check to see if she is comfortable and whether she needs anything at that particular point in time. She asks me one favor. "Please stop that beeping. It's driving me nuts and I can't rest." So I look at the machine, dumbfounded,

and worried that the patient is going to think I am incompetent because I cannot even work a simple machine. No theory from a classroom is going to teach me how to make the machine stop beeping. To make things worse, every facility has different machines. As nursing students, we go from one facility to another, trying to get accustomed to the equipment and technologies of each one. I assume that things will get easier once I have steady employment in a facility. If that particular facility changes its technologies, I would hope that there would be an in-service on the new technology. But what do I do now, as a nursing student?

Thinking Outside the Box: Possible Courses of Action

- Press the buttons on the machine, and hope that the beeping goes away.
- Seek out someone who does know how to work the machine and have that person fix it so I don't do more damage.

- Find someone who knows how to work the machine, have that person fix it, and then have the person explain to me how to fix it so I can do it next time.

Evaluating a Good Outcome: How Do I Define Success?

- Personal integrity is maintained (if I can't fix it, I feel stupid, and that's an insult to my integrity).
- Professional integrity remains intact (if I can't fix it, I will feel incompetent as a nurse—if I can't even fix a machine, how am I supposed to help a person?).

- The patient expresses relief that the beeping has stopped and she is now able to rest.

Personal Learning: Here's to the Future!

Although this does not seem like a huge or very troublesome problem, every nursing student can probably attest to feeling this way at least once. The first few times it happened to me, I just asked someone to fix it for me, thinking it was a one-time problem. Then I realized that this is something that I was facing over and over again. So I asked someone to show me how to fix the problem if it should occur again. I understood what to do and knew how to do it. Then we switched hospitals and I was confused once again. In today's environment of ever-changing technology,

I realized that it is not just the students who feel this way. Nurses, too, have these same feelings. We all learn new things every day, whether it's from a patient, another nurse, a doctor, or a technical specialist. We just need to know that it's okay to ask questions. Moreover, not knowing how to work with a piece of equipment does not mean that you are incompetent with people. Learning in the health care field is an ongoing process.

Michele Jordan, Georgetown University

REFLECTION ON QUALITY AND SAFETY COMPETENCIES

Do you agree with the criteria that the nursing student used to evaluate a successful outcome? Why or why not? What *knowledge, skills,* and *attitudes* do you need to develop to continuously improve the quality and safety of care for patients like Ms. Hao? Was professional integrity affirmed? Explain.

Patient-Centered Care: How can you deliver thoughtful, patient-centered care for patients while feeling overwhelmed by their equipment?

Teamwork and Collaboration/Quality Improvement: Who on your team is most likely to help you? What communication and interpersonal skills do you need to improve to ensure that you function as a competent and confident

member of the patient-care team? What does quality care for Ms. Hao "look like"?

Safety/Evidence-Based Practice: What does the evidence point to as "best practice" for Ms. Hao? If you stop the machine from beeping in response to her requests, will you be silencing critical alarms? What safety needs does she have and how can you meet them?

Informatics: Can you identify the essential information that must be available in Ms. Hao's electronic record to support safe patient care and coordination of care? Can you think of other ways to respond to or approach the situation? What else might the nursing student have done to ensure a successful outcome?

BOX 43-1 | HEALTHY PEOPLE 2020 GOAL: REDUCE THE PREVALENCE AND SEVERITY OF DISORDERS OF HEARING AND BALANCE; SMELL AND TASTE; AND VOICE, SPEECH, AND LANGUAGE

Overview

At least 1 in 6 Americans currently has a sensory or communication impairment or disorder. Even when they are temporary or mild, such disorders can affect physical and mental health. An impaired ability to communicate with others or maintain good balance can lead many people to:

- Feel socially isolated
- Have unmet health needs
- Have limited success in school or on the job

An impaired sense of smell or taste can lead to poor nutrition or the inability to detect smoke, gas leaks, or foods that are unsafe to eat.

Why Are Hearing and Other Sensory or Communication Processes Important?

Communication and other sensory processes contribute to our overall health and well-being. Protecting these processes is critical, particularly for people whose age, race, ethnicity, gender, occupation, genetic background, or health status places them at increased risk. The *Healthy People 2020* objectives are designed to ensure that all Americans, from birth through old age, will benefit from scientific advances in prevention, diagnosis, and treatment of hearing and other sensory or communication disorders. For example:

- One to 3 out of every 1,000 children is born with hearing loss. Through early diagnosis and intervention, these children can develop speech and language skills on schedule with their peers.
- Autism spectrum disorders, which often influence a child's ability to use language, affect 1 out of 110 8-year-old children. Researchers are investigating better ways to predict risk for autism in hopes of offering earlier treatment
- Obesity, diabetes, hypertension, malnutrition, Parkinson's disease, Alzheimer's disease, and multiple sclerosis are accompanied or signaled by chemosensory (smell and taste) problems. Diagnosis of chemosensory disorders may lead to earlier, more effective treatment of related diseases and conditions.
- Approximately 7.5 million people in the United States have trouble using their voices. People in occupations that stress the vocal cords, such as teaching and singing, may need preventive and rehabilitative services. Substantial progress has been made in the development of alternative and augmentative communication devices that help people with severe disorders communicate.

Reprinted from HealthyPeople.gov. (2013). Hearing and other sensory or communication disorders. Available at http://www.healthypeople.gov/2020/topicsobjectives2020/overview.aspx?topicid=20

Arousal Mechanism

To receive stimuli and respond appropriately, the brain must be alert or aroused. The **reticular activating system (RAS)**, a poorly defined network that extends from the hypothalamus to the medulla, mediates arousal. The optimal arousal state of the RAS is a general drive state called **sensoristasis**. Nerve impulses from all the sensory tracts reach the RAS, which then selectively allows certain impulses to reach the cerebral cortex and be perceived. The mesencephalic portion of the RAS appears to be the center of the system. Stimulation of this area produces the most pronounced and long-lasting effects on the cerebral cortex (Fig. 43-1). With its many ascending and descending connections to other areas of the brain, the RAS serves to monitor and to regulate incoming sensory stimuli, thus maintaining, enhancing, or inhibiting cortical **arousal**. States of arousal or awareness are described in Box 43-2 (on page 1634).

The body quickly adapts to constant stimuli. In addition, the repeated stimulus of a continuing noise, such as city traffic, or a noxious odor eventually goes unnoticed. Therefore, a stimulus must be variable or irregular to evoke a response. This phenomenon is termed **adaptation**. Impulses that are not acted on when received may be used at a later date in response to the same or similar stimuli. The memory process involves the storage of that material. For example, thought and memory are used when a new sensory experience occurs and the person uses a response based on previous knowledge and experience.

DISTURBED SENSORY PERCEPTION

When patients are admitted to a health agency, they are confronted with stimuli that are different in quality and quantity from those to which they are accustomed. For example, a patient confined to bedrest may receive many fewer stimuli, whereas one undergoing multiple diagnostic tests may

FIGURE 43-1. Nerve impulses from all the sensory tracts reach the reticular activating system (RAS), which then selectively allows certain impulses to reach the cerebral cortex and to be perceived.

BOX 43-2 STATES OF AROUSAL/AWARENESS

Conscious States

Delirium	Disorientation, restlessness, confusion, hallucinations, agitation, alternating with other conscious states
Dementia	Difficulties with spatial orientation, memory, language; changes in personality
Confusion	Reduced awareness, easily distracted, easily startled by sensory stimuli, alternates between drowsiness and excitability; resembles minor form of delirium state
Normal consciousness	Aware of self and external environment, well-oriented, responsive
Somnolence	Extreme drowsiness, but will respond normally to stimuli
Minimally conscious states	Part consciousness; sleep–wake cycles present; some motor function, including automatic movements; inconsistently follows commands
Locked-in syndrome	Full consciousness; sleep–wake cycles present; quadriplegic, auditory and visual function preserved; emotion preserved

Unconscious States

Asleep	Can be aroused by normal stimuli (light touch, sound, and the like)
Stupor	Can be aroused by extreme and/or repeated stimuli
Coma	Cannot be aroused and does not respond to stimuli (coma states can be further subdivided according to the effect on reflex responses to stimuli; see Glasgow Coma Scale, Chapter 25)
Vegetative State	Cannot be aroused. Sleep–wake cycles, postures or withdraws to noxious stimuli, occasional nonpurposeful movement, random smiling or grimacing.

receive a greater-than-normal level of sensory input. These and other typical experiences are likely to result in disturbed sensory perceptions experienced by the patient. Being sensitive to how visual stimuli, noises, and touch are stimulating the patient, combined with paying attention to the patient's need for privacy and for social interaction, can significantly reduce disturbances in sensory perception.

Severe sensory alterations can occur, especially in certain areas, such as the critical care or intensive care units (termed intensive care unit [ICU] psychosis). See the accompanying

RESEARCH IN NURSING

BRIDGING THE GAP TO EVIDENCE-BASED PRACTICE

Sleep and Delirium Outcomes

Critically ill adults are vulnerable when admitted to the intensive care unit (ICU) because patients are bombarded with unfamiliar sounds, bright lights, and interruptions, creating a potentially hostile environment. Instead of getting quieter, ICUs may in fact be getting noisier over time. Experts report that sound levels, or decibels (dB), all exceed recommended levels for hospital care.

Related Research

Always, A., Halm, M. A., Shilhanek, M., & St. Pierre, J. (2013). Do earplugs and eye masks affect sleep and delirium outcomes in the critically ill? *American Journal of Critical Care, 22*(4), 357–360. **doi:10.4037/ajcc2013545**

The PICO (*p*roblem, *i*ntervention, *c*omparison, *o*utcomes) question that this review addresses is: What effect do the interventions of earplugs and eye masks have on sleep and delirium outcomes in critically ill adults? Authors searched CINAHL and MEDLINE using the key words *earplugs, eye masks, sleep quality, sleep deprivation, sensory overload,* and *delirium,* limiting the search to original research studies. While sound- and light-masking interventions such as earplugs and eye masks are promising noninvasive and low-cost techniques that may improve objective sleep variables as well as subjective sleep experiences of adults in critical care settings, the findings of this review were inconclusive. The authors recommended more studies to evaluate their effectiveness as well as to explore the usefulness of interventions such as lowering voices and closing patients' doors to decrease conversation-related noise at nursing stations; reducing/eliminating overhead paging; dimming lights and enforcing unit-based quiet times; minimizing unnecessary interruptions and clustering patient care activities; and addressing "squeaky" equipment maintenance in a timely manner. Other environmental enhancements include soundproofing with carpet and ceiling tiles, as well as use of nocturnal lighting sources without blue light to maintain circadian light cycles.

Relevance to Nursing Practice

As nurses following in Florence Nightingale's tradition of emphasizing healing spaces, we have the power to offer optimal healing environments for our patients every day by (1) creating healing spaces as we reduce environmental stressors, provide positive diversions, and connect patients to nature; (2) promoting relationships by ensuring that patients have access to their support network; and (3) fostering collaboration by offering patients options and choices that normalize environmental sights and sounds within their treatment and care.

For additional research, visit thePoint.

Research in Nursing box. Factors contributing to severe sensory alteration include sensory overload, sensory deprivation, sleep deprivation, and cultural care deprivation.

 CONSIDER Ori Soltes, the young man in the ICU. The nurse would need to assess Mr. Soltes closely for underlying reasons for his confusion. Although the possible causes are numerous and most likely multiple in nature, the nurse would need to address the possibility of sensory deprivation and overload contributing to the patient's confusion. •

Box 43-3 provides an overview of sensory deprivation and sensory overload with related nursing interventions.

Sensory Deprivation

Sensory deprivation results when a person experiences decreased sensory input or input that is monotonous, unpatterned, or meaningless. With decreased sensory input, the RAS is no longer able to project a normal level of activation to the brain. As a result, the person may hallucinate simply to maintain an optimal level of arousal. Factors placing a patient at high risk for sensory deprivation include the following:

- An environment with decreased or monotonous stimuli (such as institutionalized patients or those confined to a small living area at home, on bedrest, or in isolation)
- Impaired ability to receive environmental stimuli (patients with impaired vision or hearing; with bandages or casts that interfere with vision, hearing, or tactile stimulation; or with affective disorders who "close out" the environment)
- Inability to process environmental stimuli (patients with spinal cord injuries or brain damage, those who are con-

fused or disoriented, or are taking prescribed or recreational drugs affecting the central nervous system)

 REMEMBER Dolores Pirolla, the wife of the older man with vision deficits who was developing hearing deficits. The nurse would incorporate knowledge of risk factors for sensory deprivation when developing the patient's plan of care. In this case, Mr. Pirolla's sensory deficits involving vision and now hearing are impacting his ability to receive environmental stimuli. Thus, the nurse would develop a plan of care with measures to ensure that the patient and his wife receive adequate stimulation from the environment. •

Sensory deprivation can lead to perceptual, cognitive, and emotional disturbances. *Perceptual responses* result from inaccurate perception of sights, sounds, tastes, smells, and body position, coordination, and equilibrium. These responses can range from mild distortions such as daydreams, to gross distortions such as hallucinations. *Cognitive responses* involve the patient's inability to control the direction of thought content. Typically, attention span and ability to concentrate are decreased. The patient may demonstrate difficulty with memory, problem solving, and task performance. *Emotional responses* typically are manifested by apathy, anxiety, fear, anger, belligerence, panic, or depression. Rapid mood changes also may occur (see Box 43-2 for additional information). In a discussion of the relationships among visual impairment, loss of hearing, and cognitive function in older adults, Wahl and Heyl (2003) found that cognitive capacity and nonimpaired sensory function were closely related to higher cortical functions.

BOX 43-3 OVERVIEW OF SENSORY DEPRIVATION AND SENSORY OVERLOAD

Sensory Deprivation
Sensory deprivation is insufficient quantity or quality of stimuli; may result from decreased sensory input or monotonous, unpatterned, and unmeaningful input.

Defining Characteristics	Contributing Factors	Patients at Risk
Physical behaviors: drowsiness, excessive yawning	*Decreased environmental stimuli:* institutionalized environment; separation from significant others and usual sources of stimuli; treatments that decrease access to stimuli, such as bedrest or isolation	Institutionalized patients, especially those in long-term care settings
Escape behaviors: eating, exercising, sleeping, running away to escape the deprived environment		Patients with communicable diseases (e.g., AIDS)
		Patients confined to bed
Changes in perception: unusual body sensations; preoccupation with somatic complaints (dry mouth, palpitations, difficulty breathing, nausea); change in body image; illusions and hallucinations	*Impaired ability to receive environmental stimuli:* impaired vision, hearing, taste, smell, touch resulting from treatments such as bandages or body casts that interfere with reception of stimuli, or as a result of depression and other affective disorders	Patients with sensory alterations (e.g., impaired vision or hearing, or patients with eye patches or body casts)
Changes in cognitive behavior: decreased attention span, inability to concentrate, decreased problem solving and task performance		Patients who are depressed
		Patients from a different culture
Changes in affective behavior: crying, increased irritability and annoyance over small matters, confusion, panic, depression	*Inability to process environmental stimuli:* spinal cord injuries, brain damage, confusion, dementia, medications that depress the central nervous system	Patients with a disturbance of the nervous system

(continued)

BOX 43-3 OVERVIEW OF SENSORY DEPRIVATION AND SENSORY OVERLOAD *continued*

Nursing Interventions

Maintain sufficient level of arousal by increasing sensory stimuli from all sensory modalities:

- Instruct the patient in self-stimulation methods: counting, singing, reading, reciting poetry.
- Structure meaningful tangible stimuli into the patient's external environment; include a variety of people, ideas, sensations; a pet may provide excellent stimulation.
  - Visual stimulation:
    Colorful sheets, pajamas, robes
    Colorful uniform tops for the nurse
    Face-to-face human contact
    Clocks, calendars, wristwatches
    Pictures, flowers, greeting card
  - Auditory stimulation:
    Call the person by name
    Conversation that communicates caring as well as orients the patient
    Reading to the patient
    Television, radio, iPod
  - Gustatory and olfactory stimulation:
    Attention to oral hygiene and properly fitting dentures
    Food of different textures, colors, temperatures, served attractively
    Smelling food before eating it and recalling pleasurable aromas from the past
    Seasoning foods or having favorite foods brought from home

- Tactile stimulation:
    Backrubs and foot soaks
    Turning and repositioning
    Passive range-of-motion exercises
    Hair brushing, combing, washing
    Hugs
    Touching arms or shoulders
- Cognitive input:
    Orient the patient to the environment.
    Encourage patient participation in self-care.
    Discuss current events or the patient's occupation, hobbies, or interests.
    Reinforce reality without arguing with a patient who is hallucinating. "No, I don't see a man standing there but the linen hamper may be confusing you."
- Emotional input: Encourage the patient to share fears, concerns, and perceptions; reassure the patient that illusions and misperceptions do occur with sensory deprivation.
- Incorporate culturally assistive, supportive, facilitative acts into nursing care.
- *Caution:* Because it can be difficult to distinguish the behavioral manifestations of sensory deprivation from sensory overload, introduce more stimulation cautiously. If the added stimulation only increases the patient's maladaptive behaviors, consider reducing sensory input because the patient may be experiencing sensory overload.

Sensory Overload

Sensory overload is excessive stimuli over which a person feels little control; the brain is unable meaningfully to respond to or ignore stimuli.

Defining Characteristics	Contributing Factors	Patients at Risk
Similar to those observed in sensory deprivation Older patients and patients who have suffered a stroke are more likely to experience confusion or agitation. Young patients are more likely to seek the comfort of their parents' embrace to block out sensory overload.	*Increased internal stimuli:* pain, pressure and discomfort of intrusive tubes (e.g., intravenous lines [IVs], catheters; endotracheal tubes; nasogastric tubes), worry about state of health or need to make treatment decisions *Increased external stimuli:* unfamiliar health care environment, such as lights, noises, sounds, odors, movement, and constant presence of strangers, many of whom touch the body; intrusive procedures such as diagnostic tests and treatments; scratchy linens *Inability perceptually to disregard or selectively ignore some stimuli:* nervous system disturbances, substances such as caffeine that stimulate the central nervous system arousal mechanism	Acutely or chronically ill patients Patients in pain Patients with intrusive monitoring or treatment equipment Hospitalized patients, especially those in critical care settings Patients with disturbances of the nervous system

Nursing Interventions

- Provide a consistent, predictable pattern of stimulation to help the patient develop a sense of control over the environment.
- Offer simple explanations before procedures, tests, and examinations.
- Establish a schedule with the patient for routine care such as eating, bathing, turning, positioning, coughing, and exercising.

- Speak calmly with the patient and move slowly; communicate confidence.
- Explore with the patient what stimuli are most distressing and develop a plan to reduce or eliminate them (e.g., incoming phone calls, visitors); earplugs or pain medication may be indicated. Noise-reducing headphones may be helpful.
- Be careful not to cause sensory deprivation.
- Identify and, wherever possible, eliminate culturally inappropriate stimuli.

Adapted from Lee, K. A. (1991). Sensory overload, sensory deprivation, and sleep deprivation. In M. L. Patrick, S. I. Woods, R. F. Craven, J. S. Rokosky, & P. M. Bruno (Eds.), *Medical-surgical nursing: Pathological concepts* (2nd ed.). Philadelphia: J. B. Lippincott.

Sensory Overload

Sensory overload is the condition that results when a person experiences so much sensory stimuli that the brain is unable to either respond meaningfully or ignore the stimuli. The person feels out of control and may exhibit all of the manifestations observed in sensory deprivation. The amount and quality of stimuli necessary to produce overload may differ greatly from one person to another and is influenced by factors such as age, culture, personality, and lifestyle.

In some patients, especially those coming from a quiet environment with unvarying stimuli, the experience of being hospitalized quickly results in sensory overload. In such patients, the brain is assaulted by the constant presence of strangers who not only demand to be spoken to, but also touch and poke at the body; by the strange sights, odors, sounds, and feels of the unfamiliar environment; by the constant presence of pain or discomfort from dressings, intravenous (IV) lines, drainage tubes, or endotracheal tubes; and by the ever-present worries about the meaning and course of the illness.

Nursing care focuses on reducing distressing stimuli and helping the patient to gain control over the environment (see Box 43-3).

 NOW consider Ori Soltes, the young man in the ICU. When assessing Mr. Soltes and his confusion, the nurse needs to be alert for factors that would contribute to sensory overload, such as bright lights, noises from the various monitoring devices, and frequent examinations. In addition, the nurse needs to assess for possible factors contributing to sensory deprivation. For example, the patient is receiving mechanical ventilation. As a result, health care team members may limit verbal communication with the patient, thus reducing some auditory stimuli that he would receive. Additionally, the patient is in bed with multiple injuries, also restricting his ability to interact with the environment. ●

Sensory Deficits

Impaired or absent functioning in one or more senses is termed **sensory deficit**. Examples of sensory deficits include impaired sight and hearing, altered taste, numbness and paralysis that result in altered tactile perception, and impaired kinesthetic sense. These deficits may be reversible or permanent, may occur gradually or all at once, and may be present at birth or evolve later. Awareness of a patient's sensory deficits is necessary to determine whether the patient is able to compensate for the deficit. Illness and hospitalization may threaten a patient's usual adaptive patterns and require new self-care abilities. Patients with evolving deficits will require assistance with coping and learning to compensate skillfully.

 THINK again of Dolores Pirolla, the wife of the man with vision and hearing deficits. The nurse needs to assess both the patient and his wife to determine how each is coping. From the description at the beginning of the chapter, Mr. Pirolla appears to be experiencing problems coping with the vision changes. As a result, both Mr. and Mrs. Pirolla are beginning to experience social isolation. The nurse would incorporate this information when developing a plan of care for the patient and his wife. ●

Sensory Poverty

Diane Ackerman (1990), poet, essayist, and naturalist, believes that we are now living in an age of **sensory poverty**. High-tech devices deliver a bewildering array of assaults on our senses every day. Yet we are learning about our world without experiencing it up close, right here, right now, in "all its messy, majestic, riotous detail." You have probably often heard the advice to stop and take time to smell the roses. But when was the last time you cradled a rose bloom, inhaled its perfume, and marveled at its color? When did you last lie on freshly mown grass and look up at the night sky mesmerized by the moon and stars? When did you last marvel at the complex aromas and flavors coming from a new culinary experience? Do you agree with Ackerman that our lives are becoming poorer as we lose the ability to be sensually present in the moment to the world around us?

FACTORS AFFECTING SENSORY STIMULATION

The amount of stimuli different people consider optimal appears to vary considerably. Factors influencing the amount and quality of stimuli needed to maintain cortical arousal include developmental considerations, culture, personality and lifestyle, stress and illness, and medication.

Developmental Considerations

Different types of sensory stimulation are needed for growth as sensory receptors, organs, and the nervous system mature. Although the newborn is capable of rudimentary perceptual discrimination at birth, many neural pathways are immature and must be stimulated to develop, become refined, and function adequately. Appropriate stimulation includes soothing, holding, rocking, and changes of position (tactile and kinesthetic sensations), singing and being talked to (auditory sensations), and changing patterns of light and shade, such as through the use of mobiles and bright objects (visual sensations). In contrast, the neonatal ICU may be a source of inappropriate sensory stimulation. To facilitate developmentally supportive care, medically fragile infants are recommended to have limited light and visual and vestibular stimulation to simulate being in the womb.

For children, engaging in developmentally appropriate play helps develop muscles and coordination, provide an outlet for surplus physical energy, develop communication skills, provide sources of learning, act as a stimulant to creativity, develop social skills, teach sex roles, provide an outlet for the release of emotional energy, and develop self-insights.

Sensory functioning tends to decline progressively throughout adulthood as the result of aging or chronic illness. Adults

Box 43-4 | SENSORY CHANGES RELATED TO AGING

The majority of older adults will experience some changes in their sensory capacity that can severely impact communication skills, as a normal part of aging. The following are common changes seen with advancing age and the disease states and injuries that occur more frequently in aging.

Vision Changes Common in Older Adults

Presbyopia: A loss of elasticity in the lens of eye leading to a decrease in the eye's ability to change the shape of the lens to focus on near objects such as fine print and decreased ability to adapt to light.

Diseases that Alter Vision Seen More Frequently as People Age

- *Cataracts:* Clouding of the crystalline lens presents as painless, progressive loss of vision; can be unilateral or bilateral.
- *Macular Degeneration:* The most common cause of legal blindness in the elderly. The development of drusen deposits in the retinal pigmented epithelium is the leading cause of central vision loss in older adults. More common in fair-haired, blue-eyed individuals. Other risk factors include smoking and excessive sunlight exposure. There are wet and dry forms of macular degeneration.
- *Glaucoma:* A potentially serious form of eye disease. The majority of cases of glaucoma are open-angle glaucoma (95%). Increased intraocular pressure causing atrophy and cupping of the optic nerve head causing visual field deficits that can progress to blindness. Vision changes include loss of peripheral vision, intolerance to glare, decreased perception of contrast, and decreased ability to adapt to the dark.
- *Diabetic Retinopathy:* End organ damage from diabetes causing retinopathy and spotty vision. Risk can be reduced by tight blood sugar control. Starts as nonproliferative and progresses to proliferative that should be treated with laser photocoagulation.
- *Hypertensive Retinopathy:* End organ damage from poorly controlled hypertension causing background and eventual proliferative retinopathy. Usually treated with laser photocoagulation and tight blood pressure control.
- *Temporal Arteritis:* Autoimmune disorder that causes inflammation of the temporal artery. It presents as malaise, scalp tenderness, unilateral temporal headache, jaw claudication, and sudden vision loss (usually unilateral). This vision loss is a medical emergency but is potentially reversible if identified immediately. The client should see an ophthalmologist, or go to the emergency room immediately if symptoms develop.
- *Detached Retina:* Can occur in patients with cataracts or recent cataract surgery, trauma, or be spontaneous. Presents as a curtain coming down across vision. Should see an ophthalmologist or proceed to the emergency room immediately.

Hearing Changes Common in Older Adults

- *Presbycusis:* Loss of high frequency, sensorineural hearing loss. Has a gradual onset, is progressive, and is bilateral. Due to gradual loss of hair cells and fibrous changes in the small blood vessels that supply the cochlea. Difficulty hearing high-pitched sounds such as *s, z, sh,* and *ch.* Background noise further aggravates hearing deficit.
- *Conductive Hearing Loss:* Involves the outer and/or middle ear. Causes of conductive hearing impairment include: cerumen impactions or foreign bodies, ruptured eardrum, otitis media, and otosclerosis.
- *Sensorineural Hearing Loss:* Involves damage to the inner ear, the cochlea, or the fibers of the eighth cranial nerve. Causes of sensorineural hearing loss include: hereditary causes, viral or bacterial infections, trauma, tumors, noise exposure, cardiovascular conditions, ototoxic drugs and Ménière's disease.

Diseases that Alter Hearing Seen More Frequently as People Age

- *Central Auditory Processing Disorder:* An uncommon disorder that includes an inability to process incoming signals and is often found in stroke patients and older adults with Alzheimer Dementia. The person's hearing is intact but their ability to process the sound is impaired.
- *Tinnitus:* Ringing in the ears may fluctuate, can be due to damage to the hair receptors of the cochlear nerve and age-related changes in the organs of hearing and balance. Patients with tinnitus should be referred to ENT.
- *Ménière's Disease:* Characterized by fluctuating hearing loss, dizziness and tinnitus. Possible causes of Ménière's disease include: hypothyroidism, diabetes and neurosyphilis.

Changes in Smell and Taste Common to Older Adults

- Common changes in smell include a decline in the sensitivity to airborne chemical stimuli with aging.
- Common changes in taste include a decreased ability to detect foods that are sweet. Most changes in taste are thought to occur due to decreased sense of smell, medications, diseases and tobacco use.

Diseases that Alter Smell and Taste Seen More Frequently as People Age

- *Burning Mouth Syndrome:* This is a sensation that one's tongue is tingling or burning. There may be several contributing factors: Vitamin B deficiencies, local trauma, gastrointestinal disorders causing reflux, allergies, salivary dysfunction and diabetes.

Changes in Peripheral Sensation Common to Older Adults

- Peripheral nerve function that controls the sense of touch declines slightly with age.
- Two-point discrimination and vibratory sense both decrease with age.
- The ability to perceive painful stimuli is preserved in aging. However, there may be a slowed reaction time for pulling away from painful stimuli with aging.

Diseases that Alter Peripheral Sensation Seen More Frequently as People Age

- *Peripheral Neuropathy:* Nerve pain in the distal extremities related to nerve damage from circulatory problems or vitamin deficiencies. Common vitamin deficiencies which impact peripheral nerves include B6, B12 and folate.

BOX 43-4 SENSORY CHANGES RELATED TO AGING *continued*

- *Diabetic Neuropathy:* End organ damage to the peripheral nerves from microvascular changes which occur with diabetes. Often leads to loss of sensation in the feet of diabetics leading to undetected trauma to the extremities which can lead to refractory infections due to poor vascular supply to the extremity. It is extremely important to teach diabetics and patients with peripheral neuropathy to provide special care to their feet.
- *Phantom Limb Pain:* The experience of pain that can range from dull ache to crushing pain where an amputated limb

once was. The sensory cortex of the brain has influence in this mechanism. This pain is often chronic and requires special interventions to control and manage the pain including electronic prosthetics, analgesics, and psychosocial support.
- *Acute Sensory Loss:* May be due to a stroke, acute nerve entrapment in the spine or compartment syndrome due to trauma to a limb. Will present with acute onset of numbness, tingling or lack of sensation and function in the effected extremity.

Reprinted with permission from Boltz, M., Capezuti, E., Fulmer, T. T., Zwicker, D., & O'Meara, A. (2012). *Evidence-based geriatric nursing protocols for best practice* (4th ed.). New York: Springer Publishing Company.

may experience the need to compensate for the loss of one type of stimulation by increasing other sources of sensory stimuli. See Box 43-4 and the accompanying Focus on the Older Adult: Sensory Functioning.

Culture

A person's culture may determine how much sensory stimulation is considered normal. For example, the amount of touching a child experiences in a Puerto Rican family may be different from that experienced by a child in a German family. Similarly, male and female roles may be culturally defined; for example, although men are expected to respond to the challenges of out-of-the-home sensory stimuli, a

woman who attempts to do so may be scorned if her place is considered to be in the home. Ethnic norms, religious norms, income group norms, and the norms of subgroups within a culture all influence the amount of sensory stimulation a person seeks and perceives as meaningful.

Moreover, sensory deprivation, sensory overload, and sleep deprivation are all related to or affected by a person's cultural practices, values, and beliefs. The nurse who is sensitive to the patient's culture attempts to determine what constitutes acceptable levels of stimuli from the patient's viewpoint. For example, certain cultures view touching as a natural and welcome custom, whereas other cultures may view it as insulting or offensive. Similarly, patients may

FOCUS ON THE OLDER ADULT

SENSORY FUNCTIONING

Age-Related Changes	Nursing Strategies
Decrease in vision	• Ensure that the patient is using corrective lenses such as contacts, glasses, and/or magnifiers. • Administer medications that enhance vision, such as medications that lower intraocular pressure in older adult patients with glaucoma. • Provide adequate lighting and clear pathways of clutter to prevent injury. • Provide enlarged print. • Encourage the patient to visit the ophthalmologist annually.
Decrease in hearing	• Ensure that the patient is using appropriate and functioning hearing assistive devices. • When communicating with the patient, use a lower tone. • Speak so that the patient can see your mouth movements.
Decreased sense of touch	• Protect the patient's skin from temperature extremes. • Assess the extremities for breaks in the skin, blisters, drainage, or open wounds. • Ensure that the patient is ambulating with assistive devices.
Sensory deprivation	• Discourage the use of sedatives. • Assess the effect of medications on the patient's central nervous system. • Provide interaction with children and pets. • Encourage the patient to participate in exercise classes and provide activity therapy. • Ensure that institutionalized older adults share meals with four people per table. • Ensure that homebound older adults have frequent visits from family and community resources such as Meals on Wheels or church volunteers.
Sensory overload	• Orient the patient to person, place, and time. • Decrease environmental noise. • Encourage the patient to participate in nursing care.

find comfort in cultural and religious symbols of care and healing that are absent in a hospital environment. Thus, nurses must be aware of the aspects of the patient's culture to deliver culturally competent care.

Personality and Lifestyle

Apart from a person's culture, different personality types demand different levels of stimulation. One person may thrive on a steady stream of fast-paced changes and excitement, whereas another may feel best when daily routines are rigidly structured and life sends no challenges necessitating changes. Lifestyle choices can dramatically influence the quantity and quality of stimuli a person receives. The nurse who elects to work in the emergency department of a large city hospital is exposed to stimuli vastly different from those of the nurse making home visits in a rural setting.

Stress and Illness

Increased sensory stimulation may be sought during periods of low stress simply to maintain cortical arousal. During high-stress periods, multiple stressors may already be overloading the sensory system, and the person desires decreased sensory stimulation. Illness, a time of stress, can affect the reception of sensory stimuli and their transmission and perception. Therefore, the stress of physical illness, pain, hospitalization, testing, surgery, or treatment may provide more stimulation than a person can process and respond to without assistance.

 THINK back to Muriel Hao, the woman who had surgery 2 days ago. Most likely, Ms. Hao is experiencing sensory overload from all of the events of the past several days. The constant beeping of the equipment is adding to this overload. ●

Medication

Medications that alert or depress the central nervous system may interfere with the perception of sensory stimuli. Narcotics and sedatives decrease awareness of sensory stimuli. Antipsychotics can influence how sensory stimuli are perceived and processed. Certain medications may also contribute to the impairment of sensory functioning by decreasing reception (e.g., captopril, an antihypertensive agent, can cause taste alteration). Examples of medications that are ototoxic and can impair auditory function if taken over a long period of time include furosemide (Lasix), some cancer chemotherapies, and aspirin. Be sure to review patients' medication records when assessing for sensory alterations.

THE NURSING PROCESS FOR SENSORY STIMULATION
Assessing

When assessing a patient for disturbed sensory perceptions, interview the patient and assess for sensory deficits and manifestations of sensory deprivation or overload. Be sure to include an assessment of the patient's envi-

ronment to determine whether it is providing adequate sensory stimulation for healthy development.

Identifying At-Risk Patients

Patients may be at risk for sensory disturbances for different reasons. Often there are *physiologic* reasons that place patients at risk. Aging, for example, is often accompanied by diminished senses. Diseases can also diminish senses. Diabetes-related neuropathies can result in a loss of sensation in limbs, rendering the diabetic unable to feel hot objects such as bath water, which can result in burns. Certain drugs affect taste. *Social and environmental* factors likewise place people at risk. Humans need appropriate human and environmental stimulation. When either or both are deficient or excessive, problems may result. *Lifestyle* factors may also place people at risk such as engaging in work or leisure activities that are potentially harmful to the eyes or ears, for example, exposure to chemicals, flying objects, and loud noises.

Assessment of the Sensory Experience

When assessing a patient's sensory experience, structure the history using the components of the sensory experience—stimulation, reception, and transmission–perception–reaction. See Focused Assessment Guide 43-1. Because patients may adapt to sensory impairments, it may be helpful to include someone the patient knows well (e.g., partner or parent) in the assessment to see if that person has noticed behavioral characteristics in the patient that suggest a sensory disturbance (e.g., "I've noticed he turns the television volume much louder than ever before."). Also, recognize that people may develop acuity in certain senses to compensate for losses in others. For example, many people who are blind have acute hearing. Begin by asking patients to evaluate their sensory functioning: "How would you rate your vision (hearing, and the like): Excellent, good, fair, poor, or bad?"

The mental status exam is included in assessments of sensory functioning. Chapter 25 provides a detailed description of how to assess levels of awareness (see also Box 43-2, p. 1634), levels of consciousness, memory, abstract reasoning, and language. The mini-mental status examination (MMSE or MMSE-2) is one of the most widely used clinical instruments for quickly detecting cognitive impairment and assessing its severity, as well as for monitoring cognitive changes over time (www.minimental.com).

STIMULATION

Assess for any recent changes in sensory stimulation, for example, reduction of stimulation from one or more sensory modalities ("Since my husband died, no one touches me anymore. It sounds crazy, but I'm hungry to be touched!") or new or unusual stimulation ("Ever since my granddaughter moved in with me, my house is always noisy. I can't stand the constant noise and her smoking."). Assess whether the type of stimulation present is developmentally

FOCUSED ASSESSMENT GUIDE 43-1

SENSORY STIMULATION

Factors to Assess	Questions and Approaches
Stimulation	"Does your current environment overly, insufficiently, or appropriately stimulate you?" "Are you bored? Why?" "Are you able to read? Watch television? Knit? Why not?" "Are there other people in your home during the day? Do you spend much time together? How do you spend the time?" "Who visits you while you are in the hospital?" Note reduction in the patterns or meaningfulness of stimulation in each sensory modality, changes in stimulation other than decreases (e.g., new or unusual stimulation), or developmental appropriateness of stimulation.
Reception	"Does anything interfere with the functioning of your senses?" "Describe any corrective devices you use for sensory impairments."
Assess for visual disturbances.	"Please read my name tag (or this page of print)." Note if the patient can correctly identify objects directly in front of the eyes as well as those requiring peripheral vision. Note eye rubbing, squinting, movements indicating faulty vision (bumping into furniture, overreaching or underreaching for objects), changes in the appearance of the eye (cataracts, swelling), and complaints of eye pain, spots, halos, or other visual disturbances.
Assess for auditory disturbances.	"Repeat the words that I will speak softly close to each ear." Note if the patient is able to hear equally well from both ears, distinguish voices, locate the direction of a sound; if the patient needs to face the person speaking and relies on lip reading; if the patient's responses to questions include blank looks, many nods, smiling, or inappropriate responses indicating faulty hearing. Note complaints of ringing or buzzing in the ears.
Assess for gustatory (taste) disturbances.	"Close your eyes, stick out your tongue, and tell me if what I place on your tongue is sweet, sour, bitter, or salty." "Have you been experiencing any strange tastes (bitter, metallic) or aftertastes lately?" Note if the patient is able to differentiate sweet, sour, bitter, or salty tastes or reports unusual, persistent taste sensations. Note deficient oral hygiene, ill-fitting dentures, braces, or anything else that might contribute to gustatory disturbances.
Assess for olfactory (smell) disturbances.	"Close your eyes and tell me what you smell." "Have you smelled odors lately that others cannot smell, or have you been especially sensitive to odors?" Note if the patient can correctly identify common odors (coffee, vanilla) or has noticed increased sensitivity to odors.
Assess for tactile (touch) disturbances.	"Close your eyes and tell me when you feel something (brush skin with cotton ball), if what you feel is dull or sharp (use both ends of a safety pin), hot or cold (use items from the food tray). Now, keep your eyes closed and tell me what I am placing in your hand (coin, cotton ball, paper clip)." Note if the patient can correctly sense touch and distinguish sharp and dull, hot and cold, and different shapes. Note if the patient reports decreased sensation in any part of the body; numbness, pins and needles, tingling; or abnormal sensitivity to pain or touch.
Assess for kinesthetic and visceral disturbances.	Note if the patient withdraws from being touched. "Have you noticed any changes in the way you perceive your body?" "Do you feel any unusual pressure or pain inside your body?" Note if the patient seems unsure of his or her body parts or body position and if the patient experiences new internal sensations (fullness, pressure, pain).

(continued)

FOCUSED ASSESSMENT GUIDE 43-1 *continued*

SENSORY STIMULATION

Factors to Assess	Questions and Approaches
Transmission–perception–reaction	"Are you aware of any problems with your nervous system?" "Have you found it difficult to communicate verbally?" Note consciousness, orientation, appropriateness of responses, ability to perform usual self-care activities, ability to follow simple commands, decision-making abilities, pathology affecting the central nervous system, or prescribed or recreational drug use that affects the central nervous system.
Behavioral manifestations of sensory deprivation or overload	
Perceptual responses	Mild to gross sensory distortions (illusions, hallucinations)
Cognitive responses	Thought disorganization, slowness of thought, decreased attention/concentration, difficulty with problem solving and task performance
Emotional responses	Rapid mood changes, anxiety, panic

appropriate. *High-risk patients* for problems related to stimulation include children in nonstimulating environments, older people, terminally ill patients, patients on bedrest, patients in isolation, and patients requiring intensive nursing in a critical care setting.

RECEPTION

Assess for anything that may interfere with sensory reception and identify any *corrective devices* the patient uses for sensory impairments (eyeglasses, contact lenses, hearing aids). If corrective devices are necessary, assess whether or not the patient is actually using them, has the proper equipment, and understands related care. For example, ask the patient, "When were your eyes last examined?" or "Are there batteries for your hearing aid?" The reception section of the Focused Assessment Guide 43-1 highlights assessment strategies for each sense. Patients at *high risk* for reception problems include people with visual, auditory, or other sensory impairments.

 CONSIDER Dolores Pirolla and her husband who has visual and hearing deficits. The nurse needs to assess the amount and type of stimulation Mr. Pirolla is receiving. In addition, the nurse needs to investigate what measures the couple uses to adapt to the progressive visual changes. Doing so

would provide a sound basis on which to build the plan of care. See Box 43-5 for sample documentation of Mr. Pirolla's assessment of sensory functioning. ●

TRANSMISSION–PERCEPTION–REACTION

Be alert for patients at high risk for transmission–perception–reaction problems, such as the patient who is confused or who has a nervous system impairment. Use everyday interactions as multiple opportunities to assess patients' abilities to transmit, perceive, and react to stimuli.

DEFINING CHARACTERISTICS OF SENSORY DEPRIVATION AND OVERLOAD

Complete the assessment of the patient's sensory functioning by assessing for specific indicators of sensory deprivation or overload (see Box 43-2, p. 1634). Observe for boredom, inactivity, slowness of thought, daydreaming, increased sleeping, thought disorganization, anxiety, panic, illusions, and hallucinations. Know the patient's usual state so that you can identify changes stemming from sensory deprivation or overload.

 THINK back to Muriel Hao, the woman who had surgery 2 days ago. The patient's complaints of being unable to rest due to the machine's beeping should alert the nurse to the

BOX 43-5   SAMPLE DOCUMENTATION OF A TARGETED ASSESSMENT

Mr. Anthony Pirolla came to the clinic with his wife, who reported a new concern about his hearing.

Chief complaint: Difficulty hearing.

Signs and symptoms: According to his wife, Mr. Pirolla frequently fails to answer her questions or answers inappropriately. She also reports that he plays the radio and television louder than before. He complains that people seem to be "mumbling" more than usual—especially in church. Patient denies ringing or buzzing in ears.

Onset/duration: Mr. Pirolla states that he's had difficulty hearing since Christmas (2 months ago)—when the whole

family came to visit. Mrs. Pirolla believes he had difficulty starting in the summer.

Predisposing factors: In his youth, Mr. Pirolla worked construction and was frequently around loud equipment. He is 77.

Effect on patient: Patient no longer enjoys going out or being with friends and has become more reclusive.

Self remedies: None.

Intervention: Referred Mr. Pirolla to the clinic's audiologist.

C. Taylor, RN

possibility of sensory overload. To confirm the suspicions, the nurse needs to review the patient's medical record to gather more data about the patient's usual state and behavior. ●

Physical Assessment

Physical examination skills related to the senses are discussed in Chapter 25. Ear and eye tests, whether performed by a physician or nurse, should be considered when planning care. Problems with the neurologic system require further assessment of the sensory experience.

Assessment of the Ability to Perform Self-Care

Alterations in sensory functioning may limit a person's ability to perform everyday activities safely. Exercise empathy by trying to imagine how you would get through a day if you lacked sight, hearing, or other senses. Ideally, this exercise will help you fashion a plan of care responsive to the needs of patients. Patients with new sensory alterations and their family caregivers need to be instructed about practical ways to modify their home environment for safety. For an interactive resource, try mysafehome. org or www.safekids.org for resources to prevent injuries in children. Additionally, recognize that patients who are out of their home environment need to be oriented to their new surroundings. Patients need to know how to call the nurse, how to use the lights and television, and how to navigate safely to the bathroom. Before leaving a patient's room, do a quick check to ensure that the environment is safe—especially for patients with sensory impairments.

Diagnosing

When assessment data point to sensory disturbances that can be treated independently by nursing interventions, nursing diagnoses are developed and labeled. The North American Nursing Diagnosis Association International (NANDA-I, 2012) recognizes the following diagnostic labels for sensory/perceptual problems:

- *Acute Confusion:* The abrupt onset of a cluster of global, transient changes and disturbances in attention, cognition, psychomotor activity level of consciousness, or sleep–wake cycle
- *Chronic Confusion:* An irreversible, long-standing, or progressive deterioration of intellect and personality characterized by decreased ability to interpret environmental stimuli or decreased capacity for intellectual thought processes and manifested by disturbances of memory, orientation, and behavior
- *Impaired Memory:* The state in which an individual experiences the inability to remember or recall bits of information or behavior skills. Impaired memory may be attributed to pathophysiologic or situational causes that are either temporary or permanent.

Disturbed Sensory Perception

Disturbed sensory perception is a state in which a person or group experiences or is at risk for a change in the amount, pattern, or interpretation of incoming stimuli. These altera-

tions may be further specified as visual, auditory, gustatory, olfactory, tactile, or kinesthetic. Sensory deprivation, sensory overload, and uncompensated sensory loss may also be used to further specify the disturbed sensory perception and in some cases may be the etiology. Note that this diagnosis was retired from the NANDA-I taxonomy in the 2012–2014 edition pending significant work to bring it to a higher level of evidence (NANDA-I, 2012, p. 490).

Common etiologies for disturbed sensory perception include the following:

- Altered environmental stimuli: excessive or insufficient
- Altered sensory reception, transmission, or integration
- Chemical alterations: endogenous (e.g., electrolytes) or exogenous (e.g., drugs)
- Psychological stress

See Examples of NANDA-I Nursing Diagnoses (on page 1644) in which disturbed sensory perception is the problem. Because disturbed sensory perceptions affect many other areas of human functioning, they serve as etiologies for multiple problem statements. Examples may include the following:

- Activity Intolerance related to impaired balance and coordination (kinesthetic alteration)
- Anxiety related to paranoia stemming from hearing impairment, sensory deprivation (specify setting), sensory overload
- Impaired Verbal Communication related to difficulty receiving, transmitting, and perceiving sensory stimuli
- Ineffective Coping related to sensory overload (multiple stressors)
- Deficient Diversional Activity related to impaired vision or hearing
- Delayed Growth and Development related to nonstimulating home environment
- Risk for Injury related to decreased or impaired sensation (specify visual, auditory, tactile, kinesthetic)
- Impaired Physical Mobility related to impaired balance and coordination (kinesthetic alteration)
- Impaired Parenting Associated with Failure to Provide Stimuli for Growth related to lack of knowledge, decreased motivation to provide for child's growth and development
- Self-Care Deficit: (specify) related to visual impairment, auditory impairment, tactile impairment
- Ineffective Role Performance related to sensory/perceptual alteration (blindness, deafness, and so forth)
- Sexual Dysfunction related to decreased sensation
- Impaired Skin Integrity related to absent tactile sensation (injury)
- Disturbed Sleep Pattern related to sensory deprivation or overload
- Impaired Social Interaction related to inability to receive and process interactional stimuli
- Social Isolation related to visual or auditory impairment
- Disturbed Thought Processes (specify illusions, hallucinations, decreased attention or concentration, and the like) related to sensory deprivation or overload

EXAMPLES OF NANDA-I NURSING DIAGNOSES

DISTURBED SENSORY PERCEPTION

Nursing Diagnoses	Related Factors	Sample Defining Characteristics
Disturbed Sensory Perception: Sensory Deficit or Excess Visual	Eye patches after surgery	"I never realized before how sight-dependent I am. I don't know what time of day it is now unless I have the radio on or smell food coming in." "It's frightening not to know who is in my room and what they are doing." Patient observed sitting in room with blank facial expression; frequently comments on how bored he or she is and how slowly time is passing; hesitant to move about room without assistance despite having been oriented repeatedly.
Auditory	Effects of aging	"You're right. I don't always hear what people are saying anymore so I try not to get involved in conversations. If people insist on talking, I just nod and hope I'm giving the right response." Able to hear moderately spoken word close to right ear; cannot hear same from left ear; often startled when someone approaches from left side. Sits close to television and radio; loud volume, no history of hearing testing.
Gustatory or olfactory	Chemotherapy	"I always seem to have a bitter taste in my mouth now and can't stomach certain foods at all that I used to enjoy, like beef, tomatoes, coffee....I also can't take sweets, and I used to be a real sweets junkie." "Sometimes the very smell of certain foods or even the thought of eating nauseates me." Patient has been receiving vincristine (cancer chemotherapeutic agent) for past 3 months; some nausea and vomiting; history of poor oral hygiene.
Tactile	Psychological stress	"I don't know why I feel this way, but I'm hypersensitive to touch. If anyone even brushes against me, I feel burning pain. Even the weight of my clothes against my skin bothers me. I'm trying to move my body as little as possible and keep it protected—but that's obviously impossible when even a breeze assaults me." Patient observed holding the body stiffly looking like he or she does not know what to do with the arms and legs; dressed only in a loose-fitting outfit; reports sitting at home all day afraid to go out.
Kinesthetic	Clinitron bed therapy	"I've been in this bed for 2 weeks now and I've lost all sense of my body...it's a curious weightless feeling that I have...sort of like floating in Jell-O. I'm no longer sure where my body begins and ends, and when I try to lift an arm or leg I feel like I'm in slow motion. I hope I'll be able to walk when I get out of here."
Disturbed Sensory Perception: Sensory Deprivation	Isolation	"One of the worst things that has happened to me since I found out I had AIDS is that everyone is afraid of me—and no one touches me. I'm so lonely. I've always needed a lot of people around." "Here in the hospital I think I'm going crazy. I can't leave this room. Everyone who comes in looks the same dressed in those yellow gowns. Lately, I've seen some bizarre things that I know can't be real. I look at the clock and it turns into a swirling sun with a sad face that keeps coming closer and closer to me and I'm terrified I'll burn up if it gets too close. That's crazy, isn't it? I'm really losing it now." Disturbed sleep for past 2 weeks; during the day, yawns excessively and catnaps; limited attention span; states he or she is unable to concentrate on anything.
Disturbed Sensory Perception: Sensory Overload	Trauma of rape and aftercare	"When is everyone going to stop touching me? First, he wouldn't stop. Now, everyone here is poking at me, looking at me, asking me hundreds of questions....Why did I have to report this and come to the hospital? Oh, please leave me alone. Get out of here, everyone."

Outcome Identification and Planning

In all settings in which nurses care for patients, optimal sensory stimulation is a priority. Nursing care focuses on the following patient outcomes. The patient will:

- Live in a developmentally stimulating and safe environment
- Exhibit a level of arousal that enables the brain to receive and meaningfully organize patterns of stimulation
- Demonstrate intact functioning of the senses: vision, hearing, taste, smell, touch, and kinesthetic and visceral awareness
- Schedule appropriate health screening exams for sensory functioning
- Maintain orientation to time, place, and person
- Respond appropriately (verbally and nonverbally) to sensory stimuli while executing self-care activities

Patients with impaired sensory functioning require individualized outcomes similar to the following. The patient will:

- Report feeling safe and in control of the environment
- Describe different types of meaningful stimuli present in the environment
- Demonstrate (describe) appropriate self-care behaviors for visual impairment, hearing impairment, or other sensory impairment
- Verbalize acceptance of the sensory deficit

Implementing

The nurse can assist patients to improve sensory functioning by teaching them and their significant others methods for stimulating the senses, teaching patients with intact and impaired senses appropriate self-care behaviors, and interacting therapeutically with patients experiencing sensory impairments. Safety is always a special concern for patients with sensory alterations. Ensure that the patient's environment is as free of danger as possible, and assist the patient to develop new self-care behaviors to compensate for sensory impairments. See the accompanying Examples of Nursing Interventions and Nursing Outcomes Classifications (NIC/NOC): Balance. Safety considerations are discussed in Chapter 26 in more detail. The nursing interventions described here relate to preventing sensory alteration, stimulating the senses, meeting the needs of vision- and hearing-impaired people, communicating with a confused person, and communicating with an unconscious person. Communication guidelines for patients with sensory deficits are also highlighted in Chapter 20.

Preventing Disturbed Sensory Perception and Stimulating the Senses

Prevention is the most effective means to manage sensory alteration. The key to prevention is to create a functional and meaningful environment with the patient's help, while keeping limitations in mind. The creation of such an environment requires careful observation, analysis, and creative planning.

Although numerous nursing measures can be considered when planning care, their appropriateness depends on the circumstances. Promote the patient's well-being by offering care that provides rest and comfort (see Chapters 33 and 34). Attempt to control patient discomfort whenever possible.

 RECALL Muriel Hao, the woman who had surgery 2 days ago. The patient verbalizes an inability to rest due to the "beeping of the machine." The initial priority is to stop the machine from beeping. The nurse needs to investigate the underlying problem related to the machine's beeping, such as a low battery or an occlusion. The nurse can then focus on comfort measures. ●

Be aware of a patient's need for sensory aids and prostheses, such as eyeglasses, contact lenses, hearing

---

EXAMPLES OF NURSING INTERVENTIONS AND NURSING OUTCOMES CLASSIFICATIONS (NIC/NOC)

EXERCISE THERAPY: BALANCE

Nursing Interventions	Nursing Outcomes
• Determine patient's ability to participate in activities requiring balance. • Evaluate sensory functions (e.g., vision, hearing, proprioception). • Provide opportunity to discuss factors that influence fear of falling. • Provide safe environment for practice of exercises. • Instruct the patient on the importance of exercise therapy in maintaining and improving balance.	• Maintains balance while sitting without back support • Maintains balance while standing • Maintains balance while walking • Maintains balance while turning 360 degrees • Posture

Adapted from Bulechek, G., Butcher, H., Dochterman, J., & Wagner, C. M. (Eds.). (2013). *Nursing interventions classification (NIC)* (6th ed., pp. 184–185). St. Louis: Elsevier/Mosby; and Moorhead, S., Johnson, M., Maas, M., & Swanson, E. (Eds.). (2013). *Nursing outcomes classification (NOC)* (5th ed., p. 97). St. Louis: Elsevier/Mosby. A full listing of nursing activities for each nursing intervention and outcomes can be found in these books.

aids, dentures, canes, and artificial limbs, ensuring that they are available as needed. Social activities help stimulate the senses and mind (Figure 43-2). Enlist the aid of family members to participate in or encourage these activities. Also encourage physical activity and exercise, which help maintain normal sensory perceptions and decrease the likelihood of sensory alteration (exercises are discussed in Chapter 32).

Provide stimulation for as many senses as possible. Varied sights, sounds, smells, body positions, and textures help provide a variety of sensations. For example, music therapy has been found to benefit selected physiologic variables such as pulse rate, respiratory rate, and mood state in patients receiving mechanical ventilation. Listening to music can ameliorate the stress response and promote nonpharmacologically induced relaxation for the study subjects. All nurses, especially critical care nurses, can confidently implement this nonpharmacologic, independent intervention to promote relaxation without worry of untoward side effects, which are sometimes caused by pharmacologic sedation. Consider cultural factors when stimulating the patient's senses and when offering nursing care, especially when caring for patients from cultures different from one's own. (See Chapter 27 for a discussion of common complementary and alternative therapies.)

Teaching About Sensory Experiences

Teaching is a significant nursing responsibility that helps prepare patients for sensory experiences. An informed patient is better able to handle fears, frustration, and confusion. Therefore, explain procedures before performing them or having the patient experience them. Explanations also help prevent patients feeling that their personal space and body are being invaded.

Allow patients experiencing perceptual and thought distortions the opportunity to acknowledge that fact. Discussing such experiences and reassuring the patient that these experiences are normal and usually temporary generally eases anxiety.

 REMEMBER Ori Soltes, the young man in the ICU who becomes confused. The nurse needs to acknowledge the patient's confusion,

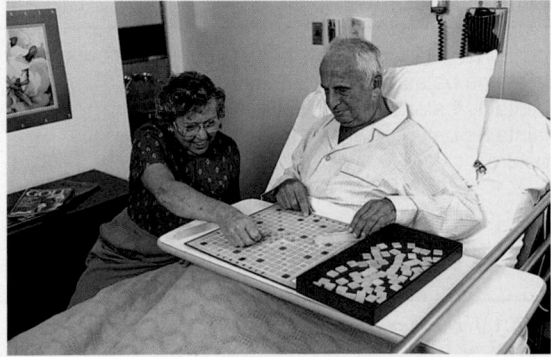

FIGURE 43-2. The nurse helps the patient find methods for stimulating the senses. Family members may participate in sensory activities.

reorienting him frequently. In addition, the patient's ability to communicate is limited because of the ventilator. Therefore, the nurse should provide the patient with alternative means to communicate, such as paper and pencil or a blackboard to write on to make his needs known. The nurse also needs to reinforce explanations about all the equipment and technologies to which the patient is being exposed to help alleviate some of his anxiety. ●

Patients and family members can be guided in sensory self-stimulation, and parents can be aided in stimulation of newborns, infants, and children. Teaching Tips 43-1 gives helpful suggestions for teaching patients about protecting and stimulating sensory function and includes suggestions that the nurse can use in a variety of situations. Table 43-1 (on page 1648) provides additional information on stimulating the senses for patients and nurses.

Promoting Health Literacy

Risk factors for inadequate health literacy include advanced age, low educational level, poverty, inability to read, learning disabilities, and lack of English proficiency. Patients may also be at risk for inadequate health literacy because of hearing or visual impairments or confusion and inability to process or remember what is heard. See the Promoting Health Literacy box on page 1649. You can also download the Joint Commission white paper, "What Did the Doctor Say?": Improving Health Literacy to Protect Patient Safety at http://www.jointcommission.org/assets/1/18/improving_health_literacy.pdf.

Meeting the Needs of Patients With Reduced Vision

Always check with the physician to learn whether a patient's visual problem is temporary, permanent, partial, or complete, and the degree to which the problem is likely to affect the patient's everyday functioning. This information is vital to developing a realistic teaching plan or plan of care.

The first priority is to teach patients self-care behaviors for maintaining vision and preventing blindness. These include:

- Do not rub the eyes.
- Avoid eyestrain, e.g., reading in poor light or viewing television or smart devices when tired.
- Avoid damage from ultraviolet rays.
- Protect eyes from foreign bodies.
- Keep eyeglasses clean, protected, and adjusted.
- Do not use nonprescription eyedrops, and seek attention for symptoms.
- Do not clean eyes or contact lenses with soiled articles.
- Use caution with aerosol sprays.
- Use caution with ammonia, lye, and so on.
- Visit your physician frequently if you are prone to eye problems.
- Know the danger signals that indicate serious eye problems: persistent eye redness; pain or discomfort,

SENSORY FUNCTIONING

Health Topic	Teaching Tip	Why Is This Important?
Hearing	• Avoid loud noise that is concentrated at the ear canal, such as with earphones. • Decrease background or loud noises. • Use ear plugs when using loud machinery, including lawn mowers, grass trimmers, or industrial equipment. • Have regular hearing assessments. Children should be assessed in school yearly. • Do not insert objects such as cotton-tipped applicators into the ear. • Do not clean inside the ear. • Have ear pain evaluated by a physician or nurse practitioner. • Be aware of the signs and symptoms of hearing loss.	Hearing loss occurring as a person ages is called presbycusis. Presbycusis involves the deterioration of nerves and structures within the inner ear. Many occupations result in hearing loss due to increased noise. Thus, the use of ear-protective devices can decrease the development of hearing loss. Instructing the patient on signs and symptoms of hearing loss and interventions to be implemented can help to slow the development of hearing loss.
Vision	• Protect the eye from damage due to ultraviolet rays with sunglasses and tinted windows. • Provide adequate light for working or reading. • Stimulate vision with colors and shapes. • Use large print to assist in readability. • Have an annual eye examination. • Do not rub the eyes. • Use cleaning products or aerosol products safely in a well-ventilated area. • Use eye shields when in contact with harmful or toxic products, such as blood or body fluids or cleaning products. • Do not use nonprescription eyedrops.	The education of the patient to maintain adequate eye function enhances the patient's quality of life. The avoidance of strain on the eye stimulates vision, thus enhancing sensory perception.
Taste (gustatory)	• Practice oral care three times per day to prevent infection and decay. • Visit the dentist biannually for dental cleaning and examination. • Notify the dentist about pain or sensitivity to hot or cold. • Provide nutritional foods that are high in fiber, and low in fat and sugar. • Enhance taste with the use of spices.	Prevention of mouth disease enhances the taste and enjoyment of foods.
Smell	• Use aromatherapy to reduce stress. • Protect the nose from noxious fumes. • Eliminate disturbing odors with adequate ventilation. • Visit the physician or nurse practitioner when experiencing nasal congestion or diminished sense of smell. • Do not wear heavy colognes or perfumes. • Enhance the sense of smell by remembering pleasant odors.	The sense of smell is important in assisting the person to relax, particularly during times of stress. It is important to evaluate any difficulty with the sense of smell and nasal congestion, since the nose lies in close proximity to the ear and the brain. Thus, the prevention of infection is a primary aspect of care.
Touch	• Protect the skin from extremes in temperature. • Provide various textures in the environment. • Provide touch such as during the bath or massage therapy. • Instruct on all aspects of invasive procedures.	Protecting the skin from temperature changes decreases damage to the skin and underlying tissues. The use of a variety of textures stimulates nerve fibers and tactile sense.
Sensory Overload	• Reduce the number and type of stimuli. • Provide periods of rest. • Provide explanation of sounds and activities within the environment. • Use relaxation techniques to enhance rest.	Sensory overload can be prevented by using these measures. As a result, the patient is able to organize stimuli to decrease anxiety and stress.
Sensory Deprivation	• Provide reading material, audiovisual stimulation, and interactive activities. • Provide stimulation through visitors, phone conversations, and e-mail. • Use therapeutic touch. • Encourage the use of assistive devices such as hearing aids and glasses. • Provide a radio and television. • Orient to time, place, and person.	Increasing sensory perception enhances the patient's responses, helping to create a meaningful environment.

Table 43-1 STIMULATING THE SENSES

SENSE	TEACHING PATIENTS	NURSING INTERVENTIONS
Vision	Surround yourself with different colors and with an environment that changes (walk through a mall, sit by a window where you see people come and go). Develop a sensitivity to changes in nature (weather patterns, dawn-to-night cycle, changing seasons, changes in a plant or animal). Use visual devices to keep oriented (watches, calendars, newspaper, television). Use crossword puzzles and games to stimulate mental activities. Create favorite scenes in your mind, paying attention to tiny details.	Wear visually stimulating and comforting colors. Keep meaningful visual stimuli such as photos, greeting cards, toys, or flowers near the patient. Position patients with impaired mobility where they can see out a window or watch local traffic on the unit.
Hearing	Decrease or eliminate distressing auditory stimuli (change bedroom, talk with family members about noise of stereos and other such equipment, use earplugs, use headphones to listen to soft music). Develop a sensitivity to different sounds (music, chirping birds, night sounds, different voices). Use the telephone to maintain contact with family and friends. Use television, radio, CDs to keep current and to stimulate mental activities. Recall favorite sounds of the past with the situations in which they were heard.	Speak in a warm and pleasant tone and communicate caring to the patient. Use your voice to orient the patient to the environment and current situation (e.g., procedure, treatment). Avoid speaking about the patient to others within the patient's hearing. Remember that patients overhearing snatches of conversation outside their room often presume it is about *them!* Decrease extraneous noise (intercom, movement of carts, loud conversations of staff); use carpets and sound-absorbing material whenever possible.
Taste	Experiment with foods of different tastes (seasonings), colors, temperature, and textures; realize that as taste buds age, things will no longer taste the same. Practice thorough oral hygiene and have regular dental examinations. Recall foods that tasted especially good in the past and the events surrounding these tastes (e.g., grandparent baking cookies or homemade bread).	Consult with the dietitian about preparing meals with varied taste sensations; serve meals attractively. Perform routine oral hygiene for patients who are unable to do this for themselves.
Smell	Consciously savor smells that are pleasant; decrease or eliminate noxious odors. Recall pleasant aromas or smells from the past and the events surrounding them (e.g., smell of the ocean when nearing the vacation house, smell of fresh pine in the house at Christmas, the body scent of a loved person or animal).	Keep the patient's room well ventilated, using opportunities when the patient is out of the room to air it out. Remove dressings, drainage, and any equipment with odors from the patient's room as quickly as possible. Encourage patients to focus on pleasant or familiar smells, such as coffee, newspaper, or flowers. Avoid wearing heavy perfumes.
Touch	Consciously surround yourself with different textures and let yourself feel and enjoy them (scratchy afghan; a puppy's moist, wet tongue; soft petal of a flower; smooth silk scarf; mug of hot chocolate). Allow these textures to evoke memories of past tactile experiences (grandchild's hug may bring back memories of hugs from own children, scrap of fabric may recall a prom dress or wedding gown or baby blanket). Recognize the need to be touched and tell someone, "I need a hug today!" Receive tactile stimulation from a pet.	Include different textures in the patient's environment (silky pillow sham from home, soft sheepskin, wooly blanket). Respect the patient's need and desire to be touched or not touched (touch the patient's forearm or shoulder, hug the patient). Use physical care (bath time, foot soaks, hair care, back massages, turning and positioning, passive range of motion) to provide tactile stimulation. Limit intrusive procedures and times when the patient needs to be uncomfortably manipulated.

GENERAL NURSING STRATEGIES IN THE HOSPITAL OR OTHER RESIDENTIAL CARE SETTING

Encourage the patient to participate in activities that require exploration of the environment (exercise, feeling, tasting, touching, moving, listening).

Use conversation to explore areas of interest to the patient.

Encourage the patient to share feelings.

Familiarize the environment by encouraging the patient to wear own clothes and keep personal items nearby.

Suggest the use of self-stimulation techniques—humming, singing, whistling, reciting, memory review, and problem solving.

PROMOTING HEALTH LITERACY

IN PATIENTS WITH HEARING DEFICITS

Patient Scenario

Mr. Rosato is 84 and until recently had no difficulty hearing. He lives in a long-term care facility because of complications from several serious diseases: diabetes, congestive heart failure, high blood pressure, degenerative joint disease. His daughter, who visits frequently, informs you, the nurse manager, that he seems to be having increasing difficulty with hearing—although he denies this. She shares that he sometimes answers questions inappropriately or asks folks to speak louder and she noticed that his television volume is always loud. She made an appointment for him with an audiologist but shares that she doesn't know the first thing about hearing disorders.

Nursing Considerations: *Tips for Improving Health Literacy*

Compliment the daughter's keen observation, report that sensory disorders are common among older adults, and tell her how important the visit with the audiologist is. Give her an information sheet about hearing disorders and tips on finding out more information about the disorder online from a credible source. Encourage her to be prepared to ask the audiologist three questions:

- What is her father's main problem?
- What do they need to do?
- Why is it important for them to do this?

What additional measures can you take to help increase health literacy in this patient and his family? What other measures would be helpful if Mr. Rosato and/or his daughter do not speak English, cannot read, or have other learning deficits?

---

especially after injury; visual disturbances; crossing eyes; a growth on or near the eyes; discharge or increased tearing; and pupil irregularities.

When communicating with patients with reduced vision, follow these guidelines:

- Acknowledge your presence in the patient's room. Identify yourself by name.
- Speak in a normal tone of voice. Remember that the blind person is unable to pick up most nonverbal cues during communication.
- Explain the reason for touching the person before doing so.
- Keep the call light or bell within easy reach of the person and place the bed in the lowest position.
- Orient the person to sounds in the environment.
- Orient the person to the arrangement of the room and its furnishings. Clear pathways for the person and do not rearrange furnishings. Clarify this fact with housekeeping personnel also.
- Assist with ambulation by walking slightly ahead of the person, allowing the person to grasp your arm.
- Stay in the person's field of vision if he or she has partial or reduced peripheral vision.
- Provide diversions using other senses.
- Indicate to the person when the conversation has ended and when you are leaving the room.

Meeting the Needs of Patients With Reduced Hearing

Temporary hearing losses are most often conductive in nature—due to a problem with the external or middle ear (wax buildup, foreign-body obstruction, infection). However, sensorineural hearing losses caused by inner ear or central nervous system problems may not be totally cor-

rectable. Health teaching to prevent hearing problems includes the following recommendations for patients:

- Avoid excessive noise.
- Do not insert sharp objects into ears.
- Do not clean the ears excessively.
- Avoid practices that can cause infection; treat infection early.
- Know the symptoms of hearing loss: asking others frequently to repeat what they said, an inability to hear at a distance, need to see the person who is talking, leaning forward or turning an ear toward the speaker, answering inappropriately, talking too loudly, inability to carry on a phone conversation, strained facial expression.

When communicating with patients who have hearing deficits or impairments, follow these guidelines:

- Orient the person to your presence before initiating conversation, such as by moving so you can be seen or by gently touching the person.
- Decrease background noises (television, radio) if possible before you speak.
- Make sure that the patient's hearing aids (if applicable) are working optimally.
- Position yourself so that the light is on your face and the person can see your lips and expressions.
- Talk directly to the person while facing him or her, or angle your chair so that your voice reaches the ear that hears best. If the person can lip-read, use simple sentences and speak in a quiet, natural manner and pace. Be aware of nonverbal communication.
- Do not chew gum, cover your mouth, or turn away when talking with the person.
- Demonstrate or pantomime ideas you wish to express, as appropriate.
- Use sign language or finger spelling, as appropriate.

• Write any statement that you cannot convey to the person in another manner.

Aids for people with reduced hearing include TDD (telecommunication devices), infrared systems, computers, voice amplifiers, amplified telephones, low-frequency doorbells and telephone ringers, closed-caption TV decoders, flashing alarm clocks, and flashing smoke detectors. The Centers for Disease Control and Prevention has numerous resources to prevent hearing loss (search for "hearing loss" at www.cdc.gov).

 CONSIDER Dolores Pirolla, the wife of the patient who has a visual deficit and is now demonstrating signs of a hearing deficit. The nurse would incorporate knowledge of the guidelines (for communicating both with people with reduced vision and hearing) when developing a teaching plan to assist Mrs. Pirolla in dealing with her husband's condition. In addition, the nurse could enlist the aid of social services to help Mrs. Pirolla obtain supportive services for her husband's visual impairment and obtain assistive devices for her husband to minimize the effects of the hearing deficit.

Communicating With a Patient Who is Confused

The patient who lacks the mental ability to process environmental stimuli may be aware of this inability and find it frustrating. This patient needs support to make adjustments to this limitation.

 ORI Soltes, the patient in the ICU who becomes confused, most likely is experiencing a high level of frustration. Due to his accident, he suddenly is thrust into an environment filled with unfamiliar sights, sounds, and activities, leading to feelings of being overwhelmed physically and emotionally. His level of frustration may be further increased by his inability to speak while receiving mechanical ventilation.

Other patients may be oblivious of this deficiency. In both instances, always protect the safety of the patient while providing optimal sensory stimulation. Nursing interventions include the following:

• Use frequent face-to-face contact to maintain the patient's social dimension (use touch when appropriate, walk arm in arm, hug, give a backrub).
• Speak calmly, simply, and directly to the patient and allow sufficient time for the patient to think before responding.
• Orient and reorient the patient to the environment, and fill the patient's personal space with as many personal objects as possible.
• Use conversation, watches, clocks, calendar, newspaper, television, radio, and other such devices to help orient the patient to time, place, and person.

• Clearly communicate that the patient is expected to perform all the self-care activities he or she can.
• Emphasize the patient's strengths rather than deficiencies, and verbally reinforce strengths.
• Offer the patient simple explanations for care, new activities, and so on.
• Vary environmental stimuli gradually while keeping the environment structured enough that the patient feels comfortable and at home.
• Use objects from the patient's past (e.g., a favorite baseball, a picture of a train, a photograph) to spark reminiscences and discussions.
• Reinforce reality if the patient is delusional.

A list of selected cognitive stimulation activities may be found in Chapter 20.

Communicating With a Patient Who is Unconscious

The following are recommended guidelines for communicating with a patient who is unconscious:

• Be careful of what you say in the person's presence. Hearing is believed to be the last sense lost; therefore, the person is often likely to hear what is being said, even if there does not appear to be a response.
• Assume the person can hear you. Talk with the person in a normal tone of voice about things you would ordinarily discuss.
• Speak to the person before touching. Remember that touch can be an effective means of communicating with the unconscious person.
• Keep environmental noises at as low a level as possible. This helps the person focus on the communication.

EVALUATING

While implementing a plan of nursing care designed to decrease excessive sensory stimuli or increase meaningful stimuli, evaluate the plan's effectiveness by observing for a decrease in the behavioral manifestations of sensory deprivation or overload. You may conclude that the plan of care is working if a patient who had begun to withdraw and spend most of the day lying in bed with a blank facial expression appears more alert and begins to initiate conversations and to take an interest in personal care. Also evaluate the patient's ability to interact appropriately with the environment while practicing necessary self-care behaviors as well as the patient's need for nursing care versus the individual's ability to manage the plan of care independently.

Ideally, the patient and family learn to manipulate the environment to promote optimal sensory stimulation for growth and development. Patients with specific sensory impairments are evaluated for their knowledge of the impairment, acceptance and management of the treatment regimen, and their ability to perform necessary self-care activities. See the accompanying concept map for Ori Soltes and the Nursing Plan of Care 43-1 for Mrs. Philomela Palikias on pages 1652–1654.

Ori Soltes, a 28-year-old man, is in the Intensive Care Unit (ICU) after a motor vehicle crash that resulted in multiple internal injuries as well as fractures. He is being monitored continuously and receiving mechanical ventilation via endotracheal tube. On the fifth day after the crash, he begins to exhibit transient episodes of acute confusion. Bilateral wrist restraints are being utilized to prevent self-extubation. In order to maintain adequate ventilation and control anxiety, intravenous sedation is prescribed as needed. His vital signs are as follows: BP 132/68 mm Hg, pulse 116 beats/minute, respirations 30 breaths/minute.

Priority 1

Nursing Diagnosis: Disturbed Sensory Perception: Sensory Overload related to excessive environmental stimuli.
Supporting Data:
• ICU environment
• Frequent examinations
• Multiple monitoring devices with alarms
• Lighted environment
• Wrist restraints
• Endotracheal intubation and mechanical ventilation
• Intravenous sedation
• BP 132/68 mm Hg, pulse 116 beats/min, respiratory rate 30 breaths/min

Priority 2

Nursing Diagnosis: Acute Confusion related to alteration in sleep–wake cycle.
Supporting Data:
• Transient episodes of confusion
• Frequent examinations
• Excessive environmental stimuli
• Restraints required to prevent self-extubation
• Critically ill with multiple monitoring modalities

Priority 3

Nursing Diagnosis: Impaired Verbal Communication related to endotracheal intubation and mechanical ventilation.
Supporting Data:
• Unable to verbalize needs due to endotracheal intubation
• Wrist restraints
• Multiple contacts with health team members

Outcome:
Patient will experience a reduction in environmental stimuli and normalization of vital signs.

Outcome:
Patient will become oriented to person, place, and time.

Outcome:
Patient will achieve alternate methods of communication.

Nursing Interventions:
• Cluster nursing interventions as tolerated to provide uninterrupted rest periods
• Eliminate nuisance alarms by maintaining appropriate alarm limits
• Dim lights when feasible
• Administer sedation as needed
• Release restraints every hour for 10 minutes while at bedside
• Communicate in soft, calm tones
• Explain all procedures prior to initiating them
• Monitor vital signs for physiologic signs of excessive stimuli
• Consider use of music therapy

Nursing Interventions:
• Reorient to person, place, and time
• Talk to patient prior to initiating touch
• Explain all procedures prior to performing them
• Encourage family to visit, talk, and provide Therapeutic Touch to the patient
• Ask family to bring in familiar objects and pictures
• Provide uninterrupted periods of sleep by clustering care activities
• Use clear, concise, and simple communication

Nursing Interventions:
• Talk directly to patient rather than talking over patient
• Establish an alternative means of communication such as picture board
• Communicate through nonverbal means, such as Therapeutic Touch
• Explain all procedures before starting
• Ascertain patient's areas of interest and talk to patient regarding these topics
• Place call bell within reach at all times

Evaluation: Ori's environment has been managed to reduce stimuli. Sedation has only been required every 4 hours. Vital signs have returned to normal.

Evaluation: Ori continues to exhibit transient periods of confusion, but with decreasing frequency. Continue interventions.

Evaluation: Ori has been unable to use picture board due to his weakened condition. Continue interventions.

- - - - - Relationship ■ Assessment ■ Nursing Diagnosis ■ Outcome Identification ■ Interventions ■ Evaluation

Concept map displaying the nursing process for Ori Soltes.

NURSING PLAN OF CARE 43-1

for Philomela Palikias

Two days ago, Mrs. Philomela Palikias delivered by cesarean birth a 32-week-old, small-for-gestational-age infant girl weighing 3 lb, 8 oz. Because of her size and respiratory distress, the infant was placed in the neonatal intensive care unit (NICU). Postpartal assessments indicate that Mrs. Palikias's physical progress is satisfactory. However, the nurses are concerned about her mental status. Mrs. Palikias arrived in the United States 3 months ago with her husband. Both speak only Greek and neither has family in the United States.

Recorded in the patient's progress notes the evening of her second postpartal day is the following nursing assessment:

12/4/15, 9 PM, nursing

Patient refused to get out of bed again this evening—demonstrates no interest in seeing baby; to date has not ambulated to NICU. Refusing to learn and participate in self-care activities—expressing breast milk or performing perineal care. Nurses throughout the day reported sudden mood changes—apathy, frustration, panic, and hostility. Unable to find someone who speaks Greek to serve as translator. Husband does not speak English but appears concerned about his wife.

—*N. Gable, RN*

NURSING DIAGNOSIS Disturbed Sensory Perception: Mixed Sensory Deprivation and Overload related to unfamiliar hospital environment (different culture) and stress of cesarean birth and infant's prematurity as manifested by patient not demonstrating interest in baby or self-care activities; limited ability to concentrate on new tasks (pericare, expressing breast milk); sudden mood changes—apathy, frustration, panic, hostility

EXPECTED OUTCOME Before discharge, the patient will:

- Demonstrate increased comfort in the hospital environment (decreased or absent mood swings—apathy, frustration, panic, hostility)

NURSING INTERVENTIONS	RATIONALE	EVALUATIVE STATEMENT
Secure assistance of an interpreter and work with the interpreter to do the following:		12/6/15 Outcome met. Patient is quiet but no longer apathetic, fearful, or hostile. Moving about in hospital with more confidence. *N. Gable, RN*
• Orient the patient to her surroundings (explaining reasons for equipment, procedures, treatment).	Sensory deprivation results from *meaningless,* unpatterned stimuli; once the patient understands her environment, she can respond to it appropriately.	
• Reassure the patient that what she is experiencing is normal given her recent stresses (moving to new country, cesarean birth of first child, infant's prematurity).	Patients experiencing strange perceptual, cognitive, and affective responses to sensory deprivation and overload often fear they are going crazy and hesitate to share their feelings.	
• Determine the patient's needs.	The patient herself is best able to voice her needs.	
Have the interpreter teach the nurse several Greek words and make recommendations about how the patient can personalize her environment, such as having her husband provide her with usual food, music, and other familiar items.	Contributing to sensory deprivation is the absence of familiar sounds (native languages, sights, tastes, or scents). Having access to familiar food and the like may reduce sensory deprivation.	

NURSING PLAN OF CARE 43-1 *continued*

for Philomela Palikias

NURSING INTERVENTIONS	RATIONALE	EVALUATIVE STATEMENT
See if the interpreter can explain usual customs regarding childbirth and aftercare in Greek.	Including culturally familiar childbirth and aftercare customs in the plan of care enhances patient well-being and cooperation in the plan of care.	
Limit the number of nurses and other personnel interacting with the patient; attempt to have the same nurse caring for her each shift.	A trusting nurse–patient relationship can develop.	
Schedule care to allow for uninterrupted periods of sleep and rest.	Sleep deprivation contributes to other sensory alterations.	

EXPECTED OUTCOME   Before discharge, the patient will:

- Resume independent self-care activities

NURSING INTERVENTIONS	RATIONALE	EVALUATIVE STATEMENT
Use services of interpreter to teach the patient the importance of ambulating and becoming independent again in self-care measures.	Regaining independence enhances the patient's sense of well-being.	12/6/15 Outcome partially met. Patient is ambulating, but she resists pericare and is fearful when expressing breast milk.
Have the interpreter write simple directions for follow-up care, times when the baby may be visited after the patient is discharged, and so on. Share these instructions with the patient's husband.	Cognitive responses to sensory deprivation and overload include decreased attention span and concentration and problem-solving ability. Written instructions and the husband's knowledge reinforce the patient's learning.	*Recommendation:* Continue teaching with assistance of interpreter. *N. Gable, RN*
See if the husband has bilingual friends or work acquaintances who might be willing to help the patient when she gets home until she has established a comfortable routine of care for the baby and is knowledgeable about community resources.	Careful discharge planning is necessary to ensure that the patient can manage new parenting responsibilities in an unfamiliar country.	

EXPECTED OUTCOME   Before discharge, the patient will:

- Demonstrate interest in her baby by visiting the NICU, holding the baby, expressing her milk, and other such activities.

(continued)

NURSING PLAN OF CARE 43-1 ·continued

for Philomela Palikias

NURSING INTERVENTIONS	RATIONALE	EVALUATIVE STATEMENT
Learn and respect cultural norms for new mothering behaviors. Assist the patient to ambulate to the unit to see the baby; if an interpreter is available, have the person explain equipment surrounding the baby and answer the patient's questions about the baby.	Nursing care that is not culturally sensitive is deficient. The patient may be refusing to visit the unit to protect herself from a barrage of frightening stimuli (sensory overload); the goal is for her to become familiar with the unit so she is able to focus on bonding with her daughter.	12/6/15 Outcome met. Patient is now visiting baby in the unit on her own. *N. Gable, RN*

SAMPLE DOCUMENTATION

Traditional Note Format

12/5/15, 10 AM, nursing

First session with interpreter and patient at 9 AM. Patient's face brightened as soon as she heard someone speak to her in Greek. Basically, patient shared she did not care too much about what was happening to her but she was terrified about the baby and afraid of what everyone was doing to the baby. Directed interpreter to orient patient to her environment, daily routine, and NICU. Patient appeared anxious when she first saw baby but looked content when able to hold her. Schedule teaching session for tomorrow AM when interpreter will come for 1 hour. Patient currently resting comfortably.

N. Gable, RN

SOAP Format

12/5/15, 9 PM, nursing

Sensory/Perceptual Alterations: Mixed Sensory Deprivation and Overload related to unfamiliar hospital environment stress of cesarean birth and infant's prematurity

S: —

O: Cried after husband left this evening; refused postpartal check; turned away from nurses.

A: Still feels overwhelmed by newness of all that is happening to her and tries to shut out what she cannot handle.

P: Continue to intervene with help of interpreter; focus on helping patient develop more control over her situation; proceed at slow pace; referral to social services for follow-up care.

N. Gable, RN

DEVELOPING CLINICAL REASONING

1. Describe the practical measures you would take to stimulate the senses of the following sensory-impaired patients. Think carefully about the special sensory needs that accompany different conditions.
   - A deaf child
   - A confused older adult
   - An adult man who has just lost his sight
   - A premature infant whose skin is extremely fragile

2. Visit a critical care unit with other students and list all the factors that contribute to sensory overload or deprivation. Try to identify how the critical care culture evolved in ways that are actually harmful to patients. Discuss which of these factors are unavoidable and which could be modified to better meet patient needs. Identify individualized nursing strategies to minimize sensory overload and deprivation.

3. Dolores Pirolla expresses concern about her husband's safety at home—especially when she is not present—because of his

increasingly limited vision. What resources can you recommend to her to "safety proof" their house?

PRACTICING FOR NCLEX

1. A nurse who is assessing an older female patient in a long-term care facility notes that the patient is at risk for sensory deprivation related to severe rheumatoid arthritis limiting her activity. Which interventions would the nurse recommend based on this finding? Select all that apply.
   a. Use a lower tone when communicating with the patient.
   b. Provide interaction with children and pets.
   c. Decrease environmental noise.
   d. Ensure that the patient shares meals with other patients.
   e. Discourage the use of sedatives.
   f. Provide adequate lighting and clear pathways of clutter.

2. A nurse is assessing a 78-year-old male patient for kinesthetic and visceral disturbances. Which techniques would the nurse use for this assessment? Select all that apply.
   a. The nurse asks the patient if he is bored, and if so, why.
   b. The nurse asks the patient if anything interferes with the functioning of his senses.
   c. The nurse asks the patient if he noticed any changes in the way he perceives his body.
   d. The nurse asks the patient if he has found it difficult to communicate verbally.
   e. The nurse notes if the patient withdraws from being touched.
   f. The nurse notes if the patient seems unsure of his body parts and/or position.

3. A nurse asks a patient to close her eyes, state when she feels something, and describe the feeling. The nurse then brushes the patient's skin with a cotton ball, and touches the patient's skin with both sides of a safety pin. Which sense is the nurse assessing?
   a. Gustatory
   b. Olfactory
   c. Tactile
   d. Kinesthetic

4. A nurse observes that a patient who has cataracts is sitting closer to the television than usual. The nurse would interpret that the etiologic basis of this sensory problem is an alteration in:
   a. Environmental stimuli
   b. Sensory reception
   c. Nerve impulse conduction
   d. Impulse translation

5. Which action would be most important for a nurse to include in the plan of care for a patient who is 85 years old and has presbycusis?
   a. Obtaining large-print written material
   b. Speaking distinctly, using lower frequencies
   c. Decreasing tactile stimulation
   d. Initiating a safety program to prevent falls

6. A patient is in the late stages of AIDS, which is now affecting his brain as well other major organ systems. The patient

confides to the nurse that he feels terribly alone because most of his friends are afraid to visit. The nurse determines that the least likely underlying etiology for his sensory problems would be:
   a. Stimulation
   b. Reception
   c. Transmission–perception–reaction
   d. Emotional responses

7. Which patient would a nurse assess as being at greatest risk for sensory deprivation?
   a. An older man confined to bed at home after a stroke
   b. An adolescent in an oncology unit working on homework supplied by friends
   c. A woman in labor
   d. A toddler in a playroom awaiting same-day surgery

8. A patient in an intensive care burn unit for 1 week is in pain much of the time and has his face and both arms heavily bandaged. His wife visits every evening for 15 minutes at 6, 7, and 8 PM. A heart monitor beeps for a patient on one side, and another patient moans frequently. Assessment would suggest that that the patient probably is experiencing:
   a. Sufficient sensory stimulation
   b. Deficient sensory stimulation
   c. Excessive sensory stimulation
   d. Both sensory deprivation and overload

9. A patient's spinal cord was severed, and he is paralyzed from the waist down. When obtaining data about this patient, which component of the sensory experience would be most important for the nurse to assess?
   a. Transmission of tactile stimuli
   b. Adequate stimulation in the environment
   c. Reception of visual and auditory stimuli
   d. General orientation and ability to follow commands

10. A nurse is diagnosing an 11-year-old 6th grade student following a physical assessment. The nurse notes that the student's grades have dropped, she has difficulty completing her work on time, and she frequently rubs her eyes and squints. Her visual acuity on a Snellen's eye chart is 160/20. Which nursing diagnosis would be most appropriate?
   a. Deficient Knowledge related to visual impairment
   b. Ineffective Role Performance (Student) related to visual impairment
   c. Disturbed Body Image related to visual impairment
   d. Delayed Growth and Development related to visual impairment

11. A nurse is caring for a male patient with a severe hearing deficit who is able to read lips and use sign language. Which nursing intervention would be best to prevent sensory alterations for this patient?
   a. Turn the radio or television volume up very loud and close the door to his room.
   b. Prevent embarrassment and emotional discomfort as much as possible.
   c. Provide daily opportunity for him to participate in a social hour with six to eight people.
   d. Encourage daily participation in exercise and physical activity.

12. In a group home in which most patients have slight to moderate visual or hearing impairment and some are periodically confused, what would be a nurse's first priority in caring for sensory concerns?
    a. Maintaining safety and preventing sensory deterioration
    b. Insisting that every patient participate in as many self-care activities as possible
    c. Emphasizing and reinforcing individual patient strengths
    d. Encouraging reminiscence and life review in groups

13. A nurse formulated the following nursing diagnosis for an 8-month-old infant: Disturbed Sensory Perception: Sensory Deprivation related to inadequate parenting. Since that diagnosis was made, both parents have attended parenting classes. However, both parents work while the infant stays with her 86-year-old grandmother, who has reduced vision. The parents provide appropriate stimulation in the evening. At an evaluation conference at the age of 11 months, the infant lies on the floor sucking her thumb and rocking her body. Her facial expression is dull, and she vocalizes only in a low monotone ("uh-h-h"). Which statement accurately reflects evaluation about the child's sensory deprivation?
    a. The infant's parents lack motivation to provide necessary stimulation.
    b. The grandmother is unable to improve the infant's care.
    c. The infant's sensory deprivation is still severe.
    d. This is normal behavior for an 11-month-old infant.

14. A nurse formulates the following diagnosis for an older female patient in a long-term care facility: Disturbed Sensory Perception: Chronic Sensory Deprivation related to the effects of aging. The patient walked out the door unobserved and was lost for several hours. Which interventions would be most effective for this patient? Select all that apply.
    a. Ignore when the patient is confused or go along to prevent embarrassment.
    b. Reduce the number and type of stimuli in the patient's room.
    c. Orient the patient to time, place, and person frequently.
    d. Provide daily contact with children, community people, and pets.
    e. Decrease background or loud noises in the environment.
    f. Provide a radio and television in the patient's room.

15. An older female patient has a severe visual deficit related to glaucoma. Which nursing action would be appropriate when providing care for this patient?
    a. Assist the patient to ambulate by walking slightly behind the person and grasping the patient's arm.
    b. Concentrate on the sense of sight and limit diversions that involve other senses.
    c. Stay outside of the patient's field of vision when performing personal hygiene for the patient.
    d. Indicate to the patient when the conversation has ended and when the nurse is leaving the room.

ANSWERS WITH RATIONALES

1. **b, d, e.** For a patient who has sensory deprivation, the nurse should provide interaction with children and pets, ensure that the patient shares meals with other patients, and discourage the use of sedatives. Using a lower tone of voice is appropriate for a patient who has a hearing deficit, decreasing

environmental noise is an intervention for sensory overload, and providing adequate lighting and removing clutter is an intervention for a vision deficit.

2. **c, e, f.** To assess for kinesthetic and visceral disturbances, the nurse would assess for perceived body changes inside and out, and changes in body parts or position. Asking if the patient is bored assesses stimulation, asking if anything interferes with his senses assesses reception, and asking about difficulty communicating assesses for transmission–perception–reaction.

3. **c.** The nurse is assessing for tactile (touch) disturbances by brushing the skin with a cotton ball and touching the skin with a safety pin. Gustatory disturbances involve taste, olfactory disturbances involve the sense of smell, and kinesthetic disturbances are related to body positioning.

4. **b.** Cataracts are interfering with the patient's ability to receive visual stimuli: altered sensory reception. The nature of incoming stimuli, the conduction of nerve impulses, and the translation of incoming impulses in the brain are not a problem here.

5. **b.** Presbycusis is a normal loss of hearing as a result of the aging process. Speaking distinctly in lower frequencies is indicated. The other choices refer to interventions for other sensory problems.

6. **d.** Emotional responses are an effect of sensory deprivation, and although they may be occurring with this patient, they are not the underlying etiology for his condition. This patient is receiving decreased environmental stimuli (**a**) (e.g., from his friends), is more than likely experiencing problems with reception because of major organ involvement (**b**), and his impaired brain function will impair impulse transmission–perception– reaction (**c**).

7. **a.** The patient confined to bedrest at home is at risk for greatly reduced environmental stimuli. All of the other patients are in environments in which environmental stimuli are at least adequate.

8. **d.** This patient's bandages may result in deficient sensory stimulation (sensory deprivation), and the monitors and other sounds in the intensive care burn unit may cause a sensory overload. All other options are incomplete responses.

9. **a.** Below-the-waist paralysis makes the transmission of tactile stimuli a problem. Although the other options may be assessed, they are indirectly related to his paralysis and of lesser importance at this time.

10. **b.** An important role for an 11-year-old is that of student. Her impaired vision is clearly disturbing her role performance as a student, as evidenced by her lower grades. Although the other options may also represent accurate diagnoses for this patient, they do not flow from the data presented.

11. **c.** Although all the options listed are appropriate, providing daily opportunities for this patient to participate in a social hour builds on his strength of being able to lip-read and provides sufficient sensory stimulation to prevent sensory deprivation resulting from his hearing loss, thereby meeting his needs.

12. **a.** Safety is a basic physiologic need that must be met before higher-level needs—such as love and belonging, self-esteem, and self-actualization—can be met.

13. *c.* Although the data show that the parents have been motivated to improve their parenting skills, it is clear from the data that the infant's sensory deprivation is still severe. The data suggest that the grandmother is not improving the infant's care, but there is nothing to suggest that she is unable to do so if shown how.

14. *c, d, f.* Even if well motivated, ignoring a patient's confusion to prevent embarrassment may be dangerous, as it was in this case in which the appropriate safety precautions were never implemented. Reducing the type of stimuli in the room and decreasing environmental noise is appropriate for a patient who is experiencing sensory overload. The other options are related to sensory deprivation and are appropriate for this patient.

15. *d.* When caring for a patient who has a visual deficit, the nurse should indicate when the conversation is over and when he or she is leaving the room, assist with ambulation by walking slightly ahead of the person and allowing her to grasp the nurse's arm, provide diversions using other senses, and stay in the person's field of vision if she has partial or reduced peripheral vision.

TAYLOR SUITE RESOURCES

Explore these additional resources to enhance learning for this chapter:

- NCLEX-Style Questions and other resources on thePoint, http://thePoint.lww.com/Taylor8e
- *Study Guide for Fundamentals of Nursing, 8th edition*
- Adaptive Learning | Powered by prepU, http://thepoint.lww.com/prepu

Bibliography

Ackerman, D. (1990). *A natural history of the senses.* New York: Vintage Books.

Always, A., Halm, M. A., Shilhanek, M., & St. Pierre, J. (2013). Do earplugs and eye masks affect sleep and delirium outcomes in the critically ill? *American Journal of Critical Care, 22*(4), 357–360.

Balas, M. S., Rice, M., Chaperon, C., Smith, H., Disbot, M., & Fuchs, B. (2012). Management of delirium in critically ill older adults. *Critical Care Nurse, 32*(4), 15–26. doi:10.4037/ccn2012480

Boltz, M., Capezuti, E., Fulmer, T. T., Zwicker, D., & O'Meara, A. (2012). *Evidence-based geriatric nursing protocols for best practice* (4th ed.). New York: Springer Publishing Company.

Bulechek, G., Butcher, H., Dochterman, J., & Wagner, C. M. (Eds.). (2013). *Nursing interventions classification (NIC)* (6th ed.). St. Louis: Elsevier.

Cox, H., Burns, I., & Savage, S. (2004). Multisensory environments for leisure: Promoting well-being in nursing home residents with dementia. *Journal of Gerontological Nursing, 30*(2), 37–45.

Crowley, A. A., Bains, R. M., & Pellico, L. H. (2005). In our community. A model preschool vision and hearing screening program: students and faculty serve a community. *American Journal of Nursing, 105*(6), 52–55.

Cutilli, C. C. (2008). Teaching the geriatric patient: Making the most of "cognitive resources" and "gains." *Orthopaedic Nursing, 27*(3), 195–200.

Guenther, U., Weykam, J., Andorfer, U., Theuerfauf, N., Popp, J., Wesley, E., & Putensen, C. (2012). Implications of objective vs. subjective delirium assessment in surgical intensive care patients. *American Journal of Critical Care, 21*(1), 12–20. doi: 10.4037/ajcc2012735

Hope, K. W., Easby, R., & Waterman, H. (2004). Finding the person the disease has: The case for multisensory environments. *Journal of Psychiatric and Mental Health Nursing, 11*(5), 554–561.

The Joint Commission. (2007). "What did the doctor say?:" Improving health literacy to protect patient safety. Available at http://www.jointcommission. org/NR/rdonlyres/F53D5057-5349-4391-9DB9-E7F086873D46/0/health_literacy_exec_summary.pdf.

Lane, K.R. & Conn, V.S. (2013). To hear or not to hear. *Research in Gerontological Nursing, 6*(2), 79–80.

Moorhead, S., Johnson, M., Maas, M. & Swanson, E. (Eds.) (2013). *Nursing outcomes classification (NOC)* (5th ed.). St. Louis: Elsevier/Mosby.

NANDA International (NANDA-I). (2012). *Nursing diagnoses: Definitions & classification 2012–2014.* West Sussex, UK: Wiley-Blackwell.

Nilforoush, M. H., Esfahani, A. A., Ishaghi, R., & Sepehmejad, M. (2012). Comparison of nursing home hearing handicap index with audiological findings: A presbycusis study. *Journal of Aging Research, vol. 2012*, Article ID 423801, 3 pages. doi: 10.1155/2012/423801

Purvis, K. B., McKenzie, L. B., Cross, D. R., & Razuri, E. B. (2013). A spontaneous emergence of attachment behavior in at-risk children and a correlation with sensory deficits. *Journal of Child and Adolescent Psychiatric Nursing, 26*(3), 165–172.

Stouffer, J. W., Shirk, B. J., & Polomano, R. C. (2007). Practice guidelines for music interventions with hospitalized pediatric patients. *Journal of Pediatric Nursing, 22*(6), 448–456.

U.S. Department of Health and Human Services. (2013). Developing Healthy People 2020. Hearing and other Sensory or Communication Disorders. Available at: http://www.healthypeople.gov/2020/topics objectives2020/overview.aspx?topicid=20

Valentjin, S. A., van Boxtel, M. P., van Hooren, S. A., Bosma, H., Beckers, H. J., Ponds, R. W., & Jolles, J. (2005). Change in sensory functioning predicts change in cognitive functioning: Results from a 6-year follow-up in the Maastricht Aging Study. *Journal of the American Geriatrics Society, 53*(3), 374–380.

44

Sexuality

JEFFERSON SMITH

Jefferson, a middle-aged man, has a history of diabetes and hypertension and is receiving numerous medications as treatment. During a routine visit to his primary care physician, Mr. Smith confides that he has been having problems "in the bedroom." He reports difficulty attaining and maintaining an erection.

PAUL ROJAS

Paul is a young adult homosexual diagnosed with AIDS. He comes to the clinic today for infusion therapy, which usually takes several hours. Mr. Rojas comments to the nurse, "You don't feel comfortable with me, do you?"

AMY LIU

Amy is a middle-aged woman who had a hysterectomy about 1 year ago for excessive uterine bleeding due to multiple uterine fibroids. She comes to the clinic for a checkup and begins to cry during the assessment. She says, "I don't feel like a woman anymore. My husband and I used to have a wonderful sexual relationship, but now I rarely want to have sexual intercourse and when I do, it hurts. My husband is being so patient, but I don't know how much longer he'll put up with me! What's wrong with me?"

LEARNING OBJECTIVES

After completing the chapter, you will be able to accomplish the following:

1. Describe male and female reproductive anatomy and physiology.

2. Describe the sexual response cycle, differentiating male and female responses.

3. Contrast different types of sexual expression.

4. Identify factors that affect a person's sexuality.

5. Perform a sexual assessment, using suggested interview questions and appropriate physical assessment skills.

6. Describe types of sexual dysfunctions and the assessment priorities for each.

7. Develop nursing diagnoses identifying a problem with sexuality that may be remedied by independent nursing actions.

8. Plan, implement, and evaluate nursing care related to selected nursing diagnoses involving problems of sexuality.

9. Assess how your personal beliefs and values about human sexuality affect your ability to deliver competent, compassionate, and respectful care to patients with sexual problems.

10. Describe effective responses to sexual harassment by patients or colleagues.

KEY TERMS

abstinence	heterosexual	sexual dysfunction
biologic sex	homosexual	
bisexual	impotence	sexual harassment
contraception	intercourse	sexual health
erogenous zones	lesbian	sexual orientation
	masturbation	
female genital mutilation	menarche	sexuality
	menopause	sexually transmitted infections (STIs)
gay	menstruation	
gender dysphoria	orgasm	
gender identity	premenstrual (tension) syndrome	transgender
gender role behavior		transsexual

A critical component of human identity and well-being, **sexuality** involves how a person exhibits and experiences maleness or femaleness physically, emotionally, and mentally. Sexuality is defined not only by a person's genitalia and hormones but also by attitudes and feelings. It can also be defined as learned behaviors in how a person reacts to one's own sexuality and by how one behaves in relationships with others. Culture profoundly influences learned behaviors involving sexuality. Sexuality is an integral part of a person's identity and is present in one's demeanor through actions, communications, and physical appearance. (See the Reflective Practice box on page 1660 for an example.)

SEXUAL HEALTH

Sexual health may be defined as the integration of the somatic, emotional, intellectual, and social aspects of sexual being, in ways that are positively enriching and that enhance personality, communication, and love. Because our sexuality is so basic to our sense of self, nurses need to value sexuality as a critical element of health and well-being in general and must be skilled in identifying and meeting problems related to sexual self-concept, body image, and sexual identity.

 THINK back to Amy Liu, the woman who reported changes in sexual desire and pain on intercourse. As a result of these changes, she reported not feeling like a woman anymore. The nurse would interpret her statements as reflecting a change in her self-concept and body image secondary to the sexual health issues. ●

Sexual identity encompasses a person's self-identity, biologic sex, gender identity, gender role behavior or orientation, and sexual orientation or preference. **Biologic sex** is the term used to denote chromosomal sexual development: male (XY) or female (XX), external and internal genitalia, secondary sex characteristics, and hormonal states. An intersex condition occurs in about 1 in every 2,000 babies, in which there are contradictions among chromosomal sex, gonadal sex, internal organs, and external genital appearance, resulting in ambiguous gender. **Gender identity** is the inner sense a person has of being male or female, which may be the same as or different from that person's biologic gender. People whose biologic sex at birth is contrary to the gender they identify with are diagnosed with **gender dysphoria**. **Gender role behavior** is the behavior a person exhibits about being male or female, which, again, may or may not be the same as biologic sex or gender identity (Pillitteri, 2012).

 CONSIDER Paul Rojas, the homosexual patient with AIDS. The nurse would need to assess his gender identity and gender role behaviors to gain a fuller understanding of his sexual identity and to provide appropriate care. ●

People experience sexual gratification in many ways; what is considered normal differs from one individual to another and among cultures. **Sexual orientation** refers to the preferred gender of a person's partner. The origins of sexual orientation are unknown, but many studies claim a

REFLECTIVE PRACTICE: CULTIVATING QSEN COMPETENCIES

CHALLENGE TO INTERPERSONAL SKILLS

During my clinical experience in the HIV/infectious disease clinic, I met Paul Rojas, a single young adult homosexual who was diagnosed with AIDS. One day he came to the clinic for infusion therapy, which usually takes several hours.

I was a 20-year-old, single white female with no personal experience with gay or lesbian friends or with individuals who are bisexual, transsexual, or transvestites.

I was confused and uncertain about how to respond to him. How should I approach him? What would we talk about during these several hours at the clinic? I was sure my instructor thought this would be a "great learning experience," but what was I supposed to learn? Usually quite self-confident, I was confused, uncomfortable, and uncertain as to how to act.

Thinking Outside the Box: Possible Courses of Action

- Hide my discomfort and simply provide the technical nursing care Paul needs; spend as little time as possible in his room.
- Refuse this assignment because I am unsure I can provide the care Paul needs.

- Talk with my instructor or another experienced nurse whom I respect about my questions and concerns.
- Share with Paul that this is my first experience working with a homosexual patient and ask him what I should know; spend extra time getting to know him and his experiences with other health care professionals.

Evaluating a Good Outcome: How Do I Define Success?

- Provide the nursing care he needs in a manner that is respectful.
- Learn from this experience how to be respectful of all patients and to interact in a way that affirms their human dignity.

- Gain knowledge about gender identity and expression through this experience.

Personal Learning: Here's to the Future!

I didn't know how to raise my questions, so I met Paul totally at a loss and did exactly what I didn't want to do: I completed the technical nursing care such as vital signs and intravenous care and then got out of the room as quickly as possible. It wasn't until almost the end of his treatment that he asked me, "You don't feel comfortable

with me, do you?" When I answered truthfully that I didn't, all of a sudden wonderful sharing began. When I look back now and think that I almost allowed my fear to prevent me from getting to know Paul and his world, I could kick myself. I hope I always remember to let patients teach me about themselves and their world.

REFLECTION ON QUALITY AND SAFETY COMPETENCIES

Do you agree with the criteria that the nursing student used to evaluate a successful outcome? Why or why not? What *knowledge, skills,* and *attitudes* do you need to develop to continuously improve the quality and safety of care for patients like Paul?

Patient-Centered Care: How would you develop a respectful and successful partnership with Paul, given your initial fears? How can you best communicate empathy and respect and use this opportunity to learn about Paul and his world? Explain how the nursing student's truthful response to the patient's question affected the therapeutic relationship.

Teamwork and Collaboration/Quality Improvement: What communication and interpersonal skills do you need

to improve to ensure that you function as a member of the patient-care team? Who might the student have turned to for help when first acknowledging her discomfort? What does quality care for Paul "look like"?

Safety/Evidence-Based Practice: What does the evidence point to as "best practice" for Paul? What safety needs does he have and how can you meet them?

Informatics: Can you identify the essential information that must be available in Paul's electronic record to support safe patient care and coordination of care? Are smart devices available for you to use to learn more about Paul and his world? Can you think of other ways to respond to or approach the situation? What else might the nursing student have done to ensure a successful outcome?

---

genetic basis. Certainly, some sexual preferences are culturally determined or may be dictated by opportunity.

Common sexual orientations are as follows:

- A **heterosexual** is one who experiences sexual fulfillment with a person of the opposite gender.
- A **homosexual** is one who experiences sexual fulfillment with a person of the same gender. Homosexual males

often use the term **gay**; homosexual females use the term **lesbian**. Heterosexuality and homosexuality can be placed at opposite ends of a continuum, with many variations in between.

- A **bisexual** is a person who finds pleasure with both opposite-sex and same-sex partners. Homosexual or heterosexual people may have bisexual relationships at times.

- Asexuality, the lack of romantic or sexual attraction to others, is sometimes listed as another category.

Transgender (often abbreviated to "trans") is an inclusive term used to describe those who feel that the sex that was assigned to them at birth incompletely describes or fails to describe them. This term includes:

- People who are **transsexual** (live as members of the sex other than the sex they were assigned to at birth)
- People who are intersex (whose reproductive or sexual anatomy does not fit the typical definition of male or female)
- People who identify outside the female/male binary
- People who have a gender expression that differs from their perceived sex, including cross-dressers and drag performance artists

For many transsexuals, the solution is to change their bodies, through surgery and hormone therapy, to match their inner feelings. A cross-dresser is a person who desires to take on the role or wear the clothes of the opposite sex in order to make the outer appearance consistent with the inner identity and gender role. Most are not interested in permanently altering their bodies since they are comfortable with their birth identities. Most cross-dressers are heterosexual, and many keep their cross-dressing hidden.

SEXUAL EXPRESSION

The methods by which people gain satisfaction through sexual stimulation are varied. Touch, smell, sight, sounds, feelings, thoughts, and fantasy can all contribute to sexual fulfillment in any form of expression chosen by people. Feelings of love for another person are closely associated with desire.

Forms of sexual stimulation include kissing, hugging, stroking, squeezing, breast stimulation, manual stimulation of the genitals, oral–genital stimulation, and anal stimulation. Sexual stimulation may be physical or psychological. Erotic stimulation through the use of films, magazines, and photographs is common. Fetishism, more often practiced by males, is sexual arousal with the aid of an inanimate object not generally associated with sexual activity. Items such as shoes, leather, rubber, and women's undergarments might be used.

On a continuum, sexual behavior ranges from adaptive to maladaptive. Adaptive responses meet the following criteria:

- Between two consenting adults
- Mutually satisfying to both
- Not psychologically or physically harmful to either
- Lacking in force or coercion
- Conducted in private

Maladaptive sexual responses are behaviors that do not meet one or more of the criteria for adaptive responses (Stuart, 2013, p. 499).

Masturbation

Masturbation is a technique of sexual expression in which an individual practices self-stimulation. It is a way for people

to learn what they prefer during stimulation and what feels good. Men masturbate by holding and stroking the shaft of the penis. Women find manual stimulation of the clitoris enjoyable, although variations of technique are numerous. Many myths and misinformation surround masturbation. The reality is that people masturbate regardless of sex, age, or marital status. People might not masturbate if they feel guilty about it or believe self-stimulation is wrong. Masturbation is not "dirty" and will not lead to blindness or insanity.

Sexual Intercourse

The act of **intercourse** (coitus or copulation) is the insertion of the penis into the partner's vagina, anus, or mouth. It usually begins by stimulation of the senses in some way, followed by a period of activity known as foreplay. "Petting" is part of foreplay; it can involve simple stroking of the breasts, arms, back, and neck without genital involvement or may lead to mutual masturbation and orgasm.

Vaginal Intercourse

The act of placing the penis in the vagina, penile–vaginal intercourse, can be accomplished in various positions. The most common position in Western cultures is the "missionary position," in which the woman lies horizontally underneath the man. (The Polynesians named this position because it was the preferred position for intercourse used by religious missionaries.) Couples may find other positions to be more stimulating and comfortable. Clitoral stimulation is difficult to achieve in the missionary position. Lying side by side, female on top, and rear entry are some examples of coital positions that enable clitoral stimulation. Sexually inhibited people may believe they need "permission" to engage in alternative sexual positions.

When the penis is pushed into the vagina, the man begins rhythmic thrusting movements of his hips to move the penis back and forth along the vaginal walls. The woman might match her partner's hip movements with movements of her own body. These movements continue until orgasm is attained by one person or both.

Simultaneous orgasms, or both people attaining orgasm at the same moment, are difficult to achieve. A preoccupation with attaining simultaneous orgasms might disrupt the ultimate intimacy and satisfaction possible during coitus.

The period after coitus is just as significant as the events leading up to it. Caressing, hugging, and kissing deepen the couple's intimacy and should be nurtured, not rushed.

Anal Intercourse

Anal intercourse, the act of inserting the penis into the anus and rectum of a partner, is another form of intercourse. Commonly practiced by gay men, it is also used by heterosexual couples. Once the penis (or any object) is placed in the rectum, it should not be introduced into the vagina without thorough cleansing because many microorganisms present in the rectum can cause vaginal infections. Care should be used to avoid injury to the delicate rectal mucosa, and lubrication is essential for comfort. Condoms are now recommended for both types of intercourse to prevent sexually transmitted infections (STIs).

Oral–Genital Stimulation

Stimulation of the genitals by the mouth and tongue might be used during foreplay or as a way to reach orgasm. Cunnilingus is stimulation of the female genitals by licking and sucking the clitoris and surrounding structures. Fellatio is stimulation of the male genitals by licking and sucking the penis and surrounding structures. One partner or both may use these techniques simultaneously (referred to in the vernacular as "*sixty-nine*"). Younger people often use oral–genital stimulation as a replacement for vaginal intercourse to reduce the incidence of pregnancy.

Abstinence

Abstinence is not having sex. It is the most effective form of birth control, preventing pregnancy 100% of the time when practiced consistently. Abstinence also prevents the transmission of STIs 100% of the time when practiced appropriately and consistently. Some STIs spread through oral–genital sex, anal sex, or even intimate skin-to-skin contact without actual penetration (genital warts and herpes can be spread this way). Therefore, only avoiding all types of intimate genital contact can prevent these STIs. Avoiding all types of intimate genital contact—including anal and oral sex—is complete abstinence. There are no side effects or health risks related to abstinence.

Alternative Forms of Sexual Expression

Alternate forms of sexual expression include the following:

*   Voyeurism is the achievement of sexual arousal by looking at the body of someone other than one's sexual partner. Some voyeurs develop complex means to spy on others that involve violations of privacy.
*   Sadism refers to the practice of gaining sexual pleasure while inflicting abuse on another person.
*   Masochism refers to gaining sexual pleasure from the humiliation of being abused.
*   Sadomasochism is the act of practicing sadism and masochism together. It might involve being tied up, biting, hitting, spanking, whipping, pinching, and other activities.
*   Pedophilia is a term used to describe the practice of adults gaining sexual fulfillment by performing sexual acts with children.

FACTORS AFFECTING SEXUALITY

Many factors influence a person's sexuality and contribute to personal feelings regarding sexuality. The brain, rather than the genitals, plays the most significant role in how people perceive themselves as sexual beings.

Developmental Considerations

The process of human development affects the psychosocial, emotional, and biologic aspects of life, which in turn affect

a person's sexuality. Biologic sex is the only distinguishing trait present at conception. From birth onward, gender, or sex, influences behavior throughout life. Table 44-1 summarizes sexuality throughout the lifespan and the nursing implications for each stage.

Culture

The manner in which a society perceives sexuality in turn influences the individual. Every culture has its own norms regarding sexual identity and behavior. To some degree, culture dictates the choice of sexual partner, duration of sexual intercourse, methods of sexual stimulation, and sexual positions. In some cultures, women might be expected merely to tolerate sex; in others, the woman's participation is encouraged. To gain an appreciation for all the ways that culture can influence sexual expression and health, talk with people from different cultures about the following questions:

*   What type of dress is appropriate for children, men, and women? How is nudity viewed?
*   What role behaviors and social responsibilities are expected of men and women?
*   Is masturbation acceptable?
*   At what age is genital sexual intimacy appropriate? With whom is it appropriate?
*   What sexual practices are accepted?
*   What are the rules for marriage? Is premarital sex, extramarital sex, or polygamy accepted?

The fact that a practice is common in a culture does not mean that it is healthy or ethical.

Female genital mutilation (FGM) includes procedures that intentionally alter or cause injury to the female genital organs for nonmedical reasons. It is a procedure that has no health benefits for girls and women and can cause severe bleeding, and problems urinating. Later in life it can cause cysts, infections, and infertility, as well as complications in childbirth and increased risk of newborn deaths. About 140 million girls and women worldwide are currently living with the consequences of FGM. In Africa an estimated 101 million girls 10 years old and older have undergone FGM. The World Health Organization (WHO, 2014) writes that "FGM is recognized internationally as a violation of the human rights of girls and women. It reflects deep-rooted inequality between the sexes, and constitutes an extreme form of discrimination against women. It is nearly always carried out on minors and is a violation of the rights of children. The practice also violates a person's rights to health, security and physical integrity, the right to be free from torture and cruel, inhuman or degrading treatment, and the right to life when the procedure results in death." There are four major types of FGM:

*   *Clitoridectomy:* partial or total removal of the clitoris and, in very rare cases, only the prepuce (the fold of skin surrounding the clitoris)
*   *Excision:* partial or total removal of the clitoris and the labia minora, with or without excision of the labia majora

Table 44-1 DEVELOPMENTAL ASPECTS OF SEXUALITY THROUGH THE LIFE SPAN

STAGE	CHARACTERISTICS	NURSING IMPLICATIONS AND TEACHING GUIDELINES
Infancy: Birth to 18 mo	• Needs affection and tactile stimulation • Boys have penile erections, and girls have orgasmic potential. • Gradually can differentiate self from others • Obtains pleasure from touching genitals • Dressed according to biologic sex	• Avoid early weaning to prevent oral deprivation. • Encourage parents to provide ample physical touch, deprivation of which may cause physical and mental underdevelopment. • Self-manipulation of genitals is normal behavior; avoid denoting this as "bad."
Toddler: Age 1–3 yr	• Establishes control over bowels and bladder • Both sexes enjoy fondling genitals. • Able to identify own gender • Develops vocabulary related to anatomy	• Allow toddler to designate his or her readiness to toilet training. Strict measures may lead to compulsive behaviors later. • Punishment of genital fondling may lead to guilt and shame regarding sexual behavior later in life. • Use proper terms for body parts.
Preschooler: Age 4–6 yr	• Becomes increasingly aware of self • Enjoys exploring body parts of self and playmates • Engages in masturbation	• Parents may cause anxiety in the child by intolerance of inconsistency of sex-role behavior. • Negative overreaction by parents to child's masturbating behavior can lead to a belief that the genitals and sex are bad and dirty.
School-aged: Age 6–10 yr	• There is attachment to the parent of the opposite sex. • Tendency toward having same-sex friends • Curiosity about sex and sharing of fears • Increasing self-awareness	• Same-sex preference for relationships is not related to heterosexual or homosexual tendencies. • Give child the information desired in a clear, factual form. May look to peers for information that may be incorrect.
Preadolescence: Age 10–13 yr	• Puberty begins for most boys and girls with development of secondary sex characteristics. • Menarche takes place. • May test behavioral limits	• Information is necessary regarding body changes to alleviate fears. This information should be given to the young person before pubertal changes begin. • Parents need to find a satisfactory middle ground for role setting. Rules that are either too rigid or too lenient can interfere with the development of self-confidence and an internal value system. • Treat body image changes with a positive attitude to prevent poor self-image.
Adolescence: Age 13–19 yr	• Primary and secondary sex characteristics develop. • Sexual fantasies are common. • Masturbation is common. • May begin to partake in sexual activity ranging from light to heavy petting to full genital intercourse • May experiment with homosexual relationships • At risk for pregnancy and sexually transmitted infections	• Parents share their beliefs and moral value systems with their children. • Teenagers may share their feelings with parents. Not taking them seriously may lead to lack of trust and a communication gap. • Teens need information regarding contraceptive measures and the potential for contracting sexually transmitted infections.
Young adulthood: Age 20–35 yr	• Premarital sex is common. • Although many young adults choose cohabitation instead of marriage, most marry and begin families before age 30 yr. • Knowledge regarding sexual response and activity increases pleasure of relationship. • May experiment with various sexual expressions • Develops own value system and respects values of other people • Many couples share financial responsibilities as well as household tasks.	• Encourage communication between partners regarding sexual needs and differences. • Teach use of abstinence and contraceptive measures to prevent unwanted pregnancies. • Counsel against promiscuous behavior to guard against sexually transmitted infections and loss of trust of partner. • Daily communication is necessary to vent stresses and work out difficulties.

(continued)

Table 44-1 DEVELOPMENTAL ASPECTS OF SEXUALITY THROUGH THE LIFE SPAN *continued*

STAGE	CHARACTERISTICS	NURSING IMPLICATIONS AND TEACHING GUIDELINES
Adulthood: Age 35–55 yr	• Bodily changes as a result of menopause. • Couples focus on quality rather than quantity of sexual experiences. • Divorce is common. • Grown children begin their own lives and sexual experiences. • Sexual satisfaction may actually increase because of loss of fear of pregnancy.	• Both men and women need positive reinforcement of what is good about themselves and their relationships. • Teach parents that empty nest syndrome (feelings of loss caused by children leaving) is common. Accentuate positive aspects of this situation. • Encourage couple to use this period as one of renewal for themselves.
Late adulthood: Age 55 yr and older	• Orgasms may become shorter and less intense in both men and women. • Vaginal secretions decrease, and period of resolution in men lengthens. • May feel need to conform to stereotypes regarding the aging process and cease sexual activity • Fear of loss of sexual abilities	• Sexual activity need not be hindered by age. • Teach couples that adaptation to bodily changes is possible with use of comfortable positions for intercourse and increased time for stimulation. • Teach alternatives to coitus, such as caressing, hugging, and stroking, when coitus is impossible because of illness or disability. • Couples who have been consistently sexually active throughout their lives may continue their intimate relationship for as long as they desire.

• *Infibulation:* narrowing of the vaginal opening through the creation of a covering seal. The seal is formed by cutting and repositioning the inner, or outer, labia, with or without removal of the clitoris.
• *Other:* all other harmful procedures to the female genitalia for nonmedical purposes, for example: pricking, piercing, incising, scraping, and cauterizing the genital area.

Religion

Some people view organized religion as having a generally negative effect on the expression of sexuality. For example, in many religions, the concept of virginity came to be synonymous with purity, and sex became synonymous with sin. In addition, many forms of sexual expression other than male–female coitus are considered unnatural by some religions. As a result of the rigid regulations and negative connotation of sex dictated by some religious groups, a number of sexual dysfunctions can be related to a person's resulting guilt and anxiety. Most major religions are re-examining their teachings on sexuality in response to challenges posed by their members. Many have recognized the importance of solid sex education within the realm of the church. There is also a new interest in the spirituality of marriage: churches are examining their role in supporting the intimate/sexual relationship of married couples.

Ethics

Healthy sexuality depends on freedom from guilt and anxiety. What one person believes is wrong might be perfectly natural and correct to another. Some individuals might feel that certain forms of sexual expression are bizarre and the people who participate in them are perverted. If the sexual expression is performed by consenting adults, is not harmful to them, and is practiced in privacy, it should not be considered a deviant behavior. Individuals should personally decide which aspects of sexual expression are comfortable for them. Frequently, all a person needs to alleviate guilt and consequently enhance sexual satisfaction is permission from a health care professional to engage in a different form of expression.

Lifestyle

Modern lifestyles greatly affect sexuality and its expression. Both men and women are exposed to stress, and many are under considerable strain to perform and function in the workplace as well as at home. Stressors might be external, such as job and financial demands, or internal, such as a competitive nature. Varied responsibilities may place a time restraint on communication between a couple as well as on the energy level and motivation for sexual satisfaction. Although some couples view sexual activity as a release from the stressors of everyday life, most place nurturing relationships and sexual expression far from the top of the list of "things to do." It is crucial to a relationship's survival that a couple set aside priority time—if not for lovemaking, then for intimate, quiet contact. Lifestyle variables can also influence the sexual expression of adolescents and young adults. Those with "time on their hands" and fewer constructive developmental opportunities (e.g., education, sports, community service) are more likely to engage in risky sexual behavior.

Menstruation

Menstruation, often referred to as a woman's "period" or menses, is a cycle during which the body prepares for the presence of a fertilized ovum. Cycles are about 28 days long but may vary from 21 to 40 days. The first menstrual period, called **menarche**, is experienced at about 12 years of age, but the age of menarche is particular to the individual and may occur anywhere between 8 and 17 years of age. **Menopause**, the cessation of a woman's menstrual activity, occurs between the ages of 45 and 55 years. The woman may experience irregular menses over time before menstruation ends.

The Menstrual Cycle

The menstrual cycle is controlled by a series of reactions that rely on feedback from the ovaries to the pituitary gland. Two cycles occur simultaneously: one in the ovaries and one in the endometrium of the uterus (Fig. 44-1).

In the ovaries, in a typical 28-day cycle, the phase from day 4 to 14 is called the follicular phase. During this phase, a number of follicles mature, but only one produces a mature ovum. At the same time, in the uterus, the endometrium is becoming thick and velvety in preparation for receiving a fertilized egg. This phase in the uterus is called the proliferation phase. Ovulation generally occurs on day 14 when the mature ovum ruptures from the follicle and the surface of

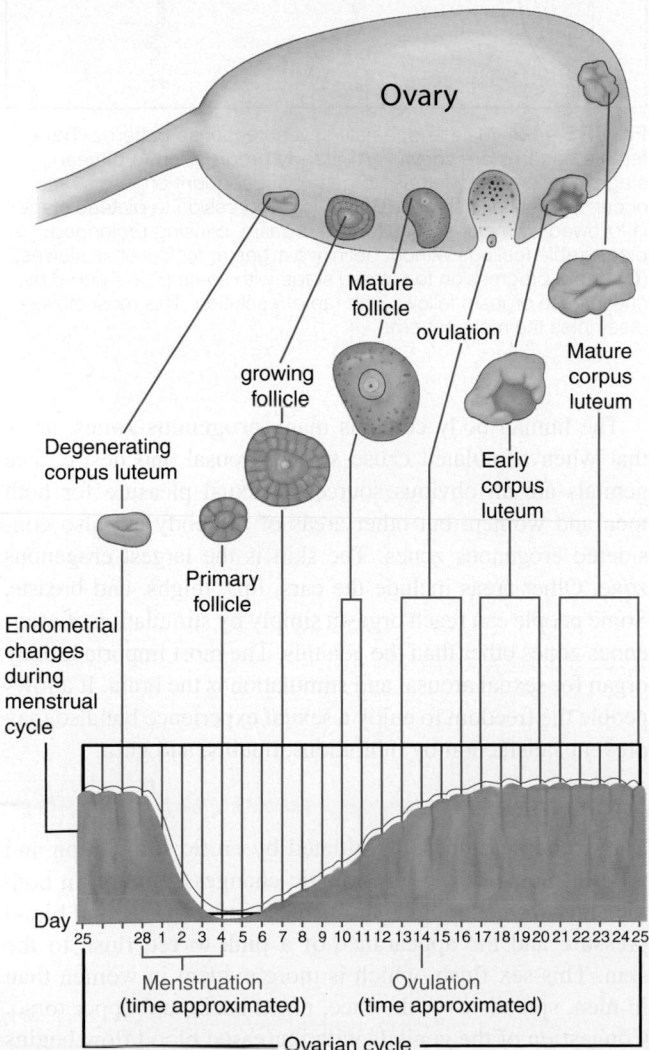

FIGURE 44-1. Schematic representation of one ovarian cycle and the corresponding changes in the endometrium.

the ovary and is swept into the fallopian tube. If sperm are present, the ovum is fertilized at this time. Some women can detect ovulation by the presence of a sharp, cramping pain over the ovulating ovary; this pain is called mittelschmerz, or middle pain, because it occurs in the middle of the cycle.

From day 15 to day 28, the phase in the ovaries is called the luteal phase. The leftover empty follicle fills up with a yellow pigment and is then called the corpus luteum, or yellow body. The purpose of the corpus luteum is to produce hormones that encourage a fertilized egg to grow. If fertilization does not occur, the corpus luteum begins to disintegrate. During the luteal phase in the ovaries, the uterus also undergoes changes. This phase is called the secretory phase. The endometrial lining thickens. However, in the absence of a fertilized egg, the corpus luteum dies and the endometrial lining disintegrates.

At day 28, menses, or the menstrual flow, begins as a result of the uterus shedding the useless portion of its endometrium. Menses lasts for 3 to 7 days, the average length of flow being 5 days. The menstrual discharge is a bloody fluid that also contains endometrial debris, mucus, and enzymes. It is odorless until exposed to the air, when the woman may notice a light, fleshy, pungent odor. Deodorized pads and tampons do little to minimize odor and can cause chemical irritation to the vulva and vagina. Good hygiene and regular bathing are much more effective during menses to prevent odor. Normal blood loss averages 30 to 80 mL. Pads and tampons should be changed frequently to prevent odor and irritation from wetness. Women using tampons should read and follow the manufacturer's suggestions to reduce the risk for toxic shock syndrome. Usually, the flow is the heaviest and is bright red on the first day or two of menses, gradually tapering off to light-brown staining. Many women experience some degree of discomfort either premenstrually or during menses.

Menstrual cycle irregularities can have many different causes, including:

- *Pregnancy or breast-feeding.* A delayed or missed period can be an early sign of pregnancy. Breast-feeding typically delays the return of menstruation after pregnancy.
- *Eating disorders, extreme weight loss, or excessive exercising.* Eating disorders (such as anorexia nervosa), extreme weight loss, and increased physical activity can disrupt menstruation.
- *Polycystic ovary syndrome (PCOS).* This common hormonal disorder can cause small cysts to develop on the ovaries and irregular menstruation.
- *Premature ovarian failure.* Premature ovarian failure refers to the loss of normal ovarian function before age 40. Women who have premature ovarian failure, also known as primary ovarian insufficiency, might have irregular or infrequent periods for years.
- *Pelvic inflammatory disease (PID).* This infection of the reproductive organs can cause irregular menstrual bleeding.
- *Uterine fibroids.* Uterine fibroids are noncancerous growths of the uterus. They can cause heavy menstrual periods and bleeding between periods (Mayo Clinic Staff, 2014).

There is no scientific rationale supporting abstinence from sexual activity during menses. Many women enjoy sex during menses owing to the increase in vascularity in the pelvic region, which heightens enjoyment. Men may also enjoy the warm wetness the menstrual flow provides to the vagina. If flow is heavy, a diaphragm can be used to hold it back during sexual activity, or a towel can be used to protect bedding. Some women who experience abdominal cramping during menses, called dysmenorrhea, find that sexual activity and orgasm relieve their discomfort.

In May 2007, the U.S. Food and Drug Administration (FDA) approved the first oral contraceptive designed to be taken 365 days a year by women who want to avoid menstruating altogether. Women who use the drug don't have regular menstrual periods although they can have breakthrough bleeding (spotting or light bleeding). While there are obvious advantages to not having menstrual periods, women should be counseled that there are no long-term safety data on these drugs. Risks are thought to be similar to those of conventional oral contraceptives: an increased incidence of blood clots, heart attacks, and stroke, especially in women who smoke. Positive benefits may include lowering the risk for ovarian cancer and endometrial cancer (Richardson, 2007).

Premenstrual (Tension) Syndrome

Menstrual cycle–related distress, commonly called **premenstrual (tension) syndrome** (PMS), reportedly occurs in 50% to 90% of the menstruating female population. PMS is characterized by the appearance of one or more of the following several days before the onset of menstruation: irritability, emotional tension, anxiety, mood changes, headache, breast tenderness, and water retention. Although it is often used to explain unusual behavior (and has been used as a legal defense), its etiology is still uncertain (both physiologic and psychogenic theories have been postulated), as are its effects on women's roles and relationships. Some literature perpetuates a twofold myth: (1) biology and physiology are destiny (many females do and should experience premenstrual distress), and (2) female biology and physiology result in psychiatric disorder, destruction, and violence. Nurses have a great role to play in researching PMS and ensuring that women and the public correctly understand its effects.

Sexual Response Cycle

The physiologic responses to sexual activity of females and males are more similar than different (Fig. 44-2). Also, the body's response is essentially the same regardless of the source of stimulation; that is, fantasy, masturbation, and sexual intercourse can all bring about the same body reactions. The sexual response cycle is not limited to the genital organs but is a total-body response that causes many physiologic changes throughout the body. The cycle has four phases: (1) excitement, (2) plateau, (3) orgasm, and (4) resolution; there is a smooth progression from one phase to the next. Although only physiologic responses are discussed here, the emotional and mental involvement of sexual response contributes a great deal to the pleasure and satisfaction of sexual activity.

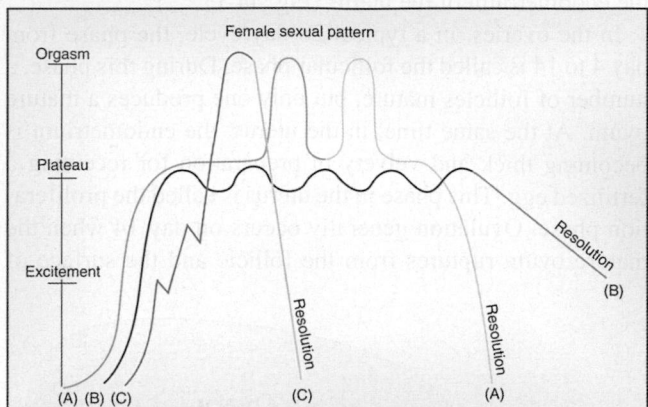

FIGURE 44-2. Male and female sexual response patterns. Three female patterns are shown: (**A**) Steady progression to plateau stage is followed by intense orgasm; subsequent orgasms may occur; resolution is slower. (**B**) Slower progression to plateau stage is followed by minor surges toward orgasm, causing prolonged pleasurable feelings without definitive orgasm; resolution is slowest. (**C**) Rapid progression to plateau stage with some peaks and dips; one intense orgasm follows with rapid resolution. This most closely resembles the male pattern.

The human body contains many **erogenous zones**, areas that when stimulated cause sexual arousal and desire. The genitals are an obvious source of sexual pleasure for both men and women, but other areas of the body are also considered erogenous zones. The skin is the largest erogenous zone. Other areas include the ears, lips, thighs, and breasts. Some people can reach orgasm simply by stimulation of erogenous zones other than the genitals. The most important body organ for sexual arousal and stimulation is the brain. It allows people the freedom to enjoy a sexual experience but also may prevent satisfaction by inhibitions, doubts, and guilt.

Excitement

The excitement phase is initiated by erotic stimulation and arousal. Some of the physiologic changes common in both men and women include an increase in heart rate and blood pressure and the appearance of a pink to red flush to the skin. This sex flush, which is more evident in women than in men, spreads over the face, neck, back, and upper torso. Congestion of the genitals with increased blood flow begins in the excitement phase and causes even more arousal. The length of the excitement phase varies greatly among people and even from one experience to another. Women usually enjoy a more prolonged period of stimulation than do men.

During the excitement phase, the woman's breasts swell and the nipples become erect and hard to the touch. Lubrication of the vagina seeps to the outside of the body along the vulvar creases and makes stimulation of the genitals more pleasurable by decreasing friction. The upper two-thirds or so of the vagina enlarges and expands. The clitoris enlarges and emerges slightly from the clitoral hood. The labia also enlarge and separate, and turn a deep rosy red with arousal.

The first obvious sign of arousal in the man is an erection of the penis caused by increased pelvic congestion of blood. The scrotum noticeably elevates, thickens, and enlarges. The skin of the penis and scrotum turns a deep reddish-purple in response to congestion and arousal. Male nipples may also harden and become erect.

Plateau

The intensity of the plateau phase is greater than that of excitement but not enough to begin orgasm. Desire and arousal continue to build and intensify. This phase varies from a few minutes to 15 to 20 minutes. In the female, the clitoris retracts and disappears under the clitoral hood. It is thought that the clitoris performs in this mysterious way as the body's protection against overstimulation. In the male, secretions from Cowper's glands may appear at the glans of the penis during the plateau phase.

Orgasm

The term **orgasm** defines the climax and sexual explosion of the tension that has been building over the preceding phases. Orgasm lasts only seconds but is an extremely intense reaction. Characteristics of the orgasm phase are the involuntary spasmodic contractions of the genital organs. The number of contractions felt by the individual depends on the intensity of the orgasm.

The orgasm phase in the female begins with a heightened feeling of physical pleasure, followed by overwhelming release and involuntary contractions of the genitals. Loss of muscular control may cause spastic contractions and twitching of the arms and legs. The number of contractions can be as few as 4 or as many as 20. Areas of the body that contract spasmodically are the uterus, anal sphincter, rectum, and urethral sphincter. It is believed that women achieve orgasm in a variety of ways. Although some women can achieve orgasm by penile thrusting in the vagina alone, most women need clitoral stimulation to reach orgasm.

During orgasm in the male, involuntary spasmodic contractions occur in the penis, epididymis, vas deferens, and rectum. The male orgasm is most often accompanied by ejaculation of semen from the urinary meatus of the penis. Ejaculation and orgasm usually, but not necessarily, occur at the same time.

Resolution

The resolution phase is characterized by a return to the normal body functioning present before the excitement phase.

Feelings of relaxation, fatigue, and fulfillment are common. Some people have a need to be held, fondled, and caressed. Physical demonstrations of affection may initiate the sexual response cycle once again. The woman is physiologically capable of immediate response to sexual stimulation. Because of this, many women can achieve multiple orgasms. The man experiences a period during which the body does not respond to continued sexual stimulation, called the refractory period. The length of the refractory period varies from a few minutes to longer, even days.

Childbearing Considerations

All sorts of questions surround childbearing, and the ability (or lack of ability) to procreate can put great pressure on a sexual relationship: Are we ready to be parents? What does it mean to be a responsible parent—especially in this age when an increasing number of prenatal interventions are available to maximize fetal outcomes (quality control)? Should we choose life partners only if genetic testing reveals a good match for reproduction? If we choose to be sexually active and not have children, what are the best means to prevent unwanted pregnancies? If we become pregnant and choose not to continue the pregnancy, what are our options? If we desperately want a child and discover one or both to be infertile, what are our options? The age of biotechnology promises "designer babies" and raises hard questions for individuals and society. People frequently look to nurses for help in sorting through how to respond to these challenges. Experienced nurses are good at detecting when a fear of pregnancy or inability to conceive is interfering with a couple's normal sexual expression or when a changing developmental stage (e.g., menopause) is interfering with normal sexual expression.

Sexually Transmitted Infections

Sexually transmitted infections (STIs) or diseases (STDs), once called venereal diseases, are infections that are spread primarily through sexual contact. They are among the most common infectious diseases in the United States today. More than 20 STIs have been identified. The Center for Disease Control and Prevention (2014) estimates that nearly 20 million new sexually transmitted infections occur every year in the United States, half among young people ages 15 to 24. Each of these infections is a potential threat to a person's immediate and long-term health and well-being, and can lead to severe reproductive health complications, such as infertility.

Table 44-2 (on page 1668) lists common types of STIs and their signs and symptoms. The annual comprehensive cost of STIs in the United States is estimated to be almost $16 billion.

According to the National Institute of Allergy and Infectious Diseases (NIAID), understanding the basic facts about STIs—the ways in which they are spread, their common symptoms, and how they can be treated—is the first step toward prevention. News releases, fact sheets, and other NIAID-related materials are available on the NIAID website

Table 44-2 SEXUALLY TRANSMITTED INFECTIONS

DISEASE	CHARACTERISTICS
Acquired immunodeficiency syndrome (AIDS)	• Human immunodeficiency virus (HIV) • Positive ELISA and Western Blot tests • Incidence high in IV drug users and homosexual and bisexual men; increasing heterosexual transmission • Fatigue, diarrhea, weight loss, enlarged lymph nodes, fever, anorexia, and night sweats
Cervical intraepithelial neoplasia (CIN) Cervical cancer	• Abnormal Pap smears • Women with multiple sex partners, women who began sexual activity before age 18, and women whose partners have multiple female partners • Asymptomatic • Possible vaginal bleeding or spotting
Chlamydia trachomatis Nongonococcal urethritis (NGU) *Chlamydia*	• The most prevalent STI to date • Intracellular bacteria • Vaginal discharge, burning on urination, urinary frequency, dysuria, and urethral soreness • Many women do not have symptoms.
Cytomegalovirus (CMV)	• A virus in the same family as herpes and Epstein-Barr • May be asymptomatic or may be confused with another disease such as pneumonia, mononucleosis, or hepatitis • Not exclusively sexually transmitted
Nonspecific vaginitis *Gardnerella vaginalis*	• Mixed anaerobic bacteria • Foul-smelling, thin, grayish-white vaginal discharge • Male partners do not have symptoms.
Neisseria gonorrhoeae "The clap" or "the drip" Gonorrhea	• Gram-negative bacteria • Both men and women may not have symptoms. • Symptoms in men: purulent penile discharge, dysuria, frequency of urination • Symptoms in women: dysuria, abnormal menses, vaginal discharge, pelvic inflammatory disease • Symptoms of pharyngitis if oral sex was practiced • May be accompanied by chlamydial infection • Detected by gonorrhea culture of cervix or penile discharge from men • Newborns exposed at birth are at risk for blindness and pneumonia. • Untreated gonorrhea can result in infertility, skin rash with lesions, and acute arthritis.
Herpes simplex virus type 1 and 2 "Cold sores" Herpes	• A DNA virus • Lesions develop mostly in oral and genital areas. • Appear as single or multiple painful vesicles, which rupture and form ulcer-like lesions; these form scabs as they heal. • First infections last about 10 to 14 days, whereas subsequent infections are shorter in duration. • Recurrences are usually preceded by prodromal symptoms of tingling and fullness.
Human papillomavirus (HPV) Condylomata acuminate Genital warts Venereal warts	• A DNA virus; vaccine now available. • Pale, soft, papillary lesions found around the internal and external genitalia and perianal and rectal areas of the body; vary in size • Profuse watery vaginal discharge, dyspareunia, intense pruritus, and vulvar irritation • Women with HPV are at risk for cervical cancer. • Male partner may or may not have lesions.
Treponema pallidum Syphilis	• A spirochete detected through serologic blood test (VDRL, RPR, STS) • Three stages to disease if left untreated *Primary:* Single painless genital lesion 10 days to 3 months after exposure *Secondary:* Generalized skin rash, enlarged lymph nodes, fever that may appear 2 to 4 weeks after appearance of primary lesion; may last for several years *Latent:* Usually no clinical symptoms present for as long as 20 years; may continue to involve and damage neurologic and cardiovascular organs; dementia, confusion, paralysis, and paresis may occur.
Trichomoniasis "Trich" *Trichomonas vaginalis*	• Protozoan with flagella • Identified on wet-mount microscopic examination of vaginal discharge • May be identified on Pap smear • Usually asymptomatic in male patients • Foul-smelling vaginal discharge, thin, foamy, and green in color, causes itching of vulva and vagina, burning on urination and dyspareunia; "strawberry" cervix may be seen on speculum examination.

Data from National Institute of Allergy and Infectious Diseases (NIAID). (2013). Sexually transmitted diseases (STDs), available at http://www.niaid.nih.gov/topics/std/Pages/default.aspx; and the Centers for Disease Control and Prevention (CDC). Sexually transmitted diseases (STDs): CDC fact sheets, available at http://www.cdc.gov/std/healthcomm/fact_sheets.htm

at www.niaid.nih.gov. NIAID recommends understanding at least five key points about all STIs in the United States today:

1. STIs affect men and women of all backgrounds and economic levels. They are most prevalent among teenagers and young adults.
2. The incidence of STIs is rising, in part because in the last few decades, young people have become sexually active earlier yet are marrying later. In addition, divorce is more common. The net result is that sexually active people today are more likely to have multiple sex partners during their lives and are potentially at risk for developing STIs.
3. Most of the time, STIs cause no symptoms, particularly in women. When symptoms develop, they may be confused with those of other diseases not transmitted through sexual contact. Even when an STI causes no symptoms, a person who is infected may be able to pass the disease on to a sex partner. That is why many doctors recommend periodic testing or screening for people who have more than one sex partner.
4. Health problems caused by STIs tend to be more severe and more frequent for women than for men, in part because the frequency of asymptomatic infection means that many women do not seek care until serious problems have developed.
   • Some STIs can spread into the uterus (womb) and fallopian tubes to cause pelvic inflammatory disease (PID), which is a major cause of both infertility and ectopic (tubal) pregnancy. The latter can be fatal.
   • STIs in women also may be associated with cervical cancer. One STI, human papillomavirus infection (HPV), causes genital warts and cervical and other genital cancers.
   • STIs can be passed from a mother to her baby before, during, or immediately after birth; some of these infections of the newborn can be cured easily, but others may cause a baby to be permanently disabled or even die.
5. When diagnosed and treated early, many STIs can be treated effectively. Some infections have become resistant to the drugs used to treat them and now require newer types of antibiotics. Experts believe that having STIs other than HIV increases one's risk for becoming infected with the HIV virus (NIAID, 2013).

Having an STI might affect one's self-concept and keep a person from becoming intimate for fear of spreading the infection.

 RECALL Paul Rojas, the homosexual patient with AIDS. The nurse would need to assess the patient's sexual practices and instruct him about sex practices to prevent the transmission of HIV/AIDS. In addition, the nurse would need to investigate the effect that this STI has had on his sexuality. ●

Sexual Dysfunction

Sexual dysfunction is a problem that prevents an individual or couple from engaging in or enjoying sexual intercourse and orgasm. Dysfunctions might occur as a result of physiologic malfunctions, conflicts with cultural norms, interpersonal problems, or any combination of these. Anxieties and fears concerning the sexual act are almost always present. Patients with severe sexual dysfunctions require intensive professional therapy from a qualified sex therapist.

Male Primary Sexual Dysfunctions
ERECTILE DYSFUNCTION
Erectile dysfunction, also called **impotence**, is the inability of a man to attain or maintain an erection to such an extent that he cannot have satisfactory intercourse. Common causes of impotence (which may be physiologic or psychological) include various illnesses, treatments for these illnesses, and personal anxieties. New medications have revolutionized treatment for erectile dysfunction.

 REMEMBER Jefferson Smith, the patient with diabetes and hypertension who is having problems with erections. The nurse would review the pathophysiologic effects of diabetes and hypertension on sexual response and would evaluate his current status, including a review of all medications that he is taking, to determine possible contributory factors. ●

PREMATURE EJACULATION
Premature ejaculation is a condition in which a man consistently reaches ejaculation or orgasm before or soon after entering the vagina. The result is that his partner usually does not have time to reach sexual satisfaction. Causes of the problem are rarely physical.

RETARDED EJACULATION
Retarded ejaculation, also called ejaculatory incompetence, refers to a man's inability to ejaculate into the vagina, or delayed intravaginal ejaculation. The causes of this problem are similar to those of impotence. When it occurs after the man has experienced normal ejaculations, the cause is most probably due to interpersonal problems.

Female Primary Sexual Dysfunctions
INHIBITED SEXUAL DESIRE
Inhibited sexual desire consists of an inhibition in sexual arousal so that congestion and vaginal lubrication are absent or minimal. Causative factors may be anxiety, negative emotions, fear, interpersonal problems, or physical factors. Orgasmic dysfunction is defined as the inability of a woman to reach orgasm. The causes are similar to those of inhibited sexual desire.

DYSPAREUNIA
Dyspareunia is painful intercourse. Although it is most often described by women, some men may also suffer

from this disorder. The cause is usually physical, although psychological problems such as fear and anxiety can cause pain.

 CONSIDER Amy Liu, the woman who had a hysterectomy and is experiencing pain on intercourse. The nurse would review the patient's history to determine if the problem is physiologic secondary to changes in the reproductive tract from surgery, or psychological, secondary to the changes in self-concept and feelings of not being a woman. •

VAGINISMUS

Vaginismus is a rare condition in which the vaginal opening closes tightly and prevents penile penetration. Vaginismus is due to involuntary spastic contractions of the muscles at and around the vaginal opening and the levator ani muscles. The cause of vaginismus may be physical, psychological, or both.

VULVODYNIA

Vulvodynia, a chronic vulvar discomfort or pain characterized by burning, stinging, irritation, or rawness of the female genitalia that interferes with sexual activity, is particularly problematic because little is known about its cause or treatment.

Other Health Conditions

A healthy body, mind, and emotions are necessary for sexual wellness. A primary sexual dysfunction can affect a person's sexual expression. Similarly, any trauma or stress that interferes with a person's ability to perform daily functions will also affect the expression of sexuality. Illness is no exception.

Diabetes Mellitus

Diabetes mellitus is a hormonal disease in which an inadequate amount of insulin is secreted by the pancreas. Although almost all hormonal disorders affect sexuality in some way, diabetes is the most prevalent and well known. Erectile dysfunction, or impotence, is a great concern among diabetic men. Treatment to date depends largely on the degree of erectile ability lost. Some men might be candidates for a penile prosthesis, which was developed in 1973. The prosthesis is surgically implanted below the base of the penis, and inflation of the device produces an erection when sexual activity is desired. Pharmacologic management (e.g., Viagra, Levitra, or Cialis) might also be indicated.

 THINK back to Jefferson Smith, the patient with diabetes and hypertension. The nurse would explore with Mr. Smith his feelings about the effect of his disorder on his sexual function and sexuality. Additional consultation with other members of the health care team would be necessary to determine the most appropriate plan for treatment of Mr. Smith's impotence. •

Diabetic women may also experience loss of capacity for orgasm (orgasmic dysfunction). Difficulty experiencing arousal and loss of vaginal lubrication have also been reported. Frequent *Monilia* infections of the vagina are also common, and can cause discomfort during coitus.

Cardiovascular Disease

Cardiovascular disease is prevalent in North America, and the sexual response cycle can greatly increase the demands on the heart and other structures. A person with a cardiovascular disease might experience much anxiety over the effect the illness will have on sexuality and sexual functioning.

HYPERTENSION

The most significant difficulty a hypertensive person faces regarding sexuality is that the medication used to control the disease frequently causes a change in sexual functioning. These sexual dysfunctions may be relieved by modifying the dose of the medication or switching to a different medication.

 CONSIDER Jefferson Smith, the patient with a history of diabetes and hypertension. The nurse would obtain a complete medication history from the patient to determine if his pharmacologic therapy is the underlying cause of his impotence or if the medication is contributing to a preexisting problem associated with his diabetes. This investigation would provide information about whether an adjustment in medication dosage might minimize or alleviate Mr. Smith's impotence. •

MYOCARDIAL INFARCTION (HEART ATTACK)

The primary goal after a myocardial infarction (MI) is to allow the heart ample time to heal. Activities of daily living, including sexual activity, should be resumed gradually, and stressors such as overexertion, alcohol consumption, and emotional upheavals should be avoided. After an uncomplicated MI, sexual activity may begin at about the third week of recovery, beginning with masturbation to partial erection in the male. Generally, this activity is gradually increased until 3 months after the MI, when sexual intercourse may be resumed. A comfortable position that places the least stress on the affected partner should be used.

Diseases of the Joints and Mobility

Joint diseases and disorders affect young and old people. Pain, fatigue, stiffness, and loss of range of motion can accompany any of the dozens of known diseases of the joints. The disease itself does not affect sexual functioning, although the manifestation of it can cause discomfort and anxiety.

Surgery and Body Image

Surgery is performed to remove diseased tissue and repair body organs, usually requiring an incision with resulting scars. The most devastating kinds of surgery are those used to remove cancerous tissue and surrounding structures. Patients are almost always distressed about a diagnosis of cancer and possible death. After surgery, patients need to adjust to major alterations in their bodies. Changes in body image also affect a person's self-perception as a sexual being.

 REMEMBER Amy Liu, the woman who had had a hysterectomy. The uterus, because it is a female reproductive organ, is often associated with childbearing and is a major component of a woman's "femaleness." The nurse would interpret the significance of the uterus to the patient's self-concept and how the surgery to remove it has affected her overall feelings of "femininity" and "femaleness." Using this information, the nurse would then correct any misconceptions that Mrs. Liu may have about this reproductive organ and develop an appropriate teaching plan. ●

Mastectomy is a surgical procedure to remove a breast and surrounding tissue. After such a surgery, a woman's return to sexual functioning depends on many factors, such as support of her partner, the value placed on the breast by the man or woman, and fear of discomfort during sexual activity.

An ostomy is a surgical opening placed on the outside of the body to allow for the passage of secretions and elimination into a closed drainage bag. Grieving over the loss of the natural means to eliminate waste, such as urine or feces, accompanies learning to live with an obvious artificial device. Many people are anxious as to how this apparatus will affect their sex lives and how accepting their partners will be of it.

Spinal Cord Injuries

Thousands of people are victims of spinal cord injuries each year as a result of various types of accidents. This type of injury almost always results in some degree of permanent disability. Such people face multiple adaptations in their lifestyles, including those related to mobility, bowel and bladder control, sexual functioning, and role expectations. The extent of sexual response that remains after a spinal cord injury depends primarily on the level and extent of the injury. Ejaculation and orgasm are most likely to remain with low spinal injuries. Women are more likely to experience orgasm than men, but they complain more about the lack of physical sensations during the excitement phase than do men. Many people find that other erogenous zones become more easily stimulated after the injury.

Chronic Pain

Many chronic illnesses are accompanied by constant pain, and a person with persistent pain might not desire any sexual contact. However, the desire for human warmth and contact does not cease because of pain. Altered or modified positions for coitus are sometimes necessary; discussing these positions with patients can be an important part of implementing the Nursing Process, reviewed later in this chapter.

Mental Illness

Various psychological and physical disorders can cause mental illness. The mind plays a powerful role in sexuality; any disruption of its functioning will no doubt cause some disturbance in sexual functioning. Even a disorder such as mild depression can affect desire and sexual functioning. Sometimes, it is difficult for the partner of a patient who has developed a mental illness to continue the sexual relationship. People afflicted with Alzheimer disease can lose the memory of any contact with a partner or spouse. At times, patients with mental illness act out in a sexual manner, such as touching themselves or removing their clothing at inappropriate times and places.

Medications

Some medications have side effects that may affect sexual functioning. These include amyl nitrates, anticonvulsants, antidepressants, antihistamines, antihypertensives, antipsychotics, antispasmodics, barbiturates, and narcotics. Recreational drugs including cocaine, ethyl alcohol, and marijuana are used by some to heighten the sexual experience. These drugs can have serious and even deadly side effects. While some use alcohol to release inhibitions and to increase sexual arousal and desire, heavy drinking can decrease libido and negatively impact sexual functioning.

THE NURSE AS ROLE MODEL

Nurses' attitudes, biases, and prejudices regarding sexuality are readily transmitted to patients through their actions, manner of speech, avoidance of certain circumstances, and types of discussion (see the accompanying box, Focused Critical Thinking Guide 44-1, on page 1672). A nurse's knowledge about sexual issues can inhibit or promote discussions of sexual health. The nurse who does not have a sound knowledge base of reproductive anatomy and physiology, sexual response, sexual expression, and other issues surrounding sexuality will be unable to assess, teach, or counsel patients with sexual concerns.

 RECALL Paul Rojas, the patient described in the Reflective Practice box. The nurse caring for Mr. Rojas needs to be comfortable with his or her own sexuality to provide nonjudgmental care. In addition, the nurse needs knowledge about sexual orientation and sexual preference to develop an appropriate, unbiased plan of care that meets Mr. Rojas's needs. ●

Nursing goals to enhance interactions with patients and to promote individual sexual health are as follows. The nurse will be able to:

- Feel comfortable as a sexual being
- Develop self-awareness regarding sexual topics
- Develop communication skills that promote discussion of sexual concerns with patients
- Identify patients with problems related to sexuality and intervene competently and comfortably to meet these needs
- Practice responsible sexual expression

FOCUSED CRITICAL THINKING GUIDE 44-1

SEXUALITY AND NONJUDGMENTAL NURSING CARE

A 33-year-old white man with AIDS who is living alone at home asks you, the visiting nurse, about the nurse who was substituting for you during your vacation. "I don't like to complain, but he was overly friendly—if you get what I mean....I wasn't comfortable with the way he was touching me and I'd rather not have help with my bath than have him back here." You have to decide how to respond.

1. Identify goal of thinking

Clarify what the patient is saying and make a judgment about the behavior behind his concern so that you can respond appropriately.

2. Assess adequacy of knowledge

Pertinent circumstances: You have been visiting the patient for the last 2 months following his discharge from a local hospital because of AIDS-related complications. Apart from his clinical picture, you know very little about the patient, who has always seemed private and reserved during your visits. You "feel sorry" that the patient is as sick as he is at this point in his life, and your instinct is to trust him. You really don't know the colleague who was substituting for you because he is a "new hire."

Prerequisite knowledge: Before you can make a judgment about the patient's concern, you need to know more about what actually happened between him and your colleague. You do not know your colleague well because he is a "new hire" and has been working in the agency for only 3 months. You have heard reports that he is gay. You know that the patient is single but do not know his sexual orientation. You need to talk with your colleague to get his description of his encounter with the patient. You also need to know more about what touch means to both the patient and your colleague because culture and individual preference can profoundly influence the meaning different people give to touch.

Room for error: Life and death do not hinge on how you respond to this patient. However, the well-being of the patient and your colleague's reputation are at stake, so the matter is grave.

Time constraints: You must make some immediate response to the patient. Because you do not have sufficient information to evaluate what happened, you should not feel pressured to make a definitive response. The patient's well-being will not be jeopardized if you postpone a complete response until you have investigated the complaint.

3. Address potential problems

The most serious obstacles to critical thinking in this situation would be false assumptions you (and the patient) might have about homosexuality in general and male homosexual nurses in particular, and the failure to reason carefully about the situation. Your tendency to "go to bat" for patients and to believe whatever a patient tells you "no matter what" may result in your unfairly and prematurely judging a colleague.

4. Consult helpful resources

Your colleague is the first resource you should consult because you need to hear his side of the event before you can think critically about what happened. When you do meet with him, he thanks you for bringing up the subject because he was similarly disturbed by his encounter with this patient. "I guess I'm a touchy-feely kind of guy and generally find that patients respond well to human touch. In the past, patients have told me how much it means to them to have someone massage their back, stroke a forearm, or greet them with a hug. Touch is certainly a big part of the 'therapeutic package' I give each of my patients. I did sense rather quickly, though, that Jim didn't like to be touched and modified my approach. My sense, from a few comments he made, is that he's probably homophobic" [afraid of homosexuals].

After listening to your colleague, you decide you need to learn more about touch, touch as a therapeutic intervention, and homophobia. You can consult the literature or local experts.

5. Critique judgment/decision

Wanting to explore the situation more fully, you responded to the patient initially by saying, "I am sorry that you felt uncomfortable by my colleague's care. I want to talk with him about his sense of what happened and will then discuss this with you when I return on Wednesday." After talking with your colleague, you are reasonably assured that he was not intending, inappropriately, to communicate anything of a sexual nature to the patient. On your return visit to the patient, you inform him about your research and judgment and say, "Touch can mean different things to different people. My sense is that Dave simply wanted to communicate that he cares. If he is going about this in the wrong way, he wants to know what he should be doing differently. We certainly don't want this to be a problem for you or any other patient. Would you like to talk more about this or to file a report?"

You initially thought you have three options: (1) to agree at the outset that your colleague has behaved in a sexually inappropriate and unprofessional manner, (2) to investigate the incident and conclude that your colleague was in the wrong, or (3) to investigate the incident and conclude that your colleague was in the right. You chose the third and are relieved when the patient seems to accept your explanation. Two months later, when you receive a similar complaint from another male patient, you are troubled. You realize now that there was a fourth option, and that this is the one you should have taken. Convinced by your colleague's sincerity and good intent, you might nonetheless have informed Dave that you need to communicate this patient's concern to your supervisor so that if future incidents are reported there will be a record of repeat complaints.

THE NURSING PROCESS FOR THE PATIENT WITH A SEXUAL HEALTH NEED

Nurses who role model good health behaviors are more effective teachers. Use the display, Promoting Health 44-1, for yourself before using it with others.

Assessing
Sexual History

The comprehensive health history should include information regarding a patient's reproductive and sexual health, depending on the circumstances in which the patient is receiving care. As a rule, three general categories of patients should have a sexual history recorded by the nurse:

• Any inpatient or outpatient receiving care for pregnancy, STI, infertility, or contraception
• Any patient experiencing sexual dysfunction
• Any patient whose illness will affect sexual functioning and behavior in any way

Information is best obtained from the patient by beginning with nonthreatening questions and progressing to more sensitive concerns (see the accompanying Focused Assessment Guide 44-1 on page 1674). Patients usually have no difficulty answering questions regarding their bodies and general reproductive issues such as, "When did your menstrual periods first begin?"

Explain to patients that this information might help you develop the plan of care and identify any sexual problems or concerns. The assessment provides an excellent opportunity to teach by helping the patient confront fears. Four general levels of sexual history are:

Level 1: Sexual history as part of a comprehensive health history—obtained by a nurse

Level 2: Sexual history—obtained by a nurse with education and training in sexuality
Level 3: Sexual problem history—obtained by a sex therapist
Level 4: Psychiatric/psychosocial history—obtained by a psychiatric nurse clinician

Each level acquires more specific information from the patient regarding sexual health and also requires the interviewer to have more sophisticated preparation and skills. The professional nurse usually performs a sexual history on level 1.

The nurse sets the tone or atmosphere for the interview. The nurse's attitudes will greatly affect the patient's response to the sexual history; patients will be more cooperative if they sense the nurse's security and ease during the interview. Privacy is essential for the sexual history; doors should be closed and no interruptions allowed. Sit close to the patient and speak in a quiet, relaxed, objective tone of voice. Use eye contact and open body posture. Explain to the patient that no one will have access to this information unless it is significant to the patient's care.

Obtain reproductive health information first, followed by the sexual health history. The best approach is to begin with general open-ended questions and progress to more specific ones. Try to use the language used by the patient because the patient might be reluctant to admit not understanding certain terms for fear of appearing ignorant or foolish. For example, the patient might use the term "come" to mean climax or orgasm.

It is useful to begin questions with phrases such as "many people like" or "many people feel." This gives patients security in knowing they are not alone in how they feel and will encourage them to talk about their problems or concerns. For example, "Many people feel that it's helpful to discuss their concerns about sex with their partner. What do you think about this?"

PROMOTING HEALTH 44-1

SEXUALITY

Use the assessment checklist to determine how well you are meeting your sexuality needs. Then develop a prescription for self-care by choosing appropriate behaviors from the list of suggestions.

Assessment Checklist

❑ almost always	❑ sometimes	❑ almost never

❑	❑	❑	1. I feel positive about my sexual identity.
❑	❑	❑	2. I have satisfying relationships with others.
❑	❑	❑	3. I accept sexual needs as a normal part of life.
❑	❑	❑	4. I am comfortable with physical actions that indicate love and belonging (such as touching and hugging).

Self-Care Behaviors

1. Avoid stereotyping typical gender roles.
2. Learn the biologic aspects of sexual functioning.
3. Ask questions about sexual needs and sexual activity when necessary.
4. Enjoy close relationships with others who love you.
5. Give a hug to someone you love.
6. Accept touch from others as a sign of caring and affection.
7. Practice safer sex (e.g., use contraceptives or condoms, and choose partner carefully).
8. Recognize how age, illness, or disability influences sexual needs and expression.

FOCUSED ASSESSMENT GUIDE 44-1

SEXUALITY

Factors to Assess	Questions and Approaches
Reproductive history	Ask women their date of menarche, date of last menstrual period, duration and length of flow in days, number of pregnancies, living children, miscarriages, abortions, method of birth control. Ask men the number of children they have fathered and method of birth control used. Ask both men and women of childbearing age if they have any concerns about their fertility and determine whether there is any interest in the new reproductive technologies and genetic testing options.
History of sexually transmitted infections	"Do you or a sexual partner have a history of sexually transmitted infections? Many people today have questions about sexually transmitted infections that they are reluctant to express. Do you have any questions? Have you noticed any signs that might indicate a problem?"
History of sexual dysfunction	"Have you ever experienced a problem such as erectile dysfunction, failure to achieve orgasm, or pain during intercourse?"
Sexual self-care behaviors	"Do you perform the breast self-exam (testicular self-exam) on a monthly basis? When was your last gynecologic (urologic) examination (Pap smear, mammogram)? Is there a family history of breast disease, ovarian cancer, testicular cancer, colon cancer? With all the attention on safer sex today and responsible parenting, many people have questions about their sexual self-care behaviors. Do you have any such concerns?" (It is important to ascertain whether patients possess the knowledge, attitudes, and skills necessary to promote their own sexual health and that of others.)
Sexual self-concept	
Sexual identity	"How do you feel about yourself as a man or woman? Is anything changing the way you feel about yourself?"
Sexual body image	"Many people have concerns about their sexual body image. Are you comfortable with your physical maleness or femaleness? Have you experienced any physical changes (e.g., baldness, weight loss or gain, impotence, menopause, mastectomy, hysterectomy, sterilization) that are troubling to you?"
Sexual self-esteem	"We all have certain expectations of ourselves. Are you comfortable with the way you are currently expressing yourself sexually and meeting your sexual needs?"
Sexual role performance	"Has anything interfered with your ability to be a spouse, sexual partner, parent (any other valued sex-related roles)?"
Sexual functioning	"It's not unusual for people with health concerns (name specific medical problem, if appropriate) to have questions related to sexuality and sexual functioning. Do you have any questions or concerns that I can help you with? Has anything (if appropriate, substitute the name of a specific disease, surgery, or medication) changed your ability to function sexually?" (Asking patients if they have questions about resuming their usual sexual activity is an appropriate part of discharge planning for many patients.)

One helpful structure for obtaining information about sexual problems follows:

- *Description of the problem:* "How would you describe the problem?"
- *Onset and cause of the problem:* "What do you think caused the problem, or what was happening when you first noticed it?"
- *Past attempts at resolution:* "What have you tried in the past to correct the problem?"
- *Goals of the patient:* "What do you wish to accomplish?"

A narrative format is generally used for recording a sexual history because it allows the interviewer to document the data in many of the patient's own words. If a patient is seeking help for a sexual problem, a more spe-

cific format is used to record information obtained by a skilled therapist.

THE BETTER MODEL

The BETTER model was created to help oncology nurses conduct sexual assessments with their cancer patients more effectively. The acronym BETTER stands for (Mick, Hughes, & Cohen, 2003):

Bring up the topic of sexuality so that patients know they can discuss sexuality openly.

Explain that you are concerned with all aspects of patients' lives affected by disease.

Tell patients sexual dysfunction can happen and that you will find appropriate resources to address their concerns.

Table 44-3 SEXUAL DYSFUNCTION AND NURSING ASSESSMENT

SEXUAL DYSFUNCTION	ASSESSMENT PRIORITIES
Male	
Erectile dysfunction (impotence)	• History of diabetes, spinal cord trauma, cardiovascular disease, surgical procedure, alcoholism • Use of certain medications such as antihypertensives, antidepressants, or illicit drugs • Determine degree of mental depression that may be present. • Obtain specific information regarding the degree of impotence, length of time of disorder, continuing life factors.
Premature ejaculation	• Assess what patient defines as his dysfunction and ability to control ejaculation. • Assess any causative relationship factors such as anxiety, guilt, lack of time, and new partner.
Retarded ejaculation	• History of neurologic disorders, Parkinson disease, or use of certain medications • Same assessment priorities as for premature ejaculation
Female	
Inhibited sexual desire	• Use of oral contraceptives or other hormonal therapy, use of alcohol or certain medications • History of sexual abuse, rape or incest, depression, or other sexual dysfunctions • Assess any other contributing or relationship factors.
Orgasmic dysfunction	• Assess knowledge regarding sexual response cycle and anatomy. • Assess the communication pattern between the patient and her partner. • Assess the usual sexual pattern and behavior between the patient and her partner. • Assess any other contributing factors.
Dyspareunia	• History of diabetes, hormonal imbalance, vaginal infection, endometriosis, urethritis, cervicitis, or rectal lesions • Use of antihistamines, alcohol, tranquilizers, or illicit drugs • Assess the patient's ability for vaginal lubrication during the sexual act. • Assess the patient's use of coital positions. • Assess the use of cosmetic or chemical irritants to the genitals, such as deodorant tampons, contraceptive creams or jellies, or condoms. • Physical assessment of internal and external genitalia • Assess any other contributing factors.
Vaginismus	• Assess knowledge regarding anatomy and sexual response. • Assess the pattern of sexual activity: how often, level of arousal, orgasm. • Assess the presence of other sexual dysfunctions. • History of sexual abuse, trauma, or rape • Assess the patient's feelings regarding her partner. • Assess any other causative factors, such as fear of pregnancy, anxiety, guilt. • Physical assessment of internal and external genitalia

Timing is important to address sexuality with each visit to let patients know they can ask for information at any time.

Educate patients about the side effects of their treatments and that side effects may be temporary.

Record your assessment and interventions in patients' medical records.

A few of the major dysfunctions and assessment priorities are briefly discussed in Table 44-3. See also Focus on the Older Adult (on page 1676).

Physical Assessment

Physical examination of the reproductive or genitourinary system is necessary for either male or female patients under the following circumstances:

- As part of a routine physical examination
- Annual women's health care examination, including a Pap smear
- Suspected STI
- Suspected pregnancy
- Workup for infertility
- Unusual lump, discharge, or appearance of the genital organs noticed by the patient
- Request for birth control
- Change in urinary function

The examiner may routinely perform a complete physical examination along with assessment of the reproductive system if the patient has not had contact with the health care system within 1 year, or if the assessment findings from a complete examination would be useful in diagnosing an ailment or complaint. See Chapter 25 for a detailed description of how to examine the female and male genitalia.

Initially, ask whether the patient has had this type of examination in the past (if this information is not evident in the patient's records). Depending on the patient's

FOCUS ON THE OLDER ADULT

NURSING STRATEGIES TO ADDRESS AGE-RELATED CHANGES IN SEXUALITY AND SEXUAL FUNCTION

Factors that contribute to sexual dysfunction in the older adult are essentially the same as those that affect performance at any age: disease or mutilating surgery of the genitourinary tract, diverse systemic diseases, and emotional disturbances coupled with societal attitudes.

Age-Related Changes	Nursing Strategies
Use of multiple medications	• Educate elderly patients, intimate partners, and family about the sexual side effects of specific medications. Sometimes a change in medication dosage or modification in the treatment regimen can reduce sexual dysfunction.
Dependence on alcohol or marijuana to cope with discomforts of aging, resulting in weakened erection, reduced desire, delayed ejaculation	• Before the patient can decide to stop using alcohol or drugs, he or she must realize the need to change his or her behavior. The nurse can assist in attitude and value clarification about substance use, sexuality, and sexual behavior. Refer the elderly patient to a counselor who can assist with sexual performance problems as well as emotional and dependence problems.
Age-related metabolic disorders such as anemia, diabetes, malnutrition, and fatigue may affect the quality of life and cause impotence.	• Symptoms may be initially discussed with the nurse. The patient may be hesitant to discuss sexual problems openly. Listen carefully. Acknowledge that sexual problems in the elderly are not unusual. Even if the nurse does not know all the answers, active listening on the nurse's part may encourage the patient to visit his or her health care provider or a counselor. Encourage elderly patients to have a thorough physical evaluation by a health care provider.
Obesity may damage cardiac and vascular integrity and reduce self-esteem, resulting in decreased sexual performance and interest.	• Encourage the patient to seek the advice of his or her health care provider and to explore weight reduction and health promotion programs.
Many elderly persons are concerned that sexual activity might increase the risk for illness or even death due to stress on the heart or blood pressure.	• Teach the patient that sexual intercourse and similar forms of sexual expression are not considered dangerous for anyone able to walk around a room and may actually offer physiological benefits.
Radical surgery or dysfunction of the genitourinary tract affects sexual capacity and libido. Extensive surgery due to malignancy may make intercourse difficult or impossible.	• Patients need support and guidance in adjusting to these changes. Provide specific suggestions for how to accommodate to the surgical changes while still maintaining a sexually satisfying relationship. Acknowledge the need for sexual expression in some form or other and provide an open, nonjudgmental response when patients display a need for warmth, close contact, and companionship. Touch is particularly important. An atmosphere of trust between the nurse and the elderly patient is essential.
Loss of a spouse	• Explore alternative forms of sexual expression with patients who are widows and widowers. Encourage them to attend a support group and become active socially. Acknowledge that human sexuality crosses a wide spectrum and that the pattern for each individual is an outcome of his or her development, experiences, and sense of personal identity. The basic pattern is not altered by age or loss of a spouse or loved one. It continues to influence one's capacity for involvement in all life activities.

Adapted from Murray, R., & Zentner, J. (2009). *Health promotion strategies through the life span.* Boston: Pearson.

knowledge base, explain the progressive steps of the examination and what the patient may feel during the examination. This will give the patient some feeling of control and security during the examination. The nurse's responsibilities during an examination of the reproductive system are as follows:

• Provide information about the examination.
• Teach the patient.

• Provide support to the patient during the examination.
• Perform the examination or assist the examiner, if appropriate, with any procedures or laboratory studies.

Keeping the patient comfortable and respecting the patient's privacy and modesty should be primary nursing considerations. Some female patients might be uncomfortable with a male examiner, or vice versa, for religious, cultural, or other reasons. The examiner can adapt to such concerns, for example, by ensuring that a female nurse is in the room when a female patient is undergoing a pelvic examination by a male physician.

Diagnosing

There are two categories of nursing diagnoses written to address problems of sexuality:

- *Ineffective Sexuality Patterns:* The state in which an individual experiences or is at risk for a change in sexual health, which results in concern regarding own sexuality. Sexual health is the integration of somatic, emotional, intellectual, and social aspects of sexual being in ways that are enriching and that enhance personality, communication, and love.
- *Sexual Dysfunction:* The state in which an individual experiences or is at risk for change in sexual function that is viewed as unsatisfying, unrewarding, or inadequate.

Related diagnoses include Rape-Trauma Syndrome, Impaired (or Risk for Impaired) Parenting, and Readiness for Enhanced Parenting (NANDA International [NANDA-I], 2012).

Ineffective Sexuality Patterns or Sexual Dysfunction as the Problem

Before a nursing diagnosis is made regarding a sexual problem, carefully review the assessment data to determine whether the situation can be corrected by independent nursing interventions. Although many problems of sexuality experienced by a patient in a health care situation are amenable to nursing action, some require the expertise of other specialties.

 AN impotent diabetic patient who would benefit from a penile implant—such as Jefferson Smith, described at the beginning of the chapter—needs medical consultation. A patient with a serious sexual dysfunction or one who practices destructive sexual expression needs intensive therapy by a clinical psychologist, sex therapist, or counselor. Appropriate referrals by the nurse should follow the identification of such problems. ●

Sexual dysfunction may be specified as erectile failure (impotence), premature ejaculation, retarded ejaculation, inhibited sexual desire, orgasmic dysfunction, vaginismus, or dyspareunia. Common etiologies for sexual dysfunction include effects of medication (specify), effects of alcohol consumption, effects of disease process (specify), history of abuse (specify rape, incest), feelings of depression, guilt, anxiety, fear of rejection, miscommunication with partner, fear of pain, effects of birth control method (specify), lack of knowledge, or effects of surgical procedure (specify).

The nursing diagnosis Ineffective Sexuality Patterns can be further specified by loss of desire (to abstinence), increased desire (to promiscuity), or change in sexual expression. Common etiologies for Ineffective Sexuality

Patterns include stress (lifestyle, job, family, finances, marital conflict), isolation from partner, effects of pregnancy (specify), feelings of depression, loss of privacy, loss of communication with partner, relationship change (new partner), effects of disease process (sexual position, frequency, mode of expression), change in body image, change in self-concept, or loss of partner. Some nursing diagnoses concerning sexuality are given in Examples of NANDA-I Nursing Diagnoses: Sexuality (on page 1678).

Ineffective Sexuality Patterns or Sexual Dysfunction as the Etiology

Changes in sexuality can affect other areas of human functioning. In the following nursing diagnoses, problems of sexuality are the etiology of another problem:

- Impaired Adjustment related to loss of sexual partner, loss of sexual body part
- Anxiety related to fear of pregnancy, loss of sexual functioning or desire, effects of disease process on sexual functioning
- Pain related to sexual position, penile penetration, effects of genital surgery, lack of vaginal lubrication
- Ineffective Coping related to effects of body image on sexual expression, change in sexual partner
- Fear related to pain during sexual intercourse, history of sexual abuse
- Anticipatory Grieving related to loss of sexual functioning, effects of surgical excision of genital body part
- Delayed Growth and Development related to sexual exploitation or abuse, sexual guilt, effects of hormonal imbalance, lack of information about sexuality
- Deficient Knowledge (specify: contraceptive methods, spread of STIs, sexual response, genital anatomy, modes of sexual expression, self-examination, effects of disease or medications) related to misinformation, sexual myths, lack of interest in learning, cognitive limitation
- Disturbed Body Image (specify: surgical excision of genital body part, loss of or gain in body weight) related to fear of rejection
- Impaired Social Interaction related to effects of marital separation or divorce
- Social Isolation related to fear of contracting STI, fear of sexual encounter

Outcome Identification and Planning

Nurses should value sexuality as an important aspect of who the patient is and how the patient is identified as a unique human. Specific patient outcomes to promote sexual health follow. The patient will:

- Define individual sexuality
- Establish open patterns of communication with significant others
- Develop self-awareness and body awareness
- Describe responsible sexual health self-care practices, identifying appropriate resources

EXAMPLES OF NANDA-I NURSING DIAGNOSES

SEXUALITY

Nursing Diagnoses	Related Factors	Sample Defining Characteristics
Sexual Dysfunction: Erectile Dysfunction	Use of antihypertensive medication	• 45-year-old man with a 3-year history of hypertension • Maintained normotensive on reserpine, 0.25 mg daily • "I have had trouble keeping an erection. My wife and I haven't made love in months. We don't talk about it anymore. I guess that part of my life is over." • Patient appears resigned and saddened.
Sexual Dysfunction: Dyspareunia	Effects of menopausal process	• 54-year-old woman whose last menses was 1 year ago • "Whenever my husband and I make love, my vagina burns and stings." • States decrease in vaginal lubrication during past several months
Altered Sexuality Patterns: Change in Sexual Expression	Loss of privacy due to hospitalization	• 23-year-old man hospitalized for past 6 weeks with injuries resulting from car crash; has been in traction for fractured right femur • "I can't take this place anymore! Everyone barges in here whenever they want to—nobody cares about my feelings—a guy can't even act like a guy around here. I wish I could be alone with my wife for a while with no interruptions."
Altered Sexuality Patterns: Loss of Desire	Change in body image due to body-altering surgery	• Surgery for bowel cancer with construction of permanent colostomy 1 month ago • "I know the colostomy was necessary to save my life, but it is so disgusting. I'll never be able to have a relationship with my husband again. It's a real turn-off to me—just imagine what he'll think—how can I expect him to want to make love to a freak?"
Alteration in Comfort: Pain	Abduction of hips in sexual positioning	• 60-year-old woman with a history of osteoarthritis for 6 years • "The act of intercourse hurts my hips so bad that I'm in pain the whole next day. I don't want to stop having intercourse with my husband, but I'm going to have to if this pain gets worse." • Patient states that the missionary position is the only position used during sex with her husband throughout their 40-year marriage.

• Practice responsible sexual expression (e.g., by 5/1/15, the patient will use rubber condoms during all sexual encounters)

Specific patient outcomes depend on the nature of the patient's problem or concern. Expected outcomes should be patient-oriented—that is, something the patient desires to do or has the ability to accomplish. For example, it is not enough to advise a method of birth control; rather, the nurse needs to know which method the patient is motivated and able to use.

Implementing
Establishing a Trusting Nurse–Patient Relationship
It is impossible to address a patient's sexuality if trust has not been developed between you and the patient (see Through the Eyes of a Student). To do so, project an objective, nonthreatening, and nonjudgmental attitude, and emphasize that the information the patient gives will be kept confidential. The nurse who is aware of one's own behavior and verbal and nonverbal cues and anticipates the patient's concerns can help the patient trust the nurse with information of an intimate nature. Be sure to establish respect for the patient and empathy before discussing sexual issues. Consider all of the patient's circumstances and life experiences using a therapeutic, not a pitying, approach. Only when you are accepted as a trusted, caring person will the patient reveal details of his or her private life, including sexual concerns.

 REVIEW the Reflective Practice display for this chapter. Note how the nursing student initially avoided interpersonal contact with the patient, performing the technical aspects of care but ignoring the patient as a person. Communication and trust did not occur until the patient asked the nursing student about the level of discomfort and the nursing student responded truthfully. •

THROUGH THE EYES OF A STUDENT

I knew it was going to happen sooner or later. Male nurses are not unheard of in this day and age, but some people just aren't yet ready for us—especially Ethel, a 68-year-old black woman with a deep religious conviction. I concluded this because she called on Jesus for help when I told her that I was her student nurse for the day, and that I would be giving her a bath.

"You're my nurse?" she said. "Help me, Jesus....No, no, you just go on and help somebody else, honey. I've already had my bath," she insisted.

Accordingly, I told her she was mistaken and that I understood her anxiety. Then I proceeded to exaggerate the truth by saying that I had done this before, when really I had given baths before, but not to members of the opposite sex. She thought *she* was having anxiety!

Next I asked my instructor, Lynn, for help. She quickly assessed the situation and tried to comfort Ethel by vouching

for my professional character and abilities, but still no go. Then I tried appealing to her logic.

"This is a hospital where male doctors examine you all the time. Why is this any different?" I asked. "Because you are not a doctor" was her logical reply.

I felt inadequate. I could not give this woman the care she needed because of my gender. Luckily, in the next bed, Michele was about to give her patient a bath. She offered to give Ethel her bath if I would help her with her patients.

Consequently, Ethel got her bath, and I learned that a nurse has to be flexible as well as willing to ask for and accept help when the patient's quality of care is at stake. This is something I hope to remember throughout my nursing career.

—Daniel E. Zirolli
Delaware County Community College, Media, Pennsylvania

Teaching About Sexuality and Sexual Health

Most nursing interventions pertaining to a patient's sexuality involve teaching to promote sexual health. Major goals of patient teaching are a change in knowledge, attitude, or behavior. In some situations, patients need help defining or redefining their sexuality and its importance to their lives. Offering information, dispelling fears, and providing positive reinforcement are some ways to help patients increase their knowledge about their bodies and sexual functioning. Patients might need assistance in modifying behaviors or learning new skills to increase the quality of sexual health and functioning. See the Promoting Health Literacy box.

Part of teaching also includes correcting sexual myths and promoting body awareness. Many people believe things about sex that they have heard from family or

friends or within their culture that are not true or are not based on scientific data. During the assessment or while providing care, take the opportunity to refute sexual myths and teach factual information (Table 44-4 on page 1680).

Patients might need assistance in becoming familiar with what they believe and feel about their sexual selves. Be helpful to patients with difficulty accepting or developing their sexuality by promoting their self-confidence and good self-concept. When patients feel comfortable about themselves and their sensual feelings, they can begin to focus on how they feel about their sexual functioning and specific sexual expressions.

Getting to know one's physical body is important to healthy sexual development. Every man and woman, sexually active or not, needs to be aware of the appearance of one's genitalia. Some people, because of their background, feel ashamed and repulsed by their bodies;

PROMOTING HEALTH LITERACY

IN PATIENTS RECEIVING THE HPV VACCINE

Patient Scenario

Mrs. Smith, mother of 15-year-old Diane Smith, was told by her daughter's high school that all girls must get the HPV vaccine. Mrs. Smith knows that Diane has been dating a boy from school for almost a year, but insists that her daughter "is not sexually active and should not have to get the vaccine." She is primarily concerned that this new vaccine is not safe.

Nursing Considerations: *Tips for Improving Health Literacy*

Tell Mrs. Smith that one in four young women between the ages of 14 and 19 is infected with at least one of the most common STIs, which include the human papillomavirus. Also, many girls between the ages of 11 and 26 get the HPV vaccine. Give both Mrs. Smith and her daughter an

information sheet about the human papillomavirus and the HPV vaccine. Encourage the mother and daughter to be prepared to ask the clinician these questions:

- What problem is the HPV vaccine trying to prevent?
- What do I need to know in order to make a good decision about getting the vaccine?
- Why does the school think it is important for all girls to get the vaccine?

What additional measures can you take to help increase health literacy in this mother and daughter? What other measures would be helpful if they did not speak English, could not read, or had other learning deficits? What other measures could you take if the daughter confided in you that she is sexually active? What additional measure would be necessary if the primary reason for refusing the HPV vaccine was religious?

Table 44-4 SEXUAL MYTHS AND FACTS TO REFUTE THEM

SEXUAL DYSFUNCTION	ASSESSMENT PRIORITIES
Each person is born with a certain amount of sexual drive, which if overdawn in youth leaves little reserve for later years.	Actually, the correlation between sexual activity and length of time it persists throughout life is just the opposite. The more consistently sexually active a person is, the longer the activity continues into the later years of life.
The need for expressing one's sexuality becomes less important in the latter half of one's life.	Physiologically, sexual desire and ability do not decrease markedly after middle age. The expression of one's sexuality, as an integral part of development, follows the overall pattern of health and physical performance.
Sexual abstinence is necessary in training for sports.	Physiologically, the achievement of orgasm is rarely more demanding than most activities encountered in daily life. The desire for sleep that often follows is most commonly due to factors other than physical exhaustion from sexual activities. There is no scientific evidence that sex "weakens" a person.
Excessive sexual activity can lead to mental illness.	The biologic significance of human sexuality has no greater effect on total development than any other necessary biologic function. There is no scientific basis for believing that one will develop a mental or physical illness with excessive or no sexual activity.
Wet dreams are indicators of sexual disorders.	Erotic dreams that culminate in orgasms are normal common physiologic phenomena in at least 85% of men. They can occur at any age after puberty. Some women also report in clinical studies that their sexual dreams culminate in orgasm. In women, this phenomenon is believed to increase with advancing age.
Because of the anatomic nature of the sex organs, women are passive and men are aggressive.	Physiologic studies disprove this myth by showing the woman to be far from passive. Maximum gratification requires each partner to be both passive and aggressive in participating mutually and cooperatively.
It is unnatural for a woman to have as strong a desire for sex as a man—women should not enjoy sex as much as men.	These myths have been reinforced by a society that has traditionally taught women that they are to suppress sexual desires to gain love, security, and society's respect, based on the assumption that it is the basic nature of women to be submissive, dependent, and subordinate. Physiologic studies indicate that, in some respects, the woman's sex drive is not only as strong but may be even stronger than that of the man.
Women who have multiple orgasms or who readily come to climax are nymphomaniacs or promiscuous.	Physiologic studies at this time suggest that we do not know women's sexual potential; these studies indicate that there is a wide range of intensity and duration of orgasmic experience, and the potential for multiple or frequent orgasms within a brief period is not at all uncommon. Therefore, women normally may have greater orgasmic capacity than men with regard to duration and frequency of orgasm.
There is a difference between vaginal orgasm and clitoral orgasm.	Physiologic misunderstanding has produced the myth of separate clitoral and vaginal orgasms rather than their interrelations. Female orgasm is normally initiated by clitoral stimulation, but because it is a total-body response, there are marked variations in intensity and timing. There is no reason to believe that the female response to the sex act is due to a vaginal rather than a clitoral orgasm.
A mature sexual relationship requires the man and woman to achieve simultaneous orgasm.	Although simultaneous orgasm may be desirable, it is unrealistic. Often, it is possible only under the most ideal circumstances and is not a determinant of sexual achievement or of satisfaction (except to someone who accepts this as dogma).
The larger penis has greater possibilities for producing orgasm in the woman.	Physiologically, there is practically no relation between the size of a man's penis and his ability to satisfy a woman sexually. Furthermore, there is little correlation between penile size and body size and their relation to sexual potency.
The face-to-face coital position is the proper, moral, and healthy one.	Knowledge of human sexual practices dispels this myth with the recognition that there is no normal or single most acceptable sexual position. Whatever position offers the most pleasure and is acceptable to both partners is correct for them. Any variation is normal, healthy, and proper if it satisfies both partners.
The ability to achieve orgasm is an indicator of a person's sexual responsiveness.	Achievement of a satisfactory sexual response is the result of numerous physical, psychological, and cultural influences. Too often, the physical fact of orgasm (or lack of orgasm) is taken to be symbolic of sexual responsiveness and seen out of context of the entire relationship between man and woman.

others feel that touching the body is dirty and might feel guilt and anxiety in stimulating themselves. Patients need assistance in improving body awareness if any of these issues are present. Patients can become accustomed to looking at their bodies by looking at nonthreatening anatomy first and then proceeding to the genitals. This can be done in the shower or with the use of a mirror. Knowing what looks normal can be of great importance so that patients can report the development of an unusual appearance later on.

After patients have developed some degree of comfort in looking at their bodies, they can progress to experiencing touch. Again, patients should progress from nonthreatening parts of the body until the genitals can be touched without stress.

A good exercise for women in developing body awareness is the use of Kegel exercises. These exercises promote good vaginal tone by localizing and strengthening the pubococcygeal muscle. A woman can locate this muscle by stopping a stream of urine midway through urination. Contracting this muscle can be repeated at any time of the day in any circumstance because its performance is undetectable. Some women who practice Kegel exercises have found that their sexual satisfaction is improved.

Promoting Responsible Sexual Expression

Patients need to know how to gain satisfactory sexual experiences while behaving responsibly in their activities. Responsible sexuality encompasses sexual expression, prevention of unwanted pregnancy, prevention of STIs, and sex education.

FORM OF SEXUAL EXPRESSION

The form of sexual expression used by patients should not inflict unwanted harm on themselves or others. When sexual expression encroaches on the rights of others, it is neither healthy nor desirable. Sexual acts that violate

another's rights are usually considered to be acts of aggression or hostility rather than stemming from sexual need or desire. Rape, in particular, is motivated by a need to dominate and humiliate the victim.

PREVENTION OF UNWANTED PREGNANCY

Contraception is a process or technique for preventing pregnancy by means of a medication, device, or method that blocks or alters one or more of the processes of reproduction in such a way that sexual union can occur without impregnation. The prevention of unwanted pregnancy must be a conscious decision. Anyone who is unprepared for pregnancy should refrain from intercourse or obtain a contraceptive method from a health care provider or from the pharmacy; it is too late to think about contraception during sexual intercourse. To practice responsible sexuality, the contraceptive method must be used consistently and according to instructions.

PREVENTION OF STIs

As described earlier, STIs are widespread. The only sure way to avoid an STI is to avoid all types of intimate genital contact. When this is impractical, there are other practices that can decrease a patient's risk for STIs (see Box 44-1). The American College of Obstetricians and Gynecologists' Committee on Health Care for Underserved Women

BOX 44-1   WHAT CAN YOU DO TO PREVENT STIs?

The best way to prevent STIs is to avoid sexual contact with others. If you decide to be sexually active, there are things that you can do to reduce your risk of developing an STI.

- Have a mutually monogamous sexual relationship with an uninfected partner.
- Correctly and consistently use a male condom.
- Use clean needles if injecting intravenous drugs.
- Prevent and control other STIs to decrease susceptibility to HIV infection and to reduce your infectiousness if you are HIV infected.
- Delay having sexual relations as long as possible. The younger people are when having sex for the first time, the more susceptible they become to developing an STI. The risk of acquiring an STI also increases with the number of partners over a lifetime.

Anyone who is sexually active should:

- Have regular checkups for STIs even in the absence of symptoms, and especially if having sex with a new partner. These tests can be done during a routine visit to the doctor's office.
- Learn the common symptoms of STIs. Seek medical help immediately if any suspicious symptoms develop, even if they are mild.
- Avoid having sex during menstruation. HIV-infected women are probably more infectious, and HIV-uninfected women are probably more susceptible to becoming infected during that time.
- Avoid anal intercourse, but if practiced, use a male condom.
- Avoid douching because it removes some of the normal protective bacteria in the vagina and increases the risk of getting some STIs.

Anyone diagnosed as having an STI should:

- Be treated to reduce the risk of transmitting an STI to a sex partner or from mother to baby.
- Discuss with a doctor the possible risk of transmission in breast milk and whether commercial formula should be substituted.
- Notify all recent sex partners and urge them to get a checkup.
- Follow the doctor's orders and complete the full course of medication prescribed. A follow-up test to ensure that the infection has been cured is often an important step in treatment.
- Avoid all sexual activity while being treated for an STI.

Sometimes people are too embarrassed or frightened to ask for help or information. Most STIs are readily treated. The earlier a person seeks treatment and warns sex partners about the disease, the less likely the disease will do irreparable physical damage, be spread to others, or in the case of a woman, be passed on to a newborn baby.

The National Institute of Allergy and Infectious Diseases (NIAID) is a component of the National Institutes of Health (NIH), which is an agency of the Department of Health and Human Services. NIAID supports basic and applied research to prevent, diagnose, and treat infectious and immune-mediated illnesses, including HIV/AIDS and other sexually transmitted infections, illness from potential agents of bioterrorism, tuberculosis, malaria, autoimmune disorders, asthma, and allergies. News releases, fact sheets, and other NIAID-related materials are available on the NIAID website at www.niaid.nih.gov.

has published a Committee Opinion on Human Immunodeficiency Virus and Acquired Immunodeficiency Syndrome and Women of Color (2008). In the United States, women of color (primarily African American and Hispanic women) comprise most new cases of HIV and AIDS among women. Most women of color acquire the disease from heterosexual contact, often from a partner who has undisclosed risk factors for HIV infection. A combination of testing, education, and brief behavioral interventions can help reduce the rate of HIV infection and its complications among women of color.

SEX EDUCATION

Sex education is critical to healthy sexual development and safe sexual behaviors. See Examples of Nursing Interventions and Nursing Outcomes Classifications (NIC/NOC): Safe Sex Activities. Information received from peers and friends is almost always inadequate and may be erroneous. Parents should be taught to answer children's questions immediately and accurately.

Considering Contraception

Unintended pregnancy remains a significant women's health issue in the United States as well as a critical social issue. *Healthy People 2020* aims to improve pregnancy planning, spacing, and preventing unintended pregnancy. One objective is to increase the proportion of intended pregnancies to 56%. The statistics that follow about contraceptive methods were obtained from Planned Parenthood Federation of America, Inc. (Planned Parenthood, 2014). Many unintended pregnancies result from the use of less effective methods of contraception, such as condoms, spermicide, or barrier methods. The past several years have seen the development of new, easier to use, and more effective methods of contraception. Nurses and nurse practitioners have a responsibility to provide information to women regarding their many contraceptive options.

Patients choose contraception for many reasons and might contact health care providers specifically to obtain information about birth control. Some people use contraception for the orderly spacing of pregnancies in a family; others may want to prevent pregnancy from occurring until a family is desired. Some people choose a permanent method to prevent pregnancy from ever occurring. Factors that affect a person's choice of a contraceptive method include age, marital status, desire for future pregnancy, religious beliefs, level of education, cost, and ease of use. Other considerations are the woman's knowledge about available methods, her perceptions of the various methods, and in many cases, her previous experience with contraception.

All contraceptive methods have advantages and disadvantages. Understanding and explaining the available methods thoroughly is a must so that patients can choose the one that will best meet their situation and needs (Box 44-2).

When choosing a contraceptive method, the patient should consider the following:

- How well will it fit into my lifestyle?
- How convenient will it be?
- How effective will it be?
- How safe will it be?
- How affordable will it be?
- How reversible will it be?
- Will it protect against STIs?

METHODS OF CONTRACEPTION

Behavioral. Abstinence is a behavioral method of contraception. There are two types of abstinence: continuous and periodic. Choosing abstinence does not mean that a

---

EXAMPLES OF NURSING INTERVENTIONS AND NURSING OUTCOMES CLASSIFICATIONS (NIC/NOC)

SAFE SEX ACTIVITIES

Nursing Interventions	Nursing Outcomes
• Instruct the patient on STIs and conception as necessary. • Discuss the patient's knowledge, understanding, motivation, and commitment level regarding various sexual protection methods. • Discuss methods of sexual protection for sexual intercourse and oral sex, including effectiveness, side effects, contraindications, and signs and symptoms that warrant reporting to a health care professional. • Discuss religious, cultural, developmental, socioeconomic, and individual considerations pertaining to sexual protection choice.	• Affirms self as a sexual being • Exhibits clear sense of sexual orientation • Uses healthy coping behaviors to resolve sexual identity issues • Reports healthy sexual functioning • Performs sexually if environment conducive • Performs sexually without coercion of partner • Describes risks associated with sexual activity

Adapted from Bulechek, G., Butcher, H., Dochterman, J., & Wagner, C. M. (Eds.). (2013). *Nursing interventions classification (NIC)* (6th ed., p. 383). St. Louis: Elsevier/Mosby; and Moorhead, S., Johnson, M., Maas, M., & Swanson, E. (Eds.) (2013). *Nursing outcomes classification (NOC)* (5th ed., pp. 504–505). St. Louis: Elsevier/Mosby. A full listing of nursing activities for each nursing intervention and outcomes can be found in these books.

BOX 44-2 KNOWLEDGE DEFICIT: CONTRACEPTIVE METHODS

Assessment Priorities

- Determine the patient's past use of contraceptive methods.
- Assess the patient's effectiveness and satisfaction with past methods.
- Assess the patient's current knowledge of contraceptive methods.
- Assess the frequency of the patient's sexual activity.
- Identify any methods that are unacceptable to the patient.
- Assess the motivation of the patient to use certain methods.
- Assess the patient's level of comfort with manipulation of genital body parts.
- Obtain a complete patient history and perform a physical examination if indicated.

Expected Outcomes

The patient will achieve the following:

- Choose a contraceptive method that the patient is motivated to use
- List the adverse effects or danger signs associated with the contraceptive method
- List the steps needed to use the contraceptive method effectively

- Use the contraceptive with every act of sexual intercourse
- Choose a back-up method
- Report back to the health care setting for follow-up as directed

Nursing Interventions

- Describe in terms at the patient's level of understanding each contraceptive method for which the patient needs information (give objective information in a matter-of-fact manner to avoid bias by nurse).
- Describe the effectiveness of each method and side effects or possible complications.
- Instruct the patient in the use of a chosen method, giving step-by-step instructions.
- Advise the patient of the importance of having a back-up method on hand.
- Instruct the patient in the use of the back-up method.
- Have the patient obtain a physical examination if indicated by the chosen contraceptive method (e.g., the pill).
- Instruct the patient to report back in a specified period for follow-up of use of method if indicated (follow-up visits to a health care facility are important, particularly if a patient elects to use the pill).

person is sexless. Most people are abstinent at some time in their lives. Abstinence can be a positive way of dealing with sexuality when it represents a well-thought-out decision regarding one's mind, body, spirit, and sexual health.

Continuous abstinence involves not having any sex with a partner at all. It is 100% effective in preventing pregnancy and STIs. However, individuals may find it difficult to abstain for long periods of time. Ending abstinence without first being prepared to protect against an unplanned pregnancy or infection might cause additional problems.

Periodic abstinence and fertility awareness methods are two methods of contraception that involve charting a woman's fertility pattern. Periodic abstinence is a method used by some sexually active women to prevent pregnancy. They become familiar with their fertility patterns and abstain from vaginal intercourse on the days they think they could become pregnant. Women who monitor their fertility to prevent pregnancy either abstain from vaginal intercourse for at least one-third of each menstrual cycle or use barrier methods during the fertile or "unsafe" period.

Three basic charting methods can be used to predict ovulation in order to plan or prevent pregnancy:

- *Temperature method:* The woman takes her temperature every morning before getting out of bed. Her temperature will rise between 0.4°F and 0.8°F on the day of ovulation and will remain at that level until her next period.
- *Cervical mucus method:* The woman observes the changes in her cervical mucus throughout the first part of the menstrual cycle, until after ovulation. Cervical mucus is normally cloudy, but a few days before

ovulation it becomes clear and slippery and can be stretched between the fingers. This indicates the most fertile phase of the cycle. The couple must abstain from vaginal intercourse or use a barrier method during this period to avoid pregnancy.

- *Calendar method:* The woman charts her menstrual cycle on a calendar. The couple must refrain from intercourse or use a barrier method during "unsafe" days.

The best approach to monitoring fertility is a combination of all three methods called the symptothermal method. Of 100 couples who use any of these methods for 1 year, 20 women will typically become pregnant. The failure rate is higher in single women. Using the methods carefully and consistently and avoiding unprotected vaginal intercourse during the fertile phase can give better results.

Coitus interruptus, the withdrawal of the penis from the vagina before ejaculation, is one of the oldest and most widely used contraceptive methods. Pregnancy cannot occur if sperm are kept out of the vagina. Of every 100 women whose partners attempt this method, 27 typically will become pregnant during the first year. Pre-ejaculate can contain enough sperm to cause a pregnancy, and pre-ejaculate or semen may spill onto the vulva.

Barrier Methods. Barrier methods include the condom, diaphragm, cervical cap, and vaginal sponge used in combination with a spermicidal agent.

Diaphragm. Diaphragm approaches have been used in various forms since ancient times. The current diaphragm is a dome-shaped device made of latex rubber that mechanically prevents semen from coming into contact with the cervix. It is also used to hold a spermicidal jelly in place against the cervix. The diaphragm is placed in the vagina before sexual activity. It fits between the pelvic notch at the front of the vagina to behind the cervix at the back. It is not felt by either the woman or her partner when correctly situated in the vagina. A diaphragm must be individually sized during a pelvic examination. The woman needs to be familiar with her body and able to handle her genitals for diaphragm placement and removal. The diaphragm must be worn during each episode of sexual activity and consistently used with a spermicidal agent. Twenty of 100 women who use the diaphragm will become pregnant during the first year of typical use; 6 will become pregnant with perfect use.

Condom. The traditional condom, or "rubber," is used by men, although it is appropriate for a woman to have a condom available for her partner's use. The condom is rolled over the erect penis and collects the semen after ejaculation occurs. If the condom does not have a nipple receptacle end, a small space should be left at the end of the condom to collect sperm (this prevents breakage). Condoms are available over the counter and have become more widely used because of the incidence of HIV/AIDS and other STIs.

A female condom is also available. The female condom is a ringed pouch that unrolls in the vagina. Advantages include the fact that the male does not need to first have an erection for the pouch to be used, and it offers significant protection from STIs.

Of 100 women whose partners use condoms, about 14 will become pregnant during the first year of typical use; 2 women will become pregnant with perfect use. The latex condom protects against STIs, including HIV. The latex condom offers better protection against STIs than any other birth control method because it blocks the exchange of body fluids that may be infected.

Cervical Cap. The cervical cap is a thimble-shaped rubber device that is placed over the cervix and may be left there for up to 3 days at a time. Its mechanism of action is similar to that of the diaphragm. Not all women can wear a cervical cap because of individual anatomic differences. There is some evidence to suggest that the cervical cap can cause cervical inflammation and increase the risk for pelvic infection.

Spermicides. Spermicides are used with barrier methods but can also be used alone. Spermicides come in creams, jellies, foams, and suppositories. Although readily available, spermicides are not as effective alone as when combined with another method, such as a diaphragm or a condom.

Vaginal Sponge. The vaginal sponge is a barrier method that contains a spermicide. The sponge acts not only as a barrier between the semen and the cervix but also as a reservoir to hold semen. The vaginal sponge carries some risk of toxic shock syndrome (TSS) and is contraindicated for use in women who have a past history of TSS. Women who use the vaginal sponge must follow package directions carefully and remove the sponge within 24 hours. The vaginal sponge is about as effective as the diaphragm.

Hormonal. Hormonal methods are based on the feedback mechanism of hormones of the menstrual cycle. Synthetic estrogens and progestin chemical compounds are used in the form of a pill, shot, or implant to prevent ovulation.

Oral Contraceptives. The oral contraceptive ("the pill") is the most common contraceptive method and the most popular method for women in their 20s. Most of the harmful side effects and dangers associated with taking the pill are related to the estrogen component. However, most pills currently available contain a small dose of estrogen. The pill also has many beneficial noncontraceptive effects. It has been shown to protect women against the development of breast, ovarian, and endometrial cancer. Taken consistently and as prescribed, the pill is almost 100% effective in guarding against pregnancy. However, its cost might be prohibitive to some women. The woman must also be motivated to take a pill every day at the same time. A health history and physical examination by a health care provider are necessary to obtain a prescription for oral contraceptives. Some women should not take the pill if they have certain physiologic disorders or diseases. Smoking increases the risks associated with oral contraceptives. Remind women who are taking the pill to take measures to protect themselves from STIs.

Norplant System. The Norplant System is a reversible, 5-year, low-dose, progestin-only contraceptive. The system consists of six matchstick-size capsules (made of Silastic tubing) that are placed just under the skin of the woman's upper arm. The average annual pregnancy rate over 5 years is less than 1%. The most common side effect is a change in the menstrual bleeding pattern, including prolonged menstrual bleeding, spotting between menstrual periods, or no bleeding at all.

Implanon. In the Implanon system, a single etonogestrel-containing rod is implanted in the woman through the use of a disposable insertion kit. Removal requires a small incision and takes about 3 minutes. The single-rod system contains 68 mg of etonogestrel in an ethylene vinyl acetate (EVA) copolymer core surrounded by an EVA membrane. The rod releases 67 mcg of etonogestrel daily. This method of contraceptive approaches 100% efficacy. The most common reason for discontinuation is weight gain.

Depo-Provera. Depo-Provera is the brand name of a progestin-only hormonal birth control system. It uses a hormone similar to progesterone, one of the hormones made by a woman's ovaries that regulates the menstrual cycle. It is called depot medroxyprogesterone acetate (DMPA). An injection of DMPA in the buttock or arm can prevent pregnancy for 12 weeks and is 99.7% effective. Protection is immediate if the injection is given on the first day of the woman's period. Irregular bleeding is the most common side effect for women using DMPA.

Of every 1,000 women who use Depo-Provera, only 3 will become pregnant during the first year of use.

Transdermal Contraceptive Patch. The transdermal contraceptive patch (Evra) supplies continuous daily circulating levels of ethinyl estradiol (20 mcg) and norelgestromin (150 mcg). The patch is applied weekly on the same day of each week for 3 weeks, followed by a patch-free week. It may be applied to any of four sites: lower abdomen, upper outer arm, buttock, or upper torso (excluding the breast). Women who use the contraceptive patch demonstrate more effective use than those using oral contraceptive pills. The patch has been found to have an overall annual probability of pregnancy (method failure plus user failure) of 0.8%. This contraceptive method has the same contraindications as oral contraceptives. The most common side effects include breast symptoms, headache, application site reactions, nausea, upper respiratory tract infection, and dysmenorrhea.

Vaginal Ring. The vaginal ring (NuvaRing) is a soft, flexible, transparent ring made of ethylene vinyl acetate copolymer. It releases approximately 120 mcg of etonogestrel and 15 mcg of ethyl estradiol daily. Each ring is inserted into the vagina and used for one cycle, which consists of 3 weeks of continuous use followed by a ring-free week. Women can insert and remove the ring themselves. It does not need to be fitted, nor does it require particular placement within the vagina. The ring works by inhibiting ovulation in much the same way as oral contraceptives. Used appropriately, the vaginal ring is 99.3% effective in protecting against pregnancy. Benefits of the vaginal ring include ease of use, self-insertion, high degree of effectiveness, and low incidence of negative or adverse effects. The most common side effects include headache, vaginal discharge, vaginitis, vaginal discomfort, foreign body sensation, coital problems, and ring expulsion.

Intrauterine Devices.

The intrauterine device (IUD) is an object that is placed by a physician or nurse practitioner within the uterus to prevent implantation of a fertilized ovum. IUDs are small devices made of flexible plastic that provide reversible birth control. IUDs usually prevent fertilization of the egg, but the precise mechanism by which it works is unknown. IUDs seem to affect the way the sperm or egg moves. It may be that substances released by the IUD immobilize sperm. Another possibility is that the IUD prompts the egg to move through the fallopian tube too fast to be fertilized. IUDs that contain copper are more effective for two reasons. The copper affects the behavior of enzymes in the lining of the uterus to prevent implantation and also causes the production of increased amounts of prostaglandin. Only 8 of 1,000 women using copper IUDs will become pregnant with perfect use.

Combination hormonal and IUD contraceptive methods include a T-shaped device with a steroid reservoir around the vertical stem (Mirena). It releases 20 mcg of levonorgestrel daily and provides contraception for up to 5 years. Fertilization is prevented because the device causes changes in cervical mucus and endometrial morphology, inhibition of sperm migration, alteration of sperm–egg binding and ovarian function, and a foreign body reaction by the uterus. Failure of implantation may occur in some women. Estradiol levels are managed within the usual range of women who are not using contraceptives. Normal function of the ovaries and fertility are restored as quickly after discontinuation as with any IUD. Efficacy approaches 100%. An additional benefit of this contraceptive method is that it controls menorrhagia in pre- and perimenopausal women. Adverse side effects peak at 3 months of use and reduce in frequency after that. The most common side effects include bleeding, depression, headache, acne, and weight changes.

Both types of IUDs have a filament string that serves two purposes. It allows for easier removal by a clinician, and it allows the woman or her clinician to check if the IUD is still in the correct position.

Emergency Contraception.

Emergency contraception, often called the "morning after" pill, is designed to reduce the risk of pregnancy after unprotected intercourse. Emergency contraception is provided in two ways:

1. Increased doses of specific oral contraceptive pills. Emergency contraceptive pills can reduce the risk of pregnancy when taken up to 120 hours after unprotected intercourse (ideally within 72 hours). Most are up to 89% effective when taken within 72 hours after unprotected sex. They are less effective as time passes.
2. Insertion of a copper IUD within 5 to 7 days after unprotected intercourse.

Planned Parenthood reports that anyone can obtain Plan B One-Step over the counter without a prescription at a drugstore or family planning clinic. All other brands of emergency contraception require a prescription from a clinician for those 16 or younger.

Sterilization.

Sterilization methods should be regarded as permanent and irreversible in both men and women. Although sterilization can sometimes be surgically reversed, the results are not always satisfactory. Sexual desire and ability are unaffected by sterilization.

Sterilization in women is accomplished by surgically severing the fallopian tubes. This procedure, known as tubal ligation, prevents the ovum from traveling down the tube. Tubal ligation is usually performed on an outpatient basis, sometimes under local anesthesia. Postoperative care and recovery time are required after a tubal ligation. Sterilization is safe and because it lasts for life is simple and convenient.

Sterilization in men is accomplished by surgically severing the vas deferens, which prevents sperm from entering the semen. The vasectomy is usually performed in a physician's office under local anesthesia. Vasectomy is the most effective birth control for men—nearly 100%

effective. The man and his partner must use an alternative form of contraception until he has produced two semen analyses with zero sperm. It usually takes about 4 to 6 weeks for all stored sperm to be eliminated from the man's ductal system.

Future Trends. Private industry remains a driving force behind contraceptive research and development. More than 100 experimental contraceptive methods are being studied around the world. The U.S. government contributes to contraceptive research primarily by funding research conducted at the National Institutes of Health.

Almost 40 million women in the United States are at risk for unintended pregnancy. Given that unintended pregnancies are as likely to end in abortion as in birth, there is a clear need to focus on the prevention of unintended pregnancy. Future trends in contraception are likely to be shaped in part by increased awareness of STIs and continuation of the AIDS pandemic. For at-risk women, the emphasis will be on a highly effective primary means of contraception used in conjunction with a barrier method, such as the condom, to prevent STIs.

Female Contraceptives. Most of the contraceptive products that will soon be available for women are refinements of products already available. New barrier methods for women will include enhanced cervical caps and vaginal sponges with microbicides to protect against STIs. New contraceptive pills, patches, and rings for women will use varied combination of hormones. Injectable progestin products might one day protect against pregnancy for up to 90 days. Oral and/or injectable vaccines may one day immunize women against pregnancy. These vaccines might produce antibodies to attack egg or sperm, or the immune system might create antibodies to a crucial type of protein molecule found on the head of sperm. Contraceptive implants designed to remain effective for 2 or 3 years, as well as biodegradable implants with efficacy of up to 18 months, are in development. Computerized fertility monitors that predict ovulation will offer couples who use fertility awareness methods of contraception a much more sophisticated and accurate charting method. Methods for permanent sterilization will expand to include chemical scarring techniques and insertion of fallopian tube chemical plugs and cryosurgery. Temporary sterilization may be effected by the use of silicone plugs.

Unisex Reversible Contraceptives. The concept of unisex reversible contraception is being explored. This method involves a group of drugs called gonadotropin-releasing hormone (GnRH) agonists and can be used to prevent the release of follicle-stimulating hormone (FSH) and luteinizing hormone (LH) from the pituitary gland. The release of FSH and LH triggers ovulation and spermatogenesis. Blocking the release of these hormones will temporarily suppress fertility for women or men. In addition, various contraceptive injections, implants, and vaccines for men are being researched.

Male Contraceptives. Methods of contraception for men continue to be explored. The challenge of developing a reversible method of contraception for men is complicated because men are always producing sperm. Because of this continuous fertility, the opportunities for reversible intervention that are permitted by women's fertility cycles are not available in men. Effective contraceptive methods for men that do not permanently impair fertility have proven elusive, but research continues. Most research has focused on a hormonal approach to decrease spermatogenesis. The major problem is that interference with steroidogenesis might also interfere with the other actions of testosterone such as sexual function, bone and muscle growth, kidney function, and protein anabolism.

Facilitating Coping With Special Sexual Needs

The nurse can help patients cope with sexual concerns generated by diseases and their treatments. See the accompanying Research in Nursing box. Offer anticipatory guidance and information to patients, stressing the importance of open communication with the patient's partner, and also include the partner in teaching.

For appropriate patients, start a discussion about possible sexual positions that can reduce pain during coitus. Show the patient drawings of possible sexual positions. Inform the patient that intercourse may be more comfortable if pain medication is taken before beginning sexual activity.

When teaching patients about medications, mention any sexual side effects that may occur to prevent anxiety and depression. Patients should alert the physician if these side effects occur because often the drug dosage can be modified or the drug changed. If patients are unaware of this, they may discontinue the medication on their own rather than sacrifice sexual functioning, if this is an important aspect of life for them.

Health Care Needs of Lesbian, Gay Male, Bisexual, and Transgender Individuals

The health and well-being of lesbian, gay male, bisexual, and transgender (LGBT) individuals has been made a priority by major federal health care agencies. The Institute of Medicine's (IOM, 2011) consensus report, *Healthy People 2020* (2011), and the U.S. Department of Health and Human Services (HHS, 2011) all highlight the need for better science-based knowledge on how best to address the existence of health disparities of LGBT individuals and the lack of compassionate services (Lim, Brown and Jones, 2013). Stigma and a range of other social and cultural factors affect the health of LGBT people as well as the ability of the health care system and providers to care for them. LGBT people come from diverse cultural backgrounds, have varied ethnic or racial identity, and differ in terms of education, age, income, and place of residence. Lesbian, gay, and bisexual people may be defined by their sexual orientation, but this definition is complex and

RESEARCH IN NURSING

BRIDGING THE GAP TO EVIDENCE-BASED PRACTICE

Sexual Health Care

Previous research has shown that nurses demonstrate a lack of attention to the impact of illness or disability on sexual health. However, in their therapeutic relationship with patients and families, nurses are in an ideal position to promote sexual health.

Related Research

McCabe, J., & Holmes, D. (2013). Nursing, sexual health and youth with disabilities: A critical ethnography. *Journal of Advanced Nursing, 70*(1), 77–86. doi: 10.1111/jan.12167

This critical ethnography study conducted in an urban pediatric rehabilitation facility explored the experiences of nurses providing sexual health care to adolescents with physical and/or developmental disabilities, with attention to the institutional and social discourses that shape these interactions. Four themes were identified (institutional space, professional interactions, engaging with sexuality, nursing experience), which revealed that nurse–patient interactions about sexual health were affected by a complex network of discourses. Key findings included:

- Even in an ambulatory setting, time and resource constraints and privacy concerns contribute to nurses' perceptions that providing sexual health care for youth with disabilities can be overwhelmingly difficult. Acute medical issues often take priority.

- In striving to maintain a therapeutic relationship with patients and families, nurses must balance the needs of patients for sexual health information with the beliefs, values, and needs of the family.
- In an effort to address sexual health, nurses often approach the topic from a biomedical perspective to frame it as an acceptable subject.

Relevance for Nursing Practice

People with disabilities demonstrate decreased sexual knowledge and sexual self-esteem, and are at increased risk of sexual abuse. Nurses occupy, and strive to maintain, the role of a caring agent. However, aspects of the clinical, institutional, and broader social environments may undermine their ability to promote sexual health. In nurses' efforts to maintain therapeutic relationships with clients, sexual health is often viewed only in medical terms to legitimize it as an appropriate topic of discussion with patients and families. This study highlights the importance of the therapeutic relationship between nurses, patients, and families and its role in supporting sexual health.

For additional research, visit thePoint.

---

variable. Sexual behavior, cultural factors, disclosure of sexual orientation and/or gender identity, prejudice and discrimination, and concealed sexual identity each present unique health challenges to this population (Box 44-3).

Other issues that affect health care delivery to the LGBT population include the following:

- *Public health infrastructure:* Efforts to research and address the health care needs of LGBT persons are hindered by an inadequate infrastructure to support and fund population-specific initiatives.

- *Access to quality health services:* Financial, structural, personal, and cultural barriers limit access to screening and prevention services and cause delays in care for acute conditions in the LGBT population.
- *Health communication:* Negative provider attitudes, lack of provider education regarding unique aspects of lesbian and gay health, and exclusion of same-sex partners in care planning seriously hamper therapeutic communication between members of the LGBT population and those who provide care.

BOX 44-3 HEALTH DISPARITIES IN THE GAY, LESBIAN, BISEXUAL, AND TRANSGENDER (LGBT) POPULATION

Healthy People 2020 (2011) identified significant LGBT health disparities and seeks much-needed collaboration from health care professionals and policy makers to address them. Among its findings are the following:

- LGBT youth are 2 to 3 times more likely to attempt suicide.
- LGBT youth are more likely to be homeless.
- Lesbians are less likely to get preventive services for cancer.
- Gay men are at higher risk of HIV and other sexually transmitted infections, especially among communities of color.
- Lesbians and bisexual females are more likely to be overweight or obese.

- Transgender individuals have a high prevalence of HIV and sexually transmitted infections, victimization, mental health issues, and suicide, and are less likely to have health insurance than heterosexual or lesbian, gay, or bisexual individuals.
- Older LGBT individuals face additional barriers to health due to isolation and a lack of social services and culturally competent providers.
- LGBT populations have the highest rates of tobacco, alcohol, and other drug use. These health issues are partly thought to be the effects of chronic stress resulting from stigmatization (IOM, 2011).

• *Educational and community-based programs:* Some government agencies, professional organizations, and health care organizations address health issues of the LGBT population, but this population still relies heavily on self-created community-based programs to address their special health care requirements.

Clearly, significant research is needed regarding the unique experience and health care needs of the LGBT population, along with increased education for health care providers. Issues of prejudice and inequitable service distribution in the health care system need to be addressed to improve the health of this population.

 THINK back to Paul Rojas, the gay patient with AIDS. The nurse needs to be acutely aware of the health care delivery system in the community to ensure that Mr. Rojas has access to the most appropriate and needed services. In addition, consultation with social services would be helpful for initiating referrals for appropriate services as Mr. Rojas's condition changes. •

Advocating Sexuality Needs of Patients

A hospital experience or institutionalization puts a strain on a person's individuality and sexual self. Illness may diminish feelings of sexual desire, and the desire for sexual interaction can signal a patient's improving health. The nurse should provide anticipatory guidance because many patients may hesitate to request help for fear of being ridiculed. Often, a patient merely desires privacy to hold and caress one's partner. The intimacy of this act often fulfills the patient's feelings of longing to be needed and loved.

There are many ways to advocate for a patient's sexual needs. Some may seem obvious and commonplace, whereas others may first require coming to terms with your own sexuality (Box 44-4).

Counseling the Patient Regarding Sexuality

Not all patients with sexual concerns need intensive therapy. Some patients benefit greatly from simply having someone listen to their concerns. Voicing their concerns allows patients to put the information into perspective and focus on what the problem is and how to solve it. When counseling patients, do not offer your own advice, because what is right for one person may be wrong for another. Also, offering false reassurances, such as, "It'll be all right," is unproductive. Rather, adopt an objective, empathic, and receptive attitude to facilitate open communication with the patient.

Abortion Counseling

Abortion remains an issue that deeply divides people. Many believe it is a woman's right to choose whether to continue a pregnancy and to take safe and legal action on a decision to terminate. Others believe that from fertilization onward, the embryo and fetus is a human being with the full respect and protection we afford adult humans; these people view abortion as always wrong. Some would allow abortion only if it is indicated for a woman's health or in cases of rape. You should examine what you believe, why you believe this, and how your beliefs are likely to influence your ability to counsel women and couples.

Counseling in Cases of Abusive Relationships and/or Rape

Nurses encounter children, adolescents, women, and sometimes men who have experienced sexual abuse or rape. The Rape, Incest and Abuse National Network (RAINN) reports that:

• **1 out of every 6 American women** has been a victim of an attempted or completed rape in her lifetime (14.8% completed rape; 2.8% attempted rape).
• **17.7 million American women** have been victims of attempted or completed rape.

Box 44-4 ADVOCATING FOR PATIENTS' SEXUAL NEEDS

• All patients should be accepted as sexual beings with the right to be treated with dignity and with sensitivity to their feelings.
• All patients have the right to some degree of privacy.
  • Anticipate the patient's desire for privacy by the simple act of drawing a curtain or closing a door.
  • Patients should be given the option of wearing their own sleepwear to promote sexual identity.
• Anticipate potentially shaming situations for the patient.
  • Give information regarding what the procedure is and why it needs to be done, and acknowledge that the patient's embarrassment is normal and understandable.
• Health care providers should not simply take for granted that patients do not mind intrusive or embarrassing procedures performed on their bodies and private parts.
• Patients have a right to question the physician regarding sexual needs or future sexual functioning.

• Anticipate these questions for the patient.
• Ask patients if they have any concerns regarding sexuality that can be answered by the nurse.
• Nurses can interface with the physician to obtain information required by the patient.
• The atmosphere in health care settings needs to allow for sexual expression between patients and their partners.
• Confidentiality is a right of every patient.
  • Do not promise confidentiality if that promise cannot be kept.
  • Allow no one access to the patient's personal records who is not directly involved in the patient's care.
  • Allow no information regarding patients to escape into idle conversation.
• All patients should be referred to formally as Mr., Mrs., Miss, or Ms., according to the patient's preference.
• Patients should be allowed to keep some personal possessions, if it is practical to do so.

- **9 of every 10** rape victims were female in 2003.
- While about **80% of all victims are white,** minorities are somewhat more likely to be attacked.
- About **3% of American men**—or **1 in 33**—have experienced an attempted or completed rape in their lifetime.
- 15% of sexual assault and rape victims are **under age 12.**

Date rape occurs when there is forced or coerced sex within a dating relationship. With acquaintance rape, the act is committed by someone known to the victim. Nearly two-thirds of all victims between the ages of 18 and 29 report that they had a prior relationship with their attacker (Center for Family Justice, 2012).

Victims of sexual assault are 3 times more likely to suffer from depression, 6 times more likely to suffer from posttraumatic stress disorder, 13 times more likely to abuse alcohol, 26 times more likely to abuse drugs, and 4 times more likely to contemplate suicide. Clearly, nurses need to be alert to evidence of sexual abuse while taking the history and conducting physical examinations. Abuse crosses all socioeconomic and ethnic groups. Become familiar with your legal and clinical responsibilities when a victim is identified. The first priority is getting the victim into a safe environment and mobilizing support for the victim and family. Multiple parties may need therapy. Be familiar with local resources and make appropriate referrals. The National Sexual Assault Online Hotline is a free, confidential, secure service that provides live help over the RAINN Web site (https://ohl.rainn.org/online/).

Evaluating

The nurse works with the patient to evaluate the effectiveness of sexual counseling or intervention. Stuart (2013) suggests considering the following three factors:

- *Sense of well-being.* Has the patient's sense of well-being improved during the treatment?
- *Functional ability.* If the person was dysfunctional, has functional ability improved or been restored?
- *Satisfaction with treatment.* Does the patient believe the treatment was helpful? Were the patient's goal and expectations met?

To evaluate the plan of care, the nurse needs to use information from the patient for most outcomes. The nurse cannot evaluate patients by observing their expression of sexuality, but the nurse can evaluate how patients are progressing toward sexuality-oriented goals by their appearance, self-confidence, and manner. For example, a patient who has expressed feelings of anxiety in the past over a sexual concern should be observably more confident and free of anxiety if the patient outcomes are being met. Ask the patient about progress toward outcomes. Some outcomes need to be "stepping stones," because not all problems are easily resolved with one-time intervention and direction.

When evaluating a patient's progress, it may help to ask: "In what ways have you been able to achieve [orgasm, increased desire, comfortable intercourse, erection]?" "What methods seemed most effective? Which were not?" "What do you think should be the next step?" Determine from this interaction with the patient whether something more needs to be accomplished. It is not enough to assume that because a set of outcomes has been met, the patient is satisfied with the results. See the Nursing Plan of Care 44-1 for Pete Manheim on pages 1690–1694.

SEXUAL HARASSMENT

Harassment is any annoying or distressing comment or conduct that is known or should be known to be unwelcome. **Sexual harassment** is unwelcome behavior that is based on one's sex or gender. This type of harassment usually occurs in the context of an asymmetrical relationship in which one person has more formal power than the other (e.g., a faculty member over a student) or more informal power (e.g., one peer over another). Sexual harassment can be directed toward people of any age, either gender, and any sexual orientation. There are two forms of sexual harassment: *quid pro quo* and environmental harassment (also called a "hostile" environment).

Quid pro quo means something given or withheld in exchange for something else. *Quid pro quo harassment* occurs when a person's employment or well-being is dependent on agreeing to unsolicited and unwelcome sexual demands. This type of harassment is typically initiated by a person in a position of authority who offers either direct or indirect reward or punishment based on the granting of sexual favors. Quid pro quo harassment is a clear abuse of power and is legally, morally, and ethically wrong.

Hostile environment harassment occurs when sex- or gender-based behaviors create a hostile, intimidating environment that hurts a person's work performance, classroom performance, or general sense of well-being. In the workplace, for example, the negative behaviors in hostile environment harassment are not directly linked to job-related consequences; instead, the employee's willingness to suffer the experience of the demeaning environment becomes a condition of employment. This type of harassment is not necessarily caused by a person with formal power. Hostile environment is sometimes difficult to identify, as it is not always easy to determine when offensive speech or behavior actually turns to true harassment. Coworkers and peers can create a hostile environment for a member of the group through the following:

- Unwelcome sexually oriented and gender-based behaviors
- Sexual bantering
- Sexual jokes
- Offensive pictures and language
- Sexual innuendoes
- Sexual behavior

Effects of Harassment

Harassment can cause feelings of helplessness, worthlessness, and guilt in the victim. This can often lead to less career satisfaction and feelings of loss of control. Anger is commonly experienced by those who have been harassed, which may lead to requests for transfer, resignation, or withdrawal from the environment where the harassment occurs. In many cases, job performance is affected due to reduced levels of concentration. Loss of job motivation and skill confidence, along with reduced job satisfaction and organizational commitment, are common.

Responding to Harassment in the Nursing Environment

Inappropriate sexual behavior by a patient may cause the nurse to respond with either passive avoidance or aggressive retaliation. An assertive response is recommended that supports the nurse in maintaining one's self-respect and encourages the patient to accept responsibility for one's behavior:

1. Be self-aware: Do not deny feelings about being harassed.
2. Confront: Provide feedback to the patient in a nonthreatening way and clearly state what behavior is or is not acceptable.

3. Set limits: Define clear and reasonable consequences that will be enforced if the behavior continues.
4. Enforce the stated limits: Maintain boundaries.
5. Report: Document the incident and submit to supervisor.

Colleagues may also be a source of harassment. The objective of employers should be to create a positive work environment that is characterized by mutually respectful behavior. Many have taken steps to eliminate hostile work environments by educating employees, developing policies against workplace harassment, and outlining guidelines for responding to sexual harassment:

1. If harassed by a coworker, confront the behavior immediately. An assertive statement is sometimes sufficient to stop the behavior.
2. If the harassment continues, document the date and time, and describe the behavior.
3. Consult your supervisor.
4. If the harassment still does not stop, file a grievance with administration.
5. Seek legal advice if all previous efforts to stop the behavior have been unsuccessful.

NURSING PLAN OF CARE 44-1

for Pete Manheim

Pete Manheim is a 13-year-old adolescent boy attending the area health clinic. He is nervous as he explains to the nurse his need for health care. He has noticed "sticky white stuff" around his penis and bedclothes on arising some mornings and fears he may be ill. Pete has also expressed concern about his lack of knowledge regarding sexuality. He has heard a lot of stories from his friends but does not feel he can talk to his parents because the subject has never been broached at home. Also, although Pete is a virgin, he is beginning to feel pressured by his friends, who boast of many sexual experiences.

After spending time in conversation with Pete, the nurse gathered the following data:

• Pete is experiencing nocturnal emissions and has little scientific knowledge about their source.

• Pete is anxious because of the stories regarding sex he has heard from his friends.
• There is no communication or dialogue at home with parents about issues of sexuality.
• Pete is having feelings of insecurity and anxiety about his present virginal status, which he feels he should change.
• Peer pressure from friends is also a concern.

The nurse will work with Pete to develop a plan of care to correct misinformation and relieve his anxiety. Planning will be directed toward correcting myths and supplying Pete with accurate information. Because Pete has a negligible knowledge base on sexuality, the plan of care will allow for ongoing sessions to augment the initial information. The nurse should outline this plan with Pete to be certain it is acceptable to him.

NURSING DIAGNOSIS Knowledge Deficit: Adolescent Sexuality Concerns related to misinformation and absent family-based sex education as manifested by self-report

EXPECTED OUTCOME By the end of the teaching session, the patient will:
• Describe the nature of nocturnal emissions

NURSING PLAN OF CARE 44-1 *continued*

for Pete Manheim

NURSING INTERVENTIONS	RATIONALE	EVALUATIVE STATEMENT
Assess patient's present knowledge base on nocturnal emission and the source of his information.	It is necessary to discover what the patient does know and to build on that knowledge.	8/1/15 Outcome met. Patient was able to differentiate between truth in sexual issues and what is myth.
Use terms that the patient has used and language at the level of the patient's understanding.	This facilitates comprehension.	*R. Gordon, RN*
Teach the patient about nocturnal emissions:	Knowledge decreases anxiety.	

• Nocturnal emissions, or "wet dreams," are normal in men of all ages, and they are particularly common in the teenage years. They are not the result of disease.
• They occur during sleep as the result of erotic dreams. The "white sticky stuff" is the result of ejaculation of semen from the penis.
• This is an involuntary action over which the male has no control.

EXPECTED OUTCOME By the end of the teaching session, the patient will:
• Differentiate sexual myths from sound knowledge

NURSING INTERVENTIONS	RATIONALE	EVALUATIVE STATEMENT
Assess what the patient has heard from peers regarding sexual information:	The nurse can then specifically address the myths to which the patient has been exposed.	8/1/15 Outcome met. Patient able to describe the source of nocturnal emissions.
Myth 1: "A large penis is better for sex than a small one."	This enables the patient to develop a positive sexual body image based on fact.	*R. Gordon, RN*
Truth: No relation exists between the size of a penis and the man's ability to perform sexually. When a penis becomes erect, it reaches sufficient size to engage in sexual intercourse.		
Myth 2: "Jerking off causes blindness. It is a dirty habit."	The patient is given permission to engage in a sexual activity of a masturbatory nature.	
Truth: Masturbation, or self-stimulation, is a natural and healthy outlet for sexual urges. Men and women of all ages masturbate. Masturbation can also teach the person what feels good and what does not. Every person has the right to masturbate if he or she wishes to do so.		

(continued)

NURSING PLAN OF CARE 44-1 *continued*

for Pete Manheim

NURSING INTERVENTIONS	RATIONALE	EVALUATIVE STATEMENT
Myth 3: "It looks bad for a guy to be a virgin—everybody's doing it" [having sex]. *Truth:* No one, whether male or female, should feel pressured into sexual activity at any age. Engaging in sexual activity carries with it a great deal of responsibility and concerns of pregnancy and spread of sexually transmitted infections (STIs). No one needs to know of another person's status if the person chooses not to discuss it.	The patient is given permission to abstain from sexual activity and not to feel pressured by friends. Almost 39% of teens have had sex by age 16 years.	

EXPECTED OUTCOME   By the end of the teaching session, the patient will:
  • List the positive aspects of abstinence in a sexual relationship

NURSING INTERVENTIONS	RATIONALE	EVALUATIVE STATEMENT
Assess the patient, including previous discussion of sexual myths and knowledge.	Giving the patient all the information necessary allows him to make an informed decision.	8/1/15 Outcome partially met. Patient able to list verbally all positive aspects of abstinence but is still undecided.
Instruct the patient on the positive aspects of abstinence, including the following:		*Revision:* Reinforce to patient that this is a personal decision that he can make for himself with a good knowledge base. Also, he does not have to make a firm decision for or against abstinence immediately. He should take time to think about this information.
• Engagement in any sexual activity should be a personal decision and not the result of pressure from friends.		
• Abstinence will guarantee protection from pregnancy and from most STIs.	Many young people think they are immune to the consequences of their actions. Therefore, it is important to stress that pregnancy and STIs are very probable results of sexual intercourse.	*R. Gordon, RN*
• People can show affection for each other without sexual involvement.	It is difficult to understand and undertake all the implications of a sexual relationship during the teenage years. The patient learns that a successful sexual relationship requires intimacy, love, and sharing; it should not be merely an outlet for sexual feelings.	
• Every person has the right to say no.	The patient has permission to refuse an activity in which he is not sure he wishes to engage.	

NURSING PLAN OF CARE 44-1 *continued*

for Pete Manheim

EXPECTED OUTCOME By the end of the teaching session, the patient will:

- Describe the correct use of rubber condoms

NURSING INTERVENTIONS	RATIONALE	EVALUATIVE STATEMENT
Assess what the patient knows about rubber condoms and their use.	Since the patient is undecided about whether to initiate a sexual relationship in the future, it is prudent to give him information to protect against pregnancy and STIs.	8/1/15 Outcome met. Patient successfully listed the steps in using a condom. *R. Gordon, RN*
Inform the patient that rubber condoms are available over the counter in drug stores. Prices vary according to type and style.	Patient should know where to purchase condoms and the variety available.	
Teach the patient the steps in using rubber condoms:	Patient should know how to use condoms safely.	
• Roll condom onto the penis as soon as it becomes erect.	Protects against sperm from secretions from Cowper's glands	
• If condom does not have a nipple receptacle end, leave a small space at end of condom to collect semen.	Provides a pocket to collect semen and prevents breakage	
• Immediately after ejaculation, remove penis and condom from vagina by holding onto base of condom.	Prevents spillage of semen into the vagina	
• Discard condom.	Condoms are not meant to be reused. A new condom is used for each act of intercourse.	
Advise the patient to use a condom with every act of intercourse. Spermicides used with the condom increase effectiveness.	To be as effective as possible, the condom should be used with every act of intercourse. The rubber condom used with spermicide is effective against pregnancy and the spread of STIs. The woman's use of a spermicide foam in the vagina increases effectiveness.	

EXPECTED OUTCOME By the end of the teaching session, the patient will:

- Express a decrease in anxiety

(continued)

NURSING PLAN OF CARE 44-1 *continued*

for Pete Manheim

NURSING INTERVENTIONS	RATIONALE	EVALUATIVE STATEMENT
Assess the patient's anxiety level by verbal and nonverbal behavior.	The patient was anxious when he came into the clinic. It is important to evaluate his level of anxiety before he leaves. If he is still anxious, reassessment should occur because the plan of care may have been unsuccessful.	8/1/15 Outcome met. Patient expressed relief that he is normal. Would like to bring a friend to next session.

Future teaching sessions to include these topics identified by patient:
- STIs, particularly AIDS
- Pregnancy—occurrence and prevention
- Sexual expression
- Further discussion of sexual myths

R. Gordon, RN

SAMPLE DOCUMENTATION

8/1/15, 11 AM, nursing
Nursing consultation with 13-year-old patient regarding anxiety about cause and source of nocturnal emissions. Patient also expressed concern about sexual myths he has heard from friends. Stated that much peer pressure exists to become sexually active. Patient admits to possessing little knowledge regarding sexual issues. Feels he cannot discuss sexuality with parents because it is not a topic that has been brought up in the past at home. Will conduct initial teaching session with patient to provide information and decrease anxiety about priority concerns. Patient is willing to return to clinic for at least three more teaching sessions to expand knowledge base of sexuality.

R. Gordon, RN

DEVELOPING CLINICAL REASONING

1. Role play with another student and perform the interview you would use to obtain a sexual history from the following individuals. Think about how you modified the interview in each situation and why. Identify what made you feel uncomfortable as either the nurse or the patient. Discuss how you can best address this discomfort:
   - A mother voices concern that her 9-year-old son is frequently playing with his penis.
   - An adult man appears distressed when he notes that he has suddenly become impotent with his partner of many years.
   - A high school girl says that her mother tells her something is wrong with her because she is attracted only to women.
   - A new resident in a long-term care facility complains that he misses his privacy and has nowhere to make love.

2. Describe how you would respond to a newly diagnosed HIV-positive woman with multiple partners who tells you that it is none of your business how she acquired the virus or what she plans to do now that she has it. Think carefully about what is at stake in terms of your response.

3. You know a patient is uncomfortable about undergoing a pelvic examination, and you ask the male physician to wait for you before he begins the examination. He tells you he can't wait and doesn't need your assistance. You know the patient wants another woman in the room. How would you respond, and what is at stake? Does it matter if the reason for the patient's request to have you present is simply preference, is linked to a history of abuse, or is related to her cultural or religious beliefs?

PRACTICING FOR NCLEX

1. A nurse is teaching parents about normal developmental aspects of sexuality in their children. Which statements from parents would warrant further teaching? Select all that apply.
   a. "When my 2-year-old son touches his genitals, I push his hand away and tell him 'No'."
   b. "I should wean my infant by 4 months and encourage him to use a sippy cup."
   c. "I should explain sexuality to my 9-year-old in a factual manner when she asks me questions about her body."
   d. "I should explain about body changes to my 11-year-old prior to them happening to alleviate her fears."
   e. "I should teach my 10-year-old about contraception and ways to avoid sexually transmitted diseases."
   f. "I should allow my teenager to establish her own beliefs and moral value system by not sharing my own beliefs."

2. A nurse is counseling an older couple regarding sexuality. Which statement from the couple should the nurse address?
   a. "We're at the age when we should consider ceasing sexual activity."
   b. "We need more time for sexual stimulation than we used to."
   c. "If we are unable to have sex we can still have an intimate relationship."
   d. "If we change our position we can still have sex and be more comfortable."

3. A nurse is performing sexual assessments of male patients in a long-term care facility. Which patients would the nurse flag as having an increased risk for erectile dysfunction? Select all that apply.
   a. A 72-year-old male with a history of diabetes
   b. A 78-year-old male who has a new partner
   c. A 75-year-old male who has Parkinson disease
   d. An 80-year-old male who is an alcoholic
   e. An 85-year-old male who takes antihypertensive medication
   f. A 76-year-old male who smokes tobacco

4. A school nurse is providing sex education classes for adolescents. Which statement by the nurse accurately describes normal sexual functioning?
   a. "Each person is born with a certain amount of sexual drive, which can be depleted in later years."
   b. "If you want to be a great athlete, sexual abstinence is necessary when you are training."
   c. "If you have a nocturnal emission (wet dream) it is an indicator of a sexual disorder."
   d. "It is natural for a woman to have as strong a desire for sex and enjoy it as much as a man."

5. The mother of an 8-year-old boy tells the nurse that she is worried because she has found her son masturbating on occasion. She asks the nurse how she should "handle this problem." What would be the best response of the nurse to this mother's concern?
   a. "Children should be taught not to masturbate because most people believe self-stimulation is wrong."
   b. "Masturbation is a means of learning what a person prefers sexually, and overreacting to it can lead to the child thinking sex is bad or dirty."
   c. "There are serious health risks associated with frequent masturbation, and the practice should be discouraged in children."
   d. "Children who masturbate demonstrate sexual dysfunction and should be seen by a child psychologist."

6. A 16-year-old female visits a local women's health clinic to obtain contraception. She asks the nurse, "What can I do to protect myself from diseases like AIDS?" Which recommendations are appropriate for anyone who is sexually active to prevent STIs? Select all that apply.
   a. Have regular checkups for STIs even in the absence of symptoms.
   b. Learn the common symptoms of STIs and seek help immediately if any develop—even if the symptom is mild.
   c. If a partner is infected, consider having sex during menstruation when the risk is greatly decreased.
   d. Douche regularly to remove any bacteria that may form in the vagina.
   e. Avoid anal intercourse, but if practiced, use a male condom.

f. Consider the fact that the younger people are when having sex for the first time, the less susceptible they become to developing an STI.

7. A patient tells the nurse that she would like to use a mechanical barrier for birth control. Which method might the nurse recommend?
   a. Diaphragm
   b. Oral contraceptive pills
   c. Depo-Provera
   d. Evra patch

8. A 17-year-old college student calls the emergency department (ED) and tells the nurse that she was raped by a professor. She wants to come to the ED but only if the nurse can assure her that they will not call her parents. What should be the nurse's first priority?
   a. Getting the patient into a safe environment and mobilizing support for her.
   b. Encouraging the student to disclose the name of the professor so that his predatory behavior will be stopped.
   c. Convincing the student to be assessed for pregnancy, STIs, or other complications.
   d. Convincing the student to tell her parents so that she can receive their support.

9. A nurse is teaching patients about contraception methods. Which statement by a patient indicates a need for further teaching?
   a. "Depo-Provera is not effective against sexually transmitted infections, but contraceptive protection is immediate if I get the injection on the first day of my period."
   b. "The hormonal ring contraceptive, NuvaRing, protects against pregnancy by suppressing ovulation, thickening cervical mucus, and preventing the fertilized egg from implanting in the uterus."
   c. "Abstinence may be an effective method of contraception and may be used as a periodic or continuous strategy."
   d. "Withdrawal is an effective method of birth control as well as an effective method of reducing the spread of sexually transmitted infections."

10. A nurse is assessing a 27-year-old female patient who visits her gynecologist. The patient tells the nurse that she has been having a vaginal discharge that "smells bad and is green and foamy." She also complains of burning upon urination and dyspareunia. What sexually transmitted infection would the nurse suspect?
    a. Human papillomavirus (HPV)
    b. Syphilis
    c. Trichomoniasis
    d. Herpes simplex virus

11. A school nurse is providing information for parents of teenagers regarding the human papillomavirus (HPV) and the recommended HPV vaccination. What teaching point would the nurse include?
    a. "HPV causes genital warts and cervical and other genital cancers."
    b. "HPV causes a single painless genital lesion and can lead to sterility."
    c. "50% of women between the ages of 14 and 19 are infected with HPV"
    d. "The HPV vaccination is only recommended for the female population."

12. A 38-year-old patient tells the nurse counselor that he can only get sexual pleasure by looking at the body of a person other than his wife from a distance. The nurse documents this data as:
    a. Masochism
    b. Pedophilia
    c. Voyeurism
    d. Sadism

13. An 18-year-old female presents at a women's health care clinic seeking oral contraceptives for the first time. She tells the nurse that she wants to have sex with her boyfriend, but doesn't know what to expect. Which statement by the nurse is not accurate?
    a. "Vaginal intercourse is most commonly performed in the missionary position."
    b. "The side by side position achieves better clitoral stimulation than the missionary position."
    c. "Achieving simultaneous orgasms is the goal of vaginal intercourse."
    d. "The period after coitus is just as significant as the events leading up to it."

14. Which patients would a nurse assess for menstrual cycle irregularities? Select all that apply.
    a. A patient who is breast-feeding
    b. A patient who is diagnosed with anorexia
    c. A patient who chooses to abstain from sexual intercourse
    d. A patient who has pelvic inflammatory disease
    e. A patient who is obsessed with exercising
    f. A patient who has a spinal cord injury

15. Which assessment question would be most appropriate for a patient who is experiencing dyspareunia?
    a. "Do you currently have a new partner?"
    b. "Have you been diagnosed with a neurologic disorder?"
    c. "Do you take anti-hypertensive medication?"
    d. "Do you use antihistamines?"

ANSWERS WITH RATIONALES

1. *a, b, e, f.* Self-manipulation of genitals is normal behavior—parents should avoid denoting this as "bad." Parents should avoid early weaning of infants to prevent oral deprivation. Parents should explain contraception and STIs to their adolescent children. Parents should share their beliefs and moral system with their children. Parents should also give their children the desired information about sexuality in a clear, factual form and give them information about body changes before they experience them to alleviate fears.

2. *a.* Sexual activity need not be hindered by age, and couples who have been consistently sexually active throughout their lives may continue their intimate relationship for as long as they desire. Nurses should teach couples that adaptation to bodily changes is possible with use of comfortable positions for intercourse and increased time for stimulation as well as teach alternatives to coitus, such as caressing, hugging, and stroking, when coitus is impossible because of illness or disability.

3. *a, d, e.* Risk factors for erectile dysfunction include history of diabetes, spinal cord trauma, cardiovascular disease, surgical procedure, alcoholism, and use of antihypertensives, antidepressants, or illicit drugs. Having a new partner may be a risk factor for premature ejaculation, and a history of Parkinson disease may predispose the patient to retarded ejaculation. Smoking is not a risk factor for impotence.

4. *d.* Physiologic studies indicate that, in some respects, the woman's sex drive is not only as strong but may be even stronger than that of the man. The more consistently sexually active a person is, the longer the activity continues into the later years of life. Physiologically, the achievement of orgasm is rarely more demanding than most activities encountered in daily life; there is no scientific evidence that sex "weakens" a person. Erotic dreams that culminate in orgasms are normal common physiologic phenomena in at least 85% of men.

5. *b.* Masturbation is a technique of sexual expression in which an individual practices self-stimulation. It is a way for people to learn what they prefer during stimulation and what feels good. The reality is that people masturbate regardless of sex, age, or marital status. People might not masturbate because they feel guilty about it or believe self-stimulation is wrong. Masturbation is not "dirty" and will not lead to blindness or insanity. Negative overreaction by parents to a child's masturbating behavior can lead to a belief that the genitals and sex are bad and dirty.

6. *a, b, e.* The best way to prevent STIs is to have regular checkups for STIs even in the absence of symptoms, learn the common symptoms of STIs and seek help immediately if they develop even if they are mild, and avoid anal intercourse, but if practiced use a male condom. It is also recommended that people avoid having sex during menstruation because HIV-infected women are probably more infectious, and HIV-uninfected women are probably more susceptible to becoming infected during that time. Women should avoid douching because it removes normal protective bacteria in the vagina. People should delay having sexual relations as long as possible, because the younger people are when having sex for the first time, the more susceptible they become to developing an STI.

7. *a.* The diaphragm is the only barrier method of contraception listed; all the other methods are hormonal.

8. *a.* While the remaining options may be indicated, the *first* priority is to ensure the safety of the woman and to get her the support she needs at this moment.

9. *d.* Withdrawal offers no protection against sexually transmitted infections.

10. *c.* Trichomoniasis causes a foul-smelling vaginal discharge that is thin, foamy, and green in color, and also causes itching of the vulva and vagina, burning on urination, and dyspareunia. HPV causes a profuse watery vaginal discharge, dyspareunia, intense pruritus, and vulvar irritation. Syphilis causes a single painless genital lesion 10 days to 3 months after exposure and generalized skin rash, enlarged lymph nodes, and fever that may appear 2 to 4 weeks after appearance of primary lesion and may last for several years. Herpes presents as single or multiple painful vesicles that rupture and form ulcer-like lesions, which form scabs as they heal.

11. *a.* HPV causes genital warts and cervical and other genital cancers. It manifests as pale, soft, papillary lesions found around the internal and external genitalia and perianal and rectal areas of the body. One in four young women between the ages of 14 and 19 is infected with at least one of the

most common STIs, which include the human papilloma-virus. The HPV vaccination is recommended for males and females.

12. **c.** Voyeurism is the achievement of sexual arousal by look-ing at the body of someone other than one's sexual partner. Masochism refers to gaining sexual pleasure from the humili-ation of being abused. Pedophilia is a term used to describe the practice of adults gaining sexual fulfillment by perform-ing sexual acts with children. Sadism refers to the practice of gaining sexual pleasure while inflicting abuse on another person.

13. **c.** Simultaneous orgasms, or both people attaining orgasm at the same moment, are difficult to achieve, and a preoccupa-tion with attaining simultaneous orgasms might disrupt the ultimate intimacy and satisfaction possible during coitus. The most common position in Western cultures is the "missionary position," in which the woman lies horizontally underneath the man. Clitoral stimulation is difficult to achieve in the missionary position. Lying side by side, female on top, and rear entry are some examples of coital positions that enable clitoral stimulation. The period after coitus is just as signifi-cant as the events leading up to it.

14. **a, b, d, e.** Causes of menstrual cycle irregularities include pregnancy or breastfeeding, eating disorders, extreme weight loss, excessive exercising, and pelvic inflammatory disease, as well as many other causes.

15. **d.** Factors contributing to dyspareunia include diabetes; hormonal imbalances; vaginal, cervical, or rectal disorders; antihistamine, alcohol, tranquilizer, or illicit drug use; and cosmetic or chemical irritants to genitals.

TAYLOR SUITE RESOURCES

Explore these additional resources to enhance learning for this chapter:

- NCLEX-Style Questions and other resources on thePoint, http://thePoint.lww.com/Taylor8e
- *Study Guide for Fundamentals of Nursing, 8th edition*
- Adaptive Learning | Powered by prepU, http://thepoint.lww.com/prepu

Bibliography

American College of Obstetricians and Gynecolo-gists' Committee on Health Care for Underserved Women. (2012). *Human immunodeficiency virus and acquired immunodeficiency syndrome and women of color.* Available at http://www.acog.org/~/media/Committee%20Opinions/Committee%20on%20Health%20Care%20for%20Underserved%20Women/co536.pdf

Anderson, J. L. (2013). Acknowledging female sex-ual dysfunction in women with cancer. *Clinical Journal of Oncology Nursing, 17*(3), 233–235.

Bulechek, G., Butcher, H., Dochterman, J., & Wag-ner, C. M. (Eds.). (2013). *Nursing interventions clas-sification (NIC)* (6th ed.). St. Louis: Elsevier/Mosby.

Center for Disease Control and Prevention. (2014). Sexually Transmitted Diseases: Data and Statistics. Available at: http://www.cdc.gov/std/stats/

Center for Family Justice. (2012). Sexual Violence Facts. Available at http://www.cwfefc.org/svfacts.html

Centers for Disease Control and Prevention (CDC). (2014). Sexually transmitted diseases (STDs). Avail-able at http://www.cdc.gov/STD/

Cholewinski, J. T., & Burge, J. M. (1990). Sexual harassment of nursing students. *Image The Journal of Nursing Scholarship, 22*(2), 106–110.

Dean, L., Meyer, I., Robinson, K., Sell, R., Sember, R., Silenzio, V., Bowen, D. J., ... Xavier, J. (2000). Lesbian, gay, bisexual, and transgender health: Find-ings and concerns. *Journal of the Gay and Lesbian Medical Association, 4*(3), 101–151.

Doll, G. M. (2013). Sexuality in nursing homes: Practice and policy. *Journal of Gerontological Nursing, 39*(7), 30–37. doi: 10.3928/00989134-20130418-01.

Hall, J. (2013). Sexuality and stroke: The effects and holistic management. *British Journal of Nursing, 22*(10), 556–559.

Healthy People 2020. (2011). *Lesbian, gay, bisexual, and transgender health.* Available at http://www.healthypeople.gov/2020/topicsobjectives2020/overview.aspx?topicid=25

NANDA International (NANDA-I). (2012). *Nurs-ing diagnoses: Definitions & classification 2012–2014.* West Sussex, UK: Wiley-Blackwell.

Higgins, A., Barker, P., & Begley, C. M. (2008). "Veiling sexualities": a grounded theory of mental health nurses responses to issues of sexuality. *Journal of Advanced Nursing, 62*(3), 307–317.

Hinchliff, S., Gott, M. (2011). Seeking medical help for sexual concerns in mid- and later life: A review of the literature. *Journal of Sex Research, 48*(2), 106–117.

Institute of Medicine, Committee on Lesbian, Gay, Bisexual, and Trans-gender Health Issues and Research Gaps and Opportunities. (2011). *The health of lesbian, gay, bisexual, and transgender people: Building a foundation for better understanding.* Washington, DC: National Academies Press.

Kazer, M. W. (2012) Issues regarding sexuality. In M. Boltz, E. Capezuti, T. Fulmer, D. Zwicker (Eds.). *Evidence-based geriatric nursing protocols for best practice* (4th ed., pp. 500–515). New York: Springer Publishing Company.

Lim, F. A., Brown, D. V., & Jones, H. (2013). Lesbian, gay, bisexual, and transgender health: Funda-ments for nursing education. *Journal of Nursing Education, 52*(4), 198–203.

Madison, J., & Minichiello, V. (2000). Recognizing and labeling sex-based sexual harassment in the health care workplace. *Journal of Nursing Scholarship, 32*(4), 405–410.

Magnan, M. A., & Norris, D. M. (2008). Nursing students' perceptions of barriers to addressing patient sexuality concerns. *Journal of Nursing Education, 47*(6), 260–268.

Mahieu, L., de Casterlé, B. D., Van Elssen, K., & Gastmans, C. (2013). Nurses' knowledge and attitudes towards aged sexuality: validity and internal consistency of the Dutch version of the Aging Sexual Knowledge and Attitudes Scale. *Journal of Advanced Nursing, 69*(11):2584–2596. doi: 10.1111

Mayo Clinic Staff. (2014). Mayo Clinic Health Information. Menstrual cycle: What's normal, what's not. Available at: http://www.mayoclinic.org/healthy-living/womens-health/in-depth/menstrual-cycle/art-20047186?pg=1

McCabe, J., & Holmes, D. (2013). Nursing, sexual health and youth with disabilities: A critical ethnogra-phy. *Journal of Advanced Nursing, 70*(1), 77–86. doi: 10.1111/jan.12167

Mick, J., Hughes, M., & Cohen, M. Z. (2003). Sexuality and cancer: How oncology nurses can address it BETTER. *Oncology Nursing Forum, 30,* 152–153.

Moorhead, S., Johnson, M., Maas, M., & Swanson, E. (Eds.) (2013). *Nursing outcomes classification (NOC)* (5th ed.). St. Louis: Elsevier/Mosby.

Morrison-Beedy, D., Jones, S. H., Xia, Y., Crean, H. F. & Carey, M. P. (2012). Reducing sexual risk behavior in adolescent girls: Results from a randomized controlled trial. *Journal of Adolescent Health, 52*(3), 314–321.

Pessagno, R. A. (2013). Don't be embarrassed: Taking a sexual history. *Nursing, 2013, 43*(9), 60–64.

National Institute of Allergy and Infectious Dis-eases. (2013). Sexually Transmitted Diseases (STDs). Available at http://www.niaid.nih.gov/topics/std/Pages/default.aspx

Pillitteri, A. (2012). *Maternal and child health nurs-ing* (6th ed.). Philadelphia: Wolters Kluwer Health/Lippincott Williams & Wilkins.

Planned Parenthood Federation of America. (2014). Birth control. Available at http://www.plannedparent-hood.org/health-topics/birth-control-4211.htm

Rawlins, S., & Smith, D. (2002). Innovative con-traception: New options in hormonal contraception. *American Journal of Nurse Practitioners, 6*(1), 9–28.

Richardson, M. (2007). By the way, doctor, is it safe to take a pill that eliminates periods? *Harvard Women's Health Watch, 8.*

Sommers, M. S., & Buschur, C. (2004). Injury in women who are raped: What every critical care nurse needs to know. *DCCN: Dimensions of Critical Care Nursing, 23*(2), 62–68.

Stuart, G. W. (2013). *Principles and Practice of Psy-chiatric Nursing* (10th ed.). St. Louis: Elsevier/Mosby.

U.S. Department of Health and Human Services (HHS). (2011). U.S. Department of Health and Human Services recommended actions to improve the health and well-being of lesbian, gay, bisexual, and transgen-der communities. Available at http://www.hhs.gov/lgbt/health.html

World Health Organization (WHO). (2014). Female genital mutilation. Available at http://www.who.int/mediacentre/factsheets/fs241/en/

45 | Spirituality

KEVIN GARGAN

Kevin, a 38-year-old divorced man on a step-down unit after treatment for a myocardial infarction, asks the night nurse, "Did you ever give much thought to whether or not there is a God?" Kevin listed his religion as Protestant but says it's been a long time since he went to church or prayed.

CHOI MIN LAI

Choi, a member of the Hmong culture from Laos, is refusing to allow physicians to perform a series of surgical repairs to correct severe deformities of his 8-year-old son's feet. "In our culture, the deformity is a sign of spiritual favor and good luck. Because of Kou's condition, a warrior ancestor whose feet were wounded in battle will no longer be spiritually trapped. You see, Kou is special."

MARGOT ZEUNER

Margot, a 75-year-old woman, is taking care of her 80-year-old husband with advanced Alzheimer disease, who was just discharged from the hospital and requires constant supervision. When visited at home, she says, "I really miss going to church and seeing everyone. They're so supportive. That was the one thing that helped to keep me going."

page 1702). A Baptist woman with a life-threatening cancer who had shared the importance of her spirituality with me recently wrote to me:

> When you made a cross on my forehead with your thumb, it felt unfamiliar—but perfect. Like a blessing with no conditions—no strings. How liberating. Affirming. Loving. And to think you did it with just your thumb. And your heart. Thank you.

SPIRITUAL DIMENSION

Humans' "spirit" dimension was first recognized in ancient cultures. One person often played the roles of both priest and physician, ministering to the spirit and the body. Over the years, however, medicine and religion evolved separately. Not until the holistic health movement took root was the person once again viewed as an integrated whole of body, mind, and spirit. Health care practitioners began again to probe the relationships among physical, psychological, social, and spiritual health. Two models are currently used to illustrate these relationships (Fig. 45-1 on page 1701). In the integrated approach, the physio-psycho-socio-spiritual model has four equal dimensions, each of which influences the other. In the unifying approach, the spiritual dimension grounds the physiologic, psychological, and sociologic dimensions. While it is interesting to interview professional healers about which model is more consistent with their experience, both demand of the nurse greater competence in identifying and meeting spiritual needs than most practicing nurses today display. National guidelines now mandate spiritual care—see the Joint Commission requirements (2008) and the National Palliative Care Consensus Project (2013).

According to Shelly and Fish (1988), three **spiritual needs** underlie all religious traditions and are common to all people:

1. Need for meaning and purpose
2. Need for love and relatedness
3. Need for forgiveness

Although nurses may differ in their beliefs about how involved they should become in meeting patients' spiritual needs, it is impossible to nurse patients well while ignoring the spiritual dimensions of health. Nurses can assist patients to meet spiritual needs by offering a compassionate presence; assisting in the struggle to find meaning and purpose in the face of suffering, illness, and death; fostering relationships (with a higher being/humans) that nurture the spirit; and facilitating the patient's expression of religious or spiritual beliefs and practices. (For an example, see the Reflective Practice box on page 1700.)

CONCEPTS RELATED TO SPIRITUALITY AND SPIRITUAL HEALTH

Spirituality, faith, religion, and the influence of these elements on everyday living and health and illness are important

Paying attention to the spiritual dimension of health and well-being is integral to holistic care. Patients facing the losses and limits related to injury, disease, or aging begin to evaluate what is important in life and often ask the "big questions": Is there a God or transcendent being? Does life have meaning and purpose? Am I dying? Is there anyone I can trust to be with me during this hard time? Nurses skilled in spiritual care are able to identify and elicit the inner resources of patients and family caregivers to promote health and healing with sensitivity to such questions. Many nurses who describe themselves as professional healers use the terms "vocation" or "calling" to describe the work of nursing. They claim to be "standing on holy ground" when they create that hospitable place where patients can expose their vulnerabilities and face their biggest concerns. We learn, with great humility, that sometimes the most important things we do are accomplished simply by being present to those we serve (see Through the Eyes of a Caregiver on

REFLECTIVE PRACTICE: CULTIVATING QSEN COMPETENCIES

CHALLENGE TO INTELLECTUAL SKILLS

During my pediatric rotation, I encountered a Hmong family from Laos whose 8-year-old son, Kou, had horribly deformed feet. It seemed as if the entire health care team was united to persuade, cajole, and if necessary force Choi Min Lai, Kou's father, and his mother to authorize a series of surgical repairs. But the parents were adamant in their refusal. In their culture, the deformity was a sign of spiritual favor and good luck. They believed that a warrior ancestor whose own feet were wounded in battle would be released from a form of spiritual entrapment because of their son's condition. This made Kou special in their community. I admired their fierce championing of their beliefs, but my heart ached for Kou because of the difficulties he would face in U.S. society if his feet were not repaired. I didn't know anything about the Hmong culture or their beliefs. As a result, I didn't know which side I should support. I also didn't know much about the legal rights of the parents to refuse a procedure that, although not lifesaving, would clearly benefit their son.

Thinking Outside the Box: Possible Courses of Action

- Remain detached from the conflict and just observe.
- Try to learn more about the family's cultural and religious beliefs to see if this information could be helpful.
- Contact the hospital attorney to find out about the legal rights of the parents to refuse a procedure that, while not lifesaving, would clearly benefit their son.
- Use my relationship with the family to try to persuade them to comply.
- Use my knowledge of Kou and his family to try to persuade the health care team to respect their wishes.

Evaluating a Good Outcome: How Do I Define Success?

- The health care team chooses a course of action that is beneficial to Kou and simultaneously respects the family's religious and cultural beliefs.
- We respect the legal rights of this family.
- My knowledge of the Hmong religion and culture is increased.
- I am faithful to my advocacy obligations.

Personal Learning: Here's To the Future!

Unfortunately, this issue was not resolved during my rotation. In fact, the conflict continued to grow. When I completed my rotation, the hospital was appealing to the court to force the parents to accept surgery. I came to believe that the rights of the parents should be respected. Their cultural community was so strong, and they clearly did not see Kou's condition as a correctable "health problem" but rather a blessing to be enjoyed. While a few other nurses felt the way I did, the physicians and the social worker felt strongly that the parents were wrong. I learned a lot about the Hmong culture, realizing that my practice will continue to surprise me as I encounter patients and families with beliefs and practices very different from mine. As a result of this experience, I hope I will keep an open mind and always be ready to learn.

REFLECTION ON QUALITY AND SAFETY COMPETENCIES

Do you agree with the criteria that the nursing student used to evaluate a successful outcome? Why or why not? What *knowledge, skills,* and *attitudes* do you need to develop to continuously improve the quality and safety of care for patients like Kou and his family?

Patient-Centered Care: How would you develop a respectful and successful partnership with Kou and his family, given that their culture is so different? How can you best communicate empathy and respect given the conflict created by their wishes?

Teamwork and Collaboration/Quality Improvement: What communication and interpersonal skills do you need to improve to ensure that you function as a member of the patient-care team when members of the team are so divided? The social worker? Other members of the health care team? What other team members can be called upon to provide needed assistance in clarifying this family's legal rights? What does quality care for Kou and his family "look like"?

Safety/Evidence-Based Practice: What does the evidence point to as "best practice" for Kou? What safety needs does he have and how can you meet them?

Informatics: Can you identify the essential information that must be available in Kou's electronic record to support safe patient care and coordination of care? Are there smart devices or online resources you can use to learn more about the Hmong culture? Can you think of other ways to respond to or approach the situation? What else might the nursing student have done to ensure a successful outcome?

concepts to understand when caring for patients. Although some use the words *spirituality, faith,* and *religion* interchangeably, there are distinctions. These and other concepts are explored in the following sections.

Spirituality

Spirituality is anything that pertains to a person's relationship with a nonmaterial life force or higher power. While one person describes spirituality in terms of coming to

The Spiritual Dimension: Integrated Approach   **The Spiritual Dimension: Unifying Approach**

FIGURE 45-1. Spiritual dimensions. No consensus exists about the role of the spiritual dimension in health. (**A**) The *integrated approach* views each of the four dimensions as equal and influencing one another. (**B**) The *unifying model* grounds the physiologic, psychological, and social dimensions in the spiritual dimension. (Redrawn from Farran, C. J., Fitchett, G., Quiring-Emblen, C. J., & Burk, J. R. [1989]. Development of a model for spiritual assessment and intervention. *Journal of Religion and Health, 28*[3], 185.)

know, love, and serve God, another speaks of transcending the limits of body and experiencing a universal energy.

Elements of spirituality include:

- Spirituality is experienced as a unifying force, life principle, essence of being.
- Spirituality is expressed and experienced in and through connectedness with nature, the earth, the environment, and the cosmos.
- People express and experience spirituality in and through connectedness with other people.
- Spirituality shapes the self-becoming and is reflected in one's being, knowing, and doing.
- Spirituality permeates life; providing purpose, meaning, strength, and guidance; and shaping the journey (Burghardt & Nagai-Jacobson, 1997).

While analyzing concepts of spirituality through a review of related literature, nurse scholar Bernice Golberg (1998) identified the following phenomena: meaning, presencing, empathy/compassion, giving hope, love, religion/transcendence, and touch and healing. All appeared to be products of relationships, some physical (presencing, touch and healing), and others emotional (meaning, empathy/compassion, hope, love, and religion/transcendence). Golberg combined these and gave spirituality the label "connection" (1998, p. 836).

Faith

Faith generally refers to a confident belief in something for which there is no proof or material evidence. It can involve a person, idea, or thing, and is usually followed by action related to the ideals or values of that belief. For example, if I have faith in my doctor, parish nurse, or healer, I am more likely to adhere to a prescribed regimen/plan of care and to experience benefits. Similarly, patients who believe

in a loving and all-powerful being who knows them and cares for them are often better able to cope with the suffering related to injury and illness. The declaration made by the World Conference of the Religions of Peace in Kyoto, Japan, in 1970 is an excellent example of a confident belief in something for which there is no proof or material evidence. Baha'i, Buddhist, Confucian, Christian, Hindu, Jain, Jew, Muslim, Shintoist, Sikh, and others discovered that the things that unite them were more important than those that divided them. They discovered that they shared:

- A conviction of the fundamental unity of the human family, of the quality and dignity of all human beings
- A sense of the sacredness of the individual person and the person's conscience
- A sense of the value of the human community
- A belief that love, compassion, unselfishness, and the force of inner truthfulness and of the spirit have ultimately greater power than hate, enmity, and self-interest
- A sense of obligation to stand on the side of the poor and the oppressed as against the rich and the oppressors
- A profound hope that good will finally prevail

Faith is a term also used to describe a cultural or institutional religion, such as Judaism, Islam, or Confucianism. An **atheist** is a person who denies the existence of a higher power; an **agnostic** is one who holds that nothing can be known about the existence of a higher power. They deserve respect for what they choose to believe, just as do those who accept a particular religious creed.

Religion

Although it is impossible for nurses to be knowledgeable about all **religions**, we are better able to meet patients' spiritual needs when we understand their religious beliefs and practices.

THROUGH THE EYES OF A CAREGIVER

My name is Janine Landry and I love nursing! I especially have a passion for emergency department (ED) nursing and I'm pleased to be employed in a faith-based community hospital. I don't feel like I have a job, but rather I look at it as an amazing opportunity to meet people from diverse cultures and beliefs. My work has enabled me to learn and grow both professionally and personally. My dream has always been to become a nurse, to have the opportunity to follow my heart and the purpose of my life—that is, to "*make a difference.*" I strive to create an environment of hope and healing and to have an impact on the people from the vulnerable population we serve. I would like to recount a true story that encompasses all that I believe in, and live, as a registered nurse.

I'll never forget the day I walked into the Grey Nuns Hospital and noticed the mission statement posted on the wall. It began with "Healing the Body, Enriching the Mind, Nurturing the Soul," and went on to express the hospital's values and beliefs, all of which I truly support. This mission statement helps to guide my decisions and actions I make every day, and in all areas in which I work. As a clinical nurse educator, I have made it my habit to instruct our newly hired staff to locate the mission statement; read, understand, and respect it; and most importantly, to live it!

In the ED, we often have repeat visitors and one particular gentleman comes to mind. Fred (not his real name) was a "high-maintenance" kind of guy who always appeared cranky. He had silky white hair, bright blue eyes, wore a constant frown on his face, and often demanded a lot of attention. Fred had a chronic condition, which resulted in him visiting us on a regular basis. At that time, I was working on the floor and I was often assigned to be his nurse. Fred was somewhat gruff when he spoke to people, and he never called me by my given name, Janine. Although I would remind him, he still chose to call me a myriad of other names.

One day while Fred was in the department awaiting admission to the medical unit, I served him his breakfast tray. He snarled and refused to eat it. I looked at him and said "Fred, you're not eating." He grumbled under his breath and said, "No, I don't want to eat this." "Fred, may I remind you that you're at the Grey Nuns Hospital, and did you know that every meal prepared here is made with love...and this breakfast was made especially for you?" "Really...it was made with love?" "Absolutely!" Not surprisingly, Fred ate all his breakfast, and later on, he ate his entire lunch. When his wife and friends came to visit him, he would tell them how amazed he was to find out that all his meals were made with love. Every time his wife and daughter would come and visit him, I would look at them and wink; this always made them smile and giggle.

A few months later, Fred was an inpatient once again. Guess which nurse was assigned to him? You're right...it was me again. While I was busy changing a wound dressing on his leg, a message came over the hospital intercom system. Fred asked, "What's that noise I hear every morning in this hospital?" "Fred, what may be noise to your ears, is known as a prayer or a reflection to others." He said "What do you call it?" "I personally call it Hope!" "Hope?" "Yes, let me explain. Do you like Neapolitan ice cream?" "Yeah!" "What's your favorite flavor?" "I like all the flavors, but I especially enjoy chocolate and my wife and daughter like the vanilla and strawberry flavors. Why do you ask?" "Imagine this; we'll compare Hope to an entire brick of Neapolitan ice cream that has three individual flavors, right?" Fred nodded and agreed. "For some people, in order to have hope, they need to taste that vanilla flavor, which represents *faith,* and depending on what their beliefs are or what they're faced with at that particular moment, having faith may require *courage;* that would be

the strawberry flavor. Most importantly, to have hope, you need *love*—a sense of love for yourself, to be able to receive love and to love others unconditionally, and for some people it also means loving God. So, just think how lucky you are Fred, knowing your favorite flavor is chocolate...that's awesome because everyone knows that chocolate and love are both really good for your heart! You can enjoy each flavor individually...and that's o.k....or you can swirl the ice cream and mix it all together to make one flavor; a delicious flavor called HOPE!"

Fred really didn't know how to respond. He looked up at me with his big bright blue eyes and a puzzled look on his face. He then asked me "Are you a tree hugger?" I said no! "Would you ever hug a tree?" I thought about it, and I said "you know, for the right reason and at the right time, yes, I guess I would hug a tree, because a tree symbolizes creation, growth, and change." Fred looked up at me and said, "If I was a tree, what type of a tree would I be?" I quickly replied "Oh...without a doubt.... you would be an ol' crabapple tree!" Fred started to laugh, it was the first time I had ever heard him laugh, and this laughter came from his toes.

A few weeks later, as I was walking in the main lobby of the hospital, I heard a familiar gruff voice calling out to me. I turned around, and sure enough it was Fred and his wife. He asked me to close my eyes and to put out my hand. When I opened up my eyes, Fred had placed the shiniest, most perfect red apple in my hand. I was speechless, but realized that we really had no need for words: our eyes spoke volumes. I'll never forget that moment.

A few months later, when Fred returned to the ED, I learned that his wife had recently passed away. Fred was depressed and acutely ill; his chronic condition had worsened and the cardiologist informed me that Fred was dying and that he was made aware of this. I quickly notified his daughter and then went to his bedside to support him, but he shouted "get out, get away from me, and leave me alone!" I respected his wishes by leaving the room; but I intentionally left the curtain slightly open so that I could continue to monitor him from the nursing desk. While I was charting, I sensed that he was watching me, so I looked up and just like the time before, our eyes silently spoke to each other.

Fred was deteriorating quickly, and his daughter hadn't arrived yet. My shift was over but I couldn't imagine leaving him alone, so I went into his room to say goodnight. Although we both knew it wasn't really "goodnight," I asked him if I could come and sit next to him, and he simply raised his finger and nodded his head. I sat next to him, and for the longest time neither one of us said anything. I held his hand and looked into his blue eyes and said, "what do you need?" His response was "this ol' tree needs a hug!" So I held him tightly in my arms for the longest time, and when his daughter arrived, I gently laid him back and said "good bye." Next, when I stood up, the most amazing thing happened: Fred looked up at me, and despite his labored breathing, he whispered, "Thank you...thank you, Janine." This was truly a precious moment for me because it was the first and only time Fred called me by my given name.

Shortly thereafter, he died. I will never forget this experience because when I walked away I was thinking about the time we had spent together, and although there were many challenging times with this gentleman, I realized that I had grown to respect him. He died with dignity, because I knew who he was, I took the time to get to know what was truly at the "core" of this man. In essence, I got to know what was in his heart...and he was truly a gift to me!

—*Janine Landry*

Self-identity as spiritual, religious

*Generally speaking, do you think of yourself as a **religious** person, or not?*
*Generally speaking, do you think of yourself as a **spiritual** person, or not?*

	Religious %	Spiritual not religious %	Neither %	DK %
U.S. general public	65	18	15	2 = 100
Unaffiliated	18	37	42	2 = 100
Atheist/agnostic	7	34	57	2 = 100
Nothing in particular	23	39	36	2 = 100
Affiliated	75	15	8	1 = 100
Christian	77	14	8	1 = 100
• Protestant	78	14	6	2 = 100
White evangelical	85	12	2	1 = 100
White mainline	68	18	13	1 = 100
Black protestant	82	15	2	2 = 100
• Catholic	73	15	12	1 = 100
White catholic	70	17	12	1 = 100
Hispanic catholic	77	11	12	1 = 100

Source: Pew Research Center survey, June 28-July 9, 2012. Combined Q97a-b.
Figures show those who think of themselves as a religious person, as spiritual but not religious, and as neither a religious nor a spiritual person. DK includes those giving no answer to Q97a. Whites and blacks include only those who are not Hispanic; Hispanics are of any race. Figures may not add to 100% due to rounding.

FIGURE 45-2. One-fifth of the U.S. public and one-third of adults under 30 are religiously unaffiliated today, the highest percentages ever in Pew Research Center polling. (Source: Pew Research Center. [2012]. "Nones" on the Rise: One-in-Five Adults Have No Religious Affiliation. Available at http://www.pewforum.org/2012/10/09/nones-on-the-rise-religion)

These can directly influence patients' responses to illness and suffering, self-care practices such as diet and hygiene, birth and death rituals, gender roles, spiritual practices, and moral codes. The beliefs and health practices of major religious traditions in the United States are briefly described in Table 45-1 (on pages 1704–1705). Figure 45-2 depicts the percentages of different religions in the United States.

The U.S. Religious Landscape Survey of 35,000 Americans by the Pew Research Center's Forum on Religion & Public Life (2012) finds that most Americans are religious and they have a nondogmatic approach to faith.

• Most Americans who are affiliated with a religion do not believe their religion is the only way to salvation. Most also believe that there is more than one true way to interpret the teachings of their religion.
• More than half of Americans rank the importance of religion very highly in their lives, attend religious services regularly, and pray daily.
• A plurality of adults who are affiliated with a religion want their religion to preserve its traditional beliefs and practices rather than either adjust to new circumstances or adopt modern beliefs and practices.

• Significant minorities across nearly all religious traditions see a conflict between being a devout person and living in a modern society.
• The relationship between religion and politics is particularly strong with respect to political ideology and views on social issues such as abortion and homosexuality, with the more religiously committed adherents across several religious traditions expressing more conservative political views.
• Americans are very similar in some basic religious beliefs. For instance, Americans are nearly unanimous in saying they believe in God (92%); large majorities believe in life after death (74%) and believe that Scripture is the word of God (63%).
• More than three quarters of American adults (78%) believe there are absolute standards of right and wrong, with a majority (52%) saying they rely primarily on practical experience and common sense for guidance regarding right and wrong. Far fewer say they rely mainly on their religious beliefs (29%), and fewer still say they rely on philosophy and reason (9%) or scientific information (5%).

(text continues on page 1706)

Table 45-1   BELIEFS AND HEALTH CARE PRACTICES OF MAJOR RELIGIOUS TRADITIONS IN THE UNITED STATES

RELIGION	BELIEFS	SELECT HEALTH CARE PRACTICES
Adventist	Believe in the person's choice and God's sovereignty. The body is believed to be the temple of the Holy Spirit.	• The taking of all narcotics and stimulants is prohibited because the body is the temple of the Holy Spirit and should be protected. Many groups prohibit meat. • Many regard Saturday as the Sabbath. • Approach to health care is holistic.
American Muslim Mission	Accept the Koran as their sacred scripture (see Islam); most stress the importance of cooperation among blacks in business and education to build self-esteem.	• Members are encouraged to obtain health care provided by members of the black community. • Major tenets involve prayer rituals, dietary restrictions (prohibitions against pork and alcohol), hygiene (extreme cleanliness), lifestyle modifications, and marital faithfulness.
Baha'i International Community	Believe in a basic harmony between religion and science	• Seek out competent medical care and pray for health • Obligatory prayers, holy days, and the 19-day fast • Permanent sterilization is prohibited, and abortion is discouraged.
Buddhism	Buddha—or "the Great Physician"—taught the Four Noble Truths to indicate the range of "suffering," its "origin," its "cessation," and the "way" that leads to its cessation. The real cause of human suffering is ignorant craving. The Noble Eightfold Path—which consists of right views, aspirations, speech, conduct, mode of livelihood, effort, mindfulness, and concentration—leads to the cessation of suffering.	• Buddhists do not outwardly proclaim healing through faith. However, spiritual peace and liberation from anxiety attained through the awakening to Buddha's wisdom may be an important factor in expediting healing and the recovery process. • Accepts modern science. The doctrine of avoidance of extremes is applied to the use of drugs, blood, vaccines. • Buddhism does not condone taking lives of any form. • Check with the patient about any special diet restrictions and the observance of holy days.
Christian Scientist	They deny the existence of health crises; sickness and sin are errors of the human mind and can be overcome by altering thoughts, not by using drugs or medicines.	• They will use orthopedic services to set a bone but decline drugs and, in general, other medical or surgical procedures. • They do not allow hypnotism or any form of psychotherapy, which alters the "Divine Mind." • A Christian Science Practitioner may be called to administer spiritual support. • Alcohol and tobacco are not used.
Church of Jesus Christ of Latter Day Saints (Mormons)	Devout adherents believe in divine healing through the "laying on of hands," though many do not prohibit medical therapy. The Church maintains an extensive and well-funded welfare system, including financial support for the sick.	• Disapprove of alcohol, tobacco, and caffeinated beverages • A special undergarment worn by some members should be removed only in an emergency.
Confucianism	Inherent in Confucianism is the appreciation of life and the desire to keep the body from untimely or unnecessary death.	• Appreciate life and desire to keep the body from untimely or unnecessary death • Historically emphasized public health solutions to impending health problems
Daoism (Taoism)	Health is a manifestation of the harmony of the universe, obtained through the proper balancing of internal and external forces. Implicit throughout the Daoist tradition is the tendency to understand salvation in the biomedical sense of health and qualitative improvement and prolongation of human life. The universal principle of the Tao is the mysterious biologic and spiritual life rhythm or order of nature.	• There is a "medicinal" concern for maintaining and prolonging human health and life (sheng). Knowing and living a natural life—following the Tao—is the secret of both health and sagehood. • Long tradition of seeking pragmatic medical techniques, along with its religious techniques of meditation and ritual for establishing a harmony of body and spirit, humanity, and nature (holistic approach)
Hinduism	Doctrine of Transmigration. Moral factors, linked with the all-embracing doctrine of "karma," are believed to be significant in promoting health or causing disease.	• Hindu medicine shows a surprising openness to new ideas, at least in respect to practical treatment. • Many Hindu dietary restrictions conform to individual sect doctrine.

Table 45-1   BELIEFS AND HEALTH CARE PRACTICES OF MAJOR RELIGIOUS TRADITIONS IN THE UNITED STATES *continued*

RELIGION	BELIEFS	SELECT HEALTH CARE PRACTICES
		• The nurse administering medications should avoid touching the patient's lips. • Certain prescribed rites are followed after death; disposal of the body is by cremation.
Islam	Allah, one God, who is only one, all seeing, all hearing, all speaking, all knowing, all willing, all powerful Must be able to practice the Five Pillars of Islam May have a fatalistic view of health	• Obligatory prayers, holy days, and fasting (Ramadan), and almsgiving • Koranic law and customs that influence birth, diet (eating pork and drinking alcohol are forbidden), care of women, death and prayer rituals • Some Muslim women are not allowed to make independent decisions; husbands may need to be present when consent is sought.
Jehovah's Witnesses	They oppose the "false teachings" of other sects; opposition often extends to modern science, including medicine.	• Blood transfusions violate God's laws and, therefore, are not allowed. • The courts have not supported the right of Jehovah's Witness parents to refuse lifesaving treatment for their children. • Use of alcohol and tobacco are discouraged.
Judaism	Formation closely bound with a divine revelation and with commitment to obedience to God's will. The Hebrew Bible is the authority, guide, and inspiration of the many forms of religion of the Jews (currently Reform, Conservative, Orthodox).	• For observant Jews: special needs in the areas of diet, birth rituals, male and female contact, and death • Treatment and procedures should not be scheduled on the Sabbath.
Native American Religions	Difficult to generalize; notion of cosmic harmony, emphasis on directly experiencing powers and visions and a common view of the cycle of life and death. Death is not the end but the beginning of new life (reincarnation or transcendent hereafter).	• Rituals mark important life changes: birth, puberty, initiation rites, death. • Medicine men and women have specialized spirits from whom they receive the mission to cure. • Common therapeutic measures: sucking, blowing, and drawing out with a feather fan
Protestantism	Worship of the one God revealed to the world through Jesus Christ. Love of neighbor is a central tenet. Other beliefs include sin, redemption, salvation, and a final accounting with God. Care of the sick is encouraged. God the author and giver of life is also the healer. Most accept modern medical science.	• Religious practices vary according to denomination; may include prayer, faith healing, "laying on of hands," and anointing. • Sacraments: baptism, communion, confirmation
Roman Catholicism	Worship of the one God revealed to the world through Jesus Christ. Love of neighbor is a central tenet. Other beliefs include sin, redemption, salvation, and a final accounting with God. Care of the sick is encouraged. God the author and giver of life is also the healer. Human life is a gift of God. Many take an antiabortion stance; most accept modern medical science.	• Importance of private devotions and Mass attendance on Sunday • Seven sacraments (importance of baptism, Eucharist, penance, and the anointing of the sick) • Dietary habits • Sexual ethical norms • Only natural means of birth control; abortion, euthanasia, and sterilization are forbidden
Unification Church	God is the living, eternal person who represents universal love and care. God created the world and humans to reflect his nature. The goal of the Unification Church is to unite Christians everywhere as one family under God.	• Most members are still healthy young adults. There is little information available on their interactions with the health care team.
Unitarian Universal Association of Churches and Fellowships	Encourage creativity, reason, and living an ethical life. No member is required to adhere to a given creed or set of religious beliefs. The inherent worth and dignity of every person is affirmed.	• Free to accept what they take to be best for their health

• The United States has largely avoided the secularizing trends that have reshaped the religious scene in recent decades in European and other economically developed nations—but not entirely. The Landscape Survey documents, for example, that the number of Americans who are not affiliated with a religion has grown significantly in recent decades, with the number of people who today say they are unaffiliated with a religious tradition (16% of U.S. adults) more than double the number who say they were not affiliated with a religion as children (7%).

Nurses who are unfamiliar with a patient's religion can gain valuable knowledge by discussions with the patient and the patient's family and spiritual adviser.

 RECALL Choi Min Lai, the father of the 8-year-old boy with foot deformities who is refusing surgical repair based on his cultural and religious beliefs. Researching information about the patient's beliefs would be essential in planning this family's care and advocating for the patient and his family. •

Never presume to know what a patient's religious beliefs or practices are just because you have learned the patient's faith tradition. Many religious groups and people work out their own set of beliefs and practices, which may or may not be compatible with the tradition at large. Also, you should not interpret the fact that a patient does not belong to an organized religion to mean that the patient has no spiritual needs; a person may be deeply spiritual yet not profess to belong to an organized religion.

Hope

Closely related to spirituality, faith, and religion, **hope** is the ingredient in life responsible for a positive outlook, even in life's bleakest moments. It enables a person both to consider a future and to work to actively bring that future into being. Hope originates in imagination but must become a valued and realistic possibility in order to energize action. Hope allows one to embrace the reality of suffering without escaping from it (false hope) or being suffocated by it (despair, helplessness, hopelessness). Hope is unique to each person. Box 42–6 on page 1619 contains a set of suggestions, developed by an interdisciplinary team for enabling hope in the terminally ill, that can apply to any situation in which people feel hopeless (Creen, 2002).

Love

Earlier, we noted that people express and experience spirituality in and through connectedness with other people. The popular musical "Les Miserables" put it well in one of its songs: "To love another person is to see the face of God." Love develops from the basic human need to love and be loved, and we cannot be spiritually whole, spiritually healthy, unless this need is met.

Spiritual Health and Healing

Defined most simply, **spiritual health** or well-being is the condition that exists when the person's universal spiritual needs for meaning and purpose, love and belonging, and forgiveness are met. O'Brien's conceptual model of spiritual well-being in illness (Fig. 45-3) identifies three empirical referents of

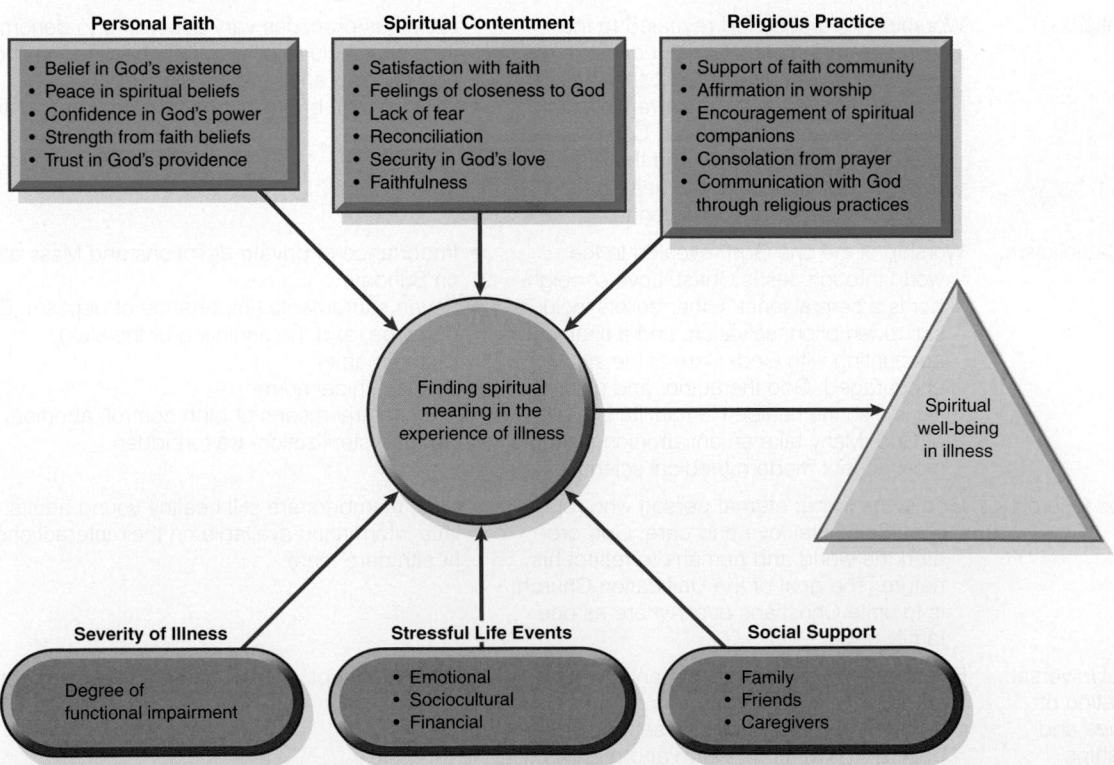

FIGURE 45-3. A conceptual model of spiritual well-being in illness. (Redrawn from O'Brien, M. E. [2003]. *Parish nursing: Healthcare ministry within the church* [p. 109]. Boston: Jones and Bartlett.)

spiritual well-being: personal faith, spiritual contentment, and religious practice. **Spiritual healing** is the movement toward integration, from brokenness to wholeness.

Spirituality and Everyday Living

Spiritual beliefs and practices are associated with all aspects of a person's life, including health and illness. According to Quinn (2002), the major wisdom traditions address the invisible Spirit—a creative, mysterious, guiding power—by creating principles and practices that:

- Cultivate love of ourselves, our neighbors, of a higher being, and of nature
- Cultivate wisdom that helps us find meaning in life; be in relationships with others; be true to ourselves; live in uncertainty and mystery; deal with suffering, sickness, and death; and honor life's transitions (birth, marriage, death)
- Cultivate awareness of the sacred dimension of life through practices such as worship, prayer, meditation, and singing
- Respect our connectedness as fellow human beings while acknowledging our differences
- Help us be generous in service to others (pp. 13–14)

Religious influences may be life affirming or life denying. Life-affirming influences enhance life, give meaning and purpose to existence, strengthen one's feelings of self-worth, encourage self-actualization, and are health giving and life sustaining. Life-denying influences restrict or enclose life patterns, limit experiences and associations, place burdens of guilt on people, encourage feelings of unworthiness, and are generally health denying and life inhibiting.

Spirituality, Health, and Illness

Spiritual beliefs are of special importance to nurses because of the many ways they can influence a patient's level of health, sense of well-being, and self-care behaviors.

Guide to Daily Living Habits

Certain practices generally associated with health care may have religious significance for a patient. For example, many religions have dietary requirements and restrictions. Acceptable birth-control practices are determined by some religious faiths, as are some types of medical treatments (refer back to Table 45-1, pp. 1704–1705).

Source of Support

Many people seek support from their religious faith during times of stress. This support is often vital to the acceptance of an illness, especially if the illness brings with it a prolonged period of convalescence or may lead to a questionable outcome. Prayer, devotional reading, and other religious practices often do for the person spiritually what protective exercises do for the body physically.

 THINK back to Margot Zeuner, the 75-year-old woman caring for her husband with advanced Alzheimer disease. Assessment reveals that

Mrs. Zeuner derived much support from her church group. The nurse, acknowledging the importance of this aspect, could work with Mrs. Zeuner to arrange for assistance at home so that she can attend church activities and continue to receive the support she needs. A referral to the church might also result in church members seeking out the Zeuners and offering assistance. ●

Box 45-1 describes how one religion, Buddhism, sees the divine grounding for all human experience, including suffering.

Source of Strength and Healing

The value of religious faith cannot be enumerated or evaluated easily. However, the effects attributable to faith are constantly in evidence to health care workers. People have been known to endure extreme physical distress because of strong faith. Patients' families have taken on almost unbelievable rehabilitative tasks because they had faith in the eventual positive results of their effort. In the accompanying Through the Eyes of a Patient box (on page 1708), a woman facing life-threatening events describes what she means by healing.

Jeff Levin (2001) synthesizes research demonstrating a positive link between health and religion in his seven principles of theosomatic medicine:

1. Religious affiliation and membership benefit health by promoting healthy behavior and lifestyles.
2. Regular religious fellowship benefits health by offering support that buffers the effects of stress and isolation.

BOX 45-1   THE CENTER POINT THAT GROUNDS US...

...I could scarcely make out the large sitting Buddha near the entrance of the house. But what caught my attention was the metal circle with spokes resembling a wheel, hanging over the Figure of the Buddha....I asked our host about the wheel. I was told it represented our eternal journey in this life and continuing into the next. Buddha's teachings say that life is suffering. We cannot avoid suffering as we move around the rim of the wheel, which represents perpetual change and the transitory nature of life. But the wheel also symbolizes wholeness or completion because the wheel revolves around the center axis that does not move. That center point represents the presence of the divine. If we remain aware of this center point, we are strengthened for whatever lies ahead.

...It is this center point that grounds us in the midst of the many changes in our lives. It is at the center point where we experience the energy and power that turns the wheel. It is at this center point that we connect with the Everywhere Spirit. When we rest in the center point, we find that we have come home again to the place from which we started. But because of the journey, it is as if we had arrived home for the first time. In our journey around the circles of life, we become new persons over and over again.

Reprinted with permission from Gregg-Schroeder, S. (1999). A transforming experience: Circles of Life. *Journal of Fellowship in Prayer*, 23–25.

THROUGH THE EYES OF A PATIENT

Seven years ago, I was faced with three life-threatening events in a period of 3 years. Those life-threatening experiences taught me that it is possible to "heal" and to live fully even when we are in the abyss of suffering. I believe everyone would benefit if we redefined "healing." Here are elements I now include in my definition.

Healing is:

• Becoming whole, a life-long journey of becoming fully human, involving the totality of our being: body, mind, emotion, spirit, social, and political context, as well as our relationships with others and with the Divine. Healing does not necessarily mean being happy or getting what we think we want out of life;, it means growth, often with pain.

• Becoming our authentic self, releasing old unreal self-images, discovering who we really are, not what we think we should be, knowing why we are here and what we really value, restoring our ability to heed our aspirations.

• Reconnecting lost aspects of ourselves, paying attention to buried feelings and places inside us that are distressed or sick, enabling us to express our self in fullness, both the light and shadow sides.

• Being open to change and new possibilities, responding to problems by changing the picture, being willing to let in more life, to open up to what may have been previously closed or destroyed for us and that which holds promise of giving us new life and fulfillment.

• Facing our fears and refusing to be injured or wounded, changing our belief systems, breaking unnecessary taboos, letting go of what is familiar, and stepping into the unknown.

• Accepting that problems, pain, and suffering are part of life and inseparable from us—not a peripheral relationship, not something isolated and avoidable—enabling us

to enter into problems and use suffering, pain, and life-threatening events to enrich our lives.

• Being empowered by the Divine; discovering meaning in our defects, disorders, problems, and disease; experiencing new degrees of creativity and life forces that we might never have imagined before our difficulty; finding that our pains and fears are transformed into relief and confidence.

• Recognizing the value and preciousness of life, knowing that every moment is unique and significant, which usually leads to greater appreciation of the wonder of our minds, bodies, and spirits and of the Divine.

• Having faith and hope—important preconditions for mental and physical health; having a belief in the Divine, the meaning of human life, and the universe; helping us to claim our capacity to create and make something new.

• Finding inner peace, contentment, and tranquility amid the realities of daily life, including its problems, changes, and chaos; experiencing a sense of fullness that makes the burdens of pain or illness lighter.

• Being forgiving of ourselves and others and being forgiven; giving ourselves and others the freedom to let go of rivalry, strife, anger, hatred, fear, and limitations.

• Feeling connected to one another, a sense of interdependence; knowing we are not isolated or autonomous, giving up the illusions of boundaries in life; taking responsibility, acting justly, and accepting that we share our humanity.

• Being loving and loved; loving one's self and wanting to love and serve others, as well as being capable of receiving love; having an ability to trust, a feeling of aliveness, and a sense of greater participation in life.

Reprinted with permission. Carol, J. (2002). What is healing? *Sacred Journey*, *53*(4), 33–35.

3. Participation in worship and prayer benefits health through the physiologic effect of positive emotions.
4. Religious beliefs benefit health by their similarity to health-promoting beliefs and personality styles.
5. Simple faith benefits health by leading to thoughts of hope, optimism, and positive expectations.
6. Mystical experiences benefit health by activating a healing bioenergy, or life force, or altered state of consciousness.
7. Absent prayer for others is capable of healing by paranormal means or divine intervention (pp. 13–14).

Source of Conflict

Sometimes religious beliefs conflict with prevalent health care practices (see Table 45-1, pp. 1704–1705). For example, the doctrine of the Jehovah's Witnesses prohibits blood transfusions. Some Navajos use a lengthy religious ceremony to cure certain diseases, such as tuberculosis. For some people, illness is viewed as punishment for sin and is therefore inevitable.

Such beliefs may require the health care worker to modify a treatment plan to accommodate the person's religion. In

some instances, acknowledgment of the patient's religious convictions and efforts by health practitioners to accommodate the patient's beliefs can result in quality health care without violating the person's religious practices. In other situations, an objective explanation of alternative treatments and the predicted consequences of each may help the patient choose acceptable therapy. Whatever the person's decision about health care, remember that each person is unique and has a right to pursue one's own convictions, even though they may differ from those of the health care provider.

Health care professionals can reduce conflict by attempting to understand how a particular religious culture influences people's thinking about basic questions of biology and ethics. Some of the major questions that religious beliefs, attitudes, and values can affect include (Davis & Zoloth, 1999):

• What is the meaning of suffering?
• How should we regard the physical body and its functions?
• What are the meaning and role of gender differences, sexuality, and reproduction?
• How are we to understand and respond to birth, aging, and death?

- What constitutes the self, and how is selfhood assessed?
- How are sin and moral culpability understood? What makes something sinful, and how is sin relieved or absolved?
- What are the tradition's specific bioethical teachings?

 REMEMBER Choi Min Lai, described at the beginning of this chapter. The nurse could use these questions to assess the family's beliefs in greater depth, providing significant data for the health care team to incorporate when discussing the possibility of surgery to repair Kou's deformities. Doing so could be helpful in minimizing the conflict between the family and health care team. ●

FACTORS AFFECTING SPIRITUALITY

Among the many factors that can influence a person's spirituality, the most important are developmental considerations, family, ethnic background, formal religion, and life events.

Developmental Considerations

Because spirituality involves the nonmaterial realm of being, a child must have developed some capacity for abstract in order to understand the spiritual self. However, this is not to say that spirituality is meaningless for children. For example, David Heller (1985) interviewed 40 children between 4 and 12 years old who were affiliated with one of four major religions (Judaism, Roman Catholicism, Protestantism, or Hinduism) and discovered that the children had definite perceptions of God. Central themes in all the children's descriptions included the following:

- Notion of a God who works through human intimacy and the interconnectedness of lives
- Belief that God is involved in self-change and growth and transformations that make the world fresh, alive, and meaningful
- Attributing to God tremendous and expansive power and then showing considerable anxiety in the face of this power
- Image of light

As the child matures, life experiences usually influence and mature the child's spiritual beliefs. With advancing years, the tendency to think about life after death prompts some people to re-examine and reaffirm their spiritual beliefs. Chapter 17 describes the stages of faith development.

Family

A child's parents play a key role in the development of the child's spirituality. What parents explicitly teach a child about spirituality and religion is generally less important than what the child learns about spirituality, life, and self from the parents' behavior.

Ethnic Background

Religious traditions differ among ethnic groups. There are clear distinctions between Eastern and Western spiritual traditions as well as among those of individual ethnic groups,

such as Native Americans. A person's culture and formal religion significantly affect whether the person's approach to religion is doing something, being someone, or continually striving for harmony.

Formal Religion

Each of the major religious groups discussed earlier in this chapter shares several characteristics:

- Basis of authority or source of power
- Scripture or sacred word
- An ethical code that defines right and wrong
- A psychology and identity, so that its adherents fit into a group and the world is defined by the religion
- Aspirations or expectations
- Ideas about what follows death

Life Events

Both positive and negative life experiences can influence spirituality, and they in turn are influenced by the meaning a person's spiritual beliefs attribute to them. For example, if two women who believe in a loving God both lose a child in a car accident, one may bitterly deny God's existence, whereas the other may spend more time in prayer, asking God to help her. Similarly, a chain of successful life experiences (marriage, promotion) may cause one person to assume success and experience no need for God, whereas for another it occasions deep gratitude and rejoicing.

 RECALL Kevin Gargan, who recently experienced a heart attack. The experience of his own mortality and the thought that he might have died now have him questioning whether or not there is a God and if yes, where he stands in relationship to God. ●

RELIGION AND LAW, ETHICS, AND MEDICINE

Christian Scientists, Jehovah's Witnesses, and members of certain faith-healing groups are among those challenging the intricate web of rights and responsibilities among individual, society, church, and state. These religious bodies are asking for protection, under the veil of religious freedom, of a right to exercise individual decisions in accordance with scriptural interpretations, even though those decisions may result in a person's own death or that of a family member, including a child. Most troubling are those cases in which treatable problems, such as bacterial meningitis, diabetes, or bowel obstruction, resulted in the death of minors whose parents chose religious means of healing over traditional medicine. (See Focused Critical Thinking Guide 45-1 on page 1710.) The American Academy of Pediatrics urges that all child abuse, neglect, and medical neglect statutes be applied without potential or actual exemption for religious beliefs.

Perhaps even more troubling for nurses are situations in which family members insist on painful care that is deemed medically futile (i.e., the likelihood of medical benefit is

FOCUSED CRITICAL THINKING GUIDE 45-1

SPIRITUALITY

A 16-year-old student approaches you, the school nurse, and confides that she is worried about her brother, who is sick and getting sicker. "My parents are Christian Scientists and have had Christian Science Practitioners in to pray for him, but he seems to be getting worse. I'm afraid he'll die if we don't get him to the hospital." Your first impulse is to visit the student's home to try to see her brother and parents. You immediately remember an article in the paper about the Supreme Court's decision to let stand a Minnesota Court of Appeals ruling upholding an award of $1.5 million to the father of a boy who died in 1989 after his mother, stepfather, and two Christian Scientist Practitioners tried to use prayer to heal his diabetes. Despite their efforts, the boy slipped into a coma and died. What is troubling you is the following comment by Stephen Carter: "By refusing to intervene in *McKown v. Lundman,* the Supreme Court has reinforced a societal message that has grown depressingly common: It is perfectly OK to believe in the power of prayer, so long as one does not believe in it so sincerely that one actually expects it to work—a peculiar fate indeed for our 'most inalienable' right" (Carter, S. L. [1996, January 31]. The power of prayer, denied. *The New York Times,* A17). You do believe in the power of prayer and are not sure how you should respond to the student's plea for help for her brother.

1. Identify goal of thinking

Clarify (1) what I believe about prayer's power to heal, and (2) what I believe about a parent's right to substitute prayer for modern medicine when a child is seriously ill. Decide how I should respond. What are my professional obligations?

2. Assess adequacy of knowledge

Pertinent circumstances: This is the first time I have encountered a family of Christian Scientists. As a school nurse, I am not responsible for my student's brother if he is not in my school and place of employment. That said, I have been asked to help and have the resources to do so.

Prerequisite knowledge: I have no knowledge of what Christian Scientists believe. Moreover, I do not know how the law in our state responds to situations like these. I do not know if any nursing or medical groups have guidelines for situations like these. I immediately get on the Internet to address these deficiencies and also contact my professional nursing organization to see what the law is and if any professional organizations have addressed this issue. I also have to find out how sick the student's brother

is and the probable consequences of his not seeking traditional medical care.

Room for error: The student's brother's very life may depend on whether or not and how I choose to respond.

Time constraints: Until I learn the exact nature of the boy's medical problems, I cannot know how urgent the need to intervene is.

3. Address potential problems

In a situation like this, the most obvious impediments to critical thinking would be (1) the unexamined belief that religion trumps all other considerations ("by golly, this country is founded on respect for religious freedom") and (2) the belief that modern medicine is owed to everyone with a life-threatening illness, no matter what other considerations are present.

4. Consult helpful resources

I decide to visit the boy's home with the student and call first to seek the parents' permission. After talking with the parents and seeing the boy, I believe that the boy is in a life-threatening situation because the parents were told that their son has diabetes. I am struck by the love and devotion of both parents and I learn via Internet research that they are doing exactly what their religion prescribes. I later consult with a local Christian Scientist group that confirms this. I learn from my professional nursing organization that there is no consensus about how society should respond in situations like these. Many believe that what these parents are doing is neglect and that if the boy dies, they should be held criminally accountable for manslaughter. Others respect their right to practice their religion. Uncertain of how I should respond, I decide to call Child Protective Services and tell them that I am willing to help if they think my relationship with the daughter would be helpful. I explain to my student what I am doing and tell her to keep me informed and to come back for help if she is not getting the assistance she needs.

5. Critique judgment/decision

Child Protective Services did intervene immediately, and the boy was hospitalized and treated against the parents' wishes. While I was happy that the boy's condition was stabilized, I did feel uncomfortable about the disrespect shown to these obviously intelligent, devout, and loving parents. I decided to learn more about how different states are responding to these challenges and to see if nursing can get involved in some way.

virtually nonexistent) because they believe that God is going to work a miracle. In these cases, simple nursing measures, such as turning or bathing patients, can become occasions of pain and torment to both the patient and nurse. Nurses are forced to administer care that they take to be cruel and abusive to patients capable of experiencing pleasure and pain. This nursing care can needlessly prolong a patient's painful dying. Unfortunately, there are no clear guidelines for drawing a line between promoting life and prolonging the dying process. Although nurses always have the moral right to withdraw from administering care that violates their personal moral code, this does not resolve the problem for the patient. More dialogue is needed on the interaction between religion and law, ethics, and medicine. Ideally, the religious freedom of patients and their families is respected, as is the moral autonomy of caregivers and the integrity of the healing professions. Nurses in these situations should seek the assistance of the ethics committee or ethics consultation service.

 CONSIDER the situation of Choi Min Lai, the father described at the beginning of this chapter. The nurse is required to respect the family's religious freedom and advocate for them while at the same time acting as a professional member of the health care team. ●

PARISH NURSING

Parish nurse programs are a relatively new movement in faith communities in many denominations. They seek to reclaim the church's role in the ministry of healing and focus again on the impact that spirituality, caring relationships, and a responsibly balanced life can have on health and wellness. Parish nurses (also called faith community nurses)

and health ministry teams work to reintegrate the healing tradition into the life of faith communities by:

- Interpreting the relationship between faith and health
- Promoting personal responsibility for health and wellness
- Serving as health counselors and educators
- Staying aware of available resources and making appropriate referrals
- Acting as advocates for people who have health needs but only limited resources
- Recruiting and training volunteers
- Visiting church members
- Initiating caring relationships with older adults, the chronically ill, and the "worried well"

Parish nurses are not visiting nurses or home health care nurses who provide direct bedside care. The key roles of the parish nurse are health educator, personal health counselor, referral agent, trainer of volunteers, developer of support groups, integrator of faith and health, and health advocate. Nurses who wish to be parish nurses must be registered and compliant with both the state or province practice act and Faith Community Nursing: Scope and Standards (American Nurses Association, 2005). Check out the International Parish Nurse Resource Center at www.parishnurses.org.

THE NURSING PROCESS

Nurses who role model good health behaviors are more effective teachers. Use the display, Promoting Health 45-1, for yourself before using it with others. Many nurses approach professional practice as more than a "job" and use the language of "sacred calling" or "vocation" to describe their career choice. Through the Eyes of a Caregiver (on page 1712) gives the prayer of one such nurse.

PROMOTING HEALTH 45-1

SPIRITUALITY

Use the assessment checklist to determine how well you are meeting your spirituality needs. Then develop a prescription for self-care by choosing appropriate behaviors from the list of suggestions.

Assessment Checklist

❑ almost always	❑ sometimes	❑ almost never

❑ ❑ ❑ 1. I am comfortable with my spiritual beliefs and values.

❑ ❑ ❑ 2. My beliefs meet my needs for love, belonging, forgiveness, and meaning and purpose.

❑ ❑ ❑ 3. I respect the belief systems of others.

❑ ❑ ❑ 4. I derive sufficient strength from my religious beliefs to meet each day's challenges, especially when confronting pain, suffering, and death.

Self-Care Behaviors

1. Explore personal values and beliefs of self and others.
2. Set aside regular periods to nurture spiritual self.
3. Explore practices that are spiritually supportive.
4. Demonstrate in interaction with others peace, inner strength, warmth, joy, caring, creativity.
5. Respect the belief systems of others.
6. Practice loving relationships with self and others.
7. Seek spiritual assistance to help cope with stress, crisis, or loss.

THROUGH THE EYES OF A CAREGIVER

The Sacred Covenant: A Nurse's Prayer

Gentle God,

You alone are the source of my strength and the center of my life;

Bless my nursing that it may always be guided by the sacred covenant of Your loving care.

Use me as Your instrument in serving the sick;

Use my eyes to look with compassion on those who are broken in body or in spirit;

Use my hands to touch with tenderness those who suffer illness or injury;

Use my lips to speak words of comfort to those who are anxious or afraid.

Dear Lord,

Let me recognize every sickroom as a tabernacle where You dwell; and

Let me not forget, as I care for the ill, that

The ground on which I am standing is holy,

The vocation to which I am called is holy.

Help me to be worthy.

Reprinted with permission from O'Brien, M. E. (2001). *The nurse's calling.* New York: Paulist Press, p. x.

Assessing

Nursing History

Because a person's spirituality and religious beliefs can influence every aspect of being, an assessment of the patient's spirituality—including beliefs and practices, the effect of these beliefs on everyday living, spiritual distress, and spiritual needs—should be included in each comprehensive nursing history. (See the accompanying Research in Nursing Box.) Many guides are available for eliciting a spiritual history, such as O'Brien (1982), Shelly and Fish (1988), and Puchalski and Romer (2000). One simple guide is Anandarajah and Hight's (2001) HOPE acronym:

H—Sources of *hope*, meaning, comfort, strength, peace, love, and connection

O—*O*rganized religion

P—*P*ersonal spirituality and practice

E—*E*ffects on medical care and end-of-life issue

Additional sample questions are listed in the Focused Assessment Guide 45-1.

If the patient reveals a spiritual problem, use interview questions to determine the specific nature of the problem, its probable causes, its related signs and symptoms, when it began and how often it occurs, how it affects everyday living, its severity and whether it can be

RESEARCH IN NURSING

BRIDGING THE GAP TO EVIDENCE-BASED PRACTICE

Spirituality and Religiosity: Definitions and Measures

Research continues to demonstrate the importance of assessing the spiritual needs of patients in order to optimize health outcomes.

Related Research

Cohen, M. Z., Holley, L. M., Wengel, S. P., & Katzman, M. (2012). A platform for nursing research on spirituality and religiosity: Definitions and measures. *Western Journal of Nursing Research, 34*(6), 795–817. DOI: 10.1177/0193945912444321

Spirituality or religiousness is important across the health trajectory, from promoting health and preventing disease to coping with illness and end of life. Research on the relationship of religiousness or spirituality to health spans more than one discipline and applies many definitions and measures. The purpose of this multidisciplinary work is to facilitate research by nurses who seek to investigate the relationship between health and religiousness or spirituality and provide evidence-based guidance for nursing practice. Senior researchers summarize the history of inquiry on this topic, discuss particular and persistent challenges posed by definitions of religion and spirituality, describe selected measures that have enjoyed wide application, and make recommendations for consideration by nurse researchers.

Relevance for Nursing Practice

Attempting to measure the degree to which a person expresses religious faith or thinks about spiritual things is challenging. The authors of this study recommend that nurse researchers:

- Be aware of the wide variety of definitions of spirituality and religiousness and the lack of consensus regarding their definitions
- Acknowledge and consider the foundation of earlier work
- Build on prior work rather than, for example, creating new instruments
- Be aware of the wide variety of measures and be guided by being clear about what they want to measure
- Consider using the Spiritual Well-Being Scale (SWBS) because it is the most widely used measure, if appropriate to the research purpose(s). This enhances the ability to compare findings across studies.
- Carefully formulate research questions and definitions
- Be clear and focus on clinically useful findings that can guide inquiry and practice.

For additional research, visit thePoint.

FOCUSED ASSESSMENT GUIDE 45-1

SPIRITUALITY

Factors to Assess	Questions and Approaches
Spiritual beliefs	"Are there particular spiritual or religious beliefs that are important to you? Have these beliefs changed recently? Is your illness challenging these beliefs? Do your religious beliefs in any way dictate a course of action that puts you in conflict with what your physicians are recommending?"
Spiritual practices	"Describe your usual spiritual practices and anything interfering with your ability to perform them. Can I help in any way to secure the aids necessary for these practices (prayer shawl, Bible, crystals, amulets, beads, icons)?"
Relation between spiritual beliefs and everyday living	"Describe ways your spiritual beliefs affect everyday living (daily schedule, diet, hygiene, sense of self and the world, relationships). Do you find this influence to be healthy (life affirming) or destructive (life denying)?"
Spiritual deficit or distress	"Are your spiritual beliefs currently causing you any distress?"
Spiritual needs	"In what ways can I and the other nurses help you to meet your spiritual needs?" "Would you like me to contact your spiritual adviser or the hospital's pastoral care minister?"
Need for meaning and purpose	"In what ways do your religious beliefs help or hinder you to understand your current situation and face it with peace and courage?"
Need for love and relatedness	"In what ways do your religious beliefs help or hinder you to meet your need to love and be loved?"
Need for forgiveness	"In what ways do your religious beliefs help or hinder you to feel at peace?"
Significant behavioral observations	Be alert to sudden changes in spiritual practices, mood changes, sudden interest in spiritual matters, and sleep disturbances—any of which may point to unresolved spiritual needs.

treated independently by nursing or needs to be referred, and how well the patient is coping.

 THINK back to Kevin Gargan, the man who experienced the heart attack. The nurse could use these questions to determine Mr. Gargan's beliefs, thereby developing a plan of care that addresses his current needs. Additionally, this assessment would provide valuable information about how the patient is coping with the current situation. ●

Nursing Observation

Because many patients find it difficult to talk about their spiritual beliefs and problems, also observe the patient's behavior for signs of spiritual distress. A family member or close friend may share significant observations:

- "He's been awfully moody since his heart attack. I can't believe how hopeless he seems now."
- "I've never seen my father so depressed. He's never in his life been away from the synagogue at Passover. I don't know how to help him."

Significant behavioral observations include sudden changes in spiritual practices (rejection, neglect, fanatical devotion), mood changes (frequent crying, depression,

apathy, anger), sudden interest in spiritual matters (reading religious books or watching religious programs on television, visits to clergy), and disturbed sleep. If you observe these behaviors, you should follow up with appropriate interview questions. Often, problems with spiritual distress do not surface until well after a patient's admission history and examination. Effective questions include the following:

- "You've been lying there so quietly. What are you thinking about?"
- "After all you've been through, you must have done a good bit of soul searching. Experiences like these are enough to shake anyone's faith—how is yours holding up?"

Diagnosing

Use each phase of the nursing process when identifying and treating spiritual problems categorized as nursing diagnoses. The NANDA International (NANDA-I, 2012) diagnoses related specifically to spirituality are:

- **Readiness for Enhanced Hope:** A pattern of expectations and desires that is sufficient for mobilizing energy on one's own behalf and can be strengthened
- **Hopelessness:** Subjective state in which an individual sees limited or no alternatives or personal choices

EXAMPLES OF NANDA-I NURSING DIAGNOSES

SPIRITUAL DISTRESS*

Nursing Diagnoses	Related Factors	Sample Defining Characteristics
Spiritual Pain	Inability to accept death of son	A 46-year-old woman, agnostic, only son died 6 months ago (lung cancer) *"I've often wondered throughout my life if there is a God—thought maybe if I had tried harder I'd have recognized him. Now, I don't care if God exists or not because if he allows this I don't want to know him."* *"My son was my whole life; there's nothing left for me to live for."* Lost 10 lb in 6 months since son died; leaves home only when necessary to purchase food, go to bank, and engage in other routine activities.
Spiritual Alienation	Separated from "faith community"	A 72-year-old Orthodox Jewish man, recently admitted to Protestant long-term care facility following 3-week hospitalization for stroke *"I guess Yahweh has written me off; first the stroke that killed half my body and then I'm abandoned here where I can't even observe the Sabbath."* *"I want to go home."*
Spiritual Anxiety	Challenged belief and value system	A 37-year-old previously healthy male executive recovering from massive myocardial infarction *"My parents were strict Methodists, but when I left home for college I stopped going to church…never gave it much thought…there was always something else to do. I started going again but it never meant much."* *"I haven't exactly done anything awful but I've also not been a saint and I find myself wondering if there is a God, what does he think of me."* *"Funny, I guess I thought I'd live forever. I sure never thought about dying and what happens after that."* Often observed lying quietly in bed awake; asked to see minister.
Spiritual Guilt	Failure to live according to religious rules	A 23-year-old, single, Baptist woman being treated for premenstrual syndrome *"I was raised in a strict Baptist home but had to leave…I needed more room to be me. I like life here at the university but there's a restlessness in me I can't describe. I've dated several men, one or two I really liked, but I always do something to mess up the relationship. It would kill my mother if she knew I lived with Gary for 3 months."* *"What it really comes down to is my own sense of betraying myself, my family, and my religion. Who am I anyway?"*
Spiritual Anger	Inability to accept illness	A 38-year-old homosexual man recently diagnosed with AIDS *"My parents are fundamentalists…all I ever heard at home was how much Jesus loves me…all the while my mom was beating the daylights out of me.…Does He love me? Does He love me so much that He had my parents throw me out when I finally told them I was gay? Does He love me so much that I got AIDS and now no one comes near me?"* Facial features are tight; body held rigidly; speech is sharp, appears angry with God, the world, himself.
Spiritual Loss	Terminal illness; anticipatory grieving; inability to find comfort in religion	A 40-year-old mother of three sons who was diagnosed with ovarian cancer 18 months ago; currently in advanced stage of disease *"I've tried hard to do it all right…I read my Bible, prayed every day, went to church each Sunday, loved my husband and kids…why is this all happening to me? Why must I lose it all? Where is God now that I need him? Some mornings I wish I could shoot myself and end it all—instead another day drags on. Who can help me?"* Cries frequently, no longer interested in everyday activities of family, no interest in praying, told family not to have pastor call anymore. *"No one can help now."*
Spiritual Despair	Feeling that no one (not even God) cares	A 92-year-old frail widow who lives alone in a two-room apartment; crippled with arthritis; has two married sons she has not seen for years. Says to community nurse who visits every week, *"No one should have to live like this. If it weren't for the neighbor who comes on Saturday with a few groceries and you, I'd be dead. I guess that would be for the best. It's been a long time since I felt like my living or dying would matter to anyone. Because I'm 92 now, I guess even God doesn't want me. Couldn't you do something to put me out of my misery?"*

*NANDA-approved nursing diagnosis label.

available and is unable to mobilize energy on own behalf

- Readiness for Enhanced Spiritual Well-Being: Ability to experience and integrate meaning and purpose in life through connectedness with self, others, art, music, literature, nature, or a power greater than oneself
- Impaired Religiosity (or Risk for Impaired Religiosity): Impaired ability to exercise reliance on beliefs and/or participate in rituals of a particular faith tradition
- Readiness for Enhanced Religiosity: Ability to increase reliance on religious beliefs and/or participate in rituals of a particular faith tradition
- **Spiritual Distress** (or Risk for Spiritual Distress): Impaired ability to experience and integrate meaning and purpose in life through one's connectedness with self, others, art, music, literature, nature, or a power greater than oneself

Spiritual distress may be further specified as spiritual pain, alienation, anxiety, guilt, anger, loss, or despair (O'Brien, 1982). Common etiologies for spiritual distress include inability to reconcile a current life situation (e.g., illness, death of loved person, divorce) with spiritual beliefs ("God is all-powerful, all-loving, all-wise, and He cares about me") or separation from the religious community or supports. Sample nursing diagnoses of spiritual distress are presented in Examples of NANDA-I Nursing Diagnoses.

Spiritual distress may affect other areas of human functioning. In the following nursing diagnoses, spiritual distress is the etiology of another problem.

- Impaired Adjustment to Illness related to inability to reconcile illness with spiritual beliefs
- Ineffective Individual Coping related to loss of religion as primary support (feels abandoned by God/higher power)
- Fear related to feeling unprepared for death and afterlife experience
- Dysfunctional Grieving: Despair related to belief that religion is meaningless
- Hopelessness related to belief that no one cares, including God/higher power
- Powerlessness related to feeling victimized by a tyrannical and arbitrary God/higher power
- Self-Esteem Disturbance related to failure to live according to dictates of religion
- Sexual Dysfunction related to values conflict
- Sleep Pattern Disturbance related to spiritual distress
- Risk for Self-Directed Violence related to feeling that life is meaningless

Outcome Identification and Planning
Enhancing Spiritual Health

Show you value spiritual health by being sensitive to the role that spiritual beliefs play in influencing both a person's thoughts about self and the world and one's interactions with the world. Your interactions with any patient

who values spirituality support the following patient outcomes. The patient will:

- Identify spiritual beliefs that meet needs for meaning and purpose, love and relatedness, and forgiveness
- Derive from these beliefs strength, hope, and comfort when facing the challenge of illness, injury, or other life crisis
- Develop spiritual practices that nurture communion with inner self, with God/higher power, and with the world
- Express satisfaction with the compatibility of spiritual beliefs and everyday living

Addressing Spiritual Distress

Goals and expected outcomes for patients in spiritual distress need to be individualized and may include a patient achieving some of the following:

- Exploring the origin of spiritual beliefs and practices
- Identifying factors in life that challenge spiritual beliefs
- Exploring alternatives given these challenges: denying, modifying, or reaffirming beliefs; developing new beliefs
- Identifying spiritual supports (e.g., spiritual reading, faith, community)
- Reporting or demonstrating a decrease in spiritual distress after successful intervention

Implementing Spiritual Care

A variety of interventions are available to help patients meet their spiritual needs. Like other nursing skills, these interventions need to be practiced before they can be used confidently, competently, and at the right moment. These interventions can be used in the home, hospital, or care center to help patients meet their spiritual needs. See Examples of Nursing Interventions and Nursing Outcomes Classifications (NIC/NOC) (on page 1716) for a list of selected spiritual support activities. When implementing spiritual care, nurses work closely with other spiritual caregivers, including chaplains and pastoral care workers. Often the most important intervention is a well-timed referral to a professional spiritual caregiver. Figure 45-4 (on page 1716) illustrates an inpatient spiritual care implementation model.

Ethical and Professional Boundaries

Before exploring spiritual care strategies, remind yourself of the importance of discussing spiritual concerns in a respectful manner and as directed by patients. While the earlier Figure 45-2 (on page 1703) shows the importance of religion to many Americans, it is also true that religion means very different things to different people. A nurse's offer to pray for a patient may be received gratefully by one and dismissed angrily by another who associates prayer with a "last resort" intervention when everything else has failed. The fact that some health care professionals confuse spiritual care with proselytizing (trying to convert others to one's own religion) is another source of concern.

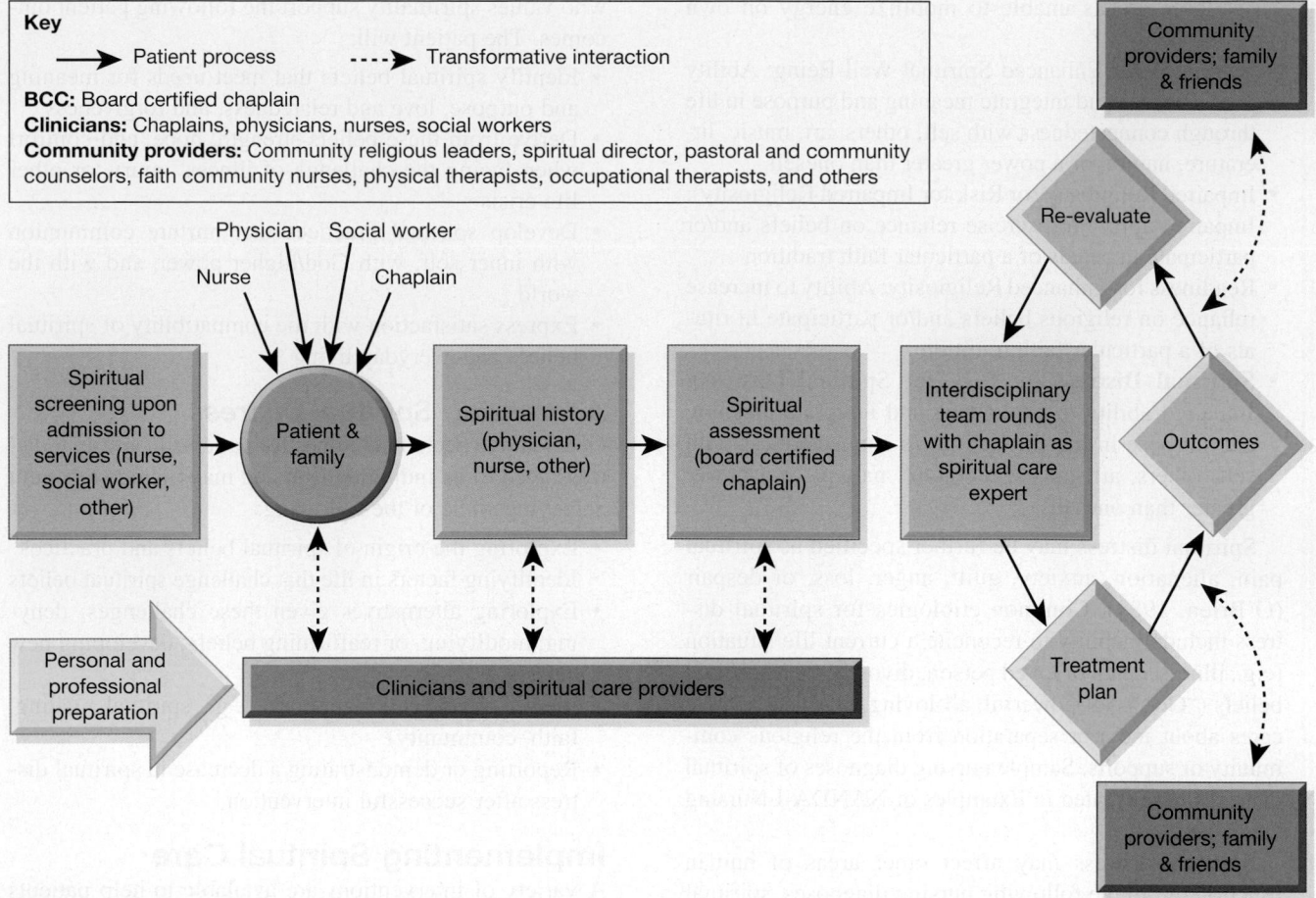

FIGURE 45-4. Inpatient spiritual care implementation model. (Reprinted with permission from Puchalski, C., Ferrell, B., Virani, R., Otis-Green, S., Baird, P., Bull, J., Chochinov, H.,...Sulmasy, D. [2009]. Improving the quality of spiritual care as a dimension of palliative care: The report of the consensus conference. *Journal of Palliative Medicine, 12*[10], 885–904.)

EXAMPLES OF NURSING INTERVENTIONS AND NURSING OUTCOMES CLASSIFICATIONS (NIC/NOC)

SELECTED SPIRITUAL SUPPORT ACTIVITIES

Nursing Interventions	Nursing Outcomes
• Be open to the patient's expressions of loneliness and powerlessness. • Encourage chapel service attendance, if desired. • Encourage use of spiritual resources, if desired. • Refer to the spiritual adviser of the patient's choice. • Use values clarification techniques to help the patient clarify beliefs and values, as appropriate. • Be available to listen to the patient's feelings. • Express empathy with the patient's feelings. • Assure the patient that a nurse will be available to support the patient in times of suffering. • Be open to the patient's feelings about illness and death.	• Quality of faith • Quality of hope • Meaning and purpose in life • Ability to love • Ability to forgive • Ability to worship • Spiritual contentment

Adapted from Bulechek, G. M., Butcher, H. K., Dochterman, J., & Wagner, C. M. (Eds.). (2013). *Nursing interventions classification (NIC)* (6th ed., pp. 352–353). St. Louis: Elsevier/Mosby; and Moorhead, S., Johnson, M., Maas, M. L., & Swanson, E. (2013). *Nursing outcomes classification (NOC)* (5th ed., p. 519). St. Louis: Elsevier/Mosby. A full listing of nursing activities for each nursing intervention and outcomes can be found in these books.

Puchalski (2006) offers the following hints about professional boundaries:

- Keep the spiritual history patient centered.
- Recognize pastoral care professionals as experts in this field and consult them appropriately.
- Proselytizing is never acceptable in professional settings. Addressing spiritual issues should not be coercive.
- More in-depth spiritual counseling should be under the direction of chaplains and other spiritual leaders.
- Praying with patients should not be initiated by the nurse unless there is no pastoral care available and the patient requests it or in situations in which the nurse and patient have a long-standing relationship or share a similar belief system. The nurse can stand in silence as the patient prays in her or his tradition. The nurse can always make a referral to pastoral care for chaplain-led prayer (p. 241).

Offering Supportive or Healing Presence

A nurse's gift of supportive presence must underlie all other types of intervention to meet the patient's spiritual needs. The aim of this intervention is to create a hospitable and sacred space ("holy ground") in which patients can share their vulnerabilities without fear. Supportive presence communicates value and respect (Fig. 45-5).

FIGURE 45-5. The nurse offers supportive presence by holding the patient's hand to show sincere concern, or simply by being present to communicate value and respect.

Chapter 20 presents basic communication skills helpful in establishing this type of presence. Box 45-2 outlines helpful steps for nurses intent on developing the art of healing presence.

The patient who senses that the nurse is sincerely concerned and committed to helping meet human needs is better able to participate in the plan of care. Patients who experience respect and affirmation from other humans find it easier to hold spiritual beliefs that meet their needs

---

BOX 45-2 STEPS FOR BEING A HEALING PRESENCE

Inasmuch as it's more art than science, you'll have your own ways of bringing healing presence into your life and the lives of others. Following is a rough order for how you might proceed.

1. Open Yourself

Begin not with the other person but with you. Become present to yourself in a way that is honest, insightful, and accepting. Open to your uniqueness, humanness, prejudices, brokenness, and wholeness. Do this by owning your life story, continually fathoming who you are in a holistic manner, and developing or utilizing a support system to which you hold yourself accountable.

2. Intend to Be a Healing Presence

Aware that healing presence doesn't just occur out of the blue, you intentionally decide to be such a presence with another. Intend to promote healing in its many forms, while being understanding of yourself as you emerge in the day-to-day intricacies of this practice.

3. Prepare a Space for Healing Presence to Take Place

Clear a space to interact with the other or others, assuring as much privacy as possible and creating an atmosphere of calm. Prepare a space also within by placing yourself out of the way and clearing away your personal expectations for what the other should be or do.

4. Honor the One in Your Care

Approach those you accompany as people with dignity and worth. Show your regard for them by honoring their individuality, equality, humanness, separateness, and sacredness. Respect their natural and unique healing capacity.

5. Offer What You Have to Give

Freely and simply make available what you have to offer, realizing it is up to the other or others to accept or not. Offer presence, loving acceptance, empathy, dependability, an unselfish focus on them, your firm belief in them, your willingness to follow their lead, and, as much as anything, hope.

6. Receive the Gifts that Come

Accept with a grateful heart what is yours to receive. This may include living your life more fully as a result of this practice. Other gifts may include uncovering your genuine self, enjoying wonderful relationships, finding personal satisfaction, realizing you have made a difference, receiving your own healing, and exploring some of life's most valuable lessons.

7. Live a Life of Wholeness and Balance

There is more to life than being a healing presence. So, live your days fully, caring for your own needs, setting appropriate boundaries, encouraging your own growth, and nurturing a loving attitude toward life, including the sacred dimension. Affirm and live out the truth of the transforming potential of healing presence. Be grateful for the possibilities.

Reprinted with permission from Miller, J. E., & Cutshall, S. C. (2001). *The art of being a healing presence: A guide for those in caring relationships.* Fort Wayne, IN: Willogreen Publishing.

for meaning and purpose, love and relatedness, and forgiveness.

Facilitating the Practice of Religion

Ways that the nurse can help the patient continue normal spiritual practices in the unfamiliar environment of the hospital or care center are as follows:

- Familiarize the patient with the pastoral and religious services and materials available within the institution.
- Respect the patient's need for privacy or quiet during periods of prayer.
- Assist the patient to obtain devotional objects and protect them from loss or damage.
- Arrange for the patient wishing to receive the sacraments to do so.
- Attempt to meet the patient's religious dietary restrictions.
- Arrange for the patient's minister, priest, or rabbi to visit if the patient so wishes.

If the patient has a conflict between spiritual beliefs and the proposed medical therapy, assist the patient in discussing this with the physician. For ill patients in the home who cannot attend services or meetings to which they are accustomed, help them find ways to meet their spiritual needs.

Nurturing Spirituality

Some patients who experience a need to get in touch with their spiritual self and to nurture their spiritual development look to the nurse for direction. Someone who lives life enmeshed in the action and noises of society may feel strangely uncomfortable when illness forces introspection. Be helpful by recommending means to develop a relationship with one's inner world (prayer, reflection, dream analysis, nature walks, enjoying art) and manifest spiritual energy in one's outer world (loving relationships, compassion, forgiveness, joy, service).

Spiritual nurturing for the patient's family caregiver(s) also is important. Recent research findings support the importance and value of caregivers' spirituality, yet this resource is often overlooked. Consider using interventions that enhance a caregiver's ability to take part in church activities to satisfy spiritual needs and to work with church groups to secure helpful services. Using clergy, prayer, forgiveness, and spiritual reading materials as resources for caregivers may also be helpful.

 KNOWLEDGE of the supportive services provided by the church group of Mrs. Zeuner, the 75-year-old woman taking care of her husband with advanced Alzheimer disease, would be important to include in the plan of care for Mrs. Zeuner and her husband. Supportive services, such as respite care, parish nursing, and meals, in addition to the emotional support provided by the group, could be extremely helpful for Mrs. Zeuner in her role as caregiver. ●

Finally, remember that, as nurses, we cannot give what we don't have. Unless our own spiritual needs are met, we will never be able to be truly present to another. Thus, the art of being a healing presence requires a lifestyle that supports our being a healing presence. Reflect on this proverb: *A happy heart is like good medicine. But a broken spirit drains your strength (dries your bones).* —*Proverbs 17:22*

The nurse can help patients to nurture their own spirituality by promoting meaning and purpose, promoting love and relatedness, and promoting forgiveness.

PROMOTING MEANING AND PURPOSE

In the book *Man's Search for Meaning,* psychiatrist Victor Frankl, who survived the horrors of the Nazi concentration camps, writes, "Once an individual's search for meaning is successful, it not only renders him happy, but also gives him the capability to cope with suffering" (1985, p. 163). To help patients searching for meaning, explore with them what has given their life meaning and purpose up to the present, sources of meaning for other people, and possible meanings for patients' current experience of illness, pain, suffering, or impending death. If a patient desires, arrange for referral to a spiritual adviser. Explore with patients spiritual practices that may give them strength and hope (e.g., prayer or reading scripture or other spiritual books). You might also want to recommend that patients read spiritual biographies or Harold Kuschner's book *When Bad Things Happen to Good People* (1983) or Kathleen Brehony's book *After the Darkest Hour: How Suffering Begins the Journey to Wisdom* (2000). Referring patients to appropriate support groups (e.g., self-help groups for people with stroke, cancer) also is helpful.

PROMOTING LOVE AND RELATEDNESS

First and foremost, always treat the patient with respect, empathy, and genuine caring. Encourage the patient to talk about relationships with others and to identify the origin of any negative beliefs about people. Box 45-3 may be a good starting point for reflection on loving kindness.

BOX 45-3 LOVING KINDNESS MEDITATION

- May you be at peace.
- May your heart remain open.
- May you awaken to the light of your own true nature.
- May you know the power of your higher self.
- May peace of mind be your only goal and forgiveness your only task.
- May you be healed of all pain and hurt.
- May you be a source of healing for others.
- May you know the inner beauty of the person you truly are.
- May you be at peace.

Source unknown.

Encourage conversation about how a patient experiences God or a higher being if that is part of the patient's spiritual beliefs. If appropriate, introduce or reinforce the belief that God is a loving and personal God who is concerned about the patient. Whenever possible, encourage and facilitate visits from the patient's family, friends, and spiritual adviser.

PROMOTING FORGIVENESS

Offer a supportive presence to the patient that demonstrates your acceptance of the patient. Explore with the patient the importance of learning to accept oneself and others, including both strengths and limitations. Explore negative feelings that make it difficult for the patient to seek forgiveness and to believe that one is forgiven.

Explore the patient's self-expectations and assist the patient to determine how realistic these are. Allow the patient to verbalize shame, guilt, and anger, and counsel about the importance of expressing negative emotions in healthy ways. Refer the patient to a spiritual adviser, if appropriate. Offer the patient examples of how not forgiving others can end up hurting only the one who cannot forgive.

Praying With Patients

Patients accustomed to regular periods of prayer but who feel too ill to pray as they would like or who enjoy praying with others may ask the nurse to pray with them or hope that the nurse will suggest this. Because there are many forms of prayer—quiet reflection, silent communion with God or higher power, reading or recitation of formal prayers, silent or loud calling on God or higher power or conversation with God or higher power, lamentations, or reading one's holy book or other religious materials—the nurse can take the lead from the patient by asking, "How would you like us to pray?" Consider the patient's religious background along with the type of prayers that have been meaningful in the past. Ask whether the patient has a particular prayer request.

A nurse unaccustomed to praying aloud or in public may find it helpful to have a Bible passage or formal prayer readily available. The prayer may also be a simple expression aloud of the patient's needs and hopes. A sample follows:

> Lord God, our Creator and Healer, I entrust Mrs. Smith and her family to your loving care. Bring peace to her mind and health and strength to her body. Be with her [as her treatment begins today, as she goes for surgery, and so on]. We remember all your blessings to us in the past and thank you. We are confident of your help now as we claim your promises.

Prayer should not block communication with the patient. Praying before a patient feels ready to pray may communicate to the patient a lack of interest in the patient's feelings. Because prayer often evokes deep feelings, the nurse should be prepared to spend time with the patient after sharing prayer to respond to these feelings.

Praying for Patients

With research suggesting links between prayer and physical, mental, and spiritual health (Levin, 2001), some have argued that health care professionals should pray for, as well as with, their patients. At the present time, no one is claiming that health care professionals are negligent if they fail to pray for patients. Prayer may, however, be an effective intervention strategy. At the very least, nurses ought to be mediators of the spiritual resources patients and their families need.

Counseling Patients Spiritually

The patient who feels that the nurse is sensitive to spiritual needs and comfortable with his or her own spirituality may choose to share spiritual concerns with the nurse rather than with a religious counselor. A nurse who feels competent to counsel the patient may assist the patient to accomplish the following:

- Articulate spiritual beliefs.
- Explore the origin of the patient's spiritual beliefs and practices.
- Identify life factors that challenge the patient's spiritual beliefs (cause spiritual distress).
- Explore alternatives given these challenges: modify lifestyle; deny, modify, or reaffirm beliefs; develop new beliefs.
- Develop spiritual beliefs that meet needs for meaning and purpose, care and relatedness, forgiveness.

To be an effective spiritual counselor, the nurse must be open to different spiritual beliefs and forms of spiritual expression, and should be supportive of the patient's efforts to nurture spiritual growth.

Contacting a Spiritual Counselor

Not every nurse feels comfortable in the role of spiritual counselor. If not, suggest that the patient talk to a pastoral caregiver or spiritual counselor. When a patient expresses a desire to speak to a spiritual counselor, help make the appropriate referral or offer to contact the patient's own spiritual adviser. Other options are to contact the health care facility's pastoral ministry department or use a referral list of clergy in the local community. If no representative of the patient's own religion can visit in the hospital at a particular time, suggest a visit from a member of the clergy from another faith. The patient, depending on the situation and the immediacy of the need, may welcome such a suggestion.

In a health care setting, you can assist the spiritual counselor by making the counselor feel welcome, directing the counselor to the patient, and ensuring that the patient is ready to receive the counselor. Preparations of the patient's room for the visit may vary, but the following are generally recommended practices:

- The room should be orderly and free of unnecessary equipment and items.
- There should be a seat for the religious counselor at the bedside or near the patient so that both can be comfortable.
- The bedside table should be free of items and covered with a clean, white cover if a sacrament is to be administered.
- The bed curtains should be drawn for privacy if the patient can't be moved to a more private setting.

Some patients and spiritual advisers may value the nurse's participation in prayers, rituals, or the administration of sacraments. By having good working relations with chaplains and pastoral caregivers, you can quickly direct them to patients most likely to benefit from their visits.

Resolving Conflicts Between Spiritual Beliefs and Treatments

Both the patient and members of the patient's family may experience conflict between a particular spiritual belief or religious law and a proposed medical treatment or health option. The patient may want assistance when conferring with the spiritual adviser about a particular procedure. The nurse's role is to help the patient obtain the information needed to make an informed decision and to support the patient's decision making. Because what the nurse says and the way it is said may powerfully influence the patient's decision, it is important to maintain objectivity. Conflicts that resist resolution may be referred to an ethics committee or consult team (see Chapter 6).

Nursing, Religion, and Conscientious Objection

In recent years, some pharmacists attracted great media attention by refusing to fill prescriptions for contraceptives. These pharmacists supported their refusals by claiming that fulfilling such a prescription would violate their religious beliefs and convictions. In this situation, the woman's right to access medications is pitted against the pharmacist's right to practice with personal integrity. Nurses can also find themselves in situations in which their professional or institutional responsibilities involve participation in activities such as abortion, assisted suicide, and counseling about birth control, which may violate their personal integrity. Nurses therefore must ensure that they can fulfill the responsibilities of their job or that they are free to exercise the

right of conscientious objection. As legislation addressing these conflicts is in a state of flux, you should be familiar with federal and state guidelines. For example, in September of 2011, the University of Medicine and Dentistry of New Jersey announced that all nurses employed in its hospital would have to help with abortion patients before and after the procedure, "reversing a long-standing policy exempting employees who refuse based on religious or moral objections." After a group of objecting nurses filed a federal lawsuit, the hospital backed down, agreeing that nurses with conscientious objections do not have to assist with pre- or postoperative care for abortions except when the mother's life is threatened and no other nonobjecting staff are available to assist (Galston & Rogers, 2012, p. 1).

Evaluating

The nurse working with a patient and family to achieve specified goals/outcomes to meet spiritual needs evaluates the plan of care in each patient interaction. Necessary to the evaluation are sensitivity to what the patient is saying and not saying and observation of the patient when alone as well as when interacting with the family and nurses.

In general, the nurse evaluates the patient's ability to accomplish the following:

- Identifying some spiritual belief that gives meaning and purpose to everyday life
- Moving toward a healthy acceptance of the current situation: illness, pain, suffering, impending death
- Developing mutually caring relationships
- Reconciling any interpersonal differences causing the patient anguish
- Verbalizing satisfaction with relationship with God/ higher being (if important to the patient)
- Expressing peaceful acceptance of limitations and failings
- Expressing the ability to forgive others and to live in the present
- Demonstrating an "interior state of peace and joy; freedom from abnormal anxiety, guilt, or a feeling of sinfulness; and a sense of security and direction in the pursuit of one's life goals and activities" (O'Brien, 1982, p. 98).

The nurse helps the patient to determine whether one's spiritual beliefs are generally life affirming or life denying and whether there is harmony between these beliefs and the patient's everyday life experiences. See Nursing Plan of Care 45-1 for Mr. Gargan.

NURSING PLAN OF CARE 45-1

for Mr. Gargan

Mr. Gargan is a 38-year-old divorced man on a step-down unit after treatment for a myocardial infarction. He owns a small car dealership. His religion is listed as Protestant. Frequently unable to sleep at night, Mr. Gargan often talks with the night nurse and once asked, "Did you ever give much thought to whether or not there is a God?" Sensing much concern behind this question, the nurse asks specific questions to determine whether the patient has spiritual needs that are not being met.

12/26/15, 2 AM

Patient again unable to sleep and initiated discussion about God. States that he was raised in a Lutheran home where everyone went to church on Sunday and tried to live according to God's commandments. Upon leaving home, he stopped going to church (was never a value for his wife) and simply has not given much thought to religion—too busy running his business. Until now, has not experienced any need for God. "But when I think how close I was to dying and that I've no idea what to expect after death—I'm actually scared. Do others feel this way?" Wants to explore religious beliefs—feels lack in his life. Said he would like to talk with hospital minister—will arrange for tomorrow.

E. Nolan, RN

NURSING DIAGNOSIS	Spiritual Distress: Anxiety related to concerns about relationship with God as manifested by self-report
EXPECTED OUTCOME	Before discharge, the patient will: • Identify his religious beliefs

NURSING INTERVENTIONS	RATIONALE	EVALUATIVE STATEMENT
Assist the patient to (1) identify the spiritual beliefs he had as a child and the origin of these beliefs, (2) evaluate these beliefs in terms of his life experiences, and (3) reaffirm, modify, or reject these beliefs or develop new spiritual beliefs.	Life experiences may challenge religious beliefs that were uncritically held as a child.	12/30/15 Outcome partially met. Patient states he has a much clearer concept of God and no longer fears that God will reject him for ignoring him for so long . . . but believes he also has a lot to learn. *E. Nolan, RN*
Assist the patient to assess whether his newly articulated spiritual beliefs are life affirming or life denying and the degree to which they meet his needs for meaning and purpose, love and relatedness, and forgiveness.	Because spiritual beliefs can exert positive (life-affirming) and negative (life-denying) influences on a person's life, individuals should have some criteria to use when evaluating their beliefs.	
Refer the patient to the hospital minister for assistance with the problem.	Patient may value speaking with a minister.	

EXPECTED OUTCOME	Before discharge, the patient will: • Reconcile his life up until the present with God

(continued)

NURSING PLAN OF CARE 45-1 *continued*

for Mr. Gargan

NURSING INTERVENTIONS	RATIONALE	EVALUATIVE STATEMENT
Reassure the patient that many people get involved in day-to-day living to the extent that they forget about God, and that in some religions, people believe that God uses illness and other stressors to invite people to rethink their spiritual beliefs. In these traditions, God is often pictured with open arms waiting to welcome a child home.	Images of a stern and unyielding God ready to strike down transgressors may contribute to a patient's spiritual distress.	12/30/15 Outcome met. "This minister has really helped. I wish I had talked to him a long time ago. I've carried so much guilt about my divorce and some other things—thought God would never forgive me. I feel so much more at peace now."
Refer the patient to a spiritual advisor for help in experiencing forgiveness if he mentions guilt feelings.	Guilt often inhibits people from seeking and experiencing the forgiveness they desire.	*E. Nolan, RN*
Communicate to the patient the importance of people accepting themselves—with all their strengths and weaknesses.	Many people have unrealistic self-expectations.	

EXPECTED OUTCOME Before discharge, the patient will:

- Verbalize that his spiritual beliefs have become a source of strength and peace rather than anxiety

NURSING INTERVENTIONS	RATIONALE	EVALUATIVE STATEMENT
Encourage the patient to compare the role of spiritual beliefs in his life before, during, and after hospitalization.	This highlights the positive and negative roles spiritual beliefs can play. It may motivate the patient to continue searching if he values his present experience.	12/30/15 Outcome met. "It's good to be able to feel more peaceful about whatever the future brings. I'm anxious to get out of here because there's a lot I want to do with God's help."
		E. Nolan, RN

EXPECTED OUTCOME Before discharge, the patient will:

- Increase night sleep to at least 6 undisturbed hours

NURSING INTERVENTIONS	RATIONALE	EVALUATIVE STATEMENT
Nurse on the 1-to-7 shift checks on the patient at the beginning of the shift to make sure he is comfortable and ready for sleep.	Nursing supervision of the patient at bedtime rules out other factors that may interfere with sleep.	12/30/15 Outcome met. Patient slept last night from midnight to 6 AM. Will continue to monitor.
		E. Nolan, RN

NURSING PLAN OF CARE 45-1 *continued*

for Mr. Gargan

NURSING INTERVENTIONS	RATIONALE	EVALUATIVE STATEMENT
Use power of suggestion to enhance sleep: *"I'm sure when I check back you'll be sound asleep."*	Suggestion has been shown to enhance the therapeutic effect of other interventions.	
If sleep remains disturbed, try relaxation exercises or guided imagery (see Chapter 41).	As spiritual anxiety decreases, sleep should improve. If sleep does not improve, other contributing factors and interventions will need to be explored.	

SAMPLE DOCUMENTATION

12/27/15, 3 PM, nursing
B. Hanks, Protestant minister, here to see patient at 1 PM. Afterward, patient said he felt "a whole lot better." Reported minister had assured him that many people in the hospital with a serious illness go through exactly what he is experiencing now—this thought seemed to decrease much of his anxiety. Minister had reinforced nurse's suggestion that he explore his religious beliefs and he has already jotted down some thoughts. "I knew you fixed bodies in hospitals but didn't know you fix souls, too." Patient looking forward to minister's visit tomorrow.

E. Nolan, RN

DEVELOPING CLINICAL REASONING

1. Assess your spiritual well-being. To what extent are you able to meet your needs for love and belonging, meaning and purpose, and forgiveness? If confronted with a life-threatening or chronic illness, would you be able to draw on religion or spirituality as a source of strength? Do you believe you need any special skills to develop to better meet the spiritual needs of your patients? Compare your responses to those of your classmates and explore reasons for differences.

2. Poll your classmates and see if they agree strongly, agree, disagree, or disagree strongly with the following statements. Discuss reasons for the differences in your answers and how this is likely to affect your professional practice:
   • Prayer has the power to heal physical, mental, and spiritual illness.
   • Nurses who do not pray for their patients are deficient professional caregivers.
   • Nurses who do not offer to pray with their patients are deficient professional caregivers.

3. How would you respond to a patient who tells you that he isn't very religious but is now wondering if there is a God, and if so, wonders where he stands in relation to God now that his life is in jeopardy? Think about how your personal experience of religion/spirituality colors your response, and determine whether your personal experience of religion/spirituality has prepared you well to respond to these queries.

PRACTICING FOR NCLEX

1. A hospice nurse is caring for a patient who is dying of pancreatic cancer. The patient tells the nurse "I feel no connection to God" and "I'm worried that I find no real meaning in life." What would be the nurse's best response to this patient?
   a. Give the patient a hug and tell him that his life still has meaning.
   b. Arrange for a spiritual adviser to visit the patient.
   c. Ask if the patient would like to talk about his feelings.
   d. Call in a close friend or relative to talk to the patient.

2. A nurse who was raised as a strict Roman Catholic stated she couldn't assist patients with their spiritual distress because she recognizes only a "field power" in each person. She said, "My parents and I hardly talk because I've deserted my faith. Sometimes I feel real isolated from them and also God—if there is a God." Analysis of these data reveals which unmet spiritual need?
   a. Need for meaning and purpose
   b. Need for forgiveness
   c. Need for love and relatedness
   d. Need for strength for everyday living

3. A nurse is performing spirituality assessments of patients living in a long-term care facility. What is the best question to assess for spiritual needs?
   a. Can you describe your usual spiritual practices and how you maintain them daily?
   b. Are your spiritual beliefs causing you any concern?
   c. How can I and the other nurses help you maintain your spiritual practices?
   d. How do your religious beliefs help you to feel at peace?

4. A patient whose last name is Goldstein was served a kosher meal ordered from a restaurant on a paper plate because the hospital made no provision for kosher food or dishes. Mr. Goldstein became angry and accused the nurse of insulting him: "I want to eat what everyone else does—and give me decent dishes." Analysis of these data reveals what finding?
   a. The nurse should have ordered kosher dishes also.
   b. The staff must have behaved condescendingly or critically.
   c. Mr. Goldstein is a problem patient and difficult to satisfy.
   d. Mr. Goldstein was stereotyped and not consulted about his dietary preferences.

5. A nurse working in an emergency department assesses how patients' religious beliefs affect their treatment plan. With which patient would the nurse be most likely to encounter resistance to emergency lifesaving surgery?
   a. A patient of the Adventist faith
   b. A patient who practices Buddhism
   c. A patient who is a Jehovah's Witness
   d. A patient who is an Orthodox Jew

6. The Roman Catholic family of a baby who was born with hydroencephalitis requests a baptism for their infant. Why is it imperative that the nurse provide for baptism to be performed?
   a. Baptism frequently postpones or prevents death or suffering.
   b. It is legally required that nurses provide for this care when the family makes this request.
   c. It is a nursing function to assure the salvation of the baby.
   d. Lack of baptism when desired may increase the family's sorrow and suffering.

7. A nurse is formulating diagnoses for patients in a hospice program who are experiencing spiritual distress. In which diagnoses is spiritual distress the etiology of another problem? Select all that apply.
   a. Ineffective Individual Coping related to loss of religion as a major support in life
   b. Powerlessness related to feeling unprepared for death and the afterlife experience
   c. Self-Esteem Disturbance related to failure to reconcile illness with spiritual beliefs
   d. Risk for Impaired Religiosity related to inability to attend church as usual
   e. Spiritual Distress related to fear of dying alone
   f. Impaired Religiosity related to inability to exercise reliance on spiritual beliefs

8. A nurse who is caring for patients on a pediatric ward is assessing the children for their spiritual needs. Which is the most important source of learning for a child's own spirituality?
   a. The child's church or religious organization
   b. What parents say about God and religion
   c. How parents behave in relationship to one another and their children, to others, and to God
   d. The spiritual adviser for the family

9. Even though the nurse performs a detailed nursing history in which spirituality is assessed on admission, problems with spiritual distress may not surface until days after admission. What is the probable explanation?
   a. Patients usually want to conceal information about their spiritual needs.
   b. Patients are not concerned about spiritual needs until after their spiritual adviser visits.

   c. Family members and close friends often initiate spiritual concerns.
   d. Illness increases spiritual concerns, which may be difficult for patients to express in words.

10. A nurse who is comfortable with one's own spirituality is caring for patients who need spiritual counseling. Which nursing action would be most appropriate for these patients?
    a. Calling the patient's own spiritual adviser first
    b. Asking whether the patient has a spiritual adviser the patient wishes to consult
    c. Attempting to counsel the patient and, if unsuccessful, making a referral to a spiritual adviser
    d. Advising the patient and spiritual adviser concerning health options and the best choices for the patient

11. A nurse performing a spiritual assessment collects assessment data from a patient who is homebound and unable to participate in religious activities. Which NANDA-I–approved diagnostic label would the nurse use when assessment data point to a spiritual problem that can be treated by independent nursing intervention?
    a. Spiritual Alienation
    b. Spiritual Despair
    c. Spiritual Distress
    d. Spiritual Pain

12. A patient states she feels so isolated from her family and church, and even God "in this huge medical center so far from home." A nurse is preparing nursing goals for this patient. Which is the best goal for the patient to relieve her spiritual distress?
    a. The patient will express satisfaction with the compatibility of her spiritual beliefs and everyday living.
    b. The patient will identify spiritual beliefs that meet her need for meaning and purpose.
    c. The patient will express peaceful acceptance of limitations and failings.
    d. The patient will identify spiritual supports available to her in this medical center.

13. A man who is a declared agnostic is extremely depressed after losing his home, his wife, and his children in a fire. His nursing diagnosis is Spiritual Distress: Spiritual Pain related to inability to find meaning and purpose in his current condition. What is the most important nursing intervention to plan?
    a. Ask the patient which spiritual adviser he would like you to call.
    b. Recommend that the patient read spiritual biographies or religious books.
    c. Explore with the patient what, in addition to his family, has given his life meaning and purpose in the past.
    d. Introduce the belief that God is a loving and personal God.

14. After having an abortion, a patient tells the visiting nurse, "I shouldn't have had that abortion because I'm Catholic, but what else could I do? I'm afraid I'll never get close to my mother or back in the Church again." She then talks with her priest about this feeling of guilt. Which evaluation statement shows a solution to the problem?
    a. Patient states, "I wish I had talked with the priest sooner. I now know God has forgiven me, and even my mother understands."
    b. Patient has slept from 10 PM to 6 AM for three consecutive nights without medication.

c. Patient has developed mutually caring relationships with two women and one man.

d. Patient has identified several spiritual beliefs that give purpose to her life.

15. Mr. Brown's teenage daughter had been involved in shoplifting. He expresses much anger toward her and states he can not face her, let alone discuss this with her: "I just will not tolerate a thief." Which nursing intervention would the nurse take to assist Mr. Brown with his deficit in forgiveness?

a. Assure him that many parents feel the same way.

b. Reassure him that many teenagers go through this kind of rebellion and that it will pass.

c. Assist the patient to identify how unforgiving feelings toward others hurt the one who cannot forgive.

d. Ask him if he is sure he has spent sufficient time with his daughter.

ANSWERS WITH RATIONALES

1. *c.* When caring for a patient who is in spiritual distress, the nurse should listen to the patient first and then ask whether the patient would like to visit with a spiritual adviser. To arrange for a spiritual adviser first may not respect the wishes of the patient. A hug and false reassurances do not address the diagnosis of spiritual distress. Talking to friends or relatives may be helpful, but only if the patient desires their visits.

2. *c.* The data point to an unmet spiritual need to experience love and belonging given her estrangement from her family and God after leaving the church. The other options may represent other needs this nurse has, but the data provided do not support them.

3. *c.* Questioning how the staff can meet patients' spiritual practices assesses spiritual needs. Asking the patient to describe spiritual practices assesses spiritual practices. Asking about concerns assesses spiritual distress, and asking about feeling at peace assesses the need for forgiveness.

4. *d.* On the basis of his name alone, the nurse jumped to the premature and false conclusion that this patient would want a kosher diet.

5. *c.* Patients who practice the Jehovah's Witness faith believe blood transfusions violate God's laws and do not allow them. The other religious groups do not restrict modern lifesaving treatment for their members.

6. *d.* Failure to ensure that an infant baptism is performed when parents desire it may greatly increase the family's sorrow and suffering, which is an appropriate nursing concern. Whether baptism postpones or prevents death and suffering is a religious belief that is insufficient to bind all nurses. There is no legal requirement regarding baptism, and although some nurses may believe part of their role is to ensure the salvation of the baby, this function would understandably be rejected by many.

7. *a, b, c.* Spiritual distress may affect other areas of human functioning. In the first three nursing diagnoses, spiritual distress is the etiology of another problem. In the last three diagnoses, spiritual distress is the problem.

8. *c.* Children learn most about their own spirituality from how their parents behave in relationship to one another, their children, others, and God/higher being. The remaining three options are less important sources of learning.

9. *d.* Illness may increase spiritual concerns, which many patients find difficult to express. The other options do not correspond to actual experience.

10. *b.* Even when a nurse feels comfortable discussing spiritual concerns, the nurse should always check first with patients to determine whether they have a spiritual adviser to consult. Calling the patient's own spiritual adviser (answer *a*) may be premature if it is a matter the nurse can handle. Answers *c* and *d* deny patients the right to speak privately with their spiritual adviser from the outset, if this is what they prefer.

11. *c.* The only NANDA-I–approved nursing diagnosis among the options is Spiritual Distress. The other options may be further specifications of the broader diagnosis Spiritual Distress.

12. *d.* Each of the four options represents appropriate spiritual goals, but identifying spiritual supports available to her in the medical center demonstrates a goal to decrease her sense of isolation.

13. *c.* The nursing intervention of exploring with the patient what, in addition to his family, has given his life meaning and purpose in the past is more likely to correct the etiology of his problem, Spiritual Pain, than any of the other nursing interventions listed.

14. *a.* Because this patient's nursing diagnosis is Spiritual Distress: Guilt, an evaluative statement that demonstrates diminished guilt is necessary. Only answer *a* directly deals with guilt.

15. *c.* This is the only nursing intervention that directly addresses the patient's unmet spiritual need concerning forgiveness. Answers *a* and *b* may make him feel better initially, but neither addresses his need to forgive. Answer *d* is likely to make him feel guilty.

TAYLOR SUITE RESOURCES

Explore these additional resources to enhance learning for this chapter:

- NCLEX-Style Questions and other resources on thePoint, http://thePoint.lww.com/Taylor8e
- *Study Guide for Fundamentals of Nursing, 8th edition*
- Adaptive Learning | Powered by prepU, http://thepoint.lww.com/prepu

Bibliography

American Nurses Association (ANA). *Faith community nursing: Scope and standards.* Silver Spring, MD: Author.

Anandarajah, G., & Hight, E. (2001). Spirituality and medical practice: Using the HOPE questions as a practical tool for spiritual assessment. *American Family Physician, 63,* 81–89.

Balboni, T., Vanderwerker, L. C., Block, S. D., Paulk, E., Lathan, C. S., Peteet, J. R., & Prigerson, H. G. (2007). Religiousness and spiritual support among advanced cancer patients and associations with end-of-life treatment preferences and quality of life. *Journal of Clinical Oncology, 25*(5), 555–560.

Bephage, G. (2008). Care approaches to spirituality and dementia. *Nursing & Residential Care, 10*(3), 134–137.

Brehony, K. (2000). *After the darkest hour: How suffering begins the journey to wisdom.* New York: Henry Holt and Company.

Bulechek, G. M., Butcher, H. K., Dochterman, J. & Wagner, C. M. (Eds.). (2013). *Nursing interventions classification (NIC)* (6th ed.). St. Louis: Elsevier/Mosby.

Borneman T, Ferrell BR, Puchalski CM. Evaluation of the FICA tool for spiritual assessment. *Journal of Pain & Symptom Management.* 2012;40(2):163–173.

Burghardt, M., & Nagai-Jacobson, M. G., (1997). In B. M. Dossey (Ed.): *Core curriculum for holistic nursing*. New York: Aspen Publishers.

Callahan, D., & Campbell, C. S. (Eds.). (1990). Theology, religious traditions, and bioethics: A special supplement. *Hastings Center Report, 20*(6), 18–19.

Carol, J. (2002). What is healing? *Sacred Journey, 53*(4), 12–17.

Carson, V. B. (1989). *Spiritual dimensions of nursing practice*. Philadelphia: W. B. Saunders.

Carson, V. B., & Koenig, H. G. (2004). *Spiritual caregiving. Healthcare as a ministry*. Chicago: Templeton Foundation Press.

Cobb, M. R., Puchalski, C. M., & Rumbold, B. R. (2012). *Spirituality in healthcare*. New York: Oxford University Press.

Coles, R. (1990). *The spiritual life of children*. Boston: Houghton Mifflin.

Creen, T. (2002). Enabling hope in the terminally ill. In R. C. Anderson et al. (Eds.). *Palliative care patient and family counseling manual* (2nd ed., pp. 16–17). New York: Aspen Publishers.

Davis, D. S., & Zoloth, L. (1999). *Notes from a narrow ridge: Religion and bioethics*. Hagerstown, MD: University Publishing Group.

Dossey, B. (Ed.). (1989). Spirituality and healing. *Holistic Nursing Practice, 3*(3), entire issue.

Fawcett, T., & Noble, A. (2004). The challenge of spiritual care in a multi-faith society experienced as a Christian nurse. *Journal of Clinical Nursing, 13*(2), 136–142.

Ferrell, B. R., & Munevar, C. (2012). Domain of spiritual care. *Progress in Palliative Care, 20*(2), 66–71.

Fowler, J. W. (1981). *Stages of faith: The psychology of human development and the quest for meaning*. San Francisco: Harper & Row.

Frankl, V. (1985). *Man's search for meaning*. New York: Washington Square Press.

Galston, W. A. & Rogers, M. (2012). Health care providers' consciences and patients' needs: The quest for balance. Governance Studies at Brookings. Available at http://www.brookings.edu/~/media/research/files/papers/2012/2/23%20health%20care%20galston%20rogers/0223_health_care_galston_rogers.pdf

Golberg, B. (1998). Connection: An exploration of spirituality in nursing care. *Journal of Advanced Nursing, 27*, 836–842.

Gregg-Schroeder, S. (1999). A transforming experience: Circles of Life. *Journal of Fellowship in Prayer*, 23–25.

Hauerwas, S. (1990). *Naming the silences: God, medicine, and the problem of suffering*. Grand Rapids: Erdmans.

Heller, D. (1985). The children's God. *Psychology Today, 19*(12), 22–27.

Hickman, J. S. (2006). *Faith community nursing*. Philadelphia: Wolters Kluwer Health/Lippincott Williams & Wilkins.

Hui, D., de la Cruz, M., Thorney, S., Parsons, H. A., Delgado-Guay, M., & Bruera, E. (2011). The frequency and correlates of spiritual distress among patients with advanced cancer admitted to an acute palliative care unit. *American Journal of Hospice & Palliative Medicine, 28*(4), 264–270.

The Joint Commission. (2008). Spiritual Assessment. In Standard FAQ Details. Available at: http://www.jointcommission.org/mobile/standards_information/jcfaqdetails.aspx?StandardsFAQId=290&StandardsFAQChapterId=29

Kirkham, S. R., Pesut, B., Meyerhoff, H., & Sawatzky, R. (2004). Spiritual caregiving at the juncture of religion, culture, and state. *Canadian Journal of Nursing Research, 36*(4), 148–169.

Koenig, H. G. (2002). *Spirituality in patient care. Why, how, when and what*. Chicago: Templeton Foundation Press.

Koenig, H. G., Lawson, D. M., & McConnell, M. (2005). *Faith in the future. Healthcare, aging and the role of religion*. Chicago: Templeton Foundation Press.

Koss-Chioino, J. D., & Hefner, P. (2006). *Spiritual transformation and healing*. Lanham, MD: Altimira Press.

Kuschner, H. S. (1983). *When bad things happen to good people*. New York: Avon.

Lazenby, M., McCorkle, R., & Sulmasy, D. (2014) *Decisions at the end of life: A spiritual sourcebook*. New York: Oxford University Press.

Levin, J. (2001). *God, faith, and health: Exploring the spirituality–healing connection*. New York: John Wiley and Sons.

Lo, B., Ruston, D., Kates, L. W., Arnold, R. M., Cohen, C. B., Faber-Langendoen, K., Pantilat, S. Z., Puchalski, ... Tulsky, J. A. (2002). Discussing religious and spiritual issues at the end of life. *Journal of the American Medical Association, 287*(6), 749–754.

Macrae, J. (1995). Nightingale's spiritual philosophy and its significance for modern nursing. *Image: The Journal of Nursing Scholarship, 27*(1), 8–10.

Miller, J. E., & Cutshall, S. C. (2001). *The art of being a healing presence: A guide for those in caring relationships*. Fort Wayne, IN: Willowgreen Publishing.

Moorhead, S., Johnson, M., Maas, M. L., & Swanson, E. (2013). *Nursing outcomes classification (NOC)* (5th ed.). St. Louis: Elsevier/Mosby.

Moorhead, S., Johnson, M., Maas, M. L., & Swanson, E. (2008). *Nursing outcomes classification (NOC)* (4th ed.). St. Louis: Elsevier/Mosby.

Murray, R. P. (2010). Spiritual care beliefs and practices of special care and oncology RNs at patients' end of life. *Journal of Hospice and Palliative Nursing, 12*(1):51–58.

NANDA International (NANDA-I). (2012). *Nursing diagnoses: Definitions & classification 2012–2014*. West Sussex, UK: Wiley-Blackwell.

Narayanasamy, A., Clissett, P., Parumal, L., Thompson, D., Annasamy, S., & Edge, R. (2004). Responses to the spiritual needs of older people. *Journal of Advanced Nursing, 48*(1), 6–16.

Narayanasamy, A., & Narayanasamy, M. (2008). The healing power of prayer and its implications for nursing. *British Journal of Nursing, 17*(6), 394–398.

National Consensus Project for Quality Palliative Care. (2013). *Clinical practice guidelines for quality palliative care* (3rd ed.). Available at http://www.nationalconsensusproject.org/Guidelines_Download2.aspx

O'Brien, M. E. (1982). The need for spiritual integrity. In H. Yura & M. Walsh (Eds.), *Human needs and the nursing process* (pp. 81–115). Norwalk, CT: Appleton-Century-Crofts.

O'Brien, M. E. (1999). *Spirituality in nursing*. Boston: Jones and Bartlett.

O'Brien, M. E. (2001). *The nurse's calling*. New York: Paulist Press.

O'Brien, M. E. (2003). *Parish nursing: Healthcare ministry within the church*. Boston: Jones and Bartlett.

O'Brien, M. E. (2007). *A sacred covenant: The spiritual ministry of healing*. Sudbury, MA: Jones and Bartlett.

Pew Forum on Religion & Public Life. (2012). The U.S. landmark religion survey. Available at http://religions.pewforum.org/pdf/report2religious-landscape-study-key-findings.pdf

Puchalski, C., Ferrell, B., Virani, R., Otis-Green, S., Baird, P., Bull, J., Chochinov, H.,...Sulmasy, D. (2009). Improving the quality of spiritual care as a dimension of palliative care: The report of the consensus conference. *Journal of Palliative Medicine, 12*(10), 885–904.

Puchalski, C., & Romer, A. L. (2000). Taking a spiritual history allows clinicians to understand patients more fully. *Journal of Palliative Medicine, 3*(1), 129–137.

Puchalski, C. M., & Ferrell, B. R. (2010). *Making healthcare whole: Integrating spirituality into patient care*. West Conshohocken, PA: Templeton Press.

Puchalski, D. M. (2006). *A time for listening and caring: Spirituality and the care of the chronically ill and dying*. New York: Oxford University Press.

Quinn, A. (2002). Spirituality and the family: What religion should I be? *Sacred Journey, 53*(4), 12–17.

Rahner, K. (1971). How to receive a sacrament and mean it. *Theology Digest, 19*, 229.

Shelly, J., & Fish, S. (1988). *Spiritual care: The nurse's role* (3rd ed.). Downer's Grove, IL: InterVarsity Press.

Smith, B. W., Ortiz, J. A., Wiggins, K. T., Bernard, J. F., & Dalen, J. (2012). *The Oxford Handbook of Psychology and Spirituality*. New York: Oxford University Press.

Sulmasy, D. P. (2006). *The rebirth of the clinic: An introduction to spirituality in health care*. Washington, DC: Georgetown University Press.

Sweat, M. T. (2005). FAQs in spiritual care. How does spiritual care begin? *Journal of Christian Nursing, 22*(2), 42.

Taylor, E. J. (2007). *What do I say? Talking with patients about spirituality*. Chicago: Templeton Foundation Press.

Taylor, C. (2012). Rethinking hopelessness and the role of spiritual care when cure is no longer an option. *Journal of Pain and Symptom Management, 44*(4), 626–630.

Walker, S., & Taylor, C. (2012). Compassion and healthcare: Luxury or necessity? In M. Cobb, B. Rumbold, and C. Puchalski (Eds.). *Spirituality in Health Care* (pp. 135–143). Oxford: Oxford University Press.

Winslow, G. R., & Winslow, B. W. (2003). Examining the ethics of praying with patients. *Holistic Nursing Practice, 17*(4), 170–178.

Glossary

A

Abduction: lateral movement of the body part away from the midline of the body

Absorption: process by which drugs are transferred from the site of entry into the body to the bloodstream

Abstinence: refraining from having sex

Accommodation: (1) ability to adjust the eye to see at various distances; (2) process by which intellectual acts are changed to handle increasingly complex information

Accreditation: process by which an educational program is evaluated and then recognized as having met certain predetermined standards of education

Acid: substance containing a hydrogen ion that can be liberated or released

Acidosis: condition characterized by a proportionate excess of hydrogen ions in the extracellular fluid, in which the pH falls below 7.35

Acquired immunodeficiency syndrome (AIDS): condition in which the body's immune system is rendered ineffective as a result of infection by the retrovirus HIV

Active euthanasia: someone other than the patient commits an action with the intent to end the patient's life, for example, injecting the patient with a lethal dose of a drug

Active exercise: joint movement activated by the person

Active immunity: antibodies against harmful effects of microorganisms or toxins that are self-produced

Active transport: movement of ions or molecules across cell membranes, usually against a pressure gradient and with the expenditure of metabolic energy

Activities of daily living: self-care activities such as eating, bathing, dressing, and toileting

Actual loss: loss that can be recognized by others as well as by the person sustaining the loss, such as loss of a limb or a spouse

Actual nursing diagnoses: problems validated by the presence of major defining characteristics and possessing four components: label, definition, defining characteristics, and related factor

Actual problems: health problems that have been validated by the presence of major defining characteristics

Acupuncture: procedure consisting of placing very thin, short, sterile needles at particular acupoints, believed to be centers of nerve and vascular tissue, along a meridian to either increase or decrease the flow of chi along the meridian, restoring the balance of yin and yang, and thereby contributing to healing

Acute illness: rapidly occurring illness that runs its course, allowing a person to return to one's previous level of functioning

Acute pain: episode of pain that lasts from seconds to less than 6 months

Adaptation: adjustment of living with other living things and environmental conditions

Addiction: a pattern of compulsive use of addictive substances for means other than those prescribed

Addictive: substance to which a person develops a psychological and physiologic dependency

Adduction: movement of a body part toward the midline of the body

Adjuvant: drugs typically used for other purposes, but also used to enhance the effect of opioids by providing additional pain relief

Adolescence: the period of time between childhood and adulthood; a time of rapid physical change, reproductive maturity, and emotional development

Advance directive: written directive that allows people to state in advance what their choices for health care would be if certain circumstances should develop

Adventitious breath sounds: abnormal breath sound heard over the lungs

Adverse drug effects: undesirable effects other than the intended therapeutic effect of a drug

Advocacy: protection and support of another's rights

Aerobic bacteria: bacteria that require oxygen to live and grow

Aerobic exercise: exercise that promotes cardiovascular fitness; it increases blood flow, heart rate, and the metabolic demand for oxygen over a period of time

Afebrile: a condition in which the body temperature is not elevated

Affective learning: changes in attitudes, values, and feelings

Ageism: attitudes that stereotype the older adult on the basis of chronologic age

Agency for Healthcare Research and Quality (AHRQ): a group of multidisciplinary experts who use research as well as a broad range of input from professional and consumer organizations and individuals to develop clinical practice guidelines

Agglutinin: an antibody that causes a clumping of specific antigens

Aggressive behavior: standing up for one's rights in a negative manner that violates the rights of others

Agnostic: person who believes that nothing can be known about the existence of a god

Albuminuria: albumin in the urine; an indication of kidney disease

Alkali: substance that can accept or trap a hydrogen ion; synonym for base

Alkalosis: condition, characterized by a proportionate lack of hydrogen ions in the extracellular fluid concentration, in which the pH exceeds 7.45

Allergic effect: immune system response that occurs when the body interprets an administered drug as a foreign substance and forms antibodies against the drug

Allodynia: characteristic feature of neuropathic pain that occurs after a normally weak or nonpainful stimuli, such as a light touch or a cold drink

Allopathy: the term generally used to describe "traditional" medical care (biomedicine), dominant for about 100 years, which spearheaded remarkable advances in biotechnology, surgical interventions, pharmaceutical approaches, and diagnostic tools

Allostasis: the process of achieving stability or homeostasis through physiologic or behavioral change

Allow natural death (AND) order: an order that no attempts are to be made to resuscitate a patient who stops breathing or whose heart stops beating

Alopecia: hair loss or baldness

Alternative care: general term used to identify various methods of nonhospital health care, including residential housing, daycare, respite care, hospice, and extended-care facilities

Alternative modalities: methods not included in the scope of conventional medical care

Alveoli: small air sacs at the end of the terminal bronchioles that are the site of gas exchange

Alzheimer disease: type of dementia in which discrete patches of brain tissue degenerate; this devastating disease eventually affects all body functions

Ambulatory care: health care settings located in areas that are convenient for people to walk into and receive care; may be provided in hospitals, clinics, or centers

Amino acid: basic building blocks used to manufacture protein and the end products of protein digestion

Ampule: glass flask containing a single dose of medication for parenteral administration

Anaerobic bacteria: bacteria that can live without oxygen

Anaerobic exercise: exercise in which the supply of oxygen is less than the demand created by contracting muscles; oxygen debt results

Analgesic drug: pharmaceutical agent used to relieve pain

Anaphylactic reaction/Anaphylaxis: severe reaction occurring immediately after exposure to a drug; characterized by respiratory distress and vascular collapse

Andragogy: the study of teaching adults

Anesthetic: agent that produces states such as loss of consciousness, analgesia, relaxation, and loss of reflexes

Angina: a temporary imbalance between the amount of oxygen needed by the heart and the amount delivered to the heart muscles

Anion: ion that carries a negative electric charge

Ankylosis: fixation or immobilization of a joint

Anorexia: lack or loss of appetite for food

Anorexia nervosa: eating disorder characterized by the denial of appetite and bizarre eating habits

Anoxia: absence of oxygen

Antagonistic effect: combined effect of two or more drugs that produces less than the effect of each drug alone

Anthropometric: measurements of the body and body parts

Antibacterial: agent that kills bacteria or suppresses their growth

Antibody: immunoglobin produced by the body in response to a specific antigen

Anticipatory loss: condition in which a person displays loss and grief behaviors for a loss that has yet to take place

Antigen: foreign material capable of inducing a specific immune response

Antimicrobial: antibacterial agent that kills bacteria or suppresses their growth

Antipyretic: agent that reduces fever

Antiseptic: substance that inhibits the growth of bacteria

Anuria: technically, no urine voided; 24-hour urine output is less than 100 mL

Anus: opening at the end of anal canal

Anxiety: vague sense of impending doom or apprehension precipitated by new and unknown experiences

Apnea: absence of breathing

Applied research (practical research): research designed to directly influence or improve clinical practice

Aromatherapy: the use of essential oils of plants to treat symptoms

Arousal: condition in which the cortical area of the brain receives and responds appropriately to stimuli

Arterial blood gas: a diagnostic test examining arterial blood; used to determine the pressure exerted by oxygen and carbon dioxide in the blood

Ascites: accumulation of fluid in the peritoneal cavity

Asepsis: absence of disease-producing microorganisms; using methods to prevent infection

Asphyxiation: stoppage of breathing or the lack of air reaching the lungs; synonym for suffocation

Aspiration: misdirection of oropharyngeal secretions or gastric contents into the larynx and lower respiratory tract

Assault: threat or an attempt to make bodily contact with another person without that person's permission

Assertiveness: ability to stand up for oneself and others using open, honest, and direct communication

Assess: to systematically and continuously collect, validate, and communicate patient data

Assimilation: process by which a person interprets information to fit the current level of cognition

Assisted suicide: the act of making a means of suicide (e.g., providing pills or a weapon) available to a patient with knowledge of the patient's intention; in assisted suicide, someone makes the means of death available but does not act as the direct agent of death

Atelectasis: incomplete expansion or collapse of a part of the lungs

Atheist: person who denies the existence of a god

Atria: upper chambers of the heart

Atrioventricular bundle: a bundle of modified heart muscle that transmits the cardiac impulse from the atrioventricular node to the ventricles, causing them to contract

Atrioventricular (AV) node: a node of specialized heart muscle located in the septal wall of the right atrium; receives impulses from the sinoatrial node and transmits them to the atrioventricular bundle

Atrophy: decrease in the size of a body structure

Attachment: active, affectionate, reciprocal relationship between two persons

Attitude: feeling or emotion, generally including a positive or negative judgment toward people, objects, or ideas

Auditory: pertaining to hearing

Aura: consists of at least seven layers of energy that surround the body and relate to the chakras

Auscultation: listening for sounds within the body

Authoritative knowledge: knowledge that comes from an expert and is accepted as truth based on a perceived level of expertise

Autocratic leadership: leadership style in which the leader assumes complete control over the decisions and activities of the group

Autologous transfusion: occurs when a patient donates one's own blood for a transfusion

Autonomic bladder: bladder no longer controlled by the brain because of injury or disease; void by reflex only

Autonomy: self-determination; being independent and self-governing

Ayurveda: a science of life that delineates the diet, medicines, and behaviors that are beneficial or harmful for life and considers that balance among people, the environment, and the larger cosmos is integral to human health

B

Bacteria: the most significant and most commonly observed infection-causing agents

Bacteriuria: condition that occurs when bacteria enter the bladder during catheterization, or when organisms migrate up the catheter lumen or the urethra into the bladder; bacteria in the urine

Bandage: piece of gauze or other material used to cover a wound

Basal metabolism: amount of energy required to carry out involuntary activities of the body at rest

Base: substance that can accept or trap a hydrogen ion; synonym for alkali

Base of support: foundation that provides stability for an object

Basic human needs: something essential to the health and survival of humans; common to all people

Basic research (pure research): research designed to generate and refine theory; the findings are often not directly useful in practice

Battery: assault that is carried out

Beliefs: special class of intellectual attitudes based primarily on faith as opposed to fact

Beneficence: principle of doing good

Bereavement: state of grieving or going through the grief process

Bereavement care: continuation of care, usually up to 1 year, for the family after loss of a loved one

Bilateral: pertaining to two sides of the body

Binder: type of bandage, usually designed to fit a large body area

Bioethics: ethics that encompass all those perspectives that seek to understand human nature and behavior, the domain of social science, and the natural world

Biofilm: a thick grouping of microorganisms

Biologic sex: term used to denote chromosomal sexual development—male (XY) or female (XX)

Biopsy: removal of a piece of tissue for microscopic examination

Bioterrorism: the deliberate spread of pathogenic organisms into a community to cause widespread illness, fear, and panic

Bisexuality: having sexual feelings for people of both sexes

Blended competencies: the set of intellectual, interpersonal, technical, and ethical/legal capacities needed to practice professional nursing

Blended family: two single-parent families joined together to form a new family unit

Blood pressure: force of blood against arterial walls

Blood typing: the laboratory examination to determine a person's blood type

Body image: how a person experiences one's body

Body language: nonverbal communication

Body mass index (BMI): ratio of height to weight

Body mechanics: efficient use of the body as a machine and as a means of locomotion

Body substance isolation (BSI): type of isolation that considers all body substances as potentially infective regardless of a person's diagnosis

Bolus: single injection of a concentrated solution administered intravenously

Bonding: process of initial emotional fusing of the mother and infant that occurs most often in the first few hours after birth and is necessary for later attachment

Bowel incontinence: the inability of the anal sphincter to control the discharge of fecal and gaseous material

Bowel movement: emptying of the intestinal tract; synonym for *defecation*

Bowel training program: program that manipulates factors within a person's control (timing of defecation, exercise, diet) to produce a regular pattern of comfortable defecation without medication or enemas

Bradycardia: slow heart rate

Bradypnea: slow rate of breathing

Breakthrough pain: temporary flare-up of moderate to severe pain that occurs even when the patient is taking around-the-clock medication for persistent pain

Bronchial sounds: those heard over the trachea; high in pitch and intensity, with expiration being longer than inspiration

Bronchodilator: medication that relaxes contractions of smooth muscles of the bronchioles

Bronchoscopy: visual examination of the trachea and bronchi

Bronchovesicular sounds: normal breath sounds heard over the upper anterior chest and intercostal area

Bruit: unusual sound, usually abnormal, heard in auscultation

Buffer: substance that prevents body fluid from becoming overly acid or alkaline

Bulimia: eating disorder characterized by episodes of gorging followed by purging; often occurs in conjunction with anorexia nervosa

Bullying: negative, often repetitive, disruptive behavior; also referred to as horizontal violence, lateral violence, and professional incivility

Bundles: evidence-based best practices that have proven positive outcomes when implemented together to prevent infection

Burnout: behaviors exhibited as the result of prolonged occupational stress

C

Calorie: measure of heat, or energy; *kilocalorie,* commonly referred to as a calorie, defined as the amount of heat required to raise 1 kg of water 1°C

Capillary filtration: passage of fluid across the wall of the capillary; results from the force of blood "pushing" against the walls of the capillaries

Capnography: a method to monitor ventilation and, indirectly, blood flow through the lungs

Carbohydrate: organic compounds (commonly known as sugars and starches) that are composed of carbon, hydrogen, and oxygen; the most abundant and least expensive source of calories in the diet worldwide

Cardiac output: volume of blood pumped from the left ventricle per minute

Cardinal signs: body temperature, pulse and respiratory rates, and blood pressure; synonym for *vital signs*

Cardiopulmonary: relating to the heart and the lungs

Cardiovascular: relating to the heart and blood vessels

Care-based approach: approach to bioethics that directs attention to the specific situations of individual patients viewed within the context of their life narrative

Caregiver burden: stress responses experienced during prolonged periods of home care by family caregivers

Caries: cavities of the teeth

Cartilage: hard, nonvascular connective tissue found in the joints as well as in the nose, ear, thorax, trachea, and larynx

Cascade iatrogenesis: downward spiral or sequence of adverse events often triggered by a medical or surgical intervention during the hospitalization of an older adult

Case management: the process of coordinating an individual's health care for the purpose of maximizing positive outcomes and containing costs

Cathartic: medication that strongly increases gastrointestinal motility and promotes defecation

Catheter: tube for injecting or removing fluids

Cation: ion that carries a positive electric charge

Center of gravity: point at which the mass of an object is centered

Centers for Disease Control and Prevention (CDC): U.S. government agency whose responsibilities include investigation, identification, prevention, and control of disease

Central venous catheter: venous access device usually introduced into the subclavian or internal jugular veins and passed to the superior vena cava just above the right atrium

Certification: process by which a person who has met certain criteria established by a nongovernmental association is granted recognition

Cerumen: wax in the external ear canals, consisting of a heavy oil and brown pigment

Ceruminal gland: gland found in the external auditory canal that secretes *cerumen*

Chakra: concentrated areas of energy aligned vertically in the body, which relate to each other as well as to specific areas of the body/ mind/spirit

Change: process of transforming, altering, or modifying something

Change agent: person who purposefully and systematically implements change

Change-of-shift report: communication method used by nurses who are completing care for a patient to transmit patient information to nurses who are about to assume responsibility for continuing care; may be exchanged verbally in a meeting or audiotaped

Channel: term used in communication theory to denote the medium selected to convey the message; the channel may target any of the receiver's senses

Chart: computerized or paper medical record containing information such as medical orders, assessments, and care; nursing documentation of plan of care, assessments, and interventions; and diagnostic/ surgery results

Charting by exception: shorthand method for documenting patient data that is based on well-defined standards of practice; only exceptions to these standards are documented in narrative notes

Cheilosis: ulceration of the lips

Chemical name: precise description of a drug's chemical composition

Chemical terrorism: the deliberate release of a chemical compound that has the potential for harming people's health

Cheyne-Stokes respirations: gradual increase and then gradual decrease in depth of respirations followed by a period of apnea

Child maltreatment: an act or series of acts of commission (abuse) or omission (neglect) by a parent or other caregiver that results in harm, potential for harm, or threat of harm to a child

Chiropractic medicine: science that investigates the relationship between structure (the spine) and function (mainly the nervous system) of the human body to restore and preserve health

Cholesterol: fat-like substance found only in animal tissues; it is important for cell membrane structure, a precursor of steroid hormones, and a constituent of bile; high serum cholesterol levels are a risk factor in the development of atherosclerosis

Chronic illness: irreversible illness that causes permanent physical impairment and requires long-term health care

Chronic pain: episode of pain that lasts for 6 months or longer; may be intermittent or continuous

Chyme: semifluid state that food is in when it leaves the stomach

Cilia: microscopic, hair-like projections that propel mucus toward the upper airway so that it can be expectorated

Circadian rhythm: rhythm that completes a full cycle every 24 hours; synonym for *diurnal rhythm*

Circumduction: moving the distal part of the limb to trace a complete circle while the proximal end remains fixed

Civil law: rule that regulates relationships among people; synonym for *private law*

Clear liquid diet: diet that contains only foods that are clear liquids at room or body temperature—gelatin, fat-free broth, bouillon, ice pops, clear juices, carbonated beverages, and regular and decaffeinated coffee and tea

Cliché: a stereotyped, trite, or pat answer

Clinical ethics: branch of bioethics concerned with ethical problems that arise within the context of caring for patients

Clinical judgment: refers to the result (outcome) of critical thinking or clinical reasoning; the conclusion, decision, or opinion a nurse makes

Clinical pathway/critical path/CareMap: case management tools used to communicate the standardized, interdisciplinary plan of care for a particular group of patients; care guidelines and outcomes are specified for each day of the patient's stay

Clinical reasoning: a specific term usually referring to ways of thinking about patient care issues (determining, preventing, and managing patient problems); for reasoning about other clinical issues (e.g., teamwork, collaboration, and streamlining work flow); nurses usually use critical thinking

Clubbing: rounding and swelling of nailbeds

Code of ethics: principles that reflect the primary goals, values, and obligations of the profession

Cognition: cerebral functioning; process of perceiving and understanding one's world

Cognitive development: learning that occurs as a result of the internal organization of an event, which forms a mental schema (plan) and serves as a base for further schemata as one grows and develops (Piaget's theory of cognitive development)

Cognitive learning: storing and recalling of new knowledge in the brain

Cognitively skilled: capable of thinking about the nature of things sufficiently to "make sense" of the world and to grasp conceptually what is necessary to achieve valued goals

Coitus: sexual activity in which the penis is placed in the vagina; synonym for *sexual intercourse*

Colic: acute abdominal pain caused by spasmodic contractions of the intestine during the first 3 months of life

Collaborative interventions: interdependent nursing actions performed jointly by nurses and other members of the health care team

Collaborative problem: actual or potential health problem that may occur from complications of disease, diagnostic studies, or the treatment regimen; the nurse works together with other members of the health care team toward its resolution

Colloid osmotic pressure: pressure exerted by plasma proteins on permeable membranes in the body; synonym for *oncotic pressure*

Colon: section of the large intestine from the cecum to the rectum

Colonization: presence of an organism residing in an individual's body but with no clinical signs of infection

Colostomy: an opening into the colon that permits feces to exit through the stoma

Comfort-measures-only order: an order written to indicate that the goal of treatment is a comfortable, dignified death and that further life-sustaining measures are no longer indicated

Common law: law resulting from court decisions that is then followed when other cases involving similar circumstances and facts arise; common law is as binding as civil law

Communication: process of sharing information; process of generating and transmitting meanings

Community: specific population or group of people living in the same geographic area under similar regulations and having common values, interests, and needs

Community-based health care: health care that is provided to people who live within a defined geographic region or who have common needs; designed to meet the needs of people as they move between and among health care settings

Complaint: legal statement of the plaintiff's claim; once filed, it initiates legal proceedings

Complementary/alternative therapies: alternative treatments used with traditional medical interventions

Compliance: act of completing what is expected of one

Comprehensive assessment: health history and complete physical examination, usually conducted when a patient first enters a health care setting; provides a baseline for comparing later assessment

Computer-based record: computer-generated patient data collection system that can be distributed among many caregivers in a standardized format, allowing them to compare and uniformly evaluate patient progress easily, or compare the progress of groups of patients with similar diagnoses

Computerized plans of nursing care: plans of patient care developed by computer software programs that enable the nurse to call up screens listing causes, goals, and related nursing interventions for nursing diagnoses and medical diagnoses

Concept: abstract images (ideas) that are formed as impressions from the environment and organized into symbols of reality

Concept mapping: instructional strategy that requires learners to identify, graphically display, and link key concepts

Conceptual framework/model: set of concepts, along with the statements that arrange the concepts into an understandable pattern

Concurrent audit: evaluation of nursing care and patient outcomes conducted while the patient is receiving care; may use direct observation of nursing care, patient interview, and chart review

Concurrent evaluation: the evaluation of nursing care and patient outcomes while the patient is receiving care, conducted by using direct observation of nursing care, patient interviews, and chart review to determine whether the specified evaluative criteria are met

Condom catheter: tube for draining urine; applied externally to the penis and connected to a collection bag

Confer: to consult with someone to exchange ideas or to seek information, advice, or instructions

Confidentiality: respecting privileged information

Congestion: presence of excessive fluids or secretions in an organ or body tissue

Conscious sedation/analgesia: analgesia used for short-term procedures in which the patient maintains cardiorespiratory function and can respond to verbal commands while the IV administration of sedatives and analgesics raises the pain threshold and produces an altered mood and some degree of amnesia

Constipation: passage of dry, hard fecal material

Consultation: process in which two or more individuals with varying degrees of experience and expertise deliberate about a problem and its solution

Consumer: the person who uses health care services (the patient)

Continent urinary reservoir: a surgical alternative that uses a section of the intestine to create an internal reservoir that holds urine, with the creation of a catheterizable stoma

Continuity of care: coordination of services provided to patients before they enter a health care setting, during the time they are in the setting, and after they leave the setting

Continuum: graduated scale

Contraception: prevention of conception or pregnancy; also used to describe methods used for birth control

Contractual agreement: pact made between two persons or parties for the achievement of mutually set goals

Contracture: permanently contracted state of a muscle

Convalescent period: stage of an illness that represents recovery from the illness (or surgery)

Coping mechanism: patterns of behavior used to neutralize, deny, or counteract anxiety

Counseling: giving guidance, assisting with problem solving

Crackles: fine, crackling sounds made as air moves through wet secretions in the lungs

Creative thinking: a process involving imagination, intuition, and spontaneity—factors that underpin the art of nursing

Credentialing: general term that refers to ways in which professional competence is maintained

Crime: offense against people or property; the act is considered to be against the government, referred to in a lawsuit as "the people," and the accused is prosecuted by the state

Crisis: (1) point at which body temperature drops rapidly to normal; (2) occurs when coping and defense mechanisms are no longer effective, resulting in high levels of anxiety, disorganized behavior, and the inability to function normally

Crisis intervention: five-step problem-solving technique to promote adaptation and improve future coping

Criteria: specified behavior; for example, the measurable criteria in a patient goal specifies how the patient must perform the desired behavior

Critical/collaborative pathway: case management plan that is a detailed, standardized plan of care developed for a patient population with a designated diagnosis or procedure; it includes expected outcomes, a list of interventions to be performed, and the sequence and timing of those interventions

Critical thinking: thought that is disciplined, comprehensive, based on intellectual standards, and, as a result, well-reasoned; a systematic way to form and shape one's thinking that functions purposefully and exactingly

Critical thinking indicators (CTIs): evidence-based descriptions of behaviors that demonstrate the knowledge, characteristics, and skills that promote critical thinking in clinical practice

Cross-matching: act of determining the compatibility of two blood specimens

Cue: significant information that is helpful in making decisions

Cultural assimilation: process that occurs when a minority group, living as part of a dominant group within a culture, loses the cultural characteristics that made it different

Cultural blindness: the process of ignoring differences in people and proceeding as though the differences do not exist

Cultural care deprivation: a lack of culturally assistive, supportive, or facilitative acts in the health care setting

Cultural diversity: diverse groups in society, with varying racial classifications and national origins, religious affiliations, languages, physical size, gender, sexual orientation, age, disability, socioeconomic status, occupational status, and geographic location

Cultural imposition: tendency of some to impose their beliefs, practices, and values on another culture because they believe that their ideas are superior to those of another person or group

Culturally competent care: care delivered with an awareness of the aspects of the patient's culture

Culture: sum total of human behavior or social characteristics particular to a specific group and passed from generation to generation or from one to another within the group

Culture conflict: situation that occurs when people become aware of cultural differences, feel threatened, and respond by ridiculing the beliefs and traditions of others to make themselves feel more secure about their own values

Culture shock: those feelings, usually negative, a person experiences when placed in a different culture

Cumulative effect: condition that occurs when the body cannot metabolize a drug before additional doses are administered

Cutaneous pain: superficial pain usually involving the skin or subcutaneous tissue

Cutaneous ureterostomy: a type of incontinent cutaneous urinary diversion in which the ureters are directed through the abdominal wall and attached to an opening in the skin

Cyanosis: bluish coloring of the skin and mucous membranes

Cyber terror: the use of high-tech means to disable or delete critical electronic infrastructure data or information

Cystoscopy: direct visual examination of the bladder, ureteral orifices, and urethra with a cystoscope

Cytologic study: study of body cells and fluids

D

Dangling: position in which the person sits on the edge of the bed with legs and feet dangling over the side of the bed

Data: information

Database: all the pertinent patient information that enables a comprehensive and effective plan of care to be designed and implemented

Data cluster: grouping of patient data or cues that points to the existence of a patient health problem

Daycare center: centers that provide care for infants, children, elderly people, and people with special health care needs

Death: termination of life

Débridement: cleaning away devitalized tissue and foreign matter from a wound

Decentralized decision-making process: autonomous, accountable professional nursing practice; a characteristic of a democratic leadership style and the heart of a self-governance model of unit organization

Decision making: purposeful, goal-directed effort applied in a systematic way to make a choice among alternatives

Deductive reasoning: cognitive process in which one examines a general idea and then considers specific actions or ideas

Deep vein thrombosis (DVT): formation of a blood clot ("thrombus") in a deep vein

Defamation of character: an intentional tort in which one party makes derogatory remarks about another that diminishes the other party's reputation; slander is oral defamation of character; libel is written defamation of character

Defecation: emptying of the intestinal tract; synonym for *bowel movement*

Defendant: the one being accused of a crime or tort

Defense mechanisms: forms of self-deception; unconscious process the self uses to protect itself from anxiety or threats to self-esteem

Dehiscence: separation of the layers of a surgical wound; may be partial, superficial, or a complete disruption of the surgical wound

Dehydration: decreased water volume in body tissue

Delegation: the transfer of responsibility for the performance of an activity to another individual while retaining accountability for the outcome

Delirium: a temporary state of confusion

Delta sleep: deep sleep, occurring during stage III and especially stage IV in NREM sleep

Dementia: organic impairment of intellectual functioning, gradually leading to interference with social or occupational functioning, memory, and often personality integration

Democratic leadership: leadership style characterized by a sense of equality between the leader and followers

Deontologic: ethical system in which actions are right or wrong independent of the consequences they produce

Dependent action: nursing action carried out at the instruction or order of an authorized health care professional other than a nurse; synonym for *physician-initiated* or *physician-prescribed intervention*

Depersonalization: subjective experience of the partial or total disruption of one's ego and the disintegration and disorganization of one's self-concept

Dermis: layer of the skin below the epidermis

Desiccation: dehydration; the process of being rendered free from moisture

Development: increase in the complexity of function and progression to skill advancement

Developmental crisis: predictable patterns of behavior and change occurring throughout the lifespan

Developmental delay: measure of development that lags behind the normal range for a given age

Developmental task: successful achievement of psychomotor, psychosocial, or cognitive skills at certain periods in life; failure to obtain the developmental task can lead to unhappiness and difficulty with later tasks

Development theory: theory to describe the orderly and predictable process of the growth and development of humans, individualized by social, biologic, and environmental factors

Diagnosis (nursing): analysis of patient data to identify patient strengths and health problems that independent nursing intervention can prevent or resolve

Diagnosis-related groups (DRGs): classification of patients by major medical diagnosis for the purpose of standardizing health care costs

Diagnostic error: failure to detect an actual unhealthy behavior or condition

Diaphoresis: an excessive amount of perspiration, such as when the entire skin is moist

Diarrhea: passage of liquid and unformed stools

Diastolic pressure: least amount of pressure exerted on arterial walls, which occurs when the heart is at rest between ventricular contractions

Dietary Guidelines: recommendations for choosing a healthy diet made by the U.S. Department of Agriculture and the U.S. Department of Health and Human Services

Diffuse pain: pain that covers a large area

Diffusion: tendency of solutes to move freely throughout a solvent from an area of higher concentration to an area of lower concentration until equilibrium is established

Digestion: gastrointestinal system's breakdown process of food into particles small enough to pass into the cells and be used by the cells

Direct transfusion: infusion of blood while it is being taken from the donor

Disaster: an emergency event of greater magnitude that requires the response of people outside the involved community

Discharge planning: systematic process of preparing the patient to leave the health care facility and for maintaining continuity of care

Discharge summary: description of where the patient stands in relation to problems identified in the record at discharge; documents any special teaching or counseling the patient received, including referrals

Discipline: specific and unique body of knowledge that uses existing and new knowledge to creatively solve problems and meet human needs within ever-changing boundaries

Disease: pathologic change in the structure or function of the body or mind

Disinfection: process used to destroy microorganisms; destroys all pathogenic organisms except spores

Distribution: movement of drugs by the circulatory system to the site of action

Disturbed sensory perception: a state in which the individual or group experiences or is at risk for a change in the amount, pattern, or interpretation of incoming stimuli

Documentation: written, legal record of all pertinent interventions with the patient—assessments, diagnoses, plans, interventions, and evaluations

Dominant group: group within a culture that has the authority to control the value system and determine the rewards of the system; usually the largest group in a society

Donor: person who donates blood or an organ to be given to another person

Do-not-hospitalize: an order specifying that a patient, usually one who is terminally ill and anticipating death, not be admitted to the hospital in the event of a worsening of condition

Do-not-resuscitate (DNR): an order specifying that there be no attempt to resuscitate a patient in the event of cardiopulmonary arrest

Dosha: the patient's basic condition; understanding dosha is central to Ayurvedic medicine

Dressing: protective covering placed over a wound

Drug: substance that modifies body functions when taken into the living organism; synonym for *medication*

Drug allergy: hypersensitivity caused by previous exposure to a medication; may occur immediately or be delayed; manifestations range from mild to severe

Drug tolerance: tendency of the body to become accustomed to a drug over time; larger doses are required to produce the desired effects

Dry powder inhalers (DPI): types of breath-activated delivery methods for inhaled medications

Dynorphin: the endorphin having the most potent analgesic effect

Dysfunctional grief: abnormal or distorted grief that may be either unresolved or inhibited

Dysphagia: difficulty in swallowing or inability to swallow

Dyspnea: difficult or labored breathing

Dysrhythmia: an abnormal cardiac rhythm

Dyssomnias: sleep disorders characterized by insomnia or excessive sleepiness

Dysuria: difficulty in voiding; may or may not be associated with pain

E

Ecchymosis: collection of blood in subcutaneous tissues that causes a purplish discoloration

Edema: accumulation of fluid in extracellular spaces

Elective surgery: surgery that is recommended but can be omitted or delayed without catastrophe

Electrocardiogram (ECG; EKG): graphic record produced by the electrocardiograph

Electroencephalograph: instrument that measures and records electric impulses of the brain

Electrolyte: substance capable of breaking into ions and developing an electric charge when dissolved in solution

Electromyograph (EMG): instrument that records muscle tone

Electronic medical record (EMR): computer-based record or data that can be distributed among many caregivers in a standardized format

Electrooculogram: recording of the electric current or potential produced by eye movements

Embolism: blocking of an artery by a blood clot or by other foreign matter brought to the site by the blood flow

Embolus: blood clot, foreign body, or air in the circulatory system; plural form is *emboli*

Emergency assessment: rapid focused assessment conducted to determine potentially fatal situations

Emergency surgery: surgery that must be performed immediately to save the person's life or a body organ

Empathy: intellectually identifying with the way another person feels

Endemic: something that occurs with predictability in one specific region or population and can appear in a different geographical location

Endogenous: infection in which the causative organism comes from microbial life harbored within the person

Endorphins: morphine-like substances released by the body that appear to alter the perception of pain

Endoscopy: direct visualization of hollow organs of the body using an endoscope (a flexible, lighted tube)

Endotracheal tube: polyvinyl-chloride airway that is inserted through the nose or the mouth into the trachea, using a laryngoscope as a guide

Enema: introduction of solution into the lower bowel

Enkephalins: opioids that are widespread throughout the brain and dorsal horn of the spinal cord and are believed to reduce pain sensation by inhibiting the release of substance P

Enteral nutrition: alternate form of feeding that involves passing a tube into the gastrointestinal tract to allow instillation of the appropriate formula

Entitlement reform: proposed legislation making changes in entitlement benefits, such as Medicare and Medicaid, paid by the government to citizens, with the goal of improving the nation's budget

Entry phase: phase of the home visit in which the nurse develops rapport with the patient and family members, mutually determines outcomes, makes assessments, plans and implements prescribed care, and provides teaching

Enuresis: involuntary urination; most often used to refer to a child who involuntarily urinates during the night

Epidermis: superficial layer of the skin

Epidural analgesia: means of providing pain relief with an opioid injection delivered by way of a catheter inserted in the midlumbar region into the epidural space

Epithelialization: stage of wound healing in which epithelial cells form across the surface of a wound; tissue color ranges from the color of "ground glass" to pink

Erection: condition that results when erectile tissue of the penis fills with blood as a result of stimulation

Erogenous zones: areas of the body that produce sexual desire and arousal when stimulated

Erythema: redness of the skin

Eschar: a thick, leathery scab or dry crust that is necrotic and must be removed for adequate healing to occur

Ethical agency: the ability to behave in an ethical way; to do the ethically right thing because it is the right thing to do

Ethical dilemma: situation that arises when attempted adherence to basic ethical principles results in two conflicting courses of action

Ethical distress: occurrence when the nurse knows the right thing to do but either personal or institutional factors make it difficult to follow the correct course of action

Ethically and legally skilled: capable of conducting oneself in a manner consistent with a personal moral code and professional role responsibilities

Ethics: system dealing with standards of character and behavior related to what is right and wrong

Ethnicity: sense of identification that a cultural group collectively has; the sharing of common and unique cultural and social beliefs and behavior patterns, including language and dialect, religious practices, literature, folklore, music, political interests, food preferences, and employment patterns

Ethnocentrism: belief that one's own ideas, beliefs, and practices are best, superior, or most preferred to those of others; using one's cultural norms as the standard to evaluate others' beliefs

Ethnopharmacology: study of the effect of ethnicity on responses to prescribed medication, especially drug absorption, metabolism, distribution, and excretion

Euphoria: unrealistic sense of well-being

Eupnea: normal respirations

Euthanasia: mercy killing; the deliberate termination of the life of a person

Evaluating: measurement of the extent to which the patient has achieved the goals specified in the plan of care; factors that positively or negatively influence goal achievement are identified, and the plan of care is terminated or revised

Evaluative statement: a judgment summarizing the nurse's findings after data have been collected and interpreted to determine patient outcome achievement

Evidence-based practice (EBP): nursing care provided that is supported by sound scientific rationale

Evidence-based practice guideline: guidelines written by a panel of experts that synthesize information from multiple studies and recommend best practices to treat patients with a disease, a symptom, or a disability

Evisceration: protrusion of viscera through an incision

Exacerbation: period in chronic illness when the symptoms of the disease reappear

Excretion: removal of a drug from the body

Exercise: active exertion of muscles involving the contraction and relaxation of muscle groups

Exogenous: infection in which the causative organism is acquired from outside the host

Expected outcome: specific, measurable criteria used to evaluate whether the patient goal has been met

Expectorant: drug that facilitates the removal of respiratory secretions

Expert witness: nurse who explains to the judge and jury what happened based on the patient's record and who offers an opinion as to whether the nursing care met acceptable standards of practice

Expiration: act of breathing out; synonym is *exhalation*

Explicit power: power obtained by virtue of a person's position

Extended-care facility: includes residential care and intermediate or skilled long-term care facility

Extended family: nuclear family and other related people

External condom catheter: soft, pliable sheath made of silicone material applied externally to the penis

Extracellular fluid (ECF): fluid outside the cells; includes intravascular and interstitial fluids

Exudate: fluid that accumulates in a wound; may contain serum, cellular debris, bacteria, and white blood cells

F

Fact witness: nurse who has knowledge of the actual incident prompting a legal case; bases testimony on firsthand knowledge of the incident, not on assumptions

Failure to thrive (FTT): physical and developmental retardation of infants or children resulting from physical or emotional neglect

Faith: (1) spiritual dimensions of a person's life regardless of religious affiliation; (2) confident belief in something for which there is no proof or material evidence

False self: a sense of self that might develop in individuals who have the emotional need to respond to the needs and ambitions that significant people, such as parents, have for them

Family: any group of people who live together and depend on one another for physical, emotional, or financial support

Fasting state: abstinence from food and fluids

Fear: a feeling of dread; a cognitive response to a known threat

Febrile: condition in which the body temperature is elevated

Fecal impaction: collection in the rectum of hardened feces that cannot be passed

Fecal incontinence: involuntary or inappropriate passing of stool or flatus

Feces: intestinal waste products

Fee for service: system in which a bill is generated and a fee is paid every time a provider does something for a patient

Feedback: verbal and nonverbal evidence that the message is received and understood

Felony: (1) crime punishable by imprisonment in a state or federal penitentiary for more than 1 year; (2) crime of greater offense than a misdemeanor

Female genital mutilation (FGM): any procedure that involves partial or total removal of the external female genitalia or other injury to the female genital organs for nonmedical reasons

Feminist ethics: type of ethical approach that aims to critique existing patterns of oppression and domination in society, especially as these affect women and the poor

Fever: elevation above the upper limit of normal body temperature; synonym for *pyrexia*

Fiber: all dietary plant material that is not digestible by the gastrointestinal tract, enzymes, and secretions

Fidelity: keeping promises and commitments made to others

Fight-or-flight response: the body preparing itself against threat, to either resist (fight) or evade (flight) the danger

Filtration: passage of a fluid through a permeable membrane whose spaces do not allow certain solutes to pass; passage is from an area of higher pressure to one of lower pressure

Fissure: a linear break on the margin of the anus

Fistula: an abnormal passage from an internal organ to the skin or from one internal organ to another

Flaccidity: decreased muscle tone; synonym for *hypotonicity*

Flatulence: excessive formation of gases in the gastrointestinal tract

Flatus: intestinal gas

Flexibility: ability to use a muscle through its entire range of motion

Flexion: the action of bending or the condition of being bent, especially the bending of a limb or joint.

Flow sheets: graphic record of abbreviated aspects of the patient's condition (e.g., vital signs, routine aspects of care)

Fluid balance: state in which water and its solutes in the body are in normal proportions and concentrations and are in appropriate body compartments

Fluid imbalance: state in which water and its solutes in the body are in improper proportions and concentrations or are improperly located in body compartments

Fluid volume deficit: deficiency in the amount of both water and electrolytes in extracellular fluid; water and electrolyte proportions remain near normal

Fluid volume excess: excessive retention of water and sodium in extracellular fluid in near-normal proportions

Flushing: red appearance of the skin

Focus charting: a documentation system that replaces the problem list with a focus column that incorporates many aspects of a patient and patient care; the focus may be a patient strength or a problem or need; the narrative portion of focus charting uses the data (D), action (A), response (R) format

Focused assessment: assessment conducted to assess a specific problem; focuses on pertinent history and body regions

Foley catheter: indwelling or retention catheter that remains in place to drain urine

Footdrop: complication resulting from extended plantar flexion

Formal teaching: planned teaching based on learner objectives

Frail-old: term for people over age 75; the fastest-growing segment of the population

Fraud: willful and purposeful misrepresentation that could cause, or has caused, loss or harm to people or property

Fremitus: vibration of the chest wall that can be palpated during the physical examination

Frequency: increased incidence of voiding

Friction: occurs when two surfaces rub against each other; the resulting injury resembles an abrasion and can also damage superficial blood vessels directly under the skin

Friction rub: crackling sounds heard in the chest cavity caused by inflamed pleura rubbing against the chest wall

Full liquid diet: diet that contains milk, plain frozen desserts, pasteurized eggs, cereal gruels, and milk and egg substitutes in addition to clear liquids; contains liquids that can be poured at room temperature

Functional health: level of health defined by one's ability to carry out usual and desired daily activities

Functional incontinence: state in which a person experiences an involuntary, unpredictable passage of urine

Fungi: plant-like organisms (molds and yeasts) that can cause infection

G

Gastric residual: feeding remaining in the stomach

Gastrostomy: opening created into the stomach

Gate control theory: theory that explains that excitatory pain stimuli carried by small-diameter nerve fibers can be blocked by inhibiting signals carried by large-diameter nerve fibers

Gay: term used to describe homosexual males

Gender dysphoria: diagnosis for a person whose gender at birth is contrary to the one with which the person identifies

Gender identity: the inner sense a person has of being male or female, which may be the same as or different from biologic gender; synonym is *sexual identity*

Gender role behavior: the behavior a person conveys about being male or female, which may or may not be the same as biologic gender or gender identity

General adaptation syndrome (GAS): biochemical model of stress describing the body's general response to stress

General anesthesia: anesthetic drugs that produce narcosis, relaxation of skeletal muscles, and reduced or absent reflex action

Generic name: name assigned by the manufacturer who first develops a drug; it is often derived from the chemical name

Genome: all the DNA in an organism, including its genes

Genomics: the study of the structure and interactions of all genes in the human body, including their interactions with each other as well as the environment.

Gerontologic nursing: nursing specialty concerned with the care of the older adult

Gerontology: study of all aspects of the aging process and their consequences

Gingivitis: inflammation of the gingivae or gums

Global self: term used to describe the composite of all the basic facts, qualities, traits, images, and feelings one holds about oneself

Glossitis: inflammation of the tongue

Glycosuria: presence of sugar in the urine

Goal: an aim or an end

Good Samaritan law: law that holds certain health practitioners blameless when undertaking to aid a person in an emergency

Gram-negative bacteria: bacteria with chemically more complex cell walls that can be decolorized by alcohol

Gram-positive bacteria: bacteria with a thick cell wall that resists decolorization (loss of color) and are stained violet

Granulation tissue: new tissue that is pink/red in color and composed of fibroblasts and small blood vessels that fill an open wound when it starts to heal

Graphic sheet: form used to record specific patient variables

Grief: emotional response to loss. *Dysfunctional grief:* distorted or abnormal grief response, including *inhibited grief* (suppression of grief reaction) and *unresolved grief* (lengthy or denied grief reaction). *Abbreviated grief:* short but genuine grief reaction. *Anticipatory grief:* grief reaction before actual loss.

Ground: conducting connection between a source of electricity and the earth

Group dynamics: study of a group's characteristics and ways of functioning

Growth: an increase in body size or changes in body cell structure, function, and complexity

Gurgles: continuous musical sounds that are audible in expiration or inspiration, or both; formerly called *rhonchi*

Gustatory: pertaining to taste

H

Half-life: the amount of time it takes for half a dose of a drug to be eliminated from the body

Halitosis: offensive breath

Hand-off: a nurse's report to another nurse or health care provider about a patient's status and progress

Healing touch (HT): uses a collection of energy techniques to assess and treat the human energy system, thereby affecting physical, emotional, mental, and spiritual health and healing

Health: state of optimal functioning or well-being

Health-belief model: what people believe to be true about themselves in relation to health

Health disparity: a specific difference that is closely linked to social, economic, and/or environmental disadvantage

Health history: a collection of subjective information that provides information about the patient's health status

Health information exchange (HIE): an electronic system that allows physicians, nurses, pharmacists, other health care providers, and patients to appropriately access and securely share a patient's vital medical information

Health insurance marketplace: federal and state system designed to help people more easily find health insurance that fits their budget and needs with a plan offering comprehensive coverage, from doctors to medications to hospital visits; insurance options can be compared based on price, benefits, quality, and other features described in plain language

Health literacy: ability to read, understand, and act on health information

Health maintenance organization (HMO): Prepaid, group-managed care plan that allows subscribers to receive all the medical services they require through a group of affiliated providers; there may be no additional out-of-pocket costs, or subscribers may pay only a small fee, called a copayment

Health problem: condition related to health requiring intervention if disease or illness is to be prevented or resolved and coping and wellness are to be promoted

Health promotion: behavior of an individual motivated by a personal desire to increase well-being and health potential

Health care–associated infection (HAI): an infection that was not present on admission to a health care institution and develops during the course of treatment for other conditions (nosocomial)

Helping relationship: interaction that sets the climate of movement of the participants toward common goals

Hematuria: blood in the urine; if present in large enough quantities, urine may be bright red or reddish brown

Hemolysis: process of freeing a red blood cell of its hemoglobin by destruction of the cell membrane

Hemoptysis: sputum-containing blood

Hemorrhage: excessive blood loss due to the escape of blood from blood vessels

Hemorrhoids: abnormally distended rectal veins

Hemothorax: blood that develops in the pleural space

Heparin lock: intravenous needle or catheter with an injection pad attached at the end

Hesitancy: delay or difficulty in initiating voiding

Heterosexuality: having sexual feelings for a person of the opposite sex

Hierarchy of needs: as defined by Maslow, certain needs are more basic than others; a person strives to at least minimally meet certain needs before attending to others

High-level wellness: functioning to one's maximum potential while maintaining balance and purposeful direction in the environment

HIPAA privacy rule: federal law enacted to ensure that health information is protected while allowing the flow of health information needed to provide and promote high-quality health care and to protect the public's health and well-being

Holism: theory and philosophy that focuses on connections and interactions between parts of the whole

Holistic health care: health care that takes into account the whole person interacting in the environment

Holistic nursing: nursing practice built on a holistic philosophy

Home health care: health care services provided in a patient's home

Home health care agency: agency eligible to receive federal funds that provides home-based health care; may be independent, hospital operated, or health department managed

Homeopathy: practice of medicine based on the belief of supporting the body while the symptoms are allowed to "run their course" to stimulate and strengthen the immune system and promote healing

Homeostasis: various physiologic and psychological mechanisms respond to changes in the internal and external environment to maintain a balanced state

Homosexuality: having sexual feelings for a person of the same sex

Hope: ingredient in life responsible for a positive outlook, even in life's bleakest moments

Horizontal violence: anger and aggressive behavior between nurses or nurse-to-nurse hostility

Hospice: a type of end-of-life care for persons who are terminally ill, characterized by the following: (1) patients are kept as free of pain as possible so that they may die comfortably and with dignity; (2) patients receive continuity of care, are not abandoned, and do not lose personal identity; (3) patients retain as much control as possible over decisions regarding their care and are allowed to refuse further life-prolonging technologic interventions; and (4) patients are viewed as individuals with personal fears, thoughts, feelings, values, and hopes

Hospitals: acute-care settings that provide various health care services, such as emergency care, inpatient care, surgery, diagnostic tests, and patient education

Host: animal or person on or within which microorganisms live

Hydration: union of a substance with water; term often is used as the opposite of dehydration, in which case it means that there is normal intracellular and extracellular water volume

Hydrometer: instrument used to determine the specific gravity of urine

Hydrostatic pressure: force exerted by a fluid against the container wall

Hypercalcemia: excess of calcium in the extracellular fluid

Hyperkalemia: excess of potassium in the extracellular fluid

Hypermagnesemia: excess of magnesium in the extracellular fluid

Hypernatremia: excess of sodium in the extracellular fluid

Hyperphosphatemia: above-normal serum concentration of inorganic phosphorus

Hyperpyrexia: high fever, above 41°C (105.8°F)

Hypersomnia: condition characterized by excessive sleeping, especially daytime sleeping

Hypertension: blood pressure elevated above the upper limit of normal

Hyperthermia: high body temperature

Hypertonic: having a greater concentration than the solution with which it is being compared

Hyperventilation: condition in which there is more than the normal amount of air entering and leaving the lungs

Hypervolemia: excess of plasma

Hypnotic: pharmaceutical agent used to induce sleep

Hypocalcemia: insufficient amount of calcium in the extracellular fluid

Hypokalemia: insufficient amount of potassium in the extracellular fluid

Hypomagnesemia: insufficient amount of magnesium in the extracellular fluid

Hyponatremia: insufficient amount of sodium in the extracellular fluid

Hypophosphatemia: below-normal serum concentration of inorganic phosphorus

Hypoproteinemia: insufficient amount of protein substances in the extracellular fluid

Hypotension: blood pressure below the lower limit of normal

Hypothermia: low body temperature

Hypotonic: having a lesser concentration than the solution with which it is being compared

Hypoventilation: decreased rate or depth of air movement into the lungs

Hypovolemia: deficiency of blood plasma

Hypovolemic shock: shock due to a decrease in blood volume

Hypoxemia: deficient oxygenation of blood

Hypoxia: inadequate amount of oxygen available to the cells

Iatrogenic infection: infection that occurs as a result of a treatment or diagnostic procedure

Ideal self: self a person would like to be or thinks one should be; includes aspirations, moral ideas, and values

Identity diffusion: failure to integrate various childhood identifications into a harmonious adult psychosocial identity

Idiosyncratic effect: unusual, unexpected response to a drug that may manifest itself by overresponse, underresponse, or response different from the expected outcome

Ileal conduit: urinary diversion in which the ureters are connected to the ileum with a stoma created on the abdominal wall

Ileostomy: opening into the small intestine allows fecal content from the ileum to be eliminated through the stoma

Illness: abnormal process in which any aspect of the person's functioning is altered (in comparison to the previous condition of health)

Imagery: using all five senses to imagine an event or body process unfolding according to a plan

Immunization: process of rendering a person immune or resistant to particular antigenic agents or bacteria

Implement: carry out the plan of care

Implied power: power obtained by force of a person's personality that might enable that person to have more power to influence others than designated leaders

Impotence: condition in which a man is unable to attain or maintain an erection to such an extent that he cannot have satisfactory sexual intercourse; synonym for *erectile failure*

Incentive spirometer: equipment to help maximize lung inflation

Incident report (or variance report): a report of any event that is not consistent with the routine operation of the health care agency that results in or has the potential to result in harm to a patient, employee, or visitor

Incision: wound made with a sharp cutting instrument

Incivility: rude, intimidating, and undesirable behavior directed at another person

Incontinence: inability to voluntarily control the discharge of urine or feces

Independent action: (1) nursing action carried out at the instruction or order of a nurse; (2) actions within the legal scope of nursing's independent domain; synonym for *nurse-initiated* or *nurse-prescribed intervention*

Inductive reasoning: cognitive process in which one identifies a specific idea or action and then makes conclusions about general ideas

Indwelling urethral catheter: catheter that remains in place for continuous urine drainage; synonym for *Foley catheter*

Infancy: period from 1 month to 1 year of age

Infection: disease state resulting from pathogens in or on the body

Inference: the judgment reached about a cue

Infiltration: escape of fluid into subcutaneous tissue

Inflammatory response: localized response of the body to injury or infection; protective mechanism that eliminates invading pathogens and allows for tissue repair to occur

Informal teaching: unplanned teaching sessions dealing with the patient's immediate learning needs and concerns

Informed consent: knowledgeable, voluntary permission obtained from a patient to perform a specific test or procedure

Inhalation: (1) act of breathing in; synonym for *inspiration;* (2) administration of a drug in solution via the respiratory tract

Initial assessment: comprehensive nursing assessment resulting in baseline data that enables the nurse to make a judgment about a patient's health status, ability to manage one's own health care, and need for nursing, and to plan individualized, holistic health care for the patient

Initial planning: planning that addresses each problem listed in the prioritized nursing diagnoses and identifies appropriate patient goals and the related nursing care

Injection: introduction of medication into the body by a syringe attached to a needle

Inpatient: person who enters a health care setting for a stay ranging from 24 hours to many years

Insomnia: difficulty in falling asleep, intermittent sleep, or early awakening from sleep

Inspection: purposeful and systematic observation

Inspiration: act of breathing in; synonym is *inhalation*

Instrumental activities of daily living (IADLs): the activities of daily living needed for independent living

Integrative care: care that uses some combination of allopathic and complementary/alternative modalities

Integument: skin

Integumentary system: skin and its appendages (i.e., hair, glands in the skin, and nails)

Intercessory prayer: involves praying for the benefit of another person to the Judeo-Christian God

Intercourse (coitus or copulation): insertion of the penis into the partner's vagina, anus, or mouth

Interdependent action: nursing action performed by the nurse in collaboration with other members of the health care team

Intermittent fever: body temperature that alternates between fever and normal or subnormal temperature

Intermittent pulse: normal pulse rhythm broken by periods of irregular rhythm

Intermittent urethral catheter: straight catheter used to drain the bladder for short periods (5–10 minutes)

Internal respiration: exchange of oxygen and carbon dioxide between the circulating blood and tissue cells

Interpersonal communication: communication that occurs between two or more people with a goal to exchange messages

Interpersonally skilled: capable of establishing and maintaining caring relationships that facilitate the achievement of valued goals while simultaneously affirming the worth of the participants in the relationship

Interstitial fluid: fluid between the cells

Intervention: any action performed to modify an expectation or to enhance outcomes

Interview: planned communication for a specific purpose (e.g., data collection)

Interviewing techniques: communication skills specifically designed to gather and validate information

Intimate partner violence (IPV): domestic violence or battering between two people in a close relationship

Intracellular fluid (ICF): fluid within the cell; synonym for *cellular fluid*

Intractable pain: severe pain that is extremely resistant to relief measures

Intradermal injection: injection placed just below the epidermis

Intramuscular (IM) injection: an injection into deep muscle tissue, usually of the buttock, thigh, or upper arm

Intraoperative phase: period lasting from admission to the operating room area to transfer to the postoperative recovery area after surgery is completed

Intrapersonal communication: communication techniques or self-talk to enhance positive interaction with the patient and family

Intravascular fluid: fluid within the vascular system; synonym for *plasma*

Intravenous (IV) infusion: injection of relatively large quantities of solution into a vein

Intravenous (IV) route: injection of a solution into the vein

Intuitive problem solving: direct understanding of a situation based on a background of experience, knowledge, and skill that makes expert decision making possible

Ion: atom or molecule carrying an electric charge in solution

Irrigation: flushing of a tube, canal, or area with solution

ISBARR communication: a process for effective hand-off communication among health care professionals about a patient's condition, standing for Identity/Introduction, Situation, Background, Assessment, Recommendation, and Read back

Ischemia: deficiency of blood in a particular area

Isokinetic exercise: exercise involving muscle contractions with resistance varying at a constant rate

Isolation: protective procedure designed to prevent the transmission of specific microorganisms; also called *protective aseptic techniques* and *barrier techniques*

Isometric exercise: exercise in which muscle tension occurs without a significant change in muscle length

Isotonic: having about the same concentration as the solution with which it is being compared

Isotonic exercise: movement in which muscles shorten (contract) and move

J

Jaundice: yellow appearance of the skin

Just culture: refers to an organization's commitment to accountability and a focus supporting universal safety in health care

Justice: process that distributes benefits, risks, and costs fairly

K

Kardex care plan: trade name for a care plan documentation system that encompasses (1) prescriptions for nursing care related to activities of daily living; (2) nursing diagnoses and related patient goals and nursing orders; and (3) the nursing care related to diagnostic measures and the medical regimen

Kegel exercises: repetitious contraction and relaxation of the pubococcygeal muscle to improve vaginal tone and urinary continence

Ketosis: an abnormal accumulation of ketone bodies that is frequently associated with acidosis

Kinesthesia: awareness of positioning of body parts and body movement

Korotkoff sounds: series of sounds that correspond to changes in blood flow through an artery as pressure is released

Kussmaul's respiration breathing: an extreme rate and depth of breathing

L

Laissez-faire leadership: leadership style in which the leader relinquishes all power to the group

Language: prescribed way of using words; a means to express thoughts and feelings

Lateral violence: verbal, emotional, or physically abusive behavior of a registered nurse toward another staff member

Law: rule of conduct established and enforced by the government of a society

Lawsuit: legal action in a court of law

Laxative: drug used to induce emptying of the intestinal tract

Leadership: ability to direct or motivate others toward the achievement of predetermined goals

Learning: increasing one's knowledge; having one's behavior changed in a measurable way as a result of an experience

Learning readiness: patient's willingness to engage in the teaching–learning process (emotional readiness) and experiential readiness to begin the challenge of learning

Lesbian: term for a homosexual female

Liability: legal responsibility for one's acts (and failure to act); includes responsibility for financial restitution of harms resulting from negligent acts

Licensure: to be given a license to practice nursing in a state or province after successfully meeting requirements

Life review/reminiscence: universal phenomenon identified by Butler as a review of one's life through one's recollections

Ligaments: tough, fibrous bands that bind joints together and connect bones and cartilage

Line of gravity: vertical line that passes through the center of gravity

Lipid: group name for fatty substances, including fats, oils, waxes, and related compounds

Literacy: ability to read and write

Litigation: process of lawsuit

Living will: advance directive specifying the medical care a person would want or refuse should that person lack the capacity to consent to or refuse treatment

Local adaptation syndrome (LAS): localized response of the body to stress, precipitated by trauma or pathology

Localized symptoms: symptoms that are limited or restricted to a discrete area

Long-term care: facilities for long-term care that provide health care and help with activities of daily living for people of any age who are physically or mentally unable to independently care for themselves

Loss: inaccessibility or change in a valued person, object, or situation. *Actual loss:* loss tangible to both the person sustaining the loss and to others. *Perceived loss:* loss tangible only to the person sustaining it. *Physical loss:* loss of life, limb, an object, person, pet, or job. *Psychological loss:* loss that affects a person's self-image. *Anticipatory loss:* loss behaviors displayed before the actual loss occurs.

Love and belonging needs: understanding and acceptance of others in giving and receiving love

M

Maceration: softening through liquid; overhydration

Macromineral: mineral that is needed by the body in amount greater than 100 mg/day

Macronutrient: essential nutrient that supplies energy and builds tissue such as carbohydrate, fat, and protein

Macroshock: electric current passing through a relatively large area of a person

Malpractice: act of negligence as applied to a professional person such as a physician, nurse, or dentist

Managed care: an organized, high-quality, cost-effective system of health care that influences the selection and use of health care services of a population

Management: the act of planning, organizing, directing, and controlling available human resources and financial resources to deliver quality care to patients and families

Masturbation: self-stimulation for sexual satisfaction

Maturational loss: the loss experienced as a result of natural developmental processes

Meaningful use: the use of certified electronic health record technology to achieve health and efficiency goals, with a financial incentive from Medicare and Medicaid

Medicaid: Title XIX (Social Security Act, 1965) to make health care available to those people with less than the minimum income who do not qualify for Medicare

Medical asepsis: practices designed to reduce the number and transfer of pathogens; synonym for *clean technique*

Medical diagnosis: statement about a specific disease process using terminology from a well-developed classification system accepted by the medical profession

Medical home: an enhanced model of primary care that provides whole-person, accessible, comprehensive, ongoing, and coordinated patient-centered care

Medical neighborhood: a patient-centered medical home and the constellation of other clinicians providing health care services to patients within it, along with community and social service organizations and state and local public health agencies

Medicare: Title XVIII (Social Security Act, 1965) to provide a measure of health coverage to all Social Security recipients

Medication: substance that modifies body functions when taken into living organisms; synonym for *drug*

Medication record: record documenting all medications administered to the patient, the nurse administering the drugs, and sometimes the reason the drug was administered and its effectiveness

Melatonin: a natural chemical produced at night that decreases wakefulness and promotes sleep

Menarche: initiation of the menstrual cycle

Meniscus: curved surface at the top of a column of liquid in a tube

Menopause: decrease of cyclic hormonal production and cessation of menses in females, usually between ages 45 and 60 years

Menstruation: periodic discharge of bloody secretions through the vagina; usually for 4–5 days each month

Mentorship: relationship in which an experienced person (the mentor) advises and assists a less experienced person

Meridian: part of an intricate structure of 72 energy circuits that nourish and support all cells and organs of the body, through which qi flows vertically in the body

Message: term used in communication theory to denote the actual physical product of the source or encoder (e.g., a speech, interview, phone conversation, chart)

Metabolic acidosis: proportionate deficiency of bicarbonate ions in the extracellular fluid

Metabolic alkalosis: proportionate excess of bicarbonate ions in the extracellular fluid

Metabolism: (1) chemical changes in the body by which energy is provided; (2) breakdown of a drug to an inactive form; also referred to as *biotransformation*

Metered dose inhaler (MDI): instrument that delivers a controlled dose of medication to narrowed airways with each compression of the canister

Micromineral: mineral or trace element that is needed by the body in an amount less than 100 mg/day

Micronutrient: vitamin or mineral needed in much smaller amount to regulate and control body processes

Microshock: electric current passing through a relatively small area of a person, usually part of the heart

Micturition: process of emptying the bladder; urination; voiding

Middle adult: the adult between the ages of 40 and 60 years; also called *middle adulthood*

Midlife crisis: realization that the halfway point in life has been reached and youthful goals may not have been achieved

Minerals: inorganic elements found in nature

Mini-infusion pump: battery-operated pump for intermittent infusion allowing medication mixed in a syringe to be connected to the primary line and delivered by mechanical pressure applied to the syringe plunger

Minimum data set: a standard established by health care institutions that specifies the information that must be collected from every patient

Minority group: group having some physical or cultural characteristic that identifies the people within the group as different from the dominant culture

Misdemeanor: crime of lesser offense than a felony and punishable by fines, imprisonment (usually for less than 1 year), or both

Mixed incontinence: symptoms of urge and stress incontinence are present, although one type may predominate

Moderate sedation/analgesia (conscious or procedural sedation): used for short-term and minimally invasive procedures

Modulation: process by which the sensation of pain is inhibited or modified

Moral development: influence of cultural effects on one's perceptions of justice in interpersonal relationships

Morals: like ethics, concerned with what constitutes right action; more informal and personal than the term *ethics*

Morbidity: frequency that a disease occurs

Mortality: number of deaths

MOLST form: stands for Medical Order for Life-Sustaining Treatment, a medical order indicating a patient's wishes regarding treatments commonly used in a medical crisis

Mourning: period during which a person learns to accept grief

Multipayer system: a health care system in which care is paid for by both private insurance companies and the government

Multispecialty practice group: organization of physicians from different specialties joined to share income, expenses, facilities, equipment, and support staff; the group practice can better provide comprehensive care

Myocardial infarction: one type of acute coronary syndrome characterized by the death of heart tissue due to lack of oxygen; also known as a heart attack

N

Narcolepsy: condition characterized by an uncontrolled desire to sleep

Narrative: descriptive record of the patient's condition; includes patient's response to interventions by health professionals and patient's progress toward goal achievement

Narrative notes: progress notes written by nurses in a source-oriented record

Nasal cannula: disposable, plastic device that delivers oxygen via two protruding prongs for insertion into the nostrils

Nasogastric (NG) tube: tube inserted through the nose and into the stomach

Nasointestinal (NI) tube: tube inserted through the nose and into the upper portion of the small intestine

National Medical Care: health care services in Canada, funded by taxes and provided to every Canadian citizen

Naturopathic medicine: a relatively new system of medicine that is not only a system of medicine but also a way of life, with emphasis on patient responsibility, patient education, health maintenance, and disease prevention

Nebulizer: instrument that disperses fine particles of medication into the deeper passages of the respiratory tract where absorption occurs

Necrosis: death of cells and tissue

Negative nitrogen balance: condition resulting in muscle wasting and decreased physical energy for movement and work (e.g., anorexia nervosa and certain cancers)

Negative-pressure wound therapy (NPWT): activity that promotes wound healing and wound closure through the application of uniform negative pressure on the wound bed, reduction in bacteria in the wound, and the removal of excess wound fluid

Negative reinforcement: an ineffective teaching strategy that uses criticism or punishment

Negativism: negative verbalizations and behaviors

Negligence: performing an act that a reasonably prudent person under similar circumstances would not do, or failing to perform an act that a reasonably prudent person under similar circumstances would do

Neonate: period from birth to 28 days of age

Nephrotoxic: capable of causing kidney damage

Neuromodulator: endogenous opioid chemical regulators that appear to have analgesic activity and alter pain perception

Neurons: nerve cells, which conduct impulses from one part of the body to another

Neuropathic pain: pain that results as a direct consequence of a lesion or disease affecting abnormal functioning of the peripheral nervous system (PNS) or central nervous system (CNS)

Neurotransmitters: substances that either excite or inhibit target nerve cells

Never events: serious but preventable surgical errors (that should never occur)

Nociceptive pain: pain from a normal process that results in noxious stimuli being perceived as painful

Nociceptors: pain receptors

Nocturia: excessive urination during the night

Nocturnal myoclonus: condition characterized by marked muscle contraction that results in the jerking of one or both legs during sleep

Noise: factors that distort the quality of a message and interfere with the communication process

Noncompliance: nonadherence to a therapeutic recommendation

Nonmaleficence: principle of avoiding evil

Nonproductive cough: forceful expiratory effort without production of mucus; also called a *dry cough*

Nonverbal communication: exchange of information without the use of words

Normal flora: microorganisms that normally inhabit various body sites and are part of the body's natural defense system

Nosocomial: something originating or taking place in the hospital (i.e., infection)

Nosocomial infection: hospital-acquired infection

NPO: nothing by mouth (Latin: *nil per os*)

Non–rapid eye movement sleep (NREM): non–rapid eye movement that characterizes four stages of sleep

Nuclear family: family unit, family of marriage, parenthood, or procreation, and their immediate children

Nuclear terrorism: intentional dispersal of radioactive materials into the environment for the purpose of causing injury and death

Nurse coach: a registered nurse who integrates coaching competencies into any setting or specialty area of practice to facilitate a process of change or development that assists individuals or groups to realize their potential

Nurse healer: a nurse who facilitates another person's growth toward wholeness (body–mind–spirit) or who assists another with recovery from illness or transition to peaceful death

Nurse-initiated intervention: independent nursing actions that involve carrying out nurse-prescribed interventions written on the nursing plan of care, as well as any other actions that nurses initiate without the direction or supervision of another health care professional and that result from their assessment of patient needs

Nurse practice act: law established to regulate nursing practice

Nursing: profession that focuses on the holistic person receiving health care services and provides a unique contribution to the prevention of illness and maintenance of health

Nursing actions: any action performed by a nurse to assist patients to meet health goals: promote wellness, prevent disease or illness, restore health, or facilitate coping with altered functioning

Nursing audit: method of evaluating the outcomes of nursing care or the process by which these outcomes are achieved using a review of patient records

Nursing care conference: formal meeting of nurses to discuss some aspect of patient's care

Nursing care rounds: procedure in which a group of nurses visit patients individually at bedside to gather information that helps to plan and to evaluate nursing care

Nursing diagnosis: actual or potential health problem that an independent nursing intervention can prevent or resolve. *Actual problem* is present. *Possible problem* may be present, but more data are needed to confirm or disconfirm the problem. *Potential problem* may occur; defining characteristics are present as risk factors.

Nursing ethics: a subset of bioethics; formal study of ethical issues that arise in the practice of nursing and of the analysis used by nurses to make ethical judgments

Nursing history: assessment of the patient by interview to identify the patient's health status, strengths, health problems, health risks, and need for nursing care

Nursing informatics: specialty that integrates nursing science, computer science, and information science to manage and communicate data, information, and knowledge in nursing practice

Nursing intervention: any treatment, based on clinical judgment and knowledge, that a nurse performs to enhance patient outcomes; there are nurse-initiated, physician-initiated, and collaborative interventions

Nursing Intervention Classification (NIC): first comprehensive, validated list of nursing interventions applicable to all settings that can be used by nurses in multiple specialties and facilitates the work of identifying appropriate interventions

Nursing order: prescribes the nursing care to be given to assist patient to meet health goals

Nursing Outcomes Classification (NOC): developed by the Iowa Outcomes Project and presents the first comprehensive standardized language used to describe the patient outcomes that are responsive to nursing intervention

Nursing plan of care: written guide to direct the efforts of the nursing team as they work with the patient to meet health goals; specifies prioritized nursing diagnoses, patient goals, and nursing orders

Nursing process: five-step systematic method for giving patient care; involves assessing, diagnosing, planning, implementing, and evaluating

Nursing research: encompasses both research to improve the care of people in the clinical setting and to study people and the nursing profession, including education, policy development, ethics, and nursing history

Nursing theory: differentiates nursing from other disciplines and activities by serving the purposes of describing, explaining, predicting, and controlling desired outcomes of nursing care practices

Nutrient: specific biochemical substance used by the body for growth, development, activity, reproduction, lactation, health maintenance, and recovery from illness or injury

Nutrition: study of the nutrients and how they are handled by the body, as well as the impact of human behavior and environment on the process of nourishment

O

Obesity: weight greater than 20% above ideal body weight

Objective data: information perceptible to the senses; may be verified by another person

Observation: conscious and deliberate use of the five senses to gather data

Occult blood: blood present in such minute quantities that it cannot be detected with the unassisted eye

Occupational Safety and Health Administration (OSHA): government agency that establishes minimum health and safety standards for workers

Occurrence charting (or variance charting): documentation when a patient fails to meet an expected outcome or a planned intervention is not implemented, including the unexpected event, the cause of the event, actions taken in response to the event, and discharge planning, when appropriate; typically used for variances that affect quality, cost, or length of stay

Official name: name by which a drug is identified in official publications

Old-old: term used to describe adults over age 75; sometimes referred to as frail-old

Older adult: refers to adults over age of 65

Olfactory: pertaining to smell

Oliguria: scanty or greatly diminished amount of urine voided in a given time; 24-hour urine output is 100 to 400 mL

Oncotic pressure: pressure exerted by plasma proteins on permeable membranes in the body; synonym for *colloid osmotic pressure*

Ongoing partial assessment: assessment that is conducted at regular intervals during care of the patient; concentrates on identified health problems to monitor positive or negative changes and evaluate the effectiveness of interventions

Ongoing planning: planning carried out by any nurse who interacts with the patient to keep the plan up to date, to facilitate the resolution of health problems, to manage risk factors, and to promote function

Opioid: more correct term for narcotic analgesics, since these drugs act by binding to opiate receptor sites in the central nervous system

Opportunist: bacteria that may potentially be harmful

Organism: a living being

Organizational communication: process of communication that involves individuals and groups to achieve established goals

Orgasm: apex of sexual activity in which rhythmic contractions of the genital organs and many other physiologic changes occur

Orthopedics: the correction or prevention of disorders of body structures used in locomotion

Orthopnea: type of dyspnea in which breathing is easier when the patient sits or stands

Orthostatic hypotension: temporary fall in blood pressure associated with assuming an upright position; synonym for *postural hypotension*

Osmolarity: concentration of particles in a solution, or a solution's pulling power

Osmosis: passage of a solvent through a semipermeable membrane from an area of lesser concentration to an area of greater concentration until equilibrium is established

Osmotic pressure: drawing power for water or the attraction for water exerted by solute particles

Osteoporosis: condition characterized by loss of calcium from bone tissue

Ostomy: general term referring to an artificial opening; usually used to refer to an opening created for the excretion of body wastes

Outcome: end product of nursing care; patient outcomes are measurable changes in patient behavior or state of health

Outcome and Assessment Information Set (OASIS): assessment instrument representing core items of a comprehensive assessment for adult nonmaternity home health care patients that forms the basis for measuring patient outcomes for the purpose of improving the quality of care provided

Outcome evaluation: evaluation that focuses on measurable changes in the health status of the patient or the end results of nursing care

Outcome identification: observation of the patient to demonstrate the resolution of the problems identified by the nursing diagnoses and general problem list, along with the time frame for accomplishing these outcomes

Outpatient: person who requires health care services but does not need to stay in an institution for those services

Overflow incontinence: involuntary loss of urine associated with overdistention and overflow of the bladder

Overhydration: above-normal amounts of water in extracellular spaces

Ovulation: discharge of ovum from the ovary at about the midpoint of each menstrual cycle

Ovum: female reproductive cell, often called an *egg*

Oxygenation: the process of providing cells life-sustaining oxygen

P

Pacemaker: another name for the sinoatrial (SA) node; initiates the transmission of electrical impulses, causing contraction of the heart at regular intervals

Pain: sensation of physical or mental suffering or hurt that usually causes distress or agony to the one experiencing it

Pain threshold: amount of stimulation required before a person experiences the sensation of pain

Pain tolerance: point beyond which a person is no longer willing to endure pain (i.e., pain of greater duration or intensity)

Palliative care: hospice care; taking care of the whole person—body, mind, spirit, heart and soul—with the goal of giving patients with life-threatening illnesses the best quality of life they can have through the aggressive management of symptoms

Palliative sedation: the lowering of patient consciousness with medication for the express purpose of limiting the patient's awareness of suffering that is intractable and intolerable

Pallor: paleness of the skin

Palpation: method of examining by feeling a part of the body with the fingers or hand

Palpitation: perception of one's own heartbeat

Paracentesis: withdrawal of fluid from a body cavity, usually from the abdominal cavity

Paralysis: absence of strength secondary to nervous impairment

Paralytic ileus: paralysis of intestinal peristalsis

Paraplegia: paralysis of the legs

Parasite: organism that lives on or in a host and relies on it for nourishment

Parasomnia: patterns of waking behavior that appear during sleep (e.g., sleep walking, sleep talking, nocturnal erections)

Parenteral: outside of intestines or alimentary canal; popularly used to refer to injection routes

Parenteral nutrition: nourishment provided via IV therapy

Paresis: impaired muscle strength or weakness

Paresthesia: numbness and tingling

Partial peripheral nutrition (PPN): nutrition prescribed for patients who require nutrient supplementation through a peripheral vein because they have an inadequate intake of oral feedings

Passive exercise: manual or mechanical means of moving the joints

Paternalism: an action that is based on what a parent would do

Pathogen: disease-producing microorganism

Patient: the person receiving care

Patient care ergonomics: practice of designing equipment and work tasks to conform to the capability of the worker in relation to patient care

Patient-controlled analgesia (PCA): method of controlling pain that involves an infusion pump that holds a vial of an IV analgesic that the patient controls and self-administers in small doses

Patient education: process of influencing the patient's behavior to effect changes in knowledge, attitudes, and skills needed to maintain and improve health

Patient goal: statement describing an expected patient outcome

Patient outcome: expected conclusion to a patient health problem, or in the event of a wellness diagnosis, an expected conclusion to a patient's health expectation

Patient Protection and Affordable Care Act (PPACA): 2010 federal legislation designed for comprehensive health reform, with an intent to expand coverage, control health care costs, and improve the health care delivery system

Patient record: a compilation of a patient's health information; the patient record is the only permanent legal document that details the nurse's interactions with the patient

Pay for performance: a strategy using financial incentives to reward providers for achieving a range of payer objectives, including delivery efficiencies, submission of data and measures to the payer, and improved quality and patient safety

Peak level: highest plasma concentration of a drug

Pedagogy: science of teaching that generally refers to the teaching of children and adolescents

Pediculosis: infestation with lice

Peer review: evaluation at the closest point to the patient and an ongoing tool to use for professional growth

Perceived loss: loss of youth, of financial independence, and of a valued environment experienced by a person, but intangible to others

Perception: conscious process of organizing and interpreting data from the senses into meaningful information

Percussion: act of striking one object against another for the purpose of producing a sound; used to assess the location, shape, size, and density of body tissues

Percutaneous endoscopic gastrostomy tube (PEG): surgically or laparoscopically placed gastrostomy tube

Performance improvement: commitment to healthier patients, quality care, reduced costs, and making a difference; accomplished by discovering a problem, planning a strategy, implementing a change, and assessing the change to see if the goal is met

Perfusion: process by which oxygenated blood passes through body tissues

Periodontitis (periodontal disease): marked inflammation of the gums that also involves degeneration of the dental periosteum (tissues) and bone

Perioperative nursing: wide variety of nursing activities carried out before, during, and after surgery

Perioperative phase: the three phases of perioperative patient care that include the preoperative, intraoperative, and postoperative phases

Peripherally inserted central catheter (PICC): type of venous access device that can be introduced into a peripheral vein and advanced as far as the superior vena cava

Peripheral parenteral nutrition (PPN): prescribed for patients who require nutrient supplementation through a peripheral vein because they have an inadequate intake of oral feedings

Peripheral resistance: restraint to blood flow created by arteriole walls in a partial state of contraction

Peristalsis: involuntary, progressive, wave-like movement of the musculature of the gastrointestinal tract

Personal health records (PHRs): information sheets that contain the individual's medical history, including diagnoses, symptoms, and medications

Personal identity: an individual's conscious sense of who he or she is

Personal protective equipment (PPE): gloves, gowns, masks, and protective eye gear designed to minimize or prevent the health care worker's exposure to infectious material

Personal space: external environment surrounding a person that is regarded as being part of that person

Petechiae: small, purplish hemorrhagic spots on the skin that do not blanch with applied pressure

pH: expression of hydrogen ion concentration and resulting acidity of a substance

Phagocytosis: engulfing of microorganisms, foreign particles, or other cells by phagocytes

Phantom pain: sensation of pain without demonstrable physiologic or pathologic substance; commonly observed after the amputation of a limb

Pharmacodynamics: process by which drugs alter cell physiology and affect the body

Pharmacogenetics: the study of how genetic variation affects an individual's response to drugs

Pharmacokinetics: movement of drug molecules in the body in relation to the drug's absorption, distribution, metabolism, and excretion

Pharmacology: study of actions of chemicals on living organisms

Pharmacotherapeutics: dynamic that achieves the desired therapeutic effect of the drug without causing other undesirable effects

Philosophy: study of wisdom, fundamental knowledge, and the processes we use to develop and construct our perceptions of life

Phlebitis: inflammation of a vein

Phlegm: thick, respiratory secretions

Physical assessment: systematic examination of the patient for objective data to better define the patient's condition and to help the nurse in planning care, usually performed in a head-to-toe format; a collection of objective data about changes in the patient's body systems

Physical dependence: phenomenon in which the body physiologically becomes accustomed to an opioid and suffers withdrawal symptoms if the opioid is suddenly removed or the dose is rapidly decreased

Physician-initiated intervention: dependent nursing actions, involving carrying out physician-prescribed orders

Physiologic needs: need for oxygen, food, water, temperature, elimination, sexuality, activity, and rest; these needs have the highest priority and are essential for survival

PIE charting: documentation system that does not develop a separate care plan; the care plan is incorporated into the progress notes in which problems are identified by number, worked up using the problem (P)–intervention (I)–evaluation (E) format, and evaluated each shift

Piggyback infusion: intermittent IV administration of medications through a primary IV line, with the additive container positioned higher than the primary IV solution

Placebo: Latin word meaning, "I shall please"; an inactive substance that gives satisfaction to the person using it

Plaintiff: person or government bringing a lawsuit against another

Plan: establish patient goals to prevent, reduce, or resolve the problems identified in the nursing diagnoses and determination of related nursing interventions

Planned change: change agent's purposeful, systematic effort to bring about change

Plan of nursing care: written guide that directs the efforts of the nursing team as the nurses work with patients to meet health goals; it specifies nursing diagnoses, outcomes, and associated nursing interventions

Plaque: invisible, destructive, bacterial film that builds up on teeth and eventually leads to the destruction of tooth enamel

Plasma: liquid constituent of blood; synonym for *intravascular fluid*

Pleurae: two-layered membranes; the visceral pleura covers the lungs, and the parietal pleura lines the thoracic cavity

Pleural effusion: fluid in the pleural space

Pleural friction rub: continuous, dry grating sound caused by inflammation of pleural surfaces and loss of lubricating pleural fluid

Pneumonia: inflammation or infection of the lungs

Pneumothorax: air in the pleural space

Podiatrist: one who treats foot disorders; synonym for *chiropodist*

Poison control center: agency that handles poison exposure and provides poison prevention teaching to the general population

POLST form: stands for Physician Order for Life-Sustaining Treatment, a medical order indicating a patient's wishes regarding treatments commonly used in a medical crisis; must be completed and signed by a health care professional, not the patient

Polyp: tumor on a stem that bleeds easily and may become malignant

Polypharmacy: the use of many medications at the same time

Polysomnography: sleep study consisting of an electroencephalographic recording of the stages of sleep and any episodes of apnea, continuous monitoring of arterial oxygen saturation, and an electrocardiographic recording to detect any cardiac dysrhythmias

Polyuria: excessive output of urine (diuresis)

Positive reinforcement: affirmation of the efforts of patients

Possible nursing diagnoses: statements describing a suspected problem for which additional data are needed to confirm or rule out the suspected problem

Possible problems: problems the patient may experience if certain trends in the patient's condition continue unreversed

Postanesthesia care unit (PACU): an area often adjacent to the surgical suite designed to provide care for patients recovering from anesthesia or moderate sedation/analgesia

Postoperative phase: period lasting from admission to the recovery area through recovery and convalescence

Postural hypotension: temporary fall in blood pressure associated with assuming an upright position; synonym for *orthostatic hypotension*

Postvoid residual (PVR): urine that remains in the bladder after the act of micturition; a synonym for *residual urine*

Power: ability to influence others to achieve a desired effect

Preceptorship: process by which an experienced person facilitates an orientee's introduction to new responsibilities through teaching and guidance

Precordium: anterior surface of the chest wall overlying the heart and its related structures

Pre-entry phase: phase of the home visit in which the nurse collects information about the patient's health care needs, gathers needed supplies, and evaluates safety factors

Preferred provider organization (PPO): a prepaid group practice that allows a third-party payer (such as an insurance company) to contract with a group of health care providers to administer services at a lower fee in return for prompt payment and a guaranteed volume of patients and services

Premenstrual (tension) syndrome (PMS): menstrual cycle–related distress; occurs a few days before the onset of menstruation

PRN orders: directives commonly written for treatment of symptoms "as needed."

Preoperative phase: period lasting from the decision that surgery is necessary until the patient is transferred to the operating room area

Presbycusis: age-related hearing loss in which there is decreased ability to distinguish higher frequencies

Presbyopia: condition of aging in which decreased elasticity of the eye lens hinders accommodation to close vision

Preschooler: period from ages 3 years to 6 years

Prescription: used by physician to convey medication plans for a patient

Pressure ulcer: any lesion caused by unrelieved pressure that results in damage to underlying tissue

Primary health care: essential health care based on practical, scientifically sound, and socially acceptable methods and technology, made universally accessible through the community's full participation and at a cost the community can afford

Primary preventive care: care directed toward health promotion and specific protection against illness

Principle-based approach: an approach to bioethics that offers specific action guides

PRN order: "as needed" order for medication

Problem-oriented medical record (POR): documentation system organized according to the person's specific health problems; includes database, problem list, plan of care, and progress notes

Process: series of actions, changes, or functions to bring about a result

Process evaluation: evaluation focusing on the nature and sequence of activities carried out by nurses implementing the nursing process

Productive cough: cough that produces respiratory tract secretions (sputum)

Profession: an occupation that meets specific criteria including a well-defined body of specific and unique knowledge, a code of ethics and standards, ongoing research, and autonomy

Professionalism: a way of being/commitment to secure the interests and welfare of those entrusted to one's care

Progress notes: any of a variety of methods of notes that relate how a patient is progressing toward expected outcomes

Proprioception: description of the sense, usually at a subconscious level, of the movements and position of the body, especially its limbs, independent of vision

Protein: vital component of every living cell; composed of carbon, hydrogen, oxygen, and nitrogen

Proteinuria: albumin in the urine; indication of kidney disease

Protocol: written plan that details the nursing activities to be executed in specific situations

Psychogenic pain: pain for which no physical cause can be identified

Psychological loss: loss caused by an altered self-image

Psychomotor learning: acquisition of physical skills

Psychosomatic disorder: physiologic alterations and illness believed to be due to psychological influences

Puberty: period during which primary and secondary sexual characteristics develop and the capability of sexual reproduction is attained

Public health agencies: local, state, provincial, or federal agencies that provide public health services to members of communities

Pulmonary ventilation: movement of air into and out of the lungs

Pulse: wave produced in the wall of an artery with each beat of the heart

Pulse deficit: difference between the apical and radial pulse rates

Pulse oximetry: noninvasive technique that measures the oxygen saturation (SaO_2) of arterial blood

Pulse pressure: difference between systolic and diastolic pressures

Purulent: containing pus

Purulent drainage: comprised of white blood cells, liquefied dead tissue debris, and both dead and live bacteria

Pyorrhea: extensive inflammation of the gums and alveolar tissues; synonym for *periodontitis*

Pyrexia: elevation above the upper limit of normal body temperature; synonym for *fever*

Pyuria: pus in the urine; urine appears cloudy

Q

Qi: represents an invisible flow of energy that circulates through plants, animals, and people, as well as the earth and sky

Qi gong: system of posture, exercise (both gentle and dynamic), breathing techniques, and visualization that regulates the qi

QSEN: stands for Quality and Safety Education for Nurses, a project for preparing future nurses with the knowledge, skills, and attitudes (KSAs) necessary to continuously improve the quality and safety of the health care systems within which they work

Qualitative research: method of research conducted to gain insight by discovering meanings

Quality assurance program: ongoing evaluation program designed and implemented to secure the excellence of health care; may involve an assessment of structure, process, and outcome standards

Quality improvement: the commitment and approach used to continuously improve every process in every part of an organization, with the intent of meeting and exceeding customer expectations and outcomes—also known as continuous quality improvement (CQI) or total quality management (TQM)

Quantitative research: research involving the concepts of basic and applied research

Quantum leadership: leadership that moves beyond the traditional modes previously experienced by all levels of workers; spawned by the impact of the information age on work and the worker

R

Race: division of human beings based on distinct physical characteristics

Radiography: examination by x-ray film

Range of motion: complete extent of movement of which a joint is normally capable

Rape: sexual violation of a person by someone who uses force, threats, and abuse

Rapid eye movement sleep (REM): stage that constitutes 20% to 25% of a person's nightly sleep; person is difficult to arouse during this stage

Rapport: feeling of mutual trust experienced by people in a satisfactory relationship

Reactive hyperemia: the body's flooding of an area with blood after it has suffered from poor circulation for a period; the occurrence of a blanchable reddening of the skin when pressure is removed

Read back: a process in which a nurse or other health care provider repeats a verbal order back to a physician to ensure that it was correctly heard and interpreted

Reality orientation: method of care used to promote awareness of reality in confused or disoriented patients

Receiver (decoder): term used in communication theory that specifies the person or object to which the message is directed

Reception: process of receiving data about the internal or external environment through the senses

Reciprocity: process allowing a nurse to apply for and be endorsed as a registered nurse by another state

Recommended dietary allowance (RDA): recommendations for average daily amounts of essential nutrients that healthy population groups should consume over time

Referral: process of sending or guiding someone to another source for assistance

Referral source: a person who recommends home health care services and supplies the home health care agency with details about the patient's needs

Referred pain: pain in an area removed from that in which stimulation has its origin

Reflective practice: occurs when the caregiver has a profound awareness of self, and one's own biases, prejudgments, prejudices, and assumptions, and understands how these may affect the therapeutic relationship

Reflex incontinence: emptying of the bladder without the sensation of the need to void

Reflex pain response: automatic response of the central nervous system to the stimulus of pain

Regional anesthesia: anesthetic drug is injected or applied topically to inhibit transmission of sensory stimuli

Regression: behavior that is more characteristic of an earlier age

Rehabilitation: process of restoring a person's highest level of possible wellness and returning that person's ability to live and to work as normally as possible after a disabling illness or injury

Rehabilitation centers: centers specializing in services for patients requiring physical or emotional rehabilitation and for treatment of any type of drug dependency

Reimbursement source: entity that pays for home health care services

Relationship: interaction of people over time

Relaxation response: an alert, hypometabolic state of decreased sympathetic nervous system arousal, which can also be viewed as the opposite of Selye's general adaptation syndrome response

Religion: organized system of beliefs about a higher power; often includes set forms of worship, spiritual practices, and codes of conduct

REM: rapid eye movement that characterizes the dream state of sleep

Remission: period in a chronic illness when the disease is present, but the person does not experience symptoms of the disease

Reporting: oral, written, or computer-based communication of patient data with the purpose of informing others

Repression: exclusion of an anxiety-producing event from conscious awareness

Research: process that uses observable and verifiable information (data), collected in a systematic manner, to describe, explain, or predict events

Reservoir: natural habitat for the growth and multiplication of microorganisms

Residual urine: urine that remains in the bladder after the act of micturition

Respiration: gas exchange between the atmospheric air in the alveoli and blood in the capillaries

Respiratory acidosis: proportionate excess of carbonic acid in the extracellular fluid

Respiratory alkalosis: proportionate deficiency of carbonic acid in the extracellular fluid

Respite care: a type of care provided for caregivers of homebound ill, disabled, or elderly patients

Rest: condition in which the body is in a decreased state of activity, with the consequent feeling of being refreshed

Restless leg syndrome (RLS): a condition in which patients are unable to lie still and report experiencing unpleasant creeping, crawling, or tingling sensations in the legs

Restraint: device used to limit movement or immobilize a client

Retention: inability to void although urine is produced by the kidneys and enters the bladder; excessive storage of urine in the bladder

Retention sutures: sutures used to provide extra support in wounds in obese patients or in wounds with increased risk of dehiscence

Reticular activating system (RAS): network of neurons in the core of the brainstem, with ascending and descending tracts to other areas of the brain that monitor and regulate incoming sensory stimuli and level of arousal

Retrospective audit: evaluation of nursing care and patient outcomes after the patient has been discharged (may use postdischarge questionnaires, patient interviews, or chart review)

Retrospective evaluation: evaluation of nursing care and patient outcomes after the patient has been discharged using postdischarge questionnaires, patient interviews, or chart review to collect data

Review of systems (ROS): physical examination of all body systems in a systematic manner as part of the nursing assessment

Risk factor: something that increases a person's chance for illness or injury

Risk nursing diagnoses: clinical judgments that an individual, family, or community is more vulnerable to develop the problem than others in the same or similar situation

Role performance: ability to successfully execute societal expectations regarding role-specific behaviors

S

Safety and security needs: person's need to be protected from actual or potential harm and to have freedom from fear

Safety event report: documentation describing any injury or potential for injury suffered by a patient in a health care agency

Sanguineous: containing or mixed with blood

SBAR: consistent, clear, structured, and easy-to-use method of communication between health care personnel; it organizes communication by the categories of: Situation, Background, Assessment, and Recommendations.

Scar: connective tissue that fills a wound area

School-age: period from ages 6 to 12 years

Science: a body of knowledge gained by observing, identifying, describing, investigating, and explaining events and occurrences that are perceived in the world

Scientific knowledge: knowledge arrived at by applying scientific methods

Scientific problem solving: systematic problem-solving process that involves (1) problem identification, (2) data collection, (3) hypothesis formulation, (4) plan of action, (5) hypothesis testing, (6) interpretation of results, and (7) evaluation resulting in conclusion or revision of the study

Scrub nurse: nurse who assists the surgeon during surgery, maintaining surgical asepsis while draping, handling instruments, and handling supplies

Scultetus binder: type of bandage with multiple tails; synonym for *many-tailed binder*

Sebaceous gland: gland found in the skin that secretes an oily substance called sebum

Secondary preventive care: care directed either to health maintenance for patients experiencing health problems or to prevention of complications or disabilities

Self-actualization: reaching of one's potential through full development of one's unique capabilities

Self-actualization needs: highest level on the hierarchy of needs, which include the need for individuals to reach their full potential through development of their unique capabilities

Self-concept: mental image or picture of self; includes body image, subjective self, ideal self, and social self

Self-esteem: person's perception of one's total being, including self-worth and body image

Self-esteem needs: need to feel good about oneself and to believe others hold one in high regard

Self-governance: employing a decentralized organizational structure for decision making; self-governance at the unit level and respect for, and acknowledgement of, professional autonomy

Semantics: study of the meaning of words

Semen: seminal plasma containing sperm

Semipermeable membrane: selectively permeable membrane that allows water to pass through it but is either impermeable or selectively permeable to solutes

Sensoristasis: arousal state of the reticular activating system; general drive state

Sensory deficit: impaired or absent functioning of one or more senses

Sensory deprivation: condition resulting from decreased sensory input or input that is monotonous, unpatterned, or meaningless

Sensory overload: condition resulting from excessive sensory input to which the brain is unable to meaningfully respond

Sensory/perceptual alteration: disturbance in the body's ability to receive or process data from its internal or external environment

Sensory poverty: condition that results when one learns about the world without experiencing it up close, right here, right now

Sensory reception: the process of receiving data about the internal or external environment through the senses

Sentinel event: an unexpected occurrence involving death or serious physical or psychological injury, or the risk thereof

Separation anxiety: condition that occurs when a child is afraid of being sent away from caregivers who are loved and who provide security

Serosanguineous drainage: mixture of serum and red blood cells

Serous: resembling blood serum; clear and watery in appearance

Serous drainage: composed of clear, serous portion of the blood and from serous membranes

Set point: level at which the hypothalamus attempts to maintain body temperature

Sexual dysfunction: condition that prevents a person or couple from engaging in or obtaining satisfaction from sexual activity

Sexual harassment: unwelcome verbal or physical advance or sexually explicit statement (e.g., leers, pats, grabs, jokes, requests for dates, and even rape) that interferes with one's ability to do one's job by making one feel humiliated, intimidated, or uncomfortable

Sexual health: the integration of the somatic, emotional, intellectual, and social aspects of sexual being in ways that are positively enriching and that enhance personality, communication, and love

Sexuality: degree to which a person exhibits and experiences maleness and femaleness physically, emotionally, and mentally

Sexually transmitted infection (or disease) (STI): disease that spreads from one person to another through intimate sexual contact

Sexual orientation: preferred gender of the partner of an individual

Shamanism: a belief that illness originates in the spirit world and usually involves a loss of power; treatment consists of first, restoring the individual's power, and second, treating symptoms

Shearing force: force created when layers of tissue move on one another

Shock: body's reaction to acute peripheral circulatory failure due to an abnormality of circulatory control or to a loss of circulating fluid

Sinoatrial (SA) node: a mass of tissue in the upper right atrium, just below the opening of the superior vena cava, that initiates the transmission of electrical impulses, causing contraction of the heart at regular intervals; also known as pacemaker

Situational crisis: change that results when a person faces an event or situation that causes a disruption in one's life

Situational leadership: theory of leadership that considers the leader's style, the work group's maturity, and the situation at hand to form a comprehensive approach to management style

Situational loss: experienced as a result of an unpredictable event, including traumatic injury, disease, death, or national disaster

Sitz bath: special type of bath that applies heated water to the pelvic or rectal area

Skin sutures: used to approximate wound tissues and skin; may be silk, synthetic, wire, or metal staples

Skin tests: tests to determine antigen–antibody reaction

Sleep: state of altered consciousness throughout which varying degrees of stimuli preclude wakefulness

Sleep apnea: a condition in which a person experiences the absence of breathing (apnea) or diminished breathing effort (hypopnea) during sleep between snoring intervals

Sleep cycle: passage through the four stages of NREM sleep (I, II, III, IV), then reversal (IV, III, II), and finally, instead of reentering stage I and awakening, entering REM sleep and returning to stage II

Sleep deprivation: a decrease in the amount, consistency, and quality of sleep; results from decreased REM or NREM sleep

Sleep hygiene: nonpharmacologic recommendations like reviewing and changing lifestyles and environment that help an individual get a better night's sleep

Small-group communication: communication that occurs when two or more nurses interact with two or more individuals, allowing the members to achieve a goal through communication

SOAP format: method of charting narrative progress notes; organizes data according to subjective information (S), objective information (O), assessment (A), and plan (P)

Social isolation: sense of aloneness because of decreasing relationships with others, resulting from attitudinal, geographic, financial, or illness-related factors

Social media: web-based technologies that allow users to create, share, and participate in dialogue in virtual communities and networks

Social self: way a person believes that others see oneself

Soft diet: regular diet that has been modified to eliminate foods that are hard to digest and to chew, including those that are high in fiber, high in fat, and highly seasoned

Solute: substance dissolved in a solution

Solvent: liquid holding a substance in solution

Somatic pain: pain originating in structures in the body's external wall

Somnambulism: sleepwalking

Sordes: accumulation of mucus and crust formation on the teeth and around the lips

Source (encoder): term used in communication theory to specify the one who prepares and sends a message to the receiver

Source-oriented record: documentation system in which each health care group records data on its own separate form

Spasticity: increased muscle tone

Specific gravity: a characteristic of urine that can be determined with manufactured plastic strips or an instrument called a urinometer or hydrometer

Sperm: male reproductive cell; synonym for spermatozoan

Spermicide: chemical agent used to destroy sperm

Sphincter: circular muscle that constricts a passage or closes a natural orifice

Spiritual beliefs: practices associated with all aspects of a person's life, including health and illness, that address the invisible "spirit"—a creative, mysterious, guiding power

Spiritual distress: an alteration in spiritual health (e.g., spiritual pain, alienation, anxiety, guilt, anger, loss, despair)

Spiritual healing: movement toward integration, from brokenness to wholeness

Spiritual health: condition that exists when the universal spiritual needs for meaning and purpose, love and belonging, and forgiveness are met

Spirituality: anything that pertains to a person's relationship with a nonmaterial life force or higher power

Spiritual need: lack of anything necessary for spiritual health (e.g., meaning and purpose, love and relatedness, forgiveness)

Spirometer: instrument used to measure lung capacities and volumes; one type is used to encourage deep breathing (incentive spirometry)

Sputum: respiratory secretion expelled by coughing or clearing the throat

Standard: acceptable, expected level of performance established by authority, custom, or consent

Standardized plan of care: prepared plan of care that identifies the nursing diagnoses, patient goals, and related nursing orders common to a specific population (e.g., normal neonates) or problem

Standard precautions: CDC precautions used in the care of all patients regardless of their diagnosis or possible infection status; this category combines universal and body substance precautions

Standards: rules or guidelines that allow nurses to carry out professional roles, serving as protection for the nurse, the patient, and the institution where health care is given

Standards for critical thinking: clear, precise, specific, accurate, relevant, plausible, consistent, logical, deep, broad, complete, significant, adequate (for the purpose), and fair

Standing order: document that details the nursing care to be implemented in specific nursing situations, frequently when a physician is not present; may expand scope of nursing responsibilities

Stat order: single order carried out immediately

Statutory law: law enacted by a legislative body

Stereognosis: the sense that perceives the solidity of objects, their size, shape, and texture

Stereotyping: assigning characteristics to a group of people without considering specific individuality

Sterilization: (1) the process by which all microorganisms, including spores, are destroyed; (2) surgical procedure performed to render a person infertile

Stertorous breathing: noisy respirations

Stimulus: agent, act, or other influence capable of initiating a response by the nervous system

Stoma: artificial opening for waste excretion located on the body surface

Stomatitis: inflammation of the oral mucosa

Stool: excreted feces

Strength (muscle): ability of the muscle to move actively against resistance

Stress: condition in which the human system responds to change in its normal balanced state

Stress incontinence: state in which the person experiences a loss of urine of less than 50 mL that occurs with increased abdominal pressure

Stressor: anything causing a person to experience stress; change in the balanced state

Stridor: harsh, high-pitched sound usually heard on inspiration when upper airways become narrowed

Structure evaluation: focuses on the environment in which care is provided; also known as an audit

Subculture: group of people with different interests or goals than the primary culture

Subcutaneous injection: injection into the subcutaneous tissue that lies between the epidermis and the muscle

Subcutaneous tissue: underlying layer that anchors the skin layers to the underlying tissues of the body

Subjective data (symptoms, covert data): information perceived only by the affected person

Subjective self: how one sees oneself; who one thinks one is

Sublingual: area in the mouth under the tongue

Sudden infant death syndrome (SIDS): sudden death of an infant under the age of 1 year when consideration of the infant's history, a postmortem examination, and investigation of the scene of the death fail to reveal a cause of death

Sudden unexplained infant death (SUID): a broad term for sudden infant deaths in which the manner and cause of death cannot readily be identified prior to an investigation

Sundowning syndrome: describes a phenomenon when a person habitually becomes confused or disoriented with darkness

Suppository: oval- or cone-shaped substance that is inserted into a body cavity and that melts at body temperature

Suprapubic catheter: catheter inserted into the bladder through a small abdominal incision above the pubic area

Surfactant: detergent-like phospholipid that reduces surface tension of the fluid lining the alveoli

Surgical asepsis: practices that render and keep objects and areas free from microorganisms; synonym for *sterile technique*

Susceptibility: degree of resistance of a host to a pathogen

Symptom: abnormality indicative of illness as experienced by the patient; synonym for *subjective data*

Syndrome (nursing diagnoses): cluster of actual or risk nursing diagnoses that are predicted to be present because of a certain event or situation

Synergistic effect: combined effect of two or more drugs is greater than the effect of each drug alone

Systematic reviews: summarized findings from multiple studies of a specific clinical practice question or topic that recommend practice changes and future directions for research; one of the strongest sources of evidence for evidence-based practice

Systemic symptoms: symptoms manifested throughout the entire body

Systolic pressure: highest point of pressure on arterial walls when the ventricles contract

T

Tachycardia: rapid heart rate

Tachypnea: rapid rate of breathing

Tactile: pertaining to touch

Tartar: hard deposit on the teeth near the gum line formed by plaque buildup and dead bacteria

Teaching: planned method or series of methods used to help someone learn

Teaching–learning process: process of patient teaching that encompasses critical steps necessary to provide teaching and to measure learning; the teaching–learning process models the nursing process

Technical competencies: skills that enable a nurse to skillfully manipulate equipment in a manner conducive to achieving a desired goal

Temperament: person's style of approaching people, situations, or events

Temperature: refers to the hotness or coldness of a substance

Tendons: strong, flexible, inelastic fibrous bands that attach muscle to bone

Teratogenic: known to have potential to cause developmental defects in the embryo or fetus

Terminal illness: illness from which there is no reasonable expectation of recovery or cure

Terminal weaning: withdrawal of life-sustaining therapy with the understanding that death may result, generally after a decision is made that the therapy in question is medically futile or disproportionately burdensome

Tertiary preventive care: care directed at helping rehabilitate patients and restore them to a maximum level of functioning after an illness

Theory: statement based on observed facts that explains or characterizes a process, an occurrence, or an event, but cannot be proved directly or absolutely as a fact

Therapeutic range: that concentration of drug in the blood serum that produces the desired effect without causing toxicity

Therapeutic touch (TT): an alternative therapy that involves using one's hands to consciously direct an energy exchange from the practitioner to the patient to facilitate healing or pain relief

Third-space fluid shift: distributional shift and trapping of body fluids into body spaces such as the pleural, peritoneal, or pericardial, or into the interstitial space (plasma-to-interstitial shift)

Thoracentesis: aspiration of fluid or air from the pleural space

Thoughtful practice: the care of a patient by a clinician who utilizes clinical reasoning and reflective practice to guide thoughtful actions and person-centered processes of care

Thrill: abnormal tremor accompanying a vascular or cardiac murmur felt on palpation

Thrombophlebitis: inflammation in a vein associated with thrombus formation

Thrombus: blood clot; plural is *thrombi*

Time-lapsed assessment: an assessment that is scheduled to compare a patient's current status to baseline data obtained earlier

Time-out: component of the universal protocol, just prior to beginning a surgical procedure, to verify the patient's identity and the correct surgical site and procedure

Toddler: period from ages 1 year to 3 years

Tolerance: occurrence of the body's becoming accustomed to an opioid and needing a larger dose each time for pain relief

Tonus: normal, partially steady state of muscle contraction

Topical application: application of a substance directly to a body surface

Tort: wrong committed by a person against another person or that person's property

Total body water (TBW): total amount of water in the body, expressed as a percentage of body weight. The term *total body fluid* also is used; fluids usually are considered to include water and electrolytes.

Total incontinence: continuous and unpredictable loss of urine, resulting from surgery, trauma, or physical malformation

Total parenteral nutrition (TPN): nutritional therapy that bypasses the gastrointestinal tract for patients who are unable to take food orally; meets the patient's nutritional needs with a highly concentrated, hypertonic nutrient solution administered intravenously through a central vein

Toxic effects (toxicities): specific groups of symptoms related to drug therapy that carry risk for permanent damage or death

Trace elements: minerals found in the body in quantities less than 5 g and needed in only small amounts (18 mg or less)

Tracheostomy: artificial opening made in the trachea through which a tracheostomy tube is inserted

Tracheostomy tube: curved tube inserted into an artificial opening made in the trachea that comes with varied angles and in multiple sizes

Trade name: drug name selected and trademarked by the company marketing the drug; also called *brand name* or *proprietary name*

Traditional Chinese medicine (TCM): healing system that believes the interaction of people with their environment is most significant in creating health

Traditional family: composed of a husband, wife, and their children, who live together in one home

Traditional knowledge: knowledge passed down from generation to generation

Transactional leadership: leadership style based on maintaining control by rewarding good behavior and punishing negative or detrimental behavior

Transcultural nursing: providing nursing care that is planned and implemented in a way that is sensitive to the needs of individuals, families, and groups representing the diverse cultural populations within our society

Transduction: activation of pain receptors

Trans fat: partially hydrogenated liquid oil; trans fat raises serum cholesterol

Transformational leadership: type of leadership in which the person creates revolutionary change and commits to the personal and professional growth of self and others

Transgender: an inclusive term used to describe those who feel that the sex assigned to them at birth incompletely describes or fails to describe them

Transient incontinence: occurrence that appears suddenly and lasts for 6 months or less and usually is caused by treatable factors, such as confusion secondary to acute illness, infection, and as a result of medical treatment, such as the use of diuretics or intravenous fluid administration

Transmission: conduction of pain sensations from the site of an injury or inflammation along clear and unclear pathways to the spinal cord and then on to higher centers

Transmission-based precautions: CDC precautions used in patients known or suspected to be infected with pathogens that can be transmitted by airborne, droplet, or contact routes; used in addition to standard precautions

Transsexual: person of a certain biologic gender with the feelings of the opposite sex

Transvestite: individual who desires to take on the role or wear the clothes of the opposite sex

Trauma: injury

Tremor: involuntary muscular movements

Trial: hearing of evidence in a legal case before a judge (and jury) with the intent of reaching a decision or verdict

Trial-and-error problem solving: method of problem solving that involves testing any number of solutions until one is found that works for that particular problem

Triglycerides: predominant form of fat in food and the major storage form of fat in the body

Trough level: the point when a drug is at its lowest concentration

Turgor: tension of the skin determined by its hydration

U

Unilateral: affecting or occurring on one side only

Universal precautions: isolation system that considers blood, body fluids containing blood, semen, and vaginal secretions of all patients as potentially infective

Unlicensed assistive personnel (UAP): individual who is trained to function in an assistive role to the licensed registered nurse in the provision of patient activities as delegated by and under the supervision of the registered professional nurse

Urge incontinence: state in which a person experiences involuntary passage of urine that occurs soon after a strong sense of urgency to void

Urgency: strong desire to void

Urgent surgery: surgery that is not an emergency, but must be done within a reasonably short time frame to preserve health

Urinary diversion: surgical creation of an alternate route for excretion of urine

Urinary incontinence: any involuntary loss of urine

Urinary retention: inability to void although urine is produced by the kidneys and enters the bladder; excessive storage of urine in the bladder

Urination: process of emptying the bladder; micturition; voiding

Utilitarian: action-guiding theory of ethics that states that the rightness or wrongness of an action depends on the consequences of the action

V

Validation: act of confirming or verifying

Valsalva maneuver: forcible exhalation against a closed glottis, resulting in increased intrathoracic pressure

Values: set of beliefs that are meaningful in life and that influence relationships with others

Values clarification: process by which people come to understand their own values and value system

Value system: organization of values ranked along a continuum of importance

Variables: factors in a research study

Variance charting: documentation method in case management that records unexpected events, the cause for the event, actions taken in response to the event, and discharge planning when appropriate

Varicosity: swollen, twisted vein

Vector: nonhuman carriers—such as mosquitoes, ticks, and lice—that transmit organisms from one host to another

Ventilation: exchange of gases

Ventricles: lower chambers of the heart

Veracity: truth telling

Verbal communication: exchange of information using words

Vesicular breath sounds: normal sound of respirations heard on auscultation over peripheral lung areas

Vial: glass bottle with self-sealing stopper through which medication is removed; may be single or multiple dose

Virulence: ability to produce disease

Virus: smallest of all microorganisms; can be seen only by using an electron microscope

Visceral: pertaining to inner organs

Visceral pain: pain originating in the internal organs in the thorax, cranium, or abdomen

Visual: pertaining to sight

Vital signs: body temperature, pulse and respiratory rates, and blood pressure; synonym for *cardinal signs*

Vitamins: organic substances needed by the body in small amounts to help regulate body processes; are susceptible to oxidation and destruction

Voiding: process of emptying the bladder; also called *micturition* or *urination*

Volume-control administration set: intermittent intravenous medication infusion diluted with a small amount of solution

Voluntary agencies: community agencies that are often funded by private donations, grants, or fund-raising and that provide a wide variety of direct services and education

W

Waist circumference: a numerical measurement of the waist, used to assess an individual's abdominal fat and establish ideal body weight

Wellness: an active process in which an individual progresses toward the maximum possible potential, regardless of current state of health

Wellness diagnosis: clinical judgment about an individual, family, or community in transition from a specific level of wellness to a higher level of wellness

Wheeze: continuous, high-pitched squeak or musical sound made as air moves through narrowed or partially obstructed airway passages

Whistle-blowing: term generally used to refer to employees who report their employers' violation of the law to appropriate law enforcement agencies outside the employers' facilities

Wound: injury that results in a disruption in the normal continuity of a body tissue

X

X-ray: high-energy electromagnetic wave capable of penetrating solid matter and acting on photographic film; synonym for *roentgen ray*

Y

Yin-yang: energy forces in Chinese teaching that must be in balance for good health; expression of strong emotions results in disharmony and imbalance between these forces

Young adult: adult between the ages of 20 and 40 years

Z

Z-track: technique used to administer medications intramuscularly that ensures that the medication does not leak back along the needle track and into the subcutaneous tissue, reducing pain and discomfort

Index